**Table 38-2.** Guidelines for Usage of Analgesics and Sedatives in Children

| Analgesics | Initial Dose | Onset | Effective Duration | Supplemental Maximum Dose | |
|---|---|---|---|---|---|
| Fentanyl | 2–3 μg/kg IV | 2 min | 30 min | Titrate to effect in 0.5 μg/kg increments | Respiratory depression (especially with rapid IV push); bradycardia; muscle rigidity<br>Have naloxone available |
| Nitrous Oxide | 30–50% mixture with $O_2$ | 1–2 min | — | — | Fail-safe system to avoid hypoxia; scavenger system<br>Contraindications: previous sedative, altered mental status, dyspnea, pneumothorax, eye injury, obstructed viscus |
| Ketamine | 1.0 mg/kg IV<br>4.0 mg/kg IM | rapid IV<br>3–5 min | 10 min<br>20 min | IV—titrate to effect<br>IM—2 mg/kg supplementation | Laryngospasm<br>Hypertension (not recommended for closed head injury patients)<br>Hypersalivation (can be controlled with atropine 0.01 mg/kg)<br>Hallucinations (can be avoided with midazolam or diazepam) |
| Morphine | 0.1 mg/kg IV | 5–10 min | 3–4 h | 0.05 mg/kg supplementation, titrate to effect | Respiratory depression (especially with rapid IV push)<br>Hypotension<br>Have naloxone available |
| Meperidine | 1.0 mg/kg IV, IM<br>1–2 mg/kg PO | rapid IV<br>10–15 min IM<br>15–30 min PO | 2–3 h | 0.5 mg/kg supplementation, max 100 mg IV, IM max 150 mg PO | Precautions as with other narcotics above<br>Can be combined with hydroxyzine, 0.5 mg/kg IM or PO<br>Have naloxone available |
| Ketorolac | 0.5–1.0 mg/kg IM, IV<br>10 mg PO (adult dose) | peak 30–60 min | 4–6 h | 0.5–1.0 mg/kg q 4–6 h<br>10 mg q 6 h | GI irritation, caution with renal impairment<br>Potential bronchospasm, anaphylactoid reaction |
| **Sedatives** | | | | | |
| Midazolam | 0.15 mg/kg IV, IM<br>0.2–0.4 mg/kg PR, intranasally<br>0.5 mg/kg PO | 2 min IV,<br>10–15 min IM, PR, intranasally or PO | 30 min IV<br>45 min IM, PR, intranasally or PO | Titrate IV dose to effect in 0.02 mg/kg increments; 0.1 mg/kg IM supplementation<br>12 mg max dose PO | Respiratory depression, apnea, hypotension (especially when combined with fentanyl)<br>Anterograde amnesia for 1–2 h |
| Methohexital | 20 mg/kg PR<br>1 mg/kg IV | 15 min PR<br>rapid IV | 20 min<br>10 min | Max PR dose 25 mg/kg | Adverse effects similar to those of pentobarbital; may lower seizure threshold in patients with known seizure disorder |
| Diazepam | 0.1 mg/kg IV<br>0.2 mg/kg PO, PR | rapid IV<br>30–60 min PO, PR | 1–2 h | Max IV dose 0.6 mg/kg over 8 h<br>Max PO dose 10 mg over 6–8 h | Adverse effects similar to those of midazolam |
| Pentobarbital | 2.5 mg/kg IV<br>2–5 mg/kg IM | rapid IV,<br>15 min IM | 30 min IV<br>2 h IM | 1.25 mg/kg (max 100 mg) IV<br>Max total IV dose 300 mg<br>100–200 mg max IM dose | Hiccups, respiratory depression, apnea, hypotension, cardiac depression |
| Chloral Hydrate | 75 mg/kg PO, PR | 30 min | 3–4 h | 2 g max dose | GI irritation, cardiac arrhythmias (rare), increased hyperbilirubinemia in premature infants |

**Table 102-1.** Formulas for Estimating Normal Weight in Children

| Age | Weight, kg |
|---|---|
| ≤ 12 months | [Age (months)]/2 + 4 |
| 1–10 years | [2 × Age (years)] + 10 |

**Table 102-3.** Recommended Schedule of Childhood Immunizations

| AGE | DPT | OPV | HIB | MMR | HepB |
|---|---|---|---|---|---|
| Birth | | | | | HepB |
| 2 months | DPT | OPV | HIB | | HepB |
| 4 months | DPT | OPV | HIB | | |
| 6 months | DPT | | HIB | | HepB |
| 15 months | | | HIB | MMR | |
| 15–18 months | DPT | OPV | | | |
| 4–6 years | DPT | OPV | | | |
| 11–12 years | | | | MMR | |
| 14–16 years | Td | | | | |

*Note:* DPT, diphtheria, pertussis, tetanus (cellular); OPV, oral poliovirus (live); HIB, *Haemophilus* influenza B conjugate; MMR, measles, mumps, rubella (live); HepB, Hepatitis B (live); Td, tetanus with diphtheria adjuvant (adult).

# EMERGENCY MEDICINE

A COMPREHENSIVE STUDY GUIDE

## NOTICE

Medicine is an ever-changing science. As new research and clinical experience broaden our knowledge, changes in treatment and drug therapy are required. The editors and the publisher of this work have checked with sources believed to be reliable in their efforts to provide information that is complete and generally in accord with the standards accepted at the time of publication. However, in view of the possibility of human error or changes in medical sciences, neither the editors nor the publisher nor any other party who has been involved in the preparation or publication of this work warrants that the information contained herein is in every respect accurate or complete, and they are not responsible for any errors or omissions or for the results obtained from use of such information. Readers are encouraged to confirm the information contained herein with other sources. For example and in particular, readers are advised to check the product information sheet included in the package of each drug they plan to administer to be certain that the information contained in this book is accurate and that changes have not been made in the recommended dose or in the contraindications for administration. This recommendation is of particular importance in connection with new or infrequently used drugs.

# EMERGENCY MEDICINE

## A COMPREHENSIVE STUDY GUIDE

American College
of Emergency
Physicians

Editor-in-Chief

## Judith E. Tintinalli, M.D., M.S.

Steven J. Dresnick, M.D. Distinguished
  Professor and Chair in Emergency Medicine
Department of Emergency Medicine
University of North Carolina at Chapel Hill
Chapel Hill, North Carolina

Associate Editors

## Ernest Ruiz, M.D.

Professor of Clinical Emergency Medicine
University of Minnesota Medical School
Head, Emergency Medicine Program
Minneapolis, Minnesota

## Ronald L. Krome, M.D.

Professor of Emergency Medicine
Wayne State University
Detroit, Michigan

*McGraw-Hill*
*Health Professions Division*

New York  St. Louis  San Francisco  Auckland  Bogotá  Caracas  Lisbon  London  Madrid  Mexico City
Milan  Montreal  New Delhi  San Juan  Singapore  Sydney  Tokyo  Toronto

*McGraw-Hill*

*A Division of The* **McGraw-Hill** *Companies*

567890 DOWDOW 998

ISBN 0-07-064879-4

This book was set in Times Roman by Quebecor/Kingsport; the editors were Jamie Kircher and Peter McCurdy; the production supervisor was Richard Ruzycka; the cover designer was José R. Fonfrias. The indexer was Irving Tullar.

R. R. Donnelley and Sons was printer and binder.

This book is printed on acid-free paper.

LIBRARY OF CONGRESS CATALOGING-IN-PUBLICATION DATA

Emergency medicine : a comprehensive study guide / American College of Emergency
    Physicians ; editor-in-chief, Judith E. Tintinalli ; associate
editors, Ernest Ruiz, Ronald L. Krome, —4th ed.
        p.      cm.
    Includes bibliographical references and index.
    ISBN 0-07-064879-4
    1. Emergency medicine.   I. Tintinalli, Judith E.   II. Krome,
Ronald L.   III. Ruiz, Ernest.   IV. American College of
Emergency Physicians.
    [DNLM: 1. Emergencies.  2. Emergency Medicine.   WB 105 E552]
RC86.7.E586      1996
616.85′27—dc20
DNLM/DLC
for Library of Congress

# CONTENTS

## SECTION 8  The Digestive System  447

## SECTION 9  Renal and Genitourinary Disorders  525

## SECTION 10  Gynecology and Obstetrics  555

## SECTION 14    Environmental Injuries    843

## SECTION 15    Endocrine Emergencies    939

# CONTRIBUTORS*

**E. Jackson Allison, M.D., MPH [210]**
Sterling Distinguished Professor, Department of Emergency Medicine
East Carolina University School of Medicine
Greenville, North Carolina

**Gregory Almond, M.D. [145]**
Chief of Service, Department of Emergency Medicine,
Metropolitan Hospital Center;
Associate Professor of Emergency Medicine,
New York Medical Center,
Valhalla, New York

**James T. Amsterdam, DMD, M.D. [205]**
Professor of Emergency Medicine, Northeastern Ohio Universities
College of Medicine;
Chairman, Department of Emergency Medicine,
Western Reserve Care System,
Youngstown, Ohio

**Robert C. Andersen, M.D. [219]**
Associate Professor of Surgery
University of Minnesota School of Medicine;
Head, Renal Transplant Service
Hennepin County Medical Center
Minneapolis, Minnesota

**David C. Anderson, M.D. [199]**
Professor and Chief
Department of Neurology, Hennepin County Medical Center,
Minneapolis, Minnesota

**Paul S. Auerbach, M.D. [164]**
Division of Emergency Medicine, Stanford University Hospital,
Stanford, California

**Tom P. Aufderheide, M.D. [85]**
Associate Professor,
Director of Research,
Department of Emergency Medicine,
Medical College of Wisconsin,
Milwaukee, Wisconsin

**Jeffrey D. Band, M.D. [125]**
Division of Infectious Diseases,
William Beaumont Hospital,
Royal Oak, Michigan

**Robert A. Barish, M.D. [75]**
Associate Professor of Surgery and Medicine,
University of Maryland School of Medicine,
Division of Emergency Medicine,
Baltimore, Maryland

**Marte E. Baro, M.D. [213]**
Department of Emergency Medicine,
Hennepin County Medical Center,
Minneapolis, Minnesota

**William Barsan, M.D. [193]**
Professor and Chief
Section of Emergency Medicine
University of Michigan Medical Center
Ann Arbor, Michigan

**Christopher W. Barton, M.D. [15, 19–21]**
Associate Professor and Head
Division of Informatics
Department of Emergency Medicine
University of North Carolina
Chapel Hill, North Carolina

**Neil Batson, NREMT-P [7]**
University of North Carolina,
Department of Emergency Medicine,
Chapel Hill, North Carolina

**Daniel G. Batton, M.D. [104]**
Chief, Neonatology
Department of Pediatrics
William Beaumont Hospital
Royal Oak, Michigan

**Phil Bendick, M.D. [255]**
Director, Peripheral Vascular Diagnostic Center
William Beaumont Hospital
Royal Oak, Michigan

**Georges C. Benjamin, M.D. [64, 67]**
Acting Commissioner of Public Health, District of Columbia;
Assistant Professor of Medicine,
Howard University,
Washington, DC;
Associate Professor of Military Medicine,
Uniformed Services University of the Health Sciences,
Bethesda, Maryland;
Clinical Instructor of Emergency Medicine,
Georgetown University,
Washington, DC

**Nicholas Benson, M.D. [3]**
Professor and Chair,
Department of Emergency Medicine,
East Carolina University School of Medicine,
Greenville, North Carolina

**William A. Berk, M.D. [12, 138]**
Department of Emergency Medicine,
Wayne State University School of Medicine;
Detroit Receiving Hospital and
University Health Center,
Detroit, Michigan

*The numbers in brackets following the contributors' names indicate the chapters written or cowritten by that contributor.

**Carol D. Berkowitz, M.D. [35, 105, 250]**
Associate Chair and Program Director,
Department of Pediatrics,
Harbor/UCLA Medical Center;
Professor of Clinical Pediatrics,
UCLA School of Medicine,
Torrance, California

**Howard Bessen, M.D. [160]**
Professor of Medicine,
UCLA School of Medicine,
Los Angeles, California;
Director, Emergency Medicine Residency Program,
Harbor-UCLA Medical Center,
Torrance, California

**Louis Binder, M.D. [124]**
Associate Professor
Emergency Medicine, Texas Tech Health Sciences Center;
Regional Academic Health Center
Office of Graduate Medical Education & Student Affairs
El Paso, Texas

**Carl L. Bose, M.D. [5]**
Professor of Neonatal/Perinatal Medicine and Emergency Medicine
The University of North Carolina-Chapel Hill
Chapel Hill, North Carolina

**George M. Bosse, M.D. [136]**
Assistant Professor, Department of Emergency Medicine,
School of Medicine,
University of Louisville,
Louisville, Kentucky

**James K. Bouzoukis, M.D. [83]**
Department of Emergency Medicine
Medical Center of Delaware
Wilmington, Delaware

**William J. Bradley, M.D.,**
Assistant Professor, Division of Emergency Medicine,
University of Virginia Health Sciences Center,
Charlottesville, Virginia

**William J. Brady, M.D. [85]**
Assistant Professor,
Division of Emergency Medicine,
University of Virginia Health Sciences Center,
Charlottesville, Virginia

**George Braitberg, M.B.B.S. [141]**
Department of Medical Toxicology,
Good Samaritan Regional Medical Center,
Phoenix, Arizona

**L. Steven Bujenovic, M.D. [261]**
Attending Physician, Department of Nuclear Medicine,
Our Lady of the Lake Regional Medical Center,
Baton Rouge, Louisiana

**Richard E. Burney, M.D. [74]**
Professor of Surgery,
The University of Michigan Medical Center,
Ann Arbor, Michigan

**Charles B. Cairns, M.D. [54]**
Assistant Professor,
Director, Colorado Emergency Medicine research Center,
Division of Emergency Medicine,
University of Colorado Health Sciences Center,
Denver, Colorado

**Donna L. Carden, M.D. [123]**
Department of Physiology and Biophysics
Louisiana State University Medical Center
Shreveport, Louisiana

**E. Martin Caravati, M.D., MPH [150]**
Associate Professor, Division of Emergency Medicine;
Associate Medical Director,
Utah Poison Control Center,
Salt Lake City, Utah

**C. Thomas Carter, M.D. [13]**
University of Virginia Health Sciences Center
Charlottesville, Virginia

**Alexander S. Cass, M.B.B.S. [221]**
Associate Professor, Urologic Surgery
University of Minnesota School of Medicine;
Head, Division of Urology
Hennepin County Medical Center
Minneapolis, Minnesota

**Michael S. Catapano, M.D. [117]**
Assistant Director, Emergency Medical Services
North Shore University Hospital;
Clinical Instructor, Department of Surgery
Cornell University Medical College
Manhasset, New York

**James A. Catto, M.D. [78]**
Department of Surgery,
William Beaumont Medical Center,
Royal Oak, Michigan

**Eugene E. Cepeda, M.D. [16]**
Neonatologist
St. John Hospital
Detroit, Michigan

**Johanna Chapel, M.D. [206–209]**
Department of Medicine,
Oakwood Hospital,
Dearborn, Michigan

**Thomas A. Chapel, M.D. [206–209]**
Clinical Professor of Dermatology,
Wayne State University,
Dearborn, Michigan

**Harold Chin, M.D. [226]**
Clinical Assistant Professor,
Department of Medicine,
University of Chicago,
Attending Physician,
Department of Emergency Medicine,
Lutheran General Hospital,
Park Ridge, Illinois

**Richard A. Christoph, M.D. [118]**
Division of Emergency Medicine,
University of Virginia Medical School
Charlottesville, Virginia

**James E. Cisek, M.D. [142]**
Residency Director, Department of Emergency Medicine,
William Beaumont Hospital,
Royal Oak, Michigan

**Richard F. Clark, M.D. [145]**
Medical Director,
San Diego Regional Poison Control Center;
Assistant Professor,
Department of Medicine,
University of California,
San Diego, California

**David M. Cline, M.D. [55]**
Clinical Associate Professor,
Department of Emergency Medicine,
University of North Carolina, Chapel Hill
Attending Emergency Physician,
Wake Medical Center
Raleigh, North Carolina

**Christine Comstock, M.D. [258]**
Assistant Professor, Obstetrics and Gynecology,
Wayne State University School of Medicine;
Director,
Division of Fetal Imaging,
William Beaumont Hospital,
Royal Oak, Michigan

**Timothy J. Crimmins, M.D. [10]**
Assistant Professor of Emergency Medicine,
University of Minnesota School of Medicine,
Department of Emergency Medicine,
Hennepin County Medical Center,
Minneapolis, Minnesota

**Natalie Cullen, M.D. [40]**
Department of Emergency Medicine,
Wright State University,
Dayton, Ohio

**Steven C. Curry, M.D. [143, 150]**
Department of
Good Samaritan Medical Center
Phoenix, Arizona

**Daniel F. Danzl, M.D. [11]**
Professor and Chair,
Department of Emergency Medicine,
University of Louisville,
Louisville, Kentucky

**Richard C. Dart, M.D., Ph.D. [163]**
Rocky Mountain Poison Center,
Denver Health and Hospitals,
Department of Public Health,
Denver, Colorado

**Daniel J. DeBehnke, M.D. [214]**
Department of Emergency Medicine,
Medical College of Wisconsin,
Milwaukee, Wisconsin

**Kathleen A. Delaney, M.D. [156]**
Department of Surgery/Emergency Medicine
University of Texas/SW Medical School
Dallas, Texas

**Robert P. Dowsett, M.D. [174]**
Department of Emergency Medicine,
University of Massachusetts,
Worcester, Massachusetts

**Steven C. Dronen, M.D. [26]**
Associate Professor,
Section of Emergency Medicine,
University of Michigan School of Medicine,
Ann Arbor, Michigan

**Constance Doyle, M.D. [172]**
Clinical Instructor, Emergency Services
University of Michigan Medical Center;
Emergency Department
Foote Hospital
Jackson, Michigan

**Mary E. Eberst, M.D. [184–189]**
Clinical Assistant Professor,
Department of Emergency Medicine,
University of North Carolina,
Chapel Hill, North Carolina

**Richard F. Edlich, M.D., Ph.D. [42–50, 197, 198]**
Distinguished Professor of Plastic Surgery and Biomedical
Engineering, University of Virginia Health Sciences Center,
Department of Plastic Surgery,
Charlottesville, Virginia

**John M. Eggleston, M.D. [46]**
Department of Plastic Surgery,
Stanford Medical School,
Palo Alto, California

**Mickey S. Eisenberg, M.D., Ph.D. [52]**
Emergency Medicine Service,
University of Washington Medical Center,
Seattle, Washington

**Charles Emerman, M.D. [119]**
Chairman of Emergency Medicine,
MetroHealth Medical Center,
Associate Professor, Case Western Reserve University
Cleveland, Ohio

**Rawden Evans, M.D., Ph.D. [89]**
Assistant Professor, Section of Emergency Medicine,
University of Michigan Medical Center,

**Martin L. Fackler, M.D. [222]**
President,
International Wound Ballistics Association,
Hawthorne, Florida

**William D. Fales, M.D. [31]**
Director of Pre-Hospital Care,
Michigan State University,
Kalamazoo Center for Medical Studies
Kalamazoo, Michigan

**Jay L. Falk, M.D. [24]**
Director, Emergency Medicine Residency Program,
Clinical Professor of Medicine,
University of Florida College of Medicine,
Orlando, Florida

**Gary G. Fifield, M.D. [213]**
Assistant Professor of Pediatrics
University of Minnesota School of Medicine;
Department of Pediatrics and Emergency Medicine
Hennepin County Medical Center
Minneapolis, Minnesota

**A. Joel Feldman, M.D. [61]**
Division of Pulmonary Medicine
William Beaumont Hospital
Royal Oak, Michigan

**Gary R. Fleischer, M.D. [108]**
Chief, Division of Emergency Medicine
Department of Medicine
Children's Hospital;
Associate Professor of Pediatrics
Department of Pediatrics
Harvard Medical School
Boston, Massachusetts

**Denise J. Fligner, M.D. [111]**
Assistant Professor, Department of Family Practice
Rush Medical College
Chicago, Illinois;
Research Director, Department of Emergency Medicine
Christ Hospital and Medical Center
Oak Lawn, Illinois

**Steven G. Folstad, M.D. [211]**
Instructor
Department of Emergency Medicine
Bowman Gray School of Medicine
Wake Forest University
Winston-Salem, North Carolina

**Phil B. Fontanarosa, M.D. [170]**
Adjunct Associate Professor of Medicine,
Division of Emergency Medicine,
Northwestern University Medical School,
Chicago, Illinois

**Marsha Ford, M.D. [158]**
Clinical Assistant Professor
Department of Emergency Medicine
University of North Carolina, Chapel Hill
Attending Emergency Physician
Carolinas Medical Center
Charlotte, North Carolina

**Scott Freeman, M.D. [2]**
Assistant Professor, Emergency Medicine,
Wayne State University School of Medicine;
Detroit, Michigan

**Susan Fuchs, M.D. [107]**
Emergency Department
Children's Hospital of Pittsburgh;
Assistant Professor of Pediatrics
University of Pittsburgh School of Medicine
Pittsburgh, Pennsylvania

**Wade R. Gaasch, M.D. [75]**
Assistant Professor of Surgery,
University of Maryland School of Medicine,
Division of Emergency Medicine,
Baltimore, Maryland

**Bassam M. Gebara, M.D. [39]**
Department of Pediatrics, William Beaumont Hospital,
Royal Oak, Michigan

**John L. Glover, M.D. [59, 60, 79]**
Chief, Department of Surgery,
William Beaumont Hospital,
Royal Oak, Michigan

**George S. Goding, Jr., M.D. [266]**
Department of Otolaryngology,
Hennepin County Medical Center;
Assistant Professor of Otolaryngology,
University of Minnesota,
Minneapolis, Minnesota

**Mark G. Goetting, M.D. [39]**
Department of Pediatrics,
William Beaumont Hospital,
Royal Oak, Michigan

**Hernan F. Gomez, M.D. [163]**
University of Michigan Medical Center
Ann Arbor, Michigan

**Susan J. Gottlieb, M.D. [244]**
Department of Psychiatry
William Beaumont Hospital
Royal Oak, Michigan

**John E. Gough, M.D. [210]**
Assistant Professor,
Assistant Medical Director,
Division of Emergency Medical Services,
Department of Emergency Medicine,
East Carolina University School of Medicine,
Greenville, North Carolina

**Daniel G. Guenin, M.D. [164]**
Division of Emergency Medicine,
Stanford University Hospital,
Stanford, California

**Cheryl H. Hack, M.D. [119]**
Assistant Professor, Wayne State University School of Medicine,
Children's Hospital of Michigan,
Detroit, Michigan

**Peter H. Hackett, M.D. [165]**
Affiliate Associate Professor, College of Health Sciences
University of Alaska;
Affiliate Associate Professor
Department of Medicine
University of Washington School of Medicine
Seattle, Washington;
Director, Air Ambulance and Staff Physician
Emergency Department
Humana Hospital
Anchorage, Alaska

**Marie-Louise Hammarskjöld, M.D. [197]**
Charles H. Ross, Jr. Chair of Multiple Sclerosis Research,
Associate Professor of Microbiology,
University of Virginia school of Medicine,
Charlottesville, Virginia

**Daniel G. Hankins, M.D. [2]**
Division of Emergency Medical Services,
Mayo Clinic and St. Mary's Hospital,
Rochester, Minnesota

**Fred Hansen, M.D., Ph.D. [98]**
Clinical Professor
Department of Emergency Medicine
University of North Carolina
Chapel Hill, North Carolina

**Wendy F. Hansen, M.D. [98]**
Assistant Professor,
Department of Obstetrics and Gynecology,
Division of Maternal-Fetal Medicine,
The University of North Carolina-Chapel Hill,
Chapel Hill, North Carolina

**Fred P. Harchelroad, Jr. M.D. [169]**
Director, Quality Assurance and Research
Assistant Professor, Emergency Medicine
Medical College of Pennsylvania—Allegheny Campus
Allegheny General Hospital
Pittsburgh, Pennsylvania

**Ann L. Harwood-Nuss, M.D. [29, 121]**
Professor, Division of Emergency Medicine,
Department of Surgery,
University of Florida
Health Science Center,
Jacksonville, Florida

**Andrew M. Hauser, M.D. [256]**
Director, Cardiac Ultrasound Laboratory
William Beaumont Hospital
Royal Oak, Michigan

**Bruce E. Haynes, M.D. [167]**
Director, EMS Authority
State of California
Sacramento, California

**Barry H. Hendler, D.D.S., M.D. [204]**
Clinical Professor of Medicine and Surgery,
Hospital of the University of Pennsylvania and Medical College
Hospitals,
Philadelphia, Pennsylvania

**Wilma V. Henderson, M.D. [138]**
Assistant Professor (Clinical-Educator)
Assistant Residency Program Director,
Department of Emergency Medicine,
Wayne State University
Detroit, Michigan

**Philip L. Henneman, M.D. [200]**
Director, Adult Emergency Department,
Harbor-UCLA Medical Center,
Associate Professor of Medicine,
UCLA School of Medicine,
Torrance, California

**Gregory L. Henry, M.D. [33, 191, 196]**
Clinical Assistant Professor, Section of Emergency Medicine
University of Michigan Medical Center;
Chief, Department of Emergency Medicine
Beyer Memorial Hospital
Ypsilanti, Michigan;
Vice President, Emergency Physicians Medical Group
Ann Arbor, Michigan

**Mark Henry, M.D. [148]**
Department of Emergency Medicine
School of Medicine
SUNY at Stony Brook
Stony Brook, New York

**Robert S. Hockberger, M.D. [57]**
Associate Clinical Professor, Emergency Medicine
UCLA School of Medicine;
Chairman, Department of Emergency Medicine
Harbor-UCLA Medical Center
Torrance, California

**Dee Hodge III, M.D. [18]**
Assistant Professor of Pediatrics and Emergency Medicine
UCLA Medical School;
Director of Pediatric Emergency Medicine
Children's Hospital of Los Angeles
Los Angeles, California

**Marion Hoelzer, M.D. [251]**
Department of Emergency Medicine,
William Beaumont Hospital,
Royal Oak, Michigan

**Gwendolyn L. Hoffman, M.D. [192]**
Program Director,
Emergency Medicine Residency,
Butterworth Hospital,
Grand Rapids, Michigan;
Associate Professor,
Department of Internal Medicine,
College of Human Medicine,
Michigan State University,
Ann Arbor, Michigan

**Robert S. Hoffman, M.D. [140]**
Director,
New York City Poison Control Center;
Assistant Professor of Emergency Medicine,
Department of Surgery/Emergency Medicine
New York University School of Medicine
Attending Physician
Department of Emergency Medical Services
Bellevue Hospital Center
New York, New York

**Jeremy J. Hollerman, M.D. [222, 259]**
Department of Medical Imaging, Hennepin County Medical
Center;
Assistant Professor of Radiology,
University of Minnesota,
Minneapolis, Minnesota

**Ronald D. Holmes, M.D. [114]**
Department of Pediatrics
Division of Pediatric Gastroenterology,
University of Michigan Medical Center
Ann Arbor, Michigan

**Edmond A. Hooker, M.D. [88]**
Assistant Professor,
Department of Emergency Medicine,
University of Louisville,
Louisville, Kentucky

**David S. Howes, M.D. [91]**
Residency Program Director,
University of Chicago Emergency Medicine Residency,
Associate Professor of Clinical Medicine,
University of Chicago
Chicago, Illinois

**D. Monte Hunter, M.D. [234, 235]**
Assistant Professor,
Department of Emergency Medicine
Department of Orthopedics,
Bowman Gray School of Medicine,
Wake Forest University,
Winston-Salem, North Carolina

**Stanley H. Inkelis, M.D. [112]**
Director, Pediatric Emergency Medicine,
Harbor-UCLA Medical Center;
Professor of Pediatrics,
UCLA School of Medicine,
University of California, Los Angeles,
Torrance, California

**Susan Isbey, M.D. [127]**
Division of Infectious Diseases
University of North Carolina at Chapel Hill
Chapel Hill, North Carolina

**Kenneth C. Jackimczyk, M.D. [246]**
Residency Director, Emergency Medicine,
Maricopa Medical Center,
Phoenix, Arizona

**Raymond Jackson, M.D., M.S. [9, 58]**
Research Director
Department of Emergency Medicine
William Beaumont Hospital
Royal Oak, Michigan

**David M. Jaffe, M.D. [107]**
Director, Division of Emergency Medicine
St. Louis Children's Hospital;
Associate Professor of Pediatrics
Washington University School of Medicine
St. Louis, Missouri

**Alvina M. Janda, M.D. [201]**
Department of Ophthalmology,
Hennepin County Medical Center,
Minneapolis, Minnesota

**Jon Jui, M.D. [27, 257]**
Department of Emergency Medicine,
Hennepin County Medical Center,
Minneapolis, Minnesota

**Rodger Keller, M.D. [175]**
Horticulturist, Matthaei Botanical Gardens
University of Michigan
Ann Arbor, Michigan

**Arthur L. Kellermann M.D. [8]**
Associate Professor and Director,
Center for Injury Control,
Emory University School of Public Health and the
Emory University School of Medicine,
Atlanta, Georgia

**Scott Kelley, M.D. [265]**
Assistant Professor of Orthopaedics,
University of North Carolina at Chapel Hill,
Chapel Hill, North Carolina

**William R. Kerns, M.D. [133]**
Clinical Instructor
Department of Emergency Medicine
Carolinas Medical Center
Charlotte, North Carolina

**Suck Won Kim, M.D. [245]**
Associate Professor of Psychiatry,
University of Minnesota Medical School,
Minneapolis, Minnesota

**Mark A. Kirk, M.D. [147]**
Medical Toxicology Fellowship Director,
Department of Emergency Medicine,
Indiana Poison Center,
Methodist Hospital of Indiana,
Indianapolis, Indiana

**Niranjian Kissoon, M.D. [103]**
Associate Professor,
Department of Pediatrics,
University of Florida Health Science Center,
Jacksonville, Florida

**Kenneth W. Kizer, M.D., M.P.H. [166]**
Department of Veterans Affairs
Under Secretary for Health
Washington, D.C.

**Steven N. Klein, M.D. [82]**
Staff Physician,
Department of Surgery,
William Beaumont Hospital,
Royal Oak, Michigan

**Sanford H. Koltonow, M.D. [249]**
Attending Physician,
William Beaumont Hospital,
Royal Oak, Michigan

**Rashmi U. Kothari, M.D. [193]**
Assistant Professor,
Section of Emergency Medicine,
University of Michigan Medical Center,
Ann Arbor, Michigan

**Robert F. Kowalski, M.D. [175]**
Attending Physician,
Department of Emergency Medicine,
William Beaumont Hospital,
Royal Oak, Michigan

**Alan J. Kozak, M.D. [199]**
Division of Infectious Diseases,
Department of Medicine,
Mary Imogene Bassett Hospital,
Cooperstown, New York

**David A. Kramer, M.D. [128]**
Director, Emergency Medicine Residency Program,
Assistant Professor,
Division of Emergency Medicine,
Emory University School of Medicine.
Atlanta, Georgia

**Gary S. Krause, M.D., M.S. [14]**
Associate Professor and
Associate Research Director,
Wayne State University School of Medicine;
Detroit Receiving Hospital and
University Health Center,
Detroit, Michigan

**Steven Kronik, M.D. [89]**
Assistant Professor
Section of Emergency Medicine,
University of Michigan Medical Center,
Ann Arbor, Michigan

**Gloria Kuhn, D.O. [97]**
Associate professor,
Department of Emergency Medicine,
Wayne State University School of Medicine,
Detroit, Michigan

**Roy M. Kulick, M.D., M.S. [38]**
Assistant Professor of Pediatrics
University of Cincinnati School of Medicine;
Associate Director, Division of Emergency Medicine
Children's Hospital Medical Center
Cincinnati, Ohio

**Donald B. Kunkel, M.D. [140]**
Medical Director,
Samaritan Regional Poison Center;
Good Samaritan Regional Medical Center,
Department of Medical Toxicology,
Phoenix, Arizona

**Tom Kunisaki, M.D. [29]**
Division of Emergency Medicine,
Department of Surgery,
University of Florida
Health Science Center,
Jacksonville, Florida

**Warren L. Kupin, M.D. [93]**
Co-Director Renal Transplantation,
Division of Nephrology and Hypertension,
Henry Ford Hospital,
Detroit, Michigan

**Myron M. LaBan, M.D. [232, 233]**
Director, Physical Medicine and Rehabilitation,
William Beaumont Hospital,
Royal Oak, Michigan

**Patricia L. Lanter, M.D. [26]**
Section of Emergency Medicine,
University of Michigan School of Medicine,
Ann Arbor, Michigan

**Harrison A. Latimer, M.D. [265]**
Division of Orthopaedics,
University of North Carolina,
Chapel Hill, North Carolina

**Frank W. Lavoie, M.D. [80]**
Associate Professor,
Division of Emergency Medicine,
University of Texas Southwestern Medical School,
Dallas, Texas

**Wesley Lee, M.D. [258]**
Associate Professor,
Obstetrics and Gynecology,
Wayne State University School of Medicine;
Division of Fetal Imaging,
William Beaumont Hospital,
Royal Oak, Michigan

**David Levy, Pharm.D.\* [23]**
Clinical Specialist—Emergency Care
Department of Pharmacy Services
Detroit Receiving Hospital and University Health Center
Detroit, Michigan

**G. Patrick Lilja [1]**
Clinical Assistant Professor
University of Minnesota School of Medicine;
Director, Emergency Department
North Memorial Medical Center
Minneapolis, Minnesota

**Christopher H. Linden, M.D. [144, 174]**
Associate Professor Medicine,
Associate Clinical Director,
Associate Director, Toxicology Service,
University of Massachusetts,
Department of Emergency Medicine
Worchester, Massachusetts

**Louis Ling, M.D. [149]**
Associate Medical Director,
Academic Affairs,
Hennepin County Medical Center,
Minneapolis, Minnesota

**Neal E. Little, M.D. [194]**
Clinical Instructor, Department of Surgery;
University of Michigan Medical School;
Attending Emergency Physician,
St. Joseph's Mercy Hospital,
Ann Arbor, Michigan

**Robert Luten, M.D. [17]**
Assistant Professor, University of Florida;
Department of Emergency Medicine
University Hospital of Jacksonville
Jacksonville, Florida

\* Deceased.

**Elizabeth Lyons, Pharm.D. [23]**
Clinical Specialist,
Emergency Medicine/Toxicology,
Wayne State University;
Detroit Receiving Hospital and
University Health Center
Detroit, Michigan

**O. John Ma, M.D. [214]**
Assistant Professor,
Department of Emergency Medicine,
Director, Carolina Air Care,
University of North Carolina,
Chapel Hill, North Carolina

**Michael E. Maddens, M.D. [62]**
Chief, Division of Geriatic Medicine,
William Beaumont Hospital,
Royal Oak, Michigan

**Brian D. Mahoney, M.D. [6, 216]**
Associate Professor of Clinical Emergency Medicine,
University of Minnesota School of Medicine,
Department of Emergency Medicine
Hennepin County Medical Center
Minneapolis, Minnesota

**Richard Malley, M.D. [108]**
Section of Pediatrics, Fellow, Emergency Medicine/Infectious
  Diseases,
Children's Hospital,
Boston, Massachusetts

**Veronica T. Mallett, M.D. [96, 101]**
Assistant Professor,
Department of Obstetrics & Gynecology,
Wayne State University,
Detroit, Michigan

**James E. Manning, M.D. [15]**
Assistant Professor
Department of Emergency Medicine
University of North Carolina
Chapel Hill, North Carolina

**Catherine A. Marco, M.D. [122]**
Instructor of Emergency Medicine
Department of Emergency Medicine
The Johns Hopkins Hospital and School of Medicine;
Attending Physician, Emergency Medicine
Francis Scott Key Medical Center
Baltimore, Maryland

**Marcus L. Martin, M.D. [169]**
Associate Professor,
Residency Program Director,
Department of Emergency Medicine,
Medical College of Pennslyvania,
Pittsburgh, Pennsylvania

**Ricardo Martinez, M.D. [8]**
Assistant Professor and Associate Director,
Center for Injury Control,
Emory University School

**William H. McCartney, M.D. [261]**
Professor of Radiology,
University of North Carolina
School of Medicine,
Chapel Hill, North Carolina

**Marshall C. McCoy, M.D. [254]**
Assistant Professor,
University of North Carolina,
Department of Emergency Medicine,
Chapel Hill, North Carolina

**James H. McCrory, M.D. [106]**
Pediatric Critical Care Medicine, The Medical Center of Central
Georgia,
Associate Professor, Pediatrics
Mercer University School of Medicine

**Cary C. McDonald, M.D. [248]**
Emergency Medicine Services Medical Director,
Wake Medical Center,
Raleigh, North Carolina;
Clinical Assistant Professor in Emergency Medicine,
Department of Emergency Medicine,
School of Medicine,
University of North Carolina,
Chapel Hill, North Carolina

**W. Kendall McNabney, M.D. [77]**
Director of Trauma Services, Truman Medical Center;
Professor and Assistant Dean for Clinical Affairs
University of Missouri—Kansas City School of Medicine
Kansas City, Missouri

**Gregory D. Mears, M.D. [7]**
Assistant Professor,
Head, Division of Emergency Medical Services,
University of North Carolina,
Department of Emergency Medicine,
Chapel Hill, North Carolina

**Frantz Melio, M.D. [240]**
Clinical Assistant Professor
Department of Emergency Medicine
University of North Carolina, Chapel Hill,
Chief, Department of Emergency Medicine,
Wake Medical Center,
Raleigh, North Carolina

**Peter Mellis, M.D. [102]**
Chippenham Medical Center,
Richmond, Virginia

**Hagop S. Mekhjian, M.D. [81]**
Professor of Medicine
Ohio State University School of Medicine
Medical Director and Associate Dean for Clinical Affairs
Ohio State University Hospital

**Terry J. Mengert, M.D. [52]**
Attending Physician and
Assistant Professor of Medicine,
Emergency Medicine Service,
University of Washington Medical Center,
Seattle, Washington

**Jeffrey S. Menkes, M.D. [223]**
Attending Physician,
Department of Emergency Medicine/Trauma,
Hartford Hospital,
Hartford, Connecticut;
Assistant Professor,
Division of Emergency Medicine,
University of Connecticut School of Medicine,
Farmington, Connecticut

**David C. Michener, Ph.D. [175]**
Assistant Curator, Matthaei Botanical Gardens
University of Michigan
Ann Arbor, Michigan

**Michael R. Mill, M.D. [63[**
Associate Professor of Surgery, University of North Carolina,
School of Medicine,
Division of Cardiothoracic Surgery,
Chapel Hill, North Carolina

**Kirk Mills, M.D. [130, 131]**
Medical Toxicologist,
Detroit Medical Center
Wayne State University,
Detroit, Michigan

**Gregory P. Moore, M.D. [246]**
Attending Physician Emergency Medicine Residency,
Methodist Hospital,
Indianapolis, Indiana

**Mary Chester Morgan, M.D., M.Sc. [238]**
Assistant Professor of Medicine,
Division of Rheumatology,
Department of Internal Medicine,
University of Pittsburgh,
Pittsburgh, Pennsylvania

**Raymond F. Morgan, M.D. [48]**
Professor and Chairman, Department of Plastic Surgery;
Professor of Orthopaedic Surgery
University of Virginia School of Medicine
Charlottesville, Virginia

**Dexter L. Morris, Ph.D., M.D. [120]**
Vice-Chairman and Assistant Professor,
Department of Emergency Medicine,
School of Medicine,
University of North Carolina,
Chapel Hill, North Carolina

**H. Arnold Muller, M.D. [173]**
Professor of Medicine
Emergency Medicine Division
Medical College of the Pennsylvania State University
Hershey, Pennsylvania

**Arthur Ney, M.D. [219, 220]**
Department of Surgery
Hennepin County Medical Center
Minneapolis, Minnesota

**James T. Niemann, M.D. [56]**
Director of Research, Department of Emergency Medicine
Harbor-UCLA Medical Center
Torrance, California

**Michael A. Nigro, M.D. [113]**
Associate Professor, Departments of Pediatrics and Neurology
Wayne University School of Medicine;
Chief, Division of Neurology
Children's Hospital of Michigan
Detroit, Michigan

**John F. O'Brien, M.D. [24]**
Assistant Director,
Emergency Medicine Residency Program,
Clinical Assistant Professor of Medicine,
University of Florida College of Medicine,
Orlando, Florida

**Allan D. Olson, M.D. [114]**
Department of Pediatrics
Division of Pediatric Gastroenterology,
University of Michigan Medical Center,
Ann Arbor, Michigan

**Stephen C. Olson, M.D. [241]**
Assistant Professor of Psychiatry,
Ohio State University School of Medicine,
Columbus, Ohio

**Harold H. Osborn, M.D. [126, 151]**
Professor and Chairman, Department of Emergency Medicine,
New York Medical College;
Chief of Service,
Lincoln Medical and Mental Health Center,
Bronx, New York

**David T. Overton, M.D. [31, 32]**
Program Director,
Emergency Medicine,
Michigan State University,
Kalamazoo Center for Medical Studies,
Kalamazoo, Michigan

**Linda Paradowski, M.D. [73]**
Division of Pulmonary Diseases,
Department of Medicine,
University of North Carolina at Chapel Hill,
Chapel Hill, North Carolina

**Monica Paraga, M.D. [154]**
Staff Physician,
Department of Emergency Medicine,
Metropolitan Hospital Center,
New York Medical College,
New York, New York

**W.F. Peacock IV, M.D [95, 202]**
The Cleveland Clinic,
Director, Clinical Operations,
Department of Emergency Medicine,
Cleveland, Ohio

**Mark D. Pearlman, M.D. [99]**
Assistant Professor
Department of Obstetrics & Gynecology
University of Michigan Medical Center
Ann Arbor, Michigan

**Thomas R. Pellegrino, M.D. [195]**
Professor and Chairman, Department of Neurology
Eastern Virginia Medical School
Norfork, Virginia

**Jeanmarie Perrone, M.D. [140]**
Professor, Department of Emergency Medicine,
Hospital of the University of Pennsylvania,
Philadelphia, Pennsylvania

**Shawna Perry, M.D. [121]**
Chief Resident
Division of Emergency Medicine,
Department of Surgery,
University of Florida Health Science Center
Jacksonville, Florida

**Robert Petrilli, M.D. [236]**
Assistant Professor,
Department of Emergency Medicine,
Bowman Gray School of Medicine,
Wake Forest University,
Winston-Salem, North Carolina

**Lawrence H. Phillips, II, M.D. [198]**
Associate Professor of Neurology,
Department of Neurology,
University of Virginia Health Sciences Center;
Department of Plastic Surgery,
University of Virginia School of Medicine,
Charlottesville, Virginia

**David Plummer, M.D. [25, 257]**
Department of Emergency Medicine,
Hennepin County Medical Center,
Minneapolis, Minnesota

**David A. Poleski, M.D. [41]**
Vice-Chief,
Department of Emergency Medicine,
Chief, Pediatrics Section,
William Beaumont Hospital,
Royal Oak, Michigan

**Nancy Pook, M.D. [40]**
Department of Emergency Medicine,
Wright State University,
Dayton, Ohio

**Stephen G. Priest, M.D. [82]**
Department of Surgery,
William Beaumont Hospital,
Royal Oak, Michigan

**Elaine S. Pomeranz, M.D. [38]**
University of Michigan Medical Center,
Assistant Professor,
Department of Pediatrics,
C.S. Mott Children's Hospital,
Ann Arbor, Michigan

**N. Heramba Prasad, M.D. [3]**
Assistant Professor and Chief,
Division of Emergency Medical Services,
Department of Emergency Medicine,
East Carolina University School of Medicine,
Greenville, North Carolina

**Mark Rabold, M.D. [159]**
Department of Emergency Medicine,
Tacoma General Hospital,
Tacoma, Washington

**Gene Ragland, M.D. [176–183]**
Chief, Emergency Medicine
St. Joseph Mercy Hospital
Ann Arbor, Michigan

**K. Venkateswara Rao, M.D. [90, 94]**
Professor of Medicine,
University of Minnesota Medical School,
Medical Director,
Renal Transplantation Program,
Hennepin County Medical Center,
Minneapolis, Minnesota

**K.P. Ravikrishnan, M.D. [65]**
Division of Pulmonology,
William Beaumont Hospital
Royal Oak, Michigan

**Earl J. Reisdorff, M.D. [171]**
Michigan State University,
Lansing, Michigan

**Nichols Relich, M.D. [37]**
Co-Director,
Neonatal Intensive Care Unit,
Department of Pediatrics,
St. John Hospital and Medical Center
Detroit, Michigan

**James Roberts, M.D. [155]**
Associate Professor, Emergency Medicine
University of Cincinnati College of Medicine
Cincinnati, Ohio

**M.K. Robbins, M.D. [73]**
Instructor
Department of Internal Medicine,
University of North Carolina,
Chapel Hill, North Carolina

**Leslie Rocher, M.D. [93]**
Director,
Division of Nephrology and Transplantation Programs,
William Beaumont Hospital,
Royal Oak, Michigan

**Gaylan L. Rockswold, M.D. [215]**
Chief of Neurosurgery, Hennepin County Medical Center;
Professor of Neurosurgery,
University of Minnesota,
Minneapolis, Minnesota

**George T. Rodeheaver, M.D. [42]**
Research Professor of Plastic Surgery
University of Virginia School of Medicine;
Director of Plastic Surgery Research
University of Virginia
Charlottesville, Virginia

**John P. Rudzinski, M.D. [226]**
Clinical Associate Professor of Surgery,
University of Illinois College of Medicine,
Rockford, Illinois;
Vice-Chairman. Department of Emergency Medicine,
Rockford Memorial Hospital,
Rockford, Illinois

**Ernest Ruiz, M.D. [212, 237]**
Professor of Clinical Emergency Medicine,
University of Minnesota
Minneapolis, Minnesota

**Douglas A. Rund, M.D. [81, 241–243]**
Professor and Chairman,
Department of Emergency Medicine,
Ohio State University,
Columbus, Ohio

**Robert Rusnak, M.D. [262–264]**
Associate Professor of Clinical Emergency Medicine,
University of Minnesota School of Medicine,
Department of Emergency Medicine
Hennepin County Medical Center
Minneapolis, Minnesota

**P.J. Ryan, M.D. [134, 135]**
Medical Director, Emergency Department
St. Luke's Medical Center
Phoenix, Arizona

**Alexander H. Sackeyfio, M.D. [244]**
Department of Psychiatry
William Beaumont, Hospital,
Royal Oak, Michigan

**Patricia R. Salber, M.D. [252, 253]**
Assistant professor of Medicine
University of California, San Francisco
San Francisco, California

**Richard F. Salluzzo, M.D. [162]**
Professor and Chairman,
Department of Emergency Medicine,
Albany Medical College,
Albany, New York

**Joseph A. Salomone III, M.D. [28]**
Associate Professor and
Associate Residency Director,
Department of Emergency Medicine,
Truman Medical Center,
University of Missouri-Kansas City
School of Medicine,
Kansas City, Missouri

**Diane Sauter, M.D. [154]**
Program Director,
Residency in Emergency Medicine,
Metropolitan Hospital Center,
Associate Professor of Emergency Medicine,
New York Medical College,
New York, New York

**Robert W. Schafermeyer, M.D. [115]**
Clinical Professor,
Department of Emergency Medicine,
University of North Carolina, Chapel Hill,
Associate Chairman,
Department of Emergency Medicine,
Carolinas Medical Center,
Charlotte, North Carolina

**Robert Schneider, M.D. [92]**
Clinical Assistant Professor,
Department of Emergency Medicine,
University of North Carolina, Chapel Hill
Residency Director, Carolinas Medical Center,
Charlotte, North Carolina

**Lawrence R. Schwartz, M.D. [168]**
Assistant Professor, Department of Emergency Medicine,
Wayne State University School of Medicine,
Detroit, Michigan

**James Seidel, M.D., Ph.D. [84]**
Chief, General and Emergency Pediatrics, Harbor-UCLA Medical Center,
Professor of Pediatrics,
UCLA School of Medicine,
Torrance, California

**Joel Seidman, M.D. [72]**
Division of Pulmonology,
William Beaumont Hospital,
Royal Oak, Michigan

**John Sessions, M.D. [76]**
Professor of Internal Medicine,
University of North Carolina,
Chapel Hill, North Carolina

**Seetha Shankaran, M.D. [16]**
Director, Neonatal-Perinatal Medicine,
Professor of Pediatrics,
Wayne State University,
School of Medicine,
Detroit, Michigan

**Stanley Sherman, M.D. [71]**
Division of Pulmonology,
William Beaumont Hospital,
Royal Oak, Michigan

**Richard O. Shields, Jr., M.D. [86]**
Department of Emergency Medicine,
Memorial Medical Center, Inc.,
Savannah, Georgia

**Robert R. Simon, M.D. [224, 239]**
Professor and Chairman,
Department of Emergency Medicine,
Cook County Hospital,
Chicago, Illinois

**Jonathan Singer, M.D. [40]**
Professor and Vice Chair,
Department of Emergency Medicine,
Wright State University,
Dayton, Ohio

**David Slobodkin, M.D. [224, 239]**
Department of Emergency Medicine,
Cook County Hospital
Chicago, Illinois

**James A. Smith, M.D. [139, 203]**
Assistant Professor of Emergency Medicine,
University of North Carolina,
Department of Emergency Medicine,
Chapel Hill, North Carolina

**Bonnie Sowa, M.D. [36]**
Clinical Assistant Professor, Division of Emergency Medicine,
Department of Pediatrics,
University of Michigan,
Ann Arbor, Michigan

**William H. Spivey, M.D. [18]***
Associate Professor of Emergency Medicine
Chief, Division of Research
Medical College of Pennsylvania
Philadelphia, Pennsylvania

**J. Stephan Stapczynski, M.D. [22, 51]**
Professor and Chair, Department of Emergency Medicine,
University of Kentucky College of Medicine,
Lexington, Kentucky

**Mark T. Steele, M.D. [215, 226–231]**
Associate Professor and Program Director,
Vice Chair and Residency Director,
Department of Emergency Medicine,
Truman Medical Center,
Kansas City, Missouri

**George L. Sternbach, M.D. [139]**
Emergency Physician
Clinical Associate Professor of Surgery
Stanford Medical Center
Stanford, California;
Emergency Physician, Seton Medical Center
Daly City, California

**Zigfrids Stelmachers, Ph.D. [247]**
Clinical Associate Professor of Psychology
University of Minnesota School of Medicine;
Crisis Intervention Center
Hennepin County Medical Center
Minneapolis, Minnesota

* Deceased.

**Robert A. Swor, D.O. [1, 217]**
EMS Coordinator,
Department of Emergency Medicine,
William Beaumont Hospital,
Royal Oak, Michigan

**Scott Syverud, M.D. [13]**
Professor and Acting Chair,
Department of Emergency Medicine,
University of Virginia,
Charlottesville, Virginia

**John Tafuri, M.D. [155]**
Department of Emergency Medicine
University of Cincinnati Hospital
Cincinnati, Ohio

**Ellen Taliaferro, M.D. [252, 253]**
Associate Professor of Surgery
University of Texas Southwestern Medical School
Executive Director, Physicians for a Violence-Free Society,
Dallas, Texas

**David Tate, M.D. [53]**
Division of Cardiology,
University of North Carolina at Chapel Hill,
Chapel Hill, North Carolina

**Thomas Terndrup, M.D. [110]**
Associate Professor, Departments of Emergency Medicine, Pediatrics
and Physiology,
Director of the Pediatric Emergency Department,
SUNY Health Sciences Center at Syracuse,
Syracuse, New York

**John G. Thacker, M.D. [42–45]**
Professor of Mechanical and Aerospace Engineering
University of Virginia
Charlottesville, Virginia

**Beverly Timerding, M.D. [235]**
Assistant Professor,
Department of Emergency Medicine,
Bowman Gray School of Medicine,
Wake Forest University,
Winston-Salem, North Carolina

**Judith E. Tintinalli, M.D., M.S. [190]**
Steven J. Dresnick, M.D. Distinguished Professor and Chair in
Emergency Medicine
Department of Emergency Medicine
University of North Carolina at Chapel Hill,
Chapel Hill, North Carolina

**Dennis T. Uehara, M.D. [225, 226]**
Clinical Associate Professor of Surgery,
University of Illinois College of Medicine,
Rockford, Illinois;
Chairman, Department of Emergency Medicine and
Medical Director, Emergency Services,
Rockford Health System,
Rockford, Illinois

**Michael V. Vance, M.D. [129, 161]**
Associate Director, Samaritan Regional Poison Center;
Department of Medical Toxicology
Good Samaritan Medical Center
Phoenix, Arizona

**Salvator Vicario, M.D. [79]**
Department of Emergency Medicine
Humana Hospital
University of Louisville
Louisville, Kentucky

**Peter Viccellio, M.D. [148]**
Vice Chairman and Residency Program Director
Department of Emergency Medicine
School of Medicine
SUNY at Stony Brook
Stony Brook, New York

**Paul T. von Oeyen, M.D. [100]**
Assistant Professor, Obstetrics and Gynecology
Wayne State University School of Medicine;
Assistant Director, Maternal-Fetal Medicine
Department of Obstetrics and Gynecology
William Beaumont Hospital
Royal Oak, Michigan

**Robert P. Wahl, M.D. [49]**
Assistant Professor,
Department of Emergency medicine,
Wayne State University,
Detroit medical Center,
Detroit, Michigan

**James S. Walker, D.O. [161]**
Associate Professor of Surgery
Director, Emergency Medicine Residency Program
Section of Emergency Medicine,
University of Oklahoma Health Science Center,
Oklahoma City, Oklahoma

**Paul M. Wax, M.D. [153]**
Director, Adult Toxicology,
Department of Emergency Medicine,
University of Rochester Medical Center,
Rochester, New York

**Joseph F. Waeckerle, M.D. [227–231]**
Clinical Professor,
University of Missiouri at Kansas City School of Medicine;
Chairman, Department of Emergency Medicine
Baptist Medical Center
Kansas City, Missouri

**Donald Weaver, M.D. [87]**
Associate Professor of Surgery, Wayne State University;
Chief, Section of General Surgery
Harper Hospital
Detroit, Michigan

**David Jay Weber, M.D., M.P.H. [127]**
Associate Professor of Medicine, Pediatrics and Epidemiology,
UNC Schools of Medicine and Public Health,
Medical Director, Hospital Epidemiology and Occupational Health
  Service,
UNC Hospitals, Chapel Hill, North Carolina

**Michael S. Weinstock, M.D. [117]**
Chief, Department of Emergency and Ambulatory Medicine,
Memorial Hospital of Rhode Island;
Clinical Associate Professor of Surgery,
Brown University School of Medicine,
Providence, Rhode Island

**Irwin D. Weisman, M.D., Ph.D. [260]**
Staff Radiologist and Section Chief, Body MRI,
Department of Medical Imaging,
Hennepin County Medical Center,
Clinical Assistant professor of Radiology,
University of Minnesota Hospitals and Clinics,
Minneapolis, Minnesota

**Robert Welch, M.D. [68]**
Assistant Professor,
Department of Emergency Medicine,
Wayne State University,
Detroit, Michigan

**Howard A. Werman, M.D. [81]**
Assistant Professor, Division of Emergency Medicine
Ohio State University
Columbus, Ohio

**Blaine C. White, M.D. [14]**
Professor, Department of Emergency Medicine,
Wayne State University,
Detroit, Michigan

**Suzanne R. White, M.D. [137]**
Wayne State University School of Medicine
Detroit, Michigan

**John G. Wiegenstein, M.D. [171]**
Director, Department of Emergency Medicine
Michigan Capital medical Center,
Lansing, Michigan

**Marcus Williams, M.D. [53, 85]**
Assistant Professor,
Division of Cardiology,
University of North Carolina at Chapel Hill,
Chapel Hill, North Carolina

**Andrew G. Wilson, Jr. [30]**
Director, Emergency Department,
Troy Beaumont Hospital
Rochester, Michigan

**Robert F. Wilson, M.D. [19–21, 218]**
Professor and Chief,
Department of Surgery, Detroit Receiving Hospital,
Wayne State University
Detroit, Michigan

**Kimberlydawn Wisdom, M.D., M.S. [69]**
Instructor, University of Michigan Medical Center,
Ann Arbor, Michigan;
Senior Staff Physician,
Henry Ford Health System,
Detroit, Michigan

**Leslie R. Wolf [157]**
Department of Emergency Medicine
University of Cincinnati
Cincinnati, Ohio

**James R. Yankaskas, M.D. [70]**
Department of Medicine,
Division of Pulmonary Diseases,
Critical Care and Occupational Medicine,
Assistant Professor, University of North Carolina
School of Medicine,
Chapel Hill, North Carolina

**Donald M. Yealy, M.D. [34]**
Associate Professor and Associate Chief,
Division of Emergency Medicine,
University of Pittsburgh School of Medicine,
Pittsburgh, Pennsylvania

**Gary P. Young, M.D. [51]**
Chief,
Department of Emergency Medicine,
Highland General Hospital,
Oakland, California

**Mark Zwanger, M.D. [66]**
Assistant Professor of Surgery
Division of Emergency Medicine
Residency Director
Thomas Jefferson University Hospital
Philadelphia, Pennsylvania

# PREFACE

This year there were more than 90 million emergency department visits nationwide. The types of emergency services provided and the conditions that require care in the emergency department continue to expand. Ambulatory care must be provided for those who utilize the emergency department for primary care, and cognitive and technical resources must be available for patients with tertiary care problems.

The way emergency physicians approach clinical care is changing. The need for improved technology and increasing efficiency is coupled with limits on resources. Whereas in the past we were satisfied with trauma treatment, today we are learning about surveillance systems and injury prevention. We are trying to balance emergency life-sustaining technologies with patients' wishes about advance directives.

The shortage of board-prepared and residency-trained emergency physicians means that generalist physicians are providing a substantial amount of emergency care, especially in rural areas.

As always, emergency medicine meets its challenges through flexibility. Our goal continues to be to assist all students, house officers, and physicians who practice in any emergency care setting to provide the best patient care possible.

JUDITH E. TINTINALLI, MD, MS

# Prehospital Care

# 1
# EMERGENCY MEDICAL SERVICES

## G. Patrick Lilja
## Robert Swor

Emergency medical services (EMS) is the extension of emergency medical care into the community. Emergency physicians must be aware of, and have input into, the prehospital care provided to their patients. To be sure, many aspects of EMS are only indirectly under medical control, but strong medical leadership is absolutely essential for a safe and effective system.

The 1966 National Highway Safety Act authorized the U.S. Department of Transportation to fund ambulances, communications, and training programs for prehospital medical services. Coincidentally, in 1967, a mobile coronary care unit to extend coronary care into the prehospital setting was put into use in Belfast, Northern Ireland. In 1973, public law 93–154 defined a goal to improve emergency medical care and EMS on a national scale. This law identified 15 elements to be addressed in an EMS system as follows: (1) manpower, (2) training, (3) communications, (4) transportation, (5) facilities, (6) critical care units, (7) public safety agencies, (8) consumer participation, (9) access to care, (10) transfer of care, (11) standardization of patient records, (12) public information and education, (13) independent review and evaluation, (14) disaster linkage, and (15) mutual aid agreements.

## STATE ROLE

The state legislatures provide laws that broadly outline what is safe and prudent for the public good. Such laws may define levels of ambulance service capability, training requirements, equipment requirements, and requirements for physician leadership and accountability. In addition, the state health department may be the lead agency in promoting and funding EMS activity.

## LOCAL ROLE IN EMS

EMS systems must be planned, organized, and operated at the local level to be effective. Each community contemplating an EMS system must identify its resources and needs and how much service it is willing or able to afford. The 15 elements of an EMS system defined by public law 93–154 can provide very helpful guidance in this process.

### Manpower

Who will provide prehospital medical care? In urban areas public safety personnel and ambulance personnel are obvious choices, but in rural or wilderness areas volunteers, park rangers, or ski patrols may be employed. The citizenry itself should not be overlooked. Public interest and participation are key ingredients in any EMS system.

### Training

Training begins with education of the private citizen. Courses in EMS system access, cardiopulmonary resuscitation (CPR), and other forms of first aid are essential. The media can be utilized to reach large populations with the minimum information necessary to participate effectively. Some communities will opt to use a dual-response system consisting of first responders followed by ambulance personnel. First responders may be firefighters, police, park rangers, or citizen volunteers. Training for first responders may include advanced Red Cross first aid or the Department of Transportation's First Responder Course. The training for ambulance personnel is usually successful completion of an emergency medical technician (EMT) course. Although various levels of EMT training have evolved in different states, the three nationally recognized levels are emergency medical technician–ambulance (EMT-A), emergency medical technician–intermediate (EMT-I), and emergency medical technician–paramedic (EMT-P). EMT-As have the necessary first aid skills, including CPR, to take care of basic and immediately life-threatening prehospital emergency conditions. Other skills include safe extrication, immobilization, and transportation of emergency victims. EMT-I training adds the additional skills of IV access, pneumatic trouser use, and esophageal airway or endotracheal intubation. EMT-P training adds drug therapy for selected prehospital conditions, interpretation of ECG rhythms, and cardiac cardioversion and defibrillation. Recently, studies have demonstrated that EMT-As trained to operate defibrillators can markedly improve cardiac arrest survival. Obviously, physicians need to be deeply involved in all training efforts and must constantly be assured that skills and equipment are being used appropriately and safely.

### Communications

The universal 911 emergency telephone number has greatly facilitated the citizen's access to emergency medical care, although many regions of the country still do not have 911 coverage. Physicians should promote this system and seek assurance that those answering the calls have the knowledge and training to properly dispatch rescue personnel and offer first aid information to the caller when appropriate. The public needs to be encouraged to use the 911 number rather than call the hospital or the physician when certain symptoms occur. Once a request for help is received, the system must assure a rapid dispatch of appropriate personnel. A system in which key information is taken by the 911 call taker and then the appropriate unit(s) for the problem is sent is known as *Priority Dispatch* and is increasingly being utilized. Ambulance personnel must be able to communicate directly or indirectly with the hospital of destination. Most importantly, ambulance personnel must be able to communicate with the physician approved to give them direction according to their standard operating procedure protocols. The overall goal of the communications system is to provide a means of early notification, prompt dispatch of the appropriate vehicles and personnel, hospital notification, and the provision of qualified medical control.

### Transportation

Ground ambulances have evolved into sophisticated and efficient mobile patient care areas where life-saving maneuvers can be performed. Federal standards provide specifications for ambulance construction. The most important aspect of design is that the attendants must be able to provide airway and ventilatory support while safely transporting the patient. Basic life support (BLS) ambulances carry equipment appropriate for attendants trained to the EMT-A level. Advanced life support (ALS) ambulances are equipped for EMT-Ps or other health care personnel capable of drug therapy and other advanced medical procedures. Ground transportation is appropriate for the majority of ill or injured patients. Air transport should be considered if time to definitive care is important and air transport will shorten this interval (see Chap. 4).

## Facilities

Emergency patients should be delivered to the hospital of their choice unless their condition can be better treated at another hospital that the system has identified as having overriding advantages under life-threatening conditions. Several systems of categorizing hospitals exist, and this process should either precede or coincide with the development of the EMS system. Prehospital personnel should not be pawns in a struggle between hospitals fighting for commercial advantage. In some areas there may be no hospital that meets system requirements for equipment and staffing. A well-functioning EMS system cannot always rely on interfacility transport to "bail out" its hospitals and medical personnel from the necessity of resuscitating critically ill or injured patients. Therefore, emergency departments capable of resuscitating and stabilizing such patients must be present or must be developed.

## Critical Care Units

Tertiary care facilities for the management of complex problems should be identified either within the system or outside it. It is not feasible for every community to support services such as a neonatal intensive care unit, burn unit, or spinal cord injury unit.

## Public Safety Agencies

It is obviously important that any EMS system have strong ties with police and fire departments. Public safety officials must have input into EMS councils, and conversely, EMS providers must have input into public safety decisions that impact on emergency medical care.

## Consumer Participation

The public must have input into the governance of its EMS system. Lay participation on councils should be provided. The public must understand what a good EMS system offers or support will dwindle. Involvement of the lay public in first aid training and in the implementation of a 911 system are important steps in constructing a successful system.

## Access to Care

A successful EMS system ensures that all individuals have access to emergency care regardless of ability to pay. A more difficult problem exists when population densities or terrain dictate longer response times for some citizens than others. EMS councils must be able to handle these inequities, which are both politically and economically difficult to adjust. EMS councils are typically advisory bodies to County Boards or other political entities. An informed, well-represented governing body will ultimately make the best decisions.

## Transfer of Care

Patients must frequently be transferred from one medical care facility to another either within the system or outside it. Transfers must be made with maximum patient safety and convenience. Many problems can be avoided when a protocol is followed that has been previously agreed to by both of the involved medical centers. The referring physician should be assured of receiving follow-up information about the patient, and the receiving physician should be assured of receiving all the important information about the patient on arrival. Proper medical support en route should be ensured by establishing radio contact with the receiving center as soon as possible and having appropriate medical personnel accompany the patient as needed.

## Standard Patient Record

Patient care is dependent on good medical records, and prehospital records are no exception. Ambulance services within a specific region should all use a similar reporting form that can be quickly and easily interpreted by receiving nurses and physicians. It is more difficult to standardize emergency department records. However, flow sheets can be used that are easily interpretable by receiving physicians and nurses. It is also wise to design record systems that lend themselves to data extraction for trauma registries and severity scoring as well as cardiac arrest outcome studies.

## Public Information and Education

The public should be well informed about the local EMS system. Consideration should be given to the following: (1) the public should understand how it stands to benefit by an excellent EMS system, (2) the public must be prepared to render first aid care, (3) the public must know how to access the system quickly, and (4) the public should understand that patients may be delivered to hospitals not of their choice under life-threatening conditions.

## Independent Review and Evaluation

Governing agencies must be assured that ongoing review of the EMS system occurs. Monitoring radio communications, review of response times, and review of run sheets are relatively mechanical methods of quality control that are easily implemented. Outcome studies of such entities as cardiac arrest and multiple trauma require considerable physician input and cooperation. The system medical director should require that such studies be conducted periodically. System access to hospital charts should be a requirement for participating hospitals, with due concern for patient privacy.

## Disaster Linkage

Disaster care is discussed later in this section (Chap. 6, "Disaster Medical Services"). The EMS system is an integral part of disaster preparedness and should be involved in planning and practice drills along with the public safety agencies and others. Public safety agencies should keep the EMS system informed of potential disaster situations or hazards that may temporarily be present. Also, hospitals must be prepared to keep the EMS system informed of their capacity to receive certain kinds of patients under disaster conditions.

## Mutual Aid Agreements

Communities should develop mutual aid agreements with their neighbors so that uninterrupted emergency care is available despite local exigencies.

## MEDICAL CONTROL

A safe and effective EMS system requires considerable physician input and surveillance to provide the best possible patient care. Emergency physicians must be involved in providing this control. Medical control consists of immediate, or "on-line," and "off-line" control (also called indirect medical control).

On-line (immediate) medical control is the provision of direct medical orders to personnel in the field either in person or by radio or phone communication. The service medical director delegates this authority to other physicians but must be assured that they understand the protocols under which the paramedics are allowed to administer care. Also, the medical director may allow ambulance personnel to carry out certain standing orders when contact with the controlling physician is not feasible in a timely fashion.

Off-line (indirect) medical control is the responsibility of the service medical director. Three main components of the off-line medical director are (1) development of protocols, (2) development of medical accountability (quality assurance), and (3) development of ongoing education. Protocol development describes those treatment procedures that prehospital personnel may perform under the medical license of the medical director. Protocols should not only address care but also specify what types of medical devices should be utilized. It is imperative that the medical director approve the medical devices utilized in the out-of-hospital environment. These protocols must be reviewed and rewritten on a regular basis to keep pace with current medical knowledge. Quality assurance requires ongoing surveillance and study of the system. It is mandatory that physicians be involved, both to review treatment and to suggest improvement in areas where deficiencies may be noted. Physicians must remember that they have the ultimate responsibility for the prehospital medical care provided. Lastly, the off-line medical director is responsible for the ongoing educational needs of the prehospital care providers under his or her direction. This means that the quality and content of the training should be directed by the medical director.

## MEDICAL BASIS FOR EMERGENCY MEDICINE SERVICES

### Emergency Cardiac Care

It is clear that advanced life support (ALS) saves lives after sudden cardiac arrest. Early studies by groups in Seattle and King County, Washington, demonstrated that as many as 26 percent of patients may be successfully resuscitated from out-of-hospital cardiac arrest. Further work in Milwaukee demonstrated a 16 percent rate of survival to hospital discharge. The overwhelming majority of survivors are from cardiac arrests that are witnessed and have an initial cardiac rhythm of ventricular fibrillation (VF). Survival is clearly related to the time from collapse of the patient to delivery of defibrillation and declines dramatically with delays of greater than a few minutes. Early literature documented 40 percent survival if treatment was within 4 min but less than 10 percent if treatment was after 10 min. There is tremendous variation in survival data, with some systems replicating these high survival rates and some large urban systems reporting very few survivors.

The documentation that survival is clearly linked to rapid defibrillation led a number of authors to train basic EMTs, who arrive first at the scene of an emergency, to recognize and treat ventricular fibrillation. Systems in King County and Iowa documented that this approach improves survival from cardiac arrest if the interval between collapse and defibrillation is short. Initial studies utilized manual defibrillators but have led to the development of automatic external defibrillators (AED), devices that evaluate cardiac rhythm and defibrillate the patient if VF is recognized. AEDs are reliable for use by personnel with minimal medical training and may be used by firefighters, police officers, and other first responders. The American Heart Association has adopted the position that first-response defibrillation should be the standard of care for all EMS systems in the United States. Because effectiveness depends on early defibrillation after cardiac arrest, citizen awareness of the signs of cardiac arrest, quick access to the EMS system, and rapid and appropriate EMS dispatch are all critical links to maximize survival.

Despite the emphasis on treatment of cardiac arrest in development of EMS systems, cardiac arrest constitutes less than 3 percent of an EMS system's volume. The most common clinical entities treated and transported by EMS systems are signs and symptoms suggestive of cardiac ischemia. Common treatment modalities include relief of ischemic chest pain with nitrates and narcotic analgesics; control of cardiac arrhythmias with antiarrhythmics; treatment of symptomatic bradydysrhythmias with external pacemakers; and treatment of left ventricular failure with diuretics and bronchodilators and, if necessary, endotracheal intubation. Most EMS authorities agree that prevention of cardiac arrest and decreasing cardiovascular morbidity through treatment of dysrhythmias, ischemic pain, and heart failure are true benefits of an ALS system. There is a lack of research to document this assertion.

An evolving role for ALS systems is to facilitate the management of the patient with an acute myocardial infarction (AMI). In addition to treating complications prior to hospital arrival, ALS units may facilitate emergency department treatment as well. The literature has documented significant emergency department time delays in the administration of thrombolytic agents for AMI. Transport by EMS units equipped with 12-lead ECG capability can decrease the time to emergency department treatment. Some EMS systems have demonstrated that the prehospital administration of thrombolytic agents is safe and decreases time to treatment. However, since no decrease in mortality has been documented, and training, equipment, and logistical costs are significant, the role of prehospital thrombolytic therapy appears limited at this time.

### Trauma Care

EMS care of the trauma patient is more controversial. There is widespread agreement that development of systems of trauma care, with rapid delivery of critically injured trauma patients to a trauma center, saves lives. Trauma systems have been designed whereby certain hospitals can be bypassed and patients delivered to a trauma center, as long as predetermined protocols, based on mechanism of injury or the patient's physiologic status, are followed.

There is less agreement on what therapy should be given by EMS providers. A markedly decreased mortality rate in war casualties was demonstrated if femur fractures were splinted prior to transportation. The landmark monograph, *"Accidental Death and Disability: The Neglected Disease of Modern Society,"* reported that 10 percent of patients with cervical spine injuries were made worse by treatment prior to hospital arrival and that careful attention to neck injuries would decrease morbidity and mortality.

Some literature reported *decreased* survival if a patient received ALS (intravenous lines and intubation) at the scene of a penetrating thoracic injury because this resulted in a delay to definitive care. Other studies have reported improved physiologic parameters and injury outcome when compared to historical controls. The most compelling literature has shown that paramedics may secure an airway, establish an intravenous line, and infuse significant volumes of fluid rapidly without delaying transport of the patient. New techniques, such as administration of hypertonic fluid, have been suggested as appropriate for field use but are still being investigated. Emphasis on rapid transport of the trauma victim and provision of supportive measures en route are well-accepted guidelines for EMS personnel.

### Medical and Pediatric Care

Besides the management of cardiac ischemia and trauma, other areas of importance to EMS systems are the management of respiratory distress, altered mental status, and pediatric emergencies. The management of respiratory distress is an important function of the EMS system. Paramedics are skilled at airway control by endotracheal and nasotracheal intubation, and appear to perform the procedures appropriately and with minimal complications. Early advanced airway measures for upper airway obstruction from burns, trauma, foreign body, or angioedema may be life-saving. Most systems administer aerosolized $\beta_2$ agonists for asthma and chronic obstructive pulmonary disease. Some systems use pulse oximetry to monitor hypoxemia. While effective, oximetry is costly and has not been widely utilized.

For patients with altered mental status, the administration of glucose for hypoglycemia and naloxone for suspected narcotic overdose can be life-saving. Control of seizures with diazepam or airway support for status epilepticus are similarly important functions.

Attention is now being focused on the care of the child in the EMS system. About 5 to 10 percent of a system's volume involves children aged 16 and under. The most common entities treated are upper and lower respiratory emergencies and trauma. Cardiac arrest in children is a rare event with a dismal outcome. The ability of paramedics to perform cardiac procedures on children is variable and often depends on the age of the child, but rates of successful intubation and intravenous access are comparable to those for adults. Endotracheal intubation and intravenous access in infants is often unsuccessful. However, many EMS systems have trained paramedics in intraosseous infusion and the rectal administration of antiepileptic drugs.

## Other Field Interventions

In addition to technical emergency medical care, EMTs and paramedics perform other invaluable functions in the care of out-of-hospital patients. A large number of EMS patients are evaluated and released without ever formally entering the health care system as we think of it. Such patients are assessed for their need for emergency medical care and their competency to refuse care. Some EMS systems have trained EMS providers to assess home situations and make social service referrals as needed. For example, a paramedic can request social service assistance for an elderly patient who has fallen and is found to have an unheated, dirty apartment. As on-scene providers, EMS professionals can assess the potential for abuse or neglect of children and the elderly or intervene in cases of domestic violence. Other innovative functions for EMS personnel are to participate in injury prevention and education, similar to the fire prevention efforts of firefighters. Finally, some EMS systems are evaluating the use of EMS providers to provide immunizations and home evaluations.

## SUMMARY

All emergency physicians deal with emergency medical services as a part of their daily practice. They should be aware of common problems encountered in the prehospital setting and approaches to these problems. The level of prehospital care given in a community is directly related to the involvement of the emergency medical community.

## BIBLIOGRAPHY

Eisenberg MS, Horwood BT, Cummins RO, et al: Cardiac arrest and resuscitation: A tale of 29 cities. *Ann Emerg Med* 19(2):179, 1990.

Gervin AS, Fischer RP: The importance of prompt transport in salvage of patients with penetrating heart wounds. *J Trauma* 22(6):443, 1982.

Kuehl S (ed): *Prehospital Systems and Medical Oversight,* 2d ed. National Association of EMS Physicians. St. Louis, Mosby, 1994.

National Academy of Sciences, National Research Council: *Accidental Death and Disability: The Neglected Disease of Modern Society.* US Dept of Health, Education and Welfare 1966.

Pionkowski RS: Resuscitation time in ventricular fibrillation—a prognostic indicator. *Ann Emerg Med* 12(12):733, 1983.

Stultz KR, Brown DD, Schug VL, Bean JA: Prehospital defibrillation performed by emergency medical technicians in rural communities. *N Engl J Med* 310:219, 1984.

Weaver WD, Hill D, Fahrenbruch CE, et al: Use of the automatic external defibrillator in the management of out-of-hospital cardiac arrest. *N Engl J Med* 319:661, 1988.

West JG, Trunkey DD, Lim RC: Systems of trauma care: A study of two counties. *Arch Surg,* 114:455, 1979.

# 2
# PREHOSPITAL DEVICES
### Daniel G. Hankins
### Scott Freeman

Immobilization of the spine and extremities are important functions of prehospital care. Devices commonly used to immobilize the spine and extremities and use of the military antishock trouser (MAST) garment are reviewed in this chapter.

## SPINAL IMMOBILIZATION

The preservation of integrity of the spinal column and spinal cord is of paramount importance in the field, along with establishment and maintenance of the airway. The first person to assess the patient immediately immobilizes the cervical spine and simultaneously performs a modified jaw thrust to open the airway, if necessary. Manual stabilization of the neck is not released until the patient has been transferred and securely strapped to a board. Whether both short and long boards are used or a long board is used alone depends on the initial position in which the patient is found by the emergency medical technician (EMT) or first responder.

Carrying boarded patients takes a heavy toll on the backs of EMTs and paramedics. Evaluation of the boarded patient is more expensive and time-consuming in the emergency department because of the need to clear the cervical spine. However, low-risk criteria for spinal injury have not been well defined for the prehospital arena. Ideal guidelines for prehospital personnel necessarily would have high sensitivity and specificity for cervical spine injuries.

## Spinal Boards and Cervical Collars

Spinal boards, either short or long, are made from plastic or wood to provide a rigid surface on which to bind the patient to ensure that no movement occurs in the cervical, thoracic, or lumbar spine. Straps are used to secure the patient for transport. Some boards are provided with firm rubber head blocks on either side of the head and straps to go across these blocks to keep the head steady between them. Blanket rolls secured to the board with tape are also effective head blocks. A popular and effective variation of the short board is the KED board (Kendrick Extrication Device), which consists of slats of rigid material bound together by heavy cloth. This board immobilizes the cervical spine, wraps partly around the patient, and is then strapped the rest of the way around for secure immobilization. The patient can be lifted by the KED board, allowing for easier extrication.

Rigid cervical collars are more accurately called *cervical extrication devices.* Multiple types are used in the field, such as the "Philadelphia collar," the "Stifneck," and the "Neck-Loc." The collars come in two asymmetric pieces, which are used and marked for "back" and "front," or as a single piece that is folded into the correct shape. By themselves, collars are not adequate for cervical immobilization but require additional lateral support to avoid movement in that direction. For adequate immobilization, the patient needs to be strapped on the back board and secured with head blocks and head straps. Once the patient is well secured to the board, the collar does not add a significant amount of stabilization and can actually be removed without compromise of the spine. It is often left in place for added protection, however. Patients with mandible or soft tissue neck injuries should probably not have a collar applied because of the potential for airway compromise, which could be masked by the collar. Newer collars have openings in the front to allow observation of the trachea and jugular veins, but this may not be adequate for observing other neck areas. Soft cervical collars are not adequate for out-of-hospital care.

## Sequence of Spinal Immobilization

Prehospital personnel are taught to have a high index of suspicion for spine trauma. If the patient is sitting in a car after an accident and is stable from respiratory and circulatory standpoints, the short spine board and rigid cervical collar are first used to safely get the patient out of the car; then the patient is moved to the long spine board. If the situation at hand is a critical one, because of the patient's condition or the threat of hazards such as chemicals, fire, or water, the patient can be extricated more rapidly.

At a noncritical scene, when the patient is still sitting in the vehicle, one EMT secures the neck with his or her hands and applies the necessary airway maneuvers, while the second EMT applies the rigid cervical collar. The short board is then slid in behind the patient and the patient is strapped to the short spine board. (Short boards are not used if the patient is not seated in a vehicle.) The first EMT maintains manual stabilization of the neck until the patient is secured to the short board. The patient can then be rotated around and slid directly on to the long board positioned on the car seat or on the ambulance cot. The MAST garment, if needed, is often already placed on the long board underneath the patient. The patient is then strapped to the long board and then to the cot. A properly boarded patient can be turned on the board or even stood on end if necessary to move the patient to the ambulance. If the patient vomits, for instance, the board can be partly logrolled up to prevent aspiration.

Because of the difference in relative size and positions of head and body, adults and children need slightly different positioning on a backboard. An adult needs more padding under the head, while a child needs more padding under the body, to maintain neutral neck position.

In more dangerous situations where rapid extrication is required, the short board is omitted. The rigid cervical collar is still used. The patient is carefully rotated out and slid on to the waiting long board.

If a patient is walking at the scene when the paramedical personnel arrive but complains of neck pain, the patient will be boarded from a standing position. If the patient is lying on the ground when the EMTs arrive, the patient will be carefully logrolled by several attendants onto a long backboard.

Radiographs can be done without difficulty through short and long boards. In general, patients should not be removed from these devices until the spine has been cleared clinically or roentgenographically. If necessary before clearing by x-ray, removal of the patient should be done carefully with a six-person lift.

## EXTREMITY IMMOBILIZATION

Most fractures encountered in the field are splinted for patient comfort and ease of transport. Air splints, or circumferential bladders that are inflated by mouth, are adequate for most distal fractures of the upper and lower extremities. In hot weather, air splints can be difficult to remove when they stick to the skin. It is better to use an air splint with a zipper and powder the inside for easy removal. The MAST garment can function as an air splint for one or both lower extremities. Other splinting possibilities include simple sling and swathe, tying the legs together with cravats to splint one injured leg with the other normal one, or using a pillow wrapped around an extremity and secured with tape. A pillow splint is comfortable and secure for the patient either out-of-hospital or in the emergency department.

## Traction Splints

Pelvic fractures and fractures of the femoral shaft are potentially life- and limb-threatening.

Stabilization of pelvic fractures is difficult. Indeed, the only effective method in the field or in the emergency department is with the MAST garment with all compartments inflated (see below). Radiographs can be performed through the shock garment.

Fractures of the femur can damage vessels and nerves when bony fragments move. Stabilization in the field is imperative to minimize blood loss and soft tissue damage. While antishock trousers are often used to stabilize femur fractures, they do limit patient assessment and cannot reduce the fracture. The femoral traction splint is the preferred device for femur fractures.

Several leg traction splint variations are available for use. The two most commonly used types are the Hare splint and the Sager splint. Other traction splints (Thomas Ring, Donway, Klippel) are less commonly used. The underlying mechanism is the application of traction by a hitch on the ankle, against resistance when the splint impinges proximally on the pelvis. The padded proximal end of the Hare splint abuts the ischial tuberosity (Fig. 2-1). The proximal end of the Sager splint rests against the pubic symphysis. These splints cannot be used if a pelvic fracture is suspected since the pressure on the pelvis may further displace a fracture and cause more bleeding. Another contraindication is the presence of a hip dislocation.

Leg traction splints may also be used for tibial shaft fractures. Traction splints should not be used for fractures near the knee, to avoid further neurovascular injury if traction is applied. Traction splints for the tibia should be reserved for angulated or displaced fractures; otherwise, an air splint or the MAST would suffice.

At the scene, clothing is removed, and the extremity assessed for injury and distal neurovascular function. If the Hare is used, the proximal half ring is placed in the crease of the buttocks against the ischial tuberosity. Traction is placed on the ankle with the padded ankle strap by one rescuer while the splint is strapped to the leg. The ankle strap is then attached to a ratcheting mechanism, and traction is tightened (Fig. 2-1). If a Sager is used, the splint is placed on the medial side of the limb up against the groin. The padded ankle hitch is applied, and traction placed until adequate. Elastic straps are then applied to hold the splint to the leg.

The Hare splint can be longer than an ambulance cot when fully extended, and care needs to be taken when closing the rear door of the ambulance. The Sager is shorter than the Hare, and one Sager can be used to splint both legs stimultaneously. The Sager is smaller and less bulky and therefore takes up less room in an ambulance or a helicopter.

## MAST

The MAST garment, a one-piece layered device made of polyvinyl fabric, is capable of sustaining internal air pressures of up to 104 mmHg and is used to reverse the signs of shock. It encloses the body from the lower rib cage to, but not including, the feet. The lower extremities are each enclosed separately, allowing access to the perineal area. Three compartments cover the abdomen and two extremities and are fastened with Velcro fasteners. Some versions of the garment allow separate inflation and deflation of these compartments. Most are inflated with a foot pump and are equipped with an interposed inflation pressure monitoring device. Internal pressures of the suit are limited by a pressure relief valve and the ability of the Velcro fastener to withstand stress.

MAST effects appear to include at least four mechanisms: (1) tamponade of bleeding in the lower body, (2) increase in peripheral resistance in the lower body, (3) selective perfusion of the upper body, and (4) an initial increase of venous return (preload) from the lower body. The fourth mechanism plays a minor role in reversing hypotension.

## Physiological Effects

### Vascular Resistance

The effect of the MAST suit on hypotension was attributed to an increase in peripheral vascular resistance by George Crile, who in-

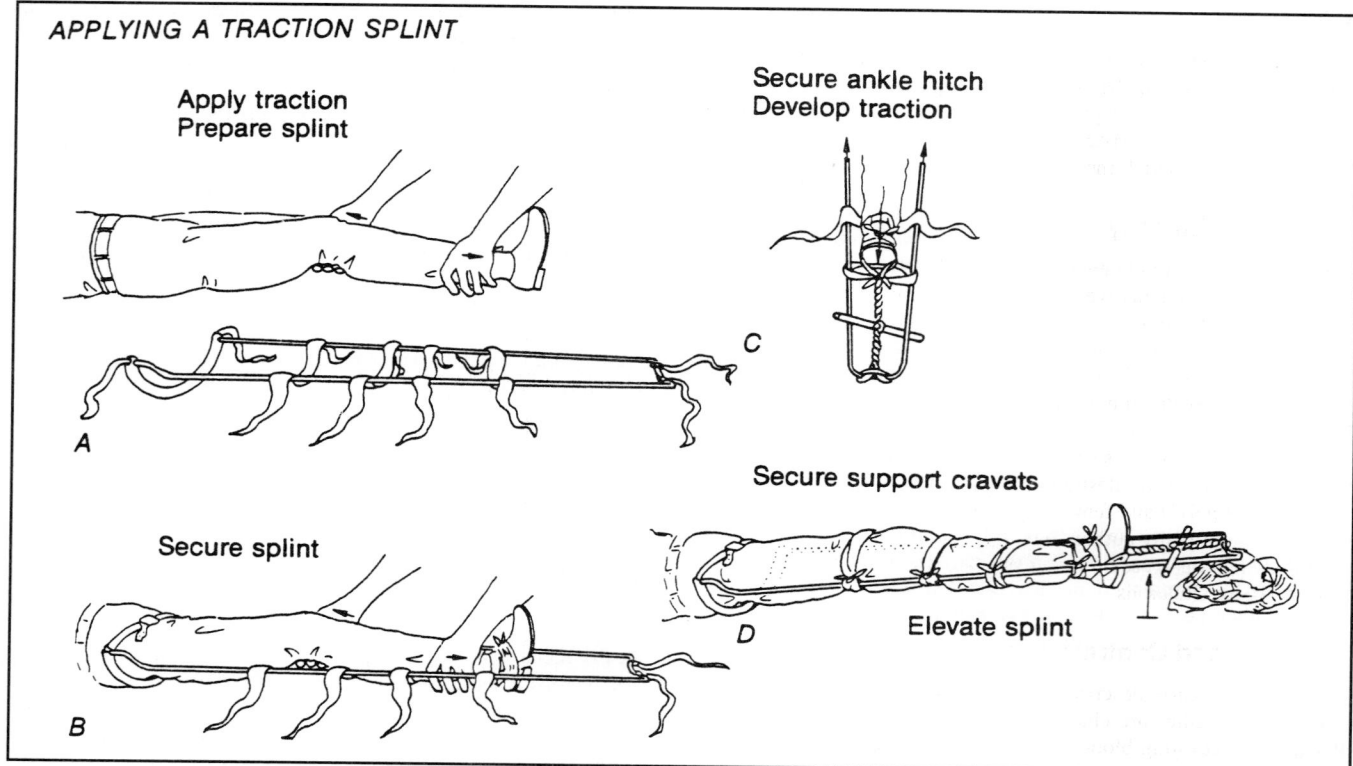

**Fig. 2-1.** Applying a traction splint. (From Caroline NL: *Emergency Care in the Streets,* 2d ed. Boston, Little, Brown, 1983, with permission.)

vented the device in 1903. Numerous authors have demonstrated increases in vascular resistance in the areas covered by the device. Some studies suggest that systemic vascular resistance increases when MAST suits are applied, and this is consistent with the observed elevation of blood pressure.

### Regional Blood Flow

Redistribution of blood flow has been demonstrated in animal experiments. In a nonshock model, flows in the carotid artery increased, while femoral artery blood flow decreased.

### Blood Pressure

The degree of blood pressure elevation is related to blood volume and inflation pressure. Blood pressure rises more with hypovolemia than with normovolemia. Several studies suggest that MAST pressures up to 60 mmHg produce the most significant increases in blood pressure and inflation pressures above this have less effect.

### Hemorrhage Control

Direct pressure is one of the traditional methods for controlling hemorrhage, and MAST slows blood loss in the areas covered by the suit. This has been attributed to decreases in vessel size and decreases in the open area of wounds. Pressure from pneumatic enclosures is also transmitted to the tissues. The pressure in the perinephric space of dogs with inflated MAST suits has been observed to be 80 percent of the suit pressure. In a shock animal model an increase in lactate was observed in the structures covered by the suit when it was inflated above systolic pressure. Centrally obtained lactate levels rose in this setting on deflation of the garment.

### Cardiac Preload

Early reports suggested that volume was displaced to the thorax when the antigravity suit was inflated. Despite this work and the earlier

suggestion that MAST suits functioned because of alterations in vascular resistance, many subsequent reports persisted in reporting that the effect of MAST suits was due primarily to an increase in preload or autotransfusion. This presumed mechanism of action was probably based on observations of the amount of fluid required to maintain blood pressure as the garment was deflated.

In an attempt to simulate the usual setting in which the MAST device is used, one team phlebotomized human volunteers and measured their blood volumes by isotope scanning before and after application of MAST. Isotope scanning allowed evaluation of the blood volume in a compartmental manner. Although the phlebotomy in this experiment amounted to 17 percent of the total blood volume, the amount displaced to the upper body was measured as less than 5 percent. The mean blood volume after phlebotomy was 4434 mL, rendering the autotransfused amount less than 222 mL for this group. Another team induced shock by phlebotomy and obtained direct measurements of the inferior vena cava flow as MAST inflation occurred. The volume of autotransfused blood in this setting was about 4 mL/kg, which, if extrapolated to humans, agrees with volumes determined to have autotransfused by noninvasive techniques. The degree of preload augmentation suggests that it is not the dominant factor in elevating blood pressure.

### Pulmonary Function

Pulmonary function can be restricted by MAST, probably because it limits diaphragmatic excursion. In normal human volunteers, inflation to 100 mmHg decreased vital capacity by 13.8 percent. A case report of a patient with traumatic quadriplegia demonstrated a larger decrease in vital capacity. At 100 mmHg MAST inflation pressure, vital capacity was decreased 42 percent with preservation of the forced expiratory volume/forced vital capacity (FEV/FVC) ratio. In one retrospective study of 25 patients requiring MAST for shock, only those with head injury (4 out of 5) showed evidence of hypercarbia.

## CNS

The effect of MAST on intracranial pressure has been examined in animal models. Even in the presence of experimentally created intracranial mass lesions, no significant changes in intracranial pressure were observed when the MAST suit was inflated. Cerebral perfusion pressure in a shock model improved after MAST inflation.

### Benefits and Efficacy

Mattox et al. prospectively evaluated the prehospital use of MAST in 911 patients. MAST suits were applied to victims of blunt or penetrating trauma with a systolic blood pressure less than 90 mmHg. Contrary to expectations, mortality was increased in the group that had MAST suits applied, especially in those with thoracic injury. Clearly, further evaluation of indications for use and benefits in trauma patients is needed.

Control of hemorrhage secondary to pelvic fracture, gynecologic hemorrhage, and gastrointestinal hemorrhage, and stabilization of fractures of the pelvis and femur have been indications for the use of MAST. Although many authors have reported use of the garment for such indications on a case-report basis, little is known about actual efficacy in these situations.

### Indications and Contraindications

It is difficult to clearly describe the indications for the use of MAST. Contemporary studies are challenging once-established views of the importance of elevating blood pressure with this device in the setting of shock. A list of relative and absolute indications and contraindications may expand as we reach a better understanding of the garment's effects. General indications for application are (1) to correct hypotension if the systolic blood pressure is below 100 mmHg in the presence of clinical shock, (2) to control pelvic or intraabdominal hemorrhage, and (3) to stabilize pelvic or femur fractures. Increases in systolic blood pressure with decreases in pulse rate have been reported when the MAST garment has been applied for treatment of septic, anaphylactic, or neurogenic shock.

Reports of termination of paroxysmal supraventricular tachycardia in both adults and children exist. When to apply MAST instead of conventional therapy is unclear.

An absolute contraindication for the use of MAST is the presence of pulmonary edema. Relative contraindications for MAST use are pregnancy, impaled objects, evisceration of the abdominal contents, and thoracic and diaphragmatic injuries. Use of MAST suits results in an increase in the vascular resistance of the lower extremities, and this may not be well tolerated by all patients.

Compartment syndromes in the lower extremity have been attributed to the use of MAST on numerous occasions. This is not a frequent complication of their use but one that is potentially serious. The length of time that MAST may be applied without the risk of developing compartment syndrome is not clear. Reports exist of compartment syndrome in untraumatized lower extremities after 140 minutes of MAST application.

### Application and Removal

The MAST garment is designed to be applied with the patient supine. The leg compartments are inflated first, then the abdominal compartment. Inflation should stop when systolic blood pressure reaches 100 mmHg or when the device itself limits further inflation. Application of the device for more than 2 h should raise concern about the development of compartment syndrome in the lower extremities. Deflation should be done in a stepwise manner that is the reverse of the inflation sequence. Deflation should be discontinued if the blood pressure falls more than 5 mmHg, and volume expansion with crystalloid or blood is necessary before further deflation. Deflation of MAST is as-

sociated with an increase in metabolic acidosis, but this should not become clinically significant.

Changes in temperature and altitude can cause pressure changes in the garment. For instance, if the garment were applied in an environment where the temperature was 38°C (100°F) and the patient were transported in an air-conditioned environment of 24°C (75°F), the suit could lose as much as 28 mmHg of pressure. Pressure within the suit rises as altitude increases and falls as altitude decreases. Extrapolation from experimental data reveals that MAST pressure changes by approximately 1.8 mmHg for each 1000-ft (350-m) change in altitude.

### BIBLIOGRAPHY

Campbell JE: *Basic Trauma Life Support: Advanced Prehospital Care.* Englewood Cliffs, NJ, Brady, 1988.

Hauswald M, Greene E: Aortic blood flow during sequential MAST inflation. *Ann Emerg Med* 15(11):1297, 1986.

Heckman JD (ed): *Emergency Care and Transportation of the Sick and Injured,* 5th ed. Rosemont, IL, American Academy of Orthopaedic Surgeons, 1993.

Johnson G, Bond R, Stack L, et al: Efficacy of military antishock trousers in compensatory and decompensatory hemorrhagic hypotension. *Circ Shock* 21:233, 1987.

Mattox K, Bickell W, Pepe P, et al: Prospective MAST study in 911 patients. *J Trauma* 29(8):1104, 1989.

McSwain NE: Pneumatic anti-shock garment: State of the art 1988. *Ann Emerg Med* 17(5):506, 1988.

Niemann J, Stapczynski J, Rosborough J, et al: Hemodynamic effects of pneumatic external counterpressure in canine hemorrhagic shock. *Ann Emerg Med* 12:661, 1983.

# 3

# RURAL EMS

## Nicholas H. Benson
## N. Heramba Prasad

## INTRODUCTION

There is no clear definition of what constitutes a rural area. The Office of Management and Budget (OMB) defines a metropolitan statistical area (MSA) as a "densely populated urban core with at least 50,000 people that is part of a county or counties comprised of at least 100,000 residents." Any region not included in the MSA can be considered rural. However, this chapter focuses on areas much less populated. Rural areas are perhaps best defined as the regions within boundaries specified by state or local officials that have a population of less than 5000. Approximately four-fifths of the country's land mass is considered rural; however, only one-fourth of the population lives in these areas.

A population of 10,000 residents may generate only one true emergency call a day. Small communities must be prepared for relatively low call volumes, unevenly distributed during the course of a year. This raises the obvious concerns of financial support and maintenance of skills by rural emergency medical services (EMS) agencies. In addition, long distances, lack of other health care resources, and inadequate communications further magnify the problems faced by rural EMS systems.

Some studies report that in rural areas transportation of the elderly with cardiac and related medical problems comprises 54 to 70 percent of all EMS calls, as compared to about 29 percent in urban areas. Routine and interfacility transfers are also more likely to occur in rural areas.

Motor vehicle crashes on rural roads may go unrecognized for a prolonged period of time in sparsely populated areas because of infrequent traffic and poor telephone facilities along the roadways. While injuries in rural areas occur as frequently as in urban areas, they tend to be more serious. The death rate from unintentional injuries is reported to be twice as high in rural as in urban communities. Death rates are inversely proportional to population density. More than half of fatal traffic collisions occur in rural areas.

The primary goals of a good EMS system include well-organized and rapid medical assistance and transportation, strong EMS physician support, quick public access, and communications. These goals should remain the same for urban as well as rural systems. The unique problems outlined above make it harder for a rural EMS system to achieve its goals.

## REGULATION AND POLICY

The issues facing state and local regulation of rural EMS providers demonstrate some of the key differences between rural and urban and suburban out-of-hospital care. The U.S. Department of Transportation's National Highway Traffic Safety Administration (NHTSA) has been responsible for development of the national standard curricula for emergency medical technicians of various levels for many years. In 1990, a contract was awarded by NHTSA for the revision of the emergency medical technician (EMT) Basic National Standard Curriculum. One of the key aspects of this revision process was to ensure review of the new curriculum by EMS personnel with strong experience in rural areas. Since so many rural providers operate at the basic life support level and are composed strictly of volunteers, this curriculum would be heavily utilized in the education of these personnel.

Every state in the nation is interested in ensuring that all of its citizens will have access to quality prehospital care. This is often easier in urban and suburban environments, where a solid tax revenue base can support paid services with strong funding of personnel, equipment, and supplies. In rural areas, there is generally heavy reliance on volunteers. Some states have adopted special statutes and regulations to increase the retention of these individuals in providing out-of-hospital care. Some state legislatures have passed statutes providing retirement benefits for persons providing volunteer EMS services for more than 25 years, death benefits, and scholarships for the children of volunteers. The state may preferentially distribute federal and state grant funds to volunteer, rural providers, rather than their urban counterparts. Also, when additional procedures or medications are considered for a level of care, for example, adding new medications for EMT–intermediates, the additional hours required for initial education and continuing education about these medications must be taken into account; the time that volunteers can deduct from their paying jobs and family lives to devote to EMS education is limited.

The Department of Transportation, in addition to curricula, also supplies federal grant funds specifically related to highway safety. Section 402 and Section 403 both supply grant funding for a variety of state-level highway safety initiatives, which include emergency medical services. In 1987 to 1988, these two sections combined distributed over $5 million dollars in funding, which was frequently augmented by individual states. These grant funds, albeit limited, are an important source for rural providers to obtain equipment and educational resources that might otherwise be unavailable.

## RESOURCE MANAGEMENT

A community of 5000 people is likely to generate approximately 500 EMS calls per year (10 percent of the population). This is an average of less than two calls per day. The urgency of these calls may vary from true emergencies to routine transfers.

Six percent of the nation's 2393 rural counties have no physicians, and one-quarter of rural residents live in federally designated health manpower shortage areas (HMSA). Soaring medical costs, combined with small patient volumes and the decline in the national economy, have resulted in the closure of over 550 hospitals in rural areas since 1981. Difficulty in recruiting and retaining health care personnel by rural health care facilities and the closure of the local hospitals put an extra burden on the rural EMS systems since in some areas they have become the only resource for nonemergent transports over long distances or for urgent primary care services such as delivering babies.

Many rural EMS providers are staffed by volunteers who are trained to the EMT–Basic (EMT-B) or EMT–Defibrillation level. They are forced to depend on donations from the community for revenue. Increasing regulations from federal agencies and insurance carriers make it difficult for the volunteer services to survive the current economic climes. Proven sources of revenue for urban EMS systems, such as the creation of EMS tax districts, billing patients for services, or "subscriber" systems, may not generate adequate income in sparsely populated areas.

Another area of concern is the availability of air medical transport services. It may take as long as 90 minutes for a helicopter, based in a tertiary care facility, to reach a remote, rural area.

Difficulty in recruiting physicians and nurses who are qualified or experienced in out-of-hospital care also results in lack of EMS medical supervision, both on-line and off-line. Without adequate physician support, many rural programs encounter suboptimal initial education and lack of focused and effective continuing education.

## MANPOWER AND TRAINING

Approximately three-fourths of rural EMS providers are volunteers. This frequently poses a problem for adequate daytime coverage, since the volunteers usually have daytime jobs. Failure to respond to calls is probably more common in rural areas than reported, especially during daytime. A well-planned mutual aid agreement with neighboring EMS agencies becomes more important in rural areas than in urban areas with full-time paid EMS services. Establishment of paid daytime coverage and volunteer nighttime coverage has been attempted in certain regions, but a recent study in eastern North Carolina showed that the problem of failing to respond to requests may not decrease. Additionally, because of prolonged EMS response times, relying on first responders to provide initial care until the arrival of EMTs is perhaps a viable alternative in rural communities compared to urbanized areas. These first responders may be police, fire personnel, or local citizens.

High turn-over rate of the rural EMTs further adds to the problem of prolonged response and transport times. Attempts to implement the strict education requirements used for urban EMS programs further decrease the retention of available volunteers. This does not mean that the quality of out-of-hospital medical care should be compromised. While designing an EMS program for a rural community, the call volume, level of care needed in an area, and appropriate educational program should be taken into consideration by the community, the EMS agency, and the EMS physician. Simply using guidelines proven to be successful in urban areas is not desirable.

In an attempt to improve retention of volunteers, certain innovative programs and incentives may be offered: use of EMS training as a desirable or necessary qualification for other occupations and the creation of new job opportunities for EMTs in other health care or educational facilities are some ways to help retain the volunteer EMT. Junior EMT programs, offered to high school students, not only serve as a ready source of new members to local volunteer squads, but also help expose the students to the field of medicine and allied health sciences at an early stage. Attempts to decrease the cost of educational programs and to increase the quality (e.g., teleconferences with the regional tertiary care centers or with established urban educational programs), establishing adequate stress management and counseling especially after major and critical incidents, provision of adequate feedback, and quality improvement programs by the sponsor hospital and the EMS medical director will also help to reduce the high turnover rate of rural EMTs.

There are currently 36 levels of EMS care in the nation, ranging from ambulance attendants to paramedics. The training requirements vary from state to state for these levels. As a general rule, the state EMS agency and the state EMS medical director establish the requirements for education. Careful planning by the squad, local medical director, and the community as to what level of care is suitable for the region will help to achieve maximum benefit. Many citizens and local physicians are totally unaware of their EMS system capabilities and are not familiar with the state guidelines under which the EMTs operate. The recently proposed Department of Transportation curriculum changes, better definition of the role of rural hospitals (designation of facilities), development of statewide surveillance system and feedback, quality assurance programs, regional/national EMS database development, and proper guidelines and support to protect the volunteer EMT from communicable diseases are other avenues that may reduce the frustrations in rural EMS.

The majority of rural EMS transportation deals with the elderly. Therefore it would seem desirable that the rural EMTs be trained in the use of semiautomatic external defibrillators (SAED) and some advanced airway techniques. However, use of SAED alone, without addressing the other problems encountered in rural EMS, may not improve survival. Capabilities to provide intravenous fluid resuscitation in a trauma victim may be necessary in certain remote areas.

## TRANSPORTATION

It is estimated that there are 35,000 ambulances in the nation. The vast majority are staffed by EMT-Bs. The design and equipment of these ambulances are regulated by state agencies. Most rural transports are by ground ambulance crews.

Volunteer systems are generally community-based. Proper planning and sharing of resources with neighboring areas is rarely undertaken. Because of this, in some areas, there is a discrepancy in the number of available ambulances and call volume.

There are over 200 air medical services programs in the country transporting an estimated 140,000 patients a year. Most of these services are based at tertiary care facilities and may not be readily available in remote and sparsely populated areas. Some services have overcome this problem by placing "satellite services" in remote locations, but low volume and high cost make this impractical for many privately owned helicopter services. Air medical services are frequently utilized for interfacility transfers of trauma victims. Only about 15 to 25 percent of trauma victims are transported directly from the scene of the motor vehicle crash. In some rural areas, this number may be as low as 7 percent. Guidelines for the rural EMT to activate the air medical transport system, defining the role of the local health care facility, and regionalization of trauma centers may improve the use of helicopters by rural EMS providers. Cost, appropriate utilization, safety of air medical transport, and patient outcome must be evaluated by the rural EMS agency and the EMS medical director.

Access to the scene of injury or illness may pose additional problems in wilderness areas. Specialized air, water, or specific geographic rescue units may be necessary. Depending on the terrain, the victim may have to be moved by these special rescue units before traditional ground or air transport can be undertaken.

While the "scoop and run" concept may be very appropriate in urban areas, advanced stabilization procedures may have to be performed at the scene by rescue and EMS personnel. In wilderness areas definitive care may be provided and the victim may not be transported to a health care facility. Thus, the protocols and training in these situations may vary greatly from conventional EMS training used in urban areas. Proper attention to these details by the EMS medical director and the supervisor of the EMS agency is necessary to avoid conflicts and frustration.

## FACILITIES

Specialized facilities for burns, hyperbaric oxygen therapy, and poisoning exist in some regions. Regionalization of trauma centers and designation of hospitals at various levels of trauma triage and stabilization have improved and expedited patient care. Many states have adapted the recommendations of the American College of Surgeons (ACS) Committee on Trauma for the establishment of trauma centers. Protocols for transfer to these facilities must be concise, clear, and explicit. Frequently, victims are transported to the local health care facility, evaluated and stabilized, and later transferred to the regional trauma center. While in most instances this is appropriate, long transportation distances cause undue delays in the definitive care of the victim. Triage criteria at the scene and at the receiving hospital should be established, and strategies to reduce time delays in ground or air transport to the regional trauma center should be explored. Establishment of scene transportation criteria in consultation with the regional trauma center will help alleviate this problem. Availability and EMS training of physicians and nurses in the local health care facility should be taken into consideration. Most rural residents and EMTs, by their own admission, have a strong tendency and desire for independence and autonomy; they tend to resent outside intervention and regulation. This may create difficulties with regionalization efforts. Public education and frank discussions may resolve the resistance to merging with neighboring communities and lead to the acceptance of regionalized health care systems.

In addition to attending to the needs of the victims, education to improve injury prevention is essential. Rural EMS providers should take an active role in trauma injury prevention programs in the community.

## COMMUNICATIONS

While most rural areas are moving toward a coordinated communication system using 911, there are still regions where this system is not available. Sparse population, remote or inaccessible service areas, poor weather and road conditions, and limited access to communications may delay detection of the need for emergency care. Installation of emergency call boxes along major roadways in rural areas, in conjunction with CB radios and cellular phones, may improve public access. A coordinated communication system such as 911 facilitates quick and appropriate response.

Appropriate training of dispatchers to provide prearrival instructions, especially in instances where there is a prolonged response time, is helpful. Not infrequently, there is only one dispatcher for police, fire, and EMS, limiting the possibility of providing prearrival instructions. Many of these dispatchers, unlike their urban colleagues, do not have the medical background necessary for providing these instructions. This is especially frustrating as the average response time to a motor vehicle crash is nearly twice as long in rural areas compared to urban areas (11 versus 6 min).

Radio "dead spots" because of limited range of the equipment or geographical barriers are also more commonly encountered in rural areas. Repeaters at 20- to 30-mile intervals will help provide adequate radio coverage of the region. The cost of equipment, training, and maintenance in relation to the low call volume and radio frequency congestion further complicate the problem. Police, fire, highway maintenance, and forestry conservation share radio spectra in many rural areas. When a special emergency radio spectrum is available, it is crowded with unnecessary and unrelated nonemergency medical licensees.

## EVALUATION

As with any type of medical care, evaluation of the quality and appropriateness of that care is always important. Although rural EMS providers may be volunteers, have less funding, and see fewer patients, the importance of providing good care in the right way at the right time is at least as important as for the nonrural areas. In fact, it may be more important, due to the longer response times and lesser number of patients than in other areas.

Distribution of the limited resources available to the rural providers is very important. Ambulances in the service area must be placed not only where the patients are likely to need them, but also where the volunteer EMTs are able to access them quickly. Frequently, this means that the ambulance is parked for the day at the home of one of the volunteers on call for that day.

Determining the level of out-of-hospital care to be provided also is a resource-based question. The number of hours of initial education and continuing education, in addition to the dollars required for equipment and supplies, vary considerably from an EMT–Basic program to an EMT–Paramedic program. As previously stated, the limited funding and heavy reliance on volunteerism are also resources that need to be carefully accounted for.

Since the early 1980s, there have been several studies reviewing the efficacy of interventions available for prehospital care. The vast majority of these have been in the urban environment, leaving questions about rural EMS efficacy very open. One recent review of the medications used in urban versus rural care in Arizona demonstrated that while 7 percent of rural emergency patient encounters received medications and 8.5 percent of urban encounters received medications, there were some differences in the use of various medications. For instance, the rural patients were more likely to receive morphine sulfate, nitrous oxide, and verapamil. Moss, et al. suggested that the longer transport times were an indication for the use of narcotics and anti-arrhythmics.

In developing rural EMS systems, medical directors and administrators need to emphasize specific interventions that will have the greatest likelihood of saving lives and reducing morbidity. A key example of this has been the growth of basic life support services offering automatic external defibrillation. In North Carolina from 1990 to 1994, there was a dramatic rise in the number of rural fire departments certified to provide automatic external defibrillation, to try to stabilize cardiac arrest patients until the transporting vehicle could arrive. This is a key example of coupling other rural resources, in this case volunteer fire departments, with rural out-of-hospital providers to maximize the delivery of care.

## PUBLIC INFORMATION AND EDUCATION

In a setting with increased response times and lower levels of out-of-hospital care, the education of the general public is extremely important. They must understand the resources available to them from their local EMS providers, when to use them, and when not to use them. Tying up scarce EMS personnel and ambulances with inappropriate calls for transportation of patients who could readily be transported by the family vehicle will potentially reduce the availability of the EMS team for more critically ill or injured patients. The general public also needs to be educated about how to access the system, since 911 is sometimes not available in these areas. Further, emergency medical dispatching, with priority dispatching of vehicles and prearrival instructions, is less available than in urban areas.

The need for increased education is also pertinent in the area of prevention. Using community resources to decrease the threat of fatal motor vehicle collisions through seatbelt awareness programs, increased visibility along rural highways, and flashing yellow beacons at dangerous intersections are some important prevention modalities.

## MEDICAL DIRECTION

Frequently, one of the chief challenges facing rural EMS is enlisting the assistance of a local physician who is interested in and knowledgeable about out-of-hospital care and willing to devote adequate time to provide off-line medical direction. Oversight of care by a licensed and involved physician is extremely important for any level of provider. The scarcity of physicians in rural environments adds to this problem. As with their urban and suburban counterparts, medical directors of rural providers need to be the champions of quality out-of-hospital care in their communities. They must be visible proponents of providing ample resources for the system and enthusiastic community support.

The arguments for and against the use of standing orders for advanced life support, rather than requiring on-line medical direction for every intervention, are as pertinent in rural areas as in nonrural areas. They may be even more pertinent, however, due to the extended distances involved and the increased likelihood of radio communication problems due to geographic obstacles, such as mountains. Added to this are concerns that the prehospital personnel will see fewer examples of serious emergencies such as acute respiratory failure, severe chest pain, or bilateral leg amputations than providers with higher call volumes. Also, physicians in the local emergency departments and primary care clinics tend to be busy, understaffed, and less able to go to a radio or a telephone to provide orders.

## TRAUMA SYSTEMS

In the mid 1990s, most rural EMS providers have access to air medical transport services to move trauma patients from rural scenes, many have access to trauma centers, and a small few are part of rural trauma systems. In many regions of the country, the trauma systems are merely a network of trauma centers, lacking any strong integration in the form of interhospital transfer criteria, field triage criteria, appropriately applied guidelines for air medical transport, and system-wide quality improvement activities.

Nevertheless, it is incumbent on the rural out-of-hospital provider to prospectively identify which patients require transport from a trauma scene directly to the closest trauma center. This requires knowledge of the capabilities of all the hospitals within reach for providing trauma care, as well as knowledge of the ground and air transport resources for these patients. The physicians, nurses, and administrative resources at the regional trauma centers must provide appropriate outreach opportunities from their centers to the smaller community hospitals and out-of-hospital personnel. Maintaining open communication and building a cooperative environment are key components to successful implementation of a rural trauma system.

## BIBLIOGRAPHY

Baker SP, Whitfield MS, O'Neill B: County mapping of injury mortality. *J Trauma* 28(6):741, 1988.

Brown LH, Prasad NH, Grimmer K: Public perceptions of a rural EMS system. *Prehosp Disaster Med* 9(4):257, 1994.

Hunt RC, Allison EJ, Yates JG: The need for improved emergency medical services in Pitt County. *N C Med J* 47(1):39, 1986.

March JA, Cassell H, Brown L, Prasad NH: Failure to respond by emergency medical services organizations. Presented at the *Rocky Mountain Emergency Medicine Conference,* Breckenridge, Colorado, January, 1994.

Moss RL, Kolaric D, Watts A: Therapeutic agents utilized in urban/rural prehospital care. *Prehosp Disaster Med,* 8(2):161, 1993.

Richless LK, Schrading WA, Polana J, et al: Early defibrillation program: Problems encountered in a rural/suburban EMS system. *J Emerg Med,* 11(2):127, 1993.

US Congress, Office of Technology Assessment: *Rural Emergency Medical Services Special Report,* OTA-H-445. Washington, DC, Government Printing Office, November, 1989.
US Department of Transportation: *National Accident Sampling System,* 1986.

# 4
# ALTERNATIVES TO GROUND TRANSPORT
### Daniel G. Hankins

## INTRODUCTION

"Stable patients who are able to be transported by ground ambulance should be transported by ground ambulance" is a generally true statement. However, other factors come into play that may change the mode of transportation best for an individual patient: accessibility, time, distance, and criticality, among others. In this chapter we deal with the place of rotor- and fixed-wing air transport, snowmobiles, and other vehicles as used for emergency medical services (EMS) transport.

The fundamental concept of this chapter is that all these modes of transport as well as the ground ambulance should be part of an *integrated EMS system.* Helicopters, fixed-wing aircraft, snowmobiles, and other vehicles are among many "tools in the EMS toolbox." Field EMS personnel at scenes, or physicians transferring patients between hospitals, should be able to select the "right tool for the right job." The proper mode of transportation for an individual patient should be used depending on the particular circumstances present. The spectrum of choice in an integrated EMS system is illustrated in Fig. 4-1. Effective implementation of all these EMS tools requires well-trained communications and dispatch personnel who can quickly assess the situation at hand and then institute the right EMS response. In addition, the entire out-of-medical care system must be medically supervised by physicians well versed in all aspects of such care.

## AIR MEDICAL TRANSPORT

A brief note about terminology is needed here: *air medical* refers to the use of aircraft for evacuation of patients, whereas *aeromedical* refers to the study of the medical effects of flight and altitude on humans.

The first air evacuation of a patient most likely occurred on November 16, 1915, during the Serbian retreat from Albania, when a French fighter pilot evacuated an injured Serbian fighter pilot in a fixed-wing aircraft.

### Helicopter (Rotor-Wing) Transport

As with many other milestones in EMS, the history of air evacuation is closely connected to the history of warfare. Igor Sikorsky's great invention, the helicopter, first flown on September 14, 1939, was used for the first rotor-wing medical evacuation in Burma in 1945. From this small start in World War II, helicopter usage blossomed extensively in the Korean war, when more aircraft were available and were of sturdier construction. It is estimated that 20,000 patients were transported by helicopter in Korea. During the Vietnamese war, the numbers markedly increased, with about 370,000 patients carried by helicopter from 1965 to 1969. These craft literally carried out Dominique-Jean Larrey's (Napoleon's chief combat surgeon) idea of "flying dressing stations" (*ambulances volantes*). Helicopters were a big factor in reducing combat-related mortality successively from World War II through Korea and then in Vietnam.

### Civilian Rotor-Wing Transport

The first hospital-based civilian program began in 1972 in Denver. Since then, some 175 to 180 programs have arisen around the country, utilizing 230 rotor-wing aircraft. Most of these programs are run by hospitals or groups of hospitals. Consortiums of hospitals with joint sponsorship of a rotor-wing service will undoubtedly become more common in the future because of the cost involved in providing the service. Helicopters are expensive to buy, ranging from $750,000 to $5,000,000. Most programs lease their helicopters from aircraft vendors who deal with multiple programs because of the high cost of purchase, the high cost of maintenance, and the cost of maintaining pilot training. For safety reasons, rotor-wing services have increasingly moved toward using two-engined helicopters with instrument flight rating (IFR), rather than single-engine helicopters with visual flight rating (VFR). The advantage of a two-engined helicopter is self-explanatory. VFR ships can only fly with good visibility, whereas an IFR craft can fly under conditions of poorer visibility. Both VFR and IFR helicopters have strict visibility limitations imposed by the Federal Aviation Administration (FAA), but the IFR ship has fewer restrictions. If the helicopter pilot unexpectedly encounters bad weather during a flight, an IFR ship has a better chance of successfully (*and safely*) completing the mission than does a VFR ship. In areas with frequent bad weather periods, some programs have elected to go even further and use *two-pilot IFR.* The addition of this more sophisticated equipment, a second pilot, and a second engine increases both initial and ongoing costs for a helicopter air medical program. Annual cost of maintaining a rotor-wing service exceeds $1 million in most circumstances.

The total number of patients transported in the United States by rotor-wing craft since 1972 is on the order of 750,000 to 1,000,000. Yearly, 100,000 to 150,000 patients are transported by helicopter in this country.

### Crew Configuration and Training

The medical crew on a rotor-wing craft can be configured in multiple ways: nurse-paramedic, nurse-nurse, nurse-physician, nurse-respiratory therapist. The literature suggests that the addition of a physician to the crew does not add a significantly higher level of care to that already rendered by a flight nurse and/or flight medic. The most frequently used crew is nurse-paramedic because of the complementary skills brought together within the flight crew by these two disciplines. Since rotor-wing missions can vary widely on the spectrum between scene flights and interfacility transports, a broad skill basis is essential in the medical crew so that they can deal with any eventuality. A comprehensive curriculum guide, developed by a number of national air medical organizations under contract from the U.S. Department of Transportation, is available to use for training medical flight crews: *Air Medical Crew National Standard Curriculum: Advanced Student Manual.* This curriculum covers all aspects of air medical care and is intended for "use by paramedics, nurses and physicians."

Knowledge of the interaction between the effects of flight and the sick and injured patient is a major difference between ground and air transport personnel. Medical flight crews need to know how the environment found on an aircraft will affect the patient's illness and how to transport the patient safely in the relatively hostile environment of

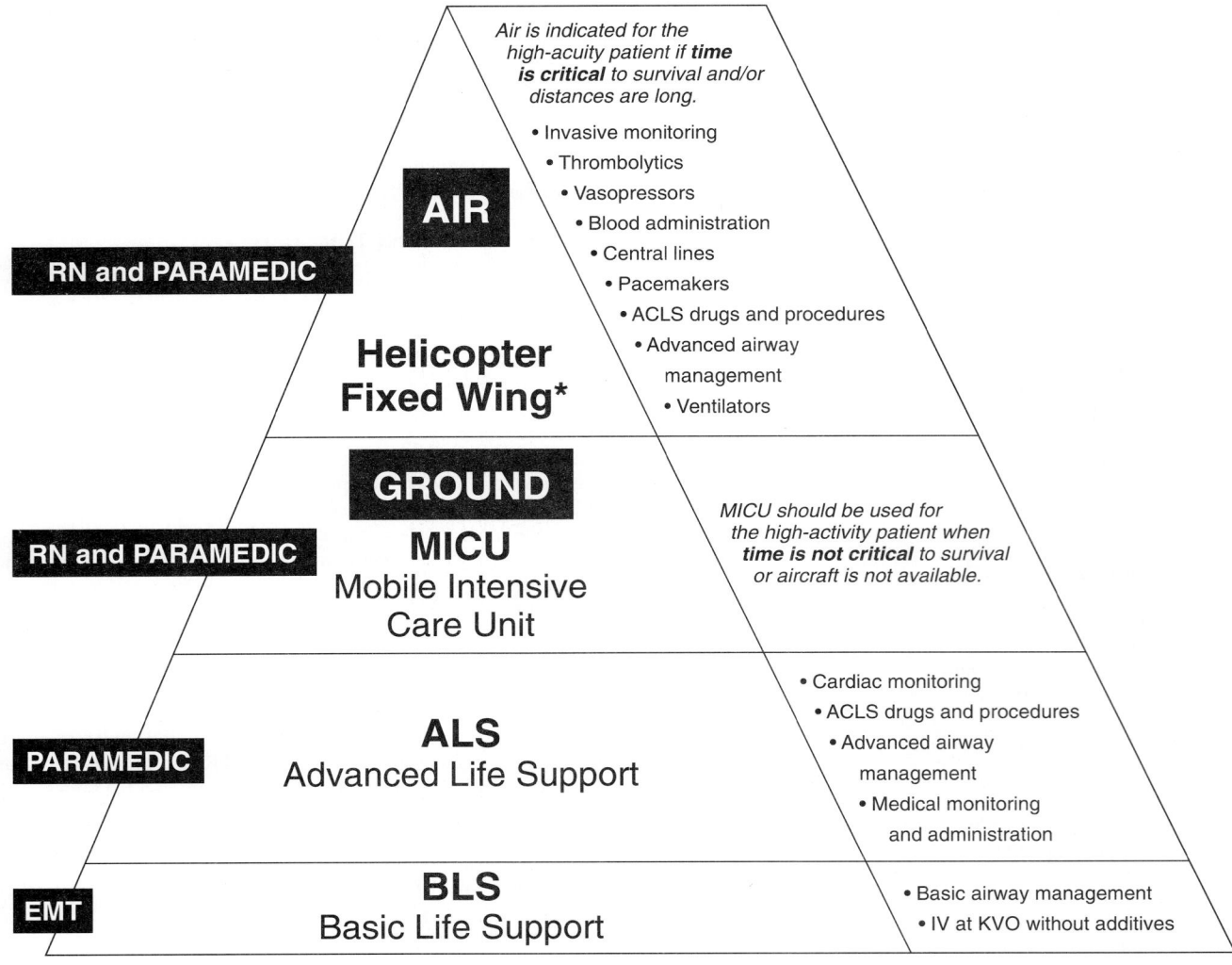

**Fig. 4-1.** The patient transport guidelines pyramid. (From North Flight EMS. *J Emerg Med Servs,* October, 1993, p. 50. Used by permission.)

that aircraft. Helicopters generally transport patients at about 2500 to 3500 ft, so low barometric pressure with barotrauma is usually not a consideration; but it could become a consideration if transportation were to occur over mountains. The noise, close quarters, vibration, and temperature changes of the cabin of a rotor-wing craft can have a marked effect on the patient's condition and can make assessment of the patient more difficult than during ground transport.

## Clinical Use of Helicopters

Helicopters are fast ambulances, cruising at 125 to 175 mph, depending on the aircraft. The usual flight range for a helicopter is 150 to 200 miles. They do not have to stop at traffic lights and are not limited by the quality of roads available. Helicopters bring sophisticated medical care to areas that otherwise might have only basic life support ground ambulance service. The air medical crews bring tertiary critical care to primary care areas and transfer patients back to the tertiary center at two to three times the speed of a ground ambulance. There is evidence that care rendered by air medical crews decreases morbidity and mortality in critically ill and injured patients. In spite of this, there is still much debate about the proper situations in which to use rotor-wing services. The two major types of helicopter missions are (1) trauma/medical scene responses, and (2) interfacility transfers. In 1993, the typical distribution of these two types

of flights for rotor-wing services was 32.5 percent scene flights and 68.5 percent interfacility flights.

## Scene Helicopter Response

The appropriate use of helicopters at trauma scenes involves a complex interplay of factors to be considered. Several questions have to be answered: How far away is the scene from the helicopter base? What resources are already responding to the patient(s)? What is the distance from the scene to the local hospital or the trauma center? How many victims are there and what is the severity of their injuries? Is there a significant amount of extrication needed before the patient can go on to definitive care?

National guidelines (see Table 4-1) have been developed to assist in making these decisions for trauma scene responses. These criteria use clinical information such as mechanism of injury, severity of injury, vital signs, and level of consciousness as one part of the equation. It has been shown that emergency medical technicians on scene are very accurate at defining which patients are critical and need air medical transport to the trauma center.

There are also logistical and operational factors to be considered. If the patient is not accessible because of location (e.g., off-road or wilderness), traffic, road conditions, or weather, a helicopter dispatch may be appropriate. Keep in mind, though, that helicopters are much

**Table 4-1.** Air Medical Dispatch: Guidelines for Trauma Scene Response

I. Clinical
  A. General
    1. Trauma victims need to be delivered as soon as possible to a regional trauma center
    2. Stable patients who are accessible to ground vehicles probably are best transported by ground
  B. Specific
    Patients with critical injuries resulting in unstable vital signs require the fastest, most direct route of transport to a regional trauma center in a vehicle staffed with a team capable of offering critical care enroute. Often this is the case in the following situations:
      1. Trauma Score <12
      2. Glasgow Coma Score <10
      3. Penetrating trauma to the abdomen, pelvis, chest, neck, or head
      4. Spinal cord or spinal column injury, or any injury producing paralysis of any extremity if any lateralizing signs
      5. Partial or total amputation of an extremity (excluding digits)
      6. Two or more long bone fractures or a major pelvic fracture
      7. Crushing injuries to the abdomen, chest, or head
      8. Major burns of the body surface area, or burns involving the face, hands, feet, or perineum, or burns with significant respiratory involvement, or major electrical or chemical burns
      9. Patients involved in a serious traumatic event who are less than 12 or more than 55 years of age
     10. Patients with near-drowning injuries, with or without existing hypothermia
     11. Adult patients with any of the following vital sign abnormalities:
        a. Systolic blood pressure <90 mmHg
        b. Respiratory rate <10 or >35 per min
        c. Heart rate <60 or >120 per min
        d. Unresponsive to verbal stimuli
II. Operational situations in which helicopter use should be considered:
  A. Mechanism of injury:
    1. Vehicle roll-over with unbelted passengers
    2. Vehicle striking pedestrian at >10 mph
    3. Falls from >15 ft
    4. Motorcycle victim ejected at >20 mph
    5. Multiple victims
  B. Difficult access situations:
    1. Wilderness rescue
    2. Ambulance egress or access impeded at the scene by road conditions, weather, or traffic
  C. Time/distance factors:
    1. Transportation time to the trauma center greater than 15 min by ground ambulance
    2. Transport time to the local hospital by ground greater than transport time to trauma center by helicopter
    3. Patient extrication time >20 min
    4. Utilization of local ground ambulance leaves local community without ground ambulance coverage

*Source:* Used by permission of the National Association of EMS Physicians.

more weather-sensitive than ground ambulances. If the weather is bad for ambulances, it is probably worse for helicopters. Since bad accidents occur with bad weather, a common complaint by ground ambulance crews is that the helicopter cannot fly when they need it the most.

Time and distance factors play a key role in electing to send the helicopter. A severe trauma or medical situation in an urban area close to a trauma center does not have the implications for the patient that the same situation would in a rural area 100 miles away from a major medical center. If the time for transport to the trauma center is greater than 15 min by ground ambulance, if the transport time to the local hospital by ground is greater than the time required for the helicopter to reach the trauma center, or if patient extrication will take longer than 20 min, then dispatch of the helicopter should be considered. In general, scene responses will occur within 25 miles of the helicopter base, although this will vary with local conditions and proto-

cols. It is likely that at distances greater than 25 miles, the patient will be transferred to the local hospital first for stabilization and then the helicopter will take the patient on to the trauma center from there. Sometimes, if the patient is extricated faster than initially thought, the ground EMS personnel will just communicate to the helicopter to divert to the local hospital rather than go to the scene.

Medical scene responses have not received as much attention in the literature as trauma scene responses. Most medical patients will be carried by helicopter as interfacility transports from one hospital to another. In rural areas, especially, it is common for helicopters to do intercepts of basic life support (BLS) ambulances that are transporting deteriorating, unstable patients or patients who have time-dependent medical conditions, such as an acute myocardial infarction needing thrombolysis.

Occasionally, the helicopter is called directly to a medical scene by BLS personnel. This may happen if the helicopter can transport the critical patient faster to the tertiary center than the ground ambulance can get the patient to the local hospital for stabilization. However, if a patient is in cardiac arrest, for instance, and the ground ambulance has a defibrillator and has secured the airway, it is unlikely that the arrival of the helicopter crew will result in any more successful resuscitation. These kinds of intercept situations must be dealt with on a local or regional level by guidelines and protocols. This reinforces the importance of an integrated EMS system in which air and ground units work smoothly together under medical direction.

One further important factor to be considered in initiating helicopter transport of a patient is whether ground transport of the patient by the local ambulance will deprive that community of vital EMS services. If the local ambulance is out of service for 5 or 6 h and emergency ambulance coverage in that area is compromised, then use of the helicopter should be strongly considered.

One other important use for helicopters is in the context of a disaster situation. Rotor-wing craft can not only bring in more-sophisticated triage and treatment personnel for better medical care at the scene, but can also give the Incident Commander a bird's-eye view of the events in order to get a better perspective of the situation. This is in addition to the usual role of the helicopter in evacuating the most seriously ill and injured back to the trauma center.

## Interfacility Helicopter Transports

The impact of Federal OBRA/COBRA legislation has made it illegal for a transferring physician to transport a patient to another medical facility with an inadequate level of care. If the patient is unstable or requires intensive care during transport, then it is not appropriate to put that patient in a BLS ambulance. A rotor-wing crew brings tertiary care to the primary care hospital and allows for safe transport of the patient, with a better chance for a good patient outcome. As a recently published position paper from the Air Medical Committee of the National Association of EMS Physicians states: "Reducing out-of-hospital time for these patients seems to be in their best interest. Ground-based out-of-hospital care providers, faced with a patient whose needs obviously exceed their abilities, may wish to access a rotor-wing air medical transport service, especially if they are distant from an appropriate medical facility." This position is strengthened by the literature, which suggests that a tertiary center can safely extend its care out to several hundred miles via rotor- or fixed-wing aircraft with no change in mortality compared with patients transported locally to that same trauma center.

## Safety

Flight programs are exceedingly safety conscious. There has been a perception in the past that helicopters are unsafe. It is probably true, however, that, per patient-mile, helicopters are safer than ground ambulances. Air medical programs must follow safety rules from the FAA. The industry itself has set forth additional stringent standards under the auspices of the Association of Air Medical Services and, more recently, the Commission on Accreditation of Air Medical Services (CAAMS). CAAMS performs site visits on request of an air medical program to certify that the program complies with strict safety and operational standards. The elevation of all services to the same industrywide set of standards ensures the greatest possibility of safe patient transport.

Weather and strikes against ground obstacles are the leading hazards. In most programs, the pilot is not told the nature of the mission until a weather check is done and the flight approved from this standpoint. The pilot does not then feel pressured into flying a mission under borderline weather conditions because of the patient's condition.

Flight crews generally wear fire-resistant clothing and many crews wear crash helmets, but safety does not just apply to the air medical crew garments. Safety involves everybody in contact with the aircraft, including, but not limited to the communications people who dispatch and do flight following, pilots, mechanics, flight crew, first responders, and ambulance personnel at the scene. It is very important to do initial (and refresher) training of ground EMS personnel on how to act around a helicopter at the scene. A helicopter can be a dangerous machine to anybody, but it is especially dangerous to the uninitiated.

Scene flights are inherently much more dangerous than landing at a regular hospital landing zone. The unfamiliar (compared to a regular hospital landing zone) landing area at a scene has more potential obstacles to strike, such as wires and trees. More material may be scattered on the ground and blown around as missiles by the rotor wash from the helicopter. EMS scenes tend to be uncontrolled, with more bystanders who have the potential of walking into a tail or main rotor. A helicopter needs at a minimum 60 ft × 60 ft for a landing zone (or 100 ft × 100 ft, depending on the helicopter model in question). This size of landing zone may be difficult to secure on a rural highway or at other accident scenes.

It is beyond the scope of this discussion to give a complete helicopter safety treatise, but several points are important. First, the craft should always be approached from the front where the pilot can see approaching personnel and can then acknowledge their presence and motion them into the helicopter. In general a flight team member will guide ground personnel into the aircraft. Second, a rotor-wing aircraft should never be approached from the rear as the tail rotor is going very fast and is virtually invisible. The tail rotor is the most dangerous area of a helicopter. Third, landings and takeoffs are the most likely times for adverse incidents to occur with a helicopter mission.

## Cost and Reimbursement

Helicopter transport is more expensive than ground transport. The average cost of a trip in 1994 by a medium-sized twin-engined helicopter at 134 knots and a 50-mile one-way travel distance is $2765.01. Reimbursement issues are complex. It is not easy to quantitate how a patient might have deteriorated if sent by ground rather than by air. It is not enough to ask the simple question: "Would the patient have died if not transported by helicopter?" Other medical factors come into play. The morbidity and quality of future life may have been positively affected by using a helicopter rather than a ground ambulance. The number of days in intensive care or duration of rehabilitation of a critical patient may be decreased because the helicopter brought the patient to the tertiary center faster and with a higher level of care than was possible with the ground ambulance. The determinants of helicopter usage must be medical, driven by national standards as described above, and not dependent on reimbursement. There is inherent conflict between the requirements of OBRA/COBRA for adequate transport and the unwillingness of other Federal agencies and third parties to pay for the service rendered.

One model from Massachusetts described in the recent literature suggests that a helicopter service may be more cost-effective than ground advanced life support (ALS) ambulance service needed to cover the same area. This study assumed about a 30-min ground ALS intercept time of a BLS service. Furthermore, the study took into account turndowns of flights because of weather or the possibility of the helicopter already being on another mission. The helicopter was still more cost-effective than the ALS ground units for similar coverage of ground surface area.

## Fixed-Wing Air Medical Transport

Whereas helicopters are for emergent care at scenes or between hospitals, fixed-wing aircraft serve a wider variety of missions, from urgent to routine care, and over greater distances. Airplane pilots do need to be a little more particular about where they land, though: they have to land at airports and they cannot do scene flights. This means that airplanes need ground ambulance connections at either end to transport the patient to and from the airport. Because of these complicating factors, fixed-wing flights generally take longer to arrange and are not used for the truly emergent patient.

There are many more fixed-wing aircraft used for air medical transport than rotor-wing craft. Rotor craft tend to be dedicated as air medical transport units, while planes are often multifunctional, being used for charter flights or business use. Unfortunately this sometimes leads to inadequate equipping and staffing of airplanes when used for air medical work. Medical fixed-wing craft need to have an adequate cargo-type door to allow adequate access for a patient on a stretcher. Removeable medical equipment modules have been developed for airplanes, to ensure presence of adequate medical equipment yet allow the aircraft to be used for other purposes for economic reasons.

Fixed-wing transports are cheaper and more practical than helicopter flights at distances over 150 miles. One study suggests that the appropriate cutoff point between rotor- and fixed-wing flights should even be 100 miles. On the average, a fixed-wing transport costs about $13 per patient-loaded mile, while a helicopter transport costs about $55 per patient-loaded mile. This is a very rough estimate because of the large number of variables (distance, aircraft type and speed, crew configuration, and the nature of the patient's condition).

Airplanes are quite variable in size and speed. Jet aircraft are faster than turboprop airplanes, which are faster than piston-driven airplanes. The appropriate aircraft to use for any one mission depends on many factors: distance; the nature of the airport at the patient's pick-up point; the weight and condition of the patient, equipment, and crew, i.e., the more critically ill the patient, the more equipment and crew may be needed. The choice of aircraft must also take into account crew and patient comfort for a trip of that distance. The cabins of fixed-wing aircraft are more spacious than those of rotor-wing craft. A larger plane that is able to be pressurized can fly above 10,000 ft, which means the plane can go faster, farther, and more comfortably. It is generally better to fly on such a craft.

Weather and distance factors play a large role in the decision to send ground, rotor-wing, or a fixed-wing craft in any particular situation. Since airplanes can fly above bad weather and are less susceptible to conditions such as ice on the wings, fixed-wing craft can often fly when helicopters cannot. Helicopters have very low tolerance to ice on the rotors, whereas airplanes often have deicing equipment. Fixed-wing planes can also fly under more difficult visibility circumstances than rotor craft because of on-board instrumentation and the possibility of ground control from an airport.

All fixed-wing services must comply with FAA rules for airplanes. Standards have been developed for air medical fixed-wing aircraft by the Association of Air Medical Services and CAAMS, just as they have been developed for helicopters. These standards deal with aircraft configuration, medical equipment requirements, medical crew configuration and training, and medical director qualifications. Recently more comprehensive guidelines have been developed for qualifications of the air medical director. These guidelines outline the scope of knowledge and practice of the medical director of an air medical program.

## Medical Direction of Air Medical Services

Active medical direction may be even more important with rotor- and fixed-wing services than with ground services; it is certainly more complicated. The air transport service medical director needs to be familiar with all aspects of flight and its effects on the sick and injured patient. The skills of the flight crew need to be more sophisticated and require more intense initial training as well as more intense ongoing education. The patients cared for are generally sicker and require more advanced interventions. Because flight crews are often far from their base of operations and acting independently out of direct voice contact, the medical director must have in place standing orders or protocols to allow the crew to intervene quickly and stabilize the patient's condition. This means that the medical director must intensely scrutinize the trip sheets and institute more stringent and complex quality improvement methods since the patients' conditions are more complex. If not already involved in the ground aspects of EMS, the air program medical director needs to coordinate with ground medical direction to integrate the ground and air EMS systems.

## OTHER MODES OF NONGROUND AMBULANCE PATIENT TRANSPORT

While the potential for transport to a medical facility by almost any vehicle exists, there are only a limited number of vehicles used within the context of the organized, formal EMS system. The bulk of out-of-hospital patient transports are done by ground, rotor-wing, and fixed-wing services. Other vehicles are often used to bring patients to these usual modes of transportation if the patient is inaccessible to them. Litter-borne patients may be carried out of remote areas. The National Ski Patrol uses toboggans pulled by snowmobiles or tracked vehicles to take the sick or injured patient to the formal EMS transport vehicle. Four-wheeled drive vehicles are often used to evacuate the patient to the EMS vehicle. Boats can be used for transport across lakes, rivers, or oceans if need be, but the patient usually gets transferred to ground, rotor-wing, or fixed-wing craft for transport to a medical facility. The local situation will dictate the appropriate vehicle needed to get the patient into the system. Cooperation is necessary among first responders, law enforcement officials, and fire and EMS personnel, along with bystanders, to use whatever resources are available to move the patient quickly and safely to the nearest appropriate medical facility.

## SUMMARY POINTS

1. Ground ambulance transports constitute the bulk of EMS system responses, but other modes of transportation are appropriate, and indeed necessary, for some patients. This may be because of severity of illness or injury, inaccessibility, time/distance factors, number of victims, or the strong need *not* to deprive a community of ground ambulance service for a prolonged period.
2. The other modes of transportation, primarily rotor- and fixed-wing craft, need to be an integral part of the total out-of-hospital care system.
3. The appropriate mode of transport for a patient must be selected by personnel familiar with *all* aspects of the integrated EMS system.
4. Cost of transport is a consideration but should be weighed in the context of the patient's medical condition and the other factors outlined in item 1 above.
5. Safety is a fundamental concern of air medical programs.
6. These other aspects of EMS along with ground ambulances require active medical direction for off-line and on-line medical control as well as for quality assurance/improvement activities.

## BIBLIOGRAPHY

Association of Air Medical Services: *Standards and Safety Guidelines.* AAMS, August, 1992.

Baxt WG, Moody P: The impact of a rotorcraft aeromedical emergency care service on trauma mortality. *JAMA* 249:3047, 1983.

Bruhn JD, Williams KA, Aghababian R: True costs of air medical vs. ground ambulance systems. *Air Med J* 12:262, 1993.

Emerman CL, Shade B, Kubincanek J: A comparison of EMT judgement and prehospital trauma triage instruments. *J Trauma* 31:1369, 1375, 1991.

Henniger S, Thompson J, Adams C: *Federal Aviation Administration: Guidelines for Integrating Helicopter Assets into Emergency Planning.* US Dept of Transportation Document DOT/FAA/RD 90/11, 1991.

Mayfield T: 1994 Annual transport statistics and transport fees survey. *Air Med J* 13:132, 1994.

National Association of EMS Physicians: Air medical dispatch: Guidelines for scene response. *Prehosp Disaster Med* 7:75, 1992.

National Association of EMS Physicians: Criteria for prehospital air medical transport: Non-trauma and pediatric considerations. *Prehosp Disaster Med* 9:140, 1994.

National Association of EMS Physicians: Medical director for air medical transport programs. *Prehosp Disaster Med* 1995, *In press*

Stone CK, Hunt RC, Sousa JA, et al: Interhospital transfer of cardiac patients: Does air medical transport make a difference? *Air Med J* 13:159, 1994.

Thomas F, Wisham J, Clemmer TP, et al: Outcome, transport times, and costs of patients evacuated by helicopter versus fixed-wing aircraft. *West J Med* 153:40, 1990.

Valenzuela TD, Criss EA, Copass MK, et al: Critical care air transportation of the severely injured: Does long distance transport adversely affect survival? *Ann Emerg Med* 19:169, 1990.

# 5

# NEONATAL AND PEDIATRIC TRANSPORT

## Carl L. Bose

Regionalized intensive care is a concept that has gained wide acceptance in many fields of medicine including neonatology, pediatric intensive care, and emergency medicine. This concept mandates that expensive, high-technology, labor-intensive therapies be limited to a few regional centers. Because patients in need of services available only in regional centers do not always present at these centers initially, interfacility transport has developed as a complement to regionalized intensive care.

The responsibility for the transport of a patient to a regional center may be assumed by either the referring hospital or the regional center. Because regional neonatal and pediatric intensive care centers often provide transport services, and because community emergency medical services are often not equipped to transport children, the interfacility transport of pediatric patients is often conducted by regional centers. However, even under these circumstances, the referring hospital has important responsibilities related to transport. These responsibilities must often be assumed by emergency personnel because the emergency department is the site of initial care. Therefore, the focus of this chapter will be the principles of stabilization and preparation of critically ill children for transport. However, since some emergency departments are also responsible for operating transport services, a brief discussion of the organization and administration of a pediatric transport program is also included.

# THE TRANSPORT ENVIRONMENT

Moving patients, particularly critically ill pediatric patients, between hospitals, or even within a hospital, invariably adds to the risks of the illness or injury because of the hazards associated with the transport environment. The principles of care provided prior to or during transport are the same as in the inpatient setting. However, the specifics can and should be influenced by the unique features of transport. Therefore, an understanding of the transport environment is essential for individuals who prepare patients for transport as well as for those who provide care during transport.

## Features

The features that may distinguish the transport environment from the inpatient setting and the effects of these features on patients and caretakers include the following:

**Excessive noise.** The acute effects of excessive noise on older pediatric and adult patients is probably minimal. By contrast, persistent sound in excess of 80 dB appears to dramatically increase the frequency of arterial oxygen desaturation in premature infants. In addition, excessive noise makes it virtually impossible to use the sense of hearing to evaluate patients during transport.

**Vibration.** Like the effects of excessive noise, the effects of vibration on patients are uncertain but are probably not of great significance. However, vibration may limit the reliability of transport equipment. Monitor artifact must be recognized, and alternative techniques for monitoring should be employed when it is present.

**Inadequate lighting.** Inadequate lighting is rarely a problem during the transport of adult patients because EMS vehicles generally have lighting designed for stretcher-bound large patients. However, task lighting for illuminating small areas and small patients is usually not available.

**Variable ambient temperature.** Although the body temperature of adult patients is rarely influenced by the range of ambient temperature encountered during transport, environmental conditions can have a dramatic influence on the body temperature of neonates and small children.

**Changes in barometric pressure.** Change in barometric pressure during ascent in nonpressurized aircraft causes expansion of gases in closed spaces (e.g., endotracheal tube cuffs, pulmonary interstitial emphysema) and a fall in the partial pressure of oxygen. These changes are rarely of sufficient magnitude to influence physiology unless the change in altitude is greater than approximately 1500 m.

**Confined space.** The confined space in transport vehicles is an obvious handicap because of the limitation on the number of caretakers and support equipment.

**Limited support services.** Similarly, the extent and precision of care are limited by the lack of support services (e.g., radiography, laboratory services).

**Motion-induced illness.** Many medical personnel develop motion-induced illnesses during transport. Symptoms are often categorized into one of two syndromes: the sopite syndrome, which is characterized by drowsiness and inability to concentrate, and the nausea syndrome. Either syndrome may impair the ability of personnel to provide skilled care.

## Precautions

An understanding of the handicaps of the transport environment and plans to minimize the impact of these handicaps are essential. Suggested guidelines include the following:

1. *Stabilize the patient carefully prior to transport.* Unless the immediate needs of the patient can be met only in the receiving hospital (e.g., severe trauma), ample time should be devoted to stabilizing the patient in the referring hospital.

2. *Anticipate deterioration.* Preparation of the patient should include not only care for the identifiable problems, but also preparation for problems which may arise during transport.

3. *Prepare the transport vehicle properly.* If repeated transport of pediatric patients is anticipated, one or more vehicles should be prepared to meet the special needs of these patients (e.g., accessory lighting, more precisely controlled thermal environment).

4. *Monitor as many physiologic parameters as possible electronically.* Because physical examination is nearly impossible during transport and because pediatric patients are often transported during dynamic changes in their physiology, electronic monitoring is essential.

# PREPARATION OF A PATIENT FOR TRANSPORT

## Decision to Transport

The decision to transport should be based on the requirements of the patient at the time of presentation and the anticipated needs during the evolution of the disease or injury. If it is determined that these needs will, at any time, exceed the resources of the hospital, then the patient should be transported as soon as possible.

## Basic Preparation

When a critically ill child arrives in the emergency department and the decision is made to transport that child to another institution, extensive preparation of the child should occur. This preparation should be completed by the referring hospital personnel, to the limits of their abilities and resources, regardless of whether they or a receiving hospital will perform the transport.

## Airway Management

The decision to intubate and mechanically ventilate a patient is usually based on objective evidence of respiratory failure. This principle still applies in patients being prepared for transport. However, the threshold for intervention should be lowered. For example, an infant with a $Paco_2$ of 50 mmHg might be observed without ventilatory support in the inpatient setting but should probably be intubated and ventilated in preparation for transport. In addition, children without respiratory failure but in whom deterioration is anticipated should be intubated in preparation for transport. This more aggressive approach to airway management is justified because, during transport, the ability to identify respiratory failure and to intubate is often impaired.

Cuffed endotracheal tubes should not be used in children less than 7 years of age. Because the distance between the thoracic inlet and the carina is extremely short in small children, the position of the tube should be confirmed with a chest radiograph as soon after insertion as possible. Soon after the initiation of mechanical ventilation, arterial blood gas analysis should be performed to ensure the appropriateness of ventilator settings. The most common error is overventilation, which may have serious consequences.

## Vascular Access

All patients should have intravascular access during transport. Critically ill patients should have at least two lines in the event that one becomes dislodged or several drugs must be administered simultaneously. Access should be through a device that includes a nonmetallic intravascular component. The metal butterfly needles often used in pediatric inpatient units are not satisfactory during transport because they frequently perforate the vessel as a result of vibration and movement.

The umbilicus is a simple site of vascular access for infants less than 1 week of age. An alternative technique for fluid and drug administration in patients in whom intravascular lines cannot be placed is intraosseous cannulation. The placement of umbilical arterial and venous catheters and intraosseous needles is discussed in detail in Chaps. 16 and 18.

In small children, intravenous lines should be infused with the use of pumps. Open "drips" should not be used, even with volumetric drip chambers, because of the risk of fluid intoxication resulting from inadvertent administration of large boluses. The amount of fluid administered should be carefully monitored and recorded.

## Special Problems of the Neonate

Stabilizing and transporting critically ill neonates present special problems because they are more dependent upon extrinsic factors to maintain homeostasis. This is particularly true when birth occurs prior to term. In fact, the complexity of care is often inversely related to birthweight and gestational age. The following aspects of care deserve special consideration:

### Thermal Regulation

Humans conserve body temperature by several mechanisms, including: (1) shunting blood from the skin and periphery to the core, (2) increasing basal metabolic rate, (3) voluntary muscle activity, (4) shivering, and (5) nonshivering thermogenesis. With the exception of nonshivering thermogenesis, all of these mechanisms are less effective in the neonate. Although older children and adults can maintain normal core body temperature in a wide range of environmental conditions, neonates, and particularly premature infants, are very limited in this regard. In addition, even in conditions in which a neonate can maintain normal body temperature, this is often accomplished at the expense of increased oxygen consumption and carbon dioxide production. These consequences are particularly onerous in infants with respiratory failure.

Whenever possible, neonates should be cared for in an environment in which core temperature remains normal and oxygen consumption is minimal. This environment is termed the *neutral thermal environment*. A neutral thermal environment is best provided by treating a neonate on or within a thermocontrolled bed especially designed for neonates. These come in two varieties: an open platform heated with an overhead radiant heat source and a closed plastic incubator heated with a convection heater. Although not satisfactory for transport, open incubators with radiant heaters are ideal for the care of critically ill neonates in the emergency department because they permit access by several caretakers. An alternative is the use of a portable overhead heat lamp and a standard crib. These devices should be used with extreme caution because they do not usually include a servocontrol mechanism. The patient's body temperature should be monitored frequently to avoid hyperthermia. The neutral thermal environment is presumed to be provided when the infant's body temperature is normal and there is a minimal gradient between the core and skin temperature.

Humans lose body heat in four ways: (1) convection, (2) conduction, (3) radiation, and (4) evaporation. Neonates, and particularly preterm infants, are particularly susceptible to heat loss because they have a relatively large surface to body mass ratio when compared to older patients. Also their skin is more permeable to water vapor, and they may have a paucity of subcutaneous tissue. In addition to providing a heat source, attempts to create a neutral thermal environment should include provisions to minimize heat loss.

1.  Infants should be thoroughly dried to avoid evaporative heat loss. This is critical after an emergent delivery. Drying should not be delayed under any circumstances. If emergent procedures are necessary, such as intubation, the infant should be coincidentally dried by another caretaker.
2.  Whenever possible, infants should be placed on a prewarmed surface to avoid conductive heat loss. The temperature of these surfaces or auxiliary heat sources (e.g., hot water bottles) should not exceed approximately 40°C (104°F) because of the risk of thermal injury.
3.  When treating an infant in an open crib or platform warmer, the room temperature should be increased to avoid convective heat loss. The infant should be located away from drafts (e.g., heat/air conditioning vents).
4.  An infant should be clothed to the extent that it does not interfere with patient care and should not be placed near cold surfaces (e.g., exterior windows) to avoid radiant heat loss. At a minimum, a hat should be placed on the head.

### Glucose Homeostasis

During fetal life, metabolic homeostasis is closely regulated by the placenta and maternal circulation. After term birth and in states of health, homeostasis is maintained by the infant's autoregulatory mechanisms. However, these mechanisms often fail during acute illness or after preterm birth. The result is increasing dependence on caretakers for normal metabolic function.

The most common metabolic abnormality in the newborn is hypoglycemia. At birth, blood glucose in the neonate is approximately 60 to 70 percent of the maternal level. Within 1 to 2 h, the level falls to approximately 40 mg/dL. This decline may be accentuated in premature infants, acutely ill infants of any gestational age, and certain other high-risk infants (e.g., infants of diabetic mothers).

Because of the risk of hypoglycemia, all neonates should receive glucose-containing fluids in preparation for and during transport. Ten percent dextrose in water ($D_{10}W$) should be used except in infants weighing less than 1000 g; $D_5W$ should be used in these infants because they are likely to develop hyperglycemia with high glucose intake.

## MONITORING DURING TRANSPORT

One of the critical aspects of care during transport is electronic monitoring. At a minimum, the following monitors should be considered:

**Heart rate and respiratory monitor.** All transported patients should be monitored with impedance ECG and respiratory monitoring. The selection of a monitor should be based on size, weight, battery life, and resistance to motion artifact. The monitor should include a screen with a graphic display of ECG and respiratory tracings. Ideally, the monitor should display pressure wave forms and digital readings of systolic, diastolic, and mean blood pressures from transduced intravascular catheters. It is not essential that the monitoring system include the capability of electrical cardioversion or pacing. The need for such a device in the care of pediatric patients is extremely rare. However, this capability should be available during the transport of patients with known arrhythmias or patients at risk for such problems (e.g., tricyclic poisoning).

**Pulse oximetry.** Continuous pulse oximetry is essential in patients with cardiorespiratory illness. Devices that display a plethysmographic waveform are ideal because they assist in identifying motion artifact.

**Body temperature monitor.** Although not essential, continuous temperature monitoring is helpful in neonates and small infants because of their predisposition to hypothermia.

**Carbon dioxide monitor.** Continuous estimation of $Pa_{CO_2}$ is helpful in patients with respiratory failure. Transcutaneous $CO_2$ monitors may be useful in young infants. However, their value in transport is limited because of the need for frequent calibration using special calibration gases. In addition, they cannot be relied upon to provide accurate absolute measurements. Rather, they are valuable only for identifying trends. Capnography, utilizing continuous in-line infrared analysis to measure end-tidal $CO_2$, is becoming increasingly popular as an alternative to transcutaneous $CO_2$ monitoring.

**Noninvasive blood pressure monitor.** Noninvasive blood pressure monitoring is advisable in patients without indwelling arterial catheters and is often useful even in those with direct monitoring.

## CONDUCT OF A TRANSPORT

The transport of a critically ill child from the emergency department in a community hospital to a regional center is rarely a scheduled event. However, the inability to anticipate the event does not mean that it should not proceed in an orderly fashion. Protocols should exist within the emergency department that outline the procedures for referral of critically ill children. These protocols should provide information about each regional center to which a patient might be referred, including:

- Special services available
- Criteria for referral
- Telephone numbers for consultation, referral, and transport
- Distance and usual response time
- Type of transport personnel and their capabilities
- Type of transport vehicles
- Protocols for preparation of patients

Whenever possible, it is also advisable to establish formal agreements with regional centers that outline the circumstances under which patients can be transported without prior administrative approval.

Once the decision has been made to transport a child, the referring hospital has certain obligations, in addition to medical care. Some of these responsibilities are mandated by the Consolidated Omnibus Budget Reconciliation Acts of 1985 and 1989. The referring physician must contact the receiving hospital and secure a receiving physician. The choice of receiving institution is critical because the referring physician is liable for the adequacy of that facility.

In preparation for transport, the referring hospital should assemble all available information pertinent to the current illness. This generally includes a copy of the emergency record, laboratory data, radiographs, and old medical records if available. The referring physician should inform the parents of the need for transfer and discuss the mechanism by which the child will be transferred. Consent to transport should be obtained from a parent or other responsible individual.

Receiving physicians will often make recommendations regarding stabilization of the patient. This information should be requested if necessary. Referring physicians are not obligated to follow these recommendations if they are considered to be medically inappropriate or beyond the capabilities of the referring hospital. However, under these circumstances, it is advisable for the referring and receiving physicians to develop an alternative plan.

A collaborative decision must also be made regarding who will assume the responsibility for transporting the patient. There are usually four options: private automobile, local ambulance service, local ambulance with personnel from the referring hospital, and service provided by the receiving hospital. The selection should be based on the appropriate balance between the needs of the patient and the resources of each type of provider. Cost should only be a consideration when more than one provider can satisfy the patient's needs.

For most critically ill pediatric patients, ideal care is provided when the emergency department of the referring hospital devotes its energy to providing emergent short-term care and the responsibility for transport is left to the regional center. This is particularly true for neonatal patients because of the special equipment and expertise required for transport. It is rarely in the best interest of critically ill patients to "pick them up and run." However, when transport services are not provided by the regional center or when time is critical, it may be appropriate for the referring hospital to provide transport. In these circumstances, it is entirely the referring hospital's responsibility to ensure the adequacy of care during transport. The converse is true if transport is conducted by the receiving hospital.

In many areas, physicians also have a choice between air and ground transportation. Again, this decision should be made collaboratively. Air transport should be reserved for situations in which reduction in the critical period of transport time is likely to reduce morbidity or mortality. In some emergencies, the critical period ends with the arrival of a transport team from a receiving hospital, because the team is able to administer the emergent therapy, at least on a temporary basis. The advantage of air transport under these circumstances is often less than when the definitive therapy is only available in the receiving hospital, in which case the time advantage includes reduced transit time for the round trip.

## ORGANIZATION OF A PEDIATRIC TRANSPORT PROGRAM

The administration and staffing of a neonatal transport program is rarely the responsibility of emergency department personnel and therefore will not be discussed in this chapter. However, programs responsible for transporting older pediatric patients often originate in the emergency department. A detailed discussion of the conduct of a pediatric transport program is beyond the scope of this book. However, this section will outline the principles of the organization of a transport program and emphasize those principles peculiar to pediatric transport. The focus will be on interhospital transport, although many of the principles also apply to prehospital and intrahospital transport.

### Administration

Components of a transport program can be divided into two general categories: medical and nonmedical components. The medical components include medical personnel, equipment, and supplies. The nonmedical components include transportation, communications, billing, and marketing. The medical components of a pediatric transport program should be supervised by an individual with training and expertise in pediatric intensive care or emergency medicine. While this individual assumes overall responsibility for the program, many management decisions may be shared with or delegated to a nurse manager or other professional. Because of the time constraints on medical professionals and their usual lack of administrative expertise, the responsibility for direction of the nonmedical components of the program is often best assumed by a member of the hospital administration.

### Transport Team Personnel

A variety of personnel might serve as attendants during pediatric transport including physicians, nurses, nurse practitioners, respiratory therapists, physician assistants, and paramedic–emergency medical technicians. The selection of a particular professional group is most often governed by practical issues such as availability, salary costs, and the requirement for training. Although it would be desirable to have a physician with expertise in pediatric emergency medicine in attendance during each transport, this is rarely practical. Utilizing physicians-in-training is an alternative. However, the competition between transport activities and other aspects of their training often makes this an unattractive alternative. An increasing number of programs now utilize specially trained nonphysician personnel exclusively.

Ideally, pediatric transport personnel would have responsibility for pediatric patients only. However, few centers have the volume of pediatric transports or the resources to support a stand-alone team for pediatric patients. More often, the responsibility for transporting infants and small children falls to teams who also transport neonatal patients. Older pediatric patients are often attended by teams who also transport adults. Both systems can result in competent patient care if special effort is devoted to preparing personnel to manage pediatric emergencies.

Training requirements for team members may vary and will depend upon their designated responsibilities during transport. For example, programs that utilize physicians may not need to train non-physicians in skills related to airway management. At least one member of the team attending every patient should include an individual who is experienced in diagnosing and managing virtually all life-threatening pediatric emergencies. It is helpful to cross-train if more than one discipline (e.g., respiratory therapy and nursing) is represented on the team. In addition, all team members should have a thorough understanding of the transport environment and should be familiar with all communication devices.

Many different training strategies have been utilized to prepare transport personnel. Common to most are didactic sessions during which cognitive knowledge is attained, laboratory sessions during which technical skills are taught, and supervised patient care. A sample curriculum is depicted in Table 5-1. This training is generally followed by participation in transport accompanied by an experienced team member.

## Vehicles

Three types of vehicles are used during interhospital transport: ground ambulances, helicopters, and fixed-wing aircraft. The choice of a vehicle for a program is often dictated by the features of the anticipated population and the relative advantages and disadvantages of each mode of transportation.

## Ambulances

Ground ambulances are available at most medical centers but may require modification for optimal transport of pediatric patients. Their disadvantage is excessive travel time between hospitals when distances are great or when terrain, road conditions, or traffic congestion require slow travel. Their advantage is relatively low operating costs compared to other forms of transportation.

## Helicopters

Helicopters provide the most rapid service when distances between hospitals are less than approximately 150 miles. When landing facilities are available at both hospitals, helicopter transportation reduces transit time by at least two-thirds compared to ground ambulance. However, noise and vibration levels are high, and it is rarely practical to stop the vehicle for the management of an emergency requiring a more stable environment. They also generally have a more confined patient care compartment compared to other vehicles. The impact of these problems can be minimized by extensive preparation of the patient prior to transport and sophisticated electronic monitoring. Because of their speed, helicopters are the vehicle of choice for programs transporting a high proportion of trauma patients for whom time to the receiving hospital is much more important than in-transit care. The major disadvantage of helicopters is the extremely high cost of operation. The purchase cost of a helicopter is usually in excess of $2.5 million; lease/operation contracts usually exceed $50,000 per month.

## Fixed-Wing Aircraft

Fixed-wing aircraft also offer the advantage of speed, which is five to six times that of ground ambulances. However, because of the requirement for transfer between airports and hospitals, this advantage is only appreciated when distances exceed approximately 120 miles. Fixed-wing aircraft are also much less costly to operate than helicopters.

## Equipment/Supplies

Equipment used to care for pediatric patients during transport is similar to that found in most emergency departments, with the exception

**Table 5-1.** Training for Pediatric Critical Care Transport Team

Certification
  Basic Life Support (Provider Class Type C)
  Pediatric Advanced Life Support
  Neonatal Resuscitation Program
Didactic training
  Respiratory failure
  Airway obstruction
  Respiratory therapies
  Congestive heart failure
  Cardiac arrhythmias
  Shock
  Sepsis and other infections
  Status epilepticus
  Near drowning
  Drug overdose
  Comatose child
  Multiple trauma
  Pharmacotherapy
  X-ray interpretation
  Aviation physiology
  Radio communications
  Vehicle safety
Technical skills training
  Endotracheal intubation
  Arterial puncture
  Central-line placement
  Intraosseous needle placement
  Thoracentesis
  Thoracostomy tube placement

that it is portable and reduced in size and weight. This is in contrast to equipment used during neonatal transport, which is usually specially designed for its unique function. The basic equipment required for pediatric transport includes the following:

Ventilator
Cardiorespiratory monitor with invasive pressure monitoring
  capability
Pulse oximeter
Intravenous pumps
Noninvasive blood pressure monitor

This equipment should be mounted to a stretcher or be fitted with devices that can be secured to the vehicle or stretcher during transport.

Supplies and small equipment should be preassembled in equipment packs. These supplies can be divided into separate packs based on those required for airway management and all other care. Suggested inventories for these two packs are included in Table 5-2.

## Communications

Reliable and rapid communications are essential for the efficient operation of a transport program. Communication systems that support transport programs are of three varieties: 911 emergency dispatch centers, communication centers within emergency departments, and communication centers dedicated solely to transport programs. Centers that support emergency medical services (EMS) as well as transport are generally more economical. This combined function also helps facilitate the integration of EMS and the transport program. However, 911 dispatch centers are usually governed by agencies other than hospitals and therefore may not be responsive to the needs of the transport program.

The dispatch center should have equipment capable of coordinating communications between the following groups: referring and receiving medical personnel, transport attendants, vehicle operators, local EMS providers, and area air traffic controllers. This may require the integration of local and long-distance telephone lines, cellular

**Table 5-2.** Content of Equipment Packs for Pediatric Critical Care Transport

**Pediatric Nursing Pack**

| | |
|---|---|
| Procedure tray, sterile | Masks |
| Intravenous catheters | Suction catheters |
| Lancets, sterile | Buretrol |
| Blood culture bottle | Disposable transducer |
| Blood collection tubes | Heimlich valves |
| IV limb boards | Thoracostomy tubes |
| Tape | Foley catheters |
| Dextrostix bottle | Blood component filter |
| Intraosseous needles | Scissors |
| Rubber bands | Hemostat |
| Safety pins | Tape measure |
| Tourniquets | Pacifier |
| Syringes | K-Y jelly |
| IV fluids | Butterfly needles |
| Transilluminator | Sterile gauze |
| Stethoscope | Stopcock |
| Nondisposable blood pressure cuffs | Extension IV tubing |
| Cotton balls | Thermometer, digital |
| Stockinette for caps | Alcohol & Betadine swabs |
| Silver thermal cap | IV extension "T" connectors |
| Ear plugs | Needles |
| Sterile gloves | ECG leads/pads |
| Yankauer suction tube | Feeding tubes |
| Replogle tube | Pediatric Medication Pack |

**Pediatric Respiratory Therapy Pack**

| | |
|---|---|
| Airway supplies | |
|   Laerdal masks | Oral airways |
|   Oxygen tubing | Pediatric ventilation |
|   Nonrebreathing mask |   bag (PEEP capable) |
|   Aerosol tubing | Laryngoscope |
|   Nasal cannula | Pediatric manual |
|   Venturi mask |   ventilation bag |
|   Pediatric trach collar | Endotracheal tubes |
| Other equipment | |
|   Benzoin applicators | Normal saline vials |
|   Wrenches | Tape |
|   Cable ties | Oxygen connectors |
|   High pressure air and | $O_2$ analyzer membrane kit |
|     $O_2$ quick connectors | $O_2$ flowmeter nipple |
|   Chemical hot packs | One-way valve |
|   Stethoscope | Septisol |
|   Pressure manometer | Tape measure |
|   Pulse oximeter sensors | Suction catheters |

telephones, UHF and VHF band radios, and radio pagers. Ideally, the centers should also have a device to record all communications.

Transport vehicles should be equipped to permit the same range of communications as the center. At a minimum, this will require the availability of both UHF and VHF band radios. Cellular telephones should also be considered in areas of the country where coverage is extensive. They offer the advantage of user friendliness and a style of communication with which more medical personnel are accustomed.

## Patient Care Protocols/Quality Assurance

Patient care protocols should be developed by the medical director of the program. These should reflect the institutional standards of care for the full range of emergencies likely to be encountered. The program should also document the techniques for training personnel and certifying competency.

During the conduct of a transport, the team should be supervised by a physician with expertise in the care of pediatric emergencies. If this individual is not in attendance, then phone or radio communication is advisable at some point during the transport.

The program should also have a systematic plan to review transports to ensure quality of care. This plan should involve all disciplines represented by the team.

## BIBLIOGRAPHY

AAP Task Force on Interhospital Transport: *Guidelines for Air and Ground Transport of Neonatal and Pediatric Patients.* Elk Grove, IL, American Academy of Pediatrics, 1993.

Bose CL: The transport environment, in MacDonald MG, Miller MK (eds): *Emergency Transport of the Perinatal Patient.* Boston, Little, Brown, 1989, pp 194–211.

Bose CL: An overview of the organization and administration of a perinatal transport service, in MacDonald MG, Miller MK (eds): *Emergency Transport of the Perinatal Patient.* Boston, Little, Brown, 1989, pp 34–75.

Hackel A: Neonatal and pediatric medical transport programs, in Shoemaker WC, Ayers SM, Grenvik A, et al (eds): *Textbook of Critical Care,* 2d ed. Philadelphia, Saunders, 1989, pp 82–87.

Klaus MH, Martin RJ, Fanaroff AA: The physical environment, in Klaus MH, Fanaroff AA (eds): *Care of the High Risk Neonate,* 4th ed. Philadelphia, Saunders, 1993, pp 114–129.

Kliegman RM: Problems in metabolic adaptation: Glucose, calcium, and magnesium, in Klaus MH, Fanaroff AA (eds): *Care of the High Risk Neonate,* 4th ed. Philadelphia, Saunders, 1993, pp 282–301.

McCloskey KA, Orr RA: Pediatric transport issues in emergency medicine. *Emerg Med Clin North Am* 9(3):475, 1991.

Schneider C, Gomez M, Lee R: Evaluation of ground ambulance, rotor-wing, and fixed-wing aircraft services. *Crit Care Clin* 8(3):533, 1992.

# 6
# DISASTER MEDICAL SERVICES
## Brian D. Mahoney

Disasters may be natural, such as earthquakes, hurricanes, volcanic eruptions, floods, or tornadoes. Or disasters may be of human origin, such as airplane or train crashes, fires, famine, leaks of hazardous materials from industrial sites or during transportation, or acts of terrorism. Contrary to popular belief, epidemics are unusual after a disaster in the developed world. A disaster may involve the destruction of a great deal of property with few human victims. In this chapter the focus is on medical disaster planning. The American College of Emergency Physicians (ACEP) defines a *medical disaster* as an occurrence "when the destructive effects of natural or manmade forces overwhelm the ability of a given area or community to meet the demand for health care." Emergency medicine is the only civilian branch of medicine in the United States that considers disaster planning and management a primary field within its domain.

Medical disaster planning primarily involves preparations for managing multiple casualty incidents. In labeling a given multiple casualty incident as a medical disaster, the key issue is not the absolute number of victims. The key is the relation between the needs of the victims and the ability of a given health care system to meet those needs using normal operating procedures. For example, in one community a head-on collision involving two cars and eight severely injured victims may require implementation of the community's medical disaster response plan. In another community such a collision could easily be managed by the normal in-place medical resources. In the daily practice of emergency medicine, maximal care is provided to a limited number of patients. In a medical disaster with multiple

**Table 6-1.** Disaster Management Team

| Title | Role |
|---|---|
| Chief executive officer (e.g., mayor or designee) | Supervision of overall operation |
| | Communication with public |
| | Direction of requests for state or federal assistance |
| Fire chief | Overall scene command |
| | Supervision of victim rescue, extrication |
| | Hazard control |
| Police | Traffic management |
| | Scene security |
| | Overall scene command in some plans |
| Emergency medical services | Victim triage |
| | Stabilization |
| | Transportation |
| Public works | Support equipment such as heavy machinery for extrication |
| | Structural safety expertise |
| Emergency manager of civil defense | Communications |
| | Extra personnel |
| | Extra equipment |
| Red Cross | Food, shelter, clothing for displaced victims |
| | Disaster welfare inquiry system |

*Source:* American College of Emergency Physicians: *Disaster Planning and Management for the Emergency Physician.* Emmitsburg, MD, Federal Emergency Management Agency, 1983. Used by permission.

casualties, changes in standard operating procedure are necessary. Instead of doing everything medically possible for one individual, field and hospital personnel strive to achieve the greatest good for the greatest number of potential survivors. For example: patients in cardiac arrest are pronounced dead, and precious resources are not spent on resuscitation attempts; patients are hospitalized only when absolutely necessary; laboratory and x-ray studies are used for critical information only; nurses have increased autonomy; and paramedics operate using standing orders, without the need for additional authorization from medical control.

A successful disaster response requires coordination of many governmental agencies and services (Table 6-1). The plan requires joint planning meetings, established lines of communication and authority, and regular coordinated multiagency drills. J. F. Waeckerle describes disasters as "unexpected, chaotic, horrendous, catastrophes. . . . One is initially horrified, then bewildered and confused about what to do, where to start." Since a medical disaster will be a time of confusion under the best of circumstances, the plan must call for following normal operating procedures as much as possible. The fewer exceptions to the rules that stressed rescuers are expected to remember, the better. Mutual aid agreements between adjacent jurisdictions should be included in the plan and practiced regularly in drills.

## PHASES OF A DISASTER RESPONSE

There are three phases to a disaster response (as taught in the ACEP course "Disaster Planning and Management for the Emergency Physician"): activation, implementation, and recovery.

### Activation

The first phase, the activation phase, has two components. The first component is notification and initial response. The first responder reports the nature of the incident, the extent of damage, the estimated number and types of injuries, the hazards for victims and rescuers, and the best access to the scene and/or routes known to be blocked. It is crucial that the first responder take the time to ascertain and relay this information to medical control before attempting to render direct medical assistance. Early, accurate information leads to the appropriate mobilization of disaster response personnel and materials. The

second component of the activation phase is the organization of an incident command post and further assessment of the scene. Typically the incident command post is set up by fire and rescue personnel, who locate it as close to the scene as safety allows, uphill and upwind of potential liquid and windborne hazards.

### Implementation

The second phase, the implementation phase, has three components. The first is search and rescue. This is usually carried out by fire and rescue personnel because of the special expertise and equipment needed in a hazardous environment. Medical providers must remember that without this expertise and equipment they may themselves become victims. The second component involves triage, stabilization, and transport. The first arriving medical providers must assess medical needs, call to mobilize medical resources, establish contact with the overall incident commander (for example, the fire or police chief), and identify hazards and a safe casualty collection point, usually uphill and upwind from the scene. As more ambulances arrive, early treatment begins but it is limited to airway control, oxygen administration, hemorrhage control, and backboarding. Triage is begun: victims are grouped by priority within the casualty collection area. The third component of the implementation phase is definitive management of scene hazards and victims. Victims are transported to hospitals for definitive care according to the priorities identified by the triage officer.

### Recovery

The first stage of the recovery phase is withdrawal from the scene, after making a systematic check for any missed victims. The second stage is the return to normal operations. Ambulances are restocked and standard operating procedures resumed. The Red Cross and the Salvation Army provide food, shelter, and clothing for displaced survivors. Concerned family members can use the Red Cross's disaster welfare inquiry system (DWIS) to locate victims.

The final stage of recovery is debriefing. A primary purpose of debriefing is to analyze the operation in order to improve future disaster responses. In addition, it plays a key part in the early identification and avoidance of potential psychological difficulties among the many rescuers.

### TRIAGE

Triage is the process of sorting and classifying patients into categories according to priority of treatment. Its aim is to do the most good for the largest number of victims.

Multiple systems of triage exist. Many of them involve a tagging system. In all of them patients are classified according to priority of need. In a typical four-category system, a patient would be classified as severe, moderate, minor, or dead or expectant death. In the severe category are patients who, given available care, have a reasonable chance of survival but without care have a markedly diminished chance of survival. This group gets the highest priority for care and transport. In the moderately injured group should be patients whose injuries will not lead to morbidity or mortality if they do not receive immediate care and transport. In the minor category are the "walking wounded," patients whose injuries will not lead to significant morbidity while they wait for treatment and transport of the two higher categories. In the fourth category are people in cardiac arrest, who are immediately pronounced dead and receive none of the scarce medical resources, and the "hopelessly wounded." Medical providers, who are accustomed to doing everything possible to save such patients on the chance that there will be a rare survivor, often have great difficulty limiting the care of patients in this category. These patients should receive supportive or palliative care until all higher-priority cases are managed. Which patients fall into which of these four categories depends on how large the medical disaster is and how thinly stretched the scarce medical resources have become. The rescuers must remember that the goal is to do the most good for the most potential survivors.

Triage is an ongoing, dynamic process. Patients' conditions are continually changing, and serial triage examinations must take place so that patients may be moved up or down in priority of treatment. Triage begins at first contact in the field. Rescuers check and correct, if possible, airway, breathing, and circulation on each victim and then rapidly move on to the next victim. Patients may or may not be tagged at this point. Only rapid life-saving maneuvers are carried out. For example, an oral airway may be placed, brief positive pressure ventilation done to see if a patient resumes spontaneous respiration, and a pressure dressing placed over a heavily bleeding wound. Cardiopulmonary resuscitation is not done.

Triage occurs again at the casualty collection point. This is usually the best time to apply triage tags. The victims are physically grouped according to priority of treatment to allow easy identification of those who should be transported first. The severe group should be collected at the location nearest to the ambulance loading area. More in-depth assessment and care may be provided according to the availability of resources. Serial examinations at the casualty collection point may lead to a change in the triage category. Triage influences the choice of a receiving hospital. Triage occurs again on arrival at the hospital. Each triage examination builds on and refines the sorting process that has already occurred.

There is some controversy over the value of triage tagging systems. Tags provide a record of critical medical interventions and prevent some redundancies in the triage survey by identifying those patients already checked. Vayer states that in many actual disasters tags are not used because they are such a marked departure from daily routine. He recommends using them as part of normal procedures, for a given period every year, in all accidents involving more than one victim. A disadvantage of tear-off tags is that they are unidirectional, allowing only for deterioration of the patient's condition. The author recommends sorting patients into physically separated groups according to degree of severity.

Each prehospital disaster plan should identify a medical response team consisting of a physician and paramedic group small enough to keep trained and up to date yet large enough that a nucleus can always be on call. The team responds to all disaster calls in a given geographic area, helping the other paramedic and medical providers to follow the philosophy and components of medical disaster management. Such medical response teams have proved valuable in actual medical disaster responses.

The members of the medical response team and their roles need to be identifiable at the scene: the best method is to use labeled vests. In reviewing the disaster response at the 1981 Hyatt Regency skywalk collapse, Orr and Robinson concluded that brightly colored overlay vests with large lettering are most effective. They reported that, initially, identification was less of a problem because rescuers recognized one another. Later, as more mutual aid providers arrived, identification became difficult. They also reported that police delayed some key personnel at the outer perimeter for lack of identification, and stated that key personnel should carry some form of disaster identification card.

## ORGANIZING THE MULTIPLE CASUALTY SCENE

The following discussion provides a framework for organizing a response to a multiple casualty incident confined to a single geographic location, for example, a fire or collapse in a single building, or an airplane crash. Modifications would be needed for larger, more diffuse multiple casualty incidents such as a tornado with multiple touchdowns, or an earthquake with multiple fires and collapses. In such cases, a response team would be required at each area of relative victim concentration.

Many systems have adapted the Incident Command System (ICS) to organize their disaster response. ICS was developed by the FIRESCOPE program in response to a series of wildfires in Southern California in 1970. It has since been taught and accepted nationally particularly by Fire services. There are seven key functions that the incident commander must manage. The ICS can be as small as one individual serving all seven functions or expand as needed by attaching divisions and task forces to each of four sections. If an incident commander is unwilling to delegate any of these seven functions, then he must assume them himself. The typical organization for the seven functions is as follows: an information officer, liaison officer, and safety officer all attached to the incident commander, and four section chiefs for finance, logistics, operations, and planning. EMS would typically fit in as a branch or division of the operations section.

Fire and rescue personnel usually provide overall incident command. They should establish an inner hazard perimeter within which emergency medical services (EMS) personnel are not allowed. Fire and rescue personnel should conduct search, rescue, and extrication of victims, bringing them out of this hazardous area. Fire personnel should establish a scene command post uphill and upwind from any hazard.

EMS personnel should gather extricated victims at the casualty collection point, which should be close enough to the disaster for easy access yet far enough away, and far enough uphill and upwind, to be free of hazard. The collection site must afford easy access to direct transportation routes to hospitals.

EMS must provide several identifiable command personnel. The EMS branch director is in overall medical control and serves as liaison to the incident commander. This person should be a physician or paramedic supervisor active in EMS and experienced in triage, resuscitation, stabilization, prehospital communications, and EMS capabilities. The EMS branch director must remember that EMS acts in support, not command, of the public safety agency in overall scene control. Ideally, a second physician, working under the EMS branch director, should have overall responsibility for triage operations. If there is only one physician, both these roles will be performed by one individual.

The EMS branch director should assign a paramedic to stay at the incident command post and act as communications liaison with the incident commander. The medical transportation officer, a paramedic supervisor, directs arriving crews in loading and transporting patients. The medical communications officer serves the transportation officer by relaying information to the regional medical control center and by relaying information back to the medical team at the scene regarding the ongoing capacity of various hospitals to handle patients.

In a large disaster extensive transport is needed. Resources to include in a regional disaster plan include metropolitan transit buses, school buses, and taxis. Many of the walking wounded will actually arrange their own transport to the nearest hospital. In general, the sicker patients are taken to the nearest capable hospital. However, the medical triage officer may elect to use helicopters and ambulances to take some patients to more distant hospitals, preserving some emergency capacity at the nearest hospital for patients who deteriorate or take longer to extricate. In smaller multiple casualty incidents, patient tracking is easier for families if all or most victims go to one or two hospitals. However, patient care must not be compromised by overloading a few hospitals.

Police need to establish an outer perimeter to ensure traffic control and deny scene access to unauthorized personnel. They must ensure crowd control and the safety of bystanders and the media, and in some cases prevent looting. Because a strong police presence is often necessary, in some systems the police chief, rather than the fire chief, is the incident commander.

Ambulance flow should be arranged in one direction. The ambulance exit route must not be blocked by other vehicles or by fire hoses too large for ambulances to drive over or that will be damaged by ambulance tires. To avoid congestion, it is often necessary to designate a staging area where ambulances and supplies are collected and then directed to the casualty collection point as needed. Unfortunately, convergence is a common phenomenon in a disaster. Uninvited rescue agencies, and large numbers of civilians, will come from surprising distances, adding to the congestion and confusion at the scene. An obstruction-free helicopter landing zone should be established close enough to be usable but far enough away so that rotor wash and noise do not interfere with the rest of the operation. If there are many victims, or the weather is inclement, a secondary casualty collection point, e.g., a school gymnasium, should be established.

A temporary morgue may be needed. The medical examiner is in charge of removal, storage, and identification of bodies. Ice arenas and refrigerator trucks are possible resources.

## COMMUNICATIONS

Communication problems are frequently identified in reviews of disaster responses. The multiple responding agencies typically do not have radios that operate on the same frequencies. Normal communications, principally the telephone, may be damaged or rapidly become overloaded. Alternatives to telephone systems include radio, cellular phones, messengers, and bullhorns. Orr and Robinson reported that in the Hyatt Regency skywalk collapse, bullhorns and messengers were necessary because of the noise of heavy extrication machinery. Hand-held radios relying on outside repeaters proved unreliable.

To avoid overloading radio channels during a disaster, paramedic radio communications to their base hospital should be limited to key information. Paramedics should be authorized by their medical director to utilize all standard operating procedures without medical control.

The regional trauma center must rapidly obtain information from all hospitals in the region regarding emergency department capacity, operating room and critical care capabilities, and hospital bed availability. This information should be regularly updated and relayed to the incident medical director and transportation officer at the casualty collection point.

## DISASTER MANAGEMENT TEAM

A disaster is a multifaceted event that requires expertise in many areas. So that personnel can adequately respond to a large, widely scattered, or prolonged disaster, a disaster management team is needed. Table 6-1 lists some key roles. In relatively small disasters, not all the personnel listed in the table may be needed, but they must be available. For large or prolonged disasters, an emergency operating center (EOC) should be provided for in the plan. Typically such a center is established in the city council offices in the nearest large city to the disaster site. The heads of each group involved in the disaster management team gather in the EOC to receive information, allocate resources, access additional supplies, and request outside assistance as needed.

## HOSPITAL

The Joint Commission on Accreditation of Health Organizations requires every hospital to have a written disaster plan, covering every department and employee in the hospital, and to test that plan twice a year. To mobilize the disaster response without overloading hospital telephone lines, a chain call system can be established. Key hospital personnel should keep telephone lists at home or in their wallets. In massive disasters, community warning sirens can be sounded, alerting the public and the hospital staff to tune in to radio and television for announcements. Emergency physicians, who are needed in large numbers as soon as a disaster occurs, should have and carry their beepers at all times. On many beeper systems, dialing a single number can sound all the beepers at once.

Many steps must be completed in a short time to prepare for a large influx of patients. The decision to institute a hospital disaster response is usually a combined medical and administrative decision. It is better to call and mobilize early than to get caught behind. However, if information from a potential disaster scene is not sufficient to merit notifying all hospital personnel, an interim response plan may be effective, in which only emergency personnel are alerted. If the early disaster information suggests a prolonged event, then everyone should be notified. However, only half should come in at once so that the entire operation does not grind to a halt in 12 to 16 hours. The importance of writing the disaster plan so that it will be as close as possible to normal operating procedures, and of following the twice-a-year drill requirement, cannot be overemphasized. When a disaster occurs, all personnel need to be able to carry out their roles automatically. It is too late to read the manual.

Hospital administration must set up a control center with adequate telephone access. It should be near but not in the emergency department.

The emergency department must be rapidly cleared. Patients ready for discharge should be discharged and those needing admission admitted. Those without a disposition whose problem is not severe should be moved to a waiting area and told to expect a long wait. *The emergency department must be adequately stocked.* All stretchers must be returned from the wards immediately; extra oxygen and crystalloid infusion equipment must be prepared. The nursing supervisors need to obtain an accurate list of beds available. Dirty rooms need rapid cleaning, and inpatients ready for discharge should be discharged immediately.

Extra security officers should be in place as soon as possible. They must secure all doors to the hospital and keep driveways clear for ambulance access. They need to control patients, concerned family, the curious, and the media.

As patients arrive at the hospital, a medical triage officer should meet them at the door and reassess their treatment priorities. Categories similar to the four prehospital categories should be employed. The severely injured must receive immediate stabilization. The moderate and minor groups need regular checks to be sure they do not deteriorate while waiting. The dead are moved to a temporary morgue, and the hopelessly injured continue to receive palliative care.

Documentation is limited to critical findings and treatments. Some plans call for the use of the prehospital disaster tag to record this limited information. Other plans include the preparation of kits containing the emergency department record, x-ray requests, laboratory slips and tubes, and wrist bands, all prelabeled with a discrete disaster number. Medical records and laboratory computers accept these numbers, which are used for patient identification until full normal registration is possible. At that point the computer will search previous medical records to match disaster numbers with the records of victims who have been patients previously. Such a prelabeled kit system can be used during normal operations, on unidentified critically ill or injured patients, so that all hospital departments are familiar with the concept. Admissions personnel are needed to log key information rapidly. Hours or days later they will be able to complete the registration process.

## PUBLIC RELATIONS

The medical disaster plan should include a section on the proper relationship with the media. Representatives of the media are present at all medical disasters. They may be a valuable resource in announcing hazards or the need for evacuation. In addition, they may be used to make a general announcement that hospital or rescue personnel should report to work. The plan should include a means to provide the media with adequate information both at the site and in the hospital. At the disaster site, regular briefings help avoid the hazard of their becoming victims while in search of more information. At the hospital, regular briefings and a room with adequate telephone access will prevent the media from invading patient care areas. A hospital public relations officer should act as liaison with the media. His or her duties are to prepare the press room, hold regular briefings, and arrange appropriate photographic opportunities. These must be carried out while balancing the public's right to know against the individual victim's right to privacy.

In their review of managing the media during a disaster, Partington and Savage warned: "If an authoritative source does not provide this information reporters will talk to anyone and may receive unreliable information from which they, not surprisingly, make erroneous deductions. It is in the interest of the hospital, therefore, to release accurate information in a responsible way."

Designated waiting areas, away from treatment areas, must be available for family members. The public relations officer or other assigned personnel must regularly update these relatives on casualty lists and patient conditions. The hospital chaplain and volunteers should be present to provide support. These waiting areas should have adequate telephone lines as well as access to food, beverages, and bathrooms.

## THE NATIONAL DISASTER MEDICAL SYSTEM

The National Disaster Medical System (NDMS) was created in 1984 to establish a mechanism to handle large numbers of casualties from a military or civilian disaster. It is a cooperative effort between the civilian hospital sector of the United States and the Department of Health and Human Services, the Department of Defense, the Federal Emergency Management Agency, the Veterans Administration, and state, regional, and local government agencies. In establishing the need for the NDMS, Mahoney et al. estimated that if the earthquake that destroyed Fort Tejon, California, in 1857 (Richter 8.3) occurred today it would cause 3000 to 14,000 deaths and from 12,000 to 55,000 injuries requiring hospitalization. No single metropolitan area or even a state could care for so many injuries. To meet the needs of an overwhelming medical disaster the NDMS is being developed to handle casualties of a magnitude of 100,000 victims arising from a massive peacetime disaster or an overseas conventional military conflict. This system builds on and replaces the Civilian Military Contingency Hospital System.

There are two component parts to the NDMS. The first part is the organization of the participating civilian hospitals and health care providers of 74 designated NDMS metropolitan areas. Each of these 74 areas is developing a system whereby large numbers of victims can be brought to that metropolitan area for definitive medical care provided by the many participating private hospitals. This system is a form of mutual aid agreement similar to that which many communities already have for local disasters. The NDMS is a mutual aid system on a national scale.

The second component of the NDMS is the development of disaster medical assistance teams (DMAT). These teams of volunteer health care providers provide their own equipment and transportation to a site of a civilian disaster in the United States. They are self-supporting so as not to be an additional burden to overstretched local resources. Theoretically there are two basic types of DMATs. The first is a 103-person clearing and staging team modeled after an Army medical clearing company. This type will provide medical care in field hospitals in the disaster area itself and aid evacuation of victims from the affected area to 1 or more of the 74 participating metropolitan areas. Several DMATs of this basic model do exist and have responded to actual disasters in the U.S. and its overseas possessions. The second type of DMAT is a 215-person mobile surgical unit modeled after a mobile Army surgical unit. These civilian DMATs will not be used in military conflicts or outside the United States.

The NDMS does not replace state, regional, or local disaster plans. It will only be used for a massive disaster. The system can be deployed if a governor asks the Federal Emergency Management Agency for federal assistance and the request is approved by presidential declaration of a major disaster. It can be deployed by the Secretary of Defense in the event of a military conflict of sufficient magnitude. In both civilian and military scenarios, the patients are transported on military medical evacuation aircraft and distributed to participating areas under the direction of the Armed Services Medical Regulating Office.

## HAZARDOUS MATERIALS INCIDENTS

Hazardous materials pose one of the greatest risks for creating massive multiple casualty incidents. The catastrophic release of methyl isocyanate at Bhopal, India in 1984 and numerous smaller events clearly show the magnitude of the risk. Thousands of hazardous chemicals are manufactured, stored, and then transported by road, water, and railroad through virtually every city and town in the United States. On a smaller scale every farm, homeowner's garage, and many businesses will have chemicals with the potential to injure many people under the right circumstances. Government has responded to these hazards through passage of the Superfund Amendments and Reauthorization Act of 1986 (SARA), and the regulations of the Environmental Protection Agency and Occupational Safety and Health Administration (OSHA). Title III of SARA, the Emergency Preparedness and Community Right-to-Know Act, and subsequent OSHA requirements mandate that responders to a hazardous materials incident have appropriate training commensurate to their role at that scene. Without this training, rescuers are at great risk to become victims themselves. The OSHA training has four increasing levels of sophistication: hazardous materials awareness, operations, technician, and specialist. All EMS personnel need the first two levels, some need the more specialized technical training, and a few need the specialist level.

A hazardous materials response team requires extensive training, equipment, and practice. This duty most often is filled by the fire department. It is unrealistic for every town to train and equip a complete hazardous materials response team. Because of the complexity of the training, specialized equipment needed, and the widespread risk of a hazardous materials incident, states may form regional response teams to supplement the local resources. It will take time for a regional team to respond and patients may present to your hospital without adequate prehospital decontamination. All emergency physicians would be wise to obtain at a minimum the hazardous materials awareness level of training.

Goals at the scene will include confining the hazard, isolating it from further entry into the hot zone, evacuation of people at risk, decontamination of those exposed, stabilization of those injured, and transporting those in need of further medical care. Rescuers must remember not to become victims themselves. This can be avoided by following training principles, including designation of a hot (contaminated), warm (where decontamination occurs), and cold area. Entry into each area must be limited to those who need to be there and who have the necessary personal protective equipment for each of these zones. Do not unnecessarily spread contamination! Do not contaminate yourself, your vehicle, or your hospital. Wear personal protective equipment, undress and decontaminate the patient at the scene if possible, remove unneeded equipment or use a BLS ambulance if possible, cocoon the patient in a blanket or body bag in the ambulance, notify the hospital of your approach, and wait in the ambulance if possible while the hospital prepares the entry floor, decontamination room, and decontamination personnel. Resources for specific information on chemical hazards include a vehicle's DOT placard, bill of lading, material safety data sheet, CHEMTREC (1-800-424-9300), your regional poison center, and the 24-hour duty officer at your state division of emergency management. Most inhalation emergencies are treated with oxygen and airway control as needed. Most skin exposures are treated by dilution and washing. Don't forget to thoroughly irrigate the eyes. Some chemicals such as sodium metal react violently with water and should instead be brushed off. For dry chemicals that create problems if inhaled, such as asbestos, a damp mopping of the skin will help to prevent the material from becoming airborne.

## MASS EVACUATION

The following is a summary of some key points in R. Leonard's review of mass evacuation. The first priority is the need to identify clearly who has the authority to order an evacuation. Often this authority rests with the fire chief. The overall disaster plan must specify the ordinance granting such authority. There are two types of evacuations—immediate, as in a toxic leak, and potential, as in a flood or hurricane. The news media can provide a valuable service in broadcasting announcements of potential mass evacuations.

There are four phases of a mass evacuation as developed by the Disaster Research Center of Ohio State University. The first phase is the warning. It is crucial that accurate, authoritative information be broadcast. The center found that people do not leave until they perceive a risk and do not evacuate if conflicting information causes doubt. Any announcements should explain the reason for evacuation, when it is to occur, and where people are to go. The second phase is withdrawal. The Disaster Research Center found that although persuading people to evacuate is often difficult, once they decide to go, they usually do so in an orderly fashion. An Environmental Protection Agency study of 500 evacuations involving 1.1 million people found that 99 percent of the people left by car. The difficult problem is in evacuating hospitals, jails, nursing homes, and mental institutions. The third phase is finding shelter. The center found that 72 percent of evacuees arrange their own shelter with friends, relatives, or motels. The other 28 percent go to public shelters (e.g., school gymnasiums, churches, and armories), where conflicts can be kept to a minimum by regular announcements on developments. The final phase is return. This is the most chaotic, as people make their own assessment of when it is safe to do so. Regular media broadcasts on continuing hazards help prevent premature return.

## MENTAL HEALTH

An often overlooked but vital part of any medical disaster plan is attention to the mental health needs of the victims, their families, and the rescuers. Wilkinson studied the psychological sequelae of 102 victims, observers, and rescuers at the Hyatt Regency skywalk collapse in Kansas City. He reported that survivors in these groups suffered repeated recollections of the disaster (88 percent), sadness (83 percent), fatigue (57 percent), nightmares (52 percent), and guilt (44 percent). Critical incident stress debriefing should be organized as soon as possible after a disaster. This will help rescuers vent their feelings and help identify individuals in need of further counseling.

## KEY POINTS

Following are the key points to remember when dealing with a disaster:

1. Do the most good for the most number of potential survivors.
2. Do not become a victim yourself.
3. Prioritize patient care, ensuring basic care for all potential survivors before organizing definitive care for lesser problems.
4. Remember that triage is an ongoing process requiring serial checks to record changes in treatment categories as patients improve or worsen.

5. Make your plan as close to day-to-day standard operating procedures as possible.
6. Remember that although limiting morbidity and mortality is the key goal in any disaster response, EMS is not in overall scene command.

---

**TEN OF AUF DER HEIDE'S PRINCIPLES OF DISASTER RESPONSE***

1. Because of the limited resources available, disaster preparedness proposals need to take cost-effectiveness into consideration.
2. Interest in disaster preparedness is proportional to how recent and how extensive the last disaster was.
3. Base disaster plans on what people are likely to do, rather than what they should do.
4. For disaster planning to be effective, it must be interorganizational.
5. The process of planning is more important than the written document that results.
6. In disasters, what are thought to be "communications problems" are often coordination problems in disguise.
7. Panic is not a common problem in disasters; getting people to evacuate is.
8. Inquiries about loved ones thought to be in the impact zone are not likely to be discouraged, but can be reduced or channeled in less disruptive ways, if the needed information is provided at a location away from the disaster area.
9. Adequate disaster preparedness requires planning with the media rather than for the media.
10. Many of the questions that will be asked by reporters are predictable, and procedures can be established in advance for collecting the desired information.

---

* *Source:* Adapted from Auf der Heide, E., *Disaster Response: Principles of Preparation and Coordination,* Mosby, St. Louis, 1989.

## BIBLIOGRAPHY

Auf der Heide, E: *Disaster Response: Principles of Preparation and Coordination.* St. Louis, Mosby, 1989.

American College of Emergency Physicians: Disaster medical services. *Ann Emerg Med* 14:1026, 1985.

American College of Emergency Physicians: *Disaster Planning and Management for the Emergency Physician.* Emmitsburg, MD, Federal Emergency Management Agency, 1983.

Leonard R: Mass evacuation in disasters. *J Emerg Med* 2:279, 1985.

Orr SM, Robinson WA: The Hyatt Regency skywalk collapse: An EMS-based disaster response. *Ann Emerg Med* 12:601, 1982.

Partington AJ, Savage PEA: Disaster planning: Managing the media. *Br Med J* 291:590, 1985.

Vayer JS, Ten Eyck RP, Cowan ML: New concepts in triage. *Ann Emerg Med* 15:927, 1986.

Waeckerle JF: The skywalk collapse: A personal response. *Ann Emerg Med* 12:651, 1983.

Wilkinson CB: Aftermath of a disaster: The collapse of the Hyatt Regency hotel skywalks. *Am J Psychiatry* 140:1134, 1983.

# 7

# MASS GATHERINGS

## Greg D. Mears
## D. Neil Batson

## INTRODUCTION

Each year over 165,000,000 people in the United States attend major sporting events (Table 7-1). Not even included in these figures are the millions who attend events in the National Hockey League, NASCAR racing, high school athletics, Olympic festivals, local and state fairs, music concerts, and religious, political, or professional gatherings.

A *mass gathering* has been defined as any collection of greater than 1000 people at one site or location. Although this specifies an exact number of people, several smaller collections share many characteristics. These include commercial airline flights, passenger trains, ferries or hydrofoils, and other situations where a large number of people are crowded into a limited area somewhat isolated from routine Emergency Medical Services (EMS). The same treatment principles can often be applied to each of these settings. Emergency physicians should understand the structure and organization of mass gatherings. Such situations have higher injury and illness rates than the general population and create unique treatment and transportation dilemmas.

Statistics have been generated from such situations and events, including the University of Nebraska Football Stadium; the Denver Mile High Stadium; the University of Arizona, Tucson; the 1984 Los Angeles Summer Olympic Games; the 1986 World's Exposition in Vancouver, British Columbia; the XV Winter Olympic Games in Calgary, Alberta; the Carrier Dome at Syracuse University; and the 1982 U.S. Rock Music Festival in Devore, California. These statistics have shown an incidence of medical problems ranging from 0.12 to 6.00 per 1000 spectators and cardiac arrests ranging from 0.3 to 4.0 per 1,000,000 spectators.

## ANATOMY OF A MASS GATHERING

A mass gathering can be classified by physical factors and administrative or operational structure that impact the EMS approach.

## Physical Factors

From a medical perspective, events are typically characterized by several major physical attributes (Table 7-2). The actual facility where the event is held is one of the major factors any plan must consider. Types of facilities include indoor and outdoor structures, such as stadiums or athletic complexes, and open terrain or outdoor amphitheater-type settings with few amenities or resources. Each facility is unique in its access routes, externally with respect to traffic and

**Table 7-1.** Attendance at Major Sporting Events 1993–1994 Season

| | |
|---|---|
| Major League Baseball (1993) | 70,256,459 |
| National Basketball Association (1993–1994) | 17,984,014 |
| National Football League (1993–1994) | 13,967,272 |
| National Collegiate Athletic Association | |
|     Men's Basketball Div I, II, and III (1993–1994) | 28,390,491 |
|     Men's Football Div I, II, and III (1993–1994) | 34,870,634 |
| Total | 165,468,870 |

*Source:* Verbal communication with Major League Baseball, Inc.; the National Basketball Association; the National Collegiate Athletic Association, and the National Football League.

**Table 7-2.** Factors Affecting Patient Volumes

| | |
|---|---|
| Setting | Outside vs. inside |
| Large numbers of attendees | Mobile vs. stationary crowd |
| Duration of event | Presence of alcohol or drugs |
| Extremes of temperature | Weather |

road access and internally with respect to aisles and seating arrangements. These can affect the ability to discover, locate, and extricate spectators from the crowd as well as transport them to a treatment site or external location.

These physical constraints are usually compounded by the second attribute, which is the size of the event or crowd. The length of the event as well as the mobility of the crowd have an effect on patient volumes. The 1984 Los Angeles Summer Olympics reported the highest medical care need in venues where spectators were allowed to move about during the events. The 1982 U.S. Rock Music Festival noted a significant increase in daily patient volume the second day of the 3-day event.

An additional attribute to consider when planning for each event is the nature of the crowd. Typically, mass gatherings are a group of young and healthy individuals. Various events, such as homecoming festivities at universities, may change the makeup of the crowd and drastically affect the medical care required. It has been shown that certain events can influence the emotional state of the crowd and therefore can require a different approach to medical care. The University of Syracuse has shown that patient volumes are tripled at concerts as opposed to athletic events. Drugs and alcohol are felt to contribute to the difference.

The temperature at the time of the event can drastically affect patient volume. Denver's Mile High Stadium has shown a significant increase in patient volumes with temperatures greater than 85°F. (29.4°C). Other seasonal weather changes, such as rain or snow, can also increase patient volumes.

The final attribute that is an important factor in any mass gathering is the normal day-to-day EMS and local medical care capabilities of the surrounding area. This may not affect the number of patients seeking medical care but can have a major influence on the treatment and transportation methods used. Limited external medical facilities may force more advanced care to be performed on site, requiring more patient care staff, supplies, and facilities.

## Operational Structure

Any medical care plan or system must be developed with the full knowledge, support, and understanding of the operational personnel and administration. Management of any large event requires a large number of support staff. These include security personnel, ushers, volunteers, and public relations personnel. Security is needed along the outside perimeter of the event or facility to control traffic and access routes as well as to maintain the security of the entrances. Security personnel are needed inside the facility to act as law enforcement and crowd control. Security officers are often the main access for notification of any medical emergency and are critical for the initial dispatch for medical assistance. Response teams often rely on security officers to clear a path through the crowds to gain access to the patient. Finally, security officers have an important role in aiding cardiac arrest victims. Security officers trained in cardiopulmonary resuscitation (CPR) are a key to the successful resuscitation of cardiac arrest victims.

Ushers and volunteers are also valuable within any mass gathering event. They can function as the starting point to access medical care and, if equipped with communications devices, can relay information for the dispatch of medical response teams. The training of ushers in CPR skills and information about medical care access can also allow for improved resource utilization.

Every mass gathering event should have a designated command

center. This should be the communications and management head-quarters of the facility. In the command center, representatives of security, ushers, public relations, parking, facility maintenance, medical operations, and athletic or program directors should be present. This will allow for a smooth exchange of information between the various branches of operations and allow for a more efficient problem-solving atmosphere should the need arise. From this command center medical response teams should be dispatched and coordinated to assure the minimal response time with maximal coverage of the entire event facility. The command center is also important in maintaining positive working relationships and optimal safety for all personnel.

Each facility should have its own unique transportation system both internally and externally. Transportation routes and methods should be developed considering the physical layout and the crowd movement and density patterns. Patient access and extrication from the crowd can be accomplished manually by stair-chair or stretcher. Once outside the crowd, transportation may be by stretcher, motorized cart, or ambulance. Transport is typically to either a treatment site or external transportation source such as an ambulance or helicopter.

Medical care is also needed for the participants or performers in the event. Often in an athletic event a physician or athletic trainer is responsible for this care, independent of spectator care. If a separate system is in place, it should complement the EMS service and cooperate in the implementation of the appropriate protocols. Communication between the two systems allows for more efficient patient care and transportation. Certain events may occur on the athletic field or performance stage and require the equipment or expertise of trained personnel.

The purpose of a medical care system at mass gatherings is not to be a disaster management system but to provide isolated medical care as needed. Many of the components required for a medical care system are designed around disaster management principles and should be incorporated into an overall disaster plan utilizing existing local and/or regional plans.

## ANATOMY OF A MEDICAL CARE SYSTEM

### Planning

The first step in designing any medical care system is to determine the level of medical care that is needed or desired. Levels of care may be transportation only, basic life support (BLS) only, treatment without transportation, advanced life support (ALS), or aggressive ALS care targeting cardiac arrest victims. The characteristics of the potential patient population must also be identified. This may be participants or performers, spectators or employees. The goal of any medical care system should be the same as that of any EMS system, that is, to provide the maximum care possible with the resources available. Spectators should expect to receive the same quality of care that they would have received if they had not attended the event. This requires the system to be cooperative, adjustable, organized, intelligent, and prepared.

If possible, the design of a medical care system should be based on known factors that can positively affect patient outcome. For instance, a response time of 3 to 5 min can positively influence the ability to resuscitate a cardiac arrest victim. Rapid airway management and early defibrillation is the cornerstone of advanced cardiac life support (ACLS) in providing positive patient outcomes, as is bystander CPR.

Medical personnel and supplies should be allocated based on the anticipated number of patients and the seriousness of the anticipated medical problems. As stated earlier, a general estimate of patient volume is from 0.12 to 6.00 patients for each 1000 spectators and 0.3 to 4.0 cardiac arrests per 1,000,000 spectators. The medical problems encountered at mass gatherings are listed in Table 7-3.

**Table 7-3.** Common Presenting Complaints

| | Relative frequency (%) |
|---|---|
| Trauma | |
| Dermal injury | 13.0–40.9 |
| Eye injury | 0.6–2.8 |
| Foreign body | 1.0–5.9 |
| Head injury | 0.6–2.0 |
| Insect bites | 0.3–3.8 |
| Musculoskeletal | 5.4–20.5 |
| Other trauma | 0.3–2.0 |
| Medical | |
| Abdominal pain | 1.8–8.8 |
| Alcohol/drug ingestion | 0.4–4.0 |
| Cardiac arrest | 0.7–1.2 |
| Chest pain | 0.6–4.0 |
| Dehydration | 1.1 |
| Diabetes | 0.6–0.7 |
| Dizziness | 0.6–6.8 |
| Epistaxis | 0.6–4.0 |
| GI complaints | 1.6–17.5 |
| Headache | 2.5–36.2 |
| Heat-/cold-related | 1.2–11.9 |
| Hyper-/Hypotension | 0.3–1.7 |
| OB/GYN | 0.3–1.2 |
| Other medical | 1.8–44.9 |
| Respiratory distress | 0.4–13.7 |
| Seizure | 0.1–0.8 |
| Syncope | 0.2–9.7 |

### Patient Care Flow

The medical care plan should address the entire flow of patient care from the occurrence of the medical problem. Ushers, volunteers, and security personnel should be equipped with adequate communications devices and trained to relay information concerning any individual in need of medical care. Those without communication devices should be informed of the location of the nearest security officer or device for contacting the command center. Training should include the ability to communicate the appropriate information in a clear, concise format. These individuals must also act as first responders in providing a path to the patient and, when necessary, providing bystander CPR.

The command center or dispatch center is responsible for dispatching the appropriate response team to the location of the patient. This dispatch center must also assist in providing adequate support with security and attempt to identify the chief complaint so that the proper personnel and equipment are supplied. The command center should provide all the necessary resources for the safe treatment and extrication of the patient. Extrication may include maintenance issues such as plumbing and electrical mishaps. The command center is also responsible for the flexibility of personnel and the positioning of the response teams around the facility to provide the best response time.

Once the response team has been dispatched, it should respond and initiate patient care. This is best accomplished by the rapid extrication of the patient from the crowd to a tunnel or open entryway. At this point, treatment can be initiated by protocol or with medical control direction. The amount of treatment provided at this point depends on the medical condition of the patient and the layout of the facility. Transport to a designated treatment site should occur as soon as possible so that a specialist can provide care at the highest level possible. Ideally, direct supervision by the medical director should be available. Staffing of the treatment facility can be variable, including nurses, physician assistants, emergency medical technicians, paramedics, Red Cross volunteers, medical students, or first responders.

A medical record should be generated based on the severity of the complaint. A form should be used to record the patient's name, age, race, gender, medical complaint, drug allergies, medical history, and the date and time of treatment and disposition. If a medical examination is performed, it should be documented with a tentative diagnosis and treatment plan complete with discharge instructions. If ALS care is provided, it is best to complete a medical record such as an ambulance trip sheet or emergency department record. Any patient requiring ALS care should be transported to a hospital for further evaluation unless the treatment facility is equipped for equivalent care. All medical records should be reviewed by the medical director.

Transportation from the event should be by the most efficient mode possible. If no access roads are available, helicopter transport may be the most appropriate option. A medical care plan should integrate the local EMS system to allow for increased transport capabilities to external hospitals if needed. This can be done by dispatching units in service within the local system to designated sites at the facility or to replace a unit that is transporting.

## Personnel

Events are often staffed by a combination of paid personnel and volunteers. The number of personnel is based on the type of care to be provided, the layout of the facility, and the size of the crowd. Response teams should be located throughout the facility to keep response times within 3 to 5 minutes. It is often very beneficial to combine security officers with medical personnel in order to provide a more safe environment and quicker response. In special situations, it may be necessary to add individuals with other special skills to the response team, such as fire fighters. Each response team should be staffed and equipped well enough to easily transport a nonambulatory patient.

Treatment facilities should be staffed with the personnel required to provide the desired care of the system. Patient numbers and medical complaints can be estimated based on the attributes previously discussed. It is the function of the medical director to determine how best to meet the demands of patient care when considering the budget of the facility. There is a great variability in the composition of nonphysician personnel who can have a direct impact on the number of physicians required. The number of physicians recommended for onsite care ranges from 1 for every 5000 to 1 for every 50,000 people. These staffing requirements should be a part of a formal contract with the facility.

## Equipment

It is the responsibility of the medical director to determine the equipment to be used within the facility and incorporate these specifications into the medical care plan. Often this is dictated by the local EMS system that provides equipment for the facility. Response teams should be equipped with basic airway and first-aid equipment. The teams must also have adequate extrication and transportation devices based on the layout of the facility. In the event of a cardiac arrest, a defibrillator should be available to be sent to the location of the patient, along with ALS personnel and advanced airway equipment. This may not be necessary if the treatment site is close by. The medical care system should have enough defibrillators to allow any location within the facility to have access to one in 5 min or less.

Equipment within the treatment sites should be based on the level of care to be provided, the number of patients anticipated, and the length of time each patient would be required to stay at the site awaiting disposition or transportation. If there is no on-site transportation, the plan should establish a system capable of transporting the patient to a hospital within 30 min of the request.

## Public Awareness

The success of any medical system is based on its planning, training, and testing. It is important to educate the public to the type of medical care that is available and how to access it. This should be done by multiple announcements before and during the event. Simple signage should direct patients to treatment sites. Training of the ushers, volunteers, concessions workers, and security personnel in the locations of these sites is also necessary.

## Quality Assurance

Drills and practice scenarios should be held yearly to make sure all participants are aware of the operations of the facility. Training in communications and knowledge of the facility layout, first aid, and CPR should be standardized. All medical records should be reviewed by the medical director and, if the volume is large, an Audit and Review committee should be involved. If an event is particularly busy or fraught with disaster, a stress debriefing session should be considered.

## SPECIAL CONSIDERATIONS

### Multiple Site Events

Mass gatherings that include multiple sites or facilities can be very complex. Events such as the Olympic Games have multiple locations that may be miles apart and even located in different climates and with different crowd attributes. Events such as these require a system designed with multiple agencies and often multiple jurisdictions. Management requires a great deal of cooperative effort and interaction. Each venue can often be considered an isolated mass gathering, but communication, supplies, and personnel must be interlinked. The same estimates stated previously can be used to predict patient volumes and complaints.

### Cardiac Arrests

The incidence of cardiac arrests in mass gatherings is higher than in the normal population. It has been postulated that, due to the natural excitement generated by competitive sports, individuals who have cardiac disease are more likely to become symptomatic. However, medical systems at mass gatherings have demonstrated much higher success rates than even the most advanced EMS systems. This is primarily due to the ability to provide early bystander CPR, airway control, defibrillation, and ALS care. Success rates have varied from 20 to 80 percent survival from documented cardiac arrest. This evidence would also support the use of automatic external defibrillators in mass gatherings where ALS support is not available in under 5 min.

### Commercial Airline In-flight Emergencies

All U.S. commercial airlines are classified by federal law as "common carriers." This status does not require the airline to provide emergency care for passengers. Passengers on board an airplane do not usually meet the criteria for a mass gathering, but the relatively large number of people in a relatively small space makes the previous discussion somewhat applicable. Many of the medical complaints generated are similar to those in mass gatherings, and the isolation from normal EMS systems and medical equipment creates unique medical situations. When a medical emergency occurs on board an aircraft, the flight attendant is left with several options. He or she has the option to evaluate the problem, ask for someone with medical experience to assist, or radio for ground medical advice. The pilot is responsible for determining if an emergency landing is needed.

Beginning August 1st, 1986, commercial airlines operating in the United States were mandated to carry a medical emergency kit. This kit can be used by any onboard physician. Contents of this kit are listed in Table 7-4.

In the 6 month period from October through March 1986, Speizer reported 8,735,000 passengers arrived at Los Angeles International Airport and 260 (0.3 per 1,000) experienced medical problems and 7 had cardiac arrests (0.8 per 1,000,000). Physician assistance on the aircraft had been noted in 20 to 63 percent of medical emergencies. It

**Table 7-4.** Medical Equipment on U.S. Commercial Aircraft

Sphygmomanometer
Stethoscope
Oropharyngeal airways (3 sizes)
Syringes and needles
Dextrose (50%, 50 mL)
Diphenhydramine (2 ampules)
Epinephrine (1:1000, 2 ampules)
Nitroglycerin tablets (10)
Standard industry-type first-aid kit

is conceivable that up to several hundred lives each year could be saved on aircraft with the availability of automatic external defibrillators and trained flight attendants.

## BIBLIOGRAPHY

Baker WM, Simone BM, Niemann JT, et al: Special event medical care: The 1984 Los Angeles Summer Olympics experience. *Ann Emerg Med* 15:185, 1986.

Carveth SW: Eight-year experience with a stadium-based mobile coronary-care unit. *Heart Lung* 3:770, 1974.

De Lorenzo, RA, Gray BC, Bennett PC, et al: Effect of crowd size on patient volume at a large multipurpose, indoor stadium. *JAMA* 7:379, 1989.

Department of Transportation, Federal Aviation Administration. Emergency Medical Equipment Final Rule-14CFR, Parts 11 and 121. Fed. Reg. January 9, 1986.

Dubin GH: *Medical Care at Large Gatherings. A Manual Based on Experiences in Rock Concert Medicine.* Rockville, MD, 1976.

Hordinsky JR, George MH: Response capability during civil air carrier in-flight medical emergencies. *Aviation, Space, and Environmental Medicine* December 1989.

Illinois State medical Society: Guidelines for the Provision of Medical Care at Large-Scale Events, March, 1984.

Ounanian LL, Salinas C, Shear CL, et al: Medical Care at the 1982 US Festival. *Ann Emerg Med* 15:520, 1986.

Pons PT, Holland B, Alfrey E, et al: An advanced emergency medical care system at National Football League games. *Ann Emerg Med* 9:203, 1980.

Sanders AB, Criss E, Steckl P, et al: An analysis of medical care at mass gatherings. *Ann Emerg Med* 15:515, 1986.

Spaite DW, Criss EA, Valenzuela TD, et al: A new model for providing prehospital medical care in large stadiums. *Ann Emerg Med* 18:825, 1988.

Speizer C, Rennie CJ, Brenton H: Prevalence of in-flight medical emergencies on commercial airlines. *Ann Emerg Med* 18:53, 1989.

Thompson JM, Savoia G, Powell G, et al: Level of medical care required for mass gatherings: The XV Winter Olympic Games in Calgary, Canada. *Ann Emerg Med* 18:385, 1991.

Weaver WD, Sutherland K, Wirkus MJ, et al: Emergency medical care requirements for large public assemblies and a new strategy for managing cardiac arrest in this setting. *Ann Emerg Med* 18:155, 1989.

# 8
# INJURY CONTROL

## Arthur L. Kellermann
## Ricardo Martinez

## INTRODUCTION

Every year, approximately one American out of every four is injured seriously enough to require medical attention. Injuries account for roughly 25 percent of all emergency department visits. Injuries are the leading cause of death among Americans from 1 to 44 years of age. Because injuries disproportionately affect the young, they account for more years of potential life lost before age 65 than all causes of cancer and all causes of heart disease *combined*.

Historically, people have considered injuries the consequence of unpredictable "accidents" or violence. We now know this is not true. Epidemiologic research has revealed that injuries, like diseases, affect identifiable high-risk groups, follow an often predictable chain of events, and are therefore preventable. The impact of those injuries that do occur can be minimized by optimal provision of acute care and rehabilitation of injured persons. This combination of strategies—prevention, acute care, and rehabilitation—has come to be termed *injury control* (Fig. 8-1)

## A PUBLIC HEALTH APPROACH

Many of our daily activities involve interaction with large amounts of energy. Every time we drive a car, hammer a nail, or iron a shirt, we are utilizing energy. As long as our capacity to control each source of energy exceeds the demands of the task, we can accomplish our objectives with little or no risk of injury. If, however, the demands of the task suddenly exceed our capacity for control (e.g., if the car hits a patch of ice) or our capacity to control the source of energy falls below the demands of the task (e.g., fatigue, intoxication, or limited visibility), an uncontrolled release of energy may occur. This moment of uncontrolled energy release is termed an *event* (Fig. 8-2) If this energy is transferred to a victim, or host, at a rate or in an amount that exceeds the body's ability to tolerate this transfer without damage, an injury will occur.

Kinetic energy, the primary agent of trauma, is usually transferred through an inanimate object, or vehicle. Examples include a speeding car, a falling rock, or a bullet. Energy can also be transferred to a host

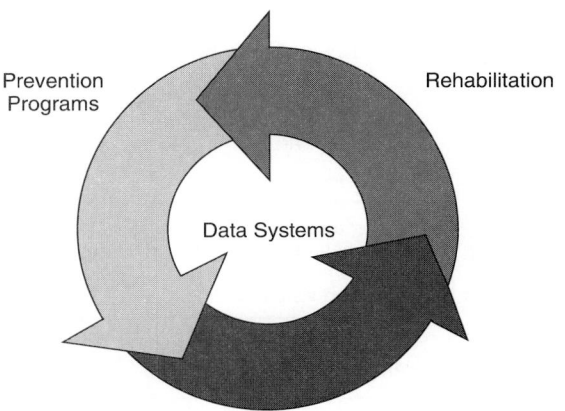

**Fig. 8-1.** Injury control.

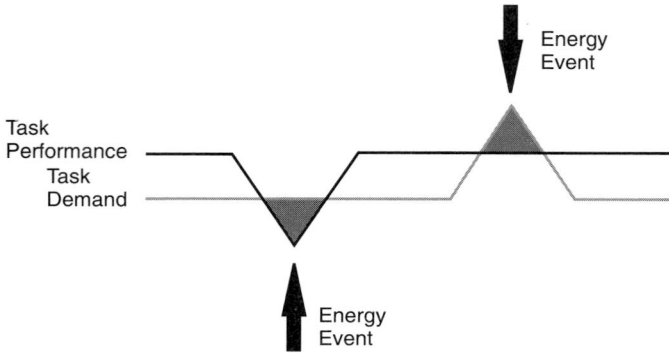

**Fig. 8-2.** How does an injury occur?

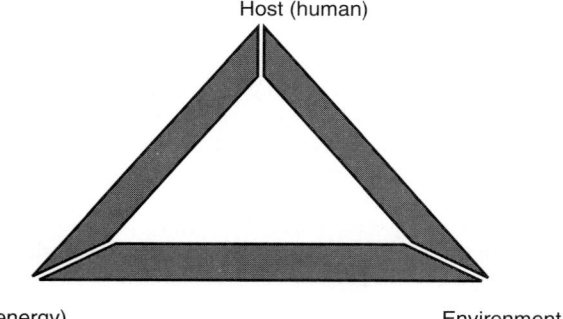

**Fig. 8-3.** The epidemiologic triangle.

by vectors, or biologic organisms such as a poisonous plant or animals that sting, bite, or kick. Finally, each injury event takes place in a physical or social environment that can independently influence the likelihood that an injury will occur or modify its severity. By viewing injuries as the result of a complex dynamic involving host, vehicle, and environment, we can understand how injuries occur and formulate strategies for their prevention (Fig. 8-3)

## The Haddon Matrix

William Haddon, the father of injury control, developed the classic approach by identifying the three principal factors of injury (host, vehicle, and environment) and subdividing each by the three temporal phases of an injury event (preevent, the event itself, and the postevent phase). The result was a "phase-factor" matrix of nine discrete cells. Examination of these cells can suggest a variety of strategies for preventing or controlling injuries. Examples of how these interventions have been applied to the control of motor vehicle–related injuries is depicted in Fig. 8-4. Since its introduction in 1972, the Haddon matrix has proven to be an invaluable tool for injury control.

## Options Analysis

Later in his career, Haddon outlined 10 generic strategies to prevent or control injuries by breaking the chain of injury causation at various points (Table 8-1). Examining this list to identify the most promising approach to dealing with a type of injury is known as *options analysis*. Certain options may be more practical to control one class of injuries, such as drowning in swimming pools, and other options may be more effective for other problems, such as burns and smoke inhalation from residential fires. The best approach is not always the most obvious one or the one most proximate to the injury event. Often a combination of approaches is more effective than any single strategy alone.

## The Injury Control Model

Haddon's approach was first applied to great effect in the control of deaths and injuries due to car crashes. Prior to his work, the Federal government poured millions of dollars into costly and largely ineffective advertising campaigns to fix "the nut behind the wheel." Little progress was made until the National Highway Traffic Safety Administration mandated changes to the design of the motor vehicles themselves (e.g., safety belts, puncture-resistant gas tanks, and shock-absorbing steering columns). Haddon's ideas also spurred work to build safer roadways and driving environments (e.g., divided highways, shock-absorbing piers in front of bridge columns, breakaway light poles).

The result of these efforts is one of the greatest public health achievements of this century. Although the number of vehicle-miles traveled in the United States has risen steadily year by year, the annual *rate* of crash fatalities per vehicle mile driven in the United States has declined dramatically. Today, our death rate due to car crashes is less than one third what it was in 1950. If the United States had not embarked on a sustained program to improve highway traffic safety, the annual toll of deaths, injuries, and costs associated with motor vehicle crashes would be billions of dollars higher than it is today.

More than a century after yellow fever was controlled by targeting the vector of transmission, Haddon's work demonstrated that many injuries could also be controlled by broadening our traditional emphasis on acute care and rehabilitation to include *preventive* efforts as well. Injury control draws on the insights and expertise of many disciplines. These include epidemiology, prevention, biomechanics, acute care, rehabilitation, law, and public administration. Prevention is attempted whenever possible. When prevention is not enough, acute care is needed to minimize further damage and halt the cascade of events that characterize major trauma. After the victim is stabilized, functional outcomes can be enhanced by optimal rehabilitation.

## PREVENTION STRATEGIES

### Active Versus Passive Countermeasures

Injury countermeasures can generally be grouped into one of two categories. *Active* countermeasures require the conscious cooperation of

| Factor | **Phase** | | |
|---|---|---|---|
| | **Preevent** | **Event** | **Postevent** |
| **Host** | • driver education<br>• alcohol and drug abuse<br>• fatigue<br>• impaired vision/hearing | • age<br>• osteoporosis | • first-aid training |
| **Vehicle** | • antilock brakes<br>• motor vehicle inspection | • tempered glass<br>• safety belts<br>• airbags | • flame-retardant fabric<br>• puncture-resistant gas tanks |
| **Environment** | • divided highways<br>• pedestrian overpasses<br>• speed limits | • breakaway poles<br>• impact-absorbing barriers | • 911 emergency number<br>• trauma care systems<br>• regional rehabilitation centers |

**Fig. 8-4.** The Haddon matrix applied to motor vehicle–related injuries.

**Table 8-1.** Options Analysis: Strategies with Examples, for Injury Control

1. Prevent creation of the hazard.
   Ban production and sale of assault weapons to civilians.
2. Reduce the amount of hazard.
   Limit water heater temperature to 125° F (47.25° C).
3. Prevent the release of a hazard that already exists.
   Put dangerous medications in "child proof" containers.
4. Modify the rate of distribution of the release of the hazard from its source.
   Require fire-safe cigarettes that cannot easily ignite furniture or bedding.
5. Separate, by time or space, the hazard from that which is to be protected.
   Construct overpasses or underpasses to eliminate crossing streams of traffic.
6. Physically separate, by barriers, the hazard from that which is to be protected.
   Equip cabs with bullet- and knife-proof partitions.
7. Modify surfaces and basic structures to minimize injury.
   Equip all new cars with driver- and passenger-side air bags.
8. Make that which is to be protected more resistant to damage.
   Issue bulletproof vests to law enforcement officers and security guards.
9. Begin to counter damage already done.
   Promote citizen training in first aid and CPR.
10. Stabilize, repair, and rehabilitate the injured person.
    Implement trauma care systems throughout the United States.

the individual to be protected each and every time they are used. Examples include manual safety belts, motorcycle helmets, and child safety seats. *Passive* countermeasures, on the other hand, require little or no cooperation but exert their protective effects automatically. Examples include air bags, automatic sprinkler systems, and spring-loaded kill switches on lawn mowers. In general, the less complex the task, and the less initiative required by the user, the greater the likelihood that the countermeasure will exert its protective effect when needed. Manual safety belts can decrease car crash fatalities by 45 to 55 percent, but they are often left unbuckled. Air bags deploy in a serious crash 100 percent of the time.

## Education

Historically, injury prevention has focused almost exclusively on "safety training." Education is still the most common strategy used in most communities and it is relatively easy to implement. Implicit in this approach is the belief that injury prevention is largely a matter of knowledge and personal responsibility. Once people are taught what to do, it is hoped that they will change their behavior and reduce their risk of injury. This is generally the first approach taken to encourage the public to accept an active countermeasure of proven efficacy. Driver's education programs, child pedestrian training, and bicycle helmet campaigns are classic examples of this strategy.

Although these campaigns are quite popular with the public and can attract large numbers of volunteers, they have not always proven to be very effective for encouraging sustained behavior change. One study evaluated the impact of a $78 million federal "alcohol safety action program." Although it was launched in dozens of communities around the United States, a subsequent evaluation revealed that the program was not successful in reducing the rate of alcohol-related fatalities among the target population.

Robertson and colleagues measured the impact of a saturation advertising campaign to promote the use of safety belts in one city served by two cable systems. One system aired over 1000 high-quality promotional spots; the other aired none. Subsequent observation revealed no difference in rates of safety belt use among subscribers of either system.

Not all public education efforts have yielded such discouraging results. A large-scale community action campaign to promote bicycle helmet use in Seattle, Washington, resulted in a sharp increase in bicycle helmet sales. Observed rates of helmet use also increased, from 6 percent to more than 38 percent. No similar increase occurred in the neighboring city of Portland, Oregon.

Thompson and colleagues have suggested that the impact of many public education campaigns is blunted by *attenuation of effect*. No matter how powerful, pervasive, and repetitive a safety message may be, there will always be some people who never encounter it. Among those who see or hear the message, some will actively reject it. Although many who encounter the message will accept it as true, some will not be sufficiently motivated to change their behavior. Among those who change their behavior, there will be some who will lapse back into old habits over time. Others will fail to follow the message on a consistent basis. Finally, not everyone who adopts the strategy will escape injury. Sometimes the amount of energy involved overwhelms even a well-conceived countermeasure. As a result of these effects, the impact of an education campaign—reduction in the rate of serious injuries or deaths—may be less than hoped.

## Enforcement

Unfortunately, research has shown that the group that has the highest risk of serious injury (i.e., young males) is also the group most resistant to behavioral change. When voluntary acceptance of a countermeasure of proven effectiveness is poor, compliance can be increased by making the countermeasure compulsory. Although "mandatory use" laws are difficult to pass, their impact can be impressive. A study of Michigan's child safety seat law indicated that injuries declined by 25 percent following passage of the law. The 55-mph speed limit is estimated to have saved 2000 to 4000 lives each year that it was in effect. Raising the minimum age to purchase alcoholic beverages in 26 states decreased nighttime fatal crashes by an average of 13 percent. After an aggressive bicycle helmet promotion program resulted in substantial improvement in helmet use rates among young children but disappointing rates among secondary students and adults, the province of Victoria, Australia, enacted legislation to make bicycle helmet use compulsory for all cyclists. A subsequent evaluation documented use rates of 95 percent among primary students and 85 to 90 percent among secondary students.

Ongoing education and aggressive enforcement are often needed to obtain maximal benefit from mandatory use laws. In Elmira, New York, an enforcement and publicity campaign to promote the state's seat belt law boosted compliance rates from 49 to 77 percent. Four months later, rates of use sagged to 66 percent but jumped to 80 percent during a reminder campaign.

Mandatory use laws are effective but are difficult to enact. People generally support measures that will limit the ability of others to injure them but resist measures intended to protect them from their own actions. Speed limits, drunk driving laws, and measures to ban the carrying of weapons on commercial aircraft enjoy broad-based support, but mandatory seat belt laws, helmet laws, and gun control often engender spirited resistance from a vocal minority who view this kind of legislation as an infringement of "personal freedom."

Political backlash can block legislation or even lead to the repeal of effective laws. Despite overwhelming evidence that motorcycle helmet laws save lives, 26 states repealed their statutes when federal incentives were relaxed in 1976. In these states, motorcycle crash fatality rates subsequently increased 40 percent.

Opponents of mandatory use laws argue that individuals should be permitted to ignore sound safety policies if they believe that the level of risk is acceptable and only they would be harmed. Unfortunately, the circle of individuals and institutions that suffer harm extends far beyond the victim. A motorcyclist or bicyclist who rides without a helmet runs an increased risk of serious head injury or death. If, however, such individuals are subsequently killed or disabled in a crash, families and loved ones will lose companionship, dependents will lose their principal source of financial support, employers will lose productivity, and insurance companies and society will be required to cover the expense of care. All of us, either directly or indirectly, bear the costs of preventable injury.

## Engineering

Many injuries can be prevented or controlled by building safer vehicles or modifying the physical environment in which injuries commonly occur. The "up front" cost of implementing a passive countermeasure is usually greater than the cost associated with education campaigns. However, engineering is usually more effective because it does not require millions of users to permanently and consistently change their behavior.

Consider the following examples. In contrast to the disappointing results of driver's education, Federal standards for motor vehicle construction saved an estimated 37,000 lives between 1975 and 1978 alone. These standards addressed such issues as passenger restraint systems, windshields, fuel tank integrity, and the flammability of interior fabric. The recent introduction of air bags has cut the nation's toll of deaths and injuries due to car crashes still further.

Construction of our interstate highway system has also saved lives. Modifications to the driving environment, such as banked curves, divided lanes of traffic, controlled ramps for ingress and egress, elimination of crossing streams of traffic, and the positioning of energy-absorbing pilings in front of fixed obstructions, have cut the death rate per 100 million vehicle-miles on interstate highways to less than half that noted on other roads.

These lessons can be applied to other hazardous products. Cigarettes cause more than half of all fatal residential house fires nationwide. Most occur when the smoker falls asleep in bed or leaves a burning cigarette on the arm of a sofa or chair. Television, radio, and print advertisements warning of the dangers of smoking in bed have had little or no impact on this problem. Promotion of smoke detectors can save lives by warning of an impending catastrophe in time to permit the occupants to evacuate the house, but they require a concerted effort to install and maintain them.

Passive engineering of the environment by installing home sprinkler systems could be a very effective strategy. These systems not only detect a fire but automatically extinguish it. Unfortunately, residential sprinkler systems are expensive and generally cannot be retrofitted into older homes. However, the cigarette itself could be modified to diminish its potential to ignite furniture or bedding. This would virtually eliminate cigarettes as a major cause of house fires. Although prototypes of this product have been available since 1984, the tobacco industry has consistently resisted efforts to require cigarettes to be "fire-safe."

Laws that require products to be designed and built in a way that diminishes their potential to cause harm can be highly effective but are extremely difficult to enact. Manufacturers often oppose such regulations out of fear that they will raise the price of their product and discourage sales. In addition to the issue of personal freedom, concerns are often raised about cost, excessive government regulation, and the impact of legislation on business competition. If efforts to regulate a hazardous product fail, product liability lawsuits may be the only avenue left to force a needed change in product design.

## PRACTICING INJURY CONTROL

### Step 1: Define the Problem

Development of effective programs to control injuries cannot occur without some understanding of the magnitude and scope of the problem. Population-based data about the incidence and impact of injury are essential to mobilize the resources necessary to achieve change. Public health surveillance data are also needed to monitor patterns and trends and evaluate the impact of injury countermeasures.

Several sources of information can be used. Death certificate data are useful to document the impact of injuries on overall rates of mor-

tality, but vital statistics will not provide information about serious, but nonfatal, injuries. Hospital discharge data and/or trauma registries can provide essential information about cases of major trauma, but both sources are institution-specific. Population-based data are needed to calculate rates of injury in defined subsets. Furthermore, hospital admission statistics and trauma registry data do not capture patients who are treated and released.

Although injuries that are managed on an outpatient basis are generally assumed to be minor, they can actually result in significant long-term disability. This is particularly true for head, back, and hand injuries. Patients who visit a hospital emergency department for injury are known to be at increased risk for recurrent injury, especially if their index visit was related to alcohol abuse or violence. Efforts to systematically identify them are therefore justified from a patient care perspective alone.

Assignment of "E-codes"—external cause of injury codes—to every injury-related emergency department visit could substantially enhance community-based surveillance efforts. Currently, several states mandate E-coding of all hospital admissions. Unfortunately, few hospitals E-code emergency department visits.

Certain types of injury can be difficult to classify in an accurate manner. Victims of assault are often unwilling to report the true nature of their injuries, much less identity the offender. For example, a woman in an abusive relationship often fears further violence, harm to her children, or abandonment more than the prospect of returning home. Sometimes the abuser is the individual at her side in the emergency department.

### Step 2: Identify Causes and Risk Factors

Once a class of injuries has been identified as important, additional research may be needed to identify factors that increase or decrease a victim's risk of injury. Information of this type is essential to fashion intervention programs. Descriptive studies are usually conducted first to determine *who* is being injured, *what* kind of injuries are involved, *where* they are occurring, *when* they are occurring, and most important, *why* they are occurring. These data can provide important clues to injury causation and often generate hypotheses that can be investigated with more analytic methods.

In some cases, the link between a risk factor and injury is so strong that no additional research is needed. For example, studies of injured drivers have demonstrated that 20 percent of all car crashes with serious injury, 50 percent of all fatal crashes, and 60 percent of all fatal single-vehicle crashes involve alcohol.

In most cases, however, it is necessary to compare the rate of injury in a group *with* the risk factor to the rate of injury in an otherwise similar group *without* the risk factor. Cohort and quasi-experimental designs are often needed to reach a definitive conclusion. When the outcome of interest is rare and exposure to the risk factor(s) of interest can be shown to precede the injury, case-control studies may also be employed. Meticulous data collection is essential to generate valid results. Efforts must also be made to control for the effects of confounding variables.

### Step 3: Develop and Test Interventions

Once the magnitude of the problem and its associated risk factors have been identified, a variety of countermeasures may be considered for implementation. Careful attention must be given to the characteristics of the target population, the feasibility of the countermeasures, their acceptability to the target population, and their cost. Pilot intervention programs are often helpful to try out various strategies. The most promising one(s) can then be selected for more widespread implementation.

Community education programs are often tried first because they are relatively easy to initiate, attract motivated volunteers, and are often invaluable for raising public awareness of an injury problem.

They are also necessary to build public support for more intrusive injury countermeasures. It is essential to take the views and values of the community into consideration at every step of the process. Citizen involvement may be crucial to a program's success and, ultimately, its survival.

Most successful programs set milestones and predefined measures of program success. For example, a program to prevent deaths and injuries in residential fires may identify selected measures of *structure* (staff hired, office space, cooperative agreements reached), *process* (number of pamphlets distributed, number of home visits made, total smoke detectors installed), or *outcome* (reductions in the rate of fire deaths, or a decline in hospital admissions due to burns and smoke inhalation).

It is not always possible to demonstrate a major impact on rates of morbidity or mortality with small-scale demonstration projects. When this is the case, surrogate measures may be employed to demonstrate program impact. For example, baseline rates of smoke detector use in a random sample of households in a target neighborhood can be compared with rates noted after a public education campaign. At the very least, telephone surveys can seek evidence of changes in knowledge, attitudes, and self-reported behavior. Self-reported changes in behavior may not predict long-term compliance, but they are better than nothing.

### Step 4: Implement Effective Interventions and Evaluate Their Impact

It is important to generate evidence that available countermeasures work. Several years ago, researchers at the Harborview Injury Prevention and Research Center studied emergency department patients who were injured in bicycle crashes and determined that bicycle helmets reduce the risk of serious head injury by as much as 85 percent. This observation prompted nationwide efforts to promote bicycle helmets and led to the passage of mandatory helmet laws in a small but growing number of states.

Once a program is initiated on a large-scale basis, evaluation data should be collected to demonstrate ongoing impact. Measures of cost-effectiveness (e.g., dollars spent per life saved, or injury prevented) are particularly important. The cost of prevention programs can be easily tracked, but the benefits of "tragedies that didn't happen" are often harder to document. Support for a program tends to wane with time, especially when no group or organization has an economic interest in seeing it continued. When money gets tight, prevention programs are often the first to go. Without careful planning and thought, worthy programs can wither and die.

## THE ROLE OF THE EMERGENCY PHYSICIANS IN INJURY CONTROL

### Patient Education

Measures to prevent or control injuries need not be implemented on a grand scale to make a difference. Emergency physicians can, and should, incorporate injury prevention into their clinical practice. The impact of these efforts could be substantial.

Special efforts should be made to correct any factors that precipitated the injury or contributed to its severity. Otherwise, the patient is likely to return with a more serious injury the next time. A child who sustains a minor head injury while riding a bike should be told to always wear a bicycle helmet. The adult who sustains minor injuries in a low-velocity motor vehicle crash should get a short lecture about the importance of safety belts.

However, any emergency department encounter may afford a "teachable moment." Injuries are the leading cause of death among Americans aged 1 to 44. Since emergency physicians are more likely to provide acute care to injured patients than any other physician group, they should have a special stake in preventing and controlling injuries. The mother who brings her child to the emergency department for evaluation of a severe otitis can leave the department with valuable information about the importance of child safety seats, bicycle helmets and four-sided fencing around her swimming pool. Emergency physicians can motivate patients to change their behavior or modify their home environment to decrease injury risk.

### Data Collection and Program Evaluation

If current trends towards capitated care continue, the emergency department will become a pivotal arena for prevention efforts and health resource utilization. Until now, the financial incentives of health care have encouraged hospitalization and intensive provision of services. The move towards capitated payment for services to large groups will substantially increase the incentive to prevent illness and injuries As the portal of entry for 40 percent of U.S. inpatients and virtually all hospital admissions due to injury, the emergency department will play a key role in monitoring system performance, controlling access to expensive inpatient care, identifying high-risk groups, and evaluating the impact of prevention programs (Fig. 8-5).

### Research

From the vantage point of the emergency department, emergency physicians are often the first to spot emerging trends. They are also

**Fig. 8-5.** Use of emergency department data to control injuries in a population.

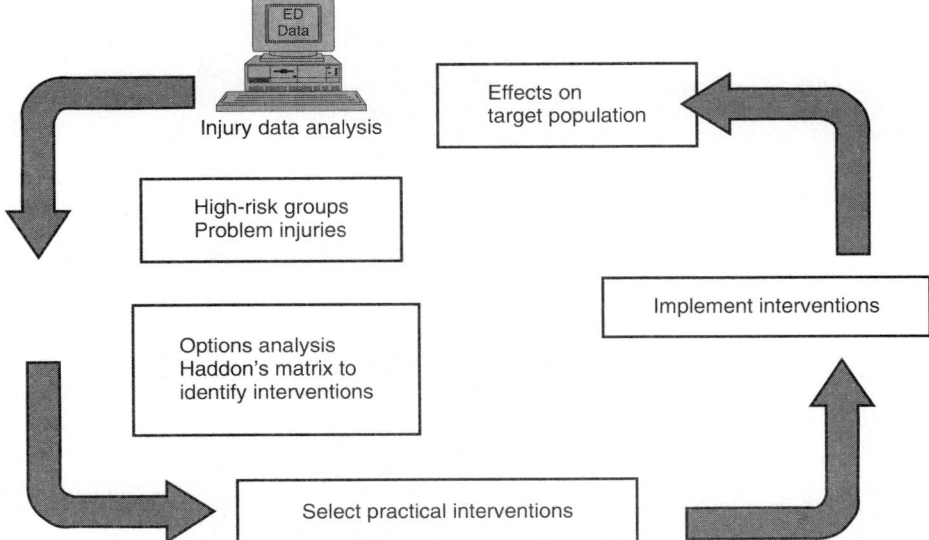

ideally positioned to conduct injury surveillance and evaluate countermeasures. A number of emergency physicians are already making important contributions to the science of injury control.

Emergency physicians should take the lead in community-based epidemiologic research. Academic emergency physicians are currently involved in research on alcohol-related trauma, drunk driving enforcement, firearm-related injuries, domestic violence, residential fires, and other issues. Emergency physicians can also make important contributions to our understanding of the biomechanics of trauma.

Evaluation research will be particularly important in the years to come. Injury control must demonstrate its value to compete successfully for a shrinking pool of health care dollars. Superficially appealing programs may not prove to be as effective as initially hoped. In order for the field to advance, we must be willing to identify our failures honestly and learn from our mistakes.

## Advocacy

Sometimes, evaluation data indicate that a countermeasure is effective but it is rarely used. When education is not enough to motivate behavioral change, passage of law to mandate use may have a major impact. The results can be impressive, particularly when they are coupled with ongoing education efforts and visible enforcement. States with mandatory motorcycle helmet laws report compliance rates as high as 98 percent.

Coalition building is essential to assemble a broad base of support. Population-based data are important, but the testimonies of health care providers, surviving family members, and disabled individuals are needed to give the statistics an emotional context. Information about the economic impact of injuries and the cost-effectiveness of the countermeasure is also helpful. Physician leadership is essential to the success of these efforts.

## CONCLUSION

Injuries are an enormous public health problem. Fortunately, substantial reductions in injury-related death and disability can be achieved through public education, dissemination of effective countermeasures, and improvements in environmental and product-related design. The success we achieved in highway traffic safety did not occur overnight, and important challenges remain. However, substantial progress can be made by applying these same principles to other types of injuries. Emergency physicians are poised to make important contributions to this rapidly growing field.

## BIBLIOGRAPHY

American College of Emergency Physicians: Guidelines for trauma care systems. *Ann Emerg Med* 22:1079, 1993.

American College of Emergency Physicians: *ACEP Policy Statement. Guidelines for Trauma Care Systems, Appendix B*. Dallas, TX, American College of Emergency Physicians, 1993, pp 1–8.

Baker SP, O'Neill B, Ginsburg M, Li G: *Injury Fact Book*, 2d ed. New York, Oxford University Press, 1992.

Baraff L: Injury prevention: Can we meet the challenge? *Ann Emerg Med* 20:1045, 1991.

Committee on Trauma Research: *Injury in America: A Continuing Public Health Problem*. Washington, DC, National Academy Press, 1985.

Dunn KA, Cline DM, Grant T, et al: Injury prevention instruction in the emergency department. *Ann Emerg Med* 22:1280, 1993.

Haddon W: The changing approach to the epidemiology, prevention, and amelioration of trauma: The transition to approaches etiologically rather than descriptively based. *Am J Public Health* 58:1431, 1968.

Haddon W: A logical framework for categorizing highway safety phenomenon and activity. *J Trauma* 12:193, 1972.

Haddon W: Energy damage and the ten countermeasure strategies. *J Trauma* 13:321, 1973.

Haddon W: Advances in the epidemiology of injuries as a basis for public policy. *Public Health Rep* 95:411, 1980.

Hargarten SW, Karlson T: Injury control: A crucial aspect of emergency medicine. *Emerg Med Clin North Am* 11:255, 1993.

Kellermann AL, Lee RK, Mercy JA, Banton JG: The epidemiologic basis for the prevention of firearm injuries. *Annu Rev Public Health* 12:17, 1991.

Kellermann AL, Rivara FP, Rushforth N, et al: Gun ownership as a risk factor for homicide in the home. *N Engl J Med* 329:1084, 1993.

Martinez R: Injury control: A primer for physicians. *Ann Emerg Med* 19:72, 1990.

Mcleer SV, Anwar RAH: The role of the emergency physician in the prevention of domestic violence. *Ann Emerg Med* 16:1155, 1987.

National Committee for Injury Prevention and Control: *Injury Prevention: Meeting the Challenge. Am J Prev Med* (suppl), New York, Oxford University Press, 1989.

Orsay EM, Turnbull TL, Dunne M, et al: Prospective study of the effect of safety belts on morbidity and health care costs in motor vehicle accidents. *JAMA* 24:3598, 1988.

Position papers from the Third National Injury Control Conference. U.S. Department of Health and Human Services, Public Health Service, Centers for Disease Control and Prevention, Atlanta, GA, 1992.

Rice DP, MacKenzie EJ, et al: Cost of Injury in the United States: A Report of Congress. San Francisco, CA: Institute for Health & Aging, University of California, and Injury Prevention Center, Johns Hopkins University, 1989.

Robertson LS: Automobile safety regulations and death reductions in the United States. *Am J Public Health* 71:818, 1981.

Robertson L: *Injury Epidemiology*. New York, Oxford University Press, 1992.

Rosenberg M, Fenley MA: *Violence in America: A Public Health Approach*. New York, Oxford University Press, 1991.

Runge JW: The cost of injury. *Emerg Med Clin North Am* 11:241, 1993.

Teret SP: Litigation for the public's health. *Am J Public Health* 76:1027, 1986.

Thompson RS, Rivara FP, Thompson DC, et al: A case control study of the effectiveness of bicycle safety helmets. *N Engl J Med* 320:1361, 1989.

Waller J: *Injury Control: A Guide to the Causes and Prevention of Trauma*. Lexington, MA, Lexington Books, 1985.

Wilson M, et al: *Saving Children: A Guide to Injury Prevention*. New York, Oxford University Press, 1991.

Withers B, Baker SP: Epidemiology and prevention of injuries. *Emerg Med Clin North Am* 2:701, 1984.

## 9

# BASIC CARDIOPULMONARY RESUSCITATION

### Raymond E. Jackson

Basic cardiopulmonary resuscitation (CPR) encompasses the concepts and techniques that form the foundation for effective emergency care. The purpose of cardiopulmonary resuscitation is to provide artificial circulation of oxygenated blood to the vital organs, especially the heart and brain, in an attempt to halt the degenerative processes associated with ischemia and anoxia until spontaneous circulation can be restored. Basic life support alone may in some instances be life-saving, but in most cases, advanced interventions are essential for the resuscitation of the patient. The critical factor in determining the success of resuscitative efforts is the time elapsed before successful restoration of effective spontaneous circulation. This, for the most part, is dependent upon use of advanced life-support techniques such as defibrillation. The immediate notification of the prehospital care system and prompt performance of basic resuscitation efforts such as closed-chest massage can extend the time window for successful defibrillation and resuscitation, providing the initial key links in the chain of survival.

In this chapter, we review the approach to the patient in extremis, discussing basic closed-chest compression technique, and summarize the initial management of the obstructed airway.

## PHYSIOLOGY OF BASIC CLOSED-CHEST COMPRESSION

### Hemodynamics

Successful resuscitation from ventricular fibrillation is dependent upon myocardial perfusion. Coronary diastolic pressure, which is the driving force for coronary blood flow during closed-chest compression, may be as high as 20 to 40 mmHg immediately after the onset of arrest, but steadily falls to below 20 mmHg. The likelihood of a successful resuscitation attempt is low with diastolic pressures below 20 mmHg. With these low pressures, coronary blood flow and myocardial perfusion are typically around 5 percent of prearrest values during closed-chest compression. There is a strong positive linear correlation between diastolic blood pressure and myocardial perfusion. Cerebral blood flow is also very low during closed-chest compression. In general, if closed-chest compression begins upon collapse of the victim, hemodynamic parameters are not as poor as depicted but deteriorate without adrenergic support.

### Mechanism of Flow Generation

How the application of force onto the thoracic cage produces movement of blood remains a subject of great interest. Liquids flow in closed systems when pressure gradients develop in them. Flow does occur during closed-chest compression, so a pressure gradient must be created by this maneuver. Two theories may explain where this pressure gradient develops during chest compressions: the cardiac pump and the thoracic pump.

The "cardiac pump" theory was first formulated by Kouwenhoven and states that the pressure gradient is developed within the heart across the valves by direct compression of the heart. Therefore, a pressure gradient from the aorta to the right atrium would be evident during the actual compression of the chest. Competent cardiac valves are an essential component of this theory.

Some investigators noted a lack of an aortic to right atrial pressure gradient and hypothesized that forward flow is generated by an intrathoracic to extrathoracic pressure gradient, the "thoracic pump" mechanism. During the compression (systolic) phase of standard closed-chest compression, all intrathoracic pressures are equal, while there is a pressure gradient from the intrathoracic to the extrathoracic arterial vessels. Only during the relaxation (diastolic) phase of the cycle does an aortic to right atrial pressure gradient develop. This pressure gradient is diastolic coronary perfusion pressure, which is the major determinant of coronary blood flow.

The relative roles of the thoracic pump and direct cardiac compression mechanisms in the generation of blood flow probably vary from patient to patient. Regardless of what mechanism is operating, increasing the rate and depth of compressions augments forward flow, though the exact formula for the proper rate and depth of compressions has not yet been determined.

## BASIC CLOSED-CHEST COMPRESSION: AN OVERVIEW OF TECHNIQUE

The application of effective CPR demands a systematic approach. The performance of the following eight maneuvers in order enables the care provider to quickly evaluate the patient's condition, determine the intensity of intervention required, and assure effective care delivery.

1. Establish unresponsiveness
2. Obtain assistance; activate the emergency medical services (EMS) system
3. Properly position the patient
4. Open the airway
5. Establish breathlessness
6. Ventilate the patient
7. Establish presence or absence of pulse
8. Perform closed-chest compression

### Establish Unresponsiveness and Obtain Assistance

The first step in assessing an individual who has collapsed is to establish the level of responsiveness by administering some sort of noxious stimulus.

If the victim is unresponsive, the initial rescuer should call for help and activate the EMS system if outside the hospital. This step is critical, since the time to the institution of advanced life support procedures is the most important determinant of ultimate outcome.

## Open the Airway

With loss of muscle tone in the obtunded patient, the tongue may fall back into the oropharynx and cause upper airway obstruction. The negative pressure generated during inspiratory efforts can force the tongue back into the oropharynx, creating a one-way valve effect and occluding the airway during inspiration. This will manifest as stridor. Three simple maneuvers are initially used to open the airway and to relieve upper airway obstruction.

The head tilt is the first maneuver that should be attempted. It is accomplished by placing one hand beneath the victim's neck and the other hand on the forehead. The neck is then flexed in relation to the thorax and the head extended in relation to the neck (the so-called sniffing position). If this maneuver is unsuccessful, the chin lift or jaw thrust should be applied. Both of these maneuvers, which should be executed along with the head tilt, effectively lift the tongue out of the oropharynx by displacing the mandible, to which the tongue is connected.

In the chin lift, the hand which had been supporting the neck is placed under the symphysis of the mandible, with the mandible lifted forward and up until the teeth barely touch. The other hand remains on the forehead. The soft tissues at the base of the tongue should not be compressed; this can increase the obstruction. If the victim has dentures, the chin lift is more effective if they remain in place.

In the jaw thrust, the rescuer, who is positioned at the head of the patient, places the hands at the sides of the victims face, grasping the angles of the mandible and lifting the mandible forward. The rescuer's elbows may rest on the surface on which the patient lies. The jaw thrust, with use of the head tilt, is the safest method for opening an airway in a patient while maintaining the integrity of the cervical spine.

## Establish Breathlessness and Begin Ventilation

After opening the airway and noting a lack of air movement or chest expansions, the rescuer should immediately begin artificial ventilations. Occasionally patients who have just lost spontaneous perfusion may have a period of agonal respirations, characterized by a rhythmic sighing. These respirations should not be mistaken for adequate ventilatory efforts, and rescue breathing should ensue.

The mouth-to-mouth method of rescue breathing is initiated by gently pinching the patient's nostrils with the thumb and forefinger. Then, after taking a deep breath, the rescuer, with open mouth around the victim's mouth making an airtight seal, forcibly exhales air into the patient's airway over 2 s. The volume delivered should not exceed 1200 mL. Larger tidal volumes, and rapid insufflation, should be avoided because of the danger of creating gastric distension and subsequent regurgitation and aspiration. Two breaths are delivered initially, allowing adequate time for exhalation. The rescuer's expired air has an $FIO_2$ of 16 to 17 percent, so resources able to deliver higher oxygen concentrations are needed as soon as possible. The rescuer watches the victim's chest to see that it rises with each forced inhalation and falls with the end of forced inhalation. Any observed impairment to air flow during rescue breathing may indicate either an obstruction in the upper airway or a serious restriction to lung expansion such as a tension pneumothorax. If lack of chest wall motion is noted or there is a large amount of resistance to flow, the oropharynx must be reinspected for an obstruction and efforts to relieve the obstruction should be executed.

With severe maxillofacial trauma, mouth-to-nose ventilation may be more effective than mouth-to-mouth. This is done by using the jaw thrust maneuver in an attempt to lift the tongue from the posterior oropharynx and sealing the mouth shut with the thumb and forefinger during inhalation. The patient's mouth is opened during exhalation to diminish the resistance to airflow. Patients with stomas or tracheostomies are ventilated by placing the mouth over the stoma or tracheostomy tube.

Mouth-to-barrier devices may be used to prevent disease transmission, though the effectiveness of these has not yet been determined.

## Relieve Foreign-Body Obstruction

Foreign bodies may cause either partial or complete airway obstruction. In 1989, upper airway obstruction was the etiology for approximately 3900 deaths. With partial obstruction, the patient may be capable of air exchange. With sufficient air exchange, the patient may cough, although there may be wheezing or stridor between coughs. As long as good air exchange continues, spontaneous coughing and breathing should be encouraged. The rescuer should not interfere with attempts to expel the foreign body. The child with partial airway obstruction and good airway exchange should not be turned upside down because this may impact a tracheal foreign body against the vocal cords.

Poor air exchange is characterized by a weak, ineffective cough, marked respiratory stridor, and respiratory distress. A patient who exhibits poor air exchange should be managed as a case of complete obstruction. With complete airway obstruction, the patient is unable to speak, breathe, or cough. If still conscious, the patient may clutch his or her neck; this is the universal distress signal. In an unconscious victim, a complete obstruction is identified by resistance to artificial ventilation and failure of the chest to rise and fall with each attempted ventilation.

## Maneuvers for Relieving Obstruction

The maneuvers recommended for relieving foreign-body obstruction are the finger sweep, back blows or chest thrusts, and manual removal of the object. The sequence in which these maneuvers in complete obstruction should be executed is as follows: check the oropharynx by performing finger sweep, attempt airway breathing, apply back blows, and apply manual thrusts. The cycle is repeated until the obstruction is cleared. If at any time the object appears in the oropharynx, it is removed manually. Back blows produce an instantaneous increase in airway pressure, which may result in either partial or complete dislodgement of the foreign body. Manual thrusts develop a lower but more sustained increase in pressure and may further assist in dislodging the object. Combining these techniques appears to be more effective than using one alone.

The back blow technique is a series of four rapid, sharp, and forcible blows delivered over the spine and between the scapulae with the heel of the hand. They may be given with the victim standing, sitting, or lying. Whenever possible, the patient's head should be lower than the chest to take advantage of gravity.

The manual thrust method (Heimlich maneuver) consists of four thrusts to the upper abdomen or lower chest. The low chest thrust develops somewhat higher flows and peak pressure. The abdominal thrust can be performed with the patient sitting or standing. The rescuer should be positioned behind the patient with arms wrapped around the victim's waist. Making a fist with one hand and placing the thumb side of the fist into the epigastrium and grasping the fist with the other hand, the rescuer delivers four quick upward thrusts. A patient who is lying prone must be placed in the supine position and the airway opened. The rescuer can be either astride or alongside the patient. The heel of one hand is placed in the epigastrium and covered with the heel of the other hand. A quick upward thrust may then be delivered. This maneuver may be self-administered by delivering a quick upward thrust to the abdomen with a fist or by leaning forward on any firm object. Rescuers must take care to avoid placing their hands over the xyphoid process. Complications of abdominal thrusts include rupture or laceration of abdominal viscera.

Chest thrusts are performed in a similar manner when the patient is lying or sitting, with the fist placed directly on the sternum. When the patient is supine, the hands should be placed over the sternum as in closed-chest compression and compressed four times. The chest thrust is useful when the rescuer's arms cannot fully reach around the patient's abdomen or when direct abdominal pressure is likely to cause complications, as in advanced pregnancy.

### Establish Pulselessness and Begin Compressions

After the initial two ventilations, the presence of a pulse is determined by placing two fingers on the carotid artery, which is located by placing the index and middle fingers on the trachea and then sliding them between the trachea and the sternocleidomastoid muscles. If there is no pulse or if the pulse is slow or weak, closed-chest compression should be started immediately. With the patient supine on a firm surface, the rescuer places two fingers of one hand over the xiphoid process and the heel of the other hand on the sternum 1 to 2 in cephalad to the xiphoid. The first hand is brought to rest on top of the hand that is on the sternum. The rescuer, positioned over the sternum with the arms straight and the elbows locked, forces the sternum straight downward 1.5 to 2 in at a rate of 80 to 100 compressions per minute. The optimum ratio of the compression phase to the relaxation phase is 1:1. With two rescuers, a ventilation is delivered after every fifth compression; with one rescuer, 2 ventilations are delivered after every 15 compressions.

## COMPLICATIONS OF CLOSED-CHEST MASSAGE

Complications of closed-chest compression include sternal and rib fractures, pulmonary contusion, and pneumothorax. Myocardial contusions, primarily of the right ventricle, may result in acute right ventricular failure. Hemorrhagic pericardial effusions have also been observed. Gastric distension, erosions, and rupture have occurred. The incidence of liver laceration is approximately 2 percent. Regurgitation and aspiration pneumonia are frequent complications. Careful performance of basic closed-chest technique can diminish, but not totally abolish, many of these complications. Stomach distension, regurgitation, then aspiration are the major complications of rescue breathing.

Late complications include development of pulmonary edema, electrolyte abnormalities, gastrointestinal hemorrhage, pneumonia, and recurrent cardiopulmonary arrest. Anoxic encephalopathy is the major cause of death in resuscitated patients.

## TERMINATING RESUSCITATIVE EFFORTS

Resuscitative efforts should be continued until ventilation and circulation are restored, the patient is transported to a hospital setting, the rescuer becomes exhausted, or a physician assumes responsibility for the patient. Success in resuscitation is time-dependent, with a dismal long-term outcome in efforts that last longer than 20 min in normothermic adults.

## BIBLIOGRAPHY

Guidelines for cardiopulmonary resuscitation and emergency care. *JAMA* 268:2171, 1992.

# 10
# THE ETHICS OF RESUSCITATION
## Timothy J. Crimmins

## INTRODUCTION

Ethics is the branch of philosophy that asks "What is right?" Medical ethics encompasses more than this, providing a standard of moral conduct that requires of physicians the highest level of professional integrity and social responsibility. The American Medical Association's Code of Ethics begins, "The physician shall be dedicated to providing competent medical services with compassion and respect for human dignity." The emergency physician should adhere to the highest standards of moral conduct, to protect and preserve life, prevent disability, and relieve suffering. The physician should be the patient's advocate and provide treatment that is in the patient's best interest.

Despite a desire to live and practice according to these laudable ethical standards, the emergency physician is often faced with dilemmas in patient care decisions when it is difficult to determine what is "right." The legal system has provided ample guidelines in the areas of consent, confidentiality, contract, and liability. Still, the emergency physician has unique ethical challenges in the area of resuscitation, when the physician's obligation towards the patient's best interest and autonomy conflict with the resources available in the community.

## RESUSCITATION

Nothing in emergency medicine arouses as much emotional turmoil as the confrontation with death and dying. In previous times death was considered the natural outcome of disease. Now emergency physicians strive to forestall the moment of death by employing a wide range of medical interventions, including cardiopulmonary resuscitation (CPR). Often the ethical mandate of the emergency physician to preserve life may conflict with the obligation to relieve suffering, prevent disability, and respect the patient's autonomy. Cardiopulmonary resuscitation should be considered as any other therapy—having indications and contraindications performed for the patient's benefit with their consent. The emergency physician should promptly institute CPR and advanced life support procedures for individuals who suffer sudden cardiac arrest or other medical emergencies in the absence of "No CPR" or DNR (do not resuscitate) orders. Cardiopulmonary resuscitation may be ethically withheld or discontinued if there is irreversible cessation of cardiac function, brain death, or imminently terminal illness. CPR need not be provided if it can be reasonably expected to be of no benefit (futility) or the patient has refused CPR through the use of advance directives (DNR orders).

### Determination of Death

Cardiopulmonary resuscitation need not be instituted if the patient is "dead." The difficulty arises in differentiating this from reversible "cardiac arrest." The Uniform Determination of Death Act states: "An individual who has sustained either irreversible cessation of circulatory and respiratory functions, or irreversible cessation of all functions of the entire brain, including the brain stem, is dead." The determination of death can be easily made if lividity, rigor, decomposition, or obviously fatal trauma is present. Sometimes, however, a trial of advanced cardiac life support is necessary to determine "irreversible cessation of circulatory and respiratory functions." The recommendations of the 1992 National Conference of the American Heart Association outline the requirements for an adequate trial of advanced life support. This trial includes endotracheal intubation, rhythm-appropriate medications, and countershocks. Persistent asystole or agonal rhythm should be present to discontinue life support, and although no specific amount of time is recommended, studies indicate that efforts are rarely successful after 25 min. Where emergency medical service (EMS) systems have advanced life support capability, some patients may be "declared dead" in the field after this trial of resuscitation. The decision to withdraw basic life support is more difficult. In some areas there may be long transport times to advanced life support. The policies to withdraw basic life support should be made by local EMS officials depending on community resources, risk to rescuers, time to advanced life support, and circumstances surrounding the cardiac arrest.

Independent brain death cannot be easily determined in the emergency setting. Although state statutes vary regarding the determination of brain death, most require serial examinations over many hours and the exclusion of the presence of certain drugs and hypothermia. These criteria are difficult to meet in the emergency department, so resuscitation of patients with apparent severe brain trauma or global ischemic injury is in order.

### Terminal Illness

Cardiopulmonary resuscitation is not indicated when the patient's death is imminent as the result of irreversible and untreatable terminal illness. Such a decision is an exercise of good medical judgement. A physician may ethically direct that resuscitation be withheld if there is no hope of a successful outcome, but this requires extensive knowledge of the patient's prior medical condition. In an emergency, resuscitation should be instituted until such time as the patient's diagnosis and prognosis are known and it can be ascertained that treatment is of no benefit.

## PATIENT AUTONOMY

Increasingly, physicians are faced with requests for "death with dignity" and "no heroics." The basis for the physician-patient relationship is the patient's consent for treatment. Competent patients may refuse medical treatment, but the emergency physician is often faced with situations involving patients with questionable decision-making capacity, vague directives, ambivalent or absent family members, or a change of mind at the time of the actual "moment of truth." Medical treatment should be instituted in the absence of clear evidence of competent patient refusal.

### No CPR (DNR) Orders

The generally accepted method for withholding CPR at the patient's prior request is through the No CPR or DNR order. The laws and local protocols for implementing No CPR orders vary with the community. Signed forms and/or bracelets have been used to identify and verify the existence of No CPR orders. No CPR or DNR orders have been defined as: "in the event of an acute cardiopulmonary arrest, no resuscitative measures will be instituted." This order does not necessarily imply terminal illness, nor is it a refusal of all medical care. Other treatments may be provided prior to cardiac or respiratory arrest. More extensive limitations of treatment can be accomplished through advance directives or hospice care plans where specific treatments can be refused. Advance directives should have been made prior to the emergency event, and appropriate justification, counselling, and documentation should be provided by the patient's personal physician. These directives should be reviewed periodically. Durable power of attorney for health care and living will laws governing decision making for the patient lacking decision making capacity provide mechanisms by which people can direct their medical care or designate a decision maker prior to losing their ability to direct their medical care. Emergency physicians should be familiar with the laws governing these matters in the state in which they practice. Patients with terminal care plans (hospice) are unique and require thoughtful consideration at critical times. An evaluation and diagnostic workup of a new problem may still be warranted. These patients certainly need ongoing medical and nursing care, as Jonsen writes: "to cure sometimes, relieve occasionally, comfort always."

The emergency physician has an obligation to aggressively resuscitate the victim of an attempted suicide and should restrain and treat those who pose an imminent danger to themselves or others, even against their will—particularly incompetent, intoxicated, or psychotic patients.

## TRIAGE

Medical triage has long been a necessity in the emergency setting. However, new constraints, primarily financial, face the physician making the emergency treatment decisions. Institutions may lack necessary resources to provide appropriate care. The emergency physician's position is unique in that he or she must evaluate all individuals presenting to the emergency department but is not obligated to treat nonemergency patient conditions. The emergency physician is sometimes forced to limit treatments and triage patients when immediately available resources are not adequate. Treatments should not be restricted on arbitrary determinations, such as the patient's cost or worth to society or the refusal by health maintenance organizations to authorize emergency treatment, or its payment.

Restrictions in treatment for financial reasons must be made at the public policy level, with the development of guidelines to limit medical care based on specific criteria that are applied to all individuals. The AMA Council on Ethical and Judicial Affairs has stated: "The organized medical staff has an obligation to avoid wasteful practice and unnecessary treatment that may cause needless expense. In a situation where the economic interests of the hospital are in conflict with patient welfare, patient welfare takes priority."

Emergency physicians should not transfer unstable patients because of financial considerations when transport may endanger the patient's well-being. Federal law should be consulted regarding patient transfers.

## SUMMARY

The emergency physician is often faced with ethical dilemmas when instituting cardiopulmonary resuscitation. Aggressive medical treatment should be used unless the patient is clinically dead, proven brain dead, or unless there is compelling evidence that no therapeutic benefit can be gained from resuscitation. Often a trial of advanced cardiac life support is necessary to determine if the patient has irreversible cessation of cardiac function. Local policies should be developed regarding the institution and discontinuation of basic life support within the community. Cardiopulmonary resuscitation may be withheld in the presence of properly executed No CPR (DNR) orders in communities that have established this process.

Emergency physicians are often obligated to triage patients in an effort to utilize available resources most effectively. This limitation of treatment to patients is ethical when there is scarcity of immediately available resources. The emergency physician has the obligation to preserve life, prevent disability, relieve suffering, and serve as the patient's advocate, providing treatment that is in the patient's best interest.

## BIBLIOGRAPHY

AMA Council on Ethical and Judicial Affairs: 1992 Code of Medical Ethics, Current Opinions, 1992.
Bonnin MJ, Pepe PE, Kimball KT, Clark PS Jr.: District criteria for termination of resuscitation in the out of hospital setting. *JAMA* 270:1457, 1993.
Jonsen A, Siegler M, Winslade W: *Clinical Ethics.* New York, Macmillan, 1982.

Kellerman AL, Hackman BB; Somes G: Predicting the outcome of unsuccessful prehospital advanced cardiac life support. *JAMA* 270:1433, 1993.

Milkes SH, Crimmins TJ: Orders to limit emergency treatment for an ambulance in a large metropolitan area. *JAMA* 254:526, 1985.

National Conference on Cardiopulmonary Resuscitation and Emergency Cardiac Care, 1992: Guidelines for cardiopulmonary resuscitation and emergency cardiac care. *JAMA* 268:2282, 1992.

# 11
# ADVANCED AIRWAY SUPPORT

## Daniel F. Danzl

Air-flow integrity, assurance of oxygenation and ventilation, and prevention of aspiration—these are the three struts underpinning the definitive text on this topic by Dailey et al. Emergency physicians are routinely confronted by the high-stakes blend of cortical and limbic airway pressures. The evolutionary villain? Our common orifice for respiration and alimentation—but then how else could you eat your own words?

This chapter reviews techniques to establish an airway and ventilate a patient after basic maneuvers have been utilized. The uses of oral and nasal airways, the bag-valve-mask unit, and various esophageal airways are discussed. The techniques of oral, nasal, and digital intubation; transillumination and fiberoptic laryngoscopy; retrograde tracheal intubation; translaryngeal insufflation; and cricothyrotomy are presented. Rapid sequence induction, neuromuscular blockade, and the role of respiratory support in cerebral resuscitation are discussed. Intubation in the setting of cervical spine trauma is presented. Finally, suctioning, extubation, and ventilator tricks of the trade are reviewed.

## ORAL AND NASOPHARYNGEAL AIRWAYS

The oral airway, or oropharyngeal tube, lifts the base of the tongue off the hypopharynx. Adult, child, and infant sizes should be available. Use the oral airway only in patients without protective airway reflexes since it stimulates the gag reflex. A short oral airway functions as a bite block and helps to prevent trismic airway occlusion of an orotracheal tube. Two components of the triple airway maneuver, mouth opening and the jaw thrust, are accomplished with the oral airway. The third, head extension, is occasionally necessary to free the base of the tongue from the posterior pharyngeal wall.

The airway is placed over the tongue once the mouth is opened. The easiest technique is to insert it after depressing the tongue with a blade. Another method is to insert the tube with the convexity caudad and then rotate it. Improper insertion will increase airway obstruction by pushing the base of the tongue backward.

A variation of the oropharyngeal tube is the S tube. It is inserted just like an oral airway, and then the patient's head is extended. Ventilation is initiated after the nose is pinched and the flange sealed against the lips.

Nasal airways, or nasopharyngeal tubes, are easier to insert than oral airways. They are better tolerated by patients who are not deeply comatose and have active gag reflexes. The tube is advanced until maximal airflow is heard. If the tip is inserted too far it may stimulate laryngospasm or enter the esophagus. Insertion of a nasal airway may be a useful temporizing maneuver in patients with seizures, trismus, or cervical spine injuries. In addition, a nasogastric tube can be passed through a nasopharyngeal tube to prevent intracranial placement in patients with cribriform plate fractures.

## THE BAG-VALVE-MASK (BVM) UNIT

The BVM unit includes a self-inflating bag, a nonrebreathing valve, and a face mask. The operator should check for adverse anatomic or pathologic facial conditions (Table 11-1). Depending on the operator's expertise, mouth-to-mask ventilation may be superior.

To deliver 100% oxygen, there must be a reservoir as large as the bag volume and an oxygen flow rate equaling the respiratory minute volume. The nonrebreathing valve at the mask or endotracheal (ET) tube allows air entry into the lungs with bag compression, while exhaled air exits through a separate port. Various sizes of transparent masks should be available.

Corrugated tubing reservoirs may be sensitive to variations in ventilatory technique and not deliver 100% oxygen. There are two more effective equipment options. Use a 2.5-L reservoir bag with an oxygen inflow of 15 L/min, or attach a demand valve to the reservoir port of the ventilating bag.

Before ventilating the patient, insert an oropharyngeal or nasopharyngeal tube and extend the stable neck. Then clamp the mask snugly to the face with your thumb and index finger on the mask, while the other fingers pull the chin upward. A major advantage of initially using a bag to ventilate via an ET tube is that you can better judge pulmonary compliance. Common errors in technique include air leaks around the mask and inadequate delivery of tidal volume.

Some alert patients with mild respiratory insufficiency who do not meet intubation criteria can be temporarily managed with continuous positive airway pressure (CPAP) through a snug-fitting face mask. This reduces the functional residual capacity and the work of breathing. Mask CPAP may thus delay or reduce the need for intubation. In patients with severe maxillofacial trauma and potential basilar skull fractures, pneumocephalus is a hazard.

## ESOPHAGEAL AIRWAYS

The esophageal obturator airway (EOA) is a prehospital ventilatory adjunct when endotracheal intubation is not a viable option. It helps prevent gastric insufflation and regurgitation during positive pressure ventilation but is not a substitute for tracheal intubation. The only advantage of the EOA is that insertion does not require laryngeal visualization.

The EOA should be inserted only in apneic, comatose adult-sized patients. Patients with upper airway obstruction, known esophageal disease, or caustic ingestions require different airway management, as do patients with massive nasal or intraoral hemorrhage.

The original EOA design is a large-bore 34-cm tube with a rounded, occluded distal tip. A snap lock connects the tube through the center of a clear plastic oronasal mask. There are sixteen 3-mm openings in the proximal half of the tube below the mask at the hypopharyngeal level.

After attaching the mask to the proximal end of the tube, the patient's mandible and tongue are pulled forward with the head held in

**Table 11-1.** Mask Ventilation Impediments

Beard ± mustache
Cervical arthritis
Edentulous
Facial fractures
Macroglossia
Mandibular surgery
Obesity
Oropharyngeal infections
Prognathism
Temporomandibular arthritis
Upper airway obstructions

a neutral position. If a neck injury is excluded, slight neck flexion will decrease the incidence of inadvertent tracheal intubation. Once the mask is sealed by hand to the patient's face, ventilation is initiated. This forces air into the trachea, which is the only unobstructed orifice. Auscultation for bilateral breath sounds ensures esophageal placement of the tube. Then the cuff is inflated with 30 to 35 mL of air. The cuff must lie below the level of the carina or partial compression of the trachea will obstruct ventilation.

One variation of the original EOA is the esophageal gastric tube airway. The distal end of this tube is patent. There are two holes in the mask. The esophageal tube attaches to one, and a nasogastric tube can be passed down the tube through a valve into the stomach. This unit allows ventilation through the second hole.

Another modification of the EOA is the tracheoesophageal airway, which includes a standard ET tube. The modified face mask has two openings: one for the ET tube and the second for oropharyngeal ventilation. When the ET tube is in the esophagus it vents the stomach and facilitates gastric decompression. Applying cricoid pressure (Sellick maneuver) while the neck is held in extension facilitates tracheal placement.

In the field, a pharyngotracheal lumen airway (PTLA) is another option when endotracheal intubation is not possible. This two-tube two-cuff airway has a large low-pressure cuff that seals the oropharynx at the proximal airway.

Another permutation is the esophageal tracheal combitube. This plastic twin-lumen tube has one lumen resembling an EOA and the other an ET tube. The combitube has a proximal pharyngeal sealing balloon (100 to 140 mL air) that functionally replaces the EOA mask. The distal balloon holds 15 to 20 mL of air. Potential advantages of the pharyngeal cuff (combitube) over an oral cuff (PTLA) include a fairly consistent inflation volume to achieve a seal and less dental trauma to the cuff.

The laryngeal mask airway is another new device that is inserted blindly into the oropharynx. The patient is ventilated through a 12-mm inside diameter (ID) tube that is connected to an oval mask with an inflatable rim.

The amount of oxygenation initially possible with the EOA is similar to that provided with an ET tube. Ventilation is less efficient. The most common complication, seen in about 10 percent of EOA insertions, is inadvertent tracheal intubation. Subsequent asphyxia will occur unless this is quickly recognized.

The incidence of esophageal rupture is unknown since most patients do not receive postmortem examinations. The probable cause of esophageal tears distal to the cuff is the increased intragastric pressure exerted against an occluded esophagus during cardiopulmonary resuscitation (CPR). Esophageal tears or perforation may also result from the direct trauma of the tube or postemesis (Mallory-Weiss syndrome).

Conscious patients may complain of shortness of breath, chest pain, and dysphagia. Physical findings include subcutaneous emphysema, pneumomediastinum, Hamman's crunch, and gastrointestinal hemorrhage. There will be an increased incidence of complications in patients who are not apneic or deeply comatose. They may vomit, aspirate, or develop laryngospasm or supraglottic obstruction.

When the patient arrives, insert a cuffed ET tube before removing the EOA. The use of esophageal airways is declining. Intubation of the trachea is rapidly becoming the prehospital technique of choice.

## OROTRACHEAL INTUBATION

The most reliable means to ensure a patent airway, provide oxygenation and ventilation, and prevent aspiration is endotracheal intubation. Many conscious patients require emergency intubation. They may be unable to clear the airway spontaneously of secretions, require mechanical ventilation, have aspirated, or lack protective airway re-

flexes. Most are lying supine on gurneys. The poignant World War I aphorism "He who looks at heaven will soon be there" still holds.

The clinical assessment of oxygenation and ventilation is unreliable in a chaotic emergency department. Oximetry is the noninvasive bedside monitoring of arterial oxygen saturation. Remember that isolated oximetry yields no clue regarding the status of alveolar ventilation. Capnography allows estimation of the $Pa_{CO_2}$ based on the waveform display of the end-tidal $P_{CO_2}$. Capnometry is the numerical display. In combination, both of these noninvasive modalities aid in determining the need for more aggressive airway interventions.

Capnography can also help verify tube placement in perfusing patients and thus prevent consequential esophageal intubation. A sudden drop in the end-tidal $CO_2$ may reflect endobronchial tube migration. When electronic capnography is unavailable, consider using disposable capnometric devices.

## Technique

Take a brief time to evaluate the upper airway anatomy. Examination of the teeth, oral cavity size, mentum-cricoid distance, mobility and posterior depth of the mandible, and neck mobility may clue the operator to anticipate a difficult airway. The normal adult mouth opening is three finger breadths. Consider asking the alert sober patient to open the mouth as widely as possible and protrude the tongue in your direction. The ease of laryngoscopy correlates well with the ability of the physician to visualize the soft palate, uvula, and faucial pillars.

While calling for an assistant, check and arrange the necessary equipment. The appropriate-size tube and an additional tube 0.5 to 1 mm in size smaller should be selected, and the cuff checked for air leaks. Selecting a tube with the proper diameter is essential (Table 11-2). The second hole at the end of the tube above the bevel is called *Murphy's eye*. This permits some airflow if the tip is occluded. Most tubes need to be cut after orotracheal intubation or they will gradually creep into the carina.

Tubes with high-volume low-pressure cuffs are best for adults. In patients younger than 6 to 8 years, use uncuffed tubes. Note that lidocaine jelly can form a clear film and eventually occlude the lumen of small pediatric tubes. Thin-walled cuffs prevent aspiration when properly inflated better than medium-walled cuffs. Microcirculation to the tracheal mucosa will be impaired if the cuff pressure exceeds 40 cm $H_2O$. After nasogastric decompression, the cuff pressure should initially be deflated to 15 to 20 cm $H_2O$, or just to the point of eliminating audible air leaks. Cuff overinflation can compromise the ET tube lumen.

Test the light on the laryngoscope and pick your blade. The straight Magill blade directly and physically lifts the epiglottis. The curved Macintosh blade rests in the vallecula above the epiglottis and indirectly lifts it off the larynx because of traction on the frenulum. Developing expertise with both blades is desirable, since they offer differing advantages, depending on the clinical setting and body habitus. The curved blade may be less traumatic and reflex-stimulating since it does not directly touch the larynx. It also allows more room for adequate visualization during tube placement. The straight blade is mechanically easier to insert in many patients who do not have large central incisors. Simply aim the tip of the blade directly at the epiglottis and lift it. Selecting the proper size blade greatly facilitates

**Table 11-2.** Approximate Adult Sizes for Endotracheal Tubes and Suction Catheters

| Patient | Endotracheal Tube Inner Diameter, mm* | Suction Catheter Size (French) Outer Diameter |
|---|---|---|
| Adult Female | 7.5–8.0 | 12–14 |
| Adult Male | 8.0–8.5 | 14 |

* Tubes of 0.5 to 1 mm smaller inner diameter are used for nasotracheal intubation.

intubation. In adults, the curved Macintosh no. 3 or 4, or the straight Miller no. 2 or 3, is most often ideal.

When all equipment is in order, the patient should be placed in the sniffing position. (*Note:* The novice laryngoscopist's most common reasons for failure—inadequate equipment preparation and poor patient positioning—occur prior to the use of the laryngoscope.)

Flexion of the lower neck with extension at the atlantooccipital joint (sniffing position) aligns the oropharyngeolaryngeal axis, allowing a direct view of the larynx. Placing a folded towel or small pillow under the occiput is often helpful.

If time permits, the patient should be oxygenated with 100% oxygen prior to intubation. Begin with the laryngoscope in the left hand and an ET tube or tonsil suction catheter in the right hand. After removal of dentures and any obscuring blood, secretions, or vomitus, the suction catheter is exchanged for the ET tube and inserted during the same laryngoscopy.

The blade is inserted into the right corner of the patient's mouth. If a curved Macintosh blade is used, the flange will push the tongue to the left side of the oropharynx. If the blade is inserted down the middle, the tongue forces the line of sight posteriorly—yet another reason for the putative "anterior larynx." After visualization of the arytenoids, lift the epiglottis directly with the straight blade or indirectly with the curved blade. The larynx is exposed by pulling the handle in the direction that it points, that is, 90° to the blade. Cocking the handle back, especially with the straight blade, risks fracturing incisors.

One can avoid the most common error, overly deep insertion of the blade, by looking for the arytenoid cartilages. If only the posterior commissure is visible, have an assistant apply pressure on the cricoid (the Sellick maneuver). Watch the cuff as it passes completely through the cords to avoid an error. Attempts at blind passage only invite anoxia. Always be willing to abort the attempt if visualization of the larynx is not successful, and resume mask ventilation. Continuous pulse oximetry during intubation can identify hypoxia quickly.

With proper technique and practice, malleable blunt-tipped metal or plastic stylets are not usually necessary. When the patient's anatomy requires it, the proximal end of the stylet may be bent 45°, but the tip should not extend beyond the end of the ET tube nor exit Murphy's eye.

One aid to intubation with direct vision is the use of a thin, flexible intubation stylet. This type of stylet can be inserted blindly around the epiglottis into the trachea. Then the ET tube is threaded over it into the trachea and the stylet removed. The Eschmann stylet (gum elastic bougie) is a common choice. Another option is to use the tip on the laryngeal tracheal anesthesia kit. With either stylet, orient the tube so that Murphy's eye is in the twelve-o'clock position.

Visualization of the larynx prior to cervical spine clearance is difficult, since alignment of the oropharyngeolaryngeal axis is not possible. One way to move the tip of the tube anteriorly is to use a slightly flexed directional-tip tube (Endotrol) coupled with a Sellick maneuver. Another is a flexible stylet, the Flexiguide, that passes through the tube and has a trigger similar to the Endotrol. The final option is to aim the tip anteriorly with Magill forceps while an assistant advances the tube.

Never force the tube through the vocal cords. Often the tube is too large, or too warm and flexible, especially with an Endotrol. Translaryngeal or directed transoral anesthesia with lidocaine can help relax the cords. There are two other options. Try performing a Seldinger maneuver. A tube can be advanced over a nasogastric tube in the trachea and passed below the cords. On occasion, lining up the bevel with the glottic opening will also succeed.

The tube should be advanced until the cuff disappears below the cords. Correct tube placement is about 2 cm above the carina. From the corner of the mouth, this is approximately 23 cm in men and 21 cm in women. The base of the pilot tube is usually at teeth level. The tube is also positioned by palpating its tip at the suprasternal notch and advancing it 2 to 3 cm.

After cuff inflation, insert an oropharyngeal airway or bite block and auscultate to verify bilateral lung expansion. Inadvertent endobronchial intubation is usually on the right side. Cut and secure the tube, being careful not to impede cervical venous return with the umbilical tape. Ideally use a modified clove-hitch knot or a commercial fixation. Avoid tying and kinking the pilot tube.

If the cuff leaks, tube replacement is possible with or without direct visualization. A length of nasogastric tubing two and one-half to three times the length of the ET tube can be inserted as a guide.

## Complications

Endobronchial or esophageal intubation will result in hypoxia or hypercarbia. Disposable capnographic devices can confirm ET tube placement. The *syringe aspiration technique* is another useful adjunct to the standard techniques for intratracheal tube confirmation. This may be especially useful in the prehospital setting. A catheter-tipped 60-mL syringe is snugly inserted through the adaptor at the proximal end of an ET tube. The tube must be at least size 7.0 ID. Resistance to aspiration reflects occlusion from esophageal collapse. If there is no resistance during aspiration, the tube is in the trachea. Commercial esophageal intubation detectors are also available. The adaptor on the detector's syringe fits over the 15-mm ET tube connector. The tube may be obstructed by a bulging cuff, secretions, kinking, or biting. Subsequent neck movement can also displace the tube.

Although they are uncommon, chronic complications of emergent endotracheal intubations do occur and may be quite debilitating. Arytenoid cartilage displacement, usually on the right, prevents the patient from phonating properly. Chordal synechiae may develop anteriorly, or commissural stenosis posteriorly. Subglottic stenosis is the most disastrous complication. Prevent tube motion in the larynx and trachea. This usually occurs in combative patients or those on ventilators.

## NASOTRACHEAL INTUBATION

Nasotracheal intubation is an essential skill that allows a flexible approach to airway management. In some locales nasotracheal intubation is a lost art. Despite the seductive pharmacologic alternative, this psychomotor skill can bail the clinician out of many difficult situations. As one example, many patients in respiratory distress may be easier to intubate in a semi-sitting position. There is always a calculated risk associated with pharmacologically extinguishing spontaneous respirations in nonfasting patients.

### Technique

Spray both nares with a topical vasoconstrictor-anesthetic. Then select a cuffed ET tube 0.5 to 1 mm in size smaller than that optimal for oral intubation. Check the tube cuff and firmly snug the tube adaptor. Despite universal precautions, secretions and blood may be expelled into the air and onto the intubator's face. Options include listening for air flow from a larger distance or through a section of IV tubing inserted into the ET tube. Alternatively, a protective filtering adaptor such as the Humid-Vent 1 (Gibeck Respiration, Sweden) can be attached to the proximal end of the ET tube.

Advance the tube, lubricated with a water-soluble (2% lidocaine, K-Y) jelly along the nasal floor on the more patent side. If the nares appear equal, try the right side. When the bevel faces the septum it helps prevent abrasions of the Kiesselbach plexus. Steady, gentle pressure or slow rotation of the tube usually bypasses small obstructions. If the right side is impassable, try the other side before resorting to a smaller tube.

In patients with intact protective airway reflexes, translaryngeal or directed transoral anesthesia often facilitates intubation. Translaryngeal anesthesia, not widely utilized in the emergency department, should always be considered when the initial intubation attempt is un-

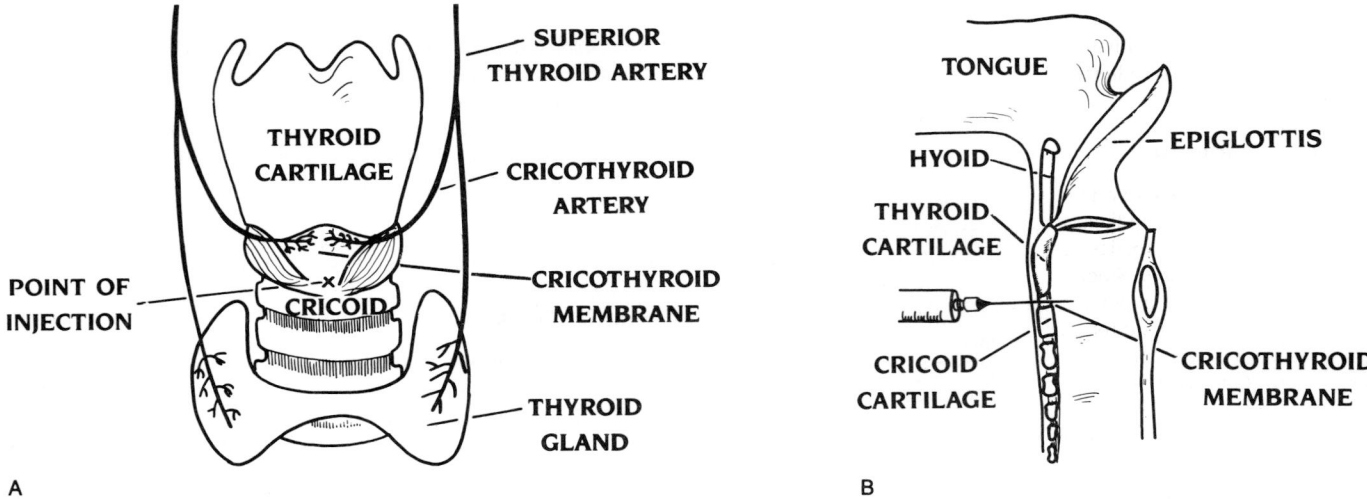

**Fig. 11-1.** Translaryngeal anesthesia via cricothyroid puncture. **A.** Anatomy—anterior view. **B.** Anatomy—cross sectional view.

successful. After palpating the superior border of the cricoid cartilage in the midline, puncture the cricothyroid membrane with a 22- to 25-gauge 0.5- to 1-in needle (Fig. 11-1). The needle should be perpendicular to the membrane in the midline, with the point of injection just cranial to the cricoid cartilage. Aspirate air, then swiftly inject 1.5 to 2.0 mL of 4% lidocaine (sterile for injection) and press the site firmly with a finger for a few seconds. Otherwise small amounts of subcutaneous emphysema would erroneously suggest laryngeal injury. In a review of 17,500 cricothyroid punctures with small-gauge needles, only eight minor complications were reported. Translaryngeal anesthesia is contraindicated if the landmarks are obscured by thyroid or tumor impingement on the cricothyroid membrane or in obese or combative patients.

Have an assistant immobilize the patient's head and initially maintain it in a neutral or slightly extended position. Stand to the side of the patient, with one hand on the tube and with the thumb and index finger of the other hand straddling the larynx (Fig. 11-2). Advance the tube while rotating it medially 15° to 30° until you hear maximal airflow through the tube. Then gently but swiftly advance the tube during early inspiration. Entrance into the larynx may initiate a cough, and most expired air should exit through the tube even though the cuff is uninflated. Look for "fogging" of the tube.

Advancement toward the carina can be observed externally. The normal distance from the external nares to the carina is 32 cm in the adult male and 27 to 28 cm in the adult female. Auscultate to verify bilateral lung expansion and cuff inflation. Secretions or blood in the tube should be removed prior to positive pressure ventilation.

If intubation is unsuccessful, carefully inspect the neck to determine the malposition of the tube. Most commonly, it is in the pyriform fossa on the same side as the nares used. A bulge will be seen and palpated laterally. Withdraw the tube into the retropharynx until breath sounds are again heard. Then redirect while manually displacing the larynx toward the bulge. If there is no contraindication, flexion and rotation of the neck to the ipsilateral side will often help while rotating the tube medially.

The other most common tube misplacement is posteriorly in the esophagus. There will be no breath sounds through the tube, and the trachea will elevate slightly. Attempt redirection after extending the patient's head and performing a Sellick's maneuver. When cervical spine pathology is suspected, use a directional tip control tube (Endotrol) or a fiberoptic laryngoscope.

When tube passage is prevented by the vocal cords, shrill, turbulent air noises will be heard. Rotate the tube slightly to realign the bevel with the cords or squirt 2 mL of 4% lidocaine (80 mg) down the tube onto the cords if translaryngeal anesthesia was omitted. The use of continuous $CO_2$ monitoring through an Endotrol during blind nasotracheal intubation can also help guide tube placement.

Congenital abnormalities in the nasopharynx, including pharyngeal bursae, may be anatomical causes of tube misplacement. With gentle technique, the obstruction can be felt and guided intubation accomplished. Hypertrophic adenoid tissue, polyps, and neoplastic lesions can also divert the tube.

### Indications

Nasal intubation is helpful in situations where laryngoscopy is difficult, neuromuscular blockade hazardous, or cricothyrotomy unnecessary. Severely dyspneic awake patients with congestive heart failure, chronic obstructive pulmonary disease, or asthma often cannot remain supine but do tolerate nasotracheal intubation in the sitting position. Nasotracheal tubes, in addition to being better tolerated by patients than oral tubes, are less traumatic to the tracheal mucosa since there is less intratracheal tube movement with head motion.

Patients often present with trismus from seizures, facial trauma, infection, tetanus, or decorticate-decerebrate rigidity. It may be impossible to align the oropharyngeolaryngeal axis in patients with arthritis, masseter spasm, temporomandibular dislocation, or recent oral surgical procedures. Agitated patients or those with a peculiar body habitus may be impossible to intubate orally.

Nasal intubation with a fiberoptic laryngoscope may be required when neoplastic lesions, lymphoid tissue, Ludwig's angina, peritonsillar abscess, or epiglottitis obstruct the pharynx. If the radiographic

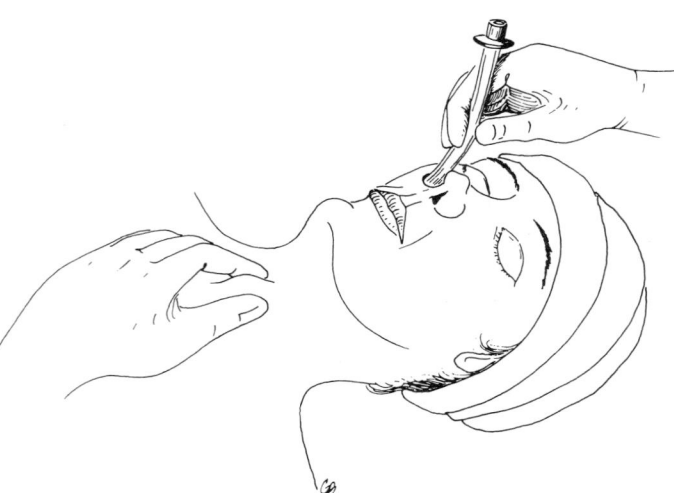

**Fig. 11-2.** Blind nasotracheal intubation while displacing the larynx to the patient's right.

status of the neck in a traumatized patient is unknown, the nasal route is one of the noninvasive alternatives to cricothyrotomy or translaryngeal ventilation.

## Contraindications

Complex nasal and massive midfacial fractures, and bleeding disorders, are relative contraindications to nasotracheal intubation. However, oral intubation impedes prompt reduction and stabilization of some maxillary fractures. Since a LeFort I fracture does not extend to the cribriform plate, it is not a contraindication. Fiberoptic guidance is preferable when feasible for LeFort II and III fractures.

The risk of inadvertent intracranial passage of a nasotracheal tube is extremely low, unlike nasogastric tube insertion. Very poor technique in the setting of obvious massive head trauma would be required. Severe traumatic nasal or pharyngeal hemorrhage may necessitate orotracheal intubation or cricothyrotomy. Contamination of the spinal fluid is a hazard with some basilar skull fractures.

## Complications

Serious complications of nasotracheal intubation are rare. In a series of 1187 patients, there was no permanent laryngeal damage. Epistaxis is seen with inadequate topical vasoconstriction, excessive tube size, poor technique, or anatomic defects. Excessive force can damage the nasal septum or turbinates. Recheck the cuff for a potential puncture by a turbinate.

Frequent suctioning, especially if epistaxis or other upper airway hemorrhage is present, will help to prevent thrombotic occlusion of the tube or a mainstem bronchus. Retropharyngeal lacerations, abscesses, and nasal necrosis have been reported.

Paranasal sinusitis, especially occurring with prolonged nasotracheal intubation or severe cranial trauma, can be an unrecognized source of sepsis. Mucopurulent nasal drainage need not be present. The risk of postintubation sinusitis correlates with the duration of intubation, which often reflects the neurologic insult. In the setting of craniofacial trauma, any subsequent CT scans should include views of the paranasal sinuses. Other factors causing sinusitis include presence of a nasogastric tube, sinus hemorrhage or fracture, and administration of glucocorticoids. As with any route of intubation, one may observe stridor on extubation, tube obstruction or displacement, subglottic stenosis or edema, cuff overinflation, or tracheobronchitis.

## DIGITAL INTUBATION

Visual landmarks may be impossible to identify because of patient positioning or anatomical disruption. Tactile digital intubation might avert cricothyrotomy when direct laryngoscopy has failed following neuromuscular blockade.

Success requires a deeply comatose patient, and even then consider inserting a molar bite-block. Lift the tongue and pull the mandible forward with a gloved hand. Insert the middle and index fingers of the other hand down the middle of the tongue. Palpate the epiglottis with the middle finger.

Then insert the ET tube, which has been shaped into a "J" configuration, with a malleable stylet. The tube slides along the middle finger which is in contact with the epiglottis. As the index finger guides the tube from behind, constant contact with the tip helps identify its position. Withdraw the stylet as resistance is felt when the tube enters the larynx.

## TRANSILLUMINATION

Transillumination with a lighted stylet or light wand can be an intubation aid and help confirm ET tube placement and positioning. This technique is of particular assistance when direct laryngoscopy is anatomically impossible. Clinicians experienced with this technique use it to facilitate "indirect visual" oral or "blind" nasotracheal intubation.

Newer instruments can be used for either nasotracheal or orotracheal intubation. Oral intubation requires a rigid light wand. For nasal intubation, remove the trocar and insert the flexible instrument into a directional tip ET tube (Endotrol). After insertion, the intubator must discriminate between the light emanating from the larynx and that from the esophagus. Usually the circumscribed "jack-o-lantern" glow arising from the larynx or trachea will not be appreciated when the distal light source is in the esophagus. It may help to shield bright ambient light from the neck.

## FIBEROPTIC ASSISTANCE

The flexible fiberoptic laryngoscope or bronchoscope is a valuable adjunct when there are anatomic or traumatic limitations that prevent visualization of the vocal cords. Clinical examples include conditions that prevent opening or movement of the mandible, congenital anatomic abnormalities, and cervical spine immobility. Fiberoptic instruments allow visualization of laryngeal structures and can enable difficult intubations, including those around expanding hematomas (Fig. 11-3). Patients in need of an immediate airway or those with ongoing hemorrhage or copious secretions are poor candidates for fiberoptic intubation because of the time and skill needed for the technique.

Directed transoral or transnasal and translaryngeal topical anesthesia is essential. Spray the nasal mucosa with a vasoconstrictor. Dual suctioning capability is needed; attach one to a tonsil suction catheter for oral blood and secretions. Tongue extrusion and anterior mandibular displacement will be helpful if the oral route is chosen. Fragile equipment is more frequently damaged transorally. The nasal route is also more ideal because the optic tip can enter the glottis at a less acute angle.

Begin by focusing the eyepiece and lubricating the flexible shaft. Immerse the lens at the tip of the laryngoscope in warm water to prevent fogging. Continuously monitor pulse oximetry and be sure that the gag reflex has been eliminated. Attach oxygen tubing to the suction port. Consider intermittent insufflation of oxygen at 10 to 15 L/min to keep the optic tip clear, while maintaining a 1 to 2 L/min supplemental flow of oxygen. Insufflation is usually a better way to clear secretions than suction.

Remove the adaptor from an ET tube that is at least 7.0 mm ID in size. To prevent barotrauma when high-flow oxygen is insufflated,

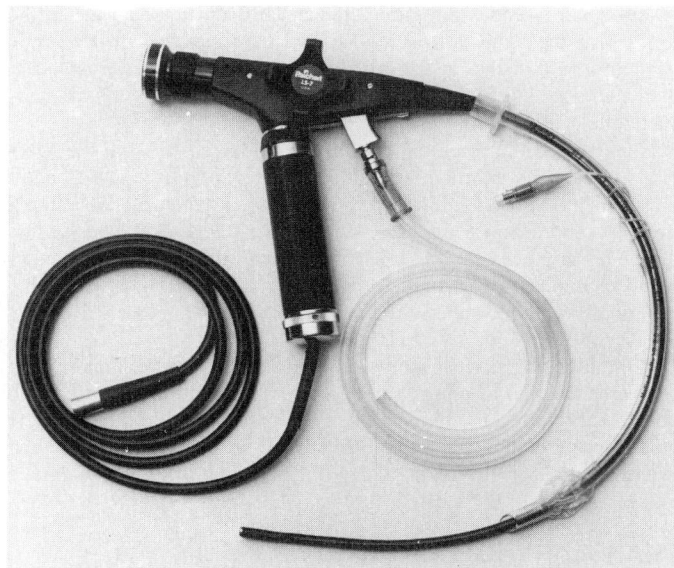

**Fig. 11-3.** Fiberoptic laryngoscope. An ET tube covers the shaft; suction or oxygen tubing is attached.

use at least a 7.5-mm (ID) tube. Then slip the lubricated ET tube over the shaft up to the handle. The distal end of the laryngoscope must extend beyond the end of the ET tube. Hold the laryngoscope with your left hand, and control the tip deflection while advancing it through the cords. The laryngoscope will function as a stylet for the tube. After the laryngoscope is in the trachea, advance the ET tube and remove the laryngoscope.

Another option is to insert a nasotracheal tube blindly into the posterior pharynx and stop about 1 to 2 cm proximal to the epiglottis. The scope is then inserted through this hollow conduit, and the fiberoptic tip can be directed into the glottis. Be careful not to pass the scope through Murphy's eye. If this occurs, it will be impossible to advance the ET tube.

The fiberoptic scope cannot be used as a stylet to guide the ET tube into the trachea. The stiffer ET tube will often deflect the thin scope tip posteriorly into the esophagus. In addition, keeping the concavity of the ET tube anteriorly toward twelve o'clock places the tube tip and Murphy's eye at three o'clock (90° to the right). The tip will then often abut the right arytenoid cartilage. Rotating the tube 90° counterclockwise lines up the tip with the upper triangular entrance into the trachea.

## RETROGRADE TRACHEAL INTUBATION

Retrograde tracheal intubation (RTI) is yet another viable option when conventional airway approaches would fail. Use the same landmarks for the cricothyroid puncture as those used for translaryngeal anesthesia. Severe maxillofacial trauma, cervical or mandibular ankylosis, and upper airway masses are some of the conditions for which RTI is potentially useful.

RTI is not impeded by the blood that obscures fiberoptically guided intubation. Insertion of a retrograde translaryngeal catheter is a less invasive option than cricothyrotomy when the neck is immobilized and nasotracheal intubation fails. This technique can be time-consuming and must be avoided in apneic patients.

Preoxygenate the patient, then administer translaryngeal anesthesia (see Fig. 11-1) via an 18-gauge needle through the caudal aspect of the membrane. Align the needle bevel with the syringe markings. This will help determine the bevel direction after cricothyroid membrane puncture. After angling the needle 30° to 45° cephalad, advance a 70- to 75-cm flexible-tip guidewire. Grasp it in the oropharynx or nares with forceps unless, with luck, it exits spontaneously. Another option when hemorrhage is present is to insert a 75-cm central venous pressure catheter and insufflate. To locate the tip, go for the bubbles. Insertion of a J-wire, which can be slowly twisted once it arrives at the oropharynx, can also be easier to locate than a straight guidewire. Clasp the guidewire securely with a hemostat at the neck.

Next, thread the proximal end of the guidewire through the Murphy's eye on the ET tube. This allows more of the ET tube to enter the trachea before the guidewire is removed. Tighten the wire like a tightrope and advance the tube. When the ET tube will pass no further, cut the guidewire or catheter flush with the cricothyroid membrane to minimize soft tissue contamination. Advance the ET tube, and finally withdraw the wire or catheter from the proximal end of the ET tube.

If the tube will not pass through the cords, try a 90° counterclockwise tube rotation to bring Murphy's eye anterior, which realigns the bevel. Another technique is to insert the guidewire end that exits the mouth into the suction port of a fiberoptic scope. The scope is then inserted over the retrograde guidewire and functions as an antegrade guide.

## TRANSLARYNGEAL VENTILATION

Percutaneous translaryngeal ventilation (PTLV) offers a temporizing alternative approach to airway management. It does not substitute for airway control with a cuffed tube. PTLV may prove valuable in the initial stabilization of patients not able to be intubated orally or nasally. In those with severe maxillofacial trauma and an unknown cervical spine status, PTLV can be initiated until cricothyrotomy is completed.

The equipment required for this technique is readily available in emergency departments. The required high-pressure oxygen source can be provided by either a 50-psi wall source with the flow meter set on flush or an oxygen cylinder without a secondary regulator valve. Demand valve devices limited to 50 cm $H_2O$ pressure (70 cm $H_2O$ = 1 psi) do not deliver sufficient tidal volume through large-bore intravenous (IV) catheters.

This technique involves puncture of the inferior aspect of the cricothyroid membrane at a caudal angle with a 12- to 14-gauge kink-resistant over-the-needle plastic catheter. Cannulae with side holes are preferable and lessen the risk of tracheal mucosal damage. After removing the needle, advance the catheter toward the carina (Fig. 11-4).

The IV catheter and three-way stopcock can be directly attached to high-pressure oxygen tubing if the edges of the stopcock are trimmed. Another convenient way to allow exhalation is to interpose a section of an 18F to 20F suction catheter with control vent between the stopcock and the tubing.

The patient is ventilated for approximately 2 full seconds or until the chest begins to rise. The valve is then released for 4 to 5 s. This simulates an I:E ratio of 1:2. If exhalation is inadequate, a second venting catheter should be inserted through the cricothyroid membrane next to the first one. Intermittently uncover the second catheter with a finger to allow exhalation. Initially ventilate at 25 psi until the correct catheter position is verified; then increase to 50 psi.

This technique differs from high-frequency jet ventilation. Rapid jet ventilation through percutaneous translaryngeal catheters has been used for emergency ventilation with pulmonary dysfunction. There are several forms of high-frequency jet ventilation, all characterized by rapid rates of ventilation (>100 respirations/min), tidal volumes less than the dead space volume, and low peak airway pressure. These characteristics increase the functional residual capacity and improve oxygenation.

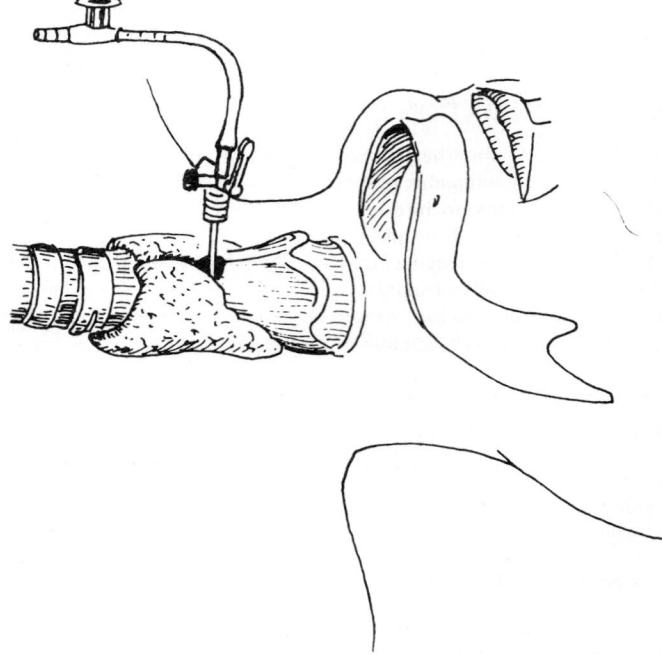

**Fig. 11-4.** Translaryngeal ventilation. A plastic IV catheter is inserted through the cricothyroid membrane. A three-way stopcock and suction catheter tubing have been attached.

## Complications

Complete expiratory obstruction of the airway complicates PTLV. Barotrauma, including air embolism, has been an experimental concern. Avoid attempts to intentionally disimpact an obstruction from below. Other complications of this technique include those reviewed with puncture of the cricothyroid membrane. If the catheter is misplaced or if exhalation is inadequate, massive subcutaneous emphysema from interstitial oxygen insufflation into tissue planes is possible. Esophageal laceration or rupture, pneumomediastinum, or pneumothorax can also occur as a result of excessive insufflation pressures.

## CRICOTHYROTOMY AND TRACHEOSTOMY

Laryngotracheobronchial injuries and total upper airway obstruction often mandate a surgical airway. Initial symptoms include cough, dysphagia, dysphonia, odynophagia, and hoarseness. Peritracheal fascial sleeves may initially maintain a patent airway until an enlarging hematoma occludes it or the distal trachea retracts into the mediastinum. More commonly, these techniques are required because less invasive means of tracheal intubation have failed. Another scenario is the patient for whom neuromuscular paralysis of spontaneous respirations could be dangerous. Cricothyrotomy carries far fewer and less serious complications than does emergency tracheostomy.

Cricothyrotomy was initially condemned in 1921 by Chevalier Jackson for its allegedly high incidence of subglottic stenosis. Most of the patients in this preantibiotic-era study had high-pressure tubes placed in the setting of acute laryngeal disease. The complication rate for patients with emergency cricothyrotomies varies widely. In a series of 147 patients undergoing the procedure, the complication rate was 8.6 percent. In another series of 38 cricothyrotomies performed in the emergency department, the complication rate was 40 percent. Technical changes dropped this rate to 23 percent at the same site in a follow-up series. Nevertheless, in several large series of tracheostomies, the complication rate ranged from 28 to 65 percent and were of greater severity.

## Indications

Indications for immediate cricothyrotomy include severe, ongoing tracheobronchial hemorrhage, massive midfacial trauma, and inability to control the airway with the usual less invasive maneuvers. Less invasive procedures may be contraindicated or impossible with mechanical upper airway obstruction, facial or cervical trauma, or uncontrollable oral hemorrhage.

Further clinical situations requiring cricothyrotomy include oral or pharyngeal edema from infection, anaphylaxis, or chemical inhalation injuries. Patients with anatomic variants, occult foreign bodies, or obstructing lesions may be impossible to intubate.

Removal of blood or vomitus may not be possible in patients with trismus or masseter spasm. In addition, cricothyrotomy may be required if blind or fiberoptic nasotracheal intubation is unsuccessful.

## Contraindications

This technique should not be used on patients who can be safely intubated orally or nasally. Emergency cricothyrotomy is relatively contraindicated in the presence of acute laryngeal disease due to trauma or infection. It should also be avoided if the patient has very recently been intubated for several days. Tracheostomy may be required in patients who develop airway obstruction after removal of an endotracheal tube in place for over 72 h.

In small children under 10 to 12 years of age, the small larynx lies much higher, at the C2-3 level rather than at the C5-6 level in adults. A 12- to 14-gauge catheter over the needle is safer than a formal cricothyrotomy or tracheostomy.

The patient must be completely immobilized because the incision site is 1.5 to 2 cm below the vocal cords and above the vascular thyroid isthmus. The esophagus is posterior and the carotid and jugular vessels lateral to the incision.

Cricothyrotomy, like blind nasotracheal intubation, can cause retraction of the distal trachea into the superior mediastinum in patients with laryngotracheal injuries. Since this is a technique of last resort, a hemorrhagic disorder is not an absolute contraindication. Hemostasis is certainly easier to achieve than with a tracheostomy. The management decision depends on operator experience and the degree of respiratory distress. Airway options include formal tracheostomy, endotracheal intubation over a flexible fiberoptic bronchoscope, insertion of a small (6- to 7-mm ID) orotracheal tube under direct vision, or low transtracheal insufflation.

## Technique

Instruments required for emergency cricothyrotomy include a curved Mayo scissors and hemostat, a dilator, a tracheal hook, and a no. 11 scalpel blade.

Have an assistant maintain cervical immobilization. After identification of the anatomic landmarks and palpation of the cricothyroid membrane, digitally stabilize the larynx. This is critical. A *vertical* 3- to 4-cm incision is made through the skin. Start at the superior border of the thyroid cartilage and incise caudally toward the suprasternal notch. Alternatively, puncture the membrane caudally with a needle, which may provide a temporizing airway and guide for the incision. The blade is then rotated to make a *horizontal* stab through the inferior aspect of the membrane after it has been repalpated (Fig. 11-5).

Stabilize the larynx by inserting the tracheal hook into the cricothyroid space and retracting upon the inferior edge of the thyroid cartilage. With the blade tip left in the larynx, scissors points or a hemostat is inserted beside the blade and spread horizontally. Then the scalpel is removed and a dilator (LaBorde, Trousseau) or hemostat is inserted and spread *vertically*. Remove the tracheal hook—it could puncture the balloon. The largest tracheostomy tube that does not injure the larynx is placed, usually a no. 4 Shiley in an adult (inner diameter 5.0 cm; outer diameter 8.5 mm). The average fiber-elastic adult cricothyroid membrane measures 9 to 10 mm by 22 to 30 mm. Do not slide the tube into the anterior mediastinum.

The cuff is then inflated and the tube securely tied. Alternatively, a small-cuffed (5-mm) endotracheal tube may be cut short and inserted. It should be electively removed after location of a curved tracheostomy tube, which is less traumatic to the posterior tracheal wall.

A vertical midline skin incision decreases the incidence of marginal vessel hemorrhage and certainly seems to help with exposure of landmarks. A vertical incision can always be extended. Horizontal incisions would be cosmetically preferable in "elective" situations. The cricothyroid membrane should be punctured interiorly and at a caudal angle, since the cricothyroid arteries anastomose superiorly over the membrane.

In patients with massive neck swelling, the hemorrhage, subcutaneous emphysema, edema, or fat may make identification of normal landmarks impossible. In such cases, more formal exposure or tracheostomy may be necessary. Tracheostomy is most often necessary in pediatric patients or those with subglottic stenosis. Airway problems caused by traumatic tracheal transection, laryngeal fracture, or a zone III hematoma cannot be managed via cricothyrotomy.

An alternative approach involves location of the hyoid bone. Estimate the distance from the angle of the mandible to the chin. Insert a blade in the midline of the neck down half of that distance from the chin. Attach a skin hook to the hyoid and vertically incise inferiorly.

Several cricotomes are commercially available. These percutaneous devices allow insertion of a needle or stylet into the trachea. A functional airway is then inserted after dilatation of the tract. There is insufficient clinical experience reported to comment on their safety, particularly in children.

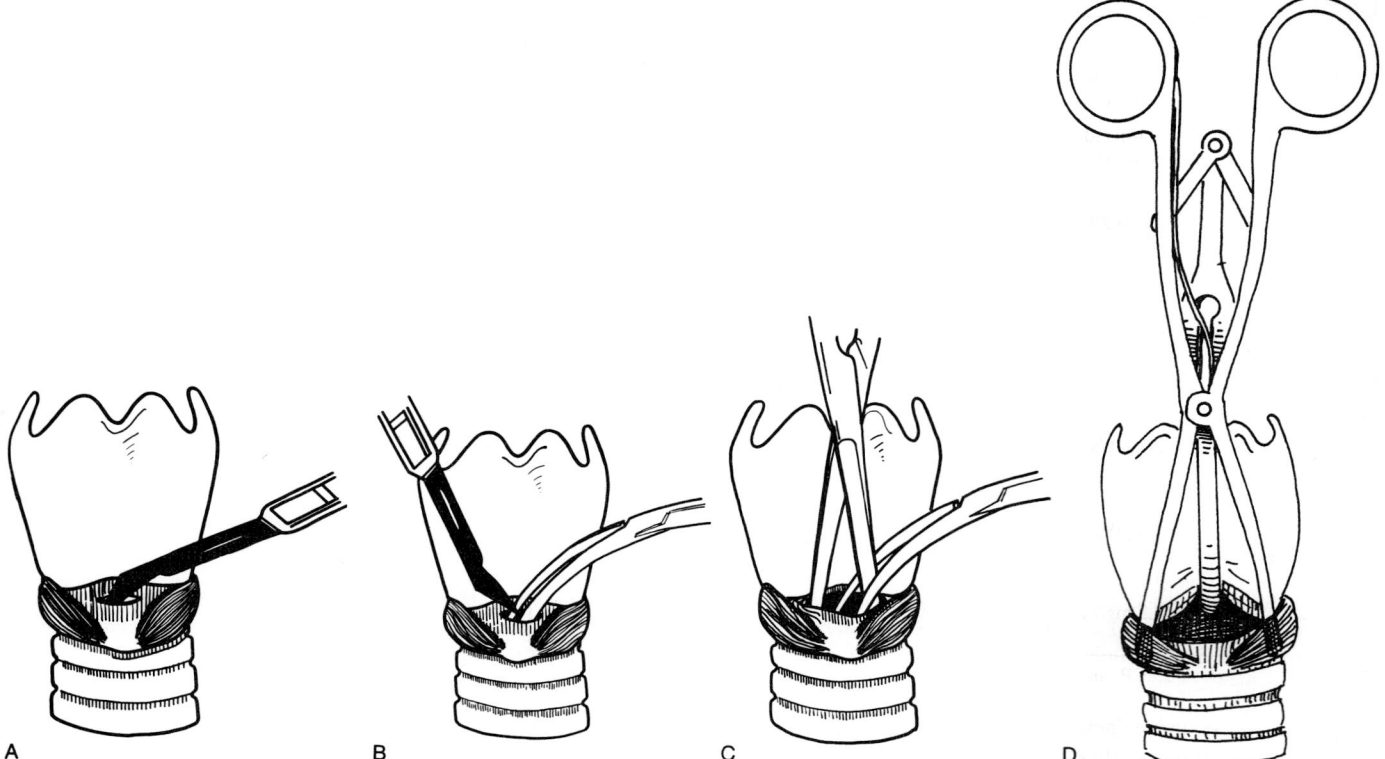

A     B     C     D

**Fig. 11-5.** Cricothyrotomy. **A.** Horizontal stab of the cricothyroid membrane following a vertical skin incision. **B** and **C.** Dilation with hemostat. **D.** Dilation with LaBorde dilator.

## Complications

Immediate complications of cricothyrotomy include prolonged execution time, excessive hemorrhage, aspiration, and unsuccessful or incorrect tube placement. The most common misplacement is superior to the thyroid cartilage through the thyroid membrane. Inferior tracheotomy placement has also been reported.

Other potential complications include mediastinal or subcutaneous emphysema or creation of a false passage into the trachea. Adjacent vascular, neural, endocrine, esophageal, or pulmonary structures may be injured. Long-term complications include dysphonia from thyroid cartilage fractures, transient dysphagia, or voice changes. Infection and perichondritis may occur.

The postoperative surgical airway management is critical. Correct head positioning, aggressive humidification, and frequent suctioning prevent acute tube occlusion. Replacement of a tube prior to epithelialization of the tract is very difficult. Secure the tube and protect it with restraints as needed. Monitor for chronic complications including infection and tracheal stenosis, which is rare with correct tube size and cuff pressure.

## RAPID SEQUENCE INDUCTION

Complex airway emergencies in select nonfasted patients may require rapid sequence induction (RSI). This couples sedation to induce unconsciousness (induction) with muscular paralysis. Intubation follows laryngoscopy while maintaining cricoid pressure to prevent aspiration. The principle contraindication is any condition preventing mask ventilation or intubation (Table 11-3).

Some agitated and combative patients can only be reasoned with pharmacologically (Table 11-4). Repeated 5-mg aliquots of haloperidol (Haldol) will control severe agitation. Droperidol (Inapsine), another butyrophenone, is a more potent and rapid onset agent. Titrate with 2.5- to 5-mg aliquots IV. Droperidol can blunt the cardiovascular response to intubation. Hypotension is rare, and there are fewer

dystonic reactions than with haloperidol. Since it is a potent antiemetic, it is ideal as a premedication or for neuroleptanalgesia.

Thiopental is a short-acting barbiturate sedative. An IV dose of 3.0 to 5.0 mg/kg will induce unconsciousness in 30 to 40 s and last about 10 min. It is the most widely used induction agent. An ultrashort-acting barbiturate is methohexital (Brevital). It is twice as potent as thiopental with half the duration of action. Avoid these cerebroprotective agents if systemic hypotension is a problem. Thiopental and methohexital are also contraindicated in status asthmaticus, and methohexital reduces the seizure threshold.

Opioids are also reversible potent induction agents. Fentanyl 2–10 μg/kg (Sublimaze) has an onset of action usually under a minute. The ideal dose is highly variable. Consider using this agent in head-injured patients. Rapid injection of high doses may cause chest wall rigidity. Alfentanil is more potent and has a more immediate onset of action. Opioids are the preferred induction choice when patients require analgesia in addition to sedation.

Another pharmacologic alternative is a short-acting benzodiazepine. Midazolam (Versed) at a dose of 0.1 mg/kg is another viable option since the antagonist flumazenil is available. If time permits, titrate with 0.5-mg increments. Finally ketamine is a potent bronchodilator to be considered in difficult hypotensive or bronchospastic

**Table 11-3.** Rapid Sequence Induction

1. Set up IV × 2 and cardiac monitor; do oximetry and capnography.
2. Check equipment; suction, airway devices; PTLV and "crico" tray.
3. Explain procedure; document neurologic status.
4. Preoxygenate (100% FiO$_2$); *no* positive pressure ventilation.
5. Consider sedation; analgesia; adjunctive lidocaine and/or atropine.
6. Defasciculate.
7. Induce with thiopental or other agent.
8. Do Sellick maneuver.
9. Give neuromuscular blocking agent.
10. Intubate trachea and release Sellick maneuver.

**Table 11-4.** Sedative/Rapid Sequence Induction Agents

| Agent | Dose | Onset | Duration | Benefits | Caveats |
|---|---|---|---|---|---|
| Haloperidol | 5-mg aliquots (adult) | minutes | Variable | Rare ↓BP | Titrate Dystonia |
| Droperidol | 2.5-mg aliquots (adult) | minutes | Variable | Rare ↓BP Antiemetic | Titrate Dystonia ↓BP |
| Thiopental | 3–5 mg/kg | 30–40 s | 10 min | ↓ICP | ↓BP Asthma |
| Methohexital | 1 mg/kg | < 1 min | 5 min | ↓ICP | ↓BP Seizures Asthma |
| Fentanyl | 2–10 µg/kg | 2 min | 30–40 min | Reversible ↓ICP Analgesia | Highly variable dose |
| Midazolam | 0.1 mg/kg | 1–2 min | 20 min | Reversible Amnesic Anticonvulsant | Apnea No analgesia |
| Ketamine | 2 mg/kg | 1 min | 5 min | Bronchodilator "Dissociative" amnesia | ↑ICP |
| Etomidate | 0.3 mg/kg | <1 min | 5 min | ↓ICP ↓IOP | Myoclonic excitation Vomiting |

*Note:* BP, blood pressure; ICP, intracranial pressure; IOP, intraocular pressure.

patients. Since ketamine increases the blood pressure, it has been popular in hypovolemic situations. However it will increase the intracranial pressure (ICP) in head trauma patients.

## NEUROMUSCULAR BLOCKADE

Neuromuscular blocking agents facilitate management of selected patients in the emergency department. The most commonly used agents are succinylcholine (Anectine), vecuronium bromide (Norcuron), pancuronium (Pavulon), and atracurium (Tracrium). Succinylcholine allows persistent depolarization to occur at the neuromuscular endplate, mimicking acetylcholine. In contrast, vecuronium, pancuronium, and atracurium are nondepolarizing curariform agents. They compete with acetylcholine at the myoneural endplate receptors. The blockade is reversible with acetylcholinesterase inhibitors (Table 11-5).

In the emergency department, neuromuscular blockade can improve mechanical ventilation and help control intracranial hypertension. Paralysis improves oxygenation and decreases peak airway pressures in a variety of disorders, including refractory pulmonary edema and respiratory distress syndrome. Patients with refractory status asthmaticus; status epilepticus; or tetanic spasms resulting from clostridial infections or a variety of toxins, including strychnine, may improve with blockade.

In addition, extremely violent, agitated patients who jeopardize aeromedical personnel or their own airway security, spinal cord integrity, or fracture stability may require pharmacologic restraint. Be certain to maintain attempts to correct hypoxia and hypovolemia, coupled with physical restraints.

For the conditions mentioned above, nondepolarizing agents are preferable to succinylcholine. Although the onset of action is delayed, there are fewer adverse cardiovascular and histaminic effects, coupled with a longer duration of paralysis.

The dosage of pancuronium is 0.10 to 0.15 mg/kg IV. After documentation of the neurologic examination, including pupil size, pre-sedation is advised unless there is a significant head injury. Muscle relaxants are neither anxiolytics nor analgesics. Omission of sedation is a common error, and patients then remain aware of their paralysis. An increased sympathetic tone can exacerbate arrhythmias. Consider pancuronium or ketamine in irreversible status asthmaticus.

Vecuronium bromide (Norcuron) is another nondepolarizing agent. This curariform drug is approximately one-third more potent than pancuronium. The duration of action is one-third to one-half as long. Vecuronium does not cause the degree of tachycardia commonly seen after pancuronium, since it has one-twentieth of the vagolytic effect. This simplifies interpretation of a tachycardia developing in the trauma patient. Hypersensitivity reactions are rare, doses are only minimally cumulative, and excretion is biliary. Despite the lack of histamine release, hypotension may occur through two other mechanisms. Sympathetic ganglia blockage occurs, and venous return is decreased from both absent muscle tone and the positive-pressure ventilation.

The usual dose of vecuronium is 0.08 to 0.1 mg/kg IV. Maximal paralysis occurs within 3 to 5 min, with full blockade lasting for 25 to 40 min.

Atracurium is another agent more suited for patients with hepatic or renal failure. Elimination is via ester hydrolysis and Hoffman degradation, a nonenzymatic process. This nondepolarizing agent's elimination half-life is approximately 20 min, versus 65 to 75 min with vecuronium. Recovery time is consistent and unaffected by anticonvulsants. Consider this agent for intubated patients requiring brief diagnostic or therapeutic procedures. Atracurium also offers advantages when continuous infusion is essential to maintain a required level of neuromuscular blockade precisely. The risk with prolonged infusion is accumulation of laudanosine, a neuroexcitatory metabolic byproduct.

The reversal of nondepolarizing muscle relaxants should not be attempted prior to some sign of motion or spontaneous recovery. Ideally, a "train of four" twitches should be elicited with a neuromuscular stimulator. Reversal requires 0.01 mg/kg of atropine IV, followed by 0.5 to 1.0 mg/kg of edrophonium IV. The onset of action is 30 to 60 s, with a duration of 10 to 30 min. This reversal may be shorter than the duration of the muscle relaxant. Edrophonium is an acetylcholinesterase inhibitor with a faster onset and fewer muscarinic side effects than the longer-acting neostigmine. Prophylactic atropine given before the cholinergic agonist edrophonium helps prevent muscarinic side effects.

When the indication for blockade is tracheal intubation, succinylcholine is the most commonly used agent. It has a more rapid onset (30 to 60 s) and shorter duration of action (average 5 to 6 min) than

**Table 11-5.** Neuromuscular Relaxants

| Agent | Intubating Dose IV | | Onset | Duration | Complications |
|---|---|---|---|---|---|
| | Adult | Child | | | |
| Succinylcholine*† | 1.5 mg/kg | 1.5–2 mg/kg | 30–60 s | 3–8 min | 1. Bradyarrhythmias<br>2. Increased intragastric, intraocular, and intracranial pressure<br>3. Hyperkalemia<br>4. Fasciculation-induced musculoskeletal trauma<br>5. Masseter spasm<br>6. Malignant hyperthermia<br>7. Prolonged apnea with pseudocholinesterase deficiency<br>8. Histamine release |
| Vecuronium | 0.08–0.1 mg/kg | 0.1 mg/kg | 1.5–4 min | 25–40 min | 1. Prolonged recovery time in obese or elderly, or if hepatorenal dysfunction<br>2. Carbamazepine and phenytoin-induced resistance |
| | 0.15–0.28 mg/kg (high-dose protocol) | 0.2 mg/kg | 1–1.5 min | 60–120 min | |
| Pancuronium | 0.1–0.15 mg/kg | 0.1–0.15 mg/kg | 1–5 min | 30–90 min | 1. Vagolytic tachyarrhythmias<br>2. Prolonged recovery in elderly or if hepatorenal dysfunction<br>3. Carbamazepine- and phenytoin-induced resistance |
| Atracurium | 0.4–0.5 mg/kg | 0.4–0.5 mg/kg | 2–5 min | 20–45 min | 1. Histamine release<br>2. Hypotension<br>3. Bronchospasm |

* Pretreat with defasciculating dose of 0.01 mg/kg vecuronium if intracranial hypertension or unstable fractures.

† Pretreat with 0.01 mg/kg atropine in children or vagotonic adults.

does vecuronium or pancuronium. After a brief fasciculation, complete relaxation occurs at 60 s with maximal paralysis at 2 to 3 min.

The dosage of succinylcholine is 1.0 to 1.5 mg/kg IV for adults and 2.0 mg/kg for children under 12 years. Be prepared to obtain an airway surgically if intubation attempts fail. Succinylcholine produces adequate intubation conditions in the emergency department, despite some significant risks (see Table 11-5).

The other alternatives for decreasing the time to intubation involve administration of a small "priming" dose (10 percent of the actual dose) of vecuronium or high-dose (0.15 to 0.28 mg/kg) vecuronium. These may prove viable alternatives in the emergency department despite their intermediate duration of action.

Approximately 2 to 3 percent of intubations prove impossible with standard techniques. Emergency physicians selecting neuromuscular blockade must anticipate difficult intubations despite time-limited assessment of the patient's physiognomy.

Before injection of succinylcholine, 0.01 mg/kg of atropine IV may attenuate the muscarinic vagal effects, especially in children and vagotonic adults. Serious arrhythmias are not rare. An additional pretreatment to consider is a subparalytic dose of 0.01 mg/kg vecuronium to prevent the initial muscle fasciculations that may cause long-bone fractures to become displaced. This is most pronounced in muscular adolescents.

Intraocular pressures also increase. In addition, increased intragastric pressure predisposes to aspiration. ICP increases are another concern with succinylcholine. This increase in ICP is greater in patients with central nervous system (CNS) neoplasms than in those with acute CNS hemorrhage or trauma. If the intubation is rapid, immediate hyperventilation may compensate. Pretreatment with vecuronium and a short-acting barbiturate can attenuate transitory intracranial hypertension, which occurs during tracheal intubation of some patients with significant head trauma.

Avoid barbiturates, including thiopental, unless the cranial trauma is isolated. There is the potential for systemic hypotension, especially with associated injuries. Topical laryngeal and/or IV lidocaine (1.5 mg/kg) may minimize the increase in the ICP.

There are other, less preventable side effects of succinylcholine. The serum potassium will transiently rise an average of 0.5 mEq/L with succinylcholine. Hyperkalemia is even more pronounced hours after muscle trauma or burns. Avoid depolarizing agents in patients with burns, muscle trauma, myopathies, rhabdomyolysis, narrow-angle glaucoma, renal failure, or neurologic disorders. Any patients with "denervated musculature" (e.g., Guillain-Barré syndrome) are particularly at risk. Genetically susceptible individuals may develop acute malignant hyperthermia. Have dantrolene sodium available.

Patients with an atypical pseudocholinesterase will require prolonged ventilatory support, as will those with burns, cirrhosis, or carcinomas who have low plasma pseudocholinesterase levels.

Effective oxygenation and ventilation during cerebral resuscitation often requires neuromuscular blockade. Autoregulation of cerebral blood flow (CBF) over a range of perfusion pressures may be impaired. As a result, CBF becomes pressure-dependent (CBF =

CPP/CVR, where CPP is cerebral perfusion pressure and CVR is cerebral vascular resistance). Autoregulation is usually intact when the CPP ranges between 50 and 130 mmHg. The CPP equals the mean arterial pressure minus the ICP. Ideally, it should be kept well over 70 mmHg.

Therefore, respiratory support of the bucking or posturing patient becomes critical. After blockade, select an $F_{IO_2}$ sufficient to maintain an arterial $P_{O_2}$ of 100 mmHg, fully saturating hemoglobin. Institute prophylaxis against atelectasis with positive end-expiratory pressure (PEEP) of up to 5 cmH$_2$O. Higher levels impair cerebral venous drainage because of the elevated intrathoracic pressure. Avoid other modalities that also increase the ICP, including excessively tight ET tube straps, tight cervical collars, or Trendelenburg positioning.

The optimal $Pa_{CO_2}$ following blockade for the individual patient with intracranial hypertension is frequently unknown. Hyperventilation will decrease cerebral blood volume while cerebral vasoconstriction is intact. Postresuscitation, cerebral vasospasm may decrease CBF, and thus overzealous hyperventilation could be harmful. Always avoid hypercapnia, generally maintaining the $Pa_{CO_2}$ around 28 to 30 mmHg.

## INTUBATION IN CERVICAL SPINE INJURY

Airway management of patients with the potential to have an unstable cervical spine injury challenges clinical judgment. There is no single best algorithm. The reported incidence of injury ranges from 1 to 12 percent. Cervical spine radiography without a thorough and reliable neurologic examination does not "clear the neck." From 20 to 30 percent of cervical spine injuries are not appreciated on a single cross-table lateral view. Spinal cord injury without radiographic abnormality (SCIWORA) is an important consideration, especially in children.

As a result, determine whether immediate airway intervention is needed. There is a large selection of airway options to consider while attempting to maintain cervical spine immobilization. The selection is far less critical than the timing. When there is evidence of a cervical cord injury or significant intracranial hypertension, consider blind nasotracheal intubation or rapid sequence induction and oral intubation. Oral intubation appears safe when achieved without hyperdistraction, flexion, or extension of the neck. Maintenance of cervical spine immobilization is the paramount issue—not the approach to secure the airway.

The need for in-line cervical stabilization should not be considered a license for axial in-line traction. In the near-hanging victim, attempting to radiographically visualize C7 by countertracting on the head and shoulders is indiscreet. Attempt to block any further increase in the ICP.

Patients not in urgent need of an airway should be neurologically and radiographically evaluated as thoroughly as is practical, given the patient's condition. The presence of systemic hypotension or intracranial hypertension guides the selection of sedatives or induction agents.

## SUCTIONING

A variety of conditions render patients unable to clear their own secretions. Aspiration usually occurs when the tone of the lower esophageal sphincter is insufficient to deal with increased intragastric pressure and protective laryngeal airway reflexes are depressed. Common iatrogenic causes include BVM ventilation, nasogastric tubes, and pharmacologic neuromuscular paralysis. Predisposing conditions include trauma, bowel obstruction, obesity, overdose, pregnancy, and hiatus hernia.

Attention to technique reduces the risk. A rigid-tip plastic tonsil suction catheter works best for large quantities of oropharyngeal secretions, including blood and vomitus. Clear the pharynx either with the tonsil suction catheter or digitally. When necessary, place the patient in a left lateral Trendelenburg position. This gets the tongue out of the laryngoscopist's way. Perform endotracheal suctioning immediately.

To suction the nasopharynx and tracheobronchial tree, use a well-lubricated, soft, curved-tip catheter. Straight catheters will usually pass into the right mainstem bronchus. If a curved-tip catheter is available, turning the head to the right in addition to catheter rotation will facilitate passage into the left bronchus.

Select a suction catheter of a size no larger than half the diameter of the tube to be suctioned. This will prevent pulmonic collapse from insufficient ventilation during suctioning. Oxygenate the patient before and after suctioning to avoid transient desaturation. Insert the catheter without suctioning, and then remove, suctioning with rotation over 10 to 15 s.

Complications of suctioning include hypoxia, cardiac arrhythmias, hypotension, pulmonic collapse, and direct mucosal injury. The magnitude of the ICP increase during endotracheal suctioning may be related to the increase in intrathoracic pressure with coughing. Consider topical laryngeal or intravenous lidocaine.

Continued airway patency is not assured after ET tube insertion. Suctioning clears clotted blood or inspissated secretions. In addition, mechanical obstruction from tumors or vascular malformations may be detected.

Endobronchial ball-valve obstruction can occur with a clot. This will impair ventilation and produce hyperinflation of individual lobes. Cuff displacement or overinflation has also resulted in ball-valve obstruction of the airway. Cuffs inflated in the field during frigid conditions will expand with warming. Recheck for unequal breath sounds or asymmetrical chest expansion. Elevated inspiratory pressures develop and exhalation is prevented, ultimately resulting in tension pneumothorax.

Deflate the cuff when tracheal ball-valve obstruction is suspected. If the tube is blocked, deflation will allow exhalation. Specific diagnosis and relief of endobronchial obstruction requires bronchoscopy.

## MECHANICAL VENTILATORY SUPPORT

Ventilators are pressure-cycled or volume-cycled. Pressure-cycling is usually limited to pediatrics and does not control the volume delivered. Most emergency departments will have volume-cycled ventilators. Other decisions regarding mechanical ventilatory support in the emergency department include the mode, $F_{IO_2}$ minute ventilation, and use of PEEP or CPAP.

There are three common ventilator modes or methods of providing the tidal volume: controlled mechanical ventilation (CMV), assist-control (A/C), and intermittent mandatory ventilation (IMV). Use the control mode for apneic patients. The A/C mode allows the patient to trigger a cycle by inhaling and lowering the air pressure, which can be adjusted by the ventilator's trigger "sensitivity" (1 to 3 cmH$_2$O). The ventilator will provide a nontriggered "controlled" breath unless one is triggered during the selected time cycle. Finally, a predetermined number of ventilator-generated tidal volumes can be assured either unsynchronized (IMV) or more commonly synchronized to patient effort (SIMV). In the emergency department, the A/C or SIMV is the preferred initial mode except with an apneic patient.

The initial $F_{IO_2}$ should be guided by the oximetry. Set the tidal volume at 10 mL/kg ideal body weight and adjust the rate accordingly. Maintain the *peak* airway pressure (PAP) below 40 to 45 cmH$_2$O to prevent barotrauma. The tidal volume can be increased up to 15 mL/kg to adjust the $Pa_{CO_2}$ unless it elevates the PAP.

PEEP or CPAP should be considered if the decreased pulmonary compliance prevents delivery of an adequate tidal volume or if hypoxemia persists despite an $F_{IO_2}$ of 100 percent. Even low levels (3 to 5 cmH$_2$O) of PEEP/CPAP usually render ventilator "sighs" (1.5 × tidal volume) unnecessary. If hypotension develops, adjust the respiratory rate and PEEP to lower the *mean* airway pressure.

## EXTUBATION

Extubations are always potentially hazardous. While patients are recovering their protective airway reflexes, they may "fight" the tube. Injection of 1 to 2 mL of 4% lidocaine (sterile for injection) down the ET tube will decrease bucking. Absorption of lidocaine via the airway yields sustained levels, while the maximum serum level is slightly lower than that from an equivalent intravenous dose.

Prior to extubation, rule out metabolic or circulatory abnormalities and check for respiratory insufficiency. Prior nasogastric decompression is advised. On command, the patient should have an inspiratory capacity of 15 mL/kg. There should be no intercostal or suprasternal reactions, and the patient's grip should be firm.

After suctioning secretions, assure adequate oxygenation of the patient with 100% oxygen. Explain the procedure to the patient. Ventilate with positive pressure, using the BVM unit to exsufflate secretions while the cuff is deflated. At the end of a deep inspiration, to prevent secretory reaccumulation, remove the tube and oxygenate by mask.

Observe the patient closely for stridor. Postextubation laryngospasm is initially treated with oxygen by positive pressure. If necessary, nebulized racemic epinephrine (0.5 mL 2.25% in 4-mL saline) often helps. Rarely, neuromuscular blockade to facilitate reintubation or cricothyrotomy is necessary.

## BIBLIOGRAPHY

Benumof JL: Management of the difficult adult airway. *Anesthesiology* 75:1087, 1991.

Dailey RH, Simon B, Young GP, Walls RM: *The Airway: Emergency Management.* St. Louis, Mosby Year Book, 1992.

Schuster DP: A physiologic approach to initiating, maintaining, and withdrawing mechanical ventilatory support during acute respiratory failure. *Am J Med* 88:268, 1990.

Storer DL: The pharmacology of airway control. *Emerg Care Q* 7:69, 1991.

Walls RM: Rapid-sequence intubation in head trauma. *Ann Emerg Med* 22:1008, 1993.

Yealy DM, Stewart RD, Kaplan RM: Myths and pitfalls in emergency translaryngeal ventilation: Correcting misimpressions. *Ann Emerg Med* 17:690, 1988.

# 12
# VASCULAR ACCESS
## William A. Berk

Obtaining access to the venous and arterial circulation is a crucial aspect of effective management of the critically ill or injured patient. Success facilitates drug, crystalloid, and blood product administration, as well as patient assessment through measurement of central venous and arterial pressures. Indications, techniques, and potential complications of establishing circulatory access are discussed in this chapter.

## VENOUS ACCESS

### Sites

The normal human anatomy has abundant peripheral veins (Figs. 12-1 and 12-2). In the arms these usually allow ready access. Leg veins are less advantageous due to the risk of precipitating phlebitis and greater technical difficulty. Internal jugular, subclavian, or femoral vein

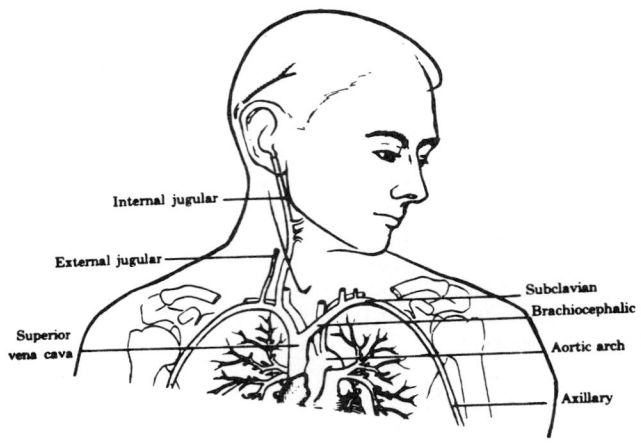

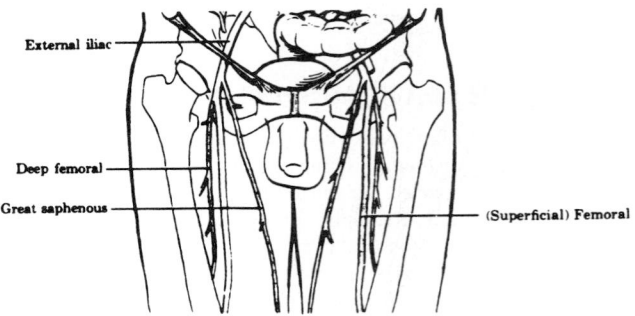

**Fig. 12-1.** Veins of torso and lower extremities.

catheterization is performed when peripheral access is impossible or when central venous pressure measurement is desired.

The cephalic vein, in both the forearm and the upper arm, is large, constant, and straight; easily catheterized, it is the time-honored choice for peripheral access. Veins of the hand are usually accessible even in obese persons but are short, tortuous, and difficult to stabilize—and thus unreliable. Veins in the antecubital fossa are excellent in emergency situations, but an armboard is necessary to prevent catheter kinking or dislodgement with movement. The large basilic vein in the upper arm is usually not visible but with practice can be catheterized by palpating the brachial artery and searching "blindly" for the medially placed vein. Puncture of the brachial artery is common but rarely of clinical significance if care is taken to prevent hemorrhage or hematoma formation; transitory paresthesias may also occur.

Veins in the legs often require cutdown for catheter placement. The superficial saphenous vein at the ankle is large, constant, and easy to isolate and cannulate. The proximal great saphenous vein in the thigh may be found reliably 5 cm below the inguinal ligament at the junction of the medial and middle third of the thigh in the supine patient. The deep femoral vein is accessible percutaneously, just medial to the femoral artery; in the pulseless patient the landmark is the junction of the median and middle third of the inguinal ligament. From the great saphenous and deep femoral veins advancement of catheters into the right atrium for central venous pressure measurement is possible.

Peripheral venous catheterization should not be attempted proximally in an extremity involved by burns or serious injury or when drainage occurs to an area that has sustained an acute serious injury, e.g., the right arm in the presence of a gunshot wound to the right chest. In all of these situations patency of the proximal veins may not be assured. Catheterization of arms in the presence of an indwelling fistula or serious neck trauma should also be avoided.

The external jugular vein can provide reliable access in both adults

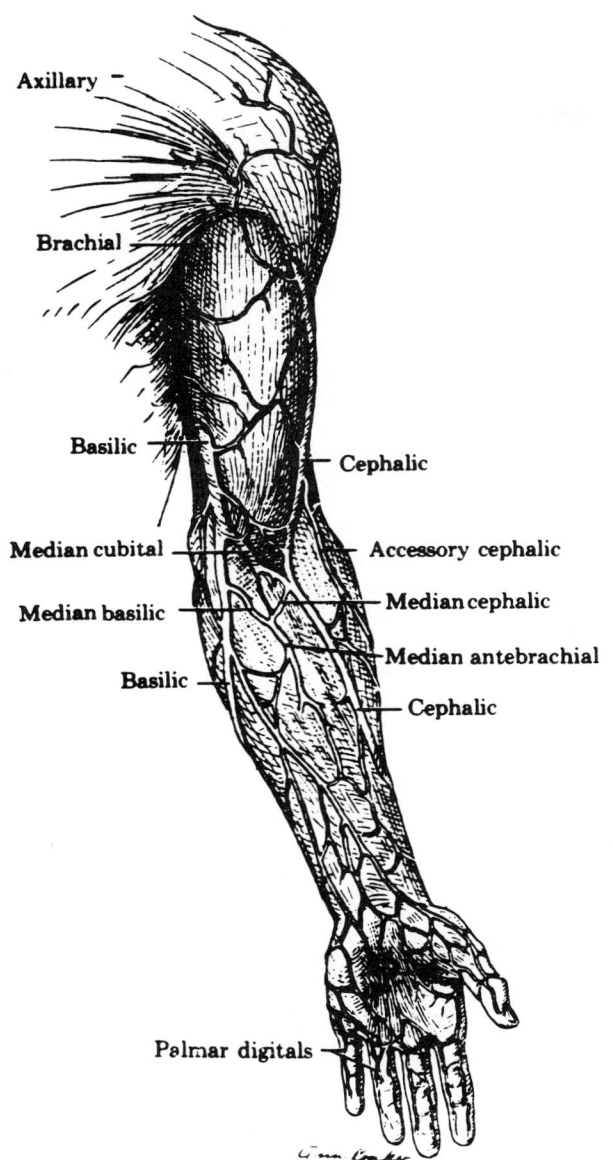

**Fig. 12-2.** Veins of upper extremity.

Axillary

Brachial

Basilic

Cephalic

Median cubital

Accessory cephalic

Median basilic

Median cephalic

Median antebrachial

Basilic

Cephalic

Palmar digitals

and children. Although readily distended by the Valsalva or Trendelenburg maneuver, scant subcutaneous support can make it difficult to catheterize. Access to central veins without the risk that attends direct internal jugular and subclavian puncture is a major advantage.

In young children intraosseous infusion provides rapid and reliable access in emergencies. A bone marrow or intraosseous infusion needle placed in the proximal or distal tibial or distal femur bone marrow can provide emergency access.

## Technique Considerations

Care must be taken to minimize the risk of local infectious complications—occurring in up to one-third of patients undergoing venous catheterization—which can rarely result in septicemia. Insertion of peripheral venous catheters should be preceded by a surgical prep and followed routinely by placement of a sterile dressing. Consideration of the indications for venous access and what constitutes appropriate and adequate access in individual patients will minimize risk and facilitate management of emergencies when they occur. If peripheral veins are small, size and visibility can be enhanced by application of hot, moist compresses for 5 min, by tapping gently on the vein before

attempting puncture, or by application of nitroglycerin ointment (0.4% for children less than 1 year old; 2% for others) over a 1-in diameter area for 2 min and then wiping off. Once access has been obtained, gentle circumferential occlusive taping may be necessary if stability of the site is tenuous, with the intravenous line looped and secondarily secured to prevent traction at the point at which the line penetrates the skin. The size of the catheter should be written on the tape dressing. When venous access is required primarily for drug administration, consideration should be given to placing a saline or heparin lock.

Complications from placement of peripheral intravenous lines include hematoma formation, phlebitis, and cellulitis. Phlebitis may occur in up to 75 percent of hospitalized patients. There is general agreement that catheters should not be left in place for longer than 3 days before replacement. Nerve and tendon damage, deep venous thrombosis, suppurative thrombophlebitis, and septicemia are rare. The unusual event of extravasation of irritative, vasoconstricting, or tissue-toxic substances such as 50% dextrose, epinephrine, phenytoin, and some drugs used for chemotherapy of malignancies may cause problems ranging from minor pain and inflammation to full-thickness sloughing of skin necessitating skin grafting.

Catheter-over-needle assemblies are now in common use and provide stable, reliable access in comparison to the steel needles they replaced. Microparticulate matter in intravenous solutions is removed by in-line micropore filters.

### Flow Rates

Infusion rate is a crucial issue in resuscitation of patients with severe hypovolemia or progressive hemorrhage. It is therefore useful to recall that fluid in a medical catheter behaves for practical purposes according to Poiseuille's law:

$$\text{Rate of flow} = \frac{\Pi \times (\text{catheter radius})^4 \times \text{pressure gradient}}{8 \times \text{dynamic fluid viscosity}}$$

The fact that flow is a function of the fourth power of the radius of the tube lumen means that the internal catheter diameter is a major limiting factor. It is important to take into account that a fluid delivery system is only as effective as its slowest component, whether this is intravenous tubing, in-line filters, or the catheter itself. Flow rates may also be affected by pressure and viscosity, the latter being an especially important consideration in relation to red blood cell transfusion. Rate of infusion is also directly proportional to catheter length, which is why a long central catheter will have a slower infusion rate than a shorter catheter of the same caliber in a peripheral vein.

Placement of two large-bore—16-gauge or greater—catheters is indicated in stable trauma patients whose injuries could cause potentially life-threatening hemorrhage or for initial therapy of medical patients with hypovolemic shock. Management of exsanguination with an 8.5F catheter with a manually operated pressure bag or a wall-mounted external pneumatic device delivers almost a liter of crystalloid per minute. A single catheter of this type is adequate for preoperative care of almost all surgically remediable injuries. Rapid infusion of larger volumes of fluid should be attended by careful monitoring for clinical signs of volume overload, especially in older patients and those with cardiovascular disease.

Volume repletion and central venous pressure measurement can be accomplished by a Y-arm catheter sheath passed percutaneously into the femoral vein. An 8.5F catheter can then be used for volume repletion, while a smaller catheter can simultaneously be inserted through the diaphragm into the right atrium for central venous pressure measurement. Femoral catheters should be left in place no longer than 48 h, since iliofemoral thrombophlebitis can result. However, with sterile technique and the use of Silastic catheters, the deep femoral system may be safely employed for a longer duration.

Pressure infusion increases flow two to three times over gravity and is superior to on-line hand-pumped bulbs. Pressure devices are available for administration of packed red blood cells. Use of a standard urologic Y irrigation set augments flow rates by reducing resistance in the tubing leading to the catheter site. For maximum infusion rates of either blood or crystalloid, use of blood administration set tubing eliminates on-line micropore filters, stopcocks, and one-way valves, which increase resistance. Addition of saline to packed red blood cell infusions decreases viscosity, increasing the speed of transfusion.

Volume repletion is effective through intravenous catheters placed distal to an inflated military antishock trouser (MAST) suit. In patients with abdominal hemorrhage, lines in the legs, as well as those in the arms, augment volume.

Warming crystalloid and blood before infusion is essential when volume resuscitation is massive. Crystalloid may be stored in a heating bath or oven, may be safely microwaved, or may be warmed with a heating coil or heat packs. Blood warming coils that allow transfusion rates of up to 500 mL/min are now available. Alternatively, cold-packed red blood cells may be warmed by diluting with an equal amount of warmed saline (up to 60°C); this will also decrease viscosity and thus enhance rate of administration. Significant hemolysis occurs with microwaving of blood but not with hot saline mixing.

## CENTRAL VENOUS PRESSURE CATHETERIZATION AND MONITORING

Central venous catheterization should be performed (1) when rapid delivery of cardiac medications to the coronary circulation is required during CPR, (2) for access when peripheral veins are inadequate, and (3) when central venous pressure measurement is desired. Determination of central venous pressure is indicated (1) when massive volume repletion is administered to elderly patients or those with heart disease, (2) when monitoring fluid administration in patients with visceral trauma and severe head injuries, and (3) when pericardial tamponade is suspected.

## Sites and Techniques for Central Venous Pressure Catheter Insertion

### Peripheral Sites

Use of peripheral veins to access the central circulation and measure central venous pressure has the indisputable advantage of avoiding the risk associated with direct puncture of the subclavian and internal jugular veins. However, low flow is inevitable, due to the long course of the catheter from extremity to superior vena cava. Peripheral sites also fail frequently due to catheter malposition and kinking. In the arm the brachial-basilic system must be used, since catheters in the cephalic system often become kinked in the plexus of veins at the shoulder. Smooth passage and correct tip positioning are more likely if the patient is sitting with his or her head angulated sharply toward the catheterized arm, the arm is held abducted, and the catheter is wire-guided. In emergency situations, however, this time-consuming approach to the central circulation is often impractical.

The external jugular vein provides ready central access, since J-wire-guided catheters pass in 75 to 90 percent of cases. Success is enhanced by introducing the wire through a 16-gauge catheter rather than through a needle; using a J-tip with no greater than a 3-mm radius; exaggerating head tilt with marked traction on the skin of the neck; and, when initial attempts with wire-through-needle techniques are met with resistance at the level of the clavicle, twisting the tip of the J wire 180° before making a second attempt.

The femoral vein can also provide central access, as mentioned above.

### Central Venous Puncture

#### Anatomy

A brief review of anatomy is warranted (Fig. 12-3). The major veins of the upper thorax are deeply and centrally placed and well protected

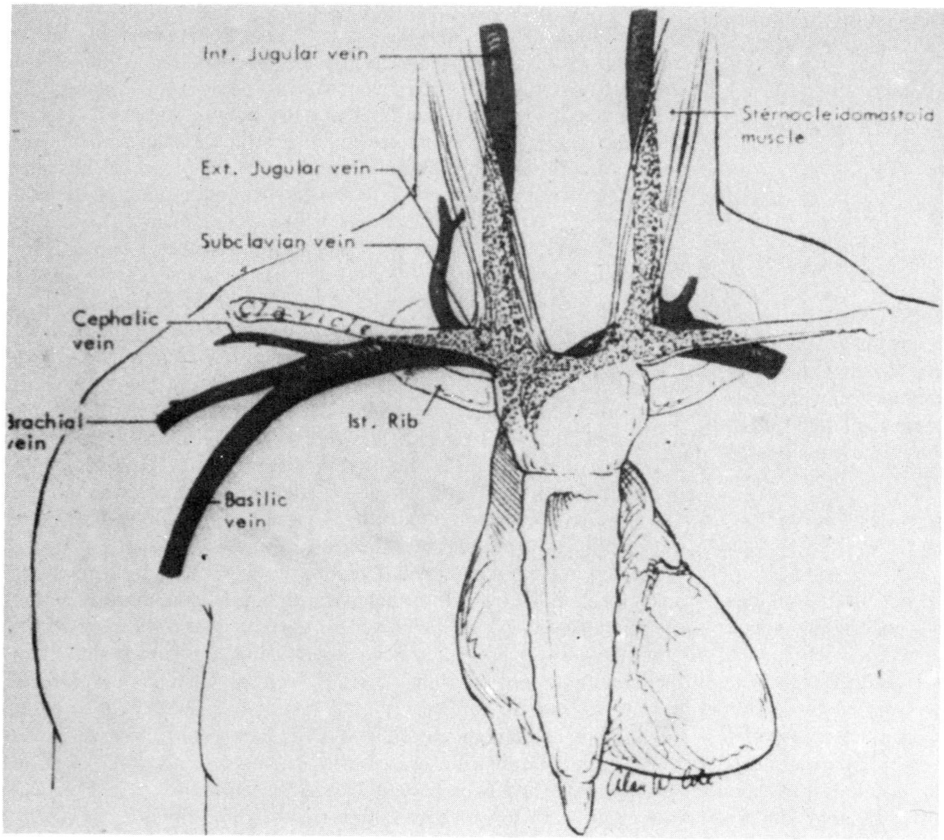

**Fig. 12-3.** Relationships of major torso veins to other anatomy.

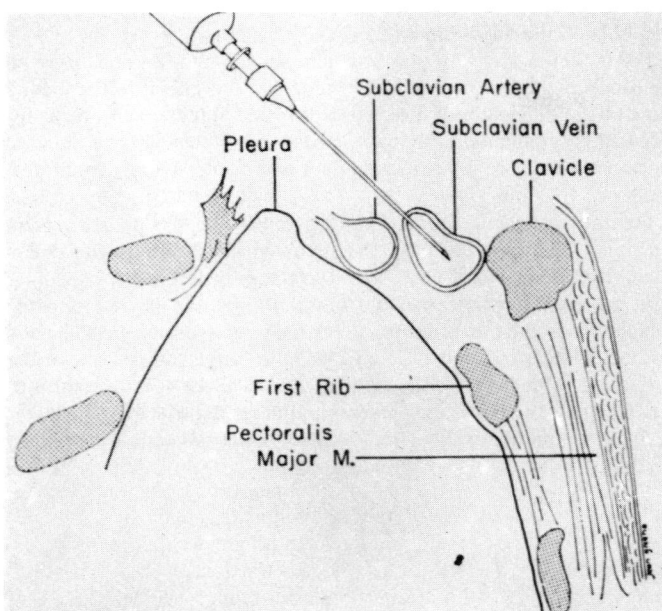

**Fig. 12-4.** Coronal section through midclavicle.

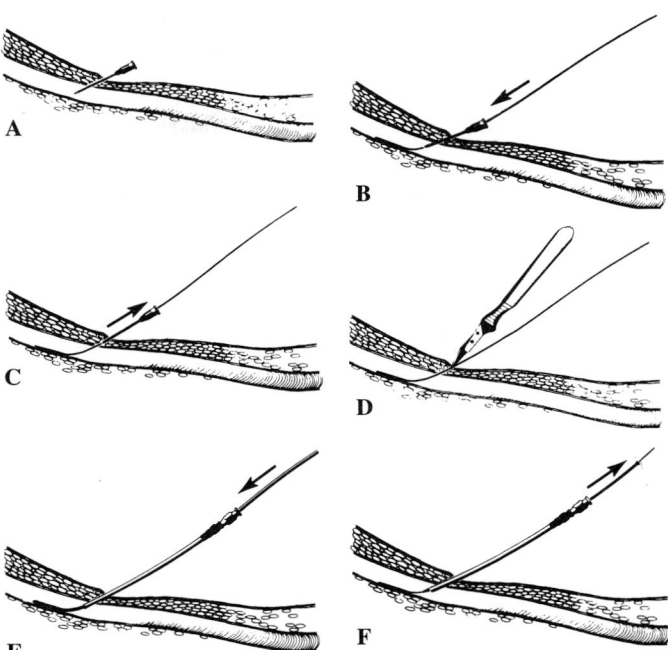

**Fig. 12-5.** Seldinger technique of catheter insertion (wire-guided). (From Conahan TJ III, Schwartz AJ, Geer RT: Percutaneous catheter introduction: The Seldinger technique. *JAMA* 237:446, 1977. Used with permission.)

by the clavicles, sternum, and strap muscles. The internal jugular veins join the subclavian veins to form the brachiocephalics (innominates), which in turn join to become the superior vena cava. The sternocleidomastoid muscle attaches separately by two heads to the sternum and clavicle; the triangle formed by these two heads and the clavicle is just above the internal jugular vein. The right internal jugular has a straight path into the superior vena cava, whereas all the other major tributaries curve. Both external jugular veins enter the subclavian veins at close to right angles. The subclavian veins lie immediately posterior to the junction of the medial and middle third of the clavicle and are anterior and inferior to the artery; the pleura are immediately posterior and inferior to the subclavian vessels (Fig. 12-4). The internal jugular vein usually lies anterolateral to the carotid.

## Equipment

Catheter-through-needle devices, whose large 14-gauge insertion needles are prone to complications and whose 16-gauge catheters allow maximum gravity-assisted flow of 100 to 150 mL/min, have been largely supplanted by wire-guided (Seldinger) catheters. Their use allows use of a small needle to place any size catheter into a vessel. An 18-gauge needle is inserted into the vein (Fig. 12-5A), a flexible wire is passed (Fig. 12-5B), and the needle is removed (Fig. 12-5C), leaving just the wire in the vein. The catheter is threaded over the wire and into the vein with a twisting motion (Fig. 12-5E). The wire is then removed, leaving only the catheter in place. If a large-bore catheter is necessary, the apparatus is used with a venodilator, which necessitates a stab for smooth skin penetration (Fig. 12-5D). In this situation the venodilator is removed with the wire, leaving the large-bore 8.5F catheter sheath in place (Fig. 12-5F).

The principal advantages of wire-guided catheters are (1) use of a small (and thus safer) needle for insertion; (2) the step-up capability with a venodilator, allowing for higher flow rates often required in trauma resuscitation; (3) the flexibility of exchanging standard intravenous catheters, central venous catheters, and Swan-Ganz catheters without repeated stabs; and (4) the use of J wires to access the central circulation from the external jugular vein.

Recent work has shown that success at internal jugular venous catheterization may be enhanced by use of a two-dimensional ultrasound. Visualization of the vein while attempting puncture reduces the number of punctures necessary for cannulation and may reduce the incidence of complications.

## Preparation—General Aspects

Before central catheterization is implemented, the physician should consider whether the situation actually requires central venous access. Many patients who require volume resuscitation can be managed with large-bore peripheral lines.

All equipment should be at the bedside, including a central venous pressure manometer. The patient should be placed in the Trendelenburg position, and the entire route of the neck should be prepped so that all three approaches are possible in case the primary approach fails. The right side is preferred over the left, since (1) the lung apex is slightly lower, (2) there is a straight relationship between the right internal jugular vein and the superior vena cava, and (3) the left-sided thoracic duct cannot be injured. With unilateral chest trauma, the attempt should be on the injured side in order to protect the uninjured hemithorax in the event of complications from the procedure. A local anesthetic should be employed in conscious patients when time permits.

After landmarks are identified (Fig. 12-6), a 5- or 10-mL syringe attached to a hollow-bore needle appropriate to the size of the guidewire should be inserted. Gentle, continuous negative pressure on the syringe should be maintained. When free flow of blood is obtained, the syringe is removed and a fingertip used to occlude the hub before wire insertion. When the catheter has been advanced over the wire to the proper depth and the wire is removed, the catheter should be sutured to the chest wall, povidone-iodine ointment placed at the needle puncture site, and a surgical dressing applied. If one approach fails, another should be performed on the same side, since a contralateral attempt could result in iatrogenic bilateral pneumothorax. A chest film should be performed immediately to verify correct catheter position and to rule out complications from the procedure.

## Technique of Commonly Utilized Approaches

The internal jugular and subclavian veins may be reliably cannulated by any of several tested approaches (Fig. 12-7A–C). Emergency

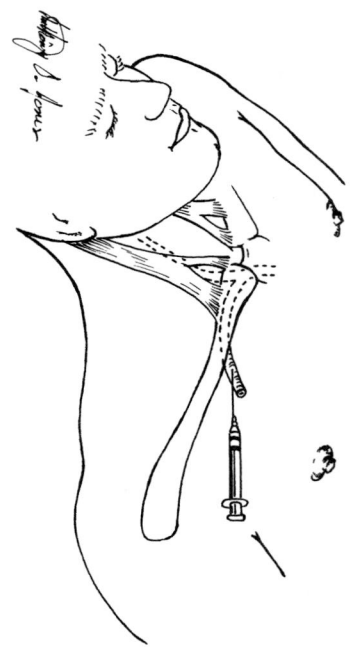

**Fig. 12-6.** Infraclavicular subclavian venipuncture.

physicians should become adept with at least two and adopt these for use as primary and backup methods. When the procedure is performed electively, preceding the approach for catheter placement with a 22-gauge needle attached to a 5- or 10-mL syringe filled with lidocaine facilitates local anesthesia and allows the operator to locate the vein.

In the *anterior approach* to the internal jugular vein, the needle should puncture the skin at the apex of a triangle formed by the tendinous and muscular heads of the sternocleidomastoid muscle. Held at a 60° angle with the plane of the skin, the needle is directed slightly lateral to the axis of the body. Blood return should be obtained within 3 cm, since the vein is very superficial here.

In the *lateral* or *posterior approach,* the head is turned slightly away from the selected side, and the needle is inserted at the posterior margin of the sternocleidomastoid muscle two to three fingerbreadths

above the clavicle and directed toward the suprasternal notch. Blood should be aspirated within 4 to 5 cm.

For the *infraclavicular subclavian approach,* the needle is inserted beneath the clavicle medial to the midpoint and lateral to the medial third of the clavicle and directed toward the suprasternal notch. Inferomedial orientation of the needle bevel facilitates entry of the wire or catheter into the brachiocephalic vein. Vessel entry occurs at a depth of 3 to 4 cm.

For the *supraclavicular subclavian approach,* the patient's head is turned slightly away from the involved side. The needle enters just above the clavicle, 1 cm lateral to the insertion of the clavicular head of the sternocleidomastoid muscle and 1 cm posterior to the clavicle. It is then directed to bisect the angle formed between the sternocleidomastoid and the clavicle, at an angle of 10° above the horizontal, with the tip pointing just caudad to the contralateral nipple. Keeping the bevel up prevents trapping of the wire or catheter against the inferior wall of the vessel. Vessel puncture occurs at a depth of 2 to 3 cm.

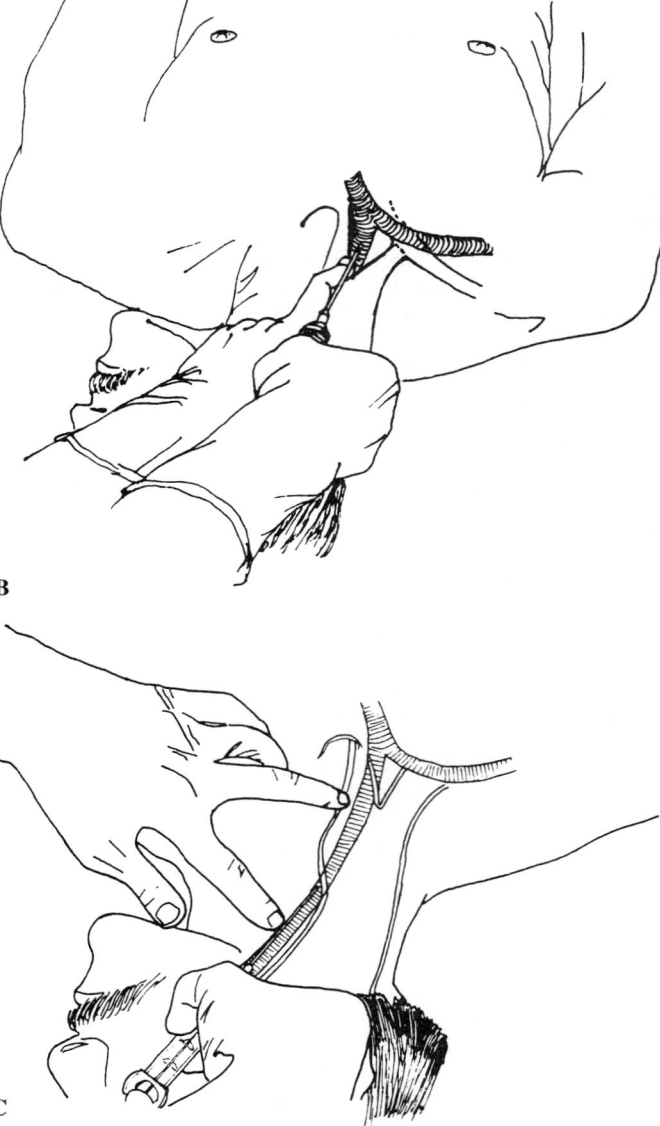

**B**

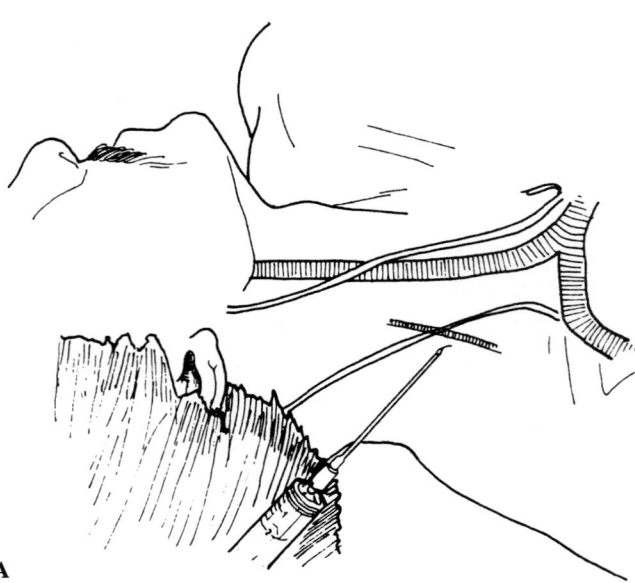

**A**

**C**

**Fig. 12-7. A.** Posterior approach for internal jugular venipuncture. **B.** Central approach. **C.** Anterior approach. (From *Textbook of Advanced Cardiac Life Support,* 2d ed. Dallas, American Heart Association, 1990, pp 149–150. Used with permission.)

## Central Venous Pressure Measurement

Central venous pressure measurement is useful mainly in assessing volume status in the acutely ill or injured patient but may also assist in the diagnosis of specific disease processes and complications. It is the product of complex interactions among (1) circulating blood volume, (2) right ventricular function, (3) intrathoracic pressure, and (4) total systemic venous resistance. Absolute measurements of central venous pressure should be evaluated in light of the presence of right- or left-sided heart disease, which produces stable and chronic elevations. A low value in a patient with heart disease usually indicates volume depletion; however, hypovolemia should still be considered when the initial measurement is high and other signs are suggestive. A fluid challenge may be attempted, with a rising central venous pressure often indicating volume overload. Thus, (1) changes in central venous pressure over time are often more helpful than a single measurement, and (2) when heart disease is present it is especially important to evaluate central venous pressure in the context of other signs of volume status.

In patients who are healthy aside from acute trauma, a low value usually reflects hypovolemia, while a high value must be presumed to indicate a specific disease process or complication—such as pericardial tamponade or tension pneumothorax—or an error in measurement. Taking these considerations into account and keeping in mind that some controversy exists, the following may be referred to for use in clinical practice:

Low: <5 cmH$_2$O
Normal: 5 to 12 cmH$_2$O
High: >12 cmH$_2$O

In addition to heart failure, pericardial tamponade, and tension pneumothorax, abnormally high central venous pressure may also be caused by pulmonary embolism, superior vena cava obstruction, or MAST suit inflation. With an initial central venous pressure reading greater than 15 cmH$_2$O, fluid challenge is seldom warranted. Potentially confounding sources of high values include the Valsalva maneuver by the patient; positive-pressure ventilation; measurement in the Trendelenburg position; an external zero point reference too low on the chest wall; a catheter tip that is outside the thorax (e.g., in the internal jugular, axillary vein); a catheter that is kinked or partially occluded by the vein wall; a catheter that has crossed the tricuspid valve and is in the right ventricle; and a stopcock that is open to IV fluid rather than the patient.

A low central venous pressure is generally due to low circulating blood volume or decreased splanchnic venous tone (e.g., anaphylaxis, spinal shock, fear, or pain). Falsely positive low measurements are secondary to having the patient in a thorax-elevated position or having the external zero reference point too high on the chest wall.

### Method of Measurement

To determine central venous pressure, the point of reference equivalent to the right atrium—the "zero point"—must be found and marked on the patient's chest wall. Although some disagreement exists on what landmark is ideal, the midaxillary line at the level of the fourth costochondral junction is frequently recommended. The manometer is filled to 20 to 25 cm with fluid by opening the three-way stopcock to the IV line leading to the source of IV solution. Then, with the patient level, supine, and breathing freely, the stopcock is opened to the patient so that fluid from the manometer runs into the patient until a steady state is reached. With the zero of the manometer at the zero reference point on the chest wall, the meniscus at end expiration gives the correct reading.

### Complications

The three most common serious complications of central vein puncture are pneumothorax, arterial puncture, and local infection. With subclavian puncture the incidence of pneumothorax is 2 to 4 percent, significantly greater than with either internal jugular approach. The incidence of arterial puncture—3 to 7 percent—is similar for all approaches. Other, less common complications include hydrothorax, hydromediastinum, air or catheter embolisms, thrombosis, arrhythmias, nerve injuries, osteomyelitis of the clavicle, catheter tip perforation of the superior vena cava (causing hydromediastinum or hydrothorax) or right atrium (causing hydropericardium), knotting with other catheters, and puncture of endotracheal tube cuffs. Care in executing the procedure and in selection of patients who will benefit from central venous catheterization will minimize occurrence of complications.

## VENOUS CUTDOWN

When percutaneous venous puncture is unsuccessful, cutdown is indicated (Fig. 12-8). The basilic vein in the antecubital fossa and the saphenous vein in the leg are most commonly utilized. The basilic vein is located two fingerbreadths above and two fingerbreadths medial to the olecranon. The saphenous vein is just anterior to the malleolus at the ankle and is also accessible in the proximal thigh three fingerbreadths below the midpoint of the inguinal ligament. Although experienced operators may be able to complete the procedure in less than a minute, in most situations 5 or 6 min is required. This means that this mode of venous access is indicated only when percutaneous access has failed or is obviously not available.

### Technique

Prep and anesthetize the skin. Make a transverse skin incision, and by blunt dissection separate the subcutaneous tissue until the vein is exposed. To avoid cannulating the artery, identify the artery and the vein before ligating or nicking a vessel. This is done by slipping a forceps or hemostat under the vessels and applying pressure; pulsatile flow will be evident in the artery. In patients with shock, this maneuver may be unsuccessful. After freeing the vein from the surrounding tissues, pass two separate sutures beneath the vein, one proximal and one distal. Leave the proximal suture untied. Tie the distal suture to occlude the vein but keep the ends of the suture long so that they can be used for applying traction to the vein. Make a nick in the vein between the proximal and distal suture. While applying traction on the vein, insert the catheter into the vein. Tie the proximal suture to secure the catheter in the vein. Suture the cutaneous incision. Care must be exercised throughout the procedure, since poor technique can result in tendon or nerve injury or extensive hemorrhage from soft tissue.

## INTRAOSSEOUS INFUSION

Obtaining vascular access in a very young child who is critically ill or injured is one of the most potentially frustrating situations an emergency physician may confront. Although peripheral venous access is fastest, in many cases it is unsuccessful. Intraosseous infusion has a very high rate of success and is faster than both cutdown and central venous catheterization in most situations.

The bone is supplied by a nutrient artery that pierces the cortex and bifurcates into ascending and descending branches, which further divide into arterioles that pierce the endosteal surface to become capillaries. The capillaries drain into medullary venous sinusoids within the medullary space, which then drain into a central venous channel. Catheter placement in the sinusoids results in ready access to the venous circulation, which studies have shown compares favorably in drug delivery to the central circulation in comparison to peripheral venous access.

### Technique

Either standard bone marrow aspiration needles or specialized intraosseous infusion needles must be used, as standard intravenous

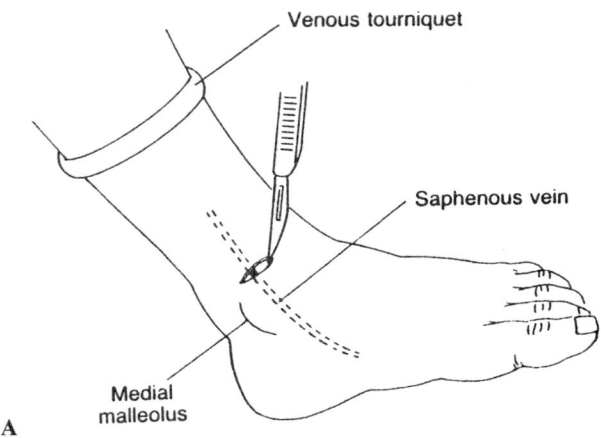

**A**

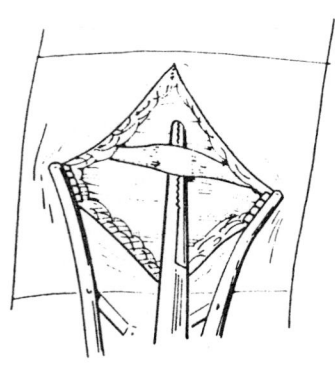

**B**

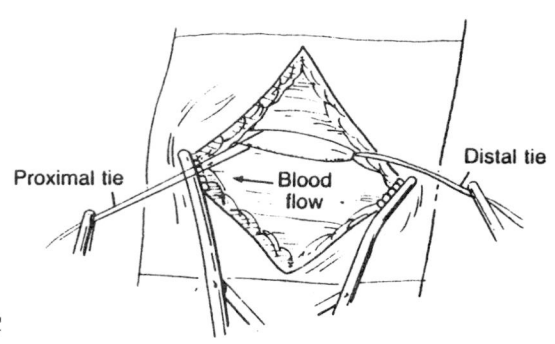

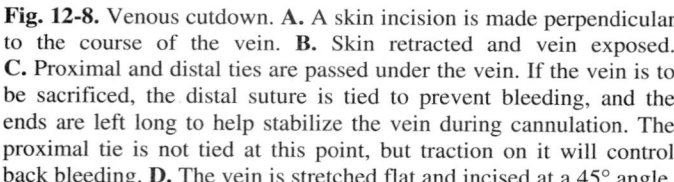

**C**

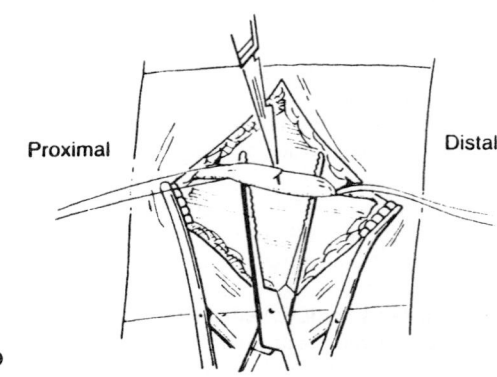

**D**

**Fig. 12-8.** Venous cutdown. **A.** A skin incision is made perpendicular to the course of the vein. **B.** Skin retracted and vein exposed. **C.** Proximal and distal ties are passed under the vein. If the vein is to be sacrificed, the distal suture is tied to prevent bleeding, and the ends are left long to help stabilize the vein during cannulation. The proximal tie is not tied at this point, but traction on it will control back bleeding. **D.** The vein is stretched flat and incised at a 45° angle.

Approximately one-third of the lumen must be exposed. Traction on the proximal tie will control back bleeding. (From Roberts JR, Hedges JR: *Clinical Procedures in Emergency Medicine,* 2d ed. Philadelphia, Saunders, 1991, p 321. Used with permission. Parts B and C first appeared in Vander Salm TJ et al: *Atlas of Bedside Procedures.* Boston, Little, Brown, 1979.)

stylets and spinal needles are likely to bend during the procedure (Chap. 18). The proximal tibia is generally considered the preferred site, but distal tibia and distal femur have also been employed. For the proximal tibia the puncture site is 1 or 2 cm distal to the midpoint between the tibial tuberosity and the medial aspect of the tibia; for the distal tibia it is the medial surface of the ankle just proximal to the medial malleolus; and for the distal femur it is the dorsal surface at the point where the condyles join the shaft of the bone.

After prepping and anesthetizing skin and periosteum if the patient is conscious, the needle is inserted with the point directed away from the joint space, distally if the site is the proximal tibia, proximally at the other two sites. The needle is grasped in the palm of the hand and directed into the bone using a twisting motion to break through the cortex. Once this has occurred, resistance decreases and crepitus is encountered as the needle enters the marrow cavity. The stylet is then removed, and aspiration with a syringe performed to obtain blood and marrow for confirmation of positioning. If shock is present, aspiration may be unsuccessful; in this situation cautious infusion of several milliliters of saline should be attempted with careful observation for extravasation. If there is none, then the needle may be assumed to be positioned in the marrow cavity.

## Complications

Infection is a major concern, but with an incidence of less than 1 percent—including both localized cellulitis and osteomyelitis—

this problem is no greater than with other modes of venous access. Infections can be avoided by limiting the duration of intraosseous infusions and in any case usually respond satisfactorily to antibiotics.

Injury of the growth plate has also been discussed as a possible complication, but there are no reports of serious morbidity arising from an injury to developing bone. Fat embolism is rare and only reported in adult patients. Tibial fractures have been reported, necessitating postprocedure x-rays when intraosseous infusion has been attempted.

## ARTERIAL CANNULATION

Arterial cannulation is indicated when arterial pressure monitoring or repeated arterial blood sampling is required, as in hypertensive crisis, cardiogenic shock treated with pressor and/or inotropic therapy, and respiratory failure. Although the radial artery is the most frequently employed site, the brachial, femoral, and dorsalis pedis arteries have also been employed in large series with little variation in occurrence of complications. In infants and neonates, the temporal or umbilical artery is often used, although radial artery cannulation is also safe in these patients. While many operators are most familiar with the radial artery site, use of the femoral artery leaves the arm clear for other procedures and in the presence of shock is less difficult to cannulate percutaneously.

## Assessment and Complications

Although catheterization of the radial artery is associated with up to a 20 percent incidence of temporary flow obstruction by Doppler study, permanent ischemic complications requiring surgical reanastomosis or amputation are quite rare. Confirmation of collateral flow through a patent ulnar artery can be obtained by performing the Allen test: while the patient clenches the wrist for 1 min, the examiner compresses the radial and ulnar vessels with thumb and forefinger. On release of ulnar compression, the patient partially extends the fingers, which are observed for rubor accentuated in comparison to the untested side. Patent ulnar circulation is indicated by return of rubor within 7 s, an equivocal result is 7 to 14 s, and longer than 14 s is considered definitely abnormal. If ulnar cannulation is contemplated, patency of the radial artery can be tested by the same test, with release of that vessel following compression.

Percutaneous cannulation of the brachial or femoral arteries may be possible when the radial pulse is absent in a hypotensive patient. The technique is similar to radial artery cannulation, although a careful groin prep, preceded by removal of hair at that site to minimize the risk of infection, is necessary.

With profound hypotension, cutdown to the radial artery may be required to cannulate the artery. This is performed through a transverse incision, with the artery punctured utilizing a technique identical to the percutaneous approach, only under direct vision. The wound should be sutured, and the catheter affixed with a silk suture.

Serious complications—infection and occlusion—are most closely related to duration of cannulation and are much more common among critically ill patients than among those undergoing monitoring as an adjunct to a surgical procedure. During a typical intensive care unit stay, the incidence of local infection can be expected to approach 20 percent, while that of generalized sepsis from primary catheter infection is 4 percent, with little site-dependent variation. Other complications include hematoma formation and hemorrhage requiring transfusion.

## Technique

The patient's nondominant extremity should be selected for radial artery cannulation. The wrist is placed in mild extension by placing a roll of gauze behind it and taping it to a splint. A sterile prep is applied and the operative area draped. Local infiltration should be performed with a small amount of lidocaine so that the pulse is not obscured. While a 20- or 22-gauge 1.25-in Teflon catheter over a needle is held in one hand, the radial pulse is palpated with the other. The skin over the radial aspect of the wrist is punctured with the needle pointing proximally and at a 45° angle with the plane of the skin. The needle is advanced into the artery until pulsations appear. The catheter is then slid off the needle into the artery. If pulsatile flow ceases, the catheter may be withdrawn until arterial flow again appears, and a second attempt may be made to advance the catheter. If this is unsuccessful, the procedure needs to be repeated. After each attempt, care should be taken to apply pressure to the site long enough to prevent hematoma formation. Once in the artery, the catheter is connected to the monitoring system and flushed through a three-way stopcock with a sterile cap. The catheter should then be secured to the skin at its hub using silk or nylon suture. Kits are available for wire-guided arterial catheterization.

If cutdown is necessary to achieve arterial puncture, exposure of the artery is performed in a manner similar to that outlined above for venous cutdown. When 1 cm of artery is visible, the vessel is isolated by passing two lengths of silk suture beneath it using a hemostat. A catheter-through-needle device is passed through the skin distal to the area of exposure and advanced into the site. The artery may then be punctured and the catheter advanced. The sutures, which are only used to control the artery, may then be removed and the skin incision closed.

## BIBLIOGRAPHY

Allen EV: Thromboangiitis obliterans: Methods of diagnosis of chronic occlusive arterial lesions distal to the wrist with illustrative cases. *Am J Med Sci* 178:237, 1929.

Dailey RH: Use of wire-guided catheters in the emergency department. *Ann Emerg Med* 12:489, 1983.

Dailey RH: External jugular vein cannulation and its use for CVP monitoring. *Emerg Med* 6:133, 1988.

Dronen SC, Yee AS, Tomlanovich MC: Proximal saphenous vein cutdown. *Ann Emerg Med* 10:328, 1981.

Dula DJ, Muller HA, Donovan JW: Flow rate variance of commonly used IV infusion techniques. *J Trauma* 21:480, 1981.

Dutky PA, Stevens SL, Maull KI: Factors affecting rapid fluid resuscitation with large bore intravenous catheters. *J Trauma* 29:856, 1989.

Gong V: Microwave warming of IV fluids in management of hypothermia. *Ann Emerg Med* 13:645, 1984.

Gurman GM, Kriemerman S: Cannulation of big arteries in critically ill patients. *Crit Care Med* 13:217, 1985.

Hedges JR, Barsan WB, Doan LA, et al: Central versus peripheral intravenous routes in cardiopulmonary resuscitation. *Am J Emerg Med* 2:385, 1984.

Iverson KV, Reeter AK, Criss E: Comparison of flow rates for standard and large-bore blood tubing. *West J Med* 143:183, 1985.

Iverson KV, Reeter A, Woods W, et al: Pressurization of IV bags: A new configuration and evaluation for use. *West J Med* 3:89, 1985.

Koski EMJ, Suhonen M, Mattila MAK: Ultra-sound-facilitated central venous cannulation. *Crit Care Med* 20:424, 1992.

Kramer DA, Staten-McCormick M, Freeman SB: Percutaneous brachial vein catheterization: An alternate site for IV access. *Ann Emerg Med* 12:238, 1983.

Mandel MA, Dauchot PJ: Radial artery cannulation in 1,000 patients: Precautions and complications. *J Hand Surg* 6:482, 1977.

Mangiante EC, Hoots AV, Fabian TC: The percutaneous common femoral vein catheter for volume replacement in critically ill patients. *J Trauma* 28:1644, 1988.

Nadeau S, Tousignant M: Use of urologic set for improved fluid administration rates. *Can Anaesth Soc J* 32:283, 1985.

Posner MC, Moore EE, Greenholz SK: Natural history of untreated inferior vena cava injury and assessment of venous access. *J Trauma* 26:698, 1986.

Rosetti VA, Thompson BM, Miller J, et al: Intraosseous infusion: An alternative route of pediatric intravascular access. *Ann Emerg Med* 14:885, 1985.

Snazajder JI, Zveibil FR, Bitterman H, et al: Central vein catheterization: Failure and complication rates by three percutaneous approaches. *Arch Intern Med* 146:259, 1986.

Tucker JF, Danzl DF, Teague E, et al: Infusion of intravenous fluids distal to pneumatic antishock trousers. *J Emerg Med* 2:79, 1984.

Wilkins RG: Radial artery cannulation and ischaemic damage: A review. *Anaesthesia* 40:896, 1985.

Youngberg JA, Miller ED: Evaluation of percutaneous cannulations of the dorsalis pedis artery. *Anesthesiology* 44:80, 1976.

# 13

# INVASIVE MONITORING AND PACING TECHNIQUES

## Scott Syverud
## C. Thomas Carter

Invasive pressure monitoring is gradually being introduced in emergency department resuscitation. Emergency physicians must have a familiarity with pacing techniques in order to treat the unstable patient with bradycardia. This chapter reviews the basics of these techniques as applied in emergency care.

## INVASIVE MONITORING TECHNIQUES

### General Considerations

Invasive pressure monitoring should never be the initial step in resuscitation. Airway assessment and stabilization and circulatory support clearly take priority. Early arterial line placement is appropriate when clinically indicated and when initial stabilization is completed. Continuous monitoring of arterial pressure is particularly helpful in pro-

longed emergency department resuscitations and in patients who require frequent adjustments in vasoactive infusions for circulatory support (i.e., hypertensive crisis, cardiogenic shock, hypothermic cardiac arrest). The arterial line also provides easy access for frequent sampling of blood gases to aid in ventilator management.

The placement of a pulmonary artery thermodilution catheter (PATC) is helpful in the diagnosis and management of a variety of critical illnesses. If possible, this procedure should be deferred until the patient reaches the more controlled and sterile environment of the intensive care unit. In many cases there may be a significant delay before a patient can be moved to intensive care or until a consultant reaches the hospital. When resuscitation management is critically dependent on hemodynamic monitoring, it may be helpful to place a PATC in the emergency department after initial resuscitation. Potential candidates include hypotensive patients with acute myocardial infarction and patients in shock, especially those with cardiopulmonary or renal disease. In such patients the information obtained with the PATC may significantly alter the physician's approach to fluid and pressor therapy.

The two essential components of any pressure monitoring system are a properly placed catheter and a functioning pressure transducer/monitor. Failure of either of these components wastes valuable time during resuscitation. Ideally, the transducer and line for pressure monitoring should be set up and ready for use prior to the patient's arrival in the emergency department. Examples of transducer systems are illustrated in Fig. 13-1. The most common error made during the

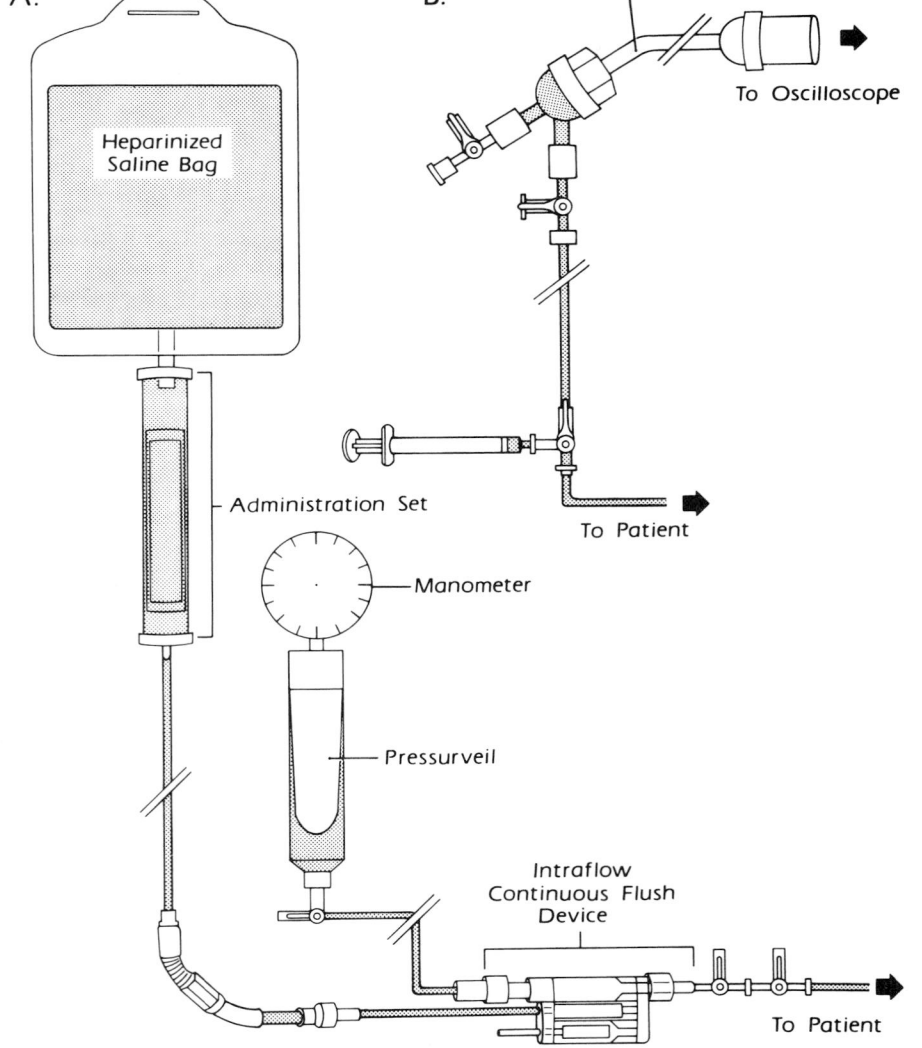

**Fig. 13-1.** Arterial pressure monitoring systems. **A.** System for continuous flush with heparinized saline connected to a mechanical pressure transducer. **B.** System for manual flush. Either system can be used with an electronic pressure transducer shown in **B.** The pressure dome should be maintained at the level of the patient's heart. (From Beal JM (ed): *Critical Care for Surgical Patients.* New York, Macmillan, 1982. Used by permission.)

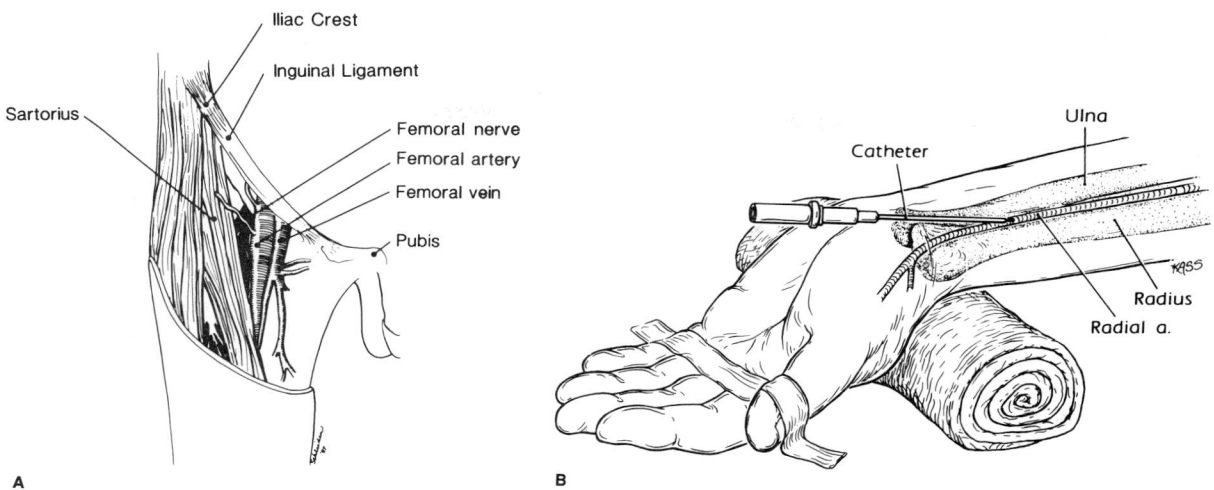

**Fig. 13-2.** Anatomic landmarks for arterial line placement. **A.** Femoral triangle. Note that the femoral artery lies lateral to the vein and midway between the pubis and the iliac crest. **B.** Radial aspect of the wrist. Note that mild extension of the wrist will aid successful placement. (From Beal JM (ed): *Critical Care for Surgical patients.* New York, Macmillan, 1982. Used by permission.)

initiation of invasive monitoring is to focus on the procedure and forget about the patient until the procedure is completed. With an unstable patient, the physician must be constantly aware of the patient's status and be ready to discontinue the procedure as circumstances dictate.

## Arterial Cannulation

Arterial lines offer several advantages over monitoring of blood pressure with an arm cuff. The line provides continuous measurement of blood pressure and can be used for easy sequential sampling of blood gases. In the setting of marked vasoconstriction or hypotension, the arterial line usually gives more accurate pressure readings than a blood pressure cuff. The radial and femoral arteries are readily accessible to rapid cannulation. Percutaneous puncture is preferred. In hypotensive patients it may be easier to cannulate the femoral artery (larger vessel, constant landmarks) than the radial artery. Cutdown on the radial artery is an alternative in such patients. Allen's test for ulnar artery patency should always be performed prior to radial arterial line placement. If the ulnar artery is occluded, a different site should be used.

Landmarks for radial and femoral artery cannulation are shown in Fig. 13-2. The catheter (usually 20 gauge, 2 in long for radial cannulation and 18 gauge, 4 in long for femoral cannulation) can be introduced by direct puncture threaded over the needle or by Seldinger technique threaded over a guide wire. Free pulsatile flow of bright red blood indicates proper placement. With marked hypotension or hypoxia, correct placement may be mistaken for venous placement (nonpulsatile dark blood returned). In all cases, connection to the transducer should reveal an arterial waveform with proper arterial placement. Failure to visualize a waveform can be due to venous placement, air in the line, a closed stopcock, or a malfunction in the transducer or monitor.

Arterial line placement is a diagnostic aid, not a treatment modality. Therapeutic procedures or definitive care (i.e., airway management, transfer to the operating room) should not be delayed solely to allow arterial line placement. Local complications of line placement include local hematoma and hemorrhage; both can usually be controlled with a pressure dressing. Arterial occlusion, thrombosis, or embolization with distal ischemia may occur; they are associated with placement in smaller vessels or in atherosclerotic vessels, with prolonged catheterization, and with use of end arteries that supply areas with poor collateral circulation. These complications can be

minimized by using the femoral or radial site, by checking for ulnar artery patency before using the radial artery , and by removing the line as soon as feasible after the patient is stabilized.

Sepsis may result from local infection at the insertion site. This complication can be avoided by proper attention to sterile technique and by frequent dressing changes with immediate removal of the catheter if evidence of site infection is detected. Early replacement of lines placed in the emergency department during resuscitation is also a rational intensive care unit policy to minimize these complications.

## Pulmonary Artery Cannulation

Pulmonary artery cannulation offers several advantages over central venous pressure (CVP) monitoring (see Chap. 18, "Vascular Access"). When the balloon tip of a PATC is properly wedged in a branch of the pulmonary artery, the pressure sensed by the catheter tip is the same as that in the left atrium. Left atrial pressure (which equals left ventricular filling pressure) is an excellent indication of the adequacy of fluid resuscitation. If this pressure is low (less than 12 mm Hg), additional fluid resuscitation is indicated. If this pressure is high (greater than 20 mm Hg), additional fluids are unlikely to improve cardiac performance; vasopressors are probably indicated for circulatory support. Although the PATC can yield a vast amount of useful diagnostic information (Tables 13-1 and 13-2), this distinction between the need for more fluids or for more pressors is its most useful application during resuscitation. CVP monitoring is less reliable than PATC, especially in the presence of valvular or pulmonary disease.

The placement technique for PATCs is discussed at length in the chapter by Kaye in McIntyre's and Levis' text. Standard catheters have two lumens, a distal one which terminates at the tip of the catheter, and a proximal one which terminates 10 to 15 cm proximal

**Table 13-1.** Hemodynamic Diagnosis of Shock States.

| Type of Shock | CO | PAO | SVR |
|---|---|---|---|
| Cardiogenic | ↓ | ↑ | ↑ |
| Hypovolemic | ↓ | ↓ | ↑ |
| Septic | ↓ or ↑ | ↓ | ↓ |
| Neurogenic | ↑ | ↓ | ↓ |
| Anaphylactic | ↓ | ↓ | ↓ |

CO, cardiac output; PAO, pulmonary artery occlusion pressure; SVR, systemic vascular resistance; (↑) increased; (↓) decreased.

**Table 13-2.** Hemodynamic Subsets in Acute Myocardial Infarction.

| Cardiac | >2 | I | | II |
|---|---|---|---|---|
| Index | <2 | III | | IV |
| (L/min/m²) | | | | |
| | | <18 | PWP | >18 |

*Note:* Initial therapy and prognosis can be determined by class. Mortality by class is 1%, 11%, 18%, and 60% for classes I–IV, respectively. Patients in class I require supportive care only. Patients in class II require treatment for pulmonary edema to lower pulmonary artery occlusion pressure (PAO). Patients in class III may improve with fluid administration. Patients in class IV require maximal circulatory support for cardiogenic shock.

to the tip (Fig. 13-3). A small balloon at the tip of the catheter helps float the catheter through the heart and also occludes a branch of the pulmonary artery to allow pulmonary artery occlusion (PAO) pressure measurement. It is the PAO pressure which best reflects the pressure in the pulmonary capillary bed and the left atrium.

In addition to the two lumens and the balloon, the PATC has a temperature sensor just proximal to the balloon. This sensor allows continuous central temperature monitoring, and measurement of cardiac output, using the thermodilution technique. After central venous access is secured (see Chap. 12, "Venous and Arterial Access in Adults"), the catheter is advanced toward the heart through an introducer sheath. The pressure waveform sensed through the distal port changes as the catheter is advanced through the heart and is used to confirm proper placement in the pulmonary artery (Fig. 13-4). Fluoroscopy can also be used to place a PATC but is rarely available in the emergency setting.

Once a PATC is in position, the clinician can rapidly measure pulmonary artery pressure, PAO pressure, cardiac output (CO), and CVP. When combined with arterial pressure measurement, these parameters can be used to calculate systemic vascular resistance. These parameters are very useful in the diagnosis and treatment of various shock states and in determining therapy in acute myocardial infarction (Tables 13-1 and 13-2). With pericardial tamponade or tension pneumothorax, the right heart pressure waveforms flatten out until CVP, atrial, ventricular, and pulmonary artery pressures are almost the same.

As with arterial cannulation, therapeutic procedures or definitive care should not be delayed solely to allow PATC placement. Complications include all the complications of central venous line placement (Chap. 12). In addition, cardiac arrhythmias and right bundle branch block may occur as the catheter traverses the heart. Other potential complications include pulmonary embolism or infarction, knotting of

the catheter, infection, and rupture of a small branch of the pulmonary artery.

## EMERGENCY PACING TECHNIQUES

### General Considerations

There is a distinct difference between *urgent* and *emergency* pacemaker placement. Urgent pacing is required in patients who are clinically stable yet may decompensate or become unstable in the near future. Provision of a standby pacer in these potentially unstable patients can be made in the emergency department using noninvasive techniques (transcutaneous pacing). If time and the clinical condition of the patient permit, all invasive cardiac pacing should be attempted in a controlled environment and should be performed by the most experienced physician available. If the patient can be stabilized with noninvasive pacing or with drug therapy, it is advised that the standard pattern of referral and consultation be used. Emergency pacing is required in those unstable patients with cardiac arrest, hemodynamically unstable bradyarrhythmias, or recurrent malignant escape rhythms who require pacing immediately. These patients cannot await the arrival of a consultant.

Since it can be instituted quickly and noninvasively, transcutaneous pacing is the technique of choice for emergent pacing. Transvenous pacing should be used for urgent pacing or after stabilization with drugs or transcutaneous pacing. Electrodes and catheters for these techniques are illustrated in Fig. 13-5.

### Transcutaneous Pacing

Transcutaneous pacing uses externally applied electrodes to deliver an electric impulse directly across the intact chest wall to stimulate the myocardium. Recent studies have demonstrated improved survival in bradyasystolic arrest patients who received pacing within 5 min of arrest onset. This observation combined with its relative ease of application has led to the application of transcutaneous pacing in prehospital settings. This technique is useful for initial stabilization of the patient in the emergency department who requires emergency pacing while arrangements for transvenous pacemaker insertion are being made.

Transcutaneous pacers differ from standard pacers in several important ways. The pulse duration of the stimulating impulse is longer and the current output higher than for standard internal leads. Muscle contraction (usually the chest wall or diaphragm) is notable during pacing, especially at higher outputs. This results in a twitching or mild bucking activity that can make assessment of cardiac output by

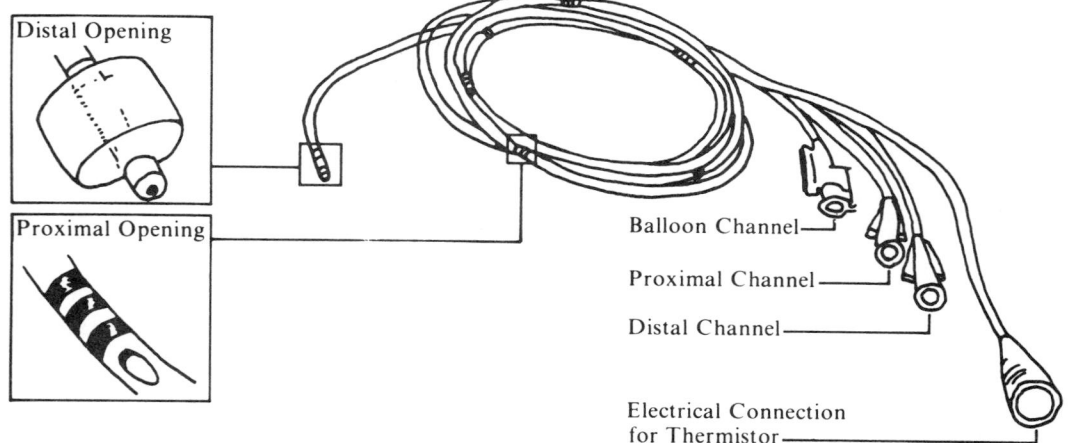

**Fig. 13-3.** Pulmonary artery thermodilution catheter (PATC). (From Beal JM (ed): *Critical Care for Surgical Patients.* New York, Macmillan, 1982. Used by permission.)

**Fig. 13-4.** Hemodynamic aspects of balloon catheter insertion into the pulmonary artery. (From Gottlieb AJ (ed): *The Whole Internist Catalog.* Philadelphia, Saunders, 1980. Used by permission.)

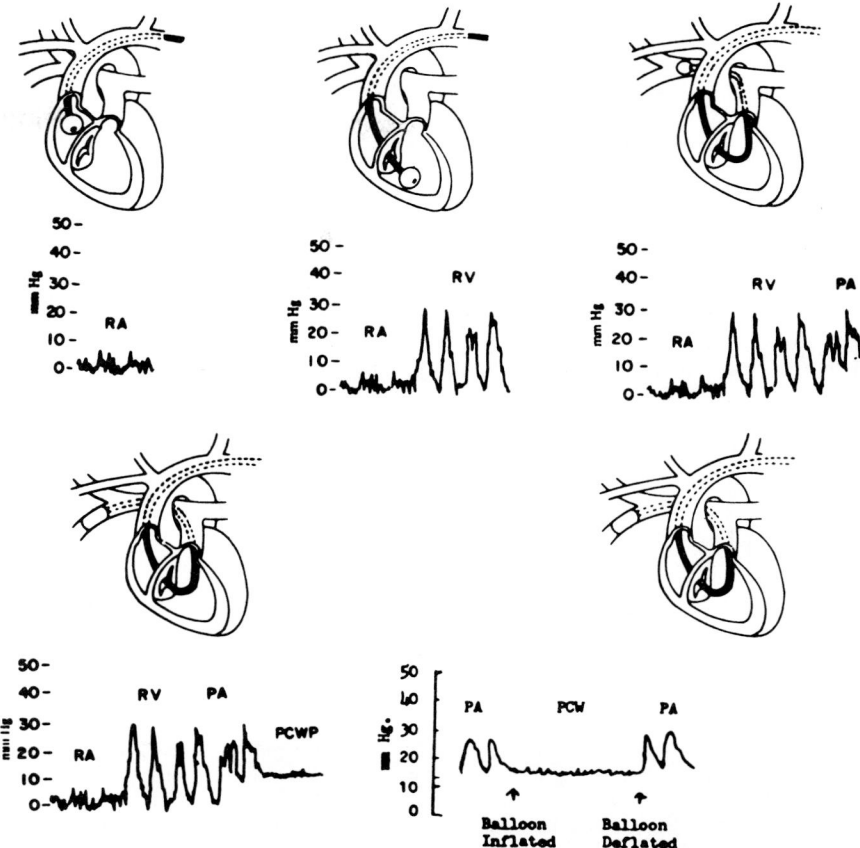

palpation of the radial, carotid, or femoral pulse unreliable during transcutaneous pacing. The higher current outputs used make cardiac monitoring with standard ECG monitors impossible due to interference from the large-amplitude pacing spike. Most transcutaneous pacing units come equipped with a monitor which automatically filters the pacing spike so that simultaneous monitoring is possible (Fig. 13-6).

The externally applied pacing electrodes are quickly and easily applied to the chest and back. There is little risk of electrical injury to health care providers during transcutaneous pacing. Chest compressions (CPR) can be administered directly over the insulated electrodes while pacing. Inadvertent contact with the active pacing surface results only in a mild shock. In the setting of bradyasystolic arrest, it is reasonable to turn the stimulating current to maximum output and then decrease the output if capture is achieved. In a patient with a hemodynamically compromising bradycardia (but not in cardiac arrest), the operator should slowly increase the output from the minimum setting until capture is achieved. Assessment of capture can be made by monitoring the electrocardiogram on the filtered monitor of the pacing unit. The hemodynamic response to pacing must also be assessed, either by blood pressure cuff or arterial catheter. Ideally, pacing should be continued at 1.25 times the threshold of initial electrical capture.

Failure to capture with transcutaneous pacing may be related to electrode placement or patient size. Patients who are conscious or who regain consciousness during transcutaneous pacing experience discomfort due to muscle contraction. Analgesia with incremental doses of morphine or sedation with a benzodiazepine makes this discomfort tolerable until transvenous pacing can be instituted. Transcutaneous pacing should be used for temporary stabilization only and should always be followed as soon as feasible by an internal pacing technique (usually transvenous).

An increasing number of defibrillators include a built-in transcutaneous pacemaker. This development ensures that pacing will be available as soon as the defibrillator reaches the patient in cardiac arrest. Previous studies have clearly demonstrated that pacing will only improve survival if it is applied very early in the course of bradyasystolic arrest.

## Transvenous Pacing

Transvenous pacing consists of endocardial stimulation of the right ventricle via an electrode introduced into a central vein. The major difficulties of transvenous pacing are venous access and proper placement of the stimulating electrode. Venous access routes most commonly used include the subclavian, internal or external jugular, femoral, and brachial. Transvenous pacing catheters can be inserted through a variety of venous introducers. A soft flexible semifloating bipolar catheter is preferred. This type of pacer is safest to use and takes advantage of any forward blood flow that may be present.

Placement of the catheter tip into the apex of the right ventricle is the key to successful transvenous pacing. Several techniques can aid successful placement. Fluoroscopic guidance is the surest method of right ventricular placement but is rarely available in the emergency department. Electrocardiographic guidance is useful in patients with narrow complexes and/or P waves when fluoroscopy is unavailable (see the chapter by Benjamin in Roberts' and Hedges' text for a description of this technique). Balloon-tipped "floating" catheters may aid placement when used in conjunction with ECG and fluoroscopic guidance or when used alone. The balloon is inflated after catheter insertion into a central vein. Forward blood flow then directs the catheter tip toward the ventricle as the operator slowly advances the catheter. As with all balloon-tipped catheters, the balloon should al-

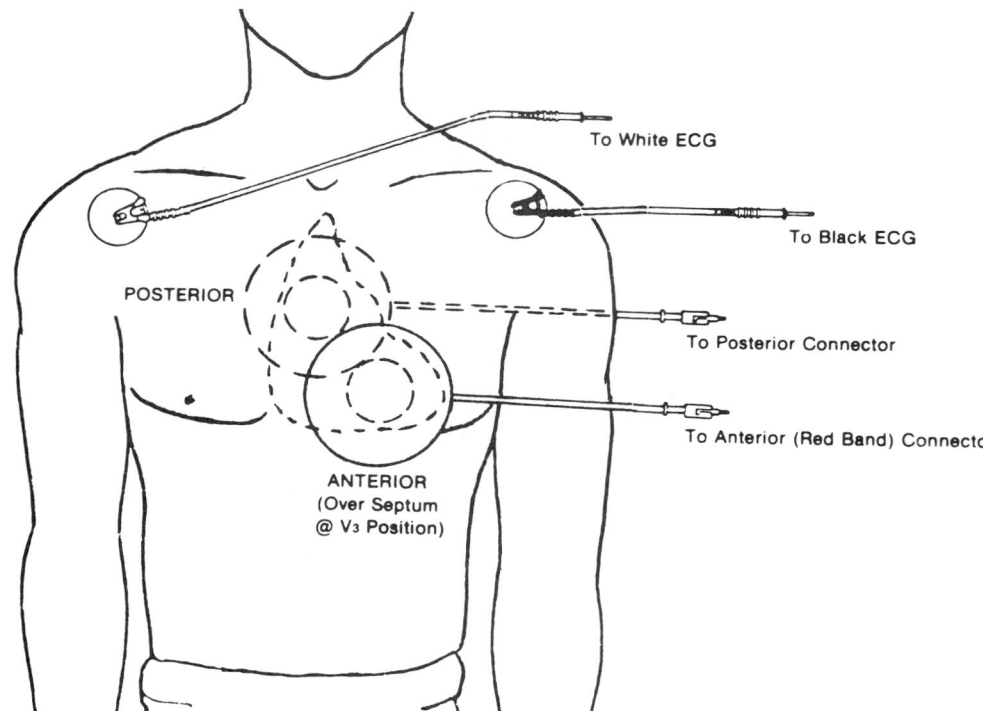

**Fig. 13-5.** Catheters and electrodes for emergency cardiac pacing. **A.** Transcutaneous. **B.** Transvenous. [From Roberts JR (ed): *Clinical Procedures in Emergency Medicine.* Philadelphia, Saunders, 1985, and from Jastremski JS (ed): *The Whole Emergency Medicine Catalog.* Philadelphia, Saunders, 1985. Used by permission.]

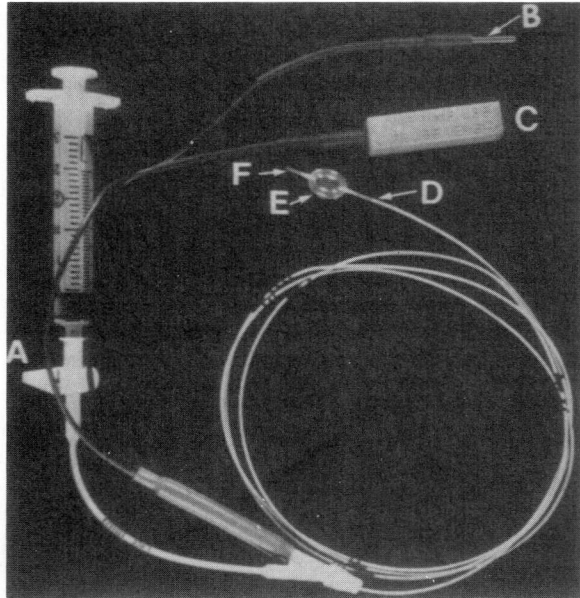

ways be deflated prior to withdrawal; the catheter should never be pulled back with the balloon inflated.

When patients have decreased or no forward blood flow (including most circumstances in which transvenous pacing would be used in the emergency department) positioning of the pacer tip within the right ventricle is difficult. Balloon-tipped catheters are not much of an aid in placement during low- or no-flow states. In a true emergency the pacemaker electrodes are connected to the power source and the catheter advanced blindly in hopes that the tip will encounter the endocardium of the right ventricle and that capture will result. In this setting a *right internal jugular* venous access route should be used. From this approach, the catheter traverses a straight line into the right ventricle and rarely curls in the atrium or deflects into the inferior vena cava.

Pacer settings vary with the clinical situation. An initial rate of 80 to 100 per minute is appropriate in most patients. Asynchronous mode (sensitivity off) should be used initially in patients requiring emergency pacing for hemodynamically unstable bradycardias. The presence or absence of capture should be assessed by ECG (Fig. 13-7). Output should initially be set at maximum (usually 20 mA) and then decreased after capture is achieved. With optimal tip position, capture should occur at less than 2 mA. Pacing should be continued at 1.5 to 2 times the threshold output required for capture. Subsequent rate and sensitivity settings should be adjusted as clinically indicated by the patient's hemodynamic status and underlying rhythm disturbance.

Chest radiographs (anteroposterior and lateral) should be obtained after patient stabilization to ensure proper tip placement and to evaluate the possibility of pneumothorax from the preceding central venous line placement. Finally, care should be taken to firmly affix the pacing catheter to the insertion site prior to patient transfer. Transvenous pacing is best used in urgent situations in which there is adequate time to utilize fluoroscopy. In the setting of cardiac arrest, transcutaneous pacing is preferred.

## AUTOMATIC AND IMPLANTABLE DEFIBRILLATORS

In William Kouwenhoven's landmark 1957 report on the first DC defibrillator, he astutely observed:

When ventricular fibrillation has been present for less than two minutes, application of this method results in survival in a high proportion of cases. . . . Effective use of closed chest defibrillation requires that the necessary equipment be available and rapidly applied.

Two recent technological developments have led to the more rapid application of defibrillation. Automatic external defibrillators allow first responders to institute defibrillation. In some cases even bystanders or family members can institute defibrillation with these devices. Implanted defibrillators allow patients with frequent malignant ventricular dysrhythmias to in effect carry their own defibrillators with them at all times. Emergency physicians need to be familiar with these devices and the special considerations associated with their use.

**Fig. 13-6.** ECG monitoring of the paced patient. Transcutaneous pacing without capture and with capture. Note the wide pacer artifact produced by the transcutaneous pacer. [From Roberts JR (ed): *Clinical Procedures in Emergency Medicine.* Philadelphia, Saunders, 1985. Used with permission.]

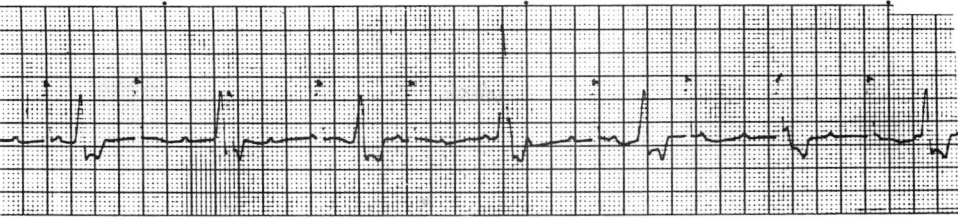

**TRANSCUTANEOUS PACING ARTIFACT WITHOUT CAPTURE**

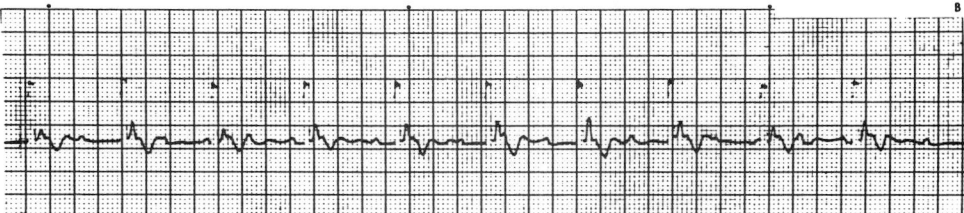

**TRANSCUTANEOUS PACING WITH CAPTURE**

## Automatic External Defibrillators

Automatic external defibrillators (AEDs) have relatively simple controls and can be applied by minimally trained providers to initiate defibrillation. AED use requires the operator to attach monitoring and defibrillation electrodes to the patient. Various models allow varying degrees of operator control. In most cases the device analyzes the cardiac rhythm and initiates defibrillation automatically after first warning the operator to stand clear prior to the actual delivery of the countershock. Some devices prompt the operator to initiate the countershock or rely on basic rhythm confirmation by the operator prior to defibrillating. As the rhythm recognition capability and reliability of these devices has improved, the need for time-consuming training of providers in rhythm recognition has decreased.

AEDs will shock patients in ventricular fibrillation several times sequentially until an organized cardiac rhythm results or until the maximum number of shocks allowed by the device's algorithm is reached. Many devices also provide a record of rhythms and events during their use, which allows the emergency physician to subsequently reconstruct the sequence of events during resuscitation.

AEDs are most effective in tiered EMS systems where AED-equipped first responders reach the patient rapidly and are backed up by the later arrival of paramedics with full advanced life-support capabilities. The failure of an AED to restore a perfusing rhythm is a poor prognostic sign often associated with long arrest times or arrest rhythms other than ventricular fibrillation. When an AED fails to resuscitate a patient in arrest, the cardiac rhythm should be identified and treated. If the rhythm is refractory ventricular fibrillation, drug therapy should be instituted while continuing further defibrillation attempts.

## Implantable Defibrillators

Over two decades have passed since the concept of an implantable defibrillator was first proposed independently by Mirowski and Schuder. Since the first human placement of an automatic implantable cardioverter-defibrillator (AICD) in 1980, over 30,000 patients have received this device, with a reduction of sudden cardiac death from 30 to 45 percent per year to less than 2 percent per year.

The AICD consists of a pulse generator and a lead system with both sensing and shocking electrodes. The pulse generator, the size of a deck of cards ($11 \times 2 \times 7.5$ cm), may be implanted in the left upper quadrant of the abdomen, deeper in the abdomen near the diaphragm, or in the chest cavity. The sensing lead system can be either a pair of screw-in epicardial pacing wires placed on the left ventricle (most common), or an endocardial lead tunnelled from the subclavian vein to the generator. The defibrillating lead system may be either two epicardial patch electrodes placed in an anteroposterior position (most common) or a transvenous spring electrode positioned in the right ventricular apex paired with an epicardial patch (implanted by thoracotomy or sternotomy) (Fig. 13-8). The patches have a radiopaque border, which may appear to be blurred, depending on the timing of the chest film.

### Function

Three generations of AICDs have been produced at the time of this writing. In the most frequently encountered second-generation device, the pulse generator continuously monitors the heart rate and the waveform configuration. If a preset heart rate is detected (e.g., 155 bpm) or if a sinusoidal waveform is detected by probability density

**Fig. 13-7.** Pacing with intermittent capture. "P" indicates paced beats. "A" indicates pacer artifact without capture.

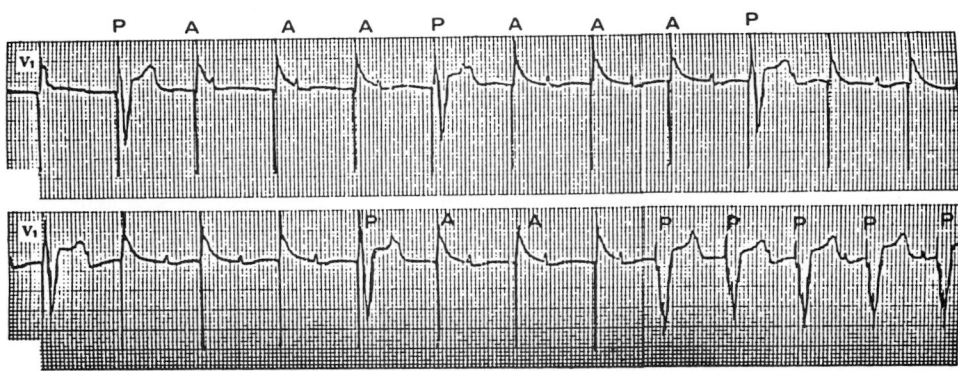

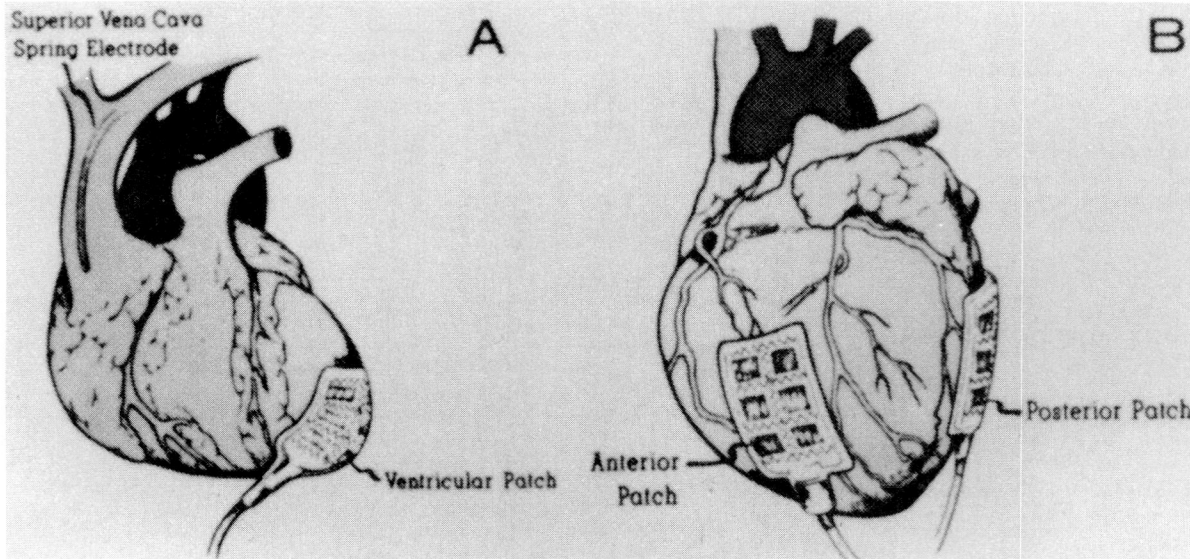

**Fig. 13-8.** Defibrillation arrangements for the AICD. **A.** Spring-patch pathway. **B.** Patch-patch pathway. (From Chapman et al, 1989. Used by permission.)

function analysis, then the device will be triggered to charge the capacitor and deliver a shock. Five to 10 s are required to detect the arrhythmia and an additional 5 to 10 s are required to charge the capacitor, with a total elapsed time of 10 to 35 s from the onset of the arrhythmia to the delivery of the first shock. A maximum of four shocks are delivered for a given rhythm. A change in the rhythm will cause the AICD to be reset in approximately 35 s. Thereafter an additional four shocks may be delivered per arrhythmia. More sophisticated third-generation devices offer additional electrical therapies, including bradycardia pacing, overdrive pacing of tachycardias, low-energy cardioversion, and higher-energy defibrillation.

## Complications

The most common reason an AICD patient presents to the emergency department is to be evaluated for the appropriateness of a previously delivered shock. Causes of inappropriate shock delivery are summarized in Table 13-3.

Complex interactions with permanent pacemakers may be encountered. These include erroneous interpretation of a pacemaker signal as a normal rhythm when the patient is in ventricular fibrillation or ventricular tachycardia, with subsequent nondelivery of shock. Also, counting of dual-chamber pacemaker spikes, or double counting of a pacemaker spike and the subsequent QRS complex, has resulted in inappropriate shocks. Inactivation of cardiac pacemaker function after AICD discharge may occur. Additional complications include accidental deactivation of the AICD by magnetic fields (stereo speakers, microwave, bingo wand), pericarditis, pericardial effusion, drug/AICD interactions changing the defibrillation threshold (e.g., amiodarone, encainide), infection (often indolent), erosions of the

**Table 13-3.** Potential Causes of Inappropriate AICD Shock Delivery

False sensing
   Supraventricular tachycardia with rapid ventricular response
   Muscular activity (shivering, diaphragmatic contraction
   Extraneous source (tapping of chest wall, vibrations, pacer
     spikes)
   Sensing T waves as QRS complex (double counting)
   Sensing lead fracture or migration
Unsustained tachyarrhythmia
AICD/pacemaker interactions
Component failure

*Source:* Adapted from Munter and DeLacey, 1994. Used by permission.

generator into surrounding tissue, atrial or ventricular wall perforation, thrombosis and pulmonary embolism, trauma from falls after discharge, battery depletion, and psychiatric trauma from frequent discharges.

## Emergency Department Evaluation and Therapy

In evaluating the patient who presents complaining of one or more AICD shocks, it is important to determine the number of shocks delivered, the activity of the patient at the time, and any prodromal symptoms of postshock trauma. Recent changes in antiarrhythmic drug dosage should be noted. Attention in the physical examination should be focused on the vital signs, the cardiovascular status, the generator pocket, and evidence of incidental trauma. The patient should be monitored during the evaluation. An ECG should be obtained and interpreted with the knowledge that ST-segment elevations or depressions due exclusively to the shock will resolve within 15 min. A chest radiograph may reveal electrode migration, displacement, or fracture. Drug levels of antiarrhythmics should be obtained, and electrolyte disturbances explored. Essential to the evaluation is a consultation with the patient's cardiologist.

Admission criteria include all unstable patients, patients with two or more shocks in a 1-week period, the presence of correctable causes of arrhythmia (e.g., electrolyte imbalances, drug toxicity, ischemia), and patients who need additional cardiology investigation for possible malfunction of the device.

When treating the patient with an AICD who presents in cardiac arrest, it can be assumed that the device delivered a full set of shocks without restoration of a viable rhythm. As with any patient in cardiac arrest, normal resuscitation measures, including external defibrillation, are indicated. If the AICD discharges while emergency personnel are performing CPR, a small electrical shock may be felt. To date no serious injuries have been reported.

Occasionally it may become necessary to temporarily deactivate the AICD, as in the case of inappropriate shock for a stable rhythm. Second-generation devices may be deactivated by placing a donut-shaped magnet over the right upper quadrant (Fig. 13-9) of the pulse generator for 30 s until the intermittent beeping ceases and a solid tone is heard. The magnet is then removed. If this does not succeed, then deactivation is attempted by placing the magnet over the opposite corner (some generators are surgically positioned upside down). Third-generation devices are only deactivated when the magnet is

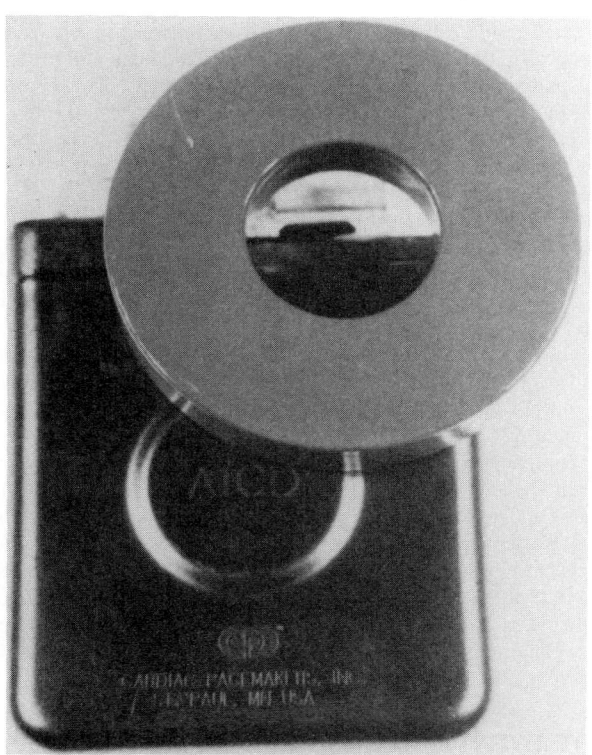

**Fig. 13-9.** Correct magnet placement to deactivate AICD. (From Chapman et al, 1989. Used by permission.)

present. This requires taping the magnet to the skin overlying the AICD. Some third-generation devices can be programmed so that they are not deactivated at all by a magnetic field.

## BIBLIOGRAPHY

### Invasive Monitoring

Barker WJ: Arterial puncture and cannulation, in Roberts JR, Hedges JR (eds): *Clinical Procedures in Emergency Medicine. 2d ed.* Philadelphia, Saunders, 1991, pp 255–268.

Forrester JS, Diamond G, Chatterjee K, et al: Medical therapy of acute myocardial infarction by application of hemodynamic subsets. *N Engl J Med* 205:1356, 1976.

Kaye W: Invasive monitoring techniques, in McIntyre KM, Levis AJ (eds): *Textbook of Advanced Cardiac Life Support.* Dallas, American Heart Association, 1983, pp 165–196.

Shoemaker WC: Monitoring the critically ill patient, in Shoemaker WC (ed): *Textbook of Critical Care Medicine.* Philadelphia, Saunders, 1984, pp 105–121.

### Pacing Techniques

Benjamin GC: Emergency transvenous cardiac pacing, in Roberts JR, Hedges JR (eds): *Clinical Procedures in Emergency Medicine,* 2d ed. Philadelphia, Saunders, 1991, pp 203–209.

Bing OH, McDowell JW, Hantman J, et al: Pacemaker placement by electrocardiographic monitoring. *N Engl J Med* 287:651, 1972.

Hazard PB, Benton C, Milnor P: Transvenous cardiac pacing in cardiopulmonary resuscitation. *Crit Care Med* 9:666, 1981.

Syverud SA: Emergency transcutaneous and transesophageal cardiac pacing, in Roberts JR, Hedges JR (eds): *Clinical Procedures in Emergency Medicine,* 2d ed. Philadelphia, Saunders, 1991, pp 177–195.

### Automatic and Implantable Defibrillators

Chapman PD: The implantable cardioverter-defibrillator, in Gibler WB, Aufderheide TP (eds): *Emergency Cardiac Care,* St. Louis, Mosby, 1994, pp 452–462.

Chapman PD, Veseth-Rogers JL, Duquette SE: The implantable defibrillator and the emergency physician. *Ann Emerg Med* 18:579, 1989.

Cummins RO: Review of the clinical experience with automatic external defibrillators. *Ann Emerg Med* 18:1269, 1989.

Kouwenhoven WB: Closed chest defibrillation of the heart. *Surgery* 42:550, 1952.

Munter WM, DeLacey WA: Automatic implantable cardioverter-defibrillators. *Emerg Med Clin North Am* 12:579, 1994.

Winkle RA, Mead RH, Ruder MA, et al: Long-term outcome with the automatic implantable cardioverter-defibrillator. *J Am Coll Cardiol* 13:1353, 1989.

# 14
# CEREBRAL ISCHEMIA

## Gary S. Krause
## Blaine C. White

The widespread availability of emergency medical services across the United States now results in about 200,000 cardiac resuscitation attempts yearly, with approximately 70,000 successful cardiac resuscitations. Only about 10 percent of the patients recover completely and are able to resume their former lifestyles. The major cause of this poor outcome is permanent neurologic injury. Discovery of effective pharmacologic tools for amelioration of brain damage by ischemia and reperfusion is dependent upon elucidation of the injury mechanisms. The crucial role of calcium and iron in the injury mechanism are outlined in this chapter, and possible therapies to ameliorate brain injury following an ischemic insult are reviewed.

Three major observations have provided the foundation for investigation of brain injury by ischemia and reperfusion: (1) morphologic studies showing that most of the structural damage occurs during reperfusion; (2) progressive hypoperfusion of the brain during reperfusion; and (3) prolonged suppression of protein synthesis. All three phenomena appear to be a result of the loss of homeostasis of two ions: calcium (causing lipolysis during ischemia) and iron (causing oxygen radical–mediated lipid peroxidation during reperfusion). Cardiac arrest resulting in ischemic-anoxic brain injury is characterized by three phases: (1) ischemia, (2) early reperfusion, and (3) late reperfusion.

## ISCHEMIC PHASE

With the onset of cardiac arrest there is a precipitous decline in brain oxygen content, which approaches zero within 6 to 12 s. The brain has very limited reserves of glucose, glycogen, or phosphocreatine; therefore, oxygen depletion leads to a sharp decline in tissue adenosine triphosphate (ATP) levels, which approach zero within 4 min. Anaerobic glycolysis and ATP depletion lead to lactic acidosis and hypoxanthine accumulation, respectively, during the ischemic phase. Since about 80 percent of the brain's ATP is used to maintain transmembrane ionic gradients for potassium, sodium, and calcium, these ionic gradients also decay rapidly. During complete ischemic-anoxia these ions equilibrate between the extra- and intracellular fluid within 5 to 10 min of the insult.

The cytosolic accumulation of calcium is now widely thought to be a major initiating event leading to cell death. The high cytosolic calcium level causes three key events: the activation of membrane phospholipase $A_2$, proteolytic cleavage of xanthine dehydrogenase, and release of excitatory neurotransmitters. Phospholipase $A_2$ cleaves a fatty acid, primarily arachidonate, from the cell membrane lipids, yielding a free fatty acid (FFA) and in the process damaging the membrane's structure. The conversion of xanthine dehydrogenase in brain endothelial cells produces xanthine oxidase, which will react with hypoxanthine to produce the oxygen free radical superoxide $(O_2^-)$ upon reperfusion.

Minimal ultrastructural injury is seen in the brain during complete ischemia. Some margination and clumping of nuclear chromatin is seen by 10 to 15 min of complete ischemia. Mitochondria may be slightly swollen, but their structure does not show major degenerative alterations for up to 30 min of complete ischemia. Similarly, some swelling of the endoplasmic reticulum (ER) may be seen during ischemia, but the polyribosomes remain appropriately associated with the ER, and disaggregation of polyribosomes does not occur during complete ischemia. Nuclear and plasma membranes show a normal, well-defined bilaminar structure without evidence of holes or general structural disintegration.

Thus, the situation at the end of 15 to 30 min of complete ischemic anoxia includes: (1) ATP levels near zero; (2) elevated hypoxanthine levels; (3) moderate lactic acidosis; (4) loss of transmembrane ionic gradients; (5) activated phospholipase with elevated FFA, especially arachidonic acid; (6) the presence of the abnormal enzyme xanthine oxidase; (7) high interstitial levels of excitatory neurotransmitters; (8) minimal injury to the high-energy capability of mitochondria; and (9) minimal and homogeneous ultrastructural changes.

## EARLY REPERFUSION

ATP levels and total adenylate charge recover rapidly during early reperfusion. If the ischemic insult has been less than 20 min, the membrane ionic gradients also recover quickly. After much longer insults of 1 to 3 h, total tissue calcium loads actually increase during reperfusion. It is felt that this reflects extensive and irreversible cell membrane injury during these very prolonged periods of ischemia.

Arachidonate is rapidly oxidized by both cyclooxygenase and lipoxygenase and returns to preischemic levels within 30 min of reperfusion. Several vasoactive substances are produced by the metabolism of arachidonate. The prostaglandins are the products of cyclooxygenase, and the leukotrienes are the products of lipoxygenase. The production of the vasodilatory prostaglandin, prostacyclin, is severely inhibited during early reperfusion. Thus, vasospastic compounds predominate in the leukotriene and prostaglandin products. While the free arachidonic acid levels rapidly return to baseline during reperfusion, leukotrienes remain markedly elevated for at least 24 h. The time course of leukotriene elevation may explain the alterations in blood flow seen in the postischemic brain.

Restoration of normal or mildly hypertensive systemic arterial pressure produces an initial brain hyperperfusion. However, within 1 h, global brain perfusion has dropped to levels of 20 to 40 percent of normal, where it remains for up to 1 to 2 days. This phenomenon is inhibited by postresuscitation treatment with calcium antagonists such as flunarizine and nimodipine, the iron chelator deferoxamine, or radical chain reaction–terminating 21-aminosteroids.

Oxygen-based free radicals produced upon reperfusion also contribute to neuronal injury, although the precise identity of the radical species responsible for initiating this damage remains unknown. Xanthine oxidase and cyclooxygenase, whose substrates are hypoxanthine and arachidonate respectively, produce $O_2^-$ as a side product. Availability of a transition metal, such as iron, is required for oxygen radical reactions, including lipid peroxidation. Iron is rapidly delocalized by reduction out of ferritin by $O_2^-$, which is present in excessive amounts during early reperfusion, and lipid peroxidation in the reperfused brain has been demonstrated by many laboratories.

Excitatory amino acid neurotransmitters appear to play a role in the injury produced by focal brain ischemia such as stroke; it is unclear if the same holds true in global brain ischemia. However, excitatory neurotransmitter uptake is inhibited by arachidonate and products of lipid peroxidation, and thus continued stimulation of receptors may contribute to neuronal damage by an as yet unidentified mechanism.

Protein synthesis is suppressed during ischemia by lack of ATP. However, even with the rapid restoration of ATP levels that accompanies reperfusion, there is a severe suppression of protein synthesis that varies with duration of ischemia, brain region, and individual proteins. Whereas most regions of the brain recover their ability to synthesize protein following a short ischemic period, protein synthesis in the selectively vulnerable regions (the pyramidal neurons of layers 3 and 5 of the cerebral cortex and $CA_1$ of the hippocampus) is depressed about 90 percent early in reperfusion and does not recover significantly. Failure of protein synthesis occurs somewhere between the end of transcription and the beginning of translation. Following a 20-min arrest and up to 8 h of reperfusion, neither brain nuclear DNA nor mitochondrial DNA shows evidence of structural damage. Although the rate of new transcription is normal during reperfusion, there is apparent retention of the newly synthesized mRNA in the nucleus. Current evidence suggests that there is a disruption in the formation of new ribosomal translation complexes. The suppression of protein synthesis in the reperfused brain may prevent the manufacture of necessary defense or repair proteins, including superoxide dismutase, glutathione transferases, NAD(P)H:quinone reductase, UDP-glucuronsyltransferases, and epoxide hydrolase.

## LATE EVENTS DURING REPERFUSION

Brain tissue ionic concentrations are indistinguishable from normal after 4 h of reperfusion following a 15-min cardiac arrest. The tissue iron has been recovered into high-molecular-weight species by 8 h of reperfusion. However, after 8 h large shifts of the concentrations of calcium, potassium, and sodium are observed. These shifts most likely reflect equilibration between the cytosol and the interstitial fluid for these ions. Electron microscopic examination of brains fixed in situ reveals in the vulnerable neurons an obvious general degradation of membrane structure with large holes in the plasmalemma. Nuclear chromatin is densely clumped, with grossly abnormal nuclear architecture. Mitochondrial architecture is well preserved. The ER is dilated and ragged, and normally arranged polyribosomes are virtually nonexistent. Histochemical evidence of lipid peroxidation can be seen by as early as 90 min following a 10-min arrest and involves 30 percent of the cells in the selectively vulnerable areas. Membrane injury by lipid peroxidation produces degradation of membrane structure to the point that the membrane becomes freely permeable to ions and the cell is irreversibly injured.

Therapy with calcium antagonists or iron chelators has produced mixed results in laboratory models. For example, in one study deferoxamine therapy following a 10-min cardiac arrest in rats produced a dramatic 100 percent increase in 10-day intact neurologic survival. However, in a 15-min cardiac arrest model in dogs, we were unable to demonstrate significant effects of therapy with deferoxamine and the calcium antagonist lidoflazine on either neurologic deficit scores or histopathologic evidence of cell death. Administration of either deferoxamine or superoxide dismutase (the scavenger enzyme for superoxide) significantly inhibits lipid peroxidation byproduct accumulation by 8 h of reperfusion. Deferoxamine retarded the loss of unsaturated fatty acids and protected tissue Na/K ratios. In these studies the calcium antagonist flunarizine had no effect on products of lipid peroxidation, ultrastructural injury, or ionic gradient decay.

Promising studies of the use of growth factors are now being done; these growth factors include fibroblast growth factor, nerve growth factor, insulin-like growth factor 1, and insulin, all of which have been shown to improve neuronal survival in the laboratory. This may be related to the role of growth factors in fundamental aspects of cell cycle control that involve regulation of the activity of initiation factors involved in protein synthesis and of transcription promoter binding factors implicated in expression of antioxidant enzymes and stress-response proteins, all of which may be important in limiting and repairing membrane damage. Future investigation of therapeutic approaches may combine iron chelators, lipid peroxidation chain-reaction terminators, and growth factors to forestall further lipid peroxidation and to stimulate repair mechanisms.

## CLINICAL IMPLICATIONS

Optimum therapy to obviate continuing injury and salvage viable brain tissue is unknown. Most therapeutic studies use animal models, use pretreatment, or contain small numbers of patients. However, a few general principles can be stated. Perfusion should be maintained at normal levels. It does not appear that intracranial pressure is increased in the postresuscitation period, and therefore therapies directed at increased intracranial pressure (hyperventilation and osmotic agents) are unneeded. Hypotension should be avoided for the obvious reasons. Oxygenation should be maintained at or near normal levels. Hyperoxia should be avoided, since it is toxic to the lungs and may increase brain damage. Prearrest hyperglycemia is associated with poor neurologic outcome, and although glucose administered postinsult has not been adequately studied, hyperglycemia should probably be avoided.

Several other therapies have been advocated, but human studies have failed to show efficacy. These therapies include pentobarbital coma, calcium antagonists, and glucocorticoids.

## BIBLIOGRAPHY

Brain Resuscitation Clinical Trial I Study Group: Randomized clinical study of thiopental loading in comatose survivors of cardiac arrest. *N Engl J Med* 314:397, 1986.

Brain Resuscitation Clinical Trial II Study Group: A randomized clinical study of a calcium-entry blocker (lidoflazine) in the treatment of comatose survivors of cardiac arrest. *N Engl J Med* 324:1225, 1991.

Calle PA, Buylaert WA, Vanhaute OA: Glycemia in the post-resuscitation period. *Resuscitation* 17(suppl):S181, 1989.

Grafton ST, Longstreth WT Jr: Steroids after cardiac arrest: A retrospective study with concurrent, nonrandomized controls. *Neurology* 38:1315, 1988.

Jastremski M, Sutton-Tyrrell K, Vaagenes P, et al: Glucocorticoid treatment does not improve neurological recovery following cardiac arrest. Brain Resuscitation Clinical Trial I Study Group. *JAMA* 262:3427, 1989.

Krause GS, Kumar K, White BC, et al: Ischemia, resuscitation, and reperfusion: Mechanisms of tissue injury and prospects for protection. *Am Heart J* 111:768, 1986.

Krause GS, Tiffany BR: Protein synthesis in the reperfused brain. *Stroke* 24:747, 1993.

Krause GS, White BC, Aust SD, et al: Brain cell death following ischemia and reperfusion: A proposed biochemical sequence. *Crit Care Med* 16:714, 1988.

Siesjo BK, Bengtsson F, Grampp W, et al: Calcium, excitotoxins, and neuronal death in the brain. *Ann NY Acad Sci* 568:234, 1989.

White BC, Grossman LI, Krause GS: Brain injury by global ischemia and reperfusion: A theoretical perspective on membrane damage and repair. *Neurology* 43:1656, 1993.

# 15
# NEWER RESUSCITATIVE TECHNIQUES

## James E. Manning
## Christopher W. Barton

## INTRODUCTION

Despite numerous advances in the science of cardiopulmonary resuscitation (CPR), the prospects for survival overall still remain dismal. The major obstacle in cardiopulmonary and cerebral resuscitation is the limited blood flow generated by the chest compressions of closed-chest CPR. Cardiac output has been reported to be between 25 and 33 percent of normal at best, and it decreases with delays in initiation of CPR. With increasing duration of arrest and progressive loss of peripheral arterial resistance, even optimally performed closed-chest CPR is unlikely to result in return of spontaneous circulation (ROSC).

Resuscitation of the patient in cardiac arrest cannot occur unless there is at least some minimal amount of blood flow to the heart. Myocardial perfusion during CPR has been shown to be directly related to the pressure gradient across the coronary vasculature. This gradient is equal to the aortic pressure minus the right atrial pressure and is termed the *coronary perfusion pressure* (CPP). Aortic pressure largely determines the CPP gradient and is dependent upon the level of residual peripheral arterial vasomotor tone. Research has shown that the CPP gradient is greatest during the relaxation phase of CPR chest compression (CPR-diastole). Both laboratory and clinical data indicate that a CPP of at least 15 mmHg is almost always required to achieve ROSC. Yet studies in humans have revealed that CPP gradients attained with standard CPR are usually in the dismal range of 1 to 8 mmHg.

The majority of research into cardiopulmonary resuscitation has focused on methods to improve artificial perfusion during cardiac arrest. In addition to the originally described "conventional" CPR technique, several alternative methods of performing closed-chest CPR have been investigated (Table 15-1). Vasoconstrictor agents have long been used as the pharmacologic adjunct to improve vital organ perfusion by increasing aortic pressure and coronary perfusion pressure. Adrenergic-mediated vasoconstriction remains the major pharmacologic intervention in all forms of cardiac arrest. Other adrenergic agents and dosages have been extensively studied, and, more recently, nonadrenergic vasoconstrictor agents have been investigated as well.

Noninvasive and invasive monitoring techniques have been examined in an effort to identify clinically useful and reliable parameters to guide resuscitative efforts (Table 15-2).

More recently, invasive perfusion techniques capable of providing near-normal artificial vital organ perfusion have also been described. Direct mechanical ventricular assistance (or actuation) and cardiopul-

**Table 15-1.** Alternative Methods of Closed-Chest CPR

Mechanical piston CPR
Simultaneous compression and ventilation (SCV-CPR)
Interposed abdominal compression (IAC-CPR)
CPR with abdominal binding
CPR with MAST
High-impulse CPR
Circumferential thoracic vest-CPR
Active compression-decompression (ACD-CPR)

**Table 15–2.** Monitoring Techniques for Assessing CPR Effectiveness

**Noninvasive**
  Ventricular fibrillation amplitude
  End-tidal carbon dioxide ($ET_{CO_2}$)
  Median frequency of ventricular fibrillation
**Invasive**
  Arterial pressure
  Coronary perfusion pressure (CPP)
  Central venous oxygen saturation

monary bypass have been reported in laboratory models and a few clinical reports. Methods to provide and augment artificial perfusion using aortic balloon catheters have recently been described in laboratory investigations.

Reperfusion-induced injury has also become a major focus of research in many fields of medicine and for numerous ischemic diseases states, including cardiac arrest, and is discussed in detail elsewhere. Cerebral resuscitation with favorable neurologic outcome after prolonged global ischemia will be the ultimate obstacle to overcome in cardiac arrest therapy. The use of pharmacologic agents capable of limiting ischemia-induced cellular damage and reperfusion-induced injury from reactive oxygen species will likely be an important form of therapy for cardiac arrest patients in the resuscitation and postresuscitation phases.

In this chapter we will briefly discuss some of the newer methods of closed-chest CPR, pharmacologic agents, monitoring methods, and invasive perfusion techniques that either influenced the latest revision of the American Heart Association advanced cardiac life support (ACLS) guidelines or are presently undergoing active investigation and hold promise for the future clinical management of cardiac arrest.

## ALTERNATIVE METHODS OF CLOSED-CHEST CPR

To understand the rationale for most of the alternative methods of closed-chest CPR that have been described, one must have at least a basic understanding of the two proposed mechanisms of blood flow during sternal CPR chest compression. The *cardiac pump theory* proposes that compression of the heart between the sternum and the spine squeezes blood out of the ventricles in a forward flow direction in a manner generally similar to normal myocardial contraction. The *thoracic pump theory* proposes that pressurization of the entire thorax, not just the heart, is responsible for blood flow and that the heart serves only as a passive or partially compressed conduit for blood flow. Net forward blood flow occurs due to competent closure of venous valves at the thoracic inlet during chest compression. The evidence for and against each theory is beyond the scope of this chapter, but it is accurate to state that the precise mechanism of blood flow during closed-chest CPR remains controversial and likely varies based on individual anatomic features. Alternative methods of performing closed-chest CPR have largely been based on efforts to exploit of one or both of the two proposed mechanisms.

### High-Impulse CPR

In 1984, Maier et al. reported a laboratory study comparing compression rates of 100 per minute and 150 per minute with the conventional rate of 60 per minute advocated prior to 1986. They observed increases in cardiac output that were roughly linear to the increase in compression rate while stroke volume remained relatively constant. Left ventricular and aortic pressure also increased in proportion to the rate of compression, while coronary blood flow plateaued at a compression rate of 100 per minute. The force of compression was also varied, with moderate to high forces generating better hemodynamics. The authors also suggested that the velocity with which the compression force was applied had a significant role in the hemodynamic effects. The importance of both compression force and velocity of

impact in the use of these rapid CPR compression rates led to the term *high-impulse CPR*. Changes in ventricular dimensions along with the consistent stroke volumes and rate-related increases in cardiac output were concluded to support the cardiac pump mechanism of blood flow. Despite laboratory evidence suggesting improved blood flow, no controlled clinical studies have been reported to evaluate resuscitation outcome in humans. However, the results of this and other laboratory studies on high-impulse CPR were partially responsible for the increase in the recommended CPR compression rate from 60 per minute to 80 to 100 per minute by the American Heart Association in 1986.

### Interposed Abdominal Compression CPR (IAC-CPR)

It was recognized in the 1980s that compression of the abdomen during cardiac arrest generated aortic pressures similar to chest compressions. The hypothesis that CPR-diastolic aortic pressure and venous return from the abdomen might be augmented by abdominal compressions led to the idea of IAC-CPR. IAC-CPR requires two persons to perform. One person performs the chest compressions of standard CPR while the other person applies a similar compression over the central abdomen during the relaxation phase of chest compression. IAC-CPR has been shown to increase CPR-diastolic aortic pressure, coronary perfusion pressure, and cardiac output in laboratory cardiac arrest models. Sack et al recently reported a randomized, controlled comparison of IAC-CPR and standard CPR in 103 in-hospital cardiac arrest patients. The use of IAC-CPR resulted in significant improvement in ROSC (51 versus 27 percent) and survival to hospital discharge (25 versus 7 percent) compared with standard CPR. Neurologic outcome was not statistically better due to the small number of patients in each group, though a trend toward improvement was seen (17 versus 6 percent). At present, the data supporting the use of IAC-CPR are not sufficient to recommend routine application. It could also be argued that IAC-CPR is physiologically very similar to high-impulse CPR with the compressions performed by two persons rather than one. However, if some method of monitoring CPR effectiveness is being utilized and standard CPR is inadequate, attempting IAC-CPR is a reasonable intervention.

### Active Compression-Decompression CPR (ACD-CPR)

Standard CPR involves a forceful or "active" chest compression phase with elastic recoil of the chest wall during the relaxation phase ('passive" decompression). A report of a successful resuscitation in which a household drain plunger was used to perform chest compression led to the conception of ACD-CPR. The ACD-CPR device consists of a circular suction cup connected to a handle with a force gauge (Fig. 15-1). With the suction cup securely attached at the midsternal chest, CPR is performed with force applied both downward (active compression) and upward (active decompression) during CPR. The principal advantage of the ACD-CPR device is that it tends to decrease the venous system pressure to a greater extent than the arterial pressures during the active decompression phase. This may increase venous return and increase the coronary perfusion pressure gradient during CPR-diastole. In the initial clinical report using the ACD-CPR device, Cohen et al. described preliminary results in 10 patients failing to respond to standard CPR and ACLS interventions. They observed higher end-tidal $CO_2$ readings and higher systolic arterial pressures with ACD-CPR compared with standard CPR, and 3 of the 10 patients rapidly had ROSC. More recently, preliminary results of a prospective randomized comparison of standard CPR and ACD-CPR in the prehospital setting revealed a trend toward increased ROSC and hospital admission with ACD-CPR. Further clinical studies are presently needed to clearly determine the value of this CPR method. Until then, the device is not approved by the Food and Drug Administration for use in the United States.

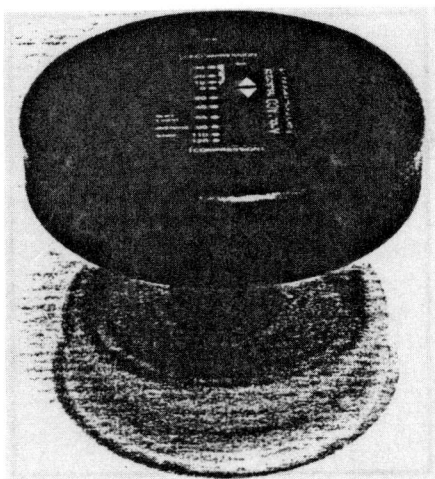

**Fig. 15-1.** The Ambu CardioPump (Ambu International Inc., Copenhagen, Denmark) is used for active compression-decompression cardiopulmonary resuscitation (ACD-CPR). The silicone rubber suction cup is positioned mid-chest at the level of the nipples. Using the circular plastic handle, the device is pushed downward during the compression phase followed by active withdrawal during the decompression phase. Force of compression and decompression is measured by the gauge located within the handle and is easily viewed by the operator during CPR. (From Lurie KG et al: *JAMA* 271:1405, 1994, with permission.)

## Circumferential Thoracic-Vest CPR

As noted above, the thoracic pump theory proposes that cyclic fluctuations in intrathoracic pressure created by CPR chest compressions are responsible for blood flow. Thus, efforts to maximize the intrathoracic pressure generated while limiting trauma to the chest would be advantageous. This led to the conception of the circumferential thoracic-vest CPR device. This involves the placement of a vest that can be pressurized around the thorax and pressurizing the thorax from all directions, as opposed to localized pressure over the lower sternum (Fig. 15-2). Halperin et al. have reported their preliminary experience in humans with a refined circumferential vest CPR device; they found significant improvements in coronary perfusion pressure and initial ROSC. In patients failing prolonged resuscitative efforts, peak CPR-systolic aortic pressure increased from an average of 78 mmHg with manual CPR to an average of 138 mmHg with vest CPR. In 34 patients randomized to receive manual CPR versus vest CPR after an average of 11 min of unsuccessful manual CPR, 8 of 17 vest CPR patients had ROSC compared with only 3 of 17 manual CPR patients. Although further investigation is needed, this appears to be a promising method of CPR.

## PHARMACOLOGIC INTERVENTIONS

### Adrenergic Therapy

Adrenergic drugs have been the primary agents studied and utilized in all forms of cardiac arrest. Epinephrine is by far the predominant adrenergic drug and remains the recommended agent. The mechanism of action of adrenergic therapy in cardiac resuscitation has been convincingly shown to be primarily α-adrenergic receptor–mediated vasoconstriction in the peripheral arterial system resulting in increased aortic pressure and, thus, increased coronary perfusion pressure. In addition to epinephrine, several other pure α-adrenergic or mixed α- and β-adrenergic agents have been studied. However, none of these agents has been shown to increase ROSC or long-term survival compared to epinephrine.

In recent years, the issue of the most appropriate dosage of adren-

ergic drugs has been the focus of intensive laboratory and clinical research. Epinephrine doses of 1 mg, which had been shown to be effective in small canine cardiac arrest experiments in the 1960s, were anecdotally reported to be successful in clinical cases. Thus, the recommended dosage of 1 mg epinephrine (equivalent to 0.01 mg/kg in the typical adult) for humans is substantially lower than the mg/kg effective dosage reported in animal models. During the 1980s, several laboratory investigations showed better CPR perfusion pressures and greater ROSC with dosages of epinephrine higher than the 0.01 mg/kg standard dose. There were also a number of anecdotal reports of patients being promptly resuscitated with "high-dose" epinephrine after failing to respond to repeated standard doses of epinephrine.

The laboratory and anecdotal clinical evidence supporting the use of higher doses of epinephrine led to large clinical trials to determine the effect of high-dose epinephrine on ROSC, survival to hospital discharge, and neurologic outcome. One of these studies was a randomized, prospective, double-blind comparison of 1 mg epinephrine versus 15 mg epinephrine versus 11 mg norepinephrine in 816 prehospital cardiac arrest patients. Although there was an increase in rate of ROSC, there was no improvement in survival to discharge or neurologic outcome with the higher adrenergic agent doses. Another multicenter randomized, controlled prehospital trial comparing 0.02 mg/kg versus 0.20 mg/kg of epinephrine showed no increase in ROSC, hospital admission rate, survival to discharge, or neurologic recovery. Although no benefit was demonstrated, no adverse results were identified with the use of high-dose epinephrine. When all laboratory and clinical data are considered, there is more scientific evidence to support the use of higher doses of epinephrine than the standard dose presently recommended. The American Heart Association has left the option of using higher doses of epinephrine open to the clinician's discretion in the clinical arena.

### Nonadrenergic Vasoconstriction

Adequate peripheral arterial resistance is crucial during closed-chest CPR in order to provide a coronary perfusion pressure high enough to promote ROSC. Although adrenergic therapy has been the pharmacologic cornerstone of this approach, there are nonadrenergic agents capable of creating arterial vasoconstriction. One such agent is endogenous angiotensin II. Little et al. have reported the use of angiotensin II in a swine cardiac arrest model and found increases in aortic and coronary perfusion pressures similar to that seen with epinephrine. The value of angiotensin II in cardiac arrest is presently unclear, but it may be a useful concurrent adjunctive agent to standard adrenergic therapy.

### Adenosine Antagonism

Release and accumulation of adenosine in ischemic tissues and adenosine's role as a depressant of cardiac pacemaker automaticity have been more clearly defined in recent years. There is limited evidence to suggest that aminophylline can reverse these effects (by acting as an adenosine antagonist) and may be useful in the treatment of bradydysrhythmias associated with myocardial ischemia. Hypothesizing that myocardial adenosine accumulation might be a contributing factor in bradyasystolic cardiac arrest refractory to standard ACLS interventions, Viskin et al. administered aminophylline, 250 mg, as a rapid intravenous bolus in 15 in-hospital bradyasystolic-arrest patients failing to respond to CPR, atropine, and epinephrine. They reported that 11 of the 15 patients had ROSC within 30 s of aminophylline administration and survived for at least 1 h. Ultimately, only 1 of the 11 responders survived neurologically intact. Although these initial results appear promising, adenosine antagonism is presently an unproven therapy. However, given the dismal prospects for survival associated with bradyasystolic arrest, a clini-

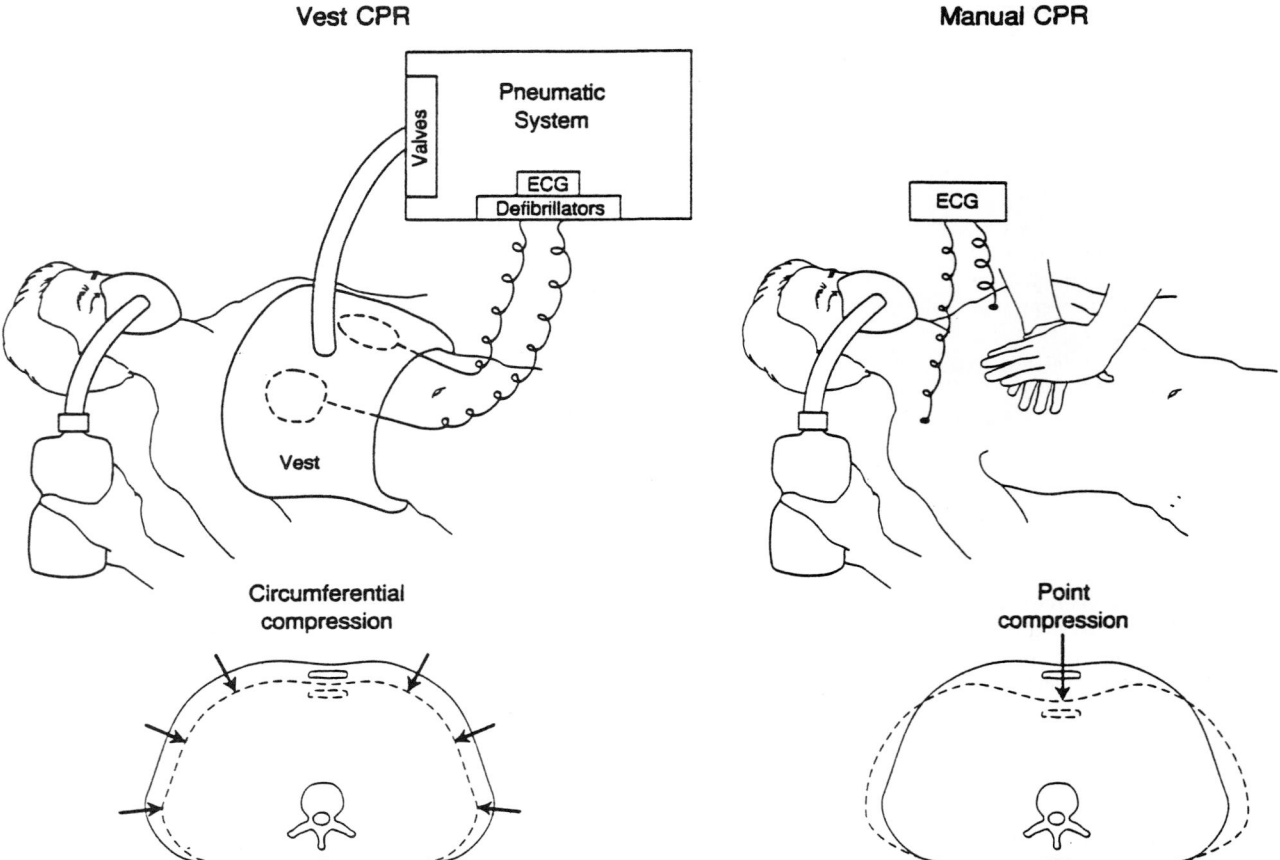

**Fig. 15-2.** A comparison of the thoracic-vest system for cardiopulmonary resuscitation (vest-CPR) with the standard manual CPR. The vest contains a bladder that is inflated and deflated by the pneumatic system. Defibrillation can be accomplished during chest compression through the flat defibrillator electrodes (dashed circles) under the vest. The ECG can be recorded through the same electrodes. The lower panels show schematic representations of transverse sections of the midthorax during vest-CPR and manual CPR. The thoracic size during chest relaxation is shown by the solid lines. The arrows indicate force applied to the thorax during chest compression. With vest inflation, there is a relatively uniform decrease in the dimensions of the thorax. With manual CPR, the sternum is displaced during compression (arrow) and the lateral thorax can bulge, thereby increasing thoracic volume and reducing the intrathoracic pressure generated during compression. (From Halperin HR et al: *N Engl J Med* 329:762, 1993, with permission.)

cian could not be faulted for administering aminophylline in such a setting, especially if there is no response to standard therapy.

### Routes for Medication Delivery

Recommended routes for administration of resuscitation drugs include intravenous, endotracheal, and intraosseous routes. Intravenous administration is considered optimal, with central venous delivery preferred over peripheral venous delivery provided that there is no time delay in gaining central venous access. Intracardiac drug injection has largely been discouraged. Central arterial administration of medications has received little attention but may be a useful alternative, especially for delivery of vasoconstrictor agents that have their effector sites in the peripheral arterial system.

Catheterization to measure arterial pressure during cardiac arrest is becoming a more accepted intervention to help guide resuscitative efforts. Thoracic aortic catheterization via a femoral artery approach allows for both pressure monitoring and homogeneous arterial drug administration. When aortic arch and central venous routes of epinephrine administration were compared in a laboratory model, aortic arch delivery resulted in a more rapid increase in CPR-diastolic aortic pressure, a greater magnitude of aortic pressure increase, and a maximal response consistently seen within 30 to 50 s of injection. The rapidity of initial and maximal aortic pressure response suggests

that adrenergic therapy could be rapidly adjusted based on a parameter reflecting vital organ perfusion. Thus, thoracic aortic catheterization allows for both rapid delivery of vasoconstrictor agents to effector sites and rapid assessment of therapeutic effect such that therapy can be rapidly titrated on an individual basis. The major limitation of this route is the need to establish central arterial access.

### TECHNIQUES FOR ASSESSMENT OF RESUSCITATIVE EFFORTS

The lack of an accurate and readily measurable parameter to guide resuscitative efforts has long frustrated clinicians and clinical investigators. Pulse quality, pupillary reactivity, serial blood gases, and the coarseness of ventricular fibrillation were the only parameters available until relatively recently, and none of these was accurate enough to allow for therapeutic adjustments on an individual case basis. Fortunately, recent technological advances have led to monitoring techniques that allow for much more accurate assessment and guidance of therapy.

### Capnometry, or End-Tidal Carbon Dioxide

Capnometry (the measurement of exhaled end-tidal carbon dioxide levels) has recently emerged as a noninvasive measure of cardiopulmonary circulation. Intensivists first used capnometry to monitor their intubated patients for instantaneous changes in expired end-tidal carbon dioxide levels ($ET_{CO_2}$). It was soon apparent that changes in $ET_{CO_2}$ levels not only signaled events such as occlusion of the endotracheal tube but also heralded changes in cardiopulmonary physiology. Soon thereafter, investigators began examining the relationship of $ET_{CO_2}$ levels to cardiac output in animal models of cardiac arrest and found a very good correlation. As cardiac output improved, $ET_{CO_2}$ levels increased, and vice versa.

End-tidal $CO_2$ measurements are affected by minute ventilation, $CO_2$ production, pulmonary transmembrane $CO_2$ diffusion, and pulmonary perfusion. Assuming that $CO_2$ production and diffusion are constant, minute ventilation and pulmonary blood flow are the variables determining $ET_{CO_2}$. If minute ventilation is held constant, $ET_{CO_2}$ will reflect the cardiac output passing through the pulmonary vasculature, which is essentially the same as systemic cardiac output. It is this principle that makes $ET_{CO_2}$ monitoring of value in the assessment of perfusion during CPR.

The use of quantitative or semiquantitative $ET_{CO_2}$ as an indicator of the effectiveness of artificial perfusion has received considerable attention in the past decade. Laboratory models of cardiac arrest demonstrated a statistically significant correlation between $ET_{CO_2}$ and coronary perfusion pressure suggesting that $ET_{CO_2}$ could serve as a useful noninvasive method to monitor the effectiveness of resuscitative efforts and to guide therapy. In one clinical study, the initial $ET_{CO_2}$ served to predict which patients would regain a pulse during the resuscitation. Those patients with an $ET_{CO_2} \geq 15$ mmHg on arrival in the emergency department had a greater than 90 percent probability of regaining a pulse, while those patients with an $ET_{CO_2} < 15$ mmHg almost never regained a pulse. In many of these patients, a sudden dramatic increase in the $ET_{CO_2}$ was noticed well before a pulse could be detected. Unfortunately, $ET_{CO_2}$ does not always correlate precisely with coronary perfusion pressure, and the relationship between the two can be affected by therapeutic changes such as adrenergic therapy. While these studies cannot be used as an endorsement for deciding when to quit or continue CPR, they do lend support to the validity of $ET_{CO_2}$ as a reflection of cardiac output. End-tidal $CO_2$ is the most accurate noninvasive method of monitoring CPR effectiveness currently available, and its use is encouraged. The most appropriate way to use $ET_{CO_2}$ is to maintain minute ventilation relatively constant while adjusting the mechanics of CPR chest compression and titrating adrenergic therapy in an effort to maximize the $ET_{CO_2}$.

## Median Frequency of Ventricular Fibrillation

It has long been recognized that the coarseness of the ventricular fibrillation waveform has a rough correlation with the duration of cardiac arrest and the prospects for successful defibrillation with ROSC. The amplitude of the ventricular fibrillation waves (measured manually) has been found to correlate statistically with ROSC, but this relationship is still a rather crude parameter. More recently, there has been an interest in measuring the median frequency (a mathematically derived computer-generated parameter of the ECG), which is a more accurate parameter of the energy of the electrical activity. Brown et al. have reported a correlation between the median frequency of ventricular fibrillation and the duration of cardiac arrest (downtime). They further suggest that median frequency can be used to predict the likelihood of successful defibrillation. Thus, median frequency could be used to help direct resuscitative efforts by guiding therapy aimed at maximizing the median frequency and by indicating when electrical countershock is likely to be effective and should be attempted.

## Invasive Hemodynamic Pressure Monitoring

Laboratory and clinical studies have demonstrated that both aortic pressure and CPP correlate strongly with coronary blood flow and ROSC. Although placement of arterial pressure catheters is a common occurrence in critical care medicine, arterial catheterization is not routinely performed in cardiac arrest patients. This is partially due to the technical difficulties associated with performing this during CPR. However, arterial pressure monitoring provides a very useful parameter to guide resuscitative efforts. The CPR-diastolic arterial pressure is the major predictor of the actual CPP. Thus, adjusting therapeutic interventions to maximize CPR-diastolic arterial pressure will result in greater CPP and improved chances of survival.

Central venous catheterization in addition to arterial or aortic catheterization allows for the accurate measurement of the CPP. Although clearly one of the most useful measurable parameters in human resuscitation, it has only been reported by a few investigators and only as an in-hospital procedure. Thus, out-of-hospital cardiac arrest patients undergoing CPP monitoring have generally been in arrest for an extended period of time. Paradis et al. reported CPP monitoring in 100 patients and found that ROSC correlated with achieving a CPP greater than 15 mmHg. However, the time intervals from onset of arrest to initial CPP readings in the 51 witnessed arrests were usually prolonged, averaging approximately 25 min. Twenty-four patients in this study had ROSC but none survived, suggesting that CPP monitoring after prolonged cardiac arrest is likely to be of limited benefit. Thus, efforts to perform invasive monitoring more rapidly upon hospital arrival or even in the prehospital setting should be pursued. The feasibility of performing prehospital invasive hemodynamic monitoring has been greatly simplified by technological advances yielding commercially available, lightweight, and portable monitoring systems that can easily be transported to the scene of out-of-hospital cardiac arrest victims.

## Central Venous Oxygen Saturation Monitoring

Rivers et al. have reported the use of central venous oximetry in evaluation of cardiac arrest patients. They found that central venous oxygen saturation yielded important information about tissue oxygen delivery/consumption balance and was predictive of ROSC. Lower venous oxygen saturations indicated a more severe oxygen delivery/consumption imbalance and were associated with higher oxygen extraction ratios and a lesser chance of ROSC. Higher venous oxygen saturations were associated with lower oxygen extraction ratios and a higher rate of ROSC. A central venous oxygen saturation of less than 30 percent resulted in a 0 percent ROSC rate, whereas a value greater than 72 percent resulted in a 100 percent ROSC rate. Impending ROSC was characterized by an abrupt or gradual increase in central venous oxygen saturation. A supranormal central venous oxygen saturation, termed *venous hyperoxia*, was frequently seen during the early phase of ROSC, followed by a return to normal levels.

## INVASIVE PERFUSION TECHNIQUES
## Direct Mechanical Ventricular Assistance

Direct mechanical ventricular assistance (DMVA) was first described by Anstadt et al. in 1965, and several laboratory studies have investigated this technique in cardiac arrest models. DMVA utilizes a cup-shaped device that fits around the ventricles and is held in place by a vacuum at the apex of the heart (Fig. 15-3). Cyclic positive and negative pressures are transmitted to a flexible diaphragm on the inner surface of the cup and result in compression and reexpansion of the ventricles, respectively. The major difference between DMVA and open-chest manual compression of the heart is the active ventricular dilatation, which enhances ventricular filling for the next compression phase. DMVA has been shown to generate higher arterial pressures and greater cardiac output than open-chest manual compression. The clinical utility of this technique in the treatment of cardiac

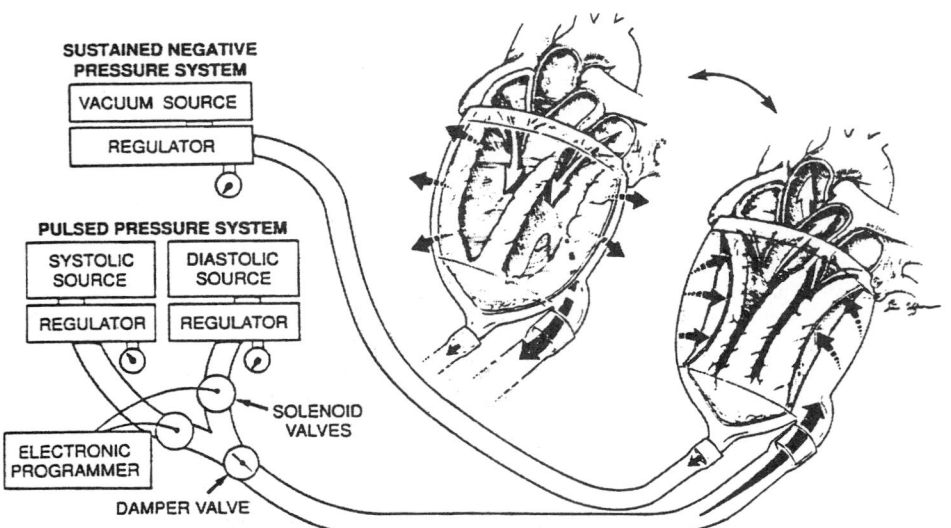

**Fig. 15-3.** Direct mechanical ventricular assistance (DMVA). Schematic diagram of DMVA drive system and cup. Note the device actuates the ventricular myocardium into systolic (right) and diastolic (left) configurations. (From Anstadt MP et al: *Resuscitation* 21:7, 1991, with permission.)

arrest has not been established. The major advantage of DMVA is that it can be sustained for an extended period of time. The major limitation of DMVA is the requirement of a thoracotomy, which largely precludes its use within an effective time frame for most victims of out-of-hospital cardiac arrest.

## Cardiopulmonary Bypass

Cardiopulmonary bypass (CPB) is an effective means of providing sustained global perfusion and has been advocated in the treatment of cardiac arrest. Several laboratory studies have demonstrated improved ROSC and neurologic recovery with CPB compared with standard ACLS interventions. There are also several case series describing the successful use of femorofemoral CPB in the treatment of cardiac arrest patients. The major advantages of CPB are that it can be performed with only a femoral vessel cutdown, artificial perfusion can be sustained for an extended period of time, and perfusion support can be gradually withdrawn. The major disadvantage is the equipment, skill, and time required to perform CPB. These factors make CPB essentially an in-hospital technique, which limits its value in the treatment of victims of out-of-hospital cardiac arrest. However, future technological advances may result in CPB devices that can more easily be used in the prehospital setting.

## Selective Aortic Arch Perfusion

Selective aortic arch perfusion (SAAP) was first described by Manning et al. as a technically less difficult invasive perfusion technique designed for use in the prehospital as well as the in-hospital setting. SAAP uses a large-lumen balloon occlusion catheter positioned in the descending aortic arch to provide selective perfusion of the heart and brain during cardiac arrest (Fig. 15-4). The SAAP catheter is inserted into a femoral artery (percutaneously or via a cutdown) and blindly advanced into the thoracic aorta. With the balloon inflated and pressure cuffs applied to the upper arms, the coronary and cerebral circulations are relatively isolated for brief perfusion. The resuscitation solution infused consists of an oxygenated blood substitute, such as a perfluorocarbon emulsion or polymerized hemoglobin solution, which might contain various agents to enhance restoration of spontaneous cardiac contraction, maintain neuronal viability, and limit both myocardial and neuronal reperfusion injury. One of the major advantages of SAAP is the ability to administer agents to combat reperfusion injury at the moment of or just prior to reperfusion.

The optimal composition of the resuscitation solution is the subject of ongoing research. Paradis et al. described fundamentally the same

technique—selective aortic perfusion and oxygenation (SAPO)—and reported improved coronary perfusion pressures and ROSC using an oxygenated bovine polymerized hemoglobin solution. Manning et al. have demonstrated improved ROSC using an oxygenated perfluorocarbon emulsion that was further enhanced when combined with aortic arch epinephrine administration. Though early laboratory results have been favorable, the efficacy of this invasive perfusion technique in human cardiac arrest has not been clarified.

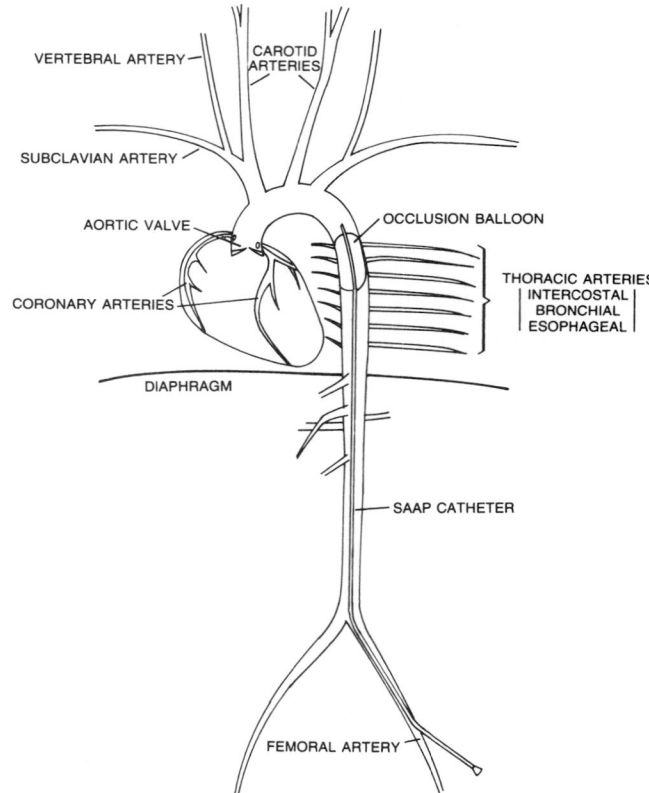

**Fig. 15-4.** Selective aortic arch perfusion (SAAP). Positioning of the SAAP balloon occlusion catheter at the end of the descending aortic arch through a femoral artery. Placement of the balloon at this level restricts flow to aortic arch vessels including coronary arteries. (From Manning JE et al: *Ann Emerg Med* 21:1058, 1992, with permission.)

# BIBLIOGRAPHY

American Heart Association, Emergency Cardiac Care Committee and Subcommittees: Guidelines for cardiopulmonary resuscitation and emergency cardiac care, III: Adult advanced cardiac life support. *JAMA* 268:2199, 1992.

Anstadt MP, Anstadt GL, Lowe JE: Direct mechanical ventricular actuation: A review. *Resuscitation* 21:7, 1991.

Brown CG, Dzwonczyk R, Werman HA, Hamlin RL: Estimating the duration of ventricular fibrillation. *Ann Emerg Med* 18:1181, 1989.

Brown CG, Martin DR, Pepe PE, et al: A comparison of standard-dose and high-dose epinephrine in cardiac arrest outside the hospital: the Multicenter High-dose Epinephrine Study Group. *N Engl J Med* 327:1051, 1992.

Callaham ML, Barton CW: Prediction of outcome of cardiopulmonary resuscitation from end-tidal carbon dioxide concentration. *Crit Care Med* 18:358, 1990.

Callaham M, Madsen CD, Barton CW, et al: A randomized clinical trial of high-dose epinephrine and norepinephrine vs. standard-dose epinephrine in prehospital cardiac arrest. *JAMA* 268:2667, 1992.

Cohen TJ, Tucker KJ, Lurie KG, et al: Active compression-decompression. A new method of cardiopulmonary resuscitation. *JAMA* 267:2916, 1992.

Halperin HR, Tsitlik JE, Gelfand M, et al: A preliminary study of cardiopulmonary resuscitation by circumferential compression of the chest with use of a pneumatic vest. *N Engl J Med* 329:762, 1993.

Little CM, Hobson JL, Brown CG: Angiotensin II effects in a swine model of cardiac arrest. *Ann Emerg Med* 22:244, 1993.

Lurie KG, Shultz JJ, Callaham ML, et al: Evaluation of active compression-decompression CPR in victims of out-of-hospital cardiac arrest. *JAMA* 271:1405, 1994.

Maier GW, Tyson GS, Olsen CO, et al: The physiology of external cardiac massage: High-impulse cardiopulmonary resuscitation. *Circulation* 70:86, 1984.

Manning JE, Murphy CA, Batson DN, et al: Aortic arch versus central venous epinephrine during CPR. *Ann Emerg Med* 22:703, 1993.

Manning JE, Murphy CA, Hertz CM, et al: Selective aortic arch perfusion during cardiac arrest: A new resuscitation technique. *Ann Emerg Med* 21:1058, 1992.

Niemann JT, Criley JM, Rosborough JP, et al: Predictive indices of successful cardiac resuscitation after prolonged arrest and experimental cardiopulmonary resuscitation. *Ann Emerg Med* 14:521, 1985.

Paradis NA, Martin GB, Rivers EP, et al: Coronary perfusion pressure and the return of spontaneous circulation in human cardiopulmonary resuscitation. *JAMA* 263:1106, 1990.

Paradis NA, Rose MI, Gawryl MS: Selective aortic perfusion and oxygenation: An effective adjunct to external chest compression–based cardiopulmonary resuscitation. *J Am Coll Cardiol* 23:497, 1994.

Rivers EP, Martin GB, Smithline H, et al: The clinical implications of continuous central venous oxygen saturation during human CPR. *Ann Emerg Med* 21:1094, 1992.

Sack JB, Kesselbrenner MB, Bregman D: Survival from in-hospital cardiac arrest with interposed abdominal counterpulsation during cardiopulmonary resuscitation. *JAMA* 267:379, 1992.

Safar P, Abramson NS, Angelos M, et al: Emergency cardiopulmonary bypass for resuscitation from prolonged cardiac arrest. *Am J Emerg Med* 8:55, 1990.

Sanders AB, Kern KB, Otto CW, et al: End-tidal carbon dioxide monitoring during cardiopulmonary resuscitation: A prognostic indicator for survival. *JAMA* 262:1347, 1989.

Viskin S, Belhassen B, Roth A, et al: Aminophylline for bradyasystolic cardiac arrest refractory to atropine and epinephrine. *Ann Intern Med* 118:279, 1993.

# 16
# NEONATAL RESUSCITATION AND EMERGENCIES

## Seetha Shankaran
## Eugene E. Cepeda

## NEONATAL RESUSCITATION

Approximately 6 percent of all newborns require life support in the delivery room or nursery, and in those neonates whose birth weights are less than 1500 g, the need for resuscitation rises to 60 percent. Personnel skilled in neonatal resuscitation should be available at every delivery. It is important to anticipate the delivery of the high-risk neonate so that the delivery room personnel may be alerted to the possible need for resuscitation.

The following factors are associated with an increased risk for neonatal resuscitation:

Maternal factors
  Inadequate prenatal care
  Age <16 to >35 years
  History of previous perinatal morbidity or mortality
  Toxemia, hypertension
  Diabetes
  Chronic renal disease
  Anemia
  Drug therapy (e.g. reserpine, lithium carbonate, magnesium, adrenergic blocking agents)
  Substance abuse
  Blood type or group isoimmunization
  Oligohydramnios
Intrapartum factors
  Abnormal presentation
  Caesarean section
  Prolonged labor or precipitous delivery
  Prolonged rupture of membranes, chorioamnionitis
  Cephalopelvic disproportion
  Forceps delivery other than outlet or vacuum extraction
  Prolapsed cord
  Cord compression
  Maternal hypotension, shock
  Analgesic or sedative drugs given within 2 h of delivery
Fetal factors
  Prematurity
  Postmaturity
  Intrauterine growth failure
  Multiple gestation
  Acidosis (fetal scalp capillary monitoring)
  Abnormal fetal heart rate per monitor
  Thick meconium in amniotic fluid
  Congenital infection
  Fetal malformation or edema diagnosed by ultrasound

The following conditions should alert nursery personnel to the possibility of apnea: previous need for resuscitation, premature infants, sepsis and/or meningitis, congenital abnormalities, respiratory distress, or seizures.

### Physiology of Asphyxia

The normal newborn is equipped with physiologic, pharmacologic, and metabolic responses to enable it to survive the hypoxia that develops as a consequence of asphyxia. Generally, brain injury only occurs when the asphyxia is severe enough to impair cerebral blood flow. Initially the injury is reversible, and only longer periods of ischemia lead to permanent damage. The pattern of injury is strongly influenced by the distribution of blood flow. During asphyxia, blood flow is redirected to the heart, brain, and adrenals at the expense of other organs, such as the kidneys and the gastrointestinal tract. Within the brain, flow is directed to the brainstem at the expense of the high cerebral structures such as the cortex. In the preterm neonate, the periventricular white matter is susceptible to injury. In the full-term or postterm neonate the gray matter regions, such as the overlying parasagittal "watershed" cortex, are more vulnerable to ischemic injury. When the asphyxial insult is severe or prolonged, hypoxic multiorgan dysfunction occurs because of the redistribution of organ blood flow and results in cardiopulmonary distress, renal failure, impaired hepatic function, seizures and encephalopathy, gastrointestinal dysfunction, and coagulopathies.

## Principles of Resuscitation

The Apgar Score (Table 16-1) is assessed at 1 and 5 min of age for every newly delivered infant. Although the scoring system has been useful in evaluating the condition of the newborn, 1 min is too long to wait to make the decision to initiate resuscitation. If the 5-min score is less than 7, additional scores are obtained every 5 min for a total of 20 min.

Perinatal asphyxia is currently defined as the presence of the following: umbilical artery acidemia (pH <7.00), 5-min Apgar score of 0 to 3, neonatal neurologic sequelae, and multiorgan dysfunction.

## Equipment

The following is a list of the equipment necessary for resuscitation.

1. Bag and mask with manometer attached, connected to a source of 100% oxygen. Oxygen should be heated and humidified. The bag should be a rubber anesthesia bag, a rebreathing bag of 500-mL capacity, or a self-inflating bag designed for newborns.
2. Rubber face masks of varying sizes 1, 2, 3, and 4.
3. Wall suction, sterile catheters, and bulb syringes.
4. DeLee suction catheter with mucus trap.
5. Laryngoscope with 0 and 1 blades.
6. Oral endotracheal tubes with stylet—sizes 2.5, 3.0, 3.5, and 4.0 mm.
7. Radiant heater with servomechanism.
8. Sterile umbilical vessel catheterization tray.
9. Glucose oxidase blood test strips.
10. A heart rate monitor with easy applicable leads.
11. Intravenous infusion equipment.
12. Transcutaneous oxygen monitor or saturation pulse oximeter.
13. Appropriate light.
14. Infant stethoscope.
15. Nasogastric tubes, 5F and 8F.
16. Clock with sweep-second hand.

**Table 16-1.** The Apgar Score

| Sign | 0 | 1 | 2 |
| --- | --- | --- | --- |
| Heart rate | Absent | <100/min | >100/min |
| Respiratory effort | Absent | Weak cry | Strong cry |
| Muscle tone | Limp | Some flexion | Good flexion |
| Reflex irritability (when feet stimulated) | No response | Some motion | Cry |
| Color | Blue: pale | Body pink; extremities blue | Pink |

## Steps to Follow During Resuscitation

### Maintain Body Temperature

Maintain infant below the level of the placenta prior to clamping the cord. When the cord is clamped, blot the infant dry with a sterile towel and place the infant under a preheated radiant warmer on a sterile table. Neonates should be placed either on the back or the left side somewhat in the Trendelenburg position, with the neck in a neutral position.

### Clear the Airway

Gently suction the nose and mouth with a bulb syringe, DeLee trap, or mechanical suction apparatus with an 8F suction catheter. A 5- to 10-s examination should be performed to determine the need for resuscitation. This examination should include an assessment of heart rate, respiratory effort, color, and muscular activity. If the infant has a lusty cry, is pink, has spontaneous respirations, and a heart rate above 120/min (Apgar > 8), no further therapy is needed.

### Initiate Breathing

If the infant is apneic or the heart rate is slow and irregular (<100 beats per minute) and the color is cyanotic (Apgar 4 to 7), administer positive-pressure ventilation with the mask over the infant's face and 100% oxygen. The respiratory rate should be maintained at 40 breaths/min with pressure applied to gently move the chest wall. In an infant who has not yet taken a breath, over 40 cmH$_2$O pressure may be necessary to expand the lungs. In mildly depressed infants, this will produce a prompt increase in heart rate and the onset of regular spontaneous respirations. If no improvement is noted in 15 to 30 s and the condition deteriorates (Apgar ≤ 4), the trachea should be intubated and assisted ventilation continued.

### Endotracheal Intubation

#### *Indications*

1. Mechanical ventilation.
2. To clear the trachea of meconium.

#### *Equipment*

Pediatric laryngoscope handle
Laryngoscope blade no. 0 for infants < 3000 g
Laryngoscope blade no. 1 for infants > 2000 g
Self-inflating bag and mask apparatus
Adapter
Scissors
Stylet
Tape
Suction apparatus
Tincture of benzoin

#### *Procedure*

1. Check that the light source on the laryngoscope blade is working. Place the infant supine and suction the mouth and oropharynx. Monitor the heart rate and color.
2. Hold the laryngoscope in the right hand and open the infant's mouth by sliding your right index finger between the infant's right upper and lower gums. Insert the laryngoscope into the infant's mouth by sliding the blade down against your index finger. Push the tongue with the blade to the left.
3. Advance the blade, and lift. You should be able to see the epiglottis. Remove your index finger, hold the blade with left hand.
4. Pass the endotracheal tube along the right side of the mouth and advance it past the vocal cords. The stylet should be gently removed while holding the tube firmly in place. The tip of the tube should not go more than 2.5 cm beyond the cords.
5. Attach the resuscitation bag to the tube and listen for breath sounds that should be equal on both the right and left chest. The

infant's oxygen saturation should improve. A chest x-ray will confirm proper placement.

6. Paint the skin with tincture of benzoin and tape the tube securely.

**Cardiac Massage**

If the heart rate is below 50 bpm with assisted ventilation, cardiac massage should be initiated by placing both hands around the infant's chest with two thumbs over the midsternum so that the sternum will be depressed two thirds of the distance to the vertebral column at 120 compressions per minute. Cardiac massage may be stopped periodically to assess improvement, and ventilation and cardiac massage should be synchronized (1:3 ratio). The chest should expand, bilateral breath sounds should be heard in the axilla, and heart rate should increase if the resuscitation is effective and the endotracheal tube is in good position. *In most instances* it is possible to obtain an adequate response with the use of external cardiac massage and assisted ventilation. If there is no response to these measures, drug therapy should be considered. Any route of access to the circulatory system is acceptable, including a peripheral vein, the umbilical vein, or an umbilical artery.

**Umbilical Artery Catheterization**

*Indications*

1. To measure arterial blood gases
2. To monitor continuous blood pressure
3. To infuse fluids

*Equipment*

2 × 2 Sponges—5
Curved hemostat
Medicine glasses—2
Scalpel blade, no. 11
Iris forceps, curved, serrated end, no teeth—2
Lacrimal probe
Needle holder
Debriding scissors
Umbilical tape 6″
Knife handle
4–0 silk suture with needle
Three-way stopcock
10-mL syringes—2
Iodine solution
3.5F catheter for infant < 1200 g
5.0F catheter for infant > 1200 g

*Procedure*

1. Immobilize the patient. Measure the distance between the umbilicus and the right shoulder.
2. Clean the umbilical stump and surrounding area with iodine solution. Drape the umbilical area but leave the head and feet uncovered.
3. Tie the base of the cord with the umbilical tape to minimize blood loss.
4. Cut the cord cleanly across its length to 1 cm with the scalpel. The arteries are small and have pin-point openings. The vein is larger and has thinner walls and a larger opening.
5. Grasp the edge of the cord with the forceps. Using the iris forceps enlarge the opening of the umbilical artery first with the tip of one arm of the forceps.
6. Insert both arms of the forceps to dilate the artery so that it will accept the catheter.
7. The length of the catheter inserted for the low position is two thirds of the distance from the umbilicus to the right shoulder and for the high position, the full measurement from the right shoulder to the umbilicus.

8. Attach the three-way stopcock and aspirate blood with a syringe. Clear the catheter with normal saline.
9. Anchor the catheter with silk suture to the umbilical stump.
10. Check the position of the catheter tip with an x-ray. It should be at the level of L4 for the low position, or between T6 and T9, which is above the diaphragm, for the high position.

Patency of the umbilical arterial line can be maintained by a continuous infusion of fluid. The catheter should be removed when the need for arterial blood gas monitoring is no longer necessary (oxygen requirement ≤ 80 percent) or complications occur.

*Complications*

Possible complications of umbilical artery catheterization are infection, thrombosis and vasospasm, and hemorrhage. Renal hypertension is a delayed complication.

**Umbilical Vein Catheterization**

The most expedient procedure for obtaining vascular access is to insert the venous catheter through the umbilicus via the umbilical vein, and the ductus venosus into the inferior vena cava. The venous catheter should be inserted 10 to 12 cm and anchored to the abdominal wall. Obtain radiographs of chest and abdomen to rule out other abnormalities and evaluate the position of the catheter.

## Drug Therapy in Resuscitation

There is a very minor role for drug therapy in resuscitation. Most resuscitative efforts in the delivery room respond to adequate support of ventilation and circulation without drug therapy.

**Dextrose**

To provide metabolic substrate and expansion of plasma volume, 10% dextrose in water ($D_{10}W$) at 100 mL/kg per day or 6 to 8 mg/kg per minute should be infused. If the Dextrostix is < 45 mg/dL, 5 mL/kg of 10 or 15% glucose solution should be infused; 25% dextrose infusions should be avoided because of the risk of rebound hypoglycemia.

**Epinephrine**

To stimulate heart rate if it is under 120/min, 0.1 mL/kg of a 1:10,000 solution may be given through the endotracheal tube or intravenously. Cardiac massage should continue following epinephrine administration.

**Naloxone**

To reverse narcotic depression, 0.01 mg/kg of a neonatal solution (0.2 mg/mL) may be administered intravenously, subcutaneously, or through the endotracheal tube. The time for peak concentration of transplacentally acquired narcotics in the fetus is 2 h, following administration of medication to the mother so that delivery of the fetus at that time would predispose the fetus to maximal depression.

**Isoproterenol**

If epinephrine has failed to raise the heart rate to at least 120 beats per minute, 1:10,000 solution or 0.05 to 0.1 μg/min may be infused.

**Bicarbonate**

In the presence of metabolic acidosis, 2 to 3 mEq/kg of sodium bicarbonate should be administered as an intravenous infusion. A continuous infusion may be necessary (not to exceed 8 mEq/kg per day) if acidosis is protracted.

**Dopamine**

Dopamine should be initiated to raise the blood pressure after adequate fluids have been administered. At low doses (2 to 5 μg/kg per minute) dopamine preserves renal and mesenteric perfusion; at higher doses (10 to 20 mg/kg per minute) it has both inotropic and vasoactive properties through α- and β-adrenergic effects.

Certain neonatal conditions require specific measures during resuscitation besides those outlined above.

## Neonatal Shock

The risk factors for shock and hypotension in the newborn infant are low birth weight, maternal sepsis, prolapsed cord, and acute onset of maternal vaginal bleeding. Clinical signs of hypovolemia are pallor, tachycardia, grunting respirations in absence of pulmonary disease, mottling of skin, poor capillary filling, thready pulse and hypotension (systolic < 45 mmHg in a 1000-g premature neonate or < 60 mmHg in a term infant), and persistent metabolic acidosis. A hematocrit should be obtained, and if anemia (hematocrit < 45 vol %) or hypotension are diagnosed, immediate plasma expansion in the form of packed RBC 5 mL/kg or whole blood, fresh-frozen plasma, Plasmanate, or 5% salt-poor albumin 10 to 20 mL/kg should be given intravenously over 10 min.

## Meconium Staining

Meconium staining of the amniotic fluid varies from 0.5 to 20 percent of all births. Aspiration of thick meconium carries a 20 to 50 percent mortality rate; however, with proper management it is almost entirely preventable. When gross meconium is noted at the time of delivery, the following procedure should be followed. After delivery of the infant's head (but before delivery of the shoulders), the nose, mouth, and pharynx should be thoroughly suctioned with a DeLee suction catheter. Repeat suctioning of the upper airway should be performed as the infant is placed under the radiant warmer. The trachea should then be visualized with a laryngoscope and meconium aspirated by direct suctioning through an endotracheal tube. Suctioning should be repeated until no more meconium is present in the trachea. The infant may then be ventilated with positive pressure as indicated. Failure to clear the trachea before assisted or spontaneous ventilation may result in dissemination of the meconium through the airways.

## Duration of Resuscitation

Resuscitation should be continued for a minimum of 30 min. Neonatal morbidity and mortality are high after 20 to 30 min of cardiac asystole and result in encephalopathy in term infants.

## Complications of Asphyxia

Infants who were successfully resuscitated at birth should have continuous monitoring of vital signs, blood gases, hematocrit, dextrose, blood pressure, fluid status, and clinical condition. Complications associated with severe asphyxia are seizures, hypoxic-ischemic encephalopathy, intracranial hemorrhage, inappropriate ADH secretion, hypocalcemia, persistent pulmonary hypertension, ischemic cardiomyopathy, hypovolemia or shock, necrotizing enterocolitis, renal failure, and coagulopathy.

## NEONATAL EMERGENCIES

### Seizures

Seizures in neonates may represent primary central nervous system (CNS) disease or a systemic or metabolic disorder. Recent data suggest that seizure activity itself may adversely affect the growing brain.

### Types of Seizures

#### Subtle

Subtle seizures occur in both preterm and term neonates. These consist of ocular movements, facial, oral, or lingual movements and respiratory manifestations, such as apnea or stertorous breathing.

#### Tonic

These are characteristic of premature infants. The seizures appear as decerebrate or decorticate posturing.

#### Multifocal Clonic

These seizures are seen in term infants. They are initially noted in one limb and migrate to another part of the body.

#### Focal Clonic

These are well localized and are accompanied by specific sharp activity on the EEG. They occur more commonly in full-term infants.

#### Myoclonic

These seizures are expressed as single or multiple jerks of flexion of the upper or lower extremities. They are rare and occur in both premature and full-term infants.

### Differentiation of Seizures

It is important to distinguish seizures from tremors or jitteriness, which may be seen in infants who have hypocalcemia, hypoglycemia, drug withdrawal, or no identifiable morbidity. Tremors are uniform fine movements that respond to sensory stimuli, stop with manual stabilization, and do not occur spontaneously. They are not accompanied by eye, oral, or lingual movements.

### Causes of Seizures

#### Hypoxic-Ischemic Encephalopathy

This is the most common cause of seizures. The seizures occur between 6 and 18 h of life. In full-term neonates the hypoxic injury may result in a cerebral hemorrhage, water-shed infarct, posterior fossa hematoma, or subarachnoid or subdural hemorrhage. In premature infants, hypoxic injury often results in periventricular-intraventricular hemorrhage. This type of seizure has a poor prognosis.

#### Metabolic Disturbances

The metabolic disturbances associated with neonatal seizures include hypoglycemia, hypocalcemia, hypomagnesemia, hyperammonemia, hypernatremia, and hyponatremia. Hypoglycemia, hypocalcemia, and hypomagnesemia are often found in premature infants with perinatal asphyxia. Hypernatremia occurs in neonates with dehydration secondary to excessive fluid losses or treatment with large doses of sodium bicarbonate. Hyponatremia may be seen secondary to inappropriate ADH secretion or acute volume overload. Inborn errors of amino acid metabolism also may present as seizures.

#### Meningitis or Encephalitis

These conditions include bacterial meningitis and encephalitis associated with TORCH complex (toxoplasmosis, rubella, cytomegalovirus infection, and herpes simplex infection) or Coxsackie B encephalitis.

#### Developmental Abnormalities

These include congenital hydrocephalus, microcephaly, and other congenital brain anomalies.

#### Drug Withdrawal

Drug withdrawal from maternal use of methadone, barbiturates, alcohol, pentazocine (Talwin), and tripelennamine (Pyribenzamine) rarely presents as seizures.

#### Pyridoxine Dependence

This condition occurs rarely but must be considered in neonatal seizures unresponsive to standard therapy.

## Maternal Anesthesia

A rare cause of seizures is inadvertent fetal scalp injection of maternal local anesthetic agents.

## Stroke

Neonatal stroke diagnosed by computed tomography (CT) has recently been described in term infants with focal motor seizures. Neonatal stroke may occur in the setting of diverse cerebrovascular disorders such as hypoxic-ischemic encephalopathy, polycythemia, acute severe hypertension, and cocaine use.

## Diagnosis of Seizures

A careful history, including intrapartum monitoring data and physical examination, are essential when considering drug withdrawal, birth asphyxia, or metabolic disorders as a cause of the seizures. A lumbar puncture with analysis of cell count, culture and Gram stain along with blood specimens for culture, sugar, calcium, magnesium, and BUN should be obtained. The skull x-ray, echoencephalogram, and EEG can be obtained after the seizures have been controlled. In a full-term infant a CT scan of the head to look for ischemic injury may be necessary as an echoencephalogram may not provide adequate visualization of the subarachnoid space or posterior fossa. Recently, positron emission tomography of the head has been utilized to evaluate the effects of asphyxia and seizures on cerebral blood flow.

## Treatment of Seizures

Repeated seizures in neonates may be accompanied by hypoventilation and apnea, resulting in hypercapnia and hypoxemia. Increase in cerebral blood flow and arterial hypertension occur with neonatal seizures. Treatment of seizures should be initiated while awaiting results of laboratory data. An intravenous access route should be established immediately and the airway maintained; assisted ventilation should be initiated if apnea persists. Hypoglycemia and hypocalcemia should be treated as stated earlier in "Neonatal Resuscitation." Hypomagnesemia is often associated with hypocalcemia and should be treated by intravenous administration of 2 to 4 mL of a 2% magnesium sulfate solution.

The anticonvulsant drugs used most frequently include phenobarbital and diphenylhydantoin. The loading dosage of phenobarbital is 20 mg/kg IV given slowly over 10 min, and the maintenance dose is 5 mg/kg per day IM or PO in two divided doses. If the initial 20 mg/kg dose of phenobarbital is not effective in controlling the seizures, additional doses of 5 mg/kg may be administered every 5 min until the seizures have ceased or the total dose of 40 mg/kg has been reached. In unresponsive cases, diphenylhydantoin may be administered with a similar loading dose followed by a maintenance dose of 3 to 5 mg/kg per day by the IV route in only two divided doses 20 min apart to avoid disturbance of cardiac function. Lorazepam is recommended for status epilepticus, as long as ventilation and blood pressure are supported. The dose of lorazepam is 0.01 mg/kg administered intravenously. Infants with pyridoxine dependence respond immediately to an intravenous injection of 50 to 100 mg of pyridoxine.

## Diaphragmatic Hernia

A failure of development of the posterolateral parts of the diaphragm at Bochdalek's foramen or retrosternally at Morgagni's foramen allows herniation of the gut into the chest cavity. Left-sided Bochdalek's hernias are more common than those on the right. The defect occurs in one out of 2200 births. Associated anomalies with diaphragmatic hernias include congenital heart disease, genitourinary anomalies, gastrointestinal anomalies, hydronephrosis, and cystic kidneys. Frequently the lungs are hypoplastic bilaterally and have abnormal pulmonary vasculature predisposing the infant to pulmonary hypertension.

Fifty percent of fetuses with diaphragmatic hernia have difficulty swallowing, and the condition is therefore associated with polyhydramnios. The diagnosis can often be made by prenatal ultrasonography.

## Clinical and Radiographic Findings

The clinical findings are localized to the respiratory and digestive tracts. The chest is large, while the abdomen is scaphoid. Bowel sounds are heard in the left chest, and the heart is displaced to the right. Dyspnea, cyanosis, retractions, and vomiting are proportional to the amount of abdominal viscera herniated into the thorax. Radiologic study will reveal air-filled loops of bowel in the chest cavity and an absent diaphragmatic margin. The heart is often displaced and the lungs are small in size.

## Management

Immediate surgical repair is a method of treatment, and the neonate should be stabilized as much as possible prior to surgery. Alternatively, the neonate can be placed on extracorporeal membrane oxygenation (ECMO) prior to repair. The infant should be intubated immediately, and little or no attempt should be made to ventilate with a mask. The endotracheal tube should be positioned above the carina. Rapid ventilatory rates and low peak inspirator pressures are used to ventilate the infant and prevent reactive respiratory acidosis and hypercarbia, which are potentially conducive to the development of pulmonary hypertension. A large-caliber 10F tube should be placed in the stomach with low continuous suction applied. An umbilical artery catheter is useful to monitor blood gases and pH. Any acidemia should be corrected and the pH maintained in the alkalotic range (pH > 7.45) if possible. Intravenous fluids should be given and the patient kept warm. Vasodilator therapy with tolazoline 2 mg/kg per hour infusion may need to be initiated (if pulmonary hypertension develops) prior to surgical repair.

The outcome of management of diaphragmatic hernia is dependent on pulmonary parenchymal and vascular hypoplasia, as well as the complex syndrome of persistent fetal circulation. The morbidity is higher when the symptoms present at birth and when the diaphragmatic hernia is detected prenatally. Morgagni hernias, if they do not affect cardiac output, generally have a better prognosis than do Bochdalek's hernias. Common complications that occur pre- and postoperatively are pneumothorax, persistent fetal circulation, overdistension of hypoplastic lungs, and chylothorax. The recent introduction of the use of ECMO for infants with persistent pulmonary hypertension after hernia repair has made a minimal impact on prognosis.

## Tracheoesophageal Fistula

A defect in the separation of the trachea from the esophagus results in a persistent channel connecting the trachea and the esophagus. There are five types of tracheoesophageal fistulas (TEF) which are descriptive of the malformation possible: (1) esophageal atresia with a distal communication between the trachea and the esophagus, the most common presentation (85 percent); (2) isolated esophageal atresia, occurring less commonly; (3) isolated TEF; (4) esophageal atresia with a proximal TEF; and (5) esophageal atresia with a double TEF.

Tracheoesophageal fistulas occur in one out of every 4500 births. One third of the affected infants weigh less than 2500 g. The incidence of associated anomalies with TEF ranges from 40 to 55 percent. The smaller the infant with TEF, the greater the number of other associated anomalies. Congenital heart malformation, vertebral anomalies, imperforate anus, and radial aplasia are common associations.

## Diagnosis

The inability to pass a catheter more than 20 cm through the gastrointestinal tract is the hallmark of esophageal atresia. An x-ray may show the air-filled proximal pouch, and if the catheter is left in place, it may coil in the proximal esophagus. Recurrent pneumonias occur in infants with an H-type (isolated TEF) fistula.

## Management

It is important to provide respiratory support by assisted ventilation if needed to correct acidosis before any surgical repair can be undertaken. A plastic sump catheter should be left in the pouch and connected to constant, low-pressure suction. The patient should be maintained in the reverse Trendelenburg or semi-Fowler position to prevent further reflux of gastric secretions through the fistula into the trachea. Intravenous fluids and antibiotics are indicated. Other coexistent problems such as a heart defect should be evaluated. Primary anastomosis is done in cases of esophageal atresia with a distal tracheoesophageal fistula.

The majority (80 percent) of infants with TEF survive. Operative mortality is low. Complications of surgery are pneumonia, atelectasis, anastomotic leak, anastomotic strictures, and (rarely) recurrent fistulas.

## Pulmonary Air Leaks

Pulmonary air leaks are a common occurrence in the neonatal intensive care unit. The air may present as a spectrum that includes pneumothorax, pulmonary interstitial emphysema, pneumomediastinum, pneumopericardium, and pneumoperitoneum.

Spontaneous pneumothorax can occur in term and postterm infants following intrapartum asphyxia and meconium aspiration. Currently, however, pneumothorax has increased in incidence with the use of continuous positive airway pressure, positive end-expiratory pressure (PEEP), mechanical ventilation, and cardiopulmonary resuscitation. Uneven ventilation caused by aspirated blood, mucus, meconium, and amniotic fluid debris can also result in an air leak. Atelectasis, poor ventilation, and air trapping are common predisposing factors. The premature, low-birth-weight infant with surfactant deficiency has a high incidence of air leaks (30 percent) as does the newborn with meconium aspiration syndrome (10 percent).

## Signs and Symptoms

The signs and symptoms of an air leak are those of respiratory distress and often present as an acute clinical deterioration. Grunting respirations and intercostal, sternal, and subcostal retractions may be seen. Cyanosis, elevated respiratory rate, and elevated heart rate are common. Auscultation of the chest will reveal decreased breath sounds on the affected side of a pneumothorax, distant heart sounds, and a shift of the mediastinum. Transillumination of the chest with a high-intensity lamp may aid in the diagnosis. A chest x-ray is diagnostic. The accuracy can be improved with a cross-table lateral film of the chest taken along with the anteroposterior and lateral views.

## Treatment

An asymptomatic pneumothorax that is less than 20 percent of the volume of the affected side may be followed clinically with no therapy and with serial radiographic studies every 4 h. Any pneumothorax with severe respiratory distress and clinical deterioration will need emergency treatment. When there is mediastinal shift and cardiovascular collapse, rapid decompression at the fourth intercostal space with a 21-gauge needle attached to a three-way stopcock and a large syringe can be life-saving.

## Thoracostomy

### *Indications*

1. To decompress tension pneumothorax, which results in decreased venous return, decreased cardiac output, and low blood pressure.
2. To relieve respiratory compromise in which there is decreased ventilation, increased work of breathing, as well as hypoxia and hypercarbia.
3. To drain pleural fluid.

### *Equipment*

Sterile towels—4
4 × 4 Sterile gauze pads—6
Curved hemostat
Scalpel
Scalpel blade, no. 15
Needle holder
000 silk suture
5-mL syringe
10F chest tube for infant <1500 g
12F chest tube for infant >1500 g
Stopcock
Chest tube drainage system
6-ft connecting tubing
Wall suction gauge
Iodine solution
Lidocaine, 1%

### *Procedure*

1. Restrain the patient in the supine position and extend the arm to 90° on the affected side. Monitor heart rate, respiratory rate, and oxygen saturation, if possible.
2. Mark the site for placement of the tube. Placement of the tube is at the 2nd or 3rd intercostal space on the midclavicular line. Posterior placement of the chest tube is at the 5th or 6th intercostal space on the anterior axillary line.
3. Clean the area with iodine solution. Infiltrate the site of insertion with lidocaine and then infiltrate the intercostal muscles and parietal pleura. Incise the skin over the rib, 1 to 1.5 cm.
4. Take the curved hemostat and with the tip in the incision enter the chest cavity just above the rib. Avoid the intercostal nerve, artery, and vein, which run on the lower edge of the rib.
5. Spread the hemostat open and slide the chest tube between the blades of the hemostat to the point where the side holes on the tube are within the pleural cavity. Connect the tube to a water-sealed vacuum system and apply 5 to 10 cm of negative pressure.
6. Increase the pressure to reduce the pneumothorax, if necessary.
7. Close the skin wound and secure the chest tube with silk suture. Verify the position of the chest tube with a chest x-ray. The lung should reexpand promptly following evacuation of the air in the pleural space.

## Omphalocele and Gastroschisis

An omphalocele is a defect in the umbilical ring which allows the intestines in a sac to protrude out of the abdominal cavity. A gastroschisis is a defect in the abdominal wall that allows the antenatal evisceration of abdominal structures, without a sac being present. There is some controversy as to the exact embryology of the two conditions.

Omphaloceles are found in one out of 6000 to 10,000 births, while gastroschisis occurs twice as frequently in the newborn population. Omphaloceles have a higher (37 percent) incidence of associated anomalies including chromosomal abnormalities. Three specific syndromes are associated with omphalocele: the upper midline pentalogy of Cantrell, Haller, and Ravitch (sternal, ventral, diaphragmatic, pericardial, and cardiac defects); the lower midline syndrome (vesicointestinal fissure); and the Beckwith-Wiedemann syndrome (macroglossia, visceromegaly, and hypoglycemia).

## Management

The emergency management of the two conditions is not different, especially when the sac in an omphalocele is ruptured. The eviscerated bowel should be wrapped in saline-soaked gauze and placed in a plastic bag to protect it from hypothermia and evaporative losses. A nasogastric tube should be inserted to decompress the intestines. Rapid infusion of 20 mL/kg of 5% Ringer's lactate may be necessary to restore vital signs, after which the infusion should be adjusted to maintain a urine output of at least 2 mL/kg per hour. Intravenous antibiotics should be administered.

Primary fascial closure is the treatment of choice and is often accomplished within hours after birth. When the defect is large, a Silastic silo may be used, but survival, nonetheless, correlates with rapid closure and removal of the prosthesis.

Complications include gastroesophageal reflux, malabsorption, diarrhea, dehydration, and failure to thrive. The mortality of omphalocele is 25 to 30 percent, largely as a result of congenital heart disease and sepsis, while death in patients with gastroschisis is associated with intestinal atresia.

## Necrotizing Enterocolitis

Necrotizing enterocolitis is a disease entity that affects the asphyxiated or stressed premature infant of less than 2000-g weight. Fullterm newborns with polycythemia or congenital heart disease and those who have had umbilical arterial or venous catheters in situ have been reported to also be at risk for necrotizing enterocolitis.

The exact cause of necrotizing enterocolitis remains unknown, and it is likely that there are multiple factors that ultimately lead to stasis, ischemia, and infection of the bowel wall. The risk factors include hypertonic feeding solutions producing damage to mucosal epithelium of the intestine, patent ductus arteriosus and episodes of apnea diverting blood flow away from the gastrointestinal tract, ischemia following exchange transfusions, and infections with *Escherichia coli, Klebsiella pseudomonas, Clostridium* species, coronavirus, rotavirus, and other enteroviruses.

### Signs and Symptoms

The signs and symptoms seen in decreasing frequency are abdominal distension, gastric distension, retention of gastric feeds, apnea, gastrointestinal bleeding, and lethargy. Other signs are abdominal tenderness, redness of abdominal wall, and the presence of reducing substances in the stool.

### Diagnosis

A supine anteroposterior and cross-table lateral and upright view will aid in the radiographic diagnosis. Nonspecific findings are distension, air-fluid levels, and separation of intestinal loops suggesting mural edema. Pneumatosis intestinalis is the radiographic hallmark, and its presence indicates gas in the bowel wall. Portal venous gas is an ominous sign, and pneumoperitoneum indicates perforation of the bowel.

### Medical Management

The medical management consists of bowel rest, with the infant receiving nothing by mouth and gastric decompression with a nasogastric tube. Cultures of blood, urine, and CSF should be obtained and systemic antibiotics administered. The blood pressure and hydration status should be maintained with liberal use of crystalloids and Plasmanate. Fluid intake may have to be increased to 200 mL/kg per 24 h and inotropic agents used if needed. Thrombocytopenia, neutropenia,

and disseminated intravascular coagulopathy are often seen in neonates who are deteriorating, and platelet transfusions should be administered if there is evidence of systemic or gastrointestinal bleeding. Respiratory support may be required, and any acidosis should be corrected. Patients with early necrotizing enterocolitis should have close clinical observations and serial x-rays to look for signs of gangrene or intestinal perforation. The medical treatment includes bowel rest for 2 weeks, with nutritional support with parenteral alimentation. The complications of necrotizing enterocolitis are bowel stricture, fistula, abscess, malabsorption, and failure to thrive.

### Surgical Management

Pneumoperitoneum related to signs of necrotizing enterocolitis is an absolute indication for surgical repair. Recent data indicate that paracentesis, indicative of intestinal gangrene prior to intestinal perforation, may be an indication for surgery. Persistent acidosis, oliguria, abdominal wall erythema, and portal vein air are associated with advanced disease. The surgical repair consists of removal of the segment of involved bowel and an enterostomy. Reanastomosis is usually performed after 4 to 6 weeks of bowel rest.

## Apnea

Apnea is the absence of respirations for a period of 20 s if it is associated with a decrease in heart rate of 80 bpm and/or accompanied by cyanosis or pallor. Apnea is categorized as *central apnea* when it is of CNS origin. There are no respiratory efforts and no gas flow in central apnea. In *obstructive apnea,* there is impaired gas flow in the presence of respiratory effort. In *mixed apnea,* there are components of both of the above. *Periodic breathing* is apnea of a few seconds duration in a 20-s span of otherwise normal breathing. In term infants, apnea is never physiologic and is usually secondary to a serious disorder.

### Pathophysiology

Apnea and periodic breathing are thought to arise from an immature respiratory center. There is an abnormal biphasic response to hypoxia with a period of tachypnea of several seconds followed by apnea. In premature babies there is a shift in the carbon dioxide curve so that higher levels of $CO_2$ are required for respiration. Airway muscle weakness as well as skeletal muscle weakness probably contribute to the problem. Lastly, it may be that the preterm infant may have problems during the sleep-waking states, much like shifts from one sleep state to another are accompanied by respiratory instability in adults.

### Clinical Presentation

Apnea may occur during any time in the neonatal period. It is always abnormal in the first day of life. After the age of 3 days in a preterm neonate, if it is not associated with any pathology, it may be called *benign apnea* of prematurity. Apnea is always abnormal in a term newborn. Siblings of children who have died of sudden infant death syndrome have periods of apnea. The pathologic conditions associated with apnea are as follows:

1. Central nervous system: Asphyxia, cerebral infarction, hydrocephalus, intracranial hemorrhage, meningitis, and seizures.
2. Cardiovascular: Congestive heart failure, patent ductus arteriosus.
3. Respiratory: Chronic lung disease, hypoxia, pneumonia, obstruction.
4. Digestive system: Necrotizing enterocolitis, overfeeding, vagal response to a nasogastric tube.
5. Other causes: Anemia, polycythemia, sepsis, temperature instability, hyponatremia, hyperkalemia, hypocalcemia, hypermagne-

semia, and high serum levels of phenobarbital, diazepam, opiates, and chloral hydrate.

## Laboratory Studies

CBC, electrolytes, calcium, glucose, blood gases, drug screen, chest x-ray, ECG, lumbar puncture, EEG, and an abdominal flat-plate film may be indicated on admission. Further workup may be necessary.

## Treatment

All infants who have benign apnea of prematurity will respond to tactile stimulation. When apnea is recurrent and sustained, specific treatment is indicated.

Theophylline, 5 to 6 mg/kg as PO or IV loading dose, followed by 2 mg/kg q 2 h as maintenance. An alternative drug is caffeine citrate, PO or IV as loading dose, with 2.5 to 5 mg/kg as maintenance dose.

Continuous positive airway pressure (CPAP) at 2 to 4 cmH$_2$O may be applied if the above drugs do not resolve the problem.

Mechanical ventilation with endotracheal intubation should be initiated if there is prolonged apnea or repeated episodes not responsive to the above medications.

## The Cyanotic Newborn

Cyanosis in the neonate may be central or peripheral. *Central cyanosis* is defined as cyanosis of the tongue, mucous membranes, and peripheral skin and indicates the presence of 5 g or more of reduced hemoglobin. *Peripheral cyanosis* is defined as a blue discoloration confined to the skin of the extremities; the arterial saturation will be greater than 94 percent. Peripheral cyanosis is common in the neonate and may persist for 2 to 3 days. It is usually due to vasomotor instability secondary to a cold environment.

## Causes of Central Cyanosis

Normal newborn infants have a P$_{O_2}$ above 50 mmHg by 5 to 10 min of age; hence it is pathologic for central cyanosis to persist beyond 20 min after birth.

### Cyanotic Heart Disease

Congenital heart disease presenting with cyanosis secondary to intracardiac right-to-left shunt includes transposition of the great vessels, tricuspid atresia, truncus arteriosus, tetralogy of Fallot and total anomalous pulmonary venous return with obstruction, pulmonary atresia, and preductal coarctation.

### Lung Disease Associated with Cyanosis

These lung disorders include hyaline membrane disease, pneumonia, meconium aspiration syndrome, and persistent fetal circulation due to pneumonia or asphyxia. Mechanical interference with lung function by air leaks (pneumothorax), diaphragmatic hernia, lobar emphysema, or mucous plugs also cause cyanosis.

### Central Nervous System Disorders

Intracerebral hemorrhage, when severe, may be associated with shock and cyanosis.

### Polycythemia

The increased viscosity and stagnation of blood may produce apparent cyanosis.

### Shock and Sepsis

Shock and sepsis result in alveolar hypoventilation.

### Methemoglobinemia

Methemoglobinemia is due to reduced oxygen-carrying capacity of the blood because of abnormal hemoglobin.

## Diagnostic Approach to Central Cyanosis

### Physical Examination

Neonates with cyanosis secondary to cyanotic heart disease rarely have respiratory symptoms other than tachypnea. A murmur may be present. Neonates with lung disease producing cyanosis have respiratory distress, grunting, tachypnea, and sternal and intercostal retractions. The cyanotic infant with CNS disturbances or sepsis has apnea, bradycardia, lethargy, and seizures. Neonates with methemoglobinemia have minimal distress in spite of their cyanotic appearance.

### Blood-Gas Profile and Response to 100% O$_2$ Breathing

The "hyperoxia test" (the response in Pa$_{O_2}$ to 100 percent oxygen breathing) may be of use in distinguishing heart disease from other causes of cyanosis. The neonate with cyanotic heart disease will not demonstrate any increase in Pa$_{O_2}$ over 20 mmHg because of the right-to-left shunting of the circulation. Most neonates with lung disease, however, will demonstrate an increase in Pa$_{O_2}$ after breathing 100% oxygen for 20 min. The neonate with persistent fetal circulation, CNS disorders, polycythemia, sepsis, and shock also will demonstrate an increase in Pa$_{O_2}$. No response will also be elicited in the neonate with methemoglobinemia. When a blood specimen is exposed to air, it turns pink in all the conditions described above except in methemoglobinemia, where the blood remains chocolate colored.

### Radiographic Examination

The chest radiograph may demonstrate pulmonary oligemia with normal heart size in tetralogy of Fallot and pulmonary or tricuspid atresia, while pulmonary vascularity is increased in transposition of great vessels, truncus arteriosus, anomalous pulmonary venous return, and hypoplastic left heart. The neonates with lung disease have radiographs that are characteristic of the underlying disease.

### Electrocardiogram and Echocardiogram

These two studies will be useful in diagnosing cyanotic heart disease. Right ventricular hypertrophy may be seen in lung disease with associated pulmonary hypertension.

## Management of Cyanotic Infants

Most of the cyanotic heart diseases are amenable to palliative or corrective surgery. Infants with severe or complete right ventricular outflow obstruction are dependent on the postnatal patency of the ductus arteriosus for maintenance of adequate pulmonary blood flow and systemic oxygenation. Short-term infusions of prostaglandin E$_1$ 0.05 to 0.1 µg/kg per minute in these infants have allowed stabilization prior to surgery.

## Congestive Cardiac Failure

Heart failure in the newborn infant is caused not only by structural heart disease but also by other systemic disorders.

## Causes of Heart Failure

These include (1) structural heart disease (most commonly transposition of the great vessels and hypoplastic left heart syndromes), (2) heart disease without structural abnormalities (myocarditis, cardiac arrhythmias, glycogen storage disease, and endocardial fibroelastosis), (3) respiratory disease with patent ductus arteriosus with left-to-right shunt, (4) anemia (hemoglobin < 3.5 g/dL), (5) polycythemia, (6) cerebral or other arteriovenous malformation, and (7) sepsis.

## Signs and Symptoms

The most frequent symptoms are feeding difficulties, tachypnea, increased sweating, tachycardia, rales and rhonchi, liver enlargement, and cardiomegaly. Less common signs and symptoms are ascites, gallop rhythm, pulsus alternans, and increase in central venous pressure. Peripheral edema is exceedingly rare. A clear distinction between right heart failure (characterized by liver enlargement, tachycardia, and dependent edema) and left heart failure (cardiomegaly, rales, tachypnea, and tachycardia) is not as obvious in the neonate as in the older child or adult.

## Management

It is essential to monitor the heart and respiratory rates and blood pressure closely. Blood gases should be performed frequently to observe onset of hypoxemia or acidosis.

### Fluid Intake

Fluid intake should be restricted to 100 mL/kg per day and adjusted according to the weight, liver size, and urine output. Electrolytes should be monitored closely. Anemia should be corrected with packed red cell transfusions.

### Posture

The neonate should be on a 10 to 30° incline with the head elevated inside the incubator.

### Digoxin

Infants with heart failure should receive digoxin unless the heart rate is below 100 bpm. The digitalizing dose of digoxin is 0.03 mg/kg PO for term neonates. For digitalization, half the calculated digitalizing dose should be given initially, a fourth of the calculated dose in 8 h, and another fourth in 8 h, with maintenance started 12 h after the last digitalizing dose. The maintenance dose is one fourth of the total digitalizing dose in two divided doses.

### Diuretics

Furosemide (Lasix) is the drug of choice with rapid response and should be used intravenously (1 to 3 mg/kg). Maintenance therapy with hydrochlorothiazide (Diuril) and spironolactone (Aldactone) to help conserve potassium may be necessary.

### Beta-Adrenergic Drugs

Neonates with severe heart failure from left-to-right shunts with cardiogenic shock and bradycardia may require β-adrenergic drugs for inotropic action. Isoproterenol (Isuprel) may be infused at 0.1 μg/kg per minute, increasing to 0.4 μg/kg per minute until the heart rate is 140 bpm. Dopamine is useful in hypotensive shock and should be infused at 5 to 15 μg/kg per minute. Both medications should be discontinued slowly while monitoring heart rate and blood pressure.

## BIBLIOGRAPHY

American Academy of Pediatrics, American College of Obstetricians and Gynecologists: Relationship between perinatal factors and neurologic outcome, in Poland RL, Freeman RK (eds): *Guidelines for Perinatal Care,* 3d ed. Elk Grove Village, IL, American Academy of Pediatrics, 1992, pp. 221–224.

Apgar V: A proposal for a new method of evaluation of the newborn infant. *Anesth Analg* 32:260, 1953.

Jain L, Ferre C, Vidyasagar D, et al: Cardiopulmonary resuscitation of apparently stillborn infants. Survival and long term outcome. *J Pediatr* 118:778, 1992.

Kanto WP, Hunter JE, Stoll BJ: Recognition and medical management of necrotizing enterocolitis, in Stoll BJ, Kliegman RM (eds): *Clinics in Perinatology: Necrotizing Enterocolitis,* Philadelphia, Saunders, 1994, pp 355–356.

Lantos JD, Miles SH, Silverstein MD, Stocking CB: Survival after cardiopulmonary resuscitation in babies of very low birth weight. Is CPR futile therapy? *N Engl J Med* 318:91, 1988.

Mizrahe EM: Consensus and controversy in the clinical management of neonatal seizures, in Volpe JJ (ed): *Clinics in Perinatology: Neonatal Neurology,* Philadelphia, Saunders, 1989, pp 485–500.

Sims DG, Heal CA, Bartle SM: Use of adrenalin and atropine in neonatal resuscitation. *Arch Dis Child* 70:F3, 1994.

Williams CE, Mallard C, Tan W, Gluckman PD: Pathophysiology of perinatal asphyxia, in Shankaran S (ed): *Clinics in Perinatology: Perinatal Asphyxia.* Philadelphia, Saunders, pp. 305–325, 1993.

# 17
# PEDIATRIC CARDIOPULMONARY RESUSCITATION
## Robert Luten

The purpose of this chapter is to review cardiopulmonary resuscitation (CPR) in children and note pertinent differences between adults and children. Some subjects that are common to both groups are discussed elsewhere.

The most striking difference between adult and pediatric arrest is etiology. The commonest cause of primary cardiac arrest in adults is coronary artery disease. Children develop cardiac arrest secondary to respiratory arrest and shock syndromes.

Age-related differences must also be considered in pediatric resuscitation. What may be an appropriate drug dose for a 6-month-old is excessive for a 1-month-old and not enough for a 5-year-old. Other aspects of resuscitation, such as endotracheal tube size, tidal volumes, cardiac compression rates, and respiratory rates, also vary with the child's age. Problems related to drug dosage and equipment selection are particular to the logistics of pediatric resuscitation and must be solved if one is to be able to resuscitate infants and children effectively. This problem is discussed below under "Drugs."

## AIRWAY

A child's airway is much smaller than an adult's and varies in size, depending upon age. Functional differences are more pronounced in the infant or young child. The airway is higher and more anterior in the child's neck than in the adult's.

When the child is in the supine position, the prominent occiput causes flexion of the neck on the chest, occluding the airway. This can be corrected by mild extension of the head to the sniffing position. Overextension or hyperextension, as is recommended for adults, causes obstruction and may kink the trachea because the cartilaginous support is poor. The sniffing position can be maintained by placing a towel or other object beneath the occiput. Despite good head position the child's hypotonic mandibular tissues may still occlude the airway posteriorly. This can be relieved by a chin lift or jaw thrust which elevates the mandible anteriorly and separates the tongue from the posterior pharyngeal wall. If these maneuvers are unsuccessful, an oral airway or endotracheal tube should be considered.

## Oral Airway

Oral airways are not widely used in pediatrics. However, they may be useful in the patient who does not respond to maneuvers to remove the mandibular tissues from the posterior pharyngeal wall. With the aid of a tongue blade they are inserted as in adults.

## Intubation

Endotracheal intubation of infants and children is felt by many to be easier than the same procedure in adults. There are, however, some differences related to patient anatomy and equipment.

Hyperextension of the neck must be avoided and the sniffing position used for intubation.

The curved (MacIntosh) blade is rarely used in children less than 4 years old for two reasons. First, because of the high and anterior tracheal opening, the floppy mandibular mass of tissue may fill the field of vision when the blade is inserted in proper position. Second, an exact-sized blade must be used to fit the curvature of the tongue. For these reasons a straight (Miller) blade is preferred.

Tracheal tube sizes vary with the patient's age. A general rule is that the correct internal diameter tube size is approximately the same size as the end of the patient's little finger. However, the child's height has been shown to be the best predictor of correct endotracheal tube size for children. Uncuffed tubes are used for children up to 7 or 8 years old, since the subglottic trachea usually narrows to form an adequate seal in this age group and cuffs are unnecessary. *One can almost always intubate with a laryngoscope blade that is too large and ventilate with a tube that is too small, but not vice versa.*

Once the child has been intubated, one person should be assigned to hold the endotracheal tube in place until it is securely fastened. Especially in small infants, minimum movements can easily displace the tube from the trachea into the esophagus.

If spontaneous ventilations are inadequate, mechanical ventilation should be instituted. For children weighing less than 10 kg, time-flow or pressure preset ventilators should be used. For time-flow ventilators, inspiratory and expiratory times are selected. For pressure ventilators, inflating pressures are determined by checking pressures necessary to inflate the lungs and cause the chest to rise. Pressures usually range from 15 to 40 mm Hg. Excess pressures can cause barotrauma. For older children, volume ventilators can be used, using a starting volume of 10 mL/kg as for adults.

## Rapid Sequence Intubation

To avoid aspiration and protect against the side effects of airway manipulation, such as elevations in intracranial pressure (ICP) and reflex bradycardia, the technique of rapid sequence intubation (RSI) is employed. This technique also provides optimal intubation conditions by producing total muscle paralysis.

The general sequence for RSI is outlined in Fig. 17-1. Tables 17-1, 17-2, and 17-3 list commonly used premedications, sedating agents, and muscle relaxants.

The first step is a period of preoxygenation to produce nitrogen washout, thus minimizing hypoxia during intubation. Premedication consists of atropine to prevent reflex bradycardia, especially if succinylcholine is used. A defasciculating dose of a nondepolarizing agent is used in children above 5 years or 20 kg if succinylcholine is given. Lidocaine should be administered to head-injured children to prevent elevations in ICP. The sedation/induction choices depend upon the patient's perfusion status and specific clinical conditions (Fig. 17-1). Cricoid pressure should be applied as soon as the patient

**Table 17-1.** Premedications Used in RSI

| | |
|---|---|
| Head trauma | Lidocaine 1.5 mg/kg (allow 1 to 2 min before paralysis) |
| 5-yr/20-kg step | |
| <20 kg/5 yr | Atropine 0.1 mg/kg |
| >20 kg/5 yr | Defasciculation with pancuronium/vecuronium for succinylcholine option |

*Source:* Adapted from Luten R (ed): *APLS Instructor Manual: The Pediatric Emergency Medicine Course,* 1994, p 235.

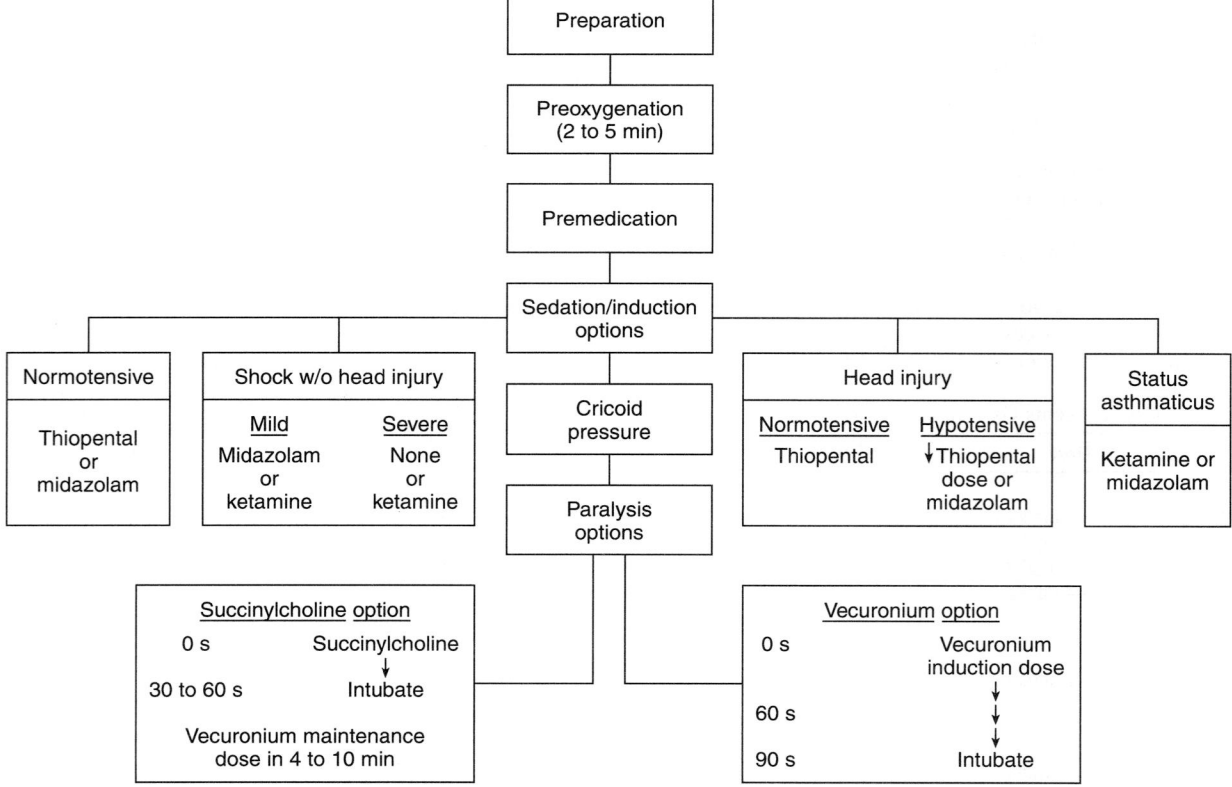

**Fig. 17-1.** Rapid sequence intubation chart. (Adapted from Luten R (ed): *APLS Instructor Manual: The Pediatric Emergency Medicine Course,* 1994, p. 234.)

**Table 17-2.** Sedation Agents Used in RSI

| Drug | Dose | Onset | Duration | Comments |
|------|------|-------|----------|----------|
| Thiopental | 3 to 5 mg/kg | 10 to 30 s | 10 to 30 min | Avoid or reduce dose in hypotension Avoid in reactive airway disease |
| Ketamine | 1 to 2 mg/kg | 1 to 2 min | 15 to 30 min | Contraindicated in presence of increased intracranial pressure |
| Midazolam | 0.1 to 0.2 mg/kg  (5 mg max) | 1 to 2 min | 30 to 60 min | Variable patient response |

*Source:* Adapted from Luten R (ed): *APLS Instructor Manual: The Pediatric Emergency Medicine Course,* 1994, p 235.

loses consciousness and maintained until the tube position is verified. Cricoid pressure prevents passive regurgitation and should be immediately released if vomiting occurs to prevent esophageal rupture. Muscle paralysis can then be obtained with the agent of choice. Succinylcholine is considered ideal for emergent RSI since it has a short onset and duration of action.

## Foreign Body Management

Controversy exists as to the safest and most effective emergency maneuvers to use with the choking child. The American Heart Association specifically discourages two common maneuvers used with adult patients: (1) the Heimlich maneuver for patients less than 1 year of age because of the potential for injury to abdominal organs, and (2) blind finger sweeps, because of the possibility of pushing the foreign body further into the airway. Serious differences of opinion exist, but current recommendations rely on the back blow and chest thrust to clear the infant's airway.

The following sequence should be followed for emergency treatment of the choking infant less than 1 year of age who cannot cough, vocalize, or breathe. (1) With the infant's torso positioned prone and head down along the rescuer's arm, or the older child draped prone and head down across the rescuer's knees, four blows are delivered to the interscapular area. (2) If the airway is still obstructed, the infant is repositioned supinely along the rescuer's arm, or the older child is placed on the floor as for external cardiac compression, and four chest thrusts (cardiac compressions) are delivered. (3) The jaw thrust is used, the mouth is inspected, and a foreign body removed if seen. (4) If obstruction persists, mouth-to-mouth or mouth-to-mouth-and-nose ventilation is attempted. (5) If obstruction persists, the sequence is repeated. The back blow and chest thrust are thought by some to potentially worsen obstruction. Future investigation may well lead to revised recommendations. For children above 1 year of age, the Heimlich maneuver as described for adults is now recommended. This can be performed with the patient standing, sitting, or lying down.

The above recommendations are directed primarily at the first responder who has neither access to nor the skills to use airway management equipment. In the emergency department one would proba-

**Table 17-3.** Paralytic Agents Used in RSI

| Drug | Dose | Onset | Duration |
|------|------|-------|----------|
| **Paralyzing agents** | | | |
| Succinylcholine | 1.0 mg/kg (>12 kg) | 30 to 60 s | 4 to 10 min |
| | 2.0 mg/kg (<12 kg) | 30 to 60 s | 4 to 10 min |
| Vecuronium | 0.2 mg/kg | 60 to 90 s | 90 to 120 min |
| Pancuronium | 0.2 mg/kg | 2 to 5 min | 120 to 150 min |
| **Maintenance dose** | | | |
| Pancuronium/ | | | |
| Vecuronium | 0.1 mg/kg ($^{1}/_{2}$ RSI dose) | | |
| **Defasciculating dose** | | | |
| Pancuronium/ | | | |
| Vecuronium: | 0.02 mg/kg ($^{1}/_{10}$ RSI dose) | | |

*Source:* Adapted from Luten R (ed): *APLS Instructor Manual: The Pediatric Emergency Medicine Course,* 1994, p 235.

bly first attempt direct laryngoscopy, visualization, and removal of the foreign body with McGill forceps.

## BREATHING

### Mouth-to-Mouth

Whether to employ mouth-to-mouth or mouth-to-mouth-and-nose ventilation depends upon the size of the patient. The rate of ventilation is shown in Table 17-4. Ventilations are done slowly to avoid the generation of high airway pressures which can overcome esophageal resistance and result in gastric distension.

### Bag-Valve-Mask

The self-inflating bag-valve-mask system is most commonly used for ventilation. Ventilation bags used for infants and children should have a minimum volume of 450 mL. There is a common misconception that children are more susceptible to pneumothoraces at high inspiratory preshan adults. In fact, pediatric lung compliance is very good, and children can tolerate high pressures. Pneumothoraces more commonly result from the administration of three to four times the required tidal volume. The tidal volume necessary to ventilate children is the same as that for adults, 10 to 15 mL/kg. It is impractical to calculate the tidal volume in emergency situations. One can start ventilating with minimal volumes and increase rapidly until adequate chest rise occurs.

### External Cardiac Compression

The brachial pulse is recommended for monitoring purposes for infants less than 1 year of age. Above this age, the carotid pulse is most easily accessible. Absence of pulses mandates external cardiac compression. Most patients should be placed on a hard surface, as are adults. With smaller infants, the wraparound technique is used.

Whether chest compressions produce blood flow by direct compression of the heart, by changes in thoracic pressure, or by both is unclear. New standards advocate compressions over the lower sternum as opposed to mid sternum since the infant heart has recently been shown to lie lower in the thoracic cage than previously believed. Whether to use two fingers, three fingers, or the heel of the hand depends upon the size of the child. Whichever method comfortably produces a compression depth of approximately one-fourth the anteroposterior diameter should be used. The rate of compressions is at least 100/min in infants and older children. The ratio of ventilations to compressions is 1:5 for both one- and two-person CPR. A pause of 1 to 1.5 s between ventilations should be allowed for adequate exhalation.

## VASCULAR ACCESS

Difficulty in obtaining rapid intravenous access is certainly one of the major differences between adult and pediatric resuscitation. Two im-

**Table 17-4.** Rate of Ventilation

| Age | Ventilation Rate, breaths/min |
|-----|-------------------------------|
| Infants and children 1–8 years | 20 (every 3 s) |
| Children over 8 years and adults | 12 (every 5 s) |

portant facts should be kept in mind. First, a significant portion of children respond to airway management alone, since most cardiac arrests in children are secondary to respiratory arrest. Time spent securing vascular access at the expense of adequate airway management is a common mistake in dealing with children, and nowhere is it more costly. Second, once a patient has been intubated, the tracheal route may be used to administer drugs such as epinephrine, atropine, and lidocaine. The dose of endotracheal epinephrine for symptomatic bradycardia or pulseless cardiac arrest is 0.1 mg/kg, 1:1000 concentration q 3–5 min. Although the doses for other drugs are not known with exactitude, they should be increased over the IV dose.

Although central access would be ideal for administration of drugs during CPR, most studies demonstrating the safety and efficacy of virtually all central venous approaches in children were done under controlled situations and mostly by experienced personnel. Therefore, the most frequently used sites are peripheral: scalp, arm, hand, or antecubital veins; the external jugular vein; femoral vein; or distal saphenous vein via cutdown. Intraosseous infusion is a quick, safe route for resuscitation drugs as well as fluid administration. This is discussed in Chap. 18, "Vascular Access."

## FLUIDS

In the face of hypotension due to volume depletion, isotonic fluid boluses of 20 to 40 mL/kg should be given *as rapidly as possible* and repeated depending upon response. In neonates or small infants, a 20-mL syringe attached to a three-way stopcock and extension tubing can be used to deliver aliquots of fluid rapidly, until the entire bolus is administered. If volume depletion has been corrected and hypotension persists, a pressor agent should be strongly considered, preferably with the aid of a central venous pressure catheter. In the normotensive patient or when the IV line is being used for drug administration only, it should be maintained at the minimum rate that will keep the vein open (KVO). Fine fluid and electrolyte calculations and adjustments can be made after the emergency treatment has been completed. Overhydration, even when IV lines are set at KVO, is a common occurrence when adult equipment is used in pediatric resuscitations. A pediatric microdrip should always be used when resuscitating children.

## DRUGS

The indications for the use of specific drugs are essentially the same for children as for adults. Particular to pediatrics, however, is the problem of drug dosage. Proper dosage in children requires knowledge of the patient's weight (Table 17-5), knowledge of the dose (usually given in milligrams per kilogram), and error-free calculation and delivery. Problems may arise in remembering the correct dose, performing calculations in the crisis situation (the most common error involves the misplacement of a decimal point and results in 10 times or one-tenth the correct dosage), and delivery of the correct dosage (because of an error in drawing up the calculated amount). Use of a chart with precalculated drug dosages can help reduce dosage errors (Table 17-6). However, estimating a child's weight accurately so that the proper dosage can be determined from the table is not easy, especially in a crisis situation, and is fraught with error. Choosing the proper size equipment for pediatric patients is similarly difficult. Valuable time can be lost in weight estimation, dosage calculations, and equipment selection.

**Table 17-5.** Body Weight Estimation Guidelines

| Age | Weight, kg | |
|---|---|---|
| Term infant | 3.5 | Birth weight (BW) |
| 6 months | 7 | $2 \times BW$ |
| 1 year | 10 | $3 \times BW$ |
| 4 years | 16 | $^1/_4$ adult weight of 70 kg |
| 10 years | 35 | $^1/_2$ adult weight |

**Table 17-6.** Essential Drugs

| Drug | Concentration | Dose |
|---|---|---|
| Epinephrine: first dose | 1:10,000 (0.1 mg/mL) | 0.01–0.02 mg/kg |
| Epinephrine: high dose | 1:1000 (1 mg/mL) | 0.1–0.2 mg/kg |
| Atropine | 1:10,000 (0.1 mg/mL) | 0.02 mg/kg |
| Sodium bicarbonate | 1 mEq/mL | 1.0 mEq/kg |

Recently, systems based on a direct measurement of a patient's length have been developed for estimating dosages and selecting equipment in pediatric emergencies. In children, length has a direct correlation with weight. It has also been shown to be one of the most accurate predictors of correct equipment sizes for pediatric patients, especially endotracheal tube sizes. The Broselow Resuscitation Tape is one length-based system currently included in the American Heart Association's Pediatric Advanced Life Support Course (PALS). It is a two-sided tape; one side displays emergency resuscitation drug dosage and the other is for equipment selection (see Figs. 17-2, 17-3, and 17-4). Fluid volumes for resuscitation as well as appropriate basic life support techniques are also displayed on the Broselow tape. To make optimal use of these systems, emergency personnel must be able to find the proper equipment rapidly. Equipment can be stored in shelves or drawers labeled by age and weight, or a system of color codes can be used in which color-coded shelves, carts, or equipment organizers correspond to specific length categories.

Drugs delivered by constant infusion and the "rule of 6" used to calculate their dosage are listed in the accompanying box; they are also contained in the Broselow tape. The pharmacology of the drugs has been well described in other sections and will not be addressed

---

**USEFUL DRUGS**

RULE OF 6 FOR MEDICATIONS DELIVERED BY CONSTANT INFUSION

Dopamine dose     = 5–20 µg/kg per min

Lidocaine dose     = 20–50 µg/kg per min

Isoproterenol dose = 0.1–1.0 µg/kg per min

Dosage of medications delivered by constant infusions is calculated in terms of micrograms per kilogram per minute. Actual calculation can be confusing and a source of lethal decimal errors. The *rule of 6* can be used for *dopamine* and *lidocaine* to simplify dosage calculation:

6 mg × wt (kg), *fill* to 100 mL with $D_5W$

The medication is mixed in an intravenous set with a measured chamber and a microdrip (1 drop/min = 1 mL/h). Rate of administration is best set by an electric pump.

**Example:** For a 10-kg infant requiring dopamine:

6 mg × 10 = 60 mg dopamine

In a measured chamber *fill* to 100 mL with $D_5W$. Weight is now factored in so that

1 mL/h = 1 µg/kg per min

5 mL/h = 5 µg/kg per min

10 mL/h = 10 µg/kg per min

For *isoproterenol* the rule of 6:

0.6 mg × wt (kg), *fill* to 100 mL with $D_5W$

1 mL/h = 0.1 µg/kg per min

5 mL/h = 5 µg/kg per min

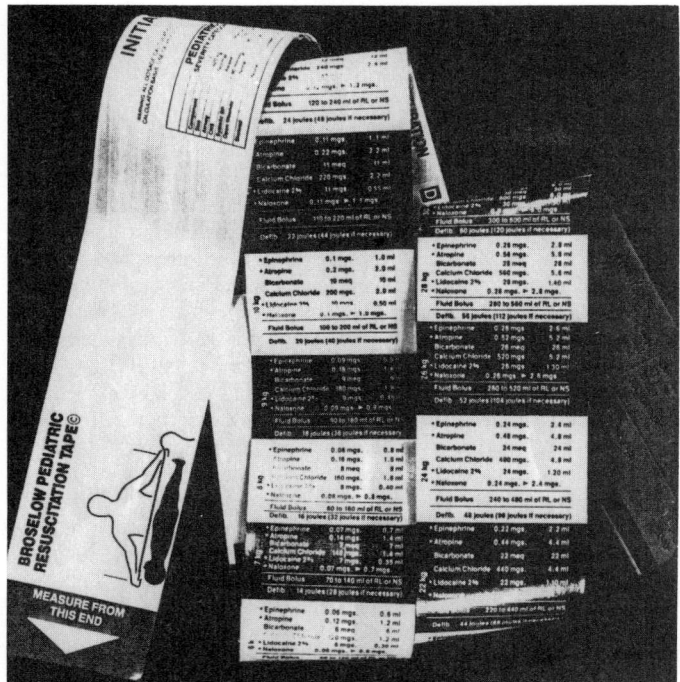

**Fig. 17-2.** The Broselow Resuscitation Tape.

| 10 kg | | | |
|---|---|---|---|
| * Epinephrine | 0.1 mgs. | 1.0 ml |
| * Atropine | 0.2 mgs. | 2.0 ml |
| Bicarbonate | 10 meq | 10 ml |
| Calcium Chloride | 200 mgs. | 2.0 ml |
| * Lidocaine 2% | 10 mgs. | 0.50 ml |
| * Naloxone | 0.1 mgs. ► 1.0 mgs. | |
| **Fluid Bolus** | **100 to 200 ml of RL or NS** | |

**Defib.     20 joules (40 joules if necessary)**

**Fig. 17-4.** Drug side of the Broselow Resuscitation Tape. One of 25 precalculated weight zones for resuscitation drugs.

here. A few peculiarities pertaining to pediatric drug use are discussed in the following paragraphs.

**Atropine and epinephrine.** Epinephrine is the one proven beneficial drug in cases of cardiac arrest. It is specifically indicated for hypoxia- or ischemia-induced *slow* rates that fail to respond to adequate oxygenation and ventilation, and pulseless arrest situations (i.e., asystole, electromechanical dissociation, and ventricular fibrillation). If the initial dose of epinephrine is not effective, 10 to 20 times that dose should be given subsequently. As of this writing, the use of high-dose epinephrine (0.1–0.2 mg/kg of the 1:1000 concentration) for resuscitation in infants and children is recommended. Thus far, the lack of adverse effects associated with the use of high-dose epinephrine in the clinical setting supports its use if there is no clinical response to a first low dose (0.01 mg/kg of 1:10,000 concentration) of epinephrine. Primary cardiac causes of slow rates are rare and may also be treated with atropine. The recommended dose is 0.02 mg/kg IV. The minimum dose is 0.1 mg, with a maximum single dose of 0.5 mg for the child and 1.0 mg for the adolescent. The dose may be repeated once, with a maximum total dose of 1.0 mg for the child and 2.0 mg for the adolescent.

**Sodium bicarbonate.** Sodium bicarbonate is no longer a first-line drug since its administration worsens acidosis when administered in the presence of inadequate ventilation *and* perfusion. It is administered only after epinephrine administration has not improved the clinical situation. An initial dose of 1 mEq/kg IV is given only after the airway has been secured, the patient hyperventilated, and CPR initiated. In the neonate or premature infant, sodium bicarbonate should be diluted 1:1 with sterile water, not saline.

**Calcium.** Because of lack of proven efficacy and possible deleterious effects, calcium has been removed from the American Heart Association standards for resuscitation. It is indicated only for hyperkalemia, hypocalcemia, and calcium channel blocker overdose.

## ARRHYTHMIAS

Arrhythmia management plays only a small role in the resuscitation of children. Since rhythm disturbances are usually secondary to respiratory arrest and not primary cardiac events, careful attention must be given to the correction of hypoxia, acidosis, and fluid balance. Ventilation and oxygenation must be accomplished first. Pulse oximetry, or arterial blood gas analysis if $P_{CO_2}$ or abnormalities are suspected, should be obtained to assess oxygen and blood gas status. An IV of 0.9% NaCl or lactated Ringer's solution should be established, and the child placed on a cardiac monitor.

A patient with an unstable cardiac rhythm or rate, coupled with evidence of poor end-organ perfusion (cyanosis, mottled skin, lethargy, etc.), requires immediate intervention. The parameters of clinical assessment and expression of instability vary with the child's age. In the neonate, blood pressure measurement is difficult, and a *heart rate* of 80 beats/min or less, coupled with evidence of poor end-organ perfusion, requires immediate intervention. In infants and children, variations in heart rate may be well tolerated clinically, and a *blood pres-*

**Fig. 17-3.** Equipment side of the Broselow Resuscitation Tape. One of seven color equipment zones.

| **C** | AIRWAY | | INTUBATION | | **D** |
|---|---|---|---|---|---|
| itraight | ORAL AIRWAY | Child | LARYNGOSCOPE | 2 Straight | ORAL AIRI |
| icuffed | B.V.M. | Child | | or curved * | B.V.M |
| 6F | O₂ MASK | Pediatric | E.T. TUBE | 4.5 mm uncuffed | O₂ MASK |
| 8F | | | STYLET | 6F | |
| | | | SUCTION CATHETER | 8-10F | |
| 8-10F | B.P. CUFF | Child | N.G. TUBE | 10F | |
| 8-10F | VASC. ACCESS | 18-22 Catheter, | URINARY CATHETER | 10F | B.P. CUFF |
| 16-20F | 21-23 Butterfly, Intraosseus Needle | | CHEST TUBE | 20-24F | VASCULAR |
| | ARM BOARDS | 8" | * Most sources recommend a straight blade for this age child. | | 21-23 Bu |
| | | | | | ARM BOAI |

SIONS     RATE 80/min    5/1 BREATH    DEPTH 1-1½"    POSITION: HEEL OF HAND. 1 FINGER WID

*sure* of 70 mmHg or less, coupled with evidence of poor end-organ perfusion is used to define instability. Figures 17-5 and 17-6 summarizes electrical and drug therapy of unstable cardiac rhythms in children.

The most common rhythms seen in pediatric arrest are the bradycardias, which lead to asystole if untreated. Outside of the code situation, by far the most common rhythm disturbance encountered is paroxysmal atrial tachycardia (SVT). It is most commonly seen in infants and usually presents as a narrow complex tachycardia with rates usually between 250 and 350 beats per minute. Treatment of the unstable patient has already been outlined. Treatment of the stable patient varies and is beyond the scope of this chapter. Adenosine (0.1 mg/kg) is the current recommended drug for SVT in children. This dose can be doubled if unsuccessful.

Sometimes it is difficult to distinguish a secondary sinus tachycardia from a primary cardiac tachycardia. Although heart rates of 150 to 200 per minute in adults are usually cardiac in origin, it is not uncommon to have compensatory sinus tachycardia as fast as 200 to 220 per minute in small infants. Children can tolerate rapid primary cardiac heart rates for long periods of time before congestive heart failure (CHF) or lethal arrhythmias develop. Differentiating primary from secondary tachycardia is critical to patient management (see Table 17-7). Note that an ECG is rarely helpful since at very fast rates, P waves are not usually distinguishable in either sinus tachycardia or SVT.

## DEFIBRILLATION AND CARDIOVERSION

Electric conversion is used on an emergency basis to treat ventricular fibrillation and symptomatic tachyarrhythmias. Ventricular fibrillation as a cause of cardiac arrest is rare in children.

**Paddle size.** Paddle size is usually 4.5 cm for infants and 8 cm for children. The paddle should be in contact with the chest wall over its entire surface area.

**Interface.** Electrode cream, electrode paste, and saline-soaked gauze pads are all acceptable. Alcohol pads are to be discouraged as serious burns may be produced. Care must be taken so that the interface substance from one paddle does not come in contact with the substance from the other paddle. This creates a short circuit, and insufficient energy may be delivered to the heart.

**Electrode position.** One paddle is placed on the right of the sternum at the second intercostal space. The other is placed in the left midclavicular line at the level of the xyphoid. The AP approach can be used but is less desirable.

**Fig. 17-5.** Asystole and pulseless arrest decision tree. IV, intravenous/IO, intraosseous; ET, endotracheal.

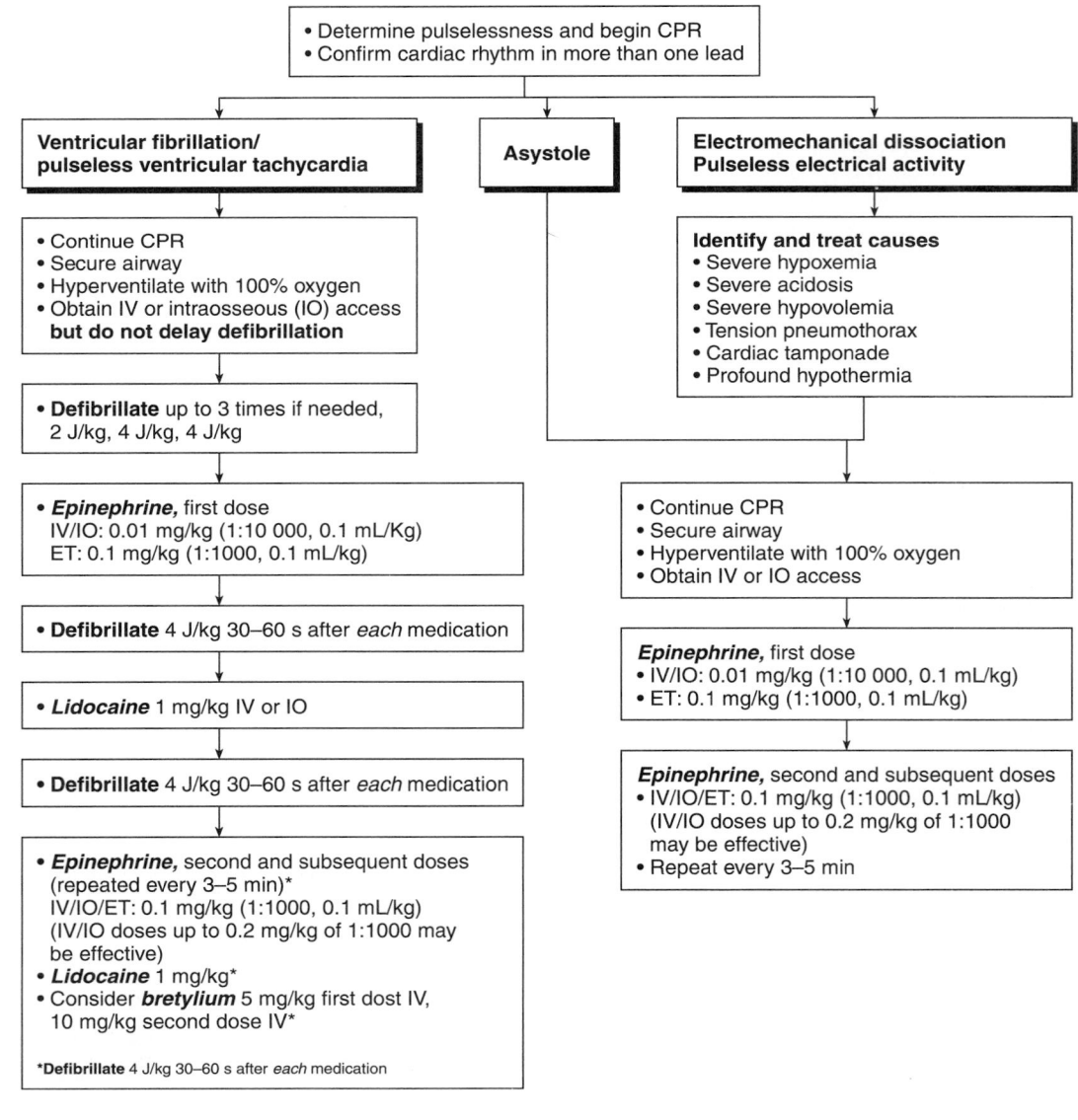

**Fig. 17-6.** Bradycardia decision tree. IV, intravenous; IO, intraosseous; ET, endotracheal.

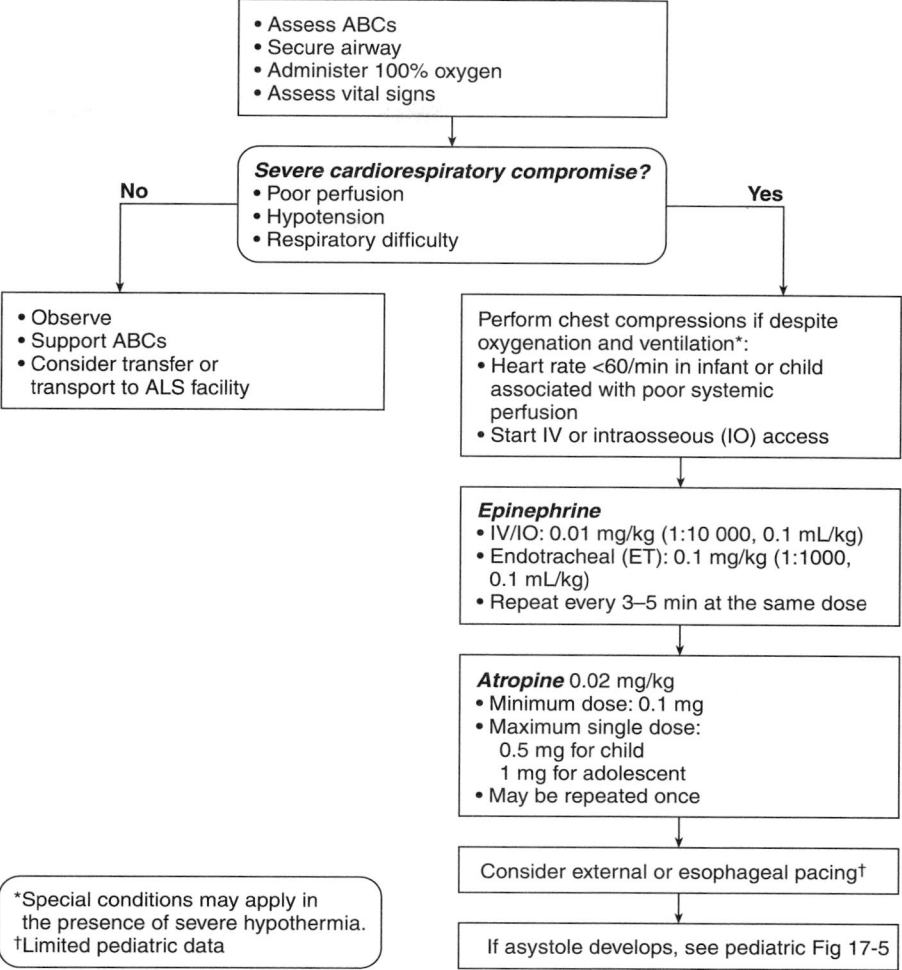

**Table 17-7.** Sinus Tachycardia vs. SVT

| Clinical Finding | Sinus Tachycardia | SVT |
|---|---|---|
| History | History usually compatible, e.g., vomiting, diarrhea, or bleeding. | In absence of known congenital heart disease, history is usually very nonspecific. |
| Physical examination | Clinical dehydration or pallor. | Patients may have rales and an enlarged liver if CHF is prolonged. The presence of a heart murmur is inconsistent. |
| Lab | Chest x-ray film shows small heart, clear lungs. Electrolytes and hematocrit usually consistent with underlying cause. | Chest x-ray film shows normal to large heart; patient may have pulmonary edema. |

**Table 17-8.** CPR

| | Infant | Child | Adult 1 Rescuer | 2 Rescuer |
|---|---|---|---|---|
| Compression/ventilation ratio | 5:1 | 5:1 | 15:2 | 5:1 |
| Cardiac compressions/minute | 100 | 80–100 | 60–80 | 60–80 |

**Defibrillation dose.** Initially, 2 J/kg should be used; if that is unsuccessful, the amount should be doubled and attempted twice at the higher energy level if necessary. If the second attempt at the higher dose is unsuccessful, epinephrine should be given, and the oxygen and acid-base status should be assessed before repeating or increasing the energy dose.

**Cardioversion.** Tachyarrhythmias are generally very sensitive to electric conversion. There are no recent published standards for cardioversion. One can either use $1/4$ to $1/2$ J/kg and double if unsuccessful, or initially place the defibrillator on the lowest possible energy setting and do the same. Of the two methods, the one that gives the lowest energy level is preferable.

## SUMMARY OF MANAGEMENT GUIDELINES

It is the age-related differences that are difficult to remember and cause major problems in pediatric resuscitation. One should not have to memorize numbers such as drug doses, tube sizes, or cardiac compression ratios. The proper organization of equipment and the posting of pediatric CPR data and equipment sheets (Tables 17-8 and 17-9) using a length-based system can eliminate the need to commit many variables to memory, thus reducing the possibility of errors. This eliminates much of the general anxiety connected with pediatric resuscitation and leaves the clinician free to apply the principles of resuscitation to the child as presented.

**Table 17-9.** Length-Based Equipment Chart

**Length, cm**

| Item | 54–70 | 70–85 | 85–95 | 95–107 | 107–124 | 124–138 | 138–155 |
|---|---|---|---|---|---|---|---|
| ET tube size (mm) | 3.5 | 4.0 | 4.5 | 5.0 | 5.5 | 6.0 | 6.5 |
| Lip-tip length (mm) | 10.5 | 12.0 | 13.5 | 15.0 | 16.5 | 18.0 | 19.5 |
| Laryngoscope | 1 Straight | 1 Straight | 2 Straight | 2 Straight or curved | 2 Straight or curved | 2–3 Straight or curved | 3 Straight or curved |
| Suction catheter | 8F | 8–10F | 10F | 10F | 10F | 10F | 12F |
| Stylet | 6F | 6F | 6F | 6F | 14F | 14F | 14F |
| Oral airway | Infant/ small child | Small child | Child | Child | Child/ small adult | Child/ adult | Medium adult |
| Bag-valve-mask | Infant | Child | Child | Child | Child | Child/adult | Adult |
| Oxygen mask | Newborn | Pediatric | Pediatric | Pediatric | Pediatric | Adult | Adult |
| Vascular access catheter/ butterfly | 22–24/23–25, intraosseous | 20–22/23–25, intraosseous | 18–22/21–23, intraosseous | 18–22/21–23, intraosseous | 18–20/21–23 | 18–20/21–22 | 16–20/18–21 |
| Nasogastric tube | 5–8F | 8–10F | 10F | 10–12F | 12–14F | 14–18F | 18F |
| Urinary catheter | 5–8F | 8–10F | 10F | 10–12F | 10–12F | 12F | 12F |
| Chest tube | 12–12F | 16–20F | 20–24F | 20–24F | 24–32F | 28–32F | 32–40F |
| Blood pressure cuff | Newborn/ infant | Infant/child | Child | Child | Child | Child/adult | Adult |

Directions for use
1. Measure patient length with centimeter tape.
2. Using measured length in centimeters, access appropriate equipment column.

*Source:* Adapted from Luten RD, Wears RL, Broselow J, et al: Length-based endotracheal tube sizing for pediatric resuscitation. *Ann Emerg Med* 21(8):900, 1992.

## BIBLIOGRAPHY

Chameides L: *Textbook on Pediatric Advanced Life Support,* 2d ed. American Heart Association, 1994.
Luten RC, Wears RL, Broselow J, et al: Length-based endotracheal tube sizing for pediatric resuscitation. *Ann Emerg Med* 21(8):900, 1992.

# 18
# VASCULAR ACCESS IN INFANTS AND CHILDREN
## William H. Spivey
## Dee Hodge III

Vascular access in children, as in adults, is necessary for fluid and drug administration, monitoring blood pressure, and obtaining blood for diagnostic studies. However, children have fewer veins available for catheterization, their veins are smaller, and they have more adipose tissue overlying the veins.

Immobilization of the child and identification of a suitable vein are essential for venous access. To accomplish immobilization, the child may be placed in a commercial papoose or wrapped in a sheet with an assistant restraining the child's legs.

Sedation may be necessary for the insertion of central lines where movement could have disastrous consequences. A local anesthetic at the puncture site and a combination of morphine 0.1 mg/kg (maximum 8 mg) and pentobarbital 4 mg/kg (maximum 100 mg) IM will provide adequate sedation for most procedures. Other sedation regimens include: midazolam, 0.1 mg/kg IV: midazolam intranasal 0.2–0.4 mg/kg; or chloral hydrate, 25–50 mg/kg PO or rectally.

## PERIPHERAL VEINS

A suitable vein can usually be found in the antecubital fossa or on the dorsum of the hand between the third and fourth metacarpals. The feet and ankles are acceptable alternatives, especially the saphenous vein on the medial aspect of the ankle. Once a vein is located, immobilize the limb by taping it to a small armboard or, in the case of an infant, by splinting with two or three tongue depressors taped together.

A 21- to 27-gauge butterfly needle may be used for venous cannulation, or a 21- to 25-gauge plastic catheter-over-the-needle may be used to provide a more secure line. When using small-gauge needles, it is helpful to first puncture the skin with a larger needle and then insert the small-gauge butterfly or plastic catheter and needle through the skin puncture. This prevents the point of the small needle from puncturing both sides of the vessel as it overcomes skin resistance. After successful cannulation, the butterfly needle or catheter is taped into position. A piece of cotton may be placed underneath to provide a better needle angle for flow.

In infants and small children a microdrip fluid chamber should be used to accurately monitor the rate of infusion and to prevent large volumes from being accidentally infused. In trauma with hemorrhagic shock a microdrip chamber should not be used.

## SCALP VEINS

Scalp veins are easily accessible in the infant under 1 year of age and provide a good route for maintenance fluid and drug administration. The infant should be immobilized and the head grasped by an assistant. Shave or clip the hair overlying the vein, large enough to accommodate the tape and the needle. The vein selected should be straight and long enough to accommodate the needle. It must also be differentiated from an artery. Arteries are generally more tortuous, pulsate, and fill from below, whereas veins fill from above.

Place a rubber band around the infant's head (Fig. 18-1) to serve as a tourniquet. After the skin has been cleansed with povidone-iodine, grasp a butterfly needle (23- to 27-gauge) by the wings and insert it approximately 0.5 cm from the intended puncture site in the direction of blood flow. In order to prevent an air embolus, the butterfly tubing is filled with saline. When the vein is entered, blood will flow back

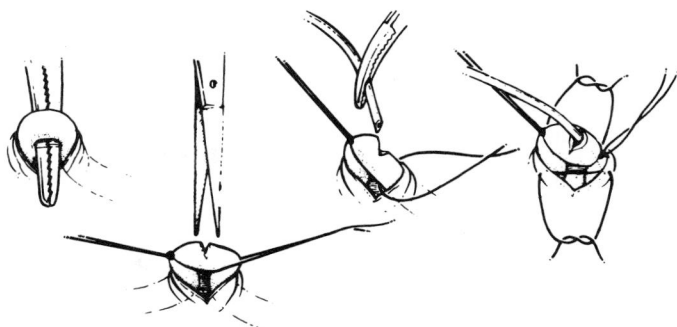

**Fig. 18-3.** After the vein has been dissected from the subcutaneous tissues, it is elevated with a hemostat and retracted with ties. A V-shaped incision is made in the vessel and the cannula inserted. The ties may be tied or a pressure dressing applied to prevent bleeding.

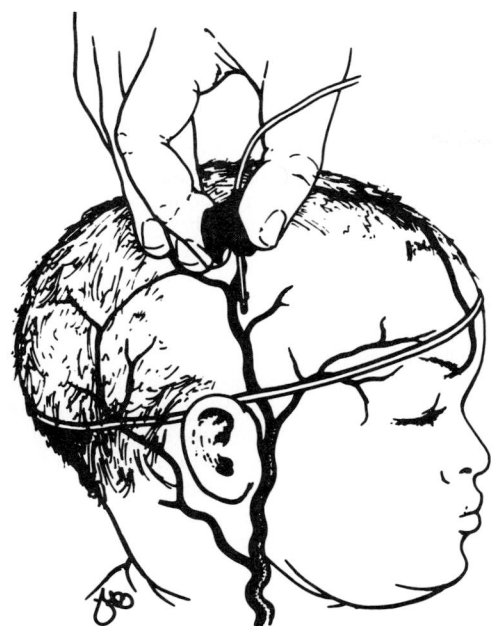

**Fig. 18-1.** A tourniquet is placed around the infant's head and the needle inserted 0.5 cm from the intended puncture site in the direction of blood flow.

into the tubing. The tourniquet is cut and 1 to 2 mL of fluid infused to establish the correct position of the needle. The needle is then taped in place with the plastic tubing, looped to prevent it from being accidentally pulled. The needle and tubing may then be covered with a small medicine cup for protection.

Complications from this procedure include local hematoma, infiltration, infection, and inadvertent arterial puncture. This procedure should be carefully explained to parents since they often become upset when hair is cut or shaved off, for whatever reason.

## VENOUS CUTDOWN

Venous cutdown catheterization is used when percutaneous attempts are not successful and rapid venous access is needed for treatment of shock or cardiac arrest.

The vein of choice for cutdown is the great saphenous vein, located between the medial malleolus and the anterior tibial tendon. Before exposing the vein, the child should be restrained and the site anesthetized with 1% lidocaine, cleansed with povidone-iodine, and draped with sterile towels. A tourniquet is not used since it increases

bleeding. A 2-cm transverse incision is made between the medial malleolus and the anterior tibial tendon, and a curved hemostat is used to spread to subcutaneous tissue along the course of the vein (Fig. 18-2). Anterior to the vein is a sensory nerve that can be spared if the vein is carefully dissected. Once the vein is isolated, two 4–0 silk ties are placed under the vein, one distal and one proximal. The distal suture may be tied and used for stabilization during insertion of the catheter, since this will permanently occlude the vein; some prefer to avoid ligation to promote recannalization of the vein when the catheter is removed.

The vein is lifted with gentle traction using the two ties, and a V-shaped incision is made in the wall with a no. 11 scalpel or fine scissors. A beveled catheter previously filled with fluid and attached to a fluid-filled syringe may then be inserted as demonstrated in Fig. 18-3. Patency is checked by aspirating blood and flushing the catheter. The proximal suture is then tied around the vein and catheter and the distal suture tied to the catheter. If the distal suture has not been tied, it may be removed.

An alternative method of cannulating the vessel, easier in the small infant, is to insert an over-the-needle plastic catheter directly into the vein once it is exposed. The vessel is elevated by holding traction on the sutures under the vessel as described above or by simply placing a hemostat under the distal end of the vessel and elevating it. The needle is then directly inserted into the vessel and the catheter advanced (Fig. 18-4). Great care must be taken to avoid through-and-through

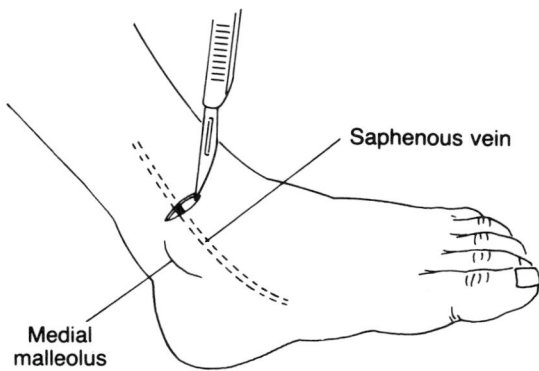

**Fig. 18-2.** A 2-cm transverse incision is made between the medial malleolus and anterior tibial tendon. The incision should extend through the skin but not into the subcutaneous tissues.

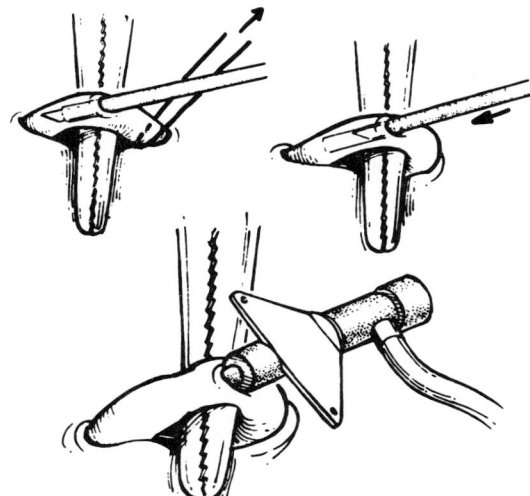

**Fig. 18-4.** The vessel is elevated with a hemostat and occluded with gentle traction from a distal tie. The needle is inserted and the sheath is advanced into the vessel. The vessel should not be tied off with this technique.

puncture of the vein. This does not require that either end of the vessel be ligated. The incision is sutured and the catheter is taped or sewn in place.

Complications of a cutdown include infection, phlebitis, laceration of a nerve, and catheter loss into a vein.

## INTERNAL JUGULAR CATHETERIZATION

Catheterization of the internal jugular vein for central venous access is preferable to using the subclavian vein in infants. The child is easier to immobilize for internal jugular catheterization, and the risk of pneumothorax is much less. Although there are several approaches to the internal jugular vein, the posterior approach and high central or anterior approach have a high success rate and fewer complications in infants and children.

In both techniques the infant is placed with head extended over the edge of the cart and rotated away from the intended puncture site. The neck is cleansed with povidone-iodine and the skin anesthetized. An 18- to 20-gauge needle and a J-shaped guidewire using the Seldinger technique is used to cannulate the vein.

In the high central approach the landmark is the apex of a triangle formed by the two heads of the sternocleidomastoid and clavicle (Fig. 18-5). The needle is inserted pointing toward the ipsilateral nipple with the syringe elevated 45° above the plane of the table. Once the vein has been entered, the syringe is removed, a guidewire is inserted through the needle, the needle is removed, and a catheter is inserted over the wire. Care must be taken never to change direction of the needle while in the neck. The razor-sharp bevel of the needle can lacerate an artery or nerve.

In the posterior approach a needle attached to a syringe is inserted at the midpoint of the lateral border of the sternocleidomastoid muscle, and is directed toward the contralateral nipple. The syringe is elevated 10° and the needle advanced, maintaining negative pressure on the syringe. Cannulation of the vessel is accomplished as described for the high central approach.

Complications of internal jugular catheterization include carotid artery puncture with hematoma, pneumothorax, thoracic duct catheterization, and damage to the cranial and cervical sympathetic nerves. By using the right side of the neck, the incidence of complications may be reduced.

## EXTERNAL JUGULAR VEIN

The external jugular vein is a good site for drawing blood when peripheral veins are not available and may be used for access to the central venous circulation. This route eliminates the danger of carotid artery puncture and pneumothorax, but the success rate of central venous catheter placement is only about 60 percent, as compared to about 80 percent for the internal jugular vein.

The child is immobilized with the head extended 15 to 20° over the edge of the bed and rotated away from the puncture site. In order to maximize the venous filling, the infant may be stimulated to cry and a finger placed over the base of the vein at the clavicle. After cleansing of the site, a 21- or 23-gauge butterfly needle attached to a syringe is inserted into the vein midway between the angle of the jaw and the shoulder (Fig. 18-6). If central venous access is required, an 18- to 20-gauge needle attached to a syringe is likewise inserted and a J-tipped guidewire passed through it. The needle is removed and a Seldinger catheter passed over the wire. Complications of this procedure include hematoma and placement of central lines outside the thorax.

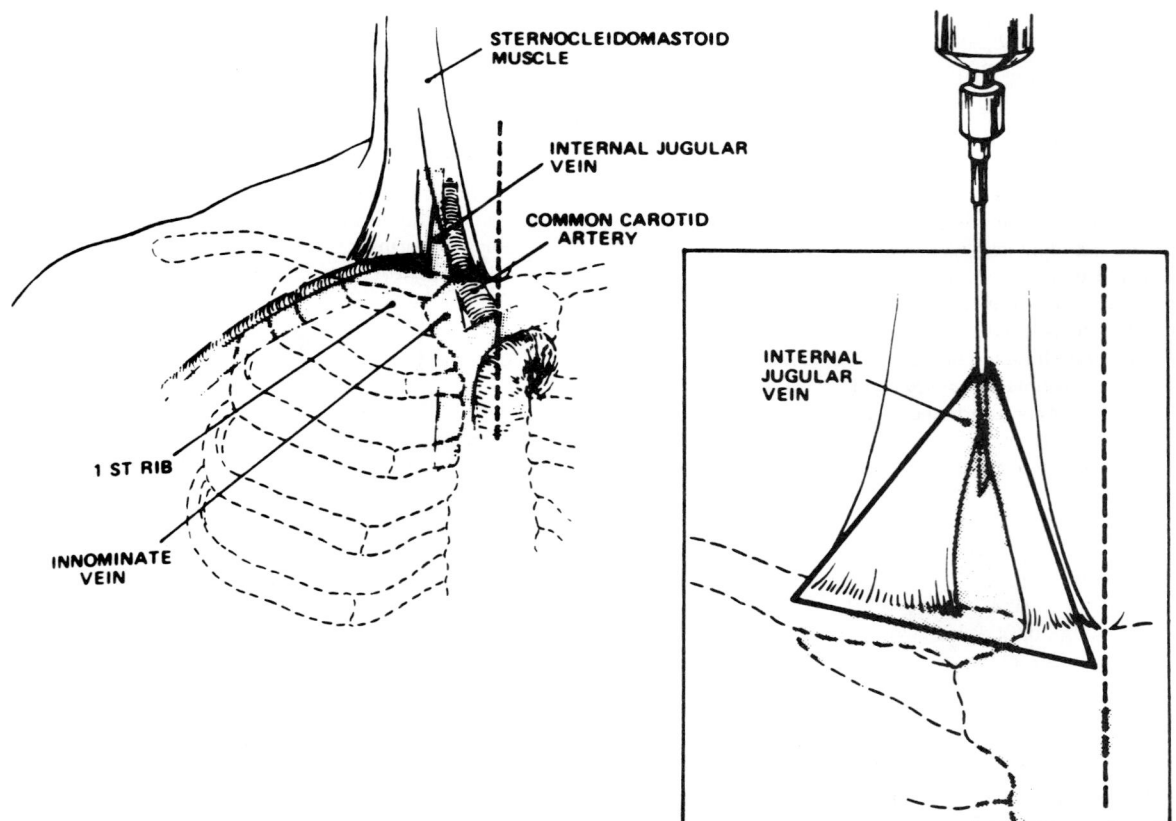

**Fig. 18-5.** The position of the internal jugular vein is demonstrated on the left. It is cannulated by inserting a needle at the apex of the triangle formed by the two heads of the sternocleidomastoid muscle and pointing it at the ipsilateral nipple with 10° elevation of the syringe. Once the vessel has entered, a guide wire is inserted and the catheter inserted over the guide wire.

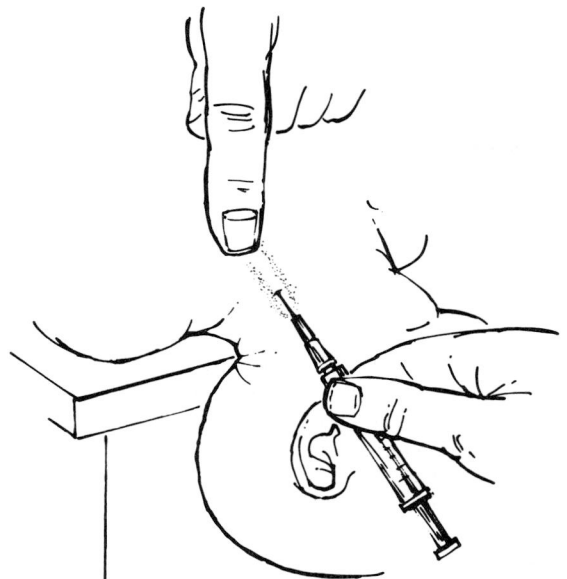

**Fig. 18-6.** Venipuncture of the external jugular vein is accomplished by immobilizing the child and extending the head 15 to 20° over the edge of the bed, with the head rotated away from the puncture site. Venous return is occluded with light pressure over the vein above the clavicle and the vein punctured distally.

## SUBCLAVIAN VEIN

This technique is indicated when emergency access to the venous circulation is required and percutaneous peripheral, femoral, or jugular access is not available. It is associated with pneumothorax, hemothorax, hydrothorax, and infection after emergency placement. It is also difficult to perform during closed-chest cardiac massage because of the motion of the chest and shoulders.

Adequate restraint is difficult unless the patient is heavily sedated. The child should be placed in the Trendelenburg position with a towel placed under the thoracic spine. The skin is cleansed and the puncture site anesthetized. A small nick is made in the skin over the medial portion of the clavicle with a scalpel. The needle is then inserted through this puncture site and advanced toward the junction of the clavicle and the first rib. When blood return occurs the catheter is then advanced into the vein (Fig. 18-7). Blood is aspirated from the catheter and fluid infused. A catheter over the needle device such as the Intramedicut cannula is commonly used and ranges from 20-gauge in newborns to 14-gauge in children over 6 years. A Seldinger-type catheter may also be used. Care must be taken not to allow air to enter the catheter and produce an air embolus. An x-ray should be obtained to confirm the position of the catheter and to check for pneumothorax.

## AXILLARY VEIN

The axillary vein may be used for central venous access when the femoral, subclavian, or internal jugular veins are not available. The incidence of pneumothorax is much lower than with the subclavian approach. Complications include infection, axillary artery puncture and nerve injury.

The child is immobilized and the arm is abducted to 45–90°. After cleansing the axillary region, the axillary artery is palpated and the needle inserted inferior and parallel to the artery. Once the vein is punctured, blood may be aspirated and catheter inserted.

Both Teflon coated over the needle catheters (18–24 gauge) and Seldinger-type catheters (3–8.5 French) may be used for this approach. If central venous pressure monitoring is desired, a catheter long enough to reach the superior vena cava should be used. Avoid

introduction of air through the cannula and check for catheter placement with an X-ray.

## FEMORAL APPROACH

The femoral vein may be used for emergency central venous catheterization. It is more accessible than the external jugular vein during cardiac arrest and has a low incidence of short-term complications. The femoral vein may be cannulated percutaneously or by cutdown. The simplest method of percutaneous catheterization is to use the Seldinger technique. The leg is externally rotated and the artery palpated. The artery lies one-half the distance between the symphysis and anterior iliac spine and 1.5 cm below the inguinal ligament (Fig. 18-8). The skin is cleansed and anesthetized and the needle inserted 0.5 cm medial to the artery into the femoral vein. When blood return is obtained, the guidewire is inserted through the needle, the needle removed, and the catheter inserted over the wire.

If the patient is in cardiac arrest, percutaneous cannulation is difficult. In this case, a 3-cm incision is made 1 to 2 cm below the inguinal ligament and the subcutaneous tissue dissected with a hemostat. When the vein is exposed, it may be cannulated under direct visualization or ligatures placed under it and cannulated as described for the great saphenous vein. Femoral cannulation may be complicated by thrombophlebitis or infection, but if it is used for only a short time, the incidence of infection is low.

## INTRAOSSEOUS ROUTE

The intraosseous route was widely used for fluid and drug administration in the 1940s but was abandoned when venous catheters were perfected. Recently the intraosseous route has been demonstrated effective for the administration of sodium bicarbonate during cardiac arrest and for emergency fluid administration. Fluids and drugs that

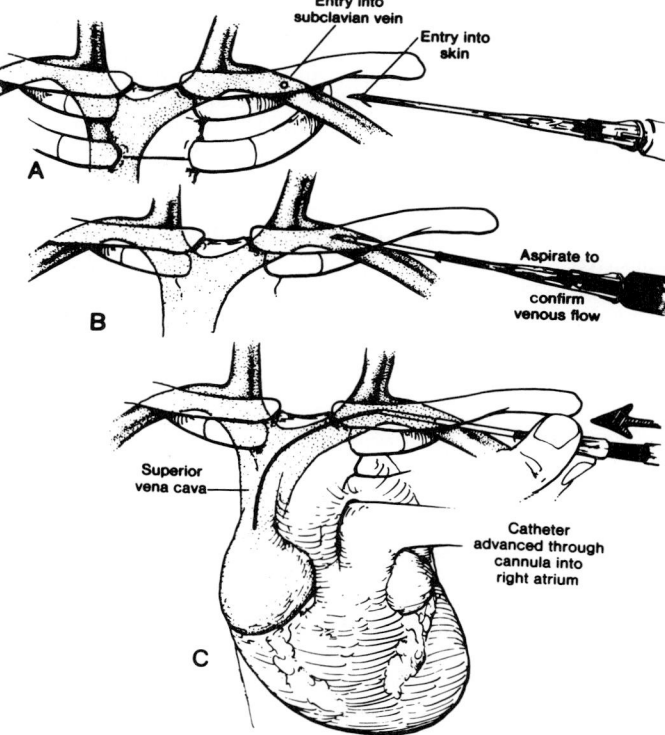

**Fig. 18-7.** The anatomic position of the subclavian vein is demonstrated in *A*. A needle is inserted at the mid-portion of the clavicle and advanced until the vein is punctured, as demonstrated in *B*. Once venipuncture is successful a catheter may be inserted through the needle or a Seldinger-type catheter may be inserted (*C*).

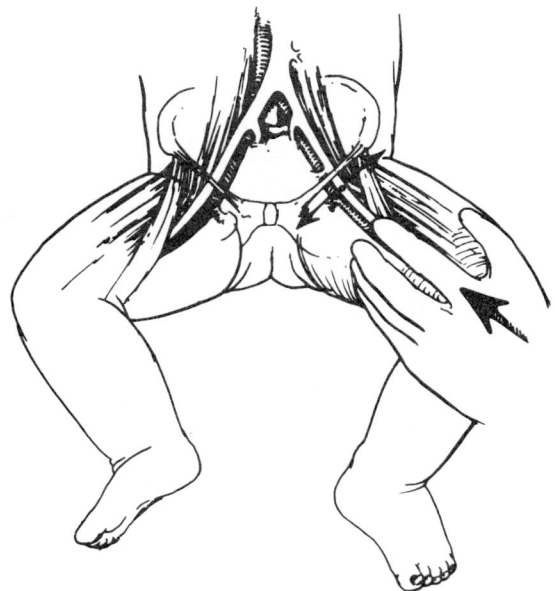

**Fig. 18-8.** The femoral vein in children lies one-half the distance between the symphysis and anterior iliac spine and 1.5 cm below the inguinal ligament.

have been administered via this route include saline, glucose, epinephrine, dopamine, sodium bicarbonate, diazepam, glucose, and antibiotics. The technique is relatively simple and is indicated when emergency venous access is required and peripheral or central routes are not available.

The bone most commonly used is the proximal tibia. The anterior tibial tuberosity is palpated with the index finger and the medial aspect of the tibia grasped with the thumb. An imaginary line is drawn between the two, and the needle is inserted 1 cm distal to the midpoint of this line. An 18-gauge spinal needle is used in infants up to age 18 months, while other children require a bone marrow needle. Using strict sterile techniques, the needle is inserted in a perpendicular or caudal direction until the needle point is felt to puncture the cortex (Fig. 18-9). The stylet is removed and blood or marrow contents aspirated to confirm position. Fluids or drugs may then be administered.

As soon as the child is resuscitated and conventional venous access obtained, the intraosseous needle should be removed and pressure applied to the puncture site. Complications include infection, fracture at the site of insertion and extravasation of drugs that may lead to

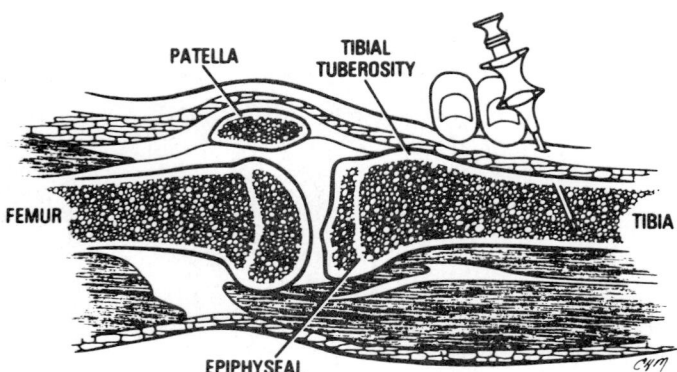

**Fig. 18-9.** The needle is inserted 2-cm distal to the tibial tuberosity on the medial aspect of the tibia. It is inserted in a caudal direction, away from the joint space.

sloughing of the skin. If sterile technique is used, the rate of infection is less than 1 percent.

## UMBILICAL VEIN

Umbilical vein access is indicated for resuscitation and stabilization of the newborn. It may be performed up to seven days after delivery. The cord is cleansed, cut to a length of 2 cm and a purse string suture placed near the junction of the skin and cord. The single large vein and two smaller arteries are identified and a catheter filled with heparinized saline is inserted into vein. The catheter, 3.5 to 5.0 French, should only be advanced 4 to 5 cm in a term infant. Further advancement may damage the liver or result in improper placement. After the catheter is placed, the purse string is tightened and fluid is infused taking care not to introduce air through the catheter.

Fluids and drugs may be administered by this route for resuscitation and maintenance afterwards. Complications include infection, air embolus, hemorrhage, vessel perforation and hepatic sclerosis from injection of sclerosing ces into the liver.

## ENDOTRACHEAL ROUTE

The endotracheal route is used when venous access cannot be obtained. It has been used for administration of epinephrine, atropine, naloxone, lidocaine, and diazepam in humans. Epinephrine and atropine have been administered most commonly, with no reports of adverse effects.

The drug is administered by injecting it directly into the endotracheal tube followed by several rapid insufflations with a bag-valve device to force the drug into the alveoli and terminal bronchioles. The optimum dose of drug has not been determined. A recent study has demonstrated that much higher doses of endotracheal epinephrine are needed to produce similar cardiovascular changes in dogs when compared to intravenous epinephrine. The current recommendation for endotracheal epinephrine is 0.1 mg/kg of the 1:1000 concentration. The endotracheal doses of other drugs should also be increased although no doses have been recommended. Prolonged duration of action may result from a depot effect in the lungs.

Adverse effects include destruction of surfactant and the development of adult respiratory distress syndrome or pneumonia, although this has not been reported in humans. Sodium bicarbonate, calcium chloride, and bretylium tosylate should not be given via this route.

## BIBLIOGRAPHY

American Heart Assn. Guidelines for cardiopulmonary resuscitation and emergency cardiac care. *JAMA* 268:2171, 1992.

Cote CJ, Jobes DR, Schwartz AJ, et al: Two approaches to cannulation of a child's internal jugular vein. *Anesthesiology* 50:371, 1979.

Hodge D, Delgado-Paredes C, Fleisher G: Intraosseous infusion flow rates in hypovolemic "pediatric" dogs (abstr). *Ann Emerg Med* 15:644, 1986.

Kanter RK, Gorton JM, Palmieri K, et al: Anatomy of femoral vessels in infants and guidelines for venous catheterization. *Pediatrics* 83:1020, 1989.

Nicholson SC, Sweeney MF, Moore RA, et al: Comparison of internal and external jugular cannulation of the central circulation in the pediatric patient. *Crit Care Med* 13:747, 1985.

Prince SR, Sullivan RL, Hacket A: Percutaneous cannulation of the internal jugular vein in infants and children. *Anesthesiology* 44:170, 1976.

Ralston SH, Tacker WA, Showen L, et al: Endotracheal versus intravenous epinephrine during electromechanical dissociation with CPR in dogs. *Ann Emerg Med* 14:1044, 1985.

Rossetti VA, Thompson BM, Miller J, et al: Intraosseous infusion: An alternative route of pediatric intravascular access. *Ann Emerg Med* 14:885, 1985.

Spivey WH, Lathers CM, Malone D, et al: Comparison of intraosseous, central, and peripheral routes of sodium bicarbonate administration during CPR in pigs. *Ann Emerg Med* 14:1135, 1985.

# 19
# ACID-BASE PROBLEMS

## Robert F. Wilson
## Christopher Barton

## DEFINING TERMS

The acidity of any solution, whether blood, interstitial fluid, or cell water, is a measure of the hydrogen ion activity of that solution. Hydrogen ion activity is directly proportional to the concentration of hydrogen ions within the solution multiplied by an activity coefficient. Thus, an equation for hydrogen activity could be derived as

$$H^+ = K_A \frac{[HA]}{[A^-]}$$

This equation assumes that the $[A^-]$ and $[HA]$ are measurements of their activities, not of their concentrations. $[HA]$ is any acid and $[A^-]$ is the conjugate base. The general equation for the acidity of any solution may now be written as

$$H^+ = K_A \frac{[acid]}{[base]}$$

The acidity of a solution is thus equal to the ratio of the activities of the acid to its corresponding base multiplied by its dissociation constant.

## pH

The concentration of hydrogen ions, even in a very acid solution, is extremely low. In a so-called neutral solution, the number of hydrogen $(H^+)$ ions equals the number of hydroxyl $(OH^-)$ ions; in water at 25°C (77°F) the number of hydrogen ions is 1/10,000,000, or $10^{-7}$ mol/L. The term *pH* refers to the negative logarithm of the hydrogen ion concentration. Thus, a solution with a pH of 1.0 has a hydrogen ion concentration of $1 \times 10^{-1}$ and is extremely acidic, whereas a solution with a pH of 13.0 has a hydrogen ion concentration of $1 \times 10^{-13}$ and is extremely alkaline.

## Henderson-Hasselbach Equation

The Henderson-Hasselbach equation states that the pH is equal to the pK (the negative log of the dissociation constant or the pH at which half of the compound is ionized) plus the log of the ratio of the concentration of a base to its related acid.

$$pH = pK + log \frac{proton\ acceptor\ (base)}{proton\ donor\ (acid)}$$

About 80 percent of the buffering for the extracellular fluid is the bicarbonate–carbonic acid system. The average normal concentration of bicarbonate is 24 mEq/L, and the average normal concentration of carbonic acid is 1.2 mEq/L. Thus, the ratio of bicarbonate to carbonic acid is normally 20:1. The log of 20 is 1.3, and adding 1.3 to 6.1 (the pK of the bicarbonate–carbonic acid system) results in 7.4, which is the normal arterial pH:

$$pH = 6.1 + log \frac{HCO_3^-}{H_2CO_2} = 6.1 + log \frac{24}{1.2}$$

$$= 6.1 + log\ 20 = 6.1 + 1.3 = 7.4$$

If the ratio of bicarbonate to carbonic acid is doubled or reduced by half, the pH changes by 0.3. The normal ratio of $HCO_3$ to $H_2CO_3$ is

20:1, and the log of 20 is 1.3. Since the log of 10 is 1.0 and the log of 5 is 0.7, whenever the ratio of $HCO_3$ to $H_2CO_3$ is reduced by one-half, the pH falls by 0.3. On the other hand, if the $HCO_3/H_2CO_3$ ratio increases from 20:1 to 40:1, the pH rises from 7.40 to 7.70.

The $H_2CO_3$ can be calculated by multiplying the $P_{CO_2}$ by 0.03. Thus, with a $HCO_3^-$ of 12 and a $P_{CO_2}$ of 40 mmHg, the $H_2CO_3$ would be 1.2, the ratio of $HCO_3^-$ to $H_2CO_3$ would be 10 (log of 1.0), and the pH would be 7.1. If the $HCO_3^-$ fell to 6 and the $P_{CO_2}$ were still 40 mmHg, the ratio of $HCO_3^-$ to $H_2CO_3$ would be 5 (log of 0.7) and the pH would be 6.8.

## Hydrogen Ion Concentrations

Some investigators prefer to use hydrogen ion concentration, rather than pH, when discussing or calculating acidity (Table 19-1). At a pH of 7.40, the hydrogen ion activity is equivalent to 40 nmol/L. The clinical relationship between $(H^+)$ (in nmol/L) and $P_{CO_2}$ and $HCO_3$ can be expressed by the following formula:

$$H^+(nmol/L) = \frac{(24)\ (P_{CO_2})}{HCO_3}$$

If a table relating $H^+$ to pH is available, it is easy to calculate pH, $P_{CO_2}$, and $HCO_3$ if two of the three are known.

Thus, if the $P_{CO_2}$ is 25 and the $HCO_3$ is 12,

$$H^+ = \frac{(24)\ (25)}{(12)} = \frac{600}{12} = 50\ nmol/L$$

A $H^+$ activity of 50 nmol/L is equivalent to a pH of 7.30 (Table 19-1).

## Intracellular pH $(pH_i)$

There are many difficulties in measuring intracellular pH, especially in humans. Measurements from human quadriceps muscle in 1978 revealed a $pH_i$ of 7.00 ± 0.06 in 13 studies. In 20 studies of human red blood cells, also in 1978, the $pH_i$ was found to range from 7.06 to 7.10. Thus, the $pH_i$ is 0.30 to 0.40 units less than the arterial pH.

To maintain a chronic stable $pH_i$, acid must be extruded from the cell relatively soon after it is formed. However, the initial handling of acid in the cell is much more complex. When responding to an acute internal acid load, the cell first recruits several relatively rapid mechanisms that consume or bind $H^+$, thereby minimizing the magnitude of the $pH_i$ decrease. Later, the $pH_i$ slowly returns toward normal as acid is extruded from the cell.

The initial mechanisms for handling an acid load include (1) physicochemical buffering, (2) cellular consumption of nonvolatile acids, and (3) the transfer of acid or alkali between the cytosol and organelles. In the broadest sense, all three are buffering mechanisms, since they reversibly consume $H^+$. In combination they neutralize more than 99.99 percent of the acid or alkali introduced into a cell. For example, the addition of $10^{-3}$ mol of $H^+$ to 1 L of cell content might lower $pH_i$ from 7.1 to 7.0, representing an increase of

**Table 19-1.** Hydrogen Ion Activity and pH

| $H^+$, nmol/L | pH |
|---|---|
| 20 | 7.7 |
| 25 | 7.6 |
| 32 | 7.5 |
| 40 | 7.4 |
| 50 | 7.3 |
| 64 | 7.2 |
| 80 | 7.1 |
| 101 | 7.0 |
| 128 | 6.9 |
| 160 | 6.8 |

only about $2 \times 10^{-8} M$ in free $[H^+]$. All the rest of the $H^+$ is "consumed" or "buffered" by the three mechanisms described above.

The conversion of a weak acid (e.g., lactic acid) to a neutral product (e.g., glucose) or to one that can readily leave the cell (e.g., $CO_2$) results in the loss of intracellular $H^+$. Internal pH can also be influenced by other reactions, such as the hydrolysis of ATP (which releases $H^+$) or phosphocreatinine (which consumes $H^+$). In one study intracellular acid loading (accomplished by increasing $P_{CO_2}$) was shown to lead to a reduction in the levels of several acidic metabolic intermediates (pyruvate, lactate, citrate, $\alpha$-ketoglutarate, maleate, glutamate, and aspartate). Intracellular acid loading also causes an elevation of glucose and glucose-6-phosphate levels. This pattern suggests that reducing $pH_i$ inhibits a step (possibly the phosphofructokinase reaction) in the glycolytic pathway. The maximum amount of $H^+$ that can be neutralized through these acidic intermediates is about 50 percent of that taken up by physicochemical buffers. There is other evidence of metabolic consumption of acid: increased lactate uptake by the isolated, perfused rat liver is associated with a rise in $pH_i$, as would be expected if lactate ions entered the cell and were converted to neutral products.

Intracellular alkalosis (produced by decreasing $P_{CO_2}$) leads to increased levels of pyruvate, lactate, and other acidic metabolic intermediates in rat brain, and these metabolic changes thereby partially neutralize the alkaline load.

Thus, physicochemical, biochemical, and organelle buffering mechanisms offer only partial and short-term solutions to acid loading. They can only minimize the decrease in $pH_i$ and are of limited capacity. The restoration of a normal $pH_i$ after an acute acid load requires the eventual extrusion of all added acid. As this extrusion proceeds, buffers release the $H^+$ which they previously consumed and are thereby restored to their initial state.

## ACID PRODUCTION, TRANSPORT, AND EXCRETION

### Carbon Dioxide (Volatile Acid)

With an average $CO_2$ production of 200 to 300 mL/min, the body's total $CO_2$ production is 288,000 to 432,000 mL/day. Since 22.4 mL $CO_2$ is equivalent to 1.0 mEq of acid, each day about 12,000 to 20,000 mEq of volatile acid is produced by the body's metabolism of carbohydrate, protein, and fat and is excreted by the lungs. Most carbon dioxide transport to the lungs from peripheral tissues is provided by plasma bicarbonate and red cell hemoglobin. Carbon dioxide present as carbonic acid in arterial blood averages about 1.2 (1.05 to 1.35) mEq/L, equivalent to a $P_{CO_2}$ of 40 mmHg.

### Nonvolatile Acid Excretion

Ordinarily the kidney excretes about 70 mEq of acid each day, but in acidotic patients, acid excretion may be increased more than tenfold. Renal tubular excretion of acid normally is accomplished by three mechanisms: (1) direct excretion of hydrogen, which accounts for only about 0.1 mEq of acid per day; (2) excretion with urine buffers, including the $NaH_2PO_4$ system, which accounts for about 20 mEq of acid per day; and (3) excretion with ammonia (produced in the distal tubal cells from glutamine and other precursors), which accounts for about 50 mEq of acid per day.

In the proximal tubule, sodium and bicarbonate are absorbed independent of the effects of aldosterone, and hydrogen is secreted into the tubular lumen in exchange for sodium ion. If the extracellular fluid volume is reduced or "contracted," increased amounts of sodium and bicarbonate are absorbed in the proximal tubule, and this may cause a "contraction metabolic alkalosis." If saline solution is given, expanding the extracellular fluid, proximal tubular absorption of sodium and bicarbonate is decreased. Sodium deficiency, increased aldosterone production, or decreased aldosterone metabolism

by the liver also increase the absorption of sodium and bicarbonate in the proximal tubule.

In the distal tubule cells, $H_2CO_3$ is dissociated into $H^+$ and $HCO_3^-$. Here $H^+$ and $K^+$ are excreted into the urine in exchange for $Na^+$. The $HCO_3^-$ which was formed in the cell and the $Na^+$ which is absorbed out of the tubule lumen move out the other side of the tubule cell into the bloodstream as $NaHCO_3$.

Anything that increases the intracellular concentration of hydrogen or potassium ions also increases the secretion of hydrogen and/or potassium ions into the distal tubular lumen and increases sodium reabsorption. When a potassium deficiency develops in the extracellular fluid, potassium ions leave tissue cells in exchange for hydrogen, resulting in an intracellular acidosis and an extracellular alkalosis. Increased potassium is also absorbed in the distal tubule in exchange for hydrogen ions, and increased hydrogen ions are then excreted in the urine. Thus, a hypokalemic alkalemic patient may put out a paradoxically acid urine.

Renal tubular acidosis may be classified as proximal or distal depending on the nephron segment primarily involved in the generation of this defect. In proximal tubular acidosis, urinary pH is increased at normal rates of bicarbonate filtration, denoting a failure of the proximal nephron to reabsorb the normal load of bicarbonate. However, when the filtered load of bicarbonate is decreased, urinary pH decreases to normal levels, indicating that the distal nephron is able to take care of the bicarbonate loads that are within the normal range.

When the distal nephron is predominately involved (distal tubular acidosis), the ability to create transepithelial pH gradients and thus to produce an acid urine is impaired at any filtered load of bicarbonate due to an intrinsic defect of the acidification capacity of the last tubule segments.

Acidification of urine by the distal nephron can be evaluated clinically by measuring urine and arterial $P_{CO_2}$ after making the urine alkaline by bicarbonate loading. The urine-blood $P_{CO_2}$ difference indicates the amount of urine $CO_2$ generation due to distal hydrogen ion secretion. When distal hydrogen ion secretion is impaired, as in distal tubular acidosis, urine $P_{CO_2}$ falls, and urine-blood $P_{CO_2}$ differences are reduced.

### Buffers

A wide variety of metabolic and respiratory factors produce or take up hydrogen ions. These changes in hydrogen ion concentration could cause wide swings in the pH if it were not for a group of substances referred to as *buffers,* which are capable of partially neutralizing acids and bases. The acid-buffering capacity of any agent or solution is determined by the number of hydrogen ions that the agent can take up for each unit change in pH. In general, for each 1000 to 10,000 mEq of acid added to the body, only about 1 mEq remains unbuffered or free to produce a change in pH. Thus, about 99.99 percent of an acid load is buffered or combined with other compounds to prevent sudden pH changes.

The average adult male has a total buffer base, or buffering capacity, of about 1000 mEq. The chief buffers in blood are the hemoglobin in red blood cells and the bicarbonate and protein in plasma. Most of the total buffering against carbon dioxide is provided by hemoglobin, but moment-to-moment buffering of the blood and interstitial fluid is provided primarily by the bicarbonate–carbonic acid system. The most important intracellular buffers are phosphate and protein. Patients with anemia, low plasma protein levels, or decreased muscle mass have a reduced buffering capacity and are apt to have wide swings in pH when they become ill or injured. In such individuals, impaired tissue perfusion of relatively short duration may cause severe acidosis.

The body generally tolerates an acid load much better than a base excess. Most of the body's buffer systems are designed to neutralize acid. Mortality and morbidity tend to be much worse in patients with alkalosis than in those with a corresponding amount of acidosis.

## Buffer Base

To recognize and quantify nonrespiratory (metabolic) acidosis or alkalosis, changes in plasma bicarbonate concentrations are traditionally evaluated. However, since bicarbonate concentration in plasma is also affected by changes in $P_{CO_2}$ (the respiratory disturbances), several $P_{CO_2}$-independent indexes of the nonrespiratory acid-base disturbance have been proposed, such as standard bicarbonate concentration or eucapnic pH (both standardized for $P_{CO_2}$ of 40 mmHg), and buffer base, either in whole blood or in plasma; base excess or deficit is a measure of the deviation of buffer base from its normal value. Conceptually all the $P_{CO_2}$-independent indicators of the metabolic acid-base disturbances are meant to parallel the differences between the sums of all strong (i.e., completely dissociated) cations and anions in plasma.

## Base Excess

An increase in the amount of buffer base present is referred to as a *base excess,* and a decrease may be referred to as a *base deficit* or a *negative base excess.*

The appropriate respiratory (ventilatory) component of the acid-base status of a patient is fairly predictable. A sudden increase of 10 mmHg in $P_{CO_2}$ (with bicarbonate staying constant) causes the pH to decrease by about 0.10 unit; whereas a sudden decrease of 10 mmHg in $P_{CO_2}$ (with bicarbonate staying constant) causes the pH to increase by about 0.13. Thus, the difference between the actual pH and the pH predicted from the $P_{CO_2}$ represents a deviation from the normal buffer base status.

The metabolic component may also be estimated because a rise in $HCO_3$ of 5.0 mEq/L (with $P_{CO_2}$ staying constant) raises the pH about 0.08, and a fall in $HCO_3$ of 5.0 mEq/L (again with $P_{CO_2}$ staying constant) lowers the pH about 0.10.

As a general rule, the base deficit (negative base excess) represents the mEq/L of bicarbonate that is required to restore the total buffer base of the extracellular fluid to normal. There are a number of ways to determine the base deficit. One can estimate it by (1) subtracting the actual bicarbonate from 26 mEq/L at a pH of 7.30 to 7.34 or 28 mEq at a pH of 7.20 to 7.29; (2) using a nomogram, (3) using a table (Table 19-2); or (4) using a technique described below, steps 1 to 3.

Thus, if the pH is 7.04, according to Table 19-2, the sum of the $HCO_3$ and buffer base should be 32 mEq/L. Thus, if the $HCO_3$ is 19.9 mEq/L, the base deficit should be about $32 - 19.9 = 12.1$ mEq/L.

If the pH is 7.47, according to Table 19-2, the sum of the $HCO_3$ and buffer base should be 23 mEq/L. Therefore, if the $HCO_3$ is 12.7 mEq/L, the base deficit should be $23 - 12.7 = 10$ mEq/L.

Another method involves three steps for estimating the metabolic component (i.e., base deficit) of an acid-base abnormality.

1. Determine the $P_{CO_2}$ variance, the difference between measured $P_{CO_2}$ and 40. Move the decimal point two places to the left.
2. Determine the predicted pH from the $P_{CO_2}$ variance: If the $P_{CO_2}$ is

over 40, subtract half of the $P_{CO_2}$ variance from the 7.40. If the $P_{CO_2}$ is under 40, add the $P_{CO_2}$ variance to 7.40.
3. Estimate the base excess (or deficit) from the pH variance: Determine the difference between the measured and predicted pHs. Move the decimal point two places to the right, and multiply by two-thirds.

**Example 1.** pH 7.04, $P_{CO_2}$ − 76 mmHg, $HCO_3$ 19.9 mEq/L.

$$76 - 40 = 36$$

$$36 \times 1/2 = 18$$

$$7.40 - 0.18 = 7.22$$

$$7.22 - 7.04 = 18$$

$$^2/_3 \times 18 = 12 \text{ mEq/L base deficit}$$

**Example 2.** pH 7.47, $P_{CO_2}$ − 18 mmHg, $HCO_3$ 12.7 mEq/L.

$$40 - 18 = 22$$

$$7.40 + 0.22 = 7.62$$

$$7.62 - 7.47 = 15$$

$$15 \times ^2/_3 = 10 \text{ mEq/L base deficit}$$

## Nonvolatile Weak Acids

In addition to $P_{CO_2}$ and plasma buffer base (BB), a third independent variable exists in body fluids, the total concentration of nonvolatile weak acids, designated as $[A_T]$. In plasma, the main constituent of $[A_T]$ is the protein (predominately albumin). The contribution of phosphate is less than one-tenth of the total $[A_T]$.

$P_{CO_2}$ and buffer base are the controlled quantities in the biological regulation of acid-base balance. However, any abnormality in the amount of nonvolatile weak acids ($[A_T]$), especially plasma proteins, will produce an acid-base disturbance. Thus, hypoproteinemia tends to cause a nonrespiratory alkalosis, and abnormally high concentrations of plasma albumin can give rise to a nonrespiratory acidosis.

If the anion gap is normal in a hypoproteinemic patient, unidentified anions must be present. This increase in unidentified anions would be missed if the plasma protein level was not known.

Plasma proteins should be measured as part of the evaluation of acid-base status. Base excess or deficit does not distinguish strong acids (e.g., lactic, keto) from weak nonvolatile acids (plasma proteins, phosphate). The existing nomograms for the estimation of buffer base are based on data obtained in blood with normal concentrations of plasma proteins. Therefore, a deficit of novolatile weak acids appears as an apparent increase in plasma buffer base.

## Carbon Dioxide Content

*Carbon dioxide content* refers to the total of all carbon dioxide present in the blood (normally 24 to 31 mEq/L). In the plasma, $CO_2$ content includes carbonic acid, bicarbonate, and carbamino compounds. The amount of carbonic acid present (averaging about 1.05 to 1.35 mEq/L) can be estimated by multiplying the $P_{CO_2}$ by 0.03. The arterial bicarbonate concentration normally is 24 mEq/L. The concentration of the carbamino compounds, which consist of various forms of $CO_2$ combined with amino groups on proteins, averages about 0.5 to 1.0 mEq/L, depending on total $CO_2$ and protein concentrations.

## EVALUATING ACID-BASE ABNORMALITIES

### Checking the Consistency and Accuracy of Laboratory Reports

#### Correlating Carbon Dioxide Content and Bicarbonate

When obtaining blood for blood gas studies in patients with complicated acute problems, additional blood for electrolyte determinations

**Table 19-2.** Estimating Base Deficit from the pH and Bicarbonate

| pH | Sum of Base Deficit and Bicarbonate | Base Deficit if Bicarbonate is 24 mEq |
|---|---|---|
| 7.00–7.09 | 32 | 8 |
| 7.10–7.19 | 30 | 6 |
| 7.20–7.29 | 28 | 4 |
| 7.30–7.34 | 26 | 2 |
| 7.35–7.45 | 24 | 0 |
| 7.45–7.49 | 23 | −1 |
| 7.50–7.59 | 22 | −2 |

should be drawn. The bicarbonate present can then be estimated from the $CO_2$ content as well as from the pH and $P_{CO_2}$.

Under ordinary circumstances, the arterial bicarbonate concentration is approximately 1.5 to 2.0 mEq/L less than the arterial $CO_2$ content reported as part of an electrolyte analysis. Since the venous $P_{CO_2}$ is normally about 6 mmHg higher than the arterial $P_{CO_2}$ and venous bicarbonate is 1.1 mEq/L higher than arterial bicarbonate, the venous $CO_2$ content is usually about 1.5 to 2.0 mEq/L higher than the arterial $CO_2$ content. Thus, if arterial blood is drawn for blood gas determinations and venous blood is drawn for electrolytes, the $CO_2$ content in venous blood should be about 3.0 to 4.0 mEq/L more than the arterial bicarbonate. One should not accept an arterial bicarbonate which is higher than a simultaneous venous $CO_2$ content.

## Correlating pH and Electrolyte Values

Correlating pH with the potassium and other electrolyte values can also help estimate acid-base status. Patients with severe acidosis tend to have high serum potassium levels, and patients with severe alkalosis tend to have low serum potassium levels. In general, a rise or fall of 0.10 in pH is associated with a corresponding fall or rise of about 0.5 (0.3 to 0.8) mEq/L in serum potassium. Thus, if the pH of a patient with a pH of 7.30 and a plasma potassium of 4.8 mEq/L were raised to 7.50, the patient's plasma potassium level would fall to about 3.8. The potassium level in serum is slightly higher than that in plasma because the clotting process releases some potassium.

## Correlating Chloride and Bicarbonate Levels

Plasma chloride and bicarbonate concentrations tend to move in opposite directions. Thus, patients who have a metabolic alkalosis (and high plasma bicarbonate levels) tend to have low plasma chloride levels, whereas those with metabolic acidosis (and low plasma bicarbonate levels) tend to have normal or elevated chloride levels. However, if there are increased amounts of unmeasured anions, such as lactate, present (causing an increased anion gap), bicarbonate may be very low and chloride may be normal or even low.

## Effect of $P_{CO_2}$ and $HCO_3^-$ on pH

With mild to moderate acidosis (pH 7.25 to 7.35), a 1.0-mmHg rise in the $P_{CO_2}$ produces a decrease of about 0.01 in pH, while a 1.0 mEq/L decrease in bicarbonate produces a pH decrease of about 0.02 (Table 19-3). Thus, a patient whose $HCO_3$ falls from 24.0 to 19.0 mEq/L and whose $P_{CO_2}$ also falls from 40 to 30 mmHg will still have a pH of approximately 7.40. This "quick and dirty" way to estimate bicarbonate from the pH and $P_{CO_2}$ can also be used as a check on the consistency and accuracy of the laboratory results, particularly if arterial bicarbonate is not 2.5 to 3.0 mEq/L less than the $CO_2$ content found on a venous electrolyte study.

**Table 19-3.** Acute pH and Bicarbonate Response to Changes in $P_{CO_2}$

| $P_{CO_2}$, mmHg | pH | $HCO_3$, mEq/L |
|---|---|---|
| 15 | 7.73 | 19 |
| 20 | 7.62 | 20 |
| 25 | 7.54 | 21 |
| 30 | 7.49 | 22 |
| 35 | 7.44 | 23 |
| 40 | 7.40 | 24 |
| 50 | 7.32 | 25 |
| 60 | 7.26 | 26 |
| 70 | 7.21 | 27 |
| 80 | 7.16 | 28 |

## Categorizing the Abnormality

### Single Disorders

Acid-base abnormalities can often be defined in terms of the pH and the relative amounts of arterial bicarbonate and carbonic acid. The normal average concentration of bicarbonate in arterial blood is 24 mEq/L, with a normal range of about 21 to 26 mEq/L. If the arterial bicarbonate is greater than 26 mEq/L and the pH is greater than 7.40, the patient is said to have a metabolic alkalosis. If the arterial bicarbonate is less than 21 mEq/L and the pH is less than 7.40, the patient is said to have a metabolic acidosis.

The $P_{CO_2}$ is normally 35 to 45 mmHg. If the arterial $P_{CO_2}$ is lower than 35 mmHg and the pH is greater than 7.40, the patient is said to have a respiratory alkalosis. In contrast, if the arterial $P_{CO_2}$ is greater than 45 mmHg and the pH is less than 7.40, the patient is said to have a respiratory acidosis.

### Mixed Disorders

In many instances, more than one acid-base problem is present at a time. For example, if a patient with chronic respiratory acidosis (pH, 7.35; $P_{CO_2}$, 50 mmHg; $HCO_3$, 26.7 mEq/L) develops pyloric stenosis and is vomiting large amounts of highly acidic fluid (which would ordinarily cause a metabolic alkalosis), the patient could develop a pH of 7.40 with a $P_{CO_2}$ of 55 mmHg and a $HCO_3$ of 32 mEq/L. This might be confusing under many clinical circumstances. However, in general, if the arterial pH is relatively normal (7.36 to 7.44) and the $P_{CO_2}$ and/or $HCO_3$ are abnormal, one can assume that a mixed abnormality is present. The mixed abnormality should also be detectable from the history and physical examination or other laboratory data. In this regard, the anion gap and buffer base may be helpful.

## Compensatory Changes

Any abnormality that disturbs the normal ratio between arterial bicarbonate and carbonic acid tends to immediately stimulate a compensatory metabolic or respiratory response—to try to bring the ratio back to 7.35 if the primary problem is an acidosis or to 7.45 if the problem is an alkalosis.

### Respiratory Compensation

**Metabolic Acidosis**

Respiratory compensation for a primary metabolic acidosis can occur very rapidly. For example, the patient who develops a metabolic acidosis with a bicarbonate of 14 mEq/L will tend to hyperventilate rather rapidly, producing a compensatory respiratory alkalosis. The $P_{CO_2}$ would have to fall to 20 mmHg to produce complete compensation to a pH of 7.40; however, the acute compensation (within 1 to 2 h) may be only about 50 percent of that, and the compensation over 24 h may be only 75 percent complete (Table 19-4).

**Metabolic Alkalosis**

Compensation for an alkalosis is seldom as good as for an acidosis. Furthermore, the compensatory hypoventilation for a metabolic alka-

**Table 19-4.** Chronic pH and Bicarbonate Response to Changes in $P_{CO_2}$

| $P_{CO_2}$, mmHg | pH | $HCO_3$, mEq/L |
|---|---|---|
| 20 | 7.47 | 14 |
| 30 | 7.45 | 20 |
| 40 | 7.40 | 24 |
| 50 | 7.37 | 28 |
| 60 | 7.35 | 32 |
| 70 | 7.33 | 36 |
| 80 | 7.32 | 40 |

losis is restricted by the hypoxemia that develops along with the hypoventilation. The $P_{CO_2}$ seldom rises above 50 to 55 mmHg to compensate for a metabolic alkalosis unless oxygen is given.

If a patient develops a metabolic alkalosis with a $HCO_3$ of 36 mEq/L, the $P_{CO_2}$ would have to rise to 60 mmHg for a complete compensation to a pH of 7.40. The acute compensation would only be about 25 to 40 percent, raising the $P_{CO_2}$ to about 45 to 48 mmHg. Even after 48 h, the respiratory compensation is often only about 60 percent complete.

### Metabolic Compensations

During acute and chronic hypocapnia and hypercapnia, the changes in $HCO_3$ are almost linear over the range of $Pa_{CO_2}$ (20 to 100 mmHg) encountered in altered pathologic states (Tables 19-3 and 19-4). Thus, you can predict to some degree what the $HCO_3$ "should be" for any $Pa_{CO_2}$. This observation leads to certain rules of thumb to characterize various acid-base abnormalities:

1. During acute hypercapnia, $HCO_3$ increases 1 mmol/L for each 10-mmHg increase in $Pa_{CO_2}$ above 40 mmHg.
2. During chronic hypercapnia, $HCO_3$ increases 4 mmol/L for each 10-mmHg increase in $Pa_{CO_2}$ above 40 mmHg.
3. During acute hypocapnia, $HCO_3$ decreases 2 mmol/L for every 10-mmHg decrease in $Pa_{CO_2}$ below 40 mmHg.
4. During chronic hypocapnia, $HCO_3$ decreases at least 5 mmol/L for every 10-mmHg decrease in $Pa_{CO_2}$ below 40 mmHg.

### Failure of Compensatory Mechanisms

Failure of compensatory mechanisms, or a combination of primary processes driving the pH in the same direction so that it rapidly falls and stays below 7.10 or rises above 7.60, is frequently lethal. Inability to compensate for an acid-base abnormality usually means a severe disturbance of ventilatory, renal, or general cellular function.

## The Anion Gap

### Definition

The concept of an anion gap in blood was described in 1939 by Gamble. It was felt that the law of electroneutrality required that the number of positive charges contributed by serum cations should equal the number of negative charges contributed by serum anions. Sodium (Na), chloride (Cl), and bicarbonate ($HCO_3$) are considered the measured ions. Potassium is ignored because its value changes so little. Thus, the concept of electroneutrality can be expressed by the simple equation:

$$Na + UC = Cl + HCO_3 + UA$$

where UC (unmeasured cations) indicates the sum of the charges of the cations other than sodium and UA (unmeasured anions) equals the sum of the charges of all of the anions other than chloride and bicarbonate.

The term *anion gap* was coined to indicate the difference between the measured sodium level and the measured chloride and bicarbonate (really $CO_2$ content) levels.

$$Anion\ gap = Na - (Cl + HCO_3)$$

The equation can also be written as

$$UA - UC = Na - (Cl + HCO_3) = anion\ gap$$

indicating that a rise in UA and/or a decrease in UC will cause an increase in the anion gap, independent of the presence or absence of an acid-base disorder. The reverse is also true. In other words, a decrease in UA and/or rise in UC will cause a decrease in the anion gap.

The "unmeasured cations" usually total about 11 mEq/L and include potassium (4 mEq/L), calcium (5 mEq/L), and magnesium (2 mEq/L).

The "unmeasured" serum anions include sulfates (1 mEq/L), phosphates (2 mEq/L), proteins (16 mEq/L), lactic acid (1 mEq/L), and other organic acids (3 mEq/L). Ordinarily, the sodium concentration is about 140 mEq/L, and the sum of the $CO_2$ content and chloride anions is about 128 mEq/L. Thus, the difference (or anion gap) between the sodium concentration and the sum of these two anions averages about 12 mEq/L. In patients with excessive acid production, the anion gap tends to be increased. On the other hand, in patients with metabolic acidosis due to loss of bicarbonate, the anion gap usually stays relatively normal.

### Unmeasured Cations and Anions

Assigning numerical values for the charges of the serum constituents is accomplished easily for sodium, potassium, bicarbonate, and chloride, but is more difficult with phosphate and protein, which can have multiple charges. Although they are measured with relative ease, calcium and magnesium are also a problem (Table 19-5). The total concentration of serum calcium and magnesium, rather than just the ionized fraction, is used in the calculation of unmeasured cations because the nonionized portions of those cations are bound to protein (especially albumin, which is a polyanion) or are complexed with bicarbonate, phosphate, sulfate, lactate, or citrate. Thus, they "cover," or balance, an equivalent number of negative charges on these anions. In other words, protein-bound and complexed calcium and magnesium contribute to the charge balance in the serum.

The difficulty in establishing the precise charge contributions of sulfate and organic acid anions arises because clinical laboratories do not measure these serum constituents on a routine basis. At least 29 acid anions are detectable in plasma; however, in normal individuals the combined contribution to the serum anions by lactate, pyruvate, acetoacetate, 3-hydroxybutyrate, and citrate is only 1.8 to 2.6 mEq/L.

Although the concentration of serum phosphate is readily measured in the clinical laboratory, it is not a simple matter to derive its charge, which is a function not only of phosphate concentration but also serum pH. Serum phosphorus concentration in mg/dL is converted to mmol/L by multiplying by 10 and dividing by 31, the atomic weight of phosphorus. At a pH of 7.4, the ratio of $H_2PO_4^{2-}$ to $H_2PO_4^-$ is about 4 to 1. Thus, 80 percent of the phosphate contributes two negative charges as $HPO_4^{2-}$, and 20 percent contributes one charge as $H_2PO_4^-$; thus, the charge contribution of phosphate in mEq/L at pH 7.4 is equal to the mmol/L of phosphate multiplied by 1.8.

Normal serum proteins are polyanions. Although their net contribution to overall charge balance is difficult to assess exactly, a normal mixture of serum proteins is about 2.3 mEq/L per gram of protein at pH 7.40. This charge reflects three variables: the type of protein, the concentration of protein, and serum pH.

Albumin contributes about 2.6 mEq/L for each g/dL, and globulin provides approximately 1.7 mEq/L for each g/dL. A 4 to 5 percent increase in the negative charge of protein for each 0.10 unit rise in pH was reported in two different studies.

**Table 19-5.** Conversion of Laboratory Values for Serum Constituents to mEq/L*

| |
| --- |
| $Ca^{2+}$ mg/dL × 10 ÷ 40 × 2 |
| $Mg^{2+}$ mg/dL × 10 ÷ 24 × 2 |
| $PO_4^-$ (mgP) mg/dL × 10 ÷ 31 × 1.8 |
| $SO_4^-$ (mmol) mmol/L × 2 |

* Conversion from mg/dL to mEq/L is done by multiplying by 10 to convert to mg/L, dividing by the molecular weight, and then multiplying by the valence.

## Etiology of Increased Anion Gap

An increased anion gap may be caused by (1) artifacts; (2) an accumulation of organic acids, such as that seen in lactic acidosis, ketoacidosis, acute renal failure, and toxic ingestions; (3) exogenous anions; (4) reduced inorganic acid excretion, such as in chronic renal failure; (5) an increase in the anionic contribution of unmeasured weak acids; (6) a decrease in unmeasured cations; or (7) a combination of these factors.

### Changes Due to Artifacts

A spurious increase in the anion gap (even in the presence of normal concentrations of the individual electrolytes) may result from excessive exposure of the serum to air. When serum placed in small measuring vessels for microautomated chemical analysis is not analyzed promptly, the percentage increases in Na, K, and Cl are similar, but $HCO_3$ decreases due to escape of $CO_2$. After 2 h, absolute increases in the concentrations of Na and Cl of $6.9 \pm 1.9$ and $4.2 \pm 1.8$ mEq/L, respectively, and a decrease in $HCO_3$ of $3.5 \pm 1.2$ mEq/L were observed. As a result, the anion gap increased $6.2 \pm 2.3$ mEq/L.

False elevations of serum Cl may result from the presence of other halide ions, as in patients intoxicated with bromide or iodide. These elevations occur because bromide and iodide interfere with both colorimetric and "ion-selective" techniques, resulting in reported values for Cl that exceed the sum of the true chloride concentration plus that of the other halide. Minimal interference with Cl measurement occurs with the use of chloridimetry, which should be used if halide poisoning is suspected.

Spurious hyperchloremia (with an equivalent apparent decrease in the anion gap) may also occur from the technical artifact caused by hypertriglyceridemia using colorimetric (but not titrimetric or potentiometric) techniques. In one prospective study every patient with a triglyceride level exceeding 1000 mg/dL had a spurious elevation of Cl ranging from 9 to 93 mEq/L. This artifact would be independent of any change induced by displacement of the water phase of the plasma (i.e., pseudohyponatremia).

If there is excess heparin in the syringe in which arterial blood is drawn, the heparin will tend to cause an acidosis and lower the pH, $P_{CO_2}$, and bicarbonate, producing a picture of metabolic acidosis with partial respiratory compensation.

### Increased Organic Acids

The organic acids most likely to increase the anion gap are lactic acid, keto acids, and a variety of other organic acids apt to increase in renal failure. Although an increase in unmeasured anions theoretically could result from increased phosphate, protein, sulfate, or organic anions, in practice, only increases in organic anions or major toxic ingestions account for large increases in the anion gap.

Patients with anion gaps greater than 35 mEq/L usually have ethylene glycol or methanol intoxication, hyperglycemic hyperosmolar coma, or lactic acidosis. In fact, such patients can have anion gaps greater than 50 mEq/L. Severe acidemia (pH < 7.00) occurs most commonly in such patients.

#### Lactic Acidosis

The causes of lactic acidosis have been divided into those due to inadequate tissue oxygenation (type A) and those due to other factors, such as diabetes mellitus, hypercarbia, tumors, etc. (type B) (Table 19-6). The presence of acidosis with an increased anion gap in a patient in severe shock most often is due to lactic acidosis.

#### Ketoacidosis and Hyperglycemic Coma

A tendency to ketoacidosis will be less apparent in patients with a good urine output. In the presence of adequate hydration with a normal or increased urine output, ketoacidosis tends to be minimal because the increased ketones are rapidly excreted. However, if extracellular fluid volume is reduced, as is usually the case, the excretion of keto anions is retarded, producing a ketoacidosis with an increased anion gap. However, if the patient maintains an adequate salt intake and preserves normal or nearly normal extracellular fluid volume, renal perfusion, and glomerular filtration rate, keto anions are excreted almost as fast as they are produced. Under these circumstances, chloride is retained by the kidney in place of ketones, a rise in the serum chloride balances the fall in the serum bicarbonate concentration, and the serum anion gap remains or becomes normal. The increase in serum chlorides will be even greater if the patient is resuscitated with 0.9% saline rather than Ringer's lactate.

Although some ketonemia probably occurs in all spontaneously occurring instances of nonketotic hyperglycemic coma, increases in neither plasma β-hydroxybutyrate nor lactate are sufficient to explain the elevated anion gap levels, which some investigators have reported to average as high as 34 mEq/L.

#### Other Organic Acids

A wide variety of organic acids may be released into the blood in increased amounts in critically ill or injured patients. These may include fatty acids, amino acids, pyruvic acid, and a large number of other acid metabolites of incomplete cell metabolism.

### Toxic Ingestions

Intoxications with cyanide, salicylate, methanol, ethylene glycol, paraldehyde, toluene, sulfur, and formaldehyde lead to the formation of acid metabolites and/or organic acids that result in an increase in the anion gap. Some of these poisonings can be suspected clinically because of the presence of an increased osmolal gap (measured serum osmolality minus calculated serum osmolality). If the patient has a high anion gap metabolic acidosis without chronic renal failure, shock, or diabetic ketoacidosis, intoxication with methanol or ethylene glycol should be the first consideration, especially if the osmolal gap is increased.

### Exogenous Anions

The influence of the poorly resorbable anion carbenicillin on the anion gap is a good example of the effect of the addition of unmeasured anion to the extracellular fluid. In addition to observing the renal tubular effects (a decrease in pH value and enhanced excretion of ammonium), some researchers detected an increase in the anion gap from the control value of 11.2 to 18.3 mEq/L. In contrast, the administration of polymyxin B, a cationic antibiotic, has been reported to cause hyperchloremia and an apparently negative anion gap.

### Reduced Inorganic Acid Excretions

In renal failure, increased quantities of sulfuric and phosphoric acid may accumulate in the bloodstream. With muscle damage a number of sulfur-containing compounds may greatly increase the anion gap.

**Table 19-6.** Classification of Lactic Acidosis

| |
|---|
| Type A (tissue hypoxia) |
|   Shock states |
|   Profound anemia |
|   Massive catecholamine excess |
| Type B (tissue oxygenation appears normal) |
|   Diabetes mellitus |
|   Liver failure |
|   Renal failure |
|   Carcinoma |
|   Seizures |
|   Alkaloses |
|   Drugs or toxins |
|   Inborn errors of metabolism |
|   Hypoglycemia |

*Source:* Adapted from Cohen RD, Woods H: Lactic acidosis revisited. *Diabetes* 32:181, 1983.

### Increased Unmeasured Weak Acids

In shock and sepsis, in particular, increased quantities of pyruvic acid, β-hydroxybutyric acid, fatty acids, citric acid, etc., may accumulate and add slightly to the anion gap. It is likely, however, that those known substances account for only a small increase in anion gap. Indeed, in sepsis, known compounds, including lactic acid, only account for 25 to 50 percent of the anion gap which develops.

### Decreased Unmeasured Cations

The unmeasured cations are relatively constant in value. However, calcium could conceivably fall from 10 to 6 mg/dL (5 to 3 mEq/L). Potassium could fall from 5.0 to 3 mEq/L and magnesium could fall from 2.5 to 1.5 mEq/L without the patient becoming extremely ill. However, these changes combined would result in a decrease of only 5.0 mEq/L in the unmeasured cations.

### Alkalemia

Alkalemia itself can induce an increase in organic acid production. However, an increased anion gap and alkalemia can coexist in the absence of a demonstrated increase in organic acids because (1) alkalemia tends to increase the net negative charge of serum proteins, and (2) certain exogenously administered anions (citrate, lactate, and acetate) can, via their metabolism, generate metabolic alkalosis and, by partial persistence in the circulation, elevate the anion gap. In the study by Gabow et al. of patients with an increased anion gap, 10 of the 42 subjects were alkalemic and 9 had a normal serum pH.

Alkalemia occurs in up to 50 percent of patients with alcoholic ketoacidosis or salicylate intoxication. Similarly, in one study 42 percent of patients with rhabdomyolysis and an increased anion gap were alkalemic. Four of seven normotensive patients with classic heat stroke had an increased anion gap. Alkalemia in alcoholic ketoacidosis, salicylate intoxication, rhabdomyolysis, and classic heat stroke is usually accounted for by enough respiratory and/or metabolic alkalosis to counteract the acidifying effect of organic acid overproduction.

Respiratory alkalosis frequently occurs in patients undergoing alcohol withdrawal. If one adds the increase in the anion gap to the actual serum bicarbonate concentration, a measure of the true extent of the metabolic alkalosis can be obtained. One can think of this value as the level of serum bicarbonate concentration that would have been present had the newly formed organic acids not titrated away a portion of the bicarbonate.

The interpretation of an increased anion gap in patients with alkalemia is complicated because alkalemia itself can increase the anion gap. Alkalemia can increase both organic acid generation and the negative charge on protein. In acute respiratory alkalosis, lactic acid production can increase modestly and thereby raise plasma lactate levels by 2 to 3 mEq/L. This increase in lactic acid production appears to result from an increased activity of phosphofructokinase, which enhances glycolysis via the Embden-Meyerhof pathway and thereby increases the conversion of glucose to lactate.

Two interrelated factors are responsible for alkalemia increasing the net negative charge on serum proteins. First, alkalemic states are often associated with a reduced blood volume and hemoconcentration. Second, proteins surrender protons when titrated in an alkaline direction, thereby uncovering additional negative charges.

Utilizing a formula derived some 30 years ago, one can anticipate that alkaline titration alone can increase the anion gap by about 0.6 mEq/L for every 0.10 rise in pH. Some investigators have reported that in humans, severe gastric alkalosis may increase the anion gap by 8 to 12 mEq/L. About 25 percent of the total increase results from increased organic acids and proteinate charge, and about 75 percent results from hemoconcentration. Before this phenomenon was emphasized in 1979, increases in the anion gap in hypotensive patients with severe gastric alkalosis were usually attributed (without confirmation) to lactic acidosis.

In summary, an anion gap greater than 30 mEq/L usually indicates the presence of an organic acidosis. Values between 23 and 30 mEq/L are also suggestive of an organic acidosis, but the nature of the retained anion frequently cannot be established. In acidotic patients with values between 16 and 22 mEq/L, uremia or mild organic acidosis may be present. If the patient is alkalemic, hemoconcentration or administration of an exogenous anion may be the cause of an increased anion gap.

## Decreased Anion Gap

An anion gap of 7 or less is unusual. The main causes of a decreased anion gap are decreased unmeasured anions, increased unmeasured cations, and various analytical errors causing falsely low sodium levels or falsely high chloride levels (Table 19-7).

### Decreased Unmeasured Anions

Hypoalbuminemia is probably the most common cause of a decreased anion gap in hospitalized patients. For each 1.0 g/dL reduction in serum albumin the anion gap will fall approximately 2.5 to 3.0 mEq/L and the standard bicarbonate (the bicarbonate that would be present if the arterial $P_{CO_2}$ were 40 mmHg) increases by an average of 3.4 mmol/L.

However, other studies present somewhat different corrections in anion gap and bicarbonate related to changes in albumin.

$$[HCO_3] = [\text{albumin, g/dL}] \, (-2.63)$$

$$[AG] = [\text{albumin, g/dL}] \, (+4.20)$$

This mechanism is the most likely explanation for the decreased anion gap frequently observed in patients with nephrotic syndrome or advanced liver disease.

Some reduction in the anion gap occurs in hypoosmolar states, presumably as a result of dilution. This change is most apparent in the syndrome of inappropriate secretion of antidiuretic hormone (SIADH). Almost 25 percent of patients with SIADH have an anion gap of less than 6 mEq/L.

### Increased Unmeasured Cations

The decreased anion gap in multiple myeloma is due to an increased serum concentration of cationic IgG paraproteins. Hypercalcemia and hypoalbuminemia can also contribute to a low plasma anion gap in patients with multiple myeloma.

### Analytical Errors

One should never assume that all reported laboratory values are correct. Among the causes of nonrandom laboratory errors leading to artifactual reduction in the anion gap, hypernatremia and hyperviscosity are the most important. When the actual serum sodium concentration exceeds 170 mEq/L, certain flame photometers yield artifactually low values. Hyperviscosity can also lead to falsely low values for

**Table 19-7.** Causes of a Decreased Anion Gap

Decreased unmeasured anions
  Hypoalbuminemia
  Dilution
Increased unmeasured cation
  IgG multiple myeloma
  Increased calcium, magnesium, or potassium
  Acute lithium intoxication
  Polymyxin B administration
Nonrandom analytical error
  Hypernatremia (severe)
  Hyperviscosity
  Bromide intoxication
  Iodide ingestion
  Hyperlipidemia

serum sodium and, hence, anion gap because the flame photometer apparatus may fail to aspirate a proper aliquot of hyperviscous serum.

Because bromide reacts very strongly with most reagents utilized to measure chloride, artifactually high values for serum chloride concentration are frequently seen in bromide-intoxicated patients. Indeed, this laboratory error may be sufficient to actually produce a negative anion gap.

Iodine, another halogen capable of accumulating in the serum, also can cause an artificial increase in serum chloride concentration and hence a decrease in the anion gap. Overestimation of serum chloride concentration also can occur in the presence of hyperlipidemia because lipids scatter light in such a way as to falsely elevate the concentration of chloride when determined by the colorimetric method.

## Ratio of Change of Anion Gap to Change in Plasma Bicarbonate

In uncomplicated increased anion gap metabolic acidosis, the decrease (change) in plasma bicarbonate should be roughly equal to the increase (change) in the anion gap (that is, $d\text{AG}/d\text{HCO}_3 = 1.0$).

Whenever the anion gap changes much more or less than the bicarbonate, one should be suspicious of a coexisting or a mixed acid-base disorder. For example, in classical diabetic ketoacidosis (DKA) and lactic acidosis, the rise in anion gap is similar, quantitatively, to the decrease in $\text{HCO}_3$. The ratio of their changes, therefore, is close to 1.0. Since excretion of the keto anions tends to reduce the anion gap while not directly affecting the $\text{HCO}_3$, some patients with DKA, whose keto anion excretion is greater than usual, may have metabolic acidosis that is substantially or even entirely of the hyperchloremic variety. The hyperchloremic acidosis so frequently observed during the treatment of DKA is also believed to be largely explainable on the same basis. In a pure hyperchloremic metabolic acidosis, the ratio is close to 0. Ratios between 0.3 and 0.7 usually, but not always, indicate a mixed acid-base disorder or a preexisting low anion gap.

In renal failure, there is no cause-and-effect relationship between the rise in anion gap and fall in the $\text{HCO}_3$, since the latter is related largely to a failure of ammonia genesis, whereas the former is related to the reduction in the glomerular filtration rate (GRF), leading to anion retention. Thus, reciprocal stoichiometry between the anion gap and $\text{HCO}_3$ should not be expected. Even in end-stage chronic renal failure, the anion gap rarely exceeds 23 mEq/L. Indeed, in patients with mild to moderate chronic renal failure (serum creatinine concentration between 2 and 4 mg/dL), the anion gap is usually normal. In patients with more severe chronic renal failure, the anion gap averages about 16 mEq/L with an average $d\text{AG}/d\text{HCO}_3$ of only 0.4.

Thus, the $d\text{AG}/d\text{HCO}_3$ ratio is helpful in the diagnosis of mixed acid-base disorder because this ratio is usually close to 1.0 in typical organic acidoses. Values greater than 1.2 or less than 0.8 suggest the presence of a mixed acid-base disorder or an independent factor affecting the anion gap.

## Urinary Anion Gap

Calculation of the urinary anion gap allows one to determine if $\text{NH}_4$ production is adequate or appropriate in patients with an acidemia. According to one group, the urinary anion gap (in mEq/L), which is determined by the difference between the UA and UC, equals Na + K − Cl. The value of potassium is included in the formula because, unlike the plasma potassium concentration, its concentration in urine is large and highly variable. The value for bicarbonate is not included because it is not easily measured in most clinical laboratories. At a urine pH of 6.8, the $\text{HCO}_3$ will generally be less than 10 mEq/L. Furthermore, if urine is more acidic (pH < 6.4), the $\text{HCO}_3$ concentration will be trivial.

The major ionic species in bicarbonate-free urine are

$$\text{Na} + \text{K} + \text{Ca} + \text{Mg} + \text{NH}_4 = \text{H}_2\text{PO}_4 + \text{SO}_4 + \text{OA}$$

**Table 19-8.** Average Daily Urinary Excretion of Cations and Anions in Four Normal Subjects on a Normal Diet*

| Cations | mEq/day | Anion | mEq/day |
|---|---|---|---|
| Na | 127 ± 6 | Cl | 135 ± 5 |
| K | 49 ± 2 | SO$_4$ | 34 ± 1 |
| Ca | 4 ± 1 | H$_2$PO$_4$ | 20 ± 1 |
| Mg | 11 ± 1 | Organic anions | 29 ± 1 |
| NH$_4$ | 28 ± 2 | | |
| Total | 219 ± 3 | | 218 ± 6 |

\* Values are shown as mean ± SE.

$$\text{Urine AG} = (N + K) - Cl = (127 + 49) - 135 = 41 \text{ mEq}$$
or
$$\text{NH}_4 = (N + K) - (Cl + 13) = (127 + 49) - (135 + 13)$$
$$= 176 - 148 = 28 \text{ mEq}$$

*Source*: Goldstein MB et al: The urine anion gap. A clinically useful index of ammonium excretion. *Am J Med Sci* 292:198, 1986.

where OA = organic anion. Excretion of phosphate, sulfate, and organic anions does not generally change importantly when acid-base status is modified. The normal mean anion gap in a 24-h collection of urine from a patient on a normal diet is approximately 40 mEq (Table 19-8).

In an acidemic patient with an acidic urine, a markedly negative anion gap (i.e., Cl much greater than the sum of Na + K) indicates a high (appropriate) level of ammonium ion ($\text{NH}_4^+$). On the other hand, finding a positive urine anion gap (Cl less than the sum of Na + K) in an acidemic patient suggests that $\text{NH}_4$ is inappropriately low.

Currently, it appears that the clinical use of urinary anion gap involves (1) the differential diagnosis (renal versus extrarenal origin) of hyperchloremic metabolic acidosis by providing an estimate of urinary ammonium levels, and (2) assessment of the cause of renal potassium wasting by providing a clue to the excretion of large amounts of nonresorbable anion resulting in a kaliuresis (Table 19-8). Examples of nonresorbable anions in an acid urine include carbenicillin, salicylate, and keto anions. Since most clinical laboratories cannot provide a measurement of urinary $\text{NH}_4$, the urinary anion gap can, in a sense, provide the clinician with a "poor man's" $\text{NH}_4$ measurement.

In general, when the cause of hyperchloremic metabolic acidosis is extrarenal, the normal kidney responds by markedly increasing the excretion of $\text{NH}_4$. In contrast, $\text{NH}_4$ excretion will be low (less than 40 to 80 mmol/day) in distal renal-tubular acidosis (RTA) or with decreased ammonia availability to the collecting tubule.

If the urinary anion gap is markedly negative (i.e., high $\text{NH}_4$ content), the differential diagnosis of a hyperchloremic metabolic acidosis includes (1) gastrointestinal alkali loss (e.g., secretory diarrhea), (2) proximal RTA with an acidic urine, (3) administration of extra chloride, and (4) high anion gap metabolic acidosis masquerading as hyperchloremic metabolic acidosis or renal origin (e.g., patients with hypoalbuminemia, halide poisoning, etc.) (Table 19-9).

If the urinary anion gap is positive or has a small negative value (e.g., representing a low rate of $\text{NH}_4$ excretion) in a patient with hyperchloremic metabolic acidosis, the different diagnosis includes (1) distal RTA, (2) reduced $\text{NH}_4$ production, and (3) acid gain plus urinary excretion of the conjugate base (e.g., ketoanionuria). If ammonium excretion is very low, urinary pH may be low (i.e., high in free $\text{H}^+$) even if the rate of distal tubular $\text{H}^+$ secretion is subnormal.

If $\text{NH}_4$ is expressed per milligram of creatinine (and factored for an average creatinine excretion of 20 mg/kg per day), one can estimate the 24-h $\text{NH}_4$ excretion from data obtained from a random specimen.

Thus, the urinary anion gap appears to be helpful in the differential diagnosis of hyperchloremic metabolic acidosis by providing an estimation of urinary ammonium levels. Highly negative values for the urinary anion gap suggest exogenous or endogenous acid loads or an extrarenal loss of alkali. Positive values are seen in patients with impaired renal ammonium excretion.

**Table 19-9.** Diagnostic Value of Urinary Anion Gap (Na + K − Cl) in an Acid Urine (pH < 6.4)

Highly negative urine anion gap (high NH$_4$)
  GI alkali loss
  Proximal RTA
  Increased Cl intake
  Hypoalbuminemia
  Halide ingestion
Positive or slightly negative urine anion gap (low NH$_4$)
  Distal RTA
  Decreased NH$_4$ production
  Ketonuria
Highly positive urine anion gap (very low NH$_4$)
  Organic aciduria

## Venous Studies

In critically ill patients with a puzzling acid-base picture or poor response to therapy, one should also analyze venous pH, P$_{CO_2}$, and bicarbonate. If, for some reason, it is difficult to obtain arterial blood or if a percutaneous sample is obtained and it is not clear whether the sample is arterial or venous, central venous blood from a subclavian or pulmonary artery catheter can be used to advantage. In patients with a normal cardiac output, arterial values can usually be obtained by adding 0.05 to the central venous pH, by subtracting 6 or 7 mmHg from the venous P$_{CO_2}$, and subtracting 1.1 mEq/L from the venous bicarbonate. However, during shock or severe heart failure, the differences between the arterial and mixed venous values may be much greater.

## METABOLIC ACIDOSIS

### Etiology

The causes of metabolic acidosis can be divided into two main groups: (1) those associated with increased production of organic acids (increased anion gap metabolic acidosis), and (2) those associated with a loss of bicarbonate or addition of chloride (normal anion gap metabolic acidosis).

### Increased Anion Gap Metabolic Acidosis

The most frequent causes of increased production of organic acids and an increased anion gap metabolic acidosis are lactic acidosis, ketoacidosis, uremia, and drug intoxication (especially methanol, ethanol, ethylene glycol, and salicylates). Ketoacidosis may be diabetic, starvation, or alcoholic (nondiabetic) in origin (Table 19-10).

The most frequent cause of an organic acidosis in critically ill or injured patients, especially those with impaired blood flow or sepsis, is lactic acidosis. The causes of lactic acidosis in turn can be divided into those associated with poor tissue oxygenation (type A) and those with normal oxygenation (type B) (Table 19-6).

The immediate precursor of lactic acid is pyruvic acid. This 3-carbon acid may be transformed into fat or amino acids, or it may be transported into michrondria, where it is incorporated into the Krebs cycle after being oxidized to acetyl-CoA. Liver and kidney cortex contain enzymes that catalyze the conversion of pyruvate back to glucose (i.e., cause gluconeogenesis).

Lactate acid, in sharp contrast to its immediate precursor, pyruvic acid, represents a metabolic dead end. Its only means of metabolic transformation is via the lactate dehydrogenase (LDH) reaction, which regenerates pyruvate and converts nicotine adenine dinucleotide (NAD) to its reduced form (NADH).

An important cause of lactic acidosis is thiamine deficiency, particularly in patients with a heavy alcoholic intake. The severity of the lactic acidosis in some of these individuals, who have usually stopped drinking 1 to 5 days earlier, has caused this problem to be referred to as acute pernicious or fulminating beriberi. A similar problem can

**Table 19-10.** Causes of High Anion Gap Metabolic Acidosis

Lactic acidosis
  Type A—decrease in tissue oxygenation
  Type B—no decrease in tissue oxygenation
Renal failure
  Acute
  Chronic
Ketoacidosis
  Diabetes
  Alcholism
  Prolonged starvation (mild acidosis)
  High-fat diet (mild acidosis)
Ingestion of toxic substances
  Elevated osmolar gap
    Methanol
    Ethylene glycol
  Normal osmolar gap
    Salicylate
    Paraldehyde
    Cyanide

occur with total parenteral nutrition (TPN) if inadequate thiamine is given with large amounts of glucose.

### Normal Anion Gap (Hyperchloremic) Metabolic Acidosis

The most frequent causes of bicarbonate loss resulting in normal anion gap (hyperchloremic) metabolic acidosis include severe diarrhea, pancreatic fistulas, RTA, adrenal insufficiency, and therapy with carbonic anhydrase inhibitors, ammonium chloride, arginine hydro-chloride, or amino acid hydrochlorides (as in TPN). The causes of normal anion gap metabolic acidosis can be further divided into those with normal or high serum potassium levels and those with hypokalemia (Table 19-11).

There are three main types of RTA: RTA I, RTA II, and RTA IV. RTA I involves failure of the distal renal tubules to excrete acid properly and RTA-II involves bicarbonate wasting in the proximal renal tubules. Both RTA I and RTA II tend to cause a normal anion gap metabolic acidosis with hypokalemia. RTA IV usually causes hyperkalemia.

## Pathophysiology

### Compensatory Changes

Any increase in the quantity of hydrogen ions in the bloodstream almost immediately results in an increase in alveolar ventilation. As a general rule, each mEq/L fall in bicarbonate tends to cause a relatively rapid 1.0- to 1.4-mmHg fall in the P$_{CO_2}$. Thus, if the bicarbonate falls to 14 mEq/L, the P$_{CO_2}$ would be expected to fall to about 26 to 30 mmHg. If the fall in P$_{CO_2}$ is less than 1.0 mmHg per mEq fall in bicarbonate, respiratory compensation is inadequate or abnormal.

**Table 19-11.** Causes of Normal Anion Gap Metabolic Acidosis

| With a tendency to hyperkalemia | With a tendency to hypokalemia |
|---|---|
| Subsiding DKA | Renal tubular acidosis—type I (classical distal acidosis) |
| Early uremic acidosis | |
| Early obstructive uropathy | Renal tubular acidosis—type II (proximal acidosis) |
| Renal tubular acidosis—type IV | |
| Hypoaldosteronism (Addison's disease) | Acetazolamide |
| | Acute diarrhea with losses of HCO$_3$ and K$^+$ |
| Infusion or ingestion of HCl, NH$_4$Cl, lysine-HCl, or arginine-HCl | Ureterosigmoidostomy with increased resorption of H$^+$ and Cl$^-$ and losses of HCO$_3^-$ and K$^+$ |
| Potassium-sparing diuretics | Obstruction of artificial ileal bladder |
| | Dilution acidosis |

Further compensation is provided during the next several days by increased renal excretion of acid.

## Muscle Function

In general, mild to moderate acidosis can increase the strength of muscular contraction. This is known as the *staircase phenomenon,* or *treppe,* in which a muscle which is rapidly and repetitively stimulated progressively increases its strength of contraction. However, a pH of less than 7.10 to 7.15 tends to impair muscular and cardiovascular function. Furthermore, if the bicarbonate is less than 5.0 mEq/L, any further reduction in bicarbonate can markedly reduce pH.

## Catecholamines and Vascular Reactivity

Acidosis increases the secretion of catecholamines. However, if the acidosis is very severe (pH < 7.00 to 7.10), it decreases the end-organ response to the catecholamines. Severe acidosis tends to cause systemic arterial vasodilation and venous constriction, increasing the tendency to capillary stasis. Severe acidosis also tends to cause pulmonary vasoconstriction with increased strain on the right heart. Beta-adrenergic receptors are particularly prone to develop rapid desensitization and uncoupling in the presence of severe lactic acidosis.

## Oxygen Delivery and Availability

Oxygen delivery to tissues is affected differently by acute and chronic metabolic acidosis. Acute acidosis shifts the oxyhemoglobin dissociation curve to the right, thereby reducing the affinity of hemoglobin for oxygen and facilitating oxygen delivery to tissues. However, acidosis for more than 12 to 36 h results in impaired erythrocyte glycolysis, reducing the intraerythrocytic concentration of 2,3-diphosphoglyceric acid (2,3-DPG), which shifts the oxyhemoglobin dissociation curve to the left, reducing the release of oxygen from hemoglobin into plasma for use by the tissues. Chronic acidosis may also make red blood cells more rigid, thereby reducing their flow through nutrient capillaries. Consequently, one should not assume that a 90 to 95 percent arterial oxyhemoglobin saturation indicates that adequate oxygen is available to the tissues.

## Diagnosis

The diagnosis of metabolic acidosis is usually based on a low pH with low bicarbonate levels. Calculation of the anion gap can help determine the cause of the metabolic acidosis. Severe metabolic acidosis, regardless of its origin, tends to cause nausea, vomiting, abdominal distress, and varying degrees of CNS dysfunction.

### Increased Anion Gap Metabolic Acidosis

The mnemonic "muksleep" is used by some students to remember the first letters of some of the more common causes of increased anion gap metabolic acidosis: methanol, uremia, ketoacidosis, salicylates, lactate, ethanol, ethylene glycol, and paraldehyde. Patients being seen in the emergency department can have any one of these problems. However, if the problem develops in the hospital, toxic drug ingestions are much less likely. Another mnemonic used is "mudpiles," where "i" represents iron or isoniazid. Other causes of increased anion gap include toluene, carbon monoxide, and cyanide.

**Lactic Acidosis**

In type A lactic acidosis, there is poor tissue oxygenation and perfusion. In type B, however, there is no evidence of decreased tissue perfusion, and the mechanism of the acidosis is unknown.

Patients with lactic acidosis may present with nonspecific findings of nausea, vomiting, restlessness, Kussmaul respirations, and stupor or coma. The serum lactic acid level (as lactate) is elevated. Other

laboratory abnormalities include hyperuricemia, hyperphosphatemia, and leukocytosis.

It is generally assumed that the development of metabolic acidosis during sepsis is secondary to lactic acidosis. However, the composition of the anion gap during severe sepsis induced by cecal perforation in rats was assessed. It was found that the lactate concentration in the septic animals was 2.2 ± 0.3 mEq/L as compared to 0.9 ± 0.2 mEq/L in the controls ($p < .001$). Only 15 percent of the increase in the anion gap in septic animals could be accounted for by increases in lactate concentration. The other measured metabolic intermediates (such as pyruvate, citrate, β-hydroxybutyrate, acetoacetate, anionic amino acids, or albumin) also could not account for the anion gap metabolic acidosis.

An increase in unmeasured strong acids in sepsis could arise from several etiologies, including renal failure and ketoacidosis. Various organic and inorganic anions from skeletal muscle can be released as a result of septic proteolysis. Elevated purine nucleotide degradation products include uric acid and free fatty acids.

**Ketoacidosis**

Ketoacidosis can be caused by either an increase in the free fatty acid load to the liver or an increased conversion of free fatty acids to keto acids. The increased free fatty acid load may be due to increased catecholamine-induced lipolysis caused by stress or, occasionally, to a high-fat diet. Increased conversion of fatty acids to keto acids may occur in diabetic ketoacidosis, in alcoholism, and, to a lesser degree, in prolonged starvation or a high-fat diet.

The most common keto acid formed is β-hydroxybutyrate, followed by acetoacetate and hydroxybutyric acid. The nitroprusside test is commonly used to document the presence of ketones in serum and urine. This test is positive with increased levels of acetoacetate or acetone, but not with β-hydroxybutyric acid. The more acidotic the patient is, the more β-hydroxybutyric acid is formed from acetoacetate. Therefore, the test may reveal little or none of the ketoacidosis present in a severely acidotic patient.

***Diabetic Ketoacidosis (DKA)***

The patient with DKA is usually an insulin-dependent diabetic who is out of control and has developed polydipsia, polyuria, and polyphagia. On physical examination, the patient tends to be hyperventilating, with acetone breath and an altered mental status. The laboratory definition of DKA is a serum glucose level greater than 300 mg/dL (16.7 mmol/L), increased serum ketones, and a pH less than 7.30.

One should not assume that ketones are absent or only minimally present if the nitroprusside test is negative or only weakly positive in patients with severe acidosis. In ketoacidosis, the retained keto anions are β-hydroxybutyrate and acetoacetate and the usual ratio of β-hydroxybutyrate to acetoacetate is 3:1 to 4:1. With increasing acidosis, the amount of β-hydroxybutyrate increases and the amount of acetoacetate decreases. Since only acetoacetate reacts with nitroprusside (the key reagent to Acetest tablets and Ketostix), the severity of the ketosis may be underestimated. This occurs typically in patients suffering concomitantly from tissue hypoxia and/or lactic acidosis.

Other laboratory findings in DKA may include leukocytosis and an increased serum osmolality and osmolal gap. Serum sodium is often low secondary to hyperglycemia. Serum potassium is often elevated due to the acidosis, in spite of total body potassium deficits of up to 10 mEq/kg of body weight.

Although elevated glucose levels are considered characteristic of DKA, they can be deceptive. Modestly elevated serum glucose levels, 150 to 250 mg/dL, can occur in alcoholic ketoacidosis and salicylate intoxication. Conversely, hypoglycemia should suggest alcoholic ketoacidosis because serum glucose levels are lower than 50 mg/dL in about 13 percent of patients with this disorder. Ketonuria may also be helpful. It occurs in almost all cases of DKA, it is common in alcoholic ketoacidosis, and it occurs in approximately 25 percent of patients with salicylate intoxication.

Depending upon the amount of hydration and ability of the kidneys to excrete the increased keto acids in the blood, there may be a wide spectrum of acid-base patterns in DKA, ranging from pure high anion gap metabolic acidosis to pure normal anion gap (hyperchloremic) metabolic acidosis. Severe dehydration tends to result in increased retention of ketones and an increased anion gap. After 4 to 8 h of therapy with saline solution, many patients will develop a hyperchloremic acidosis because of retention of chloride in excess of sodium and because of excretion of ketones by the kidneys.

### Alcoholic Ketoacidosis

Except for alcohol, the patient has generally fasted for at least 24 to 36 h. Patients tend to be dehydrated and malnourished, with epigastric pain, ethanol odor, and altered mental status. The increased anion gap is usually due to β-hydroxybutyrate. Laboratory studies usually reveal ketones, high normal or low glucose levels, elevated amylase levels, and hyperuricemia. A variable ethanol level may be present.

### Starvation Ketosis

The patient has a history of starvation and is usually cachectic, hypoglycemic, and ketotic. There is accelerated gluconeogenesis with depletion of liver glycogen stores, hypoinsulinemia, and lipolysis. In prolonged starvation (4 to 6 weeks), ketogenesis serves to supply ketones for the brain.

### High-Fat Diets

A diet with a high fat content may cause a mildly elevated anion gap due to ketosis from increased β oxidation of free fatty acids in the liver.

### Renal Failure

In acute renal failure, the GFR is decreased. As a consequence, organic acids, phosphates, and sulfates (from endogenous metabolism) are retained, producing a metabolic acidosis with a high anion gap. In chronic renal failure, ammonia excretion is diminished, causing a further increase in anions. The anion gap in uremic acidosis is usually less than 24 mEq/L, and there is a poor correlation between the change in anion gap and the change in $HCO_3$.

Severe muscle damage may greatly increase the tendency to renal failure. The resulting myoglobinuric renal failure can produce a severe metabolic acidosis with a strikingly increased anion gap level. At least part of this acidosis is caused by the metabolism of large amounts of the sulfur-containing amino acids released from myoglobin.

### Toxic Ingestions

Whenever one sees a patient with a metabolic acidosis of unknown etiology, the anion and osmolar gaps should be evaluated. Methanol, ethylene glycol, salicylate, and paraldehyde poisoning can cause metabolic acidosis with a high anion gap. Ethylene glycol and methanol can also cause an increased osmolar gap.

### Methanol

Methanol, also known as wood alcohol, is a clear liquid found in solvents, shellacs, and varnishes. It is sometimes ingested by alcoholics as a substitute for ethanol. The usual lethal dose is 30 mL of absolute methanol, but deaths have been reported after ingestion of as little as 6 mL. Peak methanol levels develop 30 to 60 min after ingestion, but there is usually a 12- to 24-h latent period before symptoms start. Classically, the patient describes cloudy, blurred, or misty vision. The person may see yellow spots or develop a central scotoma or blindness, which may or may not be reversible. These symptoms are caused by formaldehyde, a metabolite of methanol. Other symptoms include nausea, vomiting, weakness, epigastric pain, headache, dizziness, and CNS depression. Examination of the eyes may disclose optic disk hyperemia, edema, and decreased pupillary reaction to light.

Laboratory studies reveal metabolic acidosis with a high anion gap and an elevated osmolar gap. The high anion gap is caused mainly by formic acid, a metabolite of methanol.

### Ethylene Glycol

This odorless substance is present in antifreeze, hydraulic brake fluid, cellophane softeners, and solvents for paints and plastics. The minimal lethal dose is 1.0 to 1.5 mL/kg. Peak ethylene glycol levels are reached after 1 to 4 h, but toxic manifestations are delayed 4 to 12 h. The three stages of toxicity are (1) CNS injury (during the first 12 h), (2) respiratory depression and cardiopulmonary failure (at 12 to 24 h), and (3) renal failure (at 24 to 72 h). The toxic effects of ethylene glycol poisoning are produced by metabolites of ethylene glycol, including glycoaldehydes, glycolic acid, glyoxylic acid, and oxalate. Glycolic acid and lactic acid are responsible for the high anion gap. Oxalate is the primary factor in renal toxicity.

The diagnosis of ethylene glycol poisoning is supported by a urine sediment with calcium oxalate crystals. The maximum production of oxalate occurs 8 h after ingestion, so there may be no crystalluria if the the patient presents earlier.

Other laboratory findings include hypocalcemia, leukocytosis, and an elevated osmolal gap that is caused by the serum concentration of ethylene glycol. The osmolal gap may be normal if it is measured many hours after ingestion when ethylene glycol is no longer present in the serum.

### Salicylates

The usual toxic dose of salicylates is 200 to 300 mg/kg, with blood levels of 160 to 500 mg/dL reported as potentially lethal. Peak levels occur 2 to 4 h after ingestion of most preparations.

The first manifestations of salicylate poisoning include tinnitus and hearing impairment. These symptoms occur at an average adult dose of 4.5 g/day. In mild toxicity, there might also be vomiting 3 to 8 h after ingestion. In moderate toxicity, symptoms include severe hyperpnea and marked lethargy or excitability. Severe toxicity is frequently manifested by coma and seizures.

Salicylates directly stimulate the respiratory center, causing respiratory alkalosis. Later an increased metabolic rate with the production of more carbon dioxide may result in respiratory acidosis. Eventually the direct toxic effect on carbohydrate metabolism produces the classic high anion gap metabolic acidosis.

### Paraldehyde

This sedative and antiseizure medication is rarely used now. The average minimal lethal blood level is approximately 500 μg/mL. Manifestations of toxicity include gastritis, renal failure, fatty changes in the liver, pulmonary hemorrhages, edema, and congestive failure. These patients have a characteristic offensive odor, mild to moderate dehydration, hypotension, and Kussmaul respirations.

The elevated anion gap is caused by acetic acid and chloracetic acid. Diagnosis is made by detection of paraldehyde in the serum and acetaldehyde in the urine and blood. When a nitroprusside reaction test is used, paralydehyde may cause a false-positive reaction for ketones, called "pseudoketosis."

### Other Substances

Severe intoxication with lithium or magnesium reduces the anion gap by increasing unmeasured cations.

### Rapid Laboratory Evaluation of Patients with High Anion Gap Metabolic Acidosis

A urine dipstick test that is positive for both ketones and glucose rapidly confirms DKA. If the test is negative for glucose, alcoholic or starvation ketoacidosis should be considered.

If there is a history of paraldehyde ingestion, and/or the urine contains acetaldehyde, paraldehyde poisoning is possible, and the finding of ketonuria may represent a false-positive reaction. A history of starvation and alcoholism suggests alcoholic ketoacidosis.

If the urine dipstick test is negative for ketones, the serum osmolality should be tested to determine whether there is an elevated osmolar gap. Causes of a high osmolar gap include ethylene glycol and methanol poisoning and DKA. If calcium oxalate crystals are found in the urine, ethylene glycol poisoning should be suspected. If there is a history of visual impairment or an abnormal funduscopic examination, methanol poisoning is the most likely cause.

When the osmolar gap is normal, the urine should be tested with ferric chloride. If a purple color develops, salicylate poisoning should be considered, although it is important to remember that the test is very sensitive. Renal failure is diagnosed when BUN and creatinine are elevated. Lactic acidosis is confirmed by an elevated lactic acid level.

If there is no renal failure or drug intoxication, an increased anion gap is usually due to ketoacidosis or lactate accumulation. In patients without uremia, drug intoxication, or DKA, an increased anion gap is usually due to lactate accumulation.

An anion gap of 30 mEq/L or more usually indicates an organic (lactic or keto) acidosis, even in the presence of uremia. With anion gaps of 20 to 29 mEq/L, 60 to 75 percent of patients will have an organic acidosis. Of those with no identified organic acidosis, changes in total proteins, phosphate, potassium, or calcium will account for about 50 percent of the increased anion gap. The etiology of the other 50 percent of the anion gap is usually apparent.

According to Gabow et al., if the anion gap exceeds 0.5 times the serum bicarbonate concentration plus 16.0, the diagnosis of an organic acidosis is justified. Thus, a patient with a $HCO_3$ of 6 mEq/L and an anion gap of 22 mEq/L probably has an organic acidosis, because the Gabow factor is 19 $[(HCO_3 \times 0.5) + 16 = (6 \times 0.5) + 16 = 3 + 16 = 19]$, which is less than the anion gap of 22. On the other hand, if the $HCO_3$ is 18 mEq/L, the Gabow factor is $(18 \times 0.5) + 16 = 9 + 16 = 25$, and the cause of the anion gap is probably not an organic acidosis.

### Normal Anion Gap Metabolic Acidosis

Normal anion gap metabolic acidosis is caused primarily by a loss of bicarbonate with little or no increase in organic acids. A mnemonic for the possible causes of normal anion gap metabolic acidosis is "used carp": *u*reteroenterostomy, *s*mall bowel fistulas, *e*xtra chloride (such as in $NH_4Cl$ or amino acid hydrochlorides), *d*iarrhea, *c*arbonic anhydrase inhibitors (Diamox and Sulfamylon), *a*drenal insufficiency, *r*enal tubular acidosis, *p*ancreatic fistula. These and other causes of normal anion gap metabolic acidosis can be subdivided into those tending to cause hyperkalemia and those causing hypokalemia (Table 19-11).

In most of these problems, a careful history and routine laboratory studies should clarify the cause.

### Treatment

The treatment of metabolic acidosis should be directed at (1) improvement of tissue perfusion and ventilation, (2) correction of the underlying problem, and (3) administration of sodium bicarbonate if needed.

### Improved Tissue Perfusion and Ventilation

Almost every type of metabolic acidosis will be improved by restoration of an adequate or increased blood volume, cardiac output, and tissue oxygenation. If there is any problem with ventilation, so that the respiratory compensation is inadequate, early ventilatory assistance should be strongly considered.

### Correction of the Primary Process

As the patient is being resuscitated, a strong effort should be made to determine the primary process causing the metabolic acidosis and correct it. An adequate resuscitation should correct any shock, but inotropic agents may occasionally be required. Sepsis may require eradication of the focus of infection plus antibiotics. For DKA, insulin and later glucose and potassium will be needed.

Treatment of toxic ingestions may require specific therapy. The treatment of severe methanol poisoning is administration of enteral or parenteral ethanol, because alcohol dehydrogenase (the enzyme that metabolizes ethanol, ethylene glycol, and methanol) has a significantly greater affinity for ethanol than for the other alcohols. Ethanol levels should be maintained at approximately 100 mg/dL. Hemodialysis is often required if the methanol blood concentration is greater than 50 mg/dL.

Ethylene glycol poisoning is treated with supportive measures (e.g., respiratory support) and administration of ethanol. If ethylene glycol levels exceed 50 mg/dL, or if renal failure is present, hemodialysis is indicated. Some authors also recommend thiamine, 100 mg IM, and pyridoxine, 100 mg IV or IM.

Therapy for salicylate poisoning consists initially of emesis with syrup of ipecac or, in a comatose patient, lavage coupled with activated charcoal. Salicylate excretion may be enhanced through alkalinization of the urine with or without concomitant diuresis. For severe poisoning (salicylate level greater than 100 mg/dL), hemodialysis is indicated.

Treatment of paraldehyde poisoning includes lavage, activated charcoal, and supportive measures. Emesis should not be promoted, since paralydehyde is locally corrosive to the gastrointestinal tract and is rapidly absorbed.

### Bicarbonate Therapy

If a severe metabolic acidosis persists after maximal efforts to improve tissue perfusion with fluid, inotropes, and vasodilators as needed, sodium bicarbonate therapy to raise the pH from less than 7.10 to at least 7.25 should be considered. Sodium bicarbonate should probably also be given if the arterial bicarbonate falls below 5.0 mEq/L because any additional decrease in bicarbonate could cause a precipitous fall in pH.

The amount of bicarbonate given should not exceed 1.0 mEq/kg at a time so as to prevent alkaline overshoot. For each 0.1 rise in pH, oxygen availability to tissue drops by about 10 percent because of the shift of the oxyhemoglobin dissociation curve to the left. Giving bicarbonate to patients with hypoxemia due to a pulmonary or right-to-left heart shunt may rapidly lower the arterial $P_{O_2}$ to dangerous levels. In patients with severe DKA, rapid bicarbonate administration can cause severe CNS changes.

Bicarbonate deficits are usually calculated using 30 to 50 percent of the body weight as the bicarbonate space. In patients with acute mild bicarbonate deficits of less than 10 mEq/L, calculations using 30 percent of the body weight as the bicarbonate space seem to provide adequate correction. For moderate bicarbonate deficits of 10 to 15 mEq/L, 40 percent of the body weight can be used as the bicarbonate space. However, in patients with severe acidosis with base deficits exceeding 15 mEq/L, the bicarbonate space involves almost the entire total body water and should be considered to be equal to 50 percent of the body weight.

Thus, in an acutely ill 80-kg man with a bicarbonate concentration of 10 mEq/L (i.e., a deficit of 14 mEq/L), one can assume a bicarbonate space of 40 percent, or 32 L. As a consequence, he would have a total bicarbonate deficit of $(80 \text{ kg} \times 0.40) \times 14 = 448$ mEq. However, only about 1.0 mEq/kg is administered at a time, over 30 to 60 min. If the patient were hemodynamically unstable, more rapid infusion of bicarbonate might be desirable.

The American Heart Association now urges restraint in the use of sodium bicarbonate during cardiopulmonary resuscitation. Experimentally, $HCO_3^-$ administered to correct severe hypoxic lactic acidosis actually increases lactate production. Part of the difficulty may be related to the fact that carbon dioxide (elaborated by the reaction of $H^+$ and $HCO_3$) diffuses rapidly across cell membranes, creating intracellular acidosis even while the extracellular acidosis is decreased.

Bicarbonate can also cause a paradoxical cerebral acidosis. The increased $CO_2$ generated by the bicarbonate readily crosses the blood-brain barrier while the bicarbonate crosses the blood-brain barrier very slowly. The increased cerebrospinal fluid $CO_2$ generates carbonic acid which causes cerebrospinal fluid acidosis in spite of an increasing alkalemia.

## METABOLIC ALKALOSIS

### Etiology

The two most frequent causes of metabolic alkalosis are excessive diuresis (with loss of potassium, hydrogen, and chloride) and excessive loss of gastric secretions (with loss of hydrogen and chloride).

### Loss of Gastric Acid

Normally the stomach makes 2 to 5 mEq of free acid per hour. This may be increased two- to fourfold in patients with an active duodenal ulcer. Thus, a patient who is vomiting large amounts of acid due to pyloric stenosis from duodenal ulcer disease is particularly apt to develop a severe metabolic alkalosis. Removal of large amounts of gastric acid with a nasogastric tube may also produce the same effect.

### Excessive Diuresis

Hypokalemia due to diuresis with excessive loss of potassium in the urine is probably the most common cause of metabolic alkalosis. Since potassium loss in urine averages 30 to 60 mEq/L, use of diuretics can easily produce a severe hypokalemia along with an excessive loss of chloride. Potassium will tend to come out of tissue cells to correct the hypokalemia, and hydrogen ions will tend to go back into the cells, causing an alkalemia. In addition, the kidney will tend to excrete hydrogen ions to conserve potassium. Diarrhea or excessive colostomy or ileostomy drainage may contain more than 25 to 50 mEq of potassium per liter and may also cause severe hypokalemia.

### Mineralocorticoids

Mineralocorticoids tend to cause metabolic alkalosis by promoting the renal absorption of bicarbonate and sodium and by increasing the excretion of potassium, hydrogen, and chloride ions. Hypokalemia can produce a vicious cycle because the depletion of potassium causes even more excretion of hydrogen ions, aggravating the metabolic alkalosis. Reabsorption of potassium appears to be independent of aldosterone, but an aldosterone deficiency markedly reduces the ability of the distal tubule to secrete hydrogen ion and reabsorb bicarbonate.

### Increased Intake of Citrate or Lactate

Patients receiving massive blood transfusions and large amounts of Ringer's lactate will tend to become alkalotic over the next 12 to 48 h. Massive transfusions of bank blood can greatly increase the quantity of citrate in the body (17 mEq from each unit of whole blood and 5 mEq from each unit of packed red blood cells). As this citrate is metabolized over the next 24 to 48 h, plasma bicarbonate levels rise proportionally, producing an increasing alkalosis. Ringer's lactate has a pH of about 5.5. However, after it is given, about half of it (L-lactate) is metabolized in the liver into bicarbonate, which tends to cause a metabolic alkalosis. The D-lactate is excreted in the urine.

### Antacids

Clinicians often attempt to prevent stress gastric ulceration and bleeding in critically ill patients by maintaining a pH inside the stomach of 5.0 or higher with antacid and/or $H_2$-receptor antagonists, such as cimetidine. In some instances, large quantities of antacid are required. Absorption of these antacids and/or removal of the excess acid that they neutralize may significantly contribute to alkalosis.

### Dehydration

One should not attempt to correct a severe metabolic alkalosis without first correcting any coexistent dehydration. Dehydration which is not severe enough to interfere with tissue perfusion may cause a "contraction alkalosis" because sodium and bicarbonate absorption in the kidney is increased. However, if the extracellular fluid is expanded, sodium and bicarbonate reabsorption in the kidney is reduced, and this may cause a "dilution acidosis."

Since the kidney is the organ responsible for excreting excess bicarbonate when the concentration is abnormally high, renal failure may make it very difficult to eliminate bicarbonate. However, if the renal failure is mild to moderate, the ability to excrete bicarbonate is still relatively well preserved.

### Excretion of Nonresorbable Anions

The various penicillins when excreted into the tubular lumen have a negative charge and are not resorbed. This causes an increased loss of hydrogen ions in the urine. Increased excretion of phosphates may cause a similar problem.

### Hypercapnia

After a period of respiratory acidosis, a compensatory rise in bicarbonate will tend to occur until the arterial pH is about 7.35. For example, with a chronic $P_{CO_2}$ of 60 to 70 mmHg, the arterial bicarbonate will tend to rise to levels of 32 to 37 mEq/L, respectively. Even after the hypercapnia is corrected, bicarbonate levels may remain elevated for some time.

### Severe Hypoproteinemia

To maintain electrical neutrality, a fall in serum proteins, especially albumin, will tend to cause a rise in bicarbonate. A fall in albumin levels from 4.5 to 1.5 g/dL can cause serum bicarbonate levels to rise by up to 9.6 mEq/L.

### Other Problems

Other situations that tend to maintain high serum bicarbonate concentrations include hypokalemia and hypochloremia. Chloride deficiency is often listed as a cause of persistently high plasma bicarbonate levels, but chloride deficiency will only raise the renal bicarbonate threshold if it is accompanied by a reduced effective arterial volume. Resistant metabolic alkalosis may also be seen with secondary hypoparathyroidism (such as with milk alkali syndrome or malignancy-induced hypercalcemia).

## Physiologic Effects

Although alkalosis tends to inhibit sympathetic nervous system activity and decrease adrenergic effects, it also tends to increase endogenous catecholamine release and accentuate adrenergic vasodilator effects.

Metabolic alkalosis reduces the amount of potassium in the blood by about 0.5 mEq/L for each 0.10 rise in pH. Ionized calcium and magnesium levels in the plasma also fall, about 4 to 8 percent for each 0.1 rise in pH. This tends to increase neuromuscular irritability and may impair cardiovascular function, particularly if the plasma ionized calcium levels fall below 1.6 to 1.7 mEq/L. The alkalosis also reduces oxygen availability by about 10 percent for each 0.1 rise in pH. Alkalosis may also cause tachyarrhythmias, probably due to potassium and/or calcium changes. The hypokalemia which develops secondary to an alkalosis may also interfere with muscle function, causing weakness and/or ileus.

Failure to compensate adequately for a metabolic alkalosis may be the first indication of an occult hypoxemia. The usual pulmonary compensation for a metabolic alkalosis is hypoventilation with slow, shallow breathing. As the $P_{CO_2}$ rises because of hypoventilation, the $P_{O_2}$ falls, but the chemoreceptors will usually not allow the arterial $P_{O_2}$ to fall much below 60 mmHg. Thus, the arterial $P_{CO_2}$ will not usually rise above 50 to 55 mmHg unless the associated hypoxemia is prevented by giving oxygen.

One should probably not allow a patient to remain severely alkalotic, even if the patient appears to be doing well otherwise. With alkalosis, there is usually some degree of cerebral dysfunction. Blood ammonia levels tend to rise in metabolic alkalosis, and this may be part of the cause of the CNS changes.

If there is a combined metabolic and respiratory alkalosis, the arterial pH can rise rapidly to above 7.55. In a study at Detroit General Hospital, we found that the mortality rate of critically ill or injured patients was increased significantly if their arterial pH rose above 7.55. Almost all patients maintaining an arterial pH above 7.70 died.

## Diagnosis

The diagnosis of metabolic alkalosis is made from laboratory studies revealing a bicarbonate level exceeding 26 mEq/L and a pH above 7.45. In most instances, there is also an associated hypokalemia and hypochloremia. Clinically, metabolic alkalosis is characterized by slow, shallow respiration (in contrast to the hyperventilation generally seen with metabolic acidosis). Determining the cause of the alkalosis can be facilitated by determining if urine chloride levels are above 20 mEq/L or below 10 mEq/L.

The causes of metabolic alkalosis are often divided into *chloride-responsive alkalosis* and *chloride-resistant alkalosis*. Chloride-responsive alkalosis is characterized by low urine chloride levels (< 10 mEq/L) and will usually respond well to saline. In chloride-resistant alkalosis urine chloride levels exceed 20 mEq/L and there is a poor response to saline alone. Chloride-resistant alkalosis is most frequently caused by increased endogenous or exogenous adrenal corticosteroids or severe hypokalemia. Bartter syndrome (hypertrophy and hyperplasia of the cells of the juxtaglomerular apparatus) and Liddle syndrome (pseudohyperaldosteronism with a clinical picture of hyperaldosteronism but normal aldosterone secretion) are interesting examples of chloride-resistant alkaloses.

## Treatment

Chloride-responsive alkalosis, such as that caused by vomiting or excessive nasogastric suction, usually responds adequately to administration of fluid and chloride. If the patient is adequately hydrated, the chloride deficit can be calculated on the basis of 20 percent of the body weight. Thus, if the patient weighs 80 kg and has a serum chloride of 60 mEq/L, the chloride deficit can be calculated as (80 kg × 20 percent) × (100 − 60) = 640 mEq/L. If the patient is severely dehydrated, one can use 60 percent of the body weight to calculate the chloride deficit.

Half the chloride deficit is corrected over a period of 4 to 12 h. Approximately one-fourth of the chloride is given as potassium chloride and three-fourths as sodium chloride. Normally, the potassium is not given faster than 20 mEq/h and is not given if serum potassium levels exceed 5.0 mEq/L.

If the patient is hypokalemic, the kidneys tend to excrete $H^+$ and retain $HCO_3^-$, and this may result in a paradoxical aciduria (excretion of acid urine in the presence of an alkalemia). If adequate chloride is administered to patients with a chloride-responsive alkalosis, the increased chloride in the glomerular filtrate allows increased sodium absorption in the proximal tubule. As less sodium is presented to the distal tubule, less $H^+$ is excreted and less $HCO_3^-$ is absorbed and the metabolic alkalosis begins to resolve.

Chloride-resistant alkalosis is usually not associated with hypovolemia. Consequently, relatively large quantities of $Na^+$ and $Cl^-$ are filtered, and increased $H^+$ and $K^+$ are excreted as the $Na^+$ is resorbed in the distal tubule. These patients tend to require large quantities of potassium to correct the alkalosis.

If the alkalosis is severe (the $CO_2$ content exceeds 40 mEq/L, the pH exceeds 7.55, or the patient has tetany), one-half of the chloride deficit is given as sodium chloride, one-fourth as potassium chloride, and one-fourth as some type of hydrochloride ($NH_4Cl$, arginine hydrochloride, or 0.1 N hydrochloric acid). Ammonium chloride theoretically should be helpful, but many of these patients have renal or hepatic problems which increase the risk of giving ammonium compounds. Arginine hydrochloride may be helpful with hepatic insufficiency but is contraindicated in severe renal dysfunction. Interestingly, some investigators feel that these chlorides may acidify the extracellular fluid but not the cells.

If hydrochloric acid (0.10 N) is used, it must be given cautiously by slow infusion into a large vein at approximately 25 to 50 mL/h. The hydrochloric acid can be administered with amino acids to provide a higher pH and "gentler" solution than HCl alone.

In some instances, acetazolamide (Diamox), which inhibits carbonic anhydrase and thereby increases renal bicarbonate excretion, may be given by mouth or through a nasogastric tube to correct a mild to moderate metabolic alkalosis.

## RESPIRATORY ALKALOSIS

### Etiology

In stressful situations such as shock, sepsis, or trauma, there is a tendency to hyperventilate and develop respiratory alkalosis with a $P_{CO_2}$ of 25 to 35 mmHg or less. If hypoxia or metabolic acidosis develops, the tendency to hyperventilation is increased even further.

### Physiologic Effects

Severe respiratory alkalosis tends to perpetuate itself. If the arterial $P_{CO_2}$ falls, cerebral vasoconstriction occurs. In fact, each 1.0-mmHg drop in the arterial $P_{CO_2}$ reduces cerebral blood flow by about 2 to 4 percent. Thus, a severe respiratory alkalosis, especially if the $P_{CO_2}$ is less than 20 mmHg, can reduce cerebral blood flow enough to cause cerebral metabolic acidosis. This cerebral metabolic acidosis will then cause the respiratory center to increase ventilation even more, producing a progressively more severe respiratory alkalosis.

The initial response to hypocapnia is a shift of hydrogen chloride and lactate ions out of the cell. In severe respiratory alkalosis, lactic acid levels may increase by 2.0 to 3.0 mmol/L. This buffering is rapid and may be complete within 15 min of the initiation of the hypocapnia. The renal compensation will also begin to take effect within 2 to 4 h after the onset of hypocapnia.

Alkalosis shifts the oxyhemoglobin dissociation curve to the left, causing hemoglobin to hold oxygen more tightly. Each rise in pH of 0.10 lowers the $P_{O_2}$ about 10 percent and reduces oxygen availability to tissues by about 10 percent.

### Diagnosis

Respiratory alkalosis is diagnosed by a rise in pH above 7.40 and a decrease in $Pa_{CO_2}$ below 35 mmHg. Occasionally, it may be difficult to differentiate hyperventilation of psychogenic origin from compensatory hyperventilation or hyperventilation due to sepsis or pulmonary emboli.

In such patients, careful continued observation of the patient and the blood gases is essential. It should be remembered that the arterial $P_{O_2}$ may be 80 mmHg or higher in 15 percent of the patients who have pulmonary emboli demonstrated on pulmonary arteriogram. Although the $P_{O_2}$ may be relatively normal initially, with continued sepsis, the $P_{O_2}$ will eventually fall.

## Treatment

The treatment of respiratory alkalosis is correction of the primary problem, and one must look particularly for underlying hypoxia, pulmonary embolism, and sepsis. If the problem is hysterical hyperventilation, treatment is best accomplished by having the patient rebreathe expired air, which has a $P_{CO_2}$ about two-thirds that in arterial blood. Not infrequently, the most convenient rebreathing device is a paper bag. Once the $P_{CO_2}$ begins to rise toward normal, the cerebral blood flow usually improves enough to correct the intracerebral acidosis and return the pattern of ventilation toward normal.

In critically ill patients who have severe respiratory alkalosis ($P_{CO_2}$ less than 20 to 25 mmHg and pH more than 7.55 to 7.60) and are not on a ventilator, sedation may be given, but very cautiously. One must be sure that the patient does not reduce ventilation to the point of developing hypoxia.

A patient on a ventilator may be placed on intermittent mandatory ventilation (IMV) and the respirator rate progressively reduced as long as (1) the $P_{CO_2}$ does not exceed 45 mmHg, (2) the pH is not below 7.35, and (3) the patient's respiratory rate is less than 30 per minute. In some instances, 60 to 300 mL of dead space may be added to the endotracheal tube or tracheostomy to increase the $P_{CO_2}$.

## RESPIRATORY ACIDOSIS

### Etiology

A $P_{CO_2}$ elevated above 45 mmHg is usually due to inadequate minute ventilation and/or increased dead space. However, increased carbohydrate metabolism may contribute to hypercarbia if pulmonary function is marginal. This is most apt to occur in patients who are on a ventilator and are receiving three or more liters of 20 to 25% glucose IV per day.

Inadequate minute ventilation is most frequently due to head trauma, chest trauma, or disease or excess sedation. The chronic hypoventilation seen in extremely obese patients is often referred to as the *pickwickian syndrome,* after an obese character in Charles Dickens' *Pickwick Papers.* Patients with severe chronic obstructive pulmonary disease (COPD) have increased dead space and frequently also have a decreased minute ventilation.

In general, a rise in the $P_{CO_2}$ stimulates the respiratory center to increase respiratory rate and minute ventilation. However, if the arterial $P_{CO_2}$ chronically exceeds 60 to 70 mmHg, as may occur in 5 to 10 percent of patients with severe emphysema, the respiratory acidosis may depress the respiratory center. Under such circumstances, the stimulus for ventilation is provided primarily by hypoxemia acting on chemoreceptors in the carotid and aortic bodies. Giving oxygen could take away the main stimulus to breathe, causing the $P_{CO_2}$ to rise abruptly to extremely dangerous levels. Consequently, one should not administer oxygen to patients with COPD without carefully watching for the development of apnea or hypoventilation.

### Pathophysiology

With a sudden severe decrease in minute ventilation, the $P_{CO_2}$ rises rapidly and the pH may fall abruptly because bicarbonate compensation by the kidney is very slow. In completely apneic patients, the arterial $P_{CO_2}$ rises by about 2.0 to 3.0 mmHg/min. A rapid increase of the arterial $P_{CO_2}$ to 60 mmHg can cause the pH to fall to about 7.22. However, over the next few hours or days, a rise in bicarbonate will gradually restore the pH to about 7.35. A high bicarbonate level in an ambulatory patient should make one suspicious of a chronic respiratory acidosis.

Acute, severe respiratory acidosis is usually accompanied by neurologic signs or symptoms. The risk of brain acidemia is higher in respiratory acidosis than in metabolic acidosis. Carbon dioxide penetrates lipid structures, such as the blood-brain barrier, very readily and can markedly decrease the pH of the brain. Bicarbonate, which is water-soluble, penetrates much more slowly. Coma can occur at a $P_{CO_2}$ exceeding 65 to 70 mmHg; however, if the respiratory acidosis develops very slowly, coma may not develop until the $P_{CO_2}$ exceeds 100 to 110 mmHg.

## Diagnosis

Respiratory acidosis, by definition, is present when the arterial $P_{CO_2}$ exceeds 45 mmHg and the pH is 7.39 or less. If the pH is less than 7.30, the respiratory acidosis is usually acute or there is a superimposed metabolic acidosis. If the carbon dioxide content of an electrolyte study is high, one should suspect a chronic respiratory acidosis or a metabolic alkalosis. If the chloride and potassium levels are normal or high, the patient is likely to have respiratory acidosis. In contrast, metabolic alkalosis is usually associated with a hypokalemia and hypochloremia.

## Treatment

Treatment of respiratory acidosis is primarily designed to improve alveolar ventilation. In general, if the minute ventilation is doubled, the $P_{CO_2}$ will be reduced by 50 percent. In patients with COPD, bronchodilators such as aminophylline or various sympathomimetic agents such as isoproterenol or adrenalin, together with careful administration of small amounts of oxygen, may substantially improve ventilation. However, ventilating assistance may be required in some patients who do not respond adequately to lesser measures, particularly if the pH falls below 7.25 to 7.30. Unfortunately, it may be extremely difficult to extubate such patients later.

In patients with a chronic respiratory acidosis, reduction of the $P_{CO_2}$ should generally proceed slowly. The minute ventilation for a 70-kg person is normally about 6 L/min, and in COPD patients it may be less than 4 L/min. In a patient with COPD and severe hypercarbia, it may be wise to start treatment with a minute ventilation of about 5 L/min and then gradually increase it according to the clinical response and changes in $P_{CO_2}$.

Rapid correction of a chronic respiratory acidosis can cause sudden development of a severe combined metabolic and respiratory alkalosis with resulting arrhythmias. A rapid rise in pH can cause an abrupt fall in ionized calcium. The resulting ionic hypocalcemia can then cause dangerous arrhythmias or seizures. In patients with a chronic respiratory acidosis, the arterial $P_{CO_2}$ should not be reduced by more than 5.0 mEq/h.

More recently, the problems with ventilation in malnourished individuals has been explored in depth. Increased carbohydrate metabolism increases carbon dioxide production and may cause a respiratory acidosis. On the other hand, administration of adequate amounts of glucose may enable previously exhausted subjects to continue work. In malnourished individuals, increased protein intake can also gradually increase muscle mass and improve the maximal ventilatory response.

## BIBLIOGRAPHY

Gabow PA, Kaehny WD, Fennessey PV, et al: Diagnostic importance of an increased serum anion gap. *N Engl J Med* 303:854, 1980.

Lane EE: in Lane EE, Walker JF (eds): *Clinical Arterial Blood Gas Analysis.* St. Louis, Mosby, 1987.

Rose BD: *Clinical Physiology of Acid-base and Electrolyte Disorders*, 4th ed. New York, McGraw-Hill, 1994.

# 20

# BLOOD GASES: PATHOPHYSIOLOGY AND INTERPRETATION

## Robert F. Wilson
## Christopher Barton

## VENTILATION

### Minute Ventilation

The minute ventilation, the total amount of new air moved in and out of the airways and lungs each minute, is equal to the tidal volume multiplied by the respiratory rate. The normal tidal volume ($V_T$) is about 500 mL, and the normal respiratory rate (f) is 12 breaths per minute. Therefore, the normal minute ventilatory volume averages about 6 L. A human being can live only for short periods with a 2-min ventilation as low as 1.5 L and with a respiratory rate as low as 2 to 4 breaths per minute unless the person's metabolism is severely depressed, such as in deep hypothermia.

The respiratory rate occasionally rises to as high as 40 to 50 breaths per minute, and the tidal volume can become almost as great as the forced vital capacity, which is about 4500 to 5000 mL or 65 to 70 mL/kg in a young adult male. However, at rapid rates a person usually cannot sustain a tidal volume greater than 40 percent of the vital capacity for more than several hours.

### Alveolar Ventilation

The main function of the pulmonary ventilatory system is to continually renew the air in the alveoli, where it is brought in close proximity to the pulmonary capillary blood. The rate at which new air reaches these areas is called alveolar ventilation ($V_A$). During normal quiet ventilation, the tidal volume fills the respiratory passageways down as far as the terminal bronchioles, with only a portion of the inspired air actually flowing into the alveoli. The new air moves from the terminal bronchioles into the alveoli by diffusion. Diffusion is caused by the motion of molecules, with each gas molecule moving at high velocity among the other molecules. The velocity of the molecules in the respiratory air is so great and the distance from the terminal bronchioles to the alveoli so short that the gases move this remaining distance in only a fraction of a second.

### Dead Space

Usually at least 30 percent of the air that a person breathes never reaches the alveoli. This portion of the upper and lower respiratory tract is called *dead space* because it is not useful for the gas exchange process. The normal dead space in a young male adult with a tidal volume of 500 mL is about 150 mL (about 1 mL/lb of body weight), or about 30 percent of the tidal volume.

The volume of the airways to the gas exchange areas is called the *anatomic dead space*. Occasionally, some alveoli are not functional because of a lack of blood flow to their capillaries. From a functional point of view, these alveoli without capillary perfusion are considered to be pathologic dead space. When the alveolar (pathologic) dead space is included, the total dead space is called the physiologic dead space. In the normal person, the anatomic dead space is nearly equal to the physiologic dead space because all alveoli are functional. However, in those with poorly perfused alveoli, the total (physiologic) dead space may be greater than 60 percent of the tidal volume.

## GAS PRESSURES

Pressure is caused by the constant impact of moving molecules against a surface. Therefore, the pressure of a gas acting on the surfaces of the respiratory passages and alveoli is proportional to the sum of the impaction forces of all the molecules striking the surface at any given instant.

In the lungs, one deals with mixtures of gases, particularly oxygen, nitrogen, and carbon dioxide. The rate of diffusion of each gas is directly proportional to its partial pressure.

The concentration of a gas in solution is determined not only by its pressure but also by the solubility coefficient of the gas. Some molecules, especially carbon dioxide, are physically or chemically attracted to water molecules while others are repelled. When molecules are attracted to water, more can become dissolved without building up excess pressure within the solution. On the other hand, those that are repelled develop excessive pressure with little solubility.

Henry's law states that both the partial pressure and the solubility coefficient determine the volume of gas dissolved in a volume of fluid. The solubility coefficients for the important respiratory gases at body temperature are oxygen, 0.024; carbon dioxide, 0.57; carbon monoxide, 0.018; nitrogen, 0.012; and helium, 0.008. Thus, carbon dioxide is more than 20 times as soluble as oxygen, and oxygen is more soluble than the other three major gases. These solubilities help determine the quantity of the gas that is dissolved in the fluids of the body, which in turn is a major factor in determining the rate at which the gas can diffuse through tissues.

When air enters the respiratory passageways, water immediately evaporates from the surfaces of these passages and humidifies the inhaled air. Water molecules, like other dissolved gas molecules, are continually escaping from the water surface into the gas phase. The pressure that the water molecules exert to escape through the surface is called the *vapor pressure* of water. At 37°C (98.6°F), this vapor pressure is 47 mmHg. Therefore, once the gas mixture is fully humidified, the partial pressure of the water vapor in the gas mixture is 47 mmHg. This partial pressure is designated $P_{H_2O}$.

## Diffusion of Gases

Major factors that affect the rate of gas diffusion in a fluid include (1) the partial pressure of the gas, (2) the solubility of the gas in the fluid, (3) the area of the surface for diffusion, (4) the distance through which the gas must diffuse, (5) the molecular weight of the gas, and (6) the temperature of the fluid.

The greater the solubility of the gas and the greater the surface area for diffusion, the greater the number of molecules that are available to diffuse for any given pressure difference. On the other hand, the greater the distance that the molecules must diffuse, the longer it takes for the diffusion to occur. Finally, the greater the velocity of the molecules, which at any given temperature is inversely proportional to the square root of the molecular weight, the greater the rate of diffusion of the gas. All these factors can be expressed in a single formula:

$$D = \frac{PAS}{d\sqrt{MW}}$$

where $D$ = diffusion rate
$P$ = pressure difference between the two ends of the diffusion pathway
$A$ = cross-section area of the pathway
$S$ = solubility of the gas
$d$ = distance of diffusion
$MW$ = molecular weight of the gas

The characteristics of the gas itself determine solubility and molecular weight, and these together are called the *diffusion coefficient* of the gas. The diffusion coefficient, which equals $S\sqrt{MW}$, determines the relative rates at which different gases at the same pressure levels diffuse. If the diffusion coefficient of oxygen is 1.0, the relative diffusion coefficients of other gases of respiratory importance are carbon dioxide, 20.3; carbon monoxide, 0.81; nitrogen, 0.53; and helium, 0.95.

The gases that are of respiratory importance are highly soluble in lipids and, consequently, are also highly soluble in cell membranes, diffusing through them with very little impediment. The major limitation to the movement of gases in tissues is the rate at which the gases can diffuse through the tissue water.

The respiratory unit is composed of a respiratory bronchiole, alveolar ducts, atria, and alveoli. A respiratory bronchiole is the largest bronchiole that has any alveoli coming directly off of it. The alveolar walls are extremely thin and are closely applied to an almost solid network of interconnecting capillaries. Because of the extensiveness of the capillary plexus, the movement of blood past the alveoli has been described as a "sheet" of flowing blood. The membrane through which gaseous exchange between the alveolar air and the pulmonary blood occurs is known as the respiratory (pulmonary) membrane.

For oxygen to get from the alveolus into the pulmonary capillary bed, it must pass through four separate layers, referred to collectively as the *alveolar-capillary,* or *respiratory,* membrane. These include:

1. A layer of fluid lining the alveolus. Called alveolar fluid, it contains surfactant that reduces its surface tension.
2. The alveolar epithelium, composed of very thin epithelial cells and a basement membrane.
3. A very thin interstitial space between the alveolar epithelium and the capillary membrane.
4. The capillary endothelial membrane and its basement membrane, which fuses with the alveolar basement membrane in many places.

The overall thickness of the respiratory membranes averages 0.63 $\mu$m. The respiratory membrane in the normal adult is approximately 160 m$^2$. Although the lungs may contain about 700 mL of blood, the total quantity in the pulmonary capillaries at any given instant is only 60 to 140 mL.

The average diameter of the pulmonary capillaries is less than 8 $\mu$m, which means that red blood cells must actually squeeze through them. Therefore, at least part of the red blood cell membrane touches the capillary wall. Where this occurs, oxygen does not have to pass through significant amounts of plasma as it diffuses from the alveolus to the red blood cell. This helps increase the rapidity of diffusion of gases between the alveolus and the hemoglobin molecules.

## Gas Diffusion through the Respiratory Membrane

The factors that determine how rapidly a gas passes through the respiratory membrane are (1) the thickness of the membrane, (2) the surface area of the membrane, (3) the diffusion coefficient of the gas in the water of the membrane, and (4) the pressure difference between the two sides of the membrane.

The thickness of the respiratory membrane occasionally increases, usually as a result of fluid in the interstitial space. Also, some pulmonary diseases cause fibrosis of the lungs, which can further increase the thickness of some portions of the respiratory membrane. Because the rate of diffusion through the membrane is inversely proportional to its thickness, any factor that increases the thickness of the membrane to more than two to three times normal can interfere significantly with oxygenation of blood; however, diffusion is rarely a problem with carbon dioxide.

The surface area of the respiratory membrane may be greatly decreased by a variety of conditions, such as atelectasis or resection of lung tissue. In emphysema, many of the alveoli coalesce, with disso-

lution of alveolar walls. The new alveolar chambers are much larger than the original alveoli, but the total surface area of the respiratory membrane available for gas diffusion is considerably decreased, causing an increase in dead space. When the total surface area of the lung is decreased to approximately one-third to one-fourth normal, exchange of gases through the membrane is impeded significantly, even under resting conditions. During strenuous exercise, even the slightest increase in dead space in patients with severe emphysema can seriously interfere with the exchange of gases.

The pressure difference across the respiratory membrane is the difference between the partial pressure of the gas in the alveoli and the partial pressure of the gas in the blood. In room air, the normal alveolar-arterial oxygen difference ($P_{A_{O_2}} - P_{a_{O_2}}$) or [$P(A - a)_{O_2}$] is 2 to 10 mmHg. The normal alveolar-arterial carbon dioxide difference ($P_{A_{CO_2}} - P_{a_{CO_2}}$) or [$P(A - a)_{CO_2}$] is zero. An increase in the $P(A - a)_{CO_2}$ implies a significant increase in dead space.

## Diffusing Capacity

The ability of the respiratory membrane to exchange gas between the alveoli and the pulmonary blood can be expressed in quantitative terms by what is known as *diffusing capacity,* defined as the volume of a gas that diffuses through the membrane each minute for a pressure difference of 1 mmHg. In the average young adult the diffusing capacity of oxygen under resting conditions averages 21 mL/min per mmHg. The mean oxygen pressure difference across the respiratory membrane during normal, quiet breathing is approximately 12 mmHg. Multiplication of this pressure by the diffusing capacity (21 × 12) gives a total of about 250 mL of oxygen diffusing through the respiratory membrane each minute; this is approximately equal to the rate at which an average adult uses oxygen under resting conditions.

During strenuous exercise, or during other conditions that greatly increase pulmonary blood flow and alveolar ventilation, the diffusing capacity of oxygen in young male adults can increase to a maximum of about 65 mL/min per mmHg, three times the diffusing capacity under resting conditions. This is caused both by opening up of previously dormant pulmonary capillaries, thereby increasing the surface area of the blood into which the oxygen can diffuse, and by dilation of pulmonary capillaries that were already open, further increasing the surface area available for diffusion.

The diffusing capacity of carbon dioxide has not been measured because carbon dioxide diffuses through the respiratory membrane so rapidly that the average difference between the $P_{CO_2}$ in the pulmonary capillary blood and in alveoli is less than 1 mmHg. Since the diffusion coefficient of carbon dioxide is 20 times that of oxygen, one would expect the diffusing capacity of carbon dioxide under resting conditions to be about 400 to 450 mL/min per mmHg and during exercise to be about 1200 to 1300 mL/min per mmHg.

The oxygen diffusing capacity can be calculated from measurement of (1) the alveolar $P_{O_2}$, (2) the $P_{O_2}$ in the pulmonary capillary blood, and (3) the rate of oxygen uptake by the blood. Because of the difficulties encountered in measuring oxygen diffusing capacity, carbon monoxide diffusing capacity is measured and then that value is used to calculate oxygen diffusing capacity. With the carbon monoxide method, a small amount of carbon monoxide is breathed into the alveoli, and the partial pressure of the carbon monoxide in the alveoli is measured from alveolar air samples. The carbon monoxide diffusing capacity can be determined by measuring the volume of carbon monoxide absorbed over time and dividing by the partial pressure of carbon monoxide in end-tidal gas.

The diffusion coefficient of oxygen is 1.23 times that of carbon monoxide. Thus, if the average diffusing capacity of carbon monoxide in young male adults is 17 mL/min per mmHg, the diffusing capacity of oxygen is 1.23 × 17, or about 21 mL/min per mmHg.

**Table 20-1.** Partial Pressure of Gases While Breathing Room Air (mmHg)

|  | Air | Inspired Air in Trachea | Average Alveolar Gas | Average Expired Gas |
|---|---|---|---|---|
| $P_{O_2}$ | 159.0 | 149.3 | 104.0 | 120.0 |
| $P_{CO_2}$ | 0.3 | 0.3 | 40.0 | 28.0 |
| $P_{N_2}$ | 597.0 | 563.4 | 569.0 | 565.0 |
| $P_{H_2O}$ | 3.7 | 47.0 | 47.0 | 47.0 |
| Total | 760.0 | 760.0 | 760.0 | 760.0 |

## ALVEOLAR GASES

### Inspired Gases

Air at sea level has an average barometric pressure of 760 mmHg and contains approximately 20.93 percent oxygen and 0.04 percent carbon dioxide, with nitrogen making up most of the remainder. Thus, the partial pressures of oxygen and carbon dioxide in the air at sea level are 159 and 0.3 mmHg, respectively (Table 20-1).

Alveolar air does not have the same concentration of gases as atmospheric air because (1) dry atmospheric air that enters the respiratory passages is humidified before it reaches the alveoli, (2) alveolar air is only partially replaced by atmospheric air with each breath, (3) oxygen is constantly being absorbed from the alveolar air, and (4) carbon dioxide is constantly diffusing from the pulmonary blood into the alveoli.

### Humidification of Inspired Air

When air enters the upper airway, it is warmed and saturated with water, reducing the total partial pressure of the inhaled gases to about 713 mmHg. Thus, the inspired oxygen pressure ($P_{I_{O_2}}$) in the trachea and bronchi falls to $713 \times 0.2093$, or 149 mmHg (Table 20-1). If the patient is breathing 60 percent oxygen (fraction of inspired oxygen $F_{I_{O_2}}$) = 0.6, the $P_{I_{O_2}}$ in the trachea or bronchi is determined as follows:

$$P_{I_{O_2}} = (P_B - P_{H_2O})F_{I_{O_2}}$$
$$= (760 - 47)(0.6)$$
$$= 427.8 \text{ mmHg}$$

where $P_B$ is barometric pressure (assumed to be 760 mmHg at sea level).

### Rate at Which Alveolar Air Is Renewed by Atmospheric Air

The functional residual capacity of the lungs, which is the amount of air remaining in the lungs at the end of normal expiration, is approximately 2500 to 3000 mL (35 to 45 mL/kg). Only 350 mL of new air is brought into the alveoli with each new tidal volume, and the same amount of old alveolar air is expired. Therefore, the amount of alveolar air replaced by new atmospheric air with each breath is only 12 to 16 percent of the total gas present in the lungs. With normal alveolar ventilation, approximately half the old alveolar gas is exchanged in 17 s. When a person's rate of alveolar ventilation is only half normal, half the gas is exchanged in 34 s, and when the rate of ventilation is twice normal, half is exchanged in about 8 s.

The slow replacement of alveolar air helps prevent sudden changes in gas concentrations in the blood. This helps to prevent excessive changes in tissue oxygenation, tissue carbon dioxide concentration, and tissue pH when ventilation is temporarily interrupted.

### Oxygen Concentration and Partial Pressure in the Alveoli

Oxygen is continually being absorbed into the blood of the lungs, and new oxygen is continually entering the alveoli from the atmosphere. The more rapidly oxygen is absorbed, the lower its concentration in the alveoli. The more rapidly new oxygen is brought into the alveoli from the atmosphere, the higher its concentration becomes. Therefore, oxygen concentration in the alveoli is controlled by the rate of absorption of oxygen into the blood and the rate of entry of new oxygen into the lung.

### Carbon Dioxide Concentration in the Alveoli

Carbon dioxide is continually formed and discharged into the alveoli and continually removed from the alveoli by ventilation. Therefore, the two factors that determine the partial pressure of carbon dioxide in the alveoli ($P_{A_{CO_2}}$) are (1) the rate of excretion of carbon dioxide from the blood into the alveoli and (2) the rate at which carbon dioxide is removed from the alveoli by alveolar ventilation.

At a normal rate of alveolar ventilation of 4.2 L/min, the $P_{A_{CO_2}}$ is usually 40 mmHg. If alveolar ventilation is doubled, the $P_{A_{CO_2}}$ is reduced to 20 mmHg. If alveolar ventilation is decreased to 2.1 L/min, the $P_{A_{CO_2}}$ rises to 80 mmHg.

### Alveolar Gas Equation

Inspired gas in the trachea has a $P_{O_2}$ of about 149 mmHg and a $P_{CO_2}$ of about 0.3 mmHg. As the water-saturated warmed air enters the alveoli, oxygen diffuses through the alveolar capillary membranes into the plasma and carbon dioxide diffuses from the blood into the alveoli. The mixed venous blood brought to the pulmonary capillaries normally has a $P_{O_2}$ of about 40 mmHg and a $P_{CO_2}$ of 46 mmHg. On the average, for each milliliter of oxygen that leaves the alveolus, 0.8 to 1.0 mL of carbon dioxide enters it. This relationship is defined as the respiratory quotient (RQ), which can be expressed as

$$RQ = \frac{\text{rate of } CO_2 \text{ output}}{\text{rate of } O_2 \text{ intake}}$$

To estimate alveolar $P_{O_2}$ ($P_{A_{O_2}}$) from the $P_{I_{O_2}}$ and $P_{A_{CO_2}}$ (which is assumed to be equal to the arterial $P_{CO_2}$), one needs a correction factor to determine how much oxygen is consumed for each 1.0 mmHg of $P_{CO_2}$ resulting from carbon dioxide that enters the alveoli. If the RQ is 0.8, the correction factor is 1.2; if the RQ is 1.0, the correction factor is 1.0.

Thus, for the usual circumstances, in which the RQ is 0.8, the alveolar gas equation is

$$P_{A_{O_2}} = (P_B - P_{H_2O})(F_{I_{O_2}})\,(P_{a_{CO_2}})(1.2)$$

In room air $F_{I_{O_2}} = 0.21$) at sea level with a $P_{a_{CO_2}}$ of 40 mmHg, the $P_{A_{O_2}}$ is expected to be

$$P_{A_{O_2}} = (760 - 47)(0.21) - (40)(1.2) = 150 - 48 = 102$$

### End-Tidal Gases

Expired air is a combination of dead space air and alveolar air, and its overall composition is determined by the proportion of each in expired air. Dead space air is expired first. Then progressively more alveolar air becomes mixed with the dead space air until all the dead space air has finally been washed out. At the end of expiration nothing but alveolar air is expired. Therefore, to collect alveolar air for study, one simply collects end-tidal gas. Determination of end-tidal carbon dioxide levels is a useful measure of the adequacy of ventilation.

## ARTERIAL BLOOD GASES

### Arterial $P_{a_{CO_2}}$

#### Alveolar Ventilation

Carbon dioxide diffuses so rapidly that the $P_{a_{CO_2}}$ usually provides an excellent index of the adequacy of overall ventilation of perfused alveoli. If the $P_{a_{CO_2}}$ is greater than normal in a patient with a normal or low arterial pH, one can assume that ventilation is reduced. However, the patient may also have increased dead space due to emphysema, pulmonary emboli, or sepsis. An elevated $Pa_{CO_2}$ in the presence of metabolic alkalosis usually reflects compensatory effort to restore arterial pH to normal. However, an elevated $Pa_{CO_2}$ in a patient with metabolic acidosis generally indicates pulmonary insufficiency.

With adequate alveolar ventilation, the $Pa_{CO_2}$ will be closely related to the arterial pH. As a rough rule, the $Pa_{CO_2}$ should fall by 5 to 10 mmHg for each 0.10 drop in pH. Thus, if the pH is 7.30, the $Pa_{CO_2}$ should be 30 to 35 mmHg or less. If the arterial pH is 7.20 or less, the $Pa_{CO_2}$ should be 25 to 35 mmHg or less.

As a rule, for each 5.0 mEq/L that the arterial bicarbonate concentration falls below 24.0 mEq/L, the $Pa_{CO_2}$ should fall at least 5 mmHg. Otherwise one can assume that the patient has impaired minute ventilation, increased dead space, or increased carbohydrate metabolism.

Arterial pH is affected by both the bicarbonate level and the $Pa_{CO_2}$, and the $Pa_{CO_2}$ can change 100 to 200 times faster than the bicarbonate level. Using this information, one can often gain some impression of the acuteness of various respiratory changes by noting the effects of the $Pa_{CO_2}$ on the pH. For each 1 mmHg of acute rise or fall in the $Pa_{CO_2}$ the pH decreases or increases by approximately 0.01, assuming the plasma bicarbonate level remains constant during that acute change.

## Dead Space

When the ventilation of an alveolar-capillary unit is normal but perfusion of the alveolar capillary is absent, the ventilation of these alveoli and their associated airways is referred to as dead space. The volume of the dead space ($V_{DS}$) and the tidal volume ($V_T$) are often expressed as a ratio ($V_{DS}/V_T$). This is determined in the pulmonary function laboratory by measuring the $Pa_{CO_2}$ in arterial blood, measuring the average expired gas ($Pe_{CO_2}$), and using the following Bohr equation:

$$\frac{V_{DS}}{V_T} = \frac{Pa_{CO_2} - Pe_{CO_2}}{Pa_{CO_2}}$$

The normal values are

$$\frac{V_{DS}}{V_T} = \frac{40 - 28}{40} = \frac{12}{40} = 0.3$$

When the physiologic dead space is increased, some of the work of ventilation is wasted because a greater fraction of ventilated air never reaches the blood.

## Carbohydrate Metabolism

If the patient has to metabolize more than 450 g of carbohydrate per day, an increased alveolar ventilation may be required to excrete the increased carbon dioxide produced. This is most frequently a problem in patients with severe chronic obstructive pulmonary disease if they are receiving 2.5 to 3.0 L of 20 to 25% glucose per day.

## Transport of Carbon Dioxide in the Blood

Under resting conditions, each 100 mL of blood transports an average of 4 mL of carbon dioxide from the tissues to the lungs. Transport of carbon dioxide is not as great a problem as transport of oxygen because, even in the most abnormal conditions, carbon dioxide can usually be transported in far greater quantities than oxygen. However, carbon dioxide in the blood does affect acid-base balance.

The carbon dioxide formed in cells diffuses out in the form of carbon dioxide rather than bicarbonate because the cell membrane is almost impermeable to bicarbonate ions. As the carbon dioxide enters the capillary, it initiates a number of almost instantaneous reactions essential for carbon dioxide transport.

A small portion of the carbon dioxide is transported to the lungs dissolved in plasma. The amount dissolved in plasma at 46 mmHg is about 2.76 mL/dL (vol%). The amount dissolved at 40 mmHg is about 2.4 mL/dL, or a difference of 0.36 mL/dL. Therefore, only about 0.36 mL of carbon dioxide is transported in the form of dissolved carbon dioxide by each 100 mL of blood. This is about 9 percent of all carbon dioxide transported.

Much of the dissolved carbon dioxide in the blood reacts with water to form carbonic acid. This reaction would occur too slowly to be of importance were it not for the fact that the enzyme carbonic anhydrase inside the red blood cells speeds up the reaction about 500-fold. The reaction occurs so rapidly that it reaches almost complete equilibrium within a fraction of a second. This allows tremendous amounts of carbon dioxide to react with red blood cell water even before the blood leaves the tissue capillaries.

In another fraction of a second, the carbonic acid formed in the red cells dissociates into hydrogen and bicarbonate ions. Most of the hydrogen ions then combine with the hemoglobin in the red blood cells because hemoglobin is a powerful acid-base buffer. At the same time, many of the bicarbonate ions diffuse into the plasma; to offset this ionic shift, chloride ions diffuse into the red blood cells. This is made possible by the presence of a special bicarbonate-chloride carrier protein in the red cell membrane that shuttles these two ions in opposite directions at rapid velocities. Thus, the chloride content of venous red blood cells is greater than that of arterial red blood cells. This phenomenon is called the *chloride shift*.

The reversible combination of carbon dioxide with water in the red blood cells under the influence of carbonic anhydrase accounts for at least 70 percent of all the carbon dioxide transported from the tissues. Indeed, when a carbonic anhydrase inhibitor (acetazolamide) is administered to an animal to block the action of carbonic anhydrase in the red blood cells, carbon dioxide transport from the tissues becomes very poor and the tissue $P_{CO_2}$ rises abruptly.

## Carbaminohemoglobin and Carbaminoproteins

Carbon dioxide also reacts directly with hemoglobin to form carbaminohemoglobin ($Hb$–$CO_2$). This reversible reaction occurs with a very loose bond, so the carbon dioxide is easily released into the alveoli, where the $P_{CO_2}$ is lower than in the tissue capillaries. A small amount of carbon dioxide (usually equivalent to about 0.5 to 1.0 mEq of bicarbonate per liter) also reacts in this same way with the plasma proteins, but this is much less significant because the quantity of these proteins is only about one-fourth to one-half the quantity of hemoglobin.

The theoretical quantity of carbon dioxide that can be carried to the lungs in combination with hemoglobin and plasma proteins is approximately 30 percent of the total quantity transported—that is, about 1.5 mL of carbon dioxide in each 100 mL of blood. However, this reaction is much slower than the reaction of carbon dioxide with water, and it is doubtful that more than 15 to 25 percent of the total quantity of carbon dioxide is transported this way.

## The Carbon Dioxide Dissociation Curve

Carbon dioxide can exist in the blood as free carbon dioxide and in chemical combinations with water, hemoglobin, and plasma proteins. The total quantity of carbon dioxide combined with the blood in all forms depends on the $Pa_{CO_2}$.

The normal blood $Pa_{CO_2}$ averages about 40 mmHg in arterial blood and 46 mmHg in mixed venous blood. Although the normal total concentration of carbon dioxide in the blood is about 50 mL/dL (vol%), only 4 mL/dL of this is actually exchanged during normal transport of carbon dioxide. Thus, the concentration of carbon dioxide rises to about 52 mL/dL after the blood passes through the tissues, and falls to about 48 mL/dL after the blood passes through the lungs.

## Effect of the Oxygen-Hemoglobin Reaction on Carbon Dioxide Transport—The Haldane Effect

An increase in the carbon dioxide level in the blood causes oxygen to be displaced from the hemoglobin, and this promotes oxygen release to tissues at the capillary level. The reverse is also true; binding of oxygen with hemoglobin tends to displace carbon dioxide as blood moves through the pulmonary capillaries. Indeed, this effect, called the *Haldane effect*, is quantitatively far more important in promoting carbon dioxide transport than the Bohr effect is in promoting oxygen transport.

The Haldane effect results because the combination of oxygen with hemoglobin causes hemoglobin to become a stronger acid. This displaces carbon dioxide from the blood in two ways: (1) the highly acidic oxyhemoglobin has less tendency to combine with carbon dioxide to form carbaminohemoglobin, thus releasing much of the carbon dioxide present in the red blood cell into the plasma, and (2) the increased acidity of oxyhemoglobin causes it to release hydrogen ions, and these in turn bind with bicarbonate ions to form carbonic acid. The carbonic acid then dissociates into water and carbon dioxide, and the carbon dioxide is released from the blood into the alveoli. Thus, in the presence of oxygen, much less carbon dioxide can bind with hemoglobin and conversely, in the absence of oxygen, considerably more carbon dioxide can be bound to the hemoglobin.

Therefore, in tissue capillaries, the Haldane effect causes increased pickup of carbon dioxide because oxygen has been removed from the hemoglobin, and in the lungs, it causes increased release of carbon dioxide because of oxygen pickup by the hemoglobin.

## Change in Blood Acidity During Carbon Dioxide Transport

The carbonic acid formed when carbon dioxide enters the blood in the tissue decreases the pH. However, the buffers of the blood prevent the hydrogen ion concentration from rising greatly. Ordinarily, arterial blood has a pH of approximately 7.40, and as the blood acquires carbon dioxide in the tissue capillaries, the pH falls to approximately 7.35. The reverse occurs when carbon dioxide is released from the blood in the lungs. In conditions of high metabolic activity, or when blood flow through the tissues is extremely sluggish, the decrease in pH in the blood as it leaves the tissues can be 0.50 or more.

## Changes in Respiratory Quotient

The value of the RQ changes under different metabolic conditions. When a person is metabolizing a mixed diet, the RQ averages about 0.8. If the patient were metabolizing only protein, the RQ would be 0.83. For carbohydrates, the RQ is 1.00, and if one is metabolizing only fats, the RQ falls to 0.7. When oxygen is metabolized with carbohydrates, one molecule of carbon dioxide is formed for each molecule of oxygen consumed. However, when oxygen reacts with fat, a large share of the oxygen combines with hydrogen atoms from the fats to form water instead of carbon dioxide. If the patient is eating enough carbohydrates to make fat, the RQ is greater than 1.0, and if the patient is making ketones but not metabolizing them, the RQ is less than 0.7.

## Monitoring Oxygenation and Ventilation

The patient who is awake, alert, comfortable, and cooperative and has normal vital signs is generally oxygenating and ventilating adequately. However, if the patient is tachypneic and/or tachycardiac and appears to be anxious and/or confused, one should suspect a problem with the patient's ventilation or oxygenation and correct it as soon as possible. In comatose patients, it is sometimes very difficult to judge how well the patient is oxygenating or ventilating without serial blood gas determinations.

Cyanosis as a sign of inadequate oxygenation is almost worthless if the hemoglobin is less than 10 g/dL. Under such circumstances, the aterial oxygen saturation ($Sa_{O_2}$) must usually be less than 65 percent, corresponding to a $Pa_{CO_2}$ of about 30 to 35 mmHg, before the patient looks cyanotic.

## Arterial $P_{O_2}$

The arterial $P_{O_2}$ ($Pa_{O_2}$) in normal, healthy young adults under ideal conditions is considered to be about 100 mmHg. However, many healthy young adults have a $Pa_{O_2}$ of only 80 to 90 mmHg. The $Pa_{O_2}$ is extremely important because it not only reflects the functional capabilities of the lungs but also determines the rate at which oxygen enters the tissue cells.

Factors that affect the $Pa_{O_2}$ include the amount of alveolar ventilation; the concentration or fraction of oxygen in the inspired gases ($Fi_{O_2}$); the functional capabilities of the lungs; and the oxyhemoglobin dissociation curve.

## Alveolar Ventilation

If the patient hyperventilates, the $Pa_{CO_2}$ tends to fall and the $Pa_{O_2}$ tends to rise. If the $Pa_{CO_2}$ falls by 1 mmHg, the $Pa_{O_2}$ rises by about 1.0 to 1.2 mmHg. The lungs can make up for some pulmonary dysfunction by hyperventilating.

## Fraction of Inspired $O_2$

Unfortunately the $Fi_{O_2}$ is often not considered adequately in evaluating the $Pa_{O_2}$. If a patient is receiving oxygen by nasal cannula, the actual delivered $Fi_{O_2}$ is usually only 25 to 30 percent. With a properly fitting face mask, the inhaled $Fi_{O_2}$ is usually less than half that delivered to the mask. The approximate $Pa_{O_2}$ values that might be expected in normal persons who are inhaling various concentration of oxygen are listed in Table 20-2.

The expected alveolar $P_{O_2}$ when the patient is given oxygen can be estimated by multiplying the actual delivered percentage of oxygen by 6. Thus, a patient getting 60% oxygen would be expected to have a $PA_{O_2}$ of about $60 \times 6$, or 360 mmHg.

## Altitude

The $Pa_{O_2}$ expected when a patient is breathing room air varies with height above sea level. The greater the altitude, the lower the $P_{O_2}$ in the air and the greater the tendency for the patient to hyperventilate (Table 20-3).

The $Pa_{O_2}$ drops about 3 to 4 mmHg for each 1000-foot rise above sea level. Up to an altitude of approximately 10,000 ft, the $Sa_{O_2}$ remains about 90 percent. However, above 10,000 ft, the $Sa_{O_2}$ progressively falls about 1 percent for each 1 mmHg drop in $P_{O_2}$, until at 20,000 ft altitude, the $Pa_{O_2}$ is about 35 mmHg and the $Sa_{O_2}$ is only about 65 percent.

When a person breathes air at 30,000 ft, where the barometric pressure is about 226 mmHg, the $Pa_{O_2}$ is only 21 mmHg. At this height above sea level, almost three-fourths of the alveolar air is nitrogen. But if the person breathes pure oxygen instead of air, most of the space in the alveoli formerly occupied by nitrogen becomes occupied by oxygen. However, even if the person is breathing 100% oxygen at 30,000 ft, the $Pa_{O_2}$ is only 139 mmHg (Table 20-4).

**Table 20-2.** Expected $Pa_{O_2}$ in Patients Inhaling Various Concentrations of Oxygen

| $Fi_{O_2}$, mmHg | 0.21 (room air) | 0.4 | 0.6 | 0.8 | 1.0 |
|---|---|---|---|---|---|
| Expected $Pa_{O_2}$, mmHg* | 100 | 227 | 370 | 512 | 655 |

* Assuming a $PA_{O_2} - Pa_{O_2}$ of 10 mmHg and a $P_{CO_2}$ of 40 mmHg.

**Table 20-3.** Changes in $P_{O_2}$ at Various Altitudes

| Altitude ft above Sea Level | Atmospheric Pressure, mmHg | $P_{O_2}$ in Air, mmHg | $P_{A_{O_2}}$ in Alveoli, mmHg | $P_{a_{O_2}}$ in Arterial Blood,* mmHg |
|---|---|---|---|---|
| 0 | 760 | 159 | 105 | 100 |
| 2,000 | 707 | 148 | 97 | 92 |
| 4,000 | 656 | 137 | 90 | 85 |
| 6,000 | 609 | 127 | 84 | 79 |
| 8,000 | 564 | 118 | 79 | 74 |
| 10,000 | 523 | 109 | 74 | 69 |
| 20,000 | 349 | 73 | 40 | 35 |
| 30,000 | 226 | 47 | 21 | 19 |

* Assuming ideal circumstances with a $P_{A_{O_2}} - P_{a_{O_2}}$ of 5 mmHg or less.

### Age

Even in healthy individuals, pulmonary changes that cause a fall in the $P_{a_{O_2}}$ occur with advancing age. On the average, the $P_{a_{O_2}}$ falls about 3 to 4 mmHg per decade after the patient reaches 20 to 30 years of age. Thus, an otherwise normal 20-year-old patient with a $P_{a_{O_2}}$ of about 90 to 100 mmHg (room air, at sea level) might be expected to have a $P_{a_{O_2}}$ of only about 75 to 80 mmHg at 80 years of age.

## Alveolar-Arterial Oxygen Differences

One method for determining the degree to which lung function is impaired is to determine the alveolar-arterial oxygen gradient $[P_{(A - a)_{O_2}}]$. Arterial blood samples can be obtained easily. If there is a technique for trapping the end-expiratory gases (which generally represent average alveolar gases), the alveolar $P_{O_2}$ ($P_{A_{O_2}}$) can be measured and the $P_{(A - a)_{O_2}}$ calculated.

If alveolar gases are not directly measured, they can be estimated by the alveolar gas equation. One can also estimate alveolar oxygen in patients with a normal cardiac output breathing room air by subtracting the $P_{a_{CO_2}}$ from 145. This is possible because $P_{A_{O_2}}$ and $P_{A_{CO_2}}$ add up to about 145 when a patient breathes room air at sea level. Since the $P_{A_{CO_2}}$ is usually the same as the $P_{a_{CO_2}}$, the $P_{A_{O_2}}$ can be estimated from the arterial gas pressure by the following formula:

$$P_{A_{O_2}} = 145 - P_{a_{CO_2}}$$

If the patient has a $P_{a_{CO_2}}$ of 40 mmHg,

$$P_{A_{O_2}} = 145 - 40 = 105 \text{ mmHg}$$

This equation can be used to determine the $P_{(A - a)_{O_2}}$. The $P_{A_{O_2}}$ is estimated from the above formula, and the $P_{a_{O_2}}$ is determined from arterial blood-gas analysis. If the $P_{a_{O_2}}$ were 90 mmHg, the $P_{(A - a)_{O_2}}$ would be 15 mmHg, which is relatively normal. A $P_{(A - a)_{O_2}}$ of 20 to 30 mmHg on room air usually indicates mild pulmonary dysfunction, and a $P_{(A - a)_{O_2}}$ greater than 50 mmHg on room air usually indicates severe pulmonary dysfunction.

**Table 20-4.** Effects of Acute Exposure to Low Atmospheric Pressure on Alveolar Gas Concentrations and on Arterial Oxygen Saturation

| Altitude, ft | Barometric Pressure, mmHg | While Breathing Air | | While Breathing 100% $O_2$ | |
|---|---|---|---|---|---|
| | | Arterial $P_{O_2}$ in Alveoli, mmHg | $P_{CO_2}$ in Alveoli, mmHg | $P_{O_2}$ in Alveoli, mmHg | Oxygen Saturation % |
| 0 | 760 | 159 | 40 | 673 | 100 |
| 10,000 | 523 | 110 | 40 | 436 | 100 |
| 20,000 | 349 | 73 | 40 | 262 | 100 |
| 30,000 | 226 | 47 | 40 | 139 | 99 |
| 40,000 | 141 | 29 | 36 | 58 | 87 |
| 50,000 | 87 | 18 | 24 | 16 | 22 |

**Table 20-5.** Relation Between Oxygen-Hemoglobin Saturation and Plasma $P_{O_2}$

| Oxygen saturation, % | 100.0 | 98.4 | 95 | 90 | 80 | 73 | 60 | 50 | 40 | 35 | 30 |
|---|---|---|---|---|---|---|---|---|---|---|---|
| $P_{O_2}$, mmHg | 677 | 100 | 80 | 59 | 48 | 40 | 30 | 26 | 23 | 21 | 18 |

## Oxyhemoglobin Saturation

### Normal Relationships

It can be seen from oxygen-hemoglobin dissociation curves that even when the $P_{a_{O_2}}$ is decreased to 59 mmHg, the arterial hemoglobin is still about 90 percent saturated with oxygen. Furthermore, if the hemoglobin level is 15.0 g/dL and the tissue removes 5.0 mL of oxygen from each 100 mL of blood, the $P_{O_2}$ of the venous blood falls to about 36 mmHg, which is only 4 mmHg below the normal value. Thus, the tissue $P_{O_2}$ often changes minimally despite a marked fall in $P_{a_{O_2}}$.

On the other hand, if the $P_{a_{O_2}}$ rises far above the upper limit of normal (90 to 100 mmHg), the oxygen saturation of hemoglobin cannot rise above 100 percent. Therefore, even if the $P_{a_{O_2}}$ should rise to 600 mmHg or more, the saturation of hemoglobin would increase only 1 to 2 percent because at $P_{a_{O_2}}$ of 100 mmHg, the arterial oxygen saturation is only 98 to 99 percent.

Under circumstances of normal body temperature [37°C (98.6°F) and pH 7.40], certain standard relations exist between the oxygen-hemoglobin saturation and plasma $P_{O_2}$ (Table 20-5)

Thus, the relation between $S_{a_{O_2}}$ and plasma $P_{O_2}$ is almost linear when the $S_{a_{O_2}}$ is 60 to 90 percent. However, as the $S_{a_{O_2}}$ rises above 90 percent, the $P_{O_2}$ begins to rise much faster than the saturation.

### Factors Affecting Oxyhemoglobin Dissociation

The best known of the factors affecting the oxyhemoglobin dissociation curve are pH, temperature, and the amount of 2,3-diphosphoglycerate (2,3-DPG) in the red blood cells.

#### pH

The more acidic the blood, the more readily hemoglobin gives up its oxygen and the higher the $P_{a_{O_2}}$ is for a particular oxyhemoglobin saturation. In contrast, alkalosis makes hemoglobin hold onto its oxygen more tightly, lowering the $P_{a_{O_2}}$ present at a particular oxygen-hemoglobin saturation. In general, a rise or fall in pH of 0.10 causes a fall or rise (i.e., an opposite change) in the $P_{a_{O_2}}$ of about 10 percent (Table 20-6).

#### The $P_{CO_2}$

A shift of the oxygen-hemoglobin dissociation curve as a result of changes in the blood levels of carbon dioxide and hydrogen ions enhances oxygenation of the blood in the lungs and enhances release of oxygen from the blood in the tissues. This is called the *Bohr effect*. As the blood passes through the lungs, carbon dioxide diffuses from the blood into the alveoli. This reduces the blood $P_{CO_2}$ and decreases the hydrogen ion concentration because of the resulting decrease in the blood carbonic acid level. Both changes shift the oxyhemoglobin dissociation curve to the left. With a shift to the left, the quantity of oxygen binding to hemoglobin at any given $P_{a_{O_2}}$ is increased, allowing greater oxygen transport to the tissues. Then when the blood reaches the tissue capillaries, exactly the opposite effect occurs. Carbon dioxide entering the blood from the tissues shifts the curve to the

**Table 20-6.** Changes in $P_{O_2}$ Produced by Changes in pH

| pH | 7.60 | 7.50 | 7.40 | 7.30 | 7.20 | 7.10 | 7.00 |
|---|---|---|---|---|---|---|---|
| $P_{a_{O_2}}$, mmHg* | 80 | 90 | 100 | 111 | 122 | 134 | 148 |

* Assuming a temperature of 37°C (98.6°F) and a hemoglobin saturation of 98.4%.

**Table 20-7.** $P_{O_2}$ Levels at Various Temperatures

| Temperature, °F | 104.0 | 102.2 | 100.4 | 98.6 | 95.0 | 86.6 |
|---|---|---|---|---|---|---|
| Temperature, °C | 40 | 39 | 38 | 37 | 35 | 32 |
| $Pa_{O_2}$, mmHg* | 117 | 111 | 105 | 100 | 90 | 76 |

* Assuming a pH of 7.40 and a hemoglobin saturation of 98.4%.

right. This displaces oxygen from the hemoglobin and delivers oxygen to the tissues at a higher $P_{O_2}$ than would otherwise occur.

### Temperature

As blood temperature increases, hemoglobin gives up oxygen more readily, raising the $P_{O_2}$ in the plasma. The opposite occurs during cooling. For each 1°C rise in temperature, the $Pa_{O_2}$ rises about 5 percent (Table 20-7). With hypothermia, the $P_{CO_2}$ falls by about the same amount.

### Exercise

During strenuous exercise, several factors can shift the oxyhemoglobin dissociation curve to the right. Exercising muscles release large quantities of carbon dioxide and other acids, increasing the hydrogen ion concentration in muscle capillary blood. In addition, the temperature of the muscle often rises as much as 3 to 4° C, and phosphate compounds are also released. All these factors acting together shift the oxygen-hemoglobin dissociation curve of the blood in the muscle capillaries considerably to the right. Therefore, oxygen can sometime be released to the muscle at a $P_{O_2}$ as high as 40 mmHg even though as much as 75 percent of the oxygen has been removed from the hemoglobin. In the lungs the shift occurs in the opposite direction, allowing pickup of extra amounts of oxygen from the alveoli.

### 2,3-DPG

Except for hemoglobin, the compound present in greatest quantity in red blood cells is 2,3-diphosphoglycerate (2,3-DPG). A normal concentration of 2,3-DPG in a red blood cell keeps the oxyhemoglobin dissociation curve shifted slightly to the right all the time. In addition, in hypoxic conditions that last longer than a few hours, the quantity of 2,3-DPG increases considerably, shifting the oxyhemoglobin dissociation curve even farther to the right. This can cause the $P_{O_2}$ in the plasma to be as much as 10 mmHg higher than it would have been otherwise. However, the presence of increased 2,3-DPG makes it more difficult for the hemoglobin to combine with oxygen in the lungs.

If the concentration of 2,3-DPG falls, as it does in stored blood or during sepsis, the hemoglobin holds onto its oxygen more tightly and the $Pa_{O_2}$ tends to fall.

## Other Methods for Evaluating Oxygenation

### $Pa_{O_2}/Fl_{O_2}$ Ratio

A quick way to estimate the impairment of oxygenation is to calculate the $Pa_{O_2}/Fl_{O_2}$ ratio. Normally, the ratio is about 500 to 600, which usually correlates to a pulmonary shunt ($Qs/Qt$) of about 3 to 5 percent. However, if a patient has a $Pa_{O_2}$ of 80 mmHg on 40% oxygen, the $Pa_{O_2}/Fl_{O_2}$ ratio is 80/0.4, or 200. A $Pa_{O_2}/Fl_{O_2}$ ratio of less than 200 corresponds with a $Qs/Qt$ of about 20 percent and generally indicates a need for ventilatory support. The usual relationship between $Pa_{O_2}/Fl_{O_2}$ ratios and the $Qs/Qt$ in patients with a normal cardiac output is tabulated as shown in Table 20-8.

### Respiratory Index

Another method for evaluating the $Pa_{O_2}$ in relation to the $Fl_{O_2}$ is to calculate the respiratory index (RI), which is the alveolar-arterial oxygen difference [$P(A - a)_{O_2}$] divided by the $Pa_{O_2}$.

The $PA_{O_2}$ can be calculated by the alveolar gas equation:

$$PA_{O_2} = P_B - (P_{H_2O})(Fl_{O_2}) - Pa_{CO_2}(CF)$$

**Table 20-8.** Interpretation of $Pa_{O_2}/Fl_{O_2}$ Ratio

| $Pa_{O_2}$ | $Fl_{O_2}$ | Ratio | $Qs/Qt$ | Abnormality |
|---|---|---|---|---|
| 240 | 0.4 | 600 | 5% | None |
| 120 | 0.4 | 300 | 10% | Minimal |
| 100 | 0.4 | 250 | 15% | Mild |
| 80 | 0.4 | 200 | 20% | Moderate |
| 60 | 0.4 | 150 | 30% | Severe* |
| 40 | 0.4 | 100 | 40% | Very severe* |

* In trauma or septic patients, ventilatory assistance and positive end-expiratory pressure (PEEP) to reduce the $Qs/Qt$ to 15 percent should be considered. The higher the $Qs/Qt$, the greater the need for ventilatory assistance and PEEP.

where CF, the correction factor, is 1.2 if RQ = 0.8 and 1.0 if RQ = 1.0.

At sea level, one can assume $P_B = 760$ and $P_{H_2O} = 47$. Thus, if the $Fl_{O_2}$ is 0.40, the $Pa_{CO_2}$ is 40, and the RQ is 0.8 then

$$PA_{O_2} = (760 - 47)(0.4) - (40)(1.2)$$
$$= (713)(0.4) - 48$$
$$= 285 - 48 = 237 \text{ mmHg}$$

One can also estimate the $PA_{O_2}$ with an $Fl_{O_2}$ of 0.30 or higher by multiplying the percentage of oxygen inhaled by 6; for example, the $PA_{O_2}$ on 40% $O_2$ is $40 \times 6$, or 240 mmHg.

Thus, if the patient has a $Pa_{O_2}$ of 80 mmHg on 40% $O_2$, the $P(A - a)_{O_2}$ could be estimated as $240 - 80 = 160$ mmHg.

A patient with an RI of 1.0 and a cardiac index of 3.0 L/min per meter has a $Qs/Qt$ of about 15 percent. If the RI is 2.0 with a cardiac index of 2.0 L/min per square meter, the $Qs/Qt$ is about 22 to 25 percent.

## Physiologic Shunting in the Lung (Venous-Arterial Admixture) ($Qs/Qt$)

Although abnormal gas diffusion or distribution in the lungs can cause abnormal blood gases, the most important cause is usually ventilation-perfusion (V/Q) mismatching. When considering ventilation and perfusion, there can be four types of alveolar capillary units: (1) If ventilation and perfusion are normal, the unit is normal. (2) If there is ventilation without perfusion, the unit is considered to be dead space. (3) If there is perfusion without ventilation, the unit is considered to be a (right-to-left) shunt. (4) If there is neither ventilation nor perfusion, the unit is silent.

The amount of physiologic shunting in the lung (or venous-arterial admixture) ($Qs/Qt$) is probably the most sensitive guide to the onset and progression of acute respiratory failure. The *shunt* refers to that fraction of blood passing through the lungs without being oxygenated. Normally, the amount for venous-arterial admixture is about 3 to 5 percent of the cardiac output. This small amount of shunting is largely due to bronchial veins draining into pulmonary veins.

Physiologic shunting is harder to determine than alveolar-arterial oxygen differences because it requires drawing both arterial and mixed venous (pulmonary artery) blood samples and determining their oxygen contents. Mixed venous samples from the pulmonary artery are preferable to those obtained from central venous pressure catheters. However, central venous blood does give a reasonable estimate of the amount of shunting present if cardiac output is relatively normal.

Although an $Fl_{O_2}$ of 1.0 was generally used in the past to determine the amount of physiologic shunting in the lung, the high $Fl_{O_2}$ in itself may cause increased shunting. Now the shunt with an $Fl_{O_2}$ of 0.4 is considered to be a better indicator of lung function.

The $Qs/Qt$ can be calculated from a modification of Berggren's formula:

$$\frac{Qs}{Qt} = \frac{Cc_{O_2} - Ca_{O_2}}{Cc_{O_2} - Cv_{O_2}}$$

**Table 20-9.** Relation between the Physiologic Shunt in the Lung($Q_S/Q_T$) and $P(A-a)_{O_2}$ While Breathing 100% $O_2$

| | | $Q_S/Q_T$, % | | |
|---|---|---|---|---|
| $Pa_{O_2}$ | $P(A-a)_{O_2}$ on 100% $O_2$ | CO = 2.5 L/min | CO = 5 L/min | CO = 10 L/min |
| 600 | 70 | 2 | 4 | 8 |
| 500 | 170 | 5 | 10 | 17 |
| 400 | 270 | 8 | 16 | 25 |
| 300 | 370 | 11 | 19 | 32 |
| 200 | 470 | 13 | 24 | 38 |
| 150 | 520 | 14 | 26 | 42 |
| 100 | 570 | 18 | 31 | 47 |
| 90 | 580 | 20 | 34 | 50 |
| 80 | 590 | 22 | 36 | 53 |
| 70 | 600 | 24 | 39 | 56 |
| 60 | 610 | 28 | 44 | 61 |
| 50 | 620 | 33 | 50 | 67 |

*Note:* CO, cardiac output

where $Cc_{O_2}$ is the pulmonary capillary oxygen content, $Ca_{O_2}$ is the arterial content, and $Cv_{O_2}$ is the mixed venous oxygen content. Thus if $Cc_{O_2}$ is 20 mL/dL, $Ca_{O_2}$ is 19 mL/dL, and $Cv_{O_2}$ is 14 mL/dL, the shunt is

$$\frac{Q_S}{Q_T} = \frac{20-19}{20-14} = \frac{1}{6} = 17\%$$

The amount of shunting in the lung can also be estimated from arterial blood alone, using an assumption that the arteriovenous oxygen difference is approximately 5 mL/dL.

In general, if cardiac output doubles, the amount of shunt associated with a particular $P(A-a)_{O_2}$ increases by about 50 percent (Table 20-9). This is partly related to the fact that if only a small amount of blood is going through the lung, the blood flow tends to go to well-ventilated alveoli. If cardiac output increases, there is increasing likelihood that some of the blood will go through less well-ventilated tissue.

Thus, if cardiac output is high, a relatively mild hypoxemia can result in a high shunt. For example, at a $P_{O_2}$ of 300 mmHg, if the cardiac output is 2.5 L/min, the shunt might be 11 percent, but at a cardiac output of 10.0 L/min, the shunt would be 32 percent. To factor in the changes due to an increased or decreased cardiac output, we have utilized the concept of *shunt index*. The shunt index (SI) is the percent shunt divided by the cardiac index. For example, at a normal cardiac index of 3.5 L/min per square meter and a shunt of 5.0 percent, the SI is 5.0/3.5 = 1.4. If a patient has a shunt of 20 percent, with a cardiac index of 2.5 L/min per square meter, the SI is 8.0. Patients with an SI above 5.0 usually require ventilatory support.

If the cardiac index is not known, the critical $Q_S/Q_T$ is about 20 to 25 percent. Above these values the patient usually has enough of a *V/Q* abnormality to warrant aggressive ventilatory support and positive end-expiratory pressure (PEEP).

## Oxygen Availability

Oxygen availability is determined by the amount of oxygen brought to the capillaries, or oxygen delivery ($D_{O_2}$), and the dissociation of oxyhemoglobin at the tissues. To a certain extent, a good heart, which can increase cardiac output appropriately, can make up for bad lungs and a low hemoglobin level. The reverse is also true. However, a combination of poor oxygenation, low hemoglobin level, and low cardiac output may be rapidly fatal.

## Oxygen Content

The oxygen content of blood is determined primarily by the hemoglobin level and the oxyhemoglobin saturation. Each gram of hemoglo-bin measured clinically, when fully saturated, can carry 1.34 mL of oxygen. "Pure" hemoglobin can carry 1.39 mL of oxygen per gram, but clinically measured hemoglobin includes about 4 percent other compounds not carrying oxygen. Thus, a patient with a hemoglobin concentration of 15.0 g/dL can carry about 20.1 mL of oxygen per 100 mL in the red blood cells when the hemoglobin is fully saturated. Although the $Pa_{O_2}$ determines the rate at which oxygen enters the tissues, it contributes very little to the total oxygen content of blood. Each mmHg of $Pa_{O_2}$ represents only 0.0031 mL of oxygen in 100 mL of blood. Thus, a patient with a normal $Pa_{O_2}$ of 100 mmHg has only 0.31 mL of oxygen dissolved in the plasma.

The oxygen content of arterial blood ($Ca_{O_2}$) can be calculated from the following formula:

$$Ca_{O_2} = [Hb]\,(1.34)\,(Sa_{O_2}/100) + (Pa_{O_2})\,(0.003)$$

Thus, in a patient with a hemoglobin concentration of 15.0 g/dL, an $Sa_{O_2}$ of 98 percent, and a $Pa_{O_2}$ of 100 mmHg:

$$Ca_{O_2} = (15)\,(1.34)\,(98/100) + (100)\,(0.003)$$
$$= 20.0 \text{ mL of } O_2 \text{ per dL of blood}$$

If the hemoglobin concentration falls to 10.0 g/dL, even if $Sa_{O_2}$ and $Pa_{O_2}$ remain the same, $Ca_{O_2}$ falls by about a third. For example,

$$Ca_{O_2} = (10)\,(1.34)\,(98/100) + (100)\,(0.003)$$
$$= 13.132 + 0.300$$
$$= 13.4 \text{ mL of } O_2 \text{ per dL of blood}$$

Even with only 10 g of hemoglobin, the red blood cells are carrying over 40 times as much oxygen as the plasma.

## Cardiac Output

Oxygen content (in milliliters per liter of blood) multiplied by cardiac output (in liters per minute) is equal to oxygen delivery ($D_{O_2}$). Thus the $D_{O_2}$ in a patient with 15.0 g of 98% saturated hemoglobin, a $Pa_{O_2}$ of 100 mmHg, and a cardiac output of 5 L/min is

$$D_{O_2} = (Ca_{O_2} \text{ per dL})\,(10)\,(\text{cardiac output})$$
$$= \{[Hb]\,(1.34)\,(Sa_{O_2}/100)$$
$$+ (Pa_{O_2})\,(0.003)\}(10)\,(\text{cardiac output})$$
$$= [(15)\,(1.34)\,(98/100) + (100)\,(0.003)](10)\,(5)$$
$$= [(19.698 + 0.3)](50)$$
$$= (19.998)\,(50) = (20)\,(50)$$
$$= 1000 \text{ mL/min}$$

The factor 10 is used to convert oxygen content from milliliters per 100 mL of blood to milliliters per liter of blood.

Since the normal oxygen consumption of an average resting adult male is about 250 to 300 mL/min, the tissue normally takes up about 25 percent of the oxygen brought to it. Thus, the oxyhemoglobin saturation ($S_{O_2}$) falls from about 98 percent in arterial blood to about 73 percent in mixed venous blood. If there is no change in oxygen consumption but cardiac output doubles to 10 L/min, the amount of oxygen removed from each liter of blood is halved, and the venous oxyhemoglobin saturation will be about 85 percent. On the other hand, if cardiac output falls to 2.5 L/min, oxyhemoglobin saturation will fall to about 48 percent.

## Oxygen Dissociation in the Tissues

The ability of blood to give up more oxygen (increasing the arteriovenous oxygen difference) as cardiac output falls is an important homeostatic defense mechanism sometimes referred to as *oxygen reserve*. Unfortunately, there is a limit to this so-called oxygen reserve because the $P_{O_2}$ in most tissues seldom falls below 26 mmHg with an oxyhemoglobin saturation of about 50 percent.

The lowest value to which the $P_{O_2}$ in capillaries can fall is about 18 to 20 mmHg because this is the usual capillary-mitochondrial gradient for oxygen. The saturation at a $P_{O_2}$ of 20 mmHg is referred to as the $S_{20}$, and this is normally about 33 percent. The only place where the $P_{O_2}$ in venous blood is normally as low as 20 mmHg is the coronary sinus and perhaps the jugular venous bulb at the base of the brain. A relatively mild degree of alkalosis can raise the $S_{20}$ by 4 to 5 percent, thereby greatly reducing oxygen availability to the myocardium. Thus, alkalosis in low flow states can be deleterious.

## Combination of Hemoglobin with Carbon Monoxide

Carbon monoxide combines with hemoglobin at the same point on the hemoglobin molecule that oxygen does. Furthermore, it binds about 230 times more strongly than oxygen does. Therefore, an alveolar carbon monoxide level of only 0.4 mmHg, which is only 1/230 that of the $Pa_{O_2}$, allows the carbon monoxide to compete equally with oxygen for combination with hemoglobin, causing half the hemoglobin in the blood to bind with carbon monoxide instead of with oxygen. An alveolar carbon monoxide level of 0.7 mmHg (about 0.1% in air) can be lethal.

Oxygen at high alveolar pressures displaces carbon monoxide from hemoglobin much more rapidly than atmospheric oxygen does. The patient can also benefit from simultaneous administration of 4 to 5% carbon dioxide which strongly stimulates the respiratory center, increasing alveolar ventilation, reducing the alveolar carbon monoxide concentration, and allowing increased carbon monoxide to be released from the blood. A 96% oxygen and 4% carbon dioxide therapy removes carbon monoxide from the blood 10 to 20 times more rapidly than would be removed by breathing room air. The half-life of Hb–CO in a patient breathing room air is 2 to 3 h; if the patient is breathing 100% $O_2$, the half-life is about 20 to 30 min.

## OTHER METHODS FOR EVALUATING BLOOD GASES

### Pulmonary Artery Catheters

A number of pulmonary artery catheters have been developed to continuously monitor mixed venous oxygen saturation ($Sv_{O_2}$). The normal $Sv_{O_2}$ is about 70 to 75%. Changes in the $Sv_{O_2}$ can provide early warning of problems with function of the lungs or cardiovascular system. If the $Sv_{O_2}$ rises to 80% or higher, either the catheter tip is wedged so that pulmonary capillary (oxygenated) blood is being analyzed or the cardiac output has risen.

A fall in $Sv_{O_2}$ below 50 to 60% is usually due to a significant decrease in cardiac output or lung function and requires urgent investigation. A change in $Sv_{O_2}$ indicates important physiologic changes, but there can be major changes in the patient's condition without corresponding changes in the $Sv_{O_2}$.

### Noninvasive Monitoring

### Pulse Oximetry

The use of pulse oximetry for monitoring oxygen saturation and pulse amplitude in the fingers, nose, or toes can provide early warning of pulmonary or cardiovascular deterioration before it is clinically apparent. This technique employs a microprocessor that continuously measures pulse rate and oxyhemoglobin saturation. The photosensor is not heated and does not require calibration. Oxyhemoglobin ($HbO_2$) is red and reduced hemoglobin (Hb) is blue, and each has a different absorption of light at their given wavelengths. Because the ratio of transmittance at each of the two wavelengths (660 nm, red; 940 nm, infrared) varies according to the percentage of $HbO_2$, pulse oximeters can be programmed to calculate and display the percentage of oxyhemoglobin saturation at each pulse.

There is a predictable correlation between noninvasive $Sa_{O_2}$ and arterial oxygen saturation over a wide range of $Sa_{O_2}$ values. Pulse oximetry has only a minimal error of 1 to 2 percent over the range of 60 to 90 percent saturation. However, a number of factors can limit the effectiveness and accuracy of pulse oximetry. These include impaired local perfusion, abnormal hemoglobin, and very high $P_{O_2}$. Carboxyhemoglobin and fetal hemoglobin falsely raise oxyhemoglobin saturation readings while methemoglobin lowers them.

## Capnography

Capnography, by providing a real-time estimate of $Pa_{CO_2}$, is a useful and accurate means of assessing ventilatory adequacy, respiratory gas exchange, carbon dioxide production, and cardiovascular status (primarily cardiac output). Although the measurement of end-tidal carbon dioxide partial pressure ($PET_{CO_2}$) underestimates $Pa_{CO_2}$ by about 1 to 2 mmHg normally, the difference is constant for a given patient provided that the dead space/tidal volume ($VD/VT$) ratio and airway resistance are not changing.

Mainstream and side stream infrared capnometers are commercially available. A mainstream capnometer connects directly to the endotracheal tube, thus providing real-time breath-by-breath analysis. The major disadvantage of this system is its size and bulk and the fact that it cannot be used in nonintubated patients. Side stream capnometers aspirate gas at the sample site. The principal advantages of this system are that it reduces mechanical dead space and can be used in nonintubated patients; however, there are many mechanical factors related to gas sampling which require much expert attention and time and which can affect the results.

Because carbon dioxide production is directly dependent on metabolic rate, there are a large number of conditions that can lower $PET_{CO_2}$. However, sudden decreases in $PET_{CO_2}$ suggest mechanical problems in the airway, hypoventilation, or increased dead space. A gradual decrease in the $PET_{CO_2}$ is usually due to changes in the lung itself. Increases in the $PET_{CO_2}$ are generally due to hypermetabolic states.

If a simultaneous $Pa_{CO_2}$ is available, one can estimate the $P(A - a)_{CO_2}$. Normally this is zero, and if it suddenly increases, one should suspect a pulmonary embolus or drastic reduction in cardiac output.

The most frequent use of $PET_{CO_2}$ is to evaluate the adequacy of ventilation. Inadvertent esophageal intubation, tracheal extubation, and endotracheal tube obstruction can be readily detected. These monitors can reduce the number of arterial blood gas determinations obtained and be very useful in weaning patients from mechanical ventilatory support. They can also be useful in determining the adequacy of circulation during CPR. In general, capnographs are relatively inexpensive, and they are reliable in a wide variety of clinical settings.

## Transcutaneous Monitoring of Oxygen and Carbon Dioxide

In 1951 it was discovered that a finger immersed in a 45°C (113°F) electrolyte solution had a $P_{O_2}$ equal to the $Pa_{O_2}$. As a consequence, electrochemical sensors have been developed to detect the $P_{O_2}$ and $P_{CO_2}$ at the surface of the skin.

Transcutaneous oxygen and carbon dioxide tension ($PTC_{O_2}$ and $PTC_{CO_2}$) are important variables for the early warning of disturbed pulmonary function or systemic circulation as well as for the evaluation of local tissue perfusion. Comparative studies indicate that $PTC_{O_2}$ and $PTC_{CO_2}$ are more sensitive indicators of circulatory changes than conventional monitoring variables such as arterial pressure, heart rate, CVP, ECG, and urine output. If tissue perfusion is severely reduced, $Ptc_{O_2}$ and $Ptc_{CO_2}$ values deviate from their relationship with arterial partial pressures and become flow-dependent, thereby providing only qualitative information on blood flow.

### Oxygen

In adults, $Ptc_{O_2}$ is nearly always substantially lower than $Pa_{O_2}$, partly because the thicker skin layer acts as a barrier to oxygen diffusion. It has been noted that heating of the skin produces major effects: (1) vasodilation of the cutaneous blood vessels; (2) right shift of the oxyhemoglobin dissociation curve, increasing the $P_{O_2}$; and (3) altered lipid structure of the stratum corneum, allowing more rapid diffusion of oxygen. Oxygen molecules which diffuse from the "arterialized" capillary bed to the skin surface are consumed at the electrode in an electrochemical reaction which alters current flow between a cathode and anode, proportional to the oxygen tension present.

### Carbon Dioxide

The transcutaneous $CO_2$ electrode is separated from skin by a thin hydrophobic membrane that is permeable to carbon dioxide. Carbon dioxide molecules diffuse through the membrane and form carbonic acid ($H_2CO_3$), which alters the pH across a conventional pH-sensitive glass electrode.

Carbon dioxide diffuses fairly rapidly through the skin. Heating the skin causes: (1) faster diffusion of carbon dioxide to the skin surface, (2) decreased solubility of carbon dioxide, and (3) increased local metabolism and carbon dioxide production. These three heating effects cause transcutaneous $CO_2$ readings to be 1.2 to 2 times greater than arterial values.

In critically ill adults, $Ptc_{O_2}$ responds rapidly to changes in $Pa_{O_2}$ and cardiac output. Its 95 percent response time is less than 2 min, even in patients with low-flow circulatory shock. In a study of high-risk surgical patients monitored perioperatively with $Ptc_{CO_2}$ sensors and pulmonary artery catheters, it was found that decreases in cardiac output, oxygen delivery, oxygen consumption, and $Ptc_{CO_2}$ were the earliest warning signs of impending circulatory deterioration.

Although transcutaneous monitoring is a noninvasive technique and can provide constant real-time monitoring, it has a number of disadvantages. If the electrode site is not changed every 2 to 6 h, there is a risk of burns from the heated electrode. There may also be skin irritation from the adhesive ring.

### Conjunctival Oxygen and Carbon Dioxide Measurements

In 1971, two researchers attached a Clark $P_{O_2}$ electrode to the anterior surface of a scleral contact lens as a means of continuously monitoring conjunctival oxygen tension ($Pcj_{O_2}$). More recently, miniaturized fiberoptic electrodes have been developed for conjunctival $Pcj_{CO_2}$ and pH monitoring.

If cardiac output is adequate, $Pcj_{O_2}$ tracks $Pa_{O_2}$ during variations in blood oxygenation. However, during hemorrhagic shock, $Pcj_{O_2}$ tracks cardiac output. If $Pa_{O_2}$ is adequate, the $Pcj_{O_2}$, like the $Ptc_{CO_2}$, follows local oxygen delivery. $Pcj_{O_2}$ does not require a heated electrode because the conjunctiva does not have a stratum corneum that impedes oxygen diffusion. Since the conjunctiva is supplied by the ophthalmic branch of the internal carotid artery, $Pcj_{O_2}$ may also reflect carotid arterial oxygen transport.

$Pcj_{O_2}$ monitoring has been used to manage patients on mechanical ventilation, during extubation, and during therapeutic interventions. Kram and Shoemaker found that abrupt alterations in $Pcj_{O_2}$ may reflect changes in ventilator mode, $Fi_{O_2}$, therapy with fluids, vasopressors and vasodilators, or endotracheal tube suctioning. A sudden drop in $Pcj_{O_2}$ may also be due to hypoxemia, pneumothorax, reduced cardiac output, or altered local perfusion.

## BIBLIOGRAPHY

Kram HB, Shoemaker WC: Transcutaneous, conjunctival, and organ $PO_2$ and $PCO_2$ monitoring in the adult, in Shoemaker WC, Ayres S, Grenvik A, et al (eds): *Textbook in Critical Care.* Philadelphia, Saunders, 1989, pp 283–291.

Plant JCD: Functional anatomy of the respiratory tract and lungs, in Wilson RF, Wilson JA (eds): *Pulmonary Function and Respiratory Failure in Critically Ill and Injured Patients.* Detroit, Wayne State University, 1974.

Shapiro BA, Cane RD: Blood gas monitoring: Yesterday, today and tomorrow. *Crit Care Med* 17:966, 1989.

# 21
# FLUID AND ELECTROLYTE PROBLEMS

### Robert F. Wilson
### Christopher Barton

Fluid and electrolyte and acid-base problems occur frequently in critically ill patients. A general approach to these problems is as follows.

1. One should never completely trust the laboratory. Some of the worst complications of fluid and electrolyte or acid-base management have occurred when aggressive therapy was based on an erroneous laboratory result. Errors may occur in obtaining the sample, labeling the sample, performing the test, or reporting the result. If the laboratory result does not seem to correlate properly with the patient's condition or other data, three things should be done: (a) The patient and the patient's record should be carefully reexamined. (b) If the laboratory result still does not seem to fit, the test should be repeated. (c) If there is still a question about the laboratory result, a sample from a normal individual should be analyzed.
2. Abnormalities should be treated at approximately the rate at which they developed since biologic systems react primarily to rate of change and not to absolute concentrations. For example, one should not rapidly correct a chronic asymptomatic abnormality. Even when an abnormality has developed rather rapidly, only half the calculated deficit should be corrected at a time. The patient is then reevaluated and the laboratory tests repeated to determine the rate and amount of correction still required.
3. The priorities for correcting multiple fluid, electrolyte, and acid-base abnormalities are as follows: first, fluid volume and perfusion deficits; second, pH; third, potassium, calcium, and magnesium abnormalities; and fourth sodium and chloride abnormalities. If blood volume and tissue perfusion are restored to normal, many electrolyte and acid-base abnormalities will correct themselves spontaneously.
4. One should not correct the pH without also evaluating potassium, calcium, and magnesium levels, and in no instance should one be corrected without considering the effect that it may have on the others. For example, acidosis is often associated with hyperkalemia and increased plasma levels of ionized calcium and magnesium. Alkalosis lowers plasma levels of potassium and ionized calcium and magnesium. If a severely acidotic patient has a low serum potassium level, one should suspect either laboratory error or severe potassium deficiency. As a general rule, if all the measured electrolyte levels are low, symptoms are apt to be less severe than if only one were decreased.

## ATOMIC WEIGHTS

Proper correction of electrolyte abnormalities may be facilitated by some knowledge of the atomic weights of the elements most likely to be involved in fluid and electrolyte problems (Table 21-1). The equivalent weight is the atomic weight divided by its usual electrical charge or valence. For example, if the plasma level of ionized calcium, which has an atomic weight of 40 and an equivalent weight of 20, is 4.0 mg/dL, the concentration of ionized calcium can be ex-

pressed as 2.0 mEq/L or 1.0 mmol/L. Magnesium sulfate is usually stocked and given in terms of grams without indicating how many mEq of magnesium are present. Knowing the atomic weights, one can readily calculate the molecular weight of $MgSo_4 \cdot 7H_2O$ as 24 + 32 + (4)(16) + (7)(18) = 246. Thus, 1 g of $MgSO_4$ contains 4.06 mmol of Mg or 8.1 mEq Mg.

## WATER

Normally about 55 to 60 percent of the body weight of an adult is water. In the newborn, there is relatively more water, usually equivalent to 70 to 80 percent of the body weight. Fat is relatively anhydrous, and muscle is about 77 percent water. Consequently, obese adult women may have less than 50 percent of their weight as water, and muscular men may have more than 60 to 65 percent of their weight as water.

## Osmolarity and Osmolality

Alterations in the amount of water present in the various fluid spaces are primarily related to the *number* of particles present in a given volume of solution, or *colligative properties*. Osmotic pressure is one of the colligative properties with which we are most concerned. The osmotic pressure of serum is largely regulated by antidiuretic hormone (ADH), which increases water reabsorption in the collecting ducts of the kidney. The most important stimuli to ADH secretion, in descending order of potency, are nausea, pain, hypovolemia, and hyperosmolarity. Hypovolemia is a much stronger stimulus to ADH secretion than hypoosmolarity is an inhibitor. Consequently, increased ADH secretion tends to perpetuate hyponatremia in hypovolemic patients.

Serum osmolarity can be measured directly by determining the freezing point of the serum. Serum osmolarity can also be calculated from the sodium, glucose, and blood urea nitrogen (BUN) levels using the following formula:

$$\text{Osmolarity} = 2(\text{Na}) + \frac{\text{glucose}}{18} + \frac{\text{BUN}}{2.8}$$

where the glucose (mg/dL) and BUN (mg/dL) are divided by their respective molecular weights divided by 10 (because we are working with deciliters and not liters).

Thus, normal serum osmolarity, which is about 275 to 295 mOsm/L, can usually be calculated as

$$S_{\text{Osm}} = 2(140) + \frac{90}{18} + \frac{14}{2.8} = 280 + 5 + 5 = 290$$

The osmotic contributions from mannitol (mg/dL ÷ 18), glycerol (mg/dL ÷ 9), and ethanol (mg/dL ÷ 4.6) can also be included. This

**Table 21-1.** Atomic and Equivalent Weights

| Element | Symbol | Atomic Weight | Equivalent Weight |
|---------|--------|---------------|-------------------|
| Calcium | Ca | 40 | 20 |
| Carbon | C | 12 | 3 |
| Chlorine | Cl | 35.5 | 35.5 |
| Hydrogen | H | 1 | 1 |
| Magnesium | Mg | 24 | 12 |
| Oxygen | O | 16 | 8 |
| Phosphorus | P | 31 | 6.2 |
| Potassium | K | 39 | 39 |
| Sodium | Na | 23 | 23 |
| Sulfur | S | 32 | 5.3 |

equation will not provide an accurate estimate of extracellular fluid (ECF) osmolality if other (unexpected or unknown) solutes are present in significant quantity. Thus, a difference or "gap" between measured and calculated osmolality of more than 10 mOsm/kg should suggest the presence of another solute, such as lactate, ethanol, methanol, etc. An osmolar gap of more than 50 mOsm/L is often fatal.

The terms osmolarity, osmolality, oncotic pressure, and tonicity are often confused. *Osmolarity* refers to the number of particles per liter of solution (e.g., plasma), whereas *osmolality* refers to the number of particles per liter of solvent (e.g., plasma water). Since plasma is about 91 to 93 percent water, osmolality reflects osmotic pressure better and is usually 7 to 9% higher than the osmolarity.

The plasma *oncotic pressure* is the difference in osmotic pressure created by the presence of protein or other relatively nonpermeable substances, assuming that the plasma is equilibrated against a solution having the same ionic composition as plasma but lacking protein. The concentration of diffusible ions is higher in the plasma by 0.43 mmol/L than in interstitial fluid. The sum of 0.43 mmol/L and the protein concentration, which is 0.8 mmol/L, determines the plasma oncotic pressure. Since each mmol/L generates 19.3 mmHg of oncotic pressure ($\Delta\pi$),

$$\Delta\pi = 1.23 \times 19.3 \text{ mmHg} = 23.7 \text{ mmHg}$$

When the extracellular osmolality is increased by solutes restricted to the extracellular fluid, the intracellular osmolality is increased by a shift of water from the cell to the extracellular fluid. The osmols which can cause a shift of water out of the cells are called "effective" osmols, and those that distribute across the cell membrane equally and therefore do not cause shift of water out of the cell may be termed "ineffective" osmols.

The osmolality produced by effective osmols is referred to as *tonicity* or *effective osmolality*. The principal extracellular electrolytes—sodium, chloride, and bicarbonate—are all effective osmols. Glucose is an effective osmol for most, but not all, cells. For example, it easily enters red blood cells, hepatocytes, and osmoreceptor cells in the brain and hence does not draw water from them. Thus, when we consider a substance as an effective osmol, it is usually in reference to muscle, the organ that represents the greatest bulk of the body's tissues.

Some solutes (e.g., urea, ethanol, methanol, and ethylene glycol) pass freely across cell membranes and do not exert a force for water movement between the two major body fluid compartments. Such noneffective solutes contribute to body fluid osmolality but not to tonicity. Tonicity cannot be measured, but it can be estimated, under normal circumstances, as follows:

$$2 \times [\text{Na}^+] + \frac{[\text{glucose}]}{18} = (2 \times 140) + \frac{90}{18} = 285 \text{ mOsm/kg H}_2\text{O}$$

If mannitol, glycerol, and sorbitol are present in the ECF, they must be included in this calculation. Urea, ethanol, methanol, and ethylene glycol, no matter how severe the azotemia or the intoxication, need not be included.

## Fluid Spaces

Total body water is normally divided into intracellular fluid (ICF) and extracellular fluid (ECF). Intracellular fluid is about 30 to 35 percent of the body weight, and ECF (which includes water in interstitial fluid, plasma, bone, connective tissue, and transcellular fluid) is about 25 to 30 percent of the body weight (Table 21-2).

## Extracellular Fluid

Some of the fluid markers (such as sodium, chloride, and bromide) used to estimate the size of the ECF space also penetrate cells to

**Table 21-2.** Size and Sodium and Potassium Content of Various Fluid Spaces

| | % Body Weight | % Total Body Na | % Total Body K |
|---|---|---|---|
| Plasma | 4.5 | 1.2 | 0.4 |
| Interstitial fluid (lymph) | 12.0 | 20.0 | 1.0 |
| Dense connective tissue and cartilage | 4.5 | 11.7 | 0.4 |
| Bone | 4.5 | 43.1 | 7.6 |
| Transcellular | 1.5 | 2.6 | 1.0 |
| Total extracellular | 27.0 | 97.6 | 10.4 |
| Total intracellular | 33.0 | 2.4 | 89.6 |
| Total body | 60.0 | 100.0 | 100.0 |

varying degrees. Thus, they overestimate the ECF. Conversely, other ECF markers (such as insulin, mannitol, and sucrose) do not penetrate certain parts of the extracellular fluid space and therefore underestimate ECF. As a result, depending on the type of marker used, the calculated ECF may vary from 27 to 45 percent of the total body water.

Normally the intracellular water (ICW) is about 55 percent of the total body water (TBW), and the exchangeable potassium ($K_e$), which is primarily in ICW, is about 80 mEq/L in the TBW. In malnutrition, ICW falls, ECF increases, and $K_e$ can fall to about 50 mEq/L in the TBW. In contrast, the total exchangeable Na ($Na_e$), which is normally about 75 mEq/L of TBW, can rise with malnutrition, trauma, or sepsis to about 95 mEq/L of TBW. Thus, the ratio of $K_e$ to $Na_e$, which is normally about 1.05 to 1.10 (80/75), can fall to about 0.55 (50/95) in severe malnutrition. In sepsis, the $K_e/Na_e$ can fall even lower.

The electrolyte concentrations in the plasma and interstitial fluid are approximately the same except for protein-bound electrolytes, such as calcium and magnesium. Cellular fluid has much more potassium, magnesium, phosphate, and protein than ECF, but it has relatively little sodium and very little calcium or chloride (Table 21-3).

## Interstitial Fluid (ISF)

### Characteristics

The ISF space is not physiologically uniform. It consists of a small liquid and large gel phase invested by a fibrous meshwork, the latter made up largely of collagen fibers that hold the cells together. The ground substance between the collagen fibers consists largely of anionic polymers, referred to as glycosaminoglycans, which bind cations selectively and limit their mobility to varying degrees. Glycosaminoglycans also limit the mobility of water, holding some of the bound water in an icelike lattice.

**Table 21-3.** The Electrolyte Concentration of Body Fluids (mEq/L)

| Solution | Seawater | Extracellular Fluid | Interstitial Fluid | Intracellular Fluid |
|---|---|---|---|---|
| Cations | | | | |
| Sodium | 425 | 142 | 144 | 10 |
| Potassium | 15 | 4.5 | 4.5 | 150 |
| Magnesium | 105 | 2 | 1.0 | 40 |
| Calcium | 35 | 4.5 | 2.5 | |
| Total | 580 | 153 | 152 | 200 |
| Anions | | | | |
| Chloride | 500 | 102 | 113 | — |
| Phosphates | 10 | 2 | 2 | 120 |
| Sulfates | 45 | 1 | 1 | 30 |
| Bicarbonate | 25 | 27 | 30 | 10 |
| Protein | — | 16 | 1 | 40 |
| Organic acids | — | 5 | 5 | — |
| Total | 580 | 153 | 152 | 200 |

Only a small part of the interstitial fluid is freely movable, and this portion is felt to have the following characteristics:

1. The ion concentrations are predictable by the Donnan equilibrium.
2. Interstitial protein is dissolved in this portion.
3. This portion exchanges water with the capillary fluid.
4. This is the route for water to move from capillaries to lymphatics.

The electrolyte concentrations of interstitial fluid, obtained primarily by the analysis of lymph fluid, probably reflect the average composition of the freely movable interstitial fluid fairly accurately.

**Donnan Equilibrium**

The concentrations of electrolytes in the interstitial fluid are different from those in the plasma because the concentration of proteins is much lower in interstitial fluid. When two solutions are separated by a membrane permeable to water and small ions, and when one of the solutions contains more nonpermeable ions than the other, the distribution of permeable or diffusible ions occurs in a predictable manner which can be calculated from the products of the diffusible cations and anions in each solution according to the requirements of the Donnan equilibrium:

$$(C^+ \text{ plasma})(A^- \text{ plasma}) = (C^+ \text{ ISF})(A^- \text{ ISF})$$

On the average, the proteinate anion concentration in plasma is 16 mEq/L and in interstitial fluids the proteinate anion is 8 mEq/L. If the concentrations of diffusible cations and anions in the plasma are 156 and 140 mEq/L, respectively, the concentrations of diffusible cations and anions in the interstitial fluid can be calculated from the equation

$$156 \times 140 = c(c - 8)$$

where $c$ is the diffusible cation concentration in the interstitial fluid and $c - 8$ is the concentration of diffusible anions. Thus, $c^2 - 8c - 21,840 = 0$, and $c = 152$ mEq/L. Thus, the concentration of diffusible anions is 144 mEq/L (Table 21-4).

## Intracellular Fluid

Intracellular fluid has much more potassium, magnesium, phosphate, and protein than ECF, but it has relatively little sodium and almost no calcium or chloride. However, the electrolyte concentration of intracellular fluid varies greatly from tissue to tissue. For example, in muscle the concentration of chloride is 2 to 3 mEq/L, and the resting membrane potential of the cell membrane is about −90 mV. In contrast, in erythrocytes the concentration of chloride is about 70 mEq/L and the cell membrane potential is only about −7 mV.

The potassium concentration in muscle cells is about 160 mEq/L, whereas in platelets it is only 118 mEq/L. The concentration of sodium in muscle cells and in red blood cells is 12 to 17 mEq/L, but the sodium concentration in leukocytes is about 34 mEq/L. Because muscle represents the bulk of the body cell mass, it is customary to use the electrolyte concentration of muscle cells as representative of the total body's intracellular electrolyte concentration.

## Daily Fluid Requirements

Daily fluid requirements include (1) basic needs for urine and insensible water loss; (2) current losses for gastrointestinal loss, sweat, or

**Table 21-4.** Distribution of Electrolytes Across the Capillary According to the Donnan Equilibrium (mEq/L)

|  | Plasma | Interstitial Fluid |
| --- | --- | --- |
| Diffusible cations | 156 | 152 |
| Diffusible anions | 140 | 144 |
| Protein anions | 16 | 8 |
| Total | 312 | 304 |

**Table 21-5.** Average Electrolyte Content of Various Body Fluids (mEq/L)

|  | Sodium | Potassium | Chloride | Bicarbonate | Volume/ Day |
| --- | --- | --- | --- | --- | --- |
| Saliva | 10–60 | 10–20 | 15–40 | 30–15 | 1000–2000 |
| Stomach | 40–100 | 5–15 | 15–20 | — | 1500–2500 |
| Bile | 130–140 | 4–6 | 95–105 | 30–40 | 50–1000 |
| Pancreas | 130–140 | 4–6 | 40–60 | 80–100 | 1000–2000 |
| Small intestine | 130–140 | 4–6 | 40–60 | 80–100 | 1000–2000 |
| Colon | 80–140 | 25–45 | 80–100 | 30–50 | 100–600 |
| Sweat | 40–50 | 5–10 | 45–60 | — | 200–1500 |

increased loss of insensible water; and (3) correction for any deficits or excesses.

## Basic Needs

Basic needs include urine loss of about 600 to 1000 mL/m² per day and an insensible water loss of about 350 to 700 mL/m² per day. In a normal 70-kg adult man, this amounts to about 1000 to 1500 mL of urine and 1000 mL of insensible water loss per day. Insensible water loss includes about 300 mL from the skin and 700 mL from the lungs per day. It is pure water of evaporation and contains essentially no electrolytes. In contrast, sweat has an electrolyte content equivalent to about 0.2 to 0.3 $N$ saline.

## Current Losses

Current losses can include (1) about 500 mL of increased insensible water loss per 1°C fever, (2) 500 to 1500 mL extra for sweating, and (3) a mL for mL loss of gastrointestinal fluid. The electrolyte content of the various fluids that may be lost from the body vary greatly; some average values are given in Table 21-5.

## Deficits

Water deficits can be estimated from weight loss, thirst, and physical signs. Severe thirst usually indicates a fluid deficit of at least 2 or 3 percent of the body weight. Soft eyes, tachycardia, severe oliguria, or organ dysfunction usually indicate severe dehydration. An adult patient who appears slightly, moderately, or severely dehydrated has lost fluid equal to 6, 8, or 10 percent of total body weight, respectively. Thus, a severely dehydrated 70-kg man has lost at least 7.0 L of fluid. An infant with mild, moderate, or severe dehydration has lost water equivalent to 5, 10, and 15 percent of total body weight, respectively.

Oliguria is generally due to hypovolemia and impaired renal perfusion causing a prerenal azotemia. Occasionally, however, oliguria may be due to renal disease or injury. Some of the tests used to differentiate these two entities are listed in Table 21-6.

In general, a urine output of 0.5 mL/kg per hour or more indicates adequate fluid repletion, except in the presence of high-output renal failure, glycosuria, or diuretics.

**Table 21-6.** Tests Differentiating Oliguria due to Renal Failure from Oliguria Due to Prerenal Azotemia

| Test | Prerenal Azotemia | Renal Failure |
| --- | --- | --- |
| FeNa = $\dfrac{U_{Na}/P_{Na} \times 100\%}{U_{Cr}/P_{Cr}}$ | <1% | >3% |
| BUN/Cr ratio ($S_{Cr} < 4.0$ mg/dL) | >20:1 | <10:1 |
| Urine osmolarity | >450 | <300 |
| Urine S.G. | >1.015 | <1.010 |

## SODIUM

The total body sodium content is normally about 40 mEq/kg of body weight or about 2800 mEq in the normal 70-kg man. Almost 98 percent is present in ECF, where the concentration is about 140 mEq/L. About one-third is fixed in bone and the other two thirds is readily exchangeable in isotopic studies. However, intracellular sodium levels are usually less than 10 to 12 mEq/L.

## Hyponatremia

### Etiology

#### General Causes

##### Dilution

The total body sodium content tends to be kept rather constant by the kidneys, and consequently the most frequent cause of hyponatremia is too much TBW, producing a dilutional hyponatremia. The tendency to retain water can be greatly increased in patients with severe trauma, sepsis, cardiac failure, cirrhosis, renal failure, or chronic malnutrition.

##### Sodium Loss

Occasionally hyponatremia is due to sodium loss. Some of the more frequent causes of sodium loss include excessive vomiting, diarrhea, and sweating. If these losses are not corrected, the ECF and urine sodium concentration will fall. However, if these losses are treated with fluids that do not contain adequate sodium, a severe hyponatremia may develop. Increased urine sodium losses occur with diuretics, adrenal insufficiency, salt-losing nephritis, cystic disease of the renal medulla, the postoliguric phase of acute vasomotor nephropathy, and after renal transplantation or relief of urinary obstruction. Other less obvious causes of increased urine sodium loss include ketoacidosis and metabolic alkalosis with hypokalemia.

##### Factitious Hyponatremia

Factitious hyponatremia may be due to severe hyperglycemia, hyperlipidemia, or hyperproteinemia. Because glucose tends to stay in ECF, hyperglycemia tends to draw water out of cells into the ECF. Each 100 mg/dL increase in plasma glucose levels decreases the serum sodium concentration by about 1.6 to 1.8 mEq/L. Thus, if the blood glucose level of a previously normal patient rose to 1100 mg/dL, the patient's serum sodium concentration would fall to about 122 to 124 mEq/L.

In "true" hyponatremia, plasma osmolarity is reduced; in "factitious" hyponatremia, plasma osmolality is usually normal or increased. Mannitol, if present in excessive quantities, can produce factitious hyponatremia in a manner and quantity almost identical to that of glucose. If 100 g of mannitol is given rapidly and almost none is excreted, theoretically its concentration in the ECF of a 70-kg man could be as high as 7.0 g or 7000 mg/L (700 mg/dL). This could lower serum sodium levels by about 11.2 to 12.6 mEq/L, but plasma osmolarity would be normal.

Normally, plasma water occupies approximately 910 to 930 mL of each liter of plasma. High levels of plasma lipids or proteins increase plasma volume, decreasing the percentage that is water. This can be important if sodium determinations are performed with flame emission spectrophotometry (FES), which measures the mass of sodium in a given volume of serum. If the serum sodium concentration measured by FES is 140 mmol/L and if serum water occupies 93 percent of the serum volume, then the concentration of sodium in serum water will be 140 mmol/L divided by 0.93, which equals 150 mmol/L, which is normal. If the plasma contained only 86 percent water, then the serum sodium reported by FES would only be 129 mEq/L even though the concentration of sodium in the serum water would actually be 150 mEq/L.

In states of hyperproteinemia (e.g., multiple myeloma) or hyper-lipidemia (familial, idiopathic, or secondary), there is an increased mass of the nonaqueous components of serum and a concomitant decrease in the proportion of serum composed of water. The serum water fraction can be estimated from the following equation:

$$S_W = 99.1 - 0.1(S_L) - 0.07(S_P)$$

where $S_W$ is the percentage of serum volume occupied by water, $S_L$ is the serum lipid concentration (g/L), and $S_P$ is the serum protein concentration (g/L). Normally, the total serum lipids (triglycerides of 40 to 150 mg/dL and cholesterol of 140 to 220 mg/dL) are about 2 to 4 g/L and serum proteins are about 60 to 75 g/L. For example, in a patient with an abnormally high serum lipid concentration of 50 g/L and a normal protein concentration (74 g/L), only 88 percent of the serum volume will be occupied by water. If the concentration of sodium in serum water were normal (150 mmol/L), then the serum sodium concentration measured by the FES would be 150 mmol/L × 0.88 = 132 mmol/L, clearly below the normal range.

Ion-selective electrodes measure sodium activity in serum water only. That activity is unaffected by the proportion of serum occupied by water. Thus, in the aforementioned case, the sodium activity in the undiluted specimen would be about 150 mmol/L, a normal value for the sodium concentration in serum water.

Hyperlipidemia is seen in 20 to 70 percent of persons with diabetes mellitus (DI) and in up to 50 percent of patients admitted to the hospital with diabetic ketoacidosis. Hyperlipidemia is more common and severe in patients with poor glucose control, and such patients are prone to ketoacidosis or hyperosmolar hyperglycemic nonketotic states. In one series, 38 percent of patients with severe diabetic ketoacidosis were found to be hyponatremic.

#### Classification by Functional ECF

The major causes of hyponatremia can be classified according to the functional ECF volume and urine sodium concentrations (Table 21-7). Once it is clear that the hyponatremia is "real" and plasma osmolality has been documented to be less than 280 mOsm/kg, one should make a clinical estimate of the ECF volume of the patient. This estimation can be assisted by looking for predisposing factors such as vomiting or diarrhea, diuretic use, and preexisting disease such as primary nephropathy, liver or heart disease, and CNS disorders. A careful review of the fluid intake and output as well as their composition over the past few days is important. The physical examination should emphasize findings that define the patient's state of hydration. Certain laboratory tests that may be useful include serum

**Table 21-7.** Causes of Hyponatremia

---

I. Hyponatremia with decreased ECF
  A. Extrarenal losses; urinary Na < 20 mEq/L
    1. Sweating, vomiting, diarrhea
    2. Third-space sequestration (burns, peritonitis, pancreatitis)
  B. Renal losses; urinary Na > 20 mEq/L
    1. Loop or osmotic diuretics
    2. Aldosterone deficiency (Addison's disease)
    3. Ketonuria
    4. Salt-losing nephropathies; renal tubular acidosis
II. Hyponatremia with normal ECF; urinary Na > 20 mEq/L
  A. Inappropriate ADH secretion
  B. Sick-cell or "reset osmostat" syndromes
  C. Physical and emotional stress or pain
  D. Myxedema, Addison's disease, Sheehan's syndrome
III. Hyponatremia with increased ECF
  A. Urinary Na > 20 mEq/L
    1. Renal failure
  B. Urinary Na < 20 mEq/L
    1. Cirrhosis
    2. Cardiac failure
    3. Renal failure
IV. Pseudohyponatremia (hyperproteinemia, hyperlipidemia, hyperglycemia)

---

electrolytes, urea nitrogen, creatinine, glucose, and osmolality and urine electrolytes and osmolality. With these data, one can usually classify the patient's hyponatremia into one of three categories: (1) hypotonic hyponatremia associated with hypovolemia, (2) hypotonic hyponatremia associated with normal or only slightly increased ECF volume, and (3) hypotonic hyponatremia associated with hypervolemia or edema.

### Hypovolemic Hyponatremia

These conditions are associated with loss of both water and sodium, with replacement with relatively more water than sodium. In hypovolemic patients with healthy kidneys not receiving diuretics, the urine sodium concentration is usually less than 20 mEq/L; however, in severe metabolic alkalosis secondary to vomiting, increased amounts of sodium are lost in the urine along with the increased urine bicarbonate.

By far the most common cause of hypovolemic hyponatremia in children is viral gastroenteritis causing vomiting and/or diarrhea. Fistulas and various types of gastrointestinal tubes occasionally cause this condition. Another cause is excessive sweating, especially in patients with cystic fibrosis and adrenal insufficiency. A similar disturbance occurs when isotonic body fluid is translocated within the body to a "third space." The unequal balance of electrolyte and water loss produces a contracted ECF and a hyponatremia that is maintained by the inability of the kidneys to excrete free water. The impairment of water excretion to defend ECF volume at the expense of tonicity is accomplished by (1) decreased glomerular filtration, (2) increased proximal tubular reabsorption of solute and water, (3) decreased delivery of fluid to the diluting segment of the nephron, and (4) the presence of ADH released by nonosmotic stimuli.

Excessive renal loss of sodium can be caused by a number of drugs, endogenous (osmotic) diuretics, mineralocorticoid deficiency, and certain primary kidney disorders. In these conditions the urine sodium concentration is greater than 20 mEq/L. Under the influence of loop diuretics, the kidneys cannot appropriately dilute or concentrate the urine. Loop diuretics can also cause volume depletion and hypokalemia. The hypokalemia, in turn, tends to cause an intracellular movement of sodium, further contributing to the hyponatremia.

Osmotic diuretics cause increased urinary losses of sodium and water, resulting in ECF volume depletion and hyponatremia. Other causes of increased urinary sodium losses in concentrations that are at least half isotonic are glucosuria associated with uncontrolled diabetes mellitus, urea diuresis after relief of urinary tract obstruction, and administration of mannitol for the treatment of cerebral edema. Hyperglycemia and mannitol also make hyponatremia worse by causing the movement of water from the intracellular space to the ECF compartment.

The combination of hyponatremia, ECF volume contraction, hyperkalemia, and renal sodium wasting without renal failure suggests the possibility of adrenal insufficiency. Decreased mineralocorticoid secretion impairs the reabsorption of sodium in exchange for potassium and hydrogen ions in the distal tubule.

Salt wasting sufficient to cause hyponatremia occurs in certain renal disorders, such as medullary cystic disease, polycystic kidney disease, and obstructive uropathy, even in the absence of any renal excretory impairment. Patients with advanced renal failure have an impaired ability to conserve sodium, but the defect is usually mild and does not cause hyponatremia unless the patient is severely sodium-restricted. Proximal renal tubular acidosis (type 2 RTA) may also cause sodium wasting, because the bicarbonate ion, which is lost in greatly increased quantities, obligates the excretion of sodium. Hyperkalemic renal tubular acidosis (type 4 RTA) is characterized by aldosterone insensitivity of the renal tubules, high aldosterone levels, hyperkalemia, metabolic acidosis, and hyponatremia. In all of these disorders the urinary sodium concentration is relatively high despite the presence of hypovolemia.

For the most part, extrarenal sodium losses are associated with a low urinary sodium concentration. Conversely, primary renal disorders and drug- and hormone-induced renal dysfunction are associated with renal salt wasting and a high urinary sodium concentration.

### Euvolemic Hyponatremia

Patients described as having a combination of euvolemia and hyponatremia usually have a slightly increased ECF volume; however, these patients are not edematous and have a near-normal total body sodium content, despite the presence of hyponatremia. If symptoms are present, they are usually CNS manifestations of hypotonicity. Urinary sodium concentration is usually greater than 20 mEq/L and may be much higher in states of ADH excess, which is the most important factor in the initiation and perpetuation of most cases of euvolemic hyponatremia.

The syndrome of inappropriate (excess) secretion of ADH (SIADH) is the most common cause of euvolemic hyponatremia in children. The chronic hyponatremia of this syndrome is sustained by a constant or intermittent secretion of ADH, which is inappropriate in relation to both osmotic and volume stimuli. The diagnostic criteria are

1. Hypotonicity and hyponatremia (plasma osmolality <280 mOsm/kg $H_2O$)
2. Inappropriately concentrated urine (urine osmolality >100 mOsm/kg $H_2O$)
3. High urine sodium concentration (except during sodium restriction)
4. No clinical evidence of hypervolemia or hypovolemia
5. Normal renal, cardiac, hepatic, adrenal, and thyroid function
6. Correctable by severe water restriction

It should be noted that if serum osmolality exceeds 300 mOsm/L, urine osmolality should exceed 600 to 1200 mOsm/L. However, if serum osmolality is less than 270 to 280 mOsm/L, there should be almost no ADH secretion and urine osmolality should be 50 mOsm/L or less.

The diagnosis of SIADH is primarily one of exclusion. The diagnosis should be considered only in the absence of hypovolemia, hypervolemia (edema), endocrine dysfunction, renal failure, and drugs which may impair water excretion. Drugs which tend to cause hypotonic hyponatremia either stimulate the release of ADH centrally or potentiate its effect on the kidney, or both. The most frequent other causes of SIADH are malignancies, pulmonary disorders, and CNS infections or other CNS disorders (Table 21-8).

SIADH is most common in children with CNS infections, and the condition is worsened by the administration of usual volumes of parenteral fluids. Because the CNS symptoms and signs caused by hyponatremia may be obscured by primary CNS disease, hyponatremia

**Table 21-8.** Causes of SIADH

| | |
|---|---|
| Central nervous system disorders | Drugs |
|   Head trauma |   Narcotics |
|   Brain tumors, brain abscesses |   Chlorpropamide |
|   Meningitis, encephalitis |   NSAIDs |
|   Subarachnoid hemorrhage |   Vincristine, vinblastine |
|   Delirium tremens |   Cyclophosphamide, phenothiazines |
| Tumors |   Monoamine oxidase inhibitors |
|   Lung cancer (especially small-cell), cancer of the pancreas, ovarian cancer |   Tricyclic antidepressants |
|      |   Thiazide diuretics |
|   Lymphoma | Endocrine disorders |
|   Thymoma |   Hypothyroidism |
| Pulmonary disorders |   Glucocorticoid insufficiency |
|   Tuberculosis | Miscellaneous |
|   Pneumonia, empyema |   Porphyria |
|   Lung abscess |   Pain, nausea |
|   Cystic fibrosis, COPD |   Idiopathic |

itself may be the first clue to the diagnosis. It is important to remember that if the serum osmolality is less than 270 to 280 mOsm/kg, the urine osmolality should be less than 50 mOsm/kg. Furthermore, SIADH is a problem of water retention, not sodium depletion; therefore, aggressive sodium administration is appropriate only to relieve neurologic symptoms. Attempts to correct the hyponatremia of SIADH with sodium-rich solutions will cause an increase in urinary sodium excretion but little change in the serum sodium.

A variant of SIADH known as "reset osmostat" is not uncommon in chronically ill or malnourished individuals. This condition identifies a clinical state of hyponatremia which is characterized by a resetting downward of the plasma osmolality at which ADH is released. These patients have a chronic hyponatremia which is usually asymptomatic. They respond to water loading by decreasing ADH secretion and by diluting the urine. Likewise, sodium loading results in an increase in ADH secretion and hypertonic urine. Other than treatment of the underlying disease, no therapy is specifically indicated to correct the hyponatremia.

Endocrine disturbances that can cause hypotonic hyponatremia include glucocorticoid deficiency and hypothyroidism. Adrenal insufficiency allows increased ADH secretion and increased water reabsorption in the renal collecting ducts. The condition resembles SIADH except that these patients respond to exogenous glucocorticoid by abruptly increasing urine volume and decreasing urine osmolality. Severe hypothyroidism causes hyponatremia by promoting increased ADH secretion.

Acute water intoxication accounts for the diagnosis of hyponatremia in a few patients with impaired free water excretion. Since infants are unable to excrete a water load with the same efficiency as older children, they are at somewhat greater risk for developing hyponatremia from water loading. Postoperative patients are also at increased risk owing to their high ADH secretion secondary to pain and stress.

Other cases of acute water intoxication have been reported secondary to ingestion of low-solute formula in infants, use of tap water enemas, and swallowing of swimming pool water. Chronic water intoxication, or "psychogenic polydipsia," is rare except in mentally disturbed patients. The renal mechanisms resulting in hyponatremia in these patients include the "washing out" of the normal renal medullary concentrating gradient.

### Hypervolemic Hyponatremia

These patients usually have TBW in great excess, often present with pulmonary or peripheral edema, and usually have impaired ability to excrete a water load. This allows water retention that is proportionately greater than sodium retention. These patients may be subcategorized into two groups: (1) generalized edematous states of congestive heart failure, cirrhosis of the liver, and the nephrotic syndrome; and (2) advanced acute or chronic renal insufficiency.

In the generalized edematous patients, hyponatremia is often the result of a decreased effective arterial blood volume. In heart failure, the decreased effective blood volume is caused by a low cardiac output, whereas in cirrhosis of the liver, the decreased effective arterial blood volume is related to decreased peripheral resistance with arteriovenous shunting and splanchnic venous pooling. The low blood volume found in the nephrotic syndrome is a result of low capillary oncotic pressure with resultant loss of fluid from the intravascular to the interstitial space. In each of these disorders, a decline in the effective arterial blood volume activates baroreceptors, leading to increased ADH release, renal water retention, dilution of ECF solutes, and hyponatremia. Furthermore, the edematous disorders are characterized by decreased glomerular filtration rate and enhanced proximal tubular reabsorption of fluid. The avid retention of sodium causes the urinary sodium concentration to be less than 20 mEq/L unless diuretics are being used.

Patients with oliguric acute or chronic renal failure may develop extreme salt and water overload through intravenous fluid administra-

tion. The decrease in glomerular filtration largely determines the extent of the impairment of water excretion. Urinary sodium concentration is variable but usually exceeds 40 mEq/L.

## Pathophysiology

The pathophysiologic changes of hyponatremia are most obvious when serum sodium levels fall below 120 mEq/L in less than 12 to 24 h. The CNS effects are usually the most obvious, but cardiovascular and musculoskeletal dysfunction may also occur.

**Central Nervous System**

As serum sodium concentrations fall, the osmotic gradient that develops across the blood-brain barrier causes water to move into the brain, causing apathy, agitation, headache, altered consciousness, seizures, and even coma. The severity of symptoms is dependent not only on the rapidity, but also the magnitude, of the fall in the serum sodium concentration. Acute hyponatremia occurring in 24 h or less and resulting in a serum sodium concentration of less than 120 mEq/L, or a rate of fall of 0.5 mEq/L or more per hour, can cause muscular twitching, seizures, and coma. The mortality rate with acute severe hyponatremia with CNS changes has been reported to be as high as 50 percent in adults. In animals in which serum sodium is reduced to 110 mmol/L in 2 h, the mortality rate is 88 percent, and there is gross evidence of brain edema. When plasma sodium is lowered slowly during several days or weeks by a combination of sodium depletion and water ingestion, patients are usually less symptomatic, but even patients with chronic hyponatremia may experience focal weakness, hemiparesis, ataxia, and a positive Babinski sign.

As hyponatremia develops, the osmotic equilibrium between brain and plasma allows movement of increased amounts of water into the brain. However, brain swelling is less than would be predicted on the basis of the osmotic shifts alone. The brain's adaptation to hyponatremia is accomplished by two mechanisms: (1) movement of interstitial fluid into the cerebrospinal fluid and (2) loss of cellular potassium and organic osmolytes. With acute hyponatremia, water moves into the brain from the plasma, causing an increase in the hydrostatic pressure of the cerebral interstitial fluid. The increased interstitial pressure accelerates the clearance of interstitial fluid into the cerebrospinal fluid, which is returned to the systemic circulation via the arachnoid villi. The movement of sodium-rich interstitial fluid out of the brain reduces brain sodium, which in turn reduces the osmotic gradient for water moving into the brain.

The loss of sodium, potassium, and chloride from the brain provides most of the protection against cerebral edema in the first hours of hyponatremia; however, when hyponatremia is sustained, the brain slowly loses other intracellular osmolytes, mainly amino acids. Losses of organic osmolytes during prolonged or severe hyponatremia are especially important in defending the brain against swelling.

The adaptive changes that protect the brain from excessive swelling also render it susceptible to dehydration during correction of the fluid and electrolyte problem. Indeed, there is often more risk of brain damage during treatment than from the hyponatremia itself. The rate of rise of brain intracellular potassium and organic osmolytes during correction of the hyponatremia is much slower than the rate of loss of these substances during the development of the problem. If correction of hyponatremia occurs more rapidly than the brain can recover solute, the higher plasma osmolality may dehydrate and injure the brain, producing what is now called the *osmotic demyelination syndrome*, or *central pontine myelinolysis* (CPM). (See section on "Complications of Therapy.")

**Cardiovascular System**

The cardiovascular response to hyponatremia depends primarily on the effective arterial blood volume, which may be increased, decreased, or normal depending on the underlying disorder. Intravascular volume is determined in part by the distribution of water between the ICF and ECF compartments. Thus, in the volume-depleted patient, hyponatremia can cause a further decrease in the intravascular volume by allowing movement of water out of the ECF compartment into the ICF space. Accordingly, shock occurs at lesser degrees of TBW depletion in hyponatremia than similar fluid deficits when the plasma is hypertonic or isotonic.

Antidiuretic hormone is one of the main factors opposing the hypovolemic effect of fluid shifts induced by hyponatremia. The ADH is released primarily as a response to the decreased effective arterial blood volume which often accompanies hyponatremic edematous disorders. Nonosmotic stimulation of ADH release overrides the hypoosmotic suppressive effect of hyponatremia, and increased ADH is present in almost all hyponatremic conditions. The function of ADH in this setting initially may seem paradoxical, because it potentiates the hyponatremic state by increasing water reabsorption by the renal tubules. ADH is also a potent vasoconstrictor, however, and even at the low ADH concentrations which are characteristic of clinical hyponatremia, it increases peripheral vascular resistance, thereby increasing blood flow to the liver and kidneys at the expense of the skin and muscle.

### Musculoskeletal System

Most patients with hyponatremia have normal muscle tone and function. However, muscle cramps and weakness can occur during strenuous exercise, especially if excess sweating is replaced with water. These symptoms usually resolve rapidly when the serum sodium concentration is corrected back toward normal.

### Renal System

The usual renal response to hyponatremia is production of dilute urine; however, this process is abrogated to some extent by the presence of increased concentrations of ADH. The amount of ADH present depends on the primary disease process and the effective arterial blood volume.

A urine sodium concentration less than 10 mEq/L usually indicates that the renal handling of sodium is intact and that the effective arterial blood volume is contracted. In contrast, a urine sodium concentration greater than 20 mEq/L often indicates intrinsic renal tubular damage or a natriuretic response to hypervolemia. The urine sodium concentration will also vary somewhat according to the ongoing gains and losses of salt and water. Urine sodium will tend to increase if the underlying disease significantly impairs renal function.

## Diagnosis

Most hyponatremia is due to dilution (a relative excess of TBW), which may be iatrogenic or due to disease (usually congestive heart failure, hepatic failure, or nephrotic syndrome). A decrease in the total body sodium due to excess diuresis, vomiting, diarrhea, or sweating is less common. The importance of each factor can usually be determined by careful review of the patient's history and intake and output of fluid.

Additional information can be obtained by comparing the sodium concentration and osmolarity of the serum and urine. A urine sodium less than 10 to 20 mEq/L in the presence of adequate renal perfusion suggests that either the ECF or the body content of sodium is low. If the urine sodium concentration is high, the patient usually has a water overload, is reacting to diuretics, or has renal disease. If the serum sodium is less than 120 to 125 mEq/L, there is often a decreased total body content of sodium as well as hemodilution. The patient may have SIADH, but this is less common.

## Treatment

### Water Restriction

Since hyponatremia is usually due to hemodilution, fluid restriction is usually the best treatment in stable asymptomatic patients. One must,

however, attempt to correct the underlying process and maintain an adequate tissue perfusion. If the effective ECF volume is depleted, too severe a water restriction program could cause complications.

### Hypertonic Saline

If the hyponatremia is severe (less than 120 mEq/L) and develops rapidly (0.5 mEq/L decrease in serum sodium levels per hour) with CNS manifestations, administration of 3% saline solution is usually indicated. The 3% saline solution (which contains 513 mEq of sodium per liter) can be given at 25 to 100 mL/h, with careful observation for fluid overload and too rapid a rise in serum sodium levels. Attention should also be given to changes in urine sodium levels. Unfortunately, hypertonic saline often only increases the serum sodium concentration transiently because much of the administered sodium is rapidly excreted in the urine. Consequently, in many patients it may be helpful to also give furosemide to reduce the amount of water present in the body.

### Calculating Sodium Deficits

Methods of calculating sodium deficits are somewhat controversial. Most authors calculate sodium deficits using TBW (60 percent of body weight) as the sodium space because sodium tends to equilibrate with TBW even though most of the sodium is in the ECF. Thus, an 80-kg man with a serum sodium of 120 mEq/L would have a total sodium deficit of (80 kg × 60%) (140 − 120) = (48)(20) = 960 mEq. This calculation may be appropriate if the patient is normovolemic. However, most patients with hyponatremia are hypervolemic, and using 60 percent of the body weight in the calculations could result in administration of too much sodium. Accordingly, sodium deficits in hypervolemic patients are usually calculated using a sodium space equivalent to 20 percent of the body weight. Thus, a hypervolemic 80-kg man with a serum sodium of 120 mEq/L would be assumed to have a sodium deficit of (80 kg × 20%) (140 − 120) = (16) (20) = 320 mEq. Nevertheless, it must be stressed that unless there is a history or other evidence of sodium loss from the body, most patients with hyponatremia have a normal or even increased total body content of sodium, and fluid restriction is often the only treatment required.

### Treatment of Pseudohyponatremia

Treatment of pseudohyponatremia, such as that due to hyperglycemia, is directed at its cause. Once an adequate urine output is obtained and insulin becomes effective, glucose levels fall and serum sodium levels will usually correct spontaneously. No matter what type of hyponatremia is present, no treatment is usually necessary if serum osmolality is normal and the patient is asymptomatic.

### Complications of Therapy

Complications with the treatment of acute hyponatremia, especially if there is no underlying CNS, hepatic, or renal disorder, are uncommon and occur in fewer than 2 percent of patients. In chronic hyponatremia, brain edema is usually not severe and little evidence exists that chronic hyponatremia itself causes brain damage. Nevertheless, these patients appear to be at greatest risk for brain injury (CPM) during the correction process. The injury reportedly occurs after the hyponatremia has been corrected and progresses in a predictable manner. These neurologic changes are believed to be due to correction of the serum sodium at a rate faster than the brain can adapt to the higher osmolality. In patients with chronic hyponatremia, other factors contributing to the CPM may include alcoholism, malnutrition, toxins, and metabolic imbalance.

Brain histology in fatal cases shows myelinolysis and demyelination of central pontine and extrapontine myelin-bearing neurons. In typical cases the neurologic findings include fluctuating levels of consciousness, behavioral disturbances, dysarthria, dysphagia, or convulsions progressing to pseudobulbar palsy and quadriparesis. Improvement may occur after several weeks of severe debilitation, but some patients are permanently impaired.

In patients with chronic severe hyponatremia, the threshold for the production of CPM is a rate of correction of sodium levels faster than 0.5 mEq/L per hour (12 mEq/L per day). In patients with acute severe hyponatremia, correction at rates exceeding 0.5 to 1.0 mEq/L per hour, with or without diuretics, does not usually cause any problems. Severe neurologic complications have occurred almost exclusively in clinically hypernatremic patients treated with hypertonic or isotonic saline without the addition of furosemide or an osmotic diuretic. Similar patients treated with the same fluids but with furosemide almost uniformly have done well. Patients with chronic hyponatremia corrected at a rate less than 0.5 mEq/L per hour have also done well.

## Hypernatremia

### Etiology

The most frequent cause of hypernatremia is a decrease in TBW because of reduced intake or excessive loss. The more common causes of hypotonic fluid losses are diarrhea, vomiting, hyperpyrexia, and excessive sweating. Less frequently, hypernatremia is due to oral lactulose, osmotic diuresis with mannitol or glycerol, or increased intake of salt (Table 21-9). The causes of hypernatremia can also be classified according to the status of the blood volume (Table 21-10).

### Decreased Water Intake

Probably the main defense against hypernatremia is thirst. Although increased ADH secretion occurs before thirst, thirst generally is a far more important defense. However, patients who are in coma or who have a stroke and cannot move to get water will be unable to obtain adequate fluids.

### Excess Water Excretion

Failure of ADH mechanisms is an important cause of hypernatremia, and it may be central or renal in origin. Neonates with immature kidneys, and adults with certain types of renal disease, such as obstructive uropathy or renal dysplasia, may be unable to excrete sodium properly. Consequently, their urine osmolality may be fixed between 200 to 300 mOsm/kg with urine sodiums of 60 to 100 mEq/kg.

### Increased Sodium Intake

The body tends to keep its total content of sodium remarkably constant, and if excessive sodium is given, the kidney will usually excrete it quite rapidly. However, if renal function is impaired, a dangerous expansion of the ECF may occur. One source of excessive sodium administration is the use of sodium-containing antibiotics, such as ticarcillin, which has an average of 5.2 mEq of sodium per gram.

**Table 21-9.** Causes of Hypernatremia

I. Loss of water
  A. Reduced water intake
    1. Defective thirst
    2. Unconsciousness
    3. Inability to drink water
    4. Lack of access to water
  B. Increased water loss
    1. Vomiting, diarrhea
    2. Sweating, fever
    3. Hyperventilation
    4. Diabetes insipidus, osmotic diuresis
    5. Thyrotoxicosis
    6. Severe burns
II. Gain of sodium
  A. Increased intake
    1. Hypertonic saline ingestion or infusion
    2. Sodium bicarbonate administration
  B. Renal salt retention (usually because of poor perfusion)

**Table 21-10.** Causes of Hypernatremia Related to Blood Volume

I. Hypovolemia
  A. Nonrenal $H_2O$ losses ($U_{Na} < 10$ mEq/L, $U_{Osm} > 400$ mOsm/L) from skin or GI or respiratory tracts
  B. Renal $H_2O$ losses ($U_{Na} > 20$ mEq/L, $U_{Osm} < 300$ mOsm/L) from diuretics, renal disease, relief of urinary obstruction, adrenal failure, osmoreceptor failure
II. Euvolemia
  A. Impaired thirst (coma)
  B. Nonrenal $H_2O$ losses (GI, skin, respiratory)
  C. Renal $H_2O$ losses due to DI, reset osmostat, relief of urinary obstruction, renal disease, osmotic diuretics
III. Hypervolemia
  A. Iatrogenic (hypertonic saline therapy)
  B. Mineralocorticoid excess ($U_{Na} > 20$ mE/L, $U_{Osm} > 300$ mOsm/L) due to hyperaldosteronism, Cushing disease, congenital adrenal hyperplasia, exogenous glucocorticoids

### Diabetic Insipidus

A particularly interesting cause of hypernatremia is DI, which results in excessive loss of hypotonic urine. Diabetes insipidus may be central in origin (due to a failure of secretion of ADH) or nephrogenic (due to renal unresponsiveness to ADH). About 30 percent of central DI is idiopathic and about 70 percent is secondary to neoplasms (25 percent), pituitary surgery (20 percent), or trauma (15 percent). Most of the remaining 10 percent is due to various granulomas (tuberculosis, sarcoidosis, eosinophilic granuloma) or local vascular problems (aneurysms, thrombosis, Sheehan syndrome). Nephrogenic DI may be primary (familial) or secondary to a wide variety of causes including hypercalcemia, hypokalemia, renal disorders, various drugs (including lithium, demeclocycline, amphotericin B, aminoglycosides, cisplatin), hematologic disorders (sickle cell disease, myeloma), malnutrition, or amyloidosis.

Traumatic DI is typically triphasic. After an initial polyuria from insufficient ADH secretion by hypothalamic cells, there is a transient second phase lasting 1 to 7 days characterized by release of previously formed hormone from the posterior pituitary and resolution of the polyuria. In the third phase, central DI returns after the released hormone has been utilized. Regeneration of cells that secrete ADH may occur weeks to months after injury. The ADH-secreting cells have their cell bodies in the hypothalamus, and these are not usually completely destroyed by trauma.

Differentiation between central and nephrogenic DI is best achieved by noting (1) the response of serum and urine osmolarity to water deprivation (trying to reach a serum osmolarity greater than 295 mOsm/L) and (2) the response to 5 units of subcutaneous aqueous vasopressin. Patients with central DI show little or no response to dehydration, but respond well to vasopressin (urine osmolarity ≥800 mOsm/L). Nephrogenic DI shows little or no response to dehydration or vasopressin.

### Pathophysiology

Because sodium does not freely penetrate tissue cell membranes, ECF and plasma volume tend to be maintained in hypernatremic dehydration until the water loss is greater than 10 percent of body weight. Although there may be rather profound dehydration in some patients with severe hypernatremia, shock is an infrequent occurrence. When the dehydration results in loss of 10 percent of body weight, skin turgor becomes reduced and the skin of the abdomen has a characteristic "doughy" feel when it is pinched between the fingers.

Acute symptomatology is seen in many patients once serum sodium concentrations exceed 158 mEq/L. Patients tend to become irritable, and infants may also have a high-pitched cry or wail alternating with periods of severe lethargy. As dehydration and hypernatremia become more severe, one may see increased muscle tone or even coma with eventual seizures. Fever can be both a contributing cause and a result of hypernatremic dehydration.

Restlessness and irritability occur when serum osmolality increases to between 350 and 375 mOsm/kg, while ataxia and tremulousness tend to occur when osmolality is between 375 and 400 mOsm/kg. When serum osmolality rises above 400 mOsm/kg, asynchronous jerks and tonic spasms are apt to occur. Death usually occurs at an osmolality above 430 mOsm/kg.

Permanent sequelae are not uncommon in children when serum sodium concentrations exceed 160 to 165 mEq/L. Up to 16 percent of children with hypernatremia develop chronic neurologic deficits as a consequence. The overall mortality of hypernatremia is above 10 percent. If the plasma osmolality exceeds 350 mOsm/kg, the incidence of severe morbidity or mortality may exceed 25 to 50 percent.

Hypocalcemia, which is frequently seen in patients with hypernatremia, may contribute to the CNS symptomatology. However, the mechanism of the hypocalcemia is unclear.

Massive brain hemorrhage or multiple small hemorrhages and thromboses may occur when hypernatremia causes enough cellular dehydration and resultant brain shrinkage to cause tearing of cerebral blood vessels. This has been observed most frequently in neonates following acute administration of a large sodium load. As a consequence, the amount of sodium bicarbonate administered to acidotic infants must be limited.

If the hypernatremia persists for more than a few days, the brain dehydration may resolve, and brain water content may return to normal or near-normal levels due to accumulation in the brain cells of amino acids known as "idiogenic osmoles," particularly taurine. The formation of these idiogenic osmoles increases intracellular osmolality, attracts water back into the brain cells, and restores their cellular volume. If the hypertonicity develops gradually, this protective mechanism tends to prevent severe brain cell shrinkage.

## Treatment

When dehydration is severe, plasma volume should first be restored with plasma-expanding fluids, such as normal saline or Ringer's lactate, which is administered until blood pressure and tissue perfusion are adequate. Once perfusion is reestablished, fluid containing 75 to 80 mEq/L of sodium (i.e., 0.45% saline) should be given until the urine output is at least 0.5 mL/kg per hour. Moderately hypotonic fluids can then be given with the aim of restoring normal hydration and bringing serum sodium concentrations down to normal in 48 to 72 h. The reduction of serum sodium concentration should not exceed 10 to 15 mEq/L per day.

The amount of water needed to correct hypernatremia can be estimated by the following equation:

$$\text{Water deficit (in liters)} = \text{TBW}\left(1 - \frac{Na_2}{Na_1}\right)$$

where $Na_1$ is the current serum sodium and $Na_2$ is the desired serum sodium. TBW is normally expected to be about 60 percent of body weight. Thus for a 70-kg man, if $Na_1$ is 160 mEq/L and $Na_2$ is 145 mEq/L, the water deficit is

$$\text{Water deficit} = (60\% \times 70 \text{ kg})\left(1 - \frac{145}{160}\right)$$

$$= (42)\left(\frac{15}{160}\right) = \frac{630}{160} = 3.9 \text{ L}$$

As general rule, each liter of $H_2O$ deficit results in a rise of serum-sodium of 3 to 5 mEq/L or 8 to 15 mOsm/L. If there is any evidence of cardiac failure, rehydration must be done more slowly and with careful attention to changes in the central venous pressure (CVP) and/or pulmonary artery wedge pressure (PAWP). If the patient has significant ongoing fluid losses, these must be included in replacement therapy.

The sodium to be given can be calculated as 80 to 100 mEq per liter of estimated fluid deficit. Maintenance sodium needs can usually be disregarded. The sodium is given primarily as chloride, but sodium lactate or acetate can be given if the patient is acidotic. In hypernatremia with an excess total body sodium, the restoration of a normal ECF volume often initiates a substantial natriuresis. However, if this does not occur promptly, sodium should be removed with diuretics, such as furosemide, while 0.45% saline is administered.

Because of the predilection of children with hypernatremia to develop hyperglycemia, glucose should probably be given only as a 2.5% solution until glucose levels fall to relatively normal levels. Calcium gluconate may also be added, depending on serum calcium content. Once an adequate urine output is established, 20 to 40 mEq of potassium chloride should be added to each liter of fluid. Potassium aids water entry into cells.

Rapid correction of hypernatremia, especially if it is chronic, can cause seizures and severe neurologic sequelae. Unless the hypernatremia is of short duration, idiogenic osmoles are presumably present in brain cells. Consequently, too rapid rehydration and lowering of serum sodium concentration can cause brain cells to swell, resulting in cerebral edema and an increased likelihood of seizures, permanent neurologic sequelae, or even death. Serum electrolyte levels should be monitored frequently to ensure that the appropriate rate of decline of serum sodium concentration occurs.

In the case of acute hypernatremia, correction of serum sodium levels can be achieved rather rapidly with little fear of cerebral edema because idiogenic osmoles will not yet be present in brain cells. However, rapid fluid administration in patients with hypernatremia due to excessive sodium administration may result in hypervolemia and pulmonary edema.

In children with acute severe sodium excess and a serum sodium concentration of more than 180 to 200 mEq/L, peritoneal dialysis using a high-glucose (7.5%), low-sodium dialysate may be lifesaving, but must be done with frequent monitoring of serum electrolyte levels.

In the case of central DI, administration of either vasopressin or 1-deamino-8-D-arginine vasopressin (dDAVP) must be undertaken carefully, and fluid intake should be regulated so that the serum sodium concentrations do not drop too rapidly.

## POTASSIUM

Elemental potassium is the major intracellular cation in the body. Total body potassium content is about 50 to 55 mEq/kg, or a total of about 3500 mEq in a young, healthy 70-kg man. However, "exchangeable potassium" measured with $^{42}K$ provides somewhat lower values, averaging about 45 mEq/kg. Over 70 to 75 percent of the total body potassium is in muscle. Thus, protein malnutrition may be associated with severe total body deficiencies in potassium. In women with severe muscle wasting, the total exchangeable body potassium content may be as low as 20 to 25 mEq/kg.

Almost 98 percent of the total body potassium is within cells where the concentration is 110 to 150 mEq/L. In contrast, the concentration of potassium in the ECF is normally only 3.5 to 5.0 mEq/L. This large $K^+$ gradient across cell membranes is critical for normal neuromuscular function.

The normal total daily potassium intake is about 50 to 150 mEq. Meat contains about 1 mEq of potassium for each gram of protein. Some of the fruits and vegetables with a high potassium content include oranges, grapefruit, tomatoes, bananas, avocados, and raisins. Of the average 100 mEq of potassium ingested daily, 5 to 10 mEq is lost in the feces and a similar amount in sweat, leaving 80 to 90 percent to be excreted by the kidneys.

# Hypokalemia

## Etiology

The most frequent causes of hypokalemia are intracellular shifts and increased losses, especially in urine (Table 21-11).

### Intracellular Shifts

#### *Increased Bicarbonate*

Potassium tends to move inside cells and hydrogen ions tend to move out whenever the pH of the ECF rises, especially if the rise in pH is due to increased bicarbonate levels. A rise in the pH of 0.10 due to increased plasma bicarbonate levels generally causes a 0.5 (0.3 to 0.8) mEq/L fall in serum potassium levels. Thus, if a patient with a serum potassium level of 4.2 mEq/L and a pH of 7.40 is given bicarbonate and the pH is raised to 7.60, the serum potassium level will tend to fall to about 3.2 mEq/L. Interestingly, immediately after an elevation in the $P_{CO_2}$, plasma potassium levels rise transiently, but then return to baseline values fairly rapidly.

#### *Loss of Gastric Acid*

Hypokalemia seen with excessive vomiting is due primarily to the metabolic alkalosis which develops and not loss of the potassium present in the vomitus, even though the potassium content of highly acid gastric juice may exceed 10 mEq/L. The alkalosis in turn causes a shift of potassium ions into cells in exchange for hydrogen ions. The mild hypovolemia which also can develop with excess loss of gastric juice stimulates an increased secretion of aldosterone, which further contributes to the potassium loss and increased absorption of sodium and bicarbonate. Hypercalcemia can also cause increased potassium loss in the urine.

During the treatment of severe diabetic ketoacidosis, as insulin begins to become effective, potassium follows glucose into the cells, and a very dangerous hypokalemia may develop rapidly unless potassium is given as soon as glucose levels begin to fall. Although the glucose movement into cells brings potassium in with it, insulin also directly increases the cellular uptake of potassium. Furthermore, as the pH rises toward normal and urine volumes increase, serum potassium levels can fall even further because of increasing shift into the cells and loss in the urine. If potassium is not given as the hyperglycemia of diabetic ketoacidosis is corrected, severe hypokalemia may develop rapidly, causing dangerous arrhythmias.

### Diuresis

Although normal kidneys conserve sodium well, potassium is much more difficult to preserve. Indeed, potassium losses in urine are almost "obligatory" and are usually directly proportional to the volume of urine. Urine potassium normally averages about 40 to 80 mEq/L.

**Table 21-11.** Causes of Hypokalemia

I. Shift into the cell
   A. Raising the pH of blood
   B. Administration of insulin and glucose
II. Reduced intake
III. Increased loss
   A. Renal loss
      1. Primary hyperaldosteronism
      2. Secondary hyperaldosteronism associated with diuretics, malignant hypertension, Bartter syndrome, renal artery stenosis
      3. Miscellaneous
         a. Hypercalcemia
         b. Liddle syndrome
         c. Magnesium deficiency
         d. Renal tubular acidosis
         e. Acute myelocytic and monocytic leukemias
   B. Gastrointestinal loss (vomiting, diarrhea, fistulas)

Even with severe acute potassium deficits, urine potassium losses will often exceed 30 mEq/L for at least several days.

Use of loop diuretics, such as furosemide (Lasix), may cause urine potassium losses to exceed 100 mEq/L. Indeed, loop diuretics are the most common cause of severe hypokalemia. Renal losses of potassium are also increased by alkalosis, hypochloremia, and hypomagnesemia. Renal tubular acidosis (type I) causes hypokalemia due to impaired hydrogen ion excretion in the distal tubule.

### Hyperaldosteronism

Adrenal mineralocorticoids, especially aldosterone, cause the kidneys to excrete potassium and chloride and retain sodium and bicarbonate. This can cause a significant hypokalemic metabolic alkalosis. The combination of hypertension and hypokalemic metabolic alkalosis can be an important clue to hyperaldosteronism. Chronic or excessive ingestion of licorice can cause hypokalemia by a similar effect.

Bartter syndrome, occurring mostly in children, is characterized by hypokalemic metabolic alkalosis, juxtaglomerular hyperplasia, hyperreninemia and hyperaldosteronism, kaliuresis, and sodium and bicarbonate retention, without hypertension or edema. Liddle syndrome is a familial type of pseudohyperaldosteronism. The electrolyte changes are characteristic of hyperaldosteronism, but aldosterone levels are normal.

The normal colon conserves about 500 mL of water a day along with significant quantities of sodium, chloride, and bicarbonate (Table 21-12). Because of the high concentrations of potassium (up to 90 mEq/L) and bicarbonate (30 to 74 mEq/L) in stool, severe diarrhea can result in the loss of large quantities of these substances, producing a hypokalemic metabolic acidosis. Correction of only the metabolic acidosis will tend to cause an even worse hypokalemia. One should anticipate potassium deficits in patients with severe diarrhea and either prevent them or institute rapid correction.

### Epinephrine Infusions

Another interesting cause of hypokalemia is infusions of epinephrine, which can cause serum potassium levels to fall by more than 0.5 mEq/L. This may be an important cause of arrhythmias in some patients with acute myocardial infarction. It is now known that $\beta_2$-adrenergic receptors are involved in the regulation of extrarenal potassium disposal. The generation of cyclic AMP activates $Na^+$, $K^+$-ATPase, which augments intracellular-extracellular exchange of $K^+$ for $Na^+$. This increases intracellular potassium levels, hyperpolarizing the cell membrane. Theophylline potentiates this tendency of epinephrine to increase potassium influx into cells.

## Physiologic Effects

Severe hypokalemia with levels below 2.0 to 2.5 mEq/L may cause muscle weakness and increase the tendency to intestinal ileus. Indeed, respiratory paralysis has been seen with levels below 1.5 to 2.0 mEq/L.

It must be remembered that severe hypokalemia can cause nephrogenic DI and severe dehydration, which must be considered when

**Table 21-12.** Daily Water and Electrolytes Delivered to and from the Normal Colon

| Fluid or Electrolyte | Delivered to Colon | | Delivered to Stool | |
| | Amount | Concentration, mEq/L | Amount | Concentration mEq/L |
|---|---|---|---|---|
| Water | 600 mL | | 100 mL | |
| Sodium | 76 mEq | 125 | 4 mEq | 40 |
| Potassium | 5 mEq | 9 | 6 mEq | 60 |
| Chloride | 36 mEq | 60 | 2 mEq | 15 |
| Bicarbonate | 44 mEq | 74 | 3 mEq | 30 |

correcting the electrolyte abnormalities. Hypokalemia tends to cause a metabolic alkalemia with increased acid excretion in the urine (paradoxical aciduria). It also increases the tendency to glycosuria.

The sensitivity of the heart to digitalis and the likelihood of digitalis toxicity with arrhythmias or an AV block is increased in the presence of hypokalemia. In patients treated with hydrochlorothiazide, there is a direct relationship between the severity of the hypokalemia, concomitant hypomagnesemia, and the incidence of ventricular ectopy. Administration of both potassium and magnesium are important parts of the treatment of arrhythmias due to digitalis toxicity.

Hypokalemia increases renal tubular production of ammonia, and this may aggravate hepatic encephalopathy in patients with advanced cirrhosis.

## Diagnosis

The diagnosis of hypokalemia is made primarily on serum electrolyte studies. However, serum potassium levels should be interpreted relative to the arterial pH. A low serum potassium level may be expected in an alkalotic patient, but hypokalemia in an acidotic patient is either a laboratory error or evidence of a severe potassium deficit. In some instances, a patient with normal blood levels can seem to be hypokalemic, particularly after cardiopulmonary bypass and with metabolic alkalosis. In patients with metabolic alkalosis, paradoxical aciduria suggests a functional hypokalemia.

On ECG, hypokalemia less than 3.0 mEq/L may cause low-voltage QRS complexes, flattened T waves, depressed ST segments, prominent P and U waves, and prolonged QT and PR intervals. A U wave (between the T and P waves) can be seen in many normal individuals in the early precordial leads ($V_1$ to $V_3$), but it is somewhat more prominent with diastolic hypertension and coronary artery disease. The U wave may become especially prominent as potassium levels fall below 2.5 mEq/L. Potassium levels below 2.0 mEq/L also tend to widen the QRS complex.

Urine potassium levels can give some indication of the duration of hypokalemia and the severity of the total body deficit. Normal urine potassium levels (40 to 80 mEq/L) suggest that the potassium deficit is acute. However, if the hypokalemia is due to metabolic alkalosis from primary aldosteronism, urine potassium levels may be high despite severe chronic hypokalemia.

One should not attempt to correct hypokalemia rapidly if the urinary potassium is very low. Urine potassium levels less than 10 mEq/L suggest a chronic and severe potassium deficit that is not apt to respond well to attempts at rapid correction.

## Treatment

Acute severe hypokalemia is treated by infusing 10 to 15 mEq of KCl per hour in 50 to 100 mL of 5% dextrose in water ($D_5W$) or 0.9 $N$ saline by IV piggyback for 3 to 4 h. The ECG should be continuously monitored during potassium infusions. As a general rule, no more than 40 mEq of potassium should ever be put in a single liter of IV fluid (except by careful IV piggyback) and no more than 40 mEq should be given per hour.

Potassium equilibrates in the TBW, and it generally takes at least 40 to 50 mEq to raise the serum potassium level by 1.0 mEq/L. Chronic deficits usually require much larger amounts of potassium to maintain any increase in serum levels, and not infrequently, much of the infused potassium is promptly excreted in the urine.

Chronic hypokalemia may be associated with very severe potassium deficits, which often exceed 300 to 500 mEq. One way to estimate total body potassium deficits is from pH-corrected plasma potassium levels. The percentage by which serum levels (corrected for pH) are below 4.2 mEq/L is twice as large as the percentage of total body potassium deficit. Thus, a serum potassium level of 2.1

mEq/L at a pH of 7.4 indicates a 50 percent reduction in serum potassium and a 25 percent deficit in total body potassium. Total body potassium ranges between 20 mEq/kg in a markedly wasted woman to 45 mEq/kg in a normal muscular man. Thus, a serum potassium of 2.5 mEq/L at an arterial pH of 7.40 in a 50-kg woman with muscle wasting indicates a 40 percent pH-corrected potassium deficit in the plasma and a 20 percent deficit in total body potassium. The calculated total body potassium deficit would then be (20 percent)(50 kg)(20 mEq/kg) = 200 mEq.

## Hyperkalemia

### Etiology

There are many causes of hyperkalemia. It is easy to hemolyze blood as it is being drawn, producing a pseudohyperkalemia. Other causes of pseudohyperkalemia include leukocytosis, especially greater than 600,000/mm$^3$, and thrombocytosis, especially greater than 10$^6$/mm$^3$. These are particularly apt to cause hyperkalemia if the blood is not analyzed within 30 min of being drawn. Excessive opening and clenching of the fist while the tourniquet is on can raise potassium levels in veins below the tourniquet by 10 to 20 percent after several minutes. The more common causes of hyperkalemia are listed in Table 21-13.

Renal failure with oliguria is the most common cause of dangerous hyperkalemiable. Normally, 90 to 95 percent of the potassium taken in is excreted in the urine. Thus, anuria can cause a severe progressive rise in serum potassium levels.

Since each kilogram of lean muscle tissue may contain over 100 mEq of potassium, breakdown of muscle from trauma or sepsis may release large quantities of potassium into the bloodstream. Occasionally, succinylcholine can raise serum potassium levels abruptly in patients with severe crush injuries or burns. A similar problem may develop with hemolysis due to transfusion reactions.

Excessive intake of potassium is an infrequent cause of hyperkalemia but can occur with IV administration of potassium-containing drugs. Aqueous (potassium) penicillin, for example, contains about 1.7 mEq of potassium per 1 million units.

**Table 21-13.** Common Causes of Hyperkalemia

Factitious
  Laboratory error
  Pseudohyperkalemia: hemolysis, thrombocytosis, leukocytosis
Metabolic acidemia (acute)
Increased intake into the plasma
  Exogenous: diet, salt substitutes, low-sodium diet, medications
  Endogenous: hemolysis, GI bleeding, catabolic states, crush injury
Inadequate distal delivery of sodium and decreased distal tubular flow
Oliguric renal failure
Impaired renin-aldosterone axis
  Addison disease
  Primary hypoaldosteronism
  Other (heparin, β blockers, prostaglandin inhibitors, captopril)
Primary renal tubular potassium secretory defect
  Sickle cell disease
  Systemic lupus erythematosus
  Postrenal transplantation
  Obstructive uropathy
Inhibition of renal tubular secretion of potassium
  Spironolactone
  Digitalis
Abnormal potassium distribution
  Insulin deficiency
  Hypertonicity (hyperglycemia)
  Beta-adrenergic blockers
  Exercise
  Succinylcholine
  Digitalis

## Physiologic Effects

As potassium levels rise above 6.0 mEq/L, cardiac conductivity and contractility may be impaired. With severe hyperkalemia, above 6.5 to 7.0 mEq/L, an intracardiac block can be produced, first in the atria, then in the AV node, and finally in the ventricles, with the heart eventually stopping in diastole. Occasionally, hyperkalemia may cause such weakness that ventilatory failure may develop. The effects of hyperkalemia are increased if the patient has hyponatremia and hypocalcemia.

## Diagnosis

One should suspect hyperkalemia in patients with oliguric renal failure, severe hemolysis, or excessive tissue breakdown. The potassium levels must also be correlated with the arterial pH. It is a bit unusual for a moderate to severe hyperkalemia to exist without acidosis.

Mild hyperkalemia brings the membrane potential closer to threshold, and conduction in the heart is initially improved. As the serum $K^+$ level rises above 5.6 to 6.0 mEq/L, the first ECG sign of hyperkalemia is usually the development of tall, peaked T waves, best seen in the precordial leads, as a result of speeded repolarization. With further increases in serum potassium levels to 6.0 to 6.5 mEq/L, impulse conduction decreases, often resulting in prolonged PR and QT intervals. At levels above 6.5 to 7.0 mEq/L, diminished P waves and depressed ST segments can occur. This finding is not specific for hyperkalemia, however, and may also be seen with massive cerebrovascular accidents and myocardial ischemia. Although ST segments are usually depressed with moderate to severe hyperkalemia, occasionally elevation resembling acute myocardial ischemia may be seen.

At serum potassium levels of 7.0 mEq/L or greater, impulses may still be conducted from the SA node to the ventricle because the intraatrial conduction fibers are less sensitive to hyperkalemia than are atrial muscle fibers. Since conduction may be delayed in the AV node, such conduction could result in an idioventricular rhythm. Delayed conduction in the interventricular conducting system can produce patterns resembling bundle branch block.

As they exceed 7.5 to 8.0 mEq/L, P waves disappear, the QRS complex widens, the S and T waves tend to merge, and the ventricular rhythm becomes irregular. At levels exceeding 10 to 12 mEq/L, a classic sine wave is usually seen.

Death from hyperkalemia is usually the result of a diastolic arrest caused by block of the distal Purkinje fibers or of ventricular fibrillation caused by reentrant circuits that develop because of prolonged ventricular conduction.

## Treatment

If serum potassium levels rise above 5.0 to 5.5 mEq/L, one must begin to look for oliguric renal failure or increased red blood cell or other tissue breakdown. Whenever possible, all potassium-containing solutions and drugs should be discontinued. Diuresis is extremely helpful. Even when renal function is severely impaired, each liter of urine usually contains at least 30 to 40 mEq of potassium per liter.

If serum potassium levels rise above 5.5 to 6.0 mEq/L and diuresis is not possible or if there is extensive tissue damage, one should consider using an ion-exchange resin. Kayexalate (sodium polystyrene sulfonate) is an ion-exchange resin that may be administered by mouth or by retention enemas. Each gram of sodium resin exchanges with and eliminates about 1.0 mEq of potassium. When given orally, 15 to 25 g of Kayexalate is given with 50 mL of a 20% sorbitol solution every 4 to 6 h. Kayexalate tends to be constipating, and the sorbitol increases the speed of evacuation of bowel contents. Rectal administration is 20 g of Kayexalate in 200 mL of a 20% sorbitol solution every 4 h. The enema should be retained at least 30 min.

In patients with fluid overload or impaired cardiac function, the absorption of sodium from Kayexalate may precipitate acute heart failure. If serum potassium levels are less than 6.5 mEq/L and there is

no ECG changes due to the hyperkalemia, treatment efforts may be slower. If serum potassium levels rise above 6.5 mEq/L, one should consider giving glucose and insulin and possibly also sodium bicarbonate. As glucose enters cells, it "pulls" potassium, magnesium, and phosphorus in with it. After an initial 50 mL of 50% IV glucose with 5 to 10 units of regular insulin, a liter of 20% glucose with 40 to 80 units of insulin may be given over the next 2 to 4 h.

Sodium bicarbonate causes an alkalosis that tends to reduce serum potassium levels. It also increases the serum concentration of sodium, which also helps oppose the potassium effects. Each ampule (50 mL of a 7.5% solution) should be given relatively slowly by continuous IV infusion over at least 10 to 20 min, depending on the urgency of the situation.

Calcium gluconate or calcium chloride is usually only given for severe hyperkalemia with levels > 7.0 to 7.5 mEq/L. Ten mL of 10% calcium gluconate contains 4.6 mEq of calcium, while a similar ampule of $CaCl_2$ contains 13.4 mEq of calcium. The calcium is also more rapidly available from the chloride than from the gluconate. One ampule is given by slow IV infusion over at least 10 to 20 min. Additional calcium is given much more slowly as needed.

If calcium has to be given to patients on digitalis, it must be done with great caution, since hypercalcemia potentiates the toxic effects of digitalis on the heart. Therefore, if calcium must be given on an emergency basis to patients taking digitalis, an ampule should be added to 100 mL of $D_5W$ and infused slowly over at least 20 to 30 min to permit a more even distribution throughout the extracellular space.

If a dangerous tachyarrhythmia develops in a hyperkalemic patient, all of the above steps may have to be done together and rapidly. Such emergency treatment must proceed rapidly according to a predetermined program (Table 21-14). If a patient is in acute oliguric renal failure, hemodialysis and/or peritoneal dialysis should be set up while the above measures are being used.

## CALCIUM

Calcium is the most abundant mineral in the human body. The total body calcium content is 15 to 20 g/kg body weight or about 1.0 to 1.5 kg in an adult of normal size. About 99 percent is in bone as the mineral apatite. The average daily calcium intake, about 800 to 1000 mg, is primarily from milk and milk products. About a third of this calcium is absorbed, primarily in the small bowel, by both active (vitamin D–dependent) and passive (concentration-dependent) absorption. Loss of calcium into the GI tract (150 to 200 mg/day) and urine (150 mg/day) usually balances the GI absorption quite closely.

### Control of Calcium Levels

Calcium homeostasis is under the control of parathyroid hormone (PTH), calcitonin, and vitamin D metabolites, especially calcitriol (1α,25-dihydroxyvitamin $D_3$).

### Parathormone

Parathormone (PTH) is secreted by the parathyroid gland, primarily in response to low ionized calcium or magnesium levels. Parathormone raises serum calcium levels primarily by stimulating osteoclasts to increase bone resorption. It has less activity in the intestine, where it works in combination with calcitriol. It also has an indirect action in the kidney through adenyl cyclase stimulation, whereby it increases calcium resorption and increases phosphorous excretion. PTH also stimulates conversion of 25-hydroxyvitamin D to the much more metabolically active 1α,25-dehydroxyvitamin $D_3$.

### Calcitonin

Calcitonin is influenced by elevations in serum calcium, epinephrine, glucagon, and gastrin. It decreases the release of calcium from bone

**Table 21-14.** Emergency Therapy of Hyperkalemia

| Therapy | Mechanism | Dose | Onset of Action | Duration of Hypokalemic Effect |
|---|---|---|---|---|
| Ca gluconate (10%) | Antagonism | 10–20 mL IV | 1–3 min | 30–50 min |
| Na bicarbonate | Antagonism and redistribution | 50–100 mEq IV | 5–10 min | 1–2 h |
| Insulin plus glucose | Redistribution | 20 U regular insulin with 50 g glucose IV over 1 h | 30 min | 4–6 h |
| Diuretics Furosemide Ethacrynic acid | Excretion | 40 mg IV 50 mg IV | With diuresis | With diuresis |
| Cation-exchange resin (Kayexalate) | Excretion | 15–50 g PO or rectally with sorbitol | 1–2 h | 4–6 h |
| Peritoneal dialysis or hemodialysis | Excretion | | Within minutes | During dialysis |

by inhibiting the activity of the osteoclasts. It also has a limited role in increasing calcium loss through the kidney.

## Vitamin D

Vitamin D can be produced nonenzymatically by ultraviolet irradiation of skin or it can be absorbed directly from the GI tract, particularly from fortified milk products. Since it is a fat-soluble vitamin, its absorption requires bile salts and micelle formation. Vitamin D is hydroxylated in the liver to 25-hydroxycholecalciferol [25-(OH)-vitamin D] and in the kidney it is further hydroxylated to either $1\alpha,25\text{-(OH)}_2$-vitamin D or $24,25\text{-(OH)}_2$-vitamin D. The synthesis of $1\alpha,25\text{-(OH)}_2$-vitamin D, which is much more potent metabolically, increases with hypocalcemia or hypophosphatemia. During hypercalcemia there is a reversal of the above sequence so that more $24,25\text{-(OH)}_2$-vitamin D, which is much less active, is formed.

## Functions

Calcium is vital to a wide variety of bodily functions, including neutrophil chemotaxis, lymphocyte activation, and membrane stability of a wide variety of cells. It is a required factor in the clotting cascade for activation or conversion of factors IX, VII, VIII, prothrombin, and fibrinogen, and it is necessary for platelet aggregation and granule release. However, very small amounts of calcium, probably less than 0.3 to 0.4 mEq/L, are needed for clotting. Calcium is also essential for the release of neurotransmitters in the central and peripheral nervous systems, and it plays a critical role in muscle depolarization.

Calcium ion influx into the depolarized myocardial cell prolongs depolarization. This is represented by the plateau or phase 2 portion of the cardiac action potential. Stimulation of skeletal muscle causes calcium ion to be released from the sarcoplasmic reticulum into the cytoplasm where it binds to and alters troponin. This alteration of troponin allows actin and myosin to interact, causing the muscle to contract.

## Ionized and Protein-Bound Calcium

Total plasma calcium levels average 8.5 to 10.5 mg/dL. The calcium present in the plasma is in three forms: protein-bound calcium (normally 4.0 to 4.5 mg/dL), complexed (non-protein-bound, nonionized) calcium (normally 0.5 to 1.0 mg/dL), and ionized calcium (normally 4.2 to 4.8 mg/dL). Increasingly, calcium levels are being reported in milliequivalents per liter, which is half of the number expressed as milligrams per deciliter. Thus, 4.4 mg/dL of ionized calcium is the same as 2.2 mEq/L or 1.1 mmol/L. The ionized calcium fraction, which normally is 2.1 to 2.4 mEq/L or 1.05 to 1.3 mmol/L, is responsible for virtually all the physiologic effects of calcium, of which the neuromuscular changes are most obvious.

On an average, each gram of protein binds 0.8 mg of calcium. Thus, if the ionized calcium is 4.4 mg/dL and the total protein (TP) is 7.0 gm/dL, the total calcium is

$$Ca_{tot} = 4.4 + (0.8)(TP) = 4.4 + (0.8)(7.0)$$
$$= 4.4 + 5.6 = 10.0 \text{ mg/dL}$$

If the albumin (alb) and globulin (glob) concentrations are unusual, one can estimate the normal total calcium (mg/dL) by the following formula:

$$Ca_{tot} = 4.4 + (1.1)(alb) + (0.2)(glob)$$

Thus, if the albumin is 3.0 g/dL and globulin is 4.0 g/dL,

$$Ca_{tot} = 4.4 + (1.1)(3.0) + (0.2)(4.0)$$
$$= 4.4 + 3.3 + 0.8 = 8.5 \text{ mg/dL}$$

Because the relationships between total calcium, ionized calcium, and the plasma proteins vary so much, these formulas provide only a gross estimation of the relationship between ionized calcium and total calcium.

## Hypocalcemia

Hypocalcemia is often defined as an ionized calcium below 2.0 mEq/L or 1.0 mmol/L. Total calcium levels, especially in the presence of hypoalbuminemia, may be very low and yet be associated with normal ionized calcium levels. Some of the more common causes of ionic hypocalcemia are shock, sepsis, renal failure, and pancreatitis (Table 21-15). Hypocalcemia is unusual in ambulatory patients except those with chronic hypoparathyroidism following surgery or in chronic renal disease.

**Table 21-15.** Causes of Hypocalcemia

Shock or sepsis
Impaired production of $1\alpha,25$-dihydroxyvitamin $D_3$
　Malabsorption
　Severe hepatic failure
　Renal failure
　Anticonvulsant therapy
Pancreatitis
Hypomagnesemia
Alkalosis
Decreased serum albumin levels
Hypoparathyroidism
　Idiopathic
　Postsurgical
　Pseudohypoparathyroidism
Osteoblastic metastases
Fat embolism syndrome

## Etiology

### Movement into "Sick" Cells

The concentration of ionized calcium in the ECF is about 1.0 mmol/L or $10^{-3}$ $M$. The concentration of ionized calcium in the cytoplasm of most cells is about $10^{-7}$ $M$. This gradient of $10^4$, or 10,000, to 1 is maintained by active metabolic processes. Any process that interferes with cell metabolism, such as shock or sepsis, will tend to reduce ionized calcium levels by allowing increased net movement of calcium across the cell membrane into the cytoplasm of the poorly functioning cells. Following trauma, serum calcium levels may be low, especially with the fat embolism syndrome, not only because of cell dysfunction and binding of calcium to free fatty acids, but also because of fatty acid inhibition of cell membrane calcium pumps.

### Pancreatitis

Acute pancreatitis is an important cause of hypocalcemia. Pancreatic lipase breaks down fat into fatty acids and glycerol. The fatty acids combine with calcium to form insoluble calcium soaps and reduce serum calcium levels. The combination of necrotic fat cells plus calcium soaps makes up much of what is recognized as the fat necrosis of pancreatitis. In addition, as protein moves into the inflammatory exudate, the resultant hypoproteinemia may cause total calcium levels to fall. Pancreatitis can also reduce PTH secretion and the response of tissues to it. If total calcium levels fall below 7.0 or 8.0 mg/dL, there is an increased chance of severe complications from pancreatitis.

### Drugs

A large number of drugs can cause hypocalcemia (Table 21-16). One of the most frequently used of these is cimetidine. This histamine receptor–blocking agent apparently lowers serum calcium levels by decreasing the synthesis or secretion of parathyroid hormone.

### Postoperative Hypocalcemia

#### Hypoparathyroidism

Currently, more than 10 percent of postparathyroidectomy patients may have hypoparathyroidism as defined by a fasting calcium of less than 8.5 mg/dL and a simultaneous inorganic phosphorus of greater than 4.5 mg/dL. Postoperative hypocalcemia can be due to hypoparathyrodism from the permanent surgical removal of parathyroid tissue, from transient ischemia of the parathyroid glands in patients who have extensive bilateral neck surgery, or because of long-term hypercalcemic suppression of the nonadenomatous parathyroid glands.

#### Hungry-Bone Syndrome

The term *hungry-bone syndrome* was coined by Albright and now indicates postparathyroidectomy hypocalcemia due to rapid remineral-

**Table 21-16.** Drugs That Can Cause Hypocalcemia

Cimetidine
Phosphates (e.g., enemas, laxatives)
Dilantin, phenobarbital
Gentamicin, tobramycin
Cisplatin
Heparin
Theophylline
Protamine
Glucagon
Norepinephrine
Citrate (blood)
Loop diuretics
Glucocorticoids
Magnesium sulfate
Sodium nitroprusside

ization of the skeleton. During this accelerated remineralization, a persistent hypocalcemia and hypophosphatemia may be severe enough to cause tetany. These patients may require vigorous calcium and vitamin D supplementation for prolonged periods of time.

In a one study, the hungry-bone syndrome was found in 13 percent of patients after parathyroid surgery. Patients were felt to have this problem if they had a fasting calcium level less than 8.5 mg/dL and a simultaneous inorganic serum phosphorus of less than 3.0 mg/dL on postoperative day 3 or later.

### Renal Failure

Hypocalcemia is a frequent finding in renal failure. This may be partially due to the resulting hyperphosphatemia, but there is also decreased production of $1\alpha,25$-$(OH)_2$-vitamin D in the kidney, which, in turn, causes decreased intestinal absorption of calcium. Secondary hyperparathyroidism with increased PTH levels often results from the chronic hypocalcemia. If PTH levels remain elevated and hypercalcemia develops in spite of cure of the renal failure by renal transplantation, the patient is said to have tertiary hyperparathyroidism.

### Phosphate Overload

Phosphate overload from nonrenal causes may also lead to hypocalcemia. This is the presumed mechanism in the acute rhabdomyolysis of hyperpyrexia and major trauma. Excessive use of phosphate cathartics and sodium phosphate enemas can cause significant hyperphosphatemia in patients with renal disease, in children with Hirsch sprung disease, and in small infants.

### Hypomagnesemia

Hypomagnesemia use of or in association with hypocalcemia may be seen in alcoholism, diuretic use, epilepsy, and renal failure. Neonatal hypomagnesemia leads to low PTH secretion, decreased responsiveness of bone cells to PTH, and decreased calcium mobilization from bone.

### Idiopathic Hypoparathyroidism

Idiopathic hypoparathyroidism is probably an autoimmune disorder in which pernicious anemia, exostoses, moniliasis, Hashimoto disease, sterility, and Addison disease may be seen. This syndrome may also be associated with cataracts, mental retardation, intracranial calcifications, and papilledema due to increased intracranial pressure.

### Nonsurgical Primary Hypoparathyroidism

Hypocalcemia with primary hypoparathyroidism has been reported from parathyroid infarction, metastases to the parathyroids, and hemochromatosis of the parathyroids.

### Pseudohypoparathyroidism

Pseudohypoparathyroidism is a familial disorder characterized by decreased end-organ responsiveness to PTH resulting in hypocalcemia, hyperphosphatemia, parathyroid hyperplasia, and excessive serum PTH concentrations. These patients usually have a very low urinary cyclic AMP excretion that only slightly increases with infusion of parathormone. This condition may be inherited as an X-linked dominant trait with variable penetrance; the male to female ratio is 2 to 1. Patients are short in stature and have round facies; brachycephaly; a short, thick neck; short, pudgy fingers and toes; and growth failure of the fourth and fifth metacarpals. Mental retardation, seizures, and subcutaneous soft tissue calcification may be seen. The skin can be dry and coarse, and the hair is often brittle.

### Vitamin D Deficiency

Hypocalcemia due to vitamin D deficiency is rare in the United States. Infants born to vitamin D–deficient mothers who lack sunlight exposure and receive no vitamin D supplementation may have rickets. Breast milk has low vitamin D content, and breast milk feeding without sunshine exposure in unsupplemented infants may result in infantile rickets.

## Physiologic Effects

Although normal ionized calcium levels are 2.1 to 2.6 mEq/L (1.05 to 1.3 mmol/L), serious physiologic changes do not usually occur until ionized levels in serum are less than 1.4 to 1.6 mEq/L (0.7 to 0.8 mmol/L). Below those levels, hypocalcemia can cause a wide variety of signs and symptoms (Table 21-17).

The severity of signs and symptoms depends greatly on the rapidity of the fall in calcium. The more acute the drop in the serum calcium, the more likely are significant pathophysiologic changes. As serum calcium levels fall, neuronal membranes become increasingly more permeable to sodium, enhancing excitation. Potassium and magnesium have an antagonizing effect on this excitation.

Decreased ionized calcium levels reduce the strength of myocardial contraction primarily by inhibiting relaxation. They also decrease the sensitivity of the heart to digitalis. Hypocalcemia should be considered in patients with refractory heart failure.

Low ionized calcium levels increase PTH secretion, which mobilizes calcium from bone and decreases renal tubular absorption of phosphate and bicarbonate. This, in turn, may cause an increased absorption of chloride, producing a tendency to hyperchloremic hypophosphatemic renal tubular acidosis. A ratio of chloride to phosphate greater than 35 to 1 in mEq/mg in the plasma is sometimes considered to be highly suggestive of hyperparathyroidism.

Increased cytoplasmic calcium activates phospholipase, which increases prostaglandin production and alters cell lipids. Increased cytoplasmic calcium also interferes with cell metabolism. Efforts by mitochondria to pump the excess calcium from the cytoplasm into the mitochondrial matrix greatly reduce adenosine triphosphate (ATP) formation. Consequently, giving calcium during shock or sepsis may transiently improve hemodynamics, but if cell metabolism does not also improve, some of the additional calcium moves into the cytoplasm within 30 to 40 min and further impairs cell metabolism.

Movement of calcium into ischemic cerebrovascular smooth muscle cells may cause persistent cerebral vasoconstriction with resultant failure of cerebral reperfusion after strokes or cardiac arrest. This may be a major cause of the poor results in management of these problems. Consequently, there has been some interest in the use of calcium blockers for cerebral resuscitation.

## Diagnosis

### Symptoms

The most characteristic initial symptom of hypocalcemia following thyroid or parathyroid surgery is parasthesias around the mouth or in the fingertips. Hypocalcemia should be suspected in any patient who is irritable and has hyperactive deep tendon reflexes following neck surgery. It should also be suspected in patients who have seizures, particularly if they have ever had thyroid surgery, even if many years previously.

### Signs

A positive Chvostek or Trousseau sign is generally considered to be good clinical evidence of hypocalcemia. A positive Chvostek sign is a twitch at the corner of the mouth when the examiner taps over the facial nerve just in front of the ear. However, it is present in about 10 to 30 percent of normal individuals. Nevertheless, eyelid muscle contraction with the Chvostek maneuver is said to be almost diagnostic of hypocalcemia.

Trousseau sign, which is generally a more reliable indicator of hypocalcemia, is positive if carpal spasm is produced when the examiner applies a blood pressure cuff to the upper arm and maintains a pressure above systolic for 3 min. The fingers are spastically extended at the interphalangeal joints and flexed at the metacarophalangeal joints. The wrist is flexed and the forearm is pronated.

### Laboratory Findings

Signs of hypocalcemia may be found with normal total serum calcium levels if the patient is very alkalotic. Each 0.1 rise in pH lowers ionized calcium levels by about 3 to 8 percent. Consequently, a very alkalotic patient may have normal total serum calcium levels with ionic hypocalcemia. Similar signs and symptoms may be caused by hypomagnesemia, strychnine, or tetanus toxin.

Decreased plasma levels of ionized calcium are diagnostic, but one should also suspect ionic hypocalcemia if the patient has decreased levels of total calcium in the presence of normal plasma proteins. Primary hypoparathyroidism is characterized by a low serum PTH concentration, hyperphosphatemia, and hypocalcemia.

### ECG

The most characteristic ECG finding in hypocalcemia is prolonged QT intervals. However, the T wave is of normal width, and it is the ST segment which is really prolonged. This finding is usually seen with total serum calcium levels less than 6.0 mg/dL.

### X-Rays

Radiologically, rickets is characterized by craniotabes, frontal skull bossing, rachitic rosary ribs, widened rib cage (Harrison groove), bowed legs, and, often, fractures. Other radiographic changes include cupping and splaying of the metaphyseal ends of long bones, widening between the metaphyses and epiphysis, bone demineralization, and thinning of cortical bone.

## Treatment

Treatment of hypocalcemia is tailored to the individual and directed toward the underlying cause. If the patient is asymptomatic, oral calcium therapy with or without vitamin D may be all that is required. Calcium lactate, calcium glubionate, calcium ascorbate, calcium carbonate, and calcium gluconate are available in oral preparations. Milk, because of the large amount of phosphate present, is not really a very good source of calcium, except in normal growing children who also need the phosphate.

Symptomatic patients following thyroid or parathyroid surgery are often treated with parenteral calcium (Table 21-18). With severe acute hypocalcemia, 10 mL of 10% $CaCl_2$ or calcium gluconate may be given IV over 10 to 20 min followed by a continuous IV drip providing 1 g of $CaCl_2$ over a period of 6 to 12 h. If the patient is not asymptomatic or if the hypocalcemia is not severe and prolonged for more than 10 to 14 days, treatment with calcium may not be required. One should not administer calcium rapidly IV to asymptomatic patients with mild to moderate hypocalcemia because it can cause severe unnecessary cardiovascular, neuromuscular, and renal complica-

**Table 21-17.** Symptoms and Signs of Hypocalcemia

| | |
|---|---|
| General | Muscular |
|   Weakness, fatigue |   Spasms, cramps |
| Neurologic |   Weakness |
|   Tetany | Skeletal |
|   Chvostek sign, Trousseau sign |   Osteodystrophy |
|   Circumoral and digital paresthesias |   Rickets |
|   Impaired memory, confusion |   Osteomalacia |
|   Hallucinations, dementia, seizures | Miscellaneous |
|   Extrapyramidal disorders |   Dental hypoplasia |
| Dermatologic |   Cataracts |
|   Hyperpigmentation |   Decreased insulin secretion |
|   Coarse, brittle hair | |
|   Dry, scaly skin | |
| Cardiovascular | |
|   Heart failure | |
|   Vasoconstriction | |

**Table 21-18.** Treatment of Hypocalcemia

| Delivery | Supplied | Elemental Ca$^{2+}$ | Adult Dose |
|---|---|---|---|
| PARENTERAL | | | |
| Ca$^{2+}$ gluconate (10%) | 10-mL ampules | 93 mg Ca$^{2+}$ (4.6 mEq) | 10–30mL in 100 mL D$_5$W over 10–15 min |
| Ca$^{2+}$ chloride (10%) | 10-mL ampules | 272 mg Ca$^{2+}$ (13.6 mEq) | 2.5–10 mL in 100 mL D$_5$W over 10–15 min |
| ORAL | | | |
| Ca$^{2+}$ gluconate tablets | 1000 mg (also 325-, 500-, and 600-mg tablets) | 92 mg Ca$^{2+}$ (4.5 mEq) | 1–4 g/day in divided doses q6h |
| Ca$^{2+}$ glubionate (Neo-calglucon) | 5 mL syrup | 23 mg Ca$^{2+}$/mL | 1–4 g/day in divided doses q6h |
| Ca$^{2+}$ lactate tablets | 650 mg | 79 mg Ca$^{2+}$ | 1–4 g/d in divided doses q6h |
| Ca$^{2+}$ carbonate | | | |
| Titralac | 5-mL solution, or 650-mg tablet | 170, 400 mg Ca$^{2+}$ | 1–4 g/d in divided doses q6h |
| Os-Cal | Tablet | 500 mg Ca$^{2+}$ | |

tions. For chronic hypoparathyroidism, use of oral calcium salts and rather high doses of vitamin D may be required.

During massive transfusions, if the blood is being given faster than 1 unit every 5 min, 10 mL of 10% calcium chloride can be given after every 4 to 6 units of blood if the patient is in shock or heart failure in spite of adequate volume replacement therapy. Calcium is seldom required during transfusions for elective surgery.

Although, in the past, the use of calcium was advocated for the resuscitation of patients with asystole or electromechanical dissociation, it has now been shown that the chances of successful resuscitation are reduced by using calcium. On the other hand, patients with bradyasystolic arrest and chronic renal failure are apt to have hyperkalemia and hypocalcemia and may benefit from calcium administration.

For the prevention of rickets, 400 IU of vitamin D is the recommended daily allowance. Treatment of established rickets may involve a daily dose of vitamin D as high as 5000 to 10,000 IU until the electrolyte and bone changes are corrected.

## Hypercalcemia

### Etiology

Hypercalcemia may be defined as a total calcium level exceeding 10.5 mg/dL or an ionized calcium level exceeding 2.7 mEq/L. This abnormality has been found in 0.3 to 5.0 percent of patients studied in various biomedical profiles. A mnemonic used to remember some of the more common causes of hypercalcemia is "Pam P. Schmidt" for *p*arahormone, *A*ddison disease, *m*ultiple myeloma, *P*aget disease, *sar*coidosis, *c*ancer, *h*yperthyroidism, *m*ilk-alkali syndrome, *i*mmobilization, excess vitamin *D,* and *t*hiazides.

### Malignancies

The most frequent cause of severe hypercalcemia is malignant neoplasms with either extensive metastases or PTH-like activity. Hypercalcemia is quite common in women with carcinoma of the breast being treated with estrogens. Hypercalcemia is also seen with increased frequency in lung cancer (especially of the squamous cell type) and renal carcinomas. Other malignancies associated with hypercalcemia but which are less frequent include multiple myeloma, pheochromocytoma, and some acute leukemias. In general, the higher the serum

**Table 21-19.** Causes of Hypercalcemia

| | |
|---|---|
| Malignancy | Granulomatous disease |
| Lung (squamous cell cancer) | Sarcoid |
| Breast | Tuberculosis |
| Kidney | Histoplasmosis |
| Myeloma | Coccidioidomycosis |
| Leukemia | Immobilization |
| Endocrinopathies | Miscellaneous |
| Primary hyperparathyroidism | Paget disease of bone |
| Hyperthyroidism | Postrenal transplantation |
| Pheochromocytoma | Recovery from acute renal failure |
| Adrenal insufficiency | Phosphate depletion syndrome |
| Acromegaly | |
| Drugs | |
| Hypervitaminosis D and A | |
| Thiazides | |
| Lithium | |
| Hormonal therapy for breast cancer | |

calcium level, especially above 14.0 mg/dL, the more likely the hypercalcemia is to be due to malignancy.

### Primary Hyperparathyroidism

The next most common cause of hypercalcemia is primary hyperparathyroidism, which accounts for 25 to 50 percent of all hypercalcemia (Table 21-19). In ambulatory care settings, primary hyperparathyroidism is the most common cause of hypercalcemia. Primary hyperparathyroidism is caused by a parathyroid adenoma in 80 percent of cases and parathyroid hyperplasia in the remaining 20 percent. With very high calcium levels and no evidence of a malignancy, an enlarged parathyroid gland can sometimes be palpated in the neck. Parathyroid carcinoma is a rare cause of hyperparathyroidism.

### Multiple Endocrine Adenomas

Parathyroid adenomas may be sporadic or familial. The familial type may be part of a multiglandular endocrinopathy, and one should look for associated pancreatic, pituitary, adrenal, and thyroid neoplasms in any patient with primary hyperparathyroidism. The combination of parathyroid, pituitary, and pancreatic islet adenomas is known as multiple endocrine neoplasia type I, or Wermer syndrome. Multiple endocrine neoplasia type IIA (Sipple syndrome) consists of hyperparathyroidism combined with pheochromocytoma and medullary cell carcinoma of the thyroid. In infants, parathyroid hyperplasia may be inherited as a familial autosomal dominant or recessive trait. It is sometimes seen in infants of hypoparathyroid mothers in response to chronic intrauterine hypocalcemia.

### Immobilization

In patients who are immobilized, the parathyroid–vitamin D axis is suppressed, and calcium may leave bone rapidly, producing hypercalcemia, at least temporarily. Urinary excretion of calcium in such patients may exceed 200 to 300 mg/day, and there is an increased tendency to nephrolithiasis. Patients with Paget disease, especially if they are at bed rest because of their pain, may have severe hypercalcemia due to rapid bone turnover. Astronauts, due to their weightlessness, may rapidly lose large amounts of calcium from their bones and develop a severe prolonged negative calcium balance.

### Hyperthyroidism

Although intestinal absorption of calcium is reduced in hyperthyroidism, up to one-third of patients with thyrotoxicosis will concurrently have hypercalcemia, which resolves with treatment of the thyroid disorder. The source of excess calcium is presumed to be bone, but the exact mechanism is not known.

### Addison's Disease

Hypercalcemia has been seen in patients with Addison's disease and adrenal crisis perhaps because of a lack of the hypocalcemic effect of corticosteroids.

### Hypervitaminosis

Hypervitaminosis A and D can cause hypercalcemia. In vitamin A toxicity, the patient will present with arthralgias, alopecia, a desquamating pruritus, and signs and symptoms of hypercalcemia. Vitamins A and D both cause increased osteoclastic resorption of bone, but vitamin D toxicity also causes increased intestinal absorption of calcium. Vitamin A toxicity usually subsides after discontinuation of vitamin A intake, but vitamin D toxicity may require treatment with corticosteroids.

### Milk-Alkali Syndrome

Milk-alkali syndrome is an uncommon cause of hypercalcemia but has been reported in patients with peptic ulcer disease who drank excessive quantities of milk together with large amounts of antacids.

### Granulomas

Many granulomatous diseases are associated with hypercalcemia. Hypercalcemia occurs in up to 17 percent of patients with sarcoidosis due to increased sensitivity to vitamin D in the intestine resulting in increased absorption of calcium. This hypercalcemia responds to corticosteroids or to vitamin D restriction. Hypersensitivity to vitamin D can also be seen in tuberculosis. There are a number of reports of hypercalcemia in patients with disseminated coccidioidomycosis, silicon granulomas, berylliosis, and histoplasmosis.

### Thiazide Diuretics

Hypercalcemia may be seen with the use of thiazide diuretics, which increase the renal tubular reabsorption of calcium and decrease plasma volume. It is one of the more common causes of hypercalcemia in ambulatory patients. Other diuretics increase urinary calcium excretion and tend to cause hypocalcemia.

### Syndromes in Infancy

Hypercalcemia may be seen in Williams syndrome, which is characterized by supravalvular aortic stenosis and elfin facies. Blue diaper syndrome, in which excessive amounts of indole derivatives cause blue urine because of an error in tryptophan metabolism, may also be associated with hypercalcemia.

## Pathophysiologic Effects

The effects of hypercalcemia can be neuromuscular, cardiovascular, gastrointestinal, renal, and skeletal. Neuromuscular changes include decreased sensitivity, responsiveness, and strength of muscular contraction and nerve conduction. This causes increasing weakness and fatigue which may progress to ataxia and altered mental status.

In mild hypercalcemic states, the heart's conduction is slowed and automaticity is decreased with a shortening of the refractory period. There is also increased sensitivity to digitalis preparations. Gastrointestinal motility is impaired but there is increased acid secretion in response to gastrin.

Loss of renal concentrating ability, as might be expected with nephrogenic DI, is the most frequent renal effect of hypercalcemia. This is a reversible tubular defect, which results in polyuria and dehydration in spite of polydipsia. Sodium, potassium, and magnesium reabsorption are reduced in the proximal tubule. Potassium wasting results in hypokalemia in up to one-third of patients. Nephrocalcinosis and nephrolithiasis are caused by the hypercalcemia and aggravated by dehydration. As the hypercalcemia persists, increasing microscopic calcium deposits in the kidney may result in progressive renal insufficiency.

With serum concentrations greater than 16 mg/dL, calcium salts may deposit in the myocardium, kidneys, lungs, subcutaneous tissue, blood vessel walls, conjunctiva, and cornea. If phosphate is given, calcium phosphate can rapidly precipitate in tissues. Hypertension is seen with increased frequency in hypercalcemic patients, probably as a result of arteriolar vasoconstriction.

## Diagnosis

Hypercalcemic patients with plasma total calcium levels below 12.0 mg/dL are usually asymptomatic, but higher levels can cause a wide variety of symptoms and signs (Table 21-20).

Patients with total calcium levels above 14 to 16 mg/dL are usually very weak, lethargic, and confused. Coma is uncommon, but calcium levels should probably be taken in any patient with coma of unknown etiology. Polyuria, in spite of polydipsia, tends to cause increasing dehydration. Weariness and weakness are common with hypercalcemia. Polyuria and polydipsia are due to impaired renal tubular reabsorption of water. Total calcium levels above 15.0 mg/dL may cause somnolence, stupor, and even coma.

A mnemonic sometimes used for the signs and symptoms of hypercalcemia is *stones* (renal calculi), *bones* (osteolysis), *psychic moans* (psychiatric disorders), and *abdominal groans* (peptic ulcer disease and pancreatitis). The most common gastrointestinal symptoms are anorexia and constipation, but these are very nonspecific.

Hypercalcemia should be suspected in patients with extensive metastatic bone disease, particularly if the primary site involves the breast, lungs, or kidneys, and in individuals with combinations of clinical problems such as renal calculi, pancreatitis, or ulcer disease. As with hypocalcemia, ionized calcium levels should be measured and/or total calcium levels should be correlated with serum proteins. If the patient is hypoproteinemic, total calcium levels may be normal or low in spite of increased ionized calcium levels.

On ECG, hypercalcemia may be associated with depressed ST segments, widened T waves, and shortened ST segments and QT intervals. Bradyarrhythmias may occur, and bundle branch patterns may progress to second-degree block and then complete heart block. Levels above 20 mg/dL may cause cardiac arrest.

The diagnosis of primary hyperparathyroidism is primarily based on two laboratory findings: (1) elevated serum calcium levels on at least three different occasions and (2) a serum PTH level which is disproportionately high for a simultaneously measured serum calcium level. A serum chloride to phosphorus ratio exceeding 35 to 1 can help confirm the diagnosis.

**Table 21-20.** Symptoms and Signs of Hypercalcemia

| | |
|---|---|
| General | Cardiovascular |
|   Malaise, weakness |   Hypertension |
|   Polydipsia, dehydration |   Arrhythmias |
| Neurologic |   Vascular calcifications |
|   Confusion |   ECG abnormalities |
|   Apathy, depression, stupor |     QT shortening |
|   Decreased memory |     Coving of ST-T wave |
|   Irritability |     Widening of T wave |
|   Hallucinations |     Digitalis sensitivity |
|   Headache | Gastrointestinal |
|   Ataxia |   Anorexia, weight loss |
|   Hyporeflexia, hypotonia |   Nausea, vomiting |
|   Mental retardation (infants) |   Constipation |
| Metastatic calcification |   Abdominal pain |
|   Band keratopathy |   Peptic ulcer disease |
|   Conjunctivitis |   Pancreatitis |
|   Pruritus | Urologic |
| Skeletal |   Polyuria, nocturia |
|   Fractures |   Renal insufficiency |
|   Bone pain |   Nephrolithiasis |
|   Deformities | |

## Treatment

Treatment of hypercalcemia is particularly important for patients with (1) calcium levels greater than 12 mg/dL, (2) symptoms, (3) inability to maintain a good fluid intake, or (4) abnormal renal function. Treatment is aimed at correcting the dehydration, promoting urinary calcium excretion, and decreasing calcium influx into the ECF from the skeletal system and gastrointestinal tract.

Patients with hypercalcemia tend to be dehydrated because high calcium levels interfere with ADH and the ability of the kidney to concentrate urine. Consequently, the initial and safest treatment is restoration of the ECF with relatively large amounts of saline. More than 5 to 10 L of normal saline may be required in the first 24 h to correct the dehydration. Some authors attempt to achieve a urine output as high as 250 mL/m$^2$ per hour to facilitate calcium excretion and ensure continued adequate hydration. In patients with cardiac or renal disease, such fluid therapy may be dangerous, and peritoneal dialysis or hemodialysis may be required.

Once the ECF has been restored and a good urine output started, a wide variety of diuretics (but not thiazides) will further increase renal excretion of calcium. Furosemide in doses of 1 to 3 mg/kg has been advocated. Up to one-third of patients with hypercalcemia have hypokalemia, and in those with malignant disease, more than half the patients may have hypokalemia. Some patients will also have hypomagnesemia. The tendency to develop hypokalemia and hypomagnesemia will be aggravated by the diuresis and should be watched for carefully and promptly corrected.

A wide variety of modalities are available to treat hypercalcemia (Table 21-21). Mithramycin is a cytotoxic drug that suppresses bone resorption and calcium release from bone. It may be particularly helpful in patients with metastatic bone disease. Small daily doses of 15 to 25 μg/kg in 5% dextrose IV over a period of 3 h for 3 days can lower serum calcium levels within 24 to 48 h; however, the mithramycin often suppresses bone resorption for only 5 to 7 days. It must be used with caution in patients with bone marrow problems, thrombocytopenia, or renal or hepatic insufficiency.

Calcitonin (Calcimar) is also an osteoclast inhibitor and is less toxic than mithramycin. The dosage is usually 0.5 to 4 MRC units per kg given IM every 12 h. The dose may be increased to a maximum of 8 MRC units per kg every 6 h. Effects are usually seen within the first 12 h, but patients often become refractory to it within 2 days. When calcitonin is used in conjunction with corticosteroids, the action of calcitonin is more prolonged.

Glucocorticoids may reduce serum calcium levels in patients with sarcoidosis, vitamin A or D intoxication, multiple myeloma, leukemia, or breast cancer. Glucocorticoids work by inhibiting bone resorption and gastrointestinal absorption of calcium. Steroids may also cause calcium to shift inside cells where it may be bound to mitochondria. The dosage of hydrocortisone in adults is 25 to 100 mg IV every 6 to 8 h. The effect of this treatment may not be apparent until after the first 12 h. If no effect is seen after 7 to 10 days, the therapy may be discontinued.

Intravenous phosphates and EDTA are rarely used now because of the rapid fall in calcium that may occur, along with tissue deposition of calcium phosphate, renal cortical necrosis, and even shock.

When possible, irradiation or resection of neoplasms producing PTH-like activity should be considered. If parathyroid hyperplasia or adenoma is suspected, it should be treated surgically as soon as possible.

## MAGNESIUM

Magnesium is a vital element in all biologic systems and is the key element in chlorophyll, the first link in the world's food chain. The total body content of magnesium averages about 2000 mEq (24 g), with about 50 to 70 percent present in bone. The majority of the remaining magnesium is intracellular, with only 1 percent present in the ECF. The serum concentration of magnesium is about 1.8 to 2.4 mg/dL or 1.5 to 2.0 mEq/L. About 25 to 35 percent of the magnesium present in the blood is protein-bound, 10 to 15 percent is complexed, and 50 to 60 percent is ionized. The concentration of magnesium intracellularly is thought to be about 40 mEq/L, making it the second most abundant intracellular cation.

The usual daily requirement is about 24 to 28 mEq (288 to 336 mg), usually from vegetables and cereals. About 40 percent is excreted in the urine and 60 percent in feces. Renal excretion protects against hypermagnesemia, but not hypomagnesemia, which will develop if intake is consistently less than 3.0 mg/kg per day.

### Hypomagnesemia

#### Etiology

A wide variety of problems can cause hypomagnesemia (Table 21-22). In adults, magnesium deficiencies are most frequently seen in alcoholics, in malnourished patients, and in patients with cirrhosis, pancreatitis, or excessive gastrointestinal fluid losses. Diarrhea is usually more of a problem (Mg$^{2+}$ content of 10 to 14 mEq/L) than upper gastrointestinal loss (1 to 2 mEq/L). Chronic hyperparathyroidism increases urinary losses of magnesium and will eventually cause hypomagnesemia.

Intravenous hyperalimentation or treatment of diabetic ketoacidosis without providing adequate magnesium, especially in a previously malnourished patient, can cause an abrupt fall in plasma magnesium levels. This is largely due to magnesium being "pulled" into cells with glucose or as new lean body mass is synthesized. Hypophosphatemia, which can also develop with IV hyperalimentation, can contribute to the hypomagnesemia.

**Table 21-21.** Treatment of Hypercalcemia

| Drug | Dose | Cautions |
|---|---|---|
| | TO TREAT DEHYDRATION | |
| Saline | Until ECF is restored | Watch for hypokalemia |
| Furosemide | 40–100 mg IV q 2–4 h | Digitalis, renal failure |
| | TO DECREASE BONE ABSORPTION | |
| Calcitonin | 0.5–4 MRC units/kg IV over 24 h (or IM q 6 h in divided doses) | |
| Mithramycin | 25 μg/kg IV | Bone marrow and renal toxicity |
| Hydrocortisone | 3 mg/kg per day IV in divided doses q 6 h | May take 3 weeks to lower Ca$^{2+}$ |
| Indomethacin | 25 mg PO q 6 h | Peptic ulcer disease, GI bleeding |

**Table 21-22.** Causes of Hypomagnesemia

| | |
|---|---|
| Gastrointestinal | Drug-induced |
|   Protein-calorie malnutrition |   Diuretics |
|   Hyperalimentation after malnutrition |   Aminoglycosides |
|   Malabsorption (diarrhea), fistulas |   Cisplatin |
|   Alcoholic cirrhosis |   Vitamin D intoxication |
|   Pancreatitis |   Digoxin |
| Renal |   Alcohol |
|   Glomerulonephritis, pyelonephritis |   Insulin |
|   Diuretic phase of acute tubular necrosis |   Citrate (blood) |
|   Hypercalcemia | Miscellaneous |
| Endocrine |   Lactation |
|   Aldosteronism |   Sweating |
|   Hyperparathyroidism, hyperthyroidism |   Hungry-bone syndrome |
| |   Burns |
| |   Sepsis |

Renal wasting of magnesium can be seen with loop diuretics, hypophosphatemia, ketoacidosis, aminoglycosides, and nephrotoxic chemotherapeutic agents.

The normal renal threshold for magnesium (1.5 to 2.0 mEq/L) is significantly decreased by cisplatin, diuretics, hypercalcemia, growth hormone, thyroid hormone, and calcitonin. Cisplatin causes dose-dependent, cumulative, reversible renal tubular injury. Even when the GFR is not diminished by cisplatin, renal magnesium wasting along with a secondary hypocalcemia and hypokalemia may develop. Potassium wasting is thought to occur as a result of impaired ATP production when magnesium is low. This in turn impairs the function of the membrane $Na^+/K^+$ transport system and causes loss of the normal $Na^+/K^+$ gradient. The accompanying hypocalcemia may be due to (1) impaired PTH release by the parathyroid gland, (2) decreased peripheral sensitivity to PTH, or (3) abnormal blood-bone calcium balance independent of PTH.

## Physiologic Effects

Magnesium is essential to a large number of vital enzymes, including membrane-bound ATPase. Consequently hypomagnesemia may result in a wide variety of neuromuscular, gastrointestinal, and cardiovascular changes (Table 21-23).

Hypomagnesemia may cause increased muscular irritability similar to that seen with hypocalcemia. It can also cause many CNS signs and symptoms, including depression, vertigo, ataxia, and seizures. In severe chronic alcoholics, delirium tremens is often associated with moderate to severe magnesium deficiencies. Cardiac arrhythmias, particularly in patients on digitalis, is often due to both potassium and magnesium deficiencies.

Some metabolic manifestations of magnesium deficiency include difficulties in treating hypokalemia, impaired PTH secretion, decreased response to thiamine, and vitamin D–resistant hypocalcemia. Other manifestations include hypothermia, hypotension, nephropathy, incomplete distal renal tubular acidosis, dysphagia, and anemia due to shortened RBC survival.

It has been noted that patients with severe acute pancreatitis and hypocalcemia usually have normal serum magnesium levels; however, their mononuclear cell magnesium content may be significantly low and their retention of magnesium with a loading test may be significantly increased. This implies that, in spite of the normal serum magnesium levels, there is an intracellular and total body magnesium deficiency. This may contribute to the severity of the pancreatitis and the pathogenesis of the hypocalcemia.

## Diagnosis

One cannot rely on plasma levels to diagnose magnesium deficiencies because it is not unusual to have total body magnesium fall rather severely before plasma levels are lowered. The diagnosis of hypomagnesemia in the presence of normal serum calcium levels is suggested by increased neuromuscular irritability (hyperreflexia, positive Chvostek or Trousseau signs, tremor, tetany, or even convulsions). Hypomagnesemia should be suspected in alcoholics, cirrhotics, and patients on IV fluids for prolonged periods. Hypomagnesemia may also develop rapidly during IV hyperalimentation, especially when anabolism begins.

The ECG changes seen with magnesium deficiencies include prolonged PR and QT intervals, widened QRS complexes, depression of ST segments, and inversion of T waves, especially in the precordial leads. The changes may be somewhat similar to those caused by hypokalemia and/or hypocalcemia, and many of these changes may be related to $Mg^{2+}$ deficiency altering cardiac intracellular potassium content.

## Treatment

Hypokalemia, hypocalcemia, and hypophosphatemia are often present with hypomagnesemia and must be monitored carefully. It must be emphasized that the physician treating a magnesium deficiency should look for and correct any associated potassium, calcium, or phosphate deficiencies.

Patients with magnesium deficiency may require more than 50 mEq of oral magnesium (6 g $MgSO_4$) per day. In chronic alcoholics with delirium tremens and in patients with severe proven hypomagnesemia, up to 8 to 12 g of $MgSO_4$ may be given intramuscularly or intravenously the first day. The first 10 to 15 mEq (1.5 to 2.0 g) of IV $MgSO_4$ can be given over 1 to 2 h. This may be followed by up to 4 to 6 g/day thereafter. If IV alimentation is being given to a hypomagnesemic patient, 12 to 16 mEq (1.5 to 2.0 g) should be added to each liter of total parenteral alimentation (TPN).

If magnesium is being given rapidly, as in the treatment of eclampsia, the deep tendon reflexes (which disappear at about 3 to 4 mEq/L) should be checked frequently, and blood levels should be measured once or twice daily. If deep tendon reflexes decrease or disappear, magnesium administration should stop, at least temporarily.

A variety of oral forms of magnesium are available for long-term treatment (Table 21-24).

## Hypermagnesemia

### Etiology

Hypermagnesemia occurs rather infrequently, except in patients with renal failure who are given magnesium-containing drugs, particularly antacids such as Maalox. Other less frequent causes include untreated diabetic acidosis and adrenal insufficiency. Hypermagnesemia may also be seen with tumor lysis, rhabdomyolysis, hyperparathyroidism, hypothyroidism, and ECF volume contraction, all of which lead to decreased magnesium clearance.

### Physiologic Effects

Progressively increasing magnesium levels above 3.0 to 4.0 mEq/L can reduce neuromuscular irritability and cause deep tendon reflexes

**Table 21-23.** Symptoms and Signs of Hypomagnesemia

| Neuromuscular | Gastrointestinal |
|---|---|
| Tetany | Dysphagia |
| Muscle weakness | Anorexia, nausea |
| Cerebellar (ataxia, nystagmus, vertigo) | Cardiovascular |
| Confusion, obtundation, coma | Heart failure |
| Seizures | Arrhythmias |
| Apathy, depression | Hypotension |
| Irritability | Miscellaneous |
| Paresthesias | Hypokalemia |
| | Hypocalcemia |
| | Anemia |

**Table 21-24.** Treatment of Hypomagnesemia

| Drug | Size and Contents | Dose |
|---|---|---|
| | PARENTERAL | |
| $MgSO_4$ (1 g = 98 mg of elemental $Mg^{2+}$) | 10% (20-mL ampules, 0.81 mEq/mL) or 50% (2-ml ampules, 4 mEq/mL) | 1–2 g $MgSO_4$ or $MgCl_2$ by continuous IV every 4–6 h prn |
| $MgCl_2$ (1 g = 118 mg elemental $Mg^{2+}$) | 20% (30-mL bottle, 1.97 mEq/mL) | |
| | ORAL | |
| MgO | 400-mg tablets (20 mEq) | 1–4 per day |
| $Mg(OH)_2$ (milk of magnesia) | 7.5% (2.9 mEq/5mL) | 5–15 mL tid |

to disappear. Increasing muscular weakness is noted with levels above 4.0 mEq/L, and levels above 5.0 to 6.0 mEq/L may cause severe vasodilation and hypotension. Levels above 8.0 to 10.0 mEq/L can cause cardiac conduction abnormalities and neuromuscular paralysis with hypotension and/or ventilatory failure and death.

## Diagnosis

Serum magnesium levels are usually diagnostic. The possibility of hypermagnesemia should be considered in patients with hyperkalemia or hypercalcemia. Hypermagnesemia should also be suspected in patients with renal failure, particularly in those who are on magnesium-containing antacids, such as Maalox.

## Treatment

The initial treatment of hypermagnesemia is similar to that used for hypercalcemia and includes dilution by administering IV fluids and then using diuretics, especially furosemide, as needed. Any acidosis should be corrected, and a slow infusion of calcium gluconate can also help to control symptoms. Peritoneal dialysis and hemodialysis are thought by some to be relatively ineffective with divalent cations, but removal of up to 700 mg of magnesium with one hemodialysis treatment has been reported.

## PHOSPHORUS (PHOSPHATE)

The normal adult man contains about 700 g of phosphorus, of which about 80 percent is present in bones. Phosphorus is essential to a wide variety of reactions, especially energy metabolism in the form of high-energy phosphates and phosphocreatine. Serum phosphorus levels drop with age from a high of 4.0 to 7.0 mg/dL in the newborn to 3.0 to 5.0 mg/dL in adults. Serum calcium and phosphorus levels are inversely proportional, and the product of their two concentrations in milligrams per deciliter usually averages about 30 to 40. The normal oral intake is about 10 to 12 mmol, with urinary excretion largely regulated by PTH.

## Hypophosphatemia

### Etiology

Because phosphorus is available in so many foods and is so easily absorbed, hypophosphatemia is unusual unless (1) oral intake is reduced, (2) there is excess loss of phosphorus, or (3) there is excessive movement of $PO_4$ from the ECF into cells (Table 21-25).

One should look carefully for hypophosphatemia in patients on TPN, with low potassium or magnesium levels, or with hypercalcemia. Hypophosphatemia is being increasingly recognized, especially in patients with IV hyperalimentation, which increases phosphate movement into cells as anabolism occurs. Phosphorus is also consumed during phosphorylation of glucose as it moves into cells. Intracellular shifts also occur in the presence of respiratory alkalosis and with the adminstration of anabolic steroids, sodium bicarbonate, epinephrine, or glucagon.

Hypophosphatemia may be seen with metabolic alkalosis, especially after prolonged antacid therapy. Antacids with calcium and magnesium bind to phosphate and impair its intestinal absorption. Metabolic or respiratory alkalosis also increases phosphate loss in the urine. Respiratory alkalosis may also increase phosphate movement into cells. Hyperparathyroidism and alcoholism are additional causes of hypophosphatemia.

Other causes of hypophosphatemia include malignancy with hypercalcemia (due to phosphaturia), renal tubular defects, hypokalemia, hypomagnesemia, and use of phosphate-binding antacids. One should also look for and prevent or rapidly correct hypophosphatemia in patients during rapid healing or anabolism. During recovery

**Table 21-25.** Conditions Associated with Hypophosphatemia

Intake
  Deficiency of dietary phosphate
  Phosphate malabsorption in dialyzed patients, alcoholics
  Overuse of phosphate-binding agents
  TPN
Redistribution
  Glucose infusion
  Treatment of diabetes mellitus
  Respiratory alkalosis
  Beta-adrenergic agents
  Increased skeletal uptake in healing phase of rickets
  Osteoblastic metastases of cancer
  Nutritional recovery syndrome
  Androgens, estrogens
  Diuretic phase of severe burns
Renal causation
  Specific phosphate transport defect
    X-linked dominant hypophosphatemia
    Autosomal dominant hypophosphatemia
  Multiple renal tubular transport defects
    Idiopathic Fanconi syndrome
    Cystinosis
    Hereditary fructose intolerance
    Galactosemia
    Wilson disease
    Oculocerebrorenal (Lowe) syndrome
  Phosphaturia due to primary or secondary hyperparathyroidism
    Primary hyperparathyroidism
    Secondary hyperparathyroidism due to hereditary vitamin D
      dependency, types I and II
    Hypocalcemia from any cause, provided parathyroid glands are
      intact
Miscellaneous
  Tumor-induced hypophosphatemia
  Posttransplantation hypophosphatemia
  Hypercalciuric nephrolithiasis

from starvation or after severe burns, the body requirement for phosphate can greatly increase. The phosphate and potassium requirement of patients who undergo a partial hepatectomy may be particularly large, especially if more than 60 percent of the liver has been resected. In general, 5.0 mmol of phosphate is used to generate 1.0 g of pro-tein; therefore, phosphate requirements may be as high as 30 to 60 mmol/day. Thus, extensive tissue repair or healing can quickly lead to severe phosphorous deficiency if there is inadequate intake.

### Physiologic Effects

The most frequent consequences of hypophosphatemia are hematologic and neuromuscular. Hypophosphatemia may be associated with depletion of ATP in platelets, red blood cells, and white blood cells, reducing their survival time and function. Platelet membrane changes may result in a bleeding tendency due to impaired aggregation. Phosphate deficiency also causes tendency for red blood cells to become rigid spherocytes, thereby impairing capillary perfusion. In addition, decreased 2,3-diphosphoglycerate (2,3-DPG) increases the affinity of hemoglobin for oxygen, thereby reducing the arterial $P_{O_2}$ and oxygen availability to tissues. Phosphate depletion in macrophages may impair chemotaxis, phagocytosis, and intracellular killing, resulting in decreased resistance to infection.

Progressive weakness and tremors may be noted as blood phosphate levels fall below 0.5 to 1.0 mg/dL. Circumoral and fingertip paresthesias may be present along with absent deep tendon reflexes. Mental obtundation, anorexia, and hyperventilation may also occur. Patients may become so weak that they cannot be weaned from a ventilator or ambulated. Myocardial function, as measured by left ventricular stroke work, may also be impaired.

## Diagnosis

Patients with diabetic or alcoholic ketoacidosis or severe malnutrition are particularly prone to develop hypophosphatemia. This problem should be looked for with particular care within 12 to 48 h of beginning treatment of diabetic ketoacidosis, within 24 to 96 h of treating alcoholic ketoacidosis, and within 5 to 10 days of beginning IV hyperalimentation.

One should not rely completely on blood phosphorus levels to rule out phosphorus deficiency. The ratio of intracellular to extracellular phosphorus concentration is approximately 100 to 1. Since 80 percent of the total body phosphorus is in bone, serum phosphorus levels may not reflect total body stores, and the magnitude of the total body deficit cannot be estimated adequately from blood levels, particularly if there are acute changes.

## Treatment

Treatment of hypophosphatemia should be primarily preventive and must be an integral part of any nutrition program. At least 7 to 9 mmol of phosphate, usually as a combination of $KH_2PO_4$ and $K_2HPO_4$ (dibasic and monobasic phosphates), should be given with each 1000 calories. In some instances, more than double that amount of phosphate may be required to bring phosphate levels up to normal. Because phosphate administration may cause a precipitous fall in serum calcium levels, calcium should also be given, usually as calcium gluconate in doses of 0.2 to 0.3 mEq/kg per day. The hazards of phosphate therapy include soft tissue calcification, hypotension, and hyperosmolality. If potassium phosphate is used, the therapy may also cause hyperkalemia.

For severe hypophosphatemia with blood levels less than 1.0 mg/dL (0.32 mmol/L) or symptoms, immediate IV replacement is required. Otherwise oral preparations can be often used.

If the hypophosphatemia is recent and uncomplicated, the initial recommended daily dose is 2.5 mg/kg. Prolonged or multifactorial hypophyosphatemia may require 5 mg/kg. Up to 25 to 50 percent more phosphorus is needed if the patient is symptomatic; however, less is required in the presence of hypercalcemia. Each dose is administered IV over 6 h, and serum phosphorus is checked after each dose. To minimize the risks of hyperphosphatemia, a total dose of no more than 7.5 mg/kg should be administered. Risks of phosphate therapy include hypocalcemia, metastatic calcification, hypotension, and hyperkalemia from the potassium salts. One should switch to oral therapy as soon as possible.

## Hyperphosphatemia

### Etiology

Hyperphosphatemia may be due to reduced renal excretion, increased phosphate movement out of cells into the ECF, or increased phosphorus or vitamin D intake (Table 21-26). Hyperphosphatemia is most apt to be seen with renal dysfunction. It may also be seen with hypoparathyroidism or any problem associated with hypocalcemia or hypomagnesemia.

### Physiologic Effects

Problems due to hyperphosphatemia are usually those due to associated renal failure, hypocalcemia, or the hypomagnesemia which is usually present.

### Therapy

Therapy is aimed at treating the underlying cause and restricting calcium phosphate intake to less than 200 mg/day. With normal renal function, $PO_4$ excretion can be increased with saline (1 to 2 L every 4 to 6 h) and acetazolamide (500 mg every 6 h). $PO_4$ absorption from the GI tract is decreased with oral $PO_4$ binders (i.e., aluminum car-

**Table 21-26.** Conditions Associated with Hyperphosphatemia

| Intake | Renal causation |
|---|---|
| Poisoning by phosphate-containing enema or laxative | Acute and chronic reduction in GFR |
| Redistribution | Hypoparathyroid state |
| Respiratory acidosis | Primary hypoparathyroidism |
| Lactic acidosis | Pseudohypoparathyroidism |
| Diphosphonate therapy | Suppression of PTH secretion |
| Chemotherapy for neoplasms | from any hypercalemic condition |
| Rhabdomyolysis | Miscellaneous causes |
| Septic shock | Hyperthyroidism |
|  | Vitamin D intoxication |
|  | Acromegaly |
|  | Cortical hyperostosis |

bonate or hydroxide 30 to 45 mL qid). These binders also absorb $PO_4$ secreted into the gut lumen and are of benefit even if no oral $PO_4$ is given. If clinically significant hypocalcemia exists, calcium should be cautiously administered. If renal failure is present, hemodialysis may be required.

## CHLORIDE

Chloride is the major anion in the extracellular fluid. It fulfills several important physiologic functions. It is an important factor in maintaining (1) urine output and concentration in the renal countercurrent mechanisms, (2) ECF volume, (3) acid-base and potassium balance, and (4) a normal anion gap.

Chloride is readily absorbed in the large and small bowel by active and passive transport mechanisms which are either sodium or bicarbonate dependent. However, there is a Cl–HCO$_3$ exchange in the small bowel. Stomach parietal cells possess the unique capacity to secrete chloride plus hydrogen (H$^+$) ions into gastric fluid. About 90 percent of the chloride ingested is excreted in the urine and the remainder is lost in the stool and in sweat.

Chloride is almost entirely extracellular, and its concentration is usually about 70 to 75 percent that of sodium. There is little chloride in bone, and virtually all chloride in the body is diffusible and metabolically active.

### The Role of Chloride in the Kidney

One should look for hypochloremia in patients who appear to be developing renal dysfunction. The activity of chloride in the kidney is extremely important in determining its ability to concentrate urine. In most of the tubule, chloride reabsorption occurs passively along with sodium transport. However, in the water-impermeable ascending thick limb of the loop of Henle, where about 20 to 30 percent of sodium and chloride is reabsorbed, chloride transport is active. This active transport of chloride apparently provides the crucial gradient needed for the "countercurrent" urine-concentrating mechanism to function properly. In the absence of ADH, this mechanism can also allow absorption of solute without water in the collecting ducts, allowing urine to be more dilute if needed.

Chloride is also significantly involved in plasma acid-base regulation. Although not directly responsible for regulation of H$^+$ ion concentration, reciprocal changes in plasma HCO$_3$ and Cl concentrations occur during renal adjustments of ECF pH, when hydrogen and chloride are secreted, and when HCO$_3$ is reabsorbed. Renal acid excretion and HCO$_3$ reabsorption can be greatly modified by insufficient quantity of readily reabsorbable anion, particularly chloride, in the glomerular filtrate.

### Normal Levels

The range for normal serum chloride is 96 to 108 mEq/L. It can be measured in serum, plasma, urine, sweat, cerebrospinal fluid (CSF), stool, and other body fluids. Serum determinations are most commonly done, but heparinized (or EDTA) plasma may be used. Hemolysis can produce pseudohypochloremia secondary to a dilutional effect by RBC water; therefore, serum should be promptly separated from red cells. As with sodium, an increase in total serum protein may produce pseudohyperchloremia as a result of water displacement. Because all of the chemical methods for analyzing chloride also pick up the other halides, the presence of bromide and iodide can falsely elevate serum chloride levels.

## Hypochloremia

### Etiology

The most frequent causes of hypochloremia (<95 mEq/L) are excessive diuresis, especially after administration of loop diuretics, and loss of highly acid gastric secretions through vomiting or nasogastric suction. Hypochloremia is usually associated with the presence of a metabolic alkalosis that can be divided into several types according to etiology (Table 21-27).

Diuretic use promotes natriuresis, kaliuresis, and chloruresis. Vomiting and external gastric drainage lead to a complex series of events. Gastric parietal cells secrete hydrogen and chloride into gastric fluid while bicarbonate is generated into the circulation. Acid-base balance is maintained by hydrogen and chloride absorption in the more distal GI tract. Metabolic alkalosis results when this balance is upset by vomiting, or any other external loss of hydrochloric acid. This alkalosis is maintained by increased renal absorption of sodium and bicarbonate due to ECF volume depletion.

Because sodium conservation and volume maintenance take precedence over acid-base and potassium balance, the kidney is influenced by aldosterone to accelerate the exchange of sodium for potassium and hydrogen ions. However, if abundant chloride is provided, the pattern is reversed, leading to bicarbonate diuresis and correction of the alkalosis.

In contrast to gastric contents, stool is normally low in chloride and rich in potassium. Diarrheal diseases, unless vomiting is a prominent feature, are associated with metabolic acidosis rather than alkalosis. An exception is found with villous adenoma of the colon and in a rare congenital disorder known as chloride diarrhea that arises from a defect in the ileal and colonic Cl–HCO$_3$ exchange mechanism. In both these situations, metabolic alkalosis is a consequence of loss of chloride augmented by ECF volume contraction.

Serious chloride depletion can occur from the skin secondary to severe sweating or severe burns. Patients with cystic fibrosis can develop metabolic alkalosis due to marked loss of chloride in sweat.

**Table 21-27.** Types of Metabolic Alkalosis

Chloride-responsive ($U_{Cl}$ < mEq/L)
  GI losses
    Vomiting, gastric drainage
    Villous adenoma
    Congenital chloride diarrhea
    Diuretics
    Cystic fibrosis
    Rapid correction of chronic hypercapnia
Chloride-resistant ($U_{Cl}$ > 20 mEq/L)
  Excess mineralocorticoid activity
  Hyperaldosteronism
  Cushing syndrome
  Bartter syndrome
  Excess licorice
  Severe K$^+$ depletion
Unclassified (variable urine chloride)
  Massive blood transfusion
  Milk-alkali syndrome
  Alkali administration
Nonparathyroid hypercalcemia
  Large doses of carbenicillin or penicillin

## Physiologic Effects

The most frequent physiologic effects of hypochloremia are those due to the metabolic alkalosis and hypokalemia with which it is usually associated. Numerous studies have implicated chloride depletion in both the generation and maintenance of metabolic alkalosis. Because chloride is the only anion other than hydrochloric acid which is readily reabsorbed with sodium, chloride depletion accelerates Na–H exchange all along the tubule. Loss of H$^+$ in the urine results in alkalosis. In addition, because low blood chloride levels impair active chloride transport and the associated sodium reabsorption in the ascending limb, more sodium is delivered to the distal nephron for H$^+$ and potassium exchange. This exchange results in increased loss of H$^+$ and potassium in the urine, making the alkalosis more severe. Thus, urine chloride levels should be evaluated in all patients with hypochloremia.

Chloride-responsive alkalosis is established and maintained by ECF volume depletion and chloride deficits. Volume depletion supplies the stimulus for sodium retention, but chloride is not available in sufficient quantity to maintain electrical neutrality. Therefore, the exchange of sodium for hydrogen and potassium ions is accelerated. There is minimal urinary chloride excretion (less than 10 mmol/L), because there is nearly complete reabsorption of filtered chloride in the sodium-avid tubule.

### Diagnosis

No signs or symptoms are specifically characteristic of hypochloremia. A history of vomiting, excessive nasogastric suction, or diuretic therapy, together with evidence of volume depletion, should signal the possible presence of hypochloremia and an associated metabolic alkalosis. Metabolic alkalosis may produce muscle weakness, neuromuscular irritability, and hypoventilation. This hypoventilation may be especially dangerous in patients already hypoxic secondary to chronic obstructive pulmonary disease (COPD).

If a patient has a metabolic alkalosis and the urinary chloride levels are low (less than 10 mEq/L), the patient is said to have a chloride-responsive alkalosis. Such patients usually have a relatively simple chloride deficit and will often respond to chloride administration alone. If urine chloride levels are 40 mEq/L or higher, the hypochloremia is probably due to dilution. If the patient is not overloaded with fluids, the hypochloremia is apt to be due to or associated with excessive corticosteroids and/or hypokalemia.

Hypochloremia with increased urine chloride can also be caused by excess mineralocorticoid activity which causes Na$^+$ and HCO$_3$$^-$ retention and increased excretion of H$^+$, K$^+$, and Cl$^-$ (Table 21-28). The ECF volume expansion results in diminished proximal tubule NaCl reabsorption and, therefore, an increased delivery of sodium to the distal tubule. The exchange of sodium for potassium and hydrogen ions is also enhanced, resulting in an even greater loss of H$^+$ and K$^+$.

It has been noted that metabolic alkalosis with severe potassium depletion may be resistant to correction with NaCl alone. Severe potassium depletion may directly alter the renal tubular handling of chloride, resulting in chloride wasting. To reverse this chloride-wasting nephropathy, at least a partial correction of the potassium deficit is required.

### Treatment

Chloride-responsive metabolic alkalosis will usually respond to IV administration of sodium chloride alone. Chloride-resistant metabolic alkalosis usually also requires potassium and in severe cases may also require hydrogen ions. Hypochloremia due to dilution from excess total body water is usually best treated by cautious dehydration.

As a general rule, deficits in total body chloride are best treated by giving one-fourth of the calculated chloride deficit as KCl and three-fourths as NaCl. The total body chloride deficit can be estimated

**Table 21-28.** Etiology of Hyperchloremia Associated with Primary Hypernatremic States

Administration of hypertonic or excess NaCl
Normal anion-gap metabolic acidosis
  GI losses of $HCO_3$
    Diarrhea
    Small bowel
    Biliary, pancreatic
    Ureterosigmoidostomy, obstructed ileal loop conduit
    $CaCl_2$, $MgCl_2$ ingestion
    Cholestyramine ingestion
  Renal losses of $HCO_3$
    Renal tubular acidosis
    Hypoaldosteronism
    Hyperparathyroidism
    Carbonic anhydrase inhibitors
  Miscellaneous
    Dilutional acidosis
    Hyperalimentation acidosis
    Sulfur ingestion
    Compounds with Cl anion
    Compensation of chronic respiratory alkalosis
Low anion-gap states
  Hypoalbuminemia
  Bromism (other halides)
Unmeasured non-Na cations

rapidly by multiplying 20 percent of the body weight by the serum chloride deficit. Thus, an 80-kg patient with a serum chloride of 60 mEq/L has a total deficit of $(80 \text{ kg} \times 20\%)(100 - 60) = 16 \times 40$ or 640 mEq.

In attempting to correct chloride deficits, one should be aware that dehydration can greatly increase the total chloride deficit. If the patient is severely dehydrated, the total additional chloride deficit may be estimated by assuming that the mild, moderate, or severe dehydration involves a 6, 8, or 10 percent loss, respectively, of body weight as ECF containing 100 mEq of chloride per liter. Thus, if an 80-kg man is severely dehydrated, one can assume that he has lost at least 8 L of ECF containing 100 mEq of chloride per liter, or 800 mEq of chloride. Since he can be assumed to have only 8 L of ECF left, the deficit in the remaining ECF is $8 \times 40$, or 320 mEq. Thus, the total chloride deficit in a severely dehydrated 80-kg man with a serum chloride of 60 mEq/L would be 800 + 320, or 1120 mEq.

If the patient has renal dysfunction so that potassium cannot be given or if the metabolic alkalosis is very severe or does not respond to NaCl plus KCl, 0.1 $N$ HCl or amino acid hydrochlorides may be useful. If 0.1 $N$ HCl is used, it should be given slowly through a central IV line.

## Hyperchloremia

### Etiology

Hyperchloremia is usually due to dehydration, administration of excessive amounts of sodium chloride, or various problems that can cause a normal anion-gap metabolic acidosis (Table 21-28). The most frequent causes of normal anion-gap acidosis are gastrointestinal losses of bicarbonate (small bowel or pancreatic fistulas or diarrhea) or renal bicarbonate losses (Table 21-28). Excess administration of chloride as saline, KCl, and amino acid hydrochlorides can also cause hyperchloremia. All of these substances readily dissociate and consume $HCO_3$, resulting in hyperchloremic metabolic acidosis. The most frequent acid-base problem seen with IV hyperalimentation is a hyperchloremic metabolic acidosis because the amino acids are provided as chlorides or hydrochlorides.

### Pathophysiology

The physiologic effects of hyperchloremia are due primarily to the underlying dehydration or metabolic acidosis. Clinically most changes in plasma chloride concentration parallel those of sodium. Primary hypernatremic states are, for the most part, predictably accompanied by hyperchloremia. In addition, changes in serum chloride accompany reciprocal changes in serum $HCO_3$. As a result, hypochloremia usually accompanies metabolic alkalosis, and hyperchloremia accompanies normal anion-gap metabolic acidosis.

The systemic effects of acute and severe metabolic acidosis are well known and include Kussmaul (slow, very deep) respirations, decreased myocardial contractility, and a drop in peripheral resistance. Bone disease associated with chronic acidosis, such as that seen in RTA, may manifest itself as stunted growth secondary to acidosis-induced bone mineral loss, as well as rickets and osteomalacia.

### Diagnosis

Clinical features of hyperchloremia are difficult to list independently because the presentation is usually a manifestation of the primary underlying disorder and associated metabolic abnormalities. Elevated serum chloride and sodium levels usually indicate dehydration. Elevated chloride levels with normal or low serum sodium levels usually indicate either excess chloride administration as KCl or amino acid hydrochlorides or excess loss of bicarbonate from the body.

Anion gap and arterial pH can be extremely helpful in determining the cause and treatment of hyperchloremia. A low anion gap (less than 10 mEq/L) can be associated with hyperchloremia in several pathologic states. When reduced concentration of unmeasured anions exists, as in cirrhosis or nephrosis with hypoalbuminemia, the normally unmeasured anion albumin is partially replaced with the measured anions chloride and $HCO_3$ so that the anion gap will tend to fall. Unmeasured non-Na cations, such as cationic proteins in multiple myeloma or severe hypercalcemia, hypermagnesemia, and acute lithium overdose obligate an increased chloride or $HCO_3$ to counterbalance their positive charge.

An overestimation of serum chloride occurs when bromide (or other halide) is present because halides interfere with all laboratory determinations of chloride. Bromism be suspected when the anion gap is very small or negative.

### Treatment

If there is excess administration of chloride or excessive losses of bicarbonate, this should be corrected. Hyperchloremia due to dehydration is best treated by slowly administering increased istonic fluids with little or no chloride. However, if too much hypotonic fluid is given too rapidly, seizures due to cerebral edema may develop.

### BIBLIOGRAPHY

Cogan G: *Fluid and Electrolytes: Physiology and Pathophysiology.* Norwalk, CT, Appleton/Lange, 1991.
Rose BD: Clinical physiology of acid-base and electrolyte disorders, 4th ed. New York, McGraw-Hill, 1994.
Schrier RW (ed): *Renal and Electrolyte Disorders,* 4th ed. Boston, Little, Brown, 1992.

# 22
# DISTURBANCES OF CARDIAC RHYTHM AND CONDUCTION
## J. Stephan Stapczynski

The interpretation and treatment of cardiac arrhythmias is basic to the practice of emergency medicine. This chapter reviews the important cardiac rhythm and conduction disturbances and their clinical significance and emergency treatment. Discussions of defibrillation, cardioversion, and artificial cardiac pacemakers are also included.

Although emphasis is appropriately placed on drug treatment of these arrhythmias, it is also important that underlying and reversible causes of rhythm and conduction disturbances—such as hypoxia, alkalosis, electrolyte abnormalities, or drug toxicity—be recognized and treated.

## THE NORMAL CARDIAC CONDUCTING SYSTEM

The heart consists of three types of specialized tissue: (1) pacemaker cells that undergo spontaneous depolarization and can initiate an electric impulse, (2) conducting cells that form the specialized conducting system and rapidly propagate an electric impulse throughout the heart, and (3) contractile cells which contract when electrically depolarized.

The sinus node is normally the dominant cardiac pacemaker unless its activity is depressed by disease or drugs. The sinus node is located near the junction of the superior vena cava and right atrium. Blood supply is from the sinus node artery, which arises from either the proximal few centimeters of the right coronary artery in about 55 percent of individuals, or from the proximal few millimeters of the left circumflex artery in the other 45 percent. The sinus node is innervated by both sympathetic and parasympathetic nerve endings which can greatly modify the discharge rate. The intrinsic sinus node discharge rate is between 90 and 100 in middle-aged adults; the usual resting heart rate is lower, reflecting the predominance of parasympathetic activity at rest.

The electric impulse generated by the sinus node spreads like ripples throughout the right and then the left atrium, activating atrial contraction. Additionally, specialized atrial conduction tracts (anterior, middle, and posterior internodal tracts) serve to propagate the electric impulse through the atria and between the sinus node and the atrioventricular (AV) node.

The atria and ventricles are insulated electrically from each other by the fibrous connective tissue of the atrioventricular ring (annulus fibrosis). Normally, electric impulses from the atria can reach the ventricles only by passing through the AV node and infranodal conducting system.

The AV node is just beneath the right atrial endocardium and directly above the insertion of the septal leaflet of the tricuspid valve. The blood supply to the AV node in 90 percent of humans is by way of a branch off the right coronary artery as it turns to form the posterior descending artery, and in the other 10 percent, comes off the left circumflex artery. This accounts for the common occurrence of AV conduction disturbances with acute inferior myocardial infarctions. The AV node is innervated by both sympathetic and parasympathetic fibers. It has two important electrophysiological characteristics: a slow conduction velocity and a long refractory period. The slow conduction velocity through the AV node allows time for atrial contraction to give an extra boost to ventricular filling, which increases stroke volume according to the Frank-Starling principle. This "atrial kick" is most important in patients with ventricular failure. The long refractory period of the AV node protects the ventricles from excessively rapid stimulation; very rapid heart rates have a reduced cardiac output and may deteriorate into ventricular fibrillation. Cells around the AV node have pacemaker potential and can pace the heart should discharges from the sinus node fail or fall below a certain rate.

Electric impulses leave the inferior pole of the AV node along the bundle of His, which travels downward along the posterior margin of the membranous portion of the intraventricular septum to reach the top of the muscular portion. The common bundle is only 1 to 2 cm in length before it divides at the crest of the muscular intraventricular septum into the right and left bundle branches (RBB and LBB). The RBB is a compact group of fibers that travels down to the apex of the right ventricle before separating into smaller branches. The LBB travels 2 to 3 cm before fanning out into a virtual sheet of fibers to cover the left ventricle. There are two relatively distinct pathways to the base of the papillary muscles, the left anterior superior fascicle (LASF) and the left posterior inferior fascicle (LPIF).

The blood supply to the RBB and LASF is from the same sources: about half the time from both the AV nodal artery and branches from the left anterior descending coronary artery, and the other half from the left anterior descending artery alone. The LPIF is supplied about half the time from the AV nodal artery and the other half by both the AV nodal artery and left anterior descending artery. Infarction in the region supplied by the left anterior descending artery is capable of affecting the RBB and LASF but very rarely the LPIF.

Accessory tracts are embryologic remnants of myocardium found in the AV annulus that can transmit electric impulses between the atria and ventricles, bypassing all or part of the AV node and infranodal system. These bypass tracts are the anatomic basis for the preexcitation syndrome.

## THE NORMAL ECG

The clinical surface ECG records the potential (voltage) differences between "neutral" ground and recording electrodes. The ECG is generated by the electrical activity of the heart and depicts the net sum of this activity recorded over time. By convention, a potential difference that points toward a recording electrode is assigned a positive deflection on the ECG, and a potential that points away from the recording electrode is assigned a negative deflection. Also by convention, routine ECG recordings are obtained with paper speed at 25 mm/s (2.5 cm/s) and signal calibration of 1.0 mV/10 mm (1.0 cm).

In Fig. 22-1, depolarization starts on the left side of the ventricular septum and initially proceeds to the right; this is recorded as a small negative deflection in the recording electrode. Subsequent depolarization involves the free walls of both ventricles, and since the left side has a much larger mass, the net sum of electrical activity is directed toward the recording electrode and a tall, positive deflection is recorded.

The P-QRS-T complex of the normal ECG represents electrical activity over one cardiac cycle (Fig. 22-2).

The P wave indicates atrial depolarization; atrial repolarization is usually obscured by the QRS complex. The normal P wave duration is less than 0.10 s (2.5 mm), and normal amplitude is less than 0.3 mV (3 mm). A P wave originating from the sinus node is directed inferiorly and to the left on the frontal plane.

The PR interval is the time between the onset of depolarization in the atria and ventricles and is commonly used as an estimation of AV nodal conduction time. For adults in sinus rhythm, the PR interval is 0.12 to 0.20 s (3 to 5 mm).

The QRS complex indicates ventricular depolarization. In general, depolarization starts on the endocardium and spreads outward to the epicardium. Despite the large amount of myocardium that must be depolarized, the specialized conducting system makes this a rapid process and the normal QRS duration is 0.06 to 0.10 s (1.5 to 2.5 mm). Any delay in conduction (such as bundle branch blocks) results in a wide QRS. Depolarizations which originate in the ventricles

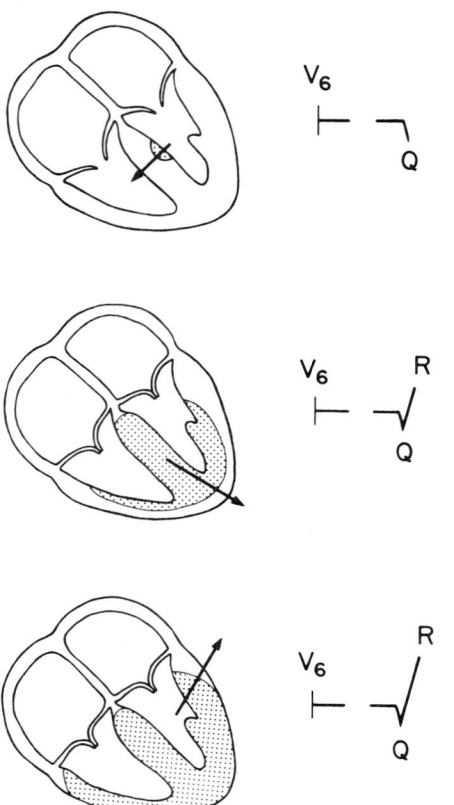

**Fig. 22-1.** Ventricular depolarization recorded in lead $V_6$.

or from a portion of the conducting system below the bifurcation of the bundle of His also have a wide QRS complex because of the slow cell-to-cell transmission (as opposed to propagation over the faster conduction system) of the electric impulse required to activate all the ventricular myocardium.

While small negative initial deflections (Q waves) are normal, large Q waves can be due to an electrically unexcitable area just under the recording electrode. An abnormal Q wave has a width of 0.04 s or greater and a height one-third that of the QRS complex.

The ST segment represents the plateau phase of ventricular depolarization. While the ST segment is usually isoelectric, small deviations, less than 0.1 mV (1 mm), are not always pathological.

The T wave indicates ventricular repolarization. Whereas depolarization is a rapid, near-simultaneous release of stored energy (like the release of a compressed spring), repolarization is a slow, asynchronous event where the metabolic machinery of each individual cell restores the transmembrane potential. Therefore, the T-wave duration is much longer and the amplitude much lower than those of the QRS complex. In general, repolarization starts on the epicardium and spreads to the endocardium. Many factors can influence this normal repolarization sequence: (1) metabolic (hypoxia, fever, drugs), (2) autonomic stimuli (abdominal pain, hyperventilation), (3) myocardial hypertrophy, (4) myocardial ischemia or inflammation, and (5) abnormal depolarization.

The QT interval represents the total duration of ventricular depolarization. While QT duration is commonly between 0.33 and 0.42 s, it does vary inversely with heart rate. The corrected interval is obtained by dividing the measured QT interval (in seconds) by the square root of the R-R interval (in seconds). The normal corrected QT interval is less than 0.47 s.

The U wave is produced by ventricular afterpotentials and can be seen as a normal component of the surface ECG, especially in leads $V_1$ and $V_2$. Afterpotentials that occur before full restoration of the transmembrane resting potential are considered early and are associated with disorders characterized by a prolonged QT interval. Early afterpotentials are exacerbated by slow heart rates. Delayed afterpotentials are seen after membrane potential is restored to the resting level and are associated with ischemia, electrolyte disorders, or sympathomimetic stimulation. Delayed afterpotentials are enhanced by faster heart rates.

## CARDIAC ARRHYTHMIAS

Cardiac arrhythmias and conduction disturbances can be classified according to a number of methods: (1) heart rate; (2) site of origin, delay, or block; (3) mechanism; or (4) ratio of atrial to ventricular depolarizations (P waves to QRS complexes). For the cardiac arrhythmias, this chapter separates them into the site of origin.

Cardiac arrhythmias may decrease cardiac output if the ventricular rate is too fast or too slow. In the normal resting adult, heart rates between 40 and 160 are usually well tolerated as physiological adapta-

**Fig. 22-2.** Normal P-QRS-T ECG pattern.

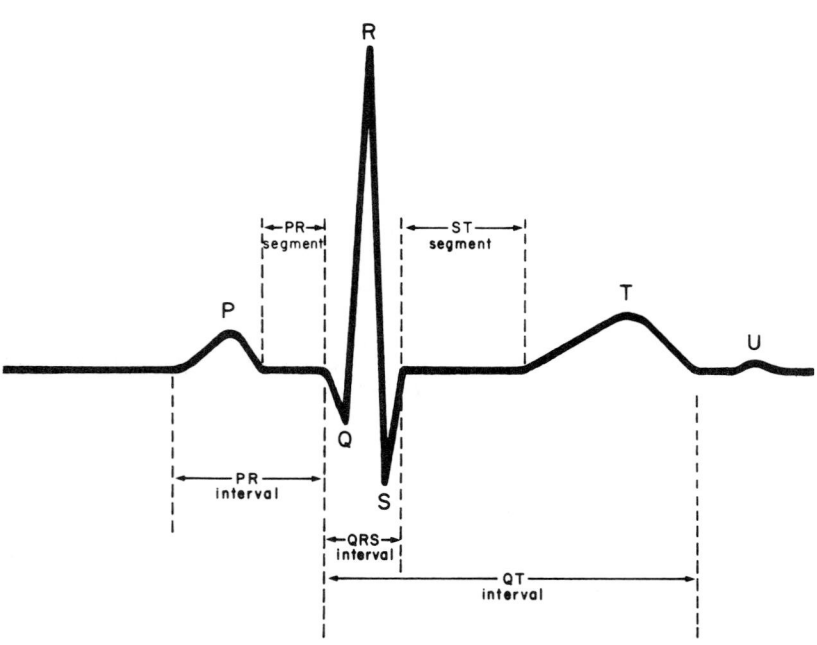

tions are able to maintain an adequate cardiac output and blood pressure. However, in adults with significant heart or peripheral arterial disease, rates below 50 or above 120 may produce ischemia in susceptible organs.

## Mechanisms of Tachyarrhythmias

Tachyarrhythmias are presumed to be caused by three mechanisms: ectopic focus, reentry, or triggered arrhythmias. While treatment would appear to be best directed by an understanding of the underlying process, uncertainty still exists over the precise mechanism of many arrhythmias, and therapy is still often empirical.

An ectopic focus is an area of the heart, away from the normal sinus node pacemaker, that acquires independent pacemaker activity and usurps the pacemaking role, resulting in single or multiple extra depolarizations. These ectopic pacemakers can be due to either (1) enhanced automaticity of subsidiary pacemaker cells (i.e., in the AV node or infranodal conducting system) or (2) abnormal automaticity of myocardial cells which seldom possess pacemaking activity (i.e., Purkinje cells). Arrhythmias due to an ectopic focus usually have a gradual onset ("warm-up period") and offset, as opposed to the abrupt onset seen with reentry or triggered mechanisms.

Reentry occurs when a closed loop of conducting tissue transmits an electric impulse around the loop, either once or repeatedly, and stimulates an atrial and/or ventricular depolarization with each pass around the circuit. Electrophysiologically, reentry requires a temporary or permanent unidirectional block in one limb of the circuit and slower-than-normal conduction around the entire circuit. Both these conditions occur when cardiac conducting tissue is stimulated during the partial refractory period (before full repolarization).

For example, the inciting impulse traveling in the normal downward direction encounters the two limbs of the reentry circuit, finds limb *a* blocked, and travels down limb *b* (Fig. 22-3). Upon reaching the bottom portion of the circuit where the two limbs rejoin, the impulse can then travel retrograde up limb *a* and reach the upper connection of the circuit. Normally, conduction is so rapid that the impulse would encounter limb *b* still refractory to stimulation, and no further propagation would occur. However, if conduction around the circuit is slow enough, limb *b* would be able to conduct the impulse again in the antegrade direction. With the right size circuit and conduction velocity, an electric impulse can be maintained traveling around the circuit in a cyclical manner. Each time the impulse passes the upper and lower limb connections, a signal can be sent out stimulating atrial and ventricular depolarizations.

Reentry can occur around anatomically defined circuits, resulting in a regular rapid rhythm such as paroxysmal supraventricular tachycardia. Conversely, reentry can also occur in a disorganized and

chaotic fashion through a syncytium of myocardial tissue, as seen, for example, in atrial or ventricular fibrillation.

Triggered arrhythmias are due to the oscillations of the transmembrane potential during or after repolarization (afterpotentials), that may reach threshold and trigger a second complete depolarization. Once triggered, this process may be self-sustaining. Triggered arrhythmias associated with early afterpotentials are enhanced by slow heart rates and usually treated by accelerating the ventricular rate with positive chronotropic drugs or electrical pacing. Triggered arrhythmias associated with delayed afterpotentials are usually seen in states of myocardial ischemia and are enhanced by fast heart rates. Treatment is usually effective with agents that have a negative chronotropic action.

The urgency with which tachyarrhythmias require treatment is guided by two considerations: (1) evidence of hypoperfusion (shock, altered mental status, anginal chest pain, or pulmonary edema) and (2) the potential to degenerate into a more serious arrhythmia or cardiac arrest. The two treatment methods most commonly used are intravenous drugs for the clinically stable patient and synchronized cardioversion for the unstable patient. Occasional tachyarrhythmias may be treated with a short period of overdrive electrical pacing in selected patients.

## Mechanisms of Bradyarrhythmias

Bradyarrhythmias can be caused by two mechanisms: depression of sinus nodal activity or conduction system blocks. In both situations, subsidiary pacemakers take over and pace the heart, and provided the pacemaker is located above the bifurcation of the bundle of His, the rate is generally adequate to maintain cardiac output.

The need for emergent treatment of bradycardias is guided by two considerations: (1) evidence of hypoperfusion and (2) the potential to degenerate into a more profound bradycardia or ventricular asystole. In general, emergent treatment is not required, unless: (1) the heart rate is below 50 and there is clinical evidence of hypoperfusion or (2) the bradycardia is due to structural disease of the infranodal conducting system (either transient or permanent) that has a risk of progressing to complete AV block. The first group of patients require immediate treatment during assessment of the etiology of the bradycardia and consideration as to whether internal carding will be required. The second group of patients do not always require immediate treatment but should be monitored closely with therapy readily available while arrangements are made for further evaluation and possible internal cardiac pacing.

Three methods are currently available for emergent treatment of bradycardias: atropine, isoproterenol, and transcutaneous cardiac pacing.

Atropine should be the initial agent, at doses of 0.5 mg IV every 5 min until the desired response is achieved or a total vagolytic dose (about 0.05 mg/kg in humans) is given. Usually, if no response is seen by a dose of 2.0 mg, further doses are not effective. The vast majority of bradycardias due to problems of either the sinus or AV node respond to atropine. Even some patients with infranodal blocks may respond, so atropine deserves consideration in most bradycardias when emergent treatment is desired.

Isoproterenol can be used when atropine is ineffective, generally as a result of disease of the infranodal conducting system. Isoproterenol is given as a constant infusion, starting at a rate of around 0.5 µg/min and increasing as required to maintain a heart rate of 60. Isoproterenol increases myocardial oxygen demand, stimulates ventricular ectopy, and produces peripheral vasodilation, making it a less attractive agent than atropine. The reported response to isoproterenol is less than that observed with atropine, although isoproterenol is usually only used in patients who fail while receiving atropine; it is difficult to say how effective isoproterenol would be if used initially.

External cardiac pacing represents a reawareness of an old concept

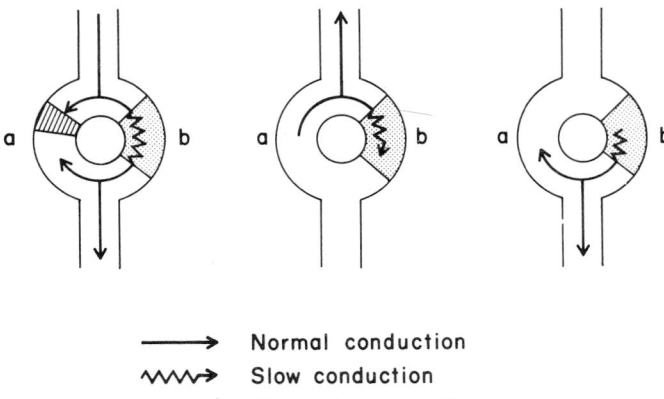

→ Normal conduction
〰→ Slow conduction
→| Blocked conduction

**Fig. 22-3.** Reentry circuit.

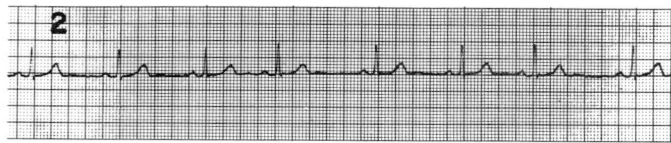

**Fig. 22-4.** Sinus arrhythmia.

and should be available in every emergency facility. External pacing is most successful when the myocardium is still responsive to electrical stimuli (pulses with each depolarization) and must be less successful when the myocardium is unresponsive (pulseless bradycardias or asystole). External pacing is discussed later in this chapter.

Internal pacing is the definitive treatment for progressive or persistent bradycardias. Emergent internal pacing is possible with the use of balloon-tipped flotation catheters, although it is often technically difficult to achieve stable placement in a patient with low cardiac output without fluoroscopic guidance.

## Supraventricular Arrhythmias

### Sinus Arrhythmia

Some variation in the sinus node discharge rate is common, but if the variation exceeds 0.12 s between the longest and shortest intervals, sinus arrhythmia is present. The ECG characteristics of sinus arrhythmia are: (1) normal sinus P waves and PR intervals, (2) 1:1 AV conduction, and (3) variation of at least 0.12 s between the shortest and longest P-P interval (Fig. 22-4).

**Clinical Significance**

Sinus arrhythmia is most commonly found in children and young adults, disappearing with advancing age. Sinus arrhythmia varies in two manners: the more common phasic (respiratory) variety and the less common nonphasic variety. In the phasic variety, the sinus node rate accelerates during inspiration and decelerates during expiration due to changes in vagal tone occurring with respiration (Bainbridge reflex). The irregularity in either the phasic or nonphasic varieties can be exaggerated by conditions which increase vagal tone. During the long intervals of sinus arrhythmia, junctional escape beats may be seen.

**Treatment**

None is required.

### Sinus Bradycardia

Sinus bradycardia occurs when the sinus node rate falls below 60. The ECG characteristics of sinus bradycardia are: (1) normal sinus P waves and PR intervals, (2) 1:1 AV conduction, and (3) atrial rate below 60 (Fig. 22-5).

**Clinical Significance**

Sinus bradycardia represents a suppression of the sinus node discharge rate, usually in response to three categories of stimuli: (1) physiological (well-conditioned athletes, during sleep, with vagal stimulation), (2) pharmacological (digoxin, narcotics, reserpine, β-adrenergic antagonists, calcium-channel blockers, quinidine), or (3) pathological (acute inferior myocardial infarction, increased intracranial pressure, carotid sinus hypersensitivity, hypothyroidism).

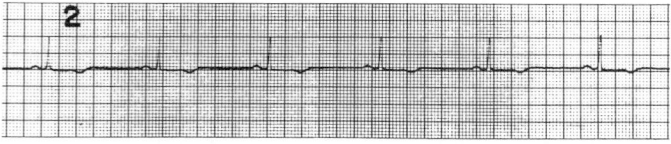

**Fig. 22-5.** Sinus bradycardia, rate 44.

**Treatment**

1. Sinus bradycardia usually does not require specific treatment unless the heart rate is below 50 and there is evidence of hypoperfusion.
2. Initial therapy should begin with atropine as previously described. Most patients will respond to one or two doses.
3. Isoproterenol can be used if atropine is ineffective.
4. External cardiac pacing can be used in the patient refractory to atropine or isoproterenol.
5. Internal pacing is required in the patient with symptomatic recurrent or persistent sinus bradycardia.

### Sinus Tachycardia

Sinus tachycardia originates from acceleration of the sinus node discharge rate. The ECG characteristics of sinus tachycardia are: (1) normal sinus P waves and PR intervals, (2) an atrial rate usually between 100 and 160, and (3) normally 1:1 conduction between the atria and ventricles (although rapid rates can occur with AV blocks) (Fig. 22-6).

**Clinical Significance**

Sinus tachycardia represents an acceleration of the sinus node discharge rate, usually in response to three categories of stimuli: (1) physiological (infants and children, exertion, anxiety, emotions), (2) pharmacological (atropine, epinephrine and other sympathomimetics, alcohol, nicotine, caffeine), or (3) pathological (fever, hypoxia, anemia, hypovolemia, pulmonary embolism). In many of these conditions, the increased heart rate is an effort to increase cardiac output to match increased circulatory needs.

**Treatment**

1. No specific treatment is usually required, but any underlying conditions should be investigated and treated.
2. Some patients with acute myocardial infarction have an "inappropriate" tachycardia and may benefit from slowing heart rate with β-adrenergic antagonists.

### Premature Atrial Contractions (PACs)

PACs originate from ectopic pacemakers anywhere in the atrium other than the sinus node. The ECG characteristics of PACs are: (1) ectopic P′ wave appears sooner (premature) than the next expected sinus beat, (2) the ectopic P′ wave has a different shape and direction, and (3) the ectopic P′ wave may or may not be conducted through the AV node (Fig. 22-7). A PAC is not conducted through the AV node if it reaches the AV node during the absolute refractory period and is conducted with a delay (longer P′R interval) during the relative refractory period. Most PACs are conducted with typical QRS complexes, but some may be conducted aberrantly through the infranodal system. The sinus node is often depolarized and "reset" so that while the interval following the PAC is often slightly longer than the previous cycle length, the pause is less than fully compensatory.

**Clinical Significance**

PACs are common in all ages and often seen in the absence of heart disease. It is generally assumed, although remains unproven, that

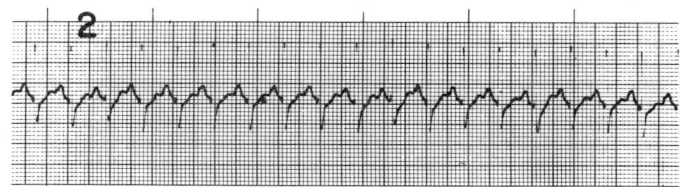

**Fig. 22-6.** Sinus tachycardia, rate 176.

**Fig. 22-7.** Premature atrial contractions (PACs). Top: ectopic P′ waves (arrows). Bottom: atrial bigeminy.

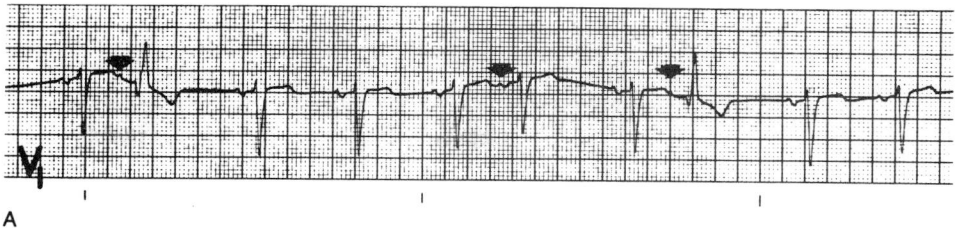

A

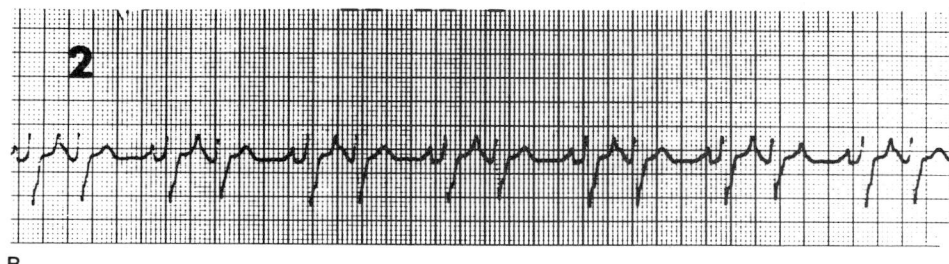

B

stress, fatigue, alcohol, tobacco, or coffee may precipitate PACs. Frequent PACs may also be seen in chronic lung disease, ischemic heart disease, or digitalis toxicity. PACs may trigger sustained atrial tachycardia, flutter, or fibrillation.

### Treatment

1. Any precipitating drugs or toxins should be discontinued.
2. Underlying disorders should be treated.
3. PACs that produce symptoms or initiate sustained tachycardias can be suppressed with quinidine, procainamide, or β-adrenergic antagonists.

## Multifocal Atrial Tachycardia (MFAT)

Multifocal atrial tachycardia (MFAT, also known as "chaotic atrial rhythm" or "wandering atrial pacemaker") is an irregular rhythm caused by at least two different sites of atrial ectopy. The ECG characteristics of MFAT are: (1) three or more differently shaped P waves, (2) varying PP, PR, and RR intervals, and (3) atrial rhythm usually between 100 and 180 (Fig. 22-8). MFAT can be confused with atrial flutter or fibrillation.

### Clinical Significance

MFAT is most often found in elderly patients with decompensated chronic lung disease, but also may complicate congestive heart failure, sepsis, or be caused by methylxanthine toxicity. Digoxin toxicity is an unlikely cause of MFAT.

### Treatment

1. Treatment is directed toward the underlying disorder. With decompensated lung disease, oxygen and bronchodilators improve pulmonary function, arterial oxygenation, and decrease atrial ectopy.
2. Specific antiarrhythmic treatment is uncommonly indicated. Standard antiarrhythmics appear to be ineffective in suppressing these multiple sites of atrial ectopy, and toxic side effects from these

agents have been reported. Likewise, attempts to slow the ventricular rate by depressing AV nodal conduction with digoxin is also difficult without producing toxic side effects. Recently, three modes of therapy have been described that may be helpful in some patients. Magnesium sulfate 2 g IV over 60 s followed by a constant infusion of 1 to 2 g/h has been shown to reduce atrial ectopy in these patients and sometimes is associated with conversion to sinus rhythm. The full antiarrhythmic effect of magnesium requires supplemental potassium to maintain serum potassium levels above 4 mEq/L. Intravenous verapamil (5 to 10 mg) slows the ventricular response in most patients, decreases atrial ectopy in some patients, and is associated with conversion to sinus rhythm in many patients. The β-adrenergic antagonists esmolol, acebutolol, and metoprolol all decrease the ventricular rate in MFAT, and metoprolol is associated with conversion to sinus rhythm in a majority of patients. However, the value of such specific antiarrhythmic treatment in MFAT is unproved.
3. Cardioversion has no effect on these multiple sites of atrial ectopy.

## Atrial Flutter

Atrial flutter is a rhythm that originates from a small area within the atria. The exact mechanism—whether reentry, automatic focus, or triggered arrhythmia—is not yet known. As studied with intracardiac electrodes, electrical activity usually begins in the inferior right atrium and propagates upward and to the left. ECG characteristics of atrial flutter are: (1) regular atrial rate between 250 and 350 (most commonly 280 and 320); (2) sawtooth flutter waves directed superiorly and most visible in leads II, III, aV$_F$; and (3) AV block, usually 2:1, but occasionally greater or irregular (Fig. 22-9). One-to-one AV conduction may occur in patients with bypass tracts or when AV nodal conduction is enhanced by drugs such as quinidine. Aberrant conduction may occur and cause atrial flutter to resemble ventricular tachycardia. Carotid sinus massage is a useful technique to slow the ventricular response, increase the AV block, and unmask flutter waves.

**Fig. 22-8.** Multifocal atrial tachycardia (MFAT).

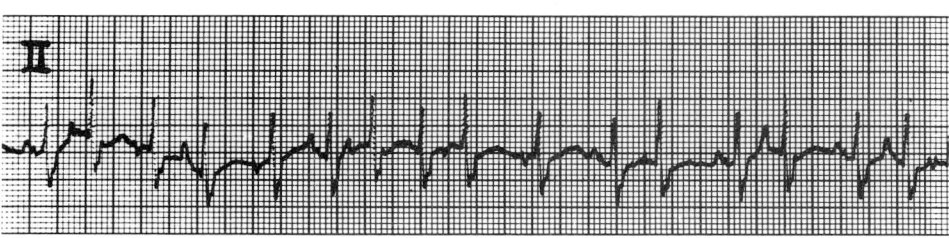

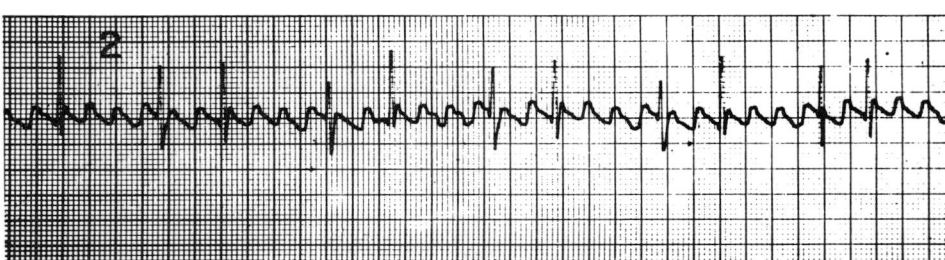

**Fig. 22-9.** Atrial flutter.

### Clinical Significance

Atrial flutter rarely occurs in patients without heart disease. It is most commonly seen in patients with ischemic heart disease or acute myocardial infarction. Less common causes include congestive cardiomyopathy, pulmonary embolus, myocarditis, blunt chest trauma, and, rarely, digoxin toxicity. Atrial flutter may be a transitional arrhythmia between sinus rhythm and atrial fibrillation.

### Treatment

1. Low-energy cardioversion (25 to 50 J) is very successful in converting more than 90 percent of cases of atrial flutter into sinus rhythm. Energies less than 10 J should be avoided as they are more likely to convert atrial flutter into atrial fibrillation than into sinus rhythm.
2. If cardioversion is contraindicated, ventricular rate control can be achieved with digoxin, verapamil, diltiazem, esmolol, or propranolol.
3. Quinidine or procainamide can be used after ventricular rate control is achieved to chemically slow or convert atrial flutter or prevent recurrence of the arrhythmia.
4. Intravenous esmolol will convert up to 60 percent of patients with new onset atrial flutter to sinus rhythm.
5. Intravenous verapamil will occasionally convert atrial flutter into sinus rhythm (up to 30 percent) or atrial fibrillation (up to 20 percent).
6. Some of the newer antiarrhythmics may also have a role in the chemical conversion of atrial flutter. For example, early reports indicate that intravenous flecainide is associated with a conversion to sinus rhythm about 40 percent of the time.

## Atrial Fibrillation

Atrial fibrillation occurs when there are multiple small areas of atrial myocardium continuously discharging and contracting. There is no uniform atrial depolarization and contraction, but instead, only a quivering of the atrial wall. While the atrial rate is usually above 400, the ventricular rate is limited by the refractory period of the AV node. The ECG characteristics of atrial fibrillation are: (1) fibrillatory waves of atrial activity, best seen in leads $V_1$, $V_2$, $V_3$, and $aV_F$; and (2) irregular ventricular response, usually around 170 to 180 in patients with a healthy AV node (Fig. 22-10). Disease or drugs (especially digoxin) may reduce AV node conduction and markedly slow ventricular response. A more rapid ventricular response may be seen in patients with bypass tracts; rates above 200 are possible. In this case, since ventricular activation occurs by way of the bypass tract,

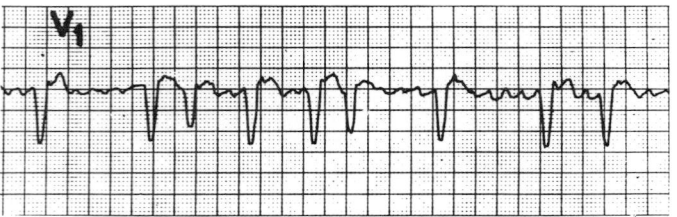

**Fig. 22-10.** Atrial fibrillation.

the QRS complex is usually wide. In addition, aberrancy—usually with a right bundle branch block configuration—is possible with rapid rates alone.

### Clinical Significance

Atrial fibrillation can occur in a paroxysmal or sustained manner. Predisposing factors for atrial fibrillation are increased atrial size and mass, increased vagal tone, and variation in refractory periods between different parts of atrial myocardium. Atrial fibrillation is usually found in association with four disorders: rheumatic heart disease, hypertension, ischemic heart disease, and thyrotoxicosis. Less common causes are chronic lung disease, pericarditis, acute alcoholic intoxication, or atrial septal defect.

In patients with left ventricular failure, left atrial contraction makes an important contribution to cardiac output. The loss of effective atrial contraction, as in atrial fibrillation, may produce heart failure in these patients. Atrial fibrillation also predisposes to peripheral venous and atrial emboli, with the risk of pulmonary and systemic arterial embolism. Up to 15 percent of patients per year in chronic atrial fibrillation have at least one embolic episode. Conversion from chronic atrial fibrillation to sinus rhythm also carries up to a 1 to 2 percent risk of arterial embolism.

### Treatment

1. Atrial fibrillation with a rapid ventricular response and acute hemodynamic deterioration should be treated with synchronized cardioversion. Over 60 percent can be converted with 100 J and over 80 percent with 200 J. Conversion to and retention in sinus rhythm is more likely when atrial fibrillation is of short duration and the atria are not greatly dilated. If initial cardioversion is unsuccessful, procainamide IV should be given to facilitate further cardioversion attempts. Maintenance of sinus rhythm can be enhanced by oral quinidine or low-dose amiodarone. Meta-analysis and decision analysis of post conversion antiarrhythmic treatment has found that the benefits of maintaining sinus rhythm with antiarrhythmics is partially offset by an increase in sudden death; presumably due to the proarrhythmic properties of these drugs.
2. In more stable patients, the first priority is to achieve ventricular rate control. Intravenous digoxin is an effective agent for this purpose, although the onset of action is slow with a mean time of over 11 hours to achieve ventricular rate control. Diltiazem 20 mg (0.25 mg/kg) IV over two minutes is extremely effective in achieving ventricular rate control with the peak response seen in two to seven minutes. An infusion of 10 mg/h is usually started after the initial dose to maintain control and a second dose of 25 mg (0.35 mg/kg) can be given at 15 minutes if rate control is not achieved. Verapamil 5 to 10 mg IV is effective in slowing the ventricular response in 60 to 70 percent of patients with atrial fibrillation and converts 10 to 15 percent into sinus rhythm. Intravenous β-adrenergic blockers (e.g., esmolol and propranolol) are effective, especially in patients with rheumatic mitral stenosis, but the depressive effects on myocardial contractility make them a poor agent to use in patients with ventricular failure.
3. Once ventricular rate control has been achieved, chemical conversion can be considered with procainamide, quinidine, or verapamil. Procainamide IV has also been used as a single agent to

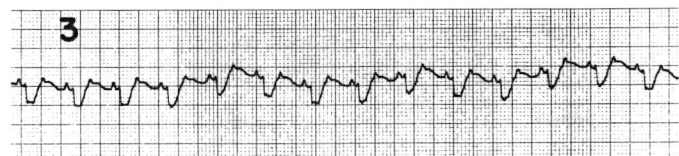

**Fig. 22-11.** Ectopic supraventricular, tachycardia (STV) with 2:1 AV conduction.

chemically convert atrial fibrillation of short duration into sinus rhythm. The intravenous administration of a number of the newer antiarrhythmias (disopyramide, pirmenol, flecainide, or amiodarone) is associated with a 40 to 70 percent conversion rate of acute atrial fibrillation to sinus rhythm. Because of the risk of intraatrial thrombi and arterial embolization, patients with atrial fibrillation of more than 2 days duration should be anticoagulated systemically for 1 to 3 weeks prior to attempts at either chemical or electrical conversion. An alternative to anticoagulation is to exclude atrial thrombi by transesophageal echocardiography; those without visible thrombi can be safely cardioverted without the need for pre-conversion oral anticoagulation.

4. Patients with a slow ventricular response not due to digitalis have AV node disease and probably a more generalized disorder of cardiac conduction (sick sinus syndrome). These patients are at increased risk for profound bradycardias or asystole following cardioversion or antiarrhythmic drug therapy.

## Supraventricular Tachycardia (SVT)

Supraventricular tachycardia is a regular, rapid rhythm that arises from either reentry or an ectopic pacemaker in areas above the bifurcation of the bundle of His. The reentrant variety is clinically the most common. These patients often present with acute, symptomatic episodes termed *paroxysmal supraventricular tachycardia* (PSVT).

Ectopic SVT usually originates in the atria with an atrial rate of 100 to 250 (most commonly 140 to 200) (Fig. 22-11). The regular P waves can be mistaken for atrial flutter or, if there is a 2:1 AV block, sinus rhythm.

Reentrant SVT constitutes the majority of patients with SVT: about 60 percent of these patients have reentry within the AV node and 20 percent have reentry involving a bypass tract. The remainder have reentry in other sites. In the normal heart, reentrant SVT at the typical rates of 160 to 200 is often tolerated for hours or days. However, cardiac output is always depressed—regardless of the blood pressure—and rapid rates may produce heart failure.

Reentrant SVT within the AV node usually is initiated when an ectopic atrial impulse encounters the AV node during the partially refractory period (Fig. 22-12). There are two functionally different parallel conducting limbs within the AV node that are connected above at the atrial end and below at the ventricular end of the node. This circuit is capable of sustained reentry when properly stimulated. In AV nodal reentry, the P wave is usually buried in the QRS complex and not visible, there is 1:1 conduction, and the QRS complex is normal.

In patients with bypass tracts, the two parallel limbs of the reentry circuit are the AV node and the bypass tract, with connections at the atrial and ventricular ends by myocardial cells. While reentry can occur in either direction, it usually occurs in a direction that goes down the AV node and up the bypass tract, producing a narrow QRS complex. In the Wolff-Parkinson-White syndrome, about 85 percent of the reentrant SVTs have narrow QRS complexes.

### Clinical Significance

Ectopic SVT may be seen in patients with acute myocardial infarction, chronic lung disease, pneumonia, alcoholic intoxication, and digoxin toxicity [where it is often associated with AV block and termed *paroxysmal atrial tachycardia* (PAT) with block]. It is commonly held that a high percentage of SVT with block, as much as 75 percent, is due to digoxin toxicity. However, not all studies have found this to be the case. The common arrhythmias of digoxin toxicity are listed in Table 22-1.

Reentrant SVT can occur in a normal heart, or in association with rheumatic heart disease, acute pericarditis, myocardial infarction, mitral valve prolapse, or one of the preexcitation syndromes.

SVT often causes a sensation of palpitations and light-headedness. In patients with coronary artery disease, anginal chest pain and dyspnea may occur from the rapid heart rate. Frank heart failure and pulmonary edema may occur in patients with poor left ventricular function. The loss of atrial contribution to cardiac output is often poorly tolerated in patients with left ventricular failure.

### Treatment

Ectopic SVT due to digoxin toxicity is treated by:

1. Discontinuing the digoxin.
2. As long as there is not a high-grade AV block, correcting any existing hypokalemia to bring serum potassium into the high-normal range in an effort to reduce atrial ectopy.
3. Digoxin-specific antibody fragments (Fab) should be considered for patients with hemodynamic deterioration or serious ventricular arrhythmias due to digoxin toxicity.
4. Atrial ectopy can be reduced by either phenytoin IV, lidocaine IV, or magnesium IV. Published reports are not adequate for determination of the response rate, risks, and benefits of each agent, so the choice is often guided by personal preference. Historically, phenytoin has been the most commonly used drug, but its response rate has not been impressive and toxic side effects are common with full loading doses (15 to 18 mg/kg IV). Lidocaine

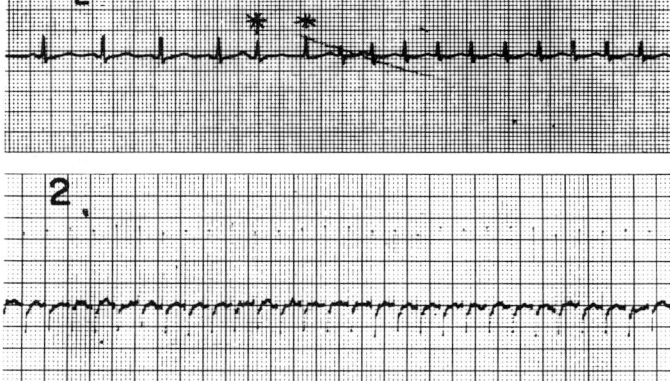

**Fig. 22-12.** Reentrant supraventricular tachycardia (SVT). Top: 2d PAC (*) initiates run of PAT. Bottom: SVT, rate 286.

**Table 22-1.** Common Arrhythmias of Digoxin Toxicity (Approximate Incidence)

| |
| --- |
| PVCs (60%) |
|   Unifocal, multifocal, bigeminy, or trigeminy |
| AV block (20%) |
|   Second-degree |
|     Mobitz I, Mobitz II |
|   Third degree |
| Ectopic SVT (20–30%) |
|   Rate 70–130 |
|     Gradual appearance and disappearance |
|     AV dissociation and/or block |
| Junctional escape beats (10%) |
| Ventricular tachycardia (10%) |
|   Bidirectional ventricular tachycardia associated with high mortality |
| Sinus bradycardia, SA block, and sinus pause (1–10%) |

has not been considered a useful agent for this arrhythmia, but a recent report indicates some benefit. Recent studies indicate that magnesium sulfate 1 g IV impressively reduces atrial ectopy due to digoxin toxicity, and perhaps this agent has a greater effect than phenytoin or lidocaine.

5. Cardioversion is not effective and is potentially hazardous.

Ectopic SVT not due to digoxin toxicity is treated by:

1. Digoxin, verapamil, diltiazem, esmolol, or propranolol to slow the ventricular rate.
2. Antiarrhythmic therapy with either quinidine, procainamide, or magnesium.

Reentrant SVT can be converted by impeding conduction through one limb of the reentry circuit; sustained reentry is then impossible and extinguishes, allowing sinus rhythm to resume ventricular pacing.

1. Maneuvers which increase vagal tone have been shown to slow conduction and prolong the refractory period in the AV node. These maneuvers can be done by themselves or after administration of drugs.
   a. Carotid sinus massage attempts to massage the carotid sinus and its baroreceptors against the transverse process of C6. Massage should be done for 10 s at a time, first attempted on the side of the nondominant cerebral hemisphere, and should never be done simultaneously on both sides. Prolonged AV block during carotid massage may occur in patients with AV node disease or who are on digoxin. Patients with carotid artery stenosis may develop cerebral ischemia or infarction from overvigorous carotid massage.
   b. Facial immersion in cold water for 6 to 7 s with the nostrils held closed ("diving reflex"). This maneuver is particularly effective in infants.
   c. Gagging.
   d. The pneumatic antishock garment (PASG) increases arterial pressure, thereby stimulating the carotid sinus. One published report has described the effectiveness of the PASG in SVT, but many other physicians have not found it to be so useful.
   e. The Valsalva maneuver done in the supine position appears to be the most effective vagal maneuver for the conversion of reentrant SVT. For maximal effectiveness, the strain phase must be adequate (usually at least 10 s) with slowing or conversion seen during the release phase.
2. Adenosine is an ultrashort-acting (20 s) agent that produces AV block and has been observed to convert over 90 percent of reentrant SVT. The initial dose is 6 mg rapid IV bolus. If no effect is seen within 2 min, a second dose of 12 mg can be given. There is no proven benefit to repeated doses or administration of more than 20 mg. Half or more of patients experience distressing, albeit transient, side effects. Because adenosine possesses no sustained antiarrhythmic effect, subsequent ectopic beats are able to initial the arrhythmia again, and early recurrences of SVT are seen in up to 25 percent of patients. The major advantage of adenosine is its ultrashort effect and its lack of hypotensive or myocardial depressive activity. Adenosine is also safe and effective in unstable patients (chest pain and/or hypotension) with reentrant SVT.
3. Verapamil, 0.075 to 0.15 mg/kg (3 to 10 mg) IV over 15 to 60 s, with a repeat dose in 30 min if necessary. Studies have found that more than 90 percent of adults with reentrant SVT will respond within 1 to 2 min to verapamil. In patients with a normal blood pressure, intravenous verapamil is almost always associated with a decrease in blood pressure, even following successful conversion of SVT. The falls in systolic and mean arterial pressures are around 20 and 10 mmHg, respectively. The drop in

blood pressure due to verapamil can be prevented and/or treated with intravenous calcium without reducing the antiarrhythmic action of verapamil. While the use of different calcium doses and salts have been reported, 90 mg of elemental calcium given IV over three to six minutes appears safe and effective (90 mg elemental calcium = 10 ml calcium gluconate 10 percent solution = 3.3 ml calcium chloride 10 percent solution). Whenever verapamil is used intravenously, calcium should be readily available. Intravenous verapamil generally is considered to be contraindicated in the hypotensive patient. Studies of intravenous verapamil in hypotensive patients with SVT report an excellent conversion rate (80 percent or better), the ventricular rate almost always slows, and rarely does the systolic blood pressure decrease without a change in ventricular rate.

4. Diltiazem 20 mg (0.25 mg/kg) IV over 2 min is reported to be 75 to 100 percent effective in converting reentrant SVT.
5. Parasympathetic tone can be increased with edrophonium. A standard treatment protocol is a 1 mg IV test dose, a wait of 3 to 5 min, followed by 5 to 10 mg IV over 60 s. Historically, edrophonium does not have the 90 percent response rate seen with verapamil.
6. Vagal tone can be enhanced by pharmacologically evaluating blood pressure with a pure peripheral vasoconstrictor; do not use agents with β-adrenergic activity. This method should be combined with carotid sinus massage. Blood pressure should be monitored frequently, and diastolic pressure should not be allowed to exceed 130 mmHg. This method should not be used if hypertension is already present.
   a. Metaraminol 200 mg/500 mL $D_5W$ or norepinephrine 4 mg/500 mL $D_5W$ can be infused at rates of 1 to 2 mL/min and titrated until the rhythm converts.
   b. Methoxamine or phenylephrine 0.5 to 1.0 mg IV over 2 to 3 min, with repeat doses as required.
7. Esmolol is an intravenous β-adrenergic blocker with an ultrashort duration of activity that can be titrated to effect. This agent can be used to control the ventricular rate in most tachycardias of supraventricular origin and is capable of converting about half of reentrant SVT. Esmolol is given as a bolus dose of 300 μg/kg over 60 s, followed by an infusion starting at 50 μg/kg per minute. If there is an inadequate response after 2 to 5 min, repeat bolus of 300 μg/kg and increases in the infusion rate in 50 μg/kg per minute increments should be done. The maximal recommended infusion rate is 300 μg/kg per minute, although most patients respond to rates of 200 μg/kg per minute or less. With aggressive dosing regimens, hypotension occurs in about half of patients but can be quickly reversed by halting the infusion.
8. Propranolol 0.5 to 1.0 mg IV slowly over 60 s, repeated every 5 min, until the rhythm converts or the total dose reaches 0.1 mg/kg. Overall, propranolol has about a 50 percent success rate in converting reentrant SVT: about 80 percent with AV nodal reentry and 15 to 20 percent with accessory tract retrograde reentry.
9. Digoxin 0.5 mg IV with repeat doses of 0.25 mg in 30 to 60 min until a response occurs or the total dose reaches 0.02 mg/kg. The chief drawback of digoxin has been its long onset of action and potential hazard in patients with accessory (bypass) tracts who develop either atrial fibrillation or flutter.
10. External noninvasive pacing has been used in a limited number of patients to terminate reentrant SVT. Asynchronous pacing with two to ten external pulses at a rate 240 to 280 (typically 40 faster than the SVT rate) with an impulse amplitude of 120 mA is effective in young, hemodynamically stable adults.
11. Synchronized cardioversion should be done in any unstable patient with hypotension, pulmonary edema, or severe chest pain. The dose required is usually small, less than 50 J.

## Junctional Arrhythmias

Traditionally, a junctional impulse is considered to be one that arises from the AV node or bundle of His above the bifurcation. While pacemaker tissue cannot be found in the AV node itself in experimental animals, the matter is not settled in humans. From its source, the impulse spreads retrograde toward the atria and antegrade toward the ventricles. Depending on the site of origin, conduction velocity, and refractory periods, the atria may be activated before, during, or after ventricular depolarization. Atrial depolarization may not be visible if retrograde conduction is blocked or atrial activation occurs simultaneously with ventricular activation and the P waves are obscured by the QRS complex. AV dissociation may occur if the rate of discharge from the junctional pacemaker is faster than the sinus node rate and the junctional impulse is blocked from retrograde conduction toward the atria.

### Junctional Premature Contractions (JPCs)

Junctional premature contractions are due to an ectopic pacemaker within the AV node or common AV bundle. The ECG characteristics of JPCs are: (1) the ectopic QRS complex is premature, (2) the ectopic P′ wave has a different shape and direction (usually inverted in leads II, III, and aV$_F$), (3) the ectopic P′ wave may occur before or after the QRS complex, (4) the P′R interval of the ectopic beat is shorter than normal, (5) the QRS complex is usually of normal shape unless there is aberrant conduction, and (6) the sinus node is usually not affected and the postectopic pause is fully compensatory (Fig. 22-13). JPCs may be isolated, multiple (as in bigeminy or trigeminy), or multifocal.

#### Clinical Significance

JPCs are uncommon in healthy hearts. They occur in congestive heart failure, digoxin toxicity, ischemic heart disease, or acute myocardial infarctions (especially of the inferior wall).

#### Treatment

1. No specific treatment is usually required.
2. Treat the underlying disorder.
3. Antiarrhythmic therapy with quinidine or procainamide may be useful if JPCs are frequent, symptomatic, or initiate more serious arrhythmias.

### Junctional Rhythms

Under normal circumstances, the sinus node discharges at a faster rate than the AV junction, so the pacemaker function of the AV junction is overridden. If sinus node discharges slow or fail to reach the AV junction, then junctional escape beats may occur, usually at a rate between 40 to 60, depending on the level of the pacemaker. Generally, junctional escape beats do not conduct retrograde into the atria so a QRS complex without a P′ wave is usually seen (Fig. 22-14).

Under other circumstances, enhanced junctional automaticity may override the sinus node and produce either an accelerated junctional rhythm (rate 60 to 100) or junctional tachycardia (rate greater than

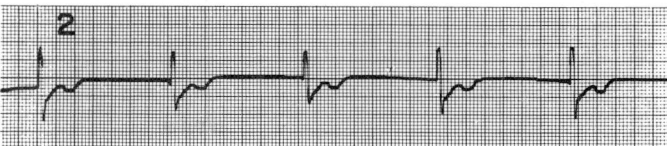

**Fig. 22-14.** Junctional escape rhythm, rate 42.

100). Usually, both the atria and ventricles are captured by the enhanced junctional pacemaker (Fig. 22-15).

#### Clinical Significance

Junctional escape beats may occur whenever there is a long enough pause in the impulses reaching the AV junction: sinus bradycardia, slow phase of sinus arrhythmia, AV block, or during the pause following premature beats. Sustained junctional escape rhythms may be seen with congestive heart failure, myocarditis, hypokalemia, or digoxin toxicity. If the ventricular rate is too slow, myocardial or cerebral ischemia may develop.

Accelerated junctional rhythm and junctional tachycardia may occur from digoxin toxicity, acute rheumatic fever, or inferior myocardial infarction. With digoxin toxicity, the rate is usually between 70 and 130. If this rhythm develops in a patient being treated with digoxin for atrial fibrillation, the ECG is characterized by regular QRS complexes superimposed on atrial fibrillatory waves. Regulation of ventricular response during digoxin therapy in a patient with atrial fibrillation should therefore raise the suspicion of digoxin toxicity.

#### Treatment

1. Isolated, infrequent junctional escape beats usually do not require specific treatment.
2. If sustained junctional escape rhythms are producing symptoms, the underlying cause should be treated. Atropine can be used to accelerate temporarily the sinus node discharge rate and enhance AV nodal conduction.
3. Accelerated junctional rhythm and junctional tachycardia usually do not produce significant symptoms. If the cause is digoxin toxicity, the drug should be discontinued. If the rate is fast and producing symptoms, it can be decreased by giving supplemental potassium to increase the serum level into the high-normal range.

## Ventricular Arrhythmias

### Premature Ventricular Contractions (PVCs)

Premature ventricular contractions are due to impulses originating from single or multiple areas in the ventricles. The ECG characteristics of PVCs are: (1) there is a premature and wide QRS complex; (2) there is no preceding P wave; (3) the ST segment and T wave of the PVC are directed opposite the major QRS deflection; (4) most PVCs do not affect the sinus node, so there is usually a fully compensatory postectopic pause or the PVC may be interpolated between two sinus beats; (5) many PVCs have a fixed coupling interval (within 0.04 s) from the preceding sinus beat; and (6) many PVCs are conducted into the atria, producing a retrograde P wave (Fig. 22-16).

Occasionally, a ventricular fusion beat occurs when a supraventricular and ventricular impulse nearly simultaneously depolarize the

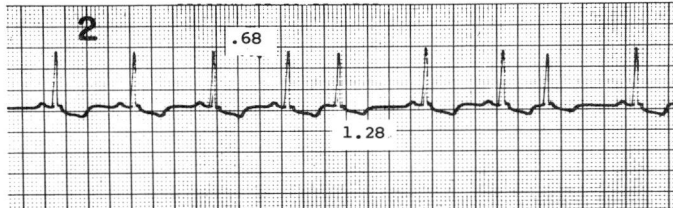

**Fig. 22-13.** Junctional premature contractions (JPCs).

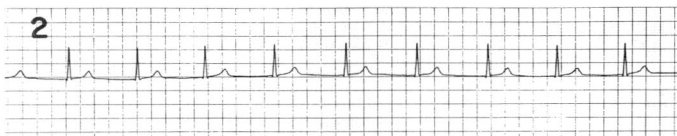

**Fig. 22-15.** Accelerated junctional rhythm, rate 61.

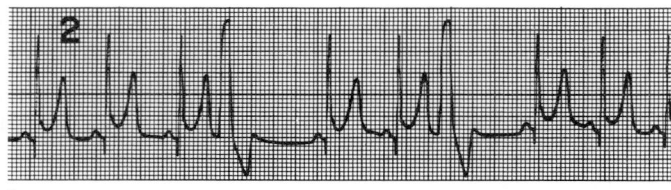

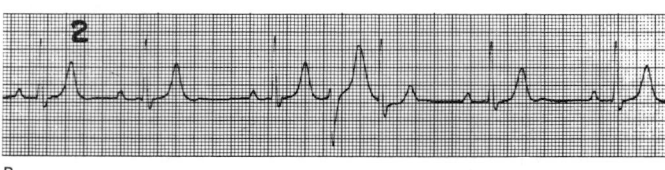

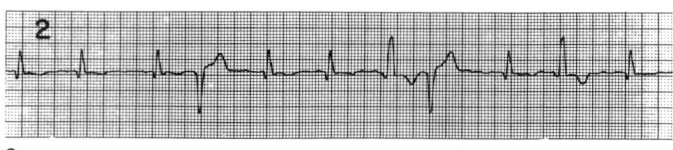

**Fig. 22-16.** Premature ventricular contractions (PVCs). Top: unifocal PVC. Center: interpolated PVC. Bottom: multifocal PVCs.

ventricles. The QRS configuration of a fusion beat contains features of the individual components.

A PVC may be confused with an aberrantly conducted supraventricular beat. Several clinical and ECG criteria can be used to help differentiate between aberrantly conducted supraventricular beats and PVCs; this is discussed in a separate section.

**Clinical Significance**

PVCs are very common, even in patients without evidence of heart disease. They occur in most patients with ischemic heart disease and are universally found in patients with acute myocardial infarction. Other common causes of PVCs include digoxin toxicity, congestive heart failure, hypokalemia, alkalosis, hypoxia, and sympathomimetic drugs.

While there is a correlation between the severity of underlying coronary artery disease and the degree of ventricular ectopy, there is disagreement as to whether ventricular ectopy itself is an independent risk factor for future morbidity or mortality. Most studies indicate that repetitive PVCs (two or more in a row) do have some associated independent risk in patients with coronary artery disease, but the evidence for other forms of ventricular ectopy is less convincing. Lown has made an attempt with his classification to quantitate the risks associated with chronic ventricular ectopy, but his classification is not universally accepted (Table 22-2).

In the setting of an acute myocardial infarction, PVCs indicate the underlying electrical instability of the heart. The patients are at increased risk for the development of primary ventricular fibrillation. Current work indicates that various degrees of PVCs ("warning arrhythmias") are not reliable predictors of subsequent ventricular fibrillation.

**Table 22-2.** Lown Grading System for Ventricular Ectopy

| Grade | |
|---|---|
| 1 | Uniform PVCs < 30/h |
| 2 | Uniform PVCs > 30/h |
| 3 | Multiform PVCs |
| 4A | Couplets (2 consecutive PVCs) |
| 4B | Triplets (3 or more consecutive PVCs) |
| 5 | R-on-T PVCs |

Although it is experimentally established that electric impulses, such as PVCs, that occur during or soon after repolarization (the so-called vulnerable period) can initiate ventricular tachycardia or fibrillation, clinical studies have found that more paroxysms of ventricular tachycardia are initiated by late-coupled PVCs than early-coupled PVCs (R-on-T phenomenon).

**Treatment**

1. Most acute patients with PVCs will respond to intravenous lidocaine, although some patients may require procainamide. In the setting of acute myocardial ischemia (unstable angina or acute myocardial infarction) many physicians would treat frequent or multiform PVCs with the goal of reducing deaths due to sudden ventricular tachycardia or fibrillation. While single studies have suggested benefit, pooled data and meta-analysis find no reduction in mortality from either suppressive or prophylactic treatment of PVCs.
2. In patients with chronic PVCs, there is no evidence that oral suppressive enhances survival. To the contrary, large randomized studies of post-infarction patients found that treatment with encainide, flecainide, or moricizine increased the incidence of cardiac arrest or arrhythmic death. Before treating chronic PVCs, the physician should consider several factors: (a) the underlying heart disease, (b) the nature of the ectopy, (c) the presence or absence of symptoms, (d) the potential side effects of oral antiarrhythmic therapy, and (e) which technique will be used to judge efficacy of therapy (usually between Holter monitoring versus electrophysiologic testing). Oral antiarrhythmic therapy requires careful monitoring.

## Ventricular Parasystole

Parasystole occurs when an independent ectopic pacemaker is protected from the influence of outside impulses ("entrance block") and competes with the dominant pacemaker to produce myocardial depolarizations. A parasystolic pacemaker can arise anywhere in the heart, but is most often located in the ventricles where it produces a rhythm that operates alongside of and is independent of the sinus node.

The ECG characteristics of ventricular parasystole are: (1) variation in the coupling interval between the preceding sinus beat and the ectopic beat, (2) common relation between the interectopic beat intervals, and (3) occurrence of fusion beats (Fig. 22-17). Usually, long rhythm strips are necessary to establish that the interectopic intervals are multiples of a common parasystolic rate.

**Clinical Significance**

Ventricular parasystole is most often associated with severe ischemic heart disease, acute myocardial infarction, hypertensive heart disease, or electrolyte imbalance. Parasystole is often self-limited and benign, but infrequently, it may lead to ventricular tachycardia or fibrillation.

**Treatment**

1. The underlying disease should be treated.
2. Antiarrhythmics are indicated in patients with symptomatic episodes or beats which initiate ventricular tachycardia.

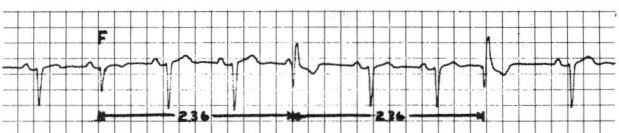

**Fig. 22-17.** The fifth and eighth ventricular complexes are premature and of similar morphology but have different coupling intervals. The second complex (marked "F") represents a fusion beat. The interectopic interval is 2.36 s. (From Heger JW, Niemann JT, Boman KG, et al: *Cardiology for the House Officer.* Baltimore, Williams & Wilkins, 1982. Used by permission.)

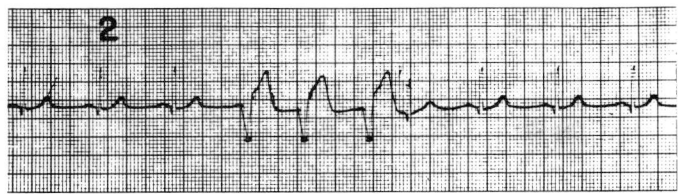

**Fig. 22-18.** Accelerated idioventricular rhythms (AIVR).

## Accelerated Idioventricular Rhythm (AIVR)

Accelerated idioventricular rhythm is an ectopic rhythm of ventricular origin occurring at rates of 40 to 100. Even though AIVR is not a tachycardia, such terms as *idioventricular tachycardia, nonparoxysmal ventricular tachycardia,* or *slow ventricular tachycardia* are sometimes used to describe this rhythm.

The ECG characteristics of AIVR are: (1) wide and regular QRS complexes, (2) rate between 40 and 100 that is often close to the preceding sinus rate, (3) most runs of short duration (3 to 30 beats) and (4) an AIVR often beginning with a fusion beat (Fig. 22-18).

### Clinical Significance

This condition is found most commonly in the setting of an acute myocardial infarction. Reports indicate that AIVR sometimes appears during successful thrombolysis of an occluded coronary. AIVR and other ventricular arrhythmias seen during this time are termed "reperfusion arrhythmias." AIVR may be seen infrequently in patients without organic heart disease. While there is some variable association with ventricular tachycardia, there is no apparent association with ventricular fibrillation. AIVR usually produces no symptoms itself. Sometimes the loss of atrial contraction and subsequent fall in cardiac output may produce hemodynamic deterioration.

### Treatment

1. Treatment is not necessary. On occasion, AIVR may be the only functioning pacemaker and suppression with lidocaine can lead to cardiac asystole.
2. If sustained AIVR produces symptoms secondary to a decrease in cardiac output, treatment with atrial pacing may be required.

## Ventricular Tachycardia

Ventricular tachycardia is the occurrence of three or more beats from a ventricular ectopic pacemaker at a rate greater than 100. The ECG characteristics of ventricular tachycardia are: (1) wide QRS complexes; (2) rate greater than 100 (most commonly 150 to 200); (3) rhythm usually regular, although there may be some beat-to-beat variation; and (4) QRS axis usually constant (Fig. 22-19). Uncommonly (about 5 percent of episodes) ventricular tachycardia may have a narrow (<120 milliseconds) QRS complex. In these cases, electrocardiographic criteria usually suggest a ventricular origin (see Aberrant versus Ventricular Tachyarrhythmias). Ventricular tachycardia can occur in a nonsustained manner—usually short episodes, lasting seconds, with spontaneous termination—or occur in a sustained fashion—longer episodes that typically require treatment.

There are several variants of ventricular tachycardia. *Ventricular flutter* is the phrase used for a regular zigzag pattern without distinguishable QRS complexes or T waves. In *bidirectional ventricular tachycardia* the QRS complexes alternate polarity as recorded in a

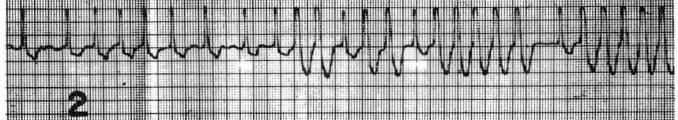

**Fig. 22-19.** Ventricular tachycardia.

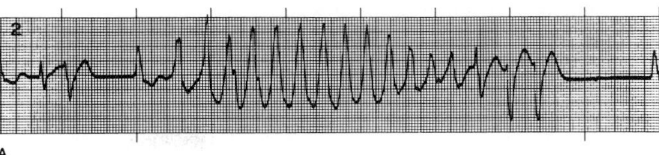

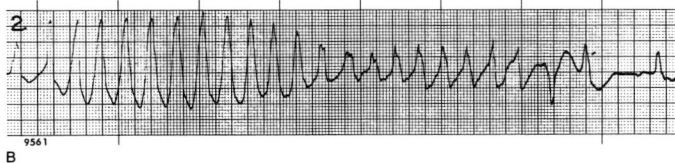

**Fig. 22-20.** Two examples of short runs of atypical ventricular tachycardia showing sinusoidal variation in amplitude and direction of the QRS complexes: "le torsade de pointes" (twisting of the points). Note that the top example is initiated by a late-occurring PVC (lead II).

single lead. In *alternating ventricular tachycardia* the QRS complexes alternate in height (but not polarity) in a single lead. (Both bidirectional and alternating ventricular tachycardia indicate serious myocardial disease and are often due to digitalis toxicity.) In *polymorphous ventricular tachycardia* the QRS complexes have many different shapes in one lead. *Atypical ventricular tachycardia* (torsade de pointes, or "twisting of the points") is where the QRS axis swings from a positive to negative direction in a single lead (Fig. 22-20). Despite the appearance, this rhythm originates from a single focus and is considered to result from a triggered arrhythmic mechanism. Atypical ventricular tachycardia usually occurs in short runs of 5 to 15 s at a rate of 200 to 240. This form of ventricular tachycardia generally occurs in patients with serious myocardial disease who have a prolonged and uneven ventricular repolarization (prolonged QT interval) (Table 22-3).

Drugs which further prolong repolarization—quinidine, disopyramide, procainamide, phenothiazines, tricyclic antidepressants—exacerbate this arrhythmia. Conventional treatment with lidocaine often is ineffective. To date, treatment for torsade de pointes consisted of accelerating the heart rate (thereby shortening ventricular repolarization) with isoproterenol (2 to 8 µg/min) while making arrangements for a ventricular pacemaker to overdrive the heart at rates of 90 to

**Table 22-3.** Etiologies and Associated Conditions in Torsades de Pointes

Familial
    Jervell-Lange-Nielson syndrome (congenital deafness)
    Romano-Ward syndrome (without deafness)
Toxins and drugs
    Antiarrhythmics: most common with classes IA, IC, and III
    Psychotropics: tricyclic antidepressants, some phenothiazines (thioridazine), tetracyclics (maprotiline)
    Organophosphate insecticides
    Liquid protein diets
Cerebrovascular disease
    Cerebrovascular accidents, intracranial hemorrhage, carotid endarterectomy
Electrolyte disorders
    Hypokalemia, hypomagnesemia, hypocalcemia
Endocrine disorders
    Hypothyroidism
Cardiac disease
    Acute rheumatic carditis, mitral valve prolapse syndrome, inflammatory myocarditis
Coronary artery disease
    Myocardial ischemia or infarction, left ventricular failure
Pacemaker malfunction
Postoperative complication

120. Temporary pacing is the most effective and safest method to treat torsades and prevent its recurrence. Recent reports have revealed that magnesium sulfate 1 to 2 g IV over 60 to 90 s followed by an infusion of 1 to 2 g/h is effective in abolishing these runs of torsade de pointes although recurrences are seen despite continued infusion. A wide variety of other agents and antiarrhythmics have reported anecdotal success, but overall efficacy has been inconsistent.

## Clinical Significance

Ventricular tachycardia is very rare in patients without underlying heart disease. The most common causes of ventricular tachycardia are ischemic heart disease and acute myocardial infarction. Less common causes include hypertrophic cardiomyopathy, mitral valve prolapse, and toxicity from many drugs (digoxin, quinidine, procainamide, sympathomimetics). Hypoxia, alkalosis, and electrolyte abnormalities exacerbate the tendency toward ventricular ectopy and tachycardia.

It is a common misconception that patients with ventricular tachycardia appear clinically unstable; this is the basis for the mistaken assumption that patients who appear stable with a wide complex tachycardia have SVT with aberrancy rather than ventricular tachycardia. This is definitely wrong. Ventricular tachycardia cannot be differentiated from SVT with aberrancy on the basis of clinical symptoms, blood pressure, or heart rate. Patients who are unstable should be cardioverted; it is effective for both arrhythmias. In patients who are stable, a 12-lead ECG should be obtained first and examined for evidence which favors one arrhythmia over another; but even then, it is often difficult to decide. Therefore, in general, it is best to treat all wide complex tachycardias as ventricular tachycardia with lidocaine or procainamide. These drugs are obviously effective in ventricular tachycardia, often surprisingly effective in SVT with aberrancy and carry little risk of harming the patient. Conversely, verapamil is harmful in most patients with ventricular tachycardia, accelerating the heart rate and the decreasing blood pressure without converting the rhythm. Adenosine appears to have little harm in patients with ventricular tachycardia and has potential merit for the treatment for wide QRS complex tachycardias. However, until further experience is gained with this agent, it cannot be recommended for routine use in this setting.

## Treatment

1. Unstable patients or those in cardiac arrest should be treated with synchronized cardioversion. Ventricular tachycardia can be converted with energies as low as 1 J and over 90 percent can be converted with less than 10 J. Rarely is more than 100 J needed. Current ACLS guidelines recommend that pulseless ventricular tachycardia be *defibrillated* (unsynchronized cardioversion) with 200 J.
2. Clinically stable patients should be treated with intravenous antiarrhythmics.
   a. Lidocaine 75 mg (1.0 to 1.5 mg/kg) IV over 60 to 90 s, followed by a constant infusion at 1 to 4 mg/min (10 to 40 µg/kg per minute). A repeat bolus dose of 50 mg lidocaine may be required during the first 20 min to avoid a subtherapeutic dip in serum level due to the early distribution phase.
   b. Bretylium 500 mg (5 to 10 mg/kg) IV over 10 min, followed by a constant infusion at 1 to 2 mg/min.
   c. Procainamide IV at a rate of less than 50 mg/min until the arrhythmia converts, the total dose reaches 15 to 17 mg/kg in normals (12 mg/kg in patients with congestive heart failure), or early signs of toxicity develop with hypotension or QRS prolongation. The loading dose should be followed by a maintenance infusion of 2.8 mg/kg per hour in normal subjects (1.4 mg/kg per hour in patients with renal insufficiency).
   d. A variety of other antiarrhythmics have been studied for the treatment of ventricular tachycardia. Most class I and III agents are effective for the acute termination of ventricular

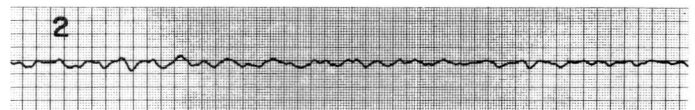

**Fig. 22-21.** Ventricular fibrillation.

tachycardia when given intravenously. Recommendations concerning their routine use will have to await further studies.

## Ventricular Fibrillation

Ventricular fibrillation is the totally disorganized depolarization and contraction of small areas of ventricular myocardium—there is no effective ventricular pumping activity. The ECG of ventricular fibrillation shows a fine to coarse zigzag pattern without discernible P waves or QRS complexes (Fig. 22-21).

Ventricular fibrillation is never accompanied by a pulse or blood pressure. In patients who are awake and responsive, the ECG pattern of ventricular fibrillation is caused by a loose lead artifact or electrical interference.

## Clinical Significance

Ventricular fibrillation is most commonly seen in patients with severe ischemic heart disease, with or without an acute myocardial infarction. Primary ventricular fibrillation occurs suddenly, without preceding hemodynamic deterioration, while secondary ventricular fibrillation occurs after a prolonged period of left ventricular failure and/or circulatory shock. Ventricular fibrillation may also occur from digoxin toxicity, quinidine toxicity, hypothermia, blunt chest trauma, severe electrolyte abnormality, or myocardial irritation caused by an intracardiac catheter or pacemaker electrode.

## Treatment

1. Current ACLS guidelines recommend immediate electrical defibrillation with 200 J. If ventricular fibrillation persists, defibrillation should be repeated immediately with 200 to 300 J for the second attempt and increased to 360 J for the third attempt.
2. If the initial three attempts at defibrillation are unsuccessful, CPR should be initiated and further electrical defibrillations done after the administration of various intravenous drugs according to ACLS guidelines.

## ABERRANT VERSUS VENTRICULAR TACHYARRHYTHMIAS

Differentiation between ectopic beats of ventricular origin and those of supraventricular origin but conducted aberrantly can be difficult, especially in sustained tachycardias with wide QRS complexes (WCT). In general, the majority of patients with WCT have ventricular tachycardia and should be approached as ventricular tachycardia, until proved otherwise. Several guidelines might help in the distinction.

1. A preceding ectopic P' wave is good evidence favoring aberrancy, although coincidental atrial and ventricular ectopic beats or retrograde conduction can occur. During a sustained run of tachycardia, AV dissociation greatly favors a ventricular origin of the arrhythmia.
2. Postectopic pause: A fully compensatory pause is more likely after a ventricular beat, but exceptions do occur.
3. Fusion beats are good evidence for ventricular origin, but again exceptions do occur.
4. A varying bundle branch block pattern suggests aberrancy.
5. Coupling intervals are usually constant with ventricular ectopic beats, unless parasystole is present. Varying coupling intervals suggest aberrancy.
6. Response to carotid sinus massage or other vagal maneuvers will

**Table 22-4.** Aberrancy versus Ventricular Ectopy

| QRS Pattern in $V_1$ | Favors | QRS Pattern in $V_6$ | Favors |
|---|---|---|---|
| rSR′ (RBBB pattern)<br>rR′ | Aberrancy | qRS | Aberrancy |
| R<br>qR<br>RS<br>Slurred downslope R | Ventricular | rS<br>S<br>qR or QR<br>R<br>qQ′ | Ventricular |
| Slurred upstroke R | Either | RS<br>Slurred R | Either |

*Source:* Wellens HJJ, Frits WHMB, Lie KI: *Am J Med* 64:27, 1978. Used by permission.

slow conduction through the AV node and may abolish reentrant SVT and slow the ventricular response in other supraventricular tachyarrhythmias. These maneuvers have essentially no effect on ventricular arrhythmias.

7. A QRS duration of longer than 0.14 s is usually only found in ventricular ectopy or tachycardia.

8. QRS morphology: Wellens et al. have studied patients with both ventricular tachycardia and SVT with aberrancy using His bundle electrocardiography. Several morphologic ECG criteria were found useful in differentiating between the two (Table 22-4).

9. Historical criteria have also been found to be useful: age of the patient over 35 and/or history of myocardial infarction, congestive heart failure, or coronary artery bypass graft strongly suggest ventricular tachycardia in patients with WCT.

## CONDUCTION DISTURBANCES

### Sinoatrial (SA) Block

The sinus node discharge must be conducted into the atria to pace the heart during sinus rhythm. If sinus node discharges are delayed or blocked in their outward propagation, then sinoatrial block is present. Sinoatrial block is divided into first-, second-, and third-degree varieties.

First-degree SA block means that the impulse is delayed in its conduction out of the sinus node into the atria—a condition that cannot be recognized on the clinical ECG.

Second-degree SA block means that some impulses get through and some are blocked. Second-degree SA block can be suspected whenever an expected P wave and the corresponding QRS complex are absent. In the variable (Wenckebach) type of second-degree SA block, the missing P wave would come after a period of progressive prolongation of the sinus node to atrium conduction time, again something undetectable on the clinical ECG. However, another ECG finding common to the Wenckebach phenomenon can be seen—progressive shortening of the P-P intervals prior to the missing P wave (Fig. 22-22). In the constant type of second-degree SA block, the sinoatrial conduction time remains constant before and after the blocked impulses. In this situation, the interval encompassing the missing beat is an exact or near-exact multiple of the cycle length (Fig. 22-23).

Third-degree SA block occurs when the sinus node discharge is

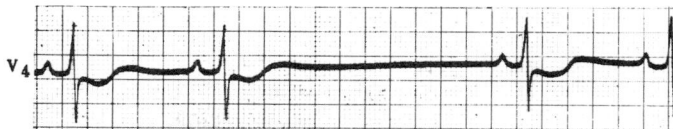

**Fig. 22-23.** Second-degree constant SA block type II (lead $V_4$).

completely blocked and no P wave originating from the sinus seen. There are three other causes of absent sinus P waves in addition to third-degree SA block: (1) sinus node failure, (2) a sinus node stimulus inadequate to activate the atria, and (3) atrial unresponsiveness.

#### Clinical Significance

Sinoatrial block usually arises from myocardial disease (acute rheumatic fever, acute inferior myocardial infarction, other causes of myocarditis) or drug toxicity (digoxin, quinidine, salicylates, β-adrenergic blockers, or calcium-channel blockers). In rare individuals, vagal stimulation can produce SA block.

#### Treatment

1. Treatment depends on the underlying cause, associated arrhythmias, and whether symptoms of hypoperfusion are present.
2. Sinus node discharge rate and sinoatrial conduction can be facilitated by atropine or isoproterenol when clinically required.
3. Cardiac pacing is indicated for recurrent or persistent symptomatic bradycardia.

### Sinus Arrest (Pause)

Sinus pause is a failure of impulse formation within the sinus node. In sinus arrest, the P-P interval has no mathematical relation to the basic sinus node discharge rate (Fig. 22-24).

#### Clinical Significance

The same conditions which produce SA block can also produce sinus arrest, especially digoxin toxicity. The combination of digoxin and carotid sinus massage is well known to be able to produce prolonged sinus arrest. Brief periods of sinus arrest may occur in healthy individuals from increased vagal tone. If sinus arrest is prolonged, AV junctional escape beats often occur.

#### Treatment

1. Treatment depends on the underlying cause, associated arrhythmias, and whether symptoms of hypoperfusion are present.
2. If sinus arrest is symptomatic, atropine will usually increase sinus node discharge rate.
3. Cardiac pacing is indicated for recurrent or persistent symptomatic bradycardia.

### Atrioventricular (AV) Dissociation

Atrioventricular dissociation is a condition in which the atria and ventricles are driven by separate and independent pacemakers. It is not a primary rhythm disturbance, but is secondary to another conduction or rhythm abnormality. There are two varieties of AV dissociation: passive (default or "escape"), and active (usurpation).

Passive AV dissociation occurs when an impulse fails to reach the AV node due to sinus node failure or block. Usually an escape rhythm takes over and paces the ventricles. When the sinus node recovers, atrial activity resumes but there may be a period during

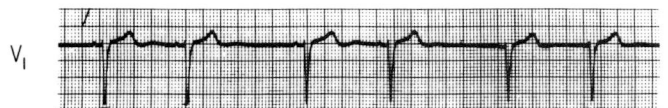

**Fig. 22-22.** Second-degree SA block type I (Wenckebach). (From Braunwald E: *Heart Disease. A Textbook of Cardiovascular Medicine.* Philadelphia, Saunders, 1980. Used by permission.)

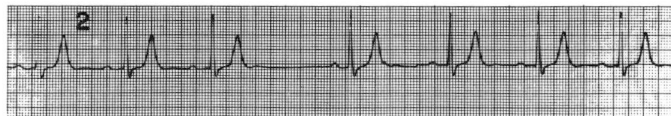

**Fig. 22-24.** Sinus pause.

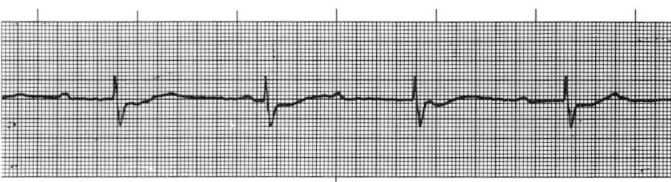

**Fig. 22-25.** Passive AV dissociation, secondary to third-degree AV block.

which the ventricles are still driven by the escape pacemaker, and the P waves and QRS complexes occur independent of each other (Fig. 22-25).

Active AV dissociation occurs when a lower pacemaker accelerates to usurp the sinus node and captures the ventricles, but the atria are still paced as before (Fig. 22-26).

In both varieties of AV dissociation, fusion beats are common. It is also common for the two pacemakers to operate with nearly identical rates, possibly as a result of mechanical or electrical influences which tend to keep them in phase with each other—a condition termed isorhythmic dissociation.

**Clinical Significance**

Passive AV dissociation occurs when the sinus node discharge rate is slowed by sinus bradycardia, sinus arrhythmia, SA block, or sinus pause. Common causes of this include: (1) ischemic heart disease (especially acute inferior myocardial infarction), (2) myocarditis (especially acute rheumatic fever), (3) drug toxicity (especially digoxin), and (4) vagal reflexes. It may also be seen in well-conditioned athletes.

Active AV dissociation occurs when the automaticity of lower pacemakers is enhanced. Common causes include myocardial ischemia and drug toxicity (especially digoxin).

**Treatment**

1. Most occurrences of AV dissociation have an acceptable heart rate and are well tolerated.
2. Therapy, if any, is directed toward the underlying cause.

## Atrioventricular (AV) Block

Clinical classification of AV block was done before modern understanding of the sites and mechanisms involved in impairing conduction between the atria and ventricles. This is unfortunate because this classification is too simple to categorize all the problems that may occur with AV conduction. However, this system is almost universally used.

First-degree AV block is characterized by a delay in AV conduction, manifested by a prolonged PR interval. Second-degree AV block is characterized by intermittent AV conduction—some atrial

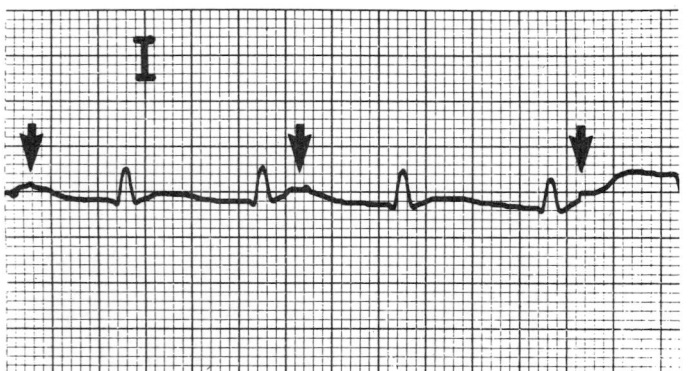

**Fig. 22-26.** Active AV dissociation. (Arrows indicate P waves.)

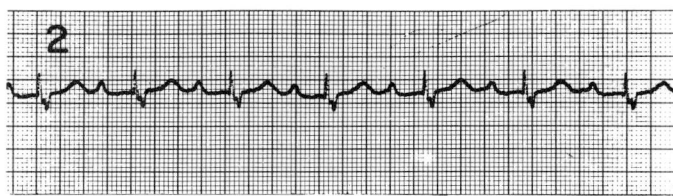

**Fig. 22-27.** First-degree AV block (PR interval = 0.3 s).

impulses reach the ventricles and others are blocked. Third-degree AV block is characterized by complete interruption in AV conduction.

Precise localization of AV conduction blocks can be made with His bundle electrocardiography. Although this method is not available for us in the emergency department, correlations can be made between the clinical ECG, the approximate location of the block, and the risk of future progression.

AV blocks can also be divided into nodal and infranodal blocks, an important distinction because the clinical significance and prognosis vary with the site. AV nodal blocks are usually due to reversible depression of conduction, often self-limited, generally have a stable infranodal escape pacemaker pacing the ventricles, and therefore do not have a serious prognosis. Infranodal blocks are usually due to organic disease of the His bundle or bundle branches, often the damage is irreversible, they generally have a slow and unstable ventricular escape rhythm pacing the ventricles, and they may have a serious prognosis depending on the clinical circumstance.

### First-Degree AV Block

In first-degree AV block, each atrial impulse is conducted into the ventricles, but more slowly than normal. This is recognized by a PR interval of greater than 0.20 s (Fig. 22-27). The AV node is usually the site of conduction delay, although it may occur at any infranodal level.

**Clinical Significance**

First-degree AV block is occasionally found in normal hearts. Other common causes include increased vagal tone (whatever the cause), digoxin toxicity, acute inferior myocardial infarction, and myocarditis. Patients with first-degree AV block without evidence of organic heart disease appear to have no significant difference in mortality compared with matched controls.

**Treatment**

1. None is usually required.
2. Prophylactic pacing in acute myocardial infarction is not indicated unless more serious infranodal conduction disturbances are present.

### Second-Degree Mobitz I (Wenckebach) AV Block

In this block there is progressive prolongation of AV conduction (and the PR interval) until an atrial impulse is completely blocked (Fig. 22-28). Conduction ratios are used to indicate the ratio of atrial to ventricular depolarizations: 3:2 indicates 2 out of 3 atrial impulses are conducted into the ventricles. Usually, only a single atrial impulse is blocked. After the dropped beat, the AV conduction returns to normal

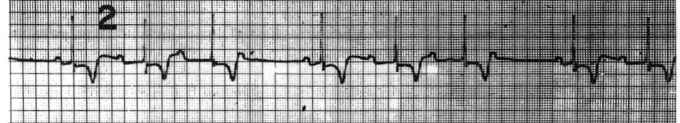

**Fig. 22-28.** Second-degree Mobitz I (Wenckebach) AV block with 4:3 AV conduction.

and the cycle usually repeats itself with either the same conduction ratio (fixed ratio) or a different conduction ratio (variable ratio). This type of block almost always occurs at the level of the AV node and is often due to reversible depression of AV nodal conduction.

The Wenckebach phenomenon has a seeming paradox. Even though the PR intervals progressively lengthen prior to the dropped beat, the increments by which they lengthen decrease with successive beats; this produces a progressive shortening of the R-R interval prior to the dropped beat (Fig. 22-28). This sign can be used to indicate that a Wenckebach phenomenon is occurring, even when the conduction delay cannot be seen, as in SA Wenckebach block.

Wenckebach block is believed to occur because each successive depolarization produces prolongation of the refractory period of the AV node. When the next atrial impulse comes upon the node, it is earlier in the relative refractory period and conduction occurs more slowly relative to the previous stimulus. This process is progressive until an atrial impulse reaches the AV node during the absolute refractory period and conduction is blocked altogether. The pause allows the AV node to recover and the process can resume.

### Clinical Significance

This block is often transient and usually associated with an acute inferior myocardial infarction, digoxin toxicity, myocarditis, or is seen after cardiac surgery. Wenckebach block may also occur when a normal AV node is exposed to very rapid atrial rates.

### Treatment

1. Specific treatment is not necessary unless slow ventricular rates produce signs of hypoperfusion.
2. 0.5 mg of atropine IV is given, repeated every 5 min as necessary, titrated to the desired effect, or until the total dose reaches 2.0 mg. Almost all cases will respond to atropine.
3. Isoproterenol is hazardous in the setting of acute myocardial infarction or digoxin toxicity and its use should be avoided.
4. Transcutaneous or transvenous ventricular demand pacing should be initiated if atropine is unsuccessful.

### Second-Degree Mobitz II AV Block

In this block, the PR interval remains constant before and after the nonconducted atrial beats (Fig. 22-29). One or more beats may be nonconducted at a single time.

Mobitz II blocks usually occur in the infranodal conducting system, often with coexistent fascicular or bundle branch blocks, and the QRS complexes are therefore usually wide. Even if the QRS complexes are narrow, the block is generally in the infranodal system.

When second-degree AV block occurs with a fixed conduction ratio of 2:1, it is not possible to differentiate between a Mobitz type I (Wenckebach) or Mobitz type II block. If the QRS complex is narrow, then the block is in the AV node or infranodal system with about

equal incidence. If the QRS complex is wide, the block is more likely to be in the infranodal system.

### Clinical Significance

Type II blocks imply structural damage to the infranodal conducting system, are usually permanent, and may progress suddenly to complete heart block—especially in the setting of an acute myocardial infarction.

### Treatment

1. Emergent treatment is required when slow ventricular rates produce symptoms of hypoperfusion. Atropine should be the first drug used, and up to 60 percent of patients will respond. Isoproterenol is effective in up to 50 percent of cases but is potentially hazardous in the setting of acute myocardial infarction or digoxin toxicity, and its use should be avoided. Transcutaneous cardiac pacing is a useful modality in patients unresponsive to atropine.
2. Most cases, especially in the setting of acute myocardial infarction, will require permanent transvenous cardiac pacing.

### Third-Degree (Complete) AV Block

In third-degree AV block, there is no atrioventricular conduction. The ventricles are paced by an escape pacemaker at a rate slower than the atrial rate (Fig. 22-30). Third-degree AV block can occur either at nodal or infranodal levels.

When third-degree AV block occurs at the AV node, a junctional escape pacemaker takes over with a ventricular rate of 40 to 60 and, since the rhythm originates above the bifurcation of the bundle of His, the QRS complexes are narrow.

When third-degree AV block occurs at the infranodal level, the ventricles are driven by a ventricular escape rhythm at a rate of less than 40. In third-degree AV block located at the His bundle level, the escape rhythm has narrow QRS complexes about half of the time. Presumably, in these cases, the escape pacemaker resides above the bifurcation of the conducting system into the separate bundle branches. Third-degree AV block located in the bundle branch or purkinje system invariably have escape rhythms with wide QRS complexes.

### Clinical Significance

Nodal third-degree AV block may develop in up to 8 percent of acute inferior myocardial infarctions where it is usually transient, although it may last for several days.

Infranodal third-degree AV blocks indicate structural damage to the infranodal conducting system, as seen with an extensive acute anterior myocardial infarction. The ventricular escape pacemaker is usually inadequate to maintain cardiac output and is unstable with periods of ventricular asystole.

### Treatment

1. Nodal third-degree AV blocks should be treated like second-degree Mobitz I AV blocks with atropine or ventricular demand pacemaker as required.
2. Infranodal third-degree AV blocks require a ventricular demand pacemaker. Isoproterenol can be used temporarily to accelerate the ventricular escape rhythm, or external cardiac pacing can be performed before transvenous pacemaker placement.

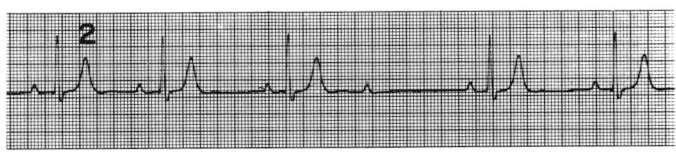

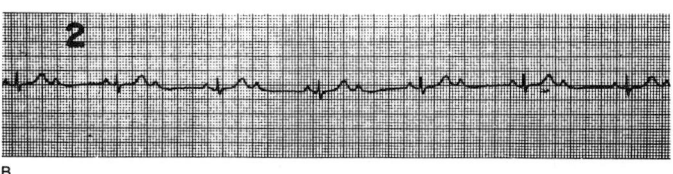

**Fig. 22-29.** Top: second-degree Mobitz II AV block. Bottom: second-degree AV block with 2:1 AV conduction.

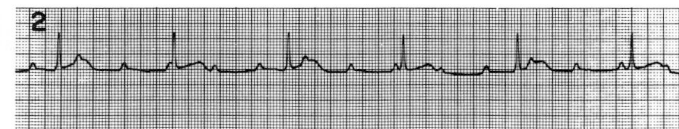

**Fig. 22-30.** Third-degree AV block.

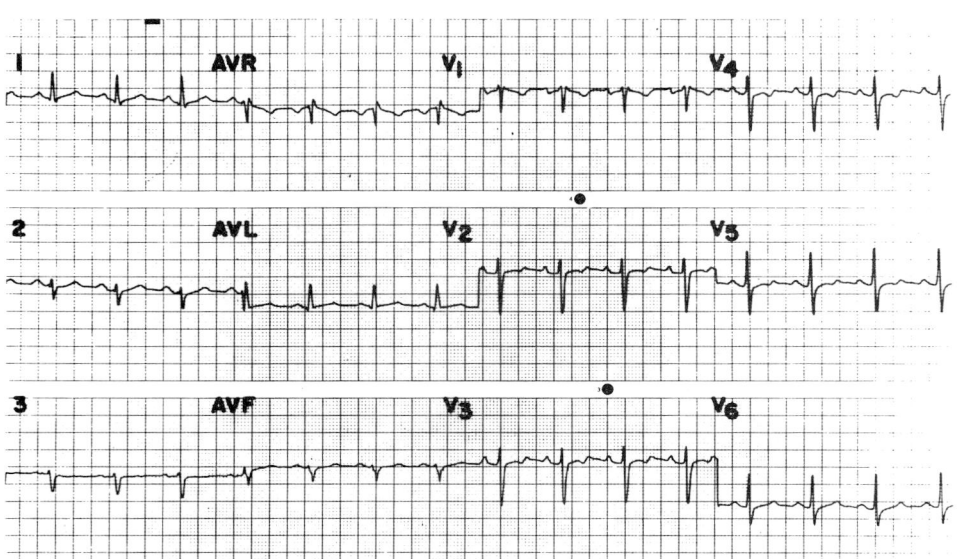

**Fig. 22-31.** Left anterior superior fascicular block (LASF block).

## FASCICULAR BLOCKS

### Unifascicular Block

Unifascicular block is a conduction block that affects one of the three major infranodal conduction pathways: right bundle branch (RBB), left anterior superior fascicle (LASF), and left posterior inferior fascicle (LPIF). A wide variety of disease processes can produce conduction block in the fascicles: ischemia, cardiomyopathies, valvular (especially aortic), myocarditis, cardiac surgery, congenital, and degenerative processes affecting the conduction tissue (Lenegre's or Lev's diseases).

In LASF block, left ventricular activation is by way of the LPIF and proceeds in an inferior-to-superior and right-to-left direction. The ECG characteristics of LASF block are: (1) normal QRS duration, (2) frontal plane mean QRS axis of less than −45°, (3) R wave in lead I greater than the R waves in leads II or III, (4) a qR complex in lead AVL, and (5) deep S wave in leads II, III, and AVF (Fig. 22-31). The LASF is small and easily affected by focal lesions. Other causes of left-axis deviation should be excluded—inferior myocardial infarction, hyperkalemia, preexcitation syndromes, or body habitus. Left ventricular hypertrophy itself does not cause an extensive left-axis deviation as seen with LASF block.

In LPIF block, left ventricular activation is by way of the LASF and proceeds in a superior-to-inferior and left-to-right direction. The ECG characteristics of LPIF block are: (1) normal QRS duration, (2) frontal plane mean QRS axis greater than 110°, (3) small r and deep S wave in lead I, (4) an R wave in lead III larger than the R wave in lead II, and (5) a qR complex in lead III (Fig. 22-32). The LPIF is broad and not affected by focal lesions; its presence indicates widespread organic heart disease. Other causes of right-axis deviation are chronic cor pulmonale, right ventricular hypertrophy, and lateral myocardial infarction.

In RBB block, ventricular activation is by way of the left bundle branch, proceeding from the left to the right ventricle. The ECG characteristics of RBB block are: (1) prolonged QRS duration (greater than 0.12 s); (2) triphasic QRS complexes (RSR′) in lead $V_1$; (3) wide S waves in the lateral leads I, $V_5$, and $V_6$; and (4) normal onset of ventricular activation in lead $V_6$ (Fig. 22-33). The frontal plane mean QRS axis is usually not deviated to the right unless there is associated right ventricular hypertrophy or LPIF block.

### Bifascicular Block

Bifascicular block refers to conduction blocks over two fascicles: (1) RBB and LASF, (2) RBB and LPIF, or (3) left bundle branch (LBB) block.

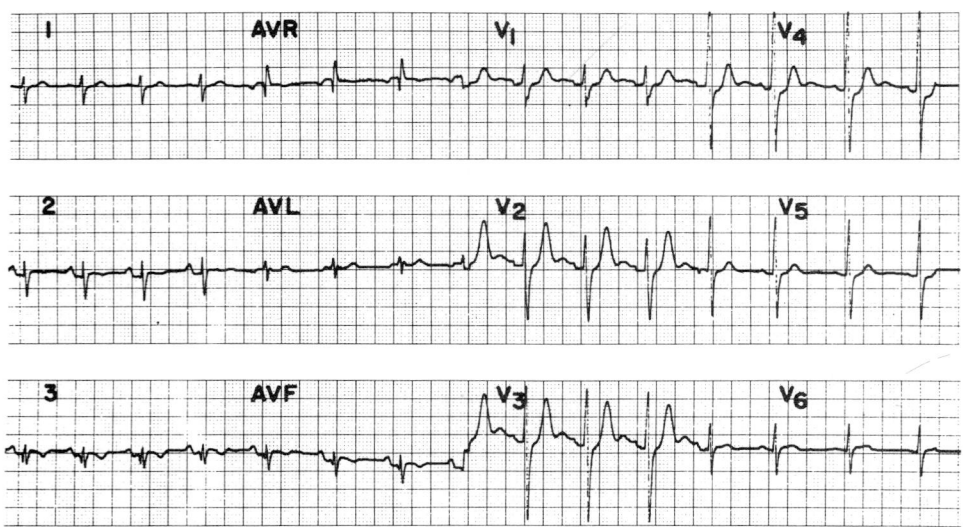

**Fig. 22-32.** Left posterior inferior fascicular block (LPIF block).

**Fig. 22-33.** Right bundle branch block (RBB block).

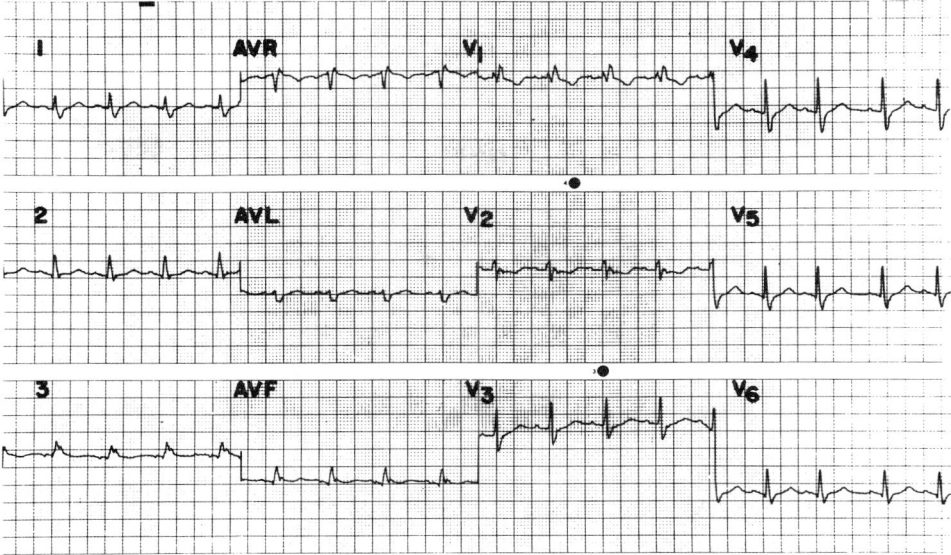

In LBB block, ventricular activation is by way of the RBB and proceeds from right to left and inferior to superior. The ECG characteristics of LBB block are: (1) prolonged QRS duration (greater than 0.12 s); (2) large and wide R waves in leads I, aV$_L$, V$_5$, and V$_6$; (3) small r wave followed by deep S wave in leads II, III, aV$_F$, and V$_1$ to V$_3$; and (4) no q waves in leads I, aV$_F$, V$_5$, and V$_6$ (Fig. 22-34).

## Trifascicular Block

Trifascicular block refers to a combination of conduction blocks in all three fascicles, either permanent or transient: (1) RBB and LASF with first-degree AV block, (2) RBB and LPIF with first-degree AV block, (3) LBB with first-degree AV block, or (4) alternating RBB and LBB block.

While bi- and trifascicular conduction blocks indicate advanced organic heart disease, long-term follow-up studies of ambulatory patients indicate that the risk of sudden progression to complete heart block and sudden death due to ventricular asystole is not high. Placement of a ventricular demand pacemaker is indicated only for symptoms due to documented bradyarrhythmias.

However, in the face of an acute myocardial infarction, the risks of complete heart block are much greater when new or preexistent bi- or trifascicular conduction blocks are present. In this setting, prophylactic placement of a ventricular demand pacemaker is indicated. This is further discussed in the chapter on acute myocardial infarction.

## PRETERMINAL RHYTHMS

Several arrhythmias may be seen during cardiac resuscitation. Ventricular tachycardia and fibrillation potentially are treatable and resuscitation may result in a functional survivor. The four other arrhythmias included here have a low successful resuscitation rate and are much less likely to yield a functional survivor. Further discussion on this is included in the chapter on cardiac resuscitation.

## Pulseless Electrical Activity (PEA)

Pulseless electrical activity is the presence of electrical complexes without accompanying mechanical contraction of the heart (Fig. 22-35). In the setting of a cardiac arrest, PEA is due to a profound metabolic abnormality of the myocardium, rendering it noncontractile. At this time, there is no clearly beneficial therapy; the best that can be recommended currently is continued cardiopulmonary resuscitation and α-adrenergic agents. Although calcium has been advocated traditionally, most studies have found no consistent benefit, and there are serious biophysiologic reasons to question the use of calcium in

**Fig. 22-34.** Left bundle branch block (LBB block).

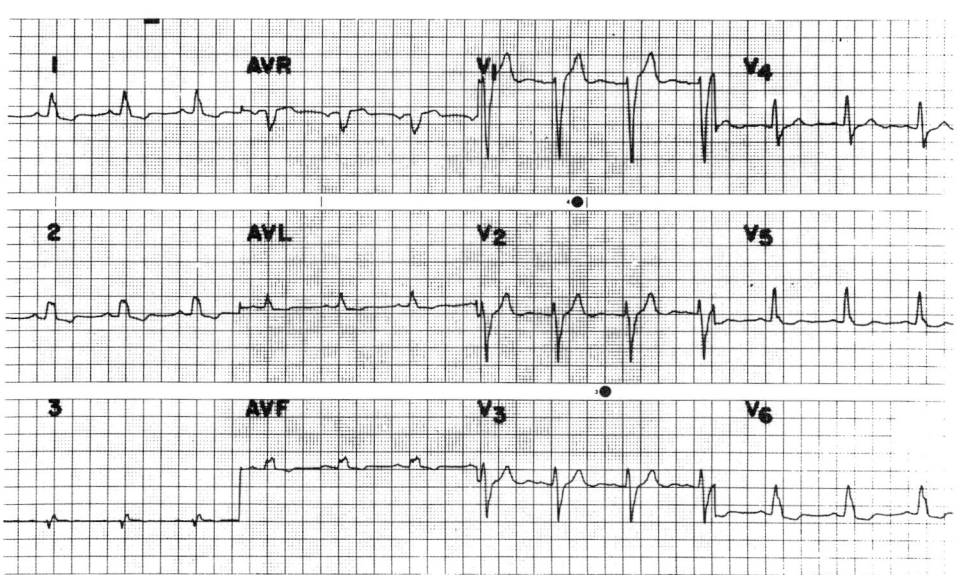

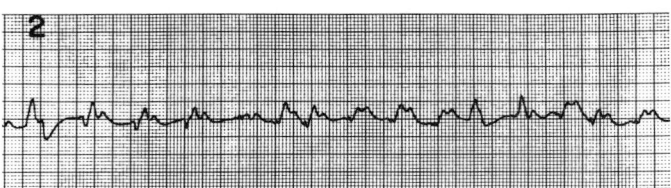

**Fig. 22-35.** Pulseless electrical activity (PEA).

the setting of cardiac arrest. Electrical pacing is, of course, not effective.

Other conditions which may mimic PEA are: (1) severe hypovolemia, (2) cardiac tamponade, (3) tension pneumothorax, (4) massive pulmonary embolus, and (5) rupture of the ventricular wall. The first three conditions are potentially treatable if recognized early.

### Idioventricular Rhythm (IVR)

An IVR is an escape rhythm of ventricular origin with very wide QRS complexes (more than 0.16 s) and a rate less than 40 (Fig. 22-36). Effective cardiac contractions and pulses may or may not be present. Idioventricular rhythm may occur as the result of complete infranodal AV block, acute myocardial infarction, cardiac tamponade, or exsanguinating hemorrhage. Treatment consists of attempting to accelerate the heart rate and enhance mechanical contractility using cardiopulmonary resuscitation and α-adrenergic agents. There is no proven benefit to the use of atropine or isoproterenol to treat IVR during cardiac resuscitation.

### Agonal Ventricular Rhythm

Agonal rhythm is the occurrence of very broad and irregular ventricular complexes at a slow rate, usually without associated ventricular contractions (Fig. 22-37).

### Cardiac Asystole (Cardiac Standstill)

Asystole is complete absence of any cardiac electrical activity. Treatment consists of attempting to stimulate electrical activity and mechanical contractions with continued cardiopulmonary resuscitation and α-adrenergic agents. Transthoracic or transvenous ventricular

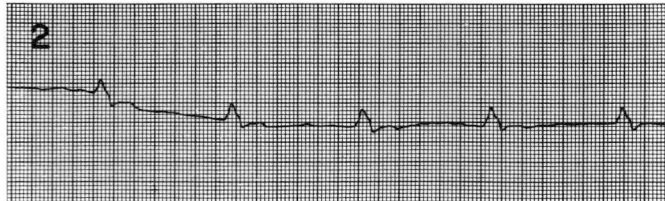

**Fig. 22-36.** Idioventricular rhythm (IVR).

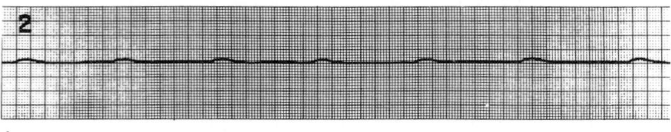

A

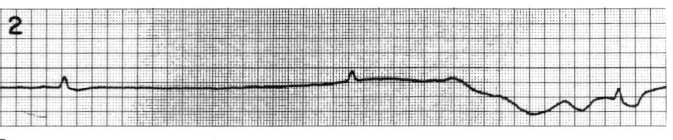

B

**Fig. 22-37.** Agonal ventricular rhythm. Top: regular. Bottom: irregular

pacing occasionally may produce electrical capture but rarely yields effective pumping action if prior agents were unsuccessful.

## TACHYCARDIA-BRADYCARDIA SYNDROME (SICK SINUS SYNDROME)

Sick sinus syndrome (SSS) is a heterogeneous disorder consisting of abnormalities of supraventricular impulse generation and conduction which produce a wide variety of intermittent supraventricular tachy- and bradyarrhythmias. The tachyarrhythmias are usually atrial fibrillation, junctional tachycardia, reentrant SVT, and atrial flutter. The bradyarrhythmias are marked sinus bradycardia, prolonged sinus arrest, and sinoatrial block usually associated with AV nodal conduction abnormalities and inadequate AV junctional escape rhythms.

### Clinical Significance

Symptoms of SSS are due to the effects of either fast or slow heart rate. Common symptoms include syncope or near-syncope, palpitations, dyspnea, chest pain, and cerebrovascular accidents.

A wide variety of cardiac disease can affect the sinus and AV node, producing the arrhythmias of SSS: ischemic, rheumatic, myocarditis and pericarditis, rheumatologic disease, metastatic tumors, surgical damage, or cardiomyopathies.

Conditions such as abdominal pain, increased intracranial pressure, thyrotoxicosis, and hyperkalemia which increase vagal tone may exacerbate the abnormalities of SSS and cause increased symptoms. Drugs such as digoxin, quinidine, procainamide, disopyramide, nicotine, β-adrenergic antagonists, or calcium-channel blockers also cause increased symptoms.

Ambulatory ECG monitoring is usually necessary for the diagnosis of SSS since a routine ECG cannot be expected to show the intermittent arrhythmias common in this syndrome. The demonstration of increased sensitivity of the sinus node to carotid sinus massage, Valsalva's maneuver, or atropine suggests sinus node dysfunction but is not conclusive proof for the diagnosis of SSS.

### Treatment

1. Symptomatic bradycardias require a permanent ventricular demand pacemaker. Because of the frequent association of AV conduction abnormalities, ventricular pacing is usually done, although atrial pacing is reasonable in selected patients.
2. Treatment of atrial tachyarrhythmias with digoxin, quinidine, disopyramide, procainamide, propranolol, or verapamil carries the risk of aggravating preexisting AV block or sinus arrest. Therefore, most patients should have pacemaker implantation before drug therapy is begun.

## PREEXCITATION SYNDROMES

Preexcitation occurs when some portion of the ventricles are activated by an impulse from the atria sooner than would be expected if the impulse were transmitted down the normal conducting pathway. Several different forms of preexcitation have been described, based on anatomic, clinical, electrocardiographic, and electrophysiological abnormalities. All forms of preexcitation are felt to be due to accessory tracts that bypass all or part of the normal conducting system. These bypass tracts have specific names (Fig. 22-38).

*James fibers* are a continuation of the posterior internodal tract and connect the atrium and proximal His bundle. Atrial impulses can therefore completely bypass the AV node to activate the ventricles. On ECG, this appears as (1) a short PR interval because the usual delay in the AV node is bypassed and (2) a normal QRS because James fibers insert directly into the infranodal conducting system and the ventricles are activated normally. When this is associated with reentrant SVT, the clinical condition is termed the Lown-Ganong-Levine (LGL) syndrome.

*Mahaim bundles* are composed of myogenic tissue, originate from

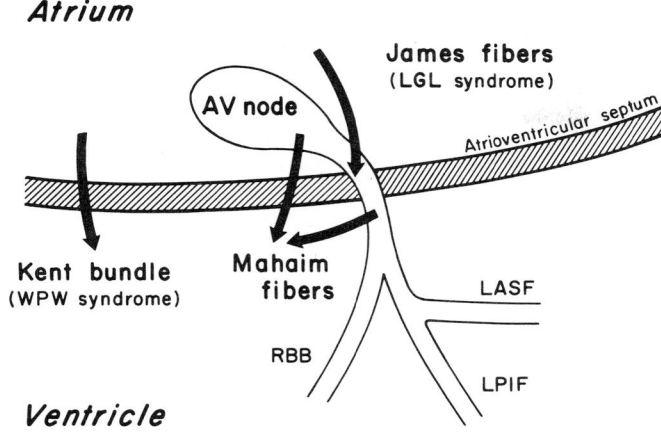

**Fig. 22-38.** Anatomic sites of bypass tracts.

either the AV node, His bundle, or bundle branches, and insert into the ventricles in the septal region. Atrial impulses pass through the AV node but then bypass all or part of the infranodal conducting system to activate the ventricles. Ventricular activation then occurs from two sources, the bypass tract and the normal conducting system, and the QRS complex represents a fusion of the two. The initial depolarization starts at the ventricular insertion of the bypass tract and is spread slowly by cell-to-cell transmission of the impulse. Subsequent depolarization by way of the faster normal conducting system then overtakes the initial depolarization and activates the bulk of ventricular myocardium. The QRS complex is basically normal with a slurred and distorted initial portion termed a delta wave. On ECG, this appears as a normal PR interval, and an initial distortion of ventricular depolarization (delta wave).

*Kent bundles* are composed of myogenic tissue and directly link the atria to the ventricles, completely bypassing the AV node and infranodal system. This is the most common form of preexcitation and is the anatomic basis for the Wolff-Parkinson-White (WPW) syndrome. On ECG, this appears as a shortened PR interval and with an initial distortion of ventricular activation (delta wave). Sometimes the bypass tract does not conduct an atrial impulse in the antegrade direction and the QRS complex is entirely normal. However, these concealed bypass tracts may conduct retrograde and be able to sustain reentrant SVT.

The WPW syndrome has been divided into types, depending on the

direction of the initial delta wave on the surface ECG. This in turn is determined by where the bypass tract (bundle of Kent) inserts into the ventricles and which portion of the ventricles is activated first. In reality, accessory tracts can insert anywhere around the AV annulus; the three types are just the most common locations.

In type A WPW, ventricular activation first occurs in the inferior-posterior region of the left ventricle and the delta wave is directed anteriorly. A positive initial deflection with a dominant R wave is seen in lead $V_1$. Q waves in leads II, III, and $aV_F$ are common (Fig. 22-39).

In type B WPW, ventricular activation first occurs in the inferior-posterior region of the right ventricle and the delta wave is directed posteriorly and to the left. A negative initial deflection and rS or QS pattern are seen in lead $V_1$ (Fig. 22-40).

In type C WPW, ventricular activation first occurs in the posterior-lateral region of the left ventricle and the delta wave is directed to the right, superiorly, and anteriorly. A positive delta wave is seen in lead $V_1$ with a negative or isoelectric delta wave in leads $V_5$ and $V_6$.

Because there is altered depolarization, repolarization is often abnormal with changes in the ST segments and T waves. The ECG changes of WPW may mimic changes seen with myocardial ischemia or infarction. Type A WPW may appear as a posterior myocardial infarction, and type B WPW may appear as an inferior myocardial infarction.

### Clinical Significance

There is a high incidence of tachyarrhythmias in patients with WPW—atrial flutter (about 5 percent), atrial fibrillation (10 to 20 percent), and paroxysmal reentrant SVT (40 to 80 percent).

Reentrant SVT occurs when an impulse is sustained around a loop composed of the bypass tract and the AV conducting system, the impulse traveling down one and up the other. Whether the QRS complex is wide or narrow depends on which limb of the circuit is used as the downward pathway to activate the ventricles. In about 80 to 90 percent of the time, reentrant SVT occurs with the impulse being conducted down the normal AV conducting system and up the bypass tract (orthodromic tachycardia). In this situation, ventricular activation occurs entirely over the normal system, the QRS complex is normal, and no delta wave is seen. Conversely, 10 to 20 percent of the time, the impulse is conducted down the bypass tract and retrograde up the AV node (antidromic tachycardia). In this case, the QRS complex is wide, and a delta wave may be visible. Reentry usually is initiated by a premature atrial contraction which encounters a bypass tract which still is refractory from the previous sinus beat, but the AV

**Fig. 22-39.** Type A Wolff-Parkinson-White syndrome.

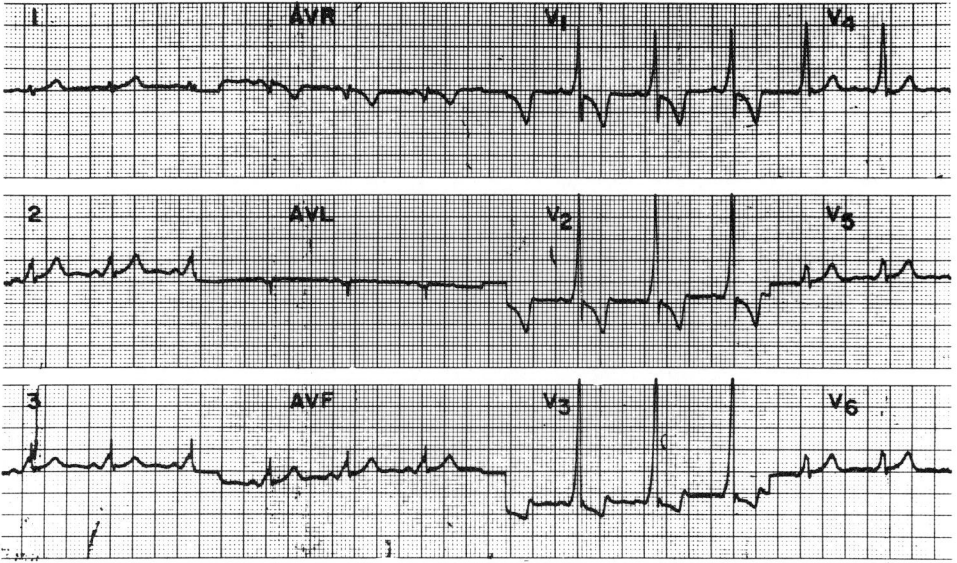

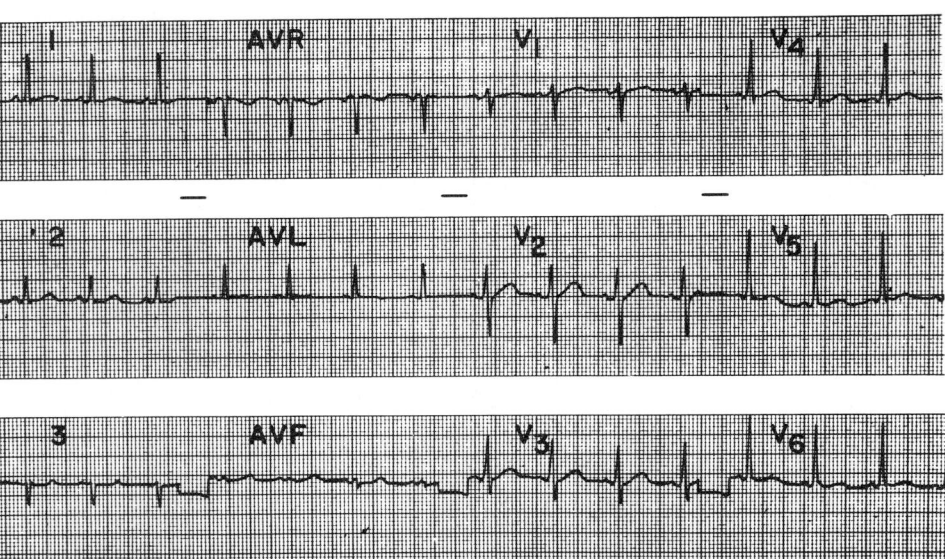

**Fig. 22-40.** Type B Wolff-Parkinson-White syndrome.

node has recovered partially and conducts the impulse more slowly than normal (Fig. 22-41). In some patients the bypass tract does not conduct antegrade during sinus rhythm and so no delta wave is seen, but it does conduct retrograde so reentrant SVT occurs. Patients with concealed bypass tracts account for about 20 percent of all patients with reentrant SVT.

If patients with WPW develop atrial flutter or fibrillation, impulses can reach the ventricles via the accessory tract, the normal conducting system, or both. Which pathway is used depends on the refractory periods of each. Most patients with WPW have longer refractory periods in their accessory tracts than in the AV node, but a minority have the opposite. In patients with short refractory periods in their accessory tracts, more atrial impulses can be conducted through the accessory tract than the AV node, so most of the QRS complexes will be wide. In atrial flutter, 1:1 AV conduction is possible with ventricular rates of 300 (Fig. 22-42). In atrial fibrillation, very rapid and irregular ventricular rates are possible. These rapid rhythms may resemble ventricular tachycardia, and excessive stimulation of the ventricles may precipitate ventricular fibrillation.

**Treatment**

1. Reentrant SVT (orthodromic, narrow QRS complex) in the WPW syndrome can be treated like other cases of reentrant SVT. Since the AV node is involved in the reentry circuit, any maneuver or drug that slows conduction through the AV node is usually effective. Verapamil or adenosine is very successful at terminating this arrhythmia in patients with WPW, but β-adrenergic blockers usually are ineffective.

2. Antidromic tachycardia (wide QRS complex) is usually associated with a short refractory period in the bypass tract, and such patients are at risk for rapid ventricular rates and degeneration into ventricular fibrillation. Stable patients should be treated with intravenous procainamide and unstable patients should be cardioverted. β-adrenergic or calcium-channel blockers should be avoided.

3. Atrial flutter or fibrillation with a rapid ventricular response is best treated with cardioversion. As an alternative, agents which prolong the refractory period of the accessory tract—such as procainamide—can be used. Lidocaine may have some utility, and experimental studies with intravenous flecainide have shown promise. In general, phenytoin, esmolol, propranolol, or verapamil have a variable effect on accessory conduction and should not be used. Digoxin is contraindicated as it may shorten the refractory period and enhance conduction over the bypass tract.

## DEFIBRILLATION AND SYNCHRONIZED CARDIOVERSION

Defibrillation and cardioversion is the technique of passing a short burst (about 5 ms) of direct electric current across the thorax to terminate tachyarrhythmias. The electric current simultaneously depolarizes all excitable cardiac tissue and terminates any areas of reentry by halting further propagation of the impulse around the reentry loop. This places all cardiac cells in the same depolarized state, and following repolarization a dominant pacemaker (usually the sinus node) paces the heart in a regular manner.

Defibrillation or cardioversion uses the same type of equipment. A device stores a known quantity of electrical energy in a storage capacitor and on command, discharges it through two paddles placed on

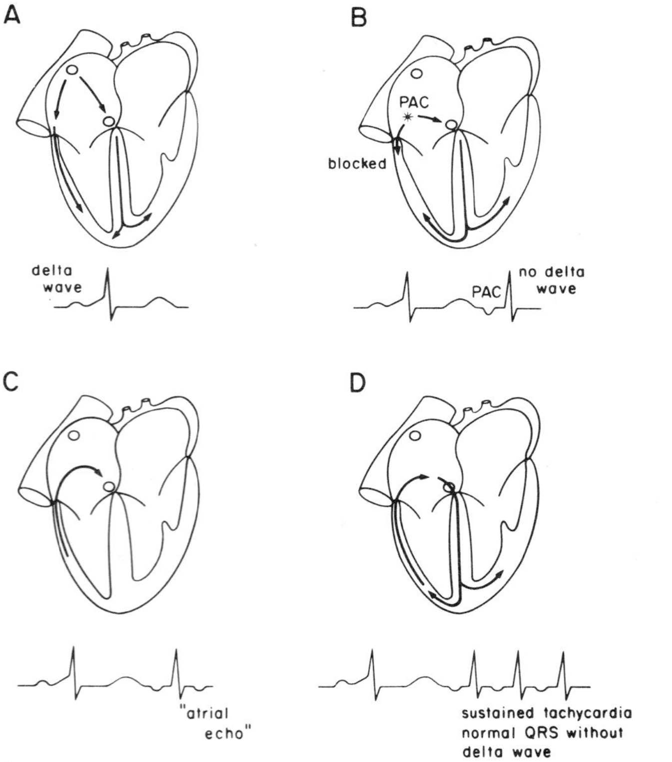

**Fig. 22-41.** Onset of reentrant SVT in Wolff-Parkinson-White syndrome.

**Fig. 22-42.** Atrial fibrillation in Wolff-Parkinson-White syndrome.

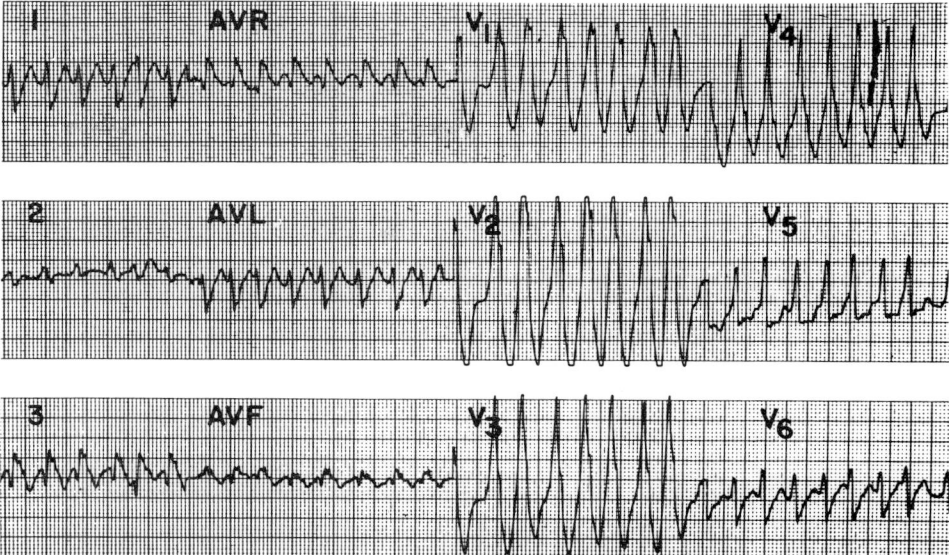

the chest wall. Usually, a rhythm monitor and a synchronizer circuit are built into the device. Paddle placement can be either anterior-posterior or apex-right parasternal. While some authors found a lower energy requirement for conversion using anterior-posterior paddles, others have not. For emergency situations, paddle placement probably does not matter.

To reduce transthorax electrical impedance and increase the amount of current passing through the heart, certain techniques are important at the paddle-chest wall interface. Electrode paste, gel, or saline pads are applied to the surface of the paddles. Firm pressure of 10 to 12.5 kg/cm$^2$ (20 to 25 lb/in$^2$) is used to achieve good electrical contact. Larger paddles, within reason, have a reduced impedance, but this does not appear to significantly influence the energy required for conversion.

Older devices had significant internal energy losses and delivered as little as 40 percent of the stored energy to the patient. This is not a problem with modern defibrillators as they deliver very close to the stored amount.

Defibrillation should be done as soon as ventricular fibrillation is diagnosed. The longer ventricular fibrillation persists, the less likely resuscitation will be successful. Current ACLS guidelines recommend 200 J for the first attempt, 200 to 300 J for the second attempt, and 360 J for subsequent defibrillations. Several studies have found that most patients can be defibrillated with 160 to 200 J. Recommendations for children are 2 J/kg (1 J/lb) in the initial attempt and 4 J/kg on subsequent attempts.

Synchronized cardioversion applies the electric current at a time during the cardiac cycle well away from the vulnerable period when there is little chance of inducing ventricular fibrillation—usually about 10 ms after the peak of the R wave. On most machines, the synchronizer circuit must be turned on each time an impulse is desired. Many devices also display by the monitor screen or a flashing light that the synchronizer circuit is detecting properly the QRS complex. Cable leads, rather than the paddles, should be used to monitor the cardiac rhythm to avoid any movement artifact that could be misinterpreted by the synchronizer circuit as the QRS complex.

Complications of defibrillation or cardioversion include:

1. Direct myocardial damage: unusual unless there are repeated shocks at high energy (more than 325 J).
2. Ventricular fibrillation: incidence is less than 5 percent with a synchronized discharge but probably greater in the presence of digoxin or quinidine toxicity, hypokalemia, or acute myocardial infarction. However, patients on maintenance digoxin therapy can be safely cardioverted using low energies (less than 50 J).
3. Systemic emboli: about 1.2 to 1.5 percent in patients with chronic atrial fibrillation.
4. ST segment changes: transient elevations or depressions, usually resolving within 5 min.
5. Bradycardias: more common in patients with inferior myocardial infarctions and those requiring multiple defibrillations-cardioversions. Usually evident during the first 5 s after shock and may occasionally persist for longer than 20 s and require external or internal pacing.
6. Tachycardias: usually sinus tachycardia, occasionally atrial flutter or fibrillation, and usually resolving spontaneously within 5 min.
7. Atrial, junctional, or ventricular ectopy: usually transient and benign.
8. Pulmonary edema: uncommon but may occur in patients with mitral or aortic valvular disease or left ventricular failure.
9. Hypotension: rare, inexplicable, and may last for several hours before spontaneously resolving.
10. Muscle damage: elevated levels of creatine phosphokinase (CPK) and lactic dehydrogenase (LDH) are common but the myocardial fractions [CPK-MB, LDH1, LDH2, and α-hydroxybutyric dehydrogenase (HBD)] are rarely abnormal.

## CARDIAC PACEMAKERS

Artificial cardiac pacemakers have two components: a power source (battery with pulse generator) and an electrode that delivers current to the heart (transvenous, epicardial, transthoracic, and transcutaneous). In permanent pacemaker placement, the power source is implanted subcutaneously, and the electrodes are run through the veins to inside the heart or through the subcutaneous tissue to the epicardial surface. In temporary pacemaker placement, the power source is external to the body and electrodes are placed in one of three ways: transvenous to an intracardiac location, transthoracic via a needle puncture through the skin into ventricular myocardium, or transcutaneous with electrodes placed on the thoracic skin.

The pulse generator can be designated to operate in either a fixed-rate mode (asynchronous or competitive) or a demand mode (synchronous or noncompetitive).

In the fixed-rate mode, the pulse generator produces an electrical

**Table 22-5.** Coding System for Permanent Pacemakers

| First Letter<br>Chamber Paced | Second Letter<br>Chamber Sensed | Third Letter<br>Mode or Response | Fourth Letter<br>Programmable Functions | Fifth Letter<br>Special Tachyarrhythmia Function |
|---|---|---|---|---|
| A = Atrium<br>V = Ventricle<br>D = Double (both) | A = Atrium<br>V = Ventricle<br>D = Double (both)<br>O = None | I = Inhibited<br>T = Triggered<br>D = Double<br>R = Reverse<br>O = None | P = Programmable<br>rate/output<br>M = Multiprogrammable<br>C = Communicating<br>O = None | B = Bursts<br>N = Normal rate<br>competition<br>S = Scanning<br>E = External |

signal at the preset rate regardless of the patient's own intrinsic cardiac rhythm. Serious arrhythmias or ventricular fibrillation may occur if the pacemaker discharges during the vulnerable period (T wave) and for this reason, fixed rate pacing is rarely done.

In the demand mode, the pulse generator has a sensing circuit which detects spontaneous cardiac activity and will discharge only if no cardiac depolarization is detected for a preset interval. Demand pacemakers may have two response modes, either inhibited or triggered. In the inhibited response mode (most commonly used), the pulse generator is inhibited by the sensed cardiac activity and does not generate an impulse. In the triggered response mode, the pacemaker detects the patient's intrinsic cardiac activity and then discharges during the absolute refractory period. On ECG, this appears as pacing spikes following each intrinsic QRS complex.

A five-letter code system is beginning to be used for pacemaker designation (see Table 22-5). The simplest type of pacemaker used—the ventricular demand inhibited response pacemaker—would be designated as VVI.

The modern permanent pacemaker is powered by a lithium battery which has an approximate lifetime of 8 to 12 years. Most units are preset for rates around 70 with a pacing interval of 0.84 s. The demand pacemaker has a built-in refractory period (0.2 to 0.4 s) during which it will not sense; this prevents it from being inhibited by its own stimulus. Most demand pacemakers have a magnetic switch which temporarily converts the pulse generator from the demand mode to the fixed-rate mode when a magnet is held over the unit. In this way the pacing rate can be quickly determined, but the magnet should be applied for only short periods to avoid initiating tachyarrhythmias. There are programmable pacemakers in which the rate and stimulus strength can be reset by noninvasive means. Since pacemaker complexity varies, the manufacturer supplies with each unit identification cards which patients should carry with them.

Temporary pacemakers are powered by 9-V radio-type batteries. On these pacemakers, there are settings for the mode (fixed or demand), rate (40 to 140), and stimulus strength (0.2 to 20 mA). During emergency pacing, initial settings should be in the demand mode with a rate around 70 and stimulus strength around 3.0 mA. The negative terminal should be connected to the distal electrode.

The transvenous intracardiac electrode may be either unipolar or bipolar. The unipolar setup has the negative electrode within the heart and the positive electrode in the chest wall. Permanent pacemakers using the unipolar setup have the positive electrode in their surface covering. Temporary pacemakers using the unipolar setup have their positive electrode connected to a needle implanted in the skin of the anterior thorax. With the bipolar setup, both electrodes are within a few millimeters of each other and both lie within the heart. Transvenous electrodes are placed most commonly into the apex of the right ventricle. Different catheters are used depending on the clinical situation. Right or semirigid catheters (No. 6 or No. 7 French) are inserted through a venous puncture or cutdown and usually require fluoroscopy for correct placement. Semifloating (No. 3 or No. 4 French) or flexible balloon-tipped catheters (No. 3 or No. 5 French) can be introduced and directed into the right ventricle without fluoroscopy using blood flow. Flexible catheters can become dislodged by patient or cardiac movement and usually are replaced with semirigid catheters within 24 h.

Transthoracic electrodes are inserted into the right ventricle through a left parasternal or subxiphoid intracardiac puncture. They are used in cardiac resuscitation when rapid placement is essential. The major disadvantage of transthoracic electrodes is that they can become dislodged with closed-chest compression. In addition, coronary artery laceration or pericardial tamponade is a hazard of percutaneous cardiac puncture. While electrical capture may be obtained in an occasional patient, it is rare to produce effective cardiac contractions with transthoracic pacing (Fig. 22-43).

Transcutaneous electrodes are self-adhesive pads which usually are placed with the negative electrode over the left anterior precordium and the positive electrode over the left infrascapular area. Transcutaneous pacing then is initiated by using the lowest current setting, which is increased until electrical capture is achieved. Most patients can be paced with 100 mA, but some may require up to 200 mA.

### Indications for Emergency Pacing

Emergency cardiac pacing is indicated either therapeutically (for symptomatic bradyarrhythmias) or prophylactically (for conduction defects which have a high risk of developing sudden complete heart block or asystole). (See Chapter 53.)

As noted before, symptomatic bradyarrhythmias should be treated with atropine and/or isoproterenol as a temporary measure to support cardiac rhythm prior to pacemaker placement. Some patients may respond adequately to atropine alone and do not require pacemaker insertion.

Most authors would recommend prophylactic placement of a pacemaker in any patient with acute myocardial infarction who has a new or age-indeterminant bi- or trifascicular block. In addition, second-degree Mobitz II and, of course, third-degree AV blocks are also indications for pacemaker insertion. Despite successful pacing, many patients with acute myocardial infarction and these serious conduction blocks have extensive left ventricular damage and a high mortality from pump failure.

### Pacemaker Malfunction

Permanent pacemaker malfunction can be categorized as either (1) failure to sense, (2) failure to pace, (3) oversensing, or (4) combinations of the first three. With current lithium batteries and reliable circuitry, most pacemaker malfunctions are due to problems with the electrodes and not the result of battery exhaustion or pulse-generator failure.

Failure to sense may occur when the voltage of the patient's own intrinsic QRS complex is too low to be detected by the sensing circuit of the pacemaker. Changing from a bipolar to unipolar setup (if possible) may help the pacemaker sense the intrinsic cardiac activity. Failure to sense may cause the pacemaker to discharge during the T wave and trigger serious arrhythmias.

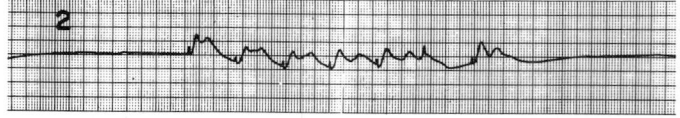

**Fig. 22-43.** Ventricular capture with transthoracic pacing.

Failure to pace may occur when tissue reaction around the electrode makes the myocardium insensitive to the electric discharge generated by the pacemaker. It is common for the pacing threshold to increase during the first few weeks after insertion, but further rises are infrequent.

Failure to both sense and pace may be due to battery exhaustion, fracture of the wires in the catheter, or displacement of the electrodes. Battery exhaustion is indicated when the pacing rate slowly decreases. With lithium batteries, such decreases usually occur years before actual battery exhaustion. Greater than a 10 percent change from the initial rate is an urgent indication for replacement. Catheter wire fracture may cause either sustained or intermittent interruption in electrical conductivity. Sudden onset of symptoms and/or bradyarrhythmias suggests catheter fracture. Catheter fractures are rarely seen on routine chest radiographs. The transvenous electrode is usually positioned in the right ventricular apex, with a characteristic appearance on chest radiograph and ECG. Displacement can be suggested when changes on radiographs or ECG occur.

Oversensing is used to describe the situation where the pacemaker senses electrical activity not associated with atrial or ventricular depolarizations; it is thus inhibited, and pacemaker impulse generation is suppressed. Causes of oversensing include physiological electrical activity (T waves, muscle potentials), external electromagnetic interference, and signals generated by the interaction of different portions of the pacing system. Unipolar electrodes are more sensitive to physiological electrical activity and electromagnetic interference than bipolar electrodes.

Under certain conditions, pacemakers may initiate tachyarrhythmias despite functioning as designed; this usually results from an intrinsic depolarization occurring during the pacemaker refractory period, therefore not being sensed, and the pacemaker firing soon thereafter and initiating a reentrant tachycardia. In this setting, maintenance of the arrhythmia does not require further participation of the pacemaker. Dual-chamber pacemakers can also induce and sustain arrhythmias. In this situation, emergent treatment requires reprogramming the pacemaker, if possible, or converting to synchronous mode by placing a magnet over the pulse generator.

## BIBLIOGRAPHY

Brugada P, Brugada J, Mont L, et al: A new approach to the differential diagnosis of regular tachycardia with a wide QRS complex. *Circulation* 83:1649, 1991.

Dreifus LS, Hessen SE: Supraventricular tachycardia: diagnosis and treatment. *Cardiology* 77:259, 1990.

Epstein AE, Hallstrom AP, Rogers WJ, et al: Mortality following ventricular arrhythmia suppression by encainide, flecainide, and moricizine after myocardial infarction. The original design concept of the cardiac arrhythmia suppression trial (CAST). *JAMA* 270:2451, 1993.

Rankin AC, Brooks R, Ruskin JN, et al: Adenosine and the treatment of supraventricular tachycardia. *Am J Med* 92:655, 1992.

Teo KK, Yusuf S, Furberg CD: Effects of prophylactic antiarrhythmic drug therapy in acute myocardial infarction. An overview of results from randomized controlled trials. *JAMA* 270:1589, 1993.

# 23
# PHARMACOLOGY OF ANTIARRHYTHMIC AND VASOACTIVE MEDICATIONS

**David Levy**
**Elizabeth Lyons**

## INTRODUCTION

This chapter discusses the actions, pharmacokinetics, indications, dosing, and adverse effect profile of antiarrhythmic and vasoactive agents that are pertinent to emergency medicine practice. Specific antiarrhythmics include procainamide, quinidine, lidocaine, various β blockers, and amiodarone. In addition, calcium channel blockers, adenosine, and digoxin are discussed. Vasoactive medications include epinephrine, dopamine, norepinephrine, isoproterenol, dobutamine, amrinone, atropine, and nitroglycerin. Vasodilating agents such as phentolamine, hydralazine, and clonidine together with other drugs used in hypertension management are discussed in Chap. 58.

## ANTIARRHYTHMIC AGENTS

Optimal therapy of arrhythmias requires knowledge of the mechanisms of action, pharmacokinetics, indications, appropriate dosing and administration, and types of adverse effects that may occur with each medication. Antiarrhythmic agents are divided into four classes based on their electrophysiologic effects and properties. Class I agents are further divided into three subgroups (see Table 23-1).

### Class I Antiarrhythmic Agents

#### Procainamide

**Actions**

Procainamide (Pronestyl) shares the same basic mechanism of action as the other class IA antiarrhythmic agents in that it suppresses automaticity by decreasing the rate and amplitude of phase 4 diastolic depolarization, prolongs the action potential duration, and reduces the speed of impulse conduction. These effects directly depress myocardial conduction, suppress fibrillatory activity in the atria and ventricles, and prevent ectopic or reentrant arrhythmias.

Procainamide, like other class IA antiarrhythmic agents, possesses dose-dependent anticholinergic activity (less than disopyramide or quinidine) that may suppress automaticity in ectopic pacemakers. Large doses of procainamide will provide extensive anticholinergic effects and may even increase automaticity (inducing a proarrhythmic effect). Class IA antiarrhythmic agents may decrease the force of myocardial contraction by inhibition of calcium transport across the cell membrane. The negative inotropic effect is more pronounced in ischemic myocardial tissue. High doses of procainamide may result in hypotension by vasodilation of the peripheral vasculature.

**Pharmacokinetics**

The onset of action of procainamide is 5 to 10 min following intravenous (IV) administration and 15 to 60 min following intramuscular (IM) injection. Procainamide has an elimination half-life of 2.5 to 4.7 h (in normal renal function) and an apparent volume of distribution (Vd) of 2 L/kg. However, in patients with congestive heart failure (CHF) and renal dysfunction, the elimination half-life may increase and the Vd may decrease (i.e., requiring smaller doses). Procainamide is metabolized to an active compound, *N*-acetyl procainamide (NAPA), in the liver via *N*-acetyltransferase. This active

**Table 23-1.** Electrophysiologic Actions of Antiarrhythmic Agents

| Class | Sub-class | Generic Name | Trade Name | Electrophysiologic Actions |
|---|---|---|---|---|
| I Fast channel blockers | Ia | Quinidine Disopyramide Procainamide | Norpace Pronestyl | ↓↓ conduction velocity ↑ action potential duration 0/↓ automaticity (↓↓ automaticity in higher doses) ↑↑ effective refractory period 0/↑ PR, QRS, and QT intervals (drug- and dose-related) |
| | Ib | Lidocaine Phenytoin Mexiletine Tocainide | Xylocaine Dilantin Mexitil Tonocard | ↓↓ phase 0 of action potential ↓ automaticity ↓↓ effective refractory period (in ischemic tissue) ↑ fibrillatory threshold ↓ repolarization period 0/↓ PR and QT intervals 0/↑ in AV nodal conduction |
| | Ic | Encainide Flecainide Propafenone Indecainide Moricizine* | Enkaid Tambocor Rhythmol Decabid Ethmozine | ↓↓ phase 0 of action potential ↓ automaticity ↓↓ conduction velocity ↑ action potential duration ↑ effective refractory period ↑ PR and QRS intervals (drug and dose-related) 0/↑ QT intervals |
| II β blockers | | Propranolol (also refer to Table 23-2) | Inderal | ↓ conduction velocity ↑ automaticity ↑ effective refractory period ↓↓ AV nodal conduction 0/↑ PR interval 0/↓ QT interval |
| III | | Bretylium | Bretylol | ↑↑ effective refractory period 0/↑ in automaticity 0/↑ in AV conduction |
| | | Amiodarone | Cordarone | ↑ fibrillatory threshold ↑ action potential duration |
| | | Sotalol | Betapace | 0/↑ PR, QRS, and QT intervals (amiodarone) |
| IV Calcium channel blockers | | Verapamil | Isoptin Calan | 0/↓ automaticity ↓/↓↓ AV nodal conduction |
| | | Diltiazem (also see text and Table 23-3) | Cardizem | ↑ AV node effective refractory period ↑ PR interval |
| Unclassified | | Digoxin Adenosine Magnesium sulfate | Lanoxin Adenocard — | 0/↓ automaticity; ↑ automaticity in high levels ↓ AV nodal ↑ AV nodal refractory period ↓ refractory period in ventricle ↑ PR interval ↓ QT interval |

* Very minimal negative inotropic effects.

metabolite has an average half-life of 7 h in patients with normal renal function. Rapid acetylators convert greater amounts of procainamide to NAPA than do slow acetylators. Plasma procainamide levels of approximately 4 to 10 μg/mL are usually required to suppress ventricular arrhythmias. Refractory arrhythmias may require levels up to 20 μg/mL (usually 10 to 15 μg/mL). Adverse effects often appear with levels greater than 12 μg/mL.

## Indications

Procainamide is a second-line agent generally used to treat and prevent recurrence of ventricular arrhythmias, specifically stable ventricular tachycardia (VT) and premature ventricular contractions (PVCs) that are not responding to lidocaine. It is infrequently used in ventricular fibrillation (VF) or pulseless VT. Procainamide may also be used for slowing or converting supraventricular tachycardias (SVT) including atrial flutter and fibrillation [especially in Wolff-Parkinson-White (WPW) syndrome], paroxysmal supraventricular tachycardia

(PSVT), paroxysmal atrial tachycardia (PAT), and paroxysmal atrioventricular (AV) junctional rhythm. Contraindications include complete AV heart block, second- or third-degree heart block (without an electrical pacemaker present), long QT intervals, and torsade de pointes. The drug should be used cautiously in patients with systemic lupus erythematosus (SLE), CHF, and hepatic or renal disease as well as in those with allergies to procaine or amide-type drugs.

## Dosing and Administration

In the past, the recommendation for IV loading of procainamide for treating ventricular arrhythmias was as a bolus injection. However, a continuous infusion has been shown to be safer (fewer adverse effects) than a bolus injection until the arrhythmia is controlled, hypotension develops, the QRS complex widens more than 50 percent, QT interval prolongation develops, or a total of 17 mg/kg (1.2 g for a 70-kg patient) has been given. The recommended infusion rate is 20 mg/min, yet in urgent situations, 30 mg/min may be given cautiously. Blood pressure and QRS complex must be monitored during IV administration. If procainamide suppresses the VT, initiate a continuous infusion at 1 to 4 mg/min to maintain the suppression. Lower doses generally are necessary for patients with CHF, hypotensive states, and hepatic or renal failure. Daily serum levels of procainamide or NAPA should be considered in patients with risk factors for impaired clearance.

Alternatively, oral therapy may be started after IV loading with procainamide (375 to 500 mg PO q 3–4 h) or a sustained-release preparation may be used (Procan SR or Pronestyl-SR in a dose of between 500 and 1000 mg q 6–8 h).

### Adverse Effect Profile

The most serious adverse effects of procainamide are from myocardial depression. Electrocardiographic changes may include prolongation of the QRS and QT interval, impairment of AV conduction, VF, and torsade de pointes. High doses or rapid infusion can cause severe hypotension. It should be initiated cautiously in patients with acute myocardial infarction (AMI) due to its potential proarrhythmic effect. Procainamide and NAPA levels should be monitored in the following patients: (1) those on procainamide longer than 24 h, (2) those on a maintenance infusion of 3 mg/min or higher, and (3) those with acute CHF or renal failure. SLE symptoms have been reported with chronic administration. Hypersensitivity reactions, characterized by angioedema, acute bronchoconstriction, vascular collapse, febrile episodes, and respiratory arrest, may occur. In addition, idiosyncratic reactions, including agranulocytosis, hepatomegaly, confusion, nausea, vomiting, urticaria, fever, maculopapular eruptions, and thrombocytopenia may develop when using procainamide.

## Quinidine (Gluconate or Sulfate)

### Actions

Quinidine is a class IA antiarrhythmic agent with essentially the same mechanism of action as procainamide. However, anticholinergic effects are more pronounced with quinidine. These anticholinergic effects may facilitate conduction across the AV node.

### Pharmacokinetics

Onset of action following IV administration is within minutes, whereas the onset for the IM and oral routes usually occurs in 1 to 3 h. Therapeutic cardiovascular effects last for the half-life of the drug, 6 to 8 h. The oral sustained-release (SR) gluconate preparation, however, can last up to 12 h. Therapeutic serum levels range between 2 and 7 µg/mL. Quinidine has an average Vd of 2 L/kg in healthy adults. It is metabolized in the liver to two active metabolites. Approximately 10 to 50 percent of a dose is excreted as unchanged drug in the urine within 24 h.

### Indications

Quinidine is effective in the treatment of atrial and ventricular arrhythmias and thus has the same indications as procainamide. Parenteral use of quinidine, however, can be considerably more dangerous. Newer agents may be safer.

### Dosing and Administration

The oral route is preferred when administering quinidine. Oral quinidine is available in three salts: sulfate (83% active drug), gluconate (62% active drug), and polygalacturonate (60% active drug). Only the gluconate and sulfate salts are available for parenteral use. IM administration is effective in acute, but not in critical, arrhythmias. IV administration should be reserved for acute symptomatic VT. The dose for quinidine varies, depending on the indication and salt used. For example, the adult dose for suppressing atrial, AV junctional, and ventricular complexes is 324 to 600 mg of extended-release quinidine

gluconate q 8–12 h, while the dose for quinidine sulfate to maintain sinus rhythm after conversion is 200 to 400 mg three or four times daily. The initial IM dose is 600 mg of quinidine gluconate, then 400 mg as often as q 2 h until desired effects are seen. Generally, the IV dosage required to abolish ventricular arrhythmias is 300 mg or less; however, 500 to 750 mg may be needed. The rate of infusion should not exceed 16 mg/min, and the ECG and blood pressure should be continuously monitored to gauge the efficacy and safety of treatment.

### Adverse Effect Profile

The adverse effect profile of quinidine is similar to that of procainamide (including a proarrhythmic effect) and includes torsade de pointes, SLE, and hypersensitivity reactions. Toxicity usually impairs therapeutic effectiveness. High serum levels of quinidine may result in cinchonism. Symptoms of cinchonism include tinnitus, blurred vision, headache, nausea, and deafness. Severe cases may lead to delirium and psychosis. Hypotension, heart failure, and hepatic disease decrease clearance. Quinidine has also been implicated in raising serum digoxin levels two- to three-fold.

## Lidocaine

### Actions

Lidocaine (Xylocaine), a class IB antiarrhythmic agent, controls ventricular arrhythmias predominantly by blocking fast sodium channels. Lidocaine decreases the slope of phase 4 depolarization and suppresses automaticity in the His-Purkinje system. The action potential duration and effective refractory period (ERP) of Purkinje fibers and ventricular muscles are also decreased, while the ratio of ERP to action potential duration is increased. Lidocaine appears to act preferentially on ischemic myocardial tissue, causing little or no effect on AV nodal or His-Purkinje conduction velocity in normal heart tissue. Lidocaine has local anesthetic effects that stabilize membranes, elevate the ventricular fibrillation threshold, and suppress ventricular ectopy in tissues during acute myocardial ischemia. It has a negligible effect on the autonomic nervous system, myocardial contractility, and peripheral vascular tone.

### Pharmacokinetics

The onset of action is 30 to 90 s following IV administration and 10 min following an IM dose. Subsequent bolus doses are generally required to attain therapeutic plasma levels early in treatment; maintenance infusions started without an initial bolus dose will not attain therapeutic levels for up to 30 min to several hours (based on disease state). Lidocaine has an approximate Vd of 1.3 L/kg in normal patients and 0.9 L/kg in patients with liver disease, CHF or in those who are hypotensive. The drug is available for IV use only because of its lack of GI absorption and its high first-pass metabolism. There is less than 10 percent excreted unchanged in the urine. The major metabolites, monoethylglycinexylidide (MEGX) and glycinexylidide (GX), possess antiarrhythmic and neurotoxic actions and are excreted renally.

Lidocaine has a short distribution half-life of 7 to 8 min following an IV bolus and 12 to 28 min following IM administration. This short distribution half-life accounts for the short duration of action after a bolus injection. The elimination half-life in healthy patients ranges from 80 to 108 min but may increase up to 7 h in patients with CHF or liver disease and is also greatly prolonged in cardiac arrest. Therapeutic serum levels range from 1.5 to 6 µg/mL; serum levels greater than 5 µg/mL may cause CNS toxicity. Not all patients require maximum serum levels.

### Indications

Lidocaine is the drug of choice for the suppression of ventricular arrhythmias and ventricular ectopy (frequent multifocal PVCs, couplets, salvos, and especially long runs of VT) in suspected acute myocardial ischemia or unstable angina. Although once popular, the *prophylactic* routine use of lidocaine is generally not recommended. Such therapy has not been shown to improve mortality following AMI. In addition, lidocaine should *not* be used to treat chronic PVCs that occur in an asymptomatic patient, as it does not prevent VF. The drug is also indicated for control of VT and VF refractory to defibrillation and epinephrine. Lidocaine should be given following successful conversion of ventricular tachyarrhythmias to normal sinus rhythm. Lidocaine can be an adjunct to procainamide for the treatment of wide-complex supraventricular arrhythmias of uncertain type (e.g., WPW syndrome).

**Dosing and Administration**

Lidocaine is given as an initial bolus dose of 1 mg/kg followed by additional bolus doses of 0.5 mg/kg q 5–10 min as needed up to a cumulative dose of 3 mg/kg. An alternative method is to give 1.5 mg/kg initially followed by 50-mg bolus doses every 5 min up to a total dose of 225 mg or 3 mg/kg. When VF is present and defibrillation and epinephrine have failed, an initial bolus of 1.5 mg/kg is recommended for all patients. Conscious patients should receive lidocaine at a rate not exceeding 50 mg/min to minimize adverse CNS effects (< 25 mg/min if infused through a central line). However, in pulseless VT or VF, lidocaine can be given by rapid IV push. IM injections are now facilitated by the availability of autoinjector devices that inject 300 mg of the 10% solution into the deltoid or the vastus lateralis muscles. Additional doses can be administered in 60 min if an IV line cannot be established. When IV lines are not available, the drug may be instilled endotracheally (ET); two to two and one-half times the IV dose up to a total volume of drug of 10 mL is recommended for optimal drug absorption.

VF and pulseless VT should be managed only with IV bolus doses. Maintenance infusions should be started at 2 mg/min and titrated up to 4 mg/min as needed (30 to 50 μg/kg per min) only upon return of perfusion (poor perfusion will hamper the drug's elimination).

Patients more than 70 years of age, those with CHF, liver disease, or impaired hepatic blood flow should have their loading dose and maintenance infusion rate lowered by 50 percent. Drug interactions that can prolong the half-life of lidocaine or increase toxicity include those that potentiate neurologic effects (e.g., procainamide, tubocurarine), drugs that undergo metabolism in the liver and increase lidocaine levels (e.g., cimetidine, propranolol), and drugs that can produce excessive cardiac depression (e.g., phenytoin). Septic shock will also produce increased cardiac depression. Since the half-life of lidocaine can be increased after 24 to 48 h in any of the above, serum levels should be obtained and infusions adjusted accordingly if therapy is used for longer than 24 h. Lidocaine toxicity may also develop in patients with renal dysfunction due to accumulation of the metabolites. Patients should be changed to oral antiarrhythmics within the first 24 h.

**Adverse Effect Profile**

Adverse effects from lidocaine usually occur when the drug is administered too rapidly in a conscious patient, when excessive doses are administered, or when a drug interaction potentiates toxicity. Symptoms of mild lidocaine toxicity that correlate with levels greater than 5 μg/mL include slurred speech, drowsiness, confusion, nausea, vertigo, ataxia, tinnitus, paresthesias, and muscle twitching. An abrupt change in mental status is classic for lidocaine toxicity and may indicate that an excessive dose was administered or that the rate of administration was excessive. Serious symptoms occurring at plasma levels greater than 9 μg/mL may include psychosis, seizures, and respiratory depression. Lidocaine is contraindicated in patients with known sensitivities to amide-type local anesthetics and those with high degrees of sinoatrial (SA) or AV block.

## Class II Antiarrhythmics: β Blockers

### General Information

**Actions**

Numerous β blockers have been introduced into the United States during the past several years. While these agents share the principal characteristic of blocking catecholamine effects on β receptors, they vary in other important properties, such as cardioselectivity, intrinsic sympathomimetic activity, α-adrenergic blocking activity, and pharmacokinetic properties (relative potency, route of elimination, distri-bution in fat and brain, and duration of action). See "Propranolol" for a basic discussion on the nonspecific β blocker (Table 23-2).

Cardioselective β-blocking (specific for the $β_1$ receptor) drugs include acebutolol, atenolol, esmolol, and metoprolol. They may be better choices for use in patients with a history of asthma, chronic obstructive pulmonary disease (COPD), or diabetes, since the blockade of $β_2$ receptors may result in adverse outcomes. The hemodynamic effects of cardioselective β blockers are similar to those of propranolol, excluding the increase in vascular resistance. At high doses, some agents lose their cardioselectivity; the exact dose at which this occurs, however, has not been clearly established.

Beta blockers with intrinsic sympathomimetic activity (ISA), such as acebutolol, carteolol, penbutolol, and pindolol, occupy the β receptor and produce a low level of stimulation. Despite this stimulation, the receptor is functionally blocked to high sympathetic tone. Theoretically, these drugs would be safer to use in patients with low cardiac output states because of their intrinsic ability to stimulate the heart. This ability may prevent acute drug-induced heart failure, but this has not been proven in clinical trials.

For information about β blockers with α-blocking actions, see the section on "Labetalol."

**Pharmacokinetics**

Refer to Table 23-2 for pharmacokinetic parameters of each of the various β blockers.

**Indications**

Indications for each of the various β-blocking agents have been similar to those of propranolol. The longer-acting agents are effective in the chronic treatment of hypertension. Cardioselective β blockers are used in patients with asthma or insulin-dependent diabetes, while drugs with intrinsic sympathomimetic activity may be better tolerated in some patients. Beta blockers (e.g., metoprolol and atenolol) can decrease mortality in AMI patients with high sympathetic tone. This fact is especially true early in the course of an AMI (within 6 h of onset), an acute anterior infarct, or a tachyarrhythmia or chest pain refractory to standard therapy. In low-risk patients receiving thrombolytics, β blockade may reduce mortality and recurrent MI if administered within 2 h of symptom onset and can lower the rate of nonfatal reinfarction and recurrent ischemia if used within 4 h. However, effects in low-risk patients and were not of sufficient magnitude to recommend routine use of β blockers following thrombolytic agents.

**Dosing**

The dosing regimens for each β blocker vary according to their potency and pharmacologic half-life. Refer to Table 23-2 for initial and maximum daily dose information. In regard to metoprolol IV dosing, recommendations are for a bolus of 5 mg q 2–5 min up to 15 mg. In patients not tolerating the full 15-mg IV dose, oral metoprolol should be given in doses of 25 to 50 mg every 6 h (depending on the degree of intolerance), starting 15 min after the last IV dose or as soon as their clinical condition allows. A similar agent, atenolol, may be given IV 5 mg over 5 min, followed by another 5-mg IV dose

**Table 23-2.** Comparison Chart for β-Blockers

| Generic Name | Trade Name(s) | Dosage Form | Receptor Selectivity | Elimination Half-life | ISA*/ MSA† | Initial Dose | Maximum Dose | Approved Indications |
|---|---|---|---|---|---|---|---|---|
| Acebutolol | Sectral | Oral | β₁ | 3–4 h (8–13 h for diacetolol) | +/+ | 400 mg/day | 1.2 g/day | HTN,‡ arrhythmias |
| Atenolol | Tenormin | IV Oral | β₁ Same | 6–9 h | 0/0 | 5 mg 50 mg/day | 10 mg 200 mg/day | Acute MI, HTN angina |
| Betaxolol | Kerlone | Oral | β₁ | 14–22 h | 0/0 | 10–20 mg/day | 20 mg/day | HTN |
| Bisoprolol | Zebeta | Oral | β₁ | 9–12 h | 0/0 | 5–10 mg/day | 20 mg/day | HTN |
| Carteolol | Cartrol | Oral | β₁ β₂ | 6–11h | +++/0 | 2.5 mg/day | 10 mg/day | HTN |
| Esmolol | Brevibloc | IV | β₁ | 9 min | 0/0 | 500 µg/kg per min load, then 25–50 µg/kg per min | 300 µg/kg per min | PSVT, sinus tachycardia kg per min |
| Labetalol | Normodyne Trandate | IV | α₁ β₁ β₂ | 5–8 h | +/0 | 20 mg IV push initially, then double the dose every 10 min | 300 mg | HTN |
| | | Oral | Same | 6–8 h | Same | 200 mg/day | 2.4 g/day | HTN |
| Metoprolol | Lopressor | IV Oral | β₁ Same | 3–7 h | 0/0 | 5 mg IV push 100 mg/day | 15 mg 450 mg/day | Acute MI, angina HTN, acute MI |
| Nadolol | Corgard | Oral | β₁ β₂ | 14–24 h | 0/0 | 40 mg/day | 320 mg/day | HTN, angina |
| Oxprenolol | Trasicor | Oral | β₁ β₂ | 1–2 h | ++/+ | 160 mg/day | 320 mg/day | HTN, angina |
| Penbutolol | Levatol | Oral | β₁ β₂ | 17–26 h | ++/0 | 20 mg/day | 80 mg/day | HTN |
| Pindolol | Visken | Oral | β₁ β₂ | 3–4 h | +++/0 | 20 mg/day | 60 mg/day | HTN |
| Propranolol | Inderal | IV | β₁ β₂ | 3–6 h | 0/++ | 1 mg | 3 mg | HTN, arrhythmias, angina, post-MI prophylaxis |
| | | Oral | Same | 5–6 h | Same | 40–80 mg/day | 480 mg/day | |
| Sotalol | Betapace | Oral | β₁ β₂ | 7–15 h | 0/0 | 80 mg/day | 640 mg/day | Arrhythmias§ |
| Timolol | Blocadren | Oral | β₁ β₂ | 4–5 h | ±/0 | 20 mg/day | 60 mg/day | HTN, post-MI prophylaxis |

* Intrinsics ympathomimetic activity

† Membrane stabilizing activity

‡ HTN, hypertension

§ Has proarrhythmic effects

*Note:* This table reflects use of β blockers for cardiovascular indication. β blockers have a variety of other uses and are available in other dosage forms under different trade names.

10 min later. In patients who tolerate the 10-mg IV dose, an oral dose of 50 mg may be initiated 10 min after the last IV dose followed by another 50-mg oral dose in 12 h. Oral metoprolol and atenolol may be given in doses of 100 mg and 50 mg, respectively, twice daily, or atenolol can be administered as a 100-mg dose daily.

**Adverse Effects**

Adverse effects are remarkably similar and include nausea, vomiting, light-headedness, mental depression, bradycardia, hypotension, bronchospasm, hyperglycemia, and pulmonary edema. Cardioselective agents cause less bronchospasm and hyperglycemia than nonselective agents. Beta blockers can also mask hypoglycemia. Some investigators feel that β blockers that are more water-soluble induce less CNS effects. These drugs are generally contraindicated in patients with heart block greater than first degree, CHF, or cardiogenic shock.

However, recent studies show that β blockers may provide some relief for CHF secondary to diastolic dysfunction. For the most part, oral β blockers as a group are very safe if used appropriately. The adverse effects are mild and resolve before it is necessary to discontinue therapy.

## Propranolol

**Actions**

In therapeutic doses, the major effect of propranolol (Inderal) is its β-adrenergic blocking activity. The drug blocks the effects of catecholamines on β receptors, inhibiting chronotropic, inotropic, and vasodilator responses to β-adrenergic stimulation. Propranolol slows the sinus rate, depresses AV conduction, decreases cardiac output, reduces blood pressure on exercise, and reduces both supine and standing blood pressures. In addition, propranolol decreases renin release and myocardial oxygen demand and protects against sudden cardiac death.

### Pharmacokinetics

The onset of action of propranolol following IV administration is within 1 min, with a half-life of elimination that varies with duration of therapy. In short-term treatment, the elimination half-life approximates 2 to 3 h, but in chronic treatment, the elimination half-life is 4 h. Propranolol is widely distributed throughout the body, undergoes extensive first-pass metabolism by the liver, and is also significantly bound to sites within the liver. For these reasons, propranolol has a low bioavailability when taken orally as compared to IV administration, making the IV dose approximately 10 times smaller than the oral dose. Several metabolites have been discovered, and they are primarily excreted in the urine and feces. In significant renal impairment, the proportion of metabolites excreted by the feces will increase. No dosage adjustments are required in renal patients. Propranolol has the highest lipid solubility of all β blockers as well as the highest protein binding (93 percent).

### Indications

Propranolol is indicated for a wide variety of supraventricular arrhythmias. These include paroxysmal atrial tachycardia, particularly those arrhythmias induced by digoxin or catecholamines or associated with the WPW syndrome; refractory sinus tachycardia; atrial flutter or fibrillation refractory to digoxin; persistent atrial extrasystoles that do not respond to conventional therapy; and tachyarrhythmias associated with thyrotoxicosis. Propranolol is less effective for ventricular than for supraventricular arrhythmias, but it can be used for ventricular tachycardias or ectopic beats due to digoxin or catecholamine toxicity.

Other indications for propranolol include the management of angina and acute myocardial ischemia or infarction because it decreases myocardial oxygen demands; management of all chronic types of hypertension either alone or in combination with other antihypertensive agents (propranolol is not indicated for hypertensive emergencies); the treatment of idiopathic hypertrophic subaortic stenosis; prophylaxis for common migraine headaches; management of familial or hereditary essential tremor; and as an adjunctive drug following an α-adrenergic blocker in controlling tachycardia due to pheochromocytoma.

### Dosing and Administration

For life-threatening arrhythmias, the IV dose of propranolol is 0.5 to 1 mg given as an IV bolus up to 5 mg at a rate not exceeding 1 mg/min. The dose may be repeated in 2 min. Since significant myocardial depression can occur when doses greater than 3 mg are given, caution should be used if additional doses are necessary. Esmolol IV infusion has been as effective as IV propranolol in reducing heart rate and has resulted in a more rapid reversal of β blockade as compared to propranolol.

### Adverse Effect Profile

The adverse effect profile for propranolol is similar to that for other nonselective β blockers. The drug is generally not given to patients with asthma or allergic rhinitis and is contraindicated in those with sinus bradycardia or advanced SA or AV block. Propranolol should also not be used in CHF or cardiogenic shock, unless these conditions are due to tachyarrhythmias. Following an AMI with the presence of heart failure, "cardiac asthma" can be aggravated with propranolol, but less so with cardioselective agents (e.g., esmolol, metoprolol, and atenolol).

## Sotalol

### Actions

Sotalol (Betapace) is a unique noncardioselective β blocker without intrinsic sympathomimetic or local anesthetic activity that also prolongs repolarization (class III antiarrhythmic activity). Sotalol is approved for use in life-threatening ventricular dysrhythmias only.

### Pharmacokinetics

Sotalol, rapidly and completed absorbed from the GI tract, does not bind to plasma proteins, forms no metabolites, and is eliminated mainly in the urine. The elimination half-life of the drug is about 12 h.

### Indications

Sotalol has been shown to be a first-line agent for suppression of life-threatening ventricular arrhythmias refractory to other antiarrhythmic agents. Clinical trials have shown sotalol to be effective in patients who have been refractory to other conventional antiarrhythmic agents. Although not approved for this indication by the U.S. Food and Drug Administration (FDA), double-blind trials have shown that sotalol can suppress SVT and atrial fibrillation.

### Dosing and Administration

The usual initial oral dosage is 80 mg bid, which can be increased to 240 mg or 320 mg/day; a therapeutic response is usually obtained at a total daily dose of 160 to 320 mg/day. There should be 2 to 3 days with QT monitoring allowed between increments. The maximum dosage is 480 to 640 mg/day; however, this dose should only be used when the potential benefit outweighs the increased risk of adverse effects. The dosing interval should be extended for renal insufficiency. Dose escalations in these patients should be done after administration of at least five to six doses and be based on the creatinine clearance. If the creatinine clearance is 30 to 60 mL/min, the dosing interval should be q 24 h; at 10 to 30 mL/min, adjusted to 36 to 48 h; and when the clearance is < 10 mL/min, the dose should be individualized.

### Adverse Effect Profile

Sotalol is well tolerated and many adverse effects are dose related; the most common are related to that of nonselective β blockade. Sotalol also can have proarrhythmic effects, particularly in those with torsade de pointes, prolonged QTc intervals, or hypokalemia, or who are taking high doses of the drug.

## Esmolol

### Actions

Esmolol (Brevibloc) possesses cardioselective β-adrenergic blocking properties, selectively blocking the β1 receptor. As with other β blockers, this drug exhibits both negative inotropic and negative chronotropic effects. Esmolol prevents excessive adrenergic stimulation on the myocardium by blocking the β1 receptors, thus producing an increase in sinus cycle length, prolongation of SA nodal recovery time, and a decrease in conduction through the AV node. Esmolol is effective for treating SVT and also possesses antihypertensive effects. These may be due to its ability to decrease cardiac output, sympathetic outflow, and renin release from the kidneys, or perhaps from the direct vasodilatory action of the drug.

### Pharmacokinetics

Within 1 to 4 min of IV loading with esmolol, both the heart rate and blood pressure decline, and the PR interval becomes prolonged on the ECG. Of all the available β-blocking agents, esmolol has the shortest duration of action. The elimination half-life is approximately 9 min, and effects of the drug completely reverse within 30 min after cessation of IV therapy. This feature makes IV esmolol a useful agent for the treatment of acute and unstable SVT, since the adverse or toxic effects disappear quickly upon discontinuation of the drug. The short duration of action also allows the drug to be titrated to effect. Although 90 percent of an administered dose is excreted renally as metabolites, the metabolites possess minimal, if any, β-blocking effects. Dosing adjustments are thus not required in patients suffering from hepatic or renal insufficiency.

### Indications

Esmolol is currently indicated to control ventricular rate for the short term when the termination of SVT is desired. It is effective to prevent or treat SVT resulting from increased sympathetic tone during or following surgical procedures. IV esmolol may also be used during surgery as replacement β-blocker therapy to prevent rebound hypertension in patients who have been receiving long-term β-blocker treatment. Esmolol can also be used to maintain normal sinus rhythm (NSR) in post-AMI patients who cannot tolerate oral medications. Esmolol is not indicated for long-term management of SVT.

### Dosing and Administration

A loading dose of esmolol is given as an IV bolus of 500 μg/kg over 1 min, followed by IV infusion starting at 50 μg/kg per min infused over 4 min. Assess for therapeutic and adverse effects immediately following the infusion. If there is no response, give another loading dose over 1 min and increase the infusion rate to 100 μg/kg per min for 4 min. If there is still no response, repeat this procedure, using the same bolus dose each time and increasing the infusion rate by increments of 50 μg/kg per min until the rate of infusion reaches 200 μg/kg per min, the desired response is achieved, or adverse effects appear. The majority of patients will respond within this dosage range. A dose-dependent action is noticed, however, and doses above 200 μg/kg per min are usually of no greater benefit. Once adequate therapeutic response is obtained, it is advisable to change infusion rates by no more than 25 μg/kg per min and not use a bolus dose. Also, avoid concentrations greater than 10 μg/mL. The use of esmolol infusions up to 24 h has been well documented. Limited data indicate that esmolol is well tolerated up to 48 h. After achieving a desired hemodynamic response, transition to alternative antiarrhythmic agents should be considered. Wean the patient off esmolol gradually.

### Adverse Effect Profile

Esmolol shares the same toxic potential and adverse effect profile as the other β-blocking agents. The most common adverse effect associated with esmolol use is hypotension, which occurs in approximately 20 to 50 percent of patients being treated for SVT. This usually occurs within 30 min of therapy initiation. Other common adverse effects include dizziness, somnolence, and nausea.

## Labetalol

### Actions

Labetalol (Normodyne, Trandate) possesses membrane-stabilizing effects and thus has some antiarrhythmic action; however, the drug is often used as an antihypertensive agent because it blocks both α- and β-adrenergic receptors. The β-adrenergic blocking effects are nonselective, while the α-blocking effects are selective for the $\alpha_1$ receptor. It appears that the β-blocking effects of labetalol are much greater than its α-blocking effects, in a ratio between 3:1 for oral and 7:1 for IV administration. Additionally, studies have found labetalol to possess some ability to stimulate rather than block the $\beta_2$ receptors.

The mechanisms by which labetalol elicits its antihypertensive effects may include any or all of the following: (1) synergistic effects resulting in hypotension when both $\alpha_1$ and $\beta_1$ receptors are blocked, (2) $\beta_2$-receptor stimulation, and (3) direct vasodilatory action. Labetalol decreases heart rate, contractility, cardiac output, cardiac work, and total peripheral resistance.

### Pharmacokinetics

Labetalol is primarily eliminated by the liver and undergoes extensive first-pass metabolism, with approximately 30 percent of the drug reaching circulation following oral administration. Geriatric patients and those with liver disease, however, may have a greater bioavailability. The onset of action of IV labetalol is within 2 to 5 min, peaks in 10 to 15 min, and lasts 2 to 4 h. Oral labetalol acts within 20 min to 2 h, peaks within 1 to 4 h, and lasts 8 to 24 h. The elimination half-life is approximately 3 to 8 h in normal individuals. Only 5 percent of the drug is excreted as unchanged drug.

### Indications

Labetalol is used in emergency medicine primarily for its antihypertensive actions. Intravenous labetalol rapidly and effectively reduces elevated pressures, causing only minimal alterations in heart rate and cardiac output. It is a good alternative for treating the hypertensive patient with myocardial ischemia. Oral labetalol may be substituted once control of blood pressure has been established. Labetalol has been used safely in pregnant patients.

### Dosing and Administration

Labetalol can be administered IV via multiple IV boluses or a continuous IV infusion. When initiating IV bolus, the clinician should start with 20 mg (0.25 mg/kg in an 80-kg patient) and repeat with 40 mg to 160 mg every 10 min until the desired effect is reached or until a total cumulative dose of 300 mg has been given. It is best to double the previous dose every 10 min, thus allowing gradual dosage increase. A smaller alternative dose would be 10 to 15 mg given every 15 m. Alternatively, labetalol may be given via continuous infusion at a rate of 0.5 to 2 mg/min until the desired response or a total cumulative dose of 300 mg has been reached. There are reports where labetalol has been used as a continuous drip over a 24-h period in severe and refractory cases. Patients receiving labetalol via the IV route should be placed in a supine position and remain supine for approximately 3 h after receiving any IV doses, since symptomatic orthostatic hypotension may occur. Following patient stabilization, labetalol may be given orally up to 2400 mg per day in two to four divided doses. Acute dosing of IV labetalol can lead to a "cumulative effect," as each dose will persist for 2 to 4 h. These patients must be under diligent observation to avoid hypotensive episodes.

### Adverse Effect Profile

Labetalol has the same adverse effects profile as the other β-blocking and $\alpha_1$-blocking agents. The most common adverse effect associated with labetalol use is orthostatic hypotension, which occurs most frequently upon initial therapy. A loss of consciousness has occurred in some patients following both IV and oral administration. Symptomatic heart failure may also occur. Adverse CNS effects that may occur include lightheadedness, drowsiness, dizziness, fatigue, lethargy, and vivid nightmares. Tingling of the scalp and skin may occur with the initiation of therapy. Occasionally, reversible elevation of the hepatic enzymes may lead to jaundice and hepatitis. Other effects include lupus-like complaints, elevated renal function tests, blood dyscrasias, and allergic reactions. Avoid the use of IV labetalol in patients with risks for intracranial bleeding as a hypotensive episode can induce CNS herniation.

## Class III Antiarrhythmic Agents

### Bretylium

#### Actions

Classified as a class III antiarrhythmic, bretylium (Bretylol) differs from lidocaine and procainamide in cardiovascular effects and electrophysiologic actions. The cardiovascular actions of bretylium are biphasic. Initially, this quaternary ammonium compound releases norepinephrine from sympathetic ganglia and the terminal nerve endings of postganglionic nerves. This effect can cause a moderate increase in blood pressure, heart rate, and cardiac output lasting approximately 20 min, especially if the drug is infused too rapidly. At 45 to 60 min, bretylium blocks the release of norepinephrine in response to sympathetic nerve stimulation by depressing the excitability of adrenergic nerve terminals. This results in a sympatholytic effect that can cause orthostatic hypotension.

Bretylium affects phase 3 (repolarization) of the action potential and markedly prolongs refractoriness, action potential duration, and the QT interval. It has also been described as an antifibrillatory agent rather than an antiarrhythmic.

#### Pharmacokinetics

The onset of action for IV bretylium in VF is within minutes but may take from 20 min up to 2 h when used for other ventricular arrhythmias. Peak effects occur in 1.5 to 6 h and last 6 to 12 h following a single dose. The drug is well absorbed following IM injection. Bretylium is eliminated primarily as unchanged drug via the kidney (70 to 85 percent) and thus may have a prolonged duration of action in patients with renal dysfunction.

#### Indications

The three indications for bretylium are (1) treatment of VF refractory to repeated countershocks and epinephrine and lidocaine bolus doses; (2) when lidocaine and procainamide have failed to control VT associated with a pulse; or (3) when adenosine and lidocaine have failed to control wide-complex tachycardias. The drug is indicated as a first-line agent when lidocaine and procainamide are contraindicated (i.e., hypersensitivity reactions).

#### Dosing and Administration

The initial dose of bretylium for VF or pulseless VT is 5 mg/kg (500 mg = 1 ampule) administered by rapid IV push. If VF persists, the dose can be increased to 10 mg/kg and repeated at 15- to 30-min intervals up to a maximum dose of 35 mg/kg. For recurrent or refractory ventricular tachyarrhythmias, 5 to 10 mg/kg should be infused over a period of 8 to 10 min. If these arrhythmias persist, repeated boluses of 5 to 10 mg/kg can be given q 1–2 h as necessary. If the IM route is used, no more than 5 mL should be injected at any one site, and injection sites should be rotated. Maintenance bolus injections with the same dosage can be given q 6–8 h. The standard dose for a bretylium infusion is 2 mg/min, with a dosing range of 1 to 2 mg/min. Consider short-term use when possible (e.g., <24 h).

#### Adverse Effect Profile

Postural hypotension is the most common adverse reaction and may occur within 15 to 30 min in as many as 60 percent of patients. If this occurs, the patient should be placed in a supine or Trendelenberg position and be resuscitated with crystalloid fluids. If hypotension persists, vasopressors may be employed, but note that these agents will increase automaticity and may negate bretylium's effects. Nausea and vomiting, along with an increase in blood pressure and heart and ventricular irritability, may also occur following a rapid IV injection in conscious patients. Bretylium should be avoided, if possible, in the setting of digoxin toxicity, since catecholamines are believed to exacerbate the toxic effects of digoxin.

### Amiodarone

#### Actions

While the exact mechanism of action has not been conclusively determined, amiodarone (Cordarone) is classified as a class III antiarrhythmic. The primary effect on cardiac tissue (including atria, ventricles, SA and AV nodes, and the His-Purkinje system) is to delay repolarization and refractoriness, especially when administered for a long period. Amiodarone slows the heart by impairing SA nodal function, depressing AV nodal conduction, modifying the automaticity of spontaneously firing fibers in the Purkinje system, and prolonging the refractory period in accessory pathways (e.g., WPW syndrome). The drug also noncompetitively antagonizes both α- and β-adrenergic responses to catecholamine, helping to contribute to the antiarrhythmic effect.

#### Pharmacokinetics

Amiodarone hydrochloride is slowly and variably absorbed following oral administration. Commercially available products yield a systemic oral bioavailability that varies from 22 to 86 percent (average, 50 percent). The variant bioavailability may be due from N-dealkylation or other metabolism in the intestinal lumen and/or GI tract, from first-pass metabolism, and/or from poor dissolution. The drug is approximately 96 percent plasma protein bound. The effect of food on absorption has not been determined. The Vd is 1.3 to 12 L/kg allowing the drug to be extensively distributed. Amiodarone is metabolized in the liver and is eliminated by biliary excretion. Peak serum concentrations may occur from 2 to 12 h (average, 3 to 7 h) after oral administration. The half-life appears to be substantially more prolonged following multiple rather than single doses. The terminal elimination half-life is 28 to 107 days. Because of the drug's slow elimination, "stopping" the drug will still allow therapeutic levels for weeks.

#### Indications

Oral amiodarone appears to be effective in the management of a wide variety of ventricular as well as supraventricular arrhythmias. However, due to the potentially life-threatening adverse effect profile, it is only used to suppress and prevent the recurrence of life-threatening ventricular arrhythmias that do not respond to documented adequate dosages of other currently available antiarrhythmic agents or when these antiarrhythmic agents cannot be tolerated.

#### Dosing and Administration

Amiodarone is a *highly* toxic drug and the lowest effective dosage should be used to minimize the risk and occurrence of adverse effects. Dosage of amiodarone must be carefully adjusted according to individual requirements and response, patient tolerance, and the general condition and cardiovascular status of the patient. The loading-dose phase of therapy should be performed in the hospital or in an environment where close monitoring can be performed (e.g., Holter monitor), especially until the risk of recurrent VT or VF has abated. Upon initiating amiodarone therapy, if possible all other antiarrhythmic agents should be gradually discontinued. In addition, ophthalmologic and pulmonary tests should be performed to obtain a baseline before amiodarone is started.

In adults, oral daily loading dosages of 800 to 1600 mg are generally required for 1 to 3 weeks (occasionally longer) until an initial therapeutic response is seen. Recommended oral doses of amiodarone to treat ventricular arrhythmias are administered once daily. However, when doses of 1 g or more are administered (e.g., during the loading-dose phase of therapy) or when intolerable adverse effects (usually GI effects) occur, a twice daily regimen with meals is suggested. Dosage reduction is essential when there is adequate control of the ventricular arrhythmias or if adverse effects become a problem. Dosages can be gradually titrated down to 600 to 800 mg daily for about 1 month and then again to the lowest effective maintenance dose. Typically, 400 to 600 mg/day are sufficient maintenance dosages.

### Adverse Effect Profile

Amiodarone exhibits several serious and potentially fatal toxicities, including pulmonary toxicity, proarrhythmic effects, and, rarely, hepatic toxicity. The likelihood of most adverse reactions appears to increase after the first 6 months of therapy and remains relatively constant beyond 1 year of therapy. Corneal microdeposits are reported in all patients with chronic administration. Additional adverse effects may include rash, skin discoloration, photosensitivity, serious neurologic effects, constipation and other GI symptoms, and others. These effects may persist for weeks or months after discontinuance. Also, thyroid function tests may appear falsely elevated or decreased.

For a variety of medications, concomitant administration of amiodarone may result in either increased levels and/or potential toxicities; such medications include digoxin, procainamide, quinidine, calcium channel blockers, β-adrenergic blocking agents, other antiarrhythmics, anticoagulants, theophylline, thyroid medications, and others.

## Class IV Antiarrhythmic Agents: Calcium Channel Blockers

There is no common functional group that characterizes calcium channel blockers as a whole. According to a classification system developed by the World Health Organization (WHO), calcium channel blockers can be broadly divided into agents that are selective or nonselective for slow, L-type calcium channels. Both of these categories can be further subdivided into three distinct classes. The selective agents include the phenylalkylamines (e.g., verapamil), dihy-

dropyridines (e.g., amlodipine, felodipine, nicardipine, nifedipine, nimodipine, nisoldipine), and benzothiazepines (e.g., diltiazem). The nonselective calcium channel blockers are diphenylpiperazines (e.g., flunarizine) and a miscellaneous category (e.g., bepridil). It has been shown that specific binding sites for calcium channel blockers have been detected in a number of tissues, including cardiac muscle, vascular and nonvascular smooth muscle, skeletal muscle, and glandular tissue. However, pharmacologic effects of each of these drugs are not apparent in all of these tissues. Pharmacokinetic differences between agents may be reflected upon disease state. See Tables 23-3 and 23-4 for more information.

### Verapamil

#### Actions

Verapamil (Isoptin, Calan), a calcium channel blocking agent, is classified as a class IV antiarrhythmic agent. In diseased tissue, verapamil decreases conduction velocity, prolongs the refractory period in the AV node, and decreases the discharge rate in the SA node. It interrupts the reentrant pathway associated with PSVT, thus causing the myocardium to return to normal sinus rhythm (NSR). In addition, verapamil can slow ventricular response in patients with atrial fibrillation and/or flutter by its action on the AV node. A decrease in heart rate and/or SA nodal block may occur in patients with SA nodal disease. Verapamil has minimal effects on normal conduction tissue.

Although verapamil has negative inotropic effects, they are often offset by the decrease in afterload. Those with severe heart failure, however, may experience a decrease in ejection fraction.

Most patients with PSVT and WPW syndrome demonstrate narrow QRS complexes of tachycardia. This indicates antegrade conduction through the AV node, with retrograde conduction over the bypass

**Table 23-3.** Comparison of Calcium Channel Blockers

| Generic Name | AML | BEP | DIL | FEL | FLU | ISR | NIC | NIF | NIM | NIS | VER |
|---|---|---|---|---|---|---|---|---|---|---|---|
| Approved, Indications | VSA CSA EH | CSA | VSA CSA AR | EH | PVD MSP | EH | CSA EH | CSA MSP RS | SAH MSP | CS A MMH CHF | VSA AR EH CSA |
| Elimination Half-Life, h | 30–50 | 33–50 | 3–6 | 10–12 | 18–19 (days) | 1.9–4.8 | 8–6 | 2–5 | 1–2 | 7–10 | 6–12 |
| Peak Levels, h | 6–9 | 2–3 | See text | 1–3 | 2–4 | 2–3 | 0.3–2 | 0.3–0.75 See text | 1–2 | 1–2 | |
| Initial Dose, mg (Oral) | 2.5–10 qd | 200 qd | See text | 10 qd | 10 qd | 2.5 bid | 10 tid | See text | 60 q4h | 10 qd | See text |
| Max. Dose, mg | 10 qd | 400 qd | See text | 20 qd | 20 tid | 10 qd | 40 tid | See text | 60 q 4 h | 40 qd | 480 qd |
| Peak Levels, h (Oral) | 6–9 | 2–9 | See text | 1–5 | 2–4 | 2–5 | 0.5–2 | See text | ≤1 | 1–15 | 1–22 |
| Heart Rate | 0/↑ | ↓/↓↓ | 0/↓ | ↑ | ↓ | ↑ | ↑ | ↑ | 0 | ↑ | 0 |
| Cardiac Output | ↑/↑↑ | 0 | 0/↑ | ↑/↑↑ | 0 | ↑↑ | ↑↑ | ↑↑ | 0 | ↑↑ | 0 |
| Peripheral Vasculature Resistance | ↓↓↓ | 0/↓ | 0 | ↓↓↓ | 0/↓ | ↓↓↓ | ↓↓↓ | ↓↓↓ | 0 | ↓↓↓ | ↓↓/↓↓↓ |
| Automaticity SA Node | 0 | ↓↓↓ | ↓/↓↓↓ | 0 | 0 | 0 | 0/↓ | 0 | 0/↓ | 0 | ↓↓/↓↓↓ |
| AV Nodal | 0 | ↓/↓↓ | ↓↓ | 0 | 0 | 0 | 0 | 0 | 0 | 0 | ↓↓↓ |

*Drug Abbreviations:* AML: amlodipine (Norvasc); BEP: bepridil (Vascor); DIL: diltiazem (Cardizem); FEL: felodipine (Plendil); FLU: flunarizine (Sibelium); ISR: isradipine (DynaCirc); NIC: nicardipine (Cardene); NIF: nifedipine (Procardia, Adalat); NIM: nimodipine (Nimotop); NIS: nisoldipine (investigational); VER: verapamil (Isoptin, Calan, Verelan).

*Other Abbreviations:* AR: Arrhythmias; CM: Cardiomyopathy; CSA: Chronic stable angina; EH: Essential hypertension; MSP: Migraine syndrome prophylaxis; MMH: Mild to moderate hypertension; PVD: Peripheral vascular disease; RS: Raynaud's syndrome; SAH: Subarachnoid hemorrhage; VSA: Vasospastic angina; 0: Minimal or no effect; ↑ or ↓: Slight effect; ↑↑ or ↓↓: Moderate effect; ↑↑↑ or ↓↓↓: Pronounced effect.

**Table 23-4.** Cardiac Medications (adenosine, atropine, bretylium, calcium)

| Generic Name (Trade Names) | Main Use(s) | Therapeutic Effects | Route(s) of Administration | Usual Dosage(s) | Side Effect(s) | Contraindications | How Supplied | Comments |
|---|---|---|---|---|---|---|---|---|
| Adenosine (Adenocard) | PSVT in the AV node; diagnostic tool to determine etiology of various supraventricular tachyarrhythmias | Exerts negative chronotropic and negative dromotropic actions on the SA and AV node. Stops PSVT by blocking AV node | *Rapid* IV push directly into vein, or most proximal IV site; each dose should be followed by a 20-mL saline flush | 6 mg over 1–2 s; give 12 mg if no response after 1–2 min—may be repeated in 1–2 min; total dose should not exceed 30 mg | Dyspnea, cough, syncope, vertigo, headache, numbness, paresthesias, dizziness, facial flushing, nausea, malaise, diaphoresis, metallic taste in mouth, retrosternal chest pain, sinus bradyarrhythmias /asystole | Second- or third-degree heart AV block or sick-sinus syndrome; adenosine is not effective in converting atrial tachyarrhythmias (e.g., atrial fibrillation or flutter) or ventricular tachycardia to normal sinus rhythm | Vials 6 mg/2 mL | Usually well tolerated since adverse effects last less than 1 min |
| Atropine | Hemodynamically unstable bradyarrhythmias (advanced second- or third-degree heart blocks, bradycardias associated with hypotension or poor tissue perfusion); asystole; acute cholinergic poisoning (organophosphates, toxic mushrooms) | Competes with acetylcholine at receptor sites at the synapse blocking the parasympathetic (vagal) response on the heart; conduction is enhanced, heart rate increases, improving cardiac output; decreases secretions (eyes, mouth, GI tract) | IV push; *rapid* IV; ET (2–2.5 × the IV dose diluted up to 10 mL per administration) | Bradycardia: 0.5 mg q 3–5 min up to 0.04 mg/kg (3 mg) Asystole: 1.0 mg q 3–5 min up to 0.04 mg/kg (3 mg) Cholinergic tox: 1.0–2.0 mg IV; additional doses of 2.0 mg can be given as needed to reverse toxic effects | Tachycardia, palpitations, bradycardia (a paradoxical reaction following a low dose of atropine), seizures, hypertension, respiratory failure, and anticholinergic symptoms, which include blurred vision, dilated pupils, headache, flushing, dizziness, drowsiness, fever, confusion, delirium, hot, dry, flushed skin, and decreased GI motility | None when used in emergency situations; *use caution* with tachycardia, myocardial infarct, when a known sensitivity to an anticholinergic drug exists (narrow angle glaucoma, GI obstructive disease, myasthenia gravis), and if an unstable cardiovascular condition exists during an acute hemorrhage | Preload syringes: 0.1 mg/mL, 5 and 10 mL 1 mg/mL, 10 mL Vials and ampoules: 0.5 mg/mL, 5 mL 0.4 mg/mL, 1 mL 0.4 mg/mL, 20 mL 0.5 mg/mL, 1 and 30 mL 0.8 mg/mL, 1 mL 1 mg/mL, 1 mL 1.2 mg/mL, 1 mL | If a dose less than 0.4 mg is given or the drug is not administered by rapid IV push, paradoxical bradycardia may occur. |
| Bretylium (Bretylol) | Refractory ventricular fibrillation or ventricular tachycardia unresponsive to lidocaine, epinephrine, and defibrillation | Raises the fibrillation threshold; initially causes rapid depletion or release of norepinephrine; an adrenergic blockade occurs following this catecholamine release. This can result in a decrease in both heart rate and arterial blood pressure; cardiac output and left ventricular filling pressure do not change | IV bolus; IV infusion as 1 g/250 mL or 2 g/500 mL in D₅W (4 mg/mL); IM alternative route (max 5 mL per site) (IM for emergency route only; use when IV access is not possible) | Ventricular fibrillation: IV push: 5 mg/kg rapid, undiluted; if fib persists, 2nd bolus of 10 mg/kg IV, up to 35 mg/kg or IV infusion at 1–2 mg/min Ventricular tachycardia: same as above, but bolus doses to be diluted and infused over 8–10 min | Hypotension and postural hypotension most frequent; bradycardia, PVCs, initial hypertension, nausea and projectile vomiting after a rapid IV bolus in the conscious patient; vertigo, dizziness, lightheadedness, and syncope are symptoms of postural hypotension | No contraindications when used to treat ventricular fibrillation or life-threatening refractory ventricular arrhythmias; may aggravate digitalis toxicity | Vials and preload syringes: 50 mg/mL, 10 mL | Consider as initial drug for cocaine-induced ventricular fibrillation; keep conscious patients supine and monitor vital signs closely; smaller doses should be given in patients being treated with catecholamine sympathomimetics. The drug was also found to be successful in reversing ventricular arrhythmias in hypothermic patients. |

| Drug | Action | Indication | Route/Administration | Dose | Adverse effects | Contraindications | Availability | Nursing considerations |
|---|---|---|---|---|---|---|---|---|
| Calcium (chloride, gluconate, gluceptate) | Essential for normal function of the nervous and muscular systems in the body; functions as an important activator in many enzymatic reactions and is required for transmission of nerve impulses; contraction of cardiac, smooth, and skeletal muscles; renal function; blood coagulation; respirations; and many endocrine secretory effects | Acute hypocalcemia (various etiologies); acute hyperkalemia; acute magnesium toxicity; acute symptoms of lead colic; to neutralize chemical burns; as an adjunct in therapy for insect and other venomous bites or stings (Portugese man-o-war, black widow spider, and others); antidote for calcium channel blocker overdose; following multiple blood transfusions over a short period of time | IV use only for chloride and gluconate salts; IV/IM for gluceptate salt (the IM route is only when the IV route is not possible; SC injection is used rarely, for local infiltration for various types of stings, bites, or hydrofluoric acid burns | Chloride: from 250 mg–1 g slow IV push (2.5–10 mL) Gluconate: 250 mg–2 g IV push or IV infusion or SC (2.5–10 mL) Gluceptate: IM: 0.44–1.1 g (2–5 mL) IV or SC; 1.1–4.4 g (5–20 mL) | Rapid IV administration may cause metallic or chalky taste, tingling or burning sensation, sense of "heat waves," peripheral vasodilation, hypotension, syncope, bradycardia and cardiac arrest (effects are using *chloride* salt; IM injections can cause mild to severe local reactions (never use *chloride* salt IM) such as burning, cellulitis and necrosis | In ventricular fibrillation and in patients with the risk of existing digitalis toxicity | Calcium chloride ampoules, vials, and syringes: 1 g/10 mL = 272 mg calcium (1.36 mEq calcium/mL) available in 10 mL Calcium gluconate vials and ampoules: 1 g/10 mL = 90 mg calcium available in 10 and 20 mL Calcium gluceptate ampoules: 1.1 g/5 mL = 90 mg calcium IM: 2–5 mL (0.44–1.1 g) IV: 5–20 mL (1.1–4.4 g) available in 5 and 50 mL | IV incompatibility with sodium bicarbonate; flush line thoroughly before and after a dose is given; if crystallization has occurred, warming may dissolve precipitation; SC or IM injections may cause severe necrosis. |
| Diltiazem (Cardizem) | Calcium channel blocker that decreases heart rate, prolongs AV nodal conduction (also has negative inotropic effect); decreases arteriolar and coronary vascular tone | Rapid conversion of paroxysmal supraventricular tachycardia, atrial fibrillation, or atrial flutter to a sinus rhythm | IV bolus over 2 min; if unsuccessful, give a second bolus dose over 2 min IV infusion: dilute 125 mg in 100 mL, 250 mg in 250 mL, or 250 mg in 500 mL | 0.25 mg/kg (20 mg in a 70-kg patient) 0.35 mg/kg (25 mg in an 80-kg patient); subsequent boluses should be individualized for each patient Continuous: 5 to 15 mg/h | Hypotension (effects generally minimal) | Hypersensitivity to diltiazem, ventricular tachycardia, sick-sinus syndrome or 2° or 3° block without a functioning pacemaker; atrial fibrillation or flutter associated with an accessory bypass tract (WPW or short PR); diltiazem and IV β-adrenergic blockers together (within a few hours); severe hypotension or cardiogenic shock | 5 mg/mL; 5 mL, 10 mL vials | Store at 2° to 8°C (36° to 45°F); do not freeze. May be stored up to 1 month at room temp (destroy after 1 month of room temp); discard unused portion of single-use vials. For an IV to oral conversion, 5 mg/h ~ 180 mg/day oral, 7 mg/h ~ 240 mg/day oral, 11 mg/h ~ 360 mg/day oral (all oral recommendations based on steady-state levels) |
| Dopamine (Intropin) | Dopaminergic receptor: renal and mesenteric vasodilation improves blood flow to the kidney to increase urine output; β1 receptor: to increase cardiac output and BP via a direct inotropic effect on myocardium; α receptor: peripheral vasoconstriction shifts blood to systemic circulation thereby increasing BP and organ perfusion | Various types of shock including cardiogenic, septic, anaphylactic, metabolic, and hypovolemic (after fluid resuscitation has failed to raise blood pressure) | IV infusion prepared in $D_5W$ or NS as: 800 mg/250 mL (3200 μg/mL) 800 mg/500 mL (1600 μg/mL) 400 mg/500 mL (800 μg/mL) 200 mg/500 mL (400 μg/mL) | Dopaminergic receptor: 1–2 μg/kg per min; β1 receptor: 2–10 μg/kg per min; α receptor: ≥10 μg/kg per min | Low-dose effects: hypotension tachycardia Moderate-dose effects: tachycardia, risk of angina, ectopic beats, ventricular dysrhythmias and ectopy, dyspnea, nausea, vomiting, headache, palpitations High-dose effects: same as moderate plus decreased kidney function and hypertension | Hypovolemic patients prior to IV fluid resuscitation; patients with pheochromocytoma | Premade IV bags: 0.8 mg/mL (100-, 250-, and 500-mL bags) 1.6 mg/mL (100-, 250-, and 500-mL bags) 3.2 mg/mL (100-, 250-, and 500-mL bags) Ampoules, vials, preload syringes: 40 mg/mL, 5 mL (200 mg) 80 mg/mL, 5 mL (400 mg) 160 mg/mL, 5 mL (800 mg) | Risk of extravasation if IV infiltrates; alkaline solutions will inactivate dopamine; flush IV line before and after if giving sodium bicarbonate; IV infusion should be titrated to desired effect and gradually tapered down when stopping infusion; monitor closely BP and ECG and drip rate. |

*(Continues)*

**Table 23-4.** Cardiac Medications—*continued*

| Generic Name (Trade Names) | Main Use(s) | Therapeutic Effects | Route(s) of Administration | Usual Dosage(s) | Side Effect(s) | Contraindications | How Supplied | Comments |
|---|---|---|---|---|---|---|---|---|
| Epinephrine (Adrenalin) | Cardiac arrest with the following conditions: ventricular fibrillation; ventricular tachycardia with no pulse; pulseless electrical activity; asystole; idioventricular rhythm; to maintain heart rate and/or arterial blood pressure | Increased contractile force of heart, SA, AV, and ventricular conduction, and heart rate (β receptor agonist effects); increased systemic vascular resistance, perfusion pressure from external chest compress. (α receptor agonist effects) | IV push in cardiac arrest (2–2.5 × the IV dose diluted up to 10 mL for ET administration) IV infusion: 1 mg in 250 mL in D₅W (4 μg/mL) | 1 mg q 3–5 min (10 mL of a IV) 1:10,000 conc) (see Comments for alternative dosing) 1–4 μg/min to titrate good BP | CNS stimulation, vomiting, nausea, headache, dizziness, tachycardia, palpitations, headache, hypertension, fatigue, muscle tremor, ventricular irritability, tachycardia, PVCs, PACs, stroke, acute MI | None when used in cardiac arrest; use with caution in pregnant patients, in those with narrow-angle (congestive) glaucoma, and when used in conjunction with local anesthetics as excessive vasoconstriction can cause sloughing of tissue | Preload syringes: 1:10,000, 0.1 mg/mL, 10 mL Ampoules, vials, and Tubex syringes: 1:1000 1 mg/mL, 1 mL, 30 mL (vials only) | Should be protected from light; can be deactivated if mixed with alkaline solutions; effects can be transient; monitor vital signs and ECG closely. (Must be diluted to 1:10,000 for IV bolus use.) |
| Esmolol (Brevibloc) | Rapid control of ventricular rate in supraventricular tachyarrhythmias (atrial fibrillation, atrial flutter); to control hypertension and tachycardia during surgery; may be effective in the management of acute MI | An ultrashort-acting selective β₁-blocking agent that blocks the negative chronotropic and negative inotropic effects; it blunts adrenergic responses during catecholamine response. Significant β₁ blockade occurs within 5 min with an elimination half-life of 9 min | IV infusion load: can give IV push or by infusion Maintenance infusion: place 5 g/500 mL in D₅W or 0.9% saline (10 mg/mL) (Note: once the desired heart rate is achieved, loading doses should be omitted and maintenance infusions should be increased by increments not exceeding 25 μg/kg per min) | Loading dose: 500 μg/kg over a 1-min period Maintenance: 50 μg/kg per min over 4 min. If there is no response, give a 2nd loading dose over 1 min and increase the maint dose to 100 μg/kg per min. If no response, repeat 3rd loading dose—same bolus dose increasing infusion rate by 50 μg/kg per min increments up to a max. of 200 μg/kg per min, desired rate is achieved, or adverse effects appear | Dose-related hypotension is common; PVCs rarely occur; others: dizziness, weakness, headache, drowsiness, burning and erythema at IV site (resolved upon DC) | Similar to other β blockers: use with caution in presence of heart failure, bronchospasm, bradycardia, AV block, and recent administration of IV calcium channel blockers | Ampoules: 10 mg/mL, 10 mL; 250 mg/mL, 10 mL | Concurrent IV morphine may increase plasma levels up to 46%. The 250-mg ampoule must be diluted prior to infusion. After stabilization, the patient can be transferred to alternative therapy (e.g., propranolol, verapamil, digoxin); the maintenance dose of esmolol should be decreased by 50% 30 min after the first dose of alternative therapy; after the second dose of the alternative therapy, clinical response should be closely monitored; if control is adequate and maintained for the first hour, DC the esmolol. |

| Drug | Indication | Action | Dose | Side Effects | Contraindications | Supply | Special Considerations |
|---|---|---|---|---|---|---|---|
| Isoproterenol (Isuprel) | Temporary adjunct therapy in hemodynamically unstable brady-arrhythmia (second- or third-degree heart blocks, brady-arrhythmias associated with hypotension or poor tissue perfusion) refractory to a vagolytic dose (0.04 mg/kg) of atropine | Increased contractile force of heart, SA, AV, and ventricular conduction, and heart rate ($\beta_1$ receptor agonist effects) Lower BP and vasodilation due to lowered peripheral vascular resistance, bronchodilation ($\beta_2$ receptor agonist effects) | IV infusion only: 1 mg/250 mL in $D_5W$ (4 µg/mL) or until PVCs appear | Hypotension, palpitations, headache, dyspnea, angina, ventricular irritability, tachycardia, PVCs, PACs, ventricular fibrillation (most of these are from an increase in myocardial oxygen requirement) | Presence of tachydysrhythmias; should not be used to raise BP in cardiogenic shock | Preload syringes, vials and ampoules: 1:5000 0.2 mg/mL, 5 and 10 mL | No longer recommended for asystole because of the vasodilation effect. |
| Lidocaine (Xylocaine) | Drug of choice for the suppression of multifocal PVCs, ventricular tachycardia, or ventricular fibrillation | Causes a membrane-stabilizing effect and raises fibrillatory threshold; also may decrease the velocity of an electrical impulse through the conduction system. Has little to no effect on the autonomic nervous system. | IV push, IM, ET (ET: 2–2.5 × the IV dose diluted up to 10 mL) IV infusion: 1 g/250 mL or 2 g/500 mL in $D_5W$ or NS (4 mg/mL) Load: 1–1.5 mg/kg (>50 mg/min for conscious) 0.5–0.75 mg/kg every 5–10 min up to a total dose of 3 mg/kg Maintenance: 2–4 mg/min titrate to effect; for acute CHF or liver failure patients, reduce loading dose by 50% and start maintenance infusion at 1 mg/min | Rapid IV push can result in any of the following in the conscious patient: euphoria, dizziness, ataxia, confusion, drowsiness, blurred or double vision, tinnitus, sensations of cold, heat, or numbness in peripheral extremities, shortness of breath, nausea or vomiting, slurred speech and dyspnea. Other effects can include muscle tremors, seizures, respiratory depression or arrest, widening of the QRS complex, bradycardia that can lead to cardiac arrest, or coma. | Hypersensitivity to amide local anesthetics; WPW syndrome; Stokes-Adams syndrome; severe degrees of SA, AV, or intraventricular heart block in the absence of a cardiac pacemaker; idioventricular or escape rhythms. | IM use: automatic injection: 300 mg/3 mL (LidoPen Auto-Injector) IM use: ampoules: 10% 100 mg/mL, 5 mL IV push: preload syringes, vials and ampoules 1% 10 mg/mL, 5 and 10 mL 2% 20 mg/mL, 5 mL IV infusion: preload syringes, vials, and ampoules: 4% 40 mg/mL, 25 and 50 mL, 10% 100 mg/mL, 10-mL vials; 20% 100 mg/mL, 5 and 10 mL Premade IV infusions: 0.2% 2 mg/mL, 500 mL; 0.4% 4 mg/mL, 250 and 500 mL; and 1 L 0.8% 8 mg/mL, 250 and 500 mL | Do not administer faster than 50 mg/min in conscious patient. Can give rapid IV push in cardiac arrest. Use with caution for bradycardia with PVCs. |

(Continues)

**Table 23-4.** Cardiac Medications—*continued*

| Generic Name (Trade Names) | Main Use(s) | Therapeutic Effects | Route(s) of Administration | Usual Dosage(s) | Side Effect(s) | Contraindications | How Supplied | Comments |
|---|---|---|---|---|---|---|---|---|
| Procainamide (Pronestyl) | Treatment of ventricular tachycardia, ventricular fibrillation, or PVCs that are refractory to lidocaine and/or bretylium. Other uses: prevent recurrence of atrial fibrillation or flutter, PSVT, or ventricular tachycardia following conversion to normal sinus rhythm. | Slows myocardial conduction velocity and decreases excitability (which may depress myocardial contractility). Fibrillatory threshold is raised and there is suppression of ventricular ectopic activity. | As a continuous IV injection given no faster than 20 mg/min until (1) arrhythmia is corrected, (2) QRS complex begins to widen, (3) hypotension develops, and (4) 17 mg/kg is administered Infusion: 1 g/250 mL or 2 g/500 mL | loading dose: 17 mg/kg  Maintenance: 1–4 mg/min titrate to effect | Precipitous hypotension may occur if IV dose is excessive or administered faster than 20 mg/min; QRS complex widening, lengthening of the PR or QT interval are possible warning signs of impending low BP; AV conduction disturbances (heart block) may follow, as may PVCs, ventricular tachycardia, or fibrillation and asystole. Other: fever, nausea, vomiting, dizziness, giddiness, psychosis with hallucinations, and seizures | Preexisting second- or third-degree heart block (without a pacemaker present), QT prolongation, or other severe conduction disturbances | For both IV push and IV infusion use: Vials: 100 mg/mL, 10 mL; 500 mg/mL, 2 mL | Drug is also used orally. Procainamide is broken down in liver to form *N*-acetyl procainamide (NAPA), which also has antiarrhythmic activity. In patients with renal failure, accumulation of NAPA occurs. This increases the potential for toxicity. |
| Verapamil (Calan, Isoptin) | Paroxysmal supraventricular tachycardia (PSVT) with narrow complexes; atrial fibrillation or flutter with rapid ventricular response | Blocks the influx and supply of calcium into cardiac muscle; this exerts a negative inotropic effect, which lowers the myocardial oxygen demand, slows conduction and prolongs the refractory period at the AV node. These AV nodal effects cause an interruption of the reentrant pathways during PSVT and help restore normal sinus rhythm. Also, by inhibiting calcium influx, the drug causes dilation of the main coronary, systemic and peripheral arteries. | IV push | Initial: 2.5 mg–5 mg over 2 min (maximum dose not to exceed 20 mg). Administer no faster than 2.5 mg/min. A repeated dose of 5 mg may be administered in 15–30 min. if response is not adequate | Symptomatic hypotension, abdominal cramps, nausea, vomiting, dizziness, or headache; prolongation of the PR interval correlates with verapamil plasma levels. PVCs, nodal escape rhythms, first-, second-, third-degree blocks, bradycardia, and asystole occur rarely; ventricular fibrillation has occurred in patients with WPW or Lown-Ganong-Levine syndrome | Hypersensitivity to verapamil, ventricular tachycardia, sick-sinus syndrome without a functioning pacemaker, second- or third-degree AV blocks; severe hypotension or cardiogenic shock. Do not administer verapamil and β-adrenergic blockers together (within a few h) since both depress myocardial contractility and AV conduction. | Ampoules, vials, and syringe 5 mg/2 mL, 2 and 4 mL Vials: 5 mg/2 mL, 5 mL | Constant ECG and BP monitoring are essential. Total dose should not exceed 20 mg (some physicians recommend 2.5-mg dose increments as opposed to 5 or 10 mg). Attempt to rule out WPW or Lown-Ganong-Levine syndrome prior to administration |

tract completing the circuit. Verapamil is safe and effective in patients with narrow-complex PSVT, even in the presence of WPW syndrome, due to the pronounced negative dromotropic effects of verapamil on the AV node. If antegrade conduction occurs over the accessory pathway, the QRS complex widens. Verapamil is contraindicated for atrial fibrillation or flutter due to WPW syndrome and in any type of wide-complex tachycardia, since it can increase rather than decrease the ventricular rate. In addition, wide-complex tachycardia could present as VT. In this case, verapamil could worsen hemodynamics because of vasodilatory and negative inotropic effects.

By inhibiting the influx of calcium, verapamil impairs the contractile processes that calcium normally activates, thereby causing dilatation of coronary and systemic arteries. Dilatation of coronary arteries improves oxygen delivery, while dilatation of the systemic arteries decreases oxygen consumption by decreasing afterload. These effects provide the myocardium with a beneficial oxygen balance in patients with vasospastic, unstable, and chronic stable angina.

### Pharmacokinetics

Verapamil elicits its hemodynamic effects within 3 to 5 min following IV administration, with effects lasting approximately 30 min. Effects on conduction begin within 1 to 2 min, peak in 10 to 15 min, and persist for 1 to 6 h. The Vd of verapamil is 4.5 to 7.1 L/kg. Verapamil undergoes first-pass metabolism in the liver and is metabolized to several metabolites. Norverapamil, an active metabolite, appears in the greatest amount. The elimination half-life of verapamil is 2 to 8 h, increasing to 4 to 12 h after 1 to 2 days of therapy.

### Indications

Verapamil is as effective as adenosine and diltiazem for terminating narrow-complex PSVT and for controlling the ventricular rate in atrial fibrillation/flutter, but not if it is associated with an accessory bypass tract, since ventricular tachyarrhythmias may be precipitated. The drug may also be used for patients presenting with narrow-complex PSVT from WPW syndrome. Diagnosis of PSVT should be confirmed by 12-lead ECG and managed with vasovagal maneuvers (e.g., the Valsava maneuver) prior to administering verapamil whenever possible.

Oral verapamil can be used for the management of vasospastic, chronic stable, and unstable angina and may also be used for the prophylaxis of PSVT. It is also used for essential hypertension.

### Dosing and Administration

When managing patients with PSVT, we recommend an IV dose of 2.5 mg given initially over 2 to 3 min and repeated in 10 min if the response is inadequate. The blood pressure should be checked immediately before and after the drug has been given. Lower initial doses of verapamil and slower administration techniques should be considered in older patients and those with hepatic dysfunction. Pretreatment with calcium chloride, gluconate, or gluceptate (500 to 1000 mg) can be given before or after verapamil infusion to prevent or reverse hypotension. Reports using calcium with verapamil have been largely anecdotal but may be most efficacious in patients whose hemodynamic status is borderline (i.e., systolic blood pressure <90 mmHg). Administration of calcium may also be considered for intentional overdose or accidentally poisoned patients who demonstrate severe bradydysrhythmias. See Table 23-4 for important information regarding different calcium salts (chloride, gluconate, and gluceptate).

For the prevention of recurrent PSVT, oral administration of verapamil, 240 to 480 mg daily, should be given in three to four divided doses. Control of ventricular rate in digitalized adults with chronic atrial fibrillation and/or flutter is 240 to 320 mg daily in three or four divided doses. Maximum antiarrhythmic effects are generally seen within 48 h after initiating a verapamil dose.

For the treatment of vasospastic, unstable, or chronic stable angina,

oral doses of verapamil can be given (80 mg q 6–8 h), with doses titrated up or down to desired clinical response. In patients with hypertension, verapamil is initiated with 80 mg three times daily and titrated to blood pressure response. Patients who are elderly and who have small stature can be started on 40 mg three times daily. Although doses of 480 mg/day have been used, efficacy with doses greater than 360 mg/day has not conclusively been proven. When switching from immediate-release tablets, the total daily dose (in mg) may remain the same. Breaking the SR tablet does not affect the therapeutic effect of verapamil SR. The SR tablets, as an initial dose of 240 mg every morning, may be used for hypertension. Titration may be accomplished with 120-mg (one-half SR tablet) increments added in the evening. Antihypertensive effects are evident within the first week.

### Adverse Effect Profile

The majority of adverse effects secondary to verapamil are related to its pharmacologic action. The incidence is increased in patients with severe heart failure, hypertrophic cardiomyopathy, and conduction disturbances. Incidence of hypotension is 5 to 10 percent with IV administration and may rarely require treatment with IV calcium salts or vasopressors. Conduction disturbances such as bradycardia, AV block, and bundle branch block occur in approximately 2 percent or fewer of patients and usually respond to a dosage reduction or discontinuation of the drug; rarely, use of atropine, cautious use of isoproterenol, or cardiac pacing may be necessary. In addition, approximately 2 percent may develop acute pulmonary edema secondary to the negative inotropic effects of verapamil. Verapamil may increase serum digoxin concentrations. Avoid the concomitant use of IV β blockers.

Noncardiac side effects with verapamil include constipation, dizziness, headache, and nausea. Other side effects, occurring in fewer than 1 percent of patients, include sleep disturbances, blurred vision, shakiness, drowsiness, confusion, dry mouth, rash, urticaria, bruising, flushing, polyuria, sexual difficulties, apnea, and muscle cramps. Several cases of hepatocellular injury accompanied by clinical signs of hepatotoxicity have also been reported. Verapamil should be given with caution to patients who are receiving agents such as β blockers, digoxin, antihypertensives, and antiarrhythmics since their effects may be additive. Cimetidine may reduce hepatic metabolism.

## Diltiazem

### Actions

The actions of diltiazem (Cardizem) on the coronary and systemic arteries resemble those of verapamil. Diltiazem, also a calcium antagonist, is a less potent vasodilator than nifedipine or verapamil. Vasodilation is predominant in the coronary arteries, allowing improved oxygen delivery, thus benefitting patients with vasospastic angina. Systemic artery dilation also reduces afterload, resulting in decreased oxygen consumption and improvement in oxygen balance in those with chronic stable angina. Diltiazem slows AV nodal conduction time and prolongs AV nodal refractoriness. It may selectively reduce the heart rate during tachycardias involving the AV node with little or no effect on normal AV nodal conduction at normal heart rates, based on frequency of use. The ventricular rate is slowed in patients with a rapid ventricular response during atrial fibrillation or atrial flutter. PSVT is converted to NSR by interrupting the reentry circuit in AV nodal reentrant tachycardias and reciprocating tachycardias (e.g., WPW syndrome). Diltiazem has no effects on sinus node recovery or the sinoatrial conduction time in patients without SA nodal dysfunction.

### Pharmacokinetics

An IV bolus dose appears to follow linear pharmacokinetics over a dosage range of 10.5 mg to 21.0 mg. The apparent Vd is 305 L. The plasma elimination of diltiazem is approximately 3 to 7 h. The drug is extensively metabolized in the liver with a systemic clearance of 65 L/h. After a continuous IV infusion, one study cited development of nonlinear pharmacokinetics over an infusion range of 4.8 to 13.2 mg/h for 24 h. As the dose is increased over this infusion range, systemic clearance decreases from 64 to 48 L/h and the apparent Vd remains unchanged (360 to 391 L). Generally, systemic clearance averaged 42 L/h and 31 L/h in patients administered continuous infusions of diltiazem at 10 mg/h to 15 mg/h, respectively, for 24 h. However, in comparison to healthy volunteers, patients with atrial fibrillation or atrial flutter had decreased systemic clearance.

Oral doses also have a 40 percent bioavailability due to first-pass effect. Oral bioavailability does increase as doses increase. The onset of action of conventional tablets is 30 to 60 min, with the peak effect occurring in 2 to 4 h. SR tablets, however, have a gradual onset of action, with a peak effect occurring in 6 to 11 h. Comparable products, a 24-h controlled drug delivery system (Cardizem-CD; Dilacor-XR), have similar absorption throughout the dosing intervals and peak serum levels occur generally between 10 and 14 h.

Diltiazem is 70 to 85 percent protein bound; 35 to 40 percent is bound to albumin and is metabolized in the liver to one active and several inactive metabolites. Approximately one-third of diltiazem is metabolized to desacetyldiltiazem, a metabolite with 25 to 50 percent of the coronary vasodilating activity of diltiazem. Diltiazem and its metabolites are excreted via glucuronide and/or sulfate conjugation.

### Indications

IV diltiazem is as effective as verapamil and adenosine for rapid conversion of PSVT to NSR and to slow ventricular rate in atrial fibrillation or atrial flutter. It should not be used in patients with a wide-complex ventricular tachyarrhythmia suggesting an accessory bypass tract (e.g., WPW syndrome).

Oral diltiazem is indicated for the treatment of vasospastic and chronic stable angina and is considered one of the drugs of choice for vasospastic angina. In patients with chronic stable angina, diltiazem is thought to be as effective as β-blocking agents and/or nitrates but is usually reserved for those who fail therapy with these agents.

Oral diltiazem is also approved for the treatment of hypertension either alone or in combination with other agents. An additive effect is commonly seen when thiazide diuretics are added to diltiazem therapy. As with other calcium channel blockers, diltiazem may be especially useful in hypertensive patients with low renin levels, who have angina, or who are African-American.

### Dosing and Administration

The IV bolus dose for control of PSVT, atrial fibrillation, or atrial flutter is 0.25 mg/kg using actual body weight (average adult dose is 20 mg) over a 2-min period. If a further response is desired, a second IV bolus of 0.35 mg/kg actual body weight can be given at the same rate (average adult dose, 35 mg). Subsequent bolus dosing should be individualized on a mg/kg basis. It should be noted that some patients may not need an initial dose greater than 0.15 mg/kg, yet duration of action may be shorter. For continued reduction of the heart rate (up to 24 h) in atrial fibrillation or atrial flutter, a diltiazem maintenance IV infusion may be started immediately following the bolus dose(s). The recommended initial rate is 10 mg/h, yet some patients may respond to a 5-mg/h dose. If needed, subsequent increases can be in 5-mg/h increments up to 15 mg/h. The infusion may be maintained for up to 24 h. Patients should have continuous ECG monitoring and frequent blood pressure checks. See Table 23-4 for IV dilution suggestions.

For patients being converted from IV to oral diltiazem, the following suggestions are based on oral steady state: 5 mg/h ~ 180 mg/day; 7 mg/h ~ 240 mg/day; 11 mg/h ~ 360 mg/day.

The oral doses and dosing intervals are variable, based on the indication and the product selected. For the treatment of vasospastic or chronic stable angina, the usual initial diltiazem dose is 30 mg before meals and at bedtime (four times daily). Most patients can be controlled with 180 to 360 mg/day in divided doses. SR products start at 60 to 120 mg/day, with optimum dosage 240 to 360 mg/day.

For patients with hypertension, diltiazem is usually given as the extended-release tablet in 60-mg or 120-mg doses twice daily. Maintenance doses are usually 240 to 360 mg/day. Doses should be titrated to clinical response in each of the above situations. Additionally, patients with hepatic and/or renal dysfunction should be dosed cautiously and may require dosage adjustments. The Cardizem-CD and the Dilacor-XR products offer 180 and 240 mg with once-daily dosing. Cardizem-CD is also available in a 300-mg strength. SR products use 60- to 120-mg strengths and are started with 120 or 180 mg daily. Some patients may respond to higher doses of up to 480 mg/day. As necessary, the optimum dose for hypertension can be titrated over a 7- to 14-day period.

### Adverse Effect Profile

Many of the adverse effects associated with diltiazem are an extension of its pharmacologic profile. Cardiovascular effects may include angina, bradycardia, asystole, CHF, AV block (first, second, or third degree), bundle branch block, PVCs, flushing, decreased blood pressure, palpitations, and peripheral edema.

Noncardiac side effects include headache (2 to 10 percent), dizziness (1 to 7 percent), asthenia (2 to 5 percent), nausea (1 to 3 percent), constipation (1 to 2 percent), rash (1 to 2 percent), vomiting, diarrhea, dry mouth, pruritus, nervousness, somnolence, insomnia, tinnitus, abnormal dreams, depression, sexual difficulties, bruising, polyuria, hyperglycemia, epistaxis, alopecia, and photosensitivity.

Diltiazem may cause a transient increase in liver function test values (e.g., AST, ALT, LDH), which may resolve despite continued therapy. However, hepatocellular toxicity has been reported in some patients. Patients receiving digoxin or β blockers may experience additive conduction disturbances. Cimetidine may increase diltiazem levels secondary to inhibition of metabolism.

## Nifedipine

### Actions

Nifedipine (Procardia, Adalat, others) is a calcium channel blocker with actions similar to other agents in this class. The coronary artery dilatation results in improved oxygen delivery benefitting patients with vasospastic angina. Systemic artery dilatation results in decreased afterload, leading to decreased oxygen consumption in patients with chronic stable angina. A reflex increase in heart rate and an increase in cardiac output may be seen with nifedipine. Unlike verapamil and diltiazem, nifedipine has little effect on the SA and AV nodal conduction clinically. Nifedipine may, however, result in a decrease in left ventricular end diastolic pressure (LVEDP) or left ventricular end diastolic volume (LVEDV) in patients with moderate to severely impaired LV function, thereby worsening their condition.

### Pharmacokinetics

Nifedipine is 45 to 75 percent bioavailable as a result of significant first-pass liver metabolism. When taken orally (conventional capsules), the onset of action is 20 min and the duration of action is 4 to 6 h. Sublingual administration or capsules chewed and swallowed results in antihypertensive effects within 2 to 3 min, lasting 2 to 3 h. Extended-release tablets (Procardia-XL, Adalat-XL) have a gradual onset of action that peaks at 6 h and persists for 24 h.

Nifedipine is metabolized in the liver to inactive metabolites. The elimination half-life of the parent drug is 2 to 5 h in patients with normal hepatic and renal function, increasing to 7 h in those with hepatic dysfunction.

### Indications

The primary use of nifedipine in emergency medicine is to rapidly lower the blood pressure in hypertensive crisis. The drug can be given sublingually or orally and is therefore particularly convenient when IV lines cannot be started and the blood pressure needs to be lowered immediately.

Approved indications for nifedipine include management of vasospastic and chronic stable angina. It is considered to be as effective as β blockers or nitrates in the treatment of chronic stable angina. Nifedipine, either alone or in combination with other antihypertensives, is indicated for the management of essential hypertension. In comparison to other classes of antihypertensives (i.e., angiotensin-converting enzyme inhibitors and β blockers), nifedipine may benefit patients with low-renin hypertension, coexisting angina, or peripheral vascular disease.

### Dosing and Administration

The initial dose of nifedipine for hypertensive crisis is 10 mg. The capsule contains liquid contents. To achieve rapid effects, the patient should chew and then swallow the capsule. If the patient is unconscious, several holes should be poked into the capsule using an 18-gauge needle, and the contents squirted below the tongue. A repeat dose can be administered 10 min later.

The dosage range for the extended-release nifedipine tablet is from 30 to 90 mg/day.

### Adverse Effect Profile

The majority of side effects occurring with nifedipine are related to its vasodilatory activity on the smooth muscle and include lightheadedness, flushing, headache, and hypotension. Nifedipine may also cause a dose-related peripheral edema in 10 to 30 percent of patients. Other cardiovascular side effects associated with the use of nifedipine include MI, CHF, and pulmonary edema. Since there have also been reported cases of reflex tachycardia, nifedipine should be used with caution in hypertensive crisis in patients who are already tachycardic. Caution should also be exercised when giving sublingual or oral doses to hypertensive patients with an intracranial bleed or an acute MI. The resultant hypotensive effects can be profound and lethal.

Noncardiac-related adverse effects include nervousness, sleep disturbances, blurred vision, nausea, somnolence, insomnia, asthenia, diarrhea, dry mouth, rash, urticaria, apnea, polyuria, sweating, sexual difficulties, and joint pain. Rarely, thrombocytopenia, leukopenia, anemia, elevated liver function tests, and bruising have occurred in patients on nifedipine. Nifedipine should be used with caution in patients with aortic stenosis, CHF, and concomitant β blocker therapy since CHF may be precipitated or exacerbated. Antihypertensive agents may enhance the hypotensive effects of nifedipine.

## Nimodipine

### Actions

Nimodipine (Nimotop) is a calcium channel blocker structurally similar to nifedipine. Like other calcium channel blockers, it inhibits the influx of calcium across the transmembrane channels, thereby inhibiting the contractile activity in the cell. The inhibition of calcium influx is seen in myocardial, vascular smooth muscle, and neuronal cells. Nimodipine has a relative selectivity for vascular smooth muscle, as opposed to the myocardium, and therefore has minimal effects on the conduction and inotropy of the myocardium. Its greatest affinity is for the CNS vasculature. It increases cerebral blood flow and may shunt blood to ischemic areas. Although inhibition of cerebral vasospasm [which often occurs following SAH (subarachnoid hemorrhage)] was initially thought to be responsible for the beneficial effects of nimodipine in SAH, angiography has not proven this. Improved collateral blood flow and prevention of large calcium influxes into neurons (causing cell destruction) may be of greater importance.

### Pharmacokinetics

Nimodipine is rapidly and well absorbed after oral administration; however, first-pass metabolism by the liver results in low and inconsistent bioavailability (3 to 30 percent). Peak concentrations occur in 30 to 60 min.

Nimodipine has a Vd of 0.94 to 2.3 L/kg and is metabolized in the liver to several metabolites, most with little or no activity. The elimination half-life following oral administration is 1.7 to 9 h.

### Indications

Nimodipine is indicated for the treatment of recent (within 96 h) SAH from ruptured congenital intracranial aneurysm in patients whose postictal neurologic condition is good (e.g., Hunt and Hess grades I to III), where it can decrease the degree of morbidity and mortality. Patients with more severe disability (Hunt and Hess grades IV to V) do not seem to benefit and may become worse with nimodipine.

### Dosing and Administration

The dose is 60 mg q 4 h for 21 days for managing patients with SAH. If oral administration is not possible, the capsules can be punctured, with the contents administered through a nasogastric tube, followed by a 30-mL saline flush.

### Adverse Effect Profile

The most common adverse effect is hypotension, which is often dose-related. In addition, edema and headache have been reported in patients with SAH. Other, less frequent, dose-related adverse effects include tachycardia, bradycardia, palpitations, flushing, hypertension, rebound vasospasm, CHF, and pulmonary edema.

Other side effects reported include thrombocytopenia, anemia, disseminated intravascular coagulation, rash, pruritus, hematoma, abdominal discomfort, constipation, elevated liver test results, depression, lightheadedness, dizziness, drowsiness, hyponatremia, and hyperglycemia.

## Nicardipine

### Actions

Nicardipine (Cardene) is a dihydropyridine calcium channel blocker structurally related to nifedipine. Like nifedipine, nicardipine inhibits the transmembrane flux of calcium into cardiac and vascular smooth muscle. The inhibition results in a decrease in the contractile activity within the myocardium and vascular smooth muscle. This agent provides selective activity on the vasculature as opposed to the myocardium. Nicardipine possesses both systemic and peripheral vasodilatory action primarily through a decrease in peripheral vascular resistance. Increases in cardiac output and cardiac index can be seen in a dose-dependent manner with nicardipine. It does not have demonstrable effects on renal blood flow or glomerular filtration rate.

Intravenous nicardipine decreases systemic vascular resistance, improves coronary artery perfusion, and increases cardiac index without raising myocardial oxygen demand or left ventricular filling pressure. Despite systemic and hemodynamic effects (hypotension and tachycardia), IV nicardipine does not have a depressant effect on the myocardium or a negative action on right or left ventricular filling pressure in patients with uncomplicated MI. However, it has been shown to produce a decrease in contractility in patients with severe heart failure.

### Pharmacokinetics

Nicardipine is well absorbed and undergoes rapid, extensive metabolism by the liver. It is highly protein bound (>95 percent) and has a Vd of 8.3 L/kg. Nicardipine is metabolized to inactive metabolites, with approximately 35 percent excreted through the bile, 60 percent renally eliminated, and less than 1 percent of the parent drug eliminated through the kidney. The onset of action of nicardipine following oral administration is approximately 20 min with a duration of action of approximately 3 h. In controlled clinical trials, the mean onset time for therapeutic IV nicardipine effects has been between 11.5 and 77 min. Based on long-term infusions of 48 h, plasma concentrations decline exponentially, with a rapid early distribution phase.

### Indications

Intravenous nicardipine is indicated for the short-term treatment of hypertension when oral therapy is not feasible or desirable. Oral nicardipine (Cardene) is indicated for chronic stable angina and essential hypertension. The drug can be used alone or in combination with other agents for both indications and appears to be equally as effective as nifedipine in treating angina and hypertension.

### Dosing and Administration

For rapid blood pressure reduction, initiate therapy at 5 mg/h. The infusion rate may be increased by 2.5 mg/h every 5 min up to a maximum of 15 mg/h or until desired blood pressure reduction is achieved. The recommendation for maintenance infusions is 3 mg/h. The initial dose of oral nicardipine is 20 mg q 8 h, titrating the dose to clinical response up to 40 mg q 8 h. When transferring from an IV dose to an oral dose, administer the first oral dose of nicardipine 1 h prior to discontinuing the IV dose. The conversion is as follows: 0.5 mg/h ~ 20 mg q 8 h; 1.2 mg/h ~ 30 mg q 8 h; 2.2 mg/h ~ 40 mg q 8 h. Dosage adjustments should be made for elderly patients or those with hepatic dysfunction.

### Adverse Effects

Adverse effects of these agents are similar to those of nifedipine and other calcium channel blockers.

## Other Antiarrhythmic Agents

### Adenosine

### Actions

Adenosine (Adenocard) is an endogenous nucleoside produced by the dephosphorylation of adenosine triphosphate (ATP). Every cell of the body contains adenosine. This compound exerts negative chronotropic and negative dromotropic actions on SA and AV nodal tissue. Adenosine terminates PSVT primarily via blockade of the AV node without altering conduction through accessory pathways, as is seen with the WPW syndrome. Reentrant SVTs not involving the AV node are not terminated by adenosine. Adenosine is a potent vasodilator; however, there is no change in systemic blood pressure following administration because it is rapidly metabolized by circulating adenosine deaminase and undergoes rapid sequestration by vascular endothelial cells.

### Pharmacokinetics

Onset of action is approximately 30 s with a duration of 60 to 90 s. The drug is rapidly metabolized in the blood, with a half-life less than 7 s. The primary routes of elimination are cellular uptake and simple or facilitated diffusion by a nucleoside transport system, metabolism to various by-products, and renal excretion of these metabolic products. The predominant final metabolite of adenosine is uric acid. Specific pharmacokinetic parameters, such as Vd, therapeutic plasma concentrations, and clearance, are difficult to assess due to the extremely short half-life of the drug.

### Indications

Adenosine (Adenocard), approved as an antiarrhythmic drug for the emergency management of PSVT involving the AV node, has been shown to be as efficacious as IV doses of verapamil or diltiazem. The drug has also been used as a diagnostic agent for distinguishing supraventricular from ventricular tachycardia as well as diagnosing broad QRS complex tachycardias. It may also detect a previously latent accessory pathway. While it is extremely effective in *initial* conversion of reentrant PSVTs, recurrence of the arrhythmia (within minutes after initial conversion) may occur. Although repeat doses of adenosine are effective, consideration of a longer-acting antiarrhythmic agent will often be necessary. This drug may be a preferable agent for treatment of PSVT in infants, children, and pregnant patients. Because adenosine shortens the action potential duration and slows the heart rate, it is contraindicated in second- or third-degree AV heart block or sick-sinus syndrome. Adenosine is not effective in converting atrial tachyarrhythmias (e.g., atrial fibrillation or flutter) or VT to NSR.

### Dosing and Administration

The initial dose for the treatment of acute PSVT is 6 mg (6 mg/2 mL) given as a *rapid* IV bolus over 1 to 2 s directly into the vein or into the most proximal port of the IV tubing on the peripheral IV site. When the latter method is used, the bolus should be followed by a 20-mL saline flush and the arm immediately elevated. This method will expedite travel of the drug to the heart and lessen the amount of drug getting caught in the IV tubing, where it rapidly breaks down. If the heart rate does not decrease within 2 min, a second bolus injection of 12 mg should be given in the same manner. A final third bolus dose may be given in 1 to 2 min if the arrhythmia persists. It is imperative that adenosine is administered *fast;* if infused too slowly, systemic vasodilation may occur, which could result in reflex tachycardia.

### Adverse Effect Profile

When adverse effects occur due to adenosine, they are minor and well tolerated because they last less than 1 min due to the drug's short half-life. The most common are dyspnea, cough, syncope, vertigo, paresthesias, numbness, nausea, and metallic taste. Cardiovascular adverse effects may include facial flushing, headache, diaphoresis, palpitations, retrosternal chest pain, sinus bradyarrhythmias (i.e., bradycardia, sinus arrest, AV block), atrial tachydysrhythmias (i.e., atrial fibrillation or flutter), PVCs, and hypotension. These adverse effects rarely require specific management. Dipyridamole and carbamazepine have been shown to enhance the negative chronotropic and dromotropic effects of adenosine and may increase the degree of toxicity. Methylxanthines and caffeine, on the other hand, compete for adenosine receptors. Therefore, asthmatics or excessive coffee drinkers may require a higher dose of adenosine to achieve a therapeutic effect.

### Digoxin

### Actions

Digoxin has three basic actions: (1) it increases the force, strength, and velocity of cardiac contractions (positive inotropic effects); (2) it slows the heart rate (negative chronotropic effects); and (3) it slows conduction velocity through the AV node.

Digoxin exerts its direct inotropic and electrophysiologic effects by binding to and inhibiting the sodium and potassium ATPase pump in the cell membrane. This action results in higher intracellular levels of sodium and causes calcium to move intracellularly in exchange for sodium. The elevated intracellular calcium concentration allows more calcium to be available to increase the rate and force of cardiac contractions.

Digoxin increases the refractory period and decreases the conduction velocity of both the SA and AV nodes but shortens the refractory period and increases conduction velocity in the atrial muscles (including atrial bypass tracts as present in WPW syndrome). The primary effect on SA and AV nodal conduction is secondary to direct enhancement of parasympathomimetic tone. ECG changes include PR interval prolongation and QT interval shortening. High doses of digoxin enhance ventricular automaticity.

Slowing of the heart results in a prolonged diastolic period, allowing a greater period for improving coronary blood and myocardial perfusion. A decrease in oxygen demand may also occur secondary to the decrease in heart rate.

### Pharmacokinetics

The onset of action is about 5 to 30 min following IV administration and 30 to 120 min for oral tablets, while peak effects occur in 1 to 4 h and 2 to 6 h, respectively. The onset of action following parenteral therapy varies based upon the rate at which digoxin is administered. In oral dosing, however, patient variability is the primary cause for variation. The large variation in peak effect can be explained by the fact that digoxin has a large Vd of 5.6 L/kg. Digoxin crosses the blood-brain barrier and the placenta, and high concentrations are found in the liver, heart, kidney, and intestines. Digoxin may also be given by oral tablets, elixir, and capsules, the bioavailability being approximately 70 percent, 80 percent, and 90 percent, respectively.

Digoxin is inactivated by hepatic degradation and is excreted unchanged in the urine. The half-life of digoxin in patients with normal renal function is 30 to 40 h and can extend to 4 to 6 days in anuric patients. Because digoxin concentrates in the tissues, serum levels of digoxin may not accurately assess the amount of drug in the body, making procedures such as dialysis or exchange transfusion ineffective.

### Indications

Digoxin is indicated to improve cardiac output in CHF and to control heart rate in atrial fibrillation, atrial flutter, and PAT. Use of digoxin in the treatment of CHF should be considered only when diuretics and vasodilators fail to improve cardiac output. Digoxin may be particularly effective in providing beneficial hemodynamic and symptomatic improvement in heart failure patients presenting with an $S_3$ gallop or "low-output" heart failure associated with depressed ventricular function. Digoxin is less effective with "high-output" heart failure, which occurs in patients with bronchopulmonary insufficiency, anemia, infection, hyperthyroidism, or arteriovenous fistulas.

### Dosing and Administration

Digoxin can be administered by oral or IV routes. The IV route is preferred when a more rapid onset of action and peak effect is desired. The IV dose is 20 to 30 percent less than an oral dose. Digoxin should not be administered by IM injection, since this route offers no advantages and can cause severe pain at the injection site.

For control of SVT, digoxin should be administered IV in a dose of 10 to 15 μg/kg (up to a total of 0.75 to 1.5 mg given over the first 24 h). This dose should be divided, with 0.25 to 0.5 mg given as the initial dose and 0.125 to 0.25 mg q 2–6 h as subsequent doses until the entire dose is administered or the heart rate is sufficiently lowered. The dose for patients with CHF without atrial fibrillation is generally lower (8 to 12 μg/kg) but can be given in a similar fashion as above until appropriate response has been achieved. Higher doses are often required to control the ventricular response to atrial fibrillation or flutter, but higher doses have more adverse effects. Cumulative doses should not exceed 1.0 mg. Loading doses should be calculated using lean body weight, since this method generally provides therapeutic effects with minimal risk of toxicity. Intravenous loading doses should be administered slowly over a 5-min period or longer, undiluted or diluted, to a fourfold or greater volume. Serum digoxin levels should not be obtained earlier than 6 to 8 h after loading because of the slow distribution of the drug.

Maintenance therapy should be adjusted according to clinical response or to maintain a serum digoxin concentration between 0.8 to 2.0 ng/mL. Dosage adjustments are necessary in renal failure, dehydration, hypokalemia, hypercalcemia, hypomagnesemia, and hypothyroidism. Drugs that interact with digoxin to cause increases in serum digoxin levels include amiodarone, verapamil, nifedipine, hydroxychloroquine, propafenone, quinidine, erythromycin, tetracycline, and anticholinergic agents. In contrast, cholestyramine, metoclopramide, kaolin-pectin, penicillamine, and dietary fiber have resulted in lower serum digoxin concentrations.

$$\text{Maintenance dose} = \frac{\text{peak body stores} \times \% \text{ daily loss}}{100},$$

where peak body stores = loading dose,
% daily loss = 14 +( 0.2 × creatinine clearance) in milliliters per minute.

### Adverse Effect Profile

When digoxin toxicity is suspected, the drug should be stopped and a serum level obtained. Digoxin serum levels do not always represent true toxicity. Toxicity may actually occur in some patients with low serum levels, since it is often the myocardial tissue level rather than serum level that determines the degree of toxicity.

Symptoms of digoxin toxicity include mental depression, confusion, headache, drowsiness, anorexia, nausea, vomiting, weakness, visual disturbances (green or yellow vision and/or halo effects), delirium, EEG abnormalities, and seizures. Patients may also present with diarrhea and abdominal discomfort. Almost any type of arrhythmia may manifest in digoxin toxicity. The most common arrhythmias include an increased number of unifocal or multiform PVCs, VT, junctional tachycardia, high-degree AV block, PSVT with block, and sinus arrest. Atrial fibrillation, bradycardia, and ventricular fibrillation may also occur. Other adverse effects may include gynecomastia, skin rash, eosinophilia, and thrombocytopenia.

While hypokalemia increases the risk of digoxin toxicity, significant digoxin toxicity itself may produce hyperkalemia due to paralysis of the transmembrane sodium-potassium pump. However, when hypokalemia develops in less severe cases of toxicity, potassium can be replaced by IV infusion, provided that there is no evidence of high-degree AV conduction block. When digoxin toxicity is associated with hyperkalemia, a corresponding intracellular deficiency of potassium exists, which may be the causative factor of subsequent arrhythmias. Treatment in this circumstance is controversial. It is not clear whether measures should be taken to decrease the total body supply of potassium (at the risk of increasing intracellular hypokalemia), to increase the total body potassium in the face of extracellular hyperkalemia, or to use measures that would ordinarily encourage movement of potassium back into cells (e.g., use of bicarbonate, glucose, and insulin). These methods may all prove useless in the absence of a functioning transmembrane sodium-potassium pump.

Lidocaine and phenytoin are antiarrhythmics that have classically been used in digoxin toxicity, but their efficacy has not been proven. Atropine and electrical pacing have been tried in cases of bradyarrhythmias, but these too have had limited success. Hemodialysis and resin hemoperfusion have been attempted in some cases of severe digoxin poisoning but have generally been unsuccessful due to the large volume of distribution of digoxin. Digoxin antibody fragments, otherwise known as Digoxin Immune FAB (fragmented antibodies) or Digibind (Burroughs-Wellcome), is available for use in treating life-threatening digoxin toxicity. This antidote is indicated for life-threatening ventricular tachyarrhythmias, sinus bradyarrhythmias, or severe AV blocks resulting from overdose or accidental pediatric ingestion of digoxin and digitalis-like glycosides that are unresponsive to conventional therapy. An additional indication for FAB, by the manufacturer, is in patients experiencing severe digoxin toxicity who have serum potassium levels greater than 5 mEq/mL. See Chap. 147 for more informational details.

## Magnesium

### Actions

Magnesium affects skeletal and smooth muscle contractility, vasomotor tone, and neuronal transmission directly via the $Na^+$, $K^+$-ATPase pump and indirectly via calcium blocking activity. It increases membrane potential, prolongs AV conduction, and increases the absolute refractory period. Hypomagnesemia can precipitate life-threatening cardiac arrhythmias, symptoms of cardiac insufficiency, and sudden cardiac death after an AMI. Resupplementation of magnesium helps to replenish intracellular potassium in hypomagnesemic, hypokalemic patients; blocks calcium to cause vasodilation; and reduces platelet aggregation. Magnesium also decreases myocardial sensitivity to and release of catecholamines, which can lead to an excessive adrenergic surge. This surge can lead to dysrhythmias, hypertension, and increased myocardial oxygen consumption.

### Pharmacokinetics

When given IV, the onset of action of magnesium sulfate is immediate and the duration of action is about 30 min. Following IM administration, the onset is about 1 h and the duration is 3 to 4 h. Magnesium is excreted by the kidney at a variable rate directly proportional to the serum concentration and the glomerular filtration rate.

### Indications

Magnesium is indicated for intractable VT/VF and torsade de pointes, regardless of prearrest serum magnesium levels. It has also been studied and shown to be useful in managing refractory PVCs, MAT, PSVT, and for ventricular arrhythmias associated with cardiac arrest and/or digoxin toxicity that occur in patients who are, or are likely to be, hypomagnesemic. Magnesium may also be considered as a prophylactic/antiarrhythmic in the post-AMI patient. Other uses for parenteral magnesium sulfate include seizures associated with toxemia/eclampsia/nephritis, hypomagnesemia (mild to severe), and hyperalimentation.

### Dosing and Administration

An IV loading dose of magnesium sulfate is administered as 1 to 2 g (8 to 16 mEq), mixed in 50 or 100 mL $D_5W$, using either the 10% (100 mg/mL) or 50% (500 mg/mL) solutions. In cardiac arrest scenarios, the IV dose can be injected over 1 to 2 min. However, if time permits, a safer method is to administer 2 to 4 g as an IV infusion over 20 to 60 min. The rate of infusion should be slowed or temporarily stopped if hypotension develops. In addition, several trials recommend the routine use of magnesium at doses of 8 to 12 g per 24 h for AMI or suspected MI. While most recommendations suggest that an IV maintenance infusion at 0.5 to 1 g/h (4 to 8 mEq) should follow for up to 24 h, the rate and duration of infusion should be based on the clinical situation and the degree of hypomagnesemia.

### Adverse Effect Profile

Hypotension is the predominant adverse effect, yet is surprisingly uncommon, even when a 1 to 2 g IV push dose is given relatively rapidly (i.e., over 1 to 2 min). Other signs of hypermagnesemia, which may begin at serum concentrations of 4 mEq/mL, include flushing, sweating, CNS depression, depression of reflexes, flaccid paralysis, depression of cardiac function, circulatory collapse, hypothermia, and fatal respiratory paralysis.

## VASOACTIVE DRUGS

## Vasoactive and Inotropic Agents

### Epinephrine

### Actions

Epinephrine is a nonselective $\alpha$- and $\beta$-adrenergic agonist. The drug increases heart rate, ventricular contractility, and peripheral vascular resistance. Epinephrine increases mean arterial pressure by stimulating $\alpha_1$-adrenergic receptors during cardiac arrest. This effect causes vasoconstriction of arterioles in the skin, mucosa, and mesenteric vasculature, redistributing blood to the heart and brain, and in turn results in improved cardiac and cerebral perfusion during resuscitation. Epinephrine also causes bronchodilation and antagonizes the effects of histamine.

### Pharmacokinetics

Both the onset of action and the duration of action of epinephrine are relatively short: 1 to 2 min and 2 to 10 min, respectively. The drug quickly becomes fixed in the tissues and is rapidly inactivated via oxidation by monoamine oxidase (MAO) and via methylation by catechol-$O$-methyltransferase (COMT). Subsequent metabolites are excreted in the urine as sulfates and glucuronides.

### Indications

Epinephrine is considered a first-line agent in the treatment of cardiac arrest and may be used in pulseless VT/VF (that has not responded to electrical countershock), asystole, and pulseless electrical activity (PEA). The drug has also been purported to "coarsen" fine ventricular fibrillation, but there is no documented evidence that this is true. Epinephrine does, however, increase the likelihood of continued hemodynamic stability in animals that have been successfully defibrillated. This effect has been attributed to the effect of epinephrine on systemic vascular resistance. Historically, the standard 1-mg dose came from the operating room practice of intracardiac injections being effective in restarting the arrested heart, but studies have shown that 1 to 3 mg of intracardiac epinephrine is effective in restarting the arrested heart. Further animal studies were performed, and their dose-response curves demonstrated that vasoactive effects of epinephrine are dose-dependent. The lower doses favored agonist effects on $\beta$-adrenergic receptors, while higher doses revealed $\alpha$-agonist effects (vasoconstriction). Over the years, it was assumed that 1 mg of epinephrine IV was equivalent and would be useful for all body weights. The dose-response curve was studied in the 1980s and early 1990s, revealing that higher doses of epinephrine (ranging from 0.045 to 0.2 mg/kg) were required to improve hemodynamics and demonstrate increased rates of spontaneous circulation. However, most trials failed to produce statistically significant improvement in survival rates to hospital discharges, compared with the standard epinephrine doses (for further information on dosing, see "Dosing and Administration," below).

Epinephrine is also used as a vasopressor to increase blood pressure and as an antidote to reverse bronchospasm due to anaphylactic and hypersensitivity reactions.

### Dosing and Administration

Current American Heart Association (AHA) Guidelines recommend that an epinephrine 1-mg IV bolus continue to be the *initial* dose in cardiac arrest. It is now recommended that the dosing frequency be increased to 3 to 5 min from a 5-min interval. The AHA recognizes that higher doses of epinephrine are acceptable, but can neither recommend nor discourage their use; however, they do say higher doses should only be used after the 1-mg dose has failed. The *intermediate* epinephrine dose suggestion is 2 to 5 mg IV push, also given every 3 to 5 min; the *escalating* regimen is 1 mg–3 mg–5 mg IV push, 3 min apart; the *high* dose reflects use of a bolus of 0.1 mg/kg every 3 to 5 min.

Epinephrine may be given via peripheral vein, via a central line, or endotracheally. The optimal dose for drug delivery is unknown; however, a dose that is at least two to two and one-half times the peripheral IV dose may be needed. Endotracheal administration is performed by placing 10 mL of a 1:10,000 solution (preload syringe) down the ET tube, and then performing several rapid ventilations to disperse the drug throughout the airways for maximal absorption. If the more concentrated epinephrine vial is used (30 mg/30 mL, 1:1000) the dose should be diluted to 10 mL.

Intracardiac administration should only be used during open cardiac massage to avoid the risk of pneumothorax, coronary artery laceration, and cardiac tamponade. External intracardiac injections will interrupt ventilations and closed chest compressions and are no longer recommended.

Although not a first-line agent, a continuous epinephrine infusion can be used for patients who are not in cardiac arrest (e.g., symptomatic bradycardia) to exert the vasopressor response. The initial dose should begin at 1 μg/min (range 2 to 10 μg/min) and be titrated to a desired hemodynamic response. Continuous IV infusions of epinephrine should be administered by central venous access to ensure prompt transport to the heart and to reduce the risk of extravasation.

### Adverse Effect Profile

Adverse effects are of minimal importance in the setting of cardiac arrest. Epinephrine does increase myocardial oxygen consumption significantly and thus can exacerbate ventricular irritability in the setting of myocardial ischemia. The α-adrenergic activity of epinephrine produces an increase in systemic vascular resistance, which could conceivably be detrimental to a failing myocardium in that increased afterload can significantly decrease cardiac output. Also, if the patient is resuscitated, hypertension, tachycardia, and arrhythmias should be anticipated. Epinephrine is not compatible in the same IV line with alkaline solutions (e.g., sodium bicarbonate) as some studies show slow catecholamine inactivation.

## Dopamine

### Actions

Dopamine (Intropin), an endogenous catecholamine and the precursor of endogenous norepinephrine, acts on dopaminergic, $\beta_1$, and α receptors. In low doses (1 to 2 μg/kg per min), dopamine acts on dopaminergic receptors, causing vasodilation of the renal, mesenteric, coronary, and intracerebral vascular beds. This effect improves organ perfusion and increases urine output. At moderate doses (2 to 10 μg/kg per min), dopamine acts on its $\beta_1$-adrenergic receptors, exerting inotropic and chronotropic effects and increasing cardiac output without marked increases in pulmonary wedge pressure. Stimulation of α receptors increases peripheral resistance, increases pulmonary wedge pressure, and decreases blood flow to the kidney. Alpha effects begin at 10 μg/kg per min and predominate above 15 μg/kg per min.

### Pharmacokinetics

Dopamine has an onset of action within 2 to 4 min and a duration of action of less than 10 min. It is used only as an IV infusion. Renal response may take 20 to 30 min. Dopamine is metabolized primarily (75 percent) to homovanillic acid (HVA) and other metabolites (including norepinephrine) by MAO and COMT and subsequently excreted in the urine. Only a fraction of the dose eliminated by the kidneys is unchanged dopamine.

### Indications

Dopamine is indicated for reversing hemodynamically significant hypotension due to myocardial infarction, trauma, sepsis, overt heart failure, renal failure, and chronic CHF when fluid resuscitation is unsuccessful (using the appropriate crystalloid or colloid solution) or not appropriate. It is also used to improve renal blood flow to increase urine output.

### Dosing and Administration

The range for low-dose dopamine is 1 to 2 μg/kg per min, while the moderate dose is 2 to 10 μg/kg per min. High dose begins at 10 μg/kg

per min and should be titrated to adequate blood pressure response. As with all vasoactive infusions, dopamine should be discontinued by tapering the dosage. Most patients can be managed on 20 μg/kg per min or less. If higher doses are needed, an IV norepinephrine infusion should be added.

### Adverse Effect Profile

Dopamine may produce dose-dependent adverse effects, including hypotension at low infusion rates, hypertension at high infusion rates, ectopic beats, headache, nausea, vomiting, angina pectoris, and tachycardia. Necrosis may occur if the infusion extravasates. Gangrene of the extremities has occurred in patients with occlusive vascular disease or diabetes as well as in those who received prolonged high-dose infusions. Monoamine oxidase inhibitors, halogen anesthetics, sympathomimetics, and phosphodiesterase inhibitors will prolong and intensify the effects of dopamine, possibly causing hypertensive and arrhythmogenic activity. Phenytoin may interact with dopamine and cause hypotension, seizures, and bradycardia. Dopamine is contraindicated in cases involving pheochromocytoma. As with epinephrine, dopamine should not be mixed with alkaline solutions in the same line.

## Norepinephrine

### Actions

Norepinephrine bitartrate (Levophed) is identical to the endogenous catecholamine synthesized in the adrenal medulla and sympathetic nervous tissue. Norepinephrine acts primarily on α receptors, inducing powerful vasoconstrictor actions on arterial and venous beds (i.e., renal and mesenteric vasoconstriction). The drug also has direct action on $\beta_1$ receptors, thus inducing inotropic and chronotropic effects. Paradoxical decreases in heart rate may result from reflex increase in parasympathetic tone. Norepinephrine differs from epinephrine in that norepinephrine has no effect on $\beta_2$ receptors.

### Pharmacokinetics

Norepinephrine is administered only as an IV infusion. The pressor effect has an onset of action within 1 to 3 min and stops within 5 to 10 min of discontinuation of the infusion. The primary elimination of norepinephrine is via uptake by adrenergic neurons and metabolism in the liver and other tissues, mainly by COMT and to a lesser extent by MAO. Norepinephrine metabolites are excreted in the urine as sulfate and glucuronate conjugates.

### Indications

Norepinephrine is used primarily as a vasopressor for the treatment of severe hypotension refractory to fluids and other pressor agents, specifically dopamine. Norepinephrine may be particularly effective when endogenous norepinephrine stores are low. This scenario may arise in patients who have been on prolonged infusions of dopamine. To a certain degree, norepinephrine increases inotropic activity and may be indicated in severe hypotension occurring during an acute myocardial infarction or septic shock. Other specific uses for norepinephrine include controlling hypotensive states during poliomyelitis, drug overdose (various phenothiazines and tricyclic antidepressants), spinal anesthesia, pheochromocytomectomy, and sympathectomy.

### Dosing and Administration

As with any vasopressor, adequate fluid or blood replacement should be corrected before starting norepinephrine. Norepinephrine should only be used as an IV infusion. The initial adult dose is 0.5 to 1 μg/min, while the pediatric dose is 2 μm²/min up to 6 μm²/min. An alternative pediatric dose is 0.1 μg/kg per min. Rates must be titrated carefully, increasing by 1 to 2 μg/min q 3–5 min until a systolic blood pressure of 80 to 100 mmHg is attained. The drug should be infused in the lowest effective dosage for the shortest period of time possible. Occasionally, high doses of norepinephrine may be necessary to reverse hypotension (e.g., 8 to 30 μg/min). Usually, the maintenance dose is 2 to 4 μg/min. Adjust the rate of flow q 3–5 min to maintain blood pressure. Once the blood pressure is adequate, the infusion may be gradually titrated down. Abrupt withdrawal may result in acute hypotension.

### Adverse Effect Profile

Large doses of norepinephrine may result in ventricular irritability, cardiac depression, decreased renal blood flow, and a reflex bradycardia. Acute hypertension may result in patients on MAO inhibitors or tricyclic antidepressants. Use norepinephrine with extreme caution in these patients. Use as large a vein as possible to minimize the risk of extravasation. If extravasation occurs, phentolamine, 5 to 10 mg in 10 to 15 mL of normal saline solution, should be infiltrated as soon as possible to prevent necrosis and sloughing. Check frequently for IV extravasation if a small vein is used. Norepinephrine is contraindicated in patients with hypotension resulting from cyclopropane or halogenated hydrocarbon anesthesia or uncorrected blood volume deficits as well as in mesenteric or peripheral vascular thrombosis.

## Isoproterenol

### Actions

Isoproterenol (Isuprel) is a synthetic sympathomimetic with *strong* $\beta_1$- and $\beta_2$-adrenergic-agonist properties. Beta$_1$ actions increase the inotropic and chronotropic activity of cardiac muscle, resulting in increased cardiac output despite a reduction in the mean blood pressure. The drop in blood pressure can be attributed to the $\beta_2$-adrenergic relaxation of smooth muscle in the splanchnic vasculature bed and alimentary tract, the lungs, and skeletal muscle, which causes peripheral vasodilation and venous pooling.

### Pharmacokinetics

After IV administration, isoproterenol has an onset of action within 1 to 5 min and a duration of action lasting 1 to 2 h. Fifty percent of the drug is eliminated unchanged in the urine, while 25 to 35 percent is metabolized primarily to 3-*O*-methylisoproterenol (which has been reported to have weak $\beta$-adrenergic blocking activity) by COMT in the lung, liver, and other body tissues and then excreted unchanged or as a sulfate conjugate.

### Indications

Isoproterenol is now indicated only for refractory torsade de pointes and immediate temporary management of hemodynamically significant bradycardias in the denervated heart of patients undergoing heart transplants. Isoproterenol is not considered the drug of choice for either of these conditions; it should be considered only as a temporary measure until pacemaker therapy is instituted. For hemodynamically unstable bradyarrhythmias, transcutaneous pacing (TCP) is the definitive treatment for this condition, since it provides better control and is a safer mode of therapy. Other agents that should be considered before isoproterenol are IV fluid challenge, atropine, and a dopamine or epinephrine infusion. The vasodilatory effects of isoproterenol have been shown to lower coronary perfusion pressure during cardiac arrest and to increase the mortality rate in experimental animals; the drug has not been shown to be efficacious in cardiac arrest or for use in hypotension.

### Dosing and Administration

Isoproterenol should be administered only via IV infusion. The infusion rate, 2 to 10 μg/min, should be titrated to the desired heart rate. The drug has been shown to be more helpful at low doses rather than high doses.

### Adverse Effect Profile

It must be emphasized that the $\beta_1$-agonist action of isoproterenol will cause an increase in chronotropic effect. This effect raises myocardial oxygen requirements and could possibly precipitate or exacerbate myocardial ischemia, inducing serious arrhythmias (e.g., VT and VF). Other adverse effects include anxiety, mild tremors, and anginal pain in patients with previously reported angina pectoris. Therefore, the drug should be avoided in patients with preexisting ischemic heart disease. Isoproterenol may also induce tachyarrhythmias in hypokalemic and digoxin-toxic patients. The primary adverse effects from $\beta_2$-adrenergic actions are facial flushing, headache, and hypotension.

## Dobutamine

### Actions

Dobutamine (Dobutrex) is a synthetic sympathomimetic agent that exerts potent inotropic and mild chronotropic activity by directly stimulating $\beta_1$-adrenergic receptors. Dobutamine also has mild $\alpha_1$-agonist activity, but the effects are balanced by the more potent $\beta_2$-agonist effects, cumulatively resulting in mild vasodilation. Doses of 2 to 20 μg/kg per min increase cardiac output, induce peripheral vasodilation, and decrease pulmonary occlusive pressures, causing minimal increase in heart rate. However, higher doses of dobutamine will accelerate the heart rate and induce arrhythmogenic effects. An increased cardiac output usually results in increased renal and mesenteric blood flow.

### Pharmacokinetics

Dobutamine has an onset of action of 1 to 2 min, but peak plasma levels may not be reached for 10 min. Its duration of action is 10 to 15 min. The plasma half-life is 2 min. Dobutamine is metabolized in the liver and other tissues by COMT and glucuronic acid, and over two-thirds of a dose is excreted as metabolites in the urine within 48 h.

### Indications

Dobutamine is used to increase inotropic activity in the short-term management of cardiac decompensation due to depressed contractility resulting either from organic heart disease or from cardiac surgical procedures. The drug should be used to increase cardiac output in the chronic CHF patient when standard therapy (diuretics, vasodilators, and digoxin) fails to improve symptoms and/or in the patient with pulmonary congestion and low cardiac output.

### Dosing and Administration

Dobutamine is administered only via IV infusion. The dosage range is 2 to 20 μg/kg per min; however, most patients can be maintained on 10 μg/kg per min or less. In some cases, very low doses (0.5 μg/kg per min) may be effective. Conversely, infusions up to 40 μg/kg per min have been used, but doses greater than 20 μg/kg per min should be used with caution because of increased risks of tachyarrhythmias. To assess the effectiveness of the drug correctly, patients should be monitored with either a Swan-Ganz catheter or a central venous pressure manometer.

### Adverse Effect Profile

The primary adverse effects of dobutamine are increased heart rate (increases greater than 5–15 bpm are uncommon), blood pressure (increases greater than 10–20 mmHg are uncommon), and ectopic arrhythmias (escape beats, unifocal and multifocal ventricular ectopic beats, and ventricular bigeminy). Less common effects include headache, paresthesias, tremors, nausea, angina, and dyspnea. Heart rate increases greater than 10 percent may induce or exacerbate myocardial ischemia.

## Amrinone

### Actions

Amrinone (Inocor) is thought to be a positive inotropic agent not related to either digitalis glycosides, catecholamines (e.g., epinephrine, dopamine, and norepinephrine), or synthetic $\beta_1$-adrenergic agonists (e.g., dobutamine and isoproterenol) and possesses potent vasodilator activity. While its true mechanism is not known, amrinone is believed to act by inhibiting cyclic adenosine monophosphate (cyclicAMP) phosphodiesterase activity, which results in increased levels of cellular cyclicAMP. Increased levels of cyclicAMP are thought to increase calcium availability to the myocardial contractile components. These actions increase myocardial contractility and force of contractions (i.e., positive inotropic effect). Some believe that the vasodilatory action is the primary mechanism responsible for increasing myocardial performance. Vasodilation resulting in conjunction with amrinone may be the result of direct action by the drug on the vessels or may be caused by a reflex withdrawal of sympathetic tone following the improvement of myocardial function. Nonetheless, the primary effect of amrinone is an increase in myocardial contractility and stroke volume with a reduction in preload and afterload.

### Pharmacokinetics

Cardiovascular effects usually begin within 2 to 5 min and generally peak within 10 min at all doses. The duration of effect is dose-related. Following a 0.75-mg/kg bolus dose the duration is about 30 min, while a 3-mg/kg dose will last approximately 2 h. Amrinone is metabolized in the liver, excreted in the urine, and has a Vd of 1.2 L/kg. In patients with normal renal function, amrinone has an elimination half-life of 3.6 h. In patients with CHF and/or hepatic or renal dysfunction, amrinone has a prolonged elimination half-life (average 5.8 h).

### Indications

Amrinone is indicated for increasing myocardial performance in the short-term management of CHF. Due to its adverse effect profile, the drug should be used only when other therapies, such as diuretics, digoxin, and vasodilators, have failed. Amrinone has been studied only in class III and IV CHF.

### Dosing and Administration

The initial dose is 0.75 mg/kg followed by a maintenance infusion at 5 to 10 µg/kg per min. Amrinone should be administered as a slow direct IV injection (undiluted) over 2 to 3 min or as a continuous infusion diluted in 0.9% or 0.45% saline. Dextrose-containing solutions may result in a loss of the drug's activity. The total daily dose should not exceed 10 mg/kg. A second IV bolus injection may be given 30 min following the first dose if desired effects have not been achieved. Adjustments in the maintenance infusion should be titrated to clinical response.

### Adverse Effect Profile

The most common adverse effects are thrombocytopenia ($<100,000/mm^3$, 2.4 percent), ventricular and supraventricular arrhythmias (3 percent), hypotension (1.3 percent), and nausea (1.7 percent). Other adverse effects, which occur in fewer than 1 percent of patients, include vomiting, anorexia, fever, chest pain, and burning at the site of injection. Although rare, hepatotoxicity with amrinone has been reported. Acute marked elevations of hepatic enzymes along with clinical symptoms may suggest a hypersensitivity reaction, which would require prompt discontinuation of the drug.

## Atropine

### Actions

Atropine sulfate, an antimuscarinic agent, increases sinus node automaticity and AV conduction by blocking vagal activity and thus has been termed a *parasympatholytic drug*. It has anticholinergic properties.

### Pharmacokinetics

The onset of action of atropine following IV, IM, and ET administration is rapid, with peak increases in heart rate occurring within 5 min. The half-life of atropine is 2 to 4 h or longer. Well absorbed and distributed throughout the body, atropine is metabolized in the liver and excreted in the urine.

### Indications

Atropine is the treatment of choice for increasing heart rate in hemodynamically unstable bradycardias (e.g., decreased heart rate with hypotension, altered mental status, "escape beats," and chest pain). Higher doses have been used in cardiac arrest, specifically, PEA, asystole, and/or pulseless idioventricular rhythm. However, efficacy has not been proven in humans. The drug reverses cholinergic medications and toxins that cause a decrease in systemic vascular resistance, heart rate, and blood pressure. Additionally, atropine may reduce nausea and vomiting that occur as a result of morphine administration.

### Dosing and Administration

The dose of atropine for hemodynamically unstable bradycardias is 0.5 mg *rapid* IV push, repeated as necessary q 3–5 min until a desired heart rate is achieved. Bolus doses of 1 mg can be given for asystole and repeated once if necessary. A total dose of 3 mg (0.04 mg/kg) results in full vagolytic blockade in humans. Atropine can be administered IV push, IM, and via the ET tube. If given via the ET tube, recommendations include a bolus of at least 1 mg at a time. No dilution is necessary when a preload syringe (1 mg/10 mL) is used. However, if the 1 mg/mL ampoules are used, dilution with up to 10 mL normal saline is recommended. It has been estimated that absorption across tracheobronchial structures appears to be good, and substantial atropine levels are achieved within 10 min of dosing.

### Adverse Effect Profile

Atropine is not indicated for bradycardia in hemodynamically *stable* patients. If administered, marked increases in heart rate can increase myocardial oxygen consumption, possibly inducing ischemia and precipitating ventricular tachyarrhythmias (including VT and VF). This is particularly true in doses greater than 0.5 mg. Doses less than 0.4 mg along with a therapeutic dose administered slowly can cause paradoxical bradycardia. This may be due to a central reflex stimulation of the vagus or a peripheral parasympathomimetic effect on the heart. There is concern by some about using atropine in AV block at the His-Purkinje level (type II AV block and third-degree block with new wide-QRS complexes). Other effects that may occur include anticholinergic symptoms (e.g., blurred vision, dry mouth, CNS stimulation, hallucinations, mydriasis, tachycardia).

## Vasodilator Agents

### Nitroglycerin

### Actions

Although the mechanism of action of nitroglycerin is not fully understood, its therapeutic benefit appears to be due to its actions on the peripheral circulation and the coronary blood flow. Nitroglycerin is a direct vasodilator that induces venodilation at low doses ($<100$ µg/min) and arteriolar vasodilation at high doses

**Table 23-5.** Nitroglycerin Chart

| Dosage Forms | Onset, min | Duration of Action | Dosing and Administration |
|---|---|---|---|
| Sublingual | 1–3 | 1–3 min | Dissolve 1 tablet under tongue; repeat q 5 min up to 3 times in 15 min if no relief |
| Translingual spray | 2 | 30–60 min | 1–2 metered dose sprays onto oral mucosa q 3–5 min up to 3 times in 15 min if no relief |
| Transmucosal tablets | 1–2 | 3–5 h | Place 1-mg tablet between lip and gum above incisors or between cheek and gum q 3–5 h while awake |
| Sustained-release tablet, capsule | 20–45 | 4–8 h | 2.5–2.6 mg tid-qid and titrate up (swallow capsules whole) |
| Topical ointment | 20–60 | 2–12 h | Apply 1–2 inches to chest wall q 4–8 h |
| Transdermal patch | 30–60 | up to 24 h | 2.5- to 15-mg patches available; start with low dose and titrate upward; apply to hair-free area and rotate sites |
| IV infusion | 1–2 | 3–5 min | Start at 5–10 µg/min, titrate in increments of 5–10 µg/min q 3–5 min to desired response; most doses range between 50 and 200 µg/min |

(>200 µg/min). Coronary artery dilation occurs throughout the dosage range.

### Pharmacokinetics

Table 23-5 describes the onset and duration of various nitroglycerin products. Nitroglycerin has a plasma half-life of 1 to 4 min and is metabolized in the liver. Oral doses undergo an extensive first-pass metabolism.

### Indications

Nitroglycerin is approved for the prophylaxis, treatment, and management of angina pectoris. Intravenous nitroglycerin is used to control hypertension associated with surgery and is also used in CHF associated with acute myocardial infarction.

### Dosing and Administration

Nitroglycerin can be administered sublingually, lingually, intrabuccally, orally, topically, or by IV infusion. The sublingual and intrabuccal tablets should not be swallowed, and the extended-release buccal tablets (transmucosal) should not be chewed or swallowed. Patients should be in a sitting or supine position immediately following sublingual, lingual, or intrabuccal administration.

An IV infusion of nitroglycerin (Tridil) should be administered via a controlled-infusion device. Since data on the incompatibility of nitroglycerin with other parenteral agents is unclear, a separate IV site for a nitroglycerin infusion should be used. Infusions should not be suddenly discontinued, since abrupt withdrawal reactions (including angina pectoris or myocardial infarction) may result. Attempts should be made to gradually wean patients off the infusion.

Specific dosing regimens are shown in Table 23-5. The dose of nitroglycerin for each patient should be titrated to individual response, using the smallest effective dose.

### Adverse Effect Profile

Most adverse effects are related to the cardiovascular actions induced by nitroglycerin. These effects include headache, dizziness, weakness, syncope, flushing, hypotension, reflex tachycardia, and occasionally bradycardia. Use in patients concomitantly using alcohol may result in hypotension; hypotension has been shown to decrease the anticoagulant effects of heparin. Also, rash has been reported with topical nitroglycerin use.

Caution is advised when using nitroglycerin in patients who are hemodynamically unstable (including those patients who are volume depleted) or who have increased intracranial pressure or severe anemia. The drug should also be used cautiously in cases of constrictive pericarditis, pericardial tamponade, and hypertrophic cardiomyopathy. Also, there have been reports involving angle-closure or open glaucoma that describe brief increases in intraocular pressure. Extended-release preparations of nitroglycerin should be avoided in patients with GI hypermotility or malabsorption syndromes.

Transdermal patches and topical ointment must be removed prior to attempting defibrillation or synchronized cardioversion. Topical nitroglycerin products alter electrical conductivity and enhance the potential for electrical arcing to occur. To avoid excessive dosing, topical products should also be removed if additional nitroglycerin is given for acute symptoms.

## BIBLIOGRAPHY

*American Hospital Formulary Service Drug Information 94.* Bethesda, MD, American Society of Hospital Pharmacists, 1994.

Cardene IV prescribing information, CI 4192-1, Wyeth-Ayerst Labs. Issued Sept. 29, 1993.

*Drugdex.* Micromedex Inc, Denver, vol 82 expires Nov. 1994.

*Drug Facts and Comparisons.* St. Louis, Lippincott, 1994.

Gilman AG, Goodman LS, Gilman A: *The Pharmacological Basis of Therapeutics,* 7th ed. New York, Macmillan, 1990.

Gonzalez ER, Ornato JP, Garnett AR, et al: Dose-dependent vasopressor response to epinephrine during CPR in human beings. *Ann Emerg Med* 18:920, 1989.

Grauer K, Cavallaro D: *Volume I, ACLS Certification Preparation,* 3d ed. St. Louis, Mosby-Year Book, 1993.

Grauer K, Cavallaro D: *Volume II, ACLS A Comprehensive Review,* 3d ed. St. Louis, Mosby-Year Book, 1993.

*Guidelines for Cardiopulmonary Resuscitation and Emergency Care: Recommendation of the 1992 National Conference.* Part III. Adult Cardiac Life Support. *JAMA* 268:2205, 1992.

# SECTION 3
# Acute Signs and Symptoms in Adults

## 24
## CHEST PAIN

Jay L. Falk
John F. O'Brien

### INTRODUCTION

Patients with acute nontraumatic chest pain are among the most challenging patients cared for by emergency physicians. They may be dramatically ill on presentation or may appear completely well, yet be at serious risk for sudden cardiac death resulting from acute coronary syndrome.

Seriously compromised patients are easily recognized. The diagnosis can usually be made from history, physical examination, electrocardiogram, chest radiograph, and arterial blood gases. Patients with acute myocardial infarction, aortic dissection, massive pulmonary embolism, spontaneous pneumothorax, pneumonia, esophageal rupture (Boerhaave's syndrome), or pericarditis with tamponade fall into this category.

Perhaps even more challenging are those with symptoms that are less severe or that have resolved at the time of examination (see Table 24-1). The cause may be benign syndromes such as dyspepsia or chest wall pain. However, the possibility of acute myocardial ischemia must always be considered. Appropriate diagnosis and disposition have become increasingly complex in the current environment, in which the pressures to provide cost-effective care intersect with the expectations of patients and their families that missing the diagnosis (when death or injury result) is completely unacceptable.

### PATHOPHYSIOLOGY OF CHEST PAIN

Stimulation of peripheral pain nerve endings results in pain perception by the brain. The location of the stimulus is interpreted by the parietal cortex. There are two categories of pain sensation: somatic and visceral. Somatic sensation results from irritation of fine pain fibers in the dermis or parietal pleura. These nerve fibers are highly concentrated, enter the spinal cord at a single level, and are precisely mapped on the parietal cortex. Accordingly, somatic pain is generally perceived as sharp, lancinating, and precisely located. Classically, chest wall or parietal pleural pain would be described in these terms. Visceral pain results from stimulation of pain fibers located in internal organs or visceral pleura. These nerves enter the spinal cord at multiple adjacent cord levels along with somatic pain nerves. Visceral pain is perceived when impulses from the internal organs and the resting potential from the somatic nerves summate in the spinal cord to reach a pain perception threshold level. Classically, visceral pain is less distinct, is usually described as being dull or aching in quality, and is less precisely located. Visceral pain may be perceived as an aching in a somatic area that shares a cord level with the involved organ. Classic examples include shoulder pain resulting from diaphragmatic irritation and arm or wrist pain resulting from myocardial ischemia. When myocardial oxygen demand exceeds supply, regional ischemia occurs, resulting

in abnormal myocardial wall tension and chemical mediator accumulation. Increased myocardial oxygen demand is caused primarily by increases in heart rate, blood pressure (mural tension), and contractility. Myocardial oxygen supply in patients with coronary disease is limited by inadequate coronary blood flow resulting from fixed lesions, vasospasm, and thrombus formation. The discomfort of myocardial ischemia is transmitted mainly via sympathetic afferents through cardiac nerves and sympathetic ganglia to the lower cervical and upper five thoracic roots of the spinal cord. These fibers synapse with the spinothalamic tract and eventually the cerebral cortex. There are also afferent somatic fibers from the upper thorax and upper extremities as well as visceral fibers from various chest structures that send information to the same cord levels. The cerebral cortex often misinterprets the origin of the pain and may thus register chest discomfort and pain radiation from any of the thoracic structures as indistinguishable from that resulting from myocardial ischemia.

### TREATMENT PRIORITY

Patients complaining of acute chest pain should be triaged to be seen with the highest priority. The First Hour program of the American Heart Association teaches us to approach every patient with acute chest pain as one who may be having an acute myocardial infarction (AMI). Prehospital advanced life support providers should treat patients with suspicious histories by IV lifeline, continuous ECG monitoring, and nasal oxygen. In the emergency department, if a physician is not *immediately* available, nursing personnel should be empowered to assess patients and provide similar precautions, including the ordering of a 12-lead ECG.

Assessment delay, including time to obtain 12-lead ECG, is unacceptable. Time goals of less than 30 min from "door to drug" have been advocated. Field 12-lead ECG by prehospital units can alert emergency department personnel that a thrombolytic candidate is en route, thus considerably shortening the time to thrombolytic drug administration.

**Table 24-1.** Etiology of Nontraumatic Chest Pain

| Cardiac causes | Pulmonary causes (cont.) |
|---|---|
| Coronary artery disease | Barotrauma |
| Stable angina | Pneumothorax |
| Unstable angina | Pneumomediastinum |
| Variant angina | Tracheobronchitis |
| Acute myocardial infarction | Musculoskeletal causes |
| Pericarditis | Costochondritis |
| Valvular/outflow disease | Intercostal muscle strain |
| Aortic stenosis | Cervical thoracic spine problems |
| Subaortic stenosis | Gastrointestinal causes |
| Mitral valve prolapse | Esophageal reflux/spasm |
| Vascular causes | Mallory Weiss syndrome |
| Aortic dissection | Biliary colic |
| Pulmonary embolus | Dyspepsia |
| Pulmonary hypertension | Pancreatitis |
| Pulmonary causes | Miscellaneous causes |
| Pleural irritation | Herpes zoster |
| Infections | Chest wall tumors |
| Inflammation | |
| Infiltration | |

## EMERGENCY DEPARTMENT EVALUATION OF PATIENTS WITH SUSPECTED AMI

### Ischemic Chest Pain

In the United States, coronary artery disease may cause as many as half of all deaths in patients aged 36 to 64 years. Approximately 1.7 million patients per year nationwide are admitted to cardiac and other intensive care units for episodes suspected to represent acute ischemic heart disease. Many more patients are evaluated in emergency departments complaining of acute chest pain. Yet the evaluation of these patients is far from precise. The rate of confirmed acute myocardial infarction in patients admitted to coronary care units is only 28 to 50 percent. Economic and other pressures tempt emergency physicians to discharge patients who have only marginal evidence of acute ischemia. The psychological, social, and financial impact on the admitted patient can be substantial and often influences decisions in borderline cases. Conversely, up to 4 to 5 percent of patients with acute myocardial infarction are inappropriately discharged from emergency departments. Missed acute myocardial infarction carries a 26 percent mortality, compared to only 12 percent for age- and sex-matched patients admitted with the syndrome. Missed myocardial infarction results in the highest dollar awards to plaintiffs resulting from emergency medicine malpractice claims.

## HISTORY

It is important to have a high index of suspicion for the presence of acute myocardial ischemia when evaluating patients in the appropriate age group and especially when risk factors are present. Risk factors include being a male or a postmenopausal female, hypertension, cigarette smoking, hypercholesterolemia, diabetes, sedentary life-style, obesity, and family history. Cocaine use has been associated with AMI even in young people with minimal or no coronary artery disease. Chronic cocaine abuse has been associated with accelerated atherosclerosis and severe coronary artery disease (CAD). Accordingly, drug history and, possibly, urine drug screening may be important in the evaluation of younger patients with chest pain.

The classic description of myocardial ischemic pain is that of a retrosternal or epigastric squeezing, tightening, crushing, or pressurelike discomfort. The patient often holds a clenched fist to the sternum in an effort to relate the experience. The pain may radiate to the left shoulder, mandible, arm, or hand. The discomfort may be associated with dyspnea, diaphoresis, nausea, lightheadedness, or a sense of profound weakness. In the elderly, these associated symptoms may predominate while the chest discomfort is minimal or absent. In cases of angina the symptoms are precipitated by exertion and relieved by rest. When episodes occur more frequently, with less exertion, are more intense or prolonged, or are new, unstable angina is defined.

Unfortunately, the description of chest discomfort characteristics is often misleading. In the multicenter Chest Pain Study Group (CPSG), only 54 percent of those who described their chest discomfort as a crushing, pressure, tightness, or heaviness had ongoing myocardial ischemia; 22 percent of those with sharp or stabbing chest discomfort were having acute ischemia. Thus, character of the pain is not a reliable discriminator for acute myocardial ischemia. The CPSG also demonstrated that chest pain lasting less than 2 min or over days is not likely to represent myocardial infarction. This allows for a large range of pain duration that may be associated with infarction. The Framingham study demonstrated that approximately one-quarter of heart attack victims did not present for medical care at the time of the event, and half of these patients could not retrospectively recall symptoms reminiscent of AMI. Thus, historical determination of chest pain etiology is too imprecise to be reliable and, when used alone, allows substantial risk for serious error.

## PHYSICAL EXAMINATION

Patients with myocardial ischemia may have perturbations of their vital signs. Hyper- or hypotension may be seen, as well as tachycardia or bradycardia. Sinus tachycardia may be reflective of increased sympathetic stimulation resulting from ischemia and decreased left ventricular stroke volume. Unexplained sinus tachycardia must always be addressed. Especially in patients who have had spontaneous relief of pain, the vital signs may be normal. Normal vital signs do not preclude the diagnosis of AMI.

Physical findings rarely contribute to the diagnosis of AMI. Patients with acute ischemia have a slightly higher incidence of abnormal heart sounds, and crackles on pulmonary examination are twice as common in patients with AMI as in those with nonischemic chest pain. However, these findings are not discriminatory. Chest wall tenderness reproducing the patient's pain has often been labeled as representing clear evidence of a musculoskeletal etiology. In one study, chest wall tenderness was present in 36 percent of chest pain patients without myocardial infarction and in 15 percent of those with acute infarction. Accordingly, neither chest wall tenderness nor a normal physical examination excludes myocardial ischemia as a diagnosis.

## ANCILLARY STUDIES

### Electrocardiography

The ECG is the most time-honored test for the evaluation of AMI. It is used to screen chest pain patients with atypical presentations, to evaluate nonischemic causes of chest pain (e.g., pericarditis), to stratify the risk of adverse outcomes among patients with suggestive chest pain, and to evaluate therapeutic intervention options. New ST-segment elevation suggesting AMI in the appropriate clinical setting is the key parameter for initiating thrombolytic therapy. However, the initial ECG is diagnostic of infarction in only 25 to 50 percent of patients subsequently confirmed to have AMI. In one study, 13 percent of initial ECGs were normal, and 26 percent showed only nonspecific changes among patients with autopsy-proven infarction. If chest pain resolves prior to obtaining an ECG in the emergency department, ischemic changes may have resolved. Accordingly, the ECG is useful if not diagnostic. *A normal ECG does not exclude AMI.* Young patients who use cocaine may have significant ischemia with ECG patterns suggestive of a "juvenile pattern." Conversely, some of these patients have ST-segment elevations resulting from coronary vasospasm. This makes selection of candidates for thrombolytic therapy perplexing in this patient population. Early cardiology consultation is indicated. The admission ECG is useful as a risk-stratification tool. Patients without evidence of AMI, ischemia, left ventricular hypertrophy, left bundle branch block, or paced rhythm have very minimal risk of developing life-threatening complications and may be safely observed in intermediate care units rather than in the more expensive coronary care units. Comparison of the initial ECG with the most recent previous ECG is also useful. Patients with new ECG changes suggestive of ischemia have substantially higher complication rates than those without.

Recently a computerized 12-lead ECG capable of near-continuous tracing acquisition and ST-segment mapping has become available. This tool has shed light on the dynamic nature of ST-segment changes over time. Application of this monitor during the emergency department evaluation of chest pain patients may capture transient ST changes that may otherwise be missed. Initial reports are encouraging, but further evaluation of this tool is needed.

A newly developed 22-lead ECG may improve the diagnostic accuracy for AMI compared to a conventional 12-lead ECG. The principle behind the 22-lead ECG is that ongoing local myocardial ischemia causes significant changes in conduction velocity in the area of hypoperfusion. This causes heterogeneous changes in conduction velocity compared to nonischemic myocardial tissue. The 22-lead

ECG uses 10 leads that are the same as the standard 12-lead ECG, with 12 others placed at specific locations on the anterior and posterior chest. The relative conduction velocity data from the 22 leads is digitized and used to calculate a temporal dispersion factor called the *ischemic index*. In one study this technique increased the diagnostic sensitivity of electrocardiography for AMI to 83 percent from 51 percent for 12-lead ECG use alone, but it is less specific than the standard technique.

## Serum Markers

An alternative diagnostic strategy is to assay for enzymatic breakdown products resulting from ischemic myocardial cellular damage. Early serum markers of AMI include myoglobin, creatine phosphokinase (CK) and its MB isoenzyme, troponin T, cardiac myosin light chains, and others. It is important to understand that these markers reflect myocardial necrosis that has already occurred. Normal serum levels of any myocardial cell breakdown product do not exclude ischemia as the etiology of acute chest pain. Rather, normal serum levels indicate only that significant tissue breakdown products have not yet been delivered to the bloodstream. If serum markers are positive, myocardial cell damage can be "ruled in." If serum markers are negative, acute myocardial ischemia cannot be "ruled out." Accordingly, serum enzyme measurements have traditionally not been relied upon in the emergency department to assist in diagnosis and disposition of patients with suspected acute ischemia. Recently, newer assays with earlier serum peaks have generated interest in "short-stay" protocols to "rule out MI," in which patients are monitored for a period of hours in an emergency department area designated as a chest pain center or clinic. Diagnostic strategies include serial ECGs and repetitive enzyme analysis, sometimes combined with other modalities such as echocardiography. Preliminary studies suggest that patients in whom the initial clinical suspicion for ischemia is low may be safely evaluated and discharged utilizing this approach, and that this can be accomplished at substantial cost savings compared to the traditional approach, which includes hospital admission. Further outcome studies are needed before this approach becomes standard practice.

Serum myoglobin is elevated as early as 1 h following myocardial infarction, with peak activity at 4 to 12 h. It is elevated in approximately 60 percent of patients with AMI at 1 h after presentation and in nearly 100 percent of cases at 3 h. Unfortunately, elevated myoglobin is not specific for myocardial cell damage; it may also be elevated in skeletal muscle injury, heavy ethanol use, renal failure, shock states, and various other clinical situations. Likewise, total CK is too nonspecific to provide useful clinical information in evaluating these patients.

CK-MB isozyme levels are specific for AMI. The percentage of patients with AMI and positive results increases over time from approximately one-third of patients at emergency department presentation to more than 90 percent of patients 3 h later. In one study of patients with AMI, 52 percent had nondiagnostic ECGs, but all had elevated CK-MB isozyme levels at 3 h.

Recent research suggests that CK-MB subform assays may increase the sensitivity and specificity for detection of myocardial cellular damage. CK-MB exists as a single form in myocardial tissue (MB-2) and is modified over time by the plasma enzyme carboxypeptidase-*N* to the more electronegative subform MB-1. Sensitive, precise, and reliable assays for MB-2 and MB-1 subforms have been validated even when CK-MB remains in the normal range. Recent release of cardiac MB isoenzyme (MB-2) results in an increase in the MB-2:MB-1 ratio even before total CK-MB levels elevate, and thus measurement of these subforms provides a technique for early detection of myocardial cell damage. Subform assays can provide rapid and reliable diagnosis of AMI within 2 to 4 h after the onset of symptoms, approximately 6 h before conventional CK-MB assays are accurate. Despite these advances, current serum markers do not identify patients with unstable angina, who remain at substantial risk if not identified. Accordingly, negative serum assays in the emergency department should not themselves constitute criteria for patient discharge.

## Echocardiography

Emergency two-dimensional echocardiography may have value in the evaluation of patients with acute chest pain, particularly those with nondiagnostic ECG changes, left bundle branch block, or paced rhythm. In the appropriate clinical setting, the finding of regional wall motion abnormalities should prompt hospital admission for presumed ischemia. Aggressive therapeutic interventions such as thrombolytic therapy may be instituted on the basis of echocardiographic findings. One prospective study showed that only 2 of 30 patients subsequently shown to have AMI would not have been admitted based on echocardiographic findings alone, and both had small, uncomplicated infarcts. Two-dimensional echocardiography may also help in identification of other cardiovascular conditions that could cause chest pain or modify the treatment of infarction (e.g., aortic dissection, pericarditis, pulmonary embolism, aortic stenosis, or hypertrophic cardiomyopathy). Finally, echocardiography can document the extent of ischemic dysfunction and thus the amount of myocardium at risk. However, the echocardiogram must be done during the episode of pain to be diagnostic. A brief period of coronary occlusion may not result in dysfunction. Further, the echocardiogram cannot consistently differentiate new wall motion abnormalities from those that may be residual from prior infarction. Transesophageal probes and Doppler flow technologies may enhance the capability of echocardiography, but issues of expense and availability of appropriately trained clinicians may limit their use in the emergency department.

## Provocative Tests

All of the above diagnostic modalities may fail to identify patients with critical coronary lesions and intermittent ischemia without infarction. Accordingly, provocative tests to elicit ischemia in appropriately selected patients with chest pain afford an opportunity to diagnose the lesion prior to loss of myocardium.

Exercise electrocardiography will show ischemic changes in 50 to 80 percent of patients who have symptomatic coronary disease, with a 10 to 15 percent false-positive rate. The accuracy of exercise testing in the general population is less clear. Negative exercise testing in patients with atypical chest pain clearly reflects a reduced chance of CAD being present. Exercise thallium testing has been demonstrated to be superior to standard exercise electrocardiography in risk assessment among patients suspected of having CAD (sensitivity of 84 percent, specificity of 87 percent). Patients with atypical chest pain and a negative, adequately performed stress thallium exercise test have a very low incidence of subsequent cardiac events. Intravenous dipyridamole, dobutamine, or adenosine with thallium imaging permits evaluation for CAD without exercise and may be used in those patients with β-antagonist or calcium channel blocker use, poor conditioning, or functional incapacity. A developing technology, positive emission tomography (PET), uses various radionuclides to further improve stress testing with dipyridamole and shows even better diagnostic accuracy compared to stress thallium exercise testing.

The role of provocative testing in the evaluation of chest pain patients in the emergency department is evolving. Low-risk patients with normal resting ECG in whom the clinical suspicion for acute ischemia is low may be stress-tested while still admitted to the emergency department. If the test is negative, these patients can be discharged with confidence. Patients in whom AMI has been ruled out with serial enzyme measurements and ECGs should be stressed prior to discharge to capture those whose pain may have represented unstable angina and who remain at risk for sudden cardiac death.

## COMPUTER-ASSISTED DECISION-MAKING

Patients with chest pain present with a multitude of individual features that, when taken in aggregate, provide the clinician with an impression as to the etiology of the pain. Computer-assisted medical decision-making developed during the past decade has been applied to the common and complex problem of identifying patients with myocardial ischemia. Several groups developed algorithms designed to weight specific historical, physical, and laboratory features in an attempt to improve upon the accuracy of the clinical diagnosis of AMI. To date, these programs have failed to improve diagnostic accuracy substantively compared to capable clinicians. They have, however, successfully improved risk stratification for admitted patients, allowing for safe step-down unit admission for patients selected by computer to be at low risk for adverse events.

Future developments in artificial intelligence utilizing neural networks that "learn" from the experience of their own databases may prove superior to clinical "judgment." Any computer-assisted technique must be rigorously tested prospectively before it replaces the traditional decision-making process.

## MAJOR CAUSES OF CHEST PAIN

A working knowledge of the clinical syndromes that cause chest pain allows the clinician to focus the clinical evaluation on those conditions that are most common among specific patient groups. The priority for emergency physicians must always be to exclude life-threatening conditions. In some patients this may require extensive testing prior to emergency department discharge. Ventilation/perfusion scanning, chest CT, or angiography may be required in selected patients. In other cases, thoughtful clinical assessment may be enough to satisfy this obligation. Chest pain in children and adolescents is very unlikely to be cardiac in origin. It is most often due to chest wall or respiratory tract causes. Anxiety may present as chest discomfort in children or adults. Adults suffering from anxiety may present with a chief complaint of chest pain. They may have multiple symptoms that lack a coherent pattern, negative physical findings, and a history of frequent medical encounters with a benign outcome. Anxiety or panic attacks must remain a diagnosis of exclusion in the emergency department.

Elderly patients who develop AMI are more likely than younger individuals to present with either nonretrosternal chest pain or no pain. Associated, nonspecific symptoms such as nausea may dominate the presentation of AMI in the elderly.

### Angina Pectoris

Typical chronic, stable angina is episodic and lasts 5 to 15 min (rarely, longer than 20 min). It is precipitated by exertion (physical or emotional) and is relieved by rest or sublingual nitroglycerin (NTG), usually within 3 min. In over 90 percent of patients, the location is retrosternal, and about 70 percent have radiation, usually to the neck, shoulders, or arms. In individual patients, the character of each attack varies little with recurrent episodes. Most patients can differentiate their usual angina from other causes of pain. "Anginal equivalents" are symptoms resulting from myocardial ischemia that do not include chest pain. Symptoms of arm or jaw aching or dyspnea precipitated by exertion and relieved by rest may be anginal equivalents. Only 50 percent of patients with spontaneous angina have ECG changes during the acute painful episode. Ambulatory ECG monitoring has demonstrated ST-segment changes consistent with ischemia in many patients who do not experience chest discomfort. So-called silent ischemia appears to be more frequent among patients with diabetes but is seen in others as well.

Most patients experiencing chronic stable angina do not seek emergency medical attention. The emergency physician must be diligent in identifying why, exactly, such a patient is in the emergency depart-ment. Anginal features defining the pattern as unstable (see below) must be sought. Many times social factors result in the hospital visit in this patient group. For example, a visiting adult child of a patient may witness an attack for the first time and insist on medical evaluation. Accordingly, emergency physicians must get a complete picture of the situation before concluding that the current episode is or is not chronic stable angina.

### Variant (Prinzmetal's Angina)

This form of angina occurs at rest. It may be precipitated by the use of tobacco or cocaine. The syndrome is defined by the presence of ST-segment elevation on the ECG during an acute attack. These changes resolve as the pain goes away. Variant angina is thought to be caused by spasm of the epicardial coronary arteries, either in patients with normal vessels (one-third) or in those with atherosclerotic lesions (two-thirds). Attacks may be complicated by tachyarrhythmias, bundle branch block, or atrioventricular nodal blocks. Variant angina is usually relieved by nitroglycerin. Patients with variant angina may go on to acute infarction, especially those with underlying obstructive coronary lesions. Accordingly, revascularization procedures may be indicated. Beta-blocker therapy may result in unopposed α vasoconstriction and is, therefore, relatively contraindicated in these patients.

### Unstable Angina

When untreated, unstable angina may rapidly progress to AMI. Patients with unstable angina are also at high risk for sudden cardiac death. Current therapy greatly reduces this risk. Accordingly, it is imperative to recognize and hospitalize these patients. Angina may be clinically categorized as unstable if it is: (1) new or of recent onset; (2) of changing character, becoming more frequent, more severe, or precipitated by less exertion, or less responsive to nitroglycerin; and (3) angina occurring at rest. Patients in the latter two subgroups are at greatest risk for early infarction and death. As delineated above, diagnostic modalities such as ECG and enzyme assays may be normal in patients with unstable angina. Accordingly, the clinician must rely on the clinical history and a high index of suspicion to make the diagnosis.

### Acute Myocardial Infarction

Ischemic pain that lasts longer than 15 min, is not relieved by nitroglycerin, or is accompanied by diaphoresis, dyspnea, nausea, or vomiting suggests the diagnosis of AMI. Longitudinal population studies indicate that 20 percent of myocardial infarctions may be clinically unrecognized.

Multicenter studies have found that up to 5 percent of patients with AMI are discharged, even from competent emergency departments. As discussed above, decision making for patients suspected of having AMI can be very complex. An overall scheme is presented in Fig. 24-1.

### Aortic Dissection

Aortic dissection is an uncommon, but not rare, cause of chest pain. The majority of cases are seen in hypertensive men in the fifth to seventh decades. The syndrome may present in patients from childhood through old age. Patients with Marfan syndrome, coarctation of the aorta, bicuspid aortic valves, and aortic stenosis are predisposed to aortic dissection. An intimal tear appears to allow for longitudinal propagation of hematoma within the aortic media. The hematoma may involved the arch (type I, 66 percent of cases) or be limited to the descending aorta (type III, 25 percent of cases). The dissection may occlude major vessels, such as the carotids, or extremities, resulting in neurologic deficits or ischemic limbs with pulse deficits. Arch dissections may occlude coronary ostia, resulting in AMI; may

**Fig. 24-1.** Disposition of patients with suspected acute myocardial ischemia.

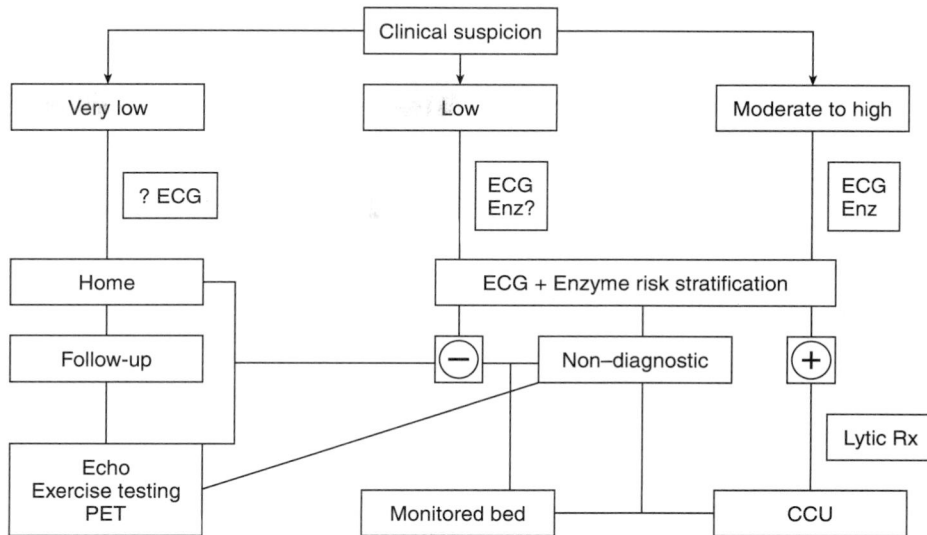

disrupt the annulus of the aortic valve, producing acute aortic regurgitation; or rupture into the pericardium, causing hemopericardium and tamponade.

A high index of suspicion will usually enable the astute clinician to make the diagnosis expeditiously. This is crucial because, if left untreated, approximately 35 percent of patients will die within 24 h while 80 percent will succumb in the first 2 weeks. Conversely, the majority of patients with acute dissection who do not present in shock or with major neurologic deficits can be salvaged with appropriate medical and surgical therapies.

The hallmark of acute aortic dissection is midline truncal pain. The pain is severe, often described as cutting, searing, ripping, or tearing. It is retrosternal and interscapular and may be felt both above and below the diaphragm. In the classic case, the pain is at its worst from the onset. Associated complications such as stroke, AMI, or limb ischemia may dominate the clinical presentation and make accurate history-taking difficult. Physical examination may reveal the diastolic murmur of aortic regurgitation (type I dissections) or pulse deficits (types I and III). Absence of these findings is the rule rather than the exception in distal dissection. Shock with hypotension may dominate the clinical presentation, while extreme hypertension may be present in other cases.

The chest radiograph is abnormal in 90 percent of cases and is characterized by dilation of the aortic shadow, a sensitive but nonspecific finding. Intimal calcification more than 6 mm within the margin of the aortic shadow is very specific but rare. Aortography remains the most definitive diagnostic tool. Contrast CT or transesophageal echocardiography are less invasive techniques that are increasingly utilized with great success. A widened aortic root and new aortic insufficiency are two echocardiographic findings that suggest dissection.

Clinical suspicion of dissection should precipitate emergent consultation with a cardiothoracic surgeon while diagnostic workup and therapeutic interventions proceed. Reduction of shearing forces on the aorta may be accomplished with negative inotropic agents (β blockade) and antihypertensive therapy. Propranolol and nitroprusside are standard agents. Urgent surgical intervention is indicated in proximal dissections and in distal dissections complicated by major vascular occlusion.

## Pericarditis

The pain of pericarditis is often acute, steady, and severe with a retrosternal location and radiation to back, neck, or jaw. Pain may be pronounced with each cardiac systole, chest motion, or respiration and is often relieved by sitting up and leaning forward. If there is associated pleuritis (pleuropericarditis), pain may be predominantly pleuritic. The presence of a pericardial friction rub supports the diagnosis. Many friction rubs are evanescent, and failure to detect a rub does not rule out the diagnosis. The ECG may show diffuse ST-segment elevation or T-wave inversions. Unlike the changes of myocardial ischemia, the changes are not limited to the distribution of a single coronary vessel. PR-segment depression is a highly specific finding. Pericardial effusion is often present and can be detected by echocardiogram. The differential diagnosis of acute pericarditis is large, and serious etiologies should be excluded prior to hospital discharge.

## Other Cardiac Conditions

Patients with hypertrophic cardiomyopathy (idiopathic hypertrophic subaortic stenosis, IHSS) and valvular aortic stenosis may experience anginal pain. In these conditions myocardial ischemia may result from inadequate blood supply to hypertrophied myocardium or from altered coronary flow. Exertional syncope and prominent systolic murmur lead to echocardiographic assessment, which is diagnostic.

Patients with mitral valve prolapse (MVP) may experience "atypical" chest pain. It tends to be poorly characterized or localized, is generally unrelated to exertion, and is episodic. Short, midsystolic mitral regurgitant murmur associated with a midsystolic click suggests the diagnosis. Echocardiography is diagnostic. Beta blockers and calcium channel blockers have been utilized successfully in patients with MVP and IHSS.

Patients with mitral stenosis often experience chest pain, most likely as a consequence of pulmonary hypertension. A history of rheumatic fever, symptoms of fatigue and pulmonary edema, and the characteristic diastolic murmur along with radiographic and electrocardiographic evidence of left atrial enlargement (straightening of the left heart border, elevated left mainstem bronchus, atrial "double density," and biphasic $p$ wave in lead $V_1$) lead to the diagnosis, which is confirmed by echocardiography.

## Pulmonary Embolus

Pulmonary embolism is an important, potentially fatal, but treatable cause of chest pain that may be very difficult to diagnose. A high index of suspicion, especially in patients with risk factors, is required. A logical approach to the workup that considers the advantages and limitations of available modalities is essential (Fig. 24-2).

Pulmonary emboli originate from venous thrombi in the lower extremities or pelvis in nearly all cases. At least one risk factor from

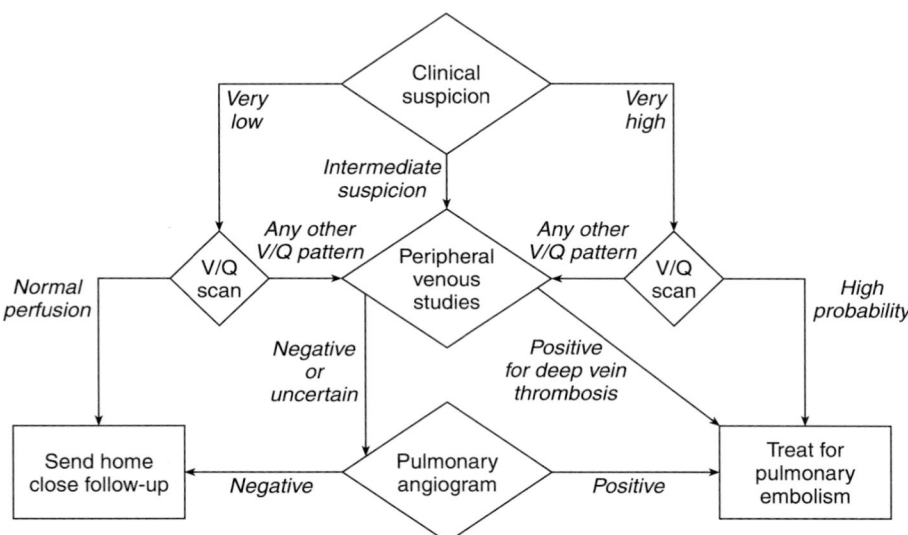

**Fig. 24-2.** Suspected pulmonary embolism.

Virchow's triad of venous stasis, vessel wall inflammation, and hypercoagulability is implicated in most patients with pulmonary embolism (Table 24-2), although as many as 20 percent of patients may have no demonstrable risk.

**Table 24-2.** Risk Factors for Venous Thrombosis/Pulmonary Embolism

General
  Age (>40 years)
  Obesity (>120% ideal body weight)
  Immobilization
  Pregnancy and postpartum state
  Surgery
Trauma
  Multiple trauma
  CNS/spinal cord injury
  Burns
  Lower extremity fractures
Medical illness
  Acute myocardial infarction
  Congestive heart failure
  Previous deep venous thrombophlebitis or pulmonary embolus
  Malignancy
  Cerebrovascular accident
  Sepsis
  Nephrotic syndrome
  Ulcerative colitis
  Varicose veins
Vasculitis
  Systemic lupus erythematosus
  Behçet's syndrome
  Homocystinuria
Acquired hematologic disorders
  Polycythemia rubra vera
  Essential thrombocytosis
Inherited disorders of coagulation or fibrinolysis
  Protein C deficiency
  Antithrombin III deficiency
  Protein S deficiency
  Dysfibrinogenemias
  Disorders of plasminogen and plasminogen activation
Drugs/medications
  IV drug abuse
  Oral contraceptives
  Oral estrogens
  Heparin
  Procainamide/hydralazine
  Chlorpromazine

The classic presentation of pulmonary embolism includes pleuritic chest pain associated with dyspnea, tachypnea, tachycardia, and hypoxemia. Unfortunately, recent studies demonstrate that many patients with pulmonary embolism may lack these symptoms and signs. Classic clinical teaching developed during an era when only the most fulminant cases could be diagnosed. Patients with more subtle presentations were overlooked. With increased awareness of the syndrome and better, less invasive diagnostic modalities, the diagnosis can be made in these patients. The key to success is maintaining a high index of suspicion in patients with risk factors for developing deep venous thrombosis (DVT).

Patients suspected of having pulmonary embolus should have a chest x-ray and ECG, primarily to rule out other conditions, since these studies are either normal or have very nonspecific abnormalities in the majority of patients with the syndrome. Hamptom's hump (triangular, pleural-based infiltrate with apex pointed toward the hilum) and Westermark's sign (dilated pulmonary vessels proximal to the embolus, with sharply demarcated cutoff and distal oligemia) are two specific but unusual chest radiographic findings in patients with pulmonary embolus. The ECG finding of an $S_1$, $Q_3$, $T_3$ pattern represents right heart strain but is present in fewer than 6 percent of patients. Sinus tachycardia and ST- and T-wave abnormalities are common but nonspecific.

Pulmonary emboli (PE) result in ventilation/perfusion mismatch and increased dead space. Patients tend to become hypoxemic and, if they are capable, tachypneic and hypocarbic. This hyperventilation may successfully maintain $Pa_{O_2}$, making calculation of alveolar-arterial oxygen $(A - a)$ gradient mandatory. Room air hypoxemia is present in more than 75 percent of cases, while abnormally widened $A - a$ gradient is present in 95 percent of cases. Accordingly, measurement of arterial blood gases and calculation of the $A - a$ gradient is a reasonable screening test for patients suspected of having pulmonary emboli.

Conversely, normal arterial blood gases do not completely exclude the diagnosis of pulmonary embolus. Accordingly, patients in whom clinical suspicion is high should be further evaluated despite this finding.

Pulmonary angiography remains the "gold standard" for diagnosing pulmonary emboli. False-negative examinations may be present in 4 to 6 percent of cases, usually as the result of inadequate studies. The invasive nature of the study, its lack of universal availability, and the definable morbidity (1 to 5 percent) and mortality (0.1 to 0.5 percent) make angiography a less attractive diagnostic test if less invasive alternatives can answer the question. Patients with pulmonary hypertension are at particular risk for complications, yet these patients are the very ones most likely to have nondiagnostic ventilation/perfusion (V/Q) scans. Pulmonary angiography remains abnormal for at least several days to 1 week following a pulmonary embolus. Accordingly, patients in whom clinical suspicion is strong and noninvasive testing is indeterminate may be anticoagulated (unless contraindications exist) until pulmonary angiography can be accomplished.

Currently, scintigraphic V/Q scanning of the lungs is the single most important diagnostic modality in the evaluation of suspected pulmonary embolus. However, few tests in medicine are as subject to inappropriate ordering and misinterpretation. The V/Q scan should be utilized as a screening test, which in some instances is diagnostic of pulmonary embolus or excludes the diagnosis. In some settings, however, it adds little to clinical assessment. The technique includes a perfusion scan, which in a normal, supine patient will have a uniform distribution of blood flow and thus radioisotope emission throughout both lungs. Any impairment of blood flow leading to a defect of 2 to 3 cm is detectable. A normal perfusion lung scan reliably excludes the diagnosis of clinically significant PE and makes further testing for PE unnecessary. An abnormal perfusion scan is not specific for PE. Atelectasis, consolidation, vasoconstriction, and other abnormalities can cause asymmetric perfusion. For this reason a ventilation scan is also performed in most situations. Patients in whom the perfusion scan is highly suggestive of PE or shows low probability or no defects obtain little increase in diagnostic accuracy with the addition of a ventilation scan. As a rule, pulmonary embolism is more likely when an area of obstructed perfusion has normal ventilation. However, this mismatch may be absent if there is concomitant decreased ventilation due to atelectasis, bronchospasm, splinting, infiltrates, effusions, or other confounding factors that may accompany pulmonary embolus.

The V/Q scan should be interpreted in a defined manner, using standard criteria that recognize perfusion defects or segmental areas of lung where perfusion is decreased relative to ventilation. V/Q scans may be categorized as high, intermediate, or low probability of pulmonary embolus or normal.

The V/Q scan must be interpreted in light of the clinical condition of each patient. The chest radiograph should be utilized to assist in its interpretation. Much of the controversy surrounding the interpretation and clinical application of the V/Q scan has been resolved following the 1990 publication of the Prospective Investigation of Pulmonary Embolism Diagnosis (PIOPED) trial, a multicenter prospective study. This study included 887 patients who were entered because of suspected PE. Of these, 252 had PE either angiographically proven or determined by an outcome classification committee. In this study patients were stratified into three categories according to their clinical likelihood of having a PE: 100 to 80 percent, 79 to 20 percent, and 19 to 0 percent likelihood. This was an effective application of Bayes theorem, which states that the probability that a positive or negative test is a "true" positive or negative is a function not only of the sensitivity and specificity of the test but also of the pretest probability that the patient has the disease. When clinicians thought the patient had a 100 to 80 percent chance of having a PE and the V/Q scan was high probability, 96 percent of the corresponding pulmonary angiograms were positive. Alternatively, if the physician's pretest probability of a PE was low (19 to 0 percent) and the V/Q scan was high probability, only 56 percent of those patients had a PE at angiogram. Parallel findings occurred for all categories. Thus the V/Q result should be taken as a diagnostic end point only when a normal scan is obtained in a patient with low prior clinical suspicion for PE or when a high-probability scan occurs in a patient with a high pretest clinical suspicion. Other studies agree with these conclusions. Despite multiple studies that attempted to show that a low-probability scan could safely be used to withhold further therapy for patients with suspected PE, it is clear that this is an inadequate approach if the physician has a significant clinical suspicion of PE.

Multiple other tests have been applied to patients suspected of having pulmonary embolism, including digital subtraction angiography, echocardiography, nuclear magnetic resonance, fiberoptic angioscopy, capnography, and radiolabeled monoclonal antibodies to thrombus. These must be considered to be developmental at best and not yet generally valuable in the diagnostic evaluation of PE.

An alternative approach to pulmonary angiography for the patient with significant clinical suspicion for PE and a V/Q lung scan that does not effectively clarify the clinical situation is to do tests looking for DVT. This approach could be used, for example, in patients with chronic obstructive pulmonary disease, in whom V/Q scan results are less reliable, and who are frequently not good candidates for pulmonary angiography. Most frequently PE is a complication of lower extremity deep venous thrombophlebitis, even though DVT is generally not clinically obvious in patients suspected of having PE. Except under unusual circumstances, the treatment of DVT parallels the treatment of PE, so that it is rarely necessary to precisely confirm the presence of PE if DVT is shown to be present. Unfortunately, the frequency of negative lower-extremity venograms in patients with pulmonary embolism proven by pulmonary angiography is about 30 percent, suggesting that a substantial number of thrombi either embolize essentially in total, are unrecognized at venography, or come from other sources. At any rate, negative lower-extremity venous vascular studies cannot reliably eliminate the possibility of PE, but positive tests are very suggestive.

Venography remains the gold standard for the diagnosis of DVT but has been supplanted by multiple other less invasive tests having similar validity, especially for proximal venous clot, which yields the highest risk for embolization. Duplex ultrasonography (Doppler flow studies with real-time ultrasound imaging), especially when combined with color flow technology, yields a sensitivity of 93 percent with 98 percent specificity for proximal DVT, with lesser efficacy for distal clot. Impedance plethysmography, which detects changes in limb volume due to temporary venous occlusion by an array of cuffs on the extremity, has similar sensitivity (93 percent) and specificity (94 percent) for proximal DVT but is also insensitive for distal clot. Phleborheography, radiolabeled plasmin scanning, and other techniques have high sensitivity and specificity in the rapid diagnosis of DVT but are quite variable in their institutional availability and reliability. Diagnosis of DVT by any technique in the setting of suspected pulmonary embolism is an indication to begin appropriate therapy.

## Musculoskeletal Causes

Chest wall pain is a common cause of chest pain among emergency department patients. It is characterized by sharp pain made worse by movement of the chest wall. Tenderness to palpation that precisely reproduces the pain of the patient's complaint is the rule. In cases of intercostal muscle strain a history of antecedent trauma or coughing is often present. In cases of costochondritis no such history is present. Tenderness localized to specific costochondral junctions suggests the diagnosis. Chest wall tenderness may be present in patients suffering from ischemic heart disease. This finding must be interpreted with all the other clinical features of the case, rather than in isolation. Chest wall pain is generally responsive to nonsteroidal anti-inflammatory agents.

## Gastrointestinal Causes

Various gastrointestinal syndromes may present as epigastric and/or lower chest discomfort (see Table 24-1). Dyspepsia syndromes and those resulting in gastroesophageal reflux cause pain described as burning or gnawing. Often the pain radiates towards the throat, and it may be associated with an acid or foul taste in the mouth and eructation. Tenderness to palpation in the epigastric or upper quadrants suggests a gastrointestinal etiology. Sometimes indigestion is just indigestion. Unfortunately, as has been discussed at length, the pain of AMI may mimic these benign syndromes.

There are no data to support the practice of a therapeutic intervention as diagnostic challenge. The episodic nature of the pain in many of these syndromes, the very strong potential for placebo effect, and the substantial impact of "negative tests" and reassurance in alleviating anxiety and pain cannot be underestimated. There are no data to prove that chest discomfort relieved by antacids is more likely to be noncardiac in origin than pain that is not so relieved. Conversely, nitroglycerin is a smooth muscle dilator that may afford relief in cases of lower esophageal spasm or biliary colic. As a rule, diagnostic decisions should not be influenced by response to a therapeutic trial. When the history, physical examination, and diagnostic workup point to a gastrointestinal etiology of the pain, the patient may be treated with antacids and H-2 blockers, with follow-up referral to an internist or gastroenterologist.

## CONCLUSIONS

Chest discomfort may be the predominant complaint in a large number of diverse syndromes seen by emergency physicians. Differentiating patients with benign syndromes from those with potentially life-threatening conditions remains a most challenging and important responsibility. Emergency physicians must be diligent in ruling out the most dangerous syndromes before assigning a benign etiology to patients at risk.

## BIBLIOGRAPHY

Eagle KA, De Sanctis RW: Diseases of the aorta, in Braunwald E (ed.) *Heart Disease,* 4th ed., Philadelphia: Saunders, 1992, p 1528.

Hackshaw BT. Excluding heart disease in the patient with chest pain. *Am J Med* 1992;(5A):46S–51S.

PIOPED investigators: Value of the ventilation perfusion scan in acute pulmonary embolus. *JAMA* 1990;263(20):2753.

Richter JE: Overview of diagnostic testing for chest pain of unknown origin. *Am J Med* 1992:(5A):41S–45S.

Rouan GW, Lee TH, Cook EF: Clinical characteristics and outcome of acute myocardial infarction in patients with initially normal or nonspecific electrocardiograms: a report from the Multicenter Chest Pain Study. *Cardiol* 1989;64:1087.

Stein PD, Terrin ML, Hales CA: Clinical laboratory, roentgenographic, and electrocardiographic findings in patients with acute pulmonary embolism and no pre-existing cardiac or pulmonary disease. *Chest* 1991;100:598.

# 25

# DYSPNEA, HYPOXIA, AND HYPERCAPNEA

## David Plummer

## DYSPNEA

*Dyspnea* is a subjective feeling of difficult, labored, or uncomfortable breathing. This common emergency department complaint is often described as "shortness of breath," "breathlessness," "not getting air all the way down," and a variety of other phrases. Dyspnea does not result from a single pathophysiologic mechanism and may result from many disorders. Two thirds of patients presenting with dyspnea have either a cardiac or pulmonary disorder. The emergency physi-

cian can usually distinguish these on the basis of history, physical examination, and occasionally, laboratory tests.

Dyspnea must be distinguished from a number of other signs and symptoms. *Tachypnea* is defined as rapid breathing. It may or may not be associated with dyspnea, and dyspnea does not require tachypnea. *Orthopnea* is dyspnea in the recumbent position. This most often results from left ventricle failure and may be associated with diaphragmatic paralysis or chronic obstructive pulmonary disease (COPD). *Paroxysmal nocturnal dyspnea* is orthopnea that awakens the patient from sleep. *Trepopnea* is dyspnea associated with only one of several recumbent positions. Trepopnea can occur with unilateral, diaphragmatic paralysis, ball valve airway obstruction, or after surgical pneumonectomy. *Platypnea* is the opposite of orthopnea and is dyspnea in the upright position. Platypnea results from the loss of abdominal wall muscular tone, and in rare cases, of right to left intracardiac shunting, such as a patent foramen ovale. *Hyperpnea* is essentially hyperventilation and is defined as a minute ventilation in excess of metabolic demand. Hyperpnea may not be associated with dyspnea, and dyspnea does not require an increased minute ventilation.

### Pathophysiology

Dyspnea has many causes (Table 25-1). Specifically, dyspnea does not require hypoxia, and hypoxic patients may not have dyspnea.

**Table 25-1.** Disorders Causing Dyspnea

| | |
|---|---|
| **Airway** | **Vascular** |
| Airway mass | Pulmonary embolism |
| Foreign body | Air embolism |
| Angioedema | Fat embolism |
| Airway stenosis | Amniotic embolism |
| Bronchiectasis | Pulmonary hypertension |
| Tracheomalacia | Veno-occlusive disease |
| **Cardiac** | Sickle cell disease |
| Left ventricular failure | Vasculitis |
| Myocardial ischemia | Arteriovenous fistula |
| Pericarditis | **Neuromuscular** |
| Pericardial tamponade | Cerebrovascular accident |
| Arrhythmia | Phrenic nerve paralysis |
| Myocarditis | Guillain-Barré |
| Cardiomyopathy | Tick paralysis |
| Intracardiac shunt | Botulism |
| Left ventricular outflow | Neuropathy |
| obstruction | **Miscellaneous** |
| Valvular disorder | Anemia |
| Hypertensive crisis | Metabolic acidosis |
| **Lung parenchymal** | Shock |
| Asthma | Low cardiac output states |
| Chronic obstructive pulmonary | Hypoxia |
| disease | Carbon monoxide poisoning |
| Pneumonia | Methemoglobinemia |
| Pneumonitis | Deconditioning |
| Pulmonary edema | Fever |
| Pulmonary contusion | Hyperthyroidism |
| Atelectasis | Hypothyroidism |
| Alveolitis | Gastroesophageal reflux |
| Pulmonary fibrosis | Psychogenic hyperventilation |
| Acute respiratory distress | |
| syndrome | |
| Sarcoidosis | |
| **Pleural and chest wall** | |
| Pneumothorax | |
| Pulmonary effusion | |
| Pleural adhesions | |
| Chest wall injury | |
| Abdominal distention | |
| Kyphoscoliosis | |
| Pectus excavatum | |
| Pregnancy | |

Dyspnea is a complex sensation that involves both objective and subjective elements. Because of its mainly subjective component, the presence or degree of dyspnea is difficult to measure. The vagus nerve supplies both efferent and afferent components to the cardiopulmonary system and provides the pathway for the majority of neurologic input that results in dyspnea. This input originates from a number of peripheral receptors that act either alone or in concert, resulting in dyspnea. Intrapulmonary parenchymal receptors, such as the pulmonary stretch and J receptors, may be stimulated by interstitial edema or change in pulmonary compliance. Airway irritant receptors are stimulated by a variety of nonspecific stimuli that may result in dyspnea. Muscle spindle receptors found in the muscles of respiration, as well as the associated Golgi tendon organ receptors, also contribute to dyspnea when stimulated. Chemoreceptors, found throughout the body, are the best studied but not necessarily the most important in the origin of dyspnea. Carotid body chemoreceptors account for hypoxic drive and act in concert with aortic body chemoreceptors. Additionally, central medullary chemoreceptors (primarily regulating hypercapnic respiratory drive) also contribute. Peripheral vascular receptors, including the right atrial and left atrial mechanoreceptor, and the pulmonary artery baroreceptor contribute to dyspnea in a poorly defined way. Input from any or all of these receptors is integrated in a complex manner in the central nervous system (CNS) at both the subcortical and cortical level. Most authors believe that dyspnea occurs when feedback from these peripheral receptors indicate that the *work of breathing is greater than would be expected by the patient's level of activity.*

## Evaluation and Clinical Features

The initial assessment of any patient with dyspnea should be directed toward identifying imminent respiratory failure on physical examination. The physician should specifically evaluate for tachypnea, tachycardia, stridor, and use of the accessory respiratory muscles, including the sternocleidomastoid, sternoclavicular, and intercostals. Other signs and symptoms of imminent respiratory failure are inability to speak due to the breathlessness and agitation or lethargy due to hypoxia. In patients with any of the above signs or symptoms, airway control and mechanical ventilation must be anticipated, and oxygen should be administered. Lesser degrees of dyspnea allow for a more detailed medical history, and possibly, laboratory tests.

A detailed medical history often identifies the primary process resulting in dyspnea. Patients can often specifically and accurately diagnose themselves. The medical history should include recent infectious and environmental exposures and the medication history.

A number of ancillary laboratory tests aid in determining the severity and specific cause of dyspnea. Pulse oximetry is a rapid but insensitive screen for disorders of gas exchange and may be normal in acute dyspnea. Arterial blood gas analysis is more sensitive, but may also be normal in the acute dyspnea and cannot evaluate the work of breathing. A chest x-ray may indicate the general category of primary disease (infiltrate, effusion, pneumothorax) but also may be normal. Spirometry with and without bronchodilator therapy can diagnose and treat dyspnea resulting from obstructive pulmonary disease. Other screening tests include electrocardiogram and hemoglobin. Uncommonly, the specific process resulting in dyspnea cannot be identified by the history, physical, and simple ancillary tests and requires specialized testing including cardiac stress testing, echocardiography, formal pulmonary function testing, computed tomography scan of the chest, or pulmonary biopsy.

## Treatment

Just as there is no single specific cause of dyspnea there is no single specific treatment. In severe dyspnea, initial treatment is maintaining the airway and oxygenation. The approach establishing the airway is described in Chapter 11. Provide supplemental oxygen with a goal of maintaining a $P_{O_2}$ of over 60 mm Hg. This can be lowered to 50 mm Hg in patients with severe COPD.

## HYPOXIA

*Hypoxia* is defined as an insufficient delivery of oxygen to the tissues. The amount of oxygen available to the tissues is a function of the arterial oxygen content and blood flow to the tissues. The arterial oxygen content, in turn, is defined as $Ca_{O_2} = Hb \times Sa_{O_2} \times 1.29$. Tissue hypoxia occurs in states of low cardiac output, low hemoglobin, or low $Sa_{O_2}$. The percent oxygen saturation of arterial hemoglobin is, in turn, dependent on the $P_{O_2}$ as described by the oxygen hemoglobin dissociation curve. *Hypoxemia* is defined as an abnormally low arterial oxygen tension. This is often used clinically to assess for hypoxia. *Relative hypoxemia* is the term used when the arterial oxygen tension is lower than expected for a given level of supplemental oxygen. This can be assessed by calculating the arterial-alveolar oxygen difference $P(A - a)_{O_2}$, where $PA_{O_2} = 145 - Pa_{CO_2}$. A normal $P(A - a)_{O_2}$ is under 20 in young healthy patients and increases with age. Although the terms hypoxia and hypoxemia are generally used interchangeably, one can occur without the other. For example, in states of low $P_{O_2}$ (hypoxemia) with concomitant polycythemia the patient may have no tissue hypoxia. Alternatively, very anemic patients may suffer tissue hypoxia despite a normal $P_{O_2}$. Hypoxemia is arbitrarily defined as a $P_{O_2}$ of less than 60 mm Hg. Note that patients with hypoxemia may not necessarily present with dyspnea, and patients with dyspnea may not have hypoxemia.

## Pathophysiology

Hypoxemia results from any combination of five distinct mechanisms.

1. *Hypoventilation*—Hypoventilation may result in hypoxemia and may be due to a wide variety of disorders. Irrespective of specific etiology, hypoxemia resulting from hypoventilation is always associated with an increased $P_{CO_2}$ and the $P(A - a)_{O_2}$ is normal.
2. *Right to left shunt*—Right to left shunting occurs when blood enters the systemic arteries without traversing ventilated lung. There is always some right to left shunting because of the direct left ventricular return of deoxygenated blood from both the coronary veins and bronchial arteries. Increased right to left shunt occurs in a variety of conditions including pulmonary consolidation, pulmonary atelectasis, and vascular malformations. Irrespective of the specific cause of the right to left shunt, there is always an increase in the $P(A - a)_{O_2}$. Additionally, right to left shunting does not increase $PA_{CO_2}$ and in fact patients suffering right to left shunt may present with an abnormally low $P_{CO_2}$. A hallmark of significant right to left shunting is its observed response to supplemental oxygen. Although a small amount of improvement is observed with supplemental oxygen, hypoxemia is never fully eliminated because of the continuing return of nonoxygenated blood to the system of circulation.
3. *Ventilation/perfusion mismatch*—Ideal pulmonary gas exchange depends on a balance of ventilation and perfusion. Any abnormality resulting in a regional alteration of either ventilation or perfusion can adversely affect pulmonary gas exchange, resulting in hypoxemia. A wide variety of etiologies may result in these regional impairments including pulmonary emboli, pneumonia, asthma, COPD, and even extrinsic vascular compression. Irrespective of the specific etiology, hypoxemia from ventilation/perfusion mismatch is associated with an increased $P(A - a)_{O_2}$ gradient and improves with supplemental oxygenation.
4. *Diffusion impairment*—Pulmonary gas exchange also depends on diffusion across the alveolar blood barrier. Any condition that influences this diffusion (acute respiratory distress syndrome, pneu-

monia, pulmonary edema) may result in hypoxemia. Irrespective of the specific cause of the diffusion impairment, the $P(A - a)_{O_2}$ is increased and hypoxemia improves with supplemental oxygenation.

5. *Low inspired oxygen*—Decreased ambient oxygen pressure results in hypoxemia. This is most commonly seen at high altitude or in nonobstructive asphyxia. The $P(A - a)_{O_2}$ is normal, and hypoxemia improves with supplemental oxygen.

There are three distinct acute compensatory mechanisms for hypoxemia. Initally, minute ventilation increases. Next, pulmonary arterial vasoconstriction decreases perfusion to hypoxic alveoli. This balances ventilation/perfusion but may also cause acute right heart failure and is ineffective with diffuse hypoxia. Lastly, sympathetic tone increases. This increases oxygen delivery by increasing cardiac output and is most easily observed as an increase in heart rate. Chronic compensatory mechanisms include an increased red cell mass and decreased tissue oxygen demands. These compensatory mechanisms appear to be activated at different levels of hypoxemia for different individuals. However, the acute compensatory mechanisms are always activated when $P_{AO_2}$ falls to less than 60 mmHg, and compensatory mechanisms fail when $P_{O_2}$ falls below 20 mmHg.

## Clinical Features

The signs and symptoms of hypoxemia are nonspecific. CNS manifestations include agitation, headache, somnolence, coma, and seizures. At $P_{ACO_2}$ values of less than 20, there is a central depression of respiratory drive. Cyanosis is not a sensitive or specific indicator of hypoxemia. Patients with chronic compensatory mechanisms may display polycythemia or alterations in body habitus (pulmonary cachexia).

## Diagnosis and Treatment

The diagnosis of arterial hypoxemia requires objective measurement. Because hypoxemia is defined as a $P_{O_2}$ of less than 60 mmHg, formal diagnosis requires arterial blood gas analysis. Pulse oximetry is useful in screening for gross alterations in $P_{AO_2}$. Although decreased oxygen saturation readings accurately predict significant hypoxemia, normal oxygen saturation readings do not rule out hypoxemia.

Irrespective of the specific cause of hypoxemia, the initial approach remains the same. The physician must ensure a patent airway and provide supplemental oxygenation with a goal of maintaining a $P_{AO_2}$ of greater than 60 mmHg.

## HYPERCAPNIA

*Hypercapnia* is arbitrarily defined as a $P_{ACO_2}$ greater than 45 mmHg. Hypercapnia is exclusively due to alveolar hypoventilation. This in turn can be due to a variety of disorders including rapid shallow breathing, small tidal volumes, underventilation of the lung, or reduced respiratory drive. It is almost never due to intrinsic lung disease, and it is never due to increased $CO_2$ production.

## Clinical Features

The signs and symptoms of hypercapnia depend on the absolute value of $P_{CO_2}$ and its current rate of change. Acute elevations result in increased intracranial pressure and patients may complain of headache, confusion, or lethargy. When severe, seizures and coma can result. Extreme hypercapnia can result in cardiovascular collapse, but this is usually only seen in acute rises of $P_{ACO_2}$ to over 100 mmHg. Chronic hypercapnia, even over 80 mmHg may be well tolerated.

## Diagnosis and Treatment

Diagnosis of hypercapnia requires arterial blood gas analysis. Pulse oximetry can be normal. Treatment of hypercapnia requires maneuvers to increase minute ventilation. This involves ensuring a patent airway and may require mechanical ventilation.

## Disposition

The disposition of hypercapnic patients depends primarily on the underlying etiology and severity. Patients with hypercapnia that causes CNS abnormality should be hospitalized. For example, asthmatics who present hypercapnic but who improve promptly and fully with bronchodilator therapy can safely be managed as outpatients. Alternatively, patients with COPD who display worsening hypercapnia despite maximal therapy require hospital admission.

## BIBLIOGRAPHY

Davies S, Ingram RP. Functional assessment of the lung and diagnostic techniques. In: *Scientific American Medicine.* New York: March 1993.

Gillespie: Concise review for primary care physicians. *Mayo Clin Proc* 69:657, 1994.

Leatherman J, Ingram RP. Respiratory failure. In: *Scientific American Medicine.* New York: July 1994.

West J. *Pulmonary Pathophysiology—the Essentials.* Baltimore: Williams & Wilkins, 1992.

# 26
# HEMORRHAGIC SHOCK
## Steven C. Dronen
## Patricia L. Lanter

## INTRODUCTION

The first record of successful treatment of hemorrhagic shock is from the early 1800s when James Blundell transfused a woman with life-threatening postpartum hemorrhage. During World War I, W. B. Cannon recognized the importance of controlling blood loss, was the first to associate acidosis and hypothermia with hemorrhage, and advocated treating hemorrhage with alkalotic intravenous fluid. He also was the first to recommend delaying fluid administration until after operative intervention. During World War II, a greater understanding was developed of the fluid shifts that accompany hemorrhage and of the need to resuscitate with both crystalloid and blood. During the Korean and Vietnam conflicts there was greater emphasis on aggressive volume replacement and rapid access to definitive care, principles that have become standards in the treatment of acute hemorrhage. The military antishock trouser garment (MAST) was also introduced as a mechanism to maintain blood pressure prior to operative intervention.

In the early 1970s, principles of hemorrhage resuscitation learned in Vietnam were widely adopted by trauma surgeons and emergency physicians in the treatment of civilian trauma victims, with a marked improvement in their overall level of care. Recently questions have been raised about some of the standard assumptions upon which treatment is based, most notably the principle of rapid early restoration of blood pressure. Recent clinical studies have also questioned the value of interventions such as MAST and aggressive fluid therapy.

## PATHOPHYSIOLOGY

Acute hemorrhage is defined as a rapid blood loss that may accompany a wide variety of medical and surgical conditions. The most common causes of significant hemorrhage include trauma, disorders of the gastrointestinal and reproductive tracts, and vascular disease. A listing is provided in Table 26-1. Hemorrhagic shock occurs when blood loss is of sufficient magnitude to overcome normal physiologic compensatory responses and compromise tissue perfusion and oxygenation.

Acute hemorrhage triggers a series of physiologic responses involving the cardiovascular, respiratory, renal, hematologic, and neuroendocrine systems. The net effect of these responses is an increase in cardiac rate and contractility, a redistribution of blood flow to preserve vital organ function, conservation of water and sodium, and control of blood loss at the site of injury.

One of the very first responses observed in animal studies of acute hemorrhage is a fall in blood pressure that cannot be accounted for simply by the initial reduction in intravascular volume. It is likely that the fall in blood pressure is caused by a sudden reduction in systemic vascular resistance, although the mechanism has not been explained. The fall in blood pressure is sensed by high-pressure baroreceptors in the carotid artery sinus and the aortic arch and low-pressure baroreceptors in the left atrium and pulmonary veins. Stimulation of the baroreceptors causes disinhibition of the medullary vasomotor center, a subsequent decrease in vagal tone, and an increase in the secretion of norepinephrine (NE). Decreased vagal tone increases heart rate and cardiac output. Norepinephrine increases heart rate and myocardial contractility, stimulates renin secretion, and causes intense vasoconstriction, especially of splanchnic and musculoskeletal blood vessels. Between 20 and 30 percent of the circulating blood volume is in the splanchnic bed providing a functional reservoir that can be used to compensate for acute blood loss.

Cardiac output typically falls during hemorrhage despite increases in myocardial rate and contractility, because of the decrease in atrial filling or preload. It is commonly taught that afterload rises during acute hemorrhage in order to maintain blood pressure. There is little evidence to support this claim. It is more likely that early in the course of hemorrhage, total systemic vascular resistance falls or remains at near-normal levels in order to facilitate flow to vital organs. There are, however, increases in regional resistance that cause redistribution of blood flow away from skin, muscle, and gut to favor the brain, heart, and kidneys.

Conservation of sodium and water during hemorrhage is mediated by an increase in the levels of aldosterone and antidiuretic hormone. Stretch receptors in the afferent arterial walls of the juxtaglomerular

**Table 26-1.** Etiologic Classification of Acute Hemorrhage

| **Trauma** | **Reproductive tract** |
|---|---|
| Solid organ injury | Vaginal bleeding |
| Pulmonary parenchymal injury | Malignancies |
| Myocardial laceration/rupture | Miscarriage |
| Vascular injury | Metrorrhagia |
| Retroperitoneal hemorrhage | Retained products of |
|   Pelvic fracture |   conception |
|   Ruptured duodenum | Placenta previa |
|   Ruptured kidney | Ectopic pregnancy |
| Fractures, esp. long bones | Ruptured ovarian cyst |
|   and pelvis | **Vascular** |
| Lacerations, esp. scalp | Aneurysms |
| Epistaxis | Dissections |
| **Gastrointestinal tract** | Arteriovenous malformations |
| Esophageal varices | |
| Ulcer disease | |
| Gastritis/esophagitis | |
| Mallory-Weiss tear | |
| Malignancies | |
| Vascular lesions (arteriovenous mal- | |
|   formations, rare congenital anomalies) | |
| Inflammatory bowel disease | |
| Ischemic bowel disease | |

apparatus (JGA) respond to a drop in blood pressure by stimulating an increase in renin secretion. Renin converts angiotensinogen to angiotensin I, which is then converted in the lung and liver to angiotensin II. The effects of angiotensin II include intense vasoconstriction of arteriolar smooth muscle and stimulation of aldosterone secretion by the adrenal cortex. Aldosterone is also secreted in response to elevation of potassium and adrenal corticotropin hormone (ACTH) levels, both of which occur during acute hemorrhage. Aldosterone increases the reabsorption of sodium and the excretion of potassium in the distal convoluted tubule. Water passively follows sodium and is therefore reabsorbed and conserved. Aldosterone also stimulates the secretion of the hydrogen ion, thus decreasing acidosis.

Osmo- and baroreceptors also regulate the release of arginine vasopressin or antidiuretic hormone (ADH), which is synthesized in the hypothalamus and stored in the posterior pituitary. Release of ADH occurs in response to both a fall in blood pressure and a decrease in sodium concentration. ADH increases the permeability of the renal distal tubule collecting ducts and loop of Henle to NaCl and water, with the net result being fluid and NaCl retention. In higher concentration, ADH is also a vasoconstrictor.

Acute hemorrhage causes local activation of the coagulation system. In response to injury, affected blood vessels contract, and activated platelets rapidly adhere to the edges of the damaged vessels. Platelets release thromboxane $A_2$, which is a potent local vasoconstrictor and further platelet activator. Platelets form an unstable jelly-like plug during the first 20 min after injury. Control of hemorrhage during this period depends upon a regional reduction in flow caused by systemic hypotension and local vasoconstriction. Vessel injury exposes collagen and releases tissue thromboplastin, causing fibrin deposition in the platelet plug and gradual formation of a stable clot. The entire process for complete fibrinous transformation takes approximately 24 h.

The compensatory mechanisms described above are quite effective at maintaining critical organ perfusion even in the face of severe hemorrhage. Animal studies demonstrate complete recovery without intervention in animals bled as much as 40 percent of their estimated blood volumes. However, if the hemorrhage is not controlled, a vicious cycle of increased myocardial work and decreased perfusion eventually develops. Progressive increases in heart rate shorten diastole, with a resultant decrease in myocardial perfusion and oxygenation, as well as cardiac filling and output. The low perfusion state increases acidemia, which in turn decreases myocardial contractility.

Eventually, cardiac output becomes inadequate to maintain cellular oxygen delivery, and characteristic changes occur. The first cellular response to hypoperfusion is an attenuation of the cell membrane and an increase in sodium influx. Adenosine triphosphate (ATP) is utilized to maintain function of the sodium-potassium pump, but during periods of low flow it cannot be regenerated in sufficient quantities through the normal oxygen-dependent pathways. As the supply of oxygen and high-energy substrates diminishes, the cells revert to anaerobic metabolism to generate ATP, resulting in accumulation of lactic acid. As ATP availability decreases, sodium continues to enter the cells, causing progressive swelling, first of the cytoplasm, then the endoplasmic reticulum, and finally the mitochondria. Eventually the cells undergo clumping of mitochondria, loss of membrane integrity, and death.

There appears to be a point of no return for individual cells as well as for the overall organism in shock. Although this point is well defined for the cell, the clinician caring for patients in shock is less able to identify this landmark. It has been suggested that a sudden and substantial decrease in oxygen consumption may be a reliable marker of irreversible shock.

## CLINICAL FEATURES

Factors that affect the clinical presentation of acute hemorrhage include the etiology, duration, and severity of hemorrhage and the patient's age and underlying medical condition. Acute hemorrhage most often accompanies blunt or penetrating trauma and is generally the presumed cause of shock in the trauma patient. Hemorrhage must be differentiated from other causes of shock associated with trauma, including cardiac tamponade (distinguished by elevated central venous pressure), tension pneumothorax (distinguished by unilaterally diminished breath sounds), and spinal cord injury (distinguished by the presence of neurologic deficits, warm skin, and a lower-than-expected pulse rate).

Hemorrhage not associated with trauma may present with a myriad of complaints depending upon the primary organ system involved. Nausea and vomiting; dizziness; syncope; pain in the chest, abdomen, or back; and rectal or vaginal bleeding are some common chief complaints.

The classic clinical features of acute hemorrhage include tachycardia, tachypnea, a narrow pulse pressure, decreased urine output, cool clammy skin, poor capillary refill, low central venous pressure, and, in the later stages, hypotension and altered mentation. Elderly patients and those with preexisting cardiac disease may show more severe signs and symptoms with less blood loss. Medications such as β blockers can mask some of the early signs and symptoms of hemorrhage. On the other hand, young athletic patients can lose considerable amounts of blood before they appear ill. In general, however, there is a somewhat predictable and orderly progression of pathophysiologic events through which the patient passes as organ and cellular perfusion deteriorates and shock develops. Blood loss less than 20 percent of circulating blood volume causes cool clammy skin, delayed capillary refill, and decreased pulse pressure. Tachycardia may be present, and generally the blood pressure is normal, although the pulse pressure may narrow. As hemorrhage progresses, with blood loss of 20 to 40 percent, patients are tachycardic and tachypneic, have postural changes in blood pressure, and may be confused or agitated. If the patient is not resuscitated and the bleeding continues, hypotension and oliguria develop, respirations quicken and become deeper, tachycardia worsens, and the skin becomes mottled. With hemorrhage exceeding 40 percent of the circulating blood volume, patients commonly demonstrate tachycardia, profound hypotension, either tachypnea or irregular respirations, markedly decreased urine output, decreased or absent peripheral pulses, pallor, and lethargy or obtundation. Death from severe hemorrhage is generally marked by respiratory arrest prior to circulatory arrest, due to fatigue of the respiratory musculature and, sometimes, bradyasystolic rhythms.

## MANAGEMENT

There are two goals in the treatment of hemorrhagic shock: control of hemorrhage and maintenance of oxygen delivery. The definitive therapy of hemorrhage is control of the source of bleeding, and generally this requires operative intervention. Thus for most patients with hemodynamic instability secondary to hemorrhage, prompt surgical consultation and intervention are mandatory. Maintenance of tissue oxygen delivery requires, first and foremost, an assessment of the adequacy of oxygenation and ventilation. Items requiring immediate evaluation include airway patency, skin color, depth and rate of respiration, presence of any mechanical obstruction to ventilation, and presence of other factors compromising ventilation including pneumothorax, hemothorax, or flail chest. Supplemental oxygen should be administered to all patients in shock and to most patients who are acutely hemorrhaging. Many patients will require endotracheal intubation and ventilatory support. Respiratory arrest caused by fatigue of the intercostal muscles and diaphragm commonly precedes cardiac arrest as a terminal event in hemorrhagic shock, and therefore it is essential that liberal guidelines for ventilatory support are applied. Tissue oxygenation also requires restoration of circulating blood volume, and it is routine to place at least two large-bore intravenous (IV) lines for infusion of crystalloid and perhaps blood. As the IV

lines are placed, initial blood samples should be drawn for type and cross matching, prothrombin time (PT), partial thromboplastin time (PTT), and a baseline complete blood count (CBC) with platelet count. All women of child-bearing age need a pregnancy test. If the shock is caused by massive gastrointestinal bleeding, liver function tests may also be helpful.

Parameters that should be routinely monitored during resuscitation of acute hemorrhage include vital signs, mentation, skin temperature, capillary refill, pulse oximetry, and urine output. There is a tendency to follow blood pressure quite closely and to gauge the adequacy of therapy by the extent to which blood pressure returns to normal levels. It is important to recognize, however, that blood pressure is an extremely crude index of the state of cellular metabolism. Also, restoration of normotension in the presence of a vascular injury may merely increase the severity of hemorrhage. Central venous pressure monitoring may be of some value in confirming the diagnosis of hypovolemia and judging the response to therapy. Swan-Ganz catheterization is usually not necessary in the acute setting except in elderly patients or those with respiratory or cardiac disease.

There has been much debate in recent years over the extent to which patients should be resuscitated prior to operative intervention, both in the prehospital setting and the emergency department. The concept of field stabilization of trauma victims has become popular despite the fact that blood loss generally cannot be controlled or corrected in the field. Standard prehospital interventions directed at restoring blood pressure, such as application of MAST and infusion of intravenous fluids, are now being subjected to careful scientific investigation.

The MAST became standard prehospital therapy in the late 1970s based on anecdotal reports of efficacy. While there is no doubt that application of the MAST often raises blood pressure, most likely through a rise in systemic vascular resistance, there is no evidence that use of MAST improves outcome. In the presence of shock and chest trauma, MAST use may increase hemorrhage severity and mortality. Thus, enthusiasm for the MAST has begun to wane except for patients with unstable pelvic fractures, for whom it may stabilize the fractures and tamponade retroperitoneal hemorrhage.

There has also been debate over the efficacy of prehospital IV line placement and fluid resuscitation. Proponents of field resuscitation state that skilled paramedics are able to place IV lines with little or no delay in transport. Opponents state that since blood loss cannot be controlled in the field, any delay in definitive treatment is excessive. Clinical studies have shown that the amount of fluid infused en route is usually minimal when compared to the total fluid requirement, and one randomized study of penetrating trauma victims has failed to show any benefit associated with preoperative fluid therapy. It is likely that prehospital fluid therapy does not affect outcome in the vast majority of cases, but it may be valuable given a specific combination of hemorrhage severity and distance from the hospital. Until conclusive data for a particular position can be obtained, it is reasonable to place IV lines once en route to the hospital whenever possible. This practice avoids potentially lethal delays in the field and grants the patients the potential benefits of prehospital fluid therapy.

It should be noted, however, that the benefits of early and aggressive fluid replacement in victims of acute hemorrhage remain unproved whether given in the prehospital setting or the emergency department. Many animal studies have shown that raising the blood pressure with either vasopressors or fluid also worsens mortality, sometimes dramatically. Investigations continue in an attempt to determine the ideal rate and volume of fluid administration as well as the appropriate therapeutic endpoint of resuscitation. At the present time the amount and type of volume expander used depends primarily on the clinical status of the patient and to a lesser extent on individual institutional preference. In most hospitals, isotonic crystalloids (0.9 % NaCl or Ringer's lactate) are the agents of choice for the initial management of acute hemorrhage. Standard therapy of the hemodynamically stable patient is rapid infusion of 20 to 40 mL/kg. If the adult patient continues to show signs of impaired perfusion after a total of 30 mL/kg (roughly 2 L), it is likely that blood loss exceeds 15 percent of the total blood volume. At this point, it is appropriate to begin red blood cell transfusions, particularly if blood loss has not been controlled. If the patient appears to be stable, it is usually possible to wait for fully cross-matched blood, but that decision must be individualized, based on the assessment of ongoing blood loss and the efficiency of the local blood bank. When in doubt, it is advisable to use type-specific blood. Several studies have shown this to be a very safe practice, and delays in providing needed oxygen-carrying capacity are potentially more harmful to the patient. Early blood therapy is particularly important in the elderly and in those with significant respiratory or cardiac disease.

More aggressive therapy is mandated in the hemorrhaging patient exhibiting any degree of hemodynamic instability or signs of end-organ hypoperfusion. These patients almost always require blood transfusions, and it is appropriate to begin type-specific blood early unless there is a prompt and persistent improvement in perfusion with saline solution alone. Type-specific blood is indicated in patients who are profoundly hypotensive on initial presentation, those who remain in shock after crystalloid infusion, and those who demonstrate rapid ongoing hemorrhage. Continued administration of crystalloid without blood may result in profound dilution of the remaining red blood cell mass, platelets, and coagulation factors. It may also disrupt clot formation in the injured vessels. Volume restored at the expense of oxygen-carrying capacity and hemostasis is of questionable therapeutic value.

The moribund patient requires even more prompt restoration of circulating red blood cell mass. In this case, type O blood should be used immediately if it is available. Type O Rh-negative blood should be given to females of child-bearing age. In most other situations type O Rh-positive blood is preferred because of its greater availability. A sample for type and cross match should always be drawn and sent before administration of type O blood.

Clotting abnormalities are commonly noted after massive transfusion (equivalent to one blood volume, or 70 to 80 mL/kg) requiring transfusion of fresh-frozen plasma (FFP). One unit of FFP and six platelet packs are often recommended for every 5 to 10 units of blood transfused. These are general guidelines, however, and transfusion of these agents is based ideally on clinical evidence of impaired hemostasis and frequent monitoring of coagulation parameters. Platelets are indicated in the actively bleeding trauma patient with a platelet count of 50,000 or less. FFP is indicated if the PT is prolonged more than 1.5 times normal (usually >18). When an underlying coagulation disorder is suspected, such as in patients taking coumadin or with evidence of severe liver disease, it may be appropriate to administer FFP without waiting for laboratory confirmation.

Autologous whole blood may be given if the hemorrhage is intrathoracic and the capabilities for autotransfusion exist (see Fig. 26-1). Autotransfusion decreases the risk of transmission of diseases such as AIDS and hepatitis and it also decreases the demand on the blood bank. There has been some discussion concerning autotransfusion in patients with intraabdominal injuries. It can be difficult to determine, especially in the emergency department, if there is fecal contamination of intraabdominal blood. Transfusion of contaminated blood has not been shown to be safe and it may be more prudent to autotransfuse blood from intraabdominal injuries only in the operating suite, after the source of blood has been discovered and the risk of transfusing contaminated blood is known.

Although isotonic saline solution is most commonly used in the initial management of hemorrhagic shock, debate continues over the fluid of choice (crystalloid vs. colloid). Albumin has fallen into disfavor, but purified protein fraction (PPF) and FFP continue to be recommended and used. Central to the issue are the effects of fluid resuscitation on the pulmonary interstitium. Proponents of protein

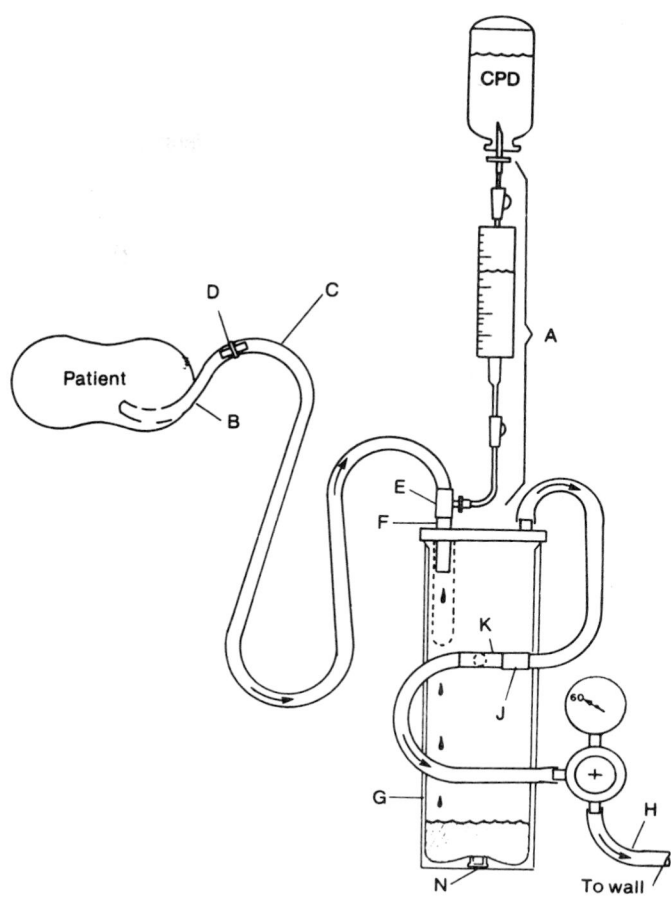

**Fig. 26-1.** Collection apparatus. A, anticoagulant volume control burette; B, chest tube; C, latex drainage tubing; D, male-to-male connector; E, end of drainage tubing with side port; F, inlet port of red liner cap attached to collection canister; G, collection liner bag; H, downstream suction hose; J, liner lid tubing connector; K, canister tee; and N, liner stem with protective cap. (From Roberts JR, Hedges JR(eds): *Clinical Procedures in Emergency Medicine,* 2d ed. Philadelphia, Saunders, 1991, p 412, with permission.)

replacement argue that saline resuscitation of hemorrhage results in a fall in intravascular oncotic pressure and a reversal of the normal gradient favoring intravascular fluid retention. Theoretically, this may lead to pulmonary edema and impaired tissue oxygenation. Colloid administration is advocated because it raises oncotic pressure in the pulmonary capillary bed. This argument ignores the fact that the pulmonary capillary endothelium permits considerable flow of fluids, including plasma proteins, between the capillaries and the interstitium. A fall in intravascular oncotic pressure is compensated for by a fall in pulmonary interstitial oncotic pressure, thereby minimizing changes in the pressure gradient. It appears likely that pulmonary capillary hydrostatic pressure (measured as pulmonary artery wedge pressure) is far more important than pulmonary capillary oncotic pressure in determining the amount of fluid flowing to the interstitium. Maintenance of the wedge pressure below 15 mmHg is probably the most important factor in preventing pulmonary edema. To date, there are few data to show that colloids are harmful, but the inability to convincingly demonstrate beneficial effects in scores of animal and clinical studies suggests that benefits are minimal. Clinicians inclined to use albumin, PPF, or FFP in the resuscitation of hemorrhagic shock should question whether the undocumented benefits of this therapy are worth the substantial increase in cost or, in the case of FFP, the risk of disease transmission.

Alternatives to the use of naturally occurring colloid preparations include synthetic colloid solutions such as hydroxyethyl starch (HES) and dextran 70. The volume-expanding properties of HES are equivalent to those of 5% albumin. These agents differ significantly from albumin, however, in that they remain predominantly in the intravascular space because of their high molecular weight and branched structure. Their plasma-expanding effects are more prolonged than those of albumin, and interstitial edema is not a significant concern.

The combination of 7.5% hypertonic saline and 6% dextran 70 (HSD) is an agent that has shown considerable promise in animal studies of acute hemorrhage. Given in small amounts HSD causes a prompt and long-lasting shift of fluid from the interstitial to the intravascular compartment, and therefore it was initially thought to be ideal for the prehospital resuscitation of hemorrhage. Thus far, clinical studies have not demonstrated an improvement in outcome with HSD, but there may be particular injury patterns (such as combined hypovolemia and head injury) in which a benefit exists.

## BIBLIOGRAPHY

Bellamy RF, Maningas PA, Wenger BA: Current shock models and clinical correlations. *Ann Emerg Med* 15:12, 1392, 1986.

Cayten CG, Murphy JG, Stahl WM: Basic life support versus advanced life support for injured patients with an injury severity score of 10 or more. *J Trauma* 35:460, 1993.

Development Task Force of the College of American Pathologists: Practice parameters for the use of fresh-frozen plasma, cryoprecipitate, and platelets. *JAMA* 271:(10), 777, 1994.

Maddox KL, Bickell WH, Pepe PE, et al: Prospective randomized evaluation of antishock MAST in postraumatic hypotension. *J Trauma* 26:779, 1986.

Martin RR, Bickell WH, Pepe PE, et al: Prospective evaluation of preoperative fluid resuscitation in hypotensive patients with penetrating truncal injury: A preliminary report. *J Trauma* 33:3, 354, 1992.

Peter RM, Hargens AR: Protein vs electrolytes and all of the Starling forces. *Arch Surg* 116:1293, 1981.

Stern SA, Dronen SC, Birrer P, Wang X: Effect of blood pressure on hemorrhage volume and survival in a near-fatal hemorrhage model incorporating a vascular injury. *Ann Emerg Med* 22:155, 1993.

# 27
# SEPTIC SHOCK
## Jon Jui

## INTRODUCTION

Sepsis is a heterogeneous clinical syndrome that can be caused by any class of microorganism. Although gram-negative and gram-positive bacteria account for the majority of sepsis cases, fungi, mycobacteria, rickettsiae, viruses, or protozoans can cause similar presentations. Microbial blood invasion is not essential to the development of sepsis.

## Epidemiology

The incidence of sepsis has continued to rise over the past 3 decades, with approximately 300,000 to 500,000 patients developing sepsis every year in the United States. About one-half of these patients develop shock, with a mortality rate ranging from 20 to 80 percent. In

**Table 27-1.** Definitions

*Infection:* Microbial phenomenon characterized by an inflammatory response to the presence of microorganisms or the invasion of normally sterile host tissue by those organisms.

*Bacteremia:* The presence of viable bacteria in the blood.

*Systemic inflammatory response syndrome* (SIRS): (The systemic inflammatory response to a variety of severe clinical insults. The response is manifested by two or more of the following conditions: (1) temperature >38°C or <36°C, (2) heart rate >90 beats per min, (3) respiratory rate >20 breaths per min or $Pa_{CO_2}$ <32 mmHg, and (4) white blood cell count >12,000/μL, <4,000/μL, or >10% immature (band) forms.

*Sepsis:* The systemic response to infection, manifested by two or more of the following conditions as a result of infection: (1) temperature >38°C or <36°C; (2) heart rate >90 beats per min; (3) respiratory rate >20 breaths per min or $Pa_{CO_2}$ <32 mmHg; and white blood cell count >12,000/μL, <4,000/μL, or >10% immature (band) forms.

*Severe sepsis:* Sepsis associated with organ dysfunction, hypoperfusion, or hypotension. Hypoperfusion and perfusion abnormalities may include, but are not limited to, lactic acidosis, oliguria, or an acute alteration in mental status.

*Septic shock:* Sepsis-induced hypotension despite adequate fluid resuscitation along with the presence of perfusion abnormalities that may include, but are not limited to, lactic acidosis, oliguria, or an acute alteration in mental status. Patients who are receiving inotropic or vasopressor agents may not be hypotensive at the time that perfusion abnormalities are measured.

*Sepsis-induced hypotension:* A systolic blood pressure <90 mmHg or a reduction of ≥40 mmHg from baseline in the absence of other causes for hypotension.

*Multiple organ dysfunction syndrome* (MODS): Presence of altered organ function in an acutely ill patient such that homeostasis cannot be maintained without intervention.

1991, sepsis was the thirteenth leading cause of death in the United States, with approximately two-thirds of the cases occurring in hospitalized patients. Recent clinical studies in patients with bacteremia indicate that gram-positive and gram-negative bacteria are the etiology of the sepsis in 35 to 40 percent and in 55 to 60 percent of the episodes, respectively. Factors that predispose to gram-negative bacteremia include diabetes mellitus, lymphoproliferative diseases, cirrhosis of the liver, burns, invasive procedures or devices, and chemotherapy. Major gram-positive bacteremia risk factors include vascular catheters, indwelling mechanical devices, burns, and intravenous drug injection. Fungemia most often occurs in immunocompromised patients.

## Definitions and Risk Categorization

In 1991, the American College of Chest Physicians and the Society of Critical Care proposed a set of definitions that could be applied to patients with sepsis and its sequelae. These definitions are contained in Table 27-1. The primary goals of this classification were (1) to provide a conceptual and practical framework of the systemic inflammatory response to infection; (2) to improve the ability of clinicians to make early bedside detection of sepsis, thus allowing early therapeutic intervention; and (3) to standardize the definition, which would allow better comparison and analysis of research protocols. Other investigators propose a complementary method of classification of sepsis based primarily on physiologic abnormalities such as the APACHE III acuity system. These investigators found that multivariate analysis using initial APACHE II score, etiology of sepsis (urosepsis or other), and treatment location before intensive care unit admission provided the greatest degree of discrimination of patients by risk of hospital death.

## PATHOGENESIS OF SEPTIC SHOCK

A focus of infection (urinary tract infection, pneumonia, cellulitis, abscess, or indwelling prosthetic device) develops, resulting in either

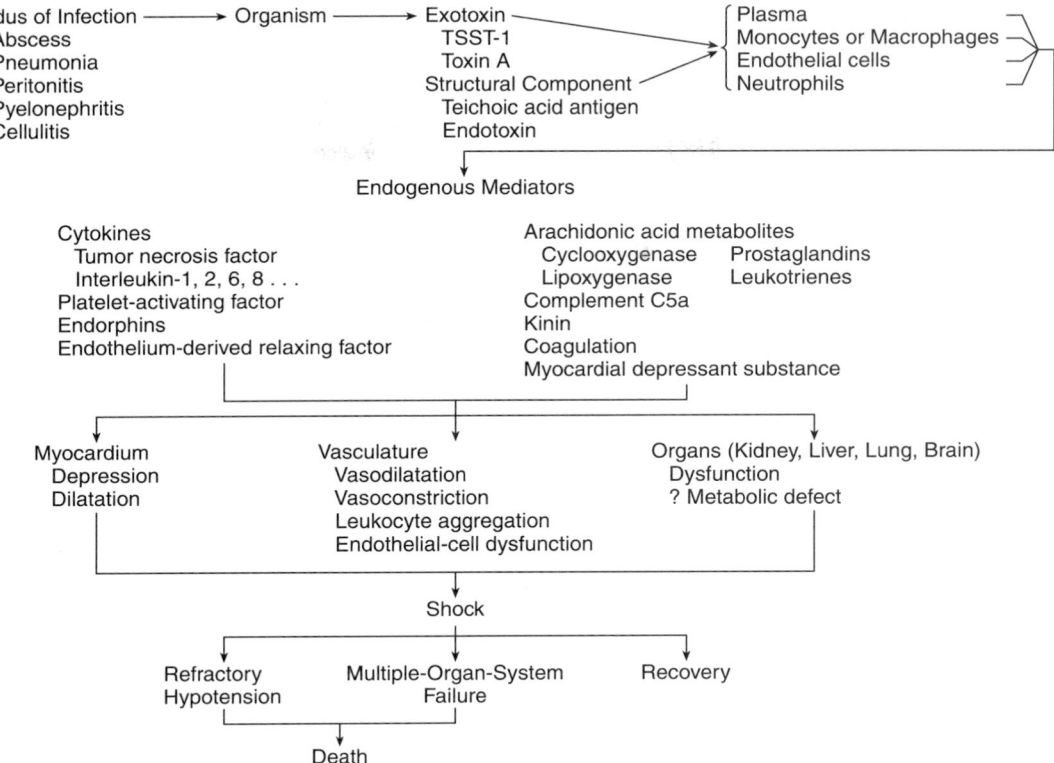

**Fig. 27-1.** Pathogenetic sequence of the events in septic shock. TSST-1, toxic shock syndrome toxin 1; Toxin A, *Pseudomonas aeruginosa* toxin A. (From Parillo JE: Pathogenetic mechanisms of septic shock. *N Engl J Med* 328:1471, 1993, with permission.)

bloodstream invasion or a proliferation of organisms at the infected site (Fig. 27-1). This focus results in release of a large amount of exogenous toxins consisting of endotoxins, exotoxins, and other components of the organism's structural components. The host's reaction to these toxins results in the release of endogenous mediators and other humoral defense mechanisms including complement, kinins, and other coagulation factors. Among the most prominent of the endogenous mediators are the cytokines [tumor necrosis factor (TNF), interleukins], platelet-activating factor (PAF), arachidonic acid metabolites, and myocardial depressant substance. Depression of myocardial function, dilation of the ventricles, and vasodilation of the vasculature ensues. These vascular and myocardial abnormalities combine to result in generalized cardiovascular insufficiency, leading to refractory hypotension and multiple organ system failure, and death.

## Molecular Pathophysiology of Sepsis

There is now compelling evidence that septic shock and its morbid consequences are the direct result of endogenous proteins and phospholipid mediators secreted by the infected individual. Molecular pathophysiology of sepsis can be divided into three phases: induction of cytokine synthesis, cytokine synthesis and secretion, and the cascade phase of sepsis.

The induction of cytokine synthesis involves the interaction of certain microbial molecules, which, when recognized by the host, results in the production of mediators that amplify and transmit the microbial signal to other cells and tissues.

Of currently available models, the pathophysiology of gram-negative infection is best understood. An individual suffering from a gram-negative infection is not only exposed to membrane-bound lipopolysaccharides (LPS) at the site of infection but is also systemically exposed to the free endotoxin on fragments of bacterial outer membrane commonly shed during bacterial growth and replication. LPS binds to LPS-binding protein, forming an LPS–LPS-binding protein complex. This complex is 1000-fold more potent than LPS alone in inducing TNF production by macrophages. The receptor for this complex is known to be the CD14 molecule and is found on monocytes, macrophages, and neutrophils. The peptidoglycan and lipoteichoic acids of gram-positive bacteria, certain polysaccharides, extracellular enzymes, and toxins elicit response in animals similar to those of LPS.

The phase of cytokine synthesis and secretion involves several regulated steps. These steps include transcision (synthesis of messenger RNA from the DNA template), translation of mRNA into protein, posttranslational processing, and secretion of protein. An example is when LPS–LPS-binding protein complex interacts with the CD14, transcription of TNF gene in vitro increases threefold, with corresponding levels of TNF mRNA increasing 100-fold. Biosynthesis and secretion of TNF, however, increase over 10,000-fold; this is primarily due to increased translational efficiency of preformed TNF mRNA as well as efficient translation of newly transcribed TNF mRNA.

The cascade portion of sepsis results from the activation and release of a central mediator [TNF, interleukin 1 (IL-1)], resulting in the secretion of various secondary mediators (IL-1, IL-6, IL-8, PAF, prostaglandins, leukotrienes); activation of neutrophils, the complement system, and vascular endothelial cells; synthesis of acute phase reactants; and onset of coagulopathy. LPS and TNF probably promote intravascular coagulation initially by inducing blood monocytes to express tissue factor, by initiating the release of plasminogen activator inhibitor-1 (PAI-1), and by inhibiting the expression of thrombomodulin and plasminogen activator by vascular endothelial cells. TNF, IL-1, and IL-6 are cytokines that have been detected in increased concentrations in patients with septic shock.

# CLINICAL FEATURES OF SEPTIC SHOCK

Hyperthermia or hypothermia, tachycardia, wide pulse pressure, tachypnea, and mental status changes are early systemic signs of infection and septic shock. Endotoxin, TNF, IL-1, and interferon-$\alpha$ have all been shown to elicit febrile responses in humans. Acute hyperventilation with respiratory alkalosis ($P_{CO_2} \leq 30$ mmHg) is an important clue for the detection of sepsis. The etiologic mechanisms of tachypnea are thought to be due either to the direct effects of endotoxins or secondary to kallikreins, bradykinin, prostaglandins, or complement activation.

The most frequent clinical mental status change in sepsis is mental obtundation. The neurologic findings are nonfocal and range from mild disorientation to confusion, lethargy, agitation, and coma. The pathophysiology is still unknown; an altered state of amino acid metabolism producing a state similar to portosystemic encephalopathy or a decrease in cerebral blood flow with secondary disruption of the blood-brain barrier are proposed mechanisms.

Ophthalmic manifestations of sepsis include retinal hemorrhages, cotton wool spots, and conjunctival petechiae. Endophthalmitis and panophthalmitis may also be present.

In the early stages of septic shock, the vasodilatory mediators predominate and patients present with warm extremities. Cardiac output and stroke volume are usually well maintained. Frequently cardiac output is increased concomitantly with tachycardia. Hemodynamic measurements show that the characteristic pattern of septic shock consists of an initial decrease in left and right ventricular ejection fractions (RVEF, LVEF), with an increase in both end-diastolic and end-systolic volume indices and normal stroke volume occurring within 24 h after the onset of septic shock. The pattern of decreased LVEF and ventricular dilation was found to be most characteristic of survivors during the initial few days of disease. In these survivors, the changes are reversible, and the ventricular function and size return to normal by 7 to 10 days after septic shock onset. Decreases in systemic vascular resistance and cardiac filling pressures are also noted. Patients with septic shock have been shown to have markedly diminished cardiac response to volume administration with only minor increments in both end-diastolic volume index (EDVI) and left ventricular stroke work index (LVSWI). Septic patients without hypotension demonstrated an intermediate response. Prognostic factors that are significant predictors of survival are an initial heart rate of <106 beats per min, a 24-h heart rate of <95 beats per min, or a systemic vascular resistance of >1529 dyne · s · cm$^{-5}$ · m$^2$, and a change over the initial 24-h heart rate with a decrease in heart rate > 18 beats per min or a decrease in cardiac index by >0.5 L/min · m$^2$. These findings also suggest that nonsurvivors have a persistence of the hyperdynamic hemodynamic profile, while the survivors' hemodynamic values return to normal by 24 h.

Myocardial depression is present in early septic shock. Studies show that the perfusion of the coronary arteries in patients with septic shock is equal to or greater than controls. These data strongly argue against the hypothesis that coronary hypoperfusion with secondary ischemic myocardial dysfunction is the cause of the myocardial depression. Significant evidence points towards the existence of one or more active circulating myocardial depressant substances (MDS). Recent molecular filtration experiments suggest that MDS is a moderate size water-soluble molecule weighing at least 10,000 to 30,000 daltons. In vitro experiments revealed that rat myocytes exposed to sera from patients in the acute phase of septic shock had significantly depressed extent and shortening of the myocyte. Furthermore, the degree of depression in vitro correlated with the amount of decrease in LVEF in vivo. This depression was not seen with sera from normal volunteers, critically ill nonseptic patients, patients with reduced ejection fractions due to structural heart disease, or patients during the recovery phase of septic shock. In a subsequent study, MDS-positive

patients had higher pulmonary artery wedge pressures and larger EDVI values than MDS-negative patients. High levels of MDS activity were found in sera from a high percentage of patients with septic shock, particularly those with the most severe cardiovascular insufficiency. Higher mean lactic acidosis and a trend for increased mortality were noted in MDS-positive patients. In vitro studies on purified preparations of IL-1, IL-2, and endotoxin produced no depression of myocyte contraction at concentrations higher than those observed in patients with septic shock. TNF at a dose of 250 units/mL did produced significant depression of myocyte shortening, with a mean decrease of 24 percent.

Sepsis remains the most common condition associated with adult respiratory distress syndrome (ARDS). ARDS is a physiologic syndrome characterized acutely by lung edema resulting from increased alveolar-capillary permeability. Recently, the concept of global microcirculatory injury has won the favor of many investigators. In the setting of trauma and sepsis, ARDS affects capillary beds throughout the body concurrently. When increased microvascular permeability presents itself in the lung, alveolar flooding occurs, causing dyspnea, hypoxemia, and abnormal opacities on chest xray. The appearance of ARDS varies from within minutes to hours of onset of sepsis. Although there are no specific and sensitive markers for ARDS, common physiologic criteria for ARDS include bilateral pulmonary infiltrates, pulmonary capillary wedge pressure (PCWP) <18 mmHG, $Pa_{O_2}/PA_{O_2}$ ratio <0.2, and static compliance <40 mL/cmH$_2$O. Clinically, severe refractory hypoxemia, noncompliant "heavy" lungs, and a chest radiograph showing bilateral pulmonary alveolar infiltrates should suggest the presence of ARDS. The hypoxemia is due to perfusion of the underventilated alveoli; the incidence of right-to-left shunting has been reported as high as 30 to 50 percent in this syndrome. Pathogenic factors implicated in the global microcirculatory injury are endotoxin, TNF-$\alpha$, IL-1, IL-6, IL-8, bacterial permeability-increasing protein, and tissue factor.

Renal manifestations of septic shock include azotemia, oliguria, and an active urinary sediment. Azotemia and oliguria are usually attributed to acute tubular necrosis (ATN). The urine in the setting of ATN contains a large number of tubular epithelial cells and coarse granular pigmented casts. The pathogenesis of the ATN in sepsis is unknown; factors associated with the development of ATN in septic shock include hypotension, dehydration, aminoglycoside administration, and pigmenturia. In patients without septic shock, renal insufficiency may occur because of glomerulonephritis or interstitial nephritis. Glomerular disease in the setting of sepsis has been reported in subacute bacterial endocarditis, pyogenic visceral abscesses, and infections at other sites. Urine sediment of glomerular disease contains red blood cells, casts (red, white, or pigmented), and protein. Renal biopsy usually shows proliferative changes. Immune complex depositions with glomerular deposits of IgG, IgM, C3, and bacterial antigens and antibody to these antigens have been reported in endocarditis and shunt nephritis. Tubulointerstitial disease has been associated with *Streptococcus pneumoniae, Strep. pyogenes, Legionella pneumophila,* salmonellosis, brucellosis, and diphtheria infections. Acute interstitial nephritis secondary to allergic reaction to methicillin has also been reported; eosinophilia and eosinophiluria are usually present in this setting. The onset of renal insufficiency secondary to tubulointerstitial disease may be acute or subacute.

Liver dysfunction is frequently seen in patients with sepsis. The most frequent presentation is cholestatic jaundice. Increases in transaminase, alkaline phosphatase (one to three times normal), and bilirubin concentrations (usually not >10 mg/dL) are frequently noted. The proposed mechanism for bilirubin elevation involves hemolysis of red blood cells and hepatocellular dysfunction due to endotoxin, cytokines, or immune complex disease. Prolonged or severe hypotension may induce acute hepatic injury or ischemic bowel necrosis.

Major blood loss secondary to upper gastrointestinal bleeding involves only a small percentage of patients with sepsis. Within 24 h of developing a severe infection, many patients with severe sepsis will develop painless 1- to 2-mm erosions in the mucosal layer of the stomach and/or duodenum. Proposed mechanisms of these ulcerations include decrease in the blood flow, hypoxia of the mucosal cells, interruption of the gastric mucosal barrier, or release of mucosal lysozyme.

Cutaneous lesions that occur as a result of sepsis can be divided into three categories: (1) direct bacterial involvement of the skin and underlying soft tissues (cellulitis, erysipelas, and fasciitis); (2) lesions that occur as a consequence of sepsis, hypotension, and/or disseminated intravascular coagulation (DIC) (acrocyanosis and necrosis of peripheral tissues); and (3) lesions secondary to infective endocarditis (microemboli and/or immune complex vasculitis).

Sepsis usually produces a neutrophilic leukocytosis with a left shift. These early changes result from demargination and release of less mature granulocytes from the marrow storage pools. One proposed mechanism of the demargination and bone marrow release is the presence of endotoxin or other similar substances and activation by complement (C3a), causing the release of neutrophil-releasing substances. The sustained neutrophilia that accompanies chronic infection is thought to be secondary to colony-stimulating factors. These glycoproteins increase granulocyte production by activating committed stem cells. Infection increases the colony-stimulating factor elaboration by macrophages, lymphocytes, and other tissues. In certain cases of sepsis, leukemoid reactions with leukocyte counts of 50,000 to 100,000 cells/µL have been reported.

Neutropenia, occurring rarely, is associated with an increased mortality. The etiologies of this neutropenia include increased peripheral utilization of neutrophils, damage to neutrophils by bacterial byproducts, or depression of marrow granulocyte production by inflammatory mediators. Both morphologic and functional changes to neutrophils have been reported in sepsis. The most commonly reported morphologic changes include the presence of toxic granulations, Dohle bodies, and vacuolization. Functional changes reported in sepsis include increased phagocytic and cytotoxic activities. Eosinophilia occurring in the presence of sepsis has been attributed to be the effect of margination or migration of these cells from the vascular space, inhibition of bone marrow release, and a decrease in marrow production. Activated complement C5a has been implicated.

Red cell number and morphologic characteristics are not usually affected by sepsis. However, red cell production and survival are decreased during sepsis. Decreased production and survival do not usually cause anemia unless the infection is prolonged. Septic patients generally possess low serum iron concentrations. Sepsis and its intermediaries cause a rapid iron flux into the liver and other parts of the reticuloendothelial cells, with the serum iron concentration decreasing by 50 percent or more within a period of hours. This effect may last for days. An attractive hypothesis is that this represents a host defense mechanism. The addition of iron to normal human serum enhances the growth of organisms. Also, iron in the reticuloendothelial system may be beneficial to the host cells in detoxifying bacterial activity.

Isolated thrombocytopenia is present in over 30 percent of cases of sepsis. Thrombocytopenia may be an early clue to bacteremia and be useful in observing the patient's response to therapy. The proposed mechanisms for the thrombocytopenia include increased platelet turnover, increased endothelial adherence, and increased destruction secondary to immunologic mechanisms. Among the immunologic mechanisms most frequently observed are the development of platelet autoantibody and the formation of immune complex to the Fc receptor.

DIC occurs in fewer than 5 percent of cases. Laboratory studies reveal thrombocytopenia, prolonged prothrombin and thrombin times, elevated fibrin and fibrinogen levels and degradation products, and decreased levels of fibrinogen and factors V and VIII. A number of hypotheses on the mechanisms of DIC have been proposed. Gram-negative infections precipitate DIC more readily than gram-positive infection. Endotoxin may massively activate clotting through interaction with factor XII of the intrinsic pathway, or by causing monocyte/macrophage release of extrinsic pathway procoagulants. Endotoxin may also cause DIC by increasing platelet adhesion and activation. TNF may suppress endothelial cell cofactor activity of the anticoagulant protein C pathway.

Hyperglycemia may suggest the presence of sepsis in diabetic patients. Proposed pathogeneses include increased amounts of catecholamines, increased cortisol and glucagon in the circulation, peripheral insulin resistance, impaired glucose utilization, and decreased insulin secretion. Hypoglycemia, with glucose levels as low as 10 to 20 mg/dL, has been reported but is a relatively uncommon manifestation of sepsis. Bacterial entities associated with hypoglycemia include *Staphylococcus aureus, Strep. pyogenes, Strep. pneumoniae, Listeria monocytogenes, Haemophilus influenzae, Neisseria meningitidis,* and Enterobacteriaceae. The presenting symptoms of hypoglycemia are mental confusion, unresponsiveness, and seizures. The proposed pathogeneses of hypoglycemia include the depletion of hepatitic glycogen and inhibition of gluconeogenesis.

Blood gas analysis performed early in the course of septic shock reveals the presence of respiratory alkalosis. Hypoxemia is often present due to ventilation/perfusion mismatches. The development of metabolic acidosis reflects inadequate tissue perfusion and increased glycolysis of peripheral tissues along with impaired hepatic clearance of lactate and pyruvate. As perfusion worsens and continues, tissue hypoxia generates more lactic acid and metabolic acidosis worsens.

## DIAGNOSIS

Septic shock should be suspected in any individual with a temperature > 38°C or < 36°C and a systolic blood pressure of <90 mmHG with evidence of inadequate organ perfusion. The hypotension should not reverse with acute plasma volume replacement of at least 1 L. Frequently the diagnosis is straightforward, with the patient presenting with hypotension or inadequate perfusion and complaints attributable to a serious infection such as pneumonia, acute pyelonephritis, or an acute abdomen. Other early clinical features of sepsis include fever or hypothermia, mental obtundation, hyperventilation, hot flushed skin, and a widened pulse pressure. In the elderly, very young, or immunocompromised patient, the clinical presentation may be atypical with no fever or localizable source of infection.

The differential diagnosis of septic shock includes the other nonseptic causes of shock. These include cardiogenic, hypovolemic, neurogenic, obstructive (pulmonary embolism, tamponade), and endocrine (adrenal insufficiency, thyroid storm) shock and anaphylaxis.

The history and physical examination with some basic laboratory or radiologic investigations will usually be successful in the initial assessment and location of the presumptive source of sepsis. Particular attention should be focused on infections in the central nervous system, (CNS) the pulmonary and intraabdominal regions, and in the skin and soft tissue, as well as on primary bacteremia.

Acute bacterial meningitis is the CNS infection most commonly associated with shock. Community-acquired meningitis with shock is usually due to *Strep. pneumoniae* or *N. meningitidis.* The majority of patients will present with nuchal rigidity and a depressed level of consciousness. Chest radiographs may show a pneumonia with secondary bacteremia due to *Strep. pneumoniae.* Disseminated meningococcemia may present only with shock without meningismus. Frequently these patients develop a " petechial rash," which is the major clue to the etiology of shock. Brain abscesses, subdural or epidural empyemas, and viral CNS infections are seldom associated with shock on the initial presentation. Shock is also unusual in neurosurgical patients with *Staph. aureus* or enteric gram-negative meningitis secondary to neurosurgical procedure or skull fracture.

The major pulmonary entity commonly leading to septic shock is acute bacterial pneumonia. The most frequent organisms are *Strep. pneumoniae, Staph. aureus,* gram-negative bacilli, and *L. pneumophila.* The physical examination and chest radiograph almost always suggest the presence of pneumonia.

Mediastinitis secondary to perforation is rare. Diagnosis of esophageal perforation is suggested by chest pain presenting in a patient with an episode of vomiting or swallowing, history of swallowing sharp or corrosive objects, or esophageal dilation. Chest radiograph may show mediastinal air; the diagnosis can usually be established by contrast esophagram.

Intraabdominal processes are the source of infection leading to septic shock in the largest proportion of patients. Acute surgical abdomen secondary to perforation of the bowel with fecal peritonitis and mesenteric ischemia are the most common clinical entities involving the bowel. Acute pancreatitis with or without infection can result in a presentation identical to septic shock. Suppurative cholangitis and empyema of the gallbladder are the primary considerations for the biliary tree.

Diagnostic imaging studies may be of significant benefit in these settings. Upright and flat plate abdominal views are useful radiologic studies for the detection of free air associated with perforation. Abdominal ultrasound is the initial procedure of choice if a biliary source of septic shock is suspected. CT of the abdomen is the imaging test of choice for pancreatic sources or other suspected intraabdominal abscesses. Angiography is necessary to diagnose mesenteric ischemia.

In women of childbearing age, septic abortion, tubo-ovarian abscess, and postpartum endometritis/myometritis are the dominating presenting infections leading to septic shock. Acute pyelonephritis from gram-negative enteric bacteria or enterococci can occasionally present with shock. Ureteric obstruction is often present.

The most common skin and soft tissue infection associated with septic shock is cellulitis due to *Staph. aureus* or *Strep. pyogenes.* Soft tissue infections secondary to gram-negative organisms are indistinguishable from those due to primary invasion by streptococci or other bacteria. Shock associated with soft tissue infections is clinically obvious and frequently associated with bacteremia. Shock associated with a generalized erythematous macular rash may represent toxic shock syndrome. Necrotizing soft tissue infections are suspect in infections in immunocompromised patients or in patients with a history of poor vascular circulation. Populations at risk for necrotizing infections are diabetics and individuals with peripheral vascular disease and poor circulation on physical examination.

Individuals without an obvious source of septic shock may have a primary bacteremia or endocarditis or noninfectious cause. The most prevalent etiologies of primary bacteremias in outpatients are *Staph. aureus, Strep. pneumoniae,* and *N. meningitidis.* Encapsulated species such as *Salmonella* or *H. influenzae* are important pathogens in individuals who are asplenic. *Pseudomonas aeruginosa* and other gram-negative bacteria are occasionally etiologies of bacteremia and endocarditis in intravenous drug users.

## Investigation

There is no reliable laboratory test for the diagnosis of septic shock. The physical examination is the foundation of investigation. Basic laboratory tests should include a complete blood count, prothrombin time, partial thromboplastin time, serum electrolytes (including magnesium, calcium, serum glucose, and phosphate), liver function tests (bilirubin, alkaline phosphate, and ALT), renal function tests (blood urea nitrogen and creatinine), arterial blood gas analysis, and urinalysis. A chest radiograph should also be a part of the basic examina-

tion. Flat and upright abdominal films are helpful in patients with a potential abdominal source and should be considered in every patient except individuals with a completely benign abdomen or an obvious alternative source. Any patient with a clinical presentation compatible with a CNS source of infection should receive a cerebrospinal fluid examination. This should be performed without delay in the emergency department. In individuals with papilledema, focal neurologic deficits, or with potential for brain abscess or epidural or subdural empyema, the lumbar puncture should be deferred until an imaging study is performed. However, if meningitis is an important consideration, empiric antimicrobial therapy should be initiated immediately.

Bacterial cultures of blood and urine should be obtained from all septic patients. At least two separate sets of blood cultures from different venipuncture sites should be obtained. Gram stain and culture of secretions from any potential site of infection should be performed. A Gram stain or other means of rapid identification of microbial etiologies is generally the only immediately available test useful in selection of antimicrobial therapy.

## THERAPY

### Initial Resuscitation

#### Fluid Replacement

Immediate attention to stabilization of the cardiovascular and respiratory systems is the priority in the management of a patient in septic shock. Immediate assessment of oxygenation and ventilation status is the first priority in the management. Oxygen by mask and consideration for endotracheal intubation should be performed immediately if the patient's airway is not secure or if respirations are inadequate. In addition, patients with hypotension not responding acutely to rapid fluid resuscitation should be intubated to avoid respiratory arrest from fatigue of the respiratory muscles due to inadequate perfusion of these muscles.

Correction or stabilization of hypotension and inadequate perfusion is the second goal of resuscitation. Rapid fluid replacement at a rate of 0.5 L (20 ml/kg in pediatrics) of normal saline or crystalloid should be administered every 5 to 10 min as needed until perfusion has been restored or clinical signs of volume overload develop; it is not unusual for the patient to require 4 to 6 L or more of crystalloid in the initial phase of resuscitation. Stabilization of the patient's mentation, blood pressure, respiration, pulse rate, skin perfusion, and central venous pressure and a urine output greater than 30 mL/h (1 mL/kg per hour in pediatric patients) are useful clinical parameters helpful in monitoring the response to these interventions. If no response to the fluid infusion is noted after 3 to 4 L of fluid or if there are signs of fluid overload (elevated central venous pressure or pulmonary edema), an infusion of dopamine is added. A PCWP of 15 to 18 mmHg with marked increases of the PCWP with additional fluids is an indication for dopamine. Often, the dose of dopamine required is 5 to 20 μg/kg per min, resulting in both β-adrenergic inotropic and α-adrenergic vasopressor activity. If the patient is still unresponsive-above a rate of 20 μg/kg per min of dopamine infusion, norepinephrine should be started to keep the mean blood pressure at least 60 mmHg. Recent data demonstrate that norepinephrine can reverse septic shock in patients unresponsive to volume replacement and dopamine. Once the blood pressure and perfusion have been stabilized by norepinephrine, the lowest dosage that maintains blood presure should be utilized to minimize the complications of vasoconstriction. Data from the canine model have suggested that the use of low-dose dopamine (1 to 4 μg/kg per min) in patients on norepinephrine increases renal blood flow and reduces renal vascular resistance. In one series, the survival rate of the norepinephrine group approached 40 percent. Vasodilators are rarely used in the emergency department but have been used in the intensive care unit in situations of severe myocardial depression, increased system vascular resistance, and adequate blood pressure. The optimal hematocrit level to be maintained is unknown; however, levels between 0.30 and 0.35 percent have been suggested.

## Empiric Antimicrobial Therapy

All patients with septic shock should receive empiric antimicrobial therapy as soon as possible. Whenever possible, samples of blood or fluids from potential sites of infection should be obtained before the initiation of antimicrobial therapy. Selection of antibiotics should be based upon the adequate coverage of all potential pathogens of the potential infection sites as well as the anticipated antimicrobial susceptibility patterns of the bacterial isolate(s).

Empiric therapy should be effective against gram-positive organisms (streptococci and staphylococci) and gram-negative bacteria. The route of administration should be intravenous in the maximum doses allowed. In adult patients without an obvious source of infection, a third-generation cephalosporin *or an antipseudomonal beta-lactamase susceptible penicillin plus* an antipseudomonal aminoglycoside (tobramycin, gentamicin, amikacin) *or imipenem alone* is an acceptable combination. In patients with a high probability of a gram-positive etiology (history of illicit drug abuse), the addition of a nafcillin or vancomycin should be added to the regime. If an anaerobic source is suspect (intraabdominal, biliary, or female genital tract location; necrotizing cellulitis, aspiration pneumonia, odontogenic infection, or an anaerobic soft tissue infection), metro-nidazole or clindamycin should be added to the regime. In patients with potential for *Legionella* species infection, the addition of eryth-romycin to the regime is recommended. In immunocompromised patients, some authorities recommend the combination of vancomycin plus a β lactam (third-generation cephalosporin or antipseudomonal β lactamase–susceptible penicillin) and an aminoglycoside as the initial combination of choice.

For neonates, the usual regime of a combination of ampicillin or extended spectrum penicillin (e.g., ticarcillin plus clavulanic acid) with an aminoglycoside is recommended. For infants 1 to 3 months of age, *H. influenzae, Strep. pneumoniae,* and *N. meningitidis* are the organisms most likely to be encountered. Combined therapy with ampicillin and cefotaxime or ceftriaxone is recommended. For children 3 months of age or older, cefotaxime or ceftriaxone has become the drug of choice.

## Removal of Source of Infection

If a focal source of sepsis is identified, removal of the nidus of infection is mandatory for successful resuscitation. Indwelling intravenous catheters should be removed and replaced. The tip should be sent for quantitative culture. Foley catheters should be replaced if obstructed. Intraabdominal or soft tissue sites of pus requires urgent drainage.

## Initial Baseline Assessment

Hemodynamic and laboratory monitoring are critical to the resuscitation of a patient in septic shock. Some clinicians advocate following the serum lactate level as a monitor of response to therapy. Arterial blood gas measurement should be repeated to monitor adequacy of ventilation and perfusion. An ECG and chest radiograph should be obtained on all patients when practical. Septic shock patients should have at least two large-bore intravenous catheters for administration of fluids and vasoactive drugs. Early placement of a central venous catheter (ideally with a Swan-Ganz catheter introducer) may help in the monitoring of fluid resuscitation. Placement of a flow-directed thermal dilution pulmonary artery wedge pressure catheter should be considered in patients requiring vasoactive therapy, where there is difficulty in assessing volume status, or when ongoing hemodynamic instability is present. Generally, the placement of this catheter can wait until the patient is in the intensive care unit.

## Other Therapies

### Therapy of Acidosis and DIC

Some investigators advocate the administration of bicarbonate for individuals with severe acidosis (pH <7.2). The efficacy of this intervention is not established. For individuals with major bleeding and evidence of DIC, replacement therapy with fresh-frozen plasma and platelets with treatment of the primary underlying infection is recommended.

### Glucocorticoids

Although some animal models have shown that high-dose glucocorticoid therapy was effective, three large clinical trials have shown no differences in mortality between steroid-treated patients and control patients. These studies also have documented the occurrence of superinfection in steroid-treated patients. Thus the primary roles of steroids are in patients with suspected or documented adrenal insufficiency. Eicosanoid inhibitors or antihistamines have not proven to be effective in the management of septic shock.

## NEW AGENTS IN THE TREATMENT OF SEPSIS

Recent advances in molecular biology and immunology have suggested that the host's inflammatory response to infection contributes substantially to the development of septic shock. Standard sepsis treatment strategies include the use of life-support procedures, antibiotics to kill invading bacteria, and surgical procedures to eradicate the nidus of infection. Despite these aggressive measures, the mortality rate of septic shock remains high. The development of new interventions is based on the premise that neutralizing bacterial toxins and the potentially harmful host mediators could stop or slow this syndrome. Researchers have targeted interventions at all three phases of the host's inflammatory responses. Interventions targeting the induction phase include all those against the endotoxin's lipopolysaccharide molecule. This category includes E5 and HA-1A monoclonal antibodies. Therapies targeting cytokine synthesis include pentoxifylline, β agonists (amrinone and dobutamine), and glucocorticoids. Therapies directed against the cascade phase of sepsis include monoclonal antibodies to TNF and IL-1 receptor antagonist, monoclonal antibodies against the neutrophil CD11/18 adhesion complex, nitric oxide synthase inhibitors, and cyclooxygenase inhibitors.

### Endotoxin

The most studied exogenous mediator is endotoxin. This macromolecule is found in gram-negative bacteria as one of the integral components of the outer bacterial LPS cell wall. The molecule can be functionally divided into three parts: a highly variable O-polysaccharide side chain that provides the heat-stable serologic specificity of gram-negative bacteria and is the basis for the O(somatic) antigen type scheme; an oligosaccharide, or R-core, region composed of approximately 10 monosaccharides; and a lipid backbone referred to as lipid A. The lipid A portion of endotoxin is responsible for the majority of the molecule's toxicity; this portion is also highly conserved and is essentially invariable and ubiquitous.

Experimental studies of the administration of endotoxin have resulted in physiologic changes paralleling those of septic shock. Administration of endotoxin in dogs results in severe hypotension. Administration of endotoxin in humans produces an increase in heart rate and cardiac index and a decrease in peripheral vascular resistance. Later hemodynamic changes include a depressed cardiac state with a dilated left ventricle. Endotoxin administration in rabbits produces DIC and bilateral renal cortical necrosis. Endotoxin administration in both animals and humans has resulted in fever.

## Polyclonal and Monoclonal Antibodies to Endotoxin

### J5

The results of the first clinical trial of J5 polyclonal core-reactive antiserum in patients with gram-negative bacteremia were reported in 1982. In this study of 191 patients, the investigators reported a significant difference between sepsis-related mortality in patients given J5 antiserum (22 percent) compared to controls (39 percent). In a subgroup of patients who required vasopressor drugs for more than 6 h, the mortality rate was 44 percent in the study group compared to 77 percent of controls. However, five subsequent clinical trials using either J5 antiserum, immune plasma, or intravenous immunoglobulin failed to show survival benefit of J5.

### E5

Monoclonal antibodies were developed to produce a more specific antiendotoxin therapy with less risk for transmission of infection. E5 is an IgM antiendotoxin monoclonal antibody produced by immunization of mice with the core LPS antigen of the E5 mutant of *Escherichia coli*. E5 is manufactured by the antibody-producing hybridoma created by the fusion of mouse spleen cells with a murine myeloma cell line. Preliminary animal studies suggest potential efficacy in septic shock. The results have been reported of the first human double-blind, placebo-controlled investigation to test the efficacy of E5 in the treatment of gram-negative sepsis. Among the 468 patients with suspected gram-negative sepsis, E5 significantly decreased 30-day mortality (30 percent versus 43 percent of the placebo) for the 137 patients (29 percent) who did not have refractory shock. E5 also significantly improved the resolution of organ failure in this subgroup of patients. No benefit was found in the 179 patients with refractory gram-negative shock or in the 152 patients with sepsis from another origin. Allergic reactions to the murine antibody were minimal.

A subsequent study was conducted to test the efficacy of E5 among 530 patients with gram-negative sepsis and organ dysfunction who were not in shock. In this study, E5 did not significantly improve survival in the 530 patients (E5 mortality, 30 percent; control mortality, 26 percent; $p = .21$). However, meta-analysis and combining data from the two trials suggest that E5 substantially decreased the time to recovery from organ dysfunction and improved survival in a subgroup of patients with gram-negative infection and organ dysfunction who were not in refractory shock. A third multicenter trial is being done.

### HA-1A

HA-1A is a human hybrid antiendotoxin antibody. The hybridoma that produces HA-1A is about 80 percent murine; the antibody itself is predominantly human. Studies of HA-1A in animals have met with varied results. A number of investigators have reported that administration of HA-1A to mice and rabbits given a lethal bacterial challenge was protective. Others, using similar models, report no protection; one investigator reported that HA-1A administration significantly decreased survival in dogs.

A human HA-1A investigation compared a single 100-mg intravenous dose of antibody to placebo. There were 543 patients enrolled in this trial. A total of 262 patients received HA-1A compared to 281 controls. Two hundred of the 543 patients had documented gram-negative bacteremia. Among the 200 patients, 105 patients received HA-1A and 95 received placebo. Active treatment produced a 39 percent decrease in 28-day mortality among the 200 patients with gram-negative bacteremia. Mortality rate for HA-1A was 30 percent (32/105); for placebo it was 49 percent (45/92). Among the 101 patients in shock, treatment with HA-1A reduced the 28-day mortality by 42 percent. Earlier resolution of organ failure was noted in actively treated patients with documented gram-negative bacteremia. HA-1A treatment did not improve survival in the 201 patients who had nonbacteremic gram-negative infections and the 342 patients

without gram-negative infections. Allergic reactions were minimal in this study. In a subsequent analysis correlating circulating endotoxin levels with clinical outcome, one-third of 82 patients tested had detectable levels of endotoxin. Mortality of the patients with detectable endotoxin who received HA-1A ($n = 27$) was 30 percent versus a 73 percent mortality in control patients. This subanalysis suggests that HA-1A provided benefit by interacting in some manner with circulating endotoxin.

Despite these favorable results, significant concerns were raised: (1) The placebo group had a higher proportion of patients with complications (DIC, acute hepatic failure, acute renal failure, and recent surgery); (2) among the 201 patients who had nonbacteremic gram-negative infections, mortality rate was somewhat higher in the HA-1A group than the placebo; and (3) the analytic plan was changed by the manufacturer after learning of interim results. When the data were analyzed using the original analytic plan, HA-1A did not show a significant effect on survival. Additionally, a second unpublished trial of HA-1A that enrolled patients with refractory shock was discontinued in January, 1993, because of concern about the relatively high mortality of nonbacteremic patients who received HA-1A compared to placebo-treated patients.

A number of conclusions can be made. Antiendotoxin core–directed antibodies have not shown a reproducible survival benefit for patients with sepsis in 10 clinical trials. However, both E5 and HA-1A may have a beneficial role in a subgroup of patients presenting with sepsis. E5 is helpful for patients who have gram-negative infection who are not in shock, regardless of whether they are bacteremic. HA-1A treatment appears to benefit individuals who have gram-negative bacteremia, regardless of whether shock is present or not. Further investigations are needed to determine if monoclonal antibody to endotoxin is an appropriate therapeutic modality for treatment of septic shock.

If antiendotoxin antibody therapy is proven to be efficacious, other questions remain. The setting where antiendotoxin antibody therapy is a therapeutic and cost-effective intervention remains to be defined. Neither E5 nor HA-1A benefitted the approximately 30 percent of individuals who did not have a gram-negative infection. The high cost of these interventions (up to $4000 per intervention) places a strain on the already limited financial resources of our health care system. A more stringent identification of patients with gram-negative bacteremia and sepsis is needed if cost-effective interventions are to become a reality. Early laboratory diagnosis of gram-negative bacteremia or endotoxemia is not currently available. Most clinical studies have focused on the factors that predict bacteremia. It is impossible to separate patients with gram-positive sepsis from those with gram-negative sepsis based upon clinical symptoms and presenting signs alone. Most helpful to the emergency department clinician is the rapid identification of the presence of gram-negative organisms from potential infections (urinary tract infections, gram-negative pneumonia, abdominal infections, gram-negative CNS infections, and soft tissue infections). The Gram stain or other rapid assays remain the most valuable tests for rapid identification of gram-negative organisms in clinical specimens. Until rapid laboratory identification of gram-negative sepsis or bacteremia is available, the use of E5, HA-1A, or other newer agents that bind and neutralize endotoxin is more likely to be effective in patients who present with a compatible syndrome and when the clinician is able to obtain clinical specimens that have gram-negative bacteria.

## Anticytokine Therapy

Cytokines are peptides that function as cellular signals to regulate the amplitude and duration of the host's inflammatory response. TNF, IL-1, and other cytokines play protective roles in the host's immune response to infection. The host's response to these cytokines consists of recruited and activated neutrophils, macrophages, and lymphocytes; increased gene expression; and release of granulocyte colony-stimulating factors. Two cytokines, TNF and IL-1, have been studied extensively in patients with sepsis. Monocytes release TNF and IL-1 when exposed in vitro to bacterial components. These two cytokines can also replicate many of the symptoms associated with septic shock.

## Tumor Necrosis Factor

TNF is a polypeptide hormone that can stimulate the release of a variety of other mediators including IL-1, IL-6, and PAF. TNF also promotes the metabolism of arachidonic acid, leading to eicosanoid formation. TNF is directly toxic to endothelial cells, increases the adhesion of polymorphonuclear leukocytes to the endothelial cells, and enhances the phagocytic activity of these cells. Finally TNF reduces the transmembrane potential of muscle cells, depresses myocardial function, and activates coagulation.

Administration of TNF to experimental animals and healthy human subjects duplicates many of the signs and symptoms of sepsis. Injection of TNF into animals results in hemodynamic collapse, multiple organ injury, and a life-threatening vascular-leak syndrome. In humans, injection of TNF produces hypotension, chills, fever, headache, and malaise synchronously with the time of the peak in serum TNF following injection. In addition, rapid and sustained activation of the common pathway of the coagulation system occurs, most likely the extrinsic pathway.

Numerous studies have reported a positive correlation between the level of serum concentrations of TNF and the clinical outcome in patients with sepsis. Significantly higher levels of TNF were found in nonsurvivors of meningococcemia, sepsis, and ARDS and in children with fatal infectious purpura. Close association of the presence of TNF and septic shock has been demonstrated. Absolute TNF levels were a significant predictive value for morbidity and mortality in patients with septic shock.

The most compelling evidence that TNF is a causal rather than simply an associative factor is contained in animal studies demonstrating that antibodies to TNF enhance survival and reduced physiologic derangements after challenge with endotoxin or live bacteria. In 1985, researchers demonstrated that in mice challenged with endotoxin treatment with polyclonal anti-TNF enhanced survival. This laboratory also reported similar results in a baboon model challenged with *E. coli*. All animals pretreated with monoclonal anti-TNF antibodies 2 h prior to infusion of high doses of bacteria survived. All control animals died. In 1990, other researchers using the baboon model reported that all six baboons treated with an infusion of monoclonal antibodies to TNF 30 min after challenge by *E. coli* survived. All six control animals died. In 1992, this group also reported that anti-TNF therapy is applicable to infections caused by gram-positive bacteria. Five control baboons infused with *Staph. aureus* died, as well as the six treated with ceftriaxone only. The six baboons treated with monoclonal antibodies to TNF and ceftriaxone all survived. Similar findings have been published for the porcine and rat models.

Human studies on the feasibility of monoclonal antibodies are currently underway. Reports from two phase 1 and one phase 2 trials have documented that administration of monoclonal antibodies was well tolerated and the serum half-life ranged from 40 to 54 h in septic patients. One team reported the use of antibody against TNF on 14 patients with severe shock. Survival of patients treated with TNF was not different from historical controls. Two large phase 2 and phase 3 double-blind trials on the role and efficacy of monoclonal antibodies with sepsis syndrome are underway. Preliminary analysis from one of the phase 3 trials has been reported. A 17 percent reduction in 28-day mortality was noted in treated patients; this difference was not significantly different from controls. There has also been a report of preliminary results of a phase 2 blind, randomized trial of recombinant human dimeric TNF receptor. Patients who received medium or high doses of human dimeric TNF receptor had worse outcomes than patients receiving placebo.

## Interleukin 1

IL-1$\beta$ is also present in the blood of patients with septic shock. Both TNF and IL-1 induce hypotension, and a combination of the two cytokines is a more potent inducer of shock than either cytokine alone. Both cytokines induce IL-6, a nonlethal cytokine that serves as an excellent marker of cytokine activity in patients with sepsis. An IL-1 receptor antagonist (IL-1ra) has been shown to block the hemodynamic consequences of *E. coli* endotoxin and heat-killed *Staph. epidermidis* in experimental animals. Human recombinant IL-1ra decreased the mortality rate of endotoxin-induced shock in rabbits and lethal *E. coli*-induced septic shock in primates. In addition, IL-1ra attenuated the decrease in mean artery blood pressure and cardiac output in the primate model.

Results are available from two human studies on the efficacy of IL-1ra in patients with septic syndrome. In a randomized phase 2 multicenter placebo-controlled trial, researchers demonstrated a 15 percent reduction in the 28-day all cause mortality rate in the IL-1ra-treated patients versus patients who received placebo. In patients with gram-negative infection, there was a strong survival trend with human recombinant IL-1ra treatment. The second trial was conducted by the IL-1ra Sepsis Syndrome Study Group. This was an open, labeled placebo-controlled phase 2 study using three doses of human IL-ra. Although numbers were too small to be definitive, there was a progressive dose-related reduction in mortality rate in patients with sepsis syndrome and septic shock due to varied infecting organisms and sites of infection. In addition, the administration of IL-1ra was associated with a survival benefit in patients presenting with septic shock at entry into the study.

In summary, most investigators feel that TNF is a key and perhaps central mediator in sepsis. To date, anti-TNF and anti-IL-1 agents have not been shown to improve outcome in the treatment of septic patients.

## The Neutrophil

Evidence suggests that the neutrophil has both beneficial and harmful effects in sepsis and septic shock. The neutrophil is a key component of the host defense. Data from neutropenic animals and humans suggest that augmented neutrophil count and function reduces the risk of infection. Studies have also shown that the neutrophil and its toxic byproducts produce tissue injury and organ dysfunction in sepsis and septic shock.

One area of intense interest is the leukocyte-endothelium interaction. This interaction appears to be a crucial step in the inflammatory cascade during sepsis. A membrane glycoprotein complex termed *CD11/CD18* has been suggested to be the primary adhesion receptor site on endothelial cells and leukocytes for this interaction and has been the target of many investigators. This complex is a cell surface receptor that regulates neutrophil-endothelial cell adhesion, the first step in the neutrophil migration to sites of infection or inflammation.

Researchers have developed monoclonal antibodies against the CD11/CD18 complex. These antibodies, both in vitro and in vivo, prevent endotoxin, TNF, and complement-induced neutrophil adhesion and injury to endothelial cells and neutrophil extravascular migration. In some animal models of sepsis and meningitis, monoclonal anti-CD 11/CD18 antibodies improved mortality rates, decreased adverse hemodynamic parameters, and decreased meningeal inflammation. In one study in rabbits, the combination of anti-CD18 antibodies and dexamethasone resulted in less meningeal inflammation and brain edema than when either agent was used alone. In a study of dogs pretreated with CD11/CD18 monoclonal antibody and challenged with TNF, animals treated with CD11/CD18 had a reduced mortality rate and better arterial oxygenation in the first 24 h; this effect was not sustained, however, and the overall survival between the two groups was not significantly different. In a subsequent study in dogs using a similar design but challenged with *E. coli,* investigators found that the CD11/CD18 monoclonal antibody worsened cardiovascular instability and decreased tissue perfusion during sepsis. Finally, these investigators studied the effects of recombinant granulocyte colony-stimulating factor in animals treated 9 days before and 3 days after bacterial challenge. This intervention revealed that granulocyte colony-stimulating factor was associated with prolonged survival, improved mean arterial blood pressure, improved cardiac function, and increased endotoxin clearance. In conclusion, studies to date suggest that efforts to inhibit neutrophil function may lead to more tissue injury and more adverse outcomes. In some patients with sepsis, colony-stimulating factor may be of benefit.

### Nitric Oxide

Nitric oxide is a low-molecular-weight, membrane-permeable gas with both harmful and beneficial effects in shock. Under normal conditions, this gas is produced in the endothelium by a calcium- and calmodulin-dependent nitric oxide synthase that converts L-arginine and $O_2$ to L-citrulline and nitric oxide. This pathway is normally well regulated by signal transduction pathways linked to cell surface receptors for vasodilators such as acetylcholine and histamine. However, inflammatory mediators induce a calcium-independent form of nitric oxide synthase that is not controlled by this mechanism. This form may give rise to abnormal amounts of nitric oxide in septic patients and patients given IL-2 for cancer treatment.

Nitric oxide functions as a neurotransmitter, regulates vascular tone, and inhibits platelet aggregation and leukocyte adhesion. At higher doses, nitric oxide has antitumor and antimicrobial activity. Nitric oxide is thought to have a beneficial role in sepsis. It is important in maintaining visceral and microvascular blood flow, acting as a counterregulatory mechanism to the vasoconstriction mediators (thromboxane and endothelin-1) released in inflammation. It prevents microvascular stasis and thrombosis by blocking platelet aggregation and leukocyte adhesion. Nitric oxide may have several harmful effects in sepsis. Overproduction of nitric oxide may be largely responsible for sepsis-induced hypotension, direct tissue injury and organ failure, and enhancement of cytokine release from phagocytic cells.

Animal studies using nitric oxide synthase inhibitors have mixed results. Researchers have reported that nitric oxide synthase inhibitors restored the responsiveness of septic vasculature to catecholamines and improved survival in endotoxin-challenged animals. Other investigators have reported opposite and harmful effects. These investigators found that the administration of a nitric oxide synthase inhibitor increased systemic and renal vascular resistance, decrease renal blood flow, increased capillary leak, decrease cardiac output, and increased mortality. In conclusion, the role of nitric oxide in septic shock warrants further investigation. To date, only nonselective nitric oxide synthetase inhibitors that block both forms of nitric oxide synthase have been extensively studied. Future research is most likely to be performed with highly selective inhibitors.

### Other Agents

#### Pentoxifylline

Pentoxifylline, a methylxanthine derivative, inhibits cytokine activation of neutrophils and the production of TNF by endotoxin-exposed monocytes. This prevents the adherence of neutrophils to endothelium and the release of toxic degranulation products. The mechanism of this action is believed to be by increasing cyclic adenosine monophosphate concentrations. Animal experiments have suggested that treatment with pentoxifylline decreases mortality rate and prevents lung injury by inhibiting migration of neutrophils through the

pulmonary capillary endothelium. Also, better survival rates and lower meningeal inflammation have been observed in animals with experimental bacterial meningitis. In healthy human volunteers, pentoxifylline inhibits the rise in TNF induced by endotoxin.

### Cyclooxygenase Inhibitors

Two principle pathways of arachidonic acid metabolism exist. The lipoxygenase pathway leads to the production of leukotrienes. Leukotrienes are potent leukocyte chemoattractants. The second pathway is the cyclooxygenase pathway. This pathway results in the release of thromboxanes and prostaglandins, which are important regulators of vascular tone.

Ibuprofen is a cyclooxygenase inhibitor. In animal models of endotoxin shock and shock from peritoneal implantation or IV infusion of bacteria, ibuprofen decreases mortality; reverses hemodynamic, metabolic, and blood coagulation abnormalities; improves pulmonary gas exchange; and attenuates the development of increases in microvascular permeability. These results are seen with ibuprofen when administered before and after the septic insult. In preliminary human studies, treatment with ibuprofen attenuates flulike symptoms and reduces fever, tachycardia, and increased metabolic rate in volunteers exposed to endotoxin. One clinical study of patients with sepsis demonstrated that ibuprofen treatment was associated with significant decreases in heart rate and minute ventilation when compared to placebo controls. In a subsequent double-blind, randomized, placebo-controlled study of 29 patients, no significant differences in hemodynamic and respiratory values or survival were demonstrated in ibuprofen-treated patients compared with controls. These investigators found that administration of ibuprofen was safe in patients with sepsis. Due to the small numbers in each group as well as the single time administration of ibuprofen, no definitive conclusions can be made from this study regarding the efficacy of ibuprofen in sepsis.

### SUMMARY

Currently, none of the therapies aimed at single targets in the inflammatory cascade has proved to be safe and effective in the treatment of septic shock in humans. In the cases of interventions that are directed at endogenous inflammatory mediators, none of the studies has produced unequivocal benefit in the treatment of sepsis. Great potential danger exists in altering the natural balance of inflammatory mediators. These mediators perform important functions such as clearing bacterial toxins and the mobilization of the host defenses that control the infection. Attempting to block the harmful effect of inflammatory mediators may compromise host defenses and ultimately worsen outcome. Successful therapeutic approaches may depend on determining which inflammatory mediators should be inhibited or augmented and when to do so.

### BIBLIOGRAPHY

Bone RC: A critical evaluation of new agents for the treatment of sepsis. *JAMA* 266(12)1686, 1991.

Natanson C, Hoffman WD, Suffredini AF, et al. Selected treatment strategies for septic shock based on proposed mechanisms of pathogenesis. *Ann Intern Med* 120(9):771, 1994.

Parrillo JE: Management of septic shock: Present and future. *Ann Intern Med* 115(6):491, 1991.

Parrillo JE: Pathogenetic mechanisms of septic shock. *N Engl J Med* 328(20):1471, 1993.

Ziegler EJ, Fisher CJ Jr, Sprung CL, et al: Treatment of gram-negative bacteremia and septic shock with HA-1A human monoclonal antibody against endotoxin. A randomized, double-blind, placebo-controlled trial. The HA-1A Sepsis Study Group. *N Engl J Med* 324(7):429, 1991.

# 28
# ANAPHYLAXIS AND ACUTE ALLERGIC REACTIONS

## Joseph A. Salomone III

## INTRODUCTION

Allergic reactions can range from mild local eruptions to severe and life-threatening multisystem systemic illnesses. The most common presenting complaints involve the dermatologic and respiratory systems, but gastrointestinal and cardiovascular involvement also occur frequently. Early recognition, rapid evaluation, and prompt intervention are necessary to prevent a potentially fatal outcome. Parenterally administered penicillin and Hymenoptera stings are the two most common etiologies of fatal anaphylaxis.

## CLINICAL IMMUNOLOGY AND PATHOPHYSIOLOGY

Hypersensitivity is an exaggerated immune system response to presented antigens. On initial contact, an antigen generally produces no obvious clinical response but sensitizes the immune system so that the next contact produces a clinical response. Immediate hypersensitivity reactions are those that manifest themselves within seconds to minutes after the presentation of the antigen, and an interaction between antigens and antibodies occurs. In humans, these reactions are mediated mostly by IgE and are responsible for attacks of extrinsic asthma, allergic rhinitis, urticaria, angioedema, and anaphylaxis.

A hapten is a small organic compound that when bound to a protein forms an antigenic complex that can stimulate immune system responses. Antigens that preferentially stimulate the immune system to produce IgE are called allergens, and most are proteins. On initial presentation, these allergens react with B-cell precursors and T cells, leading to formation of T helper cells and activated B cells. In turn, memory B cells and plasma cells are created, and the plasma cells then produce specific IgE antibodies.

IgE binds to specific receptors on mast cells and basophils. When antigen binds to the IgE on these cells, it triggers the release of mediators that are responsible for the local and systemic reactions that occur. These biologic mediators cause increased vascular permeability, vasodilation, bronchial constriction, smooth muscle contraction, increased mucous gland secretions, and attraction of inflammatory cells. Clinical manifestations thus depend on the site or sites affected by these mediators. Histamine, bradykinins, platelet-activating factor, heparin, protease, and leukotriens ($C_4$, $D_4$, and $E_4$ or SRS-A) are some of the mediators that are released.

Classically, four types of hypersensitivity reactions are described. However, current research and improved understanding of the complex immune system have defined overlapping and coexisting mechanisms of hypersensitivity. Type I hypersensitivity is an IgE-mediated, and possibly IgG-mediated, reaction to allergens. The binding of allergens to antibodies present on the surface of mast cells and basophils results in the reactions described above.

Type II reactions involve IgG and IgM antibody reactions to antigens on cell surfaces and involve complement activation and phagocytosis by killer cells. The most frequent clinical manifestations involve blood transfusion reactions, hemolytic anemias, idiopathic thrombocytopenic purpura (ITP), and Goodpasture syndrome. Type II reactions appear to be the least common cause for drug-related allergic reactions.

Type III reactions are caused by soluble immune or antigen-antibody complexes that in turn activate the complement system and platelets to form platelet aggregates and IgE complexes. This type of reaction can occur after tetanus toxoid administration in sensitized individuals. Other clinical manifestations include poststreptococcal glomerulonephritis, serum sickness, and systemic lupus erythematosus.

Type IV reactions are cell-mediated reactions not involving complement or antibodies. This reaction is called *delayed hypersensitivity* and results from the migration of specifically activated T lymphocytes to the area of antigen presentation. Clinical manifestations do not occur for 24 to 48 h after exposure and include the local reactions seen with skin tests for *Candida,* tuberculosis, and *Trichophyton.*

Persons who exhibit hypersensitivity reactions often have a history of atopic symptoms, as well as a familial history of allergy. The duration and quantity of exposure to the precipitating antigen can affect the severity of reaction. Compounds may have similar haptens and thus cause similar sensitization and reactions. Examples of this include the cross reactivity occasionally seen between penicillins and cephalosporins, or sulfonamides and sulfonylurea drugs.

## ANAPHYLAXIS

The term *anaphylaxis* was coined by Portier and Richet in 1902 and literally means "removal of protection." Today anaphylaxis describes the clinical syndrome of severe hypersensitivity reaction characterized by cardiovascular collapse and respiratory compromise. A wide variety of substances are now known to produce anaphylactic reactions. Table 28-1 contains a partial list of some of the more common causative agents.

### Clinical Features

The symptoms associated with anaphylaxis may begin within seconds of exposure to an allergen or may be delayed for up to 1 h. However, the typical response begins within minutes of exposure and primarily involves the cardiovascular and respiratory systems. The skin and gastrointestinal tract are also commonly involved, and widespread involvement of many organ systems may occur at the same time.

The clinical symptoms of anaphylaxis can vary widely. In patients who have previously suffered from an anaphylactic reaction, an "aura" of impending disaster may occur that warns them of the oncoming reaction. Cutaneous manifestations include generalized erythema, pruritus, progressive urticaria, and angioedema. Angioedema most often involves the head, neck, face, and upper airways. Flushing, chills, and diaphoresis may occur. A vague tightening sensation in the throat and chest progressing to laryngeal and bronchial spasm, manifested as hoarseness, stridor, and wheezing, may progress to se-

**Table 28-1.** Common Causes of Anaphylaxis and Anaphylactoid and Allergic Reactions

Drugs
    Penicillins and related antibiotics
    Aspirin
    Trimethoprim-sulfamethoxazole
    Vancomycin
    Nonsteroidal anti-inflammatory agents
Foods and additives
    Shellfish
    Soybeans
    Nuts
    Wheat
    Milk
    Eggs
    Monosodium glutamate
    Nitrates and nitrites
    Tartrazine dyes
Other
    Hymenoptera stings
    Insect parts and molds
    Radiographic contrast material

vere respiratory distress. Patients with a previous history of reactive airway disease often have more severe bronchospasm. Nausea, abdominal cramps, vomiting, and diarrhea are frequent complaints. Light-headedness may be the initial manifestation of impending cardiovascular collapse, with resultant tachycardia, hypotension, and typical manifestations of shock. Cardiac dysrhythmias and profound ischemia may occur, which may precipitate a myocardial infarction.

Patients with a prior history of allergies may be at increased risk for severe anaphylactic reactions. The use of β-blocking agents, particularly in patients at increased risk for anaphylaxis, may predispose patients to more severe reactions. Further, patients who are taking β blockers and develop anaphylaxis may be refractory to standard epinephrine doses. Drugs such as cimetidine that delay the clearance of β blockers should also be avoided since they may prolong the activity of the β blocker and complicate treatment.

## Diagnosis

The diagnosis of anaphylaxis is often obvious, but in the early stages the potential severity of the reaction may be underestimated. The differential diagnosis will vary depending on whether the predominant symptomatology occurs in a single organ system. Pulmonary embolism, acute myocardial infarction and cardiac dysrhythmias, airway obstruction, tension pneumothorax, acute asthma, hereditary angioedema, volume depletion, and vasovagal reactions are just a few conditions that may need to be considered in the differential diagnosis. There is no specific diagnostic or laboratory examination for anaphylaxis. For the broad differentiation, the following measurements may be indicated: a complete blood count, serum glucose, electrolytes, BUN, creatinine, and urinalysis. Additionally, arterial blood gas measurements may be required to evaluate ventilatory status.

## Emergency Department Care

Treatment begins with attention to the airway. A high flow of oxygen via face mask and immediate administration of epinephrine are indicated. If signs of shock are present, intravenous administration of 0.3 to 0.5 mg of a 1:10,000 solution is preferred. If immediate intravenous access cannot be obtained, injection into the venous plexus at the base of the tongue may provide the most rapid access. Endotracheal administration is also an alternative to intravenous access if the airway has been established. Subcutaneous administration of 0.3 to 0.5 mg of a 1:1000 solution is indicated if there is no significant circulatory compromise. Immediate endotracheal intubation may be required, but may be extremely difficult if angioedema or severe laryngospasm is present. Transtracheal jet insufflation or cricothyrotomy may be necessary to control the airway.

If the reaction may be due to intravenous solutions, administration should be discontinued. If the patient has sustained a recent bite or sting, or received an injection, a tourniquet may be placed proximal to the site to prevent further dissemination of the allergen. To avoid potential injury to the limb, this tourniquet should probably only remain until therapy has begun.

Cardiac monitoring should be initiated, and an ECG obtained in patients with previous cardiac history or ischemic symptoms. Hypotensive patients should be placed in a head-down position or, at a minimum, have their legs elevated unless respiratory status prevents such positioning. Intravenous fluid therapy with Ringer's lactate or normal saline should be established. Large volumes of crystalloid, 2 to 4 L, may be required in the hypotensive patient. Military antishock trousers (MAST) may be beneficial in the initial management of hypotension in both the prehospital setting and the emergency department. Because of the increased vascular permeability, pulmonary edema may develop with or without fluid administration. Patients with severe symptomatology may benefit from central venous pressure (CVP) or Swan-Ganz monitoring.

Administration of antihistamines may be beneficial. Diphenhydramine, 50 mg intravenously, is the most commonly utilized and may be repeated every 6 to 8 h. Currently, the addition of $H_2$-blocker therapy is also generally accepted. Cimetidine, 300 mg IV, should be given and may be repeated every 6–8 h. Inhaled bronchodilators, such as aerosolized albuterol, 0.5 mL in 3-mL saline, can be useful in managing bronchospasm. These can be administered either intermittently or continuously. Aminophylline, initial bolus of 4 to 6 mg/kg followed by a maintenance infusion, may be required for management of severe bronchospasm. Intravenous glucocorticoids, such as methylprednisolone, 125 mg, may prevent or lessen delayed reactions. Refractory hypotension may require dopamine, levoterenol, or epinephrine infusions. Patients on β blockers may require large and repeated doses of epinephrine. Glucagon, 5 to 15 μg/min IV, may be beneficial for refractory hypotension associated with β blockers. General anesthesia and neuromuscular blockade may be required to assist ventilation in patients with severe respiratory distress.

## Admission Indications

Patients should be advised to be alert for any recurrence of symptoms and to return to the Emergency Department if there is no response to outpatient therapy. However, all patients with significant generalized reactions should be observed for at least 24 h. Delayed reactions and reoccurrence of symptoms are possible, particularly as the effects of previously administered treatment decrease. Patients may benefit from repeated doses of antihistamines and glucocorticoids over the next several days, and these should be prescribed. Oral doses of antihistamines every 4 to 6 h and oral glucocorticoids such as prednisone, 40 mg/day, should probably be given for at least 72 h.

## Follow-up

All patients with allergic reactions selected for discharge should have follow-up in 24 to 48 h to evaluate outpatient therapy. All patients should be referred to an allergy specialist and advised to carry some form of self-administered epinephrine and antihistamines. Several prefilled syringe kits are available, such as Epi-pen and Ana-kit.

## ANAPHYLACTOID REACTIONS

Anaphylactoid reactions are nonimmunologically mediated systemic reactions that clinically appear very similar to anaphylaxis. Although no immunologic basis is identified, many of the same mediators are involved in these reactions. The most common agent responsible is radiographic contrast media. Other implicated agents include nonsteroidal anti-inflammatory agents, thiamine, and codeine. Recent research has found complement activation or immune-complex-mediated reactions for many agents previously thought to cause anaphylactoid reactions. Treatment is the same as for anaphylaxis.

## URTICARIA AND ANGIOEDEMA

Urticaria, or hives, is a cutaneous IgE-mediated reaction marked by the development of pruritic, erythemic wheals of varying size that generally disappear quickly. Erythema multiforme is a more pronounced urticarial variant, characterized by typical target lesions. Angioedema is also an IgE-mediated reaction characterized by edema formation in the dermis, most generally involving the face and neck. These manifestations may accompany many allergic reactions.

As with all allergic manifestations, a detailed history of exposures, ingestions, medications, infections, and family history should be obtained. If an etiologic agent can be identified, future reactions may be avoided. Treatment of these reactions is generally supportive and symptomatic, with attempts to identify and remove the offending agent if it can be identified. Epinephrine, antihistamines, and steroids are most often tried. Oral antihistamines and steroids for several days may be beneficial. The addition of an $H_2$-receptor agonist, such as cimetidine, may also be useful in more severe cases. Cold compresses to affected areas may be soothing. Referral to an allergy specialist is indicated.

Angioedema of the tongue, lips, and face can occur from use of angiotensin-converting enzyme (ACE) inhibitor antihypertensives. This manifestation is rarely life-threatening but can be severe and frightening for the patient. Management is supportive, with $H_1$ and $H_2$ antihistamines, and steroids may be indicated, although the angioedema may be refractory to medical management. Immediate withdrawal from the ACE inhibitor is indicated, and replacement with another antihypertensive as needed. All patients should have close follow-up.

Hereditary angioedema is an autosomal dominant disorder with a characteristic complement pathway deficiency. Reactions often involve the upper respiratory tract and gastrointestinal tract. Minor trauma often precipitates a reaction. Many of the typical treatments of allergic problems, such as epinephrine, steroids, and antihistamines, have been tried, but their effectiveness is not clearly demonstrated.

## OTHER COMMON ALLERGIC PROBLEMS

### Food Allergy

Hypersensitivity reactions to ingested foods are generally due to IgE-mediated reactions to food components or additives. IgE-coated mast cells lining the gastrointestinal tract react to presented allergens in ingested foods and produce clinical findings associated with the release of biologic mediators, as previously described. Non-IgE-mediated food allergy reactions have also been described. Dairy products, eggs, and nuts are some of the most commonly implicated foods.

A detailed history will provide the best clues to food allergy, with particular attention to other allergic history and prior reactions. Diagnosis is often difficult since the offending food or foods may only occasionally produce symptoms, depending on the amount ingested and other foods present.

Symptoms of food allergy include swelling and itching of the lips, mouth, and pharynx; nausea; abdominal cramps; vomiting; and diarrhea. Cutaneous manifestations such as angioedema and urticaria, as well as systemic findings of anaphylaxis, can occur. Treatment for mild reactions is supportive, with the administration of antihistamines to lessen symptomatology. More severe reactions or anaphylaxis are managed as previously described under "Anaphylaxis." Referral to an allergy specialist is indicated.

### Insect Sting Allergy

Insect stings can produce significant and sometimes fatal reactions, particularly in sensitized patients. Approximately 100 patients die annually from insect sting reactions, making insect sting the second most common cause of fatal anaphylaxis. True stinging insects belong to the order Hymenoptera, which includes three families: Apoidea (honeybee), Formicoidea (fire ants), and Vespidae (wasps, yellow jackets, hornets). The venoms of each family are unique, although all have similar types of components, mostly proteins. This difference accounts for the limited cross-reactivity seen. The usual reaction to these stings includes localized pain, pruritus, swelling, and redness. Sensitized individuals may have exaggerated local reactions with or without systemic manifestations. Systemic reactions run from mild nausea and malaise to urticaria, angioedema, or anaphylaxis.

Diagnosis depends on clinical history, with particular attention to past reactions, and an examination to locate the site of the sting. Occasionally, the site of envenomization is overlooked, and predominance of reaction in one organ system can lead to misdiagnosis. Treatment is symptomatic and supportive. Mild local reactions can be managed with application of ice and oral antihistamines. More generalized reactions or local reactions of head and neck may benefit from a short steroid course. Severe reactions are managed as outlined under "Anaphylaxis." Patients with severe reactions should be advised to carry self-administered epinephrine and antihistamines. A referral to an allergy specialist is indicated.

### Drug Allergy

Although adverse reactions to drugs are a common clinical problem, true immunologically mediated hypersensitivity reactions probably account for less than 10 percent of these problems. Since most drugs are small organic molecules, they are generally unable to stimulate the immune system alone. However, when a drug or metabolite becomes protein-bound, either in serum or on cell surfaces, this drug-protein complex can become an allergen and stimulate immune system responses. Thus, the ability of a drug or its metabolites to sensitize the immune system depends on the ability to be bound to tissue proteins. Approximately 300 patients yearly die of anaphylactic drug reactions. Penicillin is the drug most commonly implicated in eliciting true allergic reactions and accounts for approximately 90 percent of all allergic drug reactions. Of those patients who had fatal anaphylactic drug reactions, over 95 percent reacted to penicillin. Only about 25 percent of patients who die of penicillin anaphylaxis had exhibited allergic reactions during previous courses of the drug. Parenterally administered penicillin was more than twice as likely to produce fatal allergic reactions as orally administered penicillin.

The clinical manifestations of drug allergy are widely varied and can involve all four types of hypersensitivity reactions. A generalized reaction similar to immune-complex or serum-sickness reactions is very common. Beginning usually in the first or second week after the administration of the drug, this reaction may take many weeks to subside after drug withdrawal. Generalized malaise, arthralgias, pruritus, urticarial eruptions, and fever are common. Drug fever may occur without other associated clinical findings and may also occur without an immunologic basis. Circulating immune complexes are probably responsible for the lupuslike reactions caused by some drugs. Cytotoxic reactions, such as penicillin-induced hemolytic anemia, can occur. Skin eruptions may include erythema, pruritus, urticaria, angioedema, erythema multiforme, and photosensitivity, and severe reactions, such as those seen in Stevens-Johnson syndrome and toxic epidermal necrolysis (see Chap. 162), may also occur. Pulmonary complications, including bronchospasm and airway obstruction, can occur. Delayed hypersensitivity reactions may be manifested as a contact dermatitis from drugs applied topically.

Diagnosis is best determined by a careful and thorough history. Treatment is supportive, with oral or parenteral antihistamines, glucocorticoids, and β-adrenergic agents, as outlined under "Anaphylaxis." Immediate drug withdrawal is important; however, reactions can continue or recur after a period of abstinence. Referral to an allergy specialist may be indicated.

## BIBLIOGRAPHY

Atkinson TP, Kaliner MA: Anaphylaxis. *Med Clin North Am* 76(4):841, 1992.

Bochner BS: Anaphylaxis. *N Engl J Med* 324(25):1785, 1991.

Levi JH, Levi R: Diagnosis and Treatment of Anaphylactic/Anaphylactoid Reactions. *Monogr Allergy* 30:130, 1992.

Rocklin RE, David J: Clinical Immunology I, in Scientific American Medicine—CD. New York, Scientific American, September 1993.

Yuninger JW: Anaphylaxis. *Ann Allergy* 67:91, 1991.

# 29
# CYANOSIS

## Ann L. Harwood-Nuss
## Tom Kunisaki

## DEFINITION

*Cyanosis* refers to the bluish color of the skin and mucous membranes that results from an increased amount of reduced hemoglobin (deoxyhemoglobin) or hemoglobin derivatives. The detection of cyanosis can be highly subjective and is not considered a sensitive indicator of the state of arterial oxygenation. In fact, cyanosis is determined by the absolute amount of reduced hemoglobin in the blood; the amount of oxygenated hemoglobin is of little influence. Standard teaching has been that cyanosis is usually present when there is 5 g or more of reduced hemoglobin in 100 mL of capillary blood. However, this figure has been questioned recently. A study by Goss et al. has demonstrated that central cyanosis can be detected when the deoxyhemoglobin concentration is 1.5 g per 100 mL or greater. The increase in the amount of reduced hemoglobin in the cutaneous vessels can result from either an increase in the quantity of venous blood in the skin, dilatation of the venules, or a decrease in the oxygen saturation in the capillary blood. In some instances, cyanosis can be detected when the arterial saturation has fallen to 85 percent; in others, it may not be detected until saturation is 75 percent. The absolute rather than the relative amount of reduced hemoglobin produces cyanosis.

Various physiologic, anatomic, and physical factors other than the amount of reduced hemoglobin may influence the diagnosis of cyanosis, making an accurate clinical detection of the degree, or even the presence, of cyanosis difficult. Physiologic factors include the oxygen content of the blood, level of tissue oxygenation, the degree of oxygen extraction, and the oxyhemoglobin dissociation curve. Anatomic factors include the status of the cutaneous microcirculation, pigmentation, and thickness of the skin. Physical factors include the lighting under which the patient is examined and the skill of the physician. The tongue is considered one of the most sensitive sites for observing central cyanosis. The earlobes, conjunctivae, and nail beds are not reliable sites.

Clinically, the presence of cyanosis must suggest the possibility of tissue hypoxia. However, the absence of cyanosis does not mean that there is no tissue hypoxia; severe states of tissue hypoxia are possible without the presence of cyanosis. Cyanosis demands a thorough clinical evaluation for possible tissue hypoxia. Additionally, unexplained cyanosis, particularly in association with normal arterial oxygen tension (Pa$_{O_2}$), should alert the physician to promptly assess for abnormal hemoglobin, such as methemoglobin.

## CENTRAL AND PERIPHERAL CYANOSIS

Cyanosis can be divided into two categories, central and peripheral. The central type is seen under conditions where arterial blood is unsaturated or an abnormal hemoglobin derivative exists. The mucous membranes and skin are both affected. In contrast, peripheral cyanosis is due to the slowing of blood flow to an area and an abnormally great extraction of oxygen from normally saturated arterial blood. Congestive failure, peripheral vascular disease, shock states, and cold exposure all create states of vasoconstriction and decrease peripheral blood flow. The differentiation between central and peripheral cyanosis may not be possible in conditions where there may be an admixture of mechanisms (see Table 29-1).

**Table 29-1.** Causes of Cyanosis

Central cyanosis
  Decreased arterial oxygen saturation
    Decreased atmospheric pressure—high altitude
    Impaired pulmonary function
      Alveolar hypoventilation
      Uneven relationships between pulmonary ventilation and perfusion
      Impaired oxygen diffusion
    Anatomic shunts
      Certain types of congenital heart disease
      Pulmonary arteriovenous fistulas
      Multiple small intrapulmonary shunts
    Hemoglobin with low affinity for oxygen
  Hemoglobin abnormalities
    Methemoglobinemia—hereditary, acquired
    Sulfhemoglobinemia—acquired
    Carboxyhemoglobinemia (not true cyanosis)
Peripheral cyanosis
  Reduced cardiac output
  Cold exposure
  Redistribution of blood flow from extremities
  Arterial obstruction
  Venous obstruction

*Source:* Braunwald E: Hypoxia, polycythemia, and cyanosis, in Wilson J, Braunwald E, Isselbacher KJ, et al (eds): *Harrison's Principles of Internal Medicine,* ed 12, New York, McGraw-Hill, 1991, pp 224–228. Used by permission.

## THE ROLE OF ARTERIAL BLOOD GAS DETERMINATION

To the clinician, the presence of cyanosis should suggest the possibility of hypoxemia. Pulse oximetry is now readily available in most emergency departments to assist the physician in the early diagnosis of hypoxemia. The continuous oxygen saturation reading is generally reliable. However, an exception is when the hemoglobin is in a state whereby it is unable to bind to oxygen (i.e., methemoglobin or carboxyhemoglobin). In such situations, the pulse oximetry will not only overestimate the oxygen saturation but will reflect a diminished response to any changes in oxygen saturation. The arterial blood gas (ABG) analysis with cooximetry is still the "gold standard" in the assessment of any patient with suspected cyanosis. In central cyanosis, the oxygen saturation of the ABG will be decreased due to the underlying hypoxia. In peripheral cyanosis, assuming normal cardiopulmonary and hemoglobin status, the oxygen saturation should be normal. If methemoglobinemia or carboxyhemoglobinemia is suspected, the ABG will show a normal Pa$_{O_2}$, a normal calculated oxygen saturation, and a decrease in the measured oxygen saturation. This is because the measure of dissolved oxygen is unaffected; hence, the normal Pa$_{O_2}$. The calculated oxygen saturation is based on the Pa$_{O_2}$, while the measured oxygen saturation actually measures the percentage of hemoglobin bound to oxygen.

Few tests are as vulnerable to errors introduced by improper sampling, handling, and storage as are blood gas analyses. One study reports a 15.8 percent incidence of preanalytic error for ABG samples from emergency departments. In contrast, a 0.1 percent incidence of error exists from samples obtained from an indwelling arterial catheter.

Special attention should be given to the following sources of preanalytic error for ABG samples:

1. Heparin is the anticoagulant of choice, but one must be cautious that the syringe be flushed with heparin and then emptied thoroughly. This will allow adequate anticoagulation of a 2- to 4-mL blood sample with assurance that the results will not be altered by the anticoagulant. Excessive heparin affects the pH, P$_{CO_2}$, and P$_{O_2}$, as well as the hemoglobin determination.
2. Air bubbles that mix with the blood sample will result in gas equi-

libration, significantly lowering the $P_{CO_2}$ values with an increase in pH and $P_{O_2}$. Any sample obtained with more than minor air bubbles should be discarded.

3. Reducing the temperature of the blood by placing the sample immediately in an ice slush will significantly deter changes in the $P_{CO_2}$ and pH for a period of several hours. If the sample is not iced immediately, changes can be significant. As a general rule, arterial blood samples should be analyzed within 10 min or cooled immediately. A delay of up to 1 h for running a cool sample will have no significant effect on the results. Failure to properly cool the sample is a common source of preanalytic error.

## DIFFERENTIAL DIAGNOSIS OF CYANOSIS

Hypoxia, anemia, and polycythemia can be diagnosed by means of hemoglobin, hematocrit, and ABG determination. The red cyanosis of polycythemia vera occurs because the increase in number of red blood cells and hemoglobin concentration results in sludging of blood flow in cutaneous capillaries and venules. Similarly, cyanosis is enhanced in chronic hypoxemia accompanied by polycythemia.

If arterial gases, hematocrit, and hemoglobin are normal, the cause of cyanosis may be due to abnormal skin pigmentation or an abnormal hemoglobin. The term "pseudocyanosis" is used to describe the blue, gray, or purple cutaneous discoloration which may mimic cyanosis. Pseudocyanosis can be caused by heavy metals [i.e., iron (hemochromatosis), gold, silver, lead, arsenic] or drugs (i.e., phenothiazines, minocycline, amiodarone, chloroquine). Chrysiasis is a specific type of pseudocyanosis, characterized by a gray, blue, or purple pigmentation of areas exposed to light. It is a rare but dose-dependent complication of gold treatment that tends to cause permanent discoloration of the skin. Another example of pseudocyanosis is argyria, which is a slate blue to gray coloration of the skin resulting from either chronic ingestion or chronic local application of silver salts or colloidal silver. The color does not blanch with pressure, in contrast to true cyanotic skin, which will blanch. Skin biopsy confirms the diagnosis. Carboxyhemoglobinemia does not cause cyanosis. Occasionally, however, carboxyhemoglobinemia does produce a cherry-red flush of the skin, retina, or mucous membranes.

Cyanosis can be caused by methemoglobinemia and sulfhemoglobinemia. Most cases are due to acquired states secondary to chemicals or medications. Benzocaine, nitrates, and nitrites may produce methemoglobinemia. The sulfonamides, phenacetin, acetanilid, and aniline may produce sulfhemoglobinemia or methemoglobinemia. The incidence of acquired methemoglobinemia secondary to industrial exposure to aniline dyes and aromatic amino and nitro compounds has decreased with improvement in occupational health standards. Hereditary methemoglobinemia is a rare genetic disorder affecting the enzyme NADH-methemoglobin reductase, resulting in structural alterations of the hemoglobin molecule. The enzyme affects the major pathway responsible for converting methemoglobin to its reduced state. This pathway plays a clinically significant role in the treatment of methemoglobinemia because it is the pathway by which the antidote, methylene blue, is able to enhance the reduction of methemoglobin. Patients with NADH-methemoglobin reductase deficiency will appear cyanotic but have compensated and are usually asymptomatic.

Although there exist a wide number of drugs that can produce methemoglobinemia, no currently used drug does so at therapeutic dose levels. Acetanilid and phenacetin are aniline derivatives and frequent causes of methemoglobinemia and sulfhemoglobinemia. Certain sulfonamides and local anesthetics may produce methemoglobinemia. Methemoglobinemia is manifest clinically by cyanosis with as little as 1.5 g of methemoglobin present in 100 mL of blood. Since methemoglobin is incapable of binding with oxygen, the symptoms of methemoglobinemia are secondary to hypoxia. The severity is related to the quantity of methemoglobin present, the rapidity of onset,

and the patient's own cardiopulmonary system. Cyanotic patients without cardiovascular or pulmonary disease should be suspected of having methemoglobinemia, especially if cyanosis is not relieved by oxygen administration. Further, the venous blood will appear chocolate brown. Spectrophotometry is required for identification of the pigment and its quantity. In acquired methemoglobinemia, no treatment is necessary unless signs of hypoxia (i.e., angina, arrhythmias, hypotension, stupor, or coma) are present. Methylene blue in a dose of 1 to 2 mg per kilogram of body weight given intravenously over 5 min in a 1% solution is the antidote for acquired methemoglobinemia. Caution should be taken whenever methylene blue is used. By itself, at high doses, it can cause hemolysis and even precipitate methemoglobinemia and possibly worsen the patient's condition.

Sulfhemoglobinemia may result from one of the oxidizing drugs. Phenacetin (APC, Empirin compound) and acetanilid (Bromo Seltzer) are the most common causative agents. Sulfhemoglobin is inert as an oxygen carrier and when present can produce deep cyanosis at a level of less than 0.5 g of sulfhemoglobin per 100 mL of blood. Unlike methemoglobin, sulfhemoglobin is irreversible. Treatment is directed towards symptomatic and supportive care as well as the identification and removal of suspected agents.

## BIBLIOGRAPHY

Curry S: Methemoglobinemia. *Ann Emerg Med* 11:4, 1982.

Familton MJG, Armstrong RF: Pseudocyanosis: Time to reclassify cyanosis? *Anaesthesia* 44:3, 1989.

Gold W: Cyanosis, in *MacBryde's Signs and Symptoms: Applied Pathologic Physiology and Clinical Interpretation.* Philadelphia, Lippincott, 1983.

Goss GA, Hayes JA, Burden JGW: Deoxyhaemoglobin concentrations in the detection of central cyanosis. *Thorax* 43:212, 1988.

Jaffe ER: Methemoglobinemia in the differential diagnosis of cyanosis. *Hosp Pract* 20:12, 1985.

Lees MH, King DH: Cyanosis in the newborn. *Pediatr Rev* 9:2, 1987.

Martin L, Khalil H: How much reduced hemoglobin is necessary to generate central cyanosis? *Chest* 97:1, 1990.

Stadie WC: The oxygen of the arterial and venous blood in pneumonia and its relation to cyanosis. *J Exp Med* 30:215, 1991.

Szaflarski NL, Cohen NH: Use of pulse oximetry in critically ill adults. *Heart Lung* 18:444, 1989.

# 30
# SYNCOPE
## Andrew G. Wilson, Jr.

Syncope and death are the same—except that in one you wake up.
Anonymous

The foregoing aphorism summarizes the clinical dilemma of syncope. Syncope is the final common pathway of a number of pathophysiological disturbances, some of which carry substantial morbidity and mortality, and most of which demonstrate few objective findings in the emergency department. The challenge, then, is to distinguish those patients who may not wake up from a subsequent episode of syncope and who require admission to the hospital from those patients who require outpatient evaluation or simple reassurance.

## DEFINITION

Syncope is a sudden, transient loss of consciousness with loss of postural tone and with spontaneous recovery. Presyncope, a warning of syncope, shares, in most part, the pathophysiology and differential diagnosis for syncope.

## INCIDENCE

Syncope as a presenting complaint accounts for 1 to 3 percent of emergency department visits and may constitute 1 to 6 percent of hospital admissions. Depending on the specific population studied, and depending upon the motivation to admit or to deny the symptom, from 15 to 50 percent of young adults experience syncope. Syncope is common among at least some elderly populations, with 6 percent per year of residents of a chronic care institution experiencing syncope.

## PATHOPHYSIOLOGY AND CLINICAL FEATURES

The fundamental pathophysiology of syncope is simple: denial of oxygen to the brain, denial of glucose to the brain, and seizure activity of the brain. While hypoglycemia and seizure are relatively straightforward, cerebral anoxia may be a final result of multiple contributing factors. For example, in an elderly patient with severe cerebral atherosclerosis who is taking antihypertensive medication and who has age-related blunting of the postural vascular reflexes, a moderate bradycardia or tachycardia or a rapid change in posture may cause syncope. A younger person without the same pathophysiologic substrate may be unaware of the same or greater changes in heart rate.

The differential diagnosis of syncope is listed in Table 30-1. The first broad distinction to make in a patient with syncope is whether the interruption in consciousness was a seizure. If a seizure is unlikely, the manifold causes of fainting must be considered. These may be grouped, with a little artifice, into four categories: seizure disorder, cardiac, peripheral vascular, and miscellaneous.

### Seizure Disorders

Syncope due to a seizure is usually abrupt in onset. While an abrupt onset is shared with a few other causes of syncope, notably cardiac causes, disorientation after the event and a slow return to a normal mental status is a useful marker for seizure. On the other hand, a prodrome, other than an aura, including sweats or nausea militate against

**Table 30-1.** Causes of Syncope

Seizure disorder
Cardiac
  Arrhythmias
    Bradycardia
    Tachycardia
  Obstruction to flow
    Left ventricular outflow—valvular, cardiomyopathy
    Right ventricular outflow—valvular, pulmonary embolism, pulmonary
      hypertension
  Ischemic: myocardial infarction
Peripheral vascular
  Vasovagal
  Orthostatic
  Drug induced
  Situational—micturition, defecation, cough, swallow
  Carotid sinus sensitivity
  Cerebrovascular—posterior circulation TIA, subclavian steal
  Neuralgias—glossopharyngeal and trigeminal
Miscellaneous
  Hypoglycemia
  Hyperventilation
  Psychogenic

a seizure. Injury, tongue biting, and incontinence of urine or feces are not useful in discriminating a "fit" from a "faint." One must realize clearly that seizure activity in association with a loss of consciousness does not define a seizure as the cause. Cerebral anoxia often produces clonic jerks and may precipitate a generalized seizure, termed *convulsive syncope.*

### Cardiac Causes

Cardiac causes of syncope fall into three groups: rhythm disturbances, ventricular outflow obstructive processes, and myocardial ischemia. Because cardiac causes of syncope are at once among the most lethal and the most remediable, identification of cardiac syncope can be crucial. Significant rhythm disturbances, when found in temporal proximity to syncope, may be suspected of causing syncope. However, proving a cause-and-effect relationship between an arrhythmia and syncope may be most difficult. The degree of arrhythmia tolerated by a given patient is dependent on many factors such as age, intravascular volume, position, and vagal tone. In general, to be considered as the cause of syncope, the heart rate should be over 150 or under 40 bpm. Any process causing acute or chronic obstruction to ventricular inflow or outflow may cause syncope. For the left ventricle, these processes include aortic stenosis (valvular or subvalvular), atrial myxoma, or mitral stenosis. For the right ventricle, pulmonary embolism and pulmonary hypertension are important considerations. Syncope in association with cardiac ischemia is usually secondary to arrhythmia or with-effort angina pectoris. Theories on the pathophysiology of the latter postulate an inability of the heart to increase output in response to demand, increased vagal tone, and hyperventilation. Cardiac syncope should be suspected in patients with structural or electrical heart disease, especially with superimposed new cardiac symptoms. Cardiac syncope may occur with the patient in any position and usually has an abrupt onset and prompt (less than 1 min) resolution.

### Peripheral Vascular Disorders

The peripheral vascular causes of syncope are the most diverse and include vasovagal syncope, orthostatic hypotension, carotid sinus hypersensitivity, and cerebrovascular circulation. The unifying concept is that, whatever the inciting phenomenon, a tendency to venous pooling of blood is increased. Pooling of blood in capacitance vessels decreases venous return, cardiac output, and, finally, cerebral perfusion, resulting in syncope. Factors such as drugs, peripheral neuropathy, and counterproductive reflexes can defeat the vascular responses needed to assume and maintain a standing position.

The most common cause of syncope is vasovagal syncope—the common faint. Vasovagal syncope is mediated by a paradoxical withdrawal of the cardiac and peripheral vascular tone required for an upright posture—the Bezold-Jarisch reflex. Normally, assumption of an upright posture causes pooling of blood in the lower extremities, resulting in decreased cardiac filling pressure, stroke volume, and arterial pressure. These changes are compensated for by increased sympathetic tone, resulting in vasoconstriction and tachycardia, and diminished parasympathetic tone. In patients with vasovagal syncope, the compensatory response is interrupted in a few minutes by a paradoxical withdrawal of sympathetic stimulation and a replacement by enhanced parasympathetic (vagal) activity. Current theory holds that this reflex is mediated by excessive activation of cardiac mechanoreceptors, which have connections to the brainstem. The excessive activation of the mechanoreceptors may be due to mechanical or chemical factors during a period of sympathetic excitation. In some patients, the mechanoreceptors may be hypersensitive. As the pathophysiology of vasovagal syncope becomes better defined, new synonyms are gaining greater currency, among these are cardioinhibitory and neurocardiogenic syncope. Clues to vasovagal syncope include the appropriate setting (fear, injury, sight of blood, illness); upright posture; and a warning period of progressive symptoms such as a feeling of warmth, light-headedness, nausea, roaring in the ears, and a dimming of vision, culminating in a loss of consciousness. After the syncopal episode, recovery should be prompt, that is, within seconds. The exception to this rule is when a well-intentioned bystander keeps the victim propped up, slowing resolution of symptoms. Although vasovagal syncope can occur at any age, be reluctant to make the diagnosis in a first episode occurring after age 40. Be reluctant, as well, to use the diagnosis as one of convenience; require the appropriate setting and warning symptoms as outlined. Because the symptoms of vasovagal syncope reflect nothing more than slowly progressive global cerebral ischemia, be wary of other conditions, such as cardiac arrhythmias, which can also occasionally have a slowly progressive onset.

Orthostatic syncope is caused by hypotension on assuming an upright position. The diagnosis may be made if the patient has symptoms in association with an orthostatic fall in systolic blood pressure of at least 25 mmHg or a fall to less than 90 mmHg. Blood pressures should be measured after the patient has been supine for 5 min, with the patient supine, sitting, immediately on standing, and after standing for 2 min. There may be multiple contributing factors to orthostatic syncope. These include intravascular volume depletion, arising after prolonged recumbency, diseases affecting control of capacitance vessels (diabetes mellitus, amyloid, Shy-Drager syndrome), and some drugs.

Drugs may cause or contribute to syncope in several ways. They may precipitate arrhythmias, aggravate orthostatic hypotension (antihypertensives), or cause volume depletions (diuretics). The clinician should seek a history of use of the medications listed in Table 30-2. The drugs most commonly associated with syncope are nitrates, diuretics, and antiarrhythmics. Drugs may be considered as etiologic agents when orthostatic hypotension with syncope is found or a drug-related arrhythmia is present (e.g., digitalis toxicity, or torsade de pointes). Usually syncope associated with overdoses or with anaphylactic reactions does not pose diagnostic difficulties.

Carotid sinus hypersensitivity is a very uncommon cause of syncope in the younger patient and accounts for fewer than 5 percent of cases in the elderly. Two types are described, vasodepressor and cardioinhibitory. The diagnosis should be suspected in elderly patients whose immediately presyncopal state is suggestive of carotid sinus stimulation, e.g., wearing a tight collar, shaving, or head turning. One should also include this possibility in elderly patients with a recurrent syncope of unknown cause. If carotid sinus hypersensitivity is suspected, carotid sinus massage may be performed at the bedside. First, ensure that there are no carotid bruits. Second, establish venous access and a cardiac monitor, with atropine available. Third, place the patient supine. Fourth, gently massage each carotid in turn while monitoring heart rate and blood pressure. A positive response is asystole of 3 s or greater, or a drop in systolic blood pressure of 50 mmHg or more. If the vasodepressor type is suggested and massage is negative in the supine position, massage may be repeated in the sitting and standing positions, with appropriate protection from fall injuries for the patient. The examiner must be aware that this is not a specific test, as about 30 percent of nonsyncopal elderly people will have a positive response.

The remaining causes of peripheral vascular syncope include syncope associated with special circumstances such as coughing, micturition, defecation, and swallowing. Causes include reflex-mediated

**Table 30-2.** Drugs Associated with Syncope

| | |
|---|---|
| Antidepressants | Diuretics |
| Antiarrhythmias | Nitrates |
| Antihypertensives | Phenothiazines |
| Beta blockers | Recreational drugs |
| Calcium channel blockers | Alcohol |
| Cardiac glycosides | Cocaine |

changes in venous pressure, heart rate, and cardiac output. The diagnosis may be made if syncope occurs during or immediately after the activity in question.

Syncope due to primary cerebral ischemia, or a transient ischemic attack, is rare. When present, it is referable to the vertebrobasilar circulation as the vertebrobasilar arteries supply the reticular activating system. Such episodes are called "drop attacks." Syncope due to anterior circulation transient ischemic attacks would require bilateral simultaneous compromise of circulation to the cerebral hemispheres and is only theoretically possible. If one entertains the diagnosis of a transient ischemic attack as the cause of syncope, focal neurologic symptoms and signs should be reported by the patient. The brainstem is a compact structure with multiple functions, and other symptoms of brainstem ischemia should be present for syncope to be ascribed to this mechanism. Cerebrovascular disease may be a contributing factor, however, to other causes of syncope, especially in the elderly.

The subclavian steal syndrome should be sought if a blood pressure difference between the arms of at least 20 mmHg is noted, or if upper extremity exercise seems to be associated with syncope. In this entity, an obstruction of the brachiocephalic or subclavian artery causes shunting of blood through the vertebrobasilar system from the normal side past the obstruction, resulting, in effect, in a brainstem transient ischemic attack.

Glossopharyngeal and trigeminal neuralgias are thought to precipitate syncope through peripheral vasodilation and bradycardia. The characteristic pain syndromes make identification of neuralgic causes of syncope possible.

## Miscellaneous

Three miscellaneous causes of syncope are worthy of mention. First is hypoglycemia, a frequent cause of coma but an unusual cause of syncope. The usual setting is that of a diabetic taking a hypoglycemic agent, usually insulin. The incidence of syncopal hypoglycemia in the absence of hypoglycemic agents is probably rare. Second is hyperventilation, a frequent cause of presyncope and sometimes a cause of syncope. Hypocarbia causes cerebral vasoconstriction and peripheral vasodilatation. Syncope, or at least presyncope, should be reproducible by a trial of hyperventilation in the emergency department. One should ascertain that hyperventilation in a given patient is psychogenic, and not secondary to an underlying cause such as pulmonary embolism. Third, psychiatric illnesses may account for syncope in a substantial number of patients. Psychogenic syncope is a diagnosis of exclusion but may be considered in planning for follow-up for patients with recurrent, unexplained syncope.

## DIAGNOSIS

The goal in the emergency department evaluation of a patient with syncope is to establish the cause so that the physician can best determine whether outpatient or inpatient management is appropriate. If a diagnosis cannot be established, then the physician must determine whether the patient is in a high-risk group and, if so, have the patient admitted for further evaluation.

The difficulty in establishing a diagnosis for a patient with syncope reflects the nature of syncope. It is, by definition, a transient phenomenon, with evanescent findings and with a plethora of underlying pathophysiologic mechanisms. Diagnostic criteria are not firmly established and have tended to change over time. Further, syncope is an interdisciplinary malady and each specialist brings the baggage of each specialty to the study of syncope. Many studies of syncope demonstrate selection bias and lack of diagnostic standardization. Therefore, only rather general statements can be made about the frequencies of various diagnoses and about the increasingly numerous and sophisticated tests that establish those diagnoses. In those patients in whom a diagnosis was established, a distillation of frequencies is as follows: vasovagal, 30 percent; cardiac (structural and electrical), 30 percent; orthostatic, 10 percent; drug-induced, 10 percent; situational, 8 percent; the remaining causes account for fewer than 5 percent each. Although a greater proportion of patients with syncope are now receiving diagnoses, even after extensive investigation 40 to 50 percent of patients do not have an etiology established. However, in those patients with a diagnosis, about half are established with the history, physical examination, and a 12-lead electrocardiogram. Further, those basic tools allow the emergency physician to place the patient in a high-risk or a low-risk group.

The history and physical examination are aimed especially at determining what happened in the event and at detecting evidence of heart disease. The syncopal event may be considered in three phases: presyncopal, syncopal, and postsyncopal. The presyncopal phase consists of the patient's position, activities, premonitory symptoms, and environment. The description of the syncopal event itself must be obtained from others. Such information as duration of unconsciousness, rapidity of recovery, seizure activity, skin color, and presence of diaphoresis should be sought from witnesses. The history of postsyncopal events should be focused on time to recovery and any residua. Other elements of the history include past history (especially of heart disease), medication history, and any directed history that may be suggested, such as bleeding or other intravascular volume loss. The physical examination should be complete but should especially note orthostatic hypotension and cardiovascular and neurologic abnormalities.

Laboratory evaluations should be directed—for example, a hemoglobin determination when there is suspicion of blood loss—and are unlikely to be of help unless a specific concern is identified by the history and physical examination.

A 12-lead electrocardiogram is a valuable test and may provide a diagnosis of ischemia, arrhythmia, or conduction abnormality in up to 10 percent of patients. Electrocardiographic evidence of underlying structural or electrical heart disease places the patient at high risk for subsequent morbidity and mortality. It is also reasonable to place the syncope patient on a cardiac monitor while in the emergency department to identify arrhythmias.

If a strong suspicion of seizure as a cause of syncope exists, an electroencephalogram and CT scan of the head may be useful. However, these tests are neither sensitive nor specific in the general syncope patient population.

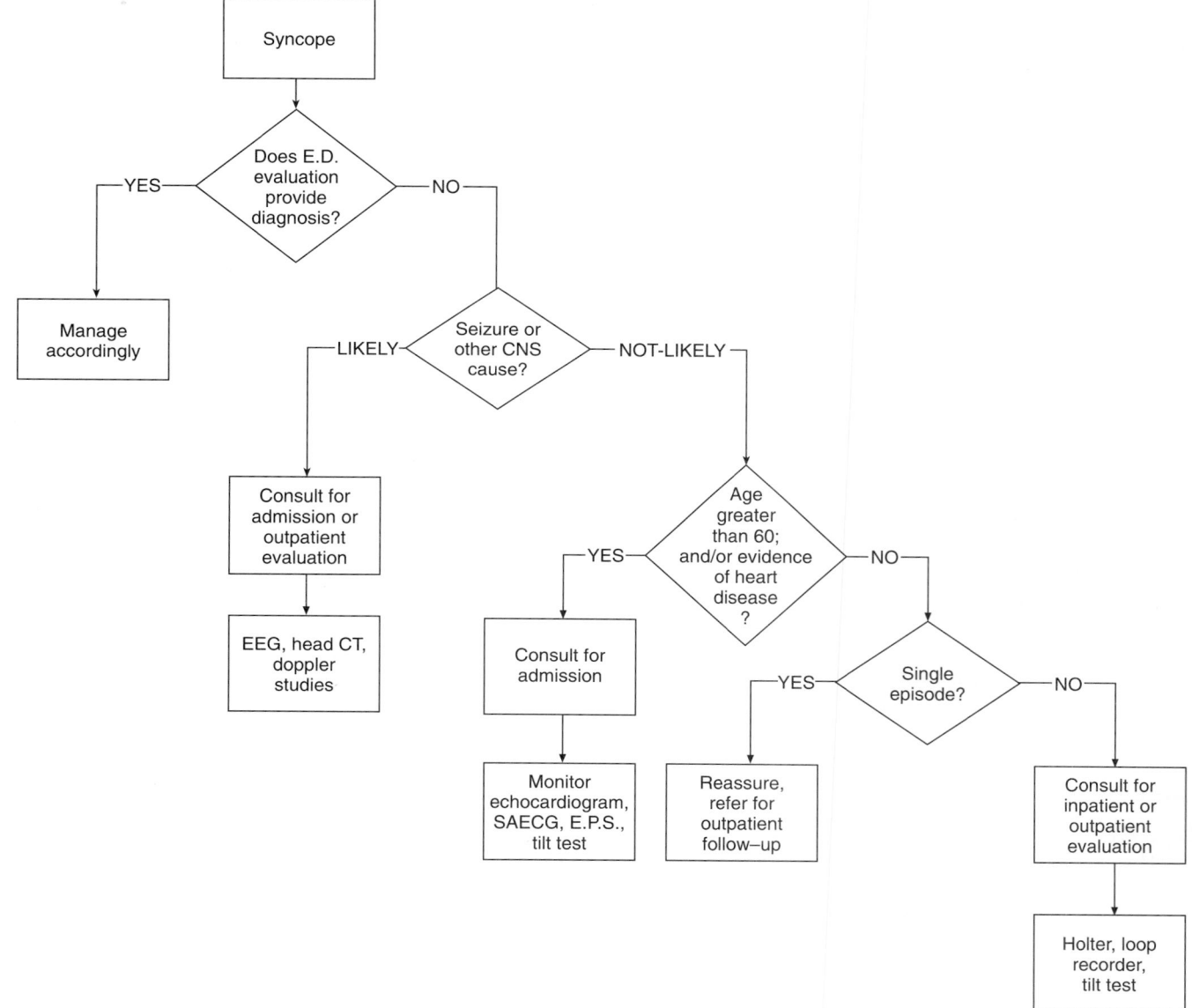

**Fig. 30-1.** Evaluation of syncopal patient.

Figure 30-1 is presented as our emergency department perspective on the referral and subsequent evaluation of syncope patients. It is impossible, with our present state of knowledge, to be specific about which subsequent tests are appropriate for which patients.

## DISPOSITION

The disposition of the patient with syncope, in the absence of a diagnosis, is directed by an assessment of subsequent risk of mortality and morbidity for that patient. Two high-risk groups emerge: the elderly (age >60) and those with heart disease and/or an established cardiac cause of syncope. Heart disease may be structural (e.g., coronary artery disease, valvular disease, cardiomyopathy, congestive heart failure) or electrical (e.g., conduction disturbances, arrhythmias). Admission should be considered for those high-risk groups. It is worth noting that there is no demonstrated benefit accruing to admission for high-risk patients, but monitoring and noninvasive and invasive testing may be expedited.

At the other end of the risk spectrum is the younger patient without heart disease, with an unknown cause of a single episode of syncope. Such patients are at no greater risk of sudden death than their age-matched cohorts. They may be reassured and referred for outpatient follow-up. The patient should be cautioned that recurrence of syncope should prompt a visit to a follow-up physician or to the emergency department.

There remains the middle group on the spectrum. This group possesses a broad range of characteristics, from young with multiple episodes to older with one or more comorbidities. Such patients must be considered individually, in consultation with their personal physicians or with consultants. For those patients in this group who are discharged, outpatient evaluation such as Holter or loop monitoring may be initiated from the emergency department.

## BIBLIOGRAPHY

Kapoor WN: Evaluation and management of the patient with syncope. *JAMA* 18:2553, 1992.

Scott WA: Evaluating the child with syncope. *Pediatr Ann* 7:350, 1991.

Sneddon JF, Camm AJ: Vasovagal syncope: Classification, investigation and treatment. *Br J Hosp Med* 5:329, 1993.

Wright K, McIntosh HD: Syncope: A review of pathophysiological mechanisms. *Prog Cardiovasc Dis* 13:580, 1971.

# 31
# ABDOMINAL PAIN

### William D. Fales
### David T. Overton

---

**IMMEDIATE LIFE THREATS**

Abdominal aortic aneurysm
Splenic rupture
Ectopic pregnancy
Myocardial infarction

---

Abdominal pain is one of the most common presenting complaints in the emergency department. In up to 42 percent of patients, however, the etiology remains obscure. Further, misdiagnosis has been reported to occur in up to 30 percent.

## TYPES OF ABDOMINAL PAIN

Three distinct types of pain response may be involved in the genesis of abdominal pain: visceral, somatic, and referred. A basic understanding of these pain responses aids the clinician in establishing a differential diagnosis.

### Visceral Pain

Visceral (splanchnic) abdominal pain results from stretching of the autonomic nerve fibers surrounding a hollow or solid viscus. Obstruction is a common cause. The pain may be described as crampy, colicky, or gaseous and is often intermittent. Pure visceral pain is felt in the midline, the exact location depending on the embryologic origin of the intraabdominal organ involved. Foregut structures (stomach, duodenum, pancreatic-biliary tree) classically are referred in the epigastrium. Midgut structures (small bowel, ascending colon) are referred to the periumbilical area. Hindgut structures (descending colon) are referred to the suprapubic area or lower back.

Despite these typical patterns, visceral pain is usually ill defined and diffuse, and the patient may be surprised to find a disparity between the location of pain and the location of tenderness on examination. Visceral pain is an early manifestation of many disorders, including appendicitis, cholecystitis, bowel obstruction, and renal colic.

### Somatic Pain

Somatic (parietal) pain occurs when pain fibers located in the parietal peritoneum are irritated by chemical or bacterial inflammation. Somatic pain is generally sharper, more constant, and more precisely localized to the area of disease. It represents the inflammation which often occurs subsequent to the obstruction of visceral pain. There is usually tenderness localized to the area of pathology, an important diagnostic feature.

### Referred Pain

Referred pain is any pain felt at a distance from the diseased organ. Thus, in a strict sense, some kinds of visceral and somatic pain are types of referred pain. Referred pain generally follows certain classic patterns. For instance, diaphragmatic irritation, due to subphrenic collections of pus or blood, often radiates to the supraclavicular area. The pain of ureteral colic often radiates to the lower quadrants, genitalia, or inner thigh.

By thorough history taking and careful, often repeated, physical examination, the clinician may use this knowledge of pain classification to more accurately distinguish causes of pain. For instance, patients with appendicitis classically report an initial phase of ill-defined discomfort localized to the periumbilical or epigastric area, which is a visceral pain corresponding to obstruction and distention of the appendiceal lumen. Tenderness at this phase is generally vague and poorly localized. Later, as the appendix becomes progressively more inflamed and irritates the surrounding parietal peritoneum, the perceived area of pain migrates to the right lower quadrant. This somatic pain is accompanied by the development of tenderness localized to McBurney's point.

## ORIGINS OF ABDOMINAL PAIN

Abdominal pain can arise from one of several origins: intraabdominal, extraabdominal, metabolic, or neurogenic.

### Intraabdominal Origin

Pain arising from intraabdominal origins can be divided into three categories: peritoneal inflammation, obstruction of a hollow viscus, and vascular disorders.

## Peritoneal Inflammation

Peritonitis is the somatic pain caused by inflammation of the peritoneum by an irritant. This irritant can be aseptic (e.g., gastric juice, bile, pancreatic juice, blood, or urine) or of bacterial origin. Peritoneal inflammation can be either primary or, more commonly, secondary. Primary ("spontaneous") peritonitis is a condition chiefly caused by *Pneumococcus, Streptococcus, Escherichia coli,* or *Mycobacterium tuberculosis.* It is most often seen in cirrhotic patients, or others with ascites. Secondary peritonitis is caused by disease or injury of the abdominal or pelvic viscera. Its microbiology parallels that of the gut flora and is often polymicrobial, involving both aerobes and anaerobes. Many causes of the acute abdomen, such as appendicitis, cholecystitis, and mesenteric infarction, eventually lead to peritoneal inflammation.

## Obstruction of a Hollow Viscus

Obstruction of the intestine, ureter, or biliary tree produces the typical colicky sensation characteristic of visceral pain. Intestinal obstruction typically leads to colicky abdominal pain, nausea, and vomiting. Vomiting tends to be more pronounced the more proximal the obstruction. There may be a decrease in rectal gas. Abdominal distention may at first be discernible only on radiograph but eventually becomes clinically evident. The most common cause is adhesions from previous surgery, but other causes, such as hernias, neoplasm, and volvulus, may also be involved.

## Vascular Disorders

Bowel infarction and aortic dissection, leakage, or rupture represent the major vascular emergencies associated with acute abdominal pain. Bowel ischemia or infarction is a difficult and often delayed diagnosis. Classically, the early symptoms are severe, diffuse abdominal pain, with a paucity of physical findings. Systemic toxicity follows, with fever, acidosis, and shock. Hematemesis and loose, bloody stools tend to be late findings. Patients are often elderly, with underlying cardiovascular disease. Mortality is high.

An expanding or leaking abdominal aortic aneurysm is a true vascular emergency. It is characterized by abdominal pain, often radiating to the back, flank, or genitalia, and eventually, hypotension and cardiovascular collapse. It is easily mistaken for the pain of renal colic, so much so that when evaluating renal colic patients, the clinician should consciously keep the possibility of an aortic aneurysm in mind.

## Extraabdominal Origin

A number of extraabdominal sources can lead to pain which is subjectively felt by the patient to arise in the abdomen. These include the abdominal wall, the pelvis, and the thorax.

Abdominal wall pain is usually traumatic in origin and may be caused by muscle strain, hematoma, or contusion. It is often accentuated by abdominal wall muscle contraction.

Intrathoracic disease, including pneumonia, pulmonary embolism, pneumothorax, and esophageal disease, may present as abdominal pain. Children with pneumonia commonly present with abdominal, rather than pulmonary, complaints. Acute myocardial ischemia may have many subtle presentations, particularly in the elderly and diabetics. Nausea, vomiting, diaphoresis, and vague abdominal distress may be the only clues to this life-threatening disorder. For this reason, clinicians should consider including an electrocardiogram in the evaluation of patients over the age of 40 with upper abdominal pain.

Pain from pelvic sources is usually reported as abdominal pain by the layperson. Disorders such as salpingitis, tuboovarian abscess, ovarian cyst torsion or rupture, or abortion commonly present with abdominal pain. Ectopic pregnancy is a common cause of acute abdominal pain in women and should be included in the differential diagnosis of these patients.

## Metabolic Disorders

A number of metabolic disorders may cause pain in the abdomen. Perhaps the most common is diabetic ketoacidosis. In this instance, it is important to rule out true, intraabdominal pathology as a factor which exacerbated the diabetes. Sickle cell crisis, porphyria, spider and scorpion bites, heavy-metal intoxication, systemic lupus erythematosus, and periarteritis nodosa can all present with abdominal pain as the predominant symptom.

## Neurogenic Causes

The preeruptive phase of herpes zoster can lead to confusing abdominal pain. Spinal disk disease and the now unusual crisis of tabes dorsalis may also present with abdominal pain.

# CLINICAL APPROACH TO THE PATIENT WITH ACUTE ABDOMINAL PAIN

With virtually any chief complaint, but with abdominal pain in particular, the clinician should keep in mind a list of immediate life threats. The initial approach to the patient should bear these in mind, with the institution of immediate resuscitative and stabilization procedures, if necessary.

## History

A detailed, careful history is the first step. The clinician should keep in mind the importance of individual patient variables (cultural, socioeconomic, educational, etc.), and confirmation of history with family or friends may be helpful.

The time of onset of pain, as well as severity at the onset, should be noted. Typically, the pain of aortic dissection, peptic ulcer perforation, and renal colic are abrupt in onset, while that of appendicitis is more gradual. The location of pain and its referral, both at the onset and subsequently, are important (see Fig. 31-1). The character of the pain (colicky, steady, sharp, burning, tearing, gnawing, aching, etc.) and its severity are helpful.

The symptoms of anorexia, nausea, and vomiting so often accompany acute abdominal distress as to limit their usefulness in distinguishing etiologies. However, persistent vomiting may result in dehydration. Diarrhea and the presence of blood in either the diarrhea or vomitus should be noted. A chronic change in bowel habits may suggest an underlying malignancy. Dysuria, frequency, or hematuria suggest a urinary source. However, inflammatory conditions such as appendicitis can produce such symptoms if the inflamed appendix is in proximity to the ureter. A thorough gynecologic history is indicated in women with abdominal pain, including a pregnancy and menstrual history and a history of sexual activity and contraception. However, it is well recognized that patients may conceal such information, so a high index of suspicion is warranted.

Cardiorespiratory symptoms such as chest pain, shortness of breath, cough, sputum, hemoptysis, and orthopnea may suggest a thoracic source of pain. Any prior occurrence of similar symptoms should be sought. Other past medical history, including operations, diseases, and drug intake, especially steroids, antibiotics, or nonsteroidal anti-inflammatory agents should be elicited.

## Physical Examination

The patient's general appearance should be noted, especially such signs as diaphoresis and pallor. Patients with visceral pain often are doubled over and tend to move about searching for a comfortable position. Patients with peritonitis, on the other hand, tend to lie still and resist movement. Jarring the bed or tapping on the heels may exacerbate their discomfort. The vital signs should be inspected. Tachycardia, hypotension, or orthostatic changes suggest volume depletion. Fever may be present in many abdominal conditions, but its absence

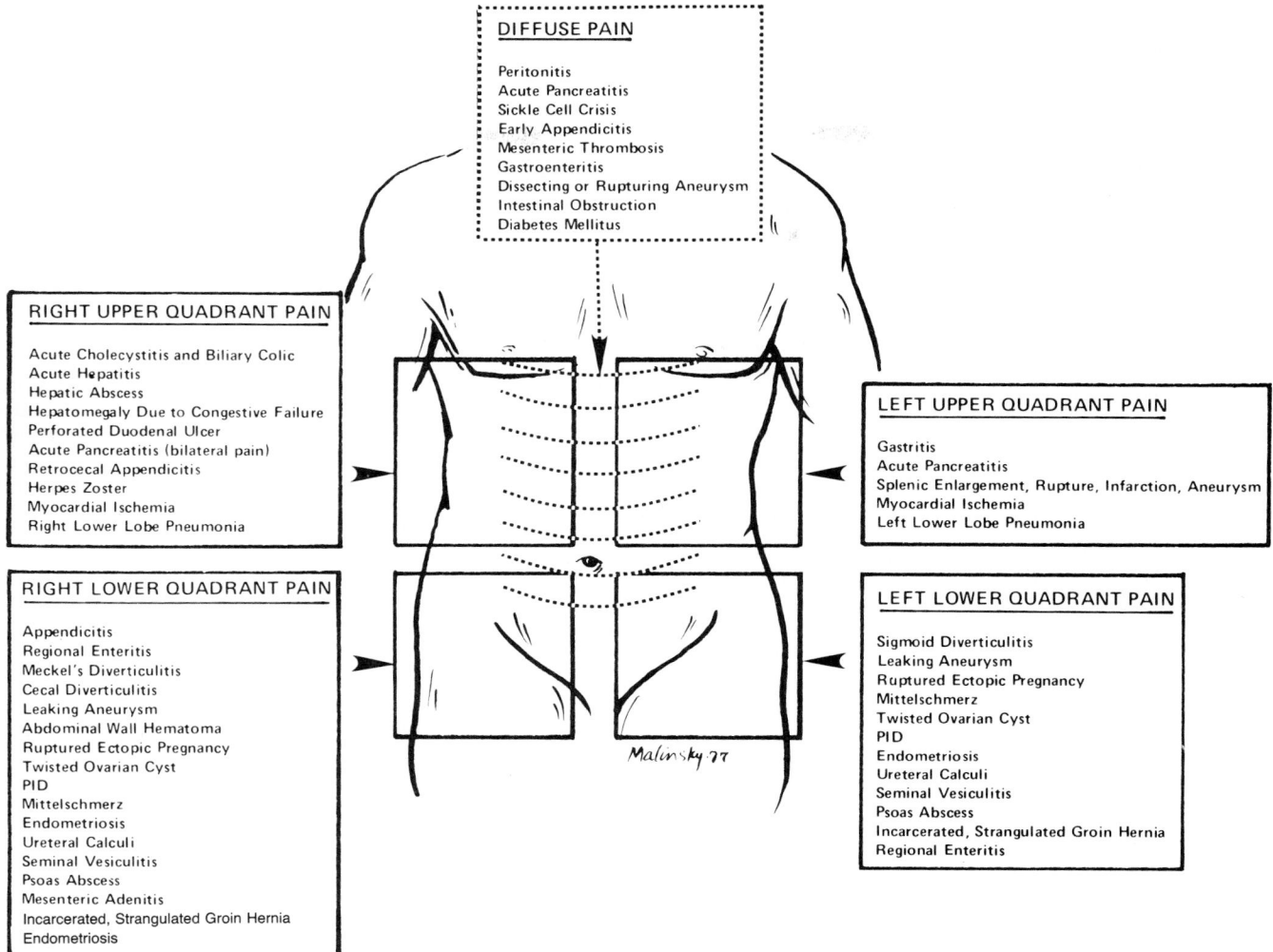

**DIFFUSE PAIN**

Peritonitis
Acute Pancreatitis
Sickle Cell Crisis
Early Appendicitis
Mesenteric Thrombosis
Gastroenteritis
Dissecting or Rupturing Aneurysm
Intestinal Obstruction
Diabetes Mellitus

**RIGHT UPPER QUADRANT PAIN**

Acute Cholecystitis and Biliary Colic
Acute Hepatitis
Hepatic Abscess
Hepatomegaly Due to Congestive Failure
Perforated Duodenal Ulcer
Acute Pancreatitis (bilateral pain)
Retrocecal Appendicitis
Herpes Zoster
Myocardial Ischemia
Right Lower Lobe Pneumonia

**LEFT UPPER QUADRANT PAIN**

Gastritis
Acute Pancreatitis
Splenic Enlargement, Rupture, Infarction, Aneurysm
Myocardial Ischemia
Left Lower Lobe Pneumonia

**RIGHT LOWER QUADRANT PAIN**

Appendicitis
Regional Enteritis
Meckel's Diverticulitis
Cecal Diverticulitis
Leaking Aneurysm
Abdominal Wall Hematoma
Ruptured Ectopic Pregnancy
Twisted Ovarian Cyst
PID
Mittelschmerz
Endometriosis
Ureteral Calculi
Seminal Vesiculitis
Psoas Abscess
Mesenteric Adenitis
Incarcerated, Strangulated Groin Hernia
Endometriosis

**LEFT LOWER QUADRANT PAIN**

Sigmoid Diverticulitis
Leaking Aneurysm
Ruptured Ectopic Pregnancy
Mittelschmerz
Twisted Ovarian Cyst
PID
Endometriosis
Ureteral Calculi
Seminal Vesiculitis
Psoas Abscess
Incarcerated, Strangulated Groin Hernia
Regional Enteritis

Malinsky '77

**Fig. 31-1.** Differential diagnosis of acute abdominal pain by location. [From Wagner DK: Approaches to the patient with acute abdominal pain. *Current Topics* (a program of the Medical College of Pennsylvania) 1:3, 1978. Used by permission.]

should not be given undue emphasis. Studies have shown that a large percentage of patients with appendicitis present with normal temperatures. High fever with shaking chills is typical of pyelonephritis and pneumonia.

The abdomen should be inspected for contour, scars, peristalsis, masses, distension, or pulsation. The Cullen sign (bluish umbilicus) and the Grey Turner sign (ecchymosis of the abdomen or flank) are unusual signs of internal hemorrhage. Auscultation should precede palpation. The diagnostic yield of abdominal auscultation is lower than that of palpation, especially in a noisy emergency environment. However, the presence and character of bowel sounds should be noted, as well as any bruits present.

Palpation is the most important physical examination modality available. It should be performed by the warmed hand in a comfortable environment. Placement of pillows under the head and knees, or having the supine patient bend the knees, may allow the abdominal musculature to relax. Palpation should be gentle, with only one or two fingers being necessary. It should begin at an area distal from the suspected location of pain. Tenderness is the patient's subjective feeling of pain exacerbated by the examiner's palpation. "Guarding" is muscular contraction in response to palpation. Involuntary guarding is the same as rigidity, which is reflex spasm of the abdominal musculature. Masses and organomegaly should be sought. Turning the patient on the right side may aid palpation of the left upper quadrant.

Certain physical signs may be of additional benefit. Murphy's sign (inspiratory arrest) is elicited with the examining fingers held under the right costal margin while asking the patient to inspire. Painful midcycle arrest of inspiration occurs when an inflamed gallbladder comes into contact with the examining fingers. The Rovsing sign is pain in the right lower quadrant upon palpation of the left iliac fossa and may be present in appendicitis. The iliopsoas sign is elicited by asking the supine patient to keep the right knee extended and flex the thigh against the resistance of the examiner's hand. Pain in the pelvis indicates irritation of the iliopsoas muscle, as in appendicitis. The obturator sign is elicited by having the supine patient flex the right knee to 90°. The examiner immobilizes the ankle and moves the knee laterally and medially, causing internal and external rotation. Pain in the pelvis also suggests appendicitis.

A genital examination is important in both males and females and should include a check for inguinal and femoral hernias. A pelvic examination is typically recommended in all postpubertal females.

During the rectal examination the entire lower pelvis should be explored with the examining finger, checking for tenderness and masses. Tenderness in the right lower quadrant may be found in acute appendicitis. The examiner should ask the patient to distinguish between the general discomfort of the examination and actual tenderness.

## Laboratory Evaluation

Laboratory evaluation, although helpful, cannot supplant a careful history and physical examination. The CBC is an integral part of the evaluation of the acute abdomen, but its limitations must be appreciated. Inflammatory conditions of surgical import such as appendicitis often have normal white blood cell counts. The hematocrit usually will not accurately reflect acute blood loss. However, serial values, together with careful clinical reevaluation, may be of value. The urinalysis may reveal hematuria, which is present in most, but not all, cases of renal colic. Pyuria suggests urinary tract infection but may be present when an inflammatory mass lies in close proximity to the urinary tract. The serum amylase level may be elevated in a number of conditions, including pancreatitis, biliary obstruction, cholecystitis, bowel obstruction, bowel infarction, salpingitis, or ectopic pregnancy, or may be of salivary origin. A pregnancy test is valuable in women of childbearing age. Improvements in technology have made urinary tests more sensitive and specific. Serum measurements of the β subunit of human chorionic gonadotropin are very sensitive and a negative value virtually excludes the diagnosis of ectopic pregnancy.

An electrocardiogram should be considered in patients over 40, especially with upper abdominal or nonspecific symptomatology. Cardiac ischemia can and does present in atypical manners, and the presence of arrhythmias, such as atrial fibrillation, is associated with intestinal infarction.

## Imaging Studies

The standard abdominal series, usually consisting of flat and upright views of the abdomen, as well as an upright view of the chest, has long been considered to be standard in the evaluation of abdominal pain. The flat plate may disclose biliary or renal calculi; air in the biliary tree; abnormal vascular calcifications, such as that of an aortic aneurysm; and abnormal gas patterns. An upright view may disclose air-fluid levels. The upright chest film may disclose free peritoneal air, or intrathoracic pathology related to abdominal pain. A right lateral decubitus view of the abdomen may also reveal free air.

A number of studies, however, have questioned the utility of standard radiographs. Several have recommended the use of the upright abdominal view only when obstruction or ileus are suspected clinically. Still others have questioned the use of abdominal x-rays at all in patients with mild, nonspecific abdominal pain, uncomplicated gastrointestinal bleeding, or suspected ureteral colic.

Barium contrast studies have traditionally had limited usefulness and availability to the emergency physician. Recently, however, increasing use of these procedures in the emergency environment has occurred. The barium enema may prove helpful in the evaluation of suspected appendicitis in patients with equivocal findings. The barium enema is the diagnostic and therapeutic procedure of choice in intussusception. It may be of further value in patients with volvulus and other cases of suspected large bowel obstruction. Complications of barium enema are rare, but include perforation and barium extravasation.

Ultrasonography is a valuable diagnostic technique in a number of causes of the acute abdomen. It is a superior imaging procedure in patients with right upper quadrant pain. Cholelithiasis, choledocholithiasis, cholecystitis, and biliary duct dilatation can all be detected, as well as solid or cystic pancreatic masses. Hydroureter can be seen. Ultrasonography is of particular value in the evaluation of lower abdominal pain in women in childbearing age groups. Intrauterine and ectopic pregnancies, ovarian and tubal pathology, and free intraperitoneal fluid can be detected. Graded compression sonography has been shown to be useful in the evaluation of suspected appendicitis with equivocal findings. Ultrasonography is also very useful in evaluating abdominal aortic aneurysms. However, in the unstable patient with an acutely leaking or expanding aneurysm, the diagnosis is clinical and the treatment immediate.

Radioisotope studies using $^{99m}$Tc-IDA have been found to be quite sensitive and specific for the cystic duct obstruction associated with acute cholecystitis. The procedure does take a number of hours to complete, making it somewhat less useful to the emergency physician.

## Laparoscopy

Laparoscopy is reported to be a useful adjunct in the evaluation of selected cases of acute abdominal pain. The difficult distinction between appendicitis and gynecologic pathology can often be made, avoiding laparotomy in a number of patients.

## Computer-Aided Diagnosis

There has been a great deal of interest in using computers to assist in diagnosing acute abdominal pain. Extensive studies, primarily in Europe, have demonstrated improved diagnostic and decision-making abilities. However, this improvement has been attributed to the more comprehensive collection of clinical data using structured forms rather than the use of artificial intelligence.

## ANALGESIA

Classic surgical teaching states that it is contraindicated to administer analgesics to patients with abdominal pain before a definitive diagnosis and plan of action is made. Recently, this viewpoint has been challenged. In the 18th edition of *Cope's Early Diagnosis of the Acute Abdomen,* Silen condemns the traditional practice of deferred analgesia in acute abdominal pain. Attard et al. demonstrated that the early administration of opiate analgesia in acute abdominal pain greatly reduced patient discomfort and did not interfere with diagnosis. Thus, upon completion of a thorough history and physical examination, the careful and judicious use of analgesics by the emergency physician is humane and appropriate.

Analgesia in acute abdominal pain is typically managed by short-acting intravenous narcotics, such as fentanyl, titrated to achieve patient comfort. Recent studies also support the use of nonsteroidal anti-inflammatory agents, either parenterally or rectally, in the treatment of renal colic.

## ABDOMINAL PAIN IN THE GERIATRIC PATIENT

While the causes of acute abdominal pain in the elderly are similar to the causes in younger adults, the relative frequencies of the various conditions differ. Conditions that are more commonly encountered in the elderly include sigmoid volvulus, diverticulitis, acute mesenteric ischemia, and abdominal aortic aneurysm. The geriatric population continues to be at risk for problems such as acute appendicitis, acute cholecystitis, peptic ulcer disease, and intestinal obstruction.

It is not uncommon for elderly patients to have delays in the diagnosis of acute abdominal disorders. They may fail to manifest the same degree of pain or tenderness, fever, vital sign abnormalities, or laboratory findings as do younger adults. Elderly patients with peritonitis may lack abdominal rigidity, fever, or leukocytosis. Further, they may fail to seek early medical attention. These delays coupled with preexisting cardiovascular, respiratory, neurologic, or other chronic disease processes contribute to a higher mortality rate from acute abdominal disorders in the elderly.

## DISPOSITION OF THE PATIENT WITH NONSPECIFIC ABDOMINAL PAIN

Despite a thorough history and physical examination and appropriate laboratory and imaging studies, a large number of patients presenting to the emergency department with acute abdominal pain will have no definite diagnosis made. The majority of these patients will have an uneventful recovery. However, some patients will worsen and require subsequent hospitalization and surgery. The emergency physician should avoid labeling nonspecific abdominal pain as "gastritis," "gastroenteritis," or other similar terms. Disposition options include discharge with scheduled out-patient follow-up in 24 h, admission for observation, or short-term observation with repeat assessment. Patients discharged from the emergency department with a diagnosis of nonspecific acute abdominal pain should be instructed to have a low threshold to return if their symptoms should worsen or fail to improve.

## BIBLIOGRAPHY

Attard AR, Corlett MJ, Kidner NJ, et al: Safety of early pain relief for acute abdominal pain. *Br Med J* 305:554, 1992.

Brewer BJ, Golden GT, Hitch DC, et al: Abdominal pain: An analysis of 1000 consecutive cases in a university hospital emergency room. *Am J Surg* 131:219, 1976.

Cordell WH, Larson TA, Lingeman JE, et al: Indomethacin suppositories versus intravenously titrated morphine for the treatment of ureteral colic. *Ann Emerg Med* 23:263, 1994.

de Dombal FT, Dallos V, McAdam WAF: Can computer-aided teaching packages improve clinical care in patients with acute abdominal pain? *Br Med J* 302:1495, 1991.

Graff L, Redford MJ, Werne C: Probability of appendicitis before and after observation. *Ann Emerg Med* 20:503, 1991.

Irwin TT: Abdominal pain: A surgical audit of 1190 emergency admissions. *Br J Surg* 76:1121, 1989.

Kauvar D: The geriatric acute abdomen. *Clin Geriatr Med* 9:547, 58, 1993.

Larsen LS, Miller A, Allegra JR: The use of intravenous ketorolac for the treatment of renal colic in the emergency department. *Ann Emerg Med* 11:197, 1993.

Lukens TW, Emerman C, Effron D: The natural history and clinical findings of undifferentiated abdominal pain. *Ann Emerg Med* 22:690, 1993.

McAdam WA, Brock BM, Armitage T, et al: Twelve years' experience of computer-aided diagnosis in a district general hospital. *Ann R Coll Surg Engl* 72:140, 1990.

Plewa MC: Emergency abdominal radiography. *Emerg Med Clin North Am* 9:827, 1991.

Silen W: *Cope's Early Diagnosis of the Acute Abdomen,* 18th ed. New York, Oxford University Press, 1991.

Stonebridge PA, Freeland P, Rainey JB, et al: Audit of computer-aided diagnosis of abdominal pain in accident and emergency departments. *Arch Emerg Med* 9:271, 1992.

Zoltie N, Cust MP: Analgesia in the acute abdomen. *Ann R Coll Surg Engl* 68:210, 1986.

# 32
# GASTROINTESTINAL BLEEDING
## David T. Overton

Gastrointestinal bleeding should be considered potentially life-threatening until proved otherwise. While most patients will volunteer complaints of hematemesis, hematochezia, or melena, gastrointestinal bleeding may have more subtle presentations. Patients with hypotension, tachycardia, angina, syncope, weakness, confusion, or even cardiac arrest may harbor occult gastrointestinal hemorrhage.

As with all true emergencies, the traditional triad of history, physical examination, and diagnosis often must be accomplished simultaneously with resuscitation and stabilization. Factors associated with high morbidity are hemodynamic instability, repeated hematemesis or hematochezia, failure to clear with gastric lavage, age over 60, and other organ system disease.

## HISTORY

A carefully performed history can often point to the source of bleeding. Symptoms of hematemesis, coffee-ground emesis, melena, or hematochezia should be sought. Classically, hematemesis or coffee-ground emesis suggests a source proximal to the ligament of Treitz. Melena suggests a source at or proximal to the right colon, and hematochezia indicates a more distal colorectal lesion. The clinician, however, should remember that exceptions to these rules occur. Weight loss or changes in bowel habits are classic symptoms of malignancy. Vomiting and retching, followed by hematemesis, is suggestive of a Mallory-Weiss tear.

A history of drug ingestion should be carefully sought, particularly of salicylates, glucocorticoids, nonsteroidal anti-inflammatory agents, and anticoagulants. Alcohol abuse is strongly associated with a number of causes of gastrointestinal bleeding, including peptic ulcer disease, erosive gastritis, and esophageal varices. Ingestion of iron or bismuth can simulate melena, and certain foods, such as beets, can simulate hematochezia. In such instances, stool guaiac testing will be negative.

A prior history of gastrointestinal bleeding should be noted. Although recurrent episodes of bleeding might appear to be from the same source, this is often not the case. A history of an aortic graft should suggest the possibility of an aortoenteric fistula.

## PHYSICAL EXAMINATION

The vital signs may reveal obvious hypotension and tachycardia or more subtle manifestations such as a decreased pulse pressure, tachypnea, or orthostatic vital sign changes. The clinician should remember that some patients can tolerate substantial volume losses with minimal or no changes in vital signs. Similarly, paradoxical bradycardia can occur in the face of profound hypovolemia.

Skin findings should be noted. Cool, clammy skin is an obvious sign of shock. Spider angiomata, palmar erythema, jaundice, and gynecomastia suggest underlying liver disease. Petechiae and purpura suggest an underlying coagulopathy. Skin findings may suggest the Peutz-Jeghers, Rendu-Osler-Weber, or Gardner syndrome.

A careful ENT examination may occasionally reveal an occult bleeding source which has resulted in swallowed blood and subsequent coffee-ground emesis or melena. The abdominal examination may disclose tenderness, masses, ascites, or organomegaly. A rectal examination is indicated, for detection of the presence of blood, its appearance (bright red, maroon, or frankly melanotic), and the presence of any masses.

## LABORATORY DATA

In patients with significant gastrointestinal bleeding, the most important laboratory test is to type and cross-match blood. Other important laboratory data include the CBC. Additionally, BUN, creatinine, electrolytes, glucose, coagulation studies, and liver function studies should be considered. The initial hematocrit level often will not reflect the actual amount of blood loss. Upper tract hemorrhage may elevate the BUN through digestion and absorption of hemoglobin. Coagulation studies, including prothrombin time, partial thromboplastin time, and platelet count, are of obvious benefit in patients taking anticoagulants or those with underlying hepatic disease. The bleeding time is necessary to evaluate qualitative platelet abnormalities.

An ECG should be considered in patients in the coronary artery disease age group. Silent ischemia can occur secondary to the decreased oxygen delivery accompanying gastrointestinal bleeding.

## RADIOGRAPHIC STUDIES

Routine abdominal radiographs are often obtained in patients with gastrointestinal bleeding. In the absence of specific indications, they

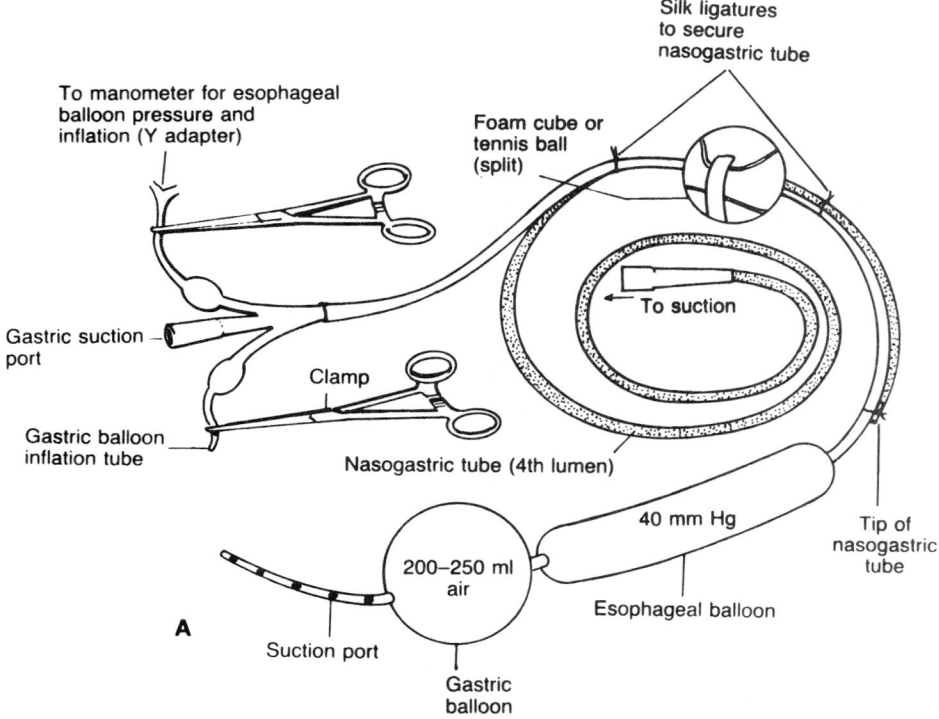

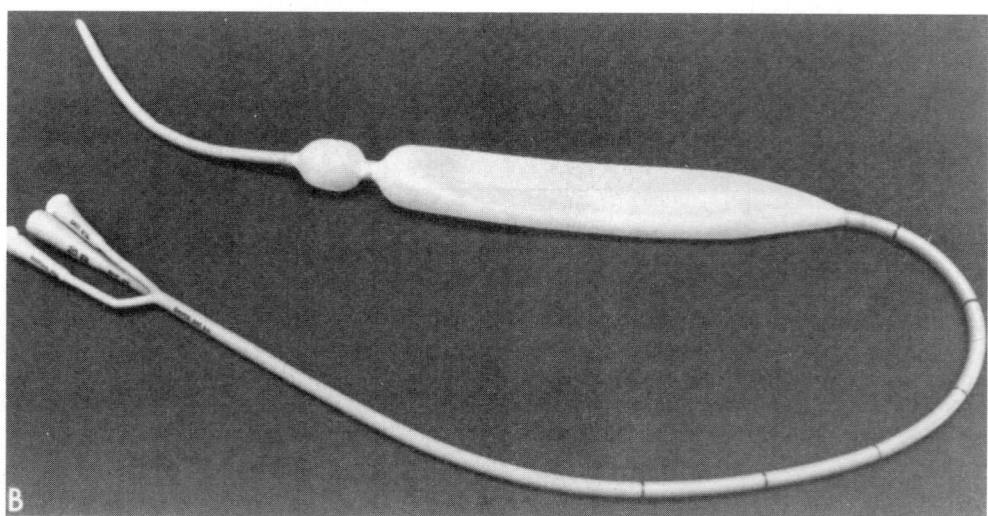

**Fig. 32-1. A.** Diagram of standard Sengstaken-Blakemore tube with nasogastric tube attached. **B.** Deflated tube. **C.** Traction is maintained on the inflated Sengstaken-Blakemore tube by taping the proximal end to the face mask of a football helmet. **D.** The pressure in the esophageal balloon should be calibrated frequently with a manometer and should not exceed a baseline of 40 mmHg. (From Roberts JR, Hedges JR (eds): *Clinical Procedures in Emergency Medicine,* 2d ed. Philadelphia, Saunders, 1991, pp 650 and 653. Used with permission.)

are of limited value. Barium contrast studies are similarly of limited value in the emergency situation. Furthermore, barium limits the use of subsequent endoscopy or angiography.

Gastrointestinal angiography can sometimes detect the site of bleeding, particularly in cases of obscure lower gastrointestinal bleeding. However, it requires a relatively brisk bleeding rate (0.5 to 2.0 mL/min) to be diagnostic. Technetium-labeled red-cell scans appear more sensitive and can localize the site of bleeding at a rate of 0.1 mL/min. Endoscopy is more accurate in most circumstances. Angiography, however, may allow intraarterial embolization, or the use of arterial vasopressors.

## MANAGEMENT

### Primary

As with any emergency situation, immediate resuscitative measures take priority. Patients with profuse upper gastrointestinal hemorrhage

may require definitive airway management to prevent aspiration of blood. Oxygen should be given and cardiac monitoring is likewise indicated. Volume replacement should be initiated with crystalloids via large-bore intravenous lines. The decision to administer blood should be based on the clinical findings of volume depletion or continued bleeding more than on initial hematocrit values. General guidelines for initiation of blood transfusion are continued active bleeding and failure to improve perfusion and vital signs after the infusion of 2 L of crystalloid. The threshold for blood transfusion is often lower in the elderly. Coagulation factors should be replaced as needed. A urinary catheter is indicated in patients with hypotension.

A nasogastric tube should be placed in all patients with significant gastrointestinal bleeding regardless of presumed source. Concerns that nasogastric tube passage may provoke bleeding in patients with varices are unwarranted. Bright red blood per rectum often unexpectedly originates from massive upper gastrointestinal sources. A negative gastric aspirate does not conclusively rule out an upper gastroin-

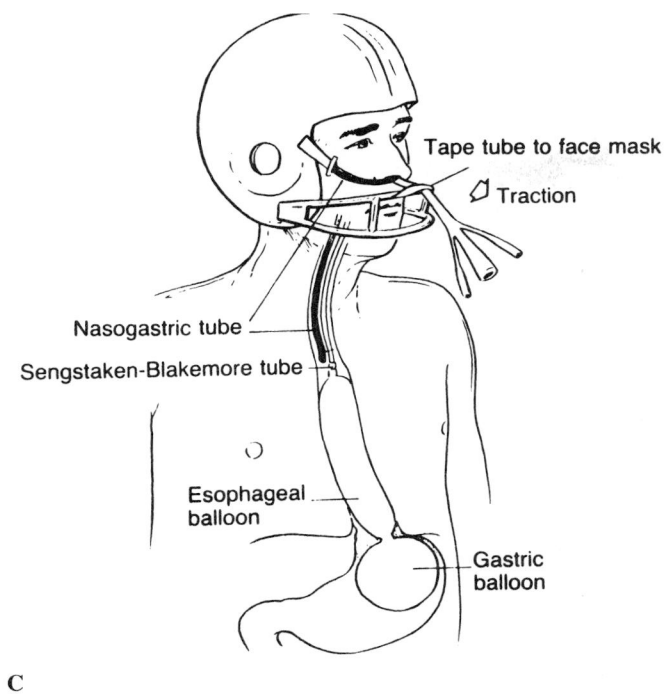

**C**

**Fig. 32-1.** (*cont.*)

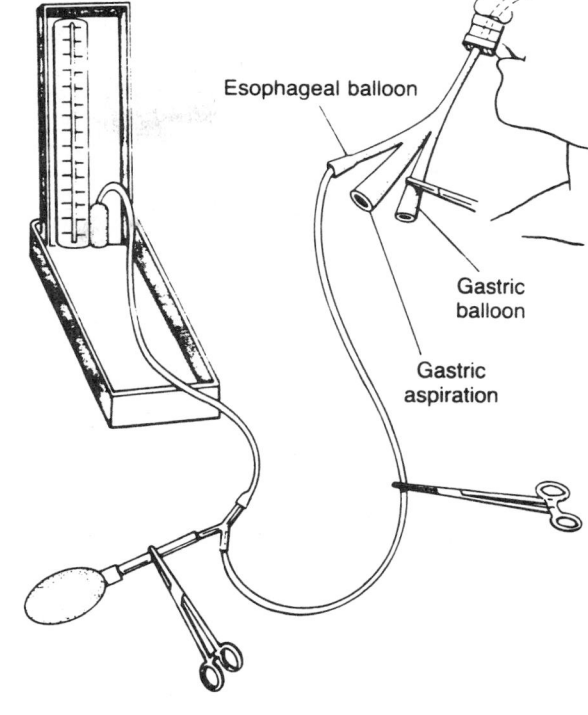

**D**

testinal cause and may result from intermittent bleeding, or pyloric spasm or edema preventing reflux of duodenal blood. Standard guaiac paper may yield falsely negative results in the presence of low gastric pH.

If bright red blood or clots are found on nasogastric intubation, gentle gastric lavage should be performed. To be effective, a large-bore tube, usually oral, must be used. Room temperature water or saline is the preferred irrigant, as iced solutions have no proved benefit and have theoretical disadvantages. The addition of levarterenol to the lavage solution is similarly of unproved benefit. Overvigorous suction should be avoided, as it may produce gastric erosions which can confuse findings on subsequent endoscopy.

## Secondary

### Endoscopy

Upper gastrointestinal endoscopy is the most accurate technique for the identification of upper gastrointestinal bleeding sites, predicting morbidity, and, with the advent of therapeutic endoscopy, is associated with improved outcomes. Ulcers larger than 1 or 2 cm are prone to rebleed, even after hemostatic therapy. Sclerotherapy of esophageal varices is the initial treatment of choice of acute variceal bleeding, and can control acute hemorrhage in up to 90 percent of patients. Sclerotherapy may decrease the duration of hospitalization and amount of blood transfused when compared with portal-caval shunting. Complications of sclerotherapy include perforation, sepsis, and portal and mesenteric venous thrombosis. Endoscopic band ligation of varices appears to be as effective as sclerotherapy, with a decreased incidence of complications.

Endoscopic hemostasis has also been used successfully in nonvariceal etiologies of upper gastrointestinal bleeding, using injection therapy, electrocoagulation, heater probes, and laser therapy.

Proctoscopy can often be diagnostic in patients with anorectal sources of bleeding. If an anorectal source such as hemorrhoids is suspected, the patient should be carefully evaluated for significant volume loss or more dangerous proximal sources of bleeding mimicking hemorrhoidal bleeding.

Sigmoidoscopy and colonoscopy can be diagnostic in other forms of lower gastrointestinal hemorrhage, such as diverticulosis or angiodysplasia, and may allow ablation of bleeding sites using the technologies noted above.

### Drug Therapy

Vasopressin has been used by both intravenous and intraarterial infusion to control gastrointestinal bleeding. Intravenous infusion has been shown to be as effective as intraarterial and is far easier to perform. Intravenous vasopressin infusion has been evaluated most extensively in the treatment of esophageal variceal bleeding. Infusion rates of 0.1 to 0.9 units/min are described, but adverse reactions are common. Hypertension, cardiac arrhythmias, myocardial and splanchnic ischemia, decreased cardiac output, and gangrene from local infiltration are all described. Although the addition of nitroglycerin to vasopressin has been shown to reduce the incidence of these side effects, the use of vasopressin should be considered an adjunct to more definitive measures.

$H_2$ antagonists remain of unproved benefit in acute upper gastrointestinal hemorrhage. There is no conclusive evidence for reduction in the rates of rebleeding, surgery, or death.

### Balloon Tamponade

Balloon tamponade with the Sengstaken-Blakemore tube or its variants can provide therapeutic benefit and presumptive diagnostic information. It can control documented variceal hemorrhage in 40 to 80 percent of patients. The device consists of gastric and esophageal balloons and, depending on the variation, may include gastric and/or esophageal aspiration ports (Fig. 32-1). The gastric balloon should be inflated first. If bleeding does not cease, the esophageal balloon should then be inflated, using a manometer to ensure that the pressure does not exceed 40 to 50 mmHg. Radiologic confirmation of proper balloon placement is suggested. The device should be kept in place

24 h after bleeding has ceased. Some authors recommend deflating the esophageal balloon for 30 to 60 min every 8 h to prevent mucosal ulceration.

Like vasopressin therapy, balloon tamponade is frequently associated with adverse reactions, often severe. Mucosal ulceration, esophageal or gastric rupture, asphyxiation from dislodged balloons, tracheal compression secondary to balloon inflation, and aspiration pneumonia have been reported. Many authors recommend routine prophylactic endotracheal intubation to prevent pulmonary complications. Because of the incidence of adverse reactions, balloon tamponade should be considered an adjunctive or temporizing measure supplementing the more definitive modality of sclerotherapy.

### Surgery

In patients who do not respond to medical therapy, and in whom endoscopic hemostasis, if available, fails, emergency surgical intervention is indicated. Surgical consultation on any patient admitted to the hospital for gastrointestinal bleeding is prudent, in case uncontrollable rebleeding occurs.

## CAUSES OF UPPER GASTROINTESTINAL BLEEDING

### Peptic Ulcer Disease

Peptic ulcer disease, including gastric, duodenal, and stomal ulcers, remains the most common etiology for upper gastrointestinal hemorrhage, encompassing approximately 50 percent of all cases. Duodenal ulcers, approximately 29 percent of the total, will rebleed in approximately 10 percent of cases, usually within 24 to 48 h. Gastric ulcers, approximately 16 percent of all cases, are more likely to rebleed. Stomal ulcers are uncommon (less than 5 percent of all upper gastrointestinal bleeds) and are present in only one third of bleeding patients with a history of prior peptic ulcer surgery.

### Erosive Gastritis and Esophagitis

Erosive gastritis, esophagitis, and duodenitis altogether are responsible for approximately 20 percent of all cases of upper gastrointestinal hemorrhage. Irritative factors, such as alcohol, salicylates, or hiatal hernia, are predisposing factors.

### Esophageal Varices

Esophageal and gastric varices result from portal hypertension, in the United States most often as a result of alcoholic liver disease. Although varices account for only about 10 percent of all cases of upper gastrointestinal hemorrhage, they are highly likely to rebleed and carry a high mortality rate. Despite this, it is interesting to note that many patients with end-stage cirrhosis never develop varices, many patients with documented varices never bleed, and many patients presenting with upper gastrointestinal bleeding and a documented history of varices will be bleeding from other sites.

### Mallory-Weiss Syndrome

The Mallory-Weiss syndrome is upper gastrointestinal bleeding secondary to a longitudinal mucosal tear in the cardioesophageal region. The classic history is repeated retching followed by bright red hematemesis, but coughing and seizures have been reported as etiologic factors.

### Other Etiologies

Stress ulcers (Cushing or Curling), arteriovenous malformations, and malignancies are other etiologies of upper gastrointestinal hemorrhage. ENT sources of bleeding can masquerade as gastrointestinal hemorrhage. An aortoenteric fistula secondary to an aortic graft is an unusual but important cause of bleeding to keep in mind. Classically, patients will present with a self-limited "herald" bleed prior to a subsequent massive hemorrhage.

## CAUSES OF LOWER GASTROINTESTINAL BLEEDING

### Lower Gastrointestinal Bleeding

The most common cause of apparent lower gastrointestinal bleeding remains upper gastrointestinal bleeding. Thus, proximal etiologies should be sought.

### Diverticulosis

Diverticulosis and angiodysplasia are the most common causes of lower gastrointestinal bleeding. Diverticular bleeding is usually painless and results from erosion into the lumen of the penetrating artery of the diverticulum. Patients are often elderly with underlying medical illnesses which contribute to morbidity and mortality. If hemorrhage does not cease spontaneously, colonoscopy with endoscopic hemostasis may be attempted. Alternatively, arteriography with vasopressin infusion or embolization may be considered. If these measures fail, emergency surgery may be necessary.

### Angiodysplasia

Arteriovenous malformations or angiodysplasia, usually of the right colon, are a common etiology of obscure lower gastrointestinal bleeding, particularly in the elderly population. They are reputed to be more common in patients with hypertension and aortic stenosis.

### Other Etiologies

Numerous other lesions may result in lower gastrointestinal hemorrhage. Carcinoma and hemorrhoids are common causes of bleeding, but massive hemorrhage is unusual. Similarly, inflammatory bowel disease, polyps, and infectious gastroenteritis rarely cause massive bleeding. A Meckel's diverticulum is an unusual but important etiology to keep in mind.

## BIBLIOGRAPHY

Collins R, Langman M: Treatment with histamine $H_2$ antagonists in acute upper gastrointestinal hemorrhage. *N Engl J Med* 313:660, 1985.

Gogel HK, Tandberg D: Emergency management of upper gastrointestinal hemorrhage. *Am J Emerg Med* 4:150, 1986.

Henderson JM, Kutner MH, Millikan WJ, et al: Endoscopic variceal sclerosis compared with distal splenorenal shunt to prevent recurrent variceal bleeding in cirrhosis: A prospective, randomized trial. *Ann Intern Med* 112:262, 1990.

Hoi H, Zuckerman MJ, Wassem C: A prospective controlled study of the risk of bacteremia in emergency sclerotherapy of esophageal varices. *Gastroenterology* 101:1642, 1991.

Lieberman D: Gastrointestinal bleeding: Initial management. *Gastroenterol Clin North Am* 22:723, 1993.

Lipper B, Simon D, Cerrone F: Pulmonary aspiration during emergency endoscopy in patients with upper gastrointestinal hemorrhage. *Crit Care Med* 19:330, 1991.

Matloff DS: Treatment of acute variceal bleeding. *Gastroenterol Clin North Am* 21:103, 1992.

Reinus JF, Brandt LJ: Vascular ectasias and diverticulosis: Common causes of lower intestinal bleeding. *Gastroenterol Clin North Am* 23:1, 1994.

Ryan P, Styles CB, Chmiel R: Identification of the site of severe colon bleeding by technetium-labeled red-cell scan. *Dis Colon Rectum* 35:219, 1992.

Steele RJ: Endoscopic haemostasis for non-variceal upper gastrointestinal haemorrhage. *Br J Surg* 76:219, 1989.

# 33

# COMA AND ALTERED STATES OF CONSCIOUSNESS

## Gregory L. Henry

Although coma is the most dramatic of the disorders of consciousness, it is only the endpoint in the continuum of altered mental status. Any disease process that can cause coma may initially present with mild alterations of, and progressively decreasing, mental status. It is often difficult or impossible to determine the direction and final outcome of a change in mental status until the most important test, time, has been applied.

In acute nervous system disease, a change in mental status is often the first sign of a severe pathologic process. It is a well-recognized rule within the neurosciences that functional change is always greater than and always precedes structural change in the brain and spinal cord. Of all the central nervous system functions, mental status is the most delicate and the most sensitive early bellwether of advancing disease.

Nothing replaces the standard approach to all emergency patients, namely, "A, B, C₃." Airway management and *b*reathing should be the first priorities of the evaluation of any patient in the emergency department. *C*ardiac status is next assessed and supported as necessary. The other two C's stand for *c*ervical spine immobilization when appropriate and *c*ompression of obvious hemorrhage. The basic rule is that in the appropriate setting a comatose patient has suffered a cervical spine injury until proved otherwise.

The principal goal of this chapter is to review classification systems for patients with altered mental status and to provide a framework for evaluating such patients in the emergency setting. The immediate duty of the emergency department, with regard to patients with altered mental status, is to divide the potentially exhaustive list of disease entities into two major groups: metabolic and toxic disease and structural, focal disease. Since the management of toxic and metabolic disease is principally medical and the management of focal disease is frequently surgical, it is important that these differentiations be made early so that correct treatment can be initiated.

The determination of structural neurologic disease is based on a focal neurologic examination. Those patients who are developing discrete, isolated lesions of motor or sensory function or specific cortical defects will have structural or anatomic damage a majority of the time.

## DEFINITIONS

A clear understanding of the terminology of altered mental status is necessary before classifying various disease entities. The physician is better served by describing in the chart exactly what he or she sees. Nonspecific terms are often misleading and not helpful for further examiners who must reassess the patient on an ongoing basis. It is much more useful to record in the chart objective findings such as the patient's ability to handle three-object retention and mathematical calculations as opposed to using terms such as "stuporous" or "lethargic." But since the following terminology has become universal in medical literature, some general understanding of the terms is needed. *Consciousness* is defined as an awareness of self and the environment. Disorders of consciousness can be divided into states where the patient appears asleep and states where the patient appears awake but is unresponsive.

## Patients Who Appear Asleep

**Sleep.** A state of nonpathologic decreased mental status from which the patient can be easily aroused to full consciousness.

**Lethargy.** Depressed mental status in which the patient may appear wakeful but has depressed awareness of self and environment globally.

**Stupor.** Unresponsiveness from which the patient can be aroused with vigorous noxious stimuli constitutes stupor. The stuporous patient, however, does not return to a normal baseline of awareness of self or environment.

**Coma.** Coma is a state of unresponsiveness, from which the patient cannot be aroused by verbal and physical stimuli to produce any meaningful response.

**Psychogenic coma.** Psychogenic coma is a state of unresponsiveness, either voluntary or involuntary, from which the patient cannot be brought to reasonable cortical response by noxious verbal or physical stimuli. These patients do, however, have normal physiologic testing and EEG responses.

## Patients Who Appear Awake but Are Unresponsive

**Abulic state.** In the abulic state (also known as *akinetic mutism* or "coma vigil"), the patient is awake with eyes open but extremely slow to respond to questions asked. The patient's frontal lobe function is so depressed, from any number of processes, that meaningful response in a normal time frame is impossible. It should be noted that these patients often do have reasonable thought processes, but because of the huge delays in their ability to process information and answer, they are often misdiagnosed in the emergency department. These patients may take several minutes to respond to any problem or question posed.

**Locked-in syndrome.** In the "locked-in" syndrome (also known as the "Count of Monte Cristo" syndrome) (M. Nortier de Villefort), patients appear absolutely motionless but their eyes are open. The lesion in the locked-in syndrome is the destruction of the ventral pontine motor tracts. The only function that these patients maintain is vertical eye movement. It is important, in all unresponsive patients who appear awake, that the examiner ask them to look up. In patients who can look up but cannot move their eyes from side to side, the diagnosis of locked-in syndrome is secured.

**Psychogenic unresponsiveness.** Also known as the *catatonic state,* psychogenic unresponsiveness is a level of unresponsiveness in which the patient appears awake and may maintain normal motor posturing and neurologic testing, but who, for voluntary or involuntary reasons, is not able to communicate with the examiner.

## Confusional States

This category covers a series of disorders in which mental status is not depressed, but in which the patient misinterprets external stimuli. These states may overlap with causes of depressed mental status and may be extremely difficult to differentiate in an emergency setting. The hallmarks of these conditions are global confusion, inability to appropriately process stimuli, or inability to make meaningful responses. Such findings are characteristic of a toxic ingestion, metabolic encephalopathy, or central nervous system infection.

## THE PATHOPHYSIOLOGY OF ALTERED MENTAL STATUS

Although the specific causes of altered mental status are legion, the pathophysiology is either bilateral cerebral cortical disease or suppression of the brainstem reticular activating formation (RAF). Cellular disorders such as lipid storage diseases or neuronal degeneration rarely present as acute changes in mental status.

## Bilateral Cortical Disease

Focal lesions in one cerebral cortex cause neurologic findings specific to that region but do not generally cause alteration of mental status. If the altered mental status is thought to be based on cortical disease, both cortices should be involved. For example, patients who have had large sections of the cerebral cortex removed by surgery can still be awake and alert. The most common causes of bilateral cortical disease altering mental status are toxins such as alcohol and illicit drugs and deficiencies of the metabolic substrates oxygen and glucose.

If the brain is deprived of its normal supply of oxygen by impairment of systemic oxygen uptake or distribution for more than about 10 s, loss of consciousness ensues. A marked decrease or increase of serum glucose can rapidly lead to changes in mental status but hyperglycemia never produces rapid onset of neurologic changes.

## Reticular Activating System Lesions

The other principal mechanism by which altered mental status is produced is through involvement of the reticular activating formation, a small grouping of fibers that traverses the brainstem to the thalamus. Through continuous stimulation of the cortex, the RAF maintains the state of wakefulness. Any sudden interruption of RAF activity affects alertness. For example, it is postulated that the mechanism by which a boxer's blow to the chin causes sudden coma is not through damage to the cortical structures but rather through torque forces on the brainstem, which interrupt RAF activity.

The reticular activating formation can be affected in three principal ways: by supratentorial pressure, by infratentorial pressure, and by intrinsic brainstem lesions.

**Supratentorial pressure.** The manner in which supratentorial lesions produce coma is by enlarging and displacing tissue. This causes compression of the opposite hemisphere, as well as deeper diencephalic and brainstem structures. By pressing on the brainstem through this remote mechanism, the RAF is also compressed. The skull has a limited area and the brain and its protective and supporting structures occupy the entire intracranial space. When additional volume accumulates in the skull, either as a discrete mass or from generalized edema, pressure is directed to the point of least resistance. The temporal lobes, which rest on the tentorium cerebelli, may be forced through the tentorial notch, compressing brainstem structures and cranial nerves. Therefore, the mechanism of coma in patients with acute supratentorial lesions such as epidural, subdural, or intraparenchymal bleeding is not due to destruction of specific cortex but rather from pressure directed toward deeper brainstem structures.

**Infratentorial pressure.** The brainstem lies below the tentorium cerebelli and is anatomically distinct from the great mass of cerebral tissue which lies above. The brainstem shares the posterior fossa with the ventricular aqueduct of Sylvius, the fourth ventricle, and the cerebellum. An increase in pressure in this area may be accompanied by movement of the posterior fossa contents upward through the tentorial notch or downward through the foramen magnum. For example, tumors involving the meninges, brainstem, and cerebellum, or acute cerebellar hemorrhage can increase pressure. This causes compression on the RAF and resultant coma.

**Intrinsic brainstem lesion.** Lesions intrinsic to the brainstem itself, such as traumatic or hypertensive pontine hemorrhage, may also compress the RAF directly.

In summary, severely depressed mental status is due to either bilateral cortical disease or involvement of the reticular activating formation. Bilateral cortical disease is almost always due to metabolic or toxic causes and generally shows no focal neurologic findings. Reticular activating formation dysfunction, on the other hand, is more likely the result of structural disease and will most frequently have focal neurologic findings.

## GENERAL APPROACH TO THE PATIENT WITH ALTERED MENTAL STATUS

### Initial Management

In the usual clinical approach to a patient, the examiner first obtains a history, then performs a physical examination and laboratory studies, and finally administers treatment. However, this sequence is not correct for patients in a coma. Coma is such a major variance from normal neurologic functioning that immediate supportive efforts are required. The A, B, $C_3$ approach must be activated. For patients who do not have an active gag reflex, mechanical airway control is urgently needed to prevent aspiration. If a cervical spinal fracture is suspected, or if the mechanism of coma is unknown, the neck must be stabilized while the airway is secured, and endotracheal intubation should be performed carefully. For patients in whom there is no obvious facial trauma and who are actively breathing, nasotracheal intubation is an excellent alternative. In patients who have had severe midfacial and oral trauma and in whom the standard approaches are contraindicated, a cricothyroidotomy or use of a retrograde wire may be necessary.

Once airway control is established, oxygenation and hyperventilation are necessary. Mild hyperventilation corrects acidosis, and lowering the $P_{CO_2}$ reduces intracranial pressure. The $P_{CO_2}$ should be lowered to approximately 25 to 30 mmHg. This level can usually be obtained by ventilating the adult patient approximately 20 to 25 times per minute.

Cardiac status should be assessed to make certain that the patient has reasonable cardiac output and that there is no reason to begin cardiac pulmonary resuscitation.

Immobilization of the cervical spine is mandatory in patients in whom trauma is suspected. The possibility of trauma always exists in patients with alcohol or drug intoxication. Aggressive neck immobilization and restraints to the body so that the head and body function as a unit is the most effective way to anticipate cervical spine injury.

Finally, obvious hemorrhage should be stopped before detailed neurologic examination is begun. One of the earliest signs of shock is apprehension and confusion. As shock worsens, mental status quickly deteriorates, and thus the patient in hemorrhagic shock may well be lethargic or comatose. Vital signs should be obtained and recorded at this point if not already done.

### Initial Treatment

As an intravenous line is being inserted, blood should be removed for laboratory analysis. Generally, enough blood should be drawn to allow for CBC, glucose, BUN, creatinine, and electrolyte analyses. Extra blood should be held for more specific studies, depending on the history and physical findings. It is generally standard to administer intravenously thiamine, 100 mg; glucose, 25 to 50 g; and naloxone, 2 to 4 mg. Newer thiamine derivatives do not produce anaphylactoid reactions when given intravenously. If glucose testing can be done immediately and hypoglycemia is not an obvious possibility, the use of glucose can be guided by test results. Nutritionally deficient patients such as alcoholics or patients receiving cancer chemotherapy should receive thiamine prior to glucose administration. Thiamine is given to facilitate carbohydrate metabolism and to prevent the unwanted complication of Wernicke syndrome.

The standard dose of glucose in adults is 25 to 50 g as a 50% solution. In the patient with an intracranial mass lesion, glucose increases the osmotic load and is potentially beneficial in reducing intracranial pressure. In the patient who is comatose because of hyperglycemia, the recommended dose of glucose is not clinically significant.

Generally, 2 mg of naloxone is given intravenously, followed by 2 mg more if no response is seen. There are no dose-related adverse affects of naloxone reported, although the possibility of an acute opiate withdrawal syndrome increases along with the dose of naloxone.

Naloxone is an effective antagonist of opiates and synthetic narcotics such as propoxyphene and pentazocine. A very large dose of naloxone may be required to overcome the endorphin receptor effects of the synthetic narcotics. Any patient who can be aroused with naloxone may become combative and disoriented, so patients should be properly restrained before naloxone is given. Unless the patient has stopped breathing, naloxone is diagnostic, not therapeutic. In cases of suspected benzodiazepine overdose, flumazenil may also be given.

## Obtaining the History

The patient is usually not a reliable source of information, so other sources must be sought. Some data may be obtained from the patient's personal effects such as medical alert tags, wallet, purse, or pill containers.

Family and friends should be contacted to provide a history. They may be able to describe previous episodes or an event that led up to the current episode. Specific questions about abnormal motor movements, food or drug ingestions, trauma, and underlying diseases should be asked. It is important to provide reassurance that the medical history obtained will remain part of the medical record and will not be inappropriately given to law enforcement officials. Families are often reluctant to discuss drug and alcohol use by the patient, fearing legal reprisals.

## General Physical Examination

Vital signs should be regularly monitored. Arrhythmias should be anticipated and treated as clinically indicated. Tachypnea should be considered a sign of inadequate oxygenation and not a sign of central nervous system damage until proved otherwise. Oxygenation and ventilation should be corrected and then mental status reevaluated. Both hypertension and hypotension should be considered to have a nonneurologic cause in a patient with shock until proved otherwise. Although systemic hypertension can be caused by an elevation in intracranial pressure, such hypertension should not initially be ascribed to a primary neurologic event. Constant cardiac monitoring of the comatose patient is useful to check for intermittent cardiac problems such as fluctuating bradycardias or ventricular arrhythmias. Although these are unusual causes of coma, they represent treatable entities from which a patient may have an excellent neurologic recovery.

As the patient is examined, signs of trauma should be carefully sought. Blood behind the tympanic membranes as well as ecchymoses in the mastoid area should be particularly noted. Any patient with these findings should be considered to have a basilar skull fracture. Careful palpation of the head may reveal cephalohematomas that are not visible at first glance. Palpation of the neck, although often advocated, is generally nonproductive in the comatose patient. It is best to assume that there is a cervical spine fracture, immobilize the neck, and perform necessary x-rays. Other general signs of trauma such as contusions, fractures, lacerations, and abrasions should also be noted.

## Skin

Needle tracks suggest IV drug use. Cyanosis suggests hypoxemia, polycythemia, or an abnormal hemoglobin. Pallor likewise may be an early indication that the patient has inadequate oxygen-carrying capacity due to loss of blood. Far advanced carbon monoxide poisoning may produce a cherry-red glow of the mucous membranes. Other more generalized skin findings such as multiple abscesses, cellulitis, uremic frost, or icterus may point to underlying conditions which may affect mental status.

## Breath

One should never assume that coma is due to alcohol merely because the odor of alcohol is detectable. The fruity fragrance of acetone or the distinct odor of anaerobic infection should be noted. Fetor hepaticus indicates advanced liver disease. A feculent odor suggests bowel obstruction while the distinctive odor of almonds may indicate cyanide poisoning.

## Cardiac Examination

Tachyarrhythmias or bradyarrhythmias can alter mental status because of decreased cardiac output. Endocarditis or arrhythmias which dislodge mural thrombi can produce cerebral emboli. Acute myocardial infarction may reduce cardiac output enough to depress consciousness. An intracranial lesion can result in static ECG changes, such as prolongation of the QT interval or ST-T changes, as well as arrhythmias. The mechanism is probably massive sympathetic outflow resulting in coronary spasm.

## Abdominal Examination

Organomegaly, ascites, bruits, and pulsatile masses should be noted to detect conditions that are causative, or present but unassociated with a decrease in mental status. For example, hepatomegaly and ascites may be present in hepatic encephalopathy. The presence of an abdominal aortic aneurysm is consistent with advanced atherosclerotic disease. Grey Turner or Cullen signs suggest retroperitoneal hemorrhage. A pelvic/rectal examination should be performed in a comatose patient to detect bleeding, masses, infection, or foreign bodies.

## Neurologic Examination

The patient should be observed for involuntary movement of all four extremities and abnormal posturing. The patient who is agitated and yet has decreased mental status may have a toxic encephalopathy. Opisthotonic contractions may be due to tetanus, strychnine poisoning, dystonic reactions, or decerebration. Seizures should be observed to determine whether they are focal or generalized.

The Glasgow Coma Scale (Table 33-1) is helpful in the individual patient only to categorize the severity of injury and need for rapid intervention in a very basic fashion. More detailed evaluation is needed to determine brain and brainstem function.

## Respiratory Pattern

The pattern and rate of respiration should be noted and recorded, as they may indicate the level of neurologic injury in the patient.

An awake patient at rest generally breathes about 12 to 18 times

**Table 33-1.** The Glasgow Coma Scale

| | EYES | |
|---|---|---|
| Open: | Spontaneously | 4 |
| | To verbal command | 3 |
| | To pain | 2 |
| No response: | | 1 |
| | BEST VERBAL RESPONSE | |
| | Oriented and converses | 5 |
| | Disoriented and converses | 4 |
| | Inappropriate words | 3 |
| | Incomprehensible sounds | 2 |
| | No response | 1 |
| | BEST MOTOR RESPONSE | |
| To verbal command: | Obeys | 6 |
| To painful stimulus: | Localizes pain | 5 |
| | Flexion-withdrawal | 4 |
| | Abnormal flexion (decorticate rigidity) | 3 |
| | Extension (decerebrate rigidity) | 2 |
| | No response | 1 |
| Total | | 3–15 |

per minute and has occasional sighing or deeper respirations as demanded by carbon dioxide levels. When the cortex is no longer functioning and the nervous system is relying on diencephalic control of breathing, *Cheyne-Stokes respirations* occur. This is a type of breathing characterized by regularly increasing depth of breaths alternating with decreasing depths of breaths then short periods of apnea. The breathing crescendoes to a peak and then decrescendoes suddenly. The apneic phase is usually short. The most frequent causes for Cheyne-Stokes respirations are bilateral metabolic hemispheric disease or structural disease of the bilateral cerebral hemispheres and basal ganglia. The principal mechanism underlying Cheyne-Stokes respirations has to do with loss of forebrain control of ventilatory stimulation.

*Hyperventilation* in the stuporous or comatose patient may be from a variety of causes. Attempts to correct hypoxia, compensation for metabolic acidosis, and brain injury itself all cause hyperventilation. Central neurogenic hyperventilation is frequently seen with midbrain involvement with destruction of those areas which normally monitor ventilatory patterns. When hyperventilation is caused by central nervous system disease it indicates upper brainstem damage.

*Apneustic breathing* is characterized by a prolonged pause at the end of inspiration, much like breath-holding. It is seen with lesions about the fifth cranial nerve. *Cluster breathing* is breathing in short bursts and is almost always associated with lesions at the level of the pons. *Ataxic breathing,* irregular breathing without pattern or regularity, is a forerunner of agonal respirations and death.

*Autisms* are involuntary neurologic acts carried out for maintenance and protection of the body. Yawning, although its mechanism is not well understood, frequently accompanies expanding lesions of the posterior fossa.

The autisms of vomiting, hiccuping, and coughing have neurogenic centers involved in their control. In the face of altered mental status, hiccuping, coughing, and vomiting may be indications of lesions involving lower brainstem centers.

## Mental Status

Mental status may be the most sensitive early indicator of nervous system disease and is the first function to be affected in a variety of lesions. The ability to respond to voice and follow commands should be recorded. If the patient cannot respond to voice, then response to firm but gentle touch must be assessed. Finally, response to noxious stimuli is recorded. There is no need to inflict pain on a patient suspected of feigning coma, since there are other more humane techniques for detecting functional disease.

## Cranial Nerves

Visual threat is an unreliable test in unresponsive patients, since reactions can be checked voluntarily in certain awake patients. Lack of response to visual threat is not certain evidence of coma. Conversely, during visual threat, when air is moved toward the cornea in a comatose patient, a blink response can be elicited.

Inspection of the ocular fundi gives the examiner the only opportunity to actually view the brain. Evidence of papilledema, hemorrhage, and spontaneous venous pulsations should be sought. Spontaneous venous pulsations in erect patients indicate normal intracranial pressure. This is often difficult to assess with comatose patients since they are recumbent. If spontaneous venous pulsations are seen when the patient is in the recumbent position, however, they clearly indicate that there is not increased intracranial pressure.

## Pupils

The size, shape, and reactivity, both direct and consensual, of each pupil should be recorded. The pupillary pathways are relatively resistant to metabolic insult. They receive their parasympathetic supply from the thalamic pretectal region and their sympathetic supply from the superior cervical ganglion which courses along the carotid artery.

Pupillary findings must be interpreted along with the entire neurologic examination. As a general rule, hemispheric disease has very little influence on pupillary function. Usually patients who are comatose from metabolic involvement of the cerebral hemispheres will have small to midrange pupils which are reactive to light. Structural lesions involving the diencephalon may cause small but reactive pupils.

Disparities in pupil size and reactivity can occur with eye trauma, ocular drugs, or previous eye surgery.

A unilateral fixed and dilated pupil should not necessarily be equated with an intracranial mass lesion. It may be the result of a cycloplegic agent instilled in one eye. An expanding aneurysm which compresses the third cranial nerve may cause an ipsilateral fixed and dilated pupil but not affect mental status. The general rule is that if a patient is alert, a dilated pupil is most likely not the result of increasing intracranial pressure. The mechanism for the fixed and dilated pupil seen with severe head injury is herniation of the uncus of the temporal lobe through the tentorial notch, which compresses the third cranial nerve. No patient with this degree of increased intracranial pressure will exhibit normal mental status.

Lesions involving the midbrain tectal regions may cause mid-sized to large pupils that may respond poorly to light. Pontine lesions frequently cause fixed pinpoint pupils that are not affected by naloxone. Anoxia, atropine, and cycloplegics may all cause dilated pupils. Pinpoint pupils that are reversible with naloxone result from narcotics. Certain narcotics, however, such as propoxyphene, may leave the pupils intact and reactive. One cannot rule out a narcotic overdose strictly on the basis of pupillary size and reactivity.

## Ocular Movements

In the awake patient, eye movements are directed by both anterior frontal lobe and posterior occipital lobe control centers which are connected to the pontine gaze centers. These gaze centers lie adjacent to the sixth cranial nerve and, in turn, direct eye movements by way of the medial longitudinal fasciculus (MLF). The MLF, which runs from the upper cervical spine through the area of the third cranial nerve, is the principal interconnection for all conjugate eye movements. Because it extends over a considerable length into the brainstem itself, testing of the MLF is the best single method for judging intactness of brainstem.

Without cortical control, most comatose patients will have roving eye movements, assuming that the brainstem is intact. Eye movements may be disconjugate or conjugate, but as long as both eyes cross the midline, there is no evidence of damage at the brainstem level.

The eyes may be abnormally deviated due to injury involving cortical gaze centers or pontine gaze centers. A general rule regarding cortical injuries is that the eyes will be directed toward a physiologically inactive lesion and away from an irritative or active focus. For example, during a seizure the eyes will be directed away from the side of the seizure focus.

To decide whether the cause of coma is a cortical or brainstem lesion, oculocephalic mechanisms must be tested. The presence of oculocephalic reflexes depends on the fact that the MLF receives constant information as to the position of the patient's head through the output of the semicircular canals. Without cortical influences, an intact brainstem maintains the eyes forward or upward when the patient is supine. This is the basis of the "doll's eye maneuver," the involuntary movement of the eyes upward and downward on passive flexion and extension of the head. In a comatose patient in whom a cervical spine injury is suspected, the test is contraindicated.

Oculovestibular or cold caloric testing is a more sophisticated method to test the integrity of the brainstem (Table 33-2). To perform

**Table 33-2.** Oculovestibular Testing for Brainstem Integrity

| Ice-Water Effect | Interpretation |
|---|---|
| Both eyes deviate and good nystagmus produced | Patient is not comatose |
| Both eyes deviate toward cold water—bilateral—no fast phase | Coma, but intact brainstem |
| No eye movement despite cold stimuli to both sides—indirectly | Brainstem—complete dysfunction from structural, metabolic, or hypothermic causes |
| Movement of only eye ipsilateral to side of stimulant but not opposite eye | Internuclear lesion |

the test, the examiner injects 50 mL of ice-cold water against the tympanic membrane. Countercurrent flow is set up in the semicircular canals, and information is transmitted to pontine gaze centers near the ipsilateral sixth nerve nucleus. The altered endolymphatic flow allows the centers to believe that the head has been rapidly turned in the opposite direction. Only four clinical responses are possible: (1) bilateral nystagmus, (2) bilateral conjugate deviation, (3) no response, and (4) unilateral eye deviation.

For the sake of the following discussion, we will assume that 50 mL of ice water has just been instilled in the right ear of a patient. If cold caloric stimulation of the right ear produces prominent nystagmus of both eyes, the cerebral cortex, MLF, and brainstem are intact. If both eyes move conjugately toward the side irrigated with cold water, and if they remain deviated in that direction, the midbrain and its brainstem reflexes are intact on that side. When cold water is instilled into the other ear, both eyes should again move conjugately toward the side of the cold-water irrigation. This assures that the entire brainstem reflex system is intact, that the pontine and midbrain structures are functioning normally, and that the brainstem is working but the correcting influences of the cortex which would cause nystagmus are not working.

If the eyes do not move in any direction despite bilateral testing, the brainstem is structurally or physiologically functionless. For example, severe hypothermia, drug overdose, or brainstem herniation can all result in absence of oculovestibular reflexes. Therefore, lack of response to cold caloric testing does not necessarily signify an irreversible process. If, however, the patient is normothermic and has no drug intoxication, a lack of any eye movement indicates a functionless brainstem.

Finally, cold water stimulation may produce an ipsilateral ocular response only. If the right ear is irrigated and the right eye moves but the left does not, an internuclear ophthalmoplegia is present. That is, the sixth cranial nerve on the side tested is functioning but is not able to transmit information to the opposite side of the brainstem. The opposite third cranial nerve which would cause the conjugate medial movement of the left eye has not been stimulated. Such a situation almost always indicates structural damage of the brainstem. This finding necessitates a rapid evaluation to determine if there is a structural problem which can be surgically corrected.

## Other Cranial Nerves

Other useful tests of the cranial nerves involve the corneal reflex and the facial muscles. The sensory portion of the corneal reflex is mediated through the fifth cranial nerve. Its efferent motor reaction is processed through the seventh cranial nerve. One must look for both the direct and consensual response to determine whether the reflex is working properly.

Facial asymmetry can only be judged in active motion. Particularly below the level of the nose, many normal people have mildly asymmetric faces. One cannot rule in or out a seventh-nerve lesion on the basis of a mild lower facial asymmetry at rest.

The eighth cranial nerve is of little localizing value in stuporous and comatose patients. Its fibers cross through the trapezoid body at the level of the lower pons and are therefore not strictly isolated to a particular side of the brainstem. Examination of the ninth, tenth, eleventh, and twelfth cranial nerves in comatose patients is likewise of little value in determining the level of functioning or underlying mechanism. Documentation of the gag response, however, is important to evaluate the risk of aspiration.

## Motor Testing

The first part of the motor examination, observation, should have already been completed. Spontaneous motor movements are generally a good sign. The ability of the muscles to move without external stimuli indicates the patient is sending some cortical instructions down the motor pathway. Any patient who can follow a command or move a body part on command is showing high-level motor system function.

Responses to stimuli help to isolate the level at which the nervous system is functioning. Abduction of the limbs or movements toward the site of noxious stimulation show motor system involvement, at least at diencephalic levels.

Decorticate posturing is hyperextension in the legs and flexion at the arms and the elbows with the hands coming in toward the center of the body. Such posturing can occur with lesions of the internal capsule and upper midbrain which interfere with the corticospinal pathways.

Decerebrate rigidity, in which the teeth are clenched and the arms and legs extended, is seen in only a few situations. It usually is caused by severe disease involving the central midbrain, leaving the lower brainstem below the central midbrain regions intact. Posterior fossa lesions causing pressure against the brainstem may also cause this type of posturing. Decerebrate posturing can also accompany postanoxic cerebral demyelinization.

Total paralysis in the comatose patient with no posturing despite the application of noxious stimuli should be considered a grave finding. This indicates that no protective brainstem mechanisms are functioning. This can be seen in severe, deep, metabolic and toxic comas but is more likely in structural lesions which affect the brainstem nuclei. To be certain that no movement is possible, stimuli must be given both above and below the foramen magnum. Patients with cervical spinal injuries may only be able to grimace or move facial musculature if their motor tracts have been severed in the cervical cord region.

## Sensory Examination

Sensory examination of the comatose patient essentially parallels the motor examination. Both the sensory or afferent fibers and the motor or efferent fibers should be tested. Hemisensory lesions as well as specific sensory levels should be sought.

## Reflex Status

Reflexes in comatose patients may be sensitive but not terribly specific. An upgoing toe can indicate lesions along the cortical spinal tract all the way from the cerebral cortex down to the motor neuron. The importance of reflex testing in the comatose patient, as in the awake patient, lies in determining the general level of the lesion by comparing responses side to side and top to bottom. Abdominal reflexes are of extremely low value and not worth testing in comatose patients.

In summary, the neurologic examination (see Table 33-3) of the patient with altered mental status has only a few areas of vital importance. Correct assessment of the level of mental status is paramount. Examination of respiratory pattern, extraocular movements, pupils, and motor function all need to be simultaneously integrated to determine the level of neurologic function. The principal goal of the neu-

**Table 33-3.** Rostrocaudal Brainstem Deterioration Secondary to Expanding Right Supratentorial Mass

| Anatomic Level | Consciousness | Respiration | Pupils | Oculovestibular | Motor |
|---|---|---|---|---|---|
| Upper diencephalon | Drowsy (dull) | Eupnea with yawns and sighs | Small, reactive | Depression of ocular checking and fast component of nystagmus | Left hemiparesis, bilat. paratonia |
| Lower diencephalon | Coma | Cheyne-Stokes (CSR) | Small, reactive | Loss of above | Left hemiparesis, decorticate |
| Mesencephalon | Coma | CSR central neurogenic hyperventilation (CNH) | Midposition fixed (MPF) | Dysconjugate response (loss of medial rectus function on horizontal gaze) | Decerebrate |
| Upper pons | Coma | CNH: ataxic | MPF | As above | Weak decerebrate |
| Lower pons | Coma | Ataxic; eupnea | MPF | None | Flaccid; areflexic |
| Medulla | Coma | Apnea | MPF | None | Same |

rologic examination is to distinguish structural, localized lesions from diffuse metabolic disease.

## LABORATORY AND X-RAY EVALUATION

The selection of laboratory and radiographic tests is guided by the history and initial evaluation. However, initial supportive therapy for the comatose patient must be done first, and an orderly approach to the laboratory can then follow.

A complete blood count is generally routine. Severe anemia or leukemias may be of diagnostic importance in coma.

Alterations in serum electrolytes, such as hyper- or hyponatremia or hypercalcemia, can cause altered mental status. Coma can result from sudden shifts in serum osmolality below 260 mOsm/L and above 330 mOsm/L. Glucose, sodium, and the alcohols are the most potent osmotically active substances generally encountered in clinical medicine. Hypoglycemia has been previously discussed.

Blood urea nitrogen (BUN), if it rises slowly, is usually not a cause of coma. Patients in whom there has been a sudden increase in BUN above 60 mg/100 mL may suffer significant alterations in mental status.

Arterial blood gases must be determined in all comatose patients. Hypoxia and hypercarbia can cause coma, and alkalosis and acidosis can change mental status.

Toxic drug screening should be ordered for those patients who have a nonfocal cause for coma and in whom no other discernible abnormal laboratory studies are found.

The indication for emergency lumbar puncture is a strong suspicion of a nonfocal infection of the central nervous system. Lumbar puncture is contraindicated in the presence of a mass lesion. In the comatose patient, in all other circumstances, lumbar puncture is at least relatively contraindicated until a CT scan is performed. In traumatic causes of coma the only immediate question of importance is the need for surgical intervention. Time is the critical factor in the salvage of brain function. Trauma Coma = CT Scan should be the rule; the sooner this can practically be done the better. When there is a strong suspicion of an operable lesion, the neurosurgeon and surgical team should be mobilized even before the CT results are known.

The EEG evaluation should be reserved for in-hospital patients who have been properly stabilized and where the usual causes of coma are ruled out. Its basic function at that point is to document lack of cortical activity.

The most important radiologic study is that of the cervical spine, to rule out fracture. A cross-table lateral view followed by anteroposterior and odontoid views are the minimum views needed. Even if the cervical spine films are found to be normal, if cervical cord injury is suspected, the neck must remain immobilized.

The CT scan has become the definitive test in the management of focal neurologic disease. In coma patients, the CT scan can detect not only intracranial lesions but fractures of the skull as well. It can detect amounts of blood as minute as 5 mL. Cervical spine films should be completed if possible, or, at the very least, a cross-table lateral

view of the spine obtained before a CT scan. If an emergency department does not have access within its hospital to CT scanning, it should have transfer arrangements available to obtain the study when focal neurologic disease entities are suspected.

## SPECIFIC CAUSES OF STUPOR AND COMA

There are literally hundreds of chemical agents and disease entities that can alter mental status. Before individual entities can be discussed it is necessary to review the most common general categories that cause coma. Two mnemonics can be useful: the word TIPS and the vowels A, E, I, O, and U (Table 33-4). If these disease entities are considered, important causes of coma will not be overlooked.

From an operational standpoint, the neurologic examination and laboratory studies divide the causes of altered mental status into toxic and metabolic diseases and supratentorial and infratentorial structural lesions that affect the reticular activating formation. It is useful, therefore, to review some specific disease entities based on this categorization. The following etiologies of coma represent a review of the more common causes encountered in the emergency department.

### Toxic and Metabolic Disorders

In most hospital emergency departments, metabolic causes dominate as the principal mechanism of coma. When toxic ingestions of drugs or other chemicals are included in this group, it is clearly the leading cause of coma in the United States. Intrinsic neurologic diseases such as Schelder leukodystrophy and other intrinsic nervous system diseases can cause coma, but they develop over a long period of time and will not usually be confused with acute decreases in mental status.

**Glucose metabolism.** In many series, the most common cause of altered mental status in the emergency department is hypoglycemia. Both hyper- and hypoglycemia may cause alterations of mental status. Diabetics are at high risk for altered mental status, not only because of abnormal glucose metabolism but also because of infection and other metabolic derangements. Hypoglycemia is not seen only in diabetics. Patients with pancreatic tumors, retroperitoneal sarcomas, and chronic alcoholics with liver disease may also present in a hypoglycemic state. Severe hypoglycemia can be induced with oral hypoglycemic agents.

**Table 33-4.** Mnemonic Aid for Coma Causes

| TIPS | Vowels |
|---|---|
| T—Trauma; all types, temperature | A—Alcohol and ingested drugs and toxins |
| I—Infection—neurologic and systemic | E—Endocrine—all types |
| P—Psychiatric and porphyria | Exocrine—liver, electrolytes |
| S—Space-occupying lesions, stroke, subarachnoid hemorrhage, shock | I—Insulin—diabetes mellitus |
| | O—Oxygen and opiates |
| | U—Uremia, renal causes including hypertensive problems |

**Liver disease.** In advanced stages of cirrhosis and other degenerative liver diseases, cellular changes are seen in the brain. These abnormal cells probably contribute to decreased mentation but have an unknown effect on the actual level of consciousness. Rapid elevations of serum ammonia levels may contribute to depressed mental status. Patients with advanced liver disease frequently have decreased liver glycogen stores, predisposing to hypoglycemia.

**Uremia.** The coma of uremia is related to changes in osmolality as the BUN rises. Cerebral water content will adjust to very gradual changes in the BUN, but coma may develop with a rapid rise in the BUN.

**Oxygen.** All portions of the cardiorespiratory system can be involved as causes of coma. Severe anemia decreases oxygen delivered to the brain. Low cardiac output due to arrhythmias or loss of myocardial contractility can cause decreased cerebral perfusion. Occasionally, older patients placed on antihypertensive medications will become lethargic. Blood pressure may have been reduced too rapidly, causing cerebral hypoperfusion. A rapid increase in $P_{CO_2}$, as with pulmonary disease, correlates closely with neurologic symptoms. With chronic hypercarbia, however, mental status does not deteriorate because the brain can become adjusted to high levels of $P_{CO_2}$.

**Endocrine disorders.** Alterations in serum sodium affect the central nervous system by changing the serum osmolality and causing shifts in intracellular brain fluid. Extreme hypothyroidism can likewise cause metabolic shifts which result in depressed mental status or even coma. Hyperthyroidism, on the other hand, usually causes an agitated and tremulous state, and coma is not seen until the patient is in severe thyroid storm or suffers a cerebral vascular accident.

**Carcinoma.** Coma can be caused by the remote effects of cancer. Hyponatremia due to inappropriate antidiuretic hormone (ADH) secretion in carcinoma of the lung, pancreas, ovary, and prostate are well recognized. Metabolic alkalosis in association with Cushing syndrome may become severe enough to alter mental status. The progressive multifocal leukoencephalopathies seen with lymphomas may first present with a depression of consciousness. Hyper- or hypocalcemia may also cause alterations in mental status.

**Poisons and toxins.** Alcohol is still the most widely used and most popular metabolic poison. Its effects are usually short-lived and it is metabolized within a matter of hours. Barbiturate comas, on the other hand, may be of extremely long duration, depending on the type of barbiturate ingested. Cases of barbiturate coma lasting several weeks followed by the return of normal mental status have been recorded. Severe metabolic acidosis from drugs such as methyl alcohol, ethylene glycol, and paraldehyde can be seen in patients who readily abuse the more traditional ethanol.

**Central nervous system infections.** Central nervous system infections and septicemia can be included in the toxic metabolic causes of coma. Meningitis can cause alterations in mental status. In bacterial meningitis, most notably tuberculous meningitis, the infecting organism can compete with the brain itself for glucose. Viral encephalitis may markedly alter consciousness and may at first present as an acute encephalopathy, followed by a rapid downhill course with depressed mental status. Severe infection anywhere in the body can also cause depressed mental status.

**Subarachnoid hemorrhage.** Subarachnoid hemorrhage is the only intracranial hemorrhage which is not focal in nature. Bleeding into the subarachnoid space quickly spreads throughout the cerebral spinal fluid. The resultant vasospasm is an initial homeostatic attempt to stop subarachnoid bleeding. This vasospasm may be partially responsible for the rapid decrease in mental status. Subarachnoid hemorrhage should be considered high on the list of diagnostic possibilities in all patients who experience headache with decreasing mental status.

**Epilepsy.** A patient who has had a seizure may present to the emergency department in postictal coma. If the underlying disease is truly idiopathic epilepsy, the patient usually has a rapid return to normal mental status without residual focal deficits. Nonconvulsive status epilepticus can cause prolonged mental status depression. Seizures lasting for more than 15 min should be suspected to be structural in nature. It is always important to check for underlying causes of seizures such as encephalitis, meningitis, metabolic abnormalities, and trauma.

**Disorders of temperature regulation.** Hypothermia below the level of 32°C can in and of itself depress neurologic functioning enough to cause coma. Hypothermia may result from underlying diseases such as myxedema or hypopituitarism, or ingested toxins. Hyperthermia above the level of 42°C may also depress mental status to the point of coma. Patients with severe hyper- or hypothermia frequently have underlying neurovascular disease and are often left with severe neurologic residues.

**Cofactor deficiency.** Wernicke encephalopathy due to carbohydrate overload and lack of thiamine can cause coma. Also, in rare instances of severe nutritional deprivation, altered mental status may be seen as the result of other minor cofactor deficiencies of cobalt, manganese, or zinc.

## Supratentorial Focal Lesions

These are localized anatomic lesions lying wholly or partially in the area above the tentorium cerebelli. They affect mental status principally by increased pressure, which compromises the reticular activating formation, and by bilateral cerebral hemisphere involvement. Such focal pressure may cause herniation of the temporal lobe (uncus) into the infratentorial space. This compresses the ipsilateral third cranial nerve, causing the uncal syndrome, with ataxic respirations, contralateral hemiparesis, and ipsilateral pupillary dilatation being the most common manifestations.

**Subdural hematoma.** In older patients, trauma victims, alcoholics, and those patients on anticoagulants, subdural hematoma is always a consideration. Even if focal neurologic findings are not present, if the patient belongs to one of these groups and has an acute change in mental status, subdural hematoma should still be considered. Subdural hematomas may compress supratentorial structures bilaterally and thus present much like dementia or progressive encephalopathy. A history of trauma, although helpful, is certainly not necessary to entertain the diagnosis of subdural hematoma. In chronic subdural hematomas, symptoms can fluctuate mildly from day to day. Laboratory tests, EEGs, and skull x-rays are of little value in diagnosis. The test of choice if the lesion is suspected is the enhanced CT scan.

**Acute epidural hematoma.** Acute epidural hematomas are almost always related to major trauma. The bleeding is usually the result of tearing of the middle meningeal artery due to skull fracture. Unlike subdural bleeding which is venous, epidural bleeding is arterial in nature and therefore progresses rapidly. The suspected epidural hematoma must be treated aggressively if the patient is to be salvaged.

**Subdural empyema.** This is a relatively rare cause of coma but must be considered in patients who have recently undergone otolaryngologic surgery, particularly related to acute sinusitis. It is occasionally seen in conjunction with acute meningitis when *Streptococcus* is the offending organism. Meningitis is not associated with focal neurologic signs. If a patient has symptoms of meningitis plus focal findings, a subdural empyema or brain abscess should be considered. Herpes simplex encephalitis, although a diffuse disease, tends to have a particular predilection for the temporal lobes. Patients thus present with temporal lobe syndromes and may appear to have a focal neurologic process.

**Cerebral vascular accidents.** The majority of thrombotic and embolic cerebral vascular accidents are not associated with coma or even significant decreased mental status. However, hemorrhagic cerebral vascular accidents are commonly associated with unconsciousness. Bleeding may be from a ruptured artery, aneurysm, or arterial venous malformation. When bleeding is the result of a hypertensive crisis, the exact site of the lesion is rarely found. If patients with severe hypertension become progressively obtunded, it is wise to stabilize the patient completely and reduce pressure to reasonable levels before attempting to localize the bleeding site.

Intraventricular hemorrhage is a particular subset of cerebral vascular accident. It is associated with an extremely poor prognosis, and death occurs within minutes to hours after pontine and medullary findings appear. The intraventricular hemorrhage does not, per se, harm brain tissue, but blood in the cerebrospinal fluid causes considerable increase in intracranial pressure. It is often very difficult to clinically differentiate intraventricular hemorrhage from pontine bleeding without the benefit of a CT scan. It is important to identify patients with acute cerebellar hemorrhage because this represents the most treatable of the intraparenchymal processes.

**Cerebral neoplasms.** It would be unusual for coma to be the first presenting sign of a cerebral neoplasm. More likely, the patient may present with a seizure followed by a prolonged postictal state. Bleeding into the tumor itself may cause symptoms indistinguishable from other types of cerebral vascular accidents. The slow enlargement of a supratentorial tumor produces brain swelling which can, over a period of time, dull mental status. Tumors in the lateral or third ventricles may obstruct outflow of cerebral fluid and cause acute downward pressure and displacement of the brainstem. In rare instances neoplasms directly infiltrate or destroy the cerebral connections of the reticular activating formation, causing irreversible coma. Almost all the findings in cerebral neoplasms, however, develop over an extended period of time.

## Infratentorial Compressive Syndromes

The infratentorial compressive causes of coma are lesions which do not originate within the brainstem itself, but which by their proximity may compress the brainstem.

**Basilar artery occlusion.** The entire brainstem is supplied continuously by the vertebral basilar system. The reticular activating formation in particular receives paramedian branches off the basilar artery. Anything which interferes with the blood supply through the vertebral basilar system can cause alteration of consciousness. Posterior circulation transient ischemic episodes are often characterized as "drop-like" attacks in which there may be a total loss of muscular tone with or without a loss of consciousness. Problems involving the posterior circulation are extremely difficult to treat but need to be separated from other entities. Thrombosis of the basilar artery causes coma and is associated without CT abnormalities in the early phases.

**Traumatic posterior fossa hemorrhage.** Severe trauma may result in bleeding below the tentorium cerebelli but without destruction of the brainstem itself. A hematoma in the posterior fossa can compress the brainstem and may be life-threatening. It is impossible to distinguish this type of hematoma from several other posterior fossa lesions on a physical examination basis alone. Since it represents a surgically correctable cause of coma it is imperative that it be diagnosed.

**Acute cerebellar hemorrhage.** Bleeding into the cerebellum is usually the result of a nontraumatic rupture of an arteriovenous malformation. Head pain and the onset of sudden vertigo with conjugate deviation of the eyes away to the opposite side of the cerebellar lesion are signs which strongly suggest acute cerebellar hemorrhage. This is the most treatable of the interparenchymal hemorrhages, and if relieved promptly, the possibility exists for good return of neurologic function.

**Pontine hemorrhage.** Pontine hemorrhage is a devastating, acute brainstem parenchymal lesion which produces coma. It is often difficult to differentiate acute pontine hemorrhage from acute cerebellar hemorrhage. These two lesions are both associated with sudden de-

**Table 33–5.** Checklist for the Patient with Depressed Mental Status

| General Examination | Neurologic Examination |
|---|---|
| Airway established | Observation |
| Breathing checked (including auscultation to rule out pneumothorax) | Respiratory pattern |
| Cardiac output assessed |   Normal |
| Cervical spine immobilized |   Cheyne-Stokes |
| Obvious hemorrhage compressed |   Hyperventilation |
| IV line started |   Apneustic breathing |
| Full vital signs (full set) |   Ataxic breathing |
| Thiamine 100 mg IV |   Agonal breathing |
| Glucose 50 mL 50% IV | Autisms |
| Naloxone 2 ampules IV, repeated if no response |   Yawning |
| The stable patient—historical features obtained including rate of onset, drugs, trauma, fever, prior episodes |   Coughing |
| |   Hiccuping |
| General physical examination—signs of trauma; i.e., Battle's sign, hemotympanum, scalp hematomas and lacerations, subcutaneous emphysema of the chest | Mental status |
| |   Responds to voice |
| |   Responds to touch |
| Obvious lesions of the abdomen, lesions of the pelvis, and long-bone injuries |   Responds to noxious stimuli |
| | Cranial nerves |
| Skin |   Visual threat |
|   Needle marks, cyanosis, pallor, rashes, dehydration |   Inspection of fundi for papilledema and hemorrhages |
| Breath and odors | Pupils |
|   Alcohol, acetone, fecal material, fetor hepaticus |   Size |
| Cardiac examination |   Reactions—direct and consensual |
|   Rhythm, gallop, rub, murmurs | Extraocular movements |
| Abdominal findings |   Oculovestibular testing |
|   Organomegaly, ascites, bruits, flank ecchymoses, rectal and pelvic examination |   Oculocephalic testing (if appropriate) |
| | Corneal reflex |
| | Facial asymmetry |
| | Motor system |
| |   Posturing |
| |   Ability of the limbs to move |
| |   Stimuli |
| | Decerebration, decortication, or true abduction by high-level centers |
| | Pathologic reflexes |

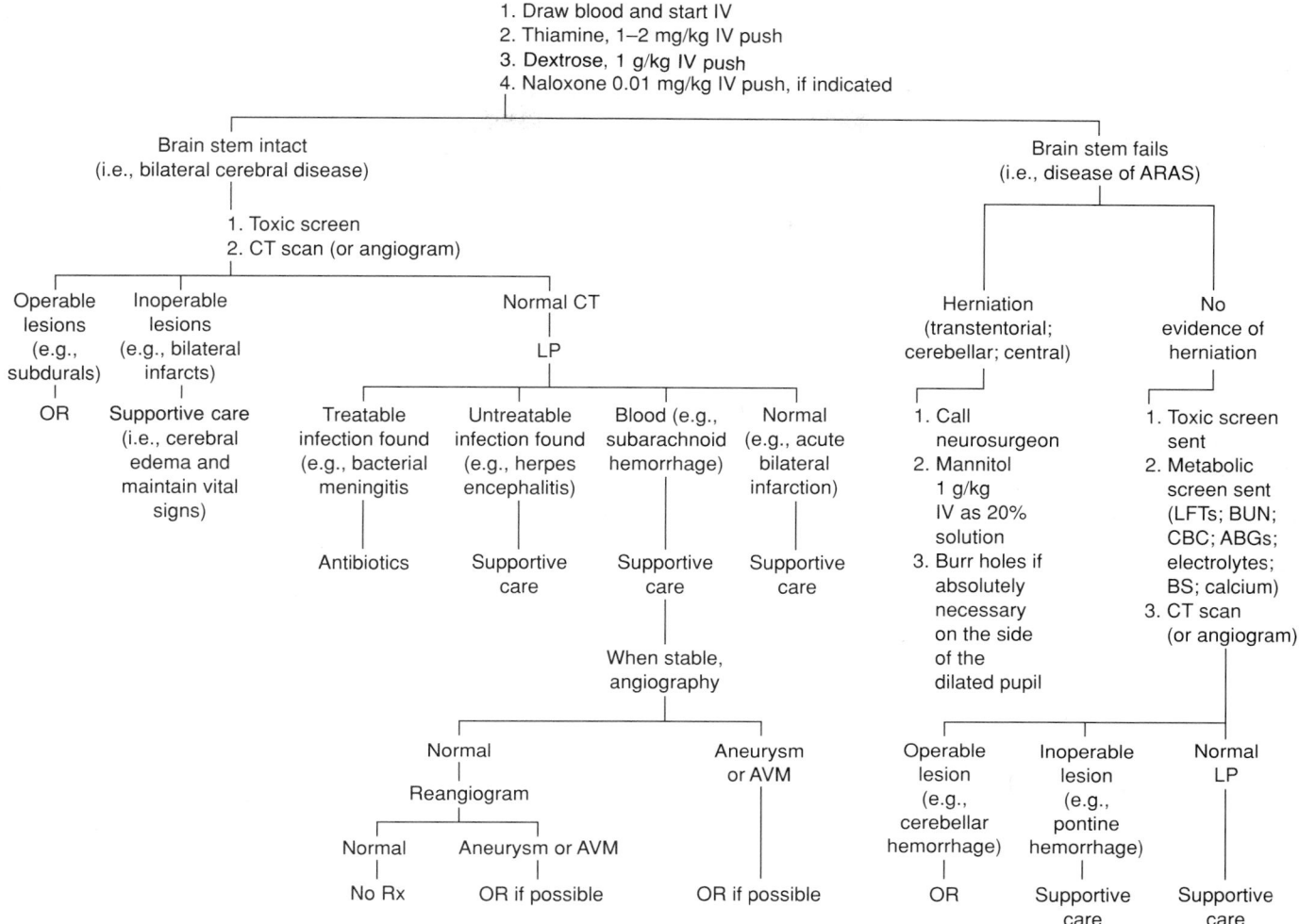

**Fig. 33-1.** Diagnosis and treatment protocol in the comatose patient. (From Samuels MA: *Manual of Neurologic Therapeutics.* Boston, Little, Brown, 1982, p. 13. Used by permission.)

creases in consciousness and ataxic breathing, pinpoint pupils, absent or abnormal ocular vestibular responses, and meningismus. Although there are some reports of successful drainage of intrapontine hematomas, the prognosis remains grave. Rapid diagnosis is crucial to separate this problem from an acute cerebellar hemorrhage, which is a surgically treatable disease.

**Brainstem tumors.** Actual parenchymal lesions of the brainstem, including angiomas, gliomas, and ependymomas, can cause brainstem compression syndromes. Most of these, however, progress slowly over a period of time and present with other localized neurologic findings before mental status is affected. Other posterior fossa tumors such as meningiomas and acoustic neuromas almost always present with cranial nerve findings before mental status is affected.

## PRACTICAL ASSESSMENT AND MANAGEMENT GUIDELINES

Up to this point we have attempted to review the basic mechanisms and etiologies of decreased mental status. Translating this into action in the emergency department should now represent little problem. Table 33-5 is a sample assessment checklist to be used for the patient with severely depressed mental status.

## X-rays and Laboratory Studies

The need for all x-ray and laboratory studies is relative. The need for the following tests will be guided by initial examination and the patient's initial response to therapy:

CBC
BUN
Electrolytes
Glucose
Calcium
Toxicology screen
Arterial blood gases
Cervical spine x-rays
Skull x-rays (for foreign body or suspected depressed fracture)
CT scan
Lumbar puncture

## Treatment Algorithm

Figure 33-1 illustrates an excellent decision-tree algorithm for the management of the comatose patient.

## BIBLIOGRAPHY

Plum F, Posner J: *Diagnosis of Stupor and Coma,* 4th ed. Philadelphia, Davis, 1984.

# 34

# SYSTEMIC ANALGESIA AND SEDATION FOR PROCEDURES IN ADULTS

## Donald M. Yealy

## INTRODUCTION

Although the tools to provide adequate pain relief and anxiolysis are available to clinicians, many procedures are accompanied by treatable or preventable discomfort. Certain groups are at higher risk for poor procedural analgesia and sedation, including patients at the extremes of age or with cognitive limits, presumably because of fears and misconceptions about analgesic use and safety. Additionally, recent investigations suggest that ethnicity influences the use of adequate analgesic regimens in emergency department patients with acute orthopaedic injuries. The root of this influence is unclear and may encompass communication and cultural biases on both the patient's and provider's behalf. The tools to combat inadequate procedural analgesia and sedation are readily available and are discussed below.

The terminology surrounding systemic analgesia and sedation are reviewed in Table 34-1. A continuum exists; light and conscious sedation are commonly provided in the emergency department, where deep sedation should be undertaken rarely and general anesthesia avoided. Patients undergoing procedures associated primarily with anxiety (i.e., imaging studies or wound repair after infiltration) are best managed using pure sedatives; in those for whom pain is anticipated and not easily treated or prevented with alternatives, systemic analgesics (alone or with sedatives) should be used. Clinicians often withhold or underuse systemic analgesics because of the fear that complications, especially oversedation, may outweigh benefits. Although absolute dosing requirements vary when treating patients,

complication phobias are not a reason to withhold therapy. Titrated doses of analgesics do not increase the risk of complications; in fact, untreated pain can increase morbidity. Dysrhythmias, myocardial ischemia, impaired host defenses, and suboptimal wound repair may result from poorly treated acute pain. Beyond this, underuse of systemic agents devalues the "complication" most feared by patients—pain and fear.

There are two absolute contraindications to providing systemic analgesia or sedation for a procedure: (1) the presence of clinical instability (e.g., hemodynamic or respiratory) that requires immediate attention, and (2) refusal by a competent patient. Endotracheal intubation and central venous catheter insertion are examples of procedures occasionally performed without systemic analgesia in an unstable patient. Even with these selected interventions, most patients can receive local anesthesia or judicious doses of a systemic analgesic to ease the discomfort without risking harm. The presence of a condition that could eventually result in instability (e.g., femur fracture or pneumothorax) is not a contraindication to analgesia for a painful procedure.

Besides drug administration, techniques such as hypnosis, distraction, and enhanced communication will reduce the perceived pain associated with a procedure. A calm, reassuring voice coupled with realistic but noninflammatory statements about the procedure and "how to relax" requires little extra effort yet reaps great benefit without risk. Allowing patients to listen to music of their choice (via headphones) will also reduce anxiety and pain perception.

## AGENTS TO PROVIDE SYSTEMIC ANALGESIA AND SEDATION

### Opioids

The opioids are the best agents available to provide rapid and reliable systemic analgesia during painful procedures (Table 34-2). These agents also relieve anxiety but offer limited amnesia. Although there are risks to systemic opioid use, these can be minimized by following some basic principles.

The best method of obtaining rapid and safe analgesia with an opioid is to administer the agent via the intravenous (IV) route in a

**Table 34-1.** The Terminology of Systemic Analgesia and Sedation

| | |
|---|---|
| **Analgesia** | Relief of perception of pain without intentional production of a sedated state. Altered mental status and sedation may be a secondary effect of medications administered for this purpose. |
| **Anxiety alleviation** | A state in which there is no change in a patient's level of awareness, only a decrease of apprehension for the situation. |
| **Conscious and light sedation** | Controlled lessening of a patient's awareness of the environment and/or pain perception while maintaining stable vital signs, an independent airway, and adequate spontaneous respirations. Light sedation refers to minimal sedative effects, while conscious sedation encompasses this and more but not to that level described for deep sedation. |
| **Deep sedation** | Profound depression of awareness to any stimuli. This state is frequently accompanied by a loss or near loss of protective reflexes and requires active attention to appropriate airway and ventilatory management and blood pressure control. |
| **General anesthesia** | A state of complete loss of consciousness, responses to verbal and painful stimuli, and protective reflexes accompanied by muscular relaxation. This state requires active airway and hemodynamic support and intensive monitoring. |

Source: Adapted from Agency for Health Care Policy and Research, Feb. 1992, and Sacchetti A, Schafermayer R, Gerardi M, et al: Pediatric analgesia and sedation. Ann Emerg Med 23:237, 1994.

**Table 34-2.** Common Agents for Systemic Analgesia in Adults

| Agents | Initial Dose | Duration | Adverse Effects |
|---|---|---|---|
| Morphine sulfate | 0.1–0.15 mg/kg IV | 3–4 h | Respiratory depression |
| Meperidine | 0.75–1.0 mg/kg IV | 2–3 h | Respiratory depression |
| Fentanyl | 0.5–1.0 µg/kg IV | 1–2 h | Respiratory depression Muscular rigidity |
| Ketamine | 0.5 mg/kg IV | 30–60 min | Hallucinations Catecholamine release Hypotension Laryngospasm Airway secretions Muscle stimulation |
| Nitrous oxide | 50:50 $N_2O:O_2$ | Minutes | Excitement Drowsiness Vertigo Avoid in: Head injury Bowel obstruction COPD Pneumothorax Air embolism Bends |
| Midazolam | 1 mg IV | 60–90 min | Respiratory depression Hypotension |
| Methohexital | 0.5–1.0 mg/kg IV | 5–10 min | Laryngospasm Respiratory depression |
| Thiopental | 1-2 mg/kg IV | 5–10 min | Laryngospasm Respiratory depression |

titrated fashion. When given to manage the pain of a procedure, incremental doses should be administered every 2 to 5 min until the patient displays mild opioid effects: miosis, somnolent but responsive to verbal stimuli, slightly impaired speech, and reporting no or minimal pain on questioning. The beginning of the procedure will help gauge the effectiveness of the analgesia; if inadequate, repeat doses should be given based on the response. Some patients who appear adequately treated during the initial stages will complain of pain at the height of the procedure (e.g., the actual relocation of a joint or probing of an abscess). Although this is sometimes unavoidable, careful titration based on the above observations should make this a tolerable and rare event.

Physicians often apply arbitrary ceiling doses to opioid analgesia regimens. Since individual needs for analgesia vary widely, fixed upper limit doses should not be employed. In practice, the true ceiling dose of any opioid is the dose that provides adequate pain relief or causes side effects, especially excessive sedation or hypotension. Failure to obtain adequate analgesia or sedation with a certain expected ceiling dose of an opioid suggests one of two things: a higher than anticipated need or failure to deliver the agent to the opioid receptors. The former is treated with more opioid unless a side effect occurs; the latter is remedied by seeking errors in drug dispensing or failure of the route of delivery (e.g., intravenous catheter disruption or infiltration).

Intramuscular (IM) and oral (PO) routes provide less reliable immediate clinical effects, limiting the ability to titrate to individual need. Intramuscular injections also cause discomfort with each dose in contrast to the "one-time" discomfort of IV insertion (which can be diminished with the use of a buffered, warmed local anesthetic wheal). Single-dose IM and PO analgesic and sedative regimens force the practitioner to estimate the optimal amount of drug used, resulting in frequent under- or overmedication. Conversely, multiple-dose regimens are impractical unless time permits prolonged pre- and postprocedure observation.

Relative contraindications to opioid analgesia include hemodynamic or respiratory compromise, altered sensorium (from injury or intoxicants), or the inability to monitor properly and manage side effects, especially respiratory depression. Patients with chronic lung, central nervous system, or heart disease (especially conduction abnormalities) and pregnant patients near term should receive these agents with caution. When used in the elderly or very young, use of smaller dose increments will help provide analgesia and avoid complications. Overall, the risk of clinically important respiratory depression with opioid use is about 1 in 1000; although the potential for a higher rate with IV use exists, close attention to titration principles and monitoring should still maintain this risk at a very low level.

Morphine (0.1- to 0.15-mg/kg IV increments) is the "gold standard" opioid; most adults will experience good pain relief at a total dose of 10 to 20 mg, with a maximal duration of effect of 3 to 4 h. Meperidine (0.75- to 1.0-mg/kg IV increments) is an alternative and has a duration of 2 to 3 h. Seizures are a rare complication seen after large doses of meperidine or in select populations (e.g., those patients with renal failure or sickle cell disease). Most adults undergoing a painful procedure will require a total meperidine dose of 1.5 to 3.0 mg/kg. Both morphine and meperidine can provide inexpensive analgesia and sedation, although the duration is often longer than needed for short outpatient procedures. Meperidine offers no clinically important advantage over morphine in most patients, although it is commonly used based on generational habits.

Fentanyl is a potent synthetic opioid congener well studied in large trials of adults and children undergoing painful procedures of short duration. An initial dose of 0.5 to 1.0 μg/kg over 60 s is optimal, with most patients requiring a total dose of 2 to 3 μg/kg. The attractive features of fentanyl are its duration of action (1 to 2 h) and low side-effect profile. When used alone in this fashion, respiratory depression is rare and often responds to temporary bag-valve-mask assistance.

Fentanyl causes little hemodynamic compromise and may be useful in those with borderline hypotension or heart failure. One rare side effect seen is truncal and jaw muscle rigidity, which, when severe, can impair ventilation. This rigidity is usually seen with high doses (>10 to 15 μg/kg) or rapid infusions of fentanyl and is not reported using the above regimen. Parenteral naloxone may reverse rigidity; if this is unsuccessful or respiratory compromise great, paralysis and endotracheal intubation are needed. Other synthetic opioids are available for procedural analgesia and sedation but offer no advantage over the aforementioned agents.

If respiratory depression occurs after any opioid, supplemental oxygen should be administered to maintain oxygen saturation at or above 95%. If verbal and physical stimuli do not increase spontaneous respirations, assisted ventilation with a bag-valve-mask device should be performed and an opioid antagonist administered. Naloxone (0.1 to 0.8 mg) is the most widely available opioid antagonist. When titrated properly, opioid reversal is rarely needed and is not a routine action after completion of a procedure.

Nausea and vomiting may be treated with intravenous antiemetics (e.g., prochlorperazine or metoclopramide, 5 to 10 mg of either for adults). Opioid-induced hypotension is usually the result of vasodilatation and responds to recumbent positioning and intravenous fluids. Pruritus (especially in the face) is common after parenteral opioids. It is usually the result of nonallergic histamine release and rarely needs treatment with an antihistamine.

## Nonopioid Analgesics

Although a variety of nonopioid analgesic agents are available for acute pain management, two (ketamine and nitrous oxide) deserve attention because of their utility during painful procedures (Table 34-2). Nonsteroidal anti-inflammatory drugs (NSAIDs) can decrease the need for opioids during certain procedures; most NSAIDs are available orally and require up to 1 h for peak effects, limiting their impact for short-duration or emergent procedures. Ketorolac can be given parenterally but is relatively costly and offers little pragmatic benefit to most patients.

Intravenous ketamine (a phencyclidine derivative), in initial doses of 0.5 mg/kg followed by incremental doses of 0.25 mg/kg as needed, produces a state of "dissociative analgesia/sedation." In this condition, patients are somnolent but responsive to verbal commands, seemingly aware but unconcerned about painful stimuli, and maintain airway reflexes well. The onset of action is rapid (15 s) with a duration of 30 to 60 min. Intramuscular ketamine (1 to 4 mg/kg) is an alternative to IV, providing analgesia and sedation within 10 to 20 min; this should be used sparingly for the reasons mentioned above.

Occasionally, recovery from ketamine sedation and analgesia is associated with hallucinations or nightmares. In the doses suggested above, these are uncommon and can be reduced by using a calm, reassuring voice in a controlled environment at the termination of treatment. The addition of a benzodiazepine attenuates this troublesome experience but should be done with caution, since increased sedation and respiratory depression can occur.

Tachycardia and increased cardiac output are common after ketamine because of its catecholamine-releasing actions. In patients with poor sympathetic tone or prolonged stress (e.g., sepsis or congestive heart failure), ketamine may cause hypotension from direct myocardial depression. Respiratory depression is rare, usually seen after high doses or when combined with other sedative agents. Also, laryngospasm has been reported in 4 percent of cases in children, usually responding to positive-pressure mask ventilation. In practice, increased airway secretions and occasional random muscular stimulation are the most common mild side effects seen with ketamine use.

Nitrous oxide:oxygen (50%:50% near sea level, maximum of 60%:40% at high elevations) mixtures provide anxiolysis and moderate analgesia when inhaled. Contrary to popular misconceptions, nitrous oxide:oxygen at this dose alone will not provide general anesthesia. Nitrous oxide:oxygen mixtures should be self-administered by the patient with a demand-valve device, allowing for patient-controlled titration. Two-tank systems are commercially available, with safety features to ensure that nitrous oxide alone cannot be delivered. Nitrous oxide:oxygen mixtures should be used in conjunction with a scavenging device to help protect the health care workers from prolonged low-level exposure.

The onset of action and duration of the 50% nitrous oxide:oxygen mixture is 30 to 60 s. Patients should be counselled about what to expect prior to the institution of therapy: the gas is colorless and sweet-smelling and may cause mild excitement, drowsiness, nausea, numbness, or a "warm, tingling" sensation. The patient can stop inhalation if any undesirable effects occur; the use of the demand valve will ensure that those who become somnolent will no longer receive the gas. Data from over 3000 applications document that 50% nitrous oxide:oxygen in these concentrations is devoid of serious side effects. It should be withheld in those with an altered sensorium or head injury, bowel obstruction, pneumothorax, or severe chronic obstructive pulmonary disease, and in suspected decompression sickness or air embolism. About 25 percent of patients will report marked pain relief with 50% nitrous oxide:oxygen, with another 40 to 50 percent reporting mild to moderate relief. For markedly painful procedures, its major utility is as an adjunct to local anesthesia or systemic analgesia.

### Sedatives and Adjuncts to Analgesics

Sedatives and adjuncts should be administered using the same dose and route principles outlined above for opioids (Table 34-2). The benzodiazepines are pure sedative agents, lacking any direct analgesic properties. Aside from their use with ketamine, the benzodiazepines are useful in two situations: to provide skeletal muscle relaxation during a procedure (e.g., orthopaedic reduction), and to help with anxiolysis and amnesia.

When used in combination with an opioid, the dose of the opioid required for adequate analgesia is lowered. If using this combination approach, it is generally safer to give the benzodiazepine first (to achieve very mild drowsiness and muscular relaxation), followed by the opioid titrated to analgesic needs. The benzodiazepines produce amnesia, primarily anterograde in nature. Although this can help improve the patient's perception of a procedure, amnesia and sedation alone should not replace analgesia.

Midazolam and diazepam are the benzodiazepines of choice for systemic sedation. The onset of action of either agent after an IV dose is 2 to 5 min. Midazolam is preferred for outpatient and emergency department procedures because of its shorter duration of action (60 to 90 min). An effective midazolam regimen in adults is 1 to 2 mg every 5 min until mild sedation or adequate muscle relaxation occurs. Diazepam (2.5- to 5-mg increments in adults) has a 2- to 4-h duration of action. When used in the elderly or in combination with an opioid, lower doses of either agent should be employed initially and close titration procedures followed to avoid respiratory or cardiovascular compromise.

The major side effects of the benzodiazepines are respiratory depression and hypotension, with the latter averted by delivering the drug slowly. Respiratory depression is dose-dependent but varies among patients and is common when using a benzodiazepine and an opioid together. Flumazenil will antagonize benzodiazepine-induced sedation and respiratory depression but has little effect on hemodynamic alterations.

Barbiturates act similarly to benzodiazepines, although through a different pharmacodynamic action, to produce sedation, anxiolysis, and amnesia with little direct analgesia. In this class, the short- and ultrashort-acting agents are alternatives to the benzodiazepines for brief procedures (e.g., cardioversion). Incremental IV titrated doses of methohexital (0.5 to 1 mg/kg) or thiopental (1 to 2 mg/kg) will produce sedation within 1 to 2 min and last for 5 to 10 min. The side effects of the barbiturates are similar to those seen with benzodiazepines, although two differences must be highlighted: (1) Airway tone can increase following barbiturate administration, limiting its use in those patients with moderate to severe reactive airway disease; and (2) the window between light sedation, deep sedation, and general anesthesia with these agents is narrow, so caution must be used when compared to presumably equipotent benzodiazepine regimens.

Propofol and etomidate are sedative agents used primarily for parenteral induction of general anesthesia or monitored deep sedation. Neither are chemically related to each other or to barbiturates and benzodiazepines, and little data are available supporting their use in the emergency department. Etomidate can suppress adrenal steroid production, but this is of little clinical significance with short-term use. Propofol displays profound and variable hypotensive and induction properties, limiting its use outside of the operative suite.

Phenothiazines and derivatives (prochlorperazine, promethazine, and chlorpromazine) are antiemetics and mild sedatives. These drugs are often erroneously used in "cocktails," or fixed regimens, to potentiate the action of an opioid. Phenothiazines do not enhance analgesia (and may counteract it) and produce nonreversible sedation. The treatment of nausea is the only indication for these agents.

## MONITORING DURING SYSTEMIC ANALGESIA AND SEDATION

After appropriate choice and administration of an agent, the single most important aspect of providing analgesia and sedation is the monitoring of each patient. Monitoring has two goals: detecting complications and ensuring adequate analgesia. Virtually all serious mishaps can be avoided with close patient monitoring during treatment.

Monitoring techniques are divided into *interactive* and *mechanical* methods. Interactive monitoring is the most important method of ensuring safe and adequate analgesia; it involves contact between the patient and the health care team. Mechanical monitoring involves the use of adjuncts to help detect complications or ease the recording of observations.

The first step of interactive monitoring involves assessing the baseline clinical status of the patient, including blood pressure, heart rate, and respiratory rate. The assessment of consciousness is based on the stimulus required to evoke a response: awake and spontaneously conversant, somnolent but responsive to verbal or painful stimuli, or unresponsive to any stimuli represent the major categories.

In adults and older children, pain should be assessed using a simple numeric scale. In clinical practice, a 1 (barely perceptible) to 10 (excruciating pain) scale is best. Verbal scales are convenient, but visual analogue scales (with end-anchoring marks only) are best for research purposes. After the initial assessment, it should be made clear to the patient what clinical actions will be taken for various subjective pain scores (e.g., a subjective pain score of >3 will be treated with analgesic agents).

After the initial assessment, ongoing interactive monitoring should take place. All patients should be continuously monitored, with documentation at 5- to 10-min intervals. Certain side effects should be specifically asked about: nausea, chest pain, dyspnea, dizziness, and auditory/visual changes. Although the clinician performing the procedure may assess the consciousness and subjective pain relief, a second provider should be available to perform the rest of the interactive monitoring steps and assist with the procedure. Continuous bedside interactive monitoring should continue for at least 20 min after the end of the procedure or the last IV dose of analgesic and until adequate recovery occurs. During the recovery phase, repeat assessment at 10- to 15-min intervals should continue until the patient is awake and conversant.

Mechanical adjuncts ease the task of interactive monitoring and detecting occult side effects but do not replace interactive monitoring. Automated blood pressure devices can eliminate the need to take repeated manual measurements but should not be used alone until a manual check confirms the accuracy. Pulse oximetry offers a noninvasive assessment of arterial oxygen saturation and heart rate. The arterial oxygen saturation should be kept above 95% throughout the procedure, with supplemental oxygen employed as needed unless contraindicated. Electrocardiographic (ECG) monitoring is another adjunct but offers little to the aforementioned devices in most patients. Currently, nasal capnometry to detect occult hypoventilation is not proved useful in addition to the steps outlined above.

## DISPOSITION

Recovery is adequate and patients are eligible for discharge only when they are awake, conversant, and ambulatory. When discharged, they should be accompanied by an adult and should not drive an automobile or operate dangerous machinery for at least 6 to 12 h. Verbal and written instructions for care must be given to the responsible accompanying person, since the systemic agents used may impair recall in the treated patient.

## BIBLIOGRAPHY

Agency for Health Care Policy and Research: *Acute Pain Management: Operative or Medical Procedures and Trauma.* Rockville, MD, US Dept of Health and Human Services, Feb, 1992.

Barsan WG, Tomassoni AJ, Seger D, et al: Safety of high-dose narcotic analgesia for emergency department procedures. *Ann Emerg Med* 22:155, 1993.

Billmire DA, Neale HW, Gregory RO: Use of IV fentanyl in the outpatient treatment of pediatric facial trauma. *J Trauma* 25:179, 1985.

Chudnofsky CR, Wright SW, Dronen SC, et al: The safety of fentanyl use in the emergency department. *Ann Emerg Med* 18:635, 1989.

Wright SW: Conscious sedation in the emergency department: The value of capnography and pulse oximetry. *Ann Emerg Med* 21:551, 1992.

Wright SW, Chudnofsky CR, Dronen SC, et al: Comparison of midazolam and diazepam for conscious sedation in the emergency department. *Ann Emerg Med* 22:201, 1993.

Zink BJ, Darfler K, Saluzzo RF, et al: The efficacy and safety of methohexital in the ED. *Ann Emerg Med* 20:1293, 1991.

# SECTION 4
# Acute Signs and Symptoms in Children

## 35
## FEVER

### Carol D. Berkowitz

Fever is the single most common chief complaint of children presenting to the emergency department, accounting for about 30 percent of pediatric outpatient visits. The physician evaluating the febrile child must differentiate the mildly ill from the seriously ill child, a challenge that may be compounded by the fact that no focus of infection is apparent. The extent of the diagnostic work-up and the institution of appropriate management, including the use of antibiotics and the need for hospitalization, must be determined. Many factors, such as clinical assessment, physical findings, age of the patient, and height of the fever, influence the evaluation and management decisions.

## PATHOPHYSIOLOGY

*Fever* is defined as a rise in deep body temperature associated with a resetting of the body's thermostat. This thermostat is located in the preoptic region of the anterior hypothalamus near the floor of the third ventricle. Exogenous fever-producing substances (pyrogens) such as bacteria, bacterial endotoxin, antigen-antibody complexes, yeast, viruses, and etiocholanolone, may stimulate the formation and release of endogenous pyrogens. Endogenous pyrogens are produced by neutrophils, monocytes, hepatic Kupffer cells, splenic sinusoidal cells, alveolar macrophages, and peritoneal lining cells and are believed to induce the synthesis of prostaglandins in the hypothalamus. Endogenous pyrogens include interleukin-1, interleukin-6, and tumor necrosis factor. The body's thermostat is then reset at a higher setting, and the patient, whose own temperature is below that of the body's thermostat, experiences a chill. Peripheral vasoconstriction, shivering, central pooling, and behavioral activity (putting on a sweater, drinking hot tea) lead to an increase in body temperature.

## CLINICAL FEATURES

The possible beneficial effects of fever have been debated for many years. Aside from these considerations, it is important to recognize that fever represents a symptom of some underlying disease, and one must determine what this disease is.

An initial question is: "What degree of temperature elevation represents a fever?" One survey conducted among pediatric training programs revealed a wide variability in the temperature considered a "fever" in infants under 2 months of age. This figure has ranged from 38° to 39.4°C (100.4° to 103°F). It is important to recognize that oral temperatures are generally 0.6°C (1°F) lower than rectal temperatures and axillary temperatures are 0.6°C (1°F) lower than oral temperatures. Temperatures taken using infrared thermometers that scan the tympanic membrane are of variable reliability and reproducibility. Body temperature normally varies from morning to evening with the body's circadian rhythm. The degree of variation, which is greater in young women and small children, is about 1.1°C (2°F).

The relationship between height of fever and incidence of bacteremia is discussed below. In general, higher temperatures are associated with a higher incidence of bacteremia. A retrospective study of hyperpyrexia reported that the incidence of meningitis was twice as high in children with fever above 41.1°C (105.9°F), compared to children with fever between 40.5° and 41.0°C (104.9° and 105.8°F). The incidence of pneumonia and bacteremia was the same in the two groups.

Other studies, many of which have also been retrospective, have had variable results and indicated that children with higher temperatures have more diagnostic studies ordered but the same incidence of different diseases.

## INFANTS UP TO 3 MONTHS

### Diagnosis

The age of the patient influences the extent of the work-up. Early studies suggested that infants under the age of 3 months were at high risk for serious life-threatening infection. Recent studies based on outpatients show that the incidence of serious bacterial infection, including bacteremia and meningitis, is about 3 to 4 percent, although serious nonbacterial infections (e.g., aseptic meningitis) are a frequent cause of fever in this age group.

The history and physical examination may provide clues to the diagnosis. A history of lethargy, irritability, or poor feeding suggests a serious infection. A history of viral illnesses in other family members suggests a similar diagnosis in the infant. The physical examination may reveal a focus of infection such as an inflamed eardrum. Inconsolable crying, or increased irritability when handled, is frequently seen in infants with meningitis. Cough or tachypnea with a respiratory rate over 40 might suggest a lower respiratory infection and the need for a chest x-ray.

Clinical assessment of the severity of illness of a young, febrile infant is problematic. Young infants lack social skills, such as the social smile, and their ability to interact with the examiner is limited. There is a report in the literature of an infant with group B streptococcal bacteremia who was judged by house staff and faculty to be clinically well. The absence of any diagnostic abnormalities on history or physical examination suggests the need for extensive laboratory tests to detect occult infection. These tests would include a complete blood count and differential, erythrocyte sedimentation rate (ESR), blood culture, lumbar puncture, chest x-ray, urinalysis and culture, and a stool culture if there is a history of diarrhea, particularly if leukocytes are noted on a stool smear. Urinary tract infections may not produce symptoms other than fever, and so a urinalysis and culture should be included routinely in the evaluation. Urinary tract infections may be associated with bacteremia in up to 30 percent of infected infants. Antibiotic therapy and hospitalization should be instituted as suggested by the results of these studies.

The recognition of occult serious infection in the well-appearing young, febrile infant is problematic. Most investigators agree that no single variable can correctly identify these infants. Combinations of variables are more helpful in the differentiation process, and these variables include factors such as age under 1 month, ESR greater than 30 mm/h, white blood cell count (WBC) at or over 15,000/mm³, polymorphonuclear cell count of at least 10,000/mm³, band cell count at or over 500/mm³, evidence of soft tissue infection, pyuria (WBC > 10/hpf), and leukocytes in the stool. The absence of these variables is usually (but not always) associated with the absence of serious illness.

## Management

The appropriate management of the young febrile infant presents another area of disagreement. There appears to be no "community standard of practice" regarding the need for hospitalization; some physicians hospitalize all febrile infants under age 3 months, and others hospitalize only those under age 1 month. Because the differentiation between a sick and well infant is so difficult, all such febrile infants need extensive septic work-ups. The decision not to hospitalize the small febrile infant must be made after careful clinical and appropriate laboratory assessment and after ensuring the reliability of follow-up.

## INFANTS OF 3 TO 24 MONTHS

### Diagnosis

Many of the considerations noted in the evaluation of the infant less than 3 months of age apply for the older infant. Patients between 3 and 24 months have been the focus of considerable research because this group appears to be at higher risk for occult bacteremia. These studies have sought to identify clinical and laboratory characteristics of bacteremic patients.

Clinical judgment appears to be more reliable in the assessment of the older infant. Characteristics that the evaluating physician should note are willingness of the patient to make eye contact, playfulness and positive response to interactions, negative response to noxious stimuli, alertness, and consolability. The toxic infant will not respond appropriately.

Again, the history and physical examination will frequently reveal the source of infection. Viral illnesses, including respiratory infections and gastroenteritis, account for the majority of febrile illnesses and usually have system-specific symptoms. Bacterial infections of the respiratory tract include most notably otitis media, pharyngitis, and pneumonia. Otitis media is generally caused by *Streptococcus pneumoniae* or *Haemophilus influenzae,* and antibiotic therapy should be directed at these organisms. Although pneumonia is commonly of viral etiology, it is appropriate to institute antibiotic therapy to ensure coverage of *H. influenzae*. The physical signs of meningitis, such as nuchal rigidity and Kernig or Brudzinski signs, may be inapparent in the child under the age of 2 years. A bulging fontanelle, vomiting, irritability that increases when the infant is held, inconsolability, or a febrile seizure may be the only signs suggestive of meningitis. Infants with aseptic meningitis should generally be hospitalized and ensured adequate long-term follow-up because they are at higher risk for subsequent neurologic and learning disabilities. The presence of petechiae on physical examination should alert the physician to the potential presence of a serious underlying infection. About 20 percent of children will have bacteremia or meningitis most frequently with *Neisseria meningitidis* or *H. influenzae*. Petechiae in association with high fever (≥ 40°C), ESR at or above 30 mm/h, and WBC of at least 15,000/mm³ are most frequently correlated with bacteremia.

Bacteremic infants may or may not have an obvious focus of infection. The height of the fever is a clue to which infants are bacteremic. Although bacteremia may be seen at lower temperatures, a temperature of over 39.5°C (103.1°F) in infants aged 3 to 24 months is associated with a higher incidence of bacteremia. Certain laboratory tests have been recommended to assist in further identifying the bacteremic patient. WBC over 15,000/mm³, band counts of at least 500/mm³, total polymorphonuclear counts at or above 10,000/mm³, and band plus polymorphonuclear counts equal to or greater than 10,500/mm³ are associated with an increased incidence of bac-

teremia, although bacteremia also occurs in the absence of these findings. The incidence of bacteremia in children 3 to 24 months with a temperature of 39.5°C (103.1°F) or over is about 5 to 6 percent. The incidence increases to 12 to 15 percent in patients with WBCs of 15,000/mm³ or over. An ESR at or above 30 mm/h has the same significance as a WBC of 15,000/mm³ or greater. The organism most commonly causing bacteremia in this age group is *S. pneumoniae*. *H. influenzae* is implicated in fewer cases of occult bacteremia since the availability of *H. influenzae* vaccine.

Is it important to perform a blood culture to detect occult bacteremia? Opinions vary on the answer to this question. It is apparent that bacteremic patients do better if they receive antibiotics early on. Many bacteremic children do have a focus of infection and so are treated anyway. Additionally, in at least 25 percent of bacteremic patients with no focus of infection the bacteremia is resolved without any antibiotics. Others develop soft tissue infections, which are then appropriately managed. The ability of oral antibiotics to prevent the development of meningitis in the bacteremic child is still unclear. The blood culture appears to be useful for following a patient who may not be returning for periodic evaluations. Therefore, from a medical and epidemiologic standpoint, blood cultures are indicated in the suspicious or high-risk infant.

## Management

Is there a role for the use of expectant antibiotics in children suspected of having occult bacteremia? Retrospective studies have all shown that early antibiotics diminished the incidence of persistent bacteremia. In a prospective randomized study comparing oral penicillin to no antibiotics, no improvement was reported in any bacteremic child who did not receive antibiotics. Other investigators report more equivocal results. Outpatient daily injections of ceftriaxone are being used by some physicians for children at increased risk of occult bacteremia. Controlled trials investigating the efficacy of this therapy have demonstrated a reduction in the incidence of meningitis in bacteremic children treated with ceftriaxone compared to those treated with oral or no antibiotics. Parenteral ceftriaxone should never be initiated without appropriate antecedent diagnostic studies. Treatment should be discontinued if cultures are negative.

An additional dilemma surrounds the management of positive blood culture results. All patients with positive blood cultures should be recalled for repeat evaluation. If they are receiving appropriate antibiotics, are clinically well, and have been afebrile, they should be instructed to complete the course of therapy. If they are afebrile and clinically well but have never been treated with antibiotics, opinions differ regarding the need for additional blood cultures and antibiotic therapy. Generally, neither is necessary unless the child has developed a specific focus of infection. However, any patient who remains febrile or does poorly even if on antibiotics should receive complete septic evaluation (CBC, blood culture, lumbar puncture, chest film, urine culture), be hospitalized, and receive parenteral antibiotics (Fig. 35-1).

## OLDER FEBRILE CHILDREN

### Diagnosis

Children over the age of 2 are easier to evaluate. They can specify their complaints and have illnesses similar to younger children, particularly upper respiratory infections and gastroenteritis. The risk of bacteremia appears lower in this age group, but the incidence of streptococcal pharyngitis is higher, especially in children between the ages of 5 and 10 and those with hyperpyrexia. Infectious mononucleosis may present with fever, tonsillar hypertrophy, and exudate, like streptococcal pharyngitis. Marked lymphadenopathy or hepatosplenomegaly would support the diagnosis. Pneumonia in this age group may be caused by *Mycoplasma pneumoniae*. These children

**Fig. 35-1.** Management of the bacteremic child; (*"Sick"—irritable, lethargic, anorexic, vomiting; †septic W/U—blood culture, lumbar puncture, chest x-ray, CBC, differential, urinalysis, urine culture; ‡focus of infection—otitis media, pneumonia, cellulitis.)

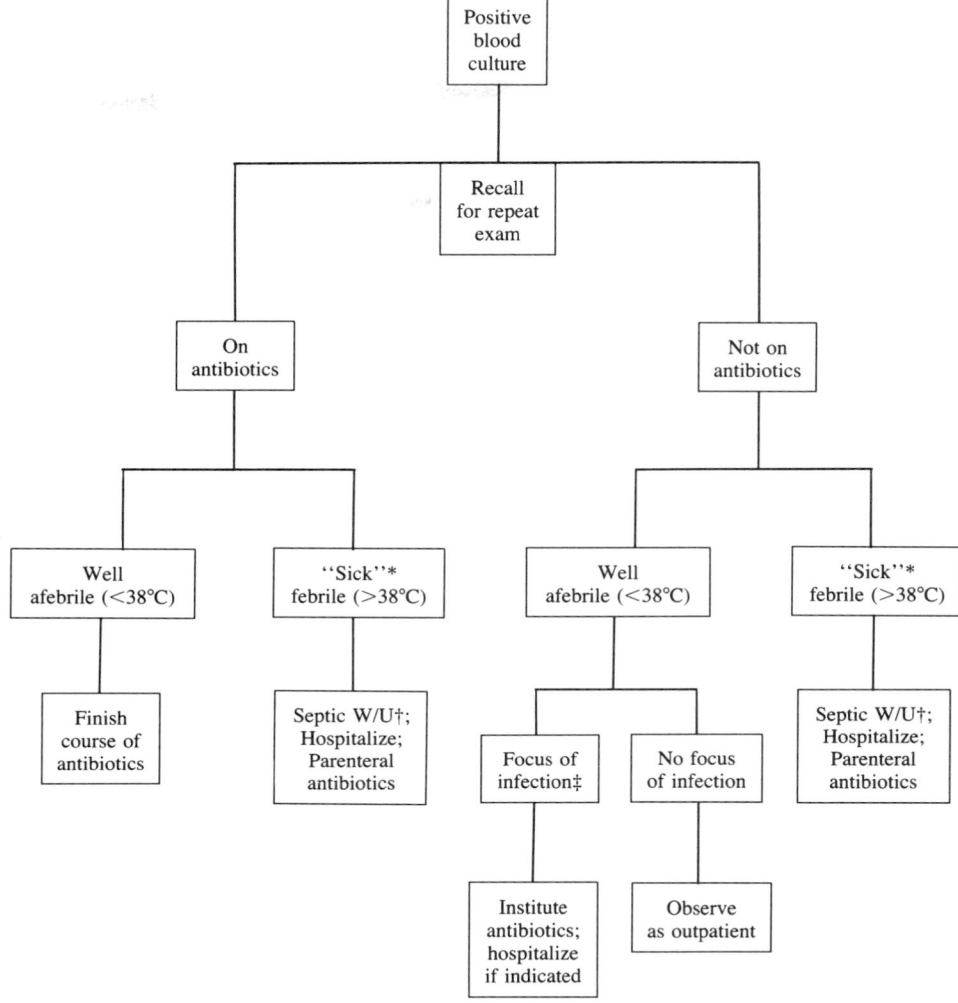

present with cough and fever. Rales may not be apparent early in the illness, although the chest film would show evidence of an infiltrate. Bedside cold agglutinins, if positive, provide a clue to the correct diagnosis. Children with pneumonia secondary to mycoplasma should be treated with erythromycin, 30 to 40 mg/kg per day (maximum dose 1 g).

## EMERGENCY DEPARTMENT CARE

### Managing the Fever

Once the issue of fever as a symptom has been addressed, it is appropriate to determine the need for fever-reducing measures.

Many parents are concerned about the harmful effects of the fever; many are aware of the risk of febrile seizures. Children who are prone to febrile seizures are not benefited by antipyretics alone because the seizure frequently occurs early in the illness, often before the parents are aware that the child is ill. Aside from febrile seizures, fever is not known to produce any harmful effects in children. Many children, however, feel uncomfortable during the fever, and so it is appropriate to institute measures directed at symptomatically reducing the fever.

The body loses heat in four ways: (1) radiation (60 percent), heat loss from the body to the air in the surrounding environment; (2) evaporation (25 percent), heat loss through the evaporation of perspiration, water, or any liquid applied to the body surface; (3) convection (10 percent), heat loss when air currents blow over the skin;

and (4) conduction (approximately 5 percent), heat loss through contact with solid surface. Heat loss through conduction is increased by the use of cooling blankets.

One can facilitate heat loss in a child using any combination of these measures. Unwrapping a bundled child increases heat loss through radiation, and rehydrating a dehydrated child will increase the heat loss through evaporation. Sponging also helps to reduce fever by evaporation. Sponging should be done slowly, using tepid water only. Very rapid cooling by sponging can result in peripheral vascular collapse, and death has been reported in the small critically ill infant. Sponging with ice water is uncomfortable and results in shivering, and sponging with alcohol carries the risk of intoxication, hypoglycemia, and coma. Vigorous rubbing of the skin induces vasodilatation and improves heat loss.

Studies have shown that sponging and antipyretics used together are more effective than either modality used alone. Acetaminophen, ibuprofen, and aspirin are equally effective and appear to work centrally to block prostaglandin synthesis. Heat is lost through peripheral vasodilatation and sweating.

Drug dosage for aspirin or acetaminophen is 10 to 15 mg/kg per dose at 4-h intervals (maximum dose 600 mg). Increasing the dose does not result in a better or more sustained effect. Administration of either drug by rectal suppository results in a slight delay in absorption. No studies have evaluated the efficacy of alternating the two drugs at 2-h intervals in an effort to avoid the recrudescence of fever. Administration of the drugs simultaneously at the usual dosage produces a reduction in temperature that is sustained for 6 h rather than 2 to 4 h. The dosage of ibuprofen is 5 mg/kg for fevers less than 39°C (102.2°F) and 10 mg/kg for fevers over 39°C (102.2°F). Ibuprofen may be given every 6 to 8 hours, with a maximum daily dose of 40 mg/kg.

The use of aspirin has been curtailed following reports linking aspirin and Reye syndrome. Aspirin should not be used in children with chickenpox or with influenza-like illnesses. The effects of aspirin are cumulative, and more than half of the reported overdoses involve therapeutic misuse. Other side effects of aspirin include gastrointestinal upset and hemorrhage and coagulation disturbances. Acetaminophen is also toxic if taken in inappropriate doses, but there is no cumulative effect, and children are less prone than adults to hepatotoxicity.

The administration of expectant parenteral antibiotics, specifically ceftriaxone, has been recommended in a recent consensus report, for children deemed to be at high risk for occult bacteremia. These are children between 3 and 36 months of age, with temperature equal to or greater than 39.5°C (103.1°F), and WBC equal to or greater than 15,000/mm³. Appropriate cultures should be obtained on these patients prior to administration of ceftriaxone, and antibiotics should be discontinued if cultures are negative.

## BIBLIOGRAPHY

Baskin MN, O'Rourke EJ, Fleisher GR. Outpatient treatment of febrile infants 28 to 89 days of age with intramuscular administration of ceftriaxone. *J Pediatr* 120:22, 1992.

Baraff LJ, Bass JW, Fleisher GR, et al. Practice guidelines for the management of infants and children 0 to 36 months of age with fever without source. *Ann Emerg Med* 22:1198, 1993.

Baraff LJ, Oslund SA, Schriger DL, Stephen ML. Probability of bacterial infections in febrile infants less than three months of age: a meta-analysis. *Pediatr Infect Dis J* 11:257, 1992.

Jones RG, Bass JW. Febrile children with no focus of infection: a survey of their management by primary care physicians. *Pediatr Infect Dis J* 12:179, 1993.

Lieu TA, Baskin MN, Schwartz S, Fleisher GR. Clinical and cost-effectiveness of outpatient strategies for management of febrile infants. *Pediatrics* 6:1135, 1992.

McCarthy P. Management of the febrile infant. Commentaries. *Pediatrics* 6:1251, 1992.

# 36
# FLUID AND ELECTROLYTE THERAPY
## Bonnie Sowa

Important differences exist in fluid and electrolyte metabolism and homeostasis between young children and adults. First, the physiologic consequences of fluid and electrolyte disturbances are more pronounced in young children; this is due to their higher metabolic rate. In young children the turnover of fluid and solute per kilogram of body weight is three times that of adults. Young children also have a higher percentage of their body weight from water, i.e., a higher percentage of total body water (TBW). In term newborns TBW accounts for 75 percent of body weight. TBW decreases to 65 percent of body weight in prepubertal children and to 60 percent in adults.

In this chapter, normal maintenance fluid and electrolyte therapy in pediatric patients are discussed. The chapter includes assessment and treatment of fluid deficits, mainly dehydration. Consideration is given to special situations that require modification of the basic guidelines of fluid and electrolyte therapy. Lastly, the use of oral rehydration for replacement of fluid deficits secondary to gastrointestinal (GI) losses are discussed.

## MAINTENANCE REQUIREMENTS

The goal of maintenance fluid and electrolyte therapy is to provide the body with water, sodium, potassium, chloride, and bicarbonate in order to maintain a state of normal homeostasis. In addition, sufficient calories are needed to prevent ketosis and minimize body protein catabolism. Normal maintenance requirements provide water and electrolytes to replace those that are lost through urine, stool, and insensible routes. Urine losses account for 50 percent of maintenance fluid requirement, and insensible water losses account for the other half. Approximately one-third of insensible losses occurs via the respiratory tract and two-thirds through the skin. Stool water losses are usually negligible.

Maintenance fluid requirements depend on the child's rate of metabolism and caloric requirements. Daily caloric requirements (which include basal metabolic expenditure plus an allowance for minimal activity) can be estimated from body weight:

| Body Weight, kg | Caloric Requirement/24 Hours |
| --- | --- |
| ≤10 | 100 kcal/kg |
| 11 to 20 | 1000 kcal + 50 kcal/kg for each kg >10 |
| >20 | 1500 kcal + 20 kcal/kg for each kg >20 |

For example, a child weighing 25 kg would have a daily maintenance caloric requirement of 1600 kcal [(100 kcal/kg × 10 kg) + (50 kcal/kg × 10 kg) + (20 kcal/kg × 5 kg) = 1600 cal].

Daily caloric requirements per kilogram of body weight decrease with increasing body size. This is due to the fact that as body size increases, a greater percentage of weight is from tissues that are metabolically inactive at rest, such as bone, muscles, and fat. Daily caloric requirements also decrease with increasing age.

There is a 1:1 relationship between calories expended and body water required. In other words, the body needs 1 mL of water for every 1 kilocalorie expended. Therefore, maintenance water requirement can be calculated in a manner similar to daily caloric requirement:

| Body Weight, kg | Water Requirement/24 Hours |
| --- | --- |
| ≤10 | 100 mL/kg |
| 11 to 20 | 1000 mL + 50 mL/kg for each kg >10 |
| >20 | 1500 mL + 20 mL/kg for each kg >20 |

Daily maintenance requirements of sodium and potassium are 2 to 3 mEq/kg per 24 h. Anions are usually given as chloride. The kidney produces the maintenance bicarbonate requirement, so in most patients additional bicarbonate does not need to be given.

Five grams of glucose per 100 kcal expended (or per 100 mL of maintenance fluid) provides approximately 20 percent of the total daily caloric expenditure and will prevent ketosis. With this caloric intake, a daily weight loss of 1 to 2 percent of body weight can occur. Newborn infants, especially premature babies, may require 10 g of glucose per 100 kcal expended (or per 100 mL of maintenance fluid) due to their higher metabolic rate.

Maintenance requirements can be provided by an intravenous solution that contains 25 mEq/L of sodium, 25 mEq/L of potassium, 50 mEq/L of chloride, and 50 g/L of dextrose. Standard intravenous solutions that meet those requirements are 5% dextrose in 0.2 or 0.25 normal saline (D₅0.2NS or D₅0.25NS) with 20 mEq/L of potassium chloride added. It should be noted that potassium should be withheld from IV therapy if there is reason to suspect renal or adrenal insufficiency and until adequate urine output has been established. Many conditions can alter a child's metabolic rate, including increased environmental temperature and humidity, artificial ventilation, fever, or intense activity. Maintenance fluid and electrolyte requirements may need to be adjusted accordingly.

## DEFICITS/DEHYDRATION

The most common mechanism for fluid deficits or dehydration in children is excessive fluid loss. These losses usually occur through the gastrointestinal tract, although they can also occur through the renal and insensible (respiratory tract, skin) routes. Severe losses can occur very quickly. It is imperative to recognize the child with a fluid deficit and treat accordingly in order to prevent cardiovascular collapse. Four areas will be discussed regarding the assessment of fluid deficits: (1) degree of dehydration, (2) types of dehydration, (3) total body potassium deficits, and (4) acid-base disturbances.

### Degree of Dehydration

The degree of dehydration is an assessment of the amount of body water that has been lost. This discussion will be confined to acute losses in which deficits occur primarily from the extracellular fluid compartment (ECF). The most accurate way of assessing the degree of dehydration is by weight. The degree of dehydration is equal to the pre-illness weight minus the presenting weight divided by the pre-illness weight. For example, if an infant usually weighs 5 kg and presents with acute gastroenteritis and a weight of 4.5 kg, she has lost 10 percent of her healthy body weight or is 10 percent dehydrated:

$$\frac{(5 \text{ kg} - 4.5 \text{ kg})}{5 \text{ kg}} = 0.10 \text{ or } 10 \text{ percent}$$

Often an accurate pre-illness weight is not available, and the degree of dehydration must be estimated clinically. Important information from the history includes intake (quantity and type of fluid), output (site, type, and amount), and other medical problems (preexisting and acute). Vital signs, including weight, temperature, heart rate, respiratory rate, blood pressure, and capillary refill time, should be taken. A complete physical examination should be performed, with emphasis on the general appearance of the child, anterior fontanelle, skin elasticity, and mucous membranes.

Estimations of dehydration are divided into three groups according to the degree of the fluid deficit: mild (<5 percent dehydration), moderate (5 to 10 percent dehydration), and severe (>10 percent dehydration). With mild dehydration there is a loss of 50 mL/kg of body weight. This estimation is usually made from the history, as physical signs are minimal or absent. The skin may be pale but usually has normal turgor and capillary refill time. Mucous membranes are usually moist and tears present. Urine output may be normal or slightly decreased. Pulse rate may be slightly increased, but blood pressure is normal.

In moderate dehydration there is a loss of 100 mL/kg of body weight. Clinical signs are much more obvious. Skin may be dry, with tenting and loss of turgor. Mucous membranes are tacky or dry. The anterior fontanelle and eyeballs will be sunken. The child will usually have an altered sensorium with lethargy, restlessness, or irritability. Oliguria, tachycardia, prolonged capillary refill time (>2 s) and weak peripheral pulses are present. Blood pressure is usually within normal limits. These patients are in the early stage of compensated shock (evidence of marked intravascular volume depletion with a normal blood pressure).

In severe dehydration there is uncompensated shock and evidence of circulatory collapse. The skin is cold, clammy, and mottled. Capillary refill time is very delayed (>3 to 5 s). Peripheral pulses may be absent, and central pulses weak. There is evidence of poor central nervous system (CNS) perfusion, with varying degrees of altered sensorium.

These signs and symptoms can occur with all types of dehydration. They reflect progressive deficits in the ECF compartment as the magnitude of dehydration increases. In general, because of their greater percentage of TBW, it takes a greater percentage of fluid loss to cause circulatory collapse in an infant and young child compared to older children and adults.

### Types of Dehydration

The type of dehydration refers to the osmolar load of the plasma relative to the degree of fluid loss. Since the main solute in plasma is sodium, serum osmolality is mainly a reflection of sodium concentration. The types of dehydration are isonatremic (isotonic), hyponatremic (hypotonic), and hypernatremic (hypertonic). Each type of dehydration is associated with special problems. Defining the type of dehydration will direct management.

The majority of pediatric patients will present with isonatremic dehydration. Serum sodium is in the normal range—130 to 150 mEq/L. There has been a proportionate loss of water and electrolytes.

In hyponatremic dehydration serum sodium is less than 130 mEq/L. The sodium deficit is greater than the water deficit. This typically occurs when sodium-poor fluids (e.g., tap water) are given to replace GI losses. With hyponatremia the ECF compartment has a proportionately lower osmolar load than the ICF compartment. Water shifts from the ECF into cells in an attempt to equalize the osmolar loads between the ECF and ICF compartments. Consequently, circulating volume decreases and the child appears more seriously ill than would be expected by the degree of dehydration. Clinical signs may overestimate the total fluid loss. Children with hyponatremic dehydration may present with CNS signs and symptoms due to the movement of water intracellularly, resulting in cerebral swelling. Seizures and coma can occur if the serum sodium is less than 120 mEq/L.

In hypernatremic dehydration serum sodium is greater than 150 mEq/L. Hypernatremia occurs when free water replacement is inadequate (incorrectly diluted formulas) or if sodium intake is abnormally high (boiled skim milk or use of baking soda as a home remedy). The increase sodium load (osmolar load) in the ECF cause fluid to shift from the ICF to ECF compartments. With severe hypernatremia serious CNS sequelae can result from the shrunken, dehydrated brain cells, including hemorrhage (from broken bridging vessels), seizures, coma, and death. However, circulating volume is maintained, and the magnitude of dehydration tends to be underestimated. As a rule, if hypernatremic dehydration is present, there must be at least a 10 percent fluid deficit present. Rapid correction of the fluid deficit with hypotonic solutions is not recommended. It may lead to a rapid shift of fluid into the cells, resulting in brain swelling and serious CNS complications. Signs and symptoms seen with hypernatremic dehydration include dry, rubbery, or doughy skin and increased muscle tone. Level of consciousness alternates between lethargy and hyperirritability.

### Potassium Deficit

Potassium deficits occur in all conditions causing water and electrolyte losses. Hypokalemia can occur with large diarrheal losses, increased renal losses (diuretics), or chloride loss with subsequent metabolic alkalosis. With chronic dehydration there is a progressive increase in intracellular potassium loss. Serum potassium accounts for only 2 percent of total body potassium and is directly affected by acid-base status. Potassium shifts between ICF and ECF compartments occur more slowly than free water shifts. Therefore, serum potassium concentration does not always reflect the intracellular concentration. Although a potassium deficit is present in all cases of dehydration, it is usually not clinically significant. However, failure to correct the deficit during rehydration therapy may produce the clinical effects of acute hypokalemia. Potassium replacement should not begin until adequate urine output is established.

## Acid-Base Disturbances

Acid-base abnormalities may occur in patients with dehydration. In infancy, most hydration disturbances produce some degree of metabolic acidosis. Mechanisms of metabolic acidosis include bicarbonate loss in stool and ketone production secondary to carbohydrate starvation. In addition, hypovolemia can lead to both decreased tissue perfusion with lactic acid production and decreased renal perfusion with decreased glomerular filtration rate and decreased hydrogen ion excretion. In most cases acidosis can be corrected by restoring circulating volume and renal function and administering glucose to decrease the production of ketones. For severe acidosis it may be necessary to provide intravenous bicarbonate (see "Therapy").

Other clinical states that lead to metabolic acidosis include diabetes, starvation, salicylism, azotemia, hypoxia, organic acidosis (aminoacidemias), and renal disease. The anion gap will be helpful in evaluating the etiology of acidosis. Metabolic acidosis caused by dehydration has an abnormal anion gap. Increased anion gap can be caused by drugs and toxins (salicylates, methanol, propylene glycol), hyperglycemic nonketotic coma, ketoacidosis, lactic acidosis, and uremia. Therapy must be aimed at treating the underlying etiology.

## THERAPY

Replacement of the fluid deficit occurs in three phases: (1) correction of shock; (2) restoration of ECF volume; and (3) replacement of ICF stores, including fluid, potassium, protein, and fat. This section will be confined to the first two phases of fluid replacement.

## Correction of Shock

The treatment of shock is directed towards preventing circulatory failure and restoring vascular volume. This phase should be instituted for any infant with a fluid deficit of 10 percent or greater or with signs of decreased circulatory volume, including tachycardia, prolonged capillary refill time (>2 s), pallor, weak peripheral pulses, and altered mental status. It is important to remember that hypotension is a very late and ominous sign of decompensated shock in infants and young children. Children may be in a shock state and still maintain normal blood pressure until they eventually decompensate.

An accurate weight (or estimation, if necessary) should be obtained on all pediatric patients. Vascular access should be started, and blood obtained for immediate analysis of electrolytes, glucose, BUN/creatinine, and pH. A rapid bedside glucose (chemstix) measurement should be done. If peripheral access cannot be obtained, percutaneous cannulâtion of the femoral or external jugular vein is an alternative. For children less than 6 years old, an intraosseous infusion needle may be placed for initial volume expansion. A venous cutdown may be attempted if the above sites are unsuccessful, but it is a time-consuming procedure even in experienced hands. All patients in shock should receive supplemental oxygen.

For correction of shock from all types of dehydration, the initial fluid bolus is the same—20 mL/kg of isotonic crystalloid (0.9% NS or lactated Ringer's solution) over 5 to 20 min. Glucose-containing solutions should be avoided as they are poor volume expanders and, in addition, bolus amounts can lead to hyperglycemia and resulting osmotic diuresis. If hypoglycemia is present, administer 0.5 to 1.0 g/kg of glucose (2 to 4 mL/kg of $D_{25}W$).

Although crystalloids provide good volume expansion and are readily available and inexpensive, if the child has underlying cardiac, pulmonary, or renal disease, 10-mL/kg boluses of colloids [salt-poor 5% albumin, fresh-frozen plasma (FFP), or synthetic colloids] should be used. These solutions are more expensive and, more importantly, carry the risk of allergic reactions and blood-borne infection.

Rapid delivery of bolus fluids can be achieved by attaching a three-way stopcock to the extension tubing of the intravenous line. A 20- to 50-mL syringe can then be used to push fluid aliquots. This method allows for rapid bolus infusion without disrupting fragile veins.

After the fluid bolus is completed, reassess the patient for changes in heart rate, skin color, capillary refill time, pulses, mental status, and urine output. If perfusion remains compromised, the fluid bolus should be repeated (20 mL/kg). For shock states attributable to dehydration alone, fluid replacement for restoration of vascular volume is the only treatment. In general, few patients require more than 40 to 60 mL/kg of isotonic crystalloid during the first hour of therapy. Some children with severe third-spacing and/or continuous on-going fluid losses may require more than 60 mL/kg of crystalloid during the first hour or two of therapy. These patients need to be monitored for signs of fluid overload (enlarged liver, pulmonary rales, or enlarged heart on chest radiograph). Serum electrolytes and glucose should be monitored closely.

## Restoration of ECF Volume

The next phase of therapy is restoration of ECF volume. The aim of this phase is correction of the fluid deficit with restoration of the fluid compartments over 24 to 48 h. Fluid therapy for this phase depends on the degree and type of dehydration present.

### Isonatremic Dehydration

For the patient with isotonic dehydration, the initial fluid boluses given are subtracted from the calculated fluid deficit. The remaining deficit is replaced over 24 h: one-half is given over the first 8 h, and the other half over the subsequent 16 h. Calculated maintenance fluids are added to the deficit replacement. For example, a 7-kg patient with 10 percent dehydration has a fluid deficit of 100 mL/kg, or 700 mL. If an initial fluid bolus of 20 mL/kg of normal saline was given, the remaining fluid deficit is 700 mL − 140 mL = 560 mL. One-half of the 560 mL, or 280 mL, is given over the first 8 h (35 mL/h). This is added to the child's maintenance fluid rate which is 30 mL/hr (7 kg × 100 mL/kg = 700 mL/24 h = 30 mL/h). Thus, the total rate of fluid administration for the first 8 h is 35 mL/h + 30 mL/h = 65 mL/h. The rate for the following 16 h is 45 mL/h (15 mL/h + 30 mL/h = 45 mL/h). The IV solution used is $D_5$0.2NS or $D_5$0.45NS. Forty mEq/L of potassium chloride should be added after adequate urine output is established.

### Hyponatremic Dehydration

In hypotonic dehydration, the water deficit is calculated and replaced as above. However, the sodium deficit is different. Most patients with hyponatremia will be at least 10 percent dehydrated. Initial fluid boluses are given as normal saline or lactated Ringer's solution, which are relatively hypertonic solutions. The remainder of the fluid deficit as well as the maintenance fluid is given as $D_5$0.45NS. Forty mEq/L of potassium chloride is added after adequate urine output is established.

If the initial serum sodium is less than 120 mEq/L or the patient has symptomatic hyponatremia (seizures), 3% saline (0.5 mEq/mL) is administered to correct the sodium deficit acutely. If the serum sodium concentration is not known, then 3 to 5 mL/kg of 3% saline is given over 5 to 10 min to bring the sodium out of the "danger zone" without overcorrecting. If the serum sodium concentration is known, then the following formula is used:

$$(\text{Desired serum Na*} - \text{present serum Na}) \times 0.6\dagger \times \text{weight (kg)}$$

Half is given slowly over 5 to 10 min. The other half is given over the next hour. Rapid correction has been associated with central pontine myelinolysis in alcoholic adults but has not been reported in children.

---

* To avoid overcorrecting, the concentration for desired serum Na is 125 mEq/L.

† Volume of distribution of freely exchangeable Na.

## Hypernatremic Dehydration

In hypertonic dehydration, rehydration therapy must address the high serum sodium concentration and the relative loss of intracellular water. The serum sodium must be lowered *slowly*. Rapid rehydration leads to rapid expansion of intracellular volume, especially in the CNS, and may cause abrupt cellular swelling and cerebral edema. However, a large proportion of the mortality and neurologic sequelae that result from hypernatremic dehydration is secondary to the initial CNS cellular desiccation. The goal is to decrease the serum sodium by approximately 10 to 15 mEq/L per day. Replacement of the fluid deficit is accomplished evenly over 48 h, or 72 h if the initial sodium is greater than 175 mEq/L. For initial serum sodium greater than 210 mEq/L, dialysis may be required.

Estimate the patient's fluid deficit. Clinically, hypernatremic patients often appear less dehydrated than they truly are because the ECF volume is preserved. They may not appear to require initial fluid boluses. However, if there is any doubt regarding the adequacy of circulation, a bolus of normal saline should be administered. The remaining fluid deficit is added to the maintenance fluid requirement for the next 48 h; this volume is administered evenly over 48 h.

For example, consider a 15-kg child with 10 percent dehydration and a serum sodium of 165 mEq/L. The fluid deficit is 100 mL/kg, or 1500 mL. The maintenance fluid requirement is 1250 mL/24 h [(100 mL/kg × 10 kg) + (50 mL/kg × 5 kg) = 1250 mL/24 h or 2500 mL/48 h]. The total 48-h fluid requirement is 4000 mL (2500 mL + 1500 mL = 4000 mL or 85 mL/h). $D_5 0.45NS$ is the fluid used, although some authors recommend $D_5 0.2NS$. After adequate urine output is established, potassium is added to the solution. Potassium will replace intracellular cation and, consequently, draw water back into the cells. Hyperglycemia can aggravate hypertonicity and is usually corrected by rehydration alone.

## Acidosis

Inadequate perfusion is the primary etiology for acidosis in the dehydrated patient. Mild to moderate acidosis is usually ameliorated by restoration of circulation, which improves renal function and oxygen/substrate (glucose) delivery to the tissues. The administration of exogenous bicarbonate should be considered if blood pH is less than 7.10 or serum bicarbonate is less than 10 mEq/L. Sodium bicarbonate, 1 mEq/kg, is added to the first hour of intravenous fluid. A repeat dose may be necessary. Always ensure adequate ventilation before administering sodium bicarbonate.

Rapid correction of plasma bicarbonate concentration should be avoided. Because compensatory mechanisms continue despite normalization of blood pH, an overcorrection can occur with resultant alkalemia. Additionally, changes in $Pa_{CO_2}$ in the CSF alter blood pH more rapidly and profoundly than do changes in arterial bicarbonate concentration; a rapid infusion of bicarbonate may correct the blood pH, but the $Pa_{CO_2}$ in the CSF may rise, consequently lowering the CSF pH and altering neurologic function.

## SPECIAL SITUATIONS

### Sepsis

Pediatric patients may be febrile (or even hypothermic) when they present with dehydration and/or shock. Upon initial presentation it may be difficult to determine whether the patient is in shock from dehydration or sepsis or both. In sepsis, peripheral vasodilatation increases the size of the vascular compartment, leading to a relative hypovolemia. Additionally, capillary permeability increases, causing further third-space fluid losses.

The treatment of septic shock is initially the same as outlined above (see "Correction of Shock"). The patient must be adequately oxygenated and ventilated, and intravenous fluids must be given to expand the vascular volume. Because sepsis frequently causes abnor-

malities of cardiac function and increased capillary permeability, adult respiratory distress syndrome (ARDS) may develop. If a patient with suspected septic shock requires resuscitation with over 40 to 60 mL/kg of crystalloid, inotropic support should be instituted. A continuous infusion of dopamine and/or epinephrine can be used. In addition, appropriate cultures should be obtained, and broad-spectrum antibiotics administered. Lumbar puncture should not be performed until the patient is hemodynamically stable.

### Trauma

Children with acute hemorrhage will generally compensate for losses up to 30 percent of their blood volume before becoming hypotensive. Other clinical parameters of circulatory status are earlier indicators of decreased vascular volume, including tachycardia, delayed capillary refill time, cool extremities, decreased pulse pressure, and altered sensorium. Hypotension is a late sign of impending circulatory failure in children. *Treatment of the pediatric trauma patient with signs of shock must begin before hypotension occurs.* Large volumes of fluid are given to replace losses. Normal saline or lactated Ringer's solution is administered as 20-mL/kg boluses. Following each bolus the patient is reassessed for changes in heart rate, blood pressure, peripheral perfusion, and urine output. If more than 40 to 60 mL/kg of crystalloid is required during the initial resuscitation, packed red blood cells, 10 mL/kg, should be administered. Sites of continuing hemorrhage should be investigated.

### Diabetic Ketoacidosis

Diabetic ketoacidosis (DKA) is a state characterized by (1) severe volume depletion of both ICF and ECF compartments, (2) osmotic imbalance between ICF and ECF compartments, (3) metabolic acidosis, and (4) caloric deficiency.

All patients in DKA have at least a 10 percent fluid deficit. Deficit replacement is similar to that used for straightforward dehydration; however, several important differences must be emphasized. Rehydration with concomitant decreasing serum glucose must be accomplished *slowly* in order to avoid rapid fluid compartment shifts resulting in cerebral edema. Sodium bicarbonate therapy should be reserved for blood pH less than 7.10 or serum bicarbonate less than 10 mEq/L; it should be administered slowly (over 1 h). Mild acidosis usually responds to adequate rehydration and insulin therapy alone and does not require supplemental sodium bicarbonate. Dehydration should be corrected initially with normal saline. Generally a large potassium deficit is present; therefore, potassium replacement should be initiated early. Careful and frequent monitoring of glucose, pH, potassium, and serum bicarbonate is essential.

### Salicylate Intoxication

In salicylate poisoning, dehydration is secondary to large fluid losses from the respiratory tract, sweating, and urine. Treatment is aimed at correction of the dehydration, hypokalemia, and metabolic acidosis. Treatment guidelines include: (1) $D_5 0.45NS$ with 25 mEq/L sodium bicarbonate at 10 to 15 mL/kg per hour for 2 h, then (2) $D_5 0.2NS$ with 20 mEq/L sodium bicarbonate and 40 mEq/L potassium chloride at 5 to 10 mL/kg per hour. The goal is to achieve active diuresis of an alkalinized urine. Aim for a urine output of 3 to 6 mL/kg per hour and urine pH >7. If severe metabolic acidosis is present, an additional 1 to 2 mEq/kg sodium bicarbonate may be administered every 1 to 2 h.

### Cystic Fibrosis

Cystic fibrosis (CF) is a hereditary disorder that occurs in 1 in 2500 Americans. Patients with cystic fibrosis have increased sweat concentrations of sodium and chloride. The initial presentation of an infant with undiagnosed CF can be hyponatremic dehydration, often associated with hypochloremic, hypokalemic metabolic alkalosis. Older children with known CF may develop hyponatremic dehydration during prolonged exposure to hot environments or from excessive physical exertion.

## Pyloric Stenosis

Pyloric stenosis is a common condition that occurs in young infants, usually males. Classically these infants present with projectile vomiting and dehydration with a hypochloremic, hypokalemic metabolic alkalosis. However, if this condition is diagnosed before there is significant dehydration, the acid-base status is normal.

Correction of the fluid deficit in these infants should be aimed at restoring intravascular volume and replacing chloride and potassium deficits. If fluid boluses are necessary, normal saline should be used. Lactated Ringer's solution should be avoided since it may worsen the alkalosis. Additional fluid should be given as $D_5 0.45NS$ with 40 mEq/L potassium chloride. Dehydration and metabolic alkalosis should be corrected prior to surgical intervention.

## Burns

In addition to airway and breathing management, fluid therapy is the cornerstone in the early care of the burned child. The percent body surface area (BSA) burned should be determined. Fluid therapy should be titrated to clinical response; i.e., adequate circulatory volume and perfusion. Urine output should be greater than 1.0 mL/kg per hour. Fluid therapy guidelines are as follows:

1. Burns less than 35 percent BSA: administer lactated Ringer's solution at 3 to 4 mL/kg per percentage BSA burned per 24 hours. Add daily maintenance fluid requirement in children with less than 20 percent BSA burned.
2. Burns greater than 35 percent BSA: administer lactated Ringer's solution at 4 mL/kg per percentage BSA burned per 24 hours.

One-half is given over the first 4 to 6 h after the occurrence of the burn, and one-fourth in the subsequent 6 h. The last one-fourth is given in the remaining 12 h. If other third-space losses (intraabdominal, long-bone fractures, etc.) occur, replacement fluids must be administered.

## Syndrome of Inappropriate Antidiuretic Hormone

With the syndrome of inappropriate antidiuretic hormone (SIADH) there is uncontrolled secretion of ADH, which results in excessive free water retention and plasma dilution. SIADH should be considered in any patient with hyponatremia and increased urine sodium excretion. Typically these patients are well hydrated. This syndrome is seen in pediatric patients with CNS infections, brain tumors, head injuries, and pulmonary disorders.

Therapy involves diagnosis and treatment of the underlying cause, as well as creating a negative water balance. Fluid intake is decreased to two-thirds maintenance or even one-half maintenance in some cases. Electrolytes and glucose are given at the usual maintenance rates (e.g., $D_5 0.33NS$ or $D_5 0.45NS$ with 20 to 30 mEq/L of potassium chloride).

## ORAL REHYDRATION

Recently the treatment of acute diarrheal illness and dehydration has focused on the use of oral rehydration solutions. Oral rehydration therapy is greatly underutilized in the United States, although it offers several advantages over IV therapy. These include lower cost, decreased hospitalization, ease of administration, and less discomfort for the child.

A number of commercial formulas are available for use in oral hydration therapy. The World Health Organization oral rehydration solution and Rehydralyte are replacement therapy solutions for patients who are acutely dehydrated. Pedialyte, Infalyte, Lytren, Resol, and Ricelyte are maintenance solutions appropriate for preventing dehydration. All of these solutions contain 2.0 to 2.5% glucose along with adequate concentrations of potassium, chloride, and base (either citrate or bicarbonate) to replace stool losses. The main difference between the rehydration and maintenance solutions is the sodium concentration. Maintenance solutions contain approximately 50 mEq/L of sodium, while the rehydration solutions have 75 to 90 mEq/L of sodium. The higher ratio of sodium to glucose maximizes intestinal absorption of water and electrolytes.

As with intravenous fluid therapy, fluid deficits and daily maintenance fluid requirement should be calculated to give the amount of solution to be administered orally over a 24-h period. Rehydration solutions are used to correct the fluid deficit, followed by a maintenance solution (or breast milk). After the first 24 h, diluted formula, low-carbohydrate juice, rice cereal, bananas, potatoes, and bread can be reintroduced. Starchy foods (rice, wheat, potatoes, and lentils) contain high concentrations of sugar polymers, which appear to increase intestinal absorption of water. Such foods should be started early during the treatment of gastroenteritis.

Contraindications to the use of oral rehydration solutions include: (1) fluid deficit of ≥10 percent dehydration, (2) excessive vomiting, (3) hypernatremia, (4) stool losses of ≥10 mL/kg per hour, and (5) noncompliance with treatment instructions.

## BIBLIOGRAPHY

Avery ME, Snyder JD: Oral therapy for acute diarrhea. *N Engl J Med* 323:891, 1990.

Ellis D, Avner E: Fluid and electrolyte disorders in pediatric patients, in Puschett J (ed): *Disorders of Fluid and Electrolyte Balance*. New York, Churchill Livingstone, 1985.

Finberg L: Oral electrolyte/glucose solutions: 1984. *J Pediatr* 105:939, 1984.

Finberg L, Kravath RE, Fleischman AR: *Water and Electrolytes in Pediatrics*. Philadelphia, Saunders, 1982.

Ichikawa I: *Pediatric Textbook of Fluids and Electrolytes*. Baltimore, Williams & Wilkins, 1990.

Silverman BK (ed): *APLS: The Pediatric Emergency Medicine Course,* 2d ed. American Academy of Pediatrics/American College of Emergency Physicians, Dallas, 1993.

Winters RW: *Principles of Pediatric Fluid Therapy*. Boston, Little Brown, 1982.

# 37
# UPPER RESPIRATORY EMERGENCIES
## Nick Relich

The diseases which cause upper respiratory tract (URT) obstruction account for a significant percentage of pediatric emergency visits. Some are very common and, ordinarily, quite benign, while others are much less common, yet are true pediatric emergencies.

The physical examination sign common to all causes of URT obstruction is inspiratory stridor. This is a harsh, raspy noise produced by the flow of air through a partially obstructed airway. Stridor on inspiration is indicative of obstruction at or above the larynx. Biphasic stridor, heard during expiration as well as inspiration, places the obstruction in the trachea, while expiratory stridor usually means obstruction below the carina. According to the American Thoracic Society's definition of respiratory sounds, stridor is a type of wheezing, that is, a continuous sound originating from the airway. In common usage, though, only isolated expiratory stridor is referred to as *wheezing;* isolated inspiratory stridor is simply called *stridor*. Throughout this chapter, stridor and wheezing will refer, respectively, to inspiratory and expiratory sounds, usually associated with prolongation of inspiratory or expiratory phases of respiration. Many other physical examination signs are present in patients with URT obstruction. The significance of these, especially in patients under 6 months of age, will be discussed before the specific disease entities are presented.

## PHYSICAL EXAMINATION

Cyanosis, while the most dramatic sign, has some inherent limitations as a diagnostic tool. It depends to a great extent on the amount of the hemoglobin in the blood and the status of the peripheral circulation. A child with severe anemia, for example, may have significant hypoxia without manifesting cyanosis. Conversely, a very young infant whose hemoglobin has not yet fallen from the normally high levels found at birth and whose peripheral circulation is normally somewhat sluggish may show varying degrees of peripheral cyanosis despite a normal $P_{O_2}$. Detection of cyanosis is sometimes quite difficult in black children. Finally, even when present, cyanosis is a late accompaniment of respiratory diseases. For all these reasons, cyanosis is of limited diagnostic value. However, when present, it is an extremely important and ominous sign.

Labored respirations consist of a triad of signs: tachypnea, chest retractions, and nasal flaring. Each of these has specific limitations that the physician must be aware of, especially in the infant less than 6 months old. As a group, however, these signs are the most valuable signs of respiratory distress. They appear early in the course of the disease and worsen as the disease worsens, thus serving as prognostic as well as diagnostic signs.

Tachypnea, an increased respiratory rate, is not specific for respiratory tract disease. It is also seen in cardiac problems, as well as diseases that cause metabolic acidosis, such as diabetic ketoacidosis and salicylate intoxication. Newborns *normally* breathe 40 to 50 times per minute. By 1 year of age, the respiratory rate is around 30 to 35, by 4 years 20 to 25, and by age 8 to 10 years it is at the usual adult rate of 12 to 15. Even with these limitations, tachypnea is an early sign of respiratory distress and correlates well with the severity of the disease.

Chest retractions and nasal flaring are much more specific for respiratory tract disorders than is tachypnea. They are both seen in respiratory tract obstruction and parenchymal lung disease. Both appear early in the course of the disease. They also correlate well with the severity of the disease, although semantically it may be difficult to distinguish "mild" from "moderate" or "moderate" from "severe" retractions or nasal flaring. Both the increased airway resistance of parenchymal lung disease and URT obstruction cause a greater than normal negative inspiratory pressure to be generated. This increased negative pressure causes the soft parts of the infant's chest, which is compliant and poorly ossified, to retract inward. Most commonly, retractions are seen in the intercostal, subdiaphragmatic, and supraclavicular spaces. If severe disease is present, the entire sternum may retract on inspiration. Nasal flaring, an outward and upward flaring of the nares on inspiration, is thought to be a primitive reflex seen in young infants, who are obligate nose breathers for the first 2 to 3 months of life. It probably is an attempt to decrease the airway resistance at the nares, which is quite high in the young infant.

Coughing is uncommon in the young infant less than 6 months old. This reflex is ordinarily not seen at this age, even in infants with large amounts of mucus in the airway. When a young infant does have a *persistent* cough, pertussis, *Chlamydia* pneumonia, or cystic fibrosis should be considered. Sneezing is more common in this age group and is much less significant. Because of the importance of nose breathing to young infants, sneezing can occur quite often, usually in the absence of any respiratory disease.

Grunting is an extremely valuable diagnostic sign. It occurs during expiration, when the glottis is partially closed, causing a delay and then a forceful, noisy expiration (the "grunt"). It seems to be the physiological counterpart of end-expiratory pressure in mechanically ventilated patients. In fact, it was through observations of neonates who grunted that continuous positive airway pressure (CPAP) and positive end-expiratory pressure (PEEP) first came to be used in the treatment of neonatal hyaline membrane disease. Grunting localizes the respiratory disease to the lower respiratory tract. That is, patients who grunt have pneumonia, asthma, or bronchiolitis. Patients with URT obstruction do not grunt. Therefore, grunting is not only specific to the airway, an early sign of disease which correlates with disease severity, but is also specific to a particular location in the respiratory tract.

Stridor is similar to grunting in its significance as a sign of respiratory distress. It appears early and correlates with the disease severity. It is specific not only for the airway but also for the URT; that is, patients with stridor have URT obstruction. Patients with pneumonia, asthma, or bronchiolitis do not have stridor. Stridor and grunting, then, are the most important signs of respiratory distress in the pediatric patient. When seeing a child who has either stridor or grunting, the physician can be confident that the disease is localized not only to the respiratory tract but to a specific part of the respiratory tract.

## STRIDOR

The causes of stridor are listed in Table 37-1. These diseases are occasionally referred to collectively as *croup syndrome*. This should not be confused with viral croup, which is a *cause* of stridor or of croup syndrome.

When confronted with a stridorous child, it is most helpful for the physician to ask two questions, the age of the patient and the duration of symptoms. The answers to these questions will narrow the differential diagnosis considerably. A child under 6 months old with a long duration of symptoms (weeks to months) characteristically has a *congenital* cause of stridor (see Table 37-1). Most of these diseases present in the newborn nursery or in the pediatrician's office and are not emergency problems.

Laryngomalacia, the most common of these, is due to a developmentally weak larynx, which collapses with each inspiration. It is a self-limited disorder, resolving completely over 6 to 12 months, although there may be exacerbations with upper respiratory infections (URI). If asked, the parent will tell you, "My child has breathed that way since birth." It is usually an incidental finding and not the reason for the emergency visit. It is a benign problem requiring no therapy.

**Table 37-1.** Differential Diagnosis of Inspiratory Stridor

| |
|---|
| Congenital* |
|     Laryngeal or tracheal webs, cysts, tumors |
|     Laryngomalacia* |
|     Vascular ring |
|     Ectopic thyroid, thyroglossal duct cyst |
|     Congenital vocal cord paralysis |
| Inflammatory |
|     Viral croup† |
|     Epiglottitis† |
|     Retropharyngeal abscess |
|     Diphtheria, tetanus |
| Noninflammatory |
|     Aspiration of foreign body into airway† |
|     Esophageal foreign body |
|     Gastroesophageal reflux |
|     Tetany, trauma, tumors |

\* Most common causes under 6 months of age.

† Most common causes over 6 months of age.

The patient over 6 months old with a relatively short duration of symptoms (hours to days) characteristically has an acquired cause of stridor. This may be inflammatory, such as viral croup or epiglottitis, or noninflammatory, such as foreign body aspiration. The remainder of the chapter deals with the most common acquired causes of stridor: epiglottitis, viral croup, foreign body aspiration, and retropharyngeal abscess.

## EPIGLOTTITIS

### Clinical

Epiglottitis is a life-threatening disease, a true pediatric emergency. The age range is 2 to 7 years old; the etiology is almost always *Haemophilus influenzae*. Classically, there is an *abrupt* onset over several *hours* of high fever, sore throat, stridor, dysphagia, and drooling. The parent can often tell you the exact time of day the child became ill. Physical examination reveals a toxic-appearing child with an ashen-gray color, very apprehensive and anxious looking, but with minimal movements. There is usually quiet breathing with little air exchange, no hoarseness, but a whispering voice. The characteristic position is sitting up with chin forward and neck slightly extended—the so-called sniffing position. Absence of a spontaneous cough can be a key historical point differentiating epiglottitis from viral croup.

Epiglottitis can also occur in teenagers and young adults, presenting with stridor, sore throat, fever, and drooling over several days, not hours. Epiglottitis should be considered at this age if the symptoms of sore throat, dysphagia, and drooling are out of proportion to the visible pharyngeal pathology. Although *H. influenzae* is the most common organism, gram-positive cocci are also common at this age. There are reports of rapid-onset URT obstruction due to traumatic epiglottitis, secondary to blind vigorous attempts, usually by the parents at home, at removal of a foreign body from the child's throat.

### Diagnosis

The *ideal* approach is to take any patient with suspected epiglottitis to the operating room, administer anesthesia, and examine the airway with a laryngoscope while the patient is anesthetized. If the diagnosis of epiglottitis is made, the patient can be intubated. If it is ruled out, the patient can be returned to the ward or the emergency department to continue the workup, secure in the knowledge that epiglottitis is *not* present. However, most hospitals do not have the luxury of 24-h availability of an in-house anesthesiologist.

Therefore, a *less than ideal but perfectly acceptable approach* is the following. A portable lateral neck x-ray is done to establish the diagnosis. The physician *must* stay with the child at all times until the diagnosis is ruled out or the airway is secured. Do *not* send the patient to the x-ray department unattended. A *portable* lateral neck x-ray is quite adequate for diagnosing epiglottitis. Once the diagnosis is made, the patient can be treated accordingly. If total airway obstruction or apnea occurs before the airway has been secured, children with epiglottitis can be bagged effectively. A bag and mask should remain with the physician at the bedside until the diagnosis is ruled out or the airway is secured.

The patient with epiglottitis who is initially seen in the office, clinic, or nontertiary emergency department should be transported to a referral hospital by ambulance *with a physician in attendance.* Oxygen should be given en route, and equipment for airway stabilization, resuscitation, and ventilatory support should be available during the transport. The referral hospital should be alerted as soon as possible. If respiratory arrest occurs during transport, suction the patient, then ventilate with bag and mask.

Lateral neck x-rays must be taken with the neck extended, or the anatomy will be impossible to see. The x-ray should be taken during inspiration. The retropharyngeal space *normally* widens during expiration, and a film taken at that time may lead to a false diagnosis of

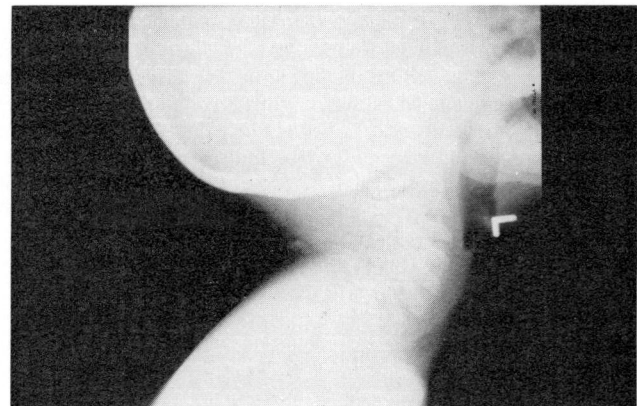

**Fig. 37-1.** A normal lateral neck x-ray.

retropharyngeal abscess. Fortunately, neither of these conditions is difficult to meet in the usual patient. The patient with epiglottitis is already in slight neck extension, and the audible stridor makes for easy timing of the film during inspiration.

A normal lateral neck x-ray is shown in Fig. 37-1. There are four things to look for in any lateral neck x-ray performed for airway problems: the epiglottis, the retropharyngeal or prevertebral space, the tracheal air column, and the hypopharynx. The epiglottis is normally tall and thin, projecting up into the hypopharynx. In epiglottitis (Fig. 37-2), it is very swollen and appears squat and flat, like a thumbprint at the base of the hypopharynx. The retropharyngeal space is normally 3 to 4 mm wide. The tracheal air column may need to be "bright-lighted" to be seen well. It should be of uniform width, without densities in the air column. Finally, the dimensions of the hypopharynx should be noted. Similarly to the gastrointestinal tract, although to a much lesser degree, the hypopharynx will distend proximal to a point of obstruction. This is illustrated by the different sizes of the hypopharynx in Figs. 37-1 and 37-2. While not specific for epiglottitis, this distension does indicate significant URT obstruction.

Until recently, attempted visualization of the epiglottis, with a tongue blade and flashlight, in the emergency department was consid-

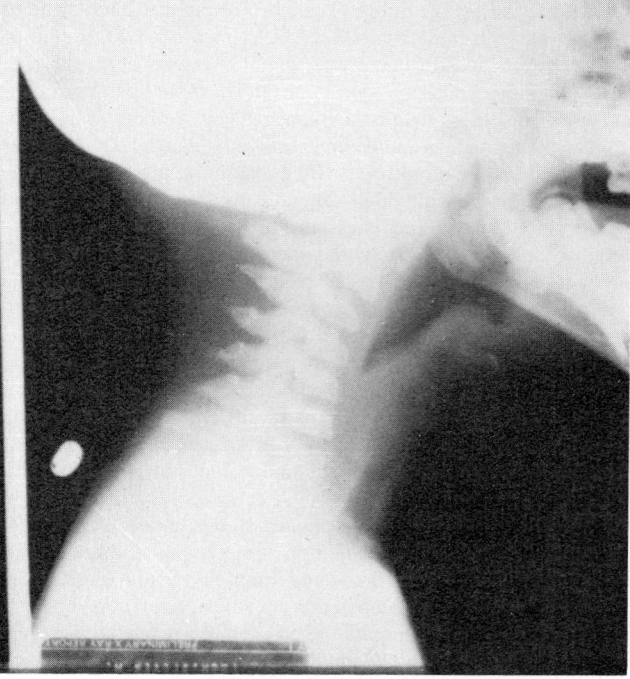

**Fig. 37-2.** Lateral neck view of a child with epiglottitis.

ered a totally unacceptable approach to diagnosis. Accepted pediatric dogma was that you should *not* attempt direct visualization of the epiglottis unless the patient is sedated *and* you are ready and able to do endotracheal intubation at that moment. The swollen, cherry-red epiglottis of the patient with epiglottitis is not as mobile as normal and does not pop up into view easily when the patient gags with a tongue blade. Also, this forceful handling of the patient will cause increased anxiety and stridor, which may cause complete obstruction of the patient's airway. However, current pediatric literature argues that direct visualization is safe and accurate. Although this remains a controversial point, it seems prudent to ensure the availability of a person skilled in intubation before attempting direct visualization.

## Airway Management

The airway may be secured either by immediate endotracheal intubation or immediate tracheostomy. The choice between these two depends on the particular institution and the 24-h availability of personnel trained in airway management. It is *mandatory* that each emergency department, along with pediatrics, anesthesia, and ENT departments, develop a protocol for managing the child with epiglottitis. Decisions concerning intubation or tracheostomy or transfer to a tertiary center must be made prior to the patient's arrival in the emergency department. It is totally unacceptable to "carefully" observe the patient in an intensive care setting for signs of deterioration. What will surely be observed is sudden and total obstruction of the patient's airway. The objective of airway management is to prevent this from occurring.

Most patients are treated with endotracheal intubation as soon as the diagnosis is made. This should be performed in the intensive care unit or operating room under controlled conditions in the sedated or anesthetized patient. We have had success using Valium (diazepam) and morphine as preintubation sedation, but some patients may require succinylcholine paralysis before intubation can be accomplished. If succinylcholine is used, the patient will have to be bagged using the endotracheal tube (ETT) until the drug effect is over, usually several minutes. Use an ETT that is one size smaller than ordinarily used for the patient's age to reduce the incidence of postintubation sequelae. Initial orotracheal intubation followed by nasotracheal intubation is the preferred method; however, orotracheal intubation alone is also well tolerated. If an oral ETT is used, an oral airway must also be inserted to prevent the patient from biting down on the ETT.

Tracheostomy has a higher morbidity in the patient with epiglottitis than does endotracheal intubation. However, in some hospitals, without adequate availability of intubation personnel, tracheostomy may be the treatment of choice. Again, these decisions should be agreed on ahead of time and made a part of the emergency department policy. Except for the patient who comes in in respiratory arrest and does not begin spontaneous ventilations after resuscitation (hypoxic brain damage) and the extremely rare patient with coexistent pulmonary edema, mechanical ventilation is not necessary. The duration of intubation is 36 to 48 h, after which time the patient can usually be extubated without visualizing the epiglottis. This should be done during day shift hours when adequate personnel are available. Once an ETT is in place, a lateral neck x-ray will not show the epiglottis. Occasionally, postextubation edema causes *mild* stridor which responds well to nebulized Vaponefrine (racemic epinephrine).

## Supportive Therapy

Supportive therapy includes IV hydration, humidification of the air to the ETT, and administration of oxygen as necessary. Because of the possibility of ampicillin-resistant *H. influenzae,* most people use cefuroxime (100 to 150 mg/kg per day). Blood cultures are positive in 80 percent of the patients. Oral antibiotics should be continued after extubation for a total of 7 to 10 days. Steroids are *not* necessary. Sedation may be required for the duration of the intubation, although verbal reassurance is often adequate, especially in the older child.

## VIRAL CROUP

This is usually a benign, self-limited disease. The age range is 6 months to 3 years; the etiology is almost always viral, usually parainfluenza virus. The male:female ratio is 1, although severe croup is more common in boys. The typical history is 2 to 3 days of a URI with a gradually worsening cough, especially at night. By the third or fourth day, there is a barking cough, stridor, and dyspnea, as well as varying degrees of anxiety. Physical examination reveals marked stridor, retractions, tachypnea, hoarseness, and mild cyanosis in room air. The patient may be fairly calm with little distress until the examination begins, at which time the patient's anxiety will increase markedly, causing a worsening of the stridor. The typical case of croup can be differentiated from epiglottitis on clinical grounds, so x-rays are not necessary in every patient. In fact, in mild croup, x-rays are usually normal. In the more severely ill child, lateral neck x-rays will show a normal epiglottis, a distended hypopharynx, and a narrowed subglottic airway. A posteroanterior (PA) chest x-ray shows a narrowed tracheal air column in the form of a "steeple" rather than the normal "square shoulder."

Treatment is symptomatic: cool mist, $O_2$ when needed, and hydration either IV or PO. Antibiotics are not needed, unless there is an associated bacterial illness (otitis media or tonsillitis). Steroids have been shown to be beneficial in croup. Ledwith et al. studied the effects of ED administration of room air mist, 0.5mL nebulized racemic epinephrine, and 0.6mg/kg dexamethasone po given within 30 min of racemic epinephrine, in 55 children with croup. Children with stridor at rest were excluded from the study. Children who did not respond to racemic epinephrine were admitted. Children who clinically improved were observed in the ED for 3 h. If, at the end of 3 h there had been no clinical relapse, that is, the child exhibited no stridor or retractions, and normal air entry, normal color, and normal level of consciousness, the child was discharged. Explicit discharge instructions on signs and symptoms of relapse were given. In this study, 30 of 55 patients were discharged and none of the 30 had an adverse outcome.

Spasmodic croup, recurrent episodes of croup, usually without a preceding URI or fever, almost always occurring at night, is thought to be due to allergy. It is very sensitive to mist. Bacterial tracheitis, a more severe form of croup, has been increasing in the past few years. Also referred to as *membranous laryngotracheobronchitis,* it is usually caused by *Staphylococcus aureus.* The patient has significantly more respiratory distress because of the purulent secretions in the airway. The clinical presentation may be similar to epiglottitis; however, the x-ray shows the typical findings of croup, or the purulent secretions in the trachea may mimic a foreign body. The best way to make the diagnosis is by direct laryngotracheobronchoscopy. This also allows removal of obstructing secretions. The patient may need intubation as well as antibiotics.

In the severely ill patient, blood gases must be monitored and endotracheal intubation or tracheostomy considered. Vaponefrine can be administered by nebulized aerosol via a face mask [intermittent positive-pressure breathing (IPPB) is *not* necessary] for acute but sometimes temporary relief of obstructive symptoms. The dose is 0.5 mL in 3 mL of normal saline. It can be repeated as needed if a good response continues to occur and no cardiac toxicity, such as arrhythmias, is seen. Because of the possibility of rebound stridor, it is recommended that the patient sufficiently ill to require Vaponefrine be admitted or watched in the ED for 6 to 12 h.

# FOREIGN BODY ASPIRATION

## Clinical

Over 3000 people die from foreign body (FB) aspiration each year, and over half of these are children less than 4 years old. FB aspiration is the most common cause of in-home accidental death in children under 6 years old. It usually occurs in the 1- to 4-year-old but may occur as young as 6 months old. The most common FBs are peanuts and sunflower seeds, but almost any conceivable type of object (metal, plastic, food, grass) may be aspirated. Under 1 year, eggshell aspiration during feeding is a common cause.

The patient may present with a variety of signs depending on the location of the FB and the degree of obstruction: wheezing, persistent pneumonia, stridor, coughing, or apnea. Recurrent stridor and/or wheezing may indicate an FB which is changing position within the airway—stridor when it is proximal and wheezing when it moves more distally. Stridor from an FB implies a location in the larynx, trachea, or mainstem bronchus. The usual location is in a mainstem bronchus, often the right, producing cough, unilateral wheezing, or stridor, and classic x-ray signs. Laryngeal and tracheal FBs are less common but *not rare,* constituting 10 to 15 percent of all FBs. The patient with persistent stridor and croup who does not improve over 5 to 7 days may have an FB in the trachea.

Classically, symptoms will occur acutely (choking, coughing, gagging) but usually subside with passage of the FB into the smaller airways. This, in turn, may lead to pneumonia, atelectasis, or wheezing. This triphasic course of symptoms—acute, latent asymptomatic period, and delayed wheezing or stridor—is classic for mainstem bronchi FBs. As many as one-third of the aspirations may *not* be witnessed or remembered by the parent. Often, there is no history of the aspiration, or it is obtained only in retrospect. The physician must have a high index of suspicion of an FB.

Upper esophageal FBs can cause stridor. They may also cause dysphagia or failure to thrive, especially with a long-term radiolucent FB, such as an aluminum "pop-top." However, even in the absence of dysphagia, the possibility of an esophageal FB should be considered in the patient with stridor.

## Diagnosis

If it is opaque, the FB can be easily seen on x-ray. However, most airway FBs are radiolucent and must be diagnosed by a change in airway appearance or dynamics. Laryngeal FBs can be outlined by air contrast on lateral neck x-rays. Tracheal FBs can also be outlined on x-rays, although this may require special technique as xerograms or laminograms. Xerograms may also be useful in outlining small nonopaque FBs in the lower airway.

Mainstem bronchi FBs will cause air trapping in the involved lung

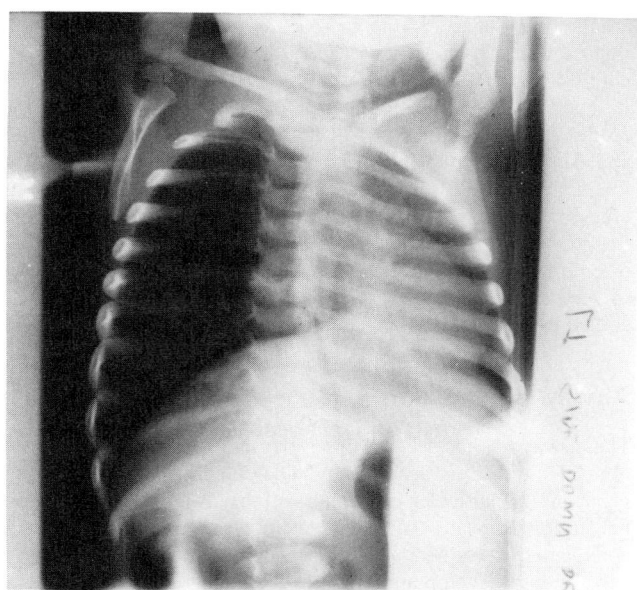

**Fig. 37-4.** Normal decubitus film with left side down.

on expiration because the bronchus constricts around the FB during expiration and obstructive emphysema occurs. This leads to hyperinflation of the obstructed lung and a shift of the mediastinum *during expiration away from the obstructed side* (Fig. 37-3). This shift can be seen on inspiratory and expiratory PA chest x-rays or fluoroscopy. If necessary, the x-ray technician can apply pressure on the epigastrium during expiration, leading to a maximal exhalation and allowing for good timing of the films. In the young or uncooperative patient, it may be impossible to obtain accurately timed inspiratory and expiratory films.

This mediastinal shift may also be seen on bilateral decubitus x-rays of the chest. Normally, the "down" hemithorax is hypoinflated with an elevated hemidiaphragm and "splinted ribs." However, the reverse occurs on the side of the FB, where there is persistent hyperinflation and no loss of volume, even when the affected lung is

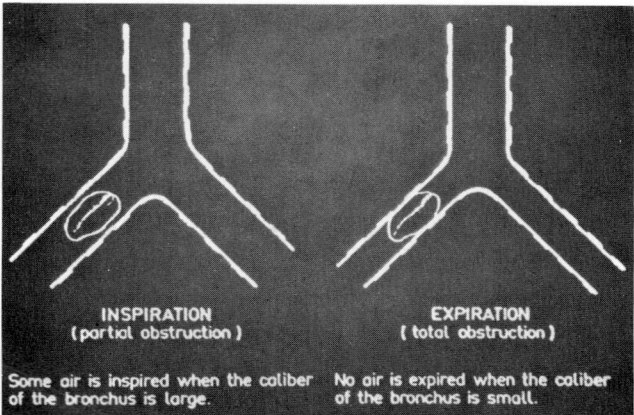

**Fig. 37-3.** Inspiratory and expiratory films in foreign body aspiration.

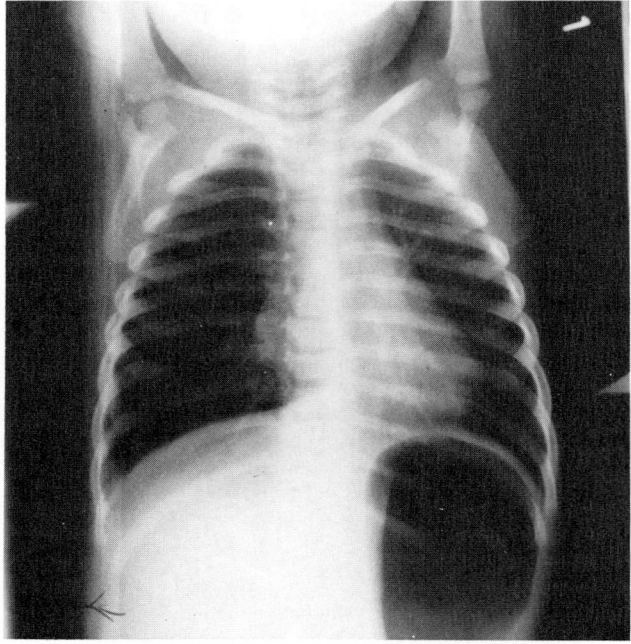

**Fig. 37-5.** Decubitus film, right side down, in foreign body aspiration.

"down" (Figs. 37-4 and 37-5). These films can be done even in young, uncooperative patients.

Most importantly, it takes some time for these findings to occur. A single negative x-ray examination does not rule out the presence of an FB. Computed tomographic scanning may be necessary for diagnosis in difficult cases. However, the most important rule is still to have a high index of suspicion. A preoperative diagnosis is made in only 60 percent of airway FBs. If you still suspect the diagnosis, even though x-rays are not confirmatory, you should probably proceed to bronchoscopy anyway.

Esophageal FBs are usually radiopaque and easy to detect on x-rays. Flat esophageal FBs, such as coins, are *almost* always oriented in the coronal plane, so that they are en face (facing forward) on a PA x-ray. Tracheal FBs are *almost* always oriented in the sagittal plane because of absent cartilage in the posterior tracheal wall. However, these "rules" do not always hold. PA *and* lateral x-rays will place the opaque FB without a doubt. Radiolucent esophageal FB may require barium swallow, xerograms, or tomograms to make the diagnosis.

## Management

Treatment of airway FBs is laryngoscopy or bronchoscopy with removal of the object in the operating room under anesthesia. This may be a difficult procedure, especially in the very young patient with tiny airways. The FB may be too cumbersome to remove whole with the bronchoscope forceps, in which case a Fogarty catheter or urine stone basket may be needed for removal. Similarly, esophageal FBs can be removed by endoscopic forceps with or without a Foley catheter. However, if the latter is used, the FB must be smooth without sharp edges and in place for less than 2 weeks and there must be no underlying esophageal disease. It is *almost* never necessary to proceed immediately to bronchoscopy. One can usually wait and schedule it electively, especially if the patient has a full stomach.

Because of the edema of the airway from the FB itself and the instrumentation necessary for removal, as well as the chemical pneumonia in cases of food aspiration (especially peanuts), the patient with an airway FB will require respiratory care for 24 to 72 h after FB removal. Antibiotics, steroids, oxygen, mist, and chest physiotherapy may all be necessary. The patient with an FB is not dramatically improved after bronchoscopic removal as is the patient with epiglottitis after intubation.

## RETROPHARYNGEAL ABSCESS

The usual age for retropharyngeal abscess formation is 6 months to 3 years. It is rare over the age of 3 because of a normal regression in the size of the retropharyngeal lymph nodes with age. It begins with a URI which localizes to the retropharyngeal lymph nodes over several days. Dysphagia and refusal to feed occur before significant respiratory distress. These children are usually toxic-appearing, febrile, and drooling and have inspiratory stridor and dysphagia. Characteristically, they assume an almost opisthotonic posture.

The diagnostic test is a lateral neck x-ray which shows a widened retropharyngeal space (Fig. 37-6). This x-ray must be done in inspiration with the neck extended or a false-positive widening will be seen. Sometimes, lucencies or actual air-fluid levels can be seen within the widened retropharyngeal space. Physical examination of the pharynx shows a retropharyngeal mass which can often be seen with a tongue blade and a flashlight. Palpation of the mass is dangerous, as it may lead to rupture of the abscess.

Treatment is high-dose IV antibiotics, usually penicillin G in doses of 100,000 units/kg per day. The most common organism is β-hemolytic *Streptococcus*. If fluctuation or severe respiratory distress occurs, an incision and drainage should be done in a controlled manner in the operating room by an experienced otolaryngologist. Complications include respiratory failure from obstruction, rupture of the abscess into the airway causing either asphyxia or bronchopneumonia, and spread of the abscess into the adjacent soft tissues of the neck.

## BIBLIOGRAPHY

Black RE, Choi KJ, Syme WC, et al: Bronchoscopic removal of aspirated foreign bodies in children. *Am J Surg* 148:778, 1984.

Bottenfield GW, Arcinue EL, Sarnaik A, et al: Diagnosis and management of acute epiglottitis—report of 90 consecutive cases. *Laryngoscope* 90:822, 1980.

Custer JR; Croup and related disorders. *Pediatr Rev* 14:19, 1993.

Fischer H: Oropharyngeal examination for suspected epiglottitis. *Am J Dis Child* 142:1261, 1988.

Hight DW, Philippart AI, Hertzler JH: The treatment of retained peripheral foreign bodies in the pediatric airway. *J Pediatr Surg* 16:694, 1981.

Kairys SW, Olmstead EM, O'Connor: Steroid treatment of laryngotracheitis: A meta-analysis of the evidence from randomized trials. *Pediatrics* 83:683, 1989.

Ledwith CA, Shea LM, Mauro RD: Safety and efficacy of nebulized racemic epinephrine in conjunction with oral dexamethasone and mist in the outpatient treatment of croup. *Ann Emerg Med* 25 (3):331, 1995.

Liston SL, Gehrz RC, Jarvis CW: Bacterial tracheitis. *Arch Otolaryngol* 107:561, 1981.

O'Neill JA, Holcomb GW Jr, Neblett WW: Management of tracheobronchial and esophageal foreign bodies in childhood. *J Pediatr Surg* 18:475, 1983.

Vernon DD, Sarnaik AP: Acute epiglottitis in children: A conservative approach to diagnosis and management. *Crit Care Med* 14:23, 1986.

Waisman Y, Klein BL, Boenning DA, et al: Prospective randomized double-blind study comparing L-epinephrine and racemic epinephrine aerosols in the treatment of laryngotracheitis (croup). *Pediatrics* 89:302, 1992.

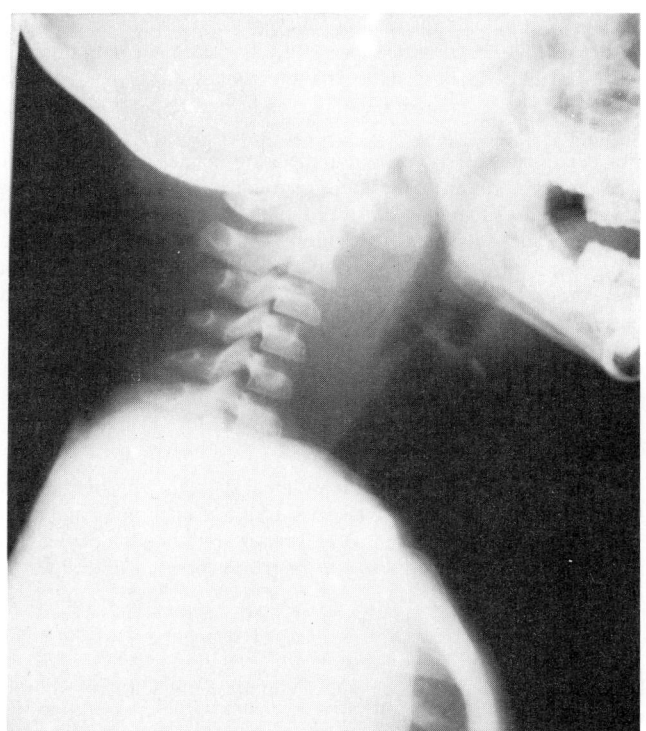

**Fig. 37-6.** Lateral neck view of a child with retropharyngeal abscess.

# 38

# PEDIATRIC ANALGESIA AND SEDATION

### Elaine S. Pomeranz
### Roy M. Kulick

Analgesia and sedation for children undergoing procedures has become a topic of great interest in the last half decade after being ignored by the medical community for years. In fact, the American College of Emergency Physicians recently published a policy statement advocating the safe use of sedatives and analgesics for children in the emergency setting. Although such guidelines were initially developed by extrapolating from studies done either in the preoperative setting or in adults, those of us practicing in this setting can now benefit from a burgeoning of the literature in this field and a tremendous growth of shared experience.

It is crucial to distinguish between analgesics and sedatives. Although decreasing anxiety with sedatives may increase the pain threshold to some extent, no amount of sedation will allow a child to comfortably undergo a painful procedure. On the other hand, analgesics are not ideal for sedation. In reality, the emergency setting frequently calls for both.

The underuse of analgesics and sedatives for children has been well documented for years. It is encouraging that this is becoming less of a problem, but a study published in 1990 still demonstrated that only 40 percent of emergency department patients of any age received analgesia for painful procedures and that pediatric patients received them only 25 percent of the time. There are several reasons for this underuse, but lack of information can no longer be considered a valid excuse. It continues to be true that the expression of pain in infants and young children is nonspecific and easily overlooked. Children are often perceived as being fragile and more vulnerable than adults to the respiratory depressant effects of many of these agents. Yet pharmacokinetic studies show that infants and young children are actually more tolerant of some of these medications. Nevertheless, the risk of respiratory depression must be anticipated when using systemic agents. To complicate matters, there is an approximately 15 percent failure rate with any of these agents, and the risk of untoward side effects increases with the dose and the number of different agents used. In addition, many drugs can occasionally cause paradoxical excitement instead of the desired effect. It is therefore understandable that so many physicians approach the matters of analgesia and sedation in children with great trepidation. However, when used correctly and with adequate monitoring, these agents can make the emergency department encounter more humane for the child, parent, and physician.

## ASSESSMENT OF PAIN IN CHILDREN

The presence or absence of pain in infants must be inferred from physiologic and behavioral responses. Physiologic responses include increases in heart rate, blood pressure, and respiratory rate. Behavioral clues include facial expression, cry, posture, and vocalization.

Preschool children understand and can begin to describe their experience of pain. Creative self-report scales have recently been developed to help young children indicate their degree of pain. These scales include, for example, line drawings of faces or a photographic scale of facial expressions ("Oucher!"). The child selects the facial expression on the analogue scale that best represents the intensity of pain. Physiologic and behavioral parameters remain important in this age group.

Older children and adolescents are better able to directly express their perception of pain intensity although self-report scales such as the linear analogue scale may still be useful.

## NONPHARMACOLOGIC APPROACHES

The emergency department is a frightening place for any sick or injured child, particularly for one in pain. The child's level of anxiety and discomfort can greatly influence the ability to perform an adequate physical examination or successfully complete a procedure. Several simple, easily applied nonpharmacologic interventions can decrease a patient's anxiety and even alter the perception of pain. However, few children will be completely anesthetized by purely behavioral techniques for a truly painful procedure. These techniques should be considered an adjunct to the appropriate use of analgesics and sedatives.

It is a challenge to establish rapport and earn a child's trust in the short time generally available in an emergency department encounter. One must take a developmentally appropriate approach to communicating with a child, considering issues such as language development, pain, separation, body image, fear of death, and autonomy. A gentle, unhurried approach is helpful. Preparation for a procedure should always include an honest, clear explanation of what is to be expected and an opportunity for questions to be addressed. To the extent that it is practical in the emergency setting, the child may be allowed to handle the equipment and practice the procedure on a doll. If, however, there is no time for this more extensive preparation, it is probably best to minimize the time the child must anticipate a painful procedure by saving the explanation until just before its performance.

Environmental alterations such as dimmed lights, a quiet room, or stereo headphones may relieve anxiety. Specific relaxation techniques such as deep-breathing exercises may be beneficial. Some children may respond to distractions such as storytelling or singing. Another technique that takes advantage of a child's unique ability to daydream or pretend is guided imagery. During guided imagery, children as young as 3 to 4 years old are encouraged to imagine they are in a favorite place or participating in their favorite activity and to describe their fantasies in great detail.

Hypnosis combines distraction, imagery, and progressive muscle relaxation. It has been used successfully to treat pain in children in many different settings including the emergency department. Formal application requires trained personnel and often requires some practice on the part of the patient.

For health care personnel to complete a procedure safely and efficiently, many children will require restraint despite all of the above efforts as well as the addition of sedation and analgesia. Manual restraint may be sufficient for quick, simple procedures such as venipuncture. Sheets or papoose boards are more appropriate for longer procedures and are usually well tolerated after an initial protest. Parents should be relieved of the responsibility of restraining a child and allowed instead to provide comfort.

## LOCAL ANALGESIA

### Infiltrative

It is important to infiltrate local anesthetics slowly, with frequent aspiration to avoid injecting into an artery. Slower infiltration and small needles also decrease the pain of infiltration. Jet injection devices are effective in minimizing the pain of injection for such procedures as lumbar puncture.

### Lidocaine

Although lidocaine is the local anesthetic most frequently used in the emergency department, it is often argued that the pain on infiltrating the skin with this drug is worse than the pain of "one quick stick" for obtaining cerebrospinal fluid or an arterial sample. Whether or not this is true is arguable, as is the myth in pediatrics of "one quick stick." One of the most common painful pediatric emergency procedures for which local anesthesia is rarely used is lumbar puncture despite the fact that recent research has shown that there is no greater risk of a "traumatic tap" (i.e., blood contaminating the spinal fluid) associated with its use.

It has been clearly demonstrated that neutralizing lidocaine's acidity by adding 8.4% sodium bicarbonate greatly diminishes the pain of infiltration. This can be accomplished by adding sodium bicarbonate to lidocaine in a ratio of 1:10. The shelf life of this mixture is approximately 1 week. Use of buffered lidocaine has now been studied in many settings and is recommended for almost all local anesthetic uses of lidocaine including digital blocks. The pain of infiltration can be reduced even further by warming the anesthetic to 40°C with an intravenous solution warmer.

Lidocaine is available in 1% or 2% solutions with or without epinephrine. Epinephrine's vasoconstricting effect makes it a helpful addition when bleeding would otherwise obscure the field and prolongs the half-life of the lidocaine by slowing absorption. However, preparations containing epinephrine should not be used on a distal extremity, nose, penis, or pinna of the ear.

The maximum recommended dose of lidocaine is 5 mg/kg for preparations without epinephrine and 7 mg/kg for preparations with.

## Bupivacaine

Bupivacaine is four times as potent as lidocaine and has a duration of action of up to 7 h. Although it is frequently used for both children and adults in the postoperative setting, its use in children has not been well studied. Commercial preparations of bupivacaine are even more acidic than lidocaine but they too can be buffered with sodium bicarbonate. They are available in 0.25% and 0.5% solutions, with and without epinephrine. The maximum recommended dose is 2 to 3 mg/kg with or without epinephrine.

## Topical

### TAC and LET

TAC is a topical anesthetic that has gained increasing acceptance for children with superficial dermal lacerations. Although the original formulation arbitrarily consisted of tetracaine 0.5%, adrenaline 1:2000, and cocaine 11.8%, one-half strength TAC appears to be equally effective and presumably has a wider margin of safety. The tetracaine component may also be eliminated.

TAC provides anesthesia equivalent to infiltrated lidocaine for superficial lacerations on the face and scalp and has several advantages. The application of TAC is painless and therefore decreases psychic trauma and encourages trust and cooperation. In addition, there is no distortion of the wound margins and there does not appear to be any increase in infection rate. However, TAC is not as effective on less vascular areas such as the extremities where supplemental infiltrated lidocaine is more likely to be required. Because the epinephrine component causes vasoconstriction, the same restrictions for lidocaine with epinephrine apply to the use of TAC.

Although rare, the potential adverse effects associated with the misuse of TAC include disorientation, hallucinations, seizures, and death, which are related to the excess systemic absorption of cocaine and tetracaine. These events have been associated with the inappropriate application of TAC on the mucous membranes of the eyes, nose, and mouth or the use of repeated applications. TAC should therefore never be used on a mucosal surface. Similarly, the inadvertent dripping of TAC onto a mucosal surface must be prevented. Its use on burns or abraded areas or on a child with a history of seizures or cardiac arrhythmias should also be avoided.

The maximal allowable dose of TAC has not been determined. However, 1.5 mL of full-strength or 3 mL of one-half strength TAC appears safe and provides adequate anesthesia for the great majority of wounds. Supplemental lidocaine can generally be comfortably infiltrated into those wounds not adequately anesthetized for suturing. The use of repeated applications of TAC is strongly discouraged. Adherence to these precautions will ensure the safe use of TAC.

TAC may be applied in the following manner:

1. Gently cleanse the wound.
2. Place the wound in a gravity-dependent position, instill TAC into the wound cavity, and allow to stand for at least 3 min.
3. Saturate a cotton ball or swab with additional TAC and hold or tape in place within the wound for 10 to 15 min prior to irrigation and suturing. The child's caretaker should apply gentle pressure to promote the even distribution of TAC throughout the wound cavity and margins.

Schillling et al. have recently shown that a topical solution of 4% lidocaine, 0.1% epinephrine and 0.5% tetracaine (LET) is equivalent to TAC for topical anesthesia to the scalp, forehead and eyebrow. It was best in those < 6 years of age.

### EMLA Cream

EMLA Cream, a mixture of 2.5% lidocaine and 2.5% prilocaine, is a topical anesthetic effective on normal intact skin. EMLA eliminates or reduces the pain associated with common emergency department procedures such as venipuncture, lumbar puncture, and skin infiltration. It is applied in a thick layer and covered with an occlusive dressing. The major disadvantage of EMLA for emergency department use is that it must be applied at least 60 min prior to the anticipated procedure to achieve adequate analgesia.

EMLA appears to be generally safe. The prilocaine component has the potential to induce methemoglobinemia, although this is extremely unlikely after single applications. EMLA should not be applied to mucosal surfaces, and it is suggested that the occlusive dressing be covered with a gauze dressing to prevent accidental ingestion in small children.

### Regional Nerve Blocks

Regional nerve blocks are described in Chapter 43 and are appropriate for children as long as the recommendations for the maximum allowable doses for the local anesthetics are adhered to.

## SYSTEMIC ANALGESIA

The American Academy of Pediatrics defines *conscious sedation* as "a minimally depressed level of consciousness that retains a patient's ability to maintain a patent airway . . . and respond appropriately to physical stimulation and/or verbal commands." This is distinguished from deep sedation and general anesthesia, for which separate guidelines for patient monitoring are suggested. The difference between conscious and deep sedation is sometimes only a matter of quantity rather than quality of drug and of individual variations in response.

Whenever a systemic analgesic or sedative is used, it is ideal to have the patient continuously monitored and under the constant observation of a physician or nurse trained in airway management, as is advocated by both the American Academy of Pediatrics and the American College of Emergency Physicians. A busy emergency department offers the advantage of having such personnel and airway equipment nearby at all times but rarely has the staffing capability to allow the physician or nurse to remain at the bedside constantly. Because the major risk that these agents pose is respiratory depression, a more practical approach would be to have such a skilled individual at the bedside whenever possible and to have the patient monitored continuously with at least a pulse oximeter. Oxygen, suction equipment, oral airways, bag and mask, and intubation equipment should be readily accessible. When narcotics are used, it is wise to have the appropriate naloxone dose (5 to 10 µg/kg) precalculated and available. When benzodiazepines are used, flumazenil should also be available.

**Table 38-1.** Suggested Strategy for Analgesia and Sedation in Children

| |
|---|
| **Analgesia for brief painful procedures (30–45 min)** |
| *Fentanyl (Sublimaze) IV |
| Nitrous oxide inhalation |
| †Ketamine IV, IM |
| **Analgesia for painful procedures 1 h or longer** |
| ‡Morphine IV |
| ‡Meperidine (Demerol) PO, IV, IM |
| Ketorolac PO, IV, IM |
| **Sedation for brief nonpainful procedures (30–45 min)** |
| Midazolam (Versed) PO, PR, intranasally, IV, IM |
| Methohexital (Brevital) PR, IM, IV |
| **Sedation for nonpainful procedures 1 h or longer** |
| Diazepam (Valium) PO, IV |
| Pentobarbital (Nembutal) IV, IM |
| Chloral hydrate PO, PR |

* May be supplemented with midazolam for synergistic sedative/analgesic effect.
† Ketamine has both sedative and analgesic properties.
‡ May be supplemented with hydroxyzine for synergistic sedative/analgesic effect.

When choosing a pharmacologic agent for a pediatric patient, important considerations include the nature of the procedure (painful or nonpainful), the desired onset and duration of action, and the route of administration most appropriate for the clinical situation. Therefore, the following discussion of individual agents is structured according to the nature and duration of the planned procedure (Table 38-1).

Suggested initial and supplemental dosages, routes of administration, timing of onset, duration of action, and risks are summarized in Table 38-2.

## Analgesia for Brief, Painful Procedures

### Fentanyl

Fentanyl, a synthetic narcotic, is well suited for use in the emergency department. It is 100 times more potent than morphine and has an almost immediate onset and a brief duration of action (approximately 30 min) when administered intravenously. Respiratory depression can be minimized by administering it slowly over 3 to 5 min. Because it is so concentrated, care should be taken not to flush any small amount that might be left over in heparin lock tubing because this could represent a significant overdose in a small child. Fentanyl was used safely and successfully in a series of 2000 children undergoing facial laceration repairs in the emergency department with the use of a pulse oximeter as a monitor for respiratory depression.

Pharmacokinetic studies suggest that fentanyl may be less likely to cause respiratory and cardiovascular depression than does morphine in young infants. It also causes less histamine release than other opiates.

As experience using fentanyl in the pediatric population has increased in the past few years, there have been reports of withdrawal problems with prolonged infusions, but short-term use has gained widespread popularity. It has proven to be especially effective when combined with midazolam for orthopedic procedures.

Oral fentanyl citrate is showing promise for use in the emergency department, but experience is currently limited.

### Nitrous Oxide

Although nitrous oxide has been used in the emergency department for over 20 years, experience with children in this setting is somewhat limited. Delivered as a 30% to 50% mixture with oxygen, it is an effective analgesic and induces a state of conscious sedation with feelings of euphoria and dissociation. Nitrous oxide is used alone, or more commonly, as an adjunct to local anesthesia for orthopedic procedures, lacerations, burns, and abrasions.

Nitrous oxide must be administered through a system that is fail safe against delivery of a hypoxic mixture. It is generally recommended that a self-administered demand valve system be used such that the patient must deliberately inhale through a mask or mouthpiece to receive the analgesic mixture. When oversedated, the mask or mouthpiece falls and the patient breathes room air leading to rapid arousal. The system should also include an oxygen analyzer and a scavenger device. The patient should be continuously monitored by using a pulse oximeter and by maintaining verbal communication.

The advantages of nitrous oxide include its rapid uptake and excretion. Peak effects are reached in 1 to 2 min and the patient is fully aroused within minutes after cessation of delivery. It has minimal respiratory or cardiovascular effects when administered in the 30% to 50% range.

A limitation to the use of nitrous oxide is that young children often have difficulty accepting or understanding the self-administered system, making it more practical for school-aged patients. Risk of aspiration is minimal. Use of nitrous oxide in the emergency setting also requires specially designed equipment and appropriately trained personnel.

Nitrous oxide is contraindicated for children who have recently received another sedative, or those with an altered mental status, dyspnea, pneumothorax, eye injuries, or suspicion of an obstructed viscus.

### Ketamine

Ketamine is considered a dissociative analgesic that also has sedative properties. Although anesthesiologists have much experience with ketamine, it has only recently become popular for children in the emergency department. It can be administered via a variety of routes, including orally. Although airway reflexes are usually protected, ketamine can cause laryngospasm. Atropine is often used as an adjunct to control associated hypersalivation, and the addition of midazolam is helpful in older children, who may otherwise be prone to unpleasant hallucinations. Ketamine raises blood pressure and intracranial pressure, so should not be used under circumstances in which this is a concern (e.g., head trauma). Moreover, it may be unsatisfactory for computed tomography (CT) due to random movements that can occur despite full sedation.

The oral use of ketamine is showing promise in the pediatric oncology population and may soon gain acceptance in the emergency department.

### Propofol

Propofol is a relatively new ultrashort-acting sedative-hypnotic, unrelated to barbiturates and benzodiazepines, which has been used most commonly in the operating room for the induction and maintenance of anesthesia. It has only recently been used outside the operating room for sedation during procedures such as CT and cardiac catheterization. Its duration of action is extremely short, requiring a continuous infusion to maintain sedation. Induction doses cause respiratory depression and significant decreases in blood pressure in a large proportion of patients. The role for propofol for sedation in the emergency department, if any, has yet to be defined.

## Analgesia for Longer, Painful Procedures

### Morphine

Morphine is still the gold standard. There is substantial experience using it, and it is easily reversed with naloxone. Unfortunately, its bioavailability is poor in oral form. Infants less than 3 months of age may be particularly susceptible to its respiratory depressant effects.

Opioids, in general, have analgesic effects at lower doses than those required for sedation. If both are desired, it is wise to combine fentanyl with midazolam (see below) or morphine or meperidine with

**Table 38-2.** Guidelines for Usage of Analgesics and Sedatives in Children

| Analgesics | Initial Dose | Onset | Effective Duration | Supplemental Maximum Dose | Precautions/ Comments |
|---|---|---|---|---|---|
| Fentanyl | 2–3 µg/kg IV | 2 min | 30 min | Titrate to effect in 0.5 µg/kg increments | Respiratory depression (especially with rapid IV push); bradycardia; muscle rigidity Have naloxone available |
| Nitrous Oxide | 30–50% mixture with $O_2$ | 1–2 min | — | —— | Fail-safe system to avoid hypoxia; scavenger system Contraindications: previous sedative, altered mental status, dyspnea, pneumothorax, eye injury, obstructed viscus |
| Ketamine | 1.0 mg/kg IV 4.0 mg/kg IM | rapid IV 3–5 min | 10 min 20 min | IV—titrate to effect IM—2 mg/kg supplementation | Laryngospasm Hypertension (not recommended for closed head injury patients) Hypersalivation (can be controlled with atropine 0.01 mg/kg) Hallucinations (can be avoided with midazolam or diazepam) |
| Morphine | 0.1 mg/kg IV | 5–10 min | 3–4 h | 0.05 mg/kg supplementation, titrate to effect | Respiratory depression (especially with rapid IV push) Hypotension Have naloxone available |
| Meperidine | 1.0 mg/kg IV, IM 1–2 mg/kg PO | rapid IV 10–15 min IM 15–30 min PO | 2–3 h | 0.5 mg/kg supplementation, max 100 mg IV, IM max 150 mg PO | Precautions as with other narcotics above Can be combined with hydroxyzine, 0.5 mg/kg IM or PO Have naloxone available |
| Ketorolac | 0.5–1.0 mg/kg IM, IV 10 mg PO (adult dose) | peak 30–60 min | 4–6 h | 0.5–1.0 mg/kg q 4–6 h 10 mg q 6 h | GI irritation, caution with renal impairment Potential bronchospasm, anaphylactoid reaction |
| **Sedatives** | | | | | |
| Midazolam | 0.15 mg/kg IV, IM 0.2–0.4 mg/kg PR, intranasally 0.5 mg/kg PO | 2 min IV, 10–15 min IM, PR, intranasally or PO | 30 min IV 45 min IM, PR, intranasally or PO | Titrate IV dose to effect in 0.02 mg/kg increments; 0.1 mg/kg IM supplementation 12 mg max dose PO | Respiratory depression, apnea, hypotension (especially when combined with fentanyl) Anterograde amnesia for 1–2 h |
| Methohexital | 20 mg/kg PR 1 mg/kg IV | 15 min PR rapid IV | 20 min 10 min | Max PR dose 25 mg/kg | Adverse effects similar to those of pentobarbital; may lower seizure threshold in patients with known seizure disorder |
| Diazepam | 0.1 mg/kg IV 0.2 mg/kg PO, PR | rapid IV 30–60 min PO, PR | 1–2 h | Max IV dose 0.6 mg/kg over 8 h Max PO dose 10 mg over 6–8 h | Adverse effects similar to those of midazolam |
| Pentobarbital | 2.5 mg/kg IV 2–5 mg/kg IM | rapid IV, 15 min IM | 30 min IV 2 h IM | 1.25 mg/kg (max 100 mg) IV Max total IV dose 300 mg 100–200 mg max IM dose | Hiccups, respiratory depression, apnea, hypotension, cardiac depression |
| Chloral Hydrate | 75 mg/kg PO, PR | 30 min | 3–4 h | 2 g max dose | GI irritation, cardiac arrhythmias (rare), increased hyperbilirubinemia in premature infants |

hydroxyzine. In fact, hydroxyzine (0.5 mg/kg orally or intramuscularly) appears to have significant analgesic effects on its own and is clearly synergistic with narcotics.

## "DPT Cocktail" (Meperidine, Promethazine, Chlorpromazine)

This combination of drugs has been extremely popular and was the most commonly cited "sedative" in a survey of pediatric emergency departments a few years ago. The reason for this may be that it has been available for a long time and that familiarity with it has led to the false belief that it is completely safe. However, it was developed for inpatient cardiac catheterization and has several drawbacks that, in the opinion of these authors, make it unsuitable for use in the emergency department. The most serious problem is the risk of respiratory depression that was as high as 13 percent in one series. The rationale behind this combination has been questioned. Moreover, DPT can only be given intramuscularly and the majority of patients sleep for more than 7 hours.

Adding to the confusion surrounding DPT is the wide range of doses used, with meperidine ranging from 1.0 to 3.0 mg/kg and promethazine and chlorpromazine ranging from 0.06 to 1.0 mg/kg. The most common combination seems to be 2 mg/kg of meperidine and 1 mg/kg each of promethazine and chlorpromazine.

## Meperidine

Meperidine is a synthetic derivative of morphine that is about one tenth as potent an analgesic when used alone and has a briefer duration of action. It is less effective in its oral form than when given parenterally, but the difference between the two routes is less than with morphine. As with other narcotics, nausea and vomiting are possible side effects although the addition of hydroxyzine as described previously decreases the frequency. Meperidine appears less likely to cause respiratory depression in neonates than does morphine.

## Nonsteroidal Anti-inflammatory Drugs (NSAIDs)

Ibuprofen and naproxen are generally used for less severe pain than are narcotics. However, a more potent formulation, ketorolac (Toradol), has recently become available. It is a potent analgesic that rivals narcotics, but has a longer duration of action and does not cause respiratory depression. Ketorolac can be given intramuscularly or intravenously in a dose of 0.5 to 1.0 mg/kg (maximum 60 mg). It may also be given orally; however, pediatric dosing recommendations for this route have not been established. The adult dose is 10 mg every 6 h. It has been used both in place of and in combination with opioid analgesics. The most common adverse effects appear to be gastrointestinal irritation and the other problems typical of NSAIDs. There have also been reports of bronchospasm and anaphylactoid reactions in adults.

## SEDATION

## Sedation for Brief, Nonpainful Procedures

### Midazolam

Midazolam is a drug well suited for use in pediatric outpatients. It is a short-acting benzodiazepine that offers great versatility in routes of administration. Although it is only supplied in vials for intravenous use, it has been given successfully via oral, rectal, intramuscular, subcutaneous, and intranasal routes.

Its intranasal administration has become popular and more than doubled parental satisfaction with emergency department suturing of children's injuries in a recent study.

Midazolam is a potent sedative and has a duration of action of only 30 to 40 min. Like the narcotics, the oral dose needed for effects equivalent to the intravenous route is much higher. Regardless of the route chosen, children require higher doses than do adults. Children given midazolam are generally awake but drowsy and disinhibited. Therefore, it is useful in rendering children cooperative for such procedures as suspected sexual abuse examinations or as a prelude to administering local anesthesia for suturing, lumbar punctures, bone marrows, etc. Midazolam is also an excellent amnestic agent, and certainly makes, for instance, the return visit for suture removal easier. It is less suitable for procedures such as CT scanning, which requires the patient to lie motionless.

Flumazenil is a benzodiazepine antagonist that is used as a reversal agent in much the same way that naloxone is used to reverse narcotics. Reversal usually occurs in 1 to 2 min, but is not always complete and is not a substitute for airway management. Experience with flumazenil is limited in children. The recommended pediatric dose is an initial dose of 0.01 mg/kg intravenously (maximum 0.2 mg), followed by 0.005 mg/kg (maximum 0.2 mg) every minute to a maximum total dose of 1 mg. However, adult doses have been used in children effectively and without untoward effect.

### Methohexital

Methohexital is frequently given per rectum to children under the age of 5 prior to general anesthesia. Although experience using it in the pediatric emergency setting continues to be limited, anesthesia experience shows that more than 90 percent of children fall asleep within

12 min of rectal administration, making it an attractive choice for the emergency department, especially when placement of an intravenous line is not desirable. Its intramuscular use has been reported but is felt by some to be unduly painful. It is available in a variety of concentrations, but the more concentrated solutions are suggested for intramuscular and rectal routes.

## Sedation for Longer, Nonpainful Procedures

### Diazepam

Diazepam, a longer-acting benzodiazepine, has been used extensively for years in children as an effective anxiolytic and amnestic agent. However, more recently, it has been largely replaced by midazolam for sedation of children in the emergency department. Midazolam causes less pain on injection, may be administered by a wider variety of routes, has a faster onset of sedation, and has a more rapid return to baseline function. For longer procedures, supplemental doses of midazolam may be administered.

### Pentobarbital

Pentobarbital is a somewhat longer-acting barbiturate that has been used to sedate children in the emergency department. Because it induces sleep, it is useful for nonpainful procedures requiring the child to be still, such as a CT scan. Although it may be administered orally, intramuscularly, or intravenously, the intravenous route allows more precise titration. Dose recommendations vary widely. However, one suggested titration schedule is to administer an initial 2.5 mg/kg (maximum 100 mg) intravenously over a few minutes followed by a 1.25 mg/kg (maximum 100 mg) supplemental dose every 5 min until the child is adequately sedated or a maximum of 5 mg/kg (maximum total dose 300 mg) is reached. Intravenous pentobarbital induces sleep within 1 min and lasts from 15 to 60 min. When administered intramuscularly, the onset is slower (15 min) and the duration is longer (2 h). Like other barbiturates, pentobarbital may cause respiratory depression and hypotension, particularly when administered by rapid intravenous push or when combined with a narcotic.

### Chloral Hydrate

Chloral hydrate has been used as a sedative for the last century with this extensive experience showing that it is unlikely to cause respiratory depression. It has been studied again recently, comparing it to some of the newer sedatives available and it continues to show good success rates. It may have its greatest success (up to 96 percent) in children 4 years of age or younger, as suggested in a study of children sedated for magnetic resonance imaging.

Chloral hydrate became the focus of controversy in the lay press when it was mentioned that one of its metabolites may be carcinogenic. As has been pointed out by authoritative experts, there is no evidence of chloral hydrate-associated carcinogenicity in human beings. Furthermore, its episodic use as in the emergency department is unlikely to be dangerous. A great advantage of chloral hydrate is that it can be given orally or rectally. The disadvantages of its use in the emergency department are its relatively slow onset of action (30 to 60 min) and its prolonged sedative effect (up to several hours).

## BIBLIOGRAPHY

Beyer JE, Wells N: The assessment of pain in children. *Pediatr Clin North Am* 36:837, 1989.

Billmire DA, Neale HW, Gregory RO: Use of IV fentanyl in the outpatient treatment of pediatric facial trauma. *J Trauma* 25:1079, 1985.

Bonadio WA: TAC—a painless alternative for wound repair. *Contemp Pediatr* 8:41, 1991.

Christoph RA, Buchanan L, Begalla K, Schwartz S: Pain reduction in local anesthetic administration through pH buffering. *Ann Emerg Med* 17:117, 1988.

Committee on Drugs, American Academy of Pediatrics. Guidelines for monitoring and management of pediatric patients during and after sedation for diagnostic and therapeutic procedures. *Pediatrics* 89:1110, 1992.

Committee on Drugs, Section on Anesthesiology. Guidelines for the elective use of conscious sedation, deep sedation, and general anesthesia in pediatric patients. *Pediatrics* 76:317, 1985.

Cote CJ: Sedation for the pediatric patient. *Pediatr Clin North Am* 41:31, 1994.

Gamis AS, Knapp JF, Glenski JA: Nitrous oxide analgesia in the pediatric emergency department. *Ann Emerg Med* 18:177, 1989.

Green SM, Nakamura R, Johnson NE: Ketamine sedation for pediatric procedures: Part I, a prospective series. *Ann Emerg Med* 19:1024, 1990.

Greenberg SB, Faerber EN, Aspinall CL, Adams RC: High-dose chloral hydrate sedation for children undergoing MR imaging: safety and efficacy in relation to age. *AJR Am J Roentgenol* 16:639, 1993.

Hawk W, Crockett K, Ochsenschlager DW, Klein BL: Conscious sedation for the pediatric patient for suturing: a survey. *Pediatr Emerg Care* 6:84, 1990.

Kohen DP: Applications of relaxation/mental imagery (self-hypnosis) in pediatric emergencies. *Int J Clin Exp Hypnosis* 34:283, 1986.

Koren G: Use of the eutectic mixture of local anesthetics in young children for procedure-related pain. *J Pediatr* 122:S30, 1993.

Mitchell AA, Louik C, Lacouture P, et al.: Risks to children from computed tomographic scan premedication. *JAMA* 247:2385, 1982.

Paris PM: Pain management in the child. *Emerg Med Clin North Am* 5:699, 1987.

Schilling CG, et al: Tetracaine, epinephrine, and cocaine (TAC) versus, Lidocaine, epinephrine, and tetracaine (LET) for anesthesia of lacerations in children. *Ann Emerg Med* 25(2): 203, 1995.

Selbst SM, Clark M: Analgesic use in the emergency department. *Ann Emerg Med* 19:1010, 1990.

Strain JD, Campbell JB, Harvey LA, Foley LC: IV nembutal: safe sedation for children undergoing sedation. *AJR Am J Roentgenol* 151:975, 1988.

Theroux MC, West DW, Corddry DH, et al.: Efficacy of intranasal midazolam in facilitating suturing of lacerations in preschool children in the emergency department. *Pediatrics* 91:624, 1993.

Wright SW, Chudnofsky CR, Dronen SC, et al.: Comparison of midazolam and diazepam for conscious sedation in the emergency department. *Ann Emerg Med* 22:201, 1993.

# 39
# HYPOGLYCEMIA IN CHILDREN

## Mark G. Goetting
## Bassam M. Gebara

Hypoglycemia is a relatively common condition in pediatrics, particularly in acutely sick infants and children. The diagnosis and treatment of hypoglycemia in the emergency department should be prompt because persistent or recurrent hypoglycemia may have permanent catastrophic effects on the brain, particularly in infants.

## DEFINITION

Hypoglycemia is defined as a serum or plasma glucose concentration less than 45 mg/dL or a whole blood glucose concentration less than 40 mg/dL (Table 39-1). The values of serum or plasma glucose concentration are 10 to 15 percent higher than those for whole blood.

## GLUCOSE HOMEOSTASIS AND PATHOPHYSIOLOGY

Plasma glucose concentration is maintained in a relatively narrow range by an elaborate regulatory system that keeps the rate of glucose

**Table 39-1.** Relation between Plasma Glucose Concentration and Hormonal or Physiologic Response

| Plasma Glucose Concentration, mg/dL | Hormonal or Physiologic Response |
|---|---|
| 70 | Activation of glucagon, epinephrine, cortisol, and growth hormone secretion |
| 55 | Intensification of glucagon and epinephrine secretion |
| 50 | Neuroelectrophysiologic changes |
| <45 | Symptoms of cerebral dysfunction and adrenergic response |

production and utilization equal. Glucose flux (production and utilization), indexed to body weight, is significantly higher in children than in adults. In the postabsorptive state, children produce and utilize glucose at a rate of 5 to 7 mg/kg per minute, compared to 1.8 to 2.2 mg/kg per minute in adults. After a 30-h fast, children decrease their glucose flux to approximately 4 mg/kg per minute. Hypoglycemia occurs when the rate of glucose utilization exceeds the rate of production. Glucose is obtained from the diet by hydrolysis of carbohydrates and is produced by glycogenolysis and gluconeogenesis. Glucose is utilized by all tissues, and certain tissues, such as brain, red blood cells, retina, and the germinal epithelium of the gonads, derive almost all of their energy from glucose metabolism. Glucose regulation depends on the availability of substrates, normal hormonal activity, normal autonomic nervous system, and functioning hepatic enzymes for gluconeogenesis and glycogenolysis (Table 39-2). Disturbances in any of these factors can produce alterations in blood glucose concentration. Risk factors for hypoglycemia in the pediatric population are listed in Table 39-3.

## Role of Hormones in Glucose Homeostasis

### Insulin

Insulin is the primary glucoregulatory hormone. It decreases plasma concentration of glucose by enhancing peripheral glucose uptake and utilization, by stimulating glycogen synthesis, and by decreasing glycogenolysis and gluconeogenesis. Insulin is a potent inhibitor of lipolysis and proteolysis, decreasing the supply of gluconeogenic substrates (glycerol, amino acids, and lactate) to the liver. The primary regulator of insulin release is the pancreatic arterial glucose level.

**Table 39-2.** Necessary Factors for Glycogenolysis and Gluconeogenesis

Substrates availability:
  Hepatic glycogen (for glycogenolysis)
  Glycerol, alanine, other amino acids, and lactate (for gluconeogenesis)
Functioning glycogenolytic and gluconeogenic enzymes
Decreased insulin and increased glucagon, epinephrine, and cortisol

**Table 39-3.** Risk Factors for Hypoglycemia in Pediatric Population

Glucose utilization is significantly higher in children than adults.
Hepatic glycogen stores are limited in infancy.
Muscle mass is small, limiting substrates for gluconeogenesis.
Infants and younger children cannot maintain normoglycemia with prolonged fasting.
Congenital deficiencies in glycogenolytic or gluconeogenic enzymes present in infancy.
Congenital deficiencies in counterregulatory hormones present in infancy.
Inborn errors of amino acid metabolism decrease substrates for gluconeogenesis.
Inborn errors of fat metabolism decrease substrates for gluconeogenesis.
Sustained or repetitive hypoglycemia retards brain growth in infants.

## Counterregulatory Hormones

The release of glucagon and epinephrine is exquisitely sensitive to small decrements in plasma glucose levels. When plasma glucose concentration decreases to approximately 70 mg/dL, glucagon and epinephrine secretion is activated. This hormonal response is markedly intensified when the plasma glucose level is 55 mg/dL. Neuroelectrophysiologic changes are evident at a plasma glucose level of 50 mg/dL. Children with hyperinsulinemia and children with insulin-dependent diabetes mellitus have a reduced glycemic threshold, to approximately 36 mg/dL, and a diminished catecholamine response to hypoglycemia.

Adrenocorticotropic hormone (ACTH), cortisol, glucagon, epinephrine, and growth hormone oppose the hypoglycemic effect of insulin by the following mechanisms:

1. Inhibiting peripheral glucose uptake (epinephrine, cortisol, and growth hormone).
2. Increasing the supply of endogenous amino acids and glycerol as substrates for gluconeogenesis (cortisol, epinephrine, glucagon, growth hormone, and ACTH).
3. Acute activation of glycogenolytic and gluconeogenic enzymes (epinephrine and glucagon).
4. Chronic induction of gluconeogenic enzymes (glucagon and cortisol).
5. Inhibiting insulin secretion from the pancreas (epinephrine).

## Hepatic Glycogenolysis and Gluconeogenesis

Glucose homeostasis is maintained by glycogenolysis in the immediate postfeeding period and by gluconeogenesis after several hours of fasting. The amount of glycogen stored in the liver and the utilization rate of glucose determine the length of time glycogenolysis can maintain glucose homeostasis. The liver of a 10-kg child contains 20 to 25 g of glycogen, which is sufficient to meet glucose requirements of 4 to 6 mg/kg per minute for 6 to 12 h. The liver of a 70-kg adult stores about 75 g of glycogen, which meets about 50 percent of the daily glucose requirements of 150 g at a utilization rate of 1.5 mg/kg per minute. When hepatic glycogen stores are depleted, the individual becomes dependent on gluconeogenesis to maintain plasma glucose concentration.

The enzymes that mediate glycogen synthesis, glycogenolysis, and gluconeogenesis are governed by insulin and the counterregulatory hormones. After meals, insulin levels peak to 50 to 100 μU/mL, causing activation of glycogen synthesis and inhibition of gluconeogenesis. In addition, insulin stimulates lipogenesis and inhibits ketogenesis. During fasting, insulin levels fall to 5 to 10 μU/mL and glucagon, epinephrine, and cortisol levels increase, causing muscle catabolism and stimulation of glycogenolysis, gluconeogenesis, lipolysis, and ketogenesis. Acetyl-CoA, which is derived from fat and ketones, becomes the primary source of energy for most tissues. In addition, acetyl-CoA activates pyruvate carboxylase enzyme, which catalyzes the conversion of pyruvate to oxaloacetate, an essential step in gluconeogenesis.

The most important endogenous amino acid for gluconeogenesis is alanine. During fasting, plasma alanine levels fall precipitously. Alanine is derived from skeletal muscle protein and de novo synthesis via transamination of lactate and glutamate. In the liver, alanine is transaminated back to lactate and enters the gluconeogenic pathway.

## Beta-Oxidation Defects of Free Fatty Acids and Hypoglycemia

Beta-oxidation of free fatty acids produces acetyl-CoA and NADH that are required to drive gluconeogenesis. Deficiencies of medium-chain acyl-CoA dehydrogenase (MCAD) and, less commonly, long- and short-chain acyl-CoA dehydrogenase (LCAD and SCAD) cause hypoglycemia due to decreased gluconeogenesis. Carnitine is an es-

sential molecule in the transfer of free fatty acids across the mitochondrial membrane for beta-oxidation. Primary carnitine deficiency is characterized by recurrent episodes of Reye-like syndrome, hypoglycemia, and low circulating concentration of ketone bodies.

## Blood, Brain, and Cerebrospinal Fluid Glucose

Glucose enters the CSF and brain extracellular fluid by a carrier-mediated transport system. The rate-limiting factor for glucose transport is the rate of movement of the carrier-glucose complex across the membrane. CSF and brain extracellular fluid glucose concentrations are dependent on plasma glucose concentration. Changes in plasma glucose concentrations are reflected in parallel changes in CSF glucose concentrations; however, because of the rate-limiting effect of the carrier-mediated transport system, these changes in CSF are delayed. After a rapid intravenous infusion of 50% glucose, the CSF glucose concentration does not reach a peak for about 2 h and does not reach equilibrium for about 4 h. There is probably a similar delay in the lowering of CSF glucose in response to acute hypoglycemia. Normal CSF glucose concentration is about 65 percent of blood glucose. Normal brain extracellular fluid glucose concentration is about 20 mg/dL and is dependent on the rate of influx of glucose into brain and the rate of glucose utilization in the brain. Under normal conditions, the rate of glucose influx is about three times the rate of brain utilization. The rate of glucose influx is dependent on plasma glucose concentration. At plasma levels below 30 mg/dL, the rate of transport can become rate-limiting for utilization, so that brain extracellular fluid glucose concentration approaches zero.

## The Brain and Hypoglycemia

Metabolism by the brain accounts for 80 percent of total basal glucose turnover in adults and for most of the endogenous glucose production in infants and young children. Glucose production correlates with brain weight. Glucose is necessary for structural protein synthesis, membrane lipids, and myelination for the growing brain. Hypoglycemia inhibits neuronal protein synthesis, alters amino acid metabolism and neurotransmitter release, causes membrane breakdown, and increases intracellular pH (Table 39-4). During hypoglycemia, alternative fuels, such as ketoacids and Krebs cycle intermediates, sustain brain metabolism at the expense of brain growth. Even during severe hypoglycemia with isoelectric EEG, the brain maintains normal cerebral oxygen metabolism for at least 10 to 20 min because of the use of alternative fuel. However, neonates are at a high risk for alternative fuel deprivation because of their limited capacity to produce ketone bodies, especially in the presence of hyperinsulinemia, which inhibits ketogenesis.

**Table 39-4.** Effects of Hypoglycemia on the Brain

| | |
|---|---|
| Cerebral metabolism | Inhibition of neuronal protein synthesis |
| | Membrane lipid breakdown |
| | Alteration in neurotransmitter release |
| | Early decrease in glucose metabolism |
| | Use of alternative fuel for brain metabolism |
| | Early presevation of brain oxygen metabolism |
| | Late decrease in brain oxygen metabolism |
| | Selective neuronal necrosis |
| | Neuronal death |
| EEG changes | Cortical slowing |
| | Seizures |
| | Burst suppression |
| | Electrical silence |
| Cerebral blood flow | Increase in cerebral blood flow |
| | Delayed hypoperfusion after glucose infusion |

Hypoglycemia may cause significant alterations in cerebral blood flow. During hypoglycemic coma, regional cerebral blood flow may increase by 300 percent, probably because of loss of autoregulation and β-adrenoreceptor stimulation. After glucose administration, a delayed hypoperfusion occurs in the cerebral cortex, with decrease in cerebral blood flow to 20 to 40 percent of normal.

Neuronal damage with severe hypoglycemia may be irreversible. Selective neuronal necrosis, and not infarction, occurs after a pure hypoglycemic insult. There is a superficial-to-deep gradient of neuronal necrosis in the cerebral cortex. The caudate, putamen, and hippocampus are vulnerable, while the brain stem, hypothalamus, and cerebellum are relatively resistant to hypoglycemia. The mechanism of neuronal necrosis may be secondary to excitotoxin release.

Severe, prolonged hypoglycemia causes permanent neurologic damage, especially in infants less than 6 months of age. However, the relationship between duration and severity of hypoglycemia and subsequent brain damage is not predictable. The effects of prolonged or repeated episodes of moderate hypoglycemia are not well studied or known.

## CLINICAL ASPECTS

Hypoglycemia occurs as a primary or secondary feature of a large number of clinical conditions. In addition, ingested substances, such as insulin, salicylates, β blockers, oral hypoglycemics, ethanol, and quinidine, can cause hypoglycemia. The symptomatology is variable and may be overshadowed by the dramatic appearance of the primary disease, such as meningococcemia. Therefore, it is prudent to assess for and treat hypoglycemia immediately. In patients suffering severe physiologic stress, hourly bedside glucose measurements are often necessary, even when the child presents initially with hyperglycemia.

Patients become symptomatic from hypoglycemia because of compensatory heightened adrenergic activity and the cerebral metabolic perturbances directly attributable to glucose deprivation. Older children usually have the same signs seen in adults (Table 39-5). Manifestations tend to be subtler and nonspecific in infants and include poor feeding, lethargy, apnea, hypotonia, and hypothermia. Infants and children with unexplained respiratory or cardiac arrest should be tested immediately for hypoglycemia.

### Management

There are three important aspects of emergency patient care: diagnosis of hypoglycemia, acquisition of germaine blood and urine specimens, and prompt restoration and maintenance of euglycemia. Clearly it is most imperative to replete the serum with glucose, but it is short-sighted to neglect the first two objectives. Discharging the patient from the emergency department with uncertainty that hypoglycemia occurred or without confirming diagnosis will necessitate expensive and uncomfortable testing at a later date.

**Table 39-5.** Clinical Signs of Hypoglycemia

| Adrenergic Excess | Neuroglycopenia |
| --- | --- |
| Anxiety | Confusion |
| Tachycardia | Ataxia |
| Perspiration | Headache |
| Nausea | Depressed consciousness |
| Tremors | Blurred vision |
| Pallor | Lightheadedness |
| Chest pain | Focal neurologic deficits |
| Weakness | Seizures |
| Abdominal pain | Strabismus |
| Hunger | Staring |
| Irritability | Paresthesias |

**Table 39-6.** Correction of Hypoglycemia

250 mg/kg dextrose IV as $D_{10}W^*$, followed by 300–500 mg/kg per hour for neonates and 200–300 mg/kg per hour for infants and children, also as $D_{10}W$.
Recheck glucose level. If less than 50 mg/dL, repeat bolus twice, rechecking after each.
If refractory:
  hydrocortisone succinate 1–2 mg/kg (maximum 100 mg) IV every 6 h.
Glucagon 0.03 mg/kg (maximum 1 mg) IV
Diazoxide 3–5 mg/kg for neonates and 1–3 mg/kg for infants and children IV over 30 min every 8 h.

* $D_{10}W$ = 100 mg/mL dextrose.

### Diagnosis

In those suspected or at risk to be hypoglycemic, bedside glucose measurement can be diagnostic within 2 min. Care is needed to ensure the testing strip is completely covered with blood and that isopropyl alcohol does not contaminate the specimen, otherwise gross errors can result. Inaccuracies with this method lead the clinician to treat children with possible signs of hypoglycemia and a whole blood glucose level less than 80 mg/dL until formal laboratory measurement is completed, as it is better to treat unnecessarily than to delay appropriate treatment.

### Specimen Collecting

After documenting hypoglycemia at the bedside, the clinician should next gather critical blood and urine specimens that will later help diagnose the cause. These include serum glucose, insulin, C-peptide, growth hormone, cortisol, ketone bodies, lactic acid, alanine, and carnitine. Blood must be placed in various tubes with some on ice, so it is helpful to plan ahead. If conservation of blood volume demands a smaller sampling, at least glucose and insulin levels should be sent. A urine sample for ketones as well as organic and amino acids can be delayed a few moments while repleting the child with glucose.

### Correction of Hypoglycemia

After specimen collection, a bolus of 10% dextrose in water ($D_{10}W$) is given intravenously or intraosseously, followed by a continuous infusion of $D_{10}W$ in an age- and weight-appropriate fashion (Table 39-6). When dosing dextrose, it is helpful to recall that $D_{10}W$ has 100 mg/mL. The extreme hypertonicity of $D_{50}W$ can easily injure a peripheral vein, causing extravasation, and therefore, it should be diluted. Also, neonates are less tolerant of a rapid osmotic load and should be given only $D_{10}W$ when possible. Hydrocortisone is useful for those who cannot achieve euglycemia despite adequate dextrose administration, especially with hypopituitarism and adrenal insufficiency. Glucagon is effective only in cases of hyperinsulinism and glucagon deficiency. Diazoxide inhibits insulin release and is also useful in endogenous hyperinsulin states. It is rarely necessary and should be given slowly, as it can produce hypotension.

### Bibliography

Pollack ES, Pollack CV: Ketotic hypoglycemia. *J Emerg Med* 11(5): 531, 1993.
Vogel C, Caraccio T, Mofenson H, et al: Alcohol intoxication in young children. *J Toxicol Clin Toxicol* 33(1): 25, 1995.

# 40

# ALTERED MENTAL STATUS IN CHILDREN

**Nancy Pook**
**Natalie Cullen**
**Jonathan Singer**

## INTRODUCTION

Altered mental status (AMS) in a child is the failure to respond to the external environment in a manner appropriate to the child's developmental level, despite verbal or physical stimulation. Alteration in mental status consists of impairment of awareness and arousal, the two components of consciousness. Patients with AMS require simultaneous stabilization, diagnosis, and treatment. The objectives of treatment are to sustain life and prevent irreversible central nervous system damage. Once the patient is resuscitated, the next objective is to establish the cause of AMS and stop disease progression.

## PATHOPHYSIOLOGY

There is a spectrum of alterations of mental status, ranging from confusion or delirium (disorders in perception) to lethargy, stupor, and coma (states of decreased awareness). A lethargic pediatric patient has decreased awareness of self and the environment. In the emergency setting, this translates to decreased eye contact with family members and nursing and physician personnel. The stuporous pediatric patient has decreased eye contact, decreased motor activity, and unintelligible vocalization. The stuporous patient can be aroused with vigorous noxious stimulation. The comatose patient is unresponsive and cannot be aroused by verbal or physical stimulation such as phlebotomy, arterial catheterization, or lumbar puncture.

Altered mental status, irrespective of the cause, is indicative of either depression of the cerebral cortex or localized abnormalities of the ascending reticular activating system. Both cerebral cortices must be affected in order to cause AMS. Classic causes of bilateral cortical impairment are toxic and metabolic states that deprive the brain of normal substrates. AMS can also be produced through dysfunction of the reticular activating system that is housed in the brainstem and midbrain. This system connects cranial nerve nuclei and extends from brainstem to thalamus. It governs respirations, cardiovascular functions, and many aspects of homeostasis, as well as daily wake/sleep cycles. Any abrupt interruption or selective destruction of the reticular activating system may result in AMS.

The pathologic conditions that effect awareness and arousal can be described using three broad pathologic categories: supratentorial mass lesion, subtentorial mass lesion, and metabolic encephalopathy.

Supratentorial mass lesions cause AMS by compressing the brainstem and/or diencephalon. Signs and symptoms of this type of lesion include focal motor abnormalities, which are often present from the onset of the altered level of consciousness. The progression of neurologic dysfunction is from rostral to caudal, with sequential failure of midbrain, pontine, and medullary function. Compromise by supratentorial lesions causes slow nystagmus toward and fast nystagmus away from a cold stimulus during caloric testing.

Subtentorial mass lesions lead to reticular activating system dysfunction, in which prompt loss of consciousness is generally the rule. There is a discrete level of dysfunction. Cranial nerve abnormalities are frequently found due to the highly packed neurologically eloquent anatomy. Abnormal respiratory patterns such as Cheyne-Stokes, neurogenic hyperventilation, and ataxic breathing are common. With brainstem injury, asymmetric and/or fixed pupils are found. No eye movements occur despite cold stimuli to both auditory canals.

Metabolic encephalopathy usually causes depressed consciousness before motor signs, which, when present, are typically symmetric. Respiratory function is involved relatively early, and abnormalities are often secondary to acid-base imbalance. Pupillary reflexes are generally preserved. Pupils may be sluggish, but the movement is intact and symmetric. Exceptions are profound anoxia and influence of cholinergics, anticholinergics, opiates, and barbiturates.

## HISTORY AND PHYSICAL EXAMINATION

Two individuals are needed to manage a pediatric patient with AMS. One individual should act as historian to perform a methodical and comprehensive interview. The key questions that must be explored are prodromal events leading to the change in consciousness, recent illnesses, the likelihood of an infectious exposure or exposure to intoxicants, and the likelihood of trauma, including abuse. The historian should make inquiries regarding antecedent fever, headache, head tilt, abdominal pain, vomiting, diarrhea, gait disturbance, palpitations, weakness, hematuria, weight loss, and rash. For infants and young children with AMS, developmental milestones need to be pursued. The past medical history, immunization, and family history are important in children of all ages. The clinician should be alert for any inappropriate responses or inconsistencies and delays in seeking care that may arouse the suspicion of child abuse. Although it may be possible to obtain a history quickly, in order to be thorough and pay attention to detail, one physician must be dedicated to obtain the history while the second physician manages the resuscitation.

One should proceed with a general examination only after cardiac and cerebral resuscitation. The objectives of the examination are to identify occult infection, trauma, toxicity, or metabolic disease. The neurologic examination should document the child's response to sensory input, motor activity, pupillary reactivity, oculovestibular reflexes, and respiratory pattern. Although several coma scales have been published, the most simplified and functional in the emergency setting is the AVPU. This is a descriptive tool, where A = alert, V = responsive to verbal stimuli, P = responsive to painful stimuli, and U = unresponsive.

Following a targeted history and a focused examination, the treating physician should anticipate and observe changes in the patient's status that may indicate improvement or deterioration. Finally, the physician must make an operational, if not specific, diagnosis of AMS.

## TREATMENT

The first priority in AMS is stabilization and reversal of acute life threats before specific diagnostic maneuvers such as lumbar puncture are undertaken. Airway, breathing, and circulation must be assured. For suspected cervical injury, spinal immobilization is mandatory and the airway is opened with the jaw-thrust maneuver.

Hypoxia must be corrected, and continuous pulse oximetry monitoring should be established. There is no contraindication to providing oxygen to children. Oxygen is obviously indicated for patients with signs of hypoxemia or hypoperfusion, but hypercapnia must be avoided. Bag-valve-mask ventilation may reverse hypercapnia, but endotracheal intubation is necessary to protect the patient from aspiration.

Fluid resuscitation is necessary in the hypotensive, comatose patient since cerebral perfusion is dependent upon adequate mean arterial pressure. A fluid bolus of 20 mL/kg of isotonic crystalloid should be quickly given. Poorly perfused patients should be reassessed, and boluses repeated up to a total dose of 60 mL/kg as necessary. Thereafter, pressors should be utilized. In the hemodynamically stable patient with either a suspected head injury, encephalitis, or meningitis, the intravenous fluids should be reduced to an hourly rate that provides two-thirds of the calculated maintenance volume. Empiric therapy may be initiated with glucose 0.25 g/kg intravenously if hypoglycemia is strongly suspected. Alternatively, blood sugar may be rapidly estimated by means of a glucose oxidase stick and glucose-containing fluids may be withheld unless indicated.

If there is clinical suspicion of opiate or clonidine overdose, a narcotic agonist may be administered. The recommended dose for naloxone is 0.1 mg/kg for individuals weighing less than 20 kg or less than 5 years of age. Beyond that age and weight, children should be given 2 mg as a starting dose. Any dose, if successful, may be repeated as necessary to maintain narcotic reversal.

Seizures should be aborted if present. Benzodiazepines are typically first-line drugs. The longer-acting anticonvulsants such as phenytoin or phenobarbital may be needed.

The treating physician must restore acid-base balance. This may be accomplished primarily by ensuring adequate hydration and compensatory ventilation. Sodium bicarbonate should be utilized sparingly and only in circumstances where the pH is $\leq 7.0$.

The clinician should control core body temperature. Maintaining euthermia is critical for minimizing metabolic demands. A child's increased body surface area hastens radiant heat loss. Heat loss may be minimized with the use of a heating lamp during resuscitation.

Septic-appearing patients or those suspected of intracranial infection should quickly receive empiric intravenous antibiotics.

## DIAGNOSIS

The differential diagnosis for AMS in children is diverse and differs slightly from the adult patient. The familiar mnemonic, AEIOU TIPS, remains a useful tool for organizing the diagnostic possibilities (Table 40-1).

**Table 40-1.** AEIOU TIPS: A Mnemonic for Pediatric Altered Mental Status

| | | | |
|---|---|---|---|
| **A** | Alcohol | **U** | Uremia |
| | Acid/base and metabolic | | Chronic renal failure |
| | disorders | | Hemolytic uremic |
| | Diabetes mellitus | | syndrome |
| | Dehydration | **T** | Trauma |
| | Hypercapnia | | General trauma with |
| | Hepatic failure | | hypovolemia |
| | Hypoxia | | Head injury |
| | Inborn errors of metabolism | | Mass lesion |
| | Arrhythmia/cardiogenic | | Cerebral edema |
| | Ventricular fibrillation | | Cerebral vascular accident |
| | Stokes-Adams attack | | Electric shock |
| | Aortic stenosis | | Decompression sickness |
| | | | Thermal |
| **E** | Encephalopathy | | Tumor |
| | Hypertensive | | |
| | Reye's syndrome | **I** | Infection |
| | Hemorrhagic shock and | | Meningitis |
| | encephalopathy syndrome | | Encephalitis |
| | | | Brain abscess |
| | Endocrinopathy | | Visceral larva migrans |
| | Addison disease | | Severe systemic infection |
| | Congenital adrenal hyperplasia | | |
| | Thyrotoxicity | | Intracerebral vascular disorders |
| | Cushing syndrome | | Subarachnoid hemorrhage |
| | Pheochromocytoma | | Venous thrombosis |
| | Hepatic porphyrias | | Arterial thrombosis |
| | | | Intracerebral and intraven- |
| | Electrolytes | | tricular hemorrhages |
| | Na, Ca, Mg, PO$_4$ | | Cerebral emboli |
| | | | Acute infantile hemiplegia |
| **I** | Insulin | | |
| | Hypoglycemia | **P** | Psychogenic |
| | Ketotic hypoglycemia | | Poisoning |
| | Hyperglycemia | | |
| | | **S** | Seizure |
| | Intussusception | | |
| **O** | Opiates | | |

**Alcohol.** In the younger pediatric patient, alcohol ingestion is typically accidental; intentional ingestion is more likely in adolescents. AMS may occur with serum levels less than 100 mg/dL. Hypoglycemia may occur concurrently.

**Acid-base and metabolic disorders.** Children with diabetes may present in ketoacidosis. The classic presentation includes weight loss, polyuria, polydypsia, polyphagia, weakness, vomiting, abdominal discomfort, Kussmaul respirations, a fruity acetone breath, and AMS. Patients with diabetic ketoacidosis (DKA) as well as many other pediatric disease states associated with a loss of circulating volume may develop inadequate perfusion. Patients with hypotonic or hypertonic dehydration may develop AMS with or without seizures. Poorly perfused patients or patients with inadequate air exchange have insufficient oxygen delivery to the brain and exhibit insomnia, somnolence, and confusion. Those patients who develop hypercapnia as a result of primary lung disease or neurologic dysfunction may also present with AMS. Those with hepatic failure present with nausea, fatigue, and behavioral alterations and may rapidly become obtunded. Patients with inborn errors of metabolism typically present early in life with poor feeding, recurrent vomiting, seizures, metabolic acidosis, lethargy, stupor, and coma.

**Arrhythmia/cardiogenic.** Ventricular fibrillation causes unconsciousness by diminished oxygen delivery to the brain. In a Stokes-Adams attack, heart block leads to loss of consciousness. Critical aortic stenosis leads to unconsciousness through decreased cardiac output.

**Encephalopathy.** Hypertensive encephalopathy may occur in pediatric patients at diastolic pressures of 100 to 110 mmHg. Reye's syndrome follows a viral illness such as influenza or varicella. Patients are afebrile, anicteric, and develop pernicious vomiting. Confusion and delirium may progress to increasing obtundation. Hemorrhagic shock and encephalopathy syndrome is a symptom complex of unknown etiology that affects previously healthy infants. The common features include a mild prodromal, nonspecific illness of several days' duration following by the onset of profuse, watery diarrhea, which becomes bloody, and seizures. Patients present poorly perfused, with profound metabolic acidosis and evidence of disseminated intravascular coagulation. Laboratory evidence of hepatic, renal, pancreatic, and myocardial dysfunction is common.

**Endocrinopathy.** AMS is a rare presentation of these disorders. Patients with Addison's disease present with nausea, vomiting, abdominal pain, weakness, malaise, hypotension, and mental status changes, including psychosis. Presumptive evidence is provided by finding hyperpigmentation, depressed sodium and blood sugar, elevated potassium, and variably increased calcium. Infants with congenital adrenal hyperplasia may present with an acute salt-losing, volume-depleted hypotensive crisis, or with virilization creating ambiguous genitalia and with cortisol insufficiency additionally manifested as hypoglycemia. Thyrotoxic infants may present with ventricular dysrhythmia. Otherwise, affected children have similarities with adults by manifesting goiter, irritability, exophthalmos, hyperthermia, high-output congestive heart failure, mania, delirium, psychosis, with apathy and decreasing levels of consciousness occurring later. Patients with pheochromocytoma may present with hypertensive encephalopathy.

**Electrolytes.** Hyponatremic children become symptomatic with plasma levels around 120 mEq/L. Manifestations include anorexia, headache, nausea, vomiting, irritability, weakness, cramps, disorientation, seizures, and AMS. Hypernatremic individuals develop muscle weakness, irritability, seizures, and AMS. Disorders of calcium, magnesium, and phosphorus present with neuromuscular signs, including weakness, tetany, seizures, and apathy.

**Insulin.** Hypoglycemia may be an end product of an endocrinopathy (adrenal insufficiency, hyperthyroidism, hypopituitarism) or the result of an exogenous substance such as ethanol, salicylate, oral hypoglycemics, and insulin. Hypoglycemia may result from a common stress pathway of decreased gluconeogenesis as seen during sepsis or Reyes syndrome. Adrenergic signs of palpitations, hunger, and sweating will often be seen at's glucose levels less than 60 mg/dL. Irritability, confusion, seizures, and coma occur at levels ≤ 40 mg/dL. Infants and children are prone to develop ketotic hypoglycemia with fasting, especially with infections in early infancy. AMS from hyperglycemia is rare in children. The most common cause of hyperosmolar central nervous system dysfunction is DKA.

**Intussusception.** Intussusception is readily diagnosed in the small percentage of younger children who present with a classic constellation of abdominal pain, vomiting, abdominal mass, and rectal bleeding. AMS may be the initial symptom and dominant concern of the physician and the parent caring for a child with intussusception. AMS persists until the bowel obstruction is reduced.

**Opiates.** Children may present with miosis, absent bowel sounds, and lethargy. Common opiates that may be present in the household include dextromethorphan, Lomotil, and Imodium. Abuse should always be suspected in children with opiate intoxication.

**Uremia.** In children with chronic renal failure, neurologic dysfunction may develop secondary to stroke, hypertension, or metabolic derangements. Encephalopathy occurs in over one-third of patients with chronic renal failure manifested by headache, irritability, cognitive derangement, and seizures. Hemolytic uremic syndrome is a pediatric disorder characterized by microangiopathic hemolytic anemia and uremia. It follows a prodrome of abdominal pain and diarrhea and is manifested by pallor, thrombocytopenia with purpura, red blood cell fragmentation, and oliguria.

**Trauma.** Trauma may occur on the cellular or global level. In the context of multisystem trauma, a hypovolemic state may create insufficient cerebral perfusion. Such hypovolemic states may be created by other "traumatic" insults, such as primary peritonitis or ruptured appendicitis with hypovolemia. Children may have transient loss of consciousness after head injury. Occasionally, a seizure may occur immediately after closed head injury, resulting in AMS from the postictal state. The signs and symptoms of acute epidural hematoma are typically posttraumatic loss of consciousness followed by a lucid interval and then rapid AMS. Acute epidural hematoma can also present with a gradual loss of consciousness associated with ipsilateral pupillary dilatation. As in adults, subdural hematomas may be acute, subacute, or chronic. Most children with subdural hematomas will have external signs of trauma. The exception are abused infants, typically less than 6 months of age, who may present without external signs of injury. Abused children who are shaken typically present with a history of vomiting, seizures, and changes in respiratory pattern associated with altered mental status. Retinal hemorrhages or a tense fontanel may suggest the diagnosis. Children with blunt head trauma are more inclined than adults to develop diffuse cerebral swelling, increased intracranial pressure, and AMS, without extracerebral or intracerebral collections of blood. Cerebral vascular accidents, including bleeding from AV malformation, though uncommon in childhood, may cause focal neurologic deficits, followed by status epilepticus and coma.

**Tumor.** Primary brain tumor and metastatic or meningeal leukemic infiltration may alter the brain's metabolism. Intracerebral tumors commonly produce focal neurologic dysfunction, but posterior fossa tumors typically block the ventricular system and create signs and symptoms of hydrocephalus. Both supratentorial and infratentorial tumors may present abruptly with AMS, fever, or meningismus after an intratumor hemorrhage.

**Thermal.** Extremes of body temperature may also lead to central nervous system dysfunction. Progressive hypothermia leads to insidious AMS. Those patients who develop body core temperatures greater than 41°C develop headache, weakness, and dizziness, followed by confusion, euphoria, combativeness, and AMS. Posturing, seizures, hemiparesis, and pupillary changes may be present.

**Infection.** Infection is more common as a cause of AMS in chil-

dren than in adults. The incidence of bacterial meningitis and septicemia is highest in early infancy and considerably higher throughout all childhood when compared to adults. Bacterial meningitis should be high on the differential list in a pediatric patient with AMS. Unless there are contraindications to lumbar puncture, examination of cerebrospinal fluid should be considered in lethargic, febrile pediatric patients (see Table 40-2). Similarly, pediatric patients may become encephalopathic due to direct invasion of the brain by multiple pathogens. Patients with encephalitis have fever, headache, and invariable signs of meningeal irritation or neurologic deficits. Herpes viruses, arbovirus, rotavirus, and Epstein-Barr virus are among the most common viral agents associated with encephalitis. Encephalitis may occur in the course of mycoplasmal illness, shigellosis, Lyme disease, or cat-scratch disease. Visceral larva migrans may produce encephalopathy in the young. A brain abscess may create signs and symptoms suggestive of encephalitis. Patients with a brain abscess present with fever and headache that precedes changes in presentation and consciousness. Affected patients may also present with generalized or focal seizure activity. Patients at risk for brain abscess include those with sinusitis, cyanotic congenital heart disease, immune deficiency states, and intravenous drug abuse. Any systemic infection associated with vasculitis or vasodepressant toxins with shock may lead to AMS secondary to cerebral hypoperfusion.

**Intracerebral vascular disorders.** Subarachnoid hemorrhage may occur following trauma or spontaneous rupture of a berry aneurysm or arteriovenous malformation. Nuchal rigidity is an inconstant finding. Venous thrombosis may follow severe dehydration or a pyogenic infection of the paranasal sinuses, mastoid, or middle ear. Periorbital edema with cranial nerve abnormalities are clues. Arterial thrombosis is uncommon in children, except in those with homocystinuria. Children with homocystinuria have a marfanoid appearance, dislocated lenses, and mental retardation. Intracerebral and intraventricular hemorrhages may follow birth asphyxia or trauma in the neonate, but in older children these may signify a congenital or acquired coagulopathy. Signs of subacute bacterial endocarditis include splinter hemorrhages, splenomegaly, microscopic hematuria, and cerebral emboli causing AMS. Acute infantile hemiplegia presents with an acute seizure, followed by hemiparesis and coma.

**Psychogenic.** Psychogenic unresponsiveness is rare in children. The patient has decreased responsiveness but has an otherwise normal neurologic examination, including occulovestibular reflexes. This may occur as a conversion reaction, an adjustment reaction, panic state, or a manifestation of malingering.

**Poisoning.** Drugs may be transferred to a fetus transplacentally. Infants and children may receive drugs through neglect, abuse, or accident. Drugs may be utilized as a suicide gesture in adolescents. AMS may be caused by exogenous intoxicants such as ethanol, ethylene glycol, methyl alcohol, paraldehyde, salicylates, anticholinergics (including antihistamines), cholinergics, opiates, tricyclic antidepressants, carbamazepine, clonidine, sedative-hypnotics, amphetamines, cocaine, nicotine, carbon monoxide, hydrocarbons, and phenothiazines.

**Seizure.** Generalized tonic-clonic major motor seizures are associated with prolonged unresponsiveness in pediatric patients. Young febrile patients who have seized should be considered candidates for intracranial infection.

## DIAGNOSTIC ADJUNCTS

Ancillary procedures for diagnosis of AMS include analysis of blood, gastric fluid, urine, and cerebrospinal fluid; electrocardiography; roentgenography; and CT scanning. Diagnostic tests should be guided by the clinical situation. Rapid estimation of blood glucose via a glucose oxidase strip is a universally accepted evaluation in pediatric patients with AMS. Electrolyte determinations, liver function studies, and renal function studies may provide additional informa-

**Table 40-2.** Procedure: Lumbar Puncture

*Relevant anatomy:* Cerebrospinal fluid is produced by the choroid plexus and circulates around the brain and spinal cord within the subarachnoid space. A spinal needle traverses the skin, subcutaneous tissue, supraspinal ligament, interspinal ligament, ligamentum flavum, dura, and arachnoid before entering the subarachnoid space surrounding nerve roots, which form the cauda equina in the lumbar region.

*Indications:* The primary indication for emergent lumbar puncture is the possibility of CNS infection. It is also indicated for suspected spontaneous subarachnoid hemorrhage.

*Contraindications:* Absolute contraindications include the presence of infection in tissues near the puncture site and increased intracranial pressure secondary to a space-occupying lesion. The presence of coagulopathy or lumbosacral deformity are relative contraindications.

*Possible complications:* The most serious complication is cardiorespiratory arrest, which may occur if a child's neck is excessively flexed. Concomitant bacteremia during the procedure may lead to seeding of infection in the subarachnoid space. Postspinal headache may rarely be seen in children. Implantation of epidermoid tumors is manifested by pain in back and lower extremities years after LP.

*Equipment needed:* Necessary equipment consists of a lumbar puncture kit with spinal needle. A 22-gauge 1 1/2 in needle is used under the age of 6 years. A 22-gauge 2 1/2 in needle is required for children age 6 to 12 years, and a 21-gauge 3 1/2 in needle is used over the age of 12. A manometer with 3-way stopcock is used to measure CSF pressure.

*Patient positioning:* An assistant is generally required to ensure proper positioning of the patient. The classic posture for lumbar puncture is lateral recumbent with spine flexed and knees drawn upward to chest with shoulders and back perpendicular to the table. An alternative for a small infant is sitting with thighs flexed toward the abdomen. It is critical to avoid flexion of the neck.

*Procedure:* The back may be cleansed with povidone-iodine surgical scrub, or povidone-iodine solution may be allowed to air-dry on the skin. Sterile draping is optional in the infant and best avoided to maximize landmark exposure and proper positioning. Local anesthesia with 1% xylocaine should be administered to all children, irrespective of age.

*Site:* The intersection of a line joining the superior portion of the iliac crest and the spine meets at the spinous process of L4. Optimal insertion is at the L3-L4 interspace but may be performed one space above or below.

*Insertion:* The spinal needle is inserted into the chosen site with the stylet in place through epidermis and dermis, then the stylet may optionally be removed through the remainder of the procedure. The clinician may not feel an increasing resistance and "pop" into the subarachnoid space in younger children.

Manometry may be performed as indicated in cooperative children who have LP performed in the lateral decubitus position. Normal relaxed pressure is 5–15 cm $H_2O$.

If the tap is bloody, one may replace the stylet and leave the needle in place. Insert a second spinal needle one interspace cephalad and collect fluid for analysis. Finally, withdraw both needles. This process minimizes red blood cell contamination in the collected fluid.

Finally, remove needle and place a bandage over the insertion site.

*Analysis:* Mandatory CSF studies include bacterial culture and Gram stain from tube 1, protein and glucose from tube 2, and cell count and differential from tube 3. Tube 4 may be sent for viral or fungal cultures, or latex agglutination in specific circumstances.

---

tion regarding the state of hydration, suspected endocrine and metabolic derangement, and liver and kidney function. If the history is consistent with a toxic ingestion or a toxidrome is identified, toxicology screening is in order. The white blood cell count and differential as an independent evaluation is rarely helpful, except perhaps in management decisions of highly febrile children less than 2 years of age. A blood culture should be obtained whenever sepsis is suspected.

Measurement of arterial blood gas or capillary blood gas with pulse oximetry may provide useful information in the setting of trauma, respiratory distress, or suspected acid-base imbalance.

It is not inappropriate to place an indwelling urinary catheter in an ill child. The initial urine specimen can be analyzed, and a portion sent for toxicologic screening.

Lumbar puncture with CSF examination should not be delayed if AMS is thought to be secondary to meningitis or encephalitis. However CT should be done first if AMS is thought to be secondary to subdural or epidural fluid collection, cavernous sinus thrombosis, lateral sinus thrombosis, cerebral hemorrhage, brain tumor, cord tumor, or brain abscess. Shock or hypotension and hypoxia should be corrected before lumbar puncture, and empiric antibiotics should be given if meningitis is suspected, but CT is necessary before lumbar puncture.

A 12-lead electrocardiogram should be obtained if there are pathologic auscultatory findings or rhythm disturbance on monitoring. An electrocardiogram may further guide therapy in the setting of a tricyclic antidepressant overdose.

Radiologic evaluation should be directed by the clinical scenario. Portable cervical spine radiography is mandatory prior to mobilization of the neck in a traumatized patient. A chest x-ray may be used to confirm or clarify examination findings and to document endotracheal tube placement. Abdominal films are indicated for the acute ingestion of radiopaque material if suspected, or if the patient exhibits signs and symptoms of an acute abdomen, including possible intussusception. Skull films are reserved for the traumatized patient in whom there is a search for a depressed fracture or a foreign body. A CT of the head may be obtained for suspected increased intracranial pressure, vascular disorder, or mass lesion.

Miscellaneous adjuncts that may be of assistance in specific instances are blood ammonia level, serum osmolality, blood alcohol level, thyroid function tests, and a blood lead level. A skeletal survey may be of significance in a potentially abused young child. Barium or air enema may be both diagnostic or therapeutic in patients with intussusception and AMS. A portable EEG may prove to be diagnostic in a case of nonmotor status epilepticus.

## DISPOSITION

All patients who present with altered mental status should receive continuing care in an area that can provide physiologic monitoring and repeated physical examinations from caretakers. In general this requires admission to an intensive care unit or transfer to tertiary care center with capabilities of pediatric intensive care. Only those patients with transient, reversible causes for AMS may be treated, monitored in the emergency department, and discharged following observation. Those patients who are discharged (such as closed head injury patients or patients with simple febrile seizure) need to receive disease-specific discharge instructions. Patients who are evaluated for AMS and discharged home should have a repeat evaluation within 24 h of discharge.

## BIBLIOGRAPHY

Avner JR: Office management of neurologic emergencies. *Pediatr Ann* 19:649, 1990.

Cantor RM: The unconscious child: Emergency evaluation and management. *Int Pediatr* 4:9, 1989.

Nass R: Rapid assessment of mental status in the infant and young child. *Emerg Med Clin North Am* 5:739, 1987.

Plum F, Posner JB: *The Diagnosis of Stupor and Coma,* 4th ed. Philadelphia, Davis, 1984.

Sabin TD: Coma and the acute confusional state in the emergency room. *Med Clin North Am* 65:15, 1981.

Siverman BK (ed): Altered level of consciousness: Overview. *APLS: The Pediatric Emergency Medicine Course,* 2d ed. Oak Grove Village, IL, American Academy of Pediatrics/American College of Emergency Physicians, 1993.

Yager JY: Coma scales in pediatric practice. *Am J Dis Child* 144:1088, 1990.

# 41
# SYNCOPE AND BREATH HOLDING
## David A. Poleski

## SYNCOPE

### Introduction

Syncope is common in children and most episodes go unreported. Syncope is a sudden, brief, and transient loss of consciousness associated with an inability to maintain normal muscle posture and tone. A reversible, short-lived impairment of cerebral perfusion occurs. Not uncommonly, seizure-like activity may follow a primary syncopal event. Other causes of altered mental status such as shock, vertigo, drug intoxication, sepsis, coma, and seizures must be excluded. The most important task is answering the clinical question "Does this represent a potentially lethal condition or one with significant morbidity?" Fortunately in most cases of pediatric syncope the answer to this question will be "No," but this is precisely the clinical dilemma. Syncope in children must be evaluated carefully because it can be the sole manifestation of a serious underlying condition.

### Incidence

The incidence of childhood syncope is undoubtedly underreported. However, at least 15 percent of children will experience an episode of syncope brought to the attention of a physician before they complete adolescence, and approximately 1 percent of pediatric admissions are for the evaluation of a syncopal episode. Vasovagal syncope is estimated to occur in 15 to 25 percent of adolescents.

### Etiology

For practical purposes the causes can be divided into cardiac, noncardiac, and unknown etiology. Cardiac causes are always worrisome; noncardiac and unknown causes are less likely to be as serious. Noncardiac causes can be further divided into neurologic, respiratory, autonomic, and metabolic etiologies.

### Cardiac Syncope

Cardiac syncope is usually caused by arrhythmias or ventricular outflow obstruction and is the most serious form of syncope in children. Historical factors suggestive of a cardiac etiology include a family history of sudden unexplained death (congenital, prolonged QT interval), prior history of Kawasaki disease (coronary artery insufficiency secondary to aneurysm formation), prior cardiac surgery (complete heart block or other arrhythmia), recent unexplained change in exercise tolerance associated with tachypnea or fever (myocarditis or cardiomyopathy), or known congenital pulmonary outflow obstruction ("tet" spell).

Syncope associated with exercise is worrisome and should bring to mind conditions such as idiopathic hypertrophic subaortic stenosis (IHSS) associated with ventricular outflow obstruction. A complete cardiac evaluation including an electrocardiogram (ECG), chest x-ray, and, if possible, an echocardiogram should be performed in the emergency department. Chest pain in an adolescent is generally not serious, but in a young child palpitations may be reported as chest pain. Particularly if a young child reports chest pain associated with dizziness, lightheadedness, or syncope, an evaluation for an arrhythmia is necessary. A single ECG in the emergency department is not enough; such children should be admitted for monitoring.

Physical findings suggestive of a cardiac etiology include a systolic ejection click, a harsh systolic ejection murmur over the base of the heart radiating to the carotids, and a palpable thrill in the suprasternal notch (all suggestive of aortic stenosis). A systolic murmur enhanced by standing or the Valsalva maneuver may be due to IHSS. Any new onset murmur heard after a child has had a syncopal event requires evaluation. In addition, a child who has the findings of congestive heart failure, myocarditis, or cardiomyopathy (tachypnea, enlarged liver, enlarged heart, rub, rales) needs a complete cardiac evaluation. Finally, recurrent syncope of unexplained etiology, even with a negative emergency department evaluation, should be referred to a pediatric cardiologist.

### Neurologic Syncope

Seizures are the primary cause of neurologic syncope. Distinguishing between a seizure disorder and the seizure-like activity that can be seen after a breath-holding spell is sometimes difficult.

In a child with syncope, the period of unconsciousness is brief, lasting only seconds, followed by a rapid recovery to normal mental status. Seizures, in contrast, result in prolonged loss of consciousness (at least several minutes) with a delay in return to the patient's normal baseline mental state. Abnormal motor activity is more likely to be seen with seizures. When associated with nonseizure syncopal episodes such as breath-holding spells, such activity is brief, lasting less than a minute. Incontinence generally does not occur with nonneurologic syncope. When present, a seizure disorder is more likely. Also a reported aura, such as an unusual taste or smell, suggests a seizure disorder.

A family history of seizures is problematic in differentiating syncope from seizures. Breath-holding spells are commonly mistaken for seizures. In addition, seizures are a common affliction, affecting about 2 percent of the population. A family history of seizures, although important, is not generally helpful in determining the etiology of a syncopal episode.

Finally, any child with a focal physical finding after a syncopal episode should be evaluated thoroughly for a seizure disorder, neurotrauma, or unsuspected central nervous system lesion or infection.

### Respiratory Syncope

Excluding breath-holding spells, which will be discussed in a separate section, the most common etiology of syncope caused by a ventilation abnormality in children is hyperventilation. This excludes syncope due to pulmonary disorders resulting in prolonged hypoxia, such as severe pneumonia or severe asthma.

Hyperventilation is something most children do at one time or another because of pain, anxiety, or, in the adolescent, as a "dare" or in an effort to hold one's breath longer. The physiology of hyperventilation causing syncope is not completely understood. Hyperventilation induces hypocapnia, which in turn results in vasoconstriction of the cerebral arteries. This seems to reduce the delivery of oxygen and glucose to the brain, thus resulting in syncope.

Prolonged, severe, frequent coughing may also result in syncope. The classic example of this phenomenon is pertussis. In an infant, the persistent coughing prevents adequate oxygenation and ventilation from occurring and is perceived as apnea; in the older child, a brief episode of syncope may be the manifestation of severe cough-induced hypoxia.

## Autonomic Syncope

Vasovagal, or vasodepressor, syncope is by far the most common cause of syncope in children, accounting for at least 50 percent of cases. Episodes of vasodepressor syncope usually occur in response to sudden emotional stress in a setting of perceived threats or injuries. The classic example is an adolescent who faints at the sight of blood or who witnesses someone undergoing a painful procedure in the emergency department. Such episodes are more likely to occur if one is tired, hungry, or just recovering from a recent illness. Environmental conditions such as crowding or a warm enclosed space also predispose to vasodepressor syncope. Prodromal symptoms include pallor, diaphoresis, and nausea. Witnesses to the event will sometimes report mydriasis. As mentioned earlier when discussing the distinctions between syncope and seizures, the event is usually sudden in onset, lasts less than 1 min, and the patient recovers a normal mental status rapidly, although symptoms such as nausea, weakness, pallor, and diaphoresis may persist. Tonic-clonic activity of very brief duration and, rarely, incontinence have been reported with vasodepressor syncope but should alert one to the possibility of a seizure disorder.

The pathophysiology of vasodepressor syncope is well described by Scott. "A decrease in peripheral vascular resistance leads to a drop in arterial pressure and cerebral perfusion. Decreased venous return results in a relatively empty ventricle. Vigorous myocardial contraction against an empty ventricle initiates a prominent vagal reflex, resulting in hypotension or bradycardia. While heart rate typically does increase prior to an episode, cardiac output does not increase in response to the fall in pressure, which may be related to decreased venous return. Bradycardia typically occurs late and is not usually a causal factor because neither atropine nor cardiac pacing is sufficient to abort the episode. Hyperventilation may also occur, aggravating the cerebral hypoperfusion."

Another form of autonomic syncope is that due to orthostatic hypotension. Upon standing there is a gravity-mediated loss of blood from the brain and thorax, with a net flow of intravascular volume to the peripheral vasculature. Venous return is reduced to the right ventricle, with a decline in ventricular filling. Reduced ventricular filling in turn is sensed by mechanoreceptors, which cause an afferent neural output interpreted by the brainstem as a hypotensive state. To correct the situation, a neurally induced increase in sympathetic output occurs, resulting in an increase in heart rate and blood pressure. In the healthy pediatric patient, orthostatic hypotension is uncommon because this reflex is unravaged by aging and subsequent degenerative coronary and neurovascular changes. However, children who are anemic (i.e., reduced oxygen-carrying capacity) or those who are hypovolemic (possibly due to a gastroenteritis or excessive sweating without adequate volume replacement) may become syncopal upon standing, even though their cardiac and neural mechanisms for compensating are intact. Any pediatric patient with a history of so-called orthostatic hypotension should be investigated thoroughly for an underlying cause such as anemia or hypovolemia and for rare pediatric problems such as degenerative vascular and neurologic diseases.

Other causes of autonomic syncope have been described. "Hair grooming" syncope, carotid sinus syncope due to wrestling, and "parade ground" syncope are reported. These probably share a common pathophysiology with vasodepressor or orthostatic syncope but have unusual triggering events.

## Metabolic Syncope

Metabolic causes of syncope in children are uncommon. Although, usually in frustration, some physicians will ascribe syncope to hypo-glycemia (not eating for a long time before the episode), hypoglycemia is a rare cause of syncope except in the insulin-dependent diabetic. Of more concern is metabolic syncope occurring as a result of drug ingestion. Alcoholism is unfortunately a major problem in adolescents, and any adolescent with a history of unexplained "black-out" spells should be questioned carefully about drug use, especially ethanol.

Syncope caused by metabolic derangements should be relatively easy to suspect by history. Unlike cardiac or vasodepressor syncope, for example, the prodrome of metabolic syncope is gradual in onset, with symptoms such as weakness, diaphoresis, confusion, and hunger. These symptoms are unrelated to position and are not usually associated with blood pressure or pulse changes.

## Hysteria

Adolescents are particularly prone to hysterical syncope. Perhaps a "swoon" would be better terminology since hysterical syncope involves no change in vital signs or temporary derangement of cerebral perfusion. A swoon occurs in front of an audience, the patient remains calm, is uninjured, and falls gracefully to the floor. Secondary gain and attention-getting are usually entwined with the swooning event. It is a diagnosis of exclusion, however, as, needless to say, histrionic adolescents can have serious cardiac arrhythmias. As usual a careful history is imperative when making the diagnosis.

## BREATH HOLDING

Breath-holding spells are a form of autonomic syncope most common in infancy and early childhood. Because they are frequently dramatic and are commonly misdiagnosed as seizures, resulting in unnecessary workup and parental anxiety, they are discussed separately.

Historically breath-holding spells have been viewed as volitional on the part of the child; a manifestational of the "spoiled brat syndrome." Children with such spells have been described as stubborn, disobedient, aggressive, and attention-seeking. Like most medical events in pediatric patients ascribed to willful behavior, breath-holding spells are not the result of a personality disorder. They are not volitional and are not associated with temperamentally difficult children. The tendency for parents to believe otherwise, however, is quite strong since most breath-holding spells are associated with an outburst of crying, anger, or pain, followed by a brief period of unconsciousness and, at times, some tonic-clonic motor activity.

Two types of breath-holding spells have been described: cyanotic and pallid. The distinction is probably not clinically significant. Each type is the result of transient cerebral anoxia. The cyanotic type occurs after vigorous crying with its consequent oxygen desaturation and is associated with vagally mediated hypotension. The pallid type is more likely to occur after a sudden unexpected fright or injury (such as a bump on the head) and is caused by a vagally mediated severe bradycardia or brief period of asystole. Cyanotic breath-holding spells are more common.

The history is paramount in helping to distinguish a breath-holding spell with a brief period of tonic-clonic motor activity from a seizure. If there is no prodrome of injury, sudden fright, vigorous crying, or painful stimuli, a seizure is more likely. On the other hand, if such prodromal stimuli are present, parents can be reassured that their child had a breath-holding spell, is not doing it on purpose, and is not a spoiled or bad child. As with uncomplicated febrile seizures, the parents need to be reassured that no brain damage has occurred and that their child should remain developmentally normal. There is a propensity for breath-holding spells to recur in children who already have had them, and a genetic predisposition to them exists. It is wise to obtain an ECG in any uncertain situation to eliminate conduction defects, such as prolonged QT interval, as a cause of the episode.

## EMERGENCY DEPARTMENT EVALUATION

Most causes of syncope can be diagnosed from the history and physical examination. When the cause is obvious, as in most cases of vasodepressor syncope and breath-holding spells, laboratory testing is not necessary. For example, when a 16-year-old is donating blood for the first time and faints, rest and reassurance are the treatment of choice.

If one suspects cardiac syncope, testing for an arrhythmia, conduction abnormality, ventricular outflow obstruction, and underlying cardiac disease is in order. An ECG and chest x-ray should be done in the emergency department. An echocardiogram and Holter monitoring may need to be arranged on an outpatient basis. A referral to a pediatric cardiologist is necessary. If an arrhythmia is strongly suspected but not seen on the ECG, the patient should be considered for admission.

In cases of suspected autonomic syncope when the history is not clear-cut, referral for tilt testing should be considered. The tilt test entails placing the patient on a tilt table and passively rotating the patient 60° to 90° from the supine position and leaving the patient upright for 5 to 10 min. Vital signs are recorded throughout the maneuver, and the patient is returned to the supine position. Since both heart rate and blood pressure have been observed to increase secondary to augmented catecholamine production just prior to vasodepressor syncope, an infusion of a catecholamine such as isoproterenol is started to mimic these conditions. The tilt is repeated with the infusion. Only a small percentage of vasodepressor-prone patients have symptoms with the passive tilt, but the yield is markedly increased with the catecholamine infusion. The sensitivity of this test in children is about 80 percent, but unfortunately it is not 100 percent specific.

Tests such as glucose, electrolytes, drug screens, and hematocrit and hemoglobin need only be done if the history and physical examination are suggestive, as in the case when pallor or orthostatic hypotension or insulin-dependent diabetes is present. Probably the most commonly performed unnecessary test is the serum glucose, perpetuating the mistaken notion that a low blood sugar is the cause of a child's problem. CT scans are seldom helpful in the emergency department. EEGs may be indicated, along with a referral to a pediatric neurologist, when tonic-clonic activity is observed or return to consciousness is prolonged after an apparent syncopal event.

## BIBLIOGRAPHY

Atkins D, Hanusa A, Sefcik MS, et al: Syncope and orthostatic hypotension. *Am J Med* 91:179, 1991.

Barron SA, Rogovski Z, Hemli Y, et al: Vagal cardiovascular reflexes in young persons with syncope. *Ann Intern Med* 118:943, 1993.

Berger TM, Porter CJ: Carotid sinus syndrome and wrestling. *Mayo Clin Proc* 68:366, 1993.

Chambers R, Clayson M, Hillis S, et al: Unexplained fainting and breathlessness. *Practitioner* 237:287, 1993.

Denniss AR, Ross DL, Richards DA, et al: Electrophysiologic studies in patients with unexplained syncope. *Int J Cardiol* 35:211, 1992.

DiMario FJ, Burleson JA: Behavior profile of children with severe breath holding spells. *J Pediatr* 122:488, 1993.

DiMario FJ, Chee CM, Berman DH: Pallid breath holding spells. *Clin Pediatr* 29:17, 1990.

Grubb PB, Temesy-Armos PN, Samdil D, et al: Tilt table testing in the evaluation of athletes with recurrent exercise-induced syncope. *Med Sci Sports Exerc* 25:24, 1993.

Hoefnagels WA, Padberg GW, Overweg J, et al: Syncope or seizure? The diagnostic value of the EEG and hyperventilation test in transient loss of consciousness. *J Neurol Neurosurg Psychiatry* 54:953, 1991.

Hoefnagels WA, Padberg GW, Overweg J, et al: Transient loss of consciousness: The value of the history for distinguishing seizure from syncope. *J Neurol* 238:39, 1991.

Koening D, Linzer M, Gontinen N, et al: Syncope in young adults: Evidence for a combined medical and psychiatric approach. *J Intern Med* 232:169, 1992.

Lewis DW, Frank LM: Hair grooming syncope seizures. *Pediatrics*

Ozme S, Alehan D, Valaz K, et al: Causes of syncope in children: A prospective study. *Int J Cardiol* 40:111, 1993.

Pavlin DJ, Links S, Rapp SE, et al: Vasovagal reactions in an ambulatory surgery center. *Ambulat Anesth* 76:931, 1993.

Perry JC, Freidman RA, Moak JP, et al: Bradycardia and syncope in children not controlled by pacing: Beta-adrenergic hypersensitivity. *PACE* 14:391, 1991.

Salins PC, Kuriokose M, Sharma SM, et al: Hypoglycemia as a possible factor in the induction of vasovagal syncope. *Oral Surg Oral Med Oral Pathol* 74:544, 1992.

Samoil D, Grubb BP, Kip K, et al: Head-upright tilt table testing in child with unexplained syncope. *Pediatrics* 92:426, 1993.

Scott SA: Evaluating the child with syncope. *Pediatr Ann* 20:350, 1991.

Sharkey AM, Clark BJ: Common complaints with cardiac implications in children. *Pediatr Clin North Am* 38:657, 1991.

# Emergency Wound Management

## 42

## THE EVALUATION OF WOUNDS IN THE EMERGENCY DEPARTMENT

**Richard F. Edlich**
**George T. Rodeheaver**
**John G. Thacker**

Traumatic wounds are one of the most common problems encountered in the emergency department. Emergency physicians treat an estimated 11 million patients with traumatic wounds annually.

When caring for wounds, the ultimate goal is to restore the physical integrity and function of the injured tissue without infection. Treatment of wounds involves a series of decisions that determine if the wound heals or becomes infected.

### PREHOSPITAL CARE

In patients with soft tissue injuries, treatment should be initiated by the paramedics under the guidance of the emergency department physician using radio and telemetered communication. The primary survey must evaluate ventilation and circulation and detect bleeding.

External bleeding almost always can be controlled by a pressure dressing. Before applying the dressing, all skin flaps that are kinked or twisted should be returned to their original position to prevent vascular compromise. Bleeding of an injured extremity that is refractory to direct pressure will stop following inflation of a sphygmomanometer placed proximal to the bleeding site. After the injured extremity is elevated for 1 min, the cuff is inflated to a pressure that is greater than the patient's systolic blood pressure. This measured level of inflation pressure can be maintained for at least 2 h without injury to the underlying vessels and nerves. Once the patient's condition has been stabilized, the secondary survey must follow.

### EMERGENCY DEPARTMENT CARE

When the patient arrives in the emergency department, treatment of life-threatening injuries continues to take precedence over management of soft tissue wounds. When a life-threatening injury warrants immediate operative intervention, soft tissue wounds can be repaired simultaneously if there is careful coordination and planning between surgical specialists and anesthesiologists.

Before inspecting the wound, the emergency physician must carefully question the patient regarding the time and mechanism of injury. The time since the accident occurred has considerable influence on surgical decisions. A delay in treatment lasting longer than 3 h is often associated with a proliferation of bacteria to a level that results in the development of infection and limits the therapeutic efficacy of antibiotics.

This research was supported by a generous gift from the Texaco Philanthropic Foundation, White Plains, New York.

### Mechanism of Injury

The divided edges of the wound are more susceptible to infection than the unwounded tissue. The resistance to infection varies with the mechanism of injury. In most soft tissue injuries, a shearing force is applied by a piece of glass, a metal edge, or a knife, resulting in a linear laceration. The resultant wound exhibits considerable resistance to the development of infection.

If a wound is caused by a collision of two bodies, the mechanism of injury is predominantly compression or tension, rather than shear. The energy requirement for tissue failure as a result of these forces is considerably greater than that for shear forces. The absorbed energy of this impact force disrupts the skin, resulting in a characteristic stellate laceration. Wounds due to compression or tension injuries are 100-fold more susceptible to infection than those caused by shear forces. While antibiotic therapy is clearly beneficial in these wounds, its efficacy is substantially less than that in wounds caused by shear forces that are subjected to a similar level of bacterial inoculum.

Disruption of the vessels in the skin and underlying tissue produces an ecchymosis. Disruption of vessels in the underlying tissue results in a hematoma. Some hematomas resorb, but those that become encapsulated usually require surgical treatment. Left untreated, such hematomas may result in permanent subcutaneous deformity. When still in the currant-jelly stage, a hematoma is best treated by incision and drainage. As further liquefaction occurs, aspiration with a large-bore needle (18 gauge or larger) may be possible.

Firearm injuries cause a considerably higher level of energy absorption per unit volume of tissue than blunt injuries. As tissues are struck by a missile, a combination of shear, tensile, and compressive forces interacts to produce a relatively reproducible amount of destruction. The severity of the wound in the body is related to the amount of kinetic energy deposited in the body. Firearm injuries are discussed in further detail in Chapter 222, "Wound Ballistics."

### Wound Contaminants

The environs in which the injury occurred may be predictive of the number of pathogens in the wound. An infective dose of bacteria may be derived from either an exogenous source (e.g., wounding instrument) or the endogenous microflora of the patient. In general, the composition of the skin microflora allows subdivision of the body into three anatomic areas (Table 42-1). Over most of the body surface, trunk, upper arms, and upper legs, the density of the bacterial population is quite low, a few thousand or less per square centimeter. The moist areas of the body, such as the axillae, perineum, toe webs, and intertriginous areas harbor millions of bacteria per square centimeter. The exposed anatomic areas (head, face, hands, and feet) of the body constitute the third anatomic region and display a bacterial density numbering in the millions per square centimeter. No error is more frequent than the habit of generalizing about the microflora in this exposed anatomic region. The dissimilarities in the density and diversity of organisms which inhabit this unique province are truly profound. Normally, the organisms are quite sparse on the palms and dorsa of the hands, numbering in the hundreds per square centimeter. The majority of organisms on the hands reside beneath the distal end of the nail plate or adjacent to the proximal or lateral nail folds. The scalp and the forehead skin also exhibit abundant bacterial growth, in the millions per square centimeter.

**Table 42-1.** Composition and Concentration of Skin Microflora

| Anatomic Site | Total Bacterial Concentrations | Ratio Aerobe:Anaerobe |
|---|---|---|
| Moister areas (axillae, perineum) | $10^4$–$10^6$ | 10:1 |
| Drier areas (trunk, upper arms, and legs) | $10^1$–$10^3$ | 5–10:1 |
| Exposed areas (head, face, hands, and feet)* | $10^4$–$10^6$ | 5–10:1 |

* Anaerobes may outnumber aerobes in the skin of the cheeks, upper back, and presternum.

In most anatomic regions, bacterial colonization of the skin is limited to the horny layer of skin, which is composed of a sloughing mass of dead cells, full of cracks which harbor bacteria. Beneath this horny layer, the stratum corneum, composed of tightly packed cells, provides an effective barrier against bacterial invasion. The horny layer of pilosebaceous appendages that line the infundibulum of hair follicles forms a receptacle for bacteria. However, these bacteria rarely descend any further than the entrance of the sebaceous ducts. Similarly, the depths of apocrine glands and sweat glands are devoid of bacteria. The organisms that reside less than 250 μm beneath the surface are within reach of topically applied antiseptic agents. As a result of topical antisepsis, sterility or near sterility can be achieved in most skin areas of the body.

Lacerations contacting the oral cavity usually are heavily contaminated with facultative species and obligate anaerobes. Within the oral cavity, the largest number of organisms is encountered in the gingival crevices plaque on the teeth. The plaque on teeth and the debris removed from the crevices are composed primarily of bacteria in the range of $10^{11}$ per gram wet weight, a number that is far greater than infective doses of bacteria ($\geq 10^6$ bacteria per gram of tissue) for most soft tissue wounds. This potential source of heavy contamination accounts for the reported high infection rate of wounds resulting from human and animal bites. Feces also possess a luxuriant microflora occurring in a concentration of $10^{11}$ per gram of passed feces. Approximately 20 to 30 percent of the net weight of stool is a solid mass of bacteria, nearly all anaerobes. Wounds contacted by human or animal fecal contaminants run a high risk of infection despite therapeutic intervention.

A careful history can also predict the likelihood of nonviable foreign bodies being in wounds. In missile injuries, clothing and missile fragments are encountered in the wounded tissue. Soil and dirt frequently are found in lacerations resulting from industrial or farming accidents. Specific infection-potentiating fractions have been identified in the soil; these fractions include its organic components as well as its inorganic clay fractions. For wounds contaminated by these fractions, only 100 bacteria are necessary to elicit infection. Their ability to enhance the incidence of infection appears to be related to their damage to host defenses. In the presence of these fractions, leukocytes are not able to ingest and kill bacteria. This deleterious effect on white blood cell function is a result of direct interaction between the highly charged soil particles and white cells. Soil infection-potentiating fractions also have considerable influence on nonspecific humoral factors. Exposure of fresh serum to these fractions eliminates its bactericidal activity. As expected, these fractions, which consist of highly charged particles, react chemically with amphoteric and basic antibiotics, limiting their activity in contaminated wounds.

The concentration of these fractions in soil can be correlated with their location. Environmental conditions in swamps, bogs, and marshes encourage the production of soil composed almost entirely (90 percent) of organic infection-potentiating fractions. The major inorganic infection-potentiating particles are the clay fractions, which reside in heaviest concentration in the subsoil rather than in topsoil.

Consequently, traumatic soft tissue injuries occurring in swamps or excavation run a high risk of being contaminated by these fractions, which predispose the wound to serious infection. Fresh water lacerations are also contaminated, usually with *Aeromonas* sp.

A corollary to these observations is that some soil constituents, such as sand grains, are relatively innocuous. The sand fraction, which has a large particle size and a low level of chemical reactivity, exerts considerably less damage on tissue defenses than the infection-potentiating fractions do. Surprisingly, the black dirt on the surface of highways also appears to have minimal chemical reactivity.

## Wound Examination

The examining medical personnel should don gloves and wear a mask when inspecting the wound. Powder-free gloves are recommended because the powder on surgical gloves (e.g., cornstarch or talc) is foreign bodies that damage the host's resistance to infection.

Powder-free gloves coated by a hydrogel polymer (Biogel, Regent Hospital Products, Greenville, SC) are easily donned by either wet or dry hands without the cornstarch lubricant. When treating wounds in patients who are infected with the human immunodeficiency virus (HIV) or whose risk profile for HIV infection is high, a double glove technique can reduce the risk of needle penetration. A new powder-free double gloving system has been developed that enhances protection against needle penetration as well as detecting the needle puncture hole (Biogel Reveal, Regent Hospital Products, Greenville, SC). It consists of a double glove system with the inner glove stained uniformly with a green dye. When the outer glove is punctured, the green glove immediately changes color at the puncture site, a warning to the emergency physician to change gloves.

The physician's visualization of the wound can be enhanced by magnification loupes. Physicians uniformly prefer a Keplerian lens system over that of the Galilean lens system. The advantages of the Keplerian lens system are its increased field of view and clearer peripheral image. This system allows the physician to visualize the exquisite details of the wound and to perform wound closure using microsurgical techniques. Examination of the injured site must begin by detecting any sensory, motor, and vascular complications or injuries to specialized ducts. When the injury occurs in an extremity, this examination can be conducted in the absence of hemorrhage if a sphygmomanometer proximal to the injury is inflated to a pressure greater than the patient's systolic blood pressure. Palpation of the bone adjacent to the wound may detect tenderness or instability consistent with an underlying bone injury. Roentgenograms of the injured site will confirm this diagnosis. Injuries requiring open reduction of fractures, neurorrhaphy, vascular anastomosis, tendon juncture, or repair of specialized ducts are best treated in the operating room, where good lighting, instruments, and assistance make the procedure safer. In the absence of these underlying injuries, wound treatment can be undertaken in the emergency department. Important considerations in wound management are also the location, configuration, and biomechanical properties of the wound.

## Wound Biomechanical Properties

The ultimate appearance and function of a scar can be predicted by the magnitude of the static and dynamic skin tensions on the surrounding skin. The static skin tensions are the forces that stretch the skin over the underlying bony framework when the body remains motionless. These inherent forces are dependent on the natural characteristics of dermal collagen fibers and on the pattern in which they are woven. Clinical evidence of these tensions is the retraction of the edges of the wounds permitting visualization of the underlying tissue.

Static skin forces differ considerably in their magnitude and direction between individuals and at various anatomic sites within the same person. In one human volunteer, the static skin tensions were

## Static Skin Tension

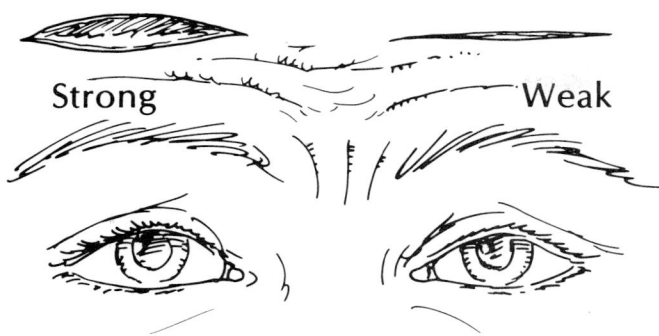

Strong       Weak

**Fig. 42-1.** The degree to which the wound edges retract can be correlated with the magnitude of static skin tensions. The wound on the right side of the patient's forehead exhibits marked retraction of its edges (≥5 mm) being subjected to strong static skin tensions. The minimal separation of the edges of the wound (<5 mm) on the left side of the patient's forehead is consistent with the presence of weak static skin tensions.

fivefold greater in his extremities than in his abdominal skin. In some regions of the body there is a directional orientation of static skin tensions. The most aesthetically pleasing scar occurs when the long axis of the scar is in the direction of the maximal skin tension. The pull of the stronger skin tensions at the ends of the wound tends to oppose the weaker forces that are perpendicular to the wound edges, thereby bringing its edges closer together. Following approximation of the wound edges, the static skin tensions continuously pull on the wound edges, resulting in the development of a visible scar. The ultimate width of the scar is proportional to the magnitude of the static skin tensions. Wounds made in skin subjected to strong static skin tensions usually heal with wide, unattractive scars. In contrast, narrow, fine scars often result from repair of wounds in skin with weak static skin tensions.

Clinical observation of the wound in the emergency department is a reliable method of predicting the ultimate appearance of the healing scar after closure. The degree to which the divided skin edges retract provides a rough estimate of the magnitude of static skin tensions. Wounds with marked retraction of their edges (≥5 mm) are subjected to strong static skin tensions and heal with wide scars (Fig. 42-1). When there is minimal separation of the wound edges (<5 mm), wound repair is accomplished with fine scars. This information should be shared with the patients as well as their families so that they can appropriately credit the aesthetic result to the biology of wound repair.

The magnitude of static skin tension per unit length of wound is influenced considerably by the configuration of the wound. In uneven, jagged-edged wounds, the perimeter of the wound is considerably longer than that of a linear incision. Consequently, the magnitude of static tensions per unit length of a jagged-edged wound is less than that of a straight laceration. Plastic surgeons have learned that meticulous reapproximation of the jagged edges of the wound yields a gratifying result with a narrow scar. Those unaware of the biomechanical principles involved in wound repair may elect to convert the jagged wound edges into a straight wound. This decision adds insult to the injury. The ill-conceived debridement eliminates the potential benefits of the long wound perimeter and leaves a lenticular-shaped defect that is considerably wider than the initial wound. Reapproximation of the edges of the debrided wound requires greater closing forces than would have been needed prior to debridement, resulting in a wide, unattractive scar. Faced with this physical deformity, the patient may seek the advice of a plastic surgeon. Six to twelve months after the injury, the plastic surgeon may elect to revise the

scar by a W- or Z-plasty. The revised incision usually yields a gratifying result, healing with a narrower scar.

Dynamic skin tensions also have considerable impact on the static skin tensions as well as on the magnitude and extent of scar formation. These changing tensions are caused by a combination of forces that are associated with joint movement or mimetic muscle contraction. The clinical significance of dynamic tensions is particularly apparent in skin of changing dimensions where elasticity is needed for normal function. In general, a linear scar intersecting the transverse axis of a joint or running perpendicular to the wrinkle lines can result in a serious contracture because the scar does not stretch or recoil like uninjured tissue.

The direction of the dynamic skin tensions can be ascertained by rather simple practical measurements (Fig. 42-2A and B). At the ends of the laceration, mark points A and B; then mark points C and D, which are perpendicular to the laceration and equidistant between points A and B. Measure first the distance between points A and B and then the distance between points C and D before and after flexion of the underlying joints or contraction of the muscles of facial expression. The dynamic skin tensions are in the direction of greatest change in dimension. Wounds with their long axes in the direction of dynamic skin tension heal with conspicuous scars that interfere with function and are aesthetically unattractive. If the long axis of the wound is perpendicular to the dynamic skin tension in a site that remains relatively stationary during muscle contraction, the magnitude of the scar formation can be predicted by the inherent static skin tensions. Unfortunately, accidental injuries often result in wounds whose axis parallels the dynamic skin tensions. In such cases, it is impera-

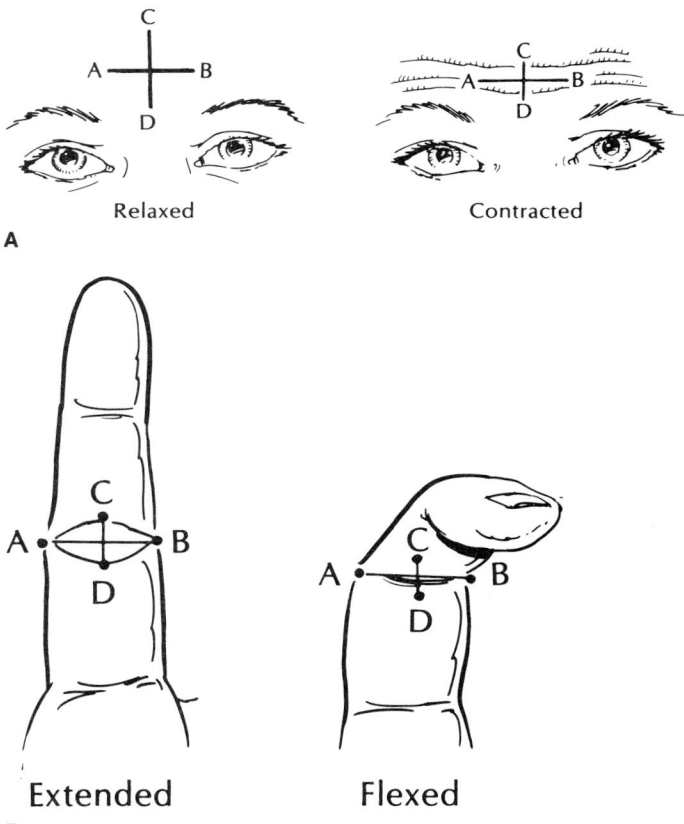

**Fig. 42-2. A.** Contraction of the frontalis muscle considerably shortens the skin in the direction of dynamic skin tensions (line CD). **B.** As the proximal interphalangeal joint flexes, the distance along the longitudinal axis of the joint shortens considerably in the same direction as the dynamic skin tension (line CD).

tive to warn the patient of the impending development, and referral to a plastic surgeon for follow-up examination and treatment is recommended. At a later date (6 to 12 months), the directional orientation of the scar can be altered by W- or Z-plasty so that the direction of a portion of the wound is perpendicular to the dynamic skin tensions.

## BIBLIOGRAPHY

Edlich RF, Rodeheaver GT, Morgan RF, et al: Principles of emergency wound management. *Ann Emerg Med* 17:1294, 1988.

Edlich RF, Crampton RS, Rockwell DD, et al: Prehospital management of the trauma patient. *EMT J* 5:186, 1981.

Thacker JG, Iachetta FA, Allaire PE, et al: Biomechanical properties—Their influence on planning surgical excisions, in Krizek TJ, Hoopes PE (eds): *Symposium on Basic Science in Plastic Surgery.* St. Louis, Mosby, 1975, vol 15, pp 72–79.

# 43

# LOCAL AND REGIONAL ANESTHESIA FOR WOUND REPAIR

**Richard F. Edlich**
**George T. Rodeheaver**
**John G. Thacker**

Cleansing bacteria and other debris from laceration followed by debridement and wound closure cannot be accomplished without either local or regional anesthesia often complemented by sedation. Assessment and treatment of laceration requires patient cooperation. The decision to use sedation, analgesia, or restraint must be individualized by the emergency physician for each patient.

Many of the principles of pain management for children are identical to those used for adults. When the patient exhibits considerable anxiety to the pain accompanying the laceration, sedation can minimize response to treatment while maintaining stable vital signs, independent airway, and adequate spontaneous respirations.

Pain control during laceration repair in the anxious patient can be achieved by *conscious sedation,* which is a medically controlled state of depressed consciousness that allows protective reflexes to be maintained, retaining the patient's ability to maintain a patent airway independently and continuously and permitting appropriate response by the patient to physical stimulation or verbal command. The use of conscious sedation must include provision of a health care professional, in addition to the physician whose responsibility is to monitor appropriate physiologic parameters and assist in supportive and resuscitative procedures as required. There must be continuous monitoring of pulse oximetry and heart rate and intermittent recording of blood pressure and respirations.

Contraindications to conscious sedation include a medical history of underlying respiratory, cardiac, or neurologic conditions, or the administration of medication with sedative effects within 24 hours before presentation. The history of recent oral intake or other known risk factors such as extreme obesity, pregnancy, or bowel motility dysfunction, require careful evaluation before administration of seda-

Our research has been supported by a generous gift from Mr. John A. McCrane, New York, New York.

tion. Conscious sedation for adults and children is described in Chapters 34 and 38.

## SELECTION OF ANESTHETIC AGENT

The selection of the anesthetic agent for infiltration anesthesia or regional nerve block is based on pharmacologic and toxicologic considerations. The pharmacodynamic properties of these agents include severity of pain elicited by the injection of the agent, onset and duration of anesthetic activity, and frequency of adequate anesthesia. The toxicologic manifestations of local anesthetic agents are almost exclusively local complications (e.g., damage to tissue defenses) because when these agents are absorbed systemically they do not affect organ systems clinically, except for the peripheral nerves. In general, the local anesthetic agents of proven merit have been the aminoesters and aminoamides. Benzocaine, the oldest of the currently available ester-type agents, is still used as a topical anesthetic agent. Procaine, tetracaine, and chloroprocaine were later developed.

### Lidocaine

Lidocaine, the first aminoamide local anesthetic agent synthesized, represented such a significant pharmacologic advance over the aminoesters that it and chemically related aminoamides have largely replaced the aminoesters. Because the free base forms of most aminoamide local anesthetic agents are poorly soluble in aqueous solutions, they are prepared as hydrochloride salts.

These aminoamide anesthetic agents are weak organic bases, comprised of charged and uncharged fractions when in solution. It is believed that the uncharged form of local anesthetic agent diffuses through the interstitial tissue and transports across the nerve membrane. The concentration of the uncharged fraction depends on the pH of the solution, with more anesthetic agent being in the uncharged form as the pH of the solution increases.

Most aminoamide local anesthetic agents are marketed as acidic solutions (pH 5.0 to 7.0) having a shelf life of 3 to 4 years. Although increasing the solution pH enhances the concentration of the uncharged form, it also increases the risk of precipitation out of solution, thereby decreasing its shelf life. Commercially prepared local anesthetic solutions containing epinephrine must also be acidified because alkaline solutions promote oxidation of catecholamines.

Because of their antibacterial and antifungal activity, antimicrobial preservatives have been added to local anesthetic solutions contained in multidose vials. The most frequently used antimicrobials are the paraben derivatives of para-hydroxybenzoate, such as methylparaben, ethylparaben, and propylparaben. The paraben derivatives are potent allergens and have been implicated in allergic reactions attributed to the local anesthetic agent. Because single-use vials do not contain these preservatives, single-use vials should not be used to dispense multiple doses of local anesthetic agents.

Clinical studies have demonstrated that the pain accompanying local anesthetic administration can be dramatically reduced by warming and buffering the local anesthetic agent. Warming and buffering the local anesthetic agent appear to act synergistically. A simple way to warm the vial or bottle of local anesthetic solution is to place it in the intravenous solution warmer heated to 40°C. Buffering the 30-mL multidose vials containing 1% lidocaine is accomplished by adding 3 mL of 4.2% sodium bicarbonate (1 mEq/mL). Using single-dose vials, the local anesthetic agent is prepared as a 10:1 dilution with a sterile solution of sodium bicarbonate (1 mEq/mL).

### Bupivacaine

When the duration of anesthesia must be prolonged, bupivacaine should be used rather than lidocaine because its duration of anesthesia is nearly four times longer than that of lidocaine. When wound closure takes longer than 2 h, consider the use of bupivacaine so that wound repair does not have to be interrupted by the additional injections of the local anesthetic agent. Like lidocaine, bupivacaine does not damage tissue defenses or potentiate infection. In addition, the pain of its subdermal injection, its onset of anesthesia, and its frequency of satisfactory anesthesia are remarkably similar to those of lidocaine. Prolonged anesthesia may not be desirable in some anatomic sites. Anesthesia of the oral cavity is such a case. Disappearance of the anesthetic effect allows the patient to resume activities requiring the use of the mouth, cheek, tongue, and lips without concern about inadvertently biting the anesthetized mucous membranes. This same principle applies to repaired fingertip injuries in which the patient must resume activities requiring normal tactile sensation.

## Epinephrine

The duration of anesthetic activity of these agents can be enhanced by the addition of the vasoconstrictor epinephrine, which slows the clearance of the agent from the tissue, thereby prolonging the duration of anesthesia. This benefit must be weighed against its deleterious effects on tissue defenses; epinephrine will damage local tissue defenses. The infection-potentiating effect of this powerful vasoconstrictor is proportional to its concentration and results from its vasoactivity. As a result of its local vasoconstrictive action, epinephrine may result in hypoxic conditions that limit white blood cell function. Consequently, the increased infection rate of epinephrine-treated wounds may result from impaired killing of bacterial contaminants by wound leukocytes in the ischemic wounds. This damage to tissue defenses argues against the use of epinephrine in potentially heavily contaminated wounds.

## TOPICAL ANESTHESIA

One method of topical anesthesia of lacerations is the use of topical solution containing 0.5% tetracaine, 0.5% epinephrine (adrenalin), and 11.8% cocaine (TAC). Advantages are anesthesia without discomfort of tissue swelling and intense vasoconstriction, resulting in a bloodless wound. TAC is most effective as a topical anesthetic agent when applied for more than 20 min before suturing. The success of anesthesia is usually evidenced by complete blanching of the skin within 1 cm of the wound edges. TAC cannot be used in lacerations involving the ear, penis, and digits because their limited vascularity may be compromised. It also cannot be used on or applied to mucous membranes because a toxic reaction to cocaine will result.

In our work, topical application of TAC resulted in an increased incidence of infection and necrosis of the wound edges. Also, the dangers of cocaine toxicity, especially in children, and the necessity of narcotic control are additional hazards to its use.

Another issue involves the medicolegal implications of TAC usage. It is not commercially available and is prepared in the hospital pharmacy for use in the emergency department. Because TAC is prepared in the pharmacy and is not distributed outside the institution, it is exempt from Food and Drug Administration (FDA) manufacturing regulations. In the absence of regulatory overview, the usual drug testing regimens, such as animal and clinical trials, have not been done. It is unclear if this lack of specific FDA approval will result in greater liability in the event that serious toxic consequences occur.

Schilling et al. have recently demonstrated in a randomized double-blind study that a topical solution of lidocaine (4%), epinephrine (0.1%), and tetracaine (0.5%) (LET) was generally equivalent to TAC in producing topical anesthesia to the scalp, forehead and eyebrow. The two agents were similar in adequacy and duration of anesthesia overall, except in children over the age of six years, who had a greater proportion of incomplete anesthesia.

Anesthesia of intact normal and diseased skin can be achieved by a topical application of a eutectic mixture of 5% lidocaine and prilocaine (EMLA), under occlusion for 60 min. This cream has been used successfully for anesthesia of split-thickness graft donor sites, venipuncture, curettage of molluscum contagiosum, cautery of genital warts, and myringotomy. This cream is not recommended for topical anesthesia of lacerations because it elicits an exaggerated inflammatory response in the wound that damages host defenses, inviting the development of infection.

## SIDE EFFECTS OF ANESTHETIC AGENTS

The side effects of local anesthetic agents administered for local anesthesia and regional nerve blocks can be divided into allergic reactions and systemic toxicity. True allergic reactions to local anesthetic agents are rare. The ester derivatives of para-aminobenzoic acid, such as procaine, were responsible for most allergic reactions; the aminoamide local anesthetic compounds have accounted for relatively few. Because the aminoamide compounds are believed to be incapable of stimulating antibody formation, true anaphylaxis should not be encountered when these compounds are used. Some patients presumed to be allergic to the amide-type compound had positive skin responses to the preservatives (e.g., methylparaben) or stabilizers added to local anesthetic agents but not to the anesthetic agent. Because the systemic clinical manifestations of a toxic response to the drug are similar to those of an allergic reaction, it may be difficult to identify a true allergic reaction. Central nervous system (CNS) stimulation by these agents manifested by tachycardia, nausea, vomiting, and seizures may be confused with IgE-mediated response or anaphylaxis. The use of vasoconstrictors, like epinephrine, with the local anesthetic agents may produce systemic effects that simulate the symptoms of anaphylaxis.

Systemic toxicity is usually due to either a rapid inadvertent intravenous injection of an excessive amount of the local anesthetic agent. Adverse reactions involve primarily the CNS and cardiovascular system and can be divided into four stages. The first adverse premonitory signs are CNS symptoms, such as dizziness, tinnitus, periorbital tingling, nystagmus, and fine skeletal muscle twitching. Such systemic reactions can be treated by discontinuing the administration of the anesthetic agent, ensuring a patent airway, providing supplemental oxygen to prevent cerebral hypoxia, and hyperventilation. Overt convulsions of the tonic or clonic type may follow. Most localized or systemic convulsions are self-limiting because of the rapid redistribution to the organ reservoirs, resulting in a decrease in blood levels. When convulsions persist, small incremental doses of diazepam are administered intravenously and repeated cautiously as needed. CNS depression may ensue in which the seizure activity ends and respiratory efforts become shallow. This stage responds to supportive measures that include maintenance of patent airway, supplemental oxygen, and hyperventilation. Signs and symptoms of cardiovascular collapse are the final stage and require treatment with intravenous fluids and a vasopressor or positive inotropic agent.

Systemic toxicity is treated best by prevention. Rapid injections of the local anesthetic agent should be avoided, and recommended drug dosages should be used. When treating a patient with a convincing history of allergy to an amide-type anesthetic agent, the emergency department physician should try a subcutaneous challenge with a local anesthetic agent different from the one causing the previous allergic reaction. An alternative approach is to inject an antihistamine, like 1% diphenhydramine hydrochlorine, into the wound, achieving anesthesia for approximately 30 min. The actual mechanism of its anesthetic activity is unclear.

## INFILTRATION ANESTHESIA

The simplest and most practical technique of anesthetizing most lacerations is infiltration anesthesia. The subcutaneous branches

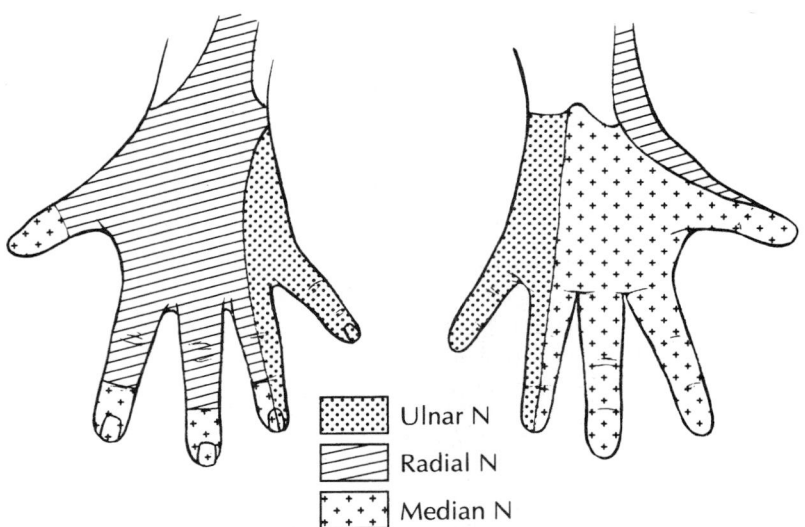

**Fig. 43-1.** The cutaneous distribution of anesthesia with block of major nerves of the wrist.

░░ Ulnar N

╱╱ Radial N

⁺⁺ Median N

of the sensory nerves to the wound are anesthetized by injecting 1% lidocaine through a 30-gauge needle into intact skin at the periphery of the wound. Injection through the cut edge of the wound is less painful, but carries the risk of disseminating bacteria throughout uninvolved tissue around the contaminated wound.

The depth and speed of injection are important determinants of the magnitude of discomfort experienced by the patient. Placement of the needle into the superficial dermis is more uncomfortable than needle passage into the subdermal area. Moreover, intradermal injections resulting in superficial wheals are significantly more painful than injections into the subdermal region. Rapid injection of a local anesthetic agent (< 2 s) always causes more pain than when the same volume of anesthetic agent is instilled over 10 s. Intracutaneous instillation of lidocaine at 37°C (98.6°F) is less painful than injection at 21°C (69.8°F). Buffering with sodium bicarbonate as a 10:1 solution of 10 ml 1% lidocaine: 1 meq/ml of sodium bicarbonate also diminishes the pain of infiltration. Full anesthesia to pinprick is produced immediately with intradermal injections and is present 5 to 6 min after subdermal injection. A reliable method of minimizing the discomfort of infiltration anesthesia is to use a syringe fitted with a 30-gauge needle and to inject the smallest amount of anesthetic agent slowly (≥ 10 s) into the deep dermal-subcutaneous tissue as the needle is slowly withdrawn.

## REGIONAL NERVE BLOCKS

When the nerve supply to the wound is superficial, a regional nerve block is a valuable clinical tool. A distinct advantage of this route of administration over infiltration anesthesia is that it does not distort the wound, facilitating reapproximation of the wound edges. Although a 30-gauge needle is ideally suited for infiltration anesthesia, larger diameter (27-gauge) needles are used for regional nerve blocks because they have a greater resistance to bending, thereby ensuring accurate deposition of the anesthetic agent near the sensory or motor nerve. The clinical value of regional anesthesia becomes especially apparent when anesthetizing lacerations of the palm of the hand or the sole of the foot. Infiltration of a local anesthetic agent into this exquisitely sensitive skin is unbearable. Fortunately, the nerve supply of these anatomic regions is susceptible to regional nerve blocks. Such blocks may be accomplished by passage of the needle through more proximal skin, which has a considerably higher threshold to pain than skin of the palm or sole. Because performance of a successful regional nerve block requires patient participation and communication, we reserve these blocks to alert mature adolescents and adults with no cognitive deficit.

## Hand Blocks

### Median Nerve

The median nerve enters the hand through the carpal tunnel, deep to the flexor retinaculum, between the tendons of the flexor digitorum superficialis and the tendon of the flexor carpi radialis. The median nerve sends cutaneous sensory fibers to the entire palmar surface and sides of the thumb, index finger, middle and lateral half of the ring finger, and the dorsum of these digits distal to their proximal interphalangeal joints (Fig. 43-1).

### Ulnar Nerve

Just proximal to the wrist, the ulnar nerve goes off a palmar cutaneous branch, which passes superficially to the flexor retinaculum and palmar aponeurosis to supply the skin of the medial side of the palm (see Fig. 43-1). It also gives off a dorsal cutaneous branch that supplies the medial half of the dorsum of the hand, the small finger, and the ulnar half of the ring finger. The ulnar nerve ends by dividing into a superficial and a deep branch. The superficial branch supplies cutaneous fibers to the anterior surfaces of the small finger and the ulnar half of the ring finger. In the small finger, the dorsal digital nerve extends to the tip of the digit. In the median nerve distribution, the volar nerve supplies the dorsum of the digit distal to the proximal interphalangeal joint (Fig. 43-2).

### Radial Nerve

The superficial branch of the radial nerve is the direct continuation of the radial nerve along the anterolateral side of the forearm and is en-

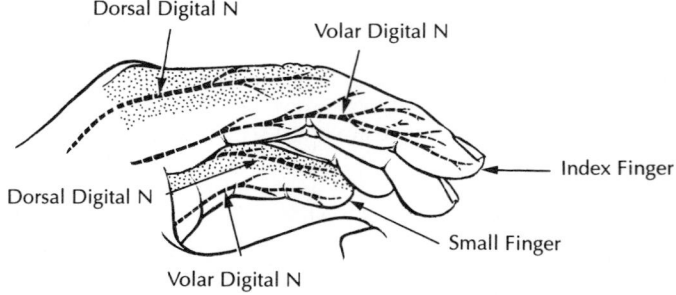

Dorsal Digital N

Volar Digital N

Dorsal Digital N

Volar Digital N

Index Finger

Small Finger

**Fig. 43-2.** The dorsal digital nerve extends to the tip of the digit in the small finger. In areas of the median nerve distribution (i.e., the ring finger), the volar nerve supplies the dorsum of the digit distal to the proximal interphalangeal joint.

**Fig. 43-3.** Regional blocks of the ulnar and median nerves.

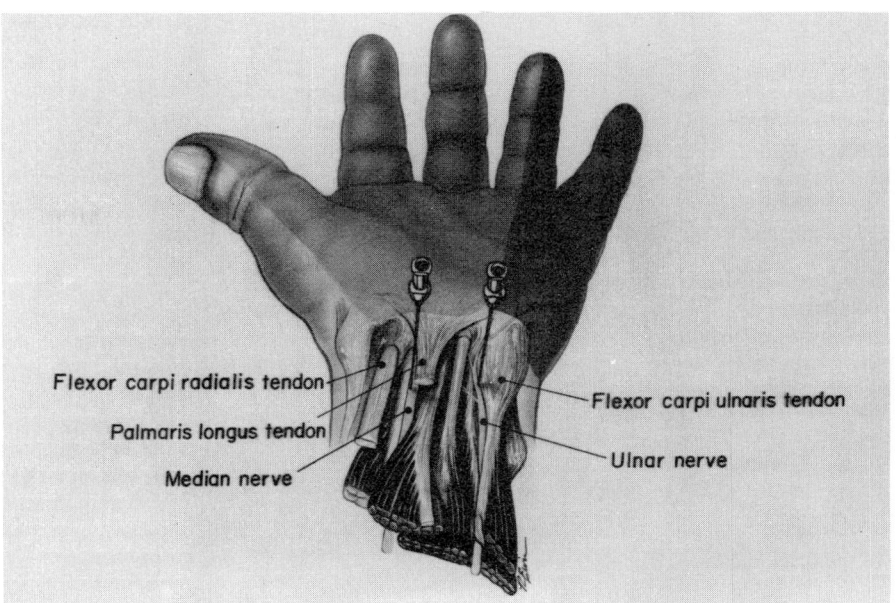

Flexor carpi radialis tendon

Palmaris longus tendon

Median nerve

Flexor carpi ulnaris tendon

Ulnar nerve

tirely sensory. It pierces the deep fascia near the dorsum of the wrist to supply skin and fascia over the lateral two thirds of the dorsum of the hand, the dorsum of the thumb, and proximal parts of the lateral one and one-half fingers (see Fig. 43-1).

## Wrist Blocks

For lacerations of the hand, regional blocks at the wrist are performed at the level of proximal volar skin crease (Fig. 43-3). The median nerve is anesthetized by inserting a 27-gauge needle perpendicular to the skin between the tendons of the palmaris longus and flexor carpi radialis muscles. A regional block of the ulnar nerve is accomplished by passing the needle between the ulnar artery and the flexor carpi ulnaris. Once inserted, the needle is moved fanwise transversely until paresthesia is elicited. When paresthesia occurs, the needle is held in place and 5 to 10 mL of 1% lidocaine with epinephrine (1:100,000) is injected slowly.

The superficial rami of the radial nerve can be blocked by raising the subcutaneous ring with 5 to 10 mL of 1% lidocaine with epinephrine (1:100,000) beginning at the level of the tendon of the extensor carpi radialis and extending around the radial border of the wrist dorsal to the styloid process (Fig. 43-4).

## Finger Blocks

### Metacarpal Block

Metacarpal blocks are used to anesthetize either the index, ring, long, or small finger (Fig. 43-5). The block is performed on each side of the affected finger by inserting a 27-gauge needle at a 90° angle to the dorsum of hand approximately 1 cm proximal to the metacarpophalangeal joint midway between each metacarpal bone. The nee-

dle is then advanced at a 90° angle to the skin until its tip is at the level of the lateral volar surface of the metacarpal head or until resistance of the palmar aponeurosis is detected. After aspirating, 3 mL of 1% lidocaine is injected slowly.

### Digital Nerve Block

Digital nerve block and metacarpal block are equally painful procedures. However, digital nerve block is more efficacious and requires significantly less time to anesthetize the injured finger. A 27-gauge needle is inserted through the skin into one side of the extensor tendon of the affected finger just proximal to the web (Fig. 43-6A). After aspirating, approximately 1 mL of 1% lidocaine is injected superficially into the subcutaneous tissue lying on the dorsal surface of the extensor tendon to block the dorsal digital nerve. The needle is then advanced toward the palm until its tip is palpable beneath the volar

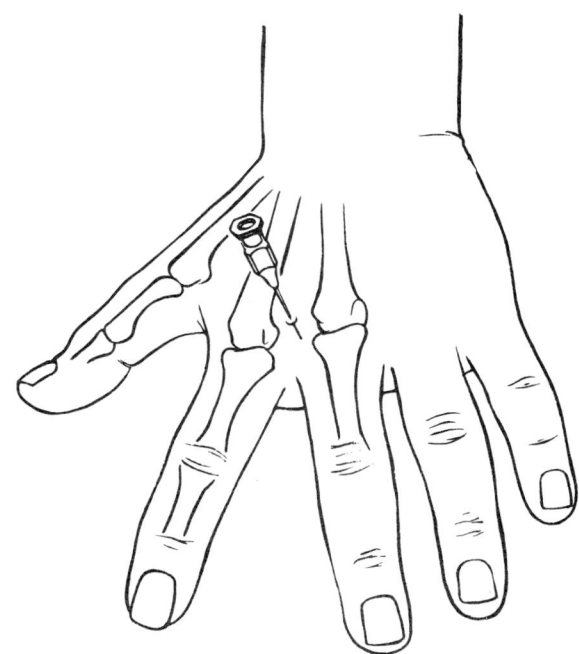

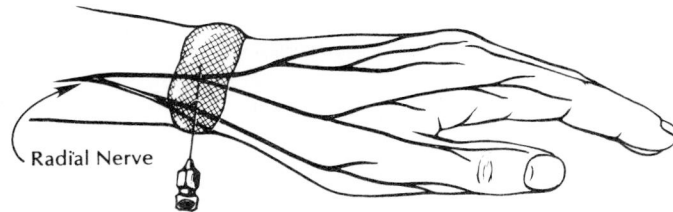

Radial Nerve

**Fig. 43-4.** Regional block of several rami of the radial nerve.

**Fig. 43-5.** Regional metacarpal nerve block.

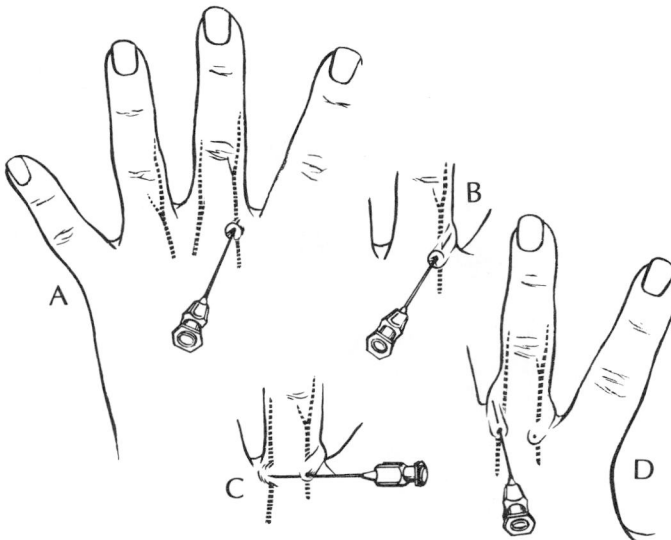

**Fig. 43-6.** Digital nerve block.

skin at the base of the finger, just distal to the web (Fig. 43-6*B*). After aspirating, another 1 mL of the anesthetic solution is injected to block the volar digital nerve.

Before removing the needle, it is redirected across the extensor tendon to the opposite side of the finger and approximately 1 mL of the anesthetic solution is injected into the tissue overlying the other dorsal digital nerve (Fig. 43-6*C*). Five minutes later, the needle is reintroduced in the anesthetized skin on the opposite side of the finger and the same technique is repeated (Fig. 43-6*D*). The total volume of the anesthetic agent should not exceed 4 mL. Epinephrine must NOT be used as an adjunct to lidocaine because it may result in irreversible ischemic injury to the finger.

## Ankle Blocks

These regional nerve blocks are used for anesthesia of surgical procedures of the foot. It is primarily an infiltration block, not requiring elicitation of paresthesia. One percent lidocaine is an excellent choice. When the injection involves regional anesthesia of all five nerves, and is circumferential, avoid the use of epinephrine. A total of 20 mL of a local anesthetic agent should not be exceeded per ankle. An ankle block should never be used in patients with peripheral vascular disease.

## Anatomy

The peripheral nerves involved in the ankle block are all derived from the sciatic nerve, with the exception of the terminal branch of the femoral nerve, the saphenous nerve (Fig. 43-7). The latter is the only branch of the femoral nerve below the knee. It becomes subcutaneous at the medial side of the knee joint and then follows the saphenous vein to a site anterior to the medial malleolus and supplies the skin over the medial malleolus. Occasionally, its innervation extends to the skin of the medial side of the foot to the first metatarso pharyngeal joint.

The remaining nerves requiring blockade are the terminal branches of the sciatic nerve, the common peroneal and tibial nerve. The common peroneal nerve divides into its terminal branches in the proximal portion of the leg, the superficial and deep peroneal nerves, while the tibial nerve divides into the posterior tibial and sural nerves.

The posterior tibial nerve is located along the medial aspect of the ankle lying between the medial malleolus and the Achilles tendon, lying just posterior and slightly deeper than the posterior tibial artery (see Fig. 43-7 and Fig. 43-9). Generally, the nerve gives off the medial calcaneus branch to the inside of the heel after which it divides into the medial and lateral plantar nerves just below the inferior margin of the medial malleolus. The medial plantar nerve supplies muscular and cutaneous branches of the sole of the foot, where

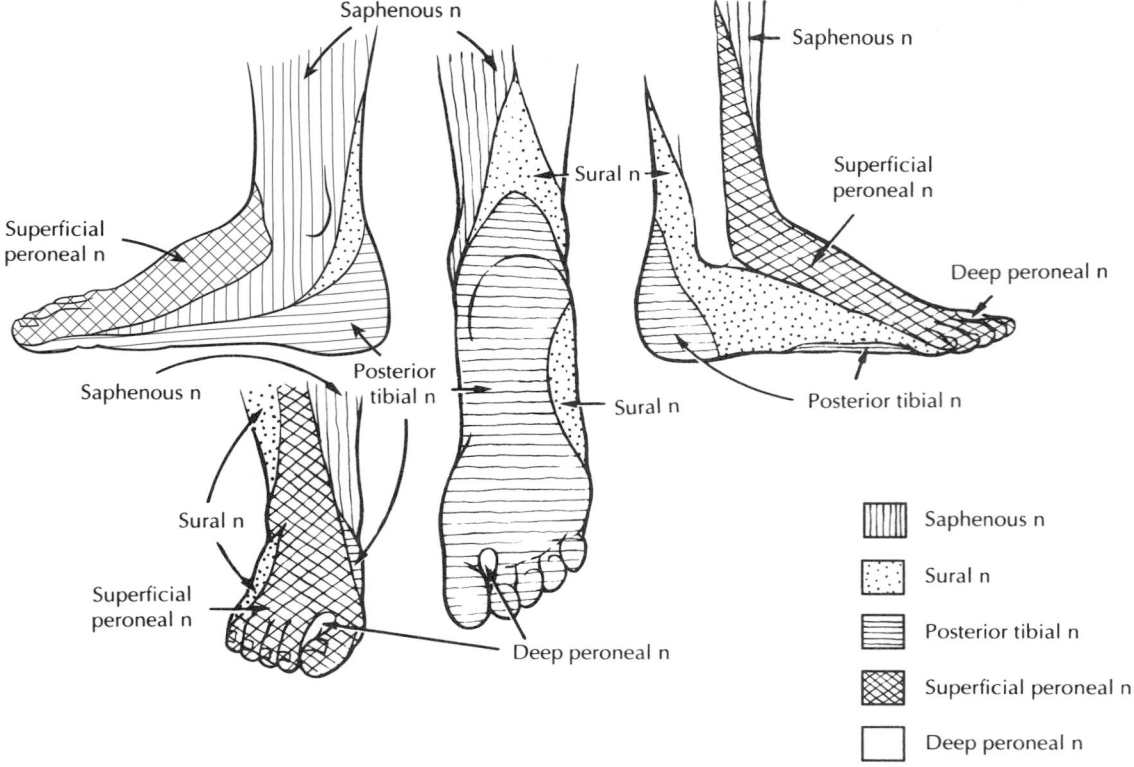

**Fig. 43-7.** Sensory innervation of the foot and ankle.

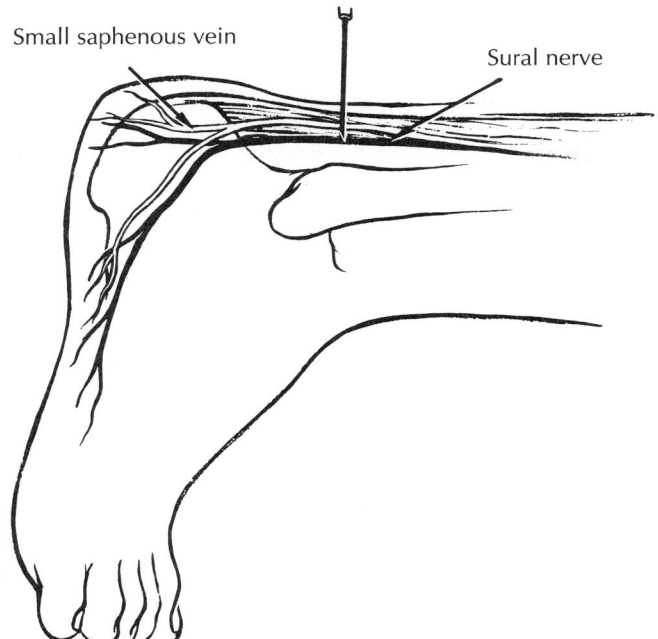

**Fig. 43-8.** Regional block of the sural nerve. Lateral view of foot.

its distribution closely resembles that of the median nerve of the hand. The lateral plantar nerve provides muscular and cutaneous branches of the sole of the foot analogous to the distribution of the ulnar nerve.

The sural nerve becomes subcutaneous somewhat distal to the middle of the leg and proceeds along with the short saphenous vein behind and below the lateral malleolus to supply the posterolateral surface of the leg, the lateral side of the foot, and the lateral side of the fifth toe (see Fig. 43-7 and Fig. 43-8). The dorsal lateral cutaneous nerve is the termination of the sural nerve.

The superficial peroneal nerve becomes the dorsal digital nerves. It descends toward the ankle in the lateral compartment entering the ankle just lateral to the extensor digitorum longus and provides the cutaneous supply to the dorsum of the foot and all five toes, except for the adjacent sides of the first and second toes (deep peroneal nerve) and lateral side of the fifth toe (sural nerve) (see Fig. 43-11). It is most commonly located lateral to the extensor digitorum longus at the level of the lateral malleolus superficially. It also supplies the peroneus longus and brevis.

The deep peroneal nerve is a continuation of the common peroneal nerve (see Fig. 43-10). A constant location is just lateral to the flexor hallucis longus at the level of medial malleolus. It approaches the anterior tibial artery from the lateral side and accompanies it through the leg; thereafter, it follows the dorsal pedis artery and first dorsal metatarsal artery through the foot, becoming cutaneous, and divides into two digital nerves along the adjacent sides of the first and second toes. It also supplies the four muscles in the anterior crural region as well as the extensor digitorum brevis.

### Technique

The posterior tibial and sural nerves are most easily blocked with the patient lying in a prone position. Once these nerves have been blocked, the patient assumes a supine position for blockade of the peroneal nerves and saphenous nerve.

The posterior tibial nerve is anesthetized as it passes behind the medial malleolus (Fig. 43-9). Lidocaine (1%) is injected through a 30-gauge needle into the subcutaneous tissue lateral to the posterior tibial artery or, should this be impalpable, immediately anterior

to the medial border of the Achilles tendon at the level with the upper border of the medial malleolus (see Fig. 43-9). Through this anesthetized skin, a 6- to 8-cm long 22-gauge needle is inserted at right angles to the posterior aspect of the tibia until it is immediately lateral to the posterior tibial artery. The direction of the needle is shifted in a mediolateral direction, often eliciting paresthesia of the posterior tibial nerve, at which time 3 to 5 mL of 1% lidocaine is injected. If paresthesia is not encountered, 5 to 7 mL of the anesthetic solution is injected against the posterior aspect of the tibia as the needle is drawn back 1 cm. The onset of anesthesia may occur in 5 to 10 min if paresthesia has been elicited, but it takes up to 30 min in its absence.

The sural nerve is located along the lateral aspect of the ankle between the lateral malleolus and Achilles tendon, lying just anterior to the short saphenous vein (Fig. 43-8). Lidocaine (1%) is injected through a 30-gauge needle into the subcutaneous tissue immediately lateral to the Achilles tendon at the cephalic border of the lateral malleolus. If no paresthesia is obtained after introducing a 6- to 8-cm long 22-gauge needle, the needle is allowed to contact the lateral malleolus, after which 5 to 7 mL of local anesthetic is injected as the needle is withdrawn.

After the patient assumes a supine position, the 30-gauge needle is inserted between the tendons of the extensor digitorum longus and extensor hallucis longus muscles to the periosteum or elicitation of paresthesia, after which 5 mL of local anesthetic is injected into this area to block the deep peroneal nerve (Fig. 43-10). From this midline skin wheal, a 6- to 8-cm 22-gauge needle is advanced subcutaneously laterally and medially to the malleoli, injecting 3 to 5 mL of anesthetic solution in each direction (Fig. 43-11). These lateral and medial approaches block the superficial peroneal and saphenous nerves, respectively.

### Toe Blocks

For laceration of the toe, digital, rather than ankle, nerve blocks are used. Epinephrine must not be used as an adjunct to lidocaine because it may result in irreversible ischemic injury to the toe. A 27-gauge needle should be introduced through the skin on the dorsal as-

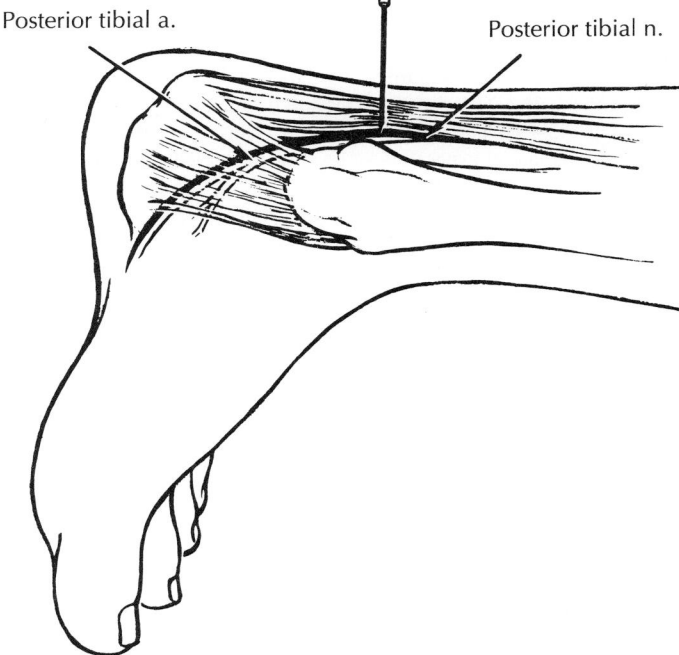

**Fig. 43-9.** Regional block of the posterior tibal nerve. Medial view of foot.

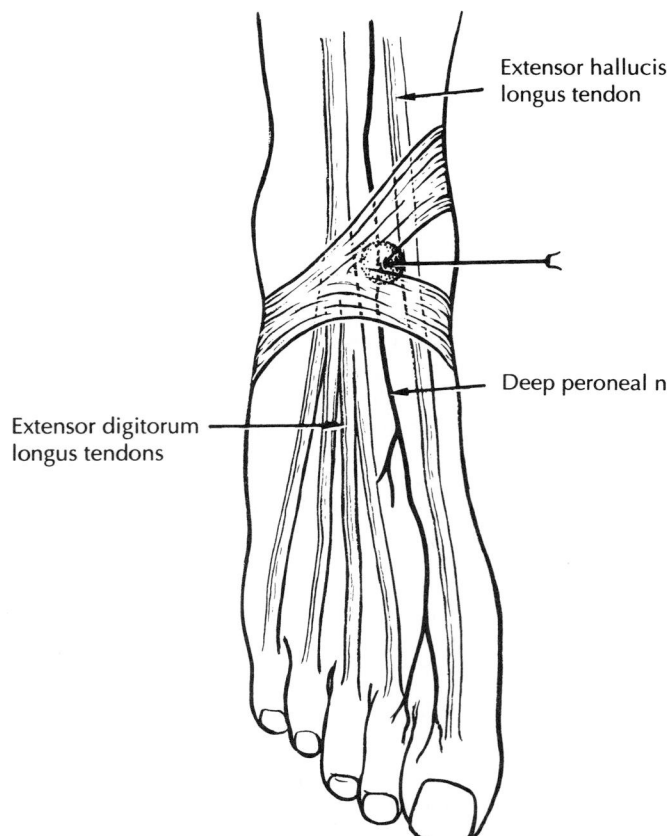

**Fig. 43-10.** Regional block of the deep peroneal nerve.

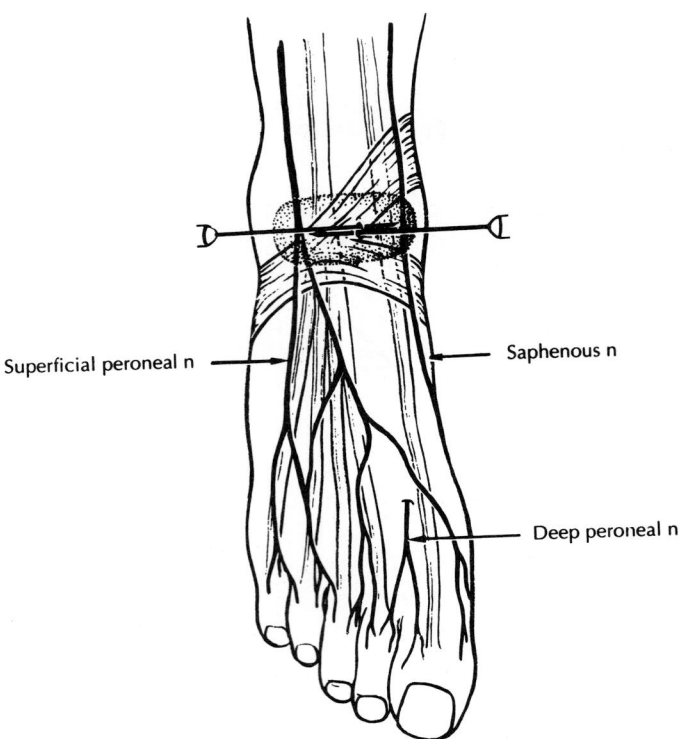

**Fig. 43-11.** Regional blocks of the superficial peroneal nerve and saphenous nerve.

pect of the base of the midpoint of the involved toe (Fig. 43-12). The needle should be angled around the bone until it induces blanching of the skin on the plantar surface. As the needle is withdrawn, approximately 1.5 mL of 1% lidocaine is injected. Before the needle is withdrawn completely from the skin, it should be redirected to the opposite side of the injured toe to inject the local anesthetic agent in a similar manner. The total volume of the injected local anesthetic agent should not exceed 3 mL.

For the hallux (great toe), a modified collar (ring) block is used (see Fig. 43-12). The 27-gauge needle is inserted through the skin on the dorsolateral aspect of the base of the toe until it blanches the plantar skin. As the needle is withdrawn, 1.5 mL of 1% lidocaine is injected into the tissues. Before the needle is removed completely from the skin, the needle is passed under the skin on the dorsal aspect of the toe and 1.5 mL of 1% lidocaine is injected as the needle is withdrawn from the skin. The needle is then introduced through the anesthetized skin on the dorsomedial aspect of the toe and advanced until it produces blanching of the plantar skin, at which time the needle is withdrawn and 1.5 mL of 1% lidocaine is injected. Usually, approximately 4.5 mL of 1% lidocaine is needed to anesthetize the hallux.

### Facial and Oral Blocks

Regional nerve blocks of the supraorbital, supratrochlear, lingual, mental, infraorbital, and greater auricular nerves are other simple and safe techniques worth remembering.

### Forehead

A regional nerve block of the forehead is accomplished with 3 to 6 mL of 1% lidocaine by raising a wheal above the nasion, after which the point of the 27-gauge needle is advanced under the skin immediately above the entire length of the eyebrow (Fig. 43-13).

### Inferior Alveolar and Lingual Nerve Block

The inferior alveolar nerve block, or mandibular block, anesthetizes the inferior teeth and gingiva on the side of the block. It often anesthetizes the ipsilateral lower lip as well. The lingual nerve is a general sensory nerve with added taste and secretory fibers from the chorda tympani. It supplies the anterior two thirds of the ipsilateral tongue, the floor of the mouth, and the gums. It enters the mouth between the medial pterygoid and the mandibular ramus. The lingual nerve can be anesthetized by using an inferior alveolar block by injecting anesthetic as the needle is removed. The block is initiated by first identifying the anterior border of the mandible (the oblique line). A 27-gauge needle is then inserted just medial to this line at a point that is approximately 1 cm above the occlusal surface of the second or third molar (Fig. 43-14). The introduction of a 27-gauge needle through the mucosa can be made painless by

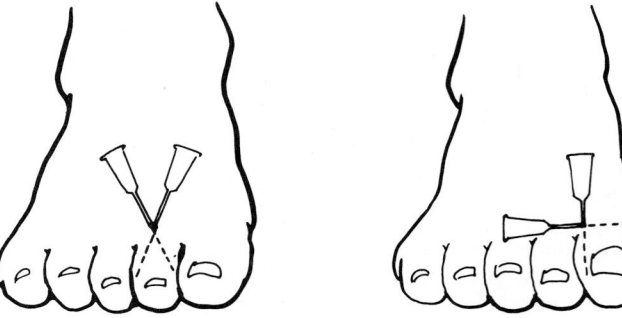

**Fig. 43-12.** (*Left*) Regional block of toe. (*Right*) Regional block of hallux (great toe).

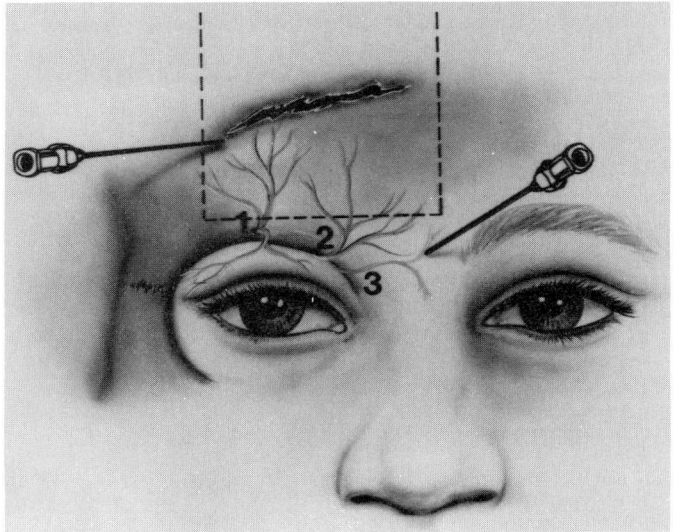

**Fig. 43-13.** Regional blocks of (1) the lateral branch of the frontal nerve, (2) the medial branch of the frontal nerve, and (3) the supratrochlear nerve. Infiltration anesthesia is an alternative approach to anesthetizing lacerations of the forehead.

the topical application of an anesthetic agent to the mucous membrane. Topical tetracaine (1%) is commonly used. After the mucosal injection site is anesthetized, the needle is slowly advanced along the medial side of the ramus to a depth of 2 cm. During the introduction of the needle, the syringe must lie parallel to the body of the mandible and the occlusal surfaces of the teeth of the lower jaw. From 2 to 4 mL of 1% lidocaine with epinephrine (1:100,000) is injected after the syringe is rotated to the premolar region of the medial side of the mandible, while the needle remains in contact with the ramus of the mandible. Alternate methods of anesthetizing the lingual nerve are by injecting anesthetic in the lateral floor of the mouth or just lingual to the premolar teeth. A regional block of the lingual nerve is the preferred route for administering anesthetics for patients with a deep laceration of the anterior tongue. It offers distinct advan-

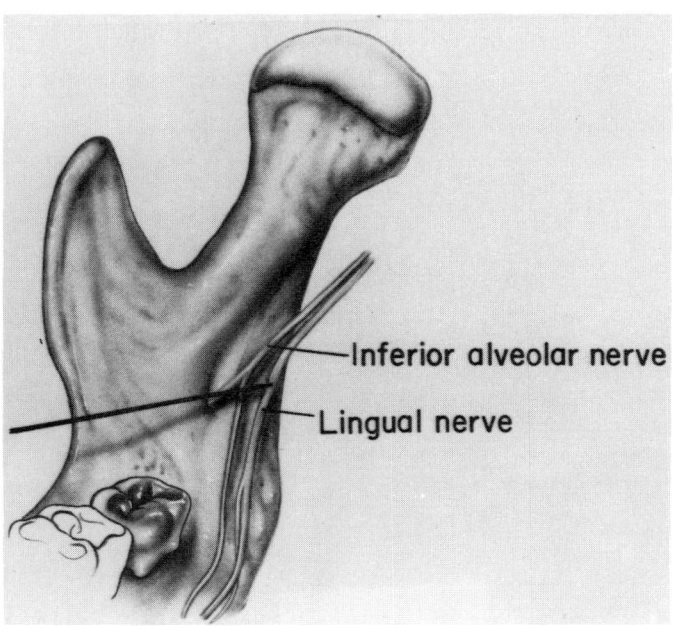

**Fig. 43-14.** Regional block of lingual nerve.

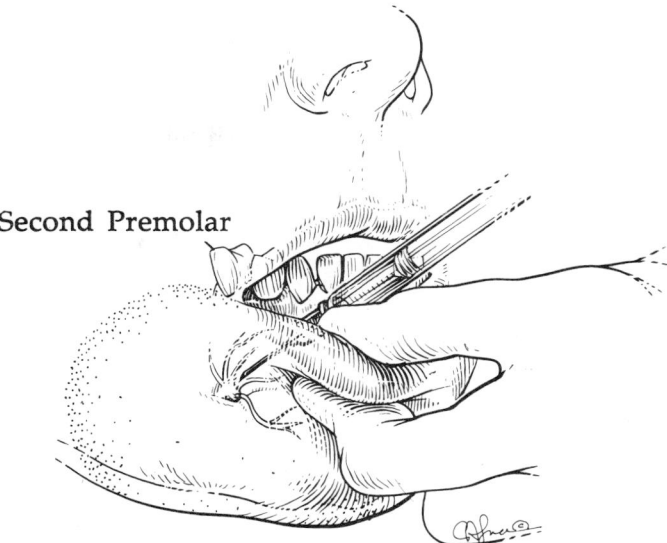

**Fig. 43-15.** Regional block of the mental nerve.

tages over infiltration anesthesia of the exquisitely sensitive moving tongue.

## Mental Nerve

The mental nerve supplies the skin and mucous membrane of the ipsilateral lower lip. A regional nerve block of the mental nerve at the mental foramen, however, is a practical method of anesthetizing lacerations of the lower lip (Fig. 43-15). A regional block of the mental nerve can be accomplished either extraorally or intraorally. In the latter case, the mucous membrane should be anesthetized by a topically applied local anesthetic agent before the needle is introduced. The mental foramen is located inside the lower lip at its junction with the lower gum, just posterior to the first premolar tooth. The needle is inserted at a point close to the mental foramen, after which 2 mL of 1% lidocaine with epinephrine (1:100,000) is injected. The needle is not introduced into the mental foramen to avoid inducing nerve injury with subsequent numbness of the lower lip.

## Infraorbital Nerve

The infraorbital nerve is the continuation of the maxillary nerve. After exiting through the orbital foramen, the infraorbital nerve divides to supply the skin of the lower eyelid, the side of the nose, the upper lip, and the mucous membrane lining the nasal vestibule. A regional nerve block of the infraorbital nerve can be accomplished either extraorally or intraorally. In the latter case (Fig. 43-16), the mucous membrane should be anesthetized by a topically applied anesthetic agent before the needle is introduced. The infraorbital nerve is identified by first palpating the midpoint of the lower border of the orbit with the tip of the long finger, after which the finger is then advanced caudad 1 cm to the site of the palpable neurovascular bundle that exits through the foramen. With the long finger remaining on the infraorbital foramen, the tips of the thumb and index finger grasp the upper lip and elevate it cephalad. A needle with syringe held in the other hand is introduced into the mucous membrane at its reflection from the upper gum until its point comes to lie under the tip of the long finger. The needle is directed parallel to the long axis of the second bicuspid tooth. The needle is not introduced directly into the infraorbital foramen to avoid nerve injury with subsequent numbness of the cheek. Regional anesthesia is accomplished by instilling 2 mL of 1% lidocaine with epinephrine

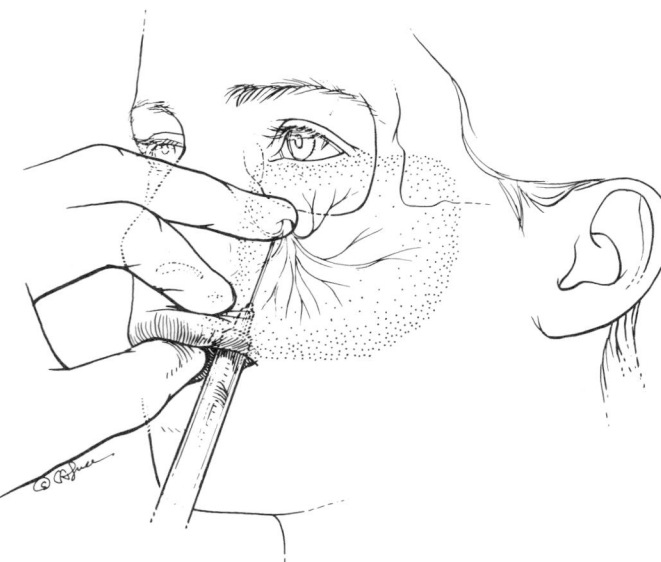

**Fig. 43-16.** Intraoral approach to regional nerve block of the infraorbital nerve.

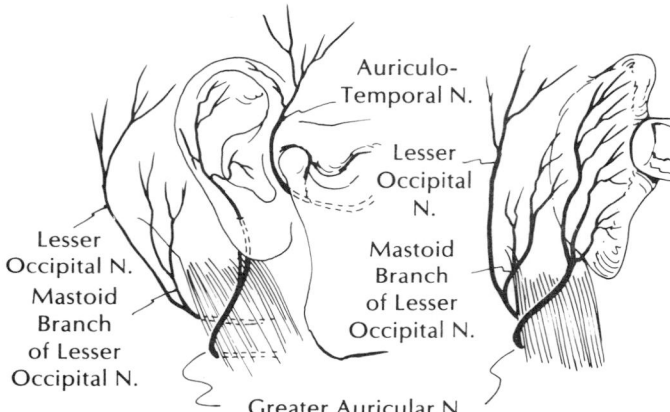

**Fig. 43-17.** Sensory nerve supply of the auricle.

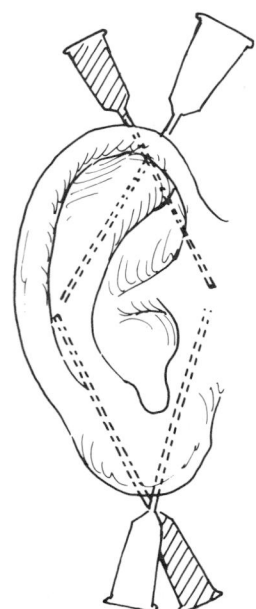

**Fig. 43-18.** Technique of regional anesthesia of the auricle.

(1:100,000). Care must be taken to avoid injecting the anesthetic agent into the facial artery and vein that are in close proximity to this nerve.

## Ear Block

The auricle is also susceptible to a regional nerve block. Its sensory supply stems mainly from the anterior and posterior branches of the greater auricular nerves, with lesser contributions from the auriculotemporal and lesser occipital nerves (Fig. 43-17). Regional anesthesia of auricle is accomplished readily by instilling the 1% lidocaine through a 27-gauge needle along its base anteriorly and posteriorly (Fig. 43-18). At times, a supplement may be needed at the posterior wall of the external auditory meatus, an area supplied by the auricular branches of the vagal nerve.

## BIBLIOGRAPHY

Altman RS, Smith-Coggins R, Ampel LL: Local anesthetics. *Ann Emerg Med* 14:1209, 1985.

Barker W, Rodeheaver GT, Edgerton MT, Edlich RF: Damage to the tissue defenses by a topical anesthetic agent. *Ann Emerg Med* 11:307, 1982.

Barfield JM, Ford DT, Homer PJ: Buffered versus plain lidocaine for digital nerve blocks. *Ann Emerg Med* 22:216, 1993.

Committee on Drugs. Guidelines for monitoring and management of pediatric patients during and after sedation for diagnostic and therapeutic procedures. *Pediatrics* 89:1110, 1992.

Dire DJ, Hogan DE: Double-blinded comparison of diphenhydramine versus lidocaine as a local anesthetic. *Ann Emerg Med* 22:1419, 1993.

Farris BL, Foresman PA, Rodeheaver GT, et al: Anesthetic properties and toxicity of bupivacaine and lidocaine for infiltration anesthesia. *J Emerg Med* 5:275, 1987.

Geant SAD, Hoffman RS: Use of tetracaine, epinephrine, and cocaine as a topical anesthetic in the emergency department. *Ann Emerg Med* 21:125, 1992.

Koop K, Trott A, Syverud S: Comparison of the digital versus metacarpal blocks for repair of finger injuries. *Ann Emerg Med* 23:1294, 1994.

Mader TJ, Playe SJ, Garb JL: Reducing the pain of local anesthetic infiltration: warming and buffering have a synergistic effect. *Ann Emerg Med* 23:550, 1994.

Powell DM, Rodeheaver GT, Foresman PA, et al: Damage to tissue defenses by EMLA® cream. *J Emerg Med* 9:205, 1991.

Schilling CG, Bank DE, Borchert BA, et al: Tetracaine, epinephrine (Adrenalin), and cocaine (TAC) versus Lidocaine, Epinephrine, and Tetracaine (LET) for anesthesia of lacerations in children. *Ann Emerg Med* 25:2, 1995. 203-208, February, 1995.

# 44

# WOUND PREPARATION

## Richard F. Edlich
## George T. Rodeheaver
## John G. Thacker

Wound preparation involves several therapeutic considerations that include hair removal, skin antisepsis, hemostasis, debridement, mechanical cleansing, antibiotics, and drains.

## HAIR REMOVAL

Hair is a source of wound contamination, and removal of hair prevents hair from becoming entangled in suture and the wound during closure. Hair removal can be minimized by clipping with scissors around the wound edges or by applying lubricant or ointments such as bacitracin to keep hair out of the wound edges. If large amounts of scalp hair must be removed for wound closure, consideration should be given to obtaining consent from the alert, oriented patient. Eyebrows should never be removed as part of wound preparation.

The infection rate in surgical wounds following razor preparation of the skin is significantly greatly than that after hair removal by electric clippers. This increased incidence of infection following razor preparation is probably related to the trauma inflicted by the razor. Wounded hair follicles provide access to and substrate for bacteria. Surgical electric clippers cut hair close to the skin surface without nicking the skin, and we now employ only electric clippers when it is necessary to remove hair. We use a surgical clipper with a disposable clipper blade assembly to remove extensive amounts of hair from the skin around the wound.[1] This clipper has no sharp edges that can contact or abrade the skin if the clipper is pressed against a soft skin surface without underlying bony support (abdomen, buttock, etc.) or if the clipper is held so that its blades are perpendicular to the skin surface. Because the blade assembly is simply detached from the power source after use and replaced with a new, clean clipper assembly for the next patient, this surgical clipper and disposable clipper blade assembly do not require cleaning and associated assembly or disassembly of the clipper blade.

Hair provides an important landmark for the precise reapproximation of the divided tissue. This is particularly true in the eyebrow, where misalignment of the wound edges may be exceedingly difficult to correct at a later date.

## SKIN ANTISEPSIS

Disinfection of the skin around the wound should be initiated without contacting the wound itself. Two groups of antiseptic agents, containing either an iodophor or chlorhexidine, exhibit activity against a broad spectrum of organisms and suppress bacterial proliferation. The superiority of one antiseptic agent over another has not been shown. Although these agents can reduce the bacterial concentration on intact skin, they appear to damage the wound defenses and invite the development of infection within the wound itself. Consequently, inadvertent spillage of these agents into the wound should be avoided.

[1] 3M Center, St. Paul, MN

This research was supported by a generous gift from the Ira W. DeCamp Foundation, New York, NY.

## HEMOSTASIS

During any wounding process, blood vessels will be divided resulting in bleeding into the wound. The magnitude of blood loss is directly related to the size of the divided vessels. Fortunately, most bleeding can be stopped by applying direct pressure to saline-soaked lint-free sponges placed within the wound. Rubbing or abrading the wound must be avoided, because this dislodges thrombi and may cause further bleeding.

Following removal of the gauze sponges, persistent bleeding from vessels whose diameter is less than 2 mm should be stopped by pinpoint electrosurgical coagulation. The use of bipolar coagulation is a more precise method of hemostasis that limits the tissue injury encountered with the more traditional monopolar coagulation. An equivalent current passed through a monopolar electrode causes approximately three times as much necrosis of the surrounding tissue as the use of bipolar coagulation. Bleeding from cut ends of large vessels whose diameter is over 2 mm can rarely be controlled by electrocoagulation. In such cases, hemostasis can be achieved easily with a suture ligature of nonreactive synthetic absorbable braided suture materials. The divided end of the vessel should be isolated over a short length and clamped with a small curved hemostat. This technique is preferred over clamping the retracted vessel along with the contiguous bloodstained tissue. In the latter case, the amount of strangulated tissue is about five times greater than with the vessel-isolating technique.

Occasionally, as with a patient with a bleeding diathesis, primary wound closure cannot be accomplished because of persistent bleeding. In such cases, the wound should be packed with type I gauze sponges and elevated, if the anatomic site of the wound allows. The wound should then be reexamined within 24 hours to determine if hemostasis is now sufficient to allow primary closure. Prior to closure, any residual hematoma should be evacuated from the wound because it can serve as a culture medium for bacteria.

## SURGICAL DEBRIDEMENT

Debridement removes tissue heavily contaminated by soil infection-potentiating fractions and bacteria and excises devitalized tissues that impair the wound's ability to resist infection. The capacity of devitalized fat, muscle, and skin to enhance bacterial infection is comparable. However, as little tissue should be debrided as possible.

Devitalized soft tissue enhances infection by acting as an anaerobic culture medium promoting bacterial growth, and by inhibiting phagocytosis. Identification of the exact limits of devitalized tissue in wounds remains a challenging problem, especially in muscle. Viability of muscle can be determined by the "4C" guidelines (color, consistency, contraction, circulation). Generations of physicians have identified nonviable muscle by its dark color, its mushy consistency, its failure to contract when pinched with forceps, and the absence of brisk bleeding from its cut surface. These clinical indicators of muscle viability are most accurate when the wound is examined 4 to 5 days after the initial operation.

The viability of skin is considerably easier to judge than that of muscle. At 24 h after injury, a sharp line of demarcation is often apparent between the devitalized and viable skin. For fresh skin wounds in which this demarcation is not precise, as little tissue should be removed as possible.

In some anatomic sites, like the trunk, debridement is best accomplished by more complete excision of the skin and deep tissues. The soft tissues are usually free of specialized tissues, such as nerves or tendons, that perform important physical functions. In these regions, heavily contaminated wounds with serpiginous defects can be converted into clean wounds by more generous tissue excisions.

The adequacy of debridement may be monitored either by forcibly packing the wound with gauze or by coloring the wound surface with a vital dye (Fig. 44-1). Complete excision of the wound, back to a

## Gauze

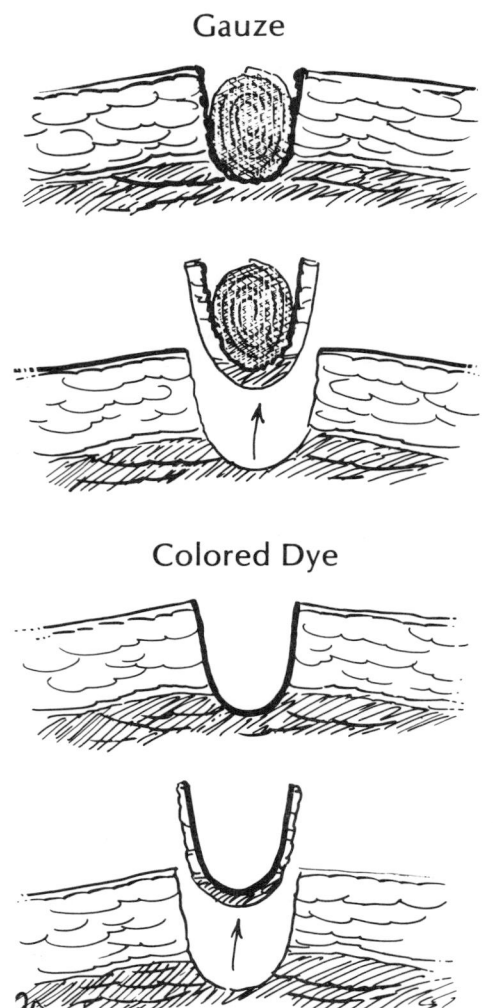

## Colored Dye

**Fig. 44-1.** Monitoring the adequacy of debridement by forcibly packing the wound with gauze (top) or by coloring the wound surface with a vital dye (bottom).

margin of normal tissue, is judged by dissecting in a plane that does not expose the gauze or the blue dye. Suturing the skin edges of the wound prior to excision may further minimize mechanical spread of the wound contaminants into uninjured tissue.

When a heavily contaminated wound contains specialized tissues, such as nerves or tendons, consultation is recommended. A specific exception to the general principle of removing all devitalized tissue is made in treating specialized tissues that perform important physical functions, regardless of their viability. Tissues like dura, fascia, and tendon may survive as free grafts without living cells if immediately covered by healthy pedicle flaps. Cells from the wound may then invade the graft as part of the healing process. If these tissues can be rendered surgically clean, they should be left in the wound.

Following debridement, the selection of wound closure technique is dependent on the level of wound contamination and the amount of residual devitalized tissue. In wounds contacted by gross pus or feces, an infective dose of bacteria often remains on the wound surface despite the most aggressive wound cleaning. Infection can be minimized by utilizing delayed primary closure. As the wound heals, it gains increased resistance to infection, permitting closure on or after the fourth postwounding day without subsequent infections.

For high-energy-depositor missile injuries, tissue injury is extensive and difficult to ascertain accurately soon after injury. In these cases, the wound should be explored in the operating theater to re-

move devitalized tissue and foreign bodies, to rule out damage to vessels and nerves, and to relieve increased compartmental pressure that may follow edema or slow bleeding into a fascia-enclosed muscle compartment. Open wound management is the method of choice.

Civilian traumatic wounds resulting from impact injuries usually contain devitalized tissue that is easily recognized. Debridement, cleansing, and antibiotic treatment usually convert these wounds into clean wounds, which are amenable to primary closure either by direct approximation of the wound edges or by coverage with a flap or graft.

Debridement of skin and underlying tissue leaves a significant soft tissue defect that resists reapproximation. As a result of strong static skin tensions on the edges of the debrided wound, repair is accomplished with a wide scar. In general, extensive wound debridement is best performed in an operating room theater with adequate lighting and surgical instruments.

## MECHANICAL CLEANSING

Mechanical forces are employed to rid the wound of bacteria and other particulate matter that are retained on the wound surface by adhesive forces. The two techniques used are irrigation and scrubbing. Low-pressure irrigation can be used for clean wounds, and high-pressure irrigation should be reserved for dirty or heavily contaminated wounds. High-pressure irrigation is defined as 7 psi, and low-pressure as 0.5 psi.

The magnitude of the hydraulic forces is a function of the relative velocities and the configuration of the particle. When subjected to the same irrigating stream, particles with a smaller frontal surface area experience less force than particles with a similar configuration, but with a greater surface area. Consequently it takes significantly smaller hydraulic pressures to rid the wound of large foreign bodies that it does to remove small particles and bacteria.

The level of hydraulic forces experienced by the particle is also increased considerably as the velocity of the irrigating stream is raised. The simplest and most practical methods of raising the velocity are to increase the pressure within the irrigating syringe and to enlarge the internal diameter of the needle or catheter.

The pressure experienced by a wound surface from fluid delivered from a 19-gauge needle and 35-mL syringe is 7 psi. In contrast, the pressure encountered by a surface irrigated by a bulb syringe is only 0.5 psi.

The bacterial removal efficiency of the irrigating stream is proportional to the pressure experienced by the wound surface. High-pressure irrigation with a 35-mL syringe attached to a 19-gauge needle operated manually by one hand effectively decreases the level of bacterial contamination. The cleansing effect of the bulb syringe irrigation is negligible because the wound bacterial concentration is not significantly affected by this low-pressure irrigation system. High-pressure syringe irrigation markedly reduces the incidence of wound infection in contaminated wounds.

Continuous high-pressure irrigation is an effective means of removing soil infection-potentiating factors in dirt from the wound. High-pressure irrigation removes 80 percent of the soil infection-potentiating factors from the wound. Changing the composition of the wound irrigant by adding chelating agents, flocculants, and dispersants or a nonionic surfactant does not significantly enhance the efficiency of removal of soil infection-potentiating factors from wounds.

In the clinical setting, high-pressure irrigation is accomplished with an inexpensive disposable irrigation assembly consisting of a 19-gauge plastic needle or catheter attached to a 35-mL syringe (Fig. 44-2). Sterile electrolyte solution (usually 1000 mL of 0.9% sodium chloride) is delivered through a one-way valve attached to the syringe barrel via standard intravenous plastic tubing. The tip of the needle, fastened to the syringe filled with saline, is placed perpendicular, and as close as possible, to the surface of the wound; then the plunger is depressed.

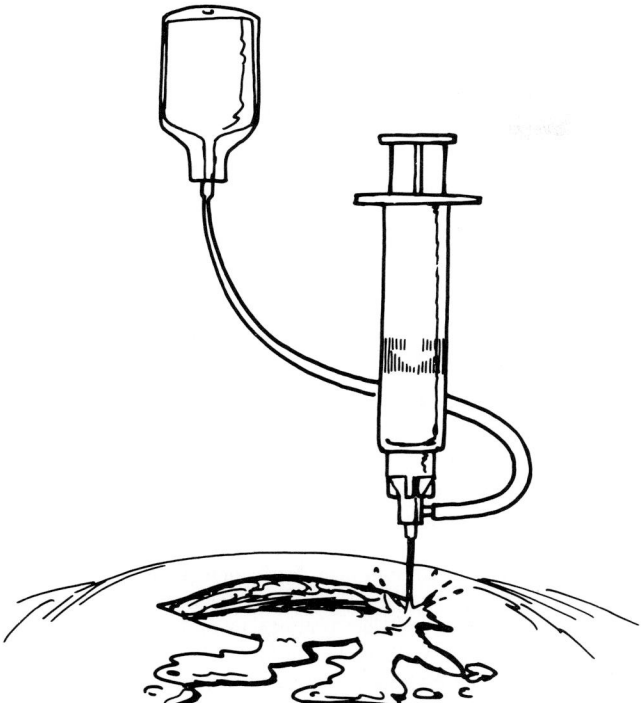

**Fig. 44-2.** High-pressure syringe irrigation assembly. Note that the needle is held as close as possible and perpendicular to the surface of the wound during wound irrigation.

The benefits of high-pressure irrigation must be weighed against potential side effects. In our studies, high-pressure irrigation does not enhance the dissemination of bacteria into soft-tissue wounds. However, the irrigation fluid disseminates into the interstices of the wound, predominantly in a lateral direction. This lateral spread occurs within the loose areolar tissue, contributing to the development of postoperative edema. Consequently, high-pressure irrigation does make the wound more susceptible to infection, so that this technique should be reserved for contaminated wounds.

The occupational risk to the emergency physician of exposure to human immunodeficiency virus or hepatitis virus by virtue of accidental splashing of the irrigant is another potential complication. Several techniques, such as cupping the gloved hand around the wound and irrigating through the space between the thumb and index finger, are recommended to reduce splatter. Recently, a cuplike device was marketed to prevent splatter while allowing irrigation with appropriate pressures. Another solution to splashing is to position the tip of the blunt-ended plastic catheter perpendicular to and in contact with the wound surface. This intimate contact of the catheter with the wound diminishes splashing and ensures that the maximum wound irrigation force is used to decontaminate the wound.

While scrubbing is an effective means of removing bacteria from wounds, tissue trauma inflicted by scrubbing impairs the wound's ability to resist infection and allows residual bacteria to elicit an inflammatory response. Sponges with a low porosity are more abrasive and exert more damage to the wound than sponges with a higher porosity. Saline solution is a very effective agent and is the most widely used. We feel that the addition of a nontoxic surfactant, poloxamer 188, to a fine-pore sponge, minimizes the tissue damage it inflicts while maintaining the bacterial removal efficiency of mechanical cleansing.

Poloxamer 188[2] is so innocuous that it can be used to soak an unanesthetized wound without discomfort to the patient. Toxic

effects and allergic reactions are very rare, and poloxamer 188 does not alter the wound's resistance to infection and healing, or the cellular components of blood. However, it exhibits no antibacterial activity.

Exposure of the wound to either Hibiclens[3] or Betadine Surgical Scrub Solution[4] (which contains detergent) causes pain or irritation and damages tissue defenses, inviting infection.

Embedded foreign debris should be removed as soon as possible.

Removal of embedded foreign particles requires either local or regional anesthesia. A natural fiber scrub brush soaked in saline or poloxamer 188 removes the embedded debris from most wounds. When the embedded particles remain in the wound despite wound cleansing in the emergency department, the patient should be transferred to the operating room to remove these particles. Power-driven abraders with stainless steel cylinders coated with tungsten carbide grit can also be used to dislodge these foreign bodies. When isolated foreign bodies are embedded deeply in the deep dermal tissue, a no. 11 scalpel blade can be used as a spud to tease or excise these particles individually. An operating room microscope enhances visualization of the particles allowing prompt, aggressive, and meticulous removal. Wound closure is accomplished with a single 8–0 monofilament synthetic nonabsorbable suture. The debrided wound is covered by fine-mesh gauze (type I) that is impregnated with bacitracin ointment. This antibiotic is reapplied every 6 h for approximately 3 to 4 days, when the gauze spontaneously separates from the underlying healing epidermis. If the foreign debris is not removed immediately, it becomes impossible to trace the paths and remove the individual particles in the depths of the dermis, resulting in a permanent traumatic tattoo.

## ANTIBIOTICS

The relative success of antibiotic therapy in the prevention of infection in wounds is influenced by the time of administration, the concentration of bacteria in the wound, the presence of soil infection-potentiating fractions, and the mechanism of injury. In laboratory and clinical studies, antibiotic therapy is significantly more effective when the drug is administered preoperatively rather than intraoperatively or postoperatively. Delay in antibiotic treatment diminishes its therapeutic merit. When there is an unavoidable delay in administering these drugs, the length of time during which the wound is left open becomes significant. Exposure causes a sequence of events that substantially limits the therapeutic value of antibiotics.

When any wound is left open, its vessels exhibit a marked increase in vascular permeability. Fluids from the intravascular space extravasate and fill the wound crater. This exudate is rich in a wide variety of proteins, including fibrinogen. Once outside the vessels, much of the protein exudate is reabsorbed and partly polymerizes to form fibrin. This resulting fibrinous coagulum surrounds the bacteria and protects them from contact with the antibiotic. The cause of this exaggerated inflammatory response in the open wound has not been defined. However, it may be related to environmental conditions. The temperature of the emergency department is usually considerably below the systemic body temperature, encouraging loss of heat from the wound. In addition, evaporation of fluid from the wound surface results in further heat loss and cooling of the tissues. A consequence of fluid heat loss from the wound is desiccation. Warming the treatment room or covering the wound with wet sponges should reduce these environmental effects. Paradoxically, the fibrinous wound coagulum, which limits the effectiveness of antibiotics, may be a crucial positive factor in the host's defense against infection. The coagulum may serve as a plug in the open mouths of lymphatics, preventing dissemination of bacteria. Occlusion of lymphatics by the coagulum then be-

[2] Calgon Corporation, St. Louis, Mo.

[3] Stuart Pharmaceuticals, Wilmington, Del.

[4] Purdue Frederick, Norwalk, Conn.

comes an obstacle to the invasion of bacteria and, in part, accounts for the resistance of an open wound to systemic sepsis. This surface coagulum may be disrupted by mechanical forces. Gentle scrubbing of the surface of the wound with a gauze sponge disturbs the fibrinous cover and allows an antibiotic to gain intimate contact with the bacteria. Consequently, the therapeutic effectiveness of antibiotics is measurably enhanced by this treatment.

The presence of wound contaminants can influence the outcome of antibiotic therapy. When the wound is contaminated by an exceedingly large number of organisms ($> 10^9$), infection will develop despite antibiotic treatment. This circumstance is encountered when the wound surface is contacted by either pus, feces, vaginal discharge, or saliva. Soil infection-potentiating fractions in wounds also have considerable influence on the efficacy of specific antibiotics. The benefit of antibiotics in the presence of these fractions is predicted by the chemical composition of the antibiotic. The basic antibiotics (e.g., gentamicin) and amphoteric antibiotics (e.g., tetracycline) are inactivated by these negatively charged fractions. The acidic antibiotics, like cephalosporins and penicillin, do not bind with these fractions and thus exert their antibacterial effect in wounds contaminated by them. Finally, impact injuries result in a demonstrable reduction in blood flow to the wound edges, limiting the access of systemically administered antibiotics. Thus the efficacy of antibiotic therapy in impact wounds is substantially less than in wounds caused by shear forces.

## Antibiotic Prophylaxis

Antibiotic prophylaxis has therapeutic merit in several clinical settings. Whenever it can be anticipated that microorganisms might gain access to the circulation of the patient, appropriate antimicrobial agents should be given immediately during and after the period of risk (Table 44-1). When pretreatment is impossible, as in the case of lacerations or infections, intravenous injection of antibiotics should be instituted as soon as possible. The intravenous route is preferred over the intramuscular route because it results in reliable antibiotic concentrations without precipitating intramuscular bleeding in the anticoagulated patient. Because bacterial endocarditis is associated with significant morbidity and mortality, its prevention by antibiotic treatment has been a universally accepted and worthwhile goal.

*Staphylococcus aureus* and *S. epidermidis* are the pathogens most often responsible for soft tissue infections resulting in bacterial endocarditis. Because most *S. aureus* isolates, whether community- or hospital-acquired, are resistant to penicillin, the current recommended regimen for preventing infective endocarditis includes either

**Table 44-1.** Indications for Antibiotic Prophylaxis in Wounds

High-risk anatomic site—i.e., forefoot, hand
Contaminated wounds
   Bodily fluids
   Organic matter or dirt
Wounds with devitalized tissue
Extensive soft tissue injury
Stellate lacerations
Lacerations >5 cm
Indwelling prosthetic devices
Endocarditis prophylaxis needed for
   Prosthetic heart valves
   Arteriovenous fistula
   Patent ductus arteriosus
   Tetralogy of Fallot
   Ventricular septal defect
   Coarctation of the aorta
   Valvular heart disease
Lymphedema
Immunocompromised patients
Peripheral vascular disease

**Table 44-2.** Suggestions for Prophylaxis of Infective Endocarditis

| Adults | Children |
|---|---|
| PATIENTS NOT ALLERGIC TO CEFAZOLIN | |
| Cefazolin 2.0 g IV | Cefazolin 30 mg/kg IV |
| *plus* | *plus* |
| Gentamicin 1.5 mg/kg IV | Gentamicin 2.0 mg/kg IV |
| Give initial dose immediately, then repeat both drugs every 8 h for five additional doses. | Give initial dose immediately, then repeat both drugs every 8 h for five additional doses. |
| PATIENTS ALLERGIC TO CEFAZOLIN | |
| Vancomycin 0.5–1.0 g IV infused slowly over 1 h | Vancomycin 20 mg/kg infused slowly over 1 h |
| *plus* | *plus* |
| Gentamicin 1.5 mg/kg IV | Gentamicin 2.0 mg/kg IV |
| Both drugs may be repeated 12 h later. | Both drugs may be repeated 12 h later. |

a penicillinase-resistant penicillin, or a cephalosporin (Table 44-2). In patients who are allergic to penicillin, vancomycin is an appropriate alternative. The addition of gentamicin produces a synergistic effect against *S. aureus* in vitro and in experimental staphylococcal endocarditis in rabbits.

The choice of an appropriate regimen to prevent bacterial endocarditis when *S. epidermidis* is the etiologic agent is complicated by the unpredictable and high frequency of multiple methicillin-resistant strains. In some institutions, these resistant strains account for 70 to 90 percent of the *S. epidermidis* causing bacterial endocarditis. There is probably no satisfactory antimicrobial regimen to prevent infective endocarditis due to methicillin-resistant *S. epidermidis,* but recent in vitro studies suggest that an aminoglycoside with a cephalosporin may be helpful. If the patient is allergic to the cephalosporin, vanocomycin can be used.

Convincing cases of hematogenous infections of arterial grafts (those appearing more than 60 days after surgery) are nearly unknown. Almost all reported infections probably originated from contamination at surgery, from contiguous areas of purulence, or from the development of a fistula between the graft and the GI tract. Even in hip arthroplasties, the sources of infection have been distant sites of established suppuration, such as tonsillitis, cholecystitis, dental abscess, pyoderma, suppurative parotitis, or cystitis, rather than procedure-induced transient bacteremia. These findings emphasize the importance of prompt and thorough treatment of distant infections in patients with indwelling prosthetic devices.

Lymphedematous patients and those with peripheral vascular disease are especially likely to develop infection. A streptococcus or, less often, a staphylococcus can be isolated from the infected tissue. Each infection produces more lymphatic destruction and edema. When a minor soft tissue laceration occurs in lymphedematous or vascular compromised tissue, antimicrobial treatment should be initiated immediately before wound closure.

Antibiotic prophylaxis should be considered for the immunocompromised patient with a wound. Primary immunodeficiency defects are defects in cellular differentiation and are classified according to whether the prominent defect is in neutrophil or T- or B-cell function. Most immunosuppression in emergency department patients is acquired secondary to disease process (e.g., malnutrition, diabetes, renal failure) or medical interventions (e.g., immunosuppressive medications). Wound infections in such patients are caused by common pathogens such as *S. aureus* and mixed bacterial species. There may, however, be a delayed onset of infection.

Antibiotic treatment of soft tissue lacerations is also advocated when the probability of infection is high (equal to or more than 10 percent). Several factors have been identified that increase the likelihood of infection. The anatomic site is one of the most important. Wounds of the forefoot are especially prone to infection, whereas facial and scalp wounds are rarely infected. The appearance of the wound is a reliable index of its risk for infections. Wounds that are judged to be dirty or contaminated exhibit a higher incidence of infection than do clean wounds. Moreover, experimental studies demonstrate that stellate lacerations with abrasions of the skin adjacent to the wound are much more infection-prone than are linear lacerations. The weakened local tissue defenses of stellate lacerations make them susceptible to the development of infection by a relatively small inoculum.

The length of the wound may be another important consideration. In our review of clinical studies, the infection rate of long wounds (5 cm or longer) was greater than that of short ones. Another indication for antibiotic treatment of a soft tissue laceration is a delay in wound cleansing and repair for 6 h or more.

Antibiotic treatment is also indicated in a patient with a wound contaminated by either saliva, feces, or vaginal secretions. Antibiotic treatment can reduce the number of bacteria in such heavily contaminated wounds, but a significant number of organisms often persists, resulting in a high incidence of infection. Consequently the most reliable method of preventing the development of infection in such wounds is open wound management.

Antibiotics must be administered to patients with wounds in which the magnitude of tissue injury is extensive and difficult to ascertain accurately soon after injury. In such cases, open wound management is the method of choice with subsequent additional debridement as dictated by the appearance of the wound. Antibiotic therapy is an adjunct to debridement, rather than a replacement. In all missile injuries, adequate blood levels of penicillin or an antibiotic (cephalosporin) with a similar spectrum of activity should be established as soon as possible after wounding to prevent streptococcal bacteremia. Streptolysin produced by the virulent streptococcal species breaks down the fibrin that has been deposited in the body in an attempt to wall off collections of bacterial pathogens.

When antibiotic treatment of soft tissue lacerations is indicated, a number of therapeutic guidelines for antibiotic usage must be considered. The immediate selection of the specific antimicrobial agent is based on consideration of the results of direct microscopic examination of a wound biopsy, the normal bacterial flora harbored in different parts of the body, and the pathogens usually encountered in various diseases or conditions. Later, the results of immediate antibiotic sensitivity testing can also influence the emergency physician's choice of antibiotic. Antibiotic sensitivity testing is performed under aerobic conditions directly on the bacterial suspension prepared from the wound biopsy specimen rather than on strains isolated from the tissue. Because soft tissue wounds are contaminated by mixtures of facultative organisms, a broad-spectrum antibiotic must be chosen. The antibiotic should be present in the wound tissue fluid in an effective concentration at the time of wound closure. Consequently, the antibiotics should be administered by an intravenous route that results in high tissue concentrations.

## DRAINS

Drainage evacuates potentially harmful collections of certain fluids, such as pus and blood, from wounds. In instances in which no definite localized fluid exists, drainage is prophylactic and its potentially harmful effects become more important. Drains act as retrograde conduits through which skin contaminants gain entrance into the wound. Placement of drains within experimental wounds exposed to subinfective inoculations of bacteria greatly enhanced the rate of infection compared with undrained controls. In our experience, both Silastic and Penrose drains dramatically increased the infection rate of soft tissue wounds. The rate of infection when the drain was brought out through the wound was similar to the rate when the drain lay entirely within the wound, suggesting a deleterious effect of the drain per se.

## BIBLIOGRAPHY

Advisory Committee on Immunization Practices (ACIP): Update of adult immunization. *MMWR* 40 (No. RR-12):1, 1991.

Custer J, Edlich RF, Prusak M, et al: Studies in the management of the contaminated wound. V. An assessment of the effectiveness of pHisoHex and Betadine surgical scrub solutions. *Am J Surg* 121:572, 1971.

Edlich RF, Thacker JG: Wound irrigation. *Ann Emerg Med* 24(1):88, 1994.

Edlich RF, Kenney JG, Morgan RF, et al: Antimicrobial treatment of minor soft tissue lacerations: A critical review. *Emerg Med Clin North Am* 4:560, 1986.

Magee C, Rodeheaver GT, Golden GT, et al: Potentiation of wound infection by surgical drains. *Am J Surg* 131:547, 1976.

Masterson TS, Rodeheaver GT, Morgan RF, et al: Bacteriologic evaluation of electric clipper for surgical hair removal. *Am J Surg* 148:301, 1984.

# 45
# METHODS FOR WOUND CLOSURE

**Richard F. Edlich**
**George T. Rodeheaver**
**John G. Thacker**

After wound cleansing, the physical integrity and function of the injured tissue must be restored. The technique of wound closure selected depends on the type of wound. Primary closure can be accomplished with clean wounds without tissue loss. For wounds with associated tissue loss, grafts or flaps are often required to close the defect. These procedures are usually performed in the operating room.

Infected or heavily contaminated wounds, and wounds resulting from high-energy-depositor missile injuries, should be left open until delayed closure can be undertaken. Wounds contaminated by pus, vaginal discharge, feces, or saliva, as well as those in which treatment is delayed longer than 6 h, should also be considered for open wound management.

Open wound management prior to delayed primary closure is accomplished by packing the wound with sterile fine-meshed gauze (type I) that is then covered by a sterile dressing. The wound should not be disturbed for the first 4 days after injury unless the patient develops an unexplained fever. Unnecessary inspection during this period increases the risk of contamination and subsequent infection. On or after the fourth day after wounding, the wound margins can be inspected. In the absence of infection and devitalized tissue, the wound edges can be approximated with minimal risk of infection.

Once it is decided to close the wound, a closure technique must be selected that allows the most accurate and secure approximation of the skin edges. Suturing is the oldest and most popular method. However, specially designed surgical tapes and staples, more recent innovations, have important roles in skin wound closure. The closure method should hold tissue in apposition until the strength of the wound is sufficient to withstand stress.

## SUTURES

Important considerations in skin closure are the type of suture, the tying technique, and the configuration of the suture loops. Selection of

This research was supported by a generous gift from Mr. Roger Milliken & Co., Spartanburg, South Carolina.

a suture material is based on its biologic interaction with the wound as well as its mechanical performance in vivo and in vitro. Sutures are divided into two general classes on the basis of their in vivo degradation: (1) Sutures that undergo rapid degradation in tissues, losing their tensile strength within 60 days, are considered "absorbable" sutures. (2) Sutures that maintain their tensile strength for longer than 60 days are "nonabsorbable" sutures. This terminology is somewhat misleading, because some so-called nonabsorbable sutures (e.g., silk, cotton, and nylon) lose some tensile strength during this 60-day interval. Silk loses approximately one-half of its tensile strength in 1 year and has no strength at the end of 2 years. Cotton loses 50 percent of its strength in 6 months, but still has 30 to 40 percent of its strength at the end of 2 years. Nylon loses approximately 25 percent of its original strength over 2 years.

Nonabsorbable sutures can be classified according to their origin. Nonabsorbable sutures made from natural fibers include silk, cotton, and linen. Metallic sutures are derived from stainless steel. There are a variety of synthetic fibers: polyamides (nylon), polyesters (Dacron), polyolefins [polyethylene, polypropylene (PP)], polytetrafluoroethylene (PTFE), and polybutester. Polybutester is a block copolymer that contains poly(butylene)terephthalate (84 percent) and poly(tetramethylene ether)glycol terephthalate (16 percent). The PTFE suture has been expanded to produce a porous microstructure that is approximately 50 percent air by volume. Nonabsorbable sutures may also be classified according to their physical configuration. Sutures constructed from one filament are called monofilament sutures (nylon, PP, polybutester, PTFE, and stainless steel); sutures containing multiple fibers are called multifilament sutures (nylon, polyester, stainless steel, silk, and cotton). Only nylon and stainless steel sutures are available as both monofilament and multifilament sutures.

Absorbable sutures are made from either collagen or synthetic polymers. Collagen sutures are derived either from the submucosa of ovine or bovine small intestine (gut suture) or from reconstituted collagen manufactured from bovine tendon collagen (collagen suture). This collagenous tissue is treated in an aldehyde solution which cross-links and strengthens the suture and makes it more resistant to enzymatic degradation. Suture materials treated in this way are called plain gut or plain collagen. If the suture is additionally treated in chromium trioxide, it becomes chromic gut or chromic collagen, which is more highly cross-linked and more resistant to absorption than plain gut or collagen. The shortcomings of collagen and gut sutures include variable strength and unpredictable absorption.

Synthetic substitutes for collagen sutures are produced from polyglactin 910 or polyglycolic acid. These high-molecular-weight polymers are extruded into thin filaments and made into braided sutures which lose their strength in tissues during a 4-week period after implantation.

Two other synthetic absorbable monofilament sutures, polydioxanone and glycolide trimethylene carbonate, retain approximately 70 percent of their breaking strength after implantation for 28 days. The chemical degradation of these synthetic absorbable sutures is by a predictable and uniform hydrolysis of their ester bonds.

All sutures compromise the local tissue defenses against infection. Several mechanisms are implicated:

1. The trauma of inserting a needle is sufficient to cause an inflammatory response.
2. Sutures tied too tightly impair blood flow and cause tissue necrosis.
3. Sutures that penetrate the intact skin provide an avenue for wound contamination via the perisutural cuff.
4. The quantity of suture and the chemical reactivity of the material affect the susceptibility to infection.

The infection-potentiating effects of suture materials are listed in Table 45-1. The infection-potentiating effect of polybutester suture has not been measured.

**Table 45-1.** Infection-Potentiating Effect of Surgical Sutures*

| Absorbable | Nonabsorbable |
|---|---|
| Synthetic absorbable | Nylon, PP, PTFE |
| Plain gut | Dacron (coated, noncoated) |
| Chromic gut | Metal |
| | Silk, cotton |

* The least reactive suture materials are listed first.

The relatively high infection rates encountered with either monofilament or multifilament stainless steel sutures may be the result of their chemical or physical configuration. Stainless steel is not generally as inert as pure polymers and undergoes degradation in vivo. In addition, metallic sutures are so stiff that patient movement induces tissue damage that impairs the wound's ability to resist infection. Sutures made of natural fibers may potentiate infection more than other nonabsorbable sutures, and should be avoided in contaminated wounds. The incidence of infection from monofilament sutures is less than that of multifilament sutures constructed from comparable materials.

There are two techniques for sutural closure of skin: percutaneous and dermal (subcuticular). Percutaneous sutures are passed through the epidermal and dermal layers of skin. Dermal, or subcuticular, sutures reapproximate the divided edges of the dermis without penetrating the epidermis. Occasionally, dermal and percutaneous sutures are used together. Either type can be used as a continuous ("running") suture or as an interrupted suture.

Percutaneous sutures of either monofilament nylon or PP are excellent for skin closure because these materials have the least effect on the wound defenses. Polybutester sutures have unique performance characteristics that may be advantageous for wound closure. With this type of suture, low forces yield significantly greater elongation than with other sutures. In addition, polybutester sutures have superior elasticity, allowing the suture to return to its original length once the load is removed. In a clinical setting in which the tied suture loops are enlarged by the edema of the wound and yet are expected to return to their original length once the edema disappears, the performance of the polybutester suture would be expected to be superior to that of other sutures. Sutures with less extensibility under low forces, like nylon, PP, polyester, or silk, will frequently lacerate or necrose the encircled tissue, thereby increasing its susceptibility to infection.

Percutaneous sutures are recommended for closure of stellate lacerations resulting from crush injuries. In these wounds, meticulous closure with percutaneous sutures approximates the skin edges more exactly than does tape. Closing these wounds is often like putting together a jigsaw puzzle, and tapes have little practical value. The more accurate approximation of skin edges by skillfully applied sutures leads to a more pleasing cosmetic result.

Because the magnitude of the damage to the local tissue defenses is related to the quantity of the suture within the wound (that is, diameter and length), we use the suture with the narrowest diameter (5–0 or 6–0) whose strength is sufficient to resist disruption of the closure. Approximating the midportion and the bisected portions of the unclosed wound with percutaneous sutures allows the least length of suture to be used in the skin closure. An interrupted dermal suture placed in each quadrant of the wound subjected to strong static and dynamic skin tensions provides sufficient strength to permit early suture removal.

It is important to mention that sutural closure of the adipose tissue beneath the skin should be avoided. Obliteration of this potential dead space between the cut edge of adipose tissue by even the least reactive suture increases the incidence of infection.

When wounds of different thickness are to be reunited, the needle should be passed through one edge of the wound and then drawn out before reentry through the other edge. This maneuver ensures that the needle is inserted at comparable levels on each side of the wound. Unless appropriate adjustment of the bite is made on the thinner side,

**Fig. 45-1.** **A.** Epithelial cells migrate downward, forming a perisutural cuff. **B.** If percutaneous sutures are not removed before the eighth day after surgery, the invasive spurs of epithelium result in needle puncture scars.

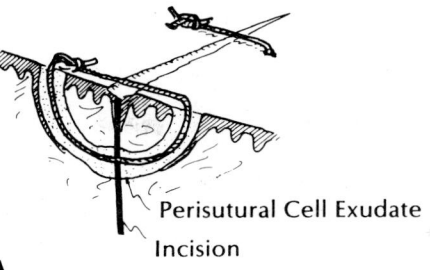

Perisutural Cell Exudate

Incision

**A**

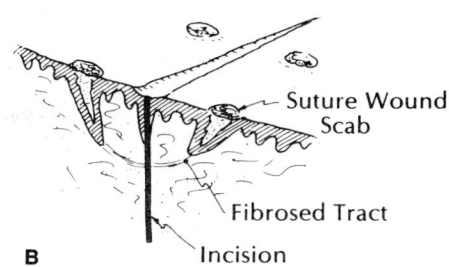

Suture Wound Scab

Fibrosed Tract

Incision

**B**

uneven coaptation of the skin will occur, resulting in a step-off scar. During reapproximation of the wound, grasping or crushing of the skin edges by forceps should be avoided.

Dermal sutures can be used alone or as adjuncts to percutaneous sutures in wounds subjected to strong skin tensions, to serve as an added precaution against disruption of the wound. Some emergency physicians prefer a synthetic absorbable suture for dermal closure, while others favor a synthetic nonabsorbable suture. When continuous nonabsorbable sutures are employed, suture removal is recommended before the eighth day after wound closure to prevent the development of needle puncture scars.

Percutaneous sutures should be avoided in favor of dermal sutures in the following circumstances: (1) in infants frightened at the prospects of suture removal, (2) when follow-up appointments will be difficult for the patient to keep, (3) when wounds are covered by casts, and (4) in patients prone to the development of keloids. When dermal closure alone is used, it is advisable to immediately apply tape skin closures to the wound edges to provide a more accurate approximation of the epidermis.

However useful, the dermal skin closure technique potentiates wound infection more than percutaneous sutures. This increased infection rate appears to be related to the large quantity of suture material that is required for a continuous dermal skin closure. Once infection develops, the collecting purulent exudate spreads preferentially between the divided edges of fat rather than penetrating the tightly sutured skin edges. By the time the infection becomes clinically apparent, it has involved the entire extent of the wound. In contrast, the localized collections of purulent discharge encountered in infected tape-closed wounds first exit between the wound edges before spreading preferentially between the divided layers of adipose tissue.

Despite the immediate aesthetically pleasing appearance of dermal skin closure, it does not improve the ultimate cosmetic appearance of the healing wound. The scar width after dermal skin closure is comparable to the scar width of wounds healing in the absence of dermal sutures. In contrast, galeal sutures limit the width of scalp scars. In fact, the use of nonabsorbable PP galeal suture reduces the postoperative stretching and depth of skin scars more than does the use of polyglycolic acid galeal suture of comparable size. Another effective method of reducing scar width is to undermine the skin edges prior to wound closure, thereby diminishing the static skin tensions. However, this benefit must be weighed against the potential damage to the skin blood supply, which may compromise the host's defenses and invite infection. Consequently, undermining the wound edges of lacerations is not recommended in the emergency department, but is reserved for elective surgery.

To prevent the development of needle puncture scars, skin sutures must be removed before the eighth day after wound closure (Fig. 45-1). Immediately following suture removal, the wound edges should be reinforced with tape skin closure to prevent wound dehiscence.

## NEEDLES

The ideal surgical needle is designed to introduce a suture that provides meticulous approximation of the divided wound edges with the least damage to tissue. All surgical needles are produced from stainless steel alloys, which have excellent resistance to corrosion. All true stainless steels contain a minimum of about 12 percent chromium, which allows a thin protective surface layer of chromium oxide to form when the steel is exposed to oxygen. High nickel maraging stainless steels have found extensive use in structural materials in many applications requiring a combination of high strength and toughness. A high nickel maraging stainless steel is composed of 7.5 to 9.5 percent nickel, 0.8 to 1.4 percent titanium, and 11 to 12.5 percent chromium. Surgical needles made of a high nickel maraging stainless steel have a greater resistance to bending and breakage than stainless steels without nickel.

Every surgical needle has three basic components: swage, body, and point. Its swage is the point of attachment of the suture. The swaging process provides a smooth juncture beneath the needle and suture. Nowadays, a laser is used to produce uniform holes in the ends of small needles, resulting in a smooth swage. Channel needles have a channel with an underlying receptacle for attachment of the suture. Laser-drilled swages should be associated with less mechanical trauma to tissues than channel swages.

Both laser-drilled and channel swages are more susceptible to bending and breakage by the needle holder jaws than the body of the needle. Physicians are warned to grasp the needle with the needle holder at a site beyond the swage. In the case of 17.5-mm long needles with laser-drilled and channel swages, the depths of the laser-drilled holes and channel swages are 1.5 mm and 6.0 mm respectively. The laser-drilled needle can be held by the needle holder jaws 3 mm from the needle end, whereas the channel swage needle is grasped 7.5 mm from the needle end (Fig. 45-2). By grasping the needle close to its end, the physician can more easily manipulate the passage of the needle through tissue. This benefit of the laser-drilled needles is accomplished without altering the needle suture attachment strength. These distinct advantages of swages produced by lasers indicate that they should eventually replace all channel swage needles.

The needle is attached to the suture by uniformly compressing the walls of the swage against the suture, creating a strong attachment force that prevents detachment of the suture from the needle without exerting considerable force on the swage. This suture attachment strength is so great that separation of the needle from the suture is most easily accomplished by cutting the suture. A newer swage requiring lower uniform forces to detach its suture, sometimes called pop-off or control release, has been developed. It was originally developed for abdominal wound closure, bolus dressings for skin grafts, and hysterectomies in which large numbers of interrupted sutures are used. Eliminating the need to cut the suture considerably reduces the length of the operation.

The body of the needle is the portion that is grasped by the needle holder. The security with which needle holder jaws grasp the needle is influenced by the presence of teeth in the needle holder jaws, the ratchet setting of the needle holder handle, and the shape of the cross-sectional area of the needle body. While the shape of the cross-sectional area of the body has a significant effect on needle holding security, the presence of teeth in the needle holder jaws and the ratchet setting of the needle holder handle are much greater determinants of needle holding security than the needle body shape.

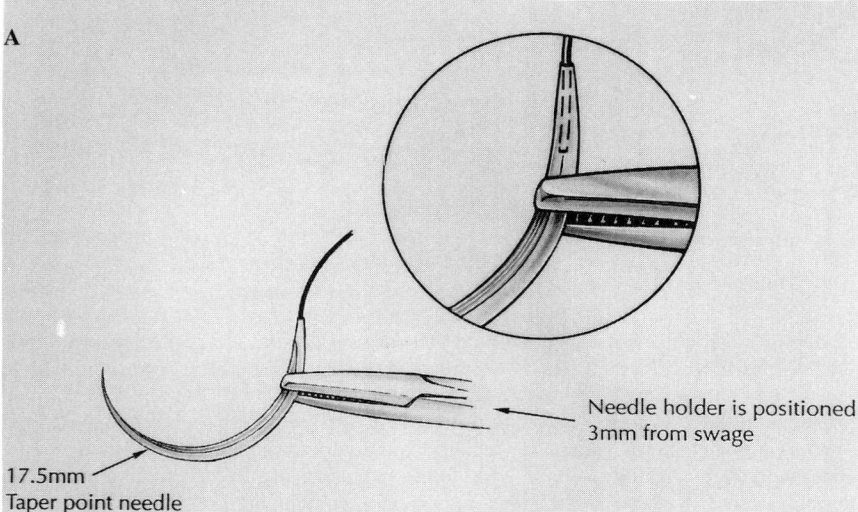

A

17.5mm
Taper point needle

Needle holder is positioned
3mm from swage

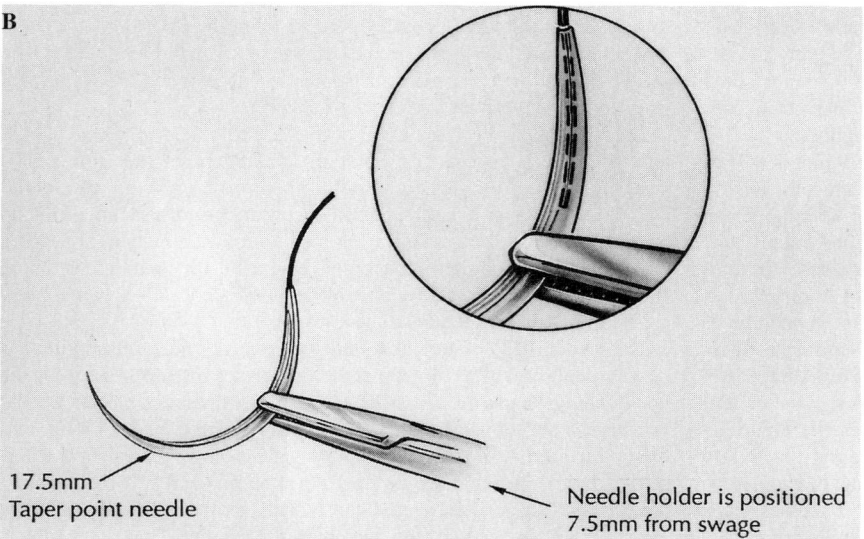

B

17.5mm
Taper point needle

Needle holder is positioned
7.5mm from swage

**Fig. 45-2. A.** Because the laser-drilled hole is 1.5 mm long, this needle can be grasped by the needle holder 3 mm from the swage (insert). Needle holder grasps the needle 3 mm from its swage. **B.** Because the length of the channel is 6.0 mm, the needle can be grasped by the needle holder 7.5 mm from the swage. **Insert.** Needle holder grasps the needle 7.5 mm from its swage.

The geometry of the body can be categorized by the shapes of cross-sectional area and geometric configuration of the length of the needle. The shape of its cross-sectional area will influence the security with which the needle holder jaws grasp the needle as well as its resistance to bending. The cross-sectional areas of the bodies of different needles have the following shapes: round, triangular, rectangular with rounded sides, and trapezoidal (Fig. 45-3). Needles with rectangular cross-sectional areas are created by either flattening the sides of the circular wire or flattening the top and bottom of the circular wire. When the top and bottom portions of the needle body are flattened, the long axis of its rectangular cross-sectional area will gain intimate contact with the faces of the needle holder jaw. This position of the needle body between the needle holder jaws is similar to that of the needle body with a trapezoidal shape. In both cases, the needle-holding security against twisting and rotation is greater than any other needle body shape (side-flattened rectangular shape, triangular, or circular). This benefit of enhanced needle-holding security must be weighed against an associated reduced resistance to bending as compared to that of the side-flattened needle bodies. We prefer side-flattened needle bodies because they exhibit greater resistance to bending than any other needle body shape. Longitudinal ribbing or grooves on the inside and outside curvatures of curved needles do not enhance needle holding security but serve as a trademark for one manufacturer.[1]

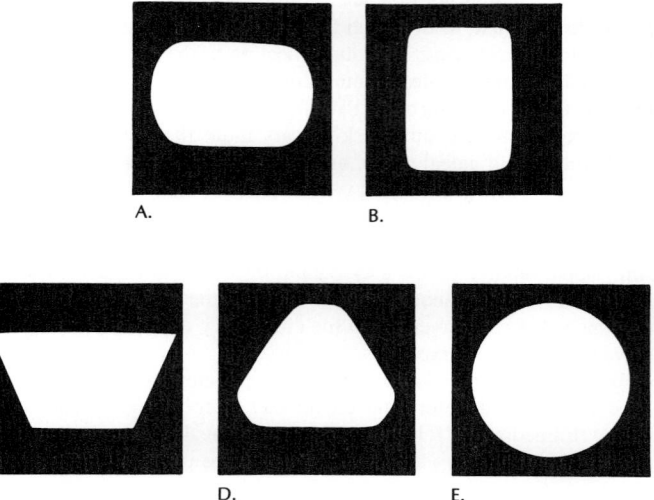

**Figure 45-3.** Cross-sectional area of body of needle. **A.** Rectangular shape created by flattening top and bottom of circular wire. **B.** Rectangular shape caused by side flattening of circular wire. **C.** Trapezoidal shape. **D.** Triangular shape. **E.** Circular shape.

[1] Ethicon, Inc., Somerville, NJ.

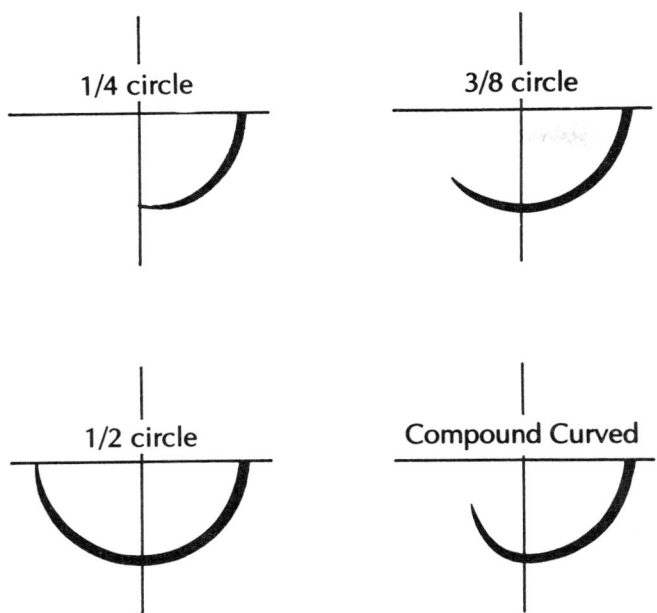

**Fig. 45-4.** Geometry of length of needle.

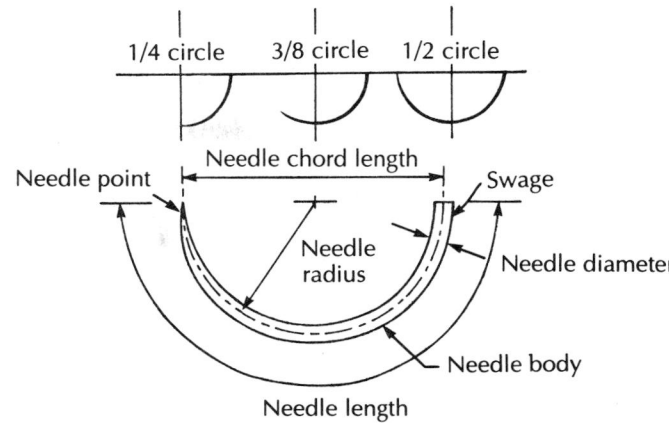

**Fig. 45-5.** Dimensions of curved surgical needle.

The geometry of the length of the needle will have considerable influence on the physician's use of a surgical needle. The curvature at the needle is described in degrees of the subtended arc. The radius of the needle is the distance from the center of the circle to the body of the needle if the curvature of the needle is continued to make a full circle. The curvature of the needle with one radius of curvature may vary from 90° (1/4), 135° (3/8), 180° (1/2), to 225° (5/8) (Fig. 45-4). A compound curved needle has two distinct radii of curvature. The tight curvature of its tip extends 35° before it assumes its regular uniform curvature in the remaining portion of the needle body (100°).

The emergency physician will use needles with a curvature of 135° to approximate divided edges of thin planar structures that are readily accessible (e.g., skin), requiring a limited arc of wrist rotation to pass the needle through the tissue. It is difficult to use the 135° needle in deeper tissues (e.g., muscle, fascia) because the limited arc of the wrist rotation involved in passing this needle is usually not sufficient to expose the needle point, which will remain buried in the tissue—a challenge for the physician to retrieve. The 180° needle is ideally suited for use in deeper tissues because a limited arc of wrist rotation will successfully pass the entire needle through the tissue, allowing adequate exposure of the needle point for easy retrieval of the needle.

The compound curved needle has been primarily used to alter the geometry of 135° needles. Its straight point readily facilitates its initial entrance through the tissue and also controls the depth. Its tight needle curvature beyond its point permits rapid, accurate needle passage at a selected depth and controlled exiting. Its design also offers a mechanical advantage over the standard needle with one radius of curvature. The compound curved needle is ideally suited for dermal skin closure.

In addition to its curvature and radius, a surgical needle can be characterized by three other measurements (Fig. 45-5). *Chord length* is the linear distance measured from the central point of the needle swage to the point of the needle. The *needle diameter* is the width of the original circular wire, utilized in the manufacturing process for the production of the needle. *Needle length* is the length of the needle measured at the center of the wire's cross section.

The point of the needle extends from the tip of the needle to the maximum cross section of the body. Each type of needle point is designed to penetrate specific types of tissue. In general, there are needles with cutting edges, taperpoint, or a combination of both. Cutting edge needles have at least two opposing edges that are designed to penetrate tough tissue.

When the cutting edge needles have three cutting edges, the position of the third cutting edge categorizes the needle as either a conventional cutting edge needle or a reverse cutting edge needle and will influence its performance. Because the apical cutting edge of the conventional cutting edge is located on the inner, or concave, surface, it cuts tissue beneath the surface and directs the needle point toward the skin (surface seeking) (Fig. 45-6). Because the physician has a tendency to apply greater force toward the concave side of the needle, there is a potential danger of dividing some tissues that ultimately will be encircled by the suture. As the needle passes through the skin, it produces a triangular defect, the apex of which is closest to the incision and is the site for the tied suture ligature. Positioning of the suture ligature at this point may predispose to skin cut-through.

In contrast, reverse cutting edge needles differ from conventional cutting edge needles in that the third cutting edge is located on the outer, convex, curvature of the needle (Fig. 45-7). This configuration offers the advantage of having the flat surface of the needle closest to the edges of the incision or wound, limiting the opportunity for tissue cutout and directing the point of the needle toward the depth of the wound (depth seeking). The hole in the skin left by the needle leaves a flattened wall of tissue for the suture to be tied against, which should resist suture pull-through.

Narrowing the point configuration of the cutting edge needle will also enhance its sharpness. The sharpness of the cutting edges can

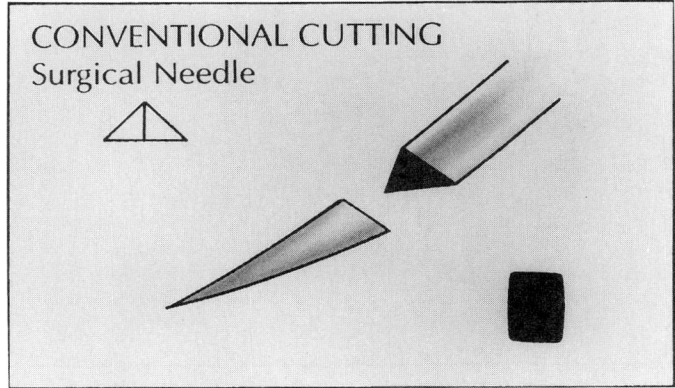

**Fig. 45-6.** Conventional cutting edge surgical needle. **Top left.** Front view of point. The point of the needle has three cutting edges, with its apical cutting edge on the inside, concave surface of the needle. **Side view.** Its apical cutting edge is positioned on the inside, concave surface of the needle. **Bottom right.** The body of the needle has a side-flattened cross-sectional configuration.

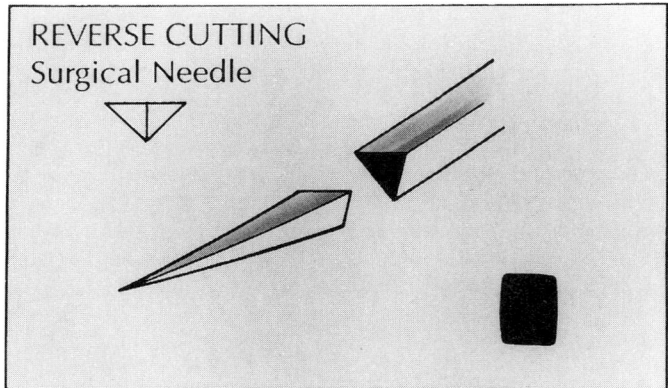

**Fig. 45-7.** Reverse cutting edge needle. **Top left.** Front view of point. The point of the needle has three cutting edges, with its apical cutting edge on the outer, convex surface of the needle. **Side view.** Its apical cutting edge is located on the outer, convex side of the needle. **Bottom right.** The body of the needle has a side-flattened cross-sectional configuration.

also be increased by reducing the angles of the cutting edges. In the reverse and conventional cutting edge needles, the shape of the needle point is triangular, with two lateral cutting edges and a cutting edge at the apex. The cutting edges of the new bevel edge needle have been developed by creating opposing concave surfaces rather than the straight planar surfaces encountered in the standard cutting edge needles (Fig. 45-8). The angles of the cutting edges at the apex and sides of the bevel cutting edges are 45° and 52.5°, respectively, rather than the 60° for the standard cutting edge needles. This decrease in the angles of the cutting edges enhances the sharpness of the needle. Coating the surfaces of the cutting edges with silicone increases their initial sharpness in tissues and maintains the sharpness after repeated passage (durability).

The taperpoint needle tapers to a sharp tip (Fig. 45-9). It spreads the tissue without cutting it. It is used in soft tissue that does not resist needle penetration, such as vessels, fascia, and muscle. It is preferred when the emergency physician wants to make the smallest hole in tissue and to avoid cutting small incisions extending from the hole periphery.

Tapercut needles combine the unique features of taperpoint and cutting edge needles (Fig. 45-10). The cutting edges of the tapercut

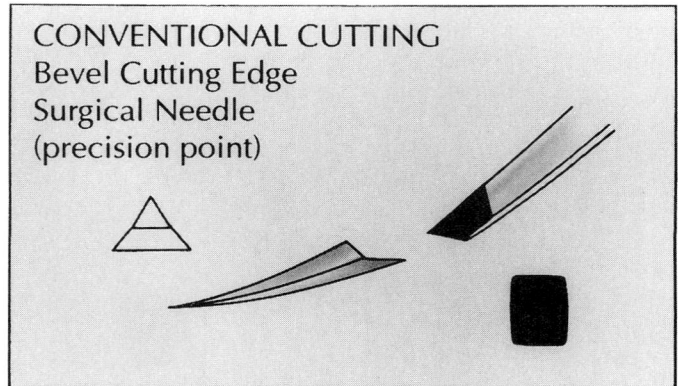

**Fig. 45-8.** Bevel conventional cutting edge needle. **Top left.** Front view of point. The opposing sides of the point of the needle have a concave geometry that reduces the angle of its cutting edges. **Side view.** The sides of the point of this bevel conventional cutting edge needle are beveled to reduce the angle of its cutting edges. **Bottom right.** The body of the needle has a side-flattened cross-sectional configuration.

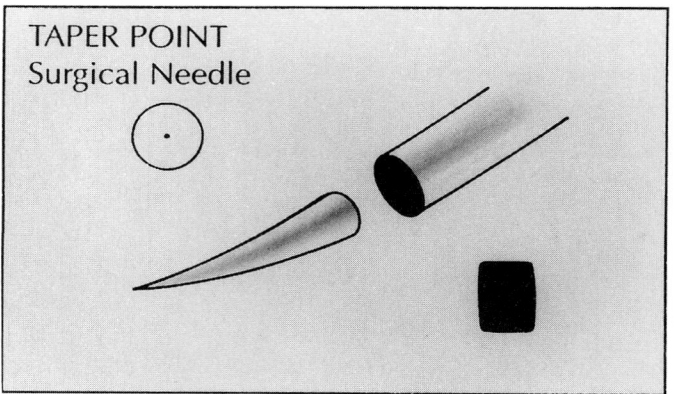

**Fig. 45-9.** Taperpoint surgical needle. **Top left.** Front view of point. The geometry of this needle tapers to a point and has no cutting edges. **Side view.** The point of this needle has a narrow taperpoint geometry. **Bottom right.** The body of the needle has a side-flattened cross-sectional configuration.

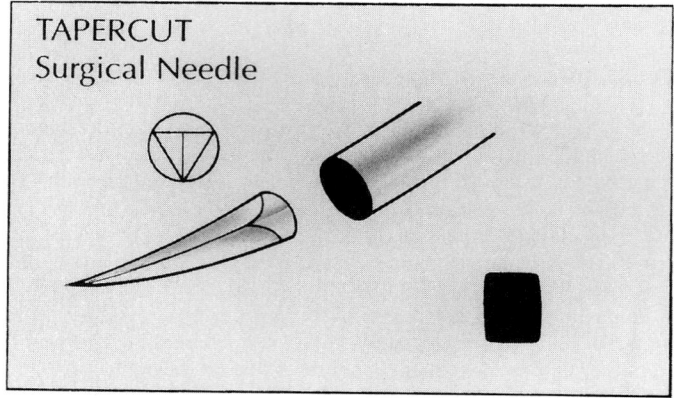

**Fig. 45-10.** Tapercut surgical needle. **Top left.** Front view of point. This tapercut needle has a short reverse cutting edge that blends into a taperpoint geometry. **Side view.** The reverse cutting edges are confined to a small portion of the tip of this needle. **Bottom right.** The body of the needle has a side-flattened cross-sectional configuration.

needle extend only a very short distance from the needle tip and blend into a round taper body. This needle provides smooth passage through oral mucous membrane, yet its round shaft without cutting edges will not cut through the deeper tissues.

Because the surgical sutures currently in use have a needle:suture ratio of approximately 2:1, the difference between the sizes of the needles and sutures leave an unfilled space at each suture hole, which may invite suture cut through thin skin. To resolve this problem, two new sutures attached to taperpoint needles have been developed. One monofilament suture made of PTFE[2] is produced with a porous microstructure that is approximately 50 percent air by volume. Its porous nature allows it to be swaged to a needle that closely approximates its suture diameter, having a needle:suture ratio of 1:1. The other suture, called Hemoseal,[3] is a monofilament polypropylene suture that has been extruded to produce a tapered swage end, which is significantly smaller than that of the remainder of the suture in order for it to be channel swaged to smaller diameter needles, with a needle:suture diameter ratio that approaches 1:1.

The biomechanical performance of surgical needles and needle holders is determined by (1) needle sharpness, (2) needle resistance to bending, (3) needle ductility, and (4) needle holder clamping mo-

[2] WL Gore & Associates, Elkins, MD.

[3] Ethicon, Inc., Somerville, NJ.

ment. Sharpness measures the force needed to pass a needle through a membrane that simulates the density of human tissue. Needle resistance to bending is measured by recording the force required to bend the needle 90°. The more critical measurement to the emergency physician is the force required to irreversibly deform the needle—the yield moment. Ductility is a measurement of the needle's resistance to breakage. The needle holder clamping moment is a measure of the force exerted by the needle holder jaws on a curved surgical needle.

Selecting the appropriate needle holder for a designated needle can be accomplished by relating the clamping moment of the needle holder at the specified ratchet setting to the yield moment for the needle placed in a measured site in the needle holder jaws. Ideally, one should use a needle holder whose clamping moment is less than that of the yield moment of the needle. Clamping a needle whose yield moment is less than the clamping moment of the needle holder will result in needle deformation.

The design of the needle holder jaw is another important consideration in the selection of a needle holder. Tungsten carbide inserts with teeth, varying from 2500 to 16,000 teeth/inch$^2$, have been incorporated into the jaws of the needle holder to enhance its needle-holding security. Teeth limit twisting and rotation of the needle, allowing accurate passage of the needle through the tissue.

However, teeth also have potential deleterious effects on suture materials and needles. Teeth can produce morphologic changes in monofilament synthetic sutures that reduce their breaking strength and can reduce needle resistance to bending or breakage. The needle holder jaw should grasp only the needle body; clamping the needle point damages the cutting edge and dulls the needle.

Smooth needle holder jaws with rounded edges do not induce structural damage to either monofilament suture or needles. However, their smooth jaw surfaces provide limited resistance to twisting or rotation of the needle between the jaws. A textured needle holder jaw metallurgically bonded with tungsten carbide particles appears to be an attractive alternative to either smooth needle holder jaws or those with teeth. Although its needle-holding security is significantly less than the jaws with teeth, it provides greater needle-holding security than the smooth jaws.

## TAPE

The superior resistance to infection of taped wounds compared with sutured wounds indicates that tape closure is a significant clinical tool. The incidence of infection of contaminated wounds whose edges are approximated even with the least reactive suture is significantly greater than the infection rate of taped wounds subjected to a comparable level of bacterial contamination. The ease with which wounds can be closed by tape varies according to the anatomic and biomechanical properties of the wound site. Linear wounds in skin subjected to minimal static and dynamic tensions are easily approximated by tape. The relatively lax skin of the face and abdomen makes it amenable to wound closure by tapes. Contrary to the usual expectation, tape closure without sutures is more easily accomplished in obese patients, and the thick cut edges of adipose tissue tend to evert the skin. The taut skin of the extremities, which is subjected to frequent dynamic joint movements, requires dermal sutures before taping. The copious secretions from the skin of the axilla, palms, and soles discourage tape adherence.

The difficulties encountered in performing sutureless tape closure of wounds subjected to strong tensions can be explained by the deformation of skin at the periphery of the wound. When the skin is cut, its inherent skin tensions retract its edges. As with any elastic membrane, the shrinkage in surface area of the skin is greatest at the wound margin, becoming progressively less as the distance from the wound increases. The extent of these changes is directly related to the magnitude of the static and dynamic forces within the skin. The use of dermal sutures prior to taping stretches the skin to its uninjured

dimensions and makes application of tape skin closures considerably easier. In wounds subjected to weak skin tension, tape skin closure can be accomplished without the use of reinforcing dermal sutures. In such cases, the tape skin closure is first attached to the skin at one wound edge. The other wound edge is then pulled toward the taped edge before the remaining portion of the tape skin closure is applied to the skin.

When tape skin closures are properly employed to close linear wounds subjected to weak tensions, cosmetic results are excellent. The discomfort of anesthetic infiltration and of suture removal, and the development of suture puncture scars, are avoided. In the child or woman with glabrous skin, tape skin closures are especially valuable for closing transverse lacerations over the brow, under the chin, or across the malar prominence.

Wound closure tapes will not adhere to wet skin. Drying with a gauze sponge sometimes does not completely remove wet exudate, and the residual fluid continues to impair tape adhesion. Compound benzoin tincture can be applied to the wound edges with applicator sticks prior to tape application. Compound benzoin tincture should not be spilled into the wound, as it increases the likelihood of infection.

## STAPLES

Skin closure by metal staples is quick and economical. Stapling is the fastest method of skin closure. An additional advantage of staples is their low level of tissue reactivity. There is uniform agreement that wounds closed by metal staples exhibit a superior resistance to infection than wounds subjected to the least reactive suture. These advantages of skin staples must be weighed against one notable drawback. The skin staple does not provide the same meticulous coaptation of lacerations with irregular skin edges that skin sutures do. The wound edges must be accurately aligned before wound closure to permit simultaneous implantation of the staple points. Because this accurate prepositioning of the wound edges is very difficult in most lacerations, staple implantation will often result in malapposition of wound edges, an invitation to the development of scar deformity. Consequently, we reserve skin staples for lacerations in anatomic sites in which the healing scar is not readily apparent (e.g., scalp).

A variety of stapling devices are commercially available for use in the emergency department. All staplers implant stainless steel staples, which assume an incomplete rectangular or arcuate shape when fully formed. The selection of a stapler by the emergency physician will be determined by its performance. Ideally, the device should be designed so that it does not obstruct the physician's view of the wound edge. Moreover, the stapler should have a prepositioning mechanism that permits the physician to hold the staple securely during its formation. The configuration of the stapler should allow the position of its cartridge to be adjusted manually to facilitate placement of the staple. In addition, the stapler should have an ejection spring that automatically releases the staple. Finally, the handling characteristics of the stapler should be such that the physician can easily implant a large number of staples without becoming fatigued.

The most recent advance in skin stapling is a disposable stapler that delivers an absorbable pin into the subcuticulous layer of tissue just below the dermis. The absorbable pin is made of an absorbable copolymer that is a synthetic polyester composed of glycolic and lactic acids. This copolymer has an extensive clinical history for absorbable devices, such as sutures, staples, and clips, demonstrating its biocompatibility and biodegradability. Activation of its movable instrument handle causes a pair of gripper blades to approximate and evert the wound edges, after which it pushes one pin into the dermis. The pin penetrates the dermis twice on both sides of the wound, thus holding the tissue together. Staple wound closure is accomplished four times faster than sutural closure of the dermis. Wounds with staple pin closure exhibit resistance to infection superior to wounds approximated by dermal sutures. Although sutures provide more immediate wound security, as measured by wound breaking strength, than dermal pins, the breaking strength of wounds subjected to either dermal pins or dermal sutures are not significantly different 14 days after wounding. Because of the low breaking strength of wounds closed by dermal pins, the dermal pin closure should be routinely reinforced by the application of microporous tapes.

## BIBLIOGRAPHY

deHoll D, Rodeheaver G, Edgerton MT, et al: Potentiation of infection by suture closure of dead space. *Am J Surg* 127:716, 1974.

Edlich RF, Becker DG, Thacker JG, et al: Scientific basis for selecting staple and tape skin closures. *Clin Plast Surg* 17:571, 1990.

Edlich RF, Thacker JG, McGregor W, et al: Past, present, and future for surgical needles and needle holders. *Am J Surg* 166:522, 1993.

Rodeheaver GT, Halverson JM, Edlich RF: Mechanical performance of wound closure tapes. *Ann Emerg Med* 12:203, 1983.

Rodeheaver GT, Thacker JG, Edlich RF: Mechanical performance of polyglycolic acid and polyglactin 910 synthetic absorbable sutures. *Surg Gynecol Obstet* 153:835, 1981.

Rodeheaver GT, Thacker JG, Owen J, et al: Knotting and handling characteristics of coated synthetic absorbable sutures. *J Surg Res* 35:525, 1983.

# 46

# TECHNICAL CONSIDERATIONS IN WOUND REPAIR

**Richard F. Edlich**
**John M. Eggleston**

The emergency physician must use several different surgical instruments to achieve wound repair. An understanding of the mechanics involved in the use of surgical instruments allows one to use them with accuracy and security, which is especially important in the management of difficult wounds.

## SURGICAL INSTRUMENTS

There are successive steps to take in the use of a surgical needle holder. First, position the surgical needle between the jaws of the needle holder 2 mm from the tips of its jaws. The needle should be placed perpendicular to the needle holder jaws 1.5 mm beyond the needle's channel or swage hole, a site that has optimal resistance to bending. The needle holder can be grasped by either the thenar grip or the thumb–ring finger grip. Each grip has notable advantages and disadvantages.

In the thenar grip, the tips of the thumb and ring finger are not inserted into the ringlets of the needle holder (Fig. 46-1). The thenar eminence and skin overlying the metacarpophalangeal joint are pressed against one ringlet, while the long, ring, and small fingers encircle the other ringlet. This position aligns the needle holder in the same direction as the longitudinal axis of the wrist and forearm, allowing the hand and needle holder to be positioned comfortably into recessed cavities (e.g., oral cavity). In addition, the needle can be released and regrasped by the needle holder without changing positions. The needle can be redirected in preparation for the next stitch

Supported by a gift from Michael L. Blumenfeld, DDS, Brookville, New York.

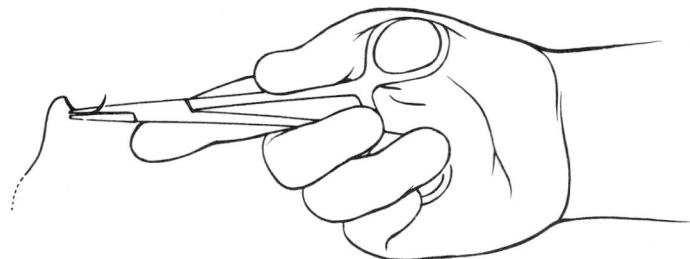

**Fig. 46-1.** Thenar grip of needle holder.

by spinning the needle holder clockwise in the palm. The disadvantage of this grip is the lack of precision when releasing the needle. When the thenar eminence applies pressure to the ringlet, it disengages the ratchet mechanism uncontrollably, causing inadvertent movement of the needle.

In the thumb–ring finger grip, the tip of the thumb is positioned in one ringlet, while the tip of the ring finger is placed in the other ringlet (Fig. 46-2). The greatest advantage of this grip is its controlled disengagement of the ratchet mechanism, permitting precise manipulation of the needle. This advantage must be weighed against the relatively large size of the physician's hand and needle holder. Because the palm of the hand is separated from the needle holder, the physician will find it difficult to position the needle holder in recessed cavities (e.g., mouth).

Curved surgical needles made of high nickel maraging stainless steels are ideally suited for closure of planar structures such as epidermis, dermis, muscle, and fascia (Fig. 46-3). Use of the compound curved needle allows the physician to pass it through the dermis with greater accuracy to a controlled depth and length of bite. Reverse cutting edge needles with precision points are used for skin and dermal closure, resulting in holes that display considerable resistance to suture tissue cut-through. Smaller diameter needles are used to approximate thin planar structures, while larger diameter needles are reserved for thicker structures. Divided muscle and fascia are approximated with taperpoint needles.

Before passing the needle through tissue, lay the free end of the suture away from you. Starting with the hand prone, introduce the needle through the tissue in a direction toward you. Because the ratchet mechanism of most needle holders is designed for right-handed individuals, most physicians prefer to hold the needle holder with the right hand, allowing them to hold tissue forceps with the left hand. The tissue forceps is held so that one arm is an extension of the thumb; the other arm is an extension of the opposing fingers. With the junction of the tissue forceps arms resting on the web space, one arm can be used to elevate a wound edge in the same manner as a skin hook, facilitating accurate passage of the curved needle (Fig. 46-4). Compressing the wound edges between the teeth of the forceps should be avoided because it crushes tissue, damaging its defenses and inviting infection.

Wound closure should be accomplished in wounds without persis-

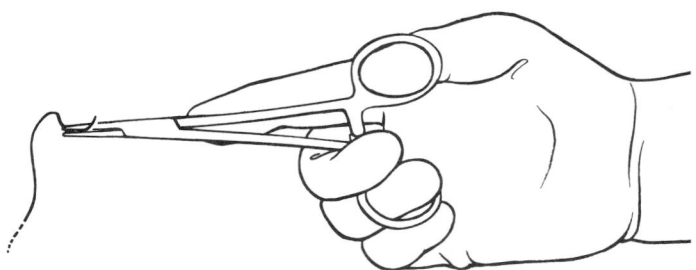

**Fig. 46-2.** Thumb–ring finger grip of needle holder.

**Fig. 46-3.** Dimensions of laser-drilled curved surgical needles with either reverse cutting edges or taper point.

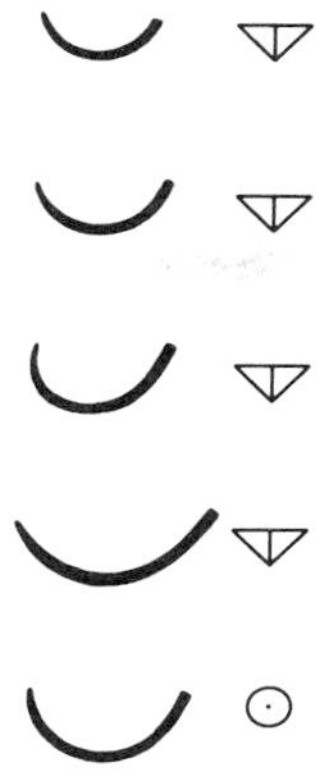

| Needle | | Diameter (mm) | Length (mm) | Radius (mm) | Degrees | Chord Length (mm) |
|---|---|---|---|---|---|---|
| | ▽ | 0.33 | 11.2 | 4.8 | 135° | 8.8 |
| | ▽ | 0.43 | 12.9 | 4.8 | 135° | 9.3 |
| | ▽ | 0.56<br>0.43 | 15.8 | 3.6<br>5.2 | | 10.2 |
| | ▽ | 0.52 | 18.7 | 8.0 | 135° | 14.7 |
| | ⊙ | 0.36 | 17.5 | 5.6 | 180° | 11.2 |

tent bleeding. Most bleeding stops after gentle compression with gauze sponges applied to the wound surface using aseptic technique. Persistent bleeding may be stopped by electrocoagulation using bipolar forceps. For larger vessels, hemostasis is best accomplished by clamping the divided ends of the bleeding vessel with the tips of curved hemostats (Fig. 46-5A). The clamped vessel can then be ligated with a 5–0 braided synthetic absorbable suture. Avoid clamping the divided vessel with contiguous adipose because the clamp will devascularize the adipose tissue, which then becomes a culture medium for bacterial growth and an invitation to the development of infection (Fig. 46-5B).

## KNOT CONSTRUCTION

The length of a suture attached to a needle is usually 18 in. (46 cm). When the suture is attached to a needle, there is a fixed end, which is attached to the needle, and a free end. The first throw of a knot is accomplished by wrapping the free end either once or twice (surgeon's knot) around the fixed end.

Formation of each throw of a knot is accomplished in three steps. The first step is the formation of a suture loop. In the second step, the free suture end is passed through the suture loop to create a throw. The final step is to advance the throw to the wound surface. For the first throw of a square, granny, or surgeon's knot square, tension is applied to the suture ends in opposite directions. With each additional throw, the direction in which tension is applied to the suture ends is reversed. The physician should construct a knot by carefully snugging each throw tightly against the preceding one. The rate of applying tension to each throw to construct a knot should be relatively slow.

The physician should apply equal and opposing tension to the suture ends in the same planes. The direction of the applied tensions will be determined by the orientation of the suture loop in relation to that of the physician's hands. When the hands lie on each side and parallel to the suture loop, tension is applied in a direction parallel to the forearms. Tension will be applied to the farther suture end in the direction away from the physician. Conversely, an equal, opposing force will be applied to the closer suture end in a direction toward the physician. After constructing the second throw of these knots, the direction of the suture ends must be reversed, with an accompanying reversal of the position of the hands. As the physician's hands move toward or away from the body, the movement of the right and left hands are in separate and distinct areas that do not cross, permitting continuous visualization of knot construction. With each additional throw, the physician must reverse the position of his or her hands.

During wound repair, knot construction involves two distinct steps. The purpose of the first step is to secure precise approximation of the wound edges by advancing either a one-throw or a two-throw knot to the wound surface. Once the throw or throws contact the wound, the physician will have a preview of the ultimate apposition of the wound edges. Ideally, the knotted suture loop should reapproximate the divided wound edges without strangulating the tissue encircled by the suture loop. If there is some separation of the wound edges, the one-throw or two-throw knot can be advanced to reduce the size of the suture loop and thereby bring the wound edges closer together.

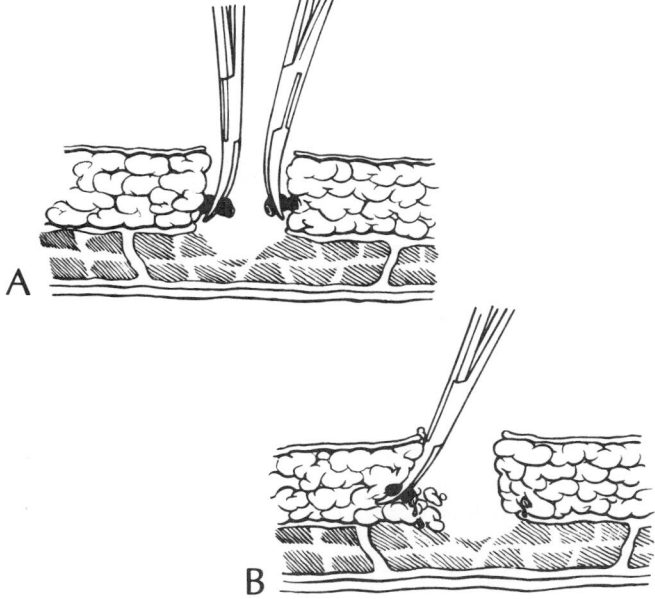

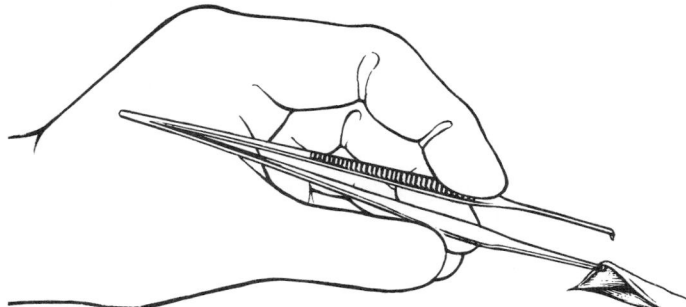

**Fig. 46-4.** While holding the tissue forceps in the left hand, the physician uses one arm of the tissue forceps to elevate a wound edge in the same manner as a skin hook.

**Fig. 46-5. A.** Clamp the divided ends of the bleeding vessel with the tips of curved hemostats. **B.** Avoid clamping the divided vessel with contiguous adipose tissue between the jaws of the curved hemostat.

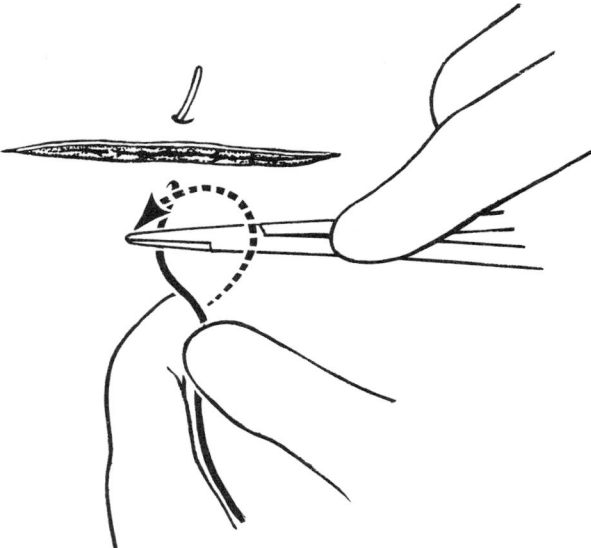

**Fig. 46-6.** *Formation of first throw; position the needle holder.* The instrument tie is performed with a needle holder held in the right hand. The left hand holds the fixed suture end between the tips of the thumb and index finger. The needle holder is positioned perpendicular to and above the fixed suture end. By keeping the length of the free suture end relatively short (<2 cm), it is easy to form suture loops (arrow) as well as to save suture material. Because the needle holder passes the free suture end through the suture loop, knot construction can be safely accomplished without detaching the needle from the fixed suture end.

## Instrument Tie Techniques

The second step in knot construction is tying of the knot, which can be accomplished by either an instrument or hand tie. An instrument tie occurs by the formation of a suture loop over an instrument, usually a needle holder. The right hand holds the needle holder, while the

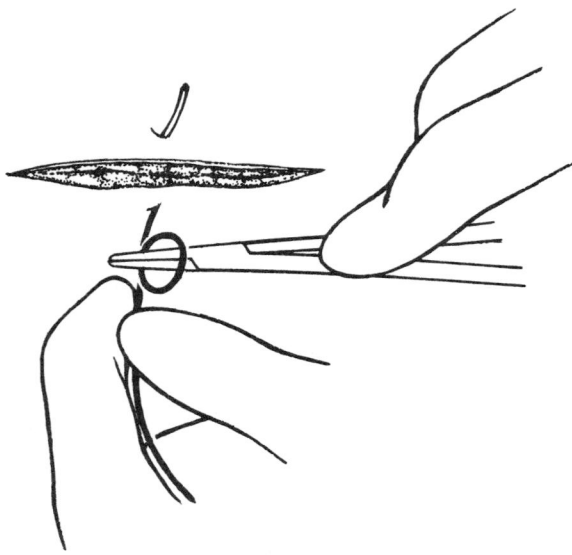

**Fig. 46-7.** *Formation of the first suture loop.* The fixed suture end held by the left hand is wrapped over and around the needle holder jaws to form the first suture loop. (If the suture is wrapped twice around the needle holder jaws, the first, double-wrap throw of the surgeon's knot square will be formed. A double-wrap, first throw displays a greater resistance to slippage than a single-wrap throw, accounting for its frequent use in instrument ties in wounds subjected to strong, static skin tensions.)

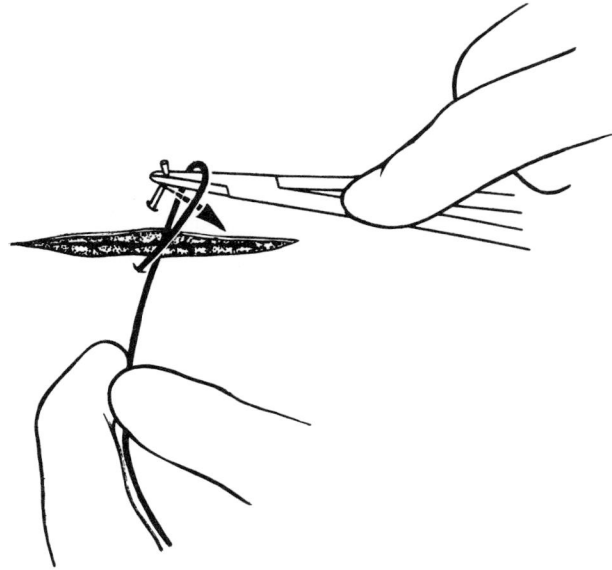

**Fig. 46-8.** *The free suture end is clamped and withdrawn through the suture loop to form the first, single-wrap throw.* The tips of the needle holder jaws grasp the suture end and withdraw it through the first suture loop (arrow). The resulting first throw will have a figure eight shape.

left hand loops the fixed suture end around the instrument. The position of the instrument in relation to the suture ends during knot construction will determine the type of knot. When the instrument is placed above the fixed suture end during the first and second throws, a square-type (1 = 1) knot will develop (Figs. 46-6 through 46-13). In contrast, a granny-type (1 × 1) knot will result when the instrument is placed above the fixed suture end for the first throw and then below the fixed suture end for the second throw. By repeating this positioning, the instrument tie is a reliable and easy method to produce multiple-throw granny knots (1 × 1 × 1), a circumstance not encountered in hand ties. Granny knots with more than two throws cannot be constructed by either the one-hand or two-hand technique, without releasing hold of both suture ends.

Instrument tying is accomplished primarily by the physician's left hand, which holds the fixed suture end. Initially the length of the

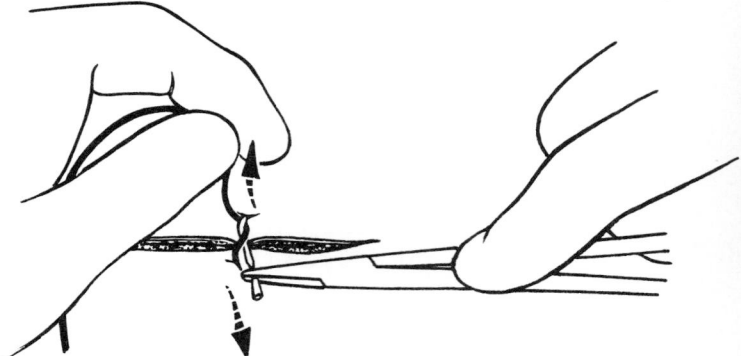

**Fig. 46-9.** *The first single-wrap throw is advanced to the wound surface.* The figure eight–shaped throw will be converted into a rectangular-shaped throw by reversing the direction of the hand movement. The left hand moves away from the physician, while the needle holder held in the right hand advances towards the physician. This single-wrap throw is advanced to the wound surface by applying tension in a direction that is perpendicular to that of the wound (arrows). Once the first throw of the square knot contacts the skin, the edges of the midportion of the wound are approximated.

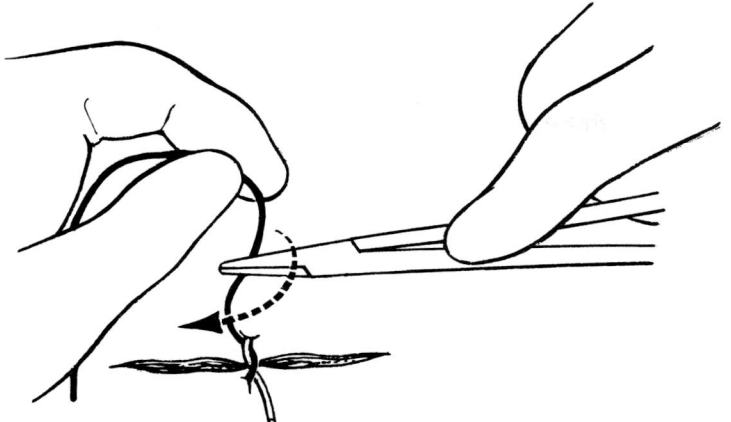

**Fig. 46-10.** *Formation of the second throw; position the needle holder.* The needle holder releases the free suture end. The right hand holding the needle holder moves away from the physician to be positioned perpendicular to and above the fixed suture ends. The second throw will be formed by the left hand as it wraps the fixed suture end over and around the needle holder jaws (arrow). If the physician were to place the needle holder beneath the fixed suture end, the ultimate knot construction would be a granny knot ($1 \times 1$).

fixed suture end held by the left hand is long (17 in), making it difficult to form knots without injuring the attending assistant. This assault can be avoided by shortening the length of the fixed suture end held by the left hand.

When tying knots with an instrument, it is difficult to apply continuous tension to the suture ends. Consequently, widening of the suture loop due to slippage is frequently encountered in wounds subjected to strong tensions. This technique, however, is ideally suited for closing a wound that is subjected to weak tensions. In this circumstance, instrument ties can be accomplished more rapidly and accurately than hand ties, while conserving considerably more suture. By using this technique, the parsimonious physician can complete 10 interrupted suture loops from one suture measuring 18 in. (46 cm). This feat would be impossible if the knots were tied by hand.

The value of instrument ties has become readily apparent in special situations in which hand ties are impractical or impossible. In microsurgical procedures, an instrument tie provides the most reliable and easiest method of knot construction. When employing suture in the recesses of the body (e.g., mouth), instruments can also form knots in sites to which the hand could never gain access.

The magnitude of the knot rundown force is influenced consider-

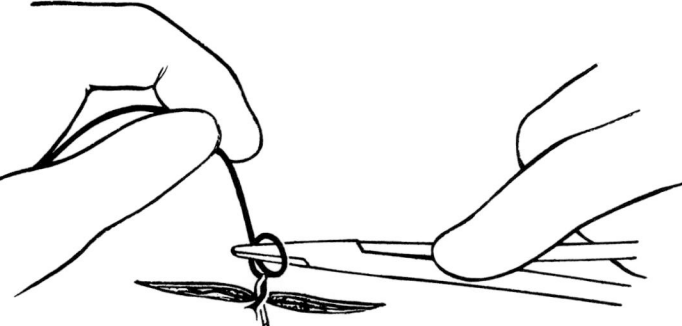

**Fig. 46-11.** *Formation of the second suture loop.* The fixed suture end held by the left hand is wrapped over and around the needle holder to form the second suture loop. With the suture wrapped around the needle holder jaws, the needle holder is moved to grasp the free suture end, after which it is withdrawn through the suture loop.

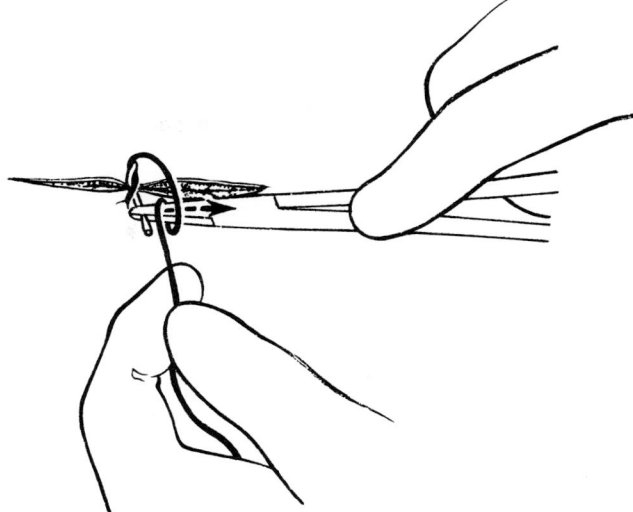

**Fig. 46-12.** *The suture end is clamped and withdrawn through the suture loop to form the second, single-wrap throw.* The tips of the needle holder jaws grasp the free suture end and withdraw it through the second suture loop (arrow). By withdrawing the free suture end through the loop, a rectangular-shaped second throw is formed. The physician will apply tension to the suture ends in a direction perpendicular to that of the wound.

ably by the configuration of two-throw knots. Knot rundown of the surgeon's knot square ($2 = 1$) generates sufficient forces to break the knot. In contrast, knot rundown of square ($1 = 1$), granny ($1 \times 1$), and slip ($S = S$, $S \times S$) knots occurs by slippage for comparable sutures. The mean knot rundown force for square knots is the greatest, followed by that for the granny knots and then the slip knots.

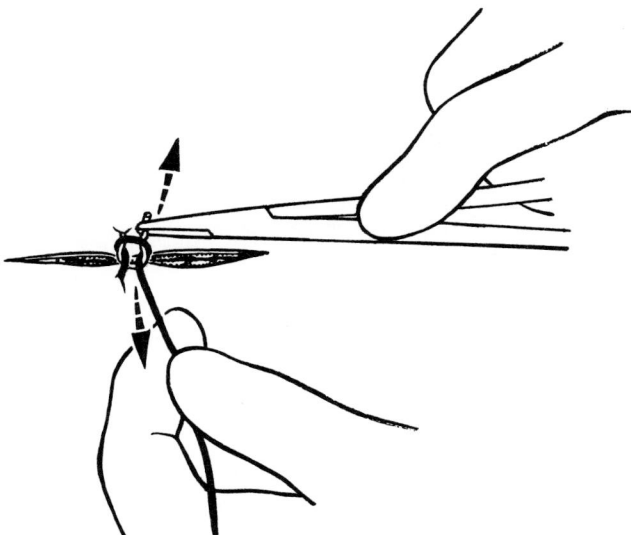

**Fig. 46-13.** *The square knot ($1 = 1$) is advanced to the wound surface.* The second throw is advanced and set against the first throw by applying tension to the suture ends in a direction perpendicular to that of the wound. Advancement of the second throw is complete when the second throw contacts the first throw and forms a square knot. Ideally, the physician should be able to advance the two-throw square knot to allow meticulous approximation of the edges. Once exact approximation of the wound edges is accomplished, the physician will construct a knot using this instrument technique, with a sufficient number of throws and 3-mm cut ears so that knot security is determined by knot breakage, rather than by slippage.

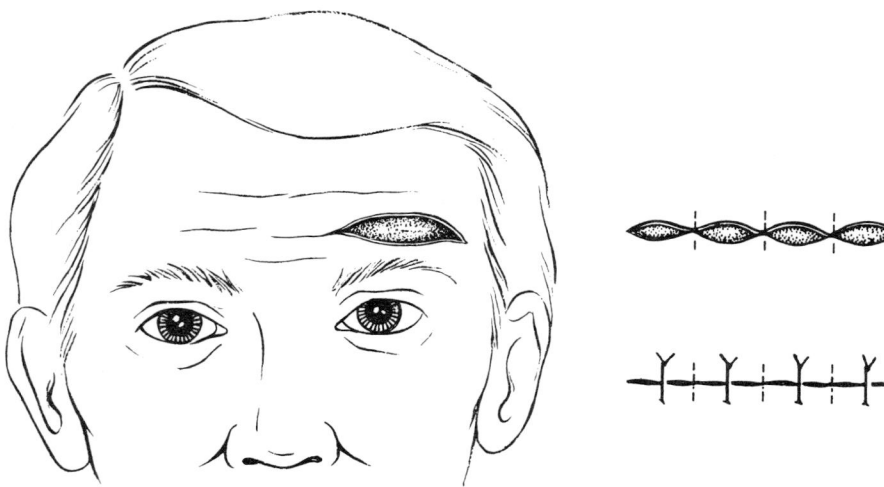

**Fig. 46-14. Left.** Linear laceration of left forehead subjected to strong static skin tensions. **Top right.** Three interrupted dermal skin sutures bring the retracted wound edges together. **Bottom right.** Four interrupted percutaneous sutures positioned between the dermal sutures provide meticulous approximation of the wound edges.

Failure of the knotted suture loop may be the result of either knot slippage or breakage, suture cutting through tissue, or mechanical crushing of the suture by surgical instruments. The knotted suture may fail by slippage, which results in untying the knot. All knots slip to some degree, regardless of the type of suture material. When slippage is encountered, the cut ends ("ears") of the knot must provide the additional material to compensate for the enlarged suture loop. When the amount of knot slippage exceeds the length of the cut ears, the throws of the knot become untied. In general, we recommend that the length of knot ears be 3 mm to accommodate for any knot slippage. Dermal sutures are, however, an exception to this rule. Because the ears of dermal suture knots may protrude through the divided skin edges, it is best to cut the dermal suture ears as they exit from the knot. It must be emphasized that more knot security is achieved in a knot without ears but with one more throw than in a comparable knot whose ear length is 3 mm.

## LACERATIONS SUBJECTED TO STRONG SKIN TENSIONS

Lacerations subjected to strong skin tensions are prone to wound dehiscence and healing with wide hypertrophic scars. These lacerations can be identified by measuring the magnitude of retraction of their wound edges and the alignment of the long axis of the wound with the wrinkle lines or transverse axis of the joint. Wounds whose edges are retracted 5 mm or more are subjected to strong static skin tensions. When the long axis of the wound is perpendicular to the wrinkle line or transverse axis of the joint, wound repair will often be accompanied by hypertrophic scar formation.

Some advocate undermining the wound edges to reduce tensions on its edges. We are reluctant to undermine the wound edges of a laceration because it reduces the blood supply to the wound, thereby damaging wound defenses and inviting the development of infection. We reserve undermining for elective surgical procedures in which the level of bacterial contamination and risk of infection are low.

In the face, muscular and fascial (galea aponeurotica) structures are approximated by using a taperpoint needle swaged to a monofilament synthetic absorbable suture and forming interrupted sutures. Galeal closure reduces the width of the scar. Closure of adipose tissue is always avoided because it enhances infection without strengthening the wound.

Dermal skin closure is recommended in these wounds to maintain their strength and prevent the development of wound dehiscence after early suture removal—within 8 days after wound closure. Because dermal sutures allow early removal of the percutaneous suture, needle puncture scars and tracts do not develop. This clinical benefit is *not* associated with a reduction in scar width.

Dermal repair is accomplished with the least number of interrupted sutures (Fig. 46-14). After an interrupted dermal suture is placed in the midportion of the wound, two additional interrupted dermal sutures are placed halfway between the wound midportion and wound corner ("divide and conquer"). These three interrupted dermal sutures markedly reduce the skin tensions on the wound, as evidenced by the reduced separation of the wound edges.

Interrupted dermal skin closure is accomplished with braided synthetic absorbable sutures attached to laser-drilled holes in compound-curved, reverse cutting edge precision-point needles (Fig. 46-15). The interrupted dermal suture is constructed so that its knot is buried (Fig. 46-16). The ears of the knot are cut flush with the knot. Interrupted percutaneous synthetic monofilament sutures are then used to close the skin edges. These sutures are positioned accurately between the dermal sutures.

## Continuous Percutaneous Suture

Continuous suture closure of skin lacerations has definite distinct advantages over interrupted suture closure. First, continuous suture closure can be accomplished more rapidly than interrupted suture closure. This time saving is related to the short time involved in constructing knotted suture loops for the continuous suture closure; there is one knotted suture at each corner of the laceration. In contrast, interrupted skin closure requires knot construction for each separate suture loop. Another advantage of the continuous suture is that

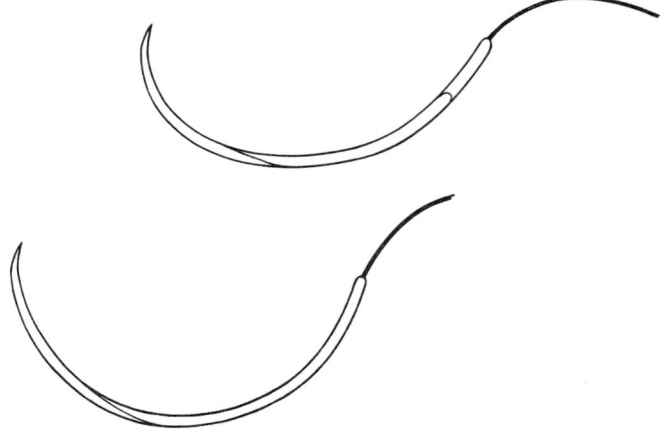

**Fig. 46-15. Top.** Compound curved needle with two distinct radii of curvature. **Bottom.** Standard curved needle with one radius of curvature.

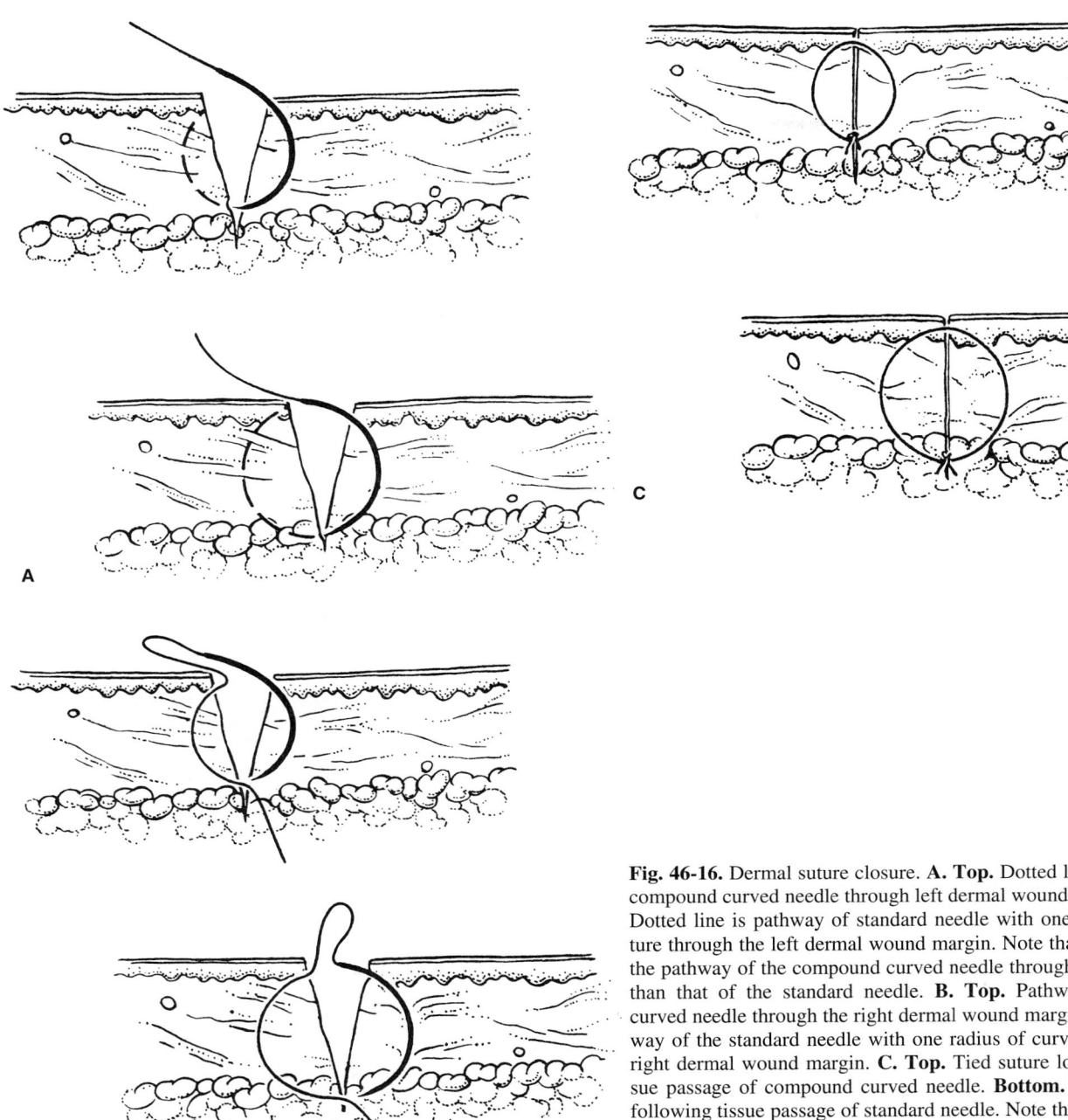

**Fig. 46-16.** Dermal suture closure. **A. Top.** Dotted line is pathway of compound curved needle through left dermal wound margin. **Bottom.** Dotted line is pathway of standard needle with one radius of curvature through the left dermal wound margin. Note that the diameter of the pathway of the compound curved needle through tissue is smaller than that of the standard needle. **B. Top.** Pathway of compound curved needle through the right dermal wound margin. **Bottom.** Pathway of the standard needle with one radius of curvature through the right dermal wound margin. **C. Top.** Tied suture loop following tissue passage of compound curved needle. **Bottom.** Tied suture loop following tissue passage of standard needle. Note that the diameter of the tied suture loop constructed by a compound curved needle is smaller than that of one constructed by a standard needle with a single radius of curvature.

it accommodates to the developing edema of the wound edges during healing. In contrast, the dimensions of the interrupted suture remain unchanged, constricting the edematous tissue within each suture loop. For either interrupted or continuous skin suture closure, we prefer a monofilament synthetic nonabsorbable suture with the lowest coefficient of friction, polypropylene, facilitating passage through tissue. These benefits of the continuous skin closure technique must be weighed against one notable disadvantage. Interrupted suture closure permits a more meticulous approximation of the wound edges than continuous suture, especially in stellate lacerations with irregular wound edges.

After interrupted dermal suture repair to reduce skin tensions, continuous suture closure of the laceration can be accomplished by two different techniques. In the first technique, the needle pathway is at a 90° angle to the wound edges and results in a visible suture that crosses the wound edges at a 45° angle (Fig. 46-17). In the other technique, the needle pathway is at a 45° angle to the wound edges so that the visible suture is at a 90° angle to the wound edges rather than at a 45° angle. In either case, the physician starts the continuous suture closure at the corner of the wound that is farthest away. In addition, the needle is passed in a direction toward the physician, rather than away from the physician. In the case of a laceration of the left arm that is in the direction of its longitudinal axis, the arm is positioned on an arm board or table with the shoulder abducted 90°. The physician should be seated in a position next to the patient's axilla, facing the patient's arm. The continuous skin suture is started in the corner of the wound closest to the axilla, and the needle is passed from the lateral side of the wound to its medial side.

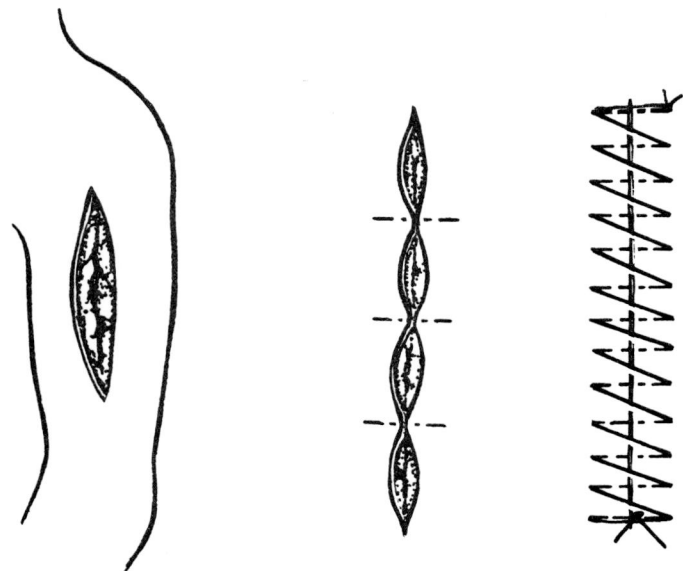

**Fig. 46-17. Left.** Linear laceration of the arm subjected to strong skin tensions, with marked retraction of wound edges. **Center.** Three interrupted dermal sutures markedly reduce the retraction of the skin edges. **Right.** Continuous percutaneous suture.

## Continuous Subcuticular Suture

The continuous dermal suture is an attractive alternative for wounds subjected to strong skin tensions, in patients prone to keloid formation, children frightened by suture removal, and those individuals who are unable to contact a health professional for suture removal. Absorbable synthetic braided or monofilament sutures are ideally suited for continuous dermal suture because they do not have to be removed. In contrast, the nonabsorbable dermal continuous suture has to exit percutaneously from the ends of the wound, as well as surfacing every 3 cm through the skin, along the length of the continuous suture, to facilitate removal. The absorbable suture is attached to

the laser-drilled hole of the compound-curved, reverse cutting edge precision-point needle. Each dermal suture is passed just beneath the dermal-epidermal junction. The suture is begun as an interrupted dermal suture with its knot buried in the subcutaneous tissue (Fig. 46-18). After cutting the one ear attached to the free suture end, the fixed suture end with attached needle is used for the continuous dermal skin closure. The next stitch is passed horizontally from the end of the wound through the superficial dermis. After exiting the dermis, the position of the next bite is identified by pulling the suture across at right angles to the wound. Accurate positioning is assured by slight backtracking of each bite. During passage of the needle, the skin is stabilized by one arm of the toothed forceps. As the small horizontal bites are taken, gentle constant traction on the fixed suture brings the wound edges together. At a point one bite from the end of the wound, a small horizontal bite is passed toward the end of the wound. The suture before this corner stitch is withheld, forming a loop for the free end of the suture that will be used in constructing the knot. After passing the suture horizontally through a small bite of dermis in the opposite wound edge, the fixed suture end and the long loop of the free suture are used to construct a five-throw square knot with no ears. The divided epidermal edges are approximated by microporous tapes to ensure a meticulous approximation of the wound edges.

Lacerations subjected to weak skin tensions do not require support by dermal sutures and can be meticulously approximated by interrupted percutaneous monofilament synthetic nonabsorbable sutures (Fig. 46-19).

## LOWER EXTREMITY LACERATIONS IN THE ELDERLY OR THIN-SKINNED PATIENT

Wounds distal to the knee heal slowly. With aging, there is a decrease in cellular growth rate and a degeneration of collagen and elastic fibers, resulting in a loss of both dermal and subcutaneous tissues and a thinning of the epidermis. Consequently, the skin loses its elasticity and appears transparent, wrinkled, thin, dry, fragile, and lacking in tensile strength. Normally, the epidermis attaches firmly to the dermis by projecting extensions of epidermis into the dermis in a

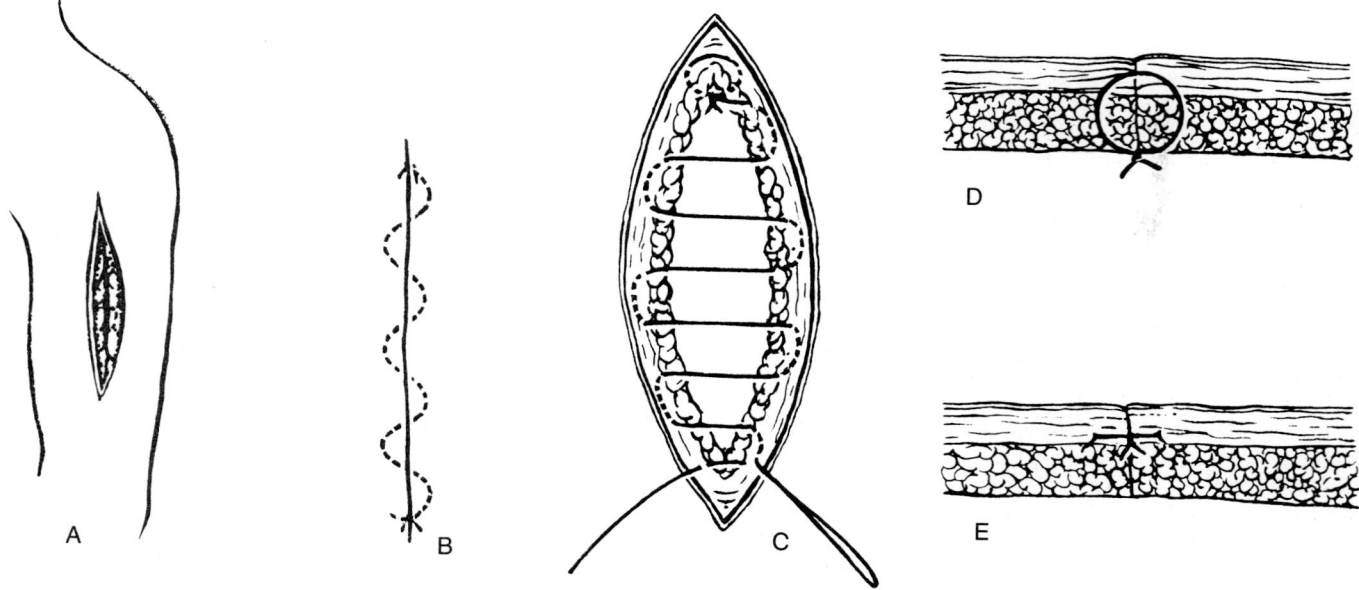

**Fig. 46-18. A.** Linear laceration of the arm subjected to strong skin tensions, with marked retraction of wound edges. **B.** Continuous subcuticular suture. **C.** Construction of continuous subcuticular suture. **D.** The subcuticular suture is begun as an interrupted dermal suture with its knot buried in the subcutaneous tissue. **E.** The subcuticular suture ends by constructing a knot located within the dermis.

**Fig. 46-19. Left.** A linear laceration of the left forehead subjected to weak static skin tensions. **Top right.** Wound repair is begun by constructing an interrupted percutaneous suture loop in the midportion of the wound. Two additional interrupted percutaneous sutures are positioned between the interrupted suture in the middle of the wound and the corners of the wound. **Bottom right.** Additional interrupted sutures are positioned between the interrupted percutaneous sutures.

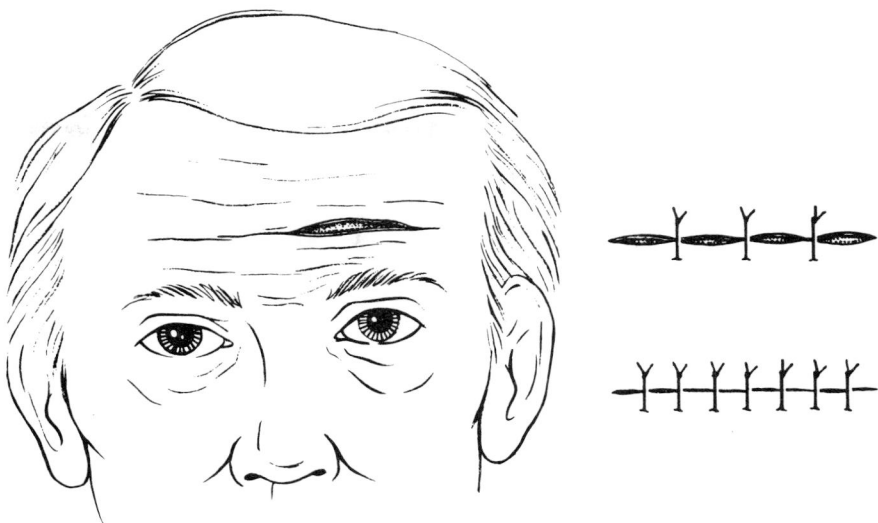

tongue-in-groove fashion (rete pegs). With aging, this dermal-epidermal junction flattens due to loss of capillaries, collagen fibers, and glycoproteins. With aging, there is also an increase in the fragility of the capillaries in the basement membrane zone, making the skin prone to subcutaneous hemorrhage or senile purpura. Due to all of these changes, aging skin tears after minor friction or shearing forces. These tears become an invitation to bacterial invasion and subsequent infection.

In the elderly, skin tears usually present as epidermal flaps. If the flap remains attached to its pedicle, it should be replaced on the dermis and approximated to adjacent tissue by skin-closure tapes (not sutures or skin staples). When the epidermal flap becomes separated from the skin, healing of the wound will be considerably delayed.

When caring for wounds with complete loss of the epidermal flap with exposure of 500 mm² or more of the dermis, coverage with a split-thickness skin graft is necessary. Skin grafts can be easily taken from anesthetized donor sites on the anterior thigh using a Weck ra-

zor with its blade spacer (Fig. 46-20A).[1] We use the thinnest of the spacers (0.008 in), allowing us to harvest a thin split-thickness skin graft. The anesthetized donor site skin is first lubricated with poloxamer 188. Traction is applied to the skin to hold it taut. The dermatome is then oscillated in the horizontal plane while moving forward with firm pressure (Figs. 46-20B and 20C). In this manner, it is possible to obtain a graft of remarkably uniform thickness, approximately 2 in wide and as long as desired. The skin graft is then meshed by cutting multiple linear slits using a no. 15 knife blade. The handle attached to the knife blade is held using a pencil grip. The donor site is then covered with fine-mesh gauze (type 1) that will spontaneously separate from the regenerated epidermal cells, usually within 14 days.

After gently washing the recipient skin site with poloxamer 188, the meshed skin graft is applied to the defect. The wound is then cov-

[1] Edward Weck & Co., New York, NY.

**Fig. 46-20. A.** A Weck razor with its blade spacer. **B.** The dermatome cuts a thin split-thickness skin graft from the donor site. **C.** The skin graft is draped over the donor site, after which it is detached from the donor site using a no. 15 knife blade.

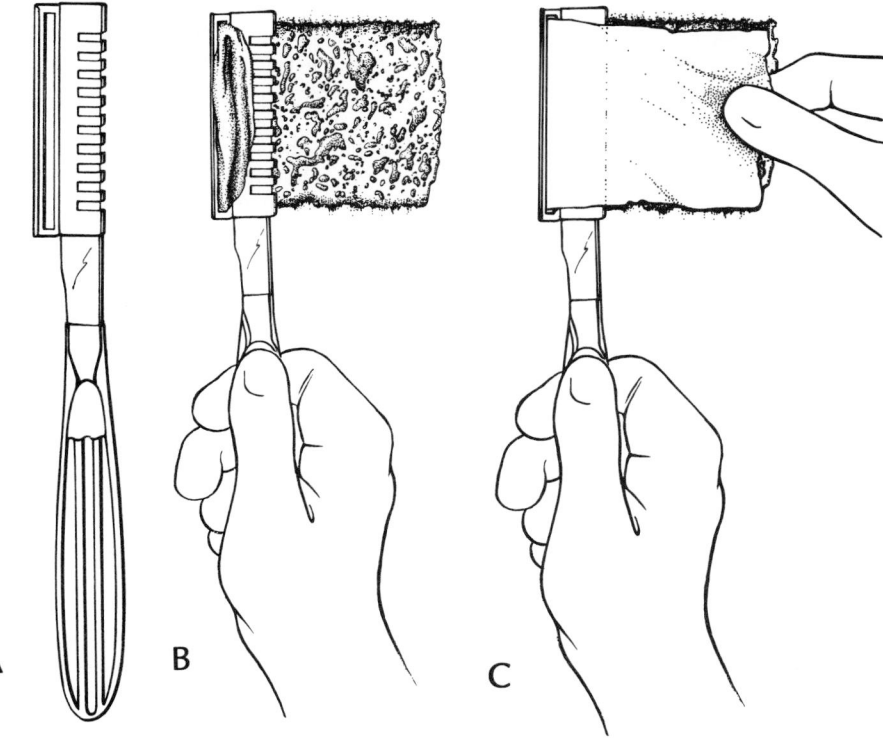

A          B                    C

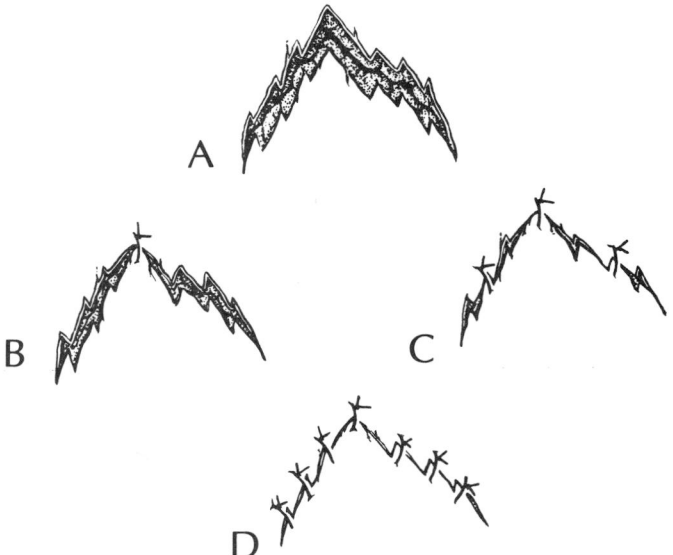

**Fig. 46-21. A.** V-shaped laceration with irregular wound edges. **B.** An interrupted percutaneous suture approximates the midportion of the wound. **C.** Two additional percutaneous sutures are used to approximate the lateral sides of the wound. **D.** Additional percutaneous sutures are positioned between the percutaneous sutures. **E.** The interrupted percutaneous sutures allow the wound to be reconstructed like a jigsaw puzzle.

ered by an Adaptik dressing followed by 4 × 4 gauze sponges. The foot, ankle, and lower leg are then covered by an Unna boot,[2] and ambulation at home is permitted. The Unna boot is changed at 5 and 14 days, with wound examination, and removed at 3 to 4 weeks.

Immediate mobilization reduces the potential risk of venous thromboembolism and eliminates the possibility of mental disorientation in elderly patients following hospitalization. Coverage of these wounds with a hydrocolloid dressing does not accelerate wound healing.

## U-SHAPED FLAPS

A U-shaped skin flap is often caused by compressive forces on skin overlying bone. The flap has abraded skin with attached subcutaneous tissues. The edges of the flap are usually irregular and fit together with adjacent wound edges, like a jigsaw puzzle. The survival of a rectangular-shaped flap is dependent on the perfusion pressure in the blood vessels of the flap. It has been demonstrated experimentally that flaps made under similar conditions of blood supply survive to the same length regardless of width. Consequently, the survival of a flap that is very wide will be comparable to flaps of similar length, regardless of width. Factors that favor survival include the following: (1) the presence of direct cutaneous arteries or veins coursing the longitudinal axis of the flap (axial pattern flap); (2) location of the flap in the head or neck, where the vascularity is excellent; (3) younger patients and those without diabetes mellitus or arteriosclerosis; (4) location above the knee and not in areas of scar or previous exposure to radiation, which, especially in the elderly, have diminished vascularity; and (5) absence of excessive tension, kinking, pressure, hematoma, or infection, which may interfere with circulation.

In any traumatic U-shaped flap, the most reliable way to determine tissue viability is examination 24 h after injury, at which time the viability is well demarcated and can be clearly ascertained. For fresh skin wounds, active bleeding from the distal and dermal margin may be present and indicates viability. The distribution of intravenously injected fluorescein dye within the tissues may be helpful. Early staining of the injured skin by fluorescein is evidence of an intact blood supply.

U-, C-, or V-shaped flaps usually heal with a trapdoor or pincushion effect that results in an elevated bulging of the tissues. Various theories to explain this phenomenon are lymphatic and venous obstruction, hypertrophy of the scar, excessive fatty and redundant tissues, beveled wound edges, and contracture of the scar. Today, most

believe that the contractive forces of the longitudinal and horizontal planes are the most important causal factors.

Because the traumatic wound is susceptible to the development of infection, it is best to reapproximate the edges of a vascularized flap with the least reactive synthetic monofilament suture using interrupted percutaneous sutures. Approximation of its irregular wound edges is like putting together a jigsaw puzzle (Fig. 46-21). The wound edges of these lacerations often have a beveled edge, rather than a perpendicular configuration (Fig. 46-22). It can be argued that this beveled edge may have a favorable influence on healing by providing a large interface between the divided edges, thereby enhancing repair. Consequently, repair of the bevel edges is advocated. This reconstruction may be time-consuming because the needle must be passed separately through one wound edge before it is passed through the other to ensure that the suture passes through the same depth on

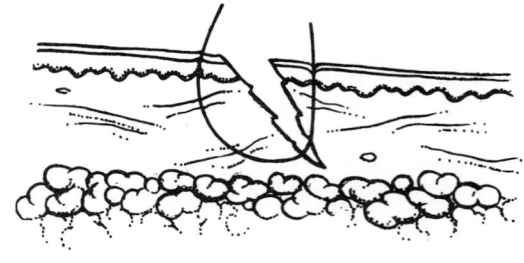

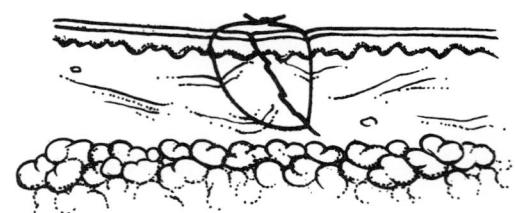

**Fig. 46-22. Top.** The edges of the V- or U-shaped laceration often have a beveled edge. Wound closure is accomplished by first passing the suture through one side of the wound, after which it is passed through the other side of the wound. This maneuver allows the suture to be passed through the same depth on either side of the wound. **Bottom.** After the knot is constructed, there is meticulous approximation of the wound edges.

[2] Beiersdorf, Inc., Norwalk, CT.

each side of the wound. This time-consuming maneuver is a worthwhile technique because it prevents malapposition of the wound edges, an unattractive scar deformity.

When a portion of the flap is devascularized, this segment should be excised. The excised flap should then be defatted, converting the flap into a skin graft that is applied to the defect and secured by a tie-over bolus dressing. After the skin graft heals without infection, the patient should be referred to a plastic surgeon for follow-up evaluation. Six months after wound closure, the plastic surgeon can correct the trapdoor deformity by performing Z- and W-plasties accompanied by peripheral undermining of the wound. It is important to undermine a section around the deformity that is greater in area than the deformity itself. For small trapdoor deformities, simple excision of the deformity resulting in a lenticular-shaped defect is an excellent alternative.

## RING TOURNIQUET SYNDROME

Acute or chronic digital swelling can leave a finger ring tightly and painfully trapped at the base of the proximal phalanx. Trauma, infections, dermatologic condition, perivenous infusions, and allergic reactions are common sources of localized digital edema or generalized swelling of the hand. As the digit expands, venous outflow from the finger is increasingly restricted by the tourniquet-like effects of the ring. Nerve damage, ischemia, and digital gangrene are frequent complications when the ring is not promptly removed. Several simple techniques may be used by the emergency physician to remove the ring, with minimal damage to the finger or, in many cases, to the ring.

The finger involved must first be assessed for major lacerations or neurovascular compromise. We routinely monitor the sensory perception of the distal phalanx using two-point discrimination. The Doppler flow meter is an excellent technique for monitoring distal digital pulses. The presence of reduced sensory perception or diminished pulses is an indication for ring cutting. In the absence of neurovascular compromise, ring-sparing techniques should be attempted initially. In any case, the patient is initially instructed to elevate the involved extremity to encourage venous and lymphatic drainage. After these measures and lubrication of the digit with poloxamer 188, the emergency physician may find that the ring will slide over intact skin with a slight pull. If not, several techniques should be considered:

**String technique.** When the digital skin is intact and neurovascular compromise is absent, the finger may be wrapped in a spiral ligature from the distal interphalangeal (DIP) joint over the proximal interphalangeal (PIP) joint and to the ring (Fig. 46-23A). Braided suture of zero gauge or larger with a taperpoint needle is recommended. Monofilament sutures should be avoided because they can tear through the skin. The wrapping is performed with enough tension so that the interstitial fluid gently moves to the proximal side of the ring, but not so tightly that the string obstructs arterial flow. The needle is then passed beneath the ring, a procedure that can virtually always be performed, and the proximal free end is thus advanced beyond the ring (Fig. 46-23B). The suture is then slowly unwound, pushing the ring on its outstretched proximal end. The ring will follow just behind the retreating coil until it has passed the PIP joint and can be readily pulled from the finger (Fig. 46-23C). Wetting the suture with poloxamer 188 can further facilitate ring removal.

**Rubber glove.** In cases where the digit is markedly swollen, a "finger" is removed from the appropriately sized, powder-free surgical glove and pulled onto the involved digit. When the rim of the glove finger nears the ring, a curved forceps, positioned proximal to the ring, is passed distally to grasp the latex and draw it between the ring and the finger. The latex is then allowed to compress the swollen finger uniformly until the ring can be passed over the finger and glove. Wetting the external glove surface with poloxamer 188 will facilitate ring removal.

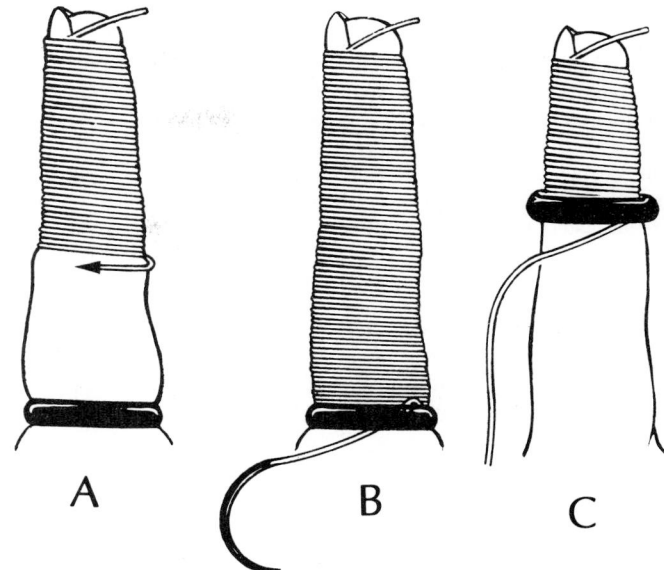

**Fig. 46-23.** String technique.

**Cutting.** When neurovascular integrity is in jeopardy or the above methods fail, the ring must be cut to arrest the progression of neurovascular compromise. The thinnest, least ornate, or most accessible portion of the ring is the ideal site for cutting. If elevation of this section is necessary for application of the ring cutter, the ring is compressed by pliers with parallel jaws at the two contralateral points 90° from the cutting site. This compression converts the ring shape from circular to elliptical. Because the long axis of the ellipse is greater than the diameter of the original circle, a space becomes apparent between the ring and underlying tissues. The finger guard of the ring cutter is passed through this space (Fig. 46-24). Compression from the sides tends to displace neurovascular bundles to the less restricted palmar region and accordingly should not compromise them.

A ring cutter has two lever arms that rotate on a fulcrum (Fig. 46-24). A finger guard on one lever arm protects the finger from injury. The other arm has a hand-turned circular saw blade that comes into intimate contact with the ring. Rotation of the saw blade will sever the ring without cutting the skin. The two ends of the divided ring are

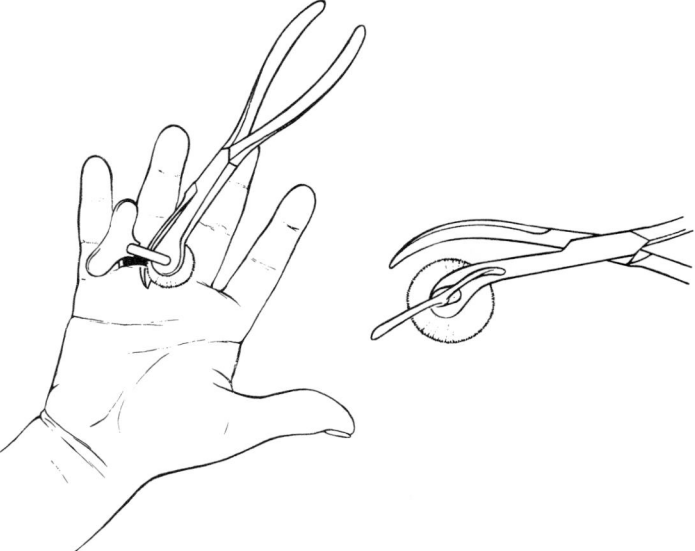

**Fig. 46-24. Left.** The finger guard of the ring cutter is passed beneath the ring. **Right.** The circular saw blade cuts the ring.

then grasped and pulled in opposite directions to open the ring and allow its removal.

When the object is too thick or tempered for this method (e.g., steel nuts or machine parts), motorized hand-held cutters with sharp-edged circular grinders[3] may be required to penetrate the material. In such cases, the rings may frequently be too strong to be bent open for removal but may be halved by making two cuts separated by 180°. To prevent metallic splintering into the hand, a silastic band or one of similar material is placed beneath the ring-cutting site.

Psychiatric patients may present with rings that have remained trapped tightly in place for extended periods of time, allowing epithelial overgrowth to cover sections of the involved ring. After local anesthesia with 1% lidocaine, surgical division of the skin bridge is performed. The ring is then cut off as described above, and the epithelialized flaps are trimmed. Wound cultures are taken to guide antibiotic therapy in the patient with cellulitis, fever, or other symptoms of systemic infection. Tetanus prophylaxis of these tetanus-prone wounds is mandatory.

After removal of a ring, neurovascular integrity must be evaluated by assessing tactile sensation and capillary refill of the finger. Deficits in either area require prompt consultation with a specialist in hand surgery.

## EMBEDDED FISHHOOK

There are many hundreds of hook patterns, which differ in size and shape according to their intended purposes (Fig. 46-25). The parts of the hook are the point, barb, bend, shank, and eye. The point of the hook is the sharpened end of a hook that penetrates the fish's mouth. Its barb is the projection extending backward from the point of a hook. The barb helps to keep the point embedded by resisting removal. A barb or barbs may be cut into the shank. These projections will anchor a soft bait such as a salmon egg or seaworm. The bend of

[3] Dremel Moto-Tool: Dremel, Division of Emerson Electric Company, Racine, Wisconsin.

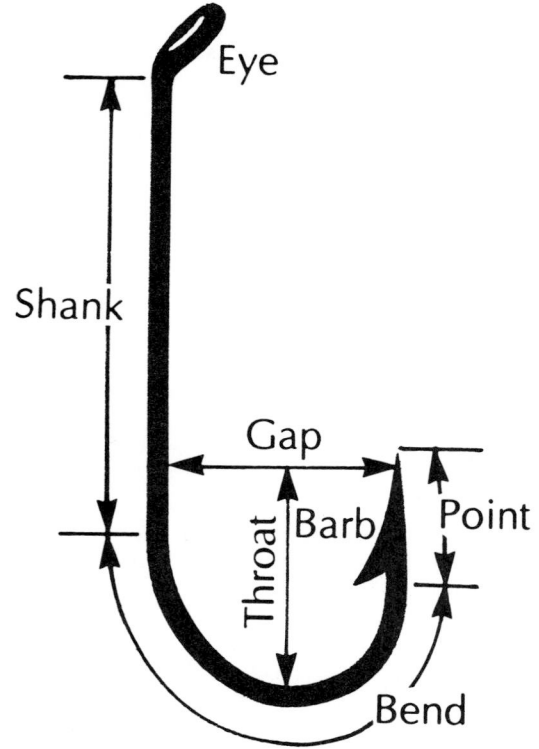

**Fig. 46-25.** Anatomy of a fishhook.

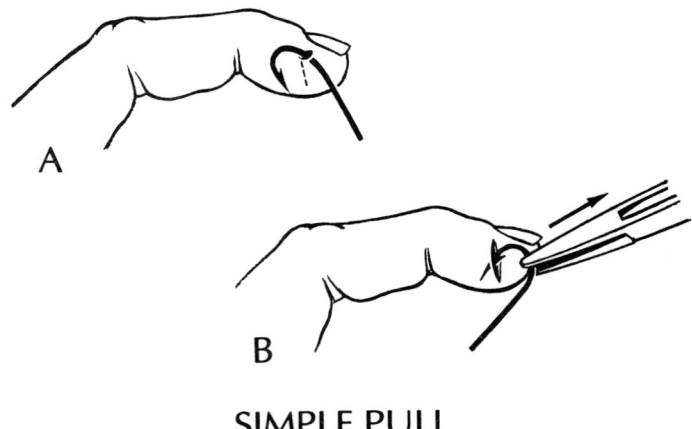

## SIMPLE PULL

**Fig. 46-26.** Simple pull technique.

the hook is the bottom or curved portion of the hook. Its shank is the upper portion of the hook that extends from the bend on the side opposite the point to the eye. The eye is a hole or loop at the end of the shank through which the line is secured.

The removal of a fishhook from the skin is a challenging procedure for the emergency physician because of the hook's barb. Appropriate strategies for hook removal depend on the type of hook involved and its anatomic location within the patient's skin—two factors that may be determined by plain radiographs if not readily apparent. Roughly half of embedded fishhook injuries occur in the hands, and over a third involve the face or head. Fishermen in warmer climates generally wear less protective clothing and are at greater risk for involvement of the trunk or proximal extremity. Four basic strategies of fishhook removal have been described. The majority of emergency department fishhook injuries require the push and clip method, while over 40 percent are removed by the less traumatic retrograde methods. These retrograde techniques should be attempted whenever possible prior to resorting to the push-and-clip method. Hook wounds do not require suture closure and should, instead, be cleaned with poloxamer 188 and approximated by sterile, microporous tape.

### Retrograde Techniques

**Simple pull.** If the hook is very superficially embedded in the epidermis or has a small barb, it may be withdrawn along its entry path using a needle holder or hemostat. When the point of the hook passes through the dermis, the barb remains embedded beneath the dermis (Fig. 46-26A). In these cases, a 1- to 2-mm incision will be needed to enlarge the entry wound on the site of the barb (Fig. 46-26B). The injury site is first cleansed with poloxamer 188, and 0.1 to 0.3 mL of 1% lidocaine is injected into the skin incision site. The incision is made with a no. 11 blade and is deepened through the dermis. The emergency physician grasps the hook with a needle holder at its bend as close to the wound as possible, and then rapidly applies traction to remove the embedded hook. As the hook is being pulled straight out, gentle pressure is applied to the shank so that the hook eye contacts the skin surface. This motion unlocks the barb from adjacent tissues and minimizes its contact with the walls of the wound track.

**String pull.** The string technique is also suited for embedded fishhooks whose barbs reside beneath the dermis (Fig. 46-27A). This method uses a strong ligature like umbilical tape or 0-gauge braided suture. It does not involve any incision, anesthesia, or surgical equipment. The physician passes the suture around the bend of the hook and then holds both ends of the suture with gloved fingers (Fig. 46-27B). The eye of the hook is then directed toward the skin as a sharp pull is applied to the suture in the direction parallel to the shank, causing removal of the embedded hook.

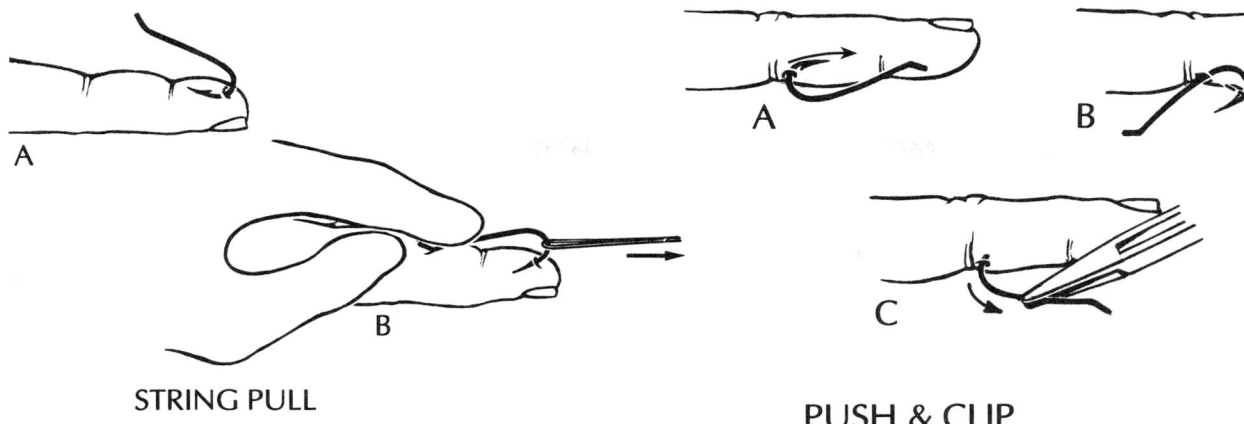

### STRING PULL

**Fig. 46-27.** String pull technique.

**Needle sheath.** This technique is used for hooks with large barbs when the barbs are buried deep beneath the dermis (Fig. 46-28A). As the hook is held in a needle holder or hemostat, a 16- or 18-gauge hypodermic needle is introduced through the entry wound and advanced along the hook's bend until the barb can be sheathed within the lumen of the needle (Fig. 46-28B). The hook and needle are then gently withdrawn together. No incision or anaesthesia is required for this procedure.

## Push-and-Clip Technique

If the fishhook is embedded deeply within a joint, cartilage, or tendon, retrograde removal of the intact hook is not recommended. Instead, the push-and-clip method is used (Fig. 46-29A). The skin around the entrance and anticipated exit site is cleansed with poloxamer 188, and the exit site is then anesthetized with 1 to 2 mL of 1% lidocaine. The middle of the hook shank is grasped with a needle holder, and the hook is advanced through the anesthetized skin (Fig. 46-29B). The point and barb of the hook are exposed, the bend of the hook is then cut with wire cutters, and the hook shank is withdrawn from the wound in a retrograde manner (Fig. 46-29C). When a hook has additional barbs on the shank, the hook is first advanced through the anaesthetized skin as described above. Then, rather than cutting the hook with wire cutters, the hook point is grasped with a needle holder and the shank of the hook is cut close to the skin to remove the hook eye. Division of the shank of the hook that is closest to the eye allows the physician to withdraw the hook from the skin with the needle holder.

Injury to the eyes is rare (<0.1 percent) but constitutes an emer-

### PUSH & CLIP

**Fig. 46-29.** Push-and-clip technique.

gency and should be immediately addressed by an ophthalmologist. Until the ophthalmologist comes to the emergency department, the patient should be seated in a semirecumbent position to minimize intraocular pressure. The patient should be instructed to not move the eye. In addition, the embedded fishhook should be shielded to prevent inadvertent contact with the hook. Pressure on the hook or on the eyelid must be avoided to prevent further injury to the eye or vitreous extrusion along the wound path.

All fishhook wounds are considered tetanus-prone and should receive appropriate tetanus prophylaxis. Antibiotic therapy is not warranted unless the eye is involved

## BIBLIOGRAPHY

### Laceration Subjected to Strong Skin Tensions

Abidin MR, Becker DR, Paley RD, et al: A new compound curved needle for intradermal suture closure. *J Emerg Med* 7:441, 1989.
Abidin MR, Towler MA, Lombardi SA, et al: Emergency physician's needle holder. *J Emerg Med* 7:581, 1989.
DuBois JJ: A technique for subcutaneous knot inversion following running subcuticular closures. *Mil Med* 5:255, 1992.
Straith RE, Lawson JM, Hipps JC: The subcuticular suture. *Postgrad Med* 29:164, 1961.

### Lower Extremity Lacerations

Payne RL, Martin ML: Skin tears . . . The epidemiology and management of skin tears in older adults. *Ostomy/Wound Management* 26:26, 1990.

### U-Shaped Flaps

Koranda FC, Webster RC: Trapdoor effect in nasolabial flaps: Causes and corrections. *Arch Otolaryngol* 111:421, 1985.

### Ring Tourniquet Syndrome

Clarke AC, Spencer RF: Ring removal from the injured or swollen finger. *Postgrad Med* 89:190, 1991.
Frary T: A few brief tips: Ring removal. *J Am Acad Physician Assist* 3:156, 1990.
Wee JTK, Chandra D: A rapid method of removal of rings impacted in fingers. *J Hand Surg* 14B:126, 1989.

### Embedded Fishhooks

Doser C, Cooper WL, Ediger WM, et al: Fishhook injuries: A prospective evaluation. *Am J Emerg Med* 9:413, 1991.
Lantsberg L, Blintsovsky E, Hoda J: How to extract an indwelling fishhook. *Am Fam Physician* 45:2589, 1992.

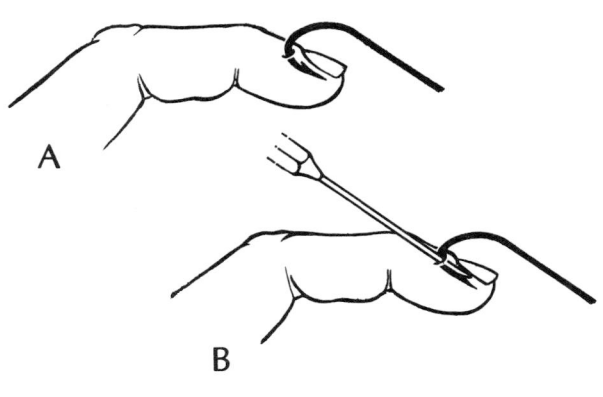

### NEEDLE SHEATH

**Fig. 46-28.** Needle sheath technique.

# 47

# SOFT TISSUE INJURIES TO THE FACE

### Richard F. Edlich

## INTRODUCTION

Facial wounds are among the most frequently encountered injuries. All wounds of the face may be divided into two basic groups: (1) injuries of the soft tissues and (2) injuries to the bone. This chapter focuses on soft tissue injuries to the face. The goals of treatment of soft tissue wounds are first to care for all injuries that are an immediate threat to life and second to repair wounds so that there is an optimal return of function and restoration of appearance.

Because facial injuries may be associated with serious injuries to other sites, emergency treatment of life-threatening conditions must take precedence over management of facial injuries. Active bleeding from soft tissue wounds of the face must be treated immediately by a pressure dressing. Because a carefully applied dressing will usually arrest bleeding, shock is not a frequent consequence of hemorrhage from facial trauma. Before applying the dressing, all kinked or twisted flaps of tissue should be returned to their original position to prevent further vascular compromise. Bleeding from the oral cavity, which is not susceptible to control by pressure, can obstruct the airway. In such cases, a patent airway can be maintained, usually by sucking blood from the patient's mouth using a Yankauer tonsil sucker. The patient should be transported immobilized and secured by a backboard. Aspiration can be prevented by turning the patient and backboard as a unit so that the patient is lying on his or her side.

Repair of facial soft tissue injuries requires an understanding of the anatomy of each special site, assessment of the aesthetic and functional deformity, and selection of the appropriate techniques for repair. Because the surgical treatment of the injury to each site of the face is dependent, in part, upon its anatomic configuration, the anatomy of the specific site will be discussed in conjunction with our surgical approaches to wound repair. The technical factors involved in wound care outlined in Section 5, "Emergency Wound Management," are applicable to soft tissue injuries of the face.

## EMERGENCY DEPARTMENT CARE

### Scalp

#### Anatomy

The scalp and forehead are parts of the same anatomic structure (Fig. 47-1). They are composed of the following five layers: (1) skin, (2) subcutaneous tissue, (3) occipitofrontalis muscle, (4) a layer of loose aponeurosis, and (5) the pericranium (Fig. 47-1A). The first layers are intimately connected and are not easily separated. The scalp skin is very thick and firmly attached to the underlying epicranial aponeurosis (galea aponeurotica) by fibrous septa. It has abundant hair follicles, sebaceous glands, and a rich network of blood vessels. The subcutaneous tissue is divided by the fibrous septa into multiple fat lobules. The septa limit vessel retraction following injury and are responsible for profuse hemorrhage.

The occipitofrontalis muscle has two pairs of muscles connected by a broad aponeurosis, the galea aponeurotica (epicranial aponeurosis). The anterior pair of muscles are the frontalis muscles, attached to the epicranial aponeurosis a little in front of the coronal suture

Our research has been supported by a generous gift from Mrs. Ruth E. Tanner, Richmond, VA.

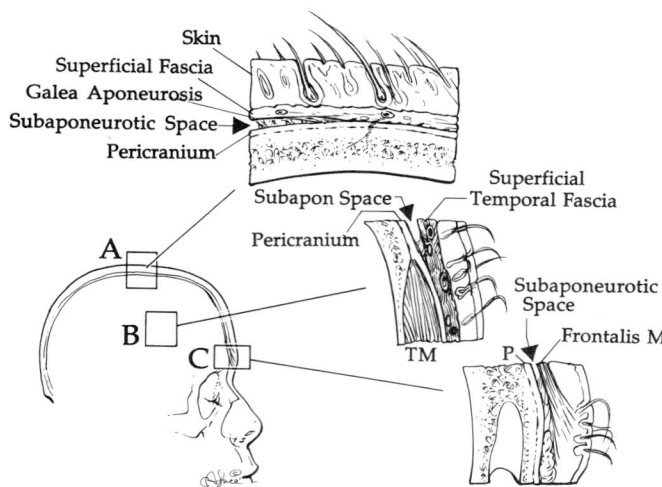

**Fig. 47-1.** Diagram of five layers of the scalp.

(Fig. 47-1C). The posterior pair of muscles (occipitalis muscles) are attached to the occipital bone above the lateral two-thirds of the nuchal line and to the mastoid process of the temporal bone. The epicranial aponeurosis is attached posteriorly to the external occipital protuberance and anteriorly to the supraorbital margin of the frontal bellies. Laterally, it blends with the fascia covering the temporalis muscle above the level of the zygomatic arch (Fig. 47-1B). It is separated from the periosteum (pericranium) overlying the skull by loose areolar tissue. This subgaleal layer permits free movement of the scalp over the cranium and is the plane where avulsion occurs in scalping injuries. This space is considered the danger zone of the scalp because hematoma and infection can spread easily through it. It is traversed by small arteries that supply the pericranium, and by the emissary veins connecting the intracranial venous sinuses with the superficial veins of the scalp. Thrombosis of the emissary veins may extend to the dural sinuses. The pericranium is adherent at the sutures and thus limits the spread of infection.

The sensory nerve supply to the entire scalp and face is supplied by branches of the trigeminal nerve, except for the skin overlying the posterior portion of the masseter muscle, which is innervated by posterior and anterior branches of the upper cervical nerves. Injuries to these sensory nerves rarely result in permanent anesthesia because of the rich overlapping system of undamaged nerves as well as nerve regeneration.

The scalp has a luxurious blood supply from five arteries on each side of the head. The occipital, superficial temporal, and posterior auricular arteries are branches of the external carotid artery, while the supraorbital and supratrochlear arteries arise from the internal carotid arteries.

### Injuries and Treatment

Soft tissue injuries of the scalp can be divided into four groups: lacerations, abrasions, contusions, and avulsions. Over half are due to motor vehicle accidents. The front-seat passenger is most commonly thrown up and forward, sustaining an impact injury to the head caused by the windshield. The construction of the windshield is a key determinant of the type of injury. Automobiles manufactured prior to 1966 had safety-glass windshields that were susceptible to penetration by the occupant's head in an angle of approximately 45 degrees in a 14-mph frontal crash. After the forward momentum had stopped, the passenger was thrown back and down into the front seat. As the victim's face returned past the lower edge of the broken windshield, it tore the brow and forehead, resulting in superiorly based U-shaped flaps. Occasionally, complete avulsion occurred and the tissue was found on the broken windshield.

High-penetration-resistant (HPR) windshields were introduced in 1966 and have changed dramatically the pattern of facial soft tissue injuries. In HPR windshields, the pane is laminated to a plastic interlayer that prevents the occupant's head from penetrating the windshield. After impact, the plastic layer stretches out, cushioning the head against it. The inner glass pane fractures into a typical mosaic pattern of breakage at the site of impact that is responsible for the characteristic soft tissue injuries consisting of numerous small, superficial lacerations and triangular avulsion flaps. Glass particles are often buried in the lacerations. These facial injuries can be avoided by the use of shoulder-lap seat belts and/or air-bag restraint systems.

Total avulsion of the scalp is an occupational hazard for personnel with long hair who work in close proximity to rotary machines. The loose areolar tissue beneath the galea aponeurotica allows the scalp to be pulled off the pericranium. Stringent safeguards have reduced the incidence of industrial accidents of this type.

It must be emphasized that eyebrows should never be clipped or shaved because their delicate contour and form are valuable landmarks for the meticulous reapproximation of the wound edges. After the wound has been cleansed and hemostasis achieved, the base of the wound should always be palpated. Physical examination is often a more accurate technique for diagnosing injuries to the underlying bone than is x-ray examination.

When the edges of a laceration of either the eyebrow or the scalp are devitalized, debridement is mandatory. When debriding these sites, the scalpel should cut at an angle that is parallel to that of the hair follicles. If the cut is made vertical to the skin surface, injury to hair follicles adjacent to the cut edge will occur and areas on both sides of the scar will be hairless.

Wound closure should be initiated first with approximation of the galea aponeurotica with buried, interrupted nonabsorbable 4–0 synthetic sutures. Galeal suture closure reduces the depth and width of the overlying skin scar. This beneficial effect of galeal sutures on scar formation is significantly more evident with nonabsorbable sutures than absorbable sutures. Another advantage of galeal suture is that it provides a barrier to the spread of superficial infection into the underlying loose areolar plane. The divided edges of muscle and fascia must also be closed with buried, interrupted, braided absorbable 4–0 synthetic sutures to prevent further the development of depressed scars.

The skin edges of anatomic landmarks should be approximated first with key stitches, using interrupted nonabsorbable monofilament 5–0 synthetic sutures (Fig. 47-2). Accurate alignment of the eyebrow, transverse wrinkles of the forehead, and the hairline of the scalp is essential. It may be necessary to have younger patients raise their eyebrows to create wrinkles, which will guide accurate placement of the key stitches.

An irregular laceration should be put together as it came apart, because it usually heals with a scar whose width is narrower than that of a linear laceration. Moreover, an irregular laceration undergoes less contraction than a linear one.

Z-plasty and flap rotation should never be considered for primary repair because there is no guarantee either that scar contracture will occur or that the repaired wound will not become infected. Scar revisions are always best accomplished when tissue healing and scar maturation are complete, 6 to 12 months after injury.

In forehead and scalp lacerations where underlying muscle and galea are divided, hematomas may form and dissect beneath the galea aponeurotica. A firm pressure dressing placed around the head can close any potential dead space, encourage hemostasis, and prevent hematoma formation. This pressure dressing should be left in place for 48 h.

Contusions of the scalp and forehead heal readily unless there is an underlying hematoma; this may become localized, with subsequent formation of an encapsulated seroma. The seroma can erode into the outer table of the skull to result in Pott's puffy tumor. A hematoma is

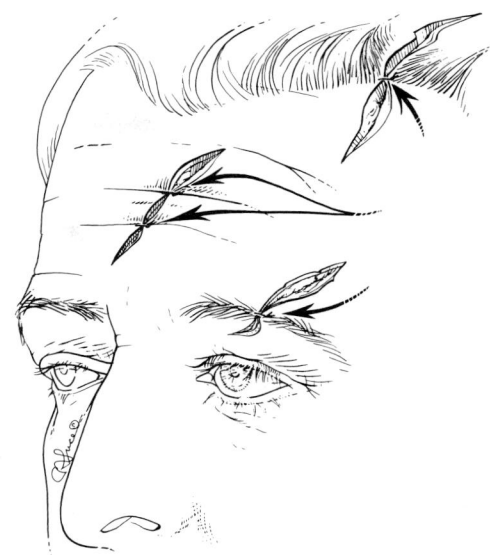

**Fig. 47-2.** Key stitches in the eyebrow.

best evacuated by an incision when still in the currant-jelly stage. As further liquefaction of the blood clot occurs, aspiration with a large-bore needle (No. 16 or larger) may be successful. After evacuation of either a hematoma or seroma, a pressure dressing should be applied to the forehead and scalp for 48 h to close the dead space and prevent reaccumulation of blood or serous exudates.

## Eyelids

### Anatomy

The upper and lower eyelids are reinforced folds of tissue which form movable curtains. From its superficial to its deep surface, the eyelid is composed of the following structures: (1) skin, (2) subcutaneous tissue, (3) orbicularis oculi muscle, (4) tarsal plate, and (5) conjunctiva. The skin of the eyelid is thinner than at any other anatomic site of the body, and has fine, downlike hairs. It is freely movable over the underlying tissues and can be picked up readily with the finger. There is normally a fold in the upper lid (supratarsal fold) under which the lower portion of the lid disappears when elevated. When the eyelids are opened, they are separated from each other by an elliptical space, the palpebral fissure. The angles of the space are the lateral and medial canthi.

The subcutaneous tissue is relatively free of fat and is penetrated by the superficial fibers of the orbicularis oculi muscle. The muscle can be divided into three parts: orbital, pretarsal and preseptal. The orbital portion forms a muscular ring extending over the orbital margin widely, interdigitating with fibers of the frontalis muscle. Contraction of this orbital portion brings the skin of the forehead and eyelids downward and shades the eyes; it is used to close the lids tightly. The pretarsal portion overlies the tarsus and divides medially into superficial and deep heads. The superficial head joins its counterpart in the opposing lid to form the medial canthal tendon, which inserts above and anterior to the anterior lacrimal crest. The deep head, after joining its counterpart, advances posteriorly to the lacrimal sac and inserts behind the posterior lacrimal crest. The preseptal part of the muscle overlies the septum orbitale and has superficial and deep fibers. Its superficial fibers insert on the orbital margin below the canthal tendon, while its deeper fibers insert on the posterior lacrimal crest just above the deep head of the pretarsal portion. The insertion of the heads of the pretarsal and preseptal parts on the posterior lacrimal crest maintains the eyelids against the ocular globe, and is responsible for the depth of the naso-orbital valley. If the medial canthal tendon is severed, reattachment of the canthal tendon posterior to the lacrimal crest is essential to reestablish the depth of the naso-orbital valley.

Both the pretarsal parts of the orbicularis oculi muscle form a raphe that is attached to the skin of the lateral canthus. The pretarsal muscles of the upper and lower lids have a tendinous insertion (lateral canthal tendon) into the orbital tubercle. The pretarsal and preseptal portions of the orbicularis oculi muscle are able to close the eyelids and are responsible for involuntary blinking. Forced closure of the eye requires the entire muscle to contract. While the temporal branch of the facial nerve innervates the major portion of the orbicularis oculi muscle, the zygomatic branch of this nerve also supplies this muscle.

The orbital septum unites the margins of the tarsal plates to the infraorbital and supraorbital margins and attaches to the medial and lateral canthal tendons. By separating the tissues of the lid from the orbital contents, it contains the orbital structures behind the lids, preventing orbital fat from herniating forward and distorting the surface contour of the lid. An intricate fascial system, known as Lockwood's suspensory ligament, is attached to the orbital walls, forming a sling beneath the eye. It attaches medially to the posterior lacrimal crest and laterally below the lateral orbital tubercle.

The upper eyelid is more movable than the lower; attached to it is the levator palpebrae superioris, which is innervated by the third cranial nerve. Together with the superior rectus muscle, it arises from the small wing of the sphenoid above and in front of the optic foramen, passes with this muscle, and finally separates from it to enter the upper lid as a fan-shaped muscle. The main insertion of the muscle is the upper part of the tarsal plate. Some of its fibers pass through the orbicularis oculi muscles to be attached to the skin of the upper eyelid and the subconjunctival fornix. The expansions of the levator palpebrae superioris, which are attached to the medial and lateral canthal ligaments, are important landmarks when attempting to locate the severed muscles. Injury to this muscle or its nerve supply results in ptosis.

Müller's muscle is a thin muscle in the upper lid which lies closely behind the levator palpebrae superioris, to which it is loosely connected by fine connective tissue fibers as far as its attachment to the superior margin of the tarsus. While the levator palpebrae superioris is striated muscle, Müller's muscle is smooth muscle, receiving innervation from the sympathetic nervous system. Stimulation of the sympathetic nerve supply of Müller's muscle results in elevation of the upper lid by 3 to 4 mm. In the lower lid, Müller's muscle arises from the sheath of the inferior rectus and is inserted on the lower border of the tarsus. Contraction of these fibers results in a lowering of the lower lid. Opening of the palpebral fissure is due to contraction of the levator palpebrae superioris and Müller's muscle in conjunction with relaxation of the orbicularis oculi.

The tarsal plate itself forms the main body of the lower half of the lid. It consists of some elastic tissue in a dense matrix of connective tissue. The upper tarsus is much larger than the lower. Its free border extends to the lid margin. Embedded in the tarsal plate are a number of simple branched alveolar glands, the meibomian glands. They open into the white line just in front of the conjunctival edge of the lid margin. In the lid margin the eyelashes are arranged in three irregular rows. Their follicles extend obliquely into the tarsal plate.

The posterior surface of the eyelid is covered by a transparent membrane, the conjunctiva. This membrane lines the lid as the palpebral conjunctiva and is reflected onto the anterior surface of the eyeball as the bulbar conjunctiva. This reflection forms a deep recess known as the fornix.

The excretory lacrimal duct system begins at the upper and lower puncta, which are positioned at the apex of the lacrimal papilla. Each punctum, which is the beginning of a canaliculus, has a diameter of 0.3 mm and is surrounded by a ring of connective and elastic tissue. The canaliculi are approximately 10 cm long and consist of a 2-cm vertical component and an 8-cm horizontal section. In the horizontal

part of the canaliculi, the lumen widens to form the ampulla, which is 2 to 3 mm at its widest diameter. In 90 percent of the population, the canaliculi join to form an internal common canaliculus before entering the lacrimal sac, which is situated in the lacrimal fossa. The lacrimal sac is the membranous extension of the nasolacrimal duct, whose length is approximately 20 mm. The nasolacrimal duct extends 3 to 5 mm above the level of the medial canthus before it becomes the osseous portion of the nasolacrimal duct. This duct opens into the anterior part of the inferior meatus of the nose. The ostium is guarded by a fold of mucosa named Hausner's valve. Tears are propelled into the excretory lacrimal duct system by gravity, the venturi effect in the inferior meatus, and the lacrimal pump.

The lacrimal pump mechanism is involved in the excretory functions of tears into the nose. The superficial and deep heads of the pretarsal muscles furnish the motor power for the lacrimal pump, closing the ampulla and shortening the canaliculi, and forcing fluid into the lacrimal sac. The preseptal muscles, through their intimate connection with the lacrimal diaphragm, also produce negative pressure in the lacrimal sac. The elasticity of the diaphragm returns it to its position of rest, and fluid is forced into the nasolacrimal duct. Closure of the eye shortens the canaliculus and exerts pressure on the lacrimal ampulla. Opening of the eye creates a vacuum within the lacrimal sac and initiates the pump mechanism.

## Injuries and Treatment

In treating eyelid injuries, major considerations are to protect the eye and to maintain vision. Preoperative examination of the eye by an ophthalmologist is mandatory. If an ocular injury is detected, treatment of the eye injury must precede repair. During wound repair, the cornea must be protected from desiccation, irritation, and trauma. Desiccation can be prevented by instilling a few drops of 0.9% saline into the conjunctival sac during wound closure. The use of a contact lens is recommended to protect the cornea from injury.

Trauma in this region can be divided into injuries to the upper and lower eyelids, to the canthal tendons, and to the lacrimal system. Injuries to the eyelids are either lacerations or avulsions. In either case, damage to the levator palpebrae superioris may be evident. The lacerations can be classified into two groups according to their depth: lacerations through the skin and lacerations through the lid margins. A superficial laceration of the skin parallel to the lid margin may require no closure, especially if it aligned with the lid fold. If the laceration is not aligned with the skin fold, approximation of the skin edges with a running, subcuticular nonabsorbable monofilament 5–0 synthetic suture is recommended. The suture should be removed 72 h after injury to avoid the development of epithelial cysts at the entrance and exits of the suture. Because the direction of this laceration is perpendicular to that of the dynamic skin tensions, wound repair will usually result in a narrow, aesthetically pleasing scar. In contrast, lacerations through skin whose direction is perpendicular to the lid margin will heal with a conspicuous scar that often develops a linear contracture causing an upward pull on the lid. A Z-plasty revision of the healing scar 6 to 12 months later will lengthen the contracture and prevent this deformity.

Closure of a laceration that extends through the entire eyelid requires a three-layer closure, with meticulous approximation of each layer (Fig. 47-3). After a protective lens is positioned in the conjunctival sac, closure should begin with a marginal nonabsorbable monofilament 5–0 synthetic suture, aligning and approximating the "gray line," which is the end of a sheet of fascia between the orbicularis oculi muscle and the tarsal plate (Fig. 47-3A). If the "gray line" is not approximated accurately, notching of the eyelid often results, with possible inversion of the eyelashes. Traction of the long untied ends of the marginal suture approximates the wound edges and aligns the anterior and posterior lid margins.

The conjunctiva and tarsal plate are then closed with interrupted,

**Fig. 47-3.** Repair of lacerations through the lid. A scleral lens has been placed in the conjunctival sac. **A.** The first suture is passed through the "grayline" of the eyelid. **B.** The conjunctiva and tarsal plate are then closed. **C.** A skin suture is tied over the long ends of the marginal suture. (See text for detail.)

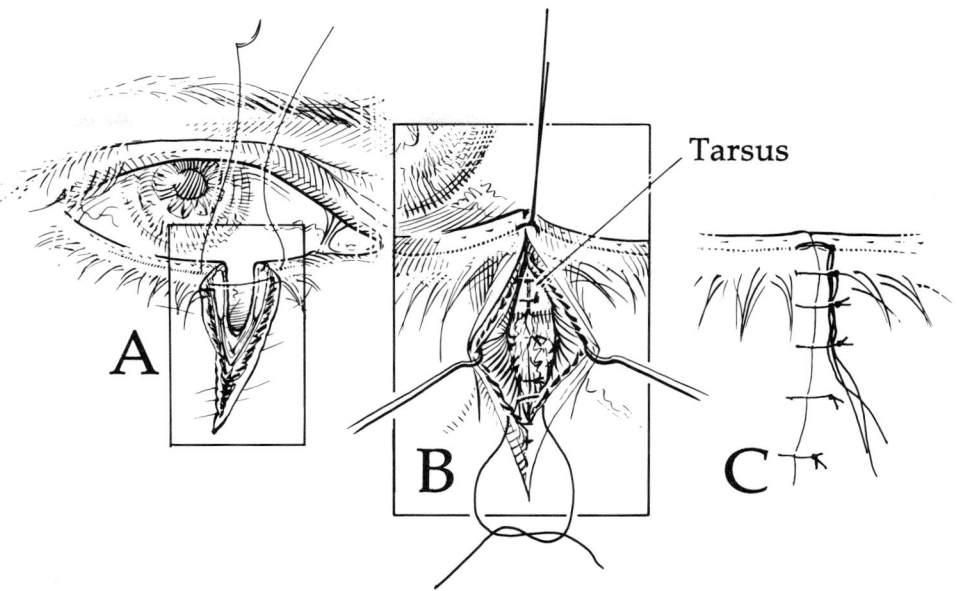

Tarsus

A    B    C

braided absorbable 6–0 synthetic sutures, whose knots are buried so that they do not abrade the cornea (Fig. 47-3B). The orbicularis oculi muscle is approximated by interrupted, braided absorbable 6–0 synthetic sutures. The eyelid skin is closed with interrupted nonabsorbable monofilament 6–0 synthetic sutures whose knots lie on the surface. A skin suture 2 mm from the lashes is tied over the long ends of the marginal suture, which prevents it from irritating the conjunctiva (Fig. 47-3C). The skin and marginal sutures are removed on the fourth postoperative day. In the following 6 months, linear contraction of the vertical scar may be encountered, resulting in a pull on the lid margin. In such cases, lengthening of the skin scar with a Z-plasty corrects the deformity.

Injuries of the lacrimal system occur most frequently in naso-orbital fractures and soft tissue lacerations. They may be difficult to diagnose because of severe ecchymosis of the eyelids. However, the location of the laceration and the physical findings can alert the emergency physician to a possible injury to this system which may be caused by a laceration medial to the punctum caused by a knife, razor, or even a coat hanger (Fig. 47-4, inset). Severance of the lower lacrimal canaliculus results in widening of the palpebral fissure. The orbicularis oculi muscle tends to enlarge the areas of the laceration and produce ectropion. Laceration of either canaliculus displaces the injured lid laterally. Proper management of injuries to this system is necessary to prevent subsequent complications, such as annoying epiphora and dacryocystitis.

While repair of injury to the lacrimal system should be done as early as possible, local edema and hemorrhage may make early operative repair difficult and even hazardous. In such cases, it is prudent to delay surgery for 12 to 24 h, by which time the bleeding will have subsided and some of the edema will have resolved. In addition, the cut ends of the canaliculus tend to evert during this time and are more easily identified. Their divided ends usually appear as small, pearly white rings.

## Nose

### Anatomy

The nose is a triangular pyramid composed of cartilaginous and osseous structures that support the overlying skin and musculature and the underlying mucosa. A median septum divides the pyramid into right and left halves that extend from the columella anteriorly to the nasal choanae posteriorly. The cephalic portion of the dorsal border of the septal cartilage is connected intimately with the cephalic portion of the lateral cartilages.

The supporting framework of the nose consists of a nasal skeleton cephalad and a cartilaginous framework caudad. The nasal skeleton is composed of the frontal processes of the maxillae laterally and the paired nasal bones and the bony nasal septum centrally. The cartilaginous framework is made up of the triangular lateral and alar cartilages laterally and the cartilaginous septum centrally. There is an overlap of about 1 cm between the nasal bones and the lateral cartilages, with an intimate fusion of the periosteum and perichondrium.

The paired, C-shaped alar cartilages form the cartilaginous support for the tip of the nose. Each alar cartilage has a medial and lateral crus. The medial crura curve downward into the columella and then diverge as they approach the base of the columella. The alar and lateral cartilages are connected by aponeurotic tissue. Muscles (procerus, nasalis, and levator labii superioris) cover the entire external surface of the bony and cartilaginous framework, except the alar car-

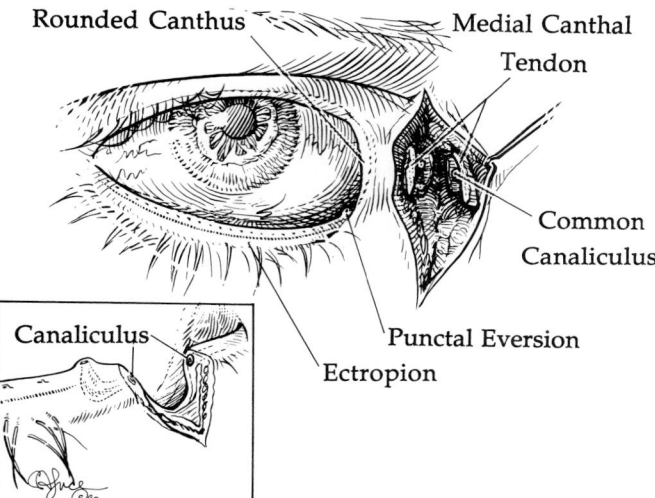

Rounded Canthus   Medial Canthal Tendon
Common Canaliculus
Punctal Eversion
Ectropion
Canaliculus

**Fig. 47-4.** The orbicularis oculi muscle exerts traction in a lateral direction on the medial canthus when the medial canthal tendon is severed. This results in a characteristic deformity with a rounded medial canthus and a decreased distance between the medial and lateral canthi. Insert: Laceration of the lower lid through the lacrimal canaliculus.

tilages where the skin is tightly bound to the cartilage. The skin covering the remaining portion of the nose is thin, supple, and mobile.

The nasal lining in the columella and vestibule is skin. The nasal vestibule is limited posteriorly by the protrusion of the lower border of the upper lateral cartilages, forming folds or internal nares. These folds extend laterally and inferiorly along the pyriform aperture outlining the posterior extent of the vestibule. The lining of the anterior part of the vestibule has thick, long hairs (vibrissae) with which are associated large sebaceous glands. The zone of the vibrissae is succeeded by the transitional zone in the vestibule lined by thick, stratified squamous epithelium. Sweat and sebaceous glands, as well as hair, are absent in the transitional zone. The mucous membrane overlying the remaining portion of the nasal canal is composed of ciliated, pseudostratified columnar epithelium.

## Injuries and Treatment

Lacerations of the nose may be limited to skin or may involve the deeper structures (sparse nasal musculature, cartilaginous framework, and nasal mucous membrane). They are repaired by accurate reapproximation of each tissue layer (Fig. 47-5).

When the laceration extends through all tissue layers, closure should begin with a marginal nonabsorbable monofilament 5–0 synthetic suture that aligns the skin surrounding the entrances of the nasal canals, to prevent malapposition and notching of the alar rim (Fig. 47-5A). Traction upon the long, untied ends of the marginal suture approximates the wound and aligns the anterior and posterior margins of the divided tissue layers. The mucous membrane should then be repaired with interrupted, braided absorbable 5–0 synthetic sutures with their knots buried in the tissue. The divided edges of the cartilage should then be approximated with interrupted, braided absorbable 5–0 synthetic sutures (Fig. 47-5B). The cut edges of the skin, with its adherent musculature, are closed with interrupted nonabsorbable monofilament 5–0 synthetic sutures (Fig. 47-5C). After wound closure, linear lacerations of the alar rim may shorten and result in notching of the rim 3 to 6 months later. A Z-plasty at the alar rim will correct this deformity.

A hematoma develops between the septal mucoperichondrium and the cartilage after either fracture or dislocation of the septum or excessive bending of the septal cartilage. Hematoma is often bilateral because the fractured septum permits passage of blood from one side to the other. If the hematoma is not detected, fibrosis may develop in the hematoma, resulting in permanent thickening of the nasal septum, with partial obstruction of the nasal airway. An untreated septal hematoma also may cause absorption of the septal cartilage, especially if infected, resulting in septal perforation and/or saddle nose deformity. Consequently, the nasal septum should be inspected for hematoma formation using a nasal speculum following any nasal injury. Packing the nose with gauze soaked in a vasoconstrictive agent (4% cocaine) limits nasal bleeding and facilitates the examination.

The presence of bluish swelling in the septum confirms the diagnosis of septal hematoma. Treatment of the hematoma is evacuation of the blood clot. Drainage of a small hematoma can be accomplished by aspiration of the blood clot through a No. 18 needle. A larger hematoma is drained through a horizontal incision through the mucoperichondrial layer along the floor of the nose. In bilateral hematomas, resection of a portion of the septal cartilage in the operating room is recommended to allow communication between both hematomas. Reaccumulation of blood can be prevented by either nasal packing or simple suction catheter drainage (scalp vein cannula and vacuum tube*). Simple suction catheter drainage is preferred over packs because subsequent pack removal is uncomfortable and may precipitate bleeding. By comparison, removal of the catheter is painless and is not accompanied by bleeding. Antibiotic treatment is

*Abbot Hospital, Inc., North Chicago, Illinois.

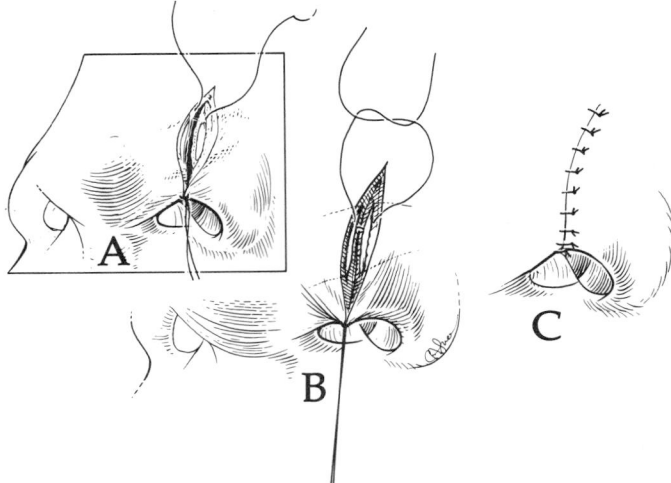

**Fig. 47-5.** Repair of a linear laceration extending through all tissue layers of the nose. **A.** A marginal suture should be placed through the alar rim to align the nasal canal. Traction should be applied to the marginal suture to align the individual tissue layers. **B.** The divided nasal mucosa and cartilage should be approximated separately. **C.** The skin edges are approximated by interrupted nonabsorbable monofilament 5–0 synthetic sutures.

recommended to prevent infection that predisposes to necrosis of cartilage.

## Lips

### Anatomy

The external surfaces of the lips have three distinct regions: the cutaneous area (skin), the vermilion, and the oral mucosa. The vermilion is a relatively thick layer of noncornified stratified epithelium that is deeply indented by vascular connective tissue papillae. Its superficial epithelial cells contain eleidin, making them translucent and permitting the underlying vascular papillae to give the vermilion its color. Glands are absent in this region, except for occasional sebaceous glands. The vermilion is continuous with a mucous membrane that covers the inner surface of the lips. Vascular connective tissue papillae of moderate length indent the epithelial cover, resulting in the pink color of the mucous membrane. Numerous glands of a mixed (mucous and serous) type and a mucous type are present in the underlying submucosal layer.

The skin meets the red-colored vermilion at the "red line." A surface prominence of paler vermilion contiguous with the skin-vermilion junction is called the "white line." Another important anatomic landmark is the junction between the red vermilion and the pink mucous membrane. Superficial landmarks unique to the skin over the upper lip are the philtral hollow, its eminences, and the associated curving of "white" and "red lines" into cupid's bows.

The orbicularis oris muscle is the voluntary muscle that surrounds the mouth. It is located between the skin and oral mucosa and is responsible for the damming of saliva and the formation of labial sounds. Lip sensation is mediated by the infraorbital and mental branches of the trigeminal nerve. The labial arteries of the upper and lower lips are branches of the facial artery that form anastomosing coronary arteries located beneath the mucosa on the inner surface of the lips, just below their free borders.

### Injuries and Treatment

The technique of closure will depend largely on the type of lip wound. There are essentially two types of wound: lacerations and avulsions. Superficial lacerations involve the skin and subcutaneous

**Fig. 47-6.** Irregular-edged vertical laceration of the upper lip. **A.** Traction is applied to the lips and closure of the wound is begun first at the vermilion-skin junction. **B.** The orbicularis oris muscle is then repaired with interrupted, braided absorbable 4–0 synthetic sutures. **C.** The irregular edges of the skin are then approximated.

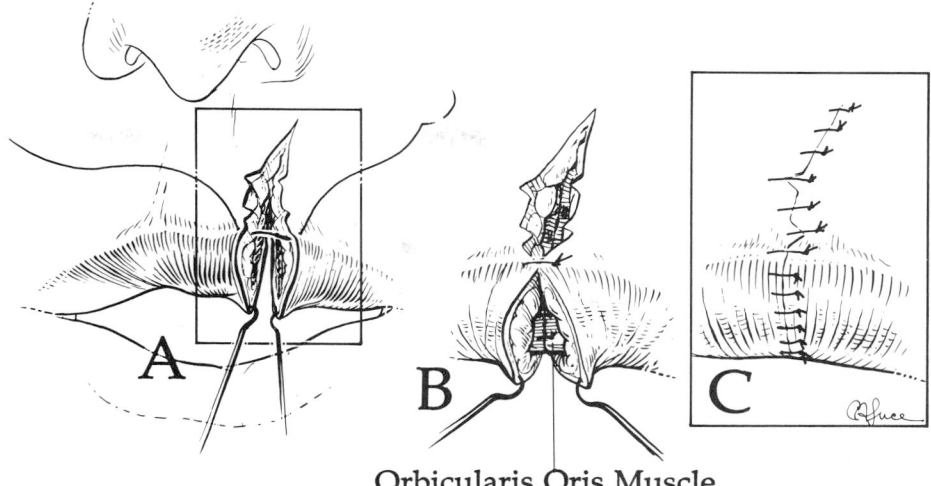

Orbicularis Oris Muscle

tissue. Deep lacerations may extend through the muscle and underlying mucosa. Bleeding may be profuse if the labial arteries are involved. Clamping the cut ends of the vessel with a hemostat and tying them with suture ligatures will control bleeding. Each tissue layer of the laceration must be reapproximated meticulously (Fig. 47-6). The vermilion-cutaneous and the vermilion-mucosal margins are important anatomic landmarks that must be apposed by key stitches to prevent the development of a "step-off" deformity that is difficult to correct at a later date.

Repair of a laceration through the lip requires a three-layered closure (Fig. 47-6). Using skin hooks, traction is applied to align the anterior and posterior borders of the laceration. Closure of the wound is begun first at the vermilion-skin junction with a nonabsorbable monofilament 6–0 synthetic suture (Fig. 47-6A). The orbicularis oris muscle is then repaired with interrupted, braided absorbable 4–0 synthetic sutures (Fig. 47-6B). The vermilion-mucous membrane junction is approximated with a braided absorbable 5–0 synthetic suture. This suture ligature is constructed so that its knot is buried in the subcutaneous tissue. The divided edges of the mucous membrane and vermilion are then closed using interrupted, braided absorbable 5–0 synthetic sutures with a buried-knot construction. The skin edges of the laceration are usually jagged and irregular, but can be fitted together as the pieces of a jigsaw puzzle using interrupted nonabsorbable monofilament 6–0 synthetic sutures with their knots formed on the surface of the skin (Fig. 47-6C). During healing, a linear wound of the lip may undergo contraction, resulting in notching of the lip. The deformity can be corrected by a Z-plasty revision of the linear scar.

## Cheeks

### Anatomy

The main boundaries of the mouth are partly osseous and partly muscular. The lateral walls are formed by the cheeks and are lined by skin and mucous membrane. Between the linings are a fat pad and facial muscles. The buccinator muscle arises from the alveolar processes of the mandible and maxilla, and the pterygomandibular raphe. It inserts into the orbicularis oris muscle and is responsible for compressing the cheeks and maintaining tone. Important structures within the cheek include branches of the facial nerve, the parotid (Stensen's) duct, and a portion of the parotid gland (Fig. 47-7).

The parotid gland is composed of superficial and retromandibular parts. The gland lies on the masseter muscle, and extends posteriorly to the sternocleidomastoid muscle and to the cartilaginous portion of the external auditory meatus. The parotid duct arises from the most prominent part of the anterior border of the gland, passes forward on the masseter muscle, and then turns around its anterior border to

pierce the buccinator muscle. It enters the vestibule of the mouth at the level of the crown of the second upper molar tooth. The course of the parotid duct is deep to a line drawn from the tragus of the ear to the mid-portion of the upper lip (line 1 in Fig. 47-7).

The facial nerve emerges from the stylomastoid foramen, after which it becomes sandwiched or enfolded between the two lobes of the parotid gland. It divides within the substance of the gland into two main subdivisions, temporofacial and cervicofacial. Branches of these subdivisions radiate out from the margins of the gland in five divisions—temporal (T), zygomatic (Z), buccal (B), marginal mandibular (M), and cervical (C)—with multiple intercommunicating, dividing, and reuniting branches (Fig. 47-7).

Knowledge of the various types of branching of the facial nerves is helpful in the identification of the severed ends of the facial nerves in a facial injury. The buccal and zygomatic branches have connections in 80 percent of the cases. The marginal mandibular branches are connected in only 5 to 12 percent.

Because the facial nerve is mainly a motor nerve governing the muscles of facial expression, facial symmetry in repose and in action (motility) is of paramount importance in detecting functional deficits. Resting tone is less important than motility in this evaluation because it is largely dependent on the smoothness of the skin surface, the thickness of the layer of subcutaneous adipose tissue, and the mass

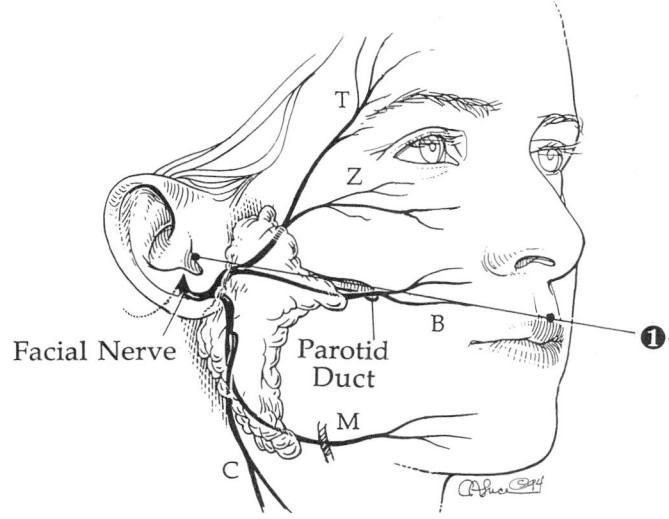

**Fig. 47-7.** The course of the parotid duct is deep to a line drawn from the tragus of the ear to the midportion of the upper lip.

and firmness of the connective tissue. In early injuries to the facial nerve or its branches in children or in patients of pyknic body type, a good resting tone with a high degree of facial symmetry is evident in the absence of muscle function.

The temporal branches innervate the anterior auricular muscles, part of the superior auricular muscles, and the muscles of the forehead, including the major portion of the orbicularis oculi muscle. Division of the temporal branch of the facial nerve results in a unilateral paralysis of the frontalis muscle. The result of this injury is asymmetry of the forehead. The muscle on the unaffected side produces the usual transverse folds across the forehead, which contrast with the smooth surface on the paralyzed side. The patient will be unable to wrinkle the forehead on the affected side. Return of function following division is always worse than that seen in the other branches.

The zygomatic branches also supply the orbicularis oculi muscles, the muscles around the nares, and the levators of the upper lip. Because of the multiple connections between the nerves that innervate the orbicularis oculi muscle, paralysis is rarely encountered. When the temporofacial subdivision of the facial nerve or both the zygomatic and temporal branches are injured, paresis of the orbicularis oculi is noted with changes in the resting tone and motility of the periocular region. The size of the palpebral fissure on the affected side will be 3 mm wider than on the uninjured side. When the tonus of lower lid on the affected side is poor, ectropion results. The inability to close the eyelids of the affected side either loosely as in sleep or firmly is evidence of abnormal motility in the periocular region.

The buccal branch of the facial nerve traverses the face along the course of the parotid duct and is usually severed if the duct has been lacerated. The buccal nerve innervates most of the muscles around the lip. Of these muscles, the orbicularis oris produces recognizable clinical signs after denervation. The orbicularis oris is a group of muscles arranged in a sphincteric fashion around the mouth. Through its action, this muscle puckers the lips, draws them inward at the commissures, or presses them against the teeth. Injury to the buccal branch limits puckering of the lips, drawing the commissures inward on the affected side. For objective grading, a decrease in the distance between the philtrum and corner of the mouth following pursing the lips is measured. Because of the numerous connections between the buccal and zygomatic branches, gradual spontaneous regeneration is frequent.

The course of the marginal mandibular branch of the facial nerve, being near the posterior facial vein, is always deep to the platysma muscle. Bleeding from this vessel is often associated with injury to the marginal mandibular branch of the facial nerve. In approximately 20 percent of patients, it is located 1 to 1.5 cm below the mandible, between the angle of the jaw and the mandibular notch. In the remaining 80 percent, the marginal mandibular branch lies on the mandible throughout its course. This nerve innervates the lower group of circumoral muscles, consisting of the triangularis, the quadratus labii inferioris, and the platysma; these muscles depress the corner of the mouth and the lower lip. Injury to this branch causes an elevation of the ipsilateral lower lip at rest and an inability to depress it. The cervical branch innervates the platysma muscle and has anastomotic neural connections with the marginal mandibular branch.

### Injuries and Treatment

Lacerations of the cheek are of great concern because they may be associated with injury to the facial nerve and/or parotid duct. An early, accurate evaluation of the integrity of the facial nerve must be made before wound closure. Facial nerve injury may be easily missed in the unconscious patient or a patient with a bandaged head. If the functions of the facial nerve are not tested soon after injury, the extent and site of injury may be missed. Damage to the cerebral cortex or corticobulbar fibers can result in upper motor neuron lesions, with loss of movement of the mimetic muscles of the lower part of the contralateral side of the face. Lower motor neuron damage to the facial nerve

can occur either intracranially, in the middle ear, or at the mastoid or stylomastoid foramen.

The site of injury to the facial nerve can be assessed accurately by assessing the functionality of its various branches. During its passage through the facial canal, it gives off several important branches: the greater superficial petrosal nerve, the chorda tympani, and the nerve to the stapedius muscle. The greater superficial petrosal nerve, which innervates tear production, can be evaluated by a modification of Schirmer's test. A strip of filter paper is hooked over the lower lid and acts as a wick. The patient is given a whiff of ammonia and the rate of flow along it is compared to that of a similar strip applied to the opposite conjunctival sac. Loss of stapedius muscle function may be detected by an acoustic impedance bridge. The chorda tympani, which supplies the anterior two-thirds of the tongue and innervates the submandibular gland, can be assessed by evaluating taste and salivary production. In cases of facial paralysis following blunt trauma, *without* soft tissue disruption, the prognosis for recovery is good and exploration is generally not needed.

Division of the submandibular glands and ducts does not require repair. The glands will drain through a fistula that usually develops after injury to the floor of the mouth. Lacerations of the cheek should be reapproximated with interrupted, nonabsorbable monofilament 5–0 synthetic sutures in a manner similar to that of putting together a jigsaw puzzle.

## Ear

### Anatomy

The external ear consists of the external auditory canal and auricle. The latter consists of a double fold of skin supported by a fibrocartilaginous framework, which in the vicinity of the lobule is replaced by fibrofatty tissue. The skin layer is more adherent laterally than medially. The configuration of the cartilage on its medial side is fairly smooth, while characteristic elevations and depressions of the auricle are noted on its lateral side. The prominent outer rim of the auricle, the helix, occasionally has a small cartilaginous tubercle, the Darwin tubercle. The helical rim terminates anteriorly in a crus that lies almost horizontally above the external auditory meatus. A second rim of the ear, the antihelix, is adjacent to and almost parallel with the helix. The antihelix diverges into superior and anterior crura, enclosing the triangular fossa. Between the helix and antihelix is a long, deep furrow, the scapha. Within the substance of, and partly surrounded by, the antihelix, a deep cavity, the concha, leads into the external meatus. The conchal cavity, composed of cymba and cavum, arises from a floor that is at least 1 cm deeper than the overlying tragus and antitragus. The most lateral point of the auricle should lie between 1.7 and 2.0 cm from the scalp. Viewed from the front, the helical rim should be visible behind the antihelix.

The auricle has a luxurious blood supply from the superficial temporal and posterior auricular arteries. The sensory nerve supply arises primarily from the anterior and posterior branches of the greater auricular nerve, with lesser contributions from the auriculotemporal and lesser occipital nerves. Regional anesthesia of the auricle is accomplished by instilling an anesthetic solution along its base anteriorly and superiorly. Since the posterior wall of the external auditory canal is supplied by the auricular branches of the vagus nerve, this site must be injected separately.

### Injuries and Treatment

Trauma to the ear can be divided into three general types: hematoma, laceration, and avulsion. A common injury in contact sports is auricular hematoma. Within hours after injury, the skin covering the anterior surface of the auricle is raised from the auricle by a hematoma or seroma, which forms in a plane between cartilage and its perichondrium. If drained, the potential space fills with serosanguineous exu-

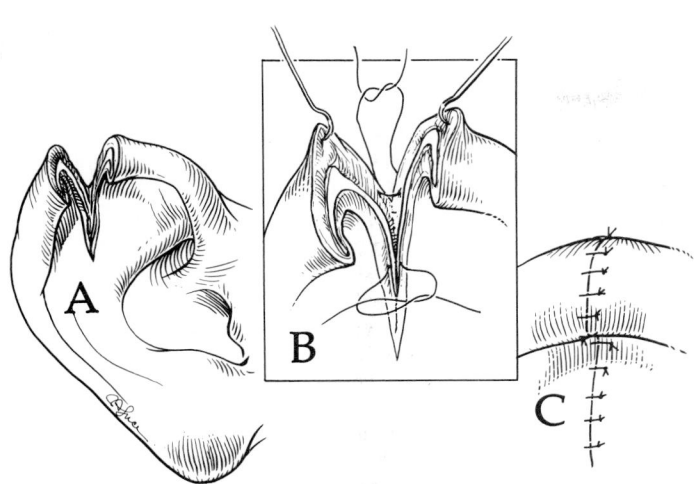

**Fig. 47-8. A.** Laceration through auricle. **B.** One or two interrupted, braided 6–0 synthetic sutures will approximate divided edges of cartilage. **C.** Interrupted nonabsorbable monofilament 6–0 synthetic sutures approximate the skin edges.

date. Unless drainage is maintained, the elevated perichondrium produces neocartilage in the tethered and scarred cauliflower ear.

For the best results, treatment should be initiated within 72 h. Many different therapeutic approaches have been proposed. Most methods for dealing with auricular hematoma depend on evacuation of the hematoma and replacing the perichondrium back on the cartilage. Hematoma drainage has been achieved by repeated aspiration, incision and drainage with pressure dressing, and suction drainage. The concept of closed suction drainage to obtain complete evacuation of the hematoma is appealing in its simplicity because no dressing is required and the patient can resume normal activities.

A laceration of the skin on the lateral aspect of the auricle should be subjected to minimal debridement because skin deficits in this site are not easily closed without distortion of the cartilage. In through-and-through lacerations, approximating the skin with minimal cartilaginous suturing will restore contour without numerous buried sutures (Fig. 47-8A, B, and C). Notching of the helical rim can be prevented by a Z-plasty, which is best performed 6 to 12 months after wound closure. Circular lacerations through the external auditory canal should be closed carefully with interrupted nonabsorbable monofilament 6–0 synthetic sutures. After wound closure, the canal should be packed tightly with an impregnated gauze. A prosthetic appliance should be worn for 4 months to prevent the development of stenosis of the canal. One of the most common injuries is laceration of the earlobe caused by traction on an earring in the pierced lobe. The repair is accomplished by resuturing the divided edges together. Incorporating a Z-plasty of the rim that will prevent notching may be performed 6 to 12 months later.

Full-thickness skin loss with intact perichondrium may be resurfaced with a postauricular, supraclavicular, or upper-eyelid full-thickness skin graft. When the perichondrium is missing, a preauricle or postauricular pedicle flap should be used to cover the defect.

## EAR LOBE CLEFTS

The most frequently encountered earlobe deformity is the complete or partial cleft caused by excessive traction on an earring in a pierced ear. Traditionally, such injuries were almost exclusively encountered in female patients but now commonly arise in both genders. Such injuries pose two major reconstructive challenges: (1) the cleft must be repaired without dimpling of the helical border of the lobule by scar retraction, and (2) continued patency of the earring canal is generally desired and must be maintained without compromise in function.

Clefts may be classified as partial or complete. A partial cleft oc-

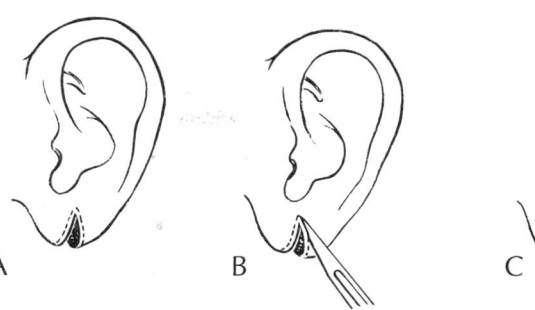

**Fig. 47-9. A.** A 1-mm margin is outlined around the wound edges. **B.** A no. 11 knife blade completely excises the cleft margins. **C.** The wound edges are approximated by interrupted percutaneous sutures.

curs when the circular canal is transformed into a linear slit that does not reach the external border of the lobe. The patient presenting with a partial earlobe cleft usually has a history of wearing heavy or dangling earrings for years, with gradual lengthening of the initial holeinto an earlobe cleft. The weight of the ear piece of a telephone on the projecting earring may commonly contribute to slow enlargement of the canal. When the cleft creates a bifid lobe, it is considered complete. Completely clefted earlobes often are partially clefted for a long time before becoming completely clefted by the application of minimal force on the earring. Less often, earlobe clefts result from an acute, sudden, forceful ripping of the earring through the lobule.

The laceration must first be cleaned with poloxamer 188, a surfactant that will remove exogenous contaminants without compromising host defenses. Manual high-pressure syringe irrigation using 0.9% saline solution is used if any gross contaminants are introduced into the cleft. Systemic antibiotic therapy has not been shown to facilitate healing, but immediate reconstruction of the lobe is indicated to minimize scar formation and allow rapid, cosmetically pleasing, and functional healing to ensue.

Strategies for repair of the earlobe cleft can be divided into two different groups: primary repair with and without the creation of an epithelialized hole in the ear lobe for the earring. The latter approach is simpler but requires subsequent repiercing of the earlobe after the wound repair.

As with any laceration to the skin of the lateral surface of the lobule, debridement of the margins of a cleft wound should be minimal because deficits in this area are difficult to close without distortion of the cartilage. Any epithelial growth over the cleft borders, however, should be removed (Fig. 47-9A). Using a sterile marking pen, a 1-mm margin is outlined around the wound, indicating the ultimate margins of the primary repair of the cleft (Fig. 47-9A). The margins are then anesthetized with 1% lidocaine administered using a 30-gauge needle. After marking the skin, a no. 11 knife blade is used to excise the cleft tissue completely to a point just above the superior aspect of the cleft (Fig. 47-9B). The edges are approximated by interrupted 6–0 polypropylene sutures (Fig. 47-9C).

Incomplete clefts are also completely excised, including the skin bridge, converting the partial cleft to a complete cleft with no epithelial lining. About 4 to 6 weeks later, the ear lobe is repierced in the most aesthetically pleasing location. If dimpling of the lobule is encountered, it can be easily corrected 6 months later by a Z-plasty of the helical rim notch.

## HOSPITAL CARE

### Scalp

The objective of treatment of avulsion injuries of the scalp is to achieve proper skin coverage of all denuded areas as soon as possible. The entire scalp can be replaced successfully by anastomosing the superficial artery and its paired vein bilaterally. By 6 months, hair growth and frontalis muscle activity can return.

Care of the amputated part requires limited treatment at the scene of injury. Any gross contaminant can be washed off, but lengthy irrigation of the part should not be undertaken because it can make identification of structures more difficult. The amputated part should be placed in a plastic bag in an ice container.

When the avulsed part is not available, treatment will depend on whether the periosteum is present. When the pericranium is intact, coverage of the exposed periosteum with a split-thickness skin graft taken either from the avulsed scalp itself or from the thigh or buttock is recommended in the operating room.

When the pericranium is destroyed, the outer table of the skull loses its blood supply and will not maintain the viability of skin grafts. In this case, coverage with pedicle flaps is recommended.

## Eyelids

Dog bites, human bites, and accidents of varying types may cause avulsion injuries of the eyelid. These avulsions may be classified according to their depth, the eyelid involved, and the size of the resulting defect. Treatment will depend on the type of injury, and whether the avulsed tissue specimen is available for reconstruction.

The levator palpebrae superioris is involved frequently in injuries to the upper lid, esp in automobile accidents and injuries from various types of machinery. In all deep transverse lacerations of the eyelid, it is important to verify levator palpebrae superioris function. If the patient cannot raise the upper lid for reasons other than edema, primary suture of the injured muscle must be undertaken in the operating room.

Medial and lateral canthal tendon deformities are usually sequelae of orbital fractures that may be associated with midfacial bone fractures and naso-orbital fractures. Zygomatic fractures are a frequent cause of dislocation of the lateral raphe and lateral canthal tendons. Deep vertical lacerations along the lateral or medial walls of the orbit may occasionally damage the lateral and medial canthal tendons. Division of the medial canthal tendon results in a characteristic deformity with a rounded medial canthus and decreased intercanthal distance (Fig. 47-4). The division of the medial canthal tendon and the inability of the orbicularis oculi muscle to maintain normal muscle tone between the medial and lateral canthal tendons causes a relaxation of the lower eyelid, eversion of the lacrimal puncta, and inadequate evacuation of tears from the lacrimal lake. Interference with the muscle power of the orbicularis oculi muscle also affects the lacrimal pump, and this further hampers the excretory system. This injury is usually complicated by an interruption of the continuity of the excretory lacrimal system.

Restoration of the integrity of the medial canthal tendon is achieved by reattachment of the divided ends of the tendon with wire sutures in the operating room. After repair of the medial canthal tendon, the continuity of the injured lacrimal system is reestablished. Complete detachment of the lateral raphe and lateral tendon results in a rounded lateral canthus and a diminution of the horizontal dimension of the palpebral fissure. Restoration of the divided ends of these structures can usually be accomplished with the same wire-fixation technique used in repair of severed medial canthal tendons.

Whenever possible, the injured canaliculus should be repaired in the operating room, even though the other remains intact. The most important principle in repairing the canalicular laceration is to reestablish canalicular patency by direct microsurgical anastomosis, suturing of the severed ends, and endocanalicular support, preferably with silicone tubing. Improper treatment leads to distortion of the structures, which may lead to chronic dacryocystitis.

## Nose

Septal perforation may follow drainage of septal hematoma, especially bilateral hematomas. Because the septum receives its blood supply from the mucous membrane, it will necrose unless the hematomas are completely evacuated. The majority of septal perforations are asymptomatic and require no further treatment. Interventions are required only in those patients with crusting, obstruction, bleeding, and whistling. Most symptomatic perforations are located at the junction of the anterior and middle thirds of the nasal septum and are greater than 0.5 cm in diameter. The more anterior and the larger the perforation, the greater the likelihood it will cause symptoms. Posterior perforations cause fewer symptoms because of the rapid humidification of the inspired air by the nasal lining and turbinates. Surgical intervention is recommended in those patients with symptomatic perforation. The surgical techniques employed include an external rhinoplasty approach, septal and intranasal mucosal flaps and a connective tissue autograft of temporalis fascia or mastoid periosteum.

When there is avulsion of components of the nose, it is best to restore the architecture with the avulsed specimen, using microsurgical techniques. If the avulsed tissue is not recovered or not suitable for replantation, the technique of reconstruction will depend on the magnitude and depth of injury.

## Lips

Tissue loss from the lip usually involves either the skin surface or all tissue layers. Defects involving all tissue layers of the lip can be further classified by location into median defects, lateral defects, and complete loss of lip. Tissue loss at the commissure is a distinct entity that deserves special consideration. Reconstruction of these lip deficits should be performed by a plastic surgeon in an operating room.

## Cheek

Once a nerve deficit is recognized, timing the repair of the extracranial peripheral branches of the facial nerve is critical. If transection has occurred, exploration and repair of the nerve should be undertaken as soon as possible in a well-vascularized bed that is free of foreign bodies, devitalized tissue, and bacteria. If the wound bed is not acceptable and/or there is loss of nerve substance, it is wiser to achieve adequate skin closure in the operating room and delay the nerve repair. The optimal time for early secondary repair is when the original wound has healed without edema, usually 2 to 6 weeks after wound closure.

Injury to the parotid duct should be suspected if clear fluid is seen emerging from a wound in the cheek. The injury can be readily identified by passing a small silicone catheter into the opening of the parotid duct. After the distal divided end of the duct is identified, the patient is transferred to the operating room for repair of the duct.

## Ear

A major auricular avulsion presents a challenging surgical problem. Microvascular surgery has played an important role in replanting ears that are amputated along with the scalp in scalping injuries. At least two ear replantations have been successful. Microvascular repair also appears to enhance survival in an incomplete ear amputation.

## BIBLIOGRAPHY

Butt WE: Auricular haematoma: Treatment options. *Aust NZ J Surg* 57:391, 1987.

Carraway JH, Mellow CG: Simple suction drainage: An adjunct to septal surgery. *Ann Plast Surg* 24:191, 1990.

Crawford JS: Intubation of obstructions of the lacrimal system. *Can J Opthalmol* 12:289, 1977.

Davis RA, Anson BJ, Budinger JM, et al: Surgical anatomy of the facial nerve and parotid gland based upon a study of 350 cervicofacial halves. *Surg Gynecol Obstet* 102:384, 1956.

Dingman RO, Grabb WC: Surgical anatomy of the mandibular ramus of the facial nerve based on the dissection of 100 facial halves. *Plast Reconstr Surg* 29:266, 1962.

Edlich RF, Kenney JG: Soft-tissue injuries of the face, in Dudley H, Carter D, Russell RCG (eds): *Operative Surgery. Part 1: Trauma Surgery.* London, Butterworth, 1989, pp 120–149.

May M, Sobol SM, Mester SJ: Managing segmental facial nerve injuries by surgical repair. *Laryngoscope* 100:1062, 1990.

Ohlsen L, Skoog T, Sohn SA: The pathogenesis of cauliflower ear. *Scand J Plast Reconstr Surg* 9:34, 1975.

Tachmes L, Woloszyn T, Marini C, et al: Parotid gland and facial nerve trauma: A retrospective review. *J Trauma* 30:1395, 1990.

Teichgraeber JF, Russo RC: The management of septal perforations. *Plast Reconstr Surg* 91:229, 1993.

# 48
# FINGERTIP INJURIES
### Richard F. Edlich
### Raymond F. Morgan

## INTRODUCTION

The fingertip is the part of the hand most frequently injured. The primary treatment consideration in fingertip injury is the functional rehabilitation of the patient. The fingertip is the end organ for touch and is richly supplied with special sensory receptors that enable the hand to perceive, relaying the shape, texture, and temperature of a manipulated object. Fingertip injuries can destroy these receptors, and the primary goal of management after fingertip injuries should be restoration of these special sensory functions whenever possible. Other management goals include (1) preservation of functional length, (2) prevention of symptomatic neuromas, (3) prevention of joint contracture, (4) short morbidity, and (5) early return of the patient to work or play. Fingertip injuries can be divided into four categories: (1) digital tip amputation with skin or pulp loss only, (2) digital tip amputation with exposed bone, (3) injury of the perionychium, and (4) fracture of the distal phalanx. Successful repair of fingertip injuries requires a knowledge of anatomy and techniques of reconstruction, and sound surgical judgment.

## ANATOMY

The glabrous skin of the palm and fingertip is specially adapted for pinch and grasp functions (Fig. 48-1). Although there are no sebaceous glands in palmar skin, eccrine sweat glands are abundant and provide pores on elevated ridges. These ridges, along with intervening valleys, make up the irregular, friction-producing surface that exhibits characteristic fingerprint patterns. The palmar skin is stabilized by numerous fibrous septa, including Clelland's and Grayson's ligaments, which anchor the skin to the underlying bone and flexor and tendon sheath. Dorsal hand skin is thinner than palmar skin and loosely adherent with little subcutaneous tissue.

The axial digital arteries and nerves pass through the subcutaneous tissue between Grayson's and Clelland's ligaments, dividing into many small branches within the pulp of the fingertip. The digital nerves trifurcate near the distal interphalangeal joint, sending a dorsal branch to the perionychium, one to the fingertip, and a third to the volar pulp. A dorsal sensory branch of each digital nerve is evident at

This research was supported by a generous gift from the Texaco Philanthropic Foundation, White Plains, New York.

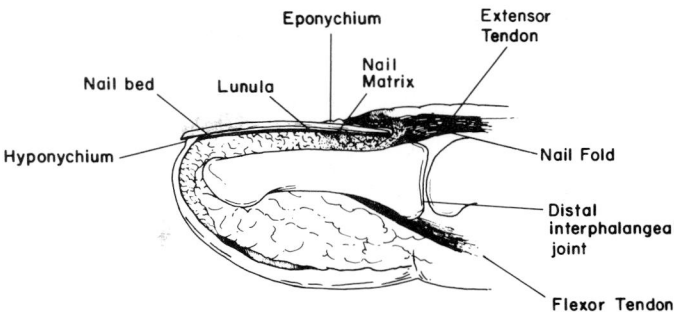

**Fig. 48-1.** The anatomy of the fingertip is shown in sagittal section.

the level of the midproximal phalanx and innervates the skin over the middle and distal phalanx. The digital nerves are volar to the arteries in the digit. The lateral bands of the extensor mechanism continue distally to insert at the dorsal base of the distal phalanx. The flexor digitorum profundus tendon inserts on the volar base of the distal phalanx.

The perionychium includes the entire complex of the nail plate, nail bed, nail matrix, and surrounding paronychium. It acts as a protective covering and assists in grasping small objects and scratching. The major part of this appendage is the hard nail plate, which is roughly flat and rectangular in shape. The nail plate is like hair, being composed primarily of protein and having a lipid content of less than 5 percent. The nail plate is intimately related to five epidermal components.

### Matrix

Most of the nail plate is produced by the nail matrix. The nail plate consists of dead cornified cells derived from the matrix. The cells of the matrix, which are similar to basilar cells, lose their nuclei, flatten, cornify, and are added to already formed nail plate. The nail matrix begins deep within the proximal nail fold beneath the eponychium and extends to the lunula of the nail, the most distal portion of the nail matrix.

### Nail Bed

The nail bed extends from the lunula to the hyponychium. There is little doubt that some material is added to the undersurface of the nail plate by the nail bed as it progresses distally, because the distal portion of the nail is thicker than the proximal portion. As additional cells are produced by the matrix, the nail plate progresses distally on the nail bed. The nail plate is loosely attached to the matrix, but densely adherent to the nail bed and eponychium. The nail bed acts as a guiding surface for the advancing nail plate. Linear ridges in the nail bed securely anchor the nail plate to the underlying epithelium. Complete longitudinal nail growth takes approximately 70 to 160 days.

The dermal component of the matrix and nail bed is unique in that it is limited by the underlying phalanx and is closely associated with its vasculature; there is no subcutaneous tissue. Consequently, the nail bed and matrix are between two relatively unyielding structures, the distal phalanx and the nail plate. These structures protect the nail bed and matrix from many moderate forces and require that the actual injuring force to the structures be significant enough to either break the bone on which the nail bed sits or deform the nail plate under which they reside.

### Proximal Nail Fold

This fold consists of two layers of epidermis. The dorsal part forms the dorsal portion of the finger epidermis, while its ventral portion overlies the newly formed nail plate. The thin membrane extending from the nail fold on to the dorsum of the nail is the eponychium. The proximal nail fold provides a protective cover for the matrix and adds a thin layer of cells to the surface of the nail. This layer of cells is derived from germinal cells located on its ventral portion and gives the nail a smooth, shiny appearance. If the proximal nail fold is absent, the nail surface will be irregular and dull.

## Hyponychium

The hyponychium is the junction of the nail bed and the fingertip skin, beneath the distal free margin of the nail plate. In this region, the nail plate leaves the underlying nail matrix and becomes a free, unattached structure. When the nail bed does not adhere securely to the nail plate, foreign material can enter over the hyponychium and be trapped between the nail bed and nail plate, becoming a source for infection. Like the nail matrix, the hyponychium requires adequate skeletal support. Without this support, the nail plate will follow an abnormally positioned nail bed and hyponychium, resulting in a hook nail deformity.

## Paronychium

The paronychium is the lateral nail fold. The nails progress distally because of confinement by these folds. If this fold has abnormal alignment, growth of the nail plate may damage the paronychium, causing irritation, pain, and infection (ingrown nail).

## EMERGENCY DEPARTMENT CARE

The majority of patients with fingertip injuries can be cared for in the emergency department as outpatients by using digital metacarpal nerve blocks. Severe injuries that required distant flaps or extensive bone fixation should be repaired in the operating room under regional block or general anesthesia. A thorough patient history and examination of the injured finger should be performed prior to initiating treatment. The etiology and time of injury will often influence the method of treatment. The age, sex, occupation, and hand dominance of the patient should also be determined. The relative importance of each finger, from the more important thumb and index finger to the less critical small finger, as well as the patient's use of the injured finger, should be considered. An office worker's nondominant small fingertip amputation should be regarded differently from a pianist's dominant index fingertip soft tissue amputation. Preoperative x-rays should be taken to identify phalangeal fractures or retained foreign bodies. Appropriate tetanus prophylaxis should be undertaken in each patient. Antibiotic treatment is usually not recommended.

Surgical repair of fingertip injuries must be performed in a bloodless field, created by a tourniquet, after wrapping with an Esmarch's bandage. The tourniquet must be calibrated, at least daily and preferably before each case. The use of a sterile, disposable tourniquet helps prevent the risk of cross-contamination. Several layers of soft cast padding are wrapped around the upper arm. The tourniquet's pneumatic cuff is applied snugly and as close to the axilla as possible. The intact skin is washed with an antiseptic solution (iodophor or chlorhexidine). Before skin antisepsis, a towel is wrapped around the distal edge of the cuff to prevent seepage of the antiseptic solutions beneath the cuff, which may result in a chemical burn.

The arm is elevated and wrapped with a disposable Esmarch's bandage to exsanguinate blood from the arm prior to inflation of the tourniquet. The tourniquet is inflated to a pressure of 250 mmHg, or 20 to 50 mmHg greater than the patient's systolic blood pressure. Slightly greater pressures are required for the person with a particularly muscular or obese arm. A pressure of 150 to 200 mmHg is recommended for children. The tourniquet may be left in place for approximately 2 h without danger of ischemia. However, most patients can tolerate the maximum cuff pressures for only 10 to 20 min before

they complain of pain. Conscious sedation will extend the limits of tourniquet use significantly.

When a minor procedure is performed on a finger, an elastic constricting wrap can be placed around the base of the digit as a tourniquet. A broad Penrose drain is safer than a rubber band or narrow catheter. The Penrose drain is wrapped around the base of the finger and clamped with a hemostat. Exsanguination of the digit prior to application of the tourniquet can be accomplished by wrapping the digit from distal end to proximal end with either a 4 by 4 in gauze sponge or a Penrose drain. Although this technique is reasonably safe for short procedures, there are distinct hazards. Because there is no practical way to standardize or measure the pressure beneath a digital tourniquet, compression of the underlying digital nerves may be excessive.

The wound should be thoroughly cleansed using fine-pore cell-size sponge soaked in poloxamer 188 (Calgon, Inc., St. Louis, MO) or normal saline. High-pressure syringe irrigation can also be used to cleanse wounds that have been contaminated. Magnification loupes are essential for visualizing the minute details of the wound that provide the landmarks for repair.

## DIGITAL TIP AMPUTATION

Amputation of the fingertip results from either impact or shear forces. Trapping of a fingertip between two objects is the most common cause of this injury, doors being the most frequent impact forces. Saws, lawn mowers, and knives provide sufficient shear forces for fingertip amputation. The age groups most frequently affected are children and young adults.

When the digital tip is amputated, the geometry of the defect dictates the various treatment possibilities. The loss may be transverse or oblique, with more volar skin loss than dorsal skin loss, or the reverse may be true. Some slicing amputations may take skin primarily from the ulnar or radial side of the digit and spare the distal tip.

### Skin or Pulp Loss Only

There are a multiplicity of techniques for management of digital tip amputations with skin or pulp loss only. Healing by secondary intention is the simplest. Two other options are replantation of the avulsed tissue as a composite graft and defatting the avulsed tissue before replantation. The use of split-thickness skin grafts has been one of the most popular methods for closure of these injuries. Some surgeons prefer more technically demanding procedures, such as cross-finger flaps or advancement flaps.

There is ample evidence that conservative management of fingertip injuries in children where there is no bone exposed is the preferred method. In children under 12, spontaneous regeneration of the fingertip occurs, usually with excellent cosmetic results. Several alternative forms of conservative treatment have been proposed. They all have in common the use of some nonadhering dressing, which is changed periodically until healing is completed. Recent studies also indicate that conservative management of fingertip injuries in adults yields results comparable to those in children, despite the fact that the regenerative potential of soft tissue in the adult is substantially less than in children.

Patients who have had skin grafts of the fingertip frequently complain about induration and fissuring of the skin, reduced sensibility in the area of the graft, and problems involving the donor site. Tenderness at the site of the graft, and cold sensitivity, are common complaints of individuals who have undergone split-thickness skin grafts. With early coverage by split-thickness skin grafts, symptomatic difficulties are likely to continue.

It is important to emphasize that there is between a 30 and 50 percent chance of having some cold intolerance and approximately 30 percent chance of having some aberration in sensitivity, regardless of what technique is used. These complications are a result of the injury and not the treatment.

## Exposed Bone

When bone is exposed in cases of digital tip amputation, the decision-making process is similar to that in cases of digital amputation of pulp alone, but with two additional considerations. Rongeuring a small protruding portion of a phalanx to shorten the fingertip and then allowing healing by secondary intention is another choice. Microsurgical replantation of the amputated part at the level of the distal interphalangeal joint is another alternative.

Conservative management of digital tip amputation with exposed bone is a valuable technique in children less than 12 years old. Their regenerative powers are so great that fingertip regeneration has been reported when the site of amputation is just proximal to the nail. Take of the amputated part as a composite graft at this same amputation site has also been reported in children less than 2 years old.

When the site of amputation is at the level of the distal interphalangeal joint, or proximal to it, microvascular replantation can be successful. Replantation of a sharply amputated single finger at this level in a child should always be considered because the future occupation of the child cannot be predicted. Amputations distal to the superficialis insertion have been found to function well after microvascular replantation because this intact flexor usually provides excellent range of motion of the digit. Because of the thumb's critical importance to hand function, even amputations distal to the interphalangeal joint should be treated by replantation if suitable vessels are found distally.

In adults, the regenerative powers of the fingertip with exposed bone are significantly less than in children. Consequently, shortening the exposed bone by rongeuring and then allowing the wound to heal by secondary intention is an attractive choice for fingertip amputations distal to the distal interphalangeal joint. As surgeons have gained more experience, they have performed fewer local and distant flaps in an effort to cover a small portion of exposed bone. Coverage of exposed bone in the distal phalanx by skin that is hypesthetic, dysesthetic, or tender may lead to a functional amputation of this part so that the patient excludes the tip of the repaired finger from activities.

As with digital tip amputation with skin or pulp loss only, regardless of the treatment modality, there is between a 30 to 50 percent chance of having some cold intolerance and approximately a 30 percent chance of having some aberration in sensitivity.

## INJURY OF THE PERIONYCHIUM

The mechanism of most nail bed injuries is impact, with the force of impact dictating the magnitude of injury. Forces that can break the durable nail plate can disrupt the nail matrix and bed. When a rela-

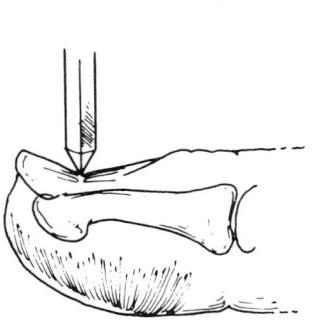
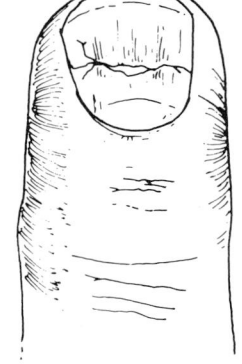

**Fig. 48-2.** A sharp object, like a nail, applies forces over a small area that usually results in a linear laceration of the nail bed or matrix.

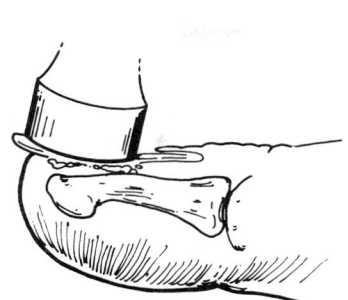
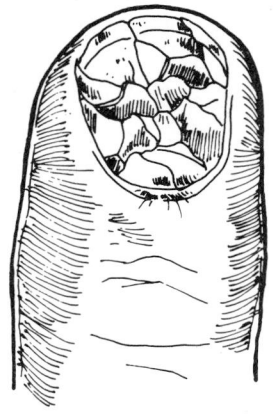

**Fig. 48-3.** A hammer applies force over a large area, resulting in multiple stellate lacerations of the nail bed and matrix.

tively sharp object, like a nail, compresses the nail between the nail and bone, a straight or tearing laceration of the nail bed or matrix occurs (Fig. 48-2). Compression of the nail by a wider object, like a hammer or door, results in stellate lacerations of the nail matrix and bed (Fig. 48-3). It is rare to have a truly sharp laceration of the nail bed. When a sharp object strikes the nail bed hard enough to perforate it, it goes through and amputates the tip. Belts or sanders are more likely to avulse portions of the nail matrix, bed, or fingertip.

If the impact forces do not contact the nail plate, they can fracture the terminal phalanx without breaking the nail plate. In such cases, the fracture often disrupts the nail bed and matrix, causing bleeding with hematoma formation beneath the intact nail. Hematomas occurring following fractures or lacerations are painful and cause the patient to seek medical treatment because of the throbbing pain.

When the nail matrix or bed sustains either a linear or stellate laceration, it will heal by scar formation. Because scar does not produce a nail, nail deformity occurs. Scar formation in the matrix results in a split or absent nail. Scars in the nail bed are followed either by a split or nonadherent nail. The magnitude of scar formation can be lessened by the meticulous repair of the injured nail matrix and bed. Because the results of late reconstruction of an injured nail are unpredictable, it is preferable to treat nail injuries as soon as possible after injury. Injuries of the perionychium can be divided into the following four groups: (1) injury with a small hematoma (less than 25 percent of the nail plate), (2) injury with a large hematoma (more than 25 percent of the nail plate), (3) injury associated with fracture of the distal phalanx, and (4) injury with avulsion of the nail bed and matrix.

The question confronting the emergency physician is whether the laceration of the matrix or bed is severe enough to require suturing to assure accurate approximation of the nail matrix or bed. The judgment is complicated by the difficulty of assessing the matrix through the nail plate because of the overlying hematoma. Thus examination of patients presenting with nail bed hematomas may require removal of the nail plates for a complete inspection of the nail beds. It is generally agreed that hematomas, which have separated over 25 percent of the nail plate from its underlying matrix or bed warrant surgical exploration.

## Small Hematoma

In an injury to the perionychium with a hematoma involving less than 25 percent of the visible nail plate, the pressure of the hematoma beneath the nail plate may cause throbbing pain, necessitating evacuation of the hematoma (Fig. 48-4). A hole must be made in the nail plate that is large enough to allow prolonged drainage. Use of a battery-powered microcautery unit is an excellent way to create the hole in the nail plate. Its heated tip passes through the nail plate, is cooled by the hematoma, and does not injure the nail bed or matrix.

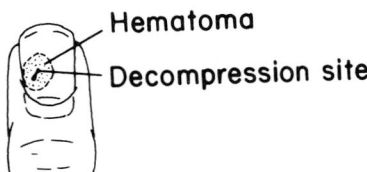

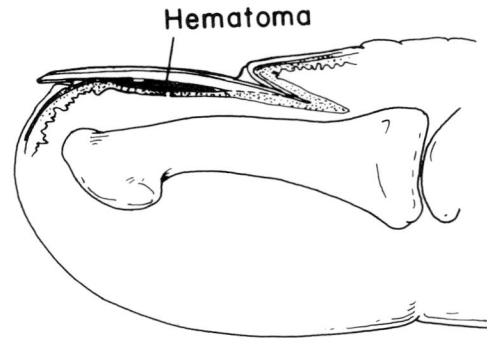

**Fig. 48-4.** A small hematoma beneath the nail plate is caused by a small laceration of the nail bed or matrix. By drilling a hole through the nail plate, decompression and drainage of the hematoma can be achieved.

A paper clip heated until red hot by either a Bunsen burner or alcohol lamp is an alternate approach. With either of these techniques, after decompression of the hematoma, the nail bed and matrix will heal with minimal scar and nail deformity. Other techniques may produce a small hole that decompresses the hematoma immediately, but does permit continued drainage, allowing formation of another hematoma.

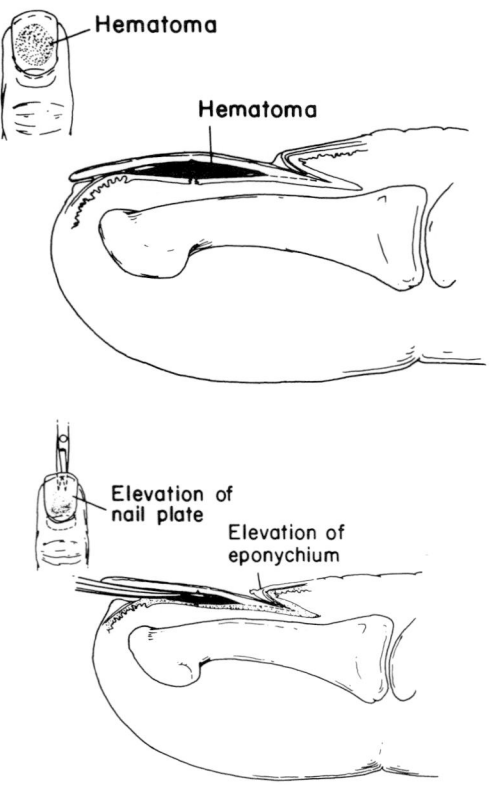

**Fig. 48-5. A.** A large hematoma involves more than 25 percent of the visible nail plate. **B.** The nail plate must be removed to permit appropriate examination and repair of the nail bed and matrix.

## Large Hematoma

If a large hematoma is present, the nail must be removed to permit examination of the injury to the nail bed or matrix (Fig. 48-5A). With appropriate anesthesia, the nail is elevated using the blades of Iris scissors (Fig. 48-5B). By opening and closing the blades of the Iris scissors, a cleavage plane is developed between the nail bed and matrix and the nail plate. Using the same technique, a similar plane is developed between the eponychium and nail plate. Once the nail plate is elevated, gentle distal traction on the nail plate will separate the plate from the proximal nail sulcus.

After washing the nail bed and matrix with a fine-pore cell-size sponge soaked in poloxamer 188 or normal saline, the nail bed and matrix are examined for lacerations. The linear and stellate lacerations are approximated with interrupted 7–0 chromic gut sutures, which are double-armed to microsurgical needles (Fig. 48-6).

Accurate approximation of the stellate laceration is comparable to putting together a jigsaw puzzle. Meticulous approximation of the lacerations of the nail bed matrix can provide surprisingly good results. Occasionally, such lacerations are associated with partial avulsion of the nail matrix from the sulcus (Fig. 48-7). In such cases, sutures should be passed from the proximal portion of the sulcus into the free margin of the nail matrix, bringing the matrix back into position beneath the nail fold. Visualization of the injured matrix may be enhanced by incisions in the proximal nail folds. The incision should be made perpendicular to the lateral curved margin of the eponychial fold (Fig. 48-8).

After the nail bed and matrix are reapproximated, the nail plate is thoroughly cleansed with poloxamer 188 saline. A hole is burned through the nail plate at a point not over the repair site to allow drainage of any blood or hematoma. The nail plate is then replaced back into the proximal sulcus to serve as a stent and protective cover of the nail bed and matrix. The nail plate is held in place by an interrupted monofilament 5–0 nylon suture attached to a precision point reverse-cutting-edge needle passed through the distal end of the nail

## BEVEL SIDE CUTTING SPATULA
## Ophthalmic Needle

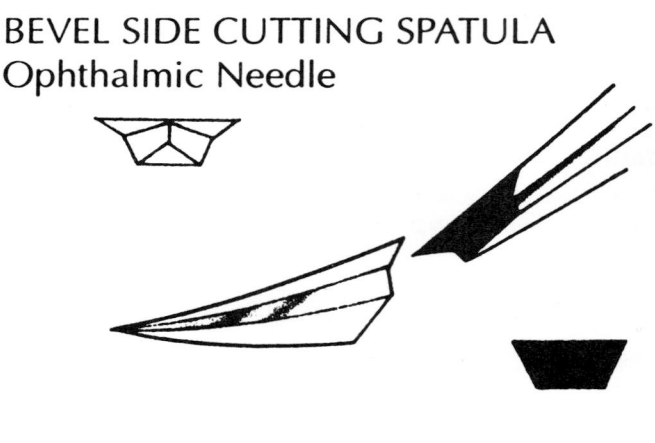

**Fig. 48-6.** Bevel side cutting spatula ophthalmic needle (*Top left;* front view of needle point). Note opposing long side cutting edges with its short apical cutting side (*Middle,* side view of needle). The concave and convex surfaces of this spatula needle are flat (*Bottom right;* cross section of needle). The trapezoidal shape of the cross section of the needle body enhances needle holding security.

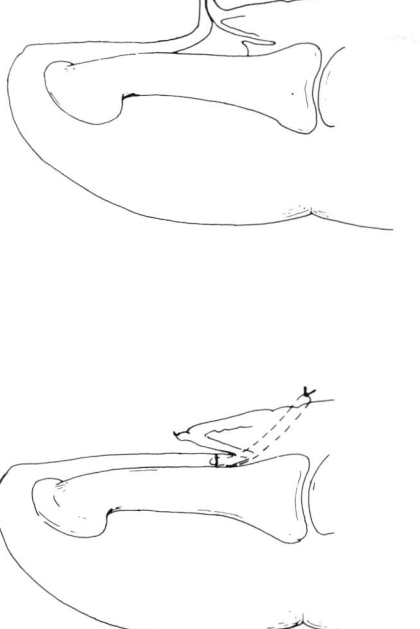

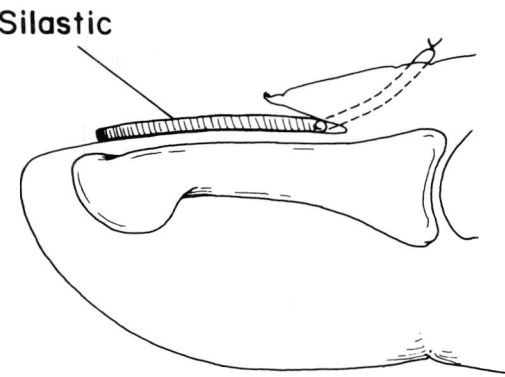

**Fig. 48-9.** A horizontal mattress suture secures the silicone (silastic) sheet to the proximal nail sulcus.

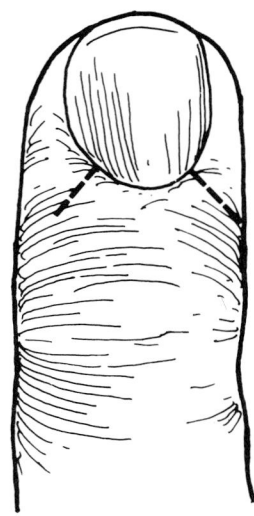

**Fig. 48-7. Top.** Partial avulsion of the nail matrix from the sulcus. **Bottom.** A horizontal mattress suture, through the proximal nail fold to the avulsed segment of the nail matrix, returns the matrix into the fold.

plate to fingertip skin. The fingertip is then dressed with nonadherent gauze, followed by a 2-in. gauze dressing. A volar splint protects the injured part, restricts movement of the distal interphalangeal joint, and alleviates pain. The dressing is removed 5 days later, and the nail checked for evidence of new hematoma formation. The volar splint remains in place for 7 to 10 days to immobilize the joint. If hematoma recurs, the hole is reopened, and the hematoma evacuated. The suture is removed from the nail 3 weeks after injury. The nail plate will frequently adhere to the nail bed and matrix for 1 to 3 months until dislodged by the new growing nail.

If the nail is destroyed or too badly damaged to be used as a splint, several synthetic substitutes have been devised. A nail-shaped sheet of 0.020-in. silicone sheet can be fabricated. A monofilament 6–0 nylon suture is passed through the proximal portion of the proximal nail

**Fig. 48-8.** Incisions in the eponychium enhance visualization and repair of injury of the nail matrix.

fold to the proximal part of the nail sulcus and then through the edge of the silicone sheet at each corner as a horizontal mattress suture to keep the silicone sheet in place (Fig. 48-9). The silicone sheet conforms to the configuration of the nail bed and matrix and keeps the nail fold open. These benefits must be weighed against the potential for erosion of bed or fold by the sheeting, mechanical interference with nail plate growth, and increased risk of infection. The use of firmer prosthetic materials, such as polypropylene, does not eliminate these problems, and these materials do not conform to the underlying tissues.

The nail bed and matrix can also be left open and covered by a nail-shaped nonadherent dressing which extends beneath the proximal nail fold and adheres adequately to the underlying tissue until healing has occurred. After dressing the wound, movement of the distal interphalangeal joint should be restricted for 7 to 10 days by the volar splint. The gauze should be removed 5 to 10 days after repair.

It should be explained to the patient that nail plate growth will take 6 to 12 months. It is also anticipated that if the injury is severe, severe nail deformity which may require surgical revision, is likely. The patient should be reminded that the leading edge of the regenerating nail plate will be irregular, and prone to catch on objects. When the nail's leading edge has extended beyond the hyponychium, it should be trimmed and filed.

### Lacerations Associated with a Fracture of the Distal Phalanx

Approximately 50 percent of nail bed injuries have an associated fracture of the distal phalanx. When a fracture of the distal phalanx occurs, there may be an associated injury to the nail matrix, often manifested by an avulsion of the nail plate out of the nail sulcus, located above the eponychium and proximal nail fold (Fig. 48-10). If a fracture of the tuft or distal phalanx is present, it must have a stable anatomic reduction. The nail bed and matrix should then be repaired, as previously described. The replaced nail plate, due to proximity to the periosteum, serves as an excellent splint to maintain fracture reduction. If stable anatomic reduction cannot be maintained, fixation with a 0.028-in. Kirschner wire is recommended (Fig. 48-11). If the fracture is not realigned accurately, nail deformity will result.

### Avulsion of the Nail Bed

The best tissue for repair of avulsions of the nail bed or matrix is the avulsed tissue. When the nail plate is avulsed, a fragment of the nail bed may remain attached to the nail plate, which can be removed from the nail plate and placed in the wound as a graft (Fig. 48-12). The nail plate should be replaced accurately, serving as a stent. All retrievable fragments unattached to the nail plate should also be re-

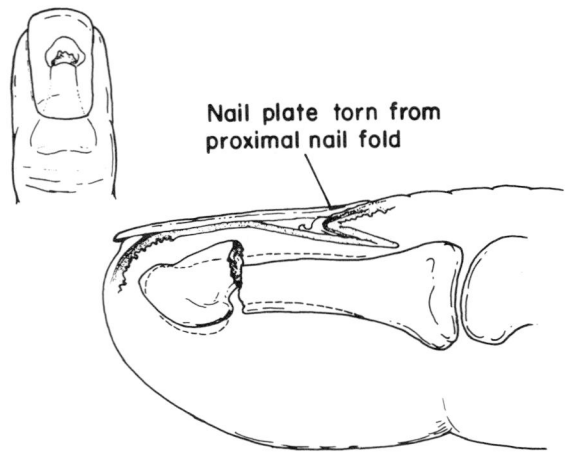

**Fig. 48-10.** A fracture of the distal phalanx may be associated with injury to the nail matrix. A manifestation of this injury is avulsion of the nail plate out of the nail sulcus.

placed as free grafts. A graft 1 cm in diameter or less will often survive by inosculation and ingrowth of circulation from the periphery, even on the bare cortex of the distal phalanx. The nail bed is one of the few areas in which cortical bone will accept a soft tissue graft. As long as bone is attached proximally to a good blood supply, grafting directly on bone is very successful. The graft should be carefully approximated to the nail bed segments using 7–0 chromic sutures attached to a microsurgical spatula needle. Skin remnants are attached to the skin with monofilament 6–0 nylon. Blood should be eliminated from beneath the graft and a pressure dressing applied to prevent accumulation of blood and serum beneath the graft.

## FRACTURES OF THE DISTAL PHALANX

Fractures of the distal phalanx heal without complications for several reasons. There are no tendons spanning the bone that deform the fracture site. In addition, the phalanx is supported dorsally by the nail plate and volarly by pulp with fibrous septa.

Fractures are common radiographic manifestations of a crushed fingertip. When a fracture of the distal phalanx has occurred, there may be an associated injury to the nail bed and matrix, which must be repaired. The excellent soft tissue support of the bone facilitates anatomic alignment of the fracture. Splinting of the fracture is neces-

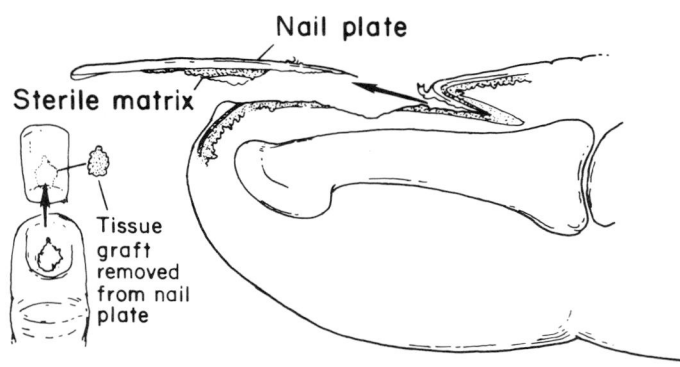

**Fig. 48-12.** Avulsion of a segment of nail bed and matrix is best treated by retrieving the avulsed tissue and replacing it as a graft. If the avulsed nail bed is not available, grafts of nail bed can be used to repair the nail bed and matrix.

sary for 10 to 14 days. When soft tissue support is lost, fixation of the fracture with Kirschner wire is required.

Because the epiphyseal plate is weaker than the insertion of the extensor tendon, an epiphyseal separation, rather than a mallet finger, results when the child is struck on the fingertip. While this injury presents clinically as a mallet finger deformity, it is usually an open fracture of the base of the proximal phalanx with the nail plate lying superficial to the eponychium. The extensor tendon inserts on the proximal fragment of the epiphyseal plate, and the flexor profundus tendon flexes the distal fragment. Closed reduction by hyperextension and placing the nail plate back under the proximal nail fold after proper cleansing is recommended.

## HOSPITAL CARE

Replantation of the sharply amputated part proximal to the nail should be considered if suitable vessels are identified distally. Patients with nail bed injuries requiring a nail bed graft are also best treated in an operating room. In the absence of retrievable avulsed nail bed and matrix, nail bed grafting is indicated to replace the avulsed tissue. If an adjacent finger has been amputated, or is so severely crushed that it has to be amputated, removal of a full-thickness nail bed graft or split-thickness nail bed graft is a good choice for coverage of the avulsion. Split-thickness nail bed grafts from the adjacent nail bed of the injured finger or from a toe nail bed provide excellent results, without causing deformities in the donor area. In harvesting a split-thickness nail bed graft, attempt is made to keep the graft so thin that the point of the knife can be seen through the graft; the thickness of such grafts varies from 0.007 to 0.01 in.

## BIBLIOGRAPHY

Shepard GH: Management of the acute nail bed avulsion. *Hand Clin* 6:39, 1990.

Van Beek AL, Kassan MA, Adson MH, et al: Management of acute fingernail injuries, *Hand Clin* 6:23, 1990.

Wu MM, Morgan RF, Thacker JG, et al: Biomechanical performance of microsurgical spatula needles for the repair of nail bed injuries. *J Emerg Med* 11:187, 1993.

Zook EG: Anatomy and physiology of the perionychium. *Hand Clin* 6:1, 1990.

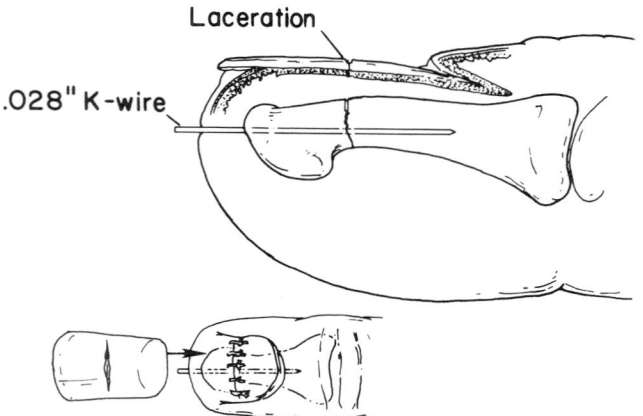

**Fig. 48-11.** Following nail bed repair, if the fracture fragments are unstable, fixation by a Kirschner wire is recommended. After stabilization, the nail plate should be returned to cover the nail bed and matrix, serving as a stent.

# 49
# PUNCTURE WOUNDS AND ANIMAL BITES

### Robert P. Wahl
### John Eggleston
### Richard Edlich

## PUNCTURE WOUNDS

The circumstances of puncture wounds are usually accidental, with the hands and soles of the feet most frequently involved. Sharp, elongated objects pierce the skin and penetrate into the deeper tissues. This results in the potential for injury to the underlying structures, foreign body retention, and development of infection. The treating physician must employ an organized and thorough approach to the evaluation and management of puncture wounds to minimize complications.

The most common sequela of puncture wounds is infection, which is reported to occur 11 to 15 percent of the time. Punctures may be predisposed to infection due to the inoculation of organisms into the deep tissues, which have a tendency to close early. Gram-positive organisms are the usual pathogens with *Staphylococcus aureus* predominating, followed by other *Staphylococcus* and *Streptococcus* species. Many other microorganisms have also been isolated from puncture wound infections, including *Aerobacter aerogenes* and *Mycobacterium fortuitum*. Violation of joint spaces can lead to septic arthritis; and penetration to relatively vascular cartilage, periosteum, and bone can lead to osteomyelitis. *Pseudomonas aeruginosa* is the most frequent etiologic agent in post–puncture wound osteomyelitis, particularly when foreign body penetration occurs through the sole of footwear, such as a tennis shoe. Because this organism is not detected in new sneakers, it has been postulated that the foam rubber material becomes colonized in the warm, humid summer months. The presence of a foreign body predisposes to both cellulitis and osteomyelitis, and failure of an infection to respond to antibiotics may be due to a foreign body.

The clinical presentation of patients sustaining puncture wounds can vary widely from simple, innocuous-appearing wounds to those grossly contaminated and infected. The treating physician needs to document the circumstances surrounding the injury completely. The historical information should include the time interval since the injury (>6 h represents a dirty wound), type and condition of the penetrating object, whether footwear was worn (plantar punctures), an estimation of the depth of penetration, whether the injury occurred indoors or outdoors, and the amount of contamination (rust, dirt, cloth contaminants). The potential for retained foreign body can be assessed in patients who remove the object by asking whether it appeared to remain intact. The patient's past medical history pertaining to immunocompromised states, diabetes mellitus, or peripheral vascular disease should be documented. In addition, the tetanus immunization status of any puncture wound patient must be determined, and appropriate treatment recommendations followed.

The treating physician should consider the likelihood of development of complications. Puncture wounds associated with the following have an increased incidence of infection: greater than 6 h from injury, larger wounds with deeper penetration, obvious contamination with foreign matter and debris, wounds occurring outdoors, wounds penetrating through footwear, and wounds in susceptible patients with underlying disease states. In addition, puncture wounds to the forefoot, distal to the metatarsal necks (Fig. 49-1), carry an increased risk of infection.

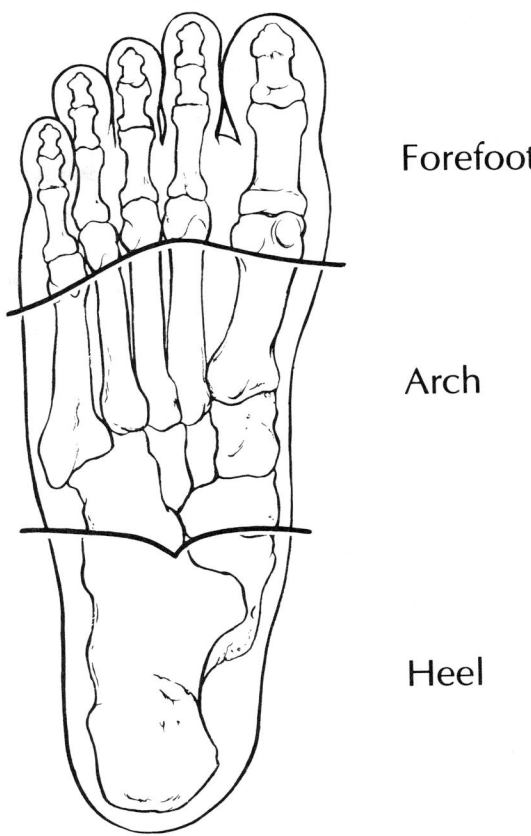

Forefoot

Arch

Heel

**Fig. 49-1.** The bony and cartilaginous structures in the forefoot region of the sole of the foot are the most prone to development of osteomyelitis after plantar puncture wounds.

On physical examination of puncture wounds, one must consider the likelihood of injury to structures beneath the skin. In hand punctures, the function of all flexor and extensor tendons, sensation to light touch and two-point discrimination, and vascular integrity must be assessed. Clinical evidence of diminished pulse, decreased range of motion, or altered sensation may indicate the presence of injury to underlying vessels, tendons, or nerves. In all puncture wounds, the location of the wound; condition of the surrounding skin with respect to the presence of any foreign matter, debris, or devitalized tissue; and the neurovascular status of the extremity distal to the site of injury should be evaluated. The presence of infection must be considered with clinical evidence of increased pain, swelling, erythema, warmth, fluctuance, decreased range of motion at joints, or evidence of drainage from a puncture wound site.

Treating physicians should maintain a high index of suspicion for the possibility of a retained foreign body. Development of an infection at a puncture wound site should prompt the search for a foreign body, which may serve as a nidus of infection. Knowledge of the type and condition of the penetrating object can heighten suspicion. Materials such as wood, glass, and plastic and thin objects such as pins and needles can easily break, leaving retained foreign bodies in the soft tissue beneath a puncture site. Wound probing with a thin, blunt instrument has been utilized to determine the depth of the wound and the presence of foreign body. However, no studies have been performed either to prove the efficacy for foreign body identification or to show decreased infection rates in probed wounds. Wound probing is probably best left to the discretion of the treating physician.

Plain film radiographs should be obtained in all infected puncture wounds and in any wound suspicious for a retained foreign body. Radiopaque foreign bodies will be identifiable in 80 to 90 percent of plain films. Radiographs will detect fragments greater than 0.5 mm in diameter, if the greatest diameter of the fragment is positioned parallel to the beam. Therefore, in general, two-view radiographs should be taken. Substances with densities close to that of soft tissue may not be distinguishable from the surrounding tissues. Many organic substances, such as wood splinters, cactus spines, thorns, and vegetable matter, may not be identified with plain film radiographs. Ultrasound has been successfully used to identify substances invisible on plain films, particularly vegetable matter. Objects as small as $1 \times 2$ mm or larger have been detected with this modality, with sensitivities as high as 95 to 98 percent and specificities from 89 to 98 percent. Ultrasound can benefit the patient by limiting exposure to radiation, which can be significant with use of fluoroscopy. CT scan may be the method of choice for the detection of retained foreign bodies not seen with other techniques, especially wood. The ability of CT to differentiate densities permits detection of substances previously "invisible" by other imaging modalities. Magnetic resonance imaging (MRI) has excellent ability to contrast between soft tissues. It may be superior to other imaging modalities in the detection of plastics; however, it cannot be used with certain substances such as metallic objects or with others such as gravel, which produces significant artifacts. Neither CT nor MRI should be used as screening examinations but as methods of last resort.

Many aspects of the treatment of puncture wounds remain controversial. Uncomplicated, clean punctures presenting less than 6 h after injury may only require wound cleansing and tetanus prophylaxis as indicated. Low-pressure irrigation (0.5 psi) of wounds is recommended to assist in cleansing of the wound for better visualization of the entrance site, as well as removal of visible foreign matter. The injection of irrigation fluid under high (7 psi) pressure into a closed wound tract may lead to displacement of foreign matter but does not disseminate bacteria deeper into the surrounding tissue.

Patients with peripheral vascular disease, diabetes mellitus, immunocompromised states, contaminated wounds, and with wounds of the forefoot (Fig. 49-1) or with deep wounds of the rest of the foot should receive intravenous antibiotics in the emergency department. A first-generation cephalosporin is often used. Debridement or "coring" of the wound tract is reserved for larger lacerations, removal of deep foreign bodies, or tract excisions if cellulitis is present. The expertise, time required for the procedure, potential tourniquet complications, and postoperative management generally dictate referral to a surgical specialist.

Attempts at debridement of infected puncture sites by superficial elliptical incision are not satisfactory to remove the nidus of infection.

The efficacy of administration of prophylactic antimicrobial agents in the management of clean puncture wounds has not been demonstrated, and their use remains controversial. In fact, it has been suggested that this practice may actually contribute to the development of secondary infections with *Pseudomonas* by altering the normal flora. Currently, there have been no definitive clinical studies guiding the decision-making regarding use of prophylactic antibiotics. Uncomplicated puncture wounds in reliable, healthy patients do not require prophylactic antibiotics. The decision to use prophylactic antibiotics should be left to the treating physician.

Infections are differentiated into cellulitis and deeper infections of bone or cartilage. Cellulitis is a localized inflammation of the skin and soft tissues surrounding the puncture wound, usually without significant drainage, and developing in 1 to 4 days. Swelling of the dorsum of the foot is often not encountered. Pain is generally noted around the puncture site, causing the patient to limit weight bearing on the affected foot. Deeper infections of bone or cartilage may also present with painful cellulitis around the puncture site that limits weight bearing on the affected foot. Most patients with deep infections, however, will also have pain and swelling involving the dorsal aspect of the affected foot even though the initial injury was on the

sole of the foot. The delay in time between the onset of symptoms due to deeper infections and the time of injury may vary from several days to 2 years.

Cellulitis of the soft tissues around the puncture wound can occur in any site in the foot. In contrast, deeper infections of the bone or soft tissue are usually identified in specific regions of the foot (Fig. 49-1). Puncture wounds involving the forefoot are the most common and carry the highest risk of infectious complications. The bones of the forefoot, a major weight-bearing region, have very little overlying soft tissues as compared with the heel and the arch of the foot. Therefore, a long wounding object is more prone to penetrate bone and cartilage in forefoot injuries, predisposing to deeper bone and cartilage infections.

When there is evidence of infection, cultures should be obtained and antimicrobial coverage should be directed at gram-positive organisms, especially *Staph. aureus*. Effective agents include penicillinase-resistant penicillins (e.g., dicloxacillin), first-generation cephalosporins (e.g., cefalexin, cefadroxil), or erythromycin for the penicillin- and cephalosporin-allergic patient. Use of fluoroquinolones (e.g., ciprofloxacin) are contraindicated in patients less than 17 years old.

Bone and joint infections are the most disastrous sequelae of puncture wounds, since they can cause severe bone and joint destruction, resulting in significant long-term morbidity. Patients with post–puncture wound osteomyelitis or septic arthritis typically have received initial management of their puncture wound and tetanus immunization, if indicated. Antimicrobial agents may have been given prophylactically or for early cellulitis. A short period of symptomatic improvement is typically followed by increasing pain, swelling, redness, drainage, or a combination of these findings. Radiographs, if taken at this time, are usually normal, and a second line of antibiotics may be administered. Partial resolution or persistence of symptoms prompts patients to seek further evaluation. It is not until an average of 3 weeks after the initial injury that radiographs are repeated and the diagnosis of osteomyelitis is made. Any patient who relapses or fails to improve after initial therapy for a puncture wound should be suspected of having osteomyelitis. Radiographs should be obtained, blood sent for an erythrocyte sedimentation rate (usually elevated), and any drainage cultured. A bone scan will be abnormal 48 to 72 h after the onset of symptoms. Broad-spectrum antibiotic coverage that includes coverage against *Staphylococcus* and *Pseudomonas* should be initiated. An acceptable regimen would consist of parenteral nafcillin and ceftazidime. Definitive management frequently necessitates operative intervention for debridement.

Although the majority of patients sustaining puncture wounds can be managed as outpatients, some require admission for parenteral antibiotic administration or operative intervention. Conditions for admission include wound infections in patients with diabetes mellitus, peripheral vascular disease, or other immunocompromised states; wounds with progressive cellulitis and lymphangitic spread; osteomyelitis; septic arthritis; and deep foreign bodies necessitating operative removal. Outpatients should be provided with instructions on rest, with non–weight bearing for plantar puncture wounds, elevation, warm soaks, and information detailing events that should prompt the patient to seek immediate medical attention, such as signs and symptoms of infection. Close follow-up must be ensured, usually within 48 h of the initial evaluation. Tetanus prophylaxis should be provided as indicated.

## High-Pressure Injection Injuries

High-pressure injection injuries constitute a unique mechanism of injury that may present as a puncture wound, usually to the hand. A material such as paint, paint thinner, grease, oil, or diesel fuel, among many others, is injected by equipment that can introduce the material under high pressure, up to several thousand psi. The type, amount, and velocity of material injected, as well as the anatomic location, will influence the degree of tissue inflammatory response, mechanical distension affecting venous outflow and arterial inflow, and dispersion of the injected material in the soft tissues and along fascial planes. Patients generally present with extremity pain and swelling, and treating physicians should carefully assess the neurovascular function. Pain control should be achieved with parenteral analgesics; digital blocks are contraindicated to avoid increases in tissue pressure with compromise of tissue perfusion. Prompt recognition and early surgical debridement provide for optimal outcome.

## HUMAN BITES

Human bites are commonly the result of fighting, passionate activity, or self-infliction, such as biting the nails. Frequent locations include the scalp and face in children; and the hand, ear, nose, forearm, breast, penis, scrotum, and vulva in adults. Occlusional bites are sustained when human teeth actually bite a part of the human anatomy. This commonly occurs to the distal portion of a digit during an altercation and may result in complete amputation. The "clenched-fist" injury (CFI) occurs at the metacarpophalangeal region of the fist as it strikes the mouth and teeth of another individual. It is these hand wounds in particular that usually result in serious sequelae, including infection, loss of function, and potential amputation if untreated or misdiagnosed. In the emergency department setting, many patients may try to conceal or even deny the true etiology of human bite wounds. Due to the serious nature of the complications, any penetrating injury in the vicinity of the metacarpophalangeal joint should be considered a CFI until proven otherwise.

Injury to the tissues results from a crushing or tearing mechanism with tissue destruction and devitalization. Underlying structures, particularly in the hand, are at risk of injury; these include the tendons, vessels, nerves, deep spaces, joints, and bone. Inoculation of these tissues and structures with the normal human aerobic and anaerobic oral flora predisposes these wounds to a high risk of subsequent infection. Many infected human bite wounds are polymicrobial, with studies reporting up to 43 percent mixed gram-positive and gram-negative organisms, and 26 to 83 percent yielding both aerobic and anaerobic bacteria. The single, most frequent aerobic organism is viridans streptococci, followed by *Staph. aureus. Haemophilus* species, among other aerobes, have also been isolated. Among anaerobes, *Bacteroides* species, *Fusobacterium* species, and anaerobic cocci (e.g., *Peptostreptococcus* species) have all been isolates and all are likely pathogenic. *Eikenella corrodens,* an aerobic gram-negative bacillus, has been isolated in up to 25 percent of wounds due to CFI and is a common cause of osteomyelitis. *E. corrodens* is susceptible to penicillin, but resistant to penicillinase-resistant penicillins, clindamycin, and metronidazole, and has variable resistance to cephalosporins.

Complications of human bite wounds are most frequently seen in hand wounds, particularly the CFI. Sequelae include localized cellulitis, lymphangitis, abscess formation, tenosynovitis, septic arthritis, and osteomyelitis. Human bites to anatomic locations other than the hand appear to have similar rates of infection as nonbite lacerations. It is noteworthy that human bites in children and bites to the face have been managed with low rates of infection, often less than 5 percent. Paronychia are frequent in children who suck their thumb and may inoculate oral flora to the region of the nail bed. In addition, several viral diseases have been transmitted by human bites. Herpetic whitlow results from contact or bites to the finger by a person infected with herpes simplex virus. Hepatitis B virus has also been transmitted after human bites from infected individuals. The most recent data available suggest that the potential risk of HIV infection through human bites appears to be negligible, likely due to the low levels of HIV present in saliva.

The clinical evaluation of human bites should identify the time interval since the injury, mechanism (i.e., occlusion versus closed-fist), location, depth of penetration, tetanus immunization status, medication allergies, and underlying medical conditions predisposing to poor wound healing. As mentioned, human bites to the hands have an increased predilection for infection. However, patients presenting less than 18 to 24 h postinjury will likely not exhibit evidence of infection. Documentation of the vascular, motor, and sensory examination is essential. Following appropriate anesthesia, careful wound exploration is necessary to determine injury to underlying structures and tissues and the potential for a foreign body. The examination of the wound in CFI must take into account the flexed position at the interphalangeal and metacarpophalangeal joints at the time of injury. The injured segment of tendon will retract proximally in the unclenched, open hand. The wound must be examined through a full range of motion at the metacarpophalangeal joint to detect extensor tendon involvement. Potential violation of the joint spaces must also be determined. Radiographs of the wound site, particularly the hand, are recommended to delineate radiopaque foreign bodies and fractures.

Patients presenting more than 18 to 24 h after injury may already exhibit evidence of infection. Physical findings frequently reveal pain, swelling, erythema, warmth, and a purulent, often malodorous discharge from the wound. Aerobic and anaerobic cultures should be obtained from the wound prior to any irrigation or cleansing of the wound. Careful examination of the wound following irrigation and cleansing should seek to determine involvement of tendons and joint spaces. Radiographs may show evidence of osteomyelitis.

An aggressive approach to the management of CFI is required. Copious wound irrigation with a 0.9% saline solution, surgical debridement of devitalized tissue, immobilization in a bulky hand dressing, and elevation to reduce edema—all play a significant role in proper treatment. Human bite wounds to the hand should initially be left open. Prophylactic antibiotics should be administered early, optimally within 3 h of presentation. Prophylactic antibiotics should be considered in human bites to locations other than the hand in high-risk situations, such as patients with asplenia, diabetes mellitus, and immune deficiency. Dicloxacillin plus penicillin is the best low-cost choice for full coverage of both aerobic and anaerobic pathogens. Oral cefuroxime or amoxicillin/clavulanic acid is an acceptable, although more expensive, alternative. Three days to a maximum of 5 days of therapy is acceptable. For the penicillin-allergic patient, erythromycin at usual doses is a reasonable alternative.

Patients with CFI presenting more than 24 h from injury usually have clinical evidence of infection. Infected wounds require systemic antibiotic administration. Mildly infected wounds, such as those showing a localized cellulitis, may be managed on an outpatient basis with close follow-up, after initial emergency department treatment as above. Moderate to severe infections manifested by fever, tachycardia, cellulitis, lymphangitis, or concern for deep tissue involvement will require parenteral antibiotic therapy. Penicillin (or ampicillin) plus a penicillinase-resistant penicillin (*Staph. aureus* coverage) or a second-generation cephalosporin (cefoxitin) provides necessary coverage. Diabetics have an increased incidence of gram-negative infection and should receive a parenteral aminoglycoside. Proper management includes copious irrigation, bulky dressings, daily dressing changes, elevation, and immobilization. Delayed primary closure or healing by secondary intention is the preferred approach for hand wound closure. Wounds in other locations, such as the face, head, and neck, have been successfully repaired with primary closure following copious irrigation and debridement. Human bite wounds other than to the hand do not appear to have as high a risk of infection, and antibiotics are considered only in high-risk patients.

Outpatient management of human bite wounds to the hand can be considered in reliable patients who present without delay (less than 18 to 24 h); exhibit no clinical evidence of infection; have no underlying injury to tendon, joint, or bone; and are otherwise healthy. The wounds must be irrigated copiously, left open to drain, placed in a bulky dressing, and elevated. Appropriate prophylactic antibiotic coverage should be initiated, with the first dose preferably within 3 h of presentation. Patients must be instructed to return in 24 h for reexamination of the wound, or sooner if infection develops. Patients presenting after more than 24 h with an established infection; wounds involving tendon, joint, or bone; and patients exhibiting systemic manifestations of infection all require hospitalization and surgical consultation for debridement. Appropriate parenteral antibiotics should be initiated in the emergency department after cultures are obtained. All patients with human bite wounds should be provided with tetanus immunization according to standard guidelines.

## ANIMAL BITES

It has been estimated that up to 1 percent of emergency department visits involve animal bites. Conservative estimates indicate that between 1 and 2 million people annually in the United States are bitten by animals. The true incidence of animal bites is difficult to determine since many victims do not report the event or seek medical attention. Bite wounds consist of punctures, lacerations, avulsions, and abrasions. Patients seek medical attention with concerns about infection, tetanus and rabies prophylaxis, and for treatment of wounds. Wound infection is the most frequent complication. Other complications are seen less frequently and include sepsis, septic arthritis, tenosynovitis, osteomyelitis, meningitis, and disfiguring wounds.

Many factors contribute to the development of infection in animal bite wounds. Characteristics of the injury, such as the type of injury, presence of foreign bodies, and anatomic location of injury; treatment factors including time delay to treatment, irrigation, debridement, and wound closure techniques; and patient characteristics, such as age and underlying medical conditions, all play an important role. Factors that appear to predict a probability of infection greater than 5 to 10 percent include full-thickness puncture, hand, or lower extremity wounds; wounds requiring debridement; wounds involving joints, ligaments, tendons, or fractures; and wounds in patients who are high-risk hosts. Treatment with antibiotics in such circumstances is recommended.

Animal bites should be considered tetanus-prone wounds, and guidelines for tetanus immunization followed. The need for rabies immunoprophylaxis must also be considered in animal bite wounds. The treating physician should document the number, type, location, and depth of all wounds, as well as the presence of any clinical evidence of infection. Wound exploration should determine involvement of any underlying structures, including vessels, nerves, tendons, soft tissue, and joint spaces. Radiographs should be obtained if there is evidence of infection or any suspicion of foreign body or bony involvement. All animal bite wounds require appropriate local wound care. Wounds must be copiously irrigated and have compromised or necrotic tissue debrided. Primary closure following appropriate wound care has been successful in wounds to the head and neck, torso, and extremities other than the hands. Puncture wounds usually heal by secondary intent. Hand wounds are best managed open initially, then followed by delayed primary wound closure in 3 to 5 days. Antibiotics should not be used as a substitute for proper local wound care.

## Dog Bites

Dogs account for 80 to 90 percent of reported animal bites in the United States. Dog bite injuries occur most frequently on the extremities (upper slightly greater than lower), followed by the head and neck, and least frequently on the trunk. Head and neck bites are more common in the pediatric age group. Infection occurs in dog bites in approximately 5 to 15 percent of cases. Factors that increase the rate of infection have been reported to include age greater than 50 years, delay in treatment greater than 24 h, hand wounds, and deep puncture.

Bite wound infections usually result from the organisms inoculated into the depth of the wound by the animal's teeth, not from the bacterial flora normally found on the patient's skin. Infections from dog bite wounds are often polymicrobial. Aerobic bacteria are present in most wounds, and anaerobic bacteria in up to 40 percent. Among the most frequent aerobes isolated are α-hemolytic streptococci, followed by *Staph. aureus* and *Pasteurella multocida* (20 to 30 percent), and *Staph. intermedius*. Other pathogenic aerobes include β-hemolytic streptococci, γ-hemolytic streptococci, *E. corrodens*, *Capnocytophaga canimorsus*, other *Pasteurella* species, and *H. aphrophilus*. The anaerobic bacteria isolated from dog bite wounds include *Actinomyces* species, *Bacteroides* species, *Fusobacterium* species, and *Peptostreptococcus* species, with less frequent occurrence of other species.

*Capnocytophaga canimorsus*, formerly known by the Centers for Disease Control and Prevention as "dysgonic fermenter-2" (DF-2), is a fastidious, thin, gram-negative bacillus that has been associated with severe infection. It was first recognized as a human pathogen in 1976. Clinically, infection with this organism may manifest as sepsis with disseminated intravascular coagulation, acute renal failure, endocarditis, peripheral gangrene, and cardiopulmonary failure. The clinical picture may be more severe in patients immunocompromised by asplenia, alcoholism, chronic lung disease, or other immunosuppression, with fatality in up to 25 percent of cases. Penicillin is the drug of choice when infection with this organism is suspected and should be used prophylactically in high-risk individuals. This bacterium is also usually sensitive to cephalosporins, tetracyclines, erythromycin, and clindamycin.

Most patients sustaining dog bite injuries can be managed as outpatients. Discharge instructions must include information about signs and symptoms suggestive of infection and assurance of follow-up within 24 to 48 h. Reliable patients who present early without evidence of infection can be treated with the local care measures mentioned above. Puncture wounds, wounds to the hand, and wounds in high-risk individuals should receive treatment with a first-generation cephalosporin (e.g., cephalexin) or an oral antistaphylococcal penicillin (e.g., dicloxacillin). Erythromycin or trimethoprim/sulfamethoxazole are acceptable alternatives in the penicillin-allergic patient. When prescribed, antibiotic therapy should be initiated as soon as possible after the patient arrives for treatment, ideally within 3 h. There is no evidence that antibiotic therapy in animal bite wounds to other anatomic locations is beneficial.

Wounds obviously infected at the time of presentation need to be cultured and have antibiotic therapy initiated. Infection developing within 24 h of injury suggests *P. multocida* as the etiology, and treatment with penicillin V potassium is recommended. Tetracycline in nonpregnant adults and erythromycin in children or pregnant adults are alternative choices. Patients with evidence of wound infection developing beyond 24 h, implicating *Staphylococcus* and *Streptococcus*, should receive dicloxacillin or cephalexin. Low-risk patients with local cellulitis only and no involvement of underlying structures can be observed closely as outpatients. Admission and parenteral antibiotic therapy are indicated in patients with infected wounds and evidence of lymphangitis, lymphadenitis, tenosynovitis, septic arthritis, or osteomyelitis; systemic signs, such as fever; or injury to underlying structures, such as tendons, joints, or bone. Intravenous penicillin G and nafcillin should be initiated pending results of wound cultures. If gram-negative organisms are suspected, an aminoglycoside should be added. A second- or third-generation cephalosporin can be given alternatively, although they are more expensive. When sepsis is suspected, broad-spectrum coverage with imipenem/cilastatin or ampicillin/sulbactam is warranted pending culture results.

## Cat Bites/Scratches

### Cat-Scratch Disease

Cat-scratch disease most often occurs in young (80 percent less than 21 years of age) immunocompetent hosts and is manifested by persistent regional lymphadenopathy in an area of the body draining lymph from a recent cat scratch or bite, usually preceded by an erythematous papule or pustule at the inoculation site. Complications, with involvement of the central nervous system, liver, spleen, bone, and skin, can be seen in up to 2 percent of affected patients. Data analysis reveals that 9.3 individuals per 100,000 population, or 22,000 people, are affected, leading to 2000 hospitalizations annually. There is a male, as well as a fall/winter seasonal predominance.

The precise etiologic agent has been difficult to elucidate. Until recently, the organism *Afipia felis* was often implicated. However, recent investigations utilizing serologic and polymerase-chain-reaction assays suggest that the bacterium *Rochalimaea henselae,* a small gram-negative rod similar to the family Bartonellaceae, may be a much more common etiologic agent of cat-scratch disease. Diagnosis traditionally requires the presence of three of the following four criteria: (1) a history of cat contact with the presence of a scratch or primary lesion, (2) a positive cat-scratch skin test antigen response, (3) negative laboratory results for other causes of lymphadenopathy, and (4) characteristic pathologic findings of lymph nodes, which may include organism detection (bacilli) via Warthin-Starry staining. Soon, serologic testing (indirect fluorescent antibody) and enzymatic immunoassay for the detection of IgG antibodies, both to *R. henselae,* may be routinely available to assist in the diagnosis.

Most patients with cat-scratch disease are not seriously ill, and spontaneous resolution is common. As a result, treatment of cat-scratch disease does not have the benefit of controlled trials to guide antibiotic therapy. Antimicrobial susceptibility testing has shown favorable minimum inhibitory concentration (MIC) values for ampicillin, second- and third-generation cephalosporins, rifampin, tetracycline, trimethoprim/sulfamethoxazole, aminoglycosides, and macrolides, among others. MIC values for quinolones were variable and were less favorable for the first-generation cephalosporins. Antimicrobial therapy for up to 28 days' duration has been described, with successful resolution of symptoms and symptom-free follow-up.

### Cat Bites

Cat bites account for 5 to 18 percent of reported animal bites in the United States. The majority of wounds are inflicted on the arm, forearm, and hand and with decreasing frequency to the head and neck, lower extremity, and trunk. Due to the long, slender fangs of cats, most bites result in puncture wounds (57 to 86 percent); the remainder are superficial abrasions (9 to 25 percent) and lacerations (5 to 17 percent). Factors related to cat bite wound infections are older age of the patient, attempting wound care at home, longer treatment delays, puncture wounds, deeper wounds, and being bitten by a "pet" cat.

The feline oral flora is more likely to contain *P. multocida* than canine oral flora, and this is the major pathogen found in wound infections due to cat bites. It is isolated from 53 to 80 percent of cultured cat bite wound infections. Wounds infected with *P. multocida* are characterized by a rapidly developing, intense inflammatory response, often within a few hours and rarely greater than 24 h after the bite. Pain and swelling are prominent. Serious bone and joint infections may be caused by *P. multocida.* Septic arthritis usually involves a single joint, with predilection for joints previously damaged by arthritis or prosthetic joints. More than half the patients with septic arthritis also have altered host defenses from glucocorticoids or alcoholism. Bacteremia may occur in the setting of serious infections with *P. multocida.*

Treatment for cat bite wounds is essentially the same as for dog bite wounds. Proper local wound care is indicated, followed by primary wound closure for most wounds that require repair. Puncture wounds and lacerations smaller than 1 to 2 cm in length should not be closed because they cannot be adequately cleaned. Delayed primary closure can be employed for wounds smaller than 1 to 2 cm in length located in cosmetically important areas. Prophylactic antibiotics should be administered to high-risk patients including those with punctures to the hand, immunocompromised patients, and patients with arthritis or prosthetic joints. Penicillin is the drug of choice for known *P. multocida* infections. Antibiotic administration when the etiology of infection is unknown is with dicloxacillin or cephalexin (similar to dog bites). Penicillin-allergic patients can be treated with erythromycin, or tetracycline in nonpregnant adults. Indications for admission are similar for dog bites; parenteral antibiotics with penicillin G and nafcillin provide necessary coverage.

## Exotic Animal Bites

Much scientific clinical data pertaining to exotic animal bite wounds and infection are lacking, and treatment regimens are often based on anecdotal case reports. The examining physician can usually adhere to the dictum that the bacteriology of the bite wound will reflect the normal oral flora of the inflicting animal, as opposed to the normal skin flora of the patient. General principles of local wound care, including irrigation and surgical debridement, wound cultures as appropriate, and tetanus and rabies prophylaxis, should be followed.

Nonhuman primate (monkey) bites are likely to be seen in animal handlers and researchers. The organisms most often encountered in the mouth of rhesus monkeys (*Macaca mulatta*) are *Neisseria* species (19.8 percent), $\alpha$-hemolytic streptococci (19.8 percent), and *H. parainfluenza* (17.2 percent). Also, *E. corrodens* remains a pathogen from primate bites. The combination of penicillin and cefoperazone has been recommended as an initial antibiotic regimen for monkey bite injuries. In addition, the potential for transmission of *Herpesvirus simiae* (B virus) must be considered. The potential consequences of B virus inoculation are grave and include local neurologic symptoms, encephalitis (91 percent), and death (68 percent). Prophylactic treatment with an antiviral agent, such as acyclovir 400 mg five times a day, can be considered when a deep penetrating wound is sustained from a macaque rhesus monkey. Following a human inoculation, the monkey should be quarantined and carefully examined for oral mucosal lesions.

The large feline carnivores, such as lions and tigers, also carry *Pasteurella* as normal oral flora, similar to domestic cats. Wound care should be the same as for other species, with an awareness for the potential for major internal injuries.

Alligator bites (*Alligator mississippiensis*) may be frequently encountered in the southeastern United States. Bite wounds can be polymicrobial, but the anaerobic organism *Aeromonas hydrophila* has been a consistent isolate noted in one study. Trimethoprim/sulfamethoxazole is considered a front-line agent for treatment, with an aminoglycoside or tetracycline as an alternative. *Bacteroides* and *Clostridium* species have also been isolated.

Bites from the common or green iguana (*Iguana iguana*), readily available in the United States as pets, are generally innocuous. These animals do not harbor the rabies virus. Local topical antiseptic wound care and verification of tetanus status is all that is needed for the emergency treatment of an iguana bite. However, bites from the venomous gila monster lizard, found in the southwestern United States, have been associated with significant morbidity including anaphylaxis, disseminated intravascular coagulation, and acute myocardial infarction.

Rat bites may be complicated by leptospirosis, a zoonosis transmitted primarily through the direct or indirect exposure of mucous membranes or abraded skin to the urine of an infected animal. The domestic rat may serve as the primary reservoir of leptospirosis in urban areas. Subclinical infections are common, and most clinical infections are self-limiting. Oral doxycycline, 100 mg twice a day for 7 days, is effective when treatment is initiated within 4 days of clinical onset of symptoms. Parenteral penicillin G, 6 million units daily for 7 days, is efficacious with more severe icteric disease. In addition, rat-bite fever may be transmitted by several small rodents, including the rat, mouse, and gerbil. The causative organisms are *Streptobacillus moniliformis* and *Spirillum minor.* Prophylactic therapy with penicillin V-K for 5 days has been recommended.

Camels can inflict serious bites as well as other associated injuries. They have enlarged canine teeth and a long neck, which allows them to reach around and bite the rider violently, and the ability to lift the rider into the air and throw him or her to the ground. The bacteriology of camel bite wounds has not been well elucidated; however, an anecdotal report of efficacy with high-dose penicillin G, gentamycin, and clindamycin has been reported in the literature.

## BIBLIOGRAPHY

Callaham ML: Wild and domestic animal attacks, in Auerbach PC, Geehr EC (eds): *Management of Wilderness and Environmental Emergencies,* 2d ed. St. Louis, Mosby, 1989, pp 683–726.

Chisholm CD, Schlesser JF: Plantar puncture wounds: Controversies and treatment recommendations. *Ann Emerg Med* 18:1352, 1989.

Dagan R, Phillip M, Watemberg NM, Kassis I: Outpatient treatment of serious community acquired pediatric infections using once-daily intramuscular ceftriaxone. *Pediatr Infect Dis J* 6:1080, 1987.

Dire DJ: Emergency management of dog and cat bite wounds. *Emerg Med Clin North Am* 10(4):719, 1992.

Edlich RF: Wound management, in *Critical Decisions in Emergency Medicine* vol 7. Dallas, American College of Emergency Physicians, 1992, pp 163–170.

Goldstein EJC: Bite wounds and infection. *Clin Infect Dis* 14:633, 1992.

Inaba AS, Zukin DD, Perro M: An update on the evaluation and management of plantar puncture wounds and *Pseudomonas* osteomyelitis. *Pediatr Emerg Care* 8:38, 1992.

Lichtenfeld NS: The pneumatic ankle tourniquet with ankle block anesthesia for foot surgery. *Foot Ankle* 13:344, 1992.

Patzakis MJ, Wilkins J, Brien WW, Carter VS: Wound site as a predictor of complications following deep nail punctures to the foot. *West J Med* 150:545, 1989.

Verdile VP, Freed HA, Gerard J: Puncture wounds to the foot. *J Emerg Med* 7:193, 1989.

Weber DJ, Hansen AR: Infections resulting from animal bites. *Infect Dis Clin North Am* 5(3):663, 1991.

Zubowicz VN, Gravier M: Management of early human bites of the hand: A prospective randomized study. *Plast Reconstr Surg* 88(1):111, 1991.

# 50
# POSTREPAIR WOUND CARE

**Richard F. Edlich**
**George T. Rodeheaver**
**John G. Thacker**

Postrepair care involves primarily wound dressing and tetanus prophylaxis.

## WOUND DRESSING

The manner in which a dressing functions is determined by its physical and chemical composition. There are eight types of absorbent cotton gauze, each type defined by the number of warp and woof threads per square inch. The degree of dressing adherence to a wound is directly related to the size of the dressing interstices. The larger the interstices, the greater the chance that the dressing will be penetrated by the granulation tissue. If debridement is the objective, the emergency physician should use a dressing with greater interstice size, at least larger than type I. Absorption of wound exudates is another important function of a dressing. The beneficial effects of absorbency are that (1) the bacteria contained within the absorbed fluid are removed; (2) the exudate itself is removed, depleting the wound of bacterial nutrients; and (3) tissue maceration is prevented. High absorbency is incompatible with nonadhesion because the serous exudate forms a powerful and adherent glue as it dries. Removal of the absorbent dressing disrupts the fibrinous scab and any granulation tissue that has become entrapped in the dressing. Absorbent dressings are therefore useful for the debridement of open wounds.

In primarily closed wounds, the dressing acts as a barrier against exogenous bacteria. Soaking dressings with serum permits passage of bacteria through the dressing. Saturation of a dressing with fluid that wets both inner and outer surfaces of the dressing is called fluid strike-through. As long as its outer surface remains dry, however, a dressing will remain an effective barrier to bacterial contamination.

The length of time that dry dressings should cover the closed wound is based on knowledge of the period during which the wound is susceptible to bacterial penetration. As sutured wounds heal, they become increasingly resistant to the development of infection from surface contamination. Swabbing the surface of the wound with either *Staphylococcus aureus* or *Escherichia coli* during the first 48 h after closure can cause localized gross infections. Contamination after the third day may not produce gross infection in the sutured wound. Thus barrier dressings are useful to protect the fresh incision from surface contamination in the first few days. Thereafter, removal of the dressings permits daily inspection and palpation of the wound. Wounds closed with tape have a greater capacity to resist infection than sutured wounds and do not need protective dressings.

Another important purpose of some dressings is to exert pressure on the underlying tissues. A pressure dressing minimizes the accumulation of intercellular fluid within the wound and limits dead space. Maximal pressure should be applied to the wound site as well as distal to it. Proximal to the wound, the pressure applied is decreased to minimize any chance of compromising the venous or lymphatic return.

A pressure dressing, by the very nature of its bulk, immobilizes what it covers. Immobilization of the site of injury is of great value—lymphatic flow is reduced, thereby minimizing the spread of the

Our clinical and experimental research has been supported by grants from the Texaco Foundation, White Plains, New York, and by a generous gift from Mr. Alex von Thelen of Charlottesville, Virginia.

wound microflora. Furthermore, immobilized tissue demonstrates the best resistance to the growth of bacteria. Whenever possible, the site of injury should be elevated above the patient's heart to limit the accumulation of fluid in the wound interstitial spaces. The injured wound with little edema proceeds more rapidly to complete rehabilitation than does the markedly edematous wound.

Dressings should also provide a physiologic environment that is conducive to epithelial migration from the wound edges across the surface of the fresh wound. When an area of epidermis is lost, water vapor begins at once to evaporate from the exposed dermal tissue. The exudate on the surface dries and becomes the outer layer of the scab, which does not prevent water from evaporating from the dermis underneath. The surface of the dermis itself progressively dries (within 18 h). This dry scab and dried dermis resist migration of epidermal cells, which must seek the underlying fibrous tissue of the upper reticular layer of dermis where enough moisture remains to support cellular viability. When the wound is covered by a dressing that prevents or delays evaporation of water from the wound surface, the scab and underlying dermis remain moist. Epidermal cells can easily migrate through the moist scab over the surface of the dermis. Under such dressings, epithelialization is more rapid and no dry dermis is sacrificed.

The dressing that delays evaporation of water vapor would seem to be ideal for coverage of primarily closed wounds and has been usefully employed in the treatment of donor sites, meshed grafts, and dermabraded skin. Unfortunately, excessive exudate may make it difficult to keep the fully occlusive dressing in place, and the moist exudate that provides an ideal medium for epidermal repair is also a suitable culture medium for the proliferation of microorganisms.

Primarily closed wounds (with the exception of those located on the face) are covered by nonwoven microporous polypropylene dressings, which are attached to surrounding skin by wide strips of microporous tape with no reinforcing fibers. In facial lacerations the development of blood clots between the edges of the sutured wounds is of more concern than the potential dangers of surface contamination. These clots will be replaced by a healing scar that can easily be avoided by swabbing the wound with half-strength hydrogen peroxide every 6 h until the wound edges are free of blood. Because hydrogen peroxide causes the sutures to lose their color, the decolorized suture becomes a sign of patient compliance with our postoperative wound care regimen.

In abraded skin, this method of suture line care is ineffective. Even if the wound is washed with hydrogen peroxide, it develops a scab that makes suture removal tedious and often painful to the patient. In such cases, we swab the wound and its adjacent edges with a water-soluble base, such as polyethylene glycol with mupirocin (Bactroban), which disrupts the wound exudates, thereby encouraging their exodus from the wound. These percutaneous sutures must be removed before the eighth postoperative day because needle puncture scars can develop. The wound edges should then be supported by sterile, microporous tape skin closures.

Abraded skin will develop permanent hyperpigmentation after exposure to the sun. Consequently, abraded skin should be protected with a sun-blocking agent for at least 6 months after injury. Photoprotection against UVA was in the past limited by the restricted range of UVA wavelengths absorbed by available sunscreen agents. Shade UVA Guard (Shering-Plough, Memphis, TN) has absorbent effect against the entire ultraviolet spectrum. This sunscreen should prove valuable in helping prevent hyperpigmentation.

## TETANUS PROPHYLAXIS

The occurrence of tetanus has markedly decreased as a result of the widespread use of tetanus toxoid. The reported incidence rate of tetanus has declined steadily since 1947, and has remained relatively constant since 1985. Tetanus occurs almost exclusively among unvaccinated, inadequately vaccinated, or immunocompromised individuals.

The incidence of tetanus increases with the age of the patient. During 1987 and 1988, 67 of the 99 U.S. patients were ≥ 50 years of age; 6 were less than 20 years. No cases of neonatal tetanus occurred because immune pregnant women transfer temporary protection against tetanus to their infants through transplacental maternal antibodies. Tetanus occurred after an identified acute injury in 74 persons. The most frequently reported injuries were puncture wounds (29 percent), followed by lacerations (18 percent) and then abrasions (13 percent). Most puncture wounds followed stepping on sharp objects.

Of the 74 patients who developed tetanus after an acute wound, 31 (42 percent) had sought medical care after the injury. Of those who did, 81 percent did not receive adequate prophylaxis. Those disappointing results are surprising, because surveys of emergency departments indicate that fewer than 5 percent of injured persons receive inadequate prophylaxis.

Complete and appropriately timed vaccination is nearly 100 percent effective in preventing tetanus. When employing tetanus prophylaxis, we employ the guidelines recommended by the Centers for Disease Control and Prevention (CDC).

Because a large proportion of adults lack protection of circulating antitoxin against diphtheria, the CDC recommends the combined preparation of Td, 0.5 mL IM. Td contains much less diphtheria toxoid than the diphtheria toxoid–containing products used in children. When treating a child or infant with a wound, decisions regarding appropriate tetanus prophylaxis should be considered as an opportunity to determine and maintain the patient's compliance with the recommended immunization schedule. When tetanus prophylaxis is indicated in a child or infant with a wound, select the appropriate vaccine that will maintain the immunization schedule and provide protection against tetanus. Documentation of the immunization record should be given to the patient. For adults who have not been immunized previously, follow-up must be arranged to complete the immunization series (Table 50-1).

## Vaccination of Persons with Hemophilia

Persons with bleeding disorders such as hemophilia have an increased risk of acquiring hepatitis B but the same risk as the general population of acquiring tetanus, diphtheria, pertussis, and *Haemophilus influenzae*. The risk of hematomas by intramuscular injections are avoided among persons with bleeding disorders by using the sub-

**Table 50-1.** Recommended Immunization Schedule for Persons ≥7 Years of Age not Vaccinated at the Recommended Time in Early Infancy

| Timing | Vaccine(s) | Comments |
|---|---|---|
| First visit | Td* | |
| Second visit (6–8 weeks after first visit) | Td | |
| Third visit (6 months after second visit) | Td | |
| Additional visits | Td | Repeat every 10 years throughout life |

* The DTP and DTaP doses administered to children <7 years of age who remain incompletely vaccinated at age ≥7 years should be counted as prior exposure to tetanus and diphtheria toxoids (e.g., a child who previously received two doses of DTP needs only one dose of Td to complete a primary series for tetanus and diphtheria).

NOTE: Td   Tetanus and diphtheria toxoids (for persons ≥7 years of age)

cutaneous or intradermal routes for vaccines that are normally administered by the intramuscular route.

If the patients receive antihemophilia or other similar therapy, intramuscular vaccination can be scheduled shortly after such therapy is administered. A narrow-gauge needle (<23 gauge) can be used for the vaccination, and firm pressure applied to the site (without rubbing) for at least 2 min.

## Use of Vaccines and Immune Globulins in Patients with Altered Immunocompetence

The development of active immunization against tetanus is diminished in immunosuppressed individuals. In such patients, passive immunization with TIG (250 units) should be instituted in conjunction with active immunization. Follow-up care should be provided to ensure that the patient has an adequate response to immunization. Serum antitoxin levels above 0.01 IU/mL have been considered protective against tetanus.

Regardless of the active immunization status of the patient, meticulous surgical care with aseptic technique that includes removal of all devitalized tissue and foreign bodies should be provided immediately for all wounds. Such care is essential as part of the prophylaxis against tetanus.

The effectiveness of antibiotics for prophylaxis of tetanus is uncertain. Proper immunization plays the most important role in tetanus prophylaxis. Recommendations on tetanus prophylaxis are based on (1) the condition of the wound, and (2) the patient's immunization history. Table 50-2 outlines some of the clinical features of wounds that are prone to develop tetanus. A wound with any one of these clinical features is considered tetanus-prone. A summary guide to tetanus prophylaxis of the wounded patient is displayed in Table 50-3. Passive immunization with tetanus immune globulin (TIG) (250 units) must be considered individually for each patient.

Recent clinical studies suggest that many elderly people are inadequately protected against tetanus and their immunologic response following a tetanus booster is delayed. It has been postulated that those who fail to seroconvert do carry a risk of developing tetanus despite the prophylaxis administered. Consequently, a more liberal approach to the use of TIG is being considered in the situation in which elderly patients with an unknown immunization history and no past military service present to the emergency department with a break in their skin barrier.

## Toxoid Side Effects and Adverse Reactions

Local reactions, generally erythema and induration without tenderness, are common after the administration of vaccines containing diphtheria, tetanus, and pertussis antigens. These reactions are most common following diphtheria and tetanus toxoids adsorbed (for pediatric use) (DTP) (40 to 70 percent of doses) and are usually self-limited and require no therapy. Fever and other systemic symptoms are less common.

Arthus-type hypersensitivity reactions, characterized by severe local reactions starting 2 to 8 h after an injection and often associated with fever and malaise, may occur, particularly among persons who have received multiple boosters of tetanus toxoid adsorbed (T). Rarely, systemic reactions, such as generalized urticaria, anaphylaxis, or neurologic complications, have been reported after administration of adsorbed tetanus toxoid, although a causal relationship has not been established. All serious adverse effects of vaccine should be reported to the Vaccine Adverse Event Reporting System (1-800-822-7967).

## Toxoid Precautions and Contraindications

A history of a neurologic reaction or a severe hypersensitivity reaction (e.g., generalized urticaria or anaphylaxis) after a previous dose is a contraindication to diphtheria and tetanus toxoids. Local side effects do not preclude continued use.

Persons experiencing severe Arthus-type hypersensitivity reactions to a dose of Td usually have high serum tetanus antitoxin levels and should not be given even emergency boosters of Td more frequently than every 10 years. There is no evidence to suggest that the diphtheria and tetanus toxoids are teratogenic.

If a contraindication to using preparations containing tetanus toxoid exists in a person who has not completed a primary immunization course of Td and who has other than a clean wound, only passive immunization should be given, using TIG.

**Table 50-2.** Clinical Features of Wounds

| Clinical Features | Tetanus-Prone Wounds | Non-Tetanus-Prone Wounds |
|---|---|---|
| Age of wound | >6 h | ≤6 h |
| Configuration | Stellate | Linear wound |
| Depth | >1 cm | ≤1 cm |
| Mechanism of injury | Missile, crush, burn, frostbite | Sharp surface (e.g., knife) |
| Signs of infection | Present | Absent |
| Devitalized tissue | Present | Absent |
| Contaminants (dirt, feces, soil, saliva) | Present | Absent |
| Denervated and/or ischemic tissue | Present | Absent |

**Table 50-3.** Guide to Tetanus Prophylaxis

| History of Adsorbed Tetanus Toxoid (Doses) | Tetanus-Prone Wounds | | Non-Tetanus-Prone Wounds | |
|---|---|---|---|---|
| | Td[a] | TIG[b,c] | Td[a] | TIG |
| Uncertain or <3 | Yes | Yes | Yes | No |
| 3 or more[d] | No[e] | No | No[f] | No |

[a] For children less than 7 years old, diphtheria and tetanus toxoids and pertussis vaccine adsorbed (For Pediatric Use DTP) are preferred to tetanus toxoid alone. Diphtheria and tetanus toxoids (For Pediatric Use DT) are recommended if pertussis vaccine is contraindicated. For persons 7 years old and older, tetanus and diphtheria toxoids adsorbed (For Adult Use Td) are preferred to tetanus toxoid alone.
[b] TIG: Human tetanus immune globulin.
[c] When TIG and Td are given concurrently, separate syringes and separate sites should be used.
[d] If only three doses of fluid toxoid have been received, a fourth dose of toxoid, preferably an adsorbed toxoid, should be given.
[e] Yes, if more than 5 years since last dose. (More frequent boosters are not needed and can accentuate side effects.)
[f] Yes, if more than 10 years since last dose.

## BIBLIOGRAPHY

Advisory Committee on Immunization Practices (ACIP): Recommendations for use of *Haemophilus* b conjugate vaccines and a combined diphtheria, tetanus, pertussis and *Haemophilus* b vaccine. *MMWR* 42 (No. RR-13):1, 1993.

Advisory Committee on Immunization Practices (ACIP): Use of vaccines and immune globulins in persons with altered immunocompetence. *MMWR* 43 (No. RR-1):1, 1994.

Committee on Trauma of the American College of Surgeons: Prophylaxis against tetanus in wound management. *Bull Am Coll Surg* 69(10):22, 1984.

Jacobs RL, Lowe RS, Lanier BQ: Adverse reactions to tetanus toxoid. *JAMA* 247:40, 1982.

# Cardiovascular Diseases

## 51
# MYOCARDIAL ISCHEMIA AND INFARCTION

**Gary P. Young**
**J. Stephan Stapczynski**

## ISCHEMIC HEART DISEASE

Ischemic heart disease and its complications cause the greatest number of deaths in the United States, approximately 700,000 each year. Over 50 percent of these deaths occur before the individual arrives at the hospital. In addition more than 1,300,000 nonfatal acute myocardial infarctions (AMIs) occur each year. Although many processes produce the imbalance between myocardial oxygen supply and demand that develops into ischemia or infarction, the most common cause by far is atherosclerosis of the epicardial coronary arteries, commonly termed coronary artery disease (CAD). CAD is a multifactorial disorder, and epidemiologic research has identified seven major risk factors for its development: age, male sex, family history, cigarette smoking, hypertension, hypercholesterolemia, and diabetes mellitus. Over the last 30 years, mortality due to CAD has declined by about 40 percent in the United States. The decline is felt to be about half due to risk factor modification in the general population and half due to improvements in the medical care of symptomatic patients with CAD.

### Pathophysiology of Myocardial Ischemia

The heart makes up 0.7 percent of the body weight in human beings, but requires 7.0 percent of the basal oxygen consumed by the body. Myocardial ischemia results from imbalance between myocardial oxygen supply and demand. Abnormalities in one or both of these factors may be present in the individual patient (Table 51-1). There are three major determinants of myocardial oxygen supply and three of myocardial oxygen demand (Table 51-2). Although the overwhelming majority of patients have fixed arterial obstruction due to atherosclerotic lesions, recent work has documented a greater incidence of coronary artery spasm than was previously appreciated.

**Table 51-1.** Etiology of Myocardial Ischemia

| |
|---|
| Decreased myocardial oxygen supply |
|   Coronary artery obstruction |
|     Fixed obstruction |
|       Atherosclerosis |
|       Miscellaneous causes |
|     Arterial spasm |
|   Decreased coronary perfusion |
|     Decreased cardiac output |
|     Systemic hypotension |
|     Severe anemia |
| Increased myocardial oxygen demand |
|   Increased myocardial inotropy |
|   Myocardial hypertrophy |
|   Tachycardia |

**Table 51-2.** Major Determinants of Myocardial Oxygen Supply and Demand

| |
|---|
| Supply |
|   Aortic diastolic pressure |
|   Coronary vascular resistance |
|   Diastolic duration |
| Demand |
|   Heart rate |
|   Wall tension |
|     Preload—left ventricular end-diastolic pressure |
|     Afterload—mean aortic pressure |
|   Contractility |

**Table 51-3.** Causes of Myocardial Ischemia without Atherosclerosis

| |
|---|
| Congenital anomalies |
| Coronary artery emboli |
| Coronary arteritis |
| Coronary trauma |
| Coronary nonatherosclerotic narrowing |
| Coronary intimal or mural thickening |
| Coronary vasomotor tone |
| Hypercoagulable in situ thrombosis |
| Mechanical obstruction |
| Myocardial oxygen supply-demand disproportion |
| Myocardial infarction with normal coronary arteries |

There are other causes of myocardial ischemia in the absence of atherosclerosis (Table 51-3).

Ischemia produces major changes in two of the important functions of myocardial cells, electrical activity and contraction. The ischemic cell has a drastically altered transmembrane action potential. For example, the ischemic ventricular myocardial cell has an action potential in which the resting potential is elevated, the rate of rise is slower, and the plateau phase is shorter (Fig. 51-1). Between normal and ischemic myocardial tissues, an electrical potential difference exists, which generates many of the arrhythmias seen with angina or AMI. Impaired myocardial contractility most importantly affects left ventricular (LV) function. Initially, there is a loss in normal diastolic relaxation, producing a decrease in ventricular distensibility and clinically manifested by an audible $S_4$. If ischemia becomes more profound, systolic contraction is lost and the affected area becomes hypokinetic or akinetic. If infarction develops, the area rapidly loses stiffness within minutes to hours and the area becomes dyskinetic,

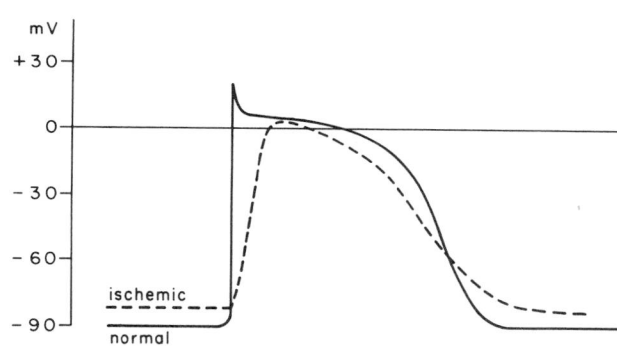

**Fig. 51-1.** Ventricular myocardial cell transmentbrane action potential.

moving paradoxically with systolic contractions. All this results in a decreased ejection fraction. To maintain cardiac output, the cardiovascular system often compensates by increasing the filling pressure to maintain an adequate stroke volume, by the Frank-Starling principle, or by increasing the heart rate, which further exacerbates myocardial ischemia.

The pathogenesis of unstable angina is thought to start with disruption of the underlying atheromatous plaque by fissuring. This results in platelet aggregation, thrombus formation, fibrin accumulation, and hemorrhage into the plaque. Although vasospasm may occur at the site of ruptured atherosclerotic plaques, it is usually not a predominant factor in unstable angina.

## Natural History of Ischemic Heart Disease

The natural history of CAD is primarily determined by two pathophysiologic factors: (1) the extent of arterial obstruction (one, two, or three vessels obstructed) and (2) the status of left ventricular function. The relationship between symptoms, clinical observations, and the natural history of CAD can be accounted for by considering these two pathophysiologic factors. Some studies have found that complex ventricular ectopy (back-to-back ventricular ectopic beats or runs of ventricular tachycardia) is an independent factor in early mortality. During recent years, the mortality from CAD has declined, primarily due to better application of medical treatment. Significant CAD can exist without clinical symptoms: such "silent" CAD has been found in 2.5 to 10 percent of various middle-aged population groups. These individuals appear to have a lower mortality than symptomatic individuals with CAD.

## ANGINA PECTORIS

### Clinical Features

Stable angina is characterized by episodic chest pain, lasting minutes (usually 5 to 15 min), provoked by exertion or stress, and relieved by rest or sublingual nitroglycerin. The pain almost always has a retrosternal component and commonly radiates to the neck, jaw, and shoulders, or down the inside of the left or both arms. Secondary symptoms—light-headedness, palpitations, diaphoresis, dyspnea, nausea, or vomiting—may accompany the pain. Auscultation of the heart may find a transient $S_4$ or apical systolic murmur indicative of mitral regurgitation. An electrocardiogram (ECG) taken during an acute attack may show changes less than half the time, usually ST segment depression or T wave inversion; less commonly, ST segment elevation is seen. Serum creatine kinase-MB isoenzyme (CK-MB) levels are not elevated. Angiography should reveal at least 50 to 75 percent reduction in the lumen of one or more coronary arteries.

Unstable (crescendo or preinfarction) angina represents a clinical state between stable angina and AMI (Table 51-4). The subgroups included in the clinical definition of unstable angina are (1) exertional angina of recent onset, usually defined as within 4 to 8 weeks; (2) angina of worsening character, characterized by increasing severity, duration, or requirement for nitroglycerin; and (3) angina at rest (angina decubitus). Unstable angina is currently felt to be due to progression in the severity and extent of coronary atherosclerosis, coronary artery spasm, or hemorrhage into nonoccluding plaques with subsequent thrombotic occlusion developing over hours to days. The

natural history of unstable angina can be partially assessed by analyzing five studies between 1956 and 1964 in which the only treatment was restriction of activities and sublingual nitroglycerin. Patients with either angina of worsening character or rest angina had a 40 percent incidence of acute infarction and a 17 percent incidence of death within a period of 3 months. A multicenter study from the 1970s found that intensive medical therapy reduced the risk of early infarction to 8 percent and the risk of early death to 3 percent. Therefore, it is important to recognize, hospitalize, and treat patients with unstable angina. Coronary angiography would be expected to reveal 90 percent or more obstruction of the lumen in at least one coronary artery.

When obtaining a history of angina less responsive to nitroglycerin, it is important to inquire about the potency of the tablets because nitroglycerin degrades over several months. If the patient has taken several tablets without the development of a local stinging or burning sensation under the tongue or a headache, the nitroglycerin is most likely old and ineffective. The sublingual spray retains its potency for more than 3 years. In unstable angina, ST segment or T wave changes may persist up to several hours after the pain episode, but there is no ECG evidence of new transmural infarction (new Q waves). Serum enzyme levels may show minor elevations without definite serial changes, especially troponin, which is elevated in about one third of unstable angina episodes, indicating the presence of a microinfarct.

Variant (Prinzmetal) angina occurs primarily at rest and without provocation. There is a tendency for attacks to recur at similar times of the day. Pain is associated with ST segment elevation that represents transmural myocardial ischemia. Painless episodes may also occur with ST segment elevation. Attacks may be associated with tachyarrhythmias, bundle branch blocks, or atrioventricular block. The current thought is that variant angina is due to spasm of the epicardial coronary arteries. When patients are studied by coronary angiography, about one third have no or insignificant atherosclerosis and about two thirds have CAD in addition to spasm. The latter may have exertional angina in addition to variant angina. Spasm is not unique to variant angina; it has been found in patients with typical angina or AMI.

## Treatment of Angina

For patients with ischemic heart disease, it is most important for the emergency physician to recognize and admit patients with AMI and unstable angina. Occasionally a patient with stable angina may present with a typical acute attack. The most important concerns are:

1. Is there a new medical problem causing exacerbation of angina?
2. Is this unstable angina?
3. Has the patient discontinued the prescribed medications?
4. Are the medications ineffective?

Sometimes, patients can be managed by adjusting or refilling medications. Ideally, this should be done with consultation of the patient's physician, and close follow-up should be arranged.

Treatment of angina should start with correction of modifiable risk factors: discontinuing smoking, controlling hypertension and diabetes, and lowering blood lipids by diet. Coexisting disorders that place stress on the heart should be treated. Medications that increase myocardial oxygen demand, such as sympathomimetics and methylxanthine derivatives, should be discontinued if possible. New-onset angina should be considered unstable angina until proven otherwise; hospital admission is advised.

A patient's primary provider usually will begin drug treatment with nitrates (Table 51-5). The primary antianginal effect of nitrates is an increase in venous capacitance, leading to a reduction in ventricular volume and pressure with improvement in subendocardial perfusion. Coronary vasodilation, improvement in collateral flow, and afterload reduction augment this primary effect. Sublingual or spray

**Table 51-4.** Canadian Cardiovascular Society Classification of Angina Pectoris

| | |
|---|---|
| Class I | No angina with normal physical activity |
| Class II | Slight limitation of normal activity |
| Class III | Marked limitation of physical activity |
| Class IV | Inability to do any physical activity without chest pain |

**Table 51-5.** Nitrates

| Agent—<br>Dosage Route | Typical<br>Dose | Action<br>Onset | Action<br>Duration |
|---|---|---|---|
| NITROGLYCERIN (NTG) | | | |
| Sublingual | 0.3–0.6 mg | 2–5 min | 10–30 min |
| Sublingual spray | 1–3 puffs | 2–5 min | 10–30 min |
| Buccal sustained release | 2.5–10 mg | 10–30 min | 1–2 h |
| Oral sustained release | 2.5–10 mg | 30–60 min | 4–6 h |
| 2% NTG OINTMENT | | | |
| Topical | 1/2–2 in<br>(7.5–15 mg) | 20–60 min | 3–6 h |
| TRANSDERMAL NTG | | | |
| Topical | 5–15 mg | | 12–24 h |
| ISOSORBIDE DINITRATE | | | |
| Sublingual | 2.5–5 mg | 10–30 min | 2–3 h |
| Oral | 5–40 mg | 30–60 min | 4–6 h |
| Oral sustained release | 40 mg b.i.d. | 1–2 h | 8–12 h |
| ISOSORBIDE MONONITRATE | 20 mg b.i.d.<br>(8 AM and 3 PM) | 1–2 h | 8–12 h |

nitroglycerin is effective for most acute attacks; relief is usually felt within 3 min or repeated every 5 min for three doses. Several long-acting forms are available to prevent anginal attacks: sublingual or oral long-acting nitrates, topical 2% nitroglycerin ointment, and prepackaged transdermal nitroglycerin delivery systems. However, there is evidence that tolerance to topical nitrates rapidly develops—sometimes within 24 h—requiring a drug-free interval overnight to reverse the tolerance that develops during the day. Intravenous nitroglycerin is a potent vasodilator, with a quick onset of action, and can be rapidly titrated to the desired response. It is standard therapy for patients with unstable rest angina, at an initial dose of 5 to 10 μg/min, increasing by 10 μg/min every 3 to 5 min, assuming hypotension

does not ensue in which case intravenous fluids may be appropriate. Headache is the most common adverse effect of nitrates.

β-Adrenergic antagonists have been shown to be useful in the treatment of angina but only moderately useful in patients with unstable angina or AMI (Table 51-6). The theoretical risk of β-blockade therapy is unopposed α-adrenergic activity precipitating coronary vasoconstriction. Thus, although β blockers alone are useful in stable exertional angina, the combination of a β blocker and a vasodilator (e.g., nitrate) is logical for patients at risk for coronary artery spasm: those with variant angina, unstable rest angina, or AMI. Nonselective agents (e.g., propranolol) inhibit β receptors in the heart, lungs, and blood vessels. Selective agents (e.g., metoprolol) preferentially inhibit $\beta_1$ receptors of the heart at low and intermediate doses. Theoretically, β blockers with intrinsic sympathomimetic activity (ISA) or partial agonist properties might be undesirable in patients with angina at low exercise levels because of less resting bradycardia. Neither cardioselectivity nor ISA seems to have any effect on antianginal activity and all β blockers appear to be equally effective in angina of effort. The β blockers are generally contraindicated in patients with congestive heart failure, atrioventricular block (AVB), variant angina, obstructive lung disease, or insulin-dependent diabetes mellitus. If given to patients with the last three diseases, selective or in some cases ISA β blockers instead of nonselective agents should be used whenever possible. In unstable angina patients who do not respond to aspirin, intravenous nitroglycerin and intravenous heparin, then the intravenous β blocker esmolol should be considered, especially in patients with tachycardia or hypertension. The dose is 500 μg/kg intravenously over 1 min followed by an intravenous infusion at 50 μg/kg/min titrated to a maximum dose of 200 μg/kg/min.

Calcium channel antagonists have been found effective for the treatment of stable angina and variant angina (Table 51-7). Several studies on the use of these agents in the treatment of unstable rest angina or evolving AMI have shown no significant effect on the risk of progression to infarction, infarct size, or mortality. The currently available calcium channel antagonists have different physiologic ef-

**Table 51-6.** β-Adrenergic Antagonists

| Agent | Brand Name | B1† | ISA† | Typical Dose | Maximum Dose |
|---|---|---|---|---|---|
| Acebutolol | Sectral | Yes | Yes | 200–600 mg b.i.d. | 1200 mg |
| Atenolol* | Tenormin | Yes | No | 50–200 mg qd | 200 mg |
| Betaxolol | Kerlone | Yes | No | 5–40 mg qd | 40 mg |
| Bisoprolol | Zebeta | Yes | No | 2.5–20 mg qd | 20 mg |
| Carteolol | Cartrol | No | Yes | 2.5–10 mg qd | 10 mg |
| Labetalol | Normodyne, Trandate | No | No | 100–600 mg b.i.d. | 2400 mg |
| Metoprolol* | Lopressor, Toprol | Yes | No | 50–100 mg b.i.d. | 400 mg |
| Nadolol* | Corgard | No | No | 40–240 mg qd | 240 mg |
| Penbutolol | Levatol | No | Yes | 20–80 mg qd | 80 mg |
| Pindolol | Visken | No | Yes | 5–20 mg b.i.d. | 60 mg |
| Propranolol | Inderal | No | No | 10–60 mg q.i.d. | 320 mg |
| Propranolol | Inderal-LA | No | No | 40–240 mg qd | 320 mg |
| Timolol* | Blocadren | No | No | 10–30 mg b.i.d. | 60 mg |
| Sotalol | Betapace | No | No | 80 mg b.i.d. | 320 mg |

\* Approved by the Food and Drug Administration for treatment of angina pectoris.

† $\beta_1$ selectivity and/or intrinsic sympathomimetic activity.

**Table 51-7.** Calcium Channel Antagonists

| Agent | Brand Name | Initial Dose | Maximum Dose (mg) |
|---|---|---|---|
| Amlodipine | Norvasc | 5 mg qd | |
| Bepridil | Vascor | 200–400 mg qd | |
| Diltiazem | Cardizem, Dilacor | 30–60 mg q.i.d., 60–120 mg b.i.d., 180 mg qd | 360 |
| Felodipine | Plendil | 5 mg qd | |
| Isradipine | DynaCirc | 2.5 mg b.i.d. | |
| Nicardipine | Cardene, Cardene SR | 20 mg t.i.d.–30 mg b.i.d. | |
| Nifedipine | Adalat, Procardia, Procardia XL | 10–20 mg t.i.d., 30–60 mg qd | 120 |
| Verapamil | Calan, Isoptin, Verelan, Isoptin SR | 80–120 mg t.i.d., 180–240 mg qd | 480 |

**Table 51-8.** Progressive Emergency Management of Unstable Angina

Oxygen
Aspirin (PO)
Nitroglycerin (SL, IV)
Heparin (IV)
Esmolol (IV)
Diltiazem (IV)

fects on the heart and blood vessels. Verapamil and diltiazem have major effects on the heart (decreased contractility and rate) and peripheral vessels (vasodilation). All of the other currently available calcium channel antagonists (nifedipine, nicardipine, isradipine, felodipine, and amlodipine) are dihydropyridines. They have predominant effects on the peripheral vessels (vasodilation) with only a small effect on the heart (decreased contractility). Nifedipine has increased mortality in small studies of unstable angina and AMI patients. Nifedipine may reverse coronary vasospasm and it should be maintained in patients already maintained on chronic nifedipine therapy. In unstable angina patients who do not respond to aspirin, intravenous nitroglycerin, intravenous heparin, and intravenous esmolol, then the calcium channel antagonist diltiazem may be considered, at a dose of 25 mg intravenous bolus over 5 min followed by a 15 mg/h intravenous infusion.

One aspirin a day, which blocks thromboxane $A_2$, a potent platelet activator and vasoconstrictor, is standard therapy to prevent ischemic cardiac events in patients with CAD or in patients at risk for developing CAD. For unstable angina, one 325-mg aspirin or two 81-mg chewable aspirins should be given to all patients as soon as possible. Its antiplatelet activity can prevent progression to an AMI. Heparin is the third-line therapy for unstable angina patients, following oral aspirin and intravenous nitroglycerin (Table 51-8). The recommended dose is an initial bolus of 5000 to 10,000 units intravenously, then a continuous infusion of 1000 to 1500 units/h. Its antithrombotic activity complements the antiplatelet activity of aspirin to prevent progression to AMI. Thrombolytic therapy has not proven beneficial for unstable angina patients.

## ACUTE MYOCARDIAL INFARCTION

### Pathogenesis

The large majority of patients with AMI have CAD. Current concepts concerning the immediate cause of AMI include the interaction of multiple factors that also cause unstable angina: progression of the atherosclerotic process to the point of total occlusion, plaque fissuring and subintimal hemorrhage at the site of an intimal plaque, platelet aggregation and thrombosis at the site of an existing narrowing, coronary artery spasm, and coronary artery embolism. Some of these processes are potentially reversible, and this has led to renewed interest in aggressive early intervention in AMI, especially antiplatelet and thrombolytic agents. The time period from the onset of symptoms to initiation of therapy is the key determinant of success. Emergency physicians commonly think of the "golden first hour" in determining the outcome of major trauma victims; it is time to consider the "first hour" in AMI as equally important. The National Heart Attack Alert Program Coordinating Committee 60 Minutes to Treatment Working Group broke this hour down into three intervals involving four "Ds": (1) door to data or ECG, (2) data to decision to treat, and (3) decision to drug administration.

### Pathophysiology

Like ischemia, infarction produces major changes in two important myocardial cell functions: electrical depolarization and contractility. The complications of AMI are caused by one or both of these events. During the first few hours, infarction is not a completed process; ar-

eas of infarction are interspersed with or surrounded by areas of ischemia or injury. The amount of infarcted tissue is a critical factor in determining prognosis, morbidity, and mortality. These ischemic areas are potentially salvageable through medical and surgical therapy.

Arrhythmias are frequent in AMI. Tachyarrhythmias and ventricular ectopy are usually caused by the electrical differences between adjacent areas of normal and ischemic myocardium. Bradyarrhythmias and AVBs are due to either increased vagal tone or ischemia and infarction directly affecting the conducting system.

The major result of impaired contractility is LV pump failure. If 25 percent of the LV myocardium is impaired, heart failure usually develops, and if 40 percent is affected, cardiogenic shock is common. AMI also causes cardiac remodeling as the remaining viable myocardium responds to the infarct. The resultant chamber enlargement and ventricular hypertrophy are physiologically adaptive. But infarct expansion, which occurs in 35 to 45 percent of transmural anterior AMIs, may cause congestive failure. The AMI patient's clinical and hemodynamic status correlates with mortality (see below). Right ventricular (RV) infarction is a common cause of hypotension in patients with an inferior AMI. The infarcted area can undergo autolysis, with distinct clinical syndromes resulting from rupture of the ventricular free wall, ventricular septum, or papillary muscles of the mitral valve, resulting in acute pulmonary edema, cardiogenic shock, and sudden death.

Stasis of the circulation can lead to venous thrombosis and pulmonary embolism. Stasis of blood within the ventricular cavity and exposure of collagen at the site of infarction can lead to development of mural thrombosis and systemic arterial embolism, particularly strokes.

### Clinical Features

The classic symptom is severe anginal pain lasting longer than 15 to 30 min, although severity and quality vary tremendously from individual to individual. As with angina, the pain may be accompanied by other symptoms such as light-headedness, dyspnea, diaphoresis, palpitations, nausea, or vomiting. Elderly patients who develop an AMI are more likely to present with either nonretrosternal chest pain or dyspnea with no pain at all compared with younger patients. In addition, the elderly are more likely to present with the nonspecific symptoms like dizziness or weakness. Longitudinal population studies indicate that up to 25 percent of myocardial infarctions are clinically unrecognized. Diabetic patients are more susceptible to such "silent" infarctions.

The physical examination may be deceptively normal. Commonly, there is a mild to moderate increase in pulse rate although inferior infarctions frequently cause bradycardia. Depending on the degree of pain and sympathetic activation, blood pressure is elevated, especially in anterior AMIs. Palpation of the apical pulse may show it to be diffuse or bulging. The loudness of $S_1$ may diminish as LV contraction is impaired. Uncommonly, the $S_2$ is paradoxically split owing to prolonged LV ejection. An $S_4$ is very common owing to decreased ventricular compliance, and a soft $S_3$ is occasionally heard. New systolic murmurs should be carefully examined. They may indicate mitral regurgitation due to papillary muscle dysfunction or rupture, ventricular septal rupture, or friction rub of pericarditis.

### Non-Q Wave versus Q Wave Infarction

The terms Q wave and non-Q wave infarction are often used to distinguish between a transmural and nontransmural (or subendocardial) infarction as determined by the presence or absence of Q waves. Autopsy studies have not found good correlation between the development of a Q wave and the presence of transmural infarction seen on pathologic examination. Non-Q wave infarction accounts for about 30 to 40 percent of AMIs. Such patients have a more frequent history

**Table 51-9.** ECG and Serum Creatine Kinase-MB Isoenzyme in the Emergency Department Diagnosis of Acute Myocardial Infarction

| | Approximate Sensitivity (%) | Approximate Specificity (%) | Approximate Positive Predictive Value* (%) |
|---|---|---|---|
| INITIAL ECG | | | |
| A. New Q waves, or ST segment elevation | 40 | 90+ | 70–80 |
| B. As in A, or new ST segment depression | 75 | 80 | 20–30 |
| C. As in A, B, or prior changes of ischemia or infarction | 85 | 75 | 5–10 |
| D. As in A, B, C, or nonspecific ST-T changes | 90 | 65 | < 5 |
| SERUM CREATINE KINASE-MB (CK-MB) LEVEL | | | |
| A. Elevated Total CK | 45 | 70 | 25 |
| B. Elevated CK-MB (electrophoresis) | 35 | 90 | 50 |
| C. Elevated CK-MB (imunochemical) | | | |
| on presentation | 50 | 95 | 85 |
| 3 h after presentation | 90 | 95 | 85 |

* Since predictive value depends on the incidence of disease in the population under study, these values are for an emergency department population of adults (age > 30 y) with a 20–30% incidence of AMI.

SOURCE: From Gibler WB, Young GP, Hedges JR, et al. *Ann Emerg Med* 19:1359, 1990.

of prior angina than do those with Q wave infarcts. They are also at risk for extending their infarct into a transmural infarction. When studied with coronary angiography soon after the onset of pain, non-Q wave infarctions have occlusion of the involved artery only about 20 percent of the time, as opposed to about an 80 percent occlusion rate for the involved artery in Q wave infarcts. The incidence of complications and mortality in AMI depends on the extent of myocardial damage and not on the existence of a Q wave. On the whole, Q wave infarctions tend to be larger (i.e., higher peak serum CK-MB levels and lower ejection fractions) and damage more myocardial tissue than non-Q wave infarctions. As a group, non-Q wave infarctions possess a lower in-hospital mortality but are more likely to be complicated by recurrent infarction or subsequent angina. As a result, the long-term mortalities of the two infarctions tend to equal out after about 3 years.

## Ancillary Tests

### Electrocardiography

The ECG diagnosis of AMI requires serial recordings, even in the emergency department. Although the ECG is the most important diagnostic test in patients with chest pain in the emergency department, only about half of all AMI patients will have diagnostic changes on their initial ECG (Table 51-9). However, a normal or nonspecific ECG does not exclude ischemia or negate the need for hospital admission; such decisions continue to be based on clinical assessment. Additional lead ECGs will increase the diagnostic yield in the evaluation of these patients in the emergency department. Besides right-sided chest leads (see below), these include the addition of lead $V_9$ (i.e., between the left scapula and the thoracic spine for posterior AMIs) as well as experimental 22-lead ECGs (e.g., for lateral AMIs involving the circumflex coronary artery).

Acute ischemia may either be confined to the subendocardial area (manifested by ST segment depression) or involve the complete transmural wall (manifested by ST segment elevation). T waves often become inverted because ischemia or infarction reverses the sequence of repolarization, causing it to occur in the endocardial-to-epicardial rather than the normal epicardial-to-endocardial direction. Because many other conditions can cause ST segment depression and T wave inversion, "ischemic" subendocardial changes are considered to be (1) horizontal or downsloping ST segments of at least 1.0 mm and (2) deep, symmetrical T wave inversions (Fig. 51-2). An important differentiating factor between ischemia and infarction is that the pain and ECG changes resolve as ischemia is relieved. Infarction eventually produces an electrically dead area of muscle, which may produce a Q wave in an overlying electrode. When they are observed in AMI, ST segment changes occur rapidly, Q waves usually require several hours to become evident, and T wave inversions are variable.

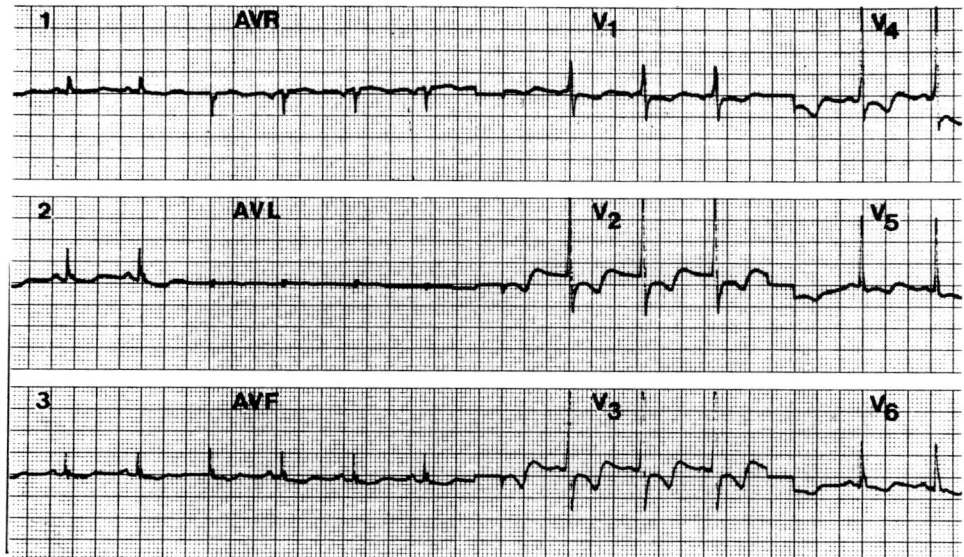

**Fig. 51-2.** Subendocardial ischemic ST-T changes.

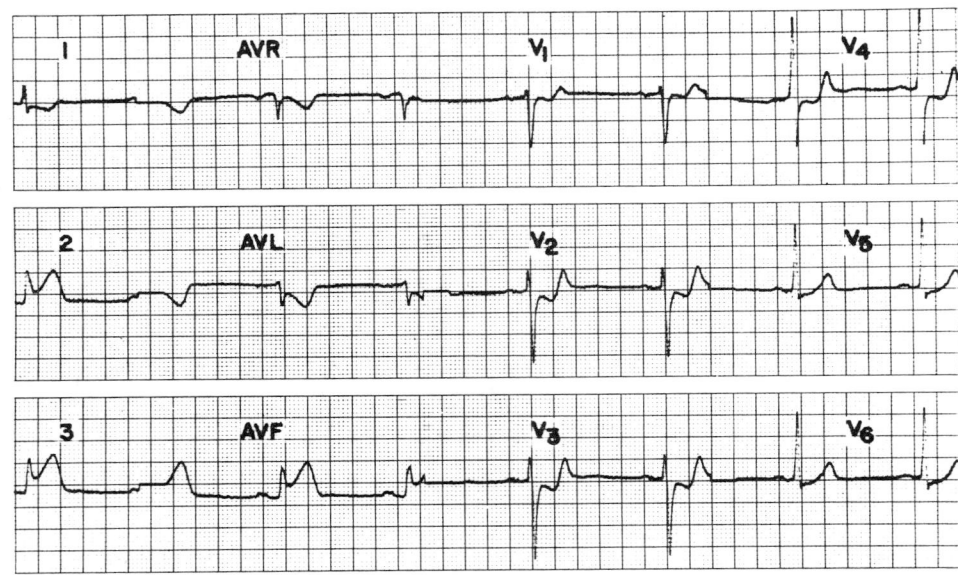

**Fig. 51-3.** Acute inferior MI.

Using abnormal Q waves and ST segment elevation on the ECG, one can localize the area of infarction:

II, III, AVF: inferior (Fig. 51-3)
$V_1$–$V_3$: anteroseptal (Fig. 51-4)
I, aVL, $V_4$–$V_6$: lateral
$V_1$–$V_6$: anterolateral
$V_{4R}$–$V_{6R}$: right ventricular (Fig. 51-5)
$V_1$–$V_2$ tall R, ST depression: true posterior (Fig. 51-6)

Right ventricular infarctions produce ST segment elevation in the right-sided chest leads, which have been shown to increase sensitivity without lowering specificity. True posterior infarctions produce a large R wave and ST segment depression in $V_1$ and $V_2$. Localization of AMI is important because the incidence and significance of complications vary with the site.

## Cardiac Enzymes

When myocardial cells are irreversibly injured, they release enzymes into the serum. The levels of commonly measured cardiac markers should not be used as criteria for "ruling out" AMI in the emergency department, but many studies show they can assist emergency physicians to avoid missing AMIs (Table 51-10).

Creatine kinase is found in high concentrations in skeletal muscle, myocardial muscle, and brain tissue. The CK-MB isoenzyme is found primarily in myocardial cells, and elevated serum levels of this enzyme are more specific for myocardial injury. Electrophoresis was the gold standard method used to measure serum CK-MB for inpatients admitted to "rule out" AMI. It is relatively insensitive and requires time for the serum level to rise sufficiently above background concentration before it can be reliably detected. Electrophoresis cannot detect the slight elevations in serum CK-MB found when patients first present to the emergency department. The first immunoassay method (immunoinhibition) was an improvement, but it still only indirectly measured the activity of CK-MB so, like electrophoresis, it required a simultaneous measurement of the total CK activity with which to compare the CK-MB activity as a ratio or index. New monoclonal antibody immunoassays can detect minimal elevations of serum CK-MB, allowing for direct measurements of the mass of CK-MB in units of ng/mL. The commercially available antibody immunoassays require only about 10 min of processing time. Studies in adults with nontraumatic chest pain and ECGs without diagnostic ischemic changes show that CK-MB immunoassays have a sensitivity of about 50 percent for AMI on emergency department presentation. With serial sampling over the next 3 h, the sensitivity increases to over 75 percent correlated with a duration of chest pain in specific

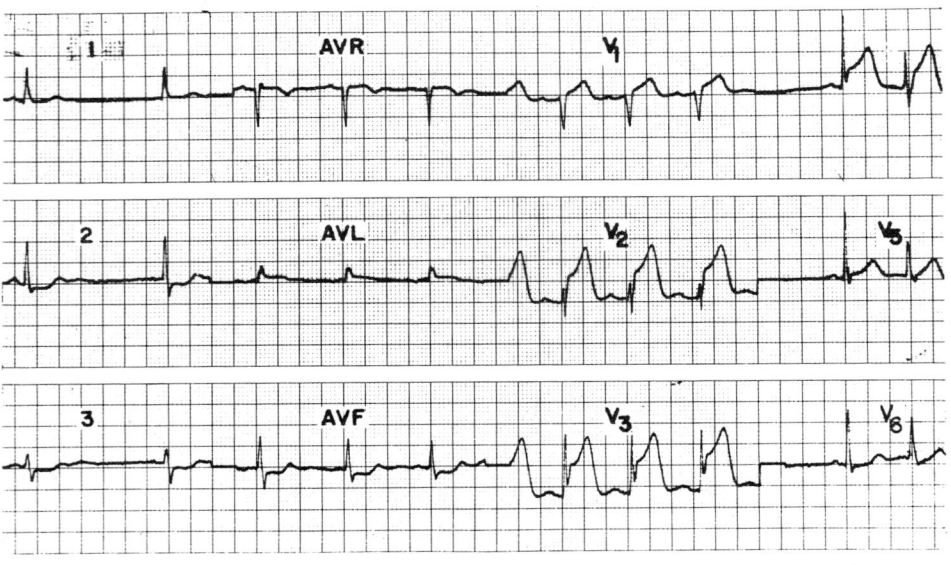

**Fig. 51-4.** Transmural ECG changes of acute myocardial infarction. Acute anterior MI.

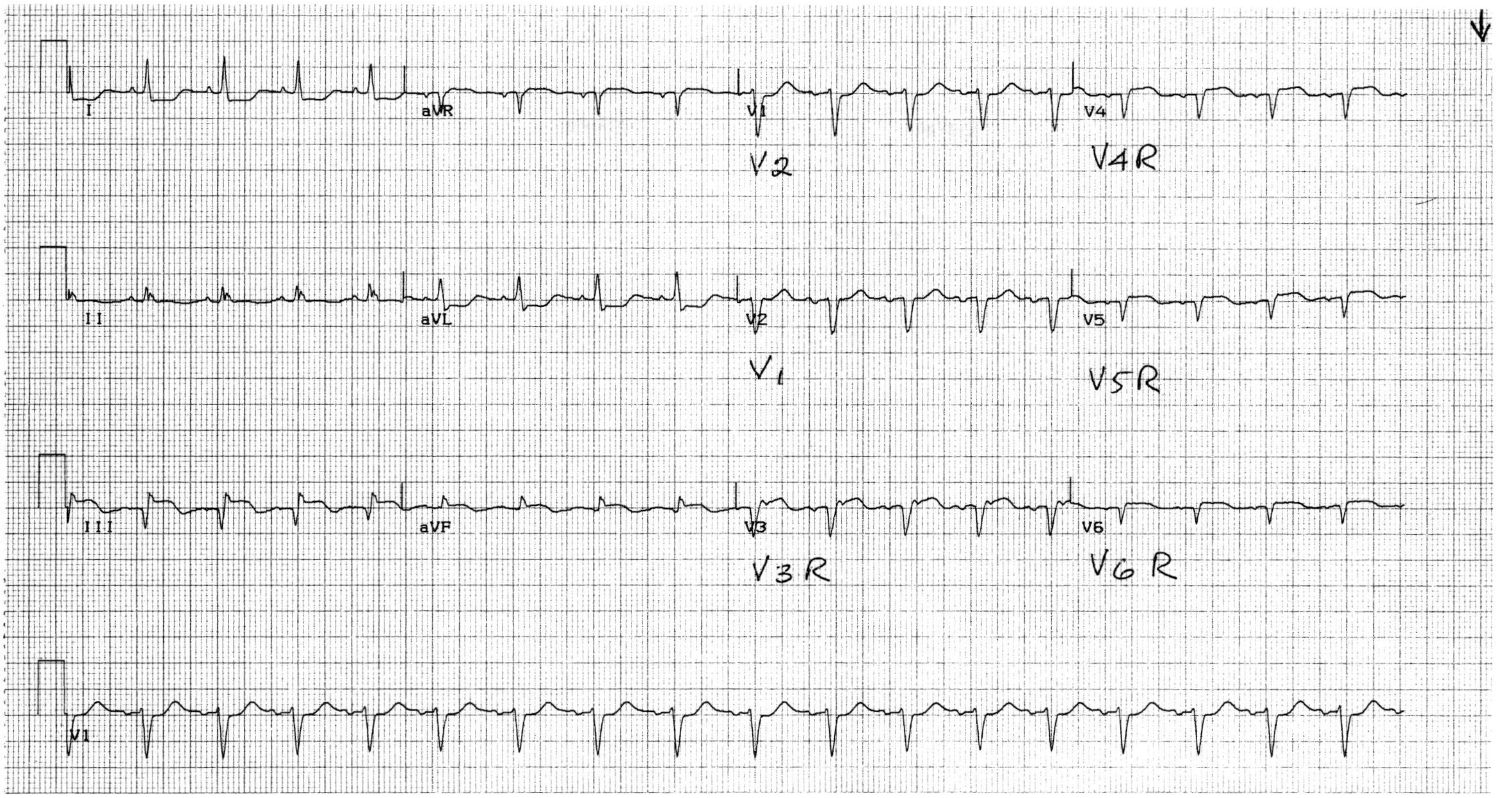

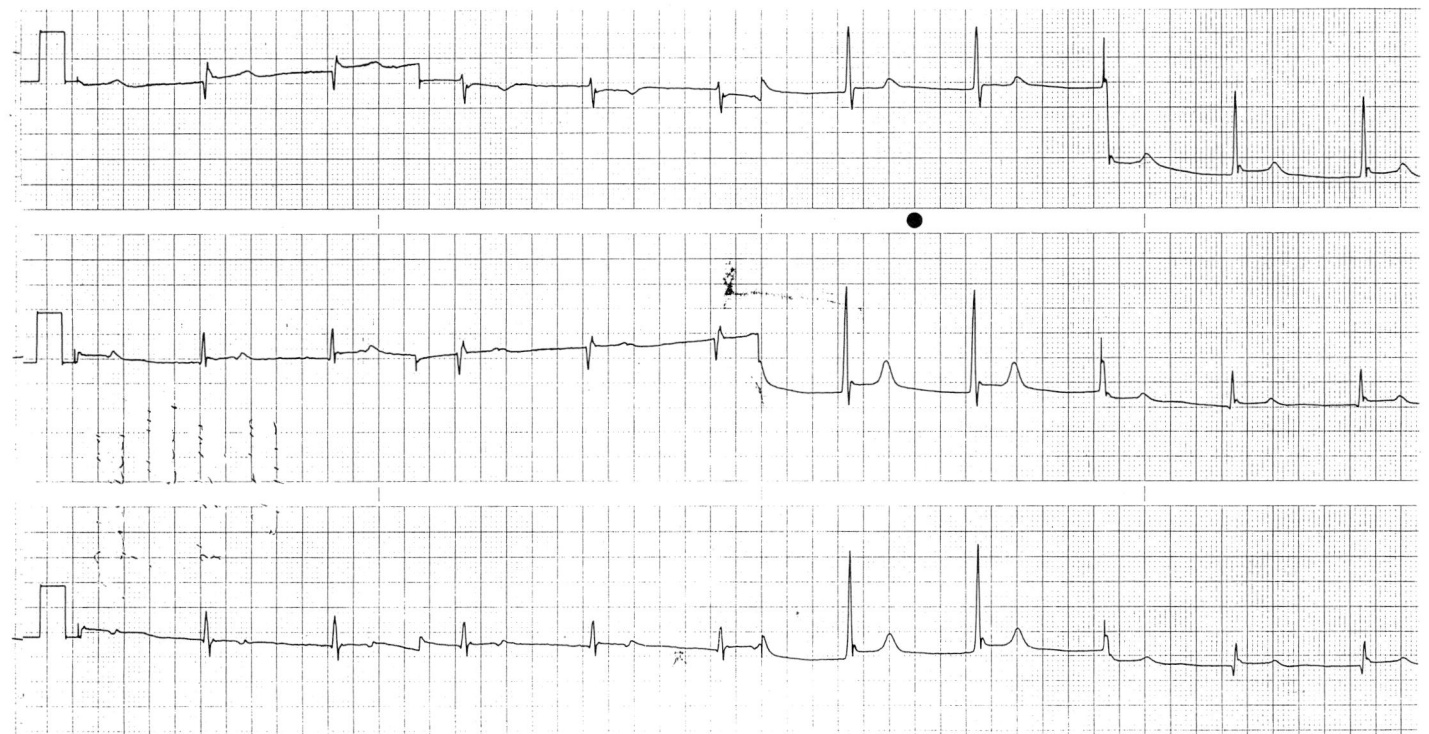

**Fig. 51-5.** Inferior infarct pattern. Right-sided leads (V$_{3R}$–V$_{6R}$) suggest right ventricular infarction. (Courtesy Ms. Lynn Evans, UNC Hospitals.)

**Fig. 51-6.** Rhythm is uncertain. Either junctional rhythm with rerograde atrial depolarization or marked first degree heart block. Tall R in lead V$_1$, ST segment elevation in the lateral leads, and Q wave in lead V$_6$ suggest posterior infarction. (Courtesy Ms. Lynn Evans, UNC Hospitals.)

**Table 51-10.** Serum Markers in Diagnosis of Acute Myocardial Infarction

| Marker | Earliest Rise | Peak | Normalize |
|---|---|---|---|
| Myoglobin | 1–2 h | 4–6 h | 1st day |
| CK-MB | 3–4 h | 12–24 h | 2nd day |
| Troponin | 3–6 h | 12–24 h | 7th day |

patients of at least 6 h and to over 90 percent in patients with a duration of chest pain of at least 9 h. Monoclonal antibody assays can also detect elevated levels of myoglobin in the serum, enabling even earlier diagnosis of AMI than CK-MB. However, unlike CK-MB, myoglobin arises from skeletal muscle like total CK so some specificity may be lost in patients with skeletal muscle trauma. Troponin can also be measured with a monoclonal antibody assay, down to levels as low as 1 ng/mL. Its advantages include more specificity than CK-MB in the setting of skeletal muscle damage (e.g., postoperative patients); more sensitivity in detecting about one third of unstable angina patients (i.e., microinfarcts); and the ability to detect myocardial damage up to one week after the event in patients presenting days after their AMI. The potential benefits of early AMI detection include better utilization of scarce resources with correct in-hospital admission decisions, prevention of discharge of AMI or some unstable angina patients with nondiagnostic ECGs, and possible early administration of thrombolytic or anti-ischemic therapy.

## Echocardiography

Soon after the onset of myocardial ischemia, muscle contraction is impaired, which can be detected by echocardiography as wall motion abnormalities. Experimentally, hypokinesis, akinesis, or dyskinesis can be seen within a few heartbeats after coronary occlusion. In selected critical care unit patients, echocardiography has a sensitivity of over 70 percent in AMI. In the few early studies in emergency department patients, echocardiography has been shown to be sensitive but not specific, where the prevalence of AMI is lower but the prevalence of CAD is higher. Echocardiography may predict which patients are more likely to have complications related to their AMIs and require critical care unit admission. Echocardiography is best used to diagnose anatomic complications of AMI that might be amenable to surgical correction in cardiogenic shock patients (i.e., septal or mitral ruptures). Echocardiography has a low sensitivity for patients with unstable angina who are pain free at the time of the study.

## Radionuclide Scans

Radionuclide scanning is not commonly available to evaluate patients in the emergency department and the early studies suggest that it has the same limitations as echocardiography. Nuclear scans are sensitive but nonspecific in detecting ischemia and infarction. In certain situations, the radionuclide scan is helpful in evaluating inpatients. Two radionuclides, technetium and thallium, are commonly used. Technetium pyrophosphate is deposited irreversibly in infarcted myocardial tissue, producing a "hot spot" on nuclear imaging. Scans first become positive within 10 to 12 h and become increasingly positive up to 24 to 72 h after onset of chest pain. Sensitivity is highest with Q wave infarctions (about 85 percent) and less with non-Q wave infarctions (about 50 percent). Thallium sestamibi is reversibly taken up by normally perfused myocardial cells; the infarcted or ischemic area appears as a "cold spot" on nuclear imaging. Thallium scanning performed within 6 h after the onset of chest pain was found to have a high sensitivity for AMI in small studies. Unfortunately, thallium scans are less sensitive in small or non-Q wave infarctions, detect less than 50 percent of patients with unstable angina, and have a low specificity (around 80 percent). In emergency department patients with chest pain, where the prevalence of AMI is low but the prevalence of CAD is high, neither echocardiography and nuclear scanning

have proven useful other than in restricted clinical research settings. In most facilities, the technical expertise required, the added cost (more than $500 for both echocardiography and nuclear scans), and the limited availability of these ancillary tests on an urgent basis restrict their routine use in the emergency department.

## Complications

### Arrhythmias

A meta-analysis of mortality at 1 month post-AMI showed a drop from over 30 percent in the 1960s to less than 20 percent in the 1980s. Most of this reduction in AMI mortality resulted from the close monitoring and treatment of arrhythmias. The out-of-hospital mortality in at least half of AMI patients is almost entirely due to arrhythmias; early assessment and treatment of these arrhythmias must first depend on their detection. All patients should be on continuous cardiac monitoring, and, equally important, the monitor must be watched by qualified personnel. The incidence of lethal arrhythmias is greatest in the prehospital phase. The site of infarction does not appear to influence the incidence of arrhythmias (Table 51-11).

Some studies have found a higher incidence of serious ventricular arrhythmias in patients experiencing an AMI who are initially hypokalemic or hypomagnesemic, especially if on prior diuretic therapy. Arrhythmias should be treated if the effect on the heart rate further exacerbates the myocardial oxygen supply and demand imbalance or has the potential to deteriorate into cardiac arrest. Experimental and clinical work indicate that the optimal heart rate is between 60 and 90 bpm in acute infarction.

Sinus tachycardia is potentially detrimental because of increased myocardial oxygen demand. It is more common with anterior AMIs. Diagnosis and therapy should be directed toward the underlying cause: increased sympathetic activity from pain, hypovolemia, hypoxia, etc. Sinus bradycardia is usually due to increased vagal tone and is common with inferior AMIs. Treatment with atropine is usually not required unless the bradycardia is complicated by hypotension or complex premature ventricular contractions (PVCs). Premature atrial contractions (PACs) are common but generally are of no significance unless they initiate more serious arrhythmias, like paroxysmal supraventricular tachycardia (PSVT) or atrial fibrillation. PSVT should be treated because the rapid rate increases oxygen demand and reduces cardiac output. The reentrant variety of PSVT should be treated with vagal maneuvers, adenosine, diltiazem, or cardioversion. Drugs that directly depress myocardial contractility (e.g., verapamil or β-adrenergic blockers) may have significant risk in the potentially unstable hemodynamics of AMI and should be used with caution. Atrial fibrillation usually occurs within the first 48 h and often in association with pericarditis or heart failure. The ventricular rate can be controlled with digoxin or diltiazem. Cardioversion is effective if the patient is hemodynamically compromised. Recurrences are common and therapy with diltiazem or procainamide infusions may be required. Atrial flutter responds readily to cardioversion, but

**Table 51-11.** Approximate Incidence of Arrhythmias in Acute Myocardial Infarction

| | Incidence (%) |
|---|---|
| Sinus tachycardia | 40–60 |
| Sinus bradycardia | 3–10 |
| Premature atrial contractions | 15–40 |
| Paroxysmal supraventricular tachycardia | 2–7 |
| Atrial fibrillation | 10 |
| Atrial flutter | 5 |
| Junctional tachycardia | 5–10 |
| Premature ventricular contractions | 80–100 |
| Ventricular tachycardia | 10 |
| Accelerated idioventricular rhythm | 8–23 |
| Primary ventricular fibrillation | 5–10 |

digoxin or diltiazem can also be used to control ventricular rate. Junctional tachycardia is caused by enhanced automaticity of the junctional pacemaker due to infarction or digoxin toxicity or dysfunction of the sinus node due to ischemia. Treatment is not necessary unless a rapid or slow rate produces hemodynamic deterioration.

Premature ventricular contractions occur in nearly all patients with AMI. The frequency or complexity of ventricular ectopy (so-called warning arrhythmias) is no longer felt to be a reliable predictor of subsequent ventricular tachycardia or fibrillation in the general population of AMI patients, in part because they occur in nearly all AMI patients. However, some physicians consider the presence of PVCs an indicator of ventricular irritability and recommend treatment with lidocaine to prevent the occurrence of ventricular tachycardia or fibrillation (see below). Ventricular tachycardia should be treated according to the hemodynamic status of the patient: if the patient is stable, intravenous lidocaine should be used; and if the patient is unstable, immediate synchronized cardioversion should be done. Accelerated idioventricular rhythm (AIVR) is usually a transient arrhythmia, with wide QRS complexes, occurring at a rate of 60 to 90/min. It is thought to arise from one of two causes: slowing of the sinus node or enhanced automaticity of ventricular tissues. Although it is usually benign, there is some variable association with ventricular tachycardia but no apparent association with ventricular fibrillation (VF). Close monitoring is advised, but specific therapy (i.e., atropine or lidocaine, respectively) is usually not indicated for AIVR. Primary VF is the sudden development of VF in the absence of shock or LV failure. Primary VF occurs in about 5 to 10 percent of patients with AMI, usually early in the course; 60 percent within 4 h and 80 percent within 12 h after the onset of symptoms. In a monitored setting, primary VF should be rapidly detected and can nearly always be successfully defibrillated. Secondary VF occurs as a terminal event after a progressive course of LV pump failure. Treatment of secondary VF is unlikely to yield long-term success. Prophylactic lidocaine therapy was recommended by more physicians to prevent primary VF in patients with definite or possible AMI during the first 24 to 48 h of hospitalization. Some studies found prophylactic lidocaine partially effective in preventing primary VF while the patient with AMI is in a monitored setting. However, meta-analysis of randomized in-hospital clinical trials showed a statistically significant increase in mortality during the treatment period in patients who received lidocaine. And meta-analysis of prehospital clinical trials with prophylactic lidocaine showed no significant mortality difference. Although the potential benefits of prophylactic lidocaine in the prehospital or emergency department setting are not proven, several points are worth noting. First, in untreated patients, the incidence of primary VF is low, about 5 to 10 percent in patients with AMI and less in patients with unstable angina. Second, primary VF should be easily detected and rapidly defibrillated in a monitored setting with a mortality of about 5 percent. Third, prophylactic lidocaine decreases the incidence of primary VF by about 90 percent. Fourth, the complications of early lidocaine are minor, and the incidence is about 5 to 10 percent. Fifth, after 24 h, serum lidocaine levels double due to decreased hepatic metabolism, particularly in elderly patients who are at risk of confusion or patients with heart failure or liver disease.

## Conduction Disturbances

Acute myocardial infarction may damage the conduction system and sometimes progress to complete (third-degree) AVB. The risk of complete AVB during an AMI depends on two major factors: (1) the site of the infarction, and (2) the occurrence of new conduction disturbances. The site of infarction is usually known, but many times the age of the conduction disturbance is not. This is reflected by the use of the term new or age-indeterminant conduction block in many studies. In addition, some studies use the term high-grade AVB, meaning that both third-degree AVB and Mobitz type II second-degree AVB

**Table 51-12.** Approximate Incidence of Complete Atrioventricular Block in Acute Myocardial Infarction

| New or Age-Indeterminant Conduction Defect | Incidence (%) |
|---|---|
| No conduction abnormality | 1–3 |
| Left anterior superior fascicular block (LASFB) | 2–4 |
| Left posterior inferior fascicular block (LPIFB) | 2–4 |
| Right bundle branch block (RBBB) | 6 |
| Left bundle branch block (LBBB) | 15 |
| RBBB and either LASFB or LPIFB | 30–40 |

are equally serious. This produces a wide variation in the reported rate of progression to AVB and yields divergent opinions as to what constitutes a high-risk situation in which prophylactic pacemaker insertion is warranted. With this in mind, data from six studies reported between 1973 and 1983 were pooled to yield the rates of progression to complete AVB with new or age-indeterminant conduction disturbances (Table 51-12). When the risk of complete AVB is above 10 to 15 percent, prophylactic pacemaker placement is probably indicated. In addition, two subgroups of patients are at particular risk. First, patients with some form of AV nodal conduction disturbance (first- or second-degree AVB) in addition to an infranodal conduction block (fascicular or bundle branch) are at increased risk for complete AVB. Second, patients with anterior infarctions are at risk for profound bradycardia if Mobitz II or complete AVB develops because the escape ventricular pacemaker is often slow and unreliable.

First-degree AVBs and Mobitz I (Wenckebach) second-degree AVBs are usually due to increased vagal tone impairing AV nodal conduction and are generally seen in inferior ischemia or infarction. Progression to complete AVB is infrequent and rarely occurs suddenly, and if it does occur, a stable infranodal pacemaker with narrow QRS complexes and a reasonable rate of about 50 is usually maintained. When treatment is necessary, these blocks usually respond to atropine. Mobitz II second-degree AVBs are usually due to structural damage to the infranodal conduction tissue and are generally seen with anterior ischemia or infarction. Complete AVB may occur suddenly, with only a slow, unstable ventricular escape pacemaker available for cardiac activity. Mobitz II blocks are an indication for prophylactic pacemaker placement. Infarctions that cause Mobitz II blocks are usually large, and even with pacemaker treatment, many patients die of pump failure.

## Left Ventricular Pump Failure and Cardiogenic Shock

Acute myocardial infarction nearly always produces impairment of LV pump function; whether this is clinically manifest depends on the extent of damage. Several classifications have been developed to correlate the extent of pump dysfunction with acute in-hospital mortality. The Killip classification is based on clinical criteria, and the Forrester-Diamond-Swan classification is based on hemodynamic measurements (Tables 51-13 and 51-14). A rough, imprecise correlation exists between clinical and hemodynamic findings. Pulmonary vascular congestion occurs when pulmonary artery wedge pressure (PAWP) rises above 18 to 20 mm Hg and is manifested by dyspnea and rales. Peripheral hypoperfusion occurs when the cardiac index falls below 2.2 to 2.5 L/min per m$^2$ and is manifested by hypotension, oliguria, mental obtundation, peripheral vasoconstriction, and tachycardia. The terms preload and afterload are often used in discussions of LV dysfunction. *Preload* is the LV filling pressure during diastole. This filling pressure can be measured directly as LV end-diastolic pressure or, more commonly, indirectly measured as PAWP. *Afterload* is the pressure against which the left ventricle pumps and is usually measured as the mean aortic pressure.

Current management of LV pump dysfunction is based on the underlying hemodynamic derangement. Pulmonary vascular congestion is traditionally treated with vasodilators, morphine, or diuretics. Of

**Table 51-13.** Killip-Kimball Classification

| Class | Approximate Incidence (%) | Approximate Mortality (%) |
|---|---|---|
| I No failure | 30 | 5 |
| II Mild failure | 40 | 15–20 |
| Bibasilar rales and $S_3$ | | |
| III Frank pulmonary edema | 10 | 40 |
| IV Cardiogenic shock | 20 | 80 |
| Systolic pressure < 90 mm Hg | | |
| Peripheral vasoconstriction | | |
| Oliguria | | |
| Pulmonary vascular congestion | | |

these three modalities, vasodilators produce the most rapid and predictable decrease in PAWP. Because of the unstable hemodynamic situation, short-acting intravenous agents that can be titrated to effect are the most appropriate agents to use: nitroglycerin, nitroprusside, or dobutamine. Sublingual, oral, and topical nitroglycerin act predominantly as venodilators, increasing venous capacitance and decreasing preload. Intravenous nitroglycerin is both a venous and an arterial dilator, but the greater effect is on the venous side until higher doses are reached (see below). Intravenous nitroprusside is a "balanced" vasodilator, with about equal effects on systemic arterial resistance and venous capacitance. However, because nitroprusside sometimes causes a deterioration in myocardial oxygen supply and demand due to a coronary "steal" syndrome, it is not routinely recommended as an afterload-reducing agent in AMI. Intravenous dobutamine is a β-adrenergic inotropic agent that also causes vasodilation so that the heart pumps better against a reduced afterload. The net result is an improvement in myocardial oxygen supply and demand. Vasodilators reliably relieve pulmonary vascular congestion, but as PAWP falls, cardiac output may also fall if the filling pressure of the LV decreases too much. Patients in heart failure usually have an elevated filling pressure, and vasodilator therapy generally improves cardiac output. Conversely, patients not in heart failure usually experience a fall in cardiac output with vasodilator therapy. Most of the clinical effect of morphine in LV pump failure is due to its general sedative actions rather than any direct effect on hemodynamics. So although morphine is still used for its sedative effect, vasodilators are more effective in reversing the abnormal pathophysiology. Furosemide is commonly thought to have a rapid venodilation action, although this has not been found in all studies, and there is evidence that intravenous furosemide acutely increases LV filling pressures for about 15 min after administration. To prevent this effect, vasodilators should be used simultaneously with intravenous furosemide. Regardless, the major effect of diuretics on pulmonary vascular congestion is to decrease the PAWP by producing a diuresis within an hour after intravenous administration of the potent loop diuretics (furosemide or bumetanide).

Depressed cardiac output should be treated by first optimizing preload, although most patients with cardiogenic shock already have an elevated PAWP. Patients without evidence of pulmonary vascular congestion can be given intravenous fluid challenges of saline cautiously (100 to 250 mL over 5 to 15 min), but once pulmonary edema develops, further therapy often requires measurement of the PAWP. Pharmacologic therapy to improve cardiac output is guided by the systolic blood pressure. If systolic blood pressure is above 100 mm

**Table 51-14.** Forrester-Diamond-Swan Classification

| Cardiac Index | Pulmonary Artery Wedge Pressure | Approximate Mortality (%) |
|---|---|---|
| I  > 2 L/min per m² | < 18 mm Hg | 3 |
| II  > 2 L/min per m² | > 18 mm Hg | 9 |
| III  < 2 L/min per m² | < 18 mm Hg | 23 |
| IV  < 2 L/min per m² | > 18 mm Hg | 51 |

Hg, cardiac output can usually be increased with afterload reduction using intravenous nitroglycerin. When systolic blood pressure is below 100 mm Hg, vasodilator therapy should be undertaken cautiously. With mild hypotension (systolic blood pressure 75 to 90 mm Hg), an inotropic agent such as dobutamine is usually effective. Experimental canine studies have found that dobutamine is a better agent in improving overall myocardial function in AMI, but unfortunately dobutamine is not a vasoconstrictor and does not adequately treat low blood pressure in frank shock. With severe hypotension (systolic blood pressure below 75 mm Hg), a vasoconstrictor is generally required to maintain vital organ perfusion. Dopamine has both ino-tropic and vasoconstrictor properties (depending on the dose) and is a good agent to use in cardiogenic shock. However, dopamine will increase myocardial work (inotropic) and increase afterload (vasoconstriction). If inotropic agents are ineffective or required for longer than a few hours, the intra-aortic balloon pump or other LV-assisting devices can be used to mechanically support the circulation while echocardiography is performed to look for mechanical complications of AMI and angioplasty is considered. Some patients require mechanical support for only a short time, allowing some myocardial recovery and resumption of adequate LV function. However, if these devices are required for longer than 24 h, many or most patients do not recover adequate LV function for weaning and may need surgical intervention for survival.

## Mechanical Defects

Cardiac rupture is a catastrophic event that presents with sudden recurrence of chest pain, hypotension, pericardial tamponade, cardiac arrest with pulseless electrical activity, and death. Patients at increased risk are those with first infarction, those with sustained hypertension after infarction, and the elderly; 50 percent of cardiac ruptures occur within the first 5 days and 90 percent within the first 14 days after infarction. Mortality is 95 percent; a few patients survive with volume replacement, pericardiocentesis for treatment of tamponade, and immediate surgery. Echocardiography is a useful diagnostic study at the bedside.

Ventricular septal rupture presents with sudden onset of pulmonary edema and a new harsh systolic murmur along the left sternal border. Septal rupture occurs about equally in anterior and inferior infarctions and is located in the muscular portion of the intraventricular septum. Diagnosis is made by Doppler flow echocardiography or the measurement of oxygen saturation in RV blood obtained via a Swan-Ganz catheter. Therapy should reflect the hemodynamic status, either dopamine to increase perfusion or afterload reduction by nitroprusside or nitroglycerin. Intra-aortic balloon pump support is often necessary while awaiting possible surgical repair.

Papillary muscle dysfunction is common, especially with inferior infarctions. The clinical presentation is usually mild, with only a transient systolic murmur, but may become severe, with florid pulmonary edema. Treatment of the ischemia and afterload reduction is usually effective. Prognosis of mild dysfunction is very good. Papillary muscle rupture is more serious, and the outcome depends on whether the whole muscle body is ruptured or only the head. Rupture of an entire muscle body is associated with a high mortality, up to 50 percent within 24 h. Rupture is usually associated with an inferior-posterior infarction and involves the posterior papillary muscle. Diagnosis of papillary muscle dysfunction or rupture may be made with echocardiography or a Swan-Ganz catheter to measure large V waves in the PAWP. Treatments similar to those mentioned for septal rupture are usually necessary.

## Thromboembolism

Prolonged bed rest and generalized circulatory stasis predispose the patient with AMI to venous thrombosis and pulmonary embolism. Other predisposing factors include previous thromboembolism, atrial fibrillation, old age, and obesity. Early ambulation and low-dose subcutaneous heparin (5000 units b.i.d.) have reduced the incidence of deep venous thrombosis.

A mural thrombosis can develop at the site of infarction. Mural thrombi occur in less than 5 percent of patients with non-Q wave or inferior infarction and in 30 to 40 percent of patients with anterior Q wave infarction. Some patients form a thrombus within 48 h; these patients usually have large infarctions with hemodynamic complications and a high in-hospital mortality. Once formed, the LV thrombus may regress, remain asymptomatic, or embolize to the systemic circulation. Most large studies report an incidence of clinically evident systemic emboli of 1 to 6 percent of all patients with AMI, although the risk in patients with mural thrombi may be as high as 30 percent. Echocardiography is a good screening tool, and if a mural thrombus is detected, full-dose anticoagulation with intravenous heparin is initiated if there are no contraindications to its use.

## Pericarditis

An acute form of pericarditis, manifested by pain and friction rub, can develop during the first 7 days postinfarction. The reported incidence is between 6 and 10 percent of all patients with AMI and is higher in patients with Q wave infarctions. The cause is the inflammation associated with necrosis of the myocardium adjacent to the pericardium. The postmyocardial infarction (Dressler) syndrome generally occurs later and is characterized by chest pain, fever, pleuropericarditis, and pleural effusion. The cause is an immunologic reaction to myocardial antigens exposed by AMI. Aspirin or indomethacin is usually recommended initially. Steroids are reserved for refractory cases because it is even more difficult to get patients off steroids, which leads to recurrent episodes.

## Right Ventricular Infarction

Infarction in the RV is now recognized as occurring in 20 to 40 percent of patients with inferior AMIs. RV infarction is due to right coronary artery obstruction, nearly always transmural, and almost always associated with LV damage. It was previously held that the RV served as a volume conduit and that RV pump dysfunction is not clinically significant. However, severe RV pump failure does cause hypotension, usually with an elevated right atrial pressure and a normal or decreased left atrial pressure. Therefore, the clinical presentation is that of hypotension, jugular venous distention, and clear lungs. In addition, most patients with hemodynamically significant RV infarction have a rise in jugular venous pressure with quiet inspiration (Kussmaul sign). RV pump dysfunction can be mimicked by occult LV failure, constrictive pericarditis, pericardial tamponade, and restrictive cardiomyopathy. Correct diagnosis of RV pump dysfunction may require simultaneous measurement of PAWP and right atrial pressure or visualization of poor RV contractions on radionuclide scanning or echocardiography. Patients with RV infarction are dependent on an elevated RV filling pressure to maintain cardiac output, and it is important to avoid or prevent decreases by the use of diuretics or nitrates. Volume infusions may produce a small improvement in cardiac output and in some patients literally liters of intravenous saline may be necessary to ensure an adequate filling pressure for the LV. An inotropic agent like dobutamine may also be indicated.

## General Treatment

All patients with documented or suspected AMI should have an intravenous line established; a 5% dextrose in water ($D_5W$) solution is generally used. Saline solutions are avoided to prevent sodium overload and pulmonary congestion, unless the blood pressure is inadequate to perfuse the coronary arteries. The cardiac monitor should be applied and observed by qualified personnel. Supplemental oxygen should be administered to all patients. Patients with a history of oxygen sensitivity or chronic obstructive pulmonary disease should be given low concentrations (2 L/min or 24%) and all other patients given higher concentrations (4 to 6 L/min or 40%). Experimentally, supplemental oxygen at a fractional ($F_{IO_2}$) of 40% inspired oxygen reduces the degree of ST segment elevation and size of the infarction. Severe hypoxia or hypercapnia often requires endotracheal intubation and mechanical ventilation with a volume-cycled respirator. Underlying acid-base disorders, especially alkalosis, should be corrected because they contribute to arrhythmias. Serum potassium should be kept above 4.0 mEq/L (10 to 40 mEq/h intravenously); magnesium may also be indicated (1 to 2 g/5 to 20 min intravenously).

With the potential liability for missing the diagnosis of an AMI, many physicians tend to overdiagnose myocardial ischemia and admit "soft" patients to the hospital as a precaution. Nationwide, this practice has led to over 1.5 million annual admissions to cardiac care units for suspected ischemia, but less than 30 percent of these patients have AMIs. Another 30 percent of these patients have either unstable or stable angina. The policy in many hospitals has been that all patients admitted because of chest pain (i.e., "rule out" AMI) have to be admitted to the cardiac care unit. Recent studies evaluating this process found that certain subgroups of these patients rarely, if ever, require cardiac care unit interventions and have a very low in-hospital mortality. Patients with AMI or unstable angina who have either ongoing pain, ECG changes, arrhythmias, or hemodynamic complications often require cardiac care unit interventions. Patients with unstable angina who have a normal or nonspecific ECG and no arrhythmias or hemodynamic complications can appropriately be admitted to a step-down or telemetry unit once their chest pain resolves. Likewise, chest pain-free patients admitted as "rule out myocardial infarction" with a normal or nonspecific ECG can be safely admitted to a step-down unit. Patients with unstable angina can be safely transferred out of the cardiac care unit after they have remained hemodynamically stable and free of ischemic pain for 24 h. Likewise, patients who have sustained a relatively uncomplicated AMI can be safely transferred 24 h after their ischemic pain has resolved. Diagnostic testing and therapeutic options (e.g., thrombolytic therapy) are being imported from the cardiac care unit to the emergency department. For example, chest pain patients with a low risk of AMI can undergo serial ECGs and serial cardiac marker testing in the "chest pain" or "cardiac" observation unit.

Pain relief is an important and humane goal. In addition, it reduces the circulatory load on the heart and decreases myocardial oxygen demand. The best treatments for pain are those that are physiologic in reducing or reversing ischemia: oxygen, aspirin, nitroglycerin, thrombolytics, anticoagulants, magnesium, β-adrenergic blockers, calcium blockers, or angiotensin-converting enzyme (ACE) inhibitors. Because such therapy takes time to provide relief, the early use of potent analgesics is often required. Intravenous morphine sulfate is the traditional treatment for the pain of AMI. Sequential small doses (4 to 6 mg) every 10 to 15 min should be used; however, complete pain relief may require up to a total dose of 15 to 20 mg of morphine. Morphine should be used with caution in patients with severe hypotension (systolic blood pressure < 80 mm Hg). In the setting of AMI, the beneficial action of morphine is predominantly sedative and analgesic, which reduces oxygen demand. Morphine produces no consistent effect on preload and may actually decrease cardiac output. Meperidine hydrochloride has effects similar to those of morphine and can also be used in patients allergic to morphine but not to meperidine.

Sublingual or intravenous nitroglycerin is both effective and safe in AMI—and more physiologic than morphine. Nitroglycerin reduces the degree of ischemia and probably reduces infarct size and decreases in-hospital mortality in AMI. Repetitive small doses (0.4 to 1.6 mg) should be given sublingually at 3- to 5-min intervals as long as systolic blood pressure remains adequate (i.e., > 100 mm Hg in most patients or > 120 mm Hg in patients with a prior history of hypertension). The response of individual patients is variable and may

**Table 51-15.** Progressive Emergency Management of Acute Myocardial Infarction

| |
|---|
| Oxygen |
| Nitroglycerin (SL, IV) |
| Aspirin (PO) |
| Thrombolytic agent(s) |
| Heparin (IV) |
| Magnesium (IV) |
| ACE inhibitor (PO) |
| β blocker (esmolol IV; oral agent) |
| Calcium blocker (diltiazem IV, PO) |

require a total nitroglycerin dose of about 20 to 30 mg for complete pain control. Nitroglycerin can be initiated at an infusion rate of 10 μg/min and increased until pain is controlled or systolic blood pressure falls by about 10 percent; most patients require between 30 and 100 μg/min. At low doses (< 30–50 μg/min), nitroglycerin acts primarily as a venodilator, reducing preload. At higher doses, its venodilator and arteriodilator effects are more balanced. Doses above 100 μg/min have been associated with a paradoxical increase in ischemia. Nitroglycerin enhances intercoronary collateral flow to ischemic areas. Approximately 2000 AMI patients have been enrolled in 10 randomized trials of intravenous nitroglycerin. If the data are pooled, the risk of death from AMI is decreased about one third. Occasionally patients with AMI have what appears to be a vasovagal reaction to nitroglycerin marked by bradycardia and hypertension. This is usually transient and responds to elevating the legs and, if required, atropine. Morphine can cause a similar reaction.

Aspirin is standard in the early management of AMI patients, either one 325-mg aspirin or two 81-mg chewable aspirins as soon as possible after arrival. Aspirin has been shown to decrease AMI mortality by 25 percent, comparable to the benefit from thrombolytic therapy. The benefit from the combination of aspirin with a thrombolytic agent is additive, reducing mortality by almost one half. Heparin is also a mandatory adjunct to thrombolytic therapy in AMI patients (Table 51-15). The recommended dose is an initial bolus of 5000 to 10,000 units intravenously, then a continuous intravenous infusion of 1000 to 1500 units/h.

Magnesium's main benefit for AMI patients is as an antiarrhythmic agent. But it is also a smooth muscle relaxant that may decrease cardiac work and may increase coronary blood flow. Of approximately 600 AMI patients entered into prophylactic magnesium trials prior to 1990, only 3 percent died in the magnesium groups versus 11 percent in the placebo groups. The 1992 LIMIT-2 trial enrolled 2316 AMI patients in a randomized trial of intravenous magnesium over the first 24 h versus placebo. At 1 month, mortality was reduced 24 percent in the magnesium group. The 1993 ISIS-4 trial in over 27,000 AMI patients failed to show a mortality reduction with a 24-h infusion of intravenous magnesium. The discrepancy between these results may reflect the 12 h delay in starting magnesium in the larger ISIS-4 trial. The mortality benefit from administering 1 to 2 g magnesium intravenously over 10 to 20 min followed by a continuous infusion of 1 to 2 g/h does not appear to be the result of its antiarrhythmic effects.

Currently available calcium channel antagonists are not recommended for early management of AMI patients. Nifedipine has been shown to increase mortality in unstable angina and AMI patients. Verapamil therapy for AMI patients has been studied in the DAVIT trials. It cannot be recommended in the peri-infarct period, but it can be beneficial in the postinfarct period in patients without heart failure. Diltiazem is the only calcium channel antagonist that has been shown to be of benefit in the peri-infarct period, not yet routine in the emergency department. Specifically, diltiazem therapy beginning 24 to 72 h after onset of chest pain in patients with non-Q wave AMIs reduced mortality. Diltiazem can also be recommended for post-AMI therapy in patients without contraindications.

The ACE inhibitors restrict conversion of angiotensin I, causing a drop in system arteriolar resistance and decreasing afterload. ACE inhibitors are the only agents shown to decrease mortality in chronic congestive heart failure patients. Multiple trials have also shown ACE inhibitors to benefit AMI patients in the postinfarct period. But the first trial of an ACE inhibitor (enalapril) begun within 24 h of AMI onset was terminated due to an excess mortality in patients older than 70 years. But the larger ISIS-4 trial and at least two similar but smaller trials of ACE inhibitors begun immediately after presentation to the emergency department showed modest benefit at 2 months (captopril therapy in 1000 patients would save five lives).

## SUMMARY

Myocardial ischemia and infarction continue to present a diagnostic and therapeutic challenge to the emergency department physician. There is no ideal method of excluding with certainty myocardial ischemia in the patients presenting with chest pain. Ischemia is even more difficult to diagnose in patients without chest pain or with atypical presentations. Additional lead ECGs and newer cardiac marker immunoassays can help the emergency department physician. Multiple therapies are available to treat the patient with an AMI. Much of their benefit depends on initiation of therapy as soon as possible after the AMI patient arrives at the emergency department. In addition to thrombolytic agents, other physiologic therapies include aspirin, heparin, nitroglycerin, magnesium, β blockers, ACE inhibitors, and calcium blockers.

## BIBLIOGRAPHY

Collaborative Group ISIS-1: Randomized trial of intravenous atenolol among 16,027 cases of suspected acute myocardial infarction. *Lancet* II:57, 1986.

Collaborative Group ISIS-2: Randomized trial of intravenous streptokinase, oral aspirin, both or neither among 17,187 cases of suspected acute myocardial infarction. *Lancet* II:349, 1988.

Collaborative Group ISIS-3: A randomized comparison of streptokinase vs tissue plasminogen activator vs anistreplase and or aspirin plus heparin vs aspirin alone among 41,299 cases of suspected acute myocardial infarction. *Lancet* 339:753, 1992.

Collaborative Group ISIS-4: Protocol for a large simple study of the effects of oral mononitrate, of oral captopril, and of intravenous magnesium. *Am J Cardiol* 68:87D, 1991.

Dell'Italia LJ, Sterling MR, Blumhardt R, et al: Comparative effects of volume loading, dobutamine, and nitroprusside in patients with predominant right ventricular infarction. *Circulation* 72:1327, 1985.

deServi S, Ghio S, Ferrario M, et al: Clinical and angiographic findings in angina at rest. *Am Heart J* 111:6, 1986.

Forrester JS, Diamond G, Swan HJC: Correlative classification of clinical and hemodynamic functions after acute myocardial infarction. *Am J Cardiol* 39:137, 1977.

Gibler WB, Young GP, Hedges JR, et al: Early detection of acute myocardial infarction in patients presenting with chest pain and myocardial infarction in patients presenting with chest pain and nondiagnostic ECGs: serial CK-MB sampling in the emergency department. *Ann Emerg Med* 19:1359, 1990.

GISSI: GISSI-3 study protocol on the effects of lisinopril, of nitrates, and of their association in patients with acute myocardial infarction. *Am J Cardiol* 70:62C, 1992.

Herlitz J, Hjalmarson A, Waagstein F: Treatment of pain in acute myocardial infarction. *Br Heart J* 61:9, 1989.

Hine LK, Laird N, Hewitt P, et al: Meta-analytic evidence against prophylactic use of lidocaine in acute myocardial infarction. *Arch Intern Med* 149:2649, 1989.

Hsia J, Hamilton WP, Kleiman N, et al: A comparison between heparin and low-dose aspirin as adjunctive therapy with tissue plasminogen activator for acute myocardial infarction. *N Engl J Med* 323:1433, 1990.

Kim YI, Williams JF: Large dose sublingual nitroglycerin in acute myocardial infarction: relief of chest pain and reduction of Q wave evolution. *Am J Cardiol* 49:842, 1982.

Lamas GA, Muller JE, Turi ZG, et al: A simplified method to predict occurrence of complete heart block during acute myocardial infarction. *Am J Cardiol* 57:1213, 1986.

Lee TH, Goldman L: The coronary care unit turns 25: historical trends and future directions. *Ann Intern Med* 108:887, 1988.

Rouan GW, Leee TH, Cook EF, et al: Clinical characteristics and outcome of acute myocardial infarction in patients with initially normal or nonspecific electrocardiograms: a report from the multicenter chest pain study. *Am J Cardiol* 64:1087, 1989.

Swedberg K, Held P, Kjekshus J, et al: Effects of the early administration of enalapril on mortality in patients with acute myocardial infarction. *N Engl J Med* 327:678, 1992.

Theroux P, et al: Aspirin, heparin, or both to treat acute unstable angina. *N Engl J Med* 319:1105, 1988.

# 52

# PREHOSPITAL AND EMERGENCY DEPARTMENT THROMBOLYTIC THERAPY

**Terry J. Mengert**
**Mickey S. Eisenberg**

## OVERVIEW

Myocardial infarction (MI) is the irreversible cellular injury and necrosis of cardiac muscle caused by prolonged ischemia. Acute MI (AMI) is the leading cause of death in the United States and most other Western industrialized countries. In 1993 alone, approximately 1.25 million Americans suffered an AMI, and nearly 500,000 of these patients died. Over one-half of the deaths occurred suddenly, within 1 h of symptom onset, and prior to the patient's hospital arrival.

Most AMIs occur secondary to a coronary artery thrombus at the site of an atherosclerotic plaque. Thrombolytic therapy is the use of one or more medications to produce rapid lysis of a thrombus or embolus. It is a crucial and life-saving intervention for the patient suffering an AMI because it directly attacks the proximate cause of the MI, the coronary artery thrombus. The early and appropriate administration of thrombolytic therapy to the AMI patient with ST-segment elevation or new left bundle branch block is now the treatment of choice and the standard of care.

Consider the following essential facts regarding thrombolytic therapy:

- Early MI mortality is decreased by as much as one-third to one-half: from 10 to 15 percent in the years immediately prior to the availability of thrombolytic therapy to 5 to 10 percent today with that therapy.
- The shorter the time interval between symptom onset and thrombolysis, the greater the reduction in mortality. Maximum benefit occurs when thrombolytic agents are administered within the first 1 to 2 h of symptom onset. For example, in GISSI-I (Gruppo Italiano per lo Studio della Streptochinasi nell' Infarcto Miocardico), the mortality reduction with streptokinase as compared to a control group was 47 percent for patients treated within 1 h of symptom onset, 22 percent for those treated between 1 and 3 h, and 18 percent for those treated between 3 and 6 h.
- Early administration of thrombolytic therapy results in improved recovery of left ventricular function, with less post-MI ventricular dilatation and remodeling.

- Though benefit is most pronounced the earlier the treatment, thrombolytic therapy still reduces mortality even when administered as late as 12 h after symptom onset.
- Approximately 20 percent of thrombosed arteries fail to reopen with lytic therapy, and approximately 15 percent of arteries that do reopen and reperfuse will subsequently close in the next several hours or days.
- Less than one-third of AMI patients in this country receive thrombolytic therapy.
- Patients deemed "ineligible" for thrombolytic therapy suffer increased morbidity and mortality.
- Unfortunately, no large randomized clinical trial has yet demonstrated improved survival in patients with cardiogenic shock treated with peripherally administered thrombolytic agents. In these patients, emergency cardiac catheterization and revascularization should be utilized if available.

## THROMBOLYTIC AGENTS AND THEIR ADMINISTRATION

The peripherally administered thrombolytic agents currently approved in this country for the AMI patient are streptokinase, anisoylated plasminogen-streptokinase activator complex (anistreplase, or APSAC), and tissue plasminogen activator (alteplase, or tPA). Though their specific mechanisms of action vary, each of these agents eventually activates plasminogen to plasmin, which then dissolves the fibrin component of the occluding coronary artery thrombus.

Streptokinase is derived from β-hemolytic streptococcal cultures (see Table 52-1 for dosing). It binds to plasminogen, resulting in a change in plasminogen's molecular configuration and activation of the plasminogen molecule. The activated plasminogen in turn converts circulating plasminogen to plasmin, with subsequent fibrin lysis and thrombus dissolution. The half-life of streptokinase is 23 min; in most patients, systemic fibrinolysis after streptokinase administration persists for up to 24 h.

Streptokinase is antigenic. In the recent GUSTO (Global Utilization of Streptokinase and Tissue Plasminogen Activator for Occluded Coronary Arteries) trial, allergic reactions occurred in 5.7 percent of patients treated with streptokinase and subcutaneous heparin. In this same group, 0.7 percent of patients suffered anaphylactic reactions and 13.3 percent had sustained hypotension. Antibodies develop approximately 5 days after streptokinase administration and persist for 6 months. Retreatment with streptokinase should not occur in this time interval. Treatment with streptokinase should also not occur within 12 months of either a streptococcal infection or APSAC therapy.

APSAC is a modified, active plasminogen-streptokinase complex (see Table 52-1 for dosing). After administration, APSAC activates other plasminogen molecules, resulting in fibrin lysis. Its half-life is 90 min. Like streptokinase, APSAC is antigenic, and its administration may result in allergic reactions, hypotension, and rarely anaphylaxis. After administration, antibodies also form to APSAC; treatment with APSAC is not recommended for 5 days to 12 months after therapy with streptokinase or APSAC or after a streptococcal infection.

Tissue plasminogen activator is a naturally occurring enzyme found in vascular endothelial cells and a number of other tissues. Commercially prepared tPA is derived from recombinant DNA technology. See Table 52-1 for several dosing regimens; in practice, the "front-loaded" regimen utilized in the GUSTO trial is recommended. Tissue plasminogen activator directly cleaves a specific peptide bond in plasminogen, converting it into active plasmin, with subsequent fibrin lysis. There is also a binding site on tPA for fibrin, which should theoretically result in clot-specific fibrin lysis and fewer bleeding complications; in practice, however, the incidence of bleeding is comparable among the different agents. The half-life of tPA is only 5 min. Unlike streptokinase and APSAC, tPA is not antigenic. In the GUSTO trial utilizing front-loaded tPA and intravenous heparin,

**Table 52-1.** Current Thrombolytic Agents and Their Dosing in the Acute MI Patient

| Drug | Dose | Comments |
|---|---|---|
| Streptokinase (SK) (Cost: $300) | 1.5 million units IV over 60 min | SK is antigenic; allergic reactions and rarely anaphylaxis (<1% incidence) may occur. Administration may cause hypotension, necessitating a slower infusion rate than that recommended. SK may not be effective if administered 5 days to 6 months after prior SK therapy or 12 months after APSAC therapy or a streptococcal infection. |
| APSAC (Anistreplase) (Cost: $1675) | 30 units IV over 2–5 min | APSAC is also antigenic and its administration may be complicated by hypotension (see above). APSAC may not be effective if administered 5 days to 12 months after prior SK or APSAC therapy or a streptococcal infection. Do not administer heparin with APSAC. |
| tPA (Alteplase) (Cost: $2200) | "Front-loaded" dosing: 15 mg IV over 2 min, followed by 0.75 mg/kg (50 mg maximum) IV over 30 min, followed by 0.5 mg/kg (35 mg maximum) IV over 60 min<br><br>"Traditional" dosing:<br>Adult patient < 65 kg:<br>total dose 1.25 mg/kg IV over 3 h, with 60% of this dose in the first hour (6–10% as a bolus over 1–2 min, and the other 50–54% of the total dose given over the remainder of the first hour), followed by 40% of the total dose given over the next 2 h of therapy.<br>Adult patient ≥ 65 kg:<br>60 mg IV over the first hour (6–10 mg as an IV bolus over the first 1–2 min) followed by 40 mg IV over the next 2 h of therapy. | Do not exceed the maximum dose of 100 mg. Unlike SK and APSAC above, tPA is not antigenic. Hypotension complicating infusion is less likely than with either SK or APSAC. Heparin should be administered concomitantly with tPA. |

the rate of allergic reactions with tPA administration was only 1.6 percent, the rate for anaphylaxis was 0.2 percent, and for sustained hypotension was 10.1 percent.

## Indications for Thrombolytic Therapy

Thrombolytic therapy should be initiated within 30 min of arrival in the emergency department of the routine AMI patient. The eligibility criteria for thrombolytic therapy are presented in Table 52-2. There are four general criteria: (1) clinical presentation consistent with an AMI; (2) ECG criteria (ST-segment elevation in two or more contiguous leads or new onset left bundle branch block); (3) absence of contraindications; and (4) absence of cardiogenic shock. The contraindications to thrombolytic therapy are presented in Table 52-3. Angiography and mechanical reperfusion, rather than a peripherally administered thrombolytic agent, are the preferred treatment modalities for those patients in cardiogenic shock, if available within 60 min of patient presentation.

When all four of the above criteria are met, the patient is *eligible* for thrombolytic therapy. Important additional considerations, however, may include patient age, location of the infarct, relative contraindications to thrombolysis, and duration of symptoms within the 12-h criterion. As with all treatment modalities, the risks and benefits of thrombolytic therapy must be considered within the framework of an individual patient's clinical presentation.

The decision to administer a thrombolytic agent should be made by the emergency physician for the "routine" AMI. Specialty consultation may only delay treatment under these circumstances and is not necessary before initiating thrombolysis. Patients who do not meet all four eligibility criteria (e.g., because symptoms have been present for > 12 h or relative contraindications to thrombolytic therapy are present) may still derive benefit from thrombolytic therapy depending, again, on a careful weighing of the risks and benefits. Under these circumstances, consultation with the physician who will assume continued definitive care of the patient (e.g., cardiologist, internist) is reasonable and appropriate before initiating thrombolysis.

## Choice of Thrombolytic Agent

The rapid administration of thrombolytic therapy is of greater importance than the specific agent used. Each of these medications is effective and has certain advantages. Streptokinase is simple to dose and is the least expensive of the three drugs, but it is antigenic and its administration may be complicated by allergic reactions and hypoten-

**Table 52-2.** Eligibility Criteria for Thrombolytic Therapy

I. **Clinical criteria**
   A. One or more of the following symptoms consistent with acute MI:
   Chest pain, pressure, aching, burning, tightness, or heaviness with or without arm, jaw, neck, shoulder, or back radiation
   Epigastric discomfort, indigestion, belching, or "heartburn"
   Nausea, vomiting, and/or diaphoresis
   Persistent dyspnea
   Miscellaneous: dizziness, lightheadedness, syncope, and/or weakness
   B. Symptom onset ≤ 12 h prior to patient presentation*
II. **ECG criteria**
   One or more of the following:
   ≥ 1 mm ST-segment elevation in ≥ 2 contiguous limb leads
   ≥ 2 mm ST-segment elevation in ≥ 2 contiguous precordial leads
   New left bundle branch block
III. **No contraindications to thrombolytic therapy***
   See Table 52-3
IV. **Patient not in cardiogenic shock†**

* Thrombolytic therapy may still be appropriate and beneficial to the AMI patient with relative contraindications or the patient with symptom duration > 12 h if the chest pain is intermittent or ST-segment elevation on the ECG is still present. Discuss relative contraindications or complicated presentations with the consulting physician (e.g., cardiologist, internist) who will assume inhospital care of the patient prior to thrombolytic therapy.

† Patients in cardiogenic shock should undergo emergent angiography and mechanical reperfusion if available. If the availability of this therapy will be delayed for ≥ 60 min, proceed with "front-loaded" tPA (tPA is less likely to exacerbate hypotension than either streptokinase or APSAC).

**Table 52-3.** Contraindications to Thrombolytic Therapy

Absolute Contraindications
 Active internal bleeding
 Altered consciousness
 Cerebrovascular accident (CVA) in the past 6 months or *any* history of
  hemorrhagic CVA
 Intracranial or intraspinal surgery within the previous 2 months
 Intracranial or intraspinal neoplasm, aneurysm, or arteriovenous
  malformation
 Known bleeding disorder
 Persistent, severe hypertension (systolic BP > 200 mmHg and/or diastolic
  BP > 120 mmHg)
 Pregnancy
 Previous allergy to a streptokinase product (this does not contraindicate
  tPA administration)
 Recent (within 1 month) head trauma
 Suspected aortic dissection
 Suspected pericarditis
 Trauma or surgery within 2 weeks that could result in bleeding into a
  closed space
Relative contraindications
 Active peptic ulcer disease
 Cardiopulmonary resuscitation for > 10 min
 Current use of oral anticoagulants
 Hemorrhagic ophthalmic conditions
 History of chronic, uncontrolled hypertension (diastolic BP > 100 mmHg),
  treated or untreated
 History of ischemic or embolic CVA > 6 months ago
 Significant trauma or major surgery > 2 weeks ago but < 2 months ago
 Subclavian or internal jugular venous cannulation

*Source:* Adapted from National Heart Attack Alert Program Coordinating Committee 60 Minutes to Treatment Working Group. NIH Publication No. 93-3278, September, 1993, p 19.

sion. APSAC is the most easily dosed of the three (30 units IV over 2 to 5 min), but it is expensive and antigenic and its administration may also be complicated by allergic reactions and hypotension. Tissue plasminogen activator is not antigenic and its use is less likely to be complicated by hypotension; however, it is the most expensive of the three agents, is somewhat complicated to dose, and requires concomitant heparin administration for optimal effectiveness.

The GUSTO investigators, in a study involving 41,021 patients with AMI from 1081 centers in 15 countries, found that front-loaded tPA with intravenous heparin resulted in a reduced mortality at 30 days posttreatment (6.3 percent mortality), as compared to streptokinase and subcutaneous heparin (7.2 percent mortality) or streptokinase and intravenous heparin (7.4 percent mortality). Subgroup analysis revealed, however, that the relatively small benefits of tPA over streptokinase were fewer or nonexistent for patients with inferior MIs, age > 75 years, or those in whom thrombolysis was not initiated until > 4 h after symptom onset.

On the basis of the above, tPA is the thrombolytic agent of choice for patients with any of the following: known allergy to streptokinase or APSAC, prior administration of streptokinase in the previous 6 months, prior administration of APSAC in the previous 12 months, prior streptococcal infection in the previous 12 months, or hemodynamic instability. On the basis of the GUSTO data, the emergency physician should consider front-loaded tPA over streptokinase in patients with anterior or lateral MIs who are < 75 years old and present within 4 h of symptom onset.

### Adjunctive Therapy to Thrombolysis

Aspirin inhibits cyclooxygenase-dependent platelet aggregation. Its immediate administration to the AMI patient results in a significant reduction in mortality, especially when used in combination with a thrombolytic agent. The oral dose is 160 to 325 mg (chewed).

Heparin should be given intravenously to patients who receive tPA

and continued in the coronary care unit for at least 72 h. Intravenous heparin is started simultaneously with tPA at a dose of 80 units/kg IV bolus followed by a continuous infusion of 15 units/kg per hour. The activated partial thromboplastin time should then be maintained at 1.5 to 2 times the control value. In the GUSTO trial, the combination of intravenous heparin with streptokinase provided no advantages over subcutaneous heparin and streptokinase. The dose of subcutaneous heparin in that trial was 12,500 units twice daily beginning 4 h after the start of thrombolytic therapy. Subcutaneous heparin was continued for 7 days or until the patient was discharged from the hospital. Heparin is of uncertain benefit with APSAC, may increase bleeding complications, and is not recommended at this time.

Other adjunctive agents useful in the AMI patient include oxygen, morphine sulfate, nitroglycerin, β-blockers, magnesium in hypomagnesemic patients, and angiotensin-converting enzyme inhibitors. See Chap. 53, "Acute Interventions in Myocardial Infarction," for the use and dosing of these medications.

## PREHOSPITAL THROMBOLYTIC THERAPY

The most comprehensive evaluation of the potential benefit of prehospital thrombolysis for patients suffering an AMI in this country was the Myocardial Infarction, Triage, and Intervention (MITI) Trial conducted in Seattle and King County, Washington. Phase II of this trial prospectively randomized 360 patients to receive either paramedic-initiated or hospital-initiated thrombolytic therapy with tPA. This study demonstrated that, on average, paramedic-initiated thrombolytic therapy was started 33 min sooner than in-hospital-delivered thrombolysis, and there were no increased complications with paramedic-initiated therapy. No significant difference was found between prehospital- and in-hospital-initiated thrombolysis in either patient mortality or infarct size, but the study was underpowered to show such a difference (mortality was 5.7 percent in the paramedic-treated group and 8.1 percent in the hospital-treated group).

The MITI study did reveal marked and significant differences in outcome for patients who received very early thrombolytic therapy, whether that therapy was paramedic- or in-hospital-initiated. The in-hospital mortality of the 82 patients treated within 70 min of symptom onset was only 1.2 percent, compared to a mortality of 8.7 percent in the 260 patients treated between 70 min and 3 h. Infarct size in the group treated within 70 min was half of that in the later-treated group.

Other clinical trials have demonstrated similar decreases in time to therapy with paramedic-initiated thrombolysis. Prehospital thrombolysis, therefore, saves time, but it remains uncertain whether it saves lives. As a result, the American College of Emergency Physician's policy on the prehospital use of thrombolytic agents states that such use is considered investigational, and routine use of prehospital-administered thrombolysis should otherwise be discouraged.

### Prehospital Electrocardiograms

While the use of prehospital thrombolysis remains controversial and investigational, a related question is whether prehospital 12-lead electrocardiograms (ECGs) are of benefit to the AMI patient's care. Technology exists to easily transmit prehospital 12-lead ECGs via cellular phones to base-station hospitals. Alternatively, prehospital 12-lead ECGs can be obtained with computer-assisted automatic interpretation. This information can then be easily relayed to a base-station hospital or a receiving hospital by telephone or radio.

Prehospital diagnosis of AMI patients eligible for thrombolytic therapy is worthwhile: it alerts the emergency department staff to the incoming patient and allows them to prepare for the patient's arrival. This is analogous to the usefulness of a medic unit notifying the emergency department of a multiple trauma patient's arrival to allow the staff to optimally prepare for timely and aggressive patient care.

The time required to take a 12-lead ECG is only several minutes, which is generally an acceptable delay in patient transport.

Obtaining prehospital ECGs as part of the prehospital evaluation of the chest pain patient is endorsed as an acceptable procedure by the American Heart Association. In their 1994 *Textbook of Advanced Cardiac Life Support,* they state that emergency medical service personnel should undertake prehospital evaluation and screening of chest pain patients by obtaining the following information:

Pain of probable cardiac origin
Patient > 30 years of age
Systolic BP < 180 mmHg
Diastolic BP < 110 mmHg
Chest pain has been present for ≥ 15 min
Patient has had no cerebrovascular accident or other serious central nervous problem in the preceding 6 months
Patient has had neither surgery nor major trauma in the preceding 2 weeks
Patient has no bleeding problems
Patient is not pregnant

When all of the above conditions apply to the patient, a 12-lead ECG should then be obtained. The ECG can be transmitted via cellular phone or a verbal report given of its computer interpretation.

## Prehospital Thrombolysis in Rural and Remote Communities

Prehospital thrombolytic therapy has only been studied in urban communities; rural settings have not been adequately evaluated. Prehospital thrombolysis seems medically reasonable in those situations in which excessive delays until arrival at the hospital occur and in those where delay is unavoidable. This is especially relevant to remote sites such as ships and offshore drilling rigs. The American College of Emergency Physician's *Guidelines for the Prehospital Use of Thrombolytic Agents* states the following:

> Prehospital administration of thrombolytic agents should be considered when the use of these agents will result in savings of at least 30 minutes in the time that thrombolytic agents can be administered in the field compared to the time required for drug administration in the hospital emergency department.

## Paramedic Training

Paramedics should receive special training in the clinical evaluation of chest pain, including an understanding of thrombosis as the cause of AMI and the importance of rapid intervention. In communities in which prehospital thrombolysis is used, paramedics must also be trained in the clinical presentation of AMI; the contraindications to thrombolytic therapy; the preparation, administration, and storage of thrombolytic agents; and the recognition and treatment of thrombolytic-related complications.

Paramedics should not be trained in the interpretation of 12-lead ECGs. Contemporary ECG machines allow sophisticated computer-assisted interpretations. These interpretations must be evaluated in the context of the patient's clinical presentation by the base-station physician or the receiving physician.

When prehospital thrombolytic therapy is a consideration, a checklist should be used in the prehospital evaluation of the chest pain patient. Figure 52-1 contains the paramedic chest pain evaluation form used in the MITI study. This sample list provides inclusion and exclusion criteria. If the appropriate boxes are checked, then the patient is eligible for prehospital thrombolytic therapy. The final decision for thrombolytic therapy must be made by the base-station controlling physician with on-line (concurrent) direction. In the MITI study, the physician had a hard copy of the 12-lead ECG with a computer interpretation, transmitted by cellular telephone, immediately at hand prior to making the decision to initiate field thrombolysis. Accurate recording of the time of onset of chest pain is crucial in evaluating the effectiveness of therapy. In communities in which prehospital thrombolysis is not used, such an extensive prehospital checklist is not indicated. The presence of ongoing chest pain in an oriented, cooperative person is a sufficient indication to obtain a 12-lead ECG.

**CHEST PAIN CHECKLIST (For Paramedic Use)**

67. CP CHECKLIST

Was Pt. Evaluated for Chest Pain?
YES ☐ NO ___
(*Complete for all patients*)

| YES | | NO |
|---|---|---|
| ☐ | Oriented, can cooperate | ___ |
| ☐ | Ongoing heart pain | ___ |
| ☐ | No terminal illness | ___ |
| ☐ | Patient consents | ___ |
| | **If all 4 boxes YES, birth year** | ___ |
| ☐ | ECG done | ___ |
| ☐ | ECG received by doctor | ___ |
| ☐ | Pain for More Than 15 Minutes and Less Than 6 Hours | ___ |
| ☐ | Age (34—74) | ___ |
| | BP Right Arm ___ /___ | |
| | BP Left Arm ___ /___ | |
| ☐ | Systolic is More Than 60 and Less Than 180 | ___ |
| ☐ | Systolic Right Arm Versus Left Arm is Less Than 20 | ___ |
| ☐ | Diastolic is Less Than 110 | ___ |
| ___ | Stroke, Seizures, Brain Surgery, Head Trauma | ☐ |
| ___ | Central Lines < 2 Wks; or Trauma < 2 Wks; or PTCA < 1 Mo. | ☐ |
| ___ | Previous Thrombolytic Rx | ☐ |
| ___ | Takes Warfarin, Coumadin | ☐ |
| ___ | Known Bleeding Problems | ☐ |
| ___ | GI Bleed in Last 2 Months | ☐ |
| ___ | Surgery in Last 2 Months | ☐ |
| ___ | Jaundice, Hepatitis, Kidney Failure | ☐ |
| ___ | Colitis, Crohn's Enteritis | ☐ |
| ☐ | Meets Criteria for Pre–Hosp TT | ___ |
| ☐ | Patient Informed<br>Kit ID #___ | ___ |
| ☐ | Thrombolytic Therapy Given<br>Amount Including Bolus ___ | ___ |
| ☐ | ASA (5gr) Given | ___ |

| TIMES | |
|---|---|
| Pain Began | ___:___ |
| Decision Time | ___:___ |
| TT Bolus | ___:___ |

**Fig. 52-1.** Chest pain evaluation checklist used by paramedics in the MITI study. (From Emergency Medical Services Division, King County Health Department, with permission.)

## INITIATING RAPID THROMBOLYSIS IN THE EMERGENCY DEPARTMENT

In the AMI patient "time is muscle." The sooner thrombolytic therapy can be initiated to the patient who is eligible for that therapy, the

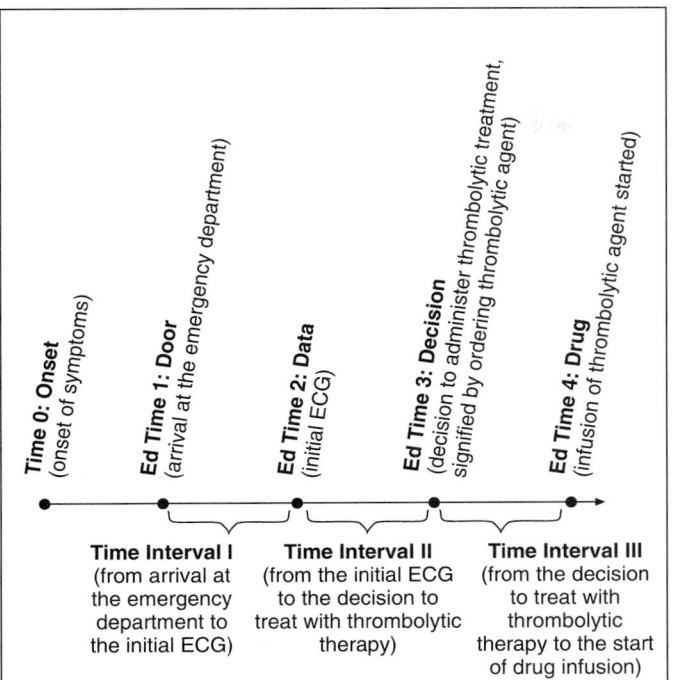

**Fig. 52-2.** Process timepoints and intervals through which the AMI patient passes until treatment in the emergency department. (From National Heart Attack Alert Program Coordinating Committee 60 Minutes to Treatment Working Group: NIH Publication No. 93-3278, September, 1993, p. 10, with permission.)

better the patient outcome in both morbidity and mortality. Currently, the average time from arrival in the emergency department to administration of thrombolytic therapy is approximately 60 to 90 min. A report from the National Heart Attack Alert Program Coordinating Committee working group on "Rapid Identification and Treatment of Patients with Acute Myocardial Infarction" recommended a time to treatment of 30 min or less.

The AMI patient passes through a well-defined and -described series of steps prior to initiation of thrombolytic therapy. These steps are outlined in Fig. 52-2 and include the following:

Onset of symptoms
Emergency department time 1: Door time—the time the patient arrives at the ED
Emergency department time 2: Data—the time the ECG is obtained
Emergency department time 3: Decision—the time the thrombolytic agent is ordered
Emergency department time 4: Drug—the time the thrombolytic agent infusion begins

Important intervals derived from the above times are also presented in Fig. 52-2 and include the following: time interval from emergency department arrival to initial ECG, time interval from initial ECG to ordering of thrombolytic therapy, and time interval from the ordering of the thrombolytic agent till its actual infusion in the patient. The sum of these three time intervals is the total "door-to-drug" time. The prospective collection of these time intervals is important in the necessary and continued improvement in the emergency department care of the AMI patient.

All factors that contribute to delays within the above time intervals should be meticulously scrutinized and every effort made to reduce them to a minimum. All patients who arrive at the emergency department, whether by ambulance or private transportation, should be rapidly and efficiently triaged. Patients with chest pain should be taken *immediately* to an intensive care bed within the emergency de-

partment. There should be no delay at registration for signatures, other data collection, or even vital sign determination. Rapid triage and admittance to an actual emergency department bed is facilitated when the emergency department is prenotified by the emergency medical services system of the arrival of a chest pain patient with worrisome ECG changes.

Figure 52-3 presents a sample algorithm/protocol for patients with symptoms and/or signs suggestive of AMI. The ECG should be obtained immediately! A reasonable goal for time interval I (emergency department arrival to initial ECG) is 5 min. Emergency department nurses should have the authority to obtain a 12-lead ECG on any patient suspected of AMI. Furthermore, ECG equipment and staff trained in its use should be available in the emergency department. Delays should never occur because emergency department staff are awaiting the arrival of an ECG technician. Once obtained, the patient's ECG must be shown immediately to a physician. For patients with fluctuating symptoms or changing clinical status, serial ECGs are helpful, especially if the initial ECG is not diagnostic.

Initial patient care that occurs simultaneously with the above includes the following: vital signs, continuous cardiac rhythm monitoring, supplemental oxygen administration, intravenous access, necessary blood sample acquisition, screening physical examination, and aspirin and nitroglycerin administration. Depending on the resources and personnel available, these important steps can be accomplished efficiently and rapidly.

Time interval II is from the initial ECG to the ordering of the thrombolytic agent. For routine AMIs, the decision to initiate thrombolytic therapy should be made by the emergency physician. Consultation with a cardiologist adds time to treatment and is unnecessary for routine cases. Specialty service consultations may be obtained for cases of shock or when the diagnosis is equivocal. The value of rapid assays for enzymes such as CK-MB, myoglobin, or troponin in facilitating the accurate diagnosis of the AMI patient is under investigation and may be of assistance in cases where the ECG is nondiagnostic.

Time interval III is the time from the decision to treat with thrombolytics to the actual administration of the drug. To minimize the duration of this interval, the thrombolytic agent should be kept in the emergency department. The staff must also be trained in the rapid reconstitution of the medicine and its proper administration.

## COMPLICATIONS OF THROMBOLYTIC THERAPY

The incidence of allergic reactions, anaphylaxis, and hypotension with the administration of streptokinase and APSAC have already been presented above. Allergic reactions should be treated with 50 mg diphenhydramine and 125 mg methylprednisolone IV. Hypotension can be treated by slowing the infusion rate of the thrombolytic agent, supplemented by intravenous crystalloid as the patient's volume status allows.

The most significant complications of thrombolytic therapy are hemorrhagic, and the most catastrophic complication is intracranial hemorrhage. In the GUSTO trial, the incidence of moderate or worse bleeding was 5.8 percent with streptokinase and subcutaneous heparin, 6.3 percent with streptokinase and intravenous heparin, and 5.4 percent with tPA and intravenous heparin. The incidence of hemorrhagic stroke in these same groups was 0.49 percent, 0.54 percent, and 0.72 percent, respectively. Note that, despite the theoretical advantage of clot-specific fibrin lysis with tPA, the risk of hemorrhagic stroke was higher with front-loaded tPA than with either streptokinase group in the GUSTO trial. This difference was statistically significant ($p = .03$).

To minimize the bleeding risks associated with thrombolytic therapy, observe the following precautions: (1) avoid all unnecessary needle sticks; (2) avoid any arterial punctures; (3) limit venous access to easily compressible sites (i.e., avoid central lines, especially in the jugular or subclavian veins); and (4) avoid both nasogastric tubes and

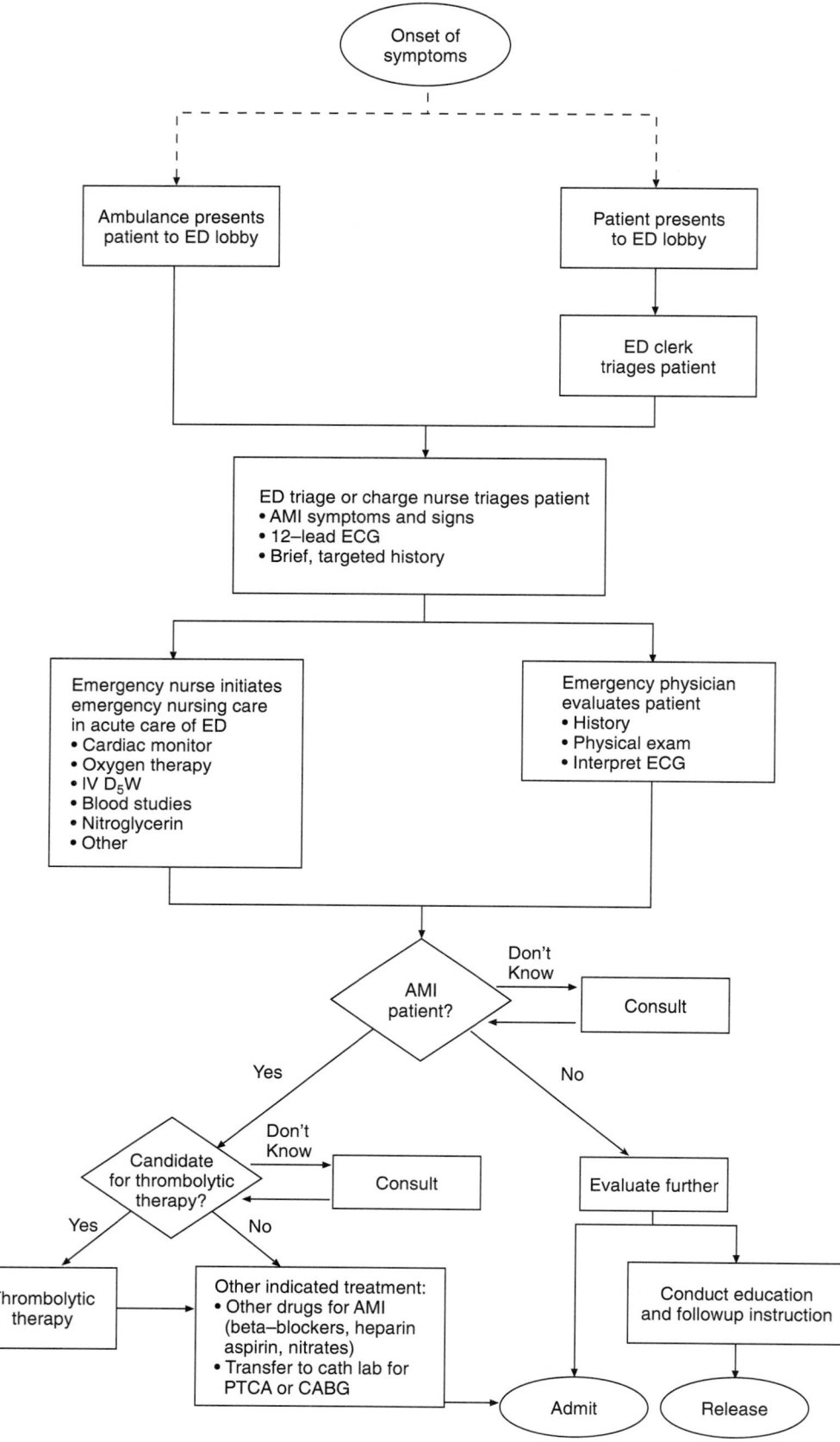

**Fig. 52-3.** Emergency department algorithm/protocol for patients with symptoms and signs of AMI. (From National Heart Attack Alert Program Coordinating Committee 60 Minutes to Treatment Working Group: NIH Publication No. 93-3278, September, 1993, p. 12, with permission.)

nasotracheal intubation. If a peripheral line has been inadvertently removed, apply at least 15 min of prolonged manual pressure to the site and monitor the site carefully for continued hemorrhage. Do not administer thrombolytic therapy to any patient with an absolute contraindication (see Table 52-3). In patients with a relative contraindication, carefully weigh the potential risks and benefits of thrombolysis in consultation with the physician who will assume inhospital care of the patient (e.g., cardiologist).

The hematocrit should be checked every 4 to 6 h after thrombolytic therapy. A fall in hematocrit > 2 percent mandates a thorough search for the source of blood loss. Most bleeding episodes (>70 percent) occur at vascular puncture sites. Also consider the possibilities of intracranial, intrathoracic, retroperitoneal, gastrointestinal, genitourinary, and/or soft tissue extremity hemorrhage.

Any site of external bleeding should be controlled with prolonged manual pressure. Significant bleeding, especially an internal site, mandates discontinuation of the thrombolytic agent, aspirin, and heparin. Replace volume with normal saline or lactated Ringer's as necessary; order type and cross-matched blood; and check thrombin time, activated partial thromboplastin time, platelet count, and fibrinogen level. Crystalloid infusion should be supplemented with red blood cell transfusion if clinically indicated. Heparin that was administered within 4 h of the onset of bleeding can be reversed with protamine. The dose of protamine is 1 mg for every 100 units of heparin that was administered as a bolus or every 100 mg that was administered as a continuous infusion in the previous 4 h. Protamine should be given slowly IV over 1 to 3 min, and the dose should not exceed 50 mg in any 10-min period.

Massive bleeding with hemodynamic compromise will necessitate coagulation factor replacement in addition to the interventions recommended above. Ten units of cryoprecipitate should be administered, and the fibrinogen level rechecked. If the fibrinogen level is less than 1 g/L, the dose of cryoprecipitate should be repeated. If bleeding continues after cryoprecipitate, or if bleeding persists despite a fibrinogen level > 1 g/L, administer 2 units of fresh-frozen plasma. If bleeding still persists after appropriate cryoprecipitate and fresh-frozen plasma, obtain a bleeding time. If it is greater than 9 min, administer 10 units of platelets followed by an antifibrinolytic agent (e.g., aminocaproic acid or tranexamic acid); if the bleeding time is less than 9 min, platelets are not necessary but an antifibrinolytic agent should still be administered in the setting of ongoing hemorrhage. The dose of aminocaproic acid (Amicar) is 5 g IV over 60 min followed by a continuous infusion of 1.0 g/h for 8 h or until bleeding stops. The dose of tranexamic acid is 10 mg/kg IV every 6 to 8 h.

Intracranial hemorrhage requires an aggressive and rapid approach. Immediately discontinue the thrombolytic agent, aspirin, and heparin. Administer protamine in the dose outlined above if the patient received heparin. The patient should also automatically receive cryoprecipitate, fresh-frozen plasma, a platelet transfusion, and an antifibrinolytic agent. Consult neurosurgery immediately.

## BIBLIOGRAPHY

American College of Emergency Physicians: Prehospital use of thrombolytic agents. *Ann Emerg Med* 23:1146, 1994.

American Heart Association, Subcommittee on Advanced Cardiac Life Support, Committee on Emergency Cardiac Care: *Textbook of Advanced Cardiac Life Support. Dallas:* American Heart Association, 1994.

Anderson HV, Wilkerson JT: Thrombolysis in acute myocardial infarction. *N Engl J Med* 329(10):703, 1993.

Benson NH, Maningas PA, Krohmer JR, et al: Guidelines for the prehospital use of thrombolytic agents. *Ann Emerg Med* 23:1047, 1994.

Califf RM, Bengtson JR: Cardiogenic shock. *N Engl J Med* 330(24):1724, 1994.

Doorey AJ: Thrombolytic therapy of acute myocardial infarction, keeping the unfulfilled promises. *JAMA* 268(21):3108, 1992.

Fuster V: Coronary thrombolysis—a perspective for the practicing physician (editorial). *N Engl J Med* 329(10):723, 1993.

Gruppo Italiano per lo Studio Della Streptochinasi nell' Infarcto Miocardico (GISSI): Effectiveness of intravenous thrombolytic treatment in acute myocardial infarction. *Lancet* 1:397, 1986.

Kereiakes DJ, Weaver WD, Anderson, et al: Time delays in the diagnosis and treatment of acute myocardial infarction: A tale of eight cities. Report from the Pre-Hospital Study Group and the Cincinnati Heart Project. *Am Heart J* 120(4):773, 1990.

Kline EM, Smith DD, Martin JS, et al: In-hospital treatment delays in patients treated with thrombolytic therapy: A report of the GUSTO Time to Treatment Substudy (abstract). *Circulation* 86(4 suppl 1):1, 1992.

Landau C, Lange RA, Hillis LD: Percutaneous transluminal coronary angioplasty. *N Engl J Med* 330(14):981, 1994.

National Heart Attack Alert Program Coordinating Committee 60 Minutes to Treatment Working Group: Emergency department: Rapid identification and treatment of patients with acute myocardial infarction. US Dept of Health and Human Services; Public Health Service; National Institutes of Health; National Heart, Lung, and Blood Institute publication no. (NIH) 93-3278, September, 1993.

Sane DC, Califf RM, Topol EJ, et al. Bleeding during thrombolytic therapy for acute myocardial infarction: Mechanisms and management. *Ann Intern Med* 111:1010, 1989.

The GUSTO Investigators: An international, randomized trial comparing four thrombolytic strategies for acute myocardial infarction. *N Engl J Med* 329(10):673, 1993.

Weaver WD, Cerqueira M, Hallstrom AP, et al (for the Myocardial Infarction Triage and Intervention Project Group): Prehospital-initiated vs hospital-initiated thrombolytic therapy: The Myocardial Infarction, Triage and Intervention Trial. *JAMA* 270(10):1211, 1993.

Weaver WD, Eisenberg MS, Martin JS, et al: Myocardial infarction triage and intervention project-phase I: Patient characteristics and feasibility of prehospital initiation of thrombolytic therapy. *Am J Cardiol* 69:991, 1992.

Weaver WD, Litwin PE, Martin JS, et al (the MITI Project Group): Effect of age on use of thrombolytic therapy and mortality in acute myocardial infarction. *J Am Coll Cardiol* 18(3):657, 1991.

# 53

# ACUTE INTERVENTIONS IN MYOCARDIAL INFARCTION

## Marcus L. Williams
## David A. Tate

## INTRODUCTION

Coronary artery disease remains the leading cause of death in the United States. In 1987 coronary disease caused 514,000 deaths. It is estimated that more than 1,500,000 persons will suffer an acute myocardial infarction (AMI) each year in the United States alone. Sixty percent will die prior to hospital arrival, and the majority of additional deaths occur during the initial hospitalization. Encouraging trends show that there has been a 47 percent reduction in age-adjusted coronary mortality rates over the past 25 years. In the past decade, with a better understanding of the pathophysiology of coronary syndromes, the diagnosis and treatment of these disorders has radically changed. The focus of therapy is on rapid reperfusion of a totally occluded coronary artery, which makes the emergency room physician's role essential in the initial management of the AMI patient.

## PATHOPHYSIOLOGY

The majority of AMIs are associated with acute thrombotic occlusion of the infarct vessel. Patients with ST elevation on a 12-lead electrocardiogram (ECG), not known to be old, in two or more contiguous leads (i.e., $\geq 1$ mV in limb leads or $\geq 2$ mV in the precordial leads) have a very high probability of acute myocardial infarction. Early coronary angiographic studies of AMI patients with these ECG findings have confirmed this observation, with greater than 90 percent having a total thrombotic occlusion. When a patient presents with ST depression consistent with a non-Q-wave myocardial infarction, the incidence of thrombosis is much lower, estimated to be 60 percent.

Acute coronary syndromes are thought to be caused by an instability of a coronary plaque. It is believed that as the atherosclerotic plaque progresses to a more mature stage of development, it predisposes the endothelial surface to rupture and tear. This can lead to small dissections within the plaque and the formation of thrombosis on the exposed intimal surface, leading to acute occlusion and myocardial ischemia. It has also been shown in animal models that with acute coronary occlusion there is a "wave front" of ischemia that progresses from the subendocardium to the epicardium over a 6-h period. This observation supports the idea that there is a window of opportunity when reperfusion of the occluded coronary artery will have its greatest benefit.

These observations have formed the basis for reperfusion strategies such as the administration of thrombolytic agents or acute angioplasty during AMI. It appears that early reperfusion does salvage ischemic myocardium and preserve left ventricular function. Clinical trials confirm that the greatest preservation of left ventricular function occurs in patients who receive their thrombolytic agent near the onset of their AMI.

## TRIAGE AND PREHOSPITAL TREATMENT

The options for treatment of the AMI patient have become more complex, raising some important issues in the prehospital management of these patients. Since a benefit has been shown with early administration of thrombolytics, it has led to several trials assessing the efficacy of thrombolytic therapy enroute to the hospital. In Seattle, the MITI trial randomized 360 patients to receive tissue plasminogen activator (tPA) either in the field or in the hospital. There was no significant difference seen, with the median time to treatment from symptom onset being 90 min for both groups. The larger European Myocardial Project (EMIP) randomized 4454 patients to infield and hospital treatment. Their median time to treatment was slightly longer at 2 h; however, those treated in the field on average received their treatment an hour earlier. There was a significant 17 percent ($p <.04$) reduction in cardiac mortality at 1 month. A recent pilot study out of Salt Lake City, the FAST-MI pilot study, showed that patients treated in the field received the thrombolytic agent in a shorter period of time with an associated decrease in peak CK and CK-MB and better preservation of left ventricular function. The prehospital treatment of the AMI patient with thrombolytics looks promising and is continuing to be studied; it will be covered in more detail in another section of this book. However, while issues centered around this therapy are being resolved, it is prudent to pretreat suspected high-probability patients with aspirin, oxygen, sublingual nitroglycerin, heparin, and intravenous β blockers when appropriate.

The administration of thrombolytics in the field is not without significant problems. In the MITI trial, of the 2472 patients screened only 27 percent had clinical criteria consistent with an AMI and were candidates for thrombolytic therapy. It is estimated that about 25 percent of all AMI patients will qualify for thrombolytic therapy, which means there is a large group of AMI patients who may require an alternative intervention such as angioplasty in order to establish prompt reperfusion. The limitations in prehospital treatment center around the ability to interpret the ECG. This is dependent on the quality of the field ECG and the training of paramedics, nurses, and physicians to interpret them. Secondly, patient characteristics play an important role in determining whether a patient is a candidate for thrombolytic therapy. The most common reasons for exclusion of patients for thrombolytic therapy have been age (over 75 years), delayed presentation (onset of symptoms greater than 6 h prior to admission), previous cerebrovascular accident, perceived inordinate bleeding risk, or nondiagnostic ECG. Many of these exclusion criteria have recently been reevaluated as discussed below.

The initial presentation and management of the AMI patient in the field can play an important role in driving further in-hospital care. If the AMI patient is not a candidate for thrombolytic therapy, attempts should be made to transfer the patient promptly to a revascularization center where primary coronary angioplasty can be considered. Even after subsequent treatment with a thrombolytic, if patients continue to have ongoing ischemia or show hemodynamic instability, they should be transferred to a major revascularization center for more aggressive management. All patients in cardiogenic shock should be transferred to a revascularization center. Patients in cardiogenic shock have an approximately 80 percent in-hospital mortality, but aggressive therapy including primary angioplasty may decrease that mortality to 50 percent. Thrombolytic therapy appears to have limited impact in this group of patients.

There are three important facets to the treatment of the AMI patient: (1) establish early coronary patency, (2) maintain that patency, and (3) protect ischemic myocardium from further injury. There are three approaches for establishing patency and/or getting adequate distal revascularization: (1) thrombolytic therapy, (2) acute primary coronary angioplasty, or (3) emergent coronary artery bypass surgery. Thrombolysis has become the most commonly used approach because of the ease and speed with which it can be done. Once the infarcted coronary artery has been opened, it is important to keep it open to protect the benefit that has been achieved; therefore anticoagulation therapy becomes important. Finally, the extent of myocardial injury is also dependent on the severity of the imbalance in myocardial oxygen demand versus supply; therefore therapy is directed at reducing this demand and the work of the heart to help protect ischemic

**Fig. 53-1.** Guideline for the management of the AMI patient. It outlines the initial decision process involved in the acute management of these patients. The guideline for management of unstable angina/non-Q-wave myocardial infarction patient is not presented. One of the most critical decision points in the acute management is whether to attempt to establish patency of the occluded coronary vessel by thrombolysis or percutaneous transluminal coronary angioplasty.

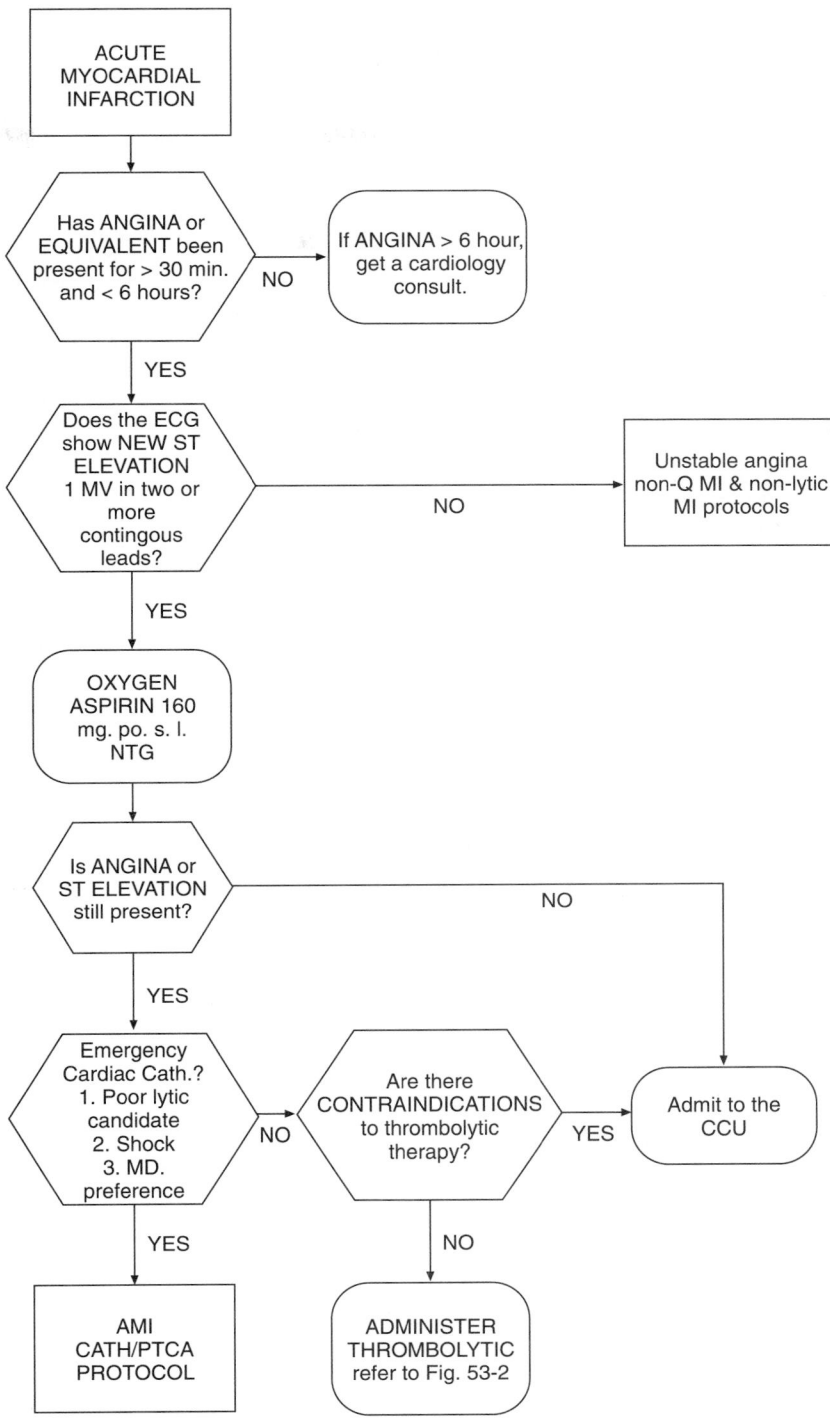

myocardium from further injury. Simple clinical guidelines are presented (Figs. 53-1 and 53-2) to map the decision and treatment processes involved in the management of the AMI patient.

## NONLYTIC PHARMACOLOGIC THERAPY

### Aspirin

Aspirin is a cyclooxygenase inhibitor that binds irreversibly and thereby inhibits platelet aggregation. During the early stages of acute coronary occlusion, the platelet forms the bulk of the clot. The ISIS-2 study randomized 18,000 patients to receive a placebo, low-dose aspirin (160 mg), streptokinase, or a combination of both aspirin and streptokinase. The administration of aspirin alone showed a significant reduction in cardiovascular deaths by 20 percent, and this benefit was additive when combined with streptokinase, yielding a 40 percent reduction in mortality. Aspirin should be considered an essential drug in the acute management of the AMI patient, independent of whether thrombolytic therapy is used. It is preferable to use 160 mg of aspirin, chewed for more rapid onset of effect.

### Nitrates

Nitrates are vasodilators that reduce cardiac preload and, to a lesser extent, afterload, which translates into lower cardiac volume; this reduces wall stress and decreases myocardial oxygen consumption. Nitrates dilate the major capacitance vessels of the coronary system and

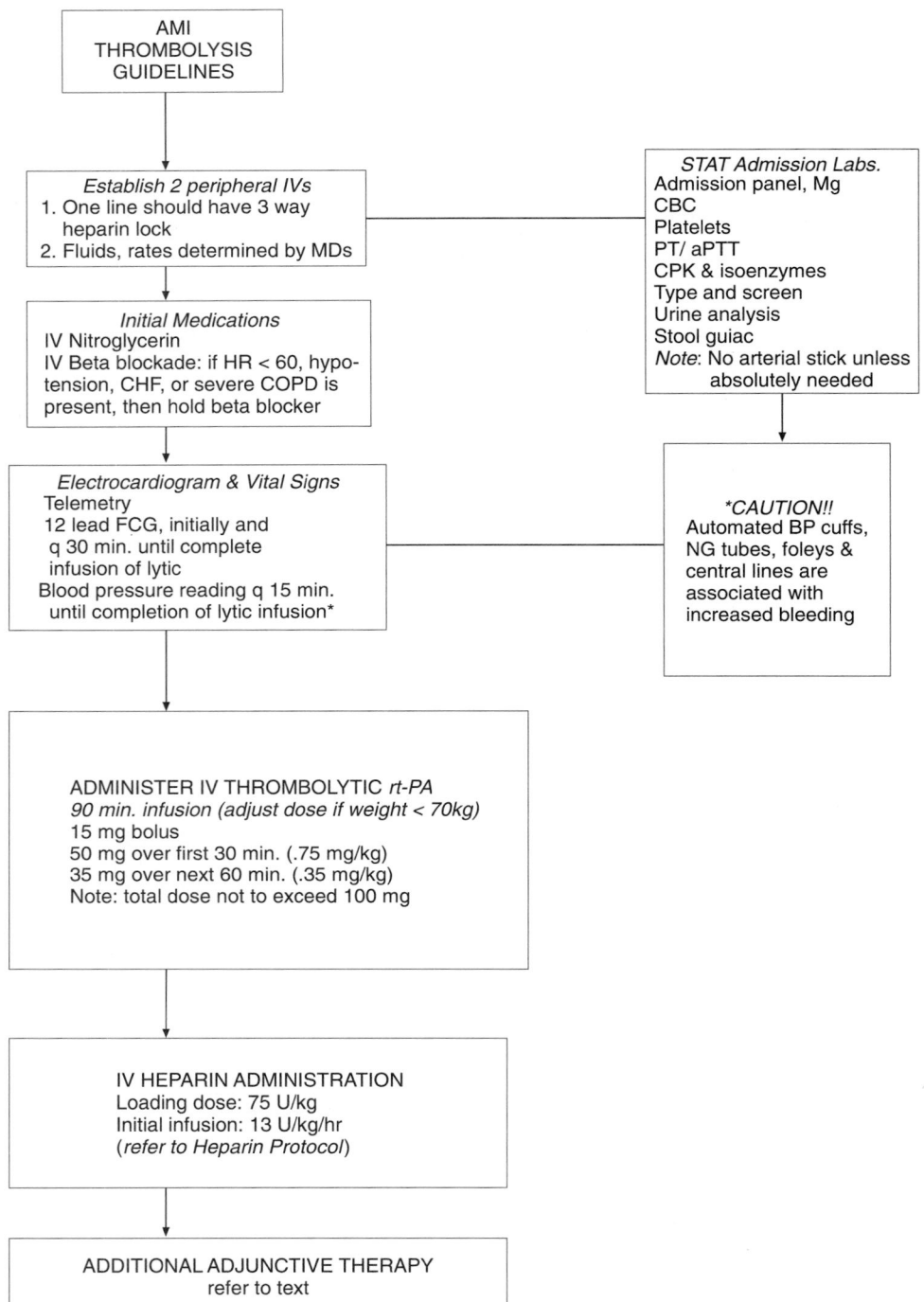

**Fig. 53-2.** Thrombolysis guideline for acute myocardial infarction. The initial medications chosen must be based on the initial presentation and hemodynamic stability of the patient. While there are several thrombolytic agents, we have chosen tPA because of the superior results in the GUSTO trial and to simplify the choices of agents in order to minimize confusion and delays in initiating treatment.

improve collateral blood flow in the myocardium. In addition, nitrates inhibit vasospasm. Based on analysis of pooled studies, clinical trials have shown a 20 to 30 percent reduction in mortality. At initial presentation, all AMI patients should receive sublingual nitroglycerin to relieve symptoms and improve coronary flow. If there is no improvement, then intravenous nitroglycerin should be started and titrated to symptoms and blood pressure. One must avoid using nitrates during hypotension, where mean systemic blood pressure drops, further worsening perfusion of the ischemic myocardium. The most recent ISIS trial, ISIS-4, which is the largest trial evaluating oral nitrates to date, presented data at the 1993 American Heart Association meeting showing no demonstrable benefit over placebo in clinical outcome when oral nitrates were used during the AMI. The benefit of oral nitrates during AMI is less certain.

## β **Blockade**

Beta blockers can reduce both the short- and long-term mortality in patients with AMI. More than 28 randomized studies involving more than 27,000 patients have demonstrated a 14 percent reduction in mortality when acute β blockade was used during the AMI (3.7 versus 4.3 percent). The ISIS-1 trial randomized 16,000 AMI patients to receive placebo or intravenous atenolol and showed a 15 percent reduction in 7-day mortality (3.9 versus 4.6 percent, $p < .05$). Almost all of this benefit was seen within the first 24 h of presentation and subsequently remained constant. Further analysis suggests that this early benefit may have been attributed to a lower incidence of cardiac rupture. The Metoprolol in Acute Myocardial Infarction (MIAMI) trial found an overall 13 percent reduction in mortality for patients given intravenous metoprolol acutely ($p = .29$). Subgroup analysis revealed a significant mortality reduction (29 percent, $p = .033$) in patients at "high risk." The factors favoring benefit from intravenous β blockade were age > 60, hypertension, diabetes, *history of heart failure,* prior infarction or angina, and diuretic use. The greatest benefits in reduction of infarct size and mortality were seen in those treated within 8 h of their initial symptoms. The TIMI-II trial showed that in 3200 patients the early use of β blockers compared to its delayed use resulted in a 37 percent decrease in recurrent ischemic events and a 50 percent reduction of reinfarction.

The mechanism is thought to be a reduction in myocardial oxygen demand caused by decrease in contractility and myocardial wall tension. Beta blockade lowers the heart rate and blood pressure, which decreases the overall workload of the heart. By slowing the heart rate, the diastolic period is prolonged and this improves coronary perfusion.

The benefit of β blockade in AMI had been shown with several classes (both cardioselective and nonselective) in prior studies. Given a choice, it is recommended that one use β blockers without intrinsic sympathomimetic activity (i.e., Lopressor, metoprolol, or Inderal). Generally accepted guidelines for the use of early intravenous β blockade include:

*Indicated/effective:*

1. Patients who are having a transmural myocardial infarction, defined by the ECG by ST elevation and new Q waves. Patients receiving thrombolytic therapy or with reflex tachycardia or systolic hypertension without signs of congestive heart failure or other contraindications to β blockers are candidates.
2. Patients with continuing or recurrent ischemic pain, and those with tachyarrhythmias such as atrial fibrillation with a rapid ventricular response.

*Uncertain efficacy/probable benefit:*

1. Patients presenting more than 6 h after symptom onset
2. Non-Q-wave AMIs

*Contraindications to β blockade:*

1. Heart rate < 60 beats/min
2. Systolic blood pressure < 100 mmHg
3. Moderate to severe left ventricular dysfunction
4. Signs of peripheral hypoperfusion
5. Type I and II second-degree AV block
6. Severe chronic obstructive pulmonary disease

*Relative contraindications to β blockade:*

1. History of asthma
2. Severe peripheral vascular disease
3. Concurrent use of calcium channel blockers (verapamil or diltiazem)
4. Difficult-to-control insulin-dependent diabetes
5. First-degree AV block

The doses of β blocker incorporated in these studies were significant, and the potential risk must be recognized. Only a subset of AMI patients will make good candidates for β-blocker therapy. The TIMI-II trial excluded more than 50 percent of its AMI patients due to contraindications.

## Calcium Channel Blockers

Calcium channel antagonists have been used extensively in patients with chronic and unstable angina. These agents have been shown to reduce coronary vasospasm, improve collateral flow, lower blood pressure, and decrease myocardial contractility. In addition, verapamil and diltiazem are excellent drugs for supraventricular tachy-arrhythmias because they control the ventricular response. However, despite these properties there has been no clear benefit shown for calcium channel antagonists in the treatment of the AMI patient.

Clinical studies show conflicting reports on the efficacy of calcium channel antagonists used during AMI. There are at least 21 trials evaluating the early administration of calcium channel antagonists for AMI, which have involved over 18,000 patients. Trials using nifedipine have shown either no benefit or a trend toward increased cardiac mortality and morbidity. The Secondary Prevention Reinfarction Israeli Nifedipine (SPRINT-2) trial, which utilized nifedipine early and then continued treatment following discharge, was stopped prematurely due to a disturbing increase in mortality among patients receiving nifedipine. The use of verapamil was evaluated extensively in the Danish Verapamil Infarction Trials (DAVIT). The DAVIT-1 study needed to exclude 52 percent of presenting patients, and of those patients randomized, only 41 percent fulfilled criteria for AMI. In those patients who fulfilled the AMI criteria, no significant difference in mortality was detected at 12 months. The largest diltiazem trial evaluated patients who received diltiazem or placebo 3 to 15 days following their AMI. The results failed to demonstrate a difference in mortality or reinfarction. Subgroup analysis did indicate a mortality benefit for patients without pulmonary congestion who received diltiazem. This benefit was offset by an increase in mortality in patients who received diltiazem and who had pulmonary congestion. The one possible exception for the use of a calcium channel antagonist may be the use of verapamil for rate control of atrial fibrillation during an AMI.

## Intravenous Magnesium

Magnesium is thought to work by inhibiting calcium influx into the ischemic myocardial cell and by more rapid regeneration of the magnesium-bound ATP, which is rapidly depleted in the ischemic myocardium. There has also been evidence of its benefit as an anti-arrhythmic. These observations have led to an interest in using intravenous magnesium to treat AMI. There have been numerous studies during the past decade evaluating the effect of intravenous magnesium given to AMI patients. The two most influential have been the Second Leicester Intravenous Magnesium Intervention Trial (LIMIT-2), and a meta-analysis of seven small randomized trials. Both reports suggested a benefit in the reduction of cardiac mortality (a 30 to 40 percent decrease in mortality) with the infusion of intravenous magnesium during the acute infarction phase, defined as the first 48 h. The benefit of intravenous magnesium remains uncertain because of the most recent report by the ISIS-4 study group at the 1993 American Heart Association meeting. Over 50,000 patients were randomized, and no clear benefit was seen for the intravenous magnesium group when compared to placebo. Currently the role for intravenous magnesium remains in question. The risk of therapy and cost in dollars is minimal, therefore in selected patients it still may be used. Patients experiencing complex ventricular arrhythmias or who have hypomagnesemia may be the best potential candidates.

## Prophylactic Lidocaine

Intravenous and intramuscular lidocaine given prophylactically (not associated with significant ventricular arrhythmias) for patients with AMI has been common practice in prior years. The goal was to reduce the incidence of life-threatening ventricular dysrhythmias, such as ventricular fibrillation and ventricular tachycardia, during the first 24 to 48 h following an AMI. There have been at least 14 randomized trials conducted, but only one has been able to show a significant reduction in ventricular fibrillation and none has demonstrated a mortality benefit. This has been attributed to the small trial sizes. An overview of the trials of prophylactic lidocaine, while limited by the unavailability of some data, indicates a reduction in ventricular fibrillation of 33 percent, but an increase of fatal asystole by 50 percent.

There was a nonstatistical trend toward an increase in overall mortality. Although no definitive conclusions can be made on the existing data, the beneficial effect of a decreasing ventricular fibrillation with prophylactic lidocaine may be out-weighed by the harmful increase in fatal asystolic events.

Certain patients may be more likely to benefit from, or be harmed by, prophylactic lidocaine. Patients presenting early (< 6 h) in the course of an acute myocardial infarction, who are less than 60 years old, are at higher risk of ventricular fibrillation and are less likely to be affected negatively by lidocaine and, therefore, may benefit. Conversely, elderly patients presenting later in their infarction are less likely to have ventricular fibrillation and more likely to develop asystolic complications relating to lidocaine therapy. In patients who demonstrate complex ventricular arrhythmias during the acute infarction phase, intravenous lidocaine is appropriate. Complex ventricular arrhythmias are defined as three or more consecutive ventricular beats at a rate greater than 120 beats per minute, ventricular fibrillation or a recent history, or frequent multiform premature ventricular contractions.

## Heparin

The independent effect of heparin on mortality reduction in the AMI patient has been hard to evaluate. When 600 patients were randomized to heparin versus no heparin in the pilot study performed prior to the ISIS-2 trial, there was a trend toward a benefit with a risk reduction of 27 percent versus 12 percent with no heparin. A twofold increase in bleeding was seen in those treated with heparin, but the data suggested that bolus intravenous heparin given early in the evolution of AMI may be a safe and effective alternative to thrombolytic therapy.

The use of postinfarction heparin has been more clearly shown to be of benefit. In addition to the risk of acute coronary thrombosis, there is the risk of developing left ventricular mural thrombus within the first 5 days of a large infarct, especially anterior infarctions. The SCATI group randomized 360 AMI patients to 12,500 units of heparin subcutaneously twice daily versus 351 patients with no heparin. While there was no difference in reinfarction rate, there was a significantly lower mortality (21 of 360 versus 35 of 351; $p < .03$).

Heparinization has become an essential adjunct to thrombolytic therapy when tPA is used because of the higher patency rates observed in those who receive it. Bleich et al. found the patency rate of tPA to be 70 percent in the heparin-treated group compared to 43 percent in the nonheparinized group. The Hart trial found a similar result, emphasizing the importance of adequate heparinization in maintaining early patency. Hsia and coworkers showed that patency correlated with activated partial prothrombin time (aPTT) prolongation in tPA-treated patients. Those patients with aPTT < 45 s had a patency of 45 percent; if > 45 s, it was 88 percent; and if > 60 s, it was 95 percent, suggesting that the higher the aPTT, the higher the patency rate in this group of patients. These findings were based on results obtained within the first 12 h. The data suggested that inadequate heparinization in the first 12 h could lead to lower patency rates in patients treated with tPA.

For streptokinase, the early reocclusion rate is much lower. The GUSTO trial showed a 90-min patency of 56 percent, compared to 81 percent for tPA. Over the next 24 h the patency rate increases for streptokinase, which is attributed to its longer half-life. The role of intravenous heparin in patients receiving streptokinase is unclear. The recent GUSTO trial found no additional benefit to using intravenous heparin when compared to subcutaneous heparin. Therefore, intravenous heparin should be reserved for patients with large anteroseptal infarction, recurrent ischemia, and other conditions that warrant higher and more constant aPTT.

An important fact when using heparin is the adequacy of heparinization, which is dependent on appropriate dosing. A study con-

**Table 53-1.** Heparin Dosing Nomogram

*Loading Dose:*  75 units/kg rounded to the nearest 100 units
*Initial Maintenance Infusion:*  13 units/kg/hour rounded to the nearest 100 units/hour
*Maintenance Infusion Adjustment:*  Measure aPTT six hours after initiating the maintenance infusion and adjust as follows:

| aPTT (sec) | Bolus (units) | Stop Infusion (minutes) | Rate Change (units/hour) | Repeat aPTT |
|---|---|---|---|---|
| <40 | 5000 | 0 | +200 | 6h |
| 40–54 | 0 | 0 | +100 | 6h |
| 55–95 | 0 | 0 | 0 | next AM |
| 96–120 | 0 | 30 | −100 | 6h |
| >120 | 0 | 60 | −200 | 6h |

*Additional Routine Monitoring:*  Hematocrit (daily)
Platelet count (every 3 days)
Guaiac all stools
Visual check for hematuria

*Note:* This heparin nomogram was developed and tested at our hospital. It was adapted from the *Arch Intern Med* 151:333, 1991. It has been accepted for publication in the *Arch Intern Med* for 1994.

ducted at the University of North Carolina Hospitals at Chapel Hill found that over 25 percent of patients' aPTT values were not within the therapeutic range during the first 24 h of therapy with intravenous heparin. A weight-based heparin nomogram was developed to minimize the time to therapeutic dosing in patients requiring intravenous heparin (see Table 53-1). Adherence to the nomogram significantly reduced the number of patients out of the therapeutic range at 24 h to 8.8 percent (a 65 percent reduction).

Heparin adjustments during the first 12 h following thrombolysis should only be to increase a low aPTT value and not to decrease a high value due to the enhanced thrombolytic effect. After 12 h, the normal adjustments as indicated by the nomogram should be followed.

## THROMBOLYTIC THERAPY FOR AMI

Early initiation of thrombolytic therapy in the appropriate patient is now considered the standard of care according to both the American Heart Association and the American College of Cardiology. Numerous studies have shown that thrombolytic therapy increases reperfusion of the occluded coronary artery, salvages ischemic myocardium, and reduces mortality. There is no clear clinical advantage of one thrombolytic agent over another. The timely administration of the thrombolytic has a more powerful impact on patient outcomes than the choice of thrombolytic. Since thrombolytic therapy has potentially very serious side effects, the appropriate selection of candidates is very important.

The specific inclusion and exclusion criteria have been used by the major clinical trials and continue to evolve. Because of these criteria, approximately 20 to 25 percent of all AMI patients presenting to the emergency room will actually receive thrombolytics. This means that for the majority of AMI patients the optimum method of reperfusion has yet to be defined. Many of the criteria mentioned are supported with very little or no scientific data.

### Patient Selection for Thrombolytic Therapy

#### Indications

The indications for treatment of AMI with thrombolytics are based on the initial ECG and the presenting symptoms. Patients with chest pain and new ST elevations on a 12-lead ECG in two or more contiguous leads (i.e., ≥ 1 mV in the limb leads or ≥ 2 mV in the precordial leads) with new Q waves have a very high probability of AMI. If the patient presents within the first 6 h of the onset of symptoms and there are no contraindications to thrombolytics, they should promptly receive thrombolytics.

## Contraindications to Thrombolysis

The most important contraindication to thrombolytic therapy is an increased risk of bleeding (Table 53-2). The most catastrophic event is an acute intracranial hemorrhage, which has an in-hospital mortality of 50 percent. The overall incidence of intracranial hemorrhage is low, at less than 1 percent in large clinical trials. Both the ISIS-3 and the GUSTO trial show that the risk of intracranial hemorrhage is twice as high for tPA compared to streptokinase. Several factors have been associated with the increased risk for intracerebral bleeds. Gore et al. showed that higher doses of tPA were associated with increase bleeding. Jaeger and coworkers found that patients with body weight < 70 kg were at increased risk of bleeding. This was attributed to the relatively higher dose to body weight ratio. Other factors associated with increased intracerebral bleeding were hypertension, prior history of cerebral vascular disease, and patients receiving anticoagulation at admission.

There are also relative contraindications (see Table 53-2), where clinical judgment must be used in weighing risk versus benefit. The relative benefit of thrombolysis is likely to be less with "small" versus "large" infarctions; inferior versus anterior infarctions; and if given relatively late. For instance, advanced age itself should not be considered a contraindication to thrombolytic therapy, but many studies have excluded patients over 75 years old, so fewer data are available in this patient population. While complications may be higher in such patients, their absolute mortality is highest so they also stand to gain the most benefit from thrombolytic therapy. This example illustrates the need to individualize the decision to use thrombolytics in patients with relative contraindications.

The most common reasons for exclusion from thrombolytic therapy in order of occurrence include delayed presentation, nondiagnostic ECG changes, age, stroke, and/or inordinate bleeding risk. Those patients who are excluded from therapy have universally higher in-hospital mortality.

**Table 53-2.** Contraindications to Thrombolysis

| Absolute | Relative |
|---|---|
| Active bleeding | Advanced age (>75 years) |
| History of cerebrovascular event* (i.e., any cva < 2 months, any hemorrhagic cva) | Puncture of a non-compressible blood vessel (<10 days) |
| Recent intracranial or spinal surgery or trauma (<2 months) | Uncontrolled hypertension (sys. BP >180 mmHg or dys. >110 mmHG) |
| Intracranial disease (i.e., neoplasm, aneurysm) | Diabetic hemorrhagic opthalmic conditions |
| Severe uncontrolled hypertension (sys. BP >180 mmHg or dia. BP >110 mmHg) | Anticoagulated (prothrombin time >15 sec.) |
| Known bleeding diathesis | Advance liver/kidney disease |
| Active internal bleeding (<10 days) | Any pathology predisposing to bleeding |
| Recent trauma, major surgery or biopsy at a non-compressible site (<10 days) | Active peptic ulcer disease |
| | Left ventricular thrombus |
| | Infectious endocarditis |
| Pericarditis | Remote embolic or thrombotic CVA or TIA events* |
| Women known to be or suspected of being pregnant | |

*There is some controversy about whether CVA and TIA should be an absolute contraindication. Remote embolic or thrombotic CVA events (> 6 months) are thought to be at a lower bleeding risk compared to recent events within the last 6 months. It is the window between 2 and 6 months after a CVA that safety has not been clarified. Patients with a remote history are safely being treated with thrombolytics at some centers.

## Late Thrombolytic Therapy

There is evidence that patients receiving thrombolytic therapy 6 h or later after onset of symptoms may still benefit clinically. The GISSI trial found a trend toward lower mortality for patients treated up to 24 h after onset of their symptoms. The Late Assessment of Thrombolytic Efficacy (LATE) trial randomized 5711 AMI patients treated with tPA between 6 h and 24 h after onset of chest pain. For patients treated within 12 h, there was a significant 27 percent reduction in mortality (8.9 percent versus 11.97 percent; $p = .023$), and a non-significant trend toward reduction in mortality was observed for those treated after 12 h (8.7 percent versus 9.2 percent; $p = NS$). However, the LATE trial showed a stroke rate twice as high in tPA-treated patients as in those receiving placebo. There were reports of increased incidence of cardiac rupture and a greater hazard of early death due to congestive heart failure. Therefore, patients who are at increased risk for intracerebral bleeding or who have very poor left ventricular function may share a higher risk of complications secondary to thrombolytic therapy. The decision to treat must be individualized based on the judgment of the clinician. Patients who present between 6 and 12 h after the onset of their symptoms are in a phase of their AMI in which it is less critically dependent on minimizing delays in treatment compared to the initial 6 h. A cardiology consultation may be appropriate before initiating late thrombolytic therapy in these patients.

## Thrombolytic Agents

There are four thrombolytic agents presently being used. They are streptokinase, tissue plasminogen activator (tPA, Activase), anisolated plasminogen streptokinase activator complex (APSAC), and urokinase. The two most commonly used agents are tPA and streptokinase. All four agents differ to some degree in their fibrin specificity, duration of action, potential allergic reactions, efficacy, and cost.

### Streptokinase

Streptokinase activates circulating plasminogen and therefore does not possess fibrin specificity. It is derived from β hemolytic streptococci and is capable of generating an antigenic response. An allergic reaction such as pruritus, rash, and low-grade fevers can occur in about 5 percent, especially in patients who have had a recent streptococcal infection. This is usually self-limiting and responds to antihistamines. Less than 0.2 percent of the time does a serious anaphylaxis episode occur.

The dose is 1.5 million units over 60 min, which produces systemic fibrinolysis that persist for up to 24 h. Antibodies may develop about 5 days after treatment and persist for 6 months; therefore, retreatment with streptokinase (or related compounds, such as APSAC) is not recommended. During the administration of streptokinase, hypotension is seen in about 15 percent of patients, which improves by decreasing the rate of infusion and by volume expansion.

Streptokinase is one of the most well studied thrombolytics available and currently the least expensive.

### Anisoylated Plasminogen Streptokinase Activator Complex (APSAC)

APSAC/Eminase is a second-generation thrombolytic agent that was developed to overcome some of the limitations of streptokinase. This drug is administered as a single bolus over 5 min and requires no prolonged infusion. Its side-effect profile is very similar to streptokinase, with a slightly lower incident of allergic reactions. It has a much longer pharmacologic half-life at 90 min so that the systemic lytic state is longer. The efficacy of this drug is similar to streptokinase. The ISIS-3 trial found that mortality was similar for APSAC, streptokinase, and tPA. APSAC did not appear to be clinically superior to the other two thrombolytics, and its advantage in the ease of administration did not translate into better outcomes. Since it costs two to three times more than streptokinase there has been no good rationale for recommending it as a first-line choice for a thrombolytic agent.

## Urokinase

Urokinase is a proteolytic enzyme produced from human fetal kidney tissue cultures. Urokinase has been approved for intracoronary administration, but its role in intravenous administration has yet to be defined. The standard dose is 3 million units (over 1 h, with 1.5 million units given as a bolus) and usually achieves systemic fibrinolysis. Allergic reactions and hypotension are very unusual with urokinase. Severe shaking chills can occasionally occur and respond to intravenous meperidine and diphenhydramine. It has similar efficacy to streptokinase, while its cost is much higher.

## Tissue Plasminogen Activator

Tissue plasminogen activator is a naturally occurring human protein without antigenic properties, which is now derived from recombinant DNA technology. The pharmacologic half life of tPA is 5 min, and it is fibrin-specific. It binds to the serine amino acid on the fibrin molecule, which activates tPA so that it converts the local plasminogen to plasmin. There is less depletion of the circulating fibrinogen compared to streptokinase. The advantages of tPA are its lack of antigenicity and the possibility of subsequent allergic reactions. It has a significantly higher early reperfusion rate when compared to streptokinase, but its reocclusion rate is higher and heparin is required to maintain the initial early patency benefit. tPA is one of the most costly thrombolytics on the market.

### tPA Dosing

There are several studies that have looked at front-loaded tPA and weight-adjusted dosing and found no increase in adverse events when compared to the traditional dosing of tPA. This was supported in the large GUSTO trial, which used front-loaded and weight-adjusted dosing. Wall's team looked at five different dosing regimens for tPA and found that the front-loaded and weight-adjusted dose given over 90 min was associated with a superior patency rate of 83 percent at 90 min and a reocclusion rate of 4 percent, with no increase bleeding risk. The TAPS investigators compared front-loaded tPA to APSAC and found the 90-min coronary patency rate was 84 percent for tPA versus 70.3 percent for APSAC ($p = .0007$), with a trend toward lower mortality and lower incidence of recurrent ischemic events and bleeding. The RAAMI investigators compared front-loaded tPA with 90-min infusion to the standard 3-h infusion for AMI and found the patency rate at 60 min was higher, at 76 percent versus 63 percent. Front-loaded tPA can be safely given, and recent data suggest that early patency may be better. Therefore, the recommended dose is a 15-mg bolus followed by 50 mg or 0.75 mg/kg, whichever is lowest, over the next 30 min, followed by 35 mg or 0.35 mg/kg, whichever is lowest, for the next hour. The total dose should not exceed 100 mg (see Fig. 53-2).

## Comparison of Thrombolytic Agents

The GUSTO trial represents the most recent and largest thrombolytic clinical trial to date. It was designed to compare four treatment strategies: streptokinase and subcutaneous heparin; streptokinase and intravenous heparin; tPA and intravenous heparin; and streptokinase plus tPA and intravenous heparin. In spite of a higher incidence of intracerebral bleeding (0.94 percent versus 0.52 percent), the mortality rate for tPA treatment group was 14 percent lower than the combined streptokinase treatment arms (6.3 percent versus 7.3 percent). The angiographic substudy within GUSTO suggested that the mortality advantage with tPA was due to significantly improved early coronary

artery patency compared to streptokinase. This is the first study to demonstrate a relationship of improved outcome to early coronary patency, lending support to the open-artery hypothesis. It appears that tPA with intravenous heparin may be slightly more efficacious when compared to streptokinase. However, this difference is small, and what is more important is administering a thrombolytic agent in a timely fashion to the appropriate AMI patient.

## INDICATIONS FOR TEMPORARY PACING

With the use of thrombolytics in the AMI patient, there is an increased bleeding risk associated with invasive procedures. Therefore, the placement of central cannulas can pose a significant bleeding risk and should only be performed with clear indications. In addition to the bleeding risk, the temporary pacemaker has been associated with the induction of arrhythmias, new right bundle branch block (7 to 25 percent), ventricular perforation (especially in right ventricular infarcts), pneumothorax, hemothorax, and infection. There has been no benefit shown in prophylactic temporary pacing; however, there are life-threatening bradyarrhythmias, ventricular tachycardias, and bundle branch blocks for which temporary pacing is indicated. Refer to Table 53-3 for generally accepted indications.

In emergent situations, the external temporary pacer can help to bridge the interval during which a central temporary pacer is placed. In nonemergent situations, the use of the external temporary pacer may be adequate. Temporary pacemakers (not external systems) can also be used to overdrive pace ventricular tachycardia and some types of atrial arrhythmias (atrial flutter) as well as medically refractory torsade de pointes (polymorphic ventricular tachycardia). When ventricular function is severely compromised, particularly in the setting of an acute right ventricular infarct, sequential AV pacing may improve output. This is attributed to the atrial augmentation and, at times, the increased heart rate, which improves cardiac output.

**Table 53-3.** Temporary Pacemaker Indications During Acute Myocardial Infarction

---

*Pacemaker therapy not required*
Asymptotic bradycardia
First-degree AV block
Second-degree AV block (Wenckebach, Mobitz type I)
Preexistent bifascicular block
Accelerated idioventricular rhythm causing AV dissociation

*Pacemaker therapy required*
Symptomatic bradyarrhythmias without escape rhythm
Second-degree AV block (Mobitz type II)*
Third-degree AV block (complete heart block)*
New RBBB & LAFB
New RBBB & LPFB
New LBBB & first-degree AV block
Alternating bundle branch block
Asystole
Atrial or Ventricular overdrive for incessant atrial flutter or ventricular
    tachycardia (i.e. torsade de pointes)
Hemodynamically unstable bradyarrhythmias†

*Pacemaker therapy controversial*
New RBBB
New LBBB

---

*Note:* This table presents the indications for a temporary pacemaker in patients having an acute myocardial infarction. Primarily, it will be patients with evolving fasicular blocks, high grade heart block and hemodynamically destabilizing bradyarrhythmias, who will need a temporary pacemaker. The potential benefit of a temporary pacemaker must be weighed against the potential complications which may occur during its placement.

*†Except in some cases of hemodynamically stable inferior wall myocardial.

† In order to maintain an adequate cardiac output, sometimes the heart rate must be increased. Also some patients are dependent on their atrial kick to maintain a good cardiac output and more stable hemodynamics.

# PERCUTANEOUS TRANSLUMINAL CORONARY ANGIOPLASTY FOR AMI

## Background and Rationale

A wealth of data, most of it from the thrombolysis literature as discussed above, is now available that emphasizes the preeminent importance of reestablishing coronary patency in the patient with AMI. The application of thrombolytic therapy to achieve this goal has led to major advances in the care of these patients. From the earliest experience with thrombolytic therapy, however, there have been concerns about its limitations. Using even the most effective thrombolytic regimens, approximately 20 percent of patients will not achieve coronary patency within 90 min. Moreover, of those in whom patency is achieved, about 40 percent will have delayed flow beyond the site of stenosis, a situation which now appears to confer a prognosis only marginally better than those who are not successfully reperfused at all. Additionally, the vast majority of patients treated with thrombolytic therapy are left with significant residual coronary stenosis, and the incidence of recurrent ischemia and infarction is substantial. Finally, thrombolytic therapy continues to be associated with a substantial incidence of bleeding complications (including intracranial hemorrhage), and, largely for this reason, a large number of patients with myocardial infarction are not eligible for thrombolytic therapy.

Given these limitations, a possible role for percutaneous transluminal coronary angioplasty (PTCA) in the treatment of acute myocardial infarction has long been considered. Angioplasty during the acute phase of myocardial infarction has been applied in three different ways, and the terminology has often been confusing. Either *immediate angioplasty* or *adjunctive angioplasty* has generally been the term used to describe angioplasty that is used in conjunction with, and immediately following, thrombolytic therapy. That is, with immediate, or adjunctive, PTCA, patients are given initial intravenous thrombolytic therapy and then taken to the cardiac catheterization laboratory for angiography and possible angioplasty if persistent occlusion and/or high-grade stenosis remains. The term *rescue angioplasty* has been applied to the use of coronary angioplasty in selected patients in whom thrombolytic therapy has been administered but has not been successful in restoring patency. Either *primary* or *direct angioplasty* has been applied to angioplasty when used as the initial reperfusion strategy, that is, utilizing mechanical revascularization instead of the administration of thrombolytic agents. The potential role for each of these approaches will be discussed in the sections below.

## Immediate (Adjunctive) Angioplasty

This strategy of utilization of angioplasty in AMI was the first to be tested in randomized clinical trials. The rationale that gave rise to these trials was compelling and rested primarily on the observation that approximately one-fourth of patients treated with thrombolytic therapy were not successfully reperfused within 90 min and, even among those who were reperfused, most were left with high-grade stenosis. It was reasonable to presume that identifying such patients with immediate coronary angiography and then proceeding to angioplasty might be of benefit. The three randomized trials were the Thrombolysis in Myocardial Infarction (TIMI) IIA trial, the European Cooperative Study Group trial, and the Thrombolysis and Angioplasty in Myocardial Infarction (TAMI) 1 trial. In all three studies, the use of immediate, adjunctive angioplasty was associated with an increased incidence of bleeding complications and a greater need for urgent bypass operation. No significant differences were found in left ventricular function, recurrent ischemia, or recurrent infarction. Finally, the European trial demonstrated a statistically significant increase in mortality with adjunctive angioplasty, and the other two trials showed a trend in that direction. These studies have caused most clinicians to abandon the routine use of immediate coronary angio-

plasty following thrombolytic therapy. However, the fact that coronary angiography and angioplasty were coupled in all three of these studies leaves unanswered the question of whether coronary angiography alone could potentially have a role in defining a more select subset of patients who might benefit from mechanical intervention. Nevertheless, these studies have appropriately dissuaded clinicians from routinely proceeding to the catheterization laboratory following thrombolytic therapy. The issue of taking a much more select group of patients to the catheterization laboratory is a complex one and is discussed next.

## Rescue Angioplasty

Rescue angioplasty refers to angioplasty used selectively in patients who have not reperfused with thrombolytic therapy. The major clinical and investigational problem with this approach has been the inability to determine by noninvasive means whether patency has been achieved. Thus, the potentially beneficial strategy of rescue angioplasty requires cardiac catheterization in all of the patients in order to determine the approximately one-quarter of them who have not been reperfused. Thus, the benefits of rescue angioplasty in the minority of patients must outweigh the risks of cardiac catheterization in the entire cohort of patients. This area is still under active investigation. The TAMI 5 trial was a double randomization to one of three thrombolytic regimens and to either immediate cardiac catheterization with possible rescue angioplasty or routine predischarge catheterization and angioplasty. In this trial of 595 patients, the immediate catheterization and potential rescue strategy was associated with improved wall motion in the infarct region and fewer adverse outcomes. A multicenter trial examining rescue angioplasty is currently in progress (Randomized Evaluation of Salvage Angioplasty with Combined Utilization of Endpoints). At the present time, the authors' opinion is that rescue angioplasty should be reserved for selected patients in whom the clinician believes a high likelihood of persistent occlusion or reocclusion is present and in whom there is a likelihood of a substantial benefit from more aggressive attempts to obtain patency. For example, although neither persistence of chest pain or persistent ST-segment elevation has correlated well with coronary patency, it would seem reasonable to consider coronary angiography with potential rescue angioplasty in the small subset of patients with very large anterior infarctions, hemodynamic instability, persistent severe chest pain, and persistent marked ST-segment elevation. With respect to the location of the infarction, patients with large, anterior infarctions probably have the most to gain from aggressive therapies, as compared to patients with inferior myocardial infarctions in whom it has been suggested that rescue angioplasty may be associated with an increased risk of adverse outcomes.

## Primary Angioplasty

Primary angioplasty, or direct angioplasty, refers to a management strategy in which emergent coronary angiography and subsequent angioplasty replaces thrombolytic therapy. This reperfusion strategy has been utilized by a number of practitioners and investigators in recent years, largely in response to the limitations of thrombolytic therapy as discussed above. While there were no randomized trials to support this practice until recently, a number of large, nonrandomized case series were compiled that suggested that primary angioplasty may be an attractive alternative to thrombolytic therapy. In the largest of these studies, by O'Keefe and colleagues, 500 consecutive patients with AMI were treated by primary angioplasty. The procedure was successful in achieving patency and reducing stenosis to less than 40 percent in 94 percent of patients. In-hospital mortality was relatively low at 7.2 percent, particularly given the broad spectrum of patients treated, including 17 percent who were older than 70 years of age and 8 percent with cardiogenic shock. In the more select subset of patients who would have met criteria for TIMI thrombolysis trials at the time, the mortality was a very impressive 1.8 percent. The incidence of significant bleeding was reported as 3 percent, and no strokes were identified. A number of smaller case series have demonstrated similar results.

These impressive nonrandomized trials prompted three randomized studies, which were published simultaneously in 1993. The largest of these was the Primary Angioplasty in Myocardial Infarction (PAMI) trial. In this multicenter study of 395 patients with AMI, patients were randomized between primary angioplasty or therapy with tPA and followed for a combined endpoint of reinfarction or death. The study showed a statistically significant difference in favor of PTCA, with reinfarction or death in 12 percent of tPA-treated patients as compared to 5.1 percent of patients treated with PTCA. In addition, there were more recurrent ischemia and more intracranial bleeding in the tPA-treated group. The second trial by Zijlstra and colleagues randomized 142 patients between therapy with angioplasty or streptokinase. This smaller trial revealed statistically significant differences with respect to recurrent ischemia, coronary patency, and left ventricular function, all favoring angioplasty. The third trial by Gibbons and colleagues involved 103 patients randomized between angioplasty and tPA. This smaller trial utilized sestamibi (a perfusion agent) to evaluate for differences in myocardial salvage. While there was no statistically significant difference in myocardial salvage demonstrated by angioplasty, this study again revealed clinical trends suggesting that angioplasty was associated with less recurrent ischemia or subsequent need for revascularization. Finally, cost analyses from both the PAMI trial and the Gibbons study suggest that primary angioplasty may result in shorter hospital stays and lower overall costs.

It should be emphasized, however, that the randomized data supporting the use of primary angioplasty for myocardial infarction remain fairly limited, with less than 1000 patients studied compared to the many thousands of patients who have been studied in randomized fashion in the thrombolysis studies. Nevertheless, both the randomized and nonrandomized studies have been impressive and suggest that primary angioplasty is a reasonable alternative to thrombolytic therapies in hospitals that are equipped with a 24-h catheterization laboratory and an experienced angioplasty team. Whether the excellent results obtained in the high-volume, very experienced centers will be broadly attainable is yet to be seen.

In the interim, the authors suggest that angioplasty be considered as an alternative to thrombolytic therapy in centers that are adequately equipped and staffed, particularly in patients at highest risk, for example, those with large anterior myocardial infarctions. In addition, we would suggest that primary angioplasty is the treatment of choice in three specific subsets. The first subset is patients who present with AMI and cardiogenic shock. The mortality in this subset of patients has long been approximately 80 percent and has not been appreciably altered with any conventional therapy, including thrombolytic therapy. Given this dismal outcome, a number of clinicians began using primary angioplasty in these patients in the mid 1980s. While only historical controls are available, several studies have suggested that an aggressive strategy of care including rapid primary angioplasty may reduce in-hospital mortality in these patients to approximately 50 percent. The second subset of patients are those who have an uncertain diagnosis or an equivocal ECG. Rapidly proceeding to coronary angiography can identify which of these patients do in fact have coronary occlusion, and angioplasty can then be utilized to reestablish coronary patency. This may frequently occur, for example, with left circumflex coronary occlusions, for which the ECG may often be nondiagnostic or may be difficult to distinguish between anterior ischemia or posterior infarction. Finally, we believe that primary angioplasty is certainly an important alternative in the large subset of patients in whom one would like to give thrombolytic therapy but who have a contraindication.

It is likely that some of the improved outcome ascribed to primary angioplasty is not due to primary angioplasty per se but to other factors inherent in this approach. The immediate coronary angiography allows a sort of invasive "triage" of patients to appropriate therapy. Patients in whom a moderate-to-large coronary artery is occluded may then proceed to angioplasty as planned. Patients who are found to have severe three-vessel coronary disease or left main coronary disease may proceed to bypass surgery. Patients who are found to have only a very small artery occluded or found to have an already patent infarct-related artery may be spared both the risks of thrombolytic therapy and angioplasty. Regardless of the acute therapy employed, it is likely that early knowledge of the coronary anatomy and documentation of patency facilitates subsequent management and risk stratification. Finally, proceeding to the catheterization laboratory for primary angioplasty also expedites other potentially beneficial interventions such as Swan-Ganz catheterization, arterial pressure monitoring, transvenous pacemakers, and intraaortic balloon pumps.

It should be emphasized that primary angioplasty for AMI is only effective if it occurs rapidly, and it must therefore be considered a team effort. The decision to proceed with angioplasty must be made by the physicians in the emergency department regardless of whether they are ultimately the proceduralists. In general, there will need to be a close working relationship and sense of trust between the physicians who are making the decision to proceed to primary angioplasty in the emergency department and those who are ultimately doing the procedure. In addition, the personnel in the emergency department must assume the role of explaining the procedure to the patient and the family and of obtaining consent. In other words, there is no time for the interventional team to reassess the decision or to go through a detailed consent. The emergency department team should also make certain that aspirin is promptly administered and that a blood specimen is sent for a type and screen. Finally, because the interventional team will not usually know the patient well and will be focused on the procedure itself, it is best if a physician and/or nurse from the emergency department accompany the patient to the catheterization laboratory to assist in other aspects of the patient's care.

## BIBLIOGRAPHY

ACC/AHA Task Force Report: Guidelines for the early management of patients with acute myocardial infarction. *J Am Coll Cardiol* 16(2):249, 1990.

AIMS Trial Study Group: Effect of intravenous APSAC on mortality after acute myocardial infarction: Preliminary report of a placebo-controlled clinical trial. *Lancet* 1:545, 1988.

Anderson HV, Wilkerson JT: Thrombolysis in acute myocardial infarction. *N Engl J Med* 329(10):703, 1993.

Antiplatelet Trialists' Collaboration: Secondary prevention of vascular disease by prolonged antiplatelet treatment. *Br Med J* 296:316, 1988.

Antman EM, Berlin JA: Declining incidence of ventricular fibrillation in myocardial infarction: Implication for the prophylactic use of lidocaine. *Circulation* 86:764, 1992.

Bleich SD, Nichols TC, Schumacher RR, et al: Effect of heparin on coronary arterial patency after thrombolysis with tissue plasminogen activator in acute myocardial infarction. *Am J Cardiol* 66:1412, 1990.

Braunwald E, Sobol BE: Coronary blood flow and myocardial ischemia, in Braunwald E (ed): *Braunwald's Heart Disease,* 3rd ed. Philadelphia, Saunders, 1988, pp 1191–1221.

Brodie BR, Weintraub RA, Stuckey TD, et al: Direct angioplasty for acute myocardial infarction: Results in candidates and non-candidates for thrombolytic therapy (abstract). *Circulation* 80(suppl 2):II-624, 1989.

Brott T, Thalinger K, Hertzberg V: Hypertension as a risk factor for spontaneous intracerebral hemorrhage. *Stroke* 17:1078, 1986.

Cairns JA, Gent M, Singer J, et al: Aspirin, sulfinpyrazone, or both in unstable angina. *N Engl J Med* 313:1369, 1985.

Carney RJ, Murphy GA, Brand TTR, et al: Randomized angiographic trial of recombinant tissue-type plasminogen activator (alteplase) in myocardial infarction. *J Am Coll Cardiol* 20:17, 1992.

Chaitman BR, Thompson B, Wittry MD, et al: The use of tissue type plasminogen activator in the elderly: Results from the thrombolysis in myocardial infarction phase I, open-label studies and the thrombolysis in myocardial infarction phase II study. *J Am Coll Cardiol* 14:1159, 1989.

Cragg DR, Friedman HZ, Bonema JD, et al: Ineligibility for intravenous thrombolytic therapy predicts high mortality after acute myocardial infarction. *Ann Intern Med* 115:173, 1991.

Danish Study Group on verapamil in myocardial infarction (DAVIT): Verapamil in acute myocardial infarction. *Eur Heart J* 5:516, 1984.

DeWood M, Spores J, Notshe R, et al: Prevalence of total coronary occlusion during the early hours of transmural myocardial infarction. *N Engl J Med* 303:897, 1980.

Ellis SG, Debowe D, Butes ER, Topol EJ: Treatment of recurrent ischemia after thrombolysis and successful repercussion for acute myocardial infarction: Effect on in-hospital mortality and left ventricular function. *J Am Coll Cardiol* 17:752, 1991.

Flaherty JT: Intravenous nitroglycerin. *Johns Hopkins Med J* 151:36, 1982.

Fung AY, Lai P, Topol EJ, et al: Value of percutaneous transluminal coronary angioplasty after unsuccessful intravenous streptokinase therapy in acute myocardial infarction. *Am J Cardiol* 58:686, 1986.

Ganz W, Geft I, Shah PK, et al: Intravenous streptokinase in evolving acute myocardial infarction. *Am J Cardiol* 53:1209, 1984.

Gasioch GM, Topol EJ: Sudden paradoxic clinical deterioration during angioplasty of the occluded right coronary artery in acute myocardial infarction. *J Am Coll Cardiol* 14:1202, 1989.

Gibbons RJ, Holmes DR, Reeder GS, et al: Immediate angioplasty compared with the administration of a thrombolytic agent followed by conservative treatment for myocardial infarction. *N Engl J Med* 328:685, 1993.

Gibson RS: Current status of calcium channel blocking drugs after Q wave and non-Q wave myocardial infarction. *Circulation* 80(suppl IV):IV-107, 1989.

Gore JM, Sloan M, Price TR, et al: Intracerebral hemorrhage, cerebral infarction, and subdural hematoma after acute myocardial infarction and thrombolytic therapy in the thrombolysis in myocardial infarction study. *Circulation* 83:448, 1991.

Graves EJ: 1987 National Hospital Discharge Survey: Annual summary, 1987. *Vital Health Stat* 13(99), 1987.

Grines CL, Browne KF, Marco J, et al: A comparison of immediate angioplasty with thrombolytic therapy for acute myocardial infarction. *N Engl J Med* 328:673, 1993.

Gruppo Italiano Perlo Studio della Streptochinssi nell'Infarto Miocardico (GISSI): Effectiveness of intravenous thrombolytic treatment in acute myocardial infarction. *Lancet* 1:397, 1986.

Gunnarsson PS, Sawyer WT, Montague D, et al: Appropriate use of heparin. Empiric versus nomogram-based dosing. *Arch Int Med* 155:526, 1995.

GUSTO (Global Utilization of Streptokinase and Tissue Plasminogen Activator for Occluded Coronary Artery): An international randomized trial comparing four thrombolytic strategies for acute myocardial infarction. *N Engl J Med* 329:673–682, 1993.

Held PH, Yusuf S, Furberg CD: Calcium channel blockers in acute myocardial infarction and unstable angina: An overview. *Br Med J* 299:1187, 1989.

Hine LK, Laird N, Hewitt P, et al: Meta-analytic evidence against prophylactic use of lidocaine in acute myocardial infarction. *Arch Intern Med* 149:2694, 1989.

Hjalmarson AKE, Herlitz J, Maleh I, et al: International beta blocker review in acute and post myocardial infarction. *Am J Cardiol* 61:263, 1988.

Holmes DR Jr, Gersh BJ, Bailey KR, et al: Emergency "rescue" percutaneous transluminal coronary angioplasty after failed thrombolysis with streptokinase: early and late results. Circulation 81(suppl 4):IV51, 1990.

Hsia J, Hamilton WP, Kleinman N, et al: A comparison between heparin and low-dose aspirin as adjunctive therapy with tissue plasminogen activator for acute myocardial infarction. *N Engl J Med* 323:1433, 1990.

Hsia J, Kleinman N, Aguire F, et al: Heparin-induced prolongation of partial thromboplastin time after thrombolysis: Relation to coronary artery patency. *J Am Coll Cardiol* 20:30, 1992.

ISIS Pilot Study Investigators: Randomized factorial trial of high-dose intravenous streptokinase, of oral aspirin and of intravenous heparin in acute myocardial infarction. *Eur Heart J* 8:634, 1987.

ISIS-1 (First International Study of Infarct Survival) Collaborative Group: Randomized trial of intravenous atenolol among 16,027 cases of suspected acute myocardial infarction: ISIS-1. *Lancet* 12:57, 1986.

ISIS-1 Collaborative Group: Mechanisms for the early mortality reduction produced by beta-blockade started early in acute myocardial infarction. *Lancet* 1:921, 1988.

ISIS-2 (Second International Study of Infarct Survival) Collaborative Group: Randomized trial of intravenous streptokinase, oral aspirin, both and neither among 17,187 cases of suspected acute myocardial infarction: ISIS-2. *Lancet* 2:349, 1988.

ISIS-3 (Third International Study of Infarct Survival) Collaborative Group: A randomized comparison of streptokinase vs. tissue plasminogen activator vs. alteplase and of aspirin plus heparin vs. aspirin alone among 41,299 cases of suspected acute myocardial infarction. *Lancet* 339:753, 1993.

Israeli Sprint Study Group: Secondary Prevention Reinfarction Israeli Nifedipine Trial (SPRINT): A randomized intervention trial of nifedipine in patients with acute myocardial infarction. *Eur Heart J* 9:354, 1988.

de Jaegere PP, Arnd AA, Bulta AH, Simons ML: Intracranial hemorrhage in association with thrombolytic therapy: Incidence and clinical predictive factors. *J Am Coll Cardiol* 19:289, 1992.

Jugdutt BI, Warnica JW: Intravenous nitroglycerin therapy to limit myocardial infarct size, expansion and complications. *Circulation* 78:906, 1988.

Kennedy JW, Ritchie JL, Davis KB, Frit JK: Western Washington randomized trial of intracoronary streptokinase in acute myocardial infarction. *N Engl J Med* 309:1477, 1983.

Kimura T, Nosaka H, Ueno K, Nobuyoshi M: Role of coronary angioplasty in acute myocardial infarction (abstract). *Circulation* 74(suppl 2):II-22, 1986.

LATE Study Group: Late Assessment of Thrombolytic Efficacy (LATE) study with alteplase 6–24 hours after onset of acute myocardial infarction. *Lancet* 342:759, 1993.

Lee L, Bates ER, Pitt B, et al: Percutaneous transluminal coronary angioplasty improves survival in acute myocardial infarction complicated by cardiogenic shock. *Circulation* 78:1345, 1988.

Lown B, Vassaux C: Lidocaine in acute myocardial infarction. *Am Heart J* 76:586, 1968.

MacMahon S, Collins R, Knight C, et al: Reduction in major morbidity and mortality by heparin in acute myocardial infarction (abstr). *Circulation* 78(suppl 2):98, 1988.

MacMahon S, Collins R, Peto R, et al: Effects of prophylactic lidocaine in suspected acute myocardial infarction. *JAMA* 260:1910, 1988.

Marco J, Caster L, Szatmary L, Fajadet J: Emergency percutaneous transluminal coronary angioplasty without thrombolysis is initial therapy in acute myocardial infarction. *Int J Cardiol* 15:55, 1987.

May GS, Furberg CD, Eberlein KA, et al: Secondary prevention after myocardial infarction: A review of short-term acute-phase trials. *Prog Cardiovasc Dis* 25:335, 1983.

Meyer J, Merx W, Schmitz H, et al: Percutaneous transluminal coronary angioplasty immediately after intracoronary streptolysis of transluminal myocardial infarction. *Circulation* 66:905, 1982.

Meyers J, Merx W, Dorr R, et al: Successful treatment of acute myocardial infarction shock by combined percutaneous transluminal coronary recanalization (PTCR) and percutaneous transluminal coronary angioplasty (PTCA). *Am Heart J* 103:132, 1982.

MIAMI (Metoprolol in Myocardial Infarction) Trial Research Group: Mortality. *Am J Cardiol* 56:156, 1985.

MIAMI (Metoprolol in Myocardial Infarction) Trial Research Group: Development of myocardial infarction. *Am J Cardiol* 56:236, 1985.

Morgan CD, Roberts RS, Haq A, et al: Coronary patency, infarct size, and left ventricular function after thrombolytic therapy for acute myocardial infarction: Results from the tissue plasminogen activator: Toronto (TPAT) placebo control trial. *J Am Coll Cardiol* 17:1451, 1991.

Multicenter Diltiazem Postinfarction Trial Research Group: The effect of diltiazem on mortality and reinfarction after myocardial infarction. *N Engl J Med* 319:385, 1988.

National Center for Health Statistics: *Monthly Vital Stat Rep* 36(13), 1988.

Neuhaus KL, Essen RV, Tebbe V, et al: Improved thrombolysis in acute myocardial infarction with front-loaded administration of alteplase: Results of the rtl-PA–APSAC patency study (TAPS). *J Am Coll Cardiol* 19:885, 1992.

O'Keefe JH Jr, Rutherford BD, McConahay DR, et al: Early and late results of coronary angioplasty without antecedent thrombolytic therapy for acute myocardial infarction. *Am J Cardiol* 64:1221, 1989.

O'Neill WW, Brodie B, Knopf W, et al: Initial report of the primary angioplasty revascularization (PAR) multicenter registry (abstract). *Circulation* 84(suppl 2):II-536, 1991.

O'Neill WW, Topol EJ, Pitt B: Reperfusion therapy of acute myocardial infarction. *Prog Cardiovasc Dis* 30(4):235, 1988.

Pitt B: Improved early infarct-related vessel patency after thrombolytic therapy. *J Am Coll Cardiol* 19(5):892, 1992.

Rothbaum DA, Linnemeier TJ, Landin RJ, et al: Emergency percutaneous transluminal coronary angioplasty in acute myocardial infarction: A 3 year experience. *J Am Coll Cardiol* 10:264, 1987.

Rude RE, Buja M, Willerson JT: Propranolol in acute myocardial infarction: The MILIS (Multicenter Investigation for the Limit of Infarct Size) experience. *Am J Cardiol* 57:38F, 1986.

SCATI Group: Randomized controlled trial of subcutaneous calcium-heparin in acute myocardial infarction. *Lancet* 1:182, 1989.

Simmons ML, Serruy PW, Brand M, et al: Early thrombolysis in acute myocardial infarction: Limitation of infarct size and improved survival. *J Am Coll Cardiol* 7:717, 1986.

Simoons ML, Arnold AER, Betriu A, et al: Thrombolysis with tissue plasminogen activator in acute myocardial infarction: No additional benefit from immediate percutaneous coronary angioplasty. *Lancet* 1:197, 1988.

Steering Committee of the Physicians' Health Study Research Group: Preliminary report: Findings from the aspirin component of the ongoing physicians' health study. *N Engl J Med* 318:262, 1988.

Teo KK, Yusuf S, Collins R, et al: Effects of intravenous magnesium in suspected acute myocardial infarction: Overview of the randomized trial. *Br Med J* 303:1499, 1991.

Thrombolysis in Myocardial Infarction (TIMI) Phase II Trial: Comparison of invasive and conservative strategies after treatment with intravenous tissue plasminogen activator in acute myocardial infarction. *N Engl J Med* 320:618, 1989.

TIMI Research Group: Immediate vs. delayed catheterization and angioplasty following thrombolytic therapy for acute myocardial infarction: TIMI II A results. *JAMA* 260:2849, 1988.

TIMI Study Group: Comparison of invasive and conservative strategies after treatment with intravenous tissue plasminogen activator in acute myocardial infarction: Results of the thrombolysis in myocardial infarction (TIMI) phase II trial. *N Engl J Med* 320:618, 1989.

Topol EJ, Califf RM, George BS, et al: A randomized trial of immediate versus delayed elective angioplasty after intravenous tissue plasminogen activator in acute myocardial infarction. *N Engl J Med* 317:581, 1987.

Van de Werf F, Arnold AER: European Cooperative Study Group for recombinant tissue type plasminogen activator (rt-PA): Intravenous tissue plasminogen activator and size of infarct, left ventricular function, and survival in acute myocardial infarction. *Br Med J* 297:2374, 1988.

Wall TC, Califf RM, George BS, et al: Accelerated plasminogen activator dose regimens for coronary thrombolysis. *J Am Coll Cardiol* 19:482, 1992.

White HD: Thrombolytic therapy for patients with myocardial infarction presenting after six hours. *Lancet* 340:221, 1992.

Wilcox RG, Hampton JR, Banks BG, et al: Trial of early nifedipine in acute myocardial infarction: The Trent Study. *Br Med J* 293:1204, 1986.

Woods KL, Fletcher S, Roffe C, Haider Y: Intravenous magnesium sulphate in suspected acute myocardial infarction: Results of the second Leicester intravenous magnesium intervention trial (LIMIT-2). *Lancet* 339:1553, 1992.

Yusuf S, MacMahon S, Collins R, Peto R: Effects of intravenous nitrates on mortality in acute myocardial infarction: An overview of the randomized trials. *Lancet* 1088, 1988.

Yusuf S, Sleight P, Held P, McMahon S: Routine medical management of acute myocardial infarction. *Circulation* 82(suppl II):II-117, 1990.

Yusuf S, Peto R, Lewis J, et al: Beta blockade during and after myocardial infarction: An overview of the randomized trials. *Prog Cardiovasc Dis* 27:335, 1985.

Zijlstra F, De Boer MJ, Hoorntje JCA, et al: A comparison of immediate coronary angioplasty with intravenous streptokinase in acute myocardial infarction. *N Engl J Med* 328:680, 1993.

# 54

# HEART FAILURE AND PULMONARY EDEMA

## Charles B. Cairns

## HEART FAILURE

The principal functions of the heart are to receive blood from the veins, send it to the lungs for oxygenation, and pump the oxygenated blood to the body. *Heart failure* occurs when there is a substantial disruption of these functions secondary to a loss of normal contractile ability. If heart failure results in abnormal fluid retention, it is commonly referred to as *congestive heart failure* (CHF). The major clinical manifestation of heart failure is shortness of breath, especially with exercise. The heart may fail when it performs excessive work for a prolonged period of time, such as in patients with hypertension and valvular heart disease. Heart failure is also seen in a variety of infectious, inflammatory, and infiltrative conditions that affect heart muscle. In the acute setting, heart failure is commonly due to a loss of heart muscle via infarction or to a loss of nourishment via ischemia. The common causes of heart failure are summarized in Table 54-1.

**Table 54-1.** Common Causes of Heart Failure and Pulmonary Edema

I. Myocardial ischemia
   A. Acute
   B. Chronic
II. Valvular dysfunction
   A. Aortic valve disease
     1. Aortic stenosis
     2. Aortic insufficiency
       a. Aortic dissection
       b. Infectious endocarditis
   B. Mitral valve disease
     1. Mitral stenosis
     2. Mitral regurgitation
       a. Papillary muscle dysfunction or rupture
       b. Ruptured chordae tendineae
       c. Infectious endocarditis
   C. Prosthetic valve malfunction
III. Other causes of left ventricular outflow obstruction
   A. Supravalvular aortic stenosis
   B. Membranous subvalvular aortic stenosis
IV. Idiopathic cardiomyopathy
   A. Hypertrophic cardiomyopathy
   B. Dilated
   C. Restrictive
V. Acquired cardiomyopathy
   A. Toxic
     1. Alcohol
     2. Cocaine
     3. Adriamycin
   B. Metabolic
     1. Thyrotoxicosis
     2. Myxedema
VI. Myocarditis
   A. Radiation
   B. Infection
VII. Constrictive pericarditis
VIII. Cardiac tamponade
IX. Systemic hypertension
X. Miscellaneous
   A. Anemia
   B. Cardiac arrhythmias

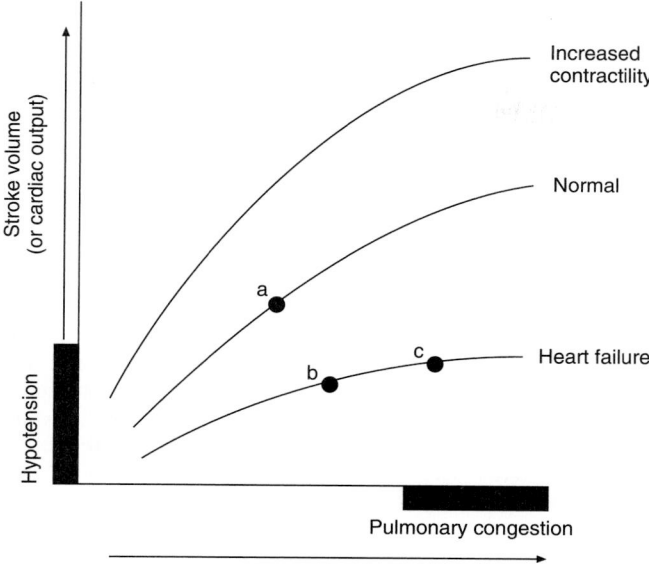

**Fig. 54-1.** Left ventricular (LV) performance (Frank-Starling) curves relate preload, measured as LV end-diastolic volume (EDV) or pressure (EDP), to cardiac performance, measured as ventricular stroke volume or cardiac output. On the curve of normal individuals (*middle line*), cardiac performance continuously increases as a function of the preload. States of increased contractility (e.g., dobutamine infusion) are characterized by an augmented stroke volume at any level of preload (*upper line*). Conversely, decreased LV contractility (commonly associated with heart failure) is characterized by a curve that is shifted downward (*lower line*). Point *a* is an example of a normal individual at rest. Point *b* represents the same individual after developing systolic dysfunction and heart failure (e.g., after a large MI): stroke volume has fallen, and the decreased LV emptying results in elevation of the EDV. Because point *b* is on the ascending portion of the curve, the increased EDV serves a compensatory role because it results in an increase in subsequent stroke volume, albeit much less so than if operating on the normal curve. Further augmentation of LV filling (e.g., increased circulating volume) in the heart failure patient is represented by point *c,* which resides on the relatively flat part of the curve: stroke volume is only slightly augmented, but the markedly increased EDP results in pulmonary congestion.

## Pathophysiology of Heart Failure

The three factors of contractility, preload, and afterload determine ventricular stroke volume. Coupled with heart rate, stroke volume determines cardiac output. Cardiac *contractility* is related to the amount of myocardial stretch, known as *preload*. Clinical measurements of cardiac stretch include the ventricular end-diastolic pressure and volume. *Afterload* is defined as the ventricular wall tension that develops during systole and reflects the resistance to outward blood flow. It is clinically estimated by the systolic arterial pressure. Many sorts of heart failure are associated with decreased contractility. The Frank-Starling relationships between stroke volume, preload, and contractility in both the normal and failing heart are illustrated in Fig. 54-1.

Heart failure can be further classified into three categories related to physiology and functional anatomy. These categories are: high versus low cardiac output, right versus left heart failure, and systolic versus diastolic dysfunction.

Heart failure can produce either low or high cardiac output states. While *low-output failure* is due to an inherent problem in myocardial contraction, *high-output failure* is due to an inability of functionally intact myocardium to keep up with excess functional demands. The causes of high-output failure are relatively few and include anemia, thyrotoxicosis, large arteriovenous shunts, beriberi, and Paget disease of the bone.

In congestive heart failure, excess fluid accumulates behind the affected chamber of the heart. In patients with left ventricular dysfunction due to either mechanical overload or infarction, excess fluid develops in the lungs. This resulting *pulmonary edema,* or congestion, is the cardinal manifestation of *left-sided heart failure.* In patients where the right ventricle is compromised (pulmonary embolus, right ventricular infarction), jugular venous distension and other signs of *right-sided heart failure* occur. Long-standing heart failure, however, usually results in compromise of both ventricles.

Systolic heart failure is characterized by an impairment of myocardial contraction, and diastolic failure by an impairment in myocardial relaxation. *Systolic failure* can occur from excessive afterload (systemic hypertension) or from damaged myocytes (infarction). *Diastolic failure* can be seen in both acute and chronic heart failure. Inhibited early diastolic relaxation as seen in myocardial ischemia is due to altered energy availability. Chronic processes such as hypertrophic cardiomyopathy increase ventricular stiffness and inhibit relaxation. Many etiologies, such as transient myocardial ischemia, can result in either systolic or diastolic failure.

Once heart failure has developed, several neurohormonal compensatory mechanisms occur. Alterations in adrenergic tone redistribute blood flow to the brain and myocardium, reducing blood flow to the skin, kidneys, gastrointestinal tract, and skeletal muscle. The reduction in blood flow to the kidneys results in increased stimulation of the renin-angiotensin-aldosterone axis and secretion of antidiuretic hormone. The end result of these processes is enhanced sodium and water retention by the kidneys, which leads to fluid overload and the clinical manifestations of CHF. Additionally, the increased adrenergic tone leads to arteriolar vasoconstriction, a significant raise in afterload, and, finally, to increased cardiac work.

## Clinical Features of Heart Failure

The clinical features of heart failure may be due to impaired perfusion or elevated venous pressures and relate to which ventricle is primarily affected (Table 54-2). Patients may present with either the chronic progressive symptoms of heart failure or with acute pulmonary edema due to sudden left-sided decompensation.

The most common symptom of left-sided heart failure is breathlessness, or *dyspnea,* particularly with exertion. When pulmonary venous pressure reaches a critical level (20 mmHg), there is movement of fluid into the pulmonary interstitium, compressing airways and alveoli. The increased resistance to airflow intensifies the work of breathing. In addition, stimulation of the juxtacapillary receptors

**Table 54-2.** Common Symptoms and Physical Findings in Heart Failure

| Symptoms | Physical Findings |
|---|---|
| **LEFT SIDED** | |
| Dyspnea | Diaphoresis |
| Orthopnea | Tachycardia, tachypnea |
| Paroxysmal nocturnal dyspnea | Pulmonary rales, wheezes |
| Fatigue | S$_3$ gallop |
| **RIGHT SIDED** | |
| Peripheral edema | Jugular venous distension |
| Right upper quadrant pain | Hepatomegaly |
| | Hepatojugular reflux |
| | Peripheral edema |

*Source:* Adapted from Coday A, Vikram J, Fifer MA: Heart failure, in Lilly LS (ed) *Pathophysiology of Heart Disease: A Collaborative Project of Students and Faculty.* Malvern, PA, Lea & Febiger, 1993, p. 159.

(J receptors) causes rapid shallow breathing. Other manifestations of pulmonary congestion include *orthopnea* and *paroxysmal nocturnal dyspnea* (PND). Orthopnea is the sensation of breathlessness while lying flat and is relieved by sitting upright. Orthopnea results from the redistribution of intravascular blood from the gravity-dependent portions of the body to the lungs. The degree of orthopnea is usually assessed by the number of pillows the patient uses at night to avoid breathlessness. PND is severe breathlessness that awakens the patient from sleep 2 to 3 hours after lying down. PND is due to the gradual reabsorption of interstitial lower extremity edema after lying down, with subsequent greater venous return to the heart and lungs.

Clinical manifestations of left-sided heart failure due to alterations in blood flow include fatigue, altered mental status, and reduced urine output (especially during the day). At night, urine output may increase due to increases in venous return. The increased urinary frequency at night is termed *nocturia*.

Right-sided heart failure causes increased systemic venous pressures and peripheral edema. Additional edema of the gastrointestinal tract causes anorexia and nausea, and right upper quadrant abdominal pain occurs as the liver becomes engorged.

Physical findings of left-sided heart failure include dusky or pale skin, diaphoresis, and cool extremities due to poor perfusion and peripheral arterial vasoconstriction. Pulmonary congestion commonly results in tachypnea (respiratory rate > 24/min) and bilateral inspiratory crackles on auscultation. Additional auscultatory findings include rhonchi and wheezing ("cardiac asthma") due to airway edema. Pleural effusions may develop, detected by dullness to percussion at the lung bases. In advanced heart failure, *Cheyne-Stokes respiration* can occur and is a respiratory pattern characterized by periods of hyperventilation separated by periods of absent breathing (apnea).

Frequently, sinus tachycardia secondary to sympathetic nervous system activity is present in heart failure patients. Cardiac auscultation may reveal a third heart sound ($S_3$), an early diastolic sound resulting from abnormal filling into the dilated ventricle. Also present may be a fourth heart sound ($S_4$), which results from forceful atrial contraction into a stiffened ventricle. Finally, *pulsus alternans* (alternating strong and weak contractions detected in the peripheral pulse) may occur in advanced heart failure.

Right-sided heart failure may result in additional physical findings due to elevated systemic venous pressures. *Jugular venous distension* (JVD) is common. Engorgement of the liver results in hepatomegaly, right upper quadrant tenderness, and the presence of the hepatojugular reflux (JVD with liver palpation). Peripheral edema accumulates in the dependent areas of the body, including the ankles and legs of ambulatory patients and the presacral region of bedridden patients.

Radiographic manifestations of left-sided CHF generally relate to the increases in pulmonary venous pressures. When the pulmonary pressures exceed 15 mmHg, hydrostatic pressure increases in the gravity-dependent edematous lower zones of the lung. Because of the higher resistance to flow in the lower regions, blood flow is selectively shunted to the upper regions and the chest radiograph shows upper zone *vascular redistribution*. As pulmonary pressures exceed 20 mmHg, interstitial edema occurs with loss of distinct vascular margins on chest x-ray. Interlobular edema results in *Kerley B lines,* which are short linear markings at the periphery of the lower lung fields on the chest x-ray. When pulmonary pressures reach 25 mmHg, alveolar pulmonary edema develops with opacification of the air spaces on x-ray. However, in patients with long-standing CHF, enhanced lymphatic drainage may minimize these radiographic findings.

Depending upon the cause of the CHF, additional radiographic findings include cardiomegaly and pleural effusions. *Cardiomegaly* is defined as a cardiothoracic ratio greater than 0.5 on a posteroanterior film. *Pleural effusions* may occur in either left- or right-sided failure but are usually the result of bilateral heart failure. High right-atrial pressure may cause azygous vein enlargement on chest x-ray.

The electrocardiogram (ECG) may reveal evidence of acute myocardial infarction or ischemia as a cause of acute decompensation in CHF. In chronic CHF, the ECG usually reveals evidence of ventricular hypertrophy, atrial enlargement, or conduction abnormalities.

In patients with dyspnea or evidence of pulmonary edema, arterial blood gases will help define the acid-base status and are necessary to quantitate the level of respiratory effort. *Hypoxia* is a frequent finding with pulmonary edema and when associated with hypercarbia and acidosis can portend impending respiratory failure.

## Treatment of Chronic Congestive Heart Failure

The treatment of heart failure involves either correction of the underlying cause of the heart failure or elimination of the symptoms. Treatment of the underlying condition may be curative in patients with readily correctable conditions such as valvular disorders, acute infections, or arrhythmias. For the remaining patients with CHF, treatment is geared toward reduction of cardiac work, control of fluid retention, and enhancement of myocardial contractility.

The reduction of cardiac work is accomplished by restriction of both physical and emotional activity coupled with pharmacologic afterload reduction. Vasodilators help to reduce the increase in afterload that occurs with the neurohormonal compensatory response to CHF. Even a modest reduction in afterload may elevate the stroke volume of the heart and reduce ventricular end-diastolic pressures.

Vasodilators can be classified by their effects—primarily on the venous bed, arterial bed, or both beds—or by their route of administration. Venodilators tend to shunt blood away from the chest to the peripherial circulation, reducing preload. Venodilators include nitroglycerin and isosorbide dinitrate. Arteriolar dilators reduce afterload and enhance stroke volume. Arteriolar dilators include hydralazine, minoxidil, and calcium channel blockers. Agents with mixed venous and arterial effects include prazosin and the angiotensin-converting enzyme (ACE) inhibitors. Intravenous agents with mixed venous and arterial dilatory effects include sodium nitroprusside and phentolamine.

The control of excess fluid retention in patients with CHF is accomplished mainly by dietary restriction of sodium intake and the use of diuretics. Diuretics reduce intravascular volume and preload by promoting the elimination of sodium and water via the kidney. However, overly vigorous reduction of preload with diuresis can result in a marked reduction of cardiac contractility. Therefore, the use of diuretics in CHF is usually restricted to those patients with evidence of pulmonary or peripheral edema.

Diuretics acting on the loop of Henle are the most potent and include furosemide, bumetanide, and ethacrynic acid. Thiazide diuretics are useful in mild CHF when renal perfusion is preserved. The most important adverse effects of these drugs are overdiuresis, with impairment of cardiac output, and electrolyte abnormalities, including hypokalemia and hypomagnesemia. Potassium-sparing diuretics, such as spironolactone and triamterene, can potentiate the action of thiazides and loop diuretics. Such combinations are useful in severe CHF, although they should not be used in patients with impaired renal function or hyperkalemia.

Enhancement of myocardial contraction via inotropic agents can be useful in patients with systolic dysfunction. Inotropic drugs increase cardiac output by shifting the Frank-Starling curve upward. Thus, for any given preload, stroke volume and contraction are augmented. The inotropic therapy of chronic CHF is mainly through the use of digitalis glycosides. In addition to enhancing contractility, digitalis reduces afterload by blunting the cardiac sympathetic response. Digitalis prolongs the refractory period of the atrioventricular node and is effective in controlling the ventricular response to atrial fibrillation. Digitalis intoxication, however, can be a life-threatening disorder characterized by atrial and ventricular arrhythmias, hyperkalemia, as well as CNS and gastrointestinal complaints.

The long-term use of other inotropic agents, such as sympathomimetic amines, is limited by a lack of oral forms and the development of drug tolerance.

In patients with diastolic dysfunction, the use of inotropic drugs is contraindicated. Diuretics may reduce pulmonary congestion and peripheral edema, and calcium channel blockers may be useful in cases of hypertension and hypertrophic cardiomyopathy.

While the use of β-adrenergic blockers is usually contraindicated in patients with significant systolic dysfunction, β blockade may be useful in counteracting the effects of excessive sympathetic stimulation. Recent studies have demonstrated a functional benefit with the use of β-adrenergic blockers, although a benefit in survival has not yet been found.

## Prognosis

Unfortunately, heart failure is a progressive, fatal condition. In the absence of a correctable underlying cause, the prognosis of patients with CHF is poor, with a 5-year mortality rate of 50 percent. Most of these deaths are due to development of refractory failure, although a large number of patients die suddenly, presumably of ventricular arrhythmias. There is no evidence, however, that these fatal arrhythmias can be prevented by the use of antiarrhythmic medications.

Recent studies have found that ACE inhibitors prolong survival in patients with heart failure and delay the onset of death in patients with impaired heart function. Combined with β-adrenergic receptor blockers, these drugs may be helpful in prolonging the life of patients with heart disease at risk for developing heart failure.

## PULMONARY EDEMA

Cardiogenic pulmonary edema is an acute, life-threatening form of left-sided heart failure. Severe hypoxia can result in this condition due to the shunting of pulmonary blood flow to hypoventilated alveoli.

## Treatment of Acute Pulmonary Edema

While attention must be given to potential precipitating causes, acute pulmonary edema is a life-threatening emergency that requires immediate improvement of systemic oxygenation.

**Oxygen.** 100% oxygen should be given by mask and arterial blood gases obtained. The patient should be seated upright in order to pool systemic blood and reduce venous return. If hypoxia persists with supplemental oxygen, then positive pressure ventilation is required. Positive end-expiratory pressure (PEEP) applied via face mask as continuous positive airway pressure (CPAP) or via endotracheal tube can be used to prevent alveolar collapse. While impedance of venous return with PEEP via the endotracheal tube can be beneficial in reducing preload, care must be taken in using the lowest possible pressure in order to avoid compromising cardiac output. If hypercarbia and acidosis are also present, then endotracheal tube ventilation is warranted.

**Vasodilators.** Nitrates are effective preload reducers. Nitroglycerin can be given via sublingual, oral, topical, or intravenous routes. For acute pulmonary edema, higher doses of sublingual nitroglycerin than those used in angina may be required (0.4 to 0.8 mg). Intravenous administration of either nitroglycerin or sodium nitroprusside can rapidly reduce preload and afterload. Because nitroprusside has the potential to induce ischemia, IV nitroglycerin is preferred in the treatment of pulmonary edemia in patients with coronary artery disease. Infusion of nitroglycerin is safer with close hemodynamic monitoring. Dosing should begin at 10 to 20 μg/min and titrated to relief of symptoms or until mean blood pressure falls 30 percent or systolic blood pressure below 90 mmHg.

**Diuretics.** Intravenous furosemide (20 to 40 mg IV) can rapidly induce a potent diuresis. While furosemide can have a venodilatory effect, use of intravenous furosemide alone may not significantly lower preload until 30 min after administration. Preload can be reduced within 5 min with concomitant administration of nitrates and furosemide.

**Inotropic agents.** In patients refractory to oxygen, nitrates, and diuretics, intravenously administered β-adrenergic agonists can be used to augment myocardial contractility. *Dopamine* is particularly useful in the setting of pulmonary edema and hypotension. At low doses (1 to 2 μg/kg per minute), dopamine increases renal and mesenteric blood flow by stimulation of dopaminergic receptors. At moderate doses (2 to 10 μg/kg per minute), dopamine increases myocardial contractility via $\beta_1$-adrenergic stimulation, and at high doses (>20 μg/kg per minute), arterial pressure is elevated due to α-adrenergic stimulation. *Dobutamine* at a dose of 2 to 20 μg/kg per minute may produce a more favorable balance between myocardial oxygen supply and demand and is the choice for treatment of pulmonary edema in normotensive patients. The administration of these drugs should be accompanied by close ECG and arterial pressure monitoring and may be optimized with pulmonary artery pressure recording. There is minimal role for digitalis in the management of acute congestive heart failure.

**Morphine.** Morphine in doses of 2 to 8 mg IV decreases afterload and produces a sedative effect, thereby reducing cardiac work. However, there are more superior vasodilators, and the value of giving sedatives to patients with acute dyspnea has been recently challenged.

**Aminophylline.** Aminophylline (200 mg IV per 20 min) can be an effective adjunct in diminishing the bronchospasm of cardiac asthma, increasing renal blood flow, and augmenting myocardial contractility.

**Phlebotomy.** Phlebotomy is a rapid, effective method of reducing circulating volume and may be particularly useful in the renal failure patient with acute pulmonary edema. The practice of rotating tourniquets has not been found to be clinically beneficial.

## BIBLIOGRAPHY

Bertel O, Steiner A: Rotating tourniquets do not work in acute congestive heart failure. *Am J Med* 80:1, 1986.

Bonow RO, Udelson JE: Left ventricular diastolic dysfunction as a cause of congestive heart failure: Mechanisms and management. *Ann Intern Med* 117:502, 1992.

Braunwald E: Heart failure, in Isselbacher KJ, et al (eds): *Harrison's Principles of Internal Medicine,* 13th ed. New York, McGraw-Hill, 1994, pp 998–1009.

Cummings RO (ed): *Textbook of Advanced Cardiac Life Support.* Dallas, American Heart Association, 1994.

Eichhorn EJ, Hjalmarson A: β-Blocker treatment for chronic heart failure: The frog prince. *Circulation* 90:2153, 1994.

Hoffman JR, Reynolds S: Comparison of nitroglycerin, morphine and furosemide in treatment of presumed prehospital pulmonary edema. *Chest* 92:586, 1987.

Katz AM: Cardiomyopathy of overload: A major determinant of prognosis in congestive heart failure. *N Engl J Med* 322:100, 1990.

Kraus PA, Lipman J, Becker PJ: Acute preload effects of furosemide. *Chest* 98:124, 1990.

Lenfant C: Report of the task force on research in heart failure. *Circulation* 90:1118, 1994.

Packer M: The neurohormonal hypothesis: A theory to explain the mechanism of disease progression in heart failure. *J Am Coll Cardiol* 20:248, 1992.

Parmley WW: Vasodilator drugs in the treatment of heart failure, in Parmley WW, Chatterjee K (eds): *Cardiovascular Pharmacology.* London, Mosby-Europe, 1994, pp 7.1–7.19.

Pfeffer MA, Braunwald E, Moye LA, et al: The effect of captopril on mortality and morbidity in patients with left ventricular dysfunction following myocardial infarction: Results of the survival and ventricular enlargement (SAVE) trial. *N Engl J Med* 327:685, 1992.

Roth A, Hochenberg M, Keren G, et al: Are rotating tourniquets useful for left ventricular preload reduction in patients with acute myocardial infarction and heart failure? *Ann Emerg Med* 16:764, 1987.

Smith TW, Kelly RA: Therapeutic strategies for congestive heart failure in the 1990s. *Hosp Pract* Nov:69, 1991.

The SOLVD Investigators: Effects of enalapril on mortality and the development of heart failure in asymptomatic patients with reduced left ventricular ejection fractions. *N Engl J Med* 327:685, 1992.

# 55
# VALVULAR EMERGENCIES AND ENDOCARDITIS
## David M. Cline

Ninety percent of valvular disease is chronic, with decades between the onset of the structural abnormality and symptoms. The emergency physician most commonly encounters patients with valvular disease after the diagnosis has been made, but will occasionally be the first to suspect valvular dysfunction based on the patient's symptoms and examination. Through chronic adaptation by dilation and hypertrophy, cardiac function can be preserved for years, which may delay the diagnosis for one to two decades until a murmur is detected on auscultation. In contrast to the more common chronic presentations, acute rupture of a cardiac valve presents with dramatic symptoms.

The four heart valves prevent the back flow of blood during the cardiac cycle, allowing efficient ejection of blood with each contraction of the ventricles. The mitral valve has two cusps, while the other three heart valves normally have three cusps. The right and left papillary muscles promote effective closure of the tricuspid and mitral valves respectively. The papillary muscles are attached to the cusps of the atrioventricular valves by tendinous cords, the chordae tendineae. Abnormalities of the valvular cusps, the papillary muscles, the chordae tendineae, or the cardiac chambers themselves can cause valvular dysfunction.

Pathophysiology of, and clinical findings for, each of the classic valvular disorders are presented below. Following these descriptions, the treatment of the disorders is presented collectively. When important differences occur in the indicated management, these recommendations are contrasted and explained.

## MITRAL STENOSIS
### Pathophysiology

Despite its declining frequency, rheumatic heart disease is still the most common cause of mitral valve stenosis. Scarring from rheumatic endocarditis causes fusion of the commissures and matting of the chordae tendineae, which interferes with valve closure. Calcification over time makes the valve less mobile. Progressive stenosis may lead to pulmonary hypertension, which may signal the need for surgery. The majority of patients eventually develop atrial fibrillation because of progressive dilation of the atria. Pulmonary hypertension may lead to pulmonary and tricuspid valve incompetence.

### Clinical Features

Even though mitral stenosis is a chronic condition, increased demands on cardiac output may precipitate acute symptoms. Conditions that prompt symptoms in mitral stenosis include exertion, tachycardia, anemia, pregnancy, infection, emotional upset, and atrial fibrillation. As with all valvular diseases, exertional dyspnea is the most common presenting symptom (80 percent of patients with mitral stenosis). Paroxysmal nocturnal dyspnea may occur with more severe disease. Hemoptysis is the second most common presenting symptom and may be massive if a bronchial vein ruptures. Other common symptoms and signs include orthopnea, premature atrial contractions, and atrial fibrillation, which is almost inevitable with the passage of time. Systemic emboli may occur and result in myocardial, kidney, central nervous system (CNS), or peripheral infarction. Embolic stroke is more frequent in the presence of atrial fibrillation. As the disease progresses symptoms of right heart failure may develop.

Signs of mitral stenosis include a middiastolic rumbling murmur, which crescendos into the $S_2$. With the onset of atrial fibrillation the presystolic accentuation of the murmur disappears. Typically the $S_1$ is loud and is followed by a loud opening "snap" that is high-pitched and heard best at the right of the apex. A prominent $a$ wave in the neck may be seen as well as an early systolic parasternal lift, which is due to right heart pressure overload. The apical impulse is small and tapping, representing an underfilled left ventricle. Systemic blood pressure is typically normal or low. Rales may be heard at the lung bases as the disease progresses. If pulmonary hypertension is present, signs may include a thin body habitus, peripheral cyanosis, and cool extremities because of low cardiac output. With pulmonary hypertension the auscultatory findings are less evident.

The electrocardiogram (ECG) may demonstrate notched or diphasic P waves and right axis deviation. On the chest radiography, straightening of the left heart border, indicating left atrial enlargement, is a typical early radiographic finding. Eventually, findings of pulmonary congestion are noted: redistribution of flow to the upper lung fields, Kerley B lines, and an increase in vascular markings. The chest radiograph is useful in assessing the degree of pulmonary congestion.

## MITRAL INCOMPETENCE
### Pathophysiology

Infective endocarditis or myocardial infarction can cause acute rupture of the chordae tendineae or papillary muscles or cause perforation of the valve leaflets. Inferior myocardial infarction due to right coronary occlusion is the most common cause of ischemic mitral valve incompetence. Rarely, trauma may cause acute mitral incompetence. Patients with acute mitral valve rupture deteriorate rapidly. Intermittent mitral incompetence can be due to ischemia which causes papillary muscle dysfunction. Rheumatic heart disease is the most common cause of chronic mitral incompetence.

Acute regurgitation into a noncompliant left atrium quickly elevates pressures and causes pulmonary edema. In contrast, in the chronic state the left atrium dilates so that left atrial pressure rises little, even with a large regurgitant flow. As an adaptation, the total stroke volume of the left ventricle increases so that effective forward flow into the aorta is maintained despite the large regurgitant volume across the mitral valve.

### Clinical Features

*Acute mitral incompetence* presents with dyspnea, tachycardia, and pulmonary edema. Usually an $S_3$ and $S_4$ will be heard. Acutely the harsh apical systolic murmur starts with $S_1$ and may end before $S_2$. Patients may quickly deteriorate to cardiogenic shock or cardiac arrest. Intermittent mitral incompetence usually presents with acute episodes of respiratory distress due to pulmonary edema and can be asymptomatic between attacks. The pronounced dyspnea may mask angina that accompanies the ischemia. Patients may have an active apical impulse, systolic thrust, and thrill at the apex. Jugular venous distension may be seen, with a prominent $a$ wave and a left parasternal lift. On chest radiography, acute mitral incompetence from papillary muscle rupture may reveal a minimally enlarged left atrium and pulmonary edema, with less cardiac enlargement than expected.

*Chronic mitral incompetence* may be tolerated for years or even decades. The first symptom is usually exertional dyspnea, sometimes prompted by atrial fibrillation. If patients are not anticoagulated, systemic emboli occur in 20 percent and are often asymptomatic. Endocarditis is still a feared complication. Signs of chronic mitral incompetence include a late systolic left parasternal lift. There is a high-pitched apical holosystolic murmur that radiates to the axilla. The first heart sound is soft and often obscured by the murmur. An $S_3$ is usually heard and is followed by a short diastolic rumble, indicating increased flow into the left ventricle. The ECG may demonstrate findings of left atrial and left ventriclar hypertrophy (LVH). On chest radiography, chronic mitral incompetence produces left ventricular and atrial enlargement that is proportional to the severity of the regurgitant volume.

## MITRAL VALVE PROLAPSE

### Pathophysiology

The etiology of mitral valve prolapse (MVP), or the click-murmur syndrome, is not known but may be congenital. Approximately 5 percent of the population has mitral valve prolapse by echocardiographic criteria. One or both of the mitral valve leaflets prolapse into the atrium during systole and this may or may not be accompanied by regurgitant flow. The presence of regurgitation, recognized clinically by a short diastolic murmur, places the patient in a higher risk group for complications. Click-murmur syndrome has unique symptoms that differentiate it from other forms of mitral regurgitation.

### Clinical Features

Most patients are asymptomatic. Symptoms include atypical chest pain, palpitations, fatigue, and dyspnea unrelated to exertion. Symptoms are more common in those who know they have the syndrome. However, there is an increased incidence of sudden death and arrhythmias in patients with MVP. Also there is an increased incidence of transient ischemic attacks under the age of 45. The classic cardiac finding is a midsystolic click. The second heart sound may be diminished by the late systolic murmur, which crescendos into $S_2$ (not present in all patients). Some patients may have pectus excavatum, a straight thoracic spine, or scoliosis. The ECG is usually normal, as is the chest radiograph unless the thoracic cage abnormalities described above are seen.

## AORTIC STENOSIS

### Pathophysiology

Congenital heart disease is the most common cause of aortic stenosis, with the presence of a bicuspid valve accounting for 50 percent of cases. Rheumatic heart disease is the second most common cause followed by degenerative heart disease or calcific aortic stenosis, which is the most common cause in patients over age 70. Blood flow into the aorta is obstructed, producing progressive left ventricular hypertrophy and low cardiac output. This produces a marked reduction in coronary blood flow.

### Clinical Features

Exercise may induce acute symptoms including syncope, dyspnea, and angina. Symptoms appear late in the course of the disease. In active persons the symptoms appear more rapidly. Dyspnea is usually the first symptom, followed by paroxysmal nocturnal dyspnea, syncope on exertion, angina, and myocardial infarction.

The most common signs include a pulse of small amplitude. The carotid pulse is the most accurate artery to assess. Blood pressure is normal or low with a narrow pulse pressure. Left ventricular hypertrophy is common. There is paradoxic splitting of $S_2$, and $S_3$ and $S_4$ are commonly present. Classically, there is a harsh systolic ejection murmur. Sudden death, usually from an arrhythmia, occurs in 25 percent of patients. Atrial fibrillation is less common than in mitral disease, but 10 percent of patients have atrial fibrillation at the time of surgery. With isolated aortic stenosis, endocarditis occurs in only 2 percent of patients. The ECG usually demonstrates criteria for LVH and, in 10 percent of patients, left or right bundle branch block. The chest radiograph is normal early, but eventually LVH and findings of congestive heart failure (CHF) are evident, if the patient does not have valve replacement.

## AORTIC INCOMPETENCE

### Pathophysiology

In 20 percent of patients the etiology is acute in nature. Infective endocarditis accounts for the majority of acute cases; aortic dissection at the aortic root causes the remainder. In acute cases, a sudden increase in back flow of blood into the ventricle raises left ventricular end-diastolic pressure, which may cause acute heart failure. Increased ventricular pressure elevates pressure in the left atrium, and pulmonary congestion results. Rheumatic heart disease and congenital disease cause the majority of chronic cases.

Syphilis, ankylosing spondylitis, and Reiter syndrome are less frequent causes. Chronic disease is more common in males than females, with a ratio of 3:2. In chronic disease, the ventricle progressively dilates to accommodate the regurgitant blood volume. Wide pulse pressures result from the fall in diastolic pressure, and marked peripheral vasodilation is seen. During exercise and tachycardia, the diastolic filling period shortens, thus decreasing the number of times per minute that regurgitation can occur. Cardiac function is therefore close to normal with exercise early in the course of the disease. In contrast, isometric exercise or stress may precipitate symptoms.

### Clinical Features

In acute disease, dyspnea is the most common presenting symptom, seen in 50 percent of patients. Many patients will have acute pulmonary edema with pink frothy sputum. Patients can complain of fever and chills if endocarditis is the cause. Patients may present with systemic emboli or a persistent sinus tachycardia. Dissection of the ascending aorta typically produces a "tearing"-like chest pain that may radiate between the shoulder blades. Sudden death is common in patients with both acute and chronic aortic incompetence.

The two major causes of acute aortic incompetence present with different signs. Elevated temperature is common with acute endocarditis. Electrocardiographic changes may be seen with aortic dissection, including ischemia or findings of acute inferior myocardial infarction, suggesting involvement of the right coronary artery. Patients commonly have signs of peripheral circulatory collapse such as sweating, marked tachycardia, tachypnea, and rales. Classically there is a high-pitched blowing diastolic murmur heard immediately after the second heart sound. There may be a third heart sound with long diastolic murmurs, and there may be a systolic flow murmur. In the acute state, the chest radiography demonstrates acute pulmonary edema with less cardiac enlargement than expected.

In the chronic state, about one-third of patients will have palpitations associated with a large stroke volume and/or premature ventricular contractions. Frequently these sensations are noticed in bed. Patients may complain of stabbing chest pain, fatigue, or dyspnea. Two-thirds of patients will have no symptoms for up to 20 years, despite hemodynamically significant lesions, defined as a diastolic blood pressure under 70 mmHg. Symptoms of left ventricular failure may present late in the course of the disease and include dyspnea, pulmonary edema, ischemic chest pain, and sweating.

In the chronic state, signs include a wide pulse pressure with a prominent ventricular impulse and this may manifest as head bobbing. "Water hammer pulse" may be noted; this is a peripheral pulse that has a quick rise in upstroke followed by a peripheral collapse. In chronic aortic incompetence, the ECG demonstrates LVH, and the chest radiograph shows LVH, aortic dilation, and possibly evidence of CHF.

## HYPERTROPHIC CARDIOMYOPATHY (IDIOPATHIC HYPERTROPHIC SUBAORTIC STENOSIS)

Hypertrophic cardiomyopathy (HCM) is known by other terms including idiopathic hypertrophic subaortic stenosis (IHSS) and asymmetric septal hypertrophy. This disorder is best described as hypertrophic cardiomyopathy and is defined by a hypertrophied, nondilated left ventricle. In 95 percent of cases, the septum is asymmetrically enlarged, but the free wall of the ventricle is also hypertrophied. The atrium is typically enlarged, and the mitral valve is thickened. Only one-fourth of patients with this disorder have a ventricular outflow obstruction sufficient to cause symptoms; therefore, "IHSS" incompletely describes this disorder. This disease is discussed in Chap. 56, "Cardiomyopathies, Myocarditis, and Pericardial Disease," and is mentioned here only to aid in its differentiation from valvular aortic stenosis.

## Clinical Features

Patients with HCM may become symptomatic at any age, but most present between age 30 and 40 years, approximately 10 years earlier than the average age of onset of symptomatic valvular aortic stenosis. Symptoms are similar to aortic stenosis, except that the patient with HCM may report that symptoms are relieved by squatting.

Signs may be absent in this disease. The classic murmur is a harsh systolic crescendo-decrescendo type heard best at the apex or the left sternal border. The Valsalva maneuver intensifies the murmur by increasing venous return, while squatting diminishes it. There is no opening snap as is commonly heard in valvular aortic stenosis. The apical impulse may be double secondary to an abrupt interruption of early systolic ejection by the asymmetric septum, which blocks outflow, as the ventricle contracts. The pulse has a brisk rise and a double peak, unlike valvular aortic stenosis in which the pulse has a slow rise and a sustained single peak.

Hypertrophic cardiomyopathy is one cause of sudden death among athletes, and all patients are at significant risk. The mechanism of sudden death is not well understood and is likely due to several mechanisms, including arrhythmias and massive myocardial infarction. Patients with HCM are at risk for endocarditis, usually involving the thickened mitral valve. Antibiotic prophylaxis is recommended for certain procedures performed in the emergency department (see Table 55-1).

## RIGHT SIDED VALVULAR HEART DISEASE

### Pathophysiology

Right sided valvular heart disease is much less common than left sided valvular disease. Drug users with endocarditis due to aggressive organisms, such as *Staphylococcus aureus,* are the largest group of patients with isolated tricuspid disease. Right ventricular failure with dilation may lead to tricuspid incompetence. Rheumatic heart disease may affect more than one valve, and tricuspid disease is frequently seen with left sided valvular disease. Rarely, blunt trauma can lead to tricuspid incompetence.

Pulmonary incompetence is most commonly due to pulmonary hypertension, and symptoms of pulmonary hypertension dominate the clinical picture. The most common cause of pulmonary stenosis is congenital tetralogy of Fallot, which is usually corrected surgically in infancy.

### Clinical Features

The most common presenting symptoms of right sided valvular disease are dyspnea and orthopnea. Because of the organisms involved, patients presenting with tricuspid incompetence in association with endocarditis are acutely ill with sepsis. As the disease progresses, signs of right sided heart failure are evident: jugular venous distension with a prominent *a* wave, peripheral edema, hepatomegaly, splenomegaly, and ascites.

In tricuspid incompetence, the murmur is soft blowing, holosystolic, and best heard along the lower left sternal border. In tricuspid stenosis, the rumbling crescendo-decrescendo diastolic murmur occurs just prior to $S_1$. This murmur is best heard along the lower left sternal border.

**Table 55-1.** Antibiotic Prophylaxis for Infective Endocarditis

| Procedure | Standard Regimen* | Alternative Regimen |
|---|---|---|
| Dental procedure known to cause bleeding Bronchoscopy with rigid bronchoscope | Amoxicillin 3.0 g orally 1 h prior to the procedure, then 1.5 g 6 h after first dose | Clindamycin 300 mg orally 1 h before procedure and 150 mg 6 h after 1st dose *or* Erythromycin ethyl-succinate 800 mg *or* Erythromycin stearate 1.0 g orally 2 h prior to procedure and one-half the dose 6 h after the first dose |
| Urethral catheterization if infection is present Urethral dilation | Ampicillin 2.0 g IV/IM plus gentamicin 1.5 mg/kg IV/IM (not to exceed 80 mg) 30 min before procedure, followed by amoxicillin 1.5 g orally 6 h after first dose | Vancomycin 1.0 g IV over 1 h plus gentamicin 1.5 mg/kg IV/IM (not to exceed 80 mg) 1 h prior to procedure and repeat 8 h later For low-risk patient, amoxicillin 3.0 g 1 h before procedure and 1.5 g 6 h after first dose |
| Incision and drainage of infected tissue | Cefazolin 1.0 g IM/IM 30 min before procedure and cephalexin 500 mg orally 6 h after first dose | Vancomycin 1.0 g IV over 1 h plus gentamicin 1.5 mg/kg IV/IM (not to exceed 80 mg) 1 h prior to procedure and repeat 8 h later |

* Includes patients with prosthetic heart valves and others at high risk. Initial pediatric doses are as follows: amoxicillin, 50 mg/kg, ampicillin 50 mg/kg, erythromycins 20 mg/kg, clindamycin 10 mg/kg, gentamicin 2 mg/kg, and vancomycin 20 mg/kg. Pediatric dose should not exceed listed adult dose.

## MULTIVALVULAR DISEASE

Multivalvular disease is common, but the presence of more than one abnormal valve makes the diagnosis of others more difficult. In addition, there may be coexisting stenosis and incompetence of diseased valves. Multivalvular and combined stenotic-incompetent valvular disease present with slightly different symptoms from the classic symptoms of single-valve disease.

### Pathophysiology

Rheumatic heart disease remains an important cause of combined aortic and mitral disease. Between 32 and 50 percent of patients with cardiac manifestations of rheumatic fever have both aortic and mitral disease. In aged patients calcification can lead to both aortic stenosis and mitral incompetence. Infective endocarditis can extend from either the mitral or aortic valve to the adjacent valve though the inflammatory process. Intravenous drug users may have multivalvular disease. Tricuspid regurgitation often occurs with right ventriclar dilation secondary to pulmonary hypertension that may be due to mitral disease or combined aortic and mitral disease.

### Clinical Features

Patients with combined valvular disease generally present at a younger age than those with a single chronic lesion. The most common symptom of combined valvular disease is dyspnea. Symptoms of multivalvular disease may resemble single-valve disease when advanced disease of one valve dominates the clinical picture. Although both syncope and angina pectoris are infrequent in patients with mitral regurgitation alone, chest pain and syncope are more common with incompetence of both the aortic and mitral valves. The presence of a chronic lesion of one valve exaggerates the effects of an acute lesion of another valve.

Physical signs are more difficult to interpret in mixed lesions. With combined aortic and mitral stenosis, the aortic systolic murmur is reduced. The mitral opening snap is infrequently audible in this setting. In regurgitant lesions of both aortic and mitral valves, the usual fall in diastolic blood pressure commonly seen with aortic incompetence may be absent. As many as 40 percent of patients with this combined valvular disease will have diastolic blood pressures above 70 mmHg.

## DIAGNOSIS OF VALVULAR HEART DISEASE

The loud background noise in the emergency department makes the accurate auscultation of subtle murmurs difficult. Despite this, the emergency physician may suspect undiagnosed valvular dysfunction on incidental cardiac auscultation. The ECG and chest radiograph may be of help but neither is confirmatory. The suspected diagnosis should be confirmed by echocardiography and/or consultation with a cardiologist. The urgency for an accurate diagnosis and appropriate referral depends on the severity of symptoms and the suspected diagnosis. For example, a patient presenting with syncope and auscultatory findings of aortic stenosis should be admitted to the hospital for observation and further evaluation.

Acute mitral or aortic incompetence are important and urgent diagnoses. Due to the severity of symptoms, it is unlikely that patients will go unnoticed in the emergency department, but the diagnosis can be difficult. Acute mitral or aortic incompetence should always be suspected in patients who present with acute pulmonary edema, especially when the heart is smaller than expected on chest radiography or when the patient does not respond to conventional therapy. When aortic dissection is suspected as the cause of acute aortic incompetence, and the patient is sufficiently stable, transesophageal echocardiography or computed tomographic scanning of the chest is useful. Angiography may still be required after CT scanning.

Emergency physicians should beware of the practice of labeling a heart murmur as "innocent." A truly innocent murmur has no abnormal symptoms or signs associated with it. The soft systolic ejection murmur begins after $S_1$ and ends before $S_2$ and the heart sounds are completely normal. The review of systems should elicit no symptoms compatible with cardiovascular disease, and a complete physical examination is normal with the exception of the flow murmur.

## EMERGENCY DEPARTMENT CARE OF SYMPTOMATIC VALVULAR HEART DISEASE

There is little that the emergency physician can do to change the structural abnormality of the diseased cardiac valve. The exception to this rule is acute mitral incompetence due to myocardial infarction. The infusion of thrombolytic therapy may reestablish blood flow to the papillary muscle, with restoration of function. The majority of treatments are directed towards symptomatic relief of the manifestations of valvular disease. However, there are certain medical treatments that can reduce the consequences of the mechanical defect. The regurgitation of aortic and mitral incompetence may be lessened by reducing afterload. In cases where the etiology of mitral incompetence is myocardial ischemia, regurgitation can be lessened by treatment with nitrates.

Pulmonary edema should be treated with oxygen, intubation for failing respiratory effort, diuretics, and nitrates if tolerated. Patients with aortic stenosis will usually have normal to low blood pressure and will not tolerate afterload reducers. In contrast, patients with mitral incompetence or aortic incompetence can benefit from intravenous nitroprusside or nitroglycerin even with normal blood pressures. Reducing afterload helps to reduce regurgitation and relieve pulmonary edema. Tachycardia reduces the regurgitant volume by reducing the time during the cardiac cycle during which back flow may

occur. Therefore, artificially lowering the pulse with a β-blocking agent may worsen symptoms.

The hypertension associated with aortic dissection should be controlled with intravenous nitroprusside and β blockade. Nifedipine has been used with success in this setting. Patients with valvular heart disease and acute pulmonary edema should be considered for Swan-Ganz catheter insertion. The presence of valvular disease, especially stenosis, may complicate the procedure of catheter insertion. In patients who do not respond to medical management, consider intraaortic balloon counter pulsation. However, this is contraindicated in wide-open aortic regurgitation.

Rapid atrial fibrillation, which may precipitate symptoms in patients with silent valvular disease, should be rate-controlled with intravenous diltiazem or digoxin. Intravenous propranolol or verapamil may be considered, but their negative inotropic action may cause more problems. Emergency cardioversion may be needed in severely compromised patients, but arrhythmia recurrence is common. The most common cause of the arrhythmia in valvular heart disease, a dilated atrium, remains unchanged by cardioversion. The danger of embolization is greater in patients with atrial fibrillation.

Hemoptysis associated with valvular heart disease most frequently accompanies pulmonary edema and is frothy pink. This form of hemoptysis does not in itself require treatment. However, if pulmonary hypertension is present, gross hemoptysis may occur from the rupture of distended bronchial veins. Mitral stenosis is the most frequent valvular heart disease associated with hemoptysis, which can be severe enough to require blood transfusion and emergency surgery.

In the event of embolization, anticoagulation should be undertaken with intravenous heparin as long as there is no evidence of CNS bleeding. This is especially needed in the setting of atrial fibrillation.

Emergency surgery should be considered in all cases of acute symptomatic valvular disease. Because stenotic lesions are slowly progressive, emergency surgery is rarely needed for stenotic defects. However, a patient with new onset of syncope in association with aortic stenosis should be considered for urgent repair. The need for emergency surgery most commonly accompanies acute regurgitant lesions of the mitral or aortic valves. Patients are acutely ill and considerable surgical risks. The urgency of these two acute regurgitant lesions leaves little time for intubation, intravenous afterload reducers, echocardiography, and assembling the surgical team for emergency valve replacement.

Patients with acute fevers should be suspected of having infective endocarditis. The evaluation and management of endocarditis are discussed below in "Infective Endocarditis." Antibiotic prophylaxis for infective endocarditis is recommended during procedures that are prone to bacteremia in patients at risk for developing endocarditis, and the American Heart Association guidelines should be followed. Patients considered at risk include those with a prosthetic heart valve, a history of endocarditis, rheumatic heart disease, acquired and congenital valvular disease, idiopathic hypertrophic subaortc stenosis, or mitral valve prolapse with a murmur. The common procedures performed by emergency physicians that require such prophylaxis are listed in Table 55-1. Endotracheal intubation does not require antibiotic prophylaxis. When a febrile patient is being evaluated for urinary tract infection, emergency physicians should consider the need for prophylaxis before using a catheter to obtain a urine specimen. However, recent data from an epidemiologic study suggest that medical and dental procedures cause only about 5 percent of endocarditis cases and that prophylaxis does not prevent all cases.

### Admission Indications

The presence of persistent symptoms in patients with valvular heart disease determines the indications for admission to the hospital. Patients with acute onset of valvular incompetence will be acutely ill and will require admission, but this will be obvious by their condition. Patients with aortic stenosis presenting with syncope on exertion should be considered for admission because of the critical limitation of blood flow that syncope usually heralds. Patients with valvular heart disease and a new symptomatic arrhythmia should also be considered for admission. Considerations for admission of patients with suspected infective endocarditis are listed below in "Infective endocarditis." Patients with intermittent symptoms from valvular heart disease can be management dilemmas. Consultation with a cardiologist may be required to determine the need for hospital admission.

### Discharge Instructions

Stable patients suspected of having valvular heart disease not previously diagnosed should be referred to a cardiologist or back to their private physician for an evaluation. The patient should be instructed to avoid strenuous exercise, work, or psychological stress–provoking activity until they have been cleared for such activity by the referral physician.

## PROSTHETIC VALVE DISEASE

Prosthetic valves are implanted in 40,000 patients per year in the United States. There are approximately 80 different types of artificial valves, each with their particular advantages and disadvantages. Patients who receive prosthetic valves are instructed to carry a card in their wallet that describes their valve. The prosthetic valves can be divided into two basic groups: the mechanical, nontissue models and the bioprostheses, using porcine, bovine, or human valves. Complications of prosthetic valves are more common in patients who have advanced heart disease, including cardiac dilation, left ventricular hypertrophy, congestive heart failure, or arrhythmias, at the time of the original operation.

### Pathophysiology

Prosthetic valves tend to be slightly stenotic, and a very small amount of regurgitation is common because of incomplete closure. Patients with mechanical valves require continuous anticoagulation. Some bioprostheses do not require anticoagulation. There are several complications that lead to dysfunction of the artificial valves. Thrombi can form on the prosthetic valve and become large enough to obstruct flow or prevent closure. The dysfunction due to thrombi can be acute or slowly progressive. Bioprostheses may gradually degenerate, undergoing gradual thinning, stiffening, and possibly tearing, which results in the valve becoming incompetent. The sutures that secure the prosthetic valve may become disrupted, leading to paravalvular regurgitation as a fistula forms at the periphery of the valve. Mechanical models may suddenly fracture or fail. These failures usually bring sudden symptoms and often are fatal before corrective surgery can be accomplished.

Systemic embolism, originating from a thrombus on the prosthetic valve, is the most important complication of mechanical models, occurring at a rate of 1 percent of patients per year. Embolism occurs less frequently with bioprostheses. Patients with artificial valves develop endocarditis at a rate of about 0.5 percent per year. Infections occur more frequently during the first 2 months after operation. The most common organisms during this period are *Staph. epidermidis* and *Staph. aureus*. Gram-negative organisms and fungi are also frequent causes of endocarditis during this early period. Late cases of endocarditis are similar to the those affecting native valves. The most frequent organism is *Streptococcus viridans,* but *Serratia* and *Pseudomonas* also occur. Patients with prosthetic valves and endocarditis may develop a ring abscess around the valve, which requires valve replacement. Patients with mechanical prostheses have an increased rate of intravascular destruction of red cells. Usually the red cell loss is easily corrected by the bone marrow, but the hemolytic anemia may be severe and indicate a paravalvular leak. Finally, patients with prosthetic valves may be particularly susceptible to hemodynamic compromise from a new arrhythmia such as atrial fibrillation.

### Clinical Features

Many patients have persistent dyspnea and reduced effort tolerance after successful valve replacement. This is more common in the presence of preexisting heart dysfunction or atrial fibrillation. Many symptoms of valvular dysfunction described in the preceding sections on specific valvular disease may occur in the setting of prosthetic valves. However, in addition to those symptoms, patients with prosthetic valves experience symptoms specific to the presence of artificial valve.

Large paravalvular leaks usually present with congestive heart failure or hemolytic anemia. Patients with new neurologic symptoms may have thromboembolism associated with valve thrombi or endocarditis. Minor embolic episodes, such as transient neurologic symptoms, amaurosis fugax, or self-limited ischemic episodes in the extremities or organs in the absence of endocarditis, are common. Patients may present with major embolic events including stroke, mesenteric infarction, or sudden death. Major bleeding due to anticoagulant therapy can also occur.

Patients with prosthetic valves usually have abnormal cardiac sounds. Mechanical valves have loud metallic-sounding closing sounds. Systolic murmurs are commonly present with mechanical models. Loud diastolic murmurs are generally not present with mechanical valves. Patients with bioprostheses usually have normal S and $S_2$, with no abnormal opening sounds. The aortic bioprosthesis is usually associated with a short midsystolic murmur. Only the mitral bioprosthesis is normally associated with a diastolic rumble.

### Diagnosis of Prosthetic Valve Dysfunction

New or progressive symptoms referable to the heart suggest a prosthetic valve disorder. Therefore, new or progressive dyspnea of any form, new onset or worsening of congestive heart failure, decreased exercise tolerance, or a change in chest pain compatible with ischemia all suggest valvular dysfunction. Severe hemolytic anemia may indicate a paravalvular leak. Persistent fever in patients with prosthetic valves should be evaluated for possible endocarditis. Changes in valve position may be noted on chest radiographs if comparison views are available. Blood studies that may be helpful include a blood count with red cell indices and coagulation studies if the patient is on warfarin. Emergency echocardiography should be requested if there is any question about valve dysfunction. Ultimately, echocardiography and/or cardiac catheterization may be required for diagnosis.

### Emergency Department Management and Admission Indications

The medical management of patients with valvular dysfunction is the same as described in "Emergency Department Care of Symptomatic Valvular Heart Disease," above. The evaluation and management of endocarditis is described in the following section. Acute prosthetic valvular dysfunction due to thrombotic obstruction has been successfully treated with thrombolytic therapy, but the diagnosis requires angiography and therefore will not be done by the emergency physician without consultation with a cardiologist.

Patients suspected of having acute prosthetic valvular dysfunction or endocarditis require admission to the hospital and evaluation for possible valve replacement. Disposition patients with worsening of symptoms can be problematic, and consultation with the patient's regular physician is needed.

# INFECTIVE ENDOCARDITIS

The preferred term, *infective endocarditis,* encompasses all types of endocarditis caused by infectious organisms and represents an infection of the endocardium occurring on the valve leaflets, the walls of the heart cavities, or the tissue surrounding prosthetic heart valves. The infection may be subacute or acute, depending on the virulence of the organism, the susceptibility of the host, and the presence of intravenous drug use. Because of the declining frequency of rheumatic heart disease, the increasing number of cardiac surgical procedures, and the increasing numbers of intravenous drug users, the nature of this disease has changed dramatically in the last twenty years.

## Pathophysiology

The cardiac valve leaflets are the portion of the heart most susceptible to infection because of their limited blood supply. Endocarditis can occur with normal valves but is more common with congenital and acquired valve disease and prosthetic valves. Bacteria and fungi gain entry to the circulation through various routes and settle on valvular tissue. A platelet-fibrin matrix forms, and further growth of the organisms enlarges to form a vegetation on the valve that makes the organisms inaccessible to normal cellular host defenses. Risk factors for infective endocarditis include congenital or acquired valvular heart disease, intravenous drug abuse, prosthetic valves, hemodialysis or peritoneal dialysis, indwelling venous catheters, postcardiac surgery, and calcific valve degeneration that occurs with increasing age. Rheumatic heart disease, although still important, is declining in frequency.

Infective endocarditis can be divided into acute and subacute forms depending on the virulence of the infecting organism. Subacute disease more commonly infects abnormal valves, while acute disease more commonly infects previously normal valves. In the acute form, devastating complications are more common and include rapid disruption of the valve leading to incompetence and heart failure. Embolism of the vegetations is responsible for many of the clinical features of the disease in both its forms. Younger patients are most likely to have acute endocarditis, while older individuals are more likely to have subacute disease. In the subacute form, anemia is common and is probably a reflection of the chronicity of the disease. Antibodies form in reaction to foreign antigen, and immune complex injury to basement membranes of the kidney may result in glomerulonephritis, which can occur in both acute and subacute disease.

Endocarditis can be further divided into left and right heart disease. Left-sided disease (aortic and mitral involvement) is the most common. The most common organisms include *Strep. viridans* (declining in frequency), *Staph. aureus* (increasing in frequency), *Enterococcus,* and fungal organisms. *Pseudomonas* and *Serratia* are important etiologic agents in intravenous drug users in certain areas of the country, especially Detroit and San Francisco, respectively. Cardiac failure is the most common cause of death in left-sided disease, but deaths due to neurologic complications are increasing. Patients with aortic involvement are more prone to ring abscess and atrioventricular block. Vegetations may embolize from the left heart causing neurologic complications, systemic infarction, or metastatic infection.

Right-sided disease is usually seen in intravenous drug abusers (60 percent) and is caused by *Staph. aureus* (75 percent), *Strep. pneumonia* (20 percent), gram-negative organisms (4 percent), and fungal organisms. Vegetations may embolize from the right heart causing pulmonary infection or infarction. The fatality rate of right-sided endocarditis is lower because the incidence of cardiac failure is less than with left-sided disease.

## Clinical Features

Acute left-sided disease presents with a picture of sepsis with or without cardiac failure. Typically, patients appear ill with fever, chills, and tachycardia and may have significant congestive failure symptoms such as dyspnea, frothy sputum, and chest pain. Patients may quickly deteriorate with acute rupture of mitral or aortic valves. Murmurs are typically those of aortic or mitral regurgitation; however, the murmur is often absent or unable to be heard over lung sounds in acute cases. Neurologic symptoms secondary to aseptic meningoencephalitis and embolization of vegetations account for about one-third of emergency department presentations. These complications most commonly are mental status changes, hemiplegia, aphasia, ataxia, or severe headache. Monocular blindness can also occur.

Patients with subacute left-sided disease present with recurrent intermittent fever and constitutional symptoms such as malaise, anorexia, or weight loss. The diagnosis is frequently missed. Patients may give a history of recurrent "flu" or report several courses of antibiotics for presumed bacterial infections such as bronchitis. The majority of patients with left-sided subacute disease have a murmur of aortic or mitral regurgitation or a change in the previous murmur at the time of their admission to the hospital. However, many admitted patients have been examined previously by a physician who did not detect the murmur. Patients may have Roth spots, which are retinal hemorrhages with central clearing. Peripheral evidence of endocarditis includes Osler nodes, tender nodules on the tips of the toes and fingers, and Janeway lesions, nontender plaques on the soles of the feet and palms of the hands. Petechiae may be seen on the conjunctiva, hard palate, neck, and upper trunk. Splinter hemorrhages may be seen in the nails of the fingers or toes. Splenomegaly is noted in 25 percent of patients. Patients may present with back pain as their only complaint.

Right-sided disease is usually acute and presents with fever and respiratory symptoms: cough, chest pain, hemoptysis, and dyspnea. Subacute presentations are unusual with right-sided disease. Murmurs are detectable in fewer than 50 percent of patients with right-sided disease. Chest radiography often reveals pulmonary effusions and multiple pulmonary infiltrates of variable size and shape. Although meningitis coexists in only 5 percent of left-sided disease, bacterial meningitis is seen in up to 30 percent of patients with right-sided disease.

## Diagnosis

The diagnosis of endocarditis is based on positive blood cultures and evidence of valvular injury or vegetations. Three separate cultures from different veins should be obtained. Aerobic, anaerobic, and fungal cultures should be obtained. Cultures should be obtained before antibiotics are started. Echocardiography is helpful but should not delay appropriate stabilizing treatments. Evidence of vasculitis or embolic events contributes to the clinical diagnosis. Nonspecific laboratory findings that support the diagnosis of endocarditis include leukocytosis, elevated C-reactive proteins, normocytic anemia, hematuria (25 to 50 percent), and pyuria.

## Emergency Department Care

The first priority in the care of patients with acute infective endocarditis is stabilization of respiratory and cardiac symptoms. For patients with mental status changes and hypoxia, or a compromised airway, intubation may be required. Cardiac decompensation is usually due to left-sided valvular incompetence and/or rupture. Acute rupture of the mitral or aortic valve should be stabilized with afterload reducers such as sodium nitroprusside, with insertion of a Swan-Ganz catheter for monitoring therapy as soon as possible. Preparation for emergency surgery should be made for patients suspected of acute valvular rupture. Aortic balloon counterpulsation may be helpful for mitral valve rupture but is contraindicated for wide-open aortic valve rupture.

The second priority is drawing three blood cultures from different sites and then starting empiric antibiotic therapy. For acute infective endocarditis, a penicillinase-resistant penicillin such as nafcillin,

1.5 g every 4 h, should be given with an aminoglycoside, chosen on the basis of local patterns of susceptibility. In areas where there is a high incidence of methicillin-resistant staphylococcus or in the case of a patient taking oral antibiotics already, use vancomycin, 1 g IV, in addition to an aminoglycoside. Patients with prosthetic valve endocarditis should be treated with antibiotics that cover *Staph. epidermidis,* usually vancomycin, 1 g IV, in addition to an aminoglycoside. Although subacute cases are frequently caused by *Strep. viridans* and this bacterium is covered by penicillin G, patients with subacute presentations who require admission should be started on a newer cephalosporin, such as ceftriaxone, 1 g IV, in addition to an aminoglycoside until cultures and sensitivities are known. For patients with subacute disease who were taking oral antibiotics for another presumed infection, consideration should be given to collecting at least seven cultures or waiting until cultures turn positive before giving intravenous antibiotics.

## Admission Indications

In general, patients with suspected endocarditis should be admitted to the hospital. The incidence of endocarditis is so high in febrile intravenous drug users that the majority of these patients should be admitted to the hospital, cultures should be drawn, and empiric therapy started.

## Ambulatory Treatment

The ambulatory treatment of culture-proven *Strep. viridans* endocarditis has recently been advocated. Patients were treated with ceftriaxone, 2 g daily IM injections for 4 weeks, and did well. This should not affect emergency medicine practice. Cultures are not usually available until some time after admission to the hospital. For patients for whom blood cultures are drawn and who are sent home, a consultation should be made to a cardiologist for evaluation and follow-up.

## NONVALVULAR INFECTIONS OF THE HEART

Nonvalvular infections of the heart involve the endocardium, the myocardium, and the pericardium. In addition, pacemakers; automatic, implantable cardioverter-defibrillators; and other cardiac devices may become infected in the subcutaneous device pocket or along the vascular tracks leading to and including the heart. Most commonly those devices become infected at the device pocket. This is more readily diagnosed because of tenderness and erythema easily noted on physical examination. Myocardial abscesses and mural endocarditis are discussed here because of their similarities to valvular endocarditis. These two conditions are difficult to diagnose because their signs and symptoms are subtle.

## Pathophysiology

Risk factors for the development of myocardial abscesses or mural endocarditis include chronic debilitating illness, immunosuppression, indwelling catheters, prolonged antibiotic therapy, and valvular endocarditis. The source of infection may be from hematogenous seeding, contiguous extension from valvular endocarditis. These two infections may coexist or one may lead to the development of the other. In the case of mural endocarditis, bacteria may seed damaged endocardium or aneurysms in the ventricular wall. In the case of myocardial abscesses, multiple areas of the myocardium may be involved, but when valvular endocarditis is the source of bacterial seeding, the paravalvular areas are usually involved. The most frequent organisms in these nonvalvular infections of the heart are *Staph. aureus, Strep. viridans,* and other organisms associated with valvular endocarditis.

## Clinical Features

The symptoms and signs may be completely nonspecific, especially with myocardial abscesses. Patients usually experience vague fevers and chills but may present with more obvious sepsis. Frequently patients are given antibiotics as outpatients for some presumed bacterial infection such as bronchitis. Patients may be suspected of having valvular endocarditis and be admitted to the hospital for IV antibiotics, yet the correct diagnosis is not made and symptoms recur after discharge. Many symptoms, including positive blood cultures, peripheral embolization, and splenomegaly, are found in both valvular and nonvalvular infections of the heart. Frequently patients have sudden fatal complications, such as myocardial rupture, tamponade, or severe peripheral embolization, and are diagnosed only at autopsy.

## Diagnosis

The diagnosis of these two conditions, myocardial abscess and mural endocarditis, is difficult. Blood cultures are positive in 75 percent of patients with myocardial abscess, but this finding is nonspecific. In cases of mural endocarditis, patients frequently have peripheral embolization and splenomegaly, but these findings do not distinguish mural from valvular endocarditis. When these conditions are found at autopsy in a previously undiagnosed patient, endocarditis is frequently the misdiagnosis. Whenever patients present with findings compatible with endocarditis, yet both physical examination and echocardiography fail to demonstrate valvular lesions, these two nonvalvular infections of the heart should be considered. Unfortunately, diagnosis with echocardiography or even cardiac angiography is difficult. Transesophageal echocardiography may offer the best results.

## Emergency Department Management

When nonvalvular infections of the heart are suspected by the emergency physician, the patient should be admitted to the hospital. Accurate structural and microbiologic diagnosis is essential to proper management, which may include surgical drainage and repair. Therefore antibiotics should be withheld until the plan for diagnostic evaluation can be initiated.

## BIBLIOGRAPHY

Cohn LH, Birjiniuk V: Therapy of acute aortic regurgitation. *Cardiol Clin* 9:339, 1991.

Dajani AS, Bisno AL, Chung KJ, et al: Prevention of bacterial endocarditis: Recommendations by the American Heart Association. *JAMA* 264:2919, 1990.

Delaney KA: Endocarditis in the emergency department. *Ann Emerg Med* 20:405, 1991.

Devereux RB, Kramer-Fox R, Brown WT, et al: Relations between clinical features of mitral valve prolapse and echocardiographically documented mitral valve prolapse. *J Am Coll Cardiol* 8:763, 1986.

Francioli P, Etienne J, Hoigne R, et al: Treatment of streptococcal endocarditis with a single daily dose of ceftriaxone sodium for 4 weeks: Efficiency and outpatient treatment feasibility. *JAMA* 267:264, 1992.

Greenberg BH: Medical therapy for patients with aortic insufficiency. *Cardiol Clin* 9:255, 1991.

Grunkemeier GL, Rahimtoola SH: Artificial heart valves. *Annu Rev Med* 41:251, 1990.

Kearney RA, Eisen HJ, Wolf JE: Nonvalvular infections of the cardiovascular system. *Ann Intern Med* 121:219, 1994.

Khan SS, Gray RJ: Valvular emergencies. *Cardiol Clin* 9:689, 1991.

Mansur AJ, Grinberg M, Lemos da Laz P, et al: The complications of infective endocarditis: A reappraisal in the 1980s. *Arch Intern Med* 152:2428, 1992.

Marti V, Subirana MT, Ballester M, et al: Successful thrombolytic therapy for prosthetic pulmonary valve thrombosis evaluated by Doppler echocardiography. *Am Heart J* 123:1065, 1992.

Samet JH, Shevits A, Fowle J, et al: Hospitalization decision in febrile intravenous drug users. *Am J Med* 89:53, 1990.

van der Meer JT, Thompson J, Valkenburg HA, et al: Epidemiology of bacterial endocarditis in the Netherlands: II. Antecedent procedures and use of prophylaxis. *Arch Intern Med* 152:1869, 1992.

# 56
# THE CARDIOMYOPATHIES, MYOCARDITIS, AND PERICARDIAL DISEASE

### James T. Niemann

## THE CARDIOMYOPATHIES

### Classification and Definition

The term *cardiomyopathy* is broadly used to describe a group of diseases that directly alter cardiac structure and impair myocardial function. Primary cardiomyopathies are those diseases that originate in the myocardium itself. By current definition, a primary cardiomyopathy is of unknown origin (idiopathic). Secondary cardiomyopathies are those that result from a systemic disease that involves the heart as part of a recognized disease process or from a variety of toxins that effect cardiac structure and function.

Three types of cardiomyopathies are recognized: (1) dilated, (2) hypertrophic, and (3) restrictive. Some secondary cardiomyopathies may present with restrictive or dilated characteristics. The cardiomyopathies, as a group, are the third most common form of cardiac disease encountered in the United States and follow coronary (ischemic) heart disease and hypertensive heart disease in prevalence.

### Dilated Cardiomyopathy

This subgroup is characterized hemodynamically by depressed myocardial systolic function or systolic pump failure. Left ventricular (LV) contractile force is diminished, resulting in a low cardiac output and increased end-systolic and end-diastolic ventricular volumes and intracavitary pressures. Cardiomegaly results from both dilatation and hypertrophy. Systemic diseases that may involve the heart and produce a dilated cardiomyopathy as part of a recognized disease process are shown in Table 56-1. The vast majority of cases are idiopathic, and a specific etiology or associated disease will be found in fewer than 15 percent of patients. With increasing use of percutaneous endomyocardial biopsy as a diagnostic tool, many patients with the presumptive diagnosis of idiopathic cardiomyopathy have been found to have active lymphocytic myocarditis, presumably of viral origin.

### Clinical Profile

As a result of systolic pump failure, the patient presents with signs and symptoms of congestive heart failure: dyspnea on exertion, orthopnea, and paroxysmal nocturnal dyspnea. Depressed ventricular

**Table 56-1.** Dilated Cardiomyopathy: Known Cause or Association

| | |
|---|---|
| *Infectious* | *Associated with neuromuscular disorders* |
| Viral | *(the muscular dystrophies)* |
| Protozoal | *Associated with collagen vascular diseases* |
| Parasitic | *Sarcoidosis* |
| *Metabolic* | *Myocardial toxins* |
| Thyrotoxicosis | Ethanol |
| Myxedema | Heavy metals |
| Acromegaly | Emetine |
| Hemochromatosis | Adriamycin |
| Glycogen storage disease | Cobalt |
| Thiamine deficiency | *Ischemia* |
| (beriberi) | |
| Hypophosphatemia | |
| *Peripartum* | |
| *Amyloidosis* | |

contractile function and dilatation may result in the formation of mural thrombi, and the patient may present with manifestations of peripheral embolization, e.g., an acute neurologic deficit, flank pain and hematuria, or a pulseless, cyanotic extremity.

Murmurs are frequently heard during cardiac auscultation and are not necessarily indicative of primary valvular disease. Ventricular dilatation and the resultant annular dilatation and displacement of the papillary muscles of the atrioventricular valves inhibit leaflet coaptation and complete valve closure. Holosystolic regurgitant murmurs of mitral and tricuspid valve origin are frequently heard at the apex or lower left sternal border in the patient with biventricular failure. On occasion an apical "diastolic rumble" may be heard and is due either to accentuated, early-diastolic atrial-to-ventricular flow (the result of mitral regurgitation and left atrial overload) or to a loud summation gallop. An enlarged, pulsatile liver may be found if tricuspid insufficiency is significant. Bibasilar rales and dependent edema are common additional findings.

The chest x-ray invariably shows an enlarged cardiac silhouette and increased cardiothoracic ratio; biventricular enlargement is common. Evidence of pulmonary venous hypertension ("cephalization" of flow, enlarged hila) is also frequent and may serve to differentiate cardiac enlargement due to myocardial failure from that due to a large pericardial effusion.

The electrocardiogram (ECG) is almost always abnormal. Left ventricular hypertrophy and left atrial enlargement are the most common findings. Q or QS waves and poor R-wave progression across the anterior precordium may produce a pseudoinfarction pattern. Atrial fibrillation and ventricular ectopy are frequently encountered rhythm disturbances.

Echocardiography in the symptomatic patient demonstrates a decreased ejection fraction, increased systolic and diastolic volumes, and ventricular and atrial enlargement.

### Therapy

Management of the patient with dilated cardiomyopathy is symptom-directed, and the prescribed therapeutic regimen almost always employs the digitalis glycosides and diuretics. Patients unresponsive to these agents may respond symptomatically after the addition of preload- and afterload-reducing agents such as the angiotensin-converting enzyme inhibitors. Chronic oral anticoagulant therapy should be used to decrease the likelihood of intracavitary thrombosis and peripheral arterial embolization, especially in patients with chronic atrial fibrillation. A thorough diagnostic evaluation should be undertaken for all patients with unexplained heart failure or cardiomegaly. Such an evaluation may reveal an underlying disease that is amenable to specific therapy in patients with secondary forms of dilated cardiomyopathy.

### Hypertrophic Cardiomyopathy

*Hypertrophic cardiomyopathy* (HCM) is a familial (autosomal dominant) or sporadic cardiac muscle disorder characterized by increased left ventricular muscle mass without associated ventricular dilatation. The diagnostic hallmarks of the disease are echocardiographic asymmetrical septal hypertrophy and histologic myocardial fiber disarray.

Hemodynamically, HCM is characterized by abnormal LV diastolic function due to reduced compliance of the hypertrophied left ventricle. This decreased compliance is reflected by an increase in LV filling pressure. Cardiac output, ejection fraction, and end-systolic and end-diastolic volumes are usually normal. During cardiac catheterization and hemodynamic monitoring, a systolic pressure gradient between the body of the left ventricle and the subvalvular outflow tract can be recorded in some patients at rest or after provocation (exercise, isoproterenol infusion). The majority of clinical symptoms in this heart muscle disease are the result of impaired diastolic relaxation and restricted LV filling.

## Clinical Profile

Severity of symptoms in most instances is related to patient age; the older the patient, the more severe the symptoms. Dyspnea on exertion is the most frequent initial complaint and is due to exercised-induced sinus tachycardia, which results in an abrupt elevated LV diastolic pressure and pulmonary venous hypertension. Additional symptoms include chest pain, palpitations, and syncope. A family history of death due to cardiac disease, frequently described as "massive heart attack" or "heart failure," is not uncommon. Complaints of paroxysmal nocturnal dyspnea and pedal edema are infrequent.

Chest pain in HCM patients is due to an imbalance between the oxygen demand of the hypertrophied left ventricle and the available myocardial blood flow. In older patients, associated atherosclerotic coronary artery disease may further limit myocardial perfusion. Precordial or retrosternal chest discomfort in HCM may mimic angina pectoris or may be "atypical." Response to nitroglycerin administration is poor and highly variable.

The HCM patient may be aware of forceful ventricular contraction and complain of an abnormal heartbeat or "palpitations." Atrial and ventricular arrhythmias are not uncommon in these patients; rapid atrial arrhythmias, especially atrial fibrillation, are particularly poorly tolerated because of the increased importance of the atrial contribution to LV filling in the poorly compliant heart and require aggressive management in the hemodynamically unstable patient.

Jugular venous pressure is usually not elevated; however, a prominent $a$ wave may be noted on close inspection of the neck veins. The upstroke of the carotid arterial pulse is rapid and frequently biphasic or bifid (pulsus bisferiens). The apical impulse is sustained and hyperdynamic, and a presystolic lift is common.

The first and second heart sounds are usually normal, and a fourth sound ($S_4$) will be heard in most patients. The characteristic systolic ejection-type murmur of HCM is heard best at the lower left sternal border or at the apex and rarely radiates to the carotid arteries. Easily performed bedside maneuvers can be used to increase the intensity and duration of the murmur (Table 56-2). Interventions that decrease LV filling and the distending pressure in the LV outflow tract or that increase the force of myocardial contraction accentuate the murmur of HCM. Such interventions include standing, the Valsalva maneuver, amyl nitrate inhalation, and isoproterenol infusion. The murmur will also be louder with the first sinus beat following a premature ventricular contraction. Maneuvers that increase LV filling (squatting, passive leg elevation, handgrip) have an opposite effect on murmur characteristics.

ECG findings of LV hypertrophy and left atrial enlargement are found in 30 percent and 25 to 50 percent, respectively, of HCM patients. Evidence of chamber enlargement is most common in patients with large gradients across the LV outflow tract. Q waves of considerable amplitude (>0.3 mV), termed *septal Q waves,* are seen in about 25 percent of patients and may be encountered in the anterior, lateral, or inferior leads. These Q waves may mimic those seen following myocardial infarction (*pseudoinfarction pattern*). The polarity of the T wave may serve as a diagnostic clue in the separation of HCM septal Q waves from Q waves due to myocardial infarction. Upright T waves in those leads with QS or QR complexes are usually found in HCM; T-wave inversion in such leads is highly suggestive of ischemic heart disease.

**Table 56-2.** Effect of Bedside Intervention on Murmur Intensity and Duration in HCM

| Increase | Decrease |
| --- | --- |
| Valsalva maneuver | Passive leg elevation in supine patient |
| Standing | Handgrip |
| Amyl nitrate inhalation | Squatting |
| β Agonists (isoproterenol infusion) | α Agonists (phenylephrine infusion) |

The chest x-ray is frequently normal, and identifiable abnormalities are largely nonspecific. Many patients do not show radiographic evidence of LV or left atrial enlargement. Evidence of pulmonary venous congestion is unusual but has been reported.

Echocardiography has played a substantial role in the diagnosis of HCM, in the correlation of the auscultatory and hemodynamic events with LV anatomic changes, and in defining inheritance patterns. The characteristic echocardiographic finding is disproportionate septal hypertrophy. Additional described echocardiographic abnormalities include normal or reduced LV end-diastolic dimensions, systolic anterior motion of the mitral valve, and midsystolic closure of the aortic valve.

## Therapy

The mainstay of medical therapy for the symptomatic patient, specifically the patient with chest pain, has been the liberal use of β blockers, which decrease LV contractility. Studies have demonstrated that calcium-blocking agents may be of value in a carefully defined population of HCM patients who do not respond to β blockade. Surgical therapy (septal muscle excision or mitral valve replacement) has not been shown conclusively to offer advantages over medical therapy. Antibiotic prophylaxis is recommended for dental procedures and potentially unsterile surgery. Several authorities discourage competitive athletics of any type, since sudden death following vigorous exertion is not infrequent in patients with HCM.

## Restrictive Cardiomyopathy

This is the least common of the clinically recognized and described cardiomyopathies. The hemodynamic characteristics of a restrictive cardiomyopathy include (1) elevated left and right ventricular end-diastolic pressure, (2) normal LV systolic function (ejection fraction > 50 percent), and (3) an abrupt and rapid rise in early-diastolic ventricular pressure following a marked decline at the onset of diastole. The rapid rise and abrupt plateau in the early-diastolic ventricular pressure tracing result in a characteristic (but not diagnostic) "square-root sign" or "dip-and-plateau" filling pattern. Simultaneously recorded left and right ventricular diastolic pressures are frequently mirror images, varying by only a few millimeters of mercury. These hemodynamic findings are similar to those reported in constrictive pericarditis, and differentiation at times may require surgical biopsy. Causes of restrictive cardiomyopathy are listed in Table 56-3. In the vast majority of cases, no specific etiology can be defined.

## Clinical Profile

In patients with advanced cardiac disease of known etiology, clinical symptoms are similar to those noted in patients with a dilated cardiomyopathy, namely, pedal edema and decreased exercise tolerance or other evidence of pulmonary venous hypertension. Chest pain, either typical for angina or atypical, is also a frequent presenting complaint, and its cause is unknown.

Findings on physical examination depend on the stage or severity of myocardial involvement. An $S_3$ and/or $S_4$ is commonly heard in the asymptomatic or minimally symptomatic patient. Gallop rhythms and systolic murmurs (due to mitral regurgitation) are usually heard in advanced cases, as are pulmonary rales, and pedal edema is present.

**Table 56-3.** Causes of Restrictive Cardiomyopathy

Idiopathic (includes endomyocardial fibrosis and Loeffler eosinophilic endomyocardial disease)
Secondary (associated with systemic disease)
    Hemochromatosis
    Amyloidosis
    Sarcoidosis
    Progressive systemic sclerosis (scleroderma)

The routine chest x-ray may be normal and, combined with symptoms and physical findings, may suggest constrictive pericarditis. In advanced cases, enlargement of the cardiac silhouette and pulmonary vascular redistribution are seen.

The ECG is frequently abnormal, but "diagnostic" changes have not been described. The most frequently reported ECG changes include chamber enlargement (ventricular and atrial) and repolarization abnormalities (nonspecific ST-T-wave changes). Low-voltage QRS complexes (<0.7 mV) have been frequently reported in patients with restrictive cardiomyopathy secondary to amyloidosis and hemochromatosis.

## Therapy

With the exception of hemochromatosis and sarcoidosis (variably responsive to chelation therapy with deferoxamine and glucocorticoid therapy, respectively), therapy for restrictive cardiomyopathy is symptom-directed and consists mainly of diuretics, digoxin, vasodilators, and antiarrhythmic agents for complicating rhythm disturbances. However, patients with amyloid cardiomyopathy may be "digoxin sensitive" (prone to toxicity) because of amyloid fibril binding of digoxin, and this medication should be used with caution in such patients.

## MYOCARDITIS

### Definition

Myocarditis is broadly but nonspecifically defined as inflammation of the heart muscle and is most frequently characterized pathologically by focal infiltration of the myocardium by lymphocytes, plasma cells, and histiocytes. Varying amounts of myocytolysis and destruction of the interstitial reticulin network are also seen. The pathologic changes have been ascribed to a number of infectious agents (Table 56-4), some of which involve the myocardium secondarily as part of a systemic disease process. Myocarditis is frequently accompanied by pericarditis.

### Clinical Profile

Fever is common, as is sinus tachycardia, which is usually "out of proportion" with respect to the extent of temperature elevation. Signs and symptoms depend on the extent of myocardial involvement and resultant depression of myocardial systolic function. In severe cases, progressive heart failure with its associated symptoms may be seen. With less extensive myocardial involvement, pericarditis and the clinical manifestations of systemic illness (fever, myalgias, headache, rigors) may overshadow clinical signs of myocardial dysfunction, and myocarditis may not be suspected. Retrosternal or precordial chest pain is a frequent presenting complaint and is most commonly secondary to associated pericardial inflammation (myopericarditis). This chest pain may mimic angina in its character. A pericardial friction rub is commonly heard in patients with myopericarditis.

The chest roentgenogram is usually normal, and reported abnormalities (cardiomegaly and pulmonary venous hypertension and/or pulmonary edema) vary with disease severity and are nondiagnostic. Reported ECG changes include nonspecific ST-T-wave changes, ST-segment elevation (due to associated pericarditis), atrioventricular

**Table 56-4.** Common Infectious Causes of Myocarditis

| Viral agents | Bacteria |
| --- | --- |
| Coxsackie B virus | *Corynebacterium diphtheriae* |
| Echovirus | *Neisseria meningitides* |
| Influenza virus | *Mycoplasma pneumoniae* |
| Parainfluenza virus | β-Hemolytic streptococci |
| Epstein-Barr virus | (rheumatic fever) |
| Hepatitis B virus | Lyme disease |
| HIV | |

block, and prolonged QRS duration. Echocardiography may reveal depressed systolic function in severe cases.

## Treatment

Current therapy in cases of idiopathic or viral myocarditis is largely supportive and symptom-directed. Myocarditis in rheumatic fever and complicating diphtheria or meningococcemia necessitates directed antibiotic therapy.

## UNEXPLAINED HEART FAILURE OR CARDIOMEGALY: DIFFERENTIAL DIAGNOSIS AND EVALUATION

Symptoms of congestive heart failure and associated cardiomegaly or evidence of cardiomegaly in the asymptomatic patient necessitates a directed evaluation. In the vast majority of instances, one of the following seven disease entities will eventually be diagnosed. Where appropriate, recognized diagnostic clues are noted.

1. *Hypertensive heart disease.* Systemic arterial hypertension affects 10 to 20 percent of the adult population. This is a disease with a high prevalence which may be diagnosed at a number of stages. The patient with a dilated cardiomyopathy and untreated cardiac failure will frequently present with an elevated blood pressure due to autonomically mediated compensatory reflexes. Isolated involvement of the myocardium as the major manifestation of systemic arterial hypertension is rare. A careful search for evidence of other end-organ damage due to arterial hypertension should be undertaken (examination of fundi, assessment of renal function, evaluation for focal neurologic changes, or history of such).
2. *Ischemic heart disease (ischemic cardiomyopathy).* Most patients with clinical signs of biventricular heart failure and cardiomegaly due to obstructive coronary arterial disease will relate a history of typical anginal pain or documented myocardial infarction(s). A few will not, and clinical presentation and physical findings in these cases will mimic those of an idiopathic dilated cardiomyopathy.
3. *Valvular heart disease.* Although the incidence of rheumatic heart disease in the United States is low, it remains a prevalent disease in underdeveloped countries and is frequently first diagnosed in recent immigrants. The growing "geriatric" population is prone to calcific aortic stenosis and mitral annular calcification. In addition, bicuspid or unicuspid aortic valve abnormalities remain as the most common congenital heart disease. All may present with congestive heart failure or incidental cardiac enlargement, and systolic and diastolic murmurs may be noted. Echocardiography is the diagnostic test of choice in the patient with suspected valvular heart disease. Hemodynamic and angiographic studies may be confirmatory.
4. *Constrictive pericardial disease.* Constrictive pericarditis frequently presents with clinical manifestations that mimic right-sided failure. A past history of pericarditis and minimal cardiac enlargement, clear lung fields, and pericardial calcification on chest x-ray are diagnostic clues.
5. *Myocarditis.* The patient with severe myocarditis may present with signs and symptoms of cardiac insufficiency. Such patients are usually young, have no significant past cardiac history, have few risk factors for atherosclerotic coronary arterial disease, and present with a recent, abrupt onset of symptoms during or immediately following a systemic or viral illness.
6. *Hypertrophic cardiomyopathy.* The patient with hypertrophic cardiomyopathy may present with a history of shortness of breath or decreased exercise tolerance. Symptoms thus mimic left heart failure. Echocardiography and, if necessary, left heart catheterization are critical diagnostic aids.
7. *Idiopathic cardiomyopathy.* This diagnosis should be considered only if the first six entities have been excluded. A careful search for potential etiologic causes should then be undertaken.

# PERICARDIAL DISEASE

The pericardium consists of a serous or loose fibrous membrane (visceral pericardium) overlying the epicardium and a dense collagenous sac (parietal pericardium) surrounding the heart. The space between the visceral and parietal pericardium may contain up to 50 mL of fluid under normal conditions, and intrapericardial pressure is normally subatmospheric. Because its layers are serosal surfaces and because of its proximity and attachments to other structures, the pericardium may be involved in a number of systemic or localized disease processes (Table 56-5). The clinical presentation of pericardial heart disease is variable and dependent on the pericardium's response to injury and how this response affects cardiac function. In this section the clinical manifestations and evaluation of acute and constrictive pericarditis are discussed.

## Acute Pericarditis

### Symptoms and Signs

The most common symptom is precordial or retrosternal chest pain, which is most frequently described as sharp or stabbing. It may be of sudden or gradual onset and radiate to the back, neck, left shoulder, or arm; referral to the left trapezial ridge (due to inflammation of the joining diaphragmatic pleura) is a particular distinguishing feature. Chest pain due to acute pericarditis may be aggravated by inspiration or movement. It may be most severe when the patient is supine and is often relieved when the patient sits up and leans forward. In most instances, these characteristics allow the pain of acute pericarditis to be distinguished from the ischemic pain of angina or acute myocardial infarction.

Associated symptoms include (1) low-grade, intermittent fever, particularly if pericarditis is infectious in origin or of the idiopathic type; (2) dyspnea, due to accentuated pain with inspiration; and (3) dysphagia, ascribed to irritation of the esophagus by the posterior pericardium.

A pericardial friction rub is the most common and important physical finding in pericarditis. A pericardial rub most closely resembles a superficial grating or scratching sound. It is best heard with the diaphragm of the stethoscope at the lower left sternal border or apex when the patient is sitting and leaning forward or in the hands-and-knees position. It may be audible only during a certain phase of respiration and characteristically is transient, i.e., heard one hour and not the next. No inference as to the amount of pericardial fluid should be drawn from the presence or absence of a pericardial friction rub.

A pericardial rub is most often triphasic in character, consisting of a systolic component, an early diastolic component occurring during the early phase of ventricular filling, and a presystolic component synchronous with atrial systole. It is less commonly biphasic, i.e., a systolic component with either an early diastolic or presystolic component. A monophasic rub is unusual (18 percent of cases) but is most often systolic.

**Table 56-5.** Common Causes of Acute Pericarditis

Idiopathic
Infectious
    Viral (especially Coxsackie virus and echovirus)
    Bacterial [especially staphylococcus, *Streptococcus pneumoniae*,
    β-hemolytic streptococci (acute rheumatic fever), *Mycobacterium
    tuberculosis*]
    Fungal (especially *Histoplasma capsulatum*)
Malignancy (leukemia, lymphoma, metastatic breast and lung carcinoma,
  melanoma)
Drug-induced (procainamide, hydralazine)
Connective tissue disease
Radiation-induced
Postmyocardial infarction (Dressler syndrome)
Uremia
Myxedema

Other common associated physical findings include fever and resting sinus tachycardia. Additional signs (paradoxical pulse, venous distension, Kussmaul sign) may result from the effects of an expanding pericardial effusion on ventricular filling.

## Diagnostic Findings

### Electrocardiogram

Serial ECGs recorded over a number of days may be diagnostic in acute pericarditis. The evolutionary ECG changes during acute pericarditis and convalescence have been divided into four stages. During stage 1, or the acute phase, ST-segment elevation (reflecting associated subepicardial inflammation and/or injury) is prominent in the precordial leads, especially $V_5$ and $V_6$, and in standard lead I. PR-segment depression may be noted in leads II, $aV_f$, and $V_4$ to $V_6$ (Fig. 56-1). In stage 2, the ST segment begins returning to the isoelectric line and T-wave amplitude decreases. T-wave inversion is rarely seen until stage 3. Stage 3 is characterized by an isoelectric ST segment and T-wave inversion in those leads previously showing ST-segment elevation. Resolution of repolarization abnormalities is the hallmark of stage 4.

If a large pericardial effusion develops during the course of acute pericarditis, additional ECG abnormalities may be noted and include low-voltage QRS complexes and electrical alternans. These phenomena are due to the "insulating" effect of pericardial fluid, which attenuates electrical signals of myocardial origin, and the pendular motion of the heart within the fluid-filled pericardial space.

Although serial ECG tracings are of diagnostic value in acute pericarditis, sequential ECG assessment is not a diagnostic luxury afforded the emergency physician. Differentiating pericarditis from the normal variant with "early repolarization" is a common problem and can be difficult when only a single 12-lead ECG is available. Acute pericarditis is a common cause of chest pain and abnormal ECGs in young adults. The ST-T-wave changes present in the early repolarization or normal variant ECG mimic those of pericarditis and have been reported in 2 percent of healthy young adults. Investigations attempting to distinguish these two conditions have yielded conflicting results. However, a simple criterion offers considerable diagnostic utility, namely, the ST segment/T-wave amplitude ratio in leads $V_5$, $V_6$, or I. Using the end of the PR segment as baseline, or 0 mV, the amplitude or height of the ST segment at its onset is measured in one of the above leads and recorded in millivolts. The height of the T wave in the same lead is measured from the baseline to the T-wave peak. If the ratio of ST amplitude (in millivolts) to T-wave amplitude (in millivolts) is below 0.25, a normal variant or early repolarization is most probable. If the ratio is above 0.25, acute pericarditis is likely. This criterion may allow differentiation of acute pericarditis (stage I) from early repolarization during emergency department evaluation (Fig. 56-1). Pericarditis alone does not cause significant cardiac rhythm disturbances.

### Radiographic Assessment

Conventional PA and lateral chest x-rays are of limited value. The cardiac silhouette may be of normal size and contour in acute pericarditis and, in some instances, the setting of cardiac tamponade. If previous chest x-rays are available for comparison, a recent increase in the size of the cardiac silhouette or an increase in the cardiothoracic ratio without radiographic evidence of pulmonary venous hypertension aids in distinguishing an expanding pericardial effusion from left heart failure. The epicardial "fat pad sign" is rarely seen on the lateral chest x-ray and has been reported in only 15 percent of cases of acute pericarditis during fluoroscopy with image intensification. If acute pericarditis is suspected on the basis of history, physical examination, or ECG, PA and lateral chest x-rays, which may demonstrate a pleuropulmonary or mediastinal abnormality, may assist in establishing an etiology, e.g., neoplastic or infectious.

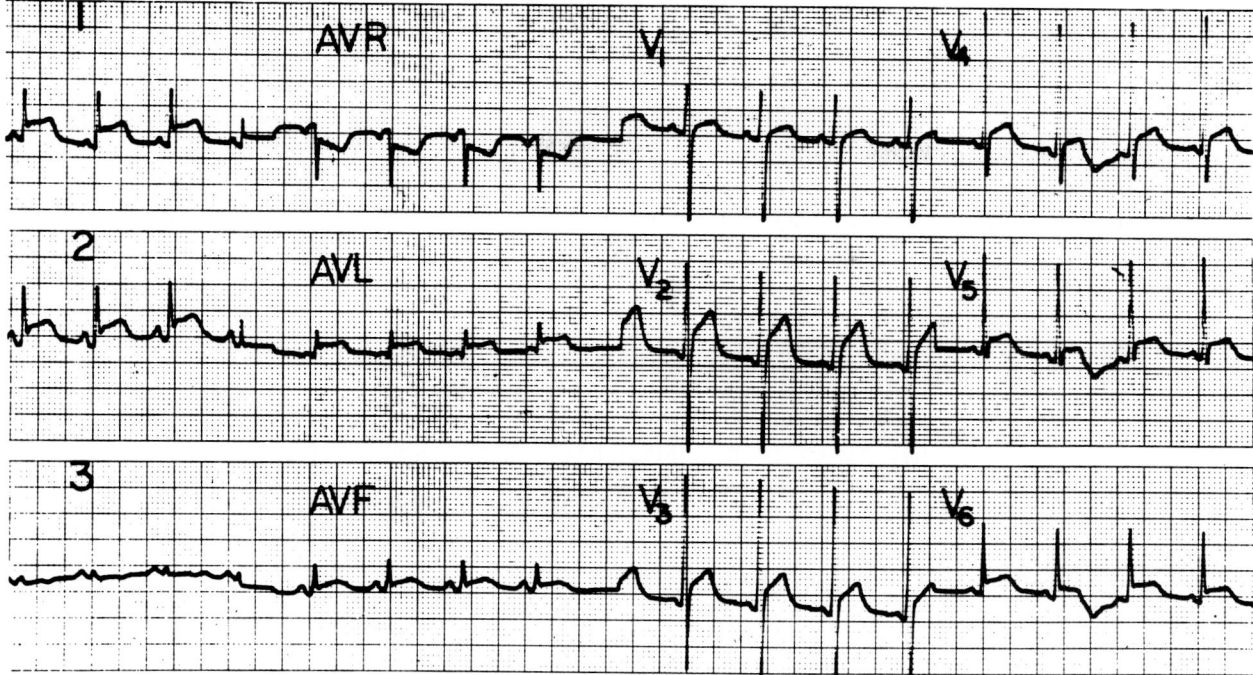

**Fig. 56-1.** This ECG was obtained from a 24-year-old male complaining of retrosternal pleuritic chest pain. A three-component pericardial friction rub was heard on examination. ECG abnormalities consistent with pericarditis are present. There is diffuse ST-segment elevation, and PR-interval depression is evident in the standard limb leads (PR interval below the isoelectric TP segment). The ST-segment/T-wave amplitude ratio in $V_6$ is approximately 0.75. (*From* Ginzton and Laks, used by permission.)

### Echocardiography

Echocardiography has become the procedure of choice for the detection, confirmation, and serial follow-up of patients with acute pericarditis and a pericardial effusion.

Normally, the pericardial sac is only a "potential" space, and the myocardium is echocardiographically in direct contact with surrounding thoracic structures. The anterior right ventricular wall is in contact with the chest wall and the posterior LV wall is in contact with the posterior pericardium and adjacent pleura. When a pericardial effusion is present, the pericardial space fills with echo-free fluid. Echocardiographically, a separation is seen between the right ventricle and the chest wall and between the left ventricle and the posterior pericardium. Quantitation of the size of the effusion is arbitrary and is determined by where the echo-free space is seen (anterior or posterior) and when in the cardiac cycle it occurs. For example, when an echo-free space is seen only posteriorly and only during systole, a "small" effusion is said to present.

### Ancillary Laboratory Evaluation

The laboratory studies listed in Table 56-6 may be of value in establishing an etiologic diagnosis. Creatine kinase (CK) and CK-MB may be elevated in acute pericarditis due to associated myocarditis.

**Table 56-6.** Ancillary Diagnostic Studies in Acute Pericarditis

CBC and differential WBC count: may suggest infection or leukemia
BUN/creatinine: may suggest a diagnosis of uremic pericarditis
Streptococcal serology (antistreptolysin O, anti-DNAse, antihyaluronidase): of
  particular value in the patient with an antecedent history of rheumatic heart
  disease or history of pharyngitis
Blood cultures (if bacterial infection suspected)
Acute and convalescent viral titers
Serological studies: antinuclear antibodies, anti-DNA titers, or RA latex
  fixation in the patient with systemic symptoms
Thyroid function studies
Erythrocyte sedimentation rate: will not facilitate an etiologic diagnosis but
  can be followed serially to assess response to therapy.

### Treatment

Most patients with idiopathic or presumed viral pericarditis will respond to nonsteroidal anti-inflammatory agents administered for 7 days to 3 weeks. If a specific etiology is identified, therapy should be directed toward the underlying disease.

## Constrictive Pericarditis

### Pathology

Constrictive pericarditis is pathologically distinct from acute pericarditis. Following pericardial injury and the resultant inflammatory and reparative process, fibrous thickening of the layers of the pericardium may occur. This fibrous reparative process is most commonly encountered after cardiac trauma with intrapericardial hemorrhage, after pericardiotomy (open-heart surgery, including coronary revascularization), in fungal or tuberculous pericarditis, and in chronic renal failure (uremic pericarditis). When the fibrous and/or collagenous response prevents passive diastolic filling of the normally distensible cardiac chambers, constriction is said to be present. Intrapericardial fluid is not required to produce such a hemodynamic effect. By its nature, constrictive pericarditis is most commonly a clinically chronic process. However, clinical manifestations may occur early if fluid also accumulates within the thickened, noncompliant pericardial sac (so-called effusive constrictive pericarditis). In the vast majority of cases of constrictive pericarditis, proved by hemodynamic assessment (see below), a specific etiology is never determined.

### Symptoms and Signs

The symptoms of constrictive pericarditis usually develop gradually and may mimic those of congestive heart failure (CHF). If symptoms develop within months of a pericardial injury, a combination of pericardial effusion and constriction should be suspected. Exertional dyspnea and decreased exercise tolerance are common patient complaints; however, orthopnea, paroxysmal nocturnal dyspnea, and chest pain are unusual. Lower extremity swelling (pedal edema) and increasing abdominal girth (ascites) are also common complaints and are the result of decreased right ventricular diastolic compliance and resultant increase in systemic venous pressure.

In most instances, physical findings and their correct interpretation will lead the clinician to suspect constrictive pericarditis. Examination of the neck veins with the torso of the patient at a 45° angle from the horizontal will reveal jugular venous distension and a rapid *y* descent of the cervical venous pulse. Elevated venous pressure is also seen in CHF, but a rapid *y* descent is infrequently encountered. The Kussmaul sign (inspiratory neck vein distension) is frequently but not invariably noted in constrictive pericarditis but rarely noted in uncompensated CHF. A paradoxical pulse is found in a minority of patients, and thus its absence does not exclude a diagnosis of constrictive pericarditis. On cardiac auscultation, an early diastolic sound, a pericardial "knock," may be heard at the apex 60 to 120 ms after the second heart sound. The pericardial knock sounds like a ventricular gallop but occurs earlier than the $S_3$ of CHF, which it may mimic. The knock is due to accelerated right ventricular inflow in early diastole and early myocardial distension, followed by an abrupt slowing of further ventricular expansion. There is usually no pericardial friction rub. Hepatomegaly, ascites, and dependent edema of varying severities are usually found.

## Diagnostic Findings

### Electrocardiogram

Diagnostic ECG changes have not been described in constrictive pericarditis. However, low-voltage QRS complexes and inverted T waves are common.

### Radiographic Assessment

Conventional PA and lateral chest x-rays most commonly demonstrate a normal or slightly enlarged cardiac silhouette, clear lung fields, and little or no evidence of pulmonary venous congestion. Pericardial calcification, which may be evident in up to 50 percent of patients with constrictive pericarditis, is seen best on the lateral chest x-ray but is not diagnostic of constrictive pericarditis.

### Echocardiography

On occasion, echocardiography may demonstrate pericardial thickening and abnormal ventricular septal motion in the patient with suspected constrictive pericarditis. However, its diagnostic utility is much less than in the patient with acute pericarditis.

## Therapy

In cases of significant constriction and impaired ventricular filling, pericardiectomy is the treatment of choice.

## BIBLIOGRAPHY

Bartman G, Sellanes M, Odell DS, et al: Discrepancy between pre- and post-transplant diagnosis of end-stage cardiomyopathy. *Am J Cardiol* 74:921, 1994.

Brockington GM, Zebede J, Pandian NG: Constrictive pericarditis. *Cardiol Clin* 8:645, 1990.

DeCastro S, d'Amati G, Gallo P et al: Frequency of development of acute global left ventricular dysfunction in HIV infection. *J Am Coll Cardiol* 24:1018, 1994.

Johnson RA, Palacios I: Dilated cardiomyopathies of the adult (parts I and II). *N Engl J Med* 307:1051, 1119, 1982.

Keren A, Popp RL: Assignment of patients into the classification of cardiomyopathies. *Circulation* 86:1622, 1992.

Maron BJ, Bonow RO, Cannon RO, et al: Hypertrophic cardiomyopathy: Interrelations of clinical manifestations, pathophysiology, and therapy (parts I and II). *N Engl J Med* 316:780, 844, 1987.

Montague TJ, Lopaaschuk GD, Davies NJ: Viral heart disease. *Chest* 98:190, 1990.

Permanyer-Miralda G, Sagrista-Sauleda J, Shabetai R: Acute pericardial disease: An approach to etiologic diagnosis and treatment, in Soler-Soler J, ed: *Pericardial Disease: New Insights and Old Dilemmas,* vol. 1. Norwell: Kluwer Academic Publishers, 1990, 193–214.

Peters NS, Poole-Wilson PA: Myocarditis: Continuing clinical and pathologic confusion. *Am Heart J* 121:942, 1991.

Report of the WHO/ISFC Task Force on the Definition and Classification of Cardiomyopathies. *Br Heart J* 44:672, 1980.

# 57
# PULMONARY EMBOLISM
## Robert S. Hockberger

Pulmonary embolism (PE) is a common and deadly disorder that can be extremely difficult to diagnose prior to autopsy. Approximately 2 to 10 percent of the 650,000 cases that occur annually in the United States are fatal, and only 10 to 30 percent of fatal cases have a correct antemortem diagnosis. There are no historical, physical, or laboratory findings that are specific for PE, and it may mimic clinically many other serious and benign medical disorders. Unfortunately, if the diagnosis of this disease is missed in the emergency department, the overall mortality, caused by recurrent emboli, increases substantially. As a result, the emergency physician must know when to suspect this disease, how to use clinical findings and the results of routine screening tests to raise or lower their index of suspicion for PE, when and how to proceed with further evaluation, and how to initiate treatment when the diagnosis of PE is confirmed or strongly suspected.

## PATHOPHYSIOLOGY
### Predisposing Factors

Vascular thrombosis and clot lysis are functions of normal homeostasis that are necessary for the repair of damaged blood vessels. Certain pathologic conditions—injury to the vascular endothelium, venous stasis, and alterations in the coagulation system—predispose an individual to clinically significant thrombosis, and its embolic sequelae, by altering the normal balance between blood clot formation and lysis. Table 57-1 lists the most commonly recognized predisposing factors for thromboembolism.

Most authorities believe that all patients with clinically significant thromboembolic disease possess at least one predisposing factor, although certain factors such as occult malignancies or alterations in the fibrinolytic system may not be apparent at the time of initial presentation. Fortunately, over 90 percent of PE occur in the presence of clinically apparent predisposing factors and, as a result, the presence or absence of such factors can be used to raise or lower one's index of suspicion for PE.

### Natural History

Pulmonary emboli may arise from pelvic vein thrombosis secondary to pelvic trauma, pelvic surgery or childbirth, or from the right side of the heart. In over 90 percent of cases, however, PE arise from the deep venous system of the lower extremities. Deep venous thrombosis (DVT) usually develops in the region of a venous valve. A thrombus normally develops over a period of minutes to hours and is then lysed within 7 to 10 days. It is during the first few days after forma-

**Table 57-1.** Predisposing Factors for Thromboembolism

Cardiopulmonary disease
    Congestive heart failure
    Myocardial infarction
    Chronic obstructive pulmonary disease
Stasis of blood flow
    Pregnancy and parturition
    Prolonged immobilization
    History of DVT or PE
    Marked obesity
Alterations in coagulation
    Malignancy
    Estrogen use
    Other*
Trauma
    Surgery within 3 months
    Lower extremity injury

* Deficiencies of antithrombin III, protein C, protein S; presence of lupus anticoagulant; and homocystinuria.

tion that embolic risk is highest. DVT confined to the veins of the calf rarely embolize. The incidence of embolization from popliteal vein thrombosis is 50 percent and approaches 70 percent for femoral vein thrombosis. Unfortunately, the clinical diagnosis of DVT of the lower extremities is unreliable and may be missed in up to 50 percent of cases.

## CLINICAL FEATURES

### Symptoms

The "classic" presentation of dyspnea associated with pleuritic chest pain and hemoptysis is rarely encountered. PE may mimic many serious and benign medical disorders (see Table 57-2) and must be considered in any patient at risk who experiences any acute nonspecific cardiopulmonary complaint, particularly dyspnea, chest pain, syncope, or shock.

The frequencies of various symptoms and signs reported in one of the largest series of patients with angiographically documented PE are shown in Table 57-3. Chest pain is the most common symptom, occurring in approximately 90 percent of patients. While the pain is usually pleuritic in nature, it may mimic the pressurelike pain of cardiac ischemia or the vague discomfort of nonspecific chest wall pain. The pain may be acute in onset or may be present for 3 to 4 days prior to presentation.

The sudden onset of unexplained dyspnea is seen in over 80 percent of patients. The absence of dyspnea should lower one's index of

**Table 57-2.** Diseases in the Differential Diagnosis of PE

| | |
|---|---|
| Skin | Pericardium |
|   Herpes zoster |   Acute pericarditis |
| Muscle | Myocardium |
|   Myositis |   Myocardial infarction |
|   Muscle strain | Intraabdominal disorders |
| Bone |   Splenic flexure syndrome |
|   Rib fracture |   Renal colic |
|   Thoracic vertebral |   Acute pancreatitis |
|     compression fracture |   Acute cholelithiasis |
|   Costochondritis |   Subdiaphragmatic abscess |
| Pleura |   Hepatitis |
|   Pleurisy | Psychiatric |
| Lung |   Hyperventilation syndrome |
|   Emphysema | |
|   Bronchitis | |
|   Asthma | |
|   Carcinoma | |
|   Tuberculosis | |
|   Spontaneous pneumothorax | |
|   Pneumonia | |

**Table 57-3.** Incidence of Symptoms and Signs in 327 Patients with Angiographically Proved Pulmonary Emboli

| Symptoms and Signs | Total Series, % |
|---|---|
| Symptoms | |
|   Chest pain | 88 |
|     Pleuritic | 74 |
|     Nonpleuritic | 14 |
|   Dyspnea | 84 |
|   Apprehension | 59 |
|   Cough | 53 |
|   Hemoptysis | 30 |
|   Sweats | 27 |
|   Syncope | 13 |
| Signs | |
|   Respirations > 16/min | 92 |
|   Rales | 58 |
|   $P_2 > S_2$ | 53 |
|   Pulse > 100/min | 44 |
|   Temperature > 37.8°C (100.04°F) | 43 |
|   Phlebitis | 32 |
|   Gallop | 34 |
|   Diaphoresis | 36 |
|   Edema | 24 |
|   Murmur | 23 |
|   Cyanosis | 19 |
| Predisposing condition | |
|   Current venous disease | 49 |
|   Immobilization | 55 |
|   Congestive heart failure and chronic lung disease | 38 |
|   Malignant neoplasm | 6 |

*Source:* Bell WR, Simon TL, DeMets DL: The clinical features of submassive and massive pulmonary emboli. *Am J Med* 62:358, 1977. Used by permission.

suspicion for PE but does not eliminate the possibility of this disease when other suggestive symptoms and signs are present. Anxiety or apprehension, probably caused by hypoxemia, occurs in approximately 60 percent of cases. PE may present as a syncopal episode, due to severe hypoxemia resulting in transient hypotension or dysrhythmia, in up to 15 percent of cases. Shock associated with distended neck veins is occasionally seen with massive PE as well as with cardiac tamponade, acute right ventricular infarction, cardiogenic shock from left ventricular infarction, and tension pneumothorax.

Less common presentations for PE include repetitive bouts of otherwise unexplained supraventricular tachyarrhythmia, the sudden onset or worsening of congestive heart failure, and sudden unexplained deterioration in patients with chronic obstructive pulmonary disease.

### Clinical Signs

Once PE migrate to the lungs and lodge in the pulmonary vasculature, platelets degranulate and release a wide variety of biologically active substances, including histamine, catecholamines, serotonin, and prostaglandins. These act to cause smooth muscle constriction of the bronchi and pulmonary arteries. Increased airway resistance and decreased total lung volume with uneven ventilation contribute to the dyspnea and tachypnea found in the majority of patients with PE. Tachypnea, defined as a respiratory rate over 16 per minute, is found in over 90 percent of patients; therefore, the presence of a normal respiratory rate should lower one's index of suspicion for PE. Localized rales, rhonchi, wheezes, or a pleural friction rub are often, but not invariably, seen.

A patient's hemodynamic response to PE depends on the extent of pulmonary vascular occlusion as well as on the patient's prior cardiovascular status. A previously healthy patient will not develop clinical signs of significant pulmonary hypertension (distended neck veins, a right ventricular heave, and a loud pulmonary component of the second heart sound) unless total pulmonary vascular obstruction approaches 40 to 50 percent. Patients with preexisting cardiopulmonary disease, however, may experience life-threatening changes in hemodynamic status with less extensive PE. Some degree of hypotension is present in up to 25 percent of PE cases, but frank shock occurs in fewer than 10 percent.

Despite the fact that over 90 percent of PE arise from DVT of the lower extremities, fewer than one-third of patients with PE will present with symptoms or signs of DVT.

## DIAGNOSIS

### Diagnostic Tests

#### Routine Screening Tests

**Arterial blood gases (ABG).** ABGs usually reflect hypoxemia caused by underperfusion of well-aerated segments of lung secondary to the emboli themselves, decrease in total lung volume secondary to diffuse bronchial constriction, inadequate respiration secondary to pain and splinting, and, occasionally, some degree of cardiac decompensation. The mean $P_{O_2}$ values among patients with documented PE in two large series were 62 and 72 mmHg, respectively; however, 10 to 15 percent of patients had a $P_{O_2}$ greater than 80 mmHg, and 5 percent had a $P_{O_2}$ greater than 90 mmHg.

The presence of an increased alveolar-arterial (A − a) oxygen gradient appears to be a more sensitive indicator of systemic hypoxemia than the $P_{O_2}$ alone. The A − a gradient at sea level is calculated using the following formula:

$$A - a \text{ gradient} = P_{A_{O_2}} \text{ (alveolar)} - Pa_{O_2} \text{ (arterial)}$$

where $P_{A_{O_2}}$ (alveolar) $= 150 - 1.2$ ($P_{CO_2}$). A normal A − a gradient $=$ (age/4) $+ 4$. Several recent studies have shown that fewer than 5 percent of patients with PE have a normal A − a gradient. Therefore, a normal A − a gradient should lower one's index of suspicion for PE.

**Electrocardiogram (ECG).** The ECG changes seen with PE are listed in Table 57-4. In the setting of clinically suspected PE, the sud-

**Table 57-4.** Electrocardiographic Manifestation: 90 Patients with Massive or Submassive Pulmonary Embolism without Prior Cardiac or Pulmonary Disease*

| Manifestation | % of Series |
|---|---|
| Normal electrocardiogram | 13 |
| Rhythm disturbances | |
|   Premature atrial beats | 2 |
|   Premature ventricular beats | 3 |
| Atrioventricular conduction disturbances | |
|   First-degree AV block | 1 |
| P pulmonale | 6 |
| QRS abnormalities | |
|   Right-axis deviation | 7 |
|   Left-axis deviation | 7 |
|   Clockwise rotation ($V_5$) | 7 |
|   Incomplete right bundle branch block | 6 |
|   Complete right bundle branch block | 9 |
|   Right ventricular hypertrophy | 6 |
|   $S_1S_2S_3$ pattern | 7 |
|   $S_1Q_3T_3$ pattern | 12 |
|   Pseudoinfarction | 11 |
|   Low voltage (frontal plane) | 6 |
| Primary RST-segment and T-wave abnormalities | |
|   RST-segment depression (not reciprocal) | 26 |
|   RST-segment elevation (not reciprocal) | 16 |
|   T-wave inversion | 42 |

* Some patients had more than one abnormality. The prevalence of none of the various electrocardiographic abnormalities differed significantly between patients with massive or submassive pulmonary embolism ($\chi^2 > .05$).

*Source:* Adapted from Stein PD, Dalen JE, McIntyre KM, et al: The electrocardiogram in acute pulmonary embolism. *Progr Cardiovasc Dis* 17:247, 1975. Used by permission.

den appearance of ECG findings of acute right heart strain correlates very highly with the presence of PE. In the setting of clinically suspected myocardial infarction, an ECG indicating multiple areas of infarction is highly suggestive of PE. The most common ECG finding in PE is nonspecific ST-T-wave changes that are transient (lasting for hours to days); comparison with previously obtained ECGs, or sequential ECGs obtained in the emergency department, may be helpful. A normal ECG, which is seen in fewer than 10 percent of cases, should lower one's index of suspicion for PE.

**Chest x-ray.** The chest x-ray is most often abnormal in PE. However, a normal chest x-ray in the setting of acute dyspnea associated with hypoxemia is highly suggestive of PE. The chest x-ray in nearly half of all patients with acute PE will show an elevated dome of one hemidiaphragm, secondary to factors mentioned previously. Other common but nonspecific radiographic findings include pleural effusions, atelectasis, and transient pulmonary infiltrates (particularly when wedge-shaped).

Two radiographic features that are uncommon but relatively specific for PE are the Hampton hump and Westermark sign. *Hampton hump* is a pleural-based density or lung consolidation with a rounded border pointing toward the hilus. *Westermark sign* refers to the presence of a dilated pulmonary outflow tract on the side of embolization with an area of decreased perfusion distal to it.

Chest x-rays are often diagnostic in conditions that mimic acute PE such as pneumonia, pneumothorax, and acute pulmonary edema. In addition, chest x-rays are essential for the correct interpretation of radionuclide studies.

### Specific Diagnostic Tests

**Venography, duplex ultrasonography, or impedance plethysmography (IPG).** Since over 90 percent of PE arise from proximal DVT of the lower extremities, a search for DVT will often preclude the need for further evaluation for PE, since both disorders require the same treatment. Venography is the "gold standard" for diagnosing DVT. Duplex ultrasonography is becoming the diagnostic modality of choice in many centers. Sensitivity and specificity approach 95 to 100 percent (see Chap. 61), but the technique is highly dependent on the skill of the technician. IPG is considered a reasonable alternative in some institutions because it is easier to perform and is less expensive. However, IPG is insensitive to infrapopliteal or partially occluding thrombi.

**Ventilation-perfusion lung scan.** The radionuclide perfusion lung scan is an extremely sensitive test that measures blood flow in pulmonary vessels as small as 50 μm in diameter. As a result, a normal perfusion scan excludes the diagnosis of PE.

Abnormal perfusion scans are not only caused by PE, however, but also by a large number of pulmonary disorders including asthma, emphysema, bronchitis, bronchiectasis, pneumonia, pleural effusions, atelectasis, congestive heart failure, pulmonary carcinoma, and congenital cysts. Therefore, in the setting of suspected PE, an abnormal perfusion scan should be followed by a ventilation scan. Normal ventilation in an area of diminished perfusion is suggestive of PE. The larger the area of ventilation-perfusion "mismatch" on lung scan, the greater the correlation with PE as documented by pulmonary angiography. Lung scans are usually classified as low, moderate, or high probability, based upon the number and size of ventilation-perfusion mismatches in comparison with chest x-ray findings. As will be discussed, patient management decisions must incorporate both lung scan results and a physician's assessment of the patient's clinical probability for having PE.

A lung scan should not be withheld from a pregnant patient for fear of fetal radiation exposure. The risk to the mother and fetus of not diagnosing PE, or the risk of anticoagulation without adequate evidence of PE, are greater than any fetal radiation risk from lung scanning. A fetus receives approximately 50 mrem of radiation exposure during a

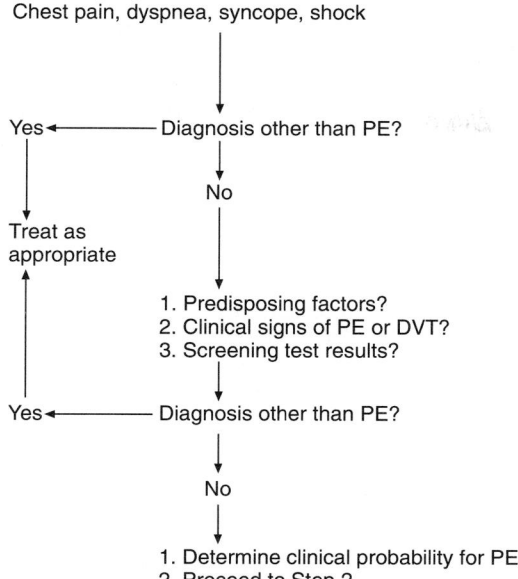

**Fig. 57-1.** Step 1: The initial evaluation of patients with symptoms suggestive of PE.

ventilation-perfusion lung scan, while the recommended maximal permissible dose for fetal gestational exposure in radiation workers is 500 mrem. Chap. 261 details ventilation-perfusion scanning.

**Pulmonary angiography.** Pulmonary angiography visualizes pulmonary vessels as small as 0.5 mm in diameter and is considered the gold standard for diagnosing PE. It is an extremely safe test in experienced hands; in one study of over 800 pulmonary angiograms performed for suspected PE, the morbidity of the test was less than 1 percent and the mortality was less than 0.01 percent. Significant complications associated with pulmonary angiography occur almost exclusively in elderly patients with severe underlying cardiopulmonary disease (congestive heart failure or chronic obstructive pulmonary disease).

**Other tests.** Radionuclide scans utilizing monoclonal antibodies directed against fibrin or platelet components, serum assays for specific fibrinopeptides, and measurement of fibrin degradation products such as D-dimer are tests for the diagnosis of thromboembolic disease currently under investigation. To date, none fulfills the dual cri-

teria of being both widely available and also sensitive and specific for the diagnosis of PE or DVT.

## Diagnostic Approach

### Step 1

PE should be suspected in all patients presenting with dyspnea, chest pain, syncope, or shock when the clinical presentation is suggestive of PE or when there is no other readily identifiable cause for the patient's symptoms (see Fig. 57-1). The determination of the clinical probability for PE should be based upon the presence or absence of predisposing factors, clinical signs for PE or DVT, and the results of routine screening tests (ABG, ECG, and chest x-ray). Patients with significant clinical findings or abnormal test results, particularly in the presence of any predisposing factors, should receive further diagnostic evaluation for PE.

### Step 2

If clinical evaluation and routine screening laboratory tests do not reasonably exclude the possibility of PE, then either duplex ultrasonography, venography, IPG, or a lung scan should be obtained (see Fig. 57-2). If duplex ultrasonography, venography, or IPG diagnose DVT, the patient should be anticoagulated and hospitalized for further care. Negative results should be followed by a lung scan. A normal lung scan, or a low-probability lung scan in the presence of low clinical probability, reasonably excludes the possibility of PE. Alternatively, a high-probability scan in a patient predetermined by the physician to have high clinical probability for PE should lead to anticoagulation and hospitalization. All other patients should have treatment decisions based on the results of pulmonary angiography.

## TREATMENT

### Stabilization

Patients clinically suspected of having PE should be placed on a cardiac monitor, have intravenous access established, and receive supplemental oxygen appropriate to their degree of distress. A patient with PE is at greatest risk for succumbing to shock or cardiac dysrhythmia during the first few hours. Early initiation of vigorous monitoring of vital signs and cardiac rhythm is essential.

Hypotension may be caused by low cardiac output secondary to right ventricular outflow obstruction or by myocardial dysfunction due to ischemia. Initial therapy should include the aggressive admin-

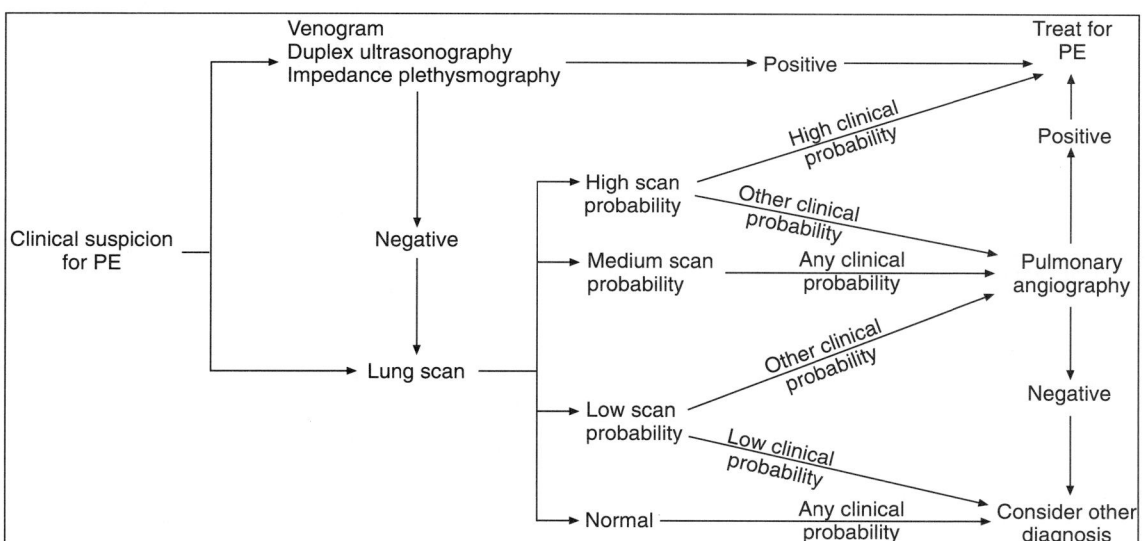

**Fig. 57-2.** Step 2: The further evaluation of patients with suspected PE.

istration of crystalloid fluids if the central venous pressure (CVP) is low or the use of vasopressors such as dopamine if the CVP is normal or high. The persistently hypotensive patient with suspected PE should be managed with Swan-Ganz catheter placement, immediate pulmonary arteriography, and early consideration of fibrinolytic therapy.

## Anticoagulation

Anticoagulation with heparin has been the cornerstone of therapy for venous thromboembolism for over 40 years. Heparin does not affect preexisting thrombi, whose dissolution depends upon the body's intrinsic fibrinolytic system, but does block new thrombus formation, which reduces the incidence of recurrent PE. One study of 516 patients with PE showed a recurrence rate of only 16 percent for anticoagulated patients, compared to a recurrence rate of 55 percent in cases where heparin was withheld because of medical contraindications; in this study, 92 percent of heparinized patients survived, compared with a 42 percent survival rate in patients who were not anticoagulated.

Patients with documented or strongly suspected PE, in the absence of absolute contraindications to anticoagulation (see Table 57-5), should receive 10,000 to 20,000 units of heparin as an intravenous (IV) bolus, followed by either continuous IV heparin (1000 units/h) or intermittent heparin (5000 units every 4 h) by the IV or subcutaneous route. While all of the aforementioned regimens are acceptable, the continuous intravenous approach, delivered by an infusion pump, is by far the most popular in the United States. The value of coagulation tests to monitor the safety and efficacy of heparin therapy is controversial, although most experts currently recommend monitoring the clotting time or partial thromboplastin time and maintaining them at 1.5 to 2.0 times the control value.

Heparin does not cross the placenta and can, therefore, be used safely in pregnant women with PE. Peripartum bleeding remains a problem, however, requiring that heparin be discontinued just prior to delivery and resumed only after postpartum hemostasis has been obtained. All cases of abnormal bleeding caused by heparin may be reversed through administration of intravenous protamine sulfate. Each milligram of protamine sulfate neutralizes approximately 100 units of heparin activity.

## Thrombolytic Therapy

The thrombolytic agents streptokinase, urokinase, and recombinant tissue plasminogen activator (rtPA) literally dissolve DVT and PE by activating the body's own fibrinolytic system. Despite extensive study, however, it has not been established that these agents alter morbidity, mortality, or recurrence rates among patients with thromboembolic disease. In addition, the incidence of bleeding complications increases when thrombolytic agents are employed.

Presently, the major indication for the use of thrombolytic therapy is in hemodynamically unstable patients with massive embolism and persistent systemic hypotension despite appropriate medical management (100% oxygen, crystalloid fluids, and pressors). The most appropriate thrombolytic agent and treatment regimen have yet to be determined. Various authors have recommended rtPA at 50 to 100 mg IV over 2 to 6 h, urokinase as an initial dose of 4400 units/kg as an IV bolus administered over 10 min, and streptokinase in a dose of 250,000 units IV administered over 30 min followed by a continuous IV infusion of 100,000 units/h for the next 12 to 24 h. Ideally, thrombolytic therapy should be administered following consultation with an intensivist and documentation of massive PE with pulmonary angiography.

## Surgery

Pulmonary embolectomy is becoming an increasingly rare surgical procedure because of the critical and unstable nature of the patients

**Table 57-5.** Contraindications to Anticoagulation

Active internal bleeding
Uncontrolled severe hypertension
Recent trauma, major surgery, or stroke
Intracranial or intraspinal neoplasm

for whom it is considered, the logistical difficulties in rapidly mobilizing the personnel and equipment necessary for cardiopulmonary bypass surgery, almost uniformly poor outcomes, and the availability of alternative thrombolytic therapy.

Vena caval clipping or ligation, or the placement of a filter in the inferior vena cava, are procedures that should be considered for patients who experience recurrent PE while on maintenance heparin anticoagulation, patients in whom anticoagulation is contraindicated (see Table 57-5), and patients with septic emboli originating in the lower extremities.

## BIBLIOGRAPHY

Calley MA, Carson JL, Palevsky HI, Schwartz JS: Diagnosing pulmonary embolism: New facts and strategies. *Ann Intern Med* 114(4):301,1991.
Goldhaber SZ: What role for thrombolysis in patients with pulmonary embolism? Guidelines for patient selection and optimum administration. *J Crit Illness* 7(2):192,1992.
Goldhaber SZ, Morpurgo M: Diagnosis, treatment and prevention of pulmonary embolism: Report of WHO/International Society and Federation of Cardiology task force. *JAMA* 268:1727,1992.
Moser KM: Pulmonary thromboembolism, in Isselbacher KJ, Braunwald E, Wilson JD, et al (eds): *Harrison's Principles of Internal Medicine,* 13th ed. New York, McGraw-Hill, 1994, pp 1214–1220.
PIOPED investigators: Value of the ventilation/perfusion scan in acute pulmonary embolism. *JAMA* 263:2753,1990.

# 58
# HYPERTENSIVE EMERGENCIES
## Raymond E. Jackson

In this chapter, we outline the approach to the diagnosis and management of hypertension in the emergency department. Hypertensive syndromes are defined and specific treatments recommended. The most useful antihypertensive medications are discussed, as well as management of complications of acute and chronic treatment.

## DEGREE OF HYPERTENSION

There are four general categories of hypertension based on presentation and the level of aggression required for treatment: (1) emergencies; (2) urgencies; (3) mild, uncomplicated hypertension; and (4) transient hypertension. An understanding of the differences in the pathophysiology of these syndromes is essential to the successful and safe management of these patients.

### Hypertensive Emergencies

A hypertensive emergency is an increased blood pressure with evidence of end-organ damage or dysfunction. The organs that are at risk for injury are the brain, the heart, and the kidneys. This now uncommon condition is experienced in only about 1 percent of all hypertensives. There are no predetermined criteria for the level of blood pressure necessary to induce a hypertensive emergency. Evidence of altered organ function, not the level of blood pressure, is the basis for the diagnosis. The most striking example of minimally elevated blood pressure inducing a hypertensive emergency is eclampsia, where hypertensive encephalopathy may occur with a blood pressure of 160/90 mmHg.

Signs and symptoms of organ dysfunction can develop progressively over hours to days. After the recognition of a hypertensive emergency, the treatment goal is to lower the blood pressure to a level which is "normal" for that patient within 30 to 60 min in a controlled, graded manner. A 30 percent reduction in 30 min is a good initial guideline. The resolution of the signs and symptoms should be used as a guide in control of pressure, although in elderly patients improvements in the signs and symptoms may lag behind the drop in pressure.

### Hypertensive Urgencies

A hypertensive urgency is an elevation of blood pressure to a level that may be potentially harmful, usually sustained at greater than 115 mmHg diastolic, without signs, symptoms, or other evidence of end-organ dysfunction. This condition is most often due to noncompliance with medications. The treatment goal is to reduce the pressure gradually within 24 to 48 h to a level appropriate for the patient. Rapid reductions in blood pressure are potentially harmful and should be avoided. Recent evidence suggests that prescribing an antihypertensive medication, regardless of emergency department blood pressure reduction, results in control of the hypertension on follow-up examinations.

### Mild, Uncomplicated Hypertension

Mild, uncomplicated hypertension is a blood pressure less than 115 mmHg diastolic without symptoms of end-organ damage. Emergency department treatment is education and encouragement to take antihypertensive medications. It should not be treated acutely but requires follow-up evaluation and care. Emergency department pressure readings cannot be the basis for the diagnosis of new-onset hypertension.

### Transient Hypertension

Transient hypertension can be seen in many conditions, such as anxiety, pancreatitis, thrombotic stroke, early dehydration, alcohol withdrawal syndromes, epistaxis, and some overdoses (pentachlorophenol, clonidine). Treatment of the underlying condition, rather than administration of antihypertensive medications, is the rule.

To emphasize, the level of blood pressure should not be the guide to treatment; rather, the golden rule of hypertension is treat the patient, not the blood pressure.

## APPROACH TO THE HYPERTENSIVE PATIENT

The initial approach to the hypertensive patient in the emergency department is the systematic exclusion of a hypertensive emergency. This is accomplished with a thorough history and physical examination directed at uncovering signs and symptoms of organ dysfunction. With the exclusion of an emergency, nonhypertensive reasons for the blood pressure elevation are sought, and, if negative, the diagnosis of an urgency is made by exclusion. The blood pressure must be taken in both arms and repeated prior to the initiation of therapy. In the elderly and for patients with a history compatible for volume depletion, as with epistaxis, the physician should check the pressure both supine and standing. A combination of decreased anxiety and regression to the mean often leads to the observation of a significant pressure decrease, making it unnecessary to intervene further.

### History

Any past history of hypertension, hypertensive complications, cardiac disease, or renal disease should be elicited. Medication history, especially of antihypertensive and monoamine oxidase inhibitors, and the history of recent compliance are important. Special attention is paid to CNS symptoms such as blurred vision, diplopia, hemiparesis, and seizures. Symptoms such as headache and dizziness are nonspecific unless they occur with grade 3 or 4 fundoscopic changes or other signs of CNS dysfunction. Symptoms of ischemic chest pain or acute congestive heart failure establish the diagnosis of an acute hypertensive cardiovascular emergency. A history of renal insufficiency may alter the diagnosis and treatment of the elevated blood pressure. Most of the above symptoms have a history of gradual onset followed by rapid progression. If the patient is pregnant, previous history of hypertension or renal disease is important as well as previous blood pressures during the pregnancy.

### Physical Examination

The blood pressure should be determined in both arms, with palpation of pulses in all extremities. The tilt test should be done on elderly patients with no signs of organ dysfunction or a history compatible with dehydration. The physical examination focuses on the neurologic, cardiac, and pulmonary evaluation, searching for signs of organ dysfunction. The abdomen should be auscultated for bruits. A fundoscopic examination is mandatory.

### Laboratory and Other Studies

A complete blood count, serum glucose, blood urea nitrogen (BUN), creatinine, electrolytes, and urinalysis should be obtained in cases of suspected hypertensive emergencies. In most cases, the clinician should use the patient's chief complaint along with the history and physical findings to guide laboratory testing. Microangiopathic hemolytic anemia is a result of ongoing medical necrosis, which exposes the red cells to subendothelial collagen and fibrin. This shears the red cells as they pass by. On viewing the peripheral smear, shistocytes and red cell fragments are apparent. Hypokalemia may be observed with high-renin forms of hypertension and in patients on diuretic therapy, increasing the risk for malignant arrhythmias. The BUN and creatinine determine the renal function and aid in the determination of the severity of the hypertensive episode as well as the choice of antihypertensive medications. The urinalysis may show proteinuria, red cells, and red cell casts.

Evidence of cardiac ischemia and left ventricular hypertrophy is determined by ECG. Signs of pulmonary edema, aortic dissection, or coarctation of the aorta may be seen on the chest x-ray. Patients with a suspected emergency should be placed on a cardiac monitor and given oxygen. A head CT scan should be obtained when the physical findings indicate cerebral ischemia or hemorrhage and in the presence of focal neurologic signs or coma.

## HYPERTENSIVE EMERGENCIES INVOLVING THE CENTRAL NERVOUS SYSTEM

### Hypertensive Encephalopathy

The most devastating complication of hypertension is hypertensive encephalopathy. Signs and symptoms include severe headache, nausea and vomiting, and altered mental status ranging from lethargy or confusion to coma. Focal findings include hemorrhage, exudates, cotton wool spots, papilledema, and sausage linking. These signs and symptoms often progress over hours and can lead to coma and death in that time span. Left untreated, the 1-year mortality for this condition is high.

Encephalopathy is secondary to cerebral hyperperfusion with loss of the integrity of the blood-brain barrier. The autoregulation of cerebral blood flow maintains a constant cerebral perfusion over a large range of mean blood systemic pressures. In normotensive patients, this range is from 60 to 125 mmHg. Flow increases with excessively high mean arterial pressures, whereas flow decreases with low mean

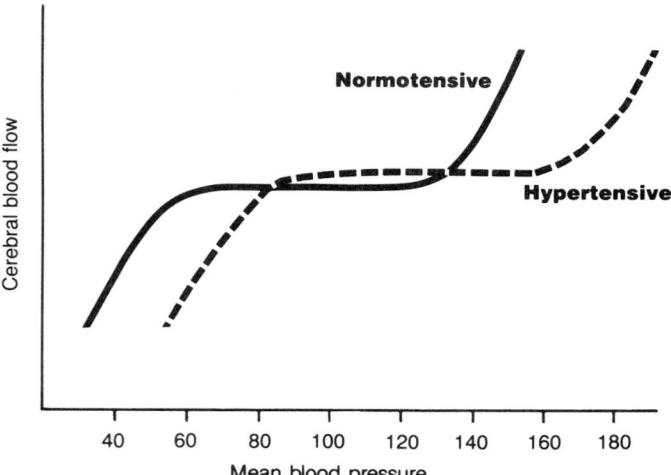

**Fig. 58-1.** Cerebral autoregulation of blood flow: changes seen with chronic hypertension.

pressures. This is demonstrated schematically in Fig. 58-1 as the cerebral autoregulation curve.

For poorly controlled hypertensive patients, partially because of changes in the structure of the cerebral arterioles, this curve shifts to the right, so that adequate cerebral blood flow is not maintained during periods of low arterial pressure that normotensive patients easily tolerate. This shift in the autoregulation curve can occur over a period of weeks to months and may be reversible with proper control of the blood pressure in younger patients.

When high blood pressure exceeds the limits of autoregulation, excessive blood flow develops and there is loss of the integrity of the blood-brain barrier at the arteriole and the glial venules. Alterations of the endothelial membrane transport mechanisms and the opening of tight junctions result in an exudation of fluid into the brain. Experimentally, symptoms of hypertensive encephalopathy seem to correlate with an increase in permeability of the blood-brain barrier, which occurs prior to the decrease in blood flow seen late in hypertensive encephalopathy. With persistent elevation in pressure, vascular necrosis occurs. This progression of pathologic findings can be witnessed in the retina with the finding of alternating areas of arteriolar constriction and dilation (sausage linking) and exudates. Late findings include generalized vasodilation, decreased blood flow, cerebral edema, and papilledema.

However, this is an oversimplified view of the dynamics of the cerebral vasculature occurring during hypertensive encephalopathy. The intracellular mechanism for the vasodilation seen has been hypothesized to be secondary to abnormal arachidonic acid metabolism and the development of oxygen-free radicals. This affects the smooth

muscle cells of the media layer by preventing the sustained contraction needed in the face of elevated pressure. It has been noted that this functional impairment persists hours after the reduction of pressure and can be partially prevented with free-radical scavengers and prostaglandin inhibitors. Without lowering the pressure, this intracellular process continues, resulting in necrosis of the media layer. Exposure of the passing blood to these necrotic structures shears the red cells, causing further disruption to flow and resulting in microangiopathic hemolytic anemia.

The treatment goal of hypertensive encephalopathy is to lower the mean arterial pressure so that the cerebral blood flow becomes normal over 30 to 60 min. Care is taken not to lower the pressure beyond the mean arterial pressure of approximately 120 mmHg.

The best agent for use in the setting of hypertensive encephalopathy is sodium nitroprusside. Intravenous labetalol is also an excellent choice. Avoid clonidine and pure β blockers.

## Hypertension and Other CNS Disorders

Differentiation of the cause-and-effect relationship between hypertension and CNS dysfunction is often very difficult. All other forms of CNS dysfunction (thrombotic stroke, intracranial hemorrhage, subarachnoid hemorrhage) are more common than hypertensive encephalopathy. The neurologic event may be the etiology of the elevation in pressure (Cushing effect) or the event may be related to the hypertension. History is often the principal means of differentiating these syndromes (see Table 58-1). The coma due to hypertensive encephalopathy is often not as dense as that with intracranial hemorrhage and may wax and wane.

In stroke, three phases of hypertensive response in previously hypertensive patients has been described. These phases occur with all forms of stroke—thrombotic, embolic, and hemorrhagic—to different degrees. The acute phase encompasses the first 4 days after the event. Approximately 90 percent of these patients are hypertensive. The hypothesized mechanism is stimulation of vasomotor centers in the pons and is independent of catecholamine and renin system involvement. Over the next 6 days, the blood pressure returns to prestroke levels without treatment, constituting the subacute phase. In the chronic phase, approximately 50 percent of previously hypertensive patients will no longer require treatment.

In the area of the stroke, there is loss of cerebral autoregulation of blood flow. Tissue blood flow then is directly pressure-dependent. With the edema accompanying the infarct, blood flow to viable tissue in the margins surrounding the ischemic area may be sensitive to small changes in pressure. This increased pressure may be a physiologic response to maintain adequate cerebral perfusion. If hypertension is not excessive, the areas of the brain not affected can maintain a proper autoregulation of flow.

Aggressive antihypertensive treatment in the face of stroke, without evidence of hypertensive end-organ damage such as malignant

**Table 58-1.** Differential Diagnosis of Hypertensive Cerebrovascular Events

| | Hypertensive Encephalopathy | Cerebral Thrombosis | Intracerebral Hemorrhage | Subarachnoid Hemorrhage | Transient Ischemia |
|---|---|---|---|---|---|
| Onset | Gradual, over 24–48 h | Acute, over 1–2 h | Rapid | Rapid | Rapid, may be recurrent |
| Neurological progression | Yes, over 24–48 h | May occur over several hours | Over minutes to hours | Rapid, in minutes | No |
| Impaired consciousness | Late | Not unless bilateral or brainstem | Usual | Usual and predominant | No |
| Other symptoms | Progressive headache, lethargy, seizures | Possible prior TIA* may occur during sleep | Sudden headache and vomiting initially | | No |
| Focal signs | Transient and migratory | Present and fixed | Present and fixed | Frequently absent | Present but brief |
| CSF findings | Pressure may be elevated | Normal unless severe edema | Frequently blood, increased pressure | Blood, increased pressure | Normal |

* Transient ischemic attack.

retinal changes (papilledema, hemorrhages, exudates), does not ameliorate symptoms, and rapid or vigorous reduction in pressure may increase ischemia by decreasing blood flow to the watershed areas. Treatment should be in a controlled manner with a short-acting agent with minimal CNS effects. The best agent is sodium nitroprusside.

With intracerebral hemorrhage, clinicians may find it difficult initially to separate the cause-and-effect relationship between the substantially increased pressure and the symptoms. The increase in the intracranial pressure associated with this event leads to a decrease in cerebral perfusion pressure, reflexively increasing the systemic blood pressure to compensate. Reducing the pressure is difficult and does not affect the incidence of rebleeding.

In the case of subarachnoid hemorrhage, nimopidine 60 mg orally every 4 h has been used to reverse the vasospasm associated with subarachnoid blood. It may improve outcome, independent of antihypertensive effects.

## PREGNANCY-INDUCED HYPERTENSION

The upper limit of normal blood pressure in the third trimester of pregnancy is 125/75 mmHg, and pressures higher than 140/90 mmHg with signs and symptoms of hyperreflexia, confusion, headache, epigastric pain, seizures, or coma should be considered an emergency. Eclampsia occurs most commonly in primagravidas and in multigravidas over the age of 35, especially those with a prior history of renal or hypertensive disease. Pregnancy-induced hypertension usually appears in the third trimester, unless a molar pregnancy is present or there is a prior history of hypertensive or renal disease.

During eclampsia, uterine blood flow decreases, necessitating monitoring of fetal heart tones. The initial emergency treatment is to lower the blood pressure with magnesium sulfate and hydralazine. Magnesium sulfate has both antihypertensive and antiepileptic properties. It is given as a 4- to 6-g bolus intravenously, followed by a 1- to 2-g/h infusion. Therapeutic levels are 6 to 8 mEq/L. Excessive magnesium sulfate administration can lead to loss of reflexes (>8 mEq/L), hypotension, and eventual respiratory arrest (>12 mEq/L). Thus, reflexes should be monitored closely, and when they disappear the infusion should be stopped. Also hydralazine, 10 to 20 mg IV push, should be given. Diazoxide decreases uterine motility and can, rarely, cause fetal hyperglycemia and hyperbilirubinemia. Sodium nitroprusside can be used, but the infusion should not be prolonged and thiocyanate levels must be monitored. Labetalol has been shown to be safe and efficacious in this setting. The definitive treatment is evacuation of the uterus. Postpartum eclampsia can develop for up to 2 weeks post partum and may be treated as above or with any other appropriate antihypertensive medication. Diuretics are contraindicated due to the volume contraction seen with pregnancy-induced hypertension. Angiotensin-converting enzyme inhibitors are also contraindicated because they cross the placenta and may depress angiotensin II levels in the fetus.

## HYPERTENSIVE CARDIOVASCULAR EMERGENCIES
### Left Ventricular Failure and Coronary Insufficiency

Alterations in left ventricular performance secondary to increased afterload is the primary mechanism by which an acute rise in pressure affects the cardiovascular system. This increases oxygen demand and may decrease coronary blood flow, which may result in angina, myocardial infarction, or acute left ventricular dysfunction with pulmonary edema.

Treatment of these syndromes is with agents that decrease both preload and afterload, thereby decreasing myocardial work and oxygen demand. Sodium nitroprusside and intravenous nitroglycerin are excellent agents, although the degree of blood pressure reduction is not as great with nitroglycerin. Because a coronary steal syndrome has been described in patients treated with sodium nitroprusside, in-

travenous nitroglycerin is an excellent first agent. Oral nifedipine has been used successfully in these situations but is not approved for this use in the United States. The physician should avoid agents that may increase myocardial oxygen demand such as diazoxide, hydralazine, and minoxidil. Beta-blocking agents and labetalol should be used cautiously in patients with a history of severe congestive heart failure. Oxygen and morphine sulfate are adjuvant therapy in this setting. Furosemide or bumetanide may be used if there is evidence of volume overload.

### Thoracic Aortic Dissection

Hypertension is the etiology for aortic dissection in about 90 percent of cases. Symptoms of chest or back pain usually begin abruptly and are severe. The location of pain varies depending on the site of dissection. The dissecting segment may involve the carotid arteries, leading to signs of acute cerebral infarction. Proximal dissection of the ascending aorta may occlude the coronary arteries, resulting in myocardial infarction, or can cause aortic insufficiency or cardiac tamponade.

The blood pressure is generally elevated but may also be normal or low. There may be discrepancies in the pulse character and blood pressure in different extremities. Any patient with acute chest pain and neurologic deficit should be evaluated for possible aortic dissection.

The agent of choice is labetalol. A combination of a β-adrenergic antagonist, such as propranolol or esmolol, and sodium nitroprusside is also very effective. The goal of the pharmacologic therapy is to reduce the blood pressure and decrease the aortic pressure wave ($dP/dt$). If the combination approach is used, propranolol should be started—1 mg IV every 5 min to a heart rate of 60 to 80. Nitroprusside is started after the first dose of propranolol. Surgery is indicated with dissections involving the ascending aorta and in cases of inadequate control of the blood pressure.

## ACUTE RENAL COMPLICATIONS OF HYPERTENSION

Deterioration of renal function in the face of an elevated pressure is considered a hypertensive emergency. Previous levels of the creatinine and BUN aid in the diagnosis. Proteinuria and the presence of red cells and red cells casts in the urine with elevation of the BUN and creatinine are diagnostic.

## CATECHOLAMINE-INDUCED HYPERTENSIVE EMERGENCY

Acute elevations of circulating catecholamines with or without hypersensitivity of adrenergic receptors can lead to acute symptomatic hypertension. Pheochromocytoma presents as episodic elevations of blood pressure, headache, flushing, and diarrhea. Use of monoamine oxidase (MAO) inhibitors prevents the metabolism of adrenergic agents and can cause hypertension if sympathomimetics are used concurrently. Tyramine is the precursor to the adrenergic compounds, and patients on MAO inhibitors who ingest tyramine-containing foods (Chianti wine, aged cheese, beer, pickled herring) develop hyperstimulation of the adrenergic receptors resulting in acute symptomatic hypertension. Hypertension may also be precipitated in these patients with over-the-counter cold preparations and diet pills. Clonidine withdrawal, especially when withdrawn concurrently with a β blocker, leads to severe hypertension. These hyperadrenergic states are best treated with an α and β blocker, such as labetalol.

## MEDICATION OPTIONS
### Overview

The ideal antihypertensive agent for a hypertensive emergency would act rapidly, in a controllable and predictable manner, with few side

## Synaptic receptors

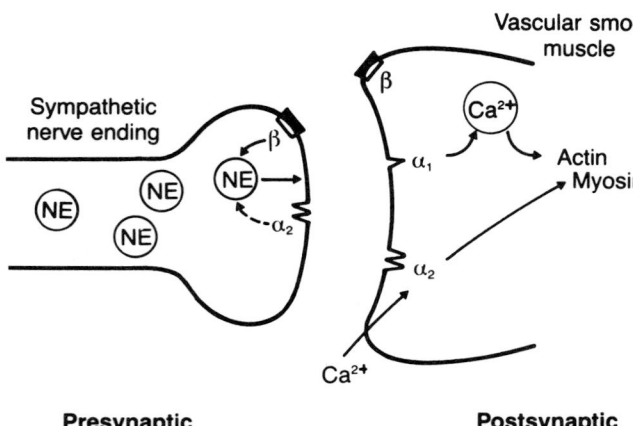

**Fig. 58-2.** Diagrammatic representation of the adrenergic receptors at the smooth-muscle synapse. ——➤, Stimulate- - -➤, inhibits.

effects; would be safe in combination with other medications and have few contraindications; and would not have adverse effects on cardiac output or myocardial, cerebral, and renal blood flows. The final common mechanism of action in the acute setting is vasodilation by alteration of the membrane receptors or intracellular messengers.

### Cellular Physiology

Postsynaptic $\alpha_1$ receptors are stimulated by synaptically released norepinephrine, causing a release of intracellular calcium stores, resulting in smooth muscle contraction. Alpha-2 receptors are found both pre- and postsynaptically. The postsynaptic $\alpha_2$ receptor is stimulated by circulating norepinephrine, causing an influx of calcium and resulting in smooth-muscle contraction. Stimulation of the presynaptic $\alpha_2$ receptor by norepinephrine prevents further release of norepinephrine (negative-feedback loop) (see Fig. 58-2). Agents that are nonspecific blockers of $\alpha$ receptors can lower pressure by smooth-muscle dilation but do not prevent the further release of norepinephrine from the nerve terminal. Agents that selectively block $\alpha_1$ receptors cause a similar decrease in pressure but allow the negative-feedback cycle to operate by not blocking the presynaptic $\alpha_2$ receptors. Stimulation of CNS $\alpha_2$ receptors decreases sympathetic outflow, resulting in bradycardia, hypotension, and somnolence.

Calcium entry into cells follows a strong concentration gradient. Once in the smooth-muscle cells, calcium binds with calmodulin, which then allows myosin and actin to bond, resulting in contraction. Small changes in intracellular calcium cause large changes in vascular tone. Calcium channel blockers vary in effect on different vessels. In general, they prevent the calcium influx seen with depolarization of the cell membrane by blocking entry through the slow channel, resulting in decreased peripheral vascular resistance.

### PRIMARY AGENTS FOR USE IN HYPERTENSIVE EMERGENCIES

The medications most commonly used for hypertensive emergencies are listed in Tables 58-2, 58-3 and 58-4.

### Sodium Nitroprusside (Nipride)

#### Actions and Pharmacology

Sodium nitroprusside, a rapidly acting arteriolar dilator and venodilator, can be used for all hypertensive emergencies, although it is not

**Table 58-2.** Antihypertensives for Initial Outpatient Treatment

| Agent | Initial Dose, mg | Times/ Day | Cautions |
|---|---|---|---|
| Hydrochlorothiazide | 12.5 | 1 | Hypokalemia, decreased plasma volume |
| Chlorthalidone | 12.5 | 1 | Hypokalemia, decreased plasma volume |
| Metoprolol (Lopressor) | 50 | 1 | May block $\beta_2$ receptors |
| Labetalol (Corgard) | 100 | 2 | May cause postural changes |
| Nifedipine (Procardia XL) | 30 | 1 | May cause hypotension |
| Captopril (Capoten) | 12.5 | 2 | May cause hyperkalemia |

the agent of choice in pregnancy-induced hypertension. It acts by reacting with cysteine to form nitrosocysteine, which is a potent activator of guanylate cyclase. Guanylate cyclase stimulates the formation of cyclic GMP, which relaxes smooth muscle. Both arterial and venous smooth muscle dilate, decreasing preload and afterload, resulting in decreased myocardial oxygen demand. Despite the lack of a direct chronotropic effect, the heart rate increases slightly secondary to a baroreceptor-mediated reflex. There is no change in cardiac output or myocardial blood flow. The dilation of small-resistance coronary vessels may lead to a "steal" syndrome in face of coronary insufficiency. Cerebral blood flow may decrease in a dose-dependent manner. There is no change in renal blood flow with treatment, and plasma renin activity is increased. Pulmonary shunting may be induced, aggravating hypoxia.

The onset of action is almost immediate, with a duration of action of 1 to 2 min, and the plasma half-life is 3 to 4 min. Nitroprusside is metabolized initially to cyanide by sulfhydryl groups in the blood and then converted to thiocyanate in the liver by rhodanase. Thiocyanate is excreted by the kidney.

### Indications

Sodium nitroprusside is an excellent agent for all hypertensive emergencies except eclampsia prior to delivery. It may be used in predelivery eclampsia if other treatments have failed and in postpartum eclampsia. It is safe for use in children.

**Table 58-3.** Selection of Medications for Various Hypertensive Emergencies

| Type of Hypertensive Emergency | First-Line Medication | Second-Line Medication | Medications to Avoid |
|---|---|---|---|
| Hypertensive encephalopathy | Nitroprusside | Labetalol | Clonidine, ACE* inhibitors |
| Acute pulmonary edema | Nitroglycerin Nitroprusside | Furosemide Morphine sulphate ACE inhibitors | Labetalol, diazoxide, hydralazine, minoxidil |
| Myocardial ischemia | Nitroglycerin | Nitroprusside Nifedipine Labetalol | Diazoxide, hydralazine, minoxidil |
| Dissecting aortic aneurysm | Labetalol Nitroprusside + propranolol | Trimethaphan | Diazoxide, hydralazine, minoxidil |
| Catecholamine crisis | Labetalol Phantolamine + propranolol | Nitroprusside + propranolol | Minoxidil |
| Pregnancy-induced hypertension | Magnesium sulfate + hydralazine Labetalol | Diazoxide Nitroprusside | Trimethaphan, furosemide, bumetanide, ACE inhibitors |

* Angiotensin-converting enzyme inhibitors.

**Table 58-4.** Medication Characteristics

| Medication | Mode of Action | Route | Onset | Duration |
|---|---|---|---|---|
| Nitroprusside | Direct arteriolar and venodilator | IV | Seconds | 1–2 min |
| Labetalol | $\alpha_1$, $\beta_1$, and $\beta_2$ blocker | IV | 5 min | 8 h |
|  | Direct arteriolar dilator | PO | 2 h | 8 h |
| Nitroglycerin | Direct arterial and venous dilator | IV | Seconds | 4 min |
| Nifedipine | Calcium channel blocker | PO | 5 min | 2–4 h |
| Hydralazine | Direct arteriolar dilator | IV | 10 min | 3–8 h |
|  |  | IM | 20 min | 3–8 h |
|  |  | PO | 30 min | 3–8 h |
| Minoxidil | Blocks calcium uptake | PO | 2 h | 12 h |
| Prazocin | Postsynaptic $\alpha_1$ blocker | PO | 2 h | > 4 h |
| Clonidine | Central $\alpha_2$ agonist | PO | 30 min | 2–4 h |
| Captopril | ACE inhibitor | PO | 30 min | 4–6 h |

## Use

A reasonable initial goal is a 30 percent reduction of the diastolic pressure in 30 to 60 min. The patient's signs and symptoms are the ultimate guide for treatment.

Fifty mg of Nipride should be mixed in 500 mL of 5% dextrose in water ($D_5W$) (100 $\mu$g/mL); the infusion is begun at 0.5 $\mu$g/kg per minute and then titrated rapidly until the desired blood pressure has been achieved. The average effective dose needed is 3 $\mu$g/kg per minute, with a range of 0.5 to 10 $\mu$g/kg per minute. Maintenance antihypertensive medication should be started concurrently with the infusion of nitroprusside. The blood pressure should be monitored every few minutes during the initial titration. An arterial line is not necessary for the institution of therapy but is necessary with long-term use. The lack of an arterial line should not delay the onset of treatment. The infusion fluid should not be used for simultaneous infusion of other medications. The infusion bottle should be covered with aluminum foil and used for no more than 24 h.

## Side Effects and Contraindications

Hypotension is the most common complication. Cyanide toxicity is rare but may occur with prolonged infusions, in infusion rates greater than 10 $\mu$g/kg per minute, or in hepatic dysfunction. Thiocyanate toxicity, manifesting as tinnitus, blurred vision, muscle weakness, changes in mental status, and seizures, is more common and seen after prolonged infusions and in patients with renal failure. Close monitoring of the infusion is required, which can present a staffing problem in many emergency departments. Nitroprusside inhibits hypoxia-induced vasoconstriction in the pulmonary vasculature and therefore may increase perfusion to nonventilated areas of the lung. The coronary steal syndrome may lead to increased myocardial ischemia. Concomitant use with clonidine has caused myocardial infarction. It is inappropriate for use in prehospital situations.

## Labetalol (Normodyne, Trandate)

Labetalol is a competitive, selective $\alpha_1$ blocker and a competitive, nonselective $\beta$ blocker. The $\beta$-blocking action is approximately 4 to 8 times the $\alpha$-blocking action. Labetalol is 6 to 10 times less potent than phentolamine as an $\alpha$ blocker. Propranolol is 1.5 to 4 times more potent as a $\beta$ blocker. The hypotensive response is a result of the $\alpha$- and $\beta$-blocking actions and a direct vasodilatory effect.

Labetalol is rapidly absorbed when taken orally, with an absorption half-life of 0.23 h for the tablets and peak plasma concentrations at 0.82 h. There exists significant first-pass hepatic metabolism, and care should be taken in oral dosing in the presence of hepatic disease. Bioavailability is only 25 percent after an oral dose but increases if taken with food or with cimetidine, and in the elderly. Elimination half-life after an oral dose is approximately 8 h.

After an intravenous dose, the distribution to peripheral tissues is rapid, with a large volume of distribution of 15.7 L/kg. Elimination half-life is 5.5 h. Onset of action after an intravenous injection is 5 to 10 min, with a duration action of 8 h. There is extensive hepatic metabolism, with less than 5 percent of the active compound excreted in the urine. It is safe for use with severe renal insufficiency without alteration of dosages.

The major hemodynamic effects are reduction of systolic arterial pressure and total peripheral vascular resistance. The reflex tachycardia associated with nonselective $\alpha$ blockade is avoided by the selective postsynaptic $\alpha_1$ blockade and the $\beta$-blocking action. Cardiac output may not change or may slightly decrease after an intravenous dose. Pulmonary artery and wedge pressures decrease. Labetalol does not reduce cerebral blood flow despite significant reduction in blood pressure. There is no change in renal blood flow or glomerular filtration rates, and angiotensin II activity is decreased with use of labetalol. Fluid retention may occur with chronic use.

Because of its nonselective $\beta$-blocking activity, labetalol decreases the forced expiratory volume $FEV_1$ in patients with asthma and chronic obstructive pulmonary disease (COPD). It may blunt the $\beta$-agonist response in the treatment of bronchospastic disease.

## Indications

Labetalol is a good intravenous medication for use in hypertensive emergencies and may be used in cases of treatment failure with sodium nitroprusside. It may be used orally for urgencies. It provides a steady, consistent drop in blood pressure and can be used in patients with cerebral vascular disease because there is no change in cerebral blood flow. Since it does not produce a reflex tachycardia, it is safe for use in the presence of coronary artery disease. It is an ideal choice for states of excessive catecholamine stimulation such as pheochromocytoma, MAO inhibitor–induced emergencies, and abrupt clonidine withdrawal. It has been used in pregnancy-induced hypertension. Use in prehospital care has not been reported.

With an intravenous bolus, blood pressure falls in 5 min, with a maximum response in 10 min, and may last for up to 6 h. The rate of fall of the blood pressure is related to the rapidity of the injection. Labetalol can be given with repeated, incremental boluses starting with 20 to 40 mg IV. If the antipressor response is inadequate, double the dose may be repeated every 30 to 60 min until adequate response is obtained or a total of 300 mg has been given. Labetalol may also be given as a continuous infusion by mixing 200 mg in 200 mL of $D_5W$ to run at 2 mg/min (2 mL/min). A 20-mg loading dose may precede the infusion. When the goal pressure is achieved, the infusion should be stopped. The initial oral dose for labetalol in hypertensive urgencies is 200 mg.

## Side Effects and Contraindications

Because of its large volume of distribution and long elimination half-life, labetalol has a prolonged action. Orthostatic hypotension occurs in 5 percent of patients. The nonselective $\beta$-blocking action of labetalol can exacerbate heart failure and induce bronchospasm. Tingling of the scalp has been noted. A paradoxical hypertensive effect can be seen when the drug is used in low doses in catecholamine-induced crisis because of the predominance of the $\beta$-blocking effect, leaving the $\alpha$ receptors unblocked for the circulating catecholamines.

## Intravenous Nitroglycerin

### Actions and Pharmacology

Nitroglycerin causes arteriolar dilation and venodilation and dilates large coronary arteries with a greater effect on capacitance vessels. Onset is almost immediate when nitroglycerin is given intravenously, with a half-life of 4 min. The mechanism of action is postulated to be formation of disulfide bonds from reduced sulfhydryl groups at a smooth-muscle nitrate receptor, resulting in an increase in cyclic GMP. Metabolism in the liver occurs by denitration by a glutathione-reductase system. The cardiac output may decrease slightly or remain unchanged.

## Indications

Intravenous nitroglycerin is the drug of choice for moderate hypertension complicating unstable angina, myocardial infarction, or pulmonary edema. It has a less deleterious effect on pulmonary gas exchange and collateral coronary blood flow than sodium nitroprusside in patients with ischemic heart disease.

## Use

Infusions should be started at 20 to 30 μg/min, then augmented by 10 μg rapidly every 3 to 5 min until symptoms are resolved or adverse effects become predominant.

## Side Effects and Contraindications

The most common side effects are headache, tachycardia, nausea, vomiting, hypoxia, and hypotension.

## AGENTS FOR USE IN HYPERTENSIVE URGENCIES

The decision to treat a hypertensive urgency in the emergency department must weigh the small potential benefit against the risk of a treatment complication. The goal in this condition is a gradual pressure reduction over the next 24 to 48 hours. Rapid reductions may lead to untoward effects regardless of the agent used. In the elderly, treatment should be initiated cautiously.

## Calcium Channel Blockers

### Nifedipine (Procardia)

#### Actions and Pharmacology

Nifedipine is a coronary and peripheral arterial dilator with no direct chronotropic effect and a mild negative inotropic effect. This results in a slight increase in heart rate but does not often cause postural hypotension. This agent undergoes extensive hepatic metabolism, and no adjustment is needed in renal insufficiency. With oral administration, the plasma level correlates to the size of the dose, but the clearance half-life of 2 to 4 h and the time to the peak level remain constant with all doses. Plasma levels of nifedipine correlate with hypotensive action. Oral administration causes a rapid surge in sympathetic activity, with an increase in plasma norepinephrine, cortisol, renin, and angiotensin I and II. There are no long-term effects on the renin-angiotensin system.

The maximal hypotensive response is observed 30 min after an oral dose. There is a slight increase or no change in glomerular filtration rate and renal blood flow and some diuretic, natriuric, and uricosuric effects. It is effective in control of pressure with renovascular hypertension. Tachycardia has been noted for 1 to 2 h after an oral dose, but in most cases it is mild.

With an oral dose, peripheral vascular resistance falls, cardiac output increases, and pulmonary capillary wedge pressures decrease in patients without congestive heart failure. Maximal *dP/dt* remains unchanged or slightly decreases. Nifedipine may improve cardiac performance with impaired ventricular function. With severe congestive heart failure, the beneficial effects seen are balanced by the small but significant negative inotropic effect, and this agent should be used with caution in these patients.

#### Indications

Nifedipine is an excellent agent for use in hypertension.

## Use

Nifedipine is primarily absorbed by the gastric mucosa. To achieve the most rapid onset of action, the patient is instructed to bite, chew, and then swallow a capsule that has been punctured. Alternatively, 10 to 20 mg may be given orally. After a 20-mg dose, the onset of hypotensive effect occurs in 5 min, with a maximal effect in 20 to 30 min that persists for up to 4 to 5 h.

### Side Effects and Contraindications

Headache, a burning sensation, flushing, and pedal and periorbital edema are observed. Postural hypotension may result if nifedipine is used concomitantly with diuretics. The effect on the cardiac index with left ventricular dysfunction is variable, and heart failure may develop. There is a negligible effect on the conduction system with therapeutic doses. There have been reports of reversible renal deterioration after a short course of nifedipine. Rebound hypertension has been described, as well as worsening of myocardial ischemia with rapid withdrawal. These symptoms can begin within 24 h of the last dose and are reversed by giving a calcium channel blocker. Nifedipine should not be used in dissection of the aorta unless a β blocker is also given.

## Direct Arteriolar Dilators

### Hydralazine (Apresoline)

#### Actions and Pharmacology

One of the first antihypertensive agents available, hydralazine acts as a direct arteriolar dilator, with onset of action within 10 min after an intravenous dose and a duration of action of 3 to 8 h. The onset of action is 20 min when hydralazine is given intramuscularly and 30 min when given orally. Hydralazine causes reflex tachycardia and increases plasma renin and catecholamines.

The plasma half-life is 2 to 4 h, but the antihypertensive effect lasts much longer than the plasma levels would indicate. Hydralazine has been detectable in the vascular walls long after being cleared from the plasma. It is metabolized by acetylation in the liver and gut walls. Approximately 50 percent of the population in the United States are "slow acetylators," and these patients have a higher incidence of hypotension and toxic complications. Hydralazine is also metabolized by ring hydroxylation and conjugation. Eighty percent of hydralazine and its metabolites are excreted within 24 h. Renal insufficiency prolongs the elimination half-life, and doses should be decreased in renal patients.

#### Indications

Pregnancy-induced hypertension is now the major indication for parenteral use. It is now used principally orally as an adjunct to other drugs.

#### Use

During eclampsia, 10 to 20 mg of hydralazine is given intravenously or 10 to 50 mg intramuscularly. The dose can be repeated in 30 min.

#### Side Effects and Contraindications

Undesirable cardiac effects prevent use of hydralazine when there is a history of coronary artery disease and in aortic dissection. This agent causes sodium and water retention and frequently causes headache, nausea, tachycardia, lethargy, and postural hypotension. Chronic oral administration can result in a lupuslike syndrome.

### Minoxidil (Loniten)

#### Actions and Pharmacology

Minoxidil is a potent oral arteriolar dilator. It acts by blocking calcium uptake through the cell membrane. The onset of action is in 2 h, with a maximal effect in 4 h and a duration of action of 12 h. Ninety percent of the drug is absorbed orally, with peak plasma levels in 1 h. Minoxidil is conjugated in the liver, and no accumulation of action is seen in renal insufficiency. It causes fluid retention and should be used with a diuretic. Reflex tachycardia is a common finding.

### Indications

Minoxidil can be used for the rapid oral control of pressure during a hypertensive urgency when other medications have failed. It is safe for use in the azotemic patient.

### Use

Ten to twenty mg should be given orally and the dose repeated in 4 h if needed. A β blocker may be needed to control symptomatic tachycardia, but an excessive hypotensive effect may result. Sodium and water retention necessitates the use of diuretics.

### Side Effects and Contraindications

Minoxidil is contraindicated with recent myocardial infarction, pheochromocytoma, congestive heart failure, and known hypersensitivity. Hirsutism may result from chronic use.

## Adrenergic Agonists

### Clonidine (Catapres)

#### Actions and Pharmacology

Clonidine, at doses used for hypertension, has potent central α₂-agonist effects. Stimulation of the postsynaptic receptors in the central nervous system results in a marked decrease in sympathetic system activity, lowering plasma catecholamine levels. While clonidine decreases basal sympathetic tone, vasomotor reflexes are not altered; thus there is little postural hypotension seen with therapeutic doses in euvolemic patients. Clonidine decreases renin secretion by a central mechanism. The net effect is a lowering of the blood pressure, bradycardia, and sedation. There is no change in renal blood flow or glomerular filtration rates. Cardiac output is decreased at rest but responds normally to exercise.

The onset of action is 30 to 60 min with oral loading, with a peak effect in 2 to 4 h. The duration of action of a single dose is 6 to 8 h. Clonidine readily passes the blood-brain barrier. Approximately 50 percent is excreted unchanged in the urine in the first 24 h. In renal failure, it is excreted in the feces. Very little is removed with dialysis.

#### Indications

Clonidine is an excellent agent for use in hypertensive urgencies. It can be used in the elderly and in renal failure. There are several unorthodox uses of clonidine, including migraine and withdrawal from opiates or nicotine.

#### Use

Oral loading is accomplished by giving 0.2 mg. Additional doses of 0.1 mg may be given hourly until the diastolic pressure is below 115 mmHg or a maximum of 0.7 mg has been given. Typically, a 0.3- to 0.4-mg dose is needed for adequate control of blood pressure. It is not necessary to discharge the patient on clonidine after its use in the emergency department.

#### Side Effects and Contraindications

Sedation and dry mouth are the most common side effects. Occasional bradycardia, especially in patients with sick sinus syndrome, has been reported. Orthostatic hypotension is not expected with therapeutic doses but may occur if used with diuretics, in hypovolemic patients, and in the elderly. Rebound and "overshoot" hypertension may be seen with rapid withdrawal from high doses of clonidine. Caution should also be used with patients on the following drugs: cyclic antidepressants, where the antihypertensive effects of clonidine may be blocked; alcohol, which enhances the sedative effects of clonidine;

β blockers, which may worsen clonidine withdrawal; and negative inotropic agents, which may cause bradyarrhythmias and disturbances when used with clonidine. Clonidine may inhibit the antiparkinsonism effect of levodopa.

## Modifiers of the Renin-Angiotensin System

### Captopril (Capoten)

#### Actions and Pharmacology

This angiotensin-converting enzyme inhibitor is a potent oral antihypertensive agent. It is rapidly absorbed after an oral dose, with an onset of action in 30 min. The peak effect is in 50 to 90 min, lasting for 4 to 6 h. Captopril is effective in congestive heart failure. No change in cardiac output or in heart rate has been observed. Captopril is not a reliable agent in patients with low renin activity. Cerebral blood flow is unchanged. The drug is metabolized rapidly and excreted in the urine. With renal insufficiency, plasma levels rise and the dose must be decreased when used chronically. Baroreceptor reflexes remain intact, and postural hypotension is rare.

#### Indications

Indications are limited to use in hypertension urgencies with known renovascular hypertension such as hypertension associated with scleroderma.

#### Use

Captopril should be administered in 25-mg doses orally three times a day.

#### Side Effects and Contraindications

Leukopenia and proteinuria may appear after chronic use. Skin rash, coughing, and loss of taste (ageusia) are not uncommon. This drug should not be used with potassium-sparing diuretics or with potassium supplements because hyperkalemia can develop. Angioneurotic edema, sometimes severe, may develop with use of this medication. Acute renal failure may occur in 1 to 2 of every 1000 patients treated. Though usually reversible with discontinuing the medication, there are reports of cases of permanent renal failure. In cases of renal artery stenosis, renal artery thrombosis has been reported.

## ADJUVANT AGENTS IN TREATMENT OF HYPERTENSION

### Loop Diuretics: Furosemide (Lasix) and Bumetanide (Burinex)

#### Actions and Pharmacology

Hypotensive effects are due to increased venous capacitance and decreased plasma volume. The diuretic effect begins within 5 min, peaks in 30 min, and last for 2 h. The drugs may decrease cardiac output but dilate renal arteries. They are usually excreted unchanged renally, but with renal impairment are cleared by biliary excretion. With renal and hepatic impairment, furosemide should be used with caution.

#### Indications

The primary use of furosemide and bumetanide is with antihypertensive agents that cause sodium and water retention. They should not be used as primary therapy of hypertensive urgencies or emergencies because volume depletion will stimulate the renin system and increase vasoconstriction.

#### Use

The initial dose of furosemide is 40 mg IV. This may be repeated with double the dose in 30 to 60 min. The initial dose of bumetanide is 1 to 2 mg.

### Side Effects and Contraindications

Hypokalemia, hypovolemia, and orthostatic hypotension are the most common acute side effects. Ototoxicity may occur with very high doses and with rapid intravenous injections of furosemide. These drugs are contraindicated in pregnancy-induced hypertension, because of the preexisting volume contraction seen with that condition.

## Propranolol (Inderal)

### Actions and Pharmacology

Propranolol is a nonselective β blocker, and the postulated mechanisms for its blood pressure reduction action includes reduced cardiac output, a readjustment to blood flow, readjustment of the baroreceptors, altered high pressure reflexes from the heart, reduced plasma renin activity, altered catecholamine synthesis, inhibited presynaptic β receptors, and a central action of an active metabolite of the agent.

### Indications

Propranolol is used primarily as adjuvant therapy with other medications. In catecholamine overdrive states (pheochromocytoma, clonidine withdrawal, and MAO inhibitor reaction), propranolol may be used in conjunction with phentolamine or sodium nitroprusside. Along with sodium nitroprusside, it is the treatment of choice for thoracic aortic dissection. It may be needed to counteract reflect tachycardia induced by many vasodilatory agents.

### Side Effects and Contraindications

The nonselective β blockade may induce bronchospasm in susceptible individuals. Left ventricular decompensation may be seen. Acute heart blocks and bradycardia have been observed. Sudden withdrawal of β blockers can precipitate angina or infarction. Because of the impaired adrenergic response seen with hypoglycemia, propanolol should be used with caution in insulin-dependent diabetics. It should not be used with clonidine, since simultaneous withdrawal from both medications may precipitate a hypertensive emergency. When used concurrently or with 1 h of verapamil or diltiazem, significant bradycardia or heart blocks may result.

## COMPLICATIONS OF THERAPY FOR HYPERTENSION

The most common complication of antihypertensive therapy is overzealous treatment for hypertensive urgencies resulting in orthostatic hypotension. Vigorous treatment of hypertension with a fixed arterial lesion may exacerbate ischemia distally. Unique complications of antihypertensive therapy include symptoms caused by abrupt withdrawal from antihypertensive medications or from overdose.

### Rapid Withdrawal

Withdrawal from antihypertensive medications that affect the adrenergic system may lead to one of five responses in the patient: (1) a small percent remain normotensive, possibly because of resetting of the "baroreceptors"; (2) the blood pressure returns to pretreatment levels over a few weeks; (3) the majority of patients have an asymptomatic return to pretreatment levels; (4) the blood pressure may "rebound" rapidly to pretreatment levels and may show signs of sympathetic overactivity; and (5) the blood pressure may "overshoot" to a pressure that may lead to a hypertensive emergency. Medications that can place the patient at risk for complications include clonidine, β blockers, and calcium channel blockers.

The mechanism of withdrawal overshoot with clonidine involves increased sympathetic discharge, increased plasma renin activity, and enhanced responsiveness of the adrenergic receptors to norepinephrine. These actions are enhanced when a β blocker is withdrawn si-

multaneously with clonidine, and with high daily doses of clonidine. Chronic use of β blockers leads to sensitization of the β receptors, which, along with the sympathetic surge seen with clonidine withdrawal, may lead to a hypertensive emergency.

Treatment depends on the symptoms. If the patient presents with sympathetic hyperactivity, the first drug of choice is labetalol. Care must be taken with the use of labetalol since low doses may exacerbate the elevation of pressure because of the predominance of the β-blocking effect. Use of phentolamine with propranolol is an adequate second choice. Sodium nitroprusside is also an excellent option. Symptoms of angina or myocardial infarction should be treated with labetalol, propranolol, or intravenous nitroglycerin.

Rapid withdrawal of β blockers and calcium channel blockers has been reported to precipitate arrhythmias, angina, and myocardial infarction.

## Angioneurotic Edema

Angiotensin-converting enzyme inhibitors are associated with angioneurotic edema, which presents as a pale swelling, usually of the face and upper airway. Swelling can be severe. Treatment includes epinephrine, antihistamines, and glucocorticoids. Close attention should be paid to the patient's airway, which can have severe compromise. Admission is generally indicated.

### BIBLIOGRAPHY

The Fifth Report of the Joint National Committee on Detection, Evaluation, and treatment of High Blood Pressure (JNCV). *Arch Intern Med* 153:154, 1993.

Calhoun DA, Oprail S: Treatment of hypertensive crisis. *N Engl J Med* 323:1177, 1990.

Gifford RW: Management of hypertensive crisis. *JAMA* 266:829, 1991.

Loyke HF: The three phases of blood pressure in stroke. *South J Med* 83:660, 1990.

Phillips SJ, Whisnant JP, and the National Blood Pressure Education Program: Hypertension and the brain. *Arch Intern Med* 152:938, 1992.

Powers WJ: Acute hypertension after stroke: The scientific basis for treatment decisions. *Neurology* 43:461, 1993.

# 59

# THORACIC AND ABDOMINAL ANEURYSMS

## John L. Glover

Physicians in emergency centers are seeing increasing numbers of patients with thoracic and abdominal aortic aneurysms because of: (1) the absolute increase in the frequency of these lesions, (2) the relative increase due to aging of the population, and (3) the frequent use of computed tomography (CT) and ultrasound for the evaluation of a variety of chest and abdominal complaints. When aneurysms are discovered, they always assume some significance for the patient; the amount varies with the size of the aneurysm, the age of the patient, and the number and type of other medical problems. A classification of the types of thoracic and abdominal aneurysms is shown in Table 59-1.

**Table 59-1.** A Classification of Thoracic and Abdominal Aortic Aneurysms

Thoracic, arteriosclerotic
    Intact
    Ruptured
Abdominal, arteriosclerotic
    Intact
    Ruptured
    Chronic, contained rupture
Dissecting aortic aneurysms
    Ascending aorta
    Descending aorta
Pseudoaneurysms and penetrating ulcer
Anastomotic aneurysms

## PATHOGENESIS

### Arteriosclerotic Aneurysms

In arteriosclerosis, arteries tend to dilate proximal to stenoses, apparently as a compensating mechanism. Greater dilatation occurs in formation of aneurysms, however, and a common definition of aneurysm is an increase in the diameter of the lumen to twice the size of that of the normal native artery proximal to the aneurysm. Arterial occlusive disease and aneurysms may, in fact, be different manifestations of arteriosclerosis, with the former being a proliferative disease of the intima and the latter a weakening of the media.

The media of the mammalian aorta is a highly organized, integrated system of fibromuscular layers, known as *fibrolamellar units,* the number of which is proportional to the aortic radius and, therefore, the tension on the arterial wall. Comparison of species shows that each fibrolamellar unit sustains a relatively constant amount of tension except those in the human infrarenal aorta, where each unit is subjected to about 60 percent more tension than in other locations. Whether this difference is evolutionary, metabolic, degenerative, or gene-linked for patients with aneurysms is not known, but it may account for the propensity for aneurysms to occur in the infrarenal location.

Another possible mechanism of the pathogenesis of aneurysms is that, in contrast to virtually all other mammals, humans have no vasa vasorum supplying the media of the aorta; tissue in the inner 300 to 600 μm obtains its oxygen and nutrition by diffusion from the lumen. Formation of arteriosclerotic plaques might interfere with this process and cause ischemia, which, in turn, could cause enough weakness to initiate aneurysmal dilatation.

Studies of enzymes in aneurysmal and nonaneurysmal aorta have shown increased levels of elastase and collagenase in the former, suggesting an endogenous mechanism causing breakdown of essential structural proteins. Three lines of evidence suggest that genetic or sex-linked factors may also be important. One is the only naturally occurring animal model of aneurysm: a mutation on the X chromosome of Blotchy mice results in aneurysms that enlarge and rupture. The second is the predominance of aneurysms in men, and the third is the studies that show an increased incidence of aneurysms in first-degree relatives of patients with aneurysms. The latter studies have obvious clinical relevance for emergency department physicians: Patients with obscure abdominal pain or acute abdominal pain without a likely clinical diagnosis should be queried about a family history of aneurysms.

### Dissecting Aneurysms

Dissecting aneurysms are different from arteriosclerotic aneurysms, and the term *dissection* should not be used to indicate rupture or pain associated with enlargement of arteriosclerotic aneurysms. In dissecting aneurysms, a tear occurs in the intima of the aorta and allows blood to "dissect" between the layers of the arterial wall, creating a true and a false lumen. The tear occurs either in the ascending aorta just above the aortic valve or at the origin of the descending thoracic aorta, in the region of the ligamentum arteriosum. Most patients are hypertensive, and the high pressures and flow cause blood to dissect both proximally and distally and over relatively long segments of aorta. The blood in the false lumen may clot or reenter the true lumen, in which case the patient may stabilize and the diagnosis may even be overlooked. If the false lumen ruptures—into the pericardium, the thorax, or the abdomen—the patient dies. Diastolic hypertension is a major factor in pathogenesis of this condition, and medical treatment evolved from knowledge that veterinarians could prevent spontaneous formation of dissecting aneurysms in turkeys being raised commercially by adding reserpine to their food. Abnormalities of connective tissue have also been implicated, and this condition has a significant association with Marfan syndrome.

### Pseudoaneurysms and Penetrating Ulcers

Recent studies have defined the pathogenesis and, to a greater extent, the natural history of a condition that was probably a significant cause of unexplained chest pain prior to good imaging techniques: *penetrating ulcer of the aorta.* Loss of a section of intima (for unknown reasons) creates an ulcer that penetrates the media and may extend beyond the confines of the aorta, causing a pseudoaneurysm (Fig. 59-1). More commonly, the aorta in the region of the ulcer changes slowly—over 2 or 3 years—and either dilates concentrically to form a fusiform aneurysm or forms a saccular aneurysm. For unknown reasons (and surprisingly), dissection hardly ever occurs; rupture is even less common. These lesions are seen most frequently in the descending thoracic aorta but may occur at any location. They are more common in patients who have aneurysms in locations other than the region of the ulcer.

### Anastomotic Aneurysms

In patients who have had vascular reconstruction, failure of healing where the graft was sewn to native artery produces an *anastomotic aneurysm,* and the most common site is the groin, where limbs of synthetic grafts are sewn to common femoral arteries. Anastomotic aneurysms may also occur in the abdomen, however, at aortic or iliac sites.

Finally, in patients who have had resection of infrarenal aortic aneurysms, the remaining segment of aorta between the renal arteries and the graft may become aneurysmal, particularly if that segment was relatively long (>2 cm).

## CLINICAL FEATURES

*Arteriosclerotic aneurysms of the abdominal aorta* have three common clinical presentations. The most common is the *incidental finding* of a painless abdominal mass with expansible pulsations or, more frequently, ultrasound (or CT) findings of an aneurysm in a patient with an unrelated problem. Patients may or may not be aware of pulsations; occasionally a patient describes "a lump" that can be felt when supine but that "goes away" when standing—in other words, tension in the abdominal wall (associated with being upright) obscures the mass, or the pulse.

Except in thin patients, aneurysms less than 5 cm in diameter are difficult to distinguish from the normal aortic pulse, and 6-cm aneurysms may not be apparent even in patients who are moderately obese.

While back pain is commonly cited as a symptom of abdominal aortic aneurysms, most patients with intact aneurysms are asymptomatic. Even grossly obvious, large aneurysms are usually painless and nontender unless they are acutely or chronically ruptured. The size of an asymptomatic aneurysm determines whether the patient should have elective surgery or serial measurements by ultrasound to

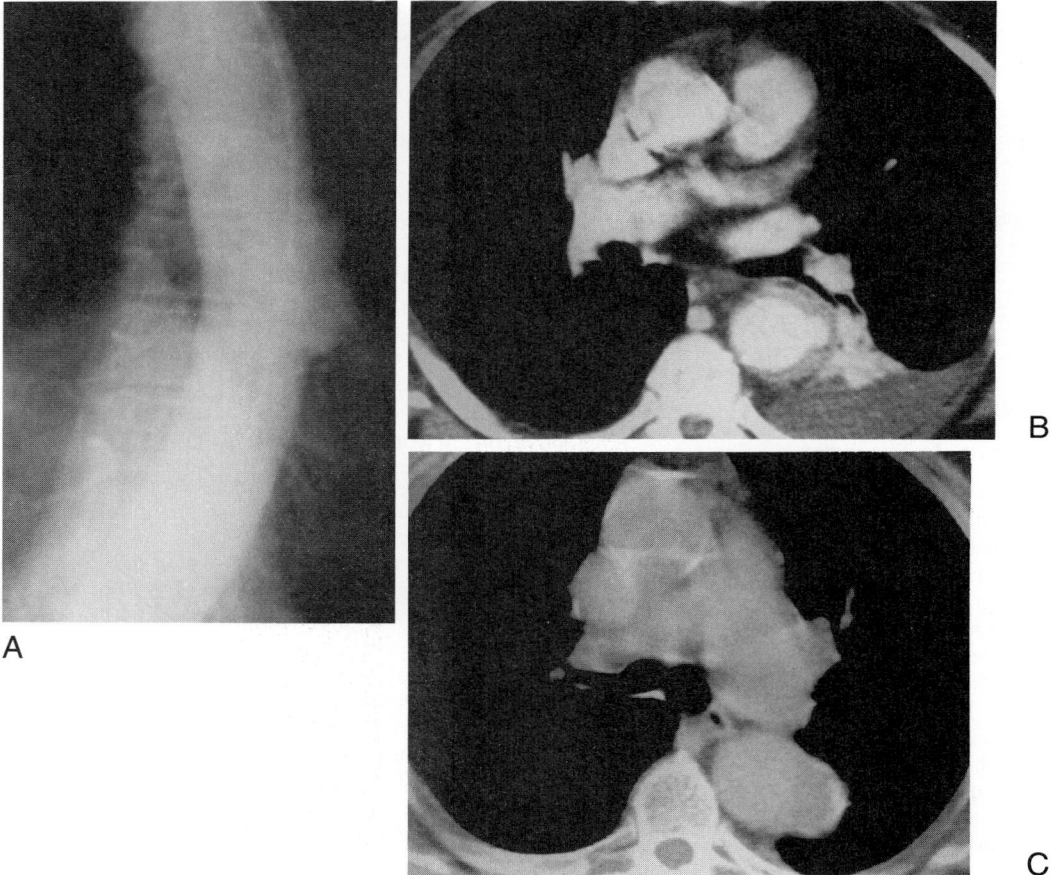

**Fig. 59-1. A.** Thoracic aortogram shows bilobed ulcer in mid-descending thoracic aorta. **B.** Contrast-enhanced CT shows upper portion of bilobed ulcer. Also seen is adjacent atelectasis and pleural effusion. **C.** CT scan after 6 years shows progression of upper portion to 5.0 cm saccular effusion. (From Harris JA et al: Penetrating atherosclerotic ulcers of the aorta. *J Vasc Surg* 19:93, 1994. Used with permission.)

monitor size and enlargement. Fusiform aneurysms 4 cm or less in *greatest transverse diameter* (either AP or lateral) virtually never rupture, whereas saccular aneurysms may. Aneurysms 5 cm or greater in diameter are at significant risk for rupture and should be treated surgically unless there are strong contraindications to surgery, such as uncorrectable heart disease or other causes of shortened life expectancy (e.g., malignancy, end-stage lung disease). For aneurysms between 4 and 5 cm in diameter, treatment is individualized according to age and other factors that affect risk. Patients with smaller lesions (e.g., 4.2 cm) are often advised to have measurements by ultrasound every 6 months, with surgery being advised if the aneurysm reaches 5 cm or enlarges more than 0.5 cm in a 6-month interval. The only factors shown to correlate with expansion are diastolic hypertension and chronic obstructive lung disease; length of the aneurysm is apparently not a factor.

The second most common presentation of abdominal aortic aneurysms is *acute rupture.* The classic history is unheralded syncope in an otherwise well patient, age 60 or more, followed by spontaneous recovery and then development of abdominal or back pain. Pain may precede syncope and even may be absent, but some type of relatively severe pain (and pain that is new for the patient) is very common. Its location, however, may vary, depending on the site of the rupture. In patients who lose relatively small amounts of blood, pain is the first symptom and syncope does not occur. The fact that a small rupture can occur in the aorta is surprising, but not infrequent. It is probably explained by the presence of layers of laminated clot in most aneurysms.

Pain in either flank or costovertebral angle is common and may cause the patient to complain of "kidney pain." Rupture into the mesentery of the left colon may cause left lower quadrant pain and tenesmus. Rupture into the right retroperitoneum may cause right hip or right lower quadrant pain.

Tenderness to palpation of an aneurysm is an ominous sign, even if the patient is stable and has had no syncope; it is an indication for an urgent evaluation for surgery. The combination of syncope with recovery and a tender, palpable aneurysm is usually indication for an emergency operation, usually with minimal or no additional studies.

The third presentation of abdominal aortic aneurysms, *chronic contained rupture,* is the most subtle and least common. The hallmark is chronic, severe pain, usually in the upper lumbar area, in a stable patient with a *nontender* aneurysm. This condition occurs when the posterior wall of the aneurysm erodes but the rupture is contained without sudden or significant loss of blood. Apparently, there is enough fibrosis to prevent blood loss, but the inflammatory process in response to erosion into adjacent structures causes unrelenting pain. The surprising clinical feature is how well the patients seem—a distinct contrast to those with acute rupture.

*Arteriosclerotic thoracic aortic aneurysms* are usually seen as abnormal contours of the aorta on chest radiographs or other imaging studies. They may involve any segment of the thoracic aorta, and some descending thoracic aneurysms extend into the suprarenal abdominal aorta. For the emergency physician, the importance of these aneurysms is recognition and referral for elective evaluation. *Rupture of thoracic aortic aneurysms* is usually catastrophic, and operative mortality is high for the few who survive long enough to get to an operating room.

The hallmark of *dissecting aortic aneurysms* is severe, tearing chest pain—precordial for dissections originating in the ascending aorta and interscapular for those originating near the ligamentum arteriosum. The path of the dissection, however, may alter the location of the pain. Dissection into the abdominal aorta may cause abdominal pain, dissection into the renal artery may cause flank pain, and dissection into an iliac artery may cause leg pain and relative ischemia. Conversely, dissection proximally, from the ligamentum into the ascending aorta, may cause chest pain. Dissection into the carotid arteries may cause a stroke or transient ischemic attack. Rarely, a patient will present with paraplegia because of interference with the blood supply to the spinal cord.

The dissection may compress the true lumen of the aorta enough to alter the pulses in the arms and/or legs. Severe chest pain in a patient with hypertension, asymmetric pulses, and no ECG changes suggestive of myocardial infarction are presumptive evidence of a dissecting aneurysm of the aorta.

Patients with *penetrating ulcers of the aorta* present most commonly with chest pain that is not typical for either myocardial infarction or dissecting aneurysm. When a pleural effusion is present, which is not uncommon, the pain may be pleuritic.

*Anastomotic aneurysms* are usually asymptomatic unless they become very large. Those that occur within the first few weeks after surgery are often associated with infection.

## DIAGNOSIS AND DIFFERENTIAL DIAGNOSIS

### Arteriosclerotic Abdominal Aortic Aneurysms

If asymptomatic aneurysms are not obvious on physical examination, ultrasound can clarify the situation easily, except in patients with extreme abdominal distension with gas (because sound is transmitted less efficiently through air than fluid or solid.) On physical examination, for example, it may be impossible to distinguish between a mass in the body of the pancreas overlying the aorta and an aneurysm, but ultrasound should separate them easily.

The biggest problem related to aneurysms is to differentiate between acute rupture of an abdominal aortic aneurysm and other conditions that can cause syncope or abdominal pain. Virtually all of these patients are old enough and have enough arteriosclerosis that cardiac arrhythmia, cerebrovascular occlusive disease, and exaggerated vagal response are major considerations in the differential diagnosis. If the patient has a palpable aneurysm, one must presume that rupture has occurred and obtain immediate surgical consultation, because the only chance for survival is to control the hemorrhage before hypotension recurs. Often, patients who appear to be stable except for slight tachycardia or postural hypotension develop sudden, refractory hypotension while being evaluated in the emergency department; these patients rarely survive even if they go to the operating room as soon as hypotension occurs. The standard explanation is that the retroperitoneal tissues and abdominal contents act as a temporary tamponade in the initial hemorrhage; then the aneurysm ruptures into the peritoneum, causing rapid blood loss and shock that is rarely reversed. Other factors, such as the duration of uncompensated fluid loss due to the initial loss of blood and the subsequent shifts of fluid, may be equally important or, in fact, the primary explanation in some patients.

Some patients with aneurysms too small to distinguish from a prominent aorta may have diffuse fullness and associated tenderness in the left side of the abdomen as a result of the retroperitoneal hematoma. This finding is usually enough to confirm the diagnosis if the patient has pain, and it certainly is if syncope occurred also.

The biggest problem in diagnosis occurs in patients whose obesity or abdominal distension prevents palpation of an aneurysm. These patients need a quick, noninvasive study to determine whether or not they have an aneurysm. Plain radiographs may show signs that suggest, but do not confirm, the diagnosis. A supine AP film may show a curvilinear calcification to the left of the lumbar spine; a lateral film may show a soft tissue bulge anterior to the lumbar spine. An abdominal ultrasound is just as quick and is more definitive, if it is available. Large amounts of gas in the bowel might prevent visualization of the aorta, but that amount of gas would be unusual in a nonintubated patient with a ruptured aneurysm, thus suggesting an alternative diagnosis. It is important to reiterate that these studies show only the presence of an aneurysm, but the presence of an aneurysm and an appropriate clinical setting are adequate reasons for an operation, because the risk of death from ruptured aneurysm far exceeds the risk of negative laparotomy for suspected rupture.

Although angiography is done frequently for elective preoperative planning in patients with aneurysms, it has no place in establishing the diagnosis of ruptured aneurysm. First of all, it might not show the rupture because layers of clot in the aneurysm might obscure a leak of contrast. Equally importantly, the time required to arrange and perform the study could be a fatal delay in treatment.

Computed tomography, on the other hand, is very useful in patients with aneurysms generally. It shows the origin and extent of the aneurysm, as well as any other relevant anatomic findings. In addition, it is very sensitive and specific for the diagnosis of rupture of an aneurysm and, in fact, is the preferred initial test for patients with chronic, contained rupture (Fig. 59-2). Its place in the emergency diagnosis of acute rupture, however, is controversial because it has the potential of delaying the diagnosis; there are many instances of patients developing hypotension while being scanned, usually with fatal outcome. Another objection is that negative tests give false security in patients with tenderness to palpation localized to the aneurysm. Such patients may be experiencing acute expansion of the aneurysm, and the usual clinical course is rupture within 24 h. CT scanning prior to rupture in such a patient might trigger the inappropriate decision to discharge the patient from the emergency center with instructions to see his or her physician the following day. Most surgeons consider tenderness to palpation localized to an abdominal aneurysm not only as a contraindication to CT scanning but also as an indication for surgery as soon as an operating room can be made available. There are instances in which CT scans are done in these circumstances, but the choice should be left to the surgeon who would assume responsibility for an emergency operation if necessary. Consequently, in the evaluation of patients in the emergency department suspected of having an arteriosclerotic abdominal aneurysm, CT scanning is indicated only for the following:

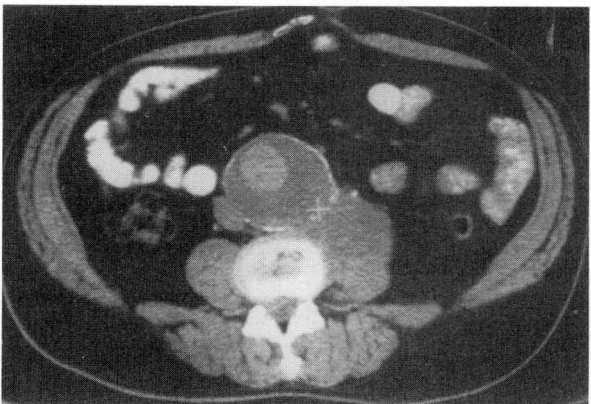

**Fig. 59-2.** Abdominal CT scan of patient showing left posterior aneurysm rupture. (From Jones CS et al: Chronic contained rupture of abdominal aortic aneurysms. *Arch Surg* 121:542, 1986. Copyright 1986, American Medical Association. Used with permission.)

1. Patients suspected of having chronic, contained rupture,
2. Stable patients who have aneurysms but are suspected to have acute abdominal conditions other than rupture,
3. Patients whom a surgeon has examined and requested CT scanning to assist in diagnosis or preoperative planning. *These patients should never be left unattended in the CT scanner.*

While diagnosis of ruptured abdominal aneurysm is easy when the patient presents in shock and with a pulsatile abdominal mass, diagnosis can be difficult in stable patients, because the signs and symptoms vary and other conditions can cause a similar picture.

Patients with aneurysms and retrocecal appendicitis or diverticulitis have abdominal pain, a palpable aneurysm, and an adjacent tender mass. They usually have fever and marked leukocytosis also, which are not common with ruptured aneurysm. In fact, any inflammatory mass can adhere to an aneurysm and cause a similar picture: benign and malignant pancreatic tumors, gastric tumors, an inflamed gallbladder, and ischemic small bowel. The fever, leukocytosis, symptoms associated with these other conditions, and the lack of postural hypotension (in most cases, but not all) are indicative of conditions other than ruptured aneurysm. CT scan can be very helpful in these patients as long as two caveats are observed: (1) a surgeon has seen the patient, and (2) the patient is not left unattended in the CT scanner.

## Other Aneurysms

*Thoracic arteriosclerotic aortic aneurysms* rarely present a problem in differential diagnosis, but their presence may be obscured by pleural effusion or atelectasis, which masks the contour of the thoracic aorta. Dissecting *aortic aneurysms* are often initially misdiagnosed as myocardial infarction. Careful attention to the history can provide helpful clues: (1) pain of dissecting aneurysms is immediately intense and tearing, (2) interscapular pain is more likely to be from dissection than infarction, and (3) pain of infarction may begin as "heaviness" that builds up gradually to crushing pain. Auscultation of the murmur of aortic insufficiency in a patient with severe, acute, chest pain usually indicates the presence of a dissecting aneurysm of the ascending aorta unless the patient was found in the past to have such a murmur. Finally, palpation of pulses in all extremities should be done *and recorded* in all patients presenting to the emergency department with chest pain suggesting myocardial infarction. Absence of a brachial pulse in a patient with sudden onset of chest pain but no pain in the arm is very suggestive of a dissection involving the aortic arch. In contrast, patients with infarction and brachial embolism nearly always have pain in the arm and decreased motor function.

Spontaneous perforation of the esophagus may also be confused with dissecting aneurysm (as well as myocardial infarction), and the initial pain may be very similar. The history of violent vomiting preceding the pain should make one think of perforation of the esophagus and look carefully for air in the mediastinum.

The course of patients with *penetrating aortic ulcers* has been described fairly recently, and the key to diagnosis is awareness of the lesion. CT with contrast is the best way to confirm its presence. Patients with *anastomotic aneurysms* in the abdomen or pelvis are usually asymptomatic but occasionally present with rupture; CT will establish the diagnosis.

## EMERGENCY DEPARTMENT CARE

Patients with abdominal and thoracic aortic aneurysms discovered incidentally need no care except prompt referral to a surgeon. The same is true for patients with penetrating aortic ulcers and unruptured anastomotic aneurysms. Patients with ruptured abdominal aneurysms and dissecting aortic aneurysms need *immediate* surgical consultation, and emergency medicine physicians must provide supportive care. Both groups require monitoring of cardiac, respiratory, and renal

function. Hypertensive patients with dissecting aneurysms require lowering of blood pressure. Patients with ruptured aneurysms require fluid resuscitation, preparation for blood replacement, and—depending on stability or the lack of it—intubation.

Presence of an incidentally found asymptomatic thoracic, abdominal, or anastomotic aneurysm is not an indication for admission, but elective outpatient evaluation should not be delayed. Patients with chronic contained rupture and penetrating aortic ulcers should be admitted to allow complete assessment and formulation of a definitive plan for treatment, which may or may not include operation within 24 to 48 h. Patients with aortic dissection require emergency admission, and those with ruptured aneurysms obviously require an emergency operation. Older patients may choose not to have surgery; those in whom the diagnosis was previously established but who were not operated on because of personal choice or because risk of elective resection was thought to be too great (or a combination of these reasons) present a dilemma. While some of these patients will survive an emergency operation, the decision must be made on an individual basis, with the patient and family participating in the process.

Recognition of other significant problems with patients who have aneurysms is important in decisions concerning the plan of treatment and the timing of surgery. Significant coronary artery disease is almost routine, and obstructive lung disease is frequent. Decreased renal function is not uncommon and may be made worse by clamping and dissection around the renal arteries during surgery or by the shock associated with ruptured aneurysms. Finally, occurrence of lung cancer is significantly increased in patients with aneurysms. Careful scrutiny of the chest radiograph and/or CT scan should be done preoperatively because presence of malignancy might cause the patient or the surgeon to decide against operation.

In spite of the associated combined conditions and the need for extensive operations, surgical treatment of aneurysms prolongs the lives of patients and allows them to resume and maintain their preoperative level of function. Physicians in emergency departments can participate in this process by recognizing aneurysms and arranging appropriate definitive treatment, be it elective, urgent, or on an emergency basis.

## BIBLIOGRAPHY

Crawford ES, Hess KR: Abdominal aortic aneurysm. *N Engl J Med* 321:1040,1989.

Harris JA, Kostaki G, Glover J, et al: Penetrating atherosclerotic ulcers of the aorta. *J Vasc Surg* 19:90, 1994.

Jones CS, Reilly MK, Dalsing MC, Glover JL: Chronic contained rupture of abdominal aortic aneurysms. *Arch Surg* 121:542,1986.

Nevitt MP, Ballard DJ, Hallett JW Jr: Prognosis of abdominal aortic aneurysms. A population-based study. *N Engl J Med* 321:1009,1989.

# 60
# MESENTERIC ISCHEMIA

## John L. Glover
## Geoffrey B. Blossom

Mesenteric ischemia is a relatively rare condition, but the incidence may be increasing in association with the advancing age of the population. It may present as an acute abdominal catastrophe or as a cause of chronic weight loss. In both circumstances, the diagnosis is usually not considered until the patient is critically ill. Consequently, morbidity and mortality are high (at least 70 percent mortality for laparotomy done for dead bowel), even though there is reasonably good understanding of the pathophysiology and the appropriate treatment. Therefore, early diagnosis is the key to improving results; and early diagnosis can be facilitated by instituting appropriate tests based on prodromal symptoms.

## ANATOMY AND PATHOPHYSIOLOGY

Knowledge of the anatomy of the intestinal blood supply is necessary to understand the pathophysiology of ischemia, especially since ischemia may be acute or chronic and may affect either the arterial or the venous supply.

Abdominal viscera are supplied with blood by three major arterial branches which arise from the anterior aspect of the abdominal aorta. The celiac trunk originates at the diaphragmatic crura. Its three main branches, the splenic, left gastric, and common hepatic arteries, supply the upper abdominal viscera and small bowel to the ligament of Treitz. The remainder of the mesenteric circulation comes from the superior and inferior mesenteric arteries. These two vessels supply a portion of the pancreatic circulation as well as the small bowel and colon. Together, the three splanchnic vessels receive 25 percent of the cardiac output at rest and contain up to one third of the total blood volume.

The venous drainage of the intestines is by the superior and inferior mesenteric veins. These vessels join the splenic vein beneath the pancreas and form the portal vein. Each drains the area supplied by its corresponding artery.

Mesenteric ischemia may be caused by (1) arterial embolism, nearly always to the superior mesenteric artery; (2) arterial thrombosis, usually due to atherosclerotic plaques; (3) venous thrombosis, often associated with a coagulopathy; or (4) insufficient arterial flow due to poor cardiac performance, the so-called low-output ischemia.

Arterial embolism accounts for 40 to 50 percent of all episodes of acute mesenteric ischemia, and the source of the embolus is nearly always the heart. In most cases, the clot is from a mural thrombus associated with a myocardial infarction; but in some cases it comes from the left atrium and is associated with acute or chronic atrial fibrillation. In the past, atrial thrombus associated with mitral valvular stenosis due to rheumatic fever was the most common source of embolism; but the decrease in rheumatic fever and the aging of the population have made mural thrombus overlying an infarcted segment of left ventricular wall or septum more common. In most cases, patients have no preexisting significant obstruction of their mesenteric vessels, and consequently there is no development of collateral circulation. When embolism occurs, therefore, it causes acute cessation of distal arterial flow. In most cases, the point of obstruction is the main trunk of the superior mesenteric artery, just beyond its right colic branch. As a result, the entire small bowel except for the most proximal jejunum becomes acutely ischemic.

Arterial thrombosis, on the other hand, is usually preceded by long periods (months at least) of relative ischemia caused by progressive stenosis at the origins of the celiac and superior mesenteric arteries. In most patients, the narrowing is due to progressive buildup of atherosclerotic plaque, but in some cases it is due to fibromuscular hyperplasia. As stenosis increases, collateral circulation develops. For example, when there is plaque at the origins of both the celiac and the superior mesenteric artery, the inferior mesenteric artery becomes very large, supplying blood through connections with the superior mesenteric, including the marginal artery which courses along the mesenteric aspect of the colon. The gradual nature of this process and the rich collateral connections make it possible to supply enough arterial flow to maintain viability under resting, basal conditions. When more blood is required, however, as when a large meal is ingested, flow becomes inadequate. The patient feels cramping abdominal pain and may vomit, expelling the source of "stress" from the intestine and possibly relieving the pain. The intermittent nature of this phenomenon and the analogy with pain related to myocardial stress generated the term "intestinal angina." This chronic situation may become acute if complete occlusion occurs or if the metabolic requirements of the intestine exceed the ability of the collateral circulation to supply adequate blood flow.

In view of the excellent arterial perfusion of the intestinal tract, it is not surprising that most instances of venous occlusion are associated with factors affecting coagulation. Some of these are hereditary disorders, such as deficiencies of antithrombin III or protein C. Others are more general, for example, dehydration, relative polycythemia, and hypercoagulable states associated with medications such as birth control pills (less common with present oral contraceptives). Venous occlusion in the presence of normal arterial flow results in massive congestion, and by the time infarction occurs, a large proportion of the blood volume is sequestered in the intestine. Consequently, large volumes of fluid are required to replenish intravascular volume, and anticoagulation is necessary to prevent further clotting.

Since the mucosa has a higher metabolic rate than the other layers of the intestine, it is the first area affected by ischemia and may be the only area affected if there is enough remaining blood flow to support the muscular layer. This situation occurs commonly in chronic intestinal ischemia, and the resulting sloughing of mucosa accounts for the presence of occult blood in the stool. Mucosal sloughing occurs in the first stages of acute ischemia from all causes. As long as the loss is patchy, or of only partial thickness, there will be no abdominal tenderness because there is no stimulation of the somatic nerve fibers which lie outside the bowel wall. When more mucosa sloughs, the combination of bacterial invasion of the muscular layer and the damaging effects of toxic products of breakdown of intestinal cells stimulates the visceral nerve endings which lie within the muscular layers of the intestine. The result is poorly localized, intermittent abdominal discomfort which makes the patient feel restless and change positions frequently. When the inflammatory process involves the full thickness of the bowel wall, the somatic nerve endings are irritated and the patient experiences constant, severe abdominal pain which is associated with abdominal tenderness. This stage usually corresponds with infarction of the full thickness of the bowel wall, and the patient must be assumed to have peritonitis whether or not perforation has occurred.

## CLINICAL PRESENTATION

The mortality rate for patients with gangrenous bowel is extremely high, and the most important factor in improving the chances for survival is to make the diagnosis before infarction occurs. This, in turn, means suspecting the diagnosis in patients with vague symptoms of abdominal distress and few, if any, clinical signs. The key to early diagnosis is to think of mesenteric ischemia in patients with abdominal pain and no obvious related problem such as previous abdominal surgery, an incarcerated hernia, or symptoms of biliary disease or ulcer. The initial presentation always involves abdominal discomfort but varies with the mechanism of mesenteric ischemia.

In acute ischemia due to embolism to the superior mesenteric artery or due to arterial thrombosis, the onset of abdominal discomfort is sudden and dramatic. With either etiology, there is pain "out of proportion to the physical findings" before peritonitis is present. The patients are nearly always over 50 and have some general evidence of cardiovascular disease. With acute ischemia due to embolism there is often atrial fibrillation or evidence of a myocardial infarction in the relatively recent past. In some cases, however, the infarction has been silent or subendocardial and the abdominal catastrophe is its first manifestation. Patients who have recently discontinued anticoagulant therapy for controlled chronic atrial fibrillation are at an increased risk for recurrent atrial thrombosis and subsequent embolization.

In patients with arterial thrombosis occurring due to progressive occlusion of the celiac and superior mesenteric arteries, one can nearly always elicit a history of unexplained weight loss over the preceding several months. It is rare, however, to elicit the classic history of intestinal angina: abdominal pain after a large meal, relieved by vomiting. More often the history is one of weight loss and "fear of food." These patients have gradually become accustomed to eating smaller and smaller meals in order to avoid abdominal pain, and this is the characteristic history for chronic mesenteric ischemia without infarction.

"Nonocclusive" intestinal ischemia usually occurs in patients hospitalized for cardiac failure, and it was much more frequent before interventional cardiology became common and measurement of cardiac output became so easy. It may still be seen in an emergency department setting in patients who are being given outpatient intensive diuretic therapy for cardiac failure and who have concurrent hypokalemia and digitalis toxicity or near toxicity.

Venous thrombosis tends to occur in younger patients because venous thrombi are associated with disorders of coagulation instead of complications of arteriosclerosis. In these patients, the onset of pain is more insidious because the occlusion is on the venous side of the circulation, and a thorough history is especially important in raising a suspicion for this diagnosis. For example, a previous spontaneous episode of venous thrombosis *either in the patient or a relative* may be a clue to protein C or antithrombin III deficiency. Other factors in the history include concurrent use of birth control pills, a history of malignancy, evidence of polycythemia (either "true" polycythemia or polycythemia secondary to other diseases), and evidence of portal hypertension. Finally, mesenteric venous thrombosis occasionally occurs during pregnancy; the large uterus may cause mesenteric vascular stasis which, in turn, may act synergistically with other factors producing hypercoagulability, such as pregnancy itself.

Other important aspects of the history and general physical examination include any evidence of cardiac or peripheral vascular disease, such as a history of symptoms of cerebrovascular disease or claudication or a history of myocardial infarction or angina pectoris. Auscultation for bruits in the neck and abdomen should be done, and the status of all peripheral pulses should be recorded. Physical evidence of chronic weight loss may be important, especially in elderly patients unable to give a good history.

Patients are usually afebrile unless infarction has been present long enough to cause peritonitis. Blood pressure is stable until sequestration of a large percentage of the blood volume causes hypovolemia, or until bacteremia occurs. These findings are not present as a rule until the patient has obvious abdominal tenderness and rigidity. The lack of abnormal vital signs except for mild tachycardia in the preinfarction stage of the disease is one of the reasons that physicians may dismiss prodromal symptoms of mesenteric ischemia as gastroenteritis.

The abdominal examination varies depending on the stage of ischemia and on whether or not infarction has occurred. Distension is not present initially but develops when ileus occurs secondary to peritonitis or to impaired motility before peritonitis occurs. If the visceral component of pain is predominant, the patient may writhe and will have difficulty localizing the pain. When the somatic component develops, patients lie still and have diffuse abdominal tenderness and rigidity. As long as some bowel is viable, bowel sounds will be active until peritonitis becomes generalized. The presence of rebound tenderness, of course, is dependent on the presence of peritoneal irritation caused by transmural inflammation of the intestine.

## DIAGNOSTIC STUDIES

A leukocytosis is present in most patients, frequently in excess of 15,000, and about half of the patients will exhibit a metabolic acidosis. Hemoglobin and hematocrit reveal hemoconcentration, and occasionally serum amylase and phosphate may be elevated, although these are nonspecific findings.

Abdominal radiographs should be obtained, primarily to look for other conditions which can have similar prodromes, such as an early bowel obstruction or gallstone ileus. Although one looks for thickening of the bowel wall, or air in it, these findings are rare and are never clear enough to make a definitive diagnosis. Air in the portal vein is a late finding indicative of dead bowel and a grim prognosis.

Duplex ultrasound may be used to diagnose chronic mesenteric ischemia, but at the current stage of development it requires expert interpretation. Furthermore, a successful examination depends on a relative paucity of gas in the abdomen, and therefore is best done after an overnight fast. However, since abdominal duplex techniques are developing rapidly, duplex ultrasound may become a useful technique even in emergency situations. The same can be said for laparoscopy, but the necessity of a general anesthetic limits its use as an early method for diagnosis in a condition with such vague and varied initial symptoms.

Arteriography, which is the mainstay of diagnosis and early treatment, should be obtained promptly in all patients who are hemodynamically stable if there is a strong suspicion of mesenteric ischemia. Embolic occlusion of the superior mesenteric artery is usually manifested by a sharp cutoff of the column of dye several centimeters from its origin, below the takeoff of the middle colic artery. Thrombosis is represented by occlusion at the origin, and nonocclusive ischemia manifests as segmental narrowing of arterial arcades. Findings in venous thrombosis are more subtle and may not be diagnostic.

If there is strong enough suspicion of the diagnosis of mesenteric ischemia to believe that angiography should be obtained, surgical consultation should be requested because the study may indicate need for an emergency operation. In addition, it may be desirable to leave a catheter in place for intraarterial infusion of vasodilating agents.

## TREATMENT

As stated previously, the challenge is to make the diagnosis of ischemia before infarction occurs. Emboli can be removed relatively easily; and the results of celiac and superior mesenteric revascularization are quite good, but cannot be done safely in the presence of generalized peritonitis. Venous infarction nearly always requires resection, but usually enough bowel can be spared to allow survival and normal nutrition if the hypercoagulability is reversed. It is crucial *to avoid laparotomy* in patients with "nonocclusive" ischemia because the anesthetic exacerbates the cause of the problem (the low cardiac output) and operative manipulation increases vasospasm and can cause ischemia to progress to necrosis. The marked differences in treatment for different varieties of ischemia point out the importance of early angiography. There is also substantial evidence that infusion of vasodilating drugs through angiographic catheters increases the amount of bowel which can be saved in cases of embolism and thrombosis, and may be therapeutic in low output ischemia.

Other adjunctive therapies are anticoagulation with heparin, decompression of dilated bowel, and use of broad-spectrum antibiotics.

Heparin, which should be started as soon as feasible after angiography, prevents propagation of thrombus in conditions of decreased arterial flow and reverses the hypercoagulability associated with venous thrombosis. Bowel decompression and antibiotics have been shown to prolong the period between ischemia and necrosis when there is marginally adequate intestinal blood supply.

Other measures include replacement of plasma volume and adequate monitoring of hemodynamic parameters. These are best accomplished in the perioperative period by placing an arterial line, a Swan-Ganz catheter, and a Foley catheter while giving appropriate fluid and electrolyte therapy.

Since all forms of intestinal ischemia may cause loss of so much intestine that life cannot be sustained, bowel with marginal viability is often left in place at the initial procedure. In such cases, a "second look" operation is done after 12 to 24 h.

Adopting an aggressive attitude toward arteriography in patients with early and vague symptoms suggestive of ischemia will undoubtedly lead to some unnecessary arteriograms, but the risk of morbidity from angiography is negligible compared to the risk of mortality from bowel which has become necrotic while physicians waited for symptoms to become clearer.

## BIBLIOGRAPHY

Batellier J, Kieny R: Superior mesenteric artery embolism: Eighty-two cases. *Ann Vasc Surg* 4:112, 1990.

Bergan JJ: Diagnosis of acute intestinal ischemia, in *Seminars in Vascular Surgery*. Philadelphia, Saunders, 1990.

Bergan JJ, Pearce WH: *The Management of Visceral Ischemic Syndrome,* 3d ed. Philadelphia, Saunders, 1989.

Boley SJ, Spraynagan S: Initial results from an aggressive roentgenological and surgical approach to acute mesenteric ischemia. *Surgery* 82:848, 1977.

Bowersox JC, Zwolak RM, Walsh DB, et al: Duplex ultrasonography in the diagnosis of celiac and mesenteric artery occlusive disease. *J Vasc Surg* 14:780, 1991.

Clavien PA, Muller C: Treatment of mesenteric infarction. *Br J Surg* 74:500, 1987.

Engelhart TC, Kerstein MD: Pregnancy and mesenteric venous thrombosis. *South Med J* 82:1441, 1989.

Fry WJ: *Mesenteric Ischemia in Current Surgical Therapy-3*, Toronto, Decker, 1989.

Kaleya RN, Boley SJ: Mesenteric ischemic disorders, in *Maingot's Abdominal Operations,* 9th ed. Connecticut, Appleton/Lange, 1989.

Serreyn RF, Schoofs PR: Laparoscopic diagnosis of mesenteric venous thrombosis. *Endoscopy* 18:249, 1986.

Sitges-Serra A, Mas X, Roquenta F, et al: Mesenteric infarction: An analysis of 83 patients with prognostic studies in 44 cases undergoing massive small bowel resection. *Br J Surg* 75:544, 1988.

# 61
# ACUTE EXTREMITY ISCHEMIA AND THROMBOPHLEBITIS
## A. Joel Feldman

## ACUTE EXTREMITY ISCHEMIA

Acute extremity ischemia is due to embolism, thrombosis, trauma, or low flow states. Embolic occlusion of a peripheral artery is the most common cause of ischemia. The clinical setting will often provide clues as to the underlying etiology. A careful history and physical examination is critical in the diagnosis and management of these patients.

### Pathophysiology

The final common pathway of all causes of ischemia is insufficient blood flow to meet the metabolic demands of the affected tissues. Skeletal muscle and peripheral nerves are most sensitive to ischemia. Cell injury and death occur both because of inadequate nutrient blood flow to maintain cellular ATP stores and membrane integrity during the period of ischemia itself and because of reperfusion injury. The latter term refers to adverse events that occur during the initial period of restoration of blood flow to the ischemic tissues. Free-radical formation occurs with reintroduction of oxygen and other metabolic substrates. Reperfusion may be subsequently blocked because of swelling of cells, sludging of red blood cells in the microcirculation, and deposition of fibrin.

The severity of the ischemic episode depends on the site of occlusion and the quality of collateral circulation around this point. Embolic occlusion frequently causes more profound ischemia than thrombotic occlusion. This is due to the suddenness of its onset and the frequent lack of well-established collateral circulation around the occlusion. Progressive thrombosis occurs in the stagnant blood column both proximal and distal to the acutely occluded site. As thrombosis progresses, sources of collateral blood supply are occluded, causing progression of ischemia. Anticoagulation can help prevent this propagation and limit the ischemic insult.

### Etiology

Embolic occlusion is the most common form of acute ischemia of the extremities. Between 75 and 80 percent of these emboli originate in the heart, although infrequently the source is a proximally located arterial lesion (arterioarterial embolus). Paradoxical embolization from the venous to the arterial circulation may occur in the setting of an atrial septal defect or patent foramen ovale.

Emboli most commonly lodge at the bifurcation of arteries and are most common in the lower extremities. In one series, 43 percent of emboli lodged at the bifurcation of the femoral artery, 18 percent at the iliac arteries, 15.5 percent in the aorta, and 15 percent at the popliteal arteries. Visceral artery embolism may occur in 7 to 10 percent of patients and is probably underdiagnosed. Estimates of cerebral vascular embolization varies from as little as 3 percent up to 15 to 20 percent. Emboli may be multiple, and the patient should be carefully examined for evidence of embolization to other extremities or to the visceral arteries.

Thrombosis can occur at a site of severe vessel stenosis (usually due to atherosclerosis) because of low flow through the stenotic area and abnormal intima. Because atherosclerosis is a systemic disease, the patient will frequently have evidence of chronic arterial occlusive disease by history and on physical examination.

The false lumen of an acute dissecting thoracic aortic aneurysm involving the abdominal aorta may occlude the blood flow to one or both legs. This diagnosis should be suspected in patients presenting with both upper and lower extremity and/or cerebral ischemia. The patient may complain of intrascapular back pain or chest pain. A widened mediastinum and/or left pleural effusion on chest x-ray further supports this diagnosis.

The patient with low cardiac output (either cardiogenic or hypovolemic) may present with acutely ischemic limbs due to inadequate peripheral perfusion rather than acute mechanical obstruction of a major artery. These patients are usually easily diagnosed because of the clinical setting of an acute myocardial infarction, blood loss, intravascular volume depletion (e.g., sepsis, dehydration), or treatment with intravenous vasopressors. Patients with severe atherosclerotic occlusive disease are at a much higher risk to develop ischemia or tissue loss in situations of low flow.

Intraarterial injection of illegal drug substances is an increasingly common problem. Injection into the arteries of the wrist, hand, or fingers results in intense burning pain, frequently followed over a period of days by extensive swelling of the hand and digital gangrene of varying degree. Vasospasm, the presence of particulate matter used to cut the drug, crystallization of the injected substance on injection, and arterial necrosis have all been implicated as causes of this injury. In our experience intraarterial injection into the femoral arteries rarely results in acute ischemia and tissue loss.

Severe venous outflow obstruction in the form of massive ileofemoral thrombosis may result in thrombosis of the capillary beds and ultimately of the larger arteries. This can result in venous gangrene. However, the clinical presentation is quite different than that of primary acute arterial ischemia.

The introduction and widespread use of various endovascular techniques for the treatment of arterial disease has resulted in an increased incidence of iatrogenically caused ischemia. The lesion may occur at the site of the treated vessel or of the access vessel (most commonly the femoral artery). A history of recent instrumentation suggests this diagnosis.

Microemboli are small collections of platelets and fibrin (platelet-fibrin emboli) and/or atheroembolic debris that originate from atherosclerotic ulcers, stenoses, or aneurysms in the aorta, iliac, femoral, or popliteal arteries. These are so-called arterioarterial emboli. The recent use of transesophageal echocardiography has heightened our appreciation of the incidence of significant atheromatous debris within the aortic arch. Microemboli may originate from an abnormal heart valve or myocardium. These small emboli do not occlude major vessels but become lodged in the smaller digital, muscular, and skin vessels causing ischemia in the small amount of tissue supplied by the occluded vessel. Clinically, this is manifested by painful, cyanotic toes (or portion of a toe), petechial skin lesions, or muscle infarcts with associated muscle tenderness and pain. These lesions may be present despite palpable pulses. Occasional massive showers of microemboli may occur. Both lower extremities can be affected. The patient's extremity may be mottled, with areas of muscle tenderness and pain, and cyanosis and pain of several toes may be present.

Upper extremity microemboli do occur but are less common. Atherosclerosis is less common in the upper extremities. Patients with upper extremity microemboli should be evaluated for atherosclerotic lesions of the proximal axillary or subclavian arteries or aortic arch, poststenotic aneurysm of the subclavian artery due to compression at the thoracic outlet, or cardiac abnormalities.

Patients who have undergone lower extremity bypass grafting may present with acute ischemia of the operated limb. This occurs due to thrombosis of their bypass graft. Manifestations are the same as for other causes of ischemia, and the initial treatment and evaluation of these patients is the same, although their treatment may differ significantly and is beyond the scope of this discussion.

Hypercoagulable states, vasculitis, and repetitive trauma to an extremity (as may occur in the workplace) may rarely cause an ischemic extremity or digit.

## Clinical Features

Pain is the most common symptom of an acutely ischemic extremity. Paresthesia, hypoesthesia, anesthesia, paresis, or paralysis result from loss of both sensory and motor nerve function. The rapidity with which these manifestations occur depends on the severity of the ischemia. The extremity is usually pale initially, though it may become cyanotic or mottled as time progresses. Pulses are absent beyond the site of arterial occlusion. Muscle palpation may elicit tenderness. However, with profound prolonged ischemia muscle cell death occurs, resulting in rigor. Much later, skin and fat necrosis occur. Microemboli are evident as areas of petechiae-like lesions of cyanosis or gangrene in the distal extremities. Microemboli to the musculature may result in extreme muscle tenderness and pain, with limited function of the affected muscle groups. Mottling of the skin of a portion or all of the extremity may be present in severe cases. Palpable pulses may be present with microembolization.

The time sequence of the various events described above is dependent on the severity of the ischemia. There is no safe interval within which revascularization always results in a functional, viable limb or beyond which salvage is not possible. In general, patients presenting with sensorimotor deficits have a severe ischemic insult and expeditious restoration of flow is needed to minimize loss of function and preserve tissue viability.

## Diagnosis

The history and physical examination are the most important parts of the initial evaluation of the acutely ischemic extremity. A history of cardiac disease (arrhythmia, myocardial infarction, valvular heart disease, etc.) favors a diagnosis of embolic occlusion. A history of claudication, rest pain, or ulceration suggests chronic peripheral vascular occlusive disease and favors thrombosis in situ of an underlying atherosclerotic lesion.

Physical examination of both the normal and symptomatic extremity is important because the former provides evidence of the patient's baseline condition. A careful sensorimotor examination is performed. The temperature and color of the skin of both extremities are noted. The presence of gangrene is important. The consistency of the limb musculature to palpation is evaluated. Of course, pulses are examined. The combination of a cardiac history and a normal asymptomatic extremity suggests an embolic occlusion. Conversely, a history of chronic occlusive disease along with an asymptomatic extremity manifesting the signs of chronic lower extremity occlusive disease suggests thrombosis.

Petechial areas of cyanosis or necrosis, cyanotic painful toes, and muscle tenderness and pain suggest microemboli. The rest of the limb may not be ischemic, and pulses may be intact.

The use of the hand-held continuous wave Doppler by an experienced individual may provide additional helpful information. Upper extremities are examined over the axillary, brachial, ulnar, and radial arteries. Lower extremities are examined over the femoral, popliteal, dorsalis pedis, and posterior tibial arteries. Note should be made of the presence or absence of a signal and of the characteristics of that signal (triphasic, biphasic, or monophasic). Complete absence of distal Doppler signals denotes profound ischemia with minimal collateralization. Such patients require urgent revascularization. The presence of distal Doppler signals denotes collateral flow. The better quality the signal, the better the collateral flow present. The Doppler examination supplements but does not supplant the history and physical examination. Management is determined by consideration of all information available.

## Management

Patients with microemboli are anticoagulated for 3 to 5 days if seen acutely (although the benefit of this is not proven). An arteriogram is performed to identify the source of emboli. In the case of lower extremity emboli, an abdominal aortic ultrasound should be obtained to determine the presence of an abdominal aortic aneurysm. If arteriography and aortic ultrasound fail to identify a likely source of microemboli, then echocardiography to evaluate a possible cardiac source is obtained. Recent studies have shown that transesophageal echocardiography (TEE) is more sensitive than transthoracic echocardiography in detecting the presence of intracavitary thrombus and valvular abnormalities. In addition, it has demonstrated a significant incidence of atherosclerotic ulcerated plaque within the aortic arch. We use TEE if other diagnostic modalities have failed to identify a source of the microemboli.

Some success has been reported in the treatment of acute extremity ischemia with thrombolytic agents (streptokinase and urokinase). Urokinase is currently our agent of choice because of its greater predictability and lower complication rate. The agent is infused through an intraarterial catheter placed in the clot. Both high- and low-dose regimens of urokinase have been described. Infusion times vary from as little as 2 to 4 h to as long as 72 h. Obviously, such therapy is contraindicated if the patient has neurologic deficits, internal bleeding, intracranial lesions, or severe ischemia. In general, we feel that surgical therapy is the treatment of choice for an embolic occlusion. Thrombotic occlusion associated with profound ischemia should likewise be treated surgically.

## ARTERIAL TRAUMA

Arterial injuries are due to either blunt or penetrating trauma. Although penetrating trauma is more common, blunt trauma is potentially more dangerous since it is not so obviously associated with vascular injury. Penetrating trauma in the civilian population is most commonly due to stab wounds or gunshot wounds. Blunt trauma is most commonly associated with motor vehicle accidents.

## Pathophysiology

The vessel may be directly injured by the penetrating implement or missile. High-velocity missiles produce widespread soft tissue damage secondary to their concussive effects. Thus, a vessel in proximity to a penetrating injury but not in its direct path may sustain significant injury. Blunt trauma may cause direct injury to the vessel or the vessel may be injured in association with long bone fractures or joint dislocations. Injury in the latter circumstance occurs because of direct vessel injury due to bone fragments or by traction on the vessel.

Arterial injury may be manifest as ischemia, with symptoms and findings similar to that of other acute arterial occlusions. There may be pulsatile bleeding, formation of a hematoma, pseudoaneurysm formation, or the injury may be entirely asymptomatic and inapparent on physical examination. Neurologic signs and symptoms may arise from direct injury to nerve structures accompanying the axial arteries or from nerve compression due to bleeding surrounding an arterial injury.

## Clinical Manifestations

Patients may present with severe ischemia distal to the level of the injury. These patients frequently will complain of ischemic rest pain to varying degrees. Mild ischemia may be asymptomatic. Of course, a pulseless extremity indicates an arterial injury. However, up to 20 percent of operatively proven arterial injuries are associated with normal pulses distal to the injury. A patient may experience parathesia or paralysis due to direct nerve injury, ischemia distal to the injury, or nerve compression due to hematoma within the neural vascular

sheath. Although pallor denotes poor skin perfusion, the causes for this may be multifactorial, and in and of itself pallor does not indicate an arterial injury. Patients with a pulsatile or expanding hematoma, pulsatile bleeding, or bruit near a site of injury are also considered to have an arterial injury.

## Diagnosis

A brief history as to the mechanism of trauma may be helpful in delineating the possibility of arterial trauma in asymptomatic patients. However, physical examination is critical. The patient's pulses are examined and noted. The color of the skin and its temperature is examined. Both sensory and motor neurologic function are assessed and documented. The site of injury in the case of a penetrating injury is identified and its trajectory established, if possible. As with acute arterial occlusion from any cause, continuous wave Doppler examination of the affected extremity may provide helpful ancillary information. Absent Doppler signals distal to the injury denote profound ischemia without significant collateralization. Urgent revascularization is mandated. The presence of a Doppler signal indicates some degree of collateral circulation or flow through the injured area.

## Management

Actively bleeding wounds should be controlled by direct pressure. Direct vessel clamping is not recommended because of the risk of further injury to the vessels and associated neurologic structures. Such patients should be taken as quickly as possible to the operating room, their wound explored directly, and identified injuries repaired. Stable patients with indications of arterial injury as discussed above should undergo biplane arteriography whenever possible. This helps to identify the specific site of injury and plan the repair. However, if this will result in an undue delay in the patient with clear ischemia, then exploration in the operating room is preferred. Emergency arteriography is contraindicated in any unstable patient. All other potentially life-threatening injuries take precedence over peripheral vascular injuries once bleeding has been controlled.

If the trajectory of a penetrating injury is thought to have passed in proximity to a neurovascular bundle, arteriography should be considered. This has been recommended in the absence of any obvious physical signs or sense of arterial injury. The yield of arteriography in such a setting is low (3 to 5 percent). Moreover, the injuries that are identified in the asymptomatic patient tend to be "minor" (e.g., intimal tears, intimal flaps, disruption of small branch vessels). Patients with such injuries have been safely observed, and surgery reserved for those who become symptomatic at a later date. This approach is not yet universally accepted. For low-velocity penetrating injuries near neurovascular structures in asymptomatic patients without physical signs of arterial injury, observation is an option. If this course is elected, outpatient follow-up is needed. Patient education about the signs and symptoms of arterial injury is necessary.

Patients with knee dislocations have a high incidence of accompanying popliteal arterial and venous injuries and arteriography should be performed in these patients.

## SYMPTOMATIC POPLITEAL ANEURYSMS

Any patient with acute ischemia of the lower leg may have a symptomatic popliteal aneurysm. Such aneurysms are among the most common of peripheral arterial aneurysms and present with either thrombosis of the aneurysmal sac or embolization of an intramural thrombus into the distal vasculature. Rupture is uncommon. These aneurysms are generally due to atherosclerosis and are more common in older males; 47 percent are bilateral, and there is a high incidence (78 percent) of associated aortic, iliac, or femoral artery aneurysms.

A popliteal mass (whether pulsatile or not) in the symptomatic leg or a pulsatile mass in the asymptomatic extremity indicates a possible symptomatic aneurysm. An arteriogram is obtained to document the diagnosis and to plan operative treatment.

## THROMBOPHLEBITIS

It is estimated that 500,000 hospital patients in the United States develop deep vein thrombosis each year, with an associated mortality of 50,000 deaths per year from pulmonary thromboembolic events. Acute venous thrombosis may occur after trauma to an extremity with prolonged periods of inactivity (such as may occur with travel) in patients with hypercoagulable states or without apparent predisposing factors. The signs and symptoms of acute venous disease vary and are related to the patient's underlying disease and the location and extent of the thrombosis.

### Pathophysiology

Virchow in 1856 first proposed the triad of conditions associated with venous thrombosis. These are stasis, mechanical injury of the vein wall, and hypercoagulability of the blood. One or more of these factors play a part in all patients with venous thrombosis. There may be a minimal or marked inflammation associated with venous thrombosis. The thrombus usually totally occludes the involved vein segments. However, it may be partially occluding in approximately 19 percent of cases, making diagnosis very difficult. Patients with partial occlusion may be asymptomatic or minimally symptomatic and may present first with a pulmonary embolus.

A postthrombotic syndrome develops in approximately 60 percent of patients with proximal deep vein thrombosis. The long-term sequelae of deep vein thrombosis are due to persistent or partial venous occlusion and damage to the valves, rendering them incompetent.

### Superficial Thrombophlebitis

In the lower extremity superficial thrombophlebitis involves the greater or lesser saphenous veins or varicosities. Redness, tenderness, and induration are present along the course of the involved vein. The differential diagnosis includes cellulitis and lymphangitis. Lymphangitis may be confused with superficial thrombophlebitis of the greater saphenous vein because the major lymphatic drainage of the leg runs along the vein. A simple continuous wave Doppler examination revealing a patent vein allows one to make the diagnosis of lymphangitis.

The diagnosis of superficial thrombophlebitis is confirmed by continuous wave Doppler examination (with a reported 94 percent accuracy rate) or by obtaining a venogram. Rarely is the latter necessary. Demonstration of flow within the examined vein excludes the diagnosis of thrombosis.

Superficial thrombophlebitis of varicosities, the lesser saphenous vein, or the distal greater saphenous vein is treated conservatively with bedrest, elevation, local heat, and analgesics as needed. Nonsteroidal anti-inflammatory drugs are useful for inflammation and pain. Thrombophlebitis of the saphenous vein in the thigh is treated conservatively unless there is some question of involvement of the saphenofemoral junction. A venous duplex examination is then obtained. If the thrombotic process involves the saphenofemoral junction or iliofemoral system, full anticoagulation and treatment as for deep vein thrombosis is indicated.

Several days of bedrest and elevation of the leg provide symptomatic relief. However, the patient should be informed that the symptoms and signs may persist, with slow improvement over a period of 3 to 6 weeks. The patient may be ambulatory during this time unless the process appears to be progressing. Patients with a recurrent episode should be carefully evaluated for an underlying hypercoagulable state or malignancy. Recurrent thrombosis of varicose veins is best treated with excision of the varicosities.

## Acute Deep Vein Thrombosis

### Clinical Features

The signs and symptoms of acute deep vein thrombosis are quite unreliable, and confirmatory testing is necessary. Again, lower extremities are most commonly involved. The classical findings of edema, warmth, erythema, pain, and tenderness are present in 23 to 50 percent of patients. Unfortunately, significant iliofemoral thrombosis can be present with minimal physical findings. Homans' sign is unreliable. The common femoral and popliteal veins are superficially located in the groin and popliteal fossa; tenderness, induration, or erythema in these areas is highly suggestive of acute thrombosis of the underlying vein.

The physical manifestations of acute deep vein thrombosis depend on the extent of thrombosis, whether it is complete or partially occluding, its location, and the extent of collateral or duplicated veins at the level of the occlusion.

### Diagnosis

A previous history of thrombotic disease, recent lower extremity trauma, treatment with estrogen, use of birth control pills, recent surgery (especially urologic, orthopaedic, or gynecologic surgery), advanced age, recent myocardial infarction, congestive heart failure, carcinoma, and obesity are all associated with an increased risk of deep vein thrombosis. Patients presenting with pain and/or edema of the lower extremities and with one or more of these factors should be evaluated by additional testing, even if the physical examination is negative.

A variety of tests are available for the diagnosis of deep vein thrombosis. The venogram remains the accepted "gold standard." This is best performed on a tilt table with the patient in a semierect or near-standing position. This distends and fills the infrapopliteal veins and markedly improves visualization of them, allowing the diagnosis of calf vein and distal popliteal vein thrombosis. Visualization of the iliac veins and inferior vena cava is limited because of dilution of dye by non-contrast-containing blood. Disadvantages of venography include its invasiveness, significant cost, x-ray exposure, and small but finite incidence of complications.

Duplex evaluation of the venous system using real time Doppler ultrasound imaging and simultaneous Doppler flow evaluation combined with color-flow mapping is a highly accurate noninvasive diagnostic modality. It currently is our procedure of choice in the diagnosis of deep vein thrombosis. A large number of series in the literature demonstrate an accuracy rate of 90 to 100 percent, depending on the population examined. Venous duplex examination can differentiate acute from chronic disease and characterize the age of the thrombus. It can assess the competence of the venous valves. Its disadvantages are the need for a skilled technician and an expensive machine to perform the test.

Impedence plethysmography (IPG) is readily and easily performed in the emergency department setting. Accuracies of 94 percent have been reported. It is insensitive to infrapopliteal or partially occluding thrombi. As collaterals develop around the occluded area the test may revert to normal. Accuracy may be decreased in patients with chronic venous disease and venous collaterals, in patients with elevated central venous pressure, in patients with severe peripheral vascular disease, and in patients with mechanical compression or obstruction of the venous system. In one study comparing duplex imaging and IPG, the overall accuracy of duplex imaging was found to be 91 percent versus 57 percent for IPG. Nonetheless, a normal study virtually excludes proximal deep vein thrombosis, and the equipment needed is relatively inexpensive compared with duplex sonography. A number of authors recommend impedence plethysmography as the initial and only diagnostic test used for deep vein thrombosis. In our institution both color-flow duplex imaging of the deep venous system and IPG have been available. Both are performed by experienced technicians. We have found the duplex scan to be more accurate and useful and it has become our diagnostic test of choice.

Continuous wave Doppler examination of the venous system is easily performed in the emergency department. Venous Doppler signals are examined in the groin, popliteal fossa, and posterior tibial veins at the medial malleolus. The presence or absence of flow, the response of flow to respiratory variation and Valsalva maneuver, and the changes in flow with compression of the musculature proximal and distal to the examined point are carefully noted. Absence of flow denotes underlying thrombosis. Absent flow variation with respiration and absent flow augmentation with Valsalva maneuver or distal compression all indicate deep vein thrombosis. The test is examiner-dependent. Overall accuracy rates of approximately 80 percent have been reported with experienced examiners. The examination is portable, inexpensive, and noninvasive. However, because of its lower overall accuracy rate, either venous duplex examination or IPG should be used to diagnose deep vein thrombosis.

## Treatment

Patients who are at high risk for deep vein thrombosis based on history or physical examination should be heparinized immediately pending the results of confirmatory tests. Other patients in whom the diagnosis is suspected undergo diagnostic testing prior to heparinization. The diagnosis is confirmed by the use of the color-flow venous duplex examination (our diagnostic test of choice), IPG, or venography.

Patients are heparinized with an initial intravenous bolus of 5000 units of heparin and placed on a continuous intravenous heparin infusion. Partial thromboplastin times are monitored q 4–6 h until they are therapeutic (1.5 to 2.5 times normal). Thereafter, the partial thromboplastin time is assessed once daily. Platelet counts are obtained daily to screen for heparin-induced thrombocytopenia. Coumadin may be started immediately. Heparin is continued for 4 to 7 days or until the prothrombin time is prolonged to an INR of 2.0 to 3.0. The patient is kept in bed with strict elevation of the legs for the first 3 to 4 days or longer if significant pain, erythema, and swelling persist. Local heat and analgesia are used as needed. Patients with no complications can be discharged after 6 to 7 days of hospitalization. Long-term anticoagulation with oral anticoagulants is continued for 3 to 6 months.

Recent studies have shown that low-molecular-weight heparin is as effective as unfractionated heparin for prophylaxis against deep vein thrombosis and in the treatment of deep vein thrombosis. Low-molecular-weight heparin has a high bioavailability after subcutaneous injection and a longer half-life than unfractionated heparin. Depending on the particular fraction used, it is possible to treat patients with acute deep vein thrombosis with once or twice daily subcutaneous injections of low-molecular-weight heparin. Coagulation parameters are not followed. The incidence of bleeding and other complications appears to be less. The efficacy is equal to and may exceed that of unfractionated heparin.

## Massive Deep-Vein Thrombosis

Phlegmasia alba dolens (milk leg) is caused by extensive iliofemoral thrombosis with swelling of the entire leg to the groin. The leg frequently has a doughy consistency but is not tensely swollen. Arterial inflow is not compromised. The leg is treated as above.

Phlegmasia cerulea dolens is due to extensive iliofemoral thrombosis involving most of the venous collateral circulation as well. The leg is tensely swollen and cyanotic. Skin bullae may be present. Swelling within the muscular compartments of the leg may cause arterial insufficiency. If all venous outflow is occluded, stasis occurs in the capillary and arteriolar beds and retrograde thrombosis of the arterial system will occur. Venous gangrene occurs in this set-ting.

The treatment consists of strict bed rest with maximum elevation of the affected extremity. Anticoagulation with heparin is instituted immediately. Treatment with fibrinolytic therapy should be considered in these patients if no contraindication exists. These patients may have intravascular volume depletion because of fluid sequestration within the affected extremity. Fasciotomy should be performed if indicated. Finally, amputation of gangrenous tissue may be necessary.

## Deep-Vein Thrombosis of the Upper Extremity

This most commonly involves the axillary and subclavian veins and is usually iatrogenic following catheterization. Effort thrombosis of the axillary or subclavian vein is seen in young persons following strenuous activity and may be more common in people who have some narrowing of the thoracic outlet.

The patient with axillary or subclavian vein thrombosis usually presents with mild swelling involving the forearm or occasionally the entire extremity. Edema is pitting and not tense. The color of the extremity is normal. Arterial flow is well preserved, and pulses are present.

The risk of pulmonary embolism in this setting is between 12 and 15 percent. Accordingly, the patient should be treated with elevation of the extremity, application of local heat, analgesia as needed, and anticoagulation, if not contraindicated by the patient's overall condition. Postphlebitic sequelae are common in these patients.

Patients with effort thrombosis of the axillary or the subclavian vein should be treated with direct catheter infusion of a thrombolytic agent into the thrombus. Following lysis of the thrombus a venogram is performed. Extrinsic compression of the vein should be surgically corrected (first rib resection, resection of a cervical rib, etc). Stenoses of the subclavian vein have been treated with balloon angioplasty.

## Thrombolytic Therapy

Thrombolytic therapy can be used to treat patients with acute deep venous thrombosis. Streptokinase combines with plasminogen to form a plasminogen-streptokinase activator complex. This, in turn, can combine with a plasminogen-fibrin complex in the thrombus to cause lysis. The activator complex may also combine with circulating plasminogen, forming plasmin and causing fibrinolysis. Urokinase, which is derived from human embryonic kidney cells, is a direct plasminogen activator. It is not antigenic and has a low pyrogenicity.

This is a useful treatment in experienced hands for appropriately selected patients. It should be considered in patients with proven venous thrombosis of the iliofemoral or above-knee venous segments of less than 4 days' duration. Some consider this the treatment of choice for phlegmasia cerulea dolens. There are a number of contraindications to its use. Patients with a history of peptic ulcer disease, severe hypertension, recent stroke, liver disease, blood dyscrasia, recent surgery, recent arterial punctures, or intracranial neoplasms are not candidates for this treatment. In addition, the efficacy of this treatment method in lowering the incidence of postphlebitic sequelae is controversial. It does result in a higher incidence of bleeding complications than standard heparin therapy.

## BIBLIOGRAPHY

Hull RD, Raskob GE, Hirsh J: Comparative value of tests for the diagnosis of venous thrombosis, in Bernstein EF (ed): *Vascular Diagnosis*. St. Louis, Mosby, 1993, p 785.

Hull RD, Raskob GE, Pineo GF, et al: Subcutaneous low molecular weight compared with continuous infusion intravenous heparin in the treatment of proximal vein thrombosis. *N Engl J Med* 328:975, 1992.

Mills JL, Porter JM: Basic data related to clinical decision making in acute limb ischemia. *Ann Vasc Surg* 5:98, 1991.

Perry MO: Vascular trauma, in Moore WS (ed): *Vascular Surgery, A Comprehensive Review*. Philadelphia, Saunders, 1991, p 500.

Quinones-Baldrich WJ: Thrombolytic therapy for vascular disease, in Moore WS (ed): *Vascular Surgery, A Comprehensive Review.* Philadelphia, Saunders, 1991, p 237.

Quinones-Baldrich WJ, Saleh S: Acute arterial occlusion, in Moore WS (ed): *Vascular Diagnosis, A Comprehensive Review.* Philadelphia, Saunders, 1991, p 578.

Strandness ED Jr: The clinical spectrum of venous disease, in Bernstein EF (ed): *Vascular Diagnosis.* St. Louis, Mosby, 1993, p 772.

# 62

# CARDIOVASCULAR PHYSIOLOGY OF AGING

## Michael Maddens

## INTRODUCTION

Because of the marked reduction in childhood and early adult mortality over the past 100 years in the United States, there has been a rapid increase in the elderly population. Between 1900 and 1990 life expectancy from birth increased 28 years. However, over the same period life expectancy in persons reaching the age of 65 increased by only 6 years. The growth in the elderly population has had a major impact on the economics of health care in this country. People over 65 years of age make up less than 15 percent of the general population in the United States, yet consume 25 percent of all prescription drugs and account for nearly 50 percent of all hospital days and one-third of all health care expenditures. The elderly account for 22 to 25 percent of emergency medical services runs and a comparable number of urgent emergency department visits. After age 75, the ratio of urgent emergency department visits is 36.6 per 100 persons per year, nearly double the rate of any other adult age group.

The prevalence of cardiovascular disease increases so much with advancing age that it may be the norm rather than the exception. However, in order to make accurate assessments and optimize therapy for elderly patients, it is important to distinguish between the

**Table 62-1.** Morphologic Changes Associated with Normal Aging

Histologic changes
  Myocardium
    Lipofuscin accumulation
    Amyloid deposition
    Increases in cell size
    Decrease in number of pacemaker cells
  Blood vessels
    Intimal cells become heterogeneous in size and spatial orientation
    Medial thickening and calcification
Macroscopic changes
  Heart
    No change in chamber size
    Slight increase in left ventricular wall thickness
    Decreased number of conducting fascicles between the main bundle and the left bundle
    Thickening of the atrial surface and atrioventricular valves
  Blood vessels
    Increased diameter and thickness of the aorta
    Increased tortuosity

SOURCE: Wei: JY, Gersh BJ: Heart disease in the elderly. *Curr Probl Cardiol* 12(1):1, 1987.

**Table 62-2.** Physiologic Changes in Cardiac Function with Normal Aging

Diminished early (passive) left ventricular filling with increased dependence on the "atrial kick" to fill the ventricle (considered secondary to an age-related decrease in left ventricular compliance)
Preserved contractility of the left ventricle
No change in resting cardiac output
Increase in end diastolic volume
Operating further up the Frank-Starling curve
Relatively greater dependence on increases in end diastolic volume relative to increases in heart rate to increase cardiac output during exercise
Decreased inotropic and chronotropic responses to catecholamines
Increase in peripheral vascular resistance
No change in ejection fraction index

physiologic changes of normal aging and the pathophysiologic changes of common diseases in the elderly. The morphologic changes of the cardiovascular system that occur as a result of normal aging have been reviewed and are presented in Table 62-1. A slight increase in the cardiothoracic ratio on chest radiographs has also been demonstrated. However, in the absence of major chest deformities it does not exceed 0.51, thus maintaining the specificity of a cardiothoracic ratio of > 50 percent for detecting cardiac pathology. Age-related physiologic changes can be divided into changes in cardiac function (summarized in Table 62-2), changes in blood vessel function, and changes in baroreceptor and endocrine homeostatic mechanisms. Particular note should be made of the increased dependence on the "atrial kick" to complete ventricular diastolic filling. This causes elderly patients to be more prone to congestive heart failure in the setting of atrial fibrillation or supraventricular tachycardia.

Changes in blood vessel function include decreased β-adrenergic–mediated vasodilatation and impaired $\alpha_1$-adrenergic responsiveness. Animal and human data suggest that although vascular smooth-muscle relaxation in response to nitrovasodilators remains intact, age-related alteration in endothelial-cell modulation of this response leads to decreased relaxation. The previously noted morphologic changes of the blood vessels are associated with increased peripheral vascular resistance and impedance, both of which contribute to an increased left ventricular workload. The nonpulsatile component of the left ventricular load, peripheral resistance, increases by 37 percent from the second to the sixth decade, while the pulsatile component, characteristic impedance (an index of aortic elasticity), increases by 137 percent over the same time span.

A wide variety of baroreceptor- and endocrine-mediated homeostatic responses have been shown to decline with advancing age. These are summarized in Table 62-3. Of particular clinical relevance is the smaller increase in heart rate with standing or tilting in the elderly. In one study it was reported that the heart rate of young patients increased by 15 beats per minute after 3 min of 60-degree head-up tilt while that of older patients (average age, 75) increased by only 6 beats per minute. Neither group experienced significant changes in blood pressure. In the face of a modest diuretic-induced sodium depletion young patients increased their heart rates even more and were able to maintain blood pressure. In contrast, elderly patients were unable to mount further heart rate increases despite significant drops in blood pressure. Thus the sensitivity of a 20-beat-per-minute heart rate

**Table 62-3.** Age-Related Changes in Baroceptor- and Endocrine-Mediated Blood Pressure Homeostatic Mechanisms

Decreased chronotropic response to standing, tilt, cough, Valsalva
Decreased carotid baroreceptor response
Little or no change in cardiopulmonary baroreceptor responses
Decreased aldosterone and renin responses to hypovolemia
Decreased antidiuretic hormone response to hypovolemia
Decreased thirst after water deprivation
Impaired natriuretic capability

increase as a clinical indicator of volume depletion declines with advancing age. The specificity of a 20-mmHg drop in blood pressure as an indicator of volume depletion also declines, partially because of the physiologic alteration in the baroreceptors but to a greater extent because of the high prevalence of other conditions which produce orthostatic hypotension (drugs, varicose veins, Parkinson disease, diabetes mellitus, and vitamin deficiency). Nonetheless, a 20-mmHg drop in systolic blood pressure within 3 min of standing has been shown to be a significant risk factor for falls and syncope.

## CARDIOVASCULAR DISEASES

### Hypertension

Hypertension is the most common cardiovascular disease in the elderly, affecting up to 50 percent of people over the age of 70. The Joint National Committee (JNC) on Detection, Evaluation and Treatment of High Blood Pressure recently redefined this condition as a systolic blood pressure greater than 139 mmHg and/or a diastolic blood pressure greater than 89 mmHg. Isolated elevation of systolic blood pressure accounts for up to half of the cases of hypertension in the elderly; it is especially prominent in the African-American population and in females. Not only does the prevalence of hypertension increase with age, but the Framingham Study has shown that the importance of a systolic blood pressure elevation also increases with age, producing a morbidity 2 to 5 times higher than that observed in the nonhypertensive elderly and a mortality 30 to 100 percent higher. Additionally, isolated systolic hypertension in this population is associated with a high incidence of carotid bruits (20 to 40 percent) and lower-extremity peripheral arterial disease. Despite its proven morbidity, studies suggest that 40 to 70 percent of elderly patients with isolated systolic hypertension are either unaware of it or not taking medication for it. Given the increased variability of blood pressure readings in the elderly and the stress of the usual emergency department visit, it is important to remember that the JNC guidelines call for multiple measurements in the seated position, with a cuff of appropriate size, after at least 5 min of quiet rest, confirmed on at least two subsequent visits, before diagnosing hypertension. Standing blood pressure should also be measured because of the high prevalence of orthostatic hypotension among the elderly. Patient evaluation should seek to exclude the relatively rare secondary causes of elevated blood pressure, such as hyperthyroidism, severe bradycardia, Paget disease, and aortic regurgitation. Evidence of end-organ damage such as retinopathy, papilledema, peripheral vascular disease, aortic aneurysms, carotid bruits, congestive heart failure, or sequelae of stroke should be documented. In the absence of such evidence and the absence of other risk factors, such as diabetes or smoking, the Canada Consensus Conference on Hypertension proposes treatment of isolated systolic hypertension only for systolic pressures greater than 200 mmHg (SBP > 200 mmHg). When target-organ damage or associated medical conditions are present, they recommend treating SBP > 180 mmHg. They suggest no treatment for SBP < 160 mmHg and the physician's discretion for SBP between 160 and 179 mmHg. The JNC V recommends treatment of isolated systolic hypertension when systolic blood pressure exceeds 159 mmHg. In any case, in the absence of acute end-organ damage (papilledema, angina, congestive heart failure) or aneurysm, there is rarely any need for immediate reductions in blood pressure. Given the previously noted baroreceptor impairments and the high prevalence of orthostatic hypotension, most elderly hypertensive patients are best served by referral to a primary care physician rather than by institution of antihypertensive therapy in the emergency department. When urgent therapy is indicated, the choice of agent is dictated by the concomitant illnesses and the side-effect profile most likely to be tolerated. It should be noted that while all classes of antihypertensive medications have been shown to be effective in lowering blood pressure in older patients, only thiazide diuretics (alone or in combination with β blockers or methyldopa) have

been used in controlled trials that have demonstrated a reduction in cardiovascular morbidity and mortality.

### Coronary Artery Disease

Coronary atherosclerotic heart disease is the most common cause of death in persons over 65 years, and the elderly account for over 50 percent of admissions to the hospital for acute myocardial infarction. Despite the high prevalence of coronary disease, only about 10 percent of the elderly population have angina pectoris. Evidence from the Honolulu Heart Study shows no difference between the elderly population and the general population in the percentage (approximately 33 percent) of clinically unrecognized myocardial infarctions ascertained by ECG changes at repeated examinations. However, with advancing age the presenting symptoms of a myocardial infarction tend to change. Beyond the age of 80, fewer than 50 percent experience chest pain, and fewer than 20 percent experience diaphoresis. Syncope, acute confusion, and stroke become increasingly more common presenting symptoms of myocardial infarction in the elderly, while the prevalence of weakness, giddiness, and vomiting are unchanged. Among elderly patients whose heart attack includes syncope as a presenting symptom, fewer than one-third have associated chest pain, but the prevalence of truly silent infarctions probably does not increase dramatically.

Risk factors for myocardial infarction and coronary heart disease mortality are similar to those seen in younger adults, though their relative importance changes. With advancing age the relative risk of hypertension increases dramatically. The relative risk of elevated total cholesterol levels declines dramatically, but high-density lipoprotein (HDL) remains significantly inversely related to coronary mortality. Smoking remains a significant risk factor in the elderly, and is associated with a 50 percent increase in coronary mortality. Diabetes mellitus remains an extremely potent risk factor, especially in older women. Electrocardiographic abnormalities associated with left ventricular hypertrophy and nonspecific ST-T changes both confer added risk for coronary artery disease. Obesity remains a powerful risk factor in elderly men and to a much smaller degree in elderly women. Physical activity, even at modest levels, has been shown to reduce mortality (both cardiac-specific and total mortality) in the elderly. Left ventricular hypertrophy is also an independent risk factor in the elderly, conferring a 1.6- to 1.67-fold increased risk for every 50 g/m increase in the left ventricular mass to height index. Use of estrogens is associated with a significant reduction in coronary mortality rates in elderly women, and there is some evidence that aspirin may reduce the risk of myocardial infarction in elderly men.

Treatment of unstable angina or acute infarction is similar to treatment in younger patients, with a few caveats. Infarctions associated with elevated CK-MB isoenzymes but a normal total CK level occur twice as often in the elderly as in younger patients. The elderly also have a higher frequency of complications, including arrhythmias, heart failure, and cardiac rupture. Most studies have shown that age itself is an independent risk factor for mortality in patients with myocardial infarction, even after controlling for other prognostic variables. Although increasing age is associated with higher complication rates from most invasive treatments for myocardial infarction, surgical repair of remediable postinfarction cardiogenic shock should not be excluded on the basis of age alone. Pooled results from major thrombolytic trials have shown a significant benefit from thrombolytic therapy; and although a decision analysis found it cost-effective, fewer than 20 percent of elderly myocardial infarction patients meet current eligibility criteria to receive it. Additionally, primary angioplasty has been reported as an effective treatment in patients over age 75. Nitrates and sodium nitroprusside must be used with additional caution in the elderly due to the age-related impairments in baroreceptor responses. It is prudent to start with an infusion rate of 5 μg/min and increase the rate by 5 μg/min every 5 min in elderly patients requiring intravenous nitroglycerin. Beta-blocker therapy in the acute phase of infarction can be undertaken cautiously, but it should be recalled that elderly patients may have a higher incidence of CNS side effects and are more likely to have contraindications to β blockade than younger patients. Lidocaine prophylaxis has recently been called into question both for prehospital and in-hospital use. Lidocaine toxicity is twice as common in patients over 70 years as it is in patients under 50. This may be due to an increased drug sensitivity as well as to the twofold increase in lidocaine half-life observed in the elderly. It has been suggested that reducing the loading dose by one-third to one-half and keeping the maintenance dose under 25 µg/kg per min is a way of avoiding toxicity.

Elderly postmyocardial infarction patients demonstrated reductions in subsequent mortality when treated with metoprolol, propanalol, or timolol, without a significant increase in side effects. The value of aspirin for secondary prevention of coronary events remains unproven. Elderly patients have up to a fourfold increase in 1-year mortality compared to younger adults, and those with non-Q-wave infarctions have been reported to have a 12 percent annual mortality rate from the third year on.

Treatment of chronic coronary artery disease is also similar to treatment in younger patients. Indications for surgical therapy remain essentially the same, but the prevalence of contraindications increases. Perioperative mortality increases progressively with advancing age (age 65: 1.9 percent; age 65 to 69: 4.6 percent; age 70 to 74: 6.6 percent; and age 75 and over: 9.5 percent). However, in elderly patients surviving surgery, 5-year survival is 87 percent (77 percent in those 75 and older), and recurrence of angina is less common than in younger patients. Survival results after angioplasty are equally favorable.

## SYNCOPE

Syncope is defined as a sudden, transient loss of consciousness characterized by unresponsiveness and loss of postural tone; recovery is spontaneous, not requiring resuscitative procedures. Among the very elderly, the 10-year prevalence of syncope is 23 percent. The yearly incidence is 6 percent, with 30 percent of patients experiencing recurrences and up to 6 percent experiencing seven or more episodes during a 2-year follow-up. Among late middle–aged adults with syncope, subsequent mortality may depend on the etiology of the episode (for example, higher mortality in cases where a cardiovascular cause is identified). However, among the elderly, no significant differences in 2-year mortality rates exist between those with cardiovascular, noncardiovascular, and unknown causes. Syncope in the elderly is associated with functional decline, as well as a substantial morbidity rate (37 percent). Morbidity includes a 10 percent incidence of major complications such as fractures, subdural hematomas, or injuries resulting from car accidents, and the iatrogenic morbidity resulting from hospitalization and diagnostic evaluation.

Any factor or combination of factors which results in a transient insufficiency in oxygen or nutrient delivery to the brain can produce syncope. Since oxygen transport capacity is directly proportional to hemoglobin content, even modest degrees of anemia may be a major contributory factor in elderly patients who have age-related physiologic declines in baroreceptor and endocrine homeostatic responses. Likewise, modest reductions in cardiac output secondary to congestive heart failure, volume depletion, or drug-induced orthostatic hypotension may also contribute. Finally, postprandial drops in blood pressure are common among the elderly and may contribute to the incidence of syncope.

Carotid sinus hypersensitivity is frequently overlooked as a cause of syncope in the elderly and should be sought by means of carotid massage during ECG monitoring. Ventricular asystole greater than 2.5 to 3 s constitutes a positive cardioinhibitory response. A systolic blood pressure decline of more than 40 to 50 mmHg or a systolic blood pressure drop below 90 mmHg is considered a positive vasode-

pressor response. While the magnitude of the physiologic vasodepressor response to carotid stimulation increases with advancing age in healthy subjects, the prevalence of frank carotid hypersensitivity is not increased in the elderly. Cardioinhibitory response is the most common (51 to 84 percent), followed by mixed response (11 to 33 percent), with pure vasodepressor response being the least common (5 to 12 percent). However a recent study demonstrated an important vasodepressar component in all 3 groups. Digitalis, propanalol, and α-methyldopa have all been reported to be associated with carotid sinus hypersensitivity. Patients with a known history of stroke or intracranial arterial disease, or who present with carotid bruits on physical examination, should be excluded.

Vasovagal syncope accounts for only 1 to 5 percent of syncopal episodes in the elderly. In most cases it probably results from initial sympathetic overstimulation of ventricular sensory receptors, resulting in a dramatic reflex reduction in peripheral vascular tone and increased parasympathetic tone, which causes bradycardia and decreased mesenteric vascular resistance.

## Evaluation and Treatment

### History and Physical Examination

Twenty-five percent of elderly syncope patients can be diagnosed by history and physical examination alone, accounting for nearly half of all cases where a cause is eventually established. History taking in the elderly patient with syncope should first establish the cognitive ability of the patient, with corroboration by family or friends whenever possible. Next, explicit details regarding the circumstances preceding the syncopal episode should be determined. These include the time of the last meal; postural changes before the episode; sensation of pain, nausea, or strong emotions before the episode; or an urge to void or defecate. Any correlation with activities that may precipitate syncope, such as exercise, coughing, swallowing, voiding, or defecating, should be sought. Simple activities such as shaving or turning the head may occasionally precipitate syncope in patients with carotid sinus hypersensitivity. A list of the patient's medications and the time of the last few doses should be noted.

The patient's description of sensations immediately preceding or during the episode, as well as eye-witness accounts, should be obtained if possible. The presence of nausea and vague abdominal distress accompanied by a flushed sensation suggests the presence of vasovagal syncope. The feeling of a prodrome or aura suggests the presence of epilepsy.

Clonic jerks may occur in the presence of cerebral hypoperfusion and do not necessarily indicate the presence of a seizure. The presence of urinary incontinence, a prolonged recovery period, or Todd's paralysis suggest the diagnosis of a seizure. Rapid onset, especially in the seated or supine position, suggests the presence of arrhythmia. A jugular venous pulse rate greater than the peripheral pulse rate, or a pulse of 20 to 40 beats per minute that is unaffected by atropine, are both suggestive of a Stokes-Adams attack. Careful note should be made of the patient's rhythm, blood pressure (including response to orthostatic stress and any concomitant symptoms), and respiratory rate. Detection of a prolonged, harsh, loud (IV, V, or VI) systolic murmur associated with a diminished second heart sound is strong evidence for significant aortic stenosis. However, many elderly patients with significant lesions have atypical murmurs and may have fairly well-preserved carotid upstrokes secondary to diminished arterial compliance. By age 50, 50 percent of people have audible ejection murmurs; by age 90, 70 percent. Due to the high prevalence of aortic ejection murmurs from hemodynamically insignificant aortic sclerosis, an echocardiogram is often required to ascertain with certainty whether sclerosis or stenosis is the cause of the murmur. The extremities should be examined for pallor, distal perfusion, clubbing, or cyanosis. After a careful neurologic examination and auscultation of the neck to determine that there are no bruits, patients without a previous history or evidence of cerebrovascular disease should have carotid sinus massage performed.

## Laboratory Evaluation

Due to the high prevalence of disease and the nonspecific presentation of many diseases in the elderly, a number of screening tests are usually performed. These include a complete blood count, creatinine and blood urea nitrogen, and a blood glucose. Some authors have questioned the diagnostic value of such tests for syncope, stating that positive findings relevant to syncope are found in fewer than 4 percent of patients.

Creatine kinase levels may be helpful in diagnosing myocardial infarction. However, 10 percent of elderly patients with syncope but without myocardial infarction and 10 percent of age-matched controls also have mildly elevated isoenzymes. The survival rate for patients with syncope and mildly elevated isoenzymes who have no other evidence of myocardial infarction is no different from the survival rate for those with syncope and normal isoenzyme levels.

An ECG should be obtained as the first laboratory test in ruling out myocardial infarction or significant arrhythmia. In over 30 percent of elderly patients with syncope caused by arrhythmia, the arrhythmia can be diagnosed on the admission ECG. Although there is a significantly increased risk of sudden death associated with frequent or complex premature ventricular complexes (PVCs), the relative risk is lower in men older than 49 compared to those 49 and younger.

Despite the relative frequency of EEG abnormalities, several series have reported the yield of new seizure diagnoses as a result of routine electroencephalography to be from 0 to 1.5 percent. Similarly, CT scanning of the brain in the absence of focal neurologic signs is generally not contributory.

Echocardiography can distinguish hemodynamically significant aortic stenosis from the more common systolic murmur produced by hemodynamically insignificant aortic sclerosis. Additionally, the echocardiogram may diagnose hypertrophic obstructive cardiomyopathy, a condition which is often missed on clinical evaluation in the elderly, even when moderate to severe.

## Ambulatory Electrocardiographic Monitoring

In elderly syncope patients, electrocardiographic monitoring for at least 24 h is the single most useful study after the history and physical examination, establishing a diagnosis in over 25 percent of patients in whom an etiology is eventually determined. Monitoring for an additional 24 to 48 h increases the yield by 60 to 80 percent, with age over 65 years, history of heart disease, male gender, and initial nonsinus rhythm all increasing the likelihood of identifying a major rhythm abnormality. However, a number of authors have reported low rates of temporal association (8 percent) of arrhythmias with symptoms of syncope or presyncope as documented by ambulatory monitoring. In one study of 1512 adult (not exclusively elderly) patients with syncope, 15 patients (1 percent) experienced syncope during ambulatory monitoring, and 241 experienced presyncope. Among those with syncope, only half the episodes were related to an arrhythmia (most commonly ventricular tachycardia); among those with presyncope, only 10 percent were related to an arrhythmia. In total, only 2 percent of studies led to a definitive diagnosis of arrhythmia. In another study although 42 percent of patients monitored for symptoms of syncope or dizziness had symptoms during monitoring, only 23 out of 41 symptomatic patients had major arrhythmia, and in only three of these cases was the arrhythmia temporally related to the symptoms reported. There was no significant difference in the incidence or type of arrhythmia between symptomatic and asymptomatic patients. Similarly, another group reported low rates of symptoms during monitoring. Fifteen percent of their subjects experienced symptoms, with 50 percent demonstrating a simultaneous causative arrhythmia. They also found a sizable number of "significant arrhythmias" among the asymptomatic group.

The significance of asymptomatic arrhythmias remains a subject of much debate. In Kapoor's study of prolonged ECG monitoring in syncope patients, mean age 56.6 ± 19.5 years, 25 percent of patients reported symptoms with corresponding arrhythmias. However, they found that frequent PVCs (more than nine per hour), or repetitive PVCs, and sinus pauses of greater than 2 s were both independent predictors of mortality. Likewise, Abdon et al. reported that 15 of 21 patients with a significant arrhythmia during an asymptomatic 24-h recording later had the same arrhythmia during symptoms. However, the likelihood of most arrhythmias increases with advancing age, increasing the chances of finding a coincidental arrhythmia with ambulatory monitoring. In a study of 13 asymptomatic active individuals 67 to 84 years old, all had at least some supraventricular and some ventricular arrhythmia; five demonstrated complex ventricular arrhythmia; and seven had complex atrial arrhythmia. In another study, major arrhythmias occurred in 13 percent of active asymptomatic elderly subjects. In a group of healthy people 60 to 85 years old screened with maximal treadmill exercise testing, 80 percent had ventricular arrhythmia, 35 percent had multiform PVCs, 11 percent had couplets, and 4 percent had ventricular tachycardia. Although 88 percent had supraventricular arrhythmia and 13 percent had paroxysmal atrial tachycardia, marked sinus bradycardia (less than 40 beats per minute) and prolonged sinus pauses (longer than 1.5 s) were each present in only 2 percent.

## Transtelephonic Monitoring

A continuous-loop ECG recorder may be a useful alternative to traditional ambulatory monitoring. The device continually records and erases cardiac rhythm. Activation of the "record" button stores in memory the preceding 64 s and the ensuing 32 s. The preserved rhythm can then be transmitted over the telephone. In this manner, patients can record rhythms accompanying their symptoms. One month of continual use is reported to cost the same as one 24-h Holter recording.

## Signal-Averaged Electrocardiography

A newer noninvasive electrocardiographic technique available to evaluate patients with syncope is signal-averaged ECG. This technique uses high-gain amplification and passband filtering of the surface ECG. Late potentials (low-amplitude potentials at the terminal portion of the QRS complex) are correlated with the likelihood of sustaining ventricular tachyarrhythmia. In one study it was found that late potentials were present in 11 of 13 patients (85 percent) with ventricular tachycardia and absent in 94 percent of patients with other causes for their syncope. In patients with recurrent syncope, late potentials had a 73 percent sensitivity and 89 percent specificity, but only a 55 percent positive predictive value for serious ventricular arrhythmia as a cause of syncope. Another study reported an 89 percent sensitivity and 100 percent specificity in predicting inducible ventricular tachycardia on electrophysiologic studies in patients with unexplained syncope. Another team reported that an abnormally low root mean square of the terminal 40 ms had an 82 percent sensitivity and a 91 percent specificity in distinguishing individuals with syncope of unknown origin who had inducible ventricular tachycardia. In a study limited to elderly syncope patients, Dabrowski et al. reported a 63 to 82 percent sensitivity and a 41 to 73 percent specificity in syncope patients with a prior myocardial infarction. In patients with no prior infarction, specificity was 60 to 80 percent, and no patient (regardless of signal-averaged ECG result) had inducible sustained monomorphic ventricular tachycardia.

## Head-Up Tilt Test

The head-up tilt test may be useful in the evaluation of syncope of unknown origin. In elderly patients with otherwise unexplained syncope, 30 to 90% will develop syncope during tilt testing, suggesting neurocardiogenic (vasovagal) syncope as the etiology. The addition of Isuprel infusions to the tilt protocol may increase the sensitivity (but less so than in younger patients) at the expense of decreased specificity and higher complication rates. Nonpharmacologically augmented tilting has been reported to produce syncope in 7% (0–100%) of elderly controls. Increased duration of tilt and the presence of an IV catheter seem to be associated with decreased specificity. In the author's experience, tilt test evaluation may be invaluable in appropriately selected individuals.

## VALVULAR HEART DISEASE

Significant aortic stenosis (AS) may be present in elderly patients in the absence of the classic *pulsus parvus et tardus* because of the increased transmission of the pulse secondary to decreased elasticity. The cause of AS in older patients is usually degenerative rather than congenital or rheumatic, as in younger patients. The male predominance seen in younger patients disappears, and the ejection click is usually absent. Severe symptomatic AS is associated with a 40 to 70 percent reduction in life expectancy among the elderly, with a 3-year survival of about 25 percent. Valve replacement is associated with a 16 percent operative mortality, but survivors usually achieve functional improvement and improved subsequent survival. Balloon angioplasty has also shown promise as a palliative treatment for elderly patients with AS. However, although symptoms improve in the majority of patients, restenosis is common.

Mitral annular calcification is almost exclusively a disease of the elderly. Over 30 percent of women and 12 percent of men over the age of 70 are affected. Fifty to seventy-five percent of patients have a systolic murmur which is usually holosystolic, crescendo-decrescendo, and radiates to the axilla, and thus can be confused with either aortic stenosis or mitral regurgitation. Although conduction abnormalities are often present, only right bundle branch block is more common than in age-matched controls. Although mitral annular calcification is associated with a higher incidence of cerebral embolic events and infective endocarditis, preventive treatment for either remains controversial.

## CONGESTIVE HEART FAILURE

Congestive heart failure increases exponentially with advancing age after the fifth decade. Special note should be made of the high prevalence of impaired diastolic function in the elderly, since 50 to 60 percent of old persons with congestive heart failure have normal or only slightly reduced ejection fractions. Treatment in these cases should be directed at improving diastolic relaxation (for example, with calcium channel blockers) rather than augmenting contractility or decreasing afterload, which may aggravate the condition.

For elderly patients with impaired systolic function (diminished ejection fraction), digoxin may improve the ejection fraction even in patients who are in sinus rhythm; however, maximum improvement is frequently seen with serum levels of 0.4 to 1.0 µg/mL. Given the increased prevalence of digoxin toxicity in the elderly, close monitoring of levels is indicated, and physicians should have a high index of suspicion for toxicity when patients on digoxin present with nonspecific complaints. Diuretics remain an integral part of treatment of congestive heart failure even at advanced age, though age- and disease-related declines in renal function may attenuate their efficacy. Most studies of angiotensin-converting enzyme inhibitors excluded persons over the age of 75. However, more than half of the patients in the CONSENSUS (Cooperative North Scandinavian Enalapril Survival Study) Trial, which showed a 40 percent reduction in mortality, were age 70 or older.

## DRUG THERAPY

A final note of caution regarding treatment of elderly individuals is warranted. The emergency physician must keep in mind that many drugs in the usual arsenal have longer half-lives or more pronounced effects in elderly patients. As a group, the elderly have decreased renal function and are less able to metabolize drugs that require hepatic oxidation or deamination. However, although mean responses change with age, the variability of responses also increases. Thus one 80-year-old may require a fraction of the usual adult dose while another requires a full dose. Where there is uncertainty, it is usually safest to start with small doses and titrate up to the desired effect or level.

## BIBLIOGRAPHY

Abdon NJ, Johansson BW, Lessem J: Predictive use of routine 24 hour electrocardiography in suspected Adams-Stokes syndrome. Comparison with cardiac rhythm during symptoms. *Br Heart J* 47:553, 1987.

Bass EB, Curtiss EI, Arena VE, et al: The duration of holter monitoring in patients with syncope. *Arch Intern Med* 150:1073, 1990.

Bayer AJ, Chadha JS, Faray RR, et al: Changing presentation of myocardial infarction with increasing old age. *J Am Geriatr Soc* 34:263, 1986.

Dabrowski A, Kubik L. Krupeinicz A, et al: Utility of signal-averaged electrocardiogram in selecting elderly patients with unexplained syncope for programmed ventricular stimulation *Cardiol Elderly* 1:311, 1993.

Fleg JL: Alterations in cardiovascular structure and function with advancing age. *Am J Cardiol* 57:33C, 1988.

Gang ES et al: Detection of late potentials on the surface electrocardiogram in unexplained syncope. *Am J Cardiol* 58:1014, 1986.

Gaggioli G, Brignole M, Menozzi C, et al: Reappraisal of the vasodepressar reflex in carotid sinus syndrome, *Am J Cardiol* 75:518, 1995.

Hackel A et al: Cardioversion and catecholamine responses to head-up tilt in the diagnosis of recurrent unexplained syncope in elderly patients. *J Am Geriatr Soc* 39:663, 1991.

Joint National Committee on Detection, Evaluation, and Treatment of High Blood Pressure: The Fifth Report of the Joint National Committee on Detection, Evaluation, and Treatment of High Blood Pressure (JNC V). *Arch Intern Med* 153:154, 1993.

Kapoor WN, et al: Syncope in the elderly. *Am J Med* 80:419, 1986.

Kapoor WN et al: Prolonged electrocardiographic monitoring in patients with syncope. Importance of frequent or repetitive ventricular ectopy. *Am J Med* 82:20. 1987.

Krumholz HM, Friesinger GC, Cook EF, et al: Relationship of age with eligibility for thrombolytic therapy and mortality among patients with suspected myocardial infarction. *J Am Geriatr Soc* 42:127, 1994.

Lew AS, Hod H, Cercek B, et al: Mortality and morbidity rates of patients older and younger than 75 years with acute myocardial infarction treated with intravenous streptokinase. *Am J Cardiol* 59:1, 1987.

Lipsitz LA: Orthostatic hypotension in the elderly. *N Engl J Med* 321:952, 1989.

Maddens ME: Isolated systolic hypertension: The rationale for treating elderly patients. *Consultant* 29:125, 1989.

Maddens ME, Lipsitz LA, We JY, et al: Impaired heart rate responses to cough and deep breathing in elderly patients with unexplained syncope. *Am J Cardiol* 60:1368, 1987.

McCaig LF: National Hospital Ambulatory Medical Care Survey: 1992. Emergency Department Summary. *Advance Data* Number 245, March 2, 1994.

McDonald A, Davidson IM, MacDonald E, et al: The effect of age on responses of human mesenteric artery rings to isosorbide dinitrate, nifedipine, and sodium nitroprusside. *Cardiology in the Elderly* 1:447, 1993.

Paciaroni E, Raffaeli S, Sirolla C, et al: Is age a predictor of mortality in patients with acute myocardial infarction? *Cardiol Elderly* 2:15, 1994.

Rich MW, Bosner MS, Chung MK, et al: Is age an independent predictor of early and late mortality in patients with acute myocardial infarction? *Am J Med* 92:F, 1992.

Rich MW: Congestive heart failure in the elderly. *Cardiology in the Elderly* 1:372, 1993.

Roelandt JRTC, Meeter K: Diagnosis and management of valvular heart disease in the elderly. *Cardiol Elderly* 1:235, 1993.

Wentink JRM, Jansen RWMM, Hoefnagels WHL: The influence of age on the response of blood pressure and heart rate to carotid sinus massage in healthy elderly volunteers. *Cardiol Elderly* 1:453, 1993.

# 63

# CARDIAC TRANSPLANTATION

## Michael R. Mill

## INTRODUCTION

Cardiac transplantation is now an established and widely practiced therapeutic procedure for patients with end-stage heart failure. The first clinically successful cardiac transplant was performed in December, 1967. Since then, advances in the immunosuppression and postoperative care of these patients have resulted in dramatically improved patient survival. This has been accompanied by a tremendous growth in the number of procedures performed. Data from the Registry of the International Society of Heart and Lung Transplantation (ISHLT) and the United Network for Organ Sharing (UNOS) reveals that 26,704 heart transplants were performed at 251 centers throughout the world between January 1, 1983, and December 31, 1993. This total includes more than 2000 heart transplants per year in the United States since 1990. The actuarial survival after transplantation reported by the Registry is 80 percent at one year, with 5-year and 10-year actuarial survivals of 65 percent and 50 percent, respectively. Given the increased number of patients undergoing transplantation and their excellent long-term survival, these patients will come to the attention of physicians in the emergency department with increasing frequency.

## TRANSPLANT RECIPIENTS

Cardiac transplantation has been applied successfully to patients of all ages, from newborns through persons in their late sixties. Heart transplantation is indicated for patients with end-stage heart failure not remedial to standard medical or surgical therapy. The etiology of heart failure in transplant recipients as reported by the ISHLT/UNOS Registry is listed in Table 63-1. The majority of adult patients have either idiopathic dilated cardiomyopathies or end-stage coronary artery disease. Many in the latter group will have undergone previous coronary artery bypass surgery. The predominant diagnoses in children undergoing transplantation are dilated cardiomyopathies and congenital heart disease. Many of the children with congenital heart disease will have undergone previous palliative or corrective operations. Patients are carefully evaluated to rule out other irreversible end-organ dysfunction and other systemic illnesses that would separately limit survival.

## CARDIAC PHYSIOLOGY AFTER TRANSPLANTATION

The physiologic basis upon which cardiac transplantation is grounded is the ability of the denervated heart to support normal circulation. The lack of sympathetic and parasympathetic innervation does, however, induce an altered physiologic state. The denervated heart has a normal sinus rhythm with a heart rate between 90 and 100 beats per minute. Denervation results in the absence of the initial centrally mediated tachycardia in response to stress or exercise. The heart remains responsive to circulating catecholamines of either endogenous or exogenous origin. The cardiac response to stress or exertion is therefore blunted. With the onset of exercise, the heart rate initially remains unchanged, then gradually increases to a level of approximately 80 percent of predicted over 10 to 15 min. After termination of exercise, this exercise-induced tachycardia will persist for approximately 20 to 30 min before slowly returning to the patient's baseline rate. Patients may complain of fatigue or shortness of breath with the onset of exercise that resolves with continued exertion as an appropriate tachycardia develops. In order to accommodate this response, patients are trained to perform warm-up exercises prior to vigorous exertion to initiate an increase in their heart rate. They are also cautioned to allow appropriate time for recovery at the end of exertion.

Cardiac hemodynamics after transplantation as measured by cardiac catheterization reveal a normal to mildly depressed cardiac output at rest. With exercise, cardiac output increases in response to increased venous return (preload) and circulating catecholamines. Maximal cardiac outputs of 80 to 100 percent of normal have been measured. Patients are able to resume normal activity levels, including vigorous exercise, following transplantation. A number of posttransplant patients have completed marathons and participated in other rigorous physical activities, and at least one such individual has competed as a professional athlete.

Cardiac denervation results in an altered response to some medications used in emergency resuscitation. In patients with supraventricular tachycardias, the lack of sympathetic innervation obviates the utility of carotid sinus massage. Atropine, which acts by abolishing reflex vagal slowing, will have no effect on heart rate in patients with symptomatic bradyarrhythmias. Conversely, denervated hearts are quite sensitive to the chronotropic effects of β-adrenergic agents such as isoproterenol, dopamine, and dobutamine. Because these are normal hearts, they are resistant to the proarrhythmic effects of these drugs. Isoproterenol is used preferentially to increase donor heart rates, because it has the greatest chronotropic effects and can be easily titrated to achieve the desired heart rate. The typical dose range is 1 to 4 µg/min administered by continuous intravenous infusion.

## EVALUATION OF THE POSTTRANSPLANT PATIENT

Electrocardiograms (ECG) obtained on transplant recipients should demonstrate normal sinus rhythm. The donor heart is implanted with its sinus node intact to preserve normal atrioventricular conduction. The technique of cardiac transplantation also results in the preservation of the recipient's sinus node at the superior cavoatrial junction. The atrial suture line renders the two sinus nodes electrically isolated from each other. Thus, ECGs will frequently have two distinct P waves (Fig. 63-1). The sinus node of the donor heart is easily identified by its constant 1:1 relationship to the QRS complex, while the native P wave marches through the donor heart rhythm independently. The presence of the two separate P waves may lead to confusion about the patient's rhythm. The ECGs may be interpreted erroneously as showing atrial fibrillation, atrial flutter, or frequent premature atrial complexes. The use of calipers aides in the definition of the two distinct P waves. Sinus node dysfunction in the posttransplant heart occurs in approximately 4 to 5 percent of patients and is manifested by either sinus bradycardia with heart rates of ≤ 50 beats per minute or sinus standstill with a junctional escape rhythm with heart rates of 60 to 70 beats per minute. This dysfunction occurs in the early postoperative period and resolves spontaneously in most patients. For patients in whom sinus node dysfunction persists, treatment consists of either theophylline, which accelerates the sinus bradycardia in some patients, or implantation of a permanent transvenous pacemaker. The type of pacemaker implanted varies depending

**Table 63-1.** Etiology of Heart Failure in Transplant Recipients

| Adult | Occurrence, % | Pediatric | Occurrence, % |
|---|---|---|---|
| Coronary artery disease | 47.2 | Congenital heart disease | 45.6 |
| Dilated cardio-myopathies | 43.5 | Dilated cardio-myopathies | 45.4 |
| Valvular | 4.2 | Retransplantation | 2.7 |
| Retransplantation | 2.3 | Miscellaneous | 6.3 |
| Congenital | 1.3 | | |
| Miscellaneous | 1.5 | | |

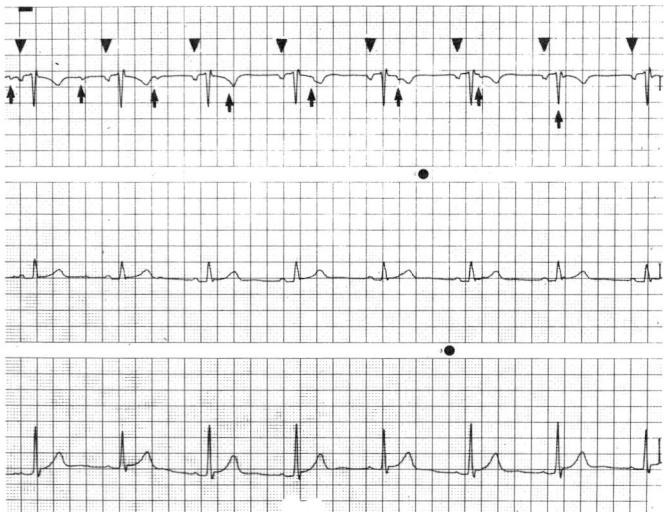

**Fig. 63-1.** Electrocardiogram demonstrating donor and recipient P waves. ▼ donor P wave; ↑ recipient P wave.

on institutional preference, but generally is either an atrial pacemaker programmed in the AAIR mode or a ventricular pacemaker programmed in the VVIR mode. Use of an atrial rate-responsive pacemaker preserves atrioventricular conduction in addition to providing physiologic rate responsiveness. Table 63-6 shows pacemaker codes.

Posttransplant chest radiographs show evidence of a prior sternotomy, but otherwise are generally normal. Some patients may have evidence of "cardiomegaly" related to the transplantation of a heart from a donor who was larger than the recipient.

Echocardiography is a useful tool for evaluating cardiac function posttransplantation. Interpretation of the echocardiogram is routine, with the exception of the evaluation of the atrial size. Because the atrial anastomoses incorporate the posterior walls of the recipient's native atria, echocardiography will show atrial enlargement, but this has no significant effect on cardiac function. Early rejection results in diastolic dysfunction, although the echocardiographic indices may be subtle and difficult to detect. Severe rejection will be accompanied by signs of biventricular enlargement with global hypocontractility and significant atrioventricular valve regurgitation.

## IMMUNOSUPPRESSION FOR CARDIAC TRANSPLANTATION

As with all types of solid organ transplantation, lifelong immunosuppression is required to prevent acute graft rejection. One of the most significant challenges of clinical transplantation is to maintain an adequate level of immunosuppression to prevent rejection while preserving adequate immunocompetence to avoid serious infectious complications. Since the mid 1980s, standard immunosuppression has employed a triple drug regimen consisting of cyclosporine (Sandimmune), prednisone, and azathioprine (Imuran). The combination of these agents has resulted in superior graft and patient survival rates, has decreased the mortality from infectious complications, and has minimized the side effects of the individual agents. In addition, many programs use induction therapy in the early postoperative period employing cytotoxic antibody preparations targeted against the T lymphocytes. The most commonly used agents include OKT3, a murine monoclonal antibody, and polyclonal preparations such as antilymphocyte serum (ALS) and antilymphocyte globulin (ALG). New immunosuppressive medications are under development, including FK-506 and rapamycin. FK-506 has recently been approved by the U.S. Food and Drug Administration (FDA) for use in liver transplantation and will become more widely available in the next several months.

**Table 63-2.** Cyclosporine–Drug Interactions

Drugs increasing cyclosporine blood levels
    Allopurinol
    Bromocriptine (Parlodel)
    Chloroquine
    Danazol (Danocrine)
    Diltiazem (Cardizem)
    Erythromycin (Erythrocin)
    Fluconazole
    Itraconazole
    Josamycin
    Ketoconazole (Nizoral)
    Methylprednisolone
    Metoclopramide
    Nicardipine (Cardene)
    Verapamil (Calan)
Drugs decreasing cyclosporine blood levels
    Carbamazepine (Tegretol)
    Phenobarbital
    Phenytoin (Dilantin)
    Rifampin (Rifadin)
    Ticlopidine
Drugs causing enhanced/additive nephrotoxicity
    Amphotericin B (Fungizone)
    Azapropazon (Prolixan)
    Cimetidine (Tagamet)
    Cotrimoxazole (sulfamethoxazole/trimethoprim) (Septra/Bactrim)
    Diclofenac (Voltaren)
    Erythromycin (Eythrocin)
    Gentamicin
    Ketoconazole (Nizoral)
    Melphalan (Alkeran)
    Ranitidine (Zantac)
    Tobramycin
    Trimethoprim
    Vancomycin (Vancocin)

Cyclosporine remains the mainstay of immunosuppressive regimens. This fungal metabolite is a potent inhibitor of T-lymphocyte activity and interferes with the generation of interleukin 2 (IL-2). It is a lipophilic substance that is metabolized in the liver by the cytochrome $P_{450}$ system. Cyclosporine is usually taken twice daily, and doses are adjusted based on serial blood levels. Target trough levels vary depending on the specific laboratory assay used. Levels are maintained in the 300 to 400 ng/dL range early after transplantation and then lowered to levels of approximately 150 ng/dL long term. The list of drugs that interact with cyclosporine (Table 63-2) continues to grow yearly, and careful consideration is required before adding or withdrawing medications for an individual patient. Such changes should always be made with the knowledge and input of the patient's transplant physician. Acute increases in cyclosporine levels may be associated with severe renal dysfunction, and acute decreases may result in the development of acute rejection.

Commonly encountered side effects of cyclosporine are listed in Table 63-3. Hypertension occurs in the majority of patients and frequently requires combination therapy to achieve adequate control. Renal insufficiency is also quite common and is mediated at least in part by the vasoconstrictive effects of cyclosporine on the proximal renal tubule. Management of cyclosporine-induced renal insufficiency requires careful monitoring, because worsening renal insuffi-

**Table 63-3.** Common Cyclosporine Side Effects

| | |
|---|---|
| Hypertension | Hyperkalemia |
| Renal insufficiency | Hypomagnesemia |
| Hirsutism | Hyperuricemia |
| Tremor | Glucose intolerance |
| Gingival hyperplasia | Seizures |

ciency results in elevated cyclosporine levels, leading to more renal dysfunction, thus creating a vicious cycle. Although early renal insufficiency is frequently reversible, some patients have developed end-stage renal disease requiring dialysis or renal transplantation.

Azathioprine is a 6-mercaptopurine derivative that acts as a false metabolite in the proliferation of bone marrow stem cells. The typical dose is 1 to 2 mg/kg per day, adjusted to maintain a white blood cell count greater than 5000/mm³. The most common side effect is bone marrow suppression manifested as neutropenia. In some patients, anemia and thrombocytopenia may be present. The most common drug interaction is with allopurinol, which may be prescribed to treat acute gouty arthritis, itself a side effect of cyclosporine therapy. If allopurinol is to be prescribed, the dose of azathioprine should be decreased by half and frequent follow-up white blood cell counts should be obtained to avoid profound bone marrow suppression.

Steroids remain an integral part of posttransplant immunosuppression. Prednisone is begun initially at high doses (0.6 to 1.5 mg/kg per day) post transplant and weaned over 6 to 8 weeks to a maintenance dose of 0.2 mg/kg per day (~15 mg/day in the average adult recipient). Many programs now attempt to wean patients off steroids in an effort to avoid the well-known deleterious effects of chronic steroid therapy. Steroid withdrawal is successful in approximately 50 percent of cases.

## REJECTION

Rejection after cardiac transplantation is a life-long risk, although the incidence of rejection decreases with time. Rejection can be divided into three types, based on mechanism of rejection and time after transplantation. *Hyperacute rejection* is mediated by preformed anti-HLA antibodies directed against the donor tissue. Hyperacute rejection results in immediate and irreversible donor heart failure and is a fatal complication unless the patient can be maintained with a mechanical assist device until a new donor heart is located. With the use of ABO blood group–compatible donors and screening of transplant candidates for elevated levels of preformed anti-HLA antibodies, hyperacute rejection is very rare in cardiac transplantation.

*Acute rejection,* the most common type of rejection encountered, occurs in approximately 75 percent of all patients at some time after transplantation. The incidence of acute rejection is greatest within the first 6 weeks post transplantation as immunosuppressive medications are weaned to chronic maintenance levels. Rejection can occur at any time after transplantation. Late episodes can usually be correlated with some change in the patient's immunosuppressive status, such as an acute illness or noncompliance with medications. Acute rejection is a cellular phenomenon resulting in the infiltration of lymphocytes into the myocardium with subsequent destruction of individual myocytes. Because most episodes of rejection do not cause clinically detectable graft dysfunction, surveillance endomyocardial biopsies are performed on a routine basis after transplantation. Biopsy specimens are examined histologically and graded according to a grading system (Table 63-4) developed by a working group of the ISHLT. Mild to moderate episodes of rejection (grades 0–2) are generally not accompanied by clinical symptoms or hemodynamic changes. Severe rejec-

tion (grade 4) can result in profound myocardial dysfunction and death. Patients with grade 2 or higher rejection are treated with augmented steroids or cytotoxic therapy, as outlined below.

*Chronic rejection* is believed to be manifested in the heart by the development of graft atherosclerosis. This antibody-mediated phenomenon is thought to result in injury to the endothelial lining of the coronary arteries, with the subsequent development of intimal hypertrophy. The lesions may be focal but are more often diffuse and concentric, involving the entire length of the epicardial and intramyocardial vessels. Because the heart is denervated, myocardial ischemia does not present with angina. Instead, recipients present with heart failure secondary to silent myocardial infarctions or with sudden death. Transplant recipients who present with new-onset shortness of breath, chest fullness, or symptoms of congestive heart failure should be evaluated for the presence of myocardial ischemia or infarction. This is done in routine fashion with ECG and serial cardiac enzymes. Echocardiography can be used to look for segmental wall motion abnormalities. If evidence for myocardial ischemia or infarction is found, cardiac catheterization with ventriculography and coronary angiography are indicated. The rate of development of graft coronary disease is quite variable, occurring months to years after transplantation; consequently, cardiac transplant programs employ annual follow-up coronary angiograms to detect its presence. The diffuse nature of graft coronary artery disease generally precludes standard methods of myocardial revascularization such as percutaneous transluminal coronary angioplasty or coronary artery bypass surgery. Retransplantation is the most effective treatment.

Although most episodes of acute rejection are asymptomatic, symptoms can occur. The most common presenting symptoms are arrhythmias and generalized fatigue. The development of either atrial or ventricular arrhythmias in a cardiac transplant recipient must be assumed to be due to acute rejection until proven otherwise. The patient's transplant center should be contacted directly so that arrangements can be made for performance of an endomyocardial biopsy. If patients are hemodynamically compromised by their arrhythmias, empiric therapy for rejection with methylprednisolone (Solu-Medrol), 1 g intravenously, may be given after consultation with the transplant center. If the diagnosis of rejection is confirmed, standard antirejection therapy should be completed. Atrial arrhythmias may respond to treatment with digoxin or calcium channel blockers. Ventricular arrhythmias may respond to lidocaine or other class I-C agents. Frequently the arrhythmias will be controlled only with antirejection therapy.

Untreated acute cardiac rejection results in progressive myocardial dysfunction. Diastolic dysfunction occurs first, followed by systolic dysfunction as the degree of myocardial damage increases. Diastolic dysfunction causes symptoms of congestive heart failure with shortness of breath, fatigue, and malaise. Progressive myocardial dysfunction results in low-output syndrome, with symptoms including nausea, vomiting, and/or diarrhea. Severe rejection leads to hypotension and circulatory collapse. Symptoms of rejection may be mistakenly attributed to a viral syndrome or gastroenteritis. Physical examination reveals signs of heart failure, including distended neck veins, an $S_3$ gallop on cardiac auscultation, rales on pulmonary auscultation, and occasionally the presence of ascites or peripheral edema. Chest x-rays show enlargement of the cardiac silhouette and pulmonary vascular congestion. Electrocardiograms may demonstrate—in addition to arrhythmias—a decrease in amplitude and widening of the QRS complex.

Patients with signs or symptoms suggestive of acute rejection should be admitted to the hospital with continuous ECG monitoring. Arrangements should be made for performance of an endomyocardial biopsy at the earliest possible time. If facilities for obtaining and interpreting biopsy specimens are not available, transfer to the nearest transplant center should be arranged. Low-output syndrome and/or hypotension should be treated with inotropic agents such as

**Table 63-4.** Standardized Cardiac Biopsy Grading System

| Grade | Histologic Description |
|---|---|
| 0 | No rejection |
| 1 | A = Focal (perivascular or interstitial) infiltrate without necrosis<br>B = Diffuse but sparse infiltrate without necrosis |
| 2 | One focus only with aggressive infiltration and/or focal myocyte damage |
| 3 | A = Multifocal aggressive infiltrates and/or myocyte damage<br>B = Diffuse inflammatory process with necrosis |
| 4 | Diffuse aggressive polymorphous infiltrate ± edema, ± hemorrhage, ± vasculitis, with necrosis |

dopamine or dobutamine while specific treatment for rejection is instituted. Treatment for rejection without biopsy confirmation is contraindicated except when the patient is hemodynamically unstable. This is especially true in patients whose symptoms are due to an occult infection because of the potential adverse consequences of high-dose steroid therapy. Empiric treatment for rejection should be employed only after consultation with the patient's transplant center.

Standard therapy for acute rejection includes intravenous methyl-prednisolone 1 g/day for 3 days. In patients with refractory rejection, treatment with specific T-cell cytotoxic agents such as OKT3, ALS, or ALG is required. Occasionally, patients have been successfully supported with mechanical assist devices for profound circulatory collapse while undergoing therapy for rejection, with resultant complete recovery of normal ventricular function.

## INFECTIOUS COMPLICATIONS AFTER CARDIAC TRANSPLANTATION

Infectious complications are fairly common after transplantation, particularly in the early posttransplant period, when the highest doses of immunosuppressive medications are employed. The infectious complications after cardiac transplantation are similar to those following all types of solid organ transplantation and those in other immunocompromised hosts. The infections most commonly encountered are listed in Table 63-5. Prophylactic regimens are employed by most transplant centers. Pretransplantation, patients are vaccinated with

**Table 63-5.** Common Infections after Cardiac Transplantation

Early posttransplant infections (first month)
  Pneumonia
    Gram-negative bacilli (GNB)
  Mediastinitis
    *Staphylococcus epidermidis*
    *Staphylococcus aureus*
    GNB
  IV lines
    *S. epidermidis*
    *S. aureus*
    GNB
    *Candida albicans*
  Urinary tract infections
    GNB
    Enterococcus
    *C. albicans*
  Skin
    Herpes simplex virus
Late posttransplant infections (after first month) and for duration of immunosuppression
  Viral
    Cytomegalovirus (CMV)
    Herpes simplex
    Variclla-zoster
    Non-A, non-B hepatitis
  Bacteria
    *Listeria*
    *Nocardia*
    *Legionella*
    *Mycobacterium*
  Fungi
    *Aspergillus*
    *Cryptococcus*
    *Candida*
    *Mucor (Phycomyces)*
  Protozoa
    *Pneumocystis carinii*
    *Toxoplasma gondii*

*Source:* Horn JE, Barlett JG, in Baumgartner WA et al (1990), p 223. Used by permission.

pneumococcal, *Haemophilus influenzae,* and hepatitis B vaccines. Perioperatively, routine antistaphylococcal antibiotics are used. Postoperatively, mycostatin mouthwash is used to prevent oral and esophageal candidiasis while the patients are on high-dose steroids and is reinstituted when augmented steroid therapy is required to treat rejection. *Toxoplasmosis gondii* can infect the transplanted heart; it may result from reactivation of a latent recipient infection or be transmitted with the donor organ. Toxoplasmosis titers are measured in all recipients and donors, and pyrimethamine is administered prophylactically for 6 weeks post transplantation if titers are elevated. Beginning approximately 2 months post transplantation, trimethoprim-sulfamethoxazole (Septra, Bactrim) is used as prophylaxis against *Pneumocystis carinii* pneumonia (PCP). Antibiotic prophylaxis for any invasive procedure (e.g., dental work, endoscopy, or surgical procedures) is recommended for the lifetime of the patient. Annual flu shots are recommended. Live attenuated virus vaccines such as those for measles, mumps, and rubella are contraindicated in transplant recipients.

Any patient with a history of solid organ transplantation who presents with symptoms of an infection must be evaluated in an aggressive and thorough manner. Appropriate stains and cultures should be obtained to allow identification of bacterial, fungal, and viral pathogens. There should be a low threshold for instituting antimicrobial therapy while awaiting culture results and for admitting patients to the hospital for further evaluation and intravenous antibiotics. Patients with evidence of pulmonary infiltrates but without productive sputum require bronchoscopy with bronchoalveolar lavage and transbronchial biopsy for definitive diagnosis. Pulmonary infections that are frequently encountered include *P. carinii, Nocardia, Legionella pneumophilia,* and *Aspergillus,* and these require special stains and studies for accurate diagnosis. Patients with gastroenteritis and nausea, vomiting, and/or diarrhea require special attention. Inability to ingest or adequately absorb immunosuppressive medications may result in the development of an episode of rejection. If there is any question about a recipient's ability to maintain adequate oral intake, the patient should be hospitalized and immunosuppressive medications should be administered intravenously.

Antibiotic therapy for documented infections should be guided by appropriate culture and sensitivities and must take into account underlying renal insufficiency and potential interactions with cyclosporine.

Of special note is the risk of cytomegalovirus (CMV) infection after cardiac transplantation. CMV is a common virus to which the majority of adults have been exposed, as demonstrated by the presence of anti-CMV IgG antibodies in the serum. Post transplantation, CMV infections can occur due either to the reactivation of latent virus in a previously infected recipient or the development of a new infection with a different viral strain transmitted with the donor organ. The latter situation is much more serious and potentially life threatening, particularly in recipients who were CMV negative prior to transplantation. Routine posttransplant surveillance for CMV infection is performed utilizing serial IgG and IgM antibody testing and throat, urine, and serum buffy coat cultures. CMV disease can occur in either a mild or severe form. Mild disease is manifested by a flulike illness with low-grade fever, fatigue, malaise, and nausea. Severe disease may include profound leukopenia; pneumonitis; gastroenteritis including epigastric pain, vomiting, and diarrhea; and hepatitis with elevated transaminases. CMV pneumonitis carries a mortality of greater than 50 percent. CMV infection typically occurs 4 to 12 weeks post transplantation. The diagnosis is made by the demonstration of cytoplasmic inclusion bodies in biopsy specimens of affected organs. Treatment includes the use of intravenous ganciclovir and, in severe cases, intravenous immunoglobulin infusions. Of particular concern is the documented increased incidence of acute rejection complicating acute CMV infections. Therefore, patients with active CMV disease must be monitored carefully for signs and symptoms of rejection. An endomyocardial biopsy should be performed if there is any suspicion of rejection.

## NONINFECTIOUS COMPLICATIONS OF CARDIAC TRANSPLANTATION

In addition to infection and rejection, cardiac transplant recipients are susceptible to all of the acute illnesses and diseases that affect the general population. These patients should be treated as any other acutely ill or traumatized patient. Patients on chronic steroids will have adrenal suppression and may need stress coverage if they are severely ill or in need of surgical intervention. Uninterrupted administration of immunosuppressive medications must be assured to avoid the development of acute rejection.

In addition to common forms of cancer, those malignancies associated with chronic immunosuppression also occur in cardiac transplant recipients. These include posttransplant lymphoproliferative disorders (PTLD), which are usually B-cell lymphomas and have been related to the Epstein-Barr virus. PTLD may occur as early as 1 month post transplantation and may present with a variety of nonspecific symptoms. If diagnosed in their early stages, they may respond to decreased levels of immunosuppression, chemotherapy, and/or radiation therapy, with long-term survival reported.

Aseptic necrosis of the femoral heads and thoracic and lumbar spine compression fractures are not uncommon manifestations of long-term steroid therapy. The development of hip pain referred to the medial thigh or knee is often indicative of early aseptic necrosis. MRI scans are the most sensitive means of detection, and patients should be referred for orthopaedic evaluation if this diagnosis is suspected.

Nonsteroidal anti-inflammatory drugs (NSAID) should be used with extreme caution in transplant patients because of the potential exacerbation of underlying renal insufficiency secondary to cyclosporine use.

## PEDIATRIC CARDIAC TRANSPLANTATION

The care and evaluation of pediatric heart transplant recipients is similar to that of adults, with a few special considerations. Rejection surveillance in infants and small children is done primarily with serial echocardiograms. Difficulties with vascular access and the need for anesthesia make serial endomyocardial biopsy procedures impractical. Acute rejection is more frequently heralded by symptoms in children than in adults. Children will present with a low-grade fever, fussiness, and poor feeding. Echocardiography will demonstrate decreased ventricular contractility, thickening of the posterior wall of the left ventricle, cardiac enlargement, and mitral and tricuspid valve insufficiency. Because the signs of rejection may be subtle and difficult to quantify, serial echocardiographic studies are required throughout the postoperative period in order to establish each patient's baseline echocardiographic characteristics.

Immunosuppression for children is based on standard triple therapy. Because of more rapid metabolism of cyclosporine, higher doses and more frequent (tid) dosing are often needed in children. Steroids are withdrawn whenever possible to avoid their deleterious effects on somatic growth.

Childhood infections are frequently encountered and should be treated according to routine practice. Live attenuated virus vaccinations are avoided. Exposure to chickenpox (varicella) is avoided if possible. If exposure does occur in a recipient without a history of previous infection, treatment with varicella immune globulin (VZIG) is indicated. Recipients who develop chickenpox are treated with intravenous acyclovir (Zovirox).

## CONCLUSION

Cardiac transplantation has resulted in successful recovery and return to an active life style for thousands of patients who would otherwise have died from end-stage cardiac disease. The success of this procedure has resulted in the development of new medical problems, including rejection and infection. Thorough and aggressive evaluation and treatment of these patients when they develop acute illnesses can lead to a successful outcome. Close communication with the patient's transplant center is essential to ensure appropriate treatment and to facilitate timely follow-up after the emergency department visit. Specially trained cardiac transplant coordinators and transplant physicians are available on a 24-h basis at all transplant centers. They should be contacted with any questions concerning appropriate patient care and whenever hospitalization is required for a transplant recipient.

## BIBLIOGRAPHY

Banner NR, Yacoub MH: Physiology of the orthotopic cardiac transplant recipient. *Semin Thorac Cardiovasc Surg* 2(3):259, 1990.

Baumgartner WA, Reitz BA, Achuff SC (eds): *Heart and Heart-Lung Transplantation.* Philadelphia, Saunders, 1990.

Billingham ME, Cary NRB, Hammond ME, et al: A working formulation for the standardization of nomenclature in the diagnosis of heart and lung rejection: Heart Rejection Study Group. *J Heart Transplant* 9:587, 1990.

Farrell TG, Camm AJ: Action of drugs in the denervated heart. *Semin Thorac Cardiovasc Surg* 2(3):279, 1990.

Hosenpud JD, Novick RJ, Breen TJ, Daily OP: The Registry of the International Society for Heart and Lung Transplantation: Eleventh Official Report—1994. *J Heart Lung Transplant* 13:561, 1994.

**Table 63-6.** NBG (NASPE*/BPEG†) Generic Pacemaker Code‡

| Position/ Category | I Chamber(s) Paced | II Chamber(s) Sensed | III Response to Sensing | IV Programmability, Rate Modulation | V Antitachyarrhythmia Function(s) |
|---|---|---|---|---|---|
| | O = None<br>V = Ventricle | O = None<br>V = Ventricle | O = None<br>T = Triggers pacing | O = None<br>P = Simple programmable | O = None<br>P = Pacing (antitachy-arrhythmia |
| Letter Codes | A = Atrium<br>D = Dual (A + V) | A = Atrium<br>D = Dual (A + V) | I = Inhibits pacing<br>D = Dual (T + I) | M = Multiprogrammable<br>C = Communicating (telemetry)<br>R = Rate modulation | S = Shock<br>D = Dual (P + S) |

Note: Positions I through III are used exclusively for antibradyarrhythmia pacing. Manufacturers may use "S" in positions I and II to indicate single chamber (A or V). A Minimum of four positions is required to describe a packmaker.

* NASPE = North American Society of Pacing and Electrophysiology.

† BPEG = British Pacing and Electrophysiology Groups.

‡ Adapted from Bernstein, A. D., Camm, A. J., Fletcher, R. D., et al: The NASPE/BPEG Generic Pacemaker Code for antibradyarrhythmia and adaptive-rate pacing and antitachyarrhythmia devices. *PACE* 10:794, 1987.

# 64
# BACTERIAL PNEUMONIAS
## Georges C. Benjamin

Bacterial pneumonia remains a leading cause of death and is responsible for about 3.3 million cases yearly and as many as 10 percent of hospital admissions in the United States. The pneumococcus accounts for up to 90 percent of all bacterial pneumonias, with *Escherichia coli, Pseudomonas aeruginosa, Klebsiella pneumoniae, Staphylococcus aureus, Hemophilus influenzae,* and group A streptococci accounting for most of the rest. Other bacteria, such as *Legionella pneumophila* and the anaerobes, are less frequent causes of pneumonia. The frequency with which each of these organisms causes disease varies from study to study.

Patients with chronic diseases such as congestive heart failure, diabetes, cancer, bronchiectasis, sickle cell anemia, acquired immunodeficiency syndrome (AIDS), and hypogamma globulinemia are at greater risk for pneumonia, as are smokers and postsplenectomy patients. Essentially all bacterial pneumonia is the result of aspiration of oropharyngeal contents. Therefore, patients with seizures, obtundation, suppressed cough reflex, and increased secretions are also predisposed to it. These and other predisposing factors are shown in Table 64-1.

Sterility of the lower airways and alveoli is due to an effective system using filtration through the upper airway, the cough reflex, mucociliary clearance, phagocytosis, and in situ bacterial killing. Cilia located in the tracheal bronchial tree are responsible for removing most infected particles greater than 5.0 μm. Particles smaller than this are removed by alveolar macrophages and local factors (surfactant, complement, IgG, IgA) that limit bacterial growth. Because of a variance in the susceptibilities of different bacterial species to these clearance mechanisms, most pneumonias are ultimately the result of a single species. This is of interest in light of the multiplicity of organisms in oropharyngeal secretions.

## LABORATORY TESTS

Laboratory tests useful in the emergency department diagnosis of bacterial pneumonia include the white blood cell count (WBC), chest ex-ray, pulse oximetry, arterial blood gas, sputum examination, blood cultures, and pleural fluid examination.

The WBC remains a useful way to document the presence of the inflammatory response from pneumonia. In healthy young patients, marked elevation usually occurs. This elevation is not diagnostic, however, and the presence of a normal count does not rule out pneumonia or suggest a viral etiology. Also, in the elderly or debilitated patient, a normal or low WBC may represent overwhelming sepsis. In these cases the presence of a left shift may be the only clue to bacterial infection.

Radiographically, bacterial pneumonias are frequently characterized as in Table 64-2. Note that these classic patterns frequently are the exception and serve only as a guide in radiographic diagnosis. Another reason to obtain a chest x-ray is to look for evidence of effusion, abscess formation, or pneumothorax. Special views such as the lateral decubitus and apical lordotic are frequently of value to further define the nature of pulmonary abnormalities. Patients with marked leukopenia or dehydration may not initially demonstrate an infiltrate. A diagnosis of pneumonia in these patients rests with a strong clinical suspicion on serial chest x-rays.

Pulmonary infarction, atelectasis, neoplasia, pulmonary edema, parenchymal scarring, and pleural thickening may all simulate pneumonitis radiographically. In these patients, clinical examination, history, and comparison with prior radiographs may aid in proper diagnosis.

Ventilation perfusion abnormality is the most common functional disorder in acute pneumonias. This is the result of sustained perfusion of poorly ventilated areas of the lung. Measurement of the oxygen content of arterial blood in patients with respiratory compromise is useful to document hypoxia and to ensure adequate oxygenation in patients on oxygen therapy. Arterial blood gases are especially important in patients with chronic lung disease because the acute hypoxia will be superimposed on an underlying ventilation perfusion mismatch. Although pulse oximetry is useful, arterial blood gases are needed to precisely measure the patient's oxygen or carbon dioxide level.

Sputum examination and culture remain the most important guides to proper antibiotic therapy. Frequently the patient is unable to generate an adequate specimen because of dehydration, obtundation, or a weak cough. Occasionally postural drainage or heated saline nebulization may be helpful to induce sputum.

Although not usually an emergency department procedure, transtracheal aspiration is frequently of value in patients who are unable to produce adequate sputum. Complications from this procedure include subcutaneous or mediastinal emphysema, cardiac arrhythmias, esophageal perforation, bleeding, and infection. Other diagnostic invasive procedures include bronchoscopy, lung biopsy, and percutaneous lung aspiration. These procedures should be done by physicians thoroughly familiar with the techniques and their complications. They are contraindicated in the patient who requires restraint, has uncorrected hypoxia, or has a coagulopathy.

Gross examination of the sputum is done first and may reveal the bloody or rusty sputum of pneumococcal pneumonia (not diagnostic, as other bacterial pneumonias may involve rusty sputum); the thick "currant jelly" sputum produced by both type 3 pneumonococcus and

**Table 64-1.** Factors Predisposing to Bacterial Pneumonia

| | |
|---|---|
| Debilitation | Chest wall disorders |
|   Alcoholism |   Myopathies and neuropathies |
|   Extremes of life |   Chest wall trauma |
|   Neoplasia |   Postoperative pain |
|   Immunosuppression | Syncope |
| Chronic diseases | Seizures |
|   Diabetes | Bronchial obstruction (tumor or |
|   Chronic obstructive pulmonary disease |   foreign body aspiration) |
|   Valvular heart disease | Pulmonary embolism |
|   Congestive heart failure | Iatrogenic invasion |
|   Leukemia |   Bronchoscopy |
|   Lymphoma |   Intubation, respiratory |
| |     support |
|   Hemoglobinopathies |   Transthoracic procedures |
| Viral infections | Stroke |

**Table 64-2.** Characteristics of Bacterial Pneumonia

| Organism | Sputum | Chest X-ray | Therapy | Complications |
|---|---|---|---|---|
| *Streptococcus pneumoniae* | Rusty, gram-positive encapsulated diplococci (type 3, thick) | Usually lobar in LLL, RLL, RML; occasionally patchy, small pleural effusion, 10% | Phenoxymethyl penicillin 500 mg PO q6h for 10 d; erythromycin 500 mg PO q6h for 10 d; azithromycin 500 mg PO on day 1 and 250 mg PO on days 2 through 5; aqueous penicillin G 20 million units/d q4–6h; procaine penicillin G 1.2 million units IM followed by phenoxymethyl penicillin 500 mg PO q6h for 10 d; vancomycin 1 g q12 h IV (penicillin-resistant); ceftriaxone 1 g qd; erythromycin lactobionate 250 mg IV q6h | Sepsis, abscess, congestive heart failure, meningitis, peritonitis, herpes labialis, septic arthritis, endocarditis, pericarditis |
| Group A streptococci | Purulent, bloody, gram-positive cocci in chains, pairs | Often lower lobes, patchy, multilobar large pleural effusion | See above | Sepsis, pleural effusion, hemoptysis |
| *Haemophilus influenzae* | Short, tiny, gram-negative, encapsulated cocci-bacilli | Patchy, frequently basilar, occasional pleural effusion | Ceftriaxone 1–2 g/d IV qd; cefuroxime 0.75–1.5 g IV q8h; amoxicillin clavulanate 500 mg PO q8h for 10 d; tetracycline 500 mg q6h for 10 d; clarithromycin 500 mg PO b.i.d. for 10 d | Septic arthritis, sepsis, meningitis, empyema |
| *Klebsiella pneumoniae* | Brown jelly, thick; short plump, gram-negative, encapsulated paired cocci-bacilli | Upper lobes, lobular bulging fissure sign, abscess formation | Cefazolin 0.25–1.0 g q8h IV; aminoglycoside (gentamicin, tobramycin, or amikacin) | Sepsis, empyema, pneumothorax, effusion, necrotizing pneumonia, hemoptysis, thick sputum |
| *Staphylococcus aureus* | Purulent; gram-positive cocci in pairs and clumps | Patchy, multicenter with early abscess formation, empyema, pneumothorax | Oxacillin 8–12 g/d IV; nafcillin 40 mg/kg per day IV 10–14 days*; vancomycin 500 mg q6h IV | Sepsis, endocarditis, empyema, necrotizing pneumonia, hemoptysis |
| *Legionella pneumophila* | Few polymorphonuclear leukocytes and no predominant bacterial species | Multiple patchy and nonsegmental infiltrates, progresses to consolidation, may cavitate, pleural effusions in 16% | Erythromycin lactobionate 250 mg IV q6; rifampin 600 mg PO qd | Shock, coma, confusion, hemoptysis, pericarditis, myocarditis, endocarditis, respiratory failure |
| *Escherichia coli* | Gram-negative cocci-bacilli | Patchy, bilateral, lower lobes | Ampicillin 6–8 g/d IV q6h; cephalosporin 9–12 g/d plus gentamicin 3–5 mg/kg per day IV q8h (tobramycin or amikacin as needed) | Sepsis, empyema |
| *Pseudomonas* | Gram-negative cocci-bacilli | Patchy, mid- and lower lung, with abscesses | Tobramycin 3–5 mg/kg per day IV; gentamicin 3–5mg/kg per day IV q8h plus carbenicillin 5–6 g q4h IV | Sepsis, empyema |

* May require 4 weeks of therapy.

*K. pneumoniae;* the green sputum caused by *P. aeruginosa, H. influenzae,* and *Streptococcus pneumoniae;* or the foul-smelling sputum of an anaerobic infection. The sputum is then Gram stained and viewed under the low-power objective to determine whether the sputum is suitable for examination and culture. If more than 10 squamous epithelial cells are present per low-power field, the specimen is contaminated and of low diagnostic value. An adequate specimen should demonstrate more than 25 polymorphonuclear leukocytes and less than 10 squamous epithelial cells per low-power field (90 percent correlation with cultures from transtracheal aspiration). In addition, a predominant bacterial form should be evident because a mixture of morphologic forms suggests oropharyngeal contamination. Such contamination frequently makes interpretation difficult. Enteric organisms are uncommon habitants in the pharynx of healthy people. However, recent viral infections, chronic obstructive pulmonary disease (COPD), chronic bronchitis, recent hospitalizations, and debilitating diseases favor colonization with gram-negative bacteria. Because of the recent increase in the incidence of tuberculosis, acid-fast bacilli smears should be done in at-risk patients.

Blood cultures are frequently of diagnostic value in patients who have presumed bacteremia, immunosuppression, or rigors, or who are seriously ill. Two to three cultures from separate sites are done when indicated.

Examination of the pleural fluid by thoracentesis, although generally not an emergency department procedure, is useful in ruling out empyema. Patients who may require a pleural biopsy should have only a diagnostic tap (10 to 20 mL) done by the emergency physician. Patients with respiratory compromise may require more extensive therapeutic drainage.

### Streptococcus pneumoniae

Pneumonococcal pneumonia is caused by *S. pneumoniae,* a gram-positive lancet-shaped, encapsulated bacterium. Based on its capsular antigens, it has been divided into at least 83 serotypes. Disease is usually caused by types 1, 3, 4, 6, 7, 8, 12, 14, 18, and 19 in adults and types 1, 6, 14, and 19 in children.

This organism is the most common cause of community-acquired bacterial pneumonia. Its peak incidence is winter and early spring, but it does occur year round. Mortality from this disease is as high as 30 percent if left untreated and less than 5 percent if treated.

Clinical disease presents as an acute shaking chill, tachypnea, and tachycardia. A single rigor lasting several minutes is so common that recurrent rigors should suggest another etiology. Sharp chest pain that causes marked splinting on the affected side occurs in 70 percent of patients. Cough may be absent in the early phases but rapidly becomes a prominent symptom. In 75 percent of patients a rust-colored sputum develops. With type 3 pneumococcus, a thick, jelly-like sputum may be present and must be differentiated from that caused by *K. pneumoniae.* Additional symptoms include malaise, anorexia, myalgias, flank or back pain, and vomiting.

On physical examination, the classic signs of consolidation, including bronchial breath sounds, egophony, and increased tactile and vocal fremitus are present. Pleural friction rubs, cyanosis, and jaundice are occasionally found. Abdominal distention from acute gastric dilatation or paralytic ileus may also develop.

The WBC generally ranges from 12,000 to 25,000 cells/mm³ but may reach 40,000/mm³. Normal or decreased WBCs are seen and suggest overwhelming infection. The chest x-ray usually demonstrates a singular infiltrate in the right middle lobe, right lower lobe, or left lower lobe. The infiltrate frequently has a lobar or segmental pattern, but patchy involvement is frequent in infants and the elderly. Occasionally bulging fissures similar to those seen with *K. pneumoniae* are noted. In 10 percent of patients a small, sterile pleural effusion is seen. Sputum culture is positive in only approximately 50 percent of cases and blood cultures in only 30 percent. This illustrates

the difficulties in establishing a definitive diagnosis. Occasionally, some patients will develop a mild perihepatitis with elevation of their liver function tests. Rhabdomyolysis has also been reported.

Untreated, this disease frequently resolves in 7 to 10 days by a clinical syndrome known as the "crisis" (prompt defervescence with diaphoresis and a rapid increase in well-being). Treated patients are often afebrile within 24 to 72 h, but in some the fever gradually decreases over 4 to 7 days. Physical signs take from 14 to 21 days to resolve, with radiographic signs resolving over another 21 days. Delayed resolution may be noted in some patients and is seen most frequently in the debilitated and the aged.

Complications include sepsis, lung abscess, congestive heart failure, meningitis, peritonitis, herpes labialis, septic arthritis, endocarditis, and pericarditis. In less than 20 percent of patients, empyema develops.

A poor prognosis is associated with type 2 and type 3 pneumococci, multilobar involvement, leukopenia, bacteremia, jaundice, splenectomized states (including sickle hemoglobinopathies), congestive heart failure, COPD, alcoholism, and diabetes.

Penicillin is still the drug of choice for pneumococcal pneumonia despite recently recognized resistant strains. The current recommendations for therapy are listed in Table 64-2. In patients allergic to penicillin, erythromycin, clarithromycin or a cephalosporin may be used. Tetracycline is not effective because of increased resistance.

### Haemophilus influenzae

*Haemophilus influenzae* is a gram-negative pleomorphic rod that exists in both encapsulated and unencapsulated forms. The capsular forms are divided into six serotypes (a through f) based on their capsular antigens. Of these, type b is found to cause 95 percent of all human infections. Both forms are able to cause pneumonia, but only the encapsulated form consistently causes bacteremia. The peak incidence of this disease occurs in winter to early spring and tends to occur in debilitated or immunocompromised patients.

The clinical presentation is one of fever, shortness of breath, and occasionally pleuritic chest pain. Lung examination may reveal rales without clear signs of consolidation. The WBC is frequently normal but may be as high as 30,000. The chest x-ray usually demonstrates patchy alveolar infiltrates, generally without effusion. Lobar consolidation does occur, but abscess formation is rare. This organism is frequently overlooked on Gram stains and diligence is required to find it and to recognize its small coccobacillary form.

Outpatient management consists of oral amoxicillin clavulanate, clarithromycin, or tetracycline (see Table 64-2). For patients requiring intravenous therapy, a third-generation cephalosporin such as ceftriaxone is now generally used.

Complications include septic arthritis, sepsis, meningitis, and, rarely, empyema. As with other serious pneumonias, the morbidity and mortality are highest in the young or compromised patient.

### Klebsiella PNEUMONIA

*Klebsiella* pneumonia is found most frequently in patients with alcoholism, diabetes, or COPD and is the most common gram-negative community-acquired pneumonia. It is a necrotizing lobar pneumonia, which is most frequently seen in the right upper lobe. In approximately 20 percent of cases empyema occurs within 24 to 48 h, along with intrapulmonary abscess formation in 4 to 5 days.

*Klebsiella* pneumonia presents as a sudden cough with rigors, shortness of breath, malaise, and often cyanosis; 80 percent of patients develop pleuritic chest pain. Pulmonary examination frequently reveals signs of consolidation and cyanosis. The WBC is elevated in 75 percent of cases. Chest x-ray frequently reveals a necrotizing lobar pneumonia in the right upper lobe. In 35 percent of cases a bulging minor fissure is seen. Occasionally, perihilar and patchy infiltrates are also seen. Sputum examination reveals a dark brown tenacious sputum, occasionally blood stained. Gram stain reveals short, plump, encapsulated gram-negative bacilli in pairs, which in poorly decolorized Gram stains can be easily confused with pneumococci. Sepsis, empyema, and pneumothorax are complications of this disease.

Initial therapy usually consists of an aminoglycoside and a cephalosporin intravenously. Attention to airway management is a must because frequently the sputum is so thick that clearance is difficult.

## OTHER GRAM-NEGATIVE PNEUMONIAS

Othe gram-negative organisms, including *E. coli, Pseudomonas, Enterobacter,* and *Serratia,* cause 10 percent of community-acquired bacterial pneumonias and as many as 50 percent of all nosocomial pneumonias. Their presence should be considered in the recently hospitalized, debilitated, or immunosuppressed patient. Therapy usually consists of intravenous carbenicillin or ticarcillin, and an aminoglycoside.

### *Legionella pneumophila*

*Legionella* is a gram-negative rod that is responsible for at least 6 percent of bacterial pneumonia. It occurs in sporadic and epidemic patterns, usually in the summer and fall. Patients presenting with legionnaires' disease generally present in one of two forms. The first known as "Pontiac fever" has an incubation period of 24 to 48 h followed by a viral-like syndrome of fever, chills, myalgia, and headache. This illness is generally brief and has a low mortality.

The second presentation is as *Legionella* pneumonia and is believed to be contracted through airborne transmission from heat-exchange systems, respiratory therapy devices, water sprays such as whirlpools and shower stalls, and cooling towers. Person-to-person spread is not felt to be the mode of transmission. Individuals at risk include those who live or work near construction sites; patients with chronic diseases such as lung disease, diabetes, or alcoholism; smokers; immunocompromised individuals; or victims of trauma. Unlike Pontiac fever *Legionella* pneumonia has a mortality rate as high as 75 percent without early treatment.

Clinical presentation includes fever, chills, headache, malaise, nonproductive cough, and shortness of breath. More than one half of patients will present with gastrointestinal symptoms of anorexia, diarrhea, nausea, or vomiting. Pleuritic chest pain and hemoptysis may also be present. Physical findings include a toxic-appearing patient with tachypnea and often a relative bradycardia. Pulmonary examination reveals diffuse fine rales progressing to frank consolidation. Mental status changes from confusion to coma may also be seen. Complications include respiratory failure, coma, shock, myocarditis, pericarditis, and endocarditis.

Laboratory studies reveal a leukocytosis with a left shift. Sputum Gram stain shows few polymorphonuclear leukocytes and no predominate organism. A serum sodium concentration of less than 130 mEq/L and hypophosphatemia are common electrolyte abnormalities. Microscopic hematuria and mild elevations of liver function tests may also be seen. Serologic testing can be performed on sputum, blood, and urine but are of limited immediate value because of the time necessary to process these tests. Direct immunofluorescence testing of the sputum has a high specificity but a low sensitivity. A rise in the blood indirect immunofluorescence titer of at least 1:128 is required for diagnosis; convalescent titers of 1:256 or greater are suggestive of recent infection. These titers usually require from 3 to 6 weeks to increase. Urine serology testing is still experimental at present. The organism can be grown from lung tissue but not from blood or sputum. Chest x-ray findings initially show a small unilateral alveolar infiltrate that later progresses to generalized bilateral patchy infiltrates. These infiltrates may go on to frank consolidation or abscess formation. Pleural effusions are seen in 16% of patients and can also

be a presenting sign. Radiographic findings are extremely slow to resolve and lag behind clinical improvement.

Erythromycin lactobionate 250 mg q6h intravenously is the drug of choice for *Legionella* infection. This is followed by oral therapy for a total of 3 weeks. Rifampin, 600 mg/d may be used in patients who do not tolerate erythromycin.

## STAPHYLOCOCCAL PNEUMONIA

Staphylococci cause 1 percent of bacterial pneumonias. Although this pneumonia occurs sporadically, it has its peak incidence during influenza and measles epidemics. Patients presenting after a viral illness with the abrupt onset of productive cough, pleurisy, multiple chills, and hectic fever are suspect for this disease. Lung examination may show fine to coarse rhonchi and rales; however, signs of consolidation are rare. The chest x-ray reveals a patchy infiltrate, which rapidly progresses to abscess formation and lobar consolidation. Empyema is common, WBCs are usually above 15,000/mm$^3$, and blood cultures are usually negative unless the pulmonary involvement is metastatic. Gram stain of the sputum reveals large gram-positive cocci in pairs and clumps.

Patients at particular risk include intravenous drug abusers, hospitalized patients, and the debilitated. Therapy includes intravenous oxacillin or nafcillin unless penicillin resistance or allergy is suspected. Vancomycin can be used in these patients.

## STREPTOCOCCAL PNEUMONIA (GROUP A)

Although a rare cause of pulmonary infection, group A streptococci can cause a rapidly progressive pneumonitis with a high mortality. The clinical syndrome is characterized by the sudden onset of fever, chills, and productive cough. In most patients pleuritic pain is a prominent symptom. Pulmonary examination usually reveals fine rales without signs of consolidation. The chest x-ray is usually consistent with a multilobar bronchopneumonia, often with a large pleural effusion. The sputum is frequently bloody and purulent. Gram stain reveals gram-positive cocci in pairs and chains. Penicillin is the drug of choice. Alternative drugs include ceftriaxone or erythromycin lactobionate.

## EMPIRICAL THERAPEUTIC GUIDELINES

In general, initial therapy is based on clinical presentation, sputum Gram stain, or culture results. The emergency department physician is often faced with a nonspecific clinical presentation or nondiagnostic Gram stain with which to initiate outpatient therapy. In this situation, an excellent choice is erythromycin 500 mg q6h for 10 to 14 days or clarithromycin 500 mg b.i.d. for 10 days with close clinical follow-up. *Hemophilus influenzae* is not covered by this approach and must be considered in patients who do not respond to therapy.

Empirical therapy for patients requiring admission is a common occurrence. Patients with community-acquired pneumonia at low risk for gram-negative pneumonia can be safely given ceftriaxone, erythromycin lactobionate, or trimethoprim/sulfamethoxazole. This approach is effective for gram-positive pneumonia, *Hemophilus* influenza, and some gram-negative pneumonias. Patients at high risk for gram-negative pneumonia or *Legionella* (diabetics, alcoholics, nursing home patients, intubated patients) should be given either erythromycin plus a third-generation cephalosporin (ampicillin sulbactam or trimethoprim/sulfamethoxazole can be substituted for the cephalosporin). An antipseudomonal penicillin plus an antipseudomonal aminoglycoside is especially useful in immunocompromised patients. If *Pseudomonas* pneumonia is suspected, an antipseudomonal penicillin such as mezlocillin or amikacin may be used. As with all therapy, local antibiotic sensitivities and resistance patterns, as well as local standards of care, should determine final antibiotic selection.

## ADMISSION GUIDELINES

Pregnant patients and those with serious underlying diseases, volume depletion, toxicity, or severe hypoxia require hospital admission. Inpatients at high risk of death have a respiratory rate of greater than 30/min, a diastolic blood pressure of 60 mm Hg or less, and a blood urea nitrogen of greater than 7 mmol/L. Social admissions include all patients who cannot care for themselves at home. Patients who, after an appropriate evaluation, are felt to be well enough for outpatient therapy should be followed up in 3 to 5 days. A chest x-ray is frequently done after 1 month to document resolution of the infiltrate.

## BIBLIOGRAPHY

Chodosh S: Examination of sputum cells. *N Engl J Med* 282:854, 1970.

Farr BM, Sloman AJ, Fisch MJ: Predicting death in patients hospitalized for community-acquired pneumonia. *Ann Intern Med* 115:428, 1991.

Fraser DW, Tsai TR, Orenstein W, et al: Legionnaires' disease: description of an epidemic of pneumonia. *N Engl J Med* 297:1189, 1977.

Sanford JP: Guide to antimicrobial therapy. Antimicrobial Therapy, Inc. Dallas, TX, 1993.

# 65

# VIRAL AND *Mycoplasma* PNEUMONIAS IN ADULTS

## K. P. Ravikrishnan

## INTRODUCTION

Pneumonia is the sixth leading cause of death in the United States. Respiratory viruses and *Mycoplasma* account for a third or more of the cases of pneumonia. The spectrum of disease caused by these agents ranges from the common cold to life-threatening pneumonia. Recently reported cases of Hantavirus pulmonary syndrome with acute overwhelming infection, respiratory failure, and death in up to 70 percent of cases, demonstrate the pathologic potential of viral infections. Predominantly two common types of lower respiratory infections are caused by viruses and *Mycoplasma*: tracheobronchitis and pneumonia. Without localizing clinical and radiographic findings, it is not easy to separate severe tracheobronchitis from pneumonia. Classic pneumonia is characterized by chills followed by high fever, cough, pleuritic chest pain, and dyspnea. Viral and *Mycoplasma* pneumonia often have atypical clinical manifestations with predominant extrapulmonary manifestations.

An understanding of pneumonia is helpful in planning management strategies. Though most often the viral and *Mycoplasma* infections are seasonal minor illnesses, their potential for causing overwhelming pneumonia and respiratory failure is well known. Epidemics should be anticipated so that the effect on the normal population and the highly vulnerable elderly, debilitated, cardiac, and pulmonary patients can be minimized. Since there is no specific treatment for most of these pneumonias, the emphasis is placed on identification of the responsible agent and supportive treatment.

## INCIDENCE AND ETIOLOGY

The spectrum of acute respiratory illnesses caused by viruses and *Mycoplasma* include pharyngitis, laryngitis, tracheobronchitis, and bronchitis. Nonbacterial agents account for over 90 percent of infectious

**Table 65-1.** Complications of Viral and *Mycoplasma* Pneumonia

1. Secondary bacterial infections
2. Recurrent pneumonia
3. Altered pulmonary function
4. Respiratory failure due to overwhelming infection
5. Bronchial hyperactivity
6. Chronic bronchitis
7. Bronchiolitis obliterans

respiratory ailments. Common complications from these infections are listed in Table 65-1. In hospitalized patients, bacteria predominate as the causative agents of pneumonia. Viral agents and *Mycoplasma* account for more than a third of cases of community-acquired pneumonia.

Increased airway reactivity from viral and *Mycoplasma* infections is well known. The inflammatory reaction and hyperreactivity to cholinergic stimulation occur during both the infectious and postinfectious phase. The mechanism of airway hyperreactivity is not clear, but patients with preexisting pulmonary diseases such as bronchiectasis and chronic obstructive pulmonary disease are prone to deterioration of pulmonary function during and after episodes of infection. This underscores the importance of prophylaxis and early management during each episode of respiratory infection.

## VIRAL PNEUMONIA

Viral infections of the respiratory tract occur commonly as epidemics in the general population or in small groups such as schoolchildren or army recruits (Table 65-2). However, sporadic cases do occur both in healthy and immunocompromised hosts. Children and debilitated older patients, especially those with underlying cardiopulmonary disorders, can become the victims of viral pneumonia or the associated secondary bacterial infections.

### Influenza and Parainfluenza Viruses

Of all the viruses, influenza and parainfluenza viruses cause the most serious respiratory infections. Influenza causes significant morbidity and mortality, either directly or secondary to bacterial superinfection. The major effect of the parainfluenza virus is in causing severe upper respiratory infections in children.

Influenza viruses are classified by their antigenic variation and are denoted by the initial place of isolation. They belong to the Orthomyxo viruses. Surface projections possess hemagglutinin and neuraminidase activity and are the antigenic determinants. Antigenic variability causes the perpetuation of infection. Horses, pigs, and birds serve as reservoirs.

### Hantavirus Pulmonary Syndrome

Hantaviruses have been isolated from rodents, predominantly in the southwestern United States. In May, 1993, an outbreak of rapidly, progressive respiratory failure was identified to be caused by Hantavirus, related to the Hantaan viruses of hemorrhagic fever. Subsequently, similar cases have been reported from areas other than the

**Table 65-2.** Common Respiratory Viruses

Influenza A and B
Parainfluenza 1 and 3
Respiratory syncytial virus*
Adenovirus
Cytomegalovirus†
Herpes simplex and zoster
Hantavirus infection‡

* Predominant infection in children.
† Infection in an immunocompromised host.
‡ Recent cluster cases of hantavirus pulmonary syndrome.

four-corner area of New Mexico, Arizona, Colorado, and Utah. The Hantavirus belongs to the Bunyaviridae family. Acute febrile illness culminates in a capillary leak syndrome leading to respiratory failure and shock. Early supportive care, hemodynamic and respiratory support, and experimental treatment with the intravenous antiviral agent, ribavirin, constitute the present approach for this deadly infection. Diagnosis depends on suspicion in patients from endemic areas and serologic confirmation with acute and convalescent serology.

### Other Viral Infections

Respiratory syncytial viruses generally cause lower respiratory infections, again usually in children. Rhinovirus (the virus of the common cold), adenovirus, Coxsackie A and B, and echoviruses cause predominantly upper respiratory infections. It is important to differentiate these infections from pneumonia, and the potential for secondary bacterial infection should be recognized. Herpesvirus and lymphocytic choriomeningitis virus also cause pneumonia in healthy and in compromised hosts. The measles virus causes predominantly mucosal inflammation leading to bronchitis and bronchiolitis. An overwhelming interstitial pneumonia from this infection can occur. Secondary bacterial infections are common following epidemics of measles, usually in debilitated infants and children.

Varicella-zoster infection causes pneumonia. Adults with chickenpox can develop an interstitial pneumonia as a complication. Although varicella pneumonia is often self-limiting, at times it is associated with severe systemic disorders, such as encephalitis and myelitis, and adult respiratory distress syndrome (ARDS) requiring ventilatory management.

Cytomegalovirus (CMV) pneumonia is a well-recognized complication among transplant recipients and in AIDS patients.

### Pathology and Pathogenesis

Influenza and viruses in general are known for their potential to cause respiratory infection rapidly after exposure, often spreading like a brush fire in the susceptible population. Droplet particles containing the virus are carried as aerosols and are deposited in the airways. Within 24 to 48 h, symptomatic disease develops. Mucosal and interstitial inflammation and impaired mucociliary clearance predispose to secondary bacterial infection. Interstitial pneumonia, either due to infection or an antigen-antibody response, occurs in a small group of patients. If pneumonia is diffuse and progressive, acute hypoxemic respiratory failure results.

### Diagnosis

Viral pneumonia is diagnosed in a patient presenting with chest pain, cough, fever, and dyspnea during the flu season. Patients usually complain of a prodrome comprising malaise, upper respiratory symptoms, and, often, gastrointestinal symptoms. Clinical findings are minimal and variable. Chest examination may reveal wheezing. Fine rales, if heard, are indicative of interstitial involvement. Chest x-ray may show patchy densities or interstitial involvement. In cases complicated by respiratory failure, there is diffuse radiographic involvement indistinguishable from other causes of ARDS.

Leukocytosis is mild (the white blood cell count is 10,000 to 15,000). Gram stain of the sputum will not demonstrate bacteria in substantial quantities. Confirmation of the diagnosis is based on the identification of viral particles and serologic studies. Secretions from the respiratory tract during this phase of pneumonia can be used for isolation of the virus. The immunofluorescent staining technique is an excellent aid in the rapid diagnosis of influenza infections. Serologic tests, though not helpful in the acute setting, are extremely useful in epidemiologic studies. Rapid diagnosis of viral, bacterial, mycoplasmal, and chlamydial infection by DNA probe and polymerase chain reaction (PCR), once they become routinely available, will be a major breakthrough in management of community-acquired pneumonias. If

secondary bacterial infection is suspected, appropriate studies should be undertaken. Fiberoptic bronchoscopy with broncho-alveolar lavage is useful in isolating the agents from the lower respiratory tract and excluding other forms of pneumonia. On occasion, a lung biopsy is necessary for definitive diagnosis.

### Management and Prophylaxis

Supportive treatment of viral pneumonia is aimed at decreasing the severity of symptoms. General management should include bed rest, analgesics, and expectorants. Older patients must guard against dehydration, and some may require parenteral fluid therapy. Patients with significant airway obstruction should be treated with bronchodilators, including theophylline and aerosolized $\beta_2$ agonists. Associated bacterial infections like the secondary staphylococcal infection should be treated with appropriate antibiotics.

Severity of respiratory functional impairment should be assessed with pulmonary function studies, arterial blood gas analysis, and close assessment of the patient's clinical status. In case of progressive respiratory difficulty, supportive respiratory care should include oxygen supplementation and, if necessary, ventilatory assistance.

Amantadine (1-adamantanamine hydrochloride) has been shown to have in vitro action against influenza A virus. This drug is useful for specific treatment and in prophylaxis. If started following exposure or within the first 48 h of infection, treatment results in reduction of clinical symptoms. This drug is advised in high-risk patients who could not be vaccinated prior to the flu season. Amantadine is given in doses of 100 to 200 mg daily. For prophylaxis amantadine should be used throughout the flu season. Side effects have been noted in 5 to 7 percent of patients taking the drug and are due to its CNS effects. Insomnia, jitteriness, difficulty in concentrating, dizziness, and rarely syncopal episodes have been described. The drug and its metabolites are excreted by the kidneys and should be used with caution in patients with renal disease.

Aerosolized ribavirin has been found to be useful against upper and lower respiratory infections caused by respiratory syncytial virus. Acyclovir is useful in the treatment of herpes viral infections.

### Influenza Vaccine

High attack rates have been noted in recent epidemics of influenza. An increase in the size of the elderly population and in the survival rates of patients with chronic pulmonary diseases such as cystic fibrosis has compelled us to be more vigorous in preventing influenza. Influenza vaccine is effective against influenza A and B viruses. Attenuated whole or split viruses are used in vaccine manufacture. The formulation of vaccine is determined by the World Health Organization (WHO) and the Centers for Disease Control and Prevention. Emphasis is on effective vaccination of the majority of the high-risk groups (Table 65-3). Current vaccines cause minimal side effects and have not been associated with Guillain-Barré syndrome.

### *Mycoplasma* PNEUMONIA

### Introduction

*Mycoplasma pneumoniae,* traditionally known to cause mild upper respiratory infection, is an important agent capable of causing pneu-

**Table 65-3.** High-Risk Patients and Groups Targeted for Influenza Vaccination

1. Adults and children with chronic cardiopulmonary disorders
2. Residents of nursing homes and other institutions
3. Healthy individuals over the age of 65 years
4. Adults and children with chronic metabolic disorders: diabetes mellitus, renal failure, anemia, immunosuppression
5. Medical personnel who have contact with high-risk patients

monia in otherwise healthy individuals. *M. pneumoniae* lacks a cell wall and this feature makes it resistant to common antibiotics which act on the cell wall. This agent is dispersed widely in the environment and accounts for nearly 25 percent of community-acquired pneumonia. It can cause extrapulmonary manifestations such as meningitis, encephalitis, pericarditis, hepatitis, and hemolytic anemia.

## Pathology and Pathogenesis

The cell structure of *Mycoplasma* is conducive to receptor attachment to host cell membranes, causing an inflammatory response in host cells. The predominant direct effect is hyperemia and polymorphonuclear leukocyte response. Host response is the production of IgG and IgM antibodies. An aggressive host response rather than the direct infection may result in predominant clinical manifestations. The exact pathogenesis of *Mycoplasma* pneumonia is not clear. Pneumonia is probably a postinfectious hypersensitivity phenomenon mediated by T lymphocytes. The delay in manifestation of pneumonia, lack of *Mycoplasma* antigen in fulminant cases, and the difficulty in identifying the agent in body fluids other than sputum, support this theory. Hence, it is likely that *Mycoplasma* infection results usually in bronchitis with the capability of an aggressive hypersensitivity pneumonia mediated by humoral and cellular mechanisms.

## Clinical Manifestations

Manifestations include upper and lower respiratory symptoms with varying severity, often associated with headache, malaise, and fever. The spectrum of disease, which is widespread, extends from a "trivial cold," pharyngitis, and bronchitis to an acute interstitial pneumonia culminating in respiratory failure.

Patients with pneumonia (fewer than 10 percent of cases) have initial upper respiratory symptoms followed by fever, chills, cough, headache, and malaise. The cough is nonproductive and often annoying and is due to bronchitis, airway obstruction, or an interstitial form of pneumonia. In some patients the cough may become chronic and may last for 4 to 6 weeks, representing a postbronchitic airway hyperreactivity phenomenon associated with significant airway obstruction. Earache is helpful in the diagnosis of *Mycoplasma* pneumonia, especially if bullous myringitis can be identified. In patients with chronic obstructive lung diseases, as with any other associated infections, there is exacerbation of airway obstruction. Manifestations of extrapulmonary involvement include musculoskeletal and gastrointestinal symptoms. Pleural involvement is rare and is manifested by pleuritic pain and in a minority of cases, pleural effusion. Splenomegaly and lymphadenopathy are rare. Central nervous system involvement could lead to aseptic meningitis and encephalitis. In uncomplicated disease, symptoms abate within a week to 10 days. Treatment reduces the duration and intensity of both respiratory and systemic symptoms.

## Complications and Extrapulmonary Manifestations

Most patients have self-limited disease and respond well to antibacterial treatment with erythromycin. Acute complications are due to hypoxemic respiratory failure leading to adult respiratory distress syndrome. Secondary bacterial infection in a small number of cases increases the morbidity. Other complications include increased airway reactivity, atelectasis, mediastinal adenopathy, pneumothorax, pleural effusion, and lung abscess.

Extrapulmonary manifestations are not necessarily complications. They may precede the pneumonia or occur during the pneumonia. Headache is often associated with pneumonia and is mild. Aseptic meningitis and (rarely) encephalitis with pleocytosis in the CSF have been described. Guillain-Barré syndrome can occur, though this is uncommon. Serologic changes are often a manifestation of infection. Rarely, hemolytic anemia results from the hemolytic potential of the cold agglutinins. Significant hemolysis is rare, and if it occurs it usually develops during the recovery phase. On rare occasions hemolysis leads to renal failure, thromboembolism, and disseminated intravascular coagulopathy. Cardiac complications result from pericarditis and myocarditis with the clinical manifestations of chest pain, congestive cardiac failure, pericardial effusion, and cardiac arrhythmia, including heart block.

## Laboratory Findings

Moderate leukocytosis (>10,000/μL) is the rule and leukopenia is rare. Exceptionally high counts over 25,000/mm³ are seen rarely. A negative tuberculin skin test, due to a transient suppression of delayed hypersensitivity, and a false-positive VDRL have been reported.

ECG changes are seen in patients with myocardial and pericardial invo. Findings of pericarditis, myocarditis, and nonspecific ST- and T- wave changes along with cardiac arrhythmias are seen occasionally.

Sputum studies help to distinguish this disease from acute bacterial infections by the lack of identifiable organisms. Specific diagnosis is dependent on isolation of the organism in the phase of acute infection or the demonstration of rise in antibody titers. These tests do not serve as an immediate tool at the time of initial presentation, yet they are very helpful in confirmation of the diagnosis. Culture and identification take 7 to 10 days. Enriched media that enhance the rapidity of growth and the detection of *mycoplasma* antigen by DNA probes and PCR hold promise for rapid diagnosis of the causative agent in the future.

## Serology

Complement-fixing antibody titers are diagnostic if there is a fourfold increase in the titers. If the initial titer is >$\frac{1}{64}$ it is highly suggestive of the infection. This IgM antibody rises at about the tenth day, peaks at 4 to 6 weeks, and could last as long as 6 months.

## Cold Agglutinins

This IgM antibody capable of fixing complement is also directed against the I antigens of the red blood cells. Titers >$\frac{1}{64}$ in the acute phase and a fourfold rise during the convalescent period are diagnostic. The hemagglutination property can be used as a bedside test, but it cannot be overemphasized that cold agglutinins are nonspecific and rise in both infectious and noninfectious disorders (Table 65-4).

## Radiology

Patchy densities to dense consolidation involving a whole lobe may be seen. An acute interstitial pneumonia, characterized by a reticulonodular pattern, is usually accompanied by significant pulmonary functional impairment, at times leading to respiratory failure, in which case the findings are indistinguishable from other causes of ARDS. Cavities, pneumatoceles, abscesses, significant pleural effusions, mediastinal adenopathy, and atelectasis have been described with clinically suspected *Mycoplasma* infection. However, these manifestations are rare and every attempt should be made to exclude an associated bacterial infection or other diagnosis if such features are present.

**Table 65-4.** Some Conditions Associated with Elevated Cold Agglutinin Titers

1. *Mycoplasma* pneumonia
2. Other viral pneumonias
3. Tuberculosis
4. Collagen vascular disorders
5. Malignancy
6. Lymphoma

## Management

Erythromycin is the drug of choice in *Mycoplasma* infections. Penicillin, which acts by destroying the cell wall of organisms, is ineffective due to the lack of a defined cell wall in these organisms. Tetracycline is also effective against *Mycoplasma* infection. Over a third of community-acquired pneumonias are caused by *Mycoplasma* chlamydia, rickettsia, viruses and *Legionella* organisms, designated as *atypical pneumonia*. Typical bacterial pneumonias, if suspected, are treated with penicillins and cephalosporins. First-line therapy for community-acquired pneumonia, if suspected to be due to an atypical organism, is erythromycin or tetracycline. The new macrolides, clarithromycin and azithromycin, have broad-spectrum bacterial coverage and are effective against atypical organisms. Their longer action and pharmacokinetics are well suited for outpatient treatment. Quinolones are not effective against *Streptococcus pneumonia* and should be avoided if *S. pneumonia* has not been excluded as the cause of pneumonia. The drug treatment reduces the duration of illness and decreases the severity of clinical symptoms during the period of illness. Treatment should be continued for 10 to 14 days, and the possibility of recurrence should be considered because *Mycoplasma* organisms can be isolated up to 12 weeks after drug treatment.

Supportive treatment should include bronchodilators, expectorants, analgesics, and antipyretics. Cough is often bothersome and may last weeks after the acute infection. Codeine-containing cough suppressants are useful in management. Patients with marked respiratory symptoms will require hospitalization.

## Chlamydial Pneumonia

The chlamydia group of organisms consists of *Chlamydia psittaci, C. trachomatis,* and the newly described TWAR strain. They are a well-known cause of urogenital tract infections and are also capable of causing an atypical pneumonia. Pneumonia occurs as a sporadic case or in small epidemics. *C. psittaci* causes infections in patients who have had contact with infected birds harboring these organisms. Clinical features are indistinguishable from other forms of atypical pneumonia. TWAR pneumonia outbreaks have been known to occur in young adults. They are characterized by a prodrome of upper respiratory infection. Pulmonary symptoms include cough, chest pain, mucoid-to-greenish sputum production, and findings of diffuse or localized parenchymal involvement. In some studies, TWAR strain accounted for pneumonia in up to 6 percent of cases. Serologic studies and special cultures are useful in confirming the diagnosis due to this group of organisms. Treatment consists of the use of erythromycin, 1 g/day for 5 to 10 days. This regimen has been inadequate in some patients with TWAR infection. They require treatment with tetracycline, 2 g/day for 7 to 10 days. The newer macrolides, clarithromycin and azithromycin, have good in vitro and in vivo activity against the *Chlamydia* TWAR organism.

## COMPARATIVE ANALYSIS OF COMMUNITY-ACQUIRED PNEUMONIA

This chapter would be incomplete without describing the differential features of common pneumonias, both typical and atypical. Table 65-5 gives a list of agents capable of causing atypical pneumonia in normal and debilitated hosts. The emergency physician is faced with the task of separating various forms of pneumonia with limited data. Initial analysis has to be thorough and complete in laying the groundwork for a definitive diagnosis, which may be possible at a later time. Separating a normal from an immunocompromised host becomes very important in the diagnosis and management. Underlying cardiopulmonary or other disorders that predispose to certain forms of bacterial pneumonia should be diagnosed appropriately. Separating pneumonia from severe laryngotracheal bronchitis is difficult at times. Once the diagnosis of pneumonia is established, the next step

**Table 65-5.** Atypical Pneumonias

1. *Mycoplasma* pneumonia
2. *Legionella* pneumonia
3. Viral pneumonia
4. *Chlamydia* pneumonia
5. Rickettsial pneumonia
6. Atypical presentation of a bacterial pneumonia

is the identification of an etiologic agent and a logical approach to management.

The spectrum of pneumonia extends from a simple, uncomplicated *Mycoplasma* pneumonia in a previously healthy individual to a complicated gram-negative pneumonia with sepsis in a debilitated elderly nursing home patient. Differentiating features are extremely helpful in distinguishing various forms of pneumonia. Physical and radiographic findings usually portray the severity of infection and do not help in defining an etiology.

Following are some of the common features that help to distinguish different forms of pneumonia:

1. Mixed bacterial infections are common in patients with chronic pulmonary disorders such as chronic bronchitis, emphysema, and bronchiectasis.
2. Anaerobic and gram-negative infections occur commonly in alcoholics and in patients prone to develop aspiration pneumonia.
3. Staphylococcal infection occurs following viral pneumonia.
4. *Legionella* pneumonia occurs in the summer months as opposed to the winter months in elderly patients.
5. A patchy, consolidative radiographic pattern with a diffuse finding of rales on examination are often the features of nonbacterial pneumonia.
6. Predominant upper airway symptoms preceding the development of pneumonia are indicative of a viral of *Mycoplasma* pneumonia.
7. Earache with bullous myringitis is a feature of *Mycoplasma* pneumonia.
8. Dense consolidation with a bulging fissure in a chest x-ray is indicative of *Klebsiella* pneumonia, especially in an alcoholic patient.
9. Elderly patients with severe constitutional and gastrointestinal symptoms and with relative bradycardia should be suspected of having *Legionella* pneumonia.
10. Chlamydia TWAR pneumonia occurs more commonly than previously recognized and often occurs as a cluster of cases in dormitories, prisons, and army barracks.

Combined features of bacterial and viral infections are indicative of concurrent bacterial infection. Travel, occupation, animal exposures, and environmental factors are helpful in diagnosing chlamydial infections, tularemia, Q fever, and especially noninfectious forms of hypersensitivity pneumonias that share the manifestations of community-acquired pneumonia. Recently described Hantavirus infection occurs in areas where there is exposure to rodents, especially deer mice, in the Southwestern United States. High leukocyte counts with polymorphonuclear leukocytosis suggest a bacterial etiology. Elevated liver enzymes with hypophosphatemia have been reported with *Legionella* infections. Multilobar involvement, especially the superior segments of lower lobes, with early findings of cavitation, should be diagnostic of anaerobic infections following an episode of aspiration. Multiple patchy lesions with a cavity or pneumatocele suggest the crucial possibility of septic pulmonary embolism, and the importance of this distinction cannot be overemphasized because of the radical difference in management. In the patient with risk factors for acquired immunodeficiency syndrome (AIDS) (i.e., homosexuals, intravenous drug addicts, patients requiring repeated transfusions), pulmonary infections with opportunistic organisms such as *Pneumocystis carinii*, cytomegalovirus, and *Mycobacterium avium-*

*intracellulare,* should be suspected. Lastly, this chapter is incomplete without emphasizing the need to rule out tuberculosis, both for epidemiologic reasons and proper patient management. A disease so common in the past still could be confusing to a young physician, since the manifestations are varied.

## BIBLIOGRAPHY

Brillman JC, Sklar DP, Davis KD, et al: Hantavirus: Emergency Department response to a disaster from an emerging pathogen. *Ann Emerg Med* 24:429, 1994.

Clyde WA Jr: Clinical overview of typical *Mycoplasma pneumoniae* infections (review). *Clin Infect Dis* 17(suppl 1):S32–6, 1993.

Dolin R, Reichman RC, Madore HP, et al: A controlled trial of amantadine and rimantadine in the prophylaxis of influenza A infection. *N Engl J Med* 307:580, 1982.

Duchin JS, Koster FT, Peters CJ, et al: Hantavirus pulmonary syndrome: A clinical description of 17 patients with a newly recognized disease. *N Engl J Med* 330:949, 1994.

Fass RJ: Aetiology and treatment of community-acquired pneumonia in adults: An historical perspective (review). J *Antimicrob Chemother* 32(supplA):17, 1993.

Glezen WP: Viral pneumonia as a cause and result of hospitalization. *J Infect Dis* 147:765, 1983.

Hall CB, McBride JT, Gala CL, et al: RIbavirin treatment of respiratory syncytial viral infection in infants with underlying cardiopulmonary diksease. *JAMA* 254:3047, 1985.

Helms CM, Viner JP, Strum RH, et al: Comparative features of pneumococcal, mycoplasmal and Legionnaires' disease pneumonias. *Ann Intern Med* 90:543, 1979.

Jacobs E: Serological diagnosis of *Mycoplasma pneumoniae* infections: A critical review of current procedures (review). *Clin Infect Dis* 17(suppl 1):S79, 1993.

LaForce FM: Antibacterial therapy for lower respiratory tract infections in adults. A review. *Clin Infect Dis* 14(suppl 2):S233, discussion S244, 1992.

Luby JP: Pneumonia caused by *Mycoplasma pneumoniae* infection (review). *Clin Chest Med* 12(2):237, 1991.

Marrie TJ, Grayston JT, Want SP, et al: Pneumonia associated with the TWAR strain of *Chlamydia. Ann Intern Med* 106:507, 1987.

Murray HW, Masur H, Senterfilt LB, et al: The protean manifestations of *Mycoplasma* pneumonia infections in adults. *Am J Med* 58:220, 1975.

Prevention and control of influenza. *MMWR* 33:253, 1984.

Ruben FL, Nguyen ML: Viral pneumonitis (review). *Clin Chest Med* 12(2):223, 1991.

Thom DH, Grayston JT: Infections with *Chlamydia pneumoniae* strain TWAR (review). *Clin Chest Med* 12(2):245, 1991.

Wijnands GJ: Diagnosis and interventions in lower respiratory tract infections (review). *Am J Med* 92 (4A):91S, 1992.

# 66
# PNEUMONIAS IN IMMUNOCOMPROMISED PATIENTS
## Mark Zwanger

Immunocompromised patients are susceptible to a wide variety of common as well as unusual pulmonary pathogens. Patients at highest risk for being immunocompromised include individuals with acquired immunodeficiency syndrome (AIDS) or congenital immune deficiencies, organ transplant recipients, and patients on chemotherapeutic or steroid medications (Table 66-1). It is essential to assess for underlying immunodeficiency in the emergency department, since the immunocompromised patient with respiratory complaints is less able

**Table 66-1.** Immunodefect, Disease Process, and Organisms to which Patients Are More Susceptible

| Immunologic Impairment | Disease Process | Organisms |
|---|---|---|
| **B-lymphocyte defect** (humoral-mediated) | Lymphoma<br>Leukemia<br>Multiple myeloma<br>Hypogammaglobulinemia<br>Agammaglobulinemia<br>Chemotherapy<br>Glucocorticoids<br>Burns | *S. pneumoniae*<br>*H. influenzae*<br>*P. aeruginosa* |
| **T-lymphocyte defect** (cell-mediated) | Lymphoma<br>AIDS<br>Carcinoma<br>Sarcoma<br>Chemotherapy<br>Renal Insufficiency<br>Glucocorticoids<br>Radiation therapy<br>Organ transplantation | Bacteria<br>  *N. asteroides*<br>  *L. pneumophilia*<br>  *M tuberculosis*<br>  *M. avium intracellulare*<br>Fungi<br>  *P. carinii*<br>  *C. neoformans*<br>  *H. capsulatum*<br>  *C. immitis*<br>  *Candida* sp.<br>Viruses<br>  Cytomegalovirus<br>  Herpes simplex<br>  Varicella-zoster<br>Protozoa<br>  *T. gondii*<br>  *S. stercoralis* |
| **Granulocyte defect** | Neutropenia<br>Myeloid metaplasia<br>Leukemia<br>Glucocorticoids<br>Chemotherapy | Gram-negative bacilli<br>  *E. coli*<br>  *K. pneumoniae*<br>  *P. aeruginosa*<br>  *S. marcescens*<br>Gram-positive bacilli<br>  *S. aureus*<br>Fungi<br>  *Aspergillus*<br>  *Mucor*<br>  *Candida* |
| **Splenic defect** | Sickle cell anemia<br>Splenectomy | *S. pneumoniae*<br>*H. influenzae* |

to ward off lung infections.

When evaluating for pneumonia in immunocompromised patients, it is useful to classify the underlying type of immunodeficiency, the temporal relationship of the disease, the onset and rapidity of disease progression, and the radiographic appearance. It is also important to note travel histories and local disease patterns within a particular geographical region and within individual hospitals.

The underlying immunodefect can suggest the type of organism responsible for the patient's pneumonia. As examples, individuals who have abnormalities in immunoglobulin synthesis are more likely to have difficulty with encapsulated bacteria; defects in neutrophil function predispose to both bacterial and fungal organisms; and cellular defects predispose to infections with opportunistic organisms (Table 66-1).

The clinical presentation and temporal relationship of the pulmonary infection assists in diagnosis. The acuity and onset of disease symptoms aids in differentiating between more routine bacterial causes of pneumonia (*Streptococcus pneumoniae, Staphylococcus aureus,* and gram-negative bacilli), which typically have an onset of less than 24 h and more subacute or chronic processes. A subacute process of several days to a week is commonly seen with most opportunistic infections, whereas a more chronic and indolent course of 1 or more weeks suggests a fungal etiology, mycobacteria, or nocardia. It is also essential to ascertain whether clinical symptoms started before or after certain treatment procedures such as radiation therapy, chemotherapy, or immunosuppressive therapy. For example, in transplant recipients, cytomegalovirus, aspergillus, nocardia, and mycobacteria pulmonary infections occur more commonly during the first 1 to 2 months after transplantation, while pneumocystis and cryptococcus are more likely causes of pneumonia at 6 months.

Although no one radiographic pattern is pathognomonic, the chest roentgenogram can suggest a particular organism as the etiologic agent causing pulmonary disease. A roentgenogram with a consolidation pattern is more likely to be from common gram-positive and -negative bacteria, legionella, nocardia, mycobacteria, aspergillus, or cryptococcus. Diffuse patterns of pulmonary infiltrates are seen with bacterial organisms, pneumocystis, disseminated histoplasmosis, miliary tuberculosis, and viral infections such as cytomegalovirus or herpes simplex. Nodular or cavitary patterns are more often caused by nocardia, *Staph. aureus,* cryptococcus, aspergillus, legionella, tuberculosis, bacterial lung abscess, and by *Rhodococcus equi* on rare occasions. Lastly, not all infiltrates are from an infectious etiology but may represent progression of the patient's basic disease process to the lungs, drug-induced pneumonitis, radiation pneumonitis, pulmonary oxygen toxicity, nonspecific pneumonitis, or pulmonary malignancy associated with immunosuppression.

History of travel and geographic distribution of organisms aid in diagnosis. Coccidioidomycosis, histoplasmosis, and blastomycosis have distinct geographical regions of predominance. Lastly, hospital and nursing home facilities typically have their own particular predilection for nosocomially acquired infections, with aspergillus and legionella the more common causes.

The following sections present an overview of the more common pneumonias in immunocompromised patients.

## *Pneumocystis carinii* PNEUMONIA

Prior to the AIDS epidemic, *Pneumocystis carinii* pneumonia (PCP) was relatively uncommon, with approximately 100 cases reported per year. Since the start of the AIDS epidemic in 1981, *P. carinii* has become the most common opportunistic infection in HIV patients, with more than 100,000 cases of PCP reported. The annual incidence of PCP in AIDS patients is approximately 30 percent, with a case-fatality rate of 20 percent per episode. Case attack rates of 20 to 40 percent are seen in patients with solid tumors and in children with acute hematologic problems.

Approximately 60 to 85 percent of HIV-infected individuals not receiving chemoprophylaxis therapy against *P. carinii* will develop PCP as their first opportunistic infection. This infection is most likely to occur when the CD4 T-lymphocyte count falls below 200 cells/mm³. The organism is an opportunistic pathogen that persists in a latent phase and can cause disease whenever the host's immune system is compromised. PCP can also occur from a new primary infection or reinfection. PCP can occur as a new primary infection or reinfection.

### Transmission and Incubation

*P. carinii* is ubiquitous in nature, although the natural habitat and mode of acquisition is unclear. It is commonly found in asymptomatic individuals and rarely causes disease except in immunosuppressive states. The infection is most likely transmitted by the airborne route. Most children have antibodies to the organism by the age of 4 years, which suggests a high incidence of exposure and subclinical infection by an early age. A slight seasonal variation, with summer greater than winter, has been noted.

Chagas noted the organism in guinea pig lungs in 1909. The first human reports of infection were described in the United States in the 1950s. The organism develops from a trophozoite into a cystic structure containing sporozoites. *P. carinii*'s life cycle is similar to that of both protozoa and fungi, and therefore its classification has been confusing; recent molecular biology studies suggest that the organism is most likely a fungus.

## Clinical Presentation

Clinical manifestations of PCP are nonspecific, range from mild to severe, and can be similar to other pneumonias. In HIV patients, PCP is usually more subacute and insidious in onset, whereas cancer and transplant patients have a more rapidly progressive clinical course. AIDS patients infected with PCP can be symptomatic for weeks prior to diagnosis.

The triad of fever, dyspnea, and cough in an HIV-infected individual should suggest PCP. A dry nonproductive cough is present in the majority of patients with PCP, with one-third of the patients reporting the production of sputum. The presence of cough in the HIV patient needs to be aggressively pursued, since this can be an initial presentation of PCP prior to radiographic evidence of PCP. Decreased exercise tolerance or exertional dyspnea is also indicative of *P. carinii* infection. The onset of respiratory symptoms aids in diagnosis, since the mean time prior to diagnosis of bacterial pneumonia is usually around 5 days, versus 21 days with PCP. Weight loss, chest pain, night sweats, chills, and fatigue can be present in PCP, but also should suggest the possibility of pulmonary tuberculosis.

Fever is noted in almost all patients, with a 2- to 3-week prodrome of fever to 39 to 40°C common. Tachypnea with a respiratory rate greater than 30 suggests a worse prognosis. Only a few rales, scattered rhonchi, or diminished breath sounds might be heard on examination since initial auscultatory findings are frequently normal or minimal. The absence of abnormal auscultatory sounds does not rule out the diagnosis of PCP.

Other clinical manifestations of immune suppression may be noted, such as oral candidiasis, hairy leukoplakia, seborrheic dermatitis, Kaposi's sarcoma, perineal herpes simplex, molluscum contagiosum, or generalized lymphadenopathy. When seen in HIV patients, these findings are suggestive of the potential development of other opportunistic infections, including PCP.

## Laboratory Studies

The white blood cell count characteristically is not elevated and shows no predominant pattern. Although leukopenia, lymphocytopenia, anemia, and thrombocytopenia occur, these findings are frequently secondary to drug therapy or manifestations of other disease processes. The T-helper cell count (CD4 lymphocyte count) is usually markedly reduced. Serum lactic dehydrogenase (LDH) is often elevated, with a rising LDH level or a value greater than 450 IU suggestive of PCP. Higher LDH levels suggest a worse prognosis, while LDH levels decrease as the infection is controlled. A low serum albumin is common and indicates a worse prognosis. An erythrocyte sedimentation rate (ESR) above 50 mm/h may be useful in helping to diagnose PCP.

While arterial blood gas abnormalities are common, a normal blood gas does not exclude the diagnosis of PCP. Hypoxia is almost uniformly present, with a $Pa_{O_2} < 70$ mmHg suggesting a worse prognosis. The majority of patients with PCP will have an elevated $P(A - a)_{O_2}$ gradient at rest. Three minutes of exercise testing at the bedside can frequently accentuate hypoxia in the symptomatic HIV-positive patient who has a normal chest radiograph. The patient should exercise while on a pulse oximetry monitor or have a repeat arterial blood gas drawn after exercise. If oxygen saturation drops by 3% or greater or if there is an increase of more than 10 mm Hg in the $P(A - a)_{O_2}$ gradient from rest, this suggests PCP as the cause.

Pulmonary function tests can be abnormal in HIV-infected patients and may be useful in the workup of a symptomatic patient with a normal chest radiograph. The diffusing capacity for carbon monoxide ($DL_{CO}$) is frequently decreased in these patients.

Gallium scans of the lung have sensitivities of 90 to 98 percent in patients with PCP but have a low specificity because of uptake by other HIV-related disease processes. Gallium scans can be useful in diagnosing PCP in the symptomatic patient who has both a normal chest x-ray and arterial blood gas. In these patients, a normal gallium lung scan has a positive predictive value of 96 percent for the patient not to have PCP. A combination of a negative gallium lung scan and a diffusion capacity greater than 80 percent virtually rules out the diagnosis of pulmonary infection from *P. carinii.* Technetium scanning of the lungs is currently undergoing investigation.

## Radiographs

The chest roentgenogram will be abnormal in 90 to 95 percent of patients. The most common radiographic finding is diffuse bilateral interstitial infiltrates extending from the hilum out into a "bat-wing" distribution (Fig. 66-1). As the infection progresses, infiltrates may involve all lung fields or produce consolidation. One-third of the patients present with an atypical appearance of asymmetric infiltrates, unilateral infiltrates, or infiltrates near the periphery of the lungs. The lung periphery and apices are frequently spared, except in patients on prophylactic aerosolized antibiotics who are likely to have disease predominantly in the upper lobes of the lungs. This pattern is thought to be a result of less of the aerosolized antibiotic reaching the upper lobes.

Radiographically, PCP can also present simulating tuberculosis with a cavitary or cystic appearance, as a solitary pulmonary nodule, as pulmonary edema, or as spontaneous unilateral or bilateral pneumothoraces. Bronchopleural fistulas, hilar lymphadenopathy, pulmonary cavitation, and pleural effusions can occur but are not common and should suggest other pulmonary disease processes. Up to 10 to 20 percent of patients with PCP infection can have a completely normal chest radiograph.

## Differential Diagnosis

The differential diagnosis for pneumonia in the immunocompromised patient includes infectious causes such as gram-positive and -negative bacterial pneumonias (streptococcus, staphylococcus, haemophilus, klebsiella, pseudomonas, *Escherichia coli,* chlamydia, legionella); mycobacterium; opportunistic organisms (pneumocystis, nocardia, protozoans); fungi; viral infections; rare and unusual pneumonias (*Pasteurella multocida, Yersinia enterocolitica, Rhodococcus equi, Paracoccidioides brasiliensis, Toxoplasma gondii, Strongyloides stercoralis,* and *Sporothrix schenckii*); and noninfectious processes such as lymphocytic interstitial pneumonitis, pulmonary hemorrhage, and drug or radiation toxicity. Concurrent pulmonary infections can occur in 10 to 20 percent of patients, and the physician should be alert for these coinfections.

## Diagnosis

Cytologic evaluation of induced sputum yields positive results for PCP inconsistently. The negative predictive value of sputum is only about 50 percent. Direct fluorescence assays using monoclonal antibodies are useful to detect *P. carinii* in sputum specimens, with assay sensitivities of near 90 percent. Sputum should also be Gram stained and examined for acid-fast bacilli and fungal organisms. Routine bacterial, fungal, and tuberculosis cultures must be done.

If sputum examination is unsuccessful for identification of the organism, fiberoptic bronchoscopy is the method of choice for the rapid diagnosis of PCP. The combination of transbronchial biopsy, bronchial brushings and washings, and bronchoalveolar lavage have a diagnostic yield for *P. carinii* of near 100 percent. Bronchoalveolar lavage alone has a sensitivity of 79 to 98 percent. For solitary lesions

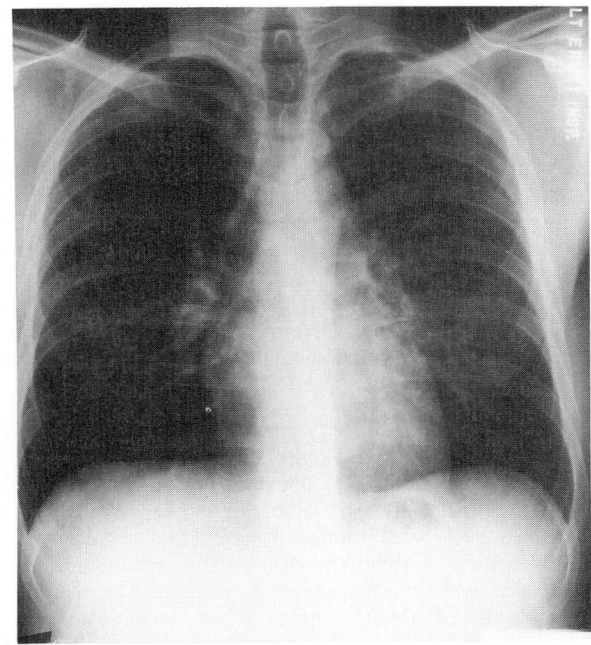

A

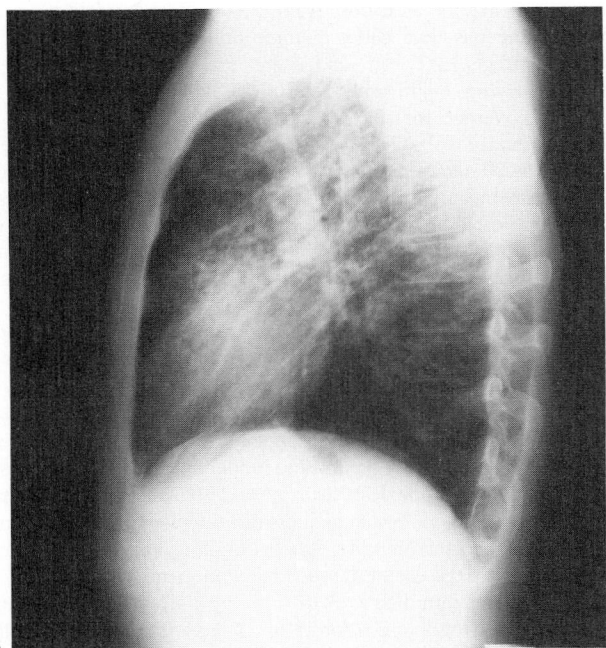

B

**Fig. 66-1.** Typical diffuse interstitial radiographic appearance of *P. carinii* pneumonia in the AIDS patient. **A.** AP view. **B.** Lateral view.

or cavitary lesions that might represent associated infections, fine-needle aspiration using computed tomography guidance assists in diagnosis. Open lung biopsy offers the greatest diagnostic yield but is expensive, time-consuming, and risks anesthesia and the complications of thoracotomy.

A general algorithmic approach to the HIV patient with pulmonary complaints is to begin with a chest radiograph and pulse oximetry. If the patient has a normal chest roentgenogram and the diagnosis of PCP is suspected clinically, arterial blood gas, exercise testing, and/or diffusing capacity of carbon monoxide should be performed. If oxygen saturation is <90 percent, or if $Pa_{O_2} < 60$ mm Hg, or if oxygen saturation falls with exercise, this suggests PCP. If oxygen saturation is >90% and the $Pa_{O_2} > 60$ mm Hg and the diagnosis is still suspected, additional studies with gallium studies, close follow-up, and a possible trial of outpatient antibiotics with trimethoprim/sulfamethoxazole are warranted.

## Treatment

Treatment of immunocompromised patients suspected of having PCP includes aggressive respiratory management and support, mechanical ventilation, antibiotics, and glucocorticoids. Patients should be admitted for treatment because they can acutely decompensate and there is a high incidence of adverse drug reactions. Oxygen therapy is guided by arterial blood gases and the results of pulse oximetry. If oxygen therapy with nasal cannula or simple face mask does not rapidly improve hypoxia, continuous positive airway pressure with a mask is useful, but is associated with potential complications of pneumothorax or pulmonary aspiration of gastric contents.

### Antibiotics

The initial drug treatment of choice is either trimethoprim/sulfamethoxazole (TMP/SMX), trimethoprim and dapsone, or pentamidine isethionate, with most studies suggesting similar efficacy and no clear preference for one regimen over the other. Because of the high incidence of adverse drug reactions with these medications, it is not uncommon for the patient to be started on one antibiotic and, because of side effects, have to be switched to another drug during therapy. Combination therapy with both TMP/SMX and pentamidine is not more advantageous than using a single antibiotic and increases the risk of side effects.

Many clinicians begin with TMP/SMX, which also provides antimicrobial coverage for some bacterial pneumonias and allows the patient eventually to be switched to oral medication. The dosage of TMP/SMX is 20 mg/kg per day of TMP and 75 to 100 mg/kg per day of SMX intravenously divided into four doses for 14 to 21 days. Estimates of side effects from TMP/SMX in AIDS patients range from 50 to 90 percent. Adverse reactions include fever, nausea, vomiting, bone marrow suppression, rash, increased liver enzymes, renal insufficiency, and electrolyte abnormalities. In the patient with a history of prior allergic reactions to sulfa drugs, renal failure, or blood cell dyscrasias (neutropenia, anemia, or thrombocytopenia), TMP/SMX should be avoided and pentamidine used.

Combination oral therapy with trimethoprim (20 mg/kg per day) and dapsone (100 mg/kg per day) appears to be as effective as the combination of TMP/SMX for mild to moderate PCP. The benefits of this combination include less toxicity and the continuation of this therapy as an outpatient. Some patients develop asymptomatic methemoglobinemia, and screening for glucose-6-phosphate dehydrogenase deficiency prior to the use of dapsone is recommended.

The dose of pentamidine is 3 to 4 mg/kg daily as a single intravenous infusion over 1 to 2 h for 14 to 21 days. The drug is instilled over a period of 1 to 2 h with frequent monitoring for hypotension. Up to fifty percent of patients on pentamidine develop adverse reactions including hypotension, tachycardia, facial flushing, pruritus, syncope, renal toxicity, elevated liver enzymes, taste disturbances, hallucinations, thrombocytopenia, rash, nausea, hypoglycemia, and pancreatitis.

Oral TMP/SMX or aerosolized pentamidine may also be used judiciously as initial therapy in patients with mild PCP, assuming close follow-up and a reliable patient.

As a last resort, trimetrexate gluconate with leucovorin rescue, difluoromethylornithine, or a combination of clindamycin and primaquine phosphate can be used in patients not responding to the more standard drug regimens.

### Glucocorticoid Therapy

Patients with PCP can be stratified into mild or severe cases based upon their arterial oxygen pressure or arterial-alveolar oxygen gradient. This distinction is important since it aids in differentiating who should receive steroids. A $P_{O_2} > 70$ mm Hg or arterial $P(A - a)_{O_2}$ gradient <35 mm Hg suggests a mild infection, and these patients have a more favorable prognosis than patients with a $P_{O_2} < 70$ mmHg or a $P(A - a)_{O_2}$ gradient >35 mm Hg who have severe pulmonary dysfunction and are more likely to have a grave prognosis.

Patients who have severe disease should be given glucocorticoid therapy as early as possible. Glucocorticoids as an adjunct in the therapy of severe PCP are clearly beneficial since they substantially reduce mortality, decrease respiratory failure, limit oxygen deterioration, and accelerate recovery. It is postulated that steroids act by reducing the lung's inflammatory response to *P. carinii* infection. Concerns about the possibility of increasing other life-threatening opportunistic infections or augmenting the spread of Kaposi's sarcoma by using steroids have not been realized, although steroid use can predispose to oral thrush and herpes infections. The following regimen is based upon the consensus recommendations of the National Institutes of Health. In patients with severe pulmonary disease, oral prednisone in the dose of 40 mg twice a day is given for days 1 through 5, 40 mg daily on days 6 through 10, and then 20 mg daily on days 11 through 21. Alternatively, intravenous methylprednisolone can be given at 75 percent of these dosages. There is currently no compelling information to suggest that steroids are beneficial in mild PCP.

## Prophylaxis

Patients with CD4 counts below 200 cells/mm$^3$ are at very high risk for developing PCP, and patients who are not on suppressive therapy and have had a prior infection with *P. carinii* have a 60 percent probability of developing a recurrent episode of PCP. These patients should be on prophylactic therapy with either oral TMP/SMX or inhaled pentamidine. Prophylactic therapy has reduced the rate of relapse by 50 to 80 percent to a recurrence rate of 6 to 16 percent.

Local side effects include cough and upper airway irritation and bronchospasm if on pentamidine. Systemic side effects are infrequent but can include hypoglycemia and pancreatitis. When on prophylaxis, these patients can develop atypical apical pneumonias and are more likely to present with disseminated *P. carinii* infection.

## Clinical Course and Prognosis

Compared to other patients with PCP, AIDS patients take longer to respond clinically and show slower radiographic improvement when treated. Since these patients can be unstable and decompensate quickly, they should be admitted for initial treatment of pneumocystis infection. Initial survival rates for PCP were approximately 57 percent. With more aggressive treatment, a wider spectrum of antibiotics available, and the use of steroids, survival rates approach 80 to 95 percent for the first PCP admission. AIDS patients may need a change in therapy if there is no clinical improvement in 4 to 5 days or if there is no radiographic improvement after 7 to 10 days. Patients needing a change in therapy usually do worse and have a higher mortality.

Respiratory failure can occur in as many as 30 percent of patients, and the need for mechanical ventilatory support is associated with a poor prognosis. Failure to respond to therapy indicates the need for reevaluation and a search for other infectious agents that might coexist. Patients who have mixed pulmonary infections and recurrent bouts of pneumonia have a worse prognosis.

Some authors suggest empirically treating patients who have clinical and radiographic features consistent with PCP and forgoing any further diagnostic studies. This approach is potentially dangerous since current recommendations include using steroids, which are lifesaving in PCP but potentially harmful in patients who have other bacterial or fungal pulmonary infections. Without a diagnosis, the treating physician will have difficulty knowing in which hypoxic patients to use steroids.

# MYCOBACTERIAL DISEASES

## *Mycobacterium tuberculosis*

Since 1986, there has been an increase in the annual incidence of tuberculosis (TB), reversing a declining rate of infection that had started in the 1950s with the advent of drugs effective in the treatment of tuberculosis. This increase parallels the development of HIV infection and is likely a consequence of HIV-positive patients either primarily developing TB or having reactivation of latent TB. The prevalence of TB in AIDS patients ranges from 2 to 20 percent. Tuberculosis is highly contagious and is spread by inhalation of infected aerosol droplets from one individual to another regardless of their immune status. The finding of acid-fast bacilli is presumptive evidence of active TB, and it should be treated until further microbiologic testing identifies the type of mycobacterium. Ultimate diagnosis depends on microbiological identification of sputum staining and slow-growing cultures.

The clinical presentation of tuberculosis in immunocompromised patients is similar to other patients who contract TB, with fever, malaise, night sweats, weight loss, chills, cough, dyspnea, productive sputum, hemoptysis, and pleuritic chest pain. Fever, tachypnea, and tachycardia are seen. Radiographic patterns can show cavitary disease of the upper lobes of the lungs, mediastinal adenopathy, or pleural effusion.

Another group of HIV patients can develop TB who are more atypical in presentation and have a greater degree of immunosuppression. On chest radiographs, these patients are less likely to show cavitary changes and instead mediastinal adenopathy, pleural effusions, or focal consolidation are seen.

Treatment involves a combination of at least two drugs and frequently more. A commonly used triple combination combines isoniazid, rifampin, and either pyrazinamide, ethambutol, or streptomycin. Increasingly, multidrug-resistant TB is being diagnosed and the quinolones or a macrolide may be of value as an additional fourth or fifth drug.

## *Mycobacterium avium-intracellulare* Complex

An unusual type of mycobacterium called *M. avium-intracellulare* complex (MAC) is commonly seen in AIDS patients who are very severely immunocompromised. MAC is the most likely organism in nontuberculous mycobacterial infections and tends to occur late in the course of HIV infection when the CD4 count is frequently less than 50 cells/mm$^3$. Less frequent pulmonary pathogens include *M. xenopi* and *M. kansasii*. In contrast to TB, which can occur at any level of immunity, these infections, while found in poultry and swine, are opportunistic in humans and are acquired from the environment rather than from person-to-person transmission. The organism is likely inhaled or invades across intestinal mucosa and may arise from infected aerosols, water, soil, or dust.

The clinical presentation includes the spectrum of asymptomatic to disseminated disease. Patients note cough, dyspnea, fever, sweats, malaise, and weakness. The chest radiographic appearance varies and can be normal or show diffuse interstitial or reticulonodular infiltrates. Apical scarring, hilar lymphadenopathy, cavitary disease, or pleural effusions are less likely. The ultimate diagnosis comes from microbiological identification of sputum cultures, blood cultures, bronchoalveolar lavage, or lung biopsy. A combination of drugs including amikacin, ethambutol, clorazimine, and rifabutin is one possible treatment regimen for MAC, with a quinolone added as needed.

# MYCOTIC INFECTIONS

## Endemic Fungi

*Histoplasma capsulatum, Blastomyces dermatitidis,* and *Coccidioides immitis* are particularly common to certain geographical regions but also occur worldwide. They have a soil-based saprophytic phase and a spore phase that can be inhaled and cause pulmonary disease.

*H. capsulatum* is endemic to the Mississippi and Ohio river valleys. The clinical presentation is usually latent reactivation of a prior exposure. The patient's symptoms may be minimal with an insidious progression, a febrile flulike state, or a full-blown life-threatening sepsis. Clinical findings include fever, weight loss, cough, dyspnea, or disseminated disease. Chest roentgenograms may show patchy nodular regions and resemble an atypical pneumonia in appearance, miliary pattern, cavitary lesions, hilar adenopathy, or appear normal. Diagnosis is made by either serology, culture, complement fixation or radioimmunoassay for antigen, or by histopathology. Drugs available for treatment include amphotericin B, ketoconazole, and the imidazoles. In AIDS patients, relapse rates are high and complete cure is unlikely.

*B. dermatitidis* is also found along the Mississippi and Ohio river valleys as well as in Wisconsin, Minnesota, and Michigan. Water activities appear to be a major risk factor. The patient may present with an asymptomatic presentation or overwhelming pneumonia. The chest radiograph can show fluffy nodules, consolidation, or hilar fibronodular disease suggesting the appearance of cancer. Diagnosis includes positive sputum examination and culture or cytologic examination of specimens for typical yeast forms. Treatment is either amphotericin B or ketoconazole.

*C. immitis* is found primarily in the southwestern United States and Mexico. The initial infection may be asymptomatic or flulike in presentation, with fever, cough, myalgias, dyspnea, headache, and nonspecific rash. The chest radiograph typically shows diffuse reticulonodular infiltrates, frequently with associated hilar lymphadenopathy. Solitary cavitation may also occur. The CBC might demonstrate eosinophilia. Spherules, characteristic cystlike spore structures, may be seen on examination of sputum, bronchoalveolar lavage, or histological specimens. Complement fixation antibody testing, immunodiffusion testing, and skin tests help in diagnosis. Amphotericin B is the drug of choice, although ketoconazole has been used for treatment.

## Cryptococcus, Aspergillus, Candida, and Mucorales

*Cryptococcus neoformans* is ubiquitous in nature and is found in soil and in high concentrations in pigeon droppings. Humans most likely acquire the organism from inhalation of spores. Isolated pulmonary disease is infrequently seen, with infections more likely presenting as meningitis or disseminated disease. Patients can present with fever, weight loss, cough, and chest pain. Severe arterial hypoxemia and a widened A − a gradient are common and can simulate PCP, making diagnosis more difficult.

Clinical clues such as the presence of a headache or meningeal signs should suggest the possibility of cryptococcus. Radiographic findings include localized or diffuse interstitial infiltrates and hilar adenopathy. The pulmonary diagnosis is based upon finding encapsulated yeast in cultures from sputum, blood, urine, or other tissues with India-ink preparations, suggesting the diagnosis. Latex agglutination test for cryptococcal antigen is highly sensitive and specific for *C. neoformans*. Amphotericin B in combination with flucytosine is currently recommended therapy.

*A. fumigatus* causes pulmonary infections in immunocompromised patients, especially after transplantation. This fungus is ubiquitous and is spread by inhalation of airborne spores. Clinically, the infection may be subacute with the patient complaining of fever, cough, dyspnea, hemoptysis, and generalized constitutional symptoms. Focal areas of consolidation with or without cavities may be seen on chest radiographs. Occasionally, a freely movable fungus ball may occur within cavitary pulmonary areas. Definitive diagnosis involves examination of bronchoalveolar lavage and transbronchial or open-lung biopsy. The organism is very resistant to treatment, and the use of intravenous amphotericin B has been less than efficacious. Surgical resection or intracavitary instillation of amphotericin B has been attempted.

*Candida* infection of the lungs is rare, and the presence of *Candida* in respiratory secretions more likely represents oropharyngeal contamination rather than pulmonary infection. Fever is frequently present, with radiographs demonstrating patchy infiltrates or nodules. *Mucor* infection is also uncommon and requires histopathologic confirmation.

## NOCARDIA AND ACTINOMYCOSIS

*Nocardia asteroides,* a bacteria, is found in soil and vegetable matter and likely infects through aerosolization. The organism may colonize only the airways without producing disease but can invade tissues and cause systemic disease. The organism is more often found in transplant recipients, patients with lymphoreticular neoplasms, and patients on chronic glucocorticoid therapy. Clinical presentation ranges from subacute infection to invasive pulmonary disease and disseminated spread. Fever, cough, chills, dyspnea, and pleurisy are seen. Radiographic patterns include consolidation, single or multiple nodules, cavitary formation, interstitial patterns, and pleural effusions. Evaluation of sputum, findings at bronchoscopy, or examination of infected tissues make the diagnosis. Trimethoprim/sulfamethoxazole or sulfonamides are usual therapy, although alternative medications include third-generation cephalosporins, imipenem, and amikacin.

Actinomycosis is an infrequent cause of pneumonia with the patient typically presenting with nonspecific constitutional findings. This is a suppurative process with extensive granulation and fibrous formation, and the diagnosis is frequently not suspected until the infection breaks through the chest wall with a draining sinus. Drug therapy includes penicillin, surgical drainage, and debridement as necessary.

## VIRAL INFECTIONS

### Cytomegalovirus

While CMV is commonly found in the respiratory tract it can either be a true pathogen causing pneumonia, as in transplant recipients (usually within 2 months after transplantation) and in patients on chemotherapy, or the virus can be a coexistent organism, as in the AIDS patient. In the HIV patient, this diagnosis should be made only after other pathogens have been excluded; culture results are positive for CMV; and when the clinical presentation includes fever, hypoxia, and pulmonary infiltrates. The radiographic pattern varies from focal nodules or infiltrates to a diffuse interstitial pattern. Treatment is with intravenous ganciclovir or foscarnet.

### Herpes Simplex and Varicella-Zoster

HSV is frequently found in oropharyngeal secretions, which raises concern as to whether the pneumonia is being caused by HSV or whether HSV is a contaminant since true HSV pneumonia is rare. Treatment is with intravenous acyclovir. Children with malignancies and transplant recipients are at risk for varicella pneumonitis. Varicella-zoster pneumonitis is diagnosed based upon the clinical presentation of chickenpox and a radiograph that shows pneumonia. Mortality is high, and immunocompromised patients with varicella pneumonitis should be treated with either vidarabine or acyclovir.

## BIBLIOGRAPHY

Anaissie E: Opportunistic mycoses in the immunocompromised host: Experience at a cancer center and review. *Clin Infect Dis* 14:S43, 1992.

Banks J: Treatment of pulmonary disease caused by opportunist mycobacteria. *Thorax* 44:449, 1989.

Barnes PF, Bloch AB, Davidson PT, et al: Tuberculosis in patients with human immunodeficiency virus infection. *N Engl J Med* 324:1644, 1991.

Bozette S, Sattler F, Chiu J, et al: A controlled trial of early adjunctive treatment with corticosteroids for *Pneumocystis carinii* pneumonia in the acquired immunodeficiency syndrome. *N Engl J Med* 323:1451, 1990.

Cameron ML, et al: Manifestations of pulmonary cryptococcosis in patients with acquired immunodeficiency syndrome. *Rev Infect Dis* 13:64, 1991.

Drabick JJ, Gasser RA, Saunders NB, et al: *Pasteurella multocida* pneumonia in a man with AIDS and nontraumatic feline exposure. *Chest* 103(1):7, 1993.

Friedman Y, Franklin C, Rackow EC, et al: Improved survival in patients with AIDS, *Pneumocystis carinii* pneumonia, and severe respiratory failure. *Chest* 96:862, 1989.

Gagnon S, Boota A, Fischl M, et al: Corticosteroids as adjunctive therapy for severe *Pneumocystis carinii* pneumonia in the acquired immunodeficiency syndrome. *N Engl J Med* 323:1444, 1990.

Greene JN, Herndon P, Nadler JP, et al: Case report: *Yersinia enterocolitica* necrotizing pneumonia in an immunocompromised patient. *Am J Med Sci* 305:171, 1993.

Guidelines for prophylaxis against *Pneumocystis carinii* pneumonia for persons infected with human immunodeficiency virus. *MMWR* 38(S5):1, 1989.

Horsburgh CR Jr: *Mycobacterium avium* complex in the acquired immunodeficiency syndrome. *N Engl J Med* 324:1332, 1991.

Katz MH, Baron RB, Grady D: Risk stratification of ambulatory patients suspected of *Pneumocystis* pneumonia. *Arch Intern Med* 151:105, 1991.

Kramer EL, Sanger JH, Garay SM, et al: Diagnostic implications of Ga-67 chest-scan patterns in human immunodeficiency virus–seropositive patients. *Radiology* 170:671, 1989.

Kramer MR, Uttamchandani RB: The radiographic appearance of pulmonary nocardiosis associated with AIDS. *Chest* 98(2):382, 1990.

Medina I, Mills J, Leonug G, et al: Oral therapy for *Pneumocystis carinii* pneumonia in the acquired immunodeficiency syndrome. A controlled trial of trimethoprim-sulfamethoxazole versus trimethoprim-dapsone. *N Engl J Med* 323:776, 1990.

Miller RF, Millar AB, Weller IVD, et al: Empirical treatment without bronchoscopy for *Pneumocystis carinii* pneumonia in the acquired immunodeficiency syndrome. *Thorax* 44:559, 1989.

National Institute of Health: Consensus statement on the use of corticosteroids as adjunctive therapy for *Pneumocystis carinii* in the acquired immunodeficiency syndrome. *N Engl J Med* 323:1500, 1990.

Pappas PG, et al: Blastomycosis in patients with the acquired immunodeficiency syndrome. *Ann Intern Med* 116:847, 1992.

Pursell KJ: Invasive pulmonary aspergillosis complicating neoplastic disease. *Semin Respir Infect* 7:96, 1992.

Rosenow EC, Wilson WR, Cockerill FR: Pulmonary disease in the immunocompromised host (parts 1 and 2). *Mayo Clin Proc* 60:473, 610, 1985.

Shelhamer JH, et al: Respiratory disease in the immunocompromised patient. *Ann Intern Med* 117:415, 1992.

Stover DE, Greeno RA, Fagliardi AJ: The use of a simple exercise test for the diagnosis of *Pneumocystis carinii* pneumonia in patients with AIDS. *Am Rev Respir Dis* 139:1343, 1989.

White DA, Zaman MK: Medical management of AIDS patients. Pulmonary disease. *Med Clin North Am* 76:19, 1992.

# 67

# ASPIRATION PNEUMONIA, EMPYEMA, AND LUNG ABSCESS

## Georges C. Benjamin

Aspiration pneumonia is an inflammation of the lung parenchyma resulting from the entrance of foreign material into the tracheobronchial tree. The clinical consequences of pulmonary aspiration of gastric contents were described in 1946 by Mendelson, who observed this complication in obstetrical patients undergoing anesthesia. Predisposing risks are depression of the cough or gag reflex, alterations in the normal physiologic handling of secretions or gastric contents, and structural alterations of the normal physiologic protective mechanisms.

## PATHOPHYSIOLOGY

The clinical and pathologic results of pulmonary aspiration depend on the pH of the aspirated material, the volume of the aspirate, the presence in the aspirate of particulate matter such as food, and bacterial contamination.

Aspiration of large particles of food or other objects that can cause upper airway obstruction is an important and easily reversible cause of mortality. This complication must be quickly recognized and treated.

### Neutral Fluids

It is generally accepted that serious injury results if the pH of the aspirate is 2.5 or less. However, many of the early pathologic changes are nonspecific and occur regardless of the pH of the aspirate. These include collapse and expansion of individual alveoli, reflex airway closure, and interstitial edema. These changes occur within seconds, producing significant ventilation-perfusion mismatch and marked hypoxia. If material with a pH greater than 2.5 is aspirated, the severity of injury depends additionally on the composition of the aspirate and the volume. The aspiration of lipid materials results in a chronic granulomatous reaction resulting in lipoid pneumonia. The consequences of aspiration of neutral, clear liquids are more easily reversible with supportive therapy; however, large-volume aspiration results in high mortality and morbidity.

### Neutral Fluids with Food Particles

Neutral fluids with food particles produce a persistent inflammatory reaction resulting in a hemorrhagic pneumonitis within 6 h after aspiration. As the pneumonitis progresses, a chronic granulomatous reaction develops which resembles the granuloma of pulmonary tuberculosis and may be visible on roentgenography.

### Acid Aspiration

The aspiration of fluids with a pH of less than 2.5 results in severe pulmonary changes analogous to those produced by a chemical burn. Volumes as low as 1 mL/kg have been shown to result in pathologic changes throughout the pulmonary parenchyma within seconds. These changes include reflex airway closure, destruction of surfactant-producing alveoli, alveolar collapse, and pulmonary capillary destruction. In the first few hours after aspiration, intrapulmonary mucosal hemorrhage, bronchial epithelial degeneration, and pulmonary edema occur. Shunting may be massive and pulmonary compliance decreases. The loss of integrity of the alveolocapillary bed results in large fluid losses that can be severe enough to require volume reple-

tion. Secondary bacterial infection results. In community-acquired aspiration, anaerobes comprise the most common bacterial isolates. In a patient who develops aspiration following hospitalization, gram-negative aerobes, including *Pseudomonas, Proteus,* and *Escherichia coli* in addition to anaerobes, are frequent isolates.

### Foreign Body Aspiration

Foreign body aspiration may represent an acute threat to life and is responsible for approximately 3000 deaths each year. Eighty percent of these cases occur in children, especially those under the age of 6. Running with food or other objects in the mouth, seizures, and forced feeding are common risk factors for this problem in children. In adults, it can result from dental or nasal surgery, unconsciousness, or poorly chewed food. Sixty percent of foreign bodies are found in the right bronchus, 19 percent in the left, and 21 percent at the larynx or cords. When complete obstruction occurs, death from asphyxiation occurs within minutes unless the condition is relieved. In these cases the patient usually is aphonic, cyanotic, and may be grabbing his or her throat. Prompt therapy with a chest or abdominal thrust is required for relief. Patients without complete obstruction present with spasmodic cough, choking, and wheezing. Physical examination may reveal fever, wheezing on the involved side, decreased breath sounds, hyperresonance on percussion, and asymmetric chest movement. Chest radiography will reveal the object if radiopaque. However, atelectasis, air trapping, or mediastinal shift on inspiratory and expiratory chest films are more commonly seen.

Therapy consists of prompt bronchoscopic removal. In some cases, tracheotomy or open thoracotomy and bronchotomy are required for removal. Patients who aspirate massive amounts of particulate matter such as dirt or sand have an increased risk for obstruction from impacted material. Bronchoscopy is indicated in severe cases; however, postural drainage with percussion has been demonstrated to be of benefit when used in a controlled setting.

Long-term complications from foreign body aspiration include bronchiectasis, hemoptysis, spontaneous perforation of the chest wall, abscess, emphysema, and pneumonia.

## CLINICAL FEATURES

Aspiration of fluid and oropharyngeal bacteria can occur in healthy persons during sleep. Pathologic aspiration also can be silent and a high index of suspicion must be maintained in order to detect this problem. Signs of hypoxemia such as tachypnea, tachycardia, and cyanosis may develop immediately or may not be present for a number of hours. Auscultation of the chest may disclose wheezing, rales, or rhonchi, and the patient may produce large amounts of frothy, bloody sputum.

Blood gas abnormalities include marked hypoxia with respiratory alkalosis. Severe aspiration may result in respiratory failure with a combined respiratory and metabolic acidosis.

Hypotension and hypovolemic shock may develop rapidly owing to the outpouring of fluid into the alveolar spaces. Although the clinical picture may resemble pulmonary edema, left ventricular function remains normal and hemodynamic monitoring usually reveals a high cardiac index with normal to low right-sided pressures.

The chest roentgenogram may show a diffuse alveolar and interstitial infiltrate or a segmental or lobar infiltrate. The lower lobe of the right lung is most frequently involved because the right mainstem bronchus courses more directly toward the right lower lobe. If the patient is in the Trendelenburg position, the infiltrates tend to involve the axillary segment of the right upper lobe and the apical segment of the right lower lobe.

Patients with chronic aspiration may have repeated bouts of pneumonia, especially involving the right lower lobe or the axillary segment of the right upper lobe.

## COMPLICATIONS

While acute respiratory failure is the most serious complication of acute pulmonary aspiration, chronic sequelae include pulmonary fibrosis, lung abscess, and empyema. The mortality due to this problem ranges from 40 to 70 percent for aspiration of fluids with a pH less than 2.5 and is higher for fluids with a pH less than 1.8. Patients who aspirate material which is grossly contaminated, as in bowel obstruction, have a mortality approaching 100 percent.

### Lung Abscess

A lung abscess is a cavitation in the pulmonary parenchyma that develops as a result of local suppuration with central necrosis, usually after the aspiration of oropharyngeal secretions. As with other forms of pneumonitis, factors that suppress the cough or gag reflexes, such as anesthesia, tooth extraction, esophageal motility disorders, strictures, or carcinoma, predispose to aspiration. Other pulmonary disorders that may lead to lung abscess formation include pneumonia, pulmonary embolism with cystic infarction, septic emboli, vasculitis, and infected cysts. The presence of periodontal disease plays an important role in the formation of anaerobic lung abscess by increasing the inoculum of organisms available for aspiration. Lung abscess is rare in edentulous people.

The flora in a lung abscess secondary to aspiration are usually polymicrobial, with as many as 60 percent exclusively anaerobes and the rest a mixture of both aerobes and anaerobes. The anaerobes include microaerophilic and anaerobic streptococci, *Fusobacterium*, and *Bacteroides*. Aerobic organisms such as *Staphylococcus aureus*, *Pseudomonas*, alpha streptococci, *Streptococcus pneumoniae*, *Proteus*, *Escherichia coli*, and *Klebsiella pneumoniae* can cause a severe necrotic pneumonitis with abscess formation. *Mycobacterium*, *Histoplasma*, *Coccidioides*, lung flukes, and *Entamoeba* can also present with abscess formation.

In patients with pulmonary aspiration, cavitation usually develops 1 or 2 weeks after the aspiration. Clinical illness is usually insidious but may present as an acute pneumonitis. Presenting signs and symptoms include a cough productive of a fetid and bloody sputum, fever, chest pain, shortness of breath, weakness, and weight loss. Oral examination usually reveals gingivitis and poor dentition. Signs of localized consolidation or cavitation may be present on pulmonary auscultation. Clubbing is rarely seen. Complete blood count usually reveals a leukocytosis with a left shift and anemia.

Diagnosis is confirmed by chest roentgenogram that demonstrates the cavity (Fig. 67-1). An air-fluid level is generally present. The most common sites for aspiration-induced abscesses are the posterior segment of the right upper lobe and the superior segments of the right and left lower lobes. A lung abscess that develops secondary to pulmonary parenchymal disease, carcinoma, opportunistic infection, or septicemia may occur anywhere in the lung.

Occasionally it may be difficult to distinguish a lung abscess from empyema on the chest roentgenogram. Schachter et al. suggest several signs that favor the diagnosis of empyema over lung abscess. These include (1) the development of an air-fluid level at the site of a previous pleural effusion, (2) a cavity with an air-fluid level that tapers at the pleural border, (3) an air-fluid level that crosses a fissure, and (4) an air-fluid level that extends to the lateral chest wall.

Sputum Gram stains are of some value in the diagnosis of aerobic infection. However, only transtracheal or transthoracic aspiration are reliable for anaerobic culture, since expectorated sputum is always contaminated with oral anaerobes. Pleural effusions are occasionally a source of positive cultures and should be cultured both aerobically and anaerobically. In patients with septic emboli, blood cultures are frequently positive.

### Hemoptysis

Hemoptysis, although usually not life-threatening, may be of concern because of the risk of airway obstruction, which initially is more life-threatening than hemorrhagic shock. Mattox defines massive hemoptysis as the expectoration of 200 mL of blood per cough, 400 mL of blood per 24 h, or hemoptysis requiring transfusion to maintain a stable hematocrit. Certain radiologic signs described by Thoms et al. are useful in identifying actual or impending hemoptysis: (1) emptying and refilling of the abscess cavity on serial films, (2) variations in the lucency and height of the air-fluid level, and (3) variable parenchymal densities representing blood clots within the cavity. Other complications include chronic lung abscess, empyema, brain abscess, and bronchopleural fistula.

### Empyema

Empyema is the collection of purulent material in the pleural space or its loculation between fissures. It generally develops secondary to hematogenous or lymphatic spread from pneumonia, or by direct extension or rupture of a lung abscess into the pleural space. Other causes of empyema include esophageal perforation and mediastinitis; rupture of a mediastinal lymph node; direct extension from vertebral osteomyelitis, retropharyngeal or subdiaphragmatic abscesses; or infection as a complication of needle aspiration, thoracostomy tubes, or thoracotomy. The common causative organisms are *Staphylococcus*, gram-negative, and anaerobic organisms.

Presenting signs and symptoms are fever and chills, pleuritic chest pain, and shortness of breath. Weight loss, fatigue, and clubbing of fingers may be present with chronic disease. On examination, dullness to percussion, decreased breath sounds, and diminished excursion of the affected hemothorax are evident.

The chest roentgenogram demonstrates an air-fluid level in the pleural space, or evidence of loculated fluid. The radiologic distinctions between empyema and lung abscess were discussed earlier. Diagnosis is made by thoracentesis with aspiration of purulent material.

Complications of empyema include empyema necessitans, bronchopleural fistula, or permanent loss of parenchyma. Empyema ne-

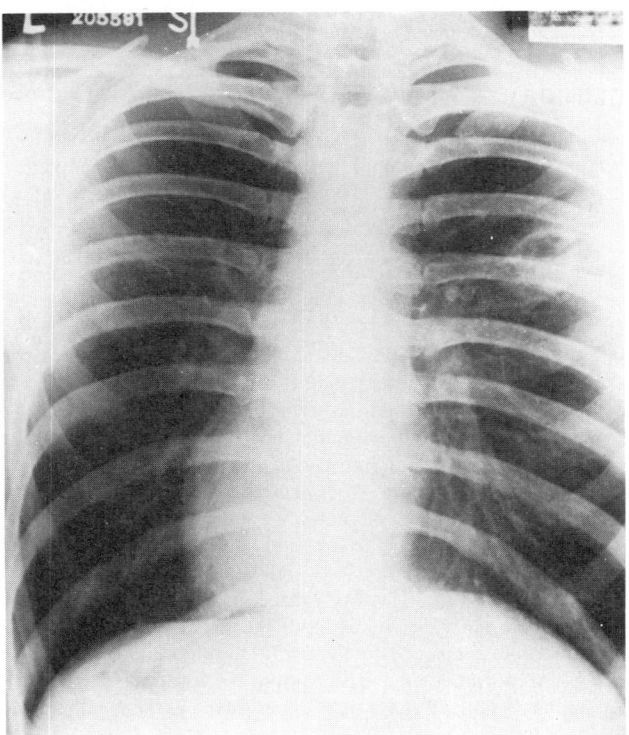

**Fig. 67-1.** Lung abscess in the superior segment of the right lower lobe.

cessitans is an encapsulated empyema that dissects into the subcutaneous tissues or through the chest wall.

An empyema may rupture into the bronchus, spreading infections throughout the tracheobronchial tree or causing airway obstruction. In chronic empyema or fibrothorax, restrictive lung disease may result.

## TREATMENT

The prevention of aspiration pneumonia is the most important consideration in the management of patients at risk. This is accomplished by particular attention to airway management. Nasotracheal or orotracheal intubation should be considered in any patient with depressed or absent gag reflexes. This is best done in adults with a high-volume, low-pressure cuffed endotracheal tube. In children and newborns, a noncuffed tube provides adequate protection in most cases. Gastric lavage is performed cautiously in the comatose or obtunded patient. Preventive measures include placing patients in the Trendelenburg position on their left sides if possible, with endotracheal intubation before lavage. The presence of a nasogastric tube does not ensure that a patient's stomach is empty. The tube may not be positioned properly to completely evacuate the stomach, or large particles may be present that cannot be removed by the nasogastric tube. Patients with an esophageal obturator airway in place must always have their airway protected prior to removal as vomiting usually occurs in this setting.

The use of nonparticulate antacids such as 0.3M sodium citrate has been shown to reduce morbidity and mortality if the pH of the gastric contents is reduced to below 2.5 and the gastric volume to below 0.4 mL/kg before aspiration occurs. Recently, $H_2$ receptor blockers such as cimetidine have been demonstrated to raise the pH of gastric contents acutely in trauma patients and may play a role in the prevention of pulmonary injury. Drugs which hasten gastric emptying such as metoclopramide may also be of value.

If pulmonary aspiration is observed, the trachea should be immediately suctioned and a sample of the aspirate checked for pH. Even in the best of circumstances, however, endotracheal suctioning cannot be expected to remove all of the aspirate.

Bronchoscopy is indicated for removal of large particles and for further clearing of the large airways. Irrigation of the tracheobronchial tree with large volumes of neutral or alkaline solution appears to have no beneficial effect and is harmful, since it may force the aspirate deeper into the terminal airways, increasing the extent of injury. Small amounts of saline may be used to clear the airway, but large volumes should be avoided.

Oxygen should always be administered. Endotracheal intubation and mechanical ventilation are indicated for hypercarbia or in the management of severe hypoxemia that cannot be corrected with oxygen by nasal cannula or face mask. Continuous positive airway pressure or positive end-expiratory pressure (PEEP) is indicated if adequate oxygenation cannot be accomplished by the above means. Both increase functional residual capacity and diminish atelectasis and interstitial edema, resulting in a reduction of ventilation and perfusion inequality. In addition, Cameron and others have shown that PEEP decreases mortality if it is begun within 6 h after aspiration.

Fluid loss into the interstitium and alveoli should be compensated for by adequate volume replacement, generally with crystalloid solution. Despite the clinical finding of wet pulmonary rales, cardiogenic pulmonary edema is usually not present in uncomplicated aspiration pneumonia. Fluid replacement should be guided by changes in central venous pressure, by urine output, and by frequent monitoring of the pulse and blood pressure. If cardiac failure is suspected, it may be necessary to monitor the pulmonary capillary wedge pressure in order to administer fluids safely and effectively.

Steroids and prophylactic antibiotics are of no value and should not be used. The patient should be monitored closely and antibiotics instituted when there is clinical evidence of infection. An antibiotic is chosen that is effective against the most likely organisms, namely selected aerobes and anaerobes. This selection is further guided by sputum culture when possible.

Follow-up supportive care includes appropriate chest physical therapy, humidification and oxygenation, and bronchodilators to treat bronchospasm.

Clindamycin is now the drug of choice for uncomplicated lung abscess, although penicillin remains useful when penicillin resistance is not an issue. Clindamycin 600 mg q 6 h IV is given until the patient has been afebrile for 5 days then switched to oral clindamycin 300 mg every 6 h for six to eight weeks. Generally, aqueous penicillin G is given 6–12 million units/day until clinical improvement occurs, followed by oral penicillin VK 500–750 mg every 6 h for up to 6 weeks. Metronidazole 500 mg every 6 h PO or cefoxitin 1–2 gm every 4 h IV are suitable alternatives. Antibiotic therapy for hospital-acquired lung abscess is guided by culture results or gram stain. Elective bronchoscopy is valuable to evaluate the presence of a tumor or foreign body, to obtain material for culture, and to facilitate drainage. Surgery is indicated for life-threatening hemoptysis, tumor, and, rarely, a residual cavity.

Patients with life-threatening hemoptysis should be placed in Trendelenburg's position, vigorously suctioned, and oxygenated. If the side of the bleeding is known, the patient should be placed with that side down. Fluid and blood must be rapidly replaced as well, and immediate consultation for bronchoscopy must be obtained, generally from a thoracic surgeon. Bronchoscopy can aid in localizing the bleeding site, can provide a route for suctioning, and the rigid bronchoscope can be used to maintain the airway. By use of a bronchoscope, the patient can be intubated with a double-lumen endobronchial tube (Carlens, Robert Shaw, or White), or selective endobronchial intubation can be done. The bleeding mainstem bronchus can then be occluded, which ensures a patent airway through the other mainstem bronchus. Both bronchoscopy and endobronchial intubation should be attempted only by trained, experienced individuals.

Empyema requires appropriate intravenous antibiotic therapy combined with tube thoracostomy with closed drainage, or by open drainage and decortication for resolution.

## BIBLIOGRAPHY

Johanson WG, Harris GD: Aspiration pneumonia, anaerobic infections, and lung abscess. *Med Clin North Am* 64,3:385, 1980.

Katz S: Primary lung abscess, in *Conn's current therapy,* Rakel RE (ed). WB Saunders, p 163, 1990.

Robertson C: A review of the use of corticosteroids in the management of pulmonary injuries and insults. *Arch Emerg Med* 2,2:59, 1985.

Strain JD, Moore EE, Markovchick VJ: Cimetidine for the prophylaxis of potential gastric acid aspiration pneumonitis in trauma patients. *J Trauma* 21,1:49, 1981.

Thoms NW, Puro HE, Arbula A: The significance of hemoptysis in lung abscess. *J Thorac Cardiovasc Surg* 59:617, 1970.

# 68
# TUBERCULOSIS
## Robert D. Welch

Despite advances in the diagnosis and treatment of many medical disorders, tuberculosis remains the leading cause of death (approximately 2.9 million per year worldwide) from a single infectious agent. The United States saw a steady decline in new cases of tuberculosis from the late 1800s until 1984, but this trend reversed in 1985 and the incidence has increased since. Factors that may be responsible for the reversal include an increase in the number of homeless persons, the human immunodeficiency virus (HIV) epidemic, drug abuse, the inability of cities and states to maintain tuberculosis control programs (many third-world countries have a higher treatment completion rate than some major U.S. cities), and a combination of the above affecting many of the same people or populations. These factors are found in many patients visiting emergency departments. This, coupled with the rapid proliferation of multidrug-resistant strains, has resulted in emergency physicians' renewed attention on the disease.

Control of the epidemic rests upon a number of factors, including: (1) recognition and treatment of the high-risk population (Table 68-1); (2) increased funding for surveillance and treatment of noncompliant patients; (3) rebuilding the health and social services structures; and (4) basic research in the pathogen, the immunologic response, and new pharmacologic therapy. Emergency physicians must be aware of local epidemiologic patterns, the common presenting symptoms, and guidelines for the isolation and treatment of potential cases.

## PATHOPHYSIOLOGY

Mycobacteria are slow-growing aerobic rods (slightly curved or straight) that have a unique multilayered cell wall. The cell wall contains a variety of lipids that account for their "acid-fast" property. Transmission occurs mainly through aerosols. After coughing, the aerosols begin to evaporate, leaving the droplet nuclei. These nuclei remain suspended for prolonged periods, making breathing the major risk factor for acquiring infection. Another less common mode of airborne transmission is by dust particles. Organisms that settle rapidly become associated with dust particles. These particles can be resuspended by small air currents. Other modes of transmission, such as by oral, GI, or skin exposure, have been described but are much less common. Persons with laryngeal infections or those with stainable mycobacteria in their saliva are the most infectious.

### Primary Infection

The initial infection results in few or no symptoms in most individuals. Infection may be caused by as few as 1 to 10 bacilli entering the alveoli. Tissue macrophages ingest the organisms where the bacilli are killed or can multiply. Organisms then travel to regional lymph nodes and, if not contained in the lymph nodes, eventually enter the thoracic duct from which they enter the bloodstream. If the latter event occurs, the bacteria disseminate to different organs, resulting in

**Table 68-1.** Patients with a High Prevalence of Tuberculosis

1. Elderly and nursing home patients
2. Immigrants from high-prevalence countries
3. HIV-infected patients
4. Alcoholics and illicit drug users
5. Residents and staff of prisons or shelters for the homeless

the potential for disease later in life. Cell-mediated immunity is activated during the first 2 to 6 weeks, and T lymphocytes release lymphokines that activate macrophages. These cells then form granulomas (tubercles), which are the pathologic feature of tuberculosis. The tubercles may undergo caseation necrosis and later calcification. The Ghon complex is calcified lung granulomas and hilar nodes. In most cases the bacteria are contained in tubercles but in some patients (such as the immunocompromised) early hematogenous spread results in disseminated tuberculosis.

Most of the disseminated organisms do not find a suitable area to proliferate, but survival is favored in areas of high oxygen content or blood flow, such as the apical and posterior segments of the upper lobe and the superior segment of the lower lobe of the lung, renal cortex, meninges, the epiphyses of long bones, and the vertebrae. Following primary infection some degree of immunity is acquired. In otherwise healthy individuals a second primary infection may result, but this occurs more frequently in high-prevalence populations. In cases of immunocompromised individuals a rapidly progressive primary infection that results in early death has been described.

### Reactivation Tuberculosis

Reactivation occurs, after a period of latency, when the host's immune system is no longer capable of containing the foci of previous hematogenous spread. The young, the elderly, or patients with other debilitating conditions are at higher risk for reactivation and disease. There is about a 10 percent lifetime risk of progressing to reactivation tuberculosis in the general population. In those with coexistent HIV infection, the incidence of reactivation rises to about 8 percent per year. This stresses the importance of cell-mediated immunity in containing infection.

## CLINICAL FEATURES
### Primary Tuberculosis

The initial infection is usually asymptomatic and only identified by a new reaction to purified protein derivative (PPD). A pneumonitis may result that is similar to a viral, bacterial, or atypical infection. Rarely, massive hilar adenopathy leads to atelectasis and bronchiectasis. Some cases proceed to what pathologically appears to be a reactivation-type infection or to a rapidly progressive severe form.

### Reactivation Tuberculosis

The majority of patients with reactivation tuberculosis will display signs and symptoms of a chronic wasting disease, but up to 20 percent will lack the typical features. Symptoms of reactivation disease include malaise, weight loss, night sweats, low-grade fever, and cough. In over 80 percent of cases pulmonary involvement is noted, and about 15 percent have extrapulmonary disease. Skin testing with PPD will be positive in 80 percent of cases. In patients with significant immunodeficiency the incidence of extrapulmonary disease is higher, as is the incidence of anergy to skin testing.

### Pulmonary Tuberculosis

Pulmonary tuberculosis is characterized by the insidious onset of chronic cough with scant sputum production and hemoptysis. Other constitutional symptoms of reactivation are typical. A wide spectrum of illness from virtually no symptoms to that of a severe destructive pulmonary disease may be seen. Physical examination of the lung generally reveals very little, and findings are only common when there is extensive pulmonary involvement. The apical and posterior segments of the upper lobe and the superior segment of the lower lobe are most commonly involved. Lesions range from small infiltrates to extensive cavitation.

## Extrapulmonary Tuberculosis

Extrapulmonary tuberculosis may result from primary infection or reactivation of infection. Common sites of extrapulmonary disease include pleura, pericardium, peritoneum, larynx, lymph nodes, meninges, genitourinary tract, gastrointestinal tract, bones and joints, and adrenal glands. There is also a miliary form. A few of these will be considered below.

### Pleural Effusion

A tuberculous pleural effusion usually occurs sometime after primary infection when a peripheral focus ruptures into the pleural space. It may also be a manifestation of a progressive primary infection of the pleura. The effusion is exudative in nature (elevated protein, low pH, and low glucose). In chronic effusions lymphocytes are the predominant cell type, but in acute disease neutrophils will be found. Acid-fast stain of the fluid is frequently nondiagnostic. Pleural biopsy reveals granulomas, thus aiding in the diagnosis. Medical treatment is usually effective and, in the case of sensitive organisms, surgical therapy is rarely needed.

### Central Nervous System

Meningitis usually occurs during the seeding of primary infection. Rupture of a subependymal lesion (Rich foci) into the subarachnoid space also results in disease. In many children the disease is acute, whereas a more indolent course is noted in adults. Early on, fever (90 to 95 percent), signs of meningeal irritation, and cranial nerve defects (30 percent) are seen. A more severe and debilitating neurologic dysfunction ensues if the condition is not treated. Typical CSF samples reveal mononuclear cells and low glucose, but early samples will have a predominance of neutrophils. Intracranial tuberculomas may be seen, and many remain asymptomatic.

### Pericarditis and Peritonitis

These are most often the result of seeding from infected nodes. Pericarditis may be a primary infection resulting from pleural extension. In pericarditis, the symptoms are typical and a rub may be heard. The diagnosis may be difficult, necessitating pericardial biopsy. Complications include tamponade and chronic constrictive pericarditis.

As in the case of pericarditis, the diagnosis of tuberculous peritonitis may be difficult. The illness is often indolent and may be confused with peritoneal fluid from cirrhosis. Fluid cultures are often negative, and peritoneal biopsy may be required.

### Miliary Tuberculosis

Miliary tuberculosis is the result of hematogenous spread either during primary infection or secondary seeding in a diseased individual. Fever, cough, weight loss, hepatomegaly, splenomegaly, lymphadenopathy, and other signs of a multisystem illness should make one suspect this entity. Laboratory abnormalities frequently seen include hyponatremia, anemia, thrombocytopenia, and leukopenia, although thrombocytosis and leukocytosis are also seen. Diagnosis may be made by bronchoscopy and bronchoalveolar lavage (BAL), bone marrow biopsy, or other organ biopsy. Treatment is the same as for other forms of tuberculosis.

### Tuberculosis and HIV

Tuberculosis (pulmonary and extrapulmonary) is an AIDS-defining illness that frequently occurs earlier than other opportunistic diseases. The incidence of tuberculosis in HIV-infected patients varies, based on the prevalence in the community, and has been found to be as high as 60 percent in Haitians with AIDS. Physicians making the diagnosis of tuberculosis should offer patients HIV testing as this may provide early diagnosis and therapy.

The incidence of extrapulmonary tuberculosis is higher in patients already diagnosed with AIDS (>70 percent) and those having less advanced HIV infections (24 to 45 percent) than in individuals not infected with HIV. Pulmonary involvement is still very common but may be difficult to distinguish from other HIV-associated lung disorders. Mortality rates range between 14 and 44 percent in coinfected patients, but the actual cause of death may have been due to other causes in some cases.

Overall response to therapy is adequate, with treatment failure rates of 0 to 16 percent and relapse rates of 0 to 15 percent. The incidence of adverse drug reactions to antituberculosis chemotherapy is higher in HIV-infected patients than in non-HIV-infected patients. Due to the number of medications taken by AIDS patients, potential drug interactions must be of concern when evaluating these patients.

## Multidrug-Resistant Tuberculosis (MDR-TB)

The increase in drug-resistant tuberculosis has become a major public health concern. In the first 3 months of 1991, the Centers for Disease Control and Prevention (CDC) found 14.2 percent of all cases examined were resistant to at least one drug and 3.5 percent were resistant to isoniazid (INH) and rifampin. In New York City, 33 percent of isolates tested were resistant to at least one drug and 19 percent were resistant to INH and rifampin. In previously treated patients the rate of resistance is much higher.

Mortality rates from the outbreak of MDR-TB investigated by the CDC between 1990 and 1992 ranged from 72 to 89 percent. The median time from diagnosis to death was 4 to 16 weeks. A review of cases treated for MDR-TB prior to the HIV epidemic revealed a treatment failure rate of 35 percent, a long-term cure rate of only 56 percent, and 22 percent died from the disease. This shows that poor outcomes are related to associated HIV infections, but delays in diagnosis, susceptibility testing, and proper therapy also contributed.

Transmission of MDR-TB to health care workers has been documented. Health care workers assigned to wards caring for MDR-TB patients have shown rates of conversion from PPD-negative to -positive of 22 to 50 percent.

## DIAGNOSIS

The diagnosis of tuberculosis presents a special challenge to emergency physicians. In the past physicians mainly considered the diagnosis when presented with a young or older patient with reactivation disease. Now one must consider the diagnosis in anyone with respiratory complaints or any extrapulmonary symptoms. The various clinical presentations along with the length of time required to culture the organism makes emergent diagnosis difficult. A heightened awareness of the disease plus potential new rapid diagnostic tests will ensure that these patients are not returned to the community without proper therapy.

### Skin Test

The Mantoux test involves the intracutaneous injection of 0.1 mL of PPD in the forearm. The test is read between 48 and 72 h after administration. Table 68-2 summarizes the American Thoracic Society's standards for interpretation of test results. All persons with a positive PPD reaction or recent conversion should be referred for possible preventative therapy, despite age.

### Chest Radiograph

The classic radiographic finding in primary infection is parenchymal infiltrates in any area of the lung (often very small) and unilateral hilar adenopathy. Calcification of the lesions may be a later finding. Reactivation tuberculosis typically appears as lesions, with or without cavitation, in the upper lobe or superior segment of the lower lobe. Miliary tuberculosis frequently shows small (1 to 3 mm) nodules

**Table 68-2.** Interpretation of PPD Skin Test

1. ≥ 5 mm is positive* in:
   a. Patients with HIV infection
   b. Patients with close contact with a tuberculosis-infected individual
   c. Patients with abnormal chest radiograph suggestive of healed tuberculosis
2. ≥ 10 mm is positive in patients not meeting the above criteria but who have other risks:
   a. Intravenous drug users
   b. High-prevalence groups (immigrants, long-term care facility residents, persons in local high-risk areas)
   c. Patients with conditions that increase the risk of progression to active disease
3. ≥ 15 mm is positive in all others
4. Detection of newly infected persons in a screening program:
   a. ≥ 10-mm increase within any 2-year period is positive if < 35 years of age
   b. ≥ 15-mm increase within any 2-year period is positive if ≥ 35 years of age
5. If the patient is anergic, other epidemiologic factors must be considered

*A positive reaction does not necessarily indicate disease.

throughout the lung fields. Pleural effusion (usually unilateral) may be the only finding. Atelectasis, fibrotic scarring, tracheal deviation, and signs of prior thoracic surgery are other findings.

HIV-infected individuals may have atypical radiographic appearances. Severely immunocompromised patients have radiographs more typical of primary infection, whereas those with a less advanced illness show signs of reactivation. Normal radiographs are seen in higher frequency in HIV-infected patients.

It must be emphasized that tuberculosis can produce virtually any type of pulmonary radiographic abnormality, and comparison with prior radiographs is of extreme importance.

## Microbiology

Staining for acid fastness (i.e., Ziehl-Neelsen stain) or a fluorochrome procedure is the quickest and least expensive method to provide a presumptive diagnosis of tuberculosis. Studies have shown 50 to 80 percent positive sputum smears in patients with pulmonary tuberculosis.

Culture is the "gold standard" for the diagnosis of tuberculosis. Sources for culture include sputum or BAL fluid, gastric lavage, body fluids, and tissue samples. Traditional cultures typically take 3 to 6 weeks for final results. New radiometric technology (BACTEC system) provides for more rapid growth (average of 9 days) and identification (5 days).

Commercially available DNA probes used on cultures can reduce identification time to as little as 1 h. The possibility of rapid identification of *M. tuberculosis* on a direct sputum sample is revolutionary for the emergency physician. Target nucleic acid amplification by the polymerase chain reaction (which requires thermocycling) or reverse transcription (euthermic) may, in the future, provide definitive results in a matter of hours.

## TREATMENT

*M. tuberculosis* develops resistance by spontaneous genetic mutation. Inadequate drug therapy or poor compliance with treatment allows for survival of these organisms. The emergence of MDR-TB prompted the CDC recommendation of treating patients with at least four drugs (and in some cases up to six drugs) until susceptibility tests are available. Beginning therapy should include INH, rifampin, pyrazinamide, and either streptomycin or ethambutol for 2 months. Options for dosing include:

1. Daily therapy for 8 weeks then 16 weeks of daily or two or three times/week. In this case treatment is continued for at least 6 months (3 months after culture conversion).
2. Daily for 2 weeks followed by two times/week for 6 weeks. INH and rifampin two times/week alone are used for the remaining 16 weeks.
3. Three times/week therapy for 6 months.

In HIV-infected patients, treatment should total 9 months and continue at least 6 months after cultures become negative.

**Table 68-3.** Dosages and Common Side Effects of Some Drugs Used in Tuberculosis

| Drug | Daily | Twice Weekly | Three Times Weekly | Some Potential Side Effects |
|---|---|---|---|---|
| INH | Adult: 5 mg/kg (max. 300 mg)<br>Children: 10–20 mg/kg (max. 300 mg) | Adult: 15 mg/kg (max. 900 mg)<br>Children: 20–40 mg/kg (max. 900 mg) | Same as twice weekly | Hepatitis, neuritis, lupus syndrome, abdominal discomfort, hypersensitivity reaction, metabolic acidosis, CNS effects |
| Rifampin | Adult: 10 mg/kg (max. 600 mg)<br>Children: 10–20 mg/kg (max. 600 mg) | Same as daily | Same as daily | Hepatitis, thrombocytopenia, drug interactions, GI disturbances |
| Pyrazinamide | Adult: 15–30 mg/kg (max. 2 g)<br>Children: Same | Adult 50–70 mg/kg (max. 4 g)<br>Children: Same | Adult: 50–70 mg/kg (max. 3 g)<br>Children: Same | Hepatitis, arthralgia, rash, hyperuricemia, GI disturbances |
| Ethambutol | Adult: 5–25 mg/kg (max. 2.5 g)<br>Children: 15–25 mg/kg (max. 2.5 g) | Adult: 50 mg/kg (max. 2.5 g)<br>Children: Same | Adult: 25–30 mg/kg (max. 2.5 g)<br>Children: Same | Optic neuritis, GI disturbances |
| Streptomycin | Adult: 15 mg/kg (max. 1 g)<br>Children: 20–30 mg/kg (max. 1 g) | Adult: 25–30 mg/kg (max. 1.5 g)<br>Children: Same | Adult: 25–30 mg/kg (max. 1 g)<br>Children: Same | 8th cranial nerve damage, renal failure, proteinuria, eosinophilia, electrolyte disorders, neuromuscular blockade |
| Amikacin | Adult: 15 mg/kg | | | Same as streptomycin |
| Kanamycin | Adult: 15 mg/kg | | | Same as streptomycin |
| Ofloxacin | Adult: 400 mg bid | | | GI disturbances, CNS disturbances, arthropathies |
| Ciprofloxacin | Adult: 750 mg bid | | | Same as oflaxacin |
| Aminosalicylic acid (PAS) | Adult: 10–12 g/day in 1–3 doses/day or 3 g qid | | | GI disturbances, hypersensitivity reaction, hematologic disturbances, goiter |
| Cycloserine | Adult: 250 mg bid to qid | | | CNS disturbances with possible seizures, hypersensitivity reactions |

**Table 68-4.** Engineering Controls to Reduce the Transmission of Tuberculosis

1. High air flow (at least six room exchanges per hour) with external exhaust
2. High-efficiency particulate air filters (HEPA)
3. Ultraviolet germicidal irritation (UVGI)
4. Negative pressure isolation rooms
5. Respiratory protection (respirators with HEPA filters) should be worn when proper controls cannot be implemented. This includes emergency transport vehicles and small rooms where cough-inducing procedures are being done.

If local INH resistance rates are less than 4 percent, an initial three-drug regimen may be adequate. When drug susceptibility results are available, therapy may be modified. The importance of directly observed therapy (DOT) cannot be overstated, and all two or three times/week regimens should be by DOT. Table 68-3 summarizes commonly used drug doses and some side effects.

Due to the appearance of untreatable disease, surgical resection is being performed, with good results.

### Emergency

Care of patients with tuberculosis begins in the prehospital setting and emergency department. All prehospital care personnel must be trained to suspect tuberculosis, institute appropriate precautions, and notify emergency departments of their suspicions. Triage workers should ask appropriate questions to detect potential cases. Patients with suspected tuberculosis should be placed in separate waiting areas, have a surgical mask placed, and be instructed to cover the mouth and nose when coughing. Prompt evaluation will ensure a minimal amount of time being spent in the ambulatory care setting.

### Admission

All hospitalized patients with suspected tuberculosis must be placed in isolation rooms until the diagnosis is certain. Admission is important in cases where social situations make it difficult to obtain a proper diagnosis and for therapy to be instituted. Hospital admission is indicated when the patient has active disease with proven MDR-TB to institute therapy and observe for drug toxicity. Other indications for admission include when the disease is of such an acute nature as to preclude outpatient therapy, the diagnosis is in question, or the patient is known to be noncompliant with treatment. Physicians need to be aware of their own state laws concerning involuntary hospitalization and treatment.

### Outpatient

The vast majority of patients are treated as outpatients. Emergency physicians must make contacts with the physician or public health services providing long-term care. Discharge instructions include home isolation procedures and sites of medication (if DOT is used) and ongoing care.

### PREVENTION

Prevention of transmission of tuberculosis in health care facilities is of extreme importance. Guidelines for prevention of transmission have been published and are available through the CDC. These recommendations include early detection and treatment of active cases, education and screening of health care workers, and engineering controls. Table 68-4 lists some controls that prevent transmission of disease. Ambulatory care facilities that frequently see tuberculosis will need isolation room availability.

### BIBLIOGRAPHY

American Thoracic Society: Diagnostic standards and classification of tuberculosis. *Am Rev Respir Dis* 142:725, 1990.

Barnes PF, Bloch AB, Davidson PT, et al: Tuberculosis in patients with human immunodeficiency virus infection. *N Engl J Med* 324:1644, 1991.

Bloom BR, Murray CJL: Tuberculosis: Commentary on a reemergent killer. *Science* 257:1055, 1992.

CDC: Guidelines for preventing the transmission of *Mycobacterium tuberculosis* in health care facilities, 1994. *MMWR* volume 23, No. RR13, October 28, 1994.

Centers for Disease Control and Prevention: Initial therapy for tuberculosis in the era of multidrug resistance: Recommendations of the advisory council for the elimination of tuberculosis. *MMWR* 421, 1993.

Iseman MD: Treatment of multidrug-resistant tuberculosis. *N Engl J Med* 329:784, 1993.

## 69

# SPONTANEOUS AND IATROGENIC PNEUMOTHORAX
### Kimberlydawn Wisdom

### INTRODUCTION

Collection of air in the pleural space causes malfunction of the thoracic pump, resulting in pulmonary and hemodynamic complications. Accumulation of air in the pleural space—*pneumothorax*—occurs in patients with or without underlying pulmonary disorders. The term *spontaneous pneumothorax* refers to the collection of air in the pleural space without any local trauma. Pneumothorax occurring spontaneously in young adults is due to the rupture of a subpleural bleb. Chest trauma or diagnostic or therapeutic procedures can also lead to pneumothorax or hemopneumothorax with resultant complications. The term *pulmonary barotrauma* is used to describe the complications resulting from increased airway pressures generated during ventilatory assistance, such as mediastinal and subcutaneous emphysema, and tension pneumothorax. Pneumothorax causes hypoxia, especially in the setting of obstructive airway disorders; immediate complications are due to the hemodynamic impact of a tension pneumothorax. Emergency thoracostomy is needed to correct the hemodynamic compromise of tension pneumothorax.

### SPONTANEOUS PNEUMOTHORAX
#### Primary Spontaneous Pneumothorax

Primary spontaneous pneumothorax occurs spontaneously in a person without underlying pulmonary disease. In reality, most individuals who develop primary spontaneous pneumothorax have a small degree of undiagnosed underlying pulmonary disease. It is more common in men than women and almost all individuals are smokers. The characteristic patient is a tall, thin man between 20 and 40 years of age. Such tall thin individuals are at increased risk due to the increased negative pressure at the apex of the lung. Pneumothorax is generally due to the rupture of a pulmonary or subpleural bleb or bulla into the pleural space but may develop when excessive mechanical stress is placed on a segment of weakened pleura. Leakage of air from the alveoli into the pleural space causes a rise in the intrapleural pressure, leading to pulmonary collapse. The recurrence rate varies from 20 to 50 percent over the next 5 years.

In many patients no underlying pathology can be determined. In some cases there is a history of deep inspiration or hyperventilation, followed by a generation of excessive intrapleural pressures such as can be induced by screaming, coughing, or the Valsalva maneuver (when smoking marijuana).

## Secondary Spontaneous Pneumothorax

Secondary spontaneous pneumothorax occurs spontaneously in a person with underlying pulmonary disease. The disease associated most commonly with secondary spontaneous pneumothorax is chronic obstructive pulmonary disease (COPD), but other lung diseases have been reported. Secondary spontaneous pneumothorax may occur in conjunction with pulmonary infection, such as staphylococcal pneumonia or tuberculosis, asthma or emphysema, pulmonary carcinoma, "honeycomb" lung disorders such as tuberous sclerosis or histiocytosis X, occupational pulmonary disease, sarcoidosis, postpulmonary irradiation, and Marfan and Ehlers-Danlos syndromes. Rarely, cyclical pneumothorax may occur in young or middle-aged females. In such cases the development of "catamenial" pneumothorax is coincident with menstruation and may be related to the presence of pelvic, pleural, or diaphragmatic endometriosis.

## Clinical Features

The two most common symptoms of both primary and secondary spontaneous pneumothorax are chest pain on the side of the pneumothorax and dyspnea. The symptoms associated with secondary spontaneous pneumothorax are more severe than the primary due to compromised pulmonary reserve. Each type of pneumothorax can be life-threatening if a tension pneumothorax develops or if there is significant hypoxia. Chest pain often occurs suddenly, sometimes at rest, and has a sharp and pleuritic character. The pain is generally anterior but it may radiate to the neck or back. Dyspnea, tachycardia, and tachypnea may be present if the degree of pneumothorax compromises pulmonary function. There may be a cough, occasionally productive of blood-streaked sputum. Subcutaneous emphysema involving the neck and chest wall may be present if air has dissected through mediastinal structures. On physical examination there may be decreased breath sounds, hyperresonance to percussion on the side of the pneumothorax, and decreased tactile fremitus. However, in some patients, especially those with emphysema, the clinical findings may be subtle. In addition, the development of pneumothorax in this group is serious and can lead to respiratory failure. In every individual with chronic obstructive pulmonary disease, pneumothorax should always be suspected as a cause for clinical deterioration.

A chest roentgenogram is necessary to confirm the diagnosis. Pneumothorax is characterized by hyperlucency and a lack of lung markings at the periphery of the lung and by the appearance of a fine line that represents the retraction of the visceral from the parietal pleura.

If a suspected pneumothorax is not visible on an inspiratory film, it may be seen on an expiratory film, since the constant volume of the pneumothorax is more evident when the size of the hemithorax decreases with expiration. A lateral decubitus film with the patient lying on the affected side may be helpful for the same reason. Tomograms are also useful in assessing emphysematous lesions.

A small amount of pleural fluid, usually represented by blunting of the costophrenic angle, is generally present. Bullae or emphysematous blebs or pulmonary infiltration may be seen on the x-ray film.

Visual estimates of pneumothorax size are inaccurate. A technique for more accurate estimation of pneumothorax size based upon measurement of interpleural distances has been described, but has not found wide acceptance of application.

Pneumothorax must be differentiated from skin folds, outlines of tubing, artifacts on the chest wall such as clothing, and bullae or cysts. Bullae and cysts have concave inner margins and rounded edges.

Hypotension, cyanosis, and marked respiratory distress may develop if the degree of pneumothorax is large, if underlying pulmonary function is poor, or if tension pneumothorax has developed (Fig. 69-1). Tension pneumothorax is characterized by severe dysp-

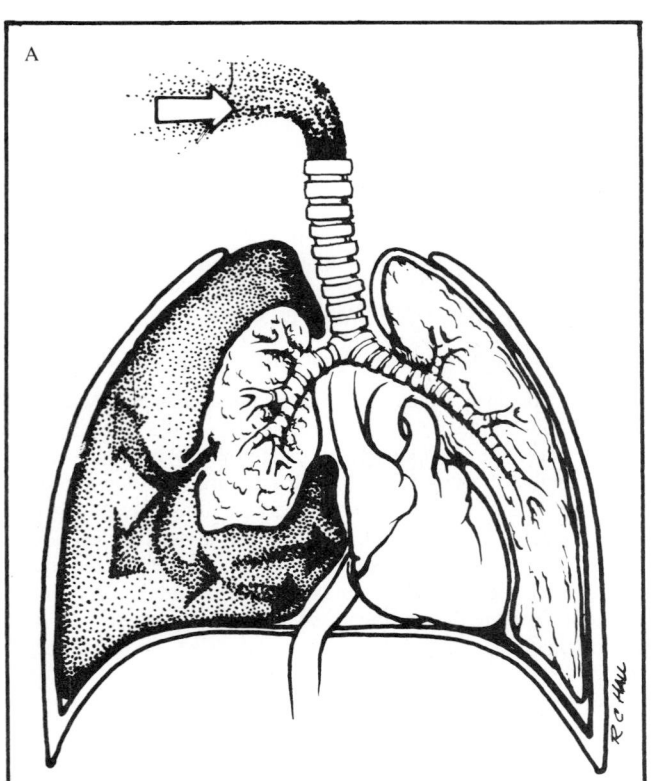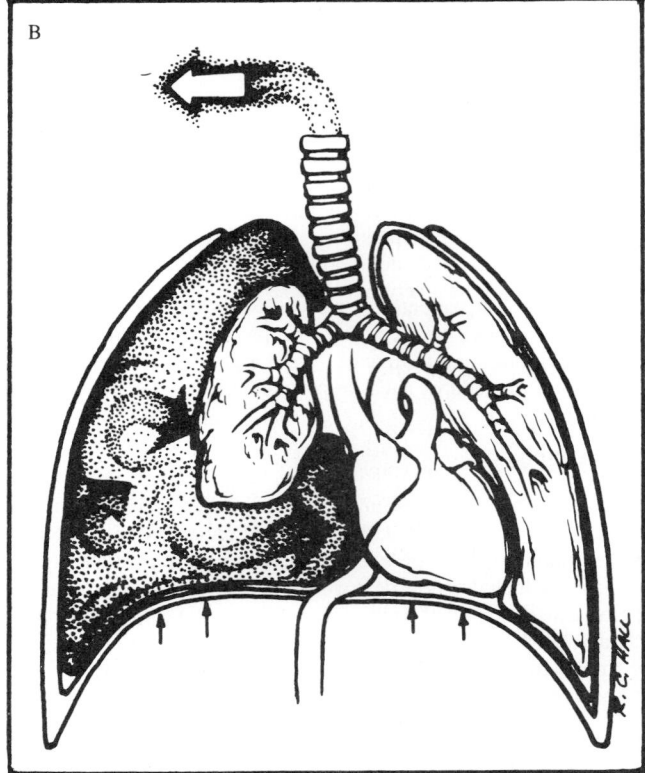

**Fig. 69-1. A.** Tension pneumothorax (inspiration). **B.** Tension pneumothorax (expiration).

nea, cyanosis, and hypotension. The chest will be hyperresonant on the side of the pneumothorax and the trachea and mediastinal structures will deviate to the opposite side. Deviation of the mediastinal structures results in kinking of the inferior vena cava and a marked decrease in venous return. Uncorrected tension pneumothorax rapidly leads to cardiorespiratory collapse. Chest x-ray is generally not necessary to make this diagnosis. Emergency thoracostomy is necessary, and procrastination to obtain a confirmatory chest x-ray can result in cardiac arrest in the patient.

## IATROGENIC PNEUMOTHORAX

Iatrogenic pneumothorax can occur secondary to procedures such as cannulation of the subclavian vein, lung inflation at high pressures, intercostal nerve block, thoracentesis, percutaneous lung biopsy, and bronchoscopy. It is the most commonly described complication of subclavian vein catheterization and generally occurs if the angle of introduction of the needle is too sharp or if the tip of the needle is directed too deeply, nicking the parietal pleura and allowing air to accumulate in the pleural cavity. It can also occur if catheterization is attempted while the patient is moving or during chest compression in CPR. It may be more common in apical procedures, as opposed to procedures generally performed at the lung bases such as thoracentesis, because airflow is greater in the apices than the bases. Consequently, subclavian vein catheterization should be approached cautiously in patients with hyperventilation or Kussmaul respirations. Simple pneumothorax can lead to tension pneumothorax rapidly in such circumstances. Chest x-ray is routinely performed immediately after subclavian vein catheterization to detect immediate pneumothorax, but delayed pneumothorax could also develop.

Lung inflation at high pressures can also lead to pneumothorax. Mouth-to-mouth or bag-mask ventilation in infants and children or even in adults can lead to pneumothorax or pneumomediastinum if excess airway pressures are generated. Pneumothorax has resulted when an oxygen cannula is inserted directly into an endotracheal tube. Oxygen is delivered at high flow rates through the cannula into the tube, but because the cannula itself nearly fills the tube lumen, adequate expiration is not possible. Lung pressures build up until pneumothorax results. The institution of mechanical ventilation or positive end-expiratory pressure can cause pneumothorax in patients with previous lung disease or can quickly lead to tension pneumothorax if there has been prior simple pneumothorax. In the latter case a thoracostomy tube is necessary before mechanical ventilation is begun.

In patients with recent subclavian vein catheterization or in those on mechanical ventilation, pneumothorax should be considered as a cause of cardiopulmonary deterioration. Intercostal nerve block for relief of pain from rib fractures or severe costochondritis should be followed by a chest x-ray to rule out iatrogenic pneumothorax.

## TREATMENT OPTIONS

### Observation

The option of observation (inpatient or outpatient) may be exercised in either primary or secondary spontaneous pneumothoraces if the pneumothorax involves less than 15 to 20 percent of the hemithorax and the patient is relatively asymptomatic. The air in the pleural space may gradually be absorbed at a rate of 1.25 percent per 24 h if the alveolar/pleural space violation is eliminated. The administration of supplemental oxygen increases the rate of absorption of pleural air.

### Tube Thoracostomy

The decision for the tube thoracostomy varies with the clinical situation, the patient's pulmonary reserve, and the treatment philosophy of the institution. Although each decision is individualized, there are general circumstances that may warrant tube thoracostomy such as

complete collapse, severe underlying lung disease, significant dyspnea, or unsuccessful simple aspiration. The technique of tube thoracostomy is discussed in Chap. 218, "Thoracic Trauma."

### Simple Aspiration

Simple catheter aspiration in pneumothorax has been described as an alternative method to tube thoracostomy in selected patients (Fig. 69-2). It may be recommended in patients with a primary spontaneous pneumothorax (particularly a first primary spontaneous pneumothorax) and moderate or even complete collapse in some cases. Two methods have been described: the nonsequential and the sequential.

In the *nonsequential* method a 14- to 16-gauge catheter is introduced into the pleural space at the level of the second or third interspace at the midclavicular line, and air is aspirated with a syringe us-

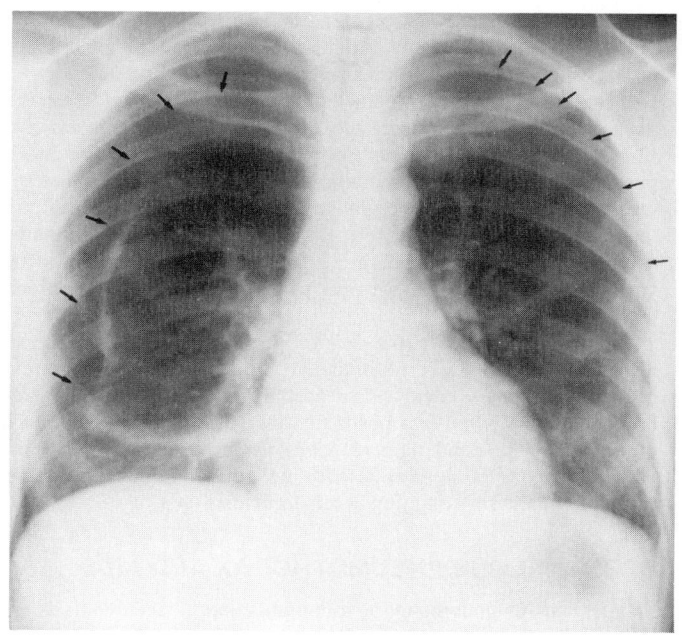

**A**

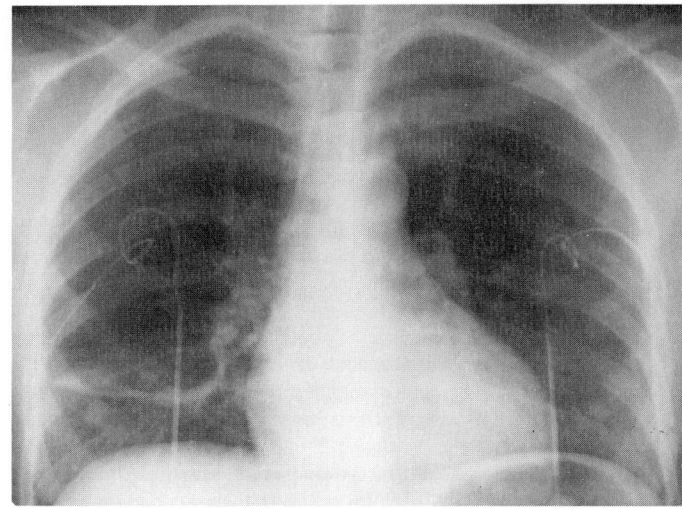

**B**

**Fig. 69-2.** Bilateral pneumothorax in an intravenous drug abuser. **A.** The catheter aspiration of the simple pneumothorax (CASP) technique was used. **B.** As shown, the catheters were successful in complete reexpansion of the lungs. (Courtesy Henry Ford Hospital.)

ing a three-way stopcock. Chest x-ray is repeated immediately after aspiration, and 6 h later is used to confirm success of the technique. Patients without evidence of pneumothorax after 6 h can be discharged with a follow-up scheduled at 24 or 48 h. Recurrence of pneumothorax at 6 h is variable, but tends to be more frequent with large pneumothoraces or with trauma.

The *sequential* method involves several steps. If the pneumothorax has not been successfully reexpanded after aspiration, a Heimlich flutter valve is attached to the catheter. If after 1 h reexpansion has been unsuccessful, then the catheter is connected to wall suction for 1 h. If a pneumothorax persists, tube thoracostomy is performed.

The catheter aspiration technique has been used successfully in patients with spontaneous pneumothorax who have no underlying pulmonary disease, have not been subject to trauma, have no hemo- or hydrothorax, who are not in any respiratory distress, and who have normal vital signs. Catheter aspiration can also be used in patients with recurrent spontaneous pneumothoraces in whom it is desirable to avoid tube thoracostomy. Admission is the practice for this latter group, especially if there is underlying pulmonary disease.

If tube thoracostomy or catheter aspiration is deferred, the patient must be frequently and carefully examined and serial chest x-ray films taken to detect the development of an increasing or tension pneumothorax. If the pneumothorax is increasing, if the patient is on mechanical ventilation, or if general anesthesia is contemplated, tube thoracostomy should be performed. If tension pneumothorax is evident, the pressure should be immediately relieved by insertion of a large-bore needle into the pleural space, followed by tube thoracostomy.

On occasion, rapid expansion of pneumothorax with excessive negative pressure may result in the development of unilateral or even bilateral pulmonary edema. This is more likely to occur if there is bronchial obstruction. It is postulated that the increase in pulmonary blood flow with rapid lung reexpansion can cause transudation of capillary fluid into the alveoli. With judicious fluid management and respiratory care this condition is self-limited.

## SPONTANEOUS PNEUMOTHORAX AND AIDS

Spontaneous pneumothorax as a complication of pneumonia is rare, but when it occurs it is usually due to organisms such as *Staphylococcus aureus, Mycobacterium tuberculosis,* or *Klebsiella,* which cause necrotizing infections. Although pneumothorax associated with *Pneumocystis carinii* pneumonia (PCP) was described over 20 years ago in malnourished and immunosuppressed infants and more recently in leukemics, it has been reported with increased frequency in the AIDS population.

The pathophysiology is not well understood. The literature reports the etiology of the pneumothorax as lymphocytic alveolar exudate, interstitial inflammation and subpleural necrosis, and cavitation with subsequent development of a bronchopleural fistula. These pathologic findings may progress to fibrosis, which predisposes the patient to pneumothorax. Usually, pneumothorax occurs with concurrent infection.

Recurrence is characteristic of pneumothorax associated with PCP, and contralateral pneumothoraces develop in approximately 50 percent of patients. Eng and associates reported one patient who had seven separate episodes. Patients with bilateral pneumothorax have also been reported.

Due to the necrotic lung surrounding the cavities these pneumothraces are extremely difficult to treat. In these special circumstances the recommendations for treatment are observation or the use of a small chest tube with a Heimlich flutter valve. The symptomatic patient should be managed with tube thoracostomy unless there are persistent or large air leaks, in which case thoracoscopy, thoracotomy, stapling of blebs, and pleurodesis may be indicated. Decisions regarding surgical intervention should be made on an individual basis.

Pneumothorax must be ruled out in an AIDS patient with prior or active PCP who presents with respiratory deterioration, and an AIDS patient who presents with a pneumothorax should be evaluated for active PCP.

## BIBLIOGRAPHY

Abolnik IZ, Lossos IS, Gillis D, Breuer R: Primary spontaneous pneumothorax in men. *Am J Med Sci* 305(5):297, 1993.

Beers MF, Sohn M, Swartz M: Recurrent pneumothorax in AIDS patients with pneumocystis pneumonia: A clinicopathologic report of three cases and review of the literature. *Chest* 98:266, 1990.

Eng RH, Bishburg E, Smith SM: Evidence for destruction of lung tissues during *Pneumocystis carinii* infection. *Arch Intern Med* 147:746, 1987.

Light RW: Management of spontaneous pneumothorax. *Am Rev Respir Dis* 148:245, 1993.

Miller AC, Harvey JE: Guidelines for the management of spontaneous pneumothrax. *Br Med J* 07:114, 1993.

Tanaka F, Masatosi I, Esaki J, et al: Secondary spontaneous pneumothorax. *Ann Thorac Surg* 55:372, 1993.

Vallee P, Sullivan M, Richardson HH, et al: Sequential treatment of a simple pneumothorax. *Ann Emerg Med* 17:936, 1988.

Wisdom K, Nowak RM, Richardson HR, et al: Alternate therapy for traumatic pneumothorax in "pocket shooters." *Ann Emerg Med* 15:428, 1986.

# 70
# HEMOPTYSIS
## James R. Yankaskas

## PATHOPHYSIOLOGY

Hemoptysis may reflect serious or relatively minor medical illnesses. This symptom produces great concern, and most patients seek medical care promptly. Prompt evaluation is necessary to ascertain whether the expectorated blood originated in the lungs or from nasopharyngeal or gastrointestinal sources and to evaluate the potential for serious recurrences. Hemoptysis may be life-threatening when associated with production of large volumes of blood, when associated with mycetomas (fungus balls) in pulmonary cavities, and when of sufficient magnitude to produce significant hypoxemia. The most important concern in massive hemoptysis is asphyxiation due to diffuse interruption of airflow and gas exchange. For clinical purposes, hemoptysis is characterized as massive or minor, based on the volume of blood expectorated. Massive hemoptysis is defined by a total volume of expectorated blood greater than 200 mL/24 h, or production of greater than 100 mL/day for 3 to 7 days. Minor hemoptysis is defined as the production of smaller quantities of blood, often as mixed blood and mucus.

Blood in the lungs can originate from bronchial capillaries, alveolar capillaries, bronchial arteries, and from pulmonary arteries. Bleeding from bronchial capillaries is most commonly associated with infection and inflammation and is typically associated with mucopurulent secretions and is minor in quantity. Hemorrhage from alveolar capillaries can be diffuse and extensive in quantity but tends to remain in the alveoli. It results in massive hemoptysis only with very severe disease, although serious respiratory compromise can occur with diffuse hemorrhage and scanty hemoptysis. Bronchial arteries, which contain blood under systemic pressure, are located adjacent to the bronchial tree and hypertrophy in the presence of chronic inflammation, particularly that associated with tuberculosis (TB) and

**Table 70-1.** Causes of Hemoptysis

| Cause | Prevalence, % |
|---|---|
| **Infectious** | |
| Tuberculosis | 2–61 |
| Bronchiectasis | 21–40 |
| Bronchitis | 5–37 |
| Fungal | 1–12 |
| Pneumonia | 1–9 |
| Abscess | 2–5 |
| **Neoplastic** | **3–24** |
| **Cardiogenic** | **0–2** |
| **Traumatic** | **0–4** |
| **Alveolar Hemorrhage** | **0–2** |
| **Other Causes** | **0–10** |
| **Unknown** | **2–19** |

bronchiectasis. Bronchial arteries are the most common source of massive hemoptysis, which is usually triggered by chronic bronchial inflammation, leading to bronchial artery hypertrophy and rupture of the fused and weakened airway/bronchial walls. These mechanisms are implicated in hemoptysis from TB, bronchiectasis, and mycetoma. The low-pressure pulmonary arteries are an uncommon source of intrapulmonary bleeding. Rarely, a tumor will erode into a pulmonary artery, producing a direct anastomosis with the bronchial tree and causing massive hemoptysis.

The diseases most commonly associated with hemoptysis, and their prevalence in different series, are listed in Table 70-1. Infectious pulmonary diseases, particularly chronic processes, cause most hemoptysis. Bronchogenic carcinoma usually causes minor bleeding, although advanced tumors can erode into bronchial or pulmonary arteries and lead to massive hemoptysis. Uncommon causes may be apparent from other symptoms (e.g., cardiogenic pulmonary edema) or reflect multisystem disease (e.g., pulmonary and renal hemorrhage in Goodpasture disease).

## CLINICAL FEATURES AND DIAGNOSIS

A *history* of underlying lung disease often provides important clues to the underlying cause. An acute onset of cough and bloody sputum, with or without fever, may indicate acute pneumonia or bronchitis. A chronic productive cough may reflect bronchitis or bronchiectasis. Fevers, night sweats, and weight loss are typical signs of tuberculosis. Anorexia, weight loss, and change in cough may reflect development of bronchogenic carcinoma, although many tumors present with a new cough and hemoptysis. Alveolar hemorrhage syndromes often present with dyspnea and minor hemoptysis, although they may be associated with renal disease and hematuria. Patients with massive hemoptysis often describe a "gurgling" or a warm sensation in the chest, that corresponds to the site of bleeding.

The *physical examination* can be useful in assessing the cause and severity of hemoptysis but is rarely a reliable means to localize the bleeding site. Fever usually indicates an infectious etiology. Tachypnea may reflect respiratory compromise from intrapulmonary blood or underlying lung disease. Blood pressure is usually not changed from baseline except in cases of very massive hemoptysis. The nasal cavity and oropharynx must be carefully examined for extrapulmonary sources of blood loss. The heart examination may reveal a diastolic murmur of mitral stenosis. The pulmonary examination may reveal fine early inspiratory crackles associated with alveolar blood; or inspiratory and expiratory crackles associated with airway secretions and blood; or wheezing associated with bronchial narrowing. The extremities may reveal cyanosis, reflecting hemoglobin desaturation, or digital clubbing, a sign associated with bronchiectasis and some bronchogenic cancers.

*Chest x-rays* (PA and lateral) are the most essential diagnostic study (an AP chest x-ray may be required for an unstable patient) and may reveal signs of underlying lung diseases, the distribution of extravascular blood in the lungs, and conditions that predispose to hemoptysis, such as mycetomas or lung masses. Essential *laboratory tests* are the hematocrit, platelet count, prothrombin time, partial thromboplastin time, arterial blood gases, and urinalysis. The initial evaluation should focus on identifying causes of massive hemoptysis that require acute intervention and stabilization. Secondary tests, such as purified protein derivative and control skin tests, and sputum bacterial, acid-fast bacilli, and fungal cultures are usually indicated.

## TREATMENT

Treatment in the emergency department depends on the severity and persistence of the hemoptysis and its likelihood of recurrence. All patients with massive hemoptysis, and some patients with minor hemoptysis and significant risk of developing massive hemoptysis in the near future, will require urgent management and hospitalization. All such patients require intravenous access, supplemental oxygen to assure adequate arterial saturation, and typing and cross-matching blood. Patients with ongoing massive hemoptysis should be positioned with the bleeding lung down, to minimize soiling of the contralateral lung. Tracheal intubation with a large diameter endotracheal tube (8F or larger) is indicated if there is respiratory failure or if the patient is unable to clear the blood from the airways. Double-lumen endotracheal tubes are rarely indicated, because the small lumen diameters limit suctioning and airway clearance. Fresh-frozen plasma should be administered to correct any blood clotting abnormalities. Cough suppression with codeine or opioids is indicated to prevent dislodging of hemostatic clots. If bleeding persists despite initial measures, the endotracheal tube should be advanced to the mainstem bronchus of the nonbleeding lung to minimize further aspiration of blood. The right mainstem bronchus is easily entered by advancing a standard orotracheal tube. The left mainstem bronchus is more sharply angled from the trachea, and selective intubation usually requires special equipment and experienced personnel. Mechanical ventilation should be instituted as necessary to support ventilation. Patients with massive hemoptysis that has subsided are at high risk of recurrence and require similar intensive management and hospital admission, usually to an intensive care unit. Consultation should be obtained with a pulmonologist and a thoracic surgeon, who may arrange for bronchoscopy, high-resolution CT scan, or bronchial artery angiography to localize the specific bleeding site. Patients with minor hemoptysis who are at high risk of developing massive hemoptysis may require emergency department observation or hospitalization. Massive hemoptysis is less common in children, but similar evaluation and management is appropriate. Patients with minor hemoptysis due to bronchitis or tumors may require sputum samples for culture and cytologic evaluation and follow-up consultation with their primary care physician or a pulmonary subspecialist.

## PATIENT DISPOSITION

The indications for admission are massive hemoptysis or the presence of diseases likely to produce it proximately (see Table 70-2). Such patients should be admitted to pulmonologists or thoracic surgeons, and usually require management in an intensive care unit. Definitive therapy may require medical treatment of infections or bronchial artery embolization. Surgery may be required for continuing massive

**Table 70-2.** Indications for Consultation/Hospitalization

Massive hemoptysis (>200 mL/24 h)
Mycetoma
Active tuberculosis
Hypoxemia requiring supplemental $O_2$
Hypercapnea
Diffuse alveolar hemorrhage

hemoptysis from a localized site or as definitive long-term therapy. If appropriate subspecialists are not available, medical stabilization is essential before considering transfer to a hospital that provides such services. Emergency department consultations with pulmonologists and thoracic surgeons may be required for patients with borderline indications for hospitalization. Patients with minor hemoptysis due to bronchitis and/or bronchogenic carcinoma should be discharged with cough suppressants for 2 to 3 days (e.g., codeine, 15 to 30 mg, q 4–6 h) and an oral antibiotic, such as ampicillin (250 mg q.i.d), amoxicillin (250 mg tid), trimethoprim/sulfamethoxazole (160 and 800 mg bid), or doxycycline (100 mg bid) to treat bronchitic organisms (e.g., *Streptococcus pneumoniae, Haemophilus influenza, Moraxella catarrhalis*). Follow-up should be obtained with internists, family physicians, or pulmonologists within a period of 7 days, with earlier return to the physician or emergency department if symptoms worsen.

## BIBLIOGRAPHY

Cahill BC, Ingbar DH: Massive hemoptysis: Assessment and management. *Clin Chest Med* 15:147, 1994.

Cohen AM, Doershuk CF, Stern RC: Bronchial artery embolization to control hemoptysis in cystic fibrosis. *Radiology* 175:401, 1990.

Johnston H, Reisz G: Changing spectrum of hemoptysis: Underlying causes in 148 patients undergoing diagnostic flexible fiberoptic bronchoscopy. *Arch Intern Med* 149:1666, 1989.

Knott-Craig CJ, Oostuizen JG, Rossouw G, et al: Management and prognosis of massive hemoptysis. Recent experience with 120 patients. *J Thorac Cardiovasc Surg* 105:394, 1993.

McGuinness G, Beacher JR, Harkin TJ, et al: Hemoptysis: Prospective high-resolution CT/bronchoscopic correlation. *Chest* 105:1155, 1994.

# 71
# ACUTE ASTHMA IN ADULTS
## Stanley Sherman

## DESCRIPTION AND DEFINITION

Asthma is a common chronic disease. While it is more common in children and young adults, onset of symptoms can occur in any decade of life. Childhood asthma often dissipates with age, but adult-onset disease is usually persistent. Despite this chronicity, the clinical course is quite variable, and only a minority suffer serious debilitation. However, despite optimal medical management, asthma *can* be a fatal disease.

While asthma is difficult to define succinctly, several concepts are central to the definition and understanding of this disease. Asthma, in contrast to other obstructive lung diseases, is defined mainly in physiologic rather than anatomic or clinical terms. *Asthma* is reversible airflow obstruction, associated with a state of increased responsiveness of the tracheobronchial tree to many different stimuli (which do not affect normal individuals). This state of increased responsiveness, manifest by widespread bronchospasm, reflects the condition of *bronchial hyperreactivity,* a concept which will be discussed later. The bronchospasm characteristic of the acute asthmatic attack is typically reversible; it improves spontaneously or within minutes or hours of treatment.

Within the spectrum of chronic obstructive lung disease, asthma may either exist as a relatively "pure" entity or coexist with chronic bronchitis, emphysema, or bronchiectasis in various combinations. In either case, patients experience dyspnea, cough, and wheezing as the major complaints. The patterns of airflow obstruction vary greatly, depending on the frequency of the acute episodes and the state of the airways between episodes. Asthma may occur sporadically or manifest as chronic airflow obstruction with episodic exacerbations.

## CLASSIFICATION

Traditionally, asthma has been classified as extrinsic or intrinsic. *Extrinsic asthma* is said to be "allergic" or immunologic in origin, occurring in atopic individuals. *Atopy* refers to the genetic predisposition to manifest immediate wheal and flare reactions to skin tests with multiple antigens, to which normal individuals do not respond. Atopic patients are usually younger and often have a history of allergic rhinitis and elevated serum levels of IgE. *Intrinsic asthma* exists when no obvious extrinsic causes are identified. Patients are typically older, nonatopic, and more likely to have a chronic course.

This timeworn division is less valuable today because understanding of the disease has evolved. A greater understanding of the complex mechanisms of bronchospasm has enabled us to view asthma as a state of bronchial hyperreactivity with many potential "triggers" (Table 71-1). An immunologic response (type I allergic reaction or immediate hypersensitivity) mediated by IgE is but one trigger, which may occur in atopic individuals (as in classic "extrinsic" asthma) as well as in nonatopic patients.

In addition, research and experience in recent years have revealed an increasing number of agents that cause asthma, either through immunologic mechanisms or by direct irritant effects. Occupational asthma has emerged as an important entity. In fact, it is estimated that as many as 5 to 10 percent of asthmatic patients (atopic and nonatopic) may have a significant trigger in the work environment. Because of the varying patterns of occupational asthma, it is difficult to correctly diagnose. Responses can be immediate, delayed 4 to 6 h following exposure, or repetitive at 24-h intervals (often in the morning).

## PATHOPHYSIOLOGY

The rapidly reversible airflow obstruction that characterizes asthma is due mainly to bronchial smooth muscle contraction. However, in addition to abnormalities in the control of airway smooth muscle, the asthmatic attack is frequently associated with mucus hypersecretion and inflammatory changes in the bronchial walls, resulting in mucosal edema. Thus, the increased airway resistance seen in the asthmatic patient usually implies a three-component response. While the focus of therapy usually centers around pharmacologic manipulation of airway smooth muscle, it is important to recognize the physiologic impairment caused by mucus production and mucosal edema. Bronchospasm can be reversed within minutes, but the airflow obstruction due to mucous plugging and inflammatory changes in bronchial walls

**Table 71-1.** Provocation of the Asthmatic Response (Triggers)

Immunologic reaction (exposure to antigen with mediator release)
Viral respiratory infections (upper and lower respiratory tract)
Changes in temperature and humidity (especially cold air)
Strong odors (perfume, etc.)
Pollutants, dusts, fumes, and other irritants (including occupational exposures)
Certain drugs and chemicals: aspirin, nonsteroidal antiinflammatory drugs, tartrazine dye (yellow dye no. 5), sulfiting agents, β-adrenergic blocking drugs
Sinus infections
Exercise
Strong emotions, laughing, coughing
Deep inspiration or forceful expiration
Gastroesophageal reflux

does not resolve for days or weeks. Failure to rapidly reverse an acute asthmatic attack strongly suggests that all three mechanisms are operative.

In addition to contributing to airflow obstruction, mucous plugging may lead to atelectasis, infectious bronchitis, and pneumonitis, with consequent impairment in gas exchange efficiency. The syndromes of allergic bronchopulmonary aspergillosis and mucoid impaction of the bronchus attest to the potential complications of mucus hypersecretion and impaired mucociliary clearance seen in some asthmatic patients.

## Bronchial Hyperreactivity

The hallmark of asthma is bronchial hyperreactivity—an extreme sensitivity of the airways to physiologic, chemical, and pharmacologic stimuli. This results in a greater degree of bronchoconstriction than seen in normal individuals. Bronchial hyperreactivity in asthmatics is, thus, an exaggerated response—an extreme irritability of airway smooth muscle to stimuli such as exercise, cold air, dust, irritants (smoke, atmospheric pollutants), inhaled antigens, histamine, serotonin, bradykinin, and various cholinergic agonists.

While the cause of bronchial hyperreactivity is not fully understood, many theories have been proposed (Table 71-2). In any case, it is important to understand the role of the autonomic nervous system in the control of airway smooth muscle, since these relationships provide the rationale for certain pharmacologic interventions in acute asthma.

The parasympathetic nervous system (PSNS) has an abundance of vagal efferent fibers ending in airway smooth muscle. Vagus nerve stimulation releases acetylcholine at postganglionic nerve endings, causing bronchospasm. Under normal conditions, a minor degree of PSNS predominance is observed, mainly in large, central airways (the main resistance airways). This tonic cholinergic activity produces a baseline bronchial smooth muscle tone, which, when abolished, produces bronchodilation. Strong emotions may lead to significant neural output from the central nervous system to airway smooth muscle (traveling through vagal efferent pathways), resulting in bronchospasm. In addition, the PSNS functions in the efferent limb of reflexive bronchoconstriction, following afferent stimulation arising from the nasopharynx, larynx, trachea, and airways. The subepithelial irritant receptors in these locations may be stimulated by mechanical pressure, dust, chemical irritants, and certain drugs. Damage to airway epithelium disrupts the tight intercellular junctions, increases the exposure of the subepithelial irritant receptors and mast cells, and sensitizes the subepithelial irritant receptors. This increased airway permeability has been cited as a possible mechanism of bronchial hyperreactivity.

Compared to the PSNS, the sympathetic nervous system (SNS) innervation of airway smooth muscle is not as abundant and is limited to smaller airways. The role of the SNS in baseline airway smooth muscle tone appears small. Direct effects are less significant than those of circulating catecholamines. β-Adrenergic stimulation pro-

**Table 71-2.** Postulated Mechanisms of Bronchial Hyperreactivity in Asthma

Decrease in baseline airway caliber
Alterations in bronchial smooth muscle (hypertrophy, hyperplasia)
Increased number of mast cells
Increased synthesis of mediators
Lowered receptor threshold
Damage to airway epithelial cells (greater exposure to subepithelial irritant receptors)
Alterations or imbalance in autonomic nervous system regulation:
  Increased parasympathetic activity
  Decreased β-adrenergic responsiveness
  Increased α-adrenergic responsiveness
  Decreased responsiveness of the nonadrenergic (purinergic) inhibitory system

motes bronchodilation of peripheral airways more than of central airways, while α-adrenergic stimulation may produce bronchoconstriction.

A third component of the autonomic nervous system consists of fibers which appear to travel with the vagus nerves to the airways. The transmitter(s) have not yet been identified. This nonadrenergic (purinergic) inhibitory system prevents bronchial smooth muscle contraction, possibly serving as the major opposition to the parasympathetic nervous system.

## Mechanisms of Bronchospasm

Physiologic reactions in the asthmatic target cells (bronchial smooth muscle cells, mast cells, mucous gland secretory cells, vagus nerve cells, and inflammatory cells) are calcium-dependent processes—i.e., activation of these cells requires mobilization of free calcium ions with a transmembranous movement to the intracellular cytoplasmic matrix. Regardless of the inciting stimulus, it appears that calcium flux represents the final common pathway for cellular response.

While the factors capable of triggering an asthmatic reaction are numerous (Table 71-1), the known mechanisms of bronchospasm are relatively few. The best known (but not necessarily the most prevalent) is the immunologic reaction. Immediate hypersensitivity (type I allergic reaction) involves IgE antibody attached to the abundant airway mast cells (scattered throughout smooth muscle bundles, in the submucosa of airways, and adjacent to submucous glands). Exposure to a specific antigen establishes a bivalent cross-linking and results in mast cell degranulation. Preformed mediators are released (histamine, eosinophil chemotactic factors of anaphylaxis, neutrophil chemotactic factors, serotonin, and others) and other mediators are rapidly synthesized and then released (leukotrienes, prostaglandins, thromboxanes, platelet-activating factor). Mediators act directly on airway smooth muscle to produce bronchoconstriction. In addition, by inciting inflammation and increasing vascular permeability, mediators may produce mucosal edema and greater airflow obstruction. They may also elicit bronchospasm indirectly, by stimulating subepithelial irritant receptors and creating a vagal-mediated reflexive response.

The autonomic nervous system may function directly in the contraction of bronchial smooth muscle. Cholinergic neural output, from the central nervous system or as part of an irritant receptor reflex, produces bronchoconstriction. Imbalance in autonomic control—reduced β-adrenergic stimulation, increased α-adrenergic stimulation, or reduced purinergic stimulation—can also result in bronchospasm.

In exercise-induced bronchospasm hyperventilation with large volumes of cold, dry air promotes a cooling of the airways, which triggers a bronchospastic response. This exercise-induced respiratory mucosal heat loss appears to involve mediator release, because the response is most consistently blocked by the prior administration of disodium cromoglycate, an inhibitor of mast cell degranulation.

In some asthmatics, bronchoconstriction may be caused by drugs which inhibit cyclooxygenase (e.g., aspirin and nonsteroidal antiinflammatory agents). The mechanism is believed to involve an alteration in the metabolism of arachidonic acid toward the lipoxygenase pathway, with production of greater amounts of leukotrienes. Leukotrienes (formerly known as the *slow-reacting substance of anaphylaxis*) comprise a family of related compounds which are potent bronchoconstrictors.

## Consequences of Airflow Obstruction

The physiologic consequences of airflow obstruction are outlined in Table 71-3. The initial abnormality is increased airway resistance, stemming from a combination of bronchoconstriction, mucosal edema, and mucus hypersecretion. These conditions result in a reduction in maximum expiratory flow rates, best determined by objective measurements of pulmonary function.

As impairment of the expiratory phase of ventilation progresses,

**Table 71-3.** Physiologic Consequences of Airflow Obstruction

Increased airway resistance
Decreased maximum expiratory flow rates
Air trapping
Increased airway pressure
   Barotrauma
   Adverse hemodynamic effects
Ventilation-perfusion imbalance
   Hypoxemia
   Hypercarbia
Increased work of breathing
   Pulsus paradoxus
   Respiratory muscle fatigue with ventilatory failure

the complete tidal volume is not exhaled, and air trapping ensues. This process, reflected in elevation of the residual volume and functional residual capacity of the lungs, has both beneficial and adverse effects on lung mechanics. Air trapping tends to maintain airway patency through a tethering effect on the airways, thus reducing airway resistance. However, an elevated residual volume places the diaphragms in a mechanically disadvantageous position and, for all the inspiratory muscles, increases the elastic work of breathing.

Increased airway resistance and air trapping combine to produce increased airway pressures, which may result in barotrauma (subcutaneous emphysema, pneumomediastinum, or pneumothorax) and may impair cardiac performance through several mechanisms.

The acute asthmatic attack also results in an uneven distribution of ventilation, which in turn results in ventilation-perfusion imbalance. While hypercarbia may be seen in extreme cases, hypoxemia is more commonly observed. Worsening of hypoxemia has been demonstrated during the early treatment of acute asthma, an effect attributed to the vasoactive nature of β-adrenergic bronchodilators (which promote increased perfusion to poorly ventilated lung zones). Since most asthmatics receive oxygen supplementation during the initial phase of treatment, this sequence is not clinically significant.

During an acute asthmatic attack, the combination of increased airway resistance, increased respiratory drive, and air trapping creates greater demands on the muscles of inspiration. Excessive contractions of these muscles (during inspiration and, for unknown reasons, during expiration also) and an increased workload contribute to the patient's sensation of dyspnea. Respiratory muscles can fatigue. When the energy supply to these muscles fails to match energy requirements, lactic acidosis ensues, followed by overt ventilatory failure. When the major muscles of inspiration, the diaphragms, begin to tire, accessory inspiratory muscles assume a greater proportion of the ventilatory work. Retraction of the sternocleidomastoids (accessory neck muscles) closely correlates with severe asthma and is not usually observed until the $FEV_1$ falls below 1.0 L.

An abnormal pulsus paradoxus (> 20 mm Hg) is associated with severe asthma. A dual mechanism has been proposed, relating to excessive negative intrathoracic pressure swings. During labored breathing, the generation of excessive negative intrathoracic pressure increases left ventricular afterload and accelerates venous return to the right heart, shifting the interventricular septum and further impairing left ventricular output. The net effect is transient reduction in cardiac output and systolic blood pressure.

## PATHOLOGY

Precise pathologic descriptions of the asthmatic lung are hampered by difficulty in determining what constitutes pure asthma. Mucous plugging of the airways is a common finding, almost universally present in fatal asthma. Within the mucus, one finds abundant eosinophils and sloughed mucosal epithelial cells. In addition, mucus may contain other characteristic elements: Charcot-Leyden crystals (crystalline structures representing coalescence of free eosinophilic granules), Creola bodies (large compact clusters of sloughed mucosal

**Table 71-4.** Asthma Mimickers

Congestive heart failure ("cardiac asthma")
Upper airway obstruction
Aspiration of foreign body or gastric acid
Bronchogenic carcinoma with endobronchial obstruction
Metastatic carcinoma with lymphangitic metastasis
Sarcoidosis with endobronchial obstruction
Vocal-cord dysfunction
Multiple pulmonary emboli (rare)

epithelial cells), and Curschmann's spirals (bronchiolar casts of sputum components). Bronchial walls demonstrate mucosal edema, thickening of the basement membranes, submucosal eosinophilic inflammatory infiltrate, smooth muscle hypertrophy, and hyperplasia of mucous glands and goblet cells. The lung parenchyma may demonstrate areas of atelectasis, secondary to mucous plugging, but destructive changes are not observed.

## CLINICAL PRESENTATION

Even though it may be difficult to define asthma precisely and to appreciate the great variability in clinical patterns, the emergency physician easily recognizes the severe asthmatic attack. The diagnosis of asthma is secure when the key elements of the database are identified and the other conditions that may mimic acute asthma are excluded (Table 71-4). In practical terms, it is not essential to distinguish between the various obstructive lung diseases, since acute management is the same, focusing on reversible components.

### History

While most patients relate a history of asthma at the onset, many will not. The patient complains of progressive dyspnea, chest tightness, wheezing, and cough. Persistent cough is often the major complaint, overshadowing the airflow obstruction and delaying recognition of the asthmatic state. The duration of acute symptomatology is important because episodes lasting more than several days are likely to be associated with significant mucosal edema and mucous plugging, factors which reduce the likelihood of successful emergency treatment and which necessitate hospitalization.

### Physical Examination

The patient presenting with a severe asthmatic attack is in obvious respiratory distress, with rapid, loud breathing. At times, wheezing may be audible without a stethoscope. The use of accessory muscles of inspiration (neck muscles are most prominent) indicates diaphragmatic fatigue, while the appearance of paradoxical respirations (inward movement of the upper abdominal wall due to inspiratory ascent of the diaphragms) reflect impending ventilatory failure. Alteration in the mental status—e.g., lethargy, exhaustion, agitation, or confusion—also heralds respiratory arrest.

Direct physical examination reveals hyperresonance to percussion, decreased intensity of breath sounds, and prolongation of the expiratory phase, usually with wheezing. Although wheezing results from the movement of air through narrowed airways, the intensity of the wheeze may not correlate with the severity of the airflow obstruction. The "quiet chest" reflects very severe airflow obstruction with air movement insufficient to promote a wheeze. A pulsus paradoxus above 20 mm Hg is also indicative of severe asthma.

### Pulmonary Function Testing

The objective demonstration of reversible airflow obstruction is central to the diagnosis. Characteristic changes in pulmonary function during acute asthma include a reduction in expiratory flow rates, such as the peak expiratory flow rate (PEFR) and forced expiratory volume in 1 s ($FEV_1$), a slight reduction in the forced vital capacity (FVC), and a ratio of $FEV_1/FVC$ of less than 75 percent (defining a state of airflow obstruction). The residual volume, functional residual capacity, and total lung capacity are increased, although the latter elevation is less pronounced. Diffusing capacity is normal. In response to bronchodilator treatment, asthmatics typically demonstrate a greater than 15 percent improvement in $FEV_1$, FVC, and PEFR.

### Chest Radiograph

Despite a low diagnostic yield in the setting of acute asthma, the chest radiograph is essential in excluding other conditions which may mimic asthma (Table 71-4) and in monitoring for associated complications. Abnormalities directly related to the asthmatic attack include pneumomediastinum, pneumothorax, atelectasis, and pneumonia. The difficulty of diagnosing pneumothorax by physical examination in the patient with acute asthma should be emphasized; the consequences of missing such a diagnosis are obvious. In the uncomplicated asthmatic, chest radiographic findings may include hyperinflation (flattening of the diaphragms, increased retrosternal air space) and increased bronchial markings, which are due to thickening of bronchial walls and which reflect an associated chronic bronchitic state.

### Additional Laboratory Investigations

With the exception of arterial blood gases (see below), other studies are not diagnostically useful. The electrocardiogram may demonstrate many nonspecific findings, such as sinus tachycardia, right ventricular strain (right-axis deviation, clockwise rotation of the heart, right atrial enlargement, right bundle branch block), and atrial or ventricular arrhythmias. Blood and sputum eosinophilia may be present, reflecting the asthmatic condition. The total white blood cell count is frequently elevated, even without overt infection.

### ASTHMA AND PREGNANCY

When asthma and pregnancy coexist (about 1 percent of all pregnancies), appropriate management is based on an understanding of the changes in respiratory physiology that accompany pregnancy, and a recognition of the hazards that the acute asthmatic attack poses for the mother and fetus.

The gradual increase in circulating progesterone during pregnancy increases central chemoreceptor sensitivity, resulting in an increase in minute ventilation (mainly tidal volume, not rate). This effect explains the frequent complaint of dyspnea during pregnancy. As a result of the increased minute ventilation, a moderate respiratory alkalosis (with appropriate renal compensation) is observed. In addition, oxygen consumption is increased during pregnancy. Pulmonary mechanics, however, are not affected by the enlarging uterus until the latter half of the pregnancy, when the functional residual capacity is reduced. Vital capacity, total lung capacity, and large airway function are unchanged.

The effect of pregnancy on the course of the asthma varies and is unpredictable. Most reports describe worsening of asthmatic symptoms in about 25 percent of cases, improvement in another 25 percent, and no change in the remaining half. Patients tend to repeat the same pattern established during preceding pregnancies.

The effect of asthma on pregnancy is also unpredictable. However, maternal complications are slightly increased. In addition, there is a greater likelihood of premature births, and the rate of perinatal mortality is twice as high. These risks correlate with the severity of the asthma. Fetal complications are due to impaired fetal oxygenation resulting from maternal hypoxemia and from the adverse effects of alkalosis on the oxyhemoglobin dissociation curve.

### Management of Asthma during Pregnancy

With few exceptions, the treatment of the pregnant asthmatic patient is no different from that of the nonpregnant asthmatic. Management should emphasize prompt and aggressive measures aimed at avoiding uncontrolled asthma and preventing hypoxemia. Most drugs used to treat asthma are safe for use during pregnancy and for nursing mothers. These include theophylline, β-adrenergic agents, corticosteroids, atropine, and most antibiotics. Caution should be exercised with the use of parenteral β-adrenergic agents near term, since these drugs may inhibit uterine contractility and occasionally produce maternal pulmonary edema. If essential for the treatment of asthma near term, β-adrenergic agonists should be administered using the aerosolized route, to minimize systemic absorption.

The use of parenteral epinephrine during the early months of pregnancy has been associated with a significant increase in fetal malformations; accordingly, this medication should be avoided. Other medications to avoid include iodides (which may cause fetal goiter and hypothyroidism), tetracycline (damage to fetal teeth, bone, and liver), and sulfonamides (interference with folic acid metabolism). Because erythromycin may interfere with theophylline metabolism (resulting in increased serum concentrations), close monitoring of serum theophylline levels is necessary when the two drugs are administered simultaneously.

### ASSESSING THE SEVERITY OF THE ASTHMATIC ATTACK

When patients present with acute asthma, the physician must assess the severity of the attack, not only to rapidly determine which patients will require hospital admission, but also to identify those at risk of respiratory failure. It is fortunate that asthmatics rarely require intubation and mechanical ventilation. However, when necessary, these measures may be lifesaving because asthmatic patients can deteriorate rapidly.

What is "severe" asthma? In the past, the term *status asthmaticus* was used to indicate the severest condition experienced by the asthmatic, short of respiratory failure. However, the term lacks precision and offers no additional insight to the treating physician. Because the meaning of status asthmaticus is likely to differ among physicians, it is best to avoid the phrase and use instead the more accurate term "severe" asthma. *Severe asthma* is a high-risk, refractory condition requiring immediate and intensive treatment to avoid respiratory failure. The patient with severe asthma has not responded with objective improvement in airflow obstruction to initial emergency treatment consisting of nebulized β-adrenergic drugs, intravenous theophylline and corticosteroids, and even nebulized anticholinergics. In terms of the mechanism of airflow obstruction, failure to rapidly improve with bronchodilator therapy indicates significant mucous plugging and mucosal edema—conditions that require many days or even weeks for complete resolution.

### Profile of the High-Risk Asthmatic

Certain characteristics of the patient and distinctive features of the acute episode enable the physician to predict a high-risk situation. Steroid-dependent patients with a labile clinical pattern (marked, rapid fluctuations in severity of bronchospasm) and a prior history of respiratory failure requiring intubation and mechanical ventilation are at greater risk of a poor outcome. Asthmatic patients who do not respond to emergency treatment are more likely to have ignored escalating symptoms for several days prior to seeking medical attention, thus allowing mucous plugging and mucosal edema to proceed unchecked. In this respect, severe asthma is often viewed as a "crisis of neglect" on the part of the patient. However, the physician often contributes to the poor outcome through inadequate assessment of the severity of the attack, delayed and suboptimal use of corticosteroids, and, during initial treatment, the use of sedation, which may lead to respiratory arrest.

### Subjective versus Objective Assessment

Both the patient and the physician often underestimate the severity of the airflow obstruction. In fact, in acute asthma, the degree of physiologic impairment correlates poorly with most signs and symptoms. While studies using objective measurements, such as the peak expiratory flow rate (PEFR), have shown that many experienced patients are more accurate than their physicians in predicting their degree of airflow obstruction, not all patients are capable of such an analysis. The perception of dyspnea is often related more to changes in inspiratory resistance and the work of breathing than to the degree of expiratory airflow limitation. Patients often have difficulty in determining when their baseline function has returned, usually underestimating the functional impairment. Nevertheless, physicians are well advised to take note of the asthmatic patient's subjective complaints.

The physician's assessment relies on physical examination findings such as increased respiratory rate, contraction of the sternocleidomastoid muscles, paradoxical respirations, the presence of pulsus paradoxus, and reduced intensity of the breath sounds with prolongation of the expiratory phase. Despite the emphasis placed on "wheezing," this sign does not correlate with the severity of the obstructive process.

Numerous studies have demonstrated that successful emergency treatment of acute asthma depends on the degree of objective improvement in pulmonary function. Measurements of the $FEV_1$ and PEFR are useful in predicting which patients are likely to require hospital admission. Physicians using objective criteria can more confidently determine who is likely to do well following discharge and who is likely to relapse.

## Warning Signs of Severe Asthma

Certain objective findings during the emergency evaluation should alert the physician to a potentially adverse outcome (Table 71-5). The performance of spirometry and measurement of PEFR have greatly enhanced the physician's ability to recognize a severe asthmatic attack. However, some asthmatics have difficulty in performing spirometry because forced expiratory maneuvers produce bronchospasm. In such cases, measurement of the PEFR may be tolerated since it does not require the forced expiration of the entire vital capacity. The correlation between these two objective measurements of airflow obstruction is good. Severe asthma is characterized by an $FEV_1$ of less than 1.0 L and a PEFR of less than 80 L/min, while a moderate impairment is associated with an $FEV_1$ of 1.0 to 1.5 L and a PEFR of 80 to 200 L/min.

Deterioration in arterial blood gases (ABGs) is a grave sign in the acutely ill asthmatic; hypoxemia ($Pa_{O_2}$ less than 60 mm Hg on room air) and hypercarbia ($Pa_{CO_2}$ greater than 45 mm Hg) portend respiratory failure (Table 71-6). While ABGs are usually drawn early in the emergency management of the acute asthmatic, this diagnostic study is clearly overused. Assessment of oxygenation status does not require ABGs. Because mild or moderate hypoxemia is nearly universal during the acute attack, one could argue that empiric oxygen supplementation be initially administered. Adequate arterial oxygen saturation ($\geq$ 90 percent) can be confirmed with pulse oximetry. The true purpose of drawing ABGs is to measure the $Pa_{CO_2}$. In this regard, ABGs do not inform the physician "how well" the patient is doing; rather, they serve to relate "how poorly" he or she is doing. Accordingly, measurement of ABGs should be reserved for the patient who

**Table 71-5.** Warning Signs of Severe Asthma

Impaired pulmonary function:
    $FEV_1 < 1.0$ L
    PEFR < 80 L/min
Hypoxemia ($Pa_{O_2} < 60$ mm Hg)
Hypercarbia ($Pa_{CO_2} > 45$ mm Hg) and acidosis (pH < 7.35)
Change in mental status: agitation, confusion, lethargy, exhaustion
Atrial or ventricular arrhythmias
Pulsus paradoxus > 20 mm Hg
Pneumothorax

**Table 71-6.** Clinical Stages of Asthma According to Arterial Blood Gases*

| Clinical Stage† | $Pa_{O_2}$ mm Hg | $Pa_{CO_2}$ mm Hg | pH |
|---|---|---|---|
| 1 | Normal (> 80) | < 35 | > 7.45 |
| 2 | Reduced (60–80) | < 35 | > 7.45 |
| 3 | Low (< 60) | 35–40 | 7.35–7.45 |
| 4 | Low (< 60) | 35–40 | < 7.35‡ |
| 5 | Low (< 60) | > 45 | < 7.35‡ |

* Clinical correlation is advised.

† Clinical stages 1 and 2 reflect "mild" disease, stage 3 is "moderate," and stages 4 and 5 indicate "severe" asthma.

‡ Reflects lactic (metabolic) acidosis related to increased work of breathing.

presents with obvious exhaustion and signs of mental deterioration or who does not improve or appears worse following initial emergency treatment. The use of ABGs outside of this framework rarely serves to alter management decisions. Arterial blood gases must be interpreted in light of the total clinical picture. For example, the physician must note whether the patient is clinically improved or worse; normocarbia is an ominous finding only if the patient is doing poorly. In the heavy smoker or the obese patient, hypercarbia may occur prematurely and not imply the same degree of risk. Fortunately, only a minority of hypercarbic episodes in acute asthmatics require mechanical ventilation; with good medical management, rapid reversibility is the rule.

Changes in mental status suggest severe physiologic impairment and, unless promptly reversed, indicate a need for intubation and mechanical ventilation. Atrial and ventricular arrhythmias may reflect multiple stresses such as hypoxemia, acidosis, and elevated levels of circulating catecholamines. A pulsus paradoxus greater than 20 mm Hg indicates severely impaired pulmonary status, usually correlating with an $FEV_1$ of less than 1.25 L. A pneumothorax in the midst of an acute asthmatic attack is a potentially fatal complication that must be managed promptly. In most instances, tube thoracostomy is desirable to prevent respiratory failure or circulatory compromise due to a tension pneumothorax. Other frequently mentioned "warning" signs such as hypertension, tachycardia, and even the "quiet" chest do not provide additional insight beyond the findings already discussed.

## TREATMENT OF ACUTE ASTHMA

The goals are simple: Improve airway function rapidly, avoid hypoxemia, and prevent respiratory failure and death. In addition, it is desirable to quickly identify those patients who require hospital admission, and avoid discharging patients who will return within hours or days. In most cases, disposition of the acute asthmatic patient can be made within 1 h.

## Indications for Hospital Admission

Criteria for hospital admission are detailed in Table 71-7. Admission decisions can and should be made early. Because bronchoconstriction is rapidly reversible with appropriate treatment, an asthmatic attack

**Table 71-7.** Criteria for Hospital Admission in Acute Asthma*

Emergency visit within the preceding 3 days
Failure of subjective improvement following treatment
Failure of posttreatment $FEV_1$ to increase by > 500 mL, or absolute value < 1.6 L
Failure of posttreatment PEFR to increase more than 15% above initial value, or absolute value < 200 L/min
Change in mental status (lethargy, agitation, exhaustion, confusion)
Failure of hypercarbia to resolve after treatment
Presence of pneumothorax

* Presence of any of these conditions warrants admission to the hospital.

of recent onset due mainly to bronchial smooth muscle contraction can be distinguished from the slowly responding episodes associated with mucous plugging and significant mucosal edema. Thus, asthmatics who do not demonstrate significant subjective and objective improvement within 30 to 60 min are likely to require many days of further intensive treatment to resolve the complex airflow obstruction. Objective assessment ($FEV_1$ or PEFR) is crucial to proper management of acute asthma.

## Basic Approach to Management

While many accepted treatment measures have a secure foundation in pulmonary physiology, few have been rigidly assessed with well-controlled double-blind studies. Nevertheless, a rational approach to the therapy of acute asthma can be constructed on the basis of current concepts of the disease process, the principles of pharmacology, and clinical experience.

Oxygen should be administered immediately to all acute asthmatics, using a nasal cannula at 2 to 3 L/min. Empiric treatment is justified because most patients will manifest some degree of hypoxemia and the potential for rapid fluctuation is great. Furthermore, in the "pure" asthmatic, the risk of oxygen-induced respiratory depression is insignificant. The adequacy of supplemental oxygen should be determined—preferably by pulse oximetry.

Because mucous plugging is prominent in patients hospitalized with acute asthma, intravenous fluids are essential for proper liquefaction and clearance of secretions. Generous fluid therapy will also benefit the many asthmatics who are dehydrated due to excessive respiratory water loss and reduced oral intake. Percussion and postural drainage may also assist in the removal of secretions, but because they are difficult to perform in the acutely dyspneic patient and can produce reflex bronchospasm, they are best avoided during early treatment.

Several measures must always be avoided in the treatment of acute asthma. Sedatives and tranquilizers are absolutely contraindicated, regardless of how "nervous" the patient appears; respiratory arrest often follows such ill-advised treatment. Mucolytic agents (acetylcysteine) are similarly contraindicated during the acute episode because they may provoke further bronchospasm. Since the benefits of iodides and glyceryl guaicolate are uncertain, these drugs should also be avoided. β-Adrenergic blocking agents (even "selective" agents) should not be used to treat arrhythmias, hypertension, or angina in the face of acute asthma. Many asthmatics respond poorly to ultrasonic nebulization and treatments with an intermittent positive pressure breathing machine (IPPB). Hydration can be achieved through the intravenous route, and airway medications can be delivered using a compressor-driven nebulizer.

## β-Adrenergic Agonists

β-Adrenergic agonists are preferred as the initial medication for the treatment of acute bronchospasm and for the stable ambulatory patient. These drugs produce greater and more rapid improvement in pulmonary function than parenteral theophylline. The addition of theophylline to β-adrenergic therapy is reserved for the more difficult cases.

### Description

β-Adrenergic receptors are divided into two types: $β_1$ and $β_2$. Stimulation of $β_1$ receptors in the heart increases rate and force of contraction, while in the small intestine motility and tone are decreased. $β_2$-Adrenergic stimulation promotes bronchodilation (in airways), vasodilation (in blood vessels), uterine relaxation, and skeletal muscle tremor.

The mechanism of bronchodilator action of β-adrenergic drugs involves stimulation of the enzyme adenylcyclase, which converts intracellular adenosine triphosphate (ATP) to cyclic adenosine monophosphate (cAMP). This action enhances the binding of intracellular calcium to cell membranes, reducing the myoplasmic calcium concentration, and results in relaxation of bronchial smooth muscle. In addition to bronchodilation, β-adrenergic drugs inhibit mediator release and promote mucociliary clearance.

The issue of tachyphylaxis with β-adrenergic agents is frequently raised. The consensus view is that if this does occur in asthmatics, the effects are not clinically significant. These drugs are metabolized by monoamine oxidase (MAO) and catechol-O-methyltransferase (COMT) to inactive compounds. In the intestine, sulfatases also inactivate these agents.

The most common side effect of β-adrenergic drugs is skeletal muscle tremor. Patients may also experience nervousness, anxiety, insomnia, headache, hyperglycemia, palpitations, tachycardia, and hypertension. Despite earlier concerns over potential cardiotoxicity, especially when these drugs are used in combination with theophylline, clinical experience has not revealed significant problems. Arrhythmias and evidence of myocardial ischemia are rare, especially in patients without prior history of coronary artery disease.

### The Aerosol Route

Aerosol therapy with β-adrenergic drugs produces superior bronchodilation and is favored over both oral and parenteral routes. The aerosol route achieves topical administration of a relatively small dose of drug, producing local effects with minimum systemic absorption and fewer side effects. Optimum deposition and retention of appropriately sized particles (1 to 5 μ in diameter) containing a bronchodilator drug is enhanced by slow inspiratory flow rates followed by prolonged (10 s or more) breath-holding. Aerosol delivery may be achieved with a metered-dose inhaler, a compressor-driven nebulizer, or an IPPB. Treatment with an IPPB device offers no advantage over compressor-driven nebulizers and may be irritating to some asthmatics. While nebulizers and inhalers are equally effective in the stable patient, the nebulizer may offer certain advantages in the acute asthmatic since the metered-dose inhaler is less effective when the respiratory pattern is rapid and shallow and the patient has difficulty coordinating actuation of the inhaler with inspiration. A spacer device attached to the inhaler can improve drug deposition when patient technique is inadequate. Even with optimum technique, however, a maximum of 15 percent of the drug dose is retained in the lungs, regardless of the aerosol method used.

### $β_2$-Adrenergic Drugs

The β-adrenergic agonists used today are analogs of naturally occurring sympathomimetics. The ideal bronchodilator in this class of drugs would possess pure $β_2$-receptor activity—bronchodilation without cardiac effects. The older catecholamine bronchodilators (isoproterenol and epinephrine) are not $β_2$-specific and have a short duration of action. Isoetharine is more $β_2$-selective, but still has a short duration of action. These drugs have nearly been replaced by newer agents produced by chemical modification of the parent compound. There are two classes of β-adrenergic drugs which share greater $β_2$ specificity (relative, not absolute), as well as longer duration of action (due to resistance to COMT and MAO) and effectiveness through the oral route (due to resistance to gut sulfatases). These include the resorcinol bronchodilators (metaproterenol, terbutaline, and fenoterol) and the saligenin bronchodilators (albuterol and carbuterol). Bitolterol represents an even newer concept in β-adrenergic therapy. This "prodrug" is inactive until hydrolyzed by esterases to the active $β_2$-specific catecholamine, colterol. Because the concentration of necessary esterases is higher in the lungs than in the heart, $β_2$ selectivity is maintained. Currently, bitolterol is available only in a metered-dose inhaler.

Table 71-8 lists the β-adrenergic bronchodilators approved for

**Table 71-8.** β-Adrenergic Bronchodilators for Acute Asthma

|  | Dose, mg | Duration, h | Dosing Interval |
|---|---|---|---|
| Subcutaneous route* | | | |
|   Epinephrine | 0.3 | 4 | 20 min × 3 |
|   Terbutaline sulfate | 0.25 | 4–6 | 20 min × 3 |
| Nebulized route | | | |
|   Isoetharine mesylate | 2.5–5.0 | 3–4 | 3 h |
|   Metaproterenol sulfate | 10–15 | 3–5 | 3 h |
| Albuterol | 2.5–5.0 | 3–4 | 1–2 h |

* Not the preferred route—should be restricted to children and young adults. Avoid in patients over 40 years old or with history of hypertension or coronary artery disease.

emergency use. Terbutaline, albuterol, and bitolterol are not available in solutions for use with compressor-driven nebulizers, although metered-dose inhalers are available. Fenoterol and carbuterol are not commercially available. Although subcutaneous injections of epinephrine and terbutaline are widely used, this mode of treatment is no more effective and is associated with more systemic side effects. The parenteral route should probably be avoided in patients over 40 years of age. Similarly, the use of continuous intravenous isoproterenol should be discouraged.

### Salmeterol

Salmeterol xinafoate is a β₂ adrenoreceptor agonist which binds with greater affinity at the β-receptor site than albuterol. Its bronchodilator effects last at least 12 h, and tachyphylaxis has not been reported with long-term use. It is an effective treatment for long-term control of asthma, especially nocturnal asthma. It is indicated for twice-daily maintenance therapy but should never be used more than twice a day or for acute exacerbations. Short-acting β₂-adrenoreceptor agonists are generally prescribed in addition for symptoms that occur despite the use of salmeterol.

### Theophylline

Until recently, intravenous theophylline has been the first-line drug for treatment of acute asthma. But this approach has been challenged by studies showing that, in acute asthma, theophylline produces less bronchodilation than β-adrenergic agents. Furthermore, theophylline in combination with inhaled β-adrenergic drugs appears to increase the toxicity but not the efficacy of treatment. Although the issue remains controversial, it is clear that nebulized β₂-adrenergic agents are the favored initial treatment for acute asthma. This is not to say that theophylline should be eliminated from the treatment program. In fact, since many severe asthmatics will require hospitalization and multidrug therapy, the addition of theophylline is rational. Theoretically, the addition of theophylline to treatment may be beneficial by providing a more sustained bronchodilator effect, contributing to small airway bronchodilation (especially when mucous plugging prevents uniform distribution of the nebulized drug), and improving respiratory muscle endurance and resistance to fatigue.

### Pharmacology

The mechanism of action of theophylline remains unknown. The majority of theophylline metabolism (90 percent) is by the liver and the remainder is excreted unchanged through the kidneys. Theophylline has numerous beneficial effects on pulmonary physiology. Bronchodilation, proportional to the serum concentration, is well recognized. In addition, theophylline increases the contractility and endurance of the diaphragm (and possibly other inspiratory muscles), improving mechanical efficiency and delaying the onset of muscle fatigue. Other actions include stimulation of mucociliary clearance, increased respiratory drive, inhibition of mediator release, increased myocardial contractility, increased gastric acid secretion, and promotion of diuresis.

The toxicity of theophylline is well described. The most common side effect is gastrointestinal disturbance (nausea, cramps, diarrhea). Also common are headache, nervousness, insomnia, and sinus tachycardia. The more serious adverse effects such as confusion, agitation, seizures, and arrhythmias are uncommon and usually associated with serum theophylline concentrations greater than 40 μg/mL. Symptomatic theophylline toxicity with a serum concentration greater than 30 μg/mL should be treated with oral charcoal (30 g every 2 h for four doses). The use of charcoal hemoperfusion should be determined on an individual basis.

### Serum Theophylline Levels

As with the beneficial effect of bronchodilation, the side effects of theophylline are related to the serum concentration. Because metabolism (hepatic clearance) of theophylline varies, the relationship between dose and serum level is unpredictable. The prudent physician will carefully monitor the serum theophylline concentration until a steady-state condition exists and also whenever events develop which are likely to alter theophylline disposition. Theophylline has a narrow therapeutic range, with a therapeutic serum concentration defined as 10 to 20 μg/mL. Some patients may benefit at levels less than 10 μg/mL. Toxicity increases in frequency at levels above 20 μg/mL but is still observed at lower levels, occasionally below the therapeutic range. In the acute setting, maintaining serum levels between 10 and 15 μg/mL is the safest approach.

Numerous factors alter theophylline metabolism by affecting hepatic oxidases. Reduced theophylline clearance (increased serum levels) is associated with liver disease, congestive heart failure, cor pulmonale, febrile viral respiratory infections, advanced age, cimetidine, erythromycin, oral contraceptives, and allopurinol. Increased theophylline clearance (decreased serum levels) is seen with cigarette smoking, phenobarbital, phenytoin, significant consumption of charcoal-broiled beef, and elimination of factors that reduce clearance.

### Theophylline Dosing

Extensive insight into the pharmacokinetics of theophylline has provided rational dosing recommendations. Because the beneficial effects are directly related to the serum concentration, it is desirable to maintain a constant therapeutic concentration of theophylline. This requires administration of a loading dose (to establish blood levels) immediately followed by a constant infusion (Table 71-9). Of course,

**Table 71-9.** Guidelines for Intravenous Theophylline in Adults

|  | Dose |
|---|---|
| LOADING DOSE* | |
|   No previous theophylline | 5 mg/kg IBW |
|   Short-acting theophylline taken < 12 h, or long-acting theophylline taken < 24 h, *and* serum levels therapeutic | None |
|   Oral theophylline as above *and* serum levels subtherapeutic | 3 mg/kg *or* ½ (desired level − observed level) mg/kg |
| MAINTENANCE INFUSION† | |
|   Patients taking oral theophylline *and* serum levels therapeutic | Same dose‡ |
|   Patients taking oral theophylline *and* serum levels subtherapeutic | Increase by 25% |
|   Patients not taking oral theophylline: | |
|     Smoking adult | 0.8 mg/kg/h |
|     Nonsmoking adult, seriously ill patient | 0.5 mg/kg/h |
|     Congestive heart failure, liver disease | 0.2 mg/kg/h |

* Loading dose should be administered in 50 mL of 5% dextrose in water over 20 to 30 min, *never as a bolus,* and *never through a central venous catheter.*
† Serum theophylline level should be monitored 24–36 h after infusion.
‡ Divide daily dose (mg) by 24 to determine the hourly infusion rate.

proper utilization of theophylline requires a knowledge of prior drug administration, as well as clinical assessment of the factors likely to alter theophylline metabolism.

## Corticosteroids

Corticosteroids are highly effective drugs in asthma; in fact, they form the cornerstone of treatment of the severe episode. While the mechanism of action is unknown, many believe that steroids produce beneficial effects by restoring β-adrenergic responsiveness and reducing inflammation. It is generally accepted that the onset of steroid effect (possibly as a result of improved β-adrenergic responsiveness) is delayed at least 6 to 8 h following intravenous administration. Many controversies remain concerning steroid use, including the basic issue of efficacy. The following recommendations represent one of many approaches, and should by no means be construed as the single standard of care.

Corticosteroids should be used immediately in all asthmatics who are currently taking, or have recently taken, these drugs. They should also be administered to patients who demonstrate any of the warning signs of severe asthma (Table 71-5) and to those who do not show objective improvement in pulmonary function (Table 71-7) after the first nebulized bronchodilator treatment. While there is considerable disagreement over what constitutes the optimum dose of corticosteroid in acute asthma, this author favors a low-dose approach utilizing an initial intravenous bolus of 60 to 80 mg of methylprednisolone (the preferred corticosteroid preparation) followed by 20 to 40 mg every 6 h until significant subjective and objective improvement is achieved (return of $FEV_1$ to at least 50% of predicted). Subsequent tapering with single morning doses of oral prednisone is attempted as the patient continues to improve. Inhaled corticosteroids are generally avoided during the initial phase of the acute episode (to minimize potential airway irritation) but are reintroduced when the corticosteroid tapering is in effect.

## Anticholinergics

Plants containing anticholinergic alkaloids have been smoked for hundreds, if not thousands, of years to treat respiratory disorders. In recent years, anticholinergics have been rediscovered as potent bronchodilators in patients with asthma and other forms of obstructive lung disease. Although comparisons of bronchodilator response between anticholinergics and β-adrenergic agonists have produced conflicting results, when the drugs are used in combination, the effects may be additive. This is probably true because the sites of action of both drugs are different: Anticholinergics affect large, central airways while β-adrenergic drugs bronchodilate smaller airways.

Anticholinergic drugs competitively antagonize acetylcholine at the postganglionic, parasympathetic effector-cell junction. This process effectively blocks the bronchoconstriction induced by vagal (cholinergic-mediated) innervation to the larger central airways. In addition, concentrations of cyclic GMP in airway smooth muscle are reduced, further promoting bronchodilation.

Earlier concerns with potential adverse effects of anticholinergics, such as mucous plugging and systemic toxicity, have not proved clinically significant, probably due to the use of the aerosol route of administration and the tendency to use small doses. Potential side effects with nebulized anticholinergics include drying of the mouth (most common), thirst, and difficulty swallowing. Less commonly, one observes tachycardia, change in mental status (restlessness, irritability, confusion), difficulty in micturition, ileus, blurring of vision, or an increase in intraocular pressure.

Because of significant systemic side effects, atropine sulfate, once the major anticholinergic nebulized in the United States, has been virtually replaced by the synthetic quarternary derivative, ipratropium bromide (Atrovent). This drug is very well-tolerated, causing far fewer systemic side effects. Ipratropium is currently available in this country only in a metered dose inhaler (18 μg/puff), but a nebulized solution may soon be released. This drug appears to be an effective bronchodilator in asthma (acute and possibly chronic) when used alone and may have additive benefits with nebulized β-adrenergics, used sequentially or in combination. The dosage range is 2 to 8 puffs every 6 h.

## Other Medications

The empiric use of a single broad-spectrum antibiotic during the treatment of acute asthma is acceptable, because secondary bacterial bronchitis is seen in many instances. Disodium cromoglycate and inhaled corticosteroids should be avoided during the acute asthmatic attack, since they are only minimally beneficial and may cause further airway irritation. Antihistamines are not beneficial in asthma.

Calcium channel blockers can inhibit the calcium-dependent reactions that lead to bronchial smooth muscle contraction, mucus secretion, mediator release, and nerve impulse conduction. These agents have been shown to prevent bronchospasm in response to exercise, hyperventilation, cold air, histamine, and various additional antigens. While the prophylactic value of calcium channel blockers has been demonstrated, these drugs have not proved to be significant or consistent bronchodilators.

Intravenous magnesium sulfate is being used with increasing frequency in the management of acute severe asthma. While the bronchodilating properties of magnesium sulfate can be helpful, it does not substitute for standard therapies. The dose is 1 to 2 g IV over 30 min.

## Mechanical Ventilation

When all efforts to relieve the severe airflow obstruction fail and the patient manifests progressive hypercarbia and acidosis or becomes exhausted or confused, intubation and mechanical ventilation are necessary to prevent respiratory arrest. Mechanical ventilation does not relieve the airflow obstruction; it merely eliminates the work of breathing and allows the patient to rest while the airflow obstruction is resolved. Fortunately, only a small percentage of asthmatics (less than 1 percent) ever require mechanical ventilation. Direct oral intubation is preferred over the nasotracheal route.

The potential complications of mechanical ventilation in the asthmatic patient are numerous. Increased airway resistance may lead to extremely high peak airway pressures (potentially resulting in frequent high-pressure alarming of the ventilator), barotrauma, and hemodynamic impairment. Due to the severity of airflow obstruction, during the early phases of treatment, the tidal volume may be larger than the returned volume; this condition leads to air trapping and increased residual volume ("intrinsic–PEEP"). These effects may be partially avoided by utilizing rapid flow rates at a reduced respiratory frequency (12 to 14 per minute), allowing adequate time for the expiratory phase. In this manner, one can achieve the major goal of ventilatory support—maintenance of an adequate arterial oxygen saturation (90 percent), without concern for "normalizing" the hypercarbic acidosis (an undesirable initial strategy). This approach is referred to as *controlled mechanical hypoventilation.* Mucous plugging is frequent, often leading to increased airway resistance, atelectasis, and pulmonary infection. Finally, an endotracheal tube may cause some asthmatics to become even more "twitchy," resulting in further bronchospasm.

## BIBLIOGRAPHY

Bone, RC: A word of caution regarding a new long-acting bronchodilator. *JAMA* 271:1447, 1994.

D'Alonzo, GE, Nathan, RA, Henochowicz, S, et al: Salmeterol xinafoate as maintainance therapy compared with albuterol in patients with asthma. *JAMA* 271:1412, 1994.

Fanta CH, Rossing TH, McFadden ER: Emergency room treatment of asthma: Relationships among therapeutic combinations, severity of obstruction and time course of response. *Am J Med* 72:416, 1982.

Green SM, Rothrock SG: Intravenous magnesium for acute asthma: failure to decrease emergency treatment duration or need for hospitalization. *Ann Emerg Med* 21:260, 1992.

Raimondi AC, Figueroa-Casas JC, Roncoroni AJ: Comparison between high and moderate doses of hydrocortisone in the treatment of status asthmaticus. *Chest* 89:832, 1986.

Turner ES, Greenberger PA, Patterson R: Management of the pregnant asthmatic patient. *Ann Intern Med* 6:905, 1980.

USDHHS PHS: *Guidelines for the Diagnosis and Management of Asthma.* National Institute of Health, 1994.

# 72

# CHRONIC OBSTRUCTIVE PULMONARY DISEASE

## Joel C. Seidman

Individuals with chronic obstructive pulmonary disease frequently present to emergency departments in severe respiratory distress and are among the most frustrating, frightening, and challenging patients encountered there. In a fearful state of mixed anxiety, intense physical effort, and disoriented fatigue, such people face a constant battle against asphyxiation. At other times, presentation is prompted by otherwise uncomplicated medical or surgical disease, which becomes more serious or catastrophic as the impact of chronic respiratory disease is unmasked.

## CAUSES AND PREDISPOSING FACTORS

The most important predisposing factor to chronic airflow obstruction is cigarette smoking. Other less well understood environmental exposures, genetic aberrations, and, probably, sustained bronchospastic airflow obstruction can cause disease in nonsmokers as well as smokers. Less is known about the roles of environmental and industrial air pollution and passive smoking than about active cigarette smoking. Some forms of industrial asthma such as byssinosis and diisocyanate-induced bronchospasm can cause irreversible airflow obstruction. Recent public communications by the Surgeon General highlight medical evidence of the serious irreversible impact of passive smoking on some individuals. Genetic disorders such as $\alpha_1$-antitrypsin deficiency and cystic fibrosis account for only a small fraction of disease. Recognition of heritable markers is of academic interest, facilitates genetic counselling, and may alter long-term clinical management (e.g. intravenous $\alpha_1$-proteinase inhibitor repletion therapy). Asthma alone, if sufficiently sustained and punctuated by repetitive endobronchial infections, may progress to chronic obstructive pulmonary disease, even in the absence of other known risk factors.

## PATHOPHYSIOLOGY

Over three decades ago, the American Thoracic Society defined the dominant clinical forms of chronic obstructive pulmonary disease as follows: (1) *pulmonary emphysema* (defined pathologically) as a condition of the lung characterized by abnormal, permanent enlargement of the air spaces distal to the terminal bronchiole, accompanied by destruction of their walls; and (2) *chronic bronchitis* (defined clinically) as a condition of excess mucus secretion in the bronchial tree, occurring on most days for at least three months in the year for at least two consecutive years. Although not included in the above definition, increased airways resistance is also a fundamental feature of either condition.

The earliest objective changes in the evolution of chronic obstructive pulmonary disease are clinically imperceptible and are measured as small increases in peripheral airways resistance or lung compliance. The slow, insidious appearance of dyspnea and hypersecretion often require several decades of disease; the sedentary life habits of many cigarette smokers result in failure to unmask exertional dyspnea; and the frequent use of denial in smokers results in suppression of symptoms or attribution of symptoms to aging, poor conditioning, obesity, or allergies. Further, the respiratory consequences of cigarette smoking are a continuum of slowly evolving and latent effects, unique to each individual, in a complex dose-response relationship. Early in disease evolution, abstinence from smoking may eliminate symptoms and result in physiologic improvement. Once well developed, however, abnormalities persist and may still progress despite abstinence.

Pathologic specimens from patients with early disease demonstrate minor metaplasia of bronchial epithelium and an increase in bronchial gland number and size. As disease evolves, such findings are exaggerated, acute and chronic inflammatory changes in the epithelium are more notable, and acinar expansion, destruction, and coalescence are seen. Elements of emphysematous disease are invariably present in concert with those of bronchitic disease, though one often predominates.

Despite recognition of causative factors, what determines the clinical onset and rate of progression of chronic airflow obstruction, and the direction toward either emphysematous or bronchitic patterns, is uncertain. Clearly, there is a great deal of variability in disease pattern and severity among individuals with seemingly similar predispositions to disease.

The central element in the pathophysiology of chronic airflow obstruction is impedance to airflow, especially expiratory airflow, due to increased resistance or decreased caliber throughout the small bronchi and bronchioles. This results from obstruction due to secretions and mucosal edema, bronchospasm, and bronchoconstriction from impaired elastance. Impedance to airflow alone accounts substantially for the abnormal physiology of the disease. Exaggerated airway resistance either reduces total minute ventilation, or increases respiratory work. To the degree that alveolar hypoventilation occurs, hypoxemia and hypercarbia result. Ventilation-perfusion mismatching occurs, so that regional relative overperfusion widens the alveolar-arterial oxygen difference, promoting hypoxemia. Increased physiologic dead space ventilation leads to alveolar hypoventilation, hypercarbia, and further hypoxemia. Even if all challenges to increased respiratory work are met, hypoxemia resulting from regional low ventilation-perfusion relationships or true physiologic right-to-left shunts cannot be overcome.

In addition to obstruction of the peripheral airways, all forms of advanced chronic airflow obstruction involve other pathophysiologic elements to complete the overall picture. Particularly in dominantly emphysematous disease, destruction and coalescence of alveolar architecture results in reduction of total "matched" alveolar-capillary surface area for diffusion of gas, while vascular destruction results in "unmatched" regions where ventilation is wasted.

Neurochemical and proprioceptive ventilatory responses in chronic airflow obstruction may be aberrant. For example, ventilatory response to hypercarbia may be blunted during sleep, and ventilatory drive and dyspnea may be exaggerated in spite of normal pulmonary inflation. The composition of muscle fiber types, breathing pattern, and resistance to fatigue of respiratory muscles are also altered in advanced chronic airflow obstruction. Finally, pulmonary arterial hypertension supervenes as chronic airflow obstruction progresses. The right ventricle transiently hypertrophies, and then dilates with the evolution of overt cor pulmonale. A low-output state in the pulmonary circulation translates into low left ventricular output. Arterial hypoxemia increases as the effects of right-to-left shunt on poorly oxygenated mixed venous blood are exaggerated. Right ventricular pressure overload is clinically poorly tolerated and associated with atrial and ventricular arrhythmias.

## COMPENSATED CHRONIC AIRFLOW OBSTRUCTION

### Clinical Features

Despite the pathophysiologic segregation of chronic airflow obstruction into categories of pulmonary emphysema, chronic bronchitis, and bronchiectasis, none of these exists as a pure entity in clinical medicine. Most patients demonstrate a mixture of symptoms and signs. The hallmark symptom is exertional dyspnea. Chronic, productive cough is common, and minor hemoptysis is frequent, especially in chronic bronchitis and bronchiectasis. Physical findings include tachypnea, accessory respiratory muscle use, and pursed-lip exhalation. Airflow obstruction causes wheezing during exhalation, especially maximum forced exhalation, and prolongation of the expiratory time. In dominantly bronchitic disease, coarse crackles are heard as uncleared secretions move about the central airways. In dominantly emphysematous disease, there is expansion of the thorax, impeded diaphragmatic motion, and global diminution of breath sounds. Weight loss is frequent due to poor dietary intake and excessive caloric expenditure for the work of breathing. Plethora due to secondary polycythemia, cyanosis, and tremor, somnolence, and confusion due to hypercarbia may be seen in advanced disease. Findings of secondary pulmonary hypertension with or without cor pulmonale may be present. The physical signs of left ventricular dysfunction are often disguised or underestimated by the seemingly more overwhelming signs of respiratory disease, or because pulmonary hyperinflation prohibits adequate auscultation.

Roentgenographic examination is often misleading. Mild chronic airflow obstruction is likely to be roentgenographically inapparent. Dominantly bronchitic disease may be associated with subtle or absent x-ray findings. On the other hand, dominantly emphysematous disease may be associated with remarkable signs of hyperaeration such as increased anteroposterior diameter, flattened diaphragms, increased parenchymal lucency, and attenuation of pulmonary arterial vascular shadows, despite only mild-to-moderate physiologic alterations. Right or left ventricular enlargement may not produce relative enlargement of the cardiac silhouette. Certainly, roentgenography is of unquestionable value in diagnosing complications such as pneumothorax, pneumonia, pleural effusion, or pulmonary neoplasia.

The most valuable tool in characterizing disease severity is pulmonary physiologic testing, including examination of lung mechanics, analysis of arterial blood gases, description of ventilatory response patterns, tests of respiratory muscle performance, metabolic assessment, and noninvasive survey of hemodynamic reserve. In clinically apparent chronic airflow obstruction, the $FEV_1$ (forced expiratory volume in 1 s) as a fraction of the FVC (forced vital capacity), also called $FEV_{1\%}$, correlates remarkably well with day-to-day functional performance, morbidity incidents, and mortality. Reduction of the FVC in the absence of restrictive ventilatory disease favors the emphysematous pattern, while improvement in the $FEV_{1\%}$ in response to bronchodilator inhalation is more commonly seen in bronchitic patients. All such studies are adaptable for use in the emergency department.

Arterial blood gas analysis can show exaggeration of the predicted normal alveolar-arterial oxygen difference as disease progresses; an increase in hypoxemia during exercise in emphysematous disease; resting hypercarbia in advanced bronchitic disease; and chronic, resting hypoxemia in all forms of advanced disease, especially with secondary pulmonary hypertension and cor pulmonale.

When ventricular function is clinically unclear, echocardiography or gated nuclear scans to estimate ejection fractions may prove invaluable. ECGs are useful to identify arrhythmias or ischemic injury but do not assess the severity of pulmonary hypertension or right ventricular dysfunction.

Other laboratory analyses may indicate advanced disease: polycythemia, with or without elevation of packed red blood cell 2,3-diphosphoglycerate (2,3-DPG) concentration, as a feature of chronic hypoxemia; elevated serum bicarbonate reflecting chronic hypercarbia and respiratory acidemia; and elevated hepatic enzymes and albuminuria indicative of high central venous pressure in cor pulmonale.

### Therapy

The appropriate and optimal management of decompensated chronic airflow obstruction in an emergency department setting requires an appreciation of chronic day-to-day therapy. Specific management limits further insults to the respiratory system, treats reversible bronchospasm, and prevents or treats complications. Seven actions comprise the core of strategy: (1) elimination of extrinsic irritants, (2) bronchodilator and glucocorticoid therapy, (3) antibiotics, (4) mobilization of secretions, (5) "respiratory" vaccines, (6) oxygen, and (7) treatment of complicating systemic disease. Cigarette smoking and other aggravating environmental factors must be limited or thoroughly eliminated.

Some combination of regular as well as symptom-guided nonsteroidal bronchodilator therapy is chronically prescribed. This may include oral theophylline or aminophylline in immediate- or sustained-release forms, oral or inhaled selective β-adrenergics, oral or inhaled glucocorticoids, and inhaled anticholinergics. The use of these agents varies with disease severity and lability, physician preference, the patient's subjective and objective response, compliance, drug cost, and availability of facilities to monitor serum concentrations of theophylline or toxicities of systemic glucocorticoid therapy.

Knowledge of certain features of the maintenance regimen are essential to the emergency physician: (1) If theophylline or aminophylline is taken, the formulation prescribed, last dose time, and total daily dose must be determined. (2) If systemic glucocorticoids are taken, the product prescribed and total daily dose, or dose as otherwise prescribed, must be known. (3) The dose and frequency of use of oxygen therapy should be identified, if only to assure continuity of therapy.

Broad-spectrum antimicrobials are frequently prescribed, and sometimes initiated independently by the patient, to treat acute mucopurulent tracheobronchitis. In mild-to-moderate bronchitis uncomplicated by pneumonia, antibiotic selection need not concur with in vitro sensitivities to assure clinical efficacy. Most commonly, tetracyclines, ampicillin or amoxicillin, sulfamethoxazole/trimethoprim, macrolides, fluoroquinolones, or first-generation cephalosporins are given; infrequently used agents include chloramphenicol and clindamycin.

Various actions are taken to mobilize respiratory secretions: assurance of generous oral fluid intake and atmospheric humidification, avoidance of antihistamine/decongestant/anticholinergic agents, and limitation of antitussive use. The efficacy of specific expectorant products is dubious.

Preventive respiratory vaccines are recommended: polyvalent (23) pneumococcal vaccine and annual trivalent influenza vaccine.

Chronic intermittent or continuous oxygen therapy is indicated if the oxygen saturation is less than 90 percent while at rest and breathing room air.

Complications of chronic airflow obstruction include those in direct consequence to respiratory disease (secondary pulmonary hypertension and cor pulmonale) or nonrelated diseases with an adverse physiologic impact upon underlying respiratory disease (left-sided heart failure, anemia, hyperthyroidism). Such problems are sometimes managed with difficulty as their treatments may aggravate bronchospasm, and vice versa.

# DECOMPENSATED CHRONIC AIRFLOW OBSTRUCTION

## Clinical Features

Tissue oxygen delivery is decreased as a result of ventilation-perfusion mismatching and alveolar hypoventilation. The former reflects intensification of bronchospastic airflow obstruction, and the latter, increased work of breathing. The end result is increasing hypoxemia and hypercarbia.

Progressive hypoxia is characterized by tachypnea, cyanosis, agitation and apprehension, tachycardia, and systemic hypertension. Signs of hypercarbia are confusion, tremor, plethora, stupor, and, finally, hypopnea and apnea. The patient complains primarily of dyspnea and orthopnea. The intensified effort to ventilate is further dramatized by sitting-up-and-forward posturing, pursed-lip exhalation, accessory muscle use, and diaphoresis. Pulsus paradoxus may be noted during blood pressure recording. Complications such as pneumonia, pneumothorax, or an acute abdomen may be neglected or minimized by the patient's generalized respiratory distress, tachypnea, or global diminution of breath sounds.

Clearly the most life-threatening feature of decompensation is critical hypoxemia where arterial saturation falls below 90 percent under ambient conditions. Correction is mandatory, even if oxygen supplementation sufficiently suppresses hypoxemic drive to require mechanical ventilation. Cyanosis alone has poor clinical correlation with hypoxia, and arterial blood gases are necessary to evaluate oxygenation and carbon dioxide retention. While pulse oximetry may identify hypoxemia, it cannot identify hypercarbia or acid-base disturbances. The finding of an arterial pH below that consistent with renal compensation for chronic respiratory acidosis implies either acute exaggeration of hypercarbia or acute metabolic acidosis.

Decompensation is usually due to worsening of airflow obstruction resulting from increased bronchospasm, superimposed respiratory infection, interference with respiratory drive, cardiovascular deterioration, smoking, noncompliance with medication, noxious environmental exposures, use of medications that prohibit bronchorrhea, and adverse responses to medication (e.g., anaphylactoid responses or institution of β-adrenergic blockade). Other respiratory pathophysiology, often with a restrictive pattern, may add to the impact of chronic airflow obstruction: pneumonia, pneumothorax, pulmonary embolism, pulmonary edema, blunt chest injury, or abdominal pain are considerations. Disordered ventilatory drive most commonly arises from misuse of oxygen therapy, hypnotics, or tranquilizers. Metabolic disturbances such as diabetic ketoacidosis, uremia, or hepatic encephalopathy may also impair ventilatory drive. Inadequate tissue oxygen delivery independent of respiratory function results from left ventricular failure, anemia, hyperthyroidism, or hyperthermia.

## Therapy

The primary goal of emergency therapy in decompensated chronic airflow obstruction is to correct tissue oxygenation. This requires the restoration of the lungs as gas exchange organs, assurance of hemodynamic efficiency, repletion of red blood cell mass where deficient, and limitation of excessive oxygen demands and carbon dioxide production.

Certain medical historical details are critical to appropriate therapy. These include the patient's current medical regimen (medications, doses, and schedule of administration), with special attention to use of theophylline, glucocorticoids, and oxygen; medication allergies; duration of symptomatic decompensation (recognizing that slow, protracted deterioration will often be slowly responsive and comparatively refractory to immediate interventions); and recent "upgrading" of therapy (recognizing that a failure to provide continued therapy of at least similar intensity will represent a "downgrading" of intervention).

The membrane gas transport capabilities of the alveolar-capillary interface in chronic airflow disease are little affected by therapies. However, the gas exchange process is facilitated by increasing the inspired partial pressure of oxygen. Oxygen is a drug with a therapeutic-toxic range. The need to increase $P_{O_2}$ must be balanced against the possibility of suppression of hypoxic ventilatory drive. If hypercarbia is present, a fixed-concentration mask with 24 to 35 percent $F_{I_{O_2}}$ should be used, with frequent reassessment of clinical response. Arterial saturation should be corrected to above 90 percent.

The application of assisted ventilation increases alveolar ventilation by accelerating the rate and depth of total ventilation, augments mean alveolar oxygen partial pressure by more effectively matching the distribution of pulmonary blood flow and alveolar ventilation, and minimizes the patient's work of ventilation. Pharmacologic bronchodilatation accomplishes similar ends by minimizing the impedance to bronchial airflow and facilitating mobilization of excessive airway secretions.

Assisted mechanical ventilation is indicated for inability to maintain oxygen saturation at 90 percent, or severe hypercarbia associated with stupor, narcosis, or acidosis. Other parameters which reflect respiratory muscle effort, extent of dead space ventilation, and the work of breathing have prognostic bearing, but none can be used to determine the need for ventilator therapy. A volume-cycled ventilator should always be used. Security of the airway should be accomplished with a cuffed endotracheal tube of generous diameter inserted orally whenever possible. Small tubes or nasotracheal tubes provide impedance to suctioning, make fiberoptic bronchoscopy more difficult, and make spontaneous ventilation with the tube in situ intolerable (because of upper airway resistive impedance). The endotracheal tube must be maintained above the carina. Excessive tidal volumes (over 15 mL/kg ideal body weight) can cause barotrauma and hypotension due to reduction of venous return and can produce a severe combined metabolic and respiratory alkalosis. Initially, high inspired oxygen concentrations should be used. In an emergency department setting, there is no clear role for the application of intermittent mandatory ventilation (IMV) or positive end-expiratory pressure (PEEP); the mode of ventilation should be assist/control (A/C).

The use of assisted mechanical ventilation in chronic airflow obstruction is a two-edged sword. Placement of an endotracheal tube, with or without assisted ventilation, impairs normal mucociliary clearance, initiates or exaggerates microbial colonization of the tracheobronchial tree, obstructs the cough mechanism, allows catheter suctioning of predominantly the right bronchial system, and injures the laryngeal and proximal tracheal supporting structures, to say nothing of the psychological impact upon the patient. It should be avoided if at all possible. In carefully selected patients, noninvasive, positive-pressure ventilation (Bi-PAP) may serve this end; the specific indications for its role in accomplishing successful outcomes remains to be defined.

Pharmacologic intervention is the most essential and least traumatic method to treat decompensated chronic airflow obstruction. Four groups of agents are used: (1) parenteral methylxanthines, (2) β-adrenergic agonists, (3) systemic glucocorticoids, and (4) inhaled anticholinergics.

## Methylxanthines

The methylxanthines, aminophylline (theophylline ethylenediamine) and theophylline, are most effective for emergency treatment when given intravenously. Historically, drug concentrations were maintained at 10 to 20 μg/mL (10 to 20 mg/L). Incremental benefit was sometimes observed at the upper region of this range, though with clearly increasing risk of major toxicities. On this account, many practitioners currently recommend a more conservative goal of 5 to 15 μg/mL (5 to 15 mg/L). Many schemes of dosing have been described, each dependent upon estimations of the patient's volume of distribution (usually approximately 0.5 times ideal body weight expressed in liters) and probable clearance rate.

The loading dose (of theophylline) to obtain an initial serum concentration of 10 $\mu$g/mL (10 mg/L) is 5 to 6 mg/kg ideal body weight in a patient currently receiving no drug. In a patient previously medicated orally with theophylline already present in serum, a mini-loading dose may be alternatively selected as: (target concentration – currently assayed concentration) $\times$ volume of distribution (i.e., 0.5 $\times$ ideal body weight in liters). With the mini-load method, the target concentration should be between 10 $\mu$g/mL (10 mg/L) and 15 $\mu$g/mL (15 mg/L).

The maintenance dose is 0.2 to 0.8 mg/kg ideal body weight per hour. Lower maintenance rates are given to patients with congestive cardiac failure or hepatic insufficiency with low clearance rates, while higher rates are given to smokers with rapid clearance. Unfortunately, no regimen suits a given patient, and the above are only guidelines. Relatively rapid determination of dosage can be obtained from the Chiou approximation of total body theophylline clearance measured during continuous, uninterrupted intravenous infusion, while two serum assays are drawn approximately 8 h apart:

$$CL = 2K_0/(C_1 + C_2) + 2VD(C_1 - C_2)/[(C_1 + C_2)(T_2 - T_1)]$$

where $CL$ = total body clearance (L/h)
$K_0$ = current infusion rate (mg/h)
$C_1$ = first serum theophylline concentration (mg/L)
$C_2$ = second serum theophylline concentration (mg/L)
$VD$ = volume of distribution (assumed to be 0.5 $\times$ ideal body weight in liters) (L)
$T_2 - T_1$ = actual time interval between blood draws (h)

Further derivation concludes:

$$K_1 = CL \times C_3$$

where $K_1$ = new infusion rate (mg/h)
$C_3$ = desired target serum theophylline concentration (mg/L)

The accuracy of this methodology assumes that theophylline clearance is constant over the short term (e.g., there has been no activated charcoal administered for toxicity), and enteric absorption of theophylline is negligible.

Maintenance theophylline infusion in a patient on chronic oral therapy is complex (whether or not a mini-loading dose has been given), particularly in attempting to account for enteric drug yet to be absorbed. A single serum assay upon arrival in the emergency department is of little value in calculating dose requirements, unless the measurement is in the toxic range. Alternatively, the already established daily dose can be administered as an intravenous infusion over 24 h. If the optimal daily dose is unknown, then the above guidelines should be used. In addition, the hourly infusion rate selected (in milligrams per hour) should be reduced for (6 – $t$) hours by $D$/6, for rapid-release formulations; and for (12 – $t$) hours by $D$/12, for sustained-release preparations (including 24-h release forms), where $t$ is the time in hours since the last oral dose taken, and $D$ is the usual oral dose. This guideline will likely minimize the risk of "summation toxicity" due to continued enteric absorption. Theophylline and aminophylline should not be given orally (unless decompensation is not severe, alimentary motility is assured, and forthcoming ambulatory care is imminent), and certainly not by rectal suppository, in an emergency setting.

## Beta-Adrenergic Agonists

Beta-adrenergic agonists produce the promptest of responses and are available in oral, parenteral, and aerosolized dosage forms. In critical settings, reliance should be placed upon parenteral or aerosolized

forms of epinephrine or, preferably, relatively selective $\beta_2$ agonists. Epinephrine 1:1000 (0.1 to 0.3 mL) or terbutaline sulfate (0.25 to 0.50 mL) may be given subcutaneously. Aerosol therapy minimizes systemic toxicity and is a favored delivery route. Isoetharine 1% 2.5 to 5.0 mg (0.25 to 0.50 mL), metaproterenol 5% 10 to 15 mg (0.2 to 0.3 mL), albuterol sulfate 0.6% (0.5% as albuterol base) 1.25 to 5.00 mg (0.25 to 1.00 mL), or bitolterol mesylate 0.2% 0.5 to 1.5 mg (0.25 to 0.75 mL) can be delivered by compressed-gas-driven nebulizer. Acceptable dose intervals for adrenergic therapies range from 1 to 4 h, depending on clinical response and signs of drug toxicity. Both parenteral and aerosol routes should not be used concurrently. Occasionally, dramatic benefit can be obtained by continuous, closely monitored, intravenous infusion of isoproterenol (0.25 to 4.0 $\mu$g/min). Continuous infusion of isoproterenol should not begin until all other adrenergic therapy (regardless of administration route) has ceased. Cardiac arrhythmias are the major hazard. Self-contained, fluorocarbon-pressurized adrenergic inhalation devices are unreliable in severe, decompensated chronic airflow obstruction and are not recommended. If prescribed, administration should be facilitated with a spacing device.

## Systemic Glucocorticoids

Systemic glucocorticoids elicit delayed bronchodilatory responses and undoubtedly attribute part of their effect to facilitation of concurrently given methylxanthine or $\beta$-adrenergics and to anti-inflammatory effects. Because of a delay of hours in onset of response, glucocorticoids should be given early. Optimally effective daily doses range between one and three times the maximal physiologic adrenal secretion rate (i.e., the equivalent of 60 to 180 mg prednisone daily). Higher doses have demonstrated dubious additional efficacy and excessive toxicity. The choice of steroid is generally not critical, though hydrocortisone should probably be avoided because of excess mineralocorticoid effect, unless primary adrenal insufficiency is concurrently present. There is no role for inhaled glucocorticoids in acute treatment.

## Anticholinergics

Although less predictable in efficacy, inhaled anticholinergic agents may be useful adjuvants superimposed upon other therapies. Historically, atropine sulfate, 1.0 to 3.5 mg, or glycopyrrolate, 0.2 to 1.0 mg, was usually administered by nebulizer. More recently, iprotroprium bromide has replaced these as agent of choice, administered by metered dose inhaler, or, as 0.02% inhalant solution, 500 $\mu$g (2.5 mL) is nebulized. The latter is miscible with albuterol inhalant solution if used promptly. Doses may be repeated as often as every 1 to 4 h.

## Further Considerations

Aggravating events other than simple "decompensation" should be identified quickly: Pneumonia, pneumothorax, pleural effusion, lobar atelectasis, pulmonary thromboembolism, and acute myocardial infarction should all be considered in the differential diagnosis.

From another perspective, the possibility of previously recognized or unrecognized chronic airflow obstruction should be considered in *any* patient over 40 years of age presenting to an emergency department with a catastrophic medical or surgical problem—and treated appropriately.

Tissue oxygen delivery must be maximized by correcting left ventricular failure or arrhythmia to improve cardiac output, replacing red blood cell mass and intravascular fluid to increase arterial oxygen content, and suppressing fever to decrease oxygen consumption. In mathematical terms, attempts should be made to optimize the mixed venous oxygen content ($C\bar{v}_{O_2}$) derived from algebraic rearrangement of Fick's equation for cardiac output.

$$C\bar{v}_{O_2} = Ca_{O_2} - \dot{V}_{O_2}/Q_T$$

where $Ca_{O_2}$ = arterial oxygen content (mL $O_2$/100 mL blood)
$\dot{V}_{O_2}$ = minute oxygen consumption (or delivery) (mL $O_2$/min)
$Q_T$ = cardiac output (mL blood/min)

Common errors encountered in emergency department care of decompensated chronic airflow obstruction include:

1. Use of parenteral or aerosolized sympathomimetics alone for sustained decompensation
2. Inadequate theophylline dosage or failure to deliver by parenteral route
3. Failure to discontinue sodium cromolyn or inhaled glucocorticoid altogether, or failure to discontinue metered-dose inhalers in patients receiving concurrent adrenergic aerosols by other means
4. Denial of systemic glucocorticoid therapy to patients already so medicated or with established "steroid-dependent" disease
5. Indiscriminate use of sedation, antihistamine/decongestants, or anticholinergics
6. Misuse of an intermittent positive pressure breathing machine (IPPB) to deliver adrenergic aerosols
7. Misuse of ultrasonic aerosols
8. Uncontrolled use of supplemental oxygen (including pressurized, high-concentration sources to drive aerosol equipment)
9. Use of pressure-cycled ventilators rather than volume-cycled machines
10. Inadvertent mechanical hyperventilation following prolonged hypercarbia (resulting in unchallenged extreme metabolic alkalosis, hypotension, arrhythmias, and seizures)
11. Failure to recognize respiratory failure or need for hospital admission.

## BIBLIOGRAPHY

American Thoracic Society: Definitions and classifications of bronchitis, asthma and pulmonary emphysema. *Am Rev Respir Dis* 85:762, 1962.

Cherniak NS (ed): *Chronic Obstructive Pulmonary Disease.* Philadelphia, Saunders, 1991.

Dantzker DR (ed): *Cardiopulmonary Critical Care,* 2d ed. Philadelphia, Saunders, 1991.

# 73
# LUNG TRANSPLANTS
### L. J. Paradowski
### M. K. Robbins

## INTRODUCTION

Since the first successful single-lung transplant in 1983 followed by the first successful double-lung transplant in 1986, lung transplantation has become a viable therapeutic modality for end-stage pulmonary disease. Currently more than 50 centers perform lung transplants in North America, and in 1993, 781 patients underwent lung transplantation worldwide. Single-lung transplantation is the more common operation and is done for emphysema, pulmonary fibrosis, and pulmonary hypertension. Double-lung transplants, or, more precisely, bilateral sequential lung transplants, are performed when it would be contraindicated to leave the native lung in place. These conditions include suppurative lung diseases, of which cystic fibrosis is the most frequent indication. Heart-lung transplants are rarely per-

formed and usually for congenital heart disease with Eisenmenger physiology. Overall, for lung transplants the median survival worldwide is 68 percent for 1 year and 60 percent for 2 years. In general, more recent transplants are yielding better survival rates as more experience is accrued.

## MANAGEMENT OF LISTED PATIENTS

Patients accepted as candidates for lung transplantation are placed on a national database maintained by the United Network for Organ Sharing (UNOS) in Richmond, Virginia. Listed patients are assigned donor lungs according to time accrued on the list, ABO blood group, and lung-to-donor size appropriateness. Cytomegalovirus (CMV) status matching is preferred but not mandatory. Unlike other types of organ transplants, there is no priority given to severity of illness. Since the availability of donor organs has not kept up with the number of potential recipients, the "wait" for lungs is currently 12 to 18 months. Some centers require patients to move into the area of their transplant center as they "move-up" on the list. These patients then receive their care at the center and participate in an exercise rehabilitation program. Other centers allow their listed patients to remain in their home town until a donor organ becomes available. Therefore, a large number of patients with end-stage lung disease awaiting lung transplant may present to the emergency department of a transplant center. Typically, the care of these patients may be influenced by their status on the list. If the patient is close to transplant, large doses of glucocorticoids (>0.2 mg/kg) are discouraged, except for brief courses, because of their unfavorable effect on airway healing. Blood transfusions are discouraged, unless for an emergency situation, to avoid the formation of preformed antibodies and possibly increase the risk of hyperacute graft rejection. If blood is deemed necessary, it should be CMV-negative to avoid infecting a CMV-negative patient. Decisions concerning intubation are very difficult since long-term mechanical ventilation (>2 weeks) may lead to respiratory muscle deconditioning, nosocomial infections, and other intensive care unit complications that may preclude successful transplantation. Communication with the transplant center physicians will allow assessment of the patient's status and the feasibility of transplantation in the near future. Patients can be intubated, ventilated, weaned, and resume their place on the list according to the protocol of their transplant center. Noninvasive positive-pressure mask ventilation (NIPPV) may be a possible method to maintain these patients without intubation while they wait for lung availability. Results of nocturnal NIPPV have been favorable, especially for patients with cystic fibrosis. Results have been mixed for patients with chronic obstructive pulmonary disease (COPD).

## MANAGEMENT OF DONORS

Emergency departments can be crucial in obtaining organs suitable for donation. Management of possibly brain-dead patients should be done to maximize possible donor retrieval. Between 20 and 30 percent of patients listed to receive lung transplant expire before an organ becomes available. If a potential organ donor is found, early contact with the local Organ Procurement Agency (OPA) can assist with evaluation and management. OPA coordinators can also facilitate discussions with families. Failure to consider and evaluate brain-dead patients for possible organ donation deprives many waiting patients of a possible life-saving organ. Organs are considered for transplantation following declaration of brain death by a physician who is not involved in the procurement process. Many donors have aspiration or chest trauma that renders the lungs unusable. Accepting centers usually require a clear chest x-ray, $Pa_{O_2} > 450$ mmHg on 100% $O_2$ and no obvious infection in the donor airways upon bronchoscopic evaluation. Attention to fluid and hemodynamic management of a possible lung donor is crucial to maintain a salvageable organ. Mechanical ventilation should maintain a $P_{O_2} > 80$ mmHg, $P_{CO_2}$ between 35 and

45 mmHg, and pH between 7.3 and 7.45. The central venous pressure should be >10 cm $H_2O$. If blood pressure cannot be maintained, fluids and dopamine can be used. Transfusions can maintain a hematocrit >30 percent. CMV-negative blood products should be used so as not to infect a CMV-negative recipient. The present cold ischemic time limit is 8 to 10 h, which may be lengthened as preservation techniques improve. This time constraint precludes HLA matching between donor and recipient prior to the transplant.

## SURGICAL TECHNIQUE

Surgical technique is similar at most centers. Single-lung transplants are done through a lateral thoracotomy incision. Double-lung transplants are performed through an anterior "clam shell" incision. A transverse incision is made in the fourth or fifth intercostal space with a transverse sternal division. Performing the operation as two separate lung transplants in a sequential manner may eliminate the need for cardiopulmonary bypass. The lung with the least perfusion on a preoperative perfusion scan is removed first. In some cases, due to severe dysfunction or lung disease, cardiopulmonary bypass may be needed. Bronchial anastomoses are secured end-to-end or by telescoping one bronchus into the other. The pulmonary veins are attached to the left atrial cuff, and the pulmonary artery anastomosis is performed last. Omentum, pulled up through an abdominal incision and wrapped around the bronchial anastomosis, may be used to provide additional blood supply to the devascularized bronchi. Lymphatics are not immediately restored, which may contribute to postoperative edema during the first few weeks.

## MANAGEMENT OF THE PATIENT AFTER LUNG TRANSPLANT

The transplant team is composed of cardiothoracic surgeons, pulmonologists, nurse coordinators, and ancillary workers such as pharmacists, physical therapists, psychologists, and social workers. A nurse coordinator is on call around the clock and has information concerning all listed and transplanted patients. Emergency department personnel should communicate directly with the nurse coordinator. The coordinator will have the patient's current medication doses, recent infection and rejection history, and a knowledge of complications for which the patient may be at risk. Initial tests for lung transplant patients presenting to the emergency department are listed in Table 73-1.

Following surgery, patients are on triple immunosuppression: cyclosporine, prednisone, and azathioprine. Major side effects of these drugs are shown in Table 73-2. Some centers use antilymphocyte globulin in the early postoperative period, avoiding the deleterious effect of steroids on bronchial healing. Alternative immunosuppressive agents such as tacrolimus (FK506) may be used instead of cyclosporine. In addition, trimethoprim-sulfamethoxazole (TMP-SMZ), acyclovir, and gancyclovir are used prophylactically to prevent *Pneumocystis carinii* pneumonia (PCP), herpes, and CMV infections, respectively. Patients learn to measure their pulmonary function ($FEV_1$ and FVC), systemic blood pressure, and temperature daily. They carry a diary with daily vital signs, present medications and doses, and hospital contact person. Patients are given guidelines concerning when to contact the nurse coordinator. Patients undergo indicated and routine bronchoscopy to diagnose subclinical rejection and infection.

**Table 73-1.** Initial Emergency Tests for Lung Transplant Patients

Chest x-ray
Arterial blood gases
Complete blood count with differential
Serum electrolytes, magnesium, and creatinine
Cyclosporine level—levels are dependent on method used by laboratory and length of time post transplant

**Table 73-2.** Drug Side Effects

Cyclosporine
  Nephrotoxicity—worsened by aminoglycosides, $H_2$-blockers, nonsteroidal anti-inflammatory drugs, trimethoprim-sulfamethoxazole, amphotericin B
  Neurotoxicity—tremors, seizures, headaches
  Hyperkalemia
  Hyperuricemia
  Hypertension
  Anorexia
  Increased bilirubin
  Cholestasis
  Gastric dysmotility
  Hirsutism
  Hypercholesterolemia
Prednisone
  Cushing syndrome
  Osteoporosis
  Adrenal suppression
  Hypertension
  Hyperglycemia
  Peptic ulcer disease
  Myopathy
  Cataracts
  Poor wound healing
  Azathioprine
Imuran (azathioprine)
  Leukopenia
  Thrombocytopenia
  Cholestatic jaundice
  Alopecia

Each transplant center has a protocol concerning bronchoscopy indications. Common warning signs of a fever (>37°C), cough, sputum, or $FEV_1$ decline > 10 percent for over 48 h would prompt a call or visit to the transplant center. Since most patients return to their home community 2 to 3 months following surgery, they may initially be treated and stabilized in their home town emergency department prior to transfer back to the transplant center.

Transplant immunosuppression induces T-cell dysfunction and creates risk for numerous infections. Despite potent immunosuppression, patients are still at high risk for acute rejection because no HLA matching is done. In the first year following transplant, many patients experience multiple episodes of rejection and infection (Table 73-3). Because of similar clinical presentations and the lack of clinical criteria to distinguish rejection from infection sensitively and specifically, patients undergo indicated bronchoscopy when they develop cough, fever, and decreased pulmonary function. It appears that transplanted lungs are exquisitely sensitive to any injury.

### Rejection

Acute rejection is very common and 3 to 6 episodes may occur in the first year. Following year 1, the frequency of acute rejection is decreased, but rejection can be seen several years following transplant. Clinically, the patient may have cough, chest tightness, fatigue, and fever (>0.5°C above baseline). Acute rejection may be manifest with frightening rapidity, causing a severe decline in patient status in only a day. Isolated fever may be the only finding; on the other hand, spirometry may show a 15 percent drop in $FEV_1$, and examination may reveal rales and adventitious sounds. Chest x-ray may demonstrate bilateral interstitial infiltrates, septal lines, and effusions. However, the chest x-ray may be normal when rejection occurs late in the course. The longer the period of time a patient is from transplant, the less classic a chest x-ray may appear for acute rejection. Infection, such as interstitial pneumonia, may present with a clinical picture similar to acute rejection.

Diagnostically, bronchoscopy with transbronchial biopsy is usually needed not only to confirm rejection but also to exclude infection.

**Table 73-3.** Frequent Time Sequence of the Most Common Problems Encountered with Lung Transplant Patients

| Time | 1 Month | 2 Months | 4 Months | ≥6 Months |
|---|---|---|---|---|
| | Bacteria | | | |
| | | CMV | | |
| | ←———————————————————— Acute Rejection ————————————————————→ | | | |
| | | | | Obliterative Bronchiolitis |

Since acute rejection is a patchy process, the sensitivity of biopsy for acute rejection is 70 percent. The histopathologic correlate of acute rejection is a perivascular lymphocytic infiltrate that is graded by the intensity of the infiltrate and its disruption of the lung architecture. If clinically indicated, i.e., infection is excluded, large doses of glucocorticoids are given (1 g IV solumedrol on day 1, followed by 500 mg solumedrol IV qd for 2 days). Treatment should result in improved symptoms and clinical parameters in 1 to 2 days. Failure to respond to glucocorticoids suggests an alternative diagnosis. Patients who have a history of seizures associated with the administration of high-dose glucocorticoids will also need benzodiazepines concurrently to prevent further seizure episodes (see "Neurologic Complications").

## Infection

In the first 3 months, bacterial infections are most common because of decreased mucociliary clearance, diminished cough reflex due to denervation, disrupted lymphatics, reperfusion injury, and heightened immunosuppression. Episodes of bronchitis and pneumonitis occur with equal frequency in both cystic fibrosis (CF) and non-CF patients. However, due to the chronic colonization of the upper airways, pseudomonads are a particular concern with CF transplant patients. Other potential sources of bacterial infection in the early postoperative phase include chronic indwelling lines and subcutaneous sites along the incision and the sternum. Bacterial bronchitis, especially >6 months after transplant, may suggest the development of obliterative bronchiolitis.

For the rest of their lives, these patients will continue to be maintained on immunosuppressive agents that induce T-cell dysfunction, and, unlike other organ transplant patients, their lung grafts are constantly exposed to airborne pathogens. Therefore, they are susceptible to a host of potential infections: fungal, viral, parasitic, as well as bacterial—particularly *Legionella* and *Mycobacteria*. *Pneumocystis carinii* pneumonia has been exceedingly rare because of prophylaxis with TMP-SMZ or aerosolized pentamidine. Mycobacterial infections either with tuberculosis or with atypical *Mycobacteria* may be extremely difficult to treat, as are fungal infections, especially those with *Aspergillus* species. Since the treatment of the above infections involves potentially toxic agents, an aggressive diagnostic approach must be taken prior to initiating therapy.

Cytomegalovirus infections are frequent following lung transplant, and the incidence of CMV disease varies with the pretransplant status of the donor (D) and recipient (R): $D^+R^- = 100$ percent, $D^+R^+ = 70$ percent, $D^-R^+ = 50$ percent, $D^-R^- = 10$ percent. CMV prophylaxis has not changed the incidence of disease, but, extrapolating from bone marrow transplant experience, ganciclovir and CMV immunoglobulin administered for up to 12 weeks after the transplant has allowed an improved mortality in these newly infected ($D^+R^-$) patients. The presentation of CMV disease may range from a flulike illness to a multisystem disease with protean manifestations, including pneumonitis, hepatitis, bone marrow suppression, gastritis, and colitis. Although the incidence of CMV disease is increased in the first few months post transplant, it may recur for the life of the patient. Key laboratory features include neutropenia and/or thrombocytopenia, conversion of anti-CMV IgM to positive, and positive CMV cultures from urine, buffy coat, or bronchoalveolar lavage. Due to persistent shedding of the CMV virus, definitive diagnosis of CMV pneumonitis requires histopathologic confirmation of viral cytopathic effects from tissue obtained by transbronchial biopsy. Treatment is

usually successful with ganciclovir or foscarnet, with or without CMV-specific immunoglobulin. Many times, treatment can be completed on an outpatient basis. Due to enhanced immunosuppression, CMV disease may temporally follow the treatment of acute rejection with high-dose glucocorticoids. Conversely, CMV disease may stimulate the immune system and precipitate an episode of acute rejection.

Primary Epstein-Barr virus (EBV) infections have been implicated as a cause of posttransplant lymphomas, and all new conversions are treated with high-dose acyclovir.

Sinusitis after transplant may require antibiotic treatment as well as surgical drainage, particularly in CF patients, since their sinuses remain colonized with bacteria and are more prone to impaired drainage due to nasal polyps.

## Other Pulmonary Complications

Immediately following lung transplantation, patients may have surgically related intrathoracic problems. If dehiscence of the airway anastomosis occurs, it is usually within the first 3 weeks and is usually managed expectantly if the underlying omentum is intact. However, this complication may be life-threatening. Bronchial stenosis at the site of the anastomosis may cause difficulty in clearing secretions and can be managed by placement of an endobronchial stent or by laser therapy. Pulmonary artery stenosis may be a cause of graft dysfunction, especially in the single-lung transplant patient. In this case, quantitative lung perfusion scan will demonstrate less than 50 percent flow to the transplanted lung and will require surgical revision. Spontaneous pneumothorax may occur within the first few weeks after discharge and usually necessitates placement of a chest tube to prevent possible infection of the pleural space. The patient will also need to be assessed for airway dehiscence. Sternal instability may suggest sternal osteomyelitis and need for surgical revision.

## Cardiac Problems

During the operation the pericardium is opened and the donor pulmonary veins are attached as an atrial cuff to the recipient's heart. Both these sites can become infected during bacteremic episodes, and therefore lung transplant patients should receive appropriate endocarditis antimicrobial prophylaxis before dental procedures, etc. Thrombosis of the pulmonary veins occurs rarely but usually within the immediate postoperative course as a cause of early graft failure.

## Gastrointestinal Complications

Gastrointestinal problems are frequent post transplant. Cyclosporine is metabolized through the hepatic $P_{450}$ enzymes and is excreted through the biliary system, which may result in complications of hepatic and biliary cholestatic disease. Cyclosporine has also been implicated in exacerbating gastric atony, which may also result from omentopexy. Azathioprine may cause pancreatitis, and steroids may be implicated in peptic ulcer disease. These effects are particularly problematic with CF patients, who already have gastrointestinal complications of their underlying disease. Reflux, dysmotility with actual bezoar formation, and distal intestinal obstruction syndrome (DIOS) have all been frequently encountered post transplant, especially with CF patients. Cholestatic symptoms have prompted cholecystectomies in many CF posttransplant patients, since acute cholecystitis is poorly tolerated in immunosuppressed patients. Hepatic cirrhosis may be unrecognized pretransplant in CF patients and its effect on morbidity and mortality posttransplant is unknown. Certainly, narcotics may exacerbate DIOS, and these patients may frequently present with signs and symptoms suggestive of small bowel obstruction. Osmotic laxatives are frequently employed both on an acute and chronic basis. If patients are unable to tolerate anything orally, their medications should be given parenterally.

## Neurologic Complications

Cyclosporine has profound effects on the neurologic system, including headaches, tremors, and seizures. Immunosuppression also increases risk of meningitis.

Seizure suppression can be obtained with intravenous diazepam or lorazepam. We discourage the use of dilantin and phenobarbital because these drugs can profoundly lower cyclosporine levels. Initial tests should include head CT and lumbar puncture, chest x-ray, complete blood count, and electrolyte and cyclosporine levels. A brain MRI may show abnormalities when the CT scan of the head is normal. Transient hypodense nonenhancing lesions with prolonged $T_2$ relaxation indicate increased water content in the cerebral white matter. These lesions resolve but may recur in different areas with new episodes of seizures. Seizures tend to occur 2 to 7 days following high-dose glucocorticoid therapy. Patients may complain of hallucinations, disorientation, and increased tremors just prior to an episode of seizures. These steroid-related seizures seem to occur primarily with CF patients who have undergone lung transplant, but they have also occurred in patients following other solid organ transplants, related to administration of high-dose steroids.

## Other Drug Side Effects

Both glucocorticoids and cyclosporine can exacerbate glucose intolerance, worsen osteoporosis, and cause myopathy and systemic hypertension. Commonly, chronic cyclosporine use at the levels employed in lung transplant immunosuppression results in some renal insufficiency by decreasing renal blood flow and by a direct effect on the renal tubules, resulting in hyperkalemia and hypomagnesemia. The major side effect of azathioprine is bone marrow suppression. Neutropenia may often result from either azathioprine or CMV infection.

Drugs that are metabolized by the hepatic P450 system will interact with cyclosporine metabolism (Table 73-4). Drugs that induce these enzymes, e.g., Dilantin, Rifampin, and phenobarbitol, may lower cyclosporine levels acutely, possibly precipitating rejection. Other drugs may retard the metabolism of cyclosporine, causing toxic levels. Those drugs that may raise cyclosporine levels include erythromycin (probably clarithromycin), ketoconazole, cimetidine, and the calcium channel blockers. These drugs are avoided unless appropriate changes in cyclosporine dosing are made in anticipation of the change in blood levels. Nonsteroidal anti-inflammatory agents should also be avoided since these drugs will act synergistically with cyclosporine to further reduce renal blood flow.

## Late Complications

### Obliterative Bronchiolitis

The most frequent cause of death in lung transplant patients after 1 year is obliterative bronchiolitis. This destructive airway process may be a form of chronic rejection similar to coronary atherosclerosis in heart transplant patients and bile duct sclerosis in liver transplant patients. Since the large airways become bronchiectatic as the small airways are obliterated, episodes of bacterial bronchitis are common. Diagnostically, the yield for bronchoscopy and biopsy is low; therefore, clinical criteria, i.e., $\geq 20$ percent fall in $FEV_1$ without any other identifiable cause, is relied upon. Typically the chest x-ray is clear of infiltrates. Current treatment is augmentation of immunosuppression and high-dose steroids, as with acute rejection. The course of disease is highly variable, with some patients stabilizing at a lower level of pulmonary function and others progressing to respiratory failure and death. Currently, obliterative bronchiolitis is the leading indication for retransplantation, with 1-year survival of only 40 percent, at this time.

## Posttransplant Lymphoproliferative Disease (PTLD)

Posttransplant lymphoproliferative disease can be a consequence of T-cell suppression with long-term cyclosporine use. The overall incidence in lung transplant patients appears to be 8 percent. The disease tends to occur with primary EBV infection following lung transplant and therefore most frequently affects adolescent patients because they are more likely to be EBV-negative at the time of transplantation. Presenting features may include: isolated lymphadenopathy, painful otitis media (secondary to tonsillar involvement), or a viral-type syndrome with malaise, fever, and myalgias. PLTD within 1 year of transplant is usually localized and can be successfully treated with reduced immunosuppression and high-dose acyclovir, with a relatively good prognosis. In contrast, PTLD after 1 year tends to be disseminated, unresponsive to treatment, and usually fatal.

The native disease has been shown to recur in the transplanted lung in patients with sarcoidosis, but with little clinical consequence. A case of giant cell pneumonitis has recurred in the transplanted lung, with dire results. However, there is no evidence that the cellular defect of cystic fibrosis recurs in the transplanted lungs.

## FUTURE GOALS

Investigative strategies to increase the availability of donor organs have been pursued through the use of cadaveric organs. Laboratory strategies on rats have shown that the lungs can be maintained without perfusion but with ventilation for several hours. The implication is that donor organs could potentially be harvested from patients who are dead on arrival or who fail resuscitation in the emergency department. Lastly, the technique of using donor lobes from living adult relatives of CF patients has been pioneered, with minimal morbidity to the donors. These patients have attained adequate levels of pulmonary function, but the technique is only applicable to small patients.

## BIBLIOGRAPHY

Armitage JM, Kormos RL, Stuart RS, et al: Posttransplant lymphoproliferative disease in thoracic organ transplant patients: Ten years of cyclosporine-based immunosuppression. *J Heart Lung Transplant* 10:877, 1991.

Egan TM, Kaiser LR, Cooper JD: Lung transplantation. *Curr Probl Surg* 26:673, 1989.

Flume PA, Egan TM, Paradowski LJ, et al: Infectious complications of lung transplantation: Impact of cystic fibrosis. *Am J Respir Crit Care Med* 149:1601, 1994.

Griffith BP, Zenati M: The pulmonary donor. *Clin Chest Med* 11:217, 1990.

Hosenpud JD, Novick RJ, Breen TJ, Daily OP: The Registry of the International Society for Heart and Lung Transplantation: Eleventh Official Report—1994. *J Heart Lung Transplant* 13:561, 1994.

Marshall SE, Kramer MR, Lewiston NJ, et al: Selection and evaluation of recipients for heart-lung and lung transplantation. *Chest* 98:1488, 1990.

Novick RJ, Kaye MP, Patterson GA, et al: Redo lung transplantation: A North American experience. *J Heart Lung Transplant* 12:5, 1993.

Trulock EP: Management of lung transplant rejection. *Chest* 103:1566, 1993.

**Table 73-4.** Cyclosporine: Drug Interactions

| Increased cyclosporine level | Decreased cyclosporine level |
|---|---|
| Diltiazem | Rifampin |
| Verapamil | Phenobarbital |
| Ketoconazole | Phenytoin |
| Fluconazole | |
| Itraconazole | |
| Erythromycin | |
| Birth control pills | |

## 74
# ESOPHAGEAL EMERGENCIES
### Richard E. Burney

### INTRODUCTION

Esophageal disease is a relatively infrequent source of emergency problems, but one that must be considered with respect to a number of more common emergency complaints, including chest pain, gastrointestinal hemorrhage, and dysphagia. While most esophageal conditions are benign, both esophageal hemorrhage and perforation carry a high morbidity and mortality if not recognized and treated promptly. Specific knowledge of the anatomy, physiology, and history of esophageal diseases, and familiarity with the diagnostic methods of identifying esophageal problems, all assist in the identification of emergency problems of esophageal origin.

### ANATOMY AND PHYSIOLOGY

The esophagus begins at the hypopharynx opposite the sixth cervical vertebra and the lower border of the cricoid cartilage; passes through three visceral compartments, the neck (cervical esophagus), the mediastinum, and the upper abdomen; and ends at the cardia of the stomach opposite the body of the eleventh thoracic vertebra. The anatomic relations of the esophagus are shown in Fig. 74-1.

The pharynx and esophagus lie immediately in front of the prevertebral fascia and are surrounded by a layer of fascia which fuses with cellular tissue of the superior mediastinum. A layer of this tissue separates laterally in the neck to unite with the prevertebral fascia, forming the retropharyngeal space of Henke. The retropharyngeal and retroesophageal space is in direct communication with the superior mediastinum, and bleeding, perforations, or abscesses in this space have a direct conduit to the superior mediastinum.

The esophagus is composed of an inner mucosal layer covering a tough, fibrous submucosal layer. There are two muscle layers surrounding the mucosal and submucosal layers. The innermost is spiral to circular while the outer is longitudinal. There is no serosa, and as a result, once the submucosa is perforated or destroyed, the perforation tends to extend into the surrounding mediastinal structures, leading to a diffuse, malignant, and often rapidly progressive and fatal mediastinitis. The striated muscle of the upper esophagus gradually gives way to the smooth muscle which forms the rest of the esophagus and the gastrointestinal tract.

The mucosa and submucosa are the layers usually involved in peptic esophagitis, which, when severe and prolonged, may result in scarring and stricture formation. Ingestion of lye and some other corrosives destroys the muscular layer to a greater or lesser degree.

### The Venous System

The submucosal plexus of veins drains to an intercommunicating plexus which surrounds the esophagus. This network anastomoses with the inferior thyroid vein in the neck, the azygous system in the thorax, and the coronary and short gastric veins (part of the portal venous system) in the abdomen. Obstruction of the portal system from such diseases as cirrhosis of the liver causes submucosal esophageal varices (Fig. 74-2).

### Deglutition and Propulsion of the Food Bolus: Physiology

A food bolus is passed from the anterior part of the tongue backward by a sequential contraction of the tongue upward against the roof of the mouth and backward against the hard and soft palate and posterior pharyngeal wall. At the same time there is a sequential contraction of the esophageal constrictor muscles from above downward. The pressure of the tongue and the contraction of the muscles of the soft palate and the superior constrictor cause an airtight closure of the nasal pharynx to the food bolus. The resulting high-pressure wave which is created by the sequential contraction of the aforementioned muscles propels food toward the esophagus.

Laryngeal muscles contract involuntarily as the bolus is passed from the front of the tongue to the middle pharynx, causing the larynx to rise and be sealed from the pharynx by the epiglottis. The cricopharyngeal muscle forms the UES and is in tonic contraction at all times, except when it relaxes as the food bolus approaches.

The bolus is then propelled caudad by a peristaltic wave which starts at the UES and is controlled by the reflex arcs of Meissner's and Auerbach's plexuses located between the inner and outer muscle layers. When the bolus reaches the distal 1 to 2 cm of the esophagus, it meets another high-pressure area, the LES, which relaxes to allow food to enter the stomach. A secondary peristaltic contraction wave starts at the level of the aortic arch, which is another area of raised pressure, and propels any leftover liquid caudad. Finally, a tertiary contraction wave may be initiated at the level of the lower one-third of the esophagus, usually by reflux of gastric contents. This may be an important mechanism for keeping the lower esophageal mucosa clear of gastric contents.

### PRESENTING SYMPTOMS
### Dysphagia
#### Definition

Dysphagia is an awareness of something wrong with the smooth pattern of swallowing, i.e., the patient mentions that food sticks, hesitates, or pauses, or that it just won't go down right. The presence of dysphagia almost always signifies esophageal pathology. It is different from "globus hystericus"—the sensation of "something always stuck in the throat"—but is akin to transfer dysphagia, which is the inability to initiate the act of swallowing and is usually due to pharyngeal muscular weakness or central nervous system disease.

#### Cause

There are two basic causes for dysphagia, either mechanical narrowing or obstruction of the lumen, or nonobstructive (Table 74-1). Mechanical problems stem from abnormality in the lumen (e.g., foreign body), in the wall (peptic stricture of the submucosa, or esophageal cancer), or extrinsic to the esophagus from encroachment by surrounding structures (goiter, enlarged subcarinal lymph nodes). Nonobstructive dysphagia can be motility-related due to intrinsic

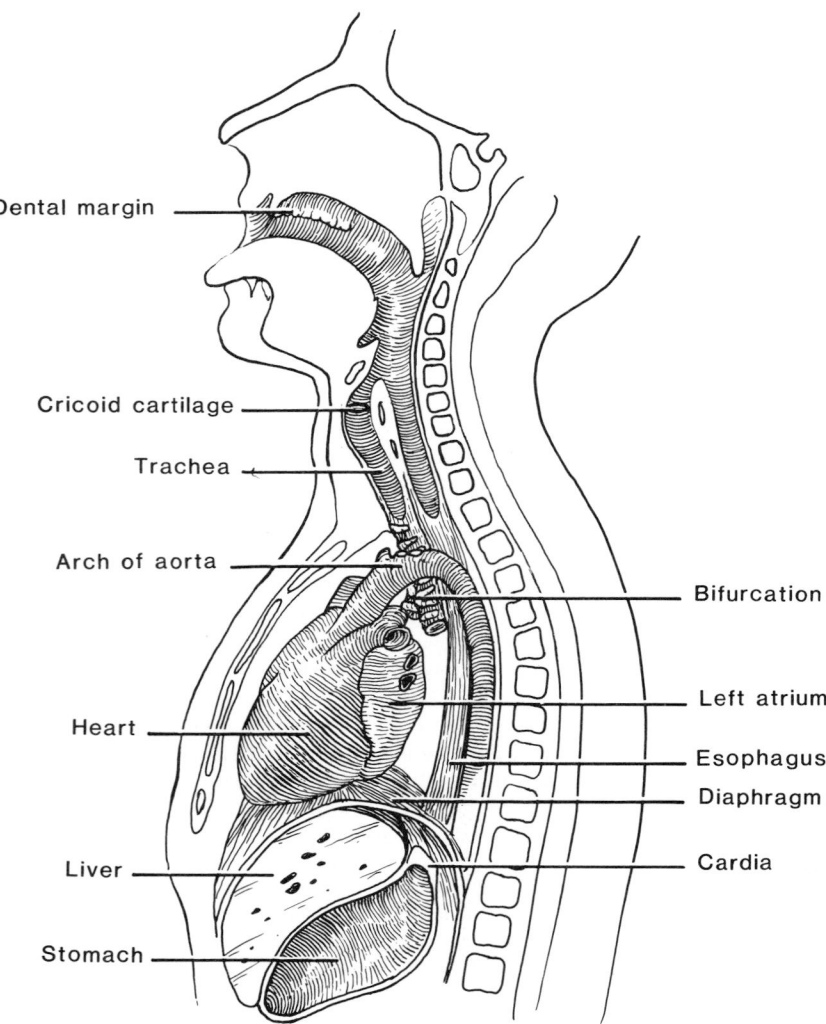

Dental margin

Cricoid cartilage

Trachea

Arch of aorta

Heart

Liver

Stomach

Bifurcation

Left atrium

Esophagus

Diaphragm

Cardia

**Fig. 74-1.** Anatomic relations of the esophagus (seen from the left side). The esophagus is about 25 cm (10 in) long. The distance from the upper incisor teeth to the beginning of the esophagus (cricoid cartilage) is about 15 cm (6 in); from the upper incisors to the level of the bronchi, 22 to 23 cm (9 in); to the cardia, 40 cm (16 in). Structures contiguous to the esophagus that affect esophageal function are demonstrated.

muscular or nervous disorders of the esophagus or pharynx, or non-motility related, due to esophageal reflux or inflammation.

## Characteristics

Dysphagia can be characterized by (1) the onset, that is, the caliber, character, and temperature of food causing it, (2) the location of the dysphagia, and (3) how it is relieved (Table 74-2).

Mechanical problems cause solid foods to stick in the esophagus. The caliber of spongy-type foods which can be swallowed decreases relentlessly over a short period of time if dysphagia is due to esophageal cancer, and more slowly if it is due to benign stricture. Fluids can usually be swallowed until the stricture is far advanced or the narrowing is suddenly blocked by a solid bolus of food or another foreign body (e.g., enteric-coated pills). Peptic stricture can produce the same symptoms, but usually the dysphagia is mild, and accompanied by heartburn due to the esophagitis. Difficulty in swallowing liquids, especially if they are cold, is a symptom of a motor disorder.

### Specific Types of Dysphagia

#### Transfer Dysphagia

Transfer dysphagia is the inability to initiate the act of swallowing (deglutition). Inflammatory lesions which are painful or cause mechanical obstruction, and neuromuscular disorders, are the usual causes for this disorder. Failure of the muscles of mastication and salivary lubrication also cause this problem, but less frequently.

Painful lesions of the tongue, oropharynx, and larynx can cause transfer dysphagia, along with odynophagia. Examples include pharyngitis of bacterial (streptococcal), viral (herpetic), and fungal (monilial) origin. The latter two occur especially in the immunocompromised patient. Parapharyngeal abscesses and tonsillitis may cause mechanical obstruction as well as odynophagia with dysphagia. Foreign bodies stuck in the throat, especially in the young and the old, and epiglottitis in the young also can lead to this symptom. Finally, cancers of the head and neck which invade the tongue and throat, and operations to cure the lesions, are an increasing cause of transfer dysphagia.

Patients with mechanical causes of transfer dysphagia tend to drool because of mechanical obstruction or pain. They are often hoarse and have a bad cough because of the laryngeal involvement. The diagnosis is made by direct laryngoscopy, except in the child with possible epiglottitis, who should be evaluated in the operating room under anesthesia.

Neuromuscular causes of transfer dysphagia include cerebrovascular accidents, polio and bulbar palsies, dermatomyositis, and polymyositis. The symptoms most associated with neuromuscular weakness are nasopharyngeal regurgitation, and cough and hoarseness due to laryngeal aspirations. A Zenker's diverticulum may also be found associated with these diseases (Tables 74-1 and 74-2).

Rare but curable, causes of transfer dysphagia in younger age

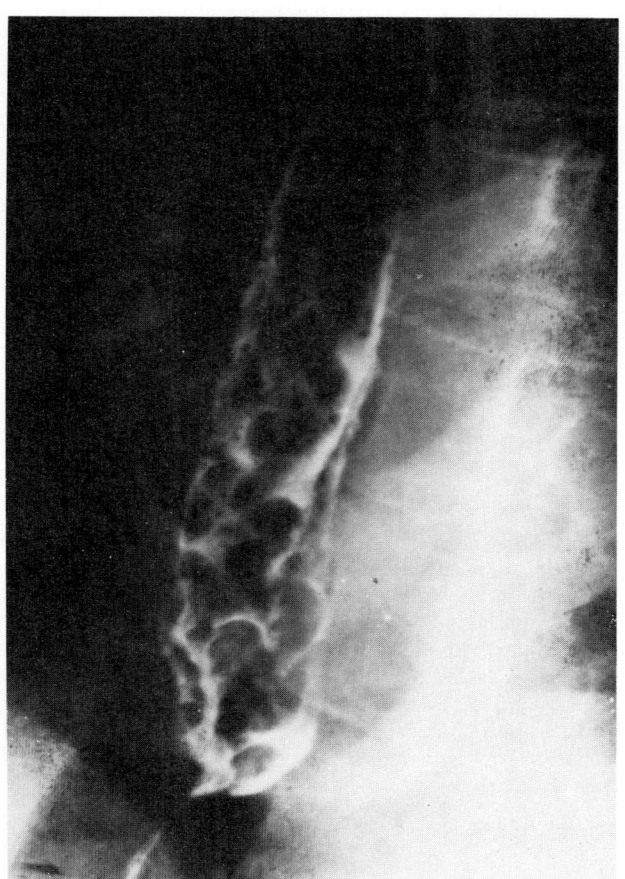

**Fig. 74-2.** Esophageal varices. Current therapy includes a vasopressin drip followed by esophagoscopy and an attempt at sclerotherapy to stop the bleeding.

groups include myasthenia gravis, thyrotoxic myopathy and lead poisoning.

## Esophageal Body Dysphagia

Mechanical causes of esophageal body dysphagia in the young include congenital stricture, swallowed foreign bodies, and vascular ring anomalies of the aortic arch. In the older patient the most com-

**Table 74-2.** Characteristics of Dysphagia

|  | Mechanical Narrowing (Tumors, Strictures) | Motility Related |
| --- | --- | --- |
| Onset | Gradual or sudden | Usually gradual |
| Progressive | Often | Usually not |
| Type of bolus | Solids (unless high-grade obstruction) | Solids and/or liquids |
| Temperature-dependent | No | Worse with cold liquids; may improve with warm liquids |
| Response to bolus impaction | Often must be regurgitated | Can usually be passed by repeated swallowing or by washing it down with fluids |
| Weight loss | Yes | No |

mon causes include hiatus hernia, reflux esophagitis, webs, rings, and cancer of the esophagus (Table 74-1). Increasingly, infections caused by herpesvirus, cytomegalovirus, and *Candida albicans* are the cause of dysphagia in the immunocompromised or immunosuppressed patient, and in the patient with AIDS.

The most important neuromuscular causes of dysphagia include achalasia, diffuse spasm, and scleroderma; achalasia-caused dysphagia is associated with esophageal retention and regurgitation of retained food. X-ray films show a dilated esophagus with a distal beak. The diagnosis is confirmed by manometry of the LES, where the pressure remains high even during swallowing.

Diffuse spasm causes dysphagia and/or pain. Segmental contractions are seen on barium swallow, and some peristaltic waves interspersed with simultaneous prolonged high-amplitude contractions are seen on manometric studies. Many patients are admitted to the coronary care unit on several occasions before a barium swallow, esophageal manometry, and coronary arteriography prove the esophageal rather than the myocardial origin of the pain.

Dysphagia associated with scleroderma usually is associated with symptoms of reflux. Aperistalsis seen on a simple barium swallow is diagnostic, but often single or multiple contractions are seen, and in such cases the barium swallow is not diagnostic.

If a patient has dysphagia, odynophagia, or esophageal colic, an emergency barium swallow, when positive, will lead to a diagnosis of mechanical or neuromuscular esophageal disease, and appropriate referral. Unfortunately, motor diseases of the esophagus, except for achalasia, may not be evident at the time of the initial barium swallow, especially diffuse esophageal spasm.

**Table 74-1.** Causes of Dysphagia

|  | Obstructive | Nonobstructive |
| --- | --- | --- |
| Acquired, infectious |  | Poliomyelitis, diphtheria, botulism, rabies, tetanus, *Candida,* herpes, cytomegalovirus |
| Congenital | Vascular abnormalities, webs |  |
| Immunologic |  | Dermatomyositis, polymyositis scleroderma, multiple sclerosis, myasthenia gravis |
| Neurologic |  | Stroke, Parkinson's, chorea, pseudobulbar palsy |
| Physical, inflammatory | Cervical spurs, stricture (caustic, reflux), Schatzki's ring | Esophagitis, spasm, peristaltic dysfunction |
| Mechanical | Foreign body, food, pills |  |
| Cardiovascular | Aortic aneurysm, left atrial enlargement, aberrant right subclavian artery |  |
| Endocrine, metabolic | Goiter | Lead poisoning, magnesium deficiency, thyrotoxicosis |
| Neoplastic | Benign and malignant tumors of esophagus, larynx, lung, pericardium, tracheobronchial tree, thyroid; metastatic disease in mediastial lymph nodes |  |
| Others | Zenker's diverticulum, paraesophageal hernia | Achalasia, spontaneous intramural hemorrhage, pharmacologic-induced |

## Odynophagia (Pain on Swallowing)

Odynophagia is defined as pain upon swallowing. It can be associated with bolus arrest (dysphagia) but may be experienced without arrest of the bolus. Odynophagia and dysphagia are the cardinal symptoms of esophageal disease.

The pain is associated with inflammation of the esophageal mucosal surface commonly seen in such conditions as gastroesophageal reflux, radiation, viral esophagitis, or trauma causing laceration or perforation.

Odynophagia appears at the time of bolus transmission and disappears when the material has left the esophagus. Therefore, unlike pain of cardiac origin, it comes with swallowing and disappears within 10 s. It may be mild or so intense that the patient refuses to swallow solids, liquids, or saliva.

## Esophageal Colic

Esophageal colic is an acute, agonizing, spasmodic, or crescendo-like pain that can mimic myocardial ischemia. (See "Chest Pain of Esophageal Origin" below.)

The pain is experienced substernally and radiates directly through to the back into the interscapular area. It may also radiate into the neck, jaw, or arms. It lasts from 5 to 10 s to hours and usually is indistinguishable from angina pectoris in terms of intensity, radiation, and relation to exercise or relief with nitroglycerin, except that it usually takes 7 to 10 min for relief instead of 2 to 3 min. It is often an associated symptom in patients with dysphagia or esophageal reflux.

## Heartburn (Pyrosis)

Heartburn is the most common symptom of esophageal disease. Unlike the first three symptoms, it is not associated with the swallowing of solids or fluids but rather with reflux of acid or alkaline contents stomach into the esophagus, altering the pH and causing inflammation and/or ulceration.

The inflammatory response depends upon the frequency and amount of acid or alkali refluxed and the rate at which it is cleared from the mucosal surface. Biopsy changes show thickening of the basal layer of the esophageal mucosa with extension of the dermal pegs to the free surface in the mildest cases of reflux esophagitis. In more severe cases the epithelial layer is obviously inflamed at esophagoscopy, and microscopically the mucosa is covered with microulcers and the lamina propria has the classic pathologic signs of inflammation.

Heartburn is perceived as a burning discomfort in the substernal area. It appears after meals, especially large ones containing fat, is worse in recumbency or with exercise, and is relieved by antacids, if only temporarily.

## Regurgitation

Regurgitation is the retrograde propulsion of fluid into the mouth. It is different from rumination, in which recently eaten food is propelled back into the mouth by a strong contraction of the abdominal wall musculature.

Regurgitation is usually due to the stomach or duodenal contents ascending through an incompetent LES. It is, therefore, associated with reflux esophagitis and heartburn. It can also be associated with the emptying of a diverticulum or with regurgitation of the retained portion of fluid in achalasia.

Regurgitation causes a bitter or acid taste in the mouth, and is usually associated with increased intraabdominal pressure resulting from bending over, lying down, or lifting heavy objects.

Regurgitation of diverticular contents or from achalasia, on the other hand, usually produces undigested, foul-tasting food, with an odor from the mouth due to the presence of putrid food. Both types of regurgitation may produce aspiration, recurrent pneumonia, and failure to thrive.

## The Bleeding Esophagus

Patients with bleeding from the esophagus may present in a variety of ways, including acute, life-threatening hematemesis, coffee-ground emesis or gastric aspirate, melena, hematest-positive stools, or anemia of chronic, occult loss, depending upon the rate and duration of bleeding. Bleeding from the esophagus, like bleeding from other parts of the gastrointestinal tract, may be classified according to the amount, source, and symptoms produced by the bleeding at presentation.

### Amount

Bleeding from the esophagus can be classified according to the amount of blood replacement needed to restore blood volume while the patient is in the emergency department.

**Mild to Moderate Blood Loss**

Mild blood loss (less than 10 percent of blood volume) is due to capillary bleeding or to sudden, nonrecurring arterial bleeding. The cause may be inflammation, infection (especially in immunosuppressed persons), or injury.

Moderate blood loss (10 to 20 percent) is due to laceration of an artery or nondistended vein. Bleeding may not stop during treatment in the emergency department. Infusion of 1 L of crystalloid, and possibly 1 to 2 units of blood, is needed to restore blood volume. Admission to the hospital for volume replacement, monitoring, and diagnostic evaluation is required.

**Major Blood Loss**

Major blood loss (20 to 40 percent) is due to a ruptured varix or an artery that has been eroded by a peptic ulcer. Vital signs are abnormal. These patients must be sent to a critical care unit. Fiberoptic endoscopy should be carried out promptly to establish the diagnosis.

Massive blood loss (more than 40 percent) can be due to a perforated artery at the base of a peptic ulcer, but is more likely due to a ruptured varix. The patient needs more than 4 units of blood in addition to the initial crystalloid replacement, and the source tends to continue bleeding. The source of bleeding should be confirmed by endoscopy in the emergency department. Surgical consultation is mandatory. Coagulation abnormalities should be sought and corrected. If esophageal varices are the cause, a vasopressin drip using 20 units in 200 mL of saline at 0.25 to 0.5 unit per minute is given. If bleeding continues, sclerotherapy or Gelfoam embolization of the left gastric vein or use of a Blakemore or similar type tube should be considered. Other methods to control esophageal bleeding are inpatient decisions.

## EXTRAESOPHAGEAL MANIFESTATIONS OF ESOPHAGEAL DISEASE

Many patients with esophageal disease present with symptoms that do not directly relate to the esophagus but which are extraesophageal manifestations (EEM) of esophageal disease.

The common EEM in the adult include chest pain, pulmonary symptoms, weight loss due to starvation, and iron deficiency anemia. The EEM in infants and retarded children include pulmonary symptoms and failure to thrive.

## Chest Pain of Esophageal Origin

Pain arising from the esophagus is the most alarming esophageal symptom since it often mimics chest pain due to mediastinitis or cardiac ischemia. Pain of esophageal origin may be the most common cause of noncardiac chest pain. It is often associated with other esophageal symptoms, such as dysphagia or reflux, although not always. There are no classic clinical features to distinguish one from the other with certainty. Relief of chest pain by antacids or repeated swallowing suggests esophageal origin. pH monitoring and manometry may be helpful confirmatory tests.

Unfortunately, precipitation of pain by exercise and relief by rest, mimicking angina pectoris, are found in patients with atypical esophageal colic due to reflux esophagitis, diffuse spasm, or irritable esophagus. Moreover, nitroglycerin relieves pain of both esophageal and cardiac origin. Pain relief in the esophageal group, however, usually takes 7 to 10 min, while pain from angina responds in 2 to 3 min and pain due to a myocardial infarction does not respond at all. Both types of patients may also have ST abnormalities on an ECG.

## Pulmonary Manifestations

Material regurgitated or refluxed into the larynx and the tracheobronchial tree can cause asthmatic-like symptoms in adults, nocturnal or early morning cough, nocturnal wheezing, hoarseness especially on arising, the need to repeatedly clear the throat, and feeling of constant pressure deep in the neck. Patients may have recurrent bouts of pneumonia with radiographic changes in the right middle lobe and superior segments of both lower lobes. Infants, retarded children and adults, and debilitated people who have suffered strokes are especially prone to aspiration pneumonia (see Chap. 67).

Aspiration may be caused by transfer dysphagia while awake, reflux from an incompetent LES, or reflux from retained food in achalasia or diverticula while asleep.

## Starvation and Failure to Thrive

Starvation and failure to thrive is seen in infants, children, and adults. In adults it is seen with increasing obstruction of the esophagus due to stricture, achalasia, or cancer, or with reflux esophagitis, especially if esophageal colic is present or the patient is mentally retarded or debilitated by a stroke.

## MANUAL SKILLS

### Nasogastric Intubation

#### Indications

A nasogastric tube should be passed for diagnostic purposes in all cases of gastrointestinal bleeding and multisystem trauma, most cases of potential esophageal injuries due to ingestion, and intestinal obstruction (Fig. 74-3). Contraindications include actual or suspected laceration or perforation of the esophagus (usual sites are at the upper weak point between the inferior constrictor and the cricothyroid muscle or at the level of LES), near-complete obstruction of the esophagus due to benign or malignant stricture, and the presence of an esophageal foreign body. The nasogastric tube must be placed orally in patients with severe midfacial trauma or rhinorrhea associated with head trauma.

A relative contraindication for placement of a nasogastric tube is a lacerated posterior larynx from whatever cause. In this case the tube should be placed under the direct visualization of a laryngoscope (after the larynx has been anesthetized with a suitable local anesthetic).

#### Anatomic Considerations

The following points should be recognized when passing a nasogastric tube (see Fig. 74-3).

1. One naris may be blocked. If so, the other naris or the mouth should be used.

2. The tip of the nose should be directed cephalad while the tip of the nasogastric tube is directed horizontally and slightly downward toward the floor of the posterior nares (not toward the roof of the anterior nares). Improper direction of the tube is the commonest cause of damage to the nasopharynx (Fig. 74-3).

3. The resistance caused by the spasmodic closure of the soft palate pressing against the superior constrictor can be overcome by having the patient swallow. Swallowing always facilitates tube passage.

4. The next level of resistance is the inferior constrictor approximately 15 to 20 cm from the ala of the nares. The tip of the nasogastric tube will catch, either on the lip formed by the cephalad surface of the cricothyroid muscle posteriorly, the pyriform fossa on either side of the larynx, or the vallecula anterior to the vocal cords or Killian's mouth. These recesses disappear with a conscious swallow with or without the use of water.

    By spasm of the constrictors, the tip may be directed anteriorly through the vocal cords into the trachea. This problem can be alleviated by two maneuvers: first by advancing the tube past this area only during the swallowing motion when the larynx rises to and is covered by the epiglottis, thus making the curve from the posterior tongue continuous with the epiglottis and the anterior lip of the esophagus (Fig. 74-3); and second by flexing the neck so that the chin is on the chest, thus directing the tip of the nasogastric tube posteriorly. Oral intubation with the patient sucking on the tube before swallowing often overcomes the problem when other maneuvers fail.

5. Insertion of the tube by way of the nasal or oral route directly into the esophagus using the Magill forceps and direct laryngoscopy may be used in the patient with an absent swallowing reflex or when it is dangerous to flex the neck, as in the unconscious trauma patient.

6. An alternative method for overcoming misdirection of the nasogastric tube is to place the second and third fingers over the tongue and direct the tips to touch the posterior pharyngeal wall. The tip of the tube is then directed over the dorsal groove formed by the approximation of the fingers.

7. The final resistance to the passage of the tube is at the proximal end of the gastroesophageal junction. This usually is overcome by slow, gentle pressure or, if this fails, by gently injecting 15 to 20 mL of water to relax the lower esophageal sphincter. Occasionally the tip may fail to pass because of a large hiatus hernia, esophageal dilation from achalasia or epiphrenic hernia, or stricture, but this is rare.

Polyethylene nasogastric tubes need not be iced before placing them. Gentle pressure should be sufficient in every case. Resistance to gentle passage indicates misdirection or obstruction. Tube placement should be confirmed by aspiration of gastric contents. If there is any question as to proper location, a radiograph should be taken.

### Endoscopy

Endoscopy using a laryngoscope is indicated for removal of foreign bodies from the hypopharynx and those lodged in the constrictor muscle and to aid direction of the tips of esophageal tubes into the esophagus. Local anesthesia must be used in the awake patient, the neck is not extended as in endotracheal intubation, the cervical vertebrae must be known to be intact, and a straight blade is more useful than a curved blade.

Flexible, fiberoptic esophagoscopy should be used for removal of foreign bodies from the esophagus. It is also used to diagnose the site of gastrointestinal bleeding before introduction of a Blakemore tube or to confirm the absence of esophageal bleeding and varices in a patient going directly to surgery for massive bleeding from a suspected gastroduodenal site.

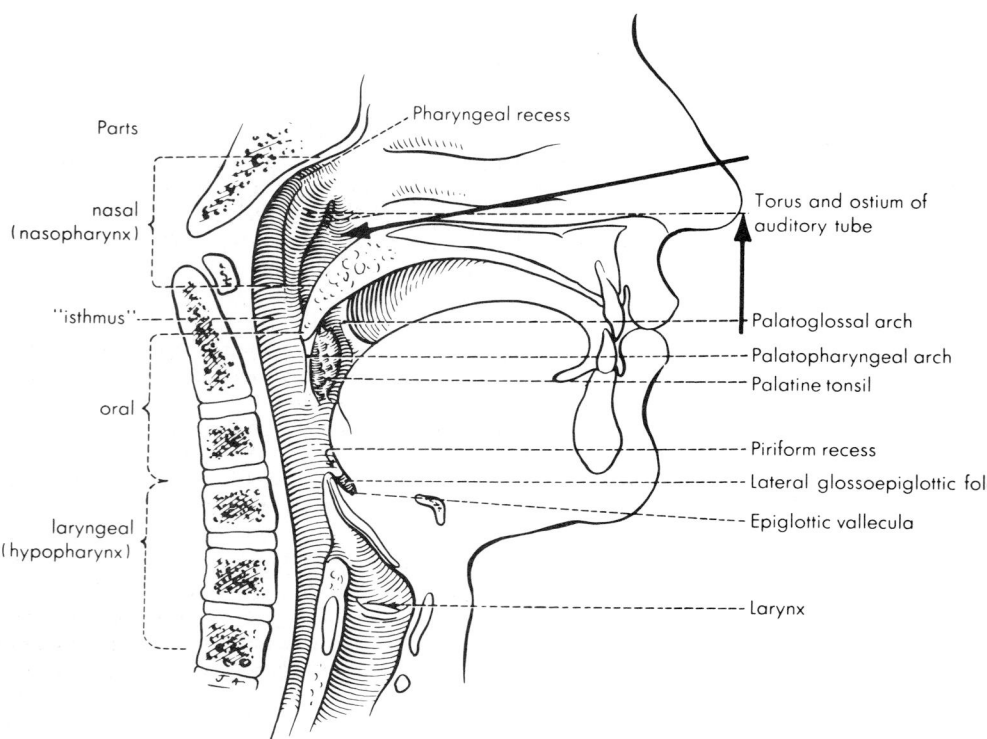

Parts

nasal
(nasopharynx)

"isthmus"

oral

laryngeal
(hypopharynx)

Pharyngeal recess

Torus and ostium of
auditory tube

Palatoglossal arch
Palatopharyngeal arch
Palatine tonsil

Piriform recess
Lateral glossoepiglottic fold
Epiglottic vallecula

Larynx

**Fig. 74-3.** Functional anatomy regarding the passage of tubes into the esophagus. The arrows indicate that the tip of the nose needs to be elevated and the tip of the tube directed along the floor of the naris in order to make the curve at the isthmus.

Both topical pharyngeal anesthesia and intravenous sedation are usually required for esophagoscopy.

### Blakemore Intubation

#### Indications

Blakemore intubation is indicated for massive or uncontrolled bleeding which is suspected to arise from the lower 10 cm of the esophagus or from the cardia of the stomach and which is not controlled by vasopressin (see discussion on the bleeding esophagus) or other measures.

Contraindications include bleeding from complete or incomplete lacerations of the esophagus or peptic ulceration with stricture.

#### Anatomic Considerations and Procedure

A complete description of how to place the Blakemore tube can be found in the package with the tube. There are, however, some precautions:

1. The tube can be placed through either the nose or the mouth.
2. The same points of obstruction found in placing nasogastric tubes obstruct passage of the Blakemore tube.
3. The oropharynx should be anesthetized prior to placement unless the patient is unconscious or lacks a gag reflex.
4. The site of bleeding must be identified by endoscopy prior to placement unless the rate of bleeding precludes it.
5. The airway must be protected by endotracheal intubation prior to placement.
6. The tip of the tube is best directed over a dorsal groove formed by the second and third fingers, which are in turn pressed loosely against the midposterior pharyngeal wall.

Endotracheal intubation should precede placing a Blakemore tube in any patient, and should be considered with any type of esophageal tube in the unconscious patient. It is necessary to release the cuff pressure while passing the tip of the esophageal tube past the level of the balloon cuff of the endotracheal tube.

## ESOPHAGEAL TRAUMA

### Etiology

Esophageal injury results from a variety of causes and agents. Because the esophagus is well protected deep in the thoracic cavity, external forces or agents are relatively infrequent causes of esophageal injury, and iatrogenic and self-induced problems predominate.

### Pathogenesis and Clinical Presentation

Esophageal injury may be partial- or full-thickness. Partialess tears occur as a result of swallowed foreign bodies or sharp objects (including tortilla chips) and heal spontaneously. They may be associated with dysphagia, odynophagia, esophageal pain, and mild upper gastrointestinal bleeding. Full-thickness injury without perforation results from ingestion of caustic substances or after injection of sclerosing agents in patients with esophageal varices. Perforation of the esophagus from penetrating trauma, foreign bodies, or instrumentation leads to mediastinitis. Early diagnosis is critical to successful treatment. If surgical repair of the perforation is made in less than 24 h, mortality is 5 percent, but if surgical treatment is delayed, mortality is as high as 75 percent.

Laceration of the mucosa and submucosa (Mallory-Weiss syndrome) and perforation of the full thickness of the thoracic and abdominal esophageal wall (Boerhaave's syndrome) are associated with a sudden, violent, and usually repeated increase in the intraabdominal pressure against a weakened esophageal wall. The cause of the sudden increase in abdominal pressure is a Valsalva movement, which usually implies a closed glottis during hiccuping, defecation, labor, epileptic attack, or lifting a heavy weight. Other causes include striking the steering wheel or compression during external heart massage. The most common cause of increased intraabdominal pressure is violent and repeated emesis.

Predisposing causes for a weakened esophageal wall include emesis in which the mucosa at the gastroesophageal junction prolapses into the esophageal lumen through the narrow hiatus and gastroesophageal junction. The mucosa becomes edematous and even bruised and inflamed after such an event. The mucosa can also be weakened by the prolonged presence of a nasogastric tube; reflux esophagitis; epiphrenic hernias; or hemorrhage into the esophageal wall.

Mallory-Weiss lacerations, are thought to occur in weakened mucosa, usually on the right posterolateral side, but Boerhaave's perforations tend to rupture on the left posterolateral side of the unsupported part of the abdominal esophageal wall. The lacerations or perforations tend to extend cephalad into the thoracic esophagus. The second most common site for both syndromes is on the right side just below the level of the azygos vein. Laceration or perforation of the cervical esophagus from flexion-hyperextension injury has also been reported as a cause of mediastinitis.

Lacerations cause usually moderate and self-limiting bleeding of the submucosal plexus of veins and arteries. They may also produce dysphagia and odynophagia and be associated with symptoms of reflux esophagitis (predisposing factor).

Perforations of the esophagus associated with Boerhaave's syndrome cause the most malignant type of mediastinitis. The force of expulsion of fluid through the perforation spreads it rapidly through the mediastinum, causing an acid burn to the mediastinal tissues and rapid spread of very virulent bacteria. The patient complains of severe abdominal pain and chest pain which often radiates into the neck. Patients rapidly develop shock and septicemia, leading to death within 48 h. There is often an associated peritonitis with air under the diaphragm, as well as air-fluid levels in the mediastinum and pyopneumothorax.

## Symptoms of Laceration and Perforation

Bleeding and dysphagia following at least one episode of previous emesis are the common signs of laceration (see the discussion of the bleeding esophagus, above). Severe and unrelenting chest and neck pain secondary to chemical and then bacterial mediastinitis, followed by shock and collapse, are the most outstanding symptoms related to perforation. The clinical and radiologic signs of perforation are related to the level of the perforation, and include pleural effusion pneumothorax and pneumomediastinum.

## Diagnosis

The most important clue to the diagnosis of esophageal injury is to suspect it from the history. All patients who swallow foreign bodies that obstruct the esophagus are at risk for laceration and perforation. This is especially true of the infant or young child who swallows small alkaline batteries which lodge for an extended time in the hypopharynx or at the level of the aortic arch. Patients who vomit blood or develop chest or abdominal pain after vomiting are especially suspect. All unconscious patients who have had instrumentation of the pharynx, larynx, or esophagus, cardiopulmonary resuscitation in the field, or instrumentation or cardiopulmonary resuscitation in the emergency department (with the exception of very routine procedures) should be suspected of having esophageal perforation.

Patients with penetrating wounds of the neck or chest and with crushing wounds to the chest must be suspected of having a lacerated or perforated esophagus. In addition, patients who have suspected splenic rupture treated nonoperatively should be observed for a late Boerhaave's rupture, since a predisposing factor to this syndrome is intramural rupture of a short gastric artery that may lead to esophageal intramural hemorrhage.

Patients with chest pain or a history outlined in the previous two paragraphs must have a chest x-ray examination for evidence of a foreign body, perforation, mediastinal fluid, or cardiac and pleural effusions.

If there is radiologic evidence of perforation on posteroanterior and lateral chest x-ray films, a water-soluble contrast study should be done to confirm the diagnosis. Esophagoscopy is only performed if a perforation is suspected but cannot be confirmed by contrast studies, or if there is upper gastrointestinal bleeding associated with a partial-thickness laceration, or if the patient with chest trauma is unconscious and a contrast study cannot be done. Anyone suspected of having a perforation should be given intravenous antibiotics immediately (e.g., cefoxitin and clindamycin), and surgical consultation obtained. Survival is inversely proportional to the length of time between perforation and operative repair.

## BIBLIOGRAPHY

Ach RD: Abdominal pain, in Blacklow RS (ed): *MacBryde's Signs and Symptoms, Applied Pathologic Physiology and Clinical Interpretation,* 6th ed. Philadelphia, Lippincott, 1983, pp 165–179.

Chest pain of undetermined origin: an overview of pathophysiology. *Am J Med* 92(5):25, 1992.

Cotton PB, Williams CB: *Practical Gastrointestinal Endoscopy,* 2d ed. Oxford, Blackwell Scientific, 1982.

Davies HA: Anginal pain of esophageal origin: Clinical presentation, prevalence and prognosis. *Am J Med* 92(5A): 5S 1992.

Fiddian-Green RG, Turcotte JG (eds): Evaluation of the bleeding patient, *and* Variceal bleeding in *Gastrointestinal Hemorrhage.* New York, Grune & Stratton, 1980, pp 3–80 and 233—328.

Han SY, McElvein RB Aldrete JS: Perforation of the esophagus: Correlation of site and cause with plain film findings. *AJR* 145:537, 1985.

Janssens, JP, Vantrappen G: Irritable esophagus. *Am J Med* 92(5A): 27S 1992.

Kim CH, et al: Discriminate value of esophageal symptoms: a study of the initial clinical findings in 499 patients with dysphagia of various causes. *Mayo Clin Proc* 68(10):948 1993.

Shackelford RT: *Surgery of the Alimentary Tract,* vol. 1, 3d ed. Philadelphia, Saunders, 1990.

Temple DM, McNeese MC: Hazards of battery ingestion. *Pediatrics* 71:100, 1983.

Terblanche J, et al: Controversies in the management of bleeding esophageal varices. *N Engl J Med* 320:1393, 1989.

# 75
# SWALLOWED FOREIGN BODIES
## Wade R. Gaasch
## Robert A. Barish

Swallowed foreign bodies, a common presentation in emergency departments, can be innocuous or life-threatening. In the United States, approximately 1500 people die yearly as a result of ingesting foreign bodies. Often thought to be confined to the pediatric population, foreign body ingestion occurs in all age groups. The pediatric age group accounts for approximately 80 percent of all cases, followed by edentulous adults, prisoners, and psychiatric patients. The presence of dentures eliminates the tactile sensitivity of the palatal surface vital to the identification of small items. A correlation exists between age groups and specific types of ingested material. Children most often ingest coins, toys, crayons, and ballpoint pen caps; adults tend to have problems with meat and bones. In addition, psychiatric patients and prison inmates may ingest such unlikely objects as spoons and razor blades.

## PATHOPHYSIOLOGY

Although most objects pass spontaneously, 10 to 20 percent require some intervention, and only 1 percent demand surgical treatment. Ingested foreign bodies may be found anywhere throughout the digestive tract, but there are several physiologic "narrow spaces" where the majority of articles tend to lodge. The pediatric esophagus has five areas of constriction where coins and other objects may become trapped: cricopharyngeal narrowing (C6), the most common site; thoracic inlet (T1); aortic arch (T4); tracheal bifurcation (T6); and hiatal narrowing (T10–11). Most pediatric obstructions occur in the proximal esophagus; the vast majority of adult impactions arise from esophageal disease in the distal esophagus.

Once an object has traversed the pylorus, it usually continues to the rectum and is passed in the stool. If, however, the object has irregular or sharp edges, it may become lodged anywhere in the gastrointestinal tract. Objects that lodge in the esophagus (not necessarily limited to sharp or irregular contour) can result in airway obstruction, stricture, or perforation with resultant mediastinitis, cardiac tamponade, paraesophageal abscess, or aortotracheoesophageal fistula. Perforation may be the result of direct mechanical erosion, as with bones, or chemical corrosion, as with button batteries.

## CLINICAL PRESENTATION

Objects lodged in the esophagus generally produce anxiety and discomfort. Adult patients often complain of retrosternal pain. Patients are likely to retch or vomit and experience dysphagia, resulting in choking, coughing, or aspiration if they attempt to wash down the object. Eventually, patients may be unable to swallow their own secretions. In the adult, the history often provides all the pertinent information necessary for diagnosis and treatment. However, this is often not true in the pediatric population. In the 16-and-under age group, symptoms include refusal to eat, vomiting (with or without hematemesis), gagging, choking, stridor ("pseudoasthma"), neck or throat pain, inability to swallow, increased salivation, and foreign body sensation in the chest.

Physical examination must include careful evaluation of the nasopharynx, oropharynx, neck, and subcutaneous tissues for air resulting from perforation of a hollow viscus. Laryngoscopy, either direct or indirect, should be done, especially when the patient complains of a sticking sensation or has ingested a bone. Although physical signs are not always present, findings consistent with foreign body ingestion in the 16-and-under age group consist of red throat, dysphagia, palatal abrasion, temperature elevation, anxiety and distress, and peritoneal signs.

## EMERGENCY DEPARTMENT MANAGEMENT

### General Care

Because the great majority of ingested foreign bodies traverse the entire gastrointestinal tract without any problems, treatment can be expectant once the object has passed through the pylorus. If, however, a foreign body obstructs the esophagus, prevention of aspiration is paramount. This can be accomplished by inserting a tube above the obstructing body to remove unswallowed fluids above the impaction.

The offending object can be located in several ways. A radiopaque object will be demonstrated on standard x-ray films of the neck or abdomen. If the foreign body is not visible radiographically, the physician must use indirect methods, such as an esophagogram, or direct visualization using fiberoptic endoscopy. If an esophagogram is performed, it cannot be followed by endoscopy because the contrast will prevent visualization of the foreign body. The use of endoscopy may enable the physician to remove the object at the time of visualization, making surgical intervention unnecessary.

Progress of the object through the gastrointestinal tract must be monitored with repeat abdominal x-ray films, usually 2 to 4 h apart. The use of metal detectors, if available, has been advocated as a means of localizing and tracking the progression of metal objects, thereby avoiding repeated radiation exposure. Abdominal examinations should be done frequently to detect early signs of developing

peritonitis should perforation occur. Virtually all symptomatic patients will require observation and esophagoscopy. If a nonfood object becomes lodged in the esophagus or is unable to pass through the pylorus, it must be removed as soon as possible, using esophagogastroscopy. Fatal lead encephalopathy has been reported in a child who ingested a lead curtain weight, which supposedly had been in the stomach for an extended time.

## Food Impaction

Meat impaction may be treated expectantly, providing the patient can manage his or her own secretions. Time and sedation will often allow the meat to pass into the stomach, but the bolus should not be allowed to remain impacted longer than 12 h. Endoscopy is the preferred method for removal. Alternatives have been suggested if endoscopy is not available.

The use of proteolytic enzymes, such as an aqueous solution of papain (e.g., Adolph's meat tenderizer), to dissolve a meat bolus has been advocated by some. This therapy is *not* recommended, however, because of the number of reported complications and because of increasing availability of and expertise in endoscopy. Several reports in the literature have described esophageal perforation secondary to the enzymatic action of the solution. Mucosal ischemia resulting from distention of the esophageal wall renders the esophagus more susceptible to enzymatic degradation. Hemorrhagic pulmonary edema has also been reported following aspiration of Adolph's meat tenderizer.

Intravenous administration of glucagon to relax esophageal smooth muscle has also been suggested as a method of treating food impaction. A test dose should be given to ensure that hypersensitivity does not exist; then the recommended dose is 1 mg. If the food bolus is not passed in 20 min, an additional 2 mg is given intravenously. An esophagogram must be performed following treatment to ensure passage.

Bell reports the successful use of nifedipine, which reduces lower esophageal sphincter pressure and the amplitude of the sphincter contractions, without changing the amplitude of contractions in the body of esophagus. By this mechanism, a bolus of food lodged in the vicinity of the gastroesophageal junction may pass. The recommended dose is 10 mg administered sublingually. Sublingual nitroglycerin has also been used successfully, but could cause hypotension.

Some authors suggest that gas-forming agents (E-Z gas) should be ingested by patients with esophageal food impactions, causing the bolus to be either forced into the stomach or regurgitated into the oropharynx, where it can easily be retrieved. Because 97 percent of adults presenting with meat impaction harbor pathologic esophageal conditions, barium swallow must be performed to confirm foreign body clearance and evaluate possible underlying disease.

## Coin Ingestion

As many as 35 percent of children with a coin lodged in their esophagus will be asymptomatic; therefore, some authors recommend that radiographs be performed on *all* children suspected of swallowing coins to determine the presence and location of the object. Coins in the esophagus lie in the frontal plane with the flat side visible on an anteroposterior radiograph; coins in the trachea lie in the sagittal plane.

The use of a Foley catheter, initially reported in the late 1960s, has been promoted as a safe and effective technique for removal when the coin has been impacted for less than 24 h. The catheter is passed down the esophagus beyond the object and the balloon inflated. As the catheter is slowly withdrawn, the object is withdrawn along with it. Retrieval of a coin by this technique is less effective after 24 h. Most clinicians prefer using the Foley catheter under fluoroscopy. Foley catheter retrieval of foreign bodies may be complicated by aspiration, and personnel and equipment for airway control must be immediately available. If endoscopic expertise is readily available, Foley catheterization retrieval should be a secondary option.

## Button Battery Ingestion

A button battery lodged in the esophagus is a true emergency because of the extremely rapid action of the alkaline substance on the mucosa. Burns to the esophagus have been reported to occur in as little as 4 h, with perforation as soon as 6 h after ingestion. Button batteries in the esophagus require emergency removal if significant morbidity is to be averted. Outcome does not appear to be affected by battery discharge state but is affected by chemical composition. Lithium cells are associated disproportionately with adverse outcome. Mercuric oxide cells tend to fragment more frequently than other cells; however, the threat of heavy metal poisoning has not been supported by the literature or clinical experience. This fact notwithstanding, blood and urine mercury levels should be measured whenever a mercury-containing cell is observed to have split while in the gastrointestinal tract.

Button ingestion can be managed along two main pathways (Fig. 75-1). If the button battery is lodged in the esophagus, its location should be documented by radiograph, then emergent endoscopic removal is mandatory. Given the widespread expertise with endoscopy, we cannot recommend alternative techniques, many of which are associated with significant complications. It should go without saying that ipecac has no place in the management of button battery ingestion. Button batteries that have passed the esophagus need not be re-trieved in the asymptomatic patient unless the cell is not passing through the pylorus after 48 h of observation. This is rarely the case unless the battery is of large diameter and the patient is under 6 y of age. In this case, endoscopic retrieval is again the preferred option. Most batteries pass completely through the body within 48 to 72 h although passage has been reported to take as long as 14 d. All patients with signs and symptoms of gastrointestinal tract injury require immediate surgical consultation. Assistance with cell identification may be obtained by calling the National Button Battery Ingestion Hotline at 202-625-3333.

## Ingestion of Sharp Objects

Management of ingested sharp and pointed foreign bodies is controversial. Objects longer than 5 cm and wider than 2 cm will rarely pass the stomach. Objects of that size and those with extremely pointed edges, such as open safety pins or razor blades, must be removed before they pass from the stomach, because 15 to 35 percent will cause intestinal perforation, usually in the ileocecal valve.

Paul and Jaffe recommend the following management for children who have swallowed sharp objects. All patients should have an initial radiograph and physical examination. If the patient is symptomatic or has ingested a sewing needle, surgical consultation for possible endoscopy and laparotomy is indicated. Children who have swallowed a sharp object (other than sewing needles) yet are asymptomatic can be managed on an expectant basis. Progression of the sharp object should be documented with serial radiographs. If progression past the stomach is not seen, a water-soluble contrast film may document gastrointestinal perforation. At the first sign of perforation, the object should be removed even if the patient remains asymptomatic. If the object does not progress through the gastrointestinal tract, surgical retrieval is indicated.

## Cocaine Ingestion

Cocaine ingestion is an increasingly widespread problem. Carriers will ingest multiple small packets of cocaine in attempts to conceal the drug. A favored packet is the condom, which may hold up to 5 g cocaine. Rupture of even one such packet may be fatal. Webb recommends surgery as the safest method of recovery to avoid the likelihood of packet rupture during endoscopic retrieval. If the packet appears to be passing intact through the intestinal tract, the clinician may choose to observe the patient and wait for the packet to be delivered spontaneously through the rectum.

## SUMMARY

Most patients who have ingested foreign bodies require nothing more than observation. Clear exceptions to this are nonfood items lodged in the esophagus and sharp or pointed items that have not yet passed the pylorus. Sharp or pointed foreign bodies that have passed the pylorus presents an ongoing risk of perforation or obstruction and mandate endoscopic or surgical consultation.

Endoscopy remains the most effective nonsurgical interventional method of foreign body management. There are three indications for surgical removal of a foreign body: (1) gastrointestinal obstruction or perforation, (2) the existence of toxic constituents, and (3) a length, size, and shape that will likely prevent the object from passing safely. Management of asymptomatic patients with prolonged passage should be approached on an individual basis.

Following removal of a foreign body from the esophagus, the patient should have a complete evaluation of esophageal function to ensure that underlying pathology did not lead to the obstruction.

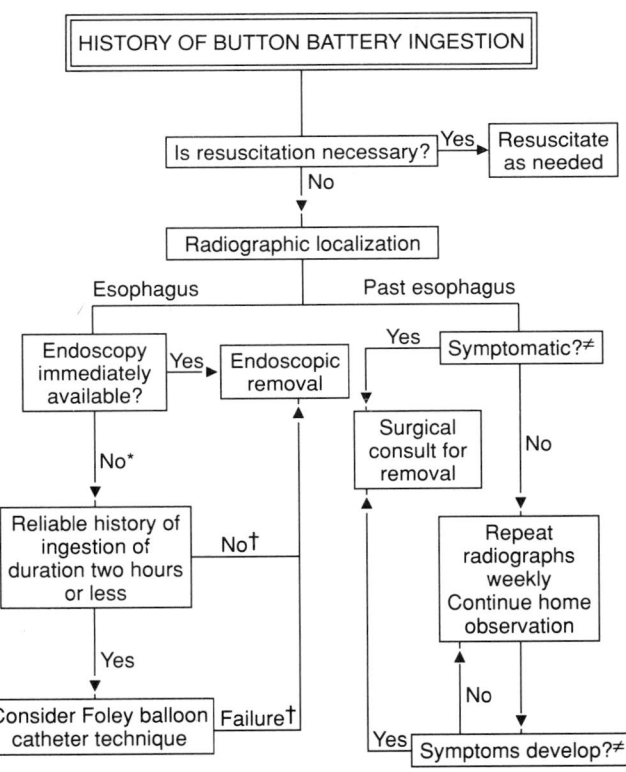

* Button batteries in the esophagus must be removed. Endoscopy should be used if available. The balloon catheter technique can be used if the ingestion is less than 2 h old, but should not be used after this because it may increase the amount of damage to the weakened esophagus.

† When the Foley technique fails or is contraindicated due to a greater than 2 h elapsed time period, the button battery should be removed endoscopically. This may require transfer of the patient.

‡ Acute abdomen, tarry or bloody stools, fever, persistent vomiting

**Fig. 75-1.** Algorithm for management of button battery ingestion. (*Adapted from* Kuhns DW, Dire DJ. Button battery ingestions. *Ann Emerg Med* 18:293, 1989.)

## BIBLIOGRAPHY

Bell AF, Eibling DE: Nifedipine in the treatment of distal esophageal food impaction. *Arch Otolaryngol Head Neck Surg* 114:682, 1988.

Binder L, Anderson WA. Pediatric gastrointestinal foreign body ingestions. *Ann Emerg Med* 13:112, 1984.

Blair SR, Graeber GM, Cruzzavala JL, et al. Current management of esophageal impactions. *Chest* 104:1205, 1993.

Caravati EM, Bennett DL, McElwee NE. Pediatric coin ingestion: a prospective study on the utility of routine roentgenograms. *Am J Dis Child* 143:549, 1989.

Litovitz T, Schmitz BF. Ingestion of cylindrical and button batteries: an analysis of 2382 cases. *Pediatrics* 89:727, 1992.

Paul RI, Jaffe DM. Sharp object ingestions in children: illustrative case and literature review. *Pediatr Emerg Care* 4:245, 1988.

Webb WA. Management of foreign bodies of the upper gastrointestinal tract. *Gastroenterology* 94:204, 1988.

# 76
# PEPTIC ULCER DISEASE
## John T. Sessions

## DEFINITION AND SELECTED ETIOLOGIC CONSIDERATIONS

Peptic ulcers are mucosal defects that develop principally in parts of the upper gastrointestinal tract bathed by acid-peptic secretions. While hospitalization for peptic ulcer is decreasing, the diagnosis must be considered in patients presenting with abdominal pain, vomiting, and/or gastrointestinal bleeding. Differences in age and sex incidences have diminished, perhaps related to increased use of cigarettes and alcohol among women and use of nonsteroidal anti-inflammatory drugs (NSAIDs) in the aging population. Infection with *Helicobacter pylori,* recently recognized as an important etiologic factor in peptic ulcer, is increased in lower socioeconomic groups and the elderly.

Peptic ulcer develops when there is an unfavorable balance between (1) factors that are protective and regenerative for gastroduodenal epithelium and (2) factors that are destructive. Included in the former are mucus and bicarbonate secretion by gastric mucosa and the pancreas, prostaglandins, and poorly understood factors of cellular regeneration and migration or restitution. Destructive factors include increased HCl secretion by an enlarged parietal cell mass (genetic, gastrinoma, partial pyloric obstruction), inflammation due to *H. pylori,* and prostaglandin depletion by NSAIDs. At present, the factors responsible for an increased frequency of peptic ulcer in patients with chronic pulmonary diseases, hepatic cirrhosis, and renal failure or transplantation are incompletely understood.

## CLINICAL FEATURES

The classic history of patients with peptic ulcer is burning epigastric pain, occurring 1 to 3 h after meals. Radiation of pain to the back occurs with more severe pain or with an associated pancreatitis. Pain may wake the patient during the night as a consequence of the circadian rhythm of gastric acid secretion and there being no food in the stomach to dilute and buffer gastric acid. Relief of the pain with taking antacids or vomiting is more reliable diagnostically than relief with eating. A pattern of daily pain for a few weeks interspersed with asymptomatic intervals of weeks or months suggests peptic ulcer as opposed to gastroesophageal reflux disease, biliary colic, the irritable bowel syndrome, or pancreatitis. Pain is a less frequent feature in elderly patients with peptic ulcer and in those associated with NSAID usage. A family history of peptic ulcer disease may reflect genetic predisposition of the disease and/or a life-style conducive to the disease, e.g., habitual excessive use of tobacco, alcohol, NSAIDs. A life-style or socioeconomic status that increases exposure to contaminated food and/or water may increase the patient's risk of chronic *H. pylori* infection of gastroduodenal mucosa and peptic ulceration.

## DIAGNOSIS AND DIFFERENTIAL DIAGNOSIS

Physical examination of a patient with mild to moderately severe peptic ulcer may well reveal only epigastric tenderness. A gastric succussion splash coupled with a history of vomiting points to delayed gastric emptying from pyloric stenosis. Physical and laboratory findings of arthritis, chronic pulmonary disease, cirrhosis, and perhaps renal insufficiency increase the likelihood of peptic ulcer disease.

Laboratory evaluation of patients seen in an emergency department setting should include a complete blood count, serum creatinine, serum calcium, and, when there has been gastrointestinal bleeding, liver chemistries and blood clotting studies. Serologic study to detect *H. pylori* infection and a serum gastrin for gastrinoma are appropriate in recurrent or severe peptic ulcer disease. Barium contrast x-ray studies (upper GI series) are effective and the preferred approach to establish a diagnosis of peptic ulcer in the patient without evidence of gastrointestinal bleeding.

## EMERGENCY DEPARTMENT CARE

The nature of this care will depend upon the manner of the patient's presentation, i.e., the certainty of diagnosis, the severity of the disease, and the nature of any complications such as bleeding, perforation, or pyloric obstruction. The pain of an uncomplicated peptic ulcer should be promptly and readily controlled with a liquid antacid (aluminum hydroxide gel, 30 to 60 mL PO hourly) and an antisecretory drug ($H_2$ receptor antagonist). A need for analgesic drugs for more than 24 h should arouse concern as to the presence of an ulcer complication or the correctness of the diagnosis. In the absence of an ulcer complication, or an extraordinary limitation in self care, outpatient care is appropriate. Patients should be given detailed written instructions including dietary strictures (no caffeine-containing beverages, e.g., coffee, tea, or most colas) and no alcoholic beverages or NSAIDs. If there is a history of frequent vomiting, weight loss, or a gastric succussion splash on physical examination, nasogastric aspiration will detect significant gastric retention. Anticholinergic drugs are not commonly used and are contraindicated in the presence of gastric or urinary retention. $H_2$ receptor antagonists (cimetidine, ranitidine, famotidine, nizatidine) are usually extremely effective in controlling ulcer pain and accelerating healing. Ulcers resistant to this treatment often respond to omeprazole, an inhibitor of parietal cell $H^+,K^+$-ATPase, the proton pump responsible for acid secretion. At present sucralfate and misoprostol are secondary drugs for treating peptic ulcer. The role of *H. pylori* in causing or perpetuating peptic ulcer is being studied intensively, and treatment regimens assessed. This problem, while important, may not be germane at present to emergency department care.

## ADMISSION INDICATIONS

Complications of peptic ulcer require special attention in the emergency department, often involving coordination of multiple hospital services and admission.

### Hemorrhage

Although most patients with bleeding ulcers present with melena, hematemesis, or both, about 5 percent present with hematochezia.

**Fig. 76-1.** Algorithm for the treatment of patients with bleeding peptic ulcers. ICU denotes intensive care unit. (From Laine and Peterson, p. 721, with permission.)

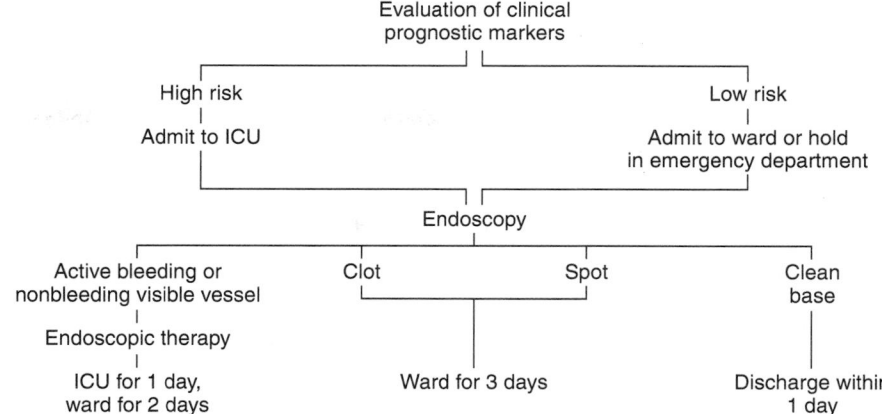

Peptic ulcer is responsible for about half of hospital admissions for upper gastrointestinal hemorrhage and requires expert, coordinated care in the emergency department by physicians, surgeons, and nurses. Factors associated with high risk from bleeding are hemodynamic instability, repeated bouts of hematemesis or hematochezia, failure to clear with gastric lavage, age over 60 years, and associated disorders of the circulatory, pulmonary, and renal systems. Prompt, adequate restoration of intravascular volume and oxygen-carrying capacity by infusion of saline and whole blood is of prime importance. Such patients should be admitted to the intensive care unit. Most rebleeding occurs within 3 days of the initial episode (Fig. 76-1). One or more large-bore intravenous lines must be established promptly, a central venous catheter being helpful for regulation of blood pressure in patients with known cerebral and cardiovascular/renal disease. The stomach should be lavaged with tap water at room temperature since iced saline or water does not improve hemostasis. Most patients should undergo endoscopy as soon as is safely possible. Early inspection of the bleeding site by fiberoptic endoscopy often improves the outcome through injection or heat coagulation of a bleeding or exposed vessel. Ulcers larger than 1 or 2 cm are prone to rebleed, even after hemostatic therapy. Finding a clean ulcer base or a red spot favor hospital discharge after 1 to 3 days and is associated with a less than 5 percent chance of rebleeding. Testing of endoscopic mucosal biopsies for urease activity (CLO test) will determine the need for medical treatment of *H. pylori*. Suppression of gastric acid secretion by oral or intravenous administration of $H_2$ receptor antagonists is usually appropriate.

## Perforation

The incidence of this complication of peptic ulcer is less than that for bleeding but more common than gastric outlet obstruction. Perforation occurs most commonly on the anterior surface of the duodenum and pylorus or the lesser curvature of the stomach. Spillage of acid contents usually causes the abrupt onset of severe pain over the upper abdomen. Subdiaphragmatic air on upright x-rays of the chest and abdomen is diagnostic. Free peritoneal air is not evident in all patients, and a perforating peptic ulcer should be considered when shock develops without an apparent cause in the elderly. If not treated aggressively, the chemical peritonitis soon becomes a bacterial one. To detect perforation, a nasogastric tube is inserted, at least 250 mL of air is insufflated, and the tube is clamped. Upright or decubitus x-rays will then demonstrate "free" air.

Treatment involves continuous nasogastric suction, prompt correction of fluid and electrolyte abnormalities, and parenteral administration of appropriate, broad-spectrum antibiotics. Timely surgical correction of the perforation continues to be the rational choice. A nonoperative approach appeared equally effective in patients under 40 years of age in a randomized trial comparing nonoperative treatment to emergency surgery.

## Pyloric Stenosis

This complication of peptic ulcer is decreasing, estimated at 1 to 2 percent of all peptic ulcer patients. Vomiting is the most frequent symptom (90 percent), followed by abdominal pain, weight loss, early satiety, and nausea. Supporting physical findings are evidences of weight loss and dehydration. An abdominal succussion splash, present in at least a fourth of the patients, is diagnostic but is confirmed by aspiration with a nasogastric tube. Hospitalization usually is necessary for correction of fluid and electrolyte abnormalities and to decompress the dilated stomach. Surgical treatment is indicated for persistent or recurrent obstruction. Use of anticholinergic drugs is contraindicated.

## BIBLIOGRAPHY

Crofts TJ, Park KGM, Steele RJ, et al: A randomized trial of nonoperative treatment for perforated ulcer. *N Engl J Med* 320:970, 1989.

Graham DY: Ulcer complication and their non-operative treatment, in Sleisenger M, Fordtran J (eds): *Gastrointestinal Disease; Pathophysiology/Diagnosis/Management,* 5th Ed. Philadelphia, Saunders, 1993, pp 698–712.

Hentschel E, Branstatter G, Dragosics B, et al: Effect of ranitidine and amoxycillin plus metronidazole on eradication of *Helicobacter pylori* and the recurrence of duodenal ulcer. *N Engl J Med* 328:308, 1993.

Laine L, Peterson WL: Bleeding peptic ulcer. *N Engl J Med* 331:717, 1994.

Peterson WL, Laine L: Bleeding peptic ulcer. Medical progress. *N Engl J Med* 331:717, 1994.

Sol AH: Gastric, duodenal and stress ulcers, in Sleisenger M, Fordtran J (eds): *Gastrointestinal Disease; Pathophysiology/Diagnosis/Management,* 5th ed. Philadelphia, Saunders, 1993, pp 580–679.

# 77

# PERFORATED VISCUS
## W. Kendall McNabney

## INTRODUCTION

In most cases, perforated viscus leads to such a profound set of symptoms and clear physical findings that recognition and subsequent treatment are straightforward when the patient presents for care. However, there are variables which contribute to a more subtle presentation either because of altered host response to inflammation or because the perforation may be walled off or does not involve the free peritoneum.

Nontraumatic perforation of the gastrointestinal (GI) tract is rare if the wall of the viscus is normal. Diligent search will reveal an etiologic factor either involving the wall or leading to rapid, marked increase in intraluminal pressures secondary to distal obstruction. The underlying process may be inflammatory, neoplastic, iatrogenic, or the result of stone formation. The presence of a self-ingested foreign body must be considered if no other obvious cause is present. Whatever organ is involved, the signs and symptoms of perforation are due first to chemical irritation of the peritoneum and then to infection or sepsis. Therefore, the chemical composition of the contents of the viscus has a significant effect on the development of chemical peritonitis, including the onset and severity.

Patients receiving glucocorticoids do not demonstrate the classic signs of perforation. Because symptoms and signs are minimal, such patients have a significant delay in treatment, and mortality approaches 80 percent. Other immunocompromised patients, such as those receiving chemotherapy, AIDS patients, and patients who have received allografts, are subject to both increased risk of perforated viscus as well as delayed recognition.

Sometimes the signs and symptoms of perforation are the first evidence of underlying disease. At other times, there is a symptomatic period relating to the disease process before signs or symptoms of perforation appear. Although most perforations of the GI tract are free into the peritoneum, they may be localized, walled off by the surrounding viscera or omentum, or occur into a limited or restricted space, such as the lesser sac. Perforations may also occur into the retroperitoneal space. Symptoms and signs, then, are generally determined by (1) the viscus involved, (2) the location of the perforation, (3) the volume and chemical composition of the leaking fluids, (4) the underlying disease, and (5) the host response mechanism.

Unless the patient has some significant contraindication, surgical intervention is indicated at the time of diagnosis. Ideally, intervention should occur before any significant contamination or sepsis has occurred, since the amount of contamination is a significant factor in survival. Emergency treatment in all suspected perforations includes (1) nasogastric suction, (2) volume replacement, (3) antibiotics consistent with local protocols, and (4) rapid surgical consultation. Use of analgesia prior to surgical consultation must be guided by the need to provide relief without masking signs or symptoms. Short-acting narcotics, such as fentanyl, are sometimes used for this purpose.

## PATHOPHYSIOLOGY

Secondary peritonitis is peritoneal infection due to perforation of a hollow viscus. The combined surface area of the peritoneum (visceral and parietal) constitutes about 50 percent of the area of the exterior body surface. Contact of intestinal contents with the peritoneum produces a sudden increase in capillary permeability, with the subsequent exudation of large volumes of plasma into the peritoneal cavity, the bowel lumen, and the bowel wall and mesentery. As much as 4 to 12 L can be shifted into this "third space" within 24 h.

Inflammation of the visceral peritoneum produces a brief period of bowel irritability and hypermotility followed by bowel atony with paralytic (adynamic) ileus and distension. The inflamed bowel no longer absorbs fluid and secretes increased salt and water into the lumen. When distension becomes sufficient to compress capillaries and prevent or compromise circulation to the inflamed area, exudation ceases. The ultimate clinical picture is one of severe hypovolemia and shock.

Fluid loss into this third space causes hypovolemia. Hypovolemia, in turn, results in inadequate cardiac output, compensatory vasoconstriction, and inadequate tissue perfusion. Oliguria, severe metabolic acidosis, and respiratory insufficiency follow if hypovolemia is not rapidly corrected. Peritonitis and septicemia may evolve into septic shock. Correction of hypovolemia is therefore mandatory.

The local response to bacterial invasion from intestinal perforation is complex. Walled off abscess formation is associated with lower mortality than generalized infection throughout the peritoneum. Bacterial contamination is generally necessary to produce fatal peritonitis. Endotoxins and exotoxins increase cell permeability and compound the already significant fluid losses into the third space.

Distal obstruction, the amount of contamination, the elapsed time prior to the institution of treatment, and the host response to infection account for the variations in the clinical response to perforation.

Sepsis and multiple organ failure still occur despite improved critical care, antibiotics, and surgical intervention.

## Perforated Ulcer

Gastric or duodenal perforations develop more commonly in benign than in malignant ulcers, although malignant gastric ulcers may also perforate. Chemical peritonitis develops in the first 6 to 8 h and is due to the effect of the gastric acid and pepsin on the peritoneum.

In general, posterior duodenal ulcers penetrate into the pancreas, rather than freely perforating into the peritoneum, and produce pancreatitis. Free perforation is prevented because of the adherence of the pancreas to the posterior duodenum. Posterior gastric or duodenal ulcers may perforate into the lesser sac, resulting in abscess formation, but this is relatively rare. Anterior ulcers generally perforate into the peritoneal cavity, although the omentum or adjacent structures such as liver or gallbladder may be adherent to the ulcer bed and limit signs and symptoms. An antecedent history of ulcer disease is not always present, and perforation may be the first manifestation. If carefully sought, though, a history of antacid use, mostly of over-the-counter preparations, will usually be found.

The pain of ulcer perforation is usually sudden and severe. The patient may even be able to give the exact time of onset. The pain is usually localized to the epigastric region, although if penetrating or posterior, it may radiate straight through to the back (not around to the back).

Significant upper GI bleeding does not accompany perforation. Whatever bleeding occurs is minimal. Chronic blood loss may occur if the ulcer has been present for a time. As a rule of thumb, massive upper GI bleeding rules out the presence of a perforated ulcer; however, a second penetrating ulcer should be considered.

## Gallbladder Perforation

Perforation of the gallbladder is associated with a high mortality, although it has decreased from 20 to 7 percent in the past 30 years. Early surgical intervention improves mortality. The highest mortalities are associated with nonoperative management. Peritonitis is the result of chemical irritation of the peritoneum as well as bacterial contamination.

Because sterile bile may cause only well-tolerated ascites, bacteria must be present to produce clinical peritonitis.

Obstruction of the cystic or common bile duct by stones produces distension of the gallbladder with eventual compromise of the vascular supply and gangrene of the wall with perforation. The stones can erode through the wall of the gallbladder, cystic duct, or common duct. Such erosions more commonly produce fistulas between the gallbladder and another portion of the GI tract than free perforation into the peritoneal cavity. Large gallstones have been found to produce obstruction of the small bowel after such fistula formation, resulting in a syndrome known as *gallstone ileus.*

Gangrene can occur in the gallbladder free of stones, and perforations have been reported in acalculous cholecystitis, especially in diabetics. In one study, perforation occurred in the absence of stones in 40 percent of patients. Acalculous cholecystitis most commonly occurs in postoperative, posttrauma, or burn patients secondary to dehydration; with hemolysis from blood transfusions; or with use of narcotics.

Those most at risk are the elderly, the diabetic, and those with a history of stones or repeated cholecystitis. Perforations have also been reported in patients with sickle cell disease or hemolytic anemias. Infection is often associated with cystic or common bile duct obstruction and stone formation. There is a male predominance of 2 or 3 to 1.

The diagnosis is difficult. Although not always present, antecedent signs and symptoms of biliary disease should be sought. Gallbladder perforation should be suspected in an elderly patient with a tender right upper quadrant mass, fever, and leukocytosis who is deteriorating clinically or who develops signs of peritonitis. The bilirubin level may be elevated, and slight elevation of the amylase level is not unusual. Nonalcoholics may give a past history of episodes of jaundice or pancreatitis, which should suggest the presence of common duct stones. Subhepatic or subphrenic abscesses may form as a result of perforation of the gallbladder. On routine x-ray, a stone may be seen free in the abdomen.

Ultrasonography should be performed in all patients suspected of having stones.

## Perforation of the Small Bowel

Nontraumatic perforations of the mid-GI tract are very uncommon. Jejunal rupture may result from certain drugs such as enteric-coated potassium tablets, which produce ulcerations of the small bowel; infections, such as typhoid or tuberculosis; tumors; strangulated hernia, either internal or external; and, rarely, regional enteritis.

In general, jejunal perforation produces a more severe chemical peritonitis than ileal rupture since the pancreatic juice that leaks out of the upper jejunum has a pH of about 8 and is rich in enzymes such as trypsin, lipase, and amylase. Fluid that leaks from lower jejunal and ileal perforations has less enzymatic activity, and the pH may also be lower. Perforations of the ileum have significant bacterial contamination. If, however, perforation is the result of obstruction, as in appendicitis followed by perforation, the clinical course is likely to be serious regardless of the level of perforation. This is because of the effect of the duration of the obstruction and the underlying inflammatory disease process. Mortality is directly proportional to degree of contamination and delay in diagnosis and treatment.

Perforations of the jejunum and ileum, especially if due to regional enteritis, may become quickly walled off, and signs of generalized peritonitis may be delayed. Free air may be detected on radiologic examination, or air may be seen in a retroperitoneal location or in the wall of the bowel. There is an elevated white blood count and a shift to the left, and the serum amylase level may also be elevated. Metabolic acidosis may be present. Tachycardia and fever are common. The abdomen may be distended. Hypoactive bowel sounds are present. Tenderness, rebound, guarding, and rigidity, usually associated with peritonitis, may all be absent, especially in the elderly. Perforations of the appendix are more likely in the extremes of age and if symptoms are prolonged prior to exploration. In patients who have equivocal physical findings, diagnostic peritoneal lavage has proven safe and accurate.

## Perforation of the Large Bowel

Nontraumatic perforations of the lower GI tract are most commonly the result of diverticulitis, carcinoma, colitis, and foreign bodies. They may result from barium enemas, colonoscopy, and sigmoidoscopy as well. Perforations of the colon produce signs and symptoms predominantly due to sepsis as opposed to chemical irritation, and therefore the abdominal symptoms are more subtle in onset.

Carcinoma of the large bowel detected by a perforation has a higher mortality than carcinoma detected because of obstruction, changes in bowel habits, or bleeding. If there is no obstruction, the more proximal the perforation, the more serious the clinical picture, probably because the fecal stream is more liquid and disseminates rapidly. An antecedent history of partial or complete obstruction,

change in bowel habits, and other findings consistent with carcinoma should be sought.

Perforation secondary to obstruction, as in carcinoma of the colon or acute diverticulitis with abscess formation, may be associated with a temporary amelioration of abdominal pain because the local distension has been relieved, although this is not common. Perforation in diverticulitis is usually the result of abscess formation, so that signs and symptoms of the abscess, and a mass, may predominate. Perforation resulting from carcinoma is the result of erosion of the carcinoma and not rupture of a normal bowel wall. This is quickly followed, however, by evidence of peritonitis, hypovolemia, and sepsis.

## CLINICAL FEATURES OF A PERFORATED VISCUS

The hallmark of perforated viscus is abdominal pain. The severity, location, and suddenness of onset are a reflection of where the perforation has occurred. Patients presenting in the emergency department may be in acute distress and want to stay in a sitting or rocking position. Patients at later stages of peritonitis want to maintain immobility, lying on one side with hips flexed.

Usually vomiting is present and follows the onset of pain. Bile in the vomitus indicates that the pylorus is open and that gastric outlet obstruction is not present. Coffee-ground vomitus may be present in patients with duodenal or gastric ulcer. A feculent drainage from the nasogastric tube, or feculent vomiting, may indicate the presence of a long-standing small bowel obstruction or the presence of dead bowel. Abdominal distension, the inability to pass gas, and constipation are all signs and symptoms of the accompanying ileus or bowel obstruction.

Fever, tachycardia, a narrowed pulse pressure, oliguria, and tachypnea are signs of hypovolemia and sepsis. A fall in blood pressure usually indicates the presence of the full-blown shock state. Aggressive fluid therapy should occur before shock develops, while the patient's vital signs, including urinary output, are monitored. Fluid correction and aggressive treatment of sepsis are a part of the resuscitation process in the emergency department, but often resuscitation cannot be completed until surgical intervention has occurred.

Marked tenderness is frequently detected on abdominal examination, usually accompanied by percussion tenderness over the area of inflammation. Rigidity is also present if generalized peritonitis has developed. Pain is aggravated by any motion of the patient, including sneezing and coughing. The patient frequently lies with hips flexed to reduce the pain by minimizing the tension in the peritoneum.

Considerable effort should be made to obtain an accurate physical examination in patients already in distress. Use of percussion tenderness as opposed to rebound tenderness gives the examiner the same indication of peritonitis but without the patient discomfort. Gentle palpation with warm hands while the patient is in a comfortable position will help measure objectivity of changes detected by repeated examinations. Bowel sounds are absent if adynamic ileus has developed as a result of the inflammation. If early obstruction is present, the bowel sounds may be hyperactive, with rushes. When the obstruction is long-standing, the bowel sounds disappear. If free air has accumulated, there may be a loss of liver dullness to percussion. Subcutaneous emphysema of the lower abdominal wall or thighs may result from perforation of the colon or rectum. The intraluminal gas spreads along neurovascular bundles and other planes to reach the subcutaneous tissues.

When a great deal of fluid is present in the peritoneum, shifting dullness may be found. Rectal and pelvic examinations are essential to determine if any pelvic or lower abdominal masses are present, or if tenderness can be elicited.

Laboratory studies may be of little help. Leukocytosis with a shift to the left is common. The blood urea nitrogen (BUN) level may be elevated if the degree of dehydration is significant. Electrolyte imbalance is frequent. Respiratory alkalosis is present early on in sepsis.

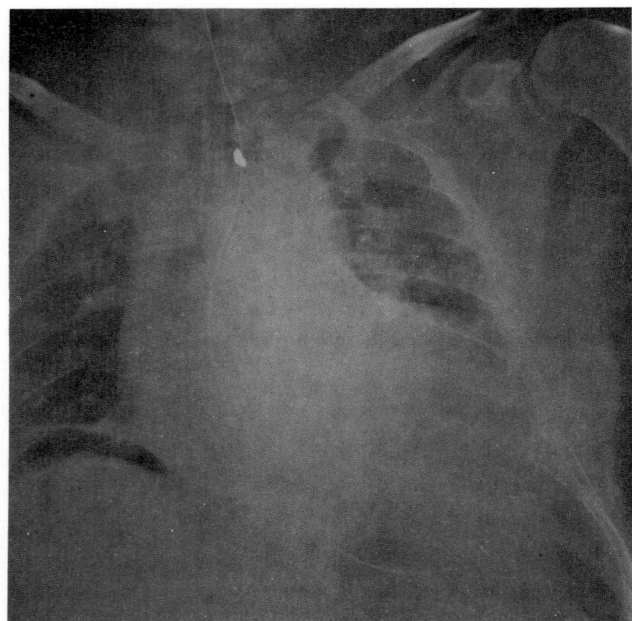

**Fig. 77-1.** Perforated viscus as shown in upright chest film. (Courtesy of Detroit General Hospital.)

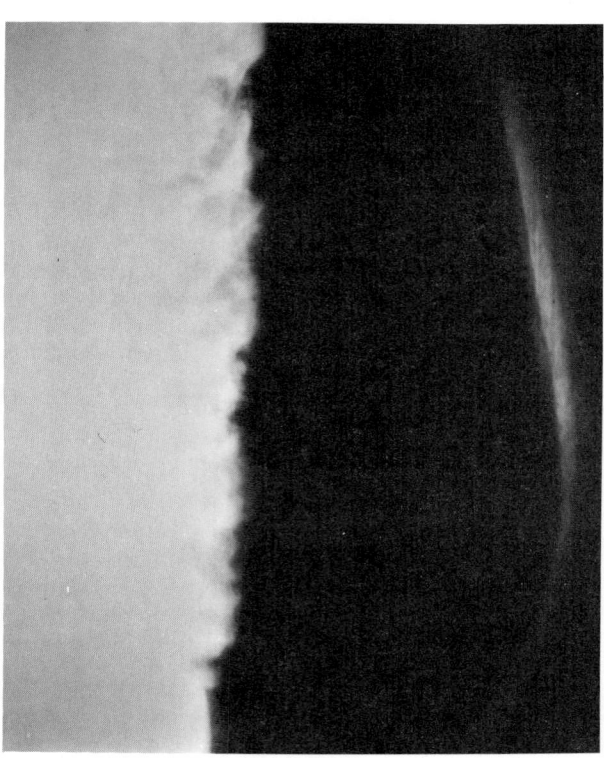

**Fig. 77-2.** Perforated viscus as shown in cross-table lateral film of abdomen. (Courtesy of Detroit General Hospital.)

Metabolic acidosis follows if the hypovolemia and sepsis are uncorrected. A mild elevation of the amylase level does not necessarily reflect pancreatitis since such elevations frequently accompany perforation, especially of the small bowel.

The elderly senile patient with multiple chronic complaints, vague history, equivocal physical findings, and no confirming laboratory findings is at high risk for delayed diagnosis and treatment. Hoffmann has reported on the utility of diagnostic peritoneal lavage (DPL) in this setting.

The open technique of DPL seems to offer the greatest degree of safety, especially when the patient has distension or has had prior abdominal operations. Lavage technique is identical to post-trauma DPL. If gas, food, bowel content, bile, or turbid or bloody fluid is detected on initial aspiration, lavage need not be done. Pus, bile, or bowel content are most consistent with free perforation. Although proven safe, this relatively simple but invasive diagnostic procedure has not achieved the same acceptable status for nontrauma as it has for abdominal trauma.

An upright chest x-ray is necessary to rule out the presence of thoracic disease and to detect free air under the diaphragm (Fig. 77–1). The leaves of the diaphragm are much more clearly demonstrated on this view. The left lateral decubitus film of the abdomen may also be helpful in detecting free air. In either case, the patient should be left in position for 10 min before obtaining the films.

Abdominal x-rays may show air-fluid levels in a stepladder pattern indicating the presence of mechanical obstruction, or simply dilated loops of bowel indicating adynamic ileus (Fig. 77-2). Air along the biliary tract may be present if a gallstone has eroded into the small or large bowel. Neighboring loops of bowel may be widely separated if the intestinal walls are edematous. Free stones may be seen.

Unquestionably, pneumoperitoneum, when present, expedites the diagnosis and treatment of perforated viscus. Since only 60 to 70 percent of perforated ulcer patients have this finding, one-third of patients with perforated viscus have potential for harmful delay of diagnosis. Most such patients will have clinical findings suggesting the diagnosis, but some will be equivocal. Insufflation of 400 to 500 mL of air into the nasogastric tube (pneumogastrography) and then clamping the tube, followed by an upright chest x-ray has been used

for equivocal cases. In Maull's series, perforated viscus patients who were diagnosed using air insufflation were operated on within 6 h of diagnosis and had an overall mortality of 9.7 percent. Failure to use insufflation led to average operative delays of 27 h and a 28 percent mortality.

The psoas shadows may be obscured by the presence of fluid in the abdomen or in the retroperitoneal space. If there is a distinct lack of gas in the intestine, dead bowel may be present.

Ultrasonography may be necessary to rule out the presence of cystic or common duct stones. CT scanning may also be helpful in identifying perforation and abscess formation by detecting masses in the mesentery or adjacent to organs. While radionuclide hepatobiliary scans can demonstrate gallbladder perforation, they are not universally available.

## TREATMENT

Vigorous fluid resuscitation, as quickly as possible, is mandatory. In general, a balanced electrolyte solution should be used. Central venous pressure (CVP) and hourly urinary output should be monitored, in addition to the pulse and blood pressure, in continuous assessment of the patient's volume status. In the presence of significant blood loss, transfusions are necessary. Nasogastric tube insertion should be done early, even if the diagnosis is only suspected. Broad-spectrum antibiotics are indicated intravenously when the diagnosis of perforation is suspected. The principles of antibiotic therapy of secondary peritonitis currently dictate that agents active against both aerobic or facultative gram-negative bacteria and anaerobes be given intravenously. Local preference, cost, and nephrotoxicity are variables that may affect the choice of several comparable monotherapy or combination therapy regimens. Because timely use of appropriate antibiotic therapy has proven efficacy, it is import to initiate treatment in the emergency department. Antibiotic treatment protocols should be determined in conjunction with the surgeon. Operative intervention is indicated as soon as volume replacement and urine output have been established, unless the risk of surgery exceeds the risk of death from perforation.

## BIBLIOGRAPHY

Ackerman NB, Sillin LF, Suresh K: Consequences of intraperitoneal bile: Bile ascites versus bile peritonitis. *Am J Surg* 149:244, 1985.

Christou NV, Barie PS, Dellinger EP, et al: Surgical Infection Society intraabdominal infection study. *Arch Surg* 128:173, 1993.

Felice PR, Trowbridge PE, Ferrara JJ: Evolving changes in the pathogenesis and treatment of the perforated gallbladder. *Am J Surg* 149:466, 1985.

Hoffmann J: Peritoneal lavage in the diagnosis of the acute abdomen of nontraumatic origin. *Acta Chir Scand* 153:561, 1987.

Koepsell TD, Inui TS, Farewell VT: Factors affecting perforation in acute appendicitis. *Surg Gynecol Obstet* 153:508, 1981.

Larmi TK, Kairaluoma MI, Junila J, et al: Perforation of the gallbladder: A retrospective comparative study of cases from 1946–1956 and 1969–1980. *Acta Chir Scand* 150:557, 1984.

Larson FA, Haller CC, Delcore R, Thomas JH: Diagnostic peritoneal lavage in acute peritonitis. *Am J Surg* 164:449, 1992.

Leijonmarck CE, Raf L: Ulceration of the small intestine due to slow-release potassium chloride tablets. *Acta Chir Scand* 151:273, 1985.

Maull KI, Reath DB: Pneumogastrography in the diagnosis of perforated peptic ulcer. *Am J Surg* 148:340, 1984.

Nadkarni KM, Shetty SD, Kagzi RS, et al: Small bowel perforations: A study of 32 cases. *Arch Surg* 116:53, 1981.

Nylander WA: The acute abdomen in the immunocompromised host. *Surg Clin North Am* 68(2): 457, 1988.

ReMines SG, McIlrath DC: Bowel perforation in steroid-treated patients. *Ann Surg* 192:581, 1980.

Rotstein DD, Meakins JL: Diagnostic and therapeutic challenges of intraabdominal infections. *Word J Surg* 14:159, 1990.

Shands JW: Empiric antibiotic therapy of abdominal sepsis and serious perioperative infections. *Surg Clin North Am* 73(2): 291, 1993.

Sievert W, Vakil NB; Emergencies at the biliary tract. *Gastroenterol Clin North Am* 17(2): 245, 1988.

Silen W: *Cope's Early Diagnosis of the Acute Abdomen,* 18th ed. New York, Oxford, 1991.

Wilson DG, Lieberman LM: Perforation of the gallbladder diagnosed preoperatively. *Eur J Nucl Med* 8:135, 1983.

# 78
# ACUTE APPENDICITIS
## James A. Catto

Appendicitis is a common cause of emergency surgery. Approximately 6 percent of the population will experience appendicitis in their lifetimes. While classically a disease of persons 10 to 30 years of age, it affects all ages. Appendicitis is most difficult to diagnose in the young, the elderly, the pregnant, and those afflicted with other diseases, such as acquired immunodeficiency syndrome or diabetes. However, it may also be difficult to diagnose in other patients, even for the most capable practitioner.

Seventy to eighty percent of appendicitis specimens reveal a nonruptured appendix; 20 to 30 percent are perforated. Of the total group, 1 percent of cases will be associated with delay of presentation, delay of recognition, error in diagnosis, and increased morbidity and mortality.

Mortality is low (0.1 to 0.2 percent) for unruptured appendicitis, but higher (3 to 5 percent) for ruptured appendicitis. There is a direct relationship between the morbidity and mortality rates associated

with acute appendicitis and delay between onset of symptoms and definitive treatment. The more common immediate morbidities include soft tissue wound infection, intraabdominal abscess, ileus, and prolonged hospitalization. Delayed morbidities may include subsequent small bowel adhesive obstruction. In women with perforation and peritonitis, infertility can result.

Other pathologic processes involving the appendix are relatively rare causes of misdiagnosis of appendicitis. They include Crohn's disease of the appendix, diverticulitis of the appendix, pinworms, inspissated barium, foreign bodies, neoplastic diseases, and mechanical complications such as intussusception and torsion. Disease entities afflicting adjacent organs are a more frequent cause of misdiagnosis. Mesenteric lymphadenitis, pelvic inflammatory disease, mittelschmerz, acute gastroenteritis, and Crohn's disease are the most common of the multitude of conditions which simulate appendicitis. Despite the newer diagnostic tests available to the clinician, no single evaluation can substitute for the diagnostic accuracy of the experienced physician.

A complete knowledge of the development of the appendix and embryologic rotation of the colon (or incomplete rotation) is essential to develop an awareness that the appendix may be anywhere within the peritoneal cavity. A healthy skepticism regarding the location of the appendix is essential to diagnosing the atypical presentations of appendicitis as seen in situs inversus viscerum, malrotation, hypermobile cecum, and the extremely long pelvic appendix.

The fact that the occurrence of appendicitis parallels the development of lymphoid tissues within the gastrointestinal tract has given rise to theories that appendicitis is caused by luminal obstruction secondary to lymphoid hyperplasia. Such theories gain credence from the fact that appendicitis often follows a flulike syndrome, an upper respiratory infection, mononucleosis, measles, bacterial enterocolitis, or some other inflammatory illness which produces generalized lymphoid hyperplasia. Other causes of luminal obstruction known to be associated with appendicitis include fecaliths, inspissated barium, seeds, pinworms, strictures, and carcinoma. Some patients present with recurrent bouts of a nonobstructive variant of appendicitis. This condition, while uncommon, is known to most clinicians.

## CLINICAL PRESENTATION

The classic presentation of (1) anorexia, (2) periumbilical pain associated with nausea or modest emesis, and (3) the development of steady pain in the right lower quadrant developing over a 24-h period is present in approximately 60 percent of cases. Anorexia and pain are the more frequent symptoms. Nausea, modest emesis, and/or diarrhea are usually described. Localized tenderness within the abdomen or pelvis is usually present. Rebound tenderness supports a diagnosis that appendicitis or some significant intraperitoneal disease is present, but need not be obvious. Rebound is muted in the obese and the elderly.

Less common is a severe, crampy, colicky presentation associated with acute appendiceal luminal obstruction secondary to a fecalith. Recurrent diarrhea associated with the pelvic location of the inflamed appendix is often misdiagnosed as acute gastroenteritis. A rectal exam may clarify the issue when localizing pain is demonstrated within the pelvis.

A high index of suspicion that all abdominal pain presentations may reflect an atypical appendicitis is necessary in evaluating the acute abdomen. Rectal and pelvic exams are essential and may demonstrate localizing tenderness within the pelvis. The results of one study of the symptoms of 53 patients over 40 years of age are listed in Table 78-1. In another study of 305 patients with appendicitis, another order of signs, symptoms, and laboratory findings, based on predicted value, was determined (Table 78-2). Other physical signs associated with appendicitis have been described. Left lower quadrant abdominal palpation may produce pain in the right lower

**Table 78-1.** Symptoms in Acute Appendicitis in Patients Over 40

| Symptom | No. | % |
| --- | --- | --- |
| Right lower quadrant (RLQ) pain | 31 | 58 |
| Nausea | 26 | 49 |
| Vomiting | 24 | 45 |
| Anorexia | 19 | 36 |
| Crampy abdominal pain | 10 | 18 |
| General pain—RLQ | 9 | 17 |
| Umbilical pain—RLQ | 6 | 11 |
| Diarrhea | 6 | 11 |
| Constipation | 5 | 9 |
| Fever | 3 | 6 |

*Source:* Adapted from Stair T, Corlette MB: Appendicitis over forty. *Ann Emerg Med* 9:77, 1980.

quadrant; this is known as Rovsing's sign. Cutaneous hyperesthesia in T10, T11, and T12 dermatomes may be present. The psoas sign is characterized by right lower quadrant pain on thigh extension while lying in the left lateral decubitus position. Internal rotation of the flexed right thigh, while supine, may produce right lower quadrant pain and is known as the obturator sign. These signs are often helpful when dealing with inflamed appendices in a more posterior position.

Appendicitis in the young taxes a physician's clinical skills in obtaining a reliable history and conducting comprehensive examination. In the less than 2 year age group, appendicitis is associated with a high degree of perforation and associated mortality. The diagnosis is evasive and must be suspected even in the absence of the classic presentation of adulthood. Irritability, emesis, and distension, while commonly present, are not very specific. The clinical presentation in young children tends to parallel that in adults. However, in children the incidence of mesenteric adenitis and acute gastroenteritis is higher than in adults.

Appendicitis in the elderly is associated with an even higher percentage of rupture than that seen in childhood, and leukocytosis is less pronounced. Diagnosis is difficult, and delay from admission to surgery tends to be longer than in other age groups.

Appendicitis occurs frequently during pregnancy (1 per 2200 pregnancies). It is associated with pain at a higher location than normally seen, but consistent with migration of the cecum from the right lower quadrant to the subcostal position during the evolution of the pregnancy. Perforating appendicitis during pregnancy carries an increased risk to the fetus and mother from septic complications. Appendectomy for nonruptured appendicitis during pregnancy seems to be well tolerated. However, the failure to identify intraabdominal pathology at appendectomy during pregnancy seems to be associated with an increased risk of abortion as the clinical presentation usually reflects some undiagnosed complication of the pregnancy.

## LABORATORY EVALUATION

In 86 percent of appendicitis cases, an elevated leukocyte count is present, and in 89 percent, an elevated absolute neutrophil count is present. In 11 percent of appendicitis cases, there will exist a normal absolute neutrophil and leukocyte count. The magnitude of leukocy-

**Table 78-2.** Predictive Factors in the Diagnosis of Appendicitis

Localized tenderness—right lower quadrant
Leukocytosis
Migration of pain
Left shift
Temperature elevation
Nausea/vomiting
Anorexia/acetone
Rebound tenderness

*Source:* Adapted from Alvarado A: A practical score for the early diagnosis of acute appendicitis. *Ann Emerg Med* 15:557, 1986.

tosis does not correlate with the histologic severity of the appendicitis. If the inflammatory process lies close to the ureter, urinalysis will often reveal microscopic hematuria.

## Radiography

Plain abdominal radiologic investigation of the abdomen thought to possess appendicitis has neither the sensitivity nor the specificity to make it a useful test. While a fecalith of the appendix, gas in the appendix, or an air fluid level in the distal small bowel may suggest appendicitis, these signs are frequently absent.

Barium enema may be useful when the results are considered along with the rest of the clinical evaluation, but is not needed if the diagnosis is already reasonably certain. Use of the test is based on the premise that the lumen of the appendix is obstructed in appendicitis. While this is usually the case, it is not necessarily true. Barium enema is available in most hospitals, is safe, and does not require special radiologic equipment or personnel. In addition, results can be interpreted by the clinician. Nonfilling of the appendix associated with spasm, thickening, or cecal indentation is suggestive, but not pathognomonic, of appendicitis. Simple nonfilling of the appendix may reflect appendicitis or luminal fibrous obliteration seen with advancing age. Visualization of the appendix with a gas collection at the tip, loculated extraluminal gas in an abscess, extravasation of barium into an abscess, or a sharp cutoff sign in a shortened appendix suggests appendicitis. Visualization of a "normal" appendix suggests the absence of appendicitis but does not exclude it. Furthermore, partial filling of the appendix may be misconstrued as complete filling. If barium enema demonstrates an abnormal location of the appendix, such as a cecum beneath the liver (incomplete rotation of the colon) or deep within the pelvis, atypical presentations of appendicitis are more likely. Diseases often confused with appendicitis, such as terminal ileitis, diverticulitis, and neoplasia of the colon, may be diagnosed by the unprepared barium enema.

## Other Diagnostic Studies

In a few selective studies, ultrasound examination was shown to have a 75 to 90 percent sensitivity and an 86 to 100 percent specificity. Visualization of the appendix as an immobile, tender, noncompressible structure is suggestive of appendicitis. Ultrasound examination is a noninvasive procedure possessing no radiation hazards and can be used in pregnancy. However, it requires special equipment, trained technicians, and physicians skilled in interpretation.

Computed tomography is not effective in detecting early appendicitis but is useful in the differential diagnosis of a right lower quadrant abdominal mass. It can differentiate between appendicitis, appendicitis with perforation and abscess, carcinoma of the cecum or appendix, appendiceal mucocele, or pseudomyxoma peritonei.

Diagnostic laparoscopy is an invasive study requiring special equipment, special surgical skills, and general anesthesia. It is relatively contraindicated in patients with abdominal distention. Visualization of an inflamed appendix is not always diagnostic of appendicitis, and identification of another cause of intraabdominal pathology does not exclude appendicitis. However, studies report high sensitivity and specificity using diagnostic laparoscopy, and the advent of therapeutic endoscopic appendectomy techniques may enhance the use of this approach for diagnosis.

Diagnostic peritoneal tap or peritoneal lavage has been studied in moderation, but has not gained wide popularity. A leukocyte-rich effusion reflects intraabdominal pathology which may include appendicitis, mesenteric adenitis, or pelvic inflammatory disease. A leukocyte-sparse effusion may be found in early appendicitis, late well-established appendicitis with chronic abscess, or early closed-loop intestinal obstructions.

Other diagnostic aids, including clinical scoring systems, computer assisted programs, radioactive isotope imaging, and barium swallow, have been evaluated. No single test exceeds the diagnostic accuracy of the experienced physician, aided when necessary by hospital admission, serial examination of the patient, and, if appropriate, surgical consultation. An experienced surgeon may then choose to utilize ultrasound examination, barium enema, or diagnostic laparoscopy to enhance diagnostic accuracy.

## TREATMENT

In the United States, surgical intervention is the treatment of choice for acute appendicitis. The patient suspected of having appendicitis should be instructed to refrain from oral consumption. Intravenous fluids should be administered to maintain current needs and to correct any deficits that may be present. A nasogastric tube may be inserted to diminish gastric distension. Antibiotics are indicated after commitment to surgical intervention has been made. The incidence of wound infection has been shown to decrease with the use of prophylactic antibiotics. Delay in operation is associated with a higher percentage of perforation and increased morbidity and mortality.

## BIBLIOGRAPHY

Alvarado A: A practical score for the early diagnosis of acute appendicitis. *Ann Emerg Med* 15:557, 1986.

Bolton JP, Craven ER, Croft RJ, et al: An assessment of the value of the white cell count in the management of suspected acute appendicitis. *BJ Surg* 62:906, 1975.

Stair T, Corbette, MB: Appendicitis over forty. *Ann Emerg Med* 9:76, 1980.

Van Dieijen-Visser MP, Go PMNYH, Brombacher PJ: The value of laboratory tests in patients suspected of acute appendicitis. *Eur J Clin Chem Clin Biochem* 29:749, 1991.

# 79
# INTESTINAL OBSTRUCTION

### Salvator J. Vicario
### John L. Glover

Intestinal obstruction is an important consideration in patients who present with abdominal complaints to the emergency department. It can be defined as an inability of the intestinal tract to allow for regular passage of food and bowel contents. In turn this can be secondary to mechanical obstruction or adynamic ileus. Adynamic ileus (paralytic ileus) is the more common entity but is usually self-limiting and does not require surgical intervention. Mechanical obstruction can be caused by either intrinsic or extrinsic factors and generally requires definitive intervention in a relatively short period of time to determine the cause and minimize subsequent morbidity and mortality.

## ETIOLOGY

Both large and small intestines may be obstructed by various pathologic processes (Table 79-1). Extrinsic, intrinsic, or intraluminal processes precipitate mechanical obstruction. Differentiating small bowel obstruction (SBO) from large bowel obstruction is important because the incidence, clinical presentation, and modes of therapy vary depending on the anatomic site of the obstruction. The small intestine is characterized by transverse linear densities that extend completely across the bowel lumen (plicae circulares). The colon is situated peripherally in the abdomen, is larger in diameter, and contains short, blunt, and thick projections (haustrae) that arise from the bowel wall and extend only partially into the lumen. Haustrae are less numerous and situated farther apart than plicae circulares.

The most common cause of SBO is adhesions following abdominal surgery. Although in most cases several months to years have passed from the time of the previous surgery, SBO may occur within the first few weeks following surgery. The second most common cause of small intestinal obstruction is incarceration of a groin hernia. This can occur in infants as well as adults and should be suspected anytime there is a complaint of a "knot" or growth in the inguinal region that fails to reduce with manipulation. Other sites that are occasionally responsible for SBO secondary to hernia include the umbilicus, femoral canal, and, rarely, the obturator foramen. Umbilical hernias are more readily apparent and occur in any age group. Obturator or femoral hernias are much less common and may present with femoral or medial thigh pain. Elderly females are particularly susceptible to these defects, and one needs to consider them as a possible cause of SBO in these patients. Finally, a defect in the mesentery itself may cause intestinal obstruction.

Other causes of SBO are much less common and are generally due to intraluminal or intramural processes. Primary small bowel lesions include polyps, lymphoma, or adenocarcinoma. An unusual cause of intraluminal obstruction is gallstone ileus. In this situation, a gallstone has eroded from the gallbladder through the bowel wall and can cause obstruction at the ileocecal valve. Besides the findings of bowel obstruction, one may note air in the biliary tree on abdominal radiographs. Lymphomas may be the leading point of intussusception and present as SBO.

Bezoars are most commonly composed of vegetable matter or pulp from persimmons. Patients who have undergone gastrointestinal pyloroplasty or pyloric resection are most susceptible to intraluminal obstruction by bezoars.

Inflammatory bowel disease may also affect the small bowel at various sites. Likewise, infectious processes including abscesses may obstruct the bowel. Radiation enteritis is also a possible cause of SBO in patients who have undergone radiation therapy.

**Table 79-1.** Causes of Alimentary Tract Obstruction

| Mechanical Causes | Duodenum | Small Bowel | Colon |
|---|---|---|---|
| Congenital | Atresia Stenosis Duodenal web Annular pancreas Congenital band | Atresia Stenosis External hernia | Atresia Stenosis Meconium ileus Imperforate anus Hirschsprung disease |
| Inflammatory | Stricture | Adhesions Regional enteritis Abscess Stricture | Granulomatous colitis Ulcerative colitis Diverticulitis Abscess Stricture |
| Neoplastic | Carcinoma Polyps | Carcinoma Lymphoma Sarcoma Leiomyoma Carcinoid | Carcinoma Sarcoma Lymphoma |
| Miscellaneous | Foreign body Hematoma Superior mesenteric artery syndrome | Foreign body Hematoma Worms Gallstone Bezoars Intussusception Hernia Volvulus | Foreign body Endometriosis Fecal impaction Intussusception Volvulus |

PARALYTIC ILEUS
Conduction defects: NA$^+$ and K$^+$ abnormalities
Peristaltic defects: as in mesenteric vascular disease and porphyria
Neural irritative states: local or general toxicity, retroperitoneal injuries

*Source:* Adapted from Schwartz GR, *Principles and Practice of Emergency Medicine,* 3rd ed, p. 1712. Malvern, PA, Lea & Febiger, 1992.

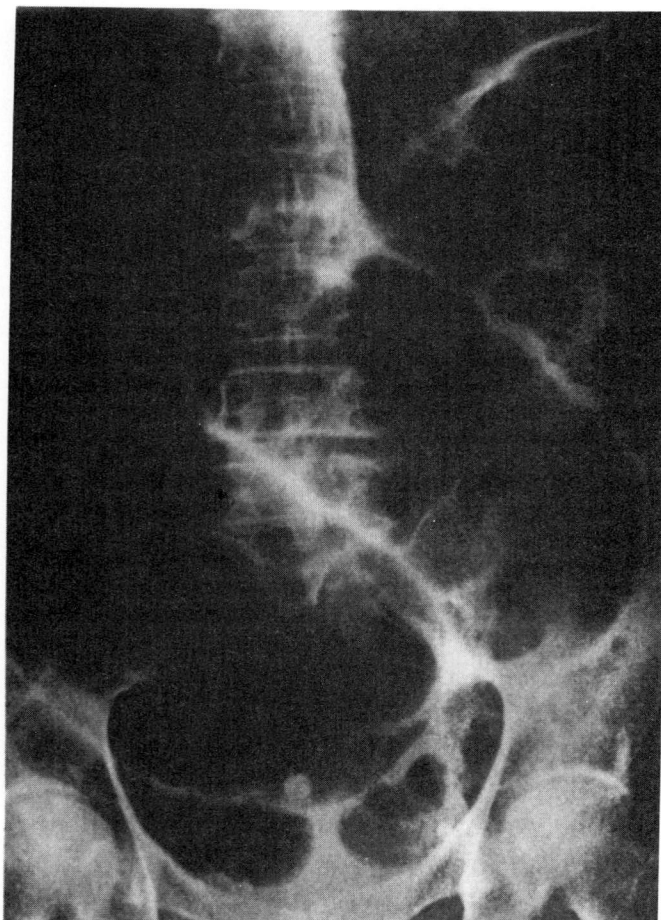

**Fig. 79-1.** Sigmoid volvulus. Note distension of large bowel and central stripe, giving a "coffee-bean" appearance.

Colonic obstruction is almost never caused by hernia or surgical adhesions. Neoplasms are by far the most common cause of large bowel obstruction. Therefore, anyone who has symptoms of colonic obstruction should be evaluated for a neoplasm. Diverticulitis may create significant secondary obstruction and mesenteric edema. Stricture formation may occur with chronic inflammation and scarring. Fecal impaction is a common problem in elderly, debilitated patients and may present with symptoms of colonic obstruction.

The next most frequent cause of large bowel obstruction after cancer and diverticulitis is sigmoid volvulus. Elderly, bedridden, or psychiatric patients who are taking anticholinergic medication are most often subject to this mechanical problem. A history of constipation may precede the volvulus and presenting symptoms. Radiographic appearance is usually classic (Fig. 79-1). Finally, although much less common, cecal volvulus may also cause large bowel obstruction.

## PATHOPHYSIOLOGY

Normal bowel contents contain gas as well as gastric secretions and food. Intraluminal accumulation of gastric, biliary, and pancreatic secretions continues even if there is no oral intake. As obstruction develops, the bowel becomes congested and there is failure of intestinal contents to be absorbed. Vomiting and decreased oral intake follow. The combination of decreased absorption, vomiting, and reduced intake leads to volume depletion with hemoconcentration and electrolyte imbalance, and ultimately can cause renal failure or shock.

Bowel distension often accompanies mechanical obstruction. Distension is due to the accumulation of fluids in the bowel lumen, an in-

crease in intraluminal pressure with enhanced peristaltic contractions, and air swallowing. When intraluminal pressure exceeds capillary and venous pressure in the bowel wall, absorption and lymphatic drainage decrease. At this stage, bacteria may enter the bloodstream, the bowel becomes ischemic, and septicemia and bowel necrosis can develop. Shock rapidly ensues. Mortality approaches 70 percent if bowel obstruction has been allowed to progress this far. With a *closed-loop obstruction* this sequence of events may occur more rapidly. In this instance, there is no proximal escape for bowel contents. Examples of closed-loop obstruction include an incarcerated hernia and complete colon obstruction in the presence of a closed ileocecal valve.

## CLINICAL FEATURES

The site and nature of the obstruction and the preexisting condition of the patient will determine the clinical presentation. Almost all patients will have abdominal pain. The pain is generally described as crampy and intermittent. Pain of mechanical SBO is often episodic, usually lasting for a few minutes at a time. In adynamic ileus, the pain tends to be less intense and more constant. If the obstruction is proximal, vomiting is usually present. The vomitus in proximal obstruction is usually bilious but is feculent in distal ileal obstruction. The pain of large bowel obstruction is usually hypogastric. Large bowel obstructions may be associated with fecal vomiting as well.

Other features that are consistently present with obstruction of small bowel or colon include the inability to have a bowel movement or pass flatus. Of course this may occur in patients with constipation of any origin and is not necessarily associated with bowel obstruction. Partial bowel obstruction, however, is often associated with regular passage of stool and flatus.

Physical findings may vary, depending on the site, duration, and etiology of the pathologic process. Early symptoms are usually associated with some abdominal distension, often impressive with colonic obstruction. This may not be readily apparent in cases of incarcerated hernia. Abdominal tenderness may be minimal and diffuse or localized and severe. Patients who have developed peritonitis will obviously have severe tenderness. The abdomen may be tympanitic to percussion. Mechanical obstruction will produce active high pitched bowel sounds with occasional "rushes." If obstruction has been present for several hours, peristaltic waves and bowel sounds may be diminished. Patients with an adynamic ileus may have some abdominal distension associated with diminished or absent bowel sounds. Careful search for localized or rebound tenderness is essential to rule out the possibility of gangrenous or perforated bowel, which requires immediate surgical intervention (Fig. 79-2).

All patients with abdominal pain or distension should be examined for signs of organomegaly or masses that may suggest a cause of the obstruction. A rectal examination may identify fecal impaction, rectal carcinoma, occult blood, or stricture. The absence of stool in the vault may aid in the diagnosis of bowel obstruction, but its presence does not eliminate a more proximal obstruction, as patients may not be able to evacuate preexisting rectal contents. A pelvic examination should be performed to identify any gynecologic pathology causing obstruction.

## LABORATORY AND RADIOGRAPHIC FINDINGS

All patients with suspected obstruction should have a flat and upright abdominal radiograph and upright chest x-ray or a lateral decubitus view if the patient cannot be upright. An abdominal radiograph can confirm the diagnosis, identify free air or masses, and localize the site to large or small bowel (Fig. 79-3A, 3B). Laboratory work should include a complete blood count and electrolyte measurements. Depending on the duration of symptoms and site of obstruction or whether there is bowel necrosis, one may find a wide range in white blood cell (WBC) counts and hemoglobin, hematocrit, and electrolyte values.

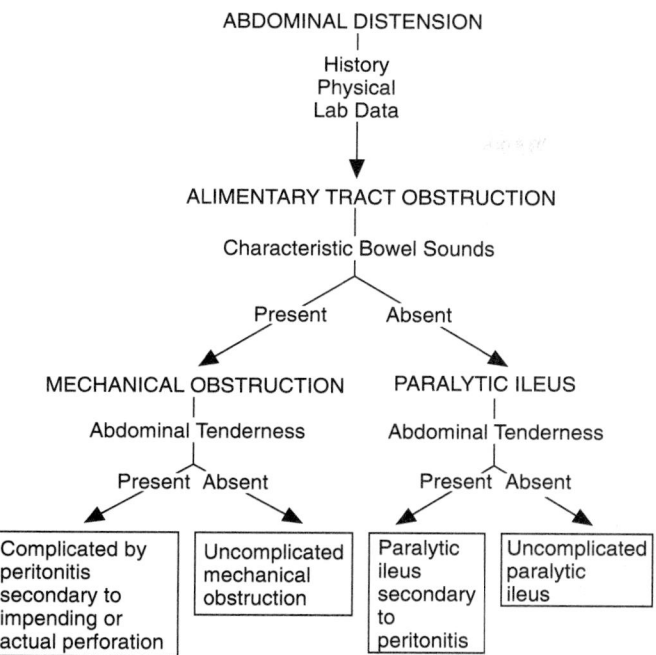

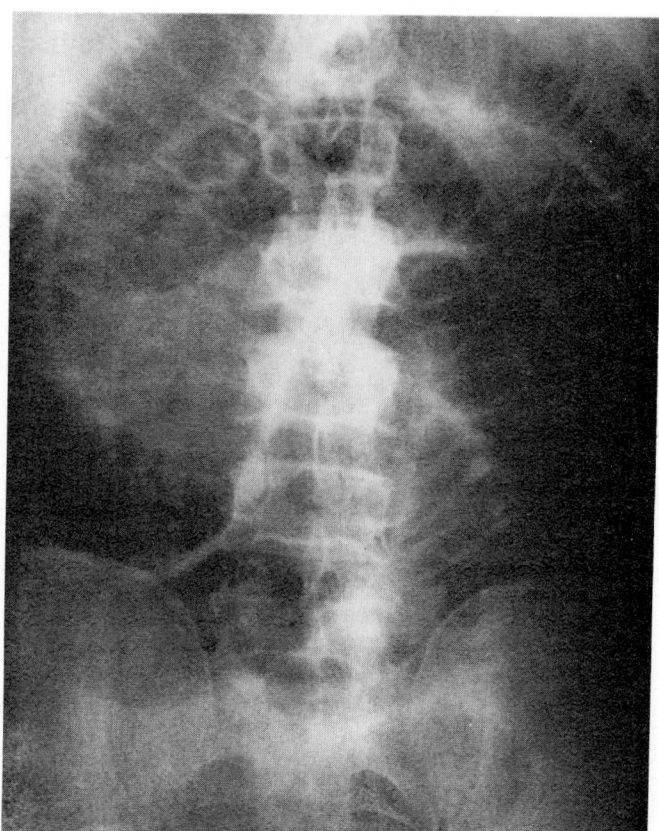

**Fig. 79-2.** Logic flow diagram emphasizing the clinical importance of abdominal tenderness in alimentary tract obstruction. (From Schwartz GR: *Principles and Practice of Emergency Medicine,* 3d ed, p 1718. Malvern, PA, Lea & Febiger, 1992, with permission.)

Patients will usually have some elevation in WBC. A white count >20,000/μL or left shift should make one suspect bowel gangrene, intraabdominal abscess, or peritonitis. Extreme WBC elevation (>40,000/μL) suggests mesenteric vascular occlusion. The serum amylase and lipase levels may be mildly elevated. Levels of serum electrolytes are usually normal or mildly reduced, depending on whether the obstruction is of short or long duration or whether there is associated emesis. The hematocrit will also elevate with ongoing obstruction and decrease in fluid volume. The BUN and creatinine will become elevated, indicating dehydration. Other indications of the severity of obstruction or secondary complications include increased urine specific gravity, ketonuria, elevated lactate levels, and metabolic acidosis.

Further investigation to determine the site or etiology of obstruction include sigmoidoscopy or barium enema. Upper gastrointestinal studies are rarely indicated. Barium enema can determine the cause and site of large bowel obstruction (Fig. 79-4). Sigmoidoscopy can identify friable mucosa, intraluminal lesions, or the dark-blue gangrenous mucosa associated with dead bowel. If the diagnosis is unclear, repeated examination, preferably by the same examiner, will be necessary.

## TREATMENT

If a true mechanical obstruction is diagnosed, then surgical intervention is usually mandatory. Prior to surgical intervention, emergency department efforts should be made to decompress the bowel with nasogastric intubation. A nasogastric tube is generally effective in removing excess bowel contents and air. Likewise, because of loss of absorptive capacity, decreased oral intake, and vomiting, most patients will require intravenous fluid replacement. Patients can be monitored prior to surgical intervention by the response of blood pressure and heart rate and measurement of urine output. Surgery should not be delayed unnecessarily by attempting to use long intestinal tubes (Baker, Cantor, or Miller-Abbott) or excessive testing. A volvulus of the sigmoid colon will usually decompress via sigmoidoscopy and insertion of a rectal tube. Should a closed-loop ob-

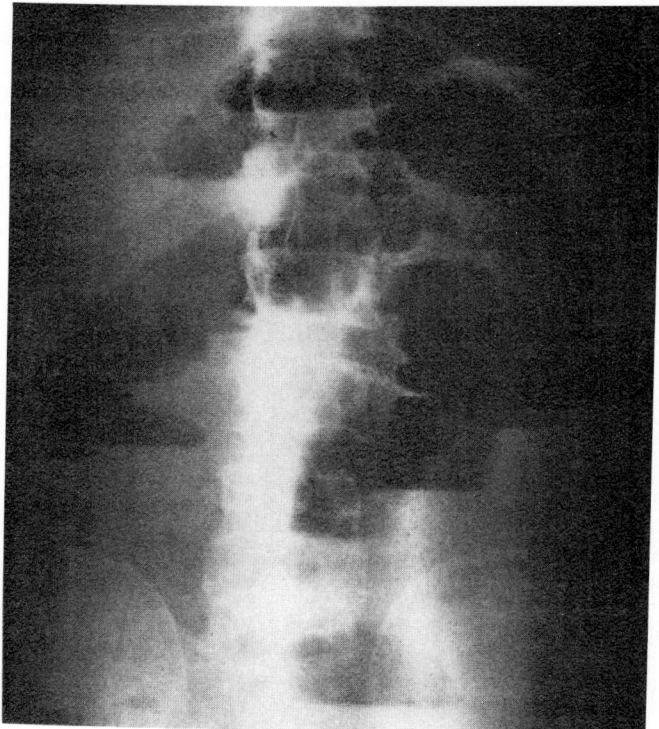

**Fig. 79-3.** *A.* Flat plate abdominal film illustrates distended loops of small bowel. *B.* Upright film demonstrates multiple air-fluid levels and "step-ladder" appearance. (From Harris JH, Harris WH: *The Radiology of Emergency Medicine,* 3d ed, p 843. Baltimore, Williams and Wilkins, 1993, with permission.)

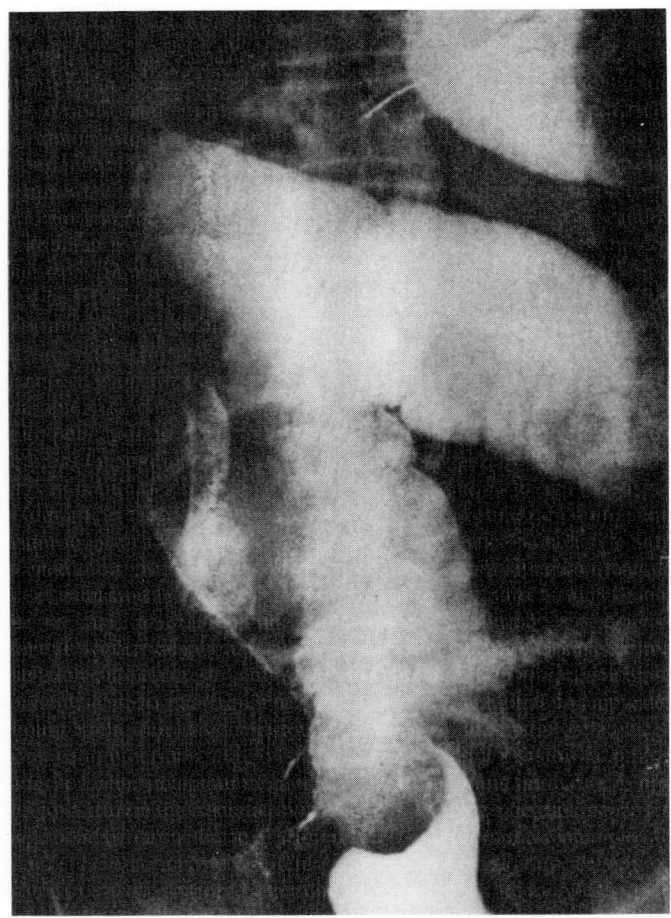

**Fig. 79-4.** Barium enema examination demonstrating incomplete filling of the sigmoid secondary to volvulus. Note the "parrot-beak" appearance of the point of the volvulus. (From Schwartz GR: *Principles and Practice of Emergency Medicine,* 3d ed, p 1720. Malvern, PA, Lea & Febiger, 1992, with permission.)

struction, bowel necrosis, or cecal volvulus be suspected, then surgical intervention should be performed without delay. All patients with mechanical obstruction will require broad-spectrum antibiotic coverage preoperatively, as the risk of infection and septicemia is significant in most conditions. If adynamic ileus is the primary problem or the diagnosis is uncertain, conservative measures, including intravenous fluids, nasogastric decompression, and observation, are generally effective in allowing the bowel to resume normal activity and function. Any medication that inhibits bowel mobility should obviously be discontinued. Radiologic examination to confirm nasogastric tube placement or long-tube location is also advised. Some authors advocate contrast radiography to distinguish partial SBO from ileus.

## PSEUDOOBSTRUCTION

Intestinal pseudoobstruction may also mimic bowel obstruction. Although any segment of bowel may be affected, low colonic obstruction is the most common clinical presentation. Large amounts of gas will be present in the large intestine. Patients may be using anticholinergic or tricyclic antidepressants, which depress motility. One must avoid the use of barium studies as the patient may be unable to evacuate the barium. Preference should be given to colonoscopy after digital rectal examination as an early intervention to rule out true ob-

struction or significant lesions. Colonoscopy will also treat the pseudoobstruction by decompression. Surgery is not helpful and may be harmful.

## BIBLIOGRAPHY

Cheadle WC, Garr FE, Richardson JD: The importance of early diagnosis of small bowel obstruction. *Am Surg* 54:565, 1988.

Dunn JT, Halls JM, Berne TV: Roentgenographic contrast studies in acute small bowel obstruction. *Arch Surg* 119:1305, 1984.

Preger L, Gronner AT, Glazer H, et al: Imaging of the non-traumatic acute abdomen. *Emerg Med Clin North Am* 7:453, 1989.

# 80
# HERNIA IN ADULTS AND CHILDREN
## Frank W. Lavoie

A *hernia* is technically defined as an *external* or *internal* protrusion of a body part from its natural cavity. Although internal herniations may be found in cerebral, diaphragmatic, hiatal, or other abdominopelvic locations, the usual use of the term is in reference to the abdominal wall and typically to external presentations. Hernias also may be *interparietal,* within the layers of the abdominal wall. Abdominal wall herniations occur both in adults and children and may be present in groin (inguinal or femoral), umbilical, anterior abdominal, pelvic, or lumbar locations.

## PATHOPHYSIOLOGY

### General Characteristics

Essential to the understanding of hernias are the anatomic characteristics of the abdominal cavity and, in particular, its fascial and aponeurotic layers. Embryologic development produces localized areas of inherent weakness in the abdominal wall. These include areas where retroperitoneal structures penetrate, as in the inguinal, femoral, and obturator canals, the sciatic foramen, and the umbilical region; and areas devoid of strong multilayer structural support, as in the anterior abdominal wall's linea alba and semilunar line. In addition, surgical incision and trauma may produce areas of abdominal wall weakness.

Herniations may include preperitoneal fat, retroperitoneal organs, and a hernia sac composed of peritoneum containing intraperitoneal structures (e.g., omentum or organs). Clinically significant herniation without a peritoneal sac is uncommon. Hernias may be complicated by inclusion of a viscus forming one wall of the hernia sac. This involves a partially retroperitoneal organ and is called a *sliding hernia.* Sliding inguinal hernias most frequently involve the colon.

The entrapment of the content of a hernia is more likely when the hernia opening is narrow. When the content can be returned to its normal cavity by manipulation, the hernia is *reducible;* when it cannot, it is *irreducible* or *incarcerated.* Incarceration may be *acute* or *chronic.* Incarceration of a single wall of a hollow viscus is known as *Richter hernia.* Incarcerated hernias are subject to inflammatory and edematous changes and are at risk for strangulation. *Strangulation* of a hernia refers to vascular compromise of the incarcerated contents. When strangulation is not relieved in a timely fashion, gangrenous changes ensue.

## Predisposing Factors

Lack of developmental maturity of anatomic structures is known to predispose to the formation of hernias, as in indirect inguinal and umbilical hernias in premature infants. Conditions that increase intraabdominal pressure, such as ascites, peritoneal dialysis, ventriculoperitoneal shunt, cystic fibrosis, and chronic obstructive pulmonary disease, are also associated with hernia. Family history, undescended testis, and genitourinary abnormalities are additional risks.

## Specific Hernia Types

**Indirect inguinal hernia.** The inguinal canal is the tract in the abdominal wall through which pass the gubernaculum, testis, and spermatic cord in males or the round ligament in females. The canal is defined by an internal ring defect in the transversalis fascia and transversus abdominis aponeurosis, lateral to the inferior epigastric vessels, and a more medial external ring defect in the external oblique aponeurosis (Fig. 80-1).

Normal passage through the inguinal canal is accompanied by peritoneal evagination known as the *processus vaginalis.* Normal obliteration of the processus occurs in infancy. Passage of contents through a persistent patent processus vaginalis along the inguinal canal leads to an indirect inguinal hernia. Congenital failure of obliteration is the etiology for all indirect inguinal hernias. Acquired myoaponeurotic defects may additionally contribute to indirect inguinal hernia in adults.

Passage of the testis is thought to enlarge the canal and increase the likelihood of inguinal hernia in males. It is more common on the right side due to later passage of the right testis. Indirect inguinal hernias not infrequently incarcerate and strangulate, particularly in the first year of life and in females.

**Direct inguinal hernia.** These are protrusions through the transversalis fascia and the external ring, medial to the inferior epigastric vessels. Direct inguinal hernias are acquired defects that do not involve passage through the inguinal canal and occur predominantly in adults; they rarely incarcerate and strangulate. Such a hernia with ipsilateral direct and indirect components may be called a *pantaloon hernia.*

**Femoral hernia.** A femoral hernia is a protrusion below the inguinal ligament and adjacent to the femoral vessels in the femoral canal. Femoral hernias are more common in women due to the different anatomic structure of the pelvis. Femoral hernias are far less common than inguinal hernias. They do frequently incarcerate and strangulate.

**Umbilical hernia.** In utero contraction of the umbilical cord insertion forms the fibromuscular umbilical ring. Incomplete development or weakness in the ring allows herniation of abdominal contents.

Congenital umbilical hernias affect 10 to 30 percent of white infants and a higher percentage of children of African descent. They are more common in females. Incarceration and strangulation of childhood umbilical hernias are very rare.

Umbilical hernias also may develop in adults. This acquired defect is more common in women and is associated with obesity, pregnancy, and ascites. Incarceration and strangulation frequently occur.

**Epigastric hernia.** An epigastric hernia involves herniation through the linea alba of the rectus sheath.

**Spigelian hernia.** Herniation at the site of the semilunar line, just lateral to the rectus muscle, through the combined aponeurosis of the transversus abdominis and internal oblique muscles is known as a Spigelian hernia. This hernia is frequently interparietal.

**Pelvic hernia.** Pelvic hernias are rare. There are *sciatic hernias,* passing through sciatic foramen; *perineal hernias,* passing between perineal muscles; and *obturator hernias,* passing through the obturator canal with the obturator vessels.

**Lumbar hernia.** Herniation rarely may occur through the inferior or superior lumbar triangles.

**Incisional hernia.** Herniation may occur through an incisional area. Infection and obesity contribute to poor wound healing, which increases the likelihood of development of incisional hernia.

**Traumatic hernia.** Traumatic herniation involving a variety of organs and locations may be observed. These usually occur without true hernia sacs.

## CLINICAL FEATURES

The majority of hernias are asymptomatic and are detected either on routine physical examination or inadvertently by the patient. Patients with incarceration frequently give a history of hernia; the patient can no longer reduce it and therefore seeks medical attention. If incarceration is acute, pain may develop suddenly. With infants, irritability may be the only presenting complaint. Incarceration may be accompanied by nausea and vomiting if partial or complete bowel obstruction has occurred. Incarcerated hernias are a leading cause of bowel obstruction, second to postoperative adhesions.

When strangulation occurs the patient may be toxic, along with signs and symptoms of bowel obstruction. In the case of Richter hernia, however, strangulation may occur without intestinal obstruction. Unrelieved strangulation may result in perforation, abscess formation, peritonitis, or septic shock.

Pain and hypesthesia along the medial aspect of the thigh to the knee are associated with obturator hernias. These patients additionally have intermittent bouts of small bowel obstruction over years.

Physical examination of the patient with a hernia may reveal an abnormal swelling. In inguinal hernias, the swelling may extend into the scrotum. The consistency of the mass varies depending upon the content of the hernia sac. If incarceration is present, the swelling is usually tender due to inflammation of the bowel wall or omentum and surrounding tissues. Tachycardia and mild temperature elevation frequently also are present.

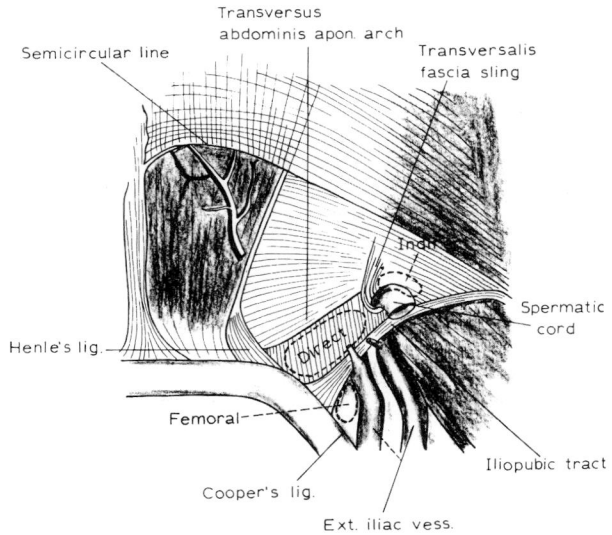

**Fig. 80-1.** The posterior inguinal wall viewed from the preperitoneal side. The peritoneum and all preperitoneal fat and lymphoid tissue have been excised, exposing the transversalis fascia. The areas through which the three common groin hernias occur are indicated, as are the transversalis fascia analogues, which are utilized in the iliopubic tract repair. [From Nyhus LM: Preperitoneal approach in the repair of inguinal hernia in adults, in Ellison EH, Friesen SR, Mulholland JH (eds): *Current Surgical Management III.* Philadelphia, Saunders, 1965, p. 465. Used with permission.]

## DIAGNOSIS

Patients frequently present to the emergency department with a complaint of groin pain. There may or may not be a history of heavy lifting. In males, palpation of the inguinal canal is easily performed by inversion of scrotal skin and passage of a digit through the external ring. Voluntary increase in intraabdominal pressure during this examination reliably detects most inguinal hernias. In females, the external ring is generally narrower and the skin of the labium majora is not easily inverted. Therefore, failure to palpate a hernial sac is not foolproof.

Groin hernias can be confused with tender lymph nodes and hydroceles. Lymph nodes are generally movable, firm, and multiple. Hydroceles may transilluminate and are not tender. Incarcerated hernias will not transilluminate and are tender. If bowel is contained in the hernia sac, bowel sounds may be heard and peristalsis may be seen. In children, retractile or undescended testes may be mistaken for hernias. Testicular torsion or tumor may be confused with incarcerated hernias.

When incarceration is acute, the white blood cell count is slightly elevated with a shift to the left. Electrolyte abnormalities and elevation of the blood urea nitrogen (BUN) level occur as a reflection of both the patient's state of hydration and the toxic state. In the elderly, laboratory studies may not be reliable indicators of the patient's state. Occasionally, as part of a diagnostic evaluation for abdominal pain, a hernia is detected on barium enema.

Upright chest films should be obtained to rule out free air under the diaphragm, which may result from perforation or dead bowel. Flat and upright films of the abdomen, including the groin, should be obtained to assess the possible presence of bowel obstruction. Loops of bowel may be seen entering a hernial sac.

Suspicion of Spigelian or pelvic hernias often necessitates use of sonography or CT scanning for diagnosis, since detection of herniation is frequently difficult and confusion with other masses is possible.

## TREATMENT

If there is a good history that the incarceration is of very recent onset, an attempt can be made to reduce the hernia. If there is any question of the duration of the incarceration, no attempt should be made so that no dead bowel is reintroduced into the abdomen. Before an attempt is made to reduce the hernia, the patient should be placed in the Trendelenburg position and given some mild sedation. A warm compress over the area may make the task easier by reducing the swelling and relaxing the abdominal musculature. Only gentle compression of the hernia should be used, and nothing should be forced back. Attempts at reduction should be limited in time and force.

If the incarceration is tender, if it cannot be reduced, or if strangulation is suspected, the patient should not be fed by mouth, and a nasogastric tube should be inserted. Intravenous fluid should be started with the thought of correcting the patient's volume and electrolyte problems.

The treatment of choice for an incarceration which cannot be reduced, or for a strangulation, is surgical. Broad-spectrum antibiotics and vigorous fluid resuscitation may be necessary, but only as a prelude to operation. Mortality is higher in the elderly when emergency surgery is required.

## DISPOSITION

Any acutely incarcerated or strangulated hernia, regardless of type or patient age, requires immediate surgical evaluation and repair.

Adult patients with reducible hernias may be discharged and referred for elective surgical repair. They should be advised to avoid conditions that increase intraabdominal pressure, such as lifting activities. Return to the emergency department should be suggested for re-currence that the patient is unable to reduce promptly. Following surgical evaluation, patients who are not candidates for operative repair occasionally may be fitted with trusses.

In children, inguinal hernias have a high risk of incarceration, particularly in the first year of life. These hernias should be electively repaired shortly after diagnosis and therefore require timely surgical consultation. Infants with inguinal hernias reduced in the emergency department should generally have repair within 24 h.

Umbilical hernias in children very rarely incarcerate. Spontaneous closure of the umbilical ring occurs in 80 percent of these children by age 3 or 4. Discharge and primary care observation is the standard of care for young children with hernias less than 2.0 cm in diameter. Children over age 4 or with larger hernias should be referred for surgical evaluation.

## BIBLIOGRAPHY

Gallegos NC, Dawson J, Jarvis M, Hobsley M: Risk of strangulation in groin hernias. *Br J Surg* 78:1171, 1991.

Nyhus LM, Condon RE: *Hernia,* 3d ed. Philadelphia, Lippincott, 1989.

Rizk TA, Deshmukh N: Obturator hernia: A difficult diagnosis. *South Med J* 83:709, 1990.

Sahdev P, Garramone RR, Desani B, et al: Traumatic abdominal hernia: Report of three cases and review of the literature. *Am J Emerg Med* 10:237, 1992.

Scherer LR, Grosfeld JL: Inguinal hernia and umbilical anomalies. *Pediatr Clin North Am* 40:1121, 1993.

Wantz GE: Abdominal wall hernias, in Schwartz SI, Shires GT, Spencer FC (eds): *Principles of Surgery,* 6th ed. New York, McGraw-Hill, 1994, pp 1517–1543.

# 81
# ILEITIS AND COLITIS
**Howard A. Werman**
**Hagop S. Mekhjian**
**Douglas A. Rund**

## CROHN'S DISEASE

Crohn's disease is a chronic inflammatory disease of the gastrointestinal (GI) tract; the exact cause is still unknown. The disease was first described by Crohn, Ginzberg, and Oppenheimer in 1932. In their initial description, the disease was thought to involve only the distal ileum. We now know that Crohn's disease can involve any part of the GI tract from the mouth to the anus. Segmental involvement of the intestinal tract by a nonspecific granulomatous inflammatory process characterizes the disease. The ileum is involved in the majority of cases. In 20 percent of cases, the disease is confined to the colon, making differentiation from ulcerative colitis, at times, a difficult clinical problem. The terms *regional enteritis, terminal ileitis, granulomatous ileocolitis,* and *Crohn disease* are used to describe the same disease process.

## Etiology and Pathogenesis

Environmental, genetic, and host factors have all been implicated as a cause of both Crohn's disease and ulcerative colitis. Atypical mycobacteria have also been considered as a possible etiology of

Crohn's disease. There are few data to support a primary causative role of psychogenic factors. Immunologic factors have received great attention recently. Several mechanisms of injury have been proposed, including autoimmune destruction of the gut mucosal cells as the result of cross-reactivity with antigens from enteric bacteria as well as nonspecific immunologic injury to the gut mucosa as the result of a chronic inflammatory process for both ulcerative colitis and Crohn's disease. Whether immune factors play a primary or secondary role in the pathogenesis of these diseases is not known. Extraintestinal manifestations suggest a role for immune complexes or an autoantibody response at various involved sites.

## Epidemiology

The peak incidence of Crohn's disease occurs in patients between 15 and 22 years of age, with a secondary peak at age 55 to 60 years. The prevalence varies from 10 to 100 cases per 100,000 population, and the incidence from 1 to 7 cases per year per 100,000 population in the United States. The incidence of Crohn's disease has been increasing over the past 20 years. The disease has a worldwide distribution but is more frequent in people of European descent. It is four times more common in Jews than non-Jews and is more common in whites than blacks. A family history of inflammatory bowel disease is present in 10 to 15 percent of patients. Ulcerative colitis, as well as Crohn's disease, may be present in other family members, and siblings of patients with Crohn's disease have a higher incidence of the disease.

## Pathology

The most important pathologic feature of Crohn's disease is the involvement of all the layers of the bowel and extension into mesenteric lymph nodes. In addition, the disease is discontinuous, with normal areas of bowel ("skip areas") located between one or more involved areas. On gross inspection, the bowel wall is thickened; subsequent luminal narrowing results in stenosis and obstruction of the intestine. The mesenteric fat often extends over the bowel wall ("creeping" fat). The appearance of the mucosa varies with the extent and severity of the disease. Longitudinal deep ulcerations are characteristic. These often penetrate the bowel wall, resulting in fissures, fistulas, and abscesses. Late in the disease, a "cobblestone" appearance of the mucosa results from the crisscrossing of these ulcers with intervening normal mucosa.

Microscopically, there is an inflammatory reaction that extends through all layers of the intestine, but which is most marked in the submucosa. This inflammatory response consists of infiltration by mononuclear cells, lymphocytes, plasma cells, and histiocytes. Fissure ulcers frequently penetrate the muscle layer. Unlike the situation in ulcerative colitis, crypt abscesses are rarely seen. Discrete granulomas consisting of epithelioid cells, giant cells, and lymphocytes are seen in 50 to 75 percent of the specimens from patients with Crohn's disease. Although the finding of granulomas is helpful, it is not essential for the diagnosis.

## Clinical Features and Course

The clinical course of Crohn's disease varies and in the individual patient is unpredictable. Abdominal pain, anorexia, diarrhea, and weight loss are present in 75 to 80 percent of cases. Occasionally, a patient with Crohn's disease may present with acute right lower quadrant abdominal pain and fever and on examination be found to have a mass in the right lower quadrant. More commonly, the patient experiences an insidious onset of recurrent abdominal pain, fever, and diarrhea which lasts for several years before the definitive diagnosis is established. Approximately 90 percent of patients develop perianal fissures or fistulas, abscesses, or rectal prolapse. In 10 to 20 percent of patients the extraintestinal manifestations of arthritis, uveitis, or liver disease may be presenting symptoms. Crohn's disease should also be considered in the differential diagnosis of patients with fever of unknown etiology.

The clinical course and manifestations of the disease appear to be related, in part, to its anatomic distribution: in 30 percent the disease involves only the small bowel, in 20 percent only the colon is involved, and in 50 percent both the small bowel and colon are involved. The recurrence rate for all patients with Crohn's disease is 25 to 50 percent within 1 year for patients whose disease has responded to medical management and is higher for those patients who require surgery. Patients with ileocolitis have the highest recurrence rate following surgery. The incidence of hematochezia and perianal disease is higher when the colon is involved, as in ileocolitis or Crohn's colitis. A slight increase in the incidence of arthritis may be associated with Crohn's colitis. With the exception of growth retardation, childhood-onset Crohn's disease seems to have a course similar to that of adult-onset disease.

Extraintestinal manifestations are seen in 25 to 36 percent of patients with Crohn's disease, and the incidence of such complications does not differ between patients with Crohn's disease and those with ulcerative colitis. Extraintestinal manifestations are divided among arthritic (19 percent), dermatologic (4 percent), hepatobiliary (4 percent), and vascular (1.3 percent) complications. Dermatologic complications include erythema nodosum and pyoderma gangrenosum. Ocular manifestations include episcleritis and uveitis. Peripheral arthropathies are commonly seen in both ulcerative colitis and Crohn's disease and tend to manifest during exacerbations of the underlying disease process. Ankylosing spondylitis can be detected in up to 20 percent of patients with inflammatory bowel disease. Symptoms may occur before, during, and after bouts of Crohn's disease or ulcerative colitis.

Hepatobiliary disease is common in patients with inflammatory bowel disease and includes pericholangitis, chronic active hepatitis, primary sclerosing cholangitis, and cholangiocarcinoma. Gallstones are detected in up to one-third of patients with Crohn's disease. The incidence of acute and chronic pancreatitis is increased in patients with Crohn's disease and ulcerative colitis.

Vascular manifestations include thromboembolic disease, vasculitis, and arteritis. Patients with thromboembolic complications have a mortality rate of approximately 25 percent. Thromboembolic disease is the result of a hypercoagulable state induced in patients with both Crohn's disease and ulcerative colitis and ranks as the third leading cause of death in patients afflicted with these conditions, behind peritonitis and malignancy. Malnutrition and chronic anemia are seen in many patients with long-standing Crohn's disease. Growth retardation can be seen in children. Hyperoxaluria is a common and potentially treatable occurrence in patients with ileal disease and steatorrhea. This results from the colonic hyperabsorption of dietary oxalate and accounts for the occurrence of nephrolithiasis in 20 to 25 percent of patients with ileal disease.

## Complications

More than three out of four patients with Crohn's disease will require surgery within the first 20 years from the onset of initial symptoms. Abscess and fissure formation are seen in approximately 30 percent of patients with Crohn's disease. Abscesses can be characterized as intraperitoneal, retroperitoneal, interloop, or intramesenteric. Patients present with abdominal pain and tenderness typical of their underlying disease but may also have fever spikes and a palpable mass. Patients with retroperitoneal abscesses may present with hip or back pain and may have difficulty ambulating. Liver abscesses have also been reported in patients with Crohn's disease.

Fistulas are the result of extension of intestinal fissures noted in patients with Crohn's disease. The most common sites are between the ileum and the sigmoid colon, the cecum, another ileal segment, or the skin. Internal fistulas should be suspected when there is a change in the patient's symptom complex including bowel frequency, amount of pain, or weight loss. Enterovesical fistulas are rare complications of Crohn's disease.

Obstruction is the result of both stricture formation due to the inflammatory process and of edema of the bowel wall. The distal small bowel is the most common site of obstruction. Symptoms include crampy abdominal pain, distension, nausea, and bloating.

Perianal complications are seen in 90 percent of patients with Crohn's disease and include perianal or ischiorectal abscesses, fissures, fistulas, rectovaginal fistulas, and rectal prolapse. These are more commonly seen in patients with colonic involvement of the disease.

While gastrointestinal bleeding is common in patients with Crohn's disease, only 2.5 percent of patients develop life-threatening hemorrhage. In patients with Crohn's disease, bleeding is the result of erosion into a vessel in the bowel wall. Toxic megacolon occurs in 6 percent of all cases of Crohn's disease and is associated with massive gastrointestinal bleeding in over half the cases. Fifty percent of all cases of toxic megacolon occur in patients with Crohn's disease. Free perforation, however, rarely occurs.

When bowel symptoms are present, malnutrition, malabsorption, hypocalcemia, and vitamin deficiency can be severe. In addition to the complications of the disease itself are complications associated with the treatment of the disease with sulfasalazine, steroids, immunosuppressive agents, and antibiotics.

Incidence of malignant neoplasms of the GI tract is three times higher in patients with Crohn's disease than for the general population.

## Diagnosis

In the majority of patients, the definitive diagnosis of Crohn's disease is established months or years after the onset of symptoms. Occasionally, the initial presenting complaint is not related to the GI tract but is an extraintestinal manifestation such as arthritis or iritis. A provisional diagnosis of appendicitis or pelvic inflammatory disease may change to Crohn's disease at the time of surgery. A careful and detailed history for previous bowel symptoms that preceded the onset of acute right lower quadrant pain may provide clues to the correct diagnosis before surgery. In addition, the absence of true guarding or rebound in patients with Crohn's disease is also noted.

A definitive diagnosis of Crohn's disease is confirmed by an upper GI series, an air contrast barium enema, and colonoscopy, performed by a consulting gastroenterologist. Oral barium studies with fluoroscopy are the most sensitive and specific for detecting ileal involvement. The classic radiographic findings in the small intestine include segmental narrowing, destruction of the normal mucosal pattern, and fistulas. The segmental involvement of the colon with rectal sparing is the most characteristic feature.

Colonoscopy is the most sensitive technique for examining patients with Crohn's colitis. This technique is useful in detecting early mucosal lesions, in defining the extent of colonic involvement, and in surveillance for the occurrence of colon cancer. Air contrast enemas are also useful in defining mucosal detail. Intraabdominal abscesses, mesenteric inflammation, and fistulas are best diagnosed using either CT scan or ultrasound.

Diseases that should be considered in the differential diagnosis of Crohn's disease include lymphoma, ileocecal amebiasis, tuberculosis, other deep chronic mycotic infections involving the GI tract, gastrointestinal tuberculosis, Kaposi sarcoma, *Campylobacter* enteritis, and yersinial ileocolitis. Fortunately, most of these are uncommon conditions and can be differentiated by appropriate laboratory tests. Yersinial ileocolitis and *Campylobacter* enteritis may cause chronic abdominal pain and diarrhea similar to Crohn's disease but can be diagnosed by appropriate stool cultures. Acute ileitis should not be confused with Crohn's disease. Patients with acute ileitis usually recover

without sequelae and should not undergo surgery. When Crohn's disease is confined to the colon, ischemic bowel disease and pseudomembranous enterocolitis as well as ulcerative colitis have to be included in the differential diagnosis.

## Treatment

The aim of therapy includes relief of symptoms, suppression of the inflammatory disease, treatment of complications, and maintenance of nutrition. In a disease that is virtually incurable and is characterized by frequent recurrences, the emphasis should be on relief of symptoms and avoidance or management of complications when they occur. The pharmacologic agents that are available for the management of Crohn's disease include symptomatic agents, anti-inflammatory agents, antibiotics, and immunomodulators.

Sulfasalazine (Azulfidine) 4 g/day has been used for many years and is an effective agent in the treatment of patients with mild to moderate active Crohn's disease. The mechanism of action is not known but is presumed to be through the topical action of 5-aminosalicylic acid, which is released by the action of colonic bacteria. Most of the toxic side effects of sulfasalazine are attributable to sulfapyridine. These include nausea, vomiting and upper epigastric distress, headache, diarrhea, anorexia, male infertility, and hypersensitivity reactions (pericarditis, pleuritis, pancreatitis, arthritis, and rash). Because of the toxicity profile associated with sulfasalazine, the 5-aminosalicylic derivative agents are now available for use either for oral or topical administration. A slow, time-dependent release mesalamine (Pentasa) 4 g/day or a pH-dependent release mesalamine (Asacol) 2.4 g/day has the primary advantage of delivery into the colon. Olsalazine (Dipentum) 1 g/day is a derivative of the sodium salt of 5-aminosalicylic acid that is converted to two 5-aminosalicylic acid molecules in the colon and has identical anti-inflammatory properties. Sulfasalazine and all the mesalamine formulations are effective primarily in colonic disease. The topical preparations have limited usefulness in the management of Crohn's disease and should be administered when the disease involves the rectum and no more than 40 cm of distal rectosigmoid.

Glucocorticoids, 40 to 60 mg/day, are reserved for the more severely affected patients and are effective primarily in small intestinal disease as well as in ileocolitis.

Immunosuppressive drugs such as 6-mercaptopurine (1 to 1.5 mg/kg per day) or azathioprine (2 mg/kg per day) are useful as steroid-sparing agents, in healing fistulas, or in patients for whom there are serious contraindications for surgery. Recent evidence suggests that they are also effective as maintenance agents. Both of these agents can be associated with leukopenia, fever, hepatitis, and pancreatitis, necessitating the need for close follow-up, particularly during the initial phase of therapy. The response to immunosuppressives should not be expected before 8 to 12 weeks following the initiation of therapy.

Metronidazole (10 to 20 mg/kg per day) has been shown to be effective in controlled therapeutic trials and it is particularly useful in patients with perianal complications and fistulous disease. Other agents such as cyclosporine, methotrexate, broad-spectrum antibiotics, and lipoxygenase inhibitors or immunoglobulin therapy must all be considered as experimental forms of therapy at this time because of insufficient experience of therapeutic efficacy in controlled clinical trials.

The role of maintenance therapy in patients with ulcerative colitis is well established. Maintenance therapy and effectiveness of various therapeutic agents in Crohn's disease is somewhat less certain. Glucocorticoids should not be used for maintaining a remission because of lack of sufficient evidence for efficacy and the potential for complications. When a patient is responsive to immunosuppression therapy, it would seem advisable to continue this in a reduced dose for the maintenance of remission. Similarly, a reduced dose of 5-aminosalicylic acid derivatives is appropriate for the maintenance of remission of colonic disease.

Diarrhea can be controlled by the use of loperamide (Imodium) 4 to 16 mg/day, diphenoxylate (Lomotil) 5 to 20 mg/day, and cholestyramine 4 g one to three times per day. The latter is particularly useful as an exchange resin in patients who have limited ileal disease or resection, no bowel obstruction, and mild steatorrhea. The mechanism of action is binding of bile acids and eliminating their known cathartic effect. The primary aim of dietary therapy is the maintenance of nutrition and the alleviation of diarrhea. Elimination of lactose from the diet is of benefit in patients with lactose intolerance. Reduction of dietary oxalate should be considered in every patient. In addition, supplementation of trace metals, fat-soluble vitamins, and medium-chain triglycerides should be considered in selected patients.

Surgical intervention is indicated in those patients with complications of the disease, including intestinal obstruction or hemorrhage, perforation, abscess or fistula formation, toxic megacolon, and perianal disease. In addition, surgery may be indicated in those patients who fail medical therapy. The recurrence rate after surgery approaches 100 percent.

## ULCERATIVE COLITIS

Ulcerative colitis is a chronic inflammatory and ulcerative disease of the colon and rectum characterized most often clinically by bloody diarrhea. The etiology, like that of Crohn's disease, remains unknown even though extensive investigations into the cause continue. Epidemiologic considerations are similar to those of Crohn's disease; the disease is more prevalent in the United States and northern Europe, and peak incidence occurs in the second and third decades of life. The incidence of ulcerative colitis is about 5 to 8 cases per 100,000 and, unlike the incidence of Crohn's disease, has not risen significantly in the past few years. First-degree relatives of patients with ulcerative colitis have a 15-fold risk of developing ulcerative colitis and a 3.5-fold risk of developing Crohn's disease.

### Pathology

Ulcerative colitis involves primarily the mucosa and submucosa. Microscopically, the disease is characterized by mucosal inflammation with the formation of crypt abscesses, epithelial necrosis, and mucosal ulceration. The muscular layer and serosa are often spared. In the usual case, the disease increases in severity more distally, the rectosigmoid being involved in 95 percent of cases. In the early stages of the disease, the mucous membranes appear finely granular and friable. In more severe cases, the mucosa appears as a red spongy surface dotted with small ulcerations oozing blood and purulent exudate. In very advanced disease, one sees large oozing ulcerations and pseudopolyps (areas of hyperplastic overgrowth surrounded by inflamed mucosa).

### Clinical Features and Course

The clinical features and course of ulcerative colitis vary but are somewhat dependent on the anatomic distribution of the disease in the colon. The disease is classified as mild, moderate, or severe depending on the clinical manifestations. Patients with mild disease have fewer than four bowel movements per day, no systemic symptoms, and few extraintestinal manifestations. Of all patients with ulcerative colitis, 60 percent have mild disease; in 80 percent of cases the disease is limited to the rectum. Occasionally, constipation and rectal bleeding are the presenting complaint. Progression to pancolitis occurs in 10 to 15 percent of patients with mild disease.

Patients with severe disease constitute 15 percent of those with ulcerative colitis. Severe disease is associated with more than six bowel movements per day, anemia, fever, weight loss, tachycardia, and more frequently extraintestinal manifestations. Patients with severe disease account for 90 percent of the mortality from ulcerative colitis. Virtually all severely affected patients have pancolitis.

Moderate disease is seen in 25 percent of patients. The clinical manifestations are less severe and patients demonstrate a good response to therapy. These patients usually have colitis extending to the splenic flexure (left-sided colitis) but may develop pancolitis.

Most commonly, ulcerative colitis is characterized by intermittent attacks of acute disease with complete remission between attacks. Such a pattern occurs in the majority of patients. In other patients, the first attack is followed by a prolonged period of disease inactivity. Infrequently, patients run a chronically active course. Factors associated with an unfavorable prognosis and increased mortality include the severity and extent of disease, a short history before the first attack, and onset of the disease after 60 years of age.

Extraintestinal complications of ulcerative colitis include peripheral arthritis, ankylosing spondylitis, episcleritis, posterior uveitis, pyoderma gangrenosum, and erythema nodosum.

### Complications

Although blood loss from sustained hemorrhage may be the most common complication of the illness, toxic megacolon is an associated clinical entity that must not be missed.

Toxic megacolon develops in advanced cases of colitis when the disease process begins to extend through all layers of the colon. The result is a loss of muscular tone within the colon and localized peritonitis. The colon begins to dilate as muscular tone is lost. If the colon continues to dilate without treatment, signs of toxicity will develop. Plain radiography of the abdomen demonstrates a long, continuous segment of air-filled colon greater than 6 cm in diameter. The distended portion of the atonic colon can perforate, causing peritonitis and septicemia. Mortality from this complication is approximately 50 percent if perforation occurs but less than 10 percent if surgery is undertaken prior to perforation.

A patient with toxic megacolon appears severely ill; the abdomen is distended, tender, and tympanitic. Severe diarrhea (more than 10 bowel movements per day) is often seen. Fever, tachycardia, and signs of hypovolemia are typically part of the clinical picture. Leukocytosis, anemia, electrolyte disturbances, and hypoalbuminemia are the supporting laboratory data.

Some of the more prominent features of toxic megacolon such as leukocytosis and peritonitis can be masked in the patient taking glucocorticoids. When such therapy is being administered, greater suspicion is required to make the diagnosis. Antidiarrheal agents, hypokalemia, narcotics, cathartics, and enemas have been implicated as precipitating factors in toxic megacolon. Medical therapy with nasogastric suction, intravenous prednisolone (60 g/day) or hydrocortisone (300 mg/day), parenteral antibiotics active against coliforms and anaerobes (ampicillin and clindamycin), and intravenous fluids should be attempted as initial therapy and in preparing the patient for possible surgery. However, prolonged medical treatment of these patients increases mortality; therefore, early surgical consultation must be sought with the aim of performing a colectomy if clinical improvement is not noted in 24 to 48 h with medical treatment.

Local complications such as small rectovaginal fistulas occur infrequently in cases of ulcerative colitis. Perirectal fistulas and abscesses are much more common in patients with Crohn's disease but occur in approximately 20 percent of patients with ulcerative colitis. Massive gastrointestinal hemorrhage, obstruction secondary to stricture formation, and acute perforation are other complications of the disease.

Clinically apparent liver disease may occur in 5 to 10 percent of patients. The manifestations of liver disease may include any of the following: pericholangitis, chronic active hepatitis, fatty liver or cirrhosis, cholelithiasis, sclerosing cholangitis, and bile duct carcinoma.

There is a 10- to 30-fold increase in the development of carcinoma of the colon in patients with ulcerative colitis. Carcinoma of the colon is the cause of 5 to 15 percent of the deaths attributed to ulcerative colitis. The major risk factors for the development of carcinoma of the colon are extensive involvement and prolonged duration of the disease. The cumulative risk of cancer after 15, 20, and 25 years is 8, 12, and 25 percent, respectively. Additional factors that increase the risk of cancer in patients with ulcerative colitis include early onset of the disease and a family history of colon cancer. The availability of fiberoptic colonoscopy allows surveillance of ulcerative colitis patients with periodic colonoscopies and biopsies to detect metaplastic change thought to predict the development of colon cancer. In patients with pancolitis, such surveillance should start 7 to 10 years after the onset of the disease.

### Diagnosis

Laboratory findings in patients with ulcerative colitis are nonspecific; they may include leukocytosis, anemia, thrombocytosis, decreased serum albumin, and abnormal liver function studies. Therefore, the diagnosis of ulcerative colitis rests on the following: a history of abdominal cramps and diarrhea, mucoid stools, stool examination negative for ova and parasites, stool cultures negative for enteric pathogens, and confirmation by sigmoidoscopic examination. The results of the latter examination are abnormal in 95 percent of the patients with ulcerative colitis. The observed pathologic changes vary depending on the severity and duration of the disease. Granularity, friability, ulceration of the mucosa, and, in more advanced cases, pseudopolyposis are quite characteristic.

Rectal biopsy is helpful in very early cases and aids in excluding amebiasis and metaplasia (see under "Pathology," above). Barium enema examination is useful in confirming the diagnosis and defining the extent of involvement of the colon. It is usually performed before biopsy as it is used to differentiate ulcerative colitis from other conditions. Colonoscopy is the most sensitive method for making the diagnosis and defining the extent and severity of the disease. In addition, in the evaluation of the patient for the development of metaplasia or colon cancer, colonoscopy is extremely useful. Barium enema examination and colonoscopy should not be performed in moderately or severely ill patients. Rigid or fiberoptic proctosigmoidoscopy can be used, however, even in the severely ill patient, provided it is done gently and without the administration of any enemas or laxatives.

The major diseases that should be considered in the differential diagnosis of ulcerative colitis include infectious colitis, Crohn's colitis, ischemic colitis, irradiation colitis, and pseudomembranous colitis. When the disease is limited to the rectum, particular attention should be paid to sexually acquired diseases that are seen frequently in the male homosexual population ("gay bowel disease"). Some of the more common diseases in this category include rectal syphilis, gonococcal proctitis, lymphogranuloma venereum, and inflammation caused by herpes simplex virus, *Entamoeba histolytica, Shigella,* and *Campylobacter.*

### Treatment

The majority of patients with mild and moderate disease can be treated as outpatients. Glucocorticoids are effective in inducing a remission in the majority of cases and constitute the mainstay of therapy in an acute attack. Long-term steroid therapy should be initiated in conjunction with a referral to a gastroenterologist. Daily doses of 40 to 60 mg of prednisone are usually sufficient and can be adjusted, depending on the severity of the disease. 5-Aminosalicylic acid enemas have been used with great success to treat patients with active proctitis, proctosigmoiditis, and left-sided colitis (less than 60 cm of active disease). Topical steroid preparations (beclomethasone, hydrocortisone, tixocortol, and budesonide) have also been successful in such patients. This therapy has also been used to maintain remission. Once clinical remission is achieved, steroids should be slowly tapered

and discontinued. There is no evidence that maintenance dosages of steroids reduce the incidence of relapses.

Sulfasalazine has been used in the treatment of acute attacks but is probably inferior to steroids, especially in the more severe cases. Its primary usefulness is in the form of adjunctive therapy and in the maintenance of a remission. Maintenance dosages of 1.5 to 2 g/day significantly reduce the recurrence rate of the disease.

In addition to sulfasalazine, the newer 5-aminosalicylic derivatives are quite effective in inducing remission as well as in maintaining it for ulcerative colitis. The main advantage of the newer agents is reduced side effects from the sulfapyridine moiety of sulfasalazine. The choice of agents available for the treatment of ulcerative colitis is very similar to those used in Crohn's disease (Pentasa, Asacol, and Dipentum). Topical glucocorticoid enemas or 5-aminosalicylic enemas (Rowasa 4 mg/60 mL per day for 3 weeks) or suppositories (500 mg twice daily) are quite effective in distal proctosigmoiditis and have lower systemic side effect profiles. In refractory cases, a combination of glucocorticoids and immunomodulators such as 6-mercaptopurine (1 to 1.5 mg/kg per day) or azathioprine (2 mg/kg per day) should be considered. The beneficial effects of these combination therapy agents will not be seen before 8 to 12 weeks, somewhat limiting their usefulness in very sick patients. For these reasons, surgical intervention with elective proctocolectomy may be necessary.

Supportive measures in the treatment of mild to moderately sick patients include the replenishment of iron stores, a nutritious diet with the elimination of lactose, and adequate physical and psychological rest. Hydrophilic bulk agents such as psyllium (Metamucil) can be used in some patients to improve stool consistency. Antidiarrheal agents should be avoided because they may precipitate toxic megacolon and because they are generally ineffective.

Patients with severe ulcerative colitis should be treated in the hospital. Intravenous steroids or ACTH, replacement of fluids, correction of electrolyte abnormalities, broad-spectrum antibiotics active against coliforms and anaerobes (ampicillin and clindamycin or metronidazole), and hyperalimentation may be considered for the individual patient. When toxic megacolon is suspected, nasogastric suction should be initiated, a surgical consultation should be obtained, and the patient should be observed by frequent examinations and flat films of the abdomen. When the diagnosis of toxic megacolon is established and the patient fails to show dramatic clinical improvement within 24 to 48 h, emergency surgery should be considered. In addition to toxic megacolon, the indications for surgery are colonic perforation, massive lower GI bleeding, suspicion of colon cancer, and disease that is refractory to medical therapy (large doses of steroids required for the control of the disease). The surgical treatment of choice is total proctocolectomy with ileostomy. Because this is not well accepted by most patients, subtotal colectomy with ileorectal anastomosis is being performed in a greater number of cases. Unlike the effects of surgery in Crohn's disease, in ulcerative colitis surgical intervention is curative.

## PSEUDOMEMBRANOUS ENTEROCOLITIS

Pseudomembranous enterocolitis is an inflammatory bowel disorder in which membranelike yellowish plaques of exudate overlay and replace necrotic intestinal mucosa. The incidence of pseudomembranous colitis has been increasing in recent years. Three different syndromes have been described: neonatal pseudomembranous enterocolitis, postoperative pseudomembranous enterocolitis, and antibiotic-associated pseudomembranous colitis. In the latter, broad-spectrum antibiotics, most notably clindamycin, cephalosporins, and ampicillin, alter the gut flora in such a way that toxin-producing *Clostridium difficile* can flourish within the colon. It should be remembered, however, that almost any antibiotic (including metronidazole and vancomycin) can lead to pseudomembranous colitis. The result is a spectrum of clinical manifestations that vary from frequent mucoid watery stools to a toxic picture that includes profuse diarrhea, crampy abdominal pain, fever, leukocytosis, dehydration, and hypovolemia. Rarely, toxic megacolon or colonic perforation may occur in patients with pseudomembranous colitis. The disease typically begins 7 to 10 days after the institution of antibiotic therapy, although in some cases symptoms may be noted within a few days of antibiotic therapy or up to 6 weeks after the antibiotic is discontinued.

The diagnosis is made by a history of antibiotic use and by endoscopy, which reveals characteristic yellowish plaques within the intestinal lumen. Lesions may be seen throughout the entire alimentary tract, although they are typically limited to the right colon. For this reason, colonoscopy may be required in some cases to establish the diagnosis. The diagnosis is confirmed by the demonstration of *C. difficile* toxin in stool filtrates by culture or by rapid enzyme-linked immunoassay techniques.

The treatment of pseudomembranous colitis includes discontinuing antibiotic therapy and instituting supportive measures such as the administration of fluids and the correction of electrolyte abnormalities. Twenty-five percent of patients will respond to such measures. For those patients with mild to moderate disease who do not respond to supportive measures, metronidazole 250 mg four times daily is the therapy of choice. Vancomycin 125 to 250 mg four times daily is an alternative regimen, although this is considerably more expensive than metronidazole.

Severely ill persons must be hospitalized. Oral vancomycin, 500 mg four times a day for 7 to 10 days, is effective in the majority of severely ill patients. The symptoms usually resolve within a few days. Rarely, emergency colectomy may be required for patients with toxic dilatation of the colon or colonic perforation.

Relapses occur in 10 to 20 percent of patients, necessitating a second course of treatment with vancomycin. Other agents that are useful in the treatment of pseudomembranous colitis include metronidazole, 500 mg four times a day, or bacitracin, 1 g per day, both administered for 7 to 10 days orally. The use of antidiarrheal agents may prolong or worsen symptoms in patients with pseudomembranous colitis and should be avoided. Steroids and surgical intervention are rarely needed for patients with pseudomembranous colitis.

## BIBLIOGRAPHY

### Crohn's Disease

Bozdech JM, Farmer RG: Diagnosis of Crohn's disease. *Hepatogastroenterology* 37:8, 1990.

Danzi M: Extraintestinal manifestations of idiopathic inflammatory bowel disease. *Arch Intern Med* 148:297, 1988.

Gran JT, Husby G: Joint manifestations in gastrointestinal disease: Pathophysiological aspects, ulcerative colitis and Crohn's disease. *Dig Dis* 10:274, 1992.

Meyers S, Sachar DB: Medical management of Crohn's disease. *Hepatogastroenterology* 37:42, 1990.

Reddy SB, Jeejeebhoy KN: Acute complications of Crohn's disease. *Crit Care Med* 16:557, 1988.

Rogers AI, Coelho-Borges S: Medical therapy in Crohn's disease. *Postgrad Med* 92(8):169, 1992.

Zenilman ME, Becker JM: Emergencies in inflammatory bowel disease. *Gastroenterol Clin North Am* 17:387, 1988.

### Ulcerative Colitis

Cole AT, Hawkey CJ: New treatments in inflammatory bowel disease. *Br J Hosp Med* 47:581, 1992.

Kirsner JB: Inflammatory bowel disease. Part II: Clinical and therapeutic aspects. *Dis Mon* 37(11):669, 1991.

Linn FV, Peppercorn MA: Drug therapy for inflammatory bowel disease: part II. *Am J Surg* 164:178, 1992.

Shanahan F, Targan S: Medical treatment of inflammatory bowel disease. *Ann Rev Med* 43:125, 1992.

### Pseudomembranous Colitis

Fekety R, Shah AB: Diagnosis and treatment of *Clostridium difficile* colitis. *JAMA* 269:71, 1993.

Fortson WC, Tedesco FJ: Drug-induced colitis: A review. *Am J Gastroenterol* 79:878, 1984.

Wilcox MH, Spencer RC: *Clostridium difficile* infection: Responses, relapses and reinfections. *J Hosp Infect* 22:85, 1992.

# 82

# COLONIC DIVERTICULAR DISEASE
## Stephen G. Priest
## Steven N. Klein

Acquired diverticular disease of the colon has become an increasingly common disorder of industrialized nations. Diverticulosis coli was first described in the early 1700s by Littre but was not identified as a pathologic entity until the mid-nineteenth century by Cruveilhier. Radiologic studies have suggested that one-third of the population will have acquired the disease by age 45 and two-thirds by age 85. Diverticula of the colon are rare in individuals under age 20.

Inflammation resulting in clinical diverticulitis has been estimated to occur in 10 to 25 percent of patients with known diverticulosis, and the incidence increases with age. Diverticulitis in the younger age group tends to be a more virulent form of the disease, with frequent complications requiring earlier surgical intervention.

Early literature indicated that the frequency of the disease was higher in men. Recent reports have shown an increased incidence in women.

## PATHOPHYSIOLOGY

Colonic diverticula are, by definition, false diverticula because they do not include all the layers of the bowel wall. They consist of mucosa and submucosa with the peritoneal covering that has herniated through a defect in the circular muscle layer of the wall. The sites of herniation are located between the mesenteric and antimesenteric taenia where intramural blood vessels penetrate the muscularis.

A pathophysiologic mechanism to explain the development of diverticular disease is not apparent. It is still unresolved whether diverticular disease is a disorder of colonic motility, a colonic muscle abnormality, a connective tissue disorder, or a normal concomitant of aging. The most common hypothesis is that acquired diverticula arise because of high intraluminal pressures in areas of relative weakness of the colonic wall. This is based upon observations that the majority of patients have diverticula located within the sigmoid colon. Laplace's law states that the tension on the wall of a hollow cylinder is proportional to the radius of the cylinder multiplied by the pressure within the cylinder. This suggests that the intraluminal pressure in the colon is greatest where the lumen is narrowest. The diameter of the colon is smallest in the sigmoid region, and thus this region of the colon is the most likely location for the development of diverticula.

The complications of diverticular disease that bring the patient to the emergency department can be divided into two broad categories: (1) inflammation and its associated complications and (2) bleeding.

Diverticulitis, or inflammation, is the most common complication of diverticular disease. It results when fecal material becomes inspissated in the neck of an acquired diverticulum, resulting in subsequent bacterial proliferation and adjacent peridiverticulitis. Fortunately, fecal contamination of the peritoneum is usually limited because perforation of a diverticulum is into the leaves of the mesentery, or because the contamination is walled off by the mobile loops of the sigmoid colon or small bowel and adjacent pelvic structures. Free perforation may occur with generalized peritonitis, but fortunately it is uncommon.

## DIAGNOSIS

The most common symptom of diverticulitis is pain. This is commonly described as a steady, deep discomfort in the left lower quadrant. Rarely, the clinical presentation may be indistinguishable from that of acute appendicitis. This may occur when the patient has a redundant sigmoid colon lying on the right side of the abdomen which becomes inflamed. Cases of diverticulitis in the cecum or ascending colon have also been reported. In patients 50 years or older, the possibility of diverticulitis should always be considered in the patient with right lower quadrant abdominal pain.

Patients will frequently complain of a change in bowel habits, either in the form of diarrhea or increasing constipation. Tenesmus is another common symptom. The involved diverticulum may irritate the bladder or ureter, causing the patient to have urinary frequency, dysuria, or pyuria. If a fistula develops between the colon and the bladder, the patient may present with recurrent urinary tract infections or pneumaturia. Paralytic ileus with abdominal distension, nausea, and vomiting may develop secondary to intraabdominal irritation and peritonitis. Small bowel obstruction may also occur if an adjacent loop of small bowel becomes kinked or narrowed in the inflammatory mass.

The patient with free perforation will often present with a history of sudden onset of abdominal pain usually beginning in the lower abdomen and then progressing to generalized abdominal involvement. The patient appears quite toxic with signs of diffuse peritonitis.

## PHYSICAL EXAMINATION

Physical examination frequently demonstrates a low-grade fever around 38°C (100.4°F). The temperature may, however, be more elevated in patients with generalized peritonitis or in those who have formed an abscess. The abdominal examination reveals localized tenderness often with voluntary guarding and localized rebound tenderness. With careful palpation, one may be able to appreciate a fullness or a mass over the involved segment of the colon. Rectal examination will often reveal tenderness on the left side. In the female patient, a pelvic examination should always be carried out to eliminate a gynecologic source of symptoms.

## LABORATORY STUDIES

Laboratory studies should include routine screening blood tests, urinalysis, and an acute abdominal series. Unfortunately, in many cases laboratory studies are not helpful in the diagnosis. Leukocytosis was seen in only 36 percent of 130 patients treated at the Lahey Clinic for acute complications of diverticular disease. The acute abdominal series may be normal or may demonstrate associated ileus, partial small bowel obstruction, colonic obstruction, free air indicating bowel perforation, or extraluminal collections of air that might indicate a walled-off abscess. Additional noninvasive studies which may be useful include abdominal and pelvic ultrasonography or a CT scan of the abdomen and pelvis. These studies may show bowel wall thickening, mesenteric inflammation, or abdominal fluid collections indicating abscess formation.

Controversy exists regarding the use of sigmoidoscopy or contrast radiographic studies in the acute inflammatory state. The general opinion is that these studies should be performed after the acute inflammatory process has subsided following conservative medical management.

## DIFFERENTIAL DIAGNOSIS

In patients over the age of 40 presenting with complaints of abdominal pain, a change in bowel habits, and urinary symptoms, a diagnosis of colonic diverticulitis should be entertained. These symptoms, however, are nonspecific, and a number of pathologic entities may present with similar signs and symptoms (Table 82-1).

### Irritable Bowel Syndrome

One-third of the patients surgically treated for diverticulitis lack microscopic inflammatory changes in the resected specimen. These patients are said to have had "painful diverticular disease," or irritable bowel syndrome. Their symptoms included diffuse crampy or colicky abdominal pain, brought on by meals or emotional upset. The passage of flatus or a bowel movement may bring relief of symptoms. Bowel habits can include alternating bouts of constipation and diarrhea. On physical examination, these patients may have a cordlike mass in the left lower quadrant corresponding to the sigmoid colon but lack signs of localized or generalized peritonitis. Laboratory studies are normal and the patient is afebrile.

### Carcinoma of the Colon

The differentiation of diverticulitis from colon carcinoma is usually not difficult. If a cancer has progressed in size to cause luminal narrowing, then a patient may present with a change in bowel habits, with either diarrhea or constipation, and/or abdominal pain which can mimic symptoms of acute diverticulitis. There may be blood mixed with the patient's stools, and weight loss. Physical examination may reveal a palpable mass, usually nontender. Fever and chills are less common, and laboratory studies may demonstrate anemia without evidence of leukocytosis.

If a patient with colonic obstruction but without symptoms of acute diverticulitis has evidence of diverticular disease on barium enema, the diagnosis could be either obstruction due to an inflamed diverticuloma or colon carcinoma with underlying diverticulosis. X-ray changes which may be helpful in differentiating between the two include the length of the segment involved and whether or not the mucosa is intact. Adenocarcinoma of the colon is a mucosal disorder that results in mucosal destruction, a short segment of involvement, and overhanging edges. Diverticular disease originates outside the lumen of the colon so that the bowel mucosa remains intact, and the segments of bowel involvement tend to be longer. If there are no signs of acute inflammation, then fiberoptic colonoscopy can be used to differentiate between diverticular disease and carcinoma.

**Table 82-1.** Differential Diagnosis for Diverticulitis

Irritable bowel syndrome
Carcinoma of the colon
Acute appendicitis
Ulcerative colitis
Crohn's disease
Pelvic inflammatory disease
Ischemic colitis
Leaking aortic aneurysm
Renal calculus
Other colonic diseases
  Amebiasis
  Lymphogranuloma venereum
  Gonorrheal proctitis
  Fecal impaction
  Foreign-body granuloma
  Endometriosis
  Collagen disease
  Postirradiation proctosigmoiditis
  Tuberculosis
  Syphilis
  Actinomycosis

## Acute Appendicitis

A redundant loop of inflamed sigmoid colon or inflamed diverticula of the right side of the colon may mimic acute appendicitis. Therefore, in patients over the age of 50, diverticulitis should always be considered in the differential diagnosis of acute appendicitis.

## Ulcerative Colitis

Inflammatory bowel disease is commonly seen in individuals under the age of 30. There does, however, exist a secondary peak in the incidence of newly diagnosed ulcerative colitis and Crohn's disease in individuals in their sixth decade. Patients with ulcerative colitis may present with frequent loose bowel movements and rectal bleeding. On physical examination, abdominal tenderness is usually absent and no masses are palpable. Difficulty again arises in the individual who has diverticulosis and concomitant ulcerative colitis. In these individuals, radiographic and endoscopic studies are most helpful.

## Crohn's Disease

Crohn's disease is a transmural disease which can cause fistulae and abscesses. Patients may present with symptoms indistinguishable from those of acute diverticulitis, and a careful history should be taken. Patients with Crohn's disease will often present with diarrhea, mucous discharge, and rectal complaints. The association of perianal disease, such as unusual fissures, fistulas, or large skin tags, is suggestive of Crohn's disease. Sigmoidoscopy and biopsy can establish the diagnosis.

## Pelvic Inflammatory Disease

Pelvic inflammatory disease may present with abdominal pain, fever, and leukocytosis, and it usually occurs in young women. A careful pelvic examination should be carried out in all female patients. A history of irregular menses, and the finding of vaginal discharge, should aid in the diagnosis.

## Ischemic Colitis

Ischemic colitis can present with a broad range of clinical manifestations. Mild transient ischemia may result in mucosal sloughing and painless rectal bleeding. If the disease progresses to gangrene, the patient develops severe abdominal pain and peritonitis. Pain may be out of proportion to physical findings. A plain film of the abdomen may reveal thumb printing in the region of the involved colonic segment. In more advanced cases, there may be gas within the bowel wall, or, if perforation has occurred, free air in the abdomen. Cautious endoscopic evaluation and contrast x-ray studies are helpful in distinguishing ischemic colitis from diverticulitis.

## MEDICAL TREATMENT

Patients who have localized pain without signs and symptoms of local peritonitis or systemic infection may be treated on an outpatient basis. Treatment consists of bowel rest and broad-spectrum oral antibiotic therapy. Patients are instructed to limit activity and to maintain a liquid diet for 48 h. If symptoms improve, low-residue foods are added to the diet. Broad-spectrum antibiotics covering both aerobic and anaerobic bacteria are given. Predominant colonic aerobes include *Escherichia coli, Klebsiella,* and *Enterobacter,* while *Bacteroides fragilis, Peptostreptococcus,* and *Clostridium* are the predominant colonic anaerobes. Common oral antibiotic agents effective against aerobic organisms include ampicillin (500 mg q 6 h), trimethoprim-sulfamethoxazole (2 tablets q 12 h), ciprofloxacin (500 mg q 12 h), or a cephalosporin, such as cefalexin (500 mg q 6 h). One of these agents is taken in combination with metronidazole (Flagyl, 500 mg q 8 h), or clindamycin (Cleocin, 300 mg q 6 h) which are utilized to treat the anaerobic organisms. Patients are instructed to contact their physicians if increasing abdominal pain, fever, or malaise occurs. Once the patient has improved, elective evaluation with contrast barium enema is performed.

## Admission Indications

If a patient has systemic signs and symptoms of infection, or localized peritonitis, then hospitalization is necessary. Again, the patient is placed on bowel rest, but in this case, nothing by mouth is given and intravenous fluids are administered. Nasogastric suction is necessary only if the patient manifests signs of bowel obstruction or an adynamic ileus. Surgical consultation should be obtained at the time of hospitalization. Intravenous antibiotics, usually ampicillin and an aminoglycoside, and clindamycin or metronidazole, are given for aerobic and anaerobic coverage.

## LOWER GASTROINTESTINAL BLEEDING AS A COMPLICATION OF DIVERTICULOSIS

In the past, most cases of massive lower gastrointestinal bleeding were attributed to diverticular disease. Over the last 20 years, however, with the development of selective mesenteric angiography and endoscopy, it has been shown that arteriovenous malformations are as common a cause of lower gastrointestinal bleeding as diverticulosis.

Nevertheless, bleeding occurs in 5 to 15 percent of the patients with diverticulosis. Diverticular bleeding is generally massive, but, fortunately, in 75 to 95 percent of the cases, bleedings stops spontaneously and can be managed with supportive therapy.

Although the majority of cases of massive lower gastrointestinal bleeding are caused by colonic diverticula or arteriovenous malformations, other etiologic factors should be considered. These include colonic tumors, inflammatory bowel disease, ischemic colitis, Meckel's diverticulum, and radiation enteritis.

## Pathogenesis

Diverticula form in areas of relative weakness created by the penetrating vasa recta. As the colonic mucosa herniates, the vasa recta are stretched and displaced over the fundus of the herniated pouch. Bleeding results when the vasa recta rupture into the diverticulum.

## Clinical Features

Lower gastrointestinal bleeding may originate from anywhere within the gastrointestinal tract. Upper gastrointestinal tract sources of bleeding must always be considered. The most common sites of upper gastrointestinal bleeding include duodenal ulcers, gastric erosions, gastric ulcers, esophageal varices, and Mallory-Weiss tears.

A careful history must be obtained, with particular attention to previous gastric or duodenal ulceration and associated abdominal, rectal, or anal symptoms. One should inquire about the onset and duration of bleeding, and whether the stools are bright red in nature and forming clots, or melanotic. Since diverticular bleeding is usually painless, the presence of abdominal pain suggests another disease process. Certain medications, and alcohol abuse, also predispose to bleeding.

## Diagnosis

Physical examination is often unremarkable. Abdominal examination may reveal a mass or tenderness suggesting causes of bleeding other than diverticula. Careful anorectal examination is necessary to ensure that fissures or hemorrhoids are not the source of bleeding. Normally, the latter do not cause serious gastrointestinal hemorrhage; however, severe hemorrhage can occur if portal hypertension is present. Proctosigmoidoscopy is necessary to identify lesions within the rectum or lower sigmoid colon that might cause bleeding, and also to ensure that no significant abnormalities within the distal bowel are present if emergent total abdominal colectomy becomes necessary. In this situation, the rectum can be saved and used for a primary anastomosis.

If anorectal causes of major lower gastrointestinal bleeding have been excluded, then a nasogastric tube should be inserted and the gastric contents aspirated to detect blood. Bilious return should be identified to be sure that an adequate sampling has been taken. Even if the nasogastric aspirate does contain bile but no gross blood, bleeding from an upper gastrointestinal source cannot be completely excluded. If there is evidence of bleeding, then an urgent esophagogastroduodenoscopy should be carried out.

### Emergency Department Care

At the time of resuscitation, blood should be drawn for type and crossmatch, CBC, coagulation profiles including bleeding time, and screening evaluations including serum electrolyte and liver function studies. Two large-bore IVs should be initiated in all patients with significant blood loss.

Once the patient is stabilized, and no obvious source of bleeding has been identified, then further studies are necessary. The next diagnostic test is a $^{99m}$Tc-labeled red blood cell scan, which can identify bleeding rates as low as 0.12 mL/min. If an area of active bleeding is identified, then selective mesenteric arteriography should be carried out. However, in order for an arteriogram to identify bleeding, the rate of blood loss must be rapid, greater than 0.5 mL/min.

If arteriography positively identifies a bleeding site, selective perfusion of vasopressin may be used in an attempt to control bleeding. If bleeding remains uncontrolled, a segmental resection of the involved colon should be carried out.

If the $^{99m}$Tc-labeled red blood cell scan is negative and bleeding stops, total colonoscopy is necessary in an attempt to identify the bleeding source. If no bleeding source is identified, but hemorrhage continues, requiring transfusions of more than 6 units of blood within 24 h, then emergency surgery should be considered. Total abdominal colectomy with ileorectal anastomosis or a temporary ileostomy is usually performed.

Fortunately, most diverticular bleeding stops spontaneously with supportive therapy. Twenty-five percent of patients will require subsequent hospitalization for recurrent bleeding. After a second bleeding episode, the risk of a third hemorrhage approaches 50 percent.

### BIBLIOGRAPHY

Freeman SR, McNally PR: Diverticulitis. *Med Clin North Am* 77(5):1149, 1993.

Milsom JW, Singh G.: Diverticulitis in young patients. *Semin colon* and *rectal surg* 1:103, 1990.

Opelka FG, Timmcke AE: Management of Bleeding Diverticulosis: Colonic diverticulitis. *Semin Colon Rectal Surg* 1, 1990.

Roberts PL, Veidenheimer MC: Current management of diverticulitis. *Adv Surg* 27:189, 1994.

# 83
# ANORECTAL DISORDERS
## James K. Bouzoukis

Anorectal disorders are varied and multiple and may also be complex, manifesting signs and symptoms of underlying serious local or systemic disorders that could be life-threatening.

### ANATOMY

The anorectum is an anatomical structure in which the entodermal intestine unites with and opens into an orifice of ectodermal origin: the anal canal. The junction of these two embryonic structures (the anorectal line) is the dentate line, which marks the anatomical beginning of the anal canal (1 to 2 cm long) and is in continuity with the perianal skin at its distal anal verge. The mucosa of the anal canal consists of stratified squamous epithelium but contains no hair follicles or sweat glands. At the anal verge (perianal region), the anoderm thickens and includes in its structure hair follicles and other cutaneous appendages. Proximal to the dentate line the rectal ampulla narrows to conform to the opening of the anal canal, and in doing so its mucosa takes on a pleated appearance, forming 8 to 14 convoluted longitudinal folds: the columns of Morgagni. Each adjacent column is connected at the dentate line by a flap of mucosa that forms a small anal crypt, normally 1 to 3 mm in longitudinal depth.

At the base of approximately one-half of these crypts is a small rudimentary anal gland that may extend centrifugally through the internal sphincter as far as the intersphincteric plane (an extension of the rectum's longitudinal muscle layer) but does not penetrate into the external sphincter. Infection and inflammation of these crypts and glands become the source of anal sepsis as characterized by the development of cryptitis, fissures, abscesses, and fistulas.

The anal wall, from its mucosal lining to the intersphincteric plane that separates the internal from the external sphincters, is a continuation of the usual layers of the wall of the colon and rectum. The innermost lining, mucosa, continues to the anal verge, undergoing a transition, just proximal to the dentate line, from rectal columnar to cuboidal to squamous epithelium. The submucosa, which normally contains the bulk of the bowel's blood vessels (and autonomic nerves), thickens considerably proximal to the dentate line, and its dilated veins in this area are referred to as the internal hemorrhoidal plexus. Likewise, the inner circular muscle layer of the rectum thickens considerably as it terminates distally in the anorectum to form the internal sphincter muscles, while the more attenuated longitudinal muscles of the rectum extend caudally, blending with fibers of voluntary skeletal muscles from the levator ani and external sphincter groups to form the intersphincteric plane (Fig. 83-1).

Additional sphincteric support is provided by an outer layer of voluntary skeletal muscles, the external sphincters, that are divided into three parts: deep, superficial, and subcutaneous. The external sphincters are actually a caudal extension of the puborectalis muscle, which interacts with the levator ani muscle that forms the pelvic floor. The puborectalis, the proximal external sphincters, and the internal sphincters form the ring of muscles that one palpates when performing a digital examination of the anorectum.

Lateral to the external sphincters and superior to the levator ani are the ischiorectal and pelvirectal spaces, where deep, life-threatening infections can occur.

### EXAMINATION OF THE PATIENT

No matter how much historical information is obtained, no definitive diagnosis can be made without a careful examination of the anus and rectum, including anoscopy and, if necessary, proctoscopy.

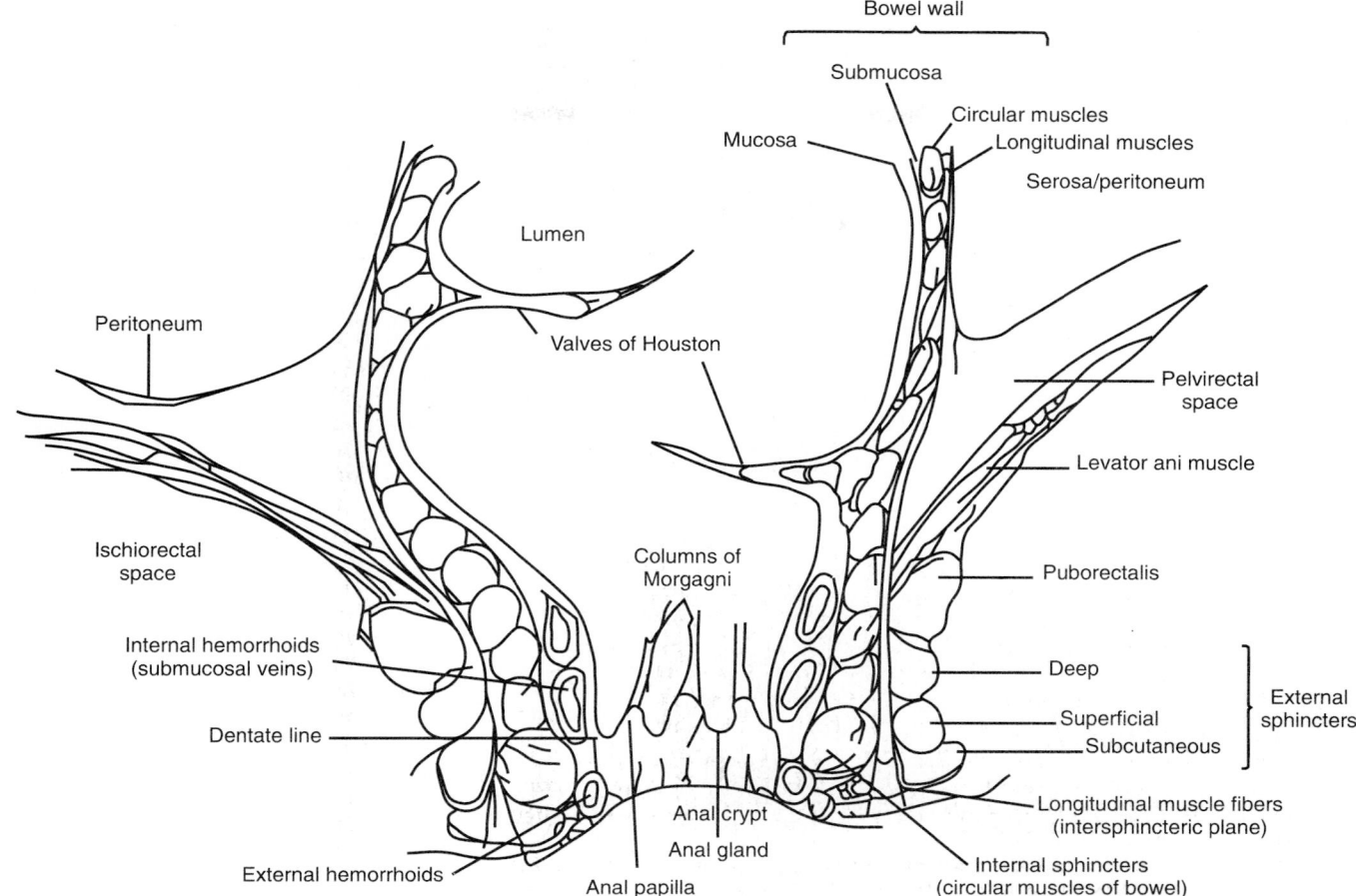

**Fig. 83-1.** Coronal section of the anorectum.

The patient should be placed in any one of three positions (Fig. 83-2). The lateral, or Sim's, position, performed with the patient lying on his or her left side with the left leg extended and the right knee and hip flexed, is probably the most commonly used approach for performing a routine digital rectal examination and is the preferred position for elderly or pregnant patients who would not otherwise tolerate the knee-chest position. In debilitated patients, one may have to perform the examination with the patient in a supine, lithotomy position. From the Sim's position, one should elevate the upper right buttock to provide better exposure of the perianal area, and, if needed, endoscopic examination of the anus and distal rectum can be performed with the patient in this position.

Examining a patient placed in the knee-chest position requires a cooperative patient who is not too ill or in too much distress. This provides for a thorough inspection of the perianal area and is convenient for anoscopy and proctoscopy. Thighs should be at right angles to the table with the feet extended over the end of the table.

The optimal position for examining and treating anorectal lesions is with the patient prone on a proctoscopic table that is tilted to place the anus in an uppermost position (Fig. 83-2C).

A digital examination should always be performed before doing any endoscopic procedure. No bowel preparation is needed to perform an anoscopic examination. After performing a digital examination and determining that the patient will tolerate passage of an anoscope, introduce a well-lubricated, lighted anoscope (Fig. 83-3); remove the obturator; and gently rotate it 360° to view the anorectum circumferentially.

It is usually difficult to perform a proper sigmoidoscopic examination in an emergency department setting. Ordinarily, the lower bowel has to be prepped; a natural bowel movement, spontaneous or induced, 1 to 2 h before examination is usually sufficient preparation. In some acute situations, such as trying to determine the source of lower GI bleeding or obtaining cultures in a case of suppurative proctitis, emergency proctoscopy may be performed. A rigid sigmoidoscope should be utilized, with the patient placed in a proctoscopic or Sim's position, depending on how hemodynamically stable the patient is. An inexperienced endoscopist should not attempt to pass the sigmoidoscope beyond the rectosigmoid junction, where the lumen is greatly angulated, because of the risk of perforation.

## HEMORRHOIDS

The anorectal area is drained by the internal and external hemorrhoidal venous systems. The internal hemorrhoidal veins, which in essence are submucosal vascular cushions that may contribute to anal continence, are located proximal to the dentate line and drain into the portal system through the superior rectals and the inferior mesenteric vein. They also communicate freely with the external hemorrhoidal veins, which are subcutaneous to the anoderm and which drain primarily through the pudendal and iliac venous systems. When these hemorrhoidal plexuses become excessively engorged, prolapsed, or thrombosed, they are referred to as hemorrhoids—one of the most common problems afflicting human beings.

Internal hemorrhoids, which course along the terminal branches of the superior rectal artery, are constant in their location, coursing longitudinally at the right posterolateral, right anterolateral, and left lateral positions (at the 2-, 5- and 9-o'clock positions when the patient is viewed prone) (Fig. 83-4). Internal hemorrhoids are not readily palpable and can best be visualized through an anoscope. External hem-

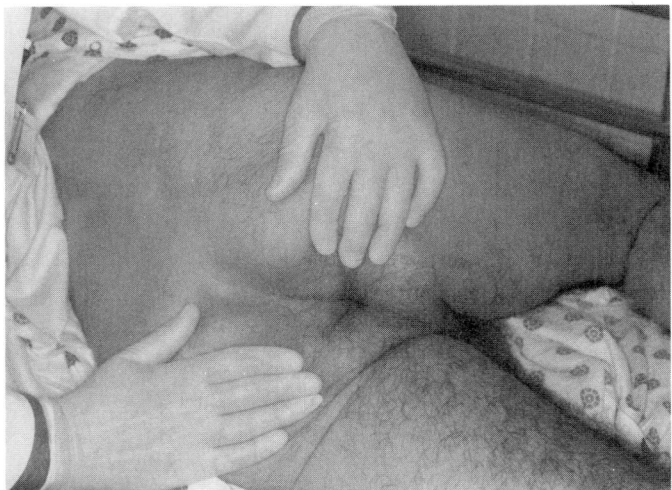

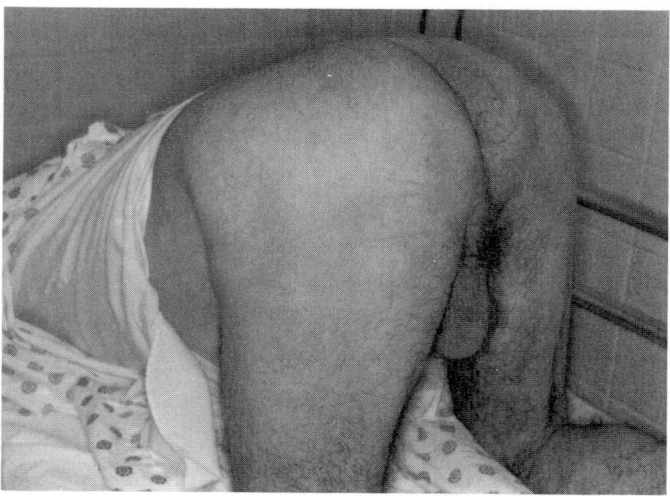

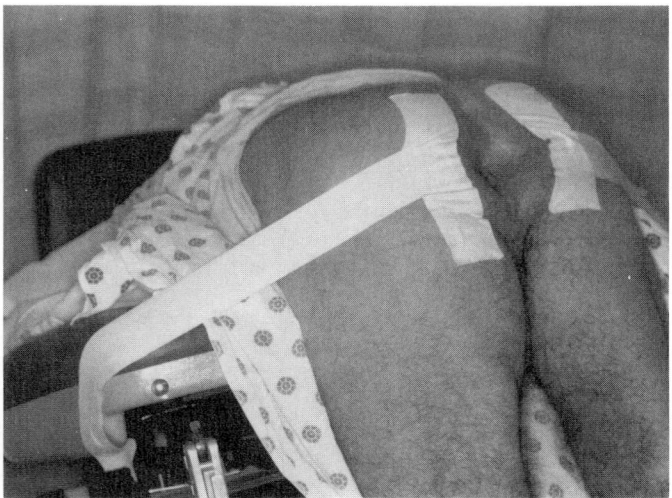

**Fig. 83-2.** Positioning the patient for anorectal examination. **A.** Lateral, or Sims' position. **B.** The knee-chest position. **C.** Position on the proctoscopic table. See the text for detailed descriptions.

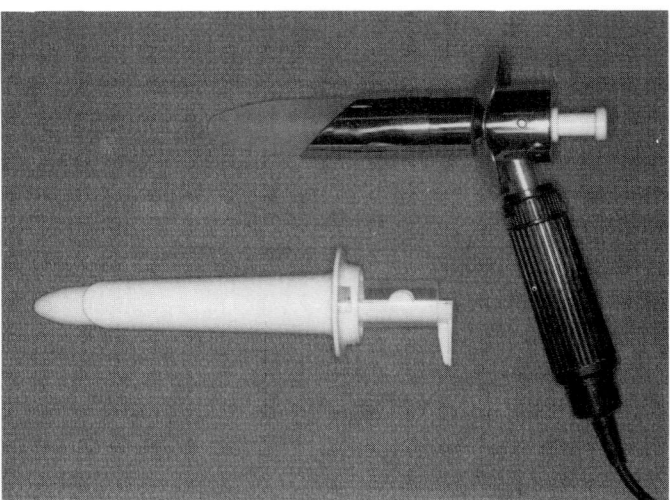

**Fig. 83-3.** Two types of anoscope. *Top:* Lighted anoscope with power source attached to handle. *Bottom:* Disposable anoscope. An extrinsic light source is required.

orrhoids are dilatation of veins at the anal verge and can be seen at external inspection.

Although the cause of hemorrhoids is not always known, there is an association with constipation and straining at stool. They are very during pregnancy and may be the result of sustained increased pressure on the venous drainage of the rectum. One of the physiologic shunts of the portal system involves the hemorrhoidal veins. Consequently, increased portal pressure, occurring as a result of chronic liver disease, may produce marked dilatation and varix formation of the hemorrhoids. The bleeding that can result is extremely difficult to control.

Tumors of the rectum and sigmoid colon, often associated with constipation, tenesmus, and incomplete evacuation, may cause hemorrhoids and must be ruled out in all cases of rectal bleeding in patients over the age of 40.

## Clinical Features

Uncomplicated internal hemorrhoids are painless, and the chief complaint is painless, bright-red rectal bleeding with defecation. Bleeding is usually limited, with the blood being found on the surface of the stool, on the toilet tissue, or dripping into the toilet bowl. Although the most common cause of rectal bleeding is hemorrhoids, other, more serious causes should be sought in all patients who present with bleeding as the chief complaint. Chronic, slow blood loss may go unnoticed but can result in a significant anemia. Pain, when present, is most severe at the time of defecation and subsides with time. Pain is usually associated with thrombosed external hemorrhoids.

As they increase in size, hemorrhoids may prolapse, requiring periodic reduction by the patient (Table 83-1). When prolapse occurs, the patient may develop a mucous discharge and pruritus ani.

If the prolapse cannot be reduced, strangulation can result. Other complications include severe bleeding and thrombosis. Both strangulation and thrombosis are extremely painful and are accompanied by

**Table 83-1.** Classification of Internal Hemorrhoids

| Degree | Symptoms |
| --- | --- |
| First | Bleeding; local, compressible swelling |
| Second | Protrude with defecation, reduce spontaneously; ± bleeding |
| Third | Protrude with defecation; must be reduced manually; ± bleeding |
| Fourth | Incarcerated |

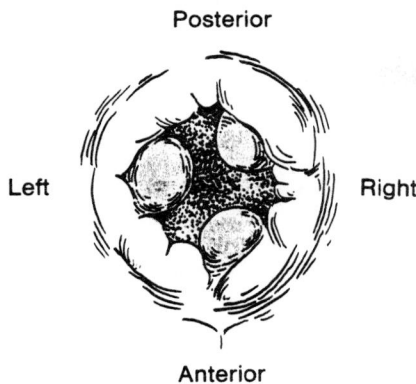

**A**

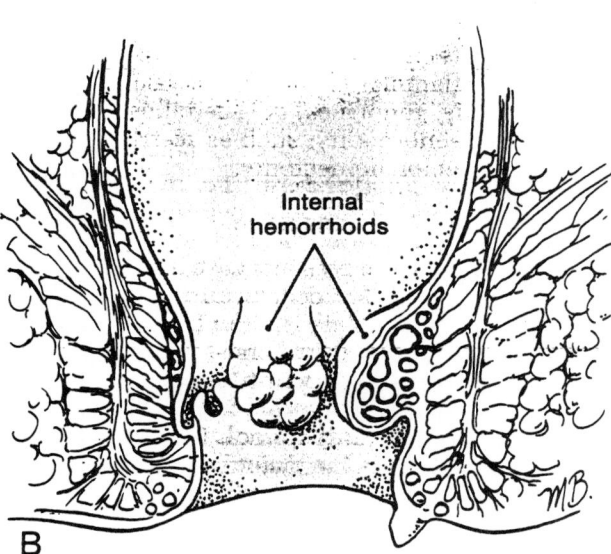

**B**

**Fig. 83-4. A.** Common sites of hemorrhoids. **B.** Protrusion of anal cushions. Internal hemorrhoids at 2, 5, and 9 o'clock. (From Barker LR, Burton JR, Zieve PD (eds): *Principles of Ambulatory Medicine,* 3d ed. Baltimore, Williams & Wilkins, 1991, p. 1262. Used by permission.)

significant edema that must be treated before surgical intervention. Ulceration of the overlying mucosa may also occur.

## Treatment

Most treatment is local and nonsurgical unless a complication is present. Hot sitz baths for at least 15 min three times a day and after each bowel movement are the most effective way to relieve pain and edema. Following the bath, the anus must be dried gently but thoroughly to avoid maceration of the perianal skin. Use of topical antibiotics, anesthetics, or steroidal creams are of limited value and may cause more harm. The patient should not sit for a prolonged period on the commode. Bulk laxatives, such as psyllium seed compounds, or stool softeners should be used after the acute phase is treated. Laxatives causing liquid stool must be avoided; this can result in cryptitis and anal sepsis. The addition of bran or other forms of roughage to the patient's diet should help ameliorate future problems.

As a rule, internal hemorrhoids bleed and, if not prolapsed, are not

palpable. External hemorrhoids thrombose. Selection of therapy for thrombosed external hemorrhoids depends on the severity of symptoms: if the thrombosis has been present less than 48 h, the swelling is not tense, and the pain is tolerable, the patient may be treated with sitz baths and bulk laxatives. Suppositories, which are placed proximal to the anorectal ring, are of no help. If, on the other hand, thrombosis is acute and recent in origin, significant relief can be provided by excising the clots. With the patient in prone position, the area of the overlying skin to be incised is infiltrated with a local anesthetic using a 30-gauge needle. While applying gentle traction to the skin adjacent to the thrombosed hemorrhoid, an elliptical incision is made in the overlying skin, exposing the thrombosed vein, which is locally excised with the elliptical flap of skin (Fig. 83-5). Because of the multiloculated clots that are invariably present, the technique of unroofing a thrombosed hemorrhoid with an elliptical incision gives far better results than the simple incision and evacuation of a clot. Bleeding is controlled by tucking the corner of a small piece of gauze into the wound and leaving it in place for a few hours. A small pressure dressing may be applied external to the gauze and removed when the patient takes the first sitz bath 6 to 12 h after the drainage procedure. Narcotics may be prescribed, but only judiciously, since they cause constipation and may produce more problems.

Surgical referral and intervention for hemorrhoids is indicated for continued bleeding; incarceration and/or strangulation; severe, unrelenting pruritus; and intractable pain. Surgical treatment can consist of sclerosing injections, the use of rubber band ligation (the current, most common form of surgical treatment), or excision. Up to 5 percent of patients undergoing rubber band ligation may develop acute thrombosis of external hemorrhoids, and immunocompromised patients treated with band ligation may develop pelvic sepsis.

## CRYPTITIS

Anal crypts are the superficial mucosal pockets that lie between the columns of Morgagni. They are formed by the puckering action of the sphincter muscles and normally flatten out during the passage of a

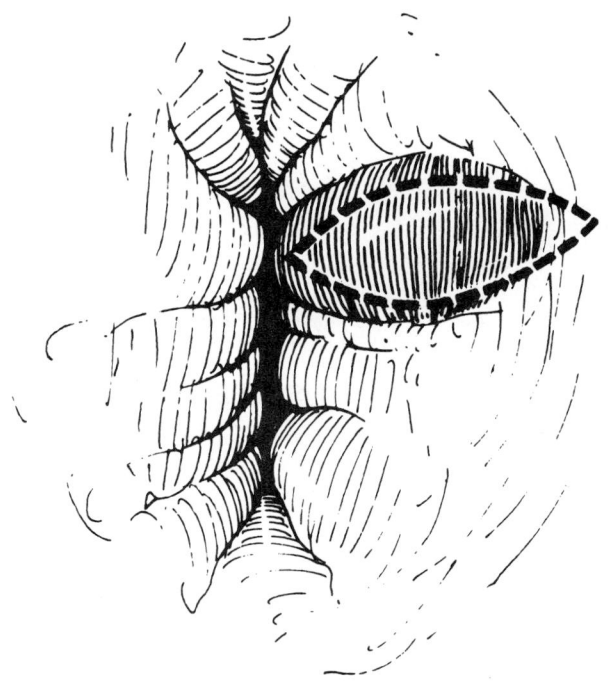

**Fig. 83-5.** Elliptical excision of thrombosed external hemorrhoid. (From Goldberg SM et al: *Essentials of Anorectal Surgery.* Philadelphia, Lippincott, 1980. Used by permission.)

stool. Sphincter spasm and superficial trauma caused by repeated bouts of diarrhea or trauma produced by evacuation of large, hard stools associated with constipation cause breakdown in the mucosal lining of the crypts. This permits infecting organisms to enter pockets and inflammation to extend into the lymphoid tissue of both the crypts and anal glands. Cryptitis could well be the common denominator for the development of such anal infections as fissure in ano, perianal and rectal abscesses, and fistula in ano.

Associated with cryptitis is the development of hypertrophied anal papillae, which lie between adjacent crypts. When hypertrophy occurs, the papillae may be palpated as small, hard nodules along the wall of the anal canal. Rarely, papillae may hypertrophy and present as a prolapsing polypoid tumor. The crypts most commonly involved are in the posterior half of the anal ring and, in most cases, in the posterior midline, the same location where anal fissures occur.

## Clinical Features

Initially, the locally inflamed crypts produce no symptoms, but as the trauma from recurrent diarrhea or passage of large, hard stools continues, the inflammation of the crypts extends to the adjacent papillae, producing an edematous swelling of the sensitive anoderm that lines this part of the canal. At this stage, the patient will experience pain with bowel movements, and if there is an associated papillitis or fissure in ano, there will also be a small amount of bleeding. Anal pain, spasm, and itching with or without bleeding are the cardinal signs and symptoms of cryptitis.

## Treatment

Treatment of anal cryptitis, which should be conservative, is based on establishing a definitive diagnosis and ruling out the possibility of more serious anorectal problems. The diagnosis can be suspected clinically from the history and the palpation of the tender, swollen crypt and its associated hypertrophied papillae. Definitive diagnosis of cryptitis is made by anoscopic examination. Gentle insertion of a hooked probe into the crypts brought into view through the anoscope will reveal the involved crypt(s) to be deeper than normal and definitely more tender.

The goal of treatment is to control the trauma of abnormal bowel movements and thus enable the inflammation to subside. Bulk laxatives and additional roughage to the diet to produce formed, soft stools combined with hot sitz baths and/or warm rectal irrigations greatly enhance healing by keeping the anus clean and the crypts empty.

Surgical intervention is indicated when the infection has progressed and there is a deep, redundant crypt that will not drain adequately on its own. In these cases, the roof (mucosal surface), as outlined by the passage of a hooked probe, should be infiltrated with local anesthetic and excised. Thus, what had been a deep pocket is converted into an open wound that should heal with proper control of bowel movements and frequent sitz baths.

## FISSURE IN ANO (ANAL FISSURE)

This disorder is the result of a linear tear of the anal canal beginning at or just below the dentate line and extending distally along the anal canal. The epithelium in this area consists of anoderm, which has a rich supply of somatic sensory nerve fibers. Consequently, anal fissures are the most common cause of painful rectal bleeding.

Anal fissures are often associated with swelling of the surrounding tissues, producing hypertrophic papillae proximally and the characteristic sentinel pile distally. The latter is frequently misdiagnosed as an external hemorrhoid when in actuality it is the result of edema and fibrosis secondary to the ulcerating fissure. In more than 90 percent of cases, anal fissures occur in the midline posteriorly. In 10 percent of women but in only 1 percent of men, it may be in the midline anteriorly. This almost constant location of anal fissures may be because of the posterior angulation of the rectum on the anus where the posterior midline of the proximal anal canal becomes the "lesser curvative" for the passage of stool. A fissure not located in the midline should arouse suspicion that another, potentially life-threatening cause may be involved. Such diagnostic possibilities include Crohn's disease, chronic ulcerative colitis, squamous cell carcinoma of the anus, adenocarcinoma of the rectum invading the anal canal, localized anal cancers such as Bowen's disease and extramammary Paget's disease, leukemia, lymphoma, syphilitc fissures, and tuberculous ulcer. Such patients must be referred for a diagnostic biopsy of the ulcer edge, culture of the anal canal, and a systemic evaluation.

Most often, the traditional midline anal fissure is caused by the trauma produced by the passage of a particularly hard and large fecal mass, but it is also seen after acute episodes of diarrhea. Fissures persist because of the severe, chronic internal sphincter spasm that occurs along with the secondary infection of its base.

## Clinical Features

Pain of the sharp, cutting variety is the most common symptom. Typically, the pain is most severe during and immediately after a bowel movement. The pain may persist for a few hours after each bowel movement, but invariably it subsides between movements, which is a distinguishing feature of fissures from other forms of painful anorectal disease. The bleeding is bright and small in quantity, usually being noticed only on the toilet paper. In infants, the presence of small amounts of bright blood on the stool or toilet paper is usually the presenting complaint for an anal fissure. Sphincter spasm and pain may be severe enough to make the patient retain stool and avoid defecation.

Diagnosis of anal fissure is usually suggested by the history; however, the anal area must be examined in all cases. With proper exposure, the sentinel pile, if present, and frequently the distal end of the fissure itself, may be seen. The mere retraction of the buttocks and the anal skin may cause considerable discomfort; sphincter spasm may be so severe that the patient will not permit digital examination. Application of a topical anesthetic may provide some relief. If the fissure can be visualized and is present in the posterior midline, rectal examination can be deferred until the patient is having less spasm and pain.

## Treatment

Treatment is aimed at providing symptomatic relief, relieving the anal sphincter spasm, and preventing stricture formation. Hot sitz baths for at least 15 min three to four times a day and after each bowel movement will relax the sphincter and provide symptomatic relief. The addition of bran to the diet will serve to prevent stricture formation by providing a bulky stool. Use of local analgesic ointments, although providing symptomatic relief, is not associated with rapid healing. Indeed, there is a risk of hypersensitivity reaction. The use of hydrocortisone-containing ointments does little to help and may even retard healing. There is one study that demonstrates that most rapid healing of the fissure occurs with sitz baths and a diet rich in bran and that healing was not aided by either an analgesic ointment or a hydrocortisone-containing ointment. Meticulous anal hygiene is imperative; following defecation, the anus must be cleaned thoroughly. Healing is by the development of granulation tissue and the reepithelialization of the ulcerated area. If healing does not occur in a reasonable amount of time, operative treatment consisting of partial sphincterotomy and excision of the fissure may be required.

## ANORECTAL ABSCESSES

Abscesses are common in the perianal and perirectal regions, as are fistulas, which are common sequelae. Almost all begin with involvement of an anal crypt and its gland. From there, the infection can progress to involve any of the potential spaces that are normally filled with fatty areolar tissue and have little inherent resistance to the progression of infection. These spaces, which can become infected alone or in combination with each other, are as follows: the perianal space, the intersphincteric space, the ischiorectal space, the deep postanal space (connecting the ischiorectal space on each side posteriorly), and the supralevator space (Figs. 83-6 and 83-7).

The perianal abscess is the most common anorectal abscess and occurs when pus spreads caudally between the internal and external sphincters to form a painful, tender, erythematous swelling at the anal verge, most often at the midline posteriorly. When it presents as a localized, superficial, fluctuant mass that is not associated with any other form of perirectal infection, it is only this type of abscess that can be adequately treated under local anesthesia in an emergency department setting.

Ischiorectal and other deep abscesses pose a different problem. The ischiorectal fossa forms a large potential space on either side of the rectum, communicating behind it through the deep postanal space, and, in males, has extensions anteriorly above the perineal membrane to the prostate. Infections in this area are insidious and extensive and can point in an area some distance from the anal verge. These abscesses can be large, and yet only a diffuse, nonfluctuant, tender "mass" is palpable either through the rectal wall or the overlying perineal skin. If only induration is present, endorectal ultrasonography and/or needle localization under anesthesia may be needed to confirm the diagnosis.

Most abscesses in the anorectal area are the result of obstruction of an anal gland that opens in the base of an anal crypt and normally drains into the anal canal. When obstruction occurs, the gland orifice is blocked, resulting in infection and abscess formation. An element of cryptitis can frequently be identified by anoscopic examination. A variety of diseases are associated with the development of fistulous abscesses, including Crohn's disease, carcinoma of adjacent organs, Hodgkin's disease, tuberculosis, and gonococcal proctitis.

## Clinical Features

Initially, the patient notices a dull, aching, or throbbing pain that becomes worse immediately before defecation, is lessened after defecation, but persists between bowel movements. The pain is increased by the increased pressure in the rectum that occurs just before defecation.

As the abscess spreads, increases in size, and comes nearer the surface, the associated pain becomes more intense. Pain will be aggravated by straining, coughing, or sneezing, which cause motion of the region. As the abscess progresses, pain and tenderness interfere with walking or sitting.

The patient appears markedly uncomfortable and may be febrile. A tender mass may be present, or there may be a tender, erythematous area with or without fluetuance. On rectal examination, a tender mass or induration is detected. Leukocytosis may be present.

## Treatment

Treatment is surgical and should be performed as soon as the diagnosis is made, before the abscesses become fluctuant. Drainage should be both early and extensive. All these abscesses should be drained in the operating room. A recent publication revealed that 32 percent of patients who had undergone a simple incision and drainage under local anesthesia were required to have a second operation because of inadequate drainage and recurrence of disease.

Isolated, simple, fluctuant perianal abscesses that are not associated with the presence of any deeper abscesses may be drained using local anesthetics in an emergency department setting. The local anesthetic should be administered with the finest-gauge needle available (30-gauge) and should be complemented with the administration of

systemic analgesia or conscious sedation. To ensure adequate drainage, a cruciate incision should be made over the fluctuant part of the abscess, and the "dog ears" resulting from the cruciate incision should be excised so as to prevent premature closure of the cutaneous wall of the abscess (Fig. 83-8). No packing is required; sitz baths should be started the next day.

As a rule, antibiotics are not necessary after an abscess has been adequately drained. On the other hand, patients whose immune system may be compromised by diabetes mellitus, AIDS, malignancies, and chemotherapy and/or those patients who have extensive cellulitis should be started on a regimen of broad-spectrum antibiotics.

## FISTULA IN ANO

An anal fistula is an abnormal tract that connects the anal canal with the skin and is lined with epithelium and granulation tissue. A fistula in ano most commonly results from a perianal or ischiorectal abscess (Fig. 83-6). It may, however, be associated with ulcerative colitis, Crohn's disease, or tuberculosis. Although anterior-opening fistulas tend to follow a simple, direct course to the anal canal (Goodsall's rule), posterior-opening fistulas may follow a devious, curving path, including some that are horseshoe-shaped.

### Clinical Features

As long as the tract remains open, there is a persistent, blood-stained, malodorous discharge. More commonly, the tract becomes blocked periodically, producing bouts of inflammation and even local, recurrent abscess formation that is relieved by spontaneous rupture. An abscess may be the only sign of fistula in ano.

### Treatment

The only definitive treatment is surgical excision. Improperly excised fistulas may result in permanent fecal incontinence.

## VENEREAL PROCTITIS

Sexually transmitted diseases (STDs) of the anorectum are not uncommon among patients who practice anal sex. The infecting organisms, for the most part, are the same ones that are transmitted with vaginal coitus; infection is transmitted and perpetuated almost entirely by men who fail to use condoms (Table 83-2). Exceptions to this occur with women whose lymphogranuloma venereum (LGV) variety of chlamydia infection extends directly to the rectum from the vagina and on occasions when there is a contamination of the anus with gonococcal-laden discharge emanating from the urethra or cervix.

As a rule, if the patient has an anorectal infection caused by one of the STDs, the assumption must be made that another STD may be present; appropriate blood tests must be obtained, and patients should be anoscoped or proctoscoped in order to obtain specimens for Gram stain as well as for viral and bacterial cultures.

### Clinical Features

Most venereal diseases involving the anorectal area manifest themselves initially with itching, seepage, and mild pain or irritation. Indeed, these mild early symptoms may heighten the sexual desire of certain patients, which could result in the rapid dissemination of the disease to other unwary and unprotected partners. Some infections may persist with mild to minimal symptoms, rendering the patient a carrier of the disease who will be detected only by epidemiologic surveys, if they are ever conducted. Most venereal infections, however, will produce significant symptoms of pain, bleeding, and discharge in addition to a bothersome pruritus that will force them to seek medical attention.

## Cryptoglandular Origin Theory

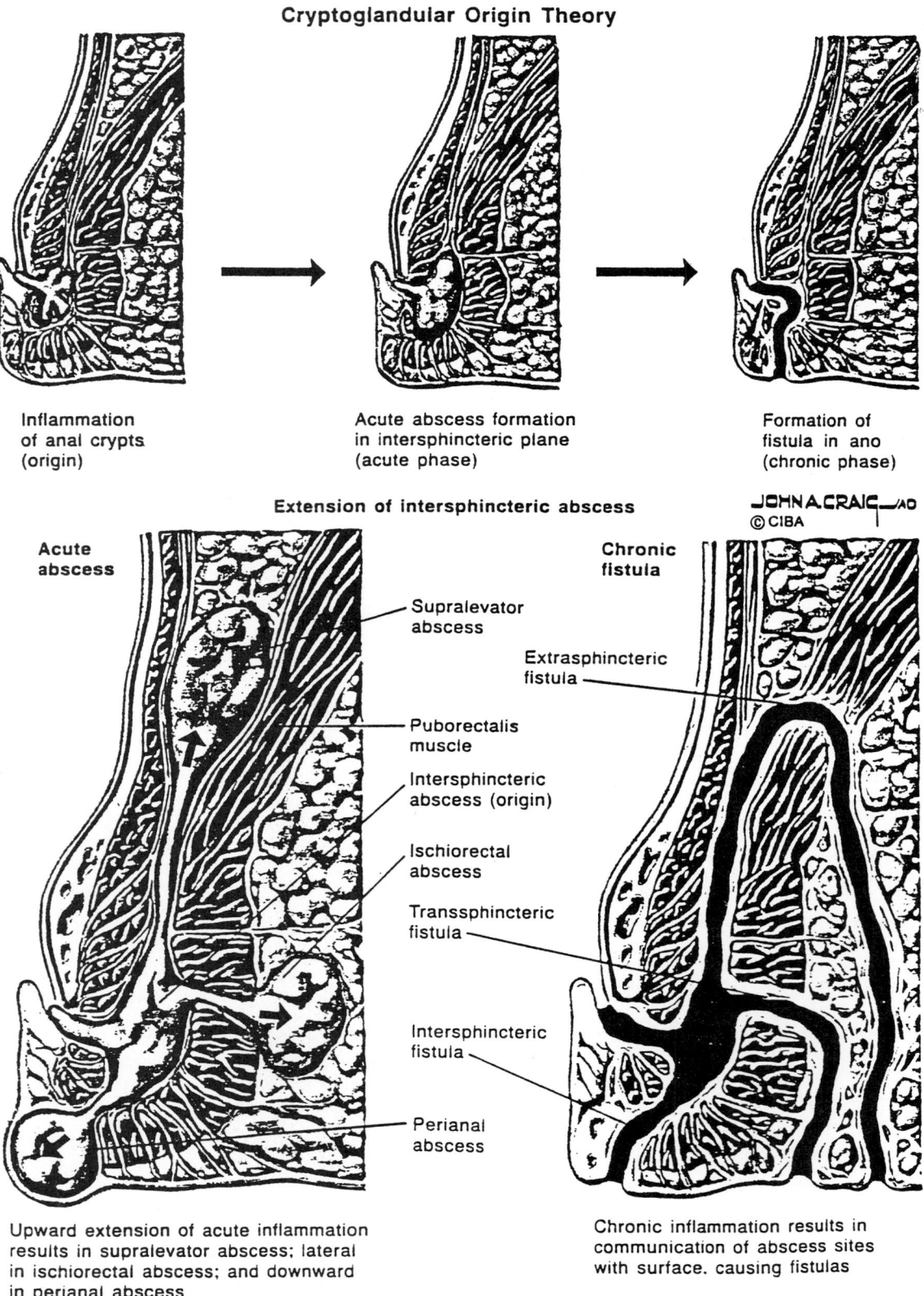

Inflammation
of anal crypts
(origin)

Acute abscess formation
in intersphincteric plane
(acute phase)

Formation of
fistula in ano
(chronic phase)

**Extension of intersphincteric abscess**

JOHN A. CRAIG _AD
© CIBA

Acute
abscess

Chronic
fistula

Supralevator
abscess

Extrasphincteric
fistula

Puborectalis
muscle

Intersphincteric
abscess (origin)

Ischiorectal
abscess

Transsphincteric
fistula

Intersphincteric
fistula

Perianal
abscess

Upward extension of acute inflammation
results in supralevator abscess; lateral
in ischiorectal abscess; and downward
in perianal abscess

Chronic inflammation results in
communication of abscess sites
with surface. causing fistulas

**Fig. 83-6.** Illustration of mechanism for anorectal abscess and fistula formation. (From Fry RD, Kodner IJ: *Clinical symposia: Anorectal disorders,* Vol. 37, No. 6. West Caldwell, NJ: CIBA Pharmaceutical Co., 1985. used by permission.)

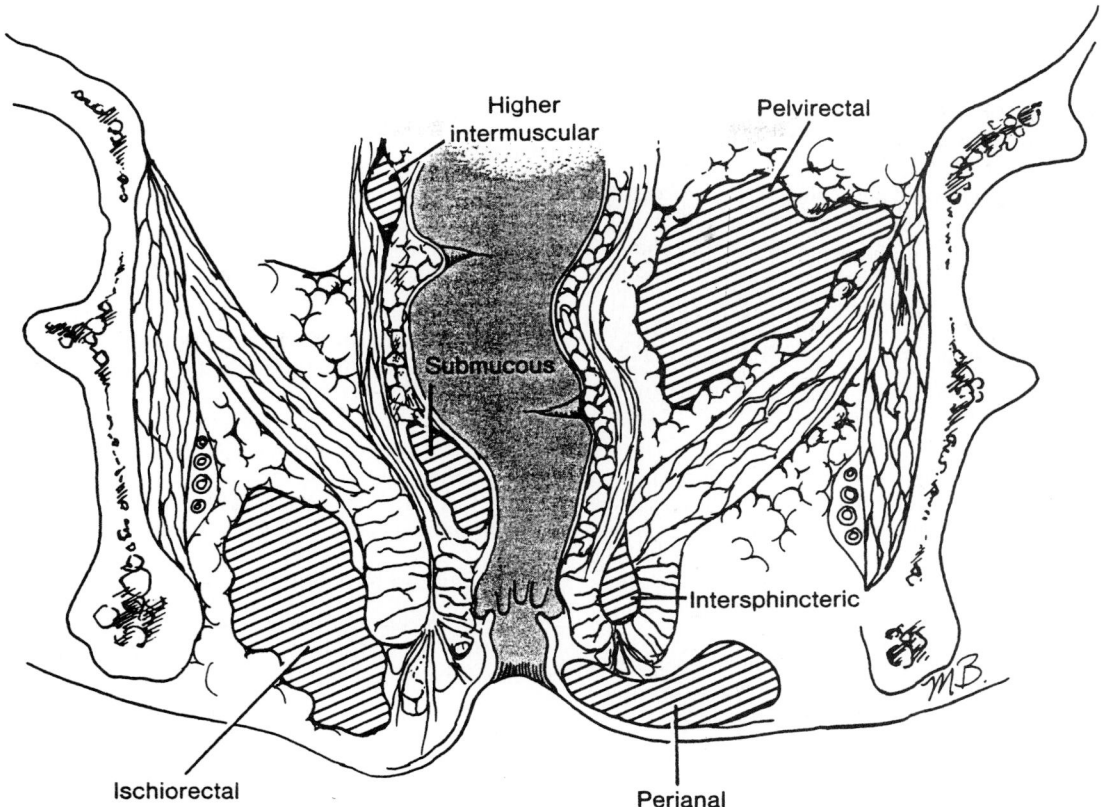

**Fig. 83-7.** Anatomical classification of common anorectal abscesses. (From Barker LR et al (eds): *Principles of Ambulatory Medicine,* 3d ed. Baltimore, Williams & Wilkins, 1991, p. 1267. Used by permission.)

**Fig. 83-8.** Technique of drainage of perianal abscess. (From Goldberg SM et al: *Essentials of Anorectal Surgery.* Philadelphia, Lippincott, 1980. Used by permission.)

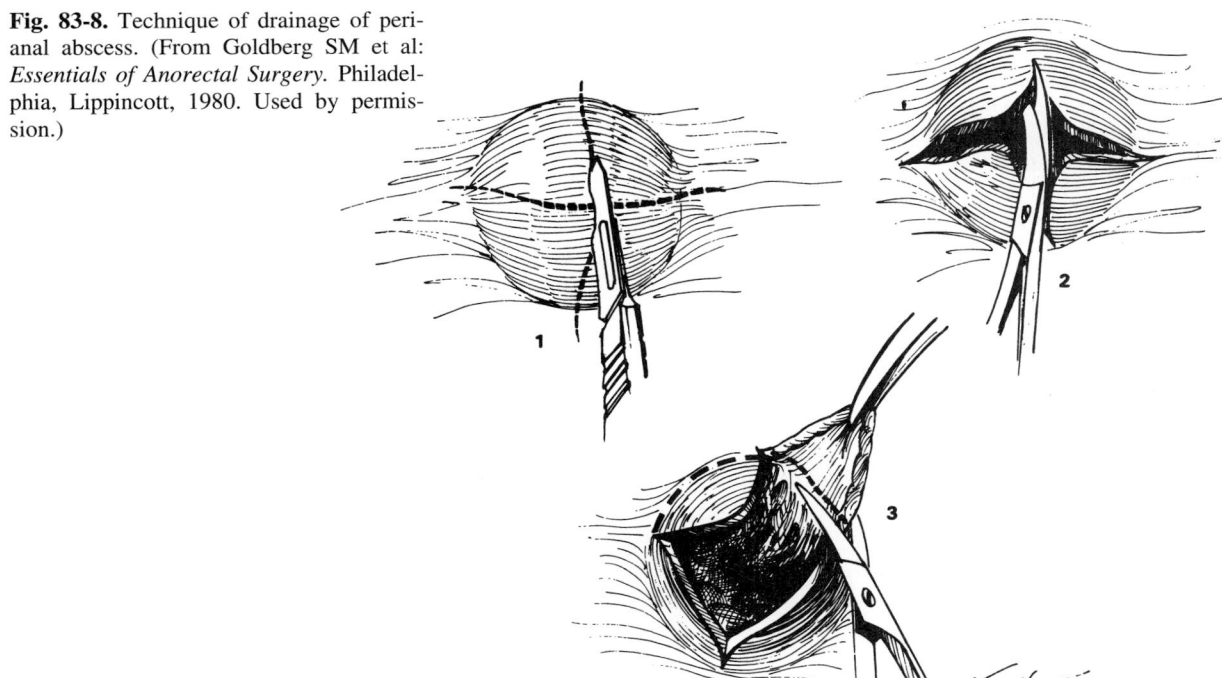

## Condylomata Acuminata

Condylomata acuminata, commonly known as anal warts, are caused by a papilloma virus and are probably sexually transmitted in more than 90 percent of cases. They begin as discreet, soft fleshy growths on the skin of the perianal area as well as on the squamous epithelium of the anal canal. Occasionally, the mucosa of the lower rectum becomes involved. Patients usually first notice the presence of a growth in the perianal areas as well as associated pruritus and varying degrees of anal pain. With time, bleeding and anal discharge become part of the symptom complex. Evaluation of a patient with condyloma acuminata must include ruling out the presence of other STDs. Because cases of squamous cell carcinoma arising in association with condyloma acuminata have been reported, multiple biopsies must be taken.

## Gonorrhea

Gonococcal proctitis occurs most commonly among homosexual men, although it may also be found among others who have had anal sex. Symptoms vary, ranging from none to severe rectal pain with profuse yellow discharge. Patients in the acute phase generally have mild anal burning and/or pruritus with some purulent seepage. Proctoscopic examination during this phase of the disease reveals marked hyperemia and edema of the rectal mucosa and diffuse inflammation with purulent discharge from the anal crypts. Unlike nonvenereal cryptitis, infection is not confined to the posterior crypt. Diagnosis is made by Gram's stain and cultures on appropriate media.

## Chlamydial Infections

*Chlamydia trachomatis* is an obligate human intracellular parasite that causes, among other conditions, both urogenital and anorectal infections. The lymphogranulomatous (LGV) variety occurs mainly in tropical and subtropical climates. Infection can involve the rectum by perirectal lymphatic invasion from vaginal seeding or from direct anorectal mucosal infections. The non-LGV chlamydial organisms may infect the rectal mucosa, although they do not cause the extensive rectal scarring and stricturing that its lymph gland–invading cousin from the tropics does. A patient with chlamydial proctitis may be asymptomatic or may present with nonspecific symptoms, including anal pruritus, pain, and purulent discharge. Bleeding may also be present.

The more severe form of proctitis occurring with this infection is usually due to the LGV type of chlamydia. In addition to rectal scarring, which is a late sequel, infection of the perirectal tissue results in perirectal abscesses and chronic fistulas.

Chlamydia may be identified by culture. The LGV forms may be distinguished from the non-LGV variety by the Frei intradermal test or the LGV complement fixation test. Treatment for LGV chlamydial infections should be maintained for at least 21 days.

## Syphilis

Chancres, the characteristic lesion of primary syphilis, usually manifest themselves at the anal verge or in the anal canal. Rarely will a chancre involve the rectal mucosa, although proctitis due to syphilis can occur in the absence of a chancre. Anal chancres may be very painful. If they are not identified and treated, they will resolve and the patient will proceed to develop secondary and tertiary syphilis. Condylomata lata, which are flatter and firmer than condylomata acuminata, appear in the perianal region as a manifestation of the secondary stage of syphilis.

## Herpes

Anorectal herpes is almost always caused by the type II herpes simplex virus (HSV-2). Infection is initially manifested by itching and

**Table 83-2.** Anorectal Sexually Transmitted Diseases

Bacteria
   *Neisseria gonorrheae*
   *Chlamydia trachomatis,* lymphogranulomatous
   *C. trachomatis,* nonlymphogranulomatous
Spirochete
   *Treponema pallidum*
Virus
   Herpes simplex type 2
   Human immunodeficiency virus
   Papilloma virus

soreness in the perianal area; this soon progresses to severe anorectal pain. Initially, the virus manifests itself as small, discreet groups of vesicles superimposed on an erythematous base. These vesicles enlarge, coalesce, and rupture, forming exquisitely tender aphthous ulcers that appear on the perianal skin, the anoderm, and even the rectal mucosa. The pain and tenesmus from these lesions may be so intense that the patient is reluctant to have a bowel movement, resulting in constipation and possibly fecal impaction.

## AIDS-Related Infections

Ironically, infection of the rectum by the human immunodeficiency virus (HIV) per se does not cause any local reaction or symptoms, but its effect on the patient inoculated with this virus is invariably devastating. Patients who have been rendered immunodeficient by the HIV virus are subject to a variety of opportunistic infections that affect the intestinal, anorectal, and other body systems. Chronic perianal infections with herpes simplex type I as well as type II are commonly seen in AIDS patients. Table 83-3 lists other, more common enteric organisms that infect AIDS patients who continue to practice anal intercourse. Severe rectal pain, diarrhea, and hematochezia are common presenting symptoms.

## Treatment

Success in the management of patients with acute venereal proctitis depends on suspecting the diagnosis, obtaining specimens to confirm the diagnosis, and initiating therapy as expeditiously as possible. Patients presenting with symptoms of anorectal pain, rectal discharge, and/or tenesmus should be considered to have proctitis until proven otherwise. These patients should have an anoscopy or proctoscopy, and a Gram's stain should be performed to document the presence of acute proctitis. In addition to the appropriate culture specimens, blood should be drawn to check for syphilis.

Antibiotic therapy should not be delayed, pending the results of cultures. Empirical therapy aimed at eradicating gonorrhea, non-LGV chlamydia, and incubating syphilis should be initiated for any patient presenting with symptoms and physical signs suggestive of acute proctitis. This therapy should be administered to all patients with acute proctitis even if there are concomitant lesions suggestive of herpetic or papilloma virus infections.

Although treatment for certain causes of venereal proctitis may be initiated in the emergency department, all patients must be referred to appropriate specialists for continued therapy and follow-up.

**Table 83-3.** Anorectal AIDS-Related Infections

Herpes simplex type 1
*Mycobactrium avium intracellulare*
Cytomegalovirus
*Salmonella enterocolitis*
*Shigella*
*Campylobacter*
*Entamoeba*
*Giardia*

# RECTAL PROLAPSE

Rectal prolapse, known as procidentia, is the circumferential protrusion of part or all layers of the rectum through the anal canal. There are three classes of rectal prolapse: (1) prolapse involving the rectal mucosa only, (2) prolapse involving all layers of the rectum, and (3) intussusception of the upper rectum into and through the lower rectum so that the apex of the intussusception protrudes through the anus.

In the first group, seen primarily in children under the age of 2, the prolapse occurs because of the loose attachment of the mucosa to the submucosal layers, and there is an associated weakness of the anal sphincter. In the second and third groups, prolapse occurs because of the laxity of the pelvic fascia and muscles in addition to a generalized weakening of the anal sphincters. In all cases, the rectum does not conform with, but lies anterior to the sacral concavity, thus obliterating the angulation that normally occurs between rectum and anus. The prolapsing mucosa of a partial prolapse rarely protrudes more than 4 cm beyond the anal verge; the mucosal folds emanate in a radial fashion from the central lumen of the prolapsed mucosa. Mucosal prolapse is frequently associated with third- and fourth-degree hemorrhoids (see Table 83-1).

Complete rectal prolapse (procidentia) occurs at the extremes of life, most commonly in elderly women. Multiparity is not a contributing factor to rectal prolapse; there appears to be a higher incidence of prolapse in women who have had a hysterectomy.

## Clinical Features

Most patients are able to detect the presence of a mass, especially following defecation or strenuous activity. In more advanced cases, this may be present when they stand or walk. Irritation to the rectal mucosa caused by recurrent prolapse results in a mucous discharge with some associated bleeding. Some patients may present because of blood-stained mucus on their undergarments, others because of fecal incontinence caused by associated anal sphincter weakness. In pediatric patients, parents often mistakenly believe that the prolapsed mucosa is hemorrhoids.

## Treatment

In young children, after appropriate analgesia and sedation, prolapse can be reduced manually by replacing the protruding mucosa proximal to the anorectal ring of sphincter muscles. Every effort should be made to prevent the child from becoming constipated, and the child should be referred for further evaluation.

Surgical intervention is generally indicated in all other age groups unless the prolapse is minimal. A variety of effective surgical procedures is available and may be used depending on the degree of prolapse and the general health of the patient. All adults should have or be referred to have a proctosigmoidoscopic examination to rule out the presence of a tumor that could have caused the intussusception. In addition, one should check for the possibility of an anterior rectal wall ulcer that may occur in patients with recurrent prolapse.

If vascular compromise appears to have occurred, reduction may be necessary on an emergency basis. Because of the risk of having reduced ischemic bowel that could perforate, these patients must be hospitalized.

# ANORECTAL TUMORS

Carcinoma of the anal area represents less than 5 percent of all large bowel malignancy. At the level of the dentate line and extending approximately 1 cm proximal is a transitional zone of epithelium connecting the squamous cell epithelium of the anoderm with the columnar epithelium of the rectum. This transition zone includes columnar, cuboidal, transitional, and squamous epithelial cells that represent the source for a variety of malignancies that arise in the anal canal (Table 83-4). For the purpose of grading malignancies, the United Nations World Health Organization has divided the anal canal into two regions: (1) malignancies of the portion proximal to the dentate line and including the transitional zone are referred to as anal canal neoplasms and (2) tumors arising in the anoderm distal to the dentate line are referred to as anal margin neoplasms.

Anal margin neoplasms have a low-grade malignant potential and are slow to metastasize. Anal canal neoplasms, on the other hand, are far more virulent, metastasize early, and have a poor prognosis. Squamous cell carcinoma of the anal canal has a much poorer prognosis than its anal margin counterpart. Anal canal malignancies metastasize not only to mesenteric lymph nodes and the portal circulation but also to the regional inguinal nodes and via the systemic circulation.

Included among the anal canal neoplasms is Kaposi's sarcoma, the most common AIDS-related malignancy. The anal canal is the third most common site for malignant melanoma (after the skin and the eye), which, when it occurs there, is usually not pigmented and frequently overlooked.

## Clinical Features

Early anal canal malignancies usually cause nonspecific symptoms such as pruritus, pain, and bleeding admixed with stool. The sensation and presence of a lump in the anal canal may be erroneously diagnosed as a hemorrhoid. As the neoplasms progress, the patient experiences anorexia, weight loss, constipation, narrowing of the caliber of the stool, and eventually tenesmus with or without bowel movement. Complete obstruction may also occur.

Anal canal tumors may produce partial rectal prolapse; hemorrhoidal dilatation and prolapse may also occur. More advanced malignancies may present as perirectal abscesses or fistulas.

Villous adenomas, which arise from the rectal columnar epithelium, frequently produce diarrhea and a profuse rectal discharge, with secondary excoriation of skin and pruritus. These patients may suffer a significant loss of electrolytes, resulting in a clinically significant hypokalemia and/or hyponatremia.

## Treatment

The anal margin neoplasms may present as persistent ulcers or as chronic dermatologic conditions such as eczema or mycotic infections. Any ulcer that fails to heal within 30 days or any discrete skin lesion that fails to improve with appropriate therapy must be biopsied to rule out the presence of malignancy.

Virtually all anorectal tumors can be detected by careful visual examination of the perianal area, digital palpation of the distal rectum and anal canal, and procto- or sigmoidoscopic examination. In one review of anal malignancies, 80 percent were in the canal and 20 percent at the anal margin. Failure to look, feel, and think would be the only reason not to suspect the presence of these curable but life-threatening lesions.

**Table 83-4.** Neoplasms of the Anal Region

Anal canal neoplasms (proximal to dentate line)
  Adenocarcinoma of the rectum
  Adenocarcinoma of anal glands and ducts
  Mucoepidermoid carcinoma
  Transitional cloacogenic (basaloid) carcinoma
  Squamous cell carcinoma of the anal canal
  Malignant melanoma
  Kaposi's sarcoma
  Villous adenoma of the rectum
Anal margin neoplasms (distal to dentate line)
  Bowen's disease
  Squamous cell carcinoma of anal margin
  Extramammary Paget's disease
  Basal cell carcinoma
  Giant solitary trichoepithelioma

## RECTAL FOREIGN BODIES

The medical literature is replete with the variety of foreign bodies that have been reported to have been inserted into the rectum (Fig. 83-9). Most foreign bodies are "low-lying," that is, in the rectal ampulla and therefore palpable through digital examination and detectable on proctoscopic examination. Any patient presenting with an intrarectal foreign body must have multiple x-rays of the abdomen taken to demonstrate not only the position, shapes, and number of foreign bodies but also the possible presence of free air. Perforation of the rectum or colon is the most frequent and most serious complication. Perforation may be either extraperitoneal or intraperitoneal; both can result in life-threatening sepsis.

### Treatment

Although many foreign bodies can be removed in the emergency department, some require surgical intervention. If the foreign body is removed in the emergency department and is of a size or shape that could cause perforation, a follow-up proctoscopic examination and x-ray studies must be performed. In questionable cases, observations for at least 12 h should be done to ensure that perforation has not occurred. Rectal and anal lacerations may be present and require repair.

Sphincter relaxation is mandatory for removal of foreign bodies. If the patient's sphincters are taut or otherwise not sufficiently relaxed, local infiltrative anesthesia must be administered to achieve proper relaxation. After the patient has been sedated and placed in the lithotomy position, local anesthetic is injected through a fine, 30-gauge needle to raise an intradermal wheal at the 6- and 12-o'clock positions. The index finger of the physician's nondominant hand is then

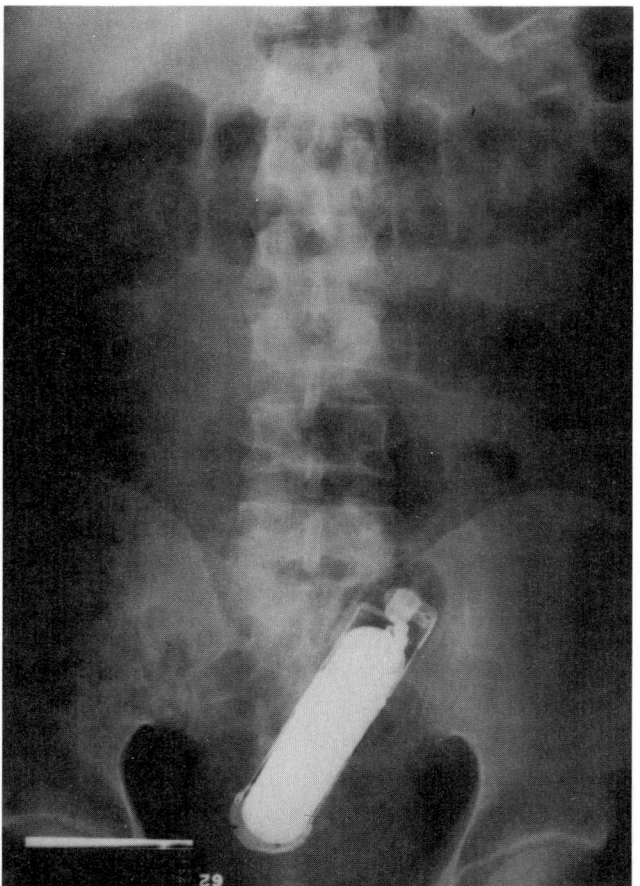

**Fig. 83-9.** Vibrator device lodged in rectum. (Courtesy of Medical Center of Delaware, Inc.)

inserted into the anal canal to act as a guide for a 1 1/2-in, larger-gauge needle through which anesthetic is injected circumferentially along the course of the internal sphincter muscles as they course along the anal canal. Five milliliters of anesthetic should suffice for each quadrant of infiltration. Large bulbar objects create a vacuumlike effect in the rectal ampulla, making it difficult to retrieve the object by simple traction. The vacuum can be overcome by passing a catheter beyond the object and injecting air. A modification of this technique is to insert Foley catheters around the foreign body and, after the vacuum is relieved by injecting air, inflate the balloons of the Foley catheters and use the catheters as traction devices to deliver the foreign body or manipulate it into a more accessible position.

If there is a risk of perforation, either by the foreign body itself or by local attempts to remove the foreign body, the patient should be prepared for emergency surgery, which includes obtaining appropriate laboratory studies, initiating intravenous therapy with crystalloid solution, passing a nasogastric tube, and administering a loading dose of broad-spectrum (second-generation cephalosporin) antibiotics.

## PILONIDAL SINUS

Pilonidal sinus has nothing to do with the anorectum, anatomically or embryologically. Pilonidal sinuses or cysts occur in the midline in the upper part of the natal cleft overlying the lower sacrum and coccyx. Because of their proximity to the anus, infected pilonidal cysts (abscesses) are sometimes mistakenly diagnosed as perirectal abscesses. An abscessed pilonidal sinus is always located in the midline (although there may be secondary fistulous openings on either side of the midline) and does not communicate with the anorectum. On the other hand, long, horseshoe-type fistulas emanating from a perirectal abscess may drain close to the location of a pilonidal sinus but not in the midline.

Although once thought to be congenital in nature, pilonidal sinus is now considered an acquired problem. The sinus is formed by the penetration of the skin by ingrowing hair, which causes a foreign body granuloma reaction. The sinus is perpetuated by the presence of the hair and repeated bouts of infection. Although pilonidal sinuses or infected pilonidal cysts occur most commonly before the fourth decade of life, a small portion of patients may develop this problem in their fourth decade. Pilonidal sinus and abscess formation should be considered a chronic and recurring disease.

Carcinoma is a rare complication of chronic, recurring pilonidal sinus disease. It is more frequent in men and is usually a well-differentiated dermal-type squamous cell carcinoma.

### Clinical Features

Depending on whether the disease presents as a cyst or a sinus, the patient generally complains of swelling, pain, or a persistent discharge. When abscess formation occurs, the patient complains of a tender mass. Although there may be more than one sinus with several tiny openings in the midline of the intergluteal cleft, the most common finding is that of a single opening from which hair is protruding. Patients usually present to the emergency department when an abscess has formed that can no longer drain.

### Treatment

Surgery is the treatment of choice. Ideally, a patient should undergo elective excision of the entire pilonidal sinus system and primary closure of skin when there is no infection present in any of the sinuses. Recent literature that suggests minimal excision, marsupialization, and packing using a local anesthetic in the emergency department is, in effect, advocating inadequate surgery that has proven to have a high failure and recurrence rate. Patients presenting with acute inflammation should have their abscess drained in the emergency department. Their wounds should be allowed to heal, and then, at least

6 weeks later, if there is no evidence of active infection, they should undergo definitive surgical excision and closure as described above.

The technique for incising and draining a pilonidal abscess is as follows: Place the patient prone on the proctoscopic table with the buttocks retracted laterally (see Fig. 83-2). The patient should be sedated or have the option of self-administering nitronox analgesia. Tuck an ABD pad between the lower gluteal cleft to prevent the prep solution from pooling at the anus or genitals. After having prepped the skin, infiltrate the area to be incised with an intradermal injection of anesthetic solution, using a fine-gauge needle. A suction apparatus should be available to aspirate the unusually foul-smelling pus that has accumulated within the abscess. Following drainage, gently break down any loculations that may be present and loosely pack the wound with iodoform gauze. Bulk dressing should then be applied and secured with tape to the patient's buttocks. The patient should be given a prescription for a strong oral analgesic and advised to begin hot sitz baths the following day. Before the sitz bath, the patient should remove the outer dressing but should not attempt to remove the packing until after having soaked in hot water for a few minutes. Ideally, one should allow the hot water current to flush the packing out of the wound. The patient should be seen in 48 to 72 h for evaluation and further advice concerning wound management.

Unless the patient is immunocompromised or there is extensive cellulitis, there is no need to obtain cultures or prescribe antibiotics for an abscess that has been adequately drained.

## PRURITUS ANI

Pruritus ani is a symptom complex that occurs secondary to a variety of anal and systemic problems. It is not in itself a specific disease process. It effects men far more often than women, and it occurs most commonly during the fifth and sixth decades of life.

There is an entity of primary or idiopathic pruritus ani, the etiology of which is unknown. To make such a diagnosis, one has to rule out the many specific, known causes of secondary pruritus ani. Even so, idiopathic pruritus ani may occur in association with or be precipitated by secondary pruritus ani. Table 83-5 lists the major categories of the various likely causes of secondary pruritus ani.

In Table 83-5, "anorectal disease" includes the various categories that have been discussed in this chapter. The pruritus that accompanies such conditions as fissures, fistulas, hemorrhoids, and prolapses occurs as a result of the perianal skin's being exposed to and macerated by constant mucous and purulent discharge. It is probably the increased perianal moisture caused by these conditions that results in itching. The itching triggers a vicious cycle of scratching, excoriation, and more itching.

Numerous dietary factors have been implicated and are associated with secondary pruritus ani, although proof of cause is lacking for most of them. Those dietary factors most commonly listed include excessive consumption of caffeine-containing liquids, such as coffee, tea, or colas, and beer, although one recent study failed to demonstrate any correlation between pruritus ani and alcohol consumption. Milk, chocolate, tomatoes, and citrus fruits are other food products that allegedly contribute to pruritus ani. Likewise, certain drugs, such as colchicine and mineral oil, have been associated with pruritus ani. Ingestion of these products can result in increased liquidity and seep-

age of fecal material, which in itself is a probable cause of pruritus ani.

Infectious agents that have to be considered as causes of pruritus ani include bacteria, viruses, fungi, spirochetes, and parasites. More common bacterial infections, such as staphylococci and streptococci, in addition to all sexually transmitted organisms, will cause pruritus, if not actual pain. Pinworms (*Enterobius vermicularis*) are the most common cause of anal pruritus in children. *Candida albicans* is commonly found on the perianal skin but is not usually associated with pruritus; the *Trichophyton* species, on the other hand, are always associated with pruritus.

Local irritants, if not the initial cause, commonly contribute to the incidence of pruritus. Fecal contamination, resulting from poor anal hygiene, is by far the most common irritant to the perianal skin. Lysozyme from intestinal mucous secretions, acting together with bacterial exotoxins to raise the stool and skin pH, will cause pruritus. Ironically, patients who compulsively clean their anus, particularly if they use perfumed toilet tissue, soaps, or detergents or hygiene sprays, cause pruritic reactions. Also, wearing of synthetic, tight-fitting underwear retains moisture that normally occurs in the perianal area, another leading cause of pruritus.

Dermatologic conditions contributing to this symptom complex include atopic dermatitis, lichen planus, psoriasis, and seborrheic dermatitis. Any of the anal margin neoplasms, particularly Bowen's disease and extramammary Paget's disease, may initially manifest itself as pruritus.

Finally, certain systemic conditions, such as diabetes mellitus, lymphoma, and certain vitamin deficiencies (vitamins A and D and niacin), because of their secondary effect on the perianal skin, will cause pruritus.

## Clinical Features

Appearance of the perianal skin will depend on the severity and chronicity of the underlying conditions that are causing the pruritus. The skin will appear normal with early, mild cases. With acute, more severe exacerbations, the perianal skin will appear reddened, edematous, and moist; frequently, there are excoriations caused by scratching. In chronic cases, the perianal skin takes on a thickened, almost leathery, depigmented appearance. The normal radiating folds of skin thicken into rugae and may include superficial fissures factitiously induced.

## Treatment

Pruritus, like any other symptom, suggests the presence of an underlying cause that should be diagnosed and treated appropriately. Thus, excision of malignancies or surgical correction of fistulas, prolapses, or hemorrhoids would be the definitive treatment for patients with those conditions.

In most cases, specific anorectal lesions are not apparent, and the patient must be referred to a proctologist or dermatologist for probable long-term management.

In the meantime, the patient should be advised to make certain dietary changes, if appropriate, and should be instructed about proper anal hygiene. Scratching of the area must be avoided; if necessary, the patient should be advised to wear gloves at bedtime, when most of the scratching is likely to occur. Patients with maceration of perianal skin should use moist cotton rather than toilet paper. Soaps should be avoided, and the patient should take sitz baths for at least 15 min two to three times a day. The skin should then be thoroughly dried either with a hair dryer or by gently blotting the area with a soft cloth. Zinc oxide ointment can provide a protective covering for the perianal skin and may enhance the healing. Fungicidal creams should be prescribed for patients with secondary fungal infections. One percent hydrocortisone cream is effective for the allergic component of

**Table 83-5.** Pruritus Ani

Anorectal disease
Dietary factors
Local infection
Local irritants
Dermatologic conditions
Systemic illness
Psychogenic factors

the inflammation. Finally, as an adjunct to providing symptomatic relief, consider prescribing hydroxyzine hydrochloride (Atarax) as an effective bedtime sedative.

## BIBLIOGRAPHY

Corman ML: *Colon and Rectal Surgery,* 3rd ed. Philadelphia, J.B. Lippincott, 1993.

Fry RD, Kodner IJ: Anorectal disorders. *Ciba Found Symp* 37:6, 1985.

Kodner IJ, Fry RD, Fleshman JW et al: Colon, rectum, and anus, in Schwartz SI (ed): *Principles of Surgery,* 6th ed. new York, McGraw-Hill, 1994, pp 1192–1306.

Zuidema GD: *Schackelford's Surgery of the Alimentary Tract,* 3rd ed. Philadelphia, W.B. Saunders, 1991.

# 84
# DIARRHEA AND FOOD POISONING
## James S. Seidel

Vomiting, diarrhea, and gastrointestinal (GI) upset are common complaints. The cause is usually food poisoning or an acute infectious illness. Diarrhea occurs in 3 to 5 billion persons worldwide and is responsible for 5 to 10 million fatalities in people of all age groups in Asia, Africa, and Latin America. In the industrialized nations, diarrheal disease is responsible for the death of more than 700 preschool children each year. It is the third most common reason for hospitalization of children in the United States. Traveler's diarrhea occurs frequently in visitors to developing nations and, if not managed properly, may persist when they return home. The causes of diarrheal illness include infection by viruses, bacteria, parasites, and fungi; enterocolitis induced by antibiotics and other drugs; inflammatory bowel disease; cystic fibrosis; endocrinopathies; acrodermatitis enteropathica; lactose intolerance; milk allergy; malignancy; obstruction (as seen in Hirschsprung disease); and extraintestinal infections such as otitis media or urinary tract infection.

Food poisoning may be caused by:

1. Toxic contaminants of food and water
   a. Heavy metals (zinc, copper, cadmium)
   b. Organic chemicals: polyvinylchlorides
   c. Pesticides
   d. Radioactive substances
   e. Alkyl mercury
2. Bacterial, fungal, viral, and parasitic contaminants of food
   a. Invasive organisms
   b. Chemical metabolites of the microorganisms
3. Toxic substances naturally present in the food: Akee fruit, mushrooms, thallophytes, fish (ciguatera, scombroid poisoning), dinoflagellates, shellfish
4. Altered host response to a food substance, e.g., foods containing tyramine, monosodium glutamate, tryptamine, etc.
5. Food intolerance: shellfish, moray eel, chili pepper

We will consider only ciguatera fish poisoning and the infectious causes of food poisoning and diarrhea.

Infectious diarrheal illness may be classified as: (1) acute (isolated cases), (2) endemic (nosocomial infections as in day-care centers and hospitals), (3) food- or water-borne, (4) associated with antibiotics, (5) traveler's, and (6) special populations (immunosupressed individuals).

## PATHOPHYSIOLOGY

*Diarrhea* may be defined as an increase in the frequency and/or liquidity of stool.

Organisms that cause diarrhea may produce (1) a noninflammatory, or secretory, diarrhea usually due to enterotoxin production; (2) an inflammatory diarrhea or dysentery due to mucosal invasion; and/or (3) enteric fever due to penetration of the mucosa and intracellular infection. The type of diarrheal syndrome found in the patient depends on the organism and the host defenses. A watery, profuse noninflammatory diarrheal syndrome may be produced by the loss of the absorptive surface of the small intestine or the actions of enterotoxin on the intestine. The diarrhea is watery and not associated with fecal leukocytes (Table 84-1). The classic example or this type of infection is cholera, in which organisms colonize the small intestine and produce an enterotoxin that causes an adenyl cyclase–mediated

**Table 84-1.** Fecal Leukocytes in Diarrheal Illness

| Present | Sometimes Present | Absent |
|---|---|---|
| *Shigella* | *Salmonella* | *Vibrio cholerae* |
| *Campylobacter* | *Yersinia* | Toxigenic *E. coli* |
| Invasive *E. coli* | *Vibrio parahaemolyticus* | Enteropathogens: |
| | *Clostridium difficile* | *E. coli* |
| | *Aeromonas* (20%) | *Bacillus cereus* |
| | *Vibrio vulnificus* | *Clostridium* |
| | *Plesiomonas shigelloides* | *perfringens* |
| | | Rotavirus |
| | | Calicivirus |
| | | Norwalk Agent |
| | | Astrovirus |
| | | *Giardia lamblia* |
| | | *Entamoeba* |
| | | *histolytica* |
| | | *Cryptosporidium* |
| | | *Isospora* |
| | | *Microspora* |
| | | *Cyclospora* |

secretory diarrhea. Large amounts of isotonic solution are lost through the bowel. Similar problems may be caused by enterotoxin-producing *Escherichia coli.* A profuse, watery diarrhea may also be produced by direct damage to the intestinal epithelium by such organisms as *Giardia lamblia, Cryptosporidium, Isospora,* Rotavirus, Norwalk agent, and Calicivirus. Diarrhea produced by enterotoxins is not usually associated with fecal leukocytes.

Invasion of the epithelium of the distal small bowel and colon may lead to an inflammatory diarrhea with the clinical findings of fever, diarrhea (often dysentery), and abdominal pain. The stool may contain blood, mucus, and sheets of fecal leukocytes. The severity of the clinical findings is dependent on the severity of damage to the intestinal lining, the extent of tissue invasion, and the presence or absence of bacteremia. Invasive organisms include *Shigella, Campylobacter, Salmonella, Yersinia,* and *E. coli.* Diarrhea caused by invasive organisms frequently has fecal leukocytes. Enteric fever is usually caused by invasive organisms such as *Salmonella typhi* and *Y. enterocolitica,* which pass through the mucosa of the intestinal tract, invade lymphatic structures and phagocytic cells, and cause systemic disease. Although the patient may be constipated at first, diarrhea is often present and the stool may contain fecal monocytes rather than polymorphonuclear cells.

Factors that may protect the host from diarrheal disease include (1) gastric acidity; (2) the normal flora of the intestinal tract, which may be altered by systemic broad-spectrum antibiotics; (3) the normal motility of the intestine, which serves to mix and help in the absorption of fluids, electrolytes, and nutrients and to maintain the distribution of the indigenous microflora of the gut; (4) the gastrointestinal mucus, which protects the lining from damage and invasion of organisms; and (5) the presence of secretory immunoglobulin and phagocytic cells, which are immune barriers.

Iatrogenic alterations of immune barriers may make the host more susceptible to severe diarrheal disease. Since diarrhea is an increase in both the volume and frequency of stool, there may be a large in-

crease in the volume of water lost. In most cases, the intestinal tract is changed from a site of absorption of water and electrolytes to one of secretion or loss of water and electrolytes. Leukocytes and blood may be present in the stool. Dehydration and electrolyte imbalance are seen frequently and are responsible for the high morbidity and mortality, particularly in the very young and very old. Interventions such as the use of broad-spectrum antibiotics and agents that inhibit motility, such as loperamide and diphenoxylate, may add to the disease process. In more chronic diarrheal illness, loss of nutrients, essential minerals, and vitamins may further compromise the patient.

## ETIOLOGY OF DIARRHEAL DISEASE

### Viral Infections

Most cases of acute diarrheal disease are caused by viral infections (Table 84-2). The most common viruses are Rotavirus, Calicivirus, Astrovirus, and Norwalk agent. Other viral organisms include enteroviruses and enteric adenovirus (serotypes 40 and 41). Clinical manifestations include watery diarrhea, nausea, and vomiting and are usually self-limiting. Infection occurs primarily in the winter and spring months and is more frequent in young children, particularly those in day-care settings.

Rotavirus has been studied most extensively, and a number of serotypes are responsible for endemic infantile gastroenteritis. It is spread from person to person through the fecal-oral route, and contamination may be associated with diaper changing. Nosocomial spread has occurred among hospitalized pediatric patients and medical personnel. Infection is sporadic and occurs primarily in infants less than 1 year of age. The incubation period is 1 to 3 days, and the typical patient has fever, vomiting, and diarrhea but may also have an upper respiratory infection or pneumonia. The diarrhea generally lasts for 3 to 10 days but may be protracted. Norwalk virus occurs in school-aged children and adults. Community outbreaks and epidemics are common. The illness is generally self-limiting and resolves in several days. Calicivirus has been isolated from infants and young children in day-care settings and produces a syndrome similar to that of Rotavirus; however, the symptoms may persist for up to 2 weeks. Astrovirus is also found in young children and the elderly, and the symptoms include fever, malaise, and watery diarrhea, which lasts several days. Enterovirus and adenoviruses have been implicated in outbreaks of acute gastroenteritis. These viruses, the clinical syndromes, and typical clinical course are shown in Table 84-2.

### Bacterial Infections

Bacterial infections are responsible for approximately 20 percent of acute infectious diarrheal illnesses (Table 84-3). Bacterial diarrhea is divided into two classes—disease caused by direct invasion and disease caused by enterotoxins.

### *Escherichia coli*

Toxigenic and invasive *E. coli* are primary agents of traveler's diarrhea. Infection is acquired by ingestion of contaminated food and water. Typically, the patient experiences mild abdominal pain and wa-

**Table 84-2.** Viral Causes of Acute Diarrhea

| Agent | Clinical Syndrome | Diarrhea | Vomiting | Fever | URI | Pneumonia |
|---|---|---|---|---|---|---|
| Rotavirus | Endemic infantile gastroenteritis | +++ | ++ | ++ | + | ± |
| Norwalk agent | Endemic gastroenteritis | +++ | +++ | + | − | − |
| | Family outbreaks | | | | | |
| Enteric type adenovirus | Intestinal "flu" | ++ | ++ | + | + | ± |
| Enterovirus | Variety of syndromes associated with mild GI upset | + | ± | ++ | + | ± |
| Calicivirus | "Flu" in children under 2, endemic gastroenteritis | ++ | + | ± | − | − |
| Astrovirus | Endemic gastroenteritis | ++ | + | + | − | − |

**Table 84-3.** Infectious Organisms Associated with Diarrheal Syndromes

| Noninflammatory | Inflammatory | Enteric Fever |
|---|---|---|
| *Vibrio Cholerae* | *Shigella* | *Salmonella* |
| *Vibrio vulnificus* | *Campylobacter* | *Yersinia enterocolitica* |
| *Aeromonas hydrophila* | *E. coli*–Invasive | *Campylobacter fetus* |
| *Vibrio parahaemolyticus* | *Salmonella* | *jejuni* |
| Rotavirus | *Clostridium difficile* | |
| Norwalk agent | *Yersinia enterocolitica* | |
| Calicivirus astrovirus | *Aeromonas* (20%) | |
| *Cryptosporidium* | *Entamoeba histolytica* | |
| *Isospora* | | |
| *E. coli* | | |
| *Microsporidan* | | |

tery diarrhea 2 to 4 days after infection. Infection may be fulminant and resemble clinical cholera but is usually self-limited and rarely associated with systemic symptoms.

The organism can cause diarrhea by three mechanisms. Enterotoxigenic strains produce heat-labile toxin, stable toxin, or both. The genes for toxin production are carried on a plasmid; thus, any serotype of *E. coli* may elaborate the toxins. The enterotoxins produced act at the cellular level, stimulating an increased production of cyclic AMP that leads to the loss of electrolytes and water into the lumen of the bowel. The enteropathogenic strains colonize the small and large intestines. They are associated with epidemics of acute diarrhea in hospital nurseries. The exact mechanism of disease is not fully understood but is thought to involve toxin production. *Escherichia coli* may also produce invasive disease and a clinical picture described below for *Shigella*.

Treatment with an antibiotic (doxycycline, trimethoprim with sulfamethoxazole, or ciprofloxacin) may be required in cases that are moderate to severe, but most patients will require only supportive therapy. Identification of enterotoxigenic organisms in the laboratory requires special techniques not widely available. Recently the 0157H7 strain of *E. coli* has been associated with outbreaks of the hemolytic uremic syndrome. These outbreaks have been associated with consumption of contaminated beef products from fast-food chains and supermarkets.

### Shigella

*Shigella* infections are common in all parts of the world and are associated with food-borne, nosocomial transmission and fecal and oral contamination. The organism is highly infectious, and ingestion of only 100 organisms may cause disease. The spectrum of illness may vary from mild—an asymptomatic carrier—to severe—a fulminant disease resulting in severe dehydration and death in the very young and old. The patient may become symptomatic 36 to 72 h after exposure. Infection is associated with abdominal pain and fever, which may reach 40° or 41°C (104° or 105.8°F) in children. Bowel movements may be explosive and associated with blood and mucus in 50 to 75 percent of these patients. Young children may present with high fever and a febrile convulsion without a history of diarrhea; the diarrhea may begin in the emergency department, often when the child is being held for lumbar puncture. *Shigella* toxin has also been associated with high fever and febrile seizurelike activity. In addition, Reiter syndrome has been associated with recent *Shigella* infection. A stool specimen should be sent to the microbiology laboratory in holding media as soon as possible. Even under the best circumstances, cultures may be negative in 30 percent of the cases and should be repeated.

*Shigella*, like *E. coli*, generally causes a self-limited disease. The largest number of bowel movements are usually within the first 24 h, and dehydration may occur in young children. Deaths have been reported in infants within 8 h after the onset of symptoms. Although

rare, bacteremia can occur with *Shigella* infections. A complete blood cell count may be helpful in differentiating *Shigella* enteritis. The white blood cell count may be low, high, or normal, and a marked left shift is common. Fecal leukocytes are usually present.

Antibiotics promptly alter the course of *Shigella* infections but are recommended only in cases of *Shigella* dysentery, infections in infants and the elderly, or institutional outbreaks of *S. flexneri*. Although many strains are sensitive to ampicillin, trimethoprim with sulfamethoxazole, ciprofloxacin, or norfloxacin are considered the treatment of choice by some as multidrug-resistant strains are emerging throughout the world. Without specific therapy the majority of patients have an uneventful recovery in 5 to 7 days. Complications of shigellosis include diarrhea and dehydration, Reiter syndrome, arthralgia, and the hemolytic uremic syndrome.

### Salmonella

Salmonella is responsible for a wide range of diseases; however, they may be divided into five clinical syndromes: (1) self-limiting enteritis, (2) enteric fever, (3) bacteremia without metastatic disease, (4) gastroenteritis, and (5) the asymptomatic carrier.

This organism is ubiqitous and is found in many animals as well as humans. Most human infections occur as a result of contamination of food and water. Eggs, egg products, chicken, and turkey are often implicated as a source of infection. Pet turtles have also been known to carry the organism.

The clinical presentation is often a self-limiting enteritis with watery diarrhea associated with abdominal pain and cramping. Infection may produce septicemia with systemic symptoms including fever, cough, and meningismus (enteric fever). There may be a relative bradycardia associated with high fever; this is most often seen with infection of *S. typhi*. Typhoid fever may present as an unremitting fever with abdominal pain, cramps, rose spots (10 to 20 percent), and meningismus. Diarrhea may be absent. Drug addicts and persons with AIDS, splenectomies, or sickle cell disease are particlarly susceptible to *Salmonella* infections. The diagnosis is based on recovery of the organism from blood, urine, and stool cultures. Febrile agglutinins may be positive, but generally this test lacks sensitivity and specificity.

Therapy depends on the clinical syndrome. Gastroenteritis is treated with replacement of fluid losses and control of nausea and vomiting. Drugs that reduce bowel motility should not be used as they may prolong the illness. Antibiotic treatment should be reserved for patients at risk for serious infection, those with enteric fever, bacteremia, or disseminated disease. Ampicillin and chloramphenicol are efficacious in the treatment of typhoid fever and bacteremia, while trimethoprim with sulfamethoxazole or ciprofloxacin should be used for nontyphoidal enteritis. Cefotaxime or ceftriaxone are preferred for meningismus or ampicillin-resistant strains. Antibiotic treatment is not recommended for the carrier state or for uncomplicated acute gastroenteritis. The carrier state may require prolonged treatment with antibiotics, which would select out resistant strains. Bacteremia and enteric fever may be accompanied by biliary disease, and, rarely, cholecystectomy may be necessary.

### Yersinia Enterocolitis

Domestic animals including household pets have been implicated in the transmission of *Yersinia* to humans. Food- and water-borne and fecal-oral transmission have also been shown to occur. Infection is associated with acute enteritis, dysentery, and fever. Mesenteric adenitis, terminal ileitis, and pseudoappendicitis may also occur. Blood is found in the stool in 25 percent of the cases, and erythema nodosum may be present, particularly in women.

*Yersinia* is difficult to isolate in the laboratory, and when infection is suspected, one should specifically request the laboratory to isolate the organism. This may take days to accomplish, and often the symptoms have subsided when the report is returned from the laboratory. Symptomatic cases may be treated with chloramphenicol, tetracycline, trimethoprim with sulfamethoxazole, or a third-generation cephalosporin, although there is no agreement about a precise treatment protocol. There is not enough experience with treatment with the quinolones to recommend them as alternative therapy.

### Campylobacter fetus sp. jejuni

*Campylobacter fetus* sp. *jejuni* was first described in 1977 as a frequent cause of diarrhea. Isolation of the organism requires special laboratory techniques, and when such isolation has been performed routinely, the organism has been shown to be more common than *Salmonella* and *Shigella* as a cause of bacterial diarrhea. A heat-labile enterotoxin and tissue invasion have been implicated in the pathophysiology. The majority of patients present with fever and bloody diarrhea; two thirds have abdominal pain, and one third have vomiting. *Campylobacter* gastroenteritis is most frequently reported in children. Water-borne infections have been reported. Erythromycin is the treatment of choice in children, and tetracycline or ciprofloxacin in adults. Parenteral treatment with gentamicin may be required to treat serious infections.

### Clostridium perfringens

*Clostridium perfringens* is a common cause of food poisoning. The organism is part of the normal flora of the colon of humans and other animals but only heat-resistant strains have been associated with enteritis. Human intestinal carriage of heat-resistant strains is in the range of 2 to 9 percent. The incubation period is 6 to 24 h, with an average of 12 h to the onset of symptoms. These include abdominal cramps and diarrhea. Constitutional symptoms such as headache, chills, and fever may occur, although they are not prominent features of clostridial food poisoning. Nausea and vomiting are not common. Meat and meat products are usually implicated in the transmission. Clostridial food poisoning is generally self-limited and requires no therapy. Antitoxin to the beta toxin has been considered useful in the treatment of necrotizing enteritis of type C *C. perfringens*.

### Clostridium difficile

An overgrowth of this organism has been associated with pseudomembranous enterocolitis, which may develop after even a short course of antibiotics. The organism releases cytotoxins that produce a profuse diarrhea that may be indistinguishable from that of severe shigellosis. Toxin A damages the mucosa of the bowel, allowing for dissemination of toxin B into the systemic circulation. If untreated, the disease is associated with high mortality. Treatment includes vancomycin, the binding of the toxin with cholestyramine, and the administration of supportive fluids.

### Staphylococcus aureus

Infections with *Staphylococcus* may occur after antibiotic therapy, with an overgrowth of the organism in the bowel and resultant enterocolitis. The enterotoxins may also contaminate food such as ham, poultry, meats, and dairy products. The organism and the enterotoxins it produces are the most common cause of food-borne disease. Vomiting and diarrhea are the most common symptoms, but abdominal cramps, headache, and prostration may occur when large amounts of toxin are ingested. The incubation period is 2 to 24 h, with symptoms appearing most often 6 to 12 h after ingestion of the toxin. The disease is generally self-limited, and supportive therapy is all that is required.

### Bacillus cereus

Bacillus cereus enterotoxins cause two clinical syndromes. They have been associated with a predominantly upper GI tract illness with vomiting that may develop 1 to 6 h after ingestion of contaminated food, particularly fried rice. A lower intestinal tract illness that resembles *C. perfringens* enteritis may also develop 6 to 24 h after ingesting a contaminated meal; *B. cereus* should be suspected if more than $10^5$ organisms are isolated from the stool. Treatment is symptomatic.

### Vibrio cholerae

Cholera is an acute infectious diarrhea caused by *V. cholerae*. The disease is transmitted by contaminated water or food. A large inoculum of the organism is required to produce disease because of the acid sensitivity of the bacteria. The illness may begin with vomiting, but production of copious watery diarrhea is the hallmark of clinical cholera. Large volumes of "rice water" stool may lead to (1) severe dehydration due to loss of isotonic fluid from the bowel, (2) acidosis due to loss of bicarbonate in the stool, and (3) hypokalemia due to potassium loss in the stool. The disease may be complicated by renal failure and hypovolemic shock. Imported cases of toxigenic *V. cholera* (0139 strain) have occurred in several states and may be seen more commonly in travelers in the future. Therapy is aimed at oral or parenteral replacement of fluids. Antibiotics may shorten the clinical course; tetracycline and trimethoprim with sulfamethoxazole are the drugs of choice.

### Vibrio parahaemolyticus

This organism has been associated with the ingestion of raw or improperly prepared seafood, particularly oysters, clams, and crabs. The spectrum of disease varies from mild gastroenteritis to explosive diarrhea associated with cramps, vomiting, and dysentery. The average incubation period is 12 h but may vary from 2 to 24 h. As is the case with cholera, symptomatic treatment is important. It is unclear if oral antibiotics are beneficial. In severe infections, however, tetracycline and chloramphenicol have been used.

### Aeromonas

*Aeromonas* is responsible for about 6 percent of bacterial diarrheal illness. It has been found in water contaminated with plant matters and is isolated from 1 to 18 percent of stool cultures. Clinical manifestations include low-grade fever and mild to moderate diarrhea, which usually lasts for more than 10 days. One third of patients will have abdominal pain, and one quarter dysenteric stools. The organism may not be routinely reported by the laboratory; thus, requests for isolation should be made in suspected cases. Treatment may not be necessary except in protracted infections, in which case either trimethoprim with sulfamethoxazole or chloramphenicol may be used. Aminoglycosides may be effective in serious infections.

### Plesiomonas shigelloides

*Plesiomonas* causes an illness very similar to *Aeromonas*. It is found in water, fish, and many animals including domestic dogs and cats. Symptomatic infection is usually self-limited but may include dysenteric stools. Diarrhea may be a particular problem in immunosuppressed individuals. Infection does not usually require antibiotic therapy.

### Vibrio vulnificus

This *Vibrio* species was first described in human illness in 1979. The organism is commonly found in the warm waters of the Gulf of Mexico, and infection is acquired by eating contaminated raw oysters and shellfish. An outbreak in Florida was associated with a 35 percent mortality rate. Persons with preexisting liver disease are particularly at risk for a bad outcome.

Venereal transmission of bacteria may occur in persons engaging in anal intercourse. Bacteria associated with enteritis include *Shigella* and *Campylobacter*. Others may cause enteritis and/or proctitis such as *Chlamydia, Campylobacter, Neisseria gonorrhoeae,* and *Treponema pallidum*. Parasites transmitted venereally include *Giardia, Entamoeba histolytica,* pinworm, *Pediculus hominis,* and *Phthirus pubis*.

## Parasites

A variety of parasitic protozoa and helminths may produce diarrhea during the course of infection. Only several, however, are important in the United States as a cause of acute diarrheal disease. (See Table 84-3.)

### Entamoeba histolytica

*Entamoeba histolytica* is found in 10 percent of the world's population, with 35 to 50 million individuals developing clinical symptoms each year. The prevalence of *E. histolytica* infection in the United States is probably between 1 and 5 percent. The majority of those infected are asymptomatic. Asymptomatic cyst passers may transmit the disease through the fecal-oral route as well as by contaminating the environment with infected cysts. The disease may also be venereally transmitted through anal intercourse. Infection may cause colitis with abdominal cramps and diarrhea, or acute amebic dysentery with profuse bloody diarrhea. Vomiting is usually absent. Approximately 5 percent of the patients with dysentery develop extraintestinal amebiasis. The liver is the most common site of amebic abscesses, but they can also develop in the lung, heart, kidney, or brain. Treatment includes the use of metronidazole, tetracycline, or, for severe infections, emetine hydrochloride or dehydroemetine plus chloroquine. Iodoquinol should also be given to eradicate the cyst stage.

### Giardia lamblia

*Giardia* is the most common intestinal parasite in the United States. Infection may be asymptomatic. Transmission is through fecal or oral contamination with infective cysts or through other contamination of water and food. Beavers have been shown to play a role in transmission through infection of mountain streams in Colorado and the northwest. Patients most often complain of abdominal pain, distension, postprandial urgency to defecate, and feeling bloated and gaseous. They may have profuse foul-smelling diarrhea. Classically the stools are floating, frothy, and foul-smelling. Diagnosis may be difficult as the cysts are only passed sporadically. Outbreaks occur commonly among travelers and in day-care centers. An antigen test of the stool is the most cost-effective method of diagnosis. The sensitivity and specificity of the newer tests are excellent. For those who do not have this test available, at least three stools should be submitted for examination for ova and parasites. If these are negative and there is a high index of suspicion, an Enterotest (string test) or duodenal aspiration may be performed to look for trophozoites, or the patient can be presumptively treated and followed for relief of symptoms. Although metronidazole has been used effectively for the treatment of giardiasis, it is not approved for use in this infection. Quinacrine hydrochloride is the drug of choice. Furazolidone may be used as an alternative to other drugs and is preferred by some for children as it comes in a liquid preparation.

### Cryptosporidium

*Cryptosporidium* is an intestinal protozoan that was described in mice in 1907. It was subsequently found to be responsible for diarrhea in a variety of animals. The first case in humans was reported in 1976 and it is now recognized as a significant pathogen in immunosuppressed patients, children in day-care, and travelers. Over 400,000 cases occurred in Milwaukee from contamination of the water supply, and beaches in New Jersey have been closed due to water contaminated with the organism. The prevalence in cases of acute diarrhea varies from 1 to 8 percent. The organism is acquired by the ingestion of infective cysts from fecal-oral contamination of food and water from human or animal sources. The infective stage is extremely resistant to various agents and may also be transmitted on fomites or contaminated environmental surfaces. Cryptosporidiosis usually presents as a profuse, watery diarrhea without gross blood. Other symptoms may include nausea, vomiting, anorexia, abdominal pain, and cramping. Diagnosis may be made by an acid-fast stain of the stool. The severity and duration of the illness depend on the immunologic status of the patient. It is usually self-limiting but may cause severe dehydration. There is no effective therapy; however, paromomycin has recently been shown to be effective in some immunosuppressed patients. In patients with AIDS, cryptosporidiosis may cause a chronic diarrheal syndrome with hepatobiliary disease and is associated with significant morbidity and mortality.

### Cyclospora parvi

*Cyclospora* resembles *Cryptosporidium* but is larger and not as acid-fast. The clinical manifestations are similar to cryptosporidiosis and no effective therapy has been found.

### Microspora

*Nosema, Encephalitozoon,* and *Enterocytozoon* are three genera that infect imunnosuppressed individuals and can cause a profuse watery diarrhea. Some investigators have questioned the pathogenicity of this organism. Treatment is symptomatic.

### Isospora belli

Like *Cryptosporidium, I. belli* is a sporozoan parasite that is probably transmitted from person to person. In normal individuals it produces a self-limiting disease consisting of mild fever, headache, diarrhea, and colicky abdominal pain. In the immunocompromised host, it produces profuse diarrhea, which may occur cyclically and is associated with significant weight loss. Diagnosis is difficult and must be made by examination of the stool by an experienced technician. Treatment with trimethoprim with sulfamethoxazole is usually successful, but relapses in AIDS patients are common.

### Dientamoeba fragilis

*Dientamoeba fragilis* is an ameboflagellate that is probably transmitted by fecal-oral contamination, although the exact mechanism is not known. Transmission in the ova of the pinworm has been suggested as a likely mode of infection. The prevalence of diarrheal disease is probably about 1 percent. The organism is not invasive and generally produces abdominal pain, anorexia, and intermittent diarrhea. Diagnosis is by examination of the stool by an experienced technician. Treatment with iodoquinol, paromomycin, or tetracycline has been successful.

### Blastocystis hominis

*Blastocystis hominis* is commonly isolated from the stool on O and P examination. There are many anecdotal reports of diarrhea attributed to this organism, but controlled studies have failed to demonstrate pathogenicity. Presence of the organism is most likely a marker for fecal-oral contamination and no treatment is usually necessary.

## Diarrhea in Immunosuppressed Individuals

Diarrhea can be particularly devastating to immunosuppressed individuals, particularly those with HIV infection. Table 84-4 lists the organisms commonly associated with diarrheal illness in these patients. Aggressive therapy to replace fluid and electrolyte losses, maintenance of positive nitrogen balance, and aggressive antimicrobial therapy are recommended.

**Table 84-4.** Organisms That Cause Gastroenteritis Associated with HIV Infection

*Salmonella*
*Shigella*
*Candida*
*Giardia lamblia*
*Cryptosporidium*
*Microspora*
*Isospora*
*Cytomegalovirus*
HIV
*Mycobacterium avium-intracellulare*
*Entamoeba histolytica*
Herpes simplex virus
*Mycobacterium tuberculosis*

## Ciguatera Fish Poisoning

Although many exogenous toxins may cause GI upset, they are too numerous to discuss in this chapter. Ciguatera fish poisoning is worth mentioning, as its prevalence is increasing in the southeastern United States. Fish whose ingestion can cause the disease are found in tropical and subtropical waters. These fish, particularly grouper, snapper, and kingfish, become sporadically poisonous when a particular dinoflagellate is present in the food chain in the late spring and summer months. The incubation period varies from 2 to 30 h after ingestion of the toxin (median 6 h). The illness may begin with vomiting and diarrhea, which are present in 78 percent of the patients. Neuromuscular and neurosensory manifestations may be particularly severe and lead to prolonged discomfort. These include myalgia of the legs and thighs, weakness, and dysesthesia and paresthesia of the perioral region and distal extremities. Occasionally patients describe a "burning" sensation of their feet or hands. Itching of various parts of the body is common and may be a late manifestation on day 2 or 3 of the illness. The disease is self-limiting, and there is no specific therapy. Symptoms generally subside in several days, but some patients have reported having sensory problems for months after the ingestion of affected fish.

## GENERAL MANAGEMENT

A complete history, including the time and onset of symptoms, travel, and the relation of symptoms to ingestion of a particular food, is important in determining the cause of the GI illness. The presence and frequency of fever may be helpful as well as the consistency, frequency, and odor of the stool. The presence of mucus or blood in the stool should also be determined. Physical examination should include all systems, as extraintestinal disease may cause GI upset and diarrhea. Particular attention should be paid to the signs of dehydration, mucous membrane, skin turgor, postural changes in blood pressure, level of consciousness, and the fontanel in young infants. Many patients with acute diarrheal disease will have abdominal tenderness, but if this is severe or persistent, the patient should be observed for a process that may require surgical intervention. Diarrheal disease can be a life-threatening emergency in the very young and the elderly.

Laboratory studies are not generally helpful in the acute management of food poisoning and infectious diarrhea. A high white blood cell count with a left shift may suggest a bacterial cause; however, this condition is not always present. In typhoid fever one may see a relatively low white blood cell count, neutropenia, or a marked shift to left. Electrolytes are indicated when dehydration is suspected, and urine specific gravity should be obtained. If a stool sample is available, a wet mount may be made by mixing a small amount of feces with normal saline or methylene blue on a slide. Microscopic examination of this preparation may show white and red blood cells, mucous strands, and trophozoites or cysts of parasitic protozoa. A guiac

**Table 84-5.** Oral Rehydration Fluids

| | Electrolyte content, mEq/L | | | |
|---|---|---|---|---|
| | **WHO** | **Pedialyte** | **Rehydralyte** | **Isolyte** |
| Sodium | 90 | 45 | 75 | 50 |
| Potassium | 20 | 20 | 20 | 25 |
| Chloride | 80 | 35 | 65 | 45 |
| Citrate | 30 | 30 | 30 | 34 |
| Glucose | 20 | 25 | 25 | — |
| Rice-syrup solids | — | — | — | 30 |

test of the stool may also reveal the presence of blood. Cultures should be sent to the laboratory in transport media when *Salmonella, Shigella, Campylobacter,* or *Vibrio* infections are suspected, because of the public health importance of these infections. An acid-fast stain of the stool may show *Cryptosporidium* or *Cyclospora.* Ova and parasite examinations may reveal *E. histolytica, Giardia, Isospora,* or *D. fragilis.*

Many prescription and over-the-counter preparations are available for the treatment of diarrhea, vomiting, and GI upset. Few have been shown to be effective in altering the course of the illness. Most infectious and noninfectious GI illnesses are self-limiting and do not require specific therapy.

Antibiotics should be reserved for patients who are febrile and toxic and only for diseases for which they have been shown to be effective. Contraindications to antibiotic therapy may exist in some uncomplicated infections, such as salmonellosis, as they prolong the carrier state.

Other medications such as diphenoxylate hydrochloride with atropine (Lomotil) or loperamide (Imodium) may provide temporary symptomatic relief and may be efficacious if the patient has uncontrollable diarrhea. These preparations and others that slow peristalsis and delay intestinal emptying may prolong the illness, as infective organisms and toxins have continued contact with the bowel. They are contraindicated in cholera. The mainstay of therapy is putting the intestinal tract at rest and maintaining hydration. Most patients can be managed with a clear liquid diet. Liquids may include clear fruit juices, sodas, gelatin dessert water, rice water, etc. The oral rehydration fluids available for infants and their electrolyte content are shown on Table 84-5. The WHO preparation was devised to treat cholera and probably contains too much sodium for use in the United States. Commonly used clear liquids may not have sufficient electrolytes to replace on-going losses (Table 84-6), and some such as apple juice and cola, have a high osmolality. The diet may be advanced to include rice, applesauce, bananas, and toast when the diarrhea has subsided. Small sips of clear liquids should be recommended when vomiting is prominent. Using Popsicles is also recommended. Feeding should begin as soon as possible to restore a positive nitrogen balance, which aids the healing of the intestinal mucosa.

Phenothiazine preparations may be used with severe vomiting but are not recommended in children because of a higher incidence of dystonic reactions. Hospitalization should be considered in the very young and old when there is evidence of dehydration.

Table 84-7 lists some of the organisms responsible for diarrhea and the drugs commonly used in treatment.

**Table 84-6.** Electrolyte-Glucose Concentrations of Clear Liquids

| Liquid | Na, mEq/L | K | HCO₃ | Glucose, g/L | Osmolarity |
|---|---|---|---|---|---|
| Cola | 2 | 0.1 | 13 | 50–150 | 550 |
| Ginger ale | 3 | 1 | 4 | 50–150 | 540 |
| Apple juice | 3 | 20 | 0 | 100–150 | 700 |
| Chicken broth | 250 | 5 | 0 | 0 | 450 |
| Tea | 0 | 0 | 0 | 0 | 5 |
| Gatorade | 20 | 3 | 3 | 45 | 330 |

**Table 84-7.** Drug Therapy for Diarrhea

| Organism | Drug | How Supplied | Dosage |
|---|---|---|---|
| *Campylobacter jejuni* | Erythromycin<br><br>*or*<br><br><br><br><br>Tetracycline (older children and adults) | Ethylsuccinate: 200-, 400 mg/5 mL, 400-mg tabs<br>Estolate: 125 mg/5 mL, 125-, 250-mg tbs<br>Salt: 125-, 250-mg tabs<br>Stearate: 125-, 250, 500-mg tabs<br>250-, 500-mg tabs<br>Syrup: 25 mg/mL<br>Drops: 100 mg/mL | 50 mg/kg (maximum 2 g) divided qid for 7–10 days<br><br><br><br><br>25–50 mg/kg divided qid (maximum 500 mg qid) 7–10 days |
| *Clostridium difficile* | Vancomycin | Oral solution: Mix to make 250 mg/5 mL or 500 mg/5 mL<br>Injectable 1-g vials | 20–40 mg/kg PO divided qid (maximum 500 mg qid) 7–10 days |
| *Entamoeba histolytica*<br>Asymptomatic cyst passers | Iodoquinol<br>*or*<br>Paromomycin | <br><br>250-mg capsules | 13 mg/kg tid × 21 days (maximum 650 mg tid)<br>7–10 mg/kg tid × 10 days |
| Passers of cysts and trophozoites | Metronidazole<br>*plus*<br>Iodoquinol<br>*or*<br>Tetracycline<br><br><br>*plus*<br>Iodoquinol | 250-mg tabs<br><br><br><br>250-, 500-mg tabs<br>Syrup: 25 mg/mL<br>Drops: 100 mg/mL<br><br>650-mg tabs | 12–17 mg/kg tid × 10 days (maximum 750 mg tid)<br>13 mg/kg tid × 21 days<br><br>2.5–5 mg/kg qid × 7 days (maximum 2g/day)<br><br><br>*plus*<br>Iodoquinol as above |
| Amebic dysentery | Metronidazole<br>*plus*<br>Iodoquinol<br>*or*<br>Dehydroemetine<br>*plus*<br>Chloroquine phosphate<br>*or*<br>Tetracycline, iodoquinol, and chloroquine | <br><br><br><br><br><br>125-, 250-mg tabs | 12–17 mg/kg tid × 10 days<br>*plus*<br>13 mg/kg tid × 21 days<br><br>1.5 mg/kg IM × 5 days (maximum 90 mg/day)<br>5 mg/kg/d × 14–21 days<br><br>Doses as listed above |
| *Escherichia coli*<br>(Only persistent infections) | Trimethoprim with sulfamethoxazole | Suspension: 40 mg TMP and 200 mg SMX/5 mL; 80/400-mg or 160/800-mg tabs | 8–10 mg/kg TMP with 40–50 mg/kg SMX divided bid (maximum 160/800 mg PO bid) 5–7 days |
| *Giardia lamblia* | Quinacrine HCl<br><br>*or*<br>Metronidazole<br><br>Furazolidone | 100-mg tabs<br><br><br>250-mg tabs<br><br>100-mg tabs<br>Suspension: 50 mg/15 mL | 7 mg/kg divided tid × 7 days (maximum 100 mg tid)<br><br>10–15 mg/kg divided tid × 7 days (maximum 250 mg tid)<br>1.5 mg/kg divided qid × 7 days (maximum 100 mg qid) |
| *Salmonella sp.*<br>(Only persistent symptomatic infections) | Ampicillin<br><br><br><br>*or*<br>Trimethoprim with sulfamethoxazole<br>*or*<br>Chloramphenicol | Suspension: 125, 250 mg/5 mL<br>Capsules: 250, 500 mg<br>Drops: 100 mg/mL<br>Chewable tabs: 125 mg<br><br>As above<br><br><br>Suspension: 150 mg/5 mL 100-, 250-mg capsules | 50–100 mg/kg divided qid × 7–14 days (maximum 500 mg qid)<br><br><br><br>As above<br><br><br>50 mg/kg divided qid for 7–14 days (maximum 500 mg qid) |
| *Shigella sp.* | Trimethoprim with sulfamethoxazole | As above | As above but × 7–14 days |
| *Shigella sp.* (resistant cases) | Ciprofloxacin HCl | 250-mg tabs | 250 mg bid × 5–7 days |
| *Yersinia enterocolitica* | Trimethoprim with sulfamethoxazole<br>*or*<br>Tetracycline<br>*or*<br>Third-generation cephalosporin | As above<br><br><br>250-, 500-mg capsules | As above<br><br><br>20–50 mg/kg divided qid × 7–10 days (maximum 500 mg qid)<br>As directed |

## BIBLIOGRAPHY

Black RE, Jackson RJ, Tsia T, et al: Epidemic *Yersinia enterocolitica* infection due to contaminated chocolate milk. *N Engl J Med* 298:76, 1978.

Communicable Disease Surveillance Center, PHLS: Surveillance of food poisoning and *Salmonella* infections in England and Wales 1170–9. *Br Med J* 281:817, 1980.

Desenclos JA, Klontz KC, Wolfe LE, et al: The risk of *Vibrio* illness in the Florida raw oyster eating population, 1981–1988. *Am J Epdemiol* 134:290, 1991.

Gorbach SL (ed): Infectious diarrhea. *Infect Dis Clin North Am* 2: 1988.

Harris JC, Dupont HL, Hornck RB: Fecal leukocytes in diarrheal illness. *Ann Intern Med* 76:697, 1972.

Kimmey M: Infectious diarrhea. *Emerg Clin North Am* 3:127, 1985.

Lawrence DN, Enriquez MB, Lumish RM, et al: Ciguatera fish poisoning in Miami. *JAMA* 244:254, 1980.

Lowenstein MS: Epidemiology of *Clostridium perfringens* food poisoning. *N Engl J Med* 286:1026, 1972.

Markell EK, Voge M, John DT: *Medical Parasitology,* 7th ed. Philadelphia, Saunders, 1991.

Ortega YR, Sterling CR, Gilman RH, et al: *Cyclospora* species—a new protozoan pathogen of humans. *N Engl J Med* 328:1308, 1993.

Rodriquez WJ, Kim HW, Arrobio JO, et al: Clinical features of acute gastroenteritis associated with human reovirus-like agent in infants and young children. *J Pediatr* 91:188, 1977.

Soave R, Johnson WD: *Cryptosporidium* and *Isospora belli* infections. *J Infect Dis* 157:225, 1988.

Tormey M, Mascola L, Kilman L, et al: Imported cholera associated with a newly developed toxigenic *Vibrio cholerae* 0139 strain—California 1993. *MMWR* 42:501, 1993.

US Department of Health and Human Services, Public Health Service: The management of acute diarrhea in children: Oral rehydration, maintenance, and nutritional therapy. *MMWR* 41:No RR-16, 1992.

# 85
# CHOLECYSTITIS AND BILIARY COLIC

### Tom P. Aufderheide
### William J. Brady

## INTRODUCTION

Biliary tract emergencies result primarily from obstruction caused by gallstones, or biliary calculi, in the gallbladder and bile ducts. The four major biliary tract emergencies related to gallstones include symptomatic cholelithiasis (biliary colic or the symptomatic presence of gallstones), cholecystitis (acute gallbladder inflammation due to obstruction of the gallbladder outlet), gallstone pancreatitis (gallstone obstruction of the ampulla of Vater with reflux of bile into the pancreas), and ascending cholangitis (acute retrograde inflammation of the bile ducts caused by complete biliary obstruction). Symptomatic cholelithiasis and acute cholecystitis are the two most frequently encountered clinical syndromes related to gallstones managed by the emergency physician.

In the United States, autopsy series have demonstrated that at least 20 percent of females and 8 percent of males over the age of 40 have gallstones. Currently, it is estimated that approximately 16 to 20 million Americans have gallstones, with 1 million new cases occurring annually resulting in 500,000 operations per year. Twenty percent of these surgical procedures are performed for acute cholecystitis. The majority (approximately 50 to 80 percent) of gallstone patients are asymptomatic. The incidence of new-onset biliary pain among patients with previously asymptomatic calculi is reportedly 10 percent at 5 years, 15 percent at 10 years, and 18 percent at 15 to 20 years. Furthermore, it appears that a minority of these patients develop complications such as acute cholecystitis. Therefore, prophylactic cholecystectomy is no longer recommended in most asymptomatic patients. Expectant management with close observation is the preferred approach to this patient group.

The typical patient who presents with symptomatic biliary tract disease is an obese female aged 20 to 40 years. Gallstones were previously thought to be rare in the pediatric population but are now recognized more frequently and are usually associated with chronic hemolytic disease and structural gastrointestinal or hepatobiliary disorders.

A number of risk factors are associated with the formation of cholesterol calculi, including increased age, female sex, parity, obesity, profound weight loss, prolonged fasting, cystic fibrosis, intestinal malabsorption syndromes, various medications (particularly oral contraceptive agents and clofibrate), and a familial tendency. Clinical characteristics that are associated with an increased risk of the development of pigment stones are Asian descent, chronic biliary tract infection, parasitic infection (e.g., *Ascaris lumbridoides*), chronic liver disease (particularly related to alcohol), and chronic intravascular hemolysis (sickle cell anemia and hereditary spherocytosis).

## PATHOPHYSIOLOGY

Bile is manufactured in and secreted from the hepatocyte and then transported to the gallbladder for storage via the canaliculi, ductiles, and bile ducts. The bile ducts become progressively larger and eventually coalesce to form the right and left hepatic ducts, which unite to form the common hepatic duct. The common hepatic duct joins with the cystic duct from the gallbladder to form the common bile duct, which then empties into the duodenum through the ampulla of Vater. The pancreatic duct often merges with the common bile duct immediately prior to entering the duodenum.

Bile, a pigmented isotonic fluid, is composed primarily of water (80 percent), bile acids (10 percent), lecithin and other phospholipids (4 to 5 percent), cholesterol (1 percent), conjugated bilirubin, electrolytes, mucus, various proteins, and medications. The major stimulus for release of bile is the gastrointestinal hormone cholecystokinin, which is secreted from the small intestinal mucosal cells when fats and amino acids enter the duodenum. Cholecystokinin causes forceful contraction of the gallbladder, relaxation of the sphincter of Oddi, increased hepatic bile production, and ultimately release of bile into the duodenum for digestion of a meal. Approximately 95 percent of bile is conserved via enterohepatic circulation.

Gallstones, crystalline structures formed from both normal and abnormal bile components, are divided into three major types: cholesterol (70 percent), pigment (20 percent), and mixed (10 percent). Cholesterol stones, the most commonly encountered gallstone, contain more than 70 percent cholesterol monohydrate. The formation of such stones is complex, involving cholesterol supersaturation of the bile, the formation of monohydrate crystals with aggregation into successively larger structures, and delayed gallbladder emptying with bile stasis. Pigment stones are subdivided into black and brown varieties. Black stones are noted in patients with advanced liver disease and hemolytic disorders, while brown stones are found commonly in patients of Asian descent, usually resulting from bacterial or parasitic infection. Both subtypes of pigment stones result from abnormal solubilization of unconjugated bilirubin coupled with the precipitation of calcium salts. The calcium content of cholesterol stones is much lower than that of pigment stones, making cholesterol stones most frequently radiolucent and pigment stones radiopaque. Anatomically, cholesterol gallstones are found in the gallbladder, cystic duct, intrahepatic ducts, and common bile duct. Brown pigment stones have a distribution similar to cholesterol gallstones, while black stones occur exclusively in the gallbladder.

The pathogenesis of symptomatic cholelithiasis involves stone migration from the gallbladder into the biliary tract with eventual obstruction. The stone, once lodged in either the cystic or common bile ducts, produces increased intraluminal pressure and distension of the hollow viscus, resulting in pain, nausea, and vomiting. Forceful, repetitive contractions of the entire biliary system may relieve the obstruction. If obstruction persists, particularly in either the cystic duct or the infundibulum of the gallbladder, acute cholecystitis may develop. The inflammatory response responsible for acute cholecystitis results from a combination of three factors: mechanical, chemical, and infectious. The mechanical factor produces the rise in intraluminal pressure and distension of the viscus, which culminates in visceral ischemia. Chemical inflammation occurs with the release of various mediators (lysolecithin, phospholipase A, and prostaglandins), resulting in direct mucosal injury. The contribution to the inflammatory response by bacterial agents is variable, occurring in 50 to 80 percent of patients with acute cholecystitis. Bacterial pathogens include enterobacteriaceae (70 percent, particularly *Escherichia coli* and *Klebsiella* species), enterococci (15 percent), bacteroides (10 percent), *Clostridium* species (10 percent), group D *Streptococcus,* and *Staphylococcus* species. The inflammatory process may progress to gangrene of the gallbladder wall, with or without perforation.

## CLINICAL FEATURES

Patients with gallstones may present in a variety of ways. Gallstones may be noted incidentally on plain film radiographs or via ultrasonography in asymptomatic patients undergoing evaluation for another medical purpose.

The most common presentation of cholelithiasis is biliary colic. Biliary colic is classically characterized by right upper quadrant or epigastric abdominal pain with radiation to the right posterior shoulder or scapula associated with nausea and vomiting. Patients may have a history of similar episodes, with both increasing frequency and intensity of the exacerbations noted over the recent past. The pain occurs quite suddenly approximately 30 to 60 min after the ingestion of a meal—a normal meal, a large meal after a period of fasting, or a fatty meal. The pain ranges from mild to severe, lasting from 1 to 6 h. Although gallstone-related pain may sometimes be constant, it is most frequently characterized by intermittent exacerbations followed by pain reduction without complete relief, as the name "colic" implies. Eventually, it may gradually subside or rapidly disappear. Patients may be left with a mild abdominal aching or soreness for 1 to 2 days after resolution of the attack. A history of chills or fever suggests that cholecystitis, cholangitis, or pancreatitis may be present. The physical examination may demonstrate mild right upper quadrant tenderness without evidence of peritoneal irritation as well as volume depletion due to protracted emesis.

Acute cholecystitis usually begins with pain similar to biliary colic, which persists beyond the typical 6 h. Associated nausea, vomiting, and anorexia are noted; a history of fever and/or chills is not uncommon. Patients may have either a history of similar attacks in the past or documented gallstones. As the inflammatory process progresses, the patient's pain changes in character and location from visceral (dull and poorly localized mid-upper abdominal) to parietal (sharp and localized right upper quadrant). The examination reveals a patient in moderate to severe distress with signs of systemic toxicity, including tachycardia and fever. The abdomen is tender in the right upper quadrant, at times with evidence of localized peritoneal irritation, distension, and hypoactive bowel sounds. Generalized peritonitis with rigidity is rare and, if found, suggests perforation. The Murphy sign—worsened pain or inspiratory arrest resulting from deep, sub-

costal palpation on inspiration—may be noted. Volume depletion is frequently found. Jaundice, usually not present, may be found in patients with prolonged biliary obstruction with late onset of inflammation or in cases of chronic intravascular hemolysis.

Acalculous cholecystitis, which occurs in 5 to 10 percent of patients with acute cholecystitis, tends to have a more rapid, malignant course. Patients frequently are elderly and have a history of diabetes mellitus. Other risk factors include multiple trauma, extensive burn injury, prolonged labor, major surgery, gallbladder torsion, systemic vasculitic states, and bacterial or parasitic infections of the biliary tract. Patients with acalculous cholecystitis are indistinguishable from those with calculous cholecystitis with two major exceptions. Acalculous cholecystitis frequently occurs as a complication of another process (e.g., multiple trauma or extensive burns), and patients frequently are gravely ill on initial presentation.

## DIAGNOSTIC STUDIES

### Biliary Colic

Laboratory studies in patients with symptomatic cholelithiasis are most often normal. The hemogram may reveal chronic anemia with or without evidence of hemolysis in patients with pigment stones. The white blood cell count is frequently within normal limits. The serum bilirubin and alkaline phosphatase may be normal or minimally elevated while the serum aminotransferases are usually normal. The serum bilirubin will be elevated in cases of hemolysis. Serum studies evaluating the pancreas, amylase, and lipase are obtained to rule out an atypical presentation of pancreatitis or coexisting gallstone pancreatitis. The urine and its sediment must be examined to exclude other causes of abdominal pain. In females, serum or urine pregnancy testing should be obtained to rule out obstetric-related causes of abdominal pain. A negative pregnancy test also enables the emergency physician to proceed safely with radiologic studies, if indicated.

Additional studies in patients with biliary colic may be performed to support the diagnosis and rule out other causes of upper abdominal pain with nausea. Plain film radiographs of the abdomen will demonstrate gallstones in only 10 to 20 percent of cases. The majority of stones are cholesterol and therefore are radiolucent. Pigment and mixed stones, if they contain at least 4 percent calcium by weight, will be radiopaque. Abdominal films are more useful in excluding other causes of pain. A chest radiograph should be obtained to rule out right lower lobe pneumonia and to look for pleural effusions, which are not uncommonly found in patients with pancreatitis. A 12-lead electrocardiogram should be obtained in all older patients to exclude myocardial ischemia or infarction.

Diagnostic studies that have the ability to demonstrate gallstones include ultrasonography and oral cholecystography. Ultrasound of the gallbladder is very accurate in the identification of calculi, demonstrating 95 percent of stones when present, and has emerged as the procedure of choice for diagnosing gallstones and related biliary obstruction. It is performed without patient preparation and is able to visualize stones as small as 2 mm in diameter. In most major medical centers, the false-negative and false-positive rates for the ultrasonographic diagnosis of gallstones is 2 to 4 percent. Additionally, ultrasound provides an evaluation of the surrounding tissues. Emergency use of ultrasound can lead to more rapid diagnosis and reduce the number of delayed or invasive diagnostic methods. Oral cholecystography remains a useful adjunctive study in patients suspected of biliary colic with a normal or equivocal sonogram.

### Acute Cholecystitis

The diagnostic evaluation of patients suspected of acute cholecystitis begins with a complete blood count. A leukocytosis with predominance of polymorphonuclear forms is most often found. Importantly, a normal white blood cell count does not rule out the possibility of cholecystitis. Additional serum and urine laboratory studies should be obtained and will reveal findings similar to those discussed for biliary colic. Ultrasonography will reveal gallstones in the vast majority of cases but may not confirm the diagnosis of acute cholecystitis. The presence of stones, a thickened gallbladder wall, distension of the gallbladder itself, pericholecystic fluid, and a positive sonographic Murphy sign have a positive predictive value in excess of 90 percent for the diagnosis of acute cholecystitis. Conversely, the absence of stones and a normal gallbladder on ultrasound make the diagnosis of cholecystitis unlikely.

Radionuclide cholescintigraphy using technetium–iminodiacetic acid analogues (e.g., HIDA and DISIDA scans) has a sensitivity approaching 100 percent for the diagnosis of acute cholecystitis. The intravenously administered radionuclide is absorbed by the hepatocyte and secreted into the biliary tract, clearly outlining the gallbladder and cystic duct in the normal patient within 1 h. Failure to demonstrate the gallbladder within this time frame is consistent with cystic duct obstruction and a diagnosis of acute cholecystitis. The use of the HIDA scan is possible in patients with a serum bilirubin less than 5 to 7 mg/dL. With serum bilirubin levels above this range, the DISIDA scan is more accurate.

The choice of imaging studies in the evaluation of patients with acute cholecystitis remains controversial. A reasonable approach for the emergency physician is initial ultrasonography followed by scintigraphic studies if necessary.

## Acalculous Cholecystitis

A more comprehensive diagnostic approach is indicated in patients with suspected acalculous cholecystitis. Ultrasound and CT scanning will demonstrate a large, tense, static gallbladder without evidence of gallstones. Radionuclide examinations reveal poor filling of the gallbladder.

## COMPLICATIONS

Fluid and electrolyte deficits due to protracted vomiting and anorexia, and upper gastrointestinal hemorrhage from emesis-related Mallory-Weiss tears, can coexist with biliary tract emergencies. Complications associated with cholelithiasis include gallstone pancreatitis, ascending cholangitis, and cholecystitis. Patients with cholecystitis may further develop a number of serious complications including gallbladder empyema and emphysematous (gangrenous) cholecystitis.

Approximately 70 percent of cases of acute pancreatitis are due to either gallstones or alcohol. Depending on the population studied, gallstones are involved in 30 to 70 percent of patients with acute pancreatitis. Of all patients with gallstones, 15 to 20 percent will develop pancreatitis as a result of biliary calculi. Gallstone pancreatitis occurs due to obstruction of the ampulla of Vater with reflux of bile into the pancreas. Patients with pancreatitis due to gallstones will present similarly to patients with pancreatic inflammation caused by ethanol, with epigastric or diffuse abdominal pain radiating to the back, associated with nausea and vomiting. Patients may manifest symptoms of both acute cholecystitis and acute pancreatitis. Management includes intravenous fluids, nasogastric decompression, analgesics, and parenteral antibiotics with subsequent surgery. In patients who present in extremis or in those who demonstrate clinical deterioration, urgent biliary decompression (surgical or endoscopic) is mandatory.

Ascending cholangitis is a life-threatening emergency with a mortality rate approaching 100 percent in untreated or improperly treated patients. The process results from complete biliary obstruction in the presence of bacteria (gram-negative organisms as well as enterococcal and various anaerobic species). As the obstruction persists, intraluminal pressure increases, resulting in reflux of bacteria into the lymphatic vessels and hepatic veins with eventual entrance into the systemic circulation. The obstruction most often is due to choledo-

cholithiasis (gallstone obstruction of the common bile duct) and less often by biliary tract strictures, surgical anastomotic strictures, various postprocedural complications, and extrinsic compression from malignancy. Patients present with jaundice, fever, right upper quadrant pain, mental confusion, and shock. The classic Charcot triad of fever, jaundice, and right upper quadrant pain is noted in only 25 percent of patients. Management includes initial volume resuscitation with vasopressor support in cases unresponsive to crystalloid infusion alone, broad-spectrum parenteral antibiotics, and rapid decompression (surgical or endoscopic) of the biliary tree.

Gallbladder empyema, a life-threatening complication of cholecystitis, results from complete obstruction of the cystic duct with bacterial infection of the stagnant bile and abscess formation within the gallbladder wall. The presentation is similar to cholangitis, with fever, right upper quadrant pain, altered mentation, and hypotension. Such patients frequently develop gram-negative sepsis and require immediate broad-spectrum antibiotic coverage, fluid resuscitation, and urgent surgical consultation for cholecystectomy. Outcome is poor without prompt, definitive care.

Gangrene of the gallbladder wall may be focal or diffuse. Focal gangrene results from segmental ischemia of the gallbladder wall caused by severe distension, acute inflammation, empyema, torsion with arterial compromise, or coexisting vasculitis. Patients with diabetes mellitus are at risk for this complication. Perforation of the wall may occur in a contained fashion (into the omentum) or free (into the peritoneal cavity).

Gangrene of the entire gallbladder, also known as *emphysematous cholecystitis,* is an uncommon complication, occurring in approximately 1 percent of patients with cholecystitis. Emphysematous cholecystitis is acalculous in 30 percent of patients. With complete cystic duct obstruction, the gallbladder wall becomes ischemic with eventual bacterial infection and gangrene. Patients, typically diabetic men, present in extremis with fever, right upper quadrant pain, and septic shock. Plain film radiographs may demonstrate air in the gallbladder itself, the gallbladder wall, or in the biliary tree because of the frequent presence of gas-forming organisms. Abdominal CT scan is the suggested imaging study. The bacteriology of either focal or diffuse gallbladder gangrene includes gram-negative, gram-positive, and anaerobic organisms. Polymicrobial infection is common. Management is similar to that of gallbladder empyema. Mortality for gangrenous cholecystitis is very high because of associated sepsis and attendant comorbidity in the typical elderly diabetic patient.

## DIFFERENTIAL DIAGNOSIS

The differential diagnosis of patients with symptomatic cholelithiasis and acute cholecystitis includes hepatitis, hepatic abscess, pancreatitis, gastritis, peptic ulcer (perforated or penetrating), appendicitis, Fitz Hugh–Curtis syndrome (gonococcal or chlamydial perihepatitis), pelvic inflammatory disease with or without tuboovarian abscess, pyelonephritis, right lower lobe pneumonia, pleuritis, and myocardial ischemia or infarction. A review of patients admitted with acute cholecystitis published in the mid-1970s revealed a misdiagnosis rate of approximately 20 percent. While the clinical impression is important in the evaluation of such patients, radiologic support (ultrasonography and/or nuclear scans) of the diagnosis is appropriate in most instances, as shown from the results of this study.

## TREATMENT

Patients with accurately diagnosed uncomplicated symptomatic cholelithiasis do not necessarily require immediate surgical intervention. Patients presenting with biliary colic and emesis are best treated with antispasmodic agents (glycopyrrolate), opiate analgesics (meperidine), and antiemetics (promethazine). Meperidine is the analgesic of choice because it produces significantly less spasm of the sphincter of Oddi as compared to other narcotic agents such as morphine. Gastric decompression with nasogastric suction may be warranted for protracted vomiting. Volume deficits and electrolyte imbalance can be corrected by isotonic intravenous fluids. With an accurate diagnosis, resolution of symptoms, correction of intravascular volume deficits, and a demonstrated ability to maintain hydration orally, the patient may be discharged from the emergency department. Prior to discharge, the case should be discussed with a surgical consultant or the patient's primary care physician to arrange for timely outpatient follow-up. Patients may be given oral narcotic-acetaminophen pain medication for the common residual abdominal aching. If the biliary colic appears to be related to a particular stimulus such as a fatty meal, this trigger is best avoided. If the symptoms do not resolve within a 4- to 6-hour period in the emergency department, the diagnosis of biliary colic must be questioned. Such prolonged pain may rather represent early, acute cholecystitis.

Ketorolac tromethamine, an injectable nonsteroidal anti-inflammatory drug (NSAID), has been shown effective in relieving the pain of gallbladder distension. This distension causes the release of prostaglandins, which are associated with the production of pain. Ketorolac inhibits the production of prostaglandins and this may explain why it is effective in this situation. It is not as effective in relieving pain in the presence of infection. When ketorolac does not relieve pain in the clinical setting of symptomatic cholelithiasis, the clinician should reconsider the diagnosis.

The patient with uncomplicated symptomatic cholelithiasis has several options for definitive treatment, including open or laparoscopic cholecystectomy, medical dissolution therapy, and gallstone lithotripsy. Open cholecystectomy with intraoperative cholangiogram provides definitive cure for patients with biliary colic. The laparoscopic technique is a relatively new approach to such patients and is rapidly replacing the traditional open cholecystectomy as the procedure of choice. Patients with frequent or severe attacks of biliary colic, a past history of any associated complications of gallstones, large biliary calculi (>2 cm in diameter), congenitally abnormal hepatobiliary system, diabetes mellitus, or a desire for rapid cure are best managed with open or laparoscopic cholecystectomy.

Medical dissolution therapy includes oral bile acid treatment as well as direct gallbladder irrigation with ether-type solvents. Indications for such an approach include small (<1.5 cm) cholesterol stones that are radiolucent. With these criteria, approximately 10 to 15 percent of gallstone patients are candidates. Oral bile acid therapy (cheno- or ursodeoxycholic acid) requires up to 2 years for complete resolution of cholelithiasis, which occurs in up to 60 percent of patients. Recurrence is not infrequent after a successful treatment regimen. Direct irrigation of the gallbladder with ether-type solvents provides a rapid means (2 to 4 h) of calculus dissolution. However, recurrence is common. A combination of medical dissolution therapy and extracorporeal shock wave lithotripsy is another option for gallstone patients. Criteria for this approach include a maximum of three cholesterol stones less than 0.2 cm in diameter that are radiolucent. This criterion applies to 15 percent of gallstone patients.

Treatment of calculous and acalculous acute cholecystitis is surgical. Basic, supportive medical therapy occurs in the emergency department prior to hospital admission and/or surgery. As with biliary colic, patients with acute cholecystitis require volume resuscitation with intravenous isotonic fluid, pain control with opiate analgesics (once the diagnosis is confirmed), and bowel rest with nasogastric suction and antiemetic agents. Antibiotic treatment is recommended despite the questionable role of acute infection in all cases of early, acute cholecystitis. In cases presenting without sepsis, single-agent therapy is adequate with a third-generation cephalosporin. Patients with obvious infection should receive broadened coverage with ampicillin, gentamicin, and clindamycin, or the equivalent. A minority of patients (usually those with either acalculous or emphysematous cholecystitis or a complication of cholecystitis) will present in septic shock and require aggressive resuscitation. All patients with acute cholecystitis must be admitted to the hospital for continued intravenous fluid therapy and antibiotics. Approximately 75 percent of patients treated medically will have a complete remission of symptoms within 2 to 7 days of hospitalization; the remainder of patients will experience either a progression of the inflammatory process or a complication of acute cholecystitis within this time frame. Most often surgery is performed 24 to 72 h after admission once symptoms have resolved. Surgical options include open or laparoscopic cholecystectomy. Patients with a toxic presentation or clinical deterioration require immediate surgery.

## BIBLIOGRAPHY

Aucott JN, Cooper GS, Bloom AD, et al: Management of gallstones in diabetic patients. *Arch Intern Med* 153:1053, 1993.

Babb RR: Acute acalculous cholecystitis: A review. *J Clin Gastroenterol* 15:238, 1992.

Carroll BA: Preferred imaging techniques for the diagnosis of cholecystitis and cholelithiasis. *Ann Surg* 210:1, 1989.

Conwell EE, Rodriguez A, Mirvis SE, et al: Acute acalculous cholecystitis in critically injured patients. *Ann Surg* 210:52, 1989.

Cooperberg PL, Jibney RG: Imaging the gallbladder. *Radiology* 163:605, 1987.

Cucchiaro G, Watters CR, Rossltch JC, et al: Deaths from gallstones: Incidence and associated clinical factors. *Ann Surg* 209:149, 1989.

Erdamar I, Avci G, Fuzun M, et al: Extracorporeal shockwave lithotripsy and litholytic therapy in cholelithiasis. *Br J Surg* 79:235, 1992.

Farrell T, Mahon T, Daly L, et al: Identification of inappropriate radiological referrals with suspected gallstones: A prospective audit. *Br J Radiol* 67:32, 1994.

Gracie WA, Ransohoff: The natural history of silent gallstones: The innocent gallstone is not a myth. *N Engl J Med* 307:798, 1982.

Grosfeld JL, Rescorla FJ, Skinner MA, et al: The spectrum of biliary tract disorders in infants and children: Experience with 300 cases. *Arch Surg* 129:513, 1994.

Johnston DE, Kaplan MM: Pathogenesis and treatment of gallstones. *N Engl J Med* 328:412, 1993.

Kelley JE, Burrus RG, Burns RP, et al: Safety, efficacy, cost, and morbidity of laparoscopic versus open cholecystectomy: A prospective analysis of 228 consecutive patients. *Am Surg* 59:23, 1993.

Lal A, Dahiya RS, Dado RC, et al: Ultrasonography versus roentgenography in suspected cases of cholecystolithiasis. *Indian J Med Sci* 46:144, 1992.

Plummer D: Principles of emergency ultrasound and echocardiography. *Ann Emerg Med* 18:1291, 1989.

Traverso LW: Clinical manifestations and impact of gallstone disease. *Am J Surg* 165:405, 1993.

Warwick DJ, Thompson MH: Six hundred patients with gallstones. *Ann R Col Surg Engl* 74:218, 1992.

# 86
# ACUTE JAUNDICE AND HEPATITIS
## Richard Owen Shields, Jr.

## JAUNDICE

*Jaundice* is the yellowish discoloration of the sclera, skin, and mucous membranes by bilirubin. The presence of carotene or long-standing hemochromatosis may also cause yellow-orange discoloration of the skin, but the sclera is not affected.

Bilirubin, a breakdown product of hemoglobin from injured or senescent red blood cells and other heme-containing proteins, is pro-

**Table 86-1.** Causes of Jaundice

Unconjugated
    Hemolytic anemia
    Hemoglobinopathy
    Transfusion reaction
    Gilbert disease
    Crigler-Najjar syndrome
    Prematurity in neonates
    Congestive heart failure
Conjugated
    Intrahepatic
        Infections
            Viral hepatitis
            Leptospirosis
            Infectious mononucleosis
        Toxic
            Drugs
            Chemicals
        Familial
            Rotor syndrome
            Dubin-Johnson syndrome
        Alcoholic liver disease
        Other
            Sarcoidosis
            Lymphoma
            Liver metastases
            Amyloidosis
            Cirrhosis
            Biliary cirrhosis
    Extrahepatic
        Gallstones
        Pancreatic tumors or cysts
        Cholangiocarcinoma
        Bile duct stricture
        Sclerosing cholangitis

duced in the reticuloendothelial system and transported on albumin to the liver. There it is conjugated mostly as the diglucuronide and excreted through the bile channels into the small intestine. An increase in the production of bilirubin or a defect in the elimination pathway may produce clinical jaundice and hyperbilirubinemia.

Hyperbilirubinemia can be divided into two subtypes: unconjugated and conjugated. *Unconjugated* hyperbilirubinemia results from an increased bilirubin load or a defect in the ability of the hepatocyte to take up and conjugate bilirubin. *Conjugated* hyperbilirubinemia results from a decrease in the ability of the liver to excrete conjugated bilirubin (cholestasis). The site of cholestasis may be either intrahepatic or extrahepatic in origin. *Intrahepatic cholestasis* is caused by decreased excretion of conjugated bilirubin, hepatocellular damage, and damage to the biliary endothelium. Obstruction of biliary outflow by a congenital defect, inflammation, a mass lesion, or gallstones produces *extrahepatic cholestasis* (see Table 86-1).

## Emergency Department Evaluation

A careful history and physical examination coupled with judicious use of the clinical laboratory frequently enable the emergency physician to arrive at a reasonable working diagnosis and decide if hospitalization is indicated. Often, more extensive diagnostic procedures are needed before the etiology of jaundice can be determined.

### History

Jaundice without other complaints and with a positive family history of jaundice suggests a hereditary cause. Viral hepatitis should be suspected in male homosexuals, patients on hemodialysis, and intravenous drug abusers, and when the history reveals raw seafood ingestion, recent blood transfusion, ear piercing, tattoos, needle puncture, foreign travel, or close contact with someone with hepatitis. Toxic

hepatitis must be considered if there is a history of exposure to toxic chemicals or the use of hepatotoxic drugs. Older patients with right upper quadrant abdominal pain, vomiting, and fever probably have extrahepatic biliary obstruction. Heavy ethanol abusers with fever and abdominal pain are likely to have alcoholic hepatitis or cirrhosis.

### Physical Examination

Jaundice can most easily be detected in the mucous membranes of the mouth and in the sclerae using natural light. The presence of ascites, edema, and spider angiomata suggests cirrhosis. Right upper quadrant tenderness, a positive Murphy's sign, or a palpable gallbladder might indicate biliary disease. Cachexia and an epigastric mass suggest a neoplastic process, while a hard, nodular liver may represent hepatic metastases. Hepatomegaly with pedal edema, jugular venous distension, and a gallop rhythm make congestive cardiac failure the likely cause of jaundice. Needle tracks should raise the suspicion of viral hepatitis.

### Laboratory

The total bilirubin level is elevated if clinical jaundice is present. With unconjugated hyperbilirubinemia, 85 percent or more of the total bilirubin is of the indirect fraction. A direct-reacting fraction of at least 30 percent (and usually higher) is present with conjugated hyperbilirubinemia. A bedside test to determine if bilirubin is conjugated is to test the urine for bilirubin. Conjugated bilirubin is water-soluble and appears in the urine at very low serum concentrations. Unconjugated bilirubin is bound to albumin and is not present in urine.

Some cholestasis is present if the serum alkaline phosphatase level is elevated to greater than three times normal. Anemia with reticulocytosis and an abnormal peripheral smear are characteristic of hemolysis. Markedly elevated aminotransferase levels are most compatible with a viral hepatitis. A prolonged prothrombin time, a low serum albumin level, and anemia suggest alcoholic hepatitis or decompensated cirrhosis.

## VIRAL HEPATITIS

Viral hepatitis produces inflammation of the liver and necrosis of hepatic parenchymal cells. The severity of illness ranges from inapparent, subclinical infections to fulminant hepatic failure. Viral hepatitis is a significant public health problem, not only because of the acute morbidity and mortality, but also because of the associated sequelae of chronic hepatitis, cirrhosis, and hepatocellular carcinoma.

Prodromal symptoms are usually constitutional and may be abrupt or insidious in onset. Nausea, vomiting, fatigue, malaise, and alterations in taste are common. Low-grade fever with pharyngitis, coryza, and headache may lead to an early misdiagnosis of upper respiratory infection or "flulike" syndrome. The majority of cases do not develop jaundice and recover uneventfully.

In icteric cases, jaundice develops 1 to 2 weeks following the onset of the prodrome and may be preceded by a few days of pruritus and dark urine. Other prodromal symptoms usually disappear during the icteric phase, but malaise and gastrointestinal symptoms frequently persist. Right upper quadrant abdominal pain may develop because of hepatic enlargement. Physical examination during the icteric phase may reveal hepatomegaly or splenomegaly. In the recovery phase, the symptoms disappear, and complete clinical and biochemical recovery is the rule in 3 to 4 months. (See Table 86-2.)

The first biochemical abnormality is an elevation of serum aminotransferase levels before the onset of the prodromal phase. The levels peak during the phase of clinical hepatitis and return to normal during recovery. The magnitude of elevation is not a reliable indicator of disease severity. Prolongation of the prothrombin time by more than a few seconds indicates extensive hepatic necrosis and a poorer prog-

**Table 86-2.** Distinguishing Features of Hepatitis Virus

| Feature | Hepatitis A | Hepatitis B | Hepatitis C | Hepatitis D | Hepatitis E |
|---|---|---|---|---|---|
| Nucleic acid | RNA | DNA | RNA | RNA | RNA |
| Incubation | 15–50 days | 45–160 days | 15–160 days | 30–180 days | 15–60 days |
| Mean | 30 days | 120 days | 55 days | ? | 40 |
| Oral-fecal | Yes | No | No | No | Yes |
| Percutaneous | Rare | Yes | Yes | Yes | No |
| Carrier state | No | Yes | Yes | Yes | No |
| Severity | Mild | Moderate-severe | Mild | Moderate-severe | Mild-moderate |
| Mortality | Very low | Low | Low | High | Moderate |

nosis, as does a persistent bilirubin level elevation to greater than 20 mg/dL. An early transient neutropenia is often followed by a relative lymphocytosis with many atypical lymphocytes. Blood glucose levels may be depressed because of poor intake, depleted glycogen stores, and decreased hepatic gluconeogenesis.

## Hepatitis A

Hepatitis A, formerly known as infectious hepatitis, is caused by a small RNA picornavirus (HAV), which is spread primarily by the fecal-oral route. Rare cases of sexual and transfusion-acquired HAV infections have been reported. Victims are usually children or adolescents. Adult victims of HAV hepatitis tend to have more severe and prolonged disease and rarely may develop fulminant hepatic failure. High-risk groups include travelers to areas with inadequate water purification systems, children in day-care centers, those institutionalized in large groups, and people who eat raw shellfish. Common-source outbreaks among people exposed to contaminated food or water are common.

About 25,000 cases are reported yearly in the United States, but this represents only a small fraction of actual cases. Nearly 50 percent of adults in the United States have serologic evidence of prior HAV infection, but most of them have no recollection of the disease. Most cases of HAV hepatitis among children are mild, anicteric, and undiagnosed. Among adults, symptomatic infection with jaundice is much more common.

The incubation period is 15 to 50 days, with viral shedding in the stool for 2 to 3 weeks prior to and up to 2 weeks after the onset of symptoms. Infants infected with HAV can shed virus for up to 12 weeks. Symptom onset is often more abrupt than with other types of viral hepatitis. If jaundice develops, it appears several days later and is usually mild. No carrier state or chronic liver disease has been described following HAV infection. Virilogic diagnosis can be made by the detection of HAV RNA or antigen in the stool, but measurement of HAV-specific antibodies in serum is much more practical and widely available. IgM anti-HAV appears in the serum during the phase of clinical hepatitis but is soon replaced by IgG anti-HAV, which persists indefinitely and confers immunity.

## Hepatitis B

Hepatitis B, formerly known as serum hepatitis, is caused by a double-stranded DNA hepadnavirus (HBV) with an inner core and an outer coat, both of which are antigenic. It is spread primarily by the percutaneous route, although in as many as 50 percent of acute cases there is no clear history of exposure. Infective particles are present in semen, saliva, and other bodily fluids as well as in blood, which accounts for at least some of the nonpercutaneous transmission of the disease.

There are more than 1 million chronic carriers of HBV in the United States alone, with about 250,000 new infections each year. About 5000 of these carriers die each year from chronic liver disease.

Certain subpopulations such as intravenous drug abusers, male homosexuals, and patients on chronic hemodialysis have a much higher carrier rate.

The incubation period of hepatitis B is 45 to 160 days, with a mean of 120 days. Most cases are inapparent and anicteric. The onset of symptoms is usually insidious and preceded, in 5 to 10 percent, by a "serum-sickness-like" illness with polyarthritis, proteinuria, and angioneurotic edema thought to be caused by circulating antigen-antibody complexes. The symptoms tend to be more prolonged and severe than with hepatitis A, but complete recovery is expected in 90 percent.

Fulminant hepatic failure develops in about 1 percent and is characterized by encephalopathy, rapidly rising bilirubin levels, and a significant coagulopathy. Complete recovery is possible, but 80 percent of those developing coma will die. About 5 to 10 percent of adult victims of hepatitis B develop chronic hepatitis or a chronic carrier state. The carrier state develops much more often in neonates and children. Patients developing chronic HBV hepatitis frequently have a relatively mild acute illness.

The identification of three distinct HBV antigens and the capability to detect viral DNA in the serum (HBV-DNA) have provided serologic methods with which to diagnose and monitor patients with HBV infection. Hepatitis B surface antigen (HBsAg) represents the outer protein coat of the viral particle. It appears in the serum of more than 90 percent of patients before the appearance of aminotransferase elevations and clinical symptoms and persists until 1 to 2 months following the icteric phase, with total antigenemia lasting about 6 months.

Antibody to HBsAg (anti-HBs) appears in the serum from 2 to 6 months following the disappearance of HBsAg. The presence of anti-HBs implies prior HBV infection or vaccination and confers immunity to subsequent infection. Anti-HBs is present in 5 to 10 percent of healthy, unvaccinated volunteer blood donors in the United States. Chronic carriers of HBV usually have persistence of HbsAg in the serum and do not develop anti-HBs.

The core of the HBV particle, called hepatitis B core antigen (HBcAg), does not appear in the serum. Anti-HBc antibody appears in the serum about 2 weeks after the appearance of HbsAg, and during the "window" between the disappearance of HBsAg and the appearance of anti-HBs, it may be the only serologic marker of recent infection. IgM anti-HBc in high titer indicates the presence of acute HBV hepatitis with high infectivity, while its persistence at low levels is found in chronic HBV hepatitis. IgG anti-HBc is also found along with HBsAg in chronic hepatitis, but its presence along with anti-HBs implies remote HBV infection.

Hepatitis B e antigen (HBeAg) is a soluble antigen found in serum containing HBsAg. Its presence implies ongoing viral replication and high infectivity. This antigen disappears in those who recover from HBV hepatitis but persists in those who develop chronic hepatitis. Antibody to the e antigen (anti-HBe) appears in the acute phase of illness and usually signifies reduced infectivity. This antibody persists for some months after HBeAg disappearance.

A fourth antigen-antibody pair, designated HBxAg and anti-

HBxAg, has recently been discovered. Their significance in monitoring HBV infection is not yet known.

The presence of HBV-DNA in the serum is the most sensitive indicator of ongoing viral replication and, therefore, of infectivity. In the typical acute HBV hepatitis, HBV-DNA is detectable in the serum in the incubation period and peaks about the time that symptoms appear. HBV-DNA is rapidly cleared from the serum in those with acute HBV hepatitis and is already undetectable in more than half of patients first seeking medical attention for the disease.

## Hepatitis C

In 1989, both radioimmune and enzyme-linked assays were developed to detect antibodies to a protein produced by a viral agent now referred to as the *hepatitis C virus* (HCV). HCV is a linear, single-stranded RNA virus with characteristics similar to the flaviviruses. Retrospective serologic studies of chronic transfusion-related hepatitis strongly suggest that HCV is the predominant etiologic agent of this disease. By early 1990, blood banks in the United States were screening all donor units for the presence of anti-HCV. This policy should significantly reduce the incidence of transfusion-related viral hepatitis.

HCV is spread primarily by the parenteral route with sexual and perinatal transmission also possible. The incubation range is 15 to 160 days, with a mean of 50 days. An estimated 175,000 new cases occur in the United States each year. The clinical course of acute HCV hepatitis tends to be milder than that with HBV. The majority of patients are asymptomatic or have only mild symptoms. Increased transaminase levels may fluctuate during the acute phase, with persistent elevations occurring in 50 percent or more. There is a marked tendency to develop chronic hepatitis, however, leading to cirrhosis and hepatocellular carcinoma more often than with HBV.

Since there are no commercially available tests for HCV antigen, serologic diagnosis of HCV infection depends on the detection of IgG anti-HCV in the serum. Unfortunately, IgG anti-HCV appears late in acute infections, between 4 and 24 weeks after the onset of symptoms, and thus is of little help in initial evaluation. IgG anti-HCV does not confirm immunity. Instead, it is a marker of chronic infection and potential infectivity. Assays for other HCV markers of more timely clinical use are under development.

## Hepatitis D

The hepatitis D virus (HDV) is an important cause of both acute and chronic viral hepatitis. This virus consists of the HDV antigen (HD-VAg) and a small, circular piece of single-stranded RNA, enclosed by a coat of HBsAg. HDV is considered a "defective" virus because it can replicate only in the presence of acute or chronic HBV infection. Thus, the mode of transmission of HDV is inextricably linked to the transmission of HBV.

Acute HDV infection can occur as a coinfection with acute HBV hepatitis or as a superinfection in HBsAg carriers. Acute coinfection is usually self-limited, with HDV being cleared as the HBV infection clears. Superinfection, however, produces a mortality rate much higher than acute infection with HBV and the development of chronic hepatitis in as many as 80 percent of cases. Chronic HDV hepatitis results in cirrhosis in 70 to 80 percent of cases and often progresses quite rapidly. Fulminant liver failure is seen more often in high-risk groups such as intravenous drug users.

Diagnosis of HDV infection is made by the demonstration of anti-HDV in the serum by radioimmunoassay. This antibody appears late and in low titer in acute infections but is persistent in high titer in chronic infections. If IgM anti-HBc is simultaneously present, the HDV is probably a coinfection with HBV. If IgM anti-HBc is absent, superinfection of HDV in chronic HBV hepatitis is likely.

No specific treatment exists for HDV infection, nor does a vaccine currently exist. Prevention of HDV infection is best achieved by immunization against HBV and by the avoidance of high-risk behaviors.

## Hepatitis E

Hepatitis E is caused by a small RNA virus of the calicivirus family. It is found sporadically and in water-borne epidemics in Asia, Africa, Mexico, and the former Soviet Union. In the United States, only imported cases have so far been reported.

While the clinical course of hepatitis E is similar to that of hepatitis A, there is a higher rate of fulminant liver failure and death. The mortality rate is usually 5 to 10 percent, but among pregnant women may be as high as 30 percent. No carrier state or chronic hepatitis has yet been reported.

Diagnosis is made by the clinical picture combined with a history of recent travel to endemic areas and negative serology for other hepatitis viruses. No serologic tests for HEV antigen or antibodies are currently commercially available in the United States.

## Hepatitis Non-A Non-B

*Hepatitis non-A non-B* (HNANB) is a term for illnesses that appear clinically to be typical viral hepatitis but in which no known viral agent can be implicated. Infections with HCV and HEV were once included in this category before these viruses were discovered. A search for know viral agents such as cytomegalovirus and Epstein-Barr virus, as well as nonviral causes for hepatitis, must be pursued before this diagnosis can be made.

## Emergency Department Evaluation and Management

When faced with a patient with suspected viral hepatitis, the emergency physician must utilize the history and physical examination as well as readily available laboratory testing to determine the etiology and to decide if hospital admission is required. Outpatient management with emphasis on rest, adequate diet, good personal hygiene, and the avoidance of hepatotoxins (e.g., ethanol) is sufficient for the majority. Discharged patients must have adequate follow-up care. Patients meeting any one of the criteria listed in Table 86-3 should be admitted for further evaluation, monitoring, and supportive care.

Every patient should have serologic testing done to confirm the diagnosis of viral hepatitis and to identify, if possible, the etiologic agent. Initial testing should include assays for HBsAg, IgM anti-HBc, IgM anti-HAV, and anti-HCV, with other studies ordered based on the history and clinical situation. Baseline coagulation studies, bilirubin, and aminotransferase levels should also be obtained.

Documented cases of viral hepatitis should be reported to the appropriate public health agency, and close personal contacts of the patient should be advised of the potential risks and offered prophylaxis if indicated (see Table 86-4).

## Prevention and Prophylaxis

Vaccines for the prevention of HAV infection have been developed and tested and found to be safe and effective. The role of these vaccines in immunoprophylaxis of HAV has yet to be clarified. The best way to prevent the transmission from persons known to have HAV hepatitis is meticulous attention to body-fluid precautions and hand

**Table 86-3.** Indications for Admission with Viral Hepatitis

Encephalopathy
Prothrombin time prolonged > 3 s
Intractable vomiting
Hypoglycemia
Bilirubin > 20 mg/dL
Age > 45 years
Immunosuppression

**Table 86-4.** Postexposure Immunoprophylaxis of Viral Hepatitis

| Source | Treatment |
|---|---|
| **HEPATITIS A** | |
| 1. Household and sexual contacts of known cases | IG, 0.02 mL/kg IM |
| 2. Day-care center, school, and custodial institution contacts of known cases if evidence of transmission | Same |
| 3. Exposure to contaminated water or food before cases begin to appear | Same |
| 4. All staff and attendees of day-care centers caring for children in diapers with any known case among children or staff | Same |
| **HEPATITIS B WITH PERCUTANEOUS OR PERMUCOSAL EXPOSURE** | |
| 1. Known HBsAg-positive | Unvaccinated: single dose HBIG ASAP, initiate vaccine series.* <br> Vaccinated: <br> Known responder: test for anti-HBs. If adequate (>10 mIU), no treatment. If inadequate: vaccine booster. <br> Known nonresponder: two doses HBIG, one ASAP, one in 30 days. <br> Response unknown: test for anti-HBs. If adequate (>10 mIU), no treatment. If inadequate: single dose HBIG STAT and vaccine booster.† |
| 2. Known HBsAG-negative | Unvaccinated: initiate vaccine series.* <br> Vaccinated: no treatment. |
| 3. Source untested or unknown | Unvaccinated: initiate vaccine series.* <br> Vaccinated: <br> Known responder: no treatment. <br> Known nonresponder: two doses HBIG, one ASAP, one in 30 days if high-risk source. <br> Response unknown: test for anti-HBs. If adequate (> 10 mIU), no treatment. If inadequate, vaccine booster.† |
| 4. Known HNANB infection | Consider single dose IG 0.06 mL/kg IM (clinical studies inconclusive). |
| **HEPATITIS B—SEXUAL EXPOSURE** | |
| Acute and chronic hepatitis B | If treatment ≤ 14 days from exposure: <br> Unvaccinated: single-dose HBIG STAT, consider vaccination.* <br> Vaccinated: test for anti-HBs; if adequate (>10 mIU), no treatment. If inadequate, single dose HBIG ASAP and vaccine booster.† |
| **HEPATITIS C, D, AND E**   No recommendations | |

*Hepatitis B vaccine is given in a three-injection series, the second injection is given 1 month after the first, and the third 6 months after the first. Each dose of Recombivax HB is 1.0 mL (10 μg) for adults, 0.5 mL (5 μg) if 11–19 years old, and 0.25 mL (2.5 μg) if <11 years old. Each dose of Engerix-B is 1.0 mL (20 μg) if ≥11 years old, 0.5 mL (10 μg) if <11 years old.

† Vaccine booster is a single injection of vaccine.

*Note:* IG, immune globulin; HBIG, hepatitis B immune globulin 0.06 mL/kg given IM; HBsAg, hepatitis B surface antigen; ASAP, as soon as possible.

*Source:* Centers for Disease Control: Hepatitis B Virus: A comprehensive strategy for eliminating transmission in the United States through universal childhood vaccination: Recommendations of the Immunization Practices Advisory Committee (ACIP). *MMWR* 40(RR-13):21, 1991.

washing. Immune globulin (IG), formerly known as gamma globulin or serum immune globulin, is a solution of antibodies, including anti-HAV, obtained by cold ethanol extraction of pooled human plasma. IG is 80 to 90 percent effective in preventing HAV hepatitis when given within 14 days of exposure.

Recommendations for postexposure prophylaxis of HAV hepatitis are based on the nature and timing of the exposure and assume that the patient being considered for prophylaxis has not developed clinical hepatitis. IG should be given to all household and sexual contacts of persons with confirmed HAV hepatitis. IG should also be given to employees and children of day-care facilities caring for children in diapers if one or more cases develop among the children or staff. In centers not enrolling children in diapers, only the classroom contacts of the index case need receive IG. School contacts of index cases in elementary or secondary schools need not be treated unless a class-

room-centered outbreak is identified. Prophylaxis for hospital staff caring for a patient with HAV hepatitis is not necessary. Prophylaxis in the situation of a common-source outbreak is not indicated unless the exposure is discovered before cases begin to appear. When indicated, IG should be given in a single intramuscular (IM) dose of 0.02 mL/kg.

IG is also used as preexposure prophylaxis for travelers to developing countries. If travel is to be completed within 3 months, a single IM injection of 0.02 mL/kg is adequate. Longer duration of travel requires modification of the dose.

In 1982, a vaccine for the prevention of HBV hepatitis was introduced that proved to be both highly effective and free of significant adverse effects. This vaccine consisted of HBsAg prepared from the pooled plasma of chronic carriers of HBV. Despite some early concern about a possible risk of contamination of the HBV vaccine with the then-unknown infectious agent causing acquired immunodeficiency syndrome (AIDS), no evidence exists linking the vaccine to AIDS. The sequential inactivation treatment used in purifying the vaccine has been shown to totally inactivate the human immunodeficiency virus (HIV). This pooled-plasma vaccine is no longer produced in the United States, having been replaced by recombinant vaccines consisting of HBsAg produced by genetically engineered yeast.

The currently recommended series of three doses of vaccine produces adequate anti-HBs response (anti-HBs ≥ 10 mIU/mL) in greater than 90 percent of adults and greater than 95 percent of infants and children. This provides virtually complete protection against subsequent HBV infection. Postvaccination testing for antibody response should be done in those people in whom knowledge of immune status is important in decision-making about subsequent care (e.g., dialysis patients, children of HBsAg-positive mothers, and those at occupational risk of needle-stick or other exposures), and should be done from 1 to 6 months after immunization is completed. This testing is not indicated after routine vaccination in infants, children, and adolescents.

The recommended site of injection is the deltoid muscle in adults and the anterolateral thigh in neonates and infants, yielding a higher rate of effective antibody response than injections in other sites. Regimens using low-dose intradermal vaccine have been tested but so far have produced unacceptably low rates of antibody response. Immunologic memory lasts for many years, even after antibody levels drop or become undetectable. The need for booster doses of vaccine has not been established and may be necessary only in those with an impaired immune status.

Vaccination against HBV was initially recommended for high-risk groups such as intravenous drug abusers, homosexual men, patients on chronic hemodialysis, household and sexual contacts of HBV carriers, infants whose mothers are HBV carriers, and selected groups of health-care providers. This strategy failed to decrease the incidence of HBV infections since it was not feasible or practical to identify and vaccinate those who practiced high-risk behaviors, and because many people not in the high-risk groups also contracted HBV.

In 1991, the Immunization Practices Advisory Committee (ACIP) of the Centers for Disease Control and Prevention (CDC) issued a document calling for the elimination of HBV transmission in the United States. In addition to vaccination of high-risk adults, the ACIP recommended: (1) routine testing of pregnant women for HBsAg to identify newborns and household contacts requiring prophylaxis or vaccination, (2) making HBV vaccine a part of routine vaccination for all children, (3) the development of multiple-antigen vaccines to reduce the cost and number of injections, and (4) vaccination of certain adolescents.

Everyone providing emergency medical care should be immunized against HBV, preferably during training programs before exposure to blood and body fluids begin. The federal Occupational Safety and Health Administration (OSHA) requires that employers provide immunization free of charge to health-care workers at risk for exposure to blood and body fluids.

Hepatitis B immune globulin (HBIG) is obtained from the plasma of donors known to have high titers of anti-HBs. Serious adverse effects from the use of HBIG are very rare, and the only contraindications to its use is a previous hypersensitivity reaction. A regimen of two doses of HBIG (each dose 0.06 mL/kg IM) following percutaneous exposure to HBsAg-positive blood is about 75 percent effective in preventing the development of HBV hepatitis, but the first dose must be given within 7 days of exposure or the HBIG becomes much less effective. An alternative regimen combines a single dose of HBIG, given as soon as possible after exposure, with the initial dose of the HBV vaccine. This regimen is at least as effective, and less expensive, than the two-dose HBIG regimen and has the added advantage of providing permanent immunity to HBV infection.

Decision-making regarding postexposure prophylaxis for hepatitis B can be complex and must take into account the relative risk that the source of exposure was HBsAg-positive and the immunity status of the exposed person. Prophylaxis should be given to newborns of HBsAg-positive mothers, sexual contacts of an HBsAg-positive partner, and persons suffering percutaneous or permucosal contacts to HBsAg-positive blood.

Persons with percutaneous exposure to blood from a patient known to have HNANB or HCV should receive a single dose of IG at 0.06 mL/kg as soon as possible after exposure, although such prophylaxis is of unproved benefit.

Measures to prevent infection with hepatitis B are sufficient to prevent HDV infection in a person susceptible to HBV infection. There is no known prophylaxis against HDV in persons with chronic HBV infection. There is also no known prophylaxis for HEV.

The current ACIP recommendations for the postexposure prophylaxis of viral hepatitis are shown in Table 86-4. These recommendations are reviewed periodically and have undergone changes over the past few years.

## TOXIC HEPATITIS

A large number of industrial chemicals and pharmaceutical agents are capable of producing hepatic injury. Although hepatic injury accounts for only a small percentage of all adverse drug effects, this etiology accounts for a significant number of hospitalizations for jaundice, especially among the elderly. Acute liver injury may be primarily cytotoxic (e.g., halothane), primarily cholestatic (e.g., anabolic steroids), or may present as a mixed form (e.g., amrinone).

Intrinsic hepatotoxins cause rapid, predictable, dose-related injury through a direct toxic effect of the agent or its metabolites on the liver. Other agents cause damage sporadically and unpredictably as a result of hypersensitivity or idiosyncratic reactions. This type of hepatic injury is not dose-related, may be delayed in onset, and may be accompanied by systemic signs and symptoms such as arthralgias, rash, fever, and eosinophilia.

Halothane, methyldopa, isoniazid, phenytoin, and other drugs may produce morphologic changes in the liver resembling those of acute viral hepatitis. Other drugs such as anabolic steroids, oral contraceptives, chlorpropamide, chlorpromazine, and erythromycin estolate may produce cholestatic changes. Massive hepatic necrosis may be produced by carbon tetrachloride, phosphorus, acetaminophen, and mushroom poisoning (e.g., *Amanita phalloides*).

Some drugs and toxins including methyldopa, vinyl chloride, arsenic, and isoniazid have been implicated in the development of chronic active hepatitis and cirrhosis.

### Halothane

Halothane hepatitis is an idiosyncratic reaction to a metabolite resulting in a combination of toxic and immunologic injury that may be mediated by genetic factors. It appears much more often in patients with multiple prior exposures to halothane and is more common in adults, especially women, and the obese. In about 25 percent, rash, fever, and eosinophilia are present. Severe icteric cases have a 20 to 40 percent mortality; even mild reactions to halothane must be recognized so that susceptible patients are not reexposed.

### Acetaminophen

Acetaminophen is a very popular nonprescription analgesic and antipyretic, as well as an increasingly common cause of hepatic injury and death when taken in accidental or intentional overdose. A toxic metabolite produces hepatic necrosis when the liver's capacity to conjugate and excrete the metabolite is overwhelmed. Liver injury may be minimized or avoided when overdose is recognized and treated as described elsewhere.

## Methyldopa

Methyldopa causes mild, usually transient elevation of aminotransferase levels in about 5 percent of those treated with this once-popular antihypertensive. In fewer than 1 percent of those treated, acute hepatitis (occasionally with cholestasis) develops, usually within the first month of therapy. A prodrome of rash, arthralgias, and lymphadenopathy may precede the onset of jaundice. Clinical improvement occurs with discontinuation of the drug, but cases of chronic hepatitis and cirrhosis have been reported. The mechanism of hepatic injury is unclear but may be a combination of immunologic and direct toxic injury.

## Chlorpromazine

Chlorpromazine induces intrahepatic cholestasis in 1 to 4 percent of those taking it, usually within 1 to 4 weeks of exposure. A prodrome of anorexia, nausea, vomiting, malaise, and pruritus may precede the onset of jaundice. Clinical recovery occurs within 4 to 6 weeks after withdrawal of the drug, with only a rare fatality reported. Chlorpromazine-induced liver injury is not dose-related and appears to be immunologically mediated.

## Treatment

During the evaluation of the patient with acute liver injury, the emergency physician must obtain a detailed history of current and recent medications as well as possible occupational and recreational exposure to drugs and chemicals. Stopping the exposure to the offending agent is vital, other treatment being nonspecific and supportive in most cases. Possible injury to other organs should be suspected as well with exposure to toxic chemicals.

## ALCOHOLIC LIVER DISEASE

More than 10 million people in the United States are alcohol abusers, and alcohol-related injuries and illnesses are major causes of death and disability. The direct and indirect costs of alcohol abuse in the United States are in excess of $100 billion per year. Alcohol is a causative or contributing factor to hundreds of diverse medical problems, but it is alcoholic liver disease that is the most important medical consequence of chronic alcohol ingestion. Within the continuum of the clinical and pathological manifestations of alcoholic liver injury, three overlapping syndromes—hepatic steatosis (fatty liver), alcoholic hepatitis, and alcoholic cirrhosis—have been described.

## Hepatic Steatosis

Most people who regularly consume even moderate amounts of alcohol develop some degree of hepatic steatosis. It is usually a benign, asymptomatic condition in which fat is deposited in the hepatocytes because of alterations in the cells redox potentials caused by the oxidation of ethanol to acetaldehyde. This change reduces the rate of oxidation of fatty acids and favors the synthesis of triglyceride.

The most common clinical finding is nontender hepatomegaly with laboratory evidence of minimal hepatic injury. Less commonly, patients with fatty liver develop a syndrome of jaundice, malaise, anorexia, and a tender, enlarged liver. Rarely, severe cholestasis or portal hypertension develops. When the patient abstains from alcohol and receives adequate nutrition, steatosis resolves in 4 to 6 weeks without residual scarring or necrosis.

## Alcoholic Hepatitis

Alcoholic hepatitis (also known as alcoholic steatonecrosis) is a syndrome characterized histologically by hepatocellular necrosis and intrahepatic inflammation. It develops in only a small percentage of chronic alcohol abusers. The clinical severity ranges from very mild illness to acute liver failure. Typically, the patient reports the gradual onset of anorexia, nausea, abdominal pain, weight loss, and weakness. Fever, dark urine, and jaundice are frequently reported.

On examination, tender hepatomegaly, low-grade fever, and jaundice are commonly noted. Laboratory evaluation usually shows elevation of the levels of serum aminotransferases in the range of two to ten times normal, with a ratio of AST to ALT of greater than 1.5. Alkaline phosphatase and bilirubin levels are usually mildly elevated, although marked elevations may occur and imply more severe disease. Anemia, leukopenia, and thrombocytopenia are common and may be caused by the toxic effects of alcohol on bone marrow or by nutritional deficits. The prothrombin time is frequently prolonged a few seconds, but prolongation greater than 8 s is a poor prognostic sign. The presence of fever and leukocytosis in the alcoholic patient mandates a thorough search for concurrent pneumonia, peritonitis, urinary tract infection, sepsis, and meningitis.

## Treatment

In-hospital treatment is mainly supportive with correction of electrolyte abnormalities, good nutrition with correction of specific deficits (e.g., folate, thiamine), rest, and abstinence from alcohol. Treatment is frequently complicated by the development of alcohol withdrawal symptoms. Symptoms of hepatic failure must be closely watched for and aggressively treated. A number of specific therapies have been advocated to speed recovery from alcoholic hepatitis or to halt the progression to cirrhosis, but at this time none is considered established. The use of glucocorticoids and anabolic androgenic steroids appear to benefit some patients. Studies of other therapies, including colchicine, penicillamine, propylthiouracil, and insulin-glucagon combinations, have shown minimal or negative results.

The histologic, biochemical, and clinical abnormalities of alcoholic hepatitis do not rapidly resolve with abstinence from drinking. Instead, from 15 to 50 percent of hospitalized patients deteriorate during the first weeks despite abstinence and nutritional support. Reported mortality is between 20 and 65 percent, with death resulting from hepatic failure with encephalopathy, gastrointestinal bleeding, and infections. Survivors face a convalescence lasting weeks to months, with a significant number developing cirrhosis.

### Emergency Department Management

Because of the difficulty of ruling out concurrent infection, the tendency toward clinical deterioration, and the significant mortality, all but the mildest cases of alcoholic hepatitis should be hospitalized. A complete blood count, prothrombin time, and levels of aminotransferases, alkaline phosphatase, bilirubin, albumin, blood urea nitrogen, creatinine, glucose, magnesium, and phosphorus should be obtained. In the febrile patient, a chest radiograph and cultures of blood, urine, and ascitic fluid are needed. If the patient has an altered mental status, occult head trauma, meningitis, hepatic encephalopathy, and hypoglycemia must be considered and aggressively treated when present.

Hydration with dextrose-containing intravenous (IV) fluids should be initiated in the emergency department at a rate to maintain an adequate intravascular volume without overloading the edematous or ascitic patient. Central venous monitoring may be necessary. Thiamine should be given in IV fluids to avoid precipitating Wernicke encephalopathy. Electrolyte abnormalities should be recognized and correction begun. Most patients will require at least supplemental potassium and magnesium.

## Alcoholic Cirrhosis

Alcoholic (Laennec's) cirrhosis is the irreversible stage of alcoholic liver disease. The liver is usually a golden yellow and may be shrunken or enlarged. Nodules of regenerating hepatocytes are separated by bands of fibrous tissue that represent scarring from previous necrosis. The normal pattern of hepatic blood circulation is disrupted, with a resultant decrease in the total blood flow through the liver as well as the shunting of blood away from the remaining functioning hepatocytes and into the systemic circulation. This portosystemic shunting and concomitant portal hypertension result in many of the clinical findings of cirrhosis as well as the associated complications.

Cirrhosis develops in only about 10 percent of chronic alcoholics and may remain unrecognized in a significant number. Genetic, nutritional, and other factors probably determine which heavy drinkers will develop cirrhosis.

## Clinical Features

A characteristic clinical feature of symptomatic cirrhosis is a general, gradual deterioration in health. Loss of muscle mass (sometimes masked by edema and ascites), weakness, easy fatigability, and anorexia are the rule. Nausea, vomiting, and diarrhea are commonly reported. Fever, usually low-grade and continuous, is much more common in alcoholic than in other types of cirrhosis and often develops in decompensated disease. Hypothermia may develop in the terminal stages. Jaundice, spider angiomata, palmar erythema, pedal edema, ascites, hepatosplenomegaly, and gynecomastia (in men) are common.

Laboratory abnormalities include elevated bilirubin and alkaline phosphatase levels, a prolonged prothrombin time, decreased albumin, anemia (from chronic disease, nutritional factors, or blood loss), leukopenia, and thrombocytopenia. Hyponatremia may be dilutional secondary to increased antidiuretic hormone activity or the result of total body sodium deficit, frequently aggravated by the injudicious use of diuretics. Hypokalemia is almost always present as a result of GI losses, secondary hyperaldosteronism, and diuretic use. Arterial hypoxemia is common in decompensated cirrhosis and may be caused by abnormal alveolar-capillary diffusion or restricted respiratory expansion secondary to massive ascites. Serum transaminase levels and alkaline phosphatase levels are only mildly elevated.

## Management

The clinical course of cirrhosis is marked by periods of relative stability interspersed with episodes of decompensation. No therapy has been shown effective in reversing the histologic changes of cirrhosis. The mainstay of outpatient management is total abstinence from alcohol, which has been shown to significantly improve 5-year survival. Other measures include salt and water restriction, the cautious use of diuretics (especially those that spare potassium), and a nutritious diet with protein restriction as needed. Emergency management may involve making alterations in diuretic dosage, correcting symptomatic anemia or fluid and electrolyte abnormalities, and recognizing and initiating treatment of the life-threatening emergencies seen in decompensated cirrhosis.

## COMPLICATIONS OF ALCOHOLIC LIVER DISEASE

### Bleeding Esophageal Varices

Bleeding esophageal varices are the most dramatic and immediately life-threatening complications of alcoholic liver disease. The mortality rate from variceal hemorrhage is high, and rebleeding is common. As many as 30 percent of all cirrhotic patients die from this complication alone. The patient usually arrives in the emergency department in hemorrhagic shock, with massive hematemesis complicated by underlying coagulation and electrolyte derangements. A significant number of patients with documented varices who develop hematemesis, however, are bleeding from other lesions, including gastric erosions, gastric or duodenal ulcers, or a diffuse gastritis. Since definitive therapy varies, emergency endoscopy should be done as soon as possible to confirm the diagnosis.

## Management

Initial management includes securing a stable airway and restoring intravascular volume. Fresh whole blood or packed red cells augmented by fresh-frozen plasma should be rapidly infused through large-bore intravenous lines to maintain adequate tissue perfusion and replace depleted clotting factors. Monitoring of central venous or pulmonary wedge pressure may be needed to guide fluid resuscitation. Transfusion of platelet concentrates may be necessary if thrombocytopenia is severe (see Table 86-5).

Control of bleeding can be attempted using pharmacologic intervention to reduce portal blood flow and/or pressure, endoscopic sclerotherapy, direct compression balloon tamponade with a Sengstaken-Blackemore or similar tube, or emergency portal decompression. All these methods have significant morbidity even in experienced hands. More detailed discussion of emergency management of variceal bleeding is described in Chap. 74, "Esophageal Emergencies."

Particular attention must be paid during emergency treatment to the evacuation of blood from the GI tract with gastric lavage, vigorous catharsis, and enemas. Otherwise, some patients in whom bleeding is controlled will die in portosystemic encephalopathy.

### Portosystemic Encephalopathy

Portosystemic encephalopathy (PSE, also referred to by the more general term of *hepatic encephalopathy*) is a complex neuropsychiatric syndrome of altered consciousness and impaired intellectual functioning seen in cirrhotics with extensive spontaneous or surgical portosystemic shunting. It is a reversible metabolic encephalopathy that apparently results from an accumulation in the blood of one or more neuroactive substances that are absorbed from the gut and not metabolized by the failing liver. Changes in permeability of the blood-brain barrier also occur, which may allow these substances enhanced access to the brain. The severity of PSE ranges from subtle changes in personality and psychomotor performance, to apathy, perseveration, sleep disturbances, and eventually to coma.

Elevated blood ammonia apparently plays a role in the pathogenesis of PSE, but the precise role has not yet been clearly defined. Elevated levels of some amino acids, short-chain fatty acids, biogenic amines, mercaptans, and false neurotransmitters have also been implicated, and it may be a synergistic effect of combinations of these substances that produces encephalopathy.

The gamma-aminobutyric acid/benzodiazepine (GABA/BZ) inhibitory neurotransmitter system on the postsynaptic membrane of neurons has also been implicated in the development of PSE. Increased GABA-ergic tone induced by barbiturates, benzodiazepines, and GABA-agonists can cause alterations in consciousness and motor control similar to that seen in PSE. An endogenous benzodiazepine-like substance has been found in the blood and cerebrospinal fluid of patients with PSE, possibly arising from bacterial activity in the gut, that may be a factor in the development of PSE. This finding has led to the experimental use of the BZ-receptor blocker flumazenil. Flumazenil has produced temporary improvement in consciousness in patients with PSE, and cases of long-term success with oral therapy have been reported. The role of flumazenil in treating PSE is promising but not yet established.

**Table 86-5.** Management of Variceal Bleeding

| |
| --- |
| Secure the airway |
| Large-bore IV Lines |
| Volume replacement with blood and plasma |
| Evacuate blood from GI tract |
| Endoscopic sclerotherapy If sclerotherapy fails or not available: |
| IV vasoconstrictors |
| Esophageal balloon tamponade |
| Portal decompression surgery |

PSE can be precipitated or exacerbated in susceptible patients by a variety of factors. Azotemia, either renal or prerenal, provides more urea to urease-producing intestinal bacteria, thereby increasing ammonia production in the gut. Gastrointestinal bleeding and high-protein diets provide large amounts of nitrogenous substrates. The careless use of analgesics, sedatives, and tranquilizers is an occasional cause of PSE in hospitalized patients. Diuretic-induced hypokalemic metabolic alkalosis results in a pH gradient favoring the passage of ammonia into cells. Other metabolic derangements such as hypoglycemia, anemia, alcohol intake, and hypoxia, as well as infection and hypotension, may also contribute. When PSE develops without precipitating cause, it is usually because of worsening liver function and implies a worse prognosis.

## Clinical Features

The patient with PSE has the stigmata of chronic liver disease including edema, ascites, spider angiomata, and hepatosplenomegaly. Fetor hepaticas, a musty odor on the breath attributed to elevated blood mercaptan levels, is often noted. Asterixis ("liver flap") is characteristic of, but not specific for, PSE. It is demonstrated most readily in the dorsiflexed wrist, but may be noted in other muscles as well. Neurologic examination may reveal a level of consciousness ranging from lethargy to coma, with variable appearance of hyperreflexia, generalized seizures, and spasticity. Occult head injury should be suspected if focal or lateralizing signs are present.

Laboratory studies reflect the underlying liver failure with jaundice, coagulopathy, and decreased albumin levels. The acid-base status and serum electrolytes must be closely monitored. Ammonia levels should be obtained from arterial samples, but absolute levels correspond poorly with the severity of PSE, and there is a 24- to 72-h lag between the rise in ammonia levels and the onset of symptoms. Serial changes in ammonia levels are more useful in monitoring the course of PSE and evaluating the effectiveness of treatment.

## Treatment

The initial treatment in the comatose patient is to maintain oxygenation and perfusion. Precipitating factors such as GI bleeding should be treated aggressively. Efforts to cleanse the gut of bacterial flora and nitrogenous substances include cathartics, enemas, and the use of poorly absorbed broad-spectrum antibiotics such as neomycin.

Lactulose is a nondigestible synthetic disaccharide that produces an acidic diarrhea, which may trap nitrogenous substances in the colon and eliminate them in the stool and suppress ammonia synthesis by gut flora. Lactulose may be given orally, through a nasogastric tube, or by enema. The usual initial oral dose is 30 mL three times a day but must be individualized.

Many other therapies have been suggested, but clinical studies have been inconclusive. With meticulous supportive care and the aggressive treatment of complications, PSE is potentially reversible, although the mortality remains very high.

## Hepatorenal Syndrome

Hepatorenal syndrome (HRS) is a syndrome of acquired renal failure without other obvious cause in patients with decompensated cirrhosis. It almost always occurs in the presence of ascites, jaundice, and portal hypertension in the hospitalized patient. This implies that iatrogenic factors may play a significant role in the pathogenesis. The mortality of HRS approaches 100 percent.

HRS probably represents a functional disturbance in the control of renal vascular tone, with a decreased glomerular filtration rate due to intense vasoconstriction and shunting of blood away from the renal cortex. This results in the production of small volumes of concentrated urine with very low sodium content, and a progressive azotemia unresponsive to attempts to expand intravascular volume.

No significant histologic changes are evident in the kidneys of patients dying with HRS. In fact, kidneys from HRS donors function normally if transplanted into recipients with normal hepatic function.

## Spontaneous Bacterial Peritonitis

Spontaneous bacterial peritonitis (SBP) is an infection of ascitic fluid without a local source of infection. The incidence of SBP increases as liver function deteriorates and is more common in cirrhotic patients with PSE and GI bleeding. The pathogenesis of SBP is thought to be the result of spontaneous bacteremia with seeding of ascitic fluid. Bacteremia in cirrhotics probably results from impaired functioning of the hepatic reticuloendothelial system, which fails to clear bloodborne organisms originating primarily from the gut. Other defects in patient defenses that predispose to bacteremia include low serum complement, abnormal neutrophil function, and decreased serum opsonic activity. These factors permit prolonged bacteremia and colonization of ascitic fluid. Low fluid protein levels result in decreased opsonic activity and complement levels, which allow SBP to develop.

SBP should be suspected in all cirrhotics with increasing ascites, worsening hepatic function, fever, chills, and abdominal pain or tenderness. More subtle symptoms such as worsening renal function, hypothermia, encephalopathy, or diarrhea may be the only signs, however. The diagnosis is established by evaluation of ascitic fluid obtained by a diagnostic paracentesis done as part of the emergency department workup.

Paracentesis can be performed using the midline infraumbilical approach or using one of the lower quadrants lateral to the rectus sheath. The lateral approach is best performed with the patient supine and slightly rotated to the side of the procedure (see Fig. 86-1). Rotation helps allow the loops of bowel floating on the fluid to move away from the procedure site. Sites of previous surgical incisions should be avoided, and a urinary catheter should be inserted to empty the bladder. The skin should be prepped and draped in a sterile fashion, and local anesthesia down to the peritoneum obtained. Traction can be applied to the skin so that, later, the holes in the skin and peri-

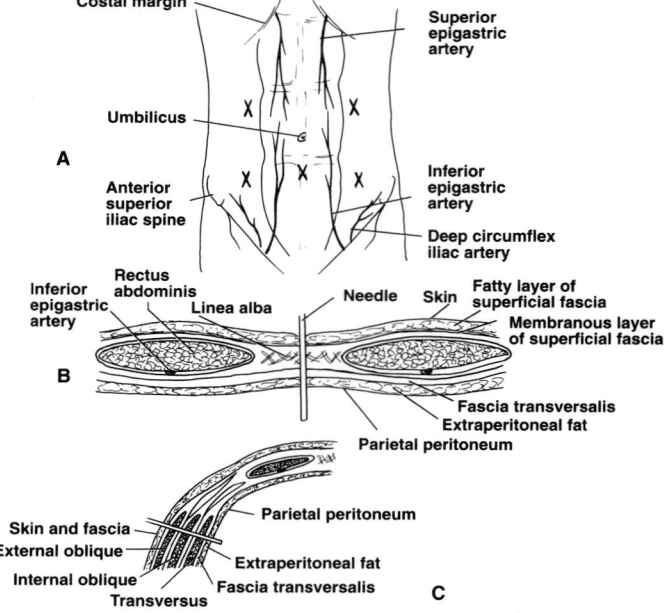

**Fig. 86-1.** Diagnostic paracentesis. **A.** Avoid the rectus sheath and arteries. **B.** and **C.** Cross-sections of anterior abdominal wall for midline and flank approaches. (Adapted from Snell R, Smith M: *Clinical Anatomy for Emergency Medicine.* St. Louis, Mosby-Year Book, 1993, with permission.)

toneum do not overlap. This may help to avoid ascitic fluid leaks. An 18-gauge needle on at least a 20-mL syringe is then inserted through the anesthetized area, holding slight constant suction until the peritoneum is entered. Penetration may be signified by a palpable "pop" and return of straw-colored fluid into the syringe. If no fluid is obtained, the needle can be cautiously advanced and rotated, maintaining suction. If this fails to produce fluid, the needle should be withdrawn and the procedure repeated. When completed, the area should be cleaned and dressed and the patient rotated to the other side.

At least 10 mL of ascitic fluid should be injected into a blood culture bottle. A total white blood cell (WBC) count with differential should also be obtained. A polymorpholeukocyte count greater than 500/mm$^3$ is highly specific for SBP, and antibiotic treatment should be immediately started. A count below 250/mm$^3$ makes SBP unlikely. A count between 250 and 500 is indeterminate, requiring treatment if the clinical picture is compatible and retapping in 12 h if not. Blood cultures are frequently positive for the infecting organism and may be positive even when the ascitic fluid culture is negative.

Ascitic fluid should also be tested for total protein, glucose, and lactate dehydrogenase (LDH). A total WBC count of > 10,000/mm$^3$, total protein of > 1 gm/dL, glucose < 50 mg/dL, or elevated LDH greatly increase the risk that the peritonitis is secondary to a localized source of infection. This mandates a vigorous search for a surgically correctable problem such as a hollow-viscus perforation or intraperitoneal abscess.

Early treatment improves survival and should be initiated in the emergency department if the clinical picture is compatible with SBP, even if laboratory results are equivocal and cultures are pending. The vast majority of SBP is caused by enteric gram-negative aerobes (e.g., *Escherichia coli*) and gram-positive aerobes (e.g., *Streptococcus* sp.). Currently, cefotaxime, a third-generation cephalosporin, appears to be the drug of choice in a dose of 1 to 2 grams every 6 h. Therapy should be modified based on sensitivity results.

Even with early detection and appropriate treatment, the mortality of SBP is high. Survivors of a first episode of SBP are at high risk for recurrent episodes. Some studies have shown that long-term selective intestinal decontamination with norfloxocin might reduce the incidence of recurrence.

## BIBLIOGRAPHY

Garcia-Tsao G: Spontaneous bacterial peritonitis. *Gastroenterol Clin North Am* 21:257, 1992.

Hoofnagle J, Bisceglie A: Serologic diagnosis of acute and chronic hepatitis. *Semin Liver Dis* 11:73, 1991.

Jones D: Hepatic encephalopathy. *J Gastroenterol Hepatol* 8:363, 1993.

Levy M: Hepatorenal syndrome. *Kidney Int* 43:737, 1993.

Zimmerman H: Update of hepatotoxicity due to classes of drugs in common clinical use: Non-steroidal drugs, anti-inflammatory drugs, antibiotics, antihypertensives, and cardiac and psychotropic agents. *Semin Liver Dis* 10:322, 1990.

# 87
# ACUTE PANCREATITIS
## Donald Weaver

The diagnosis of acute pancreatitis rests primarily on clinical grounds. The severity of the disease may range from mild pancreatic edema to frank necrosis and hemorrhage. No clinical findings are pathognomonic, and the symptoms depend largely on the amount of glandular destruction. In the mildest form, patients present with epigastric pain, abdominal distension, nausea, vomiting, and hyperamylasemia. Refractory hypotensive shock, blood loss, and respiratory failure may accompany the most severe forms. In 1977 Ransom and Posterbach proposed a schema to grade the severity of acute pancreatitis (Table 87-1). They found that the rate of serious morbidity and mortality was 14 percent in patients with fewer than three positive findings, and 95 percent in patients with three or more positive findings.

## Etiology

Acute pancreatitis is most often due to alcohol abuse or gallstones (Table 87-2). The incidence with which each is associated with pancreatitis depends largely on the age of the population and the reporting institution. Patients over the age of 50 who present in a community hospital setting most often have "biliary pancreatitis," while younger patients presenting to large inner-city emergency departments almost always have alcoholic pancreatitis.

## Pathophysiology

A complete understanding of the pathophysiology of acute pancreatitis is lacking. The common-channel concept of Opie dominated the literature for years, but anatomic studies of cadavers have shown that only a fraction of patients with pancreatitis have a true common channel. Moreover, in fatal cases, careful dissection at postmortem examinations rarely discloses an impacted stone in the ampulla of Vater. In animal experiments, neither the anastomosis of bile ducts to the pancreatic duct nor the injection of bile into the pancreatic duct without pressure produces pancreatitis. Only when trypsin or bacteria are added to bile and the mixture is injected under pressure can consistent experimental pancreatitis be produced.

A vascular insult is important either as a cause or perpetuator of acute pancreatitis. The hyperlipemic serum sometimes seen in patients following a drinking binge may be responsible for peripancreatic vascular sludging and relative pancreatic ischemia. Small-microsphere injections (8 to 20 U) result in profound pancreatitis because of plugging of the terminal arterioles. The acinar and ductal injury which then results leads to extravasation of proteolytic enzymes, and this may be responsible for the progression of the inflammatory state. More recently, the role of oxygen free radicals elaborated by ischemic cellular injury in the pancreas has been impli-

**Table 87-1.** Criteria for Projecting the Outcome from Acute Pancreatitis

| On Admission | 48 H Later |
| --- | --- |
| Age over 55 | Change in HCT (falling) decreased more than 10 percent |
| Blood sugar > 200 mg/dL | Rise in BUN over 5 mg/dL |
| WCB > 16,000/mm$^3$ | ↓ CA$^{2+}$ below 8 mg/dL |
| SGOT > 250 Sigma-Fankel units/L | ↓ Arterial P$_{O_2}$ below 60 mmHg |
| | Rapid fluid sequestration over 6 L |
| LDH > 700 IU/L | Base deficit over 4 mEq/L |

**Table 87-2.** Etiologic or Contributing Factors in Acute Pancreatitis

| Drugs and toxins | Viral infections |
|---|---|
| Ethanol and methanol | Mumps |
| Organophosphates | Hepatitis A, B, C |
| Scorpion venom | Infectious mononucleosis |
| Azathioprine and | Coxsackie group B |
| mercaptopurine | Rubella |
| Valproic acid | CMV |
| Estrogens | EBV |
| Metronidazole | HIV |
| Nitrofurantoin | Varicella |
| Furosemide | Echovirus |
| Sulfonamides | Adenovirus |
| Cimetidine | Pregnancy—any trimester, postpartum |
| Erythromycin | Collagen vascular disease |
| Acetaminophen | Systemic lupus erythematosus |
| Salicylates | Polyarteritis nodosa |
| Biliary tract disease | Infection |
| Trauma, penetrating or blunt | Typhoid fever |
| Penetrating peptic ulcer | *Salmonella typhimurium* |
| Postoperative | infection |
| Following ERCP | Scarlet fever |
| Obstruction secondary to | Streptococcal food poisoning |
| neoplasms, diverticula, | Dysentery |
| roundworms, benign polyps | Ascariasis |
| Perisphincteric fibrosis | Clonorchiasis |
| Cystic Fibrosis | MTB |
| Metabolic disturbances | Mycoplasma |
| Hyperlipidemia (Frederickson | MAI |
| types I, IV, and V) | Legionella |
| Hypercalcemia | Leptospirosis |
| Diabetes mellitus, diabetes | *Campylobacter* |
| ketoacidosis | |
| Uremia | |
| Hemochromatosis | |
| Hereditary pancreatitis | |

cated as a contributing factor to glandular injury in acute pancreatitis. Alcohol increases pancreatic ductal permeability, and this may result in a similar escape of proteolytic enzymes.

Alcoholic pancreatitis may result from duodenal inflammation that produces some degree of pancreatic duct obstruction, with increased ductal pressure. The latter may occur secondary to sphincter of Oddi spasm or pancreatic hypersecretion.

Hyperparathyroidism has been associated with an increased incidence of pancreatitis, but the mechanism by which this occurs is unknown.

Patients with primary hyperlipemias (Frederickson types I, IV, and V) are susceptible to acute pancreatitis, but patients with pancreatitis may develop transient secondary hyperlipemia because of the release of an inhibitor of lipoprotein lipase during the attack of pancreatitis.

Various drugs, such as methyl alcohol, thiazide diuretics, and phenformin, can produce pancreatitis (Table 87-3). Inflammation and infection, such as mumps or hepatitis, can also result in pancreatitis. Penetrating posterior duodenal and gastric ulcers may involve the

**Table 87-3.** Drugs Reported to be Associated with the Occurrence of Acute Pancreatitis

| | |
|---|---|
| Oral contraceptives | Donidine |
| Estrogens | Salicylates |
| Phenformin | Indomethacin |
| Azathioprine | Dextropropoxyphene |
| Glucocorticoids | Calcium |
| Rifampin | Warfarin |
| Tetracyclines | L-Asparaginase |
| Isoniazid | Paracetamol |
| Thiazides | Ethacrynic acid |
| Furosemide | |

head of the pancreas, producing a local pancreatitis. Once the pancreas becomes edematous and swollen, especially if there is significant involvement of the head, partial obstruction of the common bile duct or even gastric outlet may occur. For these reasons elevation of the bilirubin level, and even clinical jaundice, may occur. Pancreatitis may also produce adynamic ileus secondary to the peritoneal irritation.

## DIAGNOSIS

### Laboratory

Since no clinical features are pathognomonic for acute pancreatitis, the diagnosis must often rest on the presence of abnormal results from laboratory tests, most often the serum amylase level in combination with the clinical findings. Amylase is a product of two genes located on chromosome 1, known as $AMY_1$ and $AMY_2$. Each organ that makes amylase expresses either one or the other, and no organ has been found that expresses both genes. The only known site to express the $AMY_2$ gene is the pancreas. All other organs, such as the fallopian tubes, ovaries, lungs, salivary glands, lacrimal glands, and endocrine glands, express the $AMY_1$ locus. Pancreatic ($AMY_2$) amylase can be separated from nonpancreatic ($AMY_1$) amylase by a variety of electrophoretic techniques. Normally there is a nearly even distribution in the serum between $AMY_1$ and $AMY_2$ amylase. Many other isoamylases can occur but result from posttranslational modifications of the major isoenzymes.

During the past decade, recognition of the multiple organ sources of amylase has resulted in less reliance on the simple measurement of the serum amylase level as an indicator of pancreatic disease. In one study, 32 percent of the patients admitted with the clinical diagnosis of acute pancreatitis made on the basis of upper abdominal pain, nausea, vomiting, and an elevated amylase level were found to have nonpancreatic hyperamylasemia. This suggests that the clinical criteria used to make the diagnosis of acute pancreatitis may be too variable.

Since the electrophoresis of serum to differentiate isoamylases is time-consuming (approximately 2.5 h), other laboratory tests have been proposed to improve the accuracy of pancreatitis diagnosis. Observations that the amylase-creatinine clearance ratio is high in patients with acute pancreatitis suggest this might be a valuable diagnostic test. The ratio is determined using the following formula:

$$\frac{\text{Amylase clearance}}{\text{Creatinine clearance}}\% = \frac{\text{urine amy.}}{\text{serum amy.}} \times \frac{\text{serum creat.}}{\text{urine creat.}} \times 100$$

The normal clearance ratio is about 3 percent, and levels of 5 percent or greater are consistent with the diagnosis of acute pancreatitis. The mechanism for the increased renal clearance of amylase may be a tubular defect in the reabsorption of amylase. Unfortunately, elevated ratios have been found with other diseases, and not every patient with acute pancreatitis has an elevated ratio.

The level of lipase, another enzyme liberated by pancreatic disease, is nearly always elevated in acute pancreatitis. Although the lipase level is a more sensitive sign of acute pancreatitis than the serum amylase level, it too lacks specificity and immediate availability. Reports that the lipase level rises later and remains elevated longer than the serum amylase level have not been confirmed, but the course of the lipase level elevation more closely follows the clinical course than does the serum amylase level.

When pancreatic hemorrhage occurs, hemoglobin may be split by the action of pancreatic enzymes, and methemalbumin is formed. The presence of this pigment in patients with acute pancreatitis indicates hemorrhagic pancreatitis. Unfortunately, the finding of methemalbumin in the serum is not pathognomonic, since it may be elevated in any condition in which there is intraabdominal or retroperitoneal bleeding.

The finding of a wheat germ protein that inhibits the activity of salivary amylase nearly 100 times more than the activity of pancreatic amylase has led to a rapid test for approximating the levels of the serum isoamylases. Analysis of serum amylase levels before and after reaction with the inhibitor allows an estimation of what portion of the amylase comes from pancreatic sources. This test holds promise as a simple way to improve the accuracy of serum amylase interpretations but is not widely used. Patients with severe edema of the pancreatic head from pancreatitis may have elevation of the bilirubin and alkaline phosphatase levels.

As with most inflammatory conditions, leukocytosis is usually present but rarely exceeds 20,000/mL in uncomplicated pancreatitis.

Low calcium levels may be detected on laboratory analysis. Persistent hypocalcemia, less than 7 mg/100 mL, is associated with a poor prognosis. Hypocalcemia may result when calcium reacts with free fatty acids and precipitates as calcium soap, but a complete explanation for this phenomenon is lacking.

## Radiography

Plain radiographs of the abdomen have little role in the diagnosis of acute pancreatitis, although calcification, when present, suggests preexisting pancreatic disease. More often their importance is to exclude other diseases which may be confused with pancreatitis. Patients with acute pancreatitis who show evidence of ileus, and air trapped in the small bowel near the inflamed pancreas, have been described as having a sentinel loop. Gaseous distension of the colon with a distally collapsed colon suggests colonic ileus (colon-cutoff sign). None of these signs is truly diagnostic. Contrast studies of the upper GI tract occasionally show narrowing or edema of the duodenum, but the routine use of this procedure or barium enema examination to confirm the diagnosis is not helpful.

Evidence of pancreatic edema or lesser sac fluid on ultrasound or CT may be indicative of acute pancreatic inflammation. Reports indicate that CT scanning may not only aid in the diagnosis of acute pancreatitis but also provide important prognostic information. The routine use of this test, however, seems unnecessary. It should be employed only for the most severe cases or when late complications are suspected.

The injection of contrast material under pressure into the duct of an inflamed pancreas is unwise. Although cases of severe pancreatitis following endoscopic retrograde cholangiopancreatography (ERCP) have been reported, these are rare, most likely because of prudence on the part of endoscopists. Nearly all patients undergoing ERCP have a mild elevation of pancreatic amylase levels following the procedure.

## TREATMENT

The mainstay of treatment for acute pancreatitis is fluid resuscitation. Recognition that profound shock may result from high-volume fluid sequestration in the retroperitoneum has lowered morbidity as resuscitation efforts have improved. Although some controversy exists about the optimum regimen of fluid replacement, most agree that the use of a balanced electrolyte solution is essential. The observation that albumin reduces the amount of pancreatic edema in a whole perfused pancreatitis model has suggested to some that colloid solution may be of benefit. Although an uncontrolled clinical trial of fresh-frozen plasma given in large amounts to patients with acute pancreatitis seemed beneficial, most believe that these measures add little if anything to standard fluid regimens except cost. Fluids should be given in volumes adequate to ensure renal perfusion. When the pancreatitis is severe, admission to an intensive care unit with maximum hemodynamic monitoring is needed. A falling hematocrit should suggest hemorrhagic pancreatitis, and in this case blood replacement is mandatory.

Although the use of the nasogastric tube is widely accepted, no controlled clinical trial has shown its value in altering the course of the disease. The theoretical advantage of reducing pancreatic stimulation and its established value in preventing vomiting, however, make the nasogastric tube a standard part of therapy. Since acute pancreatitis is a self-limiting disease under most circumstances, attention to fluid needs, treatment of pain, and the prevention of vomiting are often sufficient treatment. A small number of patients may develop a severe systemic illness, complicated by acidosis, renal failure, severe hypocalcemia, and respiratory failure.

Acute pancreatitis is not a bacterial disease in its early stages, and the initial use of antibiotics is unwarranted. Sepsis, when it occurs, results from secondary infections and is usually encountered late in the course of the disease. The exception to this is when pancreatitis is complicated by biliary tract infection in the presence of choledocholithiasis. In this case, ampicillin and third-generation cephalosporins are indicated.

The use of a variety of medications, such as anticholinergic drugs, apoprotein, and cimetidine, has been proposed to hasten the usual recovery from pancreatitis; however, none has been shown in controlled clinical trials to alter the course of the disease.

Peritoneal lavage should be considered for patients who fail to respond to initial supportive measures. The rationale for this approach is that the dilution or removal of "toxic" shock factors released by pancreatic necrosis may be beneficial to the patient. Although the precise mechanism by which peritoneal lavage benefits patients with acute pancreatitis is speculative, more than anecdotal observations by a number of clinicians have validated its usefulness in severe cases.

The role of surgery in the treatment of acute pancreatitis is limited. Patients whose clinical course deteriorates despite maximum supportive efforts should undergo laparotomy to ensure that another more treatable condition has not been missed and to debride and drain devitalized pancreatic tissue. Patients with gallstone pancreatitis and choledocholithiasis may benefit from early biliary tract decompression.

Acute pancreatitis can be considered to be a disease of limited duration. Failure to show significant improvement by the end of a week should lead the physician to suspect a complication such as pancreatic abscess, pseudocyst, or pancreatic ascites.

Pancreatic abscess or pseudocyst should be considered in any patient with an abdominal mass, an elevated serum amylase level, an elevated serum bilirubin level, and leukocytosis.

Pseudocysts may rupture spontaneously while the patient is under observation in the emergency department with catastrophic results. Erosion into the upper gastrointestinal tract or an adjacent vessel with massive bleeding has occurred.

Pancreatitis may be a difficult diagnosis to establish. It presents as an acute surgical abdomen, and repeated observation and surgical consultation are often necessary to determine the indicated treatment.

## BIBLIOGRAPHY

Steinberg W, Tenner S: Acute pancreatitis. *N Engl J Med* 330: 1198, 1994.

# 88
# COMPLICATIONS OF GENERAL AND UROLOGIC SURGICAL PROCEDURES

## Edmond A. Hooker

Outpatient surgical procedures are becoming more commonplace, and, with increasing pressure for cost containment, admitted patients are being discharged earlier in their postoperative course. As a result, more patients are presenting to the emergency department with postoperative fever, respiratory complications, genitourinary complaints, wound infections, vascular problems, and complications of drug therapy. This chapter reviews the complications common to all surgical procedures as well as procedure-specific complications.

The operating surgeon should be called when one of his or her patients appears in the emergency department with a surgical complication. This is not just courtesy, but provides continuity of care important for one patient's well-being.

## SYMPTOMS

Fever is a common presenting complaint (Table 88-1). A mnemonic for the common causes of postoperative fever is the "five Ws": Wind (atelectasis, pneumonia), Water (UTI), Wound, Walking (deep vein thrombosis), and Wonder drugs (drug fever, pseudomembranous colitis). Fever during the initial 24 h is usually caused by atelectasis; however, necrotizing streptococcal and clostridial infection also occur in the surgical wound early in the postoperative course. Respiratory complications, pneumonia and atelectasis, and intravenous catheter-related problems such as thrombophlebitis are the predominant causes of fever in the 24- to 72-h time period.

Urinary tract infections become evident 3 to 5 days postoperatively. Seven to ten days postoperatively, clinical manifestations of wound infections develop. Deep venous thrombosis can result in fever any time but usually not until the fifth postoperative day. Antibiotic-induced pseudomembrane colitis occurs up to 6 weeks postoperatively. A stepwise approach to fever in the postoperative patient is presented in Table 88-2.

## RESPIRATORY COMPLICATIONS

Respiratory complications occur in many surgical patients and range from atelectasis and pneumonia to pneumothorax or pulmonary embolism.

**Table 88-1.** Causes of Postoperative Fevers in the General Surgical Patient

| | |
|---|---|
| Atelectasis | Pseudomembranous colitis |
| Pneumonia | Hepatitis |
| Urinary tract infections | Peritonitis |
| Skin and soft tissue injury | Pulmonary embolism |
| Thrombophlebitis (septic and sterile) | Transfusion reaction |
| Deep vein thrombosis | Thyrotoxicosis |
| Intraabdominal abscesses | Pheochromocytoma |
| Unrelated bacterial infection | Adrenal insufficiency |

**Table 88-2.** Evaluation and Management of Postoperative Fever

History
  Presenting signs and symptoms
  Onset of symptoms, time since procedure
  Procedures performed and complications
  Medications
  History of blood transfusion
Physical
  Particular attention to
    Operative sites and contiguous areas
    Sites of catheters and invasive monitors
    Signs of deep venous thrombosis and pulmonary embolism
    Decubiti
    Lungs
Laboratory
  Complete blood count with differential
  Chest radiograph
  Gram stain and culture of wound exudate
  Urinalysis (culture if infected)
  Sputum gram stain and culture
  Blood cultures
  Chest radiographs
  If diarrhea present, consider culture and *C. difficile* toxin
  Further tests as indicated (e.g., computerized tomography, radionucleide studies, venography, arteriograms)
Treatment
  If source identified, start antibiotics. Admission based on condition of patient.
  If no source identified, consider admission, change and culture all catheters, stop all medication that might be causing fever.

## Atelectasis

Atelectasis, the collapse of pulmonary alveoli, is very common. Contributing factors include inadequate clearance of secretion following general anesthetics, decreased intraalveolar pressure, and postoperative pain, which results in hypoventilation. While atelectasis can occur following any procedure, it frequently occurs following upper abdominal and thoracic surgery. The presentation varies from an isolated fever to tachypnea, dyspnea, and tachycardia.

Evaluation includes a chest radiograph, pulse oximetry, and a complete blood count (CBC). Chest radiographs may be normal or show platelike linear densities, triangular-shaped densities, or lobar consolidation. Mild hypoxemia from ventilation-perfusion mismatch is common, but hypercarbia is uncommon. Patients with mild atelectasis and no evidence of hypoxemia may be managed as outpatients with pain control and increased deep breathing. Admission is indicated for aggressive pulmonary toilet and supplemental oxygenation in debilitated patients, patients with underlying lung disease, patients with hypoxemia, or those in whom the diagnosis is in question.

## Pneumonia

Pneumonia usually presents between 24 and 96 h postoperatively. Predisposing factors include prolonged ventilatory support and atelectasis. Presenting symptoms include dyspnea, chest pain, productive cough, fever, and tachypnea. Postoperative pneumonia is likely to be polymicrobial. After cultures are obtained of sputum and blood, parenteral antimicrobial therapy with an aminoglycoside and an antipseudomonal penicillin should be administered. Admission is generally indicated.

## Pneumothorax

Pneumothorax can occur as a complication of thoracic wall surgery, breast biopsies, laparoscopic abdominal surgery, abdominal paracentesis, feeding tube insertion, thoracic surgery, central venous catheter insertion, endoscopic procedures, and tracheostomy. The pathophysiology varies with these different procedures, but clinical features are similar. Patients complain of chest pain, shoulder pain, or dyspnea. Physical findings can include tachypnea, hyperresonance to percussion, and decreased breath sounds on the affected side. Diagnosis is confirmed by chest x-ray, with expiratory views.

## Pulmonary Embolus

Pulmonary embolism (PE) may present any time during the postoperative period. A lower extremity or pelvic thrombus dislodges and migrates to the pulmonary vasculature. The presenting signs and symptoms vary depending on the size of embolus and the underlying cardiopulmonary status of the patient. Patients present with varying degrees of dyspnea, chest pain, cough, and anxiety. Hemoptysis is usually seen only late in the patient's course and with massive PE. The patient may have essentially normal vital signs or be tachypneic and tachycardiac.

Diagnosis of PE is difficult because of the poor sensitivity of noninvasive tests. While hypoxemia and a widened alveolar-arterial $(A - a)$ oxygen gradient are frequently found in larger emboli, the patient may have normal oxygen content and a normal $A - a$ gradient. Diagnosis requires venous Doppler ultrasonography, ventilation-perfusion scan, or pulmonary angiography. Patients with low clinical suspicion, normal vital signs, good oxygenation, and a low probability scan can be discharged, provided other causes of their symptoms have been addressed.

## GENITOURINARY COMPLICATIONS

The most common postoperative genitourinary (GU) complication is urinary tract infection (UTI). However, patients may present with acute urinary retention and acute renal failure (ARF).

### Urinary Tract Infection

Urinary tract infections can occur after any surgical procedure; however, there is an increased incidence in patients who have instrumentation of the genitourinary tract or bladder catheterization. The etiology is direct contamination of the urinary bladder, most commonly with *Escherichia coli*. Other organisms isolated include *Staphylococcus aureus, S. epidermidis, Proteus mirabilis, Klebsiella, Pseudomonas* and enterococci. Oral antibiotics are appropriate for most infections; however, elderly or debilitated patients and patients with evidence of sepsis require admission for parenteral antibiotics.

### Urinary Retention

Acute urinary retention occurs in about 4 percent of all surgical patients, whereas almost 60 percent of patients undergoing urethral surgery will have an episode of retention. It is postulated that urinary retention occurs as the result of catecholamine stimulation of α-adrenergic receptors in the bladder neck and urethral smooth muscle. Increased incidence of urinary retention is likely to occur in elderly males, with excessive fluid administration during surgery, and with the use of spinal or epidural anesthesia.

Patients with urinary retention present with lower abdominal discomfort, urinary urgency, and inability to void. The diagnosis is confirmed by placement of a Foley catheter. The bladder can be safely drained quickly without clamping as there appears to be no foundation for the fears of hematuria, postobstructive diuresis, and hypotension. For patients with normal renal function and no anatomic obstruction, continued catheter drainage is not necessary. For patients with retention after GU procedures, the urologist must be consulted before disposition. Prophylactic antibiotics can be given if the GU tract has been instrumented, if retention is prolonged, or if the patient is at risk for infection.

### Acute Renal Failure

Acute renal failure (ARF) is classified according to the primary cause: prerenal, intrinsic, and postrenal. Volume depletion is the most common prerenal cause. Intrinsic causes include acute tubular necrosis (ATN) and drug nephrotoxicity. Obstructive uropathy is the cause of postrenal ARF. Patients with ARF present with either oliguria or anuria, and, depending on the degree of ARF, may present with signs of uremia and electrolyte abnormalities.

Patients should be examined for signs of hypovolemia and have a urinary catheter placed. Indwelling urinary catheters must be irrigated or replaced. If the patient is hypotensive, a fluid bolus is given to determine if the cause is prerenal. In the patient with urinary outlet obstruction, the urinary catheter will be both diagnostic and therapeutic. If there is doubt about the cause of the renal failure, central venous pressure and pulmonary capillary wedge pressure can be helpful. The presence of postobstructive uropathy above the urinary bladder can be confirmed using abdominal ultrasound. When no prerenal or postrenal cause can be identified, then there is likely to be an intrinsic cause of ARF.

## WOUND COMPLICATIONS

Wound complications are frequent and include hematomas, seromas, infections, necrotizing fasciitis, and dehiscence. The patient's surgeon should be notified of all wound complications.

### Hematomas

Wound hematomas result from unrecognized inadequate hemostasis. The patient presents with pain, pressure, and swelling within the wound. Patients with wound hematomas may be febrile and have sanguineous or serous wound drainage. Making the differentiation between hematoma and wound infections can be difficult. A few sutures are removed to allow the hematoma to drain, and cultures are obtained. If there is no evidence of infection and hemostasis can be maintained, the patient can be discharged. In patients with a hematoma of the neck or who have undergone vascular surgery, extreme caution and consultation is appropriate.

### Seromas

A seroma, a collection of serous fluid, is usually the result of inadequate control of lymphatics during dissection but can also occur under split-thickness skin grafts and areas with large dead spaces (axilla, groin, neck, pelvis). The patient presents with painless swelling below the wound or graft, and needle aspiration will yield a serous fluid. Aspiration confirms the diagnosis and alleviates the problem, although it may have to be repeated later.

### Infection

Systemic factors (extremes of age, poor nutrition, diabetes) contribute to wound infections; however, local factors (necrotic tissue, poor perfusion, foreign bodies, hematomas) are of greatest significance. In nontraumatic, uninfected operative wounds, in which the respiratory, alimentary, and genitourinary tract were not entered, infection rates are low. In these cases, the infecting organism is usually from the skin but can originate from remote infected sources (e.g., urinary tract infection). If there is a remote source, the organism is probably the same in both infections. Wounds associated with entering the respiratory, alimentary, or genitourinary tract or secondary to trauma have a higher risk of infection.

Presenting signs and symptoms of wound infections include increasing pain, erythema, swelling, drainage, and tenderness at the incision site. Wounds not involving the perineum and not associated with entry into the GI or biliary tract are most often infected with *S. aureus* or streptococci. Such wounds can be safely managed with drainage, culture of the wound, irrigation, loose packing with gauze, and outpatient antibiotics. Wounds involving the perineum, or associated with the GI or biliary tract, often are infected with multiple organisms, including gram-negative bacteria and anaerobes. Parenteral broad-spectrum antibiotics are administered, and admission is necessary.

## Necrotizing Fasciitis

Necrotizing fasciitis is a feared complication. The cause is direct contamination of the wound with group A streptococci or *S. aureus*. The wound is usually extremely painful, erythematous, swollen, and warm without sharp margins. Early clinical differentiation from cellulitis can be difficult. The presence of marked systemic toxicity and pain out of proportion to local findings indicates fasciitis. In more advanced cases, there may be deep pain with patchy areas of surface hypesthesia, crepitation, or bullae. Treatment is antibiotics and immediate surgical debridement.

## Wound Dehiscence

Wound dehiscence can be superficial or can extend into the deeper fascial planes. Dehiscence is caused by either inadequate closure or intrinsic host factors such as malnutrition, glucocorticoid use, or diabetes. The patient may present with serosanguineous fluid leaking from the wound. Dehiscence of abdominal incisions has the potential for evisceration. If evisceration is not present, conservative management using abdominal binders is appropriate. However, if there is any uncertainty, operative exploration is indicated.

## VASCULAR COMPLICATIONS

Postoperative vascular complications include thrombophlebitis and deep venous thrombosis (DVT). Superficial thrombophlebitis usually occurs in the upper extremities, secondary to prolonged cannulation of the vein or infusion of irritating fluids. Deep venous thrombosis is secondary to stasis, endothelial damage, and hypercoagulopathy.

## Superficial Thrombophlebitis

Superficial thrombophlebitis is usually aseptic. The patient complains of redness and warmth of the affected vein. If there is no evidence of surrounding cellulitis or lymphangitis, the patient is treated with local heat and elevation. Suppurative superficial thrombophlebitis is characterized by erythema, palpable tender cord, lymphangitis, and pain. Suppurative thrombophlebitis requires excision of the affected vein.

## Deep Venous Thrombosis

Superficial thrombophlebitis of the lower extremities is most frequently secondary to stasis in varicose veins. When lower extremity superficial thrombophlebitis is seen, the possibility of concurrent DVT must be considered. Swelling of the extremity is the most specific physical sign and its presence requires diagnostic evaluation. Doppler ultrasonography is generally the preferred diagnostic test. Patients with normal color-flow studies should be treated with elevation and bed rest. Repeat color-flow Doppler should be performed in 3 days if symptoms persist but sooner if symptoms worsen.

## COMPLICATIONS OF DRUG THERAPY

Many different medicines have been reported to cause drug fever (Table 88-3). The mechanisms proposed are hypersensitivity reactions, pyogenic effect, and disturbed thermoregulation. In patients in whom no source for the fever can be found, it is appropriate to consider stopping medications known to cause drug fever.

Many antibiotics can cause diarrhea; however, the greatest concern in the postoperative patient is pseudomembranous colitis (PMC). PMC is due to the toxin produced by the bacterium *Clostridium difficile*. PMC is related to antibiotic use, which destroys the normal enteric bacterial flora, allowing an overgrowth of the *C. difficile*. Even short courses of antibiotics have been associated with PMC. The patient presents with watery, and sometimes bloody, diarrhea, elevated

**Table 88-3.** Medications Associated with Drug Fever

| | |
|---|---|
| Allopurinol | Methyldopa |
| Amphetamine | Metoclopramide |
| Amphotericin B | Nifedipine |
| Antihistamines | Nitrofurantoin sodium |
| Asparaginase | Nomifensine |
| Azathioprine | Oxprenelol |
| Barbiturates | Para-aminosalicylic acid |
| Benztropine | Penicillins |
| Bleomycin sulfate | Phenytoin sodium |
| Carbamazepine | Procainamide |
| Cephalosporins | Propylthiouracil |
| Chlorpromazine | Prostaglandin $E_2$ |
| Cimetidine | Quinidine sulfate |
| Clofibrate | Rifampin |
| Cocaine derivatives | Ritodrine |
| Folate | Salicylates |
| Haloperidol | Streptokinase |
| Hydralazine hydrochloride | Streptomycin sulfate |
| Ibuprofen | Sulfonamides |
| Interferon | Tetracycline |
| Iodides | Thioridazine |
| Isoniazid | Tolmetin |
| Levamisole | Triamterene |
| Lincomycin | Trifluoperazine |
| Lysergic acid | Vancomycin hydrochloride |
| Mebendazole | |

temperature, and crampy abdominal pain. The diagnosis is usually made by detecting *C. difficile* cytotoxin in the stool; however, up to 27 percent of patients with culture-proven PMC will have a negative assay for toxin. In cases of suspected PMC, empirical therapy, using either oral vancomycin, oral metronidazole, or intravenous metronidazole, is indicated.

## COMPLICATIONS OF BREAST SURGERY

Breast biopsy is a common procedure. While complications are infrequent, patients can develop minor wound infections and hematomas. Rarely, pneumothorax has been reported. Wound hematomas frequently require operative control for proper evacuation and hemostasis.

Mastectomies have about a 10 percent complication rate. Early complications include wound infection, necrosis of skin flaps, and the accumulation of seromas. The most common late complication is lymphedema of the arm. This occurs in 5 to 10 percent of women undergoing level I or level II dissection but is generally easily managed by nighttime elevation and minor activity restriction.

## COMPLICATIONS OF GASTROINTESTINAL SURGERY

Patients who have undergone any gastrointestinal (GI) surgery may present with intestinal obstruction, intraabdominal abscess, pancreatitis, cholecystitis, fistulas, and tetanus. Certain procedures such as anastomoses, gastric surgery, gastrostomy tubes, biliary tract surgery, stomas, colonoscopy, and rectal surgery have specific complications.

### General Considerations

#### Intestinal Obstruction

Ileus, a functional obstruction of the bowel, is postulated to be the result of stimulation of the splanchnic nerves leading to neuronal inhibition of coordinated intrinsic bowel wall motor activity. It is expected after any operation in which the peritoneal cavity is violated. Following gastrointestinal surgery, small bowel tone usually returns to normal within 24 h, gastric function within 2 days, and colonic function within 3 days. While ileus can also occur following nongastrointestinal procedures, it is usually secondary to anesthetic agents, and function returns to normal after 24 h. Prolonged ileus can be caused by peritonitis, intraabdominal abscess, hemoperitoneum, pneumonia, electrolyte imbalance, sepsis, and medications.

Presenting symptoms of ileus include nausea, vomiting, obstipation, constipation, abdominal distension, and abdominal pain. When these symptoms are present in the first few days after surgery, they are most often due to adynamic ileus. The symptoms of adynamic ileus are often mild and respond to nasogastric suction, bowel rest, and intravenous hydration. However, in cases of prolonged ileus, the physician must always look for an underlying cause. Evaluation of the patient with suspected ileus includes abdominal radiographs to identify air-fluid levels, chest x-ray, CBC, electrolytes, and urinalysis for secondary causes of ileus.

Mechanical ileus of the bowel is most often secondary to adhesions. Small bowel obstruction above the ligament of Treitz is associated with frequent bouts of bilious emesis. In cases of more distal obstruction, pain and distension become more severe, the frequency and volume of vomiting decrease, and emesis becomes more feculent. Abdominal radiographs demonstrate multiple air-fluid levels and a paucity of gas in the colon; however, with high obstruction, above the ligament of Treitz, there may be no air-fluid levels. In the emergency department, differentiating between functional ileus and mechanical bowel obstruction can be difficult. Both disorders result in varying degrees of abdominal pain, distension, nausea, vomiting, and constipation. Once the diagnosis of obstruction is confirmed or suspected, surgical consultation is indicated.

## Intraabdominal Abscess

Intraabdominal abscess is caused most frequently by preoperative contamination, spillage of bowel contents during surgery, contamination of a hematoma, or from postoperative anastomotic leaks. Patients may present with abdominal pain, nausea, vomiting, ileus, abdominal distension, fever, chills, anorexia, and abdominal tenderness. If the diagnosis is suspected, CT or ultrasound of the abdomen is required. The patient should receive broad-spectrum antibiotics. Although some abscesses are amenable to percutaneous drainage, many patients will require surgical exploration.

## Pancreatitis

Pancreatitis following abdominal surgery is secondary to direct manipulation or retraction of the pancreatic duct. It most commonly occurs following gastric resection, biliary tract surgery, and endoscopic retrograde cholangiopancreatography (ERCP). Clinical presentation will vary from mild nausea, vomiting, and abdominal discomfort to intractable vomiting, leukocytosis, and left pleural effusion. Severe hemorrhagic presentation can cause lumbar pain, accompanied by blue-gray discoloration of the skin in the flank area (Turner sign), or similar changes around the umbilicus (Cullen sign). While the serum amylase level rises in acute pancreatitis, it is also elevated in patients with severe cholecystitis, renal insufficiency, intestinal obstruction, perforated ulcer, or ischemic bowel. A serum lipase measurement may help to identify those with true pancreatitis, although it may be elevated in a patient with a perforated viscus. Abdominal radiographs may show localized ileus in the region of the pancreas (sentinel loop). Computed tomography is useful in defining pancreatic fluid collections or abscesses. Generally, treatment of the postoperative pancreatitis is similar to the treatment of nonoperative pancreatitis: bowel rest, antiemetics, and nasogastric suction.

## Cholecystitis

Patients may present during the postoperative period with biliary colic, acute calculous cholecystitis, or acute acalculous cholecystitis. The etiology of these disorders in the postoperative period is not clear. Ultrasonography of the gallbladder and pancreas should be obtained to aid in the diagnosis.

Acalculous cholecystitis is of particular concern in the postoperative period. While it may present at any time, it seems to be more common in elderly males. Signs and symptoms are similar to calculous cholecystitis, but ultrasound fails to reveal gallstones. Liver function studies and neutrophil count may be normal. Important findings on ultrasonography include gallbladder enlargement, wall thickening, and pericholecystic fluid collection. Hepatobiliary scintigraphy may be helpful. Early diagnosis is critical because early operative intervention can reduce morbidity and mortality.

## Fistulas

Enterocutaneous fistulas can occur almost anywhere in the GI tract and are usually the result of technical complications or direct bowel injury. High-output fistulas can result in electrolyte abnormalities and volume depletion. Fistulas involving the proximal GI tract are frequently high output and are of the greatest concern. Sepsis is the other major complication. Most patients require admission, although many fistulas will ultimately close spontaneously.

## Tetanus

While most cases of tetanus in the United States occur after minor trauma, there have been numerous reports of tetanus following general surgical procedures. *C. tetani* is found in the GI tract of 1 percent of the population. During gastrointestinal surgery there is spillage of *C. tetani*. Proliferation of the organism is facilitated by the presence of devitalized tissue, blood clots, and surgical suture. Incubation can take from 1 to 54 days, at which time the toxin leads to clinical tetanus. The classic symptoms of tetanus, trismus and opisthotonos, may not be manifest at initial presentation. Patients may present with nonspecific symptoms of abdominal discomfort, fever, and abdominal wall rigidity. Diagnosis is based on physical examination and a history of inadequate immunization.

## Specific Considerations

### Anastomosis

Anastomotic leaks occur most frequently after esophageal and colonic surgery and least frequently after gastric and small intestinal anastomoses. The cause of anastomotic leak is mainly related to surgical technique.

Intrathoracic esophageal anastomotic leaks usually manifest within 10 days of surgery. The presentation is dramatic, with fever, chest pain, tachypnea, tachycardia, and possibly shock. Chest x-ray may reveal a pneumothorax with pleural effusion. Disruption can be confirmed by contrast esophagography, using a water-soluble contrast agent. Even with immediate reoperation, morbidity and mortality are high.

The signs and symptoms of gastric anastomotic leaks include abdominal pain, fever, leukocytosis, gastric outlet obstruction, hyperamylasemia, hyperbilirubinemia, peritonitis, and shock. Plain radiographs may reveal pneumoperitoneum or air-fluid levels. The patient should have immediate volume resuscitation, parenteral broad-spectrum antibiotics, and nasogastric tube drainage. Immediate surgery is required.

Small-intestinal anastomoses infrequently leak because of the excellent blood supply and rapid healing of the area. However, if a leak occurs, the patient will usually present with local abscess formation or peritonitis. Treatment is immediate reoperation.

Colorectal anastomoses are prone to disruption because of the large number of pathogenic bacteria, propensity for colonic distension, and single thin layer of circular muscle to support sutures. The patients will usually present 7 to 14 days postoperatively with evidence of intraabdominal or pelvic abscess. Computed tomography can be helpful in diagnosis. Patients should receive broad-spectrum parenteral antibiotics, nasogastric tube drainage, and adequate fluid resuscitation in preparation for surgery.

## Gastric Surgery

Patients who have undergone partial or complete gastrectomy can present with a few distinct syndromes: dumping syndrome, alkaline reflux gastritis, afferent loop syndrome, and post vagotomy diarrhea. While these complications are rare, the symptoms can be disabling.

Dumping syndrome can occur either early or late after a meal. While the exact etiology of dumping symptoms is unclear, it occurs when the pylorus is either bypassed or removed. The hyperosmolar chyme contents of the stomach are dumped into the jejunum, resulting in rapid influx of extracellular fluid and an autonomic response.

Patients experience nausea, epigastric discomfort, palpitations, abdominal colic, diaphoresis, and, in some cases, dizziness and syncope. Patients with early dumping symptoms experience diarrhea, while those with late dumping symptoms, 2 to 4 h postprandial, usually do not. The late dumping syndrome is felt to be due to a reactive hypoglycemia. The mainstay of treatment is dietary modification, eating small dry meals, and separating solids from liquids. If this is unsuccessful, parenteral treatment with octreotide acetate, a synthetic somatostatin hormone, has been effective in some cases. In refractory cases, pyloroplasty can be tried. Most of these patients do not require admission.

Patients with alkaline reflux gastritis will present with continual burning epigastric pain, which is aggravated by meals and unrelieved by vomiting. The syndrome is caused by reflux of bile into the stomach. Diagnosis is made by endoscopic examination.

Patients with afferent loop syndrome will also present with severe epigastric pain 1 to 2 h after eating, which is relieved by vomiting. The vomitus will be bilious, without food. The syndrome occurs in patients who have undergone gastroenterostomy (Bilroth II) reconstruction after partial gastrectomy. Diagnosis is made by contrast radiography or endoscopy. Operative reconstruction is required.

Although most patients undergoing truncal vagotomy will have increased bowel movements, 5 to 20 percent of patients will have diarrhea. The exact etiology is not clear. Patients will present with diarrhea that is variable in its occurrence and not associated with food intake. It is often unpredictable and explosive, which can lead to weight loss and malnutrition as well as severe social complications. The incidence of the diarrhea decreases with time, and treatment is mostly symptomatic.

## Gastrostomy Tubes

The percutaneous endoscopic gastrostomy (PEG) tubes have become the preferred procedure for placement of gastrostomy tubes. While overall complications rates are low, reported complications include wound infections (including necrotizing fasciitis), hemorrhage, peritonitis, aspiration, granulation tissue buildup, wound dehiscence, septicemia, diarrhea, peritube leakage, pneumoperitoneum, and tube obstruction. Inflammation of the wound edges is expected secondary to local trauma from the tube and gastric acid leakage. The most common problem encountered by the emergency physician is a nonfunctioning tube or a completely dislodged tube.

When evaluating an obstructed G-tube, it is important to determine if the original PEG tube is in place (there will be no side port to inflate a balloon). If the original PEG tube is in place, the tube either must be removed endoscopically or cut and allowed to pass. While controversy still exists, the latter procedure is inexpensive, easy to perform, and eliminates the need for admission. Endoscopic removal is recommended for patients with suspected or potential obstructive disease of the GI tract, such as pyloric stenosis, intestinal pseudo-obstruction, and intestinal stricture (e.g., radiation, ischemia, and inflammatory bowel disease). If the tube is cut, an abdominal radi-

**Table 88-4.** Complications of Cholecystectomy

Bile leak
Bile duct structure
Bleeding
Bowel injury
Intraabdominal abscess
Myocardial infarction
Pancreatitis
Pulmonary complication
Retained and common duct stones
Umbilical hernia
Wound infection

ograph should be obtained 1 week later to confirm passage of the internal component. For further discussion, see Chap. 263.

## Biliary Tract Surgery

More than half of all cholecystectomies are now performed laparoscopically. There are complications seen after both open and laparoscopic cholecystectomy (Table 88-4) and complications related to the laparoscopic technique (Table 88-5). Patients are likely to present to the emergency physician with nonspecific abdominal symptoms.

The evaluation of a patient who presents after cholecystectomy complaining of abdominal pain depends on the clinical condition of the patient. If there are signs of peritoneal irritation or fever, an injury to the biliary system is likely. The patient should have a CT scan of the abdomen in addition to CBC, electrolytes, liver function tests, and an amylase blood test. Endoscopic retrograde cholangiopancreatography (ERCP) will be required to identify the site of the injury; however, a collection of bile can be seen in a CT scan. Depending on the ERCP results, reoperation may be necessary. Small collections of bile may only require observation or percutaneous drainage.

Patients presenting soon after cholecystectomy with pain, pancreatitis, and/or jaundice may have retained common duct stones. If the CT scan does not reveal an intraabdominal collection of fluid, an ERCP should be performed. Endoscopic sphincterotomy is usually an effective means of dealing with retained stones. Patients presenting late after cholecystectomy with fever, pain, and jaundice may have bile duct stricture. Diagnosis requires ERCP. While stents are usually tried at first, surgical repair may be necessary.

## Stomas

The two most common stomas placed are the ileostomy and colostomy. Problems with these stomas can be quite debilitating. Most complications are related to technical errors where the stomas are placed; however, there can be problems of new disease within the stoma (e.g., Crohn disease, cancer). Possible complications include

**Table 88-5.** Complications Related to Use of Laparoscopic Techniques

Related to pneumomediastinum
    Cardiac arrhythmias during procedure
    Subcutaneous emphysema
    Pneumothorax
    Pneumomediastinum
    Peritoneal insufflation
    $CO_2$ embolization
Related to insertion of needle and trocar
    Gastrointestinal tract injuries
        Laceration
        Intestinal burns
    Genitourinary tract injuries
    Major vessel injuries
    Hernias from trocar site
    Wound infections

ischemia and stomal necrosis, peristomal skin irritation, peristomal hernia, and stomal prolapse.

Ischemia and stomal necrosis are manifest very early in the postoperative course. The cause is inadequate blood supply to the stoma. Normally the stoma is pink, without any evidence of cyanosis. Any evidence of compromised blood flow requires surgical reevaluation.

Peristomal maceration and skin destruction are most likely secondary to a poor seal of the stomal appliance. Consultation with an enterostomal therapist for a properly fitting appliance is indicated.

Prolapse can occur with both ileostomies and colostomies. The cause is usually inadequate fixation of the intraabdominal portion or too large an abdominal wall opening. Patients present with the stoma protrusion, with or without pain. The stoma must be examined to determine viability. The stoma should be pink and painless. Attempted reduction should be made, if the tissue is viable, followed by consultation with the surgeon. Definitive therapy will require surgical revision.

Parastomal hernias are secondary to too large an abdominal wall opening. As with any hernia, determine if the hernia is incarcerated, attempt reduction, and consult the surgeon. Definitive therapy will require local reconstruction of the orifice.

## Colonoscopy

Potential complications of colonoscopy include hemorrhage, perforation, retroperitoneal abscess, pneumoscrotum, pneumothorax, volvulus, postcolonoscopy distension, bacteremia, and infection.

Hemorrhage is the most common complication and can be secondary to the polypectomy procedures, biopsies, laceration of the mucosa by the instrument, or tearing of the mesentery or spleen. If the bleeding is intraluminal, the patient will present with rectal bleeding. Patients with mesenteric or splenic injury will present with signs of intraabdominal bleeding. Treatment of intraluminal bleeding depends on the magnitude of hemorrhage. Signs of intraabdominal bleeding will require emergency laparotomy.

Perforation of the colon with pneumoperitoneum usually is manifested immediately but can take several hours to manifest. Perforation is usually secondary to intrinsic disease of the colon (e.g., diverticulitis) or to vigorous manipulation during the procedure. Most patients will require immediately laparotomy; however, in some patients presenting late (1 to 2 days later) without sign of peritonitis, expectant management may be appropriate.

## Rectal Surgery

Patients who have undergone hemorrhoidectomy frequently have problems with postoperative urinary retention, the management of which has been previously discussed. Three other problems that can occur are constipation, rectal hemorrhage, and rectal prolapse.

The management of constipation in the patient who has undergone rectal surgery is no different from that of any other patient with constipation. Gentle rectal examination is indicated, and enemas can still be used. Posthemorrhoidectomy rectal hemorrhage can occur immediately postoperatively but also at 7 to 10 days postoperatively. The cause of delayed bleeding is most likely sepsis in the pedicle. The patient may present with minimal bleeding or massive hemorrhage. While ligation of the affected vessel is needed, a temporary tamponade with a Foley catheter may be helpful.

Patients may present with mucosal prolapse or complete rectal prolapse. Mucosal prolapse occurs when the surgeon has not removed all redundant mucosa during hemorrhoidectomy and is much more common than rectal prolapse. Local treatment by a surgeon is usually corrective. Rectal prolapse can occur after any anorectal surgical procedure and probably is related to injury to the puborectalis muscle. The patient will present with the sensation of protrusion and may complain of pain. The treatment is reduction and surgical consultation.

Infection following anorectal surgery is surprisingly uncommon.

The patient usually presents complaining of increasing pain and fever. Examination of the area is necessary to reveal an abscess or cellulitis. Fournier gangrene may follow anorectal surgery. If this is suspected, broad-spectrum parenteral antibiotics are given immediately. The patient requires immediate surgical debridement.

## COMPLICATIONS OF UROLOGIC SURGERY

In the patient who has undergone a urologic procedure, the expected complications of infections and urinary retention have been discussed. However vasectomies and extracorporeal shock-wave lithotripsy (ESWL) deserve some special mention.

### Vasectomies

Vasectomies are mainly performed on an outpatient basis. While most are without complication, problems that occur include postoperative hemorrhage, scrotal discomfort and edema, and epididymitis. Early postoperative bleeding is secondary to damage to the deferent artery, and the patient presents with a large scrotal hematoma. The bleeding is unlikely to stop spontaneously, and surgical exploration is indicated.

Some scrotal discomfort and some swelling is expected after vasectomy. The swelling is caused by disruption of lymphatics. As long as there is no evidence of uncontrolled bleeding, the patient can be treated with analgesics, scrotal support, and ice packs.

Epididymitis is reported to occur in 0.4 to 6.1 percent of cases and is probably the result of epididymal engorgement from ligation of the vas. Patients present with pain and swelling of the scrotum. Diagnosis is made on physical examination, and treatment includes nonsteroidal anti-inflammatory drugs, scrotal support, and ice packs.

### Extracorporeal Shock-Wave Lithotripsy

Extracorporeal shock-wave lithotripsy (ESWL) has radically changed the management of large urinary calculi. Hematuria and some degree of pain are expected after the procedure. Other problems that occur less frequently include perirenal hematomas, ureteral obstruction, and infections.

The perirenal hematoma is secondary to subcapsular renal hemorrhage. Most will be subclinical; however, when there is enough blood sequestered under the capsule, the patient will present with flank pain and evidence of blood loss. Diagnosis is made with CT or renal ultrasonography. Usually only supportive care and bed rest are necessary.

Ureteral obstruction after ESWL is caused by either a solitary fragment or an accumulation of calculi known as Steinstrasse. Patients with obstruction present with pain, nausea, and vomiting. Diagnosis is made by intravenous pyelogram (IVP). Treatment is based on the presence of severe pain, fever, sepsis, nausea or vomiting, or failure to resolve the obstruction. Often, the fragments will pass spontaneously, and intervention is unnecessary.

Urinary tract infection (UTI) after ESWL is prevented mostly by preoperative intravenous antibiotics and postoperative oral antibiotics. However, in the presence of ureteral obstruction, patients may develop UTI or urosepsis. The patient will present with evidence of obstruction as well as fever, nausea, and vomiting. Patients with urosepsis and obstruction require antibiotics and surgical intervention to relieve the obstruction.

## BIBLIOGRAPHY

Aronson MP, Chelmow D, Pearson JW: Intraoperative and postoperative complications of gynecologic surgery, in DeCherney AH, Pernoll ML (eds): *Current Obstetrics and Gynecology Diagnosis and Treatment.* E. Norwalk, CT, Appleton and Lange 1994, pp 867–883.

DuFrayne FJ, Crooks GW, Goldman DR: Postoperative gastrointestinal dysfunction, in Goldman DR, Brown FH, Guarnieri DM (eds): *Perioperative Medicine,* 2d ed. New York, McGraw-Hill, 1994, pp 675–681.

Fuchs GJ: Renal stones: Extracorporeal shock wave lithotripsy, in Krane RJ, Siroky MB, Fitzpatrick JM (eds): *Clinical Urology.* Philadelphia, Lippincott, 1994, pp 289–302.

Hiyama DT, Zinner MJ: Surgical complications, in Schwartz SI et al (eds): *Principles of Surgery,* 6th ed. New York, McGraw-Hill, 1994, pp 455–487.

Talbot GH, Glackman SJ: Approach to the patient with postoperative fever, in Goldman DR, Brown FH, Guarnieri DM (eds): *Perioperative Medicine,* 2d ed. New York, McGraw-Hill, 1994, 511–521.

# 89

# LIVER FAILURE AND TRANSPLANTATION

## Steven Kronick
## Rawden Evans

## DEMOGRAPHICS, INDICATIONS, AND SURVIVAL

Worldwide, there are approximately 7000 liver transplantations performed yearly, with nearly half of these operations done in the United States. At present the number of transplantations performed is limited only by the availability of organ donors. Before the 1980s, 1-year survival after liver transplantation was approximately 30 percent. Improvements in surgical techniques, immunosuppression protocols, and patient selection have increased survival significantly. Taking all clinical indications, survival at 1 year averages 78.6 percent and at 3 years 72.2 percent. Today, transplantation is the treatment of choice for end-stage liver disease (ESLD) and is considered an effective means to improve quality of life as well as survival.

The majority of patients receiving transplantation suffer from cirrhosis and the complications of hepatic portal circulatory hypertension. In the United States, alcoholic liver disease is currently the most common indication for liver transplantation. Though controversial, experience has shown that a majority of properly selected patients with alcoholic liver disease do well after transplantation and remain abstinent. Other indications for transplantation include ESLD caused by viral and autoimmune hepatitis, primary biliary cirrhosis, and primary sclerosing cholangitis. Metabolic derangements causing ESLD in adults include Wilson disease, hemachromatosis, and α-antitrypsin deficiency; in pediatric patients they include hereditary oxalosis and Crigler-Najjar syndrome. A variety of conditions can result in hepatic vein obstruction or thrombosis, resulting in Budd-Chiari syndrome and acute or chronic forms of liver failure. The experience with transplantation for malignant liver disease has been generally disappointing. There have been no studies showing significant improvement in survival of patients with hepatocellular carcinoma or cholangiocarcinoma undergoing liver transplantation. Transplantation in patients with isolated or "incidental" hepatic tumors remains controversial. Acute or fulminant liver failure is also seen in toxic ingestions, acetaminophen overdose being the principal cause in the United States. Other agents that have been associated with fulminant hepatitis include *Amanita phalloides* mushroom toxin, isoniazid, phenytoin, methyldopa, valproic acid, and the halothane-like anesthetics.

Age is not a major criterion for patient selection. Patients over 60 years of age appear to do as well after transplantation as their younger counterparts. Transplantation over the age of 70 is unusual, but physiologic age is more important than chronologic age. There are both quality-of-life and severity-of-disease indications for liver transplantation. Quality-of-life factors include intractable pruritus, metabolic bone disease and fracture, recurrent biliary sepsis, xanthomatous neuropathy, intractable ascites, encephalopathy, variceal bleeding, and incapacitating fatigue. Severity-of-disease factors include hepatorenal syndrome, recurrent spontaneous bacterial peritonitis, serum albumin < 2.5 g/dL, prothrombin time (PT) prolonged > 5 s, or serum bilirubin > 5.0 mg/dL in chronic liver disease and > 10 mg/dL in cholestatic liver disease.

## MANAGEMENT OF THE PRETRANSPLANT PATIENT

The success of liver transplantation as the treatment of choice for ESLD has created a large, unmet demand at a time when organ donor numbers are falling. The emergency physician is far more likely to encounter acutely ill pretransplant patients than those posttransplant. Since ESLD is by definition a decompensated condition, management of the pretransplant patient is in many ways more difficult and challenging than that of the posttransplant patient. It is of paramount importance that the pretransplant patient have ready access to a primary care provider well versed in the management of ESLD and its many complications.

The clinical manifestations of ESLD are the net result of circulatory changes accompanying portal hypertension combined with the metabolic derangements of hepatocellular isolation and/or dysfunction. Common emergent presentations include infection, circulatory collapse, variceal hemorrhage, refractory ascites, and portosystemic (hepatic) encephalopathy.

Regardless of the underlying pathology, essentially all forms of ESLD become complicated by portal hypertension and the metabolic consequences of collateral blood flow bypassing the liver. When superimposed on hepatocellular disease and dysfunction, the synthesis of albumin and coagulation factors is affected, resulting in loss of plasma oncotic pressure and coagulopathy. Normally one-fifth of the resting cardiac output is taken by the hepatic circulation, and fully 80 percent of hepatic blood flow is derived from the splanchnic portal circulation. Portal hypertension ultimately results in the formation of ascites and gastroesophageal varices, which predispose the patient to a variety of life-threatening conditions.

The circulatory and metabolic changes that characterize ESLD promote an edematous state and formation of ascites, which is accompanied by a loss of effective blood volume. There is generalized vasodilation of the peripheral circulation, often with a paradoxical vasoconstriction in the renal circulation. Activation of the renin-angiotensin system promotes aldosterone secretion, and aldosterone clearance is diminished by liver disease. Chronically elevated aldosterone levels stimulate renal sodium retention. Water metabolism is further complicated by the inability of the kidney to produce a dilute urine. Delivery of glomerular filtrate to the diluting segment of the nephron is reduced, and ADH secretion is high, promoting back-diffusion of water in the distal nephron. The net effects of these circulatory and humoral changes are increased total body water with a decreased effective circulating volume plus a tendency to hyponatremia and potassium depletion.

Important complications of ascites include dyspnea and fatigue, spontaneous bacterial peritonitis, hydrothorax, and ruptured umbilical hernia. The latter is rare but carries a high morbidity and mortality. Related management issues include intravascular volume depletion, azotemia, electrolyte imbalances, encephalopathy, and renal failure (hepatorenal syndrome).

The occurrence of ascites in ESLD is prognostically unfavorable. Dietary sodium restriction is the mainstay of treatment but often fails secondary to noncompliance. The aldosterone antagonist spironolactone (Aldactone) is a commonly used diuretic in ESLD because of the permissive role of aldosterone in the formation of ascites and the potassium-sparing properties of this useful drug. A starting dose of 100 mg/day can be increased slowly in 100- to 200-mg increments to a maximum of 400 to 600 mg/day. If the diuretic response to spirono-lactone is inadequate and/or hyperkalemia develops, a loop diuretic such as furosemide (Lasix) can be carefully added. In refractory ascites some clinicians may use the thiazide-like diuretic metalazone (Zaroxolyn) as a last resort to medical management. Any significant change in diuretic therapy should be followed up after a short interval to ensure against dangerous changes in intravascular volume, renal function, or electrolyte imbalance.

High-volume paracentesis often becomes a necessary therapy for refractory and symptomatic ascites accompanying ESLD. Fear of secondary cardiovascular collapse and acute renal failure has been allayed in part by the successful application of paracentesis in large series of patients. As much as 6 to 8 L of ascitic fluid can be drained over a 60- to 90-min interval with the concomitant peripheral infusion of albumin (6 to 8 g/L of ascites collected). Many believe that an albumin infusion is unnecessary when peripheral edema is present, as mobilization of edema fluid is capable of attenuating intravascular volume loss. High-volume paracentesis should be avoided in the presence of significant renal insufficiency and coagulopathy.

Spontaneous bacterial peritonitis (SBP) is a relatively common complication of ESLD and ascites. The liver is an important component of the reticuloendothelial system and normally functions to help clear bacteria from the circulation. Portosystemic shunting of blood increases the likelihood of persistent bacteremia, and ascitic fluid is a culture media relatively isolated from immune surveillance. The classic presentation of SBP includes fever and chills, abdominal pain, diminished bowel sounds, diffuse rebound tenderness, hypotension, and encephalopathy. However, the diagnosis of SBP should be considered whenever a patient with ESLD presents with an acute functional decline, as the classic signs and symptoms of SBP may be absent. The presumptive diagnosis can be made by abdominal paracentesis. At least 10 mL of ascitic fluid should be reserved for culture and can be processed in the same manner as a peripheral blood culture. A total WBC count greater than $1000/\mu L$ or granulocytes in excess of $250/\mu L$ is consistent with the diagnosis of SBP. The most common infecting organisms are *Escherichia coli, Streptococcus pneumoniae,* and *Klebsiella.* Approximately three-fourths of isolates are intestinal organisms. Adequate antibiotic coverage can be achieved with cefotaxime or ampicillin plus an aminoglycoside (e.g., gentamicin). Aminoglycosides should be avoided when possible, especially in the presence of known renal insufficiency. Alternative antibiotics include cephalothin or mezlocillin.

Umbilical hernia is a common complication of ascites. Hernia rupture is a rare event that may accompany localized pressure necrosis or trauma. Volume depletion, shock, and infection are the principal dangers of hernia rupture, which requires aggressive management to avoid excess morbidity and mortality.

Significant pleural effusion accompanies ascites in approximately 10 percent of cases. So-called cirrhotic pleural effusion or hepatic hydrothorax occurs most commonly on the right side and, when severe, may cause respiratory compromise. The principal therapy is management of ascites and therapeutic thoracentesis as indicated clinically.

Hepatorenal syndrome is often a fatal complication of ESLD. Despite the preservation of renal tubular concentrating capacity and enhanced sodium retention, systemic circulatory changes result in a diminished glomerular filtration rate (GFR) and a clinical picture indistinguishable from prerenal azotemia. However, this condition does not respond to the administration of fluids and other efforts to expand circulatory volume. Liver transplantation has been found to be the only effective therapy.

Portal hypertension results in shunting of portal blood into the systemic circulation at several anatomic sites. Gastroesophageal varices form at the anastomosis of the left gastric vein and the azygous vein in the upper stomach and lower esophagus. These varices are superficial, thin-walled, and poorly supported, which predisposes to hemorrhage. Variceal hemorrhage carries an overall mortality of 50 percent,

and two-thirds of survivors have recurrent hemorrhage. In this patient population, bleeding from peptic ulcer disease and esophagogastritis are also common, accounting for approximately 50 percent of acute upper gastrointestinal tract bleeding. The presentation of variceal hemorrhage is often dramatic. Initial management includes airway protection and hemodynamic stabilization. Large-bore IV access is secured and fluid resuscitation begun. Blood remains the best volume replacement, and fresh-frozen plasma and cryoprecipitate are often indicated to manage coagulopathy. Because of the often tenuous hemodynamic status of patients with ESLD, resuscitation is best carried out in an intensive care setting with access to invasive hemodynamic monitoring.

Optimal management of variceal hemorrhage is controversial. In many centers endoscopic sclerotherapy is used acutely, and success rates of 70 to 90 percent are reported. Intravenous vasopressin is often recommended as a temporizing measure, though its efficacy remains unproven. Vasopressin decreases splanchnic blood flow and hepatic portal blood pressure, which in theory diminishes variceal bleeding. Bolus therapy consists of diluting 20 U of vasopressin in 100 mL of 5% dextrose in water and administration over 10 to 15 min. Boluses can be repeated three to four times at 2- to 4-h intervals. Alternatively, a continuous infusion at 0.3 to 0.9 U/min can be used. A potential complication of vasopressin is compromise of the coronary circulation in the presence of coronary artery disease. Balloon tamponade is an additional emergency therapy for documented hemorrhage from gastroesophageal varices. Use of the Sengstaken-Blakemore tube requires a degree of experience and careful monitoring. The main immediate complications of this therapy are airway compromise and aspiration. Prophylactic intubation should be performed prior to the use of balloon tamponade.

Hepatic or portosystemic encephalopathy is a frequently encountered complication of ESLD. This condition represents the metabolic and neurologic consequence of the splanchnic circulation effectively bypassing the liver. Oversimplifying, a variety of neuroactive metabolites from the intestine accumulate in the systemic circulation and adversely affect central nervous system (CNS) function. These substances include ammonia, mercaptans, short-chain free fatty acids, and a number of amino acid products that act as "false" neurotransmitters, as well as the neuroinhibitory substance γ-aminobutyric acid (GABA). The resultant encephalopathy is characterized as a reversible, episodic disturbance of mentation, consciousness, and motor function. Asterixis, or hepatic flap, is an early motor manifestation that appears as an involuntary jerking recovery of an extremity held actively in a posture. Typically asterixis is elicited by requesting the patient to hold his or her hands outward and fully extended at the wrists. Recognition of new or worsening encephalopathy is important because there is often an acute underlying process that has caused the altered CNS function. Common precipitants include infection, gastrointestinal bleeding, volume depletion and dehydration, electrolyte disturbances, and medication side effects. Medications normally metabolized by the liver, such as narcotics and benzodiazepines, can have an exaggerated and prolonged effect. Management of hepatic encephalopathy depends on dietary protein restriction and the elimination of toxic substance accumulation in the gut. The antibiotic neomycin, taken orally as 1 g qid, decreases intestinal bacteria number and reduces toxic substances generated by bacterial protein degradation. Use of neomycin is sometimes limited by oto- and nephrotoxicity. The cathartic lactulose traps ammonia within the lumen of the gut by decreasing intestinal pH and stimulates bacterial uptake of ammonia into fixed bacterial proteins. A dose of 50 mL is given orally every hour until the bowels move and then the dose is titrated to promote two to three stools daily.

## TRANSPLANT PROCEDURE

The liver transplantation can be divided into three phases: preoperative, operative, and postoperative. The preoperative phase involves organ harvest from donor and preparation of recipient. The operative phase is also divided into three parts: the procurement, the anhepatic, and biliary reconstruction phases.

The preoperative phase is typically short as the procedure is dependent on donor availability. Most patients undergo bilateral subcostal incision with upper midline extension to the xiphoid process. The donor liver is placed in the recipient after venovenous bypass (used in most centers). Vessels undergo reanastomosis in the following order: suprahepatic vena cava, partial infrahepatic vena cava, and hepatic artery followed by portal vein. The partially closed infrahepatic vena cava is closed after the liver is perfused to allow air, acidotic, hyperkalemic blood and preservation fluid to wash out. Normal color and consistency return to the organ in approximately 15 min.

The postanhepatic phase completes the transplant with anastomosis/reconstruction of the biliary system. If the recipient's system allows, the preferred method for reconstruction is an end-to-end choledochocholedochostomy (Fig. 89-1). The use of a T-tube biliary drain varies by center. If the anatomy does not allow choledochocholedochostomy, the patient undergoes Roux-en-Y hepaticojejunostomy.

Typically, the donor liver takes the place of the diseased liver (orthotopic). Occasionally, the donor liver is placed in the right paravertebral gutter (heterotopic).

## POSTOPERATIVE COMPLICATIONS

### Immediate

The immediate postoperative period is complicated by the postoperative complications expected with an operation of this technical difficulty and magnitude. Hemorrhage and infection (both intraabdominal and within the wound) occur. Fifteen percent of patients require exploratory laparotomy for postoperative bleeding, and although exploration improves survival, a source is identified in only 50 percent of these patients. Patients with significant bleeding frequently require transfusion and correction of their coagulopathy before exploration and evacuation of hematoma.

### Acute Nonfunction/Cholestasis

Approximately 5 to 10 percent of all patients develop primary nonfunction of the allograft, which is felt to be associated with preservation damage prior to transplantation but may be immunologically mediated. Liver function tests quickly rise to between 5 and 10,000, and there is little or no bile production. By definition, acute nonfunction occurs both within 96 h after the operation and with a patent hepatic artery and portal vein. It also has three of the following four features: (1) bile output is less than 20 mL in 12 h; (2) the bilirubin becomes greater than 10 mg/dL or rises more than 5 mg/dL; (3) PT/PTT (partial thromboplastin time) ratio is greater than or equal to 1.5; and (4) factors V and VIII are less than 25 percent of normal. Fifteen percent of patients develop "nonspecific cholestasis syndrome," or "delayed function," which is defined as a progressive rise in serum bilirubin past the third postoperative day without any identifiable cause. The cause is generally felt to be the result of ischemic injury to the liver in the course of harvest and preservation. It is analogous to acute tubular necrosis in kidneys. General synthetic function is preserved, but no bile is produced. Serum bilirubin may rise to greater than 30 mg/dL over a 2- to 3-week period. Biopsy distinguishes this syndrome from rejection.

### Bile Leak/Obstruction/Stricture

Biliary complications account for significant postoperative morbidity. The incidence of obstruction or stricture ranges from 10 to 30 percent. Biliary obstruction is heralded by three typical presentations. The most common is intermittent episodes of fever and fluctuating liver function tests. The second presentation is a gradual worsening

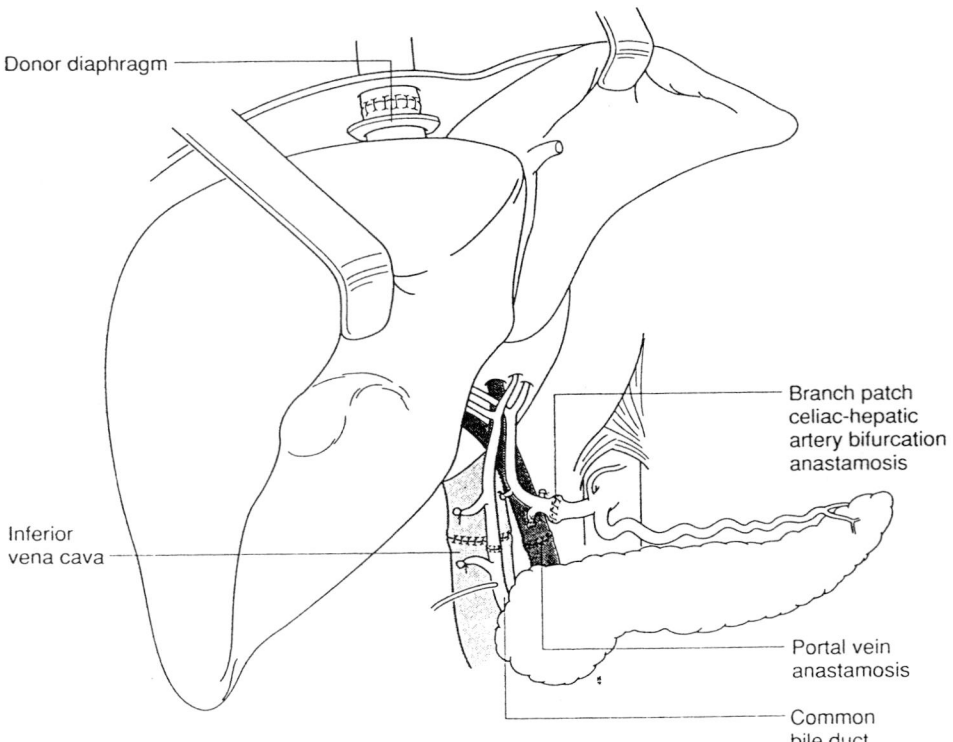

Donor diaphragm

Inferior vena cava

Branch patch celiac-hepatic artery bifurcation anastamosis

Portal vein anastamosis

Common bile duct

**Fig. 89-1.** End-to-end choledochocholedochostomy. If the recipient's system permits, this is the preferred method for reconstruction of the biliary system, the last part of the operative phase in liver transplantation.

of liver function tests without symptoms. Finally, obstruction may present as acute bacterial cholangitis with fever, chills, abdominal pain, jaundice, and bacteremia. The presentation can be difficult to distinguish clinically from rejection, hepatic artery thrombosis, cytomegalovirus (CMV) infection, or a recurrence of a preexisting disease (especially hepatitis).

Mortality is 5 to 20 percent, depending on the series and the center. The most common site of obstruction is at the site of the anastomosis at the level of the choledochocholedochostomy. Obstruction is generally secondary to some technical feature or kinking or more likely is due to ischemia, as the blood supply to and around the anastomosis comes solely from the hepatic artery. A patient with hepatic artery thrombosis is at significant risk for obstruction or leak. Any stricture/obstruction/leak should therefore prompt an evaluation of the patency of the hepatic artery. There are other factors that influence the rate of biliary complications. After transplant, there is a change in bile composition that may promote the formation of sludge or stones. Also, the presence of the T-tube postoperatively may serve as a foreign body, promoting bacterial colonization, or as the focus for the deposition of biliary sludge.

Nonanastomotic strictures have been associated with hepatic artery thrombosis as well as with chronic ductopenic rejection, extended graft preservation times, and the use of ABO-incompatible grafts. These strictures tend to be intrahepatic and develop over several months. Extrinsic processes such as a mucocele within the donor cystic remnant or loculated collections of blood, bile, or ascites can compromise the biliary tree and cause obstruction. Other sources of obstruction include papillary dysfunction or ampullary stenosis. Primary sclerosing cholangitis may recur. Depending on the etiology, temporary relief may be provided with balloon dilatation and placement of a stent. If multiple strictures are seen without the presence of vascular compromise, ischemic preservation injury is generally responsible, especially cold ischemic times greater than 13 h.

When a biliary complication is suspected, all patients should have a complete blood count (CBC) with platelet count and differential; serum chemistries including liver function tests as well as amylase and lipase levels; cultures of blood, urine, bile, and ascites, if present; chest x-ray; and abdominal ultrasound. Diagnosis begins with abdominal ultrasound with Doppler flow studies. Ultrasound rules out the presence of fluid collections, screens for the presence of thrombosis of the hepatic artery or portal vein, and identifies any dilatation of the biliary tree. On ultrasound, however, the intrahepatic ductal system rarely appears dilated appreciably, even in the presence of complete obstruction. Patients often require cholangiography for complete evaluation. Those patients with a choledochocholedochostomy are best served by endoscopic retrograde cholangeopancreatography (ERCP) because it permits both a radiographic diagnosis and the potential for nonoperative intervention. Patients who have Roux-en-Y hepaticojejunostomy or those who cannot have ERCP must have percutaneous cholangiography.

Initial episodes of obstruction may be treated with balloon dilatation, with a catheter or nasobiliary drain left in place for 48 h. All patients should receive broad-spectrum antibiotics against gram-negative and -positive enteric organisms. Early recurrences (<6 months) of a stricture may be treated with repeat balloon dilatation and stent placement. Late recurrence (>6 months) are typically treated as an initial occurrence. Surgical revision is required for those patients with strictures that are not accessible to a stent or a balloon or who have recurrent sepsis. The surgical revision for patients with a choledochocholedochostomy is generally conversion to a choledochojejunostomy. Extrinsic causes for compressive stricture are best treated by removing the inciting cause.

The most common late biliary complication is cholestasis due to the deposition of sludge. Ursodeoxycholic acid may help by increasing the solubility. Ampullary stenosis or dysfunction may be present and may respond to endoscopic sphincterotomy.

Biliary leakage is associated with a 50 percent mortality. It occurs most frequently in the third or fourth postoperative week. The high mortality may be related to the high incidence of concomitant hepatic artery thrombosis, infection of leaked bile, or the difficulty of bile repair in an area where the tissue is inflamed. Bile leak may also occur after the removal of the T-tube, which typically takes place 3 to 6 months after surgery. Immunosuppression may prevent scarring of the tract. Early bile leakage is generally more dangerous than late bile leak and requires surgical revision. Most late bile leaks are associated with removal of the T-tube and resolve spontaneously. Late bile leaks are treated with hospitalization, intravenous antibiotics, and, on occasion, placement of a biliary stent, which is inserted in a retrograde fashion into the common duct endoscopically. Patients most often present with peritoneal signs and fever, but these signs may be masked due to concomitant use of steroids and immunosuppressive agents.

## Vascular Complications

Vascular complications are rare but are associated with high morbidity, mortality, and graft failure. Hepatic artery thrombosis is the most common vascular complication. The incidence reported is between 5 and 40 percent and tends to be higher in pediatric patients. Children are usually treated with aspirin prophylactically. Contributors include technical factors at the time of operation, size of the hepatic artery (less than 3 mm), flow rate of arterial blood past the anastomosis, and the presence of a hypercoagulable state, including poor endogenous production of naturally occurring anticoagulants or the rapid increase in production of factors V and VIII after transplantation. If it occurs, thrombosis of the artery is frequently within the first 3 postoperative weeks. The incidence increases in patients with a complex interposition graft and in those who require intraoperative revision of the anastomosis.

The presentation is signalled by elevated PT and transaminase levels and little or no bile production, but this complication may also present as acute graft failure, liver abscess, unexplained sepsis, or as a biliary tract problem (leak, obstruction, abscess, or breakdown of the anastomosis). Hepatic artery thrombosis is ominous, and treatment typically requires retransplantation. Untreated, it can lead to acute hepatic encephalopathy, hemorrhage-associated coagulopathy, or progressive multiorgan failure. Occasionally, if diagnosed early, immediate thrombectomy and revision of the anastomosis may preclude need for retransplantation. Pediatric patients have a much more varied presentation, ranging from no symptoms to focal intraparenchymal abscess to isolated bile leak to fulminant failure.

Duplex ultrasonography (Doppler ultrasound with real-time scanning) has a sensitivity of 92 percent.

Portal vein thrombosis is less common and affects 2 to 3 percent of patients. Factors that predispose to thrombosis are the size of the native portal vein and the rate of flow through the anastomosis. One factor that may decrease flow through the anastomosis is the formation of collaterals. The presence of a splenorenal shunt will decrease flow; such shunts are usually interrupted at the time of operation. The diagnosis is suggested by variceal hemorrhage or other signs of portal hypertension. Initially, an attempt is made at treating the complication, but retransplantation may be required.

Thrombosis of the vena cava is rare and occurs in fewer than 1 percent of patients. The low incidence is due to the large diameter of the vessel. When present it is most likely due to technical problems at the site of the anastomosis. It typically presents with bilateral lower extremity edema or genital swelling. The diagnosis is made by physical examination, duplex sonography, and phlebography of the inferior vena cava. Treatment is anticoagulation. If the thrombosis is infrahepatic, an attempt may be made at balloon angioplasty. Hepatic vein thrombosis is also rare but may occur in the patient with preexisting Budd-Chiari syndrome.

## Intraabdominal Sepsis

Intraabdominal sepsis is seen in 5 percent of patients. It commonly presents with diffuse peritonitis and stems from localized abscess, infection of ascitic fluid, leakage of infected bile, or leakage of enteric contents. Abscesses are found in the area of the transplant graft but can be seen between loops of bowel. Mortality with intraabdominal sepsis is high (60 percent). Surgical drainage is preferred, but percutaneous techniques are often attempted in view of the frailty and the immunosuppression in this population.

## REJECTION

Allograft rejection occurs in two somewhat discrete syndromes: acute and chronic. Acute allograft rejection may become evident within 2 to 3 days after transplantation but is most commonly seen at 7 to 14 days. The frequency of acute rejection varies from 40 to 80 percent, often depending on the effectiveness of preoperative immunosuppression induction. After several months the incidence of acute rejection decreases steadily, but it may be triggered at any time by tapering of immunosuppressive agents. Though frequently subtle in presentation, a syndrome of acute rejection includes fever, liver tenderness, lymphocytosis, eosinophilia, liver enzyme elevation, and a change in bile color or production. In the perioperative period the differential diagnosis must include infection, acute biliary obstruction, or vascular insufficiency. The diagnosis can be made with certainty only by hepatic ultrasound and biopsy, which usually requires referral back to the transplant center for management and follow-up. Acute rejection is managed primarily by high-dose glucocorticoid bolus followed by a rapid taper over 5 to 7 days. Secondary therapy includes the infusion of antilymphocyte globulin ($OKT_3$), which is accompanied by a variety of potential side effects best managed at an experienced transplant center.

Chronic allograft rejection occurs in approximately 5 percent of cases and is the major cause of late graft failure. The primary manifestation of chronic rejection is persistently abnormal liver function tests and an indolent, but progressive, increase in bilirubin secondary to cholestasis. Significant loss of hepatic synthetic function is often not evident until late in the course of rejection. The diagnosis is made by biopsy, which characteristically shows mononuclear portal inflammation, arteriopathy, centrilobular cholestasis, and a decrease in interlobular bile ducts.

## INFECTION

### General Considerations

The vast majority of liver transplantation patients have at least one episode of infection at some time after their transplantation, and many have more than one episode. Infections or their complications are said to account for 88 percent of deaths. The greatest risk to the patient appears to be in the first 2 months. The types of infection seen in the first 4 weeks and the second 4 weeks vary. After the first 6 months the rate of infection decreases, but due to the patient's heavily immunocompromised state, vigilance for infection must be continued. There are many challenges to the diagnosis of infection in the posttransplant patient. One notable challenge is that illness secondary to infection may be insidious or subtle and may not present until it is life-threatening. The operation is a technically difficult one and predisposes the patient to infection, particularly in the immediate postoperative period. Many of the drugs that the patient is required to take are either toxic and cause fever, making infection seem likely, or modulate the immune system and mask signs of infection. Finally, rejection may resemble infection, but misdiagnosis is disastrous.

During the first postoperative month, intraabdominal infections, including cholangitis, peritonitis, and liver and other intraabdominal abscesses, predominate. Presentation is marked by fever, abdominal pain and distension, ascites, and occasionally jaundice. Work-up should include CBC with differential, liver function tests, urinalysis, chest x-ray, abdominal ultrasound, and blood and fluid cultures. If there are headaches, seizures, mental status changes, or localizing signs, the patient should undergo CT scan of the head and lumbar puncture if no clear etiology is seen on CT scan. Evaluation may include ultrasound, CT scan, T-tube cholangiography, ERCP, liver biopsy, and cultures of blood, urine, or aspirated fluid. Other advanced tests used to localize infection include gallium and indium scans and bone marrow biopsy for culture (especially for *Mycobacterium tuberculosis* and fungi). The organisms responsible tend to be enterococci, gram-negative aerobes, anaerobes, *Staphylococcus aureus,* coagulase-negative staphylococci, and *Candida* species. Patient may also present with pneumonia or urinary tract infection related to intubation or indwelling bladder catheterization while hospitalized. Typically, cultures should be held for fungi, viruses, CMV, *Nocardia* sp., and *M. tuberculosis.* Shell vial cultures should be obtained if there is any suspicion of CMV disease.

The first month tends to be overshadowed with reactivation of preexisting infection (hepatitis) and CMV and bacterial infection. Bacterial infection is frequently associated with the vascular or biliary anastomosis, especially hepatic artery thrombosis, but also portal vein thrombosis. Ischemia may lead to bile leak and abscess or deep soft tissue infection. Offending agents are enterococci, gram-negative coliforms, anaerobes, and *Candida* species. Gut flora often reflux into the biliary system and lead to colonization, which is usually not a problem unless bile leak or obstruction occurs.

After the first month, the incidence of bacterial infections decreases and the incidence of opportunistic infection increases, but the consideration for bacterial illness should remain high. Community-acquired pneumonia is most likely due to *Strep. pneumoniae* and *Haemophilus influenzae.* Meningitis shows a high preponderance of *Listeria monocytogenes* as well as *Strep. pneumoniae, Staph.* aureus, and gram-negative bacilli. Viral infection peaks in the second month. Protozoal infection increases for several months.

### Fungal Infections

The incidence of fungal infection is not high, but the majority occur in the first 2 months after transplant. The incidence of fungal disease is continuing to decrease, but mortality remains high. *Candida* species are responsible for up to 75 percent of fungal illnesses. The diagnosis is by culture or biopsy, and the fungus may be difficult to isolate. Disseminated infection is present when infection is found in two or more sites and is associated with even higher mortality. Viral and bacterial illness are often seen concurrently. The second most common fungal illness is aspergillosis, which has a mortality of 75 percent. Infection occurs by inhalation of spores. The primary site of infection is the lungs, but the fungus may affect multiple organs. It has a propensity for vascular invasion and tissue erosion, which may lead to localized necrosis, infarction, or hemorrhage, predisposing the organism to dissemination. Other fungal illnesses seen are mucormycosis, cryptococcosis, (in CNS and lungs), histoplasmosis, and coccidioidomycosis.

### Viral Infections

Viral illnesses tend to present within the first few months. The most common agent, and the most common cause of infection after transplantation, is cytomegalovirus (CMV), a herpes virus. It is reported to occur in between 23 and 85 percent of all liver transplant patients. Despite its high incidence and morbidity, it rarely is fatal or has a significant effect on graft survival. It generally occurs within the first 3 months, with the peak incidence in the third and fourth weeks. Later occurrence is generally related to the need to increase immunosuppression for treatment of a prolonged episode of rejection. CMV can cause primary infection, or the infection can be a reactivation. Infection has three basic effects. First, it can produce a mononucleosis-like syndrome with spiking fever, arthralgias, malaise, neutropenia, atypical lymphocytes, thrombocytopenia with mild or moderate elevation in transaminase levels, and specific organ involvement. Jaundice is rare. Second, CMV is frequently associated with opportunistic infection, which may be due to an additional immunosuppressive effect of its own. Finally, there is an increased propensity for allograft rejection thought to be due to an immunomodulating effect of CMV on class I and II HLA expression.

The patient may present with a pneumonitis that, when present, is characterized by bilateral interstitial infiltrates that may lead to adult respiratory distress syndrome. Diagnosis of CMV pneumonitis may require bronchoalveolar lavage or tissue biopsy, but chest x-ray appearance and the clinical picture may be suggestive enough for diagnosis. CMV pneumonitis may be seen in conjunction with *Pneumocystis carinii* pneumonia. CMV hepatitis may present like rejection, with fever, malaise, anorexia, abdominal pain, hepatomegaly, and liver dysfunction. Liver biopsy is frequently needed for diagnosis but still may not be able to distinguish CMV disease from rejection. Disseminated CMV disease is associated with high mortality. Disseminated disease is frequently associated with an increase in immunosuppression, especially treatment with OKT3.

There are three patterns of infection. The patient at greatest risk is the seronegative recipient of a liver from a seropositive donor. Disease may also be caused by reactivation of latent virus that replicates after the initiation of immunosuppression—typically in the seropositive recipient of a liver from a seronegative donor. Finally, a seropositive recipient may receive a liver from a seropositive donor, which may produce either reactivation or superinfection, although it is clinically impossible and irrelevant to distinguish between them.

Effective treatment depends on rapid diagnosis. Diagnosis has been traditionally based on histology and culture. Standard fibroblast tube cell culture, however, can require 10 to 14 days for incubation. Serologic markers are too insensitive in the immunosuppressed patient, and electron microscopy is cumbersome. The shell vial technique can detect the presence of CMV after 16 h of incubation. It is an indirect immunofluorescence testing method that uses a monoclonal antibody directed at an early antigen of the virus. Early detection and high antigenemia correlate positively with the severity of the infection.

Other viruses may cause illness in the posttransplant patient. Up to 34 percent of all transplant patients develop herpes simplex virus (HSV) infection, and half of these present within the first 3 weeks. Mucocutaneous or genital disease is generally due to reactivation of latent infection. It is generally not severe, and diagnosis can be made with Tzanck smear or viral culture. HSV may also produce esophagitis, colitis, hepatitis, or disseminated disease. Varicella zoster is less common, tends to occur within the first 6 months posttransplant, and is generally self-limited. Diagnosis is by Tzanck smear or culture. Epstein-Barr virus (EBV) can cause primary infection in children or the more common reactivated infection in adults. The disease can be self-limited and cause a mononucleosis-like syndrome with fever, tonsillitis, and lymphadenopathy, or it may progress to a polymorphous multiorgan B-cell infiltrative process with high mortality. Finally, it may produce a localized solid tumor. Adenovirus and enterovirus may cause systemic illness but are uncommon.

Parasites are not common. *P. carinii* pneumonia may present concomitantly with CMV or by itself. Diagnosis may require bronchoalveolar lavage or transbronchial biopsy. Prophylaxis with trimethopim/sulfamethoxazole for the first 3 months has greatly reduced its incidence. *Toxoplasma gondii* is also uncommon but may cause a meningoencephalitis or single or multiple mass lesions. Infection causes fever, mental status changes, focal neurologic findings, seizures, or visual changes.

## Management of Infection

In general, culture and sensitivity results are used to guide antibacterial therapy, but therapy must often be empirically based. For skin and superficial wounds, likely offending organisms are gram-positive cocci, especially *Staph. aureus*, and treatment should be with a penicillinase-resistant penicillin (e.g., nafcillin or oxacillin) or a first-generation cephalosporin (e.g., cefazolin), unless there is a suspicion for methicillin-resistant organisms or sensitivity to β-lactams, in which case vancomycin should be used. Local wound debridement may be necessary. Nosocomial pneumonia is likely due to gram-negative organisms such as *E. coli, Enterobacter* sp., or *Pseudomonas* sp. and should be treated with a broad-spectrum penicillin (e.g., cefoxitin, cefotetan, cefotaxime, ceftriaxone, ceftazidime). Community-acquired pneumonia should be treated as such, with the proviso that opportunistic infection may also be present. Intraabdominal infection may be due to enterococci, gram-negative bacilli, or anaerobes. Triple coverage may be necessary empirically, with ampicillin or vancomycin plus an aminoglycoside to treat enterococci; a broad-spectrum penicillin or second- or third-generation cephalosporin to treat gram-negative organisms; and piperacillin, cefoxitin, cefotetan, clindamycin, or metronidazole to treat anaerobes. Penicillins with β-lactamase inhibitors (e.g., sulbactam and clavulanic acid) have broad coverage against gram-positive cocci, gram-negative bacilli, and anaerobes. Meningitis is frequently due to *L. monocytogenes,* and patients with suspected meningitis should be treated with a third-generation cephalosporin and ampicillin.

The mainstay of fungal treatment has been on amphotericin B. Complications of treatment include local irritation, fever, nausea, rigors, and nephrotoxicity. Oral azole agents may be used for superficial infection or maintenance of treatment after a course of amphotericin B.

Viral therapy depends on the disease syndrome and the offending agent. CMV disease is treated with ganciclovir (a nucleoside analogue), which is only available intravenously. Mean duration of treatment is 16 days, with a dose of 5 mg/kg IV bid, adjusting the dose for renal insufficiency. Its toxic effects include reversible neutropenia in 25 to 67 percent, skin rashes, anemia, thrombocytopenia, liver dysfunction, and mild CNS effects. Foscarnet has been used but causes considerable nephrotoxicity. Varicella and HSV disease are typically treated with acyclovir, which has renal excretion, and the dose must be adjusted for renal insufficiency. Acyclovir is generally nontoxic but may cause nephrotoxicity at high doses or CNS effects (delirium, tremors, or EEG changes). EBV is typically treated with a reduction in the immunosuppression regimen.

Treatment of choice for *P. carinii* pneumonia is co-trimoxazole, with pentamidine reserved as an alternative therapy if co-trimoxazole is not tolerated. Toxoplasmosis is treated with pyrimethamine and sulfadiazine or clindamycin.

## COMPLICATIONS OF IMMUNOSUPPRESSIVE AGENTS

Therapeutic immunosuppression is accompanied by a number of side effects and complications. Common and most life-threatening are the variety of infections that occur with the suppression of cell-mediated immunity. The agents of immunosuppression also have a number of nonspecific toxicities that complicate their use. Combined toxicities can produce or worsen preexisting renal insufficientcy, hypertension, and hyperglycemia. Hypertension is perhaps the best example of combined toxicity. Elevated cyclosporine levels cause renal arteriolar constriction, reducing glomerular blood flow and stimulating the renin-angiotensin system, resulting in elevated blood pressure. Glucocorticoids promote renal salt and water retention, which further aggravate hypertension. A headache syndrome often indistinguishable from migraine is common in transplant recipients and usually develops within the first 2 months of immunosuppression. The important differential diagnosis must include infectious causes and malignancy when headache first presents and usually requires a head CT scan with subsequent biochemical analysis of cerebrospinal fluid.

*Azathioprine* interferes with purine synthesis and metabolism, which in turn inhibits RNA and DNA synthesis and function. Both B-cell and T-cell responses to antigenic stimulation become suppressed, which limits the proliferation of effector lymphocyte clones. Generalized myelosuppression is a common side effect resulting in leukopenia and, to varying degrees, thrombocytopenia and anemia (megaloblastic). Other observed toxicities include hepatitis, cholestasis, hepatic vein thrombosis, pancreatitis, dermatitis, and alopecia. Prolonged use also predisposes to malignancies such as squamous cell carcinoma of the skin and lip, cervical carcinoma, and lymphoproliferative disease.

*Glucocorticoids* act primarily by inhibiting T-cell and macrophage function. In addition to immune suppression, long-term use of glucocorticoids suppresses endogenous adrenal function, produces Cushing syndrome, and causes hypertension, glucose intolerance, osteoporosis, avascular necrosis of the hip, cataracts, pancreatitis, peptic ulcer disease, delayed wound healing, behavioral disorders, and malignancies.

*Cyclosporine* and *FK506* interfere with signal transduction in T cells, inhibiting the release of mitogens that stimulate immune cell proliferation. Nephrotoxicity is a common and usually reversible side effect manifested by elevated serum creatinine levels, hypertension, hyperkalemia, hyperurecemia, and gout. Other side effects include headache, hirsutism, gingival hyperplasia, hyperglycemia, hypomagnesemia, hypercholesterolemia, hypertriglyceridemia, hepatotoxicity, and hemolytic-uremic syndrome. Unlike other immunosuppressive agents, blood levels of cyclosporine and FK506 can be monitored along with serum creatinine to avoid serious toxicity.

There are a number of drug-drug interactions that can promote toxicity in transplant recipients. Cyclosporine is metabolized by the cytochrome $P_{450}$ system of the liver. Drugs that induce $P_{450}$ activity can lower circulating cyclosporine levels. Common examples include carbamazepine, nafcillin, phenobarbital, phenytoin, rifampin, valproic acid, and isoniazide. Other drugs decrease $P_{450}$ activity and can potentially increase cyclosporine level into a toxic range. Examples of these drugs include diltiazem, verapamil, erythromycin, ketoconazole, fluconazole, and cimetidine. Commonly prescribed nonsteroidal anti-inflammatory agents inhibit prostaglandin synthesis and should be used with caution in the presence of known renal insufficientcy because of the role of prostaglandins in regulating glomerular blood flow. Cyclosporine and related drugs may increase uric acid levels and precipitate gout. Allopurinol decreases uric acid production and is commonly prescribed as a gout-preventive. However, allopurinol also interferes with the degradation of 6-mercaptopurine, which can greatly potentiate the effects of azathioprine, and the two drugs should not be used together.

## PSYCHIATRIC DISORDERS

Psychiatric problems seen in the liver transplant patient are likely reactive, infectious, or metabolic. Delirium is generally self-limited. Haloperidol is effective for the acute episode. Depression is not uncommon and may accompany a steroid taper. Depression and anxiety can result from emotionally coping with the transplant process or as side effects to medication. Antidepressants have been used with some success.

## INCIDENTAL PROBLEMS

### Immunization

Immunization is important in the transplant patient because the prevention of even a common illness may be life-saving. All live virus or bacterial vaccines (polio, measles, mumps, rubella, yellow fever,

BCG) are contraindicated. Vaccines consisting of denatured protein, carbohydrate, or killed virus are safe (e.g., DPT, which consists of toxoid and inactivated bacteria; inactivated polio; *H. influenzae* Pittman type; and heptavax are all safe).

### Antibiotic Prophylaxis

Invasive procedures involving the graft are invariably preceded by intravenous antibiotic prophylaxis. For procedures that do not involve the graft, the use of prophylactic antibiotics varies by center. The typical regimen is amoxicillin, 3 g PO 1 h prior to the procedure, or clindamycin, 600 mg 1 h prior and 6 h after the procedure. For patients unable to take either antibiotic, erythromycin stearate may be used, 1.5 g PO 1 to 2 h prior and 500 mg 30 min after the procedure, but care must be taken with its use as it can interact with metabolism of cyclosporine and FK506.

### Surgery

Patients who require surgery for problems other than those related to the graft should have them performed. Preoperative evaluation should include tests of coagulation. Immunosuppression should not be stopped, and stress doses of steriods may be required.

### Bone Disease

Skeletal complications have always been responsible for significant morbidity and, because of increased survival times, are becoming more prevalent. Immobility, poor nutritional status, decreased muscle mass, steroids, and immunosuppressive drugs all cause osteopenia and osteonecrosis. The first 3 to 6 months post transplant are accompanied by accelerated bone loss (mostly trabecular). After 6 months, bone mineral density increases for several years, which is thought to be due to the normalization of hepatic function from the cholestatic state. Fractures are common in the first year postoperatively, particularly at sites of trabecular bone (vertebrae and ribs), although long bone and pelvic fractures are also seen. Fractures should be treated in the standard fashion.

### Neurologic Complications

It is reported that between 27 and 90 percent of all liver transplantation patients have a neurologic complication at some time during their posttransplant course. Structural lesions account for a portion of these complications, with noninfectious lesions being more common than infectious ones. Cerebrovascular events such as intracranial hemorrhage, infarction, subarachnoid hemorrhage, and subdural hematoma account for the majority of noninfectious lesions. Greater than 90 percent of these patients have a coexisting coagulopathy, and the median time for occurrence is about 1 month. Only one-third present with focal findings. Most present with seizure or encephalopathy. Other noninfectious structural problems include anoxic-ischemic encephalopathy, central pontine myelinolysis, cyclosporine toxicity, and malignancy. Infectious sources likely to cause a structural problem include *Aspergilla, Candida,* and *Cryptococcus* sp. Besides infection, other nonstructural neurologic complications include heptatic encephalopathy, electrolyte derangements, and drug toxicity.

### BIBLIOGRAPHY

Atterbury CE, Groszmann RJ: Approach to the patient with cirrhosis and portal hypertension, in Kelley WN (ed): *Textbook of Internal Medicine,* 2d ed. Philadelphia, Lippincott, 1992.

Campbell DA Jr, Ham JM, Turcotte JG, et al: Hepatic transplantation, in Greenfield LJ (ed): *Surgery: Scientific Principles and Practice.* Philadelphia, Lippincott, 1993, pp 524–541.

Hay JE: Bone disease in liver transplant recipients. *Gastroenterol Clin North Am* 22(2):337, 1993.

Howard RJ: Infection in the immunocompromised patient. *Surg Clin North Am* 74:609, 1994.

Lake JR: Changing indications for liver transplantation. *Gastroenterol Clin North Am* 22:213, 1993.

Lewis WD, Jenkins RL: Biliary strictures after liver transplantation. *Surg Clin North Am* 74(4):967, 1994.

Neuberger J, Lucey MR (eds): *Liver Transplantation: Practice and Management.* London, BMJ Publishing, 1994.

Ringe B: Quadrennial review of liver transplantation. *Am J Gastroenterol* 89(suppl):18, 1994.

Singh N, Yu VL, Gayowski T: Central nervous system lesions in adult liver transplantation recipients: Clinical review with implications for management. *Medicine* 73(2):110, 1994.

Wiesner RH, Marin E, Porayko MK, et al: Advances in the diagnosis, treatment, and prevention of cytomegalovirus infections after liver transplantation. *Gastroenterol Clin North Am* 22(2):351, 1993.

Zetterman RK: Primary care management of the liver transplant patient. *Am J Med* 96(suppl 1A):10, 1994.

## 90
# EMERGENCY RENAL PROBLEMS
### K. Venkateswara Rao

In the discipline of nephrology, there are many clinical disorders that require emergency medical care. They include acute renal failure, hyperkalemia, metabolic acidosis, metabolic alkalosis, hyponatremia, hypertonic dehydration, hypercalcemia, hypophosphatemia, renal stone disease, and accelerated or malignant hypertension. In addition, as patients with end-stage renal failure are currently kept alive with dialysis and renal transplantation, problems peculiar to such patients are also encountered in the emergency department. Problems included under the latter category are clotting or infection of the vascular access, pulmonary edema, uremic encephalopathy, pericarditis, cardiac arrhythmias, coronary ischemia, gastrointestinal bleeding, peritonitis, and allograft dysfunction.

Discussion in this chapter will be limited to acute renal failure and rapidly progressive glomerulonephritis. Problems associated with chronic dialysis are discussed in Chap. 94.

## ACUTE RENAL FAILURE

*Acute renal failure* is a constellation of clinical findings associated with sudden impairment in renal function leading to excessive accumulation of nitrogenous waste products in the serum. Depending on the amount of urine produced in a 24-h period, acute renal failure is classified as (1) oliguric form (< 500 mL) and (2) nonoliguric form (> 500 mL).

### Etiology

The causes of acute renal failure can be broadly divided into (1) prerenal, (2) renal, and (3) postrenal. Table 90-1 lists some of the causes of acute renal failure under the three categories.

### Differential Diagnosis

The history and physical examination may provide important clues as to the etiology of acute renal failure. A history of acute abdominal pain with nausea and vomiting may point toward a prerenal cause, while oliguria associated with suprapubic discomfort and increased area of dullness by percussion over the bladder area suggest obstructive uropathy.

The diagnostic studies listed in Table 90-2 can be completed within an hour or two of the patient's arrival in the emergency department and require only a small amount of urine for analysis. They are innocuous and pose no danger to the patient's health. An intravenous pyelogram, renal angiography, and kidney biopsy may provide additional diagnostic information but are invasive and can cause significant morbidity. Therefore, they are not used routinely in the evaluation of acute renal failure and should be reserved for specific situations only.

## Management

### Postrenal Failure

In patients with a postrenal cause of acute renal failure, an appropriate channel for urinary drainage should be established. The exact procedure employed may vary depending on the level of obstruction. For example, a Foley catheter may be adequate for obstruction arising from a benign prostatic hypertrophy, whereas a percutaneous nephrostomy tube is required for ureteral occlusion. Once the patient's medical status is optimized, definitive surgery for the correction of the obstructive lesion should be considered.

For the patient with acute anuria, obstruction is the major consideration. If no urine is obtained after proper urethral catheterization, ultrasonography and urologic consultation should be obtained on an emergency basis.

### Prerenal Failure

In those patients in whom a prerenal cause is suspected, every effort should be made to restore the effective intravascular volume. In states of volume depletion, isotonic fluids (normal saline, plasma, or Ringer's solution) should be administered at a rapid rate. When cardiac failure is contributing to prerenal azotemia, the intravascular volume should be reduced to enhance cardiac performance. Surgical correction of the underlying problem (e.g., segmental bowel resection for infarction, peritoneovenous shunt for massive ascites, valve replacement for left ventricular outflow tract obstruction, pericardiectomy for constrictive pericarditis) should be considered when the patient's medical status is stable.

### Renal Failure

Acute tubular necrosis (ATN) resulting from an ischemic injury or a nephrotoxic agent (i.e., rhabdomyolysis) is the most common cause of intrinsic renal failure. Other parenchymal diseases such as acute glomerulonephritis or allergic interstitial nephritis are less frequent causes. The history, physical examination, and simple laboratory tests may provide useful clues in distinguishing one form of intrinsic renal disease from another. The acute onset of oliguria, hypertension, pulmonary edema, and a telescopic urine sediment (red cells, white cells, protein, red blood cell casts) would suggest glomerulonephritis as the primary cause of acute renal failure. In these situations, the physician should avoid the use of nephrotoxic agents such as aminoglycosides or nonsteroidal anti-inflammatory agents, which are potentially toxic. Azotemia can be managed with dialysis until the patient regains adequate renal function.

The principles of management of patients with established renal failure are discussed in the following paragraphs.

#### Diet

The diet should be high in calories (3000 to 4000), low in protein (40 to 60 g), low in sodium (2 to 3 g), and low in potassium (60 to 80 mEq). Fluids should be restricted to 500 mL + urine output. In patients who cannot eat, sufficient caloric intake should be ensured with tube feeding. If the gastrointestinal tract is not functioning, the food calories should be provided by intravenous hyperalimentation. Adequate calorie intake will prevent tissue breakdown and minimize the daily rise in serum urea nitrogen level.

**Table 90-1.** Causes of Acute Renal Failure

| Prerenal | Renal | Postrenal |
|---|---|---|
| Reduction in cardiac output | Vascular | Lower urinary tract |
|   Congestive heart failure |   Thrombosis of renal vasculature |   Phimosis |
|   Acute pulmonary edema |   Systemic vascular disorders [thrombotic thrombocytopenic |   Meatal stenosis |
|   Valvular heart disease |     purpura (TTP), disseminated intravascular coagulation | Urethral stricture |
|   Myocardial dysfunction |     (DIC), scleroderma, malignant hypertension, etc.] |   Blood clots |
|   Pericardial tamponade |   Preferential reduction in renal cortical blood flow (e.g., |   Stones |
| Hypovolemia |     nonsteroidal anti-inflammatory drugs) |   Bladder tumors |
|   Fluid loss from skin, kidney, GI tract, or | Glomerular |   Prostatic hypertrophy |
|     hemorrhage |   Primary glomerular diseases (e.g., rapidly progressive |   Cancer of prostate |
|   Redistribution of intravascular fluids, as |     glomerulonephritis, poststreptococcal nephritis) |   Neurogenic bladder |
|     in peritonitis, pancreatitis, hepatic fail- |   Glomerular involvement in systemic disease (e.g., lupus | Upper urinary tract (usually re- |
|     ure, anaphylaxis, and septic shock |     erythematosus, bacterial endocarditis, systemic vasculitis) |   quires bilateral involvement) |
| | Tubulointerstitial |   Papillary necrosis |
| |   Ischemic acute tubular necrosis |   Calculi |
| |   Toxic tubular damage from antibiotics, pigments, |   Tumors (intrinsic or |
| |     radiographic dyes, anesthetics, and other chemicals |     extrinsic) |
| |   Drug-induced allergic interstitial nephritis (e.g., sulfonamides, |   Retroperitoneal fibrosis |
| |     penicillin, allopurinol) | |
| |   Intraparenchymal obstructive lesions (e.g., myeloma kidney, | |
| |     acute uric acid nephropathy, ethylene glycol poisoning) | |

**Table 90-2.** Laboratory Studies Aiding in the Differential Diagnosis of Acute Renal Failure

| Test Employed | Prerenal | Renal | Postrenal |
|---|---|---|---|
| Urine sodium (mEq/L) | <20 | >40 | >40 |
| $FE_{Na}(\%)$* | <1 | >2 | >2 |
| Renal failure index† | <1 | >2 | >2 |
| Urine osmolality (mosm/L) | >500 | <300 | <400 |
| Urine/serum creatinine ratio | >40: 1 | <20:1 | <20:1 |
| Serum urea nitrogen/creatinine ratio | >20: 1 | ≈10:1 | <10:1 |
| Kidney size by ultrasonic exam | Normal | Normal | May be increased |
| Radionuclide scan | Poor uptake, delayed<br>  excretion | Good uptake but marked delay<br>  in excretion | Good uptake but minimal<br>  or no excretion |

* Fractional excretion of sodium $(\%) = \dfrac{\text{urine sodium/serum sodium}}{\text{urine creatinine/serum creatinine}} \times 100$

† Renal failure index $= \dfrac{\text{urine sodium}}{\text{urine creatinine/serum creatinine}} \times 100$

### Diuretics

The benefit of diuretics in the management of established acute renal failure is limited, although in a rare instance they may augment diuresis and thus convert an oliguric form of renal failure into a nonoliguric form. Hyperoncotic solutions, such as mannitol, may cause an acute rise in blood volume in an oliguric patient and lead to massive pulmonary edema. One should be aware that rapid infusion of large doses of furosemide may cause ototoxicity. These drugs should be used with extreme caution in patients with intrinsic renal failure.

### Dialysis

Both hemodialysis and peritoneal dialysis are effective in supporting the patient with renal failure until the kidneys regain their function. The choice of hemodialysis or peritoneal dialysis is made on an individual basis, considering the available facilities, hemodynamic stability, and the status of the patient's abdomen. In recent years, slow, continuous hemofiltration and hemodialysis have been tried in patients with hemodynamic instability resulting from cardiogenic or septic shock.

Intermittent dialysis aids in the removal of nitrogenous waste products and excess fluid volume and will improve the patient's blood pressure. Dialysis also helps in the correction of metabolic acidosis and hyperkalemia, which, if untreated, can lead to cardiac instability and death. Most patients with acute renal failure require 3 to 4 h of hemodialysis every other day.

### Drugs

Dopamine in low concentrations (1 to 3 μg/kg per min) may improve renal cortical blood flow and is frequently used in the early phase of acute renal failure. At 4 to 6 μg/kg per min, dopamine begins to exert a β-adrenergic effect, increasing the heart rate and contractility. Other drugs that are renally excreted (e.g., digoxin, magnesium compounds, sedatives, and narcotic analgesics) should be used with caution. The usual therapeutic doses of such drugs may cause serious side effects as they can accumulate in excess concentration.

### Other Measures

Procedures that disrupt the host defense barriers (skin and mucosa) should be avoided if possible to prevent the risk of microbial infection. In situations where prolonged urinary drainage or intravenous infusion is required, changing the catheters and infusion devices every 4 or 5 days may reduce the chance of infection. Extrarenal complications developing in the setting of acute renal failure, such as sepsis, GI bleeding, and pericardial tamponade, should be anticipated and promptly treated.

## Prognosis

Prognosis primarily depends on the cause. Recovery can be expected in most instances of prerenal and postrenal acute renal failure. Of the patients suffering from intrinsic renal failure, a majority of those with toxin-induced acute renal failure (aminoglycosides, radiographic contrast agents, myoglobinuria) should regain renal function. However, the prognosis is poor in patients with posttraumatic and postsurgical acute tubular necrosis. Elderly patients with involvement of multiple organ systems have a poor outcome compared to young individuals who were healthy before the onset of acute renal failure. Most patients regain renal function within 2 to 3 weeks following the acute insult; however, rare cases have been reported in which recovery occurred after a lag of 6 months.

## Prevention

At the present time, 60 to 70 percent of patients with established acute renal failure die during the course of the illness. Therefore, every effort should be made to prevent the development of renal failure. Such measures include identification of high-risk patients, avoidance of nephrotoxic agents, and adequate hydration with intravenous fluids prior to angiographic studies and major surgical procedures. Among the high-risk patients are older individuals (60 years old and above), those undergoing cardiovascular or gastrointestinal operations, and those developing acute renal failure in association with multiorgan dysfunction or a systemic disease such as diabetes, lupus, or scleroderma. Expansion of intravascular volume with the use of crystalloid or colloidal solutions before, during, and after a major surgical procedure has reduced the incidence of ischemic ATN in the perioperative period.

## RAPIDLY PROGRESSIVE GLOMERULONEPHRITIS

Rapidly progressive glomerulonephritis (RPGN) is a syndrome with the following clinical features: (1) inflammation of the glomeruli, usually manifest by hematuria with or without red cell casts in the urine; (2) rapid decline in renal function leading to azotemia; (3) oliguria or anuria (a frequent finding); and (4) massive proteinuria, edema, and hypertension (may be absent in some patients). Histologically, this entity is characterized by circumferential crescents involving more than 50 percent of the glomeruli in the renal biopsy specimen. The exact cause of the crescent formation (i.e., parietal epithelial cell proliferation of Bowman's capsule) is unclear, although an immunologic basis due to the presence of antiglomerular basement membrane (anti-GBM) antibodies and circulating immune complexes has been proposed in the pathogenesis of this disorder. The term *Goodpasture syndrome* is used when the rapidly progressive anti-GBM glomerulonephritis is preceded by pulmonary hemorrhage and clinical hemoptysis. On occasion, acute poststreptococcal glomerulonephritis, IgA nephropathy, mesangiocapillary glomerulonephritis, and systemic vasculitis may present with clinical and histologic features similar to those of idiopathic RPGN.

The differential diagnosis of RPGN with glomerular inflammation includes (1) lupus nephritis, (2) polyarteritis nodosa, (3) hypersensitivity angiitis, (4) Wegener granulomatosis, (5) anaphylactoid purpura, (6) scleroderma renal disease, (7) thrombotic thrombocytopenic purpura, (8) hemolytic uremic syndrome, and (9) malignant hypertension. Most of these disorders can be diagnosed on the basis of the patient's history, physical findings, and routine laboratory studies (peripheral blood smear, platelet count, chest x-ray, etc.) and, ultimately, the renal biopsy.

The principles of therapy are similar to those employed in other settings of acute renal failure. Once the patient's clinical status is stable, a renal biopsy should be performed. The specific therapy is directed at the cause. Most patients with crescentic poststreptococcal glomerulonephritis recover their renal function spontaneously within a few weeks. Plasmapheresis in conjunction with immunosuppressive drug treatment was shown to be beneficial in some patients with anti-GBM nephritis and Goodpasture syndrome. Isolated case reports have appeared in the literature documenting the resolution of idiopathic RPGN following massive doses of intravenous steroids.

In idiopathic RPGN, despite the available treatment protocols and other supportive measures, the prognosis for survival and recovery of renal function remains poor. Sepsis is the leading cause of death in those patients who are treated aggressively with plasmapheresis and cytotoxic agents. Despite the initial improvement in clinical and radiologic findings, approximately 50 percent of patients receiving the cytotoxic agents die from sepsis in the second or third week. Those who survived but lost their renal function have tolerated the dialysis well, and many of them have subsequently received renal transplants. Recurrence of RPGN in the renal allografts is extremely rare.

## BIBLIOGRAPHY

Agmon Y, Brezis M: Acute renal failure: A multifactorial syndrome: Pathogenesis and prevention strategies. *Contrib Nephrol* 102:23, 1993.

Chow SL, Lins RL, Daeleman Sr, et al: Outcome in acute renal failure. *Nephrol Dial Transplant* 8:101, 1993.

Corwin HL, Bonventre JV: Acute renal failure. *Med Clin North Am* 70:1037, 1986.

Kihara M, Ikeda Y, Shibata K, et al: Slow hemodialysis performed during the day in managing renal failure in critically ill patients. *Nephron* 67:36,1994.

Miller TR, Anderson RJ, Linas SL, et al: Urinary diagnostic indices in acute renal failure. A prospective study. *Ann Intern Med* 89:47, 1978.

Stevens ME, McConnell M, Bone JM: Aggressive treatment with pulse methyl prednisolone or plasma exchange is justified in rapidly progressive glomerulonephritis. *Proc Eur Dialysis Transplant Assoc* 19:724, 1982.

# 91
# URINARY TRACT INFECTIONS
## David S. Howes

*Urinary tract infection* (UTI) is defined as significant bacteriuria in the presence of symptoms. It affects an estimated 20 percent of women at some point during their lifetime and accounts for a significant number of emergency department visits. Controversial aspects of the diagnosis and management of apparent lower UTI in adult women will be discussed. In the elderly, UTI is a major cause of nosocomial gram-negative sepsis, and 1 to 3 percent of patients with pyelonephritis die.

## NATURAL HISTORY

The natural history of UTI varies with age and sex (Fig. 91-1). In neonates a UTI is part of the syndrome of overwhelming gram-negative sepsis. The incidence of UTI in preschool children is approximately 2 percent, with the incidence in girls at least 10 times greater than in boys. In school-age children the incidence rises to 5 percent, almost exclusively girls.

Bacteriuria is rare in males under the age of 50 and symptoms of dysuria or urinary frequency are usually due to infection of the urethra or prostate. However, in men older than 50 years the incidence of UTI rises because of prostatic obstruction or subsequent instrumentation.

Dysuria in females is a common clinical problem and symptoms increase with age and sexual activity. Most UTIs are common in otherwise healthy young women possibly due to sexual contact. The incidence of infection in postmenopausal women is high; multiple factors are responsible for this and will be discussed.

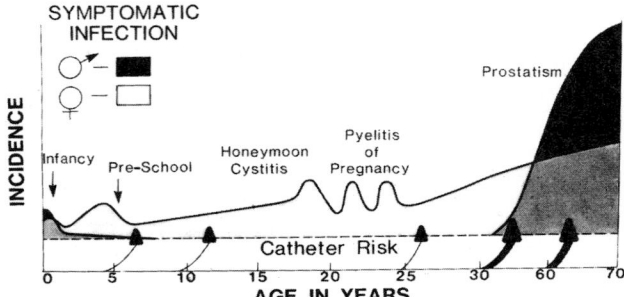

**Fig. 91-1.** Natural history of urinary tract infections.

**Table 91-1.** Etiologic Agents in Uncomplicated Urinary Tract Infection

| Organism | Incidence |
|---|---|
| *Escherichia coli* | > 80% |
| *Klebsiella* | |
| *Proteus* sp. | 5–20% |
| *Enterobacter* | |
| *Pseudomonas* | |
| Group D streptococci | |
| *Chlamydia trachomatis\** | < 5% |
| *Staphylococcus saprophyticus\** | |

\* Much more common in the "dysuria-pyuria" syndrome where sterile or low colony count culture results are obtained.

The infecting organisms are generally those found colonizing the perineum, and in women with a traditional "positive" culture of $10^5$ colony-forming units (CFU) per mL, *Escherichia coli* is responsible for approximately 90 percent of infections. However, one third to one half of cases of dysuria are characterized by sterile or low bacterial colony count culture results. This formerly was termed the "acute urethral syndrome" and was not felt to represent true UTI. In fact, further study revealed that many of these patients had low-grade or early *E. coli, Staphylococcus saprophyticus,* or *Chlamydia trachomatis* infections. Therefore, the definition of UTI based on early studies that reported only upper tract disease may be inappropriate. Such studies established that a colony count of at least $10^5$/mL is necessary to indicate the presence of "significant bacteriuria." Current research suggests that with regard to lower UTI, in the presence of symptoms, a colony count of $10^3$/mL or greater may represent significant bacteriuria, which merits treatment.

The majority of UTIs in women recur either because of relapse or reinfection. Relapse is caused by the same organism; when symptoms recur in less than 1 month this represents treatment failure. When symptoms recur in 1 to 6 months it is generally due to reinfection. Reinfection is usually from a different enteric organism or a different serotype of the same organism and may represent a defect in the defense mechanisms of the host. If a patient has a cluster of infections of more than three recurrences in 1 year, a more complete workup may be warranted to look for the presence of tumor, tuberculosis, renal calculi, structural abnormalities, or associated systemic illness such as diabetes mellitus.

A UTI during pregnancy poses special problems. If untreated, asymptomatic bacteriuria (ABU) may progress to symptomatic UTI. UTI and pyelonephritis have a high incidence in the third trimester and may lead to preeclampsia, sepsis, or miscarriage. This is the single area in which treatment of ABU is definitely indicated.

## BACTERIOLOGY

UTI should be thought of as either complicated, that is, occurring in patients with underlying renal or neurologic disease; or uncomplicated, occurring in patients in which no defect can be demonstrated. Most uncomplicated UTIs are caused by gram-negative aerobic bacilli from the gut, the vast majority due to *E. coli* (Table 91-1). As we will discuss in the management section, these coliform bacteria respond to a wide variety of antimicrobial agents. Anaerobic organisms do not grow well in urine and are rarely pathogenic. Complicated UTIs are more often caused by unusual pathogens that may be resistant to multiple antibiotics. These infections will ultimately require management by a urologist or nephrologist.

## NORMAL HOST DEFENSE MECHANISMS

Urine is generally a good culture medium depending on its pH and chemical constituents. Factors unfavorable to bacterial growth are a low pH (5.5 or less); a high concentration of urea; and the presence of organic acids derived from a diet including fruit juice and methio-

nine, a breakdown of protein food, which enhances acidification of the urine. A thin film of urine remains in the bladder after voiding. An intact bladder mucosa removes organisms from the film, probably by the production of organic acids by the mucosal cells and not by antibody formation or phagocytosis. Incomplete bladder emptying renders this mechanism ineffective and is responsible for the increased frequency of infection in patients with a neurogenic bladder and postmenopausal women with bladder or uterine prolapse. The latter group also has a lack of estrogen, which causes marked changes in the vaginal microflora, including loss of lactobacilli and increased colonization by *E. coli.*

Frequent and complete voiding has been associated with the reduction of recurrence of UTI. Investigators have shown that the concentration of bacteria in the bladder may increase tenfold after sexual intercourse due to a "milking action" of the female urethra during intercourse. The use of a diaphragm and spermicide is also associated with recurrence in some patients, probably because the spermicide enhances vaginal colonization with *E. coli.* It is suggested that prompt voiding after intercourse may lessen the frequency of UTI. A large urinary flow also dilutes the bacterial inoculum that occasionally occurs.

Alternatively, susceptibility may have a genetic basis, that is, women who do not secrete blood group antigens (nonsecretors) have a high incidence of recurrent infection. This appears to be due to the presence of specific uroepithelial cell *E. coli*-binding glycolipids that promote fecal coliform colonization of the vagina.

If the mechanisms of the lower urinary tract fail and ascending infection of the urinary tract occurs, renal defense mechanisms are called into play. Local antibodies are produced in the kidney and kill bacteria in the presence of complement. Local leukocytosis and phagocytosis also help eradicate bacteria.

## CLINICAL FEATURES

The clinical symptoms of UTI in an adult are dysuria, frequency, and lower abdominal pain. In females, a history of vaginal discharge should be sought and a pelvic examination is strongly advised to rule out vaginitis, cervicitis, or pelvic inflammatory disease as the cause of dysuria. Fever, chills, and malaise may also be present.

Flank pain and costovertebral angle tenderness can be associated with cystitis because of referred pain. However, when these are found clinically, one should assume that pyelonephritis is present.

In the male, dysuria with discharge indicates urethritis. A Gram stain of the discharge may reveal gram-negative intracellular diplococci, which is diagnostic of gonococcal urethritis. If the Gram stain is inconclusive, the diagnosis is most likely nonspecific urethritis, which is mainly chlamydial infection. In either case, a VDRL test and a culture for gonorrhea should be obtained. It should be emphasized to the emergency department triage personnel that UTI in young adult males is extremely rare; therefore, a urine specimen should be obtained at the direction of the physician after the examination has been performed. This may enhance the likelihood of a positive urethral swab in the male patient with minimal discharge. On the other hand, several authors have demonstrated that the presence of urinary leukocytes was more sensitive than urethral Gram stain in detecting patients who were later found to have chlamydial infection as confirmed by culture. Finally, if bacteriuria is present and is not clinically associated with urethritis or prostatitis, then treatment, followed by urologic referral, is indicated.

## DIAGNOSIS

If UTI is suspected, the first step in establishing the diagnosis is the careful collection of urine for a urinalysis and potentially for culture. The midstream voiding specimen is as accurate as urine obtained by catheterization if the patient is given and follows careful instructions. Instruct the woman to remove her underwear, sit facing the back of the toilet, spread the labia with one hand, cleanse from front to back with povidone-iodine swabs or liquid soap, pass a small amount of urine into the toilet, and then urinate into a sterile cup. Instruct the man to carefully cleanse the urethral meatus, retracting the foreskin if uncircumcised, and obtain a midsteam specimen as described above.

If the sample is properly collected, it should contain no or few epithelial cells. The many sources of contamination include material in the collection bottle, menses, vaginal discharge, urethral or periurethral tissue, and organisms multiplying in the urine after collection. Bacteria in urine double each hour at room temperature; therefore urine should be refrigerated if not sent directly to the laboratory. In addition to special care in cleansing, the use of a tampon also helps women to obtain a clean-cup specimen if menstruation or profuse discharge is present.

Catheterization is indicated if the patient cannot void spontaneously, is too ill or immobilized, or is extremely obese. It may also be performed as part of a urologic evaluation and to relieve obstruction. However, routine catheterization should be avoided because 1 to 2 percent of patients develop UTI after a single catheter insertion, according to Kunin. This seems to be a problem especially if done just prior to delivery.

Although blood or bile may be detected by gross examination of the urine, visual inspection or the smell of the urine is generally not helpful in determining infection. Cloudiness is usually not due to white blood cells (WBC) or bacteria but large amounts of protein or crystals. Malodorous urine may be caused by diet or medication ingestion and is not a reliable sign of infection.

Current emphasis is on the detection of pyuria and bacteriuria in the initial examination of the urine. The assessment of pyuria is imperfect. Variables include the method of centrifuging the specimen, the amount of supernatant in which the sediment is resuspended, and the final volume of urine under the cover slip that is examined. Laboratories that use a WBC counting chamber diminish some of this variability and increase accuracy in assessing both centrifuged and uncentrifuged urine. Stamm has used the latter technique and defined pyuria as the presence of 8 leukocytes or more per mL of uncentrifuged urine. This figure roughly corresponds to 2 to 5 leukocytes per high-power field (HPF) in a centrifuged specimen.

Both Komaroff and Stamm feel that this low-level pyuria is clinically important. Other authors have suggested that, in women, pyuria is significant only if there are more than 10 WBC/HPF, and only if bacteria are present on the microscopic examination. Though this is more likely to be true with typical coliform infection, lower degrees of pyuria with or without bacteriuria may be significant, especially with regard to infection with *Chlamydia.*

As knowledge of UTI in adult women evolves, it is clear that women with symptoms and low-grade pyuria (fewer than 10 WBC/HPF) do have significant bacteriuria that will symptomatically and bacteriologically respond to antimicrobial therapy. In the past, these women were not treated initially and their cultures often did not establish more than $10^5$ CFU/mL. Sensitivity to causes of lower UTI

other than typical coliforms has brought the designation of the "dysuria-pyuria syndrome" (also referred to as the "acute urethral syndrome"), which almost always benefits from treatment. It is in this subgroup of women that the urinalysis may well be more useful than the urine culture, which is often misleading, especially as reported in standard microbiologic laboratories. In addition, a positive urinalysis would dictate more immediate management interventions than would awaiting a urine culture.

In men, more than 1 to 2 WBC/HPF can be significant in the presence of bacteria. Again it must be remembered that urethritis and prostatitis are far more likely causes of pyuria in young males who are sexually active and complain of dysuria, whether or not a urethral discharge is present.

Bacteriuria is also felt to be a sensitive tool for detection of UTI in the symptomatic patient. The presence of any bacteria on a Gram stain of uncentrifuged urine is significant. In a clean specimen this correlated to a high degree with culture results. This statement is also true if more than 15 bacteria per HPF are found in a centrifuged specimen. Both of these methods will fail to detect low colony count UTI or infection caused by *Chlamydia.* False positives occur when vaginal or fecal contamination is present.

Several authors have advocated the use of the nitrate urine test. Although a positive nitrate reaction has a very high specificity, its sensitivity is low, rendering it much less useful as a screening examination.

More recently, the presence of leukocyte esterase in the urine has been evaluated as an indicator of the presence of pyuria. Initial reports of high sensitivity supported use of this test as a screening tool for pyuria. However, Propp found an unacceptable rate of false negative results for low-level pyuria (6 to 20 WBC/HPF) in an emergency department setting.

When the clinical presentation suggests UTI, a positive leukocyte esterase test supports the diagnosis, and treatment should be initiated. If the test is negative, a microscopic examination should be performed to detect lower levels of clinically significant pyuria.

Unfortunately, we are still left with women who complain of dysuria, have no pyuria or demonstrable pathogen on culture, and who do not respond to antimicrobial treatment. The absence of pyuria in these patients is useful because it indicates that antimicrobial treatment is probably unnecessary. Presuming that vulvovaginitis or cervicitis has been excluded, causes of this dysuria may include inflammation of the urethra from physical trauma or due to the use of chemical agents, such as spermicides, cleansing douches, or other feminine hygiene products.

In a symptomatic patient who has fewer than 2 to 5 WBC/HPF, other causes of false negative pyuria should be considered. These include ingestion of large amounts of fluids, which wash out the bladder and produce a dilute urine, and, more likely, old or leftover medication, or a drug belonging to another person, being taken by the patient on a self-directed basis. It should be remembered that, in the case of an obstructed kidney, pyuria may be intermittent or absent.

Although the classical definition for diagnosis of UTI has been a count of $10^5$/mL or more from a midstream catch, lower colony counts are important and current emphasis is on the detection of pyuria. Most authors agree that a urine culture must be obtained in the following settings: acute pyelonephritis; subclinical pyelonephritis (which should be especially suspected in those patients with underlying urinary tract disease, diabetes mellitus, immunocompromised state, recent instrumentation, prolonged symptoms before seeking care, three or more infections in the past year, or a history of acute pyelonephritis in the recent past); any patient who needs to be hospitalized; those patients who have a chronic indwelling catheter; and all children and adult males. If the patient is symptomatic, a single positive culture is significant. For asymptomatic bacteriuria two or three positive cultures are necessary before treatment is undertaken, with the rejoinder that treatment is always indicated in pregnancy.

## TREATMENT

The selection of antibiotics depends on the suspected bacteriology of the infection, the patient's compliance, potential drug toxicity, and cost. In uncomplicated UTI *E. coli* is the offending microorganism in the vast majority of cases. This and other typical coliform pathogens remain susceptible to a variety of agents: trimethoprim, cotrimoxazole, nitrofurantoin macrocrystals, and the quinolones (Table 91-2).

Most authorities have, until recently, recommended treating the first episode of UTI with a 7- or 10-day antibiotic regimen. Trimethoprim alone or in combination with sulfamethoxazole (cotrimoxazole) is generally recommended because these are cheap and effective (Table 91-3). Nitrofurantoin is also effective though compliance with frequent dosing is a problem. Because of increased bacterial resistance, extended-spectrum penicillins (e.g., amoxicillin) and cephalosporins have become less acceptable alternatives. In cases of treatment failure or in the host with a structural or immunologic defect, use of amoxicillin with clavulanic acid or one of the quinolones may be considered. Concern about the emergence of resistant organisms and expense preclude indiscriminate use of the latter agents. The urine should be bacteria free in 24 to 48 h with substantial relief of symptoms within the same time period. The offer of 1 to 2 days of an oral bladder analgesic, such as phenazopyridine (Pyridium), is considerate when urination is painful for the patient.

Recently, multiple investigational reports of shorter treatment regimens for uncomplicated infections in nonpregnant adult women have been published. Single-dose treatment appears to offer a number of advantages. Cost and side effects are substantially reduced, compliance improves, and the development of resistant strains of bacteria is less likely.

These reports have also generated concern. The entity of subclinical pyelonephritis has become increasingly apparent during studies of what was felt to be uncomplicated lower UTI. Detection of this entity requires sophisticated differentiation based on analysis of immunofluorescent antibody results or analysis for β-glucuronidase and lactate dehydrogenase isoenzymes. At this time these tests are principally useful as research tools and are not helpful in the routine clinical arena.

Because of this, single-dose or short-term (e.g., 3-d) regimens have limitations. In several series, a disturbing number of patients with apparent simple cystitis exhibited tissue invasion as demonstrated by the presence of antibody-coated bacteria (ACB), that is, unsuspected or subclinical pyelonephritis. This group had a poor response to short-term therapy when compared to patients who received traditional 10- or 14-day treatment and had positive ACB. Because ACB testing is justifiable only in research settings, this raises questions about the efficacy of short-term therapy in episodic care settings.

On the other hand, several authors suggest that single-dose treatment may as reliably identify patients with subclinical pyelonephritis as available diagnostic tests. This is because a single-dose or a short course of antibiotics is less likely to eradicate bacteriuria in the patient with tissue invasion. In practice, they suggest that all women with urethrocystitis symptoms be given a single dose or brief course of cotrimoxazole with the expectation of cure in the vast majority. The few patients with recurrence of symptoms, pyuria, and bacteriuria will be promptly identified as having complicated infection necessitating more prolonged therapy.

In certain emergency department settings, especially those serving indigent populations where there is delay in seeking care, the incidence of subclinical pyelonephritis may approach 70 percent of patients. In this circumstance, single-dose or short-term therapy is difficult to justify. This is especially important because acute pyelonephritis following single-dose therapy has been reported. Therefore, before an emergency department physician decides to use

**Table 91-2.** Guidelines to Outpatient Management of Uncomplicated UTI

| Type of Patient | Presumed Type of Infection | Clinical Characteristics | Antimicrobial Regimens | Comments |
|---|---|---|---|---|
| Adult female | Lower | Few prior episodes with brief duration of symptoms and no risk factors for subclinical pyelonephritis | 1. Cotrimoxazole, 2 double-strength tablets *or* 2. Cotrimoxazole, 1 double-strength tablet bid × 3 d 3. Ciprofloxacin or ofloxacin, 200–500 mg bid x 3 d | Singe-dose or brief-duration regimen Good follow-up available No culture needed |
| Adult female | Lower/upper | Risk of subclinical pyelonephritis: prolonged symptoms, relapse or recurrent UTI, diabetes mellitus, urinary tract abnormalities, recent pyelonephritis, indigent patients | 1. Cotrimoxazole, 1 double-strength tablet bid 2. Trimethoprim, 200 mg bid 3. Nitrofurantoin macrocrystals, 50–100 mg qid 4. Cefadroxil, 500–1000 mg bid 5. Amoxicillin, 250–500 mg tid *or* Amoxicillin with clavulanic acid, 250–500 mg tid *or* Ciprofloxacin or ofloxacin, 200–500 mg bid (if resistant organism suspected) | 10-d course advised Consider culture Coliforms typical |
| Adult male | Lower/upper | Suspect underlying anatomic abnormality; R/O urethritis, prostatitis | Same as above | Same as above |
| Adult female | Lower | Stuttering symptoms, new sexual partner or partner with urethritis, signs and symptoms of cervicitis, pyuria without bacteriuria | 1. Doxycycline, 100 mg bid 2. Cotrimoxazole, 1 double-strength tablet bid 3. Sulfamethoxazole, 1 g bid 4. Erythromycin, 500 mg qid ( in allergy or pregnancy-related cases and will only eradicate *Chlamydia*) | 10-d course Culture for gonococcus advisable |

**Table 91-3.** Cost Comparison of Urinary Antimicrobial Agents

| Generic Name | Cost of 10-d Course, $* | Brand Name | Cost, $* |
|---|---|---|---|
| Trimethoprim | 15.19 | Proloprim | 39.69 |
| Sulfamethoxazole | NA | Gantanol | 27.99 |
| Cotrimoxazole DS | 10.29 | Bactrim DS | 29.69 |
| Amoxicillin | 10.59 | Amoxil | 11.29 |
| Doxycycline | 14.09 | Vibramycin | 78.49 |
| Nitrofurantoin macrocrystals | 27.19 | Macrodantin | 36.49 |
| Amoxicillin with clavulanic acid | NA | Augmentin | 62.49 |
| Ciprofloxacin | NA | Cipro | 66.19 |
| Ofloxacin | NA | Floxin | 76.69 |

* The prices given are retail prices in the Chicago metropolitan area in June 1994 obtained by telephone survey by the author.

a brief course of treatment, the patient's ability to follow up within 1 week must be ensured. If follow-up compliance is not expected, or the epidemiologic risk of subclinical pyelonephritis is great, then the patient should be placed on a conventional regimen. Three-day regimens are as effective as 10-day regimens in those patients who do not demonstrate ACB, but the efficacy in patients with possible tissue invasion is likely to be lower than a conventional prolonged course of therapy.

One should be suspicious that *Chlamydia* is responsible for symptoms in the following settings: a woman with a recent, new sexual partner; a partner with urethritis; examination findings of cervicitis; or when there is low-grade pyuria with no bacteria seen on urinalysis. A 10-day course of sulfonamides or doxycycline is the preferred treatment. Although erythromycin is very effective for chlamydial infections, it is ineffective against coliform bacteria. Therefore, it cannot be recommended as empirical therapy.

For recurrent infection, culture and sensitivity tests are essential. The infection is often due to a new serotype of *E. coli,* or it may be due to newly resistant organisms that develop as a result of antibiotics excreted into the gastrointestinal tract. Empirical therapy for recurrent infections includes cotrimoxazole, nitrofurantoin macrocrystals, or the quinolones. However, successful management depends on sensitivity testing. Again, it must be emphasized that these patients need referral in the setting of chronic, recurrent infection. The institution of chronic, suppressive therapy should be left to a specialist.

Aggressive therapy is warranted for pregnant women with pyuria or bacteriuria, whether or not associated symptoms are present. Most clinicians prefer a cephalosporin for outpatient treatment. Cotrimoxazole may be considered except near term and in those with glucose-6-phosphate dehydrogenase deficiency. All regimens should be continued for 14 days. Inpatient management is stressed for suspected pyelonephritis because the incidence is higher in pregnancy, and maternal and fetal morbidity is substantial. Urine culture is mandatory.

Adjunctive therapy should include plenty of fluids to enhance diuresis, fruit juices containing vitamin C to acidify the urine, a proper diet, and frequent voiding (at least every 2 h) to diminish tissue contact with bacteria. Women should be reminded that postintercourse voiding may be helpful in reducing recurrent infection.

Once the infection is eradicated, management should be directed toward prevention of reinfection. This is designed to prevent ascending kidney infection. Up to 80 percent of women who have had a UTI develop recurrence. Because many factors are involved in reinfection and some of these are correctable, continuity of care is essential.

## PYELONEPHRITIS

On occasion, it may be difficult to distinguish lower from upper UTI. Classically, acute pyelonephritis is characterized by shaking chills and fever, flank pain, and costovertebral angle tenderness following several days of dysuria and frequency. The urine will often demonstrate WBC casts and clumps as well as bacteria.

Factors associated with pyelonephritis include pregnancy, prolonged symptoms prior to seeking care, three or more infections in the past year, immunocompromised state, and diabetes mellitus. Less often one may find congenital or acquired anatomic urinary tract abnormality, neurogenic problems that result in incomplete bladder emptying, recent urinary tract instrumentation, renal calculi and nephrocalcinosis, prostatic hypertrophy, or prostatitis present.

Young, otherwise healthy females with uncomplicated acute pyelonephritis may be candidates for outpatient management. A popular regimen at our institution is referred to as "treatment by [the rule of] twos." While in the emergency department, the patient is given 2 L of intravenous fluid, 2 Tylenol #3 capsules, and 2 g ceftriaxone. If the fever drops by 2° and the patient is able to retain 2 glasses of water, an outpatient prescription for cotrimoxazole DS, 2 times per day for 2 weeks, is given. The patient is to be followed up in 2 days, for a progress check. A recent study showed that outpatient therapy for selected patients was as safe and effective and considerably less expensive than in a comparable group of patients treated on an inpatient basis.

The decision to admit a patient with acute pyelonephritis is based on age, host factors, and response to initial emergency department interventions. Fluid replacement and parenteral antibiotics are necessary if the patient is vomiting or dehydrated. Unremitting fever and loss of vasomotor tone mandate inpatient therapy. For initial management in an otherwise healthy host with no prior or recent history of UTI, the typical offending bacteria would include *E. coli* as well as other coliform bacteria. Recent recommendations favor a single intravenous agent such as trimethoprim-sulfamethoxazole, 160 and 800 mg, q12h; a third-generation cephalosporin, for example, ceftriaxone, 1 g q12h; or an aminoglycoside, such as, gentamicin, 1.5 mg/kg, q8h. The selection of which drugs to use depends on cost considerations and on local sensitivity patterns.

Younger patients without complicating factors have the least morbidity or mortality. Despite appropriate intervention, 1 to 3 percent of patients with acute pyelonephritis die. Factors associated with an unfavorable prognosis are old age and general debility, renal calculi or obstruction, a recent history of hospitalization or instrumentation, diabetes mellitus, evidence of chronic nephropathy, sickle cell anemia, underlying carcinoma, or intercurrent cancer chemotherapy. In this type of patient it is imperative that broad-spectrum antibiotic coverage to include *Pseudomonas* species be provided. A urologic or infectious disease consultation should be considered as part of the initial management of such patients.

Complications of acute pyelonephritis include acute papillary necrosis with possible ureteric obstruction, septic shock, and perinephric abscesses. Adequate fluid hydration must be emphasized in these settings.

## BIBLIOGRAPHY

Avorn J, Monane M, Gurwitz JH, et al. Reduction of bacteriuria and pyuria after ingestion of cranberry juice. *JAMA* 271:751, 1994.

Fihn SD, Johnson C, Roberts PL, et al. Trimethoprim-sulfamethoxazole for acute dysuria in women: a single-dose or 10-day course. *Ann Intern Med* 108:350, 1988.

Komaroff AL. Acute dysuria in women. *N Engl J Med* 310:368, 1984.

Kunin CM, Van Arsdale White L, Tong HH. A reassessment of the importance of "low-count" bacteriuria in young women with acute urinary symptoms. *Ann Intern Med* 119:454, 1993.

Leibovici L, Greenshtain S, Cohen O, et al. Predictors of bacteremia and resistant pathogens in urinary tract infections. *Arch Intern Med* 152:2481, 1992.

Lipsky BA. UTIs in men: epidemiology, pathophysiology, diagnosis, and treatment. *Ann Intern Med* 110:138, 1989.

McCabe JB, Hamilton GC. Single-dose antibiotic therapy of UTI: Is it appropriate in the emergency department? *Ann Emerg Med* 13:432, 1984.

Propp DA, Weber D, Ciesla ML. Reliability of a urine dipstick in emergency department patients. *Ann Emerg Med* 18:560, 1989.

Safrin S, Siegel D, Black D. Pyelonephritis in adult women: inpatient versus outpatient therapy. *Am J Med* 85:793, 1988.

Stamm WE, Hooton TM. Management of urinary tract infections in adults. *N Engl J Med* 329:1328, 1993.

Stamm WE, Running K, McKevitt M, et al. Treatment of the acute urethral syndrome. *N Engl J Med* 304:956, 1981.

Strom BL, Collins M, West SL, et al. Sexual activity, contraceptive use, and other risk factors for symptomatic and asymptomatic bacteriuria: a case control study. *Ann Intern Med* 107:816, 1987.

# 92
# MALE GENITAL PROBLEMS
## Robert E. Schneider

One of the most anxiety-provoking problems presenting to an emergency department is the male with acute genital pain. The extensive sensory innervation of this area produces severe symptoms, and the close relationships of the abdominal and genital sensory afferent pathways in the male account for the common association of abdominal pain with some acute genitourinary disorders.

## ANATOMY
### Penis

The penis is composed of three cylindrical bodies: the two corpora cavernosa, which form the main bulk of the penis, and the corpus spongiosum, which surround the urethra (Fig. 92-1). The corpora cavernosa are the major erectile bodies, extending distally from the pubic rami and capped by the glans penis. These two cylindrical structures are encased in a thick tunic of dense connective tissue, the tunica albuginea. All three cylinders are collectively covered by a thinner Buck's fascia, which fuses with Colles's fascia at the level of the urogenital diaphragm.

The blood supply is primarily from the internal pudendal artery, which branches to form the deep and superficial penile arteries. Lymphatic drainage is into the deep and superficial inguinal nodes.

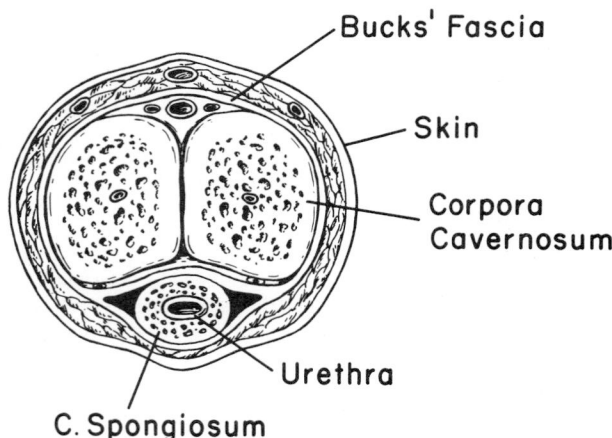

**Fig. 92-1.** Cross section of the penis.

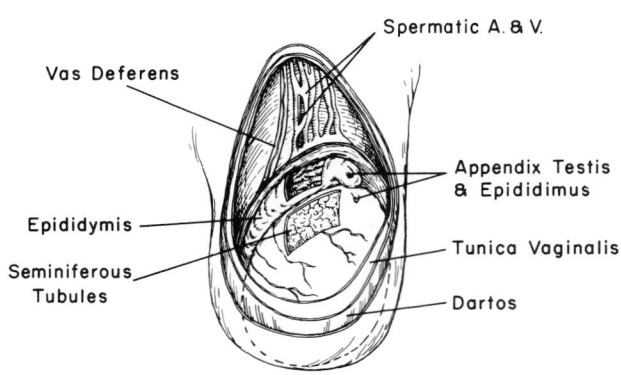

**Fig. 92-2.** Anatomy of the scrotum and the testis.

### Scrotum

The prepubertal scrotal skin is thin and thickens with subsequent hormonal stimulation. Immediately beneath the skin are the smooth muscle and elastic tissue layers of the dartos fascia, the continuous conjoined Camper and Scarpa fascial layers of the abdominal wall (Fig. 92-2). This fused layer extends into the perineum as Colles' fascia. The blood supply is primarily derived from branches of the femoral and internal pudendal arteries. Lymphatics from the scrotum drain into the inguinal and femoral nodes.

### Testes

The testes usually lie in an upright position with the superior portion tipped slightly forward and outward. The average size is between 4 and 5 cm in length and approximately 3 cm in width and depth. The overall volume is about 25 mL. Each testis is encased in a thick fibrous tunica albuginea except posterolaterally, where it is in tight apposition with the epididymis. The enveloping tunica vaginalis anchors each testis and epididymis to the posterior scrotal wall. Inferiorly, the testis is anchored to the scrotum by the scrotal ligament (gubernaculum). A lack of proper fixation leaves both structures at risk for torsion. The posterior (visceral) leaf of tunica vaginalis is contiguous with the tunica albuginea testis. A potential space exists between this visceral leaf and the anterior (parietal) tunica vaginalis. Any traumatic or inflammatory event will impede the normal parietal tunica vaginalis from absorbing viscerally secreted fluid, resulting in a hydrocele (Fig. 92-3).

The blood supply is by the internal spermatic, differential, and external spermatic arteries, which travel together in the spermatic cord. Venous return is primarily by the internal spermatic, epigastric, internal circumflex, and scrotal veins. The lymphatics drain toward the external, common iliac, and periaortic nodes.

The epididymis is a single, fine, tubular structure approximately 4 to 5 m long compressed into an area of about 5 cm. The function of the epididymis is to promote sperm maturation and motility. Vestigial embryonic structures, the appendix epididymis and the appendix testis, which have no known physiologic function, are often associated with the testes and epididymis. The appendix epididymis, a remnant of the epigenitales, is found attached to the head of the epididymis, or globus major. The appendix testis, a pear-shaped structure of müllerian duct origin, is usually situated on the uppermost portion of the testis at the junction of the testis and the globus major.

The vas deferens, a prominent part of the adnexa of the scrotal contents, is a distinct muscular tube that is easily palpable within the scrotal sac. It extends cephalad in the spermatic cord from the tail of the epididymis (globus minor), traveling the inguinal canal and crossing medially behind the bladder over the ureters to form the ampullae of the vas, where it joins with the seminal vesicles to form the paired ejaculatory ducts in the prostatic urethra.

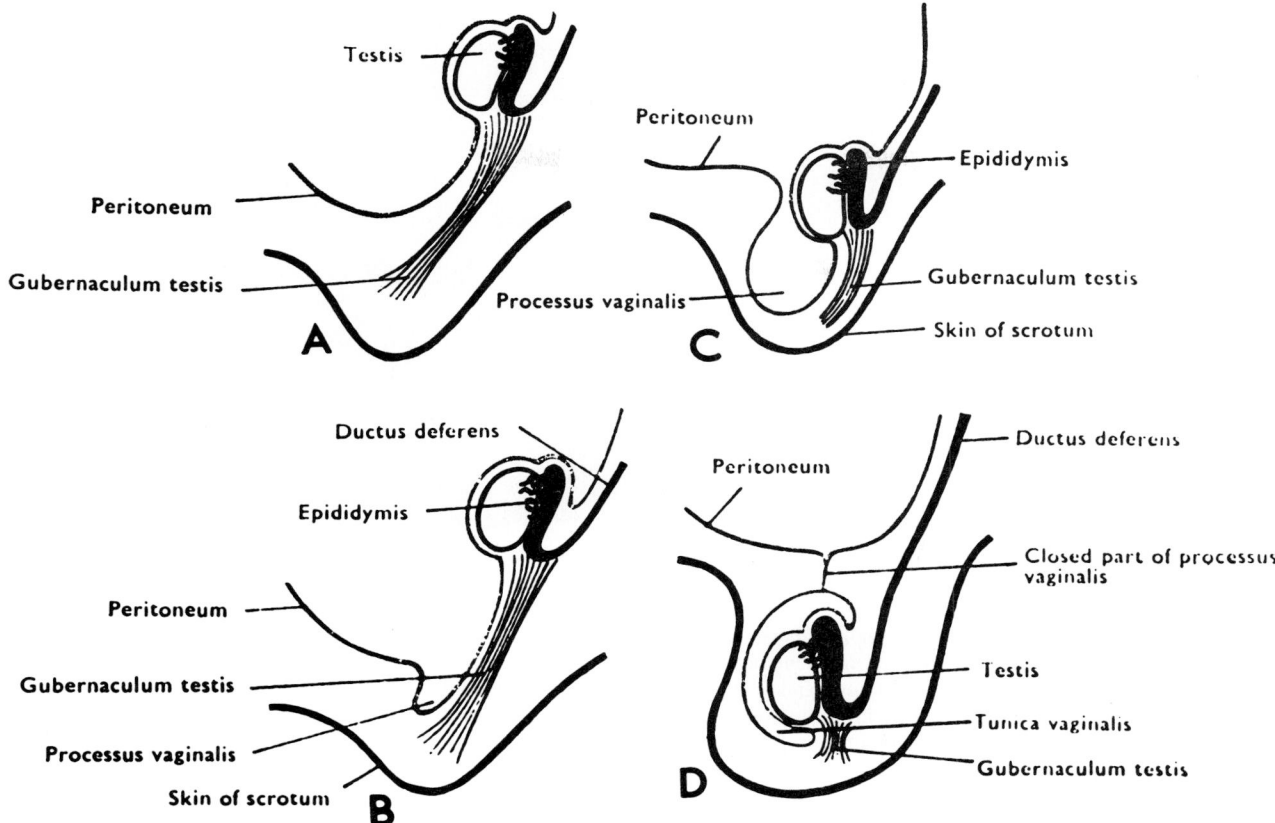

**Fig. 92-3.** Embryonic retroperitoneal testis descends into the scrotum and invaginates into the tunica vaginalis which anchors it to the posterior scrotal wall. Note the potential space in the tunica vaginalis for development of a hydrocele.

## Prostate

The prostate originates from the urogenital sinus at approximately the third month of embryonic life. It is continually enlarging and in the young male is approximately 10 to 15 g, often not definable on rectal examination. As a man matures, the prostate may enlarge dramatically, resulting in significant outlet obstruction. The hyperplastic adenoma envelops the urethra between the bladder neck and the urogenital diaphragm. Positioned just anterior to the rectal ampulla, its posterior surface is readily palpable on rectal examination.

## PHYSICAL EXAMINATION

Physical examination should be carried out with the patient in both the supine and upright positions in a well-illuminated, warm room. If the scrotum is contracted despite proper room temperature, a warm towel placed over the genitalia permits the scrotum and testes to descend and be comfortably examined.

Examination should always begin with visual inspection. In uncircumcised males, the foreskin should be fully retracted to inspect the glans, coronal sulcus, and preputial areas for ulceration or malignant lesions. The location of the urethral meatus and presence of discharge should be noted. The penile shaft should be carefully palpated for plaques, cysts, or early abscesses.

The supine or modified lithotomy position is more comfortable for both the patient and the examiner and allows a more thorough examination of each testis, epididymis, the prostate, seminal vesicles, and rectal ampulla. During the critical evaluation of a scrotal mass, patient relaxation and cooperation in the supine position are paramount. Testicular nodularity or firmness should be considered carcinoma until proven otherwise. The epididymis usually lies on the posterolateral aspect of the testis and, if not inflamed or involved with other pathologic entities, has a soft, fleshy feel similar to that of the earlobe. Many males experience pain and tenderness with palpation of a normal globus major (head), body, and globus minor (tail) of the epididymis. All males experience some discomfort during palpation of a normal prostate. The supine position helps prevent an infrequent vasovagal response to the scrotal or prostate examination. The prostate has a heart-shaped contour with its apex located more distally, abutting the urogenital diaphragm (anatomic soft spot). The consistency of the normal prostate has the same resiliency as the cartilaginous tip of the nose, while suspicious carcinogenic areas feel more like the bony prominence of the chin. The posterior lobe is small and thin, allowing palpation of the median raphe that distinguishes the two lateral lobes. A normal rectal examination does not exclude outlet obstruction secondary to an obstructing median bar or large intravesical prostate. The seminal vesicles, lying just superior to the prostate, cannot normally be distinguished unless there is inflammation, induration, or enlargement.

Examination of the inguinal canals for hernias and the scrotal spermatic cords for varicoceles is best done in the upright position, with the patient straining at the appropriate time. When the patient is upright, it should be determined whether the testes are aligned along a vertical or horizontal axis. Horizontally aligned testes are at risk of torsion, and these patients should be referred to a urologist.

The differential diagnosis of hematuria or pyuria in a properly collected urine specimen is listed in Table 92-1. The uncircumcised male patient should retract his foreskin and wash the glans penis with plain tap water before collecting a midstream specimen. Failure to do so will result in preputial contamination. The often described three-cup specimen used to localize male lower urinary tract infections is time-consuming and requires patient compliance, both factors that tend to limit its usefulness in the emergency department.

**Table 92-1.** Etiology of Hematuria and Pyuria

Genitourinary trauma
    Blunt or penetrating
    Urethral instrumentation
Tumor
Stones
Sloughed papillae
    Sickle cell anemia
    Nonsteroidal anti-inflammatory drugs (NSAIDs)
    Diabetes mellitus
Infection
    Pyogenic
    Tuberculous

## COMMON GENITOURINARY DISORDERS

### Scrotum

Because the scrotal skin is loose and elastic, dramatic enlargement of the scrotum may occur secondary to either scrotal or testicular pathologic conditions.

### Scrotal Edema

Simple isolated scrotal edema is uncommon and usually occurs secondary to insect or human bites, contact dermatitis, or, in young boys, secondary to idiopathic scrotal edema. Contiguous scrotal and penile edema occurs in older men in conjunction with lower extremity edema in fluid overload states (congestive heart failure), hypoalbuminemia, and generalized anasarca.

### Scrotal Abscess

The important distinction with a scrotal abscess is whether the phlegmon is localized to the scrotal wall, i.e., simple hair follicle abscess, or involves and even perhaps originates from infection in one of the primary intrascrotal organs, i.e., testis, epididymis, bulbous urethra. This distinction can be very difficult late in the course of the disease process when a scrotal mass may be the only discernible finding.

A simple hair follicle scrotal wall abscess can be managed by incision and drainage. Oftentimes wound care can be simplified by circumferential excision of the entire roof of the abscess. This allows access for wound care and sitz baths and assures healing from the base outward. Antibiotics are rarely needed in an immunocompetent male.

Contiguous involvement of the scrotal skin by an inflammatory mass in the testis or epididymis is best evaluated by ultrasound. A retrograde urethrogram will delineate the integrity of the urethra. Definitive care of any complex abscesses should be directed by a urologist.

### Fournier's Gangrene

Fournier's gangrene is a polymicrobial, synergistic infection of the subcutaneous tissues that originates from one of three sites: skin, urethra, or rectum. This infectious process typically begins as a benign infection or simple abscess that quickly becomes virulent, especially in an immunocompromised host, and leads to end-artery thrombosis in the subcutaneous tissue that promotes widespread necrosis of previously healthy tissue (Fig. 92-4).

The diabetic male seems to be most at risk. Prompt recognition of Fournier's gangrene in its early stages should prevent extensive tissue loss that accompanies delayed diagnosis. Aggressive fluid resuscitation; gram-positive, gram-negative, and anaerobic antibiotic coverage; and wide surgical debridement in conjunction with pre- and postoperative hyperbaric oxygen therapy are the mainstays of treatment. Urologic consultation is often required when periurethral abscess is the inciting event or when other etiologies have secondarily invaded the urinary tract and supravesical urinary drainage is needed. It is imperative that emergency medicine physicians maintain a very

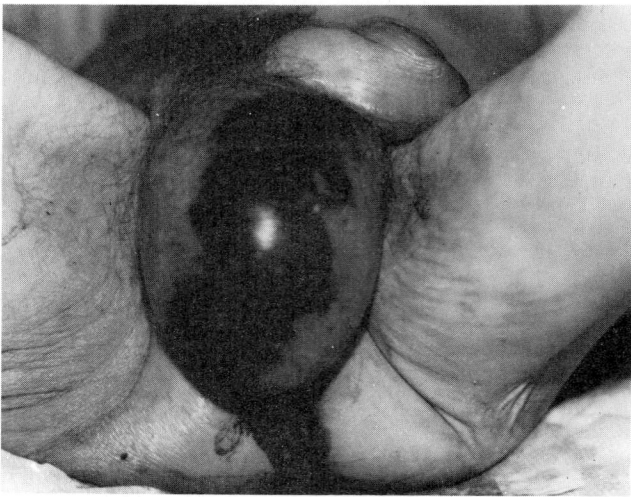

**Fig. 92-4.** A patient with idiopathic gangrene of the scrotum. Note the sharp demarcation of gangrenous changes and the marked edema of the scrotum and the penis.

high index of suspicion for this entity in immunocompromised patients who present complaining of scrotal, rectal, or any genitalia pain out of proportion to their physical examination findings. Surgical consultation is strongly recommended in all such patients, rather than deciding on symptomatic treatment and discharge from the emergency department.

### Penis

### Balanoposthitis

Balanitis is inflammation of the glans penis. Posthitis is inflammation of the foreskin. Balanoposthitis is inflammation of both the glans and foreskin. When foreskin retraction is attempted, the glans and apposing prepuce appear purulent, excoriated, malodorous, and tender. When recurrent, it can be the sole presenting sign of diabetes. Treatment consists of cleansing the area with mild soap, assuring adequate dryness, application of antifungal creams (nystatin or clotrimazole), and possibly circumcision. If secondary bacterial infection is present, a broad-spectrum antibiotic, usually a cephalosporin, should be prescribed.

### Phimosis

Phimosis is the inability to retract the foreskin proximally and posterior to the glans penis. Causes include infection, poor hygiene, or previous preputial injury with scarring. Scarring at the tip of the foreskin can occlude the preputial meatus, infrequently causing urinary retention. Hemostatic dilation of the preputial ostium relieves the urinary retention until definitive dorsal slit or circumcision can be done.

### Paraphimosis

Paraphimosis is the inability to reduce the proximal edematous foreskin distally over the glans penis into its naturally occurring position (Fig. 92-5). The resulting glans edema and venous engorgement can progress to arterial compromise and gangrene.

Paraphimosis is a true urologic emergency. If the surrounding tissue edema can be successfully compressed, the foreskin may be reduced, as demonstrated in Fig. 92-5. If arterial compromise is suspected or has occurred, local infiltration of the constricting band with 1% plain lidocaine followed by superficial vertical incision of the band will decompress the glans and allow foreskin reduction. This procedure should be done by an emergency medicine physician unless a urologist is immediately available.

**Phimosis**

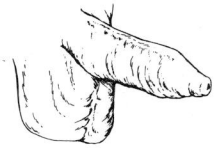

**Paraphimosis**

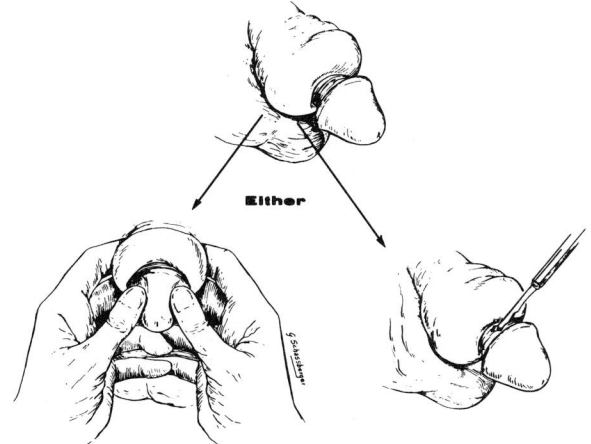

**Fig. 92-5.** Phimosis and paraphimosis. (The lower figure depicts the method of reduction.)

## Entrapment Injuries

Various objects can be placed around the penis, initially occluding the venous, and subsequently the arterial, blood supply. String, metal rings, and wire have been wrapped around the penis for sexual, experimental, or accidental reasons. One of the most insidious objects that can become entrapped behind the coronal ridge is human hair, usually found in young circumcised boys aged 2 to 5 years (Fig. 92-6). The child presents with swelling of the glans. The offending hair may be invisible within the edematous coronal sulcus. If the hair has been chronically occluding, the urethra and dorsal nerve supply of the penis may be partially or completely involved. Removal of the offending object requires ingenuity and care. Urethral integrity (retrograde urethrogram) and distal penile arterial blood supply (Doppler) must be assured prior to emergency department discharge.

## Fracture of the Penis

An acute tear or rupture of the penile tunica albuginea is rare but easily diagnosed. The penis is acutely swollen, discolored, and tender. The history is of trauma during intercourse or other sexual activity, when a sudden "snapping sound" occurs. Even though the urethra is infrequently injured, a retrograde urethrogram may be necessary to assure urethral integrity. Surgical treatment consists of hematoma evacuation and suture apposition of the disrupted tunica albuginea.

## Peyronie's Disease

The patient complains of either gradual or sudden onset of dorsal penile curvature with erections; it is painful and may preclude successful vaginal penetration during intercourse. Examination of the dorsal penile shaft will disclose a thickened plaque involving the tunica albuginea of the corpora bodies without urethral involvement. Reassurance and urologic referral are warranted. Peyronie's disease of the

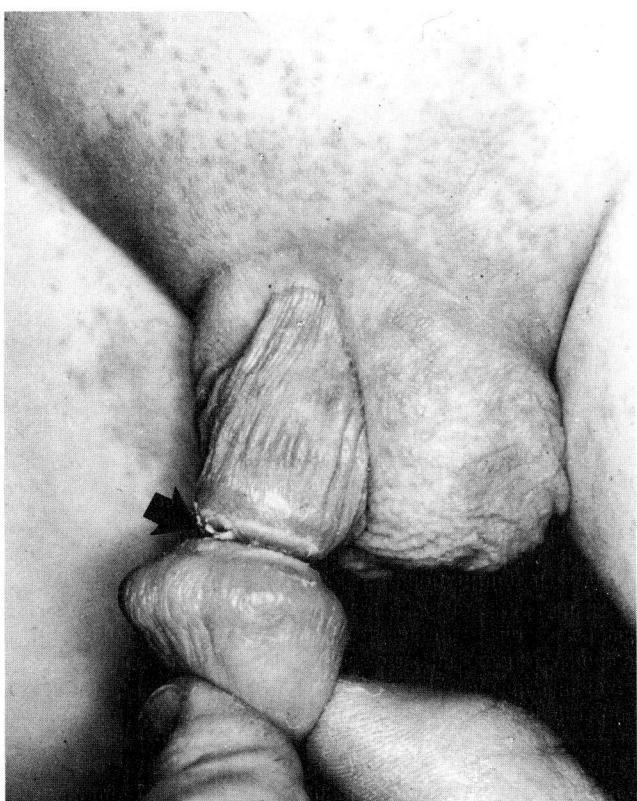

**Fig. 92-6.** Hair is entrapped behind the cocona (arrow), constricting and progressively amputating the glans.

penis has been noted in association with Dupuytren's contractures of the hand.

## Priapism

Priapism is a painful, hard, pathologic erection in which both corpora cavernosa are engorged with stagnant blood. Even though the glans penis and the corpus spongiosum urethra are characteristically soft and uninvolved, urinary retention may occur. Infection and impotence are other common complications.

Priapism is commonly labeled reversible or nonreversible depending upon etiology and the response to medical treatment. Table 92-2 lists the etiology and treatment of priapism. Regardless of etiology,

**Table 92-2.** Causes and Treatment of Priapism

**Reversible causes**
A. Sickle cell anemia
    Treatment: Terbutaline, 0.25–0.5 mg subcutaneously in the deltoid
    muscle; packed red blood cell transfusion; hyperbaric oxygenation
B. Iatrogenic injection of $PGE_1$, papaverine, or phentolamine for
    impotence
    Treatment: Terbutaline, 0.25–0.5 mg subcutaneously in the deltoid
    muscle; aspirate 30–90 mL corporal blood, then inject 30–90 mL
    of 10 mg neosynephrine in 500 mL normal saline
C. Leukemic infiltration
    Treatment: Terbutaline, 0.25–0.5 subcutaneously in the deltoid
    muscle; specific chemotherapy
**Nonreversible causes**
A. Idiopathic
B. High spinal cord lesion
C. Medication (phenothiazines, desyrel)
    Treatment of all nonreversible causes: Terbutaline, 0.25–0.5 mg
    subcutaneously in the deltoid muscle; corporal aspiration,
    neosynephrine instillation; heparin irrigation; shunt surgery

initial therapy is terbutaline, 0.25 to 0.5 mg subcutaneously in the deltoid area. Neither sedation nor ice water enemas are effective. Reversible priapism may respond to medical treatment, while nonreversible priapism usually does not respond to medical treatment and requires surgery. Urologic consultation is necessary for both reversible or nonreversible forms.

## Carcinoma

Carcinoma of the penis is a rare disease occurring in about 1 out of every 100,000 malignancies reported, usually appearing in the fifth or sixth decade in an uncircumcised male. Carcinoma may appear as a nontender ulcer or warty growth beneath the foreskin in the area of the coronal sulcus or glans penis. It is often hidden by an inflamed phimotic foreskin.

## Testes and Epididymis

### Testicular Torsion

The differential diagnosis of acute scrotal pain includes testicular torsion, torsion of the appendix testis, appendix epididymis, and epididymitis. Testicular torsion must be the primary consideration (Fig. 92-7). While the peak incidence of intravaginal torsion occurs at puberty in conjunction with maximal hormonal stimulation, it may occur at any age.

Torsion of the testis or spermatic cord results from bilateral maldevelopment of fixation between the enveloping tunica vaginalis and the posterior scrotal wall. Characteristically, the at-risk testis is aligned along a horizontal rather than a vertical axis. The axis of alignment can only be determined with the patient in an upright position, and even then the determination may be difficult.

Frequently there is a history of an athletic event or strenuous physical activity just prior to the onset of scrotal pain. However, a fair number occur during sleep. Unilateral cremaster muscle contraction results in testicular torsion. The pain usually occurs suddenly, is severe, and is usually felt in either lower abdominal quadrant, the inguinal canal, or the testis. While the pain may be constant or intermittent, it is not positional in nature as testicular torsion is primarily an ischemic event that becomes inflammatory only after the testis has infarcted.

Once the diagnosis is considered, urologic consultation and surgical exploration are necessary. Radionuclide imaging can be a helpful diagnostic study, but availability and reader sensitivity make this a time-intensive procedure in a very time-dependent condition. The often quoted 4-h warm ischemia time for testicular salvage comes from controlled animal studies and cannot be extrapolated to clinical medicine. There are no readily available clinical or laboratory parameters to judge either the degree or the duration of testicular ischemia. Therefore, no matter how long the patient has been symptomatic and no matter what the presenting physical examination suggests, if testicular torsion cannot be excluded by history and physical examination, emergency scrotal exploration is the definitive diagnostic test and procedure of choice.

While awaiting transportation of the patient to the operating room, the emergency medicine physician should attempt manual detorsion of the affected testis. Most testes torse in a lateral to medial fashion. Therefore, detorsion should initially be done in a medial to lateral motion. It must be explained to the patient that detorsion is a painful procedure and while local anesthesia of the affected spermatic cord can initially make the patient more comfortable, it also removes the important endpoint of the detorsion maneuver, i.e., relief of pain. Detorsion is done in a manner similar to opening a book (Fig. 92-8). If one were to stand at the patient's feet, the patient's right testis would be rotated in a counterclockwise fashion (Fig. 92-9); the patient's left testis in a clockwise fashion (Fig. 92-10). Any relief of pain is a positive endpoint. A worsening of the patient's pain would dictate that detorsion be done in the opposite direction. Successful detorsion converts an emergent procedure to an elective one, but one that must be done to correct a potential bilateral anatomic disaster. The timing of the surgical correction should depend on the patient's compliance and responsibility.

Increasingly, young boys are being evaluated in emergency departments complaining only of nonspecific abdominal pain. They are initially diagnosed as having a viral syndrome or gastroenteritis only to return 1 to 2 days later with surgically proven testicular torsion. Whether or not these patients had undisclosed testicular torsion at their initial evaluation is not known, but emergency medicine physicians must think about testicular torsion in the differential diagnosis of any male presenting with a complaint of abdominal pain!

### Torsion of the Appendages

The appendages of the epididymis and testis have no known physiologic function. These pedunculated structures are, however, capable of torsion and in prepubertal boys probably torse more often than the testes. If the patient is seen early, the pain is more intense near the head of the epididymis or testis, and an isolated tender nodule can often be palpated. When the involved appendage is brought close to the thin, prepubertal scrotal skin, a blue reflection may be seen when light shines upon it. This "blue dot sign" is pathognomonic of torsion of the appendix testis or epididymis. If the diagnosis can be absolutely assured and confirmed by color Doppler ultrasound showing normal intratesticular blood flow to the involved testis, immediate surgery is not necessary, since most appendages will calcify or degenerate over 10 to 14 days and cause no harm. If late in the process and testicular swelling is present, or if the color Doppler ultrasound is equivocal, then urologic consultation and surgical exploration may be necessary to exclude testicular torsion.

### Epididymitis

The onset of pain in epididymitis or epididymo-orchitis is usually more gradual than that of testicular torsion due to its inflammatory etiology. Bacterial infection is the most common cause and tends to be age-dependent. In young boys with documented epididymitis or

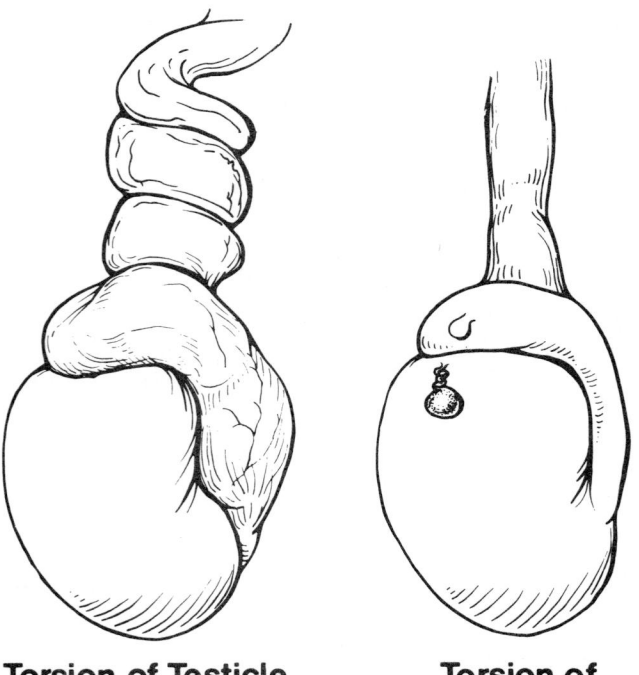

**Torsion of Testicle**          **Torsion of Appendix Testis**

**Fig. 92-7.** Diagrams of testicular torsion and torsion of the appendix testis.

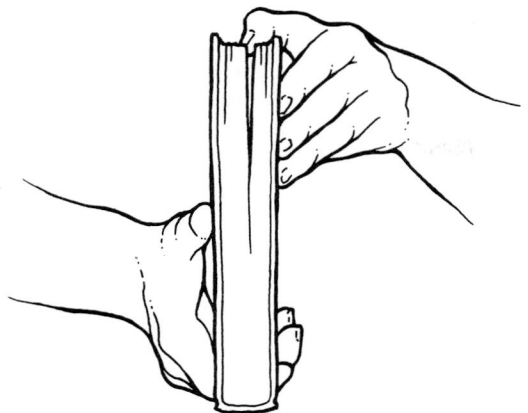

**Figs. 92-8, 92-9, 92-10.** Testicular detorsion. This procedure is best done standing alongside the foot of the patient's bed. The torsed testis is detorsed in a fashion similar to opening a book (Fig. 92-8). That is, the patient's right testis is rotated counterclockwise (Fig. 92-9), the left testis is rotated clockwise (fig. 92-10).

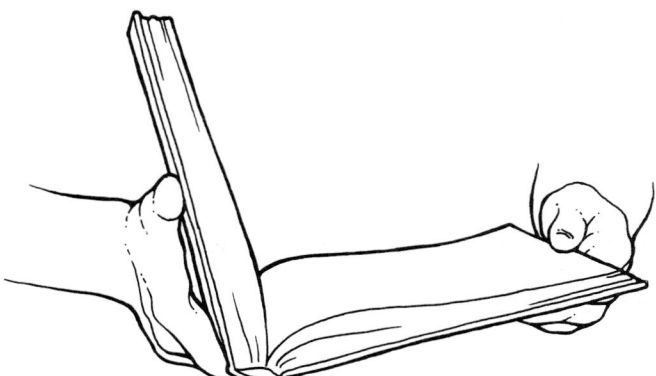

**Fig. 92-9.** (See legend to Fig. 92-8.)

**Fig. 92-10.** (See legend to Fig. 92-9.)

epididymo-orchitis, congenital anomalies of the lower urinary tract in addition to chemical epididymitis secondary to retrograde reflux of sterile urine into the globus minor (tail of the epididymis) must be considered. In patients less than 40 years of age, epididymitis is primarily due to sexually transmitted diseases (STDs) or their complications, i.e., urethral stricture. In gay men with epididymitis or epididymo-orchitis, fungal infection of the lower urinary tract in addition to the more common STD organisms must be considered. In patients over 40 years of age, epididymitis is caused by common urinary pathogens such as *Escherichia coli* and *Klebsiella*. These patients will most often have pyuria on urinalysis, but the absence of white cells or bacteria does not exclude the diagnosis. Older men with epididymitis due to infected urine must be evaluated for the cause of their lower urinary tract infection, i.e., benign prostatic hypertrophy (BPH) or urethral stricture disease. Oftentimes the answer may be found by passing a 14F or 16F Foley or Coudé catheter into the bladder. Easy passage precludes a stricture. A large residual urine should alert the physician to outlet obstruction as the cause of the patient's infection.

Epididymitis causes lower abdominal, inguinal canal, scrotal, or

**Table 92-3.** Etiology and Treatment of Epididymitis and Epididymo-orchitis

| Etiology | Treatment |
|---|---|
| Chemical | Tetracycline, NSAID |
| Gonococcal | Ceftriaxone (Rocephin), tetracycline, NSAID |
| *Chlamydia* | Ceftriaxone (Rocephin), tetracycline, NSAID |
| *E. coli* | Trimethoprim/sulfamethoxazole (Bactrim, Septra), NSAID |
| *Klebsiella* | Trimethoprim/sulfamethoxazole (Bactrim, Septra), NSAID |
| *Candida* | Fluconazole (Diflucan), NSAID |

DOSAGES

Tetracycline 500 mg q.i.d. × 10 days or doxycycline 100 mg b.i.d. × 10 days
Ceftriaxone (Rocephin) 125–250 mg IM
Trimethoprim/sulfamethoxazole DS (Bactrim, Septra) 1 tablet b.i.d. × 10 days
Fluconazole (Diflucan) 400 mg loading dose then 200 mg daily × 10 days

testicular pain alone or in combination. The retrograde progression of infection from the prostatic urethra to the epididymis explains the location and progression of pain. Patients with epididymitis are more prone to lower urinary tract irritative voiding symptoms and may note transient relief of their pain in the recumbent position with scrotal elevation, due to the inflammatory nature of the disease. Initially, isolated firmness and nodularity of the affected globus minor is noted on examination. As the disease progresses, the sulcus between the epididymis and testis becomes obliterated, and the inflammatory epididymal mass may become contiguous with the testis, producing a large, tender scrotal mass (epididymo-orchitis) that cannot be differentiated from testicular torsion or carcinoma. At this stage the patient may appear toxic and require admission for IV antibiotic therapy (see Table 92-3). Adjunctive diagnostic modalities such as radionuclide imaging or color Doppler ultrasound are no more helpful here than with testicular torsion.

Admission criteria for epididymitis include fever with elevated white blood cell count and subjective toxicity, all of which can be indicative of epididymal or testicular abscess formation. A urologist will dictate inpatient management, which should include: (1) absolute bed rest for the first 24 to 48 h, with scrotal elevation and ice application (10 to 15 min every 4 to 6 h) to the involved testis/epididymis; (2) nonsteroidal anti-inflammatory drugs (NSAIDs); (3) intravenous antibiotics based on etiology (Table 92-3); and (4) narcotics for pain control, with concomitant stool softeners. These measures will prevent further progression of the inflammatory process. Once the bedridden patient is pain-free, he should begin ambulation with a scrotal supporter, being careful not to lift heavy objects or strain when having a bowel movement, both of which will increase intraabdominal pressure and exacerbate the inflammatory cycle. Any significant deviation from this plan will prolong the recovery period. Outpatient management is identical to inpatient management except that oral antibiotics are prescribed initially for 10 to 14 days. A urologist will need to reevaluate the patient in 5 to 7 days then ultimately decide when the patient may return to work depending on their job description, i.e., a sedentary worker would be able to return sooner than a laborer.

## Orchitis

Isolated orchitis, or inflammation of the testicle, is quite rare. It usually occurs in conjunction with other systemic diseases, such as mumps, other viral illnesses, or syphilis. Orchitis usually presents as bilateral testicular tenderness and swelling over a few days' duration. Treatment is symptomatic and disease-specific with urologic follow-up.

## Testicular Malignancy

Any asymptomatic testicular mass, firmness, or induration is the hallmark of testicular carcinoma. Ten percent of tumors will present with pain secondary to acute hemorrhage within the tumor. Metastatic tes-

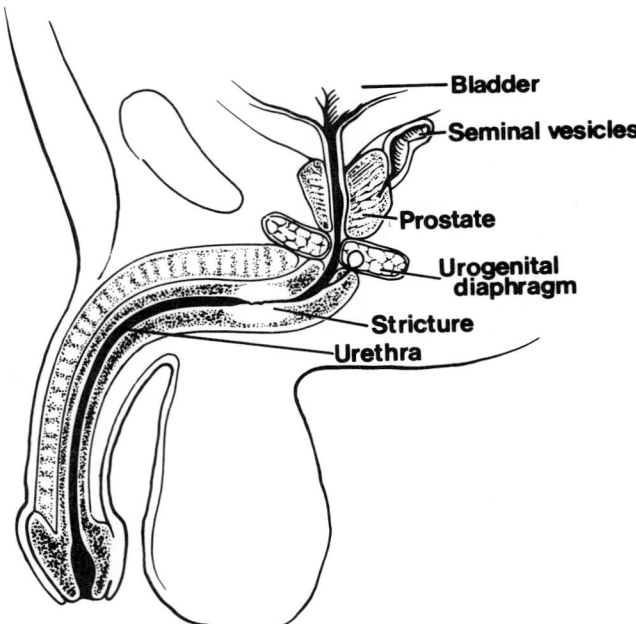

**Fig. 92-11.** Stricture of the bulbous urethra.

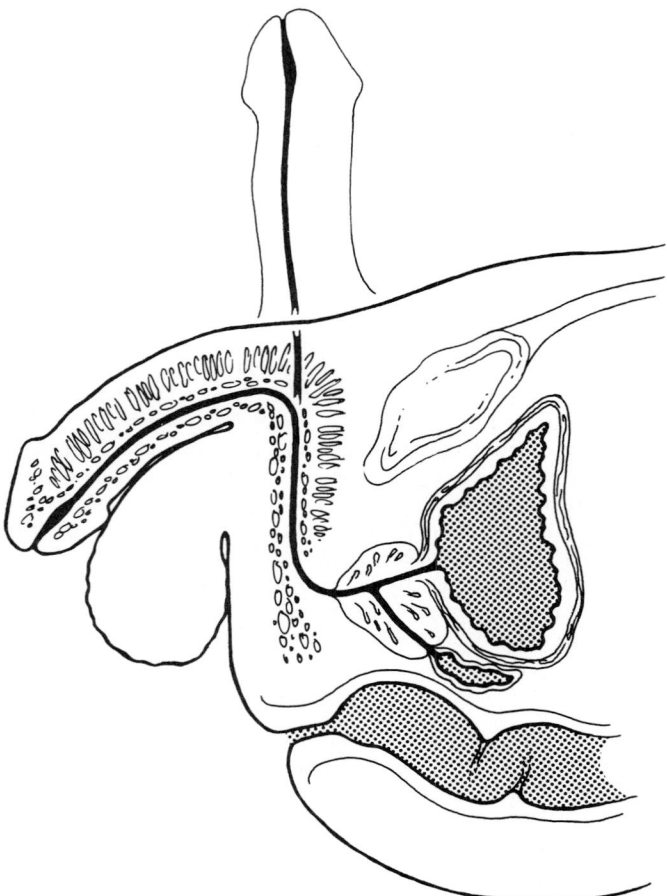

**Figs. 92-12 and 92-13.** Foley catheter placement. Holding the penis upright (Fig. 92-12) will help eliminate urethral folding (Fig. 92-13, *top*) and reduce external sphincter spasm (Fig. 92-13, *bottom*), both of which can impede catheter placement.

ticular tumors can be insidious and must be suspected in any male with unexplained supraclavicular lymphadenopathy, abdominal mass, or chronic nonproductive cough that appears resistant to antibiotic or other supportive therapy. Testicular examination may be diagnostic. While not a urologic emergency, any unexplained testicular mass must be approached as a tumor, with urgent urologic referral.

### Urethra

#### Urethral Stricture

Urethral strictures are becoming more prevalent secondary to the rising incidence of STDs. Increasingly, in teenagers and young adults, gonococcal and chlamydial infections have resulted in bulbous urethral obstruction (Fig. 92-11), while trauma and urethral instrumentation are less common and tend to be localized to areas where a traumatic event has occurred. In the older population, postendoscopy meatal stenosis or localized urethral strictures are more common.

If a patient requires measurement of his residual urine, has difficulty voiding, or is in urinary retention, and a 14F or 16F Foley or Coudé catheter cannot be easily placed into the bladder, the differential diagnostic possibilities include urethral stricture, voluntary external sphincter spasm, bladder neck contracture, or BPH. If time permits, retrograde urethrography can be done and will define the location and extent of a urethral stricture. Only endoscopy can confirm a bladder neck contracture or the extent of an obstructing prostate gland. Suspected voluntary external sphincter spasm can be overcome by holding the penis upright and encouraging the patient to relax his perineum and breathe slowly during the procedure (Figs. 92-12 and 92-13).

When a urethral stricture is encountered, copious anesthetic lubrication (Anestacon) is placed intraurethrally after the foreskin has been controlled with a folded 4 × 4. This latter maneuver is especially important in uncircumcised patients (Fig. 92-14 and 92-15). A 12F or 14F Coudé catheter may negotiate the strictured area, since this

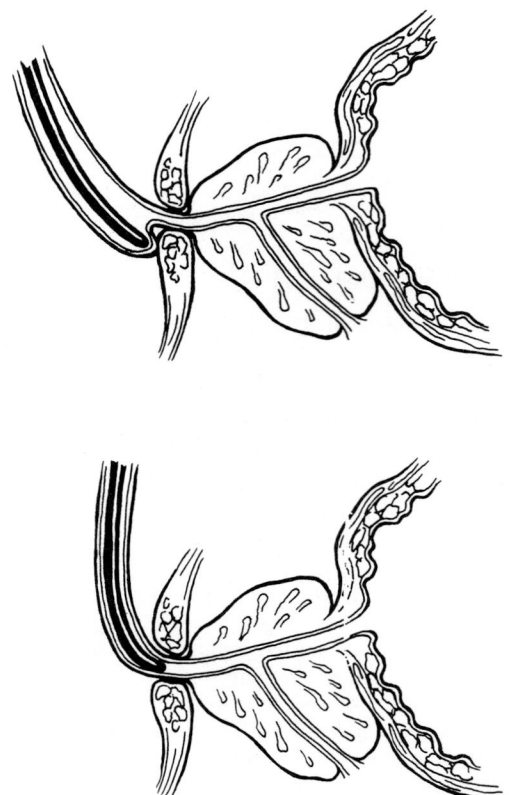

**Fig. 92-13.** (See legend to Fig. 92-12.)

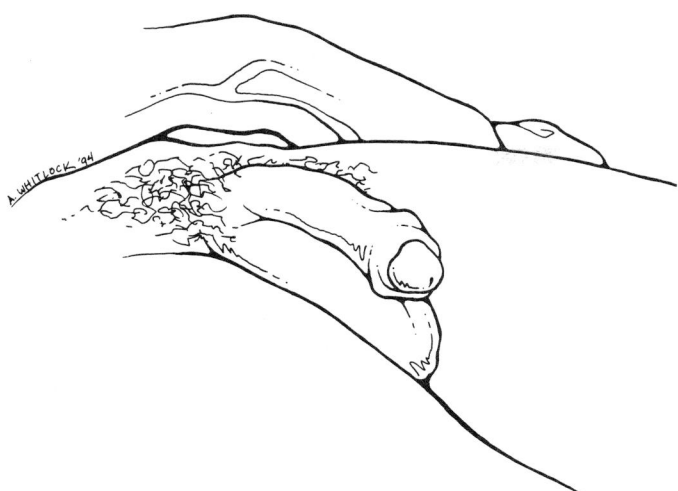

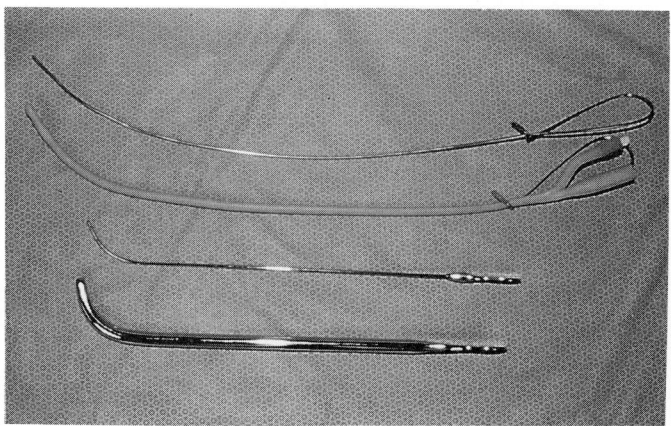

**Fig. 92-17.** Catheter guides and urethral sounds should only be used by a urologist.

**Figs. 92-14, 92-15, 92-16.** Foley catheter placement. Improper foreskin retraction and immobilization leads to difficulty with catheterization. The uncircumsized patient's (Fig. 92-14) foreskin should be fully retracted and immobilized with a folded 4 × 4 (Fig. 92-15) to allow passage of a straight (Fig. 92-16, *bottom*) or a Coudé (Fig. 92-16, *top*) catheter.

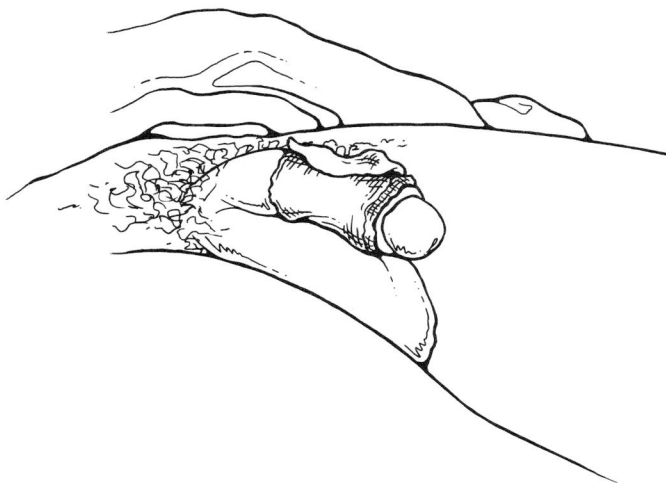

**Fig. 92-15.** (See legend to Fig. 92-14.)

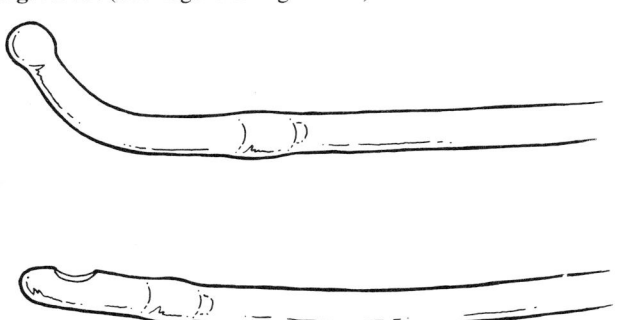

**Fig. 92-16.** (See legend to Fig. 92-14.)

catheter has an angled bend near its tip (Fig. 92-16). If there are previous false passages from attempts at dilation or unsuccessful instrumentation, passage of the Coudé catheter may be difficult. Further urethral manipulation may create new false passages, leading to unnecessary hemorrhage and possible gram-negative bacteremia. If two or three gentle attempts to pass the catheter fail, urologic consultation

is indicated. Under no circumstance should a catheter guide or urethral sound be used by anyone other than a urologist (Fig. 92-17).

In an emergency situation, suprapubic cystostomy, utilizing the Seldinger technique, can be performed with the least amount of morbidity. The infraumbilical and suprapubic area is prepped with povidone-iodine (Betadine) solution. A 25- to 27-gauge spinal needle is used to locate the bladder (Fig. 92-18). This step is especially important in cases of previous lower abdominal surgery where normal anatomic relationships may be distorted. The Cook peel-away introducer cystostomy kits are readily available and utilize the Seldinger technique, which allows easy access to the bladder with a balloon catheter for temporary drainage. After the bladder has been accessed with a syringe and needle (Fig. 92-18), the syringe is removed and a guidewire is passed through the needle into the bladder (Fig. 92-19). The needle is then removed and the fascial dilator with an overlying 14F to 18F peel away sheath is passed over the wire into the bladder (Fig. 92-20). The wire and dilator are then removed leaving the hollow peel-away sheath (Fig. 92-21). An appropriate-sized Foley balloon catheter is passed through the peel-away sheath into the bladder, urine is aspirated from the catheter to assure proper placement, and the balloon is inflated with 10 mL of water (Fig. 92-22 and 92-23). The sheath is then removed from the bladder and peeled away leaving the indwelling catheter, which should be withdrawn until it snugly approximates the cystostomy site (Figs. 92-24 and 25). Appropriate urologic follow up is necessary in 2 to 3 days.

## Urethral Foreign Bodies

Patients of all ages, but especially young children, may be victims of innocent urethral exploration or attempts to heighten sexual experiences utilizing a variety of foreign bodies such as bobby pins; long, thin paint brushes; or ball point pens. Bloody urine combined with infection and slow, painful urination should suggest a possible foreign body in the lower urinary tract. An x-ray of the bladder and urethral areas may disclose the presence of a foreign body.

Foreign bodies often require endoscopic removal or even open cystotomy. Occasionally a gentle milking action of the proximal end of the urethral foreign body by an experienced examiner will allow its retrieval from the distal urethral meatus. Even then, retrograde urethrography or endoscopic confirmation of an intact, nontraumatized urethra is indicated.

## Urinary Retention

Obstructive uropathy causes a wide expanse of signs and symptoms. Overt urinary retention represents one end of the spectrum, while symptoms of insidious overflow incontinence will often fool an unsuspecting examiner. Prior to acquiring a detailed genitourinary his-

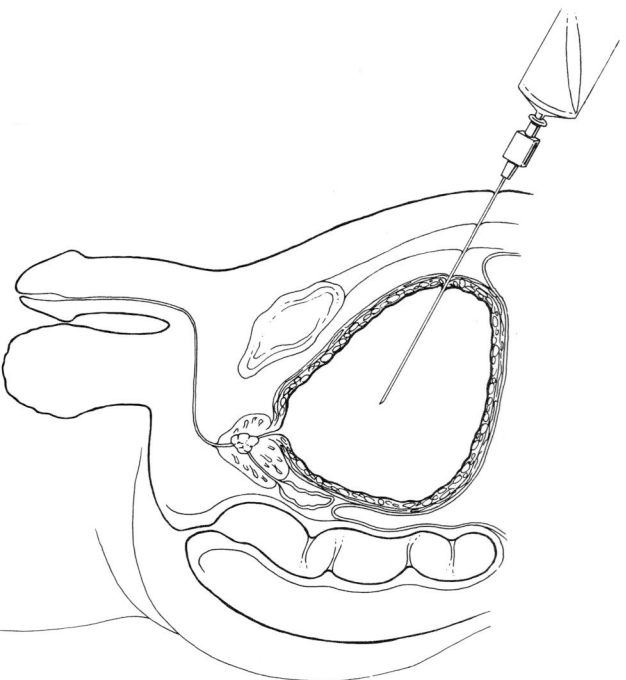

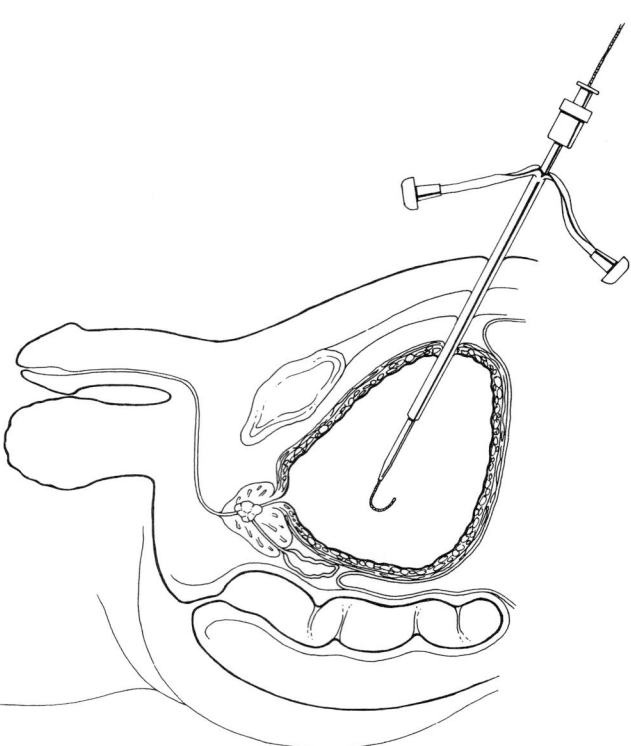

**Figs. 92-18 through Fig. 92-25.** Suprapubic cystostomy. Bladder position is verified with a syringe and needle (Fig. 92-18). Guidewire is passed through the needle (Fig. 92-19) into the bladder. Needle is removed and fascial dilator with overlying peel-away sheath is passed over guidewire into the bladder (Fig. 92-20). Guidewire and dilator are removed (Fig. 92-21). Balloon-tipped catheter is passed through the peel-away sheath (Fig. 92-22). Aspiration of urine assures bladder placement, then balloon is inflated (Fig. 92-23), sheath is pulled up out of the bladder and peeled away (Fig. 92-24). Catheter is withdrawn to assure apposition of Foley balloon to cystostomy site (Fig. 92-25).

**Fig. 92-20.** (See legend to Fig. 92-18.)

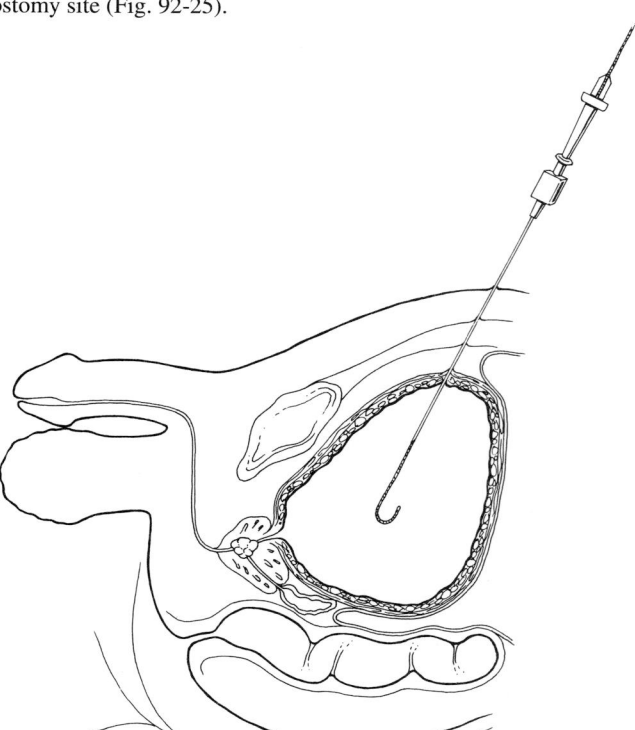

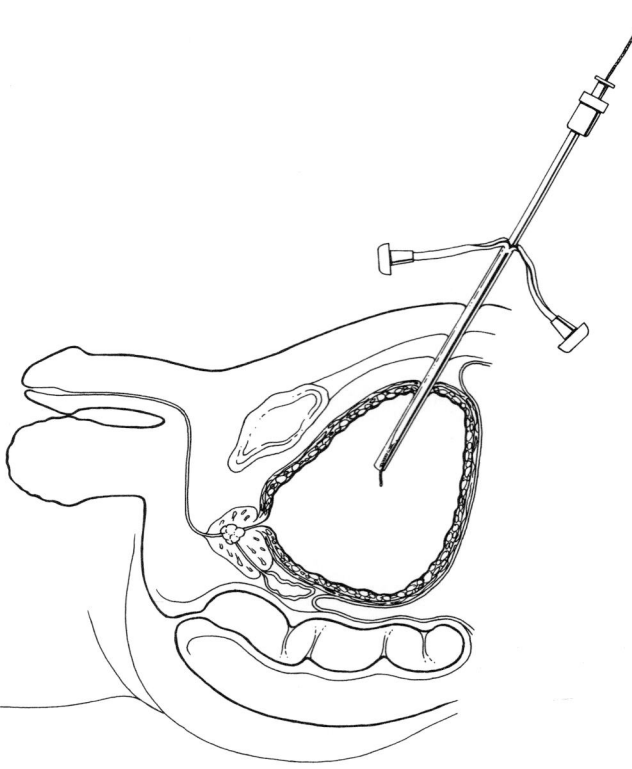

**Fig. 92-21.** (See legend to Fig. 92-18.)

**Fig. 92-19.** (See legend to Fig. 92-18.)

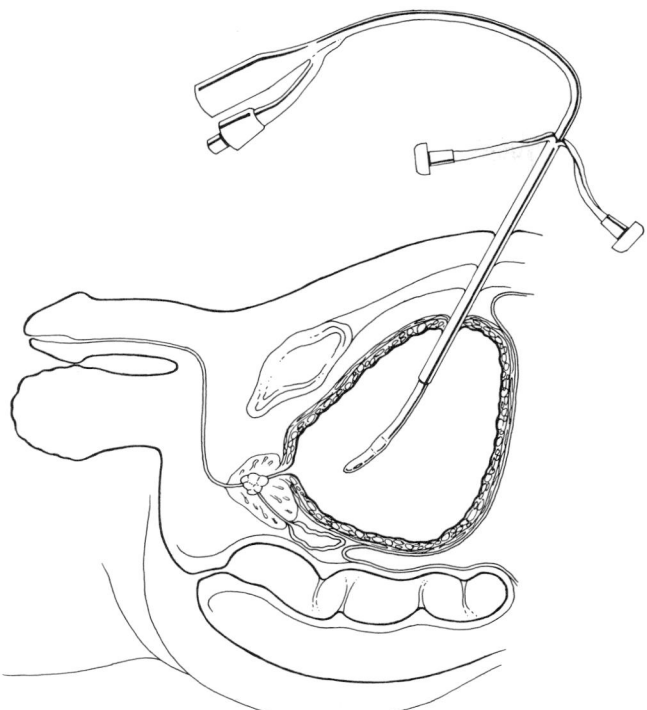

**Fig. 92-22.** (See legend to Fig. 92-18.)

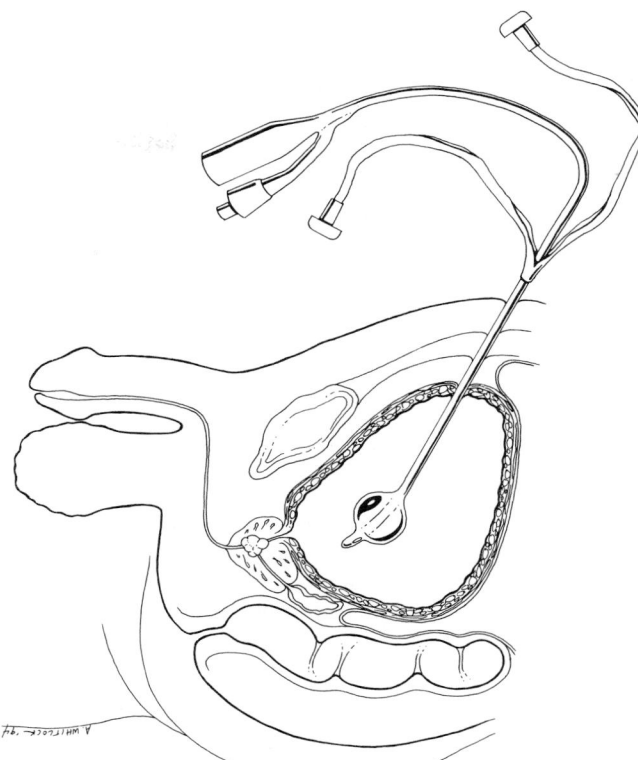

**Fig. 92-24.** (See legend to Fig. 92-18.)

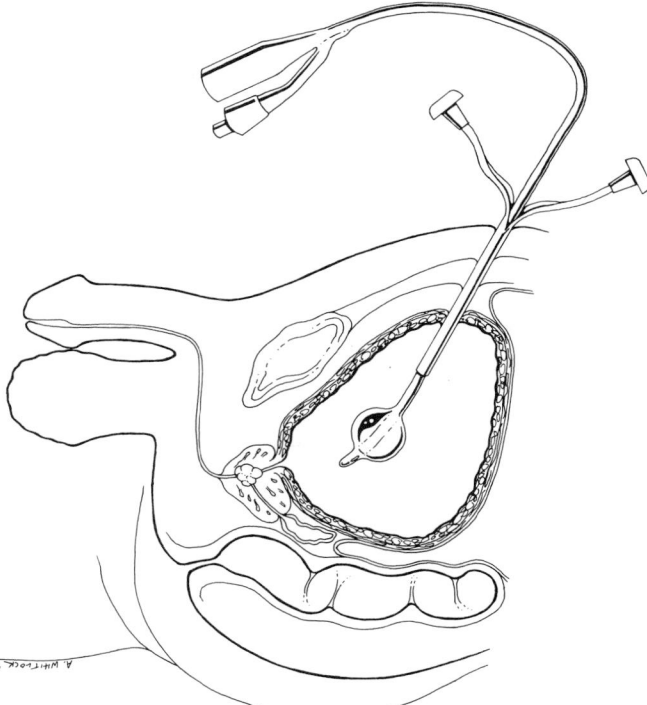

**Fig. 92-23.** (See legend to Fig. 92-18.)

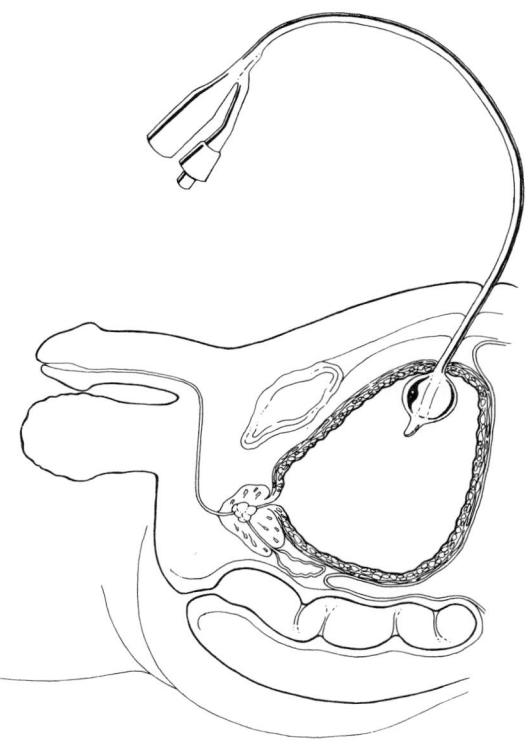

**Fig. 92-25.** (See legend to Fig. 92-18.)

tory, questions regarding chronic systemic medical illnesses or carcinomas that have as sequelae sensory or motor neurogenic side effects or complications must be addressed. A detailed medication history, including over-the-counter cold and dietary medications, will often reveal the ingestion of a sympathomimetic agonist that has secondarily caused outlet obstruction due to its muscle-constricting effect on the abundant fibers in the bladder neck. Inconvenient, and therefore infrequent, voiding during a prolonged car trip by a vacationing pa-

tient with borderline obstructive symptoms may be just enough to result in urinary retention.

A thorough voiding history begins with questions regarding problems holding or initiating the urinary stream, voiding completely with one continuous stream rather than starting and stopping of the stream, a feeling of complete bladder emptying as opposed to incomplete emptying and postvoid residual, and the relative frequency of nocturia. Most men do not void as well or completely empty their bladders when sitting down to urinate, which happens most often during the night. Infrequent ejaculation may lead to secondary prostatic congestion and subsequent spurious symptoms of irritation and outlet obstruction. Unless specific questions are asked about the latter circumstances, these easily treatable causes of obstructive symptoms can be missed.

The most difficult evaluation involves the patient with silent prostatism. Historically, voiding symptoms have gradually worsened over the years, but at such a pace that the patient often makes adjustments and then perceives each worsening state as "normal" for him. The ultimate result is retention, with a large palpable bladder and often 1600 to 2000 mL residual urine. An intact sensory examination, anal sphincter, and bulbocavernosus reflex differentiate chronic outlet obstruction from the sensory or motor neurogenic bladder and spinal cord compression.

Intraurethral causes of urinary retention are the same as those of outlet obstruction (Table 92-4). Appropriate physical examination requires inspection of the meatus for stenosis, palpation of the entire urethral length for masses or fistulas consistent with urethral stricture disease or abscess formation, lower abdominal examination for palpation of a suprapubic mass, and rectal examination to evaluate anal sphincter tone and the size and consistency of the prostate. Outlet obstruction due to a large intravesical prostate can result in a palpably normal prostate on rectal examination. Similarly, rectal examination in a patient in urinary retention may initially reveal a spuriously enlarged, nodular prostate that will shrink considerably once bladder decompression is achieved.

Most patients with bladder outlet obstruction are in distress, and passage of a urethral catheter alleviates both their pain and their urinary retention. Copious intraurethral lubrication must be used, and if attempts at passage of a straight 16F Foley catheter fail, a 16F Coudé catheter should be passed. Be certain to pass either catheter to its fullest extent, obtaining a free flow of urine, and only then inflate the catheter balloon. This will prevent balloon inflation in the prostatic urethra. If the catheter drainage holes become obstructed with lubricating jelly, gentle irrigation with sterile saline or water will quickly establish urinary drainage. Spontaneous, complete drainage of a distended bladder can be accomplished rapidly without the need for repeated clamping of the catheter. Occasionally, when a bladder has been chronically distended, bladder mucosal edema develops. Rapid decompression following catheter placement may result in transient gross hematuria. The transient hematuria is usually self-limited, of little consequence, and responds to orally induced diuresis. Postmicturitional or bladder decompression syncope is rare and should be treated symptomatically.

The catheter should be left indwelling and connected to a portable leg drainage bag. The patient or his family must be instructed in the care and drainage of this simple device. Belladonna and opium (B and O) suppositories, one every 4 to 6 h, can be prescribed to alleviate the constant urge to urinate secondary to bladder spasm, which frequently accompanies an indwelling catheter. The initiation of antibiotic therapy depends on the presence or absence of infected urine and on how long the catheter will be left indwelling. Since infection tends to be universal after 5 to 7 days of permanent drainage, appropriate antibiotic therapy should be started when the catheter is inserted. Trimethoprim alone without sulfa (Trimpex or Proloprim) is a good choice, 100-mg tablets once or twice daily. The patient or a family member should be instructed on Foley balloon deflation, should it become necessary to remove the catheter.

If urinary retention has been chronic or insidious, postobstructive diuresis may occur secondary to osmotic diuresis or interstitial tubular dysfunction. Postobstructive diuresis may occur in the presence of normal BUN and creatinine levels and may become an emergency if the patient suddenly becomes hypovolemic or hypotensive without warning. Thus, close monitoring of urine output is essential, with appropriate fluid replacement. For these reasons, all patients with chronic or insidious obstructive voiding symptoms and urinary retention should either be observed for 4 to 6 h or be admitted, with particular attention paid to hourly intake, urinary output, vital signs, and urine and serum electrolytes. Osmotic diuresis will dissipate or the dysfunctional tubules will recover within 24 to 48 h. In all cases of urinary retention, consultation and follow-up with a urologist for a complete genitourinary evaluation are necessary.

## BIBLIOGRAPHY

Bertram RA, Webster GD, Carson CC: Priapism: Etiology, treatment and results in series of 35 presentations. *Urology* 26:229, 1985.

Caldamone AA, Valvo JR, Altebarmakian VA, et al: Acute scrotal swelling in children. *J Pediatr Surg* 19:581, 1984.

Cattolica EV: Preoperative manual detorsion of the torsed spermatic cord. *J Urol* 133:803, 1985.

Clayton MD, Fowler JE, Sharifi R, et al: Causes, presentation and survival of fifty-seven patients with necrotizing fasciitis of the male genitalia. *Surg Gynecol Obstet* 70:49, 1990.

Coldiron B, Jacobson C: Common penile lesions. *Urol Clin North Am* 15(4):671, 1988.

Docimo SG, Rukstalis DB, Rukstalis MR, et al: Candida epididymitis: Newly recognized opportunistic epididymal infection. *Urology* 41:280, 1993.

Ganti SU, Sayegh N, Addonizio JC: Simple method for reduction of paraphimosis. *Urology Urotech* 26, 1986.

Likitnukul S, McCraken GH, Nelson JD, et al: Epididymitis in children and adolescents. *Am J Dis Child* 141:41, 1987.

Lindsey D, Stanisic TH: Diagnosis and management of testicular torsion: Pitfalls and perils. *Am J Emerg Med* 6:42, 1988.

Melekos MD, Hans WA, Markou SA: Etiology of acute scrotum in 100 boys with regard to age distribution. *J Urol* 139:1023, 1988.

Muschat M: The pathological anatomy of testicular torsion: An explanation of its mechanism. *Surg Gynecol Obstet* 54(5):758, 1932.

O'Brien WM: Percutaneous placement of a suprapubic tube with peel away sheath introducer. *J Urol* 145:1015, 1991.

O'Brien WM, O'Connor KP, Lynch JH: Priapism: Current concepts. *Ann Emerg Med* 18:980, 1989.

Puyor JL, Watson LR, Day DL, et al: Scrotal ultrasound for evaluation of subacute testicular torsion: Sonographic findings and adverse clinical implications. *J Urol* 151:693, 1994.

Schanta TR, Finnerty DP, Rodriguez AP: Treatment of persistent penile erection and priapism using terbutaline. *J Urol* 141:1427, 1989.

**Table 92-4.** Etiology of Outlet Obstruction

Meatal stenosis
Urethral stricture
Bladder neck contracture
Benign prostatic hyperplasia

# 93
# THE RENAL TRANSPLANT PATIENT

### Leslie Rocher
### Warren Kupin

## INTRODUCTION

Over 250 centers currently perform renal transplants, with multiorgan transplantation being performed at approximately 150 centers. In 1993, 15,283 patients received cadaveric organ transplants: 8168 kidney, 3406 liver, 2289 heart, 653 lung, and 767 pancreas allografts. Current 1-year success rates using cyclosporine as the mainstay of the immunosuppression protocol range between 70 and 80 percent for all organs, with heart-lung having the lowest and kidney having the highest survival, respectively.

The immunosuppressive protocols employed in renal transplantation and the potential metabolic and infectious complications encountered are similar to those in other organ transplants. In addition, as a consequence of the total number of renal transplants performed over the past 5 years (45,000) compared to extrarenal transplants (28,000), the probability is high that the emergency physician will encounter a renal rather than an extrarenal transplant recipient. In this chapter we will focus on a review of transplant immunology, the immunosuppressive medications used, recognition and treatment of allograft rejection, posttransplant infectious complications, and evaluation of potential organ donors in the renal transplant recipient.

## EVALUATION OF ORGAN DONORS

The number of potential recipients continues to exceed the organ donor supply. Presently, 25,000 recipients are on the waiting list for a cadaveric kidney transplant. The average waiting time has been increasing steadily and is approximately 520 days for kidneys. Dialysis therapy is available for potential renal transplant recipients, and fewer than 5 percent of potential renal transplant recipients expire prior to transplantation.

The emergency physician can play an important role in the early recognition of potential transplant donors. The most common sources for transplant organs in 1993 included victims of motor vehicle accidents (26 percent) and gun shot wounds (17 percent) and persons with head trauma (11 percent) and cerebrovascular accidents (33 percent). Although the majority of cadaver donors are usually recognized after admission to the intensive care unit (ICU), many potential donors present to the emergency department but do not survive long enough for transfer to the ICU. It has been estimated that with early recognition and initiation of appropriate supportive care, the emergency department has the potential to double the number of current cadaver donors. This number is based on the presentation of critically ill heart-beating patients to the emergency room and may be an underestimation if techniques for harvesting organs from non-heart-beating donors become further refined.

Initially, the primary candidacy of any potential donor is based solely on the establishment of clinical brain death. Fulfillment of the criteria for establishing brain death requires evaluation by a neurologist. The criteria for establishing brain death have been standardized and include cerebral and brainstem unresponsiveness, absent activity on the EEG for approximately 30 min, and a negative blood toxicology for CNS depressant drugs. This latter criteria is essential since drug-induced comatose states may be reversible but can mimic brain death.

The age range of potential organ donors has been expanded to include both younger and older individuals, from 4 to 65 years old. In younger donors, for example, both kidneys may be removed *en bloc* to be transplanted into a single adult recipient, while older donors (> 60 years old) have now become an important resource of cadaveric organs. Results obtained from this donor pool are comparable to organs from younger donors. Do not exclude a potential donor because of age until a complete assessment is made.

Obtaining a comprehensive past medical history is the next essential step in determining the candidacy of a potential donor. Cadaveric donors should have no history of long-standing hypertension or diabetes mellitus, preexisting renal disease, malignancy (except for primary brain tumors), documented systemic infection, or a perforated abdominal viscus. A history obtained from the patient's family or physician should be focused on any known history of intravenous drug abuse or homosexuality. The potential risks of occult HIV infection in these high-risk subgroups exclude them from organ donation even if the HIV test is negative. Slight elevation of the serum creatinine is acceptable if the underlying etiology can be ascribed to volume depletion. A renal biopsy is occasionally performed in selected cases (at the time of donor nephrectomy) to determine the viability of the allograft prior to transplantation.

Most institutions have a coordinator on call for the assessment of potential organ donors. In addition, the responsibility of discussing organ donation with the family is a sensitive issue, and these individuals often assume this role for the physicians. The emergency physician should be acquainted with the local programs available for organ transplantation.

## IMMUNOLOGY OF TRANSPLANTATION

The recipient of a whole-organ allograft is always at risk to reject the transplant and must therefore maintain immunosuppression indefinitely. For the renal transplant recipient, immunosuppression is maintained as long as a renal allograft continues to function, because dialysis may serve as an extended treatment of end-stage renal failure if the transplant fails.

There are three major types of rejection observed in whole-organ transplantation: hyperacute, acute, and chronic. Although *hyperacute rejection* carries the highest risk of fulminant graft loss within the first 48-h posttransplant, its appearance seems to be applicable uniquely to renal transplantation, as compared to transplantation of other solid organs. This form of rejection is mediated either by preformed antibodies to human leukocyte antigens (HLA) in the host directed to the donor HLA antigens or by transplantation across different incompatible blood groups. Blood group antibodies are present from birth, whereas HLA antibodies do not normally exist but are acquired as a consequence of previous blood transfusions or pregnancies. Hyperacute rejection may be prevented by avoiding ABO-incompatible donor-recipient transplant matches and by performing a pretransplant crossmatch to detect the presence of HLA antibodies. The crossmatch involves mixing patient serum with donor lymph nodes to determine if lympholytic antibodies are present in the potential recipient. A positive crossmatch precludes renal transplantation, but exceptions may be made in liver and heart transplants. If hyperacute rejection occurs, it does so within a few minutes to hours after surgery and causes irreversible allograft destruction. Hyperacute rejection now complicates fewer than 0.5 percent of organ transplants as a result of the use of sensitive crossmatch techniques.

*Acute rejection* is the most common form of rejection. It typically develops from 1 week to 3 months after transplant surgery. Acute rejection may also occur after the first posttransplant year if noncompliance with immunosuppression is present. Approximately 25 percent of late graft losses are due to noncompliance. Acute rejection is the result of disparity between donor and host in the major histocompatibility antigen system (HLA) in humans. This system is extremely polymorphic as evidenced by over 100 known HLA antigens. It is, therefore, not generally possible to completely match donor and recipient for these antigens in the case of cadaver donors. The HLA system encodes two classes of cell-surface structures that usually serve to distinguish self from nonself immunologically and also serve to present processed foreign antigen to appropriate host cells to initiate an immune response. The genetic code for these two classes of molecules resides on the short arm of the sixth chromosome. Class I antigens are found on virtually all nucleated cells and are composed of a heavy chain glycoprotein noncovalently linked to $\beta_2$-microglobulin. In clinical practice, relevant class I antigens are termed *HLA-A* and *HLA-B*. Every person codominantly expresses both parental HLA antigens on each cell, or two HLA-A and two HLA-B antigens. Class II antigens are much more restricted in their distribution and are found on B lymphocytes, activated T lymphocytes, macrophages, and cytokine-stimulated endothelial cells and tissue parenchymal cells. Class II antigens are composed of an alpha and a beta glycoprotein chain. In clinical practice the relevant class II antigen system is termed *HLA-DR*. As with class I antigens, each individual codominantly expresses both parentally inherited class II antigens. In general, it is believed that class II antigen disparity is the primary stimulus of the host immune response to an allograft and that class I antigens of donor parenchymal tissue serve as a major target for killer T lymphocytes of host origin.

In current clinical practice, six HLA antigens can be routinely identified (two each at HLA-A, -B, and -DR loci). HLA-C (class I) and HLA-DQ and HLA-DP (class II) antigen loci have been identified, but the individual antigens have been less well characterized and, therefore, these antigens are not used clinically for HLA matching. The more well matched the donor recipient pair for the HLA system, the better the chance of long-term successful engraftment. This is best demonstrated in the renal-transplant recipient who has a mean duration of graft function of 8 years with a cadaver donor (average HLA match, one to two antigens); 10 to 12 years with a semi-identical HLA-matched kidney (as from a parental donor, three of six antigens matched, one haplotype match); and 25 years with an HLA-identical match (HLA-identical sibling, six of six antigens plus two haplotypes matched). The fact that even recipients of HLA-identical sibling kidneys require immunosuppression provides strong argument that other inherited histocompatibility antigen systems, not encoded on the sixth chromosome, are also clinically relevant. Only recipients of grafts from identical twins are spared the need for immunosuppression. Distribution of renal transplants in the United States is based on matching, with the highest priority given to six antigen-matched kidneys. Transfer of renal allografts between states is mandated by law if a perfectly matched recipient is found, due to the superior long-term results of these transplanted organs.

*Chronic rejection* is the least well understood of the three forms of rejection and is characterized by a progressive loss of allograft function with or without the development of marked proteinuria. The degree of HLA matching and the number of early acute-rejection episodes appear to be the most sensitive predictors for the development of this form of rejection. Its course is, however, much more indolent than acute rejection and, once started, is more difficult to interrupt as intervention with short-term intense immunosuppression does not seem to confer benefit.

## CLINICAL PRESENTATION AND THERAPY OF ACUTE REJECTION

Of the three forms of rejection described above, diagnosis and treatment of acute rejection is the most critical. Without timely recognition and intervention, allograft function may deteriorate irreversibly in a few days.

The renal transplant recipient, when symptomatic from acute rejection, will complain of vague tenderness over the allograft (in the left or right iliac fossa, a heterotopic location in contrast to the orthotopic location of liver or heart transplants). The patient also may describe

**Table 93-1.** Causes of Renal Allograft Dysfunction: The Differential Diagnosis of an Elevated Serum Creatinine

Acute rejection
Prerenal azotemia from volume contraction
Drug-induced renal dysfunction
    Cyclosporine
    Trimethoprim-sulfamethoxazole
    Nonsteroidal anti-inflammatory drugs
    Aminoglycosides
Urologic complication
    Ureteral obstruction
    Compression of ureter by lymphocele
    Urine leak
Transplant glomerulonephritis
    Recurrent disease
    De novo glomerulonephritis
Urinary tract infection/pyelonephritis
Systemic infection
    CMV disease
    Sepsis
Vascular complication
    Renal artery stenosis
    Transplant renal vein thrombosis
Chronic rejection

decreased urine output, a rapid weight gain (from fluid retention), a low-grade fever, and a generalized malaise. Physical examination may disclose worsening hypertension, allograft tenderness, and peripheral edema. *The absence of these symptoms and signs, however, does not exclude the possibility of acute rejection.* With improved methods of maintenance immunosuppression (see below), the only clue may be an asymptomatic decline in renal function, as assessed by a rising serum creatinine level. Therefore, even small asymptomatic changes in serum creatinine cannot be dismissed as unimportant and must be investigated. Even a change in creatinine from 1.0 mg/dL to 1.2 or 1.3 mg/dL may be important. When such changes in creatinine are reproducible, a careful workup consists of a complete urinalysis, a renal ultrasonography, and a trough level of cyclosporine, in addition to a careful history and examination. It is critical to interpret changes in renal function in the context of prior data (e.g., trends of recent serum creatinine levels, recent history of rejection, or other causes of allograft dysfunction). The evaluation should proceed in a manner to consider the multiple etiologies of decreased renal function in the renal transplant recipient as outlined in Table 93-1. The two most common causes, apart from acute rejection causing an increase in creatinine, are volume contraction and cyclosporine-induced nephrotoxicity.

Treatment of allograft rejection generally is divided into two phases. The first is high-dose glucocorticoids, typically methylprednisolone 250 to 500 mg intravenously, for 3 to 4 consecutive days. Occasionally, oral steroids may be increased to 100 to 200 mg per day and rapidly tapered toward maintenance levels. If allograft function remains unimproved or partially improved, a biopsy is often done to assess if rejection is ongoing. If ongoing rejection is documented, second phase therapy is initiated with antibody preparations directed toward lymphocytes, most commonly with OKT3, a murine monoclonal antibody directed to the CD3 receptor present on all circulating T lymphocytes. Such therapy is highly immunosuppressive and has multiple potential toxicities, including fever, pulmonary edema, hypotension, diarrhea, headache, and aseptic meningitis. It is, therefore, undertaken only after adequate exclusion of other causes of persistent allograft dysfunction and with careful monitoring under rigorous protocols defined by the transplant service at each institution.

## MAINTENANCE IMMUNOSUPPRESSION

Not all patients experience episodes of acute allograft rejection as discussed above. Oral daily maintenance of immunosuppression is used to prevent such episodes and to mitigate emergence of chronic rejection. Patients are instructed to remain absolutely rigorous and faithful in dosing of these medications. Interruption of maintenance immunosuppression for even one day may be sufficient to induce an episode of acute rejection. Currently, three drugs are used as maintenance immunosuppression: cyclosporine, azathioprine, and glucocorticoids. Transplant immunosuppression regimens are administered in a manner analogous to cancer chemotherapy where multiple agents interfering with the rejection cascade at different physiologic sites are used. The backbone agent of all protocols used in solid organ transplantation is either cyclosporine or FK506. In addition, azathioprine and glucocorticoids are routinely added to enhance the degree of immunosuppression and avoid the need for high doses of any single drug. Newer immunosuppressive agents in clinical trials include rapamycin, mycophenolic acid, brequinar sodium, and deoxysperguanidine.

Since FK506 has only recently been approved for use and it resembles cyclosporine in immunologic activity, familiarity with the characteristics of cyclosporine will be applicable to both agents.

Cyclosporine is a cyclic 11-amino acid fungal metabolite introduced into clinical transplantation in the late 1970s and made generally available in 1983. It is a potent inhibitor of T-lymphocyte activity and interferes with the generation of interleukin 2 (IL-2), a necessary factor for propagation of the immune response to the whole-organ allograft. It is highly lipophilic and its metabolism is almost exclusively hepatic through the cytochrome $P_{450}$ system. Typical doses vary substantially but are usually 3 to 6 mg/kg per day as a single dose or in two divided doses. The therapeutic level of cyclosporine is very dependent on the type of assay used and is commonly 75 to 200 ng/mL. Many drugs are known to potentiate the metabolism of cyclosporine and thus to increase to the required dose of the immunosuppressant. Other drugs inhibit its metabolism and therefore may promote high cyclosporine drug levels. Table 93-2 lists some of these drugs. A sudden increase in cyclosporine levels is often accompanied by a decrease in renal function, which is usually hemodynamically mediated and reversible if recognized. A sudden decrease in cyclosporine drug levels may open the door to an episode of acute rejection. It is therefore incumbent on any physician treating a patient receiving cyclosporine to check that any addition or withdrawal of drugs or changes in drug dosages does not potentially affect cyclosporine metabolism. If a drug from Table 93-2 must be added, deleted, or its dosage changed, the patient and the transplant center should be informed of the potential consequences of the maneuver, and a follow-up trough cyclosporine level should be obtained in the near future.

Common side effects of cyclosporine include hypertension, hirsutism, and tremulousness. It may produce hyperkalemia, hypomagnesemia, and hyperuricemia. Attacks of gouty arthritis have been attributed to the drug. Less common are glucose intolerance, gingival hyperplasia, and seizures. The most common serious toxicity of the drug is renal insufficiency; this is a particularly vexing problem in the renal transplant recipient in whom this may be confused with acute rejection. In recipients of heart and liver transplants, the drug has caused end-stage renal failure requiring dialysis or renal transplant. In general, however, cyclosporine nephrotoxicity is a prerenal, vasospastic process that reverses upon lowering of the drug dose. Clearly, a fine line exists between drug-induced renal dysfunction and underimmunosuppression from too low a drug level.

Azathioprine is a derivative of 6-mercaptopurine and interferes with the purine metabolism of rapidly proliferating cells. It is typically given at doses of 1 to 2 mg/kg per day. Its primary toxicity is bone marrow suppression, particularly of neutrophils, but it may also cause anemia and thrombocytopenia. There are no drug levels available in clinical practice, and the white blood cell count is surveyed frequently, with the dose adjusted to avoid neutropenia. The most important drug interaction is with allopurinol, which inhibits xanthine oxidase–mediated degradation of 6-mercaptopurine, thereby dramatically potentiating the effect of azathioprine. There are case reports of profound and prolonged cytopenias after unmonitored use of allopurinol with azathioprine and consequent secondary fatal superinfections.

Glucocorticoids are also an integral part of posttransplant immunosuppression in most patients. The relevant action of glucocorticoids in these patients is mediated by interference with synthesis of IL-1 and IL-6. The numerous toxicities of this class of drugs are recognized widely and include hypertension, glucose intolerance, acne, osteopenia, cataract formation, salt retention, obesity, hyperlipidemia, mood swings, myopathy, impaired wound healing, peptic ulcer disease, alopecia, and a dampened febrile response to infection. Typical maintenance doses 3 months after surgery are 10 to 20 mg/day. Occasionally, alternate-day prednisone or even steroid withdrawal may be prescribed in well-matched donor-recipient pairs. It is hoped that, with the introduction of more potent alternatives to currently available immunosuppression, routine use of steroids may be avoided in the future.

The sum effect of maintenance immunosuppression used in the prevention of allograft rejection and intermittent high-dose immunosuppression used to treat acute rejection is a variable depression in cell-mediated immunity and a consequent increase in the risk of opportunistic infections. It is also believed that the vigor of immunosuppression is proportionally associated with an increased risk of malignancy.

## POSTTRANSPLANT INFECTIOUS COMPLICATIONS

Infections after transplantation are a common and feared complication. Predisposing factors include ongoing immunosuppression in all patients and the presence of diabetes mellitus, advanced age, obesity, and other host factors in some. Table 93-3 displays the broad array of potential infections stratified by the time after transplant they are most apt to occur.

Prophylaxis of infections is becoming an increasingly important part of transplant protocols. Pretransplant patients are generally vaccinated with pneumococcal vaccine and often with hepatitis B vaccine. Post transplant, most recipients receive trimethoprim-sulfamethoxazole for up to 12 months after surgery to minimize the risk of *Pneumocystis carinii* pneumonia and urinary tract infections. Several protocols exist using either acyclovir, ganciclovir, or immune globulin to minimize the risk of cytomegalovirus infection, depending on patient risk factors and specific transplant center preferences. Nystatin is frequently prescribed during the early transplant period, when glucocorticoid doses are at their highest, to prevent oral candidiasis. Prophylaxis for dental procedures is also prescribed. It should be recognized that some vaccines are contraindicated in the posttransplant period because live attenuated viruses still are potentially too virulent in this population. Such vaccines include the oral poliovirus vaccine and measles, mumps, and rubella vaccines.

The most common life-threatening infection in recipients of solid organs, and even more so in the case of bone marrow graft recipients,

**Table 93-2.** Cyclosporine (CsA) Drug Interactions

Drugs augmenting CsA metabolism (dropping CsA levels)
   Phenobarbital
   Phenytoin
   Rifampin
   Isoniazid
Drugs interfering with CsA metabolism (increasing CsA levels)
   Ketoconazole
   Verapamil
   Diltiazem
   Fluconazole
   Erythromycin
   Cimetidine

**Table 93-3.** Infectious Complications of Whole-Organ
Transplantation

FIRST MONTH POSTTRANSPLANT

*Bacterial*
Wound infection
Pneumonia
Urinary tract infection
Line-related sepsis
*Viral*
Herpes simplex
*Fungal*
Candidal pharyngitis, esophagitis, cystitis

SECOND TO SIXTH MONTHS POSTTRANSPLANT

*Bacterial*
Pneumonia: pneumococcal and other community acquired pneumonitis
Urinary tract infection
Nocardial infection
Listeriosis
*Viral*
Cytomegalovirus, EBV, HSV, varicella zoster
Adenovirus
Hepatitis A, B, C
Papovavirus
*Fungal*
Aspergillosis
Candidal pharyngitis, esophagitis, cystitis
*Other opportunistic infection*
*Pneumocystis carinii* pneumonia, tuberculosis, toxoplasma

BEYOND SIXTH MONTH POSTTRANSPLANT

*Bacterial*
Pneumonia: pneumococcal and other community acquired pneumonitis
Urinary tract infection
Listeriosis
*Viral*
Cytomegalovirus chorioretinitis
Varicella zoster
Hepatitis C, B
*Fungal*
Cryptococcal
*Other opportunistic infection*
*Pneumocystis carinii* pneumonia

is cytomegalovirus (CMV). Exposure to this double-stranded DNA herpes virus is very common; most people over the age of 35 exhibit detectable IgG antibody to CMV antibody levels. After initial infection of a nonimmunocompromised patient, the virus enters a latent phase and is present in virtually all organs. Hence, an allografted kidney, heart, or liver may transmit the virus. In a transplant recipient without prior CMV immunity, receipt of an organ from a serologically positive donor makes the risk of a primary CMV infection high. This infection may manifest with daily fever and malaise in its mildest form. Progressively more serious disease manifestations include leukopenia, hepatopathy (elevated transaminase enzymes), enteropathy (epigastric pain and diarrhea), and pneumonitis. The mortality associated with CMV pneumonitis exceeds 50 percent. CMV infection occurs most commonly 4 to 12 weeks after transplant surgery. Thus a patient presenting with a febrile illness at that time should have as part of their assessment a complete blood count, chest x-ray, and measurement of liver function tests. Serologic conversion to detectable anti-CMV IgG antibody levels and detectable anti-CMV IgM antibody levels occurs well after the initial presentation and is not immediately helpful in the emergency room setting. During active CMV infection, immunosuppression is maintained at the minimum possible level, and if liver, gut, or pulmonary involvement is documented, intravenous ganciclovir therapy, often in conjunction with immune globulin, is prescribed.

The initial presentation of a potentially life-threatening infectious illness may be quite subtle in transplant recipients. The transplant recipient receiving glucocorticoids may not mount an impressive febrile response. A nonproductive cough with little or no findings on physical examination may be the only clue to emerging *P. carinii* pneumonia or CMV pneumonia. The threshold for obtaining chest x-rays in the evaluation of these patients should be quite low. Central nervous system (CNS) infections are much more common in transplant recipients than other patients. Common etiologies include *Listeria monocytogenes* and cryptococci. Therefore complaints of recurrent headaches with or without fever should be investigated vigorously, first with a structural study to exclude a mass lesion (CNS lymphomas occur with increased frequency, too) and then with a lumbar puncture. Finally, a significant subset of renal-transplant recipients have undergone intentional splenectomy in an effort to improve allograft survival. While this procedure is no longer routinely practiced, these patients, as in other postsplenectomy patients, are at particularly high risk for overwhelming sepsis due to encapsulated bacteria such as the pneumococci or meningococci. Appropriate vaccines are critical in this subpopulation.

## NONINFECTIOUS COMPLICATIONS OF RENAL TRANSPLANTATION

The list of potential noninfectious complications after organ transplantation is imposing, as illustrated in Table 93-4. However, it should be remembered that the quality of life in the vast majority of recipients is very acceptable, and most are able to return to the same level of activity as they had before their organ failure.

Several of the complications listed in Table 93-4 merit discussion. Malignancies may occur in 4 to 6 percent of transplant recipients, depending on the intensity of immunosuppression to which they are

**Table 93-4.** Noninfectious Complications of Renal Transplantation

Malignancy
Cutaneous (squamous cell, basal cell, melanoma)
Lymphoma (B cell and non-B cell, CNS lymphoma)
Cervical and uterine carcinoma, Kaposi's sarcoma, carcinoma of retained native kidneys
Cardiovascular
Hypertension
Ongoing/accelerated atherosclerosis (prominent in diabetics)
Transplant renal artery stenosis
Musculoskeletal
Aseptic necrosis (particularly of femoral head and knees)
Idiopathic polyarthralgia syndrome
Osteopenia
Gout
Electrolyte
Hypercalcemia, hyperkalemia, renal tubular acidosis, hypomagnesemia, hyperuricemia
Endocrine/Metabolic
Glucose intolerance
Hyperlipidemia
Hematologic
Post transplant erythrocytosis, anemia, thrombocytopenia, leukopenia
Genitourinary
Reflux, impotence, sexual dysfunction
Nervous system
Pseudotumor cerebri, CNS lymphoma, neuropathy
Gastrointestinal
Pancreatitis, peptic ulcer disease, diverticulitis, fecal impaction, ileus, hepatitis (non-infectious)
Immune
Recurrent glomerulonephritis, de novo glomerulonephritis
Psychiatric
Depression, mania
Other
Recurrence of original disease

subjected. Lymphomas comprise the second most frequent form of malignancy secondary to chronic immunosuppression. These cancers are primarily B cell in origin and related directly to Epstein-Barr virus reactivation. Isolated CNS disease or small bowel involvement is common, and so lymphoma should be considered in the differential diagnosis of a transplant patient with new onset of seizures or bowel obstruction. In the cyclosporine era, posttransplant lymphomas often occur within the first postoperative year, which is significantly earlier than expected compared to the past use of noncyclosporine regimens. Careful monitoring with routine skin, node, breast, and prostate examinations, Papanicolaou smears, mammograms, sigmoidoscopy, and chest x-rays are warranted. Patients are advised to use sun screens. Smoking should be particularly discouraged.

Cardiovascular complications may result from immunosuppression as well as from usual risk factors, as in the hyperlipidemic diabetic renal transplant recipient.

Aseptic necrosis of the hips and knees is most common in renal transplant recipients who have had lengthy therapy with glucocorticoids and who also had secondary hyperparathyroidism associated with chronic renal failure before transplantation. The presentation of aseptic necrosis of the hips often shows referred pain to the knees or to the medial thigh. An MRI scan is the most sensitive roentgenographic study for this lesion.

Finally, the individual with systemic illness, such as diabetes mellitus or autoimmune disease, is at greater risk of progression or recurrence of underlying disease activity despite a renal transplant and its attendant immunosuppression.

## BIBLIOGRAPHY

Braun WE: Long-term complications of renal transplantation. *Kidney Int* 37:1363, 1990.

Carpenter CB: Immunosuppression in organ transplantation. *N Engl J Med* 322:1224, 1990.

Cerilli GJ: *Organ Transplantation and Replacement.* Philadelphia, Lippincott, 1988.

Flye MW: *Principles of Organ Transplantation.* Philadelphia, Saunders, 1989.

Morris PJ: *Kidney Transplantation: Principles and Practice, 2d ed.* New York, Grune & Stratton, 1984.

Rocher LL: Approach to the patient with renal transplant, in Kelley WN (ed): *Textbook of Internal Medicine.* Philadelphia, Lippincott, 1989.

Terasaki PI: *Clinical Transplants 1988.* California, The Regents of the University of California, 1988.

Williams GM, Burdick JF, Solez K: *Kidney Transplant Rejection: Diagnosis and Treatment.* New York, Marcel Dekker, 1986.

# 94
# EMERGENCIES IN CHRONIC DIALYSIS PATIENTS
## K. Venkateswara Rao

Patients with chronic progressive renal failure are treated initially with diet and medications. In the later stages they are supported by intermittent dialysis (hemodialysis or peritoneal dialysis). The indications for initiation of chronic dialysis are (1) uremic symptoms, even in the absence of high serum urea nitrogen level (e.g., nausea, vomiting, mucosal erosions, increased fatigue, pruritus, and insomnia); (2) uncontrolled hypertension due to salt and water retention; (3) hyperkalemia, requiring the use of ion-exchange resins; (4) fluid overload and congestive heart failure; (5) uremic pericarditis; (6) rapidly progressing uremic peripheral neuropathy; and (7) uremic encephalopathy. Medical emergencies commonly encountered in uremic patients before or after the initiation of dialytic therapy discussed in this chapter include uremic pericarditis, cardiovascular instability, neurologic problems, gastrointestinal disorders, peritonitis, and problems with vascular access.

## UREMIC PERICARDITIS

The classic symptom is chest pain, which is partially relieved by sitting up and leaning forward. A pericardial friction rub may not be heard in all instances or it may be heard intermittently. Low-grade fever and atrial arrhythmias (paroxysmal atrial tachycardia, atrial flutter–atrial fibrillation) are common accompaniments. Echocardiography often demonstrates a pericardial effusion. The pericardial fluid may impede venous return, leading to congestive heart failure and hypotension. The tamponade is relieved by pericardiocentesis. Instillation of glucocorticoids into the pericardial sac after the pericardiocentesis has been recommended to prevent relapses. Regular dialysis at frequent intervals using minimal doses of heparin will reduce the uremic load and aid in the resolution of pericarditis. It is the preferred form of therapy at most dialysis centers. The definitive treatment, however, is the creation of a pericardial window or an anterior pericardiectomy.

## CARDIAC ARRHYTHMIAS AND CARDIAC ARREST

The etiology of cardiac arrhythmias in uremic patients is multifactorial and includes such diverse causes as hyperkalemia, hypocalcemia, hypokalemia, hypermagnesemia, coronary ischemia, metastatic calcification of the cardiac conduction system, and toxic effects of prescribed drugs such as digitalis and quinidine. The most frequent arrhythmia encountered during dialysis is hypokalemia-induced ventricular irritability manifest by premature beats and ventricular fibrillation. This can be prevented by monitoring the patient's serum potassium level and adjusting the potassium concentration in the dialysate solution.

The most common cause of cardiac arrest in uremic patients is hyperkalemia. The treatment should include administration of calcium gluconate, followed by infusion of 50 mL of 50% glucose along with 20 units of regular insulin and infusion of 50 to 100 mEq of IV sodium bicarbonate. Hemo- or peritoneal dialysis using a lower concentration of $K^+$ in the dialysate is the most effective way to reduce the potassium level and should be employed as soon as possible.

## ALTERATIONS IN BLOOD PRESSURE
### Hypertension

In about 90 percent of uremic patients the hypertension is related to excess intravascular volume secondary to salt and water retention. Only a minority of patients (approximately 15 percent) have renin-dependent hypertension. When patients present with hypertensive crisis with encephalopathy or pulmonary edema, the blood pressure should be lowered immediately with an intravenous infusion of sodium nitroprusside and subsequently by removing the excess fluid volume with ultrafiltration dialysis. The usual measures employed in the treatment of pulmonary edema, such as phlebotomy or intravenous diuretics, are not practical in patients with renal failure. Other drugs that can be used to lower the blood pressure acutely are sublingual nifedipine and intravenous hydralazine. In those patients who have renin-dependent hypertension, the use of angiotensin-converting enzyme (ACE) inhibitors such as enalapril or lisinopril has minimized the need for bilateral nephrectomy, which used to be a common practice a decade ago. Calcium channel blockers such as nifedipine or amlodipine are also prescribed for the routine management of hypertension in dialysis patients.

## Hypotension

A sudden drop in blood pressure is a common complication during dialysis and, if not promptly treated, can lead to cardiac arrest. Subjective symptoms such as muscle cramps, nausea, yawning, and mental confusion may precede the actual hypotension in most patients but not in all. Treatment is the rapid infusion of isotonic saline. In rare instances the use of vasopressors may be required.

## NEUROLOGIC PROBLEMS

### Dialysis Disequilibrium

Symptoms of increased intracranial pressure, manifest by nausea, vomiting, headache, and mental confusion, can develop soon after or within a few hours of a dialysis treatment. It is common after the first dialysis but can also occur on a rare occasion even in patients treated with chronic dialysis. The raised intracranial pressure is the result of osmotic shift of fluid from the bloodstream into cerebrospinal fluid (CSF), because of higher CSF urea content relative to plasma. During dialysis, the plasma urea concentration is lowered quickly, but the concentration of urea in the CSF stays high because of the blood-brain barrier. After a few hours, the osmotic gradient between plasma and CSF gets equilibrated, and the symptoms of raised intracranial pressure will gradually resolve.

Diagnosis is based on the history and measurement of BUN levels both before and after the first dialysis. It should be differentiated from other causes of raised intracranial pressure such as subdural hematoma, cerebrovascular accident, and brain tumor. Therapy is purely symptomatic. Reassurance, bed rest, and administration of analgesics and antiemetics will alleviate the symptoms within a few hours. Patients usually return to their normal state of health the next day following dialysis. Dialysis disequilibrium does not occur following peritoneal dialysis because of the slower pace at which the urea is removed from plasma.

### Subdural Hematoma

Both spontaneous and posttraumatic subdural hematomas have been observed in patients treated with chronic hemodialysis. A history of trauma may or may not be elicited, as patients tend to ignore simple events such as a fall from bed or tripping over an object. The risk increases in uremic patients because of the defective platelet function and the use of heparin during dialysis.

Diagnosis is based on the history, alteration in mental status, and computed tomographic (CT) scanner confirmation of a subdural hematoma. Focal neurologic signs (such as dilated pupils, hemiplegia, or monoplegia) may not be present in all cases. The treatment consists of evacuation of the hematoma and relief of the pressure on vital intracranial structures. Preventive measures should include cautious heparinization, adjustment of pro-time levels, and avoidance of falls.

### Other Neurologic Problems

Uremic patients may present to the emergency department with seizures, coma, or mental obtundation. The evaluation should comprise a complete review of the medications; physical examination; measurement of plasma calcium, magnesium, electrolytes, BUN, and blood glucose; and an emergency head CT scan. Therapy is directed at the cause. Most patients require in-hospital management, except in cases of seizures induced by hypoglycemia.

## GASTROINTESTINAL DISORDERS

Upper gastrointestinal bleeding may result from uremic gastritis, peptic ulcer disease, or excess anticoagulation. The management does not differ from that in nonuremic patients. However, caution should be exercised in using large doses of magnesium-containing antacids.

Since magnesium is normally excreted by the kidney, abnormal levels could accumulate in the plasma of the uremic patient, leading to mental obtundation and respiratory depression.

Bowel obstruction symptoms are not uncommon, as the patients are receiving phosphate-binding antacids. The plain abdominal x-ray may demonstrate a nonspecific bowel gas pattern with a large amount of stool in the colon. The treatment measures should include fecal disimpaction, tap water enemas, and oral laxatives such as sorbitol and mineral oil. Phosphate-containing enemas such as Fleet's Phospho-soda (Na biphosphate) should be avoided. Since most of the phosphate-binding antacids [Amphojel, Basaljel (Al carbonate), aLternaGEL (Al hydroxide)] induce bowel constipation, it is a good practice to prescribe a stool softener such as 200 mg of docusate sodium (Colace or Pericolace) daily.

Diverticulitis and bowel perforation are common problems in patients who have polycystic kidney disease. Such patients also have a high incidence of spontaneous intracerebral bleeding following the rupture of a congenital berry aneurysm.

## PROBLEMS PECULIAR TO PERITONEAL DIALYSIS

Peritoneal dialysis is a reasonable alternative to certain individuals who have end-stage renal failure. The ideal patient would be one with a smaller body frame, good eyesight, and the ability to comprehend and follow the sterile technique while connecting the peritoneal bag and the peritoneal catheter. This modality of therapy would also be suitable for elderly patients who have cardiac dysfunction and those who otherwise have to travel several hundred miles to the nearest hemodialysis center.

Because of the lack of need for heparinization and the gentle nature of the dialytic process, the risks of hypotension, subdural hematoma, and dialysis disequilibrium are minimal in patients receiving peritoneal dialysis.

Technical problems such as diminished outflow from the peritoneal cavity can lead to abdominal distension and symptoms of fluid overload. The causes include fibrin thrombi occluding the indwelling trocar, intraabdominal pockets of fluid collection secondary to adhesions from a prior surgical procedure, or distended bowel loops from constipation. The management is directed at the cause. When conservative measures such as changing the body position, use of laxatives, and instillation of heparin into the peritoneal catheter fail, exploratory laparotomy and replacement of the trocar may become necessary.

Infection of the peritoneal membrane is the most frequent and critical complication in patients receiving chronic peritoneal dialysis. The symptoms may be subtle and include abdominal discomfort, pain during inflow, and fever. Physical examination may reveal abdominal tenderness, particularly around the catheter site, and decreased bowel sounds. Laboratory evaluation should include CBC and analysis of peritoneal fluid for cell count, gram stain, protein, culture, and sensitivity. A bag of drained dialysate should be used for culture and analysis. A variety of microorganisms (bacterial, fungal, and parasitic) have been found after culturing the fluid from the peritoneal cavity of dialysis patients. The mainstay of therapy is the infusion of an appropriate antimicrobial agent into the peritoneal cavity. Depending upon the results of gram stain, usually vancomycin 2 gm plus gentamicin 30 to 40 mg or tobramycin 30 to 40 mg are given. To avoid fibrin formation 1000 units of heparin are added to the infusion. Antibiotic administration should be guided by consultation with the nephrologist. In patients who have associated bacteremia, intravenous antibiotics are recommended. The incidence of peritonitis can be reduced by educating the patient on the use of sterile technique while connecting and disconnecting the catheter and proper cleaning of the exit site with an antiseptic solution. If a patient experiences recurrent bouts of peritonitis, tunnel infection, or intraabdominal abscess, the catheter should be changed. Appropriate surgical drainage of intraabdominal abscess is also warranted to prevent relapse.

Other, less critical problems observed in peritoneal dialysis patients are leakage of fluid around the trocar and accidental contamination of the catheter tip prior to its connection with the dialysate bag. A reasonable approach under these circumstances would be to advise the patient to stop further dialysis and have the medical personnel in the dialysis center assess the problem as soon as possible. Stopping the peritoneal dialysis for 1 or 2 days should not have any serious adverse effects.

## PROBLEMS RELATED TO VASCULAR ACCESS

During the past three decades a variety of vascular access devices have been tried to facilitate the flow of blood between the patient and the dialyzer and accomplish the dialytic process. These devices are of two basic types: (1) external shunts and (2) internal shunts. The former category includes (1) a Scribner shunt (two plastic tubes, one in the radial artery and the other in the cephalic vein, connected together on the outside with a Teflon piece); (2) a Thomas shunt (a device similar to the Scribner shunt, but usually placed in the groin, connecting the femoral artery and saphenous vein segments); and (3) Hemasite, a small button-shaped titanium body with a puncturable rubber septum that allows the entry of dialysis needles during the treatment and seals off when the needles are removed. Hemasite access devices are placed either in the upper arm or in the anterior thigh near the groin.

The best of all the internal access shunts is the Brescia-Cimino fistula, in which the radial artery is anastomosed to an adjacent vein. If a patient has inadequate veins, alternative devices such as a bovine heterograft (a specially treated carotid artery segment from the cow) or a Gore-Tex graft (made from a synthetic material) should be tried. These internal grafts are interposed between the artery and the vein in the patient's forearm. Occasionally they are placed in the upper arm.

The most frequent complications associated with the external shunts are clotting and infection. When the shunt is acutely clotted, the vascular surgeon must be notified immediately. Irrigation of the cannula with heparinized saline should be avoided as it may cause the clot to spread and increase the risk of pulmonary or peripheral embolization. Declotting procedures using a Fogarty balloon catheter are normally accomplished by the surgeon in the operating suite. However, in some instances, instillation of urokinase, 5000 to 10,000 units, into the arterial and venous parts of the clotted shunt may dissolve the clot and prevent the need for further intervention.

Infection of the cannula site is a significant problem in the hemodialysis patient. Coagulase-positive staphylococci and *S. epidermidis* are frequently cultured from the exit site. Physical examination may reveal local inflammation, tenderness over the cannula tips, and purulent drainage at the exit sites. Soon after obtaining cultures from the exit site and blood, antibiotics should be given, selecting a drug that is effective against penicillinase-resistant organisms (e.g., oxacillin, vancomycin, or cephalosporins). The most dreaded complications associated with the external shunt infection are septic pulmonary embolism and brisk hemorrhage resulting from dislodgement of the cannula tip. An alternative site for dialysis, such as a Quinton subclavian catheter or peritoneal dialysis, should be considered while the patient is being treated for cannula infection. Clotting and infection are rare in patients with the Brescia-Cimino fistula but common in those with bovine and Gore-Tex fistulas. Other problems encountered with these devices are (1) stricture of the arterial or venous segment leading to poor blood flow and inefficient dialysis; (2) aneurysmal dilatation with the threat of rupture; (3) ischemia of the fingertips from steal syndrome; and (4) prolonged bleeding of the puncture sites. To control the bleeding at the puncture sites, one should apply firm pressure. If pressure is unsuccessful, other measures, such as the placement of topical thrombin and neutralization of excess anticoagulation with protamine sulfate or aqueous vitamin K, should be considered. Aneurysms and strictures require surgical repair by an experienced vascular surgeon. When a bovine or Gore-Tex fistula clots, the declotting procedure should be left to the surgeons in the operating room.

To reduce the incidence of the above complications, patients are instructed to (1) practice good cannula care [cleaning the cannula tips with povidone-iodine (Betadine) and applying a sterile dressing], (2) avoid having any blood drawn from the fistula site, and (3) avoid taking blood pressure measurements on the arm containing the vascular access device. Patients should also be educated to seek emergency care as soon as these problems arise, since life-sustaining dialysis treatment cannot be provided without a functioning vascular access shunt.

## BIBLIOGRAPHY

Comty CM, Shapiro FL: Cardiac complications of regular dialysis therapy, in Drukker W, Parsons FM, Maher JF (eds): *Replacement of Renal Function by Dialysis.* The Hague, Martinus Nijhoff, 1983, pp 596–610.

Giacchino JL, Geis WP, Buckingham JM, et al: Vascular access: Long term results, new techniques. *Arch Surg* 114:403, 1979.

Nolph KD, Bowen FST, Farrell PC, et al: Continuous ambulatory peritoneal dialysis in Australia, Europe and the United States. *Kidney Int* 23:3, 1983.

Vaziri ND: Topical thrombin and control of bleeding from the fistula puncture sites in dialyzed patients. *Nephron* 24:254, 1979.

Wolfe RA, Port FK, Hawthorne VM, et al: A comparison of survival among dialytic therapies of choice: In-center hemodialysis versus continuous ambulatory peritoneal dialysis at home. *Am J Kidney Dis* 15:443, 1990.

# 95
# UROLOGIC STONE DISEASE
## W. F. Peacock, IV

Stones form throughout the urinary tract; however, the most common presentation occurs when renal stones migrate down the ureter. Primary bladder stones are much rarer.

## RENAL AND URETERAL STONES
### Pathophysiology

The precise cause of urinary stone formation is unknown. Stones are three times more common in males, usually in the third to fifth decades. There is an increased incidence from genetic predisposition, and some hereditary diseases (e.g., renal tubular acidosis, hyperparathyroidism, cystinuria) increase the frequency of kidney stones.

Lifestyle factors augment stone growth. Increasing water intake results in a decreased incidence of calculi. Patients in mountainous, desert, or tropical regions, and those in sedentary jobs, suffer a higher frequency of stone disease. There is also an increased incidence during the warmest 3 months of the year for any geographic location.

Theories regarding urinary calculi formation include urinary supersaturation of solute followed by crystal precipitation, or a decrease in the normal urinary proteins inhibiting crystal growth. Urinary stasis from physical anomaly, neurogenic bladder, catheter placement, and the presence of a foreign body (e.g., surgical suture) may provide the environment for urolith growth.

Approximately 75 percent of calculi are composed of calcium, occurring in conjunction with oxalate, phosphate, or a combination of both. This may result from increased urinary excretion of a given solute. Calcium excretion is elevated in conditions such as high dietary calcium intake, immobilization syndrome, or hyperparathyroidism. Oxalate excretion is enhanced in patients with inflammatory bowel disease and as a result of small bowel bypass surgery.

Ten percent of stones are magnesium-ammonium-phosphate (struvite). These are associated with infection by urea-splitting bacteria and are the most common cause of staghorn calculi. Staghorn calculi are large stones—essentially a cast of the renal pelvis. Antibiotics are ineffective in curing "infection stones" as there is poor penetration into the calculus. Uric acid causes 10 percent of uroliths, with cystine, and other infrequent stones, completing the remainder.

The majority (90 percent) of urinary calculi are radiopaque. Calcium phosphate and calcium oxalate stones have a density similar to bone. Magnesium-ammonium-phosphate (struvite) calculi are slightly less radiodense, followed by cystine, which is only partly radiodense. Uric acid and matrix stones are essentially radiolucent.

With acute obstruction, after an initial rise of renal blood flow and intraureteral pressure, both parameters decline. Concurrently, there is a proportional increase in renal blood flow to the contralateral kidney. These effects are reversible in acute unilateral obstruction. After 5 to 14 days of continuous blockage, there is increasing deterioration of ipsilateral renal function. Relief of the obstruction after 8 weeks results in the rapid increase in renal blood flow, with at least a partial reversal of the functional deficits. When the time of obstruction exceeds 16 weeks, only slight functional recovery of the affected kidney is expected. The contralateral kidney is usually able to maintain excretory requirements throughout the course. Therefore, serologic evaluation of renal function (BUN and creatinine) does not demonstrate a discernible adverse effect.

Passage of crystals through the urinary tract may be slowed or halted by areas of anatomic narrowing or bending. Progressing proximal to distal, common areas of impaction include the renal calyx; ureteropelvic junction, where the ureter passes over the pelvic brim and arches over the iliac vessels; and the ureterovesical junction (UVJ). The UVJ has the smallest diameter of the urinary tract and is a common location for impacted stones. The posterior pelvis in women, especially where the ureter is crossed anteriorly by the pelvic blood vessels and broad ligament, may slow the passage of a calculus.

Children under 16 years of age constitute approximately 7 percent of all cases of renal stones. Unique to this age group is a 1:1 sex distribution. The most common etiologies in this age group are metabolic abnormality (50 percent), urologic anomalies (20 percent), infection (15 percent), and immobilization syndrome (5 percent). The remainder are diagnosed as idiopathic.

In patients with a history of a kidney stone, up to a third suffer recurrence within 1 year. This is because the underlying abnormality that created the first stone persists.

## Clinical Features

Uroliths may be asymptomatic until there is at least partial obstruction of the urinary tract. The typical episode occurs while sedentary or at rest. Patients complain of the acute onset of severe pain, which can be associated with diaphoresis, nausea, and emesis. During extreme presentations, the patient is anxious, pacing or writhing, and may be unable to hold still or converse. Symptoms can be remarkably episodic due to intermittent obstruction of the urinary tract. If the stone passes or the obstruction is otherwise relieved, the patient has immediate relief of his or her symptoms.

Typically pain originates in either flank, ipsilaterally radiating anteroinferiorly around the abdomen and toward the ipsilateral testicle or labia majora. The radiating pattern is the result of autonomic nerve fibers serving both the kidney and respective gonad. Atypical pain referral patterns to the hip, thigh, or knee have rarely been reported. As the stone progresses to the midureter, anterior abdominal pain may radiate back toward the flank. With passage to near the bladder, the patient can develop urinary frequency and urgency.

Children may present in similar fashion to adults; however, 20 to 30 percent may have only painless hematuria.

The patient is frequently cool and diaphoretic; fever is unusual. Its presence should prompt a thorough investigation for urinary tract infection, pyelonephritis, or other causes of febrile illness. There are usually elevations of blood pressure and heart rate secondary to extreme discomfort.

A complete physical examination is warranted. Special attention should be given to the abdominal and cardiovascular examinations so that potential catastrophes mimicking acute renal colic are excluded. Rarely, a leaking abdominal aortic aneurysm or incarcerated hernia may be confused with renal colic. A right ureteral stone could resemble cholecystitis. Specifically in males, epididymitis or testicular torsion should be excluded. In females of childbearing age, ectopic pregnancy is a consideration. Mild tenderness may be noted over the site of the impacted stone, but true peritoneal findings suggest an alternative diagnosis. There is frequently pain with fist percussion over the ipsilateral costovertebral angle.

## Diagnosis

### Laboratory Tests

All patients with suspected renal colic require a urinalysis. An initial dipstick is an expedient method to aid in limiting the differential diagnosis. This should always be followed by a complete urinalysis, which usually demonstrates microscopic hematuria. There is no correlation between the amount of hematuria and the degree of urinary tract obstruction. Some patients demonstrate gross hematuria, but in 10 percent urinary blood is absent. While moderate pyuria can occur without infection, urinary pus indicates the need for a thorough investigation to exclude infection. Urinary crystals may indicate the etiology of the present attack, and a urinary pH exceeding 7.6 suggests infection by urea-splitting organisms. An alkaline urine is also seen in renal tubular acidosis or following ingestion of large amounts of alkali.

A complete blood count may demonstrate leukocytosis. This finding may represent demargination, but very high white cell counts can suggest infection.

### Kidney-Ureter-Bladder X-Ray

While the kidney-ureter-bladder (KUB) radiograph can assist in localizing a radiopaque stone, its greatest utility is in the exclusion of other pathologies. It is difficult to determine if a radiopaque body is a phlebolith, represents bowel contents, or is truly an obstruction within the urinary tract on this x-ray. However, the KUB can be helpful in patients with dye allergy, when ultrasound and renal scanning are unavailable, or in follow-up of known radiopaque stones. In some patients the clinical presentation is so typical that a KUB and urinalysis are all that is needed to verify the diagnosis. Oblique films may assist in localizing suspicious calcifications, and tomography may improve the utility of plain films.

### Intravenous Pyelogram (IVP)

The "gold standard" for diagnosis of renal colic is the IVP. It is usually preceded by a scout film to localize stones that might be obscured by the presence of radiocontrast dye. In contradistinction to other diagnostic modalities, the IVP yields information regarding renal function as well as anatomic morphology.

Prior to obtaining an IVP, the patient should be closely questioned regarding the presence of allergy to radiocontrast media. Appropriate materials for managing acute anaphylaxis should be readily available for the unexpected allergic reaction. A history of dye allergy should prompt the selection of an alternative diagnostic modality. "Desensitization" protocols exist but are not sufficiently rapid for use in the emergency department.

In patients at risk for pregnancy, a negative pregnancy test should be obtained before performance of an IVP. To decrease ionizing radiation exposure, pregnant patients and children are preferentially evaluated by diagnostic ultrasound.

Radiocontrast agent nephrotoxicity is most likely in patients with preexisting renal insufficiency or diabetes mellitus. Other predisposing factors may include dehydration, hypovolemia, hypotension, advanced age (>70 years), multiple myeloma, hyperuricemia, hypertension, a history of IV radiocontrast media within 72 h, and those with cardiovascular disease and on diuretics. In patients at risk for this complication, the administration of radiocontrast media should be deferred until normal renal function is assured by the measurement of blood urea nitrogen (BUN) and creatinine. Additionally, maintaining adequate urine output, by the administration of intravenous fluids prior to radiocontrast media, may decrease the risk of renal injury.

While still causing nephrotoxicity, the newer nonionic contrast agents appear to result in a lower frequency of kidney damage. However, because of markedly increased cost, their ultimate use is yet to be defined for urologic stone disease.

When performing the IVP, intravenous fluid is administered to ensure the patient is hydrated and will sustain adequate urinary flow throughout the procedure. In debilitated patients unable to tolerate IV fluids, an alternative diagnostic procedure may be considered. During injection of the contrast media, there is frequently an increase in the pain of ureteral obstruction, as well as nausea, vomiting, or flushing. This should be anticipated and pain medication made available.

After radiocontrast media are administered, an initial scout radiograph is obtained, followed by repeat films at 5, 10, and 20 min. The first, and most reliable, indication of the presence of obstruction is a delay in the appearance of the nephrogram. Adjuncts to diagnosis include distension of the renal pelvis, calyceal distortion, dye extravasation, or hydronephrosis. Since the ureter is a peristaltic structure, it is usually not completely seen on any one radiograph. Visualization of the entire ureter is suggestive of an obstruction. Frequently, the location of a radiolucent obstructing stone can be determined by a ureteral dye column cutoff. Occasionally extravasation of dye is noted. This should be considered evidence of an obstruction that has decompressed into the perinephric tissue. These patients are at risk for the formation of a urinoma.

A postvoiding film is useful to identify stones at the UVJ or distal ureter that are otherwise obscured by a full bladder. Multiple delayed films may not be required diagnostically but can assist in precise location of the obstruction. Additionally, tomograms may aid in obstruction localization.

A falsely negative IVP infrequently occurs when there is a radiolucent, partially obstructing stone. Further diagnostic evaluation, using ultrasound or another modality, should be undertaken when the examination and clinical history are strongly suggestive of renal colic despite a negative IVP.

## Ultrasound (US)

In patients who are not candidates for IVP, US may assist in the diagnosis of ureteral obstruction. US is not a functional test and provides anatomical information only. It is useful in the detection of hydronephrosis and larger stones; however, it may miss smaller (<5 mm) ureteral stones. US is helpful in diagnosing obstruction and localizing stones in the proximal and distal aspects of the ureter. Unfortunately, it does a poor job of visualizing midureteral stones. Renal size can be accurately determined, and with Doppler scanning, renal blood flow information can be obtained.

Limitations to US include its operator and equipment dependence. Body habitus (e.g., obesity) may interfere with obtaining quality scans. Lastly, since there is a time delay until the onset of pyelocaliectasis, even after total obstruction, ultrasound may miss obstructive signs in the early phase of renal colic.

## Renal Scan

This may be a useful alternative in patients with allergy to radiocontrast media. It is an excellent functional test but does not provide the anatomic detail of IVP, US, or computed tomography.

## Computed Tomography

This diagnostic procedure is rarely indicated in the emergency evaluation of urologic stones. However, it is useful when a renal or perinephric abscess is suspected or when the differential diagnosis is unclear.

## Differential Diagnosis

Critical to the treatment of these patients is to ensure that a catastrophe mimicking renal colic is not missed. This can be difficult as the patient's discomfort may interfere with the usual history and physical examination.

The most critical alternative diagnosis to consider is the dissecting or rupturing abdominal aortic aneurysm (AAA). Renal colic and AAA may have a similar presentation. Vital signs should be noted. Hypotension is not a feature of renal colic. The abdominal examination should focus on the presence of mass, focal tenderness, and abnormal pulsation, or bruit, near vascular structures. Focal abdominal tenderness is an unusual finding in renal colic. Distal extremity pulses should be evaluated. If a dissection/rupture is suspected, an emergency vascular surgical consultation should be obtained. The patient should not be sent for IVP until AAA has been excluded from the differential.

Pyelonephritis may cause flank pain. However, the prodrome is less acute, and the discomfort not as severe as in renal colic. Fever is not a finding of kidney stones, and the urinalysis of renal colic does not demonstrate bacteriuria or pyuria. If renal obstruction is suspected concurrently with pyelonephritis, obstruction must be excluded by IVP or alternative test. Antibiotics will have poor penetration into an obstructed kidney; however, they should be started in the emergency department. Emergency urologic consultation is required for prompt obstruction relief.

Papillary necrosis is most frequently seen in patients with sickle cell disease, diabetes, nonsteroidal analgesic abuse, or infection. The urinalysis may appear to represent infection, with hematuria and pyuria. The IVP can demonstrate sloughed renal papillae as a lucency within the renal pelvis. Urologic consultation and hospitalization are usually required.

Renal infarction from vascular dissection or arterial embolus presents with acute flank pain. Urinalysis may demonstrate hematuria, and an IVP will show absent renal function of the affected kidney. Emergency angiography is indicated. In renal vein thrombosis there may be increased kidney size, with decreased function indicated by IVP. Urinalysis shows proteinuria and microscopic hematuria. All of these conditions require emergency urologic consultation.

Ectopic pregnancy can occur with similar symptoms, but the presentation does not have equal acuity. History, physical examination, and a pregnancy test generally exclude this diagnosis. Salpingitis is excluded by a more insidious onset and by pelvic examination.

A number of other diagnoses can be confused with renal colic, but history and physical examination usually eliminate them from consideration. Gastroenteritis or bowel obstruction presents with abdominal pain and vomiting. However, the less acute presentation and migratory discomfort generalized to the entire abdomen are rarely confused with the consistently unilateral findings of renal colic.

Importantly, generalized abdominal tenderness does not characterize the presentation of kidney stones. Appendicitis shares the unilateral presentation with renal colic, but the subacute prodrome usually excludes urolithiasis. The onset of biliary tract disease can be similar to renal colic; however, right upper quadrant abdominal tenderness makes renal stones unlikely.

Finally, musculoskeletal strain may mimic acute colic in the location of pain, but muscle injury is characterized by worsening of discomfort with evocative maneuvers, such as straight leg raising. Patients with colic usually writhe in pain, whereas patients with muscle injury are immobile to prevent pain.

## Extracorporeal Shock Wave Lithotripsy (ESWL)

With the advent of the newer generation of extracorporeal shock wave lithotriptors, more patients are receiving this treatment as outpatients. ESWL fractures stones into small particles using focused sound waves. The resulting "sludge" is passed in the urine. When there are large fragments, an acute episode of renal colic occurs. The presentation is identical to de novo episodes of renal colic.

Treatment and disposition decisions are identical to routine renal colic. An IVP is rarely indicated as the diagnosis is already established. The usual caveats regarding the differential diagnosis and concurrent infection should be considered.

## Emergency Department Care

In routine cases, the diagnosis is clinical. Testing is performed to confirm renal colic while excluding other diagnoses. A rapid dipstick urine test for heme may provide sufficient information, coupled with clinical findings, to initiate analgesic therapy. Pain medication should not be delayed pending test results. Adequate analgesia frequently requires large doses of titrated intravenous narcotics, such as morphine, or its equivalent. Additional doses are frequently necessary. Narcotics may be accompanied by nonsteroidal anti-inflammatory drugs (NSAIDs) but should not be their replacement. The time of onset of NSAIDs is much slower than that of the intravenous narcotics. Additional analgesia is frequently required at the time of injection of radiocontrast media for an IVP.

A complete urinalysis, to exclude infection, is always required. An IVP is usually performed. This confirms the suspected diagnosis and assures the presence of two anatomically normal kidneys. In patients for whom the diagnosis is clinically very evident or already established (recent IVP or ESWL), a KUB may suffice in localizing a migrating stone. In the undiagnosed patient who is not a candidate for IVP, ultrasound is an appropriate diagnostic adjunct.

While the patient is in the emergency department, all urine should be collected and strained for the identification of any passed stones. All collected stones should be retained for pathologic analysis.

In cases complicated by urinary tract infection (UTI), routine cultures of urine and blood are indicated. Antibiotics should be started promptly while the patient is in the emergency department, and emergency urologic consultation obtained. Appropriate intravenous antibiotics include an antipseudomonal cephalosporin, ticarcillin/clavulanate, antipseudomonal penicillin with an antipseudomonal aminoglycoside, a fluroquinolone, or imipenem cilastatin.

Abdominal CT is indicated if suspicion of a perinephric abscess exists. When diagnosed with concurrent obstruction, cultures, intravenous antibiotics, and emergency urologic consultation are indicated. Appropriate intravenous antibiotics include penicillinase-resistant synthetic penicillins, first-generation cephalosporins, or vancomycin.

## Drug-Seeking Behavior

Drug seekers may present with factitious episodes of renal colic. They can be remarkably inventive in the complexity of their ruse. A history of multiple medical allergies to nonnarcotic analgesics and radiocontrast media is frequently given. They may report having a known radiolucent stone and simulate hematuria by placing blood in their urine. The vital signs may suggest this behavior if changes in blood pressure and heart rate do not match the extreme discomfort demonstrated. When the clinician is unsure, it is better to give analgesia than deprive a patient suffering from true renal colic.

**Table 95-1.** Admission Indications

Hospitalization required:
    Infection with concurrent obstruction
    Solitary kidney and complete obstruction
    Uncontrolled pain
    Intractable emesis
    Large stone
Hospitalization discussed with urologist:
    Renal insufficiency
    Severe underlying disease
    IVP with extravasation/complete obstruction
    Multiple visits

## Admission Indications

Admission indications are summarized in Table 95-1. Hospitalization with emergent urologic evaluation is indicated for patients with acute obstruction in the presence of concurrent infection. Antibiotics directed at the usual urinary pathogens should be initiated in the emergency department.

Admission and emergent urologic consultation are also required if there is absence of a kidney. Patients with a solitary kidney become functionally anephric with complete obstruction and may require urinary drainage.

Inpatient management is needed in patients with severe pain controlled only by intravenous medication. Additionally, patients with emesis preventing oral intake require hospitalization for intravenous fluids.

Patients with renal impairment are candidates for admission with urologic consultation for consideration of a drainage procedure. Such patients have little functional renal reserve and may not withstand additional insult. When there is severe concurrent underlying disease, such as angina or chronic obstructive pulmonary disease, or in the fragile elderly, the patient may be unable to tolerate the stress of renal colic and a lower admission threshold is indicated.

When the IVP demonstrates complete obstruction or dye extravasation, the admission decision requires individualization determined by the clinical scenario. These patients may be discharged provided that urologic follow-up is available within 48 h, there is no evidence of infection, and efficacious oral pain medications are tolerated.

Finally, patients who have previously been diagnosed and managed as outpatients require a lower admission threshold. A careful history and physical examination are indicated to ensure that the diagnosis is correct, but a repeat IVP is probably unnecessary.

A useful predictor for the necessity of admission is the size and contour of a stone. When visualized, either radiographically or by ultrasound, the probability of spontaneous passage of a urolith can be predicted. Stones with diameters less than 4 mm will pass in 75 percent of cases. While 4- to 6-mm stones pass in 50 percent, only 10 percent of stones exceeding 6 mm pass spontaneously. Bizarrely shaped or irregular stones with spicules and sharp edges will have a lower pass rate.

The location of the stone at diagnosis is also predictive of spontaneous passage. Rates of passage for the proximal, middle, and distal ureter are approximately 20, 50, and 70 percent, respectively, regardless of stone size. Therefore patients with large, irregular stones or with proximal locations of their stones should have a higher admission rate. Finally, with complete obstruction there is a lower rate of spontaneous passage than if the blockage is partial.

## Discharge Instructions

Unilateral renal obstruction has minimal acute or permanent effects. Discharge is appropriate in patients with smaller rounded stones, in the absence of infection, and when pain is controlled by oral analgesics. Patients may be given a urinary strainer with instructions to save anything that is passed. Alternatively, urinating into a glass jar allows visualization of any urolith. Patients need to be counseled to return promptly for fever, vomiting, or uncontrolled pain, and they should receive a prescription for oral narcotics. Follow-up with a urologist should be arranged within 5 days.

Patients whose stones pass in the emergency department require no further treatment. Elective urologic consultation should be arranged so that the etiology of the stone can be determined and a prophylactic strategy arranged.

## VESICAL STONES

### Pathophysiology

Vesical calculi may occur at any age and are endemic in some developing countries. In western industrialized countries 90 percent occur in males, 80 percent of whom are over 50 years old. Calculi are associated with outflow obstruction or neuropathic bladder disease in 70 percent of cases. Urinary tract infection, vesical diverticula, and the presence of foreign bodies (e.g., sutures, catheters, or implants) also predispose to bladder calculi.

Calcium oxalate is the most common constituent of bladder stones, but urate and struvite stones occur. Although stones are usually solitary, exceptional cases of more than 100 stones in one patient have been reported. Calculi may be of any size; stones in excess of a kilogram have been removed.

Complications include chronic bladder irritation, fistula formation, and urethral obstruction. Pericystitis occurs in chronic cases and can result in adherence of the bladder to the adjacent pelvic fat. Bladder perforation is a rare complication.

### Clinical Features

Bladder calculi may be asymptomatic, especially in patients with underlying prostatic obstruction. Typical symptoms are intermittent dysuria and terminal hematuria. The greatest discomfort usually occurs at the end of micturition, as the stone impinges upon the bladder neck. In bladder outlet obstruction there is interruption of the urinary stream, with frequency and urgency commonly reported.

There may be associated dull, aching, low abdominal pain, unrelated to urination, that is exacerbated by exercise and abrupt movement. Pain is usually referred to the penile tip or scrotum by the second and third sacral nerves. Occasionally there is referred pain to the low back or heel.

With passage of the calculus, urethral obstruction can occur. Pain is referred to the rectum or perineal area or to the site of urethral impaction. The patient reports interruption of urinary flow, followed by pain and urgency.

Physical examination is useful in excluding alternative considerations but is of little help in diagnosing a bladder calculus. Rarely, exceptionally large stones may be palpated during the rectal, vaginal, or abdominal examination.

Other forms of cystic pathology can mimic vesical stones. These include foreign body, carcinoma, neurogenic bladder, bladder diverticula, or fistula.

### Emergency Department Care

Urinalysis may demonstrate hematuria, pyuria, or bacteria. If there is coexistent infection, the complete blood count may show leukocytosis.

Plain radiographs reveal vesical stones in approximately 50 percent of patients. While ultrasound may demonstrate bladder stones, cystoscopic examination is the most accurate method of detection. Referral for definitive care is required. Bladder calculi require emergency therapy when they result in urinary obstruction or there is associated infection.

Acute urethral obstruction requires either the successful removal of the stone or the placement of a catheter. Very distal stones may be able to be gently milked from the penis or removed by forceps. All others require emergent urologic consultation. If there is coexistent infection, antibiotics should be started in the emergency department. Any patient demonstrating signs of sepsis or urinary infection, or in whom obstruction cannot be relieved, requires hospitalization for definitive care.

## BIBLIOGRAPHY

Ashworth M: Endemic bladder stones. *Br Med J* 301:826, 1990.

Davies MG, O'Brion E, O'Sullivan BJ: A bladder full of stones—a case report. *Irish Med J* 84:28, 1991.

Drach GW: Urinary lithiasis: Etiology, diagnosis, and medical management, in Walsh PC, Retik AB, Stamey TA, Vaughan ED (eds): *Campbell's Urology,* 6th ed, vol 3. Philadelphia, Saunders, 1992.

Ibrahim AIA, Shetty SD, Awad RM, Patel KP: Prognostic factors in the conservative treatment of ureteric stones. *Br J Urol* 67:357, 1991.

Juul N, Brons J, Torp-Pederson S, Fredfeldt KE: Ultrasound versus intravenous urography in the initial evaluation of patients with suspected obstructing urinary calculi. *Scand J Urol Nephrol* 137(suppl):45, 1991.

Katzberg RW: New and old contrast agents: Physiology and nephrotoxicity. *Urol Radiol* 10:6, 1988.

Kelleher JP, Plail RO, Dave SM, et al: Sequential renography in acute urinary tract obstruction due to stone disease. *Br J Urol* 67:125, 1991.

Mission RT, Cutler RE: Radiocontrast-induced renal failure. *West J Med* 142:657, 1985.

Morse RM, Resnick MI: Ureteral calculi: Natural history in an era of advanced technology. *J Urol* 145:263, 1991.

Pickworth FE, Dubbins PA, Choa RG: Case report: Limey urine. *Clin Radiol* 45:345, 1992.

Stewart DP, Kowalski R, Wong P, Krome R: Microscopic hematuria and calculus-related ureteral obstruction. *J Emerg Med* 8:693, 1990.

Van Arsdalen KN, Banner MP, Pollack HM: Radiographic imaging and urologic decision making in the management of renal and ureteral calculi. *Urol Clin North Am* 17:171, 1990.

# Gynecology and Obstetrics

## 96
# GYNECOLOGIC EMERGENCIES
### Veronica Mallett

In evaluation of gynecologic emergencies in women, particularly women of reproductive age, a delay in or improper management of the patient may compromise care and jeopardize future reproductive capabilities. Although there are several gynecologic *urgencies* that warrant expeditious management, there are only three life-threatening gynecologic *emergencies:* (1) ruptured ectopic pregnancy, (2) ruptured hemorrhagic ovarian cyst, and (3) ruptured tuboovarian abscess. If these are kept constantly kept in mind, diagnostic failures should not occur and proper management of the similar-presenting but less concerning gynecologic urgencies will be enhanced.

The objective of this chapter is to provide a suggested approach to the evaluation and management of the more common and important urgent and emergency gynecologic problems occurring in women of reproductive age. The chapter will focus on early pregnancy-related problems, ectopic pregnancy, adnexal accidents, abnormal genital bleeding conditions, and pelvic inflammatory disease (PID).

## EARLY PREGNANCY COMPLICATIONS AS CAUSES OF GYNECOLOGIC PAIN AND BLEEDING

A most useful dictum is that, until proved otherwise, amenorrhea is a normal result of pregnancy and abnormal uterine bleeding is a complication of pregnancy. The possibility of an ectopic pregnancy must be considered in every patient who presents with a clinical scenario that includes lower abdominal or pelvic pain or abnormal uterine bleeding. A spontaneous abortion, infected abortion, hemorrhagic corpus luteum of pregnancy, and uterine incarceration are additional early pregnancy complications that frequently present to the emergency department (ED).

## ABORTION

### Pathophysiology

About 15 to 20% of all known pregnancies end in what is known as a clinically recognized abortion. This incidence is increased with increasing maternal age, parity, and paternal age.

The causes of spontaneous abortion are divided into two categories, fetal and maternal. The major cause of abortion is by far genetic, with over 50% of abortuses having chromosomal anomalies, predominately of chromosomal number, with fewer involving structural abnormalities of individual chromosomes. Maternal factors include uterine abnormalities, incompetent cervix, intrauterine adhesions, progestin deficiency, and serious medical problems such as diabetes and hyperthyroidism.

### Clinical Features

To firmly establish the possibility of a pregnancy in the woman with pelvic pain and/or bleeding, a brief but accurate gynecologic and menstrual history that provides the following information must be obtained.

**Last menstrual period (LMP).** Not only the LMP, but also the timing of two or more immediate past periods should be ascertained to determine the intervals between "normal" menses. Any regularly menstruating woman whose LMP is greater than 4 weeks prior to the current date is very likely to be pregnant. If the LMP is determined to be normal and the patient is less than 4 weeks past the menses, the possibility of a pregnancy complication is highly unlikely, as spontaneous abortion and ectopic pregnancies do not present clinically before the first missed menses. If the stated LMP was lighter and shorter than normal, pregnancy must also be considered, since implantation can be associated with normal "menstrual" flow.

Most spontaneous abortions also occur prior to 8 or 9 weeks of gestation; however, abortion can occur up to the 20th week of gestation. The aborting patient initially experiences minimal intermittent or continuous spotting that progresses to very heavy bleeding with the passage of clots and gestational tissue. Volume is best assessed by determining the number of pads used per day. A soaked pad suggest 20 to 30 mL blood loss.

The pain associated with the abortive process usually occurs after bleeding has commenced and is very characteristically midline and cramping in nature, as opposed to the acute, severe, and unilaterally localized pain of an ectopic pregnancy or ruptured ovarian cyst.

The abdominal examination of the aborting patient is usually unremarkable, with the possible finding of midline suprapubic tenderness to deep palpation. On pelvic examination, a patient with a threatened abortion will be found to have a closed cervical os and minimal bleeding. In a women with an actively progressing abortion, however, the bleeding will be profuse and accompanied by the passage of blood clots and products of conception through an obviously dilated cervical opening. The uterus will usually be enlarged to a size compatible with gestational dates unless significant tissue sloughage has occurred. In the case of a complete abortion, the uterus may be found to be small and firm shortly after all tissue has been passed. The adnexal examination is unlikely to be abnormal, although slight tenderness and palpation of a fullness on the side of the corpus luteum of pregnancy is common. It should be noted that a complete abortion is unlikely to occur beyond week 7 of gestation. Ultrasound has been used with relative reliability to determine if the uterus is empty if in doubt.

In a full-blown abortive situation, the proper diagnosis is easy to determine. However, in earlier stages of the abortion process, a definitive diagnosis can be difficult and is easily confused with an ectopic pregnancy. An ultrasound examination can help to rule out an ectopic pregnancy if an intrauterine gestational sac is seen and may even be predictive of a possible abortion if absent heart tones or irregular margins of the sac are seen. However, the rare case of a twin intrauterine and ectopic pregnancy should also be considered. When the diagnosis of an intrauterine pregnancy is uncertain, intrauterine instrumentation must be avoided until an accurate diagnosis can be made. Most patients with early pregnancy bleeding problems have normal pregnancy outcomes.

### Treatment

Threatened abortion is defined as any uterine bleeding from a gestation of less than 20 weeks. If the diagnosis of a threatened abortion is made, the patient may be sent home for continued expectant management and close follow-up by her obstetrician.

Discharge instructions should include bed rest, no intercourse, and no tampon use. The patient should instructed to return to the ED if bleeding or cramping intensify, if orthostatic symptoms develop, or if there is fever or chills. If the diagnosis is complete abortion, the patient should be followed up at the physician's office within 2 weeks of the event. Discharge instructions should include instructions for the patient to return if excessive bleeding, foul smelling menstrual blood, discharge, or fever ensues.

Incomplete or inevitable abortion usually requires operative intervention with suction curettage. The time frame for performance of the procedure is dependent on the amount and rate of uterine bleeding. Missed abortion defined as fetal death before the 20th week of gestation or blighted ovum is not an operative emergency and can be scheduled accordingly.

## RETAINED PRODUCTS OF CONCEPTION

Retained gestational tissue following a spontaneous or induced abortion can serve as a nidus for an infection that is usually polymicrobial in etiology. Continued bleeding, cramping pain, fever, nausea, and generalized malaise usually accompany a postabortive endometritis. On examination, a purulent, hemorrhagic cervical discharge is seen associated with a boggy, tender, and enlarged uterus. Significant adnexal tenderness may also be elicited if the myometrium, parametrium, and fallopian tubes are involved in the process. In severe cases where uterine perforation has occurred, an infected tender mass compatible with an abscess may be palpated in the adnexae or in the cul-de-sac. Patients with postabortive endometritis require hospitalization, intensive parenteral antibiotic therapy, and repeat dilatation and curettage in an effort to prevent abscess formation and development of septic pelvic thrombophlebitis.

## ECTOPIC PREGNANCY

Ectopic pregnancy is defined as any pregnancy occurring outside the uterine cavity. It can result from a fertilized ovum implanted in the abdomen, fallopian tube, cervix, ovary or peritoneal surface. There are 70,000 ectopic pregnancies reported annually. In the past, incidence of ectopic pregnancy was reported as 4.5/1000. The current incidence is closer to 20/1000 pregnancies. Although changing etiologic factors are partly responsible, previous inconsistencies in reporting, improved diagnostic tools and an increase in acquired risks for the disease are some of the factors thought to contribute to the increase. Factors most commonly associated with ectopic pregnancy are assisted reproduction, in vitro fertilization, tubal surgery or tubal occlusion, and DES exposure.

### Diagnosis

With recent technological advances the diagnosis of ectopic pregnancy can be made more accurately and earlier in gestation. As in the past, death is most often due to delay in diagnosis leading to rupture of the tube and hemorrhage. Even with the current diagnostic methods available, the diagnosis is missed 50% of the time, at first office visit, and 36% of the time at first emergency department visit.

The clinical presentation of ectopic pregnancy is variable. The physician cannot rely on history and clinical findings as the only criteria, as they are often nondiscriminatory, particularly prior to the time bleeding and distention of the tube have occurred. The most common symptom associated with ectopic pregnancy is abdominal pain, followed by amenorrhea and vaginal bleeding. Women rarely present with dizziness and syncope. Clinical signs include abdominal and adnexal tenderness, adnexal mass, and varying uterine size. Over 70% of the time the uterus is normal size, but one can sometimes be led astray when the uterus is enlarged. The usual presentation is a uterus which is softened but not as enlarged as expected for gestational age.

These symptom characteristics are indeed altered by the presence of a combined gestation. The incidence of combined gestation is most often quoted as 1/30,000. However this number is thought to be increasing secondary to the increased numbers of assisted reproduction. In fact, recent estimates place the incidence at 1 to 8:100 in an in vitro fertilization program to 1:4000 in the general population. Classical presentation of combined gestation is abdominal pain, adnexal mass, peritoneal irritation, and enlarged uterus.

Other clinical scenarios in which one might think of combined gestation are a fundus compatible with dates in a person believed to have an ectopic; absence of bleeding following removal of an ectopic; and hemoperitoneum following a pregnancy termination.

Differential diagnosis of a single ectopic gestation includes acute salpingitis, torsion, gastroenteritis, threatened or incomplete abortion or endometriosis. PID is the most common condition confused with ectopic pregnancy. Up to 20% of patients with ectopic pregnancy may have temperatures up to 38°C (100.4°F). PID is, however, rare in pregnancy, occurring less than 1% of the time.

### Human Chorionic Gonadropin (hCG)

All currently used qualitative pregnancy tests are dependent on the ability to detect in serum or urine human chorionic gonadotropin, a glycoprotein hormone produced by trophoblast. In a normal intrauterine gestation, the hCG level increases by 66% every 2 days. A patient in whom hCG levels fall, plateau, or fail to reach a predicted slope has an abnormal pregnancy. The absolute value of a single hCG is not useful to determine the location of a pregnancy. However, ectopic gestations have a lower increase in hCG titer. Up to 15% of ectopic gestations have been reported to have a normal doubling time, and 10% of viable pregnancies will have an abnormal doubling time. The current monoclonal antibody technology allows detection of hCG within 2 to 3 days postimplantation. Serial hCG levels help to assess the viability of pregnancy and can be used to signal the optimal time for ultrasonography. In addition, after medical treatment with either an abortifacient or systemic methotrexate falling hCG levels help determine the effectiveness of treatment.

### Progesterone

Testing of single serum progesterone has recently emerged as a controversial tool for the evaluation of potential ectopic pregnancy. This tool has been used as an absolute value to determine the diagnosis of normal or ectopic pregnancy or as a mechanism for assigning risk by using a discriminatory cutoff to distinguish a normal from an abnormal pregnancy. Use of this diagnostic tool is attractive as only one measure need be obtained. Stovall et al. performed receiver–operator characteristics curve analysis on 1120 patients and compared them to hCG doubling times as predictors of ectopic pregnancy. Their data indicate that serum progesterone is a better predictor than hCG doubling time. Of note, however, is that the lowest progesterone level associated with a normal pregnancy is 5.1 ng/mL. This finding demonstrates the difficulty one has in using only serum progesterone to determine rather than predict the diagnosis. Normal intrauterine gestation is reported to exist in the presence of a low progesterone. Thus, this test should only be used to assign risk of an abnormal pregnancy and not as sole diagnostic criteria.

### Ultrasound

Further localization of the pregnancy can then be attempted with a real-time ultrasound examination of the pelvis, the findings on which will be greatly dependent on the gestational age and the type of sonographic approach used. In general, real-time sonography using an abdominal transducer can find an interuterine gestational sac by the fifth week, a sac with an embryonic or fetal pole by the sixth week, and an embryonic mass with cardiac motion by the seventh week.

The recent use of high resolution transvaginal US has improved the accuracy of diagnosis and decreased the gestational age at which an ectopic pregnancy can be diagnosed.

Timor-Tristsh, in a study of 145 patients, found the sensitivity of diagnosing ectopic pregnancy with transvaginal sonography to be 100%. The specificity was 98.2% with a positive predictive value of 98%. The negative predictive value in this study was 100%. Depending on the skill of the examiner, resolution of the probe and size and location of the ectopic pregnancy, pregnancies can be detected at as little as 31 to 32 days post-LMP. The minimal hCG titer that a sac should always be seen is unclear but an experienced transvaginal sonographer should be able to visualize a viable intrauterine pregnancy at > 2000 hCG mIU/ml. Transabdominal transducer can visualize a pregnancy at 6500 MIU/ml. Color doppler allows even better visualization of an ectopic gestation. It is important to remember that ultrasound is still considered diagnostic of an ectopic only when the sac is visible outside the uterus.

## Culdocentesis

Whenever ectopic pregnancy is suspected culdocentesis may be used to determine whether intraperitoneal hemorrhage is present. If a significant hemorrhage has occurred, cervical motion tenderness may be present accompanied by cul-de-sac fullness or bulging. With or without such a finding, however, culdocentesis should be considered in all patients with a suspected ectopic pregnancy. Culdocentesis is negative if clear fluid is aspirated and positive if nonclotting blood is aspirated. Culdocentesis is not used to determine whether or not a tubal pregnancy has ruptured, since culdocentesis is positive in the majority of ectopics, ruptured or unruptured (85% and 65%, respectively). Failure to aspirate blood on culdocentesis is nondiagnostic and may represent technical difficulties. The presence of blood does not guarantee a diagnosis of ectopic pregnancy and may represent a false positive tap from a ruptured corpus luteum in about 5% of cases.

## Dilation and Curettage and Laparoscopy

After identifying an abnormal pregnancy with either progesterone, serial hCG or ultrasound, curettage can be used to identify villi, rendering the diagnosis of ectopic gestation remote.

## Treatment

Management of the unstable patient with ectopic pregnancy is aimed toward hemodynamic support. Oxygen should be administered and volume resuscitation started immediately. The patient should be given type-specific blood as indicated. Immediate gynecologic consult for surgical management is the obvious next step. With the increased use of tubal conservation procedures the risk of repetitive ectopic pregnancy is increased.

Management of the stable patient varies depending on the degree of suspicion and the possible gestational age. Patients who have a low degree of suspicion and have just missed a menses may be followed as outpatients with serial quantitative hCG measurements or serum progesterone. Not every patient in this situation needs an ultrasound. Even if the diagnosis is delayed 48 to 72 hours little harm is done because rupture of such a small pregnancy is not life-threatening. Once the hCG value has reached the critical value for your institution ultrasound can be obtained if indicated.

## Surgical Treatment

Operative laparoscopy has virtually replaced laparotomy for the first-time treatment of ectopic pregnancy. This has occurred not only to reduce morbidity but also to preserve fertility and reduce cost. Tubal conservation procedures, linear salpingectomy or segmental resection are an attempt to preserve fertility. Unfortunately, these conservative treatments have led to the occurrence of repetitive ectopic gestations.

In addition, persistent ectopic pregnancy or the continued growth of the trophoblast after incomplete removal by conservative surgery complicates 5 to 20% of tubal operations. Occasionally this persistent tissue grows and tubal rupture occurs requiring salpingectomy for hematasis.

More recently, systemic methotrexate, discussed below, has been used to treat this condition.

## Medical Treatment

### Systemic Methotrexate

Methotrexate has been used for years in the treatment of gestational trophoblastic disease. Its mechanism of action is through inhibition of spontaneous synthesis of purines and pyrimidines, thus interfering with DNA synthesis and the multiplication of cells.

Stable patients with unruptured ectopic gestation of less than 4 cm in diameter by ultrasound are eligible for treatment.

Numerous dosing regimens have been published. However, current practice is to use single dose treatment (50 mg/m$^2$) which is accompanied by fewer side effects. Patients are followed on post therapy doses 2, 4 and 7 with serial qualitative hCG titer mengo. If there is a < 15% decline in hCG between day 4 and 7, a second dose is given. High doses of methotrexate can cause bone marrow suppression, acute and chronic hepatotoxicity, stomatitis, pulmonary fibrosis, alopecia and photosensitivity. These side effects are rarely seen in the dosing schedules used in the treatment of ectopic pregnancy.

To ensure the patient remains unruptured, care should be taken to minimize pelvic exams. Transient pelvic pain frequently occurs three to seven days after the start of methotrexate therapy. This pain is presumably due to tubal abortion and normally lasts less than four to twelve hours. Distinguishing between this pain and the pain of tubal rupture can be difficult. Observation in the hospital may be required when in doubt. Surgical intervention is required in the case of tubal rupture leading to interabdominal hemorrhage. Rupture remote from administration has been reported but was accompanied by a plateau or rise in hCG titer. Patients with rise titers should be observed constantly for rupture.

## INCARCERATED UTERUS

An uncommon complication of a late 1st-trimester pregnancy, but one that can be associated with pelvic pain and other signs and symptoms of a threatened abortion, is an incarceration of a pregnant uterus. Laceration occurs only in patients who have an introverted and retroflexed uterus as a neonal anatomic variant or as a result of endometriosis or retrouterine adhesions. Normally the uterus rises out of the pelvis as it enlarges as a result of a pregnancy and is safely beyond the bony confines of the pelvic walls by 12 to 13 weeks of gestation. However, if anteversion of such a uterus does not occur during the expansion process, the uterus may become trapped with the bony pelvis. Clinically, the patient will note progressively severe pelvic and rectal pressure, and because of marked anterior displacement of the cervix to a position behind the pubic symphysis, urinary retention may also be noted. The diagnosis is easily made by noting the cervical displacement and by an inability to mobilize the uterus on a combined abdominal-vaginal examination.

Treatment of this condition must be fairly immediate, to both deviate urinary retention and prevent a certain spontaneous abortion. Placing the patient in a knee–chest position may spontaneously, or with appropriate pressure applied through the rectum, correct the problem. If needed, repositioning can be accomplished under a general or regional anesthetic.

## NON-PREGNANCY-ASSOCIATED CAUSES OF PELVIC PAIN

In the initial evaluation of a woman with lower abdominal or pelvic pain, there is a tendency for physicians to quickly assume a gynecologic etiology for the presenting symptoms. The prudent physician, however, should first always approach each such patient with the thought of ruling out nongynecologic conditions as the source of the problem. The following common causes of pain may, with varying degrees of likelihood, falsely suggest a gynecologic problem: (1) lower lobe pneumonia, (2) cholecystitis, (3) pancreatitis, (4) gastric or duodenal ulcers, (5) gastroenteritis, (6) colitis, (7) ileitis, (8) diverticulitis, and, most commonly, (9) appendicitis. A few moments of initial history-taking will usually correctly rule out these causes or at least minimize their priority in an eventual differential diagnosis. Having done so, one can then proceed to the consideration of specific problems.

## ADNEXAL ACCIDENTS (NON-PREGNANCY-ASSOCIATED) AS CAUSES OF PELVIC PAIN

### Clinical Features

The most common noninfectious causes of pelvic pain are rupture or torsion of a cyst or a solid ovarian, tubal, or uterine mass. With the exception of rupture of a persistent corpus luteum cyst, all such adnexal accidents occur in patients whose menstrual cycles have been normal, and, except for the pain itself, any other associated localizing or systemic symptoms are unlikely. Most such problems occur in reproductive-age women who commonly have ovarian endometriomas, benign cystic teratomas ("dermoid cysts"), dysfunctional follicular cysts, or serous or mucinous cystadenomas.

Ovarian enlargement due to cystic or neoplastic processes is usually asymptomatic as a result of poor afferent innervation of ovarian tissue. The patient may experience pelvic and abdominal discomfort due to ovarian pressure on adjacent visceral organs. When ovarian rupture occurs, acute pain is caused by the irritation of pelvic peritoneum, from spillage of ovarian contents. Only in the case of dermoid tumor is this catastrophic, causing a chemical peritonitis.

Confronted with such an acute pelvic problem, there are few specific diagnostic modalities that will be helpful to the ED physician. Most importantly, a complication of pregnancy or an infectious process must be ruled out. Aside from pregnancy testing, other laboratory and routine radiologic studies are of no value. An emergent ultrasound evaluation of the pelvis may be revealing if an adnexal mass cannot be palpated on pelvic examination.

### Patient Disposition

If the cyst is detected, but unruptured, the patient should be referred for observation and follow-up. If the cyst has ruptured and there is no evidence of hemorrhage, the patient should be discharged with analgesics.

## OVARIAN TORSION

### Clinical Features

Ovarian torsion is an uncommon event and will not occur unless limited enlargement has developed. In such a circumstance the enlarging ovarian mass may stretch the mesovarium to the point where the ovary effectively becomes a pedunculated structure that may acutely twist on its pedicle. When torsion occurs, the ovarian blood supply is compromised, causing painful progressive anoxic degeneration of the ovary and eventual gangrenous necrosis. Torsion of tubal masses (hydrosalpinx, pyosalpinx) and pedunculated uterine leiomyomata ("fibroids") may also cause acute pelvic pain.

### Diagnosis

Patients with this condition usually describe sudden onset of acute, severe, unilateral, lower abdominal and pelvic pain. Up to two thirds of patients describe associated nausea and vomiting often leading to a missed diagnosis of appendicitis. In addition, many patients will re-

count previous intermittent episodes of similar pain. Pelvic exam reveals a unilateral tender adnexal mass.

### Treatment

Laparoscopic treatment by adnexal conservation or removal is the treatment of choice.

## MITTELSCHMERZ

### Clinical Features

Adnexal pain in the reproductive-age patient may be due to *mittelschmerz* ("middle pain") which is unique to ovulatory cycles. The key to the diagnosis of mittelschmerz is the relationship of the timing of the pain to the menstrual cycle. In a woman with typically regular 28- to 33-day cycles, the pain associated with ovulation will usually occur between cycle days 14 to 16, be unilateral in location, be mild to moderate in severity, and often last less than a day. The pain may also be accompanied by light midcycle endometrial spotting. Although the source of the pain has not exactly been determined, it is thought to be due to follicular fluid irritation of the periovarian visceral peritoneum at the time of ovulation.

### Diagnosis and Treatment

No diagnostic studies are helpful in evaluating the possibility of mittelschmerz, and treatment is symptomatic, with analgesics or nonsteroidal antiinflammatory agents.

### Patient Disposition

Patients should be told the pain will resolve spontaneously and instructed to keep a menstrual calendar noting the timing of the pain to confirm the diagnosis.

## ENDOMETRIOSIS

When the tissue that characterizes the normal epithelial lining of the uterine cavity, the endometrium, is found in ectopic locations, it is called endometriosis. Most commonly, endometriosis is found on or in the ovaries. All pelvic tissues, however, are subject to endometriosis growth, including the uterine serosal surface, fallopian tubes, ovarian fossae, uterosacral ligaments, cul-de-sac peritoneum, and the utero-vesical peritoneal fold.

### Diagnosis

The diagnosis of endometriosis should be considered in any reproductive-aged women complaining of any one or combination of the following signs and symptoms: acute adnexal pain, premenstrual pelvic pain, worsening dysmenorrhea, and deep dyspareunia. The most serious complication is rupture of an ovarian endometrioma. The approach is that directed at acute adnexal accidents.

### Treatment and Patient Disposition

The diagnosis of endometriosis of any extent or variety cannot be made by any combination of historical, examination, laboratory, or radiographic studies. Visual inspection of the disease either at laparoscopy or laparotomy is necessary to confirm the clinical suspicion. Therefore, unless the clinical circumstances warrant immediate operative diagnostic or therapeutic intervention by the gynecology team, the emergency physician should offer the patient analgesia and refer her to a gynecologist for definitive diagnosis and management.

## ABNORMAL GENITAL BLEEDING (NONPREGNANCY)

When abnormal bleeding occurs, pregnancy complications such as an ectopic pregnancy, an abortion, or a ruptured corpus luteum cyst will probably be the first considerations. Once these have been ruled out, it is then necessary to systematically consider pathologic and traumatic causes of lower genital tract and uterine bleeding. Except for trauma, the bleeding is usually painless.

Trauma to the vulva and vagina from a variety of causes may result in profuse bleeding and hypotension. Patient stabilization with intravenous fluids is the first priority, and a thorough pelvic examination will easily indicate the bleeding source. In most cases, hemostasis and other indicated surgical procedures will require an anesthetic and the assistance of a gynecologist.

If the bleeding is determined not to be of vulvar, vaginal, rectal, or bladder origin, attention must then be given to the following pathologic causes of uterine cervix or corpus bleeding: (1) erosion of the cervical vasculature by an invasive cervical carcinoma, (2) endometrial carcinoma, (3) endometrial polyps, and (4) submucosal leiomyomata. Pelvic exam will aid in identification of the bleeding source, i.e., if multiple myoma is palpable or a large cervical lesion is visible.

Management of these conditions requires gynecologic consultation after stabilization of the patient.

If pathologic and pregnancy-related causes of uterine bleeding have been eliminated, it is then possible to ascribe the cause of uterine bleeding to that of anovulatory dysfunctional uterine bleeding (DUB). Fortunately, most DUB problems do not require emergency treatment and are comfortably dealt with in an office or clinic setting. Virtually all severe cases of DUB occur in adolescent girls shortly after the onset of menstruation. Bleeding is occasionally severe enough to cause hemorrhagic shock. The ED management of such a patient should follow these suggested steps in an expeditious and overlapping manner:

1. Ascertain the adolescent perimenarcheal status of the patient and historically rule out a pregnancy. A lack of pain and profuse, tissue-free blood loss dramatically reduces the possibility of a ruptured ectopic pregnancy or spontaneous abortion.
2. Localize the bleeding source to the uterine cavity and assure normal uterine and adnexal anatomy with a pelvic examination.
3. Stabilize the patient with intravenous fluids or blood or bloodcomponent transfusions as needed. Obtain the following minimum laboratory studies: (a) complete blood count including platelet count; (b) blood type and Rh factor for a transfusion cross match; (c) pregnancy test; and (d) coagulation profile. Coagulopathies, particularly platelet function disorders, may first manifest as severe perimenarcheal bleeding.
4. Administer 20 mg of conjugated estrogen intravenously slowly over 10 to 15 min. Acute intravenous estrogen therapy causes vasospasm of the uterine arterial vasculature and initiates several coagulation-related functions that often dramatically decrease the uterine bleeding. Oral estrogen of up to 25 mg can have some effect.
5. Seek emergency gynecologic consultation for continuing hormonal or surgical management.

## OLDER WOMEN WITH DYSFUNCTIONAL UTERINE BLEEDING

More commonly patients do not present with acute blood loss but report a history of prolonged heavy bleeding now complicated by systemic symptoms, i.e., lightheadedness and patagia. Physical exam is usually unremarkable with the exception of vaginal bleeding.

### Treatment

If the patient is hemodynamically stable, treatment with the combination oral contraceptive pill; four pills a day for seven days, will arrest the bleeding; alternate doses of progesterone 20 to 30 mg per day for 7 days is useful in patients in whom estrogen is contraindicated.

### Patient Disposition

The patient should be told to expect to resume menses after stopping either regimen, take iron for anemia and follow-up with a gynecologic as soon as possible.

## PELVIC INFLAMMATORY DISEASE

Pelvic inflammatory disease (PID) is the most common serious infection among reproductive-age women in the United States. It is defined as an ascending infection arising from the cervix causing endometritis, salpingitis, and/or peritonitis. An estimated 2.5 million physician visits occur annually for acute salpingitis, resulting in 250,000 hospitalizations and 150,000 surgical procedures for complications of this disease. The disease causes tubal occlusion in 11% of women after their first episode. Over 25% of women are infertile after two episodes and 50% are infertile after greater than two episodes. Long-term sequelae of salpingooophoritis may include chronic pelvic pain, dyspareunia, infertility due to tubal occlusion or pelvic adhesions, tuboovarian abscess, and an increased risk of tubal ectopic pregnancies. The seriousness of the acute and chronic problems associated with PID makes it mandatory to recognize the diagnosis as early as possible in order to institute early, appropriate, and intensive antibiotic therapy.

### Etiology

The etiology of PID is polymicrobial, involving sexually and nonsexually transmitted organisms. *Neisseria gonorrhoeae* and *Chlamydia trachomatis* are the major offenders residing first in the cervical canal, then colonizing higher organs through an ascending infection. Secondary invaders are predominately anaerobes, including *Bacteroides* sp., *Peptococcus* and *Peptostreptococcus,* and *E. coli.*

### Pathophysiology

Primary PID is a result of spread of bacteria from the lower genital tract to the normally sterile endometrium and endosalpinx. These bacteria must first bypass the natural barriers to infection, the cervix through its mucus and small diameter canal, the endometrium through the monthly sloughing, and the utero–tubojunction via ciliary action.

Risk factors for the development of PID include (1) a history of previous gonococcal salpingitis, (2) frequent sexual activity with multiple partners, (3) adolescence, and (4) use of an intrauterine contraceptive device. As with other sexually transmitted diseases, single, sexually promiscuous, non-white, poor women are most commonly affected. Dilatation and curettage, endometrial biopsy, hysterosalpingography, tubal insufflation, and cautery or cryotherapy of the cervix may also predispose to the development of endometritis and salpingitis.

### Protective Factors

Pregnancy offers the best protection as the decidua effectively seals off the uterus from bacterial invasion. However, PID in pregnancy, although rare, can occur because the uterine cavity is not completely sealed until 12 weeks gestation. Infection prior to this time must be aggressively treated to prevent fetal loss. Barrier contraception offers some protection through obvious means as well as through the bactericidal effect of spermicide. Oral contraceptives also offer protection to the user possibly by increasing the density of cervical mucous.

### Diagnosis

Acute salpingitis may present with a variety of clinical manifestations including lower abdominal pain, adnexal and cervical motion tenderness, fever and generalized malaise. The discharge of pus from the tubes onto adjacent peritoneal surfaces or around the liver may cause a more localized pain of pelvic peritonitis (Fitz-Hugh–Curtis syn-

**Table 96-1.** Criteria for Clinical Diagnosis of Acute PID

All three of these conditions must be present:
  Abdominal direct tenderness with or without rebound tenderness
  Tenderness with motion of cervix and uterus
  Adnexal tenderness
One of these conditions must be present:
  Gram stain of endocervix—positive for gram-negative, intracellular
    diplococci
  Temperature greater than 38°C (100.4°F)
  Leukocytosis greater than 10,000/mm³ (μL)
  White blood cells and bacteria in peritoneal fluid collected by culdocentesis
  or laparoscopy
  Inflammatory mass documented by pelvic examination and/or sonogram

*Source:* Adapted from Hager WD et al: Criteria for diagnosis and grading of salpingitis. *Obstet Gynecol* 61:113, 1983. Used by permission.

drome). Gastrointestinal symptoms of nausea and anorexia are not uncommon and may suggest appendicitis or viral gastroenteritis. Onset frequently occurs shortly after a menstrual flow, but uterine bleeding abnormalities are uncommon. Minimal criteria for diagnosis of PID includes abdominal direct tenderness, adnexal tenderness, cervical motion tenderness, temperature greater than 38°C and leukocytosis (see Table 96-1). Laboratory studies should include Gram stain to detect gram-negative diplococci, gonococcal and chlamydial cultures, CBC with diff and urine or serum hCG. The finding of unilateral or bilateral adnexal or cul-de-sac masses strongly suggests the presence of a tuboovarian or pelvic abscess.

Of 814 patients with clinically diagnosed acute PID, or with clinically suspected PID, only 65% were confirmed to have the disease at the time of laparoscopy. Remember not every non-white young women with pain and fever has PID. PID uncomplicated by abscess formation is treated with antibiotics. Treatment goals include eradication of infection and preservation of tubal function. Inpatient parenteral (intravenous) antibiotic therapy should be considered for patients who exhibit any of the following criteria: (1) diagnosed or suspected pyosalpinx or tuboovarian abscess, (2) temperature greater than 38°C (100.4°F), (3) pregnancy, (4) nausea and vomiting that prevent the use of oral antibiotics, (5) upper peritoneal signs, (6) presence of an IUCD, (7) failure to respond to oral antibiotics within 48 h, (8) uncertain diagnosis, (9) WBC greater than 12,000, (10) presence of adnexal mass, and (11) primary fertility.

The CDC's (Table 96-2) most current treatment schedules should be used. The presence of penicillinase producing gonorrhea (PPNC) dictates the use of ceftriaxone 250 mg/m. For those communities in which PPNG is not a problem, follow CDC guidelines. Ambulatory treatment should be reserved for patients with suspected gonorrheal cervicitis, chlamydial cervicitis, or the mildest forms of salpingitis. In all such cases, the treatment regimen must include a 10- to 14-day course of a tetracycline derivative to cover chlamydia and the patient must be reevaluated after 2 days of such therapy. Other outpatient treatment for gonorrhea includes: erythromycin 500 mg P.O. × 7 (safe in pregnancy), cefixime 400 mg P.O. (single dose), ciprofloxacin 500 mg P.O. (single dose) or ofloxacin 400 mg P.O. (single dose). Alternative to outpatient treatments for chlamydia are azithromycin 1.0 g m P.O. (single dose), ofloxacin 300 g P.O. qid × 7 days, and erythromycin 500 mg P.O. bid × 7 days (safe in pregnancy) sulfisoxazole 500 mg P.O. qid for 10 days (inferior to other regimens). Failure to respond to oral outpatient therapy mandates hospitalization and parenteral antimicrobial therapy.

### Patient Disposition

Discharged patients should be instructed that they must be seen within 48 hours. Instructions to return prior to 48 hours should include worsening pain or fever and inability to ingest antibiotics.

Other outpatient treatments for gonorrhea include ofloxacin 400 g P.O. XI. Patient education about the scope and severity of the problem along with close follow-up are key.

**Table 96-2.** CDC Recommended Treatment for Acute PID–1993

*Outpatients*
  Cefoxitin 2 g IM plus probenecid, 1g orally *or*
  ceftriaxone 250 mg IM *or*
  equivalent cephalosporin
  *plus*
    Doxycycline 100 mg orally 2 times a day for 10–14 days *or*
    *Regimen B:* Ofloxacin 400 mg PO bid for 14 d *plus* either clindamycin
      450 mg PO qid or metronidazole 500 mg PO bid for 14 d.
*Inpatients*
  Recommended regimen A
    Cefoxitin 2 g IV every 6 hours *or*
    Cefotetan 2 g IV every 12 hours
    *plus*
    Doxycycline 100 mg every 12 hours orally or IV for at least 48 hours
    After hospital discharge, doxycycline 100 mg PO bid for 10–14 days
  Recommended regimen B
    Clindamycin 900 mg IV every 8 hours
    *plus*
    Gentamicin loading dose IV or IM (2 mg/kg) followed by a maintenance
      dose (1.5 mg/kg) every 8 hours for at least 48 hours
  After hospital discharge, doxycycline 100 mg orally 2 times a day for
  10–14 days. Continuation of clindamycin, 450 mg orally, 4 times a day
  for 10–14 days may be considered.

*Source:* Adapted from *MMWR* 42:1, 1993.

## HEMORRHAGIC CORPUS LUTEUM

The corpus luteum of pregnancy usually persists until the 8th week or so of gestation and frequently is palpable as a 3- to 4-cm adnexal-ovarian mass associated with a normal intrauterine pregnancy. Rupture of the luteal cyst or hemorrhage into the corpus luteum may occur in early pregnancy and cause a clinical picture indistinguishable from that of a ruptured ectopic pregnancy, in terms of the patient's menstrual history and physical examination. An ultrasound examination demonstrating an intrauterine pregnancy will clearly distinguish between the two entities.

More common than a ruptured corpus luteum of pregnancy, however, is the rupture of a persistent corpus luteum in a nonception menstrual cycle. In normal circumstances, the corpus luteum of an ovulatory cycle undergoes spontaneous luteolysis 2 weeks after ovulation. For reasons poorly understood, the corpus luteum may persist for an interval greater than 2 weeks. In such a case, the patient usually will experience amenorrhea for an additional 1 to 3 weeks, after which luteolysis occurs and a heavy menstrual flow results. If the corpus luteum persists and the cyst ruptures, the clinical presentation again could be very similar to that of an ectopic pregnancy or spontaneous abortion. HCG determinations and ultrasonography will be required for differentiation between the possible diagnoses.

Acute rupture of a corpus luteum cyst with consequent hemoperitoneum, in either a pregnant or nonpregnant state, usually requires surgical intervention and ovarian cystectomy. Outpatient management in suspected cases is contraindicated, although expectant management on an inpatient basis may be feasible if, in the judgement of the consultant gynecologist, the clinical picture warrants close observation only.

## BIBLIOGRAPHY

Carson SA, Buster JE: Ectopic pregnancy. *N Engl J Med* 329(16):117, 1993.
Centers for Disease Control and Prevention. 1993 sexually transmitted diseases treatment guidelines. *MMWR* 1993; 42(RR14):1–102.
Grimes DA, Cates W JR: Family planning and sexually transmitted diseases. In: Holmes KK, Mardh P-A, Sparling PF, Wiesner PJ, eds: *Sexually Transmitted Diseases,* 2nd ed. New York: McGraw-Hill, 1990:1087–95.
Stovall TG, Ling FW: Some new approaches to ectopic pregnancy. *Cont Ob/Gyn* 35, 1992.
Stovall TG, Ling FW: Single-dose methotrexate: An expanded clinical trial. *Cont Ob/Gyn* 168:1759, 1993.

# 97
# VULVOVAGINITIS
## Gloria Kuhn

Vulvovaginitis is the most common reason women seek medical attention and accounts for 10 million visits to physicians per year in the United States.

The most common causes of acute vulvovaginitis include (1) infections with *Gardnerella, Candida albicans, Trichomonas,* and herpes simplex virus type 2; (2) contact vulvovaginitis; (3) local response to a vaginal foreign body; and (4) atrophic vaginitis. Recent studies have shown that bacterial vaginosis is the most common form of infection (30 to 35 percent) followed closely by candidiasis (20 to 25 percent) and finally trichomoniasis (10 percent). A mixed infection is seen in 15 to 20 percent of patients.

Candidal and atrophic vaginitis may occur in virgins and after menopause, but other forms of vulvovaginitis are generally found only in sexually active women. A detailed gynecologic history, pelvic examination, and routine use of both normal saline and potassium hydroxide (KOH) slide preparations for microscopic evaluation of vaginal secretions will, in most instances, provide a diagnosis. Secretions should be checked for pH with nitrazine paper because this is a clue to the type of infection present.

## NORMAL

In the female of child-bearing age, estrogen causes the development of a thick vaginal epithelium with a large number of superficial cells serving a protective function and containing large stores of glycogen. This glycogen is used by the normal flora consisting of lactobacilli and acidogenic corynebacteria to form lactic and acetic acids. The resulting acidic environment favors the normal flora and discourages growth of pathogenic bacteria. Lack of estrogen or a dominance of progesterone results in an atrophic condition with loss of the protective superficial cells and their contained glycogen and loss of the acidic environment. Normal vaginal secretions may vary in consistency from a thin, watery material to one that is thick, white, and opaque. The quantity may also vary from scant to a rather copious amount. This material is odorless and produces no symptoms. The normal vaginal pH varies between 3.5 and 4.1. Alkaline secretions from the cervix before and during menstruation or semen, which is alkaline, reduce acidity, predisposing to infection. Before menarche and after menopause, the vaginal pH varies between 6 and 7. Because of scant nerve endings in the vagina, the patient usually does not have symptoms until both the vagina and vulva are involved in a disease process.

## *Candida* VAGINITIS

*Candida* species are a common cause of vaginitis. *C. albicans* is present as part of the normal vaginal flora in up to 50 percent of healthy, asymptomatic women, and therefore this infection is not considered a sexually transmitted disease. Immunity to candidal infections is primarily cell mediated. The growth of this organism is held in check by the normal vaginal flora, and infection usually occurs only when the normal balance is upset. Conditions that inhibit growth of normal vaginal flora (systemic antibiotics), diminish the glycogen stores in vaginal epithelial cells (diabetes mellitus, pregnancy, use of birth control pills, and the postmenopausal state), or increase the pH of vaginal secretions (menstrual blood or semen) may cause colonization by *Candida,* which is an opportunistic organism, and subsequent symptomatic infection. Tight-fitting undergarments may also contribute to the problem because of increased temperature, moisture, and local irritation.

**Table 97-1.** Treatment Regimens for Monilial Vulvovaginitis

| Agent | Dose |
| --- | --- |
| Nystatin (Mycostatin) | One vaginal tablet × 7–14 d, 1 g cream bid × 7–14 d |
| Clotrimazole (Gyne-Lotrimin, Mycelex-G) | 100 mg vaginal tablet × 7 d, 1% cream 5 g intravaginally × 7–14 d |
| Miconazole (Monistat) | 100 mg vaginal suppository × 7 nights 200 mg vaginal suppository × 3 nights 2% cream 5 g intravaginally × 7 nights |
| Terconazole (Terazol) | 80 mg vaginal suppository × 3 nights 0.4% cream intravaginally × 7 nights |
| Butoconazole (Femstat) | 2% cream 5 g intravaginally × 3 nights |

Clinical symptoms include leukorrhea, severe vaginal pruritus, and, occasionally, dysuria and/or dyspareunia. Gynecologic examination may reveal vulvar erythema and edema, vaginal erythema (20 percent), and an occasional thick "cottage cheese" discharge seen most often in pregnant patients. Often the onset of symptoms will coincide with menses or coitus.

The diagnosis of *Candida* vaginitis is made by microscopically examining a sample of vaginal secretions on a KOH slide preparation. Two drops of 10% KOH are applied to dissolve vaginal epithelial cells, leaving yeast buds and pseudohyphae intact. The sensitivity of KOH preparation is 80 percent, but the specificity is 100 percent.

Most treatment regimens are 80 to 90 percent effective in relieving symptoms but recurrence of infection is common. Three- and 7-day treatment regimens are superior to single-dose therapy. Creams, tablets, and vaginal suppositories are all available, but creams provide ease of use when there is extensive involvement of the vulvar area. The cream may be inserted intravaginally and also applied to vulvar tissue for symptomatic relief. Although nystatin, a polyene antibiotic derived from *Streptomyces noursei,* is effective, the imidazole drugs have become the mainstay of therapy and should be used whenever disease recurs. There are currently five members of this group (Table 97-1). They can be used safely during pregnancy but only when absolutely necessary during the first trimester. Treatment of recurrent fungal vulvovaginitis should include topical therapy immediately before or during menstrual flow for a minimum of two cycles following a full course of therapy.

Patients with recurrent infections should have documentation of infection by culture and should be evaluated for predisposing causes, especially diabetes mellitus, use of antibiotics, pregnancy, and human immunodeficiency virus (HIV) infection. Treatment of sexual partners is not necessary unless candidal balanitis is present.

## *Trichomonas* VAGINITIS

Trichomoniasis is almost always a sexually transmitted disease. The causative organism is a flagellated protozoa that may live quiescently in the paraurethral glands and from this nidus of infestation cause overt infection in the susceptible vagina. *Trichomonas vaginalis* may survive up to 24 h in tap water, in hot tubs, in urine, on toilet seats, and in swimming pools, but the usual sequence of events begins with the deposit of a large inoculum of organisms contained in the alkaline semen at time of intercourse. Up to 25 percent of women harboring the organisms are asymptomatic, and only about 10 percent of men infested with the organisms will have any symptoms at all.

The vaginal discharge, which may vary in character, is present in 50 to 75 percent of patients, but the classic yellow, frothy discharge is present in only 20 to 30 percent. Other symptoms include vulvovaginal soreness and irritation (25 to 50 percent), dysuria (25 percent), a disagreeable odor (25 percent), and lower abdominal discomfort (10 percent). The pH is greater than 4.5. Pruritus, pain, dyspareunia, dysuria, and a sense of vulvovaginal fullness may be intense or mild. Intermenstrual or postcoital spotting may occur. Symptoms may be more severe before, during, or after the menstrual period when the vaginal pH is more alkaline. The infection may cause changes on the Pap smear, which are inflammatory but not premalignant.

Gynecologic examination reveals the classic "strawberry cervix" secondary to diffuse punctate hemorrhages in only 2 percent of patients, but diffuse erythema of the vaginal vault is seen in 80 percent of cases.

The diagnosis of *Trichomonas* vaginitis is made through use of the "hanging drop" slide test. A cotton swab is used to obtain a specimen of secretions from the vaginal vault (not the endocervix) and is placed within a drop of normal saline on a glass slide. Microscopic examination reveals many polymorphonuclear leukocytes and motile, pear-shaped, flagellated trichomonads that are slightly larger than the leukocytes. The sensitivity of the test is 50 to 70 percent, but the specificity is 100 percent.

Treatment in the nonpregnant patient is best accomplished with a single 2-g oral dose of metronidazole (Flagyl). Metronidazole, 500 mg, b.i.d for 7 days, is recommended for treatment failures. Because metronidazole is an acetaldehyde dehydrogenase inhibitor, concomitant alcohol ingestion may precipitate an Antabuse-like reaction. Thus, alcohol should be avoided for 24 h following ingestion of the drug. Up to 90 percent of infected males are asymptomatic; thus, all male consorts should be referred for therapy. Failure of the asymptomatic male partner to seek treatment is probably responsible for the high recurrence rate of this infection. Metronidazole is a folic acid inhibitor and, therefore, is not recommended for use in the first trimester of pregnancy.

Pregnant patients with severe symptoms may be treated with clotrimazole, which has some activity against trichomonads and is recommended as the first line of therapy in pregnancy (100 mg/day for 14 days). If symptoms persist, metronidazole can be given as the 2-g, single dose after the first trimester. During lactation, the 2-g single-dose regimen is recommended, with discontinuation of breast-feeding for 24 h.

## BACTERIAL VAGINOSIS

Symptomatic bacterial vaginosis, also known as *Gardnerella* vaginitis, *Haemophilus* vaginitis, *Corynebacterium* vaginitis, and nonspecific vaginitis, is the clinical result of alterations in the vaginal microflora that promote the synergistic activity of aerobic *Gardnerella vaginalis* and vaginal anaerobes. Presence of the gram-negative rod designated *G. vaginalis* is not necessarily indicative of disease. The Centers for Disease Control and Prevention (CDC) states that for the disease to be diagnosed, three or four of the following criteria should be present: (1) homogeneous discharge, (2) pH of discharge greater than 4.5, (3) positive amine odor test, or (4) presence of clue cells.

The gram-negative rod is found in 40 percent of asymptomatic women and in children with no prior sexual contact. Males can harbor the organism in the urethra and serve as a potential source of infection.

When symptomatic, patients have mild pruritus and a copious vaginal discharge which has a disagreeable fishy odor. Gynecologic examination is usually normal except for occasional mild vaginal erythema and the presence of a thin, frothy gray-white vaginal discharge.

The diagnosis of *Gardnerella* vaginitis is often made from the wet-mount saline preparation, which shows pathognomonic *clue cells* (clusters of bacilli clinging to the surface of desquamated epithelial cells). Addition of 10% KOH to vaginal secretions will result in the release of a fishy odor (positive amine test). Often, the diagnosis must be suspected from the typical presentation accompanied by the absence of *Candida* and *Trichomonas* on microscopic examination.

Treatment for asymptomatic infection is not recommended by the CDC. Symptomatic patients may be treated with metronidazole 500 mg orally b.i.d for 7 days. Alternatively, clindamycin 300 mg orally b.i.d for 7 days may be used. Treatment of the male sex partner has not been shown to be beneficial.

In pregnancy, recent studies have suggested that bacterial vaginosis may be a factor in premature rupture of membranes and premature delivery. Until this is confirmed, routine treatment of the pregnant patient is not recommended. If it is necessary to treat the patient, clindamycin, 300 mg orally bid for 7 days is used because metronidazole is contraindicated in the first trimester of pregnancy.

## GENITAL HERPES

Genital herpes is a sexually transmitted infection caused by a DNA-containing virus specific to humans beings. There are two antigenic groups (HSV-1 and HSV-2). Initially, HSV-1 caused oral lesions and HSV-2 genital lesions, but that is no longer true, as up to 30 percent of genital lesions have been found to be due to HSV-1 in some studies. Generally it is felt that 85 to 90 percent of genital infections are caused by HSV-2. Symptomatic genital herpes is the most frequent cause of painful lesions of the lower genital tract in American women. It has been associated with cervical cancer, although a causative role has not been proved. Neonatal infection with high mortality and morbidity after passage through an infected birth canal has been seen. Although the actual prevalence is not known, it may be one of the most frequent sexually transmitted diseases. It is a recurrent disease with no cure at this time.

Initial presentation occurs 1 to 45 days (mean 5.8 days) after exposure. Usually initial infection is more severe and lasts longer than subsequent recurrences. There may be both local and systemic manifestations. The lesions begin as painful fluid-filled vesicles or papules which progress to well-circumscribed, occasionally coalescent, shallow-based ulcers. They then heal by reepithelialization of mucous membranes or by crusting by the epidermal surface. Symptoms peak in 8 to 10 days and decrease over the next week. Ulcers last 4 to 15 days with total healing in 21 days. Lymphadenopathy is usually present, and when the deep inguinal nodes are involved, severe pelvic pain may result. Urethritis is usually present, causing severe dysuria, which may cause urinary retention. Initial disease involves the cervix in over 80 percent of cases. Pharyngitis and secondary spread of lesions to other body sites, usually below the waist, have been reported in up to two thirds of patients. Systemic symptoms such as fever, malaise, headache, and myalgias are common. Hepatitis, aseptic meningitis, and autonomic nervous system dysfunction can occur. Aseptic meningitis has been seen more frequently with HSV-2 than with HSV-1 infection and has been reported in about 30 percent of patients. Sacral autonomic nervous dysfunction is rare but can result in decreased cutaneous sensation and bladder and bowel dysfunction. After the attack is over, the inactive virus resides in the dorsal root of the sacral ganglia. Under various stimuli both exogenous and endogenous, the virus travels down the sensory nerve root to the lower genital area where it replicates and becomes symptomatic.

Recurrent episodes are usually milder than the initial disease, and the patient usually does not have systemic symptoms. A recurrence may be heralded by genital tingling. Genital lesions are fewer, smaller, and more often unilateral. Lesions may be ulcerations or resemble a fissure or excoriations. Recurrences tend to occur in the same location and have the same appearance from episode to episode. Symptoms last 4 to 8 days, and the lesions have usually disappeared by 10 days. Frequency of attacks and intervals between attacks are highly variable. The average number of symptomatic recurrences is 5 to 8 per year. Asymptomatic infections, defined as culture-positive viral shedding in the absence of symptoms or lesions, have been documented.

Approximately 25 percent of initial presentations occur in women with preexisting antibody to HSV. These initial episodes tend to be less severe and resemble recurrent infections. These may, in fact, represent recurrent infections in patients who had previous asymptomatic infections. Clinically it is impossible to distinguish between HSV-1 and HSV-2 infections, but HSV-1 usually causes milder ini-

**Table 97-2.** Treatment Regimen for Genital Herpes Simplex Infection

| Episode | Acyclovir Treatment Regimen |
|---------|----------------------------|
| First genital | 200 mg PO 5 times/d 7–10 d or until clinical resolution |
| First rectal | 400 mg orally 5 times/day 10 d or until clinical resolution |
| Severe disease | 5–10 mg/kg body weight IV q8h 5–7 d until clinical resolution |
| Recurrent | 200 mg orally 5 times/day 5 d or 400 mg orally tid 5 d or 800 mg orally bid 5 d |
| Suppression | 400 mg orally bid |

tial disease, results in recurrence less frequently, and the recurrent episodes are milder and less frequent.

Diagnosis is suspected by clinical presentation and confirmed by culture. The virus can be isolated from vesicle fluid and the base of a wet ulcer. Intact vesicles, if present, should be unroofed and the fluid cultured directly. These cultures will be positive in 85 to 95 percent of cases. Scrapings of an ulcer may be taken for a Pap smear or Tzanck preparation. A Tzanck smear stained with either Wright or Giemsa stain is positive if multinucleated giant cells are present, as they are in up to 50 percent of cases. Antibody testing is usually of no value, as even if the test is positive, it does not denote active disease.

Treatment is not curative. Systemic acyclovir provides partial control of the signs and symptoms and accelerates healing of lesions, but it does not affect the frequency or severity of recurrences. Topical treatment with acyclovir is not effective and should not be used. Patients with severe disease may need hospitalization and intravenous therapy. In recurrent episodes, treatment should be instituted during the prodrome or within 2 days of onset of lesions if treatment is to be beneficial. Most immunocompetent patients do not benefit from therapy because it can seldom be initiated soon enough. For patients with frequent recurrences (six or more episodes per year) daily suppressive therapy can be used but should be discontinued after 1 year to allow assessment of the patient's rate of recurrent episodes. Daily suppressive therapy reduces frequency of recurrences by at least 75 percent. Patients who are HIV positive may have frequent infections and may benefit from increased dosages of acyclovir. Although the dosage is controversial, regimens of 400 mg orally 3 to 5 times a day have been found helpful (Table 97-2). Severe disease or treatment failure in the HIV-positive patient may necessitate hospitalization and alternative therapy. An infectious disease expert should be consulted. The safety of acyclovir therapy during pregnancy has not been established. In pregnant patients with life-threatening disease such as encephalitis, pneumonitis, or hepatitis, intravenous acyclovir may be used. It should not be used for recurrent episodes or as suppressive therapy. Pregnant women treated with the drug should be reported to the Burroughs Wellcome registry, which is kept in cooperation with the CDC (1-800-722-9292, ext. 58465). Although acyclovir-resistant strains have been isolated, they have not been associated with treatment failures among immunocompetent patients.

## CONTACT VULVOVAGINITIS

Contact dermatitis results from the exposure of vulvar epithelium and vaginal mucosa to either a primary chemical irritant or an allergen. In either case, characteristic local erythema and edema occur. Severe reactions may progress to ulceration and secondary infection. Common irritants and/or allergens include chemically scented douches; soaps; bubble baths; deodorants; perfumes; dyes and scents in toilet paper, tampons, and pads; feminine hygiene products; topical vaginal antibiotics; tight slacks and panty hose; and tight elastic underwear.

Clinically, patients report local swelling and itching or a burning sensation. The gynecologic examination reveals an erythematous and edematous vulvovaginal area. Local vesiculation and ulceration are seen more commonly with allergens or when primary irritants are used in strong concentrations. Vaginal pH changes may promote colonization and infection with *C. albicans*, thus obscuring the primary cause.

The diagnosis of contact vulvovaginitis is made by ruling out an infectious cause and by identifying the offending agent. Most cases of mild vulvovaginal contact dermatitis resolve spontaneously when the causative agent is withdrawn. For patients with severe painful reactions, cool sitz baths and wet compresses of dilute boric acid or Burow's solution may afford relief. Topical corticosteroids such as hydrocortisone acetate (Cortef), fluocinolone acetonide (Synalar), or triamcinolone acetonide (Aristocort) relieve symptoms and promote healing. Oral antihistamines should be avoided because they may actually dry the vaginal mucosal membrane and result in further irritation and discomfort.

## VAGINAL FOREIGN BODIES

Children and adolescents may insert objects intravaginally during periods of genital exploration or sexual stimulation. In young girls the most commonly inserted foreign bodies are rolled up pieces of toilet paper, toys, and small household objects. In adolescents it is often a forgotten tampon or diaphragm. Foreign objects left in place for more than 48 h can cause severe localized infections due to *Escherichia coli*, anaerobes, or overgrowth of other vaginal flora. Patients present with a foul-smelling and/or bloody vaginal discharge. The only treatment necessary for vaginitis secondary to foreign bodies is removal of the object. In most cases, the patient's associated vaginal discharge and odor will disappear without further therapy within several days.

## PINWORMS

Pinworms (*Enterobius vermicularis*) may migrate from the anus to the vagina in children and cause intense pruritus. Pruritus is often most intense during the night when gravid females pass through the gastrointestinal tract to lay eggs on the perineal skin. Cellophane tape can be used to obtain material for a slide that can be looked at microscopically for presence of ova, which are large and double walled in appearance. The child and family members need treatment with an antiparasitic agent, pyrantel pamoate (11 mg/kg, maximum 1g) as a single dose; or mebendazole, 100 mg as a single oral dose.

## ATROPHIC VAGINITIS

During menarche, pregnancy, lactation, and after menopause, the vaginal epithelium lacks the stimulation of estrogen. The maturation of the vaginal and urethra mucosa depends on the presence of estrogen and can be altered by the absence of estrogen or the presence of antiestrogenic factors such as hormones, drugs, or diseases. Menopause results in a vaginal mucosa that is attenuated, pale, and almost transparent as a result of decreased vascularity. The vagina loses its normal rugae. The squamous epithelium atrophies, the glycogen content of the cells decreases, and the vaginal pH increases. The mucosa is only three or four cells thick and is less resistant to minor trauma or infection. Marked atrophic changes can cause atrophic vaginitis. The vaginal epithelium is then thin, inflamed, and even ulcerated. Bleeding may occur. There may be a thin, scant, yellowish or pink discharge with an alkaline pH. The cervix atrophies and retracts and may become flush with the apex of the vault. The upper one third of the vagina constricts and the entire vagina becomes shorter in length and loses its elasticity. The vaginal pH increases, which may permit the growth of bacteria not normally found in the vagina and can lead to the development of a clinical vaginal infection with a copious purulent discharge. Lactobacilli and corynebacteria, normally present, are diminished, whereas coliforms, gut anaerobes, and pyogenic cocci are frequent isolates. Unless estrogenic replacement therapy is used, *Candida* and *Trichomonas* infections are rare. The changes seen vary widely from one patient to another. A Pap smear of the cervix and vagina is mandatory in the face of bleeding to rule out carcinoma. A wet preparation will show erythrocytes, leukocytes, and round or oval parabasal cells. A sulfa-containing cream should be used if there is a secondary infection, and an estrogen cream should be applied for 2 to 3 weeks. Estrogen creams should not be prescribed for any patient with a past history of cancer of any of the reproductive organs. Atrophic vaginitis is usually not seen in patients who are on systemic estrogen replacement therapy. Patients should be referred for follow-up to monitor therapy and for the results of the Pap smear.

## BIBLIOGRAPHY

Abramowicz M: Drugs for sexually transmitted diseases, In *Medical Letter on Drugs and Therapeutics.* Medical Letter Inc, pp. 1–6, 1994.

Bergman A, Brenner PF: In: Mishell DRJ (ed). *Menopause Physiology and Pharmacology.* Chicago: Year Book Medical Publishers, 1987.

Copeland L: ed. *Textbook of Gynecology.* Philadelphia: WB Saunders, 1993.

Hinman A: *1993 Sexually Transmitted Diseases Treatment Guidelines.* Atlanta: Centers for Disease Control and Prevention. Epidemiology Program Office, 1993.

Larsen B: Vaginal flora in health and disease. *Clin Obstet Gynecol* 36; 1993.

Pokorny SF: Prepubertal vulvovaginopathies. *Pediatric and Adolescent Gynecology* 19:39, 1992.

Sparks J: Vaginitis. *J Reprod Med* 36:745, 1991.

# 98
# PROBLEMS IN PREGNANCY

## Wendy F. Hansen
## Alfred R. Hansen

## INTRODUCTION

Pregnant women present to emergency departments with the same disorders and diseases as other patients. However, the emergency physician must now meet the additional challenge of pregnancy and all that it encompasses.

This chapter reviews physiologic changes in pregnancy, drugs in pregnancy, diagnostic imaging, pregnancy and co-existing diseases, selected pregnancy-related problems and perinatal infections.

## PHYSIOLOGIC CHANGES IN NORMAL PREGNANCY

These changes can give rise to a constellation of symptoms as well as alterations from "normal" in vital signs, in the results of common laboratory tests, and in the responses to some therapeutic interventions. Such alterations must be recognized and understood if one is to diagnose and effectively manage problems in pregnancy.

## Cardiovascular Changes

Cardiac output increases from 30 to 50 percent to 6.2 L/min.
Central venous pressure is unchanged.
Pulmonary capillary wedge pressure is slightly decreased to 7.5 mmHg.
Blood volume increases by 45 percent.
Plasma volume increase is greater than red cell mass; mean hemoglobin range is 10.2 to 11.6 g/dL.
Systemic vascular resistance decreases to 1210 dyne·cm·sec$^{-5}$
Heart rate increases by 15 to 20 beats per minute.
A systolic decrease of 5 to 10 mmHg and a diastolic decrease of 10 to 15 mmHg in arterial blood pressure occur during pregnancy.

Venal caval compression occurs in 10 to 15 percent of all pregnant women when they lie flat on their backs. Symptoms include dizziness, sweating, nausea, and, if prolonged, fetal bradycardia. All pregnant women should be counseled, examined, transported, and operated on in a lateral tilt position.

Blood pressure must increase by 30 mmHg systolic or 15 mmHg diastolic to be classified as hypertension in preeclampsia. When evaluating blood pressure it is important to look at the rise from the second trimester nadir. Often a diastolic of 80 mmHg is abnormal for the pregnant woman.

Cardiac output is very dependent on maternal position and is at maximum in the left lateral tilt position. This is extremely important in the management of clinical shock and maternal resuscitation.

## Pulmonary Changes

Respiratory rate is unchanged.
Tidal volume is increased 30 to 40 percent.
Vital capacity is unchanged.
Functional residual capacity is decreased.
Normal arterial blood gas values in pregnancy: pH, 7.40 to 7.45; $P_{O_2}$, 95 to 105 mmHg; $P_{CO_2}$, 28 to 32 mmHg; bicarbonate, 18 to 31 mEq/L.

The mucosa of the nasopharynx becomes edematous and hyperemic. Nasal stuffiness and epistaxis are common.

Every woman in the third trimester of pregnancy exhibits a mild respiratory alkalosis, and most feel a substantial degree of breathlessness. A $P_{CO_2}$ of 40 mmHg in a pregnant woman with asthma indicates retention.

## Renal Changes

Glomerular filtration rate increases by 50 percent.
Serum creatinine decreases to 0.5 to 0.75 mg/dL.
Serum blood urea nitrogen decreases to 9 to 10 mg/dL.
Serum uric acid levels decrease 2.0 to 3.0 mg/dL up until 24 weeks.
Late in pregnancy, levels are similar to nonpregnant states.

A creatinine level of > 1.0 mg/dL is abnormally elevated in pregnancy. Drugs that are excreted by the kidney need special dosing in pregnancy; magnesium sulfate and aminoglycosides are prime examples.

## Gastrointestinal Changes

There is decreased gastric tone and motility, decreased gastric emptying time, and decreased tone of the gastroesophageal sphincter. There is also decreased motility of the small bowel. There is no change in absorption of nutrients, except enhanced absorption of iron. The liver does not enlarge during pregnancy, and blood flow to the liver is essentially unchanged. Serum levels of bilirubin, aspartate and alanine aminotransferase, and lactate dehydrogenase are unchanged. There is increased absorption of colonic water. Gallbladder residual volumes are twice normal and the rate of gallbladder emptying is slower.

Many clinical signs and laboratory levels commonly found in normal pregnancies are suggestive of liver disease in the nonpregnant state. The increased levels of estrogen cause spider angiomata and palmar erythema. Laboratory changes are also seen: serum albumin decreases to 3.0 g/dL; serum alkaline phosphatase increases 100 to 400 percent; and fibrinogen increases to 400 to 580 mg/dL.

The blood sedimentation rate is markedly increased in pregnancy secondary to the increased fibrinogen and thus has no clinical value in pregnancy.

Aspiration during intubation or general anesthesia is a serious threat to the pregnant woman.

Nausea and vomiting of pregnancy complicates up to 70 percent of pregnancies; heartburn and esophageal reflux are common.

Constipation and engorged hemorrhoids are common and often troublesome.

## Coagulation Changes

Bleeding time, prothrombin time, partial thromboplastin time, and thrombin clotting times are unchanged.
Factors VII, VIII, IX, and X are increased.
Lower extremity venous distension increases markedly, with venous flow velocity reduced by half in the third trimester.

Risk of thromboembolism compared to nonpregnant controls is 1.8 during pregnancy and 5.5 in the postpartum period. Thromboembolism remains the number one cause of maternal mortality.

## Hematologic Changes

The leukocyte count increases in pregnancy to a mean of 10,000 per µl but may be as high as 15,000 per µl. There is also a small left shift composed mostly of bands. Lymphocytes are unchanged. This normal leukocytosis often hinders the diagnosis of appendicitis and cholecystitis.

## Metabolic Changes

Pregnancy is a diabetogenic state with increased peripheral resistance of glucose. Cholesterol, triglycerides, and free fatty acid levels increase. The woman with type I diabetes mellitus will often find that insulin requirements increase dramatically in early pregnancy. Pregnancy may indeed be an underlying cause for ketoacidosis.

## Uterine Changes

The uterus increases in size from an average of 60 g to 1000 g and can accommodate a 4500-g fetus. Uterine blood flow increase to 500 to 800 mL/min, accounting for 8 to 15 percent of cardiac output.

Average blood loss from delivery is 500 mL and from Cesarean section is 1000 mL. After delivery, increased uterine blood flow that was necessary to sustain a pregnancy is now redistributed to other organs and accounts for the minimal anemia seen after a normal delivery.

## Diagnosis of Pregnancy

The ability to diagnose pregnancy accurately has very important implications in the emergency department, especially in the woman of childbearing age with abdominal pain. Every experienced emergency department physician has discovered pregnancy in spite of a contrary menstrual history: thus the diagnosis is dependent on the laboratory test. The diagnosis of pregnancy has been made considerably easier with the advent of the enzyme-linked immunoassay (ELISA) that is specific to the β subunit of human chorionic gonadotropin (HCG). As these tests have evolved, their sensitivity has improved and, depending on the manufacturer, can detect HCG levels as low as 20 mIU. The urine pregnancy test can be completed in 5 min and does not require sophisticated laboratory equipment or personnel. Therefore it is the most common type of pregnancy test used in office settings and emergency departments. Beta-HCG is detectable 9 to 11 days after ovulation and reaches about 100 mIU at the time of the first missed menses. Although a negative qualitative urine test does not absolutely rule out ectopic pregnancy, if a properly done ELISA is negative, the diagnosis is extremely unlikely.

Serum pregnancy tests are divided into qualitative or quantitative. Qualitative serum pregnancy tests are only slightly more sensitive (10 mIU) and offer little advantage over those done on urine. Quantitative assays are available that are able to measure HCG at levels less than 5 mIU. These assays require a more sophisticated laboratory and approximately 2 h to complete. Serial quantitative measurements are especially useful in following those women at risk for ectopic pregnancy and those with suspected abnormal first trimester pregnancies. Beta-HCG should increase at least 66 percent every 48 h in the first 6 weeks of pregnancy. An abnormal rise in serial HCGs almost always heralds an abnormal pregnancy and necessitates further evaluation of the pregnancy.

A single measurement can be useful when trying to answer the very important question: at what range of serum β-HCG level should a gestational sac be seen on transvaginal ultrasound? This level is referred to as the *discriminatory zone*. The discriminatory zone is dependent on many factors: the type of assay used by each individual laboratory, the technical capability of the ultrasound equipment, and whether transvaginal or transabdominal techniques are used. These factors make it impossible to set a "gold standard." Rather, each individual hospital/clinical team must establish its own. The gestational sac is the first embryologic structure seen on transvaginal ultrasound and can be seen as early as 5 weeks from the last menstrual period. Documentation of an intrauterine gestational sac can be important in the emergency department because there is only a 1:4000 to 1:15,000 chance that an ectopic pregnancy coexists with an intrauterine pregnancy. Over the next week a yolk sac, fetal pole, and, lastly, cardiac motion will become evident on ultrasound. The demonstration of cardiac motion is particularly reassuring in the evaluation of patients at risk for spontaneous abortion, since the chance of fetal demise decreases from about 15 percent to 2 to 3 percent.

## Gestational Age Determination

Knowing the approximate gestational age is important in understanding the specific risks of drugs, infections, and diagnostic imaging to both the mother and fetus. In addition, the risks of specific complications and their management is dependent on gestational age. A term gestation is considered to be 40 weeks from an accurate last menstrual period (LMP) based on a 28-day cycle. Although it has been well documented that 50 percent of women are unsure of their LMP, a careful history including recent use of oral contraceptives and menstrual cycle regularity and length is important. Uterine size estimates can also be helpful. There are two important landmarks when sizing a uterus: (1) at 12 weeks' gestation the uterus is just rising out of the pelvis, and (2) at 20 weeks' gestation the uterus should be at the level of the umbilicus. When both a known LMP and uterine size are in agreement, an accurate estimation of gestational age can be made. When the LMP is unknown or LMP and sizing of the uterus are in disagreement, an ultrasound is appropriate.

Ultrasound prior to 20 weeks' gestation can be quite accurate in the determination of fetal age. A variety of fetal biometric measurements such as crown-rump length, biparietal diameter, femur length, and abdominal circumference are used in determining fetal age. As pregnancy progresses, the accuracy of ultrasound to determine fetal age decreases markedly, so that after 28 weeks the error of measurement is ± 3 weeks.

## DRUGS IN PREGNANCY

The emergency physician often has to prescribe drugs in the treatment of various problems encountered in pregnancy or is faced with a woman already on a medication who coincidentally learns she is pregnant. A few key principles should be kept in mind. Virtually all drugs cross the placenta to some degree with the exception of large molecules such as heparin and insulin. Lipid-soluble drugs readily cross the placenta, and water-soluble substances less well. Our knowledge base is continually changing, and access to an up-to-date reference is needed.

Many variables affect whether a drug will have a teratogenic effect: gestational age at exposure, susceptible stage of development, dosage, length of exposure, and individual genetic susceptibility. Often drugs are ingested in the earliest stages of gestation before a woman is even aware of pregnancy, and the physician is later confronted by anxious inquiries regarding the potential harmful effects of the ingestion on the embryo. The very nature of embryogenesis allows an analysis of the situation that many find comforting. *Embryogenesis* begins at conception and extends over the next 18 days. During this time an exposure is thought to cause an "all or none" effect. So few cells exist early on that irreparable damage to some cells is lethal to the entire embryo. If repair is possible, the embryo continues on with no organ-specific malformation. The second stage of gestation is termed *organogenesis* and extends from day 18 (after conception) to day 60. This is the time of greatest sensitivity to potential teratogens and is when most gross anatomic malformations are seen. The third stage is from day 60 onward and is referred to as the *fetal period*. Exposure at this time causes abnormal cell growth and differentiation. The evaluation of an effect of a drug on a fetus is a complex issue, and obstetric consultation is often needed. The Food and Drug Administration (FDA) lists five categories of labeling for drug use in pregnancy.

**Category A.** Controlled studies in women fail to demonstrate a risk to the fetus in the first trimester (and there is no evidence of a risk in later trimesters), and the possibility of fetal harm appears remote.

**Category B.** Either animal-reproduction studies have not demonstrated a fetal risk but there are no controlled studies in pregnant women, or animal-reproduction studies have shown an adverse effect (other than a decrease in fertility) that was not confirmed in controlled studies in women in the first trimester (and there is no evidence of a risk in later trimesters).

**Category C.** Either studies in animals have revealed adverse effects on the fetus (teratogenic or embryocidal, or other) and there are no controlled studies in women, or studies in women and animals are not available. Drugs should be given only if the potential benefit justifies the potential risk to the fetus.

**Category D.** There is positive evidence of human fetal risk, but the benefits from use in pregnant women may be acceptable despite the risk (e.g., if the drug is needed in a life-threatening situation or for a serious disease for which safer drugs cannot be used or are ineffective).

**Category X.** Studies in animals or human beings have demonstrated fetal abnormalities, or there is evidence of fetal risk based on human experience, or both, and the risk of the use of the drug in pregnant women clearly outweighs any possible benefit. The drug is contraindicated in women who are or may become pregnant.

## Antimicrobials

Antibiotics should be used as needed in the management of certain diagnosis. Choosing the right antibiotic is dependent not only on the infectious complication and maternal allergy status but also on gestational age. Penicillins, cephalosporins, nitrofurantoin, macrolides (erythromycin, azithromycin), and clindamycin can be used at any time in pregnancy. Erythromycin estolate is contraindicated in pregnancy because of drug-related hepatoxicity. Aminoglycosides have varying toxicity. There have been no reports of congenital abnormalities or fetal ototoxicity from gentamycin. However, kanamycin and streptomycin are contraindicated. Metronidazole use in pregnancy remains controversial. The Centers for Disease Control and Prevention (CDC) and FDA consider metronidazole to be contraindicated during the first trimester; however, its use thereafter is acceptable. Antituberculosis drugs such as isoniazid, para-aminosalicylic acid (PAS), and ethambutol have shown no teratogenic effects in pregnancy and should be used if needed. Sulfa drugs can be used in pregnancy but should be avoided near term because of their potential toxicity to the newborn. Trimethoprim/sulfamethoxazole is generally contraindicated in pregnancy because of its theoretical teratogenicity. Tetracyclines are highly bound to calcium in developing bones and teeth, causing a brown discoloration of teeth, hypoplasia of the enamel, and inhibition of bone growth. Tetracyclines should be avoided in pregnancy. Quinolones (ciprofloxacin, norfloxacin) have been shown to cause an abnormality in cartilage formation in animals and are considered contraindicated in pregnancy.

## Antivirals

Acyclovir (Zovirax) is used frequently by women for both primary and recurrent genital herpes. An acyclovir registry has now collected over 300 prenatal exposures, and no increase in malformations has been found. Acyclovir should be used for life-threatening maternal illnesses such as varicella pneumonia. Its use for recurrent herpes remains controversial, and certainly discussion with the patient concerning risks and benefits should be undertaken prior to prescription.

## Antihypertensive Agents

Two classes of antihypertensive agents are contraindicated in pregnancy. Ganglionic blockers are not well tolerated by the pregnant woman and pose a risk of meconium ileus to the fetus. Angiotensin-converting enzyme (ACE) inhibitors are currently widely used in the treatment of hypertension. Both animal studies and clinical experience have demonstrated abnormal fetal and neonatal renal function, which has been irreversible in some instances. Both of these drugs should be discontinued either prior to a planned pregnancy or once pregnancy is diagnosed.

Alpha methyldopa is the antihypertensive drug that is most thoroughly studied for both its teratogenic potential and in long-term follow-up. It is known to be safe and continues to be a first-line drug in the treatment of hypertension during pregnancy.

Other drugs that have enjoyed recent widespread use in pregnancy include β blockers (propanolol and labetolol), calcium channel blockers such as nifedipine, and vasodilators such as prazosin and hydralazine. Diuretics are not generally recommended in pregnancy and are contraindicated in the management of hypertension associated with preeclampsia. If a woman presents on long-term diuretics for hypertension, they may be continued depending on other factors.

## Anticonvulsants

The management of epilepsy in the pregnant patient appears to be a dilemma, since all of the anticonvulsants—dilantin, carbamazepine, valproic acid, primodone, phenobarbital, and trimethadone—have been associated with various congenital malformations. However, seizures represent such a risk to the mother and fetus that the primary clinical concern must be prevention, utilizing the most effective drug regimen possible. Thus, the preferred drug for pregnant women with epilepsy is the drug that best controls her seizures. There is no single drug of choice. An association between folic acid deficiency and congenital malformations has been established and in part may be responsible for the teratogenesis of anticonvulsants. Therefore a multivitamin preparation with 1 mg of folic acid is recommended before conception or when the diagnosis of pregnancy is made.

### Corticosteroids

All the corticosteroids cross the placenta to some degree. Prednisone and prednisolone are partially inactivated by the placenta, and fetal levels are about 10 percent of maternal levels. These drugs should be used when indicated for the control of maternal disease such as asthma, lupus, and certain dermatologic conditions. Recent studies show no teratogenic effects.

### Anticoagulants

Heparin is the drug of choice for pregnant women requiring anticoagulation. It is a large molecule, negatively charged, and does not cross the placenta. Hematologic consultation should be obtained before giving low-molecular weight heparin. Warfarin, or Coumadin, crosses the placenta and is a known teratogen, causing an embryopathy in one-third of fetuses exposed during the first trimester.

### Analgesics

Acetaminophen, propoxyphene, codeine, demerol, and morphine have no known teratogenic effect and should be used for the control of severe pain in pregnancy. Caution is advised in the use of narcotics as there are numerous case reports of neonatal withdrawal symptoms when these drugs are used in large amounts over a long period of time and late in pregnancy. Aspirin has no known teratogenic effect and can be used if needed. It should be limited to short courses.

### Antiemetics

Meclizine, dimenhydrinate (Dramamine), diphenhydramine (Benadryl), trimethobenzamide (Tigan), and the phenothiazines have no known teratogenic effects and can be used in pregnancy.

### Over-the-Counter Preparations

Vitamins and multiple vitamin preparations are safe in all stages of pregnancy.

Compounds for the symptomatic relief of upper respiratory symptoms are plentiful and often contain two or three drugs in combination. Pregnant patients should first be counseled to use alternative supportive measures such as humidifier, rest, and fluids and to avoid medications if possible. Most expectant mothers will appreciate that the slight amelioration of their cold symptoms is a minimal benefit to be weighed against the slight but real potential to harm their babies and will elect to do without nonessential medications. When necessary, preparations with phenylpropanolamine should be used, while those containing pseudoephedrine should be avoided, following a recent case-controlled study reporting an increased risk of fetal gastroschisis. When decongestion is the primary goal, topical nasal sprays or drops should be used when possible.

### Nonsteroidal Anti-Inflammatory Drugs (NSAIDs)

NSAIDs are not teratogenic. They have been used in pregnancy both as tocolytic agents and for the control of pain in certain clinical situations. Their use has been associated with decreased amniotic fluid throughout gestation and with closure of the fetal ductus arteriosus when used in the third trimester. Both these effects are reversible once the drug is discontinued. If NSAIDs are deemed necessary, they should be used for short durations (48 to 72 h) and not after 32 weeks' gestation. Consultation with an obstetrician/gynecologist should be initiated.

### Live Viral Vaccines

Risks from vaccination are largely theoretical, and the benefits of immunization usually outweigh the potential risks. Live viral vaccines should not be given in pregnancy except when exposure is highly probable and the threat of the disease is greater than that of the immunization, as with yellow fever. Measles, mumps, and rubella (MMR) is a live viral vaccine and should not be given in pregnancy because of its theoretical risk. Ideally, MMR should be given at least 3 months prior to pregnancy or in the immediate postpartum period. Data from over 700 women who inadvertently received MMR within 3 months before or during pregnancy have not shown any teratogenic effects. The inactivated viral vaccines include influenza, rabies, and hepatitis B and should be given in pregnancy when indicated. Pneumococcal vaccine is an inactivated bacterial vaccine and should be given in pregnancy as needed. Guidelines for the administration of tetanus toxoid or diphtheria and tetanus toxoids (Td) are unchanged in pregnancy. Specific immune globulins including hepatitis B, rabies, and tetanus should be given to the pregnant woman for postexposure prophylaxis. Varicella prophylaxis guidelines are summarized in Table 98-1.

## DIAGNOSTIC IMAGING

Imaging studies provide an invaluable aid in the evaluation and management of both medical and surgical problems. The pregnant woman poses a special situation in two ways. First, the anatomic and physiologic changes of normal pregnancy influence the usual interpretation of a study and certainly limit the efficacy of some. Second, the pregnant woman is really two patients. Therefore, a primary goal is to match the best diagnostic test for the mother with the least harmful effect to the developing embryo and fetus.

What is the actual fetal risk? The major factor determining the degree of risk to the fetus in an imaging technique is the amount of ionizing radiation involved in the test. Exposure to ionizing radiation occurs with plain x-ray films, angiography, fluoroscopy, nuclear medicine, and computed tomography (CT). Nonionizing studies include magnetic resonance imaging (MRI) and ultrasound.

Most information on hazards from radiation comes from animal studies and on fetuses exposed by the atomic bombs dropped on Japan. The most recent evidence suggests that 10 rad is a threshold for human teratogenesis, and the fetus appears to be most vulnerable at 8 to 15 weeks' gestation. The American College of Radiology's position states that there is no single diagnostic test that results in radiation doses that threaten the well-being of the developing embryo or fetus. However, cumulative doses from multiple procedures may enter the harmful range.

The radiation doses involved in commonly used diagnostic tests are given in Table 98-2.

A common nuclear medicine imaging study used by the emergency department physician is the ventilation/perfusion scan. Total fetal exposure to xenon 133 and technetium 99m is about 0.5 rad, and they can be used safely in pregnancy. Fetal exposure from other studies using technetium 99 range from 0.03 to 0.06 rad/mCi and are safe in pregnancy. Because the excretion of these radionuclide particles is often via the maternal bladder, which is close to the fetus, hydration and frequent voiding need to be encouraged.

The two nonionizing imaging studies used frequently are ultrasound and MRI. Ultrasound has been studied extensively over the past 25 years and has no known teratogenic effect. There is much less experience with MRI, but thus far there are no known harmful effects.

**Table 98-1.** Infection in Pregnancy

| | Transmission | Prevention | Maternal Symptoms | Diagnosis | Fetal Effects | Treatment |
|---|---|---|---|---|---|---|
| Cytomegalovirus (CMV) | Close contact with secretions | Universal precautions | 60% asymptomatic; 40% mononucleosis-like syndrome | Serology antibody IgM, IgG | Congenital CMV: 40% transmit infection to the fetus, only 10–15% are affected long term; counseling and diagnosis are complex, involving ultrasound, amniocentesis, and fetal blood sampling. | None available |
| Toxoplasmosis | Eating raw or improperly prepared meat of infected animals; inhaling or ingesting oocysts excreted by domestic cats | Avoid handling litter of infected animals; avoid raw meat | 60–90% fever, chills, headache, malaise, lymphadenopathy | Serology antibody IgM, IgG | 10% will have congenital toxoplasmosis; counseling and diagnosis are complex | Use of spiramycin, pyrimethamine, or Sulfonamides is controversial |
| Rubella | By droplets, direct contact, or articles contaminated with nasopharyngeal secretions | | Rash, malaise low-grade fever; many are subclinical | 1. Detection in acute and convalescent sera of a rise in rubella antibody 2. Rubella IgM antibodies are detectable up to 4 weeks after the rash | Congenital rubella syndrome (CRS); infection in the first trimester is associated with high incidence of CRS | No treatment for acute disease |
| Varicella chickenpox | 80–90% attack rate via respiratory secretions droplets, direct contact; communicability is 2 days prior to vesicular eruption until vesicles crust over | | Fever, chills, malaise, arthralgias, vesicular rash; cough and dyspnea may herald varicella pneumonia | 1. Clinical signs or symptoms. 2. Laboratory markers for both antigen and antibodies exist 3. Tzanck smear of vesicles | A congenital varicella syndrome occurs rarely in 3–5%; more common when infection occurs in first trimester | 1. Determine immunity status; 80% of women with a negative history have serologic evidence of immunity 2. If testing cannot be done or patient is seronegative, administer varicella zoster immune globulin vaccine; dosage 125 unit 10/kg to a maximum of 5 vials should be given within 96 h of exposure 3. The use of acyclovir for uncomplicated chickenpox remains controversial 4. Admit all women with respiratory symptoms and varicella |
| Human parvovirus (B19) ("fifth disease," "erythema infectiosum") | Respiratory secretions, "hand to mouth"; attack rate is 20–50% with prolonged exposure, 5% with casual exposure | | 80% have a reticular rash on the trunk and peripheral arthropathies; 20% are asymptomatic | Parvovirus-specific antibody IgM/IgG by Centers for Disease Control & Prevention; also available at State Health Department | Increased spontaneous abortion with infection in first and second trimesters Rarely attacks erythroid precursors with resultant fetal anemia and hydrops | None available |
| Hepatitis B | Parenteral and sexual contact | Universal precautions | Nausea, malaise, fatigue, jaundice | Elevated amino transferase levels; hepatitis panel | Affects neonates of infected mother | 1. Exposure by percutaneous or mucus membrane in nonimmunized women: administer hepatitis B immune globulin (HBIG) 0.06 mL/kg; two injections 1 month apart followed by vaccination series series. 2. Exposure by sexual contact: HBIG—0.06 mL/kg single dose within 14 days of contact, followed by vaccination series s 3. Acute infection: supportive care |

**Table 98-2.** Radiation Exposure to the Uterus/Fetus

| Dosage, rad | Procedure |
| --- | --- |
| 0.00005 | Chest radiography (two views) with shielding of the maternal abdomen. |
| 0.686–1.398 | Intravenous pyelogram full series; in the case of a suspected stone a one-shot pyelogram should be used when a renal ultrasound is inconclusive or unavailable |
| .1 | Kidney, ureter, bladder—single abdominal film |
| 0.051–0.126 | Lumbar spine series (three films) |
| 0.168–0.359 | Lumbosacral spine series (three films) |
| 0.007–0.02 | Mammography—diagnostic for suspected breast cancers |
| 0.01 | Cerebral angiography |
| 0.056 | Upper gastrointestinal series |
| 1.9–3.9 | Barium enema |
| <0.1 | Head computed tomography (CT) |
| <0.2 | Chest CT |
| 5.0 | Abdominal CT |
| 7.0 | Lumbar spine CT |
| 0.50 | Pelvimetry CT |

## PREGNANCY AND COEXISTING DISEASES

Pregnant women with problems that may be reasonably straightforward in the nongravid state may constitute special diagnostic difficulties. The challenge to the emergency physician is to determine which of these processes are self-limiting and which require immediate intervention.

The most common infections in pregnant women are upper respiratory (URI) and urinary disorders. The clinician should be alert to the fact that alterations in anatomy and in immune function make the pregnant woman more susceptible to fulminant pneumonias and serious urinary tract infections. In addition, when a serious septic process occurs there is a significant risk of preterm labor and birth.

## Upper Respiratory Infections

Ear, nose, and throat infections including otitis media, sinusitis, and pharyngitis are common reasons for pregnant women to seek medical care. The symptoms and signs in pregnancy are no different than in the nonpregnant patient. A throat culture or rapid antigen detection should be done when one or more signs of group A streptococcal pharyngitis (tonsilar exudates, anterior cervical lymphadenopathy, fever, absence of cough) are present. Antibiotic treatment should be instituted for positive tests, for those with two or more signs, or for those patients with low probability but poor follow-up. Over-the-counter preparations containing pseudoephedrine should be avoided. Supportive measures with fluids, rest, humidifier, and lozenges should be encouraged. Topical decongestants can be used for symptomatic relief. Treatment for sinusitis and otitis is similar to that for the nonpregnant patient, but avoiding tetracyclines. If a URI becomes protracted and is accompanied by fever or a mucopurulent drainage, antibiotic therapy should be started using a penicillin or cephalosporin.

## Pneumonia

Pneumonia can be a life-threatening complication in pregnancy. The incidence of pneumonia, depending on the population studied, is between 1 in 1287 and 1 in 2288 of pregnancies. The most common pathogens are *Streptococcus pneumoniae* and *Haemophilus influenzae,* although virtually all pathogens have been reported. Certain infectious agents, including varicella, other viruses, and tuberculosis, have greater virulence and severity in pregnancy. The major factor accounting for this increased maternal susceptibility is the alteration in the maternal immune response seen in the second and third trimester. Cell-mediated cytotoxicity by lymphocytes is diminished, and there is a decrease in the number of helper (T4) T lymphocytes.

Although no congenital abnormalities have been associated with pneumonia in pregnancy, a potential risk to the fetus exists when it is accompanied by high fever and hypoxemia. Preterm labor has also been reported in women with pneumonia and is hypothesized to be the result of the phospholipases, proteases, and prostaglandins released by bacteria inducing increased uterine activity.

The clinical features of bacterial pneumonia in pregnancy are the same as in the nonpregnant woman. Supportive therapy for pneumonia should include hydration, aggressive use of antipyretics, and supplemental oxygen. Antibiotic therapy depends on the clinical presentation. If the onset is abrupt, with fever, chills, purulent sputum, and an infiltrate on chest x-ray, antibiotic therapy should target pneumococcus or *H. influenzae.* Conversely, if the clinical presentation is more indolent, with lower fever, less toxicity, mucoid sputum, and an interstitial or patchy infiltrate, antibiotic therapy should target *Mycoplasma, Legionella,* and/or *Chlamydia.*

Influenza and varicella pneumonias are the most common viral pathogens reported. Uncomplicated influenza A usually manifests as high fever, headache, malaise, and cough and usually resolves in 3 days. If symptoms persist longer than 5 days in a pregnant women, pneumonia should be suspected. When present, the pneumonia may be a primary influenza infection of the lung parenchyma or a secondary bacterial infection. The most common secondary bacterial pathogens are *Staphylococcus aureus,* pneumococcus, *H. influenzae,* and certain gram-negative organisms. Antibiotic choice should be targeted accordingly. A primary severe influenza pneumonia can be treated with amantadine and inhaled ribavirin.

Primary varicella (chickenpox) is thought to occur in about 0.7 in 1000 pregnancies. Varicella pneumonia, a serious complication of primary varicella, is believed to be more severe and have a significantly higher mortality rate in pregnancy, with reported mortality ranging from 11 to 35 percent. Varicella pneumonia usually presents 2 to 5 days after the onset of fever, rash, and malaise. Symptoms include cough, shortness of breath, pleuritic chest pain, and hemoptysis. Chest x-ray shows diffuse miliary or nodular infiltrates. Because of the high mortality rate, any pregnant woman with varicella and a cough should receive aggressive management, including hospitalization for evaluation and treatment with intravenous acyclovir once the diagnosis is made.

## Cystitis

Urinary tract infections are the most common medical complication in pregnancy. Acute cystitis is characterized by dysuria, sometimes with gross hematuria, frequency, and suprapubic discomfort, in the absence of any systemic symptoms. Laboratory urinalysis shows white blood cells and bacteria, and invariably a urine culture grows greater than 100,000 colonies per milliliter. The most common organisms encountered are *Escherichia coli, Klebsiella pneumoniae, Proteus mirabilis,* and group B streptococci. These are often sensitive to ampicillin, nitrofurantoin, or sulfisoxazole. The usual duration of treatment is 7 to 10 days, and the recurrence rate is only 1 to 2 percent. Little information exists about the efficacy of the shorter courses of treatment in the pregnant woman.

## Pyelonephritis

The most common serious urinary tract infection in pregnancy is pyelonephritis, affecting 1 to 2.5 percent of all pregnant women. Symptoms and signs include shaking chills, dysuria, frequency, fever, flank pain, and costovertebral tenderness. More seriously ill patients appear toxic, and the presence of significant vomiting and abdominal pain sometimes may initially suggest a gastrointestinal source. The laboratory findings of pyuria, bacteriuria, and marked leukocytosis usually make the diagnosis apparent. Urine cultures should routinely be obtained to guide therapy, and blood cultures are recommended in at least the more seriously ill patients since about 10 percent of pyelonephritis patients will have a documented bacteremia.

Pyelonephritis in pregnancy necessitates admission. Intravenous antibiotic therapy should be instituted immediately. Cephalosporins are now the first choice for single-agent therapy. If sepsis is present, gentamycin may be added with careful monitoring of serum levels. Initial reports suggested that preterm labor was more common in pyelonephritis; however, many recent reports negate this finding. If a woman presents with sepsis or complaining of abdominal pain after 20 weeks' gestation, admission to a labor and delivery suite to rule out preterm labor is indicated. Fever will defervesce in the vast majority of women in 2 days and in 97 percent by 4 days. If a patient is seen who remains febrile after 4 days of treatment with an appropriate antibiotic for a suspected case of uncomplicated pyelonephritis, then a renal ultrasound to rule out a stone, renal abscess, or anatomic malformation should be obtained. The recurrence rate of pyelonephritis in pregnancy is 10 to 20 percent, and suppression with a low-dose antibiotic for the remainder of the pregnancy is often recommended.

There have been numerous case reports describing an adult respiratory distress syndrome in women presenting with pyelonephritis. The pulmonary process is thought to be mediated by a gram-negative endotoxin. Women presenting with such a picture should be considered critically ill and admitted to an intensive care setting.

## Asthma

About 4 percent of pregnancies are complicated by asthma. About one-third of pregnant women with preexisting asthma worsen, one-third improve, and one-third remain the same. When asthma is well controlled, a woman can enjoy pregnancy with no increased risk to herself or her fetus.

Mild asthma in pregnancy can usually be controlled by an inhaled $\beta_2$ agonist used as necessary when episodes of wheezing occur. Many experienced patients can anticipate circumstances that provoke attacks and use their inhalers prophylactically before challenges such as cold exposure or exercise. The inhaled $\beta$ agonists provide the cornerstone of the therapeutic regimen and can be used up to every 4 h when exacerbations occur. Chronic, moderately severe asthma may require the addition of inhaled steroids to the regimen, and there is no evidence that these agents are harmful to the fetus. Short courses of high-dose systemic steroids should be used when any significant degree of respiratory impairment remains after optimizing the use of inhaled agents. Concomitant respiratory infections should always be considered, especially pneumonia or significant bronchitis. Chest radiographs should be obtained without delay, and the appropriate antibiotic started.

Pregnant patients presenting to the emergency department with severe exacerbations of asthma require special attention because of the hazards to the fetus resulting from any significant maternal hypoxia. Arterial blood gases and measures of peak flow rates can assist in the evaluation of the patient's clinical course. Although the pulmonary system undergoes significant physiologic changes, pulmonary function tests are not significantly changed by pregnancy. Supplemental oxygen at rates adequate to maintain maternal arterial oxygen saturation at greater than 95% should be administered. Intensified therapy with inhaled $\beta_2$ agonists and the early introduction of systemic steroids should be implemented without delay. Fetal monitoring should be considered in conjunction with an obstetric consultation when the gestation has progressed to the point of potential fetal viability.

## Thromboembolism

Thromboembolism is increased in pregnancy and is the leading cause of maternal mortality. This increased risk is greatest in the postpartum period and is reported to be 5.5 times that in nonpregnant controls. Thromboembolism in pregnancy can be difficult to diagnose as many of the signs and symptoms are part of the normal physiologic changes of pregnancy.

Signs and symptoms of deep venous thrombosis include muscle pain, palpable cord, tenderness, swelling, positive Homans' sign, and dilated superficial veins. Doppler ultrasound is the diagnostic study of choice when deep venous thrombosis is suspected. Available blood assays for thrombosis include fibrinopeptide A and the fibrin degradation product, D-dimer. Although they are not specific and may be elevated in hematomas or inflammatory exudates, if negative, they essentially rule out deep venous thrombosis.

Tachypnea is the hallmark of pulmonary embolism. Other signs and symptoms include dyspnea, pleuritic pain, anxiety, cough, tachycardia, and low-grade fever. Workup should be the same as for the nonpregnant patient and include electrocardiogram, arterial blood gases, lung ventilation/perfusion scan, and chest radiograph. Again, if an assay for fibrin split products is negative, this essentially excludes the possibility of pulmonary embolism.

Anticoagulation with heparin is the mainstay of treatment for deep venous thrombosis and pulmonary embolism in pregnancy. Experience with fibrinolytic agents (streptokinase and urokinase) in pregnancy is limited to a few case reports, and their safety for both mother and fetus remains unknown. These agents should be avoided for the first 10 days postpartum because of the risk of hemorrhage from the placental implantation site.

## Acute Abdominal Pain in Pregnancy

Pregnant women presenting to an emergency department for acute abdominal pain pose a special challenge. By virtue of the pregnancy, the differential diagnosis lengthens to include ectopic pregnancy, preterm labor, placental abruption, chorioamnionitis, preeclampsia, a degenerating leiomyomata, and torsion of an adnexa. In addition, the pregnant uterus shifts the normal anatomy. This limits the clinician's ability to perform and evaluate the traditional abdominal examination and limits the diagnostic value of certain imaging tests. Lastly, the biggest danger to the pregnant woman is the fear and reluctance by many physicians to take a pregnant woman to the operating room.

### Appendicitis

Historically, appendicitis in pregnancy has been a difficult diagnosis to make, but if the diagnosis is delayed, appendicitis has serious maternal and fetal morbidity. Appendicitis presents with the same signs and symptoms as in the nonpregnant state: anorexia, nausea, vomiting, abdominal pain, fever, and leukocytosis. However, the enlarging uterus displaces the appendix gradually upward as gestation progresses, so that the classic finding of pain at McBurney's point is no longer as reliable because the appendix may be in the midline or displaced to the right upper quadrant. In addition, normal pregnancy is accompanied by an increased leukocyte count and mild left shift, which adds to the uncertainty. When the diagnosis of appendicitis is entertained but equivocal, the woman should be admitted for serial examinations and leukocyte counts. Although the diagnosis of appendicitis is largely a matter of clinical judgment, the exclusion of other diagnoses is often helpful. Ultrasound is useful in excluding ectopic pregnancy, degenerating leiomyomata, gallstones, and adnexal torsions. Laboratory studies will help sort out preeclampsia and its variants. Continuous external fetal monitoring can exclude preterm labor, while amniocentesis is the "gold standard" for chorioamnionitis.

Having a low threshold of suspicion for considering the diagnosis and obtaining obstetric and surgical consultations are absolutely necessary, since a delay in diagnosis puts both the mother and fetus at risk. Suppurative appendicitis allowed to progress to rupture, peritonitis, or abscess formation most often results in premature birth or abortion. Preterm labor will often follow a laparotomy. The episodes are nearly always transient and can be easily controlled by tocolytic therapy. Thus, in the balance, most would accept a negative laparotomy rate of 50 percent in the management of acute appendicitis in pregnancy.

## Cholecystitis

Gallbladder disease remains the second most common nonobstetric surgical condition in pregnancy. Acute cholecystitis requiring surgery occurs in about 1 in 1000 pregnancies. The clinical presentation and management of acute cholecystitis is the same as in the nonpregnant patient. The most common symptoms are colicky right upper quadrant pain, nausea, vomiting, and fever with leukocytosis. The gallbladder is usually not palpable. Ultrasound of the right upper quadrant is safe and highly valuable in the diagnosis of cholecystitis. The differential diagnosis should consider preeclampsia including the HELLP syndrome (*h*emolysis, *e*levated *l*iver enzymes, *l*ow *p*latelet count), viral hepatitis, pyelonephritis, and appendicitis. Medical management includes hydration, antibiotics, nothing by mouth, and analgesia. Cholecystectomy should be considered as recurrent attacks in pregnancy are common. The ideal time for planned surgery is the second trimester, as there is a decreased chance of preterm birth and the enlarged uterus has not yet displaced the liver.

## PREGNANCY-ASSOCIATED PROBLEMS

### Bleeding in Pregnancy

Bleeding at any time in pregnancy is worrisome to both the woman and physician as it often heralds a serious complication. The differential diagnosis and the management of bleeding in pregnancy are dependent on gestational age and clinical presentation.

### First-Trimester Bleeding

First-trimester bleeding occurs in about 40 percent of all pregnant women. In one-half of these women, the bleeding proceeds to a spontaneous abortion. In another 2 percent bleeding is a sign of an ectopic pregnancy. Other causes of first-trimester bleeding include leiomyomas, molar pregnancies, subchorionic hemorrhage, passage of a gestational sac and/or fetus in a multifetal pregnancy, and cervical or vaginal lesions. While the etiology of the bleeding is obviously important in determining the long-term viability of the pregnancy, several of the diagnoses in the differential will fall under the purview of the obstetrician providing continuing care for the patient. The most important task for the emergency physician is to accurately diagnose ectopic pregnancy. Other important tasks are to assess for spontaneous abortion, to assess the need for Rh-immune globulin, and to provide counsel and appropriate follow-up.

### Rh-Immune Globulin (RHIG, RhoGAM)

The Rh blood group system is the most common and most important cause of isoimmunization in pregnancy. The incidence of Rh-negative blood is largely race dependent, with widely varying incidences in different geographic locations. About 15 percent of white Americans and 5 to 8 percent of black Americans are Rh negative. Rh isoimmunization occurs with the transplacental hemorrhage (TPH) of fetal Rh-positive red blood cells into the circulation of an Rh-negative mother. Since the Rh(D) antigen is fully expressed on the fetal red cells by 30 days' gestation and 75 percent of pregnant women have evidence of some transplacental hemorrhage during the course of their pregnancy, the emergency physician must be alert to the need to treat Rh-negative women presenting with spontaneous abortions. First-trimester spontaneous abortion carries a 2 to 3 percent risk of isoimmunization for the unsensitized Rh-negative woman. Other obstetric complications that increase the risk of TPH are placental abruption, ectopic pregnancy, and antepartum hemorrhage.

Anti-D immune globulin (RhoGAM) was studied extensively in the 1960s and became the standard of care in the United States in 1968. The exact mechanism by which Rh antibody given passively prevents Rh immunization is unknown. The most likely hypothesis is one termed *central inhibition*, where fetal erythrocytes coated with anti-D are filtered out of the circulation by the spleen and lymph nodes. The increase in local concentrations of this D antigen–antibody D complex appears to suppress the primary immune response by interrupting the commitment of B cells to producing IgG. The standard dose of RhoGAM in North America is 300 μg intramuscularly. RhoGAM should always prevent isoimmunization unless it is given after the immune response has begun or in an inadequate amount. 300 μg of RhoGAM should cover 15 mL of fetal erythrocytes entering the maternal circulation. If a larger TPH is suspected, further testing utilizing the Kleihauer-Betke test (quantitative measurement of fetal blood in maternal blood) should be done. If for any reason a mother does not receive RhoGAM within 72 h of delivery, she should receive RhoGAM as soon as possible, up to 14 to 21 days after delivery. The current recommendation is that every Rh-negative unimmunized woman who presents with antepartum bleeding (threatened abortion) should receive 300 μg of RhoGAM IM.

### Ectopic Pregnancy

The incidence of ectopic pregnancy has increased over the past 20 years and accounts for about 2 percent of all pregnancies. This increased incidence is attributed to three major factors. First, the increased incidence of sexually transmitted diseases has caused an increased number of diseased fallopian tubes—a primary etiologic factor in ectopic pregnancies. Second, the increase in tubal sterilization as a primary means of contraception has caused a paradoxic increase in ectopic gestations. Virtually 50 to 75 percent of all pregnancies following tubal sterilization are ectopic. Lastly, recent technologic advances have allowed a much earlier diagnosis. In the past some of these ectopic pregnancies spontaneously resolved as tubal abortions.

All women of reproductive age presenting to an emergency department with abdominal or pelvic pain should have a pregnancy test. If the pregnancy test is positive, ectopic pregnancy must be considered early in the differential diagnosis. Ninety percent of women with ectopic pregnancies will have abdominal or pelvic pain as well as vaginal bleeding. Virtually all women with an ectopic pregnancy will have a positive urine pregnancy test, and about one-fifth of these patients will present to the emergency department with a ruptured ectopic pregnancy. Signs and symptoms generally seen are varying degrees of abdominal and/or pelvic pain, vaginal bleeding, a positive pregnancy test, and hemodynamic alterations. Culdocentesis is often helpful in these situations as a rapid means of diagnosing a hemoperitoneum. A ruptured ectopic pregnancy is a true emergency. Stabilization and immediate surgical intervention are indicated.

However, the majority of patients present a more subtle picture, with some pain and/or vaginal bleeding and a positive pregnancy test. Here the diagnosis is often more difficult. A complete blood count, serial quantitative HCGs, and transvaginal ultrasound can be helpful in making the diagnosis. The ability to follow-up with the patient and her desire for future fertility should all be considered in her management. The advent of specialized laparoscopic techniques has enabled a more conservative surgical approach, preserving tubal function in women who wish to maintain future fertility. Special protocols now exist that allow for the medical management of ectopic pregnancies utilizing methotrexate.

## Spontaneous Abortion

Spontaneous abortion occurs in about 15 to 20 percent of all clinically recognized pregnancies. The most common cause of spontaneous abortion is genetic, accounting for about 50 percent of all losses. However, the fact that such a large fraction of wasted pregnancies involves faulty genetic materials does not necessarily imply that one or both parents carry a "faulty gene," since 90 percent of patients who have a spontaneous abortion go on to have a normal child. Other causes of spontaneous abortion include uterine abnormalities, infections, drugs, and maternal diseases. Conventional teaching has separated the clinical presentation into one of the following categories: threatened abortion, inevitable abortion, incomplete abortion, complete abortion, and missed abortion. Threatened abortion is defined as any uterine bleeding at less than 20 weeks' gestation, without cervical dilation or effacement. An inevitable abortion is defined as uterine bleeding from a gestation less than 20 weeks, with cervical dilation but without expulsion of any placental or fetal tissue through the cervix. With an incomplete abortion there has been some but not complete passage of fetal and placental tissue. Completed abortion is one where there has been spontaneous and complete expulsion of all products of conception. A missed abortion is one in which the fetus dies in utero, but the products of conception are retained. These categories describe the natural history of a spontaneous abortion. Studies using transvaginal ultrasound in early pregnancy have clearly shown that in the vast majority of spontaneous abortions fetal demise has occurred very early in gestation, prior to the development of cardiac activity. Since the most common time for a woman to present with symptoms of cramping and bleeding is 8 to 12 weeks' gestation, fetal demise antedates spontaneous abortion, often weeks before. Fetal cardiac activity on ultrasound (seen in the 6th postmenstrual week) is a major milestone in the first trimester. Once seen, the spontaneous abortion rate decreases to 2 to 3 percent.

History is important in the differential of first-trimester bleeding, as spontaneous abortion is usually accompanied by both vaginal bleeding and uterine cramping. On speculum examination a threatened abortion will show a closed cervix that will not admit a ring forcep, whereas an inevitable or incomplete abortion will show a dilated cervix that admits a ring forcep. The differential between complete and incomplete abortion has sometimes been based on a detailed look at the products of conception, when available, and more recently by ultrasound. An incomplete abortion often requires cervical dilatation and evacuation of the remaining products of conception, as it may lead to continued pain, bleeding, and septic complications. A completed abortion will show a well-defined endometrial stripe within the uterus and may negate any need for dilatation and curettage. RhoGAM should be given to all Rh-negative unsensitized women who present with first-trimester bleeding.

## Septic Abortion

Septic abortion is defined as any type of abortion that is accompanied by uterine infection. All patients with this diagnosis should have a complete blood count and urinalysis and be considered for blood cultures, chest x-ray, and blood coagulation studies and chemistries. Admission is necessitated, and IV antibiotic therapy should be instituted immediately. This is often accomplished with a combination of ampicillin, gentamycin, and clindamycin. Other regimens that offer broad-spectrum coverage may also be effective. After adequate levels of antibiotics are obtained (about 2 h), uterine evacuation should be done in the operating room.

## Second- and Third-Trimester Bleeding

Vaginal bleeding in the late second and early third trimester is often from a placenta previa or placental abruption. Other diagnoses that need to be entertained are preterm labor, preterm cervical dilation, in-competent cervix, and cervicovaginal lesions or tumors. When a woman presents with bleeding of unknown etiology, a speculum examination is a safe and appropriate first step. Vaginal digital examination is contraindicated until an ultrasound can be completed to rule out placenta previa.

## Placental Abruption

Placental abruption is the separation of a normally implanted placenta prior to the birth of the fetus. The incidence is reported to be between 1 in 86 and 1 in 200 live births. The source of the separation lies in the small arterial vessels in the decidua of the uterus that are abnormal and prone to rupture. In some cases the bleeding may originate from fetal and/or placental vessels. As bleeding accumulates between the placenta and decidua, there is premature separation of the placenta. As the bleeding continues, the separation continues, and the part of the placenta that is involved is unable to exchange $O_2$, $CO_2$, and nutrients for the fetus. The bleeding may in part dissect between the fetal membranes and decidua and out of the cervix and into the vagina. Occasionally, when the separation is central, the bleeding will be completely concealed. The cause of abruption is unknown. However, we do know that certain women are at high risk: those who smoke, have hypertension, or use cocaine. Trauma is an uncommon but important cause of abruption, accounting for about 2 percent of all clinically recognized abruptions.

The classic presentation is vaginal bleeding with pain. It is important to note that the amount of vaginal bleeding in no way correlates with the amount lost from the maternal circulation or the amount concealed within the uterus. The abdominal pain is nonspecific, varying from mild, like the pain of early labor, to sudden, sharp, and acute. It may settle in the lower abdomen or in the back. Uterine contractions are almost always present but may be difficult to evaluate secondary to a hypertonic uterus. The differential diagnosis includes uterine rupture, placenta previa, and degenerating leiomyomas.

Placental abruption may present in a variety of stages. When vaginal bleeding is present and the separation is minimal and there is no concealed hemorrhage, no uterine tenderness, and no fetal or maternal compromise, hospitalization is warranted. If the patient is at term, delivery is effected; if preterm, close observation with an expectant approach is possible. This minimal abruption is often referred to as a *marginal sinus abruption.*

The separation is considered moderate when concealed hemorrhage, uterine tenderness, and fetal distress are present and maternal compromise is not yet present. In these instances delivery should be effected immediately. Moderate abruptions are very likely to progress to severe. Severe abruption is characterized by extensive concealed hemorrhage, uterine tenderness, maternal compromise with coagulopathy, and fetal death. A median blood loss of 2500 mL, most of which is concealed within the uterus, has been reported in severe abruptions with fetal death. If severe abruption with fetal death is present, maternal resuscitation and stabilization are the primary goals. Close attention to fluids, blood, and blood component replacement is mandatory. Transfer to a labor and delivery unit, which can both effect delivery and support the serious maternal condition, is needed.

## Placenta Previa

Placenta previa is another major cause of third-trimester bleeding, occuring in the range of 1 in 250 births. It is defined as an implantation of the placenta over the internal cervical os. There are three clinically recognized variants: total placenta previa, in which the entire cervical os is covered by the placenta; partial placenta previa is a partial covering of the cervical os by the placenta; and a marginal placenta previa is a placenta that is implanted at the margin of the cervical os. The classic clinical presentation is third-trimester painless, vaginal bleeding, which may or may not be accompanied by uterine irritability. Bleeding occurs because of separation of the placenta from the lower uterine segment during the third trimester as this area gradually thins out. The mechanism of bleeding from a placenta previa is similar to that of a partial placental abruption. Digital examinations are contraindicated in placenta previa; the diagnosis is made by ultrasound. Transvaginal ultrasound is safe in making the diagnosis of placenta previa. The management of placenta previa is dependent on the gestational age of the fetus. When the pregnancy is remote from term, expectant management with betamethasone, tocolysis if needed, and close observation can be initiated. The goal is to maintain the fetus in a healthy intrauterine environment without jeopardizing the mother. When placenta previa is diagnosed at term or amniocentesis demonstrates fetal lung maturity, delivery is accomplished via cesarean section.

## Preeclampsia

Preeclampsia is a major cause of maternal and fetal morbidity and mortality. Preeclampsia occurs in about 7 percent of all pregnancies and is most often seen in primigravidas. Other predisposing factors include a family history of preeclampsia/eclampsia, diabetes mellitus, multiple gestation, preexisting hypertension, or renal disease. Although the etiology of preeclampsia remains unknown, we do know that it is accompanied by endothelial cell injury, increased platelet activation, and platelet consumption in the microvasculature.

Preeclampsia can present with a wide spectrum of symptoms and signs, from the classical clinical triad of hypertension, proteinuria, and edema to the more unusual presentation where abdominal pain with hematologic and hepatic laboratory abnormalities are of primary concern. The HELLP syndrome represents such an unusual presentation.

Severe preeclampsia has been traditionally defined by the following criteria: blood pressure $\geq$ 160/110 mmHg, proteinuria $\geq$ 5g/24 h (3+ to 4+ dipstick), oliguria $\leq$ 500 mL/24 h, epigastric pain, cerebral or visual disturbances, or pulmonary edema. The laboratory abnormalities used for the diagnosis of HELLP syndrome include a platelet count < 100,000/$\mu$l, hemolysis defined as an abnormal blood smear (burr cells, schistocytes), lactic dehydrogenase > 600 IU/L, bilirubin $\geq$ 1.2 mg/dL, and SGOT > 72 IU/L. There is little agreement as to whether HELLP represents a separate entity or is merely a variant of preeclampsia. The vast majority of women with HELLP syndrome present with a chief complaint of epigastric or right upper quadrant pain, nausea, or vomiting. They are often misdiagnosed as having gastritis, cholecystitis, hepatitis, or a primary hematologic abnormality. The diagnosis is most commonly delayed when a woman is multiparous, remote from term, and the hypertension and proteinuria are unimpressive. Once the diagnosis is made, maternal stabilization is the primary goal. Magnesium sulfate, 4 to 6 g in 100 mL of fluid as a loading dose over 20 min, should be given and followed by a maintenance infusion of 2 g in 100 mL of fluid per hour to prevent seizures. Guidelines for administration are summarized in Table 98-3. Secondly, diastolic blood pressure of 110 mmHg should be treated with an antihypertensive agent. Both hydralazine and labatelol IV are commonly used. Careful attention should be given to fluid balance and urine output while arrangements are being made for admission or transfer to a tertiary care center. Obstetric management is based on the severity of preeclampsia and on the gestational age of the fetus; if term or near term, delivery is indicated. The management of preeclampsia remote from term continues to be a challenge and one filled with controversy.

## Preterm Labor

Preterm labor is defined as labor occurring prior to the completion of 36 weeks of gestation. Preterm labor occurs in 8 to 10 percent of all births and is responsible for 60 percent of the perinatal morbidity and mortality in neonates without congenital anomalies. Causes of preterm labor include infection, uterine abnormalities, incompetent

**Table 98-3.** Magnesium Sulfate (MgSO$_4$)

| | |
|---|---|
| *Indications:* | Seizure prophylaxis in preeclampsia<br>Tocolysis for preterm labor |
| *Dosage:* | Loading dose 4–6 g/IV over 20 min in 100 mL of IV fluid<br>Maintenance dose 2 g/h, range 1–3 g<br>Mixture 20 g in 500 mL IVF |
| *Side effects:* | Common: flushing, warmth, headache, blurred vision, nausea, dizziness<br>Overdosage: loss of deep tendon reflexes, respiratory compromise, cardiac arrest |
| *Antidote:* | Calcium gluconate 10%, 10 mL IV over 3 min |
| *Therapeutic level:* | Anticonvulsant level 4–6 mEq/L<br>No known therapeutic level exists for preterm labor |
| *Contraindications:* | Myasenthia gravis, maternal cardiovascular disease |
| *Precautions:* | Renal impairment including oligruia in preeclampsia necessitating reduced dosage as MgSO$_4$ is renally excreted<br>Pulmonary edema and cardiac depression have been reported when used with nifedipine, $\beta$-agonists and corticosteroids |

cervix, leiomyoma, exposure to diethylstilbestrol, overdistension as in multiple gestations or polyhydramnios, and premature placental separation. Although many causes have been identified, the etiology of preterm labor in the individual patient is most often unknown. The two most common risk factors identified by epidemiologic studies are previous preterm birth and the presence of a multifetal gestation.

Early symptoms of preterm labor are often difficult to recognize by both the patient and physician. Preterm labor is defined by either cervical change in response to regular uterine contractions, or contractions greater than 6 to 8 per hour that do not resolve with bedrest and hydration. Other early symptoms include a dull, low back pain or sense of intermittent pressure, lower abdominal pain, intestinal cramping with or without diarrhea, and a change in vaginal discharge. The relatively nonspecific nature of these symptoms often requires a conservative approach, with extended close observation, external monitoring to document uterine contractions, and serial cervical examinations. Since the diagnosis of early preterm labor can best be made by following the progress of the patient, any women for whom the diagnosis is seriously considered should be admitted to a labor and delivery unit.

Once labor is identified, the decision to initiate tocolysis must be made. The relative contraindications to tocolysis include preeclampsia, chorioamnionitis, advanced labor, fetal maturity, fetal distress, and maternal hemodynamic instability. Tocolysis of idiopathic preterm labor has been shown to prolong pregnancy and decrease the incidence of preterm birth. Most clinicians treat preterm labor with tocolytic agents at 34 weeks or less and approach the management of preterm labor between 34 and 37 weeks individually. A common initial step is maternal hydration, as preterm uterine contractions will often resolve; however, excessive hydration is to be avoided. Intravenous magnesium sulfate remains the tocolytic agent of choice for instituting therapy in the emergency department. Guidelines for its administration are summarized in Table 98-3. Once stabilized, the patient should be transferred to the appropriate hospital where adequate neonatal support is available.

## Preterm Premature Rupture of Membranes

Premature rupture of membranes (PROM) is defined as rupture of membranes prior to the onset of labor. The definition is not dependent on gestational age, and rupture of membranes prior to term is called preterm PROM. The cause of preterm PROM is not well understood, although there is good evidence that inflammation from infections affecting the membranes can precipitate PROM. Other potential etiologies include polyhydramnios, incompetent cervix, and placental abruption. When PROM occurs, labor is likely to ensue. Generally the closer the patient is to term, the sooner labor is likely to begin. Over 90 percent of term patients and 50 percent of preterm patients will be in labor within 24 h, and more than 85 percent of preterm patients will be in labor within 1 week. The diagnosis of PROM is made with a combination of history and physical examination. The differential diagnosis includes urinary incontinence, excess vaginal discharge, and, rarely, bloody show. Digital cervical examination in patients who are preterm should be avoided to minimize the risk of introducing infection. Speculum examination should be undertaken to confirm the diagnosis. Confirmation is often made by identifying a pool of fluid in the posterior fornix of the vagina. The pH of the vagina is usually 4.5 to 6.0 and that of amniotic fluid is 7.1 to 7.3. Nitrazine paper should change to a dark blue color. Nitrazine, however, will also turn dark blue with blood, semen, and with certain infectious discharges. A swab from the posterior fornix or pooling should also be smeared on a slide and allowed to dry for examination under the microscope. The finding of a "ferning" pattern is virtually diagnostic for the presence of amniotic fluid. If after completion of these simple bedside tests the diagnosis remains unclear, admission for observation and serial ultrasound examinations to assess amniotic fluid volume changes should be considered. All patients with a diagnosis of preterm PROM should be hospitalized. The only exception to this rule is when preterm PROM occurs prior to viability—less than 24 weeks' gestation. These situations require extensive counseling concerning prognosis, and different options should be presented to the patients. Delivery in preterm PROM is usually induced with the identification of chorioamnionitis or fetal distress. If labor spontaneously ensues, tocolytics are generally not used except in rare instances. At present there is great controversy regarding the benefit of prophylactic antibiotics in the management of preterm PROM. The presence of premature rupture of membranes most often results in preterm delivery, and hospitalization should occur where the proper neonatal support is available.

## Postpartum Problems

### Endometritis

The incidence of postpartum endometritis is usually less than 3 percent after a vaginal delivery but rises dramatically (5 to 10 times higher) when cesarean section is performed. The mechanism of infection is thought to be from ascending cervicovaginal flora. Bacteria adhere to the decidua, establishing an endometritis. This may progress into the myometrium and parametrium, establishing an endomyoparametritis. Most of these infections are polymicrobial and have ascended from the lower genital tract. Numerous organisms have been implicated including gram-negative aerobes, group A, B, and D streptococci, gram-positive and -negative anaerobes, *Chlamydia, Mycoplasma hominis, Ureaplasma urealyticum,* and others. When infection ensues in the first 48 h following delivery, group A and B *Streptococcus, Staphylococcus,* and *Clostridium* should be considered as primary etiologic agents. When infection has a delayed presentation from 48 h to 6 weeks, *Chlamydia* and *Mycoplasma* should be considered as primary etiologies. The clinical diagnosis is based on symptoms of fever, malaise, lower abdominal pain, and foul-smelling lochia. A complete physical examination is needed in order to differentiate this from pyelonephritis and other postpartum infections. Speculum examination will often, but not always, reveal a purulent discharge. The uterine fundus is tender on abdominal examination, and there is often cervical motion tenderness on vaginal examination. Laboratory studies should include a complete blood count and urine culture. Cervical/uterine cultures should be done although they have limited clinical value. Blood cultures are warranted in patients appearing septic.

Endometritis necessitates admission for the administration of broad-spectrum antibiotics intravenously. Mild endometritis, most often seen after a vaginal delivery, usually responds to a second- or third-generation cephalosporin, to a penicillin/β-lactamase inhibitor combination, or to clindamycin and gentamycin. For more severe cases, a combination of ampicillin, gentamycin, and clindamycin is commonly used.

### Mastitis

Mastitis is a cellulitis of the periglandular breast tissue that most commonly occurs in lactating women. Incidence figures are not well documented. It often begins in the second or third postpartum week but can happen at any time. It is characterized by the classic signs of localized inflammation in the affected breast (pain, induration, erythema, and warmth), with axillary adenopathy, and systemic signs and symptoms including significant fever, chills, and diffuse myalgias. Cultures of breast milk do not assist in the clinical management. The most common organisms found are *Staphylococcus aureus,* streptococci A and B, and *H. influenzae.* Treatment is on an outpatient basis, with a β lactamase–resistant penicillin (dicloxacillin) or a first-generation cephalosporin (cephalexin). The patient should be instructed to continue to nurse on the affected breast and counseled that this will not harm the baby. Most symptoms resolve within 48 h of treatment. Only rarely does abscess formation complicate mastitis. When this does occur, incision and drainage is needed.

## PERINATAL INFECTIONS

Many viral and bacterial infections in the nonpregnant state are self-limiting and of little consequence, whereas these same infections in the pregnant state are of great consequence to the mother, fetus, or neonate. A prime example is cytomegalovirus (CMV). Although often asymptomatic in the woman, it poses a significant threat to the fetus.

Fetal infection can occur once an organism has invaded the maternal bloodstream. Microorganisms in the blood may be carried within lymphocytes or neutrophils, may be attached to erythrocytes, or may be independent as they pass transplacentally. Once the organism has invaded the fetus, a variety of effects may be manifested in utero: spontaneous miscarriage, malformation, stillbirth, growth delay, or prematurity. Postnatally, the infection may be present at birth or may manifest itself weeks, months, or even years later. Two common scenarios in the emergency department are a pregnant health care worker who presents with a specific infectious exposure or a pregnant woman with a nonspecific rash. All the potential problems associated with each perinatal infection are impossible to predict. However, the emergency physician must have a practical approach to the diagnosis, potential risks to the mother and fetus, preventive measures and treatment. Guidelines for such an approach are summarized in Table 98–1. Lastly, since the incidence of human immunodeficiency virus infection is increasing, a separate section summarizing our current knowledge and treatment recommendations is included.

## Human Immunodeficiency Virus

The incidence of HIV infection is increasing in the reproductive-age female through heterosexual transmission. The virus does cross the placenta, although transmission rate to the fetus is only 15 to 25 percent. The virus is not teratogenic. Although we do not understand all the factors involved in transmission, we do know that the lower the CD4 count and the greater the viremia the greater the chance the baby will be infected. A CD4 count of less than 300 cells per microliter also increases the likelihood of maternal infectious complications during pregnancy.

A recent prospective randomized placebo-controlled trial of AZT (zidovudine) in pregnancy has shown a significant reduction in perinatal transmission to 8.5 percent. Therefore all women who have HIV infection, regardless of their CD4 count, should begin AZT at 14 weeks' gestation or as soon as pregnancy is diagnosed. Although AZT does cross the placenta it is not teratogenic. The dosage is 100 mg 5 times/day or 200 mg 3 times/day. Identification of pregnancy in a woman previously diagnosed with HIV is apt to happen in an emergency department. Conversely, HIV should be considered in the pregnant woman who presents with an atypical infection. Follow-up of these women in a prenatal clinic with the resources available to meet their complex needs should be a primary goal.

## BIBLIOGRAPHY

ACOG Technical Bulletin: *Ectopic Pregnancy,* no. 150, December 1990.

ACOG Technical Bulletin: *Hepatitis in Pregnancy,* no. 174, November 1992.

ACOG Technical Bulletin: *Perinatal Viral and Parasitic Infections,* no. 177, February 1993.

ACOG Technical Bulletin: *Preterm Labor,* no. 133, October 1989.

ACOG Technical Bulletin: *Rubella and Pregnancy,* no. 171, August 1992.

ACOG Technical Bulletin: *Premature Rupture of Membranes,* no. 115, April 1988.

Bowman JM: Hemolytic disease, in Creasy RK, Resnik R (eds): *Maternal-Fetal Medicine, Principles and Practice,* 3d. ed. Philadelphia, Saunders, 1994.

Briggs GG, Freeman RK, Yaffe SJ: *Drugs in Pregnancy and Lactation,* 4th ed. Baltimore, Williams & Wilkins, 1994.

Cefalo RC, Moos MK: *Preconceptional Health Care: A Practical Guide,* 2d ed. St. Louis, Mosby-Year Book, 1995.

Lucas MJ, Cunningham FG: Urinary tract infections complicating pregnancy, in Cunningham G (ed): *Williams Obstetrics,* 19th ed, supplement no 5, February/March. Norwalk, CT, Appleton/Lange, 1994.

Mishell DR: Abortion, in Herbst AL, Mishell DR, Stenchever MA, Droege-mueller W (eds): *Comprehensive Gynecology,* 2d ed. St. Louis, Mosby-Year Book, 1992.

National Asthma Education Program: *Management of Asthma During Pregnancy: Executive Summary.* NIH Pub. No. 93–32 79A, March 1993.

Niebyl J: Drugs in pregnancy and lactation, in Gabbe SG, Niebyl JR, Simpson JL (eds): *Obstetrics: Normal & Problem Pregnancies,* 2d ed. New York, Churchill Livingstone, 1991.

Remington JS, Klein JO (eds): *Infectious Diseases of the Fetus and Newborn Infant,* 3d ed. Philadelphia, Saunders, 1990.

Rodrigues J, Niederman MS: Pneumonia complicating pregnancy. *Clin Chest Med* 4:679, 1992.

Twickler DM, Clarke G, Cunningham FG: Diagnostic imaging in pregnancy, in Cunningham G (ed): *Williams Obstetrics,* 18th ed, supplement no. 18, June/July. Norwalk, CT, Appleton/Lange, 1992.

U.S. Public Health Service Task Force: Recommendations on the use of zidovudine to reduce perinatal transmission of human immunodeficiency virus. *MMWR* 43:1, 1994.

# 99

# BLUNT ABDOMINAL TRAUMA DURING PREGNANCY

## Mark D. Pearlman

Trauma during pregnancy is the most frequent cause of nonobstetrical maternal death and in some geographic settings may be the most frequent cause of all maternal deaths. The three major causes of maternal injury are vehicular accidents, falls, and penetrating objects. Diagnosis and treatment of the injured gravida follows the same general guidelines as management of the nonpregnant trauma victim, but several critical differences exist. Marked changes occur in almost every organ system of the gravida's body, and a basic understanding of these changes is a prerequisite to initiating treatment and interpreting diagnostic tests. This chapter will review those aspects of trauma care which are peculiar to the gravid trauma patient.

## ANATOMIC AND PHYSIOLOGICAL CHANGES ASSOCIATED WITH PREGNANCY

Treatment priorities require an understanding of the anatomic and physiological changes of pregnancy. In addition, pathological states which are unique to pregnancy such as abruptio placentae or amniotic fluid embolism may be initiated by injury and must be considered both diagnostically and therapeutically. After initial maternal stabilization, diagnosis and treatment of the second patient (fetus) must be considered.

### Cardiovascular Changes

*Cardiac output* increases during the first 10 weeks of pregnancy (up to 1.0 to 1.5 L/min) and then maintains this increased level throughout pregnancy. In the supine position late in pregnancy, the inferior vena cava can be occluded by the enlarging uterus and cardiac output falls dramatically as a result of decreased preload. By displacement of the gravid uterus off the inferior vena cava, cardiac output can increase by 25 percent late in pregnancy. This can be accomplished by either placing the patient in the left atrial decubitus position, placing a 6-in. wedge under the right hip, or manual displacement of the uterus to the left.

*Heart rate* normally increases during pregnancy. This physiological tachycardia reaches a maximum of 15 to 20 beats above baseline late in the third trimester. Tachycardia as a sign of hypovolemia must be interpreted with caution in the pregnant trauma victim.

Both *systolic and diastolic blood pressure* in normal pregnancy fall by 10 to 15 mmHg in the second trimester, with a gradual increase to prepregnancy levels toward the end of pregnancy.

*Electrocardiographic* changes are influenced by displacement of the heart by the enlarging uterus. This is demonstrated by a left-axis deviation of 15° as well as flattened or inverted T waves in lead III. Supraventricular ectopy is also more frequent during pregnancy.

### Hematologic Changes

*Blood volume* expands by a maximum of 45 percent at term. Red blood cell mass does not increase to the same degree as does plasma volume; therefore, *dilutional "anemia"* is a normal physiological finding in pregnancy. This increase in plasma volume allows a greater red blood cell loss to take place without the usual signs of hypovolemia. Fluid replacement estimates may need to be increased when considering the pregnant trauma patient.

A moderate *leukocytosis* is seen during normal pregnancy, as high as 18,000 in the second and third trimester, and as high as 25,000 during labor.

*Coagulation factors* are affected by pregnancy: fibrinogen and factors VII, VIII, IX, and X are all increased. However, bleeding time, clotting time, prothrombin time, and partial thromboplastin time are unchanged. These coagulation alterations (a result in part of elevated estrogen levels) increase the risk of formation of venous thrombosis. In addition, the release of thromboplastic materials from traumatic abruptio placentae can initiate a fulminant coagulopathy (DIC).

*Erythrocyte sedimentation rate* is elevated in normal pregnancy (average ESR = 78 mm/h).

### Pulmonary Changes

*Tidal volume* increases by approximately 40 percent, and *residual volume* decreases by approximately 25 percent. *Respiratory rate* changes little.

*Arterial blood gases* are affected by the increased tidal volume and decreased residual volume resulting in a reduced alveolar and arterial $P_{CO_2}$; $P_{CO_2}$ averages 30 torr. Normal pH is maintained by increased bicarbonate excretion by the kidney.

## Gastrointestinal Changes

*Decreased gastric motility* and *decreased gastric emptying time* both predispose to an increased risk for aspiration, especially in those patients requiring general anesthesia or with an altered sensorium.

*Cephalad displacement of the intraabdominal contents* by the gravid uterus seems to have a protective effect on these organs in blunt abdominal trauma. However, in penetrating trauma of the upper abdomen, intestinal injury is almost assured.

*Signs of peritoneal irritation* are less reliable in the gravida in comparison to those of the nonpregnant trauma victim. Rebound tenderness and rigidity are often diminished, delayed, or absent in pregnant women. This is presumably due to the gradual stretching of the peritoneum and abdominal musculature by the gravid uterus.

The placental component of *alkaline phosphatase* results in levels which are increased two to three times those of nongravid levels near term.

## Urinary System Changes

*Dilatation of the renal pelves and ureters* (right > left) occurs from 10 weeks' gestation to 6 weeks' postpartum.

The *bladder* is displaced both superiorly and anteriorly, becoming an abdominal organ around the twelfth week of gestation and rendering it more susceptible to injury.

*Decreased serum creatinine and BUN* (0.5 and <10 mg/dL, respectively, in late pregnancy) occur as a result of increased renal blood flow and increased glomerular filtration rate.

## Reproductive Organ Changes

The *uterus* increases in size from a 7-cm, 70-g organ to a 36-cm, 1000-g organ at term.

*Blood flow to the uterus* increases from 60 to 600 mL/min at term, predisposing to massive blood loss if the uterine vasculature is disrupted.

## MATERNAL INJURIES

In a prospective series by Crosby of 411 pregnant victims of serious automobile accidents, there were 16 fatalities (3.4 percent). Of these fatalities, 7 died of head injuries, 6 died of exsanguination from internal injuries, and 3 died of pelvic fractures associated with retro- or intraperitoneal hemorrhage. In addition, 7 other women suffered life-threatening injuries, including 5 pelvic fractures and 2 liver or spleen ruptures. The pattern and severity of injury depend on several factors, including speed, restraint system, direction of impact, and the victim's position in the vehicle. In most clinical settings, a majority (80 percent +) of injuries are of a minor nature. However, serious fetal injury or death can occur in the face of an apparent minor maternal injury.

## Seat Belt Injuries

In 1971 Crosby and Costiloe published a series of severely injured pregnant women and focused specifically on whether two-point restraint systems were protective or deleterious to the pregnancies. In this study, seat belts protected against death of the mother, and death of the mother was the leading cause of fetal death. In addition, abruptio placentae was not increased as a result of seat belt use. However, in a separate animal study of trauma during pregnancy, it appeared that decelerative-type injuries where the pregnant subject is in two-point restraint are at increased risk for abruptio placentae compared to three-point restraint. It is apparent that the use of 3-point restraint

systems during pregnancy reduces the risk of both fetal and maternal injury.

## Pelvic Fracture

Fracture of the maternal pelvis may be associated with life-threatening intra- or retroperitoneal hemorrhage; bladder, urethral, or ureteral laceration; fat embolism; vaginal lacerations; lumbar plexus injury; fetal skull fracture; and maternal death. Retroperitoneal hemorrhage is common following major trauma to the pelvis. Hypovolemic shock is frequently associated with injuries of this type as the retroperitoneum has a volume capacity of at least 4 L.

In general, pelvic fracture does not preclude an attempt at vaginal delivery. Pelvic deformity following pelvic fractures may interfere with normal passage of the fetus through the pelvic inlet during labor and delivery. However, cesarean section is necessary only 5 to 10 percent of the time as a result of pelvic fracture. Recent pelvic fracture is not a contraindication to vaginal delivery.

## Intraabdominal Injuries

The enlarged gravid uterus and the contained amniotic fluid together act as a hydraulic shock absorber and has a protective affect on intraabdominal organs during blunt abdominal trauma. Life threatening hemorrhage as a result of trauma is most often found in the retroperitoneum during pregnancy, however, intraperitoneal hemorrhage should *always* be considered in the gravid victim of abdominal trauma. Splenic rupture, injury to the kidney, and liver laceration remain the three most common intra-abdominal injuries.

## Uterine Rupture

Up to the twelfth week, the uterus is protected by the bony pelvis. After the twelfth week, it becomes an abdominal organ and is more vulnerable to injury. Uterine rupture resulting from trauma during pregnancy is an infrequent event, complicating <1 percent of traumatic events during pregnancy. In general, uterine rupture occurs as a result of direct and intense uterine impact. Crosby (1968) noted tremendous increases in intrauterine pressure (up to 550 mmHg) in restrained pregnant baboons subjected to experimental impacts. This is 10 times the pressure observed during normal labor. During abrupt deceleration, the uterus is thrown against the anterior abdominal wall, causing it to flatten and elongate. Rapid deceleration may cause an increase in intrauterine pressure great enough to produce uterine rupture. Asymmetry of the uterus, signs of peritoneal irritation, the presence of maternal shock, difficulty palpating the uterine fundus, and ultrasound or x-ray visualization of the fetus free in the abdominal cavity all suggest the diagnosis.

## Abruptio Placentae

Abruptio placentae occurs when the placenta prematurely separates from the uterine wall, and is the most common cause of fetal/neonatal loss resulting from trauma. The common presenting signs and symptoms include vaginal bleeding (78 percent), abdominal pain (66 percent), uterine irritability (17 percent), tetanic uterine contractions (17 percent), and fetal death (15 percent). Abruptio placentae complicates 1 to 5 percent of minor trauma and 20 to 50 percent of major/life threatening trauma. The mechanism of abruptio placentae in this type of injury is due to compression of the elastic uterus around the relatively inelastic placenta, causing a shearing of the placenta away from the underlying decidua basalis. A simultaneous increase in the intraamniotic pressure may propagate this shearing effect. In a decelerative-type injury, hyperflexion of the torso over the pregnant uterus is prevented to a great degree by a shoulder harness. In unusual circumstances, abruptio placentae can occur without direct uterine impact (e.g., a hard fall on the buttocks). The mechanism for this may result from the impact causing a sudden shortening and widening of the uterus setting up a waveform within the amniotic fluid resulting in disruption of the placenta from the underlying decidua. In addition to the bleeding from the separated uteroplacental site, release of thromboplastic materials into the maternal circulation predisposes to the development of DIC. In the presence of vaginal bleeding, uterine tenderness, or tetanic uterine contractions following trauma, fibrinogen levels, PT, PTT, and a platelet count should be obtained. A peripheral smear should also be examined for the presence of schistocytes.

## Fetomaternal Hemorrhage

The human placenta is a hemochorial system, that is, the fetal and maternal blood circulations are normally separate. Fetomaternal hemorrhage (FMH) is a condition where fetal blood is found in the maternal circulation, and some degree of FMH frequently occurs following delivery, amniocentesis, and spontaneous vaginal bleeding. Fetomaternal hemorrhage following trauma was first described in a case report by Bickers and Wennberg. Since that initial report, Rose, Pearlman, and Goodwin have studied the incidence, volume, and significance of FMH following trauma. All three studies identified a four- to fivefold increase in incidence of FMH in pregnant trauma victims compared to uninjured controls regardless of severity of injury. In addition, the volume of FMH was several-fold higher in the injured group.

The most important unfavorable consequence of FMH is isoimmunization, the development of maternal antibodies against the $Rh_o(D)$ antigen on the surface of the Rh-positive fetal cells. These maternal IgG antibodies can cross the placenta and may cause fetal red blood cell hemolysis in the current or future pregnancies. $Rh_o(D)$ immune globulin (Rhogam) has been utilized for the last two decades to protect $Rh_o(D)$-negative gravidas against the possible exposure to $Rh_o(D)$-positive blood and the development of anti-$Rh_o(D)$ antibodies. Events which increase the risk of FMH (e.g., bleeding during pregnancy, amniocentesis, chorionic villus sampling, and delivery) are generally followed by prophylaxis with Rh immune globulin in $Rh_o(D)$-negative women. Based on the available data, trauma which occurs during pregnancy should be added to this list of events.

Calculating the volume of the FMH following trauma is important in those rare instances of massive FMH because a standard dose of $Rh_o(D)$ immune globulin (300 μg) will only protect against FMH ≤ 30 mL of whole blood. Administration of this standard dose of $Rh_o(D)$ immune globulin in the face of a larger bleed may not adequately protect the gravida against Rh isoimmunization. The Kleihauer-Betke assay is a test to identify and quantitate FMH. In this test a phosphate acid buffer is added to a peripheral smear of a pregnant (or recently pregnant) woman's blood. The phosphate buffer elutes adult hemoglobin from red blood cells (RBC), whereas the fetal hemoglobin is resistant to elution and remains within the RBC. A hemoglobin counterstain is then applied to the smear, and the ratio of maternal (ghost) RBCs to fetal (stained) RBCs is counted. By multiplying this ratio by the estimated maternal blood volume, an estimate of the volume of FMH can be made. For example, if 1000 maternal cells are counted and 3 fetal cells are seen, and if the estimated maternal blood volume is 5 L, the calculated FMH is $^3/_{1000} \times 5000 = 15$-mL bleed. Fetal blood volume does not reach 30 mL until approximately 16 weeks, so the use of Kleihauer-Betke or similar quantitative assays would be unnecessary in these early gestations if 300 μg of Rh immune globulins is administered empirically to Rh-negative women following trauma.

In summary, FMH occurs frequently following trauma during pregnancy (8 to 30 percent), and the $Rh_o(D)$-negative gravida should be protected against isoimmunization by the administration of Rh immune globulin. Beyond 16 weeks' gestation, a Kleibauer-Betke assay can be considered to quantitate the volume of the transfusion so that the appropriate dose of Rh immune globulin is administered and so

that the rare episode of massive FMH is recognized, allowing appropriate intervention.

## Predicting Outcome

A number of investigators have retrospectively evaluated the predictive value of different trauma scoring systems (injury severity scoring, abbreviated injury scores, trauma score, Glasgow coma score, and Champion trauma score). While some of these studies have suggested that these scoring systems can reliably predict pregnancy outcome, none have been tested in a prospective, clinically relevant design. Furthermore, the use of continuous fetal monitoring has been shown in prospective studies to reliably predict fetal outcome. If immediate adverse events (e.g., abruptio placentae, ruptured membranes, fetal death) do not occur, then pregnancy outcome appears to be good.

## EVALUATION AND MANAGEMENT

Because fetal survival depends wholly on maternal integrity, maternal stabilization is of primary importance. Maternal shock is associated with fetal mortality approaching 80 percent. During the initial stage of evaluation, concentration should be entirely directed toward maternal status. The steps in the initial examination of a seriously injured trauma victim should be no different than in a nonpregnant trauma victim with the following exceptions: (1) in positioning the injured gravida of greater than 20 weeks' gestation, the left lateral tilt position is preferred as the uterus lies directly over the inferior vena cava, subsequently decreasing venous return; and (2) the physiological hypervolemia of pregnancy often allows 30 to 35 percent blood loss before the usual signs of hypovolemia develop, and aggressive fluid replacement, 50 percent above nonpregnant needs, is necessary. Maternal vital signs and fetal heart tones must be obtained at intervals. There are no specific studies regarding use of MAST in pregnancy.

Maternal and fetal resuscitation are best accomplished by restoring the circulating blood volume.

Vasopressors decrease uterine blood flow and therefore decrease fetal oxygen delivery. Where vasopressors are required to maintain maternal vital signs, ephedrine is the drug of choice in our institution. However, no drug should be withheld if needed to save the life of the mother regardless of the known or unknown fetal risk. If excessive bleeding is occurring from an already emptied uterus (i.e., postpartum or postabortal), dilute intravenous oxytocin or intramuscular ergonovine are both useful.

Once the patient is adequately oxygenated and her circulating volume has been restored, maternal evaluation and assessment of fetal condition should follow. The obstetric portion of the abdominal examination must be included in the general physical examination. Uterine tenderness or irritability, tetanic contractions, and vaginal bleeding are all suggestive of abruptio placentae. Uterine size should be assessed by measuring the fundal height (pubic symphysis to the top of the fundus). The fundal height is a rough estimate of gestational age (centimeters = gestational age in weeks), which allows some indication of fetal viability if delivery is necessary. Fetal heart tones should be auscultated with a Doppler instrument (after 10 weeks' gestation) or with a fetoscope (after 18 weeks' gestation). A pelvic examination is mandatory to assess trauma to the genital tract, dilatation and effacement of the cervix, the presenting fetal part, and the station of the presenting part (relationship of the presenting part to the ischial spines). The presence of amniotic fluid must be sought. Nitrazine paper (turns blue with amniotic fluid, pH >7) and "ferning" (dried amniotic fluid under a microscope reveals a fern pattern) are both highly reliable for diagnosing ruptured membranes.

Radiographs that are clinically necessary should be obtained. CT scanning of the pregnant abdomen has been used without fetal complication. Open diagnostic peritoneal lavage, using a supraumbilical approach, can also be used. Appropriate laboratory studies, including clotting studies, should be obtained when evaluating severe maternal trauma.

## Cardiotocodynamometry

In a prospective study, Pearlman et al. evaluated the sensitivity and specificity of a 4-h cardiotocodynamometry monitoring period for predicting immediate adverse outcomes following trauma during pregnancy beyond the twentieth week of gestation. Adverse outcomes in this study included abruptio placentae, fetal death, preterm delivery, or rupture of the amniotic membranes. When eight or more uterine contractions per hour at any time during the first 4 h of monitoring was used as threshold criterion, over 10 percent of pregnancies suffered immediate adverse outcomes. More importantly, when this frequency of contractions was *not* found in the first 4 h of monitoring, no episodes of immediate adverse outcomes were identified. A 4-h monitoring period appears to be a highly sensitive test for predicting immediate adverse outcome. In addition, monitoring appears to be more sensitive than ultrasound for predicting abruptio placentae in this setting (100 percent vs. 50 percent). Subjects who did not suffer immediate adverse outcomes and who were discharged after the monitoring period had pregnancy outcomes comparable to noninjured controls.

Based on the results of this and other studies, all pregnant women beyond 20 weeks' gestation with direct or indirect abdominal trauma should undergo at least 4 h of cardiotocographic monitoring. Monitoring should begin as soon as the gravida's vital signs are stable. The presence of uterine contractions, fetal brady- or tachycardia, or loss of fetal beat-to-beat variability requires immediate obstetrical consultation.

Additional indications for emergent obstetrical consultation include vaginal bleeding; abdominal tenderness, pain, or cramping; evidence of maternal hypovolemia; absence of fetal heart tones; suspected leakage of amniotic fluid; and sonographic evidence of fetal injury or suspicious retroplacental structure.

## CARDIAC ARREST AND POSTMORTEM CESAREAN SECTION

Nearly 200 cases of successful postmortem cesarean section have been reported in the literature. Several factors have been suggested to be important in predicting the chance of fetal survival:

1. Gestational age >28 weeks (or fetal weight >1000 g).
2. Interval between maternal death and delivery
   *a.* <5 min—excellent
   *b.* 5–10 min—good
   *c.* 10–15 min—fair
   *d.* 15–20 min—poor
   *e.* >20 min—unlikely
3. Maternal cause of death—if unrelated to *chronic* hypoxia, fetal chances are improved.
4. Fetal status prior to maternal death.
5. Quality of maternal resuscitation.

When postmortem cesarean section is performed, the abdomen should be opened as rapidly as possible, and the infant delivered through a "classical" (vertical) uterine incision. Neonatology consultation and attendance during the procedure should be attempted. Informed consent from the next of kin should be obtained if possible, but implied consent can be assumed if the next of kin is not available.

Cardiac arrest during pregnancy presents a difficult clinical and ethical challenge. The lives of two patients are at stake, and decisions made for one patient may adversely affect the other. There is evidence that early thoracotomy and open-chest massage may improve both maternal and fetal outcome. In addition, timely emergency cesarean section has been shown to improve both maternal venous return and cardiac output during cardiopulmonary resuscitation and to

increase the likelihood of intact neonatal survival. On the basis of this, it is suggested that if there is no response to Advanced Cardiac Life Support efforts in several minutes following maternal cardiac arrest, both of these methods should be seriously considered.

## BIBLIOGRAPHY

Agran PF, Dunkle DE, Winn DG, et al: Fetal death in motor vehicle accidents. *Ann Emerg Med* 16:1355, 1987.

Buchsbaum HJ: *Trauma in Pregnancy.* Philadelphia, Saunders, 1979.

Crosby WM, Costilloe JP: Safety of lap belt restraint for pregnant victims of automobile collisions. *N Engl J Med* 284:632, 1971.

Crosby WM, Snyder RG, Snow CC, et al: Impact injuries in pregnancy. 1: Experimental studies. *Am J Obstet Gynecol* 101:100, 1968.

Fildes J, Reed L, Jones N, et al: Trauma: The leading cause of maternal death. *J Trauma* 32(5):643, 1992.

George ER, Vanderkwaad T, Scholten DJ: Factors influencing pregnancy outcome after trauma. *Am Surg* 58(9):594, 1992.

Goodwin TM, Breen MT. Pregnancy outcome and fetomaternal hemorrhage after noncatastrophic trauma. *Am J Obstet Gynecol* 162:665, 1990.

Hoff WS, D'Amelio LF, Tinkoff GH, et al: Maternal predictors of fetal demise in trauma during pregnancy. *Surg Gynecol Obstet* 172:175, 1991.

Pearlman MD, Tintinalli JE: Evaluation and treatment of the gravida and fetus following trauma during pregnancy. *Obstet Gynecol Clin N Am* 18(2):371, 1991.

Pearlman MD, Tintinalli JE, Lorenz RP. A progressive controlled study of outcome after trauma during pregnancy. *Am J Obstet Gynecol* 162:1502, 1990.

Pearlman MD, Tintinalli JE, Lorenz RP. Blunt trauma during pregnancy. *N Engl J Med* 323:1609, 1990.

Rolbin SH, Levinson G, Shinder SM, et al: Dopamine treatment of spinal hypotension decreases uterine blood flow in pregnant ewes. *Anesthesiology* 51:36, 1979.

Rose PG, Strohm PL, Zuspan FP: Fetomaternal hemorrhage following trauma. *Am J Obstet Gynecol* 153:844, 1985.

Rothenberger D, Quattlebaum FW, Zabel J, et al: Diagnostic peritoneal lavage for blunt trauma in pregnant women. *Am J Obstet Gynecol* 129:479, 1977.

Rothenberger D, Quattlebaum FW, Perry JF, et al: Blunt maternal trauma: A review of 103 cases. *J Trauma* 18:173, 1978.

Williams JK, McClain L, Rosemary AS, et al: Evaluation of blunt abdominal trauma in the third trimester of pregnancy: Maternal and fetal considerations. *Obstet Gynecol* 75:33, 1990.

# 100
# EMERGENCY DELIVERY
## Paul T. von Oeyen

The necessity for emergency delivery outside a hospital obstetric unit is relatively uncommon (1 in 695, or 0.14 percent in Weir's large series) but is an event met with extreme anxiety by medical personnel as well as parents. Despite careful planning, precipitous labor can result in the need for delivery either at home, in transit, or in the emergency department of a hospital without an obstetric unit. Precipitous labor is often unpredictable and can occur in nulliparous teenagers, who may not recognize periodic lower abdominal cramping as labor, as well as in experienced multiparas. Other reasons for emergency delivery include inadequate preparations (including inability to make arrangements for sudden care of other children), lack of transportation, remote geographic location, fear of arriving at the hospital too early or in false labor, fear of delivery in transit, and premature labor. The issue of purposeful out-of-hospital delivery is the source of continuing heated controversy, although such delivery is fortunately still statistically quite rare, and will not be dealt with here.

## TRANSPORT OF MATERNAL PATIENTS

The current emphasis on maternal transport of high-risk pregnancies to tertiary perinatal centers rather than transport of newborns increases the importance of proper preparedness for emergency delivery in transit. The regionalization of obstetric and newborn care, and especially the establishment of neonatal intensive care centers in the 1960s and 1970s, resulted in a marked decline in neonatal mortality. Although regional centers at first operated largely for neonates, several studies have clearly established the desirability of maternal over neonatal transports. This is especially true for the premature neonate weighing less than 1500 g and born prior to 34 weeks' gestation. Maternal transports can result in improved neonatal mortality and neonatal morbidity when measured in terms of lower hospitalization costs and length of stay. Maternal transports in general are faster and less expensive than neonatal transports. Clearly, the human uterus is the best transport incubator.

Reasons for maternal transport include placental bleeding, pregnancy-induced hypertension, fetal abnormalities, multiple gestation, diabetes mellitus, and other maternal medical problems, but by far the most common indications for transfer to tertiary perinatal centers are preterm labor and preterm premature rupture of membranes. This creates the necessity to be prepared for emergency delivery and resuscitation of premature infants in transit. Delivery while en route by air or ground transportation should be relatively rare if adequate communication and proper consultation are performed. Clearly, in-utero transport should not be attempted if there is maternal or fetal cardiovascular instability or if cervical dilatation has not been arrested by tocolytic agents.

Maternal-transport vehicles should carry sterile delivery packs, intravenous solutions and tubing, medications for both maternal and neonatal use, neonatal-resuscitation equipment, and monitoring equipment for both mother and baby (see Tables 100-1 and 100-2). The transport team should be familiar with the use and side effects of the β-adrenergic drugs terbutaline and ritodrine, used for treatment of preterm labor, as well as magnesium sulfate, used for treatment of pregnancy-induced hypertension and also for preterm labor.

In general, ground ambulance appears to be the most efficient means of transportation up to a 50- or 60-mile radius. However, helicopter transport has been advocated in some densely populated urban areas even for short distances because of concern over emergency-transport delays caused by traffic congestion. Fixed-wing aircraft are most useful for transports in rural settings with transport distances greater than 100 miles where the additional speed more than adequately makes up for the time lost between hospital and airport.

Air transport, however, also brings up the issue of potential additional hazards to the fetus because of the altitude during flights as well as safety issues for emergency flights occurring in stressful conditions and sometimes hazardous weather. The small ambulance types of aircraft utilized for maternal transport are pressurized to an

**Table 100-1.** Medications for Emergency Delivery

| | |
|---|---|
| Oxytocin, 10 units/mL | Epinephrine, 1:1000 |
| Methylergonovine (Methergine), | Diazepam, 10 mg |
| 0.2 mg/mL | Lidocaine (Xylocaine), 1% |
| Magnesium sulfate, 50% | Sodium bicarbonate, 50 mEq |
| (5 g/10 mL) | Prochlorperazine (Compazine), |
| Magnesium sulfate, 10% | 10 mg/2 mL |
| (2 g/20 mL) | Diphenhydramine (Benadryl), |
| Calcium gluconate, 10 mL | 50 mg |
| Hydralazine, 20 mg/mL | Naloxone (Narcan), 0.4 mg/mL |
| Ephedrine sulfate, 0.05 g | Dimenhydrinate (Dramamine), |
| Sodium amytal, 250 mg | 50 mg |
| Terbutaline sulfate, 1 mg/mL | Sterile water for injection |

**Table 100-2.** Equipment and Supplies for Emergency Delivery

| | |
|---|---|
| Sterile gloves | Plasma |
| Doptone stethoscope | IV tubing |
| Ultrasound gel | Alcohol sponges |
| Blood pressure cuff with stethoscope | Adhesive tape |
| Surgical scissors | Adhesive bandages |
| Rubber bulb syringe | Ambu bag |
| Plastic airway | Towels |
| Padded tongue blade | Hemostats |
| Reflex hammer | Cord clamps |
| Elastic tourniquet | Gauze sponges, 4 × 4 |
| Syringes | Umbilical tape |
| Needles | Neonatal laryngoscope |
| Angiocaths | Neonatal endotracheal tubes |
| Lactated Ringer's solution, 1000 mL | Neonatal Ambu bag |
| Dextrose, 5% in 1000 mL of water | |

altitude equivalent of 5000 to 8000 ft, but accidental decompression may expose the fetus to hypoxia during transport. This could be especially deleterious to the fetus already partially compromised by pregnancy-induced hypertension, or by placental infarction or abruption. Adequate oxygen supplies for face mask or nasal administration should be available for use during high-altitude transports as well as for emergency resuscitation.

## PREPARATION FOR EMERGENCY DELIVERY

The same basic equipment as that needed for maternal transports should be available in the emergency department for emergency delivery (see Tables 100-1 and 100-2).

Any pregnant woman arriving in an emergency department who is beyond 20 weeks' gestation and appears to be actively contracting should be rapidly evaluated with a bimanual pelvic examination to assess cervical dilatation, and maternal vital signs and fetal heart rate should also be checked. An exception to this is the gravida with active vaginal bleeding, who should be evaluated with ultrasound to rule out placenta previa before pelvic examination is attempted. Also, if there is suspicion of ruptured membranes, the patient should be evaluated with sterile speculum, with Nitrazine paper and ferning tests done to confirm ruptured membranes unless delivery appears imminent. The speculum examination should afford a view of the cervix to estimate the dilatation of the cervix and allow collection of specimens for culture (in particular for group B streptococcus and *Neisseria gonorrhoeae*, if the history is unknown or there has been no prenatal care). Occasionally a pregnant woman who denies knowledge of the pregnancy will present to the emergency department. This is seen most often in the teenage years, but any woman between 12 and 45 who presents to the emergency department with vaginal bleeding or abdominal pain should be evaluated for possible pregnancy whether or not she exhibits an obviously enlarged abdomen. A Doppler fetoscope should be available for confirmation of fetal life, although the inability to detect fetal heart tones does not rule out the possibility of a viable pregnancy.

Bimanual examination should be performed with sterile gloves and lubricant with the patient in the dorsal lithotomy position. Stirrups are not necessary as an adequate examination can be made with the mother's feet drawn close to her perineum on the examining table with her knees flexed and abducted. The cervix should be checked for dilatation and effacement and the presenting part (i.e., vertex or breech) identified. Prolapse of the cord should be excluded. The pregnant woman should not be left lying flat on her back for long, however, as the weight of the pregnant uterus can compress the major vessels, resulting in supine hypotension syndrome and decreased uterine perfusion.

Prenatal records should be quickly perused, if available. Gestational age can be determined from the last normal menstrual period (LMP), if this is known, and the due date (estimated date of confinement, or EDC) can be calculated by using Naegele's rule (add 9 months and 7 days to the date of the LMP). If ultrasound examination is readily available, it may be useful for making a reasonable estimate of potential fetal viability in a premature pregnancy of uncertain dates, but third trimester ultrasound measurements are unreliable for accurate dating (± 3 to 4 weeks). Between 20 and 35 weeks, there is a rough correlation between the gestational age and the height of the uterine fundus measured in centimeters from the pubic symphysis.

If the cervix is 6 cm or more dilated in a woman experiencing active contractions, further transport even for short distances may be hazardous and preparations should be made for emergency delivery. An intravenous line should be established with lactated Ringer's solution, if there is time before delivery, in order to be prepared for the administration of medications, fluids, or blood products immediately post partum if this becomes necessary. Minimal blood testing should include hemoglobin or hematocrit measurement (or a complete blood cell count), hepatitis B surface antigen (HBsAG), blood typing (if unknown), and a clotted tube of blood to be available for emergency cross matching if necessary. If possible, urine should be tested for protein and glucose.

Maternal temperature, blood pressure (between contractions), and heart rate should be evaluated at least every 1 to 2 h. In the absence of continuous electronic monitoring, the fetal heart rate should be evaluated by Doppler fetoscope or a fetal stethoscope every 15 min prior to complete cervical dilatation (10 cm) and every 5 min during the second stage of labor (complete dilatation to delivery). The normal fetal heart rate is between 120 and 160 beats per minute and can be differentiated from the maternal heart rate if necessary by simultaneous manual assessment of the radial pulse. The fetal heart rate should be counted for at least a 30-s period following a contraction. If bradycardia is detected, the mother should be given oxygen and an intravenous fluid bolus and positioned on her side. This will maximize uterine blood flow and fetal oxygenation as well as possibly relieve cord compression. If bradycardia is associated with tetanic contractions and delivery is not imminent, consideration should be given for the administration of tocolytic agents to relax the uterus, such as terbutaline 0.25 mg subcutaneously or magnesium sulfate 4 to 6 g intravenously over 15 to 20 min. If uterine tenderness, severe back pain, or excessive vaginal bleeding is also present, the possibility of placental abruption should be considered.

If membranes are intact, there is generally no reason to rupture them artificially until actual delivery. Amniotomy may result in prolapse of the umbilical cord if the baby's head is not well-engaged in the pelvis. Bladder distension should be avoided, and if it occurs and the mother is unable to spontaneously void, straight catheterization is indicated.

Around the time the cervix has become fully dilated, the gravida will feel a nearly uncontrollable urge to bear down with a Valsalva maneuver to expel the baby. The cervix should be checked to ensure full dilatation before allowing the mother to "push." If the cervix can still be palpated, serious laceration may occur from her uncontrolled expulsive efforts. Although important throughout labor, constant reassurance and emotional support are especially crucial at this point. Suggesting an alternative behavior, such as focusing on breathing and panting through the contractions, may help the mother to follow instructions and stay in control of expulsive efforts. A lateral position may also be helpful.

Once full dilatation has been established, expulsive efforts will most likely occur spontaneously. However, the inexperienced mother may need to be coached with instructions to take a deep breath at the start of each contraction, and with breath held, exert downward pressure as if having a bowel movement. Indeed, expulsion of feces during the second stage of labor is quite common, and the perineum should be frequently cleansed with a mild soap solution. The mother should not, however, be encouraged to push beyond the duration of each uterine contraction, which can be judged by direct palpation.

## EMERGENCY DELIVERY PROCEDURE

As the baby's head descends, imminent delivery can be anticipated by bulging of the perineum and the appearance of the fetal scalp at the introitus. At this point, no attempt should be made to delay delivery, but a controlled delivery is important in preventing both fetal and maternal injury. Either a traditional dorsal lithotomy or lateral Sims' position may be used for the actual delivery. The lateral Sims' position has the advantage of slower descent and lessening tension in the perineal tissues, and this may allow easier delivery without an episiotomy. On the other hand, with the dorsal lithotomy position the less-experienced attendant may be better able to visualize and manually control the delivery process and perform episiotomy as necessary. If the dorsal lithotomy position is chosen, the mother should be tilted slightly to one side to lessen vena caval compression and brought to the edge of the bed or stretcher, or the buttocks raised on pillows, to allow room for delivery of the baby's head and shoulders. The mother's legs should be widely separated and supported with her knees flexed.

With each contraction the vaginal outlet bulges to accommodate a greater portion of the fetal head, and this process may be aided by gentle digital stretching of the perineum. Episiotomy may be performed at this time if necessary to allow delivery without spontaneous lacerations. A local anesthetic should be injected just prior to episiotomy with 5 to 10 mL of 1% lidocaine (Xylocaine) in a syringe with a small-gauge needle. If a local anesthetic is unavailable, an episiotomy may be cut with minimal pain when the perineum is most stretched, taking care to protect the infant's head with gloved fingers. A midline perineal incision should be made, taking care not to extend into the rectum.

As the head emerges, the palm of one hand should be placed over the head to assist with the normal extension of the head and at the same time prevent the head from suddenly popping out of the vagina. At this point the mother is asked not to push in order to minimize the trauma associated with uncontrolled expulsive efforts. The best method to inhibit the overwhelmingly strong desire to bear down when the fetal head is distending the perineum is generally reassurance and asking the mother to pant or breathe through her nose.

With expulsive efforts under control, and one hand on the infant's crowning head, the second hand draped with a sterile cloth can be used to gently lift the infant's chin posterior to the maternal anus. This facilitates further extension and a slow, controlled emergence of the baby's head (modified Ritgen. maneuver; see Fig. 100-1). As the

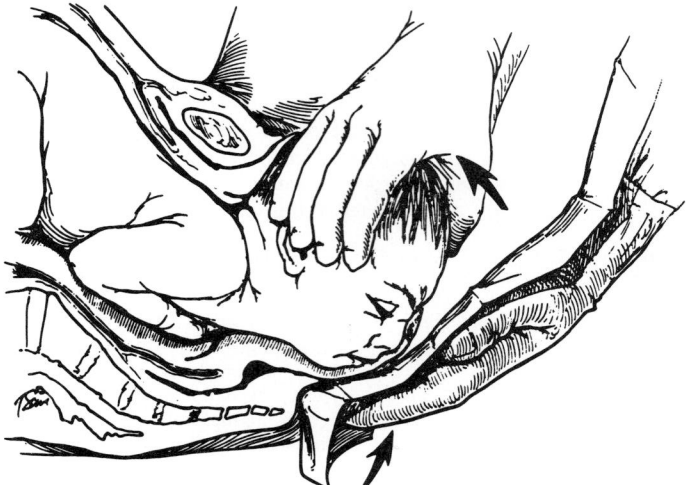

**Fig. 100-1.** Modified Ritgen maneuver. Palm of hand on infant's head while second hand draped with sterile cloth gently lifts the infant's chin. (From Cunningham et al., p. 382. Used by permission.)

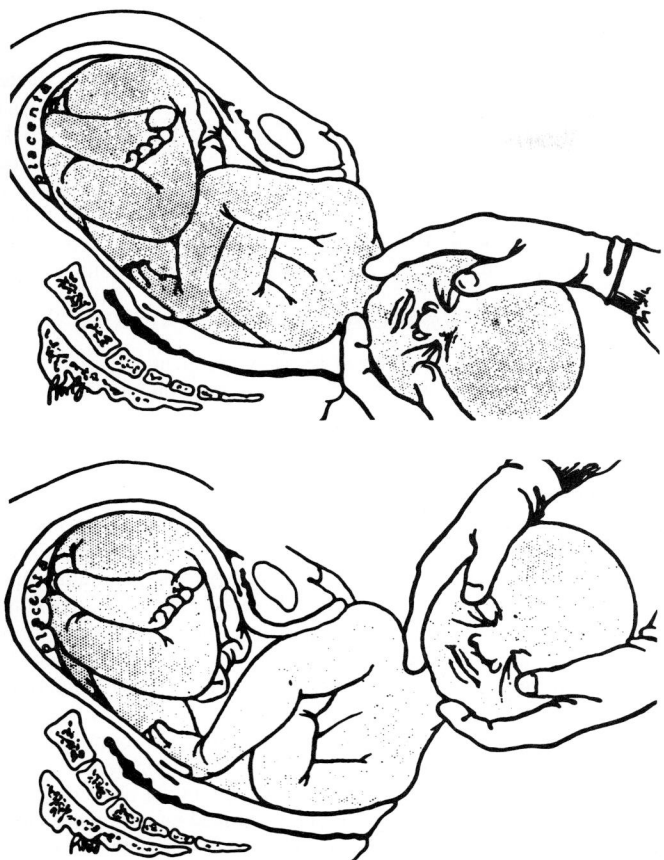

**Fig. 100-2.** Delivery of shoulders. **Top:** Gentle downward traction to ease anterior shoulder under pubic symphysis. **Bottom.** Delivery of anterior shoulder completed; gentle upward traction to deliver posterior shoulder. (From Cunningham et al., p. 384. Used by permission.)

head is delivered, usually with the face down, it tends to restitute to one or the other lateral positions.

The baby's neck region should be palpated immediately after delivery of the head to check for a nuchal cord, which may be found about 25 percent of the time. If the cord is relatively loose, it can be slipped out of the way over the baby's head. If the cord is tight, two clamps should be placed close together on the most accessible portion of the cord (usually anteriorly) and the cord cut in between. The cord can then be unwound if there are multiple loops.

Before the delivery of the shoulders and thorax is continued, the baby's face should be wiped off and the mouth and nose aspirated with a soft rubber bulb syringe to clear the airway. This is especially important to prevent meconium aspiration if there has been meconium staining of the amniotic fluid. If no bulb syringe is available, the mouth should be scooped out with the finger as well as possible. Squeezing the nose between the fingers and stroking the upper neck from the larynx toward the mandible may also be helpful.

Attention should now be turned toward delivery of the shoulders. This can be facilitated by placing both hands on either side of the baby's head, and a gentle downward traction will ease the anterior shoulder under the pubic symphysis (see Fig. 100-2). Care should be taken not to use undue force, as this may result in brachial plexus injury. If there is resistance, an assistant should be asked to employ suprapubic pressure (not fundal pressure) to avoid impaction of the shoulder behind the symphysis. When the anterior shoulder is visible, gentle upward traction will deliver the posterior shoulder. Care should be taken not to let the posterior shoulder pop out uncontrolled,

as this may result in a laceration of the anal sphincter and into the rectum (third-degree perineal laceration).

The baby will be very slippery, especially if there is thick vernix (white, cheesy desquamated skin). The posterior hand should slide down onto the posterior shoulder as it is delivered and then behind the back of the neck to support the baby's head. The anterior hand should then be brought along the baby's back as the body delivers spontaneously. Placing the index finger between the lower legs, and the third finger and thumb around each leg, ensures a safe grip. The baby should not, however, be held by its heels upside down. The body can easily be cradled in the same arm that is gripping the legs, and the other hand can be used to further wipe the body off and suction out the mouth and pharynx as needed.

If the baby is breathing spontaneously and is close to term, there is no need to rush cutting the cord. The baby can be dried off, wrapped in a warm blanket, and placed on the mother's abdomen to help minimize heat loss. The cord should be doubly clamped before cutting with a sterile scissors. If sterile scissors are unavailable, it is better to leave the cord uncut until sterile instruments can be found.

An immediate assessment of the baby with Apgar scoring should be done to determine the need for resuscitation. See Chap. 16 for details of neonatal resuscitation.

## Management of Shoulder Dystocia

Shoulder dystocia during emergency delivery should be a rare event. Nevertheless, because of the risk of resulting fetal or maternal trauma including fetal brachial plexus injury or fetal death, it is important for anyone who may be involved in emergency delivery to have some preexisting practical knowledge of its management. In this situation time is of the essence; the emergency physician does not have the luxury of waiting for expert help to arrive or of being talked through management procedures over the telephone. The following paragraphs will try to outline some practical methods for dealing with shoulder dystocia, but a comprehensive discussion of this or other complicated obstetric procedures is beyond the scope of this chapter, which cannot be a substitute for the major obstetrical texts and direct obstetrical experience and teaching.

Shoulder dystocia involves the impaction of the anterior fetal shoulder behind the pubic symphysis with subsequent arrest of delivery after the expulsion of the fetal head. Occasionally the posterior shoulder may also become lodged against the sacrum, further compounding the impaction. It is usually caused by a large, macrosomic infant whose shoulder girdle is relatively large compared to the size of the fetal head.

Shoulder dystocia should be recognized when the standard maneuver of mild downward traction on the fetal head with the mother pushing fails to result in the emergence of the anterior shoulder under the pubic symphysis. Typically, the fetal head is pulled tightly to the perineum, the so-called turtle sign. At this point, what is most important is to recognize the shoulder dystocia and call for assistants who can be directed to help in the following maneuvers even if they are inexperienced. The baby's mouth and nose should be cleared and the maternal bladder drained if distended.

The first step in dealing with shoulder dystocia is to position the mother for maximum room and maneuverability. The maternal perineum should be at the end of the examining table and the maternal legs should not be in stirrups but sharply flexed toward the abdomen in the McRoberts maneuver. If the mother cannot hold her legs flexed in this position with her hands, assistants may be required to help, one on each side. A generous episiotomy, extending through the anal sphincter if necessary, should be cut, preferably with adequate local anesthesia. At this time *suprapubic,* not fundal, pressure should be applied by an assistant. Shoulder dystocia is likely to be further aggravated by fundal pressure, but suprapubic pressure can help dislodge the anterior shoulder impacted behind the pubic symphysis.

If these measures fail, manual rotation of one or both shoulders toward the anterior surface of the fetal chest should be attempted to try to produce a smaller shoulder-to-shoulder diameter and displace the anterior shoulder from behind the pubic symphysis. A variation of this, the Woods corkscrew maneuver, consists of progressively rotating the posterior shoulder 180 degrees in a corkscrew fashion, resulting in the release of the impacted anterior shoulder. Of course, any maneuvering in the birth canal may be difficult with a large, macrosomic infant filling it. At the same time, suprapubic pressure may be applied but at a 45° lateral angle in the direction of the attempted rotation of the anterior shoulder.

If the corkscrew maneuver fails, the next step should be to attempt to deliver the posterior arm. A large proctoepisiotomy is likely to be necessary to accomplish this. The operator's hand follows the shaft of the humerus to the elbow. The forearm is grasped or, if it is not possible to do so, pressure is applied on the antecubital fossa in order to flex the forearm to within reach. The forearm is then swept across the baby's chest and face and out through the introitus. If gentle traction while the patient pushes does not now result in delivery, a corkscrew maneuver can again be attempted, but this time the posterior arm can also be used to rotate the posterior shoulder across the chest toward the pubic symphysis, allowing the anterior shoulder to dislodge from under the pubic symphysis and deliver through an oblique pelvic diameter.

Almost all shoulder dystocias will have been reduced by now (all of these maneuvers together taking only a few minutes). If the baby still cannot be delivered, intentional fracture of the anterior clavicle or humerus is still preferable to a brachial plexus injury from severe downward traction, a prolonged period of hypoxemia, or fetal death. If general anesthesia and cesarean section delivery are immediately available, it may be possible to flex the fetal head and slowly push it back into the vagina, while a cesarean section is performed, the Zavenelli maneuver.

## PRETERM DELIVERY

Since preterm labor is a common cause for unexpected childbirth, emergency deliveries frequently involve premature infants. It is very important to deliver a premature infant in a slow, controlled fashion, because the premature baby has greater fragility and may be more susceptible to rupture of intracranial blood vessels as well as superficial bruising. For this reason, it may be best to avoid artificial rupture of the membranes with preterm delivery and to allow delivery to occur *en cul,* or with the membranes intact. In spite of the premature infant's smaller head size, an episiotomy should be liberally performed to prevent prolonged pounding of the infant's head against a resistant perineum as well as sudden popping of the head out of the introitus. Premature infants should be dried off quickly to reduce their rapid heat loss. The cord should be rapidly clamped and cut so the infant can be quickly assessed for resuscitation. Any ventilation assistance that may be required should be performed with a small Ambu bag, taking care to avoid higher pressures that would result in pneumothorax.

Premature babies are more often in breech presentation than term infants are. Although the procedure of choice for premature breech delivery is by cesarean section, this may not be possible in an emergency situation. As much as possible, the breech infant should be allowed to deliver spontaneously, at least until the level of the umbilicus has been reached. A warm towel should be placed on the baby's lower back and buttocks, and with gentle handling of the baby's pelvic bones and back (not abdomen!) one shoulder should be rotated anteriorly and delivered by lowering the infant's entire body. The remaining shoulder may be delivered by rotating the infant in the reverse direction and again lowering the body. Alternatively, if trunk rotation does not occur smoothly, the posterior shoulder may be delivered first by raising the infant's body and then slowly sweeping a fin-

ger across the perineum from the back of the infant's shoulder across the chest, gently releasing the arm.

After the shoulder and arms are delivered the back usually rotates spontaneously in the direction of the symphysis. If not, manual rotation of the body should be performed to place the back under the symphysis. An assistant should apply pressure suprapubicly to help maintain flexion of the baby's head. As the neck appears, a finger can be placed over the baby's maxilla or, if done gently, into the baby's mouth, to flex the head for delivery and avoid entrapment in the cervix. The breech infant is more likely to require resuscitation.

## MANAGEMENT IMMEDIATELY POSTPARTUM

The placenta should be allowed to separate spontaneously, unless there is considerable active bleeding. Pulling on the cord risks cord rupture or the possible catastrophe of inversion of the uterus. The usual signs of placental separation are a gush of blood and lengthening of the cord. As the placenta is expelled, the membranes may be teased out by rotating the placenta and twisting the membranes.

After the placenta is out, the uterus should be massaged to help it to contract and remain firm. Oxytocin, 10 units, may be given slowly intravenously (or mixed in the intravenous bag), or by intramuscular injection if no intravenous line is available, to help maintain uterine contraction. Uterine atony often results after precipitous labor (total labor less than 3 h). Excessive bleeding calls for vigorous uterine massage, an increased amount of intravenous crystalloid solutions, and additional oxytocin or methylergonovine (Methergine). Bleeding sites for lacerations should also be identified and controlled with clamps or direct pressure. Episiotomy or laceration repair should await the availability of an experienced practitioner or obstetrician.

It should be emphasized that the infant should be thoroughly dried and wrapped in warm towels or blankets to minimize heat loss. Meconium should be suctioned out immediately after delivery of the head and before the infant takes its first breath. If personnel skilled in neonatal intubation are present, the infant with thick meconium should be intubated and suctioned under direct laryngoscopy. If a warm isolette is not available, the infant can be kept in close contact with the mother to conserve heat.

The goal of every delivery, including in the emergency situation, is a safe delivery with minimal trauma to the mother and without injury to the infant. Usually this can be accomplished even with minimal equipment if the attending individual(s) have the basic knowledge and skills for the mechanics of delivery and can give emotional support to the mother during the process. If need be, the basic points of delivery can be reviewed with a consultant by telephone in order to accomplish a safe outcome to both mother and baby.

## BIBLIOGRAPHY

American Academy of Pediatrics Committee on Fetus and Newborn, American College of Obstetricians and Gynecologists Committee on Obstetrics: *Maternal and Fetal Medicine, Guidelines for Perinatal Care,* 3d ed, 1992.

Bowes WA: Delivery of the very low birth weight infant. *Clin Perinatol* 8:183, 1981.

Crenshaw C, Payne P, Blackmon L, et al: Prematurity and the obstetrician: A regional neonatal intensive care unit is not enough. *Am J Obstet Gynecol* 147:125, 1983.

Cunningham FG, MacDonald PC, Gant NF, et al (eds): *Williams Obstetrics,* 19th ed. Norwalk, CT, Appleton/Lange, 1993.

Elliot JD, O'Keeffe DF, Freeman RK: Helicopter transportation of patients with obstetric emergencies in an urban area. *Am J Obstet Gynecol* 143:157, 1982.

Gianopoulos JG: Emergency complications of labor and delivery. *Emerg Med Clin North Am* 12:201, 1994.

Parer JT: Effects of hypoxia on the mother and fetus with emphasis on maternal air transport. *Am J Obstet Gynecol* 142:957, 1982.

Weir PE, Beischer NA: Birth before arrival in hospital. *Med J Aust* 2:31, 1980.

# 101

# COMMON COMPLICATIONS OF GYNECOLOGIC PROCEDURES

## Veronica T. Mallett

With the advent of same-day surgery and the increasing necessity to discharge patients within 3 days of a major procedure, postsurgical gynecologic patients are presenting to emergency departments with increasing frequency. The objective of this chapter is to provide an overview of the common complications of gynecologic procedures likely to lead to an emergency department visit and the diagnostic and therapeutic approach to these patients.

## COMMON COMPLICATIONS OF ENDOSCOPIC PROCEDURES

### Laparoscopy

Gynecologic laparoscopy, both diagnostic and therapeutic, involves the use of a rigid endoscope, which is inserted usually through a small subumbilical incision bluntly into the abdominal cavity. Prior to the insertion of the laparoscope, the abdomen is insufflated with nitrous oxide or carbon dioxide gas administered through a small-diameter verres needle.

Laparoscopy can be used to diagnose existing pelvic disease and to perform simple and complex gynecologic surgeries. The most common surgical procedure in the United States today is female sterilization, and more than 60 percent of sterilizations are performed through the laparoscope. With advanced technology and increased operator skill, the laparoscope is currently used for laser ablation of endometriosis and pelvic adhesions, sharp lysis of adhesions, linear salpingostomy or salpingectomy for the treatment of ectopic pregnancy, laser ablation of small myomata, oophorectomy, cystectomy, laparoscope-assisted vaginal hysterectomy, and retropubic urethropexy.

All these procedures have the same potential complications, but the more complicated surgeries carry considerably more risk. The major complications associated with the use of the laparoscope are (1) thermal injuries to the bowel; (2) bleeding at the site of tubal interruption or sharp dissection; and (3) rarely ureteral and/or bladder injury, large bowel injury, and pelvic hematoma or abscess.

Of these complications the most serious and dreaded is that of thermal injury to the bowel. This injury occurs most commonly in the terminal ileum, although injuries to the rectosigmoid and colon have been reported. Various series have reported the incidence of electrothermal injuries to be in the range of 0.5 to 3.2 per 1000 cases. The injury that goes unrecognized presents the most serious problem. These patients generally appear 3 to 7 days postoperatively, depending upon the degree of necrosis, with signs and symptoms of peritonitis, including bilateral lower abdominal pain, fever, elevated white cell count, and direct and rebound tenderness. X-rays may show an ileus or free air under the diaphragm. Although gas has been used to insufflate the abdomen, it should be absorbed totally within 3 postoperative days. Patients who have increasing pain after laparoscopy, either early or late, have a bowel injury until proved otherwise. If thermal injury is a serious consideration and cannot be distinguished from other causes of peritonitis, it is best to err on the side of early laparotomy.

Traumatic bowel injury is less problematic than thermal injury. This is because it is usually caused by the very small diameter verres needle and is recognized when the needle is withdrawn. Peritonitis

rarely develops following this complication, and hospital revisits are uncommon.

Bleeding may occur with any laparoscopic procedure, but due to direct visualization, it is usually arrested during the original procedure.

Infection has not been a frequent or particularly serious complication of laparoscopy. Excluding minor incisional infection, pelvic infection is reported in fewer than 1 per 1000 cases. When pelvic infection does occur, it is probably secondary to a subacute coexisting infection present prior to the procedure or secondary to the introduction of skin contaminants. Its presentation is not unique. Broad-spectrum antibiotic treatment provides a rapid response.

Infection dehiscence and herniations of the laparoscopic abdominal incision are rare but have been reported. Infection is usually treated with drainage. Dehiscence usually involves protrusion of the omentum and, in rare cases, the small bowel through the opening. Immediate wound reclosure is usually sufficient, provided no bowel injury has occurred and there is no evidence of infection.

### Hysteroscopy

Hysteroscopy involves the direct investigation of the interior of the uterine cavity using a rigid or flexible fiberoptic instrument. It can be carried out in an office procedure using the contact or flexible hysteroscope or under IV sedation or general anesthesia using the panoramic hysteroscope. It is used for both diagnostic and therapeutic purposes. Indications for use include investigation of any intrauterine pathology, i.e., endometrial polyps, submucous myomata, and foreign bodies. Therapeutic applications include directed biopsies, removal of small myomata, endometrial ablation using laser for menorrhagia, and division of small uterine septae or synechiae.

Complications of hysteroscopy fortunately are rare; they include: (1) reaction to the distending media, (2) uterine perforation, (3) cervical laceration, (4) anesthesia reaction, (5) intraabdominal organ injury, (6) infection, and (7) postoperative bleeding.

Postoperative bleeding will be the most likely cause of hospital revisit. Surgical procedures that could result in postoperative uterine bleeding include lysis of adhesions, resection of myomata, and YAG laser obliteration of the endometrium. After hemodynamic stabilization of the patient, an intrauterine tampon such as a pediatric foley generally can control this problem. Occasionally reexploration to cauterize a bleeding area is necessary. Rarely, abdominal control of the bleeding is required.

Infection as a result of the hysteroscopic procedure is uncommon; considering the number of cases done, the most severe infection, tuboovarian abscess, has rarely been reported. Treatment should be commensurate with presentation and symptoms.

Damage to intraabdominal contents has been reported. The seriousness of these complications ranges from the inconsequential rupture of a hydrosalpinx to damage to the bowel at the time of intrauterine biopsy, uterine perforation, or laser ablation. These are not common and generally are eliminated by the concomitant use of laparoscopy. Should injury go unrecognized, it would present as described.

Uterine perforations are mentioned only because they are a relatively common complication associated with the procedure but seldom require more than observation.

## COMPLICATIONS RELATED TO MAJOR ABDOMINAL PROCEDURES

Those complications that would lead to an emergency department visit would, by their nature, present more than 3 days postoperatively. Late-onset complications include, but are not confined to, wound infection and related morbidity, phlebitis (superficial and deep), urinary tract infection, ileus and bowel obstruction, and ureteral or bladder injury.

## Wound Infection

### Clinical Features

Wound infection may occur as late as several months following surgery, but more than 90 percent of the cases present within the first 2 weeks. The first sign is usually fever followed by tachycardia and varying degrees of increased tenderness. As the infection progresses, the wound may be fluctuant or firm. The incision is swollen, erythematous, edematous, and tender. There may be spontaneous purulent drainage from the wound. Initial management consists of opening the wound and probing with a cotton-tipped swab to ensure the fascia is intact, then allowing the wound to drain. If the patient has been discharged with staples in place, the wound opens easily after staple removal. If the staples have been removed, gentle probing will open the wound. Aerobic and anaerobic wound cultures should be obtained for use if the patient does not respond rapidly. Once a wound infection has been opened or drained, care is directed toward debridement and packing with saline-soaked gauze or half-strength peroxide.

### Patient Disposition

Rarely are antibiotics required unless there is an underlying cellulitis. Readmission is common practice, at least for observation and patient teaching.

## Wound Hematoma

### Clinical Features

Hematomas are a common complication of wound closure that are more frequent in transverse than vertical incisions. The wound itself may swell and be painful, but in general, the smaller hematoma can and should be managed expectantly. If there are any signs of infection, the wound should be managed accordingly. The patient should be instructed to return if signs of infection develop.

## Wound Seroma

### Clinical Features

Wound seromas are relatively uncommon in the gynecologic incision, with the exception of groin dissection. It is, by definition, a collection of serous fluid, which may drain spontaneously. In general, it is the presence of drainage, not fever or pain, that brings the patient to the emergency department. If the wound remains intact after gentle probing, the seroma can be watched and usually will disappear. Wound infection precautions should be given.

## Dehiscence and Evisceration

### Clinical Features

Dehiscence is a failure of normal healing and locally means disruption of any layers of a surgical incision. Clinically, dehiscence connotes disruption of all layers, including fascia but not peritoneum. Evisceration occurs when there is complete breakdown of the healing processes through all levels of the abdominal wall, with the omentum or bowel presenting through the incision.

### Diagnosis

The classic sign of impending wound disruption is the sudden outpouring of serosanguinous blood from the abdominal incision. Most often this occurs between postoperative days 5 and 8. The patient may describe a "pop" or tearing sensation. About one-third of the cases of wound dehiscence will be associated with evisceration. When evisceration has occurred, the abdomen should be covered with moist sterile towels and supported with tape to prevent further extrusion of the gut.

### Patient Disposition

The patient should be taken directly to the operating room for closure. In those cases in which there is a sudden appearance of blood but no bowel, it is best to follow the same procedure because evisceration usually is imminent.

## Ureteral Injury

### Clinical Features

Operative injury to the ureter results from one of three types of trauma: crushing, transection, and ligation. Each type of injury may be either partial or complete. This complication occurs more often during the performance of abdominal hysterectomy than in any other pelvic surgery. Unilateral ureteral injury usually is discovered within 48 to 72 h postoperatively but may go undiscovered for up to 2 to 3 weeks. Occasionally, permanent and complete occlusion will lead to renal atrophy without symptoms.

### Diagnosis

In most instances, ureteral injury produces symptoms of fever, flank pain, and costovertebral angle tenderness. These symptoms may indicate pyelitis, but if the patient has unexplained or persistent fever, persistent abdominal distension, unexplained hematuria, or especially escape of a watery discharge, an intravenous pyelogram (IVP) should be obtained. Further indications for an IVP include oliguria or the appearance of a lower abdominal or pelvic mass following pelvic surgery. If the diagnosis is made 2 to 3 weeks postoperatively, percutaneous nephrostomy with delayed repair is the treatment of choice.

## MISCELLANEOUS COMPLICATIONS OF MAJOR GYNECOLOGIC PROCEDURES

### Cuff Cellulitis

#### Clinical Features

Cuff cellulitis refers to infections of the contiguous retroperitoneal space immediately above the vaginal apex and including the surrounding soft tissue. It is a common complication following both abdominal and vaginal hysterectomy. It usually produces a fever between postoperative days 3 to 5 and thus, generally, will delay discharge of the postabdominal hysterectomy patient. The postvaginal hysterectomy patient conceivably will have been discharged, as such patients are being discharged within 12 h postoperatively. These women present with a complaint of fever and lower quadrant pain. Pelvic tenderness and induration are prominent during the bimanual examination. A vaginal cuff abscess may be palpable.

#### Patient Disposition

The treatment of choice is readmission, drainage, and intravenous antibiotics.

### Urinary Retention

Voiding difficulties in the healthy female are uncommon. However, many women experience either an inability to void or incomplete emptying of the bladder during the postoperative period.

#### Clinical Features

Inability to void is more frequent after operations that involve the urethra and bladder neck, i.e., anterior repair or any modification of the retropubic urethropexy. Most problems with voiding following any of these procedures resolve with time and without medication.

#### Patient Disposition

If mechanical obstruction is not suspected to be a factor, intermittent straight catheterization is the treatment of choice. The patient should be instructed to attempt to void on a timed schedule, with an interval of less than 3 h. She should be discharged with instructions for self-catheterization should she be unable to void and be reassured that voiding function will return in time.

## Postconization Bleeding

### Clinical Features

Treatment of high-grade squamous intraepithelial lesions of the cervix may be treated by LEEP (loop electrocautery), laser vaporization, or cold knife care. The most common complication associated with these procedures is bleeding. If delayed hemorrhage occurs, it usually occurs 7 days postoperatively. Bleeding following this procedure can be rapid and severe.

### Patient Disposition

Visualization of the cervix is the key to controlling such bleeding. Application of Monsel's solution is a reasonable first step if it is easily available. Usually, however, suturing of the bleeding arteriole is necessary. Quite often, the patient must be taken to the operating room for repair secondary to poor visualization.

## Induced Abortion

There are three major methods for termination of pregnancy: instrumental evacuation by the vaginal route, stimulation of uterine contraction, and major surgical procedures. Vacuum evacuation of the uterus has been associated with immediate and delayed complications. Immediate complications include uterine perforation, hemorrhage, and cervical laceration. Delayed complications of all methods of abortion include retention of products of conception, causing bleeding, infection, and possibly thrombophlebitis.

The majority of immediate complications will be arrested at the time of the abortion; however, uterine perforation, if unrecognized, could be complicated further by injury of intraabdominal contents with the suction. If this should occur and go unrecognized, the patient will present with the appropriate signs of organ injury. The organ most commonly injured is the bowel; however, the ureter has been in-jured as a consequence of this mishap. Management of these complication was discussed previously.

Advanced gestation abortion may result in injury to the uterus and infundibulopelvic or ovarian artery from the large dilators used in these procedures. If performed in a freestanding clinic, catastrophic blood loss could result in a true emergency. Resuscitation, replacement of blood loss, and emergency surgery are essential in the prevention of maternal mortality. If a patient with an injury of this nature is being transferred, pretransfer notification of the gynecology service may save valuable time.

Retained products of conception and a resulting endometritis are far more common complications.

### Clinical Features

The patient usually will present 3 to 5 days posttermination with complaints of excessive bleeding, fever, and abdominal pain. She may not present for up to 2 weeks. Pelvic examination reveals a subinvoluted tender uterus with foul-smelling blood vaginally. An elevated white blood count is common.

### Patient Disposition

Treatment must include evacuation of intrauterine contents and intravenous antibiotic therapy. Triple antibiotic therapy is the standard; however, there is increasing evidence that ampicillin with sulbactam (Unasyn) is equally as effective. If the patient has pain, bleeding, or both, but unaccompanied by fever, ectopic pregnancy must be ruled out. The presence of villi on the pathology report (if available) confirms the presence of an intrauterine gestation but cannot rule out the rare occurrence of both ectopic and intrauterine gestations.

## BIBLIOGRAPHY

Brooks P: Complications of operative hysterorscopy: How safe is it? *Clin Obstet Gynecol* 35:256, 1992.

Daly JW: Dehiscence, evisceration and other complications. *Clin Obstet Gynecol* 31:754, 1988.

# Pediatrics

## 102
## NORMAL CHILD DEVELOPMENT

### Peter Mellis

### INTRODUCTION

Children account for approximately 30 percent of visits in most emergency departments. The majority have minor or self-limited illness, which may optimally be cared for in a nonacute setting. However, the differentiation of the critically ill pediatric patient from the larger number of less ill children with similar complaints represents one of the most important and challenging diagnostic skills for the emergency physician. The key to mastering this process of identifying the ill child is a knowledge of child development as applied to the emergency setting.

### GENERAL PRINCIPLES OF THE DEVELOPMENTAL APPROACH

Although there are many specific aspects of the developmental approach, a few general principles are applicable to all age groups of children and their families.

### Communicate with the Child

Children are best approached in a positive and gentle manner, with an awareness that the first impression sets the tone for the encounter. Review the emergency record for patient name and age so that an introduction and a developmentally structured interaction may be planned. An awareness of the child's age-related communication skills and perspective will result in a more meaningful evaluation. Whenever possible, look at the child from his or her own eye level. Use the child's motor skills, vocabulary, and specific life experiences as reference points. Hunger, discomfort, fear of separation or pain, and feelings of loss of control should be directly addressed. Recognize that the emergency department is a strange and threatening environment and, whenever possible, isolate the child from the sights and sounds of other patient care experiences that may heighten their own anxiety. Most importantly, be honest with children regarding expectations for their experience so that trust can be established.

### Communicate with the Family

Assess and treat the child in the context of his or her family, avoiding separation whenever possible. Emergency department policy should encourage parental accompaniment of children to the clinical area. It is optimal to consider that there are two patients, child and parent(s), each with expectations that must be addressed. Caregivers have essential historical information and, in the case of infants and toddlers, are physically necessary to the performance of a meaningful physical assessment. At all ages, children watch their parents for cues with re-spect to how to respond to the medical staff. Parents who understand and accept the sequence of events involved in emergency care become allies in enlisting their child's cooperation. Whenever possible, parents should be encouraged to remain present during procedures, maintaining visual and physical contact from a sitting position. Appropriate exceptions include parental discomfort and critical illness. Finally, because parents are intimately familiar with their child's range of verbal and nonverbal behavior, the examiner must take the phrase "this is not my child" as parental concern for abnormal level of consciousness. This reliance on parental knowledge is particularly applicable to the assessment of the child with developmental delay.

### Assess by Means of Observation

Every effort should be made to gain information regarding the young child prior to directly interacting with him or her. Infants and young children communicate a normal level of consciousness through age-appropriate motor and social responses to their environment. Observe the child's behavior from a distance, preferably without his or her awareness. This can often be accomplished while obtaining the history from the caretakers. Antipyretic therapy and satisfying hunger are often crucial to achieving this period of optimal observation. Often more is learned regarding neurologic status from a brief period of observation than from the traditional physical examination. Nonemergent uncomfortable examination components and procedures should be performed last.

### Obtain Meaningful Vital Signs

Normal ranges for pulse, respirations, and blood pressure vary significantly with age and must be interpreted in the context of the child's activity at the time. Anxiety, pain, fever, and crying will increase all values, and these states should be documented if present. Optimal vital signs are obtained without eliciting an adverse reaction to the examiner, for example, respirations taken by observing abdominal movements, heart rate auscultated through clothing. If fever is a concern, temperature should be obtained rectally in infants and uncooperative children as the oral, axillary, and tympanic routes are less reliable. Weight is a pediatric vital sign because of dosing considerations and the importance of growth as an indicator of chronic disease in children (Table 102-1). Appropriate scales and growth charts should be available in the emergency department. For resuscitation purposes, estimates of weight are frequently inaccurate, and length-based resuscitation resources (e.g., Braselow tapes) are recommended.

### GROWTH AND DEVELOPMENTAL STAGES

The process of development is not unique to children, but the pace at which change occurs and the implications for patient care are maximal during this period of life. *Developmental stages* are described with associated age ranges, but these are best viewed as a sequence of events with significant individual variation in rate of progression. For purposes of facilitating patient care in the emergency department, two aspects of each developmental stage must be considered. *Physical aspects* include growth and physiologic parameters unique to a given developmental stage, a knowledge of which is essential to provide excellent care. *Neurologic aspects* include motor, language, and social/psychological milestones that impact on both patient assessment and responses during acute illness or injury. These milestones and

**Table 102-1.** Formulas for Estimating Normal Weight in Children

| Age | Weight, kg |
|---|---|
| ≤ 12 months | [Age (months)]/2 + 4 |
| 1–10 years | [2 × Age (years)] + 10 |

their related strategies are summarized in Table 102-2. Based on a knowledge of these, the examiner is well equipped to proceed with a developmentally *age-specific approach.*

## Early Infancy (0 to 6 Months)

### Physical Aspects

Rapid growth rate is a characteristic feature of the young infant, for whom the major work is eating. After a 5 to 10 percent loss over the first 3 days of life, term infants regain birth weight by 10 days of age. A 20- to 30-g/day weight gain is the best overall sign of health. Normal infants double their birth weight by 5 months. Young infants have a high surface area to body mass ratio with a proportionally large head, resulting in a high rate of heat loss and risk of hypothermia. The normal anterior fontanelle is slightly depressed when the child is upright. Young infants are obligate nose breathers and may experience partial airway obstruction with abnormal positioning or viral upper respiratory tract infections. Normal neonates may exhibit periodic breathing, or 5- to 10-s pauses followed by tachypnea, due to immature central control of respiration. Both cardiac output and minute ventilation are relatively rate-dependent in early infancy. Heart rate > 180 and respiratory rate > 60 should be considered abnormal. Blood pressure is well maintained by compensatory mechanisms at this age, with hypotension a very late finding in shock. The pulmonary vascular bed dilates over the first 6 weeks of life, so that congenital heart lesions resulting in a left-to-right shunt, for example, ventricular septal defect, will present after this age. Finally, the primary series of immunizations, including diphtheria, pertussis, tetanus (DPT), oral poliovirus (OPV), and *Haemophilus* influenza B (HIB), are completed by 6 months of age (Table 102-3).

### Neurologic Aspects

Motor development is the major indicator of neurologic health and proceeds in a cephalocaudal fashion. Neonates demonstrate involuntary "primitive" reflexes, such as the suck, grasp, and Moro (startle) responses, which may be elicited to demonstrate muscle tone and should always be symmetric. By 1 month of age infants can lift their heads, follow a moving object, and demonstrate a social smile. By 4 months head control is steady, the child will reach for and grasp objects with the whole hand, a cooing response may be elicited, and rolling over has begun. During this period normal infants learn trust from their parents and will respond positively to the gentle examiner. This is the period of least parental confidence, and many "inappropriate" emergency department visits are made because of lack of knowledge and a need for reassurance.

### Age-Specific Approach

Assessment is optimally made by direct interaction using a pleasant, confident tone of voice and smiling face directed towards the infant. Observation of muscle tone, spontaneous activity, eye contact, responsive smile, and recognition of parents is most important. Examination of the infant is best performed in the parent's lap, with use of brightly colored or pleasant sounding objects to elicit a motor response. Feeding the infant or eliciting the sucking reflex with a finger will often result in greater cooperation. Optimal examination is done in order of least to most invasive interactions, i.e., observation, auscultation, and palpation, being careful to avoid uncomfortable procedures such as ear and throat examination until the child's level of consciousness is established. Parental confidence should be directly

**Table 102-2.** Developmental Stages and Emergency Department Assessment Strategy

| Stage | Milestone | Strategy |
|---|---|---|
| Early infancy (0–6 months) | Motor: lifts head, reaches<br>Verbal: cooing<br>Social: responsive smile | Observation<br>Examine in parent's arms<br>Direct approach |
| Late infancy (6–18 months) | Motor: reaches/obtains, sits, walks<br>Verbal: jargon, few words<br>Social: stranger anxiety/dependence | Observation<br>Examine in parents arms<br>Indirect approach |
| Toddler (18–36 months) | Motor: walks well, scribbles<br>Verbal: speaks in phrases<br>Social: stranger anxiety/autonomy | Observation<br>Indirect approach |
| Preschool (3–5 years) | Motor: runs well, colors<br>Verbal: speaks in sentences<br>Social: magical thinking | Indirect or direct approach<br>Explain briefly just prior to procedures |
| School age (5–12 years) | Motor: schoolwork, sports<br>Verbal: concrete reasoning<br>Social: task-oriented | Direct approach<br>Explain in detail prior to procedures |
| Adolescence (12–17 years) | Motor: adult<br>Verbal: abstract reasoning<br>Social: autonomy, rebellion | Direct approach<br>Confidentiality<br>Treat as adult |

reinforced. Young infants should be carefully monitored during procedures involving conscious sedation or abnormal positioning because of the risk of airway compromise. Finally, the motor abilities of young infants result in a limited potential for self-inflicted accidental injury. Whenever the observed injury is developmentally inconsistent with the stated mechanism, the potential for child abuse must be investigated.

## Late Infancy (6 to 18 Months)

### Physical Aspects

The normal infant triples his or her birth weight by 1 year of age, but the rate of growth slows during this period. The primary teeth begin to erupt by 6 months of age, with an average rate of acquisition of one per month. Head size, center of gravity, and surface area to mass ratio remain large in comparison to the adult. The anterior fontanelle is closed by 18 months of age. The first DPT booster is given by 18 months of age (Table 102-3).

### Neurologic Aspects

The normal infant sits with minimal support, transfers objects from hand to hand, and babbles by 6 months. By 9 months of age the infant

**Table 102-3.** Recommended Schedule of Childhood Immunizations

| AGE | DPT | OPV | HIB | MMR | HepB |
|---|---|---|---|---|---|
| Birth | | | | | HepB |
| 2 months | DPT | OPV | HIB | | HepB |
| 4 months | DPT | OPV | HIB | | |
| 6 months | DPT | | HIB | | HepB |
| 15 months | | | HIB | MMR | |
| 15–18 months | DPT | OPV | | | |
| 4–6 years | DPT | OPV | | | |
| 11–12 years | | | | MMR | |
| 14–16 years | Td | | | | |

*Note:* DPT, diphtheria, pertussis, tetanus (cellular); OPV, oral poliovirus (live); HIB, *Haemophilus* influenza B conjugate; MMR, measles, mumps, rubella (live); HepB, Hepatitis B (live); Td, tetanus with diphtheria adjuvant (adult).

is crawling, pulling to a standing position, and verbalizing with non-specific jargon. By 12 months the infant has a mature pincer-type grasp, begins to walk, and acquires specific words. The developmental combination of mobility and grasp results in increasing risk of toxic and foreign-body ingestion. Between 9 and 12 months a strong sense of "stranger anxiety," related to fear of separation from parents, is acquired and complicates every aspect of physical assessment. Conversely, the failure of an older infant or toddler to recognize and preferentially respond to parents suggests significant disease.

### Age-Specific Approach

Assessment of the older infant and toddler begins with observation, preferably without the child's awareness of the examiner's presence. The child should be undressed in order to obtain a meaningful respiratory rate and to observe the work of breathing. Spontaneous motor activity, such as sitting and pulling up, and purposeful responses to parental overtures, such as reaching for objects and smiling, are indicators of a normal level of consciousness. The child should see the examiner approach gradually and engage his or her caretakers first. The entire examination requiring any degree of cooperation is best performed while the child is held on the parent's lap or shoulder so that perception of separation is avoided. As for younger infants, the examination proceeds from least to most invasive interactions. Procedures in this age group require adequate physical restraint. Although parental restraint is acceptable for nonpainful examination procedures, parents should not be asked to immobilize their child for invasive procedures. Caretakers should be encouraged to remain present to reassure their child during procedures if it is their desire to do so. The high level of anxiety at this age frequently results in persistently uncooperative behavior despite adequate analgesia. Sedation for procedures may require a significantly higher per kilogram dose of anxiolytic/analgesic drug to achieve the desired effect.

### Toddler (18 to 36 Months)

#### Physical Aspects

Decelerating growth rate and decreased appetite are seen during this period, although the head approaches its adult size. The 20 primary teeth are in place by 36 months, and dental caries are common. High center of gravity, mobility, and curiosity lead to increasing risk for head and orthopedic injuries. The toddler's open growth plates are far more likely to sustain epiphyseal fracture than ligamentous injury. Traction injuries to the arm will frequently result in subluxation of the annular ligament of the radial head, i.e., "nursemaid's elbow."

#### Neurologic Aspects

By 18 months of age most children can walk well, feed themselves, follow simple commands, and use four to six words to indicate their desires. Stranger anxiety peaks at this age but remains important throughout the toddler period. By 24 months most children can run, climb stairs, and speak with three-word phrases, although only 50 percent of speech is intelligible to nonfamily members. Toddlers understand far more than their spontaneous speech would indicate and learn by imitating the behavior of their family members. When given opportunity to draw, the toddler will scribble with a brief attention span. Parents consistently underestimate the mobility and problem-solving ability of the toddler, resulting in a peak risk for falls and ingestions at this age.

#### Age-Specific Approach

An examination strategy of indirect observation followed by direct interaction in the safety of the parent's arms should be followed, as described for the older infant. The examiner should encourage the parent to have the toddler walk and follow commands as an important component of the assessment for acute systemic or neurologic disease. Allow the child a favorite object, such as a doll or blanket, for comfort during the examination. Talk to him or her in simple language about what you will do and offer to let them touch or hold the examination instruments in order to gain their trust. Older toddlers may indicate the site of pain specifically, but many will be unable to communicate localized pain or tenderness. As described above, perform the physical assessment in order of least to most invasive examination components. As for the older infant, restraint is routinely indicated for painful procedures and a higher per kilogram dose of anxiolytic/analgesic drug may be required. Because of likelihood of epiphyseal fracture, the young child with tenderness over the growth plate following injury should be immobilized with a splint, even if x-ray films are negative.

### Preschool Age (3 to 5 Years)

#### Physical Aspects

Growth rate slows significantly during this period, and appetite decreases further. Children develop a more lean body habitus. The incidence of injuries increases with increasing activity. The preschool child is no longer restrained in a car seat and is at risk for defined injury complexes from improperly fitting lap and shoulder belts. A DPT booster is given shortly before beginning school, between the ages of 4 and 6 years (Table 102-3).

#### Neurologic Aspects

Preschool children develop progressive autonomy in terms of mobility and self-care. Attraction to books, drawing, and coloring is common. Expressive language skills expand rapidly, and children this age are often able to identify site(s) of specific complaint. However, a strong sense of fear of pain remains, and the level of anxiety remains high in the emergency setting. Preschool children live in the present and have limited sense of time and history, so that prior symptoms are frequently forgotten. Self-centered "magical" reasoning is the rule, so that many preschool children believe that emergency department care is punishment for misbehavior. This is occasionally reinforced by parents who state they will "have the doctor give you a shot," which should be discouraged.

#### Age-Specific Approach

Many preschool children may be directly approached and examined in the traditional systematic fashion. However, some will require the indirect approach described for the toddler, and the nearby presence of the parent is typically essential for cooperation. The examiner should always talk directly with the preschooler to establish rapport and confirm the general complaint. Identification of recent positive experiences such as birthdays or favorite cartoon characters is frequently helpful in gaining cooperation. However, the preschool child should be expected to identify only his or her current complaint, and reliance on parental history should remain. Cooperation during the physical examination is likely, although less comfortable components are still best performed at the end. The performance of painful procedures requires a careful approach. It is always best to be honest regarding discomfort, but information should be given immediately before performing the procedure to minimize the effects of fantasy regarding pain and causality as well as delaying tactics. Comfort and distraction by the parent is frequently effective for minor procedures; however, restraint as for the toddler is typically necessary. Rewards such as verbal praise and a sticker for bravery often significantly enhance the memory of the experience for the child and family.

## School Age (5 to 12 Years)

### Physical Aspects

The school years represent the slowest period of growth in childhood, and the body habitus is typically slender. The primary teeth are loosening and the secondary teeth erupt. The lymphatics reach maximal dimensions relative to body size by 6 years of age. There is increased physical activity including organized sports during this period, and injuries become common.

### Neurologic Aspects

The school-age child experiences rapid language growth and maturing motor ability. Concrete reasoning ability emerges with an ability to understand cause and effect. The child is increasingly aware of his or her body and develops a sense of modesty. Task-oriented behavior is common, and school and sports activity are typically the central events of the child's life. School-age children are eager to please and often reluctant to express their fears of pain and death.

### Age-Specific Approach

The direct examination approach is typically successful for the school-age child. Parental accompaniment and respect for modesty should be maintained. Historical information should be elicited from child as well as parent. An effort to inquire as to school or extracurricular interests will enhance rapport. Change in school performance is a helpful indicator of chronic disease. Painful procedures are best preceded by explanations to both parent and child, given well in advance with honesty regarding discomfort. The child should be given some degree of choice in the manner in which the procedure is completed, such as a comfortable position, in order to minimize the sense of loss of control.

## Adolescence (12 to 17 Years)

### Physical Aspects

The teen years mark a second period of rapid growth, beginning at age 10 years in girls and 12 years in boys. Secondary sexual development begins shortly after beginning the growth spurt, with menarche starting between 10 and 16 years in girls. Sexual activity and drug use are common during adolescence, and many teens are parents themselves, complicating both the differential diagnosis and issues of maturity and reliability in carrying out the follow-up plan.

### Neurologic Aspects

Abstract reasoning ability progressively develops during adolescence, paired with a self-centered world view and self-consciousness regarding appearance. Feelings of immortality and denial of the consequences of risky behavior are common. Loss of autonomy is the greatest fear of the adolescent, and mistrust of and rebellion toward authority is normal. Previously well-controlled chronic disease frequently becomes unstable as a result of these developmental issues. Psychiatric disease and suicidal behavior are increasingly recognized in this age group. The parents of teenagers are frequently angered by these changes and may project these feelings on the emergency department staff.

### Age-Specific Approach

The traditional history and physical examination with respect for modesty is effective in the assessment of adolescents. The examiner should communicate to the teenager that he or she will be treated "like an adult." Choices must be allowed, such as parental presence during the examination, with proper limit-setting regarding cooperative behavior. The parent's concerns must be addressed individually and, if necessary, in private. Confidentiality should be stressed, particularly as the law requires with respect to pregnancy and sexually transmitted disease.

## SUMMARY: THE DEVELOPMENTAL APPROACH IN THE EMERGENCY DEPARTMENT

Knowledge and application of the principles of child development gives the emergency physician powerful tools for the care of the acutely ill child. Significant illness in children is frequently indicated by altered mental status, which can be detected only if the normal is known to the examiner. A developmental approach to pediatric assessment allows the examiner to plan a strategy for optimal examination, establish the child's level of consciousness based on age-appropriate motor and social behavior, enhance patient and parent satisfaction, and, in the process, reduce the anxiety and decibel level in the emergency department.

## BIBLIOGRAPHY

Algraneti PS: *The Pediatric Patient: An Approach to History and Physical Examination.* Baltimore, Williams and Wilkins, 1992.

Committee on Infectious Diseases, American Academy of Pediatrics: *Report of the Committee on Infectious Diseases,* 22d ed. Elk Grove Village, IL, American Academy of Pediatrics, 1991.

Ilingsworth RS: *The Normal Child,* 10th ed. New York, Churchill Livingstone, 1991.

# 103
# COMMON NEONATAL PROBLEMS
## Niranjan Kissoon

The assessment of the neonate in the emergency department is more difficult than that of the older child or the adult. Symptoms are usually vague and nonspecific. Signs are usually subtle and even when recognized may not be helpful in pinpointing the exact diagnosis. For example, respiratory distress may be due to primary respiratory or cardiac disease, generalized sepsis, abdominal pathology, or metabolic derangements. Examination of the neonate is time-consuming and requires special skills in the approach to the infant as well as to the anxious parent.

The prerequisites for the proper evaluation of neonates are a great deal of patience as well as an appreciation for the marked variations in normal vegetative functions in this population. Many visits are initiated because of parental concerns relating to feeding patterns, weight gain, stool frequency, color, and consistency, and breathing patterns. Physicians involved in the care of neonates in the emergency department should therefore be knowledgeable of patterns of normal vegetative functions in this population.

## NORMAL VEGETATIVE FUNCTIONS
### Feeding Patterns

During the first few weeks of life, feeding is usually dictated by the infant, with a specific pattern established by 1 month in 90 percent. Most bottle-fed infants will want six to nine feedings per 24 h by the first week of life, while breast-fed infants may require feeding every 2 to 4 h. Parents usually need reassurance that their infant is obtaining adequate nutrition because of the wide variation in the intakes of normal infants compared to one another.

## Weight Gain

While it is difficult to judge the exact caloric intake of breast-fed infants and feeding frequency varies widely, intake is adequate if the neonate is gaining weight appropriately and appears content between feeds. Intake is satisfactory if infants are no longer losing weight by 5 to 7 days and are gaining 10 to 30 g/kg per day by 12 to 14 days of age.

## Stool Patterns

The number, color, and consistency of bowel movements vary greatly in the same infant and between infants regardless of diet or environment. Stool frequency may vary from one to seven times per day, with loose stools frequent in breast-fed infants. Infrequent bowel movements do not necessarily mean constipation, since breast-fed infants may occasionally go 5 to 7 days without a bowel movement. Stool color is of no significance unless blood is present.

## Breathing Patterns

In the first month of life breathing patterns vary widely. Normal full-term infants have episodes during sleep when periodic breathing occurs. This is manifested as an interruption of respiration two or more times within a 20-s period. It is, however, not associated with heart rate or color changes and has no prognostic significance.

## REASONS FOR EMERGENCY DEPARTMENT VISITS

A review of presenting complaints in our pediatric emergency department, a tertiary care referral center, over a 6-month period indicates the spectrum most likely to be seen by the emergency physician (Table 103-1). Complaints in neonates are usually not single but can more correctly be referred to as "symptom complexes." These reflect the nonspecific nature of signs and symptoms in the neonate and the similar presentation of many commonly seen diseases of diverse etiology.

## CRYING/IRRITABILITY/LETHARGY

This group of symptoms is fairly common yet difficult to treat even in the presence of an identifiable cause. Most neonates will exhibit varying degrees and periods of crying during a 24-h period. However, those infants who present with an episode of acute inconsolable crying should be observed closely for an underlying cause (Table 103-2).

**Table 103-1.** Common Presenting Complaints

Crying/irritability/lethargy
(See Table 103-2)
Gastrointestinal tract symptoms
  Feeding difficulties
  Regurgitation
  Vomiting
  Diarrhea
  Abdominal distension
  Constipation
Cardiorespiratory symptoms
  Rapid breathing
  Cough and nasal congestion
  Noisy breathing and stridor
  Apnea/periodic breathing
  Blue spells/cyanosis
Jaundice
Eye discharge/redness
Diaper rash/oral thrush
Fever and sepsis
Sudden infant death

**Table 103-2.** Conditions Associated with Uncontrollable Crying and/or Irritability and/or Lethargy in Neonates

Intestinal Colic
Traumatic conditions
  Battered child syndrome (fractures, burns, etc.)
  Falls (skull or extremity fractures)
  Open diaper pin
  Strangulation of digit or penis
  Corneal abrasion or foreign body
Infections
  Meningitis
  Generalized sepsis
  Otitis media
  Urinary tract infection
  Gastroenteritis
Surgical
  Incarcerated hernia (umbilical or inguinal)
  Testicular torsion
  Anal fissure
Improper feeding practices

## Intestinal Colic

The most common cause of crying is intestinal colic. This usually occurs in normal, healthy, thriving babies in the second or third week of life and persists until 3 months of age. Episodes commonly occur in the late afternoon or evening and begin with screaming episodes with drawing up of knees, as if the infant is in pain, and usually passage of flatus. Intestinal colic is not known to have any grave clinical significance or long-term effects.

The diagnosis is usually made when there is no evidence of physical illness (normal growth and development) and if the bouts of crying are episodic in nature. However, a careful history, physical examination, and appropriate laboratory investigations will enable the emergency physician to diagnose colic and exclude the serious conditions listed in Table 103-2. In doubtful situations, admission for observation or return for reassessment is reasonable. More often than not, parents have visited several physicians and are angry, frustrated, or dissatisfied with the advice and care given. While colic cannot be treated or cured in the emergency department, reassurance that all is well and follow-up are essential in all cases.

The emergency physician may be helpful in the following ways:

1. Suggesting changes in care-taking styles such as increased carrying and rocking, decreased interfeed intervals and use of pacifier.
2. Changes in environment, for example background music, rides in car and stroller, etc.
3. Suggesting a trial of feeding change in refractory cases. Changes in feeds is helpful if the infant has other manifestations such as visible peristalsis, persistent regurgitation and symptoms following cows milk protein. Removal of cows milk from the diet of the mother of a breast-fed baby may be tried. However, a switch to formula or change of formula is not indicated.

## Abuse and Trauma

Traumatic conditions, though less common, are frequently overlooked in the neonate. A careful history (inconsistent or implausible history) may lead the physician to strongly suspect the diagnosis of child abuse, while physical examination may reveal unexplained injuries (bruises of varying ages, skull fractures, extremity fractures, cigarette burns, etc.). If the diagnosis is suspected, the child should be admitted for protection and further investigations. In many cases, children with intracranial injuries as a result of whiplash injuries (shaken baby) will present with subtle, non-specific signs, seizures, coma or respiratory insufficiency. An examination of the eye, though difficult, is essential since the presence of retinal hemorrhage especially in the absence of external signs of trauma suggests a whiplash injury due to severe shaking. The examination of the eye is also useful to rule out an eyelash in the eye or a corneal abrasion as reasons for the infant's symptoms. Congenital glaucoma, though rare, may also present with irritability and crying. The piercing of the skin with an open diaper pin as well as strangulation of integuments with hair are not uncommon reasons for distress in the neonate.

## Infections

Infections in the neonate will manifest as a variety of symptoms and signs such as feeding difficulties, fever, jaundice, or respiratory distress. Neck rigidity and Kernig's and Brudzinski's signs are usually absent in the neonate with meningitis. A septic neonate may present with a normal or subnormal temperature rather than fever. Urinary tract infections in neonates are often associated with nonspecific signs such as irritability, diarrhea, or poor feeding, and diagnosis is established by urine culture rather than urinalysis. There is general consensus that all neonates with possible sepsis should be hospitalized and given broad-spectrum antibiotic therapy pending results of appropriate cultures (urine, blood, cerebro-spinal fluid, etc.).

## Surgical Lesions

Surgical lesions such as incarcerated hernia (umbilical or inguinal) as well as testicular torsion require prompt diagnosis and surgical referral. The most common signs are irritability and crying, followed by poor feeding, vomiting, constipation, and abdominal distension. Physical examination may reveal a red, edematous, tender lump at the site of the hernia or testicular torsion. These findings are very easy to overlook when irritability is the only symptom and the neonate has not been undressed fully for examination. Anal fissures may also present at this age and may be difficult to diagnose. Most can easily be seen if the bottom of a small test tube is inserted into the anal verge and the fissure is examined through the bottom glass surface.

## Improper Feeding Practices

Improper feeding practices may result in an irritable infant with periods of inconsolable crying. This usually results from overfeeding with inadequate burping during feeds. The infant subsequently swallows large amounts of air resulting in bowel distension and occasionally respiratory distress. Instruction in proper feeding practices usually alleviates the problem.

## GASTROINTESTINAL TRACT SYMPTOMS

### Feeding Difficulties

Most visits for feeding difficulties are due to parental perception that the infant's food intake is inadequate. The neonate's pattern of intake is not fully established until about 1 month of age. If weight gain is satisfactory and the infant is satisfied after feeds, intake is adequate. Parents can usually provide accurate information of the intake of the bottle-fed infant. The weighing of the breast-fed infant before and after feeds is not advised, since weights may be inaccurate. In addition, weighing may have adverse psychological effects on the mother whose infant is doing poorly.

Rarely, anatomic abnormalities can cause difficulty in feeding and swallowing. A careful history usually pinpoints these difficulties as occurring from birth. These infants appear malnourished and dehydrated. The most likely causes are esophageal obstruction (stenoses, strictures, laryngeal clefts, cleft palate) and double aortic arch compressing the esophagus or trachea. Infants with a recent decrease in intake, who were feeding normally previously, have an acute disease, usually an infection.

## Regurgitation

Regurgitation of small amounts is common in the neonate and is due to reduced lower-esophageal sphincter pressure and relatively increased intragastric pressure. Parents may confuse regurgitation with vomiting. Vomiting results from forceful contraction of the diaphragm and abdominal muscles, whereas regurgitation is independent of any effort and probably represents the ultimate degree of gastrointestinal reflux. If the neonate is thriving, parents can be reassured that regurgitation is of no clinical significance and will decrease as the infant grows. Infants who are not thriving or having respiratory symptoms should be investigated for anatomical causes of regurgitation or chronic aspiration.

Regurgitation rarely results from pathological processes such as intrinsic compression of the esophagus or occasionally compression of the trachea in which case it is usually accompanied by stridor and cough. Dysphagia, irritability, anemia due to chronic blood loss, and malnutrition are sequelae of chronic regurgitation with esophagitis, but this condition is rare. Investigations such as scintigraphy, pH monitoring, endoscopy and biopsy are utilized to confirm the diagnosis of reflux esophagitis. Such invasive investigations are not justified in patients who are healthy. Such infants usually respond well to thickening of feeds. Postural therapy, with the infant's upper body elevated after feeds, can be added if thickening of feeds alone does not solve the regurgitation.

## Vomiting

Vomiting usually results from a variety of causes and rarely presents as an isolated symptom. During the first few weeks of life, vomiting is uncommon and often is confused with regurgitation. Vomiting from birth is most likely due to an anatomic abnormality such as a tracheoesophageal fistula, upper gastrointestinal obstruction, or midgut rotation. More commonly, acute vomiting may be part of the symptom complex of some diseases (Table 103-2), especially increased intracranial pressure, and infections (sepsis, urinary tract infections, gastroenteritis).

Projectile vomiting is usually seen in infants with pyloric stenosis and usually assumes its characteristic pattern after the second and third week of life. This condition usually occurs in firstborn males and is characterized by projectile vomiting at the end of feeding or shortly thereafter. The vomitus does not contain bile or blood. Examination of these infants should be done with the infant relaxed and the stomach empty. Prominent gastric waves may be seen going from left to right. A firm olive mass may be felt by palpating under the liver edge. Malnutrition and dehydration may be evident. Hospitalization is necessary for rehydration and surgical referral.

In any infant who is vomiting, signs of dehydration and candidiasis of the mouth should be sought. Hepatobiliary disease (e.g., jaundice), urinary tract, and central nervous system disease can also cause vomiting. Vomiting due to inborn errors of metabolism may present with hypoglycemia and metabolic acidosis. Infants who are vomiting should be admitted for evaluation and therapy.

## Diarrhea

Diarrhea is associated with the excessive loss of fluid and electrolytes in stools. The complaint of diarrhea in the neonate in many cases reflects ignorance of the marked normal variation in stool frequency and consistency. Where the infant is feeling well and gaining weight appropriately, the only treatment necessary is to reassure parents that all is well.

Diarrhea may be associated with systemic diseases such as generalized sepsis, otitis media, and urinary tract infections. This entity, termed *parenteral diarrhea,* is nonspecific and does not contain blood or mucus. Infectious diarrhea, on the other hand, is usually associated with fever and is mostly of viral etiology, with rota and enteroviruses being most common. Bacterial causes (*Escherichia coli, Salmonella, Shigella*) and parasitic causes (*Giardia, Entamoeba histolytica*) are rare in neonates. Causes of bloody diarrhea in the neonate include necrotizing enterocolitis, bacterial enteritis, antibiotic-associated diarrhea, milk allergy, and rarely, intussusception. In the absence of other signs of infection, a bleeding diathesis should also be suspected. Close attention to hydration and nutritional status as well as fluid and electrolytes is mandatory. Infants who are moderately or severely dehydrated should be admitted for treatment, while those with mild dehydration can be followed closely as outpatients if parents are reliable and follow-up ensured.

Necrotizing enterocolitis usually presents with other signs of sepsis (jaundice, lethargy, fever, poor feeding, abdominal distension, and discoloration). Abdominal radiography may demonstrate pneumatosis intestinalis. True milk allergy presents with abdominal distension, explosive bloody diarrhea, and, in severe cases, shock. Intussusception usually occurs in the older infant and toddler but can also occur in the neonate, with abdominal distension, feeding difficulty, and a mass in the right upper quadrant.

## Abdominal Distension

Abdominal distension is normal in the neonate and is usually due to lax abdominal musculature and relatively large intraabdominal organs. It may also be accentuated by excessive gas within the bowel. In the majority of cases, if the infant is comfortable and feeding well and the abdomen is soft, there is no need for concern. Abdominal distension may also occur in association with bowel obstruction, constipation, or as a result of ileus due to sepsis or gastroenteritis. Congenital organomegaly (hepatomegaly, splenomegaly, renal enlargement) undetected in the perinatal period may also present as abdominal distension.

## Constipation

Infrequent bowel movements in neonates do not necessarily mean that the infant is constipated. The breast-fed infant may on occasion go without a bowel movement for 5 to 7 days and then pass a normal stool. However, if the infant has never passed stools, the possibility of intestinal stenosis or atresia, Hirschsprung's disease, and meconium ileus or plug should be considered.

Constipation occurring after birth but within the first month of life suggests Hirschsprung's disease, hypothyroidism, or anal stenosis. The diagnosis of Hirschsprung's disease is supported by absence of feces on rectal examination and abrupt change in bowel luminal size on barium enema and is confirmed by rectal biopsy demonstrating absence of ganglion cells. Hypothyroidism is manifested as feeding problems, a weak, hoarse cry, hypothermia, hypotonia, and peripheral edema.

## CARDIORESPIRATORY SYMPTOMS

The neonate is prone to respiratory problems (Table 103-1) for a variety of reasons. Anatomic reasons that are disadvantageous are the barrel-shaped chest, flattened diaphragm, limitation of diaphragmatic movement by abdominal compression, smaller airway diameter, and higher closing volumes. In addition, the high compliance of the chest wall, low compliance of the infant lung, and less fatigue-resistant fibers in the diaphragm and intercostal muscles are also significant contributory factors. Cardiorespiratory symptoms are also more common in this age group, since structural and functional abnormalities of the airway and heart are more likely to present at this time.

Cardiorespiratory symptoms in neonates are nonspecific and may be due to primary organ failure (cardiovascular or respiratory) or secondary to a variety of systemic diseases such as sepsis and metabolic acidosis, abdominal pathology, and severe meningitis. Regardless of

**Table 103-3.** Causes of Rapid Breathing in the Neonate

Pneumonia
    Bacterial
    Viral
    *Chlamydia*
    Aspiration
Bronchiolitis
    ness to other organ systems
    Septicemia
    Central nervous system, e.g., meningitis
    Abdomen, e.g., distension, gastroenteritis
    Metabolic acidosis
Congenital diseases:
    Respiratory disease
    (1) Delayed presentation of diaphragmatic hernia
    (2) Tracheoesophageal fistula
    (3) Lobar emphysema
    (4) Tracheal stenosis, webs
    Heart disease
    (1) Cardiac failure, e.g., hypoplastic left heart, critical coarctation of aorta, aortic stenosis, patent ductus arteriosus
    (2) Cyanotic disease, e.g., transposition of great arteries
    (3) Vascular ring
    Neuromuscular disease
    (1) Infantile botulism
    (2) Muscle weakness

etiology, the concern is, first, the assessment and stabilization of airway, breathing, and circulation; and second, establishing the diagnosis.

## Rapid Breathing

Rapid breathing can be due to minor problems such as abdominal distension or life-threatening illnesses such as sepsis. Rapid breathing or grunting should always be considered a medical emergency. Admission for investigations, monitoring, and therapy should be considered in all but the mildest cases. When a cause cannot be identified on initial presentation, a full sepsis workup (full blood count, blood culture, urinalysis, chest x-ray, and cerebrospinal fluid examination) should be done and broad-spectrum antibiotic therapy instituted (Table 103-3).

### Pneumonia

Bacterial pneumonias (pneumococcal, streptococcal, staphylococcal) as well as viral pneumonias may present as a period of fussiness, stuffy nose, and decreased appetite followed by an abrupt onset of high fever (<39°C), nasal flaring, grunting, retractions, tachypnea, and tachycardia. *Chlamydia* pneumonia usually occurs after 3 weeks of age and is accompanied by conjunctivitis in 50 percent of cases. The infants are tachypneic, afebrile, and have a prominent cough. Chest examination reveals rales but few wheezes. Chest x-ray shows hyperinflation with diffuse patchy infiltrates. Aspiration pneumonia is more likely to occur in infants with a tracheoesophageal fistula, or swallowing dysfunction, and in debilitated infants. Following aspiration, symptoms such as tachypnea and cough usually occur within 1 h and are seen within 2 h in almost all cases. Infants with pneumonia should be admitted for monitoring and institution of antibacterial therapy (Table 103-4) as indicated.

### Bronchiolitis

Acute bronchiolitis usually presents in infancy as a serous nasal discharge accompanied by sneezing. These symptoms are followed by fever (38.5 to 39°C), diminished appetite, cough, dyspnea, irritability, and, commonly, periods of apnea. Apnea is more common in infants and usually presents in the first 3 days of the illness. Physical exami-

**Table 103-4.** Antibiotic Therapy for Infections

| Indications | Drugs* |
|---|---|
| Pneumonia (bacterial) | Ampicillin (100 mg/kg per day q 6 h) |
| Generalized sepsis | and |
| Necrotizing enterocolitis | Gentamicin (7.5 mg/kg per day q 8 h) |
| Bacterial meningitis | *or* |
| Gonococcal infections | Cefotaxime (200 mg/kg per day q 6 h) |
| Urinary tract infections | Length of therapy depends on infection being treated. |
| Bronchiolitis (RSV) | Ribavirin (nebulized) 20 mg/mL water for 12–18 h/day for 3–7 days. |
| Conjunctivitis (bacterial) | Sodium sulamyd 10% or topical erythromycin, 2 drops to each eye, q 4 h for 5–7 days. Erythromycin 40 mg/kg per day q 6 h for 14 days |
| Pneumonia (chlamydial) | Erythromycin 40 mg/kg per day q 6 h for 14 days. |
| Oral thrush | Oral nystatin suspension 100,000 units q 4–6 h after feeds for 7–14 days. |
| *Candida* dermatitis | Nystatin/amphotericin cream to affected area q 4–6 h for 7–14 days. |

nation reveals a rapid respiratory rate (<60 breaths per minute), cyanosis, air hunger, hyperinflation, intercostal and subcostal retractions, and palpable liver and spleen due to hyperinflation of the lungs. Prolonged expiration, wheezes, and fine rales are present. Chest x-rays usually reveal hyperinflation with atelectasis. Since in many cases it is difficult to differentiate bronchiolitis from reactive airway disease, a trial of bronchodilators in the emergency department is reasonable. However, in infancy, admission for monitoring and therapy is required (Table 103-4) in all but the mildest cases.

## Illness Involving Other Organ Systems

The search for pathology in other organ systems is mandatory since the presence of respiratory symptoms may divert attention from the underlying significant problem. For example, generalized sepsis, meningitis, gastroenteritis, and metabolic acidosis may present with respiratory distress as the predominant symptom.

## Congenital Diseases

### Respiratory Disease

Occasionally, H-type tracheoesophageal fistula may present in the first month of life or later with recurrent pneumonia, respiratory distress after feeds, and problems handling mucus. Tracheal stenosis may present initially with noisy breathing or high-pitched cry and tremendous respiratory difficulty even after mild upper respiratory infections. Similarly, neonates with chronic respiratory insufficiency, e.g., bronchopulmonary dysplasia, may present in respiratory failure even after mild upper respiratory infections.

### Heart Disease

Rapid breathing due to cardiac disease is usually not associated with significant retractions and use of accessory muscles. As a general rule, the well-developed neonate who presents with unexplained cyanosis and tachypnea should be suspected of having congenital cardiac disease. In neonates with transposition of the great arteries and ventricular septal defect or critical coarctation of the aorta, congestive cardiac failure may be the presenting feature. Signs of heart failure may be very subtle but are life-threatening and require emergent referral. Dyspnea, hepatomegaly, cyanosis, and cardiomegaly are present, and peripheral pulses are weak.

### Neuromuscular Disease

Any form of muscle weakness may be associated with shallow breathing and an increase in respiratory rate as a compensatory mechanism.

## Cough and Nasal Congestion

Cough may be a prominent feature of most of the primary respiratory conditions listed in Table 103-3. It may also be the initial presentation of a variety of congenital anomalies including cleft palate, laryngotracheomalacia, laryngotracheal cleft, tracheal webs, tracheoesophageal fistula, tracheal hemangiomas, and vascular rings. Although congenital malformations resulting in cough and nasal congestion are more likely to occur in the neonate, in most instances, cough is due to a viral upper respiratory infection and may be associated with sneezing and nasal congestion. It may also be a prominent feature of bronchiolitis, and *Chlamydia* and *Pertussis* infections. Treatment of the underlying condition is the therapy of choice. Cough suppressants should be used with extreme caution in neonates. Nasal congestion is best treated with instillation of saline drops when necessary.

## Noisy Breathing and Stridor

Noisy breathing is a common presenting complaint in the neonate and is usually benign. Stridor is usually due to congenital anomalies (webs, cysts, atresia, stenosis, clefts, hemangiomas) extending anywhere from the nose to the trachea and bronchi. Infants who were intubated in the neonatal period are prone to develop subglottic stenosis. Infection (croup, epiglottitis, abscess) as a cause of stridor in the neonate is rare. Stridor worsening with cry suggests laryngomalacia or subglottic hemangioma; stridor and feeding difficulties suggest vascular ring, laryngeal cleft, or tracheoesophageal fistula; stridor with hoarseness suggests vocal cord paralysis. Laryngomalacia is the most common cause of stridor in the neonate. It is characterized by noisy, crowing inspiratory sounds which usually improve during the first year of life.

## Apnea and Periodic Breathing

Periodic breathing, which may occur in normal neonates, should be differentiated from apnea. However, periodic breathing may precede apnea and both may occur in the same patient. *Apnea* is defined as a cessation of respiration for 10 to 20 s with or without bradycardia and cyanosis. It signifies critical illness and warrants prompt investigation and admission.

Apnea may be precipitated by any of the disease conditions listed in Table 103-3 and usually indicates respiratory muscle fatigue and impending respiratory arrest. Resuscitation including airway support and ventilation should be followed by a thorough search for the inciting condition. If no obvious cause is found, the neonate should be assumed to be septic. Cultures should be obtained and broad-spectrum antibiotics started.

## Cyanosis and Blue Spells

The infant with cyanosis and blue spells usually presents a diagnostic challenge since these findings may be due to a variety of disorders. If breathing is rapid but not labored, the most likely cause is cyanotic congenital heart disease with right-to-left shunting. Methemoglobinemia, though rare, may present similarly. Irregular or shallow breathing may be associated with sepsis, meningitis, cerebral edema, or intracranial hemorrhage and may also be accompanied by cyanosis. If breathing is labored (grunting, indrawing), pulmonary disease (pneumonia, bronchiolitis) is likely. Infants with cyanosis should be admitted for monitoring and further investigation.

## JAUNDICE

Jaundice (Table 103-5) is a yellowish-green pigmentation of the skin and sclera due to excess bilirubin. It may appear at varying times during the neonatal period and requires a complete diagnostic evaluation. Jaundice during the first 24 h rarely presents to the emergency de-

**Table 103-5.** Causes of Jaundice in Neonates

| | |
|---|---|
| <24 h | ABO, Rh incompatibility |
| | Sepsis |
| | Congenital infections (rubella, toxoplasmosis, cytomegalic inclusion disease) |
| | Secondary to bruising |
| 2–3 days | Physiologic |
| 3 days–1 week | Septicemia |
| | Syphilis, toxoplasmosis, cytomegalic inclusion disease |
| >1 week | Septicemia, congenital atresia of bile ducts, serum hepatitis |
| | Congenital hemolytic anemias (sickle cell anemia, spherocytosis) |
| | Hemolytic anemia due to drugs (e.g., in glucose-6-phosphate dehydrogenase deficiency) |
| | Rubella, herpetic hepatitis |
| | Hypothyroidism |
| | Breast-milk jaundice |

partment (ED). The commonest causes of jaundice seen in the ED are physiologic, secondary to sepsis, breast-milk jaundice, and, occasionally, hemolysis due to autoimmune congenital causes.

Physiologic jaundice is due to the breakdown of fetal red blood cells, and bilirubin rises at a rate of <5 mg/dL per 24 h with a peak of 5 to 6 mg/dL during the second to the fourth day of life, returning to <2 mg/dL by 5 to 7 days. The septic infant with hyperbilirubinemia will also have other features of sepsis, i.e., vomiting, abdominal distension, respiratory distress, and poor feeding. Jaundice associated with breast-feeding may start as early as the third to fourth day and reaches a peak of 10 to 27 mg/dL by week 3. Cessation of breast-feeding causes rapid decline in 2 to 3 days. This is thought to be due to the presence of substances which inhibit glucuronyl transferase in breast milk.

A proper history and physical examination will provide a clue to the causes of jaundice. The well-looking child who is gaining weight and feeding well is unlikely to be septic. Laboratory evaluation should include full blood count for anemia, smear for hemolysis, direct and total bilirubin, a reticulocyte count, and Coombs' test. In addition, admission, appropriate cultures, and antibiotics are appropriate for neonates who are unwell and have any of the signs or symptoms listed in Table 103-6. In all cases, arrangements should be made for monitoring of bilirubin and hemoglobin levels. While most well infants can be monitored out of hospital, infants who are anemic or those with bilirubin levels approaching transfusion levels (approximately 20 mg/dL) should be admitted.

## EYE DISCHARGE AND REDNESS

Most commonly, the neonate with red eye will be suffering from conjunctivitis. While the commonest cause of conjunctivitis in the neonate is chemical, due to silver nitrate, this rarely presents to the emergency department. For the first 2 weeks of life, the commonest causes of conjunctivitis are chlamydial infection, *Neisseria gonorrhoeae,* and gram-negative bacilli (*Escherichia coli* and *Pseudomonas*). In neonates older than 2 weeks of age, these infections along with other viral infections (herpes) and staphylococcal and streptococcal species should be considered.

**Table 103-6.** Signs and Symptoms of Neonatal Sepsis

| | |
|---|---|
| Temperature instability | Fever, hypothermia |
| CNS dysfunction | Lethargy, irritability, seizures |
| Respiratory distress | Apnea, tachypnea, grunting |
| Feeding disturbance | Vomiting, poor feeding, gastric distension, diarrhea |
| Jaundice | |
| Rashes | |

Gonococcal conjunctivitis begins after an incubation period of 2 to 5 days with a mild inflammation accompanied by a serosanguineous discharge which becomes purulent within 24 h. *Chlamydia trachomatis* has an incubation period of 5 to 14 days and is associated with a thick, purulent discharge in an afebrile and alert infant. It may also accompany pneumonia in the neonate greater than 3 weeks of age.

The neonate with a red eye and irritability may also be suffering from a corneal irritation or abrasion usually due to an eyelash. Acute glaucoma, though rare, will present as a red, teary eye. In these instances, the cornea may be stained or cloudy, the anterior chamber shallow and intraocular pressure increased. Prompt ophthalmological referral of all suspected cases of glaucoma is mandatory. Infectious causes should also be treated (Table 103-4).

## DIAPER RASH AND ORAL THRUSH

*Candida* diaper dermatitis is an erythematous plaque with a scalloped border, sharply demarcated edge, and studded by satellite lesions. It usually occurs in the moist, occluded diaper area and intertriginous zones. It usually results from the action of organisms harbored in the gastrointestinal tract. Treatment consists of an anticandidal agent with each diaper change or four times daily. Protection of the area with zinc oxide paste overlying the cream will prevent friction. In addition, an oral course of treatment is usually warranted to prevent colonization of the gut (Table 103-4).

Oral lesions are white, flaky plaques covering the tongue, lips, gingiva, and mucous membranes. These lesions are common in debilitated infants and in those on antibiotics. Oral lesions may affect oral intake because of pain and discomfort. Treatment of ill infants consists of treating the underlying pathology, oral antifungal therapy, and an anesthetic gel prior to feeding. Cool liquids may prevent discomfort and pain.

## FEVER AND SEPSIS

Fever (Table 103-6) is most commonly due to infectious causes. Most infections occurring in the first 5 days of life are acquired by vertical transmission from the mother. Bacterial infections are usually caused by group B streptococci (30 percent), *E. coli* (30 to 40 percent), other gram-negative enteric organisms (15 to 20 percent), and gram-positive cocci (10 percent). Viral infections are also common and are most likely due to enteroviruses (Coxsackie and echovirus) acquired at the time of delivery or respiratory syncytial viruses acquired postnatally. Neonates with presumed sepsis should be admitted and started on broad-spectrum antibiotics after a full sepsis workup.

## SUDDEN INFANT DEATH

Neonates may occasionally present in cardiorespiratory arrest. Although sudden infant death syndrome should be considered, catastrophic deterioration is more likely to be due to infectious causes (septicemia, meningitis), trauma (intracranial bleed, child abuse), and inborn errors of metabolism (medium-chain acyl dehydrogenase deficiency).

In most cases, cardiopulmonary resuscitation is unsuccessful since the myocardium has suffered severe hypoxic ischemic damage. The physician's role in these cases is to provide supportive care for the family. In most cases, this entails reassurance that all appropriate efforts were made to save their child's life and that the infant has been treated with dignity. Other personnel (chaplain, social worker, family physician, etc.) may also be required to provide support.

When the cause of death is not known, physicians should obtain appropriate samples (blood, urine, skin biopsy, etc.) and obtain permission for an autopsy. This is very important because of the genetic implications of metabolic disease. A postmortem protocol for sudden neonatal deaths should be available in all EDs.

## BIBLIOGRAPHY

Baraff LJ, Bass JW, Fleisher GR, et al: Practice guidelines for the management of infants and children 0 to 36 months of age with fever without source. *Pediatrics* 92:1, 1993.

Behrman RE, Vaughan VC: *Nelson, Textbook of Pediatrics,* 14th ed. Philadelphia, Saunders, 1992.

Fleisher G, Ludwig S: *Textbook of Pediatric Emergency Medicine,* 3rd ed. Baltimore, Williams & Wilkins, 1993.

*Report of the Committee on Infectious Diseases,* American Academy of Pediatrics, 1991; 141 Northwest Point Boulevard, P.O. Box 927, Elk Grove Village, Illinois 60009-0927.

# 104
# THE NICU GRADUATE
## Daniel G. Batton

The graduate of the neonatal intensive care unit (NICU) may be a frequent visitor to the emergency department and often requires rehospitalization during the first few months following discharge. Most NICU graduates are low-birthweight infants who may have a variety of complications related to prematurity. These infants should be evaluated based upon *postconceptional* age, not chronologic age. For example a 32-week-gestation premature infant with an 8-week chronologic age since birth is evaluated as a term infant.

Premature infants are usually discharged from the hospital at a postconceptional age of 35 to 40 weeks, although a few infants will be much older. The normal respiratory rate at this age is 30 to 40 per minute, although an infant with bronchopulmonary dysplasia may breathe 60 to 70 times per minute. The heart rate ranges from 120 to 160 beats per minute but can be considerably lower during quiet sleep. Most laboratory values will be similar to adult values, although the hematocrit can be as low as 20 to 25 percent because of physiologic anemia. Neurodevelopmental milestones most appropriate for a given infant are those corresponding to the postconceptional age. When caring for the NICU graduate, attention must be paid not only to the presenting signs and symptoms but also to general problems related to prematurity.

## GENERAL CONSIDERATIONS
### Cold Stress

Following hospital discharge, premature infants remain susceptible to cold stress when exposed to lower environmental temperatures primarily because of decreased subcutaneous tissue. Infants who are cold-stressed are not capable of responding by shivering but rather attempt to maintain body temperature by increasing their metabolism of brown fat, which results in heat production. However, this increases oxygen consumption and can lead to hypoglycemia. If this compensatory increase in metabolic rate is insufficient to overcome the low environmental temperature, then body temperature will fall. A normal body temperature, however, does not eliminate the possibility of cold stress since body temperature may be maintained at a considerable metabolic expense. The best way to avoid cold stress is to provide an adequate environmental temperature for the infant who is being evaluated in the emergency department. If the room temperature cannot be adjusted appropriately, a heat lamp should be available. Commercial heat lamps are available which have automatic timers and can be adjusted to provide varying amounts of heat. These should be standard equipment in emergency departments which treat infants and children.

### Hypoglycemia

Premature infants are at risk of developing hypoglycemia with an acute illness. This may be due in part to increased glucose consumption, cold stress, poor enteral intake during the illness, or suboptimal glycogen stores. Since hypoglycemia can have severe consequences, glucose testing is necessary for all premature infants presenting with an acute illness. If the blood sugar is less than 45 mg percent, intravenous glucose therapy [10% dextrose in water ($D_{10}W$) at 100 mL/kg per day] should be initiated.

### Hypertension

Longitudinal studies of convalescing premature infants have demonstrated that systemic hypertension may develop in as many as 9 percent. The possible causes include thromboembolic renal artery occlusion following umbilical artery catheterization and bronchopulmonary dysplasia. Although the normal range is age-dependent, a systolic blood pressure greater than 120 mmHg or a diastolic pressure greater than 75 mmHg warrants consideration of systemic hypertension.

### Fractures

Because of decreased bone mineralization (osteopenia) related to prematurity, fractures of the long bones and ribs are not uncommon in premature infants during their initial hospitalization. Usually by the time of hospital discharge, bone mineralization has improved to such an extent that new fractures are uncommon, but there may be evidence of healing fractures on x-ray examination. This should be kept in mind if fractures are incidentally noted on an x-ray because of the confusion this may create with child abuse. Comparison of current x-rays with previous films may help to clarify the issue.

### Failure to Thrive

The establishment of consistent weight gain with oral feedings is a standard criterion for discharge from the hospital for most premature infants. However, this does not ensure that the pattern of weight gain will continue following discharge. Failure to thrive may occur either because of an ongoing chronic disease (i.e., bronchopulmonary dysplasia, malabsorption, or central nervous system disease) or because of dysfunctional parenting. NICU graduates should be consuming approximately 150 mL/kg per day of a standard formula if not breast feeding and should be consistently gaining approximately 20 g/day. A comparison of the current weight with the discharge weight (which parents usually remember) allows for a quick evaluation of this problem. Any infant with failure to thrive requires a thorough diagnostic evaluation and often hospitalization for accurate documentation of caloric intake.

### Immunizations

The recommendation by the American Academy of Pediatrics is to immunize premature infants on the same schedule as normal full-term infants. However, because of a prolonged hospitalization and complicated follow-up, it is possible immunizations might be missed. Inquiry about the immunization status may uncover such a situation. Although it may not be desirable to immunize an infant during an acute illness, appropriate recommendations for follow-up should be made.

## ACUTE RESPIRATORY DETERIORATION IN INFANTS WITH BRONCHOPULMONARY DYSPLASIA

Many infants are discharged from the NICU with ongoing pulmonary disease, most commonly bronchopulmonary dysplasia (BPD). BPD is

**Table 104-1.** Causes of Acute Respiratory Deterioration in Infants with Bronchopulmonary Dysplasia

Respiratory infection
Aspiration
    Gastroesophageal reflux
    Incoordinate suck/swallow
Bronchospasm
Pulmonary edema
Dehydration
    Gastroenteritis
    Diuretic therapy
Anemia
Cor pulmonale

usually a sequela of prematurity, hyaline membrane disease, and mechanical ventilation, although it may be associated with other conditions. Features of BPD include tachypnea, hypercarbia, suboptimal oxygenation, and sometimes reactive airway disease. In some cases, pulmonary hypertension, pulmonary edema, and cor pulmonale are prominent. The cornerstones of therapy for bronchopulmonary dysplasia are oxygen and nutrition. It is essential to take a medication history as chronic diuretics or bronchodilators are used in selected patients, although their value remains poorly defined. Systemic glucocorticoids are being used more commonly as chronic therapy and can lead to adrenal suppression.

Acute deterioration in patients with BPD is usually manifested by an increase in respiratory rate, an increase in respiratory effort, a decrease in oxygenation, and poor feeding. The most common causes of an acute respiratory deterioration in infants with BPD are listed in Table 104-1. A careful history can usually delineate the likely etiology. For example, infants with infectious causes usually have a history of an upper respiratory infection for a few days preceding the development of respiratory distress and may have fever. Sudden respiratory deterioration is usually due to aspiration, either from gastroesophageal reflux or to a poorly coordinated suck/swallow reflex. Exposure to cigarette smoke or other environmental pollutants may precipitate acute bronchospasm. An increase in pulmonary edema is usually accompanied by the development of peripheral edema and excessive weight gain.

Dehydration is an important cause of acute respiratory deterioration since many infants possess an altered myocardial compliance (Starling curve shifted to the right), making cardiac output more dependent on end-diastolic filling. Therefore, if an infant becomes dehydrated secondary to either vomiting and diarrhea or to aggressive diuretic therapy, cardiac output will decrease and secondary respiratory deterioration will follow. When evaluating and treating an infant with BPD with respiratory distress, there is often a temptation to use diuretics. However, one must be sure the infant is not already hypovolemic since in that case diuretics make the infant worse.

Anemia may also exacerbate respiratory distress in an infant with BPD and is suggested by the presence of pallor on examination. Acute cor pulmonale can develop secondary to hypoxemia from any of the above-mentioned causes, and deterioration can be very rapid. The only effective way to treat acute cor pulmonale in infants with BPD is to treat the hypoxemia and its underlying cause.

The usual evaluation of an infant with acute respiratory deterioration includes a complete blood count, arterial blood gas determination, and a chest x-ray. However, the chest x-ray can be difficult to interpret because of the presence of chronic abnormalities. Therefore, it is essential to compare the current x-ray with previous films to identify acute changes. Therapy should be directed toward the specific cause of deterioration, but oxygenation is the cornerstone of treatment. Although BPD infants often have chronic $CO_2$ retention, there is no evidence that respiratory drive is decreased with oxygen administration. Therefore, oxygen should be used liberally while definitive diagnosis and treatment are debated. Some infants may re-

quire a brief course of glucocorticoids during acute respiratory deterioration. It is most important to recognize how quickly infants with BPD can deteriorate during an acute infection, particularly one due to respiratory syncytial virus. Infants often require rehospitalization for close observation, as many will worsen to the point of requiring mechanical ventilation.

## APNEA AND HOME APNEA MONITORS

Most infants resolve their apnea of prematurity before discharge and do not require apnea monitoring at home. However, home monitoring is sometimes utilized for premature infants with severe apnea or if apnea persists beyond 38 weeks' postconceptional age. Infants may be brought to the emergency department because of an actual apneic episode or because the parents were not sure of the significance of an alarm. Studies have demonstrated that the majority of alarms at home are not associated with a change in cardiorespiratory status and probably represent monitor dysfunction, such as loose leads. However, caution must be exercised before attributing an alarm to a mechanical problem with the monitor.

All episodes associated with cyanosis or bradycardia; directly observed episodes of apnea; and any episode requiring intervention, such as stimulation or mouth-to-mouth resuscitation, should be thoroughly evaluated and require admission. A recurrence of apnea in a premature infant who was discharged home apnea-free warrants admission and a thorough search for the cause. The differential diagnosis (Table 104-2) includes respiratory infection (especially respiratory syncytial virus or pertussis), sepsis, gastroesophageal reflux and aspiration, aspiration with feedings, anemia, and metabolic problems such as hypoglycemia. Other, more unusual causes include seizures, cardiac arrhythmias, and posthemorrhagic hydrocephalus. Therapy is directed to the specific cause.

## POSTHEMORRHAGIC HYDROCEPHALUS

Premature infants who have had an intraventricular hemorrhage may develop posthemorrhagic hydrocephalus in the newborn period. This can progress during the initial hospitalization, in which case the infant will usually be discharged with a ventriculoperitoneal (VP) shunt in place, or the hydrocephalus may develop gradually following discharge. Such infants can present to the emergency department because of progressive hydrocephalus, if unshunted, or shunt obstruction or infection. Infants presenting with infection usually have nonspecific signs such as poor feeding, lethargy, irritability, fever, and vomiting similar to those of any other child presenting with central nervous system infection. Infants with obstructed shunts most often present with a tense fontanelle and a history of vomiting, although the infant usually does not appear particularly ill. A comparison of the current head circumference with the head circumference at discharge (if available) is helpful in evaluating for progressive hydrocephalus. Cranial ultrasound can also rapidly determine the size of the ventricles if the anterior fontanelle remains open. Shunt infections usually require removal of the foreign body, although successful treatment without removal has been reported for *Staphylococcus epi-*

**Table 104-2.** Most Common Causes of Apnea and Bradycardia at Home in NICU Graduates

Respiratory infection
    Respiratory syncytial virus or pertussis
Sepsis
Gastroesophageal reflux and aspiration
Aspiration with feedings
Anemia
Hypoglycemia
Seizures
Cardiac arrhythmias
Posthemorrhagic hydrocephalus

*dermidis* infections. For both shunt infections and hydrocephalus neurosurgical consultation is required.

## THE EXPECTED HOME DEATH

Some infants are discharged from the NICU with lethal conditions for which further medical intervention is futile, and the parents are expecting the child to die at home. In many cases the parents are instructed to take the infant to the emergency department to be pronounced dead by a physician. The parents should be given a letter at the time of the original hospital discharge by their physicians delineating the infant's problems to provide guidance to the emergency physician facing such a situation.

This is a very traumatic time for the parents, and a futile resuscitation effort is not indicated and can prolong the parents' agony. However, it is very important to request autopsy permission to completely delineate the infant's problems and to provide optimal counseling for future pregnancies.

## BIBLIOGRAPHY

Abman SH, Bradley AW, Lum GM: Systemic hypertension in infants with bronchopulmonary dysplasia. *J Pediatr* 104:928, 1984.

Ballard RA: *Pediatric Care of the ICN Graduate*. Philadelphia, Saunders, 1988.

Berger LR, Schaefer AR: The premature infant goes home. *Am J Dis Child* 139:200, 1985

Consensus Statement: National Institutes of Health Consensus Development Conference on Infantile Apnea and Home Monitoring, Sept 29 to Oct 1, 1986. *Pediatrics* 79:292, 1987.

Groothuis JR, Gutierrez KM, Lauer BA: Respiratory syncytial virus infection in children with bronchopulmonary dysplasia. *Pediatrics* 82:199, 1988.

Klaus MH, Fanaroff AA: *Care of the High-Risk Neonate*, 3d ed. Philadelphia, Saunders, 1986.

Martin RJ, Miller MJ, Waldemar AC: Pathogenesis of apnea in preterm infants. *J Pediatr* 109:733, 1986.

Mutch L, Newdick M, Lodwick A, Chalmers L: Secular changes in rehospitalization of very low birth weight infants. *Pediatrics* 78:164, 1986.

Rush MG, Hazinski TA: Current therapy of bronchopulmonary dysplasia. *Clin Perinatol* 19:563, 1992.

Sauve RS, Singhal, N: Long-term morbidity of infants with bronchopulmonary dysplasia. *Pediatrics* 76:725, 1985.

# 105
# SUDDEN INFANT DEATH SYNDROME
## Carol D. Berkowitz

## SUDDEN INFANT DEATH SYNDROME

Sudden death may affect persons of any age, but it is especially devastating when it affects previously healthy individuals. Between 5000 and 10,000 infants (1 to 2 per 1000 live births) succumb yearly to sudden infant death syndrome (SIDS), also known as "crib death."

The term *SIDS* was officially designated in 1963 to describe a syndrome of unexpected death in infants under 1 year of age for which no pathologic cause could be determined by a thorough postmortem examination. The syndrome is the leading cause of death of infants between 1 month and 1 year.

An understanding of SIDS is essential for the emergency physician so that he or she can recognize the syndrome, initiate resuscitation, manage the infant who has experienced an apparent life-threatening event (ALTE, previously termed *"near miss" SIDS*), and counsel the family of the victim.

## PATHOPHYSIOLOGY

Over 70 different theories for SIDS have been proposed, including suffocation from sleeping with the parent, milk allergy, and thymic enlargement (status thymicolymphaticus). The main disturbance appears to be with the infant's ventilatory response, and SIDS and infantile apnea appear related, although the exact nature of this relation is uncertain. Death is due to respiratory rather than cardiac arrest, and some potential SIDS victims may be successfully resuscitated with ventilation alone. Arrhythmias probably occur only as a terminal event, and syndromes such as prolonged QT interval or Wolff-Parkinson-White syndrome are very rare associations. Prospective studies monitoring normal infants showed no antecedent arrhythmias in infants who eventually succumbed to SIDS. Conversely, approximately 2 percent of premature and low-birthweight infants experienced bradycardia (<50 beats per minute) without apnea 1 week after discharge.

Information implicating ventilation disturbances and hypoxemia has been obtained from two sources: autopsies of infants who succumbed to SIDS, and studies of those who experienced an ALTE but survived. This latter group represents infants who were found limp, cyanotic, pale, and lifeless, without any respiratory effort, but who were successfully resuscitated.

Autopsies of some SIDS victims reveal pathologic changes initially felt to be indicative of long-standing hypoxemia. These changes include smooth muscle thickening in small pulmonary arteries, right ventricular hypertrophy, hematopoiesis in the liver, increase in periadrenal brown fat, adrenal medullary hyperplasia, and abnormalities of the carotid body. The only marker now reported with regularity is brainstem gliosis.

Recently, much attention has been given to SIDS and sleeping in the prone position. Epidemiologic studies indicate that the incidence of SIDS is lower in countries where infants sleep supine or in the side-down position, and that a reduction in the incidence of SIDS follows a reduction in prone sleeping. Concerns about aspiration in infants sleeping in the supine position are unfounded. Two mechanisms linking SIDS to prone sleeping are noted. With prone sleeping, infants will assume a face-down position, particularly in response to a cold stimulus on the face. This may result in upper airway obstruction. However, upper airway obstruction has not been observed in clinical trials; rather, it has been noted that infants rebreathe expired air and experience hypercarbia. Because of these observations related to the prone position, the American Academy of Pediatrics now recommends a supine or side sleeping position in normal infants.

The link between child abuse, SIDS, and ALTE has also received renewed interest. Familial cases of SIDS raise the possibility of abuse. Some investigators report that 10 percent of SIDS cases are due to abuse. Some children with ALTE have been purposefully asphyxiated, and in some cases the complaints have simply been fabricated. These problems are referred to as *Munchausen syndrome by proxy* (see Chap. 25, "Spectrum of Child Abuse and Neglect"). Child abuse is the diagnosed cause of death in 2000 cases a year. The presence of bruises, long bone fractures, rib fractures, internal hemorrhages, evidence of physical neglect, or trauma around the nares suggests abuse. Rib fractures in infants are not induced by cardiopulmonary resuscitation. A history inconsistent with the usual events surrounding a SIDS death may also raise the suspicion of abuse. An interesting report on death-scene investigations revealed that in 23 of 26 infant studied, circumstantial evidence of accidental death was present. It is beyond the scope of the emergency department physician to conduct such investigations. However, more and more communities are convening Child Death Review Boards to assure the full evaluation of sudden and unexpected death in children. It is important, however, to be aware of the possible role of accidental or intentional trauma in some SIDS victims.

## SIDS and Apnea

Four groups of infants who appear at increased risk of SIDS have been identified: (1) term infants who have had a life-threatening episode of apnea, or ALTE; (2) premature infants of low birthweight; (3) siblings of infants who have succumbed to SIDS; and (4) infants of substance-abusing mothers.

Studies of infants with ALTE may reveal (1) hypoventilation ($P_{CO_2} > 45$ mmHg) and chronic hypoxemia, (2) a depressed ventilatory response to $CO_2$ breathing, (3) prolonged sleep apnea (>15 s, associated with cyanosis or pallor), (4) bouts of frequent short apnea, (5) increased periodic breathing (characterized by repeated 3-s pauses in breathing followed by normal breathing for less than 20 s with bradycardia), (6) obstructive apnea, and (7) mixed obstructive and central apnea.

Southall has described three separate components associated with respiratory abnormalities in infants.

First, there is central apnea, in which immaturity, tumor, head injury, infection, or congenital malformation leads to primary failure of respiratory center control. In addition, peripheral chemoreceptors act in an abnormal manner, particularly in response to hypercarbia and hypoxia. The dive reflex may contribute to apnea on a central basis. Young monkeys receiving a cold or wet stimulus to the face in the area of the trigeminal nerve stop breathing. This situation may be analogous to the young infant lying in a regurgitated feeding. Alternatively, this stimulus may lead to a face-down sleeping position and airway obstruction.

Airway obstruction is a second component. Obstructive apnea may occur in response to nasal occlusion, as with an upper respiratory infection, and is noted with tonsillar enlargement, hypotonia of the hypopharynx, or glossoptosis. It is a contributing factor in about 5 percent of ALTE episodes. It is detected by the presence of increased chest-wall movement, with bradycardia and decreased $P_{O_2}$ (by surface oximeter). It is a contributing component to SIDS in infants with upper respiratory infection.

The third and most significant component is expiratory apnea. Prolonged expiratory apnea is associated with sudden atelectasis. Ventilation perfusion inequalities, hypoxia, and sudden cyanosis within 5 to 10 s occur. There is a rapid loss of consciousness. These episodes may occur even in the face of nasotracheal intubation. In older children, they may occur with crying, as cyanotic breath-holding spells.

Acute hypoxic episodes are felt to occur in 80 percent of SIDS cases.

## EPIDEMIOLOGIC FACTORS

The diagnosis of SIDS is confirmed by autopsy, but there are many clinical and epidemiologic features that characterize the syndrome. Although the overall incidence is between 1 and 2 per 1000 live births, there is variation among different ethnic groups, with an incidence of 0.51 per 1000 among Asian Americans and 5.93 per 1000 among Native Americans. Victims range in age from 1 month to 1 year, with peaks at $2\frac{1}{2}$ months and at 4 months. The infant frequently has been premature or small for gestational age, and there is a higher incidence of SIDS among infants with residual bronchopulmonary dysplasia. One study reported that 11 percent of premature infants with bronchopulmonary dysplasia subsequently died of SIDS.

The syndrome is rare in the first month of life, probably because the neonate has a better anaerobic capacity for survival, and with a gasp may be able to raise his or her arterial $P_{O_2}$ over 20 mmHg and continue breathing. Of the infants who are otherwise healthy, 30 to 50 percent have some acute infection, usually of the upper respiratory tract, at the time of the event. Infection with respiratory syncytial virus has been associated with apnea, particularly in premature infants and those with an antecedent history of apnea. Otitis media and gastroenteritis have also been associated with SIDS. Infected infants tend to be older than noninfected infants, and males outnumber females in the infected group by 2:1. The sex ratio is equal in the noninfected group. There is a disproportionate number of babies from the lower socioeconomic group, although this is true for deaths in infancy from all causes. Mothers frequently are under 20 years and unwed, smoke, use drugs, and have made few prenatal and postpartum visits. SIDS is more likely to occur during the winter months and when the infant is asleep.

## CLINICAL FEATURES

A number of scenarios may confront the physician in the emergency department. These scenarios mirror the range of problems that may be broadly categorized under the heading "SIDS" or "ALTE."

Some infants are completely well appearing at the time they are examined, and the parents relate a history of cessation of respiration. The physician must then determine if the event represented an episode of apnea, was severe enough to be life-threatening, or represents a different disorder.

The sequence of events prior to the episode may be a clue to the cause. If the infant stiffened or exhibited clonic movements, the cessation of respiration may have been postictal apnea following a seizure. With a seizure, an infant is frequently awake before becoming apneic. Gastroesophageal reflux may lead to apnea and also may occur in the awake infant following a feeding. A history of an upper respiratory infection followed by paroxysmal cough with an apneic episode would be suggestive of pertussis. Hypoglycemia may also be associated with apnea, with or without a seizure. The differential diagnosis also includes infection (sepsis or meningitis) and cardiomyopathy. Infantile botulism may be the cause in 5 to 10 percent of SIDS victims.

The evaluation of the healthy-appearing infant with a history of apnea is problematic. Occasionally parents may have misinterpreted acrocyanosis, postprandial regurgitation, or color changes with stooling as an episode of apnea. The parents should be carefully questioned about what they did to revive the baby, for example, stimulation or mouth-to-mouth resuscitation. No resuscitative efforts suggest a benign event. Conversely, the need for mouth-to-mouth resuscitation bespeaks a more serious event. The finding of irregular respiration or poor muscle tone on physical examination would assist in the diagnosis of an ALTE.

Some infants who have experienced an ALTE have not been fully resuscitated in the field. They should receive the benefit of vigorous cardiopulmonary resuscitation, unless signs of irreversible death (livedo reticularis, blood pH of 6, box-car venous pooling in the fundi) are apparent. Frequently the heart will resume beating after prolonged arrest. The infant heart is a remarkably resistant organ and may be revived after irreversible brain damage.

## DIAGNOSIS

The evaluation of the infant who has experienced an ALTE should include a complete history, particularly of the event itself, and take into account the perinatal and epidemiologic factors associated with SIDS and ALTE. A history of other infant deaths in the family should be obtained because of the familial incidence of SIDS. Familial cases of SIDS suggest the possibility of inborn errors of metabolism or child abuse, as noted above. Initial reports suggested that siblings of SIDS victims are at increased risk (about 10-fold) for subsequent SIDS. More recent studies show at most a twofold increase in the incidence of SIDS among SIDS siblings.

The physical examination should be complete, with special emphasis on the neurologic evaluation and the presence of any injuries. The initial laboratory assessment should include a complete blood cell count; determination of levels of serum electrolytes, blood sugar, calcium, phosphate, and magnesium; and a 12-lead ECG. A septic workup including blood culture, cerebrospinal fluid analysis, urine culture, and chest x-ray is indicated in most cases, although studies have shown a negligible yield in the absence of associated findings such as fever. In the infant with ALTE, stool should be sent for clostridial culture and botulinum toxin testing, especially if hypotonia is present. Other studies should be obtained if suggested by the history and physical examination; these include determination of serum ammonia, sleep and awake EEGs, skull x-rays, barium swallow, and CT scan.

## TREATMENT

Initial treatment in the emergency department involves continued resuscitation of the infant, if necessary, and stabilization. In general, all ALTE victims and infants with a history of apnea and/or cyanosis should be admitted to the hospital. The evaluation of these infants is designed to rule out treatable causes of apnea and to determine if, in the absence of these other causes, the infant is at risk for SIDS, an event reported in from 20 to 100 percent of infants with an ALTE.

Apnea monitoring should be carried out in the hospital. Most hospitals are able to obtain pneumograms, which give evidence of abnormalities related to periodic breathing or episodes of apnea. Polysomnography measures the amount of air flowing in at the mouth and nose and can detect obstructive apnea; the test is complicated and is generally done in a sleep laboratory. Certain tertiary care centers are equipped to evaluate responses to $CO_2$ breathing and diminished $F_{I_{O_2}}$.

## HOME MONITORING

Two major treatment modalities are recommended for infants who have experienced an ALTE or are at risk for SIDS. Xanthine derivatives such as caffeine and theophylline are used frequently in treating apnea of prematurity because of their central excitatory effect. Their use is associated with the normalization of the respiratory pattern in over 80 percent of such children. Their efficacy in the prevention of SIDS is unclear. A pragmatic approach to the use of theophylline would be to limit it to infants with abnormal pneumograms. Reversal of these abnormalities with theophylline would be an indication for its use. Theophylline is given at 6 mg/kg per day, and a serum level of 5 to 15 mg/mL should be maintained.

Home apnea monitoring is the second modality which can be offered. Three groups have been defined in a National Institutes of Health Consensus Statement in 1986 as being candidates for home monitoring. Group 1 consists of term infants with unexplained apnea of infancy, usually manifested by a life-threatening episode and/or abnormal pneumogram. The absence of an abnormal pneumogram does not preclude home monitoring. The second group consists of preterm infants who have continued to manifest apnea beyond term (i.e., after 40 weeks postconception). The third group consists of subsequent siblings of two or more SIDS victims, but not of one SIDS victim. Twins of SIDS victims were reported in the past to have a 20-fold increase in their risk for SIDS. More recent studies suggest their chance is the same as for nontwin siblings. Additional candidates for home monitoring include infants with bronchopulmonary dysplasia, especially if oxygen-dependent, and infants who require tracheostomy for airway support.

Home-monitoring devices usually measure chest-wall movement and heart rate. The detection of bradycardia is particularly important in infants with an obstructive component because chest-wall movement is not diminished with obstructive apnea. Parents must be instructed in equipment maintenance, interpretation of the alarm, and cardiopulmonary resuscitation. Home monitoring does not mean simply supplying a family with a mechanical device. It involves the development of a medical team to support the family, interpret any episodes of apnea, and decide when home monitoring can be discontinued. Technicians who are available 24 h a day to maintain the equipment are also required.

Emergency physicians are frequently consulted about monitor alarms. Infants are brought to the emergency department because of alarm triggering. The physician must be able to differentiate the false alarm from a true episode. The need for vigorous stimulation or mouth-to-mouth resuscitation again suggests a serious episode. If there is concern about equipment malfunction, technical assistance should be obtained from the monitoring company.

The use of home monitors has increased dramatically in recent years. The estimated cost of monitoring (including initial assessment) ranges from $3000 to $5000 per infant, with monthly rental and maintenance costs ranging from $150 to $300. Although parental anxiety is frequently reduced, the reduction in the incidence of subsequent SIDS in monitored infants is questioned. Recent reports have shown a mortality as high as 50 percent in infants on home monitoring. In many cases, technical errors and parental noncompliance contributed to the infant's demise. There were, however, some infants who simply failed to respond to aggressive cardiopulmonary resuscitation.

The decision to discontinue monitoring is usually made by the infant's primary physician. In general, most infants remain on a monitor for 6 to 8 months. Criteria for discontinuing the monitor include 2 to 3 months with no episodes requiring stimulation or resuscitation, 3 months without apnea of 20 s or more, no apnea associated with an upper respiratory infection or immunization, and an improvement in any neurologic problem for which the monitoring was instituted (e.g., apnea associated with seizures.)

## THE SIDS VICTIM

The management of the nonresuscitatable SIDS infant and his or her family is equally challenging for the physician. The emergency department physician is confronted by the distraught mother who had fed her infant several hours earlier, went to check the sleeping infant, and found the baby cold, blue, and lifeless. Frequently, valiant though unsuccessful efforts are carried out in the emergency department, or the infant is revived briefly, only to succumb after several hours in the intensive care unit.

The major responsibility of the physician is then to notify, counsel, and educate the family. In most jurisdictions, victims of sudden and unexplained deaths must be referred to the coroner's office, where an autopsy is performed at the coroner's discretion. Some jurisdictions have infant death teams that fully evaluate the circumstances surrounding the unexpected death of young infants. If the physician believes the infant is a victim of SIDS, the family should be so advised but told that the final confirmation awaits the autopsy report. The emergency physician should assure the family about their lack of responsibility for the infant's death and assuage their feelings of guilt. He or she should then serve as a facilitator maintaining contact with the family to advise them of the autopsy results. The hospital chaplain or social worker may provide additional support, but the physician's empathy is especially supportive to the family. Most communities have organizations for parents of SIDS victims, and information about these organizations can be obtained from the National Foundation for Sudden Infant Death, 101 Broadway, New York, New York 10036. Parents should be referred to these organizations.

## BIBLIOGRAPHY

American Academy of Pediatrics Task Force on Infant Position and SIDS: Positioning and SIDS. *Pediatrics* 89:1120, 1992.

Bass M, Kravath RE, Glass L: Death-scene investigation in sudden infant death. *N Engl J Med* 315:100,1986.

Carroll JL, Loughlin GM: Sudden infant death syndrome. *Pediatr Rev* 14:83, 1993.

Chiodini BA, Thach BT: Impaired ventilation in infants sleeping facedown: Potential significance for sudden infant death syndrome. *J Pediatr* 123:686, 1993.

Emery JL: Child abuse, sudden infant death syndrome, and unexpected infant death. *Am J Dis Child* 147:1097, 1993.

Goyco PG, Beckerman RC: Sudden infant death syndrome. *Curr Prob Pediatr* 13:299, 1990.

Klonoff-Cohen HS, Edelstein SL, Lefkowitz, ES, et al: A case-control study of routine and death scene sleep position and sudden infant death syndrome in southern California. *JAMA* 273:790, 1995.

# 106
# HEART DISEASE
## James H. McCrory

The incidence of congenital heart disease is only 8 per 1000 live births. The incidence of acquired pediatric heart disease is also relatively rare. This low incidence rate contrasts sharply with the prevalence of cardiovascular disease in the adult population, in which the mortality from heart disease is almost 50 percent. Because of low incidence and age-related differences in presentation, recognition of heart disease in infants and children remains a challenge for the primary care physician.

Congenital heart disease is usually classified on the basis of presence or absence of cyanosis or on the nature of the anatomical defect (shunt, obstruction, transposition, or complex). The common acquired conditions include complications secondary to rheumatic fever and to severe chronic anemias, as well as myocarditis, pericarditis, endocarditis, and supraventricular tachycardia (SVT).

There are six common clinical presentations of pediatric heart disease: cyanosis, congestive heart failure, pathologic murmur in an asymptomatic patient, abnormal pulses, hypertension, and syncope. Table 106-1 lists the most common lesions in each category. Evaluation of a murmur is an elective diagnostic workup which can be done on an outpatient basis. Referral to a pediatrician or pediatric cardiologist, with an electrocardiogram (ECG) and chest x-ray, are indicated when the murmur appears to be more than an innocent flow murmur (i.e., grade VI or louder, holosystolic or diastolic in timing, and radiating away from the heart). This chapter will focus on those conditions producing cardiovascular symptomatology and presenting in the

**Table 106-1.** Clinical Presentation of Pediatric Heart Disease

| | |
|---|---|
| Cyanosis | TGA, TOF, TA, TAt, TAVR |
| Congestive heart failure | See Table 106-3 |
| Murmur/asymptomatic pt. | Shunts: VSD, PDA, ASD |
| | Obstructions |
| | Valvular incompetence |
| Abnormal pulses | |
| Bounding | PDA, AI, AVM |
| Decreased | Coarctation, HPLV |
| Hypertension | Coarctation |
| Syncope | |
| Cyanotic | TOF |
| Acyanotic | Critical AS |

*Note:* AI, aortic insufficiency; AS, aortic stenosis; ASD, atrial septal defect; AVM, arteriovenous malformation; HPLV, hypoplastic left ventricle; PDA, patent ductus arteriosus; TA, truncus arteriosus; TAt, tricuspid atresia; TAVR, total anomalous venous return; TGA, transposition of the great arteries; TOF, tetralogy of Fallot; VSD, ventricular septal defect.

emergency department. These conditions require immediate recognition, therapeutic intervention, and prompt referral to a pediatric cardiologist.

## CONGESTIVE HEART FAILURE
### Recognition

The first task confronting the physician in the emergency department is to recognize congestive heart failure and to differentiate it from more common conditions, such as pneumonia or sepsis. The distinction between pneumonia and congestive heart failure in infants requires a high index of clinical suspicion and is a difficult one to make. Pneumonia can cause a previously stable cardiac condition to decompensate, so that both problems can present simultaneously. The common symptoms and signs of an infant presenting in congestive heart failure are outlined in Table 106-2.

Although hepatomegaly appears long before ascites, anasarca, or peripheral edema in right-sided failure in infants, it is usually a late sign. Hepatomegaly exists when the liver is more than 2 cm below the right costal margin in the absence of downward displacement by hyperexpanded lungs. In hepatomegaly, the liver border is rounded rather than sharp.

Both increased pulmonary blood flow in left-to-right shunts and pulmonary edema decrease lung compliance and thus result in tachypnea, which is the cardinal sign of left-sided failure in infants. Although the work of breathing is increased in congestive heart failure, the tachypnea is usually effortless because of the lack of airway obstruction. Since feeding is an infant's primary form of exertion, dyspnea and sweating during feeding can often be elicited in the history.

In addition to hepatomegaly and tachypnea, excessive fluid retention can be appreciated by weight changes in response to fluid restriction and diuresis, although such changes are not helpful for initial recognition. An important age-related difference is the fact that peripheral edema, jugular venous distension, and rales are unusual and late signs in infants.

Cardiomegaly evident on chest x-ray is universally present except in constrictive pericarditis. A cardiothoracic index greater than 0.6 is abnormal. Heart size can be difficult to judge on the posterior-anterior view because of the thymic shadow but can be readily assessed on the lateral view. The primary radiographic signs of cardiomegaly on the lateral chest x-ray are an abnormal cardiothoracic index and lack of retrosternal airspace due to the heart's directly abutting against the sternum. On the posterior-anterior view, the thymic shadow can be distinguished from the cardiac silhouette by the "sail sign," if present, and by the scalloped border that is produced by compression of the thymus against the rib cage.

### Differential Diagnosis

Once congestive heart failure is recognized, age-related categories simplify further differential diagnosis (Table 106-3). In the first few minutes of life, congestive failure occurs from a variety of noncardiac origins such as asphyxia, acidosis, hypoglycemia, hypocalcemia,

**Table 106-2.** Recognition of Congestive Heart Failure in Infants

| | Right-Sided Failure | Left-Sided Failure | Both |
|---|---|---|---|
| Cardinal signs | Hepatomegaly | Tachypnea Dyspnea and sweating on feeding Rales | Cardiomegaly Failure to thrive Tachycardia |
| Unusual signs | Jugular venous distension Peripheral edema | | |

**Table 106-3.** Differential Diagnosis of Congestive Heart Failure Based on Age of Presentation

| Age | Spectrum | |
|---|---|---|
| 1 min | Noncardiac origin: anemia, acidosis, hypoxia, hypoglycemia, hypocalcemia, sepsis | Acquired |
| 1 h | | |
| 1 day | | |
| | PDA in premature infants | |
| 1 week | HPLV | |
| 2 weeks | Coarctation | Congenital |
| 1 month | VSD | |
| 3 months | Supraventricular tachycardia | |
| 1 year | Myocarditis | Acquired |
| | Myocardiopathy | |
| | Severe anemias | |
| 10 years | Rheumatic fever | |

For meaning of acronyms, refer to Table 106-1.

anemia, and sepsis. In critically ill premature neonates, patent ductus arteriosus is the most common cause of congestive heart failure. Among full-term newborns, a hypoplastic left ventricle is the most common cause in the first week, and coarctation of the aorta in the second week of life. Transposition of the great arteries presents within the first 3 days of life, either with cyanosis or congestive heart failure.

Ventricular septal defects (VSD) complicated by transposition of the great arteries, truncus arteriosus, aortic stenosis, or coarctation can present with failure at any time during the first few weeks. Large, uncomplicated VSDs can present with congestive heart failure. Onset of the failure is usually insidious between 1 and 3 months of age, when the left-to-right shunt increases as the pulmonary vascular resistance decreases to normal from high fetal values.

Clinical assessment also involves estimation of the degree of severity of the congestive heart failure. For example, depending on the size of the defect, a VSD may present in a variety of ways, ranging from mild tachypnea to chronic compensated congestive heart failure accompanied by growth failure. The onset of failure with a VSD is insidious because of the gradual increase in the amount of the left-to-right shunt produced by the gradual decrease in pulmonary vascular resistance during the first 2 months from high fetal values. Small VSDs present as a holosystolic murmur in an asymptomatic patient and can be hemodynamically insignificant even though the murmur may be louder than that of a large VSD.

In contrast to the gradual onset of failure with a VSD, coarctation of the aorta can present with abrupt onset of congestive heart failure precipitated by a delayed closure of the ductus arteriosus during the second week of life. The severity of the symptoms is directly proportional to the degree of obstruction and can vary from mild tachypnea to cardiogenic shock. Milder degrees of coarctation, on the other hand, present later in life with hypertension and diminished pulses in the lower extremities.

Onset of congestive heart failure after 3 months of age usually signifies acquired heart disease as opposed to congenital heart disease. The exception to this rule occurs when pneumonia, subacute bacterial endocarditis, or other complicating factors cause a previously stable congenital lesion to decompensate. Before 2 years of age, myocarditis, cardiomyopathies, and severe anemias are the most common diseases in the differential diagnosis. The peak incidence of rheumatic fever is between 8 and 12 years of age.

**Myocarditis.** Myocarditis is often preceded by a viral respiratory illness and needs to be differentiated from pneumonia. As with pneumonia, the infant often presents in distress with fever, tachypnea, and tachycardia. Chest x-ray shows a cloudy lung field, either from inflammation or pulmonary edema. Cardiomegaly with poor distal pulses and prolonged capillary refill, however, distinguish it from a common pneumonia. Once cardiomegaly is discovered, admission and an echocardiogram are indicated. The latter will show a dilated, poorly contracting left ventricle with a low ejection fraction (10 to 55 percent), and possibly a pericardial effusion. Parents need to be made aware that sudden death can occur due to a lethal dysrhythmia. Congestive failure is usually initially treated with inotropic infusions, such as dopamine and dobutamine, along with fluid restriction, diuresis, and oxygen. Intubation and mechanical ventilation often become necessary during the hospital phase of the illness. In severe cases, failure of improvement in left ventricular function in 1 to 6 weeks can lead to cardiac transplantation.

**Pericarditis.** Usually, pericarditis presents as cardiomegaly discovered on a chest x-ray. Clinical signs such as chest pain, muffled heart sounds, and a rub may be present. An echocardiogram is performed on an urgent basis to distinguish a pericardial effusion from a dilated myocardiopathy (myocarditis) or a hypertrophied one. The most common etiology is in association with a Coxsackie viral myocarditis. Bacterial pericarditis from *Haemophilus influenzae* was uncommon even before the availability of the Hib vaccine. When pericarditis accompanies rheumatic fever, lupus, or chronic renal failure, it is usually a secondary finding and does not produce the main symptomatology that brings the patient to the emergency department.

Since diagnostic pericardiocentesis can be complicated by hemorrhage, cardiac tamponade, and arrest, it is usually deferred to a pediatric cardiologist or intensivist with the backup of a cardiovascular surgeon. A pericardiocentesis with an 18-gauge catheter over a needle is indicated in the emergency department, however, if an infant or child with a large heart goes into arrest or decompensates (loses consciousness, muscle tone, and distal pulses). As in adults, the needle is placed in the subxiphoid region and aimed towards the left shoulder. As little as 30 to 50 mL of pericardial fluid can cause tamponade and arrest in a child.

**Cor pulmonale.** If an infant presents in pure right-sided congestive failure, the primary problem is most likely to be pulmonary. Hepatomegaly and anasarca may be present, but in early stages lid edema is often the first noticeable sign. Moreover, the lid edema is likely to be appreciated by the parents more than the physician, and has to be elicited by the question, "Do your child's eyes look puffy?" A positive response should be believed. If the underlying problem is bronchopulmonary dysplasia (BPD) resulting from prematurity and infantile respiratory distress syndrome, the infant may already be on home oxygen and diuretics, and the parents aware of the diagnosis. Upper airway obstruction from hypertrophied adenoids and tonsils can also produce cor pulmonale, presenting as edema or anasarca. The clinical features of airway obstruction, however, are subtle: a careful history will reveal continuous mouth breathing while awake and sleeping, with or without snoring. Sleep studies and tonsillectomy are in order. Cor pulmonale from upper airway obstruction in infants usually responds to diuresis and oxygen alone, without the need for digoxin.

## Initial Stabilization

The degree of severity of congestive heart failure outlined above dictates the types of therapeutic interventions necessary for the initial stabilization phase. The infant who presents with mild tachypnea, hepatomegaly, and cardiomegaly simply needs to be seated upright in a comfortable position and be kept in a neutral thermal environment to avoid the metabolic stresses imposed by either hypothermia or hyperthermia. If the work of breathing is appreciably increased by an increased pulmonary blood flow, 1 to 2 mg/kg of furosemide parenterally is indicated. If pulmonary edema is present, then the hypoxemia can usually be corrected by fluid restriction, diuresis, and an increased $F_{IO_2}$, although continuous positive airway pressure is sometimes necessary.

Severe degrees of congestive heart failure can present with signs of low cardiac output or cardiogenic shock. Aggressive management is often necessary for secondary derangements, including respiratory insufficiency, acute renal failure, lactic acidosis, disseminated intravascular coagulation, hypoglycemia, and hypocalcemia.

For definitive diagnosis and treatment of congenital lesions presenting in congestive failure, cardiac catheterization followed by surgical intervention is often necessary. Stabilization and improvement of left ventricular function can often first be accomplished with inotropic agents. Digoxin is used in milder forms of congestive failure. Initial digitalization is performed intravenously, giving one-half the daily dosage, then $1/4$ and $1/4$ at 6 to 8 hour intervals. Maintenance digoxin consists of $1/8$ the daily dosage given intravenously or orally at 12-h intervals. For full-term infants up until 2 years of age, the dosage is 0.03 to 0.05 mg/kg per day. Hence, 0.02 mg/kg would be the appropriate first digitalizing dose to be given in the emergency department.

At some point, congestive heart failure progresses to cardiogenic shock, in which distal pulses are absent and end-organ perfusion is threatened. In such situations, continuous infusions of inotropic agents such as dopamine or dobutamine are indicated instead of digoxin. The initial starting range is 5 to 10 μg/kg per minute. The "Rule of Six" simplifies the necessary calculations. Six milligrams per kilogram of body weight of either dopamine or dobutamine are placed in a microdrip chamber and filled to 100 mL with 5% dextrose in water ($D_5W$) or normal saline. One milliliter per hour equals one microgram per kilogram per minute, so that it is administered via a pump initially at 5 mL per hour (=5 μg/kg per min). Prior to starting a continuous inotrope infusion, acid-base balance should be checked and corrected with 1 to 2 mEq/kg of bicarbonate as necessary, and cautious volume expansion with 10 mL/kg of normal saline also performed if necessary.

## SUPRAVENTRICULAR TACHYCARDIA

With the exception of SVT, arrhythmias are uncommon in the pediatric age group. In infants, SVT presents with a 4- to 24-h history of poor feeding, tachypnea, pallor, and lethargy. In the older child, palpitations and chest pain can be prominent in the symptomatology. Physical examination reveals thready pulses and a tachycardia that can be too rapid to be counted accurately. Depending on the time since onset of SVT, other physical signs can vary from congestive heart failure to cardiogenic shock with pending arrest. Low cardiac output is secondary to inadequate ventricular diastolic filling time.

An ECG rhythm strip shows an unvarying ventricular rate between 220 and 360, as opposed to a range of 150 to 200 in adults with SVT. The QRS complexes are narrow and regular. P waves are absent or abnormal.

SVT must be distinguished from sinus tachycardia, which is the most common tachyarrhythmia in children. In sinus tachycardia, P waves are present. The normal range for heart rate in newborns is 120 to 200. Under age 5, it is not unusual to find a sinus tachycardia up to a rate of 200, due to fever, stress, or hypovolemia. The latter requires prompt recognition and adequate volume expansion.

Digoxin has been the time-honored standard of medical management of SVT in infants. Since it takes 4 to 6 h before the rhythm converts, however, it is used more for chronic management than acute conversion. Dosage is the same as for congestive heart failure listed above.

Verapamil is contraindicated in infants following case reports in 1985 describing cardiac decompensation and arrest associated with its use in this age group. Intravenous adenosine (0.1 mg/kg) is now the standard treatment in most pediatric cardiology centers. Because the half-life of adenosine is a matter of seconds, it is administered as a rapid bolus via a peripheral intravenous line. Two syringes can be inserted into the intravenous port simultaneously to minimize any lag time in delivery of the medication: the first syringe contains the adenosine, and the second contains 5 to 10 mL of saline flush. Both syringes can be sequentially emptied in less than 5 seconds. A brief (3 to 10 seconds) period of asystole is sometimes seen before return of a normal sinus rhythm. If necessary, the dosage can be doubled, tripled, or quadrupled to convert the rhythm (maximum dosage: 12 mg).

Vagal maneuvers to convert SVT can be attempted but are usually not successful until after the first dose of digoxin. The diver's reflex, which is elicited by submersing the face in ice water, usually produces the greatest vagal tone. An alternative to submersion is to place the ice water in a plastic bag which can be lowered briefly on the infant's face.

Cardioversion with 0.25 to 1 W·s per kilogram is indicated in infants and children presenting in profound cardiogenic shock with pending arrest.

## CONGENITAL LESIONS THAT PRODUCE SYNCOPE

### Tetralogy of Fallot

Most cyanotic lesions usually are recognized in the first few days of life before the infant is discharged from the newborn nursery. Failure of hypoxemia to resolve on $F_{IO_2}$ 1.00 distinguishes an intracardiac shunt from pulmonary disease.

Tetralogy of Fallot is a common cyanotic lesion that may escape detection in the nursery. It is therefore important for the emergency medicine physician to recognize this lesion, as well as to recognize and treat hypercyanotic spells. The degree of cyanosis is directly proportional to the severity of the pulmonary stenosis. In fact, cyanosis may be subtle or absent at rest and clinically obvious only when the infant is active or crying.

The other cardinal features on physical examination are the holosystolic ventricular septal defect (VSD) murmur in the third intercostal space at the left sternal border and the diamond-shaped systolic murmur of pulmonary stenosis in the second intercostal space at the left sternal border. The history may reveal exercise intolerance relieved by squatting. The main radiographic findings are a boot-shaped heart with decreased pulmonary vascular markings. A right-side aortic arch is present in 25 percent of tetralogies. Right ventricular hypertrophy with right axis deviation are the primary ECG abnormalities.

Dynamic obstruction below the pulmonary valve can lead to an acute increase in the right-to-left shunt and produce a *hypercyanotic spell* or *syncope with cyanosis*. Prolonged or recurrent syncope due to tetralogy of Fallot can be a life-threatening emergency, so that referral after initial stabilization is indicated for further diagnostic evaluation and possible urgent surgical intervention.

Initial medical management of a hypercyanotic spell includes placing the infant in the knee-chest position, maximizing the $F_{IO_2}$, and administering intravenous morphine. The infant should be made comfortable and kept quiet. The knee-chest position can be maintained while the infant is held upright in the parent's arms and the parent is seated. If the infant is aggravated by a face mask after consciousness has returned, then the parent can administer oxygen blown by the infant's face at a high flow rate. Direct manipulation of the infant is limited to establishing an intravenous line for medications. Morphine in the dosage of 0.1 mg/kg can relieve the hyperdynamic spell. If the syncope does not respond to this therapy, the dose of morphine can be repeated before considering usage of propranolol.

Because of the high mortality and CNS morbidity associated with hypercyanotic spells, surgical intervention is indicated. The two options are total repair, which requires heart-lung bypass, or a palliative shunt between the aorta and the pulmonary artery. Since many physicians consider that administration of propranolol is a contraindication to bypass surgery, initiation of this form of therapy should be done in coordination with the pediatric cardiologist and the cardiovascular surgeon.

## Critical Aortic Stenosis

Critical aortic stenosis is a noncyanotic lesion that can be life-threatening and may present at any age. In an older child, exercise intolerance with easy fatigability and chest pain can be present in the history. Prominent physical findings are a systolic ejection click and a diamond-shaped murmur that radiates to the neck and can be accompanied by a suprasternal thrill. Left ventricular hypertrophy with strain can be present on ECG, and the chest x-ray may show poststenotic dilatation of the aorta, although neither of these signs is consistently present.

*Syncope without cyanosis* due to critical aortic stenosis can portend a sudden life-threatening arrhythmia. The patient should be kept strictly at rest, using sedation if necessary. Immediate referral for further diagnosis and possible urgent surgical repair is indicated.

## SUBACUTE BACTERIAL ENDOCARDITIS PROPHYLAXIS PRIOR TO PROCEDURES

Prophylactic treatment is recommended for patients with congenital heart malformations and rheumatic fever with valvular disease who are undergoing surgical or dental procedures and instrumentations involving mucosal surfaces. Timing of the medication should be such that an effective serum level will be present during the 15 min after the mucosal manipulation, when the transient bacteremia occurs. Amoxicillin 50 mg/kg (maximum 2 g) is given 1 h before the procedure and 25 mg/kg (maximum 1.5 g) 6 h later. For patients with valvular disease, 2 mg/kg of gentamicin is given IV or IM 30 min before the procedure and 8 h later, in addition to the amoxicillin. Erythromycin 20 mg/kg PO (maximum 800 mg E.E.S. or 1 g stearate) can be given 2 h before the procedure, with half the dose given 6 h later.

## EVALUATION OF FEVER IN AN INFANT WITH KNOWN HEART DISEASE

Finally, infants and children with known heart disease are prone to the same accidents and illnesses as other children. When they present to the emergency department for febrile illnesses, they are most likely to be hemodynamically stable and capable of handling the illness. Any signs of congestive heart failure are an indication for an admission. Otherwise, a blood culture should be drawn before administration of oral or parenteral antibiotics and discharge home, to rule out early bacteremia and subacute bacterial endocarditis. A follow-up visit or phone call in 24 to 72 h is also indicated.

## BIBLIOGRAPHY

Epstein ML, Kiel EA, Victorica BE: Cardiac decompensation following verapamil therapy in infants with supraventricular tachycardia. *Pediatrics* 75:737, 1985.

Fyler DC (ed): *Nadas' Pediatric Cardiology.* Philadelphia, Hanley and Belfus, 1992.

Gewitz MH, Vetter V, Silverman BK: Cardiac emergencies, and the patient with a heart murmur, in Fleisher G, Ludwig S (eds): *Textbook of Pediatric Emergency Medicine* 3d ed. Baltimore, Williams & Wilkins, 1993, pp. 533–572.

Talner NS: Congestive heart failure in the infant: A functional approach. *Pediatr Clin North Am* 18(4):1011, 1971.

Till J, Shinebourne EA, Rigby ML, et al: Efficacy and safety of adenosine in the treatment of supraventricular tachycardia in infants and children. *Br Heart J* 62:204, 1989.

# 107
# OTITIS AND PHARYNGITIS IN CHILDREN

**Kimberly S. Quayle**
**Susan Fuchs**
**David M. Jaffe**

## OTITIS MEDIA AND EXTERNA

### Otitis Media

Otitis media, defined as inflammation of the middle ear, is one of the most common pediatric diagnoses. Acute otitis media (AOM) (acute suppurative, purulent, bacterial) is associated with signs and symptoms of inflammation of the middle ear, such as otalgia, otorrhea, fever, or recent onset of irritability. Otitis media with effusion (OME) (secretory, nonsuppurative, serous, mucoid) is a relatively asymptomatic collection of fluid in the middle ear. The duration (not the severity) of OME can be divided into acute (<3 weeks), subacute (3 weeks to 3 months), and chronic (>3 months). The most important distinction between OME and AOM is that the signs and symptoms of acute infection (otalgia, otorrhea, and fever) are lacking in OME, but hearing loss may be present in both conditions.

### Acute Otitis Media (AOM)

Infants and young children are at greatest risk for the development of otitis media, with the peak incidence occurring between 6 and 13 months. By 3 years, more than two thirds of children have had at least one episode of AOM and one third have had three or more episodes. The incidence is higher in males, Native Americans, Alaskan and Canadian Eskimos, children who attend daycare, those exposed to tobacco smoke, and children with cleft palate or other craniofacial anomalies (e.g., Down syndrome). The incidence is lower in breast-fed infants.

Middle ear effusion may persist for weeks to months after an episode of AOM. Antibiotic therapy generally sterilizes the effusion but does not clear it from the middle ear space. After the first episode of AOM, 70 percent of children still have a middle ear effusion at 2 weeks, 40 percent at 1 month, 20 percent at 2 months, and 10 percent at 3 months.

#### Etiology

Bacteria are the most common cause of AOM and can be isolated in a pure culture from the middle ear exudate in 60 to 75 percent of cases. These organisms colonize the nasopharynx and enter the middle ear via the eustachian tube. *Streptococcus pneumoniae* and *Haemophilus influenzae* are still the most common pathogens (*Strep. pneumoniae* 30 to 40 percent, *H. influenzae*—primarily nontypable strains—25 to 45 percent), and *Moraxella* (formerly *Branhamella*) *catarrhalis* the third most common organism (5 to 15 percent). Of importance is a major change in the increased prevalence of β-lactamase-producing *M. catarrhalis* (70 to 100 percent) and *H. influenzae* (30 to 40 percent), which will affect antibiotic therapy decisions. *Strep. pyogenes* (group A) and *Staphyloccocus aureus* are each found in 2 percent of cultures. However, in infants 6 weeks or less, gram-negative enteric bacilli and *S. aureus* account for 10 to 20 percent of isolates. Although viruses are rarely recovered from middle ear effusions, recent studies have shown an increased risk of OME following an upper respiratory tract infection due to respiratory syncytial virus, adenovirus, and influenza virus A or B.

## Pathophysiology

Abnormal function of the eustachian tube appears to be the dominant factor in the pathogenesis of middle ear disease. Two types of tube dysfunction may result in otitis media: obstruction and abnormal patency. Obstruction can result from persistent collapse of the eustachian tube due to increased tubal compliance, an inadequate active opening mechanism, or both. Infants and younger children are prone to eustachian tube obstruction because the cartilage which supports the eustachian tube is less stiff than in adults. In addition, an upper respiratory tract infection or allergies can obstruct the eustachian tube and decrease its function. The obstructed eustachian tube prevents equilibration of air pressure between the middle ear and the atmosphere and creates conditions favorable to the development of purulent or sterile effusions. The other type of dysfunction is abnormal patency, which may allow reflux of nasopharyngeal secretions.

## Clinical Findings

Classic signs and symptoms of AOM include ear pain (otalgia), otorrhea, and fever; however, ear pulling and irritability may be the only clues in an infant. The most important diagnostic tool is the pneumatic otoscopic examination. Before adequate visualization of the external canal and tympanic membrane (TM) can be obtained, cerumen must be removed from the canal by blunt curettage, or by irrigation with warm water. The presence or absence of discharge, and position, color, and degree of translucency and mobility of the TM must be assessed. The light reflex is of no diagnostic value. The normal eardrum is translucent and pearly gray but may become reddened with crying. The eardrum should be freely mobile in response to positive and negative pressure by the pneumatoscope; however, retracted TMs have reduced mobility. The TM of AOM is usually opaque, hyperemic, and sometimes bulging, and bony landmarks (long and short process of the malleus) are not easily discernible. However the most significant sign is the loss of or decrease in mobility of the TM.

Tympanometry is a noninvasive diagnostic technique which is used to determine the compliance of the TM and the middle ear. A fixed tone at a given intensity is delivered through a probe snugly placed in the external ear canal, as the air pressure in the canal is varied from positive to negative. The tympanogram is a recording of the acoustic compliance of the middle ear, and patterns obtained are useful in distinguishing a normal ear from one with an effusion. Acoustic reflectometry is a technique that in the uncooperative infant or child is easier to perform than tympanometry and provides similar information about the presence of middle ear fluid.

Aspiration of the middle ear is the most definitive method of verifying the presence and type of middle ear effusion and infecting organism; however, its use for this purpose in the emergency department setting is rarely practical. It may be beneficial in (1) children with overwhelming sepsis, (2) immunologically deficient children, (3) neonates, (4) children with persistent symptoms of AOM after more than 48 to 72 h on antimicrobial therapy, or (5) otitis media with confirmed or potential suppurative complications. Diagnostic tympanocentesis may be performed by inserting an 18-gauge spinal needle or catheter over a needle, attached to a syringe, through the inferior portion of the TM. The aspirate should be cultured in blood culture broth and on blood and chocolate agar plates. When therapeutic drainage is required, a myringotomy should be performed. The incision should be made in the lower half of the TM and should be large enough to allow adequate drainage and aeration of the middle ear. Myringotomy may relieve unusually severe otalgia, either at initial examination or at any time during the course of the disease. In addition, it should be performed when a suppurative complication (meningitis, facial paralysis, mastoiditis) is present.

## Treatment

Selection of the appropriate antibiotic is based on several factors: (1) knowledge of the likely etiologic agent or recovery of a specific pathogen from middle ear fluid, (2) the efficacy of certain antibiotics against the organism responsible for AOM, (3) antibiotic penetration into middle ear fluid, and (4) a history of drug allergy. Amoxicillin (30 to 40 mg/kg per day divided tid) or ampicillin (50 to 100 mg/kg per day divided qid) for 10 days is still the drug of choice for the treatment of AOM, because of its in vitro and in vivo activity against Strep. pneumoniae and most strains of H. influenzae. However, if β-lactamase-producing H. influenzae or M. catarrhalis are suspected or documented, appropriate antibiotics include trimethoprim-sulfamethoxazole (TMP-SMZ) (Bactrim, Septra) (8 and 40 mg/kg per day, respectively, divided bid), erythromycin and sulfisoxazole in combination (Pediazole) (40 to 50 and 100 to 160 mg/kg per day, respectively, divided qid); cefaclor (40 mg/kg per day divided tid), or amoxicillin/clavulanate potassium (Augmentin) (40 mg/kg per day divided tid). In children in whom the aforementioned medications have failed, cefuroxime axetil (Ceftin—30 mg/kg per day divided bid), cefixime (Suprax—8 mg/kg per day once daily or 4 mg/kg per day divided bid), ceftibuten (Cedax—9 mg/kg per day once daily), cefprozil (Cefzil—30 mg/kg per day divided bid), cefpodoxime (Vantin—10 mg/kg per day divided bid), or loracarbef (Lorabid—30 mg/kg per day divided bid) can be used, as all are active against β-lactamase-producing organisms. In infants 6 weeks of age or less, cefaclor (30 to 40 mg/kg per day divided bid or tid) is preferred because of the potential presence of gram-negative enteric bacilli or S. aureus as pathogens. If the child is allergic to penicillin, erythromycin and sulfisoxazole in combination, TMP-SMZ or clarithromycin (Biaxin—15 mg/kg per day divided bid) are recommended.

When deciding which antibiotic to use, there are several issues to consider: (1) cefaclor efficacy is lower than that of amoxicillin-clavulanate, cefuroxime axetil, or cefixime; (2) the efficacy of cefixime against Strep. pneumoniae is less than that of the other cephalosporins, but it is one of the preferred agents when a β-lactamase producing organism is suspected; (3) in some areas of Europe, 20 to 40 percent of pneumococcal isolates are resistant to TMP-SMX.

There has also been an increase in pneumococci resistant to penicillin (and amoxicillin) in Spain, Paris (France), and other European countries. The specific isolates responsible (serotypes 6, 9, 14, 15, 19, and 23) have also been found with increasing incidence in the western United States and Alaska. Of more concern is the recent emergence of highly resistant strains of Strep. pneumoniae (which resulted in the development of meningitis despite amoxicillin or amoxicillin-clavulanate therapy). These isolates are also resistant to TMP-SMX, erythromycin, all cephalosporins, and ciprofloxacin. If these bacteria cause bacteremia or other serious infections, vancomycin with or without rifampin is the treatment of choice.

Although there have been several studies looking at a shorter duration of treatment of AOM, including the use of a single injection of ceftriaxone, further studies including long-term follow-up are needed.

In the numerous trials of antibiotics in the treatment of otitis media, adverse reactions requiring the discontinuation of the drug have occurred in fewer than 5 percent of patients. With ampicillin, amoxicillin, and amoxicillin-clavulanate, diarrhea is the most common side effect, followed by rash. TMP-SMZ can also cause diarrhea and skin rash (including Stevens-Johnson syndrome), but the major concern is the development of neutropenia and thrombocytopenia. In addition, a patient with glucose 6-phosphate dehydrogenase deficiency should not receive sulfonamides. Erythromycin often causes gastrointestinal symptoms including abdominal cramps, nausea, vomiting, and diarrhea. Cefaclor, besides the possible cross-sensitivity in patients with pencillin allergy, can cause a serum sickness-like reaction consisting of a rash, arthralgia or arthritis, and fever.

Additional therapy including antipyretics and analgesics may be helpful in alleviating some of the acute symptoms. A topical analgesic (Auralgan) instilled into the external ear canal often provides some relief from otalgia, but it should not be used when a TM perforation is present. Decongestants, antihistamines, or glucocorticoids have no demonstrable role in the treatment of AOM. With appropriate antimicrobial therapy, most children with AOM are significantly improved within 48 to 72 h. Persistent or recurrent pain or fever after 48 to 72 h indicates a need for reexamination of the child and the possible selection of another antimicrobial agent. Reasons for response failure include a resistant organism, noncompliance, and host-related structural or immunologic abnormalities.

Children with an uncomplicated course should be reexamined within 10 to 14 days of the completion of antibiotic therapy. At this time, some children have a persistent (but asymptomatic) middle ear effusion. Two further treatment options exist: (1) "watchful waiting" (no treatment) in children who have asymptomatic OME, with reexamination 6 weeks later or until the middle ear is normal; or (2) treatment for 10 days with another antimicrobial agent that is effective against possible resistant bacteria; then reexamination.

### Recurrent AOM (RAOM)

Many children have repeated episodes of AOM (recurrent AOM). RAOM is defined as three or more episodes of AOM over a 6-month period. Some develop symptoms and a new ear effusion, often associated with an upper respiratory tract infection, after a previous effusion has resolved, while others develop symptoms of AOM with no documented resolution of a previous effusion. There is a correlation between these "otitis-prone" children with the onset of AOM before 1 year of age. Other risk factors include day-care attendance and genetic susceptibility: a sibling or parent with a history of severe or recurrent AOM. Due to the risk of long-term sequelae such as hearing loss and speech impairment, prevention of further episodes is desirable. A more thorough physical examination, laboratory or x-ray studies should be performed to rule out sinusitis, allergies, immune deficiencies (C3 and C5 deficiency), submucous cleft palate, or a tumor of the nasopharynx. If none of these are present, several methods of prevention are available. These include (1) prophylaxis with antibiotics: amoxicillin (20 mg/kg per day qhs), sulfisoxazole (50 mg/kg per day qhs), TMP/SMZ (4/20 mg/kg per day qhs), or erythromycin (20 mg/kg per day for penicillin-allergic patients ≥2 years); or (2) myringotomy with tympanostomy tube insertion. Patients receiving prophylaxis should be reevaluated every 1 to 2 months, and the need for continuation reconsidered in 3 to 6 months.

### Persistent AOM

Persistent AOM is defined as the persistence of AOM within 6 days of initiating therapy or the recurrence of signs and symptoms within a few days of completing a 10-day course of antibiotics. This condition may be caused by the same pathogen (relapse) or a new bacterial species (reinfection). Ideally, tympanocentesis for culture and identification of the organism should be performed, although this is not always feasible. A search for a suppurative complication of OM (mastoiditis) or a concurrent infection (meningitis) should be done before changing antibiotic therapy. If these are not present, another medication can be prescribed, taking into account the spectrum of the initial choice (specifically, coverage of β-lactamase-producing organisms), as well as the antibiotic resistance patterns in the community. The patient should be followed closely, with a recheck in 2 to 3 days and again after 10 to 14 days.

### Chronic Suppurative Otitis Media (CSOM)

This is the persistence (>6 weeks) of a chronic purulent ear discharge in the presence of a nonintact tympanic membrane. It is thought to be a sequela of partially treated or untreated AOM or RAOM. *Pseudomonas aeruginosa,* gram-negative bacilli, and *S. aureus* are the most common causative organisms, although anaerobes have also been cultured. It is thought that they gain access to the middle ear through the perforated TM and become pathogens in the middle ear. A thorough examination is imperative, as chronic ear drainage can be

a manifestation of a cholesteatoma (which requires surgery). In the absence of a cholesteatoma, recent studies suggest that the following steps result in a more rapid improvement in ear drainage and a decreased need for tympanomastoid surgery: (1) Parenterally administered broad-spectrum, antipseudomonal antibiotics [ticarcillin, ticarcillin/clavulanate (Timentin), mezlocillin, or ceftazidime (Fortaz, Tazicef or Tazidime)] either on an inpatient or an outpatient basis; and (2) daily cleansing and aspiration of the external and middle ear followed by instillation of ear drops (Cortisporin suspension—polymyxin B, neomycin, and hydrocortisone; or Coly-Mycin—colistin, neomycin, and hydrocortisone).

### Complications and Sequelae of Otitis Media

The complications and sequelae of otitis media predominantly involve the middle ear and adjacent structures within the temporal bone, but in rare instances, intracranial complications may occur. The aural or intratemporal complications and sequelae include hearing loss, perforation or retraction pocket of the TM, tympanosclerosis, adhesive otitis media, ossicular discontinuity and fixation, chronic suppurative otitis media, cholesteatoma, mastoiditis, petrositis, labyrinthitis, and facial paralysis. Suppuration in the middle ear or mastoid, or both, may extend into the intracranial cavity producing the following intracranial complications: meningitis, extradural abscess, subdural empyema, focal encephalitis, brain abscess, and lateral (sigmoid) sinus thrombosis. These complications are uncommon except in neglected cases.

### Otitis Media with Effusion (OME)

OME is the collection of fluid in the middle ear, without acute clinical signs and symptoms, which often follows an episode of AOM. Hearing loss is by far the most prevalent complication and morbid outcome of OME. The extent of hearing loss is dependent on the volume of the effusion rather than the physical properties of the effusion. Audiometry is of limited value as a diagnostic method for the identification of OME, but it can be helpful in the evaluation of the effect of middle ear disease on hearing. The relation between persistent or episodic conductive hearing loss and impairment in the cognitive linguistic and speech development of children has been reported. However, the degree and duration of the hearing loss required to produce such deficits have not been defined.

Other factors that should be considered in addition to hearing loss when deciding whether to treat OME include (1) occurrence in young infants, as they are unable to communicate their symptoms and may have suppurative disease, (2) an associated acute purulent upper respiratory infection, (3) permanent conductive/sensorineural hearing loss, (4) vertigo, (5) alterations in the tympanic membrane: severe atelectasis and/or a deep retraction pocket in the posterosuperior quadrant or the pars flaccida, (6) middle ear changes such as adhesive otitis or ossicular involvement, (7) persistence of the effusion for more than 3 months (chronic OME), or (8) occurrence of the episodes so close together that the child has OME for 6 out of 12 months. A thorough search for an underlying cause (sinusitis, allergy, submucous cleft, tumor) should be attempted before treatment is begun. If an antimicrobial treatment has not been tried recently, it should be tried now. Because bacteria that cause OME are similar to those found in AOM, although *H. influenzae* is more common than *Strep. pneumoniae*, the antibiotics used are the same. Amoxicillin is the drug of choice except in chronic OME, in which erythromycin-sulfisoxazole, trimethoprim-sulfamethoxazole, amoxicillin/clavulanate potassium, cefuroxime axetil, or cefpodoxime proxetil should be used. The other nonsurgical methods available, including oral combinations of decongestants and antihistamine, topical intranasal or systemic glucocorticoids, and immunotherapy, have not been shown to be effective in clinical trials. If antibiotic therapy fails, the situation warrants referral to a pediatric otolaryngologist for evaluation for surgical therapy such as myringotomy with the insertion of tympanostomy tubes. Myringotomy with tympanostomy tube placement improves the conductive hearing loss for longer periods of time than myringotomy alone. Tympanostomy tubes remain in place for a few weeks to several years, with an average of 6 months. Possible complications of myringotomy tubes are scarring (tympanosclerosis), localized atrophy, persistent perforation, and the rare development of a cholesteatoma. For children ≥4 years who have recurrent chronic otitis media with effusion and who have had one or more myringotomy and tympanostomy tube operations in the past, adenoidectomy is a reasonable option. The presence of upper airway obstruction, recurrent acute/chronic adenoiditis or both would be another indication to consider adenoidectomy.

## Otitis Externa

External otitis (OE) is any inflammatory condition of the auricle, external ear canal, or outer surface of the tympanic membrane. It can be caused by infection, inflammatory dermatoses, trauma, or combinations of the three.

### Etiology and Pathophysiology

The flora of the ear canal are the same as those of normal skin. They include *Staphylococcus epidermidis,* diphtheroids, β-hemolytic streptococcus, *Staphylococcus aureus,* anaerobes, and fungi. Compromise of any of the protective features of the ear canal (shape and cerumen) can lead to OE due to colonization and invasion by pathogenic organisms, especially gram-negative enteric bacteria, pseudomonads, and fungi. Causes include (1) high environmental temperature and humidity, (2) hyperhydration and maceration of epithelial tissue in the canal, (3) absorption of moisture by the stratum corneum, (4) lack of cerumen through blocked gland ducts and/or mechanical removal (scratching), (5) obstruction of gland ducts by edema and keratin debris, (6) invasion by exogenous or endogenous organisms through breaks in the damaged epithelial surface, and (7) trauma.

### Clinical Findings

The mildest form of OE is characterized by itching or a sense of fullness in the ear. As it progresses, increasing pain, itching, redness, swelling, tenderness of the canal, and cheesy discharge occur. Inward pressure on the tragus, or pulling the auricle up and back, usually results in discomfort. If the TM can be visualized, it is often red, thick, and covered with the flat vesicles or areas of desquamating epithelium. In some cases, the pain is intense and constant, aggravated by any motion of the jaw or external ear. The regional lymph nodes may be enlarged and tender. When otomycosis is present (either as primary or secondary cause), intense itching is usually more prominent than pain.

### Differential Diagnosis

The hardest part of the diagnosis is to distinguish between OE and OM. Ideally, clinical inspection of the TM with a pneumatic otoscope will help establish the diagnosis; however, the TM of a child with OE may be as red and distorted as one with OM, although mobility of the TM is normal or slightly decreased in OE. In addition, visualization of the TM may be difficult because of edema of the canal in OE. Tympanometry can be helpful if the canal is clear and a tight seal for the earpiece can be formed without too much discomfort. Parotitis, periauricular adenitis, mastoiditis, dental pain, and temporomandibular joint dysfunction should be considered when the discomfort is poorly localized and the ear canal and TM appear normal. In addition, pain can be referred from pharyngitis or tonsillitis, but this pain is often made worse by swallowing or eating. Foreign bodies in the ear can also cause OE.

### Treatment

Cleansing of the ear canal is the most important part of therapy. For mild infections, dry mopping using a small tuft of cotton attached to a wire applicator is sufficient and may be curative. If the canal is inflamed, edematous, and occluded by debris, cleansing can be done with gentle suctioning; a soft plastic infant feeding tube (with an opening at the tip) attached to a DeLee trap can be used. If there is no perforation of the TM, irrigation with warm hypertonic (3%) saline or 2% acetic acid in Burow's solution (Otic Domeboro) is helpful. Acidified isopropyl alcohol (equal parts vinegar and alcohol) can also be used, followed by drying with suction, compressed air, or a hair dryer. The use of cotton swabs to clean the ears should be strongly discouraged.

Acetic acid ear drops are the easiest and least expensive way to eliminate the infecting agent. A 2% solution is effective and available commercially in aqueous (Otic Domeboro) or propylene glycol (Vosol, Orlex) solutions. These drops should be used three to four times a day for at least 1 week. However, when OE is accompanied by a TM perforation, burning or stinging will occur with the use of acid or alcohol-containing medication, so an antibiotic preparation containing neomycin, polymyxin B, and hydrocortisone (Cortisporin Otic suspension) is less irritating. Another option is the use of Cortisporin ophthalmic suspension, which is free of both acid and alcohol. Ophthalmic gentamicin or tobramycin are alternative drugs; however, when these agents are administered systemically, they have ototoxic properties, although hearing loss due to their topical use has not been documented. Otic chloramphenicol should be avoided because of the risk of aplastic anemia. Swimming should be prohibited during the course of treatment. After brief showers (with infrequent hair washing), drops should be instilled into the ear.

The basic treatment of otomycosis is similar to that for acute bacterial OE, with cleansing followed by 2% acetic acid or M-cresyl acetate (25%) preparations. Patients who do not respond can be treated with topical ophthalmic suspensions of miconazole, nystatin, or amphotericin B. Glucocorticoids are present in many topical otic preparations, but their value is unproven. Topical benzocaine and lidocaine may be useful to reduce the itching, but they are inadequate for the relief of moderate to severe pain, for which oral analgesics may be required.

Children who fail to respond to treatment within 48 h must be reevaluated. Examination should confirm the presence of a clear, dry, and patent canal, free of foreign bodies, and an intact TM. Evidence of other conditions, including cellulitis, abscess formation, or underlying dermatoses requires specific treatment, depending on the condition.

Patients with progressive, unresponsive, or severe infection may require parenteral (IV) therapy. Cultures of canal secretions should be taken and a combination of an aminoglycoside (gentamicin or tobramycin) and an antipseudomonal penicillin (ticarcillin or piperacillin) started. If the clinical findings and course of the illness suggest an infection due to *S. aureus,* a penicillinase-resistant penicillin (nafcillin or vancomycin) should also be given.

## PHARYNGITIS

Pharyngitis, infection of the pharynx and the tonsils, is a very common pediatric problem. It is estimated that $300 million are spent annually in its diagnosis and treatment. Despite physicians' long-standing familiarity with pharyngitis, there remains wide variability in approach. Controversies and new developments pertain to (1) selection of patients for throat culture and antibiotic treatment, (2) use of new rapid diagnostic tests for group A β-hemolytic streptococcus (GABHS), (3) increased incidence of serious systemic streptococcal disease, and (4) occurrence of bacteriologic and clinical failure with penicillin treatment of GABHS.

## Nonstreptococcal Pharyngitis

### Etiology

Many organisms—viral, bacterial, fungal, and even protozoal—have been associated with pharyngitis; however, only a relatively few are of practical significance to the emergency evaluation of pharyngitis in the immune competent child. Common viral isolates include adenovirus, Epstein-Barr virus (see below), influenza virus, parainfluenza virus, and enteroviruses. In one series, viral isolates were obtained from 37 percent of children with nonstreptococcal pharyngitis. *Chlamydia* and *Mycoplasma* have been implicated as common pharyngeal pathogens in adults. While only 3 percent of children and adolescents with pharyngitis as the major manifestation of illness were found to have *Mycoplasma pneumoniae*, pharyngitis was present in 32 percent of children with pneumonia caused by *M. pneumoniae*. A recent study of *Chlamydia trachomatis* in adolescents with and without pharyngitis found a prevalence of only 2 percent among symptomatic adolescents, and 0 percent among those asymptomatic. Recent studies have suggested *Arcanobacterium haemoliticum* (formerly *Corynebacterium haemoliticum*) might be a cause of non-GABHS tonsillopharyngitis, with or without a scarlatiniform rash. Erythromycin is the treatment of choice; however, no prospective therapeutic studies are available. Among bacterial pathogens, GABHS is clearly the most important, accounting for nearly half of all pharyngeal infections in patients between the ages of 5 and 15 years. GABHS pharyngitis is unusual in children under 3 years of age, and rheumatic fever is vanishingly rare in this age group.

### Differential Diagnosis

The few non-GABHS organisms that occasionally require specific diagnosis are *Corynebacterium diphtheriae, Neisseria gonorrhoeae,* and Epstein-Barr virus. Despite the many etiologic possibilities, in school-age children the diagnostic task is most often reduced to distinguishing GABHS, which requires specific antibiotic therapy, from nonstreptococcal pharyngitis.

*Diphtheria* is a rare but serious cause of pharyngitis in developed countries. Immunization in infancy with an alum-precipitated toxoid combined with pertussis antigen and tetanus antigen (DPT) has been effective in nearly eliminating diphtheria in childhood, but it can occur in crowded conditions in which there are socioeconomic barriers to immunization. Morbidity occurs because of both infectious and toxic reactions. Infectious invasion and spread occurs with enough tissue necrosis to produce a pseudomembrane that can progress to cause airway obstruction. The *C. diphtheriae* bacteria also produce an exotoxin that can cause widespread organ damage, including myocarditis and cardiac arrhythmia, neuritis with both bulbar and peripheral paralysis, nephritis, and hepatitis. Diagnosis must be clinical in order to expedite effective therapy; however, the bacteria can be grown on Loeffler's media. Treatment is directed both at killing the bacteria and neutralizing the exotoxin. Therefore, both antibiotic (penicillin or erythromycin) and horse-serum antitoxin must be given.

*Neisseria gonorrhoeae* is an infrequent but important cause of pharyngitis in sexually active adolescents. Gonococcal pharyngitis in younger children strongly suggests child sexual abuse. Gonococcal pharyngitis may be either asymptomatic or cause very mild symptoms with occasional exudative tonsillitis and/or cervical lymphadenopathy. Pharyngeal throat swabs should be plated on Thayer-Martin medium to recover the organism. Rectal and vaginal or urethral cultures as well as serum to test for syphilis should be obtained whenever gonorrhea is suspected or documented. Gonoccocal pharyngitis in children and adolescents should be treated with ceftriaxone (125 mg IM once). Children who cannot tolerate ceftriaxone may be treated with spectinomycin (40 mg/kg IM once). Children 9 years or older should also receive oral doxycycline (100 mg bid for 7 days) for presumptive *Chlamydia* infection. Children 8 years or younger should receive erythromycin (40 mg/kg per day in divided doses).

*Epstein-Barr virus* (EBV) is a herpesvirus that is a common cause of infection in childhood and adolescence. While EBV has been associated with a variety of clinical syndromes, most children infected with EBV are asymptomatic or have only mild nonspecific symptoms. EBV can cause isolated tonsillopharyngitis and pharyngitis as a manifestation of infectious mononucleosis (IM). Clinically, the classic IM syndrome begins with malaise, fatigue, and sore throat. Fever and adenopathy are the most common signs. Splenomegaly and hepatomegaly are also present in the majority of infected children, while skin rash, enanthem, eyelid edema, and jaundice occur much less commonly. Pharyngitis occurs in nearly all children with IM. The appearance of the throat can resemble that of bacterial GABHS disease. Dual infection with EBV and GABHS has also been documented. Classic IM is much less common in children under the age of 2 years, when EBV tends to cause a nonspecific febrile illness. However, recently IM has been reported to occur in toddlers more commonly than was once thought. These younger children most often have a syndrome characterized by fever, tonsillitis, lymphadenopathy, and hepatosplenomegaly.

The laboratory can be helpful in establishing the diagnosis of IM. There is an increase in both the proportion and the absolute number of atypical lymphocytes in the peripheral blood smear (generally ≥50 percent lymphocytes and ≥10 percent atypical lymphocytes). Liver transaminase levels show moderate elevation (generally AST is <600 U/dL). The heterophil antibody is present (and can be demonstrated by rapid slide test methods) in over 90 percent of children over the age of 5 with IM, but in only 75 percent between the ages of 2 and 4, and in fewer than 30 percent under the age of 2. EBV-specific serologic testing can provide information as to the likelihood of acute, postacute, old quiescent, and reactivation-type infection. These determinations are made on the basis of the presence of specific patterns of IgM and IgG antibodies to viral capsid antigen, and IgG responses to EBV early antigen, and to the Epstein-Barr nuclear antigen.

IM is generally a benign, self-limited, though somewhat prolonged, illness. In general, treatment involves nonspecific supportive modalities (fluids, acetaminophen, and rest). Fatal complications are rare. Mortality can be caused by neurologic complications (meningoencephalitis, Guillain-Barré syndrome), splenic rupture and hemorrhage, and bacterial and fungal sepsis. Immunocompromised children may have unusual susceptibility to fulminant EBV infection. Airway obstruction secondary to tonsillar hypertrophy can also occur. This complication responds rapidly to glucocorticoid administration (dexamethasone 1 mg/kg to 10 mg maximum; then 0.5 mg/kg every 6 h) and rarely requires intubation. Airway obstruction is the only complication for which the use of steroids is widely accepted.

## Streptococcal Pharyngitis

GABHS pharyngitis is the most common treatable cause of pharyngitis in children. The peak months of infection are January to May, but because of the high frequency of occurrence in school-age children, the beginning of school in the fall is also associated with GABHS pharyngitis in many areas. The peak ages are 4 to 11 years, with GABHS infection being uncommon under the age of 3 years.

### Diagnosis

No set of symptoms or signs is completely specific for GABHS. Nonetheless, there are findings which are typically, but not exclusively, associated with GABHS. Generally, the infected child experiences sudden onset of sore throat and fever. The tonsils and pharynx appear markedly red and have a moderate to large amount of exudate. The soft palate and uvula are also red and may have petechiae. The anterior cervical lymph nodes are enlarged and tender. The presence of a scarlatiniform rash and pharyngitis is virtually diagnostic of GABHS. Headache, vomiting, abdominal pain, meningismus, and torticollis can occur as well. These are of little diagnostic importance but must be recognized as possibly attributable to GABHS. The presence of significant coughing or rhinorrhea or both suggests an alternative diagnosis. Diagnostic accuracy on the basis of clinical findings alone is reported at about 50 to 75 percent for children thought to have GABHS and 75 to 85 percent for children thought not to have GABHS. There is general agreement that clinical diagnosis alone would result in an unacceptably high rate of misdiagnosis.

The mainstay of laboratory diagnosis is still the throat culture, although rapid antigen-detection techniques are gaining popularity in pediatric offices and emergency departments. The tonsil or posterior pharyngeal wall should be swabbed vigorously. In many centers, the swab is sent to the laboratory in appropriate culture medium for further handling. The sample is plated on a blood agar culture medium with neomycin and nalidixic acid added. Colonies which show β-hemolysis are identified as group A by bacitracin disk tests, fluorescent antibody staining, or latex agglutination. The rate of false-negative results from single throat culture is about 10 percent. Recovery rates are maximized by good swabbing technique, multiple cultures (rarely actually performed), and incubation in a carbon dioxide-enriched environment. Positive cultures may indicate either an acute GABHS infection or the carrier state. Rates of GABHS carriage vary with season but have been reported as high as 15 percent. There is imperfect correlation between the amount of growth (generally reported on a scale of 1+ to 4+) and the likelihood of true infection. Chronic carriers of GABHS are not at increased risk for developing true GABHS pharyngitis or suppurative and nonsuppurative (rheumatic fever and nephritis) sequelae, nor do they pose an increased risk for disease transmission.

Incubation of throat cultures takes 24 to 48 h, during which time management must occur with uncertainty as to the diagnosis. Antigen detection procedures are often available in emergency departments and practitioners' offices. The tests involve extraction of group A carbohydrate antigen from a throat swab and then combining the antigen with a latex agglutination, coagglutination, or enzyme-linked immunosorbent assay. Recently a chemiluminescent DNA probe test has also become commercially available. These tests provide rapid, direct detection of *Strep. pyogenes* cRNA from throat swabs. The nonculture tests take 10 to 30 min to perform and are generally more expensive per test than direct plate culturing. Sensitivity under controlled laboratory conditions using the culture as the "gold standard" ranges from 85 to 90 percent, and specificity ranges from 98 to 100 percent. Unfortunately, when measured in the field under less well-controlled circumstances, sensitivity has been as low as 50 percent. In other words, the false-positive rate is low, but the false-negative rate may be unacceptably high. Any emergency department or office planning to use a rapid diagnostic test must assess the performance of the test on site. A safe and commonly used approach is to obtain swabs for both throat culture and rapid test simultaneously. Children with positive rapid tests are treated for GABHS. If the test is negative, the throat culture is processed and the children are managed according to an acceptable strategy while awaiting throat culture results.

## Management

The objectives of treatment for GABHS are (1) to prevent rheumatic fever, (2) to prevent suppurative complications (peritonsillar abscess and cellulitis, suppurative cervical lymphadenitis, and retropharyngeal abscess), and (3) to hasten clinical recovery. GABHS is highly sensitive to penicillin, and there has been no evidence of development of resistance in vitro despite decades of use. A single dose of intramuscular penicillin G benzathine—600,000 units if the patient is ≤27 kg (60 lb) and 1.2 million units if >27 kg—is effective but causes

significant local discomfort in over 50 percent of recipients. A preparation containing 900,000 units of penicillin G benzathine and 300,000 units of penicillin G procaine (CR Bicillin 900/300, introduced in 1976) is effective for children who weigh ≤ 27 kg, and significantly reduces the magnitude and frequency of local reactions. Oral penicillin V is a popular alternative. A regimen of 250 mg three times daily for 10 days effectively eradicates infection and prevents rheumatic fever. Variable levels of compliance have been reported. Improvements in compliance can be achieved with careful parent education at the time of discharge. If compliance or follow-up are problematic, the intramuscular route should be used. Alternatives to penicillin for children with penicillin allergy include erythromycin, cephalosporins, clindamycin, and azithromycin.

An increased number of apparent treatment failures with penicillin has been reported. GABHS remains susceptible to penicillin in vitro. Alternative explanations for these findings may be children who are carriers of GABHS and develop a viral pharyngitis, patients who reacquire the organism from a family member or another close contact, or patients who are noncompliant with the prescribed penicillin. Other proposed mechanisms include development of GABHS penicillin tolerance and the production of β-lactamases from other normal pharyngeal flora. The evidence does not support the diminished efficacy of penicillin therapy for GABHS pharyngitis. These reports of the proposed therapeutic failures have prompted many recent studies comparing the efficacy of penicillin with other antibiotics. In general, penicillin remains the recommended antibiotic of choice based on past experience, cost, and historically successful prevention of rheumatic fever.

The overall incidence of rheumatic fever has been declining in the developed countries and is now approximately 0.6 per 100,000 in the continental United States, although it has recently been reported to be much higher in Hawaii. A number of scattered outbreaks of acute rheumatic fever were reported in the United States during the latter part of the 1980s. There is ample justification for adherence to the American Heart Association's recommendations that one of the above antibiotic regimens for documented GABHS pharyngitis must be provided. Antibiotic treatment begun within 9 days of the onset of infection is effective in preventing rheumatic fever.

Poststreptococcal glomerulonephritis is a nonsuppurative complication of GABHS disease that is not preventable with antibiotic therapy. Its occurrence is related to infection with nephritogenic strains of streptococci.

Research has also clearly demonstrated the beneficial effects of early antibiotic therapy on reduction of signs and symptoms of GABHS pharyngitis. In addition, because it is recommended that children with GABHS receive antibiotics for 24 h prior to returning to school or day care, early treatment benefits both the children and their parents, especially parents who work outside the home. Based on these considerations, many strategies for testing and treatment have been proposed, ranging from treating all children with pharyngitis with antibiotics to withholding antibiotics from all pending culture results. Cost-effectiveness studies employing decision-analysis methods have been performed to compare some of these strategies. The best strategy for a given institution depends on the local prevalence of GABHS, the availability and accuracy of rapid antigen testing, and the ability to follow up successfully on untreated children found to have positive cultures. A widely accepted strategy that incorporates the latest technology is to perform rapid antigen testing on all children with pharyngitis and to treat all positives. In addition, children with classic clinical findings or a scarlatiniform rash should be treated regardless of the result of rapid testing. Those with a negative rapid test and equivocal or atypical clinical features for GABHS should have a throat culture sent, but treatment may be withheld pending culture results. Positive culture results indicate the need for treatment. It is not necessary to reculture to test for eradication of GABHS in asymptomatic children. Children with recurrent or persistent symptoms and those with previously documented rheumatic fever do require reculturing. Children with persistent positive cultures in this context can be treated with a different antibiotic. Although the asymptomatic carrier state need not be treated, a combination of penicillin and rifampin has been shown to be effective in eradicating GABHS in carriers.

Some authors have suggested that early treatment of GABHS pharyngitis due to the availability of a positive nonculture test may lead to more frequent recurrences, possibly secondary to suppression of the immune response. Other studies have not supported this view. An intentional delay in the initiation of penicillin therapy for GABHS pharyngitis is not recommended at present.

Indications for tonsillectomy remain uncertain and controversial. One study showed that for children with many recurrent episodes of pharyngitis (seven or more episodes in 1 year, five or more annually for 2 years, or three or more annually for 3 years) tonsillectomy reduces the incidence of pharyngitis for the subsequent 2 years compared with nonsurgical management. However, 5 of 6 children in the nonsurgical groups experience significant improvement as well. Decision as to tonsillectomy for such children should be individualized to account for various considerations of risks, benefits, and quality of life, including the quality of available anesthetic and surgical services, impact of recurrent illness versus surgery on the child and parents, school performance, and comparative costs to the family.

Symptomatic therapy for both GABHS and nonstreptococcal pharyngitis includes acetaminophen for analgesia. A throat spray (e.g., Chloraseptic) can be used before meals and bedtime if further analgesia is required. Lozenges should be avoided in children under 5 years because of the possibility of aspiration. Recent outbreaks of pharyngitis caused by groups G and C streptococci have been reported. Although the acute clinical syndromes associated with these organisms are identical to that of GABHS pharyngitis, they are not known to cause preventable nonsuppurative sequelae. Nonetheless, by analogy to GABHS, treatment of children with pharyngitis caused by group G streptococci with the same penicillin regimens as in GABHS is recommended to hasten clinical recovery. Indications for treatment of group C-associated pharyngitis have not been established.

Recent resurgence of invasive GABHS infections has been noted. Serious illnesses include septicemia, toxic shocklike syndrome, pneumonia, cellulitis, and lymphangitis. These systemic infections may produce an extraordinarily virulent syndrome progressing rapidly to shock and death. Data suggest an appearance of new serotypes of GABHS but also an increased strain-associated virulence rather than virulence related to a given serotype. The pathogenetic mechanism by which these virulent strains produce severe disease is not well understood.

## BIBLIOGRAPHY

### Otitis

Baquero F, Loza E: Antibiotic resistance of microorganisms involved in ear, nose and throat infections. *Pediatr Infect Dis J* 13:S9, 1994.

Bluestone CD: Modern management of otitis media. *Pediatr Clin North Am* 36:1371, 1989.

Bluestone CD, Klein JO, Paradise JL, et al: Workshop on effects of otitis media on the child. *Pediatrics* 71:639, 1983.

Fliss DM, Leiberman A, Dagan R: Medical sequelae and complications of acute otitis media. *Pediatr Infect Dis J* 13:S34, 1994.

Marcy SM: Infections of the external ear. *Pediatr Infect Dis J* 4:192, 1985.

McCracken GH: Management of acute otitis media with effusion. *Pediatr Infect Dis J* 7:442, 1988.

Paradise JL, Otitis media in infants and children. *Pediatrics* 65:917, 1980.

Pichichero M: Assessing the treatment alternatives for acute otitis media. *Pediatr Infect Dis J* 13:S27, 1994.

Ruuskanen O, Heikkinen T: Otitis media: Etiology and diagnosis. *Pediatr Infect Dis J* 13:S23, 1994.

Stool SE, Berg AO: Clinical practice guideline, otitis media with effusion in young children. Rockville, MD: Agency for Health Care Policy and Research. (Publication 94-0622), 1994.

### Pharyngitis

1989 STD Treatment Guidelines: *MMWR* 38(suppl):58, 1989.

American Academy of Pediatrics: Gonococcal infections, in Peter G, (ed): *1994 Red Book: Report of the Committee on Infectious Diseases, 23d ed.* Elk Grove Village, IL, American Academy of Pediatrics, 1994, pp 195–202.

Bisno AL: Acute rheumatic fever: Forgotten but not gone. *N Engl J Med* 316:476, 1987.

Broughton RA: Infections due to *Mycoplasma pneumoniae* in childhood. *Pediatr Infect Dis* 5:71, 1986.

Denny FW: Effect of treatment on streptococcal pharyngitis: Is the issue really settled? *Pediatr Infect Dis* 4:352, 1985.

DuBois D, Ray VG, Nelson B, et al: Rapid diagnosis of group A strep pharyngitis in the emergency department. *Ann Emerg Med* 15:157, 1986.

Ferrieri P, Kaplan EL: Invasive group A streptococcal infections. *Infect Dis Clin North Am* 6:149, 1992.

Gerber MA: Critical appraisal of the clinical relevance of rapid diagnosis in pediatrics. *Diagn Microbiol Infect Dis* 3:39S, 1985.

Gerber MA: Culturing of throat swabs: End of an era? *J Pediatr* 107:85, 1985.

Gerber MA, Markowitz M: Management of streptococcal pharyngitis reconsidered. *Pediatr Infect Dis* 4:518, 1985.

Gerber MA, Randolph MF, Chanatry J, et al: Antigen detection test for streptococcal pharyngitis: Evaluation of sensitivity with respect to true infections. *J Pediatr* 5:654, 1986.

Gerber MA, Randolph MF, DeMeo KK, et al: Lack of impact of early antibiotic treatment for streptococcal pharyngitis on recurrence rates. *J Pediatr* 117:853, 1990.

Gerber MA, Randolph MF, Martin NF, et al: Community wide outbreak of group G streptococcal pharyngitis. *Pediatrics* 87:598, 1991.

Gerber MA, Spadaccini LJ, Wright LL, et al: Twice-daily penicillin in the treatment of streptococcal pharyngitis. *Am J Dis Child* 139:1145, 1985.

Grose C: The many faces of infectious mononucleosis: The spectrum of Epstein-Barr virus infection in children. *Pediatr Rev* 7:35, 1985.

Haggerty RJ: Sore throats and tonsillectomy. *N Engl J Med* 298:453, 1978.

Howie JGR, Foggo BA: Antibiotics, sore throats and rheumatic fever. *J R Coll Gen Pract* 35:223, 1985.

Huss H, Jungkind D, Amadio P, et al: Frequency of *Chlamydia trachomatis* as the cause of pharyngitis. *J Clin Microbiol* 22:858, 1985.

Kaplan EL: Benzathine penicillin G for treatment of group A streptococcal pharyngitis: A reappraisal in 1985. *Pediatr Infect Dis* 4:592, 1985.

Karpathios T, Drakonaki S, Zervoudaki A, et al: *Arcanobacterium haemoliticum* in children with presumed streptococcal pharyngotonsillitis or scarlet fever. *J Pediatr* 121:735, 1992.

Levin RM, Grossman M, Jordan C, et al: Group A streptococcal infection in children younger than three years of age. *Pediatr Infect Dis* 7:581, 1988.

Lieu TA, Fleisher GR, Schwartz JS: Clinical performance and effect on treatment rates of latex agglutination testing for streptococcal pharyngitis in an emergency department. *Pediatr Infect Dis* 5:655, 1986.

Markowitz M, Gerber MA, Kaplan EL: Treatment of streptococcal pharyngotonsillitis: Reports of penicillin's demise are premature. *J Pediatr* 123:679, 1993.

Meier FA, Centor RM, Graham L, et al: Clinical and microbiological evidence for endemic pharyngitis among adults due to group C streptococci. *Ann Intern Med* 150:825, 1990.

Paradise JL, Bluestone CD, Bachman RZ: Efficacy of tonsillectomy for recurrent throat infection in severely affected children. *N Engl J Med* 310:674, 1984.

Pichichero ME, Disney FA, Talpey WE, et al: Adverse and beneficial effects of immediate treatment of group A beta-hemolytic streptococcal pharyngitis with penicillin. *Pediatr Infect Dis J* 6:635, 1987.

Pichichero ME, Margolis PA: A comparison of cephalosporins and penicillins in the treatment of group A beta-hemolytic streptococcal pharyngitis: A meta-analysis supporting the concept of microbial co-pathogenicity. *Pediatr Infect Dis J* 10:275, 1991.

Poses RM, Cebul RD, Collins M, et al: The accuracy of experienced physicians' probability estimates for patients with sore throats. *JAMA* 254:925, 1985.

Randolph MF, Gerber MA, DeMeo KK, et al: Effect of antibiotic therapy on the clinical course of streptococcal pharyngitis. *J Pediatr* 106:870, 1985.

Schwartz RH, Hayden GF, Wientzen R: Children less than three-years-old with pharyngitis. *Clin Pediatr* 25:185, 1986.

Steed LL, Korgenski EK, Daly JA: Rapid detection of *Streptococcus pyogenes* in pediatric patient specimens by DNA probe. *J Clin Microbiol* 31:2996, 1993.

Sumaya CV, Ench Y: Epstein-Barr virus infectious mononucleosis in children. I. Clinical and general laboratory findings. *Pediatrics* 75:1003, 1985.

Sumaya CV, Ench Y: Epstein-Barr virus infectious mononucleosis in children. II. Heterophil antibody and viral-specific responses. *Pediatrics* 75:1011, 1985.

Turner JC, Fox A, Fox K, et al: Role of group C beta-hemolytic streptococci in pharyngitis: Epidemiologic study of clinical features associated with isolation of group C streptococci. *J Clin Microbiol* 31:808, 1993.

Wheeler MC, Roe MH, Kaplan EL, et al: Outbreak of group A streptococcus septicemia in children; clinical, epidemiologic, and microbiological correlates. *JAMA* 266:533, 1991.

# 108
# SKIN AND SOFT TISSUE INFECTIONS

## Richard Malley
## Gary R. Fleisher

This chapter will discuss several of the more common skin and soft tissue infections of childhood. The diseases will include conjunctivitis, impetigo, sinusitis, and cellulitis. Because of its particular severity, orbital/periorbital cellulitis will be highlighted in a section separate from the general discussion of cellulitis; however, the pathophysiology and clinical manifestations which are shared will not be repeated.

## CONJUNCTIVITIS

### Definition

Conjunctivitis is an inflammation of the conjunctivae, the membranes that line the surface of the eye. This inflammation may be the result of infection, allergy, or mechanical or chemical irritation. Keratoconjunctivitis involves the cornea as well as the conjunctivae.

### Etiology

The etiology of infectious conjunctivitis differs between the newborn and the older child (Table 108-1). In the newborn, pathogens that re-

**Table 108-1.** Etiology of Infectious Conjunctivitis

| Frequency | Neonate | Child |
|---|---|---|
| Very frequent | *Chlamydia trachomatis* | Adenoviruses<br>*Haemophilus* species |
| Moderately frequent | *Streptococcus pneumoniae*<br>*Streptococcus fecalis*<br>  (enterococcus)<br>*Neisseria gonorrhoeae* | *Streptococcus pneumoniae* |
| Infrequent | *Haemorphilus influenzae*<br>Herpes simplex<br>*Staphylococcus aureus* | *Neisseria gonorrhoeae*<br>*Neisseria meningitidis*<br>*Chlamydia trachomatis*<br>Herpes simplex<br>*Staphylococcus aureus*<br>*Corynebacterium diphtheriae* |

side in the birth canal play a major role in ocular infections. *Chlamydia trachomatis* is the most frequent, but *Neisseria gonorrhoeae* poses the greatest threat to the integrity of the eye. Later in childhood, the respiratory tract pathogens predominate, particularly *Haemophilus* species. Trachoma, a recurrent chlamydial conjunctivitis seen in tropical regions, will not be discussed.

### Epidemiology

Conjunctivitis is the most common ocular infection of childhood. It may occur at any age. Neonates acquire most infections during passage through colonized birth canals; in older children, respiratory tract pathogens spread from person to person. Conjunctivitis is usually a sporadic disease, but epidemics of viral illness may occur.

### Pathophysiology

Pathogens introduced into the conjunctival sac may proliferate and produce hyperemia and an inflammatory exudate. This exudate may be purulent, fibrinous, or serosanguinous. With certain organisms, corneal involvement (keratitis) may also occur.

### Clinical Findings

Older children with conjunctivitis may complain of photophobia, ocular pain or pruritus, a sensation of a foreign body in the eye, crusting of the eyelids, or conjunctival erythema. Infants and young children are usually brought by their parents for "pink eye" or crusting. The duration of symptoms with infectious conjunctivitis is most often 2 to 4 days but may be longer in cases which are untreated or resistant to therapy.

As with any ocular complaint, the physician should perform a thorough examination of the structure and function of both eyes including, when age appropriate, examination of visual acuity, visual fields by confrontation, extraocular muscle function, periorbital area, eyelids (with eversion), conjunctivae, cornea with fluorescein staining, pupillary reflex, anterior chamber, and fundus. Erythema and increased secretions characterize conjunctivitis. Chemosis may be seen. Intense erythema and purulent discharge are more common with an infectious rather than an allergic cause. The cornea does not stain with fluorescein in children with conjunctivitis unless an associated keratitis has developed, as with herpes simplex or adenoviruses. Most importantly, visual acuity is normal.

Fever and/or other systemic symptoms do not occur with isolated conjunctivitis. However, conjunctivitis may be only one manifestation of a viral upper respiratory tract infection, in which case the temperature may be elevated.

### Diagnosis

The diagnosis of infectious conjunctivitis rests primarily on the clinical examination. A Gram stain, which should be performed in neonates or in confusing cases, usually shows more than five white blood cells per oil immersion field and, in many cases, bacteria. The finding of gram-negative intracellular diplococci presumptively identifies *N. gonorrhoeae* in the first few weeks of life. Conjunctival scrapings and/or cultures may be performed in selected circumstances to diagnose *C. trachomatis* or specific viral and bacterial pathogens.

### Differential Diagnosis

The differential diagnosis of the "red (or pink) eye" includes conjunctivitis, orbital/periorbital infection, foreign body, corneal abrasion, uveitis, and glaucoma. Periorbital and orbital infections cause obvious swelling and tenderness around the eye and/or loss of ocular mobility. Foreign bodies should be visible on direct examination, often only following eversion of the upper eyelid. Thus, the differential diagnosis usually revolves around four conditions: conjunctivitis, corneal abrasion, uveitis, and glaucoma (Table 108-2). Both uveitis

**Table 108-2.** Differential Diagnosis of the "Red Eye"

| | Conjunctivitis | Corneal Abrasion | Uveitis | Glaucoma |
|---|---|---|---|---|
| History | URI | Trauma, contact lens | JRA, sarcoid, trauma | Prematurity, Marfan's syndrome, homocystinuria |
| Visual acuity | Normal | Normal or decreased | Normal or decreased | Decreased |
| Ocular exam | | | | |
|   External | Watery or purulent discharge | Watery discharge | Watery discharge | Watery discharge |
|   Cornea | Usually normal; staining if keratitis | Staining | Normal or band keratopathy | Cloudy, staining |
|   Anterior chamber | Normal | Normal | Cells, hypopyon, hyphema | Normal or shallow |
| Pupil | Normal | Normal | Small | Fixed |
| Intraocular pressure | Normal | Normal | Variable | Increased |

*Note:* URI = upper respiratory infection; JRA = juvenile rheumatoid arthritis.

and glaucoma are uncommon. The erythema in these conditions is concentrated around the limbus, and the discharge consists primarily of tears. Additionally, the vision is decreased in glaucoma, and the cornea may be cloudy. A corneal abrasion is easily identified by the uptake of fluorescein.

Finally, conjunctivitis may be only one manifestation of a systemic disorder, such as measles and Kawasaki disease.

## Complications

Conjunctivitis is generally self-limited, with the notable exceptions of herpes simplex and *N. gonorrhoeae*. The potential complications are corneal ulceration and scar formation leading to visual impairment.

## Management

Bacterial and viral conjunctivitides are far and away the most common cause for the complaint of a red eye in childhood. Once the diagnosis of conjunctivitis is established on the basis of diffuse injection, purulent discharge, and normal vision (Table 108-2), infectious and noninfectious causes are next separated. Allergic conjunctivitis is usually distinguished by chronicity, seasonality, pruritus, and associated symptoms of allergic rhinitis; if the physician is uncertain, a Gram stain can be done (Table 108-3).

In approaching infectious conjunctivitis (Fig. 108-1), the physician must decide whether the ocular disorder is one manifestation of a systemic illness such as measles or is occurring in relative isolation. Isolated conjunctivitis may be due to various viruses and bacteria, of which herpes simplex and *N. gonorrhoeae* are particularly severe, or to *C. trachomatis,* especially in the first 3 months of life.

Fluorescein staining should always be performed in an effort to identify the dendritic corneal ulcerations characteristic of herpetic disease. If they are identified, treatment is with acyclovir or other antiviral agents under the supervision of an ophthalmologist. Because *N. gonorrhoeae* is usually acquired during passage through the birth canal, infants under 1 month of age must always be tested for this

pathogen with a Gram stain and culture. If gram-negative intracellular diplococci are seen on smear, a single intramuscular injection of ceftriaxone (125 mg) is indicated.

Infants beyond 1 month of age and older children with an obvious clinical diagnosis of conjunctivitis do not routinely require smears or cultures. In patients under 3 months of age, treatment is instituted with erythromycin (50 mg/kg per day) orally for *C. trachomatis* (Table 108-4). Older children require only topical antibiotic instillation into the conjunctival sac. A child who has unusually severe disease or who fails to respond to therapy within 48 h may benefit from a laboratory investigation. Appropriate studies in the infant under 1 month of age would include a Gram stain and bacterial culture and either a scraping or culture for *C. trachomatis*. Older children require only a Gram stain and bacterial culture. Diagnostic tests for herpes simplex are not usually rewarding in the absence of corneal ulceration; culture for adenoviruses may be helpful in persistent or severe hemorrhagic infections to avoid unnecessary additional testing, but there is no specific treatment. All children with conjunctivitis should be reevaluated within 48 h. Failure to improve warrants further investigation and continued, careful follow-up.

## IMPETIGO

### Definition

Impetigo is a superficial bacterial infection of the skin confined to the epidermis. Deeper spread to the dermis leads to ecthyma. There are two varieties of impetigo: impetigo contagiosa and bullous impetigo.

**Table 108-3.** Differential Diagnosis of Allergic and Infectious Conjunctivitis

| | Allergic | Infectious |
|---|---|---|
| History | | |
|   Pruritus | Yes | No |
|   Chronic | Yes | No |
|   Recurrent | Yes | No |
|   Seasonal | Yes | No |
|   Sneezing, rhinorrhea | Yes | Variable |
| Exam | | |
|   Discharge | Watery | Watery or purulent |
|   Chemosis | Present | Usually absent |
|   Fluorescein | Negative | Negative, except keratitis |
| Lab | | |
|   Gram stain | Negative | White cells, bacteria |

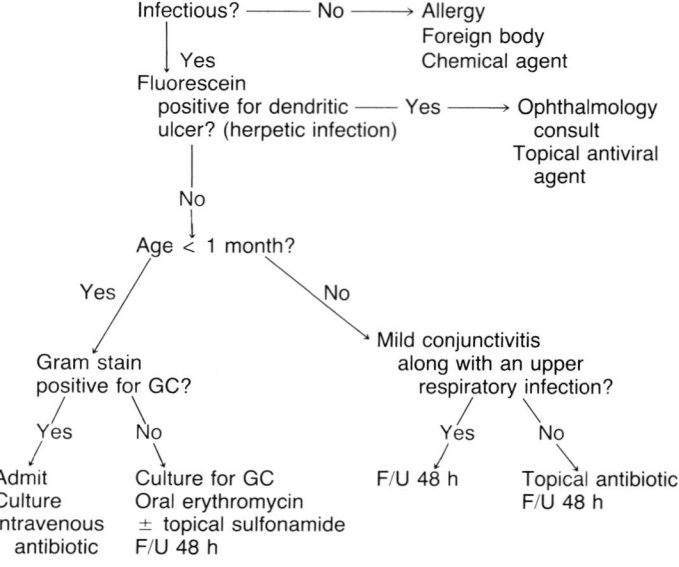

**Fig. 108-1.** Approach to the child with an isolated, infectious conjunctivitis. F/U: follow-up; GC: gonorrhea culture.

**Table 108-4.** Treatment of Conjunctivitis by Pathogen

| | |
|---|---|
| Viruses | |
| Herpes simplex | Trifluridine, vidarabine, or acyclovir, topically (neonates may also have systemic infection) |
| Other | Supportive |
| *Chlamydia* | |
| *Chlamydia trachomatis* | Erythromycin, 50 mg/kg per day orally, for 14 days |
| Bacteria | |
| *Neisseria gonorrhoeae* | Child: ceftriaxone 125 mg intramuscularly once |
| | Adult: ceftriaxone 250 mg intramuscularly once |
| *Neisseria meningitidis* | Child: penicillin, 50,000 units/kg per day, intravenously, for 7 days |
| | Adult: penicillin, 10 million units/day, intravenously, for 5 days |
| *Haemophilus influenzae,* *Streptococcus pneumoniae,* and others | Topical antibiotic ointments: sulfonamide, erythromycin, etc. |

## Etiology

Traditionally, group A β-hemolytic streptococcus (GABHS) was considered the major pathogen in impetigo contagiosa. However, recent studies have suggested that *Staphylococcus aureus* can often be the primary infecting agent and that therapy which does not include coverage for this organism is significantly less effective. In particular, in bullous impetigo, the primary pathogen is *S. aureus.*

## Epidemiology

Impetigo is the most common skin infection seen in the emergency department. The prevalence is greatest in young children, particularly those under the age of 6 years. Impetigo may occur sporadically or, occasionally, in epidemics. Conditions favoring epidemic spread include warm weather, overcrowding, and poor hygiene. Bullous impetigo is less common than impetigo contagiosa.

## Pathophysiology

The intact epidermis forms a relatively impervious barrier to bacteria. The development of impetigo follows a breach in the integument; this may be an obvious abrasion or an inconspicuous insect bite. Bacteria then invade the skin and elaborate toxins, such as streptolysins, which promote local spread.

## Clinical Findings

The chief complaint of children with impetigo is most often that of sores on the body. There are no associated systemic manifestations such as fever or malaise. Regional lymph nodes may be minimally enlarged.

The typical lesion of impetigo contagiosa begins as an erythematous papule. Small vesicles may follow transiently, but rapid progression to crusted lesions occurs. These crusts, which are initially honey-colored and fine in consistency, may appear on any area of the body; between the upper lip and the nose is a very characteristic site. The lesions enlarge over days to weeks, and the crusts become thicker. Erythema is mild. No induration is present.

In bullous impetigo, the characteristic skin lesions are superficial bullae filled with purulent material. The bullae range in size from 0.5 to 3 cm and have minimal, if any, surrounding erythema.

## Diagnosis

The diagnosis of impetigo rests with the visual appearance of the lesions. Rarely are laboratory tests needed.

In cases where the diagnosis of impetigo is uncertain, Gram stain of the lesions is helpful, showing abundant polymorphonuclear leukocytes and gram-positive bacteria. Local culture may be obtained from patients whose disease does not respond to standard therapy. If performed, the peripheral white blood cell count is normal.

## Differential Diagnosis

Several dermatologic disorders may resemble either impetigo contagiosa or bullous impetigo. These include tinea corporis, nummular eczema, small burns or abrasions, allergic contact dermatitis, eczema herpeticum (with underlying atopic dermatitis), and scalded skin syndrome.

## Complications

Impetigo may spread locally or, in the case of streptococcal infections, lead to remote, nonsuppurative sequelae. Occasionally, impetigo may progress to cellulitis or lead to lymphadenitis in the regional nodes. The attack rate for acute poststreptococcal glomerulonephritis has been as high as 1 percent in certain epidemics; however, the disease is unusual following sporadic skin infections.

## Management

The treatment of impetigo is oral antibiotic therapy or an appropriate topical antibiotic for limited eruptions. A first generation oral cephalosporin such as cephalexin (50 mg/kg/day) or erythromycin (50 mg/kg/day) provides effective oral therapy. Mupirocin is the only topical agent with proven efficacy. Combination topical and systemic therapy is unnecessary. Vigorous scrubbing, in addition to topical or systemic antibiotic agents, offers no advantage; routine cleanliness is sufficient.

Antibiotic therapy hastens the resolution of impetigo and limits suppurative complications. Although the incidence of glomerulonephritis may be reduced, it has not been possible to demonstrate this effect with certainty in clinical studies due to the low incidence of this disease.

## SINUSITIS

### Definition

Sinusitis is an inflammation of the paranasal sinuses: maxillary, ethmoid, frontal, or sphenoid. This inflammation may be on the basis of infection or allergy; it may be acute, subacute, or chronic.

### Etiology

The major pathogens in acute bacterial sinusitis in childhood are *Streptococcus pneumoniae* and *Haemophilus influenzae.* Wald and colleagues studied the etiology of infectious sinusitis using culture of material obtained by aspiration. Bacteria were recovered from 79 aspirates performed on 50 children as follows: 22 *S. pneumoniae,* 15 *Moraxella catarrhalis,* 15 *H. influenzae* (nontypable), 1 group A streptococcus, 1 group C streptococcus, 1 α-hemolytic streptococcus, 1 *Eikenella corrodens,* 1 *Peptostreptococcus,* and 1 *Moraxella.* Similar clinical investigations in adults have been in general agreement, finding nontypable *H. influenzae* and *S. pneumoniae* in 60 to 70 percent of the cases. Although *Staphylococcus aureus* and anaerobic organisms are isolated occasionally, they rarely play a role in acute infections in childhood. Severe sinusitis is not a common illness in children, but mild or subacute disease may occur more frequently

### Pathophysiology

The ethmoid and maxillary sinuses are present at birth, but the frontal and sphenoid sinuses do not become aerated until 6 or 7 years of age.

The sinuses are lined primarily by ciliated columnar epithelium and connect with the nasopharynx via narrow ostia. Normally, the epithelium is coated by a double layer of mucus: a viscid gel layer superficially and a more fluid layer underneath. Resistance to infection depends on the patency of the ostia, the function of the ciliary mechanism, and the quality of the secretions.

Obstruction of the ostia results either from mucosal swelling or, less commonly, mechanical obstruction. By far the most frequent offenders are viral upper respiratory infection and allergic inflammation. Less common causes include cystic fibrosis, trauma, choanal atresia, deviated septum, polyps, foreign body, and tumor.

Factors that impair normal mucociliary function include viral infections, cold or dry air, certain chemicals or drugs, and, rarely, inborn errors of motility. Alterations of the mucus occur in asthma and cystic fibrosis.

The bacteria that cause sinusitis often colonize the nasopharynx of healthy children. Disruptions in one or more of the barriers described above allow these organisms to ascend through the ostia and multiply within the sinuses.

## Clinical Findings

The spectrum of sinusitis has not been completely defined as it relates to clinical manifestations. However, there are two major types of infection which can usually be distinguished on clinical grounds: acute, severe sinusitis, and mild, subacute sinusitis (Table 108-5).

Acute, severe infections of the sinuses are infrequent during childhood. Such patients often have a history of headache and an elevated temperature. Findings include fever, localized swelling and/or erythema, and facial tenderness. A mucopurulent discharge usually accompanies severe sinusitis but may also indicate a nasal foreign body when unilateral.

Mild, subacute sinusitis is encountered more commonly than the severe form during childhood. This type of infection usually manifests as a protracted "cold." Rather than improving in 3 to 7 days, these children persist with the symptoms of an upper respiratory infection beyond 2 weeks. They have a nasal discharge, which may be serous or mucopurulent. Fever is infrequent.

Bacterial infection of the sinuses must be contrasted with congestion of brief duration found in association with some viral upper respiratory infections. Such congestion per se does not constitute a purulent infection.

## Diagnosis

The diagnosis of sinusitis is usually made on clinical grounds without any laboratory or radiographic studies. In older children and adolescents, transillumination of the maxillary or frontal sinuses may provide assistance. Absence of light transmission has been shown to correlate with the recovery of pathogens on aspiration.

Standard radiographs, including anteroposterior, lateral, and occipitomental views should be obtained in patients with an uncertain clinical diagnosis and in cases of severe sinusitis. The most diagnostic findings for purulence are an air-fluid level or complete opacification. Mucosal thickening greater than 4 mm is usually indicative of infection but may accompany viral upper respiratory disease, particularly in the first year of life. A normal radiograph suggests, but does not prove, that a sinus is free of disease.

**Table 108-5.** Signs and Symptoms in Children with Sinusitis

|  | Acute, Severe Disease | Mild, Subacute Disease |
| --- | --- | --- |
| Headache | +++ | ++ |
| Fever | +++ | + |
| Facial tenderness | ++ | — |
| Facial swelling | ++ | — |
| Nasal discharge | +++ | ++++ |

Several studies have shown that ultrasonography may be useful for the diagnosis of sinusitis, but there is not sufficient experience to recommend this modality for routine use. The anatomy of the paranasal sinuses is superbly defined by computed tomography (CT). However, the cost of CT does not justify its substitution for plain radiography, except in cases where complications are suspected.

Ultimate confirmation of infection within the paranasal sinuses rests with demonstration of organisms by Gram stain and quantitative culture of aspirated secretions. Aspiration is not routinely indicated but can easily be performed in selected cases of maxillary sinusitis in the outpatient setting via the intranasal route. The presence of organisms on Gram stain and a count of at least $10^4$ colony-forming units point to bacterial infection. Appropriate circumstances for aspiration include (1) life-threatening complications, (2) immunosuppressive conditions, (3) clinical unresponsiveness, and (4) unusually severe disease.

## Differential Diagnosis

Sinusitis may cause local swelling, facial pain, or nasal discharge. Other causes of swelling include superficial infection (cellulitis), trauma, cold injury, and allergic edema. Facial pain may be neurogenic, odontogenic, or related to the temporomandibular joint. Nasal discharge, particularly unilateral, should lead to a suspicion of a foreign body within the nares.

## Complications

The proximity of the paranasal sinuses to the brain sets the scene for the occurrence of life-threatening complications from sinusitis; however, the use of antibiotics has reduced the incidence of such complications. Infection may spread from the sinuses to surrounding structures through the diploic veins, which have no valves, or by erosion through bone.

The most commonly encountered complications are periorbital cellulitis and orbital cellulitis/abscess. Periorbital infection causes swelling around the eye, while intraorbital accumulation of pus may be recognized on the basis of proptosis and decreased ocular motion. Infection may also produce osteomyelitis of the surrounding bone; in the frontal region this is referred to as Pott's puffy tumor. Less commonly, complications follow intracranial extension and may include epidural, subdural, or brain abscess; meningitis; and cavernous sinus thrombosis. Meningitis rarely follows sinusitis; it more commonly occurs after bacteremia. Focal intracranial involvement can be demonstrated by CT.

## Management

In deciding upon appropriate therapy, the first step is to differentiate bacterial sinusitis from nasal congestion accompanying viral upper respiratory tract disease. Although the latter resolves spontaneously or may be treated with decongestants, sinusitis requires therapy with antibiotics (Table 108-6). Mild, subacute infections respond well to oral therapy for 10 to 14 days; as for otitis media, amoxicillin (40 mg/kg per day) remains the first-choice antimicrobial (Fig. 108-2). Failure to improve with amoxicillin therapy suggests infection with pathogens that are often resistant to this drug, such as *M. catarrhalis* or *H. influenzae*, or perhaps with penicillin-resistant *S. pneumoniae*. A second course of treatment with erythromycin/sulfisoxazole, newer oral second and third generation cephalosporins such as cefprozil or cefpodoxime, or amoxicillin/clavulanic acid should then be instituted; aspiration for culture may be useful for those patients in whom the infection still persists after a second course of therapy.

Acute, severe sinusitis may result in life-threatening complications and requires intravenous antibiotic therapy directed at *S. pneumoniae*, amoxicillin-resistant *H. influenzae*, and less commonly *S. aureus*. Cefuroxime (100 mg/kg per day) or ceftriaxone (75 mg/kg per day)

**Table 108-6.** Antibiotic Therapy for Sinusitis

|  | Acute, Severe Sinusitis | Mild, Subacute Sinusitis |
| --- | --- | --- |
| Initial | Cefuroxime, 100 mg/kg per day IV *or* Ceftriaxone, 75 mg/kg per day IV *or* Ampicillin/sulbactam, 200 mg/kg of Ampicillin per day IV | Amoxicillin, 40 mg/kg per day PO |
| Persistent | Antibiotics as above plus surgical drainage | Cefprozil, 30 mg/kg per day PO *or* Erythromycin/sulfisoxazole; 40 mg/kg per day of erythromycin PO |
| Penicillin allergic | Cefuroxime, 100 mg/kg per day IV | As for persistent cases |

**Table 108-7.** Etiology of Cellulitis

|  | Most Likely | Less Likely |
| --- | --- | --- |
| IMMUNOCOMPETENT HOST |  |  |
| Trunk/extremity | *Staphylococcus aureus* *Streptococcus pyogenes* | *Haemophilus influenzae* |
| Face* (periorbital/buccal); unimmunized | *H. influenzae* | *S. aureus* *S. pneumoniae* |
| Face* (periorbital/buccal); immunized | *S. aureus* *S. pneumoniae* | *H. Influenzae* |
| Any site/animal bite | *S. aureus* | *Pasteurella multocida* |
| Any site/human bite | Anaerobic organisms | *S. aureus* |
| IMMUNOCOMPROMISED HOST |  |  |
| Any site | *S. aureus*, gram-negative rods | Anaerobic organisms |

\* Definitive epidemiology awaits further studies since the advent of widespread immunization against *H. influenzae* type B.

represent single-drug regimens effective for this disease; ampicillin/sulbactam (200 mg/kg per day) is an alternative for the nonallergic patient. Failure of severe disease to respond promptly to antibiotic therapy or the occurrence of complications indicates the need for surgical consultation in regard to drainage procedures.

## CELLULITIS

### Definition

Cellulitis is an infection of the skin and subcutaneous tissues. It extends below the dermis, differentiating it from impetigo, but does not involve muscle (pyogenic myositis) or bone (osteomyelitis). Any region of the body may be involved, but two divisions are important in regard to predicting the most likely pathogens: (1) the trunk and extremities and (2) the face (buccal and periorbital cellulitis).

### Etiology

The organisms that play an important role in the immunocompetent host under normal circumstances include *Staphylococcus aureus, Streptococcus pyogenes* (group A β-hemolytic streptococcus), and *Haemophilus influenzae* (Table 108-7). In general, *S. aureus* is the most common and *H. influenzae* the least among the three major pathogens, particularly in children immunized against *H. influenzae* type B. However, in certain anatomic locations, particularly for young or unimmunized children, *H. influenzae* remains an important consideration. Additionally, unusual organisms may cause cellulitis in immunocompromised hosts or following their introduction in special types of wounds (Table 108-7).

### Epidemiology

Cellulitis is a frequent infection, particularly in the warm weather. The precise incidence is unknown; however, in a study at an urban children's hospital, this infection accounted for 1 of every 500 visits. Children of any age may develop cellulitis, but, as noted above, disease due to *H. influenzae* has become rare, affecting mainly infants under the age of 6 months.

### Pathophysiology

Cellulitis may occur either when a pathogen is directly inoculated into the subcutaneous tissue or following an episode of bacteremia. The majority of infections involve local invasion after a breach in the integument. The organisms responsible are usually *S. aureus* and *S. pyogenes*. In contradistinction, *H. influenzae* disseminates hematogenously.

### Clinical Findings

The child with cellulitis manifests a local inflammatory response at the site of the infection, including erythema, edema, warmth, and tenderness. There may be a history of a preceding wound or a complaint related to loss of function, such as limp with an infection of a lower extremity. Fever is unusual except in infections due to *H. influenzae* (Table 108-8).

Inspection of the area of cellulitis usually shows intense erythema. A violaceous hue suggests *H. influenzae* but has been reported with other pathogens including *Streptococcus pneumoniae*. Red streaks may radiate proximally along the course of the lymphatic drainage, and the regional nodes may enlarge.

### Diagnosis

The diagnosis of cellulitis is made by inspection. Laboratory studies including a WBC count, blood culture, and aspirate culture are ob-

**Table 108-8.** Usual Clinical and Laboratory Features of Children with Cellulitis

| Characteristic | *H. influenzae* | *S. aureus* |
| --- | --- | --- |
| Age | <3 yrs | Any |
| Fever | Yes | No |
| Color of lesion | Violaceous | Erythematous |
| Location | Cheek, periorbital | Trunk, extremity |
| Preceding wound | No | Yes |
| WBC count | >15,000/mm³ | <15,000/mm³ |
| Bacteremia | Yes | No |

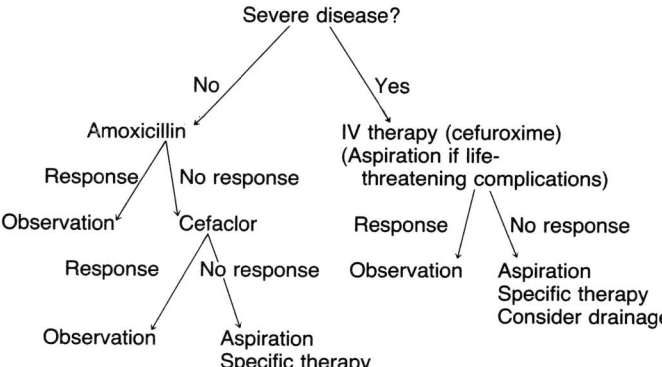

**Fig. 108-2.** Approach to sinusitis in the immunocompetent child.

tained for specific indications: immunocompromise, fever, severe local infection, facial involvement, and failure to respond to therapy.

The WBC count is normal in most cases of infection due to *S. aureus* or *S. pyogenes,* which are locally invasive. On the other hand, cellulitis due to *H. influenzae* results from bacteremia and is usually accompanied by a polymorphonuclear leukocytosis. In one study of children with cellulitis, the WBC count was over 15,000/mm³ in 3 of 4 children infected with *H. influenzae,* and 0 of 19 infected with *S. aureus* or *S. pyogenes.* Among 194 patients with *H. influenzae* cellulitis reported in the literature as reviewed in 1983, the WBC count was greater than 15,000/mm³ in 84 percent, with a mean of 20,850/mm³.

The blood culture is usually negative in infections due to *S. aureus* and *S. pyogenes.* On the other hand, *H. influenzae* as a rule causes a bacteremic infection.

Aspirate cultures are best obtained close to the center of an infected lesion, as the periphery may consist primarily of edema fluid devoid of organisms. The needle should be sufficiently large to permit the evacuation of purulent material—22 gauge for the face and 19 gauge for the trunk and extremities. Using a 5- or 10-mL syringe prefilled with 1 mL of sterile, nonbacteriostatic saline, the needle is directed into the subcutaneous tissue to a depth of approximately 0.5 to 1.0 cm, and aspiration is attempted. If there is no return, the saline is injected and reaspirated. The material obtained is used for culture and Gram stain.

## Differential Diagnosis

Cellulitis must be differentiated from other causes of erythema and edema, including trauma and allergic reaction. Allergic edema is not tender and usually only mildly erythematous. Traumatic lesions may be easily distinguished when there is a history of injury and absence of fever. Cold injury, especially on the cheeks ("popsicle panniculitis"), may be confused with cellulitis.

## Complications

Cellulitis due to *S. aureus* and *S. pyogenes* may at times spread locally or involve the regional lymph nodes; distant foci occur only rarely. Bacteremic *H. influenzae* infections are more likely to spread hematogenously, involving the central nervous system, epiglottis, joints, or pericardium.

## Management

The treatment of cellulitis is the administration of systemic antibiotic therapy. Although most patients respond rapidly to oral antistaphylococcal agents, the clinician must identify those individuals who require broad-spectrum or intravenously administered drugs (Fig. 108-3).

Obviously, signs of sepsis are indicative of hematogenous dissemination and demand treatment as an inpatient. Additionally, children under 6 months of age and those with impaired immunity are unable to contain local bacterial infections and will benefit from intravenous therapy.

Among otherwise healthy children over 6 months of age, only those who are clinically ill-appearing, or in whom bacteremic disease is suspected, need to be admitted to the hospital. Prior to the advent of the *Haemophilus* vaccine, physicians could identify patients at risk for invasive *Haemophilus influenzae* disease fairly reliably on the basis of anatomic location, presence of fever, and a WBC count greater than 15,000/mm³. Although the incidence of this disease has dropped considerably, it is important to remember that young infants are still at some risk of being infected with this organism.

The usual therapy for patients discharged from the emergency department is an antistaphylococcal antibiotic, such as dicloxacillin or cephalexin. Broad-spectrum therapy is recommended presumptively for patients who are immunocompromised or suspected to have bacteremia, pending a definitive isolate (Table 108-9).

## PERIORBITAL/ORBITAL CELLULITIS

### Definition

Cellulitis as previously defined may involve the tissues anterior to the orbital septum (periorbital cellulitis) or within the orbit (orbital cellulitis).

### Etiology

*S. aureus, S. pneumoniae,* and *H. influenzae* are the principal etiologic agents. Orbital infections are most often caused by *S. aureus.*

### Epidemiology

Children under the age of 3 years are more likely to become bacteremic than those who are older; thus, they experience the highest incidence of periorbital disease. Orbital cellulitis may occur at any age.

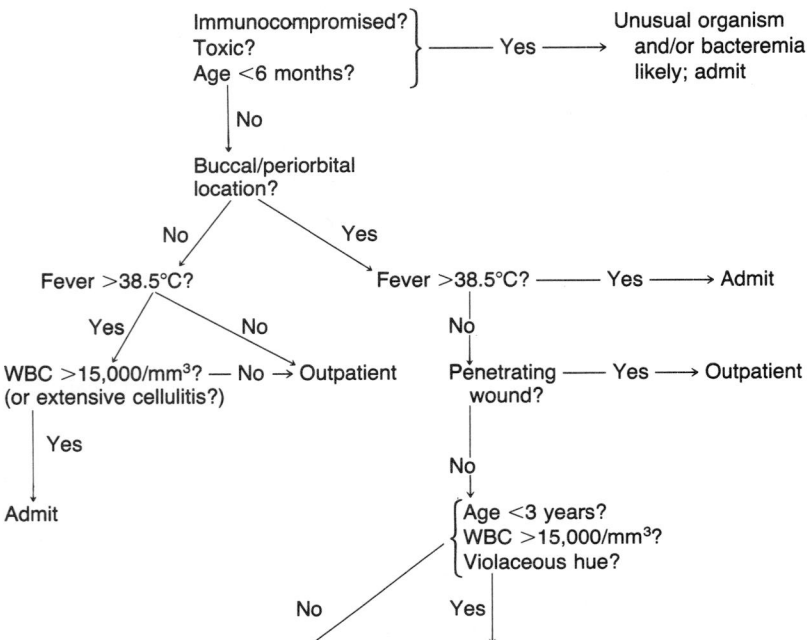

**Fig. 108-3.** Approach to the child with cellulitis.

**Table 108-9.** Initial Antibiotic Therapy for Cellulitis

|  | Drug | Dose | Route |
|---|---|---|---|
| **Presumptive** | | | |
| **Immunocompetent** | | | |
| 1. Extremity | | | |
|   a. Afebrile | Dicloxacillin | 50–100 mg/kg per day | PO |
| | *or* | | |
| | Cephalexin | 50–100 mg/kg per day | PO |
|   b. Febrile/leukocytosis | Ampicillin/sulbactam | 200 mg/kg as ampicillin per day | IV |
| | *or* | | |
| | Cefuroxime | 100 mg/kg per day | IV |
| | *or* | | |
| | Ceftriaxone | 75 mg/kg per day | IV |
| 2. Buccal/periorbital | As above | As above | As above |
| **Immunocompromised** | | | |
|   Any site | Oxacillin | 150 mg/kg per day | IV |
| | *or* | | |
| | Cefazolin | 100 mg/kg per day | IV |
| | ***and*** | | |
| | Gentamicin | 5–7.5 mg/kg per day | IV |
| | *or* | | |
| | Tobramycin | 5–7.5 mg/kg per day | IV |
| **Specific Organism** | | | |
| *Streptococcus pyogenes* | Penicillin | 100,000 units/kg per day | PO *or* IV |
| *Staphylococcus aureus* | Dicloxacillin | 50–100 mg/kg per day | PO |
| | *or* | | |
| | Oxacillin | 150 mg/kg per day | IV |
| *Haemophilus influenzae* | | | |
|   Ampicillin-sensitive | Ampicillin | 200 mg/kg per day | IV |
|   Ampicillin-resistant | Cefuroxime | 100 mg/kg per day | IV |
| | *or* | | |
| | Ceftriaxone | 75 mg/kg per day | IV |

## Pathophysiology

Organisms reach the periorbital area either hematogenously or by direct extension from the ethmoid sinus. In the case of orbital disease, contiguous spread is most common.

## Clinical Findings

Orbital and periorbital cellulitis cause the periorbital area to appear red and swollen. The periorbital edema is usually more prominent with preseptal infections. Proptosis or limitation of extraocular muscle function indicates orbital involvement. Fever is more common with periorbital cellulitis.

## Diagnosis

Periorbital and orbital cellulitis are distinguished from noninfectious disorders on the basis of the clinical findings and the WBC count. Leukocytosis occurs frequently with cellulitis, more often with bacteremic preseptal infections. A blood culture is often positive.

Computed tomography is performed when orbital involvement is likely. An inflammatory mass is easily demonstrated when present using this modality.

## Differential Diagnosis

As for cellulitis in other regions, allergic and traumatic causes for edema must be considered. Additionally, tumors and metabolic disease may cause swelling, discoloration, and/or proptosis. Thyrotoxicosis usually occurs in adolescents. The most likely tumor is metastatic neuroblastoma. Pseudotumor occurs rarely.

## Complications

Periorbital cellulitis may serve as a focus for metastatic bacterial disease; of particular concern is the occurrence of meningitis. Orbital cellulitis may evolve into a subperiosteal abscess; this condition threatens the integrity of the eye and should be considered a surgical emergency. Intracranial extension may occur rarely.

## Management

Admission and treatment with intravenous antibiotics is the rule. Blood cultures should always be done, and an aspirate culture is indicated for any ill child. In a child under 6 months of age, strong consideration of a lumbar puncture is indicated whenever infection with *H. influenzae* is suspected. Beyond 6 months of age, in the immunized child, although the possibility of meningitis remains, a decision regarding a lumbar puncture can be based on the clinical status and examination of the patient. Presumptive therapy of periorbital or orbital cellulitis is directed against *S. aureus* and *H. influenzae* (Table 108-9). Surgical drainage may be necessary with abscess formation or sinusitis.

## BIBLIOGRAPHY

Adams WG, Deaver KA, Cochi SL, et al: Decline of childhood *Haemophilus influenzae* type b (Hib) disease in the Hib vaccine era. *JAMA* 269:221, 1993.

Barton LL, Friedman AD: Impetigo: A reassessment of etiology and therapy. *Pediatr Dermatol* 4:185, 1987.

Barton LL, Friedman AD, Sharbey AM, et al: Impetigo contagiosa VII: Comparative efficacy of oral erythromycin and topical mupirocin. *Pediatr Dermatol* 6:134, 1989.

Fleisher GR, Heger P, Topf P: *Hemophilus influenzae* cellulitis. *Am J Emerg Med* 3:274, 1983.

Gigliotti F, Hendley JO, Morgan J, et al: Efficacy of topical antibiotic therapy in acute conjunctivitis in children. *J Pediatr* 104:623, 1984.

Hammerschlag MR: Conjunctivitis in infancy and childhood. *Pediatr Rev* 5:285, 1984.

Laga M, Naamara W, Brunham RC, et al: Single-dose therapy of gonococcal ophthalmia neonatorum with ceftriaxone. *N Engl J Med* 315:1382, 1986.

Sandstrom KI, Bell TA, Chandler SW, et al: Microbial causes of neonatal conjunctivitis. *J Pediatr* 105:706, 1984.

Vichgamond P, Brown Q, Jackson D: Acute bacterial conjunctivitis: Bacteriology and clinical implications. *Clin Pediatr* 25:506, 1986.

Wald ER, Reilly JS, Casselbrant M, et al: Treatment of acute maxillary sinusitis in childhood: A comparative study of amoxicillin and cefaclor. *J Pediatr* 104:297, 1984.

Wald ER, Byers C, Guerra N, et al: Subacute sinusitis in children. *J Pediatr* 115:28, 1989.

# 109
# BACTEREMIA, SEPSIS, AND MENINGITIS IN CHILDREN
## Peter Mellis

For the emergency physician who frequently cares for the young child with complaint of fever, the identification and treatment of potentially life-threatening systemic infectious disease represents a continuing challenge. The purpose of this chapter is to provide an overview of the presentation and management of bacteremia, sepsis, and meningitis in the pediatric patient in the emergency department. Although each will be discussed separately, it must be kept in mind that these entities represent different points along a spectrum and may occur concurrently as a result of progression of disease.

## BACTEREMIA

### Pathophysiology

From birth to 3 years of age, children are at increased risk for blood-borne bacterial disease due to immaturity of the reticuloendothelial system. The term *bacteremia* refers to the presence of a positive blood culture without reference to clinical symptomatology. The risk of bacteremia decreases with age, with infants in the first 3 months of life having the highest incidence. The term *occult bacteremia* (OB) refers to the presence of a positive blood culture in a febrile child who looks well, with no major focus of infection on examination. Children ages 3 to 36 months are at risk for OB, with an estimated incidence of 5 percent of children with rectal temperatures of 39°C or higher. The most common organism responsible is *Streptococcus pneumoniae*, which accounts for 85 percent of OB and produces a low-titer bacteremia that carries a 5 percent risk of progression to meningitis. *Haemophilus influenzae* type b (HIB) accounts for 10 percent of OB but carries a 25 percent risk of progression to meningitis. The impact of the HIB vaccine on OB has not yet been investigated, but this organism is likely to play a lesser role in the face of adequate immunization. Other organisms such as *Neisseria meningitidis*, *Salmonella* sp., and group A streptococci contribute a significant minority of cases but with a high rate of subsequent invasive disease. Recent series have indicated that OB carries a 20 percent risk of persistent bacteremia and a 10 percent risk of progression to a major focus of infection, such as meningitis, pneumonia, epiglottitis, or septic arthritis. The pathophysiologic mechanisms for progression to complicating focal infection have not been elucidated.

### Clinical Features

The presentation of OB includes fever and either no other signs of infection or signs of minor infection, such as viral upper respiratory infection, otitis media, or gastroenteritis. Children with OB appear well when examined following appropriate antipyretic therapy and in the comfort of the parent's arms. During this period of "optimal observation," such children are observed to be alert and interact appropriately with their parents without lethargy or irritability. A rectal temperature below 39°C correlates well with low risk of a positive blood culture. Similarly, the incidence of a positive blood culture rises incrementally with rectal temperatures above 39°C. By definition, however, it is impossible to specifically distinguish children with OB from those without bacteremia by clinical features alone.

### Diagnosis

Occult bacteremia may be only presumptively identified on the basis of the above clinical features and supportive laboratory evidence. In the setting of a well-appearing child with a temperature ≥ 39°C and a white blood count (WBC) in the 5000 to 15,000/µL range, the incidence of OB is 2 to 3 percent. A WBC > 15,000/µL is positively and progressively correlated with an increased risk of OB, but this choice of threshold will fail to identify 25 percent of cases. Other widely available tests, such as erythrocyte sedimentation rate and C-reactive protein, have failed to provide significantly greater sensitivity or specificity. Rapid antigen techniques, such as latex agglutination and enzyme-linked immunosorbent assay (ELISA), lack the sensitivity necessary to detect the low-titer pneumococcal bacteremia. Thus, the diagnosis of OB remains problematic for the emergency physician. The differential diagnosis includes systemic and focal viral infections and minor focal bacterial infection without bacteremia.

### Treatment

#### Emergency

Recent studies have conclusively demonstrated that ceftriaxone, a third-generation cephalosporin given in a dose of 50 mg/kg IM, is effective in markedly reducing the risk of progression from OB to a potentially life-threatening focal complication. In contrast, oral amoxicillin has not been shown to reduce the rate of complications from OB but reduces the duration of fever in those who do not develop complications. Studies utilizing oral third-generation cephalosporins have not yet been performed.

Recommended emergency department management for febrile children 2 to 36 months of age with temperatures ≥ 39°C would thus include the following: (1) physical examination to exclude clinical suspicion for meningitis or sepsis and identification of any minor focus of infection; (2) obtaining a WBC as a screen for OB; (3) consideration of other diagnostic laboratory tests to identify subtle sources of infection, i.e., chest film for tachypnea or significant cough and catheterized urine culture and urinalysis for males < 6 months or females < 2 years old with no respiratory symptoms or if there is a history of prior urinary tract infections; (4) for those children with WBC > 15,000/µL, a blood culture should be obtained and ceftriaxone, 50 mg/kg IM, given if no other major source of infection is identified warranting alternative therapy.

#### Outpatient

Follow-up within 24 h and clear instructions regarding indications for early return are the cornerstone of management of the well-appearing febrile infant, as no combination of clinical and laboratory assessment is sufficiently predictive of OB. Communication with the patient's primary physician to facilitate such follow-up represents optimal management. In the absence of a primary physician, consideration should be given to performing such follow-up in the emergency department, with repeat daily doses of ceftriaxone until (1) the patient is afebrile, (2) the blood culture is sterile, or (3) a complication requiring admission is identified. In all cases, the parent should be instructed to return with the child to the emergency department immediately for lethargy or irritability.

## Admission

Patients with a persistent febrile illness with identified bacteremia should be managed according to their clinical appearance on follow-up and the specific organism isolated. Patients who look ill or have either *H. influenzae* or *N. meningitidis* isolated on blood culture are at risk for bacterial sepsis and should have a complete reassessment, including lumbar puncture, and be treated as inpatients.

## SEPSIS

### Pathophysiology

Sepsis is a clinical syndrome defined by bacteremia with clinical evidence of invasive, systemic infection; it can progress with variable rapidity to circulatory failure. Sepsis can occur in isolation or with focal bacterial disease such as meningitis. The pathophysiology of sepsis is related to (1) colonization with a pathogen, usually nasopharyngeal; (2) invasion of the blood by encapsulated bacteria and release of inflammatory mediators, e.g., endotoxins; and (3) host defense response failure. This process results in systemic manifestations that are clinically detectable. Circulatory consequences may include alteration in systemic vascular tone and decreased myocardial contractility. Neurologic effects include decreased cerebral perfusion pressure and abnormal temperature homeostasis. Sepsis may also result in a microvascular angiopathy and disseminated intravascular coagulopathy involving the kidneys, lungs, and skin.

Host defense risk factors for sepsis include impaired splenic function, i.e., congenital absence, surgical removal, or functional impairment in sickle hemoglobinopathy, as well as the more rare primary or acquired humoral and cellular immunodeficiency states. The presence of an indwelling foreign body or obstruction to drainage of a body cavity represent additional risk factors.

The likely pathogens for sepsis demonstrate an age-related distribution. In the first month of life, group B streptococcus and *Escherichia coli* dominate and are capable of causing an explosive sepsis syndrome, which may increasingly be recognized in emergency departments with the trend to early newborn discharge. The risk presented by these organisms falls dramatically by the third month of life. In infancy and early childhood, *H. influenzae* type b and *N. meningitidis* predominate as pathogens for sepsis. *S. pneumoniae* is more likely to cause focal disease but may also result in sepsis syndrome, particularly with sickle cell disease. In school-age children, *N. meningitidis* predominates as the cause of sepsis, but group A β-hemolytic streptoccocus has increasingly been implicated. At all ages, Rocky Mountain spotted fever, caused by *Rickettsia rickettsii* acquired following tick bite in endemic areas of the United States, must not be overlooked as a seasonally important cause of sepsis.

### Clinical Features

The sepsis syndrome may present with either a subtle or obvious, rapidly progressive clinical picture. Neurologic symptoms most frequently include altered mental status with irritability, confusion, or lethargy. Poor feeding, lack of spontaneous motor activity, and hypotonia are common findings. Hyperpyrexia, defined as a rectal temperature > 41.1°C, may occur, although this is not specific for sepsis. Hypothermia may occur, particularly in the infant under 3 months of age, and is a grave finding. Tachypnea and retractions may reflect hypoxia or the development of metabolic acidosis. Early septic shock is accompanied by findings of tachycardia at rest, bounding pulses with a high pulse pressure, warm distal extremities, and brisk capillary refill. Progressive hemodynamic compensation is evidenced by classic findings of shock: weak distal pulses, delayed capillary refill, altered sensorium, and hypotension. Cutaneous findings may include petechiae, which may progress to coalescent purpura over hours to days.

## Diagnosis

Sepsis represents a *clinical* diagnosis of exclusion pending cultures and treatment because of the potential for rapid progression of disease. Obvious septic shock rarely presents a problem of diagnosis, but rather of management. In more subtle cases, the combination of altered mental status and abnormal vital signs should suggest to the emergency physician the possibility of sepsis. Because of the characteristically nonspecific presentation, febrile or ill-appearing infants under the age of 1 month should be considered septic until proved otherwise. No laboratory test is diagnostic, although a WBC > 20,000/μL is not unusual. The presence of a WBC in the "normal" range in the setting of an ill-appearing child is not reassuring. A WBC < 5000/μL or platelet count < 150,000/μL is a grave prognostic sign, particularly for disease due to *N. meningitidis*. Cultures of the blood, urine, CSF, and diarrheal stool, if present, should be obtained to identify a primary focus of infection and guide future therapy. Gram-stained smears made from CSF and petechial scrapings may provide immediate diagnostic information regarding the identity of the organism.

The differential diagnosis for the "septic-appearing" child includes infectious, cardiac, metabolic, and traumatic disease. Major focal bacterial infections, such as meningitis and pericarditis, and systemic viral disease may present with findings of fever, altered mental status, and cardiorespiratory compromise. The young infant with congenital heart disease may present in cardiogenic shock with respiratory distress and signs of poor perfusion. Toxic ingestion and congenital metabolic disease may present with altered mental status as the major complaint. Finally, child abuse with head or abdominal injury may present with altered mental status, temperature instability, and signs of poor perfusion without historical or cutaneous evidence of trauma.

## Treatment

### Emergency

Stabilization must take priority over completion of the diagnostic workup. Restoration of oxygenation and perfusion are the first priorities in the initial management of sepsis. The ill-appearing child should be provided with high-flow oxygen, and monitoring of heart rate, respirations, and oxygen saturation should be initiated. Attention to airway patency should continue throughout the assessment, with particular emphasis during procedures. Secure vascular access should be obtained early and, in the setting of signs of poor perfusion, fluid resuscitation performed with 20-mL/kg boluses of normal saline with serial reassessments. In such cases, an indwelling Foley catheter should be placed to ensure adequate urine output of 1 to 2 mL/kg per hour. In young infants in particular, hypoglycemia should be identified early by bedside testing and corrected with 25% dextrose in 0.5-g/kg bolus(es). If the patient is judged to have advanced respiratory or circulatory failure or neurologic compromise with potential for loss of airway control, endotracheal intubation and mechanical ventilation are indicated. If serial fluid bolus therapy does not restore evidence of adequate perfusion, inotropic support with dopamine in the setting of normal blood pressure or epinephrine in hypotensive states is indicated (Table 109-1).

The diagnostic evaluation of the septic-appearing infant in the emergency department should include cultures of the blood, urine, and CSF. Diarrheal stool should be stained for white blood cells and cultured if present. A complete blood count, electrolyte panel, and blood glucose measurements are routinely indicated. A chest x-ray and arterial blood gas measurement are indicated for signs of respiratory distress or critical illness. Liver functions tests, coagulation stud-

**Table 109-1.** Supportive Drug Therapy for Sepsis and Meningitis

| Drug | Dose | Indication |
|---|---|---|
| Oxygen | High flow | Poor perfusion |
| Normal saline | 20 mL/kg per dose IV bolus | Poor perfusion, repeat serially |
| 25 % Dextrose | 2 mL/kg per dose IV bolus | Hypoglycemia |
| Lorazepam | 0.1 mg/kg per dose IV over 1 min bolus | Seizures |
| Phenytoin | 15 mg/kg IV over 10 min | Persistent seizures |
| Phenobarbital | 5–10 mg/kg IV over 10 min | Persistent seizures |
| Dopamine | 10 μg/kg per min IV | Poor perfusion despite fluid boluses, titrate to effect |
| Epinephrine | 0.1 μg/kg per min IV | Hypotension despite fluid boluses, titrate to effect |
| Dexamethasone | 0.15 mg/kg IV | Suspected bacterial meningitis, give early |

ies, and fibrin split product analysis should be considered for the critically ill child.

Antibiotic therapy should be initiated in the emergency department as soon as possible and never withheld pending lumbar puncture if the patient is initially unstable. Antibiotic selection is made according to the likely age-related pathogens. In the first month of life, ampicillin, 100 mg/kg, and gentamicin, 2.5 mg/kg IV, are indicated. Children 2 months and older should receive a parenteral third-generation cephalosporin such as cefotaxime or ceftriaxone, 50 mg/kg IV. For infants in the second month of life, the combination of ampicillin and a third-generation cephalosporin as above represents optimal empirical therapy (Table 109-2). In endemic areas during the summer and early fall, chloramphenicol, 25 mg/kg IV, should be considered for children with potential exposure to Rocky Mountain spotted fever. In every case, care must be taken to monitor the patient following antibiotic administration, as the abrupt lysis of large numbers of organisms may result in endotoxic shock in a previously stable child.

## Admission

All ill-appearing or febrile infants in the first month of life should be admitted until sepsis is excluded by negative cultures. Well-appearing febrile infants in the 1 to 2 months age range should have a complete laboratory evaluation for sepsis and be admitted if clinical or laboratory evidence for sepsis exists. Children aged 3 months or older require laboratory evaluation for sepsis and admission if ill-appearing. In all cases, follow-up must be possible for an outpatient plan to be justified. Disposition decision-making for the possibly septic child must also include choice of the appropriate pediatric inpatient unit. The stable child with limited suspicion for sepsis may be admitted to a pediatric floor unit for antibiotic therapy pending culture results.

**Table 109-2.** Antibiotic Therapy for Sepsis and Meningitis

| Age | Antibiotic | Dose |
|---|---|---|
| < 1 month | Ampicillin | 100 mg/kg IV |
| | *plus* | |
| | gentamicin | 2.5 mg/kg IV |
| 1–2 months | Ampicillin | 100 mg/kg IV |
| | *plus* | |
| | cefotaxime | 50 mg/kg IV |
| | *or* | |
| | ceftriaxone | 50 mg/kg IV |
| > 2 months | Cefotaxime | 50 mg/kg IV |
| | *or* | |
| | ceftriaxone | 50 mg/kg IV |

The child with evidence of cardiorespiratory or neurologic compromise should be admitted to a pediatric intensive care unit because of the risk of progression of disease. If transfer of such a patient is necessary, a pediatric transport team should be utilized.

## MENINGITIS
### Pathophysiology

In most cases, meningitis occurs as a complication of a primary bacteremia. The inflammatory response to the products of bacterial multiplication may result in alteration of the permeability of the blood-brain barrier, with extension of infection and inflammation to the brain itself. The resulting brain edema, increased intracranial pressure, decreased cerebral blood flow, and vascular thrombosis produce neuronal injury. Less commonly, meningitis occurs via the hematogenous route from a distant primary focal infection, direct extension from adjacent infection, or following head injury with cribriform plate fracture. The incidence of meningitis is highest between birth and 2 years of age, with age-related peak risks during the neonatal period and between 3 and 8 months. Host-defense factors resulting in impaired splenic function or immunodeficiency are equally associated with increased risk for sepsis and meningitis.

The pathogenic organisms responsible for bacterial meningitis parallel those responsible for sepsis. In the neonatal period, group B streptococcus and *E. coli* predominate. During infancy and the preschool years *H. influenzae* type b, *S. pneumoniae,* and *N. meningitidis* are the likely pathogens. *S. pneumoniae* and *N. meningitidis* are most commonly implicated in school-age children, with much lower risk of *H. influenzae* type b disease beyond 12 years of age.

### Clinical Features

Because the presenting symptoms are subtle and overlap with those of less serious infection, a high index of suspicion for meningitis is crucial. Two modes of presentation are seen. The most common pattern is an insidious progression of a febrile illness over several days. Less commonly, a fulminant progression to septic shock and meningitis may occur over hours, most commonly caused by *N. meningitidis.*

Symptoms and signs of bacterial meningitis are dependent on patient age and duration of illness. No single complaint or physical finding is specific. However, the finding of a change in the child's state of alertness by parents or examiner constitutes a reasonable basis for suspicion for meningitis. Infants typically present with nonspecific symptoms including lethargy, poor feeding, and vomiting. Although common, fever is not universally present at the time of diagnosis. Signs of "paradoxical irritability" despite being held and comforted by the parent, decreased level of consciousness, hypotonia, bulging fontanelle, or respiratory distress may be seen. Children will usually complain of headache, photophobia, nausea, and vomiting. As for infants, signs of lethargy and confusion are primary indicators for suspicion of meningitis, and fever may not be consistently present. Nuchal rigidity and the classic findings of the Kernig sign, neck pain elicited with passive knee extension, and the Brudzinski sign, involuntary lower extremity flexion elicited with passive neck flexion, are helpful only if positive. Seizures occur early in the course of 25 percent of patients with bacterial meningitis and, if generalized, are not associated with adverse outcome. Focal neurologic findings, including focal seizures, and presentation with obtundation or coma suggest an adverse outcome. Pretreatment with oral antibiotics is associated with an altered presentation, characterized by less consistent findings of fever or altered level of consciousness and longer duration of symptoms before diagnosis.

### Diagnosis

On the basis of reasonable clinical suspicion, a lumbar puncture must be performed to make or exclude the diagnosis of meningitis. A

WBC is not an adequate screen for meningitis. Approximately 10 percent of lumbar punctures will identify meningitis when performed with an appropriate index of suspicion. CSF should be obtained for culture and sensitivity, measurement of protein and glucose levels, and for cell count and Gram stain, which should be rapidly performed. CSF pleocytosis with a leukocytic predominance and CSF glucose level less than 50 percent of blood glucose are considered positive screening tests for bacterial meningitis. The Gram stain will frequently identify the offending organism. The child with signs and symptoms strongly suggestive of meningitis but with normal initial CSF studies should undergo repeat lumbar puncture as an inpatient in 6 to 8 h as the CSF may appear normal during early stages of the disease. If prior treatment with antibiotics has occurred, a lower threshold for performing a lumbar puncture should be maintained and rapid antigen techniques such as latex agglutination for specific bacterial antigens are indicated. A CBC, electrolyte panel, blood glucose measurement, and blood and urine cultures should be obtained before performing the lumbar puncture. Although blood cultures are positive in over 80 percent of cases when obtained early in the course of meningitis, these should not be relied upon for sole diagnostic purposes unless patient instability precludes early lumbar puncture. Indications for deferring lumbar puncture in the emergency department include cardiorespiratory compromise or risk of increased intracranial pressure. In such cases, antibiotic therapy should be given in the emergency department and lumbar puncture performed as soon as possible in the inpatient setting.

The differential diagnosis for bacterial meningitis includes the same spectrum of systemic disease as described for sepsis. Aseptic meningitis refers to evidence of meningeal inflammation with negative CSF cultures. Most frequently, this is due to viral meningeal infection, but other causes such as tuberculosis or syphilis should be considered. Parameningeal infection or brain abscess may rarely mimic the presentation and laboratory features of meningitis.

## Treatment

### Emergency

As for the clinically septic child, treatment for meningitis begins with stabilization of oxygenation, ventilation, and perfusion. Provision of supplemental oxygen and monitoring of heart rate and oxygen saturation during lumbar puncture is often appropriate, with careful attention to prevention of airway compromise. The child with meningitis is often septic and may require vigorous initial isotonic fluid bolus therapy to restore systemic and central nervous system (CNS) perfusion. However, subsequent fluids should be provided at maintenance rates to minimize brain edema. Neurologic complications are frequent and must be treated aggressively to prevent secondary CNS injury. Seizures are treated with IV lorazepam, 0.1 mg/kg, and, if necessary, phenytoin, 15 mg/kg, or phenobarbital, 5 to 10 mg/kg, along with correction of any underlying metabolic disorder. Suspicion of increased intracranial pressure should prompt endotracheal intubation, hyperventilation, and IV mannitol, 1 g/kg, if hemodynamic stability permits (see Table 109-1).

Empirical antibiotic therapy for the likely age-related pathogens should be initiated as soon as possible in the emergency department. Deferred lumbar puncture or CT scanning should not delay antibiotic administration when clinical suspicion exists. In the first month of life, ampicillin, 100 mg/kg, and gentamicin, 2.5 mg/kg IV, are indicated. Children 2 months and older should receive a parenteral third-generation cephalosporin such as cefotaxime or ceftriaxone, 50 mg/kg IV. For infants in the second month of life, the combination of ampicillin and a third-generation cephalosporin represents optimal empirical therapy (see Table 109-2).

Steroid therapy has been shown to significantly decrease the incidence of neurologic complications in bacterial meningitis due to *H. influenzae* and *S. pneumoniae,* presumably due to an anti-inflammatory effect. Current guidelines are to administer dexamethasone, 0.15 mg/kg IV, either before or immediately after the initial antibiotic dose to children 6 weeks of age or older unless there is clear laboratory and epidemiologic evidence of aseptic meningitis.

Prophylaxis of contacts to eliminate carriage of organisms from the upper respiratory tract is indicated following identification of an index case of meningitis caused by organisms capable of causing epidemic disease. For *H. influenzae* disease, a regimen of rifampin, 20 mg/kg (maximum 600 mg), once per day for 4 days is indicated for (1) household members if there is a home contact aged less than 4 years old, and (2) day-care center staff and enrollees resembling households, defined as children < 2 years of age with contact of 25 h per week or more. For *N. Meningitidis* disease, a regimen of rifampin, 10 mg/kg (maximum 600 mg), twice per day for 2 days is indicated for all household members, day-care center contacts, and medical personnel who have had direct physical exposure to the index case prior to antibiotic therapy.

### Admission

All patients with identified or presumed meningitis should be admitted for supportive care, monitoring for complications, and antibiotic therapy, if indicated. As for sepsis, the disposition decision for the child with meningitis must also include choice of the appropriate pediatric inpatient unit. The stable child may be admitted to a monitored isolation bed on a pediatric floor unit for antibiotic therapy pending culture results. The child with evidence of cardiorespiratory or neurologic compromise should be admitted to a pediatric intensive care unit because of the risk of progression of disease. If transfer of such a patient is necessary, a pediatric transport team should be utilized for referral to a tertiary care center.

## BIBLIOGRAPHY

Baker MD, Bell LM, Avner JR: Outpatient management without antibiotics of fever in selected infants. *N Engl J Med* 329:1437, 1993.

Baraff LJ, Bass JW, Fleisher GR, et al: Practice guideline for the management of infants and children 0 to 36 months of age with fever without source. *Pediatrics* 92:1, 1993.

Baraff LJ, Oslund S, Prather M: Effect of antibiotic therapy and etiologic microorganism on the risk of bacterial meningitis in children with occult bacteremia. *Pediatrics* 92:140, 1993.

Baskin MN, O'Rourke EJ, Fleisher GR: Outpatient treatment of febrile infants 28 to 89 days of age with intramuscular administration of ceftriaxone. *J Pediatr* 120:22, 1992.

Feigin RD, McCracken GH, Klein JO: Diagnosis and management of meningitis. *Pediatr Infect Dis J* 11:9 (suppl) 785, 1992.

Odio CM, Faingezicht I, Paris M, et al: The beneficial effects of early dexamethasone administration in infants and children with bacterial meningitis. *N Engl J Med* 324:1525, 1991.

Rothrock SG, Green SM, et al: Pediatric bacterial meningitis: Is prior antibiotic therapy associated with an altered clinical presentation? *Ann Emerg Med* 21:146, 1992.

# 110

# VIRAL AND BACTERIAL PNEUMONIA IN CHILDREN

## Kathleen Connors
## Thomas E. Terndrup

## INTRODUCTION

Pneumonia is defined pathologically as an inflammation of lower tract lung tissue. Clinically, pneumonia is defined by the presence of pulmonary infiltrates on a chest radiograph, usually associated with a combination of clinical signs, such as cough, fever, chest pain, tachypnea, and a variety of abnormal auscultatory findings. Most commonly, pneumonia is caused by an infectious agent, although aspiration of irritants and interstitial inflammation is also referred to as such. This chapter will not discuss other entities associated with the diagnosis of pneumonia such as interstitial processes, foreign body aspiration, chemical inflammation, *Mycobacterium tuberculosis,* and certain protozoal infections causing pneumonia (e.g., *Pneumocystis carinii*).

The incidence of pneumonia in children decreases as a function of age. An estimated frequency of 4.0 percent in preschool children decreases gradually to a frequency of approximately 0.9 percent in 10 year olds. Seasonal variation is typified by parainfluenza occuring predominantly in the fall, respiratory syncytial virus (RSV) in the winter, and influenza in the spring. Bacterial pneumonia is more common in the winter, when indoor crowding promotes respiratory transmission of microbes. The mortality of childhood pneumonia is very low in industrialized nations (i.e., less than 1 percent), but accounts for up to 25 percent of deaths in children less than 5 years of age in developing countries.

## PATHOPHYSIOLOGY

The majority of pneumonias are acquired through aspiration of infective particles into the lower respiratory tract. There are a number of protective mechanisms preventing infection from aerosolized infective particles. Aerosolized particles are filtered in the nasal cavities or are entrapped and cleared by the normal mucous and ciliated epithelium of the upper respiratory tract. Aspiration is further prevented by laryngeal reflexes and coughing. In the lower respiratory tract, alveolar macrophages and various immune mechanisms prevent further invasion by infectious agents. These defense mechanisms include macrophages ingesting and killing bacteria, activation of complement and antibodies that neutralize bacteria, and particles being transported from the lung by lymphatic drainage. Abnormalities in any of these protective mechanisms predispose patients to acquired pneumonia. Anatomic abnormalities of the respiratory tract, immune deficiencies, neuromuscular weakness, airway abnormalities that predispose the child to aspiration, and alterations in quantity or quality of mucus secretion (e.g., cystic fibrosis) also predispose patients to acquired pneumonia. Passively acquired maternal antibodies may further prevent respiratory tract infection by pneumococcal and *Haemophilus influenzae* infections.

Suppression of the normal respiratory physiologic and anatomic defenses may occur secondary to a preceeding viral infection of the upper respiratory tract. In 50 percent or more of cases in children, co-existence of viral and bacterial pathogens has been demonstrated. Alternatively, the invading virus may spread distally to involve the lower respiratory tract and cause a viral pneumonia. Viral-induced injury to the normal defense mechanisms may allow pathogenic bacteria to infect the lower respiratory tract. Bacteria that cause pneumonia include many of the same organisms that colonize the child's upper airway. In addition, organisms that are transmitted person-to-person by airborne droplet spread may cause pneumonia. Less commonly, bacterial and certain viral microbes (e.g., herpes simplex virus, varicella, rubella, rubeola, and Epstein-Barr virus) may cause pneumonia through hematogenous spread or extension of a contiguous infection.

Parenchymal invasion by bacteria results in an acute inflammatory response that includes: exudation of fluid, deposition of fibrin, and infiltration of the alveoli with fluids and polymorphonuclear leukocytes, soon followed by macrophages. Accumulation of excess alveolar fluid creates the characteristic consolidation seen on chest radiograms. Viral agents, mycoplasma, and chlamydia typically cause inflammation characterized by a predominantly mononuclear infiltrate involving submucosal and interstitial tissues.

## Microbiology

The predominant pathogens that cause pneumonia in pediatric patients are a function of the patient's age, the presence of underlying disease(s), the vaccination status, and attendance in day-care. Clustering of cases of pneumonia due to a particular microbe are common, so it is helpful to be aware of recent local outbreaks. The most common etiologic agents causing pneumonia according to age groups is shown in Table 110-1.

Most children with pneumonia (60 to 90 percent) are infected by viral agents. In newborns, viral agents causing pneumonia include rubella, cytomegalovirus (CMV), and herpes simplex virus (HSV). Respiratory syncytial virus (RSV), parainfluenza virus, and adenovirus are the most common viral isolates in those between 1 and 6 months of age. Influenza virus and enteroviruses are isolated less frequently in this age group. Children between 6 months and 4 years with nonbacterial pneumonia are most often infected with adenovirus, parainfluenza, viruses, and Epstein-Barr virus (EBV). There are at least 14 other viral agents isolated in children with pneumonia, including influenza, rhinoviruses, enteroviruses, measles, varicella, rubella, HSV, and EBV.

The newborn age group is the only group in whom bacterial infections are more common than viral agents as the leading cause of pneumonia. The majority of infections in this age group are caused by aspiration of the maternal genital organisms present during labor and delivery. The predominant pathogen is group B streptococcus,

**Table 110-1.** Common Organisms Causing Pediatric Pneumonia

| Age Group | Organism(s)* |
|---|---|
| Newborn | Group B streptococci<br>Gram-negative bacilli<br>*Listeria monocytogenes*<br>Herpes simplex<br>Cytomegalovirus<br>Rubella |
| 0.5 to 4 months | Viruses<br>*Chlamydia trachomatis*<br>*Streptococcus pneumoniae*<br>*Haemophilus influenzae*<br>*Staphylococcus aureus* |
| 4 months to 4 years | Viruses<br>*S. pneumoniae*<br>*H. influenzae*<br>*Staph. aureus* |
| 5 years to 17 years | *Mycoplasma*<br>Viruses<br>*S. pneumoniae* |

* Listed from top to bottom by greatest to lowest frequency of occurrence.

followed by *Escherichia coli, Klebsiella* species, and other gram-negative enteric bacilli from the Enterobacteriaceae group. Other less commonly encountered organisms include nontypeable *H. influenzae*, other streptococci (group A and α-hemolytic species), *Enterococcus, Listeria monocytogenes, Bordetella pertussis,* and anaerobic bacteria. Between 1 and 3 months of life these organisms cause pneumonia much less frequently. Recent reports documenting the emergence of serious group A streptococcal infections have included pneumonia in young children. Infants between 3 weeks and 3 months may develop infections with *Chlamydia trachomatis.* Chlamydial infections often coexist with viral infections.

In the preschool age group the most common bacterial pathogen encountered is *Streptococcus pneumoniae. H. influenzae* type b (HIB) is encountered nearly as frequently. Children who attend day-care, where colonization rates are high, are more likely to be infected with HIB. Widespread vaccination of children against HIB infection may reduce the incidence of infection with this organism. Sixty percent of *Staphylococcus aureus* pneumonias occur in children less than 1 year old. Other bacteria that are isolated less commonly include group A streptococcus, *Moraxella catarrhalis, Bordetella pertussis,* and *Neisseria meningitidis.* Once children reach school age, *Mycoplasma pneumoniae* is the most frequent bacterial cause of pneumonia. *Chlamydia pneumoniae* is estimated to be the cause of up to 19 percent of adolescent pneumonias.

In all age groups, gram-negative bacilli including *Pseudomonas* should be considered in patients who have recently been hospitalized. Anaerobic infections should be considered in children with neurologic or anatomic defects that predispose them to aspiration. Unusual causes of bacterial pneumonia in children include *M. tuberculosis, Legionella* pneumonia, *C. psittaci, Francisella tularensis,* and rickettsial infections. Children with progressive or unresponsive pneumonia should be evaluated for evidence of these microorganiams. The immunocompromised host is susceptible to all of the infections listed above, as well as opportunistic infections such as *P. carinii,* CMV, and fungal diseases.

## CLINICAL FEATURES

Clinical findings of pneumonia are highly variable and are dependent upon the specific respiratory pathogen, the severity of the disease, underlying illnesses, and the patient's age. Older children typically have cough, fever, rigors, dyspnea, tachypnea, chest pain, increased sputum production, and other nonspecific symptoms, such as congestion, sore throat, and poor appetite. Infants frequently lack these classic symptoms and present with a variety of nonspecific findings. Pneumonia may occur in association with a sepsis syndrome in infants. Nonspecific symptoms and signs of pneumonia in infants include fever without a localizing source, apnea, poor feeding, abdominal pain, vomiting or diarrhea, hypothermia, grunting, bradycardia, lethargy, and shock. Sputum production is uncommon in nontracheostomized children less than 8 years of age.

Some historical features may provide clues as to the etiologic agent of pneumonia. Viral pneumonia is typically slow in onset and often preceded by upper respiratory symptoms, often with an exanthem. The onset of lower respiratory tract symptoms is usually gradual, compared to patients with bacterial pneumonia who tend to have sudden, more severe disease at the onset of illness. In older children, fever is often accompanied by chills and pleuritic chest pain. Pneumonia due to *Staph. aureus* is notorious for being particularly rapid in the progression of clinical findings. Patients with *B. pertussis* pneumonia typically develop a mild cough, conjunctivitis, and coryza (i.e., rhinitis), which last 1 to 2 weeks. A severe, paroyxsmal cough followed by an inspiratory whoop and emesis is characteristic of pertussis infections.

A history of maternal pelvic or conjunctival chlamydial infection is present in up to 50 percent of cases in which the infant develops *C. trachomatis* pneumonia. Chlamydia pneumonia in adolescents is usually insidious in onset and often includes complaints of sore throat and dysphagia. Mycoplasma infections generally present with the gradual onset of malaise, fever, and headache. A hacking, nonproductive cough usually begins 3 to 5 days after the onset of illness and is present in up to 98 percent of children. Patients with underlying disorders such as sickle cell anemia seem to manifest an increased severity of disease, regardless of the microbiologic etiology of pneumonia.

The severity of pneumonia may be judged by some historical features. Infants with poor feeding and lethargy may have more severe disease and often require hospital admission. A patient with a history of immunosuppressive therapy, primary immune deficiencies, or a history suggestive of an immune deficiency may have more severe pneumonia, often caused by unusual pathogens. Children with underlying illness such as congenital heart disease or chronic pulmonary disease are often more severely compromised by pneumonia. Infants and children with suspected chlamydial, *B. pertussis,* and *M. tuberculosis* pneumonia are prone to complications and should generally be hospitalized during initiation of therapy.

The findings upon physical examination in patients with pneumonia vary with the patient's age, microbial etiology, and the severity of the infection. Tachypnea is the most frequent sign of pneumonia in children and may be an otherwise isolated finding in febrile children. Tachypnea is also a nonspecific symptom and may occur secondary to fever, anxiety, metabolic disease, cardiac disease, or other respiratory problems. Auscultation of the lungs may reveal localized rales, wheezing, and decreased air entry in the affected area. Auscultatory findings are less reliable in children less than 1 year old because transmission of breath sounds over the much smaller pediatric chest makes localization difficult. In younger children, decreased breath sounds rather than rales are often heard, as the involved areas tend to be ventilated poorly. Grunting respirations may also be present, particularly in infants. Dullness to percussion is a less common finding and tends to indicate an effusion or extensive pneumonia. Abdominal distension and pain may be present secondary to a paralytic ileus or diaphragmatic irritation in lower lobe pneumonias. More severe pneumonia is associated with deterioration of the patient's mental status; the use of accessory muscles; and the presence of retractions, nasal flaring, splinting, and cyanosis.

The physical examination is usually abnormal in childhood pneumonia. Children with viral pneumonia are more likely to have diffuse findings on chest examination and will often have a component of airway disease producing wheezing, prolonged expiration, and hyperinflation. Bacterial pneumonia tends to produce localized findings on chest examination. Patients with bacterial pneumonia also tend to appear relatively toxic and are almost always febrile. Infants with chlamydial infection are usually afebrile, have a distinct staccato cough (i.e., short, abrupt onset), and diffuse rales on auscultation. They rarely appear systemically ill. Mycoplasmal infection may produce a pharyngitis, and rales are present in approximately 75 percent of patients. A variable rash that may be papular, vesicular, urticarial, or erythema multiforme–like is present in about 10 percent of patients with mycoplasma pneumonia.

## DIFFERENTIAL DIAGNOSIS

Initially it is important to differentiate pneumonia from noninfectious pulmonary conditions, such as congestive heart failure, atelectasis, and primary and metastatic tumors, and from congenital abnormalities, such as pulmonary hypoplasia or congenital lobar emphysema. The wide variety of conditions that may simulate pneumonia include radiologic imaging problems (i.e., poor inspiration, prominent thymus), recurrent or acute aspiration, atelectasis, tumors, collagen vascular disorders, allergic alveolitis, chronic pulmonary diseases (e.g., cystic fibrosis, asthma), and congenital abnormalities. A thorough history and physical examination usually help to exclude many of these conditions. Differentiating the various microbiological etiologies of pneumonia is often more difficult.

Although an occasional patient with pneumonia who is dehydrated may have a normal x-ray, the chest radiograph generally confirms or refutes the diagnosis of pneumonia. Radiographically, viral pneumonias tend to appear as diffuse interstitial infiltrates, frequently with hyperinflation, peribronchial thickening, and areas of atelectasis. Viral-positive/bacterial-negative children had more negative chest x-rays than other patients in a study of 128 Scandanavians. The gram-negative bacteria that cause pneumonias in the newborn tend to be very destructive and result in pneumatocele formation. *S. pneumoiae* and HIB typically cause lobar or segmental consolidation. Pneumatocele formation and a combination of pneumothorax and empyema are highly suggestive of *Staph. aureus* infection. *C. trachomatis* infections usually lead to hyperexpansion and diffuse alveolar or perihilar interstitial infiltrates. Radiographic patterns for *M. pneumniae* are variable. Lower lobe streaky or patchy infiltrates are the most common findings, but many other patterns are possible, incluing lobar infiltrates in 10 to 25 percent of cases. Pleural effusions have been reported in as many as 20 percent of mycoplasma cases in adults.

In children with bacterial pneumonia, blood cultures are positive 10 to 30 percent of the time. In pneumococcal disease, they are positive in about 10 percent of cases. *Staph. aureus,* HIB, and group A streptococcal pneumonia have a higher incidence (up to 90 percent for HIB) of positive blood cultures. Sputum cultures may also help in identifying the causative organism but are difficult to obtain from nontracheostomized children, particularly those less than 8 years of age. Cultures of the nasopharynx for viral pathogens, chlamydia, pertussis, and mycoplasma will often reveal the etiologic agent in patients with pneumonias caused by these organisms. These tests may provide useful information for the primary management of the child and should be considered if the test is available and the disease is suspected. Fluorescent antibody tests for *C. trachomatis* and *B. pertussis* are preferable to culture in some settings.

Rapid viral antigen tests exist for a number of organisms but are not widely available on a stat basis, except for RSV identification. Bacterial antigen testing is available in some centers but has a poor sensitivity and specificity in diagnosing the etiology of a pneumonia. Serologic testing can be done for viruses, mycoplasma, parasites, and fungi in persistent or puzzling cases. Skin testing for tuberculosis should also be considered in patients not responding to traditional therapy or with apical, cavitary pneumonias. More invasive diagnostic procedures such as endotracheal cultures, percutaneous lung puncture, bronchoalveolar lavage, or open lung biopsy may be necessary in patients with severe disease that is unresponsive to empiric therapy.

The white blood count (WBC) is usually elevated with a left shift in bacterial pneumonia, most notably in pneumococcal disease. Typically viral, chlamydia, and pertussis pneumonias will produce lymphocytosis. However, it is not unusual for viral pneumonia to initially provoke a significant polymorphonuclear cell response. An exception to this guideline is in children with sickle cell disease or other hemoglobinopathies, where leukemoid reactions (i.e., extreme leucocytosis) may occur. In patients with mycoplasmal pneumonia, the total WBC and differential count are usually normal, but the erythrocyte sedimentation rate may be elevated. Chlamydial infections or parasitic infections often produce an eosinophilia.

A pulse oximetry measurement to screen for hypoxia is useful in all patients with pneumonia and any degree of respiratory distress. Capnometry and arterial blood gases are helpful in assessing a patient with impending respiratory failure. Cold agglutinins have been demonstrated to be positive in 72 to 92 percent of patients with *M. pneumoniae* infection. Cold agglutinins may also be positive in viral infections and are less consistently positive in young children. To perform the bedside test for cold agglutinins, place several drops of blood in a blue-stopper coagulation profile tube and place in ice-water for 15 to 30 s. The presence of floccular agglutination is considered a positive test, and the agglutination should disappear upon rewarming.

## EMERGENCY DEPARTMENT CARE

All patients with pneumonia should be assessed for hypoxia, and oxygen provided if tachypnea and desaturation ($O_2$ saturation $\leq 92\%$) are evident. Additional respiratory support should be provided as dictated by the patient's clinical condition. Hydration status should be assessed, and supplemental fluid administered if needed. Children with consolidation on chest radiograph should generally have a blood culture obtained. The performance of other laboratory tests in children with pneumonia depends upon their clinical presentation. In addition to antimicrobial therapy, children should receive supportive measures, which include maintenance of hydration and humidification of air or oxygen.

In patients requiring hospital admission for suspected bacterial pneumonia, intravenous antibiotics should be administered. Empiric coverage should be guided predominantly by the age of the patient. In the newborn, ampicillin (150 to 300 mg/kg per day) in combination with either an aminoglycoside (gentamicin 2.5 mg/kg per dose) or a third-generation cephalosporin (cefotaxime, 100 to 150 mg/kg per day) is preferred. The ampicillin provides coverage against *Listeria* and enterococcus species. In children over 3 months of age, a cephalosporin alone (cefuroxime, cefotaxime, ceftriaxone) is usually sufficient. In children who are unresponsive to this therapy or with a suggestive clinical presentation, mycoplasma and chlamydial infections should be considered. Appropriate coverage for these infections would include erythromycin (50 mg/kg per day) or tetracycline, the latter in children over 9 years of age. If the clinical presentation is suspicious for staphylococcal pneumonia, then additional coverage (nafcillin, 150 mg/kg per day) should be added.

Children with fulminant viral pneumonias, such as varicella in the immunocompromised host, may require treatment with acyclovir. Lymphocytic interstitial pneumonia in HIV-positive children should include a combination of prednisone and zidovudine. Bone marrow and solid organ transplant patients with CMV pneumonia may require ganciclovir and gammaglobulin. In a recent report, ceftazidime or ceftriaxone eradicated noscomial pneumonia in 90 percent of cases, but ceftazidime had improved efficacy against *P. aeruginosa*. Children with cystic fibrosis often develop acute infectious exacerbations secondary to *Pseudomonas* and *Staph. aureus,* often with reduced antimicrobial resistance to standard antibiotics.

## ADMISSION INDICATIONS

Suggested criteria for admission of children with pneumonia include hypoxia ($O_2$ saturation $\leq 92\%$), respiratory distress, toxic appearance, dehydration, age less than 3 months, impaired immune function, and infections unresponsive to oral therapy. The presence of underlying disease and the ability of the caregivers should also be considered. Children found to be bacteremic with pneumonia should be hospitalized. Age less than 1 year or the finding of a pleural effusion or pneumatocele suggests a pathogen other than *S. pneumoniae* (particularly HIB or *Staph. aureus*). These infections can be rapidly progressive and are not well tolerated, so strong consideration should be given to hospitalizing these patients. Infants with suspected chlamydial, *B. pertussis,* or *M. tuberculosis* infections should be admitted for observation and to begin presumptive therapy. Children with complications from pneumonia should be hospitalized. Children discharged with a diagnosis of pneumonia should generally have clinical follow-up arranged within 24 to 48 h.

## AMBULATORY TREATMENT

Most children with uncomplicated pneumonia can be managed as outpatients. If a bacterial etiology is suspected, the patient should be placed on an appropriate antibiotic. The choice of oral antibiotic should be based on the considerations discussed above regarding the most likely etiologic organisms, considering the age and clinical presentation of the patient. For outpatient treatment, amoxicillin (40 mg/kg per day) is preferred for children between 3 months and 4 years. Alternatively, daily intramuscular ceftriaxone may be used, while some authors feel benzathine penicillin G should not be used for childhood pneumonia. After 4 years of age and in penicillin-allergic children, erythromycin (40 mg/kg per day) is the preferred initial agent. Recent data indicate similar cure rates, fewer side effects, and reduced termination of therapy with clarithromycin, compared to erythromycin. If viral pneumonia is suspected, no specific antibiotic therapy is warranted. Symptomatic treatment should include fever control and hydration. In the vast majority of cases in which pneumonia is diagnosed, antibiotic therapy is employed because bacterial disease cannot be ruled out with certainty. Patients with viral pneumonia often have a mixture of airway and airspace disease. If the patient has prominent airway disease (bronchiolitis-like) symptoms, bronchodilator therapy should be considered. In RSV pneumonia, ribavirin therapy should be considered for selected children.

## FOLLOW-UP INTERVAL

Routine follow-up should be performed by a primary care provider within 1 to 2 days. The duration of therapy varies with the clinical response, predisposing host factors, and suppurative complications. Ten days of antimicrobial treatment should suffice for most uncomplicated cases. Parenteral therapy, if initiated, should be continued until clinical improvement occurs. Whenever pneumonia is complicated or prolonged, roentgenographic follow-up is recommended to assure complete resolution, which may take 4 to 6 weeks or longer.

Most viral pneumonias will resolve spontaneously without specific therapy. Complications are similar to those for bronchiolitis and include dehydration, bronchiolitis obliterans, and apnea. Apnea is commonly seen in very young infants with RSV, chlamydial or pertussis infections. Pleural effusions can occur with viral pneumonias but are not common. Indications for admitting patients with RSV pneumonia are the same as for RSV bronchiolitis.

Uncomplicated bacterial pneumonia usually responds rapidly to antibiotic therapy. A delay in improvement or a worsening condition after therapy has begun should prompt an evaluation for possible complications. Complications of bacterial pneumonia include pleural effusions, empyemas, pneumothorax, pneumatoceles, dehydration, and development of additional infectious foci. Pneumococcal pneumonias will be accompanied by pleural effusions in 10 percent of cases. Pneumonia due to HIB will be complicated by pleural effusions in 25 to 75 percent of cases. Other foci of infection are frequently seen with HIB and can include meningitis, septic arthritis, epiglottitis, soft tissue infections, and otitis media. Pneumonias secondary to *Staph. aureus* have a high rate of complications including empyemas (80 percent) and pneumatoceles (40 percent). Mycoplasmal pneumonia can rarely be complicated by pleural effusions, meningitis, encephalitis, arthritis, and hemolytic anemia.

## DISCHARGE INSTRUCTIONS

Caregivers of all children released to home from the emergency department with a diagnosis of pneumonia should receive and understand discharge instructions. Specific advice on when to return to the emergency department or primary care provider, dosage and interval of medication(s), and signs of worsening respiratory distress should be given. Caregivers of children who are unable to ingest adequate

fluids or prescribed antibiotics should be instructed to return these patients for further care.

## BIBLIOGRAPHY

Bassetti D, Cruciani M, Solbiati M, et al: Comparative efficacy of ceftriaxone versus ceftazidime in the treatment of nosocomial lower respiratory tract infections. *Chemotherapy* 37:371, 1991.

Chien SM, Pichotta P, Siepman N, Chan CK: Treatment of community-acquired pneumonia. A multicenter, double-blind, randomized study comparing clarithromycin with erythromycin. Canada-Sweden Clarithromycin-Pneumonia Study Group. *Chest* 103:697, 1993.

Feigin RD, Cherry JD: *Textbook of Pediatric Infectious Diseases,* 3d ed. Philadelphia, Saunders, 1992.

Friis B, Eiken M, Hornsleth A, Jensen A: Chest x-ray appearances in pneumonia and bronchiolitis: Correlation to virological diagnosis and secretory bacterial findings. *Acta Paediatr Scand* 79:219, 1990.

Korppi M, Heiskanen-Kosma T, Jalonen E, et al: Aetiology of community-acquired pneumonia in children treated in hospital. *Eur J Pediatr* 152:24, 1993.

Lerman SJ: Benzathine penicillin G for the treatment of infants and children with pneumonia. *Pediatr Infect Dis J* 9:683, 1990.

Novotny W, Faden H, Mosovich L: Emergence of invasive group A streptococcal disease among young children. *Clin Pediatr* 31:596, 1992.

Wesley AG: Prolonged after-effects of pneumonia in children. *S African Med J* 79:73, 1991.

# 111
# PEDIATRIC URINARY TRACT INFECTIONS AND VULVOVAGINITIS
## Denise J. Fligner

## URINARY TRACT INFECTIONS IN CHILDREN

Urinary tract infection (UTI) is an important problem in pediatrics. UTI in young children is associated with significant later morbidity, including renal insufficiency and hypertension; the majority of damage occurs before 5 years of age. The goals of diagnosis are to provide relief for acute symptoms, to prevent damage to the upper urinary tract, and to identify those children at risk for late complications.

### Pathophysiology

#### Etiology

Bacteria usually enter the urinary tract system following colonization of the urethral meatus with perineal flora. In infants, UTI may be secondary to bacteremia. Gram-negative enteric bacteria are thus the most common organisms found in UTI after the neonatal period. *Escherichia coli* accounts for 80 percent of acute, uncomplicated infections. Other pathogens include *Klebsiella* and *Enterobacter* species. *Enterococci, Proteus* species, and *Pseudomonas* are more likely with recurrent infections and in children receiving antibiotic prophylaxis for chronic infections.

#### Incidence

The incidence of UTI varies with age and sex. In infants younger than 3 months, the rate of bacteriuria is 1 percent. In febrile infants (temperature > 38.1°C) the rate increases tenfold and ranges from

7 to 17 percent. Infection is two to three times more common in boys than girls, and 80 to 90 percent of male infant UTI occurs in uncircumcised boys. Sepsis associated with UTI is reported in 10 to 35 percent of infants.

Past 3 months of age, girls are at many times greater risk of both bacteriuria and symptomatic infection, and this risk persists in adults. School-age girls have a 1 to 2 percent prevalence of bacteriuria, compared to less than 0.1 percent prevalence in boys. The cumulative risk of UTI in girls is 3 to 5 percent.

## Complications

Reflux nephropathy, or renal scarring, previously termed *chronic pyelonephritis,* is the major preventable cause of renal insufficiency in childhood. The main determinants of renal scarring in children are vesicoureteral reflux (VUR), obstruction, UTI during the first year of life, and delay in diagnosis and treatment. Almost half of children less than 1 year of age with UTI will have VUR or other significant abnormalities. In boys, this is usually a structural abnormality. In girls with a first UTI, 25 to 30 percent have significant reflux. VUR predisposes the child with UTI to renal scarring, which progresses which each subsequent infection. After 5 years of age, the likelihood of progressive damage from reflux decreases.

## Clinical Features

Infants and young children present with nonspecific complaints including unexplained fever, irritability, vomiting, diarrhea, feeding problems, and failure to thrive. Older children may complain of abdominal pain. Toilet-trained children may develop enuresis or urge incontinence (dribbling) and complain of dysuria and frequency. Constipation is frequently present. Importantly, UTI may occur concurrently with both gastrointestinal and respiratory infection.

Findings on physical examination are usually minimal. There may be suprapubic or abdominal tenderness; flank pain suggests upper urinary tract infection but is not specific for pyelonephritis. The external genitals of all children who present with dysuria or other symptoms of UTI should be specifically examined for vulvovaginitis in girls and urethritis in boys.

## Diagnosis

The diagnosis of UTI requires urine culture. Presumptive diagnosis based on clinical symptoms or urinalysis is unreliable. Confirmation of UTI by culture has critical importance in children under 5 years of age because of the prognostic implications of UTI in this age group.

### Specimen Collection

Specimen collection for culture in infants and young children is problematic. Bag specimens are easily contaminated by fecal and skin flora, even following proper cleansing of the perineum. In addition, the specimen usually remains in contact with the perineum for an undetermined length of time, allowing for overgrowth of bacteria. A negative culture from bag urine reliably excludes UTI. Positive bag urine cultures and indeterminate results are unreliable in the diagnosis of UTI and must be confirmed by a suprapubic or catheterized specimen. In young children, if antibiotics are to be started pending culture results, it is crucial that urine for culture first be obtained by bladder catheterization or suprapubic aspiration. In older children, a midstream clean-catch specimen obtained following careful cleansing of the genitals is adequate. The specimen should be plated immediately or else refrigerated at 4°C (39.2°F) to prevent bacterial overgrowth.

### Urinalysis

Urinalysis results should not be used as a screen for determining the need for culture. The presence of leukocytes in spun urine is suggestive of UTI but not diagnostic. Pyuria (>10 white blood cells per high-power field of spun urine) can be found in gastroenteritis, vulvovaginitis, appendicitis, and other acute abdominal conditions. Pyuria is also common in the sexually transmitted diseases. Of greater concern, pyuria is often absent in culture-positive bacteriuria; in infants with culture-proven UTI, fewer than half have pyuria.

However, microscopic examination of fresh, unspun urine for bacteria can provide a rapid, reliable estimate of probable culture results. One bacterium per high-power field seen in unspun urine correlates well with growth of greater than $10^5$ colonies on urine culture.

### Culture Results

The definition of a positive culture depends on the method of collection. In fresh urine obtained from a midstream clean-catch specimen, the presence of $10^5$ colonies of a single organism per milliliter of urine is diagnostic. The probability of infection with one positive culture is 80 percent; with two separately collected positive cultures it is 90 percent. Colony counts between $10^4$ and $10^5$ are uninterpretable and should be repeated. Colony counts less than $10^4$ or the presence of two or more organisms indicates contamination. Several factors may lower the colony count in the presence of significant infection. These factors include dilution, low urine pH and specific gravity, recent antibiotic therapy, fastidious organisms, inappropriate culture techniques, bacteriostatic agents in the urine, and complete obstruction of the ureter.

The presence of greater than $10^3$ colonies per milliliter of urine in a catheterized specimen or any bacteria in a suprapubic specimen indicates infection.

## Differential Diagnosis

Dysuria can be the presenting complaint in urethral, vulvar, and vaginal inflammation. Vulvovaginitis is a far more common cause of dysuria than is UTI. Dysuria due to vulvar inflammation can often be distinguished by older adolescents and adults as being external, in contrast to the deeper discomfort that occurs with UTI. Dysuria from UTI is usually associated with urinary frequency.

Pyuria and dysuria with negative urine cultures is frequently seen with *Neisseria gonorrhoea, Chlamydia trachomatis,* and *Trichomonas* in both sexes. In adolescent boys, sterile pyuria is strongly suggestive of sexually transmitted urethritis.

## Treatment

### Emergency Department Care

Following proper collection of a specimen for culture, treatment of the symptomatic patient may be started pending culture results.

### Indications for Admission

Hospitalization and parenteral therapy are preferred for infants under 3 months of age; children who appear toxic, febrile, or unable to tolerate oral therapy; and when pyelonephritis is suspected. Parenteral ampicillin alone or in combination with an aminoglycoside is used initially. Antibiotic therapy should be adjusted once culture results and sensitivities are known.

### Outpatient Treatment

In the afebrile, nontoxic patient, outpatient therapy can be instituted with oral antibiotics. Amoxicillin (50 mg/kg per day in three doses), sulfisoxazole (150 mg/kg per day), or trimethoprim/sulfamethoxazole (TMP/SMX: 6 to 8 mg/kg per day TMP, 30 to 40 mg/kg per day SMX in two doses) are reasonable choices. Since resistance develops rapidly to amoxicillin and sulfonamides, TMP/SMX or trimethoprim alone are preferred for suspicion of pyelonephritis, recurrences, and prophylaxis. The flouroquinolones are neither approved by the FDA nor currently recommended for routine therapy in childhood UTI. Flouroquinolones may be of value in selected children with recurrent UTI due to multiply resistent organisms, in particular *Pseudomonas* species.

### Duration of Therapy

Upper urinary tract infection should be treated for 10 days. Treatment for 3 to 5 days in uncomplicated UTI is usually adequate in children with radiologically normal urinary tracts and probably decreases the occurrence of antibiotic complications such as candidiasis and diarrhea. Single-dose therapy is not recommended in children. Though the cure rate at 48 h is comparable to conventional therapy, the recurrence rate at 10 days appears to be unacceptably high.

### Prophylaxis

Continued antibiotic prophylaxis following treatment is recommended in children with recurrent UTI, children under 5 to 7 years of age with VUR, and children awaiting radiologic evaluation following a first UTI. A single nightly dose of TMP/SMX (1 to 2 mg/kg TMP, 5 to 10 mg/kg SMX) is effective. Asymptomatic bacteriuria does not require treatment in the child with a radiologically normal urinary tract.

### Follow-Up

Children with UTI should be seen within 48 h to assess the clinical response. Routine culture at this time is of questionable value. Additional cultures should be done following cessation of therapy to exclude persistent bacteriuria or recurrence. The risk of recurrence after the first infection is 30 percent and increases to 75 percent in children with three or more previous infections. Children with a documented UTI need periodic examination and culture of the urine.

## Radiologic Evaluation

The majority of children should have radiologic evaluation of the urinary tract system within 2 to 4 weeks following the first documented UTI. Specifically this includes all children under 5 years of age, all boys, and all school-age girls with recurrent infection. The goals of radiographic evaluation are to diagnose structural abnormalities of the urinary tract system, to determine the presence and severity of VUR, and to assess the renal parenchyma for scarring.

Voiding cystourethrography (VCUG) and ultrasonography are currently recommended for initial screening. VCUG is done initially to evaluate VUR and to delineate structural abnormalities of the lower urinary tract. Ultrasonography can delineate structural abnormalities of the upper tract but provides no functional information. If either test is abnormal, further testing to identify renal cortical involvement is necessary. Intravenous pyelography has been the standard test for evaluation of the upper urinary tract and to detect renal scars; nuclear renal scanning (renal cortical scintigraphy) provides the same information and may be of value in the diagnosis of acute pyelonephritis.

## PEDIATRIC VULVOVAGINITIS

### Pathophysiology

Vulvovaginitis is a common problem in females of all ages. Estrogen effects are a major determinant of susceptibility to vulvovaginitis; therefore, the likely causes vary with physiologic age and stage of pubertal development. The neonate shows the effects of intrauterine maternal estrogen stimulation. In the prepubertal girl, unestrogenized vulvar skin is thin, easily inflamed, and unprotected by the adult labial fat pads and pubic hair. The vulva is vulnerable to trauma, contact irritants, and bacterial contamination from both proximity to the anus and typical childhood hygiene. Puberty moves the spectrum of vulvovaginitis towards infections that prefer estrogenized vaginal epithelium. The causes of vulvovaginitis in adolescent girls are similar

to those of adult women and are likewise effected by sexual experience. This section focuses on vulvovaginitis in prepubertal and peripubertal girls; the diagnosis and treatment of adult vulvovaginitis (Chap. 97) and sexually transmitted disease (Chap. 120) apply to sexually active adolescents and are not reviewed here. Table 111-1 lists the causes of pediatric vulvovaginitis.

## Clinical Features

Vulvar inflammation can cause redness, itching, and burning. Squirming and an awkward walk may be seen in younger children. Dysuria is a common symptom and more often caused by vulvovaginitis than by UTI. A complaint of vaginal discharge suggests a specific infectious etiology, though a persistent, foul, or bloody discharge also occurs with retained foreign bodies. On examination, inflammation of the vulva and distal vagina should be distinguished from a primary vaginitis without prominent vulvar symptoms.

## Diagnosis by Age and Pubertal Status

### The Infant

A physiologic vaginal discharge commonly occurs in newborn girls during the first 2 weeks of life due to intrauterine estrogen stimulation. The discharge may become slightly bloody secondary to maternal estrogen withdrawal. During this time, the infant's estrogenized vagina is also susceptible to candidiasis and less commonly to trichomoniasis, which are acquired from the mother during vaginal delivery. *Trichomonas* may rarely cause a persistent urethritis or vaginitis after estrogen levels decrease. Vaginal or rectal infection with *C. trachomatis* may also be acquired perinatally, though most children are culture negative by 18 months of age. Maternally transmitted condyloma may appear up to 1 year of age and generally resolve without treatment.

### The Prepubertal Girl

#### Approach to the Child

The general appearance, hygiene, and pubertal stage according to Tanner classification should be noted, and the child examined for signs of systemic illness and dermatologic disorders. Thorough inspection of the perineum and external genitals provides sufficient examination for most children with symptoms of vulvovaginitis. Young

**Table 111-1.** Causes of Pediatric Vulvovaginitis

Vulvitis and nonspecific inflammation
    Nonspecific vulvovaginitis: poor hygiene, local irritants
    *Enterobius vermicularis* (pinworms)
    *Candida albicans* and other yeasts
Vaginal infections
    Respiratory: group A and B *Streptococcus, Streptococcus pneumoniae, Neisseria meningitidis, Haemophilus influenzae**
    Skin: *Staphylococcus aureus**
    Enteric: *Shigella, Yersinia, Escherichia coli**
Sexually transmitted infections
    Vaginitis: *Neisseria gonorrhoea, Chlamydia trachomatis, Trichomonas vaginalis, Gardnerella vaginalis**
    Vulvitis: Condylomata acuminata, herpes simplex
Vulvar skin disease and systemic illness
    Childhood exanthems: measles, chicken pox, scarlet fever
    Generalized skin disorders: seborrheic and atopic dermatitis
    Infestations: scabies, pediculosis, molluscum contagiosum
Noninfectious causes
    Trauma
    Sexual abuse
    Foreign body: toilet paper wads, tampons
    Structural anomalies of the genitourinary tract

* Can be found as normal vaginal flora in asymptomatic children.

girls may be more comfortably examined while sitting on their parent's lap with their legs placed outside the parent's legs. The child's perineum is then easily exposed by having the parent recline slightly and spread their own legs. The perineal skin, perianal area, labia majora and minora, and periurethral area are observed for signs of inflammation and trauma. The hymen and distal vagina are inspected by outward traction on the posterior labia majora. Signs of sexual abuse should be specifically looked for, and the shape, width, and any irregularities of the hymen noted. If sexual abuse is suspected or vaginal discharge is present, specimens should be collected for microscopic examination and cultures; however, a discharge is found in only half the children with this complaint. Specimens are collected by gentle swabbing with a saline-moistened calcium alginate swab, which is smaller and less abrasive than cotton swabs. Aspiration of vaginal secretions for culture is often better tolerated than swabbing and can be aided by instilling a few drops of nonbacteriostatic saline. The cooperative child should be further examined in a prone knee-chest position, which allows visualization of the upper vagina and often the cervix. Vaginoscopy is indicated acutely for vaginal bleeding, suspicion of foreign body, and trauma. Vaginoscopy for persistent symptoms following treatment may be referred to the pediatric gynecologist. Bimanual abdominal rectal examination is helpful to assess for masses or foreign bodies and to milk any discharge from the vagina.

### Vulvitis

#### Nonspecific Vulvovaginitis

Nonspecific vulvovaginitis, the most common condition in the prepubertal age group, is defined by lack of any identifiable pathogen or etiology. On examination, the vulva is erythematous and swollen with secondary inflammation of the distal vagina. Discharge is usually scanty. Excoriations and, in severe cases, ulcerations may be present. Cultures, when done, grow mixed vaginal and enteric flora. Multiple factors contribute to inflammation of the vulva. Management consists of eliminating local and chemical irritants and improving hygiene by the use of absorbent cotton underpants, loose clothing, bland soaps, front-to-rear wiping after bowel movements, and handwashing. For severe inflammation, cool sitz baths or wet compresses will provide relief within 2 to 3 days. Amoxicillin may be tried for cases that persist after 3 to 4 weeks of conservative therapy.

#### Enterobius vermicularis

*Enterobius vermicularis* should be routinely tested for in girls with vulvitis since 20 percent of infestations have an associated vulvovaginitis characterized by prominent nocturnal itching. Treatment is a single mebendazole chewable tablet (100 mg) administered to the affected child and all household members; treatment is repeated in 2 weeks.

#### Candidiasis

Candidiasis is far less common than nonspecific vulvovaginitis in prepubertal girls, and antifungal treatment should be based only on microscopic diagnosis. Factors associated with prepubertal candidiasis include recent antibiotic therapy, diabetes mellitus, underlying skin disorders, and exogenous estrogen exposure.

### Specific Vaginal Infections

#### Respiratory and Enteric Pathogens

Respiratory and enteric pathogens develop primarily or concurrently with infection at another site. Transmission occurs through autoinoculation, and handwashing should be stressed for treatment and prevention. A bloody discharge suggests *Shigella* or group A *Streptococcus;* both can occur without signs of infection at another site. Diagnosis is by culture, and treatment is an antibiotic appropriate to the organism.

#### Foreign Bodies

Foreign bodies, most commonly wads of toilet paper, also cause a persistent, foul, or bloody discharge and are found in 4 percent of symptomatic children. Vaginoscopy is required for diagnosis and to assure complete removal.

#### Candida, Trichomonas, and Gardnerella vaginalis

*Candida, Trichomonas,* and *Gardnerella vaginalis,* the three primary causes of vaginitis in adults, are all unusual in prepubertal girls because the unestrogenized vaginal epithelium is relatively resistant to these organisms. Typical clinical and microscopic features are usually adequate for diagnosis; unclear or persistent cases may require culture.

### Sexually Transmitted Infections

#### Prepubertal Gonorrhea

Prepubertal gonorrhea presents as a vaginitis rather than the endocervicitis typical past puberty. The primary symptoms are dysuria, purulent vaginal discharge, and, less commonly, abdominal pain. Culture is mandatory for diagnosis and documentation since nongonococcal *Neisseria* can also cause infection. Asymptomatic infection is usual and has been found in one-third of children residing in the household of an infected child. In culture-proven gonorrhea, all household members should have cultures of the vagina (urethra in boys), rectum, and pharynx.

#### Other STDs

*Gonorrhea, Chlamydia, Trichomonas,* genital herpes, and condylomata acuminata usually indicate sexual contact. *Gardnerella* can be cultured from asymptomatic girls, but symptomatic infection is found more commonly in girls who report sexual abuse. Though nonsexual transmission of most sexually transmitted pathogens has been suggested, their presence should prompt a thorough investigation into possible sexual abuse of the child.

## The Peripubertal Girl

Pubertal girls and adolescents are more likely than younger girls to have an infectious cause for vulvovaginitis, though nonspecific cases and retained foreign bodies also occur in this age group. The onset of sexual activity increases the incidence of sexually transmitted infections and the occurrence of pelvic inflammatory disease. A speculum examination should be performed in most adolescents; it may be omitted in the young virginal girl with physiologic discharge or candidiasis. Bimanual examination is necessary to assess for pelvic tenderness. The examination offers a good opportunity to discuss proper hygiene, the virtues of safe sexual practices, and contraception.

### Physiologic Vaginal Discharge

The onset of pubertal estrogenic influence precedes menarche by up to a year; the timing corresponds roughly to breast bud development. Estrogen results in a physiologic discharge, often termed *leukorrhea,* which is composed of mucus and normal vaginal epithelial cells without leukocytes. The discharge is mucoid or gray-white, odorless, and generally nonirritating. The amount increases prior to menarche, and minor irritation can result from copious discharge, especially if nonabsorbent underpants are worn. Yellow staining of the underpants, a common complaint, is due to the protein content, which discolors when heated during washing. No treatment is necessary, but reassurance should be given that this is a healthy sign of puberty and absorbent cotton underpants advised if the discharge is copious or irritating.

### Vaginitis and Sexually Transmitted Disease

Candidiasis occurs in the pubertal girl both before and after menarche and is the most common cause of pruritic vulvovaginitis in premenarchal pubertal girls. *G. vaginalis* deserves mention because it is found in the normal vaginal flora of asymptomatic girls. A diagnosis of bacterial vaginosis associated with *G. vaginalis* is reserved for symptomatic patients and requires a gray-white vaginal discharge with a characteristic fishy odor (positive "whiff" test when KOH is added) in addition to clue cells on microscopic examination. Asymptomatic patients do not require treatment. Both bacterial vaginosis and *Trichomonas* are suggestive of sexual activity, so that any adolescent with *Trichomonas* or bacterial vaginosis should also have cultures for gonorrhea and *Chlamydia*.

## Treatment

### Emergency Department Care

The management of any girl with vulvar complaints should include instruction on general hygienic measures covered in the section on nonspecific vulvovaginitis. Conservative therapy will result in improvement in the vast majority of children. Specific infections are additionally treated with an antibiotic appropriate to the organism cultured.

Sexually transmitted infections should be treated in accordance with the current guidelines provided by the Centers for Disease Control and Prevention. In general, adolescents and children weighing over 40 kilograms are treated with adult regimens. Children under 8 years of age with culture-proven *C. trachomatis* should be treated with erythromycin, 50 mg/kg per day for 10 days. Older children may receive a standard course of doxycycline. All children with suspected or proven STD should be referred for further evaluation of sexual abuse.

## BIBLIOGRAPHY

### Urinary Tract Infections

Andrich MP, Majd M: Diagnostic imaging in the evaluation of the first urinary tract infection in infants and young children. *Pediatrics* 90:436, 1992.

Lohr JA, Portilla MG, Geuder TG: Making a presumptive diagnosis of urinary tract infection by using a urinalysis performed in an on-site laboratory. *J Pediatr* 122:22, 1993.

Schlager TA, Lohr JA: Urinary tract infection in outpatient febrile infants and children younger than 5 years of age. *Pediatr Ann* 22:505, 1993.

Zelikovic I, Adelman RD, Nancarrow PA: Urinary tract infections in children. An update. *West J Med* 157:554, 1992.

### Pediatric Vulvovaginitis

Jenny C: Sexually transmitted diseases and child abuse. *Pediatr Ann* 21:497, 1992.

Pokorny SF: Prepubertal vulvovaginopathies. *Obstet Gynecol Clin North Am* 19:39, 1992.

Vandeven AM, Emans SJ: Vulvovaginitis in the child and adolescent. *Pediatr Rev* 14:141, 1993.

# 112
# ASTHMA AND BRONCHIOLITIS
## Stanley H. Inkelis

## ASTHMA

Asthma is a disorder of the tracheobronchial tree characterized by bronchial hyperirritability and airway inflammation with subsequent obstruction to airflow after exposure to any one of many stimuli. Examples of these stimuli include extrinsic allergens, viral respiratory infections, vigorous exercise, cold air, cigarette smoke, and air pollutants. Narrowing of the airways is dynamic and improves either spontaneously or as a result of therapy. The symptom that is most characteristic of asthma is wheezing. However, the often-quoted statement, "all that wheezes is not asthma," is certainly true and emphasizes the importance of the differential diagnosis which will be addressed later in this chapter. Asthma may occur, on the other hand, without evidence of overt wheezing and is often missed in children who are diagnosed as having recurrent pneumonia, recurrent or chronic bronchitis, or recurrent colds with chest congestion. Because misdiagnosis and undertreatment occur frequently, some authors feel that a more appropriate statement may be, "most things that wheeze, plus some things that do not, are asthma."

## Epidemiology

Asthma is one of the leading causes of chronic illness in children, with a prevalence rate of nearly 10 percent. This prevalence rate is increasing, as evidenced by a 29 percent rise from 1980 to 1987. The severity of asthma also appears to be increasing. From 1979 to 1987, there was a 4.5 percent per year increase in hospital admissions in children less than 18 years of age. The greatest increase occurred in children less than 5 years old, particularly in African-American children in this age group.

In a group of 100 patients with status asthmaticus admitted to a children's hospital between February and June 1988, demographic data indicated that these patients tended more often to be young, male, and African-American than did other patients admitted to the same hospital. Forty-five percent of these patients also had sinusitis, otitis, or pneumonitis. Although there was no increase in mortality in asthmatic patients in this study, many others have reported an increase in the number of deaths from asthma over similar time periods. For example, the death rate from 1980 to 1987 increased by 31 percent. Children at risk of dying from asthma are those who (1) have been intubated for asthma; (2) have had two or more hospitalizations for asthma in the past year; (3) have had three or more emergency department visits for asthma in the past year; (4) have had an emergency department visit or hospitalization for asthma in the past month; (5) have a past history of syncope or hypoxic seizure related to an asthma exacerbation, (6) are dependent on glucocorticoids or recently withdrew from them, (7) have increased use of β agonists, (8) are of lower socioeconomic status with poor access to health care, especially those of this group who are African-American, and/or (9) have psychosocial issues that may prevent delivery of care.

In children dying of asthma, the assessment of the severity of their illness by both patient and physician is often inadequate. In addition, compliance with medication schedules is poor in these patients, and there is frequently a delay in the initiation of therapy for progressively worsening illness.

Children who have had near-fatal episodes of asthma need appropriate treatment to maximize their lung function. In addition, they need careful monitoring and adjustment of medications to prevent acute exacerbations. Children who are old enough should monitor their peak expiratory flow at home and be given specific instructions to increase their treatment and summon help if there is a decrease in their peak expiratory flow rate of more than 30 percent. Those children with asthma and concomitant psychological disturbance should be referred to a therapist for counseling.

Although there has been an increase in morbidity and mortality in recent years, the prognosis for asthmatic children in general is very good. About half of these children will be free of symptoms by the time they are adults.

## Etiology

The etiology of asthma is multifactorial. Immunologic, infectious, endocrine, and psychological factors play a role in the development of asthma in different individuals. Rather than being one disease, asthma may, in fact, be a number of diseases that have in common the physiologic finding of reversible obstructive airway changes.

Asthma has been categorized as *extrinsic* (atopic or IgE-mediated), *intrinsic* (not IgE-mediated, usually triggered by infection), and *mixed* (IgE- and infection-induced). These distinctions are probably artificial since both allergic and nonallergic groups have almost identical immune mediator–induced mucosal injury from similar stimuli. Moreover, Burrows et al., in a recent study, found a strong association across all age groups between the prevalence of asthma and serum IgE levels, suggesting that asthma is almost always associated with an IgE-related reaction and therefore has an allergic basis. Based on this information and that of others, it is more useful to categorize asthma according to "triggers" that set off an attack than to use the aforementioned classifications.

Viral respiratory infection is the most common precipitant of asthma in children younger than 2 years of age. These infections are most commonly caused by respiratory syncytial virus (RSV), rhinovirus, parainfluenza, and influenza viruses. Viral infections cause airway inflammation, increase bronchial hyperreactivity, and may decrease β-adrenergic receptor function. Although bacterial infections are not usually associated with wheezing in children, sinusitis often causes exacerbation of asthma and, when treated, results in improvement of the asthma. *Mycoplasma pneumoniae* infections often cause wheezing. *Chlamydia pneumoniae* has also been recently reported as a cause of wheezing in children.

Allergens are the most important trigger of asthma in children older than 2 years of age. The dust mite is the most common allergen provoking an asthmatic exacerbation, followed by the aeroallergen, *alternaria,* and cats. Pollens, dander, molds, and foods also cause bronchial hyperirritability.

Exercise-induced asthma (EIA) is seen in nearly 100 percent of children with asthma. It may also be the only manifestation of asthma in some children, especially those with allergic rhinitis. There is no relationship between the degree of EIA and the severity of asthma, and the response to exercise in an individual child may be variable. The type of exercise influences the extent of the airway obstruction. For example, running causes more severe symptoms than bicycling, whereas swimming rarely causes bronchial hyperactivity. As ventilation increases with exercise, airways are cooled by the loss of water to the relatively dry air. It is postulated that mast cells respond to this cooling by releasing mediators that induce bronchoconstriction.

Irritants such as cigarette smoke, smoke from burning wood, and air pollution also trigger asthma. Parental smoking of tobacco increases airway responsiveness in early infancy and over time affects lung growth and function.

Other triggers of asthma include gastroesophageal reflux, drugs such as aspirin, nonsteroidal anti-inflammatory medications, β-blocking medications, food additives and sulfites, endocrine factors, weather, and psychological factors. A careful history should be obtained to evaluate possible triggers of asthma in children.

## Pathophysiology

Most of the information available regarding the pathology of asthma comes from postmortem examination. The lungs are hyperinflated and pale and are difficult to collapse with pressure. Numerous tenacious mucous plugs exude from the larger and middle-sized bronchi. On microscopic examination, sloughing of mucosal cells, edema of the bronchial mucosa, and hyperplasia and hypertrophy of bronchial and bronchiolar smooth muscle are seen. Often, there is infiltration of the submucosa by eosinophils. All of these factors lead to airway obstruction, which is thought to be initiated by a series of inflammatory events in the airway.

In the past, bronchial smooth muscle hyperreactivity has been considered the main reason for the pathologic findings associated with asthma. Hyperreactive airways play a major role in the pathology of the asthmatic patient, particularly in the new-onset asthmatic or in the early phase of an asthmatic attack. Bronchial smooth muscle hyperreactivity is characteristic of this disease. The smooth muscle lining of the respiratory tract is under autonomic control, with sympathetic fibers causing bronchodilation (β$_2$ receptors) and parasympathetic fibers causing bronchoconstriction. The exact cause of airway hyperreactivity is unknown. In addition to neurogenic factors and changes in intrinsic airway smooth muscle responsivity, recent evidence suggests that all asthmatic patients have airway inflammation, including those with mild asthma, indicating that inflammation plays a key role in airway hyperresponsiveness. Moreover, patients who are treated for airway inflammation appear to have less airway hyperresponsiveness. Certainly, in patients with chronic asthma, inflammation of the airways plays an equal or greater role in the pathologic changes. Biopsies of bronchial tissue as well as bronchoalveolar lavage have demonstrated an increased proportion of inflammatory cells, particularly eosinophils and lymphocytes.

The eosinophil is the inflammatory cell most characteristic of asthma. These cells release proteins that are toxic to airway epithelial cells. The most cytotoxic of these proteins are major basic protein and eosinophil cationic protein. In one study, the number of peripheral blood eosinophils and levels of eosinophils and eosinophil cationic protein in bronchoalveolar lavage fluid correlated with the severity of asthma. In addition, intraepithelial eosinophils were present only in patients with asthma.

Neutrophil infiltration is not commonly found in asthmatic patients. T lymphocytes are commonly found in the airways of asthmatic patients, and there is strong evidence that they play an important role in generating airway inflammation. For example, mediators released from T lymphocytes may affect the eosinophils and their function in airway inflammation.

Numerous inflammatory mediators contribute to pathologic findings in the asthmatic patient. IgE-sensitized mast cells, which are antigenically stimulated, begin a reaction that results in the release of preformed mediators, including histamine, chemotactic factors, proteases, and platelet-activation factor (PAF). Metabolism of membrane phospholipids is also activated to release arachidonic acid, which is metabolized to form the generated mediators, leukotrienes, thromboxanes, and prostaglandins. These mediators are responsible for bronchial hyperreactivity, edema, and mucus formation as well as chemotaxis for other inflammatory cells, which release more mediators and continue the inflammatory process. Macrophages and epithelial cells also play a role in mediator release.

The early phase of an asthmatic attack is characterized by bronchoconstriction secondary to release of histamines and leukotrienes. Chemotactic factors, PAF, and other mediators bring on inflammatory cells, which cause the late phase of an asthmatic attack. This phase begins 2 to 8 h later and is characterized by airway hyperreactivity lasting for days to weeks.

The combination of mucosal edema, bronchospasm, and mucous

plugging results in airway obstruction which leads to increased airway resistance and gas trapping. Varying degrees of obstruction, atelectasis, and decreased compliance cause ventilation-perfusion mismatch. Hypoxia occurs because of perfusion of inadequately ventilated portions of the lung. Early in severe asthma, carbon dioxide tensions are usually below normal because of compensatory hyperventilation. As the obstruction increases, the number of alveoli being adequately ventilated and perfused decreases, giving rise to $CO_2$ retention. A "normal" $P_{CO_2}$ of 40 mmHg in the setting of asthma may be an indication of respiratory muscle fatigue and impending respiratory failure.

Acidosis results from both hypoxia and hypercapnia. Along with hypoxia, acidosis leads to pulmonary vasoconstriction, pulmonary hypertension, right heart strain, and, occasionally, cardiac failure.

Infants with asthma have more severe respiratory symptoms and are more vulnerable to respiratory failure. The anatomic and physiologic reasons for this are (1) increased peripheral airway resistance, (2) decreased elastic recoil pressure and early airway closure, (3) deficient collateral channels of ventilation, and (4) an unstable rib cage and mechanically disadvantaged diaphragm.

## Clinical Features

Wheezing is the hallmark of asthma and is present in almost every child presenting to the emergency department with this disorder. The notable exceptions to this are (1) the child who is in extreme respiratory distress and is so "tight" that there is not enough movement of air to produce audible wheezing and (2) the child who has a persistent nonproductive cough or who coughs and becomes short of breath with exercise. In the latter case, many of the patients will have findings characteristic of asthma on pulmonary function testing and will respond to bronchodilator therapy.

Attacks of asthma may be acute or may be of gradual onset. Exposure to allergens or bronchial irritants causes the acute attack of asthma which is due to spasm and inflammation of the small and medium airways. Viral upper respiratory infections usually cause attacks of slower onset with a gradual increase in frequency and severity of cough and wheezing over a few days.

Other signs and symptoms in addition to wheezing and cough associated with asthma include tachypnea, shortness of breath with prolonged expiration and use of accessory muscles of respiration, cyanosis, hyperinflation of the chest, tachycardia, abdominal pain, a feeling of "tight chest," poor exercise tolerance, "recurrent chest colds," "recurrent" or "chronic" bronchitis, or "recurrent pneumonia."

## History

A brief, well-directed history focusing on the exacerbation should be obtained. The following questions should be asked:

When did the wheezing begin?
How bad is it? Is it getting worse?
What medications is the child taking?
Does the child take the medications all the time or only with an acute attack?
When was the last dose taken?
Has there been any improvement with the medications?
Has the child ever been on steroids?
Has the child been in the emergency room before?
Hospitalized before? How long ago and when admitted?
What was the response to hospitalization?
Was the child in an intensive care unit?
Has the child ever lost consciousness or been intubated or on a ventilator due to asthma?
Does the child have a cold, cough, fever?
Are there any suspected triggers that may have set off this attack?

## Physical Examination

On physical examination the chest is hyperinflated and hyperresonant to percussion. A barrel chest deformity suggests chronic, severe asthma. Expiratory wheezes are prominent; occasionally inspiratory wheezes will be heard as well. Musical rales may be present. The child usually is restless with tachypnea and tachycardia and may, if severely obstructed have significant accessory muscle use, including severe intercostal and tracheosternal retractions with nasal flaring. The child's overall alertness may be diminished. If the child is in extreme respiratory distress, wheezing may be absent, as noted above. To make breathing easier, the child may assume a hunched-over, tripod-like sitting position. Cyanosis may be apparent. Pulsus paradoxus may be present and will increase as airway obstruction increases. If there is a fall in systolic blood pressure of >20 mmHg during inspiration, moderate to severe obstruction is present. However, it is often difficult to assess pulsus paradoxus because of the rapid heart rate in children. The liver and spleen may be palpable because of hyperinflation of the lungs and downward movement of the diaphragm. Successful treatment will produce color improvement and wheezing as air begins to move through the lungs.

## Laboratory and X-ray Findings

Most asthmatic children have normal blood counts; however, an elevated white blood cell count does not necessarily indicate infection. Both the "stress" of an acute asthma attack and the injection of epinephrine may cause leukocytosis. Blood eosinophilia above 250 to 400 cells/mm$^3$ is common in asthmatic children, with the total eosinophil count being preferred to estimation from differential white counts. Eosinophils in the sputum and nasal secretions are usually present, as well. Sputum cultures are not very helpful in children. Polymorphonuclear leukocytes and bacteria on a nasal smear in an allergic child are suggestive of sinusitis.

A chest x-ray should be taken on every child under 1 year of age with the first episode of wheezing or a history of persistent symptoms of asthma, such as "chronic cough" or "chronic bronchitis" (if no x-ray was taken previously) to rule out foreign body aspiration, heart disease, parenchymal disease, and congenital anomaly.

Strong consideration should be given to obtaining a chest x-ray in children over 1 year of age with a first wheezing episode. However, the need for an x-ray in children over 1 year of age with first episodes of wheezing is controversial. The results of one study of 371 children over 1 year of age presenting with their first episode of wheezing suggest that routine chest x-rays in children of this age are not necessary since evaluation of vital signs [respiratory rate $\geq$60, pulse $\geq$160, and/or temperature $\geq$38.3°C (100.9°F)] and pretreatment auscultation (localized rales and/or localized decreased breath sounds) provide sufficient information to reveal which patients will have abnormal radiographic findings that might influence therapeutic decisions. Vital signs and auscultatory findings noted above are helpful in determining which children need chest x-rays. Children who fail to respond to therapy, have increasing respiratory distress, or who are clinically suspected of having a wheezing illness other than asthma should also have a chest x-ray taken. Although the chest x-ray may be normal in an acute attack of asthma, the lungs are usually hyperinflated with flattening of the diaphragms and increased bronchial markings. The AP diameter is increased on lateral view. In addition, there may be patchy areas of infiltrate or atelectasis and, less commonly, pneumomediastinum and pneumothorax. Routine chest x-ray is not necessary, however, for the known asthmatic with an uncomplicated attack.

Pulmonary function tests are useful determinants of response to therapy in the asthmatic child. The forced expiratory volume ($FEV_1$) or peak expiratory flow rate (PEFR) are the most reliable measurements of the degree of airway obstruction. The $FEV_1$ is the volume of air expired in 1 s from maximum inspiration. The spirometer measures $FEV_1$ and may be used in most children aged 6 and older with some coaching. The PEFR is the maximum flow rate that can be obtained during a forced expiration starting with full inflation of the lungs (total lung capacity). The peak flow meter measures PEFR and may be used for some coordinated 2- and 3-year-old children but, because the test is so effort-dependent, it usually is more reliable for children 5 years of age or older. Because the $FEV_1$ correlates well with the PEFR, many physicians have chosen to use peak flow meters for adults as well as children. Some studies suggest that subjective measurements, such as those for dyspnea and wheezing, by physicians and patients may be inaccurate. In addition, by the time wheezing is detected with a stethoscope, the PEFR is already decreased by 25 percent or more. Consequently, measurements of the PEFR in those children who are able to perform the test in conjunction with clinical evaluation is very helpful in identifying patients needing admission or close outpatient follow-up. Predicted PEFR values (liters/min) for normal children are based on height (Table 112-1). In some cases where a peak flow meter is used at home, the child may have a "personal best" PEFR taken during a well period. A PEFR of ≥90 percent of the predicted value or personal best is considered normal, <80 percent is abnormal, and <50 percent indicates severe obstruction. If the PEFR is less than 60 percent of the predicted level after aggressive emergency department therapy, admission should be strongly considered since these patients are more likely to fail outpatient therapy. In patients with a PEFR of less than 25 percent of predicted, hypercarbia is likely. Rapid and aggressive treatment is indicated, and admission is warranted. Selected patients with poor PEFRs may be treated as outpatients if close, frequent follow-up can be arranged or if a holding area is available.

Pulse oximetry is a useful noninvasive method of following a child's oxygen saturation ($Sa_{O_2}$). It limits the necessity of measuring arterial blood gases (ABGs) to titrate and taper oxygen therapy. Since hypoxia commonly occurs in asthmatic patients, often with limited clinical manifestations, all patients with asthma should have their $Sa_{O_2}$ measured with a pulse oximeter on presentation to the emergency department and then monitored periodically while receiving treatment. Those children with severe asthma should be monitored continuously. An initial $Sa_{O_2}$ of 91 percent or less helps predict which children will have a poor outcome (admission to the hospital or relapse necessitating a return visit to the emergency department). Peak expiratory flow rate and initial $Sa_{O_2}$ are useful in determining the severity of an acute asthmatic attack, but the initial $Sa_{O_2}$ may be a better predictor of outcome in those not initially admitted to the hospital.

Arterial blood gases are indicated in the severely ill asthmatic child who does not respond to bronchodilator therapy and/or in whom

**Table 112-1.** Predicted Average Peak Expiratory Flow for Normal Children and Adolescents, Male and Female

| Height, in | L/min | Height, in | L/min |
|---|---|---|---|
| 43 | 147 | 56 | 320 |
| 44 | 160 | 57 | 334 |
| 45 | 173 | 58 | 347 |
| 46 | 187 | 59 | 360 |
| 47 | 200 | 60 | 373 |
| 48 | 214 | 61 | 387 |
| 49 | 227 | 62 | 400 |
| 50 | 240 | 63 | 413 |
| 51 | 254 | 64 | 427 |
| 52 | 267 | 65 | 440 |
| 53 | 280 | 66 | 454 |
| 54 | 293 | 67 | 467 |
| 55 | 307 | | |

*Source:* From Polger G, Promedhat V: *Pulmonary Function Testing in Children: Techniques and Standards.* Philadelphia, Saunders, 1971.

**Table 112-2.** Differential Diagnosis of Wheezing

| | |
|---|---|
| Asthma | Cystic fibrosis |
| Bronchiolitis | Heart disease |
| Foreign body aspiration | Vascular ring |
| Pneumonitis | Tracheoesophageal fistula |
|   Viral | Stenosis: tracheal and bronchial |
|   *Mycoplasma pneumoniae* | $\alpha_1$-antitrypsin deficiency |
|   *Chlamydia pneumoniae* | Bronchiectasis |
|   Chemical | Mechanical obstruction |
|   Hypersensitivity |   Lymph gland enlargement |
| Croup |   Neoplasm |
| Epiglottitis |   Bronchogenic cysts |
| Anaphylaxis | |
| Gastroesophageal reflux | |

hypercarbia is suspected. ABGs should be obtained from the radial or brachial artery in children. They are not indicated in the child with uncomplicated asthma. Measurement of a PEFR less than 25 percent of the predicted level is helpful in determining which children are hypercarbic and therefore need arterial blood gas monitoring. Unfortunately, the PEFR is difficult to obtain in small children, and the need for a blood gas must be based on the clinical severity. The $P_{CO_2}$, which is usually low during the early part of an asthmatic attack, begins to rise as the obstruction increases. When the $P_{CO_2}$ is >35 mmHg, it is an indication for concern, and blood gases should be monitored frequently. The blood pH usually remains normal until the buffering capacity of the blood is superseded.

## Differential Diagnosis

Although most children who wheeze have asthma, there are many other etiologies that should be considered before the child is given the diagnosis of asthma. Early in the course of a wheezing illness, the definitive diagnosis is difficult to determine. A thorough history, complete physical examination, and, often, response to therapy help in differentiating other illnesses from asthma (Table 112-2).

Bronchiolitis and infantile asthma are very similar in their clinical presentation, and their differentiation provides a challenge for even the best of clinicians. In fact, in some situations, it may be impossible to clinically differentiate between the two. The most important differential clue to infantile asthma is a history of recurrent episodes of wheezing and/or coughing in an infant, regardless of age. Other clinical features suggesting asthma are a postive family history of asthma or allergy, physical evidence of atopic disease in the patient, sudden onset of wheezing without preceding infection, markedly prolonged expiration, and rapid reversibility of bronchospasm with sympathomimetic therapy.

Acute bronchiolitis usually occurs in children between 2 and 6 months of age (but may occur until age 2 years) in the winter and spring months. There are often other family members with an upper respiratory infection (URI) and the infant's illness begins with signs of a URI. There is usually no history of associated atopic disease in the patient or family.

Some physicians are reluctant to diagnose asthma in a child less than 1 year of age and label children who have recurrent episodes of coughing and wheezing with diagnoses such as asthmatic bronchitis, wheezy bronchitis, and recurrent bronchiolitis. There is good evidence, however, that approximately 30 percent of children with asthma are symptomatic in their first year of life. Since acute viral bronchiolitis is rarely a recurrent condition, infants with recurrent attacks (three or more episodes of "bronchiolitis") should be considered asthmatic and treated as such.

The relationship between bronchiolitis and the subsequent development of asthma is very intriguing. Considering that 25 to 50 percent of children with bronchiolitis develop asthma later in life, bronchiolitis may constitute the first attack of asthma in these children. It is not clear whether the airways of some children are genetically hyperactive, thus predisposing them to bronchiolitis, or the first viral infection and resultant epithelial damage sensitize irritant receptors and lead to hyperactive airways.

It is known that respiratory syncytial virus (RSV) and other viruses are potent stimulants of wheezing in the individual prone to asthma. This suggests that bronchiolitis may be the first attack of asthma in the atopic child and that these children may be more likely to wheeze if infected with RSV or other viruses. A recent study determined that infants with diminished lung function before the age of 6 months and prior to any lower respiratory illness were more likely to have a wheezing lower respiratory illness in their first year of life than those infants with normal lung function.

In most patients with RSV infection of any kind, IgE is bound to exfoliated nasopharyngeal epithelial cells. The persistence of cell-bound IgE in patients with RSV-induced bronchiolitis or asthma, in contrast to those patients with mild upper respiratory tract infection or pneumonia from RSV, may explain the recurrent episodes of wheezing that occur in infants after RSV-induced bronchiolitis. Other studies have demonstrated pulmonary function abnormalities in symptom-free children years after their episode of bronchiolitis, indicating that these children are left with residual parenchymal or airway lesions that may predispose them to chronic obstructive lung disease. Mild bronchiolitis, on the other hand, does not seem to be associated with abnormal pulmonary function. It is probable that environment, genetic predisposition, and lung injury, either individually or in combination, play roles in the development of wheezing in children.

Infants with bronchopulmonary dysplasia often have hyperreactive airways and are more likely to have a positive family history of asthma. They are predisposed to developing bronchiolitis or asthma with respiratory infections. Infants with bronchopulmonary dysplasia may be identified by a previous history of prematurity complicated by the respiratory distress syndrome for which they required mechanical ventilation. Their chest x-rays show evidence of chronic lung disease not seen in the infant with wheezing due to bronchiolitis or asthma alone. These children often present with mild illness that rapidly progresses to severe respiratory distress with tachypnea and cyanosis. Occasionally, the cause of the wheezing and respiratory embarrassment in these children is from pulmonary edema and may present a confusing clinical picture.

Recurrent food aspiration from gastroesophageal reflux or tracheoesophageal fistula usually presents with a history of frequent vomiting after feeding and associated coughing and choking. Foreign bodies in the trachea, bronchus, or esophagus may be differentiated from bronchiolitis in that severe coughing, cyanosis, and respiratory distress usually develop suddenly in a well child who has recently been eating peanuts, popcorn, coins, seeds, etc. Often, the wheezing will be unilateral. A chest x-ray may identify the foreign body if it is radiopaque. If it is not, one may see hyperinflation on the affected side of an expiratory film. Since expiratory films are difficult to obtain in small children, bilateral, lateral decubitus films are very helpful. Normally, the dependent lung against the table will have less volume than the other lung because of its immobility. However, if a foreign body is present on the side closest to the table, air trapping persists and hyperinflation is evident.

Bronchial stenosis is commonly manifest by wheezing and recurrent lower respiratory infection. This disorder can be diagnosed by bronchoscopy.

Children with cystic fibrosis on initial presentation may be difficult to differentiate from those with bronchiolitis or asthma. If there is a history of recurrent wheezing, pneumonitis, and respiratory distress in an infant who is failing to thrive, one must strongly consider this diagnosis.

Congestive heart failure from congenital heart disease or viral myocarditis may present in a fashion similar to bronchiolitis or asthma, especially with a palpable liver and spleen confusing the issue. A history of normal growth and development and the absence of a heart murmur makes the diagnosis of bronchiolitis or asthma more likely. The chest x-ray in congestive heart failure will usually demonstrate a large heart. Infants with heart disease sometimes go into congestive heart failure with viral infections and may present with both conditions at once.

Vascular rings, mediastinal cysts, and tumors may compress the trachea or a bronchus. If one suspects a vascular ring but cannot see compression of the trachea on chest x-ray, a barium swallow may demonstrate constriction of the esophagus at the site of the ring. A mediastinal cyst or tumor will be apparent as a mass on chest x-ray.

Salicylate intoxication or other metabolic disorders may mimic bronchiolitis or asthma clinically because of the rapid respiratory rate. These disorders may be diagnosed by asking specifically about salicylate ingestion from aspirin or from other salicylate-containing products such as Pepto-Bismol, and by obtaining measurements of arterial blood gas, salicylate levels, and serum electrolytes, especially if no wheezing is present.

Pneumonitis, typically from infection with viruses, *M. pneumoniae*, or *C. pneumoniae*, or chemical pneumonitis from exposure to hydrocarbons may cause wheezing in children.

Croup, epiglottitis, and other causes of upper airway obstruction usually present with inspiratory wheezing (stridor) but rarely with expiratory wheezing. If there is doubt about the diagnosis, chest and lateral neck x-rays may be helpful. If one is seriously considering the diagnosis of epiglottitis, however, one should follow the hospital protocol for this disease and, above all, never leave the patient unattended by a physician, especially if the child is going for an x-ray.

## Treatment

### Theory

The treatment of asthma is aimed at decreasing smooth-muscle spasm (early phase) and airway inflammation (late phase). Smooth muscle spasm or bronchial hyperreactivity is assisted by increasing levels of cyclic AMP (cyclic adenosine 3′, 5′-cyclic phosphate) and is opposed by cyclic GMP (cyclic guanosine monophosphate). Elevation of cyclic AMP causes smooth muscle relaxation (bronchodilation) and may inhibit the release of mediators from airway mast cells, while elevation of cyclic GMP causes constriction of smooth muscle (bronchoconstriction). Sympathomimetics increase levels of cyclic AMP by activating the enzyme adenyl cyclase, which catalyzes ATP to cyclic AMP. Methylxanthines were originally thought to increase cyclic AMP by inhibiting the enzyme phosphodiesterase, which degrades cyclic AMP. Although there are a number of proposed theories, currently the mechanism of action of theophylline is unknown.

Sympathomimetic (adrenergic) agents, which are often the first-line medication used in the treatment of asthma, exert their activity by combining with receptors on cell surfaces. The two types of adrenergic receptors are $\alpha$ and $\beta$. Usually, drugs affecting $\alpha$-adrenergic receptors are associated with excitatory functions while drugs affecting $\beta$-adrenergic receptors are associated with inhibitory functions (e.g., muscle relaxation). Stimulation of $\alpha$-adrenergic receptors by agents such as norepinephrine decreases the amount of available cyclic AMP, and stimulation of $\beta$-adrenergic receptors increases the amount of available cyclic AMP. Consequently, adrenergic drugs which stimulate $\beta$ receptors are useful in treating the asthmatic patient. The $\beta$-adrenergic system has two groups of receptors: the $\beta_1$ receptors, which control heart rate, myocardial contractility, and lipolysis; and the $\beta_2$ receptors, which control bronchiolar and arteriolar dilatation. Therefore, adrenergic drugs with more $\beta_2$-selective activity, such as albuterol and terbutaline, affect bronchodilation without affecting an increase in heart rate and myocardial contractility that occur with epinephrine and isoproterenol, which stimulate both $\beta_1$ and $\beta_2$ receptors.

Levels of cyclic GMP are controlled by the parasympathetic nervous system. Vagal stimulation or cholinergic drugs increase produc-

**Table 112-3.** Estimation of Severity of Acute Exacerbations of Asthma in Children

| Sign/Symptom* | Mild | Moderate | Severe |
|---|---|---|---|
| Respiratory rate (see Table 112-4) | Normal to 30% increase above the mean | 30 to 50% increase above the mean | Increase over 50% above the mean |
| Alertness | Normal | Normal | May be decreased |
| Dyspnea† | Absent or mild; speaks in complete sentences | Moderate; speaks in phrases or partial sentences | Severe; speaks only in single words or short phrases |
| Pulsus paradoxus | <10 mmHg | 10–20 mmHg | 20–40 mmHg |
| Accessory muscle use | No intercostal to mild retractions | Moderate intercostal retraction with tracheosternal retractions; use of sternocleidomastoid muscles | Severe intercostal retractions, tracheosternal retractions with nasal flaring |
| Color | Good | Pale | Possibly cyanotic |
| Auscultation | End expiratory wheeze only | Wheeze during entire expiration and inspiration | Breath sounds becoming inaudible |
| Oxygen saturation | >95% | 90–95% | <90% |
| $P_{CO_2}$ | <35 mmHg | <40 mmHg | >40 mmHg |
| PEFR | 70–90% predicted or personal best | 50–70% predicted or personal best | <50% predicted or personal best |

*\* For discussion of these parameters, see text. Within each category, the presence of several parameters, but not necessarily all, indicates the general classification of the exacerbation.*

*† Parents or physician's impression of degree of child's breathlessness.*

*Source:* This table was adapted from the National Asthma Education Program (NAEP) Expert Panel Report, publication No. 91-3042.

tion of the enzyme guanylate cyclase, which increases the concentration of cyclic GMP. Atropine and other anticholinergic drugs block cholinergic (muscarinic) receptors. This prevents the binding of acetylcholine and decreases the availability of cyclic GMP. The side effects associated with atropine limit its use. Ipratropium bromide, a derivative of atropine, has minimal side effects and is becoming a much more used medication in the treatment of asthma.

Glucocorticoids and cromolyn sodium are agents used to treat the airway inflammation. The mechanism of action of glucocorticoids is not entirely understood, but it is known that they inhibit the release of mediators from macrophages and eosinophils. In addition, they reduce microvascular leakage, decrease the number of inflammatory cells coming to the lung by effecting the chemotactic response, reduce eosinophilia in the peripheral blood, and increase the number of β-adrenergic receptors available for response to β agonists. Cromolyn sodium appears to stabilize mast cells and prevent release of mediators.

## Emergency Department Care: Acute Exacerbations

The severity of acute asthma exacerbations should be assessed as quickly as possible, and treatment should be instituted accordingly. Initial evaluation should include a combination of parameters that are helpful in determining the severity of airway obstruction. These parameters include pulsus paradoxus, accessory muscle use, color, quality

of wheezing, oxygenation, and peak expiratory flow rate (Tables 112-3 and 112-4). Table 112-3 and most of the other tables in this chapter have been taken from the Expert Panel Report of the National Asthma Education Program of the National Heart, Lung, and Blood Institute, which developed *Guidelines for the Diagnosis and Management of Asthma*. This report was developed to enhance the early recognition of asthma, including early determination of disease severity, and to determine appropriate therapeutic interventions for asthma. In general, the following recommendations for care of the child with asthma is in agreement with these guidelines.

Most children presenting to the emergency room with asthma have an acute episode of airway obstruction that can be reversed relatively easily with bronchodilators. Nebulized β₂ agonists are the initial bronchodilators of choice (Fig. 112-1). They provide equal or better bronchodilation and fewer systemic side effects than parenteral therapy. The nebulized β₂ agonist most commonly used is albuterol (0.5% solution) because it has the most β₂ selectivity with the longest duration of action. It should be given at 0.15 mg/kg (0.03 mL/kg) to a maximum dose of 5 mg diluted in 3.0 mL of saline solution and administered every 20 min by nebulization for up to six doses (minimum dose, 1.25 mg/dose). If there is little or no improvement after six doses, consider continuous nebulized albuterol using 0.5 mg/kg per hour (maximum 15 mg/h) (Table 112-5). Hospitalization is likely at this point unless marked improvement is evident. Albuterol should be delivered with an oxygen flow of 6 to 7 L/min, and the pulse

**Table 112-4.** Respiratory Rates (Breaths/Minute) of Normal Children, Sleeping and Awake

| Age | Sleeping | | | Awake | | | Mean Difference Between Sleeping and Awake |
|---|---|---|---|---|---|---|---|
| | No. | Mean | Range | No. | Mean | Range | |
| 6–12 months | 6 | 27 | 22–31 | 3 | 64 | 58–75 | 37 |
| 1–2 years | 6 | 19 | 17–23 | 4 | 35 | 30–40 | 16 |
| 2–4 years | 16 | 19 | 16–25 | 15 | 31 | 23–42 | 12 |
| 4–6 years | 23 | 18 | 14–23 | 22 | 26 | 19–36 | 8 |
| 6–8 years | 27 | 17 | 13–23 | 28 | 23 | 15–30 | 6 |

*Source:* Waring WW: The history and physical examination, in Kendig. Cherniak (eds): *Disorders of the Respiratory Tract in Children,* Philadelphia, Saunders, 1983, p 63.

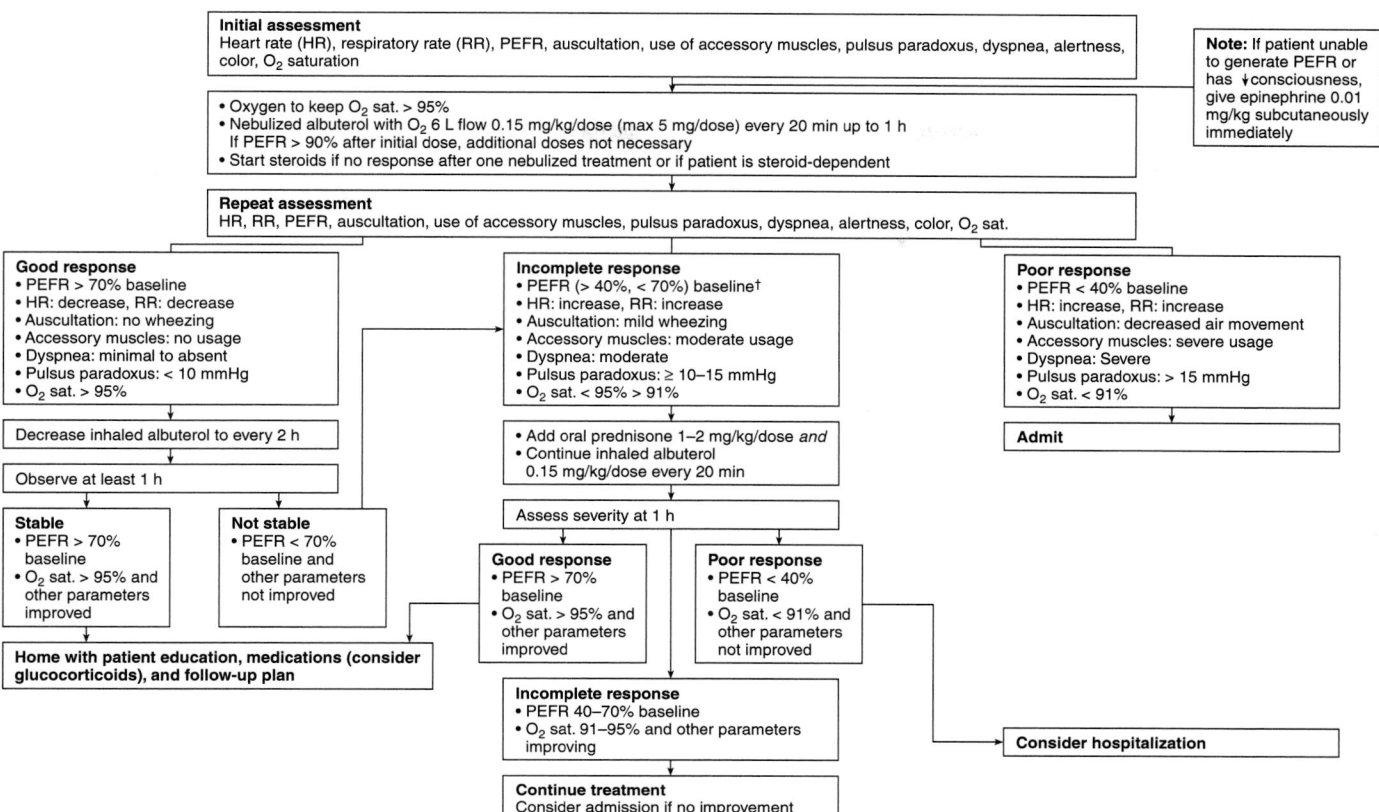

**Initial assessment**
Heart rate (HR), respiratory rate (RR), PEFR, auscultation, use of accessory muscles, pulsus paradoxus, dyspnea, alertness, color, $O_2$ saturation

**Note:** If patient unable to generate PEFR or has ↓consciousness, give epinephrine 0.01 mg/kg subcutaneously immediately

• Oxygen to keep $O_2$ sat. > 95%
• Nebulized albuterol with $O_2$ 6 L flow 0.15 mg/kg/dose (max 5 mg/dose) every 20 min up to 1 h
  If PEFR > 90% after initial dose, additional doses not necessary
• Start steroids if no response after one nebulized treatment or if patient is steroid-dependent

**Repeat assessment**
HR, RR, PEFR, auscultation, use of accessory muscles, pulsus paradoxus, dyspnea, alertness, color, $O_2$ sat.

**Good response**
• PEFR > 70% baseline
• HR: decrease, RR: decrease
• Auscultation: no wheezing
• Accessory muscles: no usage
• Dyspnea: minimal to absent
• Pulsus paradoxus: < 10 mmHg
• $O_2$ sat. > 95%

**Incomplete response**
• PEFR (> 40%, < 70%) baseline†
• HR: increase, RR: increase
• Auscultation: mild wheezing
• Accessory muscles: moderate usage
• Dyspnea: moderate
• Pulsus paradoxus: ≥ 10–15 mmHg
• $O_2$ sat. < 95% > 91%

**Poor response**
• PEFR < 40% baseline
• HR: increase, RR: increase
• Auscultation: decreased air movement
• Accessory muscles: severe usage
• Dyspnea: Severe
• Pulsus paradoxus: > 15 mmHg
• $O_2$ sat. < 91%

Decrease inhaled albuterol to every 2 h

Observe at least 1 h

• Add oral prednisone 1–2 mg/kg/dose *and*
• Continue inhaled albuterol 0.15 mg/kg/dose every 20 min

**Admit**

Assess severity at 1 h

**Stable**
• PEFR > 70% baseline
• $O_2$ sat. > 95% and other parameters improved

**Not stable**
• PEFR < 70% baseline and other parameters not improved

**Good response**
• PEFR > 70% baseline
• $O_2$ sat. > 95% and other parameters improved

**Poor response**
• PEFR < 40% baseline
• $O_2$ sat. < 91% and other parameters not improved

**Home with patient education, medications (consider glucocorticoids), and follow-up plan**

**Incomplete response**
• PEFR 40–70% baseline
• $O_2$ sat. 91–95% and other parameters improving

**Consider hospitalization**

**Continue treatment**
Consider admission if no improvement

*Therapies are often available in a physician's office. However, most acutely severe exacerbations of asthma require a complete course of therapy in an emergency department.
†PEFR % baseline refers to the norm for the individual, established by the clinician. This may be % predicted based on standardized norms or patient's personal best.
Courtesy of NAEP, used by permission.

**Fig. 112-1.** Acute exacerbations of asthma in children, emergency department management. (Used with permission of NAEP.)

should be monitored to keep it less than 180. In some asthmatic patients, higher doses of continuous nebulized albuterol may be helpful. In a recent study, Katz et al. demonstrated that continuous nebulized albuterol given at doses of 3 to 5 mg/kg per hour appeared to be safe and was not associated with cardiotoxicity.

The use of albuterol by metered-dose inhaler with a spacer (MDI-spacer) has been advocated by some authors because of the familiarity of patients with this method, ease of use, and decrease in therapist time. Recent studies have demonstrated that $\beta_2$ agonists delivered by MDI-spacers are as effective as those delivered in the nebulized form for the treatment of asthma exacerbations if the dose administered by MDI-spacers for the acute asthma attack is increased appropriately. Nebulizers deliver less drug to the lungs (1 to 5 percent) than MDI-spacers (21 percent) because drug is left in the tubing, is lost to the atmosphere, and is retained in the nebulizer.

In a recent study by Kerem et al., the response of children 6 to 14 years of age to inhaled albuterol after administration by MDI-spacer was compared with the response after administration by nebulizer, using a dose ratio of 1:5. The MDI-spacer medication was administered as follows: children weighing less than 25 kg received 6 puffs of 100 µg per puff; between 25 and 35 kg, 8 puffs; and those children more than 35 kg in weight received 10 puffs. All of the puffs were given in rapid sequence. Nebulized albuterol was administered at 0.15 mg/kg to a maximum of 5 mg. The researchers found that MDI-spacers and nebulizers are equally effective in delivering $\beta_2$ agonist to children with acute asthma. It is not known, however, if small children or children with severe asthma do as well with MDI-spacers as with nebulizers.

It should be remembered, however, that nebulized and MDI medications are dependent on patient cooperation and inspiratory effort.

When administering nebulized drugs to the very young child, the drug must be delivered properly so that the patient's airways are receiving it. The child resisting an inhalation treatment may not be receiving adequate medication. Also, in children with severe obstruction, the nebulized drug may not get to as much of the bronchial tree as will a systemic medication, which will reach it through the bloodstream. In such cases, particularly if the patient is hypoventilating, apneic, or has decreased consciousness, parenteral adrenergics are indicated. Aqueous epinephrine, 1:1000, may be administered subcutaneously at a dose of 0.01 mL/kg up to a maximum dose of 0.3 mL. This dose may be repeated twice at 20-min intervals with monitoring of respiratory status and heart rate. Terbutaline (1 mg/mL), which is more $\beta_2$-specific, may be given subcutaneously in place of epinephrine at a dose of 0.01 mL/kg (up to 0.25 mL). The dose may be repeated at 20-min intervals if no adverse effects occur. If there is improvement in airway obstruction in the very severe asthmatic with the use of parenteral adrenergics or if the child is intubated, nebulized $\beta_2$ agonists should be started.

Close monitoring of the pulse, respiratory rate, auscultatory findings in the chest, use of accessory muscles, oxygen saturation, and PEFR should be done before and after each treatment with adrenergic agents and should be recorded in the chart. The decision to repeat or withhold these agents should be based on the above clinical findings rather than rigidly following a protocol.

Anticholinergics are effective bronchodilators but until recently have been associated with many undesirable side effects. With the introduction of ipratropium bromide (Atrovent), a derivative of atropine, side effects are negligible. In several studies of patients treated with nebulized ipratropium bromide in combination with nebulized $\beta_2$ agonists, the two drugs provide more bronchodilation than a

**Table 112-5.** Dosages of Drugs in Acute Exacerbations of Asthma in Children

| Drug | Available Form | Dosage | Comment |
|---|---|---|---|
| **INHALED β₂ AGONIST** | | | |
| ***Albuterol*** | | | |
| Metered-dose inhaler | 90 μg/puff | 2 inhalations every 5 min for total of 12 puffs, with monitoring of PEFR or FEV₁ to document response | If not improved, switch to nebulizer. If improved, decrease to 4 puffs every hour. |
| Nebulizer solution | 0.5% (5 mg/mL) | 0.1–0.15 mg/kg/dose up to 5 mg every 20 min for 1–2 h (minimum dose 1.25 mg/dose) | If improved, decrease to 1–2 h. If not improved, use by continuous inhalation. |
| | | 0.5 mg/kg/h by continuous nebulization (maximum 15 mg/h) | |
| ***Metaproterenol*** | | | |
| Metered-dose inhaler | 650 μg/puff | 2 inhalations | Frequent high-dose administration has not been evaluated. Metaproterenol is not interchangeable with β₂ agonists albuterol and terbutaline. |
| Nebulizer solution | 5% (50 mg/mL) | 0.1–0.3 mL (5–15 mg). Do not exceed 15 mg. | |
| | 0.6% unit dose vial of 2.5 mL (15 mg) | As above 5–15 mg. Do not exceed 15 mg. | |
| ***Terbutaline*** | | | |
| Metered-dose inhaler | 200 μg/puff | 2 inhalations every 5 min for a total of 12 puffs | |
| Injectable solution used in nebulizer | 0.1% (1 mg/mL) solution in 0.9% NaCl solution for injection<br>Not FDA approved for inhalation. | | Not recommended as not available as nebulizer solution. Offers no advantage over albuterol, which is available as nebulizer solution. |
| **SYSTEMIC β AGONIST** | | | |
| ***Epinephrine HCl*** | 1:1000 (1 mg/mL) | 0.01 mg/kg up to 0.3 mg subcutaneously every 20 minutes for 3 doses. | Inhaled β₂ agonist preferred. |
| ***Terbutaline*** | (0.1%) 1 mg/mL solution for injection in 0.9% NaCl. | Subcutaneous 0.01 mg/kg up to 0.3 mg every 2–6 h as needed. Intravenous 10 μg/kg over 10 min loading dose. Maintenance: 0.4 μg/kg/min. Increase as necessary by 0.2 μg/kg/min and expect to use 3–6 μg/kg/min. | Inhaled β₂ agonist preferred. |
| ***Theophylline*** | Aminophylline (80% anhydrous theophylline) | Loading dose:* If theophylline concentration known: every 1 mg/kg aminophylline will give 2 μg/mL increase in concentration. | |
| | | Loading dose:* If theophylline concentration is unknown:<br>No previous theophylline: 6 mg/kg aminophylline<br>Previous theophylline: 3 mg/kg aminophylline | |
| | | Constant infusion rates: Infusion rates to obtain a mean steady-state concentration of 15 μg/mL. | |
| | | *Age*<br>1–6 months<br>6 mo–1 year<br>1–9 years<br>10–16 years | 0.5 mg/kg/h aminophylline<br>1.0 mg/kg/h aminophylline<br>1.5 mg/kg/h aminophylline<br>1.2 mg/kg/h aminophylline |
| **GLUCOCORTICOIDS** | | | |
| Outpatients | Oral prednisone, prednisolone, or methylprednisolone | 1–2 mg/kg/day in single or divided doses. | Reassess at 3 days as only a short burst may be needed. No need to taper dose. |
| Emergency department or hospitalized patients | Methylprednisolone IV or PO | 1–2 mg/kg/dose every 6 h for 24 h then 1–2 mg/kg/day in divided doses q 8–12 h | Length depends on response. May only need a few days. |

* Check serum concentration at approximately 1, 12, and 24 h after starting the infusion.

$\beta_2$ agonist alone. Ipratropium bromide may be combined with albuterol in patients 5 years of age or older who do not respond satisfactorily to albuterol alone. If the child is severely ill, ipratropium bromide may be added to the first dose of albuterol. A recent study by Schuh et al. demonstrated significant improvement in patients with severe asthma (baseline $FEV_1$ < 50 percent predicted) receiving three continuous doses of nebulized ipratropium bromide and three continuous doses of nebulized albuterol when compared with patients receiving one dose of ipratropium plus three doses of albuterol and those receiving albuterol alone with no ipratropium. The children in the ipratropium/albuterol group were also less likely to be hospitalized. The dosage of ipratropium bromide in children is 250 µg/dose in 2 mL of normal saline. Its use in children less than 5 years of age has not been established but it may be beneficial. Ipratropium in conjunction with albuterol should be considered in the severely ill asthmatic child less than 5 years old who is not responding to $\beta_2$ agonists alone.

Theophylline does not increase bronchodilation in patients optimally treated with β agonists. Therefore, theophylline is no longer recommended in the management of the acutely ill asthmatic child in the emergency department. However, there continues to be controversy regarding its usefulness in the inpatient setting, especially in selected cases. In situations where theophylline is used in the hospitalized asthmatic child, it may be started in the emergency department (see "Emergency Department Care: Status Asthmaticus").

Glucocorticoids are potent anti-inflammatory medications that are particularly useful in the inflammatory or late phase of asthma (2 to 8 h into the attack). Treatment with glucocorticoids early in the course of an asthma exacerbation prevents progression of the illness, lessens the need for emergency department visits and subsequent hospitalizations, and reduces morbidity. Moreover, glucocorticoids have been shown to improve oxygenation, decrease airway obstruction, and work synergistically with β agonists to improve bronchodilation in acute asthmatic attacks. Therefore, the question is when to start glucocorticoids rather than who deserves them. Clearly, however, not every child with a mild attack of asthma needs glucocorticoids to reverse the attack.

If a child presents to the emergency department with an infrequent acute attack of mild asthma and responds quickly to $\beta_2$ agonists (within 1 h), glucocorticoids are probably not necessary. They should be given early to children with an acute attack of asthma in the following cases: (1) a child with an infrequent acute attack of mild asthma who does not respond to inhaled $\beta_2$ agonists after 1 h of treatment (Table 112-3), (2) a child with a moderate attack of asthma who does not respond after one treatment with an inhaled $\beta_2$ agonist, (3) a child with a severe attack of asthma, (4) a child who is well known to the treating physician or the hospital or has a history of frequent emergency department visits or hospitalizations, (5) a child who is known to respond for a short period of time to bronchodilators but who subsequently develops wheezing again and returns to the emergency department for further therapy or to be admitted for status asthmaticus, (6) a child who has a second attack of asthma requiring an emergency department visit within a period of 1 week while on bronchodilators at home and who has responded on both emergency department visits to $\beta_2$ agonists, (7) a child with a viral upper respiratory infection who may or may not have symptoms of asthma when presenting to the emergency department but who is known to have rapid progression of symptoms once an attack begins, (8) a child who is chronically on glucocorticoids or who has needed frequent short-term bursts in the past, and (9) a child who has a history of respiratory failure.

Prednisone or prednisolone at 1 to 2 mg/kg per day, given in single or divided doses, is not associated with toxicity and does not cause adrenal suppression. Liquid preparations have made administration to small children easier. Some children, however, prefer crushed tablets mixed with apple sauce, yogurt, or other tasty treats. Steroid bursts

for 5 days or less, if done no more than four times per year, do not require tapering, since there is no adrenal suppression. Occasionally, after a viral illness, steroids may be required for 7 to 10 days. If they are needed for longer than 5 days or if the child has had four or more bursts per year, they should be tapered over 10 to 14 days. If a child is receiving chronic steroid treatment, he or she should be given high doses of prednisone or prednisolone for acute exacerbations and returned to a maintenance dose when the acute exacerbation is resolved. Steroids may be given orally, except in the severely ill child, since intravenous administration does not offer additional benefit.

Prior to prescribing steroids, the physician should inquire about exposure or potential exposure to varicella. If a child presents to the emergency department with varicella and wheezing, he or she should be treated aggressively with $\beta_2$ agonists. If steroids are needed, infectious disease consultation should be obtained immediately and the decision regarding the use of steroids should be discussed. Hospitalization is recommended for these children. It is known that varicella-susceptible individuals receiving glucocorticoids are at much higher risk of developing severe or fatal varicella, particularly in those patients with a malignancy or underlying immunosuppression. It is not known, however, if there is higher risk of developing severe varicella from glucocorticoid-induced immunosuppression in asthmatic patients. Presently, steroid therapy should not be withheld in patients with significant asthma who have been exposed to varicella. The lower dose (1 mg/kg per day) should be used and the child should be reassessed in 2 to 3 days. The physician caring for the patient should consider giving varicella-zoster immune globulin if the patient has been exposed within 72 h and/or starting acyclovir with the initial onset of lesions. If the patient has not been exposed but chicken pox is prevalent in the community, attempts to prevent exposure should be made. When the varicella vaccine is licensed, patients with asthma should be targeted for early vaccination.

After an acute attack of asthma, all children should be sent home with steroids, if needed, and an inhaled or oral $\beta_2$ agonist for 1 to 2 weeks to prevent further exacerbation of their symptoms (for dosages see "Treatment of Chronic Asthma"). Children who are already on a regimen of medication may need intensification of therapy and close monitoring. Cromolyn sodium should be continued at home in those patients with acute exacerbations and should be started in those patients with frequent recurrent attacks of asthma.

## Emergency Department Care: Status Asthmaticus

Status asthmaticus may be defined as severe, persistent wheezing and dyspnea that fail to respond to usually effective outpatient therapy. Respiratory failure may occur in patients with status asthmaticus; this makes this disorder a true medical emergency. Hospitalization is mandatory for these patients (Fig. 112-2).

All patients with status asthmaticus are hypoxic and some are hypercapneic. Consequently, all patients should be monitored with a pulse oximeter. Arterial blood gas levels should be obtained to determine baseline $P_{O_2}$, $P_{CO_2}$, and pH, particularly in patients whose PEFR is less than 25 percent of predicted. These should be repeated frequently if one does not have an available pulse oximeter or if the $P_{CO_2}$ is high until the patient's clinical condition improves. Humidified oxygen should be administered immediately to every child with status asthmaticus. The pulse oximeter should be maintained at or above 95-percent saturation and/or the $P_{O_2}$ should be maintained between 70 and 90 mmHg. Mist tents are not indicated, both because water does not reach the lower airway in any significant way, and because mist irritates the airways of many asthmatics.

Many children with status asthmaticus become dehydrated. This is the result of several factors, including decreased fluid intake, excessive work of breathing, and pulmonary insensible water loss. When

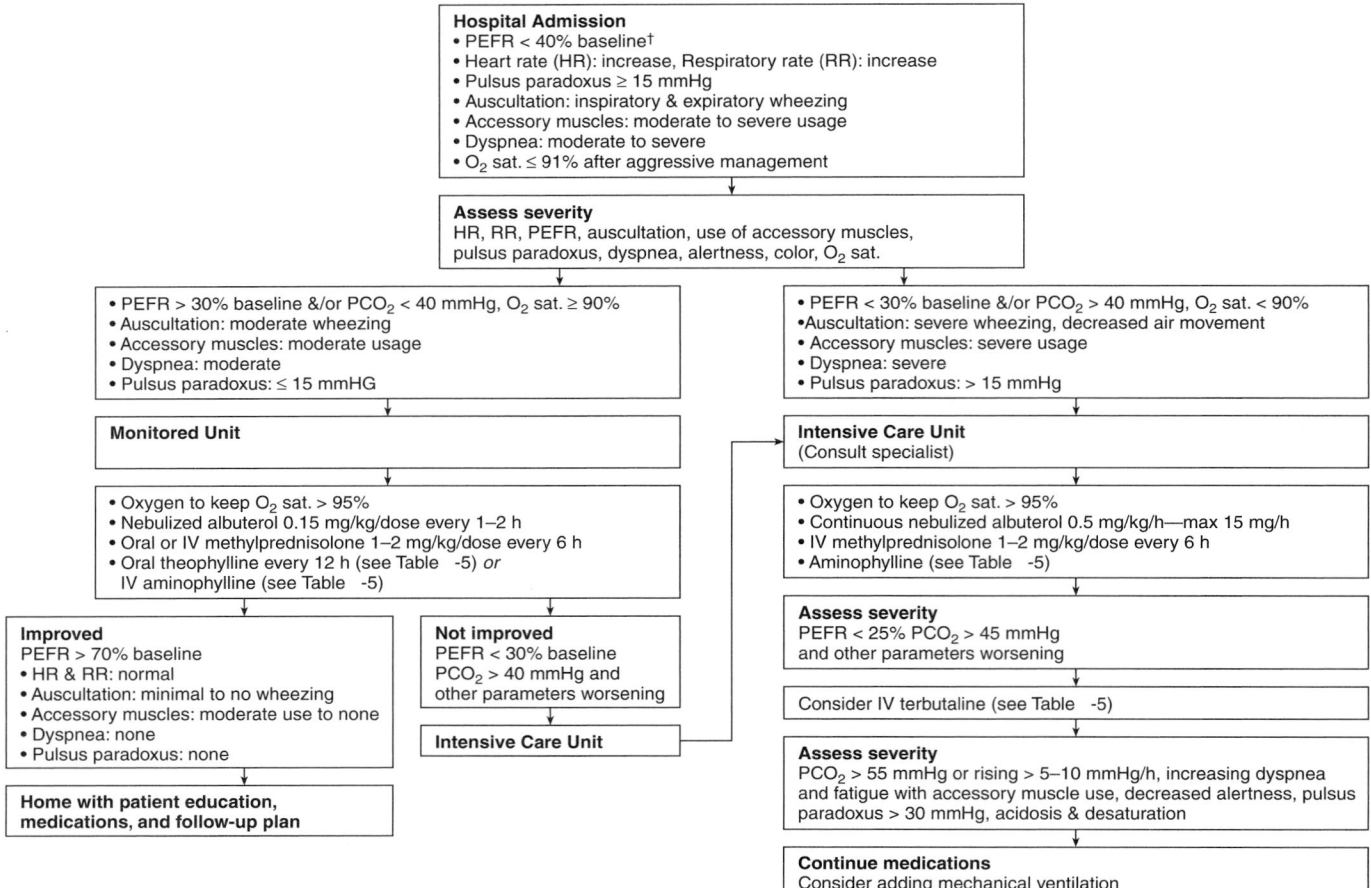

**Hospital Admission**
• PEFR < 40% baseline†
• Heart rate (HR): increase, Respiratory rate (RR): increase
• Pulsus paradoxus ≥ 15 mmHg
• Auscultation: inspiratory & expiratory wheezing
• Accessory muscles: moderate to severe usage
• Dyspnea: moderate to severe
• O₂ sat. ≤ 91% after aggressive management

**Assess severity**
HR, RR, PEFR, auscultation, use of accessory muscles,
pulsus paradoxus, dyspnea, alertness, color, O₂ sat.

• PEFR > 30% baseline &/or PCO₂ < 40 mmHg, O₂ sat. ≥ 90%
• Auscultation: moderate wheezing
• Accessory muscles: moderate usage
• Dyspnea: moderate
• Pulsus paradoxus: ≤ 15 mmHG

**Monitored Unit**

• Oxygen to keep O₂ sat. > 95%
• Nebulized albuterol 0.15 mg/kg/dose every 1–2 h
• Oral or IV methylprednisolone 1–2 mg/kg/dose every 6 h
• Oral theophylline every 12 h (see Table   -5) *or*
  IV aminophylline (see Table   -5)

**Improved**
PEFR > 70% baseline
• HR & RR: normal
• Auscultation: minimal to no wheezing
• Accessory muscles: moderate use to none
• Dyspnea: none
• Pulsus paradoxus: none

**Not improved**
PEFR < 30% baseline
PCO₂ > 40 mmHg and
other parameters worsening

**Intensive Care Unit**

**Home with patient education,
medications, and follow-up plan**

• PEFR < 30% baseline &/or PCO₂ > 40 mmHg, O₂ sat. < 90%
• Auscultation: severe wheezing, decreased air movement
• Accessory muscles: severe usage
• Dyspnea: severe
• Pulsus paradoxus: > 15 mmHg

**Intensive Care Unit**
(Consult specialist)

• Oxygen to keep O₂ sat. > 95%
• Continuous nebulized albuterol 0.5 mg/kg/h—max 15 mg/h
• IV methylprednisolone 1–2 mg/kg/dose every 6 h
• Aminophylline (see Table   -5)

**Assess severity**
PEFR < 25% PCO₂ > 45 mmHg
and other parameters worsening

Consider IV terbutaline (see Table   -5)

**Assess severity**
PCO₂ > 55 mmHg or rising > 5–10 mmHg/h, increasing dyspnea
and fatigue with accessory muscle use, decreased alertness, pulsus
paradoxus > 30 mmHg, acidosis & desaturation

**Continue medications**
Consider adding mechanical ventilation

†PEFR % baseline refers to the norm for the individual, established by the clinician. This may be % predicted based on standardized norms or % patient's personal best.
Courtesy of NAEP, used by permission.

**Fig. 112-2.** Acute exacerbations of asthma in children, hospital management.

hydrating children with status asthmaticus, it must be taken into account that they have increased secretion of antidiuretic hormone, and there is danger of overhydration and subsequent pulmonary edema. Consequently, fluid administration must be carefully monitored. Hydration in excess of maintenance is usually unnecessary and may be harmful.

Nebulized albuterol or other $\beta_2$ agonist should be administered every 20 min or continuously if necessary (see "Emergency Department Care: Acute Exacerbations").

Theophylline has not proved to be of benefit in the emergency department treatment of asthma. Its use for severely ill hospitalized patients is controversial. Most recent studies suggest that the routine addition of theophylline to inhaled $\beta_2$ agonists and glucocorticoids provides little or no additional benefit and that there is significant risk of adverse effects associated with its use. Consequently, theophylline should not be used routinely for patients with status asthmaticus but should be considered on an individualized basis. Theophylline may stimulate respiration centrally, increase diaphragmatic contractility, enhance mucociliary clearance, and inhibit late-phase inflammation, which may benefit selected patients. Its use should be considered in children who fail to respond adequately to albuterol and steroids and for children who are already taking oral theophylline for maintenance therapy. In these cases, theophylline may be started in the emergency department.

Aminophylline (85% theophylline) should be administered as a loading dose of 6 mg/kg (lean body weight) diluted in 25 to 50 mL of

saline given intravenously over a period of 20 min. If the child is a known asthmatic who has taken a dose of oral theophylline at home within 4 to 6 h prior to arriving at the hospital, the loading dosage of aminophylline should be adjusted by deducting the amount given in the past 4 to 6 h from the ordinary bolus of 6 mg/kg of aminophylline. One study suggested that even if the child has taken theophylline within 6 h of arriving at the hospital, a loading dose of 6 mg/kg may be given with few side effects. If a recent theophylline level is known, one may calculate the loading dose with the knowledge that, as a general rule, 1 mg/kg of theophylline will raise the serum concentration by approximately 2 μg/mL. The loading dose can thus be calculated with the following formula:

$$\text{Loading dose (mg)} = \frac{\text{desired level} - \text{measured level}}{2} \times \text{kg}$$

Another approach, advocated by some physicians, is to give 6 mg/kg of aminophylline to patients who have not taken a recent dose of theophylline and 3 mg/kg to patients who have taken a recent dose.

A theophylline level should be obtained prior to the administration of aminophylline if the child has been on an oral theophylline preparation. The loading dose should be followed by a constant maintenance infusion of aminophylline of 1.0 to 1.2 mg/kg per hour for children 1 to 9 years old, 0.8 to 1.0 mg/kg per hour for children 10 to 16 years, and 0.6 to 0.8 mg/kg per hour for children over 16 years. This will usually maintain serum concentrations of approximately

10 μg/mL. If there is significant fever, liver disease, or heart failure, the maintenance infusion should be reduced by 50 percent. Because infants, particularly those under 6 months of age, are erratic in their clearance rate of theophylline, a formula for infants less than 1 year of age is useful.

$$\text{Dose (mg/kg per day)} = 0.3 \times \text{age in weeks} + 8$$

It is extremely important to measure serum theophylline levels because of the variable clearance rates from one patient to the next. If, after the initial theophylline level is obtained, the patient continues to have significant wheezing, the dose of aminophylline can be increased until a theophylline level of 15 μg/mL is reached. Levels should also be measured whenever toxicity is suspected on the basis of symptoms such as gastrointestinal upset, CNS irritability, and headaches. Theophylline should be delivered by a constant infusion pump. If constant infusion cannot be delivered safely, boluses of aminophylline at 5 mg/kg every 6 h (or an amount which will give a serum concentration of 10 to 15 μg/mL) should be administered over a period of 30 min.

Intravenous glucocorticoids should be started in the child with status asthmaticus. The beneficial effects of steroid therapy, i.e., decreasing inflammation, facilitating recovery from hypoxia, increasing cyclic AMP, and possibly restoring β-adrenergic responsiveness to adrenergic drugs in patients who have become unresponsive to these drugs, outweigh the remote possibility of adverse effects from short-term glucocorticoid use. Hydrocortisone (Solu-Cortef) or methylprednisolone (Solu-Medrol) may be administered. The dosage of hydrocortisone is 4 to 6 mg/kg every 6 h for 48 to 72 h. Methylprednisolone may be administered at 1 to 2 mg/kg every 6 h for 48 to 72 h. When intravenous steroids are discontinued, the patient should be maintained on oral prednisone at 1 to 2 mg/kg per day in two divided doses for a total of 5 days or more if clinically indicated.

Ipratropium bromide may be used in patients with status asthmaticus (see "Emergency Department Care: Acute Exacerbations"). Further studies need to be conducted to determine the frequency of use in those patients not responding to three doses.

Sedation is contraindicated in patients with status asthmaticus. Antibiotics should not be used routinely. If bacterial infection is suspected, attempts should be made to identify the causative organism; the patient should be started on a broad-spectrum antibiotic while the culture results are pending.

Occasionally, the patient with status asthmaticus develops respiratory failure. Clinical signs and symptoms of respiratory failure are decreased or absent breath sounds, severe retractions and use of accessory muscles, cyanosis on 40% oxygen, depressed level of consciousness, decreased response to pain, and poor skeletal muscle tone. Arterial blood gas levels are the final determinant of respiratory failure and must be monitored frequently in the distressed child. Respiratory failure may be defined as a $P_{O_2}$ <50 mmHg on 100% inhaled $O_2$, or $P_{CO_2}$ >50 mmHg. The child with a rapidly rising $P_{CO_2}$ (e.g., from 35 to 40 mmHg in 1 h) who is receiving optimal therapy and is tiring, should be considered to be in respiratory failure and treated as such.

In a child whose arterial $P_{CO_2}$ is rising rapidly but is less than 55 mmHg and whose arterial $P_{O_2}$ is more than 60 mmHg on oxygen, continuously nebulized albuterol should be administered in an attempt to avert the need for mechanical ventilation. The dosage of albuterol is 0.5 mg/kg per hour. An alternative to albuterol is continuously nebulized terbutaline at 4 mg/h.

Some studies advocate the use of intravenous albuterol to avert the need for mechanical ventilation. At the present, albuterol is not available for intravenous use in the United States, but it is available in Canada and Europe. If intravenous albuterol is used, the dosage is 10 μg/kg over 10 min, followed by 0.2 μg/kg per minute. This should

be increased by 0.1-μg/kg increments every 15 min as needed and titrated according to response. Potassium levels should be obtained, since hypokalemia occurs frequently in patients receiving intravenous albuterol. Supplementary potassium is often needed with this treatment. If albuterol is not available, terbutaline may be used instead. The dose is 10 μg/kg over 10 min, followed by 0.2-μg/kg per minute increments titrated according to clinical response. The usual infusion rate is between 3 and 6 μg/kg per minute. The pulse with all of these medications should not be higher than 180. Continuous delivery of an intravenous β2 agonist will ordinarily be administered in a properly equipped intensive care unit. If admission to the intensive care unit is delayed, initial therapy may be undertaken in the emergency department, but only with continuous cardiac monitoring and a constant infusion pump.

Intravenous isoproterenol was used in the recent past to avert mechanical ventilation. It is no longer recommended because β2 agonists are more specific, they decrease $P_{CO_2}$ more rapidly, and they have fewer side effects than intravenous isoproterenol.

If medical therapy fails to control respiratory failure, mechanical ventilation is required. Any child with a $P_{CO_2}$ rising at 5 to 10 mmHg/h during aggressive therapy, a $P_{CO_2}$ greater than 55 mmHg after 1 to 2 h of aggressive therapy, or a $P_{O_2}$ less than 50 mmHg on 100% inspired oxygen should be started on assisted ventilation. If a child has a $P_{CO_2}$ of more than 65 mmHg initially, immediate intubation should be strongly considered. Ketamine, because of its bronchodilating property, may be used as an inducing agent. Other standard medications used for rapid-sequence induction are also satisfactory for this procedure. Rapidly changing lung compliances make the use of a volume respirator preferable. An initial tidal volume of 10 mL/kg should be used with a short inspiratory time and an expiratory time as long as possible. A Swan-Ganz catheter should be placed if there is right heart strain, low pulse pressure, or low urine output. The patient may be given diazepam or midazolam for sedation and pancuronium bromide or other nondepolarizing agent for muscle relaxation. These medications will help with synchronization of respiration with the ventilator. Parenteral and inhaled medication should be continued throughout the period of ventilation.

## Management of Complications

Atelectasis occurs in 10 percent and pneumomediastinum occurs in 5 percent of children hospitalized with asthma. Treatment of atelectasis and pneumomediastinum should be conservative; they will usually resolve with drug therapy. Percussion and postural drainage are helpful for the resolution of atelectasis. Pneumomediastinal air is absorbed over 7 to 10 days.

Pneumothorax occurs rarely in children with asthma. When it does occur, a pneumothorax may be small and cause minimal respiratory compromise or it may be large or under tension, causing significant respiratory distress. A small pneumothorax may be managed conservatively and will often respond to the treatment of asthma. A large pneumothorax or tension pneumothorax will require placement of a chest tube.

## Admission Indications

There are no definitive criteria for hospitalization of children with asthma. Certainly, the child with respiratory failure or significant respiratory distress, hypoventilation, apnea, alteration of consciousness, hypotension, severe hypoxia, and/or hypercarbia needs admission to a pediatric intensive care unit (Figs. 112-1 and 112-2). Admission should be strongly considered for children with any of the following criteria: (1) persistent respiratory distress after albuterol and glucocorticoid treatments; (2) a return visit within 24 h to the emergency department; (3) an $Sa_{O_2}$ of ≤91 percent on room air on arrival and

≤94 percent after treatment; (4) a PEFR of <60 percent of predicted after treatment; (5) persistent vomiting of medications; (6) underlying high-risk illness, e.g., bronchopulmonary dysplasia, congenital heart disease, cystic fibrosis, and neuromuscular disease; and (7) near-fatal experiences with previous asthma exacerbations, i.e., previous intubations or history of respiratory failure. Admission should also be considered for children who may not quite meet the above criteria but who have a history of poor medication compliance at home and poor or difficult access to medical care or advice because of lack of a telephone or transportation. Observing the child with a significant exacerbation in the emergency department for approximately 1 h after the last bronchodilator treatment is advisable. This action may decrease the chance of a return visit within a few hours.

## Ambulatory Treatment of Chronic Asthma

An attempt should be made to determine the environmental factors that may trigger an attack of asthma. Some of these factors include allergens such as animal dander, pollen, house dust, molds, and foods; irritants such as smoke, perfumes, and aerosol spray products;

**Table 112-6.** Classification of Asthma by Severity of Disease*

| Characteristics | Mild | Moderate | Severe |
|---|---|---|---|
| **Pretreatment** | | | |
| Frequency of exacerbations | Exacerbations of cough and wheezing no more often than 1–2 times/week. | Exacerbation of cough and wheezing on a more frequent basis than 1–2 times/week. Could have history of severe exacerbations, but infrequent. Urgent care treatment in hospital emergency department or doctor's office <3 times/year. | Virtually daily wheezing. Exacerbations frequent, often severe. Tendency to have sudden severe exacerbations. Urgent visits to hospital emergency departments or doctor's office >3 times/year. Hospitalization >2 times/year, perhaps with respiratory insufficiency or, rarely, respiratory failure and history of intubation. May have had cough syncope or hypoxic seizures. |
| Frequency of symptoms | Few clinical signs or symptoms of asthma between exacerbations. | Cough and low-grade wheezing between acute exacerbations often present. | Continuous albeit low-grade cough and wheezing almost always present. |
| Degree of exercise tolerance | Good exercise tolerance but may not tolerate vigorous exercise, especially prolonged running. | Exercise tolerance diminished. | Very poor exercise tolerance with marked limitation of activity. |
| Frequency of nocturnal asthma | Symptoms of nocturnal asthma occur no more often than 1–2 times/month. | Symptoms of nocturnal asthma present 2–3 times/week. | Considerable, almost nightly sleep interruption due to asthma. Chest tight in early morning. |
| School or work attendance | Good school or work attendance. | School or work attendance may be affected. | Poor school or work attendance. |
| **Pulmonary function** | | | |
| Peak expiratory flow rate (PEFR) | PEFR >80% predicted. Variability† <20%. | PEFR 60–80% predicted. Variability 20–30%. | PEFR <60% predicted. Variability >30%. |
| Spirometry | Minimal or no evidence of airway obstruction on spirometry. Normal expiratory flow volume curve; lung volumes not increased. Usually a >15% response to acute aerosol bronchodilator administration, even though baseline near normal. | Signs of airway obstruction on spirometry are evident. Flow volume curve shows reduced expiratory flow at low lung volumes. Lung volumes often increased. Usually a >15% response to acute aerosol bronchodilator administration. | Substantial degree of airway obstruction on spirometry. Flow volume curve shows marked concavity. Spirometry may not be normalized even with high-dose steroids. May have substantial increase in lung volumes and marked unevenness of ventilation. Incomplete reversibility to acute aerosol bronchodilator administration. |
| **After optimal treatment is established** | | | |
| Response to and duration of therapy | Exacerbations respond to bronchodilators without the use of systemic glucocorticoids in 12–24 h. Regular drug therapy not usually required except for short periods of time. | Periodic use of bronchodilators required during exacerbations for a week or more. Systemic steroids also usually required for exacerbations. Continuous around-the-clock drug therapy required. Regular use of anti-inflammatory agents may be required. | Requires continuous, multiple around-the-clock drug therapy including daily steroids, either aerosol or systemic, often in high doses. |

* Characteristics are general; because asthma is highly variable, these characteristics may overlap. Furthermore, an individual may switch into different categories over time.

† Variability means the difference either between a morning and evening measure or among morning peak flow measurements each day of a week.

and climate. If these environmental stimuli are identified, their removal may "cure" the child's asthma.

More often than not, the physician is unable to identify a precipitating environmental factor and must resort to medication to control a child's asthma. Mild or intermittent asthma with symptoms less than one or two times per week (Table 112-6) may be controlled with inhaled $\beta_2$ agonists such as albuterol or terbutaline. The use of one of these medications three or four times a day as needed may be the only treatment necessary to control symptoms. Aerosolized adrenergics are particularly recommended for children with exercise-induced asthma. Two inhalations may provide more bronchodilation and fewer side effects than the oral preparations of these medications. Since metered-dose inhalers are often used improperly, it is important to instruct patients in their use. Even after instruction, some older children have difficulty with metered-dose inhalers. In these children and especially those who are 3 to 5 years of age, spacers or holding chambers have provided an easy way to take advantage of aerosolized $\beta_2$ agonists. Since this method of delivery is preferred, it is worth trying the MDI-spacer in children as young as 1 year of age. Oral $\beta_2$ agonists may be used in place of the inhaled form if the young child is unable to use the MDI-spacer. Because metered-dose inhalers are occasionally abused, parents and patients must be warned about this tendency.

Several medications can be used alone or in combination to control symptoms in children with moderate chronic asthma. These children have more than two asthmatic episodes per week or occasional nocturnal asthma. Their symptoms may last for several days and may require either more than one medication or occasional emergency department therapy or hospitalization. This group of patients should be taking $\beta_2$ agonists two to four times a day on an as-needed basis, as well as a daily medication. Cromolyn sodium is the preferred agent because of its anti-inflammatory properties and an effectiveness equal to that of theophylline in controlling symptoms with fewer associated side effects. Theophylline, however, continues to be favored by many allergists as the first-line medication for these children. Because of its side effects, particularly behavioral ones, it should be considered an alternative to cromolyn sodium. It is especially beneficial for nocturnal asthma. Often these medications work well in combination with cromolyn sodium, particularly after an acute attack of asthma in a child who needs the sustained bronchodilating effect of theophylline and the anti-inflammatory effect of cromolyn sodium. Inhaled glucocorticoids provide excellent anti-inflammatory therapy. They should be used after a trial of cromolyn sodium for children whose symptoms are not controlled by cromolyn sodium and who continue to need a $\beta_2$ agonist more than three or four times a day or who continue to have nocturnal symptoms. There is concern about the long-term safety of inhaled steroids in children, especially regarding the potential to decrease linear growth and decrease concentrations of plasma cortisol. Consequently, if inhaled steroids are needed, it may be possible after a prolonged period of control to reduce the dosage or replace the inhaled glucocorticoid with cromolyn sodium. Short-burst oral steroids are sometimes needed to control symptoms of an acute exacerbation (see "Emergency Department Care: Acute Exacerbations").

Children with daily or continuous symptoms, a limited activity level, and frequent exacerbations have chronic severe asthma. These children require daily therapy with a $\beta_2$ agonist three to four times a day as needed and inhaled glucocorticoids (beclomethasone, triamcinolone, or flunisolide). Beclomethasone at 2 to 4 puffs two to four times per day is a reasonable starting dose. Cromolyn sodium and/or theophylline may be added if there is no significant improvement or nocturnal symptoms persist. Oral steroids may be necessary in younger children who cannot use an MDI-spacer. The switch to inhaled steroids should begin as soon as possible, since there are fewer side effects associated with them than with oral preparations. In chil-

dren with intractable symptoms, oral steroids should be considered and should preferably be given as an alternate-day dose. In any case of difficult-to-manage asthma, especially in a child in whom chronic steroids may be indicated, consultation with an allergist should be obtained. Those with asthma and concomitant psychological disturbances should be referred to a therapist for counseling.

Cromolyn sodium stabilizes mast cells and prevents the release of mediators and thus decreases inflammation. It also decreases bronchial hyperresponsiveness. Cromolyn sodium is primarily used as a prophylactic antiasthmatic medication. It may also be used acutely before exercise to block exercise-induced asthma. Cromolyn sodium is available in three preparations: 20-mg dry powder cap-

**Table 112-7.** Dosages for Therapy in Childhood Asthma

| $\beta_2$ Agonists | |
|---|---|
| *Inhaled:* examples: albuterol, metaproterenol, bitolterol, terbutaline, pirbuteral | |
| Mode of administration | |
| Metered-dose inhaler | 2 puffs q 4–6 h |
| Dry powder inhaler | 1 capsule q 4–6 h |
| Nebulizer solution* | Albuterol 5 mg/mL; 0.1–0.15 mg/kg in 2 mL of saline q 4–6 h, maximum 5.0 mg |
| | Metaproterenol 50 mg/mL; 0.25–0.50 mg/kg in 2 mL of saline q 4–6 h, maximum 15.0 mg |
| *Oral* | |
| Liquids | |
| Albuterol | 0.1–0.15 mg/kg q 4–6 h |
| Metaproterenol | 0.3–0.5 mg/kg q 4–6 h |
| Tablets | |
| Albuterol | 2- or 4-mg tablet, q 4–6 h |
| | 4-mg sustained-release tablet q 12 h |
| Metaproterenol | 10- or 20-mg tablet q 4–6 h |
| Terbutaline | 2.5- or 5.0-mg tablet q 4–6 h |
| **Cromolyn sodium** | |
| MDI | 1 mg/puff; 2 puffs bid-qid |
| Dry powder inhaler | 20 mg/capsule; 1 capsule, bid-qid |
| Nebulizer solution | 20 mg/2-mL ampule; 1 ampule bid-qid |
| **Theophylline** | |
| Liquid | |
| Tablets, capsules | |
| Sustained-release tablets, capsules | |
| Dosage to achieve serum concentration of 5–15 μg/mL | |
| **Glucocorticoids** | |
| *Inhaled†* | |
| Beclomethasone | 42 μg/puff, 2–4 puffs bid-qid |
| Triamcinolone | 100 μg/puff, 2–4 puffs bid-qid |
| Flunisolide | 250 μg/puff, 2–4 puffs bid |
| *Oral‡* | |
| Liquids | |
| Prednisone | 5 mg/5 mL |
| Prednisolone | 5 mg/5 mL |
| | 15 mg/5 mL |
| Tablets | |
| Prednisone | 1, 2.5, 5, 10, 20, 25, 50 mg |
| Prednisolone | 5 mg |
| Methylprednisolone | 2, 4, 8, 16, 24, 32 mg |

\* Premixed solutions are available. It is suggested that the per/kg dosage recommendations be followed.

† Consider use of spacer devices to minimize local adverse effects.

‡ For acute exacerbations, doses of 1–2 mg/kg in single or divided doses are used initially and are then modified. Reassess in 3 days, as only a short burst may be needed. There is no need to taper a short (3- to 5-day) course of therapy. If therapy extends beyond this period, it may be appropriate to taper the dosage. For chronic dosage, the lowest possible alternate-day A.M. dosage should be established.

sules, 20-mg solution for nebulizer use, and a metered-dose inhaler at 1 mg/puff to be administered at 2 mg (2 puffs) per dose (Table 112-7). Each preparation should be administered four times per day and may be reduced to two to three times per day if the child remains stable on the four times per day regimen. If cromolyn sodium is used for exercise-induced asthma, 2 puffs of the metered dose inhaler should be administered just prior to exercise.

As noted above, theophylline is considered by some to be the oral bronchodilator of choice in the outpatient management of chronic asthma. In most cases, however, it should be considered an alternative therapy. Theophylline comes in many forms. Depending on the specific theophylline preparation chosen and individual patient clearance, it may be given every 6 h, every 8 h, or every 12 h. Sustained-release preparations, those given every 8 to 12 h, are recommended because they decrease fluctuations in serum concentrations and increase compliance. In children who clear theophylline rapidly, sustained-release theophylline should be given every 8 h. Nocturnal symptoms may be controlled with a single evening dose.

The initial dose for most children is 12 to 14 mg/kg per day. Depending on individual differences in metabolism, smaller or larger doses may be needed to maintain serum concentration between 5 and 15 µg/mL. In many cases, children do very well at levels of 5 to 10 µg/mL. Levels greater than 15 µg/mL rarely have to be exceeded to gain good control. Children less than 6 months and over 9 years of age should be started on the lower-end dose because of their slower clearance rate of theophylline. Infants less than 6 months of age have erratic clearance rates of theophylline, and their serum theophylline levels should be checked in 24 h and then monitored accordingly (see formula in "Emergency Department Care: Status Asthmaticus"). Any child receiving theophylline should always be observed for signs of toxicity such as nausea, vomiting, restlessness, irritability, and seizures. If any of these signs appear, theophylline levels should be obtained and the medication stopped. If a child has a fever for longer than 24 h, theophylline should be reduced by half. It should not be given with erythromycin, cimetidine, or ciprofloxacin because of their effect on the clearance of theophylline.

Oral β agonists (albuterol and terbutaline) may be used alone or in combination with other bronchodilators or anti-inflammatory medications, particularly if the child continues to be symptomatic on only one medication. Albuterol is the most commonly used oral β agonist in children. It is available as a liquid (2 mg/5 mL), with a starting dose of 0.1 to 0.15 mg/kg per dose three times a day not to exceed 6 mg, or as a tablet (2 mg and 4 mg), with starting doses for children 6 to 12 years of 2 mg three or four times a day; for children over 12 the dose is 2 to 4 mg three or four times a day. Albuterol is also available in a longer-acting form known as a Repetab, which may be used in children older than 12 years of age at a dose of 4 to 8 mg every 12 h. Terbutaline is available as 2.5- and 5-mg tablets. The dose for children from 12 to 15 years of age is 2.5 mg three times a day. For adolescents over age 15, the dose is 5 mg three times a day. Terbutaline tablets are not currently recommended for children less than 12. If tachycardia, nervousness, tremors, palpitations, or nausea develop in patients taking β2-adrenergic drugs, the dose should be reduced.

Small infants who respond well to nebulized therapy but not as well to oral medication may benefit from a home nebulizer.

## Exercise-Induced Asthma (EIA)

Wheezing with exercise is common in asthmatic children, in those with other allergic conditions, and in some children with no allergic manifestations (see "Etiology"). It occurs less frequently in the child whose asthma is well controlled. An inhaled β2 agonist (e.g., albuterol) or cromolyn sodium given 15 to 30 min before exercise controls symptoms in most children with EIA (see "Ambulatory Treatment of Chronic Asthma"). Those children who continue to experience symptoms may increase the dosage of albuterol to 4 puffs before exercise or use both albuterol and cromolyn sodium. Some children may need to repeat these medications as needed if exercise continues for more than 2 h.

## Discharge Instructions/Follow-up Interval

Children who respond satisfactorily to medications for their acute exacerbation may be discharged (see Fig. 112-1) with appropriate medications (see "Emergency Department Care: Acute Exacerbations," "Ambulatory Treatment of Chronic Asthma," and Table 112-7), which should be taken for 5 to 7 days after the exacerbation. Typically a β-agonist and glucocorticoid are prescribed. If cromolyn sodium already is given at home, it should be continued. It is important that the child or the parents are given instructions on how to administer the medications and that they understand the instructions. Parents whose children do not have a primary care physician should be given the telephone number of the emergency department for questions that may arise regarding their child's asthma. They should be instructed to call their physician or return to the emergency department if their child has rapid breathing or more difficulty breathing, or if wheezing increases and is not controlled with medication. If there is significant respiratory distress, cyanosis or apnea, or a change in the level of consciousness, parents should be instructed to call for paramedic assistance. If the child is having difficulty taking the medications, the physician should be contacted. Follow-up should be arranged in 24 to 72 hours, depending on the severity of the exacerbation.

In addition to the above measures, parents should be instructed to be aware of precipitating triggers, such as infection. Beta agonists are recommended early, i.e., at the start of a cold for children who wheeze every time they get a cold. Instructing patients and parents about home monitoring with a peak flow meter and at what PEFR percentage of personal best they should seek medical attention is also helpful in preventing serious exacerbations.

## Other Therapeutic Modalities

A number of medications are being tested for their effectiveness in the treatment of asthma. Calcium channel blockers have been studied but have not up to now demonstrated proven benefit. Magnesium sulfate causes bronchodilation and is considered an adjunct to β2-agonist therapy by some, but its effects have not been studied in children. Nedocromil sodium (Tilade) is an anti-inflammatory with clinical effectiveness similar to cromolyn sodium. Troleandomycin potentiates the anti-inflammatory effects of steroids and may prove useful in chronic asthmatic patients on high-dose corticosteroid therapy.

## BRONCHIOLITIS

*Bronchiolitis* is the term used to describe a clinical syndrome in infancy characterized by rapid respiration, chest retractions, and wheezing. It typically occurs during the winter and spring months, more often in male than female infants less than 2 years of age, with the greatest frequency between the ages of 2 and 6 months. Morbidity and mortality are highest in very young children, especially those less than 2 months of age, and in those infants with a history of prematurity, underlying cardiopulmonary disease, bronchopulmonary dysplasia, or immunosuppression. The mortality rate in these high-risk children with bronchiolitis is approximately 1%.

### Etiology

The most common cause of bronchiolitis is the respiratory syncytial virus (RSV). It is the etiologic agent in approximately 75 percent of infants admitted to the hospital with this disorder. Other organisms that cause bronchiolitis are parainfluenza virus, influenza virus, mumps virus, adenovirus, echovirus, rhinovirus, *Mycoplasma pneumoniae,* and *Chlamydia trachomatis.* Adenovirus, particularly types 3, 7, and 21, may cause a more destructive form of bronchiolitis, known as bronchiolitis obliterans, a chronic, obstructive lung disease.

## Pathophysiology

The most important pulmonary lesion associated with bronchiolitis is bronchiolar obstruction characterized by submucosal edema, peribronchiolar cellular infiltrate, mucous plugging, and intraluminal debris. These pathologic changes lead to narrowing of the lumens of small bronchi and bronchioles, increasing airway resistance, and concomitant wheezing. The obstruction is not uniform throughout the lungs, so that some of the small bronchi and bronchioles are affected while others are not. However, normal exchange of gases in the lung is impaired. Hypoxia is the major result of abnormal gas exchange in which alveoli are poorly ventilated but remain well perfused (ventilation-perfusion imbalance). Compensation for the hypoxia results in hyperventilation, which is a more sensitive indicator of reduced oxygen tension than is cyanosis. Carbon dioxide retention does not occur in mild cases of bronchiolitis, but in more severe cases where larger numbers of alveoli are obstructed, hypercapnia and respiratory acidosis ensue. Carbon dioxide retention is associated with respiratory rates of greater than 60 and increases in proportion to the increasing rate.

## Clinical Features

Bronchiolitis usually occurs in children in contact with family members who have an upper respiratory infection. It also occurs more frequently in children exposed to parental cigarette smoke. The infant is first noted to have signs of upper respiratory infection, such as runny nose and sneezing, accompanied by a low-grade fever, 38 to 39°C (100 to 102°F), and decreased appetite. Lower respiratory symptoms develop over a few days and include dyspnea, tachypnea, intercostal retractions, wheezing, and cyanosis. In more severely affected patients, the symptoms may develop more rapidly, within a few hours. Apnea may occur, especially in children less than 6 months of age.

On examination of the patient with bronchiolitis, one will typically see a tachypneic infant in mild to severe respiratory distress, with respirations ranging from 60 to 80 per minute, flaring of the alae nasi, and using the accessory muscles of respiration with intercostal and subcostal retractions. Cyanosis may not be present, but significant abnormalities of gas exchange may develop in the absence of cyanosis. Respirations are shallow because of the persistent distension of the lungs by trapped air. Diffuse, fine sibilant and/or musical rales are often present, and the expiratory phase of breathing may be prolonged with audible wheezing. Barely audible breath sounds are a sign of impending respiratory failure. The liver and spleen may be palpated below the costal margins, suggesting hepatosplenomegaly; however, their position is secondary to downward displacement of the diaphragm from pulmonary hyperinflation. Signs of dehydration are often present, usually caused by inadequate oral fluid intake secondary to respiratory distress.

It is during the first 48 to 72 h after the onset of cough and dyspnea that the infant is most critically ill. Improvement typically occurs quickly after this time and the infant is usually fully recovered within a few days. The course is often prolonged in infants with underlying disease.

## Laboratory and X-ray Findings

The chest x-ray in bronchiolitis shows hyperinflation of the lungs and an increased AP diameter on lateral view. There are sometimes small areas of atelectasis which may mimic pneumonitis. The white blood cell count and hemoglobin level are usually within the normal range. Pulse oximetry and blood gases frequently reveal hypoxia, which correlates with the respiratory rate. Carbon dioxide retention occurs infrequently in children with bronchiolitis but is present in those infants in severe respiratory distress. Since hypoxia commonly occurs in children with bronchiolitis, often with limited clinical manifestations, all children with bronchiolitis should have their $Sa_{O_2}$ measured with a pulse oximeter on presentation to the emergency department and then monitored periodically while receiving treatment. Infants with moderate to severe bronchiolitis should have their $Sa_{O_2}$ monitored continuously. Arterial blood gases should be obtained in those children with severe bronchiolitis.

Viral cultures are positive in the majority of infants with bronchiolitis, with RSV being by far the most frequently identified. Fluorescent monoclonal antibody testing on specimens from nasal washings or deep nasopharyngeal swabs is a useful way of rapidly detecting the presence of RSV. This study is especially important for those children hospitalized with bronchiolitis who may nosocomially spread the illness to others, particularly those with underlying disease. It may also be helpful in influencing the use of ribavirin therapy for this illness (see "Emergency Department Care," below).

## Differential Diagnosis

See "Asthma: Differential Diagnosis."

## Emergency Department Care

The treatment of bronchiolitis in the emergency department is primarily supportive and should be based on the child's clinical condition. The infant with mild bronchiolitis (alert, playful, feeding well with good hydration, respiratory rate <50, and no subcostal retractions) and no significant associated illness, such as bronchopulmonary dysplasia or congenital heart disease, may be managed conservatively as an outpatient with careful observation and small frequent feedings. Almost all other children with bronchiolitis are hypoxic, especially when they are asleep.

Consequently, the most important therapy for bronchiolitis is humidified oxygen at an $F_{I_{O_2}}$ of 28 to 40%. This should be delivered by mask, hood, or tent, since nasal prongs may produce reflex bronchoconstriction. Pulse oximetry and arterial blood gases are useful in monitoring those patients in moderate to severe respiratory distress (respiratory rate >60). Mist has not proved helpful since almost no moisture reaches the lower respiratory tract to liquefy secretions.

Children with bronchiolitis should be given a trial of $\beta_2$ agonists in all but the mildest cases of this disease. Although the use of bronchodilators for bronchiolitis is still controversial, most recent studies have confirmed their beneficial effects. Nebulized albuterol should be given at 0.15 mg/kg per dose for up to three doses at 20-min intervals. The child should be examined after each dose to determine the need for further medication. If the child responds, it suggests that he or she has reversible bronchospasm and should be followed for future wheezing episodes. A trial of aerosolized albuterol with an MDI-spacer (2 puffs q 4 h) or oral albuterol after discharge should be considered in the child who responds to nebulized albuterol. The dose is 0.1 to 0.15 mg/kg per dose three times a day. If there is some improvement with nebulized albuterol but the child is still having significant wheezing and especially if admission is likely, continuous albuterol may be indicated. If the child is atopic or there is a strong family history of asthma, this may be the first attack of asthma and the child should be treated accordingly, especially if the child requires admission. Subcutaneous epinephrine or terbutaline may be indicated in selected children with bronchiolitis and respiratory failure (see "Asthma: Emergency Department Care: Acute Exacerbations").

Racemic epinephrine may have some beneficial effect in the treatment of bronchiolitis. A recent study by Sanchez et al. compared racemic epinephrine, 0.1 mL/kg of a 2.25% solution, to 0.03 mL/kg (0.15 mg/kg) of albuterol and found that racemic epinephrine was superior to albuterol in treating bronchiolitis. Further studies are needed to confirm these findings, but racemic epinephrine should be considered in children with bronchiolitis who do not respond to albuterol.

Glucocorticoids have been studied extensively in bronchiolitis and have not been shown to alter the course of this disease. In children with recurrent episodes of bronchiolitis, which is probably infantile asthma, or in children with an atopic history or strong family history of asthma, glucocorticoids should be considered in the acute management.

Ipratropium bromide (Atrovent) given with albuterol does not appear to provide any additional benefit to the use of albuterol alone. Theophylline has also been extensively studied and it is not beneficial in the treatment of bronchiolitis.

Many children with bronchiolitis become dehydrated because of decreased fluid intake secondary to the excessive work of breathing and pulmonary insensible water loss. Intravenous fluids ($D_5$ one-fourth normal saline solution with added KCl) must be administered to these children, but should be given with some caution as pulmonary edema may occur with overaggressive fluid therapy. Hydration in excess of replacement and maintenance is unnecessary.

Routine administration of antibiotics has not proved beneficial in bronchiolitis. If the child is desperately ill, or if the infant's clinical condition suddenly deteriorates, one should consider bacterial infection superimposed on viral infection. In this case, a broad-spectrum antibiotic such as cefuroxime may be useful. Prior to administering the antibiotic, tracheal secretions should be examined by Gram stain and by culture, and blood cultures should be obtained. Recently, two forms of inpatient therapy have been used to alter the course of the very ill child with bronchiolitis. Ribavirin, an antiviral agent, administered by aerosolization, has been shown to decrease morbidity due to RSV infections, and extracorporeal membrane oxygenation (ECMO) has been used successfully in children with bronchiolitis whose condition deteriorates despite maximal ventilator management.

Ribavirin is recommended for hospitalized children with RSV infection at high risk for complications due to underlying disease (e.g., cardiopulmonary disease), severely ill infants, and for all children mechanically ventilated for RSV infection. It should also be considered in very young infants (less than 6 weeks of age) or those children with underlying conditions such as multiple congenital anomalies who may be at increased risk of progressively worsening disease.

The use of RSV immune globulin for children at high risk for severe illness from RSV infection has recently been studied. It appears that this form of therapy is a safe and effective means of RSV prophylaxis in young, high-risk children.

Sedation should be avoided because of its effect on suppression of the respiratory drive unless the child is intubated with assisted ventilation and closely monitored.

Frequent reassessment in the emergency department is essential. Small infants may become unstable in a short period of time and develop respiratory failure (see "Asthma: Emergency Department Care: Status Asthmaticus"). Continuous positive airway pressure (CPAP) may be started prior to mechanical ventilation if time permits. Intubation with mechanical ventilation is necessary for the child in frank respiratory failure, if CPAP fails, or if there are frequent apneic spells.

## Admission Indications/Discharge Instructions/ Follow-up

One may consider managing a child with bronchiolitis as an outpatient if the child is well hydrated, drinking fluids well, is not cyanotic, appears comfortable, and is not in visible respiratory distress (respiratory rate <60). Since hypoxia is a common finding in bronchiolitic children pulse oximetry and/or arterial blood gases should be obtained in all instances. Children who are not drinking fluids well, are having apneic episodes or have a history of apnea, and/or appear to be in respiratory distress should be admitted. Occasionally, children with severe bronchiolitis develop respiratory failure. These infants and those with frequent episodes of apnea may need endotracheal or nasotracheal intubation for ventilatory support and admission to the intensive care unit. Infants with a past history of respiratory distress syndrome resulting in bronchopulmonary dysplasia, complex congenital heart disease, or other significant underlying disease who develop bronchiolitis need close observation and should, in almost all cases, be hospitalized.

If the social situation is such that following instructions and giving adequate home care seem unlikely, or if parental anxiety is so great that the parents are having trouble coping with their child's illness, the child should be admitted. If one chooses to discharge a patient with mild bronchiolitis, parents should be given detailed instructions regarding hydration and increasing respiratory distress. Children who respond to albuterol should continue taking this medication at home (see "Emergency Department Care"). All these children should be called or seen again 12 to 24 h after their presentation to the emergency department.

## BIBLIOGRAPHY

### Asthma

Barnes PJ: A new approach to the treatment of asthma. *N Engl J Med* 321:1517, 1989.

Bosquet J, Chanez P, Lacoste JY, et al: Eosinophilic inflammation in asthma. *N Engl J Med* 323:1033, 1990.

Burrows B, Martinez FD, Halonen M, et al: Association of asthma with serum IgE levels and skin-test reactivity to allergens. *N Engl J Med* 320:271, 1989.

Furukawa CT: Stepping up the treatment of children with asthma. *Pediatrics* 92:144, 1993.

Geelhoed GC, Landau LI, Le Soüef PN: Evaluation of $Sa_{O_2}$ as predictor of outcome in 280 children presenting with acute asthma. *Ann Emerg Med* 23:1236, 1994.

Jones JF; FDA Varicella Warning. *Pediatrics* 90:479, 1992.

Katz RW, Kelly W, Crowley MR, et al: Safety of continuous nebulized albuterol for bronchospasm in infants and children. *Pediatrics* 92:666, 1993.

Kerem E, Levison H, Schuh S, et al: Efficacy of albuterol administered by nebulizer versus spacer device in children with acute asthma. *J Pediatr* 123:313, 1993.

Larsen GL: Asthma in children. *N Engl J Med* 326:1540, 1992.

National Asthma Education Program Expert Panel. *Guidelines for the Diagnosis and Management of Asthma.* National Heart, Lung and Blood Institute, National Asthma Education Program Expert Panel REport. *J Allergy Clin Immunol* 88:425, 1991.

Schuh S, Johnson DW, Callahan S, et al: Efficacy of continuous ipratropium in severe asthma. *Pediatr Res* 37:148A, 1994.

Shapiro GG: Childhood asthma: Update. *Pediatr Rev* 13:403, 1992.

Smith L: Childhood asthma: Diagnosis and treatment. *Curr Probl Pediatr* 23:271, 1993.

Strauss RE, Wertheim DL, Bonagura VR, et al: Aminophylline therapy does not improve outcome and increases adverse effects in children hospitalized with acute asthmatic exacerbations. *Pediatrics* 93:205, 1994.

Tinkelman DG, Reed CE, Nelson HS, et al: Aerosol beclomethasone dipropionate compared with theophylline as primary treatment of chronic, mild to moderately severe asthma in children. *Pediatrics* 92:64, 1993.

### Bronchiolitis

Klassen TP, Rowe PC, Sutcliffe T, et al: Randomized trial of salbutamol in acute bronchiolitis. *J Pediatr* 118:807, 1991.

Sanchez I, De Koster J, Powell RE, et al: Effect of racemic epinephrine and salbutamol on clinical score and pulmonary mechanics in infants with bronchiolitis. *J Pediatr* 122:145, 1993.

Schuh S, Johnson D, Canny G, et al: Efficacy of adding nebulized ipratropium bromide to nebulized albuterol therapy in acute bronchiolitis. *Pediatrics* 90:920, 1992.

# 113
# SEIZURES AND STATUS EPILEPTICUS IN CHILDREN
## Michael A. Nigro

Approximately 2 percent of the United States population has some form of epilepsy. Many more experience seizures in association with febrile illnesses or other acute problems. In children aged 0 to 9 years, the prevalence is 4.4 cases per 1000, and in those 10 to 19 years, the prevalence is 6.6 cases per 1000. Simple febrile convulsions constitute a separate category, with an incidence of 3 to 4 percent in children.

These numbers alone do not reveal the most important features of the seizure phenomenon—the increased morbidity and mortality that are a direct result of seizures, their cause, or their treatment. Epidemiologic studies indicate an overall mortality two to three times higher in epileptic patients than in nonepileptics. The earlier the onset of seizures and the more deprived the social environment, the higher the morbidity and the mortality.

Typically a patient with seizures arrives at the emergency department with one of the following:

1. The initial or a recurrent seizure
2. Status epilepticus
3. Complications of medication
4. A history of seizures with an acute, underlying disease—e.g., sickle cell anemia, metabolic disease, or febrile illness—that needs treatment

Emergency care should include (1) safely stopping the seizure, (2) identifying and correcting immediately treatable or reversible causes, and (3) initiating appropriate diagnostic studies and arranging follow-up. If management is difficult, the patient should be admitted. There are significant enough differences in the treatment of children that unless the physician is experienced in pediatric management or able to readily obtain pediatric consultation, the child should be transferred to a pediatric facility. Treatment and diagnostic studies may be complex, and time is important in reducing morbidity.

## DEFINITION

A *seizure* is an episodic, involuntary alteration in motor activity, behavior, sensation, or autonomic function. It represents an abrupt change in brain function. The term *epilepsy* indicates recurring seizures without a simple discernible and reversible cause. Physiologically, a seizure is an abnormal, sudden, and excessive electric discharge of neurons (gray matter) which propagates down the neuronal processes (white matter) to affect end organs in a clinically measurable fashion.

The International Classification of Epileptic Seizures is accepted as the contemporary standard (see Table 113-1).

## THE FIRST SEIZURE

The first seizure in a child usually causes some degree of panic in the parents, and an accurate account of seizure and preseizure events may not be obtainable. If it lasts seconds to minutes, and if others in the family have experienced seizures, an emergency visit may not be made. Unless the child is in status epilepticus, or seizures recur in the emergency department, the physician can defer immediate anticonvulsant treatment and concentrate on defining the cause and the risk of recurrence.

Hauser and co-workers categorized seizure recurrence for all ages according to the presumed cause. Of their patients, 73 percent were categorized as having idiopathic seizures, and 27 percent as having remote symptomatic seizures. Idiopathic seizures recurred in 17 percent of the patients by 20 months after the initial seizure, and in 26 percent of the patients by 36 months after the first seizure, but the recurrence rate was greater in patients with generalized spike-wave EEGs, and in patients with siblings who had had seizures. In patients with prior neurologic insult (cerebrovascular accident, meningitis, etc.) the recurrence rate was 34 percent by 20 months after the initial seizure.

Immediate diagnostic evaluation (see Table 113-2) can be initiated in the emergency situation, and if the seizure was brief and appears to be idiopathic, the decision to initiate anticonvulsant therapy can be deferred until the appropriate neurologic assessment is completed. The causes of the first seizure vary, but idiopathic seizures account for 26.3 to 47 percent of the children with seizures seen, depending on the study cited. Secondary seizures occur for a variety of reasons (e.g., inflammatory, structural, metabolic, or secondary to general illness).

In any group of seizure patients, there is a subgroup in whom the seizure is a symptom of an underlying disorder and is not due to idiopathic epilepsy. In such cases correction of the primary problem makes seizure recurrence unlikely. Thus, the primary goal must be to

**Table 113-1.** International Classification of Epileptic Seizures

Partial seizures (seizures beginning locally)
  Partial seizures with elementary symptomatology (generally without impairment of consciousness)
    With motor symptoms (includes Jacksonian seizures)
    With special sensory or somatosensory symptoms
    With autonomic symptoms
    Compound forms
  Partial seizures with complex symptomatology (generally with impairment of consciousness)
    With impairment of consciousness only
    With cognitive symptomatology
    With affective symptomatology
    With "psychosensory" symptomatology
    With "psychomotor" symptomatology
    Compound forms
  Partial seizures secondarily generalized
Generalized seizures (bilaterally symmetric without local onset)
  Absences (petit mal)
  Bilateral massive epileptic myoclonus
  Infantile spasms
  Clonic seizures
  Tonic seizures
  Tonic-clonic seizures (grand mal)
  Atonic seizures
  Akinetic seizures
Unclassified epileptic seizures

*Source:* Gastaut H: Clinical and electroencephalographical classification of epileptic seizures. *Epilepsia* 11:102, 1970. Used by permission.

**Table 113-2.** Diagnostic Studies in Seizure Patients*

| Study | Neonatal Seizure | First Seizure in Children | Status Epilepticus | Recurring Breakthrough (nonstable) |
|---|---|---|---|---|
| CBC with differential | X | X | X | — |
| Random blood sugar | X | X | X | X |
| Electrolytes | X | X | X | X |
| Creatinine | X | — | X | — |
| Magnesium | X | X | X | — |
| Calcium | X | X | X | X |
| BUN | X | X | X | — |
| Blood gases | X | — | X | — |
| Serum ammonia | X† | — | — | — |
| Urine and serum amino acid screen | X† | X† | — | — |
| TORCH titers | X† | — | — | — |
| Lumbar puncture | X† | X† | X† | — |
| Anticonvulsant levels | — | — | X | X |
| EEG | X | X | X† | — |
| Echoencephalogram (real time cerebral ultrasound) | X† | — | — | — |
| CT scan | X† | X† | X† | X† |
| MRI scan | X† | X† | X† | X† |
| Chest x-ray | X† | X† | X† | X† |
| Skeletal (x-ray) survey | X† | — | — | — |
| Cardiac/pulmonary evaluation | X† | — | X | — |
| Evaluation for superimposed medical problems, infectious disease | X | X | X† | X |

\* X, diagnostic studies to be performed; —, studies need not be performed.
† When history or physical examination warrants it.

uncover disorders that are readily identifiable and reversible. Symptomatic seizures of hypoglycemia, hypocalcemia, and electrolyte imbalance can be treated immediately; there is little risk of recurrence, and they usually do not require anticonvulsant use. Seizures occurring as a result of intracranial infections and craniocerebral trauma may require only immediate or short-term anticonvulsant use. Symptomatic seizures of systemic lupus erythematosus (SLE), sickle cell anemia, leukemia, arteriovenous malformations, and neoplasms may be the heralding symptoms of a complex, yet treatable, underlying disease. Seizures have been reported in children following topical application of N,N-diethyl-m-toluamide (DEET) and lindane (Kwell).

If the initial seizure is prolonged or classified as status epilepticus, appropriate therapy and diagnostic workup must be initiated (Tables 113-2, 113-3, or 113-6). If several seizures occur, or if the initial seizure is prolonged or occurs in a patient at higher risk for recurrence (such as one with prior neurologic insult), anticonvulsant therapy can be initiated immediately (Table 113-3). For tonic, tonic-clonic, clonic, or partial seizures, pheonobarbital is used most often,

and the initial doses need not be the higher, loading doses required in status epilepticus (Table 113-6). Phenytoin is the second most commonly used drug in this situation. Carbamazepine is considered equal to phenytoin in anticonvulsant properties but has a different spectrum of potential side effects. Felbamate was introduced in 1993 as an adjunct antiepileptic drug (AED). Felbamate is indicated in the treatment of complex partial epilepsy. Common side effects include anorexia and insomnia, which usually subside after 2 to 3 months. In mid 1994 severe hematologic and hepatic abnormalities associated with felbamate resulted in withdrawal of the drug from most patients and careful surveillance in the select few continuing to use it. There are significant potential drug-drug interactions, especially with phenytoin. Gabapentin was also introduced in 1993 as an add-on AED in the treatment of complex partial epilepsy. Its major benefits are that it does not interact with other AEDs and is excreted unmetabolized.

Absence (petit mal) seizures rarely require emergency care, and an EEG should be obtained for confirmation before one starts drugs

**Table 113-3.** Initial and Maintenance Doses in the First Seizure (*Nonstatus* Partial and Tonic, Clonic, and Tonic-Clonic Seizures of Childhood)

| Drug | Initial Dose, mg/kg | Maintenance Dose, mg/kg per 24 h | Doses/Day | Therapeutic Level, μg/mL Total | Free | Half-Life, h |
|---|---|---|---|---|---|---|
| Phenytoin (Dilantin) | 8 | 4–8* | 2–3 | 10–20 | 1.2–2.1 | 24 ± 12 |
| Phenobarbital | 6 | 3–8 | 1–2 | 15–20 | NA | 60 ± 20 |
| Carbamazepine (Tegretol) | 5 | 10–40 | 2–4 | 6–12 | NA | 20 ± 5 |
| Primidone (Mysoline) | 5 | 10–20 | 2–4 | 5–12 | NA | 12 |
| Valproic acid (Depakene/Depakote) | 10 | 20–60 | 2–4 | 50–130 | 10–25 | 6–12 |
| Ethosuximide (Zarontin) | 20 | 20–30 | 2–3 | 50–100 | NA | 30 |
| Clonazepam (Clonopin) | 0.05 | 0.1–0.3 | 2–4 | NA | NA | 18–50 |
| Acetazolamide (Diamox) | 10 | 10 | 1–2 | NA | NA | 24–42 |
| Felbamate (Felbatol) | 15 | 45 | 3 | NA | NA | 19.4 |
| Gabapentin (Neurontin) | 5 | 20–30 | 3 | NA | NA | 5–7 |

\* Up to 12 mg/kg in infants.
*Note:* NA = not applicable.

that are more specific, namely, ethosuximide, valproate, and acetazolamide.

## FEBRILE SEIZURE

Febrile seizure is a unique and common form of seizure in childhood. Although various types occur (tonic, tonic-clonic, clonic), the characteristics of a simple febrile seizure separate it from other symptomatic and idiopathic seizure disorders. The National Institutes of Health Consensus Development Conference of Febrile Seizure defined it as "an event in infancy or childhood usually occurring between three months and five years of age, associated with fever but without evidence of intracranial infection or defined cause." Typically, these seizures are generalized and last less than 10 min (some physicians say 15 to 20 min is more typical), and there is no postictal focal neurologic deficit. The EEG usually does not reveal paroxysmal (epileptic) activity, and there often is a family history of similar seizures. Typically a rapid rise in temperature, usually above 38.8°C (101.8°F), occurs at the onset of the illness and, on occasion, recurs several times in the course of the illness. Three to four percent of young children experience febrile seizures, and of these, 30 to 40 percent have recurrences, especially when the first seizure occurs under 1 year of age. The mortality from simple febrile seizures is extremely low.

### Evaluation

The first febrile seizure warrants the most concern, because the benign nature of the illness has not been established. More concern regarding intracranial infection is justified with the febrile-seizure child before the propensity for recurring simple febrile seizures has been established. The initial evaluation concentrates on serious causes, such as meningitis, encephalitis, and sepsis or bacteremia. Lumbar puncture is warranted with the first febrile seizure or whenever intracranial sepsis appears likely. If a cause it not found and the child is ill, admission, workup, and therapy are warranted. Underlying diseases should be diagnosed. Toxic encephalopathy with fever as a symptom should be identified and treated. An EEG can be done electively, and, although its benefits are arguable, it can be helpful in identifying the child who is at greater risk of recurrent seizure.

### Treatment

Therapy for the cause of the fever is the main goal. If a child appears well after experiencing a single febrile seizure, anticonvulsant therapy can be deferred, the child can be evaluated electively, and the family and attending physicians can decide whether anticonvulsants will be used. Phenobarbital at therapeutic levels (15 to 30 µg/mL) may reduce febrile seizure frequency. A recent study indicated no significant benefit from phenobarbital prophylaxis and a 6-point loss in full-scale I.Q. in lower functioning children. At this time, prophylaxis for febrile seizures remains an unresolved issue. If the child is ill, has had recurring seizures with this febrile illness, or has had several seizures with prior febrile illnesses, administration of phenobarbital can be initiated and maintained until the child improves and a decision is reached regarding the use of long-term anticonvulsants. There are subgroups of febrile seizure patients who warrant long-term anticonvulsant (phenobarbital) use, including the child (1) with a preexisting neurologic deficit, such as mental retardation or cerebral palsy, (2) with repeated seizures in the same febrile illness, (3) under 1 year of age, (4) with prior nonfebrile seizures and siblings or parents with epilepsy, or (5) with more than three febrile seizures in 6 months. When parents request phenobarbital prophylaxis, having been informed of the risks and benefits, it is reasonable to treat the child.

The protocol to follow when treating a child with febrile seizure is as follows:

1. Administer a loading dose of phenobarbital (15 mg/kg) orally, intravenously, or intramuscularly, followed by 4 to 6 mg/kg per day to attain therapeutic levels of 15 to 30 µg/mL.
2. Interrupt the fever gradually with tepid baths (use no alcohol) and acetaminophen or ibuprofen.
3. Identify the source of infection and do a lumbar puncture if meningitis or encephalitis is suspected, or if unexplained febrile seizure occurs for the first time.
4. Arrange for follow-up studies with the child's family physician.
5. Admit the ill child without an easily treatable problem or one in whom recurrent seizures have occurred within several hours or 1 day.
6. Obtain an EEG when appropriate. An EEG may be helpful (if definitely abnormal) as a further indication of a convulsive disorder.

Phenobarbital is the most effective medication for febrile seizures. Phenytoin is considered ineffective. Rectally or orally administered diazepam has been used successfully but is not in standard use in the United States. Rectal diazepam administration is initiated by a clinical nurse specialist in consultation with the parents, instructing them in dosage, administration, and monitoring. Usual dosage is 0.2 to 0.5 mg/kg as a single dose. Valproic acid has been effective, but its relative toxicity increases its risk, which contraindicates its use in the prevention of febrile seizure.

## NEONATAL SEIZURES

Seizures in the neonate are difficult to identify and often require aggressive therapy. All neonates experiencing seizures should be considered to be at serious risk from the underlying disorder and the effect of unremitting seizures and also to be at increased risk of epilepsy. Electroconvulsive activity should be of as much concern as the outward clinical signs of seizure. Prompt, effective anticonvulsant therapy and other specific therapies lessen the impact of short-term detrimental effect on long-term neurologic functioning. In many instances, the seizure itself is less important for its immediate effects than it is as an indicator of significant underlying disease (e.g., galactosemia, meningitis) that will ultimately have more effect on the morbidity and mortality.

The difference in seizure presentation is due to the predominantly inhibitory brain of newborns and the particular illnesses to which they are subject. Multifocal or fragmentary seizures occur more commonly at this age, and clonic or tonic movements independently affect the limbs simultaneously or fleetingly. Progressive migratory partial seizures (jacksonian) are rarely seen at this age. Autonomic seizures manifest as variable changes in respiration (tachypnea, depression, or apnea), temperature, and color (cyanosis), and also as cardiac arrhythmias and pupillary changes. Myoclonic seizures usually have hypoxic or metabolic causes and indicate a poor prognosis unless the cause is easily identifiable and readily reversible (e.g., hypocalcemia, hypoglycemia). Myoclonic seizures can, however, be refractory in metabolic disorders such as urea cycle defects and nonketotic hyperglycinemia. Unilateral (partial or focal) seizures may be associated with structural lesions, and permanent neurologic deficit may be associated with them. The causes of neonatal seizures are diverse, but the majority of the seizures are attributable to a few well-defined causes.

### Evaluation

Common neurologic nonepileptic problems encountered in the newborn are hyperexcitability in the tremulous infant, and nonepileptic cerebral manifestations of sepsis, cardiac disease, and hypoxia. Benign myoclonus is also seen. Respiratory immaturity with apnea is a particularly difficult problem at this age.

The workup includes early assessment for treatable causes. Sepsis and metabolic derangements are frequent causes of neonatal seizures.

The highest incidence of neonatal seizures is in infants with hypoxia/ischemia, sepsis, or hypoglycemia.

Complex hereditary metabolic disorders—e.g., urea cycle defects with hyperammonemia; maple syrup urine disease; and methylmalonic acidemia—usually become evident days or weeks after feedings with protein are initiated. Others may appear symptomatic in utero or soon after delivery, e.g., nonketotic hyperglycinemia, in which the mother reports fetal hiccoughs, and soon after birth the infant is flaccid, exhibiting myoclonic seizures. Seizures in these metabolic disorders are a signal that significant CNS impairment may be present.

Some of these disorders may be completely controlled or the effects may be reversed with appropriate dietary manipulation (galactosemia) or coenzyme replacement (pyridoxine dependency, biotin dependency, subtypes of methylmalonic acidemia).

In evaluating the infant, the cause of the seizures may be readily apparent. The dysmorphic newborn could have a chromosomal defect (trisomy, deletion) or be identifiable only by the combination of unusual features (Cornelia de Lange syndrome). Neurocutaneous diseases infrequently cause seizures in the newborn but are readily identifiable by certain signs, e.g., encephalotrigeminal hemangiomatosis in Sturge-Weber syndrome, or achromic patches in tuberous sclerosis. Cutaneous herpes with seizures may be an indication that herpes simplex encephalitis is present. Chorioretinitis is a clear sign of an intrauterine infection which could cause seizures (e.g., herpes, toxoplasmosis, cytomegalovirus, rubella). Cerebral imaging is warranted in neonates to help define cerebral hemorrhage and structural abnormalities. Ultrasound may be sufficient for diagnosis in some cases but MRI is the best study for migrational defects of the central nervous system (e.g., lissencephalia, heterotopias, agenesis of the corpus callosum). Single photon emission tomography (SPECT) and positron emission tomography (PET) are helpful in defining epileptic foci but are not indicated for emergency evaluation and treatment.

## Treatment

There are several factors influencing treatment in the neonate: (1) variations in the metabolic half-lives of drugs; (2) associated etiologic conditions (e.g., hypoxia prolongs the half-life of many drugs and may affect the renal or gastrointestinal clearance rate); and (3) greater difficulty in identifying the end point of seizure control in neonates.

Effective seizure control is obtained by rapidly achieving therapeutic blood levels of the anticonvulsant chosen. Newborns have different rates of metabolism and excretion of anticonvulsants from older infants and children. In infants less than 7 days old, the half-life of phenobarbital, the drug of first choice, is 100 h, and after 28 days of continuous therapy, the half-life of the drug is reduced to 60 to 70 h.

In the presence of hypoxia with tissue acidosis and renal and hepatic compromise, anticonvulsant half-lives may be increased, with toxic levels reached more readily.

Blood levels of phenobarbital of 16 to 40 μg/mL are necessary to achieve seizure control in the majority of cases. Levels of 40 to 80 μg/mL have been maintained in resistant cases with inconsistent benefit. Dosages of phenobarbital of 3 to 4 mg/kg per day maintain mid to high therapeutic levels and prevent toxicity.

Phenytoin is the second drug of choice in treating neonatal seizures and has the disadvantage of requiring intravenous use to obtain and maintain therapeutic levels. Loading doses vary from 15 to 20 mg/kg, and maintenance dosages of 8 to 12 mg/kg per day are satisfactory and not likely to produce toxicity. Pyridoxine (vitamin $B_6$) 100 mg/day is empirically used when no reasonable cause of the seizure is found. The only reasonable determinant of its effectiveness is a cessation of seizure activity. The electroencephalogram does not immediately improve with intravenous pyridoxine use.

In status epilepticus of the neonate, diazepam or lorazepam must be used with caution since its half-life may be prolonged, and respiratory depression superimposed on an immature and possibly compromised respiratory apparatus should be anticipated. Diazepam may exaggerate hyperbilirubinemia by uncoupling the bilirubin-albumin complex and should be used with caution in jaundiced babies.

Treatment principles in the management of neonatal seizures are as follows:

1. Identify and correct treatable causes (hypocalcemia, hypoglycemia, electrolyte imbalance).
2. Identify and treat associated problems such as sepsis, hyperbilirubinemia, acidosis, etc.
3. Initiate anticonvulsant therapy with appropriate loading doses, and carefully observe blood levels to adjust the maintenance dosage (see Table 113-4).

## INFANTILE SPASMS

Infantile spasms are a unique form of seizures. The onset is typically between 3 and 9 months of age and may begin as late as 18 months. Concurrently, the child exhibits a regression in development. The spasms are very brief, lasting a split second, often with flexion or extension of the head and trunk. They occur singly or repeatedly in bursts of 5 to 20 spasms at a time, usually occurring several times per day and more often upon arousal from sleep or with sudden auditory or physical stimulation. The EEG is abnormal in virtually every case (hypsarrhythmic in 50 percent). Mental retardation is as high as 85 percent of patients with this disorder. Parents are often frustrated because medical professionals fail to diagnose these spasms as seizures.

There are many causes of infantile spasm (secondary type) including migrational defects, prior CNS trauma, hypoxia, neurocutaneous disorders, and infectious and metabolic disorders. The idiopathic type is the most alarming because it affects children with no prior neurologic disorder.

Early diagnosis and aggressive management with adrenocorticotropic hormone (ACTH) within a month of onset result in an optimum response. Since there is an urgency to this problem, hospitalization, neurologic referral, appropriate diagnostic workup, and initiation of treatment must be rapidly conducted. Aggressive management with steroids or anticonvulsants, careful monitoring of the EEG, and identification of side effects make this therapeutic problem beyond the scope of emergency care with one exception: recognizing the problem.

## HEAD TRAUMA AND SEIZURES

Head trauma can result in seizures of three types: immediate seizures, early posttraumatic seizures, and late posttraumatic seizures. Immediate seizures result from impact and presumably are due to traumatic depolarization of neurons. The risk of recurring seizures in these pa-

**Table 113-4.** Drug Regimen for Neonatal Seizures

1. Vitamin $B_6$ (pyridoxine), 50 mg IV (up to 100 mg/day)—used in the absence of an obvious cause of seizures
2. Glucose, 2 mL/kg (25% solution) bolus—given to infants stressed with proven hypoglycemia or when merely suspect
3. Calcium gluconate, 4 mL/kg IV
4. Magnesium—magnesium sulfate, 50%, 0.2 mL/kg IM—given to infants with a proven deficiency
5. Phenobarbital loading
   - Premature infant    20 mg/kg IV
   - Full-term infant    15 mg/kg IV
6. Phenytoin (Dilantin), loading dose, 15 mg/kg IV
7. Diazepam (Valium) for continuous s, 0.2 mg/kg IV, repeat twice if necessary (see text)
8. Lorazepam, 0.05 mg/kg IV (may repeat twice if necessary)
9. Clonazepam (Klonopin), 0.1 mg/kg NG if high therapeutic levels of phenobarbital and phenytoin (Dilantin) are ineffective

tients is minimal unless there are more serious prognostic factors such as prolonged coma and penetrating head injury. Anticonvulsants are sometimes used because of the unknown potential for immediate recurring seizures. In the patient who recovers rapidly, chronic anticonvulsant use is usually not indicated. An exception would be a patient with a prior seizure history or a family history of epilepsy.

Early posttraumatic seizures occur within the first week after trauma, and epilepsy results in 20 to 25 percent of these patients. These early seizures are presumed to result from the focal effects of contusions or lacerations and the associated hypoperfusion, which causes ischemia and related metabolic changes.

Treatment of immediate and early posttraumatic seizures requires the correction of neurologic problems (depressed fracture, hematoma), the reduction of cerebral edema, proper oxygenation (airway maintenance, correction of shock), and the careful administration of anticonvulsants. With immediate and early posttraumatic seizures when impaired consciousness already prevails, it is important to avoid the use of significant sedative medication (barbiturates or diazepam) if possible. Phenytoin may be used successfully with relative safety (see Table 113-3). The dosage is determined by the clinical presentation; rapid loading is warranted to obtain immediate therapeutic levels in the patient in whom repeated seizures are occurring or likely to recur, especially when a seizure may further aggravate associated medical or surgical conditions.

Immediate posttraumatic seizures warrant anticonvulsant therapy for initial control, while long-term management of immediate seizures remains controversial.

Late posttraumatic seizures occur after 1 week and may be seen as late as 10 years after the trauma. Structural changes such as atrophy with cicatrix and permanent local vascular changes, altered dendrite branching, and presumably modified neurotransmitter function account for the development and permanence of these seizures. Of these seizures, 40 percent are focal or partial seizures and 50 percent are temporal lobe seizures, indicating the predilection for traumatic injury and known epileptogenic properties of this structure. The risk of recurring seizures in this group is reported to be as high as 70 percent.

Early and late posttraumatic seizures warrant long-term anticonvulsant therapy in view of the risk of immediate and later recurrence. Late-onset posttraumatic seizures are most likely to recur, and long-term anticonvulsant therapy is necessary. Patients at greater risk for chronic posttraumatic seizures include those with depressed skull fractures, posttraumatic amnesia more than 24 h after the trauma, dural penetration, acute intracranial hemorrhage, early posttraumatic epilepsy, and a foreign body in a cerebral wound. The more severe the seizure and the later the onset, the less likely remission will occur.

Emergency management of seizures related to trauma should emphasize neurosurgical assessment, the rapid, careful administration of nonsedative anticonvulsants, the interruption of the seizures, and the stabilization of the general medical condition.

## BREAKTHROUGH SEIZURES IN THE KNOWN EPILEPTIC

When seizures recur in a known epileptic, something has occurred to alter the balance of the excitation-inhibition complex, and the seizure threshold has been lowered. Complete seizure control is not always possible. The child with mental retardation, cerebral palsy, and complex partial seizures with or without secondary generalization is most likely to have recurring seizures. Tonic-clonic (grand mal) seizures are the most dramatic and often lead to emergency treatment. The usual causes of seizure breakthrough can be summarized as follows:

1. Lowered anticonvulsant blood levels.
    a. Due to noncompliance. This is a common cause, most often in the preteen or teen who has been given the responsibility for self-medication.
    b. Related to intercurrent infection. Anticonvulsant levels fall during acute infections (viral or bacterial) with or without fever. Quite often the child's seizure recurrence is an indication of the infection before the acute problem is evident, e.g., with varicella or otitis media.
    c. The interaction of different drugs. An example is the reduction of the phenytoin level by the induction of parahydroxylators when barbiturates are used concomitantly (see "Problems of Anticonvulsant Use").
2. Change in habits.
    a. Altered sleep patterns because of trips, holidays, or parties.
    b. A job, exams, or an emotional stress. In the active teen, this may lead to seizures. If a pattern develops, knowledge of the pattern is quite helpful in defining treatment.
    c. Alcohol use. This can lower the seizure threshold and can also increase noncompliance.
    d. The use of illicit drugs or prescription drugs that lower the threshold. Examples are neuroleptic agents, lindane (Kwell), theophylline, PCP, LSD, and certain anesthetic agents (e.g., ethrane).
3. Complicating factors of epilepsy management.
    a. Toxic levels of drugs. An example is phenytoin intoxication, which can increase seizure frequency. Carbamazepine in therapeutic dosage has been found to infrequently increase seizures.
    b. The use of phenytoin in some myoclonic epilepsies.
    c. Valproic acid. Its use in complex partial seizures with secondary generalization has been reported to increase the partial (focal) seizure.
    d. Anticonvulsant-induced osteomalacia with hypocalcemia (ricketts). This uncommon problem may increase the seizure frequency and typically occurs after 5 to 7 years' use.
    e. Downregulation of benzodiazepine receptor sites with decreasing antiepileptic response (e.g., clonazepam, nitrazepam).
4. The progression of the underlying cause. Examples are subacute focal (Rasmussen) encephalitis, neoplasm, arteriovenous malformation, and degenerative disease (ceroid lipofuscinosis). Blume and co-workers reported that 16 of 38 children undergoing cerebral resection for intractable seizures were found unexpectedly to have a cerebral tumor.
5. The vagaries of epilepsy. An unprovoked episode of seizures may occur in a well child with adequate therapeutic levels of anticonvulsants.
6. Superimposed head trauma may precipitate seizures.

When a child known to have epilepsy presents with recurring seizures, several steps may minimize the treatment time and disclose the reason for the breakthrough. The physician should first assess the obvious factors: the airway and the vital signs. Next, if the patient is having seizures at the time, the physician should test for the levels of anticonvulsants, electrolytes, calcium, and glucose and should obtain a complete blood cell count with differential. An intravenous catheter should be inserted if the child is not alert, so that medication can be administered if necessary. If the patient if febrile, a source of infection should be sought.

Once these procedures have been completed, anticonvulsant management is initiated. Assume the anticonvulsant levels are low and give a partial loading dose. If the patient is compliant, give the daily dose of phenobarbital or phenytoin orally if the patient is able to swallow, or intravenously if not. If the patient is known to be noncompliant or if the levels of the anticonvulsant are found on testing to be significantly below the therapeutic range, give the daily dose twice (e.g., in the child on 60 mg of phenobarbital, give 60 mg initially and repeat the dose if the seizures recur despite levels in the low therapeutic range).

If the anticonvulsant levels are within a high therapeutic range and the child is well without an obvious source of infection or other cause of breakthrough, then one can decide if another anticonvulsant is necessary. One may decide to wait and see if there is a trend toward increased seizure frequency, warranting additional medication, or if this is a solitary episode, warranting observation, monitoring of drug levels, and follow-up. If the levels are within the high therapeutic range and seizures recur, additional anticonvulsants are warranted in appropriate loading doses (Table 113-3).

Recurring or frequent tonic, tonic-clonic, and clonic seizures warrant loading doses that produce therapeutic levels rapidly. Phenobarbital and phenytoin can be given orally or intravenously to achieve therapeutic levels. Primidone (Mysoline) and carbamazepine (Tegretol) are not typically used as emergency drugs or given in large loading doses because of their side effects. Valproic acid (Depakene) or its enteric-coated form, divalproic acid (Depakote) is usually given orally; the enteric-coated form may be used with less likelihood of abdominal discomfort and nausea. Liquid valproate (60 mg/kg with equal amounts of saline) has been used rectally to achieve therapeutic levels rapidly in patients in status epilepticus. It can be given this way in patients temporarily unable to swallow.

Seizures which begin with focal features, partial or complex partial (temporal lobe, psychomotor), may appear less dramatic and typically warrant a slower modification of drug therapy unless the seizures are prolonged or postical Todd's paralysis occurs. If the patient requires additional drugs, phenobarbital, phenytoin, and carbamazepine can be used interchangeably, although the last cannot be loaded rapidly without producing uncomfortable side effects. Patients with petit mal (generalized absence) epilepsy rarely are brought to the emergency room, since the seizures are not alarming to the parents. If some injury occurs because of the absence spells, or if the parent is unusually concerned and brings the child for emergency treatment, determining the blood levels of anticonvulsants is most useful. Addition of another anticonvulsant can be initiated, for example, ethosuximide (Zarontin), valproate, clonazepam (Klonopin), or acetazolamide (Diamox).

Most often the epileptic patient can be sent home and modification of the drug regimen can be carried out by the attending physician. Following the initial evaluations, modification of drug therapy, and treatment for any superimposed problems, the emergency physician should (1) arrange for follow-up evaluations by the attending physician, (2) emphasize the need for compliance, and (3) provide continued treatment for infections.

## STATUS EPILEPTICUS

Status epilepticus represents a state of "epileptic seizure that is so frequently repeated or so prolonged as to create a fixed and lasting epileptic condition." This definition applies to continuous seizures lasting at least 30 min. More specific classification is listed in Table 113-5.

About 5 to 10 percent of children with epilepsy and 60,000 to 100,000 total epileptics experience one bout of status grand mal (SGM). This condition is a neurologic emergency which could be fatal. The longer the SGM persists, the greater the morbidity and the mortality and the more difficult it is to control the seizures. In patients with no neurologic sequelae, the mean duration of SGM is $1\frac{1}{2}$ h. Neurologic sequelae result when SGM lasts an average of 10 h. The mean duration of SGM in patients who die is 13 h.

### Effects of SGM

Experimental models in animals provide evidence of the neurologic effects of SGM. Selective permanent cell damage in the hippocampus, amygdala, cerebellum, thalamus, and middle cerebral cortical layers develops after 60 min of seizure activity. Even with artificial ventilation and correction of existing metabolic derangements, most changes still occur. This cell death results from the increased metabolic demands and the exhaustion of the continuously firing neurons.

In addition, there are secondary effects which probably exaggerate the adverse effects of SGM. After unremitting SGM, the cerebral $P_{O_2}$ and amounts of cytochrome A and cytochrome $A_3$ reductase decrease, enhancing the risk of cell damage. Increases in calcium, arachidonic acid, arachidonal diglycerol, prostaglandin, and leukotriene levels in the neurons exaggerate or cause cerebral edema and cell death. Increased levels of cyclic AMP and increased release of prolactin, growth hormone, ACTH, cortisol, insulin, glycogen, epinephrine, and norepinephrine may contribute to the progression of cell damage with the loss of physiologic responsiveness.

Late secondary effects include lactic acidosis, elevated cerebrospinal fluid pressure, hyperglycemia (followed later by hypoglycemia), dysautonomia with hyperthermia, diaphoresis, dehydration, hypertension followed by hypotension, and eventually shock. In addition, excessive muscle activity leads to myolysis, myoglobinuria, and renal failure. Neuropathologic studies indicate nucleovacuolation and ischemic nerve cell damage leading to neuronal dissolution.

### Treatment

Treatment is best initiated when the type of seizure is identified. To obtain the most effective and rapid cessation of status epilepticus, the following specific therapeutic goals must be reached.

1. Specific delineation of the type and subtype of status epilepticus so that appropriate treatment can be chosen. For example, tonic-clonic generalized status epilepticus is very responsive to diazepam or phenytoin; noncontinuous clonic or tonic-clonic seizures may be refractory to diazepam.
2. Identification and treatment of the reversible precipitating cause of status epilepticus, e.g., cerebral infection, trauma, electrolyte disturbance, brain abscess, hypoglycemia.
3. Rapid cessation of status epilepticus to prevent secondary effects that both prolong the seizures and cause irreversible neuronal damage.
4. Full support of medical systems to prevent unwarranted complications of the seizures or the treatment, e.g., respiratory depression, arrhythmia, aspiration pneumonia, shock, myoglobulinuria.

In treating the patient with continuous grand mal or tonic-clonic seizures, the end point is clear: the cessation of seizures. The amount of diazepam necessary to stop the seizures has been derived from studies that confirm one significant point—complications usually occur in markedly ill patients with complex disorders or with prior use of high dosages of other hypnotic drugs. The safety of diazepam to a maximum dose of 2.6 mg/kg over the course of treatment has been

**Table 113-5.** Classification of Status Seizures

  I. Primary generalized convulsive status grand mal (continuous and noncontinuous)
    A. Tonic-clonic status
    B. Myoclonic status
    C. Clonic-tonic status
 II. Secondary generalized convulsive status (continuous and noncontinuous)
    A. Tonic-clonic status with partial onset
    B. Tonic status
III. Simple partial status
    A. Partial motor status including EPC*
    B. Partial sensory status
    C. Partial status with vegetative or autonomic symptoms
    D. Partial status with cognitive symptoms
    E. Partial status with affective symptoms
IV. Complex partial status
 V. Absence (petit mal) status

* Epilepsia partialis continua.
*Source:* Modified from Delgado-Escueta AV, Bajorek JG: Status epilepticus: Mechanisms of brain damage and rational management. *Epilepsia* 23(suppl 1):S29, 1982. Used by permission.

substantiated. Smith and co-workers described an effective dose of diazepam as 0.08 to 2.72 mg/kg in infants and young children with an average effective dose of 0.68 mg/kg. Many authors recommend initial doses of 1 mg per year of age with a maximum total dose of 5 mg in infants and 10 mg in children. Eckert reported maximum doses in adolescents as 35 mg in brief periods and 100 mg in 24 h.

A starting diazepam dose of 0.2 to 0.5 mg/kg, given at a rate of 1 mg/min and repeated as needed to a maximum of 2.6 mg/kg, is recommended to stop continuous tonic-clonic and clonic seizures. This higher dose is rarely used since most patients stop seizing at lower doses and additional drugs such as phenytoin may be employed. Care must be taken to ensure adequate ventilation.

Rapid-acting benzodiazepines remain the drugs of choice in SGM. Lorazepam and diazepam are used with equal effectiveness. Diazepam is effective in 80 percent of cases within 5 min of administration. To maintain the seizure-free state, one must use a long-term anticonvulsant. Therefore, after diazepam causes the seizures to cease, a phenytoin loading dose of 15 mg/kg is administered with maintenance dosages of 5 to 8 mg/kg per day to maintain therapeutic blood levels of 10 to 20 µg/mL. Phenobarbital 15 mg/kg can be used instead of or in addition to phenytoin.

Currently lorazepam is used with greater frequency in the treatment of SGM. Efficacy and side effects are equal for diazepam and lorazepam. Theoretically, lorazepam is better than diazepam because of its pharmacokinetic properties, exhibiting a slower onset of action (latency) but a longer duration of action, allowing for a more prolonged seizure-free interval following initial infusion. In an open study by Lacey and co-workers, lorazepam was administered to 31 children exhibiting status epilepticus. The initial dose was 0.05 mg/kg, with 20 patients receiving two injections and 1 receiving three injections. The median dose was 0.05 mg/kg, with a total median accumulative dose of 2.0 mg. The median latency was 10 min; control lasted at least 3 to 6 h in 83 percent of the patients and 24 h in nearly 50 percent of the patients. In a double-blind randomized trial by Leppik and co-workers, 78 adult patients were treated with either lorazepam (4 mg) or diazepam (10 mg). Latency (2 to 3 min), efficacy (76 to 89 percent), and adverse effects (12 to 13 percent) did not differ significantly in both groups. Midazolam, a more rapid acting benzodiazepine, is currently being evaluated for its safety and effectiveness in the management of SGM.

The following 10 steps should be followed when treating continuous SGM (tonic-clonic status epilepticus) (Table 113-6):

1. Assess basic functions immediately and maintain blood pressure, airway, and pulse.
2. Obtain blood to be tested for levels of anticonvulsants, electrolytes, BUN, calcium, and glucose, and for a complete blood cell count with differential while inserting an IV catheter for fluid administration.
3. Administer IV a bolus of 25% glucose, 2 mL/kg.
4. Administer IV diazepam, 0.2 mg/kg, and repeat up to a total dose of 2.6 mg/kg or early signs of respiratory depression. Alterna-

tively, administer IV lorazepam, 0.1 mg/kg over 2 min, repeating in 15 min and 30 min if necessary.

5. Administer IV phenytoin, 15 mg/kg, after diazepam is infused, at a maximum rate of 25 mg/min.
6. Administer IV phenobarbital, 15 mg/kg, if phenytoin is ineffective. When the patient requires step 6, transfer to the intensive care unit is warranted.
7. If seizures persist, give additional 10 mg/kg of phenobarbital to reach levels of 60 µg/mL.
8. Administer rectally paraldehyde, 0.3 mL/kg, mixed with an equal amount of mineral oil, if step 6 is ineffective.
9. Under intensive care monitoring, administer pentobarbital 2 mg/kg bolus, followed by maintenance of 1 to 2 mg/kg per hour to effect 3.8 s of electroencephalographic burst suppression.
10. In noncontinuous SGM, administer clonazepam (Klonopin) through nasogastric tube in a single dose of 0.2 to 0.6 mg/kg initially followed by 0.1 to 0.4 mg/kg per day maintenance.

Noncontinuous status epilepticus can be more difficult to treat since the end point is more elusive. Rapidly acting drugs such as diazepam and lorazepam are less effective, and a more sustained effect is necessary. Often noncontinuous status epilepticus is not responsive to appropriate therapeutic levels of phenytoin and phenobarbital. Large doses (0.2 to 0.6 mg/kg) of clonazepam via nasogastric tube may be used to produce the desired effect of rapid cessation of noncontinuous seizures, and the anticonvulsant effect maintained by additional drugs (phenytoin, phenobarbital) and clonazepam (0.1 to 0.3 mg/kg per day).

Paraldehyde administered rectally can be very effective in noncontinuous status epilepticus. Paraldehyde should be administered only with glass syringes and rubber tubing in view of its degradation to toxic forms in the presence of certain plastics.

Absence (petit mal) status is a much simpler form of status epilepticus to deal with since it is exquisitely responsive to diazepam given intravenously. It rarely happens that a patient requires emergency care for this form of epilepsy.

Epilepsia partialis continua is a serious neurologic condition, although it does not appear threatening at firse. The patient exhibits repeated continuous or minimally interrupted clonic jerking of one side of the body and usually one part of an extremity for days, weeks, or months. It is typically due to encephalitis or cerebrovascular accident or associated with heterotopias and indicates a relatively poor prognosis. Initial management is similar to that of noncontinuous SGM.

## DIFFERENTIAL DIAGNOSIS OF SEIZURES

It is necessary to identify nonepileptic paroxysmal disorders to prevent confusion with epilepsy. The differential diagnosis of seizures must take into account many disorders that can produce loss of consciousness, unusual movements, impaired awareness, or bizarre behavior. Many of these disorders are age-specific.

**Table 113-6.** Doses for Status Epilepticus in Children

| Drug | Recommended Loading Dose | Route | Repeat | Rate | Maximum Dose |
|------|--------------------------|-------|--------|------|--------------|
| Diazepam (Valium) | 0.2 mg/kg | IV | 3 times | 1 mg/min | 5 mg 0–2 years 10 mg 2 years and older |
| Lorazepam | 0.05 mg/kg | IV | 2 times | over 2 min | 0.2 mg/kg |
| Phenobarbital | 15.0 mg/kg | IV | 0 | | 400 mg |
| Phenytoin (Dilantin) | 15.0 mg/kg | IV | 0 | 1 mg/kg per min | 1000 mg |
| Paraldehyde* | 0.3 mL/Kg | Rectal | q 4 h | | 15 mL |
| Clonazepam (Klonopin) | 0.3 mg/kg | NG | 1 time | | 10 mg |
| Valproic acid (Depakene*) | 60.0 mg/kg | Rectal | 0 | | |
| Lidocaine | 2.0 mg/kg | IV | | 5–10 mg/kg per h | |

* See text.

In the newborn, the problems partly reflect the intrauterine experience. Jitteriness or hyperexcitability appears as high-amplitude tremulousness easily brought out by passive movement of the extremities or jarring of the crib. The drug-withdrawn infant is irritable and tremulous and may have diaphoresis, vomiting, and diarrhea; in addition, seizures may occur. Sepsis, hypoglycemia, and hypocalcemia may produce nonepileptic paroxysmal activity in addition to seizures. Hyperekplexia, or startle disease, mimics tonic and clonic seizures. Near-miss sudden death syndrome (SIDS) remains a multifactorial condition in which seizures are part of the differential diagnosis and might be considered part of the cause.

In the older infant it is more common to see cyanotic and pallid breath-holding spells, which typically occur following an abrupt trauma (fall, minor spanking) or a verbal reprimand. The infant gives a sudden cry followed by prolonged inhalation or exhalation, resulting in no air exchange, and a Valsalva maneuver, often with bradycardia. A brief tonic nonepileptic seizure often occurs. Drug intoxication manifested by hyperkinesis, impaired awareness, or altered behavior (hallucinations) is usually accidental at this age. In adolescence, phencyclidine (PCP) intoxication mimics complex partial seizures and may result in seizures with more severe overdoses.

Congenital heart disease can produce paroxysmal events at all ages. Abrupt mental-status changes may occur in patients with pulmonary hypertension, aortic stenosis, tetralogy of Fallot, atresia of the ventricles, cardiac rhabdomyomas, etc. Acquired cardiomyopathy may result in decreased cardiac output (Adams-Stokes disease) or cerebrovascular accident. The prolonged Q-T syndrome and neurocardiogenic syncope may cause nonepileptic seizures or syncopal episodes. They should be evaluated for when epilepsy is unsubstantiated or the more obvious problems of diaphoresis, light headedness, and skin color/temperature changes precede or accompany unconsciousness.

Hyperkinetic movement disorders can be difficult to differentiate from complex partial seizures. Sydenham chorea is infrequently seen today, and drug-induced chorea (ethosuximide, carbamazepine, diphenhydramine hydrochloride) and lupus-induced chorea are likewise very uncommon. Tourette syndrome is more frequently seen, but rarely does the child appear acutely ill. Kinesogenic chorea is a movement disorder brought on by action and mimics complex partial seizures.

Immediate posttraumatic migraine may recur after relatively minor injury and cause confusional states mimicking concussion or complex partial seizures.

In the adolescent, syncope due to stretching and yawning or following hair combing (vasovagal) is more common. Many children experience syncope when standing in church.

Pseudoseizures represent a particular problem for the treating physician because the "seizures" appear to represent a significant threat to the patient's safety, and vigorous anticonvulsant therapy is often initiated. Unfortunately, pseudoseizures often occur in patients with documented epilepsy. Secondary gain should become evident in these cases. The "seizures" are atypical in that the patient may waken fully in the interictal phase and require repeated large doses of anticonvulsants even to the point of protracted drug-induced depression. Another form of pseudoseizures consists of those described by the parent and never observed by other witnesses.

To distinguish pseudoseizures from true epileptic spells, a bedside technique may be dramatic and diagnostic, and prevent overtreatment. One method is to gently insert a nasopharyngeal tube and observe the patient's response. The pseudoseizure patient will become responsive immediately. Experience dictates referral for patients with a diagnosis of pseudoseizure, or even hospitalization, to prevent recurrences, provide family education, and lessen the likelihood of inappropriate treatment.

Simple sleep myoclonus and night terrors are of concern to parents. They are, however, easily distinguished from nocturnal seizures.

Preventing misdiagnosis and mistreatment is an essential part of the emergency management of seizures and related disorders.

## PROBLEMS OF ANTICONVULSANT USE

Unwanted features of anticonvulsants may be seen soon after the drug is initiated or may develop weeks, months, or years later. These problems may turn up during evaluation for other illnesses (e.g., macrocytic anemia) or be the basis for emergency treatment.

Immediate side effects often subside in time. Lethargy occurs more often with barbiturates, is usually dose-related, and subsides with chronic use and half-life stabilization. Irritability and changes in cognition can persist and be so significant that a nonbarbiturate anticonvulsant must be substituted. Rashes may occur within days or weeks of initiation of therapy but must be differentiated from concurrent viral exanthem. Pruritic and/or morbilliform rashes usually require cessation of medication. Stevens-Johnson syndrome, with bullous skin lesions affecting mucous membranes, is a serious potential reaction. There is a risk of serious sequelae—blindness, esophageal stenosis, or loss of life.

With valproic acid use, hepatic failure may occur within days or up to 2 years after first use. The drug reaction results in alteration of behavior, increasing lethargy, and vomiting. Levels of liver enzymes may be minimally to markedly elevated, and hyperammonemia with or without symptoms of hepatic failure may be found. Immediate cessation of valproate, hospitalization, and observation are necessary if symptomatic hepatic reaction is evident. In the asymptomatic patient with enzyme-level elevations, a reduction of the dosage and careful observation are warranted. Gastrointestinal side effects are common with initial use of valproic acid and may be so severe that more serious hepatic problems are considered. These side effects can be avoided by a more frequent dosage schedule, by taking the drug with meals, and by avoiding carbonated beverages and citric juices, or alternatively by using the enteric-coated form. Pancreatitis secondary to valproate use also has been reported.

Toxicity due to overdosage at any time can produce some readily identifiable symptoms and signs. Phenytoin toxicity occurs when serum levels exceed 25 μg/mL in most patients (above 20 μg/mL in some). Nausea, dysarthria, diplopia, and ataxia are seen early, with progression to impaired levels of consciousness and decerebrate posturing. Virtually all anticonvulsants produce ataxia and lethargy with significant overdosage. Cardiopulmonary monitoring during high-dose drug use in status epilepticus should be employed since cardiac collapse or respiratory depression can occur. Burning in the limb used for the infusion of phenytoin has also been reported. Using a free-flowing, well-positioned needle and a short tubing distance and infusing at a rate of 1 mg/kg per min or less lessens the likelihood of phenytoin side effects. Chronic phenytoin use can result in folate deficiency with macrocytic anemia, acquired osteomalacia (increased vitamin D turnover), neutropenia (often transient), peripheral neuropathy, lupus-like syndromes, and myasthenic weakness.

Valproate-induced thrombocytopenia is a significant side effect warranting lowering or discontinuation of the drug. Lower carnitine levels due to valproate metabolism may be a contributing factor of valproate hepatotoxicity.

Drug interactions may be quite dramatic. Valproate and aspirin can result in a bleeding diathesis. Antihistamines used in conjunction with barbiturates can be very sedating, warranting smaller doses of the antihistamine. When erythromycin is used, particular care must be exercised since the carbamazepine levels may rise to toxic levels rapidly. Toxicity is greater when carbamazepine and lithium are used together, and blood levels may be in the therapeutic range. Total phenytoin levels are typically reduced when valproic acid is also used, but free phenytoin usually remains therapeutic. It is essential to measure free phenytoin when valproate is used concurrently. When barbiturates are used concomitantly with phenytoin, increased parahydroxylation can cause enhanced metabolism of phenytoin so that therapeutic levels fall, resulting in seizure breakthrough. Hyperbilirubinemia and hypoalbuminemia can affect anticonvulsant binding and blood levels.

Movement disorders (e.g., chorea) can result after several weeks' or months' use of ethosuximide and rarely with carbamazepine. The movements may be profound and usually respond promptly to the cessation of use of the drug and the use of diphenhydramine (Benadryl), 12.5 to 25 mg given intravenously. Clonazepam and diazepam can cause acute bladder dysfunction with urinary retention.

Many problems of dose-related toxicity can be avoided by maintaining therapeutic blood levels. Blood level determinations should be done randomly to determine compliance and at times of increased seizure frequency or when signs of toxicity develop. In some patients, side effects develop at therapeutic levels. Idiosyncratic effects cannot be predicted, but families must be made aware that significant side effects can develop with little warning, and evaluation by a physician is recommended before a drug is dismissed. Obtaining the patient's history, consulting with the primary physician or consultant, and reviewing readily available drug information in the package insert or *Physicians' Desk Reference* make emergency evaluation and treatment of anticonvulsant drug reactions simpler.

## ERRORS IN EMERGENCY MANAGEMENT OF SEIZURES

After the patient arrives for treatment, the initial assessment may be incomplete, resulting in inappropriate or inadequate therapy. Not identifying treatable infections, electrolyte imbalance, child abuse, and accidental trauma can lead to rapidly progressive deterioration and demise, or may make seizure control difficult. By not ascertaining anticonvulsant levels in the patient with epilepsy, the physician loses an opportunity to determine if the anticonvulsant is ineffective or simply at too low a level.

If the emergency physician communicates with the primary physician, unnecessary studies, and drugs which either were ineffective or produced some side effects, can be avoided. Additionally, it is important to consult with the patient's physician when prescribing nonanticonvulsants which might interfere with anticonvulsants or produce unwanted side effects.

In the aggressive treatment of seizures (status epilepticus and recurring breakthrough seizures), inadequate loading doses or improper drug selection may prolong the seizures and worsen the prognosis. Excessive dosage can result in respiratory depression or hypotension and, in rare instances, can exacerbate the seizures. If nonepileptic paroxysmal disorders are not recognized, the patient is put at the additional risk of unnecessary medication and inadequate treatment of the real disorder.

The emergency physician cannot deal with all the problems facing the patient with epilepsy. Follow-up care by the primary physicians or appropriate consultants ensures better compliance and, one hopes, lessens emergency situations in the future.

## BIBLIOGRAPHY

Berg AT, Shinnar S, Hauser WA, et al: A prospective study of recurrent febrile seizures (see comments). *N Engl J Med* 327(16):1161, 1992.

Blume BT, Gerven JP, Kaufmann JCE: Childhood brain tumors presenting as chronic uncontrolled focal seizures. *Ann Neurol* 12:538, 1982.

Commission on Classification and Terminology of the International League Against Epilepsy: Proposal for revised clinical and electroencephalographic classification of epileptic seizures. *Epilepsia* 22:489, 1981.

Delgado-Escueta AV, Treiman DM, Walsh GO: The treatable epilepsies (first of two parts). *N Engl J Med* 308:1508, 1983.

Delgado-Escueta AV, Treiman DM, Walsh GO: The treatable epilepsies (second of two parts). *N Engl J Med* 308:1576, 1983.

Dieckmann RA: Rectal diazepam for prehospital pediatric status epilepticus. *Ann Emerg Med* 23:216, 1994.

Eckert C: Neurologic Emergencies, in *Emergency-Room Care,* ed 4. Boston, Little, Brown, 1981, pp. 409–420.

Farwell, JR, Lee YJ, Hertz DG, et al: Phenobarbital for febrile seizures—effects on intelligence and on seizure recurrence. *N Engl J Med* 322:364, 1990.

Gross TV, Shinnar S: Convulsive status epilepticus in children. *Epilepsia* 34(suppl 1):12, 1993.

Hauser WA, Anderson VE, Levenson RB, et al: Seizure recurrence after a first unprovoked seizure. *N Engl J Med* 307:522, 1982.

Lacey DJ, Singer WD, Horwitz SJ, et al: Lorazepam therapy of status epilepticus in children and adolescents. *J Pediatr* 108:771, 1986.

Leppik IE, Derivan AT, Homan RW, et al: A double blind study of lorazepam and diazepam in status epilepticus. *JAMA* 249:1452, 1983.

Maytal J, Novak GP, King KC: Lorazepam in the treatment of refractory neonatal seizures. *J Child Neurol* 6(4):319, 1991.

Millichap JG, Colliver JA: Management of febrile seizures: Survey of current practice and phenobarbital usage. *Pediatr Neurol* 7(4):243, 1991.

Nypaver MM, Reynolds SL, Tanz RR, Davis AT: Emergency department laboratory evaluation of children with seizures: Dogma or dilemma? *Pediatr Emerg Care* 8(1):13, 1992.

Rivera R, Segnini M, Baltodano A, Perez V: Midazolam in the treatment of status epilepticus in children (see comments). *Crit Care Med* 21(7):955, 1993.

Seizure temporally associated with use of DEET insect repellant—New York and Connecticut. *MMWR* 38:678, 1989.

Smith BT, Masotti RE: Intravenous diazepam in the treatment of prolonged seizure activity in neonates and infants. *Dev Med Child Neurol* 13:630, 1971.

Tassinari CA, Daniele O, Michelucci R, et al: Benzodiazepines: Efficacy in status epilepticus. *Adv Neurol* 34:465, 1983.

# 114
# GASTROENTERITIS
## Ronald D. Holmes
## Allan D. Olson

Gastroenteritis is a major public health problem; up to one-fifth of all acute-care outpatient visits to hospitals are by families with infants or children affected by acute gastroenteritis. Acute diarrhea is the most prominent symptom of gastroenteritis in infants and children. Most enteric infections are self-limited, but excessive loss of water and electrolytes, resulting in clinical dehydration, may occur in 10 percent and is life-threatening in 1 percent. Pathogenic viruses, bacteria, or parasites may be isolated from nearly 50 percent of children with diarrhea. Viral gastroenteritis is the most common cause of acute infectious diarrhea and accounts for the vast majority of cases. Bacterial pathogens may be isolated in 1 to 4 percent of cases. Parasitic infestations are the least common but may be pervasive in day-care settings.

## PATHOPHYSIOLOGY

A number of factors contribute to the excessive water losses and increased frequency of stools due to gastrointestinal infections. These factors include decreased digestion and malabsorption of nutrients, active secretion of fluids and electrolytes into the intestinal lumen, and intestinal dysmotility, which shortens intestinal transit time.

Viral pathogens cause acute gastroenteritis by tissue invasion and a directly cytopathic effect to small intestinal villous cells. As a consequence, there are villous damage and decreased intestinal absorption of nutrients, electrolytes, and water, resulting in watery diarrhea in volumes that may exceed 50 mL/kg body weight per day (normal less than 5 mL). The villous injury reduces the total cell population of mature, villous-tip absorptive enterocytes, which are replaced by immature crypt secretary cells. Disaccharidase leveles are decreased, and total mucosal glucose-coupled sodium transport is diminished. The end result is a decrease in intestinal water absorption. The volume of fluid delivered from the lumen of the damaged small intestine exceeds the colon's limited ability for fluid absorption, and the net result is watery diarrhea. Distension of the intestinal lumen associated with excessive secretion of fluids initiates peristaltic motor complexes and increases the rate of intestinal transit. Increased transit rate decreases the digestion and absorption and contributes to an increase in stool water loss and stool frequency.

Bacteria cause diarrhea by a variety of mechanisms, including production of enterotoxins and cytotoxins and damage to the mucosal absorptive surface. Enteric infections with *Esherichia coli* are prototypic for understanding several of these pathogenic processes. Enterotoxigenic *E. coli* (ETEC) and enteropathogenic *E. coli* (EPEC) adhere to the mucosa and produce enterotoxins or damage the microvilli, respectively. Certain strains of enteroinvasive *E. coli* (EIEC) invade the colonic mucosa, resulting in inflammation and an illness similar to shigellosis. Enterohemorrhagic *E. coli* (EHEC) has emerged as a cause of outbreaks of bloody diarrhea in the United States. EHEC (*E. coli* 0157.H7) typically produces a hemorrhagic colitis with little inflammation and may produce verotoxins that have been implicated in causing hemolytic-uremic syndrome (HUS) in children. *Vibrio cholerae* and ETEC are the classic bacterial organisms that produce an enterotoxin, causing watery diarrhea. The toxin of *V. cholerae* activates adenylate cyclase, resulting in increased intracellular levels of cyclic adenosine $3',5'$-monophosphate (cGMP) levels, respectively, resulting in secretory diarrhea.

Inflammatory diarrhea occurs when organisms invade the bowel wall and produce colitis or dysentery, resulting in bloody and mucousy diarrhea. *Shigella, Campylobacter, Salmonella,* and enteroinvasive *E. coli* cause this type of diarrhea. Antibiotic-associated diarrhea and colitis due to cytotoxigenic *Clostridium difficile* causes a similar pattern of diarrhea.

Parasitic infestations may cause diarrhea by a variety of mechanisms similar to those discussed for viral gastroenteritis. Brush border damage occurs with *Giardia lamblia* infestation, and intestinal motility is increased as part of an adaptive response to expel the organisms. The myoelectric and motor abnormalities resulting in increased motility are similar to those induced by viral infections.

In summary, diarrhea may be the result of the host's response to the offending organism to prevent attachment to epithelial surfaces and invasion of enterocytes. The concept of intestinal secretion as a final common pathway of diarrhea production has been replaced by a broader pathophysiologic mechanism including maldigestion and malabsorption, damage to the brush border, and altered intestinal motility.

## CLINICAL FEATURES

Enteric infections causing diarrhea are spread by the fecal-oral route, with contaminated food, water, fomites, or direct inoculation as the vehicles of transmission. Rotaviruses, Norwalk viruses, the enteric adenoviruses, calicivirus, and astroviruses are the most commonly recognized viral pathogens in children. Of these, rotavirus is the most common, typically occurring in the cooler months of the year (October through April), and infects every child in the United States by age 4 years. This virus causes potentially lethal dehydration in 0.75 percent of children under 2 years of age. Older children and adults have acquired immunity against the rotaviruses and are less likely to develop the severe dehydrating syndrome. Symptomatic enteric adeno-

virus (EAd) infection with serotypes 40 and 41 causes diarrhea that is associated with concurrent respiratory symptoms. Infections occur throughout the year with no clear peaks and may be responsible for 5 to 20 percent of hospitalizations for childhood diarrhea. Outbreaks of EAd infection occur second only to rotavirus infection in prevalence. As with rotavirus infection, nearly half the infected children may be asymptomatic. A majority of children are seropositive for EAd by 4 years of age.

Outbreaks of diarrhea due to infections with caliciviruses and astroviruses are less common and are associated with day-care center exposure. Astrovirus may account for as many as 7 percent of the cases of diarrhea in day-care centers, but it is most common as both an epidemic and endemic cause of diarrhea in infants less than 18 months of age. Norwalk virus infection is also implicated in causing epidemic gastroenteritis. In addition to developing nausea, vomiting, diarrhea, and abdominal cramps, affected children and adults may have headache, fever and chills, and myalgias. Vomiting is more prevalent in children, while diarrhea is more common in adults.

The major bacterial enteropathogens in the United States are *Campylobacter jejuni, Shigella* species, *Salmonella* species, *Yersinia enterocolitica, C. difficile,* and *Aeromonas. E. coli* is the most common bacterial organism causing diarrhea in children around the world but is less common in the United States. Diarrhea due to *E. coli* may be watery (ETEC, EPEC) or present as a dysentery-like disease (EHEC). EHEC infections due to *E. coli* serotype 0157:H7 are associated with causing HUS.

*Giardia lamblia* is a common cause of diarrhea in infants and young children in day-care centers. As many as 50 percent of infected children may be asymptomatic. *Cryptosporidium* infestations occur in a similar epidemiologic pattern. Although *Cryptosporidium* was first recognized as an opportunistic pathogen in immunocompromised children, it is now recognized as a cause of protracted watery diarrhea in otherwise healthy children. *Entamoeba histolytica* causes diarrhea, proctitis, dysentery, or hematochezia; symptomatic infection in children results from exposure by travel to a geographic locale endemic for the organism or in adolescents through sexual transmissions.

Infants and children who attend day-care centers are at risk of acquiring a variety of enteric infections. In some areas, *G. lamblia* is the most common cause of diarrhea, but outbreaks of *Shigella, Campylobacter, C. difficile, Salmonella,* and *Cryptosporidium* are frequently reported. The attack rate during outbreaks may range from 30 to 100 percent. Shigellosis is particularly contagious.

## DIAGNOSIS/DIFFERENTIAL DIAGNOSIS

The approach to diagnosis and successful treatment involves careful history and selective laboratory testing (Fig. 114-1). Various cultures and immunoassays of stool for the presence of the enteric pathogens are now well established in most hospital laboratories. Routine stool culture for bacterial pathogens now includes *C. jejuni, Y. enterocolitica,* and *Aeromonas* in addition to *Salmonella* and *Shigella;* subculturing for *E. coli* serotypes or stool assays for *C. difficile* toxin activity are available. Enzyme immunoassays also are available to test stool for the presence of rotavirus, enteric adenovirus, and astrovirus.

Most children present with a nonspecific gastroenteritis and not dysentery. In these cases the clinician must assess the likelihood of defining a treatable etiology and, as a consequence, the indication for doing a stool culture. If the patient is febrile, has abrupt onset of diarrhea occurring more than four times per day, or blood in the stool, the illness is more likely to have been caused by a bacterial pathogen and stool cultures are indicated. The likelihood of identifying bacterial pathogens is increased if the patient's stool or accompanying exudate contains polymorphonuclear leukocytes (PMNs). A fresh stool sample must be collected to be stained for fecal leukocytes by methylene blue stain. A loopful of mucus or bloody exudate from the stool spec-

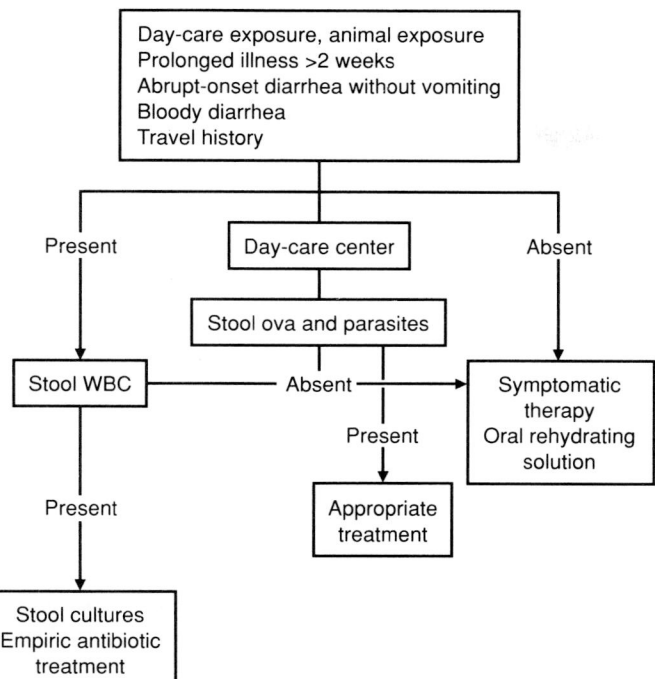

**Fig. 114-1.** Approach to diagnosis and treatment. Empiric antibiotic treatment may occasionally be justified for inflammatory diarrhea (see text).

imen is mixed with a drop of nonbacteriostatic saline or methylene blue stain on a clean slide, placed under a cover slip, and examined under high-dry magnification. More than five PMNs seen in several high-dry fields is positive. The stool should also be tested for occult blood using a modified guaiac test (Hemoccult). The positive test for fecal leukocytes correlates 90 percent of the time with the presence of bacterial enterocolitis if there are no anal fissues or perianal skin lesions that could provide a source of blood and a falsely positive test.

Stool cultures should also be obtained if there is a history of seafood ingestion or ingestion of poorly cooked ground meat, prior antibiotic treatment, or day-care center exposure even if fecal leukocytes or blood is not seen. If there has been a history of unexplained fever or abdominal pain, exposure to a sick pet with diarrhea, or signs and symptoms suggesting appendicitis or mesenteric adenitis, then a culture for *Y. enterocolitica* and other pathogens should be obtained. Any child presenting with a dysentery-like illness should have stool sent for culture and, if indicated, examination for ova and parasites regardless of the results of fecal leukocyte smear. A swab of mucus or bloody exudate from the stool, which has been collected in a cup, should be placed in transport medium, such as Culturette II, and sent to the laboratory. *Shigella* is a fastidious pathogen and is more likely to be recovered from a swab than from a fresh stool specimen. In cases of persistent or recurrent diarrhea, especially with weight loss or day-care center exposure or in immunocompromised children, at least three fresh stool samples should be collected in fixative and examined for *G. lamblia, E. histolytica,* and *Cryptosporidium.* Infants and children who present with bloody or mucousy diarrhea after having received antibiotics may have antibiotic-associated pseudomembranous colitis due to infection with cytotoxigenic *C. difficile,* and anaerobic stool cultures and assay of stool for toxin activity should be obtained. Finally, serologic testing or sigmoidoscopy for confirming *E. histolytica* infection may be necessary.

Watery diarrhea is usually a sign of viral gastroenteritis but may also be caused by infections with enterotoxigenic bacteria such as *V. cholerae* and *E. coli.* Bacterial toxins may also be ingested directly in food. *Staphylococcus aureus* produces five distinct heat-stable toxins

**Table 114-1.** Diagnosis of Enteric Infection

| Watery diarrhea | Bloody diarrhea (dysentery) |
|---|---|
| *Vibrio cholerae* | *Shigella* |
| *Escherichia coli* (toxigenic) | *Salmonella* |
| Staphylococcal food poisoning | *E. coli* (enteroinvasive) |
| *Bacillus cereus* | *Campylobacter jejuni* |
| Rotavirus | *Yersinia* |
| Norwalk-like viruses | *Clostridium difficile* |
| Adenovirus (enteric) | *Aeromonas* |
| *Giardia* | *Entamoeba histolytica* |
| *Cryptosporidium* | Enteric fever |
| Astrovirus | *Salmonella* |
| Calicivirus | *Yersinia* |
| | *Campylobacter fetus* |

in improperly stored meats, poultry, and dairy products. *Bacillus cereus* also produces a heat-stable toxin typically ingested with boiled or fried rice. Although *Shigella* is considered a prototype organism causing dysentery, it can also produce a toxin that causes watery diarrhea, encephalopathy, and/or convulsions. Table 114-1 lists the causes of enteric infections in children presenting with symptoms of watery diarrhea, bloody diarrhea, or enteric fever.

While viral gastroenteritis is the most common cause of vomiting and/or diarrhea in children presenting to the emergency department, other more serious gastrointestinal conditions must also be considered. In addition, vomiting and diarrhea may be a nonspecific presentation for other infectious disease such as otitis media or urinary tract infections or other more serious conditions. Intussusception, malrotation, increased intracranial pressure, and metabolic acidosis, among others, should also be considered.

## EMERGENCY DEPARTMENT CARE

Most cases of acute diarrhea are self-limited, and little more than oral rehydration therapy is required. Certain infections require antibiotics to reduce morbidity and reduce the risk of contagion. The use of antimotility agents is contraindicated in acute infectious diarrhea.

The most important part of the evaluation of acute gastroenteritis begins with the evaluation of the child's state of hydration (Table 114-2) and should also rule out other more serious causes of vomiting and diarrhea. Signs of mild dehydration may be minimal and include dryness of the oral mucosa and decreased tearing. Severe dehydration with decrease in capillary refill, lethargy, and hypotension requires immediate emergency fluid therapy and hospitalization for parenteral rehydration. BUN, although often elevated, may not correlate with the degree of hydration. Severely dehydrated children are often acidotic with pH less than 7.35. However, the majority of children with diarrhea and dehydration can be treated with oral rehydrating glucose-electrolyte solutions, even if they are vomiting. Oral rehydration therapy capitalizes on the fact that glucose-coupled sodium and water absorption remain sufficiently intact during most infections, despite

**Table 114-2.** Clinical Criteria for Estimating Extent of Dehydration

| | Estimated Body Weight Loss, % | | |
|---|---|---|---|
| **Parameter** | **5** | **5–10** | **>10** |
| Skin turgor | Slight decrease | Decreased | Very decreased |
| Oral mucosa | Dry | Very dry | Parched |
| Tears | ± Decreased | Absent | Absent |
| Fontanelle | Normal | Depressed | Sunken |
| Heart rate | ± Increased | Increased | Marked tachycardia |
| Blood pressure | Normal | ± Decreased | Decreased |
| Urine output | Mild oliguria | Oliguria | Oliguria-anuria |
| Level of consciousness | Irritable | Lethargic | Unresponsive |

*Source:* From Bonadio WA, Hennes HH, Machi J, et al: Efficacy of measuring BUN in assessing children with dehydration due to gastroenteritis. *Ann Emerg Med* 18:755, 1989.

**Table 114-3.** Recommendations for Using Oral Glucose-Electrolyte Solutions

Treatment of Acute Dehydration

Oral rehydration solution:
1. Give volume equal to estimated fluid deficit (e.g., 5% dehydration = 50 mL/kg deficit).
2. Usually 40–50 mL/kg is given over 4 h.
3. Reevaluate clinical status and therapy after 3–4 h.

Prevention of Dehydration or Maintenance of Hydration after Rehydration

Oral maintenance solution:
1. Daily volume should not exceed 150 mL/kg per day.
2. Supplement with water, breast milk, or lactose-free formula to satisfy thirst.
3. Do not delay refeeding more than 24 h.

significant impairment of $Na^+Cl^-$ uptake. Rehydration solutions contain 75 to 90 mEq of sodium per liter. The glucose concentration is 2.0 to 2.5% and does not exceed the sodium concentration in millimolar units by more than 2:1.

The osmolality of commercial rehydration solutions is 310 mOsm/L. In contrast, other clear fluids such as soft drinks, juices, and sherbet are largely carbohydrate-based and have osmolalities ranging from 510 to 1225! The routine use of such highly osmolar sugar-based solutions to treat acute diarrhea will predictably amplify net small intestinal fluid secretion and increase diarrhea.

Rehydration solutions should be used for rapid rehydration of dehydrated infants, regardless of initial serum osmolality, with the estimated fluid deficit replaced over 4 to 6 h. After the calculated deficit has been replaced, maintenance solution is given to replace ongoing gastrointestinal losses. Maintenance solutions contain 40 to 60 mEq of sodium per liter and a concentration of 2.0 to 2.5% glucose. The carbohydrate may be provided as a glucose solution or a rice-based solution. Rice-based oral maintenance fluids have been shown to decrease stool volume through increased intestinal absorption of rice carbohydrates. The daily volume of maintenance solutions should not exceed 150 mL/kg per day. Breast milk or infant formula should be used if additional fluid is needed to satisfy thirst. In general, reintroduction of food may begin after 4 to 6 h of rehydration and never delayed more than 24 h. These guidelines are for patients of all ages. The recommendations for use of oral glucose-electrolyte solutions are outlined in Table 114-3.

Rapid IV hydration within the emergency department is becoming a popular option for mildly to moderately dehydrated children. Between 30 and 50 mL/kg of Ringer's lactate may be given over 3 h. Serum electrolytes must be measured in all patients since children with hypernatremic dehydration should not receive rapid rehydration. Following rehydration many children may be discharged home on maintenance oral hydration fluids.

If the child has had diarrhea lasting longer than 10 to 14 days, has a significant fever or systemic complaints, or has inflammatory cells in the stool, then empiric antimicrobial treatment may be indicated after obtaining a stool sample for bacterial culture. Therapy should provide coverage for the usual dysenteric agents (*Shigella* and *Salmonella*), and either ampicillin or trimethoprim/sulfamethoxazole are reasonable choices. Erythromycin is usually given for *Campylobacter*.

Antibiotic therapy does not affect the clinical course in most cases of acute gastroenteritis and is contraindicated in some infections. Patients with uncomplicated *Salmonella* gastroenteritis should not be given antibiotics unless they appear septic or are bacteremic, have a hemoglobinopathy, or have an underlying chronic gastrointestinal disease. However, infants less than 6 months of age are generally treated with antibiotics because of their overall risk of bacteremia or suppurative disease. In these cases ampicillin, chloramphenicol, or trimethoprim/sulfamethoxazole may be used. *Shigella* dysentery responds to treatment with trimethoprim/sulfamethoxazole (8 to 10 mg/kg trimethoprim plus 40 to 50 mg/kg sulfamethoxazole per day divided every 12 h) or ampicillin (50 to 100 mg/kg per day divided every 6 h to a maximum of 2 to 4 g/day). The usual clinical course of shigellosis with antibiotic therapy is shortened, and the period of fecal shedding may be reduced. Most cases of *C. jejuni* will spontaneously resolve without antibiotics, but early administration of erythromycin ethylsuccinate (50 mg/kg per day in four equal doses) may reduce the duration of diarrhea and fecal excretion of the organism. Mild to moderate cases of *Y. enterocolitica* enteritis resolve spontaneously, but infants less than 3 months of age and children with severe diarrhea may be treated with chloramphenicol or trimethoprim/sulfamethoxazole. The efficacy of antibiotics in altering the course of this infection has not been proved.

Most cases of antibiotic-associated colitis caused by *C. difficile* resolve spontaneously if antibiotics are discontinued. Infants and children with protracted diarrhea that has not improved after discontinuing antibiotics may benefit from receiving cholestyramine (240 mg/kg per day divided into three equal doses). Cholestyramine is an anion exchange resin that absorbs *C. difficile* cytotoxin. Debilitated patients, children with underlying gastrointestinal disorders, immunocompromised children, and children with severe bloody diarrhea should be treated orally with vancomycin (10 to 40 mg/kg per day divided every 6 h) or metronidazole (15 to 40 mg/kg per day in three divided doses).

The use of antimotility agents is problematic in infants and young children. Loperamide is commonly used to treat both acute and chronic diarrhea and acts by inhibiting secretion in the small intestine and by decreasing intestinal motility. However, clinical trials have failed to show clear beneficial effects. Loperamide poisoning may result in toxic dilatation and paralytic ileus in young infants.

## ADMISSION INDICATIONS

All infants who appear toxic should be admitted. Patients with circulatory compromise, 10 to 15 percent dehydration, inability to drink, intractable vomiting, or altered consciousness should be given a rapid infusion of normal saline or Ringer's lactate, 20 mL/kg, regardless of the serum osmolality, and admitted. Infants who are less ill but whose families may not be able to precisely follow the guidelines for oral rehydration should also be admitted.

Infants who are malnourished and present with acute diarrhea require special attention. They more often need to be admitted to the hospital. Malnutrition in general is a risk factor for the development of persistent diarrhea. In addition, malnourished infants are more likely to develop metabolic acidosis accompanied by an increase in the anion gap and renal dysfunction. This increased anion gap acidosis is due to the accumulation of unmeasured anions, lactate, protein, and phosphate and is accompanied by normochloremia. This is in contrast to most well-nourished infants who develop hyperchloremic acidosis due to fecal loses of bicarbonate. The latter group of infants can be expected to improve with oral therapy.

Infants and children with protracted bloody diarrhea who may have a gastrointestinal infection due to *E. coli* 0157:H7 or other verotoxin-producing *E. coli* serotypes represent another high-risk group because of the strong association with the development of HUS. The risk factor most frequently identified in outbreaks has been exposure to foods of bovine origin such as undercooked ground meat and unpasteurized milk. Person-to-person transmission, especially in child day-care centers, is also a well-recognized risk factor for childhood HUS. Therefore, any child who presents with acute bloody diarrhea and laboratory evidence of hemolytic anemia, thrombocytopenia, azotemia, and/or elevated serum creatinine should be admitted.

## DISCHARGE INSTRUCTIONS

Infants and children who are not dehydrated or who have responded well to oral or intravenous hydration may be discharged on oral glucose-electrolyte solutions. Rehydration feeds should be continued for at least 4 to 6 h before the child is switched to a maintenance glucose-electrolyte or rice carbohydrate-electrolyte solution and allowed to resume his or her usual diet. Breastfeeding should be routinely continued, and formula-fed infants may resume their usual formula within 24 h. The family should be instructed to return to the emergency department or to their own physician if the child is unable or unwilling to drink the rehydration solution or maintenance solution, begins to vomit, or shows signs of dehydration, i.e., decreasing urine output or tearing, or if there is a decrease in the child's level of activity or state of alertness.

## AMBULATORY TREATMENT

In general, reinstatement of food should begin after the 4- to 6-h rehydration phase is completed and never delayed more than 24 h. Breastfeeding should be routinely continued in infants with acute gastroenteritis. Infants who have been receiving formula feedings and who are not dehydrated may rapidly return to their feeding. Recent studies have shown that the introduction of full-strength formula or unrestricted diet immediately following rehydration is associated with decreased duration of diarrhea, positive nitrogen balance, and increased weight gain. There is no need to give dilute formula or lactose-free feedings. Older infants may resume their usual diet.

## FOLLOW-UP INTERVAL

Infants and small children should be reevaluated within 24 h, especially if the child continues to have diarrhea. The family should be instructed to telephone their primary care provider and he or she should decide if a visit is necessary. If the family does not have a primary care physician, then the family should contact the emergency department.

## BIBLIOGRAPHY

American Academy of Pediatrics Committee on Nutrition: Use of oral fluid therapy and posttreatment following enteritis in children in a developed country. *Pediatrics* 75:358, 1985.

Lebaron CW, Furutan NP, Lew JF, et al: Viral agents of gastroenteritis: Public health importance and outbreak management. *MMWR* 39:1, 1990.

Moineau G, Newman J: Rapid intravenous rehydration in the pediatric emergency department. *Pediatr Emerg Care* 6:186, 1990.

O'Loughlin E, Scott R, Gall D: Pathophysiology of infectious diarrhea: Changes in intestinal structure and function. *J Pediatr Gastroenterol Nutr* 12:5, 1991.

Rosenton G, Freeman M, Standard AL, Weston N: Warning: Use of lomotil in children. *Pediatrics* 51:132, 1973.

# 115
# PEDIATRIC ABDOMINAL EMERGENCIES
## Robert W. Schafermeyer

Evaluation of abdominal emergencies in childhood presents a diagnostic challenge to the emergency physician. Some diseases are common to adults and children and others are age-specific, such as congenital anomalies, volvulus, and Hirschsprung's disease. One must understand the differential diagnoses of the presenting symptoms, recognize the clinical manifestations of the more common and life-threatening diseases, and be sensitive in approaching the infant and child.

One can classify abdominal disease processes in several ways. Is the child febrile or afebrile? Does the disease appear to be obstructive or nonobstructive, abdominal or extraabdominal in nature? Is it due to a local process, or is it a systemic process? Does the child appear healthy and happy or sick and septic?

The child's age influences the presenting signs and symptoms significantly. The spectrum of pathologic gastrointestinal conditions of a 2-day-old infant is vastly different from that of a 2-week-old, and both are quite different from that of a 2-year-old.

## HISTORY

The infant or young child cannot give a complete history, but if the child is verbal, one should try to get historical information from him or her and then obtain and listen carefully to what the parent or care giver says. Find out an accurate chronology of events, whether fever has been a part of the illness, the quality and location of pain, feeding and bowel habits, and the quality and quantity of vomiting and bowel losses. Inquire whether bleeding has been present in vomitus or stools. The clinicians must ask about weight changes. A history of prematurity, necrotizing enterocolitis, congenital anomalies, inborn errors of metabolism, cystic fibrosis, intussusception, or sickle cell anemia are all associated with abdominal complications.

Unfortunately, because a child either is too young or too frightened to speak for him- or herself or has not been under continuous observation, trauma as a factor in the development of a GI emergency may be missed in the battered or abused child. The parent or care giver may mislead and confuse the physician by evasion and lies. Trauma must always be considered by the physician evaluating the pediatric patient presenting with what appears to be an abdominal emergency.

## EVALUATION

Children vary greatly in their ability to cooperate with a physical examination. One should take a few moments to gain the confidence of the child before any painful examination or procedures occur. Allowing the child to rest or be on the care giver's lap may help. Remove clothing to avoid missing an incarcerated hernia, petechiae, visible masses, or peristalsis. Look first, then feel. Consider some nontouch maneuvers and observations such as the child's responses during coughing, walking, climbing onto the table, or jumping up and down.

The child can be invited to self-palpate or palpate with the physician. Start in the least painful areas. Also evaluate extraabdominal areas such as the pharynx, mucous membranes, neck, lung fields, inguinal regions, femoral triangles, testes, and scrotum. Failure to do so may result in delayed or missed diagnoses. Never omit the rectal examination and guaiac test. The diagnosis of Hirschsprung's disease, volvulus, or intussusception will be missed without them.

The most important studies include a urinalysis, a complete blood count and differential, and a test of the stool for occult blood. Other tests, ultrasound, and x-ray evaluation should be guided by history, physical examination, how ill the child appears, and the differential diagnoses. Electrolyte and amylase studies, a pregnancy test, and chest and abdominal x-rays may be useful in certain cases.

Once the history, physical examination, and laboratory studies are performed, one should have a list of differential diagnoses. If the child is critically ill, resuscitation and evaluation must be simultaneous. Early consultation must be part of the child's care. If the child is ill but stable and the findings are equivocal, then the patient should be admitted for observation and reassessment.

## KEY SYMPTOMS

The important gastrointestinal signs and symptoms are pain, vomiting, diarrhea, constipation, bleeding, jaundice, and masses.

## Pain

Abdominal pain can be a manifestation of a variety of disease states not necessarily related to the intestinal tract. The origin of the pain may be extraabdominal, such as one might see in the 3- to 6-year old with tonsillitis or pneumonia. Therefore, a careful general physical examination is necessary. One should distinguish between two types of pain, peritonitic and obstructive:

1. Peritonitic pain tends to be exacerbated by motion and thus keeps the patient relatively immobile, as, for example, in appendicitis.
2. Obstructive pain is usually spasmodic and associated with restlessness and motion, as, for example, with intussusception.

In the very young (up to 2 years of age), pain is usually described by the care giver in general terms, such as fussiness, irritability, and inconsolableness. With severe peritonitic pain, the care giver may state that the child is very irritable or lethargic or seems to be grunting as if in pain. Peritonitis or pain from intussusception may present as lethargy or an altered level of consciousness. Between 2 and 6 years of age, pain of GI origin is usually referred to the periumbilical region, and diagnosis requires correlation of the patient's observations and the physician's visual and tactile evaluation. The youngster with pain of peritonitic origin walks with obvious discomfort and prefers to lie still. In contrast, the youngster with obstructive pain may be unable to remain immobile on the examining table. The etiologies of pain vary significantly with age (Table 115-1). Every emergency physician must be familiar with and recognize the life-threatening causes of pain (Table 115-2). The clinician must provide appropriate supportive therapy while completing the diagnostic evaluation and/or consultation.

## Vomiting

Vomiting is a common childhood problem and may be a specific or nonspecific manifestation of a benign process or a serious, life-threatening illness or injury. Vomiting or regurgitation may be a manifestation of a relatively minor problem (e.g., a nervous parent, poor feeding habits, or gastroesophageal reflux) or it may be a sign of a more serious illness. Bilious vomiting is always a serious manifestation in an infant or a child. Vomiting may be a sign of obstructive or nonobstructive gastrointestinal diseases, or of infections or metabolic disorders (Table 115-3).

Vomiting (bilious or not) is a classic symptom of mechanical intestinal obstruction in the child. In the early phases of illness, before the child has developed electrolyte abnormalities (e.g., in the child with pyloric stenosis) or before the child has reached the stage of harboring gangrenous bowel (e.g., internal volvulus), the child's general condition may appear to be good. The child may be hungry immediately after vomiting and even feed vigorously. One must not ignore

**Table 115-1.** Etiology of Pain

| Under 2 Years | 6–11 Years |
|---|---|
| Appendicitis | Appendicitis |
| Colic | Diabetic ketoacidosis |
| Congenital anomalies | Gastroenteritis |
| Gastroenteritis | Henoch-Schönlein purpura |
| Incarcerated hernia | Incarcerated hernia |
| Intussusception | Inflammatory bowel disease |
| Malabsorption | Obstruction |
| Malrotation | Peptic ulcer disease |
| Metabolic acidosis | Pneumonia |
| Obstruction | Renal stones |
| Sickle cell pain crises | Sickle cell syndrome |
| Toxins | Streptococcal pharyngitis |
| Urinary tract infection | Torsion of ovary or testicle |
| Volvulus | Toxins |
| | Urinary tract infection |
| **2–5 Years** | **Over 11 Years** |
| Appendicitis | Appendicitis |
| Diabetic ketoacidosis | Cholecystitis |
| Gastroenteritis | Diabetic ketoacidosis |
| Hemolytic uremic syndrome | Dysmenorrhea |
| Henoch-Schönlein purpura | Ectopic pregnancy |
| Incarcerated hernia | Gastroenteritis |
| Intussusception | Incarcerated hernia |
| Malabsorption | Inflammatory bowel disease |
| Metabolic acidosis | Obstruction |
| Obstruction | Pancreatitis |
| Pneumonia | Peptic ulcer disease |
| Sickle cell pain crises | Pneumonia |
| Toxins | Pregnancy |
| Urinary tract infection | Renal stones |
| Volvulus | Sickle cell syndrome |
| | Torsion of ovary or testicle |
| | Toxins |
| | Urinary tract infection |

the possibility of a serious underlying intraabdominal pathologic condition merely because the vomiting child appears to be systemically well.

The emergency physician must evaluate the child's circulatory and volume status and administer normal saline at 20 ml/kg for any child in shock or dehydrated. A one-time dose of an antiemetic can be given safely to children over 6 months of age. The child with shock or severe dehydration will need consultation. For children who appear systemically well after about 2 h, 30 ml of clear liquids or infant rehydration solution can be provided at 15- to 30-minute intervals.

## Diarrhea

Diarrhea is an increased number of watery stools over a defined period of time. An infant may have a formed or semiformed stool after each feeding and this could be normal. There are several mechanisms that can cause diarrhea in the child, including osmotic, secretory, and transit disorders. Viral and bacterial pathogens cause the majority of episodes of diarrhea. Some tumors, such as neuroblastomas, secrete hormones that can increase stool water content.

When the presenting symptom is diarrhea, one must quantitate the

**Table 115-2.** Life-Threatening Causes of Pain

| | |
|---|---|
| Appendicitis | Metabolic acidosis |
| Congenital anomalies | Peptic ulcer disease: complications |
| Diabetic ketoacidosis | Pneumonia |
| Ectopic pregnancy | Sepsis |
| Hemolytic-uremic syndrome | Toxins |
| Incarcerated hernia | Trauma |
| Intussusception | Volvulus |

**Table 115-3.** Causes of Vomiting

| Newborn (0–3 Months) | Under 2 Years |
|---|---|
| Congenital anomalies | Appendicitis |
| Congenital adrenal hyperplasia | Congenital adrenal hyperplasia |
| Gastroesophageal reflux | Diabetic ketoacidosis |
| Gastroenteritis | Foreign body |
| Hirschsprung's disease | Gastroenteritis |
| Hydrocephalus | Head trauma |
| Inborn errors of metabolism | Hirschsprung's disease |
| Incarcerated hernia | Hydrocephalus |
| Kernicterus | Incarcerated hernia |
| Malrotation | Intussusception |
| Meconium ileus | Malrotation |
| Meningitis | Meningitis |
| Necrotizing enterocolitis | Metabolic acidosis |
| Obstruction: anatomic causes | Neurologic diseases |
| Obstruction: renal system | Obstruction |
| Pneumonia | Pneumonia |
| Pyloric stenosis | Pyloric stenosis |
| Sepsis | Sepsis |
| Toxins | Toxins |
| Urinary tract infection | Urinary tract infection |
| Volvulus | Volvulus |

**Over 2 and Adolescents**

| | |
|---|---|
| Appendicitis | Neurologic diseases |
| Diabetic ketoacidosis | Pancreatitis |
| Foreign body | Peritonitis |
| Gastroenteritis | Pneumonia |
| Head trauma | Pregnancy |
| Hirschsprung's disease | Sepsis |
| Incarcerated hernia | Toxins |
| Meningitis | Urinary tract infection |
| Metabolic acidosis | |

number and volume of stools, consistency, and the presence of blood. Ascertain the norm for the child, since there is great individual variability in frequency and type of stools. Associated symptoms or the presence of diarrheal illness in other members of the family helps in establishing the diagnosis. Dehydration and electrolyte imbalance should be assessed and treated. Diarrhea may represent fluid expelled around an anatomic obstructive mass, such as an impaction, or functional obstruction, as in Hirschsprung's disease (absence of parasympathetic ganglia cells in the muscle layers of the colon). Bloody diarrhea may be infectious or a manifestation of a systemic disease (e.g., hemolytic-uremic syndrome; Table 115-4).

Treatment of diarrhea will vary depending on cause. A suspicion of Hirschsprung's or Crohn's disease warrants surgical consultation. Malabsorption, hemolytic-uremic syndrome, cystic fibrosis, or persistent diarrhea with weight loss and failure to thrive warrants pediatric consultation. Other causes may only require 24 h of rehydration solution and avoiding fatty or high carbohydrate containing foods for 2 or 3 days. Stool cultures are warranted in children with bloody diarrhea, diarrhea for more than 5 days, or toxic appearance or to track an epidemic form of illness.

## Constipation

Constipation is infrequent, dry, hard stools that may result from defects in filling or emptying the rectum.

Constipation may be a sign of a pathologic or functional process. Eventually, watery stool works its way around the impaction causing diarrhea. Thus, rectal examination is very important in the evaluation of both constipation and diarrhea.

Causes of constipation are quite different in the infant and older child. In infancy, one must consider causes such as maternal drugs, congenital gastrointestinal anomalies, cystic fibrosis, Hirschsprung's disease, poor intake, and anal fissure. One should note abdominal

**Table 115-4.** Causes of Diarrhea

Anatomic: Hirschsprung's disease
Dietary: allergy, malabsorption, overfeeding
Infectious: bacterial, parasitic, toxic, viral
Inflammatory: Crohn's disease, hemolytic-uremic syndrome, ulcerative colitis
Malabsorption: cystic fibrosis, enzyme deficiencies, celiac disease
Systemic: endocrinopathy, immunodeficiencies
Obstructive: fecal impaction

shape and girth, presence of bowel sounds and masses, and check the anal area. Check rectal tone and stool for occult blood. If a bowel obstruction is suspected, surgical consultation is necessary. If no systemic cause or serious illness is suspected, dark thick molasses or corn syrup can be added to the diet. Finally, if the child is listless or hypotonic, one should consider infantile botulism (see Table 115–5).

In the older child one should not automatically think that the cause is functional. Constipation is seen in children who are anorexic or who have cerebral palsy, neuromuscular disease, dehydration, hypercalcemia, hypokalemia, hypothyroidism, or depression or who have ingested drugs such as diuretics, antihistamines, anticholinergics, or narcotics. A thorough history and physical examination, including rectal, are necessary. An empty rectal vault does not rule out constipation. If there are signs of bowel obstruction, tumor, or serious illness, one should consult an appropriate specialist.

Acute constipation is treated by increased oral fluids and possibly a stool softener or milk of magnesia. Chronic constipation is treated in three separate steps, and follow-up with a primary care specialist is important. The steps are cleanout, maintenance, and behavior modification.

## Bleeding

Bleeding may be a sign of GI inflammation, duplication, foreign body infection, or systemic illness, or it may be nothing more than an anal fissure or milk allergy. GI bleeding in the newborn, either vomited or per rectum, may be the result of swallowed maternal blood. The laboratory can differentiate between maternal and fetal blood by the Kleihauer-Betke test or hemoglobin electrophoresis. Rarely hemorrhagic states cause GI bleeding in the newborn. Small amounts of blood in the stool of an infant, if fresh, may be a manifestation of anal fissures, which are easily identified. In children 2 to 10 years of age,

**Table 115-5.** Acute and Chronic Constipation

NONORGANIC

| Miscellaneous | Drugs |
|---|---|
| Anorexia nervosa | Anticholinergics |
| Functional | Antihistamines |
| Limited fluid intake | Diuretics |
| Minimal bulk diet | Opiates |
| Prolonged immobilization | Phenothiazine |
| Psychogenic | Thorazine |
| | Vincristine |

ORGANIC

| Gastrointestinal | Metabolic |
|---|---|
| Anal fissure | Dehydration |
| Anal stricture/stenosis | Hypercalcemia |
| Chagas disease | Hypokalemia |
| Cystic fibrosis | Hypothyroidism |
| Hirschsprung's disease | Renal tubular acidosis |
| Obstruction | Neuromuscular |
| Tumor | Amyotonia congenita |
| Volvulus | Myotonic dystrophy |
| Infectious | Spina bifida |
| Infantile botulism | Spinal cord disease or injury |
| | Tumors |

painless bleeding of small to moderate amounts of fresh blood usually mixed through the stool might be an indication of benign GI polyps, or bloody diarrhea may indicate a bacterial infection or inflammatory bowel disease.

The presence of small to moderate amounts of blood in the stool of an infant (particularly associated with vomiting) must lead the physician to consider malrotation of the midgut. This is a life-threatening condition that requires immediate investigation and surgical consultation because volvulus of the midgut can lead to midgut gangrene if the problem is not identified and corrected early in its course.

Major painless upper GI bleeding in the infant or child is most commonly the result of bleeding varices secondary to portal hypertension. Major painless lower GI bleeding in the infant or child is frequently ascribable to a Meckel's diverticulum.

Frequently, the cause of minimal to moderate amounts of blood in the stool of an infant or a child may never be identified. Repeated episodes of bleeding require GI studies, endoscopic evaluation, and Meckel's isotope scanning (Table 115-6).

## Jaundice

Jaundice is an ominous sign, since it represents hepatic dysfunction. It might represent sepsis, congenital infection (TORCHS), or postnatal viral hepatitis. It might represent a minor ABO incompatibility or a major ABO or Rh factor incompatibility, with the possibility of kernicterus or death. It may represent the first signs of cystic fibrosis, galactosemia, or other hepatic enzyme deficiencies, or it could be the harbinger of an anatomic problem such as biliary atresia, a choledochal cyst, or even pyloric stenosis. All jaundiced patients must be evaluated promptly and consultation obtained (Table 115-7).

## Masses

The presence of a mass could be the first sign of a congenital anomaly or a tumor (e.g., Wilms' tumor or neuroblastoma). It could be a pyloric "olive" or the intussusception mass if associated with vomiting or a guaiac-positive stool. If the child has an acute surgical or obstructive abdomen, resuscitation and prompt surgical consultation are necessary. Otherwise, emergency evaluation should be followed by pediatric consultation and admission (Table 115-8).

**Table 115-6.** Causes of GI Bleeding

| Under 2 Months | Under 2 Years | Over 2 Years |
|---|---|---|
| | UPPER GI BLEEDING | |
| Bleeding diathesis | Bleeding diathesis | Esophageal varices |
| Swallowed maternal blood | Foreign body | Foreign body |
| Vascular malformation | Gastroenteritis | Gastroenteritis |
| | Traumatic hemobilia | Traumatic hemobilia |
| | Vascular malformation | Mallory-Weiss tear |
| | | Peptic ulcer disease |
| | | Vascular malformation |
| | LOWER GI BLEEDING | |
| Congenital duplications | Anal fissure | Allergy |
| Intussusception | Congenital duplication | Colitis |
| Meckel's diverticulum | Gastroenteritis | Gastroenteritis |
| Necrotizing enterocolitis | Hemolytic-uremic syndrome | Hemolytic-uremic syndrome |
| Swallowed maternal blood | Henoch-Schönlein purpura | Henoch-Schönlein purpura |
| Vascular malformation | Inflammatory bowel disease | Inflammatory bowel disease |
| Volvulus | Intussusception | Meckel's diverticulum |
| | Meckel's diverticulum | Polyps |
| | Milk allergy | |
| | Polyps: benign, familial | |

**Table 115-7.** Causes of Bilirubin Abnormalities

| Unconjugated | Conjugated |
|---|---|
| ABO or Rh incompatibility | Anatomic defect: biliary, hepatic |
| Autoimmune hemolytic anemia | Hemolytic-uremic syndrome |
| Hepatic: Crigler-Najjar syndrome, Gilbert's disease | Hepatic abscess |
| Hypothyroidism | Hepatitis: congenital, acquired |
| Sepsis | Hepatitis: TORCHS |
| Sickle cell anemia | Inflammatory bowel disease |
| G-6-PD deficiency | Metabolic: cystic fibrosis, galactosemia, etc. |
| | Sepsis |
| | Sickle cell anemia |
| | Toxins |
| | Urinary tract infections |
| | Wilson's disease |

## DIAGNOSIS AND MANAGEMENT OF SELECTED EMERGENCIES

### GI Emergencies in Infants in the First Year of Life

#### Malrotation with and without Volvulus

Volvulus is a major life-threatening complication of malrotation. The complications of malrotation occur most commonly in the first year of life, although malrotation can give rise to symptoms at any time in a person's life. It is the most urgent of GI emergencies in infants and children because of consequent gangrene of the total midgut. The time interval from the first symptom to the development of total midgut gangrene may be only a few hours.

**Pathophysiology**

During gestation, at approximately 6 weeks of age, the elongating intestines prolapse into the yolk sac. Upon reentry at 10 weeks, the midgut undergoes a 270° counterclockwise turn around the superior mesenteric artery. Usually, the duodenum and the cecum become fixed by peritoneal bands, and the small intestine has a broad mesenteric attachment along its base. Abnormal rotation and inadequate fixation can occur during gestation. Incomplete rotation or malrotation can leave the cecum high in the abdomen, with its peritoneal attachments crossing the duodenum in an obstructing manner. The mesentery fails to fan out, and the midgut is suspended and its entire vascular supply travels along a narrow pedicle.

**Clinical Features**

The presenting symptoms are usually vomiting (ultimately becoming bilious), with or without abdominal distension, and streaks of blood in the stool. An infant with symptoms of obstruction or bilious vomiting must receive prompt surgical consultation and active resuscitation. The most dramatic presentation in a newborn is the sudden onset of an acute abdomen and shock, with a rigid and discolored abdomen associated with bilious or bloody vomiting and bloody stools, indicating the presence of gangrenous bowel. On physical examination, the infant may appear pale and have grunting respirations, and approximately one-third of the infants will appear jaundiced. The vast majority of cases present within the first month of life. In the older child the pain is usually constant, not colicky. This symptom

**Table 115-8.** Causes of Abdominal Masses

Hepatomegaly
Splenomegaly
Gastrointestinal duplication
Neuroblastoma
Sacral teratoma
Wilms' tumor
Pyloric stenosis
Intussusception mass

complex usually occurs in a previously healthy child. However, there may have been minor episodes in the past of vomiting or abdominal discomfort. The child suspected of harboring a malrotation with possible midgut volvulus should have flat and upright abdominal x-rays. The presence of a loop of bowel overriding the liver is suggestive of the diagnosis. Occasionally an upper GI examination may reveal an abnormal location of the ligament of Treitz.

Intussusception, duodenal stenosis, or atresia can produce a clinical picture similiar to midgut volvulus.

### Treatment

An infant with systoms of obstruction or bilious vomiting must receive prompt surgical consultation and active resuscitation. Intravenous fluid should be started immediately, and a nasogastric tube placed. Blood should be typed and crossmatched. Any child with vomiting or bloody stools who is identified as having an incompletely rotated bowel requires urgent laparotomy to prevent the development of midgut volvulus and total midgut gangrene.

## Incarcerated Hernia

### Clinical Features

An incarcerated hernia will not be detected unless the infant or child is totally undressed at the time of examination. The symptoms include irritability, poor feeding, vomiting, and an inguinal or scrotal mass. The differential diagnosis of an inguinal or scrotal mass most frequently includes hydrocele of the cord or the scrotum, undescended testicle, torsion of the testicle, torsion of the appendix testis, inguinal lymphadenopathy, inguinal node abscess, orchitis, and inguinal or scrotal trauma. The incidence of incarceration of inguinal hernias is highest in the first year of life. In both boys and girls, the incarcerated sac may contain small or large bowel. In girls, an ovary may be present in the sac.

### Treatment

In most instances, provided the child is examined gently and his or her confidence obtained, it is possible to achieve manual reduction of the incarcerated hernia (if it has been present for only a short period of time) without the use of sedation. When this maneuver is unsuc-

cessful, most cases can be successfully reduced following the administration of intramuscular meperidine (up to 2 mg/kg of body weight in the first year of life). Quite often, as a result of the relaxation induced by the meperidine, the hernia spontaneously reduces. In the absence of spontaneous reduction, one should attempt to reduce the hernia. The few patients who do not respond to these maneuvers must undergo surgical reduction.

Once the hernia is reduced, the patient should be referred for surgical repair on an elective basis. If it was a difficult reduction, the child should be admitted to an observation unit for 6 to 12 h.

## Intestinal Obstruction

### Clinical Features

Intestinal obstruction presents in infants and young children in the classic manner, with symptoms of pain (manifested by irritability); vomiting; abdominal distension; and, later, absence or diminution of bowel movements. The differential diagnosis of intestinal obstruction in the newborn and infant includes intestinal atresia or stenosis, meconium ileus (newborn only), incarcerated inguinal hernia, malrotation, malrotation with volvulus, volvulus around a congenital intraabdominal band, duplication cysts of the intestinal tract, imperforate anus, and Hirschsprung's disease.

### Diagnosis and Treatment

Flat and upright films of the abdomen, show dilated loops of bowel with air-fluid levels (Fig. 115-1). Such an appearance on the plain x-ray film warrants a barium enema examination with a Hirschsprung's catheter, which helps to differentiate between Hirschsprung's disease, malrotation, and colonic stenosis and also separates lower large bowel obstruction from upper small bowel obstruction.

Once intestinal obstruction has been diagnosed, the patient should be prepared for surgical intervention by having an intravenous line and a nasogastric tube placed.

## Pyloric Stenosis

The child with a history of nonbilious projectile vomiting must be considered to have pyloric stenosis. The disorder affects approximately 1 in 150 male and 1 in 750 female patients. It occurs more fre-

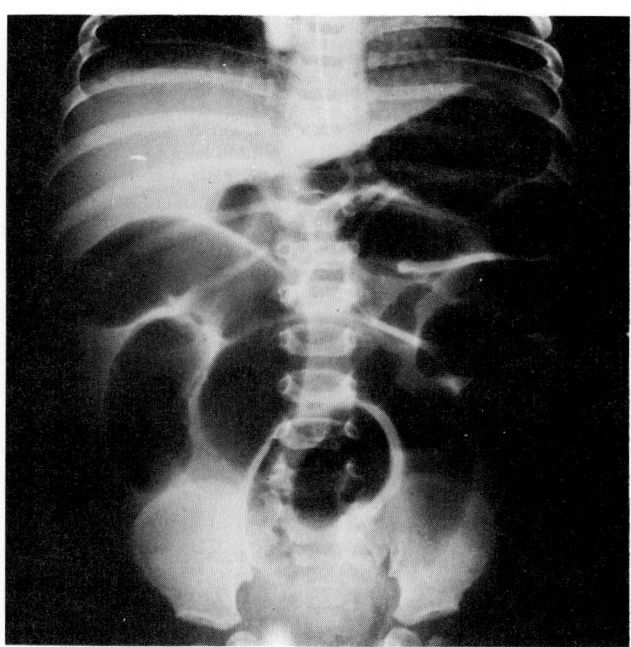

A                                                              B

**Fig. 115-1.** Mechanical intestinal obstruction. **A.** Upright film. **B.** Flat film.

quently in firstborn males, and a familial incidence is noted in approximately 50 percent of patients. It is caused by diffuse hypertrophy and hypoplasia of the smooth muscle that narrows the antrum of the stomach to a small channel that can be easily obstructed.

### Clinical Features

Onset is rare before the age of 1 week, and the disorder usually begins in the second or third week of life. It seldom develops after the third month of life. Initially, the infant may only regurgitate small amounts of milk, making it difficult to distinguish the cause of vomiting from simple regurgitation, gastric reflux, or milk intolerance. Vomiting usually becomes projectile within a week of onset of symptoms, and the vomitus is never bile-stained although it may occasionally have streaks of blood. Vomiting occurs just after or near the end of feeding, and afterwards the infant will refeed hungrily unless the child has become malnourished or dehydrated.

Vomiting eventually becomes projectile in nature. Constipation usually is noted because the infant is not retaining enough formula and becomes dehydrated.

Physical examination usually demonstrates a hungry infant who has failed to gain weight over the past several weeks or has lost weight. Jaundice occurs in 1 to 2 percent of cases. If one undresses and then feeds the infant, peristaltic waves can sometimes be seen passing from left to right across the upper abdomen, just prior to an episode of vomiting. Palpation of a pyloric tumor—the "olive"—is pathognomonic. If it is present, one can be sure of the diagnosis. The olive is usually felt near the lateral margin of the right rectus muscle just below the liver edge. Palpation of the olive is very dependent upon the amount of hypertrophy of the pylorus and the skill of the clinician.

In advanced cases, the physical examination will reveal dehydration and lethargy. The child may appear moribund, with decreased elasticity of the skin and loss of subcutaneous tissue. The eyes may be sunken, and the child has the appearance of an old person.

### Diagnosis

If the olive is palpated, further studies are not necessary. If no olive is palpated, abdominal ultrasonography is recommended. Accuracy is dependent on the use of a high-resolution machine and an experienced sonographer. While false-positives are rare, false-negatives can occur in up to 20 percent of cases, often due to bowel gas interference. If the diagnosis is highly suspected and ultrasonography is negative, an upper GI series can be performed. This usually demonstrates delayed gastric emptying and indentation of the antrum by the pyloric olive. The pyloric channel is narrowed and appears like a "string." If pyloric stenosis is not noted, the radiographer can evaluate the infant for gastroesophageal reflux. The major risk from the upper GI series is the potential for aspiration. The barium should be removed after the x-ray to prevent aspiration.

### Treatment

Once the diagnosis of pyloric stenosis has been confirmed or is highly suspected, surgical consultation should be obtained. Surgery is the treatment of choice, and the procedure is very safe.

Oral intake should be restricted and an intravenous line started. Dehydration and electrolyte abnormalities must be corrected before surgery. Much of the reduced morbidity and mortality from surgery for this disease can be attributed to improved preoperative status. Extensive and protracted vomiting in pyloric stenosis may lead to hypokalemia and hyponatremia. More striking decreases occur in chloride concentration and an increase in pH and carbon dioxide content. This constitutes the characteristic changes of hypochloremic alkalosis. Initial administration of 5% dextrose in normal saline or normal saline to which potassium chloride is added gradually and successfully replaces the calculated deficits of potassium chloride and sodium

## Intussusception

Intussusception occurs when a portion of the alimentary tract is telescoped into another segment. It is the most common cause of intestinal obstruction between 3 months and 6 years of age and is rare under 3 months of age. The male:female ratio is 4:1.

### Pathophysiology

The causes of most intussusceptions are unknown. There is a seasonal incidence that seems to follow peak viral illness seasons. In some patients, recognizable causes for intussusception are found, such as Meckel's diverticulum, intestinal polyp, duplication, lymphosarcoma, or as a complication of Henoch-Schönlein purpura. Rarely, tumors or foreign bodies may cause intussusception. Ileocolic intussusceptions are the most common. The upper portion of the bowel invaginates into the lower portion, bringing the mesentery with it. Constriction of the mesentery obstructs venous return with engorgement of the intussusceptum. With edema and bleeding there may be bloody stools, with mucus giving rise to the characteristic "currant jelly" stool.

### Clinical Features

The classic patient is a robust, 6- to 18-month-old infant without prior difficulty. Suddenly, the child appears to be in pain. The youngster may be playing quietly in the playpen and suddenly stop playing, begin to cry, and even roll around in discomfort. Just as suddenly, the pain ceases, and the child appears to be as happy and content as before the onset of pain. Episodes may recur at more frequent intervals, with the duration of the painful attacks increasing. Some children become very still, listless, and pale, and appear to be in a shocklike state due to the visceral pain. Vomiting is rare in the first few hours but usually develops after 6 to 12 h. The classic "currant jelly" stool associated with intussusception is a late manifestation of the disease complex and is present in only 50 percent of cases. Its absence should not delay evaluation for intussusception in the patient. However, a positive stool guaiac test is present in almost every case. Fever can occur and even rise to 41°C (106°F). Respirations may be shallow and grunting in nature.

Examination between attacks may reveal the oft-described sausage-shaped tumor mass of intussuscepted bowel in the right side of the abdomen. If this mass is felt in the epigastrium, the long axis is usually horizontal. At least one-third of patients do not have a palpable mass, but the absence of a mass must not delay further investigation. An ileoileal intussusception may have a less typical presentation, with symptoms and signs suggestive of intestinal obstruction.

### Diagnosis

The presumptive diagnosis of intussusception is made on the basis of the history and may be seriously considered as a result of a telephone description of the child's problem by the care giver. The apparent well-being of the child in the absence of clinical findings should not mislead the physician. An x-ray examination of the abdomen may show a mass or filling defect in the right upper quadrant of the abdomen (Fig. 115-2A). Even in the presence of normal plain x-ray films, the history described demands a barium enema examination, which demonstrates the classic "coiled spring" (Fig. 115-2B). The barium enema examination is not only a diagnostic tool in the management of this disease, but is frequently curative. If it is obtained in the first 12 to 24 h of the developing intussusception, up to 80 percent of cases can be corrected by barium enema alone. When barium enema does not resolve the intussusception, surgical intervention is indicated. If the barium enema reduces the intussusception, the parents should be warned a 5 to 10 percent recurrence rate, usually within the first 24 to 48 h following barium enema reduction.

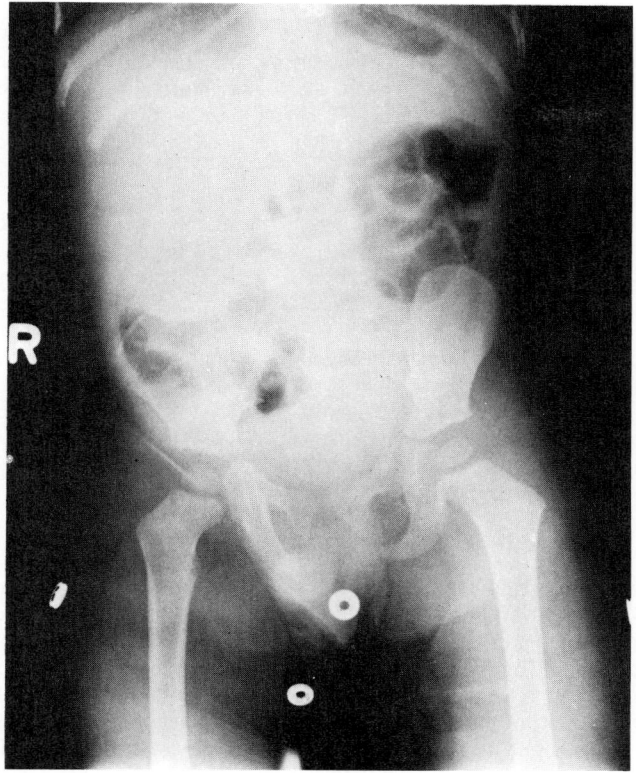

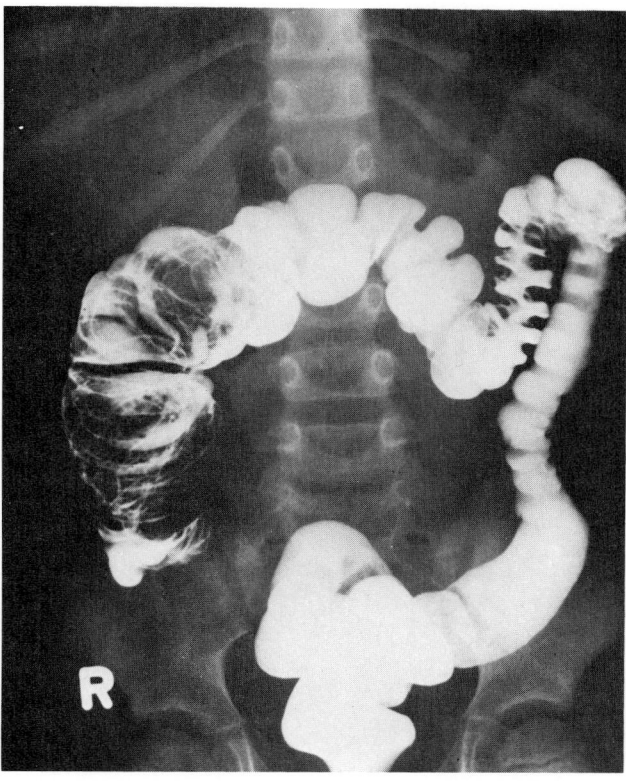

A

B

**Fig. 115-2.** Intussusception. **A.** Plain film showing a filling defect in the right upper quadrant. **B.** With barium enema, showing a "coiled spring" in the ascending colon.

## GI Emergencies in Children 2 Years and Older

### Appendicitis

#### Clinical Features

While appendicitis can occur under age 2, the presentation is usually one of peritonitis or sepsis because of the delay in diagnosis. Over age 2, appendicitis becomes a more important part of the differential diagnoses of abdominal pain. The classic progression of symptoms associated with appendicitis applies equally to children and adults. The events involve early anorexia followed by the development of mild to moderate periumbilical pain and then vomiting and the movement of the pain to the right lower quadrant of the abdomen. The youngster should be observed walking into the examining room; in most instances the child appears to be in discomfort as he or she moves along. This discomfort associated with motion can be exacerbated by asking the youngster to jump up and down before he or she lies down on the examining table. On inspection of the patient, the physician may find limited motion of the lower abdomen due to inflammation of the peritoneum, and depending on the duration of the symptoms, there may be abdominal distension. Palpation may reveal the presence of tenderness in the right lower abdominal quadrant. The position of the appendix may vary greatly, and thus tenderness on examination may vary. Guarding and rebound tenderness may or may not be present in this area. The longer the duration of the symptoms, the greater the possibility of finding a right lower quadrant mass representing localized perforation with the development of an appendiceal abscess. A rectal examination should be performed in order to detect the presence of a low-lying, intrapelvic, acutely inflamed appendix or to palpate a mass. The child may have a mild fever and an elevated white blood cell count in the range of 11,000 to 20,000. When there is doubt in the overall symptom complex, an x-ray may reveal the presence of an appendicolith (Fig. 115-3).

#### Diagnosis

Symptoms consistent with appendicitis together with the presence of an appendicolith warrant the clinical diagnosis of appendicitis and laparotomy. Intravenous fluids should be given and surgical consultation obtained.

The following signs and symptoms make the diagnosis of acute appendicitis difficult:

1. The temperature may be normal.
2. The white blood cell count may be normal.
3. The child may not be anorexic and may actually request food.
4. A heavily built child may manifest minimal right lower quadrant tenderness and minimal tenderness on rectal examination.
5. Gastroenteritis is not infrequently associated with appendicitis. Thus, a child presenting with a several-day history of vomiting and diarrhea, perhaps even with siblings suffering from the same problem, should not have the diagnosis of appendicitis discounted on this basis. Intensification of pain in the presence of a history of gastroenteritis should suggest an acutely inflamed appendix secondary to gastroenteritis.
6. Appendicitis has been identified in children under 1 year of age and is not uncommon in the second year. The incidence of perforation in this age group is much higher because of the difficulty of making the diagnosis and the confusion with gastroenteritis.

#### Treatment

Once the diagnosis of appendicitis is strongly considered or confirmed, surgical consultation should be obtained. The child should receive any appropriate supportive therapy. If the child is febrile, rectal acetaminophen may be given. The child should not receive any oral fluids or food. Start an intravenous line and administer fluid boluses if the child shows signs of sepsis or shock. Closely monitor the

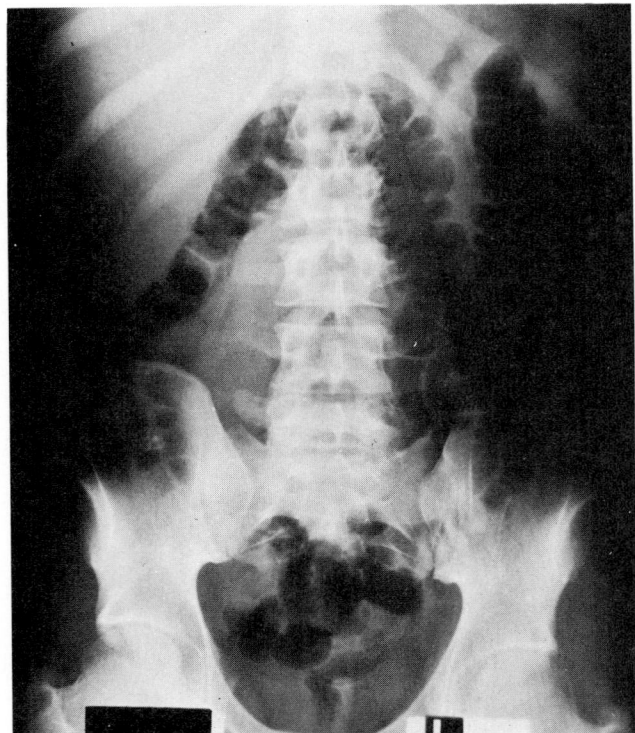

**Fig. 115-3.** Appendicitis; appendicolith in the right lower quadrant.

child's vital signs and give pain medication parenterally after consultation with the surgeon.

If the diagnosis is possible but not probable, surgical consultation should be obtained and the child observed until either resolution of the illness or need for laparotomy is determined.

## Meckel's Diverticulum

A Meckel's diverticulum can cause a variety of signs and symptoms, such as bleeding, peritonitis, intussusception, and intestinal obstruction. The presence of gastric mucosa in the diverticulum may give rise to an ulcer in the adjacent ileum, which may cause symptoms such as painless rectal bleeding. Bleeding is brisk and usually bright red. The ulcer may perforate and cause peritonitis. Isotope scanning reveals the presence of a Meckel's diverticulum containing gastric mucosa in up to 50 percent of the cases. A negative scan does not eliminate the diagnosis.

Acute inflammation in a Meckel's diverticulum may simulate acute appendicitis or may initiate intussusception. Finally, the vitellointestinal remnant attaching the apex of a Meckel's diverticulum to the intraabdominal umbilical region may be the focus around which volvulus of the small bowel or an internal hernia develops, each of these giving rise to intestinal obstruction. One should consult with an appropriate surgeon for evaluation and management of these patients.

## Colon Polyps

Single polyps or multiple or classic familial polyposis may give rise to painless bright-red lower intestinal bleeding. Most commonly the polyp is single, or perhaps there are two or three. Single polyps are usually benign (juvenile), with no propensity for malignant degeneration. Frequently, the parent describes what is obviously a prolapsed polyp, easily palpated on rectal examination. It is rare for bleeding originating from a polyp to be life-threatening. Familial polyposis is rare and is a premalignant syndrome. The child should be referred to a pediatric surgeon for care of these conditions.

## Other Causes of GI Bleeding

Blood represents local irritation or erosion in the majority of children. What appears to be a small amount of blood on the stool or diaper of a healthy child is probably due to an anal fissure or could be related to food substances that have a red or melanotic coloration. A stool test for occult blood and a gentle rectal examination may be all that is needed in the healthy child

On the other hand, if the child is sick- or ill-appearing or shocklike or has petechiae, one must consider vascular malformation, Meckel's diverticulum, intestinal duplication or sepsia. In adolescents, one must consider stress ulceration, peptic ulcer disease, and inflammatory bowel disease. Sepsis, severe gastroenteritis, Henoch-Schönlein purpura, and hemolytic-uremic syndrome should also be part of the differential diagnoses.

In the infant, a coagulation survey should be included in the evaluation if the child is ill or shocklike or has a family history of a clotting disorder. Also remember that GI bleeding could be the presentation of intussusception or volvulus.

## Intraabdominal Masses

Every child should have a careful abdominal examination because intraabdominal masses grow silently at first until they cause obstruction, bleeding, or hemorrhage into the tumor or until a parent sees a mass protruding in the abdomen. The child should be supine with his or her head turned toward the parent and one should carefully palpate all quadrants of the abdomen. If a mass is palpated, the child should be referred to a pediatric surgeon and diagnostic imaging studies obtained. A careful rectal examination, especially if the child has constipation or a gait abnormality, must be done to check for a presacral teratoma and for ovarian masses; both of these tumors can show calcifications on plain film x-rays in approximately 50 percent of cases.

Neuroblastomas can arise from adrenal glands or along the sympathetic chain. They often cross to the midline, and the best cure rate is obtained in the child under 1 year of age. CT scan is the best way to evaluate this tumor. Wilms' tumor is an intrarenal tumor initially and should be considered in the child with hematuria. Ultrasound and CT scan help define this tumor. Bone scan is also needed. Rhabdomyosarcoma occurs in the pelvis or anywhere there is striated muscle, and it is highly malignant.

In girls over the age of menarche, one must consider pregnancy, and if there is lower quadrant pain, one must consider ectopic pregnancy. One should obtain a serum pregnancy test and consider the use of pelvic, intravaginal ultrasound.

## Foreign Bodies in the GI Tract

It is safe to generalize that anything that reaches the stomach will eventually traverse the GI tract and be spontaneously evacuated per rectum. Nails, open safety pins, pieces of glass, and coins are examples of objects that have traveled the intestinal tract completely. It may take weeks for a coin, for example, to complete the trip to the anus. Any foreign body caught in the esophagus must be removed by esophagoscopy. (See Chap. 75.) Very rarely is surgical removal of a foreign body in the stomach or distal to the stomach warranted. Occasionally, a long, thin foreign body may not traverse the duodenum and may need to be removed surgically. Round objects almost always pass spontaneously.

## Portal Hypertension

Portal hypertension is rare in children but is one of the common causes of major upper GI hemorrhage. Extrahepatic portal thrombosis, parenchymal liver disease associated with fibrocystic disease, and biliary cirrhosis in the youngster with congenital biliary atresia surviving as a result of portal enterostomy are examples of conditions that can result in portal hypertension and esophagogastric varices.

## BIBLIOGRAPHY

Andrassy RJ, Mahour GH: Malrotation of the midgut in infants and children. *Arch Surg* 116: 158, 1981.

Boyle JJ: Gastrointestinal bleeding, in Ludwig S, Fleisher GR (eds): *Textbook of Pediatric Emergency Medicine,* 2d ed. Baltimore, Williams & Wilkins, 1988, pp 171–179.

Fleisher GR: Diarrhea, in Ludwig S, Fleisher GR (eds): *Textbook of Pediatric Emergency Medicine,* 2d ed. Baltimore, Williams & Wilkins, 1988, pp 133–137.

Puri P, O'Donnell B: Appendicitis in infancy. *J Pediatr Surg* 13:173, 1978.

Ruddy RM: Abdominal pain, in Ludwig S, Fleisher GR (eds): *Textbook of Pediatric Emergency Medicine,* 2d ed. Baltimore, Williams & Wilkins, 1988, pp 70–77.

Schnaufer L, Mahboubi S: Abdominal emergencies, in Ludwig S, Fleisher GR (eds): *Textbook of Pediatric Emergency Medicine,* 2d ed. Baltimore, Williams & Wilkins, 1988, pp 936–965.

Singer J: Jaundice: Conjugated hyperbilirubinemia, in Ludwig S, Fleisher GR (eds): *Textbook of Pediatric Emergency Medicine,* 2d ed. Baltimore, 1988, pp 205–209.

Watkins JB: Jaundice: Unconjugated hyperbilirubinemia, in Ludwig S, Fleisher GR (eds): *Textbook of Pediatric Emergency Medicine,* 2d ed. Baltimore, Williams & Wilkins, 1988, pp 201–204.

# 116
# THE DIABETIC CHILD
## David A. Poleski

## INTRODUCTION

Type I, or insulin-dependent, diabetes mellitus (IDDM) is an increasingly common disease in childhood. Diabetic ketoacidosis (DKA) remains the leading cause of death in pediatric diabetes. Life expectancy for patients developing the disease under age 20 is reduced by one-third. Morbidity from the complications of retinopathy, nepropathy, neuropathy, premature coronary and peripheral vascular disease, and stroke significantly impairs patients' life-styles. Meticulous attention to the diagnosis and treatment of IDDM on the part of emergency physicians is important in the effort to reduce the morbidity and mortality of IDDM.

## INCIDENCE

IDDM affects 1 in 300 children, making it the most common endocrine disorder of childhood. Males and females are equally affected, with a mean age of onset of $12\frac{1}{2}$ for males and 11 for females. New cases are more common in winter and summer months, although this seasonal variation is not noted in patients presenting under 5 years of age. Socioeconomic factors do not appear to play a role in the incidence of IDDM.

## ETIOLOGY

Type I diabetes is probably an autoimmune disease. Its onset is associated with the appearance of circulating islet-cell antibodies and autoreactive T lymphocytes. Factors involved in triggering the autoimmune destruction of pancreatic insulin-secreting β cells remain to be delineated. Viruses, particularly rubella, CMV, Epstein-Barr, mumps and coxsackie have all been implicated as triggering agents. In addition a genetic predisposition for acquiring IDDM exists. Ninety percent of patients diagnosed with IDDM carry the HLA antigens HLA-DR3, HLA-DR4, or both. In addition, individuals with the HLA-B7 or HLA-DR2 antigens seem to be protected from IDDM. Other etiologic factors may be involved, but all the puzzle pieces are not yet in place.

## DIAGNOSIS

The diagnosis of IDDM is relatively easy. The triad of polyuria, polydipsia, and polyphagia is the classic presentation. In children and particularly infants, (DKA) and coma are frequent presenting findings. Symptoms which occur prior to the onset of polyuria, polydipsia, polyphagia, and DKA include anorexia, weight loss, malaise, nocturia, erratic behavior, and changes in school performance. These are nonspecific, and usually only serendipity allows the diagnosis of IDDM to be made early in the development of the disease. Glycosuria associated with elevated serum blood glucose values will establish the diagnosis. Glucose tolerance tests in children are of little value and may be detrimental, particularly if elevated serum glucose levels are already present.

## DIABETIC KETOACIDOSIS

DKA is a common complication of childhood diabetes, accounting for 14 to 31 percent of hospitalizations related to diabetes. Mortality is reported to be as high as 15.4 percent, although the actual incidence is probably lower. Treating DKA costs over $1 billion annually and accounts for 160,000 hospital admissions. Emergency physicians must be prepared to recognize and treat DKA effectively and expeditiously.

The details of the physiology of DKA are reviewed comprehensively elsewhere. A brief summary is necessary to understand treatment and to avoid pitfalls in management.

DKA develops because of a relative lack of insulin and because of increased activity of the counterregulatory hormones glucagon, cortisol, growth hormone, and epinephrine. Glycogen is mobilized, contributing to the rise in glucose levels; proteolysis and muscle breakdown result in increased amino acid levels; and lipolysis results in increased free fatty acids. Ketone bodies (acetoacetate and β-hydroxybutarate) increase, resulting in ketosis and metabolic acidosis. The hallmarks of DKA are thus hyperglycemia, metabolic acidosis, and ketosis.

Hyperglycemia leads to increased serum osmolality and a subsequent osmotic diuresis. Depending on the duration and extent of the hyperglycemia significant dehydration and possibly shock can result from the diuresis. Infants, whose fluid intake is dependent on their parents, are more apt to develop dehydration and shock than older children, who can compensate by increasing their oral intake at least for a period of time. In addition to volume contraction induced by the osmotic diuresis other important metabolic disturbances are the increased loss of sodium, potassium, and phosphate. Potassium loss may impair cardiovascular function if severe, and phosphate depletion may result in reduced oxygen transport by red blood cells due to diminished levels of 2,3-diphosphoglycerate. Hyperglycemia also may play a role in the development of cerebral edema by leading to the increased production of "idiogenic osmoles." Renal function is impaired as GFR drops due to the osmotically induced hypovolemia.

Ketoacidosis results from increased production in the liver of acetoacetate and β-hydroxybutarate, both of which are strong organic acids. β-hydroxybutarate predominates in the serum (by a 3:1 ratio), but acetoacetate is the one measured by commonly available techniques. Measurement of serum ketones during the management of DKA is thus misleading and of little clinical value. The metabolic acidosis produced by increased ketone body production (and by hypoperfusion if fluid loss is advanced) results in a compensatory respiratory alkalosis manifested clinically in advanced stages by Kussmaul respirations. In addition, severe acidosis depresses myocardial function and may contribute to arrhythmias or cardiovascular collapse. Acidosis also can cause paralytic ileus and gastric distension and may account for the abdominal pain and vomiting which frequently accompany DKA.

The diagnosis of DKA should be suspected in any patient with polyuria, polydipsia, hyperventilation, acetone-smelling breath, and lethargy. Abdominal pain and vomiting can also be presenting complaints. In young children the diagnosis can be more difficult, and in particular in children under 2 years of age DKA can mimic bacterial sepsis. The diagnosis should be apparent, however, once laboratory results are available. Infection is frequently the stress precipitating DKA, and a thorough search for sources of infection must be performed.

## Treatment of DKA

Volume replacement is the mainstay of treatment for DKA. The average deficit is 100 to 150 mL/kg. If possible the fluid deficit should be calculated by comparing the patient's weight on presentation to the emergency department with a known recent weight. If such an estimate is not possible, assume a deficit of 10 percent unless the patient is in shock. Given the importance of fluid replacement in DKA therapy, it is better to overestimate rather than underestimate the amount of fluid loss.

In most cases initial replacement should be a 20 mL/kg bolus of normal saline given over 1 h. If shock is present (rapid pulse, capillary refill greater than 2 sec, obtundation, orthostatic blood pressure changes in the older child, and in the extreme case a falling blood pressure), modify initial therapy by repeating 20 mL/kg boluses until the shock state is corrected. Reevaluate the patient's hydration state and clinical condition frequently, preferably every 30 min. After the initial resuscitation is completed, the calculated remaining deficit should be replaced over 24 to 36 h and will average a rate of infusion approximately 1.5 times maintenance needs per hour. Use 0.45% NaCl as the maintenance and replacement fluid. Once the blood glucose is 250 mg/dL $D_5$ 0.45% NaCl should be substituted. Urinary output during the first 6 h should be measured and replaced with 0.45% NaCl. Oral fluids can be started as soon as nausea and vomiting are no longer clinical problems.

The net effect of adequate fluid resuscitation includes improved renal perfusion with a subsequent increased urinary excretion of glucose and drop in serum glucose levels. In addition peripheral perfusion is improved with partial correction of the metabolic acidosis.

Fluid resuscitation and correction of metabolic derangements in DKA should not be carried out too rapidly in order to avoid the complication of cerebral edema (see "cerebral edema," below).

Once fluid resuscitation has commenced and hyperglycemia (greater than 250 mg/dL on a Dextrostix) has been verified, insulin therapy should be started. Low-dose continuously infused short-acting (regular) insulin is now the method commonly used, although frequent IM injections will also work. The dose recommended is 0.1 unit/kg per hour. Continuously infused insulin has the advantage of smoother and more predictable correction of the metabolic abnormalities associated with DKA. The insulin should be mixed in normal saline (NS) with a concentration of 1 unit per 5 mL of saline. Infusions must be made with an IV infusion pump to avoid inadvertent administration of excess insulin. An initial bolus of 0.1 unit/kg IV of insulin is no longer recommended since this may exacerbate preexisting and unsuspected hypokalemia. Before administering the insulin infusion, approximately 50 mL of the solution should be run through the intravenous tubing in order to saturate the insulin binding sites of the tubing. With the infusion running, glucose determinations should be made hourly and once levels have declined to 250 mg/dL, 5% glucose should be added to the maintenance and replacement fluid ($D_5$ 0.45 NS). If the glucose level has fallen below 250 mg/dL before the patient's pH has reached 7.30, continue both the insulin infusion and

5% glucose until the acidosis has resolved. This may require titrating the amount of insulin versus the amount of infused dextrose to maintain a glucose level between 200 and 250 mg/dL. Once a pH of 7.30 is reached and the glucose is below 250, subcutaneous short-acting insulin can be started. This should be given about 1 h prior to discontinuing the insulin infusion. Ideally this should be done by the physicians who will be providing the child's long-term follow-up care since meticulous monitoring is needed and is unfortunately difficult to provide in a busy emergency department.

As important, if not more important, as insulin therapy in DKA is the monitoring and correction of electrolyte imbalances. $Na^+$ and $K^+$ are both lost in the urine with the osmotic diuresis induced by hyperglycemia, which results in total body depletion of these electrolytes. The loss of $Na^+$ is not as clinically significant as that of $K^+$. Sodium levels should be monitored, but fluid resuscitation with normal saline or 0.45% NS will ordinarily prevent problems with rapid osmolar shifts due to hypo- or hypernatremia. The management of potassium disturbances with DKA is much more critical. Serum $K^+$ does not reflect total body potassium levels since most potassium is intracellar. The acidosis of DKA exacerbates the problem by causing additional shifting of $K^+$ from the intracellar to extracellular space. This results in high serum $K^+$ levels even in the face of total body deletion. Patients with DKA should have cardiac monitoring to detect hypo- or hyperkalemia pending the results of serum potassium levels. Once the serum level is known, decisions regarding the amount and rate of replacement can be made. If the pH is 7.10 or less and the $K^+$ normal or reduced, replacement should begin immediately since hypokalemia will be exacerbated as the pH improves and can cause life-threatening cardiac dysfunction. If the $K^+$ level is high (greater than 6.0), however, replacement should be withheld so that iatrogenic hyperkalemia is not induced with its potential for cardiac complications as well. Once the $K^+$ level is normal and the pH is improving, therapy can begin. Forty mEq of KCL added to each liter of maintenance fluid given at the calculated maintenance replacement rate on an infusion pump is sufficient. Some clinicians recommend replacing potassium with potassium phosphate (20 mEq/L) and potassium chloride (20 mEq/L). This approach has the theoretical but as yet unsubstantiated clinical advantages of maintaining the level of 2,3-diphosphoglycerate which is important in the transfer of oxygen to the tissues. Phosphate and calcium levels should be measured at some point in the management of DKA but are seldom of concern to the emergency physician.

Finally, the issue of bicarbonate therapy in the treatment of DKA needs to be addressed. As yet no convincing evidence exists that bicarbonate therapy affects the outcome of DKA. Classically, arguments favoring bicarbonate use have pointed out that myocardial function and ventilatory effort are impaired when the pH falls below 7.1. At least in children these considerations do not appear to be clinically significant. On the other hand, use of bicarbonate may contribute to the complications of DKA treatment, although again the clinical relevance of these problems is still unclear. Bicarbonate therapy can result in a paradoxical CNS acidosis which may alter CNS function; a shift of the oxyhemoglobin dissociation curve to the left with impaired tissue oxygenation, worsening hypokalemia; and possibly in hypernatremia contributing to rapid osmolar shifts which may play a role in the development of cerebral edema. Since there is no convincing evidence of the benefit of bicarbonate therapy, it is probably best avoided except in life-threatening situations. These would include cardiac arrhythmias due to hyperkalemia or cardiac dysfunction due to severe acidosis.

Laboratory tests necessary in the management of DKA are glucose, electrolytes, urinalysis, venous pH (which accurately correlates which arterial pH and is easier to obtain in children), BUN, and creatinine. Serum acetone can be obtained but is usually unnecessary. The degree of ketosis can be estimated by calculating the anion gap which will be due primarily to the ketone bodies and lactate. It is advisable to check glucose, electrolytes (particularly potassium), and venous pH on an hourly basis and adjust therapy accordingly. Cardiac monitoring until the dangers of potassium-induced cardiac problems are passed is recommended. If the stress inducing DKA is not apparent from the history and physical examination, a CXR, blood cultures, lumbar puncture, and complete blood count should be considered to look for occult sources of infection. If serious infection is suspected, antibiotics should be started pending the results.

## Cerebral Edema

Although rare, cerebral edema can be a fatal complication of DKA in children. Increasing evidence suggests that subclinical cerebral edema exists in most children with DKA. For reasons that are not clear some patients develop malignant edema, which will lead to death in over 90 percent of cases. The etiology of this complication is not well understood. Overly aggressive fluid resuscitation with its attendant rapid osmotic shifts has been implicated, but cerebral edema has occurred without such therapy. Hyponatremia, bicarbonate therapy resulting in paradoxical CSF acidosis, cerebral hypoxia, and elevated intracellar potassium levels due to insulin therapy have also been implicated. The complication usually occurs when the child appears to be improving, about 6 to 10 h after treatment has started. Typical symptoms are abrupt mental status changes with progression to coma. Additional symptoms can include sudden and severe headache, incontinence, opththalmoplegia, and vomiting. Treatment attempts have been discouraging. Intubation with hyperventilation to reduce intracranial pressure should be performed. Mannitol 1 to 2 g/kg may help. Fluid restriction should be instituted. Until more is understood about this complication, the slowest correction of fluid deficits and metabolic derangements associated with DKA consistent with patient well-being is the prudent course to follow.

## HYPOGLYCEMIA

In children the initial treatment of a hypoglycemia episode depends on the clinical presentation. In those with mild symptoms, such as dizziness, diaphoresis, or weakness, oral supplements including candy, table sugar, or commercially prepared glucose supplements are adequate. When hypoglycemia leads to significant mental status changes such as unconsciousness or seizures, treatment consists of administering 0.5 mL/kg of $D_{50}W$ or 1.0 mL/kg of $D_{25}W$ intravenously. If IV access cannot be obtained, glucagon 0.5 mg IM can be given to children under 6 years of age or 1 mg IM to those 6 years old or older. In children with already depleted glycogen stores, glucagon may not work; in all cases, efforts to establish IV access should continue. In children under 3 years of age, intraosseous infusions may be used for glucose infusions if IV access cannot be obtained and glucagon is unsuccessful. Once normal mental status is regained, oral glucose supplements or a regular meal can be given.

Important to note is the growing concern for overtreatment of hypoglycemia. If serious symptoms such as coma or seizures are not present, treatment with a maintenance infusion of $D_{10}W$ is preferable to repeated boluses of $D_{25}W$ or $D_{50}W$ to avoid unnecessary hyperglycemia. Overtreatment can also occur if one doesn't recall that approximately 10 min will elapse between initial glucose therapy and the time the patient begins to feel better. It is during this time frame that excessive amounts of glucose are frequently administered.

Whenever possible, hypoglycemia should be verified by Dextrostix or serum glucose determinations prior to treatment. Treating presumed hypoglycemia can delay the diagnosis of other entities in diabetic children with altered mental status, such as sepsis, meningitis, toxic overdoses, and head injuries.

The etiology of the hypoglycemic episode should always be sought. Insulin excess is most common, but consider also dietary indiscretion, such as missed meals or prolonged overnight fasting, concurrent drug use particularly alcohol, sulphonomides, sulphonylureas

and propranolol, gastroparesis, and a change in baseline physical activity such as an increase in exercise intensity.

## OTHER CONSIDERATIONS

With the increasing realization that IDDM is an autoimmune disease, interest is growing in starting treatment with immunosuppressive drugs, particularly cyclosporine, as soon as the diagnosis of new-onset IDDM has been made. As tempting as this idea is, the treatment is still experimental and is not currently recommended in newly diagnosed emergency department cases.

Interest is growing in providing outpatient management for children with newly diagnosed insulin-dependent diabetes. If a child is stable, not acidotic, able to tolerate oral fluid intake, has reliable social support, and can follow up with physicians comfortable with outpatient management of new onset disease, the emergency physician should try to arrange for this option.

The acute treatment of known childhood diabetics in the emergency department is primarily concerned with the management of hypoglycemia and DKA. Long-term day-to-day management of childhood diabetes is complicated and requires a good long-term physician-patient relationship. Emergency department physicians are not in a position to provide this and should make efforts to coordinate any decisions about care with the patient's primary physician. Follow-up with the patient's primary doctor should always be assured prior to emergency department discharge.

## BIBLIOGRAPHY

Bland GL, Wood VD: Diabetes in infancy: diagnosis and current management. *J Natl Med Assoc* 83:361, 1991.

Chase HP, Crews KR, Gary S: Outpatient management vs. in-hospital management of children with new onset diabetes. *Clinical Pediatrics* p 450, August, 1992.

Chase HP, Garg SK, Jelley DH: Diabetic ketoacidosis in children and the role of outpatient management. *Pediatr Rev* 11:297, 1990.

Chase HP, Garg SK, Jelley DH: Diabetic ketoacidosis in children and the role of outpatient management. *Pediatr Rev* 11:297, 1990.

Duck SC, Wyatt D: Factors associated with brain herniation in the treatment of diabetic ketoacidosis. *J Pediatr* 113:10, 1988.

Ginsberg-Fellner F: Insulin-dependent diabetes mellitus. *Pediatr Rev* 11:239, 1990.

Plotnick L: Insulin-dependent diabetes mellitus. *Pediatrics in Review* 15:137, 1994.

Krane EJ: Diabetic ketoacidosis. *Pediatr Clin North Am* 34:935, 1987.

Rosenbloom AL, Riley WJ, Weber FT, et al: Cerebral edema complicating diabetic ketoacidosis in childhood. *J Pediatr* 96:357, 1980.

Rosenbloom AL, Schatz DA: Diabetic ketoacidosis in childhood. *Pediatr Ann* 23:284, 1994.

Schatz DA: Hypoglycemia in childhood diabetes. *Pediatr Ann* 23:289, 1994.

Scibilia J, Finegold D, Dorman J: Why do children with diabetes die? *Acta Endocrinol* 113(suppl):326, 1986.

Swift PG, Hearnshaw JR, Botha JL, et al: A decade of diabetes: Keeping children out of the hospital. *BMJ* 307:96, 1993.

Silverstein JH, Johnson S: Psychosocial challenge of diabetes and the development of a continuum of care. *Pediatr Ann* 23:300, 1994.

# 117
# PEDIATRIC EXANTHEMS
## Michael S. Weinstock
## Michael S. Catapano

Rashes with diverse etiologies can look alike. The emergency physician's task is to obtain an accurate history regarding prior immunizations, potential human or animal contacts, and recent environmental exposure. This, along with the signs and symptoms either preceding or presenting with the exanthem, helps to determine the diagnosis. The various etiologic agents and associated exanthems are noted in Table 117-1.

## BACTERIAL

### Bullous Impetigo

Bullous impetigo, or staphylococcal impetigo, is a local skin infection caused by phage group II staphylococci. The staphylococci produce an epidermolytic toxin that acts locally to cause separation of the skin at the granular layer, giving rise to bullae. The infection occurs primarily in newborn infants and young children. The characteristic skin lesions of bullous impetigo are superficial, flaccid, thin-walled bullae that occur most often on the extremities but can occur anywhere. They range in size from 0.5 to 3 cm. They can arise from normal skin or may have a thin, red halo. The bullae are filled with a clear, pale-to-yellow fluid and rupture easily, leaving a moist, denuded base that dries rapidly with a shiny coating. Extensive areas of skin may be involved if untreated.

The clinical appearance of the lesions usually makes diagnosis easy. However, single lesions or extensive involvement may not be as typical. Staphylococci cultured from fluid from aspirated bullae will establish the diagnosis.

Systemic antistaphylococcal antibiotics, usually oral, along with local wound cleansing and topical antibiotics (such as neosporin) are effective in eradicating the infection. Prognosis for complete recovery is good.

### Impetigo Contagiosum

Impetigo is a superficial pyoderma caused by infection with group A, β-hemolytic streptococci, although staphylococci may also be cultured. It is a common skin infection, primarily affecting young children, especially in warm, humid conditions. Impetigo can arise at the site of insect bites or superficial cutaneous trauma; sometimes there is no apparent predisposing skin lesion. Fever and systemic signs are uncommon.

The skin lesions start as small erythematous macules and papules. These develop into discrete, thin-walled vesicles which become pustular and quickly rupture (see Fig. 117-1). As the vesicles rupture, a yellow fluid forms an exudate, which dries to form a stratified golden, yellow crust that accumulates. The crusts can be readily removed, leaving a smooth, red surface. The crusts can spread the infection to other parts of the body. Initially, the lesions are discrete, but they may enlarge and become confluent. Local adenopathy may be present. The infection occurs most frequently on the face, neck, and extremities.

The diagnosis of impetigo can be readily made on the basis of the typical clinical appearance. Cultures are generally not necessary. Systemic antibiotic therapy must be combined with wound scrubbing and cleansing and application of neosporin or mupirocin ointment for optimal results. Effective antibiotics include benzathine penicillin and oral antibiotics such as penicillin V, erythromycin, cephalosporin, and dicloxacillin.

### Erysipelas

Erysipelas, or St. Anthony's fire, is cellulitis and lymphangitis of the skin caused by group A, β-hemolytic streptococci. It is frequently accompanied by fever, chills, malaise, headache, and vomiting.

The rash is characterized by local redness, heat, swelling, and a raised, indurated border. There is marked involvement of the superficial dermal lymphatics. The rash starts as an erythematous plaque that rapidly enlarges by peripheral extension. At first, it is scarlet, hot, brawny, swollen, and tender. The edge is raised and sharply demarcated. The rash can vary in appearance from a transient hyperemia to intense inflammation, vesiculation, and bullae. The face is the most frequent site. A skin wound, fissure, or ulcer may act as a portal of entry.

Diagnosis is made on clinical grounds, although aspiration of the leading edge of the lesion will frequently demonstrate streptococci. A brief course of parenteral penicillin is usually warranted because of the rapid advancement of the infection, the acutely toxic state of the patient, and the possibility of suppurative complications. Rapid clinical response is usually obtained. Erythromycin may be used in patients unable to take penicillin.

### Mycoplasma Infections

*Mycoplasma pneumoniae* infections are a common cause of pneumonia, upper respiratory infections, and bronchitis in children between 5 and 19 years of age. The most frequent presenting clinical findings in

**Table 117-1.** Differential Diagnosis of Exanthems

| Vesiculopustules | Maculopapules | Urticaria | Petechiae |
|---|---|---|---|
| Drug eruption | Drug eruption | Varicella (urticaria around vesicle) | Drug eruption |
| Herpes simplex | Secondary lues | Coxsackie A5, A9 | Bacterial endocarditis |
| Variola | Scarlet fever | Infectious hepatitis | Echovirus |
| Vaccinia | Echovirus 9, 16 | Mononucleosis | Coxsackie A5, A9 |
| Varicella | Coxsackie A5, A9, A16, B5 | *Mycoplasma pneumoniae* | Mononucleosis |
| Generalized zoster | Reovirus 2 | Hepatitis | Rubella |
| Rickettsialpox | Erythema infectiosum | | Thrombocytopenia with many acute infections |
| Coxsackie A and B | Gianotti-Crosti syndrome | | |
| Reovirus 2 | Rubella | | |
| *Mycoplasma pneumoniae* | Rubeola | | |
| Echovirus 4 | Hepatitis | | |
| Contagious ecthyma (orf) | Infectious mononucleosis | | |
| | Arbovirus (dengue) | | |
| | Rickettsioses | | |

*Source:* From Burnett JW, Crutcher WA: Viral and rickettsial infections in Moschella SL, Hurley, HJ: *Dermatology,* Philadelphia, Saunders, 1985, vol 1, chap 12, pp 673–738.

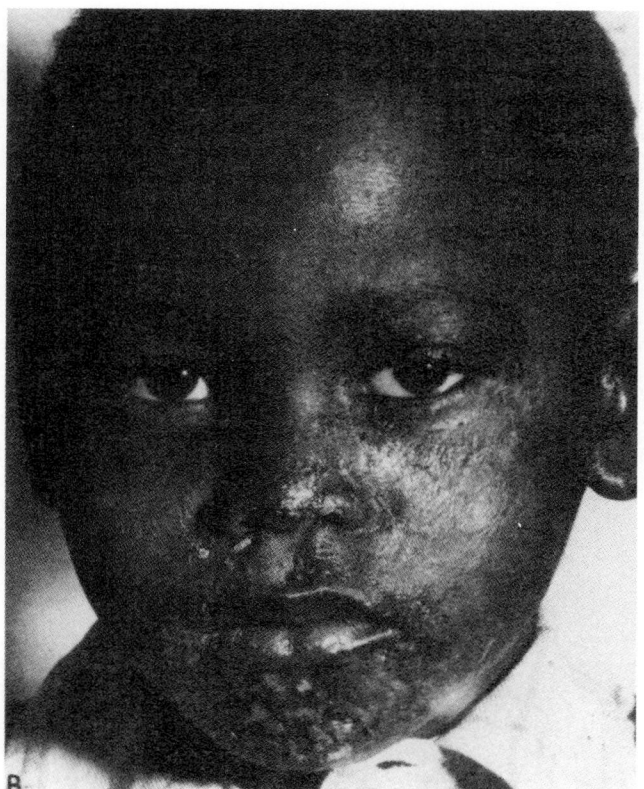

**Fig. 117-1.** Impetigo contagiosum. (*From* Marples RR, Leyden JL: Bacterial infections, section I, Fundamental cutaneous microbiology in Moschella SL, Hurley HJ (eds): *Dermatology,* Philadelphia, Saunders, 1985, vol I, chap 11, pp. 590–642, with permission.)

children and adults are fever, cough, sore throat, malaise, headache, chills, and rash. An erythematous maculopapular rash, the most frequent presentation, is located on the trunk and may be discrete or confluent. However, the most frequently reported exanthem is consistent with *Erythema multiforme* and Stevens-Johnson syndrome, with lesions occurring primarily on the trunk, legs, and arms. The rash occurs most commonly during the febrile period. An enanthem of generalized ulcerative stomatitis or pharyngitis-tonsillitis associated with the exanthem is common. The diagnosis can be confirmed by the use of either serum cold agglutinins or several specific antibody tests.

*Mycoplasma* responds to several antimicrobials, including erythromycin, tetracycline, chloramphenicol, and aminoglycosides. Infection with *M. pneumoniae* should be suspected in patients with pneumonia and a rash.

### Scarlet Fever

Scarlet fever is an acute febrile illness, primarily affecting young children, caused by group A, β-hemolytic streptococci. Recently group C streptococci have been implicated as well. Clinical manifestations include acute onset with fever, sore throat, headache, vomiting, and abdominal pain followed by a distinctive exanthem in 1 to 2 days.

There are both an exanthem and an enanthem associated with scarlet fever. They are caused by an erythrogenic toxin elaborated by the streptococcal organism. The tonsils and pharynx are red and covered with exudate, although occasionally pharyngeal findings are minimal. The tongue has a white coating through which red and hypertrophied papillae project, creating the appearance of a "white strawberry tongue." The white coating disappears by day 4 or 5, and the tongue acquires a bright-red appearance, the "red strawberry tongue."

Bright-red or hemorrhagic spots may be seen on the soft palate or anterior pillars of the tonsillar fossae.

The exanthem of scarlet fever begins 1 or 2 days after the onset of the illness. It starts on the neck, axillae, and groin, spreading to the trunk and extremities. The rash is red and finely punctate, consisting of 1- to 2-mm papules giving the rash a characteristic rough, sandpaper feel. It is sometimes easier to identify the rash by palpation. The rash blanches with pressure. Linear petechial eruptions, Pastia's lines, are often present in the antecubital and axillary folds. There is facial flushing with circumoral pallor. A branny desquamation occurs at 2 weeks, yielding fine flakes of dry skin.

The diagnosis of scarlet fever is readily made on clinical grounds. Throat swabs usually culture group A, β-hemolytic streptococci, although group C may be cultured as well. Treatment with antibiotics is necessary to reduce the incidence of rheumatic fever and nephritis and will probably ameliorate the course of the disease. Penicillin is the antibiotic of choice with erythromycin also being effective for those who are penicillin-allergic.

### Staphylococcal Scalded-Skin Syndrome

The staphylococcal scalded-skin syndrome (SSSS) is a febrile illness of neonates and young children characterized by a generalized, confluent superficial exfoliation of skin. It is also called Ritter's disease or dermatitis exfoliativa neonatorum. SSSS is caused by the action of an epidermolytic toxin, exfoliatin, elaborated by phage group II *Staphylococcus aureus.* The staphylococci do not occur in the involved skin but rather in a distant, separate focus such as the pharynx, nose, conjunctiva, skin wounds, or even septicemia. Exfoliation causes the skin to separate at the granular layer, resulting in a superficial exfoliation.

The illness starts with fever, malaise, irritability, and skin tenderness. There is a diffuse macular erythroderma of the face, neck, axillae, and groin with rapid extension. The palms, soles, and mucous membranes are spared. Within 1 to 3 days there is wrinkling of the skin or separation in response to gentle stroking, a positive Nikolsky's sign. Large, flaccid, thin-walled bullae appear which rupture spontaneously. The epidermis separates in large sheets leaving moist, glistening denuded areas, which quickly dry and undergo a flaky desquamation. Healing occurs without scarring unless secondary infection occurs.

The diagnosis of SSSS can usually be made clinically. Cultures are not necessary. SSSS can be distinguished from toxic epidermal necrolysis (TEN) by biopsy of exfoliated skin. In SSSS the cleavage plane is at the granular layer, while in TEN the skin separates at the dermal-epidermal junction or within the dermis.

Therapy for SSSS includes parenteral antistaphylococcal antibiotics, fluid resuscitation, temperature regulation, and wound care. Topical antibiotics are of no benefit, and steroids should not be used. Staphylococci should be eliminated from the focus of infection, ending toxin production. Prognosis for complete recovery is good.

### RICKETTSIAL

### Rocky Mountain Spotted Fever

Rocky Mountain spotted fever (RMSF) is an infectious disease caused by *Rickettsia rickettsii* which is transmitted by ticks. The prominent clinical manifestations of RMSF can be directly related to the primary pathologic lesion in the endothelial cells lining small blood vessels where the rickettsia multiply. Rash, headache, mental confusion, terminal heart failure, and shock are manifestations of the generalized vasculitis.

The incubation period is from 2 to 12 days with either a sudden or gradual onset of symptoms. Peak severity usually occurs within 1 to 2 weeks. Headache, fever, toxicity, rash, and myalgia are the major clinical features. The rash (Fig. 117-2), a pathognomonic feature of

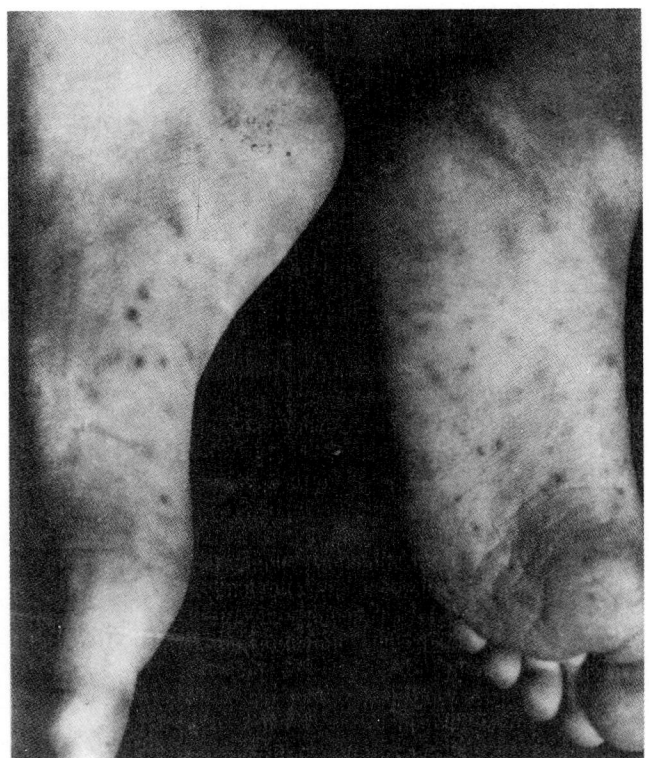

**Fig. 117-2.** Rocky Mountain spotted fever. (*From* Burnett JW, Crutcher WA: Viral and rickettsial infections, in Moschella SL, Hurley HJ (eds), *Dermatology,* Philadelphia, Saunders, 1985, vol 1, chap 12, pp. 673–738, with permission.)

the disease, usually appears on the second or third day. The initial lesions first appear on the wrist and ankles spreading rapidly to the extremities and trunk. These lesions also are found on the palms and soles of the patient. Initially, lesions are small, erythematous macules which blanch on pressure. They rapidly become maculopapular and petechial.

Laboratory diagnostic confirmation is difficult during the early phase of the disease, frequently mandating treatment based on clinical criteria. Serologic tests are used to confirm the diagnosis of RMSF. Some laboratory data may be helpful in establishing the presumptive diagnosis early, such as leukopenia and thrombocytopenia.

Specific therapy consists of tetracycline or chloramphenicol. In seriously ill children 100 mg/kg per 24 h of chloramphenicol up to 3 g total dose is advised. As improvement is noted, therapy can be changed to 50 mg/kg per 24 h in four divided doses orally. Treatment can be terminated 2 or 3 days after fever returns to normal for 24 h. The mortality of RMSF in the United States has held steady for a decade at 3 to 6 percent of identified cases despite treatment.

## VIRUSES

### Enteroviruses

Enteroviruses are an exceedingly common cause of illness and exanthem in young children. Enteroviruses are small, single-stranded RNA viruses belonging to the picornavirus group and consist of polioviruses and nonpolioviruses (coxsackievirus and echovirus). There are many types of coxsackieviruses and echoviruses that have been associated with illnesses. They usually occur in epidemics and are most prevalent in the summer and early fall. Transmission usually occurs by fecal-oral route and possibly by the respiratory route.

The clinical manifestations of infection with coxsackieviruses and echoviruses are extensive. The spectrum of disease includes nonspecific febrile illness, upper respiratory infection, parotitis, croup, bronchitis, pneumonia, bronchiolitis, vomiting, diarrhea, abdominal pain, hepatitis, pancreatitis, conjunctivitis, pericarditis, myocarditis, orchitis, nephritis, arthritis, meningitis, and encephalitis.

Similarly, the associated skin manifestations include an array of exanthems. Diffuse macular eruptions, morbilliform erythema, vesicular lesions, petechial and purpural eruptions, rubelliform rash, roseola-like rash, and scarlatiniform eruptions have been reported.

Strict clinical-virologic associations have been difficult to demonstrate. A single clinical syndrome can be associated with many types of coxsackieviruses and echoviruses. On the other hand, some types of coxsackieviruses and echoviruses have been associated with multiple illnesses and exanthems.

Hand, foot, and mouth disease is an acute infectious illness, caused by enteroviruses, that primarily affects children. Initial manifestations include fever, anorexia, malaise, and sore mouth. Oral lesions appear 1 to 2 days later and cutaneous lesions shortly thereafter. The oral lesions begin as vesicles on an erythematous base which ulcerate. The vesicles are usually 4 to 8 mm in size, and are very painful. They are located on the buccal mucosa, tongue, soft palate, and gingiva. The exanthem starts as red papules which change to gray vesicles about 3 to 7 mm in size. They are found on the palms and soles but may occur on the dorsum of the feet and hands and on the buttocks, as well. They may be oval, linear, or crescentic and may run parallel to skin lines. They heal in 7 to 10 days.

Herpangina is a febrile disease of children associated with many types of coxsackieviruses and echoviruses. The onset is acute with fever to 40°C, headache, sore throat, dysphagia, anorexia, and, occasionally, stiff neck. In the pharynx, there are one or more yellowish-white 2-mm vesicles with hyperemic borders. They are located in the posterior pharynx on the tonsils, uvula, soft palate, and anterior faucial pillars. The vesicles will usually ulcerate, leaving a shallow, gray-yellow crater 2 to 4 mm in size. The lesions persist for 5 to 10 days.

Boston exanthem is caused by echovirus 16. It is an acute illness with fever, anorexia, pharyngitis, and lymphadenopathy. An enanthem similar to herpangina may be present. The exanthem begins as small, discrete, pink macules that develop into papules. It appears on the face and chest, spreads centrifugally, and may involve the palms and soles. As in roseola, the rash may appear with defervescence of the fever.

Infection due to echovirus 9 is prevalent and produces a typical enteroviral illness. Clinical manifestations include fever, headache, nausea, vomiting, abdominal pain, cough, coryza, pharyngitis, and nuchal rigidity. The exanthem is rubelliform, a maculopapular rash beginning on the face and neck or extending to the trunk and feet and sometimes the palms and soles. Occasionally, there are lesions on the buccal mucosa and soft palate that resemble Koplik's spots. Petechiae may occur. The appearance of this rash and the presence of nuchal rigidity makes this illness occasionally mimic meningococcemia. The exanthem persists for about 5 days.

Infection with coxsackievirus A9 is a common cause of exanthem. It is an acute febrile illness with a discrete erythematous maculopapular rash that begins on the face and neck and extends to the trunk and extremities. Aseptic meningitis may occur. The rash may also be vesicular or urticarial.

The clinical differentiation of enteroviral disease is difficult. Since there is no specific therapy for enteroviral infection, it is more important to consider bacterial diseases in the differential diagnosis in order to exclude treatable causes of sepsis, meningitis, myocarditis, and pneumonia. Symptomatic therapy for enteroviral infections includes adequate hydration, antipyretics, and viscous lidocaine gel for painful oral lesions.

## Erythema Infectiosum

Erythema infectiosum (fifth disease) is an acute, febrile illness with a unique exanthem. Outbreaks of erythema infectiosum occur primarily in the spring. During epidemics, the attack rate is highest in children 5 to 15 years of age, but all age groups can be affected. The illness is caused by infection with human parvovirus, a single-stranded DNA virus.

The abrupt appearance of the rash is frequently the first manifestation of erythema infectiosum. It begins with a characteristic fiery red rash on the cheeks. The rash is a diffuse erythema of closely grouped tiny papules on an erythematous base. The edges are slightly raised. The erythema is most intense below the eyes and extends over the cheeks in a pattern reminiscent of butterfly wings; it is sometimes referred to as a *slapped-cheek appearance.* There is circumoral pallor as well as sparing of the eyelids and chin. The facial rash fades after 4 to 5 days. Approximately 1 to 2 days after the appearance of the facial rash, a nonpruritic macular erythema or erythematous maculopapular rash occurs on the trunk and limbs. It is at first localized to the deltoid areas, trunk, and forearms but usually extends to involve a large area. This stage of the exanthem may last 1 week. A distinctive aspect of the rash is that it fades with central clearing, giving a reticulated or lacy appearance. The palms and soles are rarely affected.

The exanthem may recur in the ensuing 3 weeks, sometimes briefly. The intensity of the recurrent exanthem varies and may be related to exposure to environmental factors such as sunlight, hot baths, and, perhaps, physical exertion or emotional upset. Associated symptoms frequently occur and may include fever, malaise, headache, sore throat, cough, coryza, nausea, vomiting, diarrhea, and myalgia. Arthralgias and arthritis can occur, but usually only in adults. These symptoms may occur before or after the onset of the rash.

There is no specific treatment for human parvovirus infection. Symptomatic therapy is all that is required. Recovery is usually complete.

## Measles

Prior to a nationwide immunization program in 1965 measles was an expected disease of childhood. It is a highly contagious, endemic myxovirus infection. It is a winter-spring disease in temperate climates, but it occurs throughout the world.

After exposure, the incubation period for the disease is about 10 days. The prodromal period lasts approximately 3 days and is characterized by upper respiratory symptoms. The onset of clinical measles is characterized by general malaise, systemic toxicity, fever, coryza, conjunctivitis, photophobia, and cough.

The exanthem develops about the fourteenth day following exposure. The rash first appears behind the ears and at the hairline of the forehead. It spreads in a centrifugal pattern from the head to the feet. It is initially erythematous and maculopapular but rapidly progresses to confluence, especially on the face. Initially the rash is red and blanches on pressure. As it fades, it takes on a copper-to-brownish hue. With healing there may be some fine desquamation. The rash generally lasts 7 days.

Koplik's spots are an associated pathognomonic enanthem. The lesions are white, 1-mm discrete spots which first appear on the buccal mucosa opposite the lower molars and then spread to involve the entire buccal mucosa. The treatment of measles is supportive.

## Infectious Mononucleosis

The diagnosis of infectious mononucleosis can be entertained in those children, adolescents and young adults who present with fever, sore throat, malaise, and fatigue accompanied by tonsillopharyngitis and lymphadenopathy.

There is strong evidence for Epstein-Barr virus (EBV) as the etiologic agent of the "mononucleosis syndrome." The age of initial (primary) infection varies and appears to depend upon socioeconomic status. The mononucleosis symptom complex is associated with the primary infection. A 2- to 5-day prodromal period of malaise and fatigue with or without fever may precede the full onset of the syndrome. The adenopathy is usually confined to the anterior and posterior cervical chain but may be generalized. There is a 5 percent incidence of a generalized erythematous maculopapular rash associated with an enanthem consisting of petechiae on the soft palate. The incidence of the rash increases to almost 100 percent in those patients taking ampicillin or its congeners. The treatment for infectious mononucleosis is supportive.

## Rubella

Rubella (German measles) is a common childhood disease with its highest incidence during the spring. The incubation period is 12 to 25 days following exposure with a 1- to 5-day prodrome of fever, malaise, headache, and sore throat.

The exanthem varies and is sometimes difficult to identify. It may present as a short-lived blush, or it may have the more common 2- to 3-day course. The exanthem begins as irregular pink macules and papules on the face spreading to the neck, trunk, and arms in a centrifugal distribution. It coalesces on the face as the eruption reaches the lower extremities and then clears in the same fashion. An enanthem of pinpoint petechiae involving the soft palate (Forschheimer's spots) may accompany the rash but is nonspecific.

Lymphadenopathy is a clinical manifestation of rubella, with the enlargement characteristically in the suboccipital and posterior auricular nodes. The clinical diagnosis of the individual case is often difficult, but the epidemic nature of the illness, along with the seasonal variation and high expression rate of the exanthem, help in establishing the diagnosis. A history of inadequate immunizations may assist in the diagnosis. There is no specific therapy.

## Varicella

Varicella, or chickenpox, is a result of infection with varicella-zoster virus, a herpes virus. In normal children it is characterized by a pruritic generalized vesicular exanthem with mild systemic manifestations. Cases generally occur in late winter and early spring. It is highly contagious in the prodromal and vesicular stage. Varicella most frequently occurs in children less than 10 years old, but it may occur at any age.

The exanthem starts on the trunk or scalp and first appears as faint, red macules. Within 24 h, the rash acquires the typical vesicular appearance of varicella. The rash consists of teardrop vesicles on an erythematous base, which then dry and crust over (see Fig. 117-3). Successive fresh crops may appear for a few days. The extent of the rash may be minimal but usually will spread centrifugally and become widespread. Palms and soles are spared. Vesicles may occur on mucous membranes and proceed to rupture and form shallow ulcers. Low-grade fever, malaise, and headache are frequently present but are usually mild. The diagnosis of varicella is usually made clinically on the basis of its distinctive rash. A Tzanck smear of the vesicle contents will demonstrate varicella giant cells with inclusion bodies.

Complications of varicella can occur, including encephalitis, pneumonia, nephritis, and infection of the vesicles with staphylococci or streptococci. Neonates born to mothers with perinatal varicella infection may develop serious illness.

Uncomplicated varicella requires no specific therapy. Acetaminophen may be used as needed, but aspirin should be avoided as it may predispose to the development of Reye's syndrome. Oral antihistamines may be useful to reduce itching. Most importantly, lesions should be cleansed regularly to prevent secondary infection. In the absence of central nervous sytem complications, the prognosis is excellent. Older children can be treated with acyclovir to lessen disease

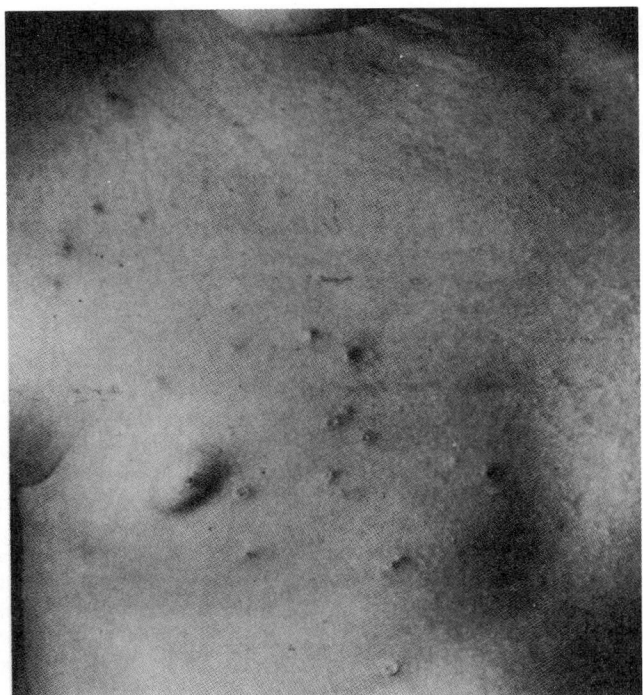

**Fig. 117-3.** Varicella. (*From* Burnett JW, Crutcher WA: Viral and rickettsial infections, in Moschella SL, Hurley HJ: *Dermatology*, Philadelphia, Saunders, 1985, vol 1, chap 12, pp. 673–738, with permission.)

severity. While limited data are available on pediatric use, no unusual toxicity or problems have been noted. The dose is 80 mg/kg/day in 4 divided doses up to 800 mg/ dose.

Immunocompromised patients with varicella require aggressive treatment with antiviral drugs such as acyclovir. Administration of varicella-zoster immune globulin (VZIG) should be considered for immunocompromised patients exposed to individuals with varicella.

### Roseola Infantum

Roseola infantum, or exanthem subitum, is a common acute febrile illness of childhood. There appears to be no seasonal preponderance to its occurrence. The etiologic agent has been identified as the human herpesvirus 6 infection.

Roseola is characterized by a febrile period of 3 to 5 days, defervescence, and the appearance of a rash for 1 to 2 days. Primarily, young children are affected, with most patients being between 6 months and 3 years. The illness begins abruptly with high fever, sometimes as high as 40.6°C. The child is usually alert and active but may be irritable, especially with very high fever. Associated symptoms are usually mild and may include cough, coryza, anorexia, and abdominal discomfort. Lymphadenopathy may be present. Febrile convulsions may occur. The fever persists for 3 to 5 days, and most often returns to normal by crisis. The child rapidly becomes well.

The exanthem in roseola usually coincides with defervescence of the fever, but it may follow a short afebrile interlude. The rash is an erythematous macular or maculopapular eruption that consists of discrete, rose or pale-pink lesions 2 to 5 mm in size. It is most prominent on the neck, trunk, and buttocks, but the face and proximal extremities may also be involved. The lesions blanch with pressure. There is no mucous membrane involvement. The rash lasts 1 to 2 days but may fade rapidly, usually without desquamation.

There is no specific treatment for roseola. Acetaminophen is useful for fever control and convulsions should be treated vigorously. Recovery is usually complete.

## ETIOLOGY UNCLEAR

### Erythema Nodosum

Erythema nodosum is an inflammatory exanthem of unknown etiology. It is probably an inflammatory reaction to a stimulus. In the past, erythema nodosum was associated with streptococcal infections, tuberculosis, sarcoid, fungal infections, *Yersinia* infections, vasculitis, inflammatory bowel disease, and leukemia. Now it is more commonly associated with drugs, especially oral contraceptives. Any age can be affected. Constitutional symptoms may be present at the onset, including fever, malaise, myalgias, and arthralgias.

Erythema nodosum presents a distinctive clinical appearance. Bilateral, very tender nodules develop symmetrically. They usually occur on the shins but can occur on the arms, thighs, calves, and buttocks. The nodules are 1 to 5 cm in diameter, and individual lesions may coalesce to form sizable areas of induration. The skin over the nodules is red, smooth, and shiny. No ulceration occurs. After a week or two, the color of the lesions changes from red to blue and may achieve a dull, purple, bruised appearance. The eruption lasts several weeks.

The diagnosis of erythema nodosum is usually readily made on clinical grounds. A thorough history and physical, and perhaps laboratory evaluation, must be performed to exclude an underlying cause. There is no known therapy to alter the course of the disease. Nonsteroidal anti-inflammatory drugs may provide relief from the sometimes significant pain associated with these lesions.

### Kawasaki Disease (Mucocutaneous Lymph Node Syndrome)

Kawasaki disease, or mucocutaneous lymph node syndrome (MLNS), is a disease of unclear etiology found predominantly in children under 9 years of age.

The diagnosis of this disorder is based on a constellation of clinical findings. The patient must exhibit a prolonged fever associated with at least four of the following: (1) conjunctivitis, (2) rash, (3) lymphadenopathy, (4) changes in the oropharynx consisting of injection of the pharynx and lips with prominent papillae of the tongue (strawberry tongue), and (5) extremity erythema and edema.

The rash has been described as erythematous, morbilliform, urticarial, scarlatiniform, or erythema multiforme-like. It has a predilection for the perineum. Additional supportive evidence which may help in the presumptive diagnosis are leukocytosis, elevation of acute-phase reactants, elevated liver function tests, arthritis, arthralgia, and irritability.

In the second phase, there is usually a sharp rise in the platelet count, desquamation of the fingers and or toes, and the most serious complication, the development of coronary artery aneurysm. A small percentage (1 to 2 percent) of patients with coronary artery anuerysm develop sudden cardiac failure, resulting in death from myocardial infarction with coronary artery thrombosis.

The differential diagnosis includes drug allergy, toxic epidermal necrolysis, staphylococcal toxin–mediated syndromes, erythema multiforme, and scarlet fever. The etiologic speculations include a hyperimmune response to a variety of infections, a viral syndrome, allergic or toxic response to pollutants, drugs, toxic agents, and a possibility of a rickettsial disease.

Treatment of Kawasaki disease is controversial and includes various antibiotics, salicylates, and steroids. Intravenous gamma globulin is now routinely recommended. Aspirin may be the most promising therapy. Bed rest, supportive therapy, and frequent monitoring are mainstays of treatment.

## Pityriasis Rosea

Pityriasis rosea is a mild inflammatory exanthem of unknown cause. The available evidence suggests a viral etiology. Pityriasis rosea affects all age groups but occurs most commonly in patients 10 to 35 years old. It tends to occur in spring and fall but not in epidemics. Pityriasis rosea is not contagious. A pityriasis rosea–like eruption has been associated with some drugs and viruses. Occasionally there are prodromal symptoms including malaise, headache, sore throat, fatigue, and arthralgia.

The rash of pityriasis rosea evolves over a period of several weeks. It begins with a "herald patch," a solitary, erythematous lesion with a raised edematous border most frequently occurring on the chest or back. It is 2 to 6 cm in diameter. About 1 or 2 weeks later, there is a widespread, symmetrical eruption of pink- or salmon-colored maculopapular lesions. The patches are oval to circinate and are covered with dry epidermis which desquamates to form a collarette of scale at the periphery. The lesions are 0.5 to 1.5 cm in diameter and are at first discrete, but can become confluent. The long axes of the patches frequently run parallel to lines of skin tension, giving rise to the Christmas tree pattern seen on the back. The eruption is generalized and chiefly affects the trunk, although it can occur anywhere. The lesions can be localized. Mucous membranes can be involved with plaques, hemorrhagic punctate spots, or ulcers. Successive crops of skin lesions can occur, and the entire illness can last 3 to 8 weeks. Healing is complete, without sequelae or evidence of organ involvement.

The diagnosis of pityriasis rosea is made by the clinical appearance. It can be confused with viral exanthem, drug eruptions, and seborrheic dermatitis. Potassium hydroxide preparation of skin scrapings will serve to distinguish pityriasis rosea from tinea corporis. A serologic test for syphilis must be done to exclude that diagnosis.

Therapy is directed at alleviating symptoms. No treatment has been shown to shorten the duration of the rash. The rash is sometimes very itchy. Oatmeal baths and oral antihistamines will provide temporary relief. Emollients will help dryness and irritation. Secondary infection must be prevented with thorough cleansing.

## BIBLIOGRAPHY

Anderson MJ, Lewis E, Kidd IM, et al: An outbreak of erythema infectiosum associated with human parvovirus infection. *J Hyg,* 93:85093, 1984.

Burnett JW, Crutcher WA: Vial and rickittsial infections, in Moschella SL, Hurley HJ(eds): *Dermatology.* Philadelphia, Saunders, 1985.

Cherry JD: Mycoplasma and ureaplasma infections, in Feigin RD, Cherry JD (eds): *Textbook of Pediatric Infectious Diseases.* Philadelphia, Saunders, 1987.

Corkey RJ et al: Diagnosis and treatment of impetigo. *J Am Acad Dermatol* 17:62, 1987.

Hurwitz S: Kawasaki disease, in Hurwitz S (ed): *Clinical Pediatric Dermatology: A Textbook of Skin Disorders of Childhood and Adolescence.* Philadelphia, Saunders, 1981, pp. 397–401.

Melish ME, et al: The staphylococcal scalded skin syndrome. *N Engl J Med* 282:1114, 1970.

Nihill MR, Feigin RD, Gruber R, Morens D: Kawasaki disease in Feigin RD and Cherry JD (eds): *Pediatric Infectious Disease,* 2d ed. Philadelphia, Saunders, 1987.

Parrono JM: Pityriasis rosea update. *J Am Acad Dermatol* 15:159, 1986.

Urbach AH, McGregor RS, Malatack JJ, et al: Kawasaki disease and perineal rash. *Am J Dis Child* 142:1174, 1988.

Yamanishi K, Okuno T, Shiraki K et al: Identification of human herpesvirus-6 as a casual agent for exanthem subitum. *Lancet* 11:1065, 1988.

# 118
# MUSCULOSKELETAL DISORDERS IN CHILDREN
**Richard A. Christoph**

## PHYSIOLOGY OF MUSCULOSKELETAL SYSTEM IN CHILDREN

The child's musculoskeletal system differs from the adult's in multiple respects, reflecting the child's active growth and development. These differences relate to the patterns of injury and illness manifested by children presenting to the emergency department. In utero, fetal positioning leads to a flexor pattern in the extremities, with external rotation of the hips and internal rotation of the tibiofibular apparatus. The ankle is in dorsiflexion, and the feet are inverted. Upon the newborn's arrival, motor development progresses predictably in a rostral to caudal direction and in a proximal to distal direction. Thus, the infant achieves head and trunk control prior to extremity control. Proficiency in movements of the upper extremity precede lower extremity control.

The joint contractures brought about by fetal positioning and motor development influence the child's gait. The child requires a broad base of support and maintains distinct flexion of hips and knees and dorsiflexion of the ankles, resulting in a high-stepping gait. The arms of the toddler are abducted at the shoulder and flexed at the elbow. The child does not develop reciprocating arm swinging until about 2 years of age.

Simultaneous with development of the central nervous system and the maturation of motor milestones and gait, the child is growing most actively in early childhood. Bone growth occurs through two types of ossification. Growth in circumference occurs at the periosteal surface, as mesenchymal cells differentiate into osteocytes, which lay down new bone in a process known as *intramembranous ossification.* Longitudinal growth is achieved through *endochondral ossification,* consisting of a proliferation and hypertrophy of cartilage cells at a physis. An organized vascular invasion of this cartilage results in delivery of mesenchymal cells to the area, which then differentiate into osteocytes, completing the transformation of cartilage to bone.

It is helpful to think of long bones as consisting of discrete anatomic areas. Long bones may have physes, or areas of growth cartilage, at both ends (e.g., tibia, femur). Other long bones (e.g., the phalanges) have a physis at only one end. The area of the long bone between a physis and the adjacent joint is the epiphysis, whereas the area of bone between a physis and a point for muscle or ligamentous attachment is referred to as an apophysis. The metaphysis of a long bone represents the area of widening, or flaring, of the long bone between its midshaft (the diaphysis) and the physis.

The long bones of children are generally less dense and more porous than the long bones of adults. The resulting increased compliance contributes to the tendency of children's long bones to respond to mechanical stress by bowing and buckling, rather than fracturing through and through, as in adult fracture patterns. The periosteum of the diaphysis and the metaphysis is thicker in children and is continuous from the metaphysis to the epiphysis, surrounding and protecting the mechanically weaker physis. This physeal weakness is related to the reduced oxygen tension found in the hypertrophic zone of the physis, a location of frequent fractures within the physis. The physis is sensitive to alterations in the blood supply to this hypertrophic zone as well as to nutritional, hormonal, and mechanical influences.

Growth of the musculoskeletal system, and its response to illness, injury, and nutrition, is also influenced by the growth of muscle and

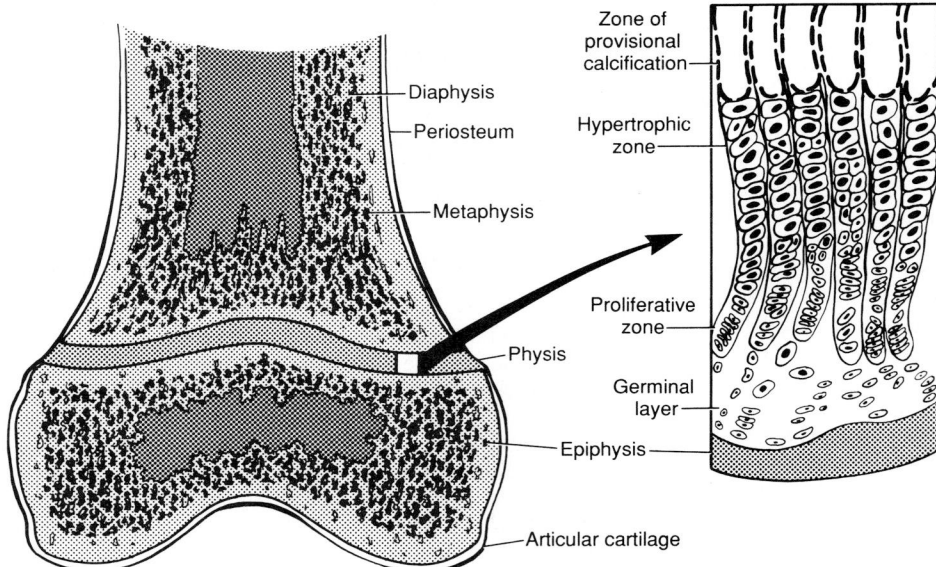

**Fig. 118-1.** Relationship between anatomic regions of a typical long bone and the physis. Detail: cellular zones of physis. (Reproduced with permission from Tolo and Wood, 1994.)

connective tissues. The ligaments of children are stronger and more compliant than in adults, often tolerating mechanical forces at the expense of apophyseal attachments or epiphyseal integrity. While the absolute number of muscle fibers is fixed at birth, the fibers of tendons can increase in number and in size. The growth of muscle through hypertrophy and the growth of tendons through hypertrophy and proliferation depend on the mechanical forces applied to them.

## CHILDHOOD PATTERNS OF INJURY

### Physeal Injuries

The weakest zone, or layer, of the physis is its third layer of cells and matrix (hypertrophic cell zone). It is particularly susceptible to shearing, bending, and tension stresses. It represents the layer of the physis that is most consistently fractured. Consequently, the reserve and proliferative cartilage cells in the first two zones of the injured physis usually remain with the epiphysis. This is relevant in that the predominant circulatory support of the cells in these two reproductive zones of the physis arises through the epiphyseal vasculature and thus is

more likely to be spared in the event of physeal injury (see Fig. 118-1).

It has been demonstrated that compression forces applied to the physis can affect bone growth. This is particularly true when compression forces are applied to the epiphyseal side of the physis. The injury to bone growth caused by compression results from interruption of the epiphyseal circulation to the reproductive cells of the physis.

Although several authors have classified injuries to the physis, the Salter and Harris classification system offers a thorough and practical classification based on the mechanism of injury, the relationship of the fracture line to the germinal (reproductive zones) layer of the physis, and the prognosis for disturbance of bone growth (see Fig. 118-2).

### Type I Physeal Fracture

In the type I physeal fracture (representing 6 percent of physeal injuries), the epiphysis separates from the metaphysis. The cleavage is through the hypertrophic cell zone of the physis. The reproductive cells of the physis remain with the epiphysis. There are no associated fragments of bones as the thick periosteal attachments surrounding

**Fig. 118-2.** Salter-Harris classification of physeal injuries. (Reproduced with permission from Tolo and Wood, 1994.)

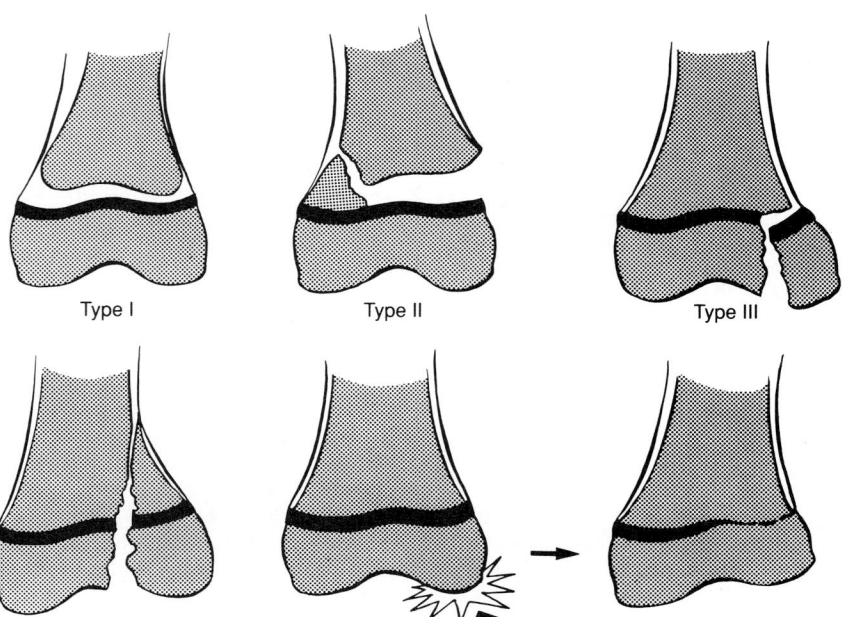

the physis remain intact. The epiphysis may, however, somewhat displace from the metaphysis. Bone growth is not usually disturbed (see Fig. 118-2).

Diagnosis is suspected clinically in a child with point tenderness over a physis. Radiographically, the only abnormality may be an associated joint effusion. Any epiphyseal displacement will usually be apparent on one or more views. In the absence of epiphyseal displacement, the diagnosis is a clinical one, supported by the appearance of the typical joint effusion.

Treatment consists of immobilization of the suspected fracture using an appropriate splint, the application of cold compresses for 48 h, and elevation. Referral to an orthopaedic surgeon is probably warranted in order to render aftercare and to assure monitoring for bone growth disturbances. Analgesia may be necessary, despite immobilization, for 24 to 72 h, after which time the child usually remains quite comfortable in the immobilization device.

## Type II Physeal Fracture

The type II physeal fracture is the most common, representing 75 percent of physeal injuries. The line of fracture extends a variable distance along the hypertrophic cell zone of the physis and then out through a piece of metaphyseal bone. The periosteum on the concave side (overlying the metaphyseal fragment) remains intact, whereas the periosteum on the convex (opposite) side of the fracture is torn away from the diaphysis while remaining adherent to the epiphysis (see Fig. 118-2). Growth is preserved since the reproduction layers of the physis maintain their position with the epiphysis and the epiphyseal circulation. Diagnosis is made radiographically by noting the triangular shaped fragment of metaphysis (Holland's sign), unassociated with discernible injury to the epiphysis.

Reduction of the fracture should be gentle and is usually easily achieved. Analgesia, with or without sedation, should be offered to the child prior to any reduction maneuvers. When using sedation and analgesics, precautions should be taken as to patient selection, premedication assessments, monitoring, and postmedication observation consistent with institutional guidelines. Overreduction of the type II fracture is usually prevented by the periosteal hinge remaining on the concave side of the fracture.

Immobilization, cold compresses, and elevation are principles of management, just as in the case of type I fractures. Referral to an orthopaedic surgeon for aftercare and observation is important, as is the provision of adequate analgesia in the initial days following the fracture.

## Type III Physeal Fracture

The hallmark of this injury is an intraarticular fracture of the epiphysis extending to the hypertrophic cell zone of the physis, with the cleavage plane continuing along the physis to the periphery (see Fig. 118-2). The injury, usually involving the proximal or distal tibia epiphysis, is caused by severe intraarticular shearing forces. The prognosis for subsequent bone growth relates to the preservation of circulation to the epiphyseal bone fragment and is usually favorable. The type III physeal fracture represents 8 percent of physeal injuries.

Diagnosis is a radiographic one and is based on the appearance of an epiphyseal fragment, unassociated with an apparent metaphyseal fracture. There may or may not be an associated periosteal injury.

Reduction of the unstable epiphyseal fragment with careful restoration of the alignment of the articular surface is critically important. Open surgical techniques are frequently necessary in order to assure the necessary anatomic reduction of the articular surface, especially with severely displaced fractures. This fracture warrants consultation with an orthopaedic surgeon in the emergency department.

Decisions regarding admission or operative open reduction will be made in consultation with an orthopaedic surgeon experienced in the management of physeal injuries. If closed reduction techniques are successfully employed by the orthopaedic consultant, aftercare instructions are similar to those offered to patients suffering from type II physeal injuries.

## Type IV Physeal Fracture

The fracture line originates at the articular surface and extends through the epiphysis, the entire thickness of the physis, and continues through the metaphysis (see Fig. 118-2). It is an injury pattern most often involving the distal humerus and represents 8 percent of physeal injuries. Future bone growth is at risk. Perfect anatomic reduction of the articular surface and of the physis is required to minimize the potential for premature bone growth arrest.

The diagnosis is made upon identification of epiphyseal and metaphyseal fragments radiographically. The fragments may or may not be variably displaced. Radiographic interpretation of fractures involving the distal humerus and elbow can be challenging in light of the dynamic nature of the ossification centers of the region.

Open surgical reduction should be performed early by an experienced orthopaedic surgeon. Internal fixation of the fragments is accomplished by using fine, smooth Kirschner wires traversing the physeal growth plate perpendicularly.

## Type V Physeal Fracture

This fortunately rare injury pattern (1 percent of physeal injuries) usually involves the knee or ankle. It is the result of severe abduction or adduction to the joint, which transmits profound compressive forces to a local segment of the physis, crushing the reproductive chondrocytes of the reserve zone and proliferative zone. Minimal or no displacement of the epiphysis occurs (see Fig. 118-2).

The diagnosis of type V physeal injuries may be very difficult initially. Often, the seriousness of the injury is underappreciated. An initial diagnosis of sprain or possible type I physeal fracture may prove incorrect in view of subsequent development of premature growth arrest. Radiographs may appear normal or may demonstrate focal narrowing of the physeal plate. An associated joint effusion is the norm, although its presence is nonspecific.

Treatment of type V physeal injuries consists of cast support of the knee or ankle, non-weight-bearing for at least 3 weeks, and close orthopaedic outpatient follow-up in anticipation of the nearly inevitable focal bone growth arrest.

## Torus Fractures

The porosity and compliance of the metaphyses of children's long bones, coupled with the relative thickness of the periosteum in this area, confer unique fracture characteristics. Compressive forces often result in a bulging or buckling of the periosteum rather than a more complete fracture line. Cortical, or *torus,* fractures are so named to describe a prominence or bulging of the bony cortex, usually involving the metaphysis.

Diagnosis is based on point tenderness over the site of the torus fracture. While a simple torus fracture will not produce a visible deformity to the shape of the extremity, soft tissue swelling routinely overlies the bone injury. In children who are not morbidly obese, the torus fracture is frequently palpable as a ridge over the metaphyseal area of the long bone.

Radiographically, the manifestation of a torus fracture may be somewhat subtle. Interpretation of radiographs is aided by following the contour of the metaphyseal flare, observing any asymmetry, bulging, or deviation of the cortical margin. With magnification, deviations in the trabecular pattern of the cortical markings can be seen to be associated with the bulging prominence of the cortical margin.

Since torus fractures are not typically associated with severe angulation, displacement, or rotational abnormalities, most can be competently managed by the emergency physician. Reduction techniques are rarely, if ever, necessary. The extremity is splinted in a position of function for 3 to 4 weeks. Aftercare can be arranged through the child's primary care physician or an orthopaedic consultant, usually in 2 weeks. Analgesia requirements in the immediate days after the injury are usually minimal following the application of the splint.

## Greenstick Fractures

Stresses and forces can be applied to the porous, compliant bones of children in such a way as to create an incomplete cortical fracture. A *greenstick* fracture is characterized by cortical disruption and periosteal tearing on the convex side of the bone, with an intact periosteum on the concave side of the fracture. Greenstick fractures are more stable and somewhat less painful than complete fractures, since the area of intact periosteum protects the child from bony crepitance.

The need for reduction is related to the degree of angulation of the fracture, the age of the child, and the anatomic location of the injury. Orthopaedic consultation may be helpful in the decision analysis regarding possible reduction and outpatient management.

## Plastic Deformities

Plastic deformities (sometimes known as bowing or bending fractures) are almost exclusively limited to the forearm and lower leg long bones. Usually this pattern of injury is noted in combination with a completed fracture of the other bone of the forearm or lower leg. The cortex of the diaphysis of the long bone is deformed, with preservation of the periosteum all along the diaphysis. They result from the compliance and porosity of the child's bones, with the associated tendency to deform (bend) rather than fracture in the traditional sense.

Diagnosis is made radiographically. Proper interpretation of the radiographs requires an awareness of the normal shape of the long bones involved, since fracture lines and disruptions in the periosteum will be absent.

Prompt orthopaedic consultation is important.

## FRACTURES ASSOCIATED WITH CHILD ABUSE

It is important to remember that all of the skeletal injuries associated with accidental trauma can also be inflicted as a result of nonaccidental injury (child battering, shaken baby syndrome, child abuse). However, certain injury patterns are encountered consistently as a result of child maltreatment, particularly multiple fractures in various stages of healing. An understanding of the different mechanisms of inflicted injury will facilitate better awareness of the patterns of injury suggesting abuse. Correlation of the child's age, motor capabilities, and the alleged mechanism of injury with the injury pattern being evaluated is fundamental to the evaluation of childhood skeletal injuries, as is the identification of coexisting cutaneous signs suggestive of abuse (suspicious bruises, burns, etc.).

**Direct Blows.** These may result in transverse, oblique, longitudinal, or greenstick/torus fractures. All of these fractures are commonly associated with accidental mechanisms and are nonspecific for child abuse. Correlation with the child's age or motor development, however, may arouse suspicions. A transverse or oblique fracture of the humerus of a 2-month-old infant is quite a different situation than an isolated similar fracture in an 8-year-old.

**Twisting Injuries.** These create spiral fractures in long bones, highly specific for child abuse in children who are not yet ambulatory. Spiral fractures in ambulatory children lose their specificity for child abuse but remain a potential manifestation of abuse and warrant careful consideration. Whereas toddlers (1 to 3 years of age) commonly suffer spiral fractures of the lower one-third of the tibia accidentally as the result of a trivial fall or by twisting themselves on a planted foot (the so-called toddler's fracture), spiral fractures of the tibia may occur with child abuse. Spiral fractures of the femur may

be accidental in toddlers but can also be seen in child abuse in this age group. Spiral femur fractures in newborns and preambulatory infants are highly suggestive of nonaccidental trauma. Correlation with the alleged mechanism of injury and a discrete but careful inspection for other evidence of abuse will prove helpful, along with a review of past injuries experienced by the child or the child's siblings.

The injury pattern correlating most closely with inflicted injury is that of metaphyseal-epiphyseal fractures. More specifically, chip fractures of the metaphyses or epiphyses, particularly in different stages of healing, are seen as the result of twisting or jiggling forces. Callus formation becomes striking during the healing process, along with remarkable new bone deposits along the periosteum. Subperiosteal hemorrhage may create an elevation of the periosteum away from the underlying bony cortex. Fragmentation of the clavicle and acromion and separation of the costochondral junctions of the ribs are especially suggestive of abuse.

**Distraction Injuries.** Distraction injuries to the long bones create hemorrhagic separation of the distal metaphyses, creating a lucency parallel and proximal to the physis. The result is a bucket-handle fracture.

**Shaking Injuries.** These create similar fractures to twisting mechanisms. In addition, retinal hemorrhages, intracranial injuries, and intraabdominal injuries may result. Spinal compression fractures, vertebral subluxations and dislocations, and anterior notching of vertebral bodies can be seen.

**Squeezing Injuries.** These create encirclement bruises and rib fractures, highly suggestive of abuse. Particular attention should be given to multiple rib fractures and rib fractures in varying stages of healing, the presence of which is classically associated with the battered child syndrome. Appreciation of this phenomenon is related to an understanding of normal bone healing and an ability to date the approximate age of any bone injuries identified in the child's workup. By looking for associated soft tissue findings, the appearance of a distinct fracture line, callus formation and calcification, and ossification of newly laid periosteal bone, the physician will be in a better position to detect discrepancies between the alleged history of the injury(s) and the radiographic evidence of injury.

## CLAVICLE FRACTURE

The clavicle, extending from the scapular acromion process to the manubrium sterni, serves as the sole skeletal connection between the upper extremity and the trunk and absorbs all medial forces imposed upon the upper arm. The clavicle consists of a double curve in the horizontal plane. The medial two-thirds convexes forward, while the lateral one-third concaves forward. The junction between the two curves represents its structurally weakest area and most frequently fractured site. The clavicle is the most commonly fractured bone in children.

Clavicle fractures may occur in the newborn as a result of shoulder compression during a difficult delivery. In the older infant, toddler, or child, the usual mechanism of fracture is a fall onto an outstretched hand or elbow or onto the side of a shoulder. Often, in younger children, the fracture is of the incomplete, or greenstick, type. A direct blow to the clavicle may also cause a fracture.

Diagnosis of clavicular fracture is facilitated by its subcutaneous location and the ease of its palpation on examination. Newborns with clavicle fractures may not be symptomatic. When they are symptomatic, it may come in the form of "pseudoparalysis," or nonuse of the ipsilateral upper extremity. Alternatively, parents or health care providers may notice the bone callus at 2 to 3 weeks of age, indicative of a fracture previously unappreciated.

Older infants and children with clavicular fractures have pain on attempted range of motion of the neck or upper extremity. Soft tissue swelling, point tenderness, and bone crepitance are indicative of the fracture site. In view of the close proximity of the clavicle with the subclavian vessels and lung, careful assessment of the circulation to the ipsilateral upper extremity and chest auscultation are important. Anteroposterior radiographs of the clavicle and shoulder are principally useful in excluding other associated skeletal injuries, particularly those involving the proximal humerus and scapular prominences. Dislocations of the sternoclavicular joint, particularly posterior dislocations of the proximal clavicle, are optimally visualized by lordotic views.

Care of the child with a clavicle fracture is principally directed toward comfort and analgesia for the child. The child's future bone growth and the modeling potential confer great healing and restorative capability to the fractured clavicle. Even displaced fractures nearly always heal well, whether or not strict anatomic reduction is accomplished in the emergency department.

"Figure-of-eight" shoulder abduction restraints are available in various sizes and can be offered to children outside infancy. Application should assure a snug, symmetrical fit without excessive tightness or pinching. As is the case with the application of any orthopaedic appliance, subsequent assessment of the child's neurovascular status in the upper extremities is mandatory. Some children, however, complain of greater discomfort with the figure-of-eight restraint than without. In such instances, the use of an upper extremity sling-and-swathe or shoulder immobilizer will offer adequate protection from the discomfort associated with shoulder and upper extremity movements.

Children with either type of immobilizing or restraint device are encouraged to wear the restraint day and night for 2 weeks, followed by daytime use for another 2 to 3 weeks. Oral analgesia sufficient to assure the child's comfort is of paramount importance. Follow-up care can be arranged through the child's primary care physician or an orthopaedic surgeon.

## SUPRACONDYLAR FRACTURES

The most common elbow fracture in childhood is the supracondylar fracture of the distal humeral metaphysis. It is an important injury pattern, not only by virtue of its frequency but also because of its associated potential neurovascular complications. Hyperextension forces, during a fall against an outstretched arm, displace the distal fragment posteriorly and proximally.

The close proximity of the brachial artery to the supracondylar fracture predisposes the artery to contusion, laceration, or entrapment by fractured fragments. Subsequent arterial spasm or compression by splints, casts, or other dressings may further embarrass the arterial blood supply to the muscles of the forearm and to the hand. A resultant forearm compartment syndrome may ensue, with the development within hours of permanent injury and disability to the function of the involved forearm and hand. This is called *Volkmann's ischemic contracture* and is presaged by (1) pain referred to the proximal forearm upon passive extension of the fingers, (2) "stocking-glove" anesthesia of the ischemic hand, and (3) rock-hard forearm swelling. Skin perfusion is usually normal despite the severe ischemic insult to the entire forearm and hand, and pulses may remain palpable at the wrist despite serious vascular compromise. The clinical suspicion of a *potential* ischemic compartment syndrome involving the forearm necessitates an immediate consultation by an orthopaedic surgeon who is prepared to offer a complete and radical forearm decompression if reduction of the fracture does not satisfactorily restore vascular integrity.

The diagnosis of a supracondylar fracture of the distal humerus is suspected when tenderness is elicited upon palpation of the distal humerus and the child complains of pain on passive flexion of the elbow. The child usually prefers to maintain the forearm in pronation. The degree of soft tissue swelling and ecchymosis of the elbow ranges from severe to subtle.

As mentioned above, neurovascular assessment of the hand and forearm is the most critical step in the evaluation of elbow injuries in children. In addition to assessments of vascular integrity, injuries to the ulnar, median, or radial nerves should be noted. Such associated injuries are common, occurring in 5 to 10 percent of children with supracondylar fractures.

Differential diagnostic considerations include fractures to the humeral condyles, intercondylar fractures, fractures of the radial head and the olecranon of the ulna, and subluxation of the radial head ("nursemaid's elbow"). The physical examination of all these conditions may be undistinguishing except for that of nursemaid's elbow.

Definitive diagnosis of supracondylar fractures rests with radiography, which usually delineates the injury. Occasionally the appearance of the fracture line is subtle. Observations of a loss of the usual anterior angulation of the capitellum or of a posterior fat pad sign, indicative of an intraarticular elbow effusion (usually of blood), may confer indirect evidence of a supracondylar fracture if the fracture line itself is inapparent. An anterior humeral line, an imaginary line drawn along the anterior margin of the distal humeral diaphysis, normally bisects the posterior two-thirds of the capitellum in the lateral view of the elbow. In subtle supracondylar fractures with loss of the normal anterior angulation of the capitellum, the anterior humeral line may bisect the anterior portion of the capitellum. In association with a posterior fat pad sign, such a loss of the normal anatomic relationships may well indicate a supracondylar fracture.

Management of a child's supracondylar fracture is begun immediately upon arrival in the department. Splinting of the affected elbow in extension is recommended in order to safeguard against development of secondary injury to the vessels, nerves, and soft tissues surrounding the fracture. Frequent reassessments of neurovascular status of the forearm and hand are important. Consultation with an orthopaedic surgeon is necessary in all cases of supracondylar fracture. In cases of neurovascular compromise, immediate fracture reduction is mandatory. Careful monitoring of neurovascular status following fracture reduction and maintenance of the elbow in extension are in order. If an ischemic volar forearm compartment is still suspected over the succeeding 6 h, surgical decompression and/or arterial exploration may be indicated.

In the absence of neurovascular compromise, therapy is influenced largely by the degree of displacement of the distal fragment, associated soft tissue swelling, and the reliability of the follow-up arrangements. Admission is indicated for all children whose supracondylar fracture is displaced, who manifest significant soft tissue swelling, or whose parents cannot assure reliable outpatient follow-up. Open reduction is indicated if closed reduction techniques are unsuccessful, especially for oblique fractures. Outpatient management is considered for the child whose fracture is nondisplaced and has minimal swelling. The orthopaedic surgeon should reexamine these children within 24 h of injury.

Lateral and medial condylar fractures, intercondylar fractures, and transcondylar fractures carry their own associated risks of neurovascular compromise. Children with these fractures typically present with moderate to severe soft tissue swelling and tenderness of the elbow, which is maintained in a moderate degree of flexion. Circulatory integrity of the forearm and hand should be assessed immediately. Peripheral nerve function, particularly ulnar nerve function, is at risk.

Immediate orthopaedic consultation is indicated as these fractures often require open reduction and carry with them risks of long-term sequelae. Neurovascular insults usually resolve nicely with appropriate management of the fracture; growth arrest is rare.

## RADIAL HEAD SUBLUXATION

This extremely common injury (nursemaid's elbow), with a peak incidence between 1 and 4 years of age, has been recognized for centuries. While a history of linear traction upon a hand or wrist is frequently elicited, it is not uncommon to receive a history of an incidental fall in which the arm, elbow, and forearm were impacted between the ground and the child's trunk. Occasionally there is no history of trauma at all, and the parents note only nonuse of the affected limb.

The child maintains the arm partially flexed at the elbow and in forearm pronation. Typically, the arm is kept close to the trunk. The child usually is found seated in the parent's lap and appears quite contented and playful but declines to actively move the affected arm.

A slow and pleasant approach to the child's examination demonstrates no tenderness to palpation of the clavicle, shoulder, humerus, elbow, forearm, wrist, or hand. By carefully avoiding movements involving the elbow and forearm, the physician will note painless passive range of motion of the shoulder, hand, and wrist. In contrast, even modest attempts to supinate the forearm or to flex or extend the elbow elicit pain and anguish.

There is seldom clinical doubt if the child's age, mechanism of injury, body positioning, and examination (nonuse as opposed to tenderness to palpation) are consistent with the diagnosis. Radiographs in such a situation are superfluous, since there are no radiographic abnormalities associated with this condition and since the examination effectively excludes other entities. Radiographs should be considered, however, if the child exhibits point tenderness, soft tissue swelling, or ecchymosis of the elbow.

Reduction is usually easily accomplished. The physician's thumb is placed over the child's radial head. The child's hand is grasped by the physician. Beginning with the child's elbow in extension and the forearm in pronation, three simultaneous maneuvers are rapidly accomplished: (1) downward pressure on the child's radial head by the physician's thumb, (2) passive *full* supination of the child's forearm, and (3) passive *full* flexion of the child's elbow. A "click" is often but not always palpated by the physician's thumb as reduction is accomplished. The child cries out for a few seconds but is usually and easily soon distracted. Observation for up to 15 min typically demonstrates a full return to normal function and use, especially if the physician notes the click. If function and use have not normalized within 15 min, a repeated attempt at reduction is recommended. Alternative diagnoses should be considered if the child's arm does not return to normal function and use following a second reduction attempt. Radiographic studies may then be indicated.

For children who recover full unrestricted use after one or two reduction maneuvers, further therapy is unnecessary. A sling may be offered to the child whose function and use have improved but are not complete. The toddler will often discard the sling within minutes or hours, however. Parents should be gently reminded to avoid lifting the child by the hand, wrist, or forearm and should be informed of the increased risk of recurrence until the child reaches 5 to 6 years of age.

## DISORDERS OF THE HIP AND LOWER EXTREMITY

### Slipped Capital Femoral Epiphysis (SCFE)

Associated with obesity and puberty, slipped capital femoral epiphysis is of multifactorial etiology, including physeal cartilage fatigue, genetic predisposition, endocrinologic factors, and trauma. There is a male to female predominance of 8:3, and it is more common in blacks than whites. Peak incidence occurs between 12 and 15 years in males and between 10 and 13 years in females. The child with SCFE may present clinically with either a chronic slip or an acute slip.

With a *chronic SCFE,* the child complains of pain in the groin referred to the anteromedial thigh and knee. The pain is dull, vague, intermittent or continuous, and is exacerbated by physical activity. It may or may not be related to a history of trivial or significant injury. If walking is observed, the lower limb is held in lateral (external) rotation and the gait is antalgic. Typically, the examiner notes that attempts at hip flexion are accompanied by lateral rotation of the thigh. Full flexion is restricted, and the child cannot touch his or her thigh to

the abdominal wall. Limb shortening of 1 to 2 cm may be noted, as well as disuse atrophy of the muscles of the proximal thigh.

*Acute SCFE* may be the result of an acute traumatic event or may represent an acute-on-chronic slip in which sudden, severe pain and inability to bear weight develop in a patient who has been experiencing weeks to months of pain in the hip-thigh-knee region. Examining a patient with a suggested acute slip elicits great pain. Marked external rotation of the thigh is noted, as well as readily apparent limb shortening. Great gentleness is required of the examining physician, and the hip should not be forced into maximum range of motion, which can aggravate the displacement of the fracture. The child is not asked to walk to observe the gait.

The differential diagnosis includes septic arthritis, toxic tenosynovitis, Legg-Calvé-Perthes disease, and other hip fractures. Differentiating SCFE from septic arthritis is usually not difficult, since the child with SCFE is not febrile or toxically ill-appearing and demonstrates no remarkable elevation in peripheral white blood cells (WBC) or erythrocyte sedimentation rate (ESR). Differentiation from the other entities requires radiographs including AP films and bilateral "frogleg" lateral radiographs.

Medial slips of the femoral epiphyses will be noted on the AP views, while the frogleg lateral films of both hips are used in comparison to detect posterior slips. In the AP view, a line drawn along the lateral (superior) aspect of the femoral neck should transect the lateral quarter of the femoral epiphysis (see Fig. 118-3). The slipped epiphysis will not be transected by the line at all or will be transected less than noted on the unaffected hip. Moderate to severe slips will be detected by this method (see Fig. 118-4), while mild slips require the interpretation of the frogleg lateral x-rays of both hips. If the diagnosis of SCFE is suspected, both types of radiographs are necessary.

Management in the emergency department consists of (1) confirmation of the diagnosis, (2) assurance of absolute non-weight-bearing, (3) orthopaedic consultation, and (4) admission to the hospital. No patient with SCFE is treated as an outpatient, even if the intent is to perform surgery the following day. The management of SCFE is operative reduction and fixation, although there exists a certain amount of discussion in the orthopaedic literature as to the optimal technical approach. Subsequent immobilization of the hip is main-

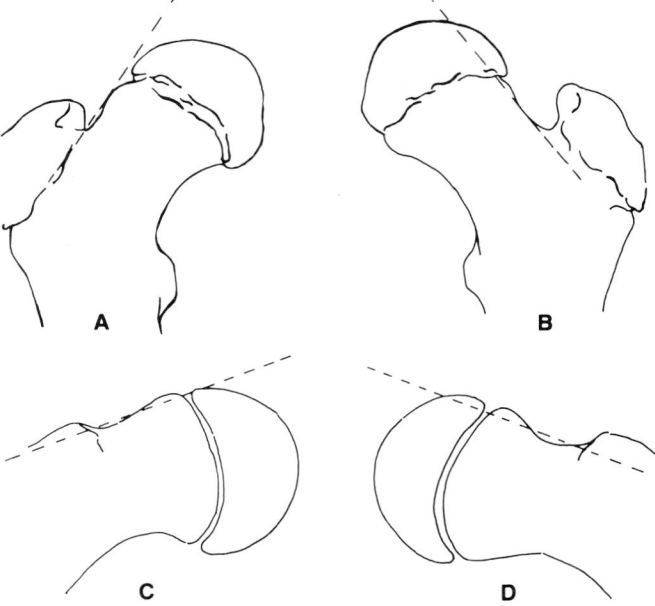

**Fig. 118-3.** Line drawn along the lateral (superior) aspect of femoral neck fails to transect the lateral quarter of the femoral head in medial SCFE seen in **A** and **C**. The normal anatomic relationship is illustrated in **B** and **D**.

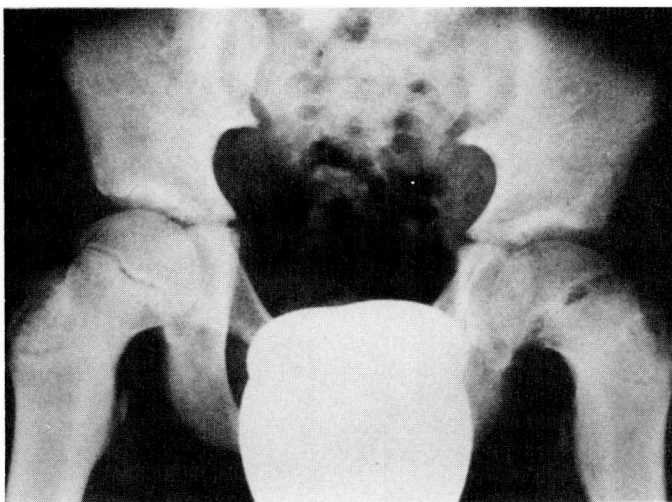

**Fig. 118-4.** AP radiograph illustrating a medial SCFE involving the left hip.

tained for at least 12 weeks, and careful observation for 1 to 2 years thereafter is necessary in anticipation of the development of this condition's most serious complication, avascular necrosis of the femoral head.

## Transient Tenosynovitis of the Hip

Acute transient tenosynovitis of the hip is the most common cause of hip pain in children less than 10 years of age (peak: 3 to 6 years). There is a boy to girl predominance that is variously described as 3:2 to 5:1. The right hip is somewhat more commonly affected than the left, and the condition is bilateral in 5 percent of cases. The etiology of the condition is not known, although trauma, viral and bacterial infection, and allergy (hypersensitization) have been proposed by authors to explain the condition.

Symptoms may be acute or gradual in onset. There may be a history of recent upper respiratory symptoms offered by the parent. Considering the age group, such an association is probably best interpreted casually. The child complains of pain in the anteromedial or anterolateral thigh and knee. The gait is antalgic. Tenderness is elicited upon palpation of the anterior hip, and range of motion is limited by the discomfort. The child's systemic temperature is normal or minimally elevated. The child does not appear toxically ill.

The peripheral WBC and ESR are usually normal. If performed, tuberculin skin tests, rheumatoid factor titers, and hemolytic streptolysin O (HSO) titers are negative. Radiographs of the hip are either normal or demonstrate mild to moderate hip effusion (see Fig. 118-5). There are no bone changes associated with the condition.

The differential diagnosis includes SCFE and other hip fractures, Legg-Calvé-Perthes disease, and suppurative arthritis of the hip. Less common differential considerations include rheumatic fever, juvenile rheumatoid arthritis, and, rarely, tuberculosis of the hip.

In the event that the peripheral WBC and ESR are substantially elevated and a hip effusion is noted on the radiograph, a diagnostic arthrocentesis should be performed to exclude suppurative arthritis. Consideration should be given in this circumstance to open irrigation of the hip joint in the operating room by an orthopaedic consultant after obtaining samples of synovial fluid for laboratory studies, Gram stain, aerobic and anaerobic cultures, and AFB stain/culture. The synovial fluid in transient tenosynovitis of the hip is clear transudative, will have negative stains for microorganisms, and will yield sterile cultures.

In the event that further differentiation of transient tenosynovitis of the hip from Legg-Calvé-Perthes disease is necessary, technetium

99m bone scan or an MRI scan will confirm the absence of avascular necrosis of the femoral head. This aspect of the diagnostic workup can be performed in the ambulatory setting.

Admission to hospital is necessary only for management of SCFE, other hip fractures, and septic arthritis of the hip. Once these diagnostic considerations are effectively eliminated, the child with suspected transient tenosynovitis of the hip can be managed as an outpatient. Weight-bearing is eliminated, and anti-inflammatory agents are recommended until the child's hip is painless and range of motion returns to normal (3 to 7 days). Some authors recommend an additional period of rest (7 to 10 days) after symptoms have resolved. Antibiotics are of no value; glucocorticoids are not recommended.

Various authors have noted an association between transient tenosynovitis of the hip and the subsequent development of Legg-Calvé-Perthes disease, ranging from 0.5 to 10 percent. It remains unclear whether the association is one of cause and effect or misdiagnosis of early Legg-Calvé-Perthes disease. Follow-up clinical evaluations of patients with a diagnosis of transient tenosynovitis of the hip should occur at 2 weeks with the child's primary care physician. Subsequent clinical elevations (possibly to include radiographs) are performed by the primary care physician at 2 months and 6 months after the initial episode.

## Legg-Calvé-Perthes Disease (Coxa Plana)

The incidence of Legg-Calvé-Perthes disease varies worldwide from 1:1200 to 1:12,500. The onset of symptoms is between 4 and 9 years in 80 percent of patients, with a range of age between 2 and 13 years. It is bilateral in 10 percent of cases.

The disease process is characterized as an avascular necrosis of the femoral head complicated by subsequent subchondral stress fracture. Resorption of areas of bone within the femoral head (rarefaction) is followed by the laying down of new bone. Collapse and flattening of the femoral head may ensue, along with the potential for subluxation. The result is a painful hip joint associated with restricted range of motion, muscle spasm, and soft tissue contractures.

Clinically, the child with Legg-Calvé-Perthes disease presents with limp and pain of weeks' to months' duration. Pain is usually mild, chronic, and dull. It is most noticeable in the groin, the anteromedial thigh, and the knee. It is exacerbated by physical activity, relieved by rest, and is associated with an antalgic limp. There are no associated systemic symptoms. Hip range of motion is restricted; there may be a flexion-abduction contracture as well. Thigh muscle atrophy, due to disuse, is common.

The radiographic findings associated with Legg-Calvé-Perthes disease depend on the stage of the disease process. During the incipient stage (1 to 3 months), the radiograph of the hip demonstrates only widening of the cartilage space of the affected hip and a smaller size

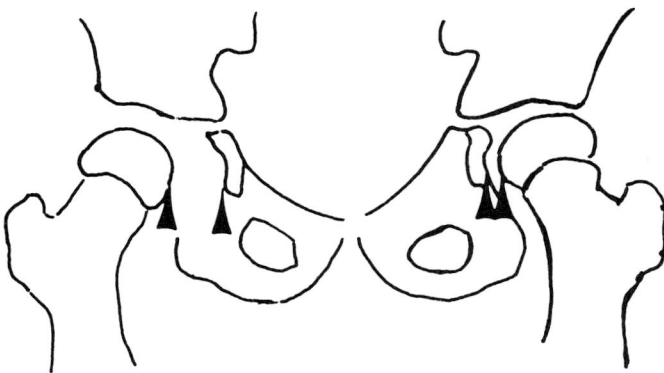

**Fig. 118-5.** Widening of the joint space, indicating an effusion, is a nonspecific finding seen in children with toxic tenosynovitis, Legg-Calvé-Perthes disease, suppurative arthritis, and hemarthrosis.

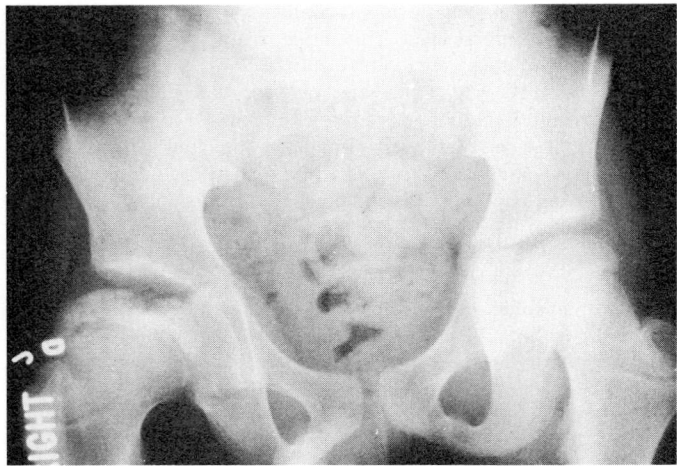

**Fig. 118-6.** Legg-Calvé-Perthes disease. The right hip illustrates joint space widening, reduced size of the ossific nucleus of the femoral head, and increased opacification of the femoral head.

of the ossific nucleus of the femoral head (see Fig. 118-6). The second radiographic sign is the appearance of the subchondral stress fracture line in the femoral head (Caffey's sign). The third radiologic finding is increased opacification of the femoral head, brought on by deposition of new bone upon avascular trabeculae, calcification of the sclerotic marrow, and by collapse and crowding of the avascular trabeculae in the dome of the epiphysis. Ultimately, deformities of the femoral head and neck become apparent, along with subluxation and extrusion of the femoral head from the acetabulum.

The other commonly employed imaging modalities include technetium 99m bone scan (see Fig. 118-7) and MRI. The scan demonstrates markedly reduced uptake of nuclide within the affected femoral head. These findings precede apparent plain film radiographic abnormalities. MRI offers superior resolution and sensitivity, with areas of low signal intensity reflecting necrotic regions within the femoral head (see Fig. 118-8). Arthrogram-like images of the cartilaginous portions of the femoral head and acetabular rim are produced. Excellent visualization is possible of deformities and flattening of the femoral head as well as subluxation or anterolateral extrusion of the femoral head from the acetabulum.

The differential diagnosis of coxa plana includes toxic tenosynovitis of the hip, which shares many similar features with early Legg-Calvé-Perthes disease. Careful review of the radiographs is necessary to exclude the findings associated with coxa plana, as mentioned previously. When in doubt, consider technetium 99m bone scan or MRI imaging studies.

The differentiation of coxa plana from acute rheumatic fever (ARF) is based on the natural history and responsiveness of ARF to salicylates. Tuberculous arthritis of the hip may mimic coxa plana. Differential screening tests should include a PPD skin test and an ESR. Unilateral tumors such as eosinophilic granuloma, osteoid osteoma, osteoblastoma, and lymphoma should be considered and excluded by laboratory studies and CT scan. Bone dysplasias are often confused with Legg-Calvé-Perthes disease. Hypothyroidism (juvenile cretinism), sickle cell disease, and Gaucher's disease should also be excluded.

Care in the emergency department involves the consideration or establishment of the accurate diagnosis and orthopaedic consultation. Treatment efforts are directed toward restoration of full range of motion of the hip and stabilization of the femoral head within the acetabulum, with resumption of normal activities as rapidly as possible. All except the most mildly affected children are hospitalized initially and treated with traction. The duration of traction and the timing of further therapy directed at containing the femoral head within the ac-

etabulum (orthotics versus surgical containment) depend on the severity of the coxa plana and the responsiveness of the hip irritability to traction therapy.

## Other Avascular Necrosis Syndromes

### Kohler's Disease of the Tarsal Navicular

This is an uncommon condition affecting boys more commonly than girls (4:1), occurring at about 5 years of age in boys and at about 4 years of age in girls. It appears to result from repetitive compressive forces applied to the tarsal navicular, the last bone of the foot to ossify in normal children. Affected children appear to have a delayed ossification of this bone during a critical phase in its growth, predisposing it to the compressive stresses of preschool ambulation.

The child presents with an antalgic limp, bearing weight on the lateral side of the foot, thus splinting the medial longitudinal arch. The child complains of local pain and tenderness over the navicular bone of the foot and often has induration over the area. There is no fever nor other constitutional symptoms. Range of motion of the other joints of the foot is intact.

Radiographically, the picture is classic. The tarsal navicular is narrowed, as seen in the lateral view of the foot and ankle, and flattened with irregular rarefaction and sclerosis. Comparison of radiographs of the contralateral foot are often helpful.

Treatment is as an outpatient using a short leg walking cast. The use of crutches to assure non-weight-bearing is recommended for the initial 3 weeks. Orthopaedic aftercare should be arranged. The prognosis is very good.

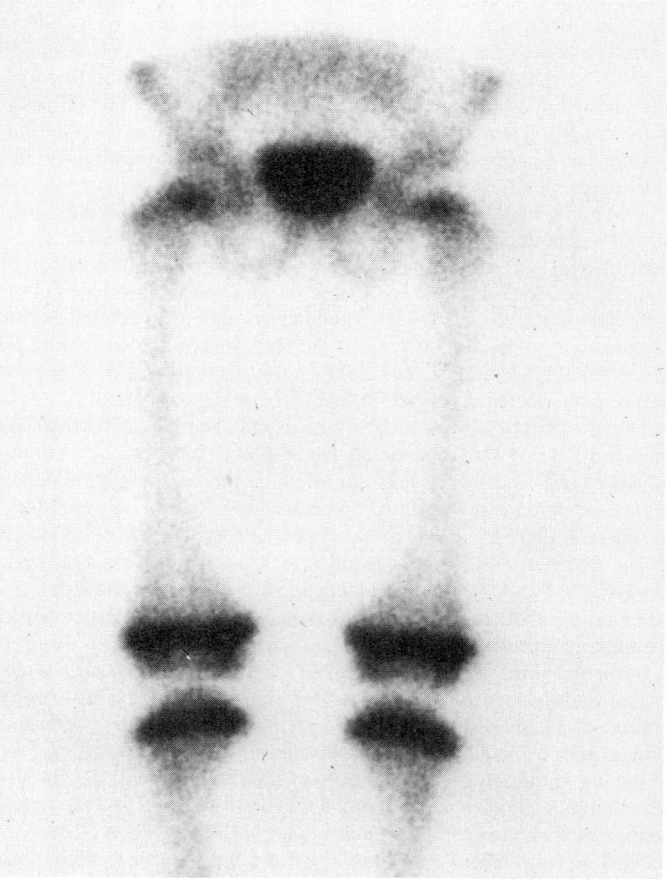

**Fig. 118-7.** Technetium 99m bone scan of patient with left-sided Legg-Calvé-Perthes disease, illustrating reduced nuclide uptake within the left femoral head.

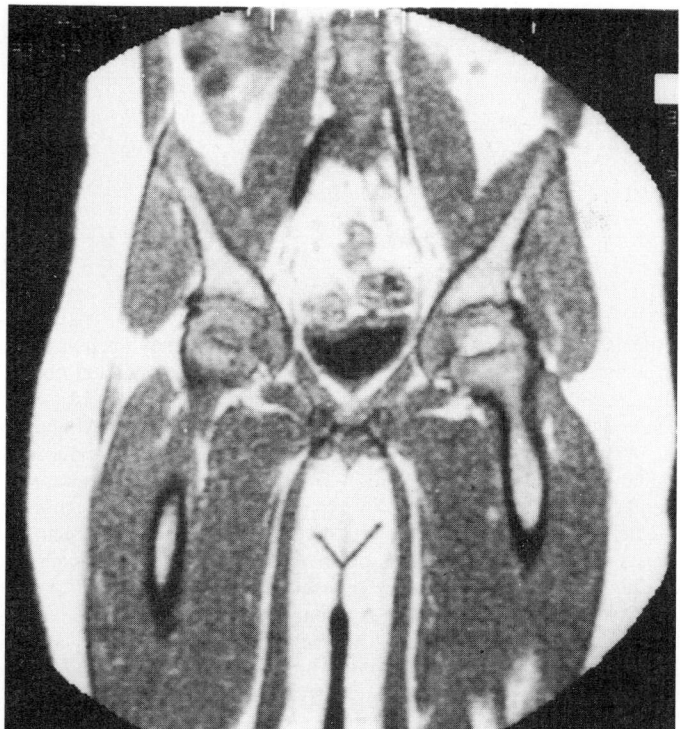

**Fig. 118-8.** MRI of patient with Legg-Calvé-Perthes disease, illustrating necrosis within left femoral head.

## Frieberg's Infarction

This condition of adolescents is seen much more commonly in girls (3:1). The usual site of involvement is the head of the second metatarsal, although other metatarsals can be affected, and it is occasionally bilateral. While its etiology is not known with certainty, it is generally presumed to be caused by a vascular insufficiency (aseptic necrosis).

Clinically, the patient complains of pain and tenderness under the affected metatarsal head. This is associated with local soft tissue swelling and restricted range of motion of the metatarsophalangeal joint. Radiographs of the foot demonstrate flattening, sclerosis, and irregularity of the metatarsal head. CT scan or $^{99m}$Tc bone scan may serve to clarify the diagnosis in selected patients whose diagnosis remains obscure.

Management is as an outpatient, utilizing a short leg walking cast for 3 to 4 weeks. Follow-up care is provided by an orthopaedist who may recommend a surgical excision of the affected area of metatarsal if conservative therapy is ineffective.

## Osgood-Schlatter Disease

This very common syndrome affects preadolescent males three times more often than females. The etiology is a traumatic stress imposed upon the proximal tibial tuberosity by a contracted quadriceps muscle mechanism. The ligamentum patellae detaches cartilaginous fragments from the tibial tuberosity without necrosis. However, an inflammatory process is established by the reparative process, resulting in a patellar tendinitis and a remarkable prominence, induration, and tenderness of the tibial tuberosity. There is no avascular necrosis of the tibial tuberosity.

The patient complains of pain and tenderness over the anterior aspect of the knee and of the tibial tuberosity. It is exacerbated by running, climbing stairs, jumping, and by kneeling. Symptoms are relieved with rest. Examination reveals thickening and tenderness of the patellar tendon, with maximum palpation tenderness over the in-

sertion point of the patellar tendon onto the tibial tubercle. The tibial tuberosity is noticeably enlarged and indurated. There is no knee effusion.

Radiographs will illustrate patellar tendon thickening and soft tissue swelling over the tibial tuberosity without knee effusion. The irregularity of the ossification of the tibial tubercle is normal for this age group and is *not* a diagnostic feature of Osgood-Schlatter disease. However, prominence of the tibial tuberosity, with or without a small free bone fragment located anterior and superior to the tibial tubercle, *is* characteristic of the disorder.

The disease is self-limited. Acute symptoms subside following restriction from excessive physical activities for a period of approximately 3 months. Severely painful knees may benefit symptomatically from the use of crutches. Contracted, taut, hypertrophic quadriceps and hamstring muscles require stretching exercises. Rarely, more aggressive strategies to assure rest of the knee are utilized, such as the use of a knee immobilizer or long leg cylinder cast. Even so, the stretching exercises of the quadriceps and hamstring groups are continued. The use of glucocorticoid injection into the patellar tendon and the para-apophyseal soft tissues is controversial and is to be discouraged.

## ACUTE SUPPURATIVE ARTHRITIS

Acute suppurative arthritis, an inflammation of a joint caused by pyogenic organisms, occurs in all age groups but is more commonly a condition affecting neonates, infants, and children less than 3 years of age. The hip is the most commonly involved joint, followed in frequency by the knee and the elbow. Any joint can be involved. Simultaneous infection of more than a single joint can occur.

Bacteria may access the joint through hematogenous transmission, from direct extension of infection from an adjacent area of infected metaphyseal bone, or via direct inoculation during arthrocentesis (or accidentally during femoral venipuncture). The etiologic organisms encountered in septic arthritis vary with the age of the child (see Table 118-1). The relative frequency of certain organisms (e.g., *Haemophilus influenzae*) has evolved as a consequence of immunization practices.

The pathophysiology of septic arthritis exemplifies the seriousness of the condition and the risks of long-term sequelae. Synovial edema and hyperemia accompany increased secretion of synovial fluid, which may be serosanguinous early on, cloudy, or frankly suppurative with polymorphonuclear (PMN) leukocyte counts ranging from 5000 to 200,000 and exceeding $50,000/\mu L^3$ after the earliest stages. Synovial fluid glucose concentration is decreased, and the protein content is elevated. The mucin string is poor to very poor. Within days, the synovial fluid becomes frankly purulent, if it was not so initially. The hyaline articular cartilages degenerate initially at points of contact between opposing articular surfaces. The synovium itself is eventually replaced by granulation tissue, and the infection invades surrounding bone, particularly epiphyseal and metaphyseal bone. Adhesions are created within the joint, which restrict motion. Subluxation or dislocation may occur in the setting of marked distension of the damaged joint capsule. In the hip joint, avascular necrosis of the femoral head ensues. Eventually, the untreated infection leads to ankylosis or total destruction of the joint.

Although systemic symptoms can be subtle in the newborn, the diagnosis is not usually in doubt in the older infant or toddler. Symptoms are acute in onset and predominantly involve pain in the affected joint. The child with a lower extremity septic arthritis walks with a severely antalgic limp or more typically cannot bear weight at all. Profound signs of constitutional and systemic illness are the rule, with high fever [40 to 40.5°C (104 to 105°F)], apprehension, irritability, anorexia, and prostration manifestly apparent. Examination of the affected joint demonstrates warmth, soft tissue swelling, and exquisite palpation tenderness. The child maintains an infected hip in 30° to

**Table 118-1.** Etiology of Suppurative Arthritis in Children

| Newborn (0–2 months) | | Infant (2–36 months) | | Child (>36 months) | |
|---|---|---|---|---|---|
| *Staphylococcus aureus* | (35–46%) | *H. influenzae*\* | (30–35%) | *Staph. aureus* | (30–45%) |
| Group B *streptococcus* | (20–25%) | *Streptococcus* sp. | (12%) | *Streptococcus* sp. | (18–26%) |
| Gram-negative bacilli | (10–28%) | *Staph. aureus* | (11%) | Gram-negative bacilli | (10–15%) |
| *Neisseria gonorrhoeae* | (5–7%) | Gram-negative bacilli | (10%) | *Strep. pneumoniae* | (7%) |
| *Haemophilus influenzae* | (2%) | Unknown or unidentified | 35%) | *N. gonorrhoeae* | 5–10%) |
| *Candida albicans†* | (7–17%) | | | | |

\* Data collected prior to implementation of *H. influenzae* B (Hib) vaccine.
† Hospital acquired.

60° of flexion, with milder degrees of abduction and external rotation.

Radiographic imaging studies are helpful but nondiagnostic. They are important in order to assure the absence of changes that would indicate an adjacent osteomyelitis, fracture, or other processes. The expected findings are those of joint effusion and distention (see Fig. 118-9). Comparison films of the contralateral joint in question are often helpful.

The differential diagnosis includes osteomyelitis, acute rheumatic fever (ARF), acute pauciarticular juvenile rheumatoid arthritis (JRA), transient tenosynovitis, cellulitis and suppurative bursitis, hemarthrosis, Legg-Calvé-Perthes disease, and SCFE (when the involved joint is the hip).

Distinguishing suppurative arthritis from an osteomyelitis involving an adjacent metaphysis is probably the most difficult problem in the differential diagnosis. Gentle examination may enable the physician to ascertain the area of greatest tenderness: osteomyelitis is most tender over the metaphysis, while septic arthritis manifests greatest tenderness directly over the joint line. Motion of the joint is much more painful and more restricted in septic arthritis compared to osteomyelitis. Osteomyelitis creates more swelling over the limb as a whole. Arthrocentesis is necessary to establish the diagnosis of suppurative arthritis. Care is necessary during the arthrocentesis to avoid contaminating a noninfected joint by introducing organisms from an infected metaphysis, cellulitis, or bursa. A sympathetic effusion from an area of metaphyseal osteomyelitis usually is serous and contains only a few thousand PMNs.

The other differential diagnostic considerations usually pose fewer problems to the clinician. Transient tenosynovitis does not manifest symptoms and signs of systemic toxicity. The peripheral WBC and ESR are normal or only minimally elevated. Occasionally, arthrocentesis is necessary to adequately exclude the diagnosis of suppurative

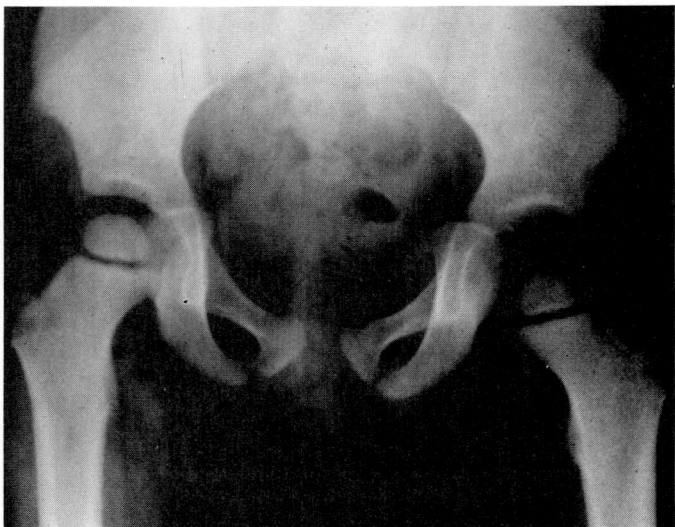

**Fig. 118-9.** Large left hip effusion in child with suppurative arthritis.

arthritis, however. JRA of the pauciarticular form may present with an isolated inflamed joint but is usually an illness of gradual onset, and the child does not appear toxically ill. The affected joint is not as tender as in septic arthritis and has better range of motion. Although the WBC is elevated and the mucin string is poor in both conditions, the Gram stain of synovial fluid in JRA is negative and its culture is sterile.

Rheumatic fever is characterized by the fleeting, migratory nature of the arthritis and may be associated with other stigmata, such as carditis, as illustrated by Jones' revised criteria for the diagnosis of ARF (see Table 118-5). There is a remarkable responsiveness of the arthritis of ARF to salicylates. The response of the arthritis to salicylates should be used as a diagnostic tool only after the diagnosis of suppurative arthritis has been excluded by arthrocentesis, with Gram stain and culture of the synovial fluid.

Cellulitis is notable for local skin erythema, induration, and tenderness. The adjacent joint has relatively preserved motion and is less tender. Lymphangitis or regional lymphadenitis is commonly encountered with cellulitis. Often the patient or examiner will note the presence of a minor abrasion, laceration, puncture, or furuncle within the cellulitis, serving as an entrance site for local invasion of bacteria.

Hemarthrosis can rarely pose a problem in the differential diagnosis of septic arthritis. In the absence of a history of trauma, a congenital or acquired coagulopathy is suspected (hemophilia A, factor IX deficiency, Von Willebrand's disease, leukemia, etc.). Henoch-Schönlein purpura may present with one or more painful joints prior to manifestation of the other cardinal symptoms of the disease (abdominal pain, nephritis, purpura). The arthralgia with this condition is migratory, however, and represents a periarticulitis rather than an actual arthritis. If the joint of involvement happens to be the hip, a diagnosis of Legg-Calvé-Perthes disease may come to mind. This condition is not, however, associated with high fever, systemic signs of illness, and prostration, and the examination and culture of the synovial fluid will easily distinguish this condition from septic arthritis.

The management of acute suppurative arthritis consists of (1) establishing the diagnosis by obtaining synovial fluid from the infected joint for Gram stain and culture as well as other microscopic and laboratory studies; (2) drainage of the infected joint of bacterial products and infectious debris [suppurative arthritis of the hip requires open surgical drainage (arthrotomy), whereas more superficial joints can frequently be drained arthroscopically or even through arthrocentesis]; (3) emergent initiation of appropriate initial antibiotic therapy (see Table 118-2); and (4) local care of the joint (support by skin traction for larger joints; splinting of the wrist, ankle, and smaller joints).

An analysis of the CSF is indicated in children suspected of suppurative arthritis or osteomyelitis caused by *H. influenzae*. This is necessary since meningitis is a frequently coexisting illness in children with influenza suppurative arthritis and since the antibiotic dosages for meningitis differ from the dosages used in suppurative arthritis. Follow-up considerations (hearing tests, cognitive tests) will also vary in the setting of coexisting meningitis.

The prognosis of suppurative arthritis is influenced by: (1) the length of time between onset of symptoms and initiation of treatment;

**Table 118-2.** Initial Antibiotic Therapy of Acute Suppurative Arthritis in Children

| Age | Suspected Organism | Antibiotics |
|---|---|---|
| **Newborn** (0–2 months) | *Staphylococcus aureus* | Methicillin or nafcillin* |
| | Group B *Streptococcus* | Ampicillin or penicillin and gentamicin |
| | Gram-negative bacilli | Cefotaxime/ceftriaxone |
| | *Neisseria gonorrhoeae* | Cefotaxime/ceftriaxone |
| | Unknown | Methicillin or nafcillin* and cefotaxime/ceftriaxone |
| **Infant** (2–36 months) | *Haemophilus influenzae* | Cefuroxime or cefotaxime/ceftriaxone |
| | *Streptococcus* sp. | Penicillin G |
| | *Staph. aureus* | Methicillin or nafcillin* |
| | Gram-negative bacilli | Cefotaxime/ceftriaxone |
| | Unknown | Methicillin or nafcillin* and cefotaxime/ceftriaxone |
| **Child** (>36 months) | *Staph. aureus* | Methicillin or nafcillin* |
| | *Streptococcus* sp. | Penicillin G, other beta lactams, clindamycin |
| | Gram-negative bacilli | Cefotaxime/ceftriaxone |
| | *N. gonorrhoeae* | Ceftriaxone or penicillin G |
| | Unknown | Methicillin or nafcillin* and cefotaxime/ceftriaxone |

* Vancomycin, if methicillinase-resistant *Staph. aureus* is suspected.

(2) the joint involved (prognosis is poorer if the hip is involved); (3) the presence of associated osteomyelitis (poorer); and (4) the age of the patient, with neonates and younger infants having a less favorable prognosis than older children due to the typically longer delay in initiation of specific treatment.

## STRUCTURAL SCOLIOSIS

Scoliosis is a lateral deviation of a series of vertebral bodies from the normal spinal axis. If progressive, structural deformities occur in the vertebral bodies and the rib cage. Scoliosis is a physical sign and is not itself a diagnosis. Eighty percent of structural scoliosis is idiopathic, i.e., it does not relate to a paralytic or neurologic etiology and there are no causative congenital vertebral anomalies.

There are three peak periods of onset of idiopathic structural scoliosis: infantile (0 to 3 years), juvenile (4 years to puberty), and adolescent (onset of puberty to physeal closure). Prevalence data has been obtained in two ways historically: school screening and chest radiographs obtained for screening of tuberculosis. The prevalence of curves of <10° is 2 to 3 percent in North America, while the prevalence of more severe curves decreases as the severity of the curve increases. While the prevalence of minor (<10°) curves is equal among boys and girls, there is a distinct female gender predilection for curves exceeding 15° to 20°. This presumably relates to the observation that curve progression is more common in girls.

Large-scale screening programs remain somewhat controversial. Overreferral to the orthopaedist is common and is to be expected. Use of a scoliometer can dramatically reduce overreferral. The potential for excessive exposure to ionizing radiation is minimized by ensuring that an experienced orthopaedic surgeon reexamines all referred patients prior to the ordering of the diagnostic scoliosis radiogram (single, standing anterior-posterior radiogram of the entire spine with the iliac crests as high as possible). Another difficulty with screening programs is parental noncompliance. Finally, the cost-effectiveness of large-scale screening programs is yet to be firmly established.

Despite the difficulties and controversies of large-scale screening programs, primary care physicians and emergency physicians are in a strong position to rapidly and easily identify scoliosis in children presenting to the emergency department for unrelated problems. Children with scoliosis do not usually complain of backache or fatigue.

Their complaints, if they have any, relate to concerns of high shoulder, prominent scapula or breast, prominent hip, asymmetry of rib cage, trunk, or flank creases, poor posture or they have noticed the curve itself.

When the diagnosis is being considered, the examination of the child and the spine should be orderly. The child is observed standing, first clothed, then unclothed (but with appropriate draping for modesty), for body habitus, posture, and alignment. Lateral deformity of the spine is usually best visualized from behind the standing child. Look for balance of the head, neck, and shoulders over the pelvis. A plumb line held over the spinous process of the seventh cervical vertebra normally should pass right over the intergluteal cleft. Lateral deviation from the midline should be noted and can be measured in centimeters.

The Adams forward bending test optimally demonstrates the degree and direction of any associated rotation of the vertebrae. The patient's knees should be straight and the feet placed together. The child bends forward at the hips with the arms dependent and the palms held in opposition. The child is inspected head-on for cervical and thoracic rotation and from the rear for thoracolumbar and lumbar rotation. The right and left posterior rib cage and the paravertebral lumbosacral muscles are inspected and compared for asymmetry. Rotational abnormalities of the vertebral bodies, associated with the lateral curvature of scoliosis, will result in one side (rib cage, paravertebral lumbar muscles) being higher than the other. In structural scoliosis, the vertebral body rotation is toward the convex side of the curve of the scoliosis and toward the elevated side of the rib cage or paravertebral lumbar muscles. This asymmetry can be quantified by use of a scoliometer, a gravity level device that measures in degrees of rotation. Scoliosis manifesting greater than 10° of vertebral rotation warrants referral to an orthopaedic surgeon.

Conservative management of scoliosis is employed for structural scoliosis manifesting less than 50° of vertebral rotation or 50° of curve when measured radiographically. Various orthotic braces (e.g., TLSO, Charleston-Bending brace) are utilized with varying success. Nonoperative candidates with more severe curves (35° to 50°) usually obtain better results using orthotic devices worn nearly continuously (23 h daily), such as the TLSO, compared to nighttime-only braces. All of these devices are fitted to a particular child's torso. They require substantial discipline of the part of the child and the parents, however. Careful follow-up care is provided by the orthopaedic surgeon, who must be particularly vigilant for progression of the scoliosis, defined as an increase in the curvature of more than 5° on two or more successive visits. Such curve progression is ominous in that it is associated with the development of more severe curvatures ultimately requiring surgical stabilization.

## SELECTED RHEUMATOLOGIC DISORDERS IN CHILDREN

### Kawasaki Syndrome

Kawasaki syndrome is a generalized vasculitis involving small and medium size arteries, with characteristic involvement of the coronary arteries. There is growing evidence to suggest that Kawasaki syndrome is caused by superantigen bacterial toxins, which stimulate large populations of T cells expressing particular T-cell receptor β chain variable-gene segments. Superantigen stimulation induces massive proliferation and expansion of the target T cells, with subsequent production of proinflammatory cytokines. Vascular endothelial cells are recruited into this inflammatory process with resulting vascular damage. Toxins elaborated by *Staphylococcus aureus* and *Streptococcus pyogenes* are known to possess superantigen properties. There is increasing evidence to suggest that these organisms elaborate superantigen toxins in children with Kawasaki syndrome.

Epidemiologically, Kawasaki syndrome affects 3000 to 5000 children annually in the United States. There is a male to female prepon-

**Table 118-3.** Diagnostic Criteria for Kawasaki Syndrome

| |
|---|
| Fever of at least 5 days' duration (100%) |
| Presence of at least four out of the following five conditions |
|   1. Bilateral conjunctivitis (85%) |
|   2. Changes of the lips and oral mucosa (90%) |
|     Dry, red, fissured lips |
|     Strawberry tongue |
|     Oropharyngeal edema |
|   3. Changes of the extremities (75%) |
|     Erythema of palms and soles |
|     Edema of hands and feet |
|     Periungual desquamation |
|   4. Polymorphous rash (80%) |
|   5. Cervical lymphadenopathy (70%) |
| Illness not explained by other known disease process |

derance of 1.5:1. The peak age of onset is 1 to 2 years, with 80 percent of patients being less than 4 years of age.

The diagnosis of Kawasaki syndrome is established by the presence of certain clinical criteria listed in Table 118-3. The fever is high, spiking, and prolonged, persisting for 1 to 2 weeks in untreated patients. The conjunctivitis is nonpurulent and bilateral and has an onset shortly after the appearance of the fever. The oropharyngeal features are prominent during the acute febrile period. The extremities, particularly the palms and soles, are often quite painful. The polymorphous rash is most commonly a raised, deep-red plaquelike eruption. Less commonly, it may be scarlatiniform, a morbilliform maculopapular rash, or even a fine pustular eruption. It is most widespread on the trunk and proximal extremities, with particular involvement of the perineum. At least one cervical lymph node measuring 1.5 cm in diameter is necessary to fill the lymphadenopathy criterion. There are a wide variety of associated findings in Kawasaki syndrome, as illustrated in Table 118-4.

The acute febrile phase of the disease lasts 7 to 14 days and is marked by the features listed in Table 118-3. The subacute phase, lasting 2 to 4 weeks, is indicated by a gradual resolution of the fever, rash, and lymphadenopathy. The irritability and conjunctival injection may persist. The characteristic desquamation of the fingers and toes occurs during this subacute phase, as does the associated symptom of arthralgia/arthritis. Thrombocytosis approaching $1,000,000/\mu L^3$ is also noted during this subacute phase, during which time the patient is at greatest risk for the development of coronary artery thrombosis. The convalescent phase begins when all clinical and associated signs and symptoms have disappeared and continues until the ESR and the platelet count return to normal (6 to 10 weeks).

An acute carditis develops in 50 percent of patients, usually manifested by a myocarditis with symptoms of tachycardia and gallop rhythms indicative of mild to severe congestive heart failure. Pericarditis, conduction disturbances, and valvular insufficiencies are less frequent manifestations of carditis.

Most seriously, coronary artery aneurysmal dilatations occur in 20

**Table 118-4.** Associated Features of Kawasaki Syndrome

| | |
|---|---|
| Cardiovascular system | Genitourinary system |
|   Coronary artery aneurysms |   Urethritis with sterile pyuria |
|   Myocarditis–pericarditis |   Proteinuria |
|   Mitral or aortic insufficiency | Pulmonary system |
|   Dysrhythmias |   Pneumonitis |
|   Peripheral ischemia |   Cough, coryza |
| Central nervous system | Gastrointestinal system |
|   Irritability |   Hydrops of the gall bladder |
|   Aseptic meningitis |   Hepatitis |
|   Anterior uveitis |   Nausea, vomiting, diarrhea |
|   Sensorineural hearing loss |   Abdominal pain |
| Hematologic system | |
|   Thrombocytosis (subacute phase) | |
|   Anemia | |

percent of untreated patients. Coronary artery involvement can be detected as early as the seventh day, with a peak frequency of coronary aneurysm formation occurring 4 weeks after the onset of illness. Untreated, the coronary artery aneurysms are quite prone to thrombosis during the subacute phase because of the hypercoagulable state created by the thrombocytosis. Sudden death can occur in 1 to 2 % of untreated patients, and the remainder are at risk for long-term consequences such as coronary artery stenosis and subsequent cardiac ischemia.

The laboratory features of Kawasaki syndrome reflect the marked inflammatory and immune activation characteristic of the disease. Such findings, however, are nonspecific. A moderate leukocytosis with a left shift, a remarkable thrombocytosis appearing during the second week of the illness, and other secondary laboratory abnormalities consistent with a diffuse systemic vasculitis may be present.

The care of the child with Kawasaki syndrome in the emergency department consists primarily of establishing the diagnosis. Patients meeting diagnostic criteria with consistent laboratory findings are usually admitted. The use of intravenous immunoglobulin (IVIG) has substantially decreased the morbidity and mortality associated with the disease. Rapid resolution of fever and the other clinical stigmata and reversal of the laboratory abnormalities occur following IVIG infusion. More importantly, the use of IVIG within the first 10 days of the illness reduces the incidence of coronary artery aneurysms to 3 to 4 percent. It also has been demonstrated to be effective in promoting the resolution of established aneurysms. A single infusion of intravenous IVIG in a dose of 2 g/kg infused over a 10-h period has been demonstrated to be the most effective regimen. Aspirin can be used as adjunctive therapy in anti-inflammatory doses of 80 to 100 mg/kg per day until the fourteenth day of the illness. The dose is then reduced to 3 to 5 mg/kg per day for its platelet antiadhesive effect during the period when the child is at risk of clotting coronary artery aneurysms due to the thrombosis. Usually, the low-dose aspirin therapy is continued until the platelet count returns to normal. However, patients exhibiting coronary aneurysms despite IVIG therapy should receive low-dose aspirin indefinitely or for at least 1 year following the resolution of the aneurysms. Echocardiography, necessary to the identification of coronary artery aneurysms, provides valuable baseline information for the child who does not initially manifest abnormalities. The echocardiogram is repeated 3 to 6 weeks after IVIG therapy in order to guide further aspirin therapy decisions.

## Henoch-Schönlein Purpura

Henoch-Schönlein purpura is a common, self-limited generalized leukocytoclastic vasculitis. Vasculitis involves primarily small vessels and is mediated by immune complexes produced through IgA and the alternate complement pathways. A variety of infectious and noninfectious stimuli appear to precipitate the immunologic mechanisms of the vasculitis.

The disorder is classically characterized by the appearance of a dermovasculitis with a propensity for the lower trunk, buttocks, perineum, and lower extremities, as is characteristic of generalized vasculitides (see Fig. 118-10). Additionally, the vasculitis includes involvement of the glomeruli, with the subsequent development of hematuria and with the potential for long-term renal sequelae. Involvement of the bowel wall confers recurrent colicky abdominal pain and frequently proceeds to the development of melena or hematochezia. Eight percent of children with severe abdominal colic caused by Henoch-Schönlein purpura experience massive gastrointestinal hemorrhage or intussusception. Arthritis, or more specifically a polymigratory periarticulitis, occurs in most affected children. Rarely, massive pulmonary hemorrhage can occur.

The clinical diagnosis is not usually obscure in those children manifesting all or several characteristics of the disorder. The child with hematuria, abdominal pain, a history of migratory periarthritis, and a palpable, purpuric tender rash on the buttock and lower extremity is not a diagnostic dilemma. Difficulty ensues upon the evaluation of

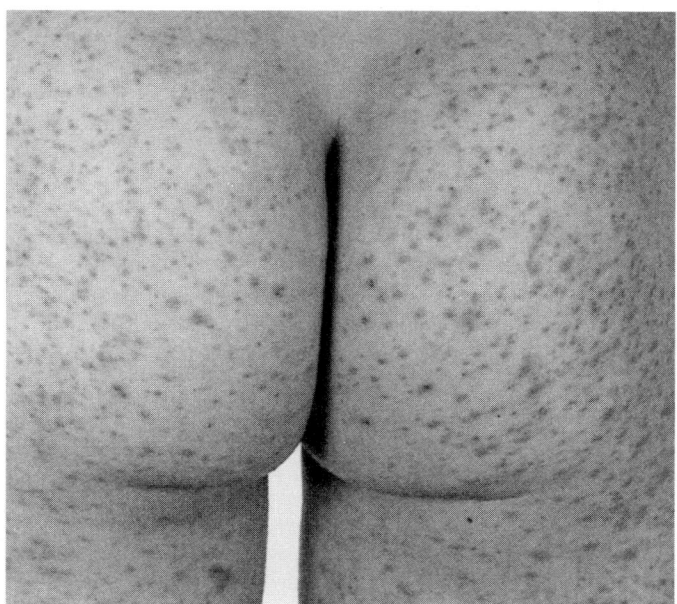

**Fig. 118-10.** Henoch-Schönlein purpura. Purpuric lesions of dependent body areas, particularly on flanks, buttocks, and lower extremities.

a child manifesting exclusively abdominal colic or apparent arthritis.

Care of the child with suspected Henoch-Schönlein purpura in the emergency department consists of establishing the diagnosis or maintaining a high index of suspicion for the diagnosis. Otherwise, emergency care is entirely supportive. Consideration of specific laboratory or imaging studies is influenced by the specific symptoms manifested by the child. For example, the child presenting exclusively with hematuria and abdominal pain may require a urine analysis and urine culture, a KUB (*k*idneys, *u*reters, *b*ladder) abdominal radiograph, assessment of renal function, and a complete blood count. Such circumstances might even serve as an indication for a renal ultrasound or an intravenous pyelogram if the clinician suspects ureterolithiasis as the cause of the child's symptoms. Similarly, a child with migratory polyarthritis might reasonably be expected to undergo an evaluation of arthritis, including plain radiographs of affected joints, complete blood count, rheumatoid factor titer, antinuclear antibody titer (ANA), and complement levels. In summary, the diagnostic evaluation in the emergency department is often influenced by the need to exclude other disease processes that share common features with this generalized vasculitis. When the entire clinical picture presents itself, however, the extent of the diagnostic workup is much reduced.

Children with Henoch-Schönlein purpura are admitted to the hospital when the diagnosis is in doubt, for observation and control of abdominal pain, for monitoring of renal function, and for fluid hydration in the setting of recurrent emesis. Children with extremely mild symptoms can be safely and expectantly observed as outpatients, as long as an experienced primary care provider is available. Arthritis, when present as an isolated symptom, is usually easily controlled with aspirin. Prednisone is not utilized in the management of arthritis when it represents the child's only symptom of active vasculitis. The child's primary care physician maintains contact with the family on a daily basis and evaluates the child in the office at frequent intervals in the initial weeks following the establishment of the diagnosis. Particular attention is directed to the development of symptoms suggestive of abdominal colic, gastrointestinal hemorrhage, intussusception, and the development of chronic renal disease. Chronic renal sequelae are reported in approximately 7 to 9 percent of children with Henoch-Schönlein purpura and do not respond well to glucocorticoid therapy.

## Acute Rheumatic Fever

An acute inflammatory disease affecting widely disparate organ systems, acute rheumatic fever (ARF) primarily affects children of school age. The incidence of ARF has steadily fallen in developed countries, although outbreaks regularly are reported in North America. It is preceded by infection with certain strains of group A β-hemolytic streptococcus (mucoid types 3, 5, and 18). Different layers of the cell wall of the streptococcal organism appear to stimulate antibody production to variable host tissues. The hallmark histologic feature of rheumatic fever is the Aschoff body, found in the connective tissue and created by edematous, fragmented collagen fibers. The connective tissue of the heart, joints, central nervous system, and subcutaneous tissues and skin are targeted by the immune reaction. The carditis is an endomyocarditis, with valvulitis primarily involving the mitral and aortic valves. The arthritis is characterized by synovial edema and periarticular swelling with joint effusions.

The child develops the disorder 2 to 6 weeks following a streptococcal pharyngitis. While nonspecific symptoms of systemic illness predominate early on, physical examination eventually reveals evidence of arthritis, carditis, choreiform movements, erythema marginatum, or subcutaneous nodules, individually or in combination. Jones' criteria for establishing a diagnosis of acute rheumatic fever are illustrated in Table 118-5. Either two major criteria or one major and two minor criteria plus evidence of an antecedent streptococcal infection are necessary to establish the diagnosis.

Arthritis (occurring in 60 to 75 percent of initial attacks) is characterized as a migratory, fleeting polyarticular arthritis primarily affecting the large joints. The carditis occurs in a third of new cases and may be mild or severe. Its presence is heralded by any combination of a new cardiac murmur, tachycardia, a gallop rhythm, a pericardial friction rub, congestive heart failure, or a hyperactive precordium. Sydenham's chorea occurs in 10 percent of cases and may have its initial appearance months following a streptococcal infection. Chorea may be the sole manifestation of acute rheumatic fever. The skin rash of acute rheumatic fever (erythema marginatum) is described as serpiginous and persists only for several days. It usually coexists with the presence of carditis in some form. Subcutaneous nodules are more rare and are located on the extensor surfaces of the wrists, elbows, and knees. The greatest morbidity and mortality is associated with the development of carditis.

Diagnostic studies are utilized to clarify the associated antecedent infection by group A streptococcus (a pharyngeal swab for culture, antistreptolysin titers, or streptozyme titers), or are employed to identify and assess the presence and extent of carditis. An ECG is obtained to assess for conduction delays or hypertrophy. A chest x-ray serves to identify cardiac dilatation or pulmonary vascular congestion or edema. Echocardiography is utilized to identify evidence of

**Table 118-5.** Revised Jones' Criteria for the Diagnosis of Acute Rheumatic Fever

| Major | Minor |
|---|---|
| Carditis | Fever |
|   New or changing murmurs |   Arthralgia |
|   Cardiomegaly, congestive |   History of previous attack of ARF |
|     heart failure |   Elevated ESR, C-reactive protein |
|   Pericarditis |   Prolonged PR interval on ECG |
| Migratory polyarthritis |   Rising titer of antistreptococcal |
| Chorea |     antibodies |
| Erythema marginatum | |
| Subcutaneous nodules | |

*Diagnosis is likely when two major criteria or one major and two minor criteria are met. Group A* Streptococcus *may be documented by a history of scarlet fever, isolation of group A* Streptococcus *from throat culture, or rising titers of antistreptococcal antibodies.*

valvulitis or valvular insufficiency and also to exclude other diagnostic considerations.

The differential diagnosis includes juvenile rheumatoid arthritis (JRA), septic arthritis, Kawasaki syndrome, viral or other forms of cardiomyopathy, leukemias, and other forms of vasculitis, including drug reactions. Rarely, tumors of the central nervous system require differentiation from ARF when the child's sole clinical manifestation is chorea.

Treatment of ARF in the emergency department is directed primarily toward the management of complicating features of carditis. In the absence of cardiac or hemodynamic instability (and such is the rule), early consultation with a pediatric cardiologist is recommended, and admission to the hospital is generally advised in the early stages until the diagnosis is confirmed. Arthritis is managed with high-dose aspirin therapy (75 to 100 mg/kg per day) in order to effect a serum salicylate level in the range of 20 to 30 mg/dL. The aspirin dose is reduced after approximately 1 week to 50 mg/kg per day for an additional 4 to 6 weeks. Significant carditis or congestive heart failure is managed with glucocorticoids, usually in the form of prednisone in a dose of 1 to 2 mg/kg per day. This is continued for 2 weeks following the resolution of symptoms and the return of the ESR to normal. The duration of glucocorticoid therapy requires a subsequent taper of the steroids over a 4 to 6 week period. Chorea can be managed with haloperidol, 0.01 to 0.03 mg/kg per day in four divided doses. All children with ARF are treated with penicillin, even if the cultures for group A streptococcus are negative. Benzathine penicillin G can be administered in a single dosage of 1.2 MU. Alternatively, procaine penicillin G, 600,000 U, can be administered daily for 10 days. Penicillin V, 25,000 to 50,000 U/kg per day divided into four doses and administered orally, is also effective. Erythromycin may be substituted for the penicillin-allergic patient. All therapy, if pursued, is administered for 10 days. Long-term prophylactic therapy against group A streptococcus is begun upon completion of the acute phase of therapy. Acceptable prophylactic regimens include benzathine penicillin G, 1.2 MU administered intramuscularly every month, penicillin V, 200,000 U administered orally twice daily, or sulfadiazine, 1 g administered orally each day. The duration of required prophylactic therapy is incompletely understood, but 5 years of prophylactic antibiotics for those children without cardiac involvement represents the minimum. Patients with manifestations of carditis are placed on life-long prophylactic antibiotic regimens.

### Juvenile Rheumatoid Arthritis

Juvenile rheumatoid arthritis (JRA) is not a single entity; rather, it encompasses a group of disorders characterized by chronic noninfectious synovitis and arthritis and is associated with a wide range of systemic manifestations. The hypothetical etiology of the arthritis is that of an autoimmune response to a number of antigens not yet completely identified.

*Pauciarticular* disease is the most common form of the disease in children. It usually involves a single large joint, typically the knee. Serology for rheumatoid factor is negative, while ANA titers are positive in 90 percent of patients. Extraarticular manifestations of this form of the disease include the development of iridocyclitis, Reiter's syndrome, and inflammatory bowel disease. Ultimate joint damage occurs only infrequently.

*Polyarticular* disease occurs in approximately a third of cases. Rheumatoid factor (RF) serology may be positive or negative, while ANA titers are positive in 25 percent of the RF-negative patients and 75 percent of RF-positive patients. There is a female preponderance, and both large and small joints may be affected. Contrary to the case in pauciarticular JRA, long-term morbidity with polyarticular disease is related to progressive joint destruction, particularly of the hips and knees.

*Systemic* JRA is the least common presentation, occurring in only

about 20 percent of children with the disease. This form is associated with the particularly high fevers commonly associated with the disease, which characteristically produces one or two fever spikes per day exceeding 39.5°C, and is often associated with shaking chills. In addition, there are other prominent extraarticular manifestations of the disease including a pale, erythematous coalescing macular rash, primarily on the trunk but also present in other areas including palms and soles. Hepatosplenomegaly, pleuritis, and pericarditis are common. Serology for RF and ANA are negative. The arthritis of systemic JRA may progress substantially, leading to joint destruction in as many as a quarter of patients.

Laboratory evaluations associated with the disease are not highly specific for JRA. Arthrocentesis is often necessary to exclude acute suppurative arthritis, particularly in pauciarticular presentations. Initially, radiographs demonstrate only soft tissue swelling and synovial effusions. The findings associated with bone and joint damage occur later.

Emergency department management focuses primarily upon excluding other diagnostic considerations, especially in children who have not previously received a confirmed diagnosis of JRA. Hospital admission is recommended for those children in whom the diagnosis is in doubt or who are to be treated empirically for suspected acute suppurative arthritis while synovial fluid cultures are pending.

Initial therapy for those with an established diagnosis includes aspirin at a dosage of 80 to 125 mg/kg per day, with careful monitoring of salicylate levels to maintain a therapeutic level between 20 and 30 mg/dL. Other nonsteroidal anti-inflammatory drugs are becoming increasingly popular.

The use of glucocorticoids should be reserved for use exclusively in those patients in whom the diagnosis is categorically certain and whose systemic JRA symptoms are proved unresponsive to aspirin. They are also utilized in the management of decompensated pericarditis or myocarditis and in the management of unresponsive iridocyclitis. Other management strategies including intraarticular glucocorticoid injections and the use of gold, chloroquine, or cytosine should be orchestrated by a pediatric rheumatologist.

### BIBLIOGRAPHY

Rowely AH, Gonzalez-Cruzzi F, Shylman ST: Kawasaki syndrome. *Adv Pediatr* 38:51, 74, 1991.

Swischuk LE: Radiographic signs of skeletal trauma, in Ludwig S, Kornberg AE (eds): *Child Abuse,* 2d ed. New York, Churchill Livingstone, pp 151–174, 1992.

Tachdjian MO: *Pediatric Orthopedics,* 2d ed. Philadelphia, Saunders, 1990.

Tolo VT, Wood B: *Pediatric Orthopedics in Primary Care.* Baltimore, Williams & Wilkins, 1994.

Warren RW, Perez MD, Wilking AP, Myones BL: Pediatric rheumatic diseases. *Pediatr Clin North Am* 41(4):783, 1994.

## 119
# EVALUATING THE HANDICAPPED OR DISABLED CHILD

### Cheryl H. Hack

There are about 7 million children in the United States who have conditions that impair their ability to function physically or mentally. Some disabilities and handicaps may be medically distinct and self-limited, such as limb deformities, hearing impairments, or spastic diplegia. Others are multidimensional, consisting of multiple medical problems such as meningomyelocele or severe mental impairment with associated severe cerebral palsy. Impaired neurologic functioning, orthopedic deformity, and chronic illness with multiple system involvement results in complex medical problems and greater likelihood that an individual will encounter difficulties and require emergency evaluation and treatment. Caring for handicapped or disabled children in the emergency department can be a difficult task due to complex ongoing medical problems, limited historical information, altered baseline functioning, and/or the need for the emergency physician to consider the impact of interventions on the course of the underlying disability or impairment.

Evaluating the child with handicapping or disabling conditions in the emergency department requires more time. Patience in obtaining a good history will assist the physician in decision-making. Knowledge of specific medical problems associated with various handicapping or disabling conditions will help to focus the history and examination. Identification of management issues will allow the physician to design interventions that benefit the child and the family in both the long and short term.

Obtaining a medical history in the emergency department can be difficult, even with a normally healthy child. Obtaining a medical history in a disabled or handicapped child provides even more challenges. A medical condition of importance may not be reported because it is under treatment and is not currently creating any difficulty for the individual (e.g., neurogenic bowel or bladder). Information regarding the use of assistive devices such as braces, hearing aides, glasses, or prosthetics may not be offered because the family does not realize that this may give the physician information needed for making treatment decisions. Directed questioning may be necessary to avoid difficulties.

While obtaining the medical history, attempt to identify all existing medical conditions. Medications currently being used can be helpful in this task. A list of medications commonly used in cerebral palsy is given in Table 119-1. Information regarding the use of assistive devices may be important in management issues. Ask specifically about bracing, hearing aids, glasses, and use of suppositories and enemas. Hearing aids in a child with external otitis media or perforated tympanic membrane must be a consideration. Braces or night splints must be considered when lacerations or skin lesions are present. Children with complex medical problems may receive a variety of medical procedures in the home setting, including suctioning, nebulizer treatments, chest percussion and drainage, clean intermittent catheterization, and fecal disimpactions. Knowledge of these home-based procedures will help in making decisions regarding hospitalization and/or further home treatment. Associated medical conditions may impact development of a differential diagnosis. Use information from the medical conditions associated with individual disorders described below to guide your questioning regarding associated medical problems.

**Table 119-1.** Medications Commonly Used in Cerebral Palsy

| Generic Name (Brand Name) | Most Common Side Effects |
| --- | --- |
| Baclofen (Lioresal) | Drowsiness, dizziness, weakness, confusion, headache, insomnia, hypotension, nausea, constipation, urinary frequency |
| Clonidine (Catapres) | Drowsiness, dry mouth, orthostatic hypotension, nausea and vomiting, anxiety, depression, sleep disturbance, nocturia, rash |
| Dantrolene (Dantrium) | Drowsiness, dizziness, weakness, diarrhea, constipation |
| Diazepam (Valium) | Drowsiness, ataxia, weakness, confusion, constipation, dysarthria, diplopia, rash, urinary retention |

## CEREBRAL PALSY

Cerebral palsy is a disorder of movement and posture due to static, nonprogressive injury sustained by the developing brain. It occurs in 2 to 4 per 1000 individuals. The movement problems manifest themselves in a variety of forms and can affect the head, trunk, and extremities in a variety of ways. Cerebral palsy is commonly classified by type, distribution, and degree of involvement. Types include spastic, dyskinetic (choreoathetoid), hypotonic, and mixed forms. Distribution relates to the involvement of the extremities. Diplegia, hemiplegia, and quadriplegia are the most common. Rarely one sees a child with monoplegia, paraplegia, or triplegia. Severity is rated subjectively as mild, moderate, or severe.

Children with cerebral palsy can have other associated medical problems as a direct effect or complication of motor dysfunction or underlying brain damage. Seizures, oral motor dysfunction, gastroesophageal reflux, constipation, urinary tract infections, pneumonia, wheezing, hearing loss, strabismus, visual impairments, scoliosis, contractures, and hip dislocation or subluxation are all seen with increased frequency in children with cerebral palsy. Children with less severe presentations have minimal associated medical problems. As the severity of impairment increases, the incidence and severity of associated problems and need for emergency medical treatment also increase.

In managing the child with cerebral palsy in the emergency department, special attention should be given to seizures, respiratory tract problems, fluid status, nutritional status, and bracing and skin problems.

### Seizures

Seizures are present in 50 percent of children with cerebral palsy. With increasing severity of cerebral palsy there are often more frequent and complex seizures. Multiple seizure types may occur in a single individual. This may cause difficulty in eliciting a complete seizure history if the physician is unaware that different seizure presentations are documented historically. Multiple anticonvulsant medications may be required to adequately control seizures. When multiple anticonvulsants are required, the physician should be alert to the possibility of multiple seizure types, interactions of the various anticonvulsant medications, and the possible fragility of seizure control. Contact with the managing neurologist is strongly advised in such cases. The treatment of medical problems should be evaluated with regard to drug-drug interactions whenever a medication is recommended. Anticonvulsant medications may affect or be affected by many other drugs. Theophylline is known to lower seizure threshold, and erythromycin may elevate drug levels into the toxic range. Further information on emergent seizure management in the child is available in Chap. 113.

### Pulmonary Problems

Respiratory tract symptoms are common, with chronic congestion and recurrent wheezing. Recurrent pneumonia has long been a recognized problem, often associated with aspiration. Respiratory tract problems are generally related to oral motor dysfunction and gastroesophageal reflux. Oral motor dyspraxia presents with exaggerated gag and retained bite reflexes, tongue thrust, and oral hypersensitivity, which can lead to choking, gagging, and aspiration. Oropharyngeal incoordination manifests early with poor feeding and failure to thrive and contributes to aspiration. Gastroesophageal reflux is often associated with esophagitis and aspiration. Pneumonia is generally due to aspiration and may be observed for resolution; however, it is frequently treated because of the tendency for bacterial superinfection. See Chap. 110 for management of pneumonia.

Wheezing is a more difficult problem. Children who were premature and had respiratory difficulties at the time of birth are known to have reactive airways and need to be treated appropriately with bronchodilators. However, some of the children may be wheezing due to reactive airways triggered by aspiration of minute quantities of saliva, food, or gastric fluid. The respiratory tract may be responding to a potential threat, and in this case treatment with a bronchodilator may not be the most desirable or most effective treatment.

Management of wheezing and aspiration in the emergent situation starts with an assessment of the contribution of aspiration. A simple, initial evaluation should investigate the effect of positioning in severely affected individuals with impaired head control. Placing the head and neck in the "sniffer" position to maximize the airway and minimize the risk of secretions pooling in the posterior pharynx may improve respiratory functioning by decreasing aspiration. Further evaluation for gastroesophageal reflux and aspiration will require multiple radiographic studies and should be done either in the outpatient setting or, if the respiratory distress is severe, on an inpatient basis following resolution of the immediate distress. Medications to decrease reflux or secretions may be helpful. If significant impairment of air movement is compromising the patient, bronchodilators may be used with caution, remembering that if the wheezing is due to aspiration there may be little to no improvement. In such cases reconsideration of treatment options is always warranted. Children will need to be hospitalized if secondary pneumonia is suspected or if respiratory compromise is evident.

## Constipation

Constipation occurs secondary to increased tone and impairment of sphincter relaxation. It may be accompanied by rectal tears, overflow diarrhea, and anorexia. Getting an accurate history is important in the diagnosis of constipation. Families frequently complain of constipation if the child cries, strains, or does not have a bowel movement daily. Constipation is hard balls of stool even if that occurs on a daily basis. There is no constipation if the stools are soft even if the child cries, appears to strain, or does not have a daily stool. Emergent management of constipation is by suppository if the problem is of brief duration or with an enema if long-standing or if fecal material can be palpated in the abdomen. Saline, fleets, or oil-based enemas may be used. If constipation is of long duration, a home program will be needed. Contact with the treating physician or a gastroenterologist will most likely be needed.

In children with recurring constipation, avoid the routine use of fleets enemas so as to prevent electrolyte abnormalities. Avoid chronic use of oral mineral oil because it causes impaired absorption of fat-soluble essential vitamins. If a home program has been developed with frequent use of these products, electrolytes should be monitored and vitamin deficiency syndromes may need to be considered.

## Growth Failure

Growth failure may be a problem in the child with cerebral palsy. Increased energy requirements accompanied by difficulty in handling food in the oral cavity combine to cause growth failure. Chronic failure to thrive decreases energy and strength to accomplish motor tasks and coordinate movement and may impair immunologic functioning. Energy requirements in the young child with cerebral palsy may be increased to 140 to 160 kcal/kg per day. Along with difficulties in growth there may be a marginal or deficient fluid load. When the child with failure to thrive and limited fluid status develops a routine gastroenteritis, dehydration and nutritional status become major difficulties. Some of these children dehydrate with minimal diarrhea and have difficulty maintaining hydration until the diarrhea resolves. Hospitalization decisions should be based on the history of diarrhea, hydration status of the patient in relation to the amount of diarrhea reported, and baseline nutritional status. The further below the 5th percentile for weight a child is, the greater the concern that the child cannot be orally hydrated if diarrhea or vomiting persist. When rapid dehydration occurs in the malnourished individual with limited hydration as the baseline, intravenous access may be a problem. If an IV cannot be placed successfully, interosseus line placement should be considered. In addition to treatment with fluid boluses, full feeds should be continued.

## Enuresis

Enuresis, or incontinence, may persist due to motor and mental difficulties. In the severely impaired child, as with infants, urinary tract infections should be considered in the uncomfortable, ill-appearing child without clear evidence of other infectious sources. An increased incidence of urinary tract infections has been observed without evidence of urinary tract abnormalities. This has been ascribed to hygiene issues in the past, though a neurogenic bladder with urinary retention should be ruled out. A urinalysis should be done, with care taken to limit external contamination. Contractures of the hips and tight adductors make it difficult at times to clean the vaginal and perineal areas. Referral for radiologic studies to rule out anomalies of the urinary tract is recommended. Most urinary tract infections can be managed on an outpatient basis. If pyelonephritis is suspected, a urology consultation and hospitalization should be considered.

## Sensory Problems

Problems with vision and hearing are common and do not generally cause any difficulty on an emergent basis. Hearing loss is present in 5 to 15 percent of children with hemiplegia. In addition there may be conductive losses in children who are bottle-fed in a supine position. Visual problems include strabismus, hyperopia, cataracts (congenital infections), retinopathy of prematurity, and cortical blindness.

## Contractures and Fractures

Contractures of the extremities are one of the most commonly perceived difficulties of children with cerebral palsy. Subluxed or dislocated hips are seen frequently and may cause pain and arthritis over time. The routine treatment for the pain is the same as for degenerative arthritis. Bracing is used for management of contractures and should be closely evaluated when wounds are sustained in braced areas. Bracing will hold the joint in a different position, and areas of skin tension will change with bracing. Placement of sutures or dressings may be affected by the brace or the altered position of an extremity without a brace. Friction from the brace could impair wound healing, increase the chance of infection, and create new wounds due to the pressure of the brace if proper assessment and attention to the brace is not part of the management. Removal of a brace may be required in early wound management unless a tension problem will complicate management more. Similar problems may occur with serial casting procedures.

Osteopenia frequently develops in bones secondary to disuse and nutritional issues. Fractures occur more easily in osteopenic bones. Children with limited movement and osteopenia may sustain fractures without excessive force being used. Lifting or moving an older child may cause fractures when osteopenia is present. Stretching and range-of-motion exercises used to prevent the development of contractures can also result in fractures if the person doing them is unaware of osteopenia and uses an aggressive stance for therapy. Fractures may present with discomfort and swelling of an extremity and should be considered in the irritable, severely impaired child. Fractures may be treated with casting if the child has and uses voluntary movement, but soft wraps may be used in the child with significantly limited voluntary movement. Displaced fractures are uncommon, and forceful activity is generally involved. Routine handling and therapy are generally not associated with this type of injury. Consultation with an orthopedic surgeon and hospitalization may be required.

## Scoliosis

Scoliosis is present in children with quadriplegia and may contribute to respiratory tract problems due to restrictive phenomena. Skin problems may also develop under braces, requiring modification of the brace. Referral for orthopedic management may be required to evaluate the brace, particularly if it is new or very old.

## MENINGOMYELOCELE (MYELOMENINGOCELE)

Meningomyelocele is the most common congenital defect of the neural tube. The spinal cord, meninges, and vertebral column are involved due to failure of the neural tube to fuse in early embryogenesis. It causes varying amounts of sensory and motor impairment based on the level of the lesion and accompanying medical problems. Incidence is 0.7 per 1000 live births in the United States. Etiology is considered to be multifactorial, although folic acid deficiency has been associated. Folic acid is currently recommended as a supplement as early as possible during pregnancy. Other neural tube defects are anencephaly, encephalocele, lipomeningocele, spina bifida occulta, sacral agenesis, and meningocele.

Children with meningomyelocele have multiple, complex medical problems due to impairment of nerves at or below the site of the lesion. There is variable impairment of sensory and motor nerves controlling voluntary and autonomic functioning. Associated medical concerns include neurogenic bowel and bladder function, contractures, scoliosis, club feet, hydrocephalus, Chiari II malformation, tethering of the spinal cord, spinal cord syrinx, vesicoureteral reflux, decubitus ulcers, constipation, encopresis, recurrent urinary tract infections, growth failure, latex allergy, gastroesophageal reflux, apnea/stridor syndrome, seizures, partial agenesis of the corpus callosum, strabismus, visual acuity impairment, precocious puberty, and osteoporosis. Individuals may also have cognitive impairments. Mild forms of cognitive impairment may affect visual motor functioning. More severe cognitive impairment has been associated with sparing of verbal skills and a "cocktail party" syndrome, in which the children may be able to carry on superficial social conversations with ease but be unable to comprehend and utilize specific information provided to them or respond to specific questions.

## Hydrocephalus

Hydrocephalus is present in 70 to 90 percent of children with thoracic or lumbar level defects and in substantial numbers of those with sacral level defects. It is routinely treated with shunt placement early in life. Concerns regarding shunt function are common in patients presenting to the acute care setting. Signs and symptoms of shunt malfunction are lethargy, irritability, nausea, vomiting, visual problems, cognitive changes, neck pain, headache, swelling along the shunt path, or seizure. Not all symptoms need be present to indicate malfunction of the shunt. The symptomatology is nonspecific and can easily be due to a variety of other problems such as sepsis, urinary tract infection, otitis media, gastroenteritis, sinus infection, or viral syndromes. A number of children with massive constipation and a shunt may complain of similar symptomatology, which resolves when the fecal backup is relieved. Evaluation for shunt malfunction should proceed only after infectious and other causes have been eliminated. Preliminary studies for a malfunctioning shunt include a shunt survey (radiographs of the skull, chest, and abdomen) to evaluate connections and the shunt position and head CT to assess ventricular size and position of the proximal end in the ventricle. If questions remain, a shunt tap should be utilized to evaluate opening pressures and assess for infection. If inconclusive, a shunt clearance study with dye or radioisotope may provide additional information regarding flow through the system. Shunt taps should be done by neurosurgical staff when they are available, unless respiratory or cardiac compromise appear to be life-threatening.

## Urinary Tract Problems

Urinary tract problems were at one time a primary cause of morbidity and mortality in children with meningomyelocele. Neurogenic bladder with chronic retention from dyssynergia, overflow incontinence, dribbling incontinence from an open bladder neck, vesicoureteral reflux, renal calculi, and urinary tract infections are common problems in this population. Children may be on prophylactic antibiotics, oxybutynin, or imipramine in an attempt to eliminate infections, minimize upper tract damage, and assist in the development of urinary continence. The side effects of the latter two are given in Table 119-2. Urinary tract colonization has been described in 60 to 70 percent of this population, and in the absence of vesicoureteral reflux treatment is reserved for those with symptomatic urinary tract infection. Use of nitrofurantoin, trimethoprim/sulfamethoxazole, or amoxicillin is advised until culture results are available, to minimize development of resistant strains of bacteria. Prior to treating an infection it is important to know what antibiotics are currently in use. If broad-spectrum antibiotics have been utilized recently, there is an increased potential for a monilial infection.

Clean intermittent catheterization is utilized to increase continence and manage urinary retention. When used with good technique, it does not increase the incidence of urinary tract infection. On rare occasions, false channels are formed with catheterization. When this occurs, special catheters such as coudé (curved tip) catheters may be used to facilitate catheterization and minimize the chance of further trauma. It is wise to question the family regarding catheterization, catheter size, and special types of catheters that may be used. Use of indwelling catheters with balloons is not recommended due to problems with latex allergies (see below).

Intractable incontinence may be present due to severe bladder neck or sphincter deficiency and/or a noncompliant, high-pressure, low-capacity bladder. Reconstructive surgery such as bladder augmentation, bladder neck sling, artificial urinary sphincter, or collagen injections to the bladder neck may be required to provide continence and an adequate bladder capacity. Bladder augmentation has been widely used to increase the bladder capacity of some children with small hyperreflexic bladders. Any individual with a bladder augmentation who presents with abdominal pain should be evaluated for rupture of the bladder. Symptoms of bladder rupture include abdominal pain, which may radiate to the shoulder; abdominal distension; and shock. This is a life-threatening event requiring vascular support, antibiotic prophylaxis, and immediate operation. If this is suspected, the urologist should be contacted immediately.

A small number of children may develop renal calculi. If a small stone is being passed, symptomatic treatment for severe pain is required. Larger stones and asymptomatic stones should be noted, and follow-up with the child's urologist is recommended.

## Chiari II Malformation

Chiari II malformation is present in the majority of children with meningomyelocele. Chiari II malformation consists of malformation of the cerebellum, hindbrain, and brainstem. Aqueductal stenosis is commonly associated. Symptomatic Chiari malformation is characterized by apnea, vocal cord paralysis, stridor, oral motor dysfunc-

**Table 119-2.** Medications Commonly Used in Meningomyelocele

| Generic Name (Brand Name) | Most Common Side Effects |
|---|---|
| Oxybutynin (Ditropan) Propantheline (Pro-Banthine) | Dry mouth, blurred vision, gastrointestinal intolerance, fever, flushing |
| Imipramine (Janimine, Tofranil) | Nervousness, sleep disorders, tiredness, mild GI disturbances, constipation, seizures, anxiety, syncope |

tion, visual dysfunction, and upper limb weakness and incoordination in the infant. In older children it presents with visual dysfunction, motor incoordination, headache, and hand weakness. Even mild cervical hyperflexion–extension injuries may result in symptoms. Of greatest concern is the young child or infant who presents to the emergency department with stridor and meningomyelocele. Suspicion of a Chiari malformation should be present, and evaluation should be ordered on an expedited basis. Stridor may be associated with vocal cord paralysis and may proceed to complete airway obstruction in a small number of patients. Evaluation is by MRI of the craniocervical junction. When significant respiratory compromise is associated with Chiari II malformation, tracheostomy may be required. For children with severe respiratory compromise, immediate hospitalization is required. If respiratory tract function is not severely impaired and the process is static by history, a case-by-case decision should be made regarding hospitalization based on availability of prompt outpatient services from neurosurgery, otorhinolaryngology, and radiology for MRI.

### Spinal Cord Tethering

Tethering of the spinal cord can occur as the child grows. Tethering may present as ataxia, loss of functional motor level, a change in urinary continence (new-onset incontinence in a child who had previously been dry on a bladder program), or new-onset orthopedic deformities of the lower extremities. For the child who presents with increasing urinary incontinence with no evidence of an acute urinary tract infection, a neurosurgical consult should be considered. This is generally not an emergency, although it should be evaluated promptly in an office setting.

### Skin Problems

Burns and pressure sores are seen in insensate areas with increased frequency. Burns occur and can be quite severe due to a lack of protective response triggered by pain. Evaluation and management of burns is covered in Chap. 168. Pressure sores are frequent due to a lack of sensation. Common areas for pressure sores are under braces and in the sacral and ischial regions. Caution should be used in evaluation of pressure sores as healthy-appearing tissue may overlie abscesses or infected tracts extending proximally toward bony structures deep to them. When infections track deep, osteomyelitis may develop, requiring hospitalization, surgical debridement, long-term intravenous antibiotic therapy and management of the skin surface.

Open areas should be carefully evaluated for evidence of tracts. Other wounds proximate to a pressure ulcer should be carefully documented with a suspicion that they may be connected by tracts. Evaluation should include probing for tracts, looking for undermined areas, obtaining radiographs to assess bony changes of osteomyelitis, and an erythrocyte sedimentation rate (ESR). If cellulitis or bone changes are identified, consider admission for institution of intravenous antibiotics and a more complete evaluation of bone involvement. Simple pressure ulcers without evidence of infection or extension can be treated successfully with local measures and pressure relief. Superficial wounds can be treated with sulfadiazine or duoderm wafers. Deeper wounds require wet-to-dry or gel dressings. Sulfadiazine, wet-to-dry dressings, and gel dressings are changed two to four times daily. Duoderm wafers are left in place for up to 3 days at a time if they remain dry and intact. Ulcers below braces require discontinuation of the bracing for 3 to 6 weeks to allow healing to occur. Ulcers on the buttocks require staying in a prone or supine position, with all pressure off the wound.

Additionally, the physician should check to ensure that a pressure relief system is intact and functioning to prevent future skin breakdown. For wheelchair users, cushions to relieve pressure are advised. Air-filled ROHO cushions, gel cushions, and foam cushions are available and utilized extensively for this purpose. Children are also instructed in wheelchair push-ups to change their position in the chair. Watches with alarms that can be set to go off every 15 to 20 min are advised to remind the individual to do a push-up.

### Bowel Problems

Neurogenic bowel is often seen, with resulting fecal incontinence, encopresis, or constipation. Many children are on a routine bowel management program in an attempt to achieve fecal continence. Bowel problems may present in the emergency department in a number of atypical ways. Children with shunted hydrocephalus often present with complaints of headache or shunt malfunction. This may be due to significant intraabdominal pressure from fecal retention, which may be transmitted via the shunt to the head. Abdominal discomfort may also be a presenting complaint, but frequently the child and family will deny any bowel problems or constipation. Even in children with daily stools, severe fecal stasis may develop due to impaired peristalsis. The child who presents with intermittent diarrhea may also have fecal stasis and buildup with overflow incontinence.

Bowel management techniques in the home include dietary manipulation, karo syrup in feeds, Senokot, Dulcolax, glycerin suppositories, or a variety of enemas. Due to the chronic nature of this difficulty, mineral oil and fleets enemas are not routinely used. This is to minimize the chance of families repeatedly using preparations that may cause vitamin deficiency or metabolic disturbances with frequent, ongoing use.

When constipation or fecal stasis is a consideration, a flat plate of the abdomen is helpful in clarifying the problem. Constipation of significant proportion can be handled by a high enema, suppository, or manual disimpaction. High enema is often the most effective. Difficulties may be encountered due to poor rectal tone and the inability of the child to retain an enema or suppository voluntarily. Families who routinely use enemas may have adapters to assist in the retention of an enema. When constipation or fecal stasis is the problem, there is generally no need for hospitalization. Following an initial clean-out procedure in the emergency department, the child can be discharged. Follow-up with the general pediatrician, a comprehensive spina bifida program with specialists knowledgeable about bowel management, or an enterostomal therapist to arrange an ongoing bowel management program is advised.

### Sexual Abuse

Sexual abuse questions may come up on occasion in children with meningomyelocele. Care must be taken in the assessment because rectal tone is often impaired and a patulous anus may result. Rectal tears and prolapse may also be present in the child with constipation.

### Latex Allergy

Latex allergy is becoming a concern in children and adults with meningomyelocele. Increasingly severe allergic-type reactions are being reported related to latex and latex-containing products. Reactions vary from mild local reactions to anaphylaxis. Children may present with local or generalized swelling, hives or edema, itching, or a rash. Runny nose or eyes, coughing, sneezing, wheezing, stridor, and difficulty swallowing or breathing may also be presenting complaints. A history of latex allergy or sensitivity should be obtained in all children with meningomyelocele prior to any examination or procedure in which latex gloves or other latex-containing supplies may be utilized. Many routine medical supplies contain latex, including frequently used supplies on the crash cart. (See Table 119-3 for a list of latex-containing supplies.) Many programs are recommending that identification bands be worn by children with meningomyelocele and latex allergy. If a severe allergic reaction is observed, the child should be discharged with an Epi-Pen, and formal testing for latex sensitivity should be done in the private physician's office. All surgeons providing care and the local anesthesiologist should be noti-

**Table 119-3.** Latex-Containing Supplies and Alternatives

| Latex-Containing Supplies | Latex-Free Alternatives or Adaptations |
|---|---|
| Airways, masks and straps | Hudson, Vital Signs airways, masks |
| Ambu bag (black reusable) | Clear bags (Respironics, Laerdal) |
| Anesthesia bags, tubing | Neoprene bag |
| Band-Aids | Sterile dressing with plastic tape |
| Blood pressure cuff | Use over clothing or stockinette, Clean Cuff (Vital Signs) |
| Bulb syringe | |
| Catheters, condom | Silicone (Mentor, Coloplast) |
| Catheters, indwelling Foley—even silicone may have a latex balloon | Silicone (Kendall, Argyle, Bard) |
| Catheter leg bags straps | Velcro, nylon (Mentor, Dale) |
| Catheters, straight | Mentor, Bard, Coloplast, MMG |
| Catheters, urodynamics | Bard, Rush, Cook |
| Catheters, rectal pressure | Cover latex balloons, use vinyl glove |
| Condoms, diaphragms | Polyurethane, tachylon Natural skin over/under latex condom |
| Crutches—axillary, hand pads | Cover with stockinette |
| Disposable diapers | Huggies, Pampers |
| Dressings—Moleskin (Johnson & Johnson), Coban (3M) | Tegaderm, Duoderm, Steri-strip, Reston foam liner, Comfeel, Xerofoam, PinCare, Bioclusive, Webrill |
| Elastic bandages, Ace wrap (brown), Esmarch | TEDS, Baxter elastic bandages, white cotton Ace wrap |
| Electrode pads | Baxter, Conmed EKG, Dantec EMG |
| Endotracheal tubes | Plastic tubes (Mallinekrodt, Sheridan, Portex) |
| Feeding nipples | Silicone (Gerber, Evenflo, MAM) |
| Foam rubber lining of braces | Line with cloth, felt |
| Gloves, sterile and exam, surgical and medical | Vinyl, neoprene, polymer gloves: Neolon, Senicare, Tru-touch, Tachylon, Tachyl, Dermaprene, Allergard |
| IV access: injection ports, Y-sites, PRN adapters, needleless systems | Use stopcock to inject medications; cover Y-sites and do not puncture; flush IV tubing before use; Abbott, Baxter, IVAC, Braun tubing; Braun, Clave needleless systems |
| IV bag ports, buretrols | Do not puncture ports to add medications; B. Braun burette |
| Jobst spandex products | Jobst has a nonlatex material |
| OR garb (masks, hats, shoe covers) | Remove elastic bands |
| Medication vials | Remove latex stoppers |
| Pacifiers | Plastic, silicone, and/or vinyl |
| Penrose drains | Jackson-Pratt, Zimmer Hemovac |
| Rubber bed pads (washable) | Disposable underpads |
| Stethoscope tubing | Cover tubing with stockinette |
| Suction catheters | Mallinekrodt, Yankauer, Davol |
| Syringes, disposable | Prepare medication in syringe right before use, or use glass syringes; Abboject, Abbott PCA vials |
| Tape, adhesive | Plastic, silk tape: Microfoam, Micropore, Transpore, Dermaclear, Dermicel, Waterproof |
| Tourniquet | Place over clothing or stockinette: VelcroPedic, Grafco tourniquets |
| Theraband strips and tubes (OT) | Cover with cloth |
| Wheelchair cushions, tires | Neoprene cushions (ROHO), cover seat with fabric, use leather gloves |

fied. This can be done by notifying the local physician or clinic responsible for the child's specialty care.

## Fractures

Fractures occur with increased frequency when the child has osteopenia. Children with fractures to the lower extremity should be evalu-ated for level of sensation. If the child is insensate and paraplegic, casting may not be required. Soft wrapping of the extremity and elevation are the preferred mode of treatment.

## Respiratory Tract Problems

Respiratory tract problems are generally not associated with meningomyelocele other than vocal cord paralysis with Chiari II malformations or the child with severe allergy to latex. Rarely, fibrotic changes in the lung have been associated with oxybutynin usage. If chronic respiratory difficulties are presented in a child on oxybutynin, discontinuation of the drug should be considered along with acute management.

## SPINAL CORD INJURY

Pediatric spinal cord injury is an acute traumatic lesion of the spinal cord and roots resulting in motor and/or sensory deficit occurring between birth and adolescence. About 1100 new pediatric cases occur each year secondary to motor vehicle accidents, sporting accidents, falls, gunshot wounds, and birth trauma.

Spinal cord injury may result in complete or partial loss of neurologic function below the level of the lesion. Pain, heterotopic bone ossification, hypercalcemia, renal calculi, and depression are frequent issues for all children with spinal cord injury. Other associated medical problems are similar to those encountered by children with meningomyelocele. Neurogenic bowel and bladder, decubitus ulcers, spasticity or hypotonicity, gastroesophageal reflux, esophagitis, aspiration, impaired sensation, ureterovesical reflux, scoliosis, contractures, and osteoporosis are common. For children with cervical or thoracic level lesions, respiratory compromise due to impaired phrenic nerves and/or abnormal innervation of abdominal musculature may be present. Autonomic dysreflexia and oral motor dysfunction may also be present. Since many of the issues are well covered in the section on meningomyelocele, this section will cover only the issues specific to spinal cord injuries.

## Autonomic Dysreflexia

Autonomic dysreflexia is dramatic paroxysmal hyperactivity of uninhibited sympathetic and parasympathetic nerves in children with spinal cord lesions proximal to thoracic level 6. It is caused by stimulation below the level of the lesion by bladder overdistension, fecal impaction, skin breakdown, or fractures. Presentation is sweating, flushing, pounding headache, hypertension, bradycardia, and piloerection above the level of the lesion. Death or cerebral vascular accident may result.

Dysreflexia is managed by eliminating the stimulus. Moving the child to a sitting position to take advantage of orthostatic hypotension, discontinuation of procedures in progress, emptying the bladder, disimpaction of the bowel, and normalizing body temperature should be used as required. When disimpaction is required, an anesthetic gel or ointment should be used to minimize afferent stimulation. If positional changes and elimination of the stimulus do not suffice, treatment may require sublingual nifedipine or IM or IV hydralazine. Nitropaste in a 1-in patch may also be applied, if available, for emergency reduction of hypertension. It should be removed immediately when blood pressure returns to normal.

## Pain

Chronic pain described as dysesthesia or paresthesia is common in adolescents with spinal cord injury but infrequent in younger children. Pain is generally managed with analgesic agents. Long-term use of narcotic analgesics is avoided. Heat, relaxation therapy, and hypnosis have also been useful adjuncts. Care must be taken in the emergency room to avoid prescribing of medications that may be abused.

## Heterotopic Bone Formation

Heterotopic bone formation may develop months after spinal cord injuries. It presents with heat, swelling, restricted motion, and pain. Commonly affected joints are the hip, knee, elbow, or shoulder. Ankylosis may develop and make routine activities impossible. This will need to be differentiated from fracture, infection, or other emergent conditions. Management is conservative, with analgesics for pain. Aspirin is sometimes used for prevention of recurrence. When heterotopic bone formation is present, the child and family should be prepared for problems with skin breakdown and secondary infection, which occur rarely.

## Respiratory Dysfunction

Respiratory dysfunction is seen in some children with cervical level lesions. Use of ventilators may be necessary either during the night or full-time. Even in those with no need for early ventilator support, respiratory difficulty may develop due to increasing spasticity of abdominal muscles or muscular fatigue. When children present with respiratory difficulty, attention must be paid to pulmonary toilet, use of assistive devices, and the presence of previous respiratory difficulties or progression of respiratory difficulties. Impaired motor control may result in reflux and aspiration, which may contribute to the difficulties being experienced. Pulmonary consultation, if available, may allow the emergency physician to adjust the ventilator and prevent hospitalization. Children with phrenic nerve stimulators may need to be hospitalized for management.

## Psychiatric and Psychological Problems

Psychiatric and psychological problems develop related to loss of independence and impairments of body image. Depression, severe uncontrolled anger, panic attacks, and temper tantrums can make care of these children difficult. Most difficulties of this type can be handled on an outpatient basis by a psychologist, social worker, or physician experienced in working with this population. For severe depression, suicidal ideation, or other emotional problems that are out of control, hospitalization and/or psychiatric evaluation may be needed.

## DEVELOPMENTAL DISABILITY (MENTAL RETARDATION)

Mental retardation is a substantial limitation in present functioning associated with subaverage intellectual capabilities and limitations in two or more adaptive skill areas (communication, self-care, home living, social skills, community use, self-direction, health and safety, functional academics, leisure, and work). It is a result of injury, disease, metabolic disorder, or other abnormality of the central nervous system occurring before the age of 18. Mental retardation occurs in 2.5 percent of the population. Etiology is known for certain syndromes associated with mental retardation, but the majority of individuals with mental retardation have no clearly identified etiology. Down syndrome, fetal alcohol syndrome, and fragile X syndrome are the most common known etiologies of mental retardation.

Dealing with the mentally retarded child in the emergency department is difficult because of the variety of medical problems that may be encountered and because the individual is often not able to clearly communicate the problem to the physician or the care provider. It is important to be aware that a child or care provider who cannot cooperate with questioning or physical examination may be mentally impaired.

Children with mental retardation have a wide variety of associated medical problems. With increasing severity of mental retardation, there is increased incidence of associated problems. Cerebral palsy, visual deficits, seizure disorders, failure to thrive, hypotonia, gastroesophageal reflux, aspiration, and psychiatric disorders have all been seen in the general population with mental retardation. Mental retardation associated with known syndromes may have diagnosis-specific medical problems such as in Down syndrome, the best known of these syndromes. Listings of diagnosis-specific medical problems can be found in Table 119-4.

## Pulmonary Problems

Respiratory tract symptoms may be seen in severely mentally retarded individuals with chronic congestion and recurrent wheezing. Aspiration pneumonia and respiratory tract problems are generally related to oral motor dysfunction and gastroesophageal reflux. Oral motor dysfunction presents with retained gag and bite reflexes, tongue thrust, and oral hypersensitivity, which can lead to choking, gagging, and aspiration. Pneumonia is generally treated due to the tendency for bacterial superinfection. (See Chap. 110 for management of pneumonia.) Wheezing is a more difficult problem. Children who were premature and had respiratory difficulties at the time of birth are known to have reactive airways and need to be treated appropriately with bronchodilators. However, some children may be wheezing due to reactive airways triggered by aspiration of minute quantities of saliva or refluxed material. The respiratory tract may be responding to a potential threat, and thus treatment with a bronchodilator may not be the most desirable treatment nor the most effective. Evaluation and appropriate management of the aspiration is essential. A simple initial evaluation should investigate the effect of positioning in severely affected individuals with impaired head control. Placing the head and neck in the sniffer position to maximize the airway and minimize the risk of secretions pooling in the posterior pharynx may improve respiratory functioning and decrease aspiration. Aspiration may come from matter in the pharynx or from gastroesophageal reflux. If aspiration is a consideration, a full evaluation will need to be considered. If the problems are not severe, the evaluation may be done on an out-

**Table 119-4.** Medical Conditions Associated with Specific Mental Retardation Syndromes

| | |
|---|---|
| Down syndrome | Atlantoaxial instability leading to spinal cord compression in the cervical region, congenital heart defects, atrioventricular canal defects, atrial septal defects, ventricular septal defects, tetralogy of Fallot, patent ductus arteriosus, pulmonary hypertension, duodenal atresia, tracheoesophageal fistula, Meckel diverticulum, Hirschsprung disease, imperforate anus, obesity, constipation, hypothyroidism, uteropelvic junction obstruction, hydronephrosis, undescended testes, hypospadius, leukemia (acute lymphocytic and nonlymphocytic), chronic serous otitis media, chronic sinus infections, tear duct infections, questionable immunologic dysfunction (thyroiditis), alopecia areata, diabetes, rheumatoid-type arthropathy, autoimmune hemolytic anemia, nystagmus, alternating esotropia, congenital cataracts, glaucoma, keratoconus, blepharitis, conductive hearing loss, obstructive sleep apnea, dental malocclusions, short stature, hypotonia resolving with age, Tourette syndrome, Alzheimer disease |
| Fragile X syndrome | Mitral valve prolapse, seizures, strabismus, frequent ear infections, and self-abusive behaviors |
| Prader-Willi syndrome | Hyperphagia, obesity, hypoventilation, cor pulmonale, NIDDM, scoliosis, strabismus, inability to vomit, decreased sensitivity to pain, seizure disorder, acanthosis nigricans, hypoxia, right sided heart failure, pulmonary hypertension, gastric perforation, obstructive sleep apnea |
| Williams syndrome | Supravalvular aortic stenosis, pulmonic stenosis, coarctation of the aorta, strabismus, joint contractures, hypertension, urethral stenosis, vesicoureteral reflux, constipation, ulcers, and hypercalcemia |
| Rett syndrome | Hyperventilation, breath-holding, air-swallowing, bruxism, ataxia, muscle wasting, poor circulation, scoliosis, seizures, and intermittent flushing |

patient basis. If wheezing is severe and there is respiratory compromise, the child should be admitted and evaluation undertaken when the respiratory status is improved. Studies must be obtained to evaluate the reason for aspiration. A multiple-texture barium swallow and scintigraphic studies of gastric functioning should be ordered.

## Gastroesophageal reflux

Gastroesophageal reflux is often present when tone is low. It may contribute to aspiration problems and can be associated with gastritis and esophagitis. Gastroesophageal reflux may present as emesis, nonspecific irritability, discomfort, or a lack of appetite and may contribute to failure to thrive. When the family complains about emesis, the physician needs to clarify their description; they may be seeing clearing of secretions from the upper airways. In the severely impaired child, "emesis" may be a stimulated gag and cough to clear secretions from the posterior pharynx. True emesis should contain stomach contents. If the child is tube-fed, this will be formula. Often the parent will describe emesis that is composed of mucousy material instead of formula or food.

Evaluation for gastroesophageal reflux is generally not required on an emergent basis, but management information may be useful. Metoclopramide can be used to improve transit time through the stomach when delayed gastric emptying is found on scintigraphic studies of gastric functioning. Ranitidine and other new blocking agents have been used to decrease the acidity of the gastric contents when gastritis or esophagitis are identified. Thickened feedings, positioning, and other techniques have been used with some success but are of questionable assistance in older individuals. In some cases, Nissan fundoplication is required for management of moderate to severe reflux not responsive to medical management.

Children with cognitive impairments may have unusual behaviors such as pica. When indigestible materials are ingested on a routine basis, bezoars may develop consisting of hair, cloth, or other materials. This may also present like reflux due to outlet obstruction. A barium swallow should identify this problem. Surgical removal may be required on an emergent basis. This problem should be evaluated for admission of a case-by-case basis.

## Seizures

Seizures are present in 30 percent of children with mental retardation. With increasing severity of mental retardation there are often increasingly complex seizures. Problems associated with epilepsy are identical to those of children with cerebral palsy described in the section earlier in the chapter. The physician should be alert to the possibility of multiple seizure types, use of multiple anticonvulsants, drug-drug interactions of anticonvulsant medications, and the possible fragility of seizure control. Contact with the managing neurologist is strongly advised in such cases. Further information on emergent seizure management in the child is available in Chap. 113.

## Psychiatric and Behavioral Problems

Psychiatric and behavioral problems combined with limited understanding of what is happening to them and an unfamiliar, overstimulating situation often lead to an uncooperative and at times combative child. The prevalence of major psychiatric disorders and attention deficit disorder is two to three times that of the general population. Stereotypy and self-injurious behavior are seen almost exclusively in the mentally retarded population, with increased incidence in children with the most severe cognitive limitations. Treatment of psychiatric and behavioral disorders is similar to treatment of these disorders in the general population.

The most worrisome problem in the emergency department is self-injurious behaviors. Self-injurious behavior is chronic, repetitive acts that may result in serious medical consequences. Self-injurious behaviors may include head-banging, chewing, hitting, and picking at various body parts. Behavior management, protective strategies, and pharmacologic intervention have all been used with variable success. When dealing with injuries sustained secondary to self-injurious behavior, use protective strategies immediately. Referral to psychiatric, psychological, or developmental services for behavior management and possible pharmacologic intervention is advised. This may be done on an outpatient basis. For children with known problems who are currently being treated for psychiatric disorders or behavioral problems, the side effects of the medications may become an issue. See Table 119-5 for a list of pharmacologic agents and their side effects.

## Down Syndrome

Congenital heart defects occur in 40 to 60 percent of children with Down syndrome. Atrioventricular canal defects, ventricular septal defects, atrial septal defects, tetralogy of Fallot, and patent ductus arteriosus are all reported in this population. Pulmonary hypertension may develop in these children, associated with chronic upper airway obstruction and left-to-right shunts. Congestive heart failure has been described even in children without known heart lesions. Mitral valve prolapse and aortic regurgitation are described in adults but not in children.

Gastrointestinal problems are common, including imperforate anus, pyloric stenosis, tracheoesophageal fistula, and Hirschsprung disease. Due to gastrointestinal malformations, hypotonia, and previous surgeries, partial bowel obstruction and constipation may present as problems in the emergency room.

Atlantoaxial instability and dislocation have been identified and are felt to be related to joint laxity. Spinal cord compression may develop, with neck pain, head tilt, torticollis, frequent staggering or falling, increased deep tendon reflexes, clonus, limb weakness, paresthesias, or hemi- or quadriplegia. Symptomatic children require immediate surgical stabilization.

Recurrent upper respiratory infections, chronic sinusitis, and chronic middle ear effusions are seen in many young children with Down syndrome. These can be treated using standard protocols but should be referred to an otorhinolaryngologist or pulmonologist when they occur repeatedly. Sleep apnea and obstructive apnea are described but are not generally problems in the emergency setting.

A variety of other medical problems may be seen on an emergent basis: hypothyroidism, thyroiditis, leukemia, and transient neonatal leukoproliferative disorder. Skin problems are seen including eczema, folliculitis, alopecia areata, and sun hypersensitivity.

## Fragile X Syndrome

Fragile X syndrome is an X-linked condition consisting of mental retardation or learning disabilities, connective tissue disorders, and sen-

**Table 119-5.** Medications Commonly Used in Mental Retardation

| Generic Name (Brand Name) | Most Common Side Effects |
|---|---|
| Diazepam (Valium) | Drowsiness, ataxia, weakness, confusion, constipation, dysarthria, diplopia, rash, urinary retention |
| Desipramine (Norpramin, Pertofrane) | Drowsiness, incoordination, weight gain, constipation, blurred vision, dry mouth, insomnia, anxiety, confusion, nightmares, delusions, psychosis, blood dyscrasias |
| Fluphenazine (Permitil, Prolixin), haloperidol (Haldol), Methyl-phenidate (Ritalin), thioridazine (Mellaril) | Extrapyramidal movement disorders, neuroleptic malignant syndrome, drowsiness, restlessness, nausea, blurred vision, rash, dry mouth, polyuria, altered glucose regulation, weight gain or loss Anorexia, insomnia, rebound, headache, tics, agitation, rash, tachycardia, hypertension, weight loss, decreased growth rate, abdominal pain |

sory integration dysfunction. It affects 1 in 1000 individuals and affects males more severely than females. There are few associated medical conditions and generally they do not cause severe problems. Mitral valve prolapse, seizures, strabismus, frequent ear infections, allergies, self-abusive behaviors (particularly biting), and hyperextensible joints are reported in some children. The major difficulties that may be encountered may be related to autistic-like behaviors and self-abusive behaviors.

## Prader-Willi Syndrome

Prader-Willi syndrome is a condition characterized by mental retardation, hypotonia, hypogonadism, and obesity. It is a sporadic multisystem disorder with an incidence of 1 in 10,000. It is due to a chromosomal deletion on the 15th chromosome. Presentation in infancy is of poor suck, hypotonia, developmental delay, and early failure to thrive. During childhood the poor eating habits change to hyperphagia and obesity, which becomes a major problem for health and life. Consequences of obesity include somnolence, hypoventilation, cor pulmonale, and non-insulin dependent diabetes mellitus. Associated problems are scoliosis, strabismus, and inability to vomit. Occasional problems may include decreased sensitivity to pain, seizure disorder, short stature, skin picking, easy bruisability, fractures from minor trauma, and acanthosis nigricans.

Obesity develops due to hyperphagia, inability to vomit, and decreased caloric requirements. Children become obsessed with food and eating. Abnormal behaviors are manifested with gorging, foraging for food, eating inedibles, and violent temper outbursts when eating is thwarted. Respiratory problems occur secondary to massive obesity. Pickwickian syndrome with hypoventilation, hypercapnia, hypoxia, and right sided heart failure have been seen in older children. Impaired breathing leads to carbon dioxide retention, acidosis, constriction of the pulmonary arterioles, pulmonary hypertension, and the chance of pulmonary embolus. Non-insulin-dependent diabetes mellitus is seen in some patients related to their obesity. Most people with diabetes can be managed with oral hypoglycemics and/or weight loss. Insulin is rarely required, and response to insulin may be unpredictable. Early atherosclerosis and glomerulosclerosis may occur secondary to the diabetes.

The inability to vomit can be of concern in the emergency department. Hyperphagia may result in food foraging, consumption of non-food materials, and toxic ingestions. In this patient population ipecac should be avoided. Ipecac toxicity can result if the patient is unable to vomit. Gastric aspiration or other techniques should be utilized.

Respiratory insufficiency with hypoventilation is frequently not responsive to hypercapnia. Medroxyprogesterone acetate may be helpful as a respiratory stimulant in some cases. Gastric perforation as a consequence of overeating is seen in rare cases.

## Williams Syndrome

Williams syndrome is a disorder of unknown etiology that presents with elfinlike facies, cardiovascular disease, infantile hypercalcemia, learning disabilities or mild to moderate mental retardation, and an outgoing personality. It appears to develop into a multisystem disease in adulthood.

Cardiovascular difficulties, endocrinologic abnormalities, urinary tract problems, gastrointestinal problems, and arthropathy are observed with increasing incidence over time. Supravalvular aortic stenosis is the most common cardiac problem. Pulmonic stenosis, coarctation of the aorta, strabismus, joint contractures, and hypertension are also reported. Hypercalcemia is seen in infants and recurs in adults. Calcium levels should be monitored. Children who present with polydypsia, polyuria, irritability, and constipation should be evaluated for hypercalcemia. Urethral stenosis, bladder diverticuli, vesicoureteral reflux, renal artery stenosis, constipation, ulcers, diverticulitits, and arthropathy are reported in adults with the syndrome.

## Rett Syndrome

Rett syndrome is a form of mental retardation occurring only in females and characterized by normal early development followed by a loss of purposeful hand use, regression in social development, progressive ataxia or spasticity, and development of mental retardation. Hand stereotypies and spontaneous noncommunicative vocalizations or laughter are typical of this syndrome. Hyperventilation, breath-holding, air swallowing, bruxism, ataxia, muscle wasting, poor circulation in the lower extremities, frequent fractures, scoliosis, seizures, and intermittent flushing have been described in association with this syndrome.

These girls may present to the emergency department with a variety of symptoms, including fainting due to apnea or hyperventilation or with severe abdominal distension due to air swallowing. Apnea has been known to last 30 to 40 s and may involve cyanosis. Screaming attacks may occur in puberty. Children need to be assessed for possible pain due to an acute abdomen, dental pain, kidney stones, or other medical causes. If no source of medical concern is identified, the child may be suffering from a screaming attack.

Seizures are seen often in this population and may be generalized, partial, or mixed. Atypical infantile spasms have also been described. Seizures may be refractory to drug therapy and individuals are at times prone to adverse reactions to their anticonvulsant medications. Some "seizures" may actually be nonepileptic paroxysmal events unresponsive to antiepileptic medications. Caution is advised in adjusting dosages. Consultation with the treating neurologist or specialist managing the child is strongly advised if seizure is the presenting problem.

## BIBLIOGRAPHY

Batshaw M (guest ed): The child with developmental disabilities. *Pediatr Clin North Am* 40:3, 1993.

Boyd J, Perrin J: Spinal cord injury, in Molnar G (ed): *Pediatric Rehabilitation*, 2d ed. Baltimore, Williams & Wilkins, 1992, pp 334–362.

David R (ed): *Pediatric Neurology for the Clinician*. Norwalk, CT, Appleton & Lange, 1992.

Gersh E: Medical concerns and treatments, in Geralis E (ed): *Children with Cerebral Palsy: A Parents Guide*. Rockville, MD, Woodbine House, 1991, pp 57–91.

Luckasson RA (ed): *Mental Retardation: Definition, Classification, and Systems of Supports*, 9th ed. Washington, American Association on Mental Retardation, 1992.

Wolraich M: *The Practical Assessment & Management of Children With Disorders of Development & Learning*. Chicago, Year Book, 1987.

# SECTION 12
# Infectious Diseases and Allergy

## 120
## SEXUALLY TRANSMITTED DISEASES

### Dexter L. Morris

Sexually transmitted diseases (STDs) are commonly encountered in emergency and urgent care settings. Although rarely immediately life-threatening, it is important to diagnose and treat them to protect the health and future fertility of the patient as well as the health of the patient's sexual contacts. Furthermore, individuals with STDs are more likely to acquire human immunodeficiency virus (HIV) infection than the general population. Thus, diagnosis of an STD suggests the need for HIV counseling and testing. This chapter discusses the major STDs with the exception of HIV, which is discussed in Chapter 122. Pelvic inflammatory disease (PID) and vaginosis are also discussed elsewhere (Chapters 96 and 97, respectively). In addition to specific antimicrobial treatment for STD patients, the end of the chapter contains important guidelines for follow-up and reporting of STDs. Treatment guidelines for STDs change frequently. The *Morbidity and Mortality Weekly Report* of the Centers for Disease Control and Prevention (CDC) is an excellent source of updates.

## CHLAMYDIAL INFECTIONS

*Chlamydia trachomatis* are obligate intracellular bacteria and have a growth cycle that alternates between two morphologic forms. Chlamydial infections present with a wide spectrum of clinical manifestations. In men, infection causes urethritis, epididymitis, and proctitis. In women, urethritis, cervicitis, and PID are common. In both sexes, the prevalence of asymptomatic infection is high, ranging from 3 to 5 percent in the general population to 15 to 20 percent among individuals attending STD clinics. Patients with gonorrhea have an even higher incidence of concomitant chlamydial infection. Untreated chlamydial infections are thought to be an important cause of infertility in women. The incubation period is 1 to 3 weeks and symptoms, if present, can range from mild burning or irritation to peritonitis.

**Diagnosis.** Although the organism can be cultured, this has a relatively low yield. Indirect methods using direct immunofluorescence, enzyme-linked immunosorbent assay (ELISA)-type assays, and DNA probes are available. Newer assays that can be performed on urine are also available.

**Treatment.** Doxycycline, 100 mg orally bid for 7 days has been the standard therapy, but now azithromycin 1 g orally in a single dose appears to be as effective. Table 120-1 lists various treatment options.

## GONOCOCCAL INFECTIONS

*Neisseria gonorrhoeae* are gram-negative diplococci that are very sensitive to antibiotics (penicillin). Recent years have seen the emergence of strains resistant to penicillin (up to 25 percent) and less commonly, tetracycline. Gonococcal infection presents usually as urethritis in men and cervicitis or PID in women. Epididymitis and prostatitis can also occur in men. Rectal infection occurs in 30 to 50 percent of women with gonococcal cervicitis and can be the only site

**Table 120-1.** Antimicrobial Therapy for Sexually Transmitted Diseases

| Disease | Recommended Treatment | Alternative(s) |
|---|---|---|
| Chlamydial infection | Doxycycline 100 mg PO bid × 7 d *or* Azithromycin 1 g PO single dose | Ofloxacin 300 mg PO × 7 d *or* Erythromycin 500 mg PO qid × 7 d |
| Gonococcal infections | Ceftriaxone 125 mg IM single dose *or* Cefixime 400 mg PO single dose *or* Ciprofloxacin 500 mg PO single dose *or* Ofloxacin 400 mg PO single dose | |
| Trichomoniasis | Metronidazole 2 g PO single dose | Metronidazole 500 mg PO bid × 7 d |
| Syphilis, 1°, 2°, early latent | Benzathine penicillin G 2.4 million units IM single dose | Doxycycline 100 mg PO bid × 14 d |
| Syphilis, late latent or unknown | Benzathine penicillin G 2.4 million units IM 3 doses 1 wk apart | |
| Herpes simplex infections | Acyclovir 200 mg (400 mg for proctitis) PO 5 times a day × 7–10 d | |
| Chancroid | Azithromycin 1 g PO single dose *or* Ceftriaxone 250 mg IM single dose *or* Erythromycin base 500 mg PO qid × 7 d | Amoxicillin 500 mg plus clavulanic acid 125 mg PO tid × 7 d *or* Ciprofloxacin 500 mg PO bid × 3 d |
| Lymphogranuloma venereum | Doxycycline 100 mg PO bid × 21 d | Erythromycin 500 mg PO qid × 21 d |

SOURCE: Adapted from Centers for Disease Control and Prevention. *MMWR* 42:RR-14, 1993.

of infection in homosexual men. *N. gonorrhoeae* can also be isolated from the pharynx, but rarely does it cause a pharyngitis. The incubation period ranges from 3 to 21 days. Disseminated infection also occurs in approximately 2 percent of untreated primary gonorrhea. This manifestation is characterized by skin lesions (tender pustules on an erythematous base, 50 to 70 percent), arthralgias, tenosynovitis, or arthritis (30 to 40 percent), and fever or general malaise (80 percent). Gonococcal infections can decrease fertility in women presumably by scarring the fallopian tubes; they also increase the chance of ectopic pregnancy by the same mechanism.

**Diagnosis.** Cervical or urethral culture on a selective medium is the standard for diagnosis, having a sensitivity of 80 to 90 percent. A Gram stain of a urethral smear showing intracellular gram-negative diplococci is sensitive and specific in men but much less useful in women. Diagnosis of disseminated gonococcal infection is more difficult with only 20 to 50 percent of blood, lesion, or joint cultures being positive. Cervical, rectal, and pharyngeal smears may improve the chance of a culture diagnosis.

**Treatment.** Ceftriaxone 125 mg intramuscularly in a single dose has been a standard treatment since the emergence of resistant organisms. Cefixime 400 mg orally, ciprofloxacin 500 mg orally, or ofloxacin 400 mg orally all in single dose are also effective. Patients should also be treated for a presumed chlamydial infection. Disseminated disease is usually treated with higher doses of ceftriaxone on an inpatient or outpatient basis depending on the particular circumstances.

## TRICHOMONAS INFECTIONS

*Trichomonas vaginalis* is a flagellated protozoan that causes urogenital infections in men and women. The prevalence is less than 1 percent in women but up to 15 percent in those attending STD clinics. Disease is most commonly characterized by vaginosis with discharge. Abdominal pain can also be present. In men, the disease is often asymptomatic but can cause urethritis. Incubation ranges from 3 to 28 days.

**Diagnosis.** Microscopic examination of wet preparations of cervical smears or spun urine samples that reveal the classic motile parasites is diagnostic.

**Treatment.** Metronidazole 2 g orally in a single dose is the usual treatment.

## GENITAL WARTS

Human papillomaviruses (HPV) are DNA viruses that cause genital warts by direct transmission. Different genotypes have also been implicated in cervical cancer, but the evidence is far from clear. The warts usually appear after an incubation period of 3 to 4 months and may coalesce to form condylomata acuminata. Although painless, their location or size may cause discomfort.

**Diagnosis.** Diagnosis is clinical with care to exclude other STDs.

**Treatment.** Cryotherapy with liquid nitrogen is recommended but is not usually performed in the emergency department.

The following diseases often present with genital lesions that may be difficult to distinguish from one another. Characteristics of the lesions and their accompanying signs and symptoms are provided in

**Table 120-2.** Clinical Feature of Genital Ulcers*

| Disease | Nature of Genital Ulcer | Incubation Period (Range) | Painful | Inguinal Adenopathy |
|---------|------------------------|---------------------------|---------|---------------------|
| Syphilis | Indurated, relatively not clean base; heals spontaneously | 2 wk or longer | No | Firm, rubbery nodes; tender |
| Herpes simplex infection | Multiple, small, grouped vesicles coalesce and form shallow ulcers; vulvovaginitis | 2–7 d | Yes | Tender bilateral adenopathy |
| Chancroid | Irregular purulent; undermined edges; not indurated; multiple ulcers | 2–12 d | Yes | Present in 50%; usually unilocular; if fluctuant, very painful; may form crater |
| Lympho-granuloma venereum | Usually not observed; small and shallow; rapid spontaneous healing | 5–21 d | No | More common in males; nodes in matted clusters; unilateral or bilateral multi-loculated |

SOURCE: Adapted from Scientific American Medicine. *Sexually Transmitted Diseases.* New York: Scientific American Medicine, December 1993.

Table 120-2. Granuloma inguinale (donovanosis) rarely occurs in the United States and readers are referred to the bibliography.

## SYPHILIS INFECTIONS

*Treponema pallidum*, a spirochete, is the causative agent of syphilis as well as yaws and pinta. It enters the body through mucous membranes or nonintact skin. It remains very sensitive to penicillin, thus diagnosis, rather than treatment, is the main difficulty in controlling this disease. The last 7 years has seen a marked increase in syphilis thought to be secondary to behavior associated with drug use. Syphilis occurs in three stages.

1. *Primary:* The initial stage of infection is characterized by a painless chancre with indurated borders on the penis, vulva, or other areas with sexual contact. The incubation period is about 21 days with lesions then disappearing after 3 to 6 weeks. There are no constitutional symptoms and the lesion may be absent.
2. *Secondary:* This stage, which occurs 3 to 6 weeks after the end of the primary stage, includes nonspecific symptoms such as sore throat, malaise, fever, and headaches. Rash and lymphadenopathy are the most common symptoms. The rash often starts on the trunk and flexor surfaces, spreading to the palms and soles. It takes on many forms but is often dull red and papular. This stage also resolves spontaneously.
3. *Tertiary (Latent):* Involvement of the nervous and cardiovascular system is characteristic of this stage, which may occur years after the initial infection. Specific manifestations range from acute meningitis, dementia, and neuropathy (tabes dorsalis) to thoracic aneurysm. Tertiary syphilis is uncommon.

**Diagnosis.** Dark-field microscopy can be used to identify treponemes from primary lesions and also from secondary lesions. Several serologic tests are available including nontreponemal tests (rapid plasma reagin, VDRL) and specific treponemal antibody tests (fluorescent treponemal antibody absorption [FTA-ABS]). Nontreponemal tests are positive about 14 days after the appearance of the chancre and false positive in 1 to 2 percent of the population. FTA-ABS tests are slightly more sensitive and specific but more difficult to perform.

**Treatment.** Given the multiple stages and manifestations of syphilis, considering the diagnosis is the most crucial part of treatment. Benzathine penicillin G 2.4 million units intramuscularly in a single dose has remained the standard of care. Doxycycline 100 mg orally bid for 2 weeks may be used for allergic individuals. Treatment of latent syphilis is usually three doses of penicillin as above, given 1 week apart.

## HERPES SIMPLEX INFECTIONS

Herpes simplex virus (HSV)-2 or HSV-1 can cause genital herpes infections by infection of mucosal surfaces or nonintact skin. Primary infections are characterized by painful pustular or ulcerative lesions occurring 8 to 16 days after contact with an infected individual (although infections can be asymptomatic). Systemic symptoms are common and include fever, headache, and myalgias. Dysuria is common and urinary retention secondary to swelling and pain is not unheard of in women. Approximately 80 percent of patients also have lymphadenopathy and aseptic meningitis can occur. The untreated illness lasts 2 to 3 weeks to complete healing. Unfortunately the virus remains latent and recurrent infections occur in 60 to 90 percent of patients. These are usually milder, unilateral, and of shorter duration.

**Diagnosis.** Clinical diagnosis of the painful vesiculopustular lesions is often possible. A smear may be taken of the lesions and stained to demonstrate large intranuclear inclusions, although this is less sensitive than direct culture. Viral cultures can be done and are positive in 1 to 4 days. New assays using ELISA and polymerase chain reactions are being developed.

**Treatment.** Treatment is with acyclovir 200 mg orally 5 times a day for 7 to 10 days for primary illness (400 mg for proctitis) and 200 mg orally 5 times a day *or* 800 mg orally bid for 5 days for recurrent episodes. Acyclovir at 5 mg/kg body weight may be given intravenously for patients requiring hospitalization.

## CHANCROID

*Haemophilus ducreyi* is a pleomorphic gram-negative bacillus that causes genital ulcers and lymphadenitis. It is much more common in developing countries but has seen a resurgence in recent years in the United States. After an incubation period of 3 to 10 days, a tender papule appears at the site of infection, followed by ulceration of the lesion. Multiple lesions may be present and coalesce. Painful inguinal adenopathy is present in up to 50 percent of patients and may include bubo formation and spontaneous rupture. There are few constitutional symptoms.

**Diagnosis.** Diagnosis can be made on clinical grounds, but other diseases such as syphilis need to be excluded. A swab of a lesion or pus from a bubo can be cultured but only with limited success.

**Treatment.** Azithromycin 1 g orally in a single dose or ceftriaxone 250 mg intramuscularly in a single dose or erythromycin base 500 mg orally qid for 7 days are all recommended treatments. Several alternative treatments are available (see Table 120-1).

## LYMPHOGRANULOMA VENEREUM

Specific serotypes of *C. trachomatis* cause this disease, which although endemic in other parts of the world, is seen only sporadically in the United States. The primary lesion can take on many forms and be confused with other STDs (See Table 120-2). Ten days to 6 months following the initial lesion, an inguinal bubo forms (unilateral in 60 percent). The buboes continue to grow, either rupturing or forming firm inguinal masses.

**Diagnosis.** Serologic tests and culture are the mainstays of diagnosis.

**Treatment.** Doxycycline 100 mg orally bid for 21 days is the usual regimen. Table 120-1 gives alternative treatments.

## GENERAL RECOMMENDATIONS FOR TREATMENT AND FOLLOW-UP

When treating patients for STDs in the emergency department, it is important to remember that many STDs occur together; follow-up and compliance for many emergency department patients is poor, and lack of treatment can contribute to infertility. For these reasons, a standardized approach is suggested for patients with suspected STDs. This should include:

1. Treating even when an STD is only suspected, especially for gonorrhea and chlamydia with emphasis on single-dose treatments
2. Obtaining a serologic test for syphilis
3. Ascertaining pregnancy status and consulting obstetrics if the patient is pregnant
4. Reporting appropriate diseases to the state health department
5. Counseling patients about prevention of STDs
6. Counseling patients about the advisability of HIV testing
7. Counseling patients about advising partner(s) to seek treatment
8. Arranging for appropriate follow-up
9. Documenting all of the above on the medical record

## BIBLIOGRAPHY

Adimora AA, Hamilton H, Holmes KK, Sparling PF: *Sexually Transmitted Diseases—Companion Handbook.* New York, McGraw-Hill, 1994.

Centers for Disease Control and Prevention: 1993 Sexually transmitted diseases treatment guidelines. *MMWR* 42:RR-14, 1993.

Scientific American Medicine SAM-CD: *Sexually Transmitted Diseases.* New York, Scientific American, December 1993.

# 121
# TOXIC SHOCK SYNDROME AND TOXIC SHOCK–LIKE SYNDROME

**Ann L. Harwood-Nuss**
**Shawna Perry**

## TOXIC SHOCK SYNDROME

Toxic shock syndrome (TSS) is a severe, life-threatening syndrome characterized by high fever, profound hypotension, diffuse erythroderma, mucous membrane hyperemia, pharyngitis, diarrhea, and constitutional symptoms. It can rapidly progress to multisystem dysfunction with severe electrolyte disturbances, renal failure, and shock. Although first described in 1978 by Todd in seven children with *Staphylococcus aureus* infections, TSS has been associated primarily with tampon use. In 1981, a nationwide epidemic of TSS associated with continuous tampon use was widely recognized among otherwise healthy young women.

The TSS case definition is given in Table 121-1. This definition was formulated in 1980 by the Centers for Disease Control and Prevention (CDC) to ensure that cases included in various surveillance studies were the same clinical entity as TSS. In the absence of a definitive laboratory marker, the strict application of the case definition is warranted but undoubtedly excludes the less severe (subclinical) cases.

Since 1980, there have been significant advances in the understanding of the clinical and epidemiologic aspects of TSS. The incidence of reported cases has declined, with a decrease in both the case fatality ratio and the proportion of cases associated with menstruation. At present, the majority of cases occur in settings not related to menstruation and cross all segments of society.

### Pathophysiology

#### Etiology and Pathogenesis

Most cases of TSS have been directly associated with colonization or infection with *S. aureus*. Approximately 67 percent of the organisms are phage type I, while 25 percent are nontypable. An exotoxin, *toxic shock syndrome toxin* (TSST-1) is produced by 20 percent of randomly tested *S. aureus* isolates. TSST-1 has been implicated as a sig-

**Table 121-1.** Criteria for Diagnosis (Must Have All)

1. Temperature >38.9°C (102°F)
2. Systolic BP <90 mmHg, orthostatic decrease of systolic BP by 15 mmHg, or syncope
3. Rash (diffuse, macular erythroderma) with subsequent desquamation, especially on palms or soles of feet
4. Involvement of three of the following organ systems clinically or by abnormal laboratory tests:
   Gastrointestinal: Vomiting, profuse diarrhea
   Musculoskeletal: Severe myalgias or twofold increase in CPK
   Renal: Increase in BUN and creatinine two times normal; pyuria without evidence of infection
   Mucosal inflammation: Vaginal, conjunctival, or pharyngeal hyperemia
   Hepatic involvement: Hepatitis (twofold elevation of bilirubin, SGOT, SGPT)
   Hematologic: Thrombocytopenia < 100,000 platelets/mm$^3$
   CNS: Disorientation without focal neurologic signs
5. Negative serologic tests for Rocky Mountain spotted fever, leptospirosis, measles, hepatitis B surface antigen, fluorescent antinuclear antibody, VDRL, and monospot; and negative blood, urine, and throat cultures

nificant factor in the production of symptoms associated with TSS, either through direct toxic effects on the host or through stimulation of secondary mediators in response to TSST-1. The biologic properties of TSST-1 include the ability to: (1) induce fever directly on the hypothalamus or indirectly via interleukin 1 (IL-1) and tumor necrosis factor (TNF) production; (2) promote T-lymphocyte "superantigenization" and overstimulation; (3) induce interferon production; (4) enhance delayed hypersensitivity; (5) suppress neutrophil migration and immunoglobulin secretion; and (6) enhance host susceptibility to endotoxins.

Ninety percent of menstrual-related cases of TSS (MRTSS) are caused by *S. aureus* strains that produce TSST-1, whereas only 40 percent of isolates from non-menstrual-related TSS (NMTSS) produce this exotoxin. Enterotoxins B and C have been identified from isolates of NMTSS, with almost identical biochemical structure to TSST-1. This explains the similarity in clinical manifestations seen with both MRTSS and NMTSS. Although an endotoxin of possibly gastrointestinal or genitourinary origin may be involved in the development of TSS associated with TSST-1 and the enterotoxins, there are no data to support its existence.

The amount of TSST-1 produced by toxigenic strains of *S. aureus* is dependent on a number of factors. Its production in MRTSS is enhanced by certain vaginal conditions: temperature of 39 to 40°C, a neutral pH, a $P_{O_2}$ of > 5%, and supplemental $CO_2$. These conditions can be met with the change in vaginal pH from acidic to neutral during menses and an increase in $O_2$ and $CO_2$ content of the vagina with the introduction of tampons or intravaginal devices. It has also been demonstrated that TSST-1 production is influenced by the concentration of magnesium, the composition of fibers used in tampons, and by a synergistic relationship between *S. aureus* and *Escherichia coli* involving tryptophan substrate production.

The most impressive aspect of the pathophysiology is the massive vasodilatation and rapid movement of the serum proteins and fluids from the intravascular to the extravascular space. Hypotension is accounted for by (1) decreased vasomotor tone, causing pooling of blood in the periphery and therein decreased central venus pressure and pulmonary capillary wedge pressure; (2) nonhydrostatic leakage of fluid into the interstitium, causing decreased intravascular volume and generalized nonpitting edema, primarily of the head and neck; (3) depressed cardiac function, including decreased wall motion and decreased shortening fraction; and (4) total body water deficits secondary to vomiting, diarrhea, and fever.

TSST-1 is a potent activator of the immunostimulant cytokines IL-1 and TNF, which appear to be pivotally involved in generating TSS. IL-1 is capable of producing hypoalbuminemia, hypoferrinemia, and proteolysis of skeletal muscle, consistent with the peripheral edema, anemia, and rhabdomyolysis seen in TSS. A potent pyrogen, TNF has been shown in animal models to induce profound acidosis, shock, and multisystem organ failure within hours of infusion. In TSS, this can result in the rapid onset of oliguria, hypotension, and low central venous pressure. The multisystem involvement seen in TSS may be a reflection of the rapid onset of hypotension and decreased perfusion, or there may be direct effects of the toxin or toxins on the parenchymal cells of different organs, yet to be elucidated.

The immunologic status of the individual may play a role in the pathogenesis of TSS. An age-related rise in anti-TSST-1 antibodies has been found in both sexes, with 70 to 80 percent having measurable antibodies by early adulthood and 90 to 95 percent by age 40. Convalescent titers are low in the majority of patients with TSS for up to 1 year after infection.

## Epidemiology

Since the CDC began surveillance of TSS in 1979, 3295 definite cases have been reported. The CDC reported a decrease from 900 cases in 1980 to 351 cases in 1988. In 1992, only 44 definite cases of TSS were reported, 51 probable cases, and 3 deaths (only 1 death was definitely due to TSS). Of the 44 definite cases, slightly less than half (20) occurred during menstruation. The decrease in cases is presumably due to changes in the composition of tampons, the general public's awareness of the risks from tampon use, and increased medical awareness and detection. Although the use of contraceptive sponges and diaphragms places the individual at risk, their exact contribution to the development of TSS is unclear.

TSS was initially a disease of young, healthy, menstruating women; 50 percent of cases reported in 1986 and 1987 were found in this group. Tampon use carried a 33 times greater risk of TSS developing in susceptible females. *S. aureus* has been isolated from the vaginas of 98 percent of women with TSS, compared to an 8 to 10 percent carrier rate in controls. It is presumed that women who develop menstrual TSS are colonized with *S. aureus* before the onset of menstruation.

The proportion of cases not associated with menstruation (NMTSS) has increased since 1980, primarily because of the decrease in the number of menstruation-related cases. The absolute number of cases of NMTSS has remained relatively constant, however. Nearly 25 percent of NMTSS cases are associated with postpartum and *S. aureus* vaginal infections. There is an increasing incidence of NMTSS in males. Men comprise one-third of patients with TSS, with a mortality rate 3.3 times that of MRTSS in women. A 50 percent mortality rate has been reported in non-TSST-1 *S. aureus* infections (i.e., enterotoxin B or C) but only 10 percent in TSST-1–producing *S. aureus* infections.

The means by which *S. aureus* enters the host in TSS are numerous and have been well documented in a wide variety of clinical settings. TSS has also been reported following influenza and influenza-like illnesses and is associated with significant mortality (43 percent). Nasal packing (nasal tampons) is also associated with TSS, with 20 to 40 percent of the adult population carrying *S. aureus* in the nasal vestibule.

## Clinical Features and Diagnosis

### Differential Diagnosis

There are other systemic illnesses that are characterized by fever, rash, diarrhea, myalgias, and multisystem involvement and that resemble TSS (Table 121-2). *Kawasaki disease* (mucocutaneous lymph node syndrome) is characterized by fever, conjunctival hyperemia, and erythema of the mucous membranes with desquamation. Although the exanthems may be quite similar, Kawasaki disease may present with target lesions resembling erythema multiforme, and the bright-red appearance of the vermillion border is not common in TSS. Further differentiation of Kawasaki disease from TSS lies in the fact that more than 99 percent of those afflicted with Kawasaki disease are under 10 years of age and that Kawasaki disease is not characterized by hypotension, renal failure, or thrombocytopenia.

*Staphylococcal scalded skin syndrome* (SSSS) is most commonly seen in children less than 5 years of age and is characterized by fever, generalized painful erythroderma, and conjunctivitis. SSSS may be distinguished from TSS by its lack of multisystem involvement. In

**Table 121-2.** Differential Diagnosis of Toxic Shock Syndrome

| | |
|---|---|
| Acute pyelonephritis | Acute viral syndrome |
| Septic shock | Leptospirosis |
| Acute rheumatic fever | Systemic lupus erythematosus |
| Streptococcal scarlet fever | Rocky Mountain spotted fever |
| Staphylococcal scarlet fever | Tick typhus |
| Staphylococcal scalded skin syndrome | Gastroenteritis |
| Legionnaires disease | Kawasaki disease |
| Pelvic inflammatory disease | Reye syndrome |
| Hemolytic uremic syndrome | Toxic epidermal necrolysis (TEN) |
| | Erythema multiforme |

contrast, *staphylococcal scarlet fever* is so similar to TSS with the full-thickness desquamation that only pathology specimens or serologic evidence of the exfoliatin toxin will differentiate the two entities. In streptococcal scarlet fever, the "sandpaper" rash is distinct from the macular "sunburn" rash of TSS.

*Rocky Mountain spotted fever,* a rickettsial infection acquired from tick bites, has a presentation similar to TSS, but the rash is usually petechial and delayed in onset. TEN (*toxic epidermal necrolysis*) resembles SSSS and occurs primarily in adults. Non-toxin-mediated, it is related to drug exposure and has a bullous component. *Erythema multiforme* can be associated with fever, pharyngeal erythema, and toxemia. The rash is multiform with symmetric involvement of the lower extremities. Immunologically mediated from a drug exposure or infectious agent, it can progress to Stevens-Johnson syndrome.

Septic shock must always be considered in the differential diagnosis of TSS. In general, the appearance of a rash and the laboratory abnormalities associated with TSS will aid in distinguishing these two entities.

## Clinical Presentation

TSS should be considered in any unexplained febrile illness associated with erythroderma, hypotension, and diffuse organ pathology, especially in menstruating women. Diagnostic criteria for TSS are listed in Table 121-1. Patients with MRTSS usually present between the third and fifth day of menses. The median time to onset of illness in postsurgical NMTSS is two postoperative days. There appears to be a spectrum of severity of TSS. Mild cases of TSS may be excluded from the CDC case definition. Mild TSS is generally characterized by fever and chills, myalgias, abdominal pain, sore throat, nausea, vomiting, and diarrhea. Hypotension is usually not present, and the illness is self-limited. Severe TSS is an acute-onset, multisystem disease with symptoms, signs, and laboratory abnormalities reflecting multiple-organ involvement. Headache is the most common complaint. Some patients may experience a prodrome consisting of malaise, myalgias, headache, nausea, vomiting, and diarrhea. Sudden onset of fever and chills occurs approximately 1 to 4 days prior to presentation. Diffuse myalgias, particularly in the proximal aspects of the extremities, abdomen, and back are reported by virtually all patients; arthralgias are also common. Profuse, watery diarrhea and repeated vomiting are reported by 90 to 98 percent of patients. Orthostatic lightheadedness or syncope may be present. Patients also complain of sore throat, headache, paresthesias, and photophobia. The patient may complain of abdominal pain, cough, or sore throat.

Physical examination reveals hypotension or an orthostatic decrease in systolic pressure of 15 mm Hg in all cases. In general, victims of TSS appear acutely ill. The initial state usually lasts about 24 to 48 h; the patient may be obtunded, disoriented, oliguric, and hypotensive. There is an overall body fluid deficit due to losses from fever, vomiting, diarrhea, and decreased systemic vascular resistance. Depressed cardiac function may also be present. Patients may show nonpitting edema of the face and extremities secondary to nonhydrostatic leakage of intravascular fluid into the interstitium. Other prominent signs may include profound muscle weakness and tenderness or abdominal tenderness. The diarrhea is usually watery and profuse, frequently with associated incontinence. One-half to three-quarters of patients have pharyngitis with a strawberry-red tongue; conjunctival hyperemia and vaginitis are also seen. Tender, edematous external genitalia, diffuse vaginal hyperemia, "strawberry" cervix, scant purulent cervical discharge, and bilateral adnexal tenderness are seen in 25 to 35 percent of patients with menstruation-related TSS.

The rash of TSS is a diffuse blanching erythroderma, classically described as painless "sunburn," which fades within 3 days of its appearance and is followed by full-thickness desquamation during convalescence, especially of the palms and soles. This CDC criterion is most often missed as it may be subtle or difficult to detect in darkly pigmented patients. Variations include patchy erythroderma and localized maculopustular eruptions. In all cases, a fine, generalized desquamation of the skin, with peeling over the soles, fingers, toes, and palms, occurs from 6 to 14 days after the onset of illness. More than 50 percent of severely ill patients experience loss of hair and nails 2 to 3 months later.

Specific focal neurologic findings rarely occur. Patients present with varying degrees of altered consciousness. Approximately 75 percent of patients have nonfocal neurologic abnormalities without signs of meningeal irritation. Confusion, disorientation, agitation, hysteria, somnolence, and seizures have been reported, consistent with a toxic encephalopathy from cerebral edema. If the clinical picture is unclear, CT scan and lumbar puncture should be performed. Figure 121-1 illustrates the temporal relationships of the major manifestations of TSS.

Abnormal laboratory values reflect the multisystem involvement in TSS. Leukocytosis with an increase in immature forms is frequently seen; lymphocytopenia has also been reported. A mild anemia with

**Fig. 121-1.** Composite drawing of major systemic, skin, and mucous membrane manifestations of toxic shock syndrome. (*From* Chesney PJ, David JP, Purdy WK, et al: Clinical manifestations of toxic shock syndrome. *JAMA* 246:741, 1981, with permission.)

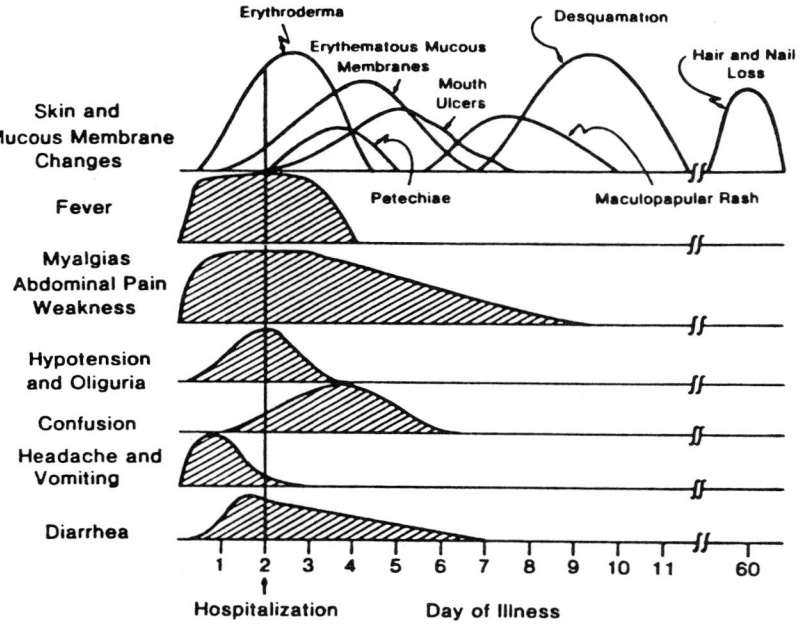

acute hypoferrinemia and abnormal peripheral smears consistent with microangiopathic hemolytic anemia or disseminated intravascular coagulation may be found. Azotemia, myoglobinuria, and abnormal urinary sediment (sterile pyuria and red blood cell casts) are seen as acute renal failure develops. Liver function abnormalities and hyperbilirubinemia are seen in approximately 3 percent of patients with clinical evidence of coagulopathy. Metabolic acidosis secondary to hypotension is also seen. Electrolyte abnormalities, including hypocalcemia, hypophosphatemia, hyponatremia, and hypokalemia, are common. Hypocalcemia will be out of proportion to the degree of hypoalbuminemia and may be difficult to correct if there is a concomitant decrease in the serum magnesium.

Acute renal failure secondary to acute tubular necrosis is a complication of TSS. It appears to be secondary to prerenal deficits, renal ischemia caused by hypotension, rhabdomyolysis, and possibly direct damage from TSST-1 mediators. Ventricular arrhythmias, bundle branch block, first degree heart block, and T-wave and ST-T-wave changes have been reported. Echocardiography of patients with TSS show wall motion abnormalities and decreased shortening fraction suggestive of toxic cardiomyopathy. Adult respiratory distress syndrome (ARDS) with refractory hypotension represents the ultimate end-organ damage secondary to TSS.

## Treatment

Management of TSS depends on its severity. The most important aspect of initial management is the aggressive management of circulatory shock. Continuous monitoring of the heart rate, respiratory rate, blood pressure, urinary output, central venous pressure, and pulmonary capillary wedge pressure is necessary. During the first 24 h, patients may require 4 to 20 L of crystalloid and fresh-frozen plasma. There have been reports of patients requiring up to 20 L of fluid in the first 24 h of hospitalization. A dopamine infusion beginning at 5 to 20 $\mu$g/kg per minute may be used if volume correction fails to restore normal arterial pressure. Large amounts of intravenous fluid and pressors to treat refractory hypotension can result in the rapid onset of pulmonary edema. ARDS may then complicate TSS and require mechanical ventilation with positive end-expiratory pressure.

Evaluation must include arterial blood gases, CBC screen with peripheral smear, serum electrolytes including $Mg^{2+}$ and $Ca^{2+}$, coagulation studies, urinalysis, and chest radiograph. Patients with abnormal coagulation profiles and evidence of bleeding require colloid replacement, fresh-frozen plasma, or transfusions. Thrombocytopenia may require platelet transfusions. An electrocardiogram and echocardiogram may also be indicated.

A focus of infection should be aggressively sought and promptly treated. Cultures of all potentially infected sites should be obtained, including blood cultures, prior to initiating antibiotic therapy. Women with tampon-related TSS should have the tampon removed. Some authors recommend irrigation of the vagina with saline or povidone-iodine solution. Early consultation with a surgeon or a gynecologist is recommended if drainage or debridement of infectious sites is warranted.

Although antimicrobial agents have not been shown to affect the outcome of the acute illness, they are recommended and have been given to most patients to eradicate the focus of toxin-producing staphylococci as well as to decrease the recurrence rate. Antibiotic selection should include an antistaphylococcal penicillin or cephalosporin with $\beta$-lactamase stability. Nafcillin or oxacillin in doses of 1 to 2 g every 4 h provides adequate antimicrobial coverage. Cefazolin, 2 g every 6 h, also provides adequate coverage, but the first-generation cephalosporins are less $\beta$-lactamase-stable than the antistaphylococcal penicillins. In penicillin-allergic patients clindamycin, vancomycin, and first-generation cephalosporins can be used. Vancomycin, trimethoprim/sulfamethoxazole, or rifampin may be used if methicillin-resistant strains are encountered. Although data

on the optimum duration of antimicrobial therapy are not available, it seems prudent to administer parenteral antibiotics for at least 3 days or until the patient clinically improves. Oral antistaphylococcal antibiotics (dicloxacillin or clindamycin in penicillin-allergic patients), should then be administered for an additional 10 to 14 days. Although prospective studies are lacking, the addition of rifampin to the oral regimen is suggested because of the ability of this drug to eradicate the carrier state. Methylprednisolone and intravenous immunoglobulin have shown improvement in TSS in animal studies, but routine use of either of these therapies is currently not recommended.

Most patients become afebrile and normotensive within 48 h of hospitalization. Initial laboratory abnormalities resolve within 1 to 2 weeks, although full anemia correction occurs in 4 to 6 weeks.

Numerous sequelae of TSS have been reported and include late onset of maculopapular rash, decreased renal function, reversible loss of hair and nails, prolonged neuromuscular abnormalities, and cyanotic extremities. Neurologic deficits are common, with 50 percent of patients exhibiting residual memory deficits, decreased ability to concentrate, and diffuse electroencephalographic abnormalities.

The exact mechanism responsible for these sequelae is not yet clear; it has been suggested that they are due to either the delayed effects of the toxin or circulating immune complexes or are drug-mediated.

Up to 60 percent of patients not treated with $\beta$-lactamase-stable antimicrobial drugs have recurrence of the disease. Most recurrent episodes of MRTSS occur by the second month following the initial episode and happen on the same day of menses as the prior attack, although some have recurred in less than 1 month and some more than 1 year later. In the majority of patients having recurrence, convalescent antibody titers are low and nonprotective. The initial episode is the most severe, although deaths have resulted from recurrences of initially mild cases of TSS.

## STREPTOCOCCAL TOXIC SHOCK–LIKE SYNDROME

In 1987, Cone et al. published a report on two patients having a clinical presentation similar to toxic shock syndrome but due to severe streptococcal infection. In 1993, the CDC responded to the rising number of similar cases and formulated a consensus definition for this apparently new, severe streptococcal infection. *Streptococcal toxic shock–like syndrome* (TSLS) is now recognized as a life-threatening infection characterized by fever, hypotension, rash, and progressive soft tissue infection caused by *Streptococcus pyogenes,* a group A hemolytic streptococcus. Similar in presentation to TSS, TSLS progresses rapidly to multisystem organ failure with shock. It is associated with a significantly higher mortality than that of TSS (30 percent versus 5 percent). Since the first report, more than 50 cases of TSLS have been reported in the United States and over 300 cases worldwide.

The CDC case definition of streptococcal toxic shock syndrome is identical to that of TSS (see Table 121-1), except that TSLS develops in association with a severe soft tissue infection and cultures from a normally sterile site (i.e., blood, pleural fluid, surgical wound) must be positive for *S. pyogenes.* Positive cultures from nonsterile sites (i.e., throat, sputum, vagina) designate a probable case of TSLS. TSLS is reported most often in healthy females (68 percent) with soft tissue infection. However, 20 percent of cases can result from pharyngitis, sinusitis, and abdominal or pelvic sources. Bacteremia is present in 50 percent of cases of TSLS; in contrast, TSS must have negative blood cultures to meet the CDC criterion.

## Pathophysiology

### Etiology

The resurgence of invasive streptococcal infection appears to be the result of the production of more virulent exotoxins from isolates of *S. pyogenes. Streptococcal pyrogenic exotoxins* (SPEs) are produced by

90 percent of group A streptococcal isolates. Three distinct exotoxins (SPEs A, B, and C) have been identified. SPE A, also known as the *scarlet fever toxin,* is the most powerful of the SPEs and has a similar molecular structure to enterotoxin B of NMTSS. SPE A displays features similar to TSS-mediated exotoxins, including pyrogenicity, superactivation of T cells, and enhanced susceptibility to endotoxin-mediated shock. SPE B is associated with a streptococcal cysteine proteinase that inhibits fibrin clot formation and causes myocardial necrosis and death in animal models. Recent studies have demonstrated an association between the lack of antibodies to SPE and the severity of disease. SPE C has been found in fewer *S. pyogenes* isolates and its role in TSLS is unclear.

## Clinical Features

### Clinical Presentation

The presentation of TSLS is remarkably similar to TSS (see "Clinical Presentation" for TSS). The major difference is that patients with TSLS have an identifiable source of infection, usually a skin or soft tissue infection that is often necrotizing. TSLS has also been caused by pharyngitis, sinusitis, and pneumonia. Patients with TSLS lack the profound CNS changes seen in TSS. The multisystem organ damage of TSLS frequently precedes the onset of hypotension, whereas hypotension is part of the initial presentation of TSS. TSLS appears to progress more rapidly than TSS, particularly in immunocompromised patients in whom death may occur within 24 h of the onset of symptoms and mortality approaches 60 percent. The macular erythroderma is delayed in onset in TSLS, but the rash ultimately progresses to desquamation and occasionally alopecia during convalescence. Laboratory values may show less liver involvement and more profound renal failure than TSS, with positive steptozyme assay and antistreptolysin O titers.

### Differential Diagnosis

The differential diagnosis is that of TSS (Table 121-2).

### Treatment

The evaluation and treatment of TSLS and TSS are the same, with aggressive management of shock and organ failure. (See "Treatment" for TSS). Frequently, drainage and debridement of necrotic areas are necessary to control infection. Early surgical consultation is appropriate. Unequivocal differentiation of TSLS from TSS is not possible until final culture results are available. Antimicrobial therapy should cover both *S. pyogenes* and *S. aureus. S. pyogenes* is sensitive to penicillin G or erythromycin for penicillin-allergic patients. These antibiotics must be included in the treatment for TSS when the causative organism is unknown.

## BIBLIOGRAPHY

Centers for Disease Control: Historical perspectives: Reduced incidence of menstrual toxic-shock syndrome—United States, 1980–1990. *MMWR* 39(25):421, 1990.

Cone LA, Woodard DR, Schlievert PM, Tomory GS: Clinical and bacteriological observations of a toxic shock-like syndrome due to *Streptococcus pyogenes. N Engl J Med* 317:146, 1987.

Freedman JD, Beer DJ: Expanding perspectives on the toxic shock syndrome. *Adv Intern Med* 36:363, 1991.

Hackett SP, Stevens DL: Superantigens associated with staphylococcal and streptococcal toxic shock syndrome are potent inducers of tumor necrosis factor-β synthesis. *J Infect Dis* 168:232, 1993.

Kain KC, Schulzer M, Chow AW: Clinical spectrum of nonmenstrual toxic shock syndrome (TSS): Comparison with menstrual TSS by multivariate discriminant analyses. *Clin Infect Dis* 16:100, 1993.

The Working Group on Severe Streptococcal Infections of the Center for Disease Control: Defining the group A streptococcal toxic shock syndrome: Rational and consensus definition. *JAMA* 269(3):390, 1993.

# 122
# HIV INFECTION AND AIDS
## Catherine A. Marco

## INTRODUCTION

The spectrum of disease caused by human immunodeficiency virus (HIV) infection is commonly encountered in the practice of emergency medicine. Emergency department presentation may vary from asymptomatic HIV infection to life-threatening complications. The acquired immunodeficiency syndrome (AIDS) has been recognized since 1981, when several cases of *Pneumocystis carinii* pneumonia (PCP) and Kaposi's sarcoma were described. AIDS was initially defined by the Centers for Disease Control and Prevention (CDC) in 1982. Since that time, recognition of the disease has improved as modes of transmission and identification of risk factors have been studied and as serologic testing has become readily available. The CDC published an updated definition of AIDS for surveillance purposes in 1987. The diagnosis of AIDS is most commonly made with laboratory evidence of HIV infection and the presence of one or more indicator diseases. Table 122-1 contains a partial list of the conditions that, together with laboratory results, are diagnostic of AIDS.

The number of patients infected with HIV is growing dramatically worldwide. Actual seroprevalence is not known, as HIV seropositivity is currently not a reportable disease. As of 1993, over 334,000 cases of AIDS had been reported in the United States. Reported cases are thought to greatly underestimate the number of actual cases. Reports of the rate of HIV infection in inner-city emergency department patients range from 4.2 to 8.9 percent. The majority of these patients have unrecognized HIV infection. Studies in suburban hospitals have shown significantly lower rates. Risk factors commonly associated with HIV infection include homosexuality or bisexuality, injecting drug use, heterosexual exposure, blood recipients prior to 1985, and maternal-neonatal transmission. Heterosexual transmission accounts for the fastest-growing segment of the HIV-infected population.

Infection with HIV may be diagnosed by several methods: detection of antibodies to HIV, detection of viral-specific antigens, isolation of the virus by culture, and assays for HIV nucleic acid. At this time, because of difficulties in assuring confidentiality and providing adequate counseling, HIV testing is rarely indicated in the emergency department. However, recognition of risk factors and referral for counseling and testing may be appropriately initiated in the emergency department.

**Table 122-1.** AIDS-Defining Conditions

Esophageal candidiasis
Cryptococcosis
Cryptosporidiosis
Cytomegalovirus retinitis
Herpes simplex virus
Kaposi's sarcoma
Brain lymphoma
*Mycobacterium avium* complex
*P. carinii* pneumonia
Progressive multifocal leukoencephalopathy
Brain toxoplasmosis
HIV encephalopathy
HIV wasting syndrome
Disseminated histoplasmosis
Isosporiasis
Disseminated *M. tuberculosis* disease
Recurrent *Salmonella* septicemia

## PATHOPHYSIOLOGY

The human immunodeficiency virus is a cytopathic retrovirus which kills infected cells. It appears to selectively attack cells involved in immune function, primarily CD4 T-lymphocyte cells. The viral genes are carried as single-stranded RNA within the viral particle. Within the host cell, the RNA template is reverse-transcribed into DNA, which becomes permanently integrated into the host's DNA. As a result of infection, immunologic abnormalities ensue, including lymphopenia, qualitative CD4 T-lymphocyte function defect, autoimmune phenomena, and circulating immune complexes. The profound defect in cellular immunity is typically manifest as a variety of opportunistic infections and neoplasms.

Transmission of HIV has been shown to occur via semen, vaginal secretions, blood or blood products, breast milk, and by transplacental transmission in utero. HIV has also been isolated from saliva, urine, cerebrospinal fluid, brain, tears, alveolar fluid, synovial fluid, and amniotic fluid. Transmission has not been documented by casual contact. The HIV is a very labile virus and is easily neutralized by heat or common disinfecting agents, such as Lysol, a 1:10 solution of household bleach, 0.3% hydrogen peroxide, 35% isopropyl alcohol, or 50% ethanol.

Progression of disease after infection varies among individuals. Antibodies may be detected within several weeks to months after exposure. A study of homosexual males showed that 5 to 10 percent of patients will develop symptoms within 3 years of seroconversion. Predictors of high rates of progression include high serum B2-microglobulin level, low CD4 T-lymphocyte count, presence of p24 antigen, and hematocrit less than 40. The mean incubation time from the time of exposure to the development of AIDS is estimated at 8.23 years for adults and 1.97 years for children under age 5. The average survival time following a diagnosis of AIDS is approximately 9 months, although newer treatments under evaluation may alter this prognosis.

Immunologic status is often evaluated with the use of the CD4 T-lymphocyte count. Lymphocytes bearing the CD4 glycoprotein cell surface marker are the primary target of HIV infection. Measurement of the CD4 T-lymphocyte count is therefore valuable in evaluating the clinical immunologic status of HIV-infected patients. As the CD4 T-lymphocyte count drops below 200 cells/$\mu$L, the risk of opportunistic infection and other complications increases dramatically, and prophylactic treatment against *P. carinii* pneumonia is generally indicated.

## CLINICAL PRESENTATIONS AND MANAGEMENT

The spectrum of disease caused by HIV infection varies greatly. Many patients with asymptomatic HIV infection may be encountered for complaints unrelated to HIV disease. Other patients may be seen with involvement of virtually any organ system, commonly with more than one concurrent problem. Because of the complexity of HIV infection, and related opportunistic infection or malignancy, many specific diagnoses cannot be made in the emergency department. Diagnostic and therapeutic maneuvers are directed toward recognition of organ system involvement, assessment of the severity of disease, and, institution of specific therapy. Patient records should be reviewed whenever they are available to determine prior and current infections, complications, and recent CD4 T-lymphocyte counts. Table 122-2 lists some of the common causative conditions of organ system involvement in HIV-infected patients. Table 122-3 contains a summary of common infections and current recommendations for therapy.

### Systemic Symptoms

Early infection with HIV may be manifest with a period of malaise, fever, arthralgias, myalgias, lymphadenopathy, and weight loss, followed by a long asymptomatic period. Once the first symptoms appear, others may occur at any time. In such cases, systemic infection and malignancy must be excluded. In addition to a complete history and physical examination, appropriate laboratory investigation may include electrolytes, complete blood count, blood cultures (aerobic, anaerobic, and fungal), urinalysis and culture, liver function tests, chest radiograph, serologic testing for syphilis, and blood tests for cryptococcal antigen and *Toxoplasma* and *Coccidioides* serologies. Lumbar puncture may also be considered if no source of fever is identified.

Although fever may indicate any of a variety of infections, including bacterial, fungal, viral, and protozoal pathogens, the most common etiologies of fever include HIV-related fever, systemic infections such as *Mycobacterium avium* complex (MAI), cytomegalovirus (CMV), Hodgkin's disease, and non-Hodgkin's lymphoma.

MAI complex causes disseminated disease in up to 50 percent of AIDS patients. It is usually associated with weight loss, diarrhea, fever, malaise, and anorexia. It may also cause pulmonary involvement. Anemia and liver function test abnormalities may be seen. Diagnosis may be made by acid-fast stain of stool or other body fluids, or by blood culture. Treatment is often ineffective, especially for disseminated disease, due to wide resistance to isoniazid and rifampin.

CMV also commonly causes disseminated disease in HIV-infected individuals and is often associated with PCP. It is the most common cause of retinitis in such patients. Gastrointestinal involvement is also common. Ganciclovir (DHPG) is commonly used as treatment. It is thought to be especially effective for patients with retinitis and colitis.

Many HIV-infected patients with fever may be managed as outpatients. Outpatient management may be attempted if the source of the fever does not dictate admission, appropriate laboratory studies have been initiated, the patient is able to function adequately at home (e.g., ambulation and sufficient oral intake), and appropriate medical follow-up can be arranged.

### Cutaneous Manifestations

Cutaneous manifestations of HIV infection are commonly encountered in the emergency department. Generalized cutaneous complaints such as xerosis (dry skin) and pruritus are common, and may be manifest prior to development of opportunistic infections. Xerosis may be treated with emollients, and if necessary, with mild topical steroids. Pruritus may respond to oatmeal baths, and if necessary, antihistamines. Exacerbation of any underlying dermatologic condition is common.

Infections including *Staphylococcus aureus* (manifest as bullous impetigo, ecthyma, or folliculitis), *Pseudomonas aeruginosa* (which may present with chronic ulcerations and macerations), herpes simplex, herpes zoster, syphilis, and scabies are commonly seen and should be treated with standard therapies.

Kaposi's sarcoma is the second most common manifestation of AIDS (second to PCP). It is usually widely disseminated and may involve mucous membranes. Since Kaposi's sarcoma is not generally associated with significant morbidity or mortality, therapy is only indicated for extensive, painful, or cosmetically disfiguring lesions. Chemotherapy with vincristine, vinblastine, or doxyrubicin, or radiation therapy may be used.

Varicella zoster eruptions are commonly seen. In the HIV-positive patient, outpatient management may be sufficient. However, in the AIDS patient, or with disseminated disease, admission is frequently indicated for therapy with intravenous acyclovir (30 mg/kg per day). Varicella immune globulin (VZIG) may be useful in patients with primary infection and visceral involvement.

**Table 122-2.** Common Conditions Causing Organ System Involvement in AIDS Patients

| | Systemic | Pulmonary | GI | Neurologic |
|---|---|---|---|---|
| **Bacteria** | | | | |
| *Staphylococcus aureus* | X | X | | |
| *Streptococcus pneumoniae* | X | X | | |
| *Clostridium perfringens* | X | | | |
| *Haemophilus influenzae* | X | X | | |
| *Shigella* species | X | | X | |
| *Salmonella* species | X | | X | |
| *Listeria monocytogenes* | X | | | |
| *Treponema pallidum* | X | | | X |
| *Neisseria gonorrhoeae* | | | X | |
| *Campylobacter jejuni* | | | X | |
| *Nocardia asteroides* | X | X | | |
| *Chlamydia* species | X | | X | |
| *Legionella* species | X | X | | |
| *M. avium complex* (MAI) | X | X | | |
| *M. tuberculosis* | X | X | | |
| Anaerobic species | X | | | |
| **Viruses** | | | | |
| Human immunodeficiency virus | X | | X | X |
| Hepatitis viruses | X | | | |
| Epstein-Barr virus | X | | | |
| Herpes simplex virus (HSV) | X | X | X | X |
| Cytomegalovirus (CMV) | X | X | X | X |
| Herpes zoster virus | X | | | X |
| Adenoviruses | X | X | X | |
| **Fungi** | | | | |
| *Aspergillus* species | X | | | |
| *Histoplasma capsulatum* | X | X | | |
| *Cryptococcus neoformans* | X | X | | X |
| *Coccidioides* | X | X | | |
| *Candida* species | X | X | X | |
| **Protozoa** | | | | |
| *Cryptosporidium* species | X | | X | |
| *Toxoplasma gondii* | X | X | | X |
| *Pneumocystis carinii* | X | X | | |
| *Isospora* species | X | | X | |
| *Entamoeba* species | X | | X | |
| *Giardia lamblia* | | | X | |
| *Strongyloides* | | | X | |
| **Malignancy** | | | | |
| Kaposi's sarcoma | X | X | X | |
| Lymphoma | X | X | X | X |
| Hodgkin's disease | X | | | |

Herpes simplex infections are common among AIDS patients and may present as either local infection or systemic involvement. Herpes simplex infections respond well to standard therapy with oral acyclovir (200 mg five times daily for 10 days). Intravenous therapy (15 to 30 mg/kg per day) may be required in extensive disease.

Molluscum contagiosum presents as small flesh-colored papules with a white core. Since cure is difficult, treatment is recommended for symptomatic lesions only. Treatment may be instituted by a dermatologist with cryotherapy or curettage.

Intertriginous infections with either *Candida* or *Tricophyton* are common, and may be diagnosed by microscopic examination of potassium hydroxide preparation of lesion scrapings. Treatment may include topical imidazole creams (such as clotrimazole, miconazole, or ketoconazole).

Seborrheic dermatitis is a common eruption, and may present as erythematous, hyperkeratotic, scaling plaques involving the scalp, face (typically in a malar distribution), ears, chest, and genitalia. Treatment with topical steroids is effective in most patients.

Human papillomavirus infections occur with increased frequency in immunocompromised patients. Treatment is cosmetic or symptomatic, and may include cryotherapy, topical therapy, or laser therapy.

Other dermatologic conditions which occur with increased frequency among HIV-infected patients include psoriasis, atopic dermatitis, and alopecia. Referral for dermatologic consultation is generally indicated.

## Neurologic Complications

Central nervous system disease occurs in 75 to 90 percent of patients with AIDS, and 10 to 20 percent of AIDS patients initially present with CNS symptoms. The most common symptoms are seizures or altered mental status, but headache, meningismus, and neuropathy also commonly occur. Emergency department evaluation should include a complete neurologic examination, and when appropriate, computed tomography and lumbar puncture. Specific CSF studies which may be of value include opening and closing pressures, cell

**Table 122-3.** Treatment Recommendations for Common HIV-Related Infections

| Organ System | Infection | Therapy |
|---|---|---|
| Systemic | MAI | No known effective therapy |
| | CMV | Ganciclovir, 7.5–15 mg/kg/d; maintenance therapy required |
| Pulmonary | *P. carinii* | TMP-SMX, 15–20 mg TMP/kg/d and 75–100 mg SMX/kg/d, PO or IV, for 3 weeks<br>*or*<br>Pentamidine, 4 mg/kg/d, IV or IM, for 3 weeks |
| | *M. tuberculosis* | Isoniazid, 5–10 mg/kg/d PO<br>*plus*<br>Rifampin, 9 mg/kg/d<br>*plus*<br>Pyrazinamide, 25 mg/kg/d PO *or* streptomycin, 0.75–1.0 mg/kg/d IM |
| CNS | Toxoplasmosis | Pyrimethamine, 25–50 mg/d PO<br>*plus*<br>Sulfadiazine, 100 mg/kg/d, for 3–6 months |
| | Cryptococcosis | Amphotericin B, 0.4–0.6 mg/kg/d; maintenance therapy required |
| Ophthalmologic | CMV | Ganciclovir, 5 mg/kg bid for 2 weeks; maintenance therapy required |
| GI | Candidiasis | Clotrimazole, 30–50 mg/d<br>*or*<br>Ketoconazole, 200–400 mg/d; maintenance therapy required<br>*or*<br>Fluconazole, 100 mg/d |
| | Salmonellosis | TMP-SMX, 10 mg TMP/kg/d and 50 mg SMX/kg/d, IV or PO<br>*or*<br>Ampicillin, 12 g/d IV; maintenance therapy required |
| | Cryptosporidiosis | No known effective therapy |
| Cutaneous | HSV | Acyclovir, 1000 mg/d PO<br>*or*<br>Acyclovir, 15 mg/kg/d IV |
| | Herpes zoster | Acyclovir, 25–30 mg/kg/d IV |
| | *Candida, tricophyton* | Clotrimazole, miconazole, or ketoconazole, topical therapy bid-tid for 3 weeks |

count, glucose, protein, Gram stain, India ink stain, bacterial culture, viral culture, fungal culture, *Toxoplasma* and *Cryptococcus* antigen, and coccidioidomycosis titer. The most common etiologies of neurologic symptoms include AIDS dementia, *T. gondii*, and *C. neoformans*.

AIDS dementia complex (also referred to as HIV encephalopathy, or subacute encephalitis) is a progressive dementia, commonly heralded by impairment of recent memory and other cognitive deficits, caused by direct HIV infection. It occurs in over one-third of AIDS patients. Zidovudine (AZT) is the recommended therapy.

Toxoplasmosis is the most common cause of focal encephalitis in patients with AIDS. Symptoms may include headache, fever, focal neurologic deficits, altered mental status, or seizures. Diagnosis may be made by a contrast-enhanced CT scan showing ring-enhancing lesions. However, because of possible false-negative CT scans, MRI or a delayed CT scan may be necessary to establish the diagnosis. Other etiologies in the differential diagnosis of ring-enhancing lesions include lymphoma, fungal infection, and cerebral tuberculosis. Often the diagnosis may be definitively established only with brain biopsy. Treatment for toxoplasmosis should be instituted with oral sulfadi-

azine (100 mg/kg per day) and pyrimethamine (25 to 50 mg/d), with folinic acid added to reduce the incidence of hematologic toxicity. Short courses of steroids may be employed. Chronic suppressive therapy is usually indicated after acute treatment.

Cryptococcal CNS infection may be seen in up to 10 percent of AIDS patients and may cause either focal cerebral lesions or diffuse meningoencephalitis. Presenting symptoms may include headache, lightheadedness, depression, seizures, or cranial nerve palsies. Diagnosis is made by India ink preparation or fungal culture, or by the presence of cryptococcal antigen in the CSF. Treatment should include intravenous amphotericin B (0.4 to 0.6 mg/kg per day). Flucytosine (75 to 100 mg/kg per day) may be added to this therapy. Sixty percent of patients may be expected to respond to therapy. Initial therapy should continue for 6 weeks, and chronic suppressive therapy is often indicated.

Other infections such as bacterial meningitis, brain abscess, CMV or herpes simplex virus (HSV) encephalitis, and neurosyphilis should also be considered in the differential diagnosis of neurologic presentations.

Disposition may be considered after appropriate evaluation is undertaken in the emergency department. Most patients with new or changed neurologic involvement should be admitted.

## Psychiatric Disorders

AIDS and its associated disease states may manifest as physiologic, neurologic, or psychiatric abnormalities, and may also involve complex psychological and social issues. Interactions with family and friends may be altered, and issues of confronting chronic illness and death may prove devastating. The most common psychiatric presentations include delirium, dementia, depression, and psychosis.

Delirium or dementia suggest the presence of a primary physiologic disease state and should be thoroughly investigated as discussed above.

Depression is common among AIDS patients, and may be initially manifested as a primary complaint or as a suicide attempt. Patients with a previous history of depression are at increased risk. Depression is often responsive to hospitalization and psychosocial intervention. Antidepressant therapy may be considered if symptoms of depression continue longer than 2 weeks. Suicidal ideation may often require inpatient psychiatric management.

AIDS psychosis is poorly understood; and the patient may present with psychiatric symptoms such as hallucinations, delusions, or other abnormal behavioral changes. The etiology is unclear.

## Ophthalmologic Manifestations

Eye complaints such as change in visual acuity, photophobia, redness, or pain are common among AIDS patients and may represent retinitis or malignant invasion of the eye or periorbital tissues.

The most common eye finding in AIDS patients is cotton-wool spots, which are probably secondary to microvascular lesions and often resolve spontaneously. No specific therapy is indicated.

Cytomegalovirus retinitis occurs in 10 to 15 percent of patients. It accounts for the majority of retinitis among AIDS patients. It may be asymptomatic or may present with photophobia, scotoma, redness, pain, or change in visual acuity. It has a characteristic appearance of fluffy white retinal lesions, often perivascular. Treatment should be initiated with ganciclovir (5 mg/kg bid) for 2 weeks, followed by long-term maintenance therapy.

## Pulmonary Complications

Pulmonary manifestations of HIV infection are one of the most common reasons for emergency department visits among AIDS patients.

**Table 122-4.** Chest Radiographic Abnormalities: Differential Diagnosis in the AIDS Patient

| Finding | Etiologies |
| --- | --- |
| Diffuse interstitial infiltration | PCP |
| | CMV |
| | MTB |
| | MAI |
| | Histoplasmosis |
| | Coccidioidomycosis |
| | Lymphoid interstitial pneumonitis |
| Focal consolidation | Bacterial pneumonia |
| | *M. pneumoniae* |
| | *P. carinii* |
| | MTB |
| | MAI |
| Nodular lesions | Kaposi's sarcoma |
| | MTB |
| | MAI |
| | Fungal lesions |
| | Toxoplasmosis |
| Cavitary lesions | PCP |
| | MTB |
| | Bacterial infection |
| | Fungal infection |
| Adenopathy | Kaposi's sarcoma |
| | Lymphoma |
| | MTB |
| | Cryptococcosis |

Common presenting complaints may include cough, hemoptysis, shortness of breath, or chest pain. Evaluation in the emergency department may include history, lung examination, pulse oximetry and arterial blood gas determination, sputum culture, Gram stain, acid-fast stain, blood cultures, and chest radiograph. Leukocytosis, productive cough, and presence of a focal infiltrate are suggestive of bacterial pneumonia. The most common etiologies of pulmonary abnormalities include PCP, *Mycobacterium tuberculosis* pneumonia (MTB), CMV, *Cryptococcus neoformans, Histoplasma capsulatum,* and neoplasm. Nonproductive cough and the presence of a diffuse infiltrative process on chest radiography suggest PCP, CMV, or Kaposi's sarcoma. Hilar adenopathy with a diffuse pulmonary infiltrate may be associated with cryptococcosis, histoplasmosis, mycobacterial pneumonia, or neoplasm. Since the chest radiograph may be normal in 5 to 10 percent of patients with PCP, a normal chest x-ray does not exclude the possibility of active pulmonary disease. Table 122-4 summarizes common radiographic findings in the AIDS patient.

Emergency department management may include supplemental oxygen, volume repletion if indicated, and, when appropriate, initiation of antibiotic therapy. Admission should be considered for patients with new-onset pulmonary symptoms and especially for those with hypoxia.

PCP is the most common opportunistic infection among AIDS patients. More than 80 percent of patients will acquire PCP at some time during their illness. It is often the initial opportunistic infection which establishes the diagnosis of AIDS. Common presenting symptoms may include cough, typically nonproductive, and shortness of breath. Chest radiography may show a diffuse interstitial infiltrate, but may be falsely negative in 5 to 10 percent of patients. Presumptive diagnosis is often assumed if there is hypoxia without any other explanation. Gallium scanning of the chest is more sensitive but may result in more false positives. Other diagnostic tests include bronchoscopy with lavage, biopsy, and culture or examination of induced sputum by indirect immunofluorescence using monoclonal antibodies. Initial therapy for PCP should be instituted with TMP-SMX

(trimethoprim, 20 mg/kg per day, and sulfamethoxazole, 100 mg/kg per day), either PO or IV for 2 to 3 weeks. Pentamidine isothionate (4 mg/kg per day) may be used as an effective alternative therapy. A majority of patients respond to therapy. Oral steroid therapy should be instituted for patients with $Pa_{O_2} < 70$ mm Hg, or alveolar-arterial gradient > 35. The usual regimen consists of oral prednisone; 80 mg for 5 days, followed by 40 mg for 5 days, followed by 20 mg for an additional 11 days. Relapses are common; 65 percent of patients will have a reinfection within 18 months. Repeat infections may be less responsive to therapy. Prophylactic therapy with an agent such as TMP-SMX, inhaled pentamidine, or dapsone may be used.

The incidence of MTB among AIDS patients is increasing. Reactivation of prior infection due to immunosuppression is common. Chest radiography may be nondiagnostic, since the typical pulmonary upper lobe involvement is less common among AIDS patients. Negative PPD tests are frequent among AIDS patients due to immunosuppression. Diagnosis may be made by sputum stain and culture or by bronchoscopy with biopsy. Triple therapy with isoniazid, rifampin, and ethambutol should be initiated. This regimen may be supplemented with pyrazinamide or streptomycin. It is currently recommended that all HIV-infected patients with positive PPD should receive prophylaxis.

## Gastrointestinal Complications

Gastrointestinal manifestations of HIV infection are common. Approximately 50 percent of AIDS patients will present with GI complaints at some time during their illness. The most common presenting symptoms include abdominal pain, bleeding, and diarrhea. Common causes include *Candida,* Kaposi's sarcoma, MAI, HSV-1 and HSV-2, CMV, *Campylobacter jejuni, Shigella, Salmonella, Giardia, Entamoeba histolytica, Cryptosporidium,* and *Isospora* species. Emergency department evaluation should focus on identification and severity of symptoms and on obtaining appropriate initial diagnostic studies. Therapy should include rehydration and initiation of antibiotic therapy when appropriate.

Oral candidiasis affects more than 80 percent of AIDS patients. The tongue and buccal mucosa are commonly involved. Differentiation from hairy leukoplakia (usually manifest as white thickened lesions on the lateral tongue borders), may be difficult, but microscopic examination on potassium hydroxide smear can confirm the diagnosis. The development of oral candidiasis is a poor prognostic sign and is predictive of progression to AIDS. Most oral lesions can be managed symptomatically on an outpatient basis. Clotrimazole troches (five times daily) are the preferred treatment. Oral ketoconazole or fluconazole may be used if clotrimazole is ineffective. Nystatin suspension is not recommended due to limited duration of application in the oropharynx.

Oral involvement with HSV, Kaposi's sarcoma, or other pathogens is also common and may usually be managed on an outpatient basis with symptomatic therapy.

Esophageal involvement may occur with *Candida,* HSV, and CMV. Esophagitis may present with complaints of dysphagia or odynophagia. Endoscopy, fungal stains, viral cultures, or biopsy may be necessary to establish the diagnosis. An air-contrast barium swallow may be obtained in the emergency department to establish the diagnosis of *Candida* esophagitis. A pattern of ulceration with plaques is typically seen. Treatment should be initiated with oral ketoconazole or fluconazole. Relapses are common and intravenous amphotericin B may occasionally be required. Herpes esophagitis may produce punched-out ulcerations without associated heaped-up plaques. Treatment with acyclovir should be initiated.

Hepatomegaly occurs in perhaps 50 percent of AIDS patients. Elevation of alkaline phosphatase is commonly seen. Jaundice is uncommon. Coinfection with hepatitis B and hepatitis C is common, especially among IV drug users. Opportunistic infection with CMV, MAI, and MTB may also cause signs of hepatitis.

Diarrhea is the most common gastrointestinal complaint and is estimated to occur in 50 to 90 percent of AIDS patients. Emergency department evaluation may include microscopic examination of stool for leukocytes, acid-fast stain, and examination for ova and parasites, as well as bacterial culture of stool and blood. Management should be directed toward repletion of fluid and electrolytes. *Cryptosporidium* and *Isospora* infection in particular are common etiologies and are associated with prolonged watery diarrhea. Salmonella also occurs commonly among AIDS patients, and may cause bacteremia. Long-term management of diarrhea not requiring specific therapy may be established with attapulgite (Kaopectate), psyllium (Metamucil), and if necessary, diphenoxylate hydrochloride with atropine (Lomotil).

## Cardiovascular Manifestations

Clinically significant cardiac disease among AIDS patients is uncommon. Findings such as pericardial effusion, cardiomyopathy, and congestive heart failure are frequently reported at autopsy but are often clinically silent.

## Renal Manifestations

Renal insufficiency among AIDS patients may be secondary to prerenal azotemia, drug nephrotoxicity, or HIV-associated nephropathy (HIVAN), which may cause chronic renal insufficiency due to focal and segmental glomerulosclerosis. Management decisions should be made in conjunction with a nephrologist.

## Sexually Transmitted Diseases

Several sexually transmitted diseases are epidemiologically associated with HIV infection. In addition to such common entities as gonorrhea, chlamydia, and herpes infections, syphilis is seen with increased frequency and may more commonly present in the secondary stage of infection. Patients with any sexually transmitted disease should be evaluated for syphilis. Empiric therapy may be instituted in cases where secondary syphilis is suspected, with intramuscular benzathine penicillin, 2.4 million units weekly for three weeks. Therapy for other sexually transmitted diseases is based on current CDC guidelines (see Chap. 120).

## IMMUNIZATIONS OF HIV-INFECTED PATIENTS

According to the U.S. Public Health Service Immunizations Practices Advisory Committee (ACIP), routine immunization schedules for DPT, Td, and MMR should be followed for HIV-infected patients Other vaccinations are generally not indicated in the emergency department. Response to vaccination may be variable among individuals. Table 122-5 summarizes the Centers for Disease Control recommendations for common immunizations.

**Table 122-5.** Immunization Recommendations for HIV-Infected Patients

| Vaccine | Asymptomatic | Symptomatic |
|---|---|---|
| DPT (to age 7) | Yes | Yes |
| Td | Yes | Yes |
| OPV | No | No |
| IPV (inactivated polio vaccine) | Yes | Yes |
| MMR | Yes | Consider vaccine |
| H. flu (HbCV) | Yes | Yes |
| Pneumococcal | Yes | Yes |
| Influenza (inactivated) | No (although not contraindicated) | Yes |

*Source:* Adapted from Centers for Disease Control, *MMWR* 38:205, 1989.

## DRUG REACTIONS

Reactions to pharmacologic therapy are common among HIV-infected patients and must always be considered as a possible etiology of new symptomatology. In a recent series, 5 percent of emergency department visits by symptomatic HIV-positive patients were related to complications of pharmacologic therapy. Table 122-6 illustrates common side effects of medications used in AIDS patients.

## ETHICAL CONSIDERATIONS

Many ethical considerations are involved in testing and treatment of HIV-infected patients. Testing for HIV in the emergency department is generally not indicated. Many departments have adopted strict policies against such testing, due to the difficulties of ensuring adequate confidentiality and counseling. This may change as the need for early identification and treatment of patients is demonstrated. Initiation of counseling and referral for testing are recommended for patients at high risk.

Resuscitation in patients with advanced AIDS is a controversial subject. Since emergency department physicians may have limited information about individual patients, their wishes, and the state of their disease, it is recommended that appropriate therapy and resuscitative measures be undertaken, unless advance directives are available.

Confidentiality regarding HIV-related diagnoses is paramount in providing appropriate patient care. Treatment without discrimination, as with all disease states, should be initiated in all patients unless they specifically request otherwise.

## PRECAUTIONS FOR HEALTH CARE WORKERS

Health care workers are often exposed to HIV-infected patients and their body fluids. Precautions in handling potentially infectious fluids are crucial to protect against occupational acquisition of HIV infection. Since HIV infection is often undiagnosed at the time of the emergency department encounter, the use of universal precautions is strongly recommended. Departments should educate employees regarding specific precautions regarding needle handling, cleaning of patient areas and equipment, and the use of gloves, gown, glasses, and masks. However, it should also be noted that the risk of acquiring HIV through occupational exposure is low. The risk of contracting AIDS after such exposure has been estimated at 0.32 percent. Approximately 80 percent of cases of documented occupational exposure have been due to needle-stick injuries. If a significant occupational exposure to a patient occurs, HIV testing of the patient, with the patient's consent, is recommended. If the patient tests positive for HIV, HIV testing of the employee is recommended at 6 weeks, 3 months, and 6 months following exposure. Prophylaxis with zidovudine may be considered after acute parenteral exposure to infected blood, although its efficacy in preventing HIV transmission is as yet unproven.

## DISPOSITION

Consultation with an infectious disease specialist, neurologist, psychiatrist, or gastroenterologist is often necessary to provide proper therapy and disposition.

Disposition decisions, as for all patients, are based on determination of the patient's ability to function as an outpatient, with special consideration regarding oral intake and ambulation; availability of adequate outpatient therapy for the specific condition; and the availability of appropriate medical follow-up. Admission is generally indicated for patients with abnormal vital signs, unexplained neurologic findings or seizures, hypoxia worse than baseline, significant volume depletion, bone marrow suppression, or any other condition causing extreme debilitation or requiring intravenous therapy.

**Table 122-6.** Common Drug Reactions Seen in the HIV-Infected Patient

| Medication | Fever | Rash | Nausea & Vomiting | Diarrhea | Constipation | Headache | Mental Status Change | Phlebitis | Neuropathy |
|---|---|---|---|---|---|---|---|---|---|
| **Antimicrobials** | | | | | | | | | |
| TMP-SMX | X | X | X | | | | | | |
| Pentamidine | | X | | | | | | | |
| Isoniazid | X | X | X | | | | | | X |
| Clindamycin | | X | | | | | | | |
| Dapsone | X | X | X | | | X | | | X |
| **Antifungal agents** | | | | | | | | | |
| Amphotericin | X | | X | | | X | | X | |
| 5-FU | | | X | X | | | | | |
| Ganciclovir | | | X | X | | | | X | |
| Clotrimazole | | | X | X | | | | | |
| Nystatin | | | X | X | | | | | |
| Ketoconazole | | | X | X | | | | | |
| **Antiviral agents** | | | | | | | | | |
| Zidovudine | | | X | | | X | X | | |
| Acyclovir | | | X | X | | X | | | |
| **Pain medications** | | | | | | | | | |
| Ibuprofen | | X | X | X | X | | | | |
| Narcotics | | | X | | X | | | | |

| Medication | ↑LFT | ↑Glucose | ↓Glucose | ↓K | ↓Mg | ↓WBC | ↓Plt | ↓Hct |
|---|---|---|---|---|---|---|---|---|
| **Antimicrobials** | | | | | | | | |
| TMP-SMX | X | | | | | X | X | |
| Pentamidine | | X | X | | | X | | X |
| Isoniazid | X | | | | | X | X | X |
| Clindamycin | | | | | | | | |
| Dapsone | X | | | | | X | | X |
| **Antifungal agents** | | | | | | | | |
| Amphotericin | | | | X | X | | | X |
| 5-FU | X | | | | | X | | |
| Ganciclovir | | | | | | X | | |
| Clotrimazole | | | | | | | | |
| Nystatin | | | | | | | | |
| Ketoconazole | X | | | | | | | |
| **Antiviral agents** | | | | | | | | |
| Zidovudine | | | | | | X | | X |
| Acyclovir | | | | | | | | |
| **Pain medications** | | | | | | | | |
| Ibuprofen | X | | | | | X | | X |
| Narcotics | | | | | | | | |

## BIBLIOGRAPHY

Centers for Disease Control: AIDS and human immunodeficiency virus infection in the United States: 1988 update. *MMWR* 37, 1988.

Centers for Disease Control: Guidelines for prevention of transmission of human immunodeficiency virus and Hepatitis B virus to health-care and public safety workers. *MMWR* 38(suppl no. S-6), 1989.

Centers for Disease Control: Heterosexually acquired AIDS—United States, 1993. *JAMA* 271:975, 1994.

Centers for Disease Control: *HIV/AIDS Surveillance Report.* May 1993.

Centers for Disease Control: Public Health Service statement of management of occupational exposure to human immunodeficiency virus, including considerations regarding zidovudine postexposure use. *MMWR* 39(RR-1), 1990.

Centers for Disease Control: Revision of the CDC surveillance case definition of acquired immunodeficiency syndrome. *MMWR* 36(suppl 1), 1987.

Cohen PT, Sande MA, Volberding PA (eds): *The AIDS Knowledge Base.* Waltham, Massachusetts, Massachusetts Medical Society, 1990.

Fischl MA, Richman DD, Grieco MH, et al: The efficacy of azidothymidine (AZT) in the treatment of patients with AIDS and AIDS-related complex: A double-blind, placebo-controlled trial. *N Engl J Med* 317:185, 1987.

Glatt AE, Chirgwin K, Landesman S: Treatment of infections associated with human immunodeficiency virus. *N Engl J Med* 318:1439, 1988.

Henderson DK: HIV in the health care setting, in Mandell GL, Douglas RG, Bennett JE, (eds): *Principles and Practice of Infectious Diseases,* 3d ed. New York, Churchill Livingstone, 1990.

Kelen GD, DiGiovanna T, Bisson K, et al: Human immunodeficiency virus infection in emergency department patients: Epidemiology, clinical presentations and risk to health care workers: The Johns Hopkins experience. *JAMA* 262:516, 1989.

Kelen GD, Fritz S, Qaqish B, et al: Unrecognized human immunodeficiency virus (HIV) infection in general emergency patients. *N Engl J Med* 318:1645, 1988.

Murray JF, Garay SM, Hopewell PC, et al: Pulmonary complications of the acquired immunodeficiency syndrome: of the second National Heart, Lung and Blood Institute workshop. *Am Rev Respir Dis* 135:504, 1987.

Sande MA, Volberding PA: *The Medical Management of AIDS.* Philadelphia, Saunders, 1993.

# 123

# TETANUS

## Donna L. Carden

Tetanus is an acute, frequently fatal disease which results from a wound infected with the organism *Clostridium tetani*. The clinical manifestations of tetanus are all secondary to an exotoxin, tetanospasmin, elaborated at the wound site by the clostridial organism and consist of generalized muscular rigidity and violent muscular contractions.

## PATHOPHYSIOLOGY

*Clostridium tetani* is an anaerobic gram-positive rod which exists in either a vegetative or sporulated form. The spores formed by the organism are extremely resistant to destruction and can survive in soil and on environmental surfaces for years. *Clostridium tetani* is usually introduced into a wound in the sporulated form where it may later germinate into the tetanospasmin-producing vegetative form if tissue oxygen tension is sufficiently low. Any factor which lowers the local oxidation-reduction potential, such as the presence of crushed, devitalized tissue or a foreign body, or the development of suppuration, favors the development of the vegetative form of *C. tetani*.

The infection caused by *C. tetani* remains localized at the site of injury, but the exotoxin is transmitted to the central nervous system by retrograde axonal transport where it is responsible for all of the clinical manifestations of tetanus. Tetanospasmin acts on the motor end plates of skeletal muscle, in the spinal cord, in the brain, and in the sympathetic nervous system. This extremely potent exotoxin prevents the release of the inhibitory neurotransmitters glycine and γ-aminobutyric acid (GABA) from presynaptic nerve terminals and, therefore, results in disinhibition of the motor and autonomic nervous systems as well as all of the clinical manifestations of the disease.

## CLINICAL FEATURES

Although safe and effective immunization exists for the prevention of tetanus, the disease is still a major health problem worldwide and is an important cause of infant mortality in developing countries. In the United States, approximately 60 cases of tetanus are reported each year, the majority of cases occurring in patients over 50 years of age who are inadequately immunized. In fact, the majority of Americans over 60 years of age lack adequate immunity to tetanus. The overall case fatality rate in the United States for the disease in 1989 and 1990 was 24 percent.

Tetanus occurs most frequently following an acute, unreported injury, most commonly a puncture wound to an extremity. However, tetanus can also develop after minor trauma, surgical procedures, otitis media, and abortion, and can develop in neonates through infection of the umbilical cord. The majority of tetanus cases in the United States occur in the rural southern states, with the states of California, Texas, and Florida responsible for the greatest number of reported cases of tetanus (17, 12, and 11, respectively).

The incubation period of tetanus, that is, the period from infection to the first appearance of symptoms, can range from less than 24 h to over 1 month. The shorter the incubation period, the more severe the disease and the worse the prognosis for recovery.

Clinical tetanus can be categorized into four forms: local, generalized, cephalic, and neonatal. The different categories of clinical tetanus are dependent upon what population of neurons are involved.

*Local tetanus* is manifested by persistent rigidity of the muscles in close proximity to the site of injury and usually resolves after weeks to months without sequelae. Local tetanus may progress to the generalized form of the disease.

*Generalized tetanus* is the most common form of the disease and usually follows unreported minor trauma. Of note is the fact that of those patients who develop tetanus and do seek medical care, the majority (>90 percent) do not receive appropriate tetanus prophylaxis. The most frequent presenting complaints of the patient with tetanus are pain and stiffness in the jaw and trunk muscles. The transition from muscle stiffness to rigidity leads to the development of trismus and the resultant characteristic facial expression, *risus sardonicus* (sardonic smile). Reflex convulsive spasms and tonic contractions of muscle groups are responsible for the development of dysphasia, opisthotonos, flexing of the arms, clenching of the fists, and extension of the lower extremities. Patients are completely conscious and alert unless laryngospasm and tonic contraction of the respiratory muscles result in respiratory compromise.

Disturbances of the autonomic nervous system, generally a hypersympathetic state, occur during the second week of clinical tetanus and present as tachycardia, labile hypertension, profuse sweating, hyperpyrexia, and increased urinary excretion of catecholamines. The autonomic complications of generalized tetanus are particularly difficult to manage and contribute significantly to the morbidity and mortality of the disease.

*Cephalic tetanus* follows injuries to the head or occasionally otitis media and results in dysfunction of the cranial nerves, most commonly the seventh. This form of tetanus has a particularly poor prognosis.

*Neonatal tetanus* is an important cause of infant mortality in developing countries and carries an extremely high mortality rate. Neonatal tetanus is uniformly associated with inadequate maternal immunization.

## DIAGNOSIS

Tetanus is diagnosed solely on the basis of clinical evidence. A reliable history of active immunization with a booster within the previous 10 years virtually eliminates tetanus as a diagnostic possibility.

There are no laboratory tests to diagnose tetanus, although serum antitoxin titers of $\geq 0.01$ IU/mL are usually protective and may be helpful retrospectively. In addition, the recovery of the *C. tetani* organism from a wound is meaningless in an immunized patient.

The differential diagnosis of tetanus is presented in Table 123-1. Strychnine poisoning most closely mimics the clinical picture of generalized tetanus.

## TREATMENT

The patient with tetanus should be managed in an intensive care unit. Respiratory compromise may require immediate neuromuscular blockade (succinylcholine) and orotracheal intubation, but tracheostomy provides the best method of prolonged ventilatory control. Environmental stimuli must be minimized in order to prevent the precipitation of reflex convulsive spasms.

Identification and debridement of the wound through which the clostridial spores were introduced are necessary to minimize further toxin production and to improve the oxidation-reduction potential of

**Table 123-1.** Differential Diagnosis of Tetanus

| |
|---|
| Strychnine poisoning |
| Dystonic reaction (phenothiazines) |
| Hypocalcemic tetany |
| Peritonsillar abscess |
| Peritonitis |
| Meningeal irritation (bacterial meningitis, subarachnoid hemorrhage) |
| Rabies |
| Temporomandibular joint disease |

the infected tissue. A wound may not be identified in up to 10 percent of patients with tetanus.

## Tetanus Immune Globulin

Human tetanus immune globulin (TIG) neutralizes circulating tetanospasmin and toxin in the wound but not toxin that is already fixed in the nervous system. Despite the fact that TIG does not ameliorate the clinical symptoms of tetanus, there is evidence that its administration significantly reduces mortality. The commonly recommended intramuscular dose of TIG is 3000 to 5000 U; however, 500 U has been shown to be equally effective and can be administered in a single injection.

## Antibiotics

Antibiotics, although of questionable utility in the treatment of tetanus, have traditionally been administered. *Clostridium tetani* is sensitive to a number of antibiotics (e.g., penicillins, cephalosporins, tetracycline, erythromycin) but parenterally administered metronidazole should be considered the antibiotic of choice. Penicillin, a centrally acting $GABA_A$, antagonist, may potentiate the effects of tetanospasmin and, therefore, should be avoided.

## Muscle Relaxants

As noted above, tetanospasmin prevents transmission at inhibitory interneurons, and so therapy of tetanus is aimed at restoring inhibition. The benzodiazepines are centrally acting inhibitory agents which have been used for this purpose. Diazepam has been extensively utilized and results in a desirable degree of sedation as well as amnesia. Lorazepam, because of its long duration of action, is the benzodiazepine of choice. Large intravenous doses of all benzodiazepines result in metabolic acidosis secondary to the propylene glycol vehicle, a complication that is avoided by administering oral benzodiazepines

**Table 123-2.** Summary Guide to Tetanus Prophylaxis in Wound Management

| History of Adsorbed Tetanus Toxoid (Doses) | Clean, Minor Wounds | | All Other Wounds[a] | |
|---|---|---|---|---|
| | Td[b], 0.5 mL | TIG, IM 250 U IM | Td[b], 0.5 mL IM | TIG, 250 U IM |
| Unknown or <three | Yes[c] | No | Yes | Yes |
| ≥Three[d] | No[e] | No | Yes[f] | No |

[a] For example, wounds >6 h old, contaminated with soil, saliva, feces, or dirt; puncture or crush wounds; avulsions; wounds from missiles, burns, or frostbite.

[b] DPT for children <7 years of age (Td if pertussis vaccine is contraindicated); Td for persons >7 years of age.

[c] The primary immunization series should be completed. Three doses total are required, with the second dose given at least 4 weeks after the first and the third dose 6 months later.

[d] If only three doses of fluid toxoid have been received, then a fourth dose of *absorbed* toxoid should be given.

[e] Yes, if routine immunization schedule has lapsed in a child <7 years of age of if >10 years since last dose.

[f] Yes, if routine immunization schedule has lapsed in a child <7 years of age or if >5 years since last dose. Boosters more frequent than every 5 years may predispose to side effects.

*Source:* Adapted, with permission, from American College of Emergency Physicians: Tetanus immunization recommendations for persons seven years of age and older, *Ann Emerg Med* 15:1111, 1986; and American College of Emergency Physicians: Tetanus immunization recommendations for persons less than 7 years old, *Ann Emerg Med* 16:1183, 1987.

or by use of the sedating agent, midazolam. Methocarbamol and baclofen have also been suggested as alternative modalities for restoring central inhibition and providing muscle relaxation. Dantrolene is a peripherally acting muscle relaxant that has been successfully employed in a limited number of cases.

## Neuromuscular Blockade

Neuromuscular blockade may be required in the treatment of tetanus for control of ventilation and muscular spasms as well as for prevention of fractures and rhabdomyolysis. Vecuronium is the neuromuscular blocking agent of choice because of its minimal cardiovascular side effects. Concomitant sedation with barbiturates or benzodiazepines is mandatory.

## Treatment of Autonomic Dysfunction

The combined $\alpha$- and $\beta$-adrenergic blocking agent labetalol has been successfully used to treat the manifestations of sympathetic hyperactivity in tetanus. However, several investigators have reported fatal cardiovascular complications in patients treated with $\beta$-adrenergic blocking agents alone. Adrenergic blocking drugs, although effective in the treatment of the autonomic dysfunction of tetanus, may precipitate dangerous myocardial depression if sympathetic activity transiently diminishes.

Magnesium sulfate, because of its ability to inhibit catecholamine release, has been advocated as a means of treating the autonomic dysfunction of tetanus. Continuous epidural block with bupivacaine has been employed recently to provide sympathetic blockade, muscle relaxation, and analgesia in the treatment of the generalized form of the disease. Morphine sulfate provides control of the sympathetic hyperactivity of tetanus without compromising cardiac output. The central $\alpha$-receptor agonist clonidine has met with initial success in managing the cardiovascular instability seen in tetanus, presumably by decreasing sympathetic tone and causing peripheral vasodilation.

## Active Immunization

Patients who have recovered from tetanus must undergo active immunization since the disease does not confer immunity. Absorbed tetanus toxoid, 0.5 mL, should be administered intramuscularly at the time of presentation and at 6 weeks and 6 months after injury. Tetanus-diphtheria (Td) should be administered to patients older than 7 years of age, and diphtheria-pertussis-tetanus (DPT) to patients younger than 7 years of age. A summary of the guidelines for active tetanus immunization is presented in Table 123-2. A summary of the management of tetanus is presented in Table 123-3.

## SUMMARY

Despite the fact that tetanus is a completely preventable disease, it remains a source of significant morbidity and mortality in the rural southern states and in urban intravenous drug abusers. The sporulated form of *C. tetani* survives in soil and on environmental surfaces indefinitely and often gains access to the host through a minor, unreported wound. Once introduced into tissue, the spores of *C. tetani* may germinate and result in the production of tetanospasmin, the exotoxin responsible for all of the clinical manifestations of tetanus. Human tetanus immune globulin (TIG) neutralizes circulating exotoxin but not tetanospasmin fixed within nervous tissue. Nevertheless, administration of TIG lowers the case fatality rate of tetanus and is an important therapeutic intervention. Because of the extreme potency of tetanospasmin, the quantity of the exotoxin necessary to produce clinical disease is insufficient to confer immunity and therefore all patients recovering from tetanus require active immunization.

**Table 123-3.** Treatment of Tetanus

| | |
|---|---|
| Respiratory management | Succinylcholine, 80 mg for emergency oral intubation; tracheostomy except in localized or mild tetanus |
| Immunotherapy | TIG 500 U IM as a single dose<br>*and*<br>Tetanus toxoid (DPT or Td depending on age), 0.5 mL IM at presentation, and 6 weeks and 6 months after presentation |
| Antibiotic therapy | Metronidazole, 500 mg IV every 6 h<br>*or*<br>Erythromycin 2 g/day |
| Muscle relaxation | Lorazepam, 2 mg IV to effect<br>*or*<br>Diazepam, 5 mg IV every 1–3 h to effect<br>*or*<br>Midazolam, 5–15 mg/h continuous IV infusion |
| Neuromuscular blockade | Vecuronium, 6–8 mg/h IV |
| Management of autonomic dysfunction | Labetalol, 0.25–1.0 mg/min continuous IV infusion<br>*or*<br>Magnesium sulfate, 70 mg/kg IV loading, then 1–4 g/h continuous infusion to maintain blood level of 2.5–4 mmol/L<br>Morphine sulfate, 0.5–1.0 mg/kg per hour<br>Clonidine, 300 µg every 8 h per nasogastric tube |

## BIBLIOGRAPHY

Blake PA, Feldman TM, Buchanan TM, et al: Serologic therapy of tetanus in the United States, 1965–1971. *JAMA* 235:42, 1976.

Bleck TP: Pharmacology, management, and prophylaxis. *Dis Mon* 37:551, 1991.

Groleau G: Tetanus. *Emerg Med Clin North Am* 10:351, 1992.

Kefer MP: Tetanus. *Am J Emerg Med* 10:445, 1992.

Weinstein L: Tetanus. *N Engl J Med* 289:1293, 1973.

# 124
# RABIES
## Louis S. Binder

Rabies is a near uniformly fatal disease and represents the most serious potential complication of an animal bite. The disease is caused by an RNA-containing rhabdovirus and is transmitted by inoculation with infectious saliva from a carnivore or bat bite, or by salivary contact with a break in the skin or mucous membrane. The disease exists primarily in wildlife, which serves as the viral reservoir in endemic areas and which represents the most important source of infection for human beings and domestic animals in the United States. The prevalence of rabies in wild carnivores varies in different geographical areas, which accounts for differences in prevalence of rabies in domestic animal population (as the virus is transferred from wild to domestic animals and subsequently to human beings).

Worldwide, rabies causes 25,000 to 50,000 deaths per year. The disease is endemic throughout Latin America, Asia, Africa, South American, Europe, the Middle East, India, and Southeast Asia. A few island countries are free of rabies: England, Australia, Japan, Hawaii, Antarctica, and parts of the Caribbean.

In the United States, the rabies virus is present in the 48 continental states and Alaska. The virus is most prevalent in the mid-Atlantic and southern Atlantic states (New York to Florida), the south central states (Arkansas, Louisiana, Oklahoma, and Texas, especially the US–Mexico border), and the Midwest (the Dakotas, Minnesota, Iowa, Missouri, and Kansas). It is rare in the Ohio River valley and the Rocky Mountain states. Skunks are the most commonly identified species in California and the Midwest. Raccoons are commonly infected in the Atlantic states and are an increasingly important source of rabies (along with bats) in New England. In domestic animals, dogs are important carriers in south Texas and the Midwest; cats are more commonly infected in the mid-Atlantic region.

One hundred and forty-eight cases of dog rabies and approximately 500 to 600 cases of domestic animal rabies were reported to the Centers for Disease Control and Prevention (CDC) in 1991. Seventeen cases of human rabies have been reported in the United States since 1980, six since 1990; ten of these were related to rabies exposure outside the United States. Nine had no definite history of animal bites or other exposure, and in nine patients the diagnosis was only made postmortem. This is greatly decreased from an average animal rate of 8000 cases of dog rabies and 22 cases of human rabies reported in 1946, reflecting the implementation and effectiveness of both immunization programs for domestic animals and public health programs to remove stray animals from the community as potential vectors in epizootic areas.

In developing countries where rabies is endemic and animal immunizations are uncommon, dogs are the primary (but not only) reservoir of disease and the principle source (over 90 percent) of human exposure. In developed countries, such as the United States, where indigenously acquired rabies in human beings has been virtually eliminated, dog and cat bites are the most common reason for implementation of postexposure prophylaxis, but the most important source of active rabies transmission is wildlife transmission (85 percent of reported animal rabies since 1970). New human rabies cases in the United States are usually associated with extramural exposure or from exposure to wild carnivores. Thus, animal bites either contracted outside the United States in an undeveloped country or domestic bites from an appropriate species of carnivore should be considered at high risk for rabies transmission.

Rabid wildlife species reported to the CDC in 1988 include skunks (38 percent), racoons (31 percent), bats (14 percent), and foxes (4 percent). Twelve percent of rabid animals reported were domestic species: cats (4 percent), cattle (4 percent), dogs (3 percent), and other livestock. In areas where the disease is endemic, up to 34 percent of animals submitted for testing are found positive for rabies, making human transmission a real possibility. In contrast, rodents (squirrels, chipmunks, hamsters, rats, mice, etc.) and lagomorphs (rabbits, hares, etc.) have never been implicated as carriers, and bites by these animals are not at risk for transmission.

Rabid animals are agitated and labile, may indiscriminately attack anything that moves, and may otherwise wander aimlessly. Feeble bark, drooling, stupor, and convulsions mark more advanced disease preceding death of the animal.

Transmission through inhalation without bite exposure (spelunkers in bat-infested caves) or from laboratory accidents is rare but has been reported. Human-to-human transmission by tissue transplantation (corneal transplants) has been reported in six cases. Although theoretically there exists a risk to health care workers of transmission of rabies virus from infected patients, no such cases have been identified. However, strict adherence to universal precautions is advised, and postexposure prophylaxis is recommended for health care providers with potentially infectious exposure to body fluids of infected patients.

## PATHOPHYSIOLOGY

Once introduced, the initial infection and multiplication occur within local myocytes for the first 48 to 96 h. Subsequently, the virus spreads across the motor end plate and ascends and replicates along peripheral nervous axoplasm to the dorsal root ganglia, the spinal cord, and the central nervous system (CNS). Following CNS replication in the gray matter, the virus spreads outward by peripheral nerves to virtually all tissues and organ systems. Viral infection of the salivary glands engenders infectivity of saliva; the infectivity of additional body fluids is less well established.

Histologically, rabies manifests the same findings as seen in other forms of encephalitis: diffuse and extensive monocellular infiltration with focal hemorrhage and demyelination, predominantly in perivascular areas in the gray matter of the CNS, basal ganglia, and the spinal cord. Negri bodies are the characteristic histologic finding for rabies, which is the site of CNS viral replication. They are eosinophilic intracellular lesions found within cerebral neurons and are highly specific for rabies. Negri bodies are encountered in only 75 percent of proven animal rabies cases; thus, although their presence is pathognomonic for rabies, their absence does not exclude rabies as a diagnostic possibility.

## CLINICAL PRESENTATION

As human rabies has decreased in the United States, the proportion of rabies patients without animal bite exposure has increased. In the majority of recent cases in the United States, no history of such exposure was identified, and rabies may be overlooked diagnostically in such patients. Because most domestic cases are now related to exposure outside of the United States, travel to a country where rabies is endemic may be an important diagnostic clue. In untreated rabid bites, the risk of contracting rabies ranges from 25 to 50 percent. Rabid hand and foot bites carry a 15- to 20-percent mortality rate; rabid head and neck bites, a 50-percent mortality rate.

Incubation periods average 20 to 90 days; periods as short as 12 days and as long as 700 days have been reported. Incubation times average 46 to 78 days for extremity bites and 25 to 48 days for head and neck bites. Variations in incubation period depend on the size of the viral inoculum, host immunity, and bite location: the more rostral the bite, the shorter both the travel distance and the incubation time for the virus.

The initial symptoms of human rabies are nonspecific: fever, malaise, headache, anorexia, nausea, sore throat, cough, and pruritus or paresthesias at the bite site (80 percent). This initial phase may last for 2 to 10 days. Subsequently, in classic, or "furious," rabies (80 percent), evidence of CNS involvement becomes apparent, with restlessness and agitation, altered mental status, painful bulbar and peripheral muscular spasms, opisthotonos, and bulbar or focal motor paresis. Alternatively, in paralytic rabies (20 percent), an ascending, symmetric, flaccid, and areflexic paralysis, comparable to the Landry-Guillain-Barré syndrome, may be seen. Hypersensitivity to sensory stimuli (light, noise, and touch) and hydrophobia may occur at this stage, the latter resulting from the sight, sound, swallowing, or even mention of water. Hydrophobia results from bulbar spasms, diaphragmatic and respiratory muscular spasms, and seizures that occur with swallowing; its presence should be clinically suggestive for the diagnosis of rabies. Progressively, lucid and confused intervals may become interspersed, autonomic hyperactivity may manifest (hyperpyrexia, mydriasis, and increased lacrimation and salivation), and brain stem dysfunction (dysphagia, optic neuritis, and facial palsies) with hyperreflexia and extensor plantar responses may occur.

Common complications include adult respiratory distress syndrome, diabetes insipidus, syndrome of inappropriate antidiuretic hormone, volume depletion, electrolyte imbalances, pneumonia, and cardiogenic hypotension and arrhythmias from rabies myocarditis.

Coma, convulsions, and apnea are the final manifestations of rabid death.

Death universally occurs in 4 to 7 days in untreated patients, which may be prolonged to 25 days if supportive care is instituted. There are three reported cases of neurologically intact survivors of rabies, who received rabies vaccine before onset of symptoms and intensive supportive care. In these patients, supportive care maintained vital functions while the patient's stimulated immune response eradicated the infection. Such recoveries, however, are exceedingly rare.

## DIAGNOSIS

The premortem diagnosis of rabies is made via detection of rabies virus antigen or antibody from saliva, serum, cerebrospinal fluid (CSF), or skin biopsy. Saliva is a potential source of rabies viral antigen or antibody detection, or viral isolation. *In unimmunized patients*, serum antibody titers become positive between days 6 and 12, and a fourfold increase of antibody titers in these patients is considered diagnostic. *In vaccinated patients*, CSF analysis for viral isolation or antibody titers suggests the diagnosis because immunization alone rarely produces detectable antibodies in the CSF. CSF titers for rabies antibody become positive between days 8 and 16, with titers of 1:200 or higher being diagnostic. Elevated CSF protein and a mononuclear pleocytosis are also seen. Finally, *rapid confirmation* of rabies infection may be possible via skin biopsy from the hair-covered area of the neck (highly innervated, hence high concentration of rabies antigen) assayed by fluorescent antibody testing. The sensitivity is 50 to 60 percent, and specificity is 80 percent; thus a positive test is helpful and confirmatory although a negative test does not rule out the diagnosis, and may be repeated later when more antigen would be present.

The definitive diagnosis of rabies in animals and human beings is made by analysis of brain tissue from biopsy or autopsy. Analysis for Negri bodies is highly specific, but carries a 25 percent false negative rate. Fluorescent antibody testing has become the procedure of choice due to low cost, speed, and reliability (90 percent sensitivity and specificity) when performed in a competent laboratory. Mouse inoculation tests and tissue culture tests are accurate and are used for confirmation or as the primary test in less sophisticated laboratories, but require weeks for results. More recently, enzyme-linked immunosorbent techniques have been used with satisfactory results compared with those of fluorescent antibody testing and tissue culture, and nested polymerase chain reaction techniques have been reported but are less well established.

The differential diagnosis includes viral or other infectious encephalitis, polio, tetanus, viral process, severe alcohol withdrawal, meningitis, brain abscess, septic cavernous sinus thrombosis, adrenergic or cholinergic poisoning, and Landry-Guillain-Barré syndrome. The clinical diagnosis of rabies is difficult to distinguish from other etiologies of acute encephalitis because routine laboratory tests are nondiagnostic; only 30 percent of patients are so diagnosed prior to the perimortem period. However, the diagnosis should be considered in patients with a picture of acute, progressive, and unexplained encephalitis. Diagnosis is more likely if a history of endemic travel or exposure is present or if hydrophobia is clinically evident.

## TREATMENT

To date, once the disease occurs, there is no successful treatment for rabies, and the care of established infection is entirely supportive. However, prior to the establishment of CNS infection, the prognosis for survival is excellent if immunization therapy is begun promptly before the patient is symptomatic. Postexposure prophylaxis has been uniformly effective when established treatment guidelines are meticulously followed. Therefore, management of a potentially rabid bite exposure consists of institution of postexposure immunoprophylaxis as early as possible (preferably before the onset of symptoms). For the rare patient with subsequent rabies, intensive supportive care should be instituted to maintain vital functions, with hope that the stimulated immune system can overcome the infection.

## POSTEXPOSURE PROPHYLAXIS

On 6th July, 1885, Louis Pasteur attempted to protect, for the first time in the history of medicine, a child bitten by a rabid dog. He prepared a modified rabies virus ("virus fixe") which he inoculated intracerebrally into a rabbit, and subsequently prepared a suspension of rabbit spinal cord. The nervous tissue suspension was used to inoculate the boy during eleven days with thirteen doses containing increasing amounts of active virus. The boy survived.

Thus was reported the first (and most dramatic) antirabies vaccine ever produced and used to induce immunity and protection against rabies in man. It has been subsequently shown that the use of hyperimmune serum (conferring passive immunity) or interferon inducer together with a vaccination regimen (conferring active immunity) yielded complete survival from rabies. Both the passive antibodies and interferon perform a critical biologic function in controlling local propagation and spread of the virus until the patient can develop active immunity from the vaccine.

Following inoculation, the rabies virus often remains latent for a period in myocytes prior to spreading to nervous tissue. Use of local cleansing (to eliminate the virus from the infection site) and local infiltration of hyperimmune serum may successfully control the spread of infection. Postexposure immunization of an infected individual can induce active antibody production and prevent CNS infection if the propagation and spread of local rabies infection can be initially controlled. Postexposure treatment must be instituted promptly because effectiveness decreases proportionately to the delay in institution of treatment.

Currently indicated pharmaceuticals for rabies prophylaxis are human rabies immune globulin (HRIG) for passive immunization and human diploid cell vaccine (HDCV) for active immunization. HRIG is antirabies gammaglobulin concentrated by cold ethanol fractionation of the plasma of hyperimmunized human donors. Neutralizing antibody content is standardized to contain 150 IU/mL. The half-life of the passive protection is 21 days, and no cases of human immunodeficiency virus (HIV) or hepatitis B transmission from HRIG administration have been reported. HDCV is an inactivated virus vaccine grown in human diploid cell tissue culture, is rich in rabies antigen, and engenders a universally excellent antibody response in recipients. HDCV induces IgM rabies-specific antibodies on day 3, IgG rabies-specific antibodies on day 7, early IgM/IgG conversion, and a 99- to 100-percent incidence of adequate titers at 42 and 90 days, respectively. Active immunity persists for at least 2 years in most vaccine recipients, with 2 to 7 percent manifesting inadequate titers beyond 2 years.

Figure 124-1 presents a clinical algorithm for the evaluation of animal exposures for rabies postexposure prophylaxis. Critical factors in the process of deciding whether to institute prophylaxis are the animal species, the nature of the exposure (whether salivary contact with wounds or mucous membrane did or did not occur), whether the animal is available for observation or rabies testing, and whether the animal has been immunized. Two or more doses of inactivated animal rabies vaccine induces adequate rabies antibody titers for at least one

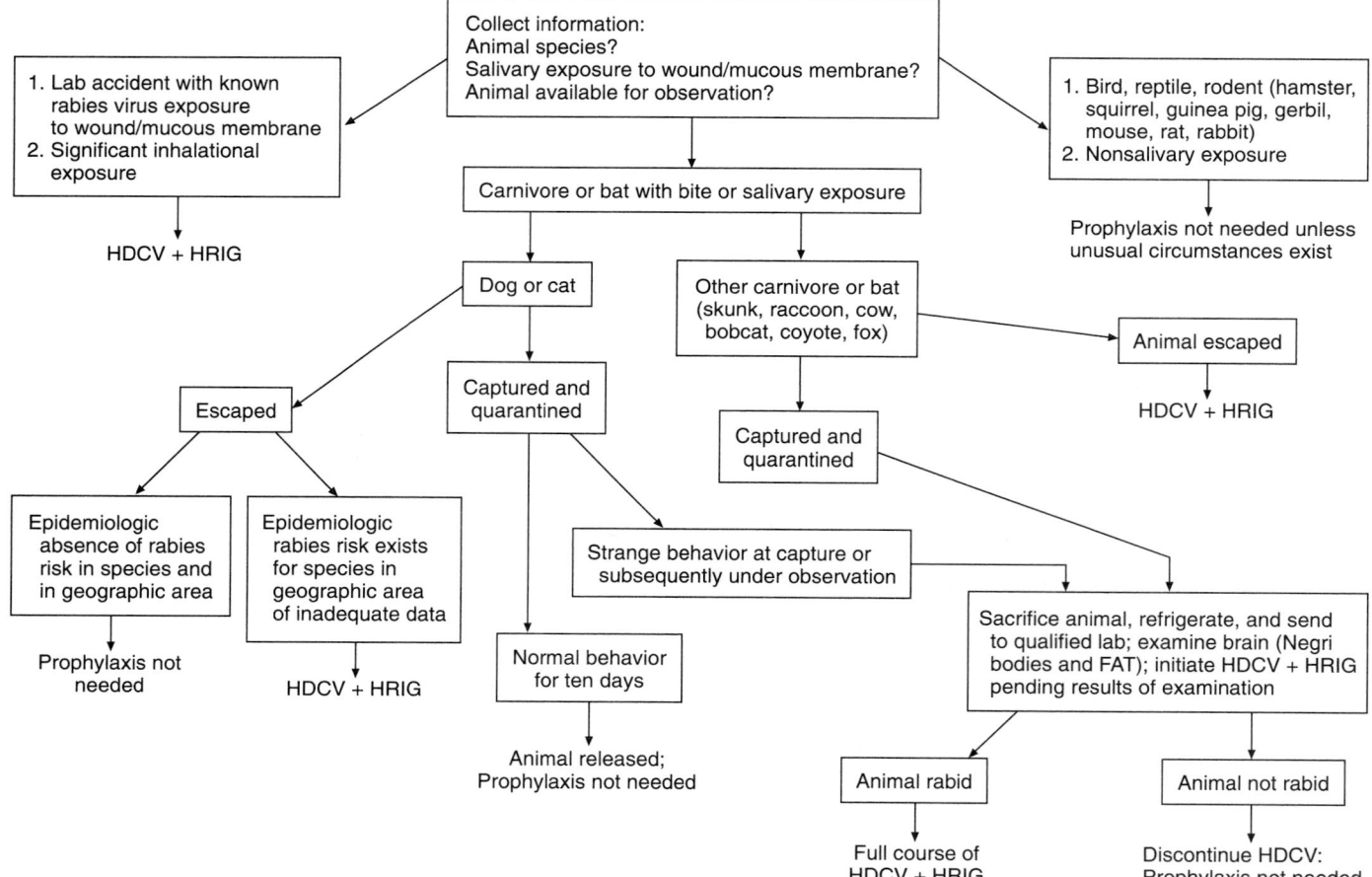

**Fig. 124-1.** Clinical guidelines for administration of rabies postexposure prophylaxis. FAT, fluorescent antibody test; HDCV, human diploid cell vaccine. HRIG, human rabies immune globulin. (Adapted from Mann JM. Rabies risk: Systematic evaluation and management of animal bites. *Comp Ther* 7:53, 1981. Used by permission.)

year and prevents canine and feline rabies during this period. In the United States, approximately 10,000 persons receive postexposure prophylaxis yearly.

Dogs and cats with normal behavior when captured may be quarantined for 10 days, which is sufficient time in these species for the disease to manifest if the animal is infected. If no signs become apparent, the animal can be considered nonrabid. The principle indication in clinical practice for the initiation of postexposure prophylaxis is a bite wound by an uncaptured dog or cat in an endemic area or a bite wound by an uncaptured bat or appropriate species of carnivore. State or local health officials should be consulted regarding the possibility of rabies in local dog, cat, rodent, and lagomorph populations before decisions on initiating postexposure rabies prophylaxis are made. The likelihood that a domestic dog or cat is infected with rabies varies from region to region; hence, the need for postexposure prophylaxis for these bites varies geographically.

Preexposure prophylaxis should be considered for persons involved in rabies animal diagnosis and control, wildlife trapping, rabies vaccine production, animal handlers, hunters, veterinarians, and travelers to areas where rabies is endemic. In the United States, approximately 18,000 persons receive rabies preexposure prophylaxis yearly. Seroconversion for antirabies antibody titers is 100 percent for a three-dose regimen (see below), and titers remain adequate for 2 years. Prophylaxis should be completed at least 30 days before anticipated exposure. Either booster doses or antibody titer determinations have been recommended every 2 years for persons with continuing risk of exposure and every 6 months for persons working with live rabies virus in research laboratories or vaccine production facilities.

## TREATMENT GUIDELINES

Treatment should be started immediately following exposure. Prompt debridement and cleansing of wounds to remove rabies virus is important in reducing the viral inoculum. Scrubbing and cleansing the wound with soap, debridement of devitalized tissue, and thorough irrigation with sterile saline solution or water should be undertaken, along with tetanus prophylaxis and prophylactic antibiotic coverage as indicated. If there is strong concern for rabies virus contamination of the wound, it should not be sutured because this promotes rabies virus replication. Such local measures reduce the incidence of subsequent rabies by 90 percent.

Human rabies immune globulin is administered only once at the onset of therapy. The dose is 20 IU/kg, with half the dose (if possible, based on volume constraints) infiltrated locally at the exposure site and the remainder administered intragluteally. HRIG can be given up to 8 days after the first dose of HDCV; beyond this time, HRIG is unnecessary due to the developing active immunity from HDCV. HRIG is packaged in 2-mL (300-IU) or 10-mL (1500-IU) vials; a 70-kg man will thus require 1400 IU from one large or five small vials. HDCV should be administered in five 1-mL doses intramuscularly as soon as possible following exposure, on days 0, 3, 7, 14, and 28. The World Health Organization also recommends a sixth dose on day 90.

Human diploid cell vaccine should be administered in the deltoid muscle rather than in the gluteal area; the anterolateral thigh is also acceptable in children. A reduced rabies antibody response has been shown with gluteal administration, presumably due to loss of rabies antigen to subcutaneous fat. Additionally, HDCV should always be administered via a different syringe and injection site than HRIG to prevent antigen/antibody complex formation and loss of immunogenicity from HDCV. Deviations from the above regimen (particularly gluteal injection of HDCV) are the chief reasons for vaccine failure.

The average cost of a course of HRIG and HDCV is $400 to $700, depending on body weight. The dismal prognosis of patients with clinical disease justifies the high cost of prevention, despite the low incidence of disease.

Preexposure prophylaxis for susceptible individuals consists of HDCV 1 mL intramuscularly on days 0, 7, and 21 or 28. Patients who have been previously immunized with rabies vaccine (either preexposure or postexposure prophylaxis with HDCV or other vaccine), who have a documented adequate rabies titer, and who have sustained another exposure or potential exposure to rabies virus should receive two doses of HDCV at days 0 and 3. Rabies antibody titers are subsequently recommended to determine the adequacy of the immune response. An HDCV booster followed by repeat titers in 2 to 3 weeks is indicated for inadequate rabies antibody titers.

Adverse reactions following the use of HRIG have been limited to local pain and low-grade fever (noted in 30 to 74 percent of recipients), which are transient and can be treated with salicylates or nonsteroidal anti-inflammatory medication. HDCV can precipitate similar local reactions in 25 percent of recipients. From 5 to 40 percent of HDCV recipients may manifest mild headache, nausea, dizziness, and myalgias, and 6 percent of booster recipients have experienced an immune complex-like reaction similar to serum sickness. Rare cases of anaphylaxis and transient neuroparalytic reactions similar to Landry-Guillain-Barré syndrome have also been reported with HDCV use. Rabies prophylaxis should not be stopped due to mild reactions, but serious neuroparalysis or anaphylaxis during treatment poses a therapeutic dilemma. Postexposure assessment of the clinical risk of rabies must be weighed against the risks of treatment, with possible choices consisting of continuation of therapy, switching to an alternative vaccine, pretreatment with antihistamine for hypersensitive patients, or discontinuation of treatment. Both the CDC and state or county health departments can provide assistance in the management of complications.

Rabies antibody titers are not recommended following immunization of healthy individuals, but are recommended following an incomplete immunization course or in immunocompromised patients. Immunosuppressant illnesses or agents (including HIV), corticosteroids, and antimalarial agents (particularly chloroquine, which may be given simultaneously for preexposure travel prophylaxis) may interfere with the development of active immunity after vaccination. If possible, withhold immunosuppressive drugs while administering vaccine, or time preexposure prophylaxis to avoid the presence of immunocompromising illness or drugs. Postvaccination titers, if indicated, should be assessed 2 to 4 weeks after immunization.

Because no fetal abnormalities have been reported and because of the possibility of rabies infection without passive and active treatment, pregnant patients may receive passive and active immunization for rabies prophylaxis.

Both animal bites and rabies are reportable entities in all states. Physicians should notify the county or state public health department of cases of rabid animals or human beings. Animal bites should be reported to the local animal control unit (usually associated with public health or police departments) so that appropriate animals are captured and quarantined for observation in a timely fashion.

Future therapies under investigation for the pre- and postexposure treatment of rabies virus exposure include the effectiveness of abbreviated immunization regimens, live recombinant virus vaccines expressing the rabies glycoprotein, a synthetic peptides vaccine (rather than live virus) to engender a solid and protective immune response, and monoclonal antibodies directed against different rabies virus antigens.

## BIBLIOGRAPHY

Baevsky RH, Bartfield JM. Human rabies: a review. *Am J Emerg Med* 11:279, 1993.

Fishbein DB. Rabies. *Infect Dis Clin North Am* 5:53, 1991.

Fishbein DB, Robinson LE. Rabies. *N Eng J Med* 329:1632, 1993.

Harrigan RA, Kauffman F. Current issues in rabies: epidemiology, clinical management, and postexposure prophylaxis. *Emerg Med Rep* 14:37, 1993.

US Public Health Service, Centers for Disease Control and Prevention. Rabies prevention—United States, 1991. Recommendations of the Immunization Practices Advisory Committee. *MMWR* 40 (RR-3):1, 1991.

# 125
# MALARIA
## Jeffrey D. Band

With the increase in international travel and the continued shift of travel to tropical locales, it is not surprising that physicians are seeing more patients with infectious diseases acquired in the tropics. Malaria, a protozoan disease transmitted by the bite of the *Anopheles* mosquito, remains one of the most significant of these. Annually, over 250 million persons develop malaria, and more than 2.5 million persons die. The incidence of malaria has been increasing in recent years despite worldwide aggressive attempts at control. Not only is the mosquito vector becoming less susceptible to a variety of insecticides, but *Plasmodium falciparum*—the parasite responsible for the most deadly form of malaria—is becoming increasingly resistant to antimalarial medications.

Malaria, especially disease due to *P. falciparum,* represents a medical emergency in any nonimmune host. Its early manifestations are largely nonspecific and can mimic other infectious diseases. Failure to rapidly diagnose infection can be disastrous. Likewise, failure to use specific antimalarial agents to which the individual strain is susceptible can result in early death. A diagnosis of malaria must be considered in any person returning from the tropics with an unexplained febrile illness. Questions regarding recent travel should become routine in emergency departments.

## ETIOLOGY

Four species of the genus *Plasmodium* infect humans: *P. vivax, P. ovale, P. malariae,* and *P. falciparum.* The organism is transmitted primarily by the bite of an infected female anopheline mosquito. This vector is most frequently found in tropical and subtropical regions below 8200 ft (2500 m) above sea level. Plasmodial sporozoites are injected into the host's bloodstream during the mosquito's blood meal and are carried directly to the liver. The hepatic parenchymal cells are invaded, and asexual reproduction of the parasite begins (preerythrocytic schizogony or exoerythrocytic stage). As thousands of daughter merozoites are formed, the parenchymal liver cell ruptures, releasing daughter merozoites back into the circulation where they rapidly invade erythrocytes (erythrocytic stage). In *P. vivax* and *P. ovale* infection, a portion of the intrahepatic forms are not released and remain dormant for months. These forms can later activate and cause clinical relapses.

The clinical manifestations of malaria first appear during the erythrocytic stage. Once merozoites enter this stage, they never reinvade the liver. Merozoites mature within the erythrocyte and take on vari-

ous morphologic forms, including the early ring forms, trophozoites, and schizonts (which represent a mass of new merozoites). Eventually, the target erythrocyte lyses, and new merozoites invade uninfected red blood cells, continuing the infection and causing clinical manifestations. Lysogeny may become regular, occurring at 2- to 3-day intervals in established and untreated infections, producing the classic periodicity of symptoms.

After several cycles, a proportion of the merozoites develop into sexual forms (gametocytes). Upon ingestion by another feeding anopheline mosquito, male and female gametocytes undergo sexual reproduction and become infective sporozoites ready for their next host.

Each species of plasmodium has specific characteristics, including typical morphologic forms and selective red blood cell tropism (Table 125-1). Many of these characteristics are responsible for important pathophysiologic consequences.

Malaria may also be transmitted by direct transfusion of infected blood or passed transplacentally from mother to fetus. In these cases an exoerythrocytic phase is absent.

## EPIDEMIOLOGY

Malaria transmission occurs in large areas of Central and South America, the Caribbean, sub-Saharan Africa, the Indian subcontinent, Southeast Asia, the Middle East, and Oceania. Certain species may predominate in a given geographic area. For example, *P. vivax* is more common in the Indian subcontinent and in Central America, while *P. falciparum* is the most prevalent form in Africa, Haiti, and New Guinea.

The risk of malaria varies considerably between regions. It is largely dependent upon the intensity of transmission in both urban and rural areas, and, for travelers, upon the itinerary and time and type of travel. From 1980 to 1990 the Centers for Disease Control reported 4585 cases of malaria among U.S. civilians. Of the more than 500 cases that occurred in 1990, 308 (57 percent) were acquired in sub-Saharan Africa; 133 (24 percent) in Asia; 58 (11 percent) in the Caribbean and Central America; 28 (5 percent) in Oceania; and only 18 (3 percent) in South America. *Plasmodium vivax* accounted for 49 percent of all cases, and *P. falciparum* for another 40 percent. Mixed infections were uncommon, representing less than 1 percent of all cases. Thus, more than half of all cases of malaria, including the majority of cases due to *P. falciparum,* are acquired from travels in sub-Saharan Africa. Yet for every traveler to sub-Saharan Africa, at least 10 travelers visit potential malarious areas of Asia and South America each year. Clearly, the intensity of exposure appears to be much higher in sub-Saharan Africa.

Resistance of *P. falciparum* to chloroquine continues to spread (Table 125-2). In addition, strains exist of *P. falciparum* that are resistant to other chemotherapeutic agents, including pyrimethamine-sulfadoxine, quinine, mefloquine, and doxycycline, and new agents,

**Table 125-1.** Characteristics of Malaria-Causing *Plasmodium* Species

| | *P. falciparum* | P. vivax | *P. ovale* | P. malariae |
|---|---|---|---|---|
| Incubation period (mean) | 8–25 days (12) | 8–27 days (14) | 9–17 days (15) | 15–30 days |
| Asexual erythrocytic cycle | 48 h | 48 h | 48 h | 72 h |
| Relapse | No | Yes | Yes | No |
| Red blood cell preference | Reticulocytes (but can infect RBCs of all ages) | Reticulocytes | Reticulocytes | Older cells |
| Morphologic characteristics | | | | |
|   Degree of parasitemia | High (multiple rings per RBC) | Low | Low | Low |
|   Ring forms and early trophozoites | Ring forms predominate; threadlike cytoplasm with double chromatic dots | Amoeboid cytoplasm | Compact cytoplasm | Compact cytoplasm |
|   Mature trophozoites | Rarely seen | Observed | Observed | Observed |
|   Schizonts | Rarely seen | Observed | Observed | Observed |
|   Gametocytes | Banana-shaped | Round | Round | Round |

**Table 125-2.** Geographic Distribution of Malaria Including Resistant Strains

| Geographic Region | Areas with Malaria | Countries with Chloroquine-Resistant *P. falciparum* (CRPF) | Countries with Fansidar-Resistant *P. falciparum* |
|---|---|---|---|
| Central America | All countries | None | None |
| Caribbean | Dominican Republic and Haiti | None | None |
| South America | | | |
|    Temperate | Argentina | None | None |
|    Tropical | All countries | All countries except Paraguay | Interior Amazon Basin |
| East Asia | China | China | South China |
| Eastern South Asia | All countries except Brunei and Singapore | All infected areas | Infected areas except Philippines |
| Middle South Asia | All countries | All countries | Afghanistan and Bhutan |
| Western South Asia and Middle East | Iraq, Oman, Saudi Arabia, Syria, Turkey, and UAE | Oman and Saudi Arabia | None |
| Northern Africa | All countries except Tunisia | Algeria | None |
| Sub-Saharan Africa | All countries except Cape Verde, Réunion, São Tomé/Príncipe, and Seychelles | Widespread | Widespread |
| Southern Africa | All countries except Lesotho and St. Helena | Widespread | None |
| Oceania | Limited to Papua New Guinea, Solomon Islands, and Vanuatu (small foci elsewhere) | Widespread | Papua New Guinea and Vanuatu |

including halofantrine and artesunate (the latter two agents are not available in the United States). Recently, strains of *P. vivax* have been isolated from patients who have failed chloroquine therapy. Prior to 1990, no strains of *P. vivax, P. ovale,* or *P. malariae* were resistant to chloroquine.

## PATHOGENESIS

After an incubation period ranging from 8 days in the nonimmune and unprotected host to several weeks or more, disease ensues. Both incomplete suppression by partially active chemoprophylaxis and incomplete immunity can markedly prolong the incubation period to months or even years. Only the asexual intraerythrocytic parasite is responsible for the symptoms and pathophysiologic consequences. The hallmark of malaria is the recurring febrile paroxysm which corresponds to hemolysis of infected erythrocytes and release of antigenic products with activation of macrophages and production of cytokines.

Hemolysis can be high with *P. falciparum* infection, since parasitemia can be overwhelming and erythrocytes of all ages are susceptible. Parasitized erythrocytes lose flexibility and are removed in the microcirculation with resultant obstruction and tissue anoxia of the lungs, kidneys, brain, and other vital organs. Noncardiac pulmonary edema, renal failure, and cerebral malaria may result. Sequestration accounts for the paucity of observed mature parasites in the peripheral smear of patients infected with *P. falciparum.*

In addition to prolonged high fever, hemolysis, and, in the case of infection with *P. falciparum,* obstruction to capillary flow, immunologic sequelae, may also occur, resulting in glomerulonephritis, nephrotic syndrome, thrombocytopenia, and polyclonal antibody stimulation.

Lastly, hypersplenism with resultant pancytopenia may occur, especially in cases of prolonged, untreated malaria.

## CLINICAL MANIFESTATIONS

Typically, patients develop a prodrome of malaise, myalgia, headache, and low-grade fevers often accompanied by chills. In some patients, headache, chest pains, cough, abdominal pain, arthralgias, or diarrhea may be prominent. The early manifestations are quite nonspecific and can easily become confused with a viral syndrome, influenza, hepatitis, and other less severe self-limited clinical entities. Illness usually progresses to severe chills followed by high-grade fevers accompanied by tachycardia, nausea, orthostatic dizziness, and extreme weakness. After several hours the fever abates and the pa-

tient becomes diaphoretic and exhausted. Over time, the paroxysms of malaria—chills and fever followed by diaphoresis—may occur at nearly regular intervals which correspond to the length of the asexual erythrocytic cycles (Table 125-1). The classic paroxysms of malaria are often lacking in malaria due to *P. falciparum.*

The findings on physical examination are also not specific for malaria. Most patients appear acutely ill with high fevers, tachycardia, and tachypnea. Splenomegaly and tender abdomen are commonly present in advanced infection. The liver may or may not be enlarged. Features quite atypical for malaria include lymphadenopathy and a maculopapular skin rash.

Laboratory features include normochromic normocytic anemia with findings suggestive of hemolysis, a normal or mildly depressed total leukocyte count, thrombocytopenia, an elevated erythrocyte sedimentation rate, and mild abnormalities in liver and renal functions. Other laboratory abnormalities include hyponatremia, hypoglycemia, and a biologic false-positive VDRL.

Complications of malaria can occur rapidly in untreated infection, especially when the agent is *P. falciparum.* Infections caused by any species of plasmodium can result in hemolysis, splenic enlargement, and occasionally splenic rupture. An immune-mediated glomerulonephritis is also common to all forms but tends to occur most often in *P. malariae* infection. With the ability to cause high parasitemia levels and sequestration with capillary sludging, *P. falciparum* infection can be fatal. Cerebral malaria—characterized by somnolence, coma, delirium, and seizures—is associated with mortality rates in excess of 20 percent. Reversible causes of encephalopathy must be excluded. The cerebrospinal fluid is usually normal with the exception of a slightly elevated opening pressure and protein concentration. A mild pleocytosis might also be present. Other life-threatening complications associated with *P. falciparum* infection include respiratory failure due to noncardiogenic acute pulmonary edema (similar to adult respiratory distress syndrome), renal failure (acute tubular necrosis), and severe metabolic abnormalities including lactic acidosis and profound hypoglycemia. Any target organ is susceptible to the effects of severe tissue hypoxia from the cytoadherence between the parasitized erythrocyte and the vascular endothelium of the host.

Persons at greatest risk for complications due to *P. falciparum* include the very young, the elderly, and pregnant women.

## DIAGNOSIS

Certain clinical and epidemiologic clues provide supportive evidence for a presumptive diagnosis. The definitive diagnosis is established

**Table 125-3.** Guidelines for Preparing Malaria Smears

1. Use scrupulously clean slides; manufacturers' precleaned slides may have residual debris.
2. Obtain a large drop of blood from the patient's finger using a blood lancet.
3. Place the cleaned surface of the slide against the drop of blood; with a quick circular motion, make a film the size of a dime. Do not mix excessively or distortion will result. The thick smear should be of such depth that newsprint would be barely legible. (Let the smear air-dry for 30 to 60 min.)
4. Obtain a small drop of blood from the patient's finger, and with a second clean slide, spread the blood gently over the slide. Air-dry the thin film, fix it with methyl alcohol, and stain it with Giemsa stain.
5. If the thin smear is negative, examine the thick smear. Once air-dried, the thick film should not be fixed prior to staining with Giemsa.

by the visualization of parasites on Giemsa-stained thick and thin blood smears. In early infection, especially infection due to *P. falciparum,* in which parasitized erythrocytes are sequestered from the bloodstream, parasitemia may be undetectable. Also, parasitemia fluctuates over time. It generally is highest during chills and as the fever is on the rise. High fevers are schizonticidal.

In highly suspicious cases, failure to detect parasitemia is not an indication to withhold therapy. Delay in the diagnosis and treatment of malaria can have disastrous results. If parasitemia is not seen in the stained thin smear, a thick smear which concentrates blood cells may provide the diagnosis. Extreme care in the preparation of slides is important, since debris may result in false-positive smears. If parasites are not visualized, repeated smears should be obtained at least twice daily for 3 days to fully exclude malaria (Table 125-3). The two major questions to be answered by the blood smear are the degree of parasitemia present (correlates with prognosis) and whether or not *P. falciparum* is responsible for infection. Most patients with *P. falciparum* infection should be managed in the hospital setting, as should any patient with more than 3 percent parasitemia. Clues to the diagnosis of *P. falciparum* infection include the presence of small ring forms with double chromatin knobs within the erythrocyte, multiply infected rings in individual red blood cells, a paucity of trophozoites and schizonts on smear, the pathognomonic crescent-shaped (banana-shaped) gametocyte, and parasitemia exceeding 4 percent. Repeated smears should be obtained twice daily to assess the efficacy of drug treatment.

## THERAPY

Therapeutic decisions are based upon the severity of the illness, the agent, and whether the patient may be infected with chloroquine-resistant *P. falciparum*. If *P. falciparum* infection can be excluded,

**Table 125-4.** Treatment Regimens for Malaria

| | | Dosage Guidelines | |
| --- | --- | --- | --- |
| **Clinical Setting** | **Drug** | **Adults** | **Children** |
| Uncomplicated infection with *P. vivax, P. ovale, P. malariae,* and chloroquine-sensitive *P. falciparum* | Chloroquine phosphate | 1-g load (600-mg base), then 500 mg (300-mg base) in 6 h, then 500 mg (300-mg base) per day for 2 days (total dose 2.5 g) | 10 mg/kg base to maximum of 600 mg load, then 5 mg/kg base in 6 h and 5 mg/kg base per day for 2 days |
| | *plus* | | |
| | Primaquine phosphate[a] | 26.3 mg load (15-mg base) per day for 14 days upon completion of chloroquine therapy | 0.3 mg/kg base for 14 days upon completion of chloroquine therapy |
| Uncomplicated infection with chloroquine-resistant *P. falciparum* | Quinine sulfate | 650 mg PO tid for 5–7 days | 8.3 mg/kg PO tid for 5–7 days[b] |
| | *plus* | | |
| | Pyrimethamine-sulfadoxine (Fansidar)[c] | 3 tablets (75 mg/1500 mg) PO × 1 dose | Over 2 months old: |
| | *plus* | | >50 kg    3 tabs |
| | | | 30–50    2 tabs |
| | | | 15–29    1 tab |
| | | | 10–14    ½ tab |
| | | | 4–9    ¼ tab |
| | Doxycycline | 100 mg PO bid for 10 days | Contraindicated in children <8 years of age |
| | *or* | | |
| | Mefloquine | 1250 mg PO × 1 | 1 tablet/10 kg PO × 1[d] |
| | *plus* | | |
| | Doxycycline[e] | See above | See above |
| | *or* | | |
| | Halofantrine[f] | 500 mg 6 h apart for 3 doses (repeat again in 1 week) | 8 mg/kg salt orally, given q 6 h for 3 doses (repeat again in 1 week) |
| Complicated infection with chloroquine-resistant *P. falciparum* | Quinidine gluconate | 10 mg/kg load over 2 h then 0.02 mg/kg per min continuous infusion until patient stabilizes and is able to tolerate PO therapy (see above) | Same as adults[g] |
| | *plus* | | |
| | Doxycycline | 100 mg IV q 12 h until tolerating PO therapy (see above) | Contraindicated in children <8 years of age |

[a] Terminal treatment of *P. vivax* and *P. ovale* only.

[b] If unable to administer with doxycycline due to patient's age, extend treatment to full 10 days.

[c] Optional; of unlikely value if acquisition in area with Fansidar resistance.

[d] Not formally approved yet by FDA in this setting.

[e] Optional; many experts feel comfortable with mefloquine alone.

[f] Although FDA approved, halofantrine is not yet commercially available in the United States. (Contact SmithKline Beecham at 1-800-366-8900.) Becoming drug of choice for self-treatment of presumptive malaria in Thai-Cambodian and Myanmar borders *if* access to medical care is not available. In these areas, may need to extend treatment to 3 days instead of 1 day.

[g] Consult an expert in pediatric infectious disease immediately for guidance.

**Table 125-5.** Adverse Effects, Precautions, and Contraindications of Antimalarial Drugs

| Drug | Minor Toxicity | Major Toxicity | Precautions/Contraindications |
|------|----------------|----------------|-------------------------------|
| Chloroquine | Nausea/vomiting, diarrhea, pruritus, postural hypotension, rash, fever, headache, dizziness | Rare; hypotension and shock after parenteral therapy; retinopathy after prolonged use | Avoid in patients with severe psoriasis and some types of porphyria |
| Mefloquine | Nausea/vomiting, cramps, diarrhea, anorexia, dizziness, headaches, bradycardia | Rare unless underlying heart disease with bradycardia or the patient is on selected cardiotoxic medications (arrhythmias, arrest); acute toxic confusional states may occur, as can seizures | Contraindicated during pregnancy and in children <15 kg.; avoid if receiving quinine, quinidine, calcium-channel blockers or beta-blockers; avoid if heart conduction disturbance or if underlying seizure disorder |
| Fansidar | GI disturbances, phototoxicity, headaches, dizziness, skin rash | Fatal cutaneous eruptions reported, agranulocytosis | Contraindicated during pregnancy and in infants or if allergic to sulfonamides or pyrimethamine |
| Doxycycline | GI disturbances, phototoxicity, vaginal candidiasis | Rare | Contraindicated during pregnancy, in children <8 years of age; may depress prothrombin time in patients receiving anticoagulants |
| Proguanil* | Generally well tolerated; may develop mouth ulcers, dizziness, or alopecia | Rare; anemia after prolonged use | Contraindicated if allergy to proguanil; best to avoid use during pregnancy and in young infants |
| Quinine or quinidine | Cinchonism (nausea and vomiting, headache, tinnitus, dizziness, visual disturbance) | Hypotension, cardiac arrhythmias, hypoglycemia, Coombs'-positive hemolysis, abortions, neuromuscular paralysis (myasthenia) | Contraindicated in cardiac disease; cautiously in pregnancy, myasthenia gravis |
| Primaquine† | Nausea, vomiting, diarrhea, cramps, methemoglobulinemia | Massive hemolysis in patients with G6PD deficiency, exacerbation of SLE or RA | Contraindicated in G6PD deficiency, pregnancy |
| Halofantrine | GI disturbances, headaches, dizziness, pruritus | Similar to mefloquine | Similar to mefloquine |

\* Not used for acute therapy.

† Terminal treatment for *P. vivax* and *P. ovale* infections only.

most persons can be managed in the ambulatory setting. Close follow-up, including repeated smears, is necessary. Patients with significant hemolysis or who have underlying severe chronic medical problems which can be aggravated by high fevers or hemolysis are best hospitalized. Infected infants and pregnant women are also best managed in the hospital.

The drug of choice for treatment of infection due to *P. vivax, P. ovale,* and *P. malariae* is chloroquine. Table 125-4 summarizes the treatment regimens for malaria. With treatment, the parasite load should decrease significantly within the first 24 to 48 h. No asexual forms of the parasite should be detectable 3 to 4 days after treatment is completed. Gametocytes, the sexual forms, may persist for several weeks after treatment and are not an indicator of treatment failure. Gametocytes do not cause disease in the human host. Chloroquine has no effect on the exoerythrocytic parasites, which may be dormant in the liver with infection due to *P. vivax* and *P. ovale.* Unless terminal treatment is administered with primaquine, clinical relapses commonly occur. Primaquine should not be used in patients with G6PD deficiency because it may induce massive hemolysis of erythrocytes. Table 125-5 summarizes the commonly described adverse effects and precautions or contraindications of the antimalarial medications. Despite treatment with both chloroquine and primaquine, persistence of infection or relapse may occur.

Treatment of *P. falciparum* infection is generally best managed in a hospital setting, particularly if the level of parasitemia exceeds 3 percent. Unless one is certain that the patient could not have chloroquine-resistant *falciparum* infection (based upon geographic exposure, Table 125-2), it is best to assume the infecting strain is resistant to chloroquine and to initiate treatment with a combination of quinine and pyrimethamine-sulfadoxine and/or doxycycline. Mefloquine is also an effective therapy for chloroquine-resistant *P. falciparum* (and the asexual erythrocyte stages of the other plasmodium species). Halofantrine, a newly approved antimalarial compound, is especially useful for self-treatment of presumptive malaria acquired in Southeast Asia or if multiple drug–resistant malaria is suspected.

Persons presenting with complications due to *P. falciparum* or with high parasitemia but unable to tolerate oral medications due to vomiting should receive intravenous medications. Supportive care is critical in these patients and includes close hemodynamic monitoring, use of judicious fluid replacement, correction of significant metabolic abnormalities, and additional support as needed (dialysis, mechanical ventilation, etc.). Exchange transfusions have been lifesaving in some patients with parasitemia in excess of 10 percent. Glucocorticoids have not been shown to be of benefit in the treatment of cerebral malaria and should not be used. Quinidine is probably the intravenous drug of choice due not only to its widespread availability but also to its enhanced activity against *P. falciparum.* Parenteral quinine is only available from the Centers for Disease Control and Prevention.

Quinine and quinidine are potent inducers of insulin release and may cause severe hypoglycemia. Sudden changes in orientation, sweating, tremor, tachycardia, or anxiety should prompt measurement of plasma glucose concentration. Cinchona alkaloids are myocardial depressants, so cardiac monitoring is needed during administration. Terminal treatment with primaquine is not needed in patients with falciparum malaria due to the absence of dormant asexual forms in the liver.

## PREVENTION

Malaria is largely preventable through use of personal protection measures and appropriate chemoprophylaxis. A recent study confirmed that travelers to malarious areas frequently do not use antimosquito measures or take antimalarial drugs. Between dusk and dawn, travelers should remain in well-screened areas, use mosquito nets if needed, and wear long-sleeved clothing. A pyrethrum-containing insect spray should be used during evening hours and before retiring to bed. Permethrin can be sprayed on clothing for additional protection and an insect repellent containing *N,N*-diethyl-metatoluamide (DEET) applied to exposed skin.

**Table 125-6.** Recommended Chemoprophylactic Regimens for Prevention of Malaria*

| Drug | Adult Dose | Pediatric Dose |
|---|---|---|
| TRAVEL TO AREA WHERE CRPF HAS NOT BEEN REPORTED | | |
| Primary drug | | |
| Chloroquine phosphate | 300-mg base (500 mg salt) PO, 1/week | 5 mg/kg base (8.3 mg/kg salt) PO, 1/week, up to adult dose |
| Second-line drugs | | |
| Doxycycline | 100 mg PO qd | >8 years of age: 2 mg/kg PO qd up to adult dose |
| TRAVEL TO AREAS WHERE CRPF HAS BEEN REPORTED | | |
| Primary drug | | |
| Mefloquine | 228-mg base (250 mg salt) PO, 1/week | >45 kg: 1 tab/week 31–45 kg: $^3/_4$ tab/week 20–30 kg: $^1/_2$ tab/week 15–19 kg: $^1/_4$ tab/week |
| Second-line drugs | | |
| Doxycycline† | See above | See above |
| Chloroquine | See above | See above |
| *plus* | | |
| Fansidar‡ | See Table 125-5 | See Table 125-5 |
| *plus* | | |
| Proguanil§ | 200 mg PO qd | >10 years: adult dose 7–10 years: 150 mg/day 2–6 years 100 mg/day <2 years: 50 mg/day |
| TRAVEL TO AREAS WHERE MULTIPLE DRUG RPF HAS BEEN REPORTED | | |
| Primary Drug | | |
| Doxycycline | See above | See above |
| Second-line drug | | |
| Halofantrine (self-treatment) | See Table 125-4 | See Table 125-4 |

* For prolonged exposure in areas with *P. vivax* or *P. ovale,* primaquine (Table 125-5) should be added at completion of prophylaxis.

† Doxycycline is the preferred second-line agent for travels where Fansidar resistance is prevalent such as the Amazon Basin area; the sub-Saharan countries listed above; and Southeast Asia, Burma, and Papua New Guinea.

‡ Fansidar may be used for unexplained febrile illnesses if medical assistance is not readily available. See a physician as soon as possible.

§ Some experts add proguanil to chloroquine prophylaxis for alternative prophylaxis in selected sub-Saharan countries (Angola, Burundi, Kenya, Malawi, Mozambique, Rwanda, Tanzania, Uganda, Zaire, Zambia).

Appropriate chemoprophylaxis depends upon where one will be traveling. If potential exposure to infected mosquitos is likely, prophylaxis is warranted even if such exposure will be brief. Table 125-6 summarizes the chemotherapeutic agents of choice. The Centers for Disease Control and Prevention maintains a 24-h malaria hotline [(404) 332-4555], which provides up-to-date information on resistance patterns in countries. Chemoprophylaxis should generally be taken for 4 weeks following the exposure.

Lastly, even with the religious use of antimosquito measures and chemoprophylaxis, malaria can be contracted or can recur. For reasons discussed earlier, malaria must be considered whenever fever occurs in someone who has traveled to a malarious area or who has received "successful" therapy in the past. Vaccines directed against various antigens of the malaria parasite are currently in development.

## BIBLIOGRAPHY

Centers for Disease Control and Prevention: *Health Information for International Travel 1993.* US Dept of Health and Human Services publication No. (CDC) 93-8280, 1993.

Lobel HO: Malaria and use of prevention measures among United States travelers, in Steffen R, Lobel HO, Waworth J, et al (eds): *Travel Medicine.* Berlin, Springer, 1989.

Szela JJ, Band JD: Traveling healthy: A guide for physicians and their patients. *Contemp Intern Med* 5:29, 1993.

Valero MV, Amador LR, Galindo C, et al: Vaccination with SPf66, a chemically synthesized vaccine, against *Plasmodium falciparum* malaria in Colombia. *Lancet* 341:705, 1993.

Weinke T, Loscher T, Fleischer K, et al: The efficacy of halofantrine in the treatment of acute malaria in nonimmune travelers. *Am J Trop Med Hyg* 47:1, 1992.

Winters RA, Murray HW: Malaria—the Mime revisited: Fifteen more years of experience at a New York City teaching hospital. *Am J Med* 93:243, 1992.

World Health Organization: *International Travel and Health—Vaccination Requirements and Health Advice.* Geneva, Switzerland, 1994.

Wyler DJ: Malaria: Overview and update. *Clin Infect Dis* 16:449, 1993.

# 126
# COMMON PARASITIC INFECTIONS
## Harold Osborn

Despite significant advances in medical knowledge and technology over the last half century, parasitic disease remains prevalent worldwide. It is estimated that 200 million people, living mostly in the rural tropics, suffer from schistosomiasis and that hookworm infects approximately a quarter of the world's population. Parasites such as *Ascaris* and *Enterobius* each infect 1 billion people.

In the United States parasitic disease is becoming increasingly recognized. In addition to the persistence of endemic parasites in this country, three factors account for this trend: (1) immigration to the United States of infected individuals from the countries of Asia, Africa, and Latin America; (2) increased travel by Americans, particularly to the underdeveloped parts of the world; and (3) the rise of parasitic infections among immunosuppressed patients, especially those afflicted with the human immunodeficiency virus (HIV-1).

*Ascaris* is said to infect 3 million people in North America; *Enterobius* infection rates among children in the United States vary from 10 to 45 percent. Serologic surveys in the United States have demonstrated that 20 to 70 percent of the population have antibodies to *Toxoplasma* and over 90 percent have antibodies to *Pneumocystis carinii.* These two parasites can cause significant morbidity and mortality when they reactivate in immunosuppressed individuals and create opportunistic infections.

Finally, *Cryptosporidium* and *Giardia* are now recognized as etiologies of traveler's diarrhea and have become major causes of diarrhea in immunocompetent individuals in the United States. Person-to-person spread of these parasites has led to diarrheal illness in day care centers and other institutions, and contamination of municipal water supplies has led to major outbreaks. In March and April of 1993, 400,000 people in Milwaukee became ill after *Cryptosporidium* contaminated the drinking water, and 54 people died as a result. Interestingly, this parasite cannot be contained by chlorination, iodination, or ozonation of the water; it must be eliminated by filtration. The federal government is now planning to spend $5.5 billion over the next 5 years to monotor the nation's water supply for this one parasite.

The agents that cause parasitic diseases belong to three major groups: helminths (worms), protozoa, and arthropods. The multicellular helminths include nematodes (roundworms), cestodes (flatworms), and trematodes (flukes). The protozoa are single-celled organisms that cause a variety of diseases ranging from malaria to amebiasis. Arthropods are classified as ectoparasites and are medically important as obligatory intermediate hosts and as mechanical vectors in many diseases. This chapter reviews diseases caused by helminths and protozoa. Malaria is discussed in Chapter 125.

## HISTORY

The recognition of parasitic disease begins with the elicitation of a careful history. Specifically, the clinician should inquire about travel to or immigration from high-risk areas. Parasites flourish in warm, moist climates where sanitation is poor and where many of the people share a low socioeconomic status and have inadequate nutrition. Children are infected with parasites more frequently than adults because of their oral behavior, poor hygiene, and inability to ward off arthropod vectors.

Parasitic disease should be considered in any patient with unexplained fever, abdominal pain, diarrhea, skin ulcers, rash, or eosinophilia. The history should include dates of travel or immigration, destination or country of origin, living conditions, and activities. Certain specific areas of the world may implicate particular parasitic agents. Hmong tribesmen, who came to this country from Indochina in large numbers in 1979 and 1980, often harbor *Paragonimus westermani* (lung fluke), whereas visitors to Leningrad or the Rockies may return with *Giardia*. The history should also include questions about sexual orientation and contacts, drug use, past illnesses, and a complete review of systems. The use of pretravel medications, including antimalarial and antidiarrheal agents, should be elicited.

The presence of risk factors can provide a clue to specific parasitic diseases (Table 126-1). Recently cases of acute Chagas disease (trypanosomiasis) and babesiosis following blood transfusions have been described in the United States and Canada. Institutionalized patients may suffer from amebiasis and can become infected with *Hymenolepis nana* (the most common tapeworm in the United States) or *Giardia* (especially day care centers). Immunocompromised hosts (those on steroids or antineoplastic agents) are susceptible to infection by *Strongyloides, Toxoplasma, Cryptosporidium,* and *P. carinii* and can develop a life-threatening hyperinfection syndrome with *Strongyloides stercoralis*. Interestingly, patients with acquired immunodeficiency syndrome (AIDS), although susceptible to *Toxoplasma, Cryptosporidium, Pneumocystis, Isospora, Microsporidium,* and *Cyclospora,* are not any more susceptible to *Amoeba* and *Strongyloides* than immunocompetent individuals. Finally, the consumption of raw food has been associated with a variety of parasitic diseases including fish, pork, and beef tapeworm.

## PATHOPHYSIOLOGY

Parasites differ in their pathogenicity and in their capacity to produce invasive or systemic disease. The subclass Coccidia, for example, in-

**Table 126-1.** Risk Factors for Parastic Disease

Blood transfusion: *Plasmodium* species, *Trypanosoma, Babesia, Toxoplasma*
Intravenous drug use: *Plasmodium* species
Homosexuality: *Entamoeba* (often seen after colonic irrigation therapy), *Giardia, Cryptosporidium*
Immunocompromised host: *Toxoplasma, Pneumocystis, Strongyloides, Cryptosporidium, Microsporidium, Isospora,* and *Cyclospora*
Institutionalization: *H. nana, Entamoeba histolytica, Giardia*
Day care centers: *Giardia, Cryptosporidium*
Livestock workers: *Cryptosporidium*
Pica: *Toxocara* (visceral larva migrans), hookworm (*Necator americanus*)
Consumption of raw food:
  Sushi, sashimi, gefilte fish—*Diphyllobothrium, Anisakis*
  Pork—*Taenia solium, Trichinella, Sarcocystis*
  Beef—*Taenia saginata, Toxoplasma, Sarcocystis*

cludes both *Toxoplasma* and *Isospora*. However, *Isospora* is unable to invade the intestinal mucosa and thus produces only an enterocolitis, whereas *Toxoplasma* crosses the intestine and produces severe systemic illness.

Sometimes different forms of the parasite differ in their ability to cause illness. The adult from of *Trichinella spiralis* remains in the intestine, while the larval form crosses and migrates to striated and cardiac muscle. Amebiasis can result in both intestinal and visceral infections. Pathogenicity may vary among different strains within a genus. Infection with *Entamoeba* can result in an asymptomatic cyst carrier state or hepatic abscesses, depending on the strain involved.

Finally, organisms differ in their virulence. The infectious dose of *Giardia* and *Cryptosporidium* is in the order of 10 to $10^3$ organisms. By contrast, the infectious dose of *Vibrio cholereae* and *Salmonella* is $10^5$ to $10^8$ organisms. This may be an important factor in the genesis of outbreaks in institutions and day care centers.

## CLINICAL FEATURES

Unfortunately, symptoms may be nonspecific and the latency period between exposure and symptom appearance may be years. Symptoms can be acute or chronic, specific or vague. Parasitic disease can present with relatively common complaints such as headache, fever, cough, and malaise or with acute, life-threatening complications such as seizures, hemoptysis, melena, and intestinal obstruction. A differential diagnosis can be made on the basis of history and knowledge of typical symptoms associated with different parasitic agents (Table 126-2)

## DIFFERENTIAL DIAGNOSIS

Diarrhea is an exceedingly common complaint and can be a manifestation of an inconsequential and self-limited problem, or it can be the hallmark of a serious chronic illness or infection with occasional life-threatening potential. Although a variety of systemic illnesses, toxins, drugs, and malabsorption syndromes can cause diarrhea, the infectious causes are of most immediate concern. Although viruses and bacteria are the most common causes of infectious diarrhea, parasites constitute a significant and increasingly more common cause as well.

The majority of diarrhea-inducing infections are noninflammatory, usually arising in the upper small bowel from the action of an enterotoxin (e.g., *Vibrio cholerae,* enterotoxigenic *Escherichia coli),* or other processes that alter the absorptive function of the villous tip (e.g., *Cryptosporidium, Giardia,* Rotavirus, Norwalk-like virus). In contrast, inflammatory diarrhea, which often presents as dysentery (bloody stools), arises in the colon from an invasive process, sometimes mediated by a cytotoxin (e.g., *Salmonella, Shigella, Campylobacter, Clostridium difficile,* and *Amoeba*).

If diarrhea has persisted for a few days, is bloody in nature (dysentery), or is accompanied by substantial fever, dehydration, or weight loss, evaluate the patient more closely (Fig. 126-1). Diarrheal illness lasting 10 days or longer and diarrhea in those with risk factors (see Table 126-1) should prompt a vigorous search for parasites. One should remember that malaria may also present with prominent gastrointestinal symptoms, including diarrhea, in as many as two thirds of cases.

A stool smear for fecal leukocytes may be helpful, although this is controversial. The presence of fecal leukocytes has been considered a sign of inflammatory diarrhea and has been used to exclude toxigenic bacteria, viruses, and most parasites. However, when studied, the presence of fecal leukocytes is neither sensitive nor specific for inflammatory etiologies.

Examination of a stool specimen for ova and parasites is the best method for detecting intestinal parasites including the cysts and trophozoites of protozoa and the larvae, eggs, or adults of helminths. Three specimens collected on different days should be examined and the stool must be free of substances like bismuth, barium, nonab-

**Table 126-2.** Symptoms of Parasitic Disease

| Symptom | Possible Cause |
|---------|----------------|
| Hemoptysis | *Ascaris, Paragonimus, Echinococcus* |
| Meningitis | *Trichinella, Toxocara, Naegleria, Acanthamoeba, Trypanosoma, Malaria* |
| Malaria | (*Plasmodium falciparum*), primary amebic meningoencephalitis |
| Urticaria | *Ascaris, Strongyloides, Dracunculus, Trichinella, Fasciola* |
| Diarrhea | Hookworm, *Strongyloides, Trichuris, Trichinella, Schistosoma, Fasciola, Fasciolopsis, Taenia, Hymenolepis, Entamoeba, Giardia, Dientamoeba, Palantidium, Leishmania donovani* |
| Abdominal pain | *Ascaris,* hookworm, *Trichuris, Schistosoma, Entamoeba, Clonorchis, Fasciola, Taenia, Hymenolepis, Diphyllobothrium, Giardia* |
| Pruritus | *Enterobius, Trichuris,* filariae (*Onchocerca volvulus*), *Dientamoeba, Leishmania* |
| Nausea and vomiting | *Ascaris, Trichuris, Trichinella, Taenia, Entamoeba, Giardia, Leishmania* |
| Seizures | *Hymenolepis, Trichinella, Paragonimus,* tapeworm (*Echinococcus, Cysticercus*) |
| Anemia | *Plasmodium* species, *Babesia,* hookworm (*N. americanus, Ancylostoma duodenale*), *Trichuris, Diphyllobothrium, L. donovani* |
| Pneumonia | *Ascaris, Strongyloides, Trichinella,* filariae (*Wuchereria bancrofti, Brugia malayi*), fluke (*P. westermani*) |
| Myocardial disease | *Trichinella, Taenia, Trypanosoma* (*T. cruzi*) |
| Conjunctivitis and keratitis | *Trichinella,* filariae (*O. volvulus*), *Taenia, Trypanosoma* |
| Jaundice | *Toxoplasma,* fluke (*Clonorchis sinensis, Opisthorchis viverrini*), *Plasmodium* species |
| Asthma | *Ascaris* |
| Skin ulcers | *Dracunculus,* hookworm (*Ancylostoma duodenale*), *L. donovani, Trypanosoma* |
| Splenomegaly | *Babesia, Toxoplasma, Plasmodium* species |
| Intestinal obstruction | *Arcaris, Strongyloides,* fluke (*Fasciolopsis buski*), *Taenia, Diphyllobothrium* |
| Eosinophilia | *Srongyloides,* hookworm, *Trichuris, Dracunculus, Fasciola, Toxocara, Ascaris, Trichinella,* filariae (*W. bancrofti, B. malayi*) *Hymnenolepis, Schistosoma,* fluke (*P. westermani, C. sinensis, Fasciolopsis leuski*), *Taenia* |
| Fever | *Ascaris, Toxocara,* hookworm, *Trichuris, Trichinella,* filariae (*W. bancrofti*), *Schistosoma,* fluke (*C. sinensis*), *Fasciola, Entamoeba, Giardia, Trypanosoma, L. donovani, Babesia, Plasmodium* species |
| Hepatomegaly | *Trypanosoma, L. donovani, Toxocara, Schistosoma,* fluke (*C. sinensis, O. viverrini, Fasciola*), tapeworm (*Echinococcus*), *Plasmodium* species |
| Edema | *Trichinella,* filariae (*W. bancrofti*) *Fasciolopsis, Trypanosoma* |

sorbable antidiarrheal agents, and mineral oil. Antimicrobial agents should be stopped at least 1 week prior to the stool collection. Fresh specimens are best, and specimens over an hour old should be preserved with formalin or polyvinyl alcohol. Multiple stool examinations are particularly important when dealing with formed stool, which usually contains fewer parasites than diarrheal specimens.

Occasionally *Giardia, Cryptosporidium,* and the larvae of *Strongyloides* may be detected by examining a duodenal aspirate or by having the patient swallow a string with a gelatin capsule (Entero-test). Recent studies suggest that detection of *Giardia* by examination of seven stool specimens is just as effective as examination of duodenal contents.

Special procedures for removing parasites include the following: warm water concentration through a filter for *Strongyloides* (Baermann test), sticky tape swab of the perianal area for *Enterobius*

(Swube test), passage of urine through a nucleopore filter for *Schistosoma hematobium* and use of an acid-fast stain to detect *Cryptosporidium, Isospora,* and *Cyclospora.*

The enzyme-linked immunosorbent assay (ELISA) technique can be used to make a serologic diagnosis of a variety of parasitic infections. In addition, the ELISA technique has been used to detect antigens of *Giardia* and *Cryptosporidia* in stool. Malaria-causing plasmodia, babesia, microfilaria of *Wucheria* and *Brugia,* and the trypanosomes that cause Chagas disease can be detected by Giemsa-stained thick and thin films of peripheral blood.

Finally, organisms that affect the central nervous system (CNS) (*Plasmodium falciparum*—cerebral malaria and *Acanthamoeba* or *Naegleria*—amoebic meningoencephalitis) can be detected by culture or microscopic examination of centrifuged cerebrospinal fluid. Pneumocystis is detected by characteristic findings on chest x-ray, elevated lactate dehydrogenase (LDH), and evidence of hypoxemia, and is confirmed by lung biopsy with special stains while *Toxoplasma* is detected by characteristic findings on computed tomography (CT) in association with elevated serum antibodies, and is rarely confirmed by brain biopsy.

## HELMINTHS

### Nematodes (Roundworms)

Nematodes are cylindrical, unsegmented, elongated white worms. Their mode of entry into the human host varies from ingestion of eggs (*Ascaris* and *Enterobius*), to penetration of the skin (*Necator, Ancylostoma,* and *Strongyloides*), to inoculation by insect bite (*Wucheria*).

### *Ascaris*

*Ascaris lumbricoides* has a worldwide distribution with an estimated 3 million Americans infected each year. Its life span untreated is 2 to 7 years. Larval invasion follows the ingestion of *Ascaris* eggs, and during this stage the parasite migrates through the lungs. Patients can present with fever, cough, dyspnea, hemoptysis, and eosinophilia. The diagnosis is made by finding eggs or occasionally the adult worm in the stool. Serologic tests including bentonite flocculation, ELISA, and indirect hemagglutination may be helpful. Treatment is with mebendazole, albendazole, or pyrantel pamoate. Intestinal obstruction may necessitate surgery, especially in children.

### *Enterobius* (Pinworm)

Adult *Enterobius* (pinworm) resides in the cecum, appendix, ileum, and ascending colon after its eggs are ingested. The gravid female migrates to the anus especially at night where it causes intense pruritus. Autoinfection with hand-to-mouth transmission is possible after scratching. Whether or not *Enterobius* can cause appendicitis has not yet been settled. A host of problems from vaginitis to enuresis have been attributed to infection with *Enterobius* but none too convincingly. Pinworm infection is most prevalent in temperate climates during the winter and fall. The diagnosis is confirmed with cellophane tape swab of the anus. All family members should be examined. Treatment is with pyrantel pamoate, albendazole, or mebendazole and should be repeated after 2 weeks. All those living in close contact with the patient should be treated.

### Hookworm

*Necator americanus* (American hookworm) prevails in the southern United States and is often seen in immigrants from warmer climates. Infection is associated with the use of human fertilizer and the lack of shoes and latrines. Because each worm can withdraw 0.03 to 0.2 mL of blood a day, infection often leads to chronic anemia. Pica and geophagy are often seen in infected children. Patients may present

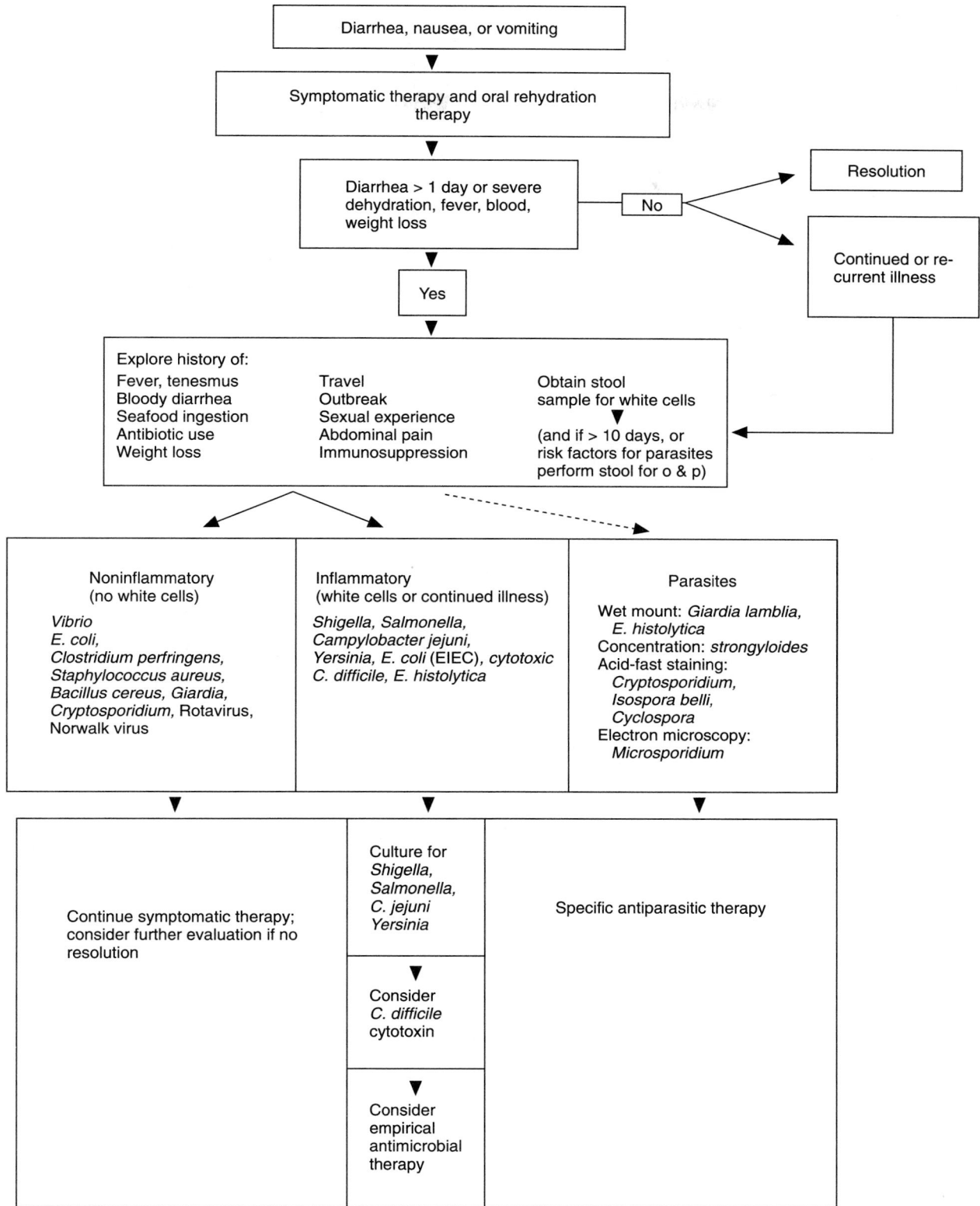

**Fig. 126-1.** Algorithm for evaluating a patient with diarrhea. (Adapted from Guerrant RL, Bobak DA. Bacterial and protozoal gastroenteritis. *N Engl J Med* 325:327, 1991.)

with cough, low-grade fever, abdominal pain, diarrhea, weakness, weight loss, heme-positive stools, and eosinophilia. The diagnosis is made by finding ova in the stool. In mild infections multiple stool specimens or concentration techniques may be necessary. The parasite burden can be estimated using Beaver's stool or Kato's slide smear method. Infections with less than 2100 eggs per gram of feces (< 50 adult worms) are usually not hematologically important, whereas infections with over 11,000 eggs per gram result in a significant anemia. Hookworm is best treated with mebendazole, albendazole, or pyrantel pamoate.

### Strongyloides (Threadworms)

Adult threadworms reside in the mucosa of the small intestine. Because entry of the parasite is through the skin, penetration can lead to allergic manifestations, pruritus, and an erythematous rash. Migration throughout the lungs can produce cough, dyspnea, and pneumonia; the intestinal phase is manifested by abdominal pain, diarrhea with mucus and blood, and eosinophilia. Larval migration in the skin produces cutaneous larva migrans. Fatalities may occur in the elderly and the immunocompromised (leprosy, nephrotic syndrome, hepatic disease, lymphoproliferative disorders, and those on steroids). *Strongyloides* is probably a hyperinfection rather than an opportunistic infection. The diagnosis is confirmed by finding larvae in the stool. Occasionally a formol-ether concentration method or duodenal aspiration may be necessary. Various stages of the parasite may be found in the sputum. An upper gastrointestinal series may reveal a deformed duodenal bulb, and *Strongyloides* may be confused with ulcer disease. Treatment is with thiabendazole or ivermectin.

### Trichuris trichiura

*Trichuris trichiura,* like *Ascaris,* is found in rural communities in the southern United States. The infection is most often acquired in childhood because the ova are deposited in the soil where children play and defecate freely. The adult worm resides in the cecum. Patients complain of anorexia, insomnia, abdominal pain (including pain in the right upper quadrant), fever, flatulence, diarrhea, weight loss, and pruritus and may have eosinophilia and a microcytic hypochromic anemia. *Trichuris* can result in colitis or rectal prolapse in children. The diagnosis is made with the finding of ova in the stool. Mebendazole or albendazole is the treatment of choice.

### Trichinella spiralis

Trichinosis is common in Mexico and the United States and results from the consumption of infected pork and, less commonly, bear and walrus meat. Autopsy studies have revealed an infection rate in human diaphragms of 4 to 5 percent. In the early stages of infection with *T. spiralis,* the patient may present with acute myocarditis, non-suppurative meningitis, bronchopneumonia, or catarrhal enteritis. The primary lesions are in striated muscle. Clinical symptoms depend on the number of worms ingested, the number of larvae produced, and the site of invasion. Patients may present with nausea and vomiting, diarrhea, fever, urticaria, periorbital edema, splinter hemorrhages, myalgia, muscle spasm, stiff neck, headache, and psychiatric disturbances. The periorbital edema is pathognomonic.

Laboratory manifestations of trichinosis include leukocytosis, eosinophilia, elevated creatine kinase, and electrocardiographic (ECG) changes. The diagnosis can be confirmed with latex agglutination, skin test, and a complement fixation or bentonite flocculation test available from the Centers for Disease Control and Prevention. A new ELISA test is very specific and sensitive after the third week of infection. Biopsy of tender muscle may be helpful after the fourth week. Since *T. spiralis* encysts in striated muscle, stool examination is not helpful after the initial gastrointestinal phase in making the diagnosis. The differential diagnosis includes staphylococcal and sal-monella food poisoning, shigellosis, and amebiasis. Mebendazole is indicated for treatment of the intestinal phase but may be ineffective after encystment. Steroids are indicated for CNS disease and myocarditis but are not advocated routinely because their use can increase the number of circulating larvae. Most cases are mild and never come to medical attention.

### Trematodes (Flukes)

Trematodes are leaflike, symmetical flatworms lacking a body cavity but possessing a ventral sucker to hold their position. They live in intermediate hosts like snails, crabs, and fish and shed their eggs from the human host in the feces (*Schistosoma, Clonorchis, Fasciola*), urine (*S. haematobium*), or sputum (*Paragonimus*).

### Schistosoma

Schistosomes penetrate the skin, creating a papular pruritic rash. The adult form resides in the venous system. Symptoms of acute disease—fever, lymphadenopathy, and hepatosplenomegaly (so-called Katayama fever)—are rarely seen. More typically patients present in the chronic stage with granulomas in the liver (portal hypertension) and bladder (obstructive hydroureter). Patients may present with diarrhea, abdominal pain, melena, hepatosplenomegaly, hematemesis, and in the late stages, ascites and liver failure. With *S. haematobium,* dysuria and hematuria may be found. The diagnosis can be confirmed by finding eggs in the feces or on rectal biopsy. Treatment is with praziquantel.

### Cestoda (Flatworms)

The cestodes are flatworms commonly referred to as tapeworms. They have a scolex or head equipped with suckers or hooks. Cestodes grow by segmentation, extending proglottids from the neck.

### Taenia

*Taenia solium* (pork tapeworm) is occasionally encountered in the United States today in immigrants or visitors from Central America and the Middle East. *Taenia saginata* (beef tapeworm) is seen more often, especially in those who consume raw beef (e.g., steak tartare). Adult worms live in the small intestine. Infected patients can be asymptomatic or present with nausea and vomiting, headache, abdominal pain, pruritus, constipation, diarrhea, and intestinal obstruction. The larval stage of *T. solium* can cause clinical disease (cysticercosis), which can be serious and sometimes fatal. *Taenia* cysts may be found in subcutaneous tissue, the eye, the brain, and the heart. Radiographs of the soft tissues may reveal curvilinear calcifications indicative of cysts, and cysts can be seen in the meninges and brain parenchyma on CT scanning. The diagnosis is made by finding gravid proglottids in the stool. An ELISA or hemagglutination reaction may be helpful, but both can be falsely negative if the cysts are calcified. Treatment of the adult (intestinal) stage is with niclosamide or praziquantel; the larval (tissue) stage is treated with albendazole.

### Diphyllobothrium

*Diphyllobothrium* (fish tapeworm) has been reported in the Pacific Northwest, Minnesota, Michigan, and other areas where raw fish (e.g., sushi and sashimi) and gefilte fish are consumed. *Diphyllobothrium* can compete with the host for vitamin $B_{12}$, and thus patients can present with pernicious anemia. Treatment is the same as for *Taenia.*

## PROTOZOA

### Amebas

Amebiasis, which is caused by *E. histolytica,* occurs world-wide and is associated with poor sanitation. Outbreaks have been reported in institutions for the mentally retarded and in the homosexual community. Amebae inhabit the cecum and large intestine, where they cause ulcers and diffuse inflammation, which can mimic ulcerative colitis. An ameboma can rarely develop in the liver and present as a liver abscess. Approximately half of all infected patients are asymptomatic. Symptoms include nausea and vomiting, anorexia, diarrhea, fever, abdominal pain, and leukocytosis. Protozoan infections, amebiasis included, do not produce eosinophilia. The diagnosis is established with stool testing including postcathartic stools and concentration and staining techniques. Stool specimens should be fixed in polyvinyl alcohol, formalin, or merthiolate-iodine-formalin. Serologic tests (ELISA and indirect hemagglutination reaction) can be helpful in the presence of extraintestinal disease. Treatment is with metronidazole or tinidazole followed by chloroquine phosphate.

### Giardia

*Giardia* is probably the most common intestinal parasite in the United States. It inhabits the duodenum and upper jejunum where the alkaline pH creates a favorable milieu. Cysts are ingested in fecally contaminated water or food or are passed by hand-to-mouth transmission. Water-borne outbreaks have become more common in the United States because the cysts are resistant to chlorination. Day care centers have been increasingly implicated in promoting giardiasis. Symptoms depend on the duration of infection at the time of presentation. Patients may complain of explosive, watery or foul-smelling diarrhea, flatus, abdominal distention, fatigue, and fever, or chronic diarrhea with weight loss or general debilitation. Stools should be examined with routine and concentration techniques. *Giardia* antigen can be detected in the stool with immunofluorescence or ELISA technique. Occasionally duodenal aspiration, string test (Entero-test), or small-bowel biopsy is necessary to make the diagnosis. The drug of choice for treatment is metronidazole.

### Trypanosoma

American *Trypanosoma* (*Trypanosoma cruzi*) causes Chagas' disease; three strains of African *Trypanosoma* cause sleeping sickness. Chagas' disease is usually transmitted by the reduviid (kissing) bug, but infection can also follow breast-feeding and blood transfusion, as has occurred in the United States. A nodular swelling or chagoma develops at the site of inoculation following a bite. The acute phase of the disease can last 2 to 3 months, and patients present with fever, headache, anorexia, conjunctivitis, and myocarditis. Infants can develop a meningocephalitis, and heart involvement can lead to congestive heart failure and ventricular aneurysms. The organism can attack the myenteric plexus of the gastrointestinal tract resulting in megacolon. Chronic infection can result in a cardiomyopathy. Laboratory abnormalities include anemia, leukocytosis, an elevated sedimentation rate, and ECG changes (PR interval, T wave changes, heart block, and arrhythmias). During the acute phase serologic tests are helpful and trypomastigotes can be seen on a peripheral smear. In the chronic phase the diagnosis is made with a complement fixation test or biopsy of the liver, spleen, or bone marrow. Treatment of Chagas' disease is with nifurtimox; treatment of sleeping sickness is with suramin sodium.

### Babesia

*Babesia* is a Protozoa which, like *Plasmodium* species, possesses an erythrocytic phase. It is transmitted by *Ixodes* ticks and occasionally by blood transfusion. Babesiosis has been reported in Europe and in the northeastern United States (especially Nantucket, Massachusetts and Long Island). Babesiosis in the northeastern United States is invariably caused by the murine species, *Babesia microti,* and is transmitted by the deer tick, *Ixodes dammini,* which also serves as a vector for Lyme disease. Patients may present with intermittent fever, splenomegaly, hemolysis, and jaundice. Infection can be fatal in splenectomized patients but is apparently not increased in incidence in immunocompromised patients. Diagnosis can be made on a Giemsa-stained peripheral smear, but occasionally *Babesia* smear can be confused for the ring forms of *P. falciparum* malaria. Babesiosis can simulate rickettsial diseases like Rocky Mountain spotted fever and Lyme disease. Treatment is with clindamycin and quinine.

### Cryptosporidium

*Cryptosporidium* is a protozoan parasite belonging to the subclass Coccidia, which also includes *Toxoplasma, Isospora, Cyclospora, Eimeria,* and *Sarcocystis. Cryptosporidium parvum* is the species that most commonly causes disease in human beings. Previously regarded only as a disease of immunodepressed individuals (especially those with AIDS), *Cryptosporidium* is now recognized as an important and increasingly common cause of diarrhea, including traveler's diarrhea, worldwide.

Like giardiasis, water-borne transmission of cryptosporidiosis has been well documented in England and the United States, most recently in Milwaukee, Wisconsin, where 400,000 people were infected in 1993, and 54 deaths occurred. Similar to *Giardia, Cryptosporidium* causes diarrhea by altering the microvillous tips of the cells lining the small intestine. *Cryptosporidium* can infect other mammals, including cows, and waste water (raw sewage) and runoff from dairies and pastures may be the source of oocysts that contaminate reservoirs and pools.

The diarrhea of cryptosporidiosis, in both immunocompetent and immunocompromised patients, is profuse and watery (cholera-like), usually without blood, fecal leukocytes, and mucus. It is occasionally associated with crampy abdominal pain, nausea and vomiting, low-grade fever, and weight loss. Although the illness is self-limited in most immunocompetent individuals (lasting several days to 2 weeks), it can be relentless and debilitating in the immunocompromised, often resulting in servere dehydration, malabsorption, weight loss, and death. Rarely *Cryptosporidium* can also cause respiratory and biliary tract disease.

The diagnosis is made by finding oocytes in the stool. Concentration of the stool specimen using formalin ether gives a higher yield. A modified Ziehl-Neelsen acid fast stain is used to visualize the oocysts. A serum ELISA for antibodies to *Cryptosporidium* is available but is useful only for epidemiologic surveys to detect the prevalence of exposure.

Treatment of severe cryptosporidiosis is mainly supportive (oral or intravenous hydration and the use of antidiarrheal agents). Treatment of the disease in immunocompromised patients is difficult and, at present, there is no accepted treatment. Recently, a somatostatin-like agent, octreotide, has been used with some success and trials with azithromycin have shown some promise.

## Protozoan Infections in the Immunocompromised Host

### Respiratory Tract

Pneumonia occurs commonly in immunocompromised patients and is often due to *P. carinii.* Because most normal children have antibodies to *P. carinii, P. carinii* pneumonia probably represents a reactivation of a latent infection. The natural habitat and mode of transmission of *P. carinii* are poorly understood. Patients present acutely with fever, dyspnea, a nonproductive cough, and scant rales. Arterial blood gases may reveal hypoxia or an increased alveolar-arterial (A-a) gradient. The serum LDH level may be elevated. Early, the chest x-ray may be normal. Later, the classical appearance is of symmetrical interstitial infiltrates in the mid and lower lung zones. *P. carinii* occurs in premature and debilitated infants, AIDS patients, those receiving organ

**Table 126-3** Commonly Used Antiparasitic Drugs

| Drug | First-Line Agent | Alternative Agent | Side Effects |
|---|---|---|---|
| Albendazole (Zental) | Tapeworm (*E. granulosus, Cysticercus*), *Ascaria,* cutaneous larva migrans, *Enterobius, Gnathostoma, Trichuris,* hookworm (*A. duodenale, N. americanus*) | *Capillaria, Trichostrongylus,* visceral larva migrans | Diarrhea, abdominal pain |
| Amphotericin B (Fungizone) | Amebic meningoencephalitis (*Naegleria*) | Leishmania (*L. braziliensis, L. mexicana*) | Fever, headache, anorexia, nausea, diarrhea, muscle and joint pain, azotemia, anemia, RTA, leukopenia |
| Bithionol (Bithin) | Fluke (*Fasciola hepatica*) | | Photosensitivity, nausea and vomiting, urticaria |
| Chloroquine | Plasmodium species (except resistant *P. falciparum*) | | Pruritus, vomiting, headache, confusion, skin eruptions, myalgias, EOM palsies |
| Clindamycin (Cleocin) | *Babesia,* chloroquine-resistant *P. falciparum* | | |
| Diethylcarbamazine (Hetrazan) | filaria (*Wuchereria bancrofti, Loa loa,* tropical pulmonary eosinophilia), visceral larva migrans | | Allergic reactions, GI symptoms |
| Iodoquinol (Yodoxin) | *Entamoeba* (*E. histolytica*), *Dientamoeba* | *Balantidium* | Rash, acne, enlarged thyroid, nausea, diarrhea, anal pruritus, rarely: optic atrophy, peripheral neuropathy |
| Ivermectin (Mectizan) | Filariae (*O. volvulus*), *Strongyloides* | | Fever, pruritus, tender nodes, bone and joint pain, headache |
| Lindane (Kwell) | | Lice, scabies | Eczema, conjunctivitis, aplastic anemia |
| Mebendazole (Vermox) | *Angiostrongylus, Ascaria, Capillaria, Enterobius,* filariae (*Mansonella perstans*) *Trichuris,* hookworm, *Trichinella* | *Leishmania,* visceral larva migrans | Diarrhea, abdominal pain, agranulocytosis |
| Mefloquine (Lariam) | | Chloroquine-resistant *P. falciparum* | Vertigo, nausea, nightmares, headache |
| Meglumine (Glucantime) | *Leishmania* | | Joint and muscle pain, nausea |
| Metronidazole (Flagyl) | Entamoeba (*E. histolytica, E. polecki*), *Dracunculus, Trichomonas, Blastocystis, Giardia* | *Balantidium* | Nausea, headache, dry mouth, reaction with alcohol, rarely: seizures, ataxia, leukopenia, pancreatitis |
| Niclosamide (Niclocide) | Fluke (*F, buski*), tapeworm (*Diphyllobothrium, Taenia, Dipylidium*) | Tapeworm (*Hymenolepis*) | Nausea, abdominal pain |
| Nifurtimox (Lampit) | *Trypanosoma* (*T. cruzi*) | | Anorexia, vomiting, sleep disorder, tremors |
| Octreotide (Sandostatin) | *Cryptosporidia, Microsporidia* (*E. bieneusi*) | | |
| Paromomycin (Humatin) | *Dientamoeba* | *E. histolytica, Giardia* | GI disturbance, rarely: eighth nerve and renal damage, GI damage |
| Pentamidine isethionate (Pentam) | *P. carinii* | *Trypanosama* (*T. brucei*), *Leishmania* | Hypotension, hypoglycemia, vomiting, blood dyscrasia, renal damage, GI disturbance |
| Praziquantel (Biltricide) | Fluke,*Schistosoma,* tapeworm (*Hymenolepis, Cysticercus*); tapeworm (*Diphyllobothrium latum, Taenia, Dipylidium, H. nana, Cysticercus cellulosae*) | | Malaise, headache, dizziness, abdominal upset, fever, eosinophilia |
| Primaquine phosphate | P. vivax, P. orale (prevention of relapse only) | | G6PD hemolysis, neutropenia, GI disturbance |
| Pyrantel pamoate (Antiminth) | *Ascaria, Enterobius,* hookworm, *Trichostrongylus, Moniliformis* | | GI disturbances, headache, dizziness, rash, fever |
| Pyrimethamine (Daraprim) | Chloroquine-resistant *P. falciparum, Toxoplasma* | | Blood dyscrasias, folate deficiency, rarely: rash, vomiting, seizures, shock |
| Quinacrine (Atabrine) | | *Giardia* | Dizziness, headache, vomiting, diarrhea, yellow skin, toxic psychosis, insomnia, rash, blood dyscrasias |
| Quinine sulfate (Quinamm) | *Babesia,* chloroquine-resistant *P. falciparum* | | Cinchonism, hemolytic anemia, blood dyscrasias, photosensitivity, hypoglycemia, arrhythmias, hypotension |
| Spiramycin (Rovamycin) | | *Toxoplasma* | GI symptoms |

**Table 126-3 (Cont.)**

| Drug | First-Line Agent | Alternative Agent | Side Effects |
|---|---|---|---|
| Sodium stibogluconate (Pentostam) | *Leishmania* | | Muscle pain, joint stiffness, nausea, diarrhea, rash, pruritus, liver and heart damage, bradycardia, rarely: hemolytic anemia, sudden death |
| Suramin sodium (Germanin) | *Trypanosoma* (African) | | Vomiting, pruritus, urticaria, paresthesias, neuropathy |
| Thiabendazole (Mintezol) | *Angiostrongylus, Strongyloides,* visceral larva migrans, cutaneous larva migrans | *Capillaria, Dracunculus, Trichostrongylus* | Nausea, vertigo, rash, leukopenia, hallucinations, erythema multiforme, Stevens-Johnson syndrome, rarely: shock, seizures |
| Tetracycline (Achromycin) | *Dientamoeba* | | |
| Tinidazole (Fasigyn) | *Amoeba* (*E. histolytica*), *Trichomonas* | *Giardia* | Nausea, vomiting, metallic taste |
| Trimethoprim-sulfamethoxazole (Septra) | *Isospora, Pneumocystis carinii, Cyclospora* | | Allergic reactions |

*Source:* Adapted from: Drugs for parasitic infections. *Med Lett* 32:23, 1990.

transplants, and those with inherited immune deficiencies. Diagnosis is usually made by obtaining tissue from lung biopsy. The specimen should be stained with methenamine–silver nitrate or toluidine blue. Serologic tests are of limited value, because so many normal individuals have antibodies to *P. carinii.* Treatment is with trimethoprim-sulfamethoxazole or pentamidine isethionate. In patients with respiratory compromise ($P_{O_2}$ < 70 mm Hg or A-a gradient > 35 mm Hg on room air) the addition of steroids has been shown to be beneficial.

## Gastrointestinal Tract

Most patients with AIDS (50 to 98 percent) either present with or later develop diarrhea that is often life-threating. Gastrointestinal disease in the immunocompromised host is often due to *Cryptosporidium, Isospora, Microsporidia,* and *Cyclospora.*

The diagnosis of *Cryptosporidium* is made with a modified Ziehl-Neelsen acid-fast stain or Kinyoun stain of the stool. A vast array of antimicrobial and antidiarrheal agents have been tried without much success in the treatment of cryptosporidiosis. Azithromycin has a limited effect in some patients. Recently octreotide has been used with some success. The high rate of recurrence and relapse in this disease is probably related more to the underlying immunodeficiency. *Isospora belli* is another protozoa that can cause significant gastrointestinal disease. As with *Cryptosporidium,* infection with *Isospora* occurs after ingestion of oocysts in contaminated food or water and following sexual contact. Symptoms may vary from acute gastroenteritis in the immunointact individual to severe, protracted diarrhea in the immunocompromised. Characteristic oocysts can be detected in the stool with acid-fast stains. Treatment is with trimethoprim-sulfamethoxazole.

*Microsporidium* is an obligate intracellular protozoan that is becoming more commonly recognized as a pathogen in patients with AIDS as well as those who are immunocompetent. Most patients present with diarrhea and a wasting syndrome, but hepatitis, peritonitis, and a keratitis have been described. Diagnosis by stool examination is difficult due to the small spore size. Immunologic detection of spores with polyclonal serum has been attempted. Definitive diagnosis usually requires intestinal biopsy and detection with transmission electron microscopy. Treatment is difficult. Patients who do not respond to standard antidiarrheal therapy can be tried on octreotide, albendazole, or metronidazole.

## Central Nervous System

*Toxoplasma* is an intracellular parasite carried by cats and other intermediate hosts that can cause significant disease in the immunocompromised patient. Infection can come from the ingestion of oocysts or undercooked meat, by placental transfer, following organ transplant, or during a blood transfusion. Acquired toxoplasmosis is usually asymptomatic. During acute infection, transient lymphadenopathy and splenomegaly may be present. Reactivation can result in encephalitis, chorioretinitis, myocarditis, and pneumonia. Symptoms of cerebral toxoplasmosis can include severe headache, seizures, confusion, and lethargy. Focal deficits may appear, and cerebellar, brain stem, and cranial nerve lesions may be seen. Making the diagnosis may be difficult. Ventricular fluid, brain tissue, or the buffy coat from a blood sample may be inoculated into test animals. The Sabin-Feldman dye test is fairly specific. An ELISA test for antibodies to *Toxoplasma* is now available but is less reliable in AIDS patients due to low titers. CT scanning may reveal characteristic intracerebral lesions with ring enhancement following the use of contrast. Magnetic resonance imaging is more sensitive than CT scanning. Treatment is with pyrimethamine plus sulfadiazine or spiramycin.

## EMERGENCY DEPARTMENT CARE

Patients with potentially life-threatening infections (cerebral malaria, pneumocystic pneumonia, amebic meningoencephalitis, CNS toxoplasmosis) should be started on antiparasitic treatment immediately (Table 126-3). Patients who are dehydrated from gastrointestinal losses or fever should receive intravenous hydration. Those who can take fluids orally can be rehydrated by mouth.

## ADMISSION INDICATIONS

Patients with diarrhea who appear severely ill, toxic, or dehydrated, those who cannot tolerate anything by mouth, and those with organ systems involved (e.g., lung, blood, CNS) should be admitted for intravenous hydration, further diagnostic evaluation, and antiparasitic drug treatment as indicated.

## AMBULATORY TREATMENT

Patients who do not require hospitalization can be treated with antiparasitic agents if a specific diagnosis is made and should be referred for follow-up. Those who can tolerate oral fluids can be reliably rehydrated with the World Health Organization oral rehydration solution. Such a solution can be prepared by adding 3.5 g sodium chloride (or $^3/_4$ teaspoon of table salt), 2.5 g sodium bicarbonate (or 2.9 g sodium citrate or 1 teaspoon of baking soda), 1.5 g potassium chloride (or 1 cup of orange juice or two bananas), and 20 g glucose (or 40 g sucrose or 4 tablespoons of sugar) to a liter (1.05 quart) of clean water. This makes a solution of approximately 90 mmol sodium, 20 mmol potassium, 80 mmol chloride, 30 mmol bicarbonate, and 111 mmol glucose per liter.

## BIBLIOGRAPHY

Cook GC: Opportunistic parasitic infections associated with AIDS: parasitology, clinical presentation, diagnosis and management. *Q J Med* 65:967, 1987.

Drugs for parasitic infections. *Med Lett* 35 (Issue 911):111, 1993.

Grant IH, Gold JWM, Wittner M, et al: Transfusion-associated acute Chagas disease acquired in the United States. *Ann Intern Med* 111:849, 1989.

Guerrant RL, Bobak DA: Bacterial and protozoal gastroenteritis. *N Engl J Med* 325:327, 1991.

Nazer H: The need for three stool specimens in routine laboratory examinations for intestinal parasites. *Br J Clin Pract* 47:23, 1993

Rosenblatt JE: Laboratory diagnosis of parasitic infections. *Mayo Clinic Proc* 69:779, 1994.

Tanowitz HB, Weiss LM, Wittner M: Diagnosis and treatment of protozoan diarrheas. *Am J Gastroenterol* 83:339, 1988.

Winter M, Tanowitz HB, Weiss LM: Parasitic infections in AIDS patients. *Infect Dis Clin North Am* 7:569, 1993.

# 127
# TICK-BORNE DISEASES
## David J. Weber
## Susan Isbey

Many diseases can be transmitted to humans by arthropod vectors. In the United States, more vector-borne diseases are transmitted by ticks than by any other agent. The incidence of tick-borne diseases, especially Lyme disease, has been increasing as a result of reforestation, movement of humans into rural areas, and increased recreational outdoor activity. Ticks can transmit infections with viruses, bacteria, rickettsia, and parasites (Table 127-1).

Ticks (phylum Arthropoda, class Arachnida, order Acarina) are obligate, blood-sucking parasites found worldwide. There are three families of ticks; two of these, the Ixodidae (hard ticks) and Argasidae (soft ticks), are known to cause human and animal disease. Starting as an egg, all ticks go through three stages during their growth: larva, nymph, and adult. Hard ticks, which require a blood meal at each stage for morphogenesis, generally remain attached to the host for hours or days at a time. Three genera of hard ticks are known to transmit disease to humans in the United States: *Ixodes, Dermacentor,* and *Amblyomma.* Soft ticks, which may have several nymphal stages, may take multiple blood meals, each meal usually lasting less than 30 min. In the United States, only soft ticks belonging to the genus *Ornithodoros* have been known to transmit disease to humans.

## PREVENTION OF TICK-BORNE DISEASES

Individuals living in endemic areas should attempt to minimize exposure to ticks by avoiding tick-infested areas, use of tick repellents, and keeping pets tick-free. Protective clothing is useful but may be impractical during hot weather. An effective preventative method is careful examination twice a day of the body, including scalp, pubic area, axillary hair, and other anatomic crevices, with prompt removal of ticks. Removal is best accomplished by grasping the head of the tick with a forceps and gently pulling until removed. Care should be taken to avoid crushing attached ticks, spraying blood from engorged ticks, and excoriating the area. Following removal, the area should be cleaned with soap and water or a disinfectant.

## LYME DISEASE

Lyme disease, the most frequently transmitted vector-borne infection in the United States, was first described in 1977 after an epidemic of oligoarticular arthritis was noted in three communities surrounding Lyme, Connecticut. The causative agent, *Borrelia burgdorferi,* was discovered in 1982. The principal vectors of *B. burgdorferi* in the United States are *I. scapularis* in the east and upper midwest and *I. pacificus* in the west. Small mammals (rodents and rabbits) serve as hosts for the ticks in the wild; deer are an important host for the adult tick.

### Epidemiology

More than 8000 cases of Lyme borreliosis were reported in 1993. Although almost all states reported cases of Lyme disease, more than 85 percent of cases were reported from the New England, mid-Atlantic, and south Atlantic regions.

The majority of infections occur during the late spring and early summer, when both *I. scapularis* nymphal stage and human outdoor activity peak. Efficient transmission of *B. burgdorferi* by its tick vector requires a minimum of 36 to 48 h of attachment. However, less than a third of patients recall having had a tick bite, probably because the adult *I. scapularis* tick is only the size of a sesame seed, and the nymph stage (responsible for as many as 50 percent of the cases) is only the size of a poppy seed.

**Table 127-1.** Major Tick-Borne Diseases In The United States

| Disease | Causative Agent | Classification | Major Vector | Region |
|---|---|---|---|---|
| Lyme disease | *Borrelia burgdorferi* | Bacteria (spirochete) | *Ixodes* | Northeast, Wisconsin, Minnesota, California |
| Rocky Mountain spotted fever | *Rickettsia rickettsii* | Rickettsia | *Dermacentor* | Southeast, west, south central |
| Tularemia | *Francisella tularensis* | Bacteria | *Dermacentor, Amblyomma* | Arkansas, Missouri, Oklahoma |
| Ehrlichiosis | *Ehrlichia chaffeensis* | Rickettsia | *Dermacentor, Amblyomma?* | South central, south Atlantic |
| Relapsing fever | *Borrelia* species | Bacteria (spirochete) | *Ornithodoros* | West |
| Colorado tick fever | Coltivirus species | Virus | *Dermacentor* | West |
| Babesiosis | *Babesia* species | Protozoa | *Ixodes* | Northeast |
| Tick paralysis | Toxin | Neurotoxin | *Dermacentor, Amblyomma* | Northwest, south |

*Source:* Adapted with permission from Spach DH et al, 1993.

**Table 127-2.** Manifestations Of Lyme Disease By Stage

| System | Localized (Stage I) | Disseminated (Stage II) | Persistent (Stage III) |
|---|---|---|---|
| Skin | Erythema chronicum migrans (ECM) | Secondary annular lesions, malar rash, diffuse erythema or urticaria, evanescent lesions, lymphocytoma | Acrodermatitis chronica atrophicans, localized scleroderma-like lesions |
| Musculoskeletal system | | Migratory pain in joints, tendons, bursa, muscle, bone; brief arthritis attacks; myositis; osteomyelitis; panniculitis | Prolonged arthritis attacks, chronic arthritis, peripheral enthesopathy, periostitis or joint subluxations below lesions of acrodermatitis |
| Neurologic system | | Meningitis, cranial neuritis, Bell's palsy, motor or sensory radiculoneuritis, subtle encephalitis, mononeuritis multiplex, myelitis, chorea, cerebellar ataxia | Chronic encephalomyelitis, spastic paraparesis, ataxic gait, subtle mental disorders, chronic axonal polyradiculopathy, dementia |
| Lymphatic system | Regional lymphadenitis | Regional or generalized lymphadenopathy, splenomegaly | |
| Heart | | Atrioventricular nodal block, myopericarditis | |
| Eyes | | Conjunctivitis, iritis, choroiditis, retinal hemorrhage or detachment, panophthalmitis | Keratitis |
| Liver | | Mild or recurrent hepatitis | |
| Respiratory system | | Nonexudative sore throat, nonproductive cough, adult respiratory distress syndrome | |
| Kidney | Microscopic hematuria or proteinuria | | |
| Genitourinary system | Orchitis | | |
| Constitutional symptoms | Minor | Severe malaise and fatigue | Fatigue |

Adapted with permission from Steer AC: Lyme disease. *N Engl J Med* 321:586–596, 1989.

## Clinical Manifestations

Lyme disease is a multisystemic disorder that is generally divided into three stages; although there may be remissions between any stage, not all stages need appear and stages may overlap (Table 127-2).

Stage I is characteristically identified by the presence of erythema chronicum migrans (ECM), an annular, erythematous lesion with central clearing, which expands from the site of the tick bite lesion. This generally occurs 7 to 10 days (range 3 to 31 days) after the bite. ECM occurs in 60 to 80 percent of cases and may be accompanied by generalized malaise and fatigue (80 percent), headache (64 percent), fever and chills (59 percent), stiff neck and arthralgias (48 percent), and constitutional symptoms. Untreated ECM and other early symptoms typically resolve spontaneously in about 4 weeks.

Stage II results from dissemination of *B. burgdorferi* from the site of primary infection to distal sites and commonly occurs within days to a few weeks after infection. Symptoms of disseminated infection include multiple secondary annular lesions, fever, adenopathy, and other constitutional symptoms. Approximately 10 percent of untreated patients develop neurologic manifestations, including headache, meningoencephalitis, or unilateral or bilateral facial nerve palsy. Patients may also develop first-, second-, or third-degree atrioventricular block, which occasionally may require temporary pacemaker placement.

Stage III, or persistent infection, is characterized by chronic arthritis, chronic central nervous system disease, and/or chronic dermatitis (rare in the United States). Characteristically the arthritis presents as brief, recurrent episodes of migratory oligoarthritis, with periods of remission longer than the exacerbations. The joints affected in decreasing order of frequency are the knee, shoulder, elbow, temporomandibular, ankle, wrist, hip, and the small joints of the hands and feet. Pain is the most common symptom, and it is unusual for any joint other than the knee to swell.

## Diagnosis and Therapy

Unfortunately, sensitive and specific diagnostic tests for Lyme infection are unavailable. For this reason, the diagnosis of Lyme disease is based on compatible clinical findings in patients with a reasonable likelihood of exposure to ticks in an area endemic for Lyme disease. Enzyme-linked immunosorbent assay (ELISA) tests have been widely used to screen for antibodies to *B. burgdorferi*, which are usually detectable within 6 weeks of infection. However, this test has not yet been standardized. Western immunoblotting has been used as confirmatory test, and criteria for positivity have been proposed. Polymerase chain reaction (PCR) tests remain experimental. The "gold standard" for diagnosis remains isolation of *B. burgdorferi* from ECM lesions, but this procedure requires special media, has low sensitivity, and is rarely clinically available.

Antimicrobial agents appear to be effective in treating Lyme disease, especially when begun early (Table 127-3). However, few controlled clinical trials have been conducted. Early disease appears to respond to a variety of agents, but the choice of drugs and duration of treatment for late Lyme disease is controversial.

The use of antibiotics prophylactically in patients in an endemic area with a history of a tick bite but without symptoms is controversial.

## ROCKY MOUNTAIN SPOTTED FEVER

Rocky Mountain spotted fever (RMSF) is the most common rickettsial disease in the United States. A clinical illness, later recognized to be RMSF, was first described in the late nineteenth century among

**Table 127-3.** Treatment Of Lyme Disease

| Disease Manifestation | Drug | Adult Dosage | Pediatric Dosage |
|---|---|---|---|
| Erythema chronicum migrans | Doxycycline | 100 mg PO 2× daily | |
| | Amoxicillin | 500 mg PO 3× daily | 25–50 mg/kg/day divided 3× daily |
| | Cefuroxime | 500 mg PO 2× daily | |
| Neurologic disease | | | |
| Bell's palsy | Doxycycline | 100 mg PO 2× daily | |
| | Amoxicillin | 500 mg PO 3× daily | 25–50 mg/kg/day divided 3× daily |
| Serious CNS disease* | Ceftriaxone | 2 g/day IV | 75–100 mg/kg/day IV |
| | Penicillin G | 20–24 million units/day IV divided 6× daily | 300,000 units/kg/day IV divided 6× daily |
| Cardiac disease | | | |
| Mild† | Doxycycline | 100 mg PO 2× daily | |
| | Amoxicillin | 500 mg PO 3× daily | 500 mg PO 3× daily |
| Serious‡ | Ceftriaxone | 2 g/day IV | 75–100 mg/kg/day IV |
| | Penicillin G | 20–24 million units/day IV divided 6× daily | 300,000 units/kg/day IV divided 6× daily |
| Arthritis | | | |
| Oral | Doxycycline | 100 mg PO 2× daily | |
| | Amoxicillin | 500 mg PO 3× daily | 50 mg/kg/day divided 3× daily |
| Parenteral | Ceftriaxone | 2 g/day IV | 75–100 mg/kg/day IV |
| | Penicillin G | 20–24 million units/day IV divided 6× daily | 300,000 units/kg/day IV divided 6× daily |

* Meningitis, encephalitis, neuropathy, encephalopathy.
† Primary AV block with PR interval <0.3 s and no symptoms.
‡ Primary AV block with PR interval >0.3 s or second degree or complete AV block.
*Note:* Oral regimens are generally given for 10 to 30 days, IV regimens for 14 to 21 days.
*Source:* Adapted with permission from *Med Lett* 34:95, 1992.

residents of the Bitter Root and Snake River Valleys of Montana and Idaho. RMSF is an important infectious disease because of its prevalence, the difficulty of clinical diagnosis, potentially fatal outcome (especially among certain populations), and lack of a widely available sensitive and specific diagnostic test during the acute stage of illness.

## Epidemiology

The etiologic agent of RMSF is *Rickettsia rickettsii,* a member of the spotted fever group of Rickettsiaceae. These organisms are small coccobacilli, which are obligate, intracellular bacteria. In the United States, the major vectors are the wood tick, *Dermacentor andersoni,* in the Rocky Mountain states and the dog tick, *D. variabilis,* in the eastern and southern states. It is unclear whether the Lone Star tick, *Amblyomma americanum,* may also be a vector.

In 1993, 456 cases of RMSF were reported to the Centers for Disease Control and Prevention (CDC). In recent years the highest incidence of cases has occurred in a band running from Virginia, North Carolina, and South Carolina horizontally to Oklahoma and Kansas. However, it is important to realize that isolated cases were reported from more than 40 states in 1993.

RMSF is a seasonal disease, with greater than 95 percent of cases occurring between April 1 and September 30. Sporadic cases of RMSF may occur throughout the year, especially when and where the winter months are warm.

The highest incidence of infection occurs in persons aged 5 to 9 years, but a substantial incidence and mortality have been noted in men older than 60 years of age in North Carolina.

## Clinical Manifestations

RMSF is a multisystem disease. Although the disease may be mild in some patients who have been treated early, most patients develop moderate or severe illness.

The usual incubation period of RMSF is 4 to 10 days (average, 7 days), although it may vary from 2 to 14 days. The onset of disease may be abrupt or gradual. Initial symptoms are nonspecific and include fever, malaise, headache that is often severe, and myalgias. Other early symptoms commonly present include nausea, vomiting, anorexia, abdominal pain, and photophobia.

Rash is the hallmark of RMSF but is absent in 5 to 15 percent of patients. So-called spotless fever occurs in higher proportions of fatal cases, older patients, and African-Americans. Characteristically, the rash appears between the third and fifth days of illness. Early in the course of disease, the rash is maculopapular in appearance and may be ignored by the patient and missed by the physician. As the rash evolves, it becomes more defined and petechial. Generally, the rash begins at the extremities, often around the wrists and ankles, and spreads centripetally to the trunk, with relative sparing of the face. As the rash progresses, it characteristically involves the palms and/or soles. Progression to skin necrosis or gangrene has been reported in 2 to 4 percent of patients.

Gastrointestinal signs and symptoms are prominent in RMSF and include nausea or vomiting, abdominal pain, and/or diarrhea. Gastrointestinal symptoms may occur early in the course of disease prior to the onset of rash and may lead to an incorrect diagnosis of gastroenteritis or acute surgical abdomen.

Pneumonitis is a common and potentially life-threatening clinical feature of RMSF. Symptoms and signs include cough, dyspnea, pulmonary edema, infiltrates visible by chest radiography, and systemic hypoxemia.

The central nervous system is the most crucial target organ in RMSF. Severe neurologic dysfunction has been noted to occur in 23 to 38 percent of patients. Clinical symptoms include confusion, stupor, ataxia, coma, and seizures. Other important clinical manifestations of RMSF include renal or cardiac dysfunction.

Most patients with RMSF will have a normal number of leukocytes but a shift to more immature forms is common (~70 percent will have >10 percent band forms). Anemia is noted in about 30 percent of patients. Mild thrombocytopenia (platelets < 150,000 cells/μL) has been noted in 30 to 50 percent of patients, and severe thrombocytopenia (platelets < 20,000 cells/μL) has been noted in 10 percent. RMSF is characterized by increased vascular permeability leading to edema and hypovolemia. Hyponatremia is noted in about 20 percent of patients. The cerebrospinal fluid (CSF) of patients with RMSF often shows an elevated protein and/or pleocytosis.

## Diagnosis and Treatment

The clinical diagnosis of RMSF frequently is difficult despite a careful history, complete physical examination, and appropriate screening laboratory studies. Early in the course of illness, especially if rash is absent, RMSF may be mistaken for a variety of disorders including viral illness (e.g., measles, rubella, hepatitis, mononucleosis, enteroviral exanthem), gastroenteritis, acute surgical abdomen, streptococcal pharyngitis, disseminated gonococcal infection, pneumonia, meningitis (especially due to *Neisseria meningitidis*), secondary syphilis, leptospirosis, typhoid fever, and encephalitis.

The emergency physician should remember the following caveats: (1) the early manifestations of RMSF are nonspecific; (2) although RMSF is associated with certain areas of the United States, cases have been reported from almost all states; (3) the rash, which is often described as the hallmark of the disease, may be absent or a late manifestation; (4) delays in diagnosis are not the fault of patients, who usually seek medical advice early, but are a result of the physician failing to consider RMSF; (5) patients are frequently unaware of a tick bite; (6) the white blood cell count is usually normal. Physicians are most familiar with features of the disease that occur in the second week of illness because this is what textbooks emphasize. Most of the laboratory manifestations that are accepted as aiding in the diagnosis, such as low sodium, low platelet count, coagulopathy, and low serum albumin, do not occur early in the disease but rather are manifestations of the second week of illness when there is significant mortality.

Early definitive diagnosis of RMSF requires demonstration of rickettsiae in biopsy samples of the rash by fluorescent antibody methods (sensitivity 70 percent, specificity 100 percent). Serologic tests are of value in confirming RMSF. However, since treatment must be initiated before antibody usually is detectable, the diagnosis of RMSF must be based on clinical symptoms and signs and on epidemiologic grounds. In general, serologic tests will not become reliably positive for 6 to 10 days after the onset of clinical illness.

Early treatment with appropriate antibiotics dramatically reduces the mortality associated with RMSF. Currently available antibiotics are all rickettsiostatic. Appropriate antibiotic therapy for the adult patient includes doxycycline, 100 mg orally twice a day; tetracycline hydrochloride, 500 mg orally four times a day; or chloramphenicol sodium succinate, 50 to 75 mg/kg per day intravenously in four divided doses. Appropriate therapy for children (i.e., <45 kg, or 100 pounds) includes doxycycline, 4.4 mg/kg orally in two divided doses on day 1, then 2.2 mg/kg per day orally in a single dose; tetracycline hydrochloride, 30 to 40 mg/kg per day in four divided doses for children older than 8 years of age; or chloramphenicol sodium succinate, 100 mg/kg per day intravenously up to a total of 3g in four divided doses, then chloramphenicol orally. Therapy is generally administered for 5 to 7 days, continuing until the patient is afebrile and clinically improved for 2 days. Antibiotics should be administered intravenously in patients with nausea, vomiting, or severe multisystem disease. Doxycycline is considered by many to be the drug of choice. Chloramphenicol has been advocated during pregnancy and for young children, where staining of the teeth and bones is of concern. Risks associated with chloramphenicol use include dose-related bone marrow depression, hemolytic anemia in patients with the Mediter-

ranean form of glucose-6-phosphate dehydrogenase deficiency, "gray baby" syndrome in premature infants and neonates, and rarely aplastic anemia. As short courses of doxycycline have not been associated with clinically apparent staining of teeth, physicians in consultation with their patients should weigh the risks and benefits of doxycycline versus chloramphenicol for children.

Successful treatment of seriously ill patients with RMSF requires meticulous attention to fluid and electrolyte balance. The loss of fluid, electrolytes, and protein from the intravascular space may lead to hypotension, oliguria, acute renal failure, and shock.

## TULAREMIA

The etiologic agent of tularemia ("rabbit skinners" disease) is *Francisella tularensis,* a small, gram-negative, nonmotile coccobacillus. Tick vectors in the United States include *A. americanum* in the southeastern and south central United States, *D. andersoni* in the west, and *D. variabilis,* which has the widest distribution of the three. Tularemia may also be transmitted by the bite of the deerfly, *Chysops discalis.* The reservoirs of *F. tularensis* include numerous small animals, especially rabbits, hares, muskrats, beavers, and some domestic animals; also various hard ticks.

### Epidemiology

More than 100 cases of tularemia were reported to the CDC in 1993. The disease is widespread throughout the United States, but the highest numbers of cases have been reported from Arkansas, Missouri, and Oklahoma. Cases occur in all months of the year; incidence may be higher in adults in early winter during rabbit-hunting season and in children during summer when ticks and deerflies are abundant.

Multiple modes of transmission have been described, including bites of infected arthropods; animal bites (coyote, squirrel, skunk, hog, rabbit, dog, and domestic cat); inoculation of skin, conjunctival sac, or oropharyngeal mucosa with blood or tissue while handling infected animals (by skinning, dressing, or performing necropsies); by fluid of infected flies, ticks, or other animals; by handling or ingestion of inadequately cooked rabbit or hare meat; by drinking contaminated water; by inhalation of dust from contaminated soil, grain, or hay, and from contaminated pelts. Laboratory infections may occur and usually present as a primary pneumonia or typhoidal tularemia.

### Clinical Manifestations

The incubation period averages 3 to 5 days (range, 1 to 21 days). Tularemia usually starts abruptly, with the onset of fevers, chills, headache, anorexia, malaise, and fatigue. Other symptoms may include myalgias, cough, vomiting, pharyngitis, abdominal pain, and diarrhea. Fever typically lasts for several days, remits for a brief interval, and then recurs.

The clinical presentation largely depends on the route of inoculation. Clinical syndromes include the following: Ulceroglandular fever (21 to 87 percent of cases) follows tick bites and animal contact. It is characterized by enlarged and tender local lymphadenopathy. A papule develops at the inoculation site and undergoes necrosis, leaving a tender ulcer with raised border. Glandular tularemia (3 to 20 percent of cases) occurs when patients present with tender regional lymphadenopathy without evidence of a local cutaneous lesion. Oculoglandular tularemia (0 to 5 percent of cases) is characterized by photophobia and lacrimation. Patients demonstrate lid edema and painful conjunctivitis with injection and chemosis. Preauricular, submandibular, and cervical adenopathy may be noted. Pharyngeal tularemia (0 to 12 percent of cases) is acquired from contaminated foods or water and is characterized by exudative pharyngitis or tonsillitis. Typhoidal tularemia (5 to 30 percent of cases) may result from any mode of transmission. Symptoms suggest multiorgan involvement and include fever, headache, chills, myalgias, pharyngitis, nausea, vomiting, diarrhea, abdominal pain, and cough. Hepatomegaly and splenomegaly may be noted. Secondary pneumonitis may occur in up to 45 percent of patients. Finally, tularemia pneumonia (7 to 20 percent of cases) may occur following inhalation of the organism. Symptoms include fever, cough, minimal or no sputum production, substernal chest tightness, and pleuritic chest pain. Physical examination is frequently nonspecific but may reveal rales, consolidation, or a pleural rub.

## Diagnosis and Treatment

The multiple clinical presentations of tularemia often lead to misdiagnosis. Glandular and ulceroglandular tularemia may be confused with pyogenic bacterial infection, cat-scratch disease, rat-bite fever, syphilis, tuberculosis, nontuberculous mycobacterial infection, toxoplasmosis, sporotrichosis, anthrax, and plague. Pneumonic tularemia is in the differential diagnosis of atypical pneumonia (viruses, *Mycoplasma, Legionella,* plague, anthrax, Q fever, psittacosis, etc.). The typhoidal form of disease may be extremely difficult to diagnose properly. The differential diagnosis includes *Salmonella* infection, brucellosis, Q fever, disseminated mycobacterial or fungal disease, rickettsial infection, malaria, endocarditis and other causes of infection without localizing signs.

The key to proper diagnosis is obtaining a history of potential exposure to *F. tularensis;* routine laboratory tests are nonspecific. The white blood cell count may be normal or elevated. Thrombocytopenia, hyponatremia, elevated liver enzymes, or myoglobinuria may be found occasionally. *F. tularensis* may be recovered from blood, lymph nodes, wounds, sputum, and pleural fluid when processed on special media. Tularemia presents special hazards to laboratory personnel, and they should always be notified if tularemia is considered. The diagnosis of tularemia is mostly confirmed with serologic studies. ELISA is the preferred diagnostic test. Acute and convalescent sera are usually required.

The drug of choice for treatment is streptomycin: 7.5 to 10 mg/kg intramuscularly every 12 h for 7 to 14 days (the alternative is gentamicin). The pediatric dose is 30 to 40 mg/kg per day intramuscularly in two divided doses for 7 days. Tetracycline and chloramphenicol have been used orally for therapy, but both are bacteriostatic and a high rate of relapses has been noted. Many other drugs (erythromycin, rifampin, cefoxitin, cefotaxime, ceftriaxone, fluoroquinolones) have demonstrated in vitro activity, but clinical studies of in vivo effectiveness are, in general, unavailable.

## RELAPSING FEVER

Relapsing fever is caused by spirochetes of the genus *Borrelia.* Vectors are various species of *Ornithodoros* ticks.

## Epidemiology

Relapsing fever is most commonly reported in remote settings in the western United States. The incidence is largely unknown. Cases may occur year-round but appear to peak in the summer months.

## Clinical Manifestations

Most patients are unaware of a tick bite, but a nonspecific 2- to 3-mm pruritic eschar may develop at the site. The incubation period is about 7 days (range, 4 to 18 days). Illness characteristically begins abruptly, with high fever, chills, tachycardia, headache, myalgias, abdominal pain, and malaise. Other common symptoms include neurologic involvement (5 to 10 percent) and rash (4 to 50 percent), which may be petechial, macular, or papular. Laboratory findings include leukocytosis and thrombocytopenia. Without treatment, three to five relapses generally occur.

## Diagnosis and Therapy

A specific diagnosis may be made rapidly by observing the spirochetes on a Giemsa- or Wright-stained smear of peripheral blood (sensitivity, 70 percent). Serologic tests on acute and convalescent sera may confirm the diagnosis, but such tests have not been standardized.

Controlled trials of specific drug therapies have not been conducted. The tetracyclines are considered the drugs of choice. Erythromycin is an alternative. Therapy is usually continued for 7 to 10 days. Severely ill patients may require hospitalization. The Jarisch-Herxheimer reaction (fever, chills, tachycardia, hypotension) may occur during therapy. Meptazinol may be effective in treating a Jarisch-Herxheimer reaction, if one occurs.

## BABESIOSIS

Babesiosis is caused by members of the genus *Babesia,* a malaria-like, intraerythrocytic protozoan parasite. The first human case was described in 1957. More than 100 cases have been reported in the past 38 years. Babesiosis is transmitted by *I. scapularis,* the same species that transmits Lyme disease. Cases have also been transmitted via blood transfusions (including platelets and frozen erythrocytes) and transplacentally.

## Epidemiology

Most cases have been reported from the islands off the northeast coast of the United States (Nantucket, Martha's Vineyard, Long Island, Fire Island) and the northeast mainland. More recently, disease has been reported from the upper midwest and west coast. Novel species of *Babesia* may be involved in cases from the west coast.

## Clinical Manifestations

The clinical manifestations of babesiosis range from subclinical illness to fulminant disease resulting in death. Seroepidemiologic studies suggest that many persons develop inapparent infection. In symptomatic persons, the incubation period ranges from 1 to 6 weeks. Although patients may present with a flulike illness, most patients with clinically apparent disease exhibit a more severe presentation. Typically, there is a gradual onset of malaise, anorexia, and fatigue that is followed by intermittent temperatures that may reach 40°C. Accompanying symptoms commonly include chills, sweats, myalgias, arthralgias, nausea, and vomiting. Less common symptoms include headache, sore throat, abdominal pain, conjunctival injection, photophobia, weight loss, and nonproductive cough. Rash is only rarely a manifestation of babesiosis.

Physical examination is usually only remarkable for fever. Splenomegaly and/or hepatomegaly are occasionally noted. Abnormal laboratory findings include mild to moderately severe hemolytic anemia due to lysis of the red cells by the parasite, elevated liver function tests (50 percent), and thrombocytopenia. The white blood cell count is usually normal, but immature leukocytes (bands) may be present.

Babesiosis usually lasts for a few weeks to several months, with prolonged recovery of up to 18 months. Splenectomized patients may develop a fulminant illness that ends in death or a prolonged convalescence. Signs and symptoms in these cases may include high fever, severe hemolytic anemia, hemoglobinuria, jaundice, ecchymoses, petechiae, congestive heart failure, pulmonary edema, renal failure, adult respiratory distress syndrome, and coma.

## Diagnosis and Therapy

Babesiosis is usually diagnosed by visualizing the parasite on Giemsa stain of thick or thin blood smears. *Babesia* species are round to oval and have blue cytoplasm and red chromatin. The ring form is more common. Multiple thick and thin smears should be examined, as only a few erythrocytes are infected early in disease. Ultimately, around 10 percent of erythrocytes are parasitized in normal hosts and up to 85 percent in asplenic persons. Babesiosis can also be confirmed by measuring babesial antibody using an immunofluorescent antibody test.

A truly effective therapy for babesiosis has not been developed. Therapy is generally reserved for seriously ill patients. Adult therapy consists of clindamycin, 300 to 600 mg every 6 h intramuscularly or intravenously, and oral quinine, 650 mg every 6 to 8 h for 7 to 10 days. Pediatric therapy includes clindamycin, 20 mg/kg per day intramuscularly or intravenously every 6 h, and quinine, 25 mg/kg per day orally every 8 h for 7 to 10 days. Exchange transfusions may be required in severe cases.

## EHRLICHIOSIS

The first human case of ehrlichiosis was described in 1987 in a report of a 51-year-old man with fever, encephalopathy, mild hepatitis, anemia, and thrombocytopenia who had rickettsia-like inclusion bodies among his circulating leukocytes. Serologic results suggested infection with *Ehrlichia canis,* but subsequent investigators have shown that the agent of human ehrlichiosis is a closely related species, now named *E. chaffeensis. Erhlichia* belong to the family Rickettsiaceae and are small, gram-negative, pleomorphic coccobacilli that primarily infect the circulating leukocytes. The primary vector is probably *D. variabilis.*

### Epidemiology

More than 250 cases of ehrlichiosis have been reported in the United States. Most cases have occurred in the south central and south Atlantic regions, especially Oklahoma, Missouri, and Georgia. Approximately 75 percent of cases have occurred in May through July. The incidence of disease increases with age, and most infections occur in men.

### Clinical Manifestations

A tick bite in the previous 3 weeks has been reported in approximately 70 percent of cases. The median incubation period is about 7 days (range, 1 to 21 days). Most patients present with a nonspecific febrile illness. Clinical features most commonly include high fever and headache, but malaise, nausea, vomiting, rigors, myalgias, and anorexia occur commonly. A rash (maculopapular or petechial) develops in approximately 35 percent of patients and rarely involves the palms or soles.

Severe complications are unusual but have included renal failure, disseminated intravascular coagulation, cardiomegaly, seizures, and death (1.3 percent).

Laboratory abnormalities are most pronounced at 5 to 7 days and include leukopenia, absolute lymphopenia, thrombocytopenia, elevated serum hepatic enzymes, and rarely CSF pleocytosis.

### Diagnosis and Therapy

The diagnosis of ehrlichiosis depends mainly on the clinical findings; serologic tests provide retrospective confirmation.

Tetracycline (or its analogues) is the drug of choice, with chloramphenicol as an alternative. Although controlled trials of therapy have not been performed, doses and duration of therapy similar to RMSF have been recommended.

## COLORADO TICK FEVER

Colorado tick fever is an acute viral illness first described in 1850. The etiologic agent is an RNA virus of the genus coltivirus. *D. andersoni* appears to be the main vector for human disease.

### Epidemiology

Colorado tick fever has been reported from the mountainous regions of several western states. Approximately 200 to 300 cases are reported annually in the United States. Most infections occur between late May and early July.

### Clinical Manifestations

Approximately 3 to 6 days (range, 0 to 14) after a tick bite, patients typically develop the sudden onset of fever, chills, severe headache, myalgias, and photophobia. The symptoms tend to persist for 5 to 8 days and resolve spontaneously. Approximately 3 days after resolution, 50 percent of patients develop a secondary phase with similar symptoms, lasting 2 to 4 days. A transient petechial or macular rash may develop.

Laboratory abnormalities may include leukocytosis and thrombocytopenia.

### Diagnosis and Therapy

The diagnosis of Colorado tick fever is usually confirmed by serologic studies. It can also be diagnosed by isolation of the virus from blood or CSF inoculated into suckling mice.

No specific therapy exists. Recovery usually takes about 3 weeks. Treatment is limited to supportive care.

## TICK PARALYSIS

Tick paralysis is a relatively uncommon tick-borne disease resulting in an ascending paralysis. The disease is of clinical importance because with prompt recognition and treatment (*which consists solely of tick removal*), it is curable, but mortality in untreated cases may be as high as 12 percent. It is caused by a venom secreted from the female tick salivary glands during feeding. The venom is most likely a neurotoxin that produces a conduction block at the peripheral motor nerve branches, resulting in a failure of acetylcholine release at the neuromuscular junction.

Cases in North America are usually caused by *D. andersoni,* but up to 43 tick species, from both Ixodidae and Argasidae families, have been implicated as causative agents.

### Epidemiology

Tick paralysis occurs during the months of heavy tick feeding (late spring to late summer) and seems to affect children more commonly than adults. The incidence is higher in girls than in boys.

### Clinical Manifestations

Symptoms develop within 4 to 7 days (median 5) after attachment by the female tick. Irritability, restlessness, and hand and feet paresthesias may initially be reported. Within 1 to 2 days the presenting symptoms are followed by a symmetric, ascending, flaccid paralysis accompanied by loss of deep tendon reflexes. In severe untreated cases, death results from bulbar and respiratory paralysis. Loss of coordination and ataxia may indicate cerebellar involvement.

### Diagnosis and Therapy

Tick discovery and removal are both diagnostic and therapeutic for this disease. Careful search must be made, with particular attention paid to the scalp. Most patients begin showing signs of recovery within hours after tick removal. Complete resolution within 48 to 72 h is the rule.

Other treatment modalities should be directed at the complications of the disease that may have occurred before tick removal, most notably respiratory support.

## BIBLIOGRAPHY

### Comprehensive Texts

Benenson AS (ed): *Control Of Communicable Diseases In Man,* 15th ed. Washington, DC, American Public Health Association, 1990.

Mandell GL, Bennett JE, Dolin R (eds): *Principles And Practice Of Infectious Diseases,* 4th ed. New York, Churchill Livingstone, 1995.

### Reviews

Fishbein DB, Dawson JE, Robinson LE: Human Ehrlichiosis in the United States, 1985–1990. *Ann Intern Med* 120:736, 1994.

Krause PJ, Feder HM: Lyme disease and babesiosis. *Adv Pediatr Infect Dis* 9:183, 1994.

Pfister H-W, Wilske B, Weber K: Lyme borreliosis: Basic science and clinical aspects. *Lancet* 343:1013, 1994.

Spach DH, Liles WC, Cambell GL, et al: Tick-borne diseases in the United States. *N Engl J Med* 329:936, 1993.

Steere AC: Lyme disease. *N Engl J Med* 321:586, 1989.

Weber K, Pfister H-W: Clinical management of Lyme borreliosis. *Lancet* 343:1017, 1994.

Weber DJ, Walker DH: Rocky Mountain spotted fever. *Infect Dis Clin North Am* 5:19, 1991.

# 128
# UNIVERSAL PRECAUTIONS
## David A. Kramer
## Judith E. Tintinalli

Health care workers, especially prehospital and emergency department personnel, are at risk for infection from contact with bodily fluids or aerosols for a number of diseases, especially AIDS, syphilis, tuberculosis, and hepatitis. This chapter reviews the pathophysiology of transmission and recommended universal precautions primarily for blood-borne pathogens and tuberculosis. The concept of universal precautions, although most often discussed in relation to HIV, is generalizable to minimizing the transmission risk from exposure to all infectious organisms found in blood and body fluids.

The critical factors for the transmission of blood-borne pathogens are serum concentration in the source patient and inoculum dose. Other factors involved in the transmission of blood-borne pathogens are loss of infectivity during transfer of inocula, and portal of entry. Exposures that ocur in the research setting usually result from contact with concentrated specimens and thus pose a greater risk than exposures in the hospital setting. The inoculation from blood transfusion is usually large, while in the clinical setting, the inoculum is usually small. Portals of entry include percutaneous injuries (needlesticks and bites), and mucocutaneous and ocular exposure.

Kelen et al. recently demonstrated that nearly two-thirds of tasks and procedures performed in the ED are associated with potential blood and body fluid contact. Most potential contacts involve blood or bloody body fluids.

## HIV INFECTION

The major modes of transmission of HIV are through sexual contact, exposure to infected blood or blood products, and perinatal exposure. Although the virus has been isolated from many body fluids, blood contact still poses the greatest risk of occupational transmission for prehospital and emergency department personnel.

A number of factors make it difficult to determine the true risk of HIV transmission to health care workers. These include variation in the seroprevalence of the virus, which depends on multiple factors, and the type of exposure involved. As a result, in 1987, the Centers for Disease Control and Prevention (CDC) published Recommendations for Prevention of HIV Transmission in Health-Care Settings. This paper detailed the use of universal precautions. The basic premise is that health care workers should consider ". . . all patients as potentially infected with HIV and/or other blood-borne pathogens and to adhere rigorously to infection-control precautions for minimizing the risk of exposure to blood and body fluids of all patients."

### Seroprevalence

Several studies have looked at the HIV seroprevalence rate among emergency department patients. Kelen and colleagues found an overall seroprevalence rate of 6.0 percent among 2544 emergency department patients at the Johns Hopkins Hospital. Of all those that they studied, 3.7 percent had unrecognized infection. This study showed that the rate of HIV infection in this population of patients had increased from the previous year. The prevalence of HIV infection continues to increase. Kelen and coworkers have also shown that even with risk factor assessment of the patient (previous blood or blood product transfusion, intravenous drug use, homosexual/bisexual activity in men, prostitution, and sex with a partner with the above risk factors), unrecognized HIV disease could not be reliably detected. Of those without the above risk factors, 1.5 percent had unrecognized HIV infection. Furthermore, they found that 14.5 percent of those recently testing HIV negative had unrecognized HIV infection.

Marcus and associates examined the seroprevalence of HIV in both inner city and suburban emergency departments. The HIV seroprevalence rate ranged from 0.2 to 8.9 percent and reflected the patient population served by the emergency departments. They found the rates highest in the 15 to 44 age group, in men, and among blacks. This did not change regardless of the rate of the particular ED.

### Risk of Acquiring HIV

Various studies have estimated the risk of becoming infected from a single percutaneous needle stick with HIV-infected blood to be approximately 0.3 percent. In 1991, Fahey and coworkers studied approximately 8000 cutaneous exposures to blood presumably infected with HIV. They found no evidence of HIV transmission. Nevertheless, this does not mean that the risk of transmission from cutaneous exposure to HIV infected blood is zero. Marcus and colleagues estimate the combined risk from both cutaneous and percutaneous contact to be about 1 in 6700 in high HIV seroprevalence areas and 1 in 96,000 in low HIV seroprevalence areas. They also point out that since cutaneous blood contact is more common than percutaneous, the annual risk of transmission from each may be about the same. This becomes more important in light of the relative efficacy of universal (barrier) precautions when used properly. If one source patient is under treatment with antiviral agents, specifically zidovudine (AZT), the source HIV plasma concentration may be decreased but the potential for disease transmission is not eliminated.

Through 1992, the CDC documented 33 cases of occupational transmission of HIV from infected blood. Twenty-eight of these were from percutaneous exposure, four from mucocutaneous exposure, and one from both. HIV transmission is more likely from percutaneous than from cutaneous contact. Various studies point out that to significantly reduce the risk of occupational HIV transmission, we need to develop improved means of preventing percutaneous exposure.

### Decreasing Risk

In view of our demonstrated inability to predict which emergency department patients have unrecognized HIV infection, universal precautions were recommended by the CDC as early as 1985. In December

1991, the Occupational Safety and Health Administration (OSHA) mandated compliance with the CDC's guidelines.

In its 1987 recommendations, the CDC stated that universal precautions "should be used in the care of *all* patients, especially including those in emergency-care settings in which the risk of blood exposure is increased and the infection status of the patient is usually unknown." The CDC stipulated six basic universal precautions:

1. Appropriate barrier precautions should be routinely used when contact with blood or other body fluids is anticipated. Wear gloves. Masks and eye protection are indicated if mucous membranes of the mouth, eyes, and nose may be exposed to drops of blood or other body fluids. Gowns should be worn if splashes of blood are likely.

2. Hands and skin should be washed immediately if contaminated. Wash hands as soon as gloves are removed.

3. Exercise care in handling all sharps during procedures, when cleaning them, and during disposal. Never recap or bend needles. Carefully dispose of sharps in specially designed containers.

4. Use a BVM to prevent the need for mouth-to-mouth resuscitation. Such devices should be readily available.

5. Health care workers with weeping dermatitis should avoid direct patient care until the condition resolves.

6. Because of the risk of perinatal HIV transmission, pregnant health care workers should strictly adhere to all universal precautions.

Unfortunately, despite the CDC recommendations and the OSHA mandate for universal precautions, many studies indicate that compliance is poor. However, Kelen and colleagues were able to demonstrate improved compliance when universal precautions were made institutional policy. Three reasons commonly given for not using indicated universal precautions in the emergency department are the urgency of the intervention, interference with performance of the procedure, and discomfort with the attire. Others have reported noncompliance because the patient did not appear to be at high risk and because they learned their skills without using universal precautions.

Kelen (1995) stresses that virtually all ED procedures and tasks require gloves, and face protection is recommended, especially for invasive procedures, such as lumbar puncture, and for examination of the bleeding patient. Barrier precautions make up only one component of universal precautions. Furthermore, universal precautions do not apply to HIV alone. They are designed to protect against other blood-borne pathogens such is hepatitis and syphilis. At this time using universal precautions is the best method available to prevent the occupational transmission of HIV and other blood-borne pathogens.

## HEPATITIS B AND C INFECTION

Epidemic infection with hepatitis B in health care workers was reported in the 1960s and 1970s and was felt to be due to new techniques such as hemodialysis, increased use of laboratory tests, and increasing numbers of immunocompromised patients who were exposure sources. Epidemic transmission to health care workers has decreased since the introduction of hepatitis B vaccine. The risk is greatest for those in hemodialysis, surgery, laboratory, and emergency medicine. All health care workers should receive hepatitis B vaccine.

There is an increased prevalence of HBsAg in hospitalized patients, providing more opportunities for exposure in health care workers. HIV-positive patients are at least 4 times more likely to be positive for HBsAg than those that are HIV negative. Some groups, especially Southeast Asian immigrants, have a high prevalance of HBsAg, increasing opportunity for infection in health care workers.

Most cases of nonA-nonB hepatitis are due to hepatitis C, and this disease can be transmitted by needlestick exposure. While health care workers appear to be at increased risk for hepatitis C, there is very limited data available. To date, there is no effective postexposure prophylaxis for hepatitis C.

## TUBERCULOSIS

The risk of tuberculosis in health care workers has increased because of resurgence of the disease, the emergence of multi-drug resistant strains, and increased susceptibility of immunocompromised or HIV+ health care workers to the disease.

Data on risk estimates are extremely limited. Factors involved with increased disease transmission from the source patient include ineffective therapy, extensive disease on radiographs, acid-fast bacilli evident on sputum smear, cough or laryngeal tuberculosis, cough-inducing procedures, and delay in disease diagnosis.

Transmission of tuberculosis to health care workers is positively correlated with the number of patients with active tuberculosis in contact with a worker, infectiousness of the source case, ventilation rate of the worker, duration of exposure, and air-exchange rate in the work environment. Workers in inner-city hospitals are at most risk. Workers without direct contact can be exposed if air from rooms with infected patients is recirculated. CDC recommendations and OSHA regulations require persons entering rooms housing patients with known or suspected tuberculosis to wear HEPA (high-efficiency particulate air) masks. Masks that are protective against tuberculosis must ensure protection from droplet nuclei that are 1–5 micron in diameter. All health care workers should be encouraged to participate in tuberculoisis screening and prophylaxis programs.

## BIBLIOGRAPHY

CDC. Recommendations for prevention of HIV transmission in health-care settings. *MMWR* 36(suppl 2S):1S, 1987.

Gerberding JL. Management of occupational exposures to blood-borne viruses. *N Engl J Med* 332:444, 1995.

Kelen GD et al: Determinants of Emergency Department procedure- and condition-specific universal barrier precaution requirements for optimal provider protection. *Ann Emerg Med* 25:743, 1995.

Henry K, Campbell S, et al. Compliance with universal precautions and needle handling and disposal practices among emergency department staff at two community hospitals. *Am J Infect Control* 22:129, 1994.

Kelen GD, DiGiovanna TA, Bisson L, et al. Human immunodeficiency virus infection in emergency department patients: epidemiology, clinical presentations, and risk to health care workers: the Johns Hopkins experience. *JAMA* 262:516, 1989.

Kelen GD, DiGiovanna TA, Celentano DD, et al. Adherence to universal (barrier) precautions during interventions on critically ill and injured emergency department patients. *J Acquir Immune Defic Syndr* 3:987, 1990.

Kelen GD, Fritz S, et al. Unrecognized human immunodeficiency virus infection in emergency department patients. *N Engl J Med* 318:1645, 1988.

Kelen GD, Green GB, Hexter DA, et al. Substantial improvement in compliance with universal precautions in an emergency department following institution of policy. *Arch Intern Med* 151:2051, 1991.

Lanphear BP. Trends and patterns in the transmission of blood borne pathogens to health care workers. *Epidemiol Rev* 16:437, 1994.

Marcus R, Culver DH, Bell DM, et al. Risk of human immunodeficiency virus infection among emergency department workers. *Am J Med* 94:363, 1993.

Menzies D, Fanning A, Yuan L, et al. Tuberculosis among health care workers. *N Engl J Med* 332(8):92–98, Jan 12, 1995.

Occupational Safety and Health Administration. Occupational exposure to blood borne pathogens: final rule. *Federal Register* 56 (Dec 6):64004, 1991.

# Toxicology

## 129
## GENERAL MANAGEMENT OF THE POISONED PATIENT
### Michael V. Vance

### INCIDENCE OF POISONING

During 1992, poison centers in the United States assisted with more than 2.4 million poisonings. Although the actual incidence of poisoning is unknown, the American Association of Poison Control Centers (AAPCC) estimates that more than 4 million poisonings occur annually in the United States.

### CHARACTERISTICS OF POISONING
#### Pediatric Poisoning

Well over half of poisonings reported to the AAPCC by participating poison centers occur in young children (1 to 5 years). Exposures in this age group are generally "accidental" (implying no harmful intent) and relatively mild. Although they represent a large number of exposures, pediatric patients account for only about 10 percent of all hospital admissions due to poisoning and only 5 percent of fatalities. Despite the almost universally accidental nature of pediatric poisoning, the emergency physician should be aware of other reasons for a child to present with a toxic exposure, including child abuse through intentional poisoning by parents, other caretakers, and even siblings. More common reasons for exposure in older children (including the preteen age group) include intentional drug experimentation/abuse and adolescent and preadolescent suicide attempts. A good rule of thumb is to consider a toxic exposure in any child over the age of 5 with normal intellectual development to be suspicious.

#### Adult Poisoning

Although adult poisoning is responsible for less than half of calls to poison centers, these result in 80 to 90 percent of hospital admissions due to toxic exposures. An increasing number of adult poisonings are accidental, due to chemical exposures in the workplace or at home; however, most are intentional. Although the motives for these intentional exposures may be very different—recreational drug abuse, suicide "gestures," or a bona fide suicide attempt—the emergency physician must recognize and be prepared to deal with the associated psychological factors in these patients. Above all, a firm but nonjudgmental approach may avoid violent verbal and even physical confrontations and may well pave the way for appropriate psychiatric intervention.

### EVALUATION OF THE POISONED PATIENT
#### History

A thorough, accurate history provides a working diagnosis and assists with management decisions for most patients in the emergency department. Unfortunately, the history in a poisoning is notoriously unreliable (pediatric patients, drug abuse, suicide attempts), whether it is obtained from the patient, friends, and family members or emergency medical service personnel. Despite the possible inaccuracies, the important historical factors include *what* poison was involved, *how much* was taken, *how* it was taken, *when* it was taken, *why* it was taken, and especially *what else* was taken (a significant number of intentional ingestions involve more than one substance, with ethanol being a common coingestant).

#### Physical Examination

A complete head-to-toe physical examination may offer supportive evidence and credence to the history, may indicate the presence of additional or entirely different substances, or may provide an exact diagnosis. The approach to the physical examination of the poisoned patient includes (1) vital signs, (2) identification of toxic syndromes, (3) evaluation for complications, and (4) evaluation for underlying disease states.

#### Vital Signs

As in any emergency department patient, physical assessment of the poisoned patient starts with the ABCs. *Airway* evaluation should include not only the usual factors indicating gross airway compromise (stridor, snoring, vomitus, etc.), but also specific evaluation of the gag reflex. If there is any question about the integrity of the airway, active airway management should be initiated as soon as possible to protect against further compromise or aspiration. *Breathing* evaluation includes not only a baseline respiratory rate but also evaluation of the quality of respirations: shallow respirations suggest the need for early ventilatory support; deep respirations suggest the presence of an underlying hypoxemia or metabolic acidosis. *Circulation* evaluation includes a baseline pulse rate and blood pressure, and any suggestion of serious poisoning should dictate continuous electrocardiographic (ECG) monitoring and serial blood pressure determinations.

#### Temperature

In addition to the usual vital signs discussed above, a baseline temperature should be obtained. This is given special emphasis because an oral or rectal temperature is frequently not obtained early—if at all—in the poisoned patient for a variety of reasons. The patient may be uncooperative, combative, or require a number of other important diagnostic or therapeutic measures on arrival in the emergency department. However, the emergency physician must recognize that environmental exposure (hot or cold) or direct toxic effects may produce a wide range of thermoregulatory and core temperature abnormalities. Hyperthermia and hypothermia frequently accompany toxic exposures and may well interfere with treatment if they are not identified and managed appropriately. Thus, despite the possible difficulty of obtaining an oral or rectal temperature in a cursing/spitting/vomiting/seizing/dying patient, its importance should not be forgotten.

#### Toxic Syndromes

Numerous toxic syndromes may be identified virtually at first glance with certain poisonings. Many, including the anticholinergic syndrome, the cholinergic syndrome, and the sympathomimetic syndrome, are described in detail in later chapters in this section. Table 129-1 lists some basic elements of the more common toxic syn-

**Table 129-1.** Toxic Syndromes (Multiple-Cause Symptom Complexes)

| Syndrome | Causes | | | Manifestations |
|---|---|---|---|---|
| **Anticholinergic** | *Belladonna alkaloids* | | | *Peripheral antimuscarinic* |
| | Atropine (hyoscyamine) | | | Dry skin and mucous membranes |
| | Belladonna alkaloid mixtures: belladonna leaf, fluid extract, tincture | | | Thirst |
| | Homatropine | | | Dysphagia |
| | Methscopolamine | | | Vision blurred for near objects |
| | Methylatropine nitrate | | | Fixed dilated pupils |
| | Plants: *Atropa belladonna, Datura stramonium, Hyoscyamus niger,* | | | Tachycardia |
| | *Amanita muscaria or pantherina* | | | Sometimes hypertension |
| | | | | Rash, scarlatiniform |
| | Scopolamine (I-hyoscine) | | | Hyperthermia, flushing |
| | | | | Abdominal distention |
| | | | | Urinary urgency and retention |
| | *Synthetic anticholinergics* | | | *Central* |
| | Adiphenine | Isopropamide | Pipenzolate | Lethargy |
| | Anisotropine | Mepenzolate | Piperidolate | Confusion to restlessness, excitement |
| | Cyclopentolate | Methantheline | Poldine | Delirium, hallucinations |
| | Dicyclomine | Methixene | Propantheline | Ataxia |
| | Diphemanil | Oxyphenonium | Thiphenamil | Seizures |
| | Eucatropine | Oxyphencyclimine | Tridihexethyl | Respiratory failure |
| | Glycopyrrolate | Pentapiperide | Tropicamide | Cardiovascular collapse |
| | Hexocyclium | | | |
| | *Incidental anticholinergics* | | | |
| | Antihistamines | Benactyzine | Phenothiazines | |
| | Tricyclic antidepressants | | | |
| **Acetylcholinesterase inhibition** | *Organophosphates* | | | |
| | | | | *Muscarinic effects* |
| | TEPP | | | Sweating, constricted pupils, lacri- |
| | OMPA | | | mation, excessive salivation, |
| | Dipterex | | | wheezing, cramps, vomiting, diar- |
| | Chlorthion | | | rhea, tenesmus, bradycardia *or* |
| | Di-Syston | | | tachycardia, hypotension *or* hyper- |
| | Co-ral | | | tension, blurred vision, urinary in- |
| | Phosdrin | | | continence |
| | Parathion | | | *Nicotinic effects* |
| | Methylparathion | | | Striated muscle: fasciculations, |
| | Malathion | | | cramps, weakness, twitching, paral- |
| | Systox | | | ysis, respiratory failure, cyanosis, |
| | EPN | | | arrest |
| | Diazinon | | | Sympathetic ganglia: tachycardia, el- |
| | Guthion | | | evated blood pressure |
| | Trithion | | | *CNS effects* |
| | | | | Anxiety, restlessness, ataxia, sei- |
| | | | | zures, insomnia, coma, absent re |
| | | | | flexes, Cheyne-Stokes respirations, |
| | | | | respiratory and circulation depres- |
| | | | | sion |
| **Cholinergic** | Acetylcholine | Betel nut | Methacholine | Same as muscarinic under anticholin- |
| | *Areca catechu* | Bethanechol | Muscarine | esterases, also nicotinic |
| | | Carbachol | Pilocarpine | |
| | | *Clitocybe dealbata* | *Pilocarpus* species | |
| **Extrapyramidal** | Acetophenazine | Mesoridazine | Thioridazine | *Parkinsonian* |
| | Butaperazine | Perphenazine | Thiothixene | Dysphonia, dysphagia, oculogyric |
| | Carphenazine | Piperacetazine | Trifluoperazine | crises, rigidity, tremor, torticollis, |
| | Chlorpromazine | Promazine | Triflupromazine | opisthotonos, shrieking, trismus, |
| | Haloperidol | | | laryngospasm |
| **Hemoglobinopathies** | Carbon monoxide | | | Headache, nausea, vomiting, dizziness, |
| | Methemoglobin | | | dyspnea, seizures, coma, death |
| | | | | Cutaneous bullae, gastroenteritis |
| | | | | Epidemic occurrence with carbon mon- |
| | | | | oxide |
| | | | | Cyanosis, chocolate blood with methe- |
| | | | | moglobin |
| **Metal fume fever** | *Fumes of oxides of* | | | Chills, fever, nausea, vomiting, muscu- |
| | Brass | Iron | Nickel | lar pain, throat dryness, headache, fa- |
| | Cadmium | Magnesium | Titanium | tigue, weakness, leukocytosis, respira- |
| | Copper | Mercury | Tungsten | tory distress |
| | | | Zinc | |

**Table 129-1.** Toxic Syndromes (Multiple-Cause Symptom Complexes) (*Continued*)

| Syndrome | Causes | | | Manifestations |
|---|---|---|---|---|
| **Narcotic** | Alphaprodine | Ethylmorphine | Normeperidine (meperidine metabolite) | CNS depression |
| | Anileridine | Ethoheptazine | | Pinpoint pupils |
| | Codeine | Fentanyl | Opium | Slowed respirations |
| | Cyclazocine | Heroin | Oxycodone | Hypotension |
| | Dextromethorphan | Hydromorphone | Oxymorphone | Response to naloxone |
| | Dextromoramide | Levorphanol | Pentazocine | Pupils may be dilated and excitement |
| | Diacetylmorphine | Meperidine | Phenazocine | may predominate |
| | Dihydrocodeine | Methadone | Piminodine | Normeperidine: tremor, CNS |
| | Dihydrocodeinone | Metopon | Propoxyphene | excitation, seizures |
| | Dipipanone | Morphine | Racemorphan | |
| | Diphenoxylate (Lomotil) | | | |
| **Sympathomimetic** | Aminophylline | Ephedrine | Methylphenidate (Ritalin) | CNS excitation |
| | Amphetamines | Epinephrine | | Seizures |
| | Caffeine | Fenfluramine | Pemoline | Hypertension |
| | *Catha edulus* (Khat) | Levarterenol | Phencyclidine | Hypotension with caffeine |
| | Cocaethylene | Metaraminol | Phenmetrazine | Tachycardia |
| | Cocaine | Methamphetamine | Phentermine | |
| | Dopamine | Methcathinone | | |
| **Withdrawal** | Alcohol | Ethchlorvynol | Methyprylon | Diarrhea, mydriasis, piloerection, hypertension, tachycardia, insomnia, lacrimation, muscle cramps, restlessness, yawning, hallucinosis |
| | Barbiturates | Glutethimide | Opioids | |
| | Benzodiazepines | Meprobamate | Paraldehyde | |
| | Chloral hydrate | Methaqualone | | |
| | Cocaine | | | Depression with cocaine |

SOURCE: Adapted from Done AK. *Poisoning—A Systematic Approach for the Emergency Department Physician.* Presented Aug. 6–9, 1979, at Snowmass Village, CO, Symposium sponsored by Rocky Mountain Poison Center. Used by permission.

dromes, and the rapid identification of such presentations saves considerable time and frustration in the evaluation and management of the poisoned patient.

Whether a toxic syndrome is readily identified or not, the primary goal of physical assessment of the poisoned patient is to identify any effects on the three vital organ systems most likely to produce immediate morbidity and mortality: the respiratory system, the cardiovascular system, and the central nervous system (CNS).

### Respiratory Complications

Airway compromise in the patient with an altered level of consciousness is as common in the poisoned patient as in patients with any other serious illness or injury. Ventilatory insufficiency frequently accompanies airway problems, as does the risk of aspiration. Other respiratory complications include the early development of noncardiogenic pulmonary edema or the later development of adult respiratory distress syndrome (ARDS); bronchospasm due to direct or indirect toxic effects may also be present.

### Cardiovascular Complications

The most common cardiovascular complication of poisoning is rhythm disturbance. *Tachyarrhythmias* are fairly common but are usually not associated with serious perfusion problems unless the patient has underlying cardiovascular disease. One exception to this is in poisoning by agents such as quinidine (sodium channel blockers), amiodarone, and satolol (class III agents), which prolong the QT interval and can produce *torsade de pointes. Bradyarrhythmias* are relatively uncommon and usually are associated with more serious underlying metabolic problems, such as hypoxia or acidosis. *Hypotension* is frequently seen and is almost always associated with decreased vascular tone either due to decreased central sympathetic outflow (benzodiazepines) or direct vasodilation (calcium channel blockers). *Hypertension* is occasionally seen and may be accompanied by serious sequelae, such as cerebrovascular hemorrhage.

### Neurologic Complications

*Altered level of consciousness* is a frequent complication of poisoning and may range from mild drowsiness to agitation, hallucinations,

coma, medullary depression, cardiopulmonary depression, and death. In addition, advanced levels of CNS depression are typically associated with many of the primary respiratory and cardiovascular complications listed above. *Seizures* are one of the most serious complications seen in the poisoned patient and may be due to underlying perfusion or metabolic problems, or due to primary drug effect. *Behavioral abnormalities,* although not as lethal as other CNS complications, are nonetheless among the greatest problems for emergency department personnel. Confused, combative patients create additional difficulties in the treatment of patients with potentially severe toxic effects of poisoning.

### Underlying Disease States

The final emphasis on physical assessment of the poisoned patient is to evaluate for the presence of underlying disease states that may increase the likelihood of complications. Patients with asthma or chronic obstructive pulmonary disease are obviously at increased risk for the respiratory complications; patients with underlying cardiovascular disease are more likely to develop severe arrhythmias. As is the usual case, the very young and very old are also more susceptible to toxic effects of poisoning.

## EMERGENCY DEPARTMENT MANAGEMENT

Management of the poisoned patient in the emergency department is directed toward a number of goals. *Decontamination* limits absorption and minimizes the extent of toxicity; *supportive care* limits the effects of the serious complications of poisoning on the primary organ systems at risk; and *definitive care* limits the severity or duration of toxicity through the use of pharmacologic antagonists (*antidotes*) or the enhanced *elimination* of the toxin itself.

### Decontamination

The vast majority of serious poisonings are due to ingestion of toxic substances. Thus, *gastrointestinal decontamination* is a common consideration in the management of the poisoned patient. Because the stomach is the first recipient of a bolus of ingested material, this organ has long received the most attention for recovery of toxic material and prevention of absorption.

One recent study using an acetaminophen model demonstrated that placing the patient in the *left lateral decubitus position* significantly decreased systemic absorption for at least 2 h by reducing the transit of the ingested medication through the pylorus and into the small intestine, where the vast majority of absorption occurs. This should be adopted as the standard position for transport of patients to the emergency department and initial emergency department management until a decision is made whether to pursue definitive gastrointestinal decontamination techniques.

For decades, *syrup of ipecac* has been the most commonly accepted method of accomplishing gastric emptying, although the routine use of ipecac has come under increased scrutiny and criticism in recent years. While ipecac has the advantages of widespread acceptance and active promotion by poison centers for use in home management, its utility in the context of serious poisoning in the emergency department is virtually nonexistent. Studies consistently show that ipecac-induced emesis only reduces absorption by about 30 percent (leaving 70 percent to be absorbed to produce toxic effects) and actually interferes with the efficacy of other methods of decontamination (such as administration of activated charcoal). In addition, the vomiting produced by ipecac may interfere with other diagnostic and therapeutic measures necessary for the well-being of the patient, and one study demonstrated that the use of ipecac significantly prolonged the time spent by poisoned patients in the emergency department. Although still showing some potential for use in the home management of poisoning in the pediatric population, in the 1990s ipecac appears to be nothing more than an interesting historical footnote in the management of poisoning in the emergency department.

*Gastric lavage* is one alternative to the use of ipecac as a method of gastrointestinal decontamination. The proper technique requires the use of a large-bore (36 to 40 French in an adult) *orogastric hose* connected to appropriate irrigation and drainage tubing, with infusion and recovery of 250- to 300-mL aliquots of fluid until the return is clear. Gastric lavage has the advantages of providing immediate recovery of gastric contents (compared with a 15- to 30-min delay with ipecac-induced emesis), control of lavage duration, and direct access for instillation of activated charcoal. Disadvantages include the invasive nature of the procedure and the technical difficulties of having a relatively alert patient accept a tube somewhat larger than his or her trachea. In experienced hands, recovery of gastric contents is at least as good as ipecac-induced emesis. However, the efficacy of gastric lavage after the first 1 to 2 h postingestion in all but the most serious presentations is questionable, and there is risk of inviting aspiration unless measures are taken to protect the patient's airway, such as endotracheal intubation or maintenance of the left lateral decubitus position, preferably with the addition of some Trendelenburg (head down) position.

*Activated charcoal* is the agent of choice for gastrointestinal decontamination in acute poisoning. Activated charcoal acts by adsorbing molecules of chemicals on its surface, thereby inhibiting their absorption and preventing systemic toxicity. In addition, technologic advances have produced a superactivated charcoal, which boasts an adsorptive surface area of 3000 $m^2$/g, approximately three times the older preparations. While ipecac or lavage may recover 30 percent of an ingested dose, studies suggest that the use of activated charcoal alone, given in timely fashion, may reduce absorption by as much as 50 percent. The dose is 1 g/kg. Disadvantages of activated charcoal include poor patient acceptance and the messy result if the patient happens to regurgitate stomach contents.

*Cathartics* are another method of gastrointestinal decontamination with a long history of endorsement by poison centers and medical personnel. In theory, cathartics (sorbitol, magnesium sulfate, magnesium citrate) speed up gastrointestinal motility, thereby shortening absorption time for chemicals in the gut. However, studies do not show that cathartics positively affect patient outcome, and the osmotically increased gastrointestinal fluid load may even *increase* systemic absorption and toxicity of some substances. Their major disadvantage is frequent liquid stools, which may become distracting to nursing and other personnel responsible for continuing care of the patient and may interfere with more appropriate evaluation and monitoring needs. In young children, dehydration and electrolyte imbalance can occur.

*Whole bowel irrigation* is gaining increasing popularity as a method to rapidly wash gastrointestinal contents through the system in an effort to reduce the potential absorption time. Some indications for this technique include packaged materials (body packers and body "stuffers" who swallow illicit drugs either to smuggle materials or to hide evidence) and sustained-release or enteric-coated medications. The technique consists of passing a gastric tube and continuously administering nonabsorbable polyethylene glycol (Go-Litely) at a rate of 1-2 L/h (500 mL/h for pediatric patients) until the objects are recovered or the effluent clear. No significant changes in serum osmolality or serum electrolytes have been reported. Disadvantages include patient handling and collection/disposal of the effluent.

Future directions in gastrointestinal decontamination will most likely see the increased use of activated charcoal in both prehospital and emergency department settings. Administration of activated charcoal prior to gastric lavage (20 to 30 min) has been shown to double the effectiveness of lavage, and the use of activated charcoal immediately following lavage, or as a primary method of decontamination, and even as a tool to enhance elimination of already absorbed toxin, continues to gain acceptance and popularity, although much of the previous literature on multiple-dose charcoal has not been based on controlled studies.

Other decontamination concerns include removal of toxic substances from the *skin*, primarily through complete removal of clothing followed by thorough soap and water wash; *eye* decontamination, using 15 to 30 min of constant irrigation for chemical exposures until a conjunctival pH of 7 is attained (perhaps even longer for alkalis) (see Chapter 201), and decontamination of special areas, which may produce increased or prolonged absorption, such as hair, skin folds, mucous membranes, and damaged skin.

## Supportive Care

Supportive care of the poisoned patient is directed toward the prevention or limitation of respiratory, cardiovascular, and neurologic complications. The initiation of standard diagnostic and therapeutic measures including administration of oxygen, establishing intravenous access, and placing the patient on a cardiac monitor should be routine in any serious poisoning.

### Management of Respiratory Complications

*Airway protection* is an essential step in the treatment of a poisoned patient. If any airway compromise (vomitus, stridor, diminished gag reflex) is present in a patient with altered level of consciousness, orotracheal or nasotracheal intubation should be accomplished as soon as possible. Correction of airway problems frequently resolves associated *ventilatory insufficiency*, but if any doubt remains, assisted ventilation should be instituted until ventilatory status may be further evaluated. *Bronchospasm* may cause significant problems in patients with underlying pulmonary disease but usually responds to standard bronchodilator therapy. *Noncardiogenic pulmonary edema* may be seen early and is due to increased alveolocapillary permeability, requiring treatment with high-flow oxygen, positive pressure ventilation, and consideration of positive end-expiratory pressure (PEEP). In contrast, true ARDS is rarely seen as an emergency department complication, but early anticipation may allow early, aggressive treatment and limit its consequences. *Aspiration* is best treated by prevention through early airway control, but if it has already occurred, it requires only simple ventilatory support. Although antibiotics and steroids are frequently used, studies do not support their efficacy and neither is recommended.

## Management of Cardiovascular Complications

*Tachyarrhythmias* are rarely associated with serious perfusion problems and usually require nothing more than cardiac monitoring. However, ventricular irritability should be aggressively managed with appropriate antiarrhythmic agents. Bradyarrhythmias are best treated with atropine but may require chronotropic agents or even pacing. *Hypotension* usually reflects decreased peripheral vascular resistance and should be treated with fluid administration; only rarely are vasopressors required. *Hypertension* that is complicated by pulmonary edema, cardiac ischemia, or encephalopathy should be controlled with direct arterial vasodilators (nitroprusside, calcium channel antagonists, etc.).

## Management of Neurologic Complications

*Coma,* or altered level of consciousness, represents no significant problems except as it relates to the respiratory and cardiovascular complications previously discussed. *Seizures,* on the other hand, are one of the most dangerous complications encountered in the poisoned patient, requiring treatment early and often. Standard anticonvulsant therapy with rapid-acting benzodiazepines and barbiturates (diazepam, pentobarbital) will control most toxin-induced seizures. Repeated or prolonged seizures should be initially controlled with paralyzing agents (pancuronium) to avoid progressive metabolic acidosis, hyperthermia, and rhabdomyolysis, although care must be taken to guard against the adverse CNS effects of electrical status epilepticus. Phenytoin is no longer regarded as efficacious for longer-term control or seizure prophylaxis in the poisoned patient, and loading with phenobarbital as a long-acting anticonvulsant is currently recommended. *Behavioral abnormalities,* including hallucinations, combativeness, and agitation, are frequently due to early stages of CNS depression (the excitation stage of anesthesia). Therefore, the use of "chemical restraints" only compounds the intoxication and may on occasion precipitate catastrophic cardiopulmonary complications. Therefore, physical restraints should be used as much as possible, although patients who continue to be unmanageable to the extent that essential diagnostic or therapeutic measures are unable to be carried out or who are in danger of developing hyperthermia and rhabdomyolysis may require sedation. Short-acting benzodiazepines (diazepam, etc.) may be used for rapid control of patients; haloperidol is effective for longer-term control.

## Diagnostic Studies

As information is being obtained via history and physical examination and supportive care is being initiated, ancillary studies may be important to confirm the presence of suspected or unsuspected toxins, to confirm the clinical status or chronic effects on organ systems, or to obtain baseline information for future comparison.

*Drug screens* rarely alter the basic management of patients because of delayed turnaround times or a limited scope of the assays. Generally, urine drug screens may assist in identifying toxins that are not clinically apparent, but their scope and quality may be extremely variable. Some institutions routinely require only a "drug of abuse" screen (barbiturates, benzodiazepines, cannabinoids, cocaine, ethanol, methadone, opiates, phencyclidine, propoxyphene, sympathomimetic amines), whereas others require a thorough screen of literally thousands of substances with gas chromatography or mass spectrometry. On the other hand, specific management of some toxins, such as acetaminophen, will be directly determined by quantitative blood levels; the emergency department physician should be familiar with time-dependent blood drug levels and their interpretation relative to the time of ingestion. Comprehensive drug screens or isolated blood levels are still controversial, and the emergency physician must weigh the poor return against the possibility of "missing" the presence of a significant toxin. In all cases, drug levels should be guided to the extent possible by history and physical findings. It is essential that emergency physicians be familiar with their own laboratories' capabilities and limitations in providing rapid, accurate drug screens. Other laboratory studies may include the usual baseline determinations, including a complete blood cell count, electrolyte levels, glucose levels, arterial blood gas levels, osmolality, and organ function (renal, hepatic, etc.). However, these studies also rarely alter the emergency department management of the poisoned patient. *Arterial blood gases* may be important in the evaluation of the oxygenation, ventilation, and metabolic status of seriously poisoned patients. However, laboratory studies should be ordered on an individual basis, depending on the exposure, the presence or absence of complications, and the overall clinical status of the patient. Similarly, ancillary studies (ECGs, x-ray studies, etc.) should also be ordered based on specific indications.

## Definitive Care

In most instances, "definitive" care of the poisoned patient is accomplished by decontamination and supportive care. However, in a number of conditions the use of an *antagonist* is indicated. Any patient presenting with an altered level of consciousness deserves a trial of two essential cellular substrates, oxygen and glucose, and the opiate antagonist naloxone if history or clinical findings suggest the presence of an opioid. There is no current justification for the empirical use of the benzodiazepine antagonist flumazenil. Additional antagonists used in the treatment of poisoning are listed in Table 129-2.

The other technique considered a part of definitive care is the enhancement of *elimination* of toxic substances already absorbed into the system. Previously, such efforts concentrated on increasing renal excretion by manipulating urinary pH. And while alkalinization is still an important technique in increasing the elimination of many drugs (salicylates, barbiturates, etc.), acidification is unlikely to remove any significant amount of total body drug burden and may contribute to renal complications from some of the chemicals supposedly undergoing "ion-trapping" by acidification (amphetamine, phencyclidine, etc.). Some studies have demonstrated the marked efficacy of activated charcoal in enhancing the elimination of certain toxins, including parent compounds and active metabolites. Repeated doses may be given every 2 to 4 h, although decreased gastrointestinal motility (anticholinergics, etc.) may require that the dosage interval be much longer. It appears that the administration of activated charcoal is as important in removing some substances such as theophylline and phenobarbital from the system as it is in preventing absorption in the first place, but the routine use of multidose charcoal in all poisonings is not recommended at present. Finally, enhancement of elimination may include extracorporeal methods. However, hemodialysis and hemoperfusion are only effective in removing chemicals found in high concentration in the vascular space. In addition, the use of these techniques is generally limited to cases involving very specific chemicals (methanol, ethylene glycol), progressive deterioration despite adequate supportive care, or the presence of renal failure.

## Disposition

While the continued care of victims of accidental poisoning is straightforward and depends on clinical condition (ambulatory discharge versus emergency department observation versus admission), the disposition of the patient with intentional exposure is frequently difficult. If the patient shows no significant toxicity, psychiatric evaluation should be a prerequisite for discharge. Above all, emergency physicians must avoid the temptation to accept the demands of an ex-

**Table 129-2.** Emergency Antidotes

| Poison | Antidote | Adult Dosage* | Comments |
|---|---|---|---|
| Acetaminophen | *N*-Acetylcysteine | Initial dose: 140 mg/kg | Most effective within 16 h |
| Arsenic | *See* Mercury | | |
| Atropine | Physostigmine | Initial dose: 0.5–2 mg IV | Can produce convulsions, bradycardia |
| Benzodiazepines | Flumazenil | Initial dose: 0.2 mg (2cc) q1 min to a total dose of 1–3 mg | Can cause seizures or VT, especially if tricyclics have been ingested |
| Carbon monoxide | Oxygen | | |
| Cyanide | Amyl nitrite; | Inhale contents of crushed pearl for 30 s; breath oxygen for 30 s | Methemoglobin-cyanide complex |
| | *then* Sodium nitrite | 10 mL of 3% solution over 3 min IV in adults | Causes hypotension. Dosage assumes normal level hemoglobin |
| | | 0.33 mL (10 mg 3% sol.)/kg initially in children | |
| | Sodium thiosulfate | 25% solution—50 mL IV over 10 min in adults; 1.65 mL/kg in children | Forms harmless sodium thiocyanate |
| Ethylene glycol | *See* Methyl alcohol | | |
| Iron | Deferoxamine | Initial dose: 10–15 mg/kg per hour IV | Deferoxamine mesylate—forms excretable ferrioxamine complex |
| Lead | Calcium disodium edetate *or* | 1 ampoule/250 mL D₅W over 1 h | 5-mL ampoule IV 20% solution. Dilute to less than 3% solution. Calcium displaced by lead |
| | Dimercaptosuccinic acid | 250 mg PO | |
| Mercury, Arsenic, Gold | BAL (British anti-Lewisite) | 5 mg/kg IM as soon as possible | Each mL BAL in oil has dimercaprol, 100 mg, in 210 mg (21%) benzyl benzoate and 680 mg peanut oil. Forms stable non-toxic excretable cyclic compound |
| | Dimercaptosuccinic acid (DMSA; succimer) | 250 mg PO | Oral, water soluble preparation of BAL |
| Methyl alcohol, Ethylene Glycol | Ethyl alcohol in conjunction with dialysis | 1 mL/kg of 100% ethanol initially in glucose solution; maintain blood level of 100 mg/100 mL | Competes for alcohol dehydrogenase; prevents formation of toxic metabolites |
| Nitrites | Methylene blue | 0.2 mL/kg of 1% solution IV over 5 min | Exchange transfusion may be needed for severe methemoglobinemia |
| Opiates | Naloxone | 0.4–0.8 mg IV in adults; up to 8–22 mg 0.01 mg/kg IV in children | Higher doses may be required for certain high-affinity substances such as propoxyphene (Darvon) and diphenoxylate (Lomotil) |
| Organophosphates | Atropine | Initial dose: 2–5 mg IV in adults; 0.05 mg/kg IV in children | Physiologic: blocks acetylcholine (at muscarinic receptor sites). Up to 5 mg IV every 15 min (or more) may be necessary in the critical adult patient |
| | Pralidoxime (2-PAM chloride) (Protopam) | Initial dose: 1 g IV in adults; 25–30 mg/kg IV in children | Specific: breaks alkyl phosphate-cholinesterase bond, regenerating acetylcholinesterase activity |

* Dosages listed may require modification according to specific clinical conditions.
SOURCE: Adapted from the American College of Emergency Physicians poster on poisoning, Dallas, TX, 1980.

cited, angry, combative, and potentially intoxicated patient who states "You can't keep me here against my will!" A patient who is under extreme emotional distress and perhaps unable to make a rational decision because of a drug or alcohol intoxication requires attention to his or her psychiatric needs.

## BIBLIOGRAPHY

Goldfrank LR, Flomenbaum NE, Lewin NA, et al. *Goldfrank's Toxicologic Emergencies,* 4th ed. East Norwalk, CT: Appleton & Lange, 1990.

Haddad LM, Winchester JF, (eds). *Clinical Management of Poisoning and Drug Overdose,* 2nd ed. Philadelphia: WB Saunders, 1990.

# 130
# TRICYCLIC ANTIDEPRESSANTS
### Kirk C. Mills

Tricyclic antidepressants (TCAs) are responsible for more intentional drug overdose-related deaths than any other group of prescribed medications. Reported mortality rates for intentional TCA overdoses range between 2 to 5 percent. This underscores the low therapeutic-to-toxic ratio that characterizes TCAs.

Currently, 10 different TCAs are available by prescription in the United States (Table 130-1), but many more varieties are available in other countries. Despite their toxicity, TCA availability is increasing

**Table 130-1.** Tricyclic Antidepressants

Amitriptyline
Amoxapine (see text for discussion)
Clomipramine
Desipramine
Doxepin
Imipramine
Maprotiline (see text for discussion)
Nortriptyline
Protriptyline
Trimipramine

**Table 130-2.** Pharmacologic Actions of Tricyclic Antidepressants

**Antagonism of Acetylcholine at Muscarinic Receptors**

| **Central Effects** | **Peripheral Effects** |
|---|---|
| Sedation | Dry mouth |
| Delirium | Mydriasis |
| Hallucinations | Blurred vision |
| Seizures* | Dry axillae |
| Abnormal speech | Sinus tachycardia |
| Tremor | Ileus |
| Respiratory depression | Urinary retention |
| Myoclonus | Hyperthermia |

**Inhibition of Amine Uptake**

| **Norepinephrine** | **Serotonin** |
|---|---|
| Tachycardia | Myoclonus |
| Early mild hypertension | Hyperreflexia |
| | Seizures* |
| | Rigidity |

| **Na⁺ Channel Blockade** | **K⁺ Efflux Blockade** |
|---|---|
| QRS prolongation | QT interval prolongation |
| PR prolongation | Torsades de pointes |
| Ventricular arrhythmias | |
| Heart blocks | |
| Bradyarrhythmias | |
| Impaired contractility/hypotension | **GABA Antagonism** |
| Seizures* | Seizures* |

$\ast$ Denotes possible explanation for seizures.
GABA, $\gamma$-aminobutyric acid

as therapeutic indications for their use expand beyond treating depression to include other psychiatric and medical conditions such as obsessive-compulsive disorder, attention deficit disorder, panic and phobia disorders, chronic pain syndromes, peripheral neuropathies, nocturnal enuresis, anxiety disorders, eating disorders, migraine headache prophylaxis, and adjunctive therapy in selected drug abstinence regimens.

Over the past 10 years a number of new antidepressants have been developed and include fluoxetine, sertraline, paroxetine, trazodone, and bupropion. These antidepressants differ from TCAs in their chemical structure, pharmacology, and toxicity. Their management is discussed in chap. 131.

## PHARMACOLOGY

Tricyclic antidepressants have a distinct chemical structure comprised of three aromatic rings: a central seven-member ring, two outer benzene rings, and an aminopropyl side chain connected to the central ring. Amoxapine differs slightly from the other TCAs in that it has an aromatic side chain. Maprotiline has an ethylene bridge across the center ring giving it a tetracyclic chemical structure. At therapeutic plasma levels there are considerable differences in pharmacologic activity among the TCAs, but these differences are lost at higher plasma levels typically seen in overdose. Therefore, all of the drugs listed in Table 130-1 should be considered as having equivalent drug toxicity when ingested in large amounts.

Tricyclic antidepressants are nonselective agents that exhibit a multitude of pharmacologic effects. Only a few of these drug-receptor interactions are responsible for their therapeutic action such as inhibition of amine uptake and antagonism of postsynaptic serotonin receptors. The remaining drug-receptor interactions explain TCA-related adverse effects and overdose toxicity. Competitive inhibition of central nervous system (CNS) histamine receptors contributes to CNS sedation. Rare cases of TCA-induced neuroleptic malignant syndrome can be attributed to their inhibition of postsynaptic dopamine receptors.

The majority of clinical findings seen in TCA overdose can be explained by the following six pharmacologic actions (Table 130-2).

**Inhibition of amine uptake.** The primary mechanism for terminating neurotransmission after neuronal release of norepinephrine, serotonin, and dopamine is by uptake of released neurotransmitters into the presynaptic nerve terminal by membrane pumps. TCAs inhibit the action of these neuronal pumps. They are more potent inhibitors of norepinephrine and serotonin uptake than they are dopamine uptake. Inhibition of neurotransmitter uptake leads to increased synaptic levels and subsequent augmentation of the neurotransmitter response. Inhibition of norepinephrine uptake is thought to produce the early sympathomimetic effects occasionally seen in some TCA overdoses and may contribute to the development of cardiac arrhythmias. Serotonin syndrome results from increased serotonin brain stem activity and has been produced by TCAs that are particularly potent serotonin uptake inhibitors. Elevated serotonin levels produce myoclonus, muscle rigidity, and hyperreflexia.

**Anticholinergic effects.** The TCAs are competitive antagonists of acetylcholine at central and peripheral muscarinic receptors. They do not antagonize acetylcholine at nicotinic receptors. Central anticholinergic symptoms vary from agitation to delirium, hallucinations, slurred speech, ataxia, sedation, and coma. Peripheral anticholinergic symptoms include dilated pupils, blurred vision, tachycardia, decreased oral and bronchial secretions, dry skin, ileus, urinary retention, increased muscle tone, and tremor.

**Inhibition of adrenergic receptors.** The TCAs are inhibitors of central and peripheral $\alpha_1$- and $\alpha_2$-adrenergic receptors. They do not inhibit $\beta$-adrenergic receptors. Inhibition of postsynaptic $\alpha$-adrenergic receptors produces hypotension secondary to vasodilation and is usually accompanied by reflex tachycardia. Inhibition of ocular $\alpha$-adrenergic receptors produces miosis. This action frequently offsets anticholinergic-induced pupillary dilation. Thus, patients with TCA toxicity can present with constricted, dilated, or midpoint-sized pupils.

**Sodium channel blockade.** Cardiotoxicity induced by TCAs is a major cause of patient mortality. Life-threatening cardiotoxicity results from TCA-induced inhibition of sodium influx through voltage-dependent sodium channels. Sodium channel blockade has previously been referred to as membrane stabilizing, quinidine-like, or local anesthetic effects. Inhibition of fast sodium channels in His-Purkinje cells and myocardial tissue leads to decreased $Na^+$ influx and delayed depolarization. This results in a prolongation of phase O of the action potential, which becomes more pronounced with rapid heart rates, hyponatremia, and acidosis. This effect expresses itself electrocardiographically (ECG) as prolongation of PR and QRS intervals. Rapid influx of sodium is linked to the release of intracellular calcium stores and subsequent myocardial contractility. Sinus tachycardia secondary to anticholinergic activity partially offsets the negative chronotropic effect of sodium channel blockade. Therefore, bradycardia is particularly worrisome when accompanied by QRS complex widening and PR interval prolongation because it indicates profound sodium channel blockade. Local changes in electrical conduction can predispose to ventricular arrhythmias by establishing reentry loops. In summary, severe sodium channel blockade culminates in depressed myocardial contractility, heart blocks, hypotension, wide QRS, and cardiac ectopy.

Alkalinization of blood (pH 7.50 to 7.55) and increasing the serum sodium concentration have been found to have an additive effect in partially overcoming sodium channel blockade. Intravenous sodium bicarbonate ($NaHCO_3$) is thought to be more effective than either hyperventilation (alkalinizes blood) or sodium chloride (increases $Na^+$) in treating TCA cardiotoxicity. One explanation for the greater effectiveness of $NaHCO_3$ is that it produces both blood alkalinization and increased serum sodium concentration. The mechanism by which blood alkalinization partially reverses sodium channel blockade remains unknown, but it does not appear to be related to enhancement of plasma TCA protein binding. It may be related to decreased affinity of TCAs towards the sodium channels.

**Potassium channel antagonist.** The TCAs block myocardial potassium channels and inhibit the efflux of potassium during repolarization. This effect is seen on the ECG as QT interval (specifically JT interval) prolongation, which is more pronounced at slower heart rates. Ironically, because most TCA overdose patients are tachycardiac, they are partially protected from severe QT interval prolongation, which is otherwise capable of producing torsades de pointes at slower heart rates.

**γ-Aminobutyric acid/Chloride channel antagonist.** Generalized seizures occur in approximately 10 to 30 percent of symptomatic patients with TCA overdose. Even therapeutic doses of TCAs can produce seizures in up to 4 percent of patients. Possible mechanisms for these seizures include TCA-induced γ-aminobutyric acid$_A$ (GABA$_A$) receptor antagonism, neuronal sodium channel blockade, central anticholinergic activity, and effects on biogenic amines. The exact etiology of these seizures remains speculative, but TCA-induced antagonism of the GABA$_A$ receptor may represent the most important mechanism. Benzodiazepines and barbiturates are potent GABA$_A$ receptor agonists. They are the anticonvulsants to use in treating TCA-induced seizures.

## PHARMACOKINETICS

All TCAs share similar pharmacokinetic properties. They are highly lipophilic, readily cross the blood-brain barrier, and reach peak plasma levels between 2 and 6 h postingestion at therapeutic doses. Gastrointestinal absorption can be prolonged due to their anticholinergic effect on the gastrointestinal tract. Bioavailability is only 30 to 70 percent due to extensive first-pass metabolism. They are highly protein bound to $\alpha_1$ acid glycoproteins. Their apparent volume of distribution is extremely large and ranges from 10 to 50 L/kg. Tissue TCA levels are commonly 10 to 100 times greater than plasma levels. Only 1 to 2 percent of the total body burden of TCAs is found in the blood. These pharmacokinetic properties explain why attempts at removing TCAs by hemodialysis, hemoperfusion, peritoneal dialysis, or forced diuresis are generally unproductive.

The TCAs are eliminated almost entirely by hepatic oxidation, which consists of N-demethylation of the amine side chain groups and hydroxylation of ring structures. Some TCAs undergo enterohepatic circulation prior to their eventual oxidation, conjugation, and renal elimination, but this does not significantly contribute to their toxicity. Tertiary amines such as amitriptyline, imipramine, doxepin, clomipramine, and trimipramine are demethylated to active metabolites (secondary amines) before their elimination. Although secondary amines such as desipramine, nortriptyline, and protriptyline are effective antidepressants, their metabolites are generally considered inactive. Amoxapine and maprotiline both have active metabolites.

The average elimination half-life of TCAs is approximately 24 h (range 6 to 36 h) at therapeutic doses, but this can increase to 72 h after overdose. Inhibition of TCA metabolism by other drugs that use the same hepatic enzymes can prolong the half-life of TCAs. This carries the risk of elevating TCA plasma levels and producing clinical TCA toxicity at therapeutic doses. Approximately 7 percent of the US population are genetically slow metabolizers of TCAs and are prone to develop higher plasma levels at any given daily TCA dose.

## TOXICITY

Therapeutic doses of TCA range from 2 to 4 mg/kg. Any dose greater than this has the potential to produce TCA toxicity. Life-threatening symptoms usually occur with ingestions of greater than 10 mg/kg in adults. Pediatric patients are particularly susceptible to TCA toxicity, especially to anticholinergic effects. Other patients at higher risk for TCA toxicity include patients who have coingested additional cardiotoxic or CNS depressive medications, geriatric patients, and patients with heart disease. Some TCAs, especially desipramine, are able to precipitate severe cardiotoxicity (e.g., wide QRS, hypotension) without producing significant anticholinergic symptoms. TCA-related fatalities are commonly associated with ingestions of greater than 1 g. Most fatalities occur within 2 h after the TCA overdose often before the patient ever reaches the hospital. Fatalities are rare after 24 h postingestion and are usually due to overdose-related complications.

Quantitative plasma TCA levels are helpful in monitoring chronic drug therapy (e.g., compliance, metabolism), but they are of limited value in assessing acute TCA overdose toxicity. Some studies have shown that if a combined plasma level of parent TCA and metabolite is greater than 1000 ng/mL patients are at greater risk to develop serious TCA toxicity. However, degree of toxicity does not always correlate with the extent of plasma TCA elevation. Patients can develop severe toxicity with plasma levels less than 1000 ng/mL. Currently, data on amoxapine and maprotiline are insufficient to determine if a meaningful correlation exists between their respective plasma levels and clinical toxicity. As always, the most important thing is to treat the patient and not the drug level.

## CLINICAL FEATURES

The clinical presentation of TCA toxicity varies tremendously from mild anticholinergic symptoms to severe cardiotoxicity secondary to sodium channel blockade. In approximately 50 percent of TCA poisonings, coingested drugs are also involved and the additional toxicity from these coingestants should be considered when evaluating these patients. Anticholinergic symptoms commonly serve as markers for TCA toxicity (e.g., dry mouth and axillae, sinus tachycardia), but they alone are rarely responsible for patient fatalities. Also, anticholinergic symptoms are not uniformly present in TCA toxicity. As an example, sinus tachycardia is the most frequent arrhythmia noted in TCA toxicity, but it is only present in approximately 70 percent of symptomatic patients.

Mild to moderate TCA toxicity may present as drowsiness, confusion, slurred speech, ataxia, dry mucous membranes and axilla, sinus tachycardia, ileus, urinary retention, myoclonus, and hyperreflexia. Mild hypertension is occasionally observed and rarely requires treatment. With increasing TCA toxicity, CNS depression progresses to coma and respiratory depression. Nontolerant individuals occasionally develop coma and respiratory depression after relatively small overdoses without obvious peripheral anticholinergic effects or QRS widening.

Serious toxicity is almost always seen within 6 h of major TCA ingestion and consists of the following symptoms: coma, cardiac conduction delays, supraventricular tachycardia, hypotension, respiratory depression, premature ventricular beats, ventricular tachycardia, and seizures. Secondary complications from serious toxicity include aspiration pneumonia, anoxic encephalopathy, and rhabdomyolysis.

Seizures are usually generalized, single, and brief in duration. The exception to this rule is seen in amoxapine and maprotiline overdoses. These agents can cause status epilepticus. Amoxapine seizures commonly occur without corresponding wide QRS complexes.

Electrocardiographic abnormalities are common, especially prolongation of the PR, QRS, and QT intervals. Other ECG abnormalities include conduction blocks, right axis deviation, and nonspecific ST segment and T wave changes. The natural progression of ECG and cardiac abnormalities occurs in the following order: sinus tachycardia, widening of the QRS complex, decreased cardiac inotropy, increased PR interval, and finally, decreased heart rate. However, not all patients will follow such an orderly progression of ECG and cardiac abnormalities. Prolongation of the QT interval is most commonly seen at therapeutic TCA doses.

Right axis deviation of the terminal 40 ms of greater than 120° has been proposed as a reliable ECG criterion to predict TCA toxicity. Although this ECG abnormality is frequently seen in TCA toxicity, it lacks the sensitivity and specificity to be of any meaningful predictive value by itself.

Prolongation of the QRS complex greater than 100 ms occurs in 20 to 50 percent of cases of TCA toxicity. Patients with QRS widening appear to be at higher risk for severe toxicity than patients without QRS widening. Unfortunately, a significant percentage of the normal population has a baseline QRS width equal to or greater than 100 ms. Therefore, QRS prolongation by itself is too insensitive and nonspecific to be used as a single clinical criterion to predict severe TCA toxicity. Nonetheless, when QRS complex widening is accompanied by other signs of TCA toxicity the clinician should assume the patient to be at high risk for developing life-threatening toxicity.

## DIFFERENTIAL DIAGNOSIS

Three main groups of drugs should be considered in the differential diagnosis of TCA toxicity. First are medications that produce seizures, wide QRS complex sinus rhythm, and anticholinergic symptoms. These include carbamazepine, phenothiazines (e.g., mesoridazine), antihistamines (e.g., diphenhydramine), quinidine, quinine, procainamide, disopyramide, and cyclobenzaprine (QRS widening is rare). Second are medications that produce seizures and wide complex sinus rhythm, but do not have anticholinergic activity. These medications include propranolol, class IC antiarrhythmic agents, cocaine, local anesthetic agents, lithium, and propoxyphene. Third are sympathomimetics that can produce narrow complex tachycardia, hypertension, and seizures but are not associated with anticholinergic symptoms.

## GENERAL MANAGEMENT PRINCIPLES

All patients should be immediately evaluated for alterations in level of consciousness, hemodynamic instability, and respiratory impairment. Patients with altered consciousness/depression require a trial of intravenous dextrose, thiamine, naloxone, and oxygen to rule out reversible causes of CNS depression. Unresponsive patients may have unrecognized head or neck trauma. Flumazenil should not be given to patients suspected of having mixed drug overdoses involving TCAs and benzodiazepines because this action may immediately precipitate generalized seizures.

Every patient requires an intravenous line, cardiac monitoring, and an ECG. Aspiration pneumonia is especially common in patients with decreased level of consciousness and can be evaluated by plain film chest radiography. Most symptomatic patients will require a urinary catheter to prevent urinary retention. A nasogastric tube is usually necessary in patients with absent bowel tones. Patients who are initially asymptomatic may rapidly deteriorate and should therefore be closely monitored for several hours.

### Gastrointestinal Decontamination

Although the best method of gastrointestinal decontamination in TCA ingestions remains undefined, a few generalizations are still possible. The risks associated with using syrup of ipecac outweigh any beneficial effects and its use cannot be recommended. Activated charcoal has been shown to effectively bind TCAs and decrease their absorption. Therefore, all patients should receive 1 g/kg of activated charcoal. Whether gastric lavage and activated charcoal is better than ac-

tivated charcoal alone remains unproven. Studies have shown that gastric lavage is most effective when it is performed within the first few hours after ingestion. Most emergency physicians opt to perform gastric lavage and give activated charcoal to patients who present relatively early after TCA ingestion. The proper method of performing gastric lavage in alert patients is to place the patient in the left lateral decubitus position to prevent pulmonary aspiration. Obtunded patients require endotracheal intubation prior to performing gastric lavage. Asymptomatic patients with reliable histories of minimal TCA ingestions can be treated with AC alone and observed for toxicity. Some authors have recommended giving repeat doses of activated charcoal to enhance TCA elimination, but these recommendations should be viewed cautiously in the setting of decreased intestinal motility. The role of cathartics in gastrointestinal decontamination remains undefined and they cannot be routinely recommended.

### Sodium Bicarbonate Therapy

Indications for $NaHCO_3$ therapy include QRS complex widening greater than 100 ms, hypotension refractory to fluid challenges, and ventricular arrhythmias. Initially, $NaHCO_3$ is administered as a bolus of 1 to 2 mEq/kg, which can be repeated until the patient improves or until blood pH equals 7.50 to 7.55. Alkalinization beyond this point can be deleterious and is therefore discouraged. Continuous infusions of $NaHCO_3$ are usually administered as 2 ampules (50 mEq/50 mL) being placed in 1 L 5% dextrose in water (hypotonic with $NaHCO_3$ added) or 1/2 normal saline (slightly hypertonic with $NaHCO_3$ added) solution and run at a rate of 2 mL/kg per hour. Adjustments in the intravenous rate are made based on blood pH measurements, serum sodium level, and the clinical response to therapy. Hypokalemia can occur with $NaHCO_3$ therapy. Intravenous potassium supplementation is usually required and serum potassium levels should be frequently measured.

### Disposition

Patients who remain asymptomatic 6 h after ingestion do not require hospital admission for toxicologic reasons. However, they may require hospital admission because of other coexisting medical or psychiatric conditions. Most patients who have intentionally ingested TCAs will also require a psychiatric evaluation.

All symptomatic patients require hospital admission to a monitored unit. Patients demonstrating signs of moderate to severe toxicity should be admitted to an intensive care unit. Suggested laboratory studies include serum electrolytes, creatinine, glucose, and creatine phosphokinase levels. In addition, a serum acetaminophen level is recommended in all overdose patients. Most symptomatic patients will require an arterial blood gas measurement. In hospitalized patients, cardiac monitoring can be safely discontinued in the setting of normal mental status, no anticholinergic symptoms (including tachycardia), and a normal or baseline ECG.

## TREATMENT OF SPECIFIC COMPLICATIONS
### Coma/Agitation

Coma from TCA toxicity is typically rapid in onset. Management of coma consists of airway protection, ventilatory support, and consideration of instituting mechanical prophylactic measures to prevent deep vein thrombosis. Agitation is secondary to central cholinergic receptor antagonism. It is commonly seen in the early stages of TCA toxicity and in previously comatose patients as they awaken. It is best controlled with reassurance, decreased environmental stimulation, and benzodiazepines. Physostigmine can be used to control agitation when other measures have failed and should only be used in agitated patients with accompanying peripheral anticholinergic symptoms and a narrow QRS complex. Physostigmine should not be used to awaken comatose patients. The adult dose of physostigmine is 0.5 to 2 mg diluted in 10 mL saline given by slow infusion over 5 min. A repeat dose can be given after 10 to 20 min if there is no improvement. Therapeutic effects of physostigmine last between 20 and 40 min. Physostigmine use is not without significant risk and can be associated with life-threatening adverse effects. Physostigmine is contraindicated in patients with reactive airway disease, urinary or intestinal obstruction, glaucoma, cardiac disease, pheochromocytoma, diabetes, and peripheral vascular disease.

## Seizures

Most seizures occur within the first 3 h after ingestion. Typically, single TCA-induced seizures do not require anticonvulsant therapy unless they are caused by amoxapine or maprotiline. These two TCAs have been reported to produce status epilepticus in patients who have not immediately received anticonvulsants. Focal seizures are atypical and require further neurologic evaluation.

Benzodiazepines (e.g., valium, lorazepam) are the anticonvulsants of choice to stop existing seizure activity. Barbiturates (e.g., phenobarbital) are indicated to treat seizures resistant to benzodiazepines and to prevent recurrent seizures. The initial intravenous dose of phenobarbital should be at least 10 to 15 mg/kg and can be repeated as needed in patients with continued seizure activity and adequate blood pressure. Phenytoin is an ineffective anticonvulsant for stopping TCA-induced seizures. Physostigmine and NaHCO$_3$ do not stop TCA-induced seizures. If seizures continue despite adequate dosing with benzodiazepines and phenobarbital, consideration should be given to paralyzing the patient with a neuromuscular blocking agent. This will stop the physical manifestations of the seizure and its secondary effects, which include metabolic acidosis, hyperthermia, rhabdomyolysis, and renal failure. It does not stop brain seizure activity. Therefore, following the induction of muscle paralysis these patients require electroencephalographic monitoring and continued anticonvulsant therapy.

## Hypotension

Hypotension should initially be treated with isotonic crystalloid fluids in increments of 10 mL/kg. In the setting of impaired cardiac contractility, pulmonary edema can develop if excessive fluids are administered. Hypotension that does improve with appropriate fluid challenges should be treated with NaHCO$_3$ (regardless of QRS width). Vasopressors should be used when hypotension is unresponsive to fluids and NaHCO$_3$ therapy. The most effective vasopressor is norepinephrine because it directly competes with TCAs at $\alpha$-adrenergic receptors. Dopamine is less effective than norepinephrine in reversing TCA-induced hypotension. In many cases dopamine administration will actually cause a lowering in systolic blood pressure due to its $\beta$-adrenergic and dopaminergic actions, which promote vasodilation. A pulmonary artery catheter should be placed in patients whose hypotension is refractory to fluid, NaHCO$_3$, and vasopressor therapy. Physicians should be cautioned that mechanical irritation of the heart during pulmonary artery catheter placement may precipitate life-threatening conduction abnormalities and ventricular arrhythmias.

Hypotension induced by TCAs represents a potentially reversible cause of cardiovascular collapse. Mechanical support of the circulation via cardiopulmonary bypass, overdrive pacing, or aortic balloon pump assistance may be warranted in patients with refractory hypotension although no studies document their effectiveness.

## Dysrhythmias

The TCAs frequently alter cardiac rate, conduction, and contractility. Asymptomatic patients with sinus tachycardia, isolated PR and QT prolongation, or first-degree atrioventricular block do not require specific pharmacologic therapy. Conduction blocks greater than first degree are worrisome because they can rapidly progress to complete heart block secondary to impaired infranodal conduction. Patients with QRS prolongation greater than 100 ms should be treated with NaHCO$_3$ therapy. This recommendation is made despite an absence of randomized controlled human trials demonstrating NaHCO$_3$ therapy benefits otherwise asymptomatic patients with QRS prolongation. Nonetheless, it has become the standard of care in treating wide complex TCA-induced dysrhythmias.

Ventricular dysrhythmias should immediately be treated with NaHCO$_3$ administration. Lidocaine is the second agent of choice in treating ventricular dysrhythmias. Excessive lidocaine administration is capable of producing seizures. Bretylium is generally considered a third-line drug for ventricular dysrhythmias. Synchronized cardioversion is appropriate in patients with unstable dysrhythmias. Torsades de pointes should initially be treated with 1 to 2 gms intravenous magnesium sulfate. Efforts should be made to rule out other causes of torsades de points. Overdrive pacing is frequently required to prevent a recurrence of this dysrhythmia. Intravenous isoproterenol may be of some benefit in treating recurrent torsades de points when overdrive pacing is not available.

The following medications are contraindicated in the treatment of TCA-induced dysrhythmias: all class IA and IC antiarrhythmic agents, $\beta$-blockers, calcium channel blockers, and phenytoin.

## BIBLIOGRAPHY

Callaham M, Kassel D. Epidemiology of fatal tricyclic antidepressant ingestion: implications for management. *Ann Emerg Med* 14:1, 1985.

Dziukas LJ, Vohra J. Tricyclic antidepressant poisoning. *Med J Aust* 154:344, 1991.

Hoffman JR, Votey SR, Bayer M, Silver L. Effect of hypertonic sodium bicarbonate in the treatment of moderate-to-severe cyclic antidepressant overdose. *Am J Emerg Med* 11:336, 1993.

Pentel PR, Benowitz N. Tricyclic antidepressant poisoning. *Medical Toxicology* 1:101, 1986.

Pentel PR, Keyler DE, Haddad LM. Tricyclic and newer antidepressants. In: Haddad LM, Winchester JF (eds). *Clinical Management of Poisoning and Drug Overdose,* 2nd ed. Philadelphia: WB Saunders, pp. 636–655, 1990.

Preskorn SH. Pharmacokinetics of antidepressants: why and how they are relevant to treatment. *J Clin Psychiatry* 54(suppl 9):14, 1993.

Slovis CM, Murray LM, Segar D. Emergency management of cyclic antidepressant overdose: an effective and organized approach. *Emergency Medicine Reports* 14:115, 1993.

# 131
# NEWER ANTIDEPRESSANTS AND SEROTONIN SYNDROME
## Kirk C. Mills

Monoamine oxidase inhibitors (MAOIs) and tricyclic antidepressants (TCAs) represent the first clinically useful antidepressants and as such are often referred to as first-generation antidepressants. However, both MAOIs and TCAs have nonselective pharmacologic actions that result in a high incidence of adverse effects and greater potential for severe toxicity in overdose. Newer antidepressants are now available that offer significant advantages over the first-generation antidepressants, including fewer adverse effects and drug interactions, no dietary restrictions, and decreased toxicity in overdose. The newer antidepressants discussed in this chapter include trazodone (Desyrel), bupropion (Wellbutrin), venlafaxine (Effexor), and the selective serotonin reuptake inhibitors (SSRIs): fluoxetine (Prozac), sertraline (Zoloft), and paroxetine (Paxil).

Newer antidepressants are commonly referred to as atypical, heterocyclic, or second-generation antidepressants to distinguish them from MAOIs and TCAs. This distinction is important because newer antidepressants are more selective in their pharmacologic activity and have drastically different toxicologic behavior than MAOIs and TCAs. As a group, the newer antidepressants are the most popular form of pharmacotherapy for the treatment of major depression. In addition, they are also commonly prescribed in the treatment of many other psychiatric disorders. Emergency physicians are increasingly challenged to evaluate patients who have taken these newer antidepressants. Questions commonly arise as to the extent of management needed to treat these overdoses. Management of these overdoses differs significantly from that of MAOIs and TCAs and will be discussed individually for each drug. However, all antidepressants, especially the MAOIs and SSRIs, have been associated with a recently recognized drug-induced disorder called serotonin syndrome, which is discussed at the end of this chapter.

## GENERAL PRINCIPLES OF NEWER ANTIDEPRESSANTS

The newer antidepressants are a heterogenous group of drugs that differ in chemical structure, pharmacokinetic properties, and adverse effect profile. However, they also share many similarities that can be summarized by the following points.

1. All of the newer agents act mainly by inhibiting presynaptic biogenic amine neuronal uptake, which allows for increased availability of serotonin, norepinephrine, or dopamine.
2. These agents do not inhibit cardiac sodium, calcium, or potassium ion channels. Overdoses are not characterized by significant cardiotoxicity.
3. They do not inhibit MAO activity and are not associated with tyramine-like reactions. Dietary restrictions are not necessary.
4. They have negligible affinity for postsynaptic cholinergic, histaminic, dopamine, adrenergic, γ-aminobutyric acid (GABA), and glutamate receptors. Therefore, they are not associated with anticholinergic or orthostatic hypotension (except trazodone) side effects.
5. Most deaths involving these agents involve mixed-drug overdoses. Although these agents are generally much safer than the MAOIs and TCAs they can still cause fatalities, especially when combined with other drugs.
6. All of the newer antidepressants are highly protein bound and have extremely large volumes of distribution. This makes it impractical to enhance elimination via hemodialysis, hemoperfusion, or forced diuresis.
7. All of the newer antidepressants are routinely missed on hospital plasma and urine drug screens. Certain speciality laboratories have the capability to measure parent drug and metabolite plasma levels, which allow for confirmation of suspected drug overdoses. However, these results are usually not immediately available to the emergency physician nor are they helpful in emergency department management and are therefore not recommended.

## TRAZODONE

Trazodone hydrochloride (Desyrel) was released in the United States in 1982 for the treatment of endogenous depression. It remains a common poisoning concern for emergency physicians. Over the past 8 years there has been a 30 percent annual increase in trazodone poisonings (exposures) reported to poison centers. In 1993 there were more than 3800 reported trazodone exposures and six trazodone-related deaths.

The average outpatient therapeutic dose for trazodone is 150 to 400 mg/d. Inpatients may receive a maximum dose of 600 mg/d. Trazodone is available as 50-, 100-, 150-, and 300-mg tablets. There is a low potential for trazodone abuse. No withdrawal syndrome is associated with its discontinuation.

### Pharmacology

Trazodone is a triazolopyridine derivative and is structurally unrelated to other antidepressant agents. Its antidepressant action is believed to be due to its ability to inhibit serotonin uptake and inhibit postsynaptic serotonin-2 receptors. Trazodone is a moderately potent nonselective α-adrenergic receptor blocker with five times greater affinity for $\alpha_1$- than $\alpha_2$-adrenergic receptors. Thus, trazodone is commonly associated with orthostatic hypotension. Sedation is a common side effect of trazodone therapy, which is believed to be secondary to inhibition central α-adrenergic and histamine receptors. Trazodone does not inhibit MAO activity and is essentially devoid of anticholinergic activity. There is no correlation between trazodone dose and serum levels with clinical response to drug therapy.

Trazodone has one active metabolite, m-chlorophenylpiperazine (m-CPP), but its contribution to trazodones's antidepressant action remains uncertain. m-CPP is more potent than trazodone at serotonin uptake inhibition, has a longer duration of action, directly interacts with multiple serotonin receptors (as an agonist and antagonist), and interacts with other neurotransmitters systems.

Trazodone is rapidly and completely absorbed following oral ingestion. Peak plasma levels occur between 0.5 and 2 h after ingestion. It demonstrates biphasic elimination kinetics with an average half-life of approximately 8 h. The majority of trazodone undergoes hepatic oxidation by the cytochrome oxidase system (P-450). Trazodone does not induce nor inhibit the P-450 metabolism of other medications.

### Adverse Effects

Dose-related adverse effects include sedation, hypotension, dizziness, dry mouth, nausea, and peripheral edema. These side effects represent an extension of trazodone's therapeutic action and can be minimized by taking the medication before bedtime. The onset of orthostatic hypotension correlates with peak trazodone blood levels and resolves over 4 to 6 h. Trazodone is not thought to be epileptogenic and is generally considered to have little effect on the seizure threshold. Important adverse effects less closely correlated to trazodone dosage include priapism, reversible liver inflammation, and possible cardiotoxicity in patients with preexisting heart disease.

Priapism is the most serious noncardiac adverse reaction produced by trazodone. The incidence of trazodone-induced priapism is approximately 1 in 1000 to 1 in 10,000 patients on routine trazodone therapy. Trazodone is the most common cause of drug-induced priapism. Other medications with α-adrenergic receptor blocking activity (e.g., antipsychotics, antihypertensive agents) share trazodone's predilection to chemically induce priapism. Any patient with a history of increased frequency, duration, or inappropriate erections should immediately discontinue trazodone therapy.

There have been a few case reports of patients experiencing liver enzyme elevation, jaundice, and abnormal liver histology in association with trazodone therapy. Resolution of liver abnormalities occurred in all three cases once trazodone exposure was discontinued.

Human and laboratory animal experimental evidence overwhelmingly proves that trazodone is far less cardiotoxic than the TCAs. However, trazodone has been occasionally reported to be arrhythmogenic, especially in patients with underlying cardiac risk factors such as conduction abnormalities or ischemic heart disease. Cardiac rhythm abnormalities reported in association with trazodone therapy include sinus arrest, sinus bradycardia, various atrioventricular blocks, complete heart block, atrial fibrillation, and ventricular dysrhythmias (premature ventricular beats, nonsustained ventricular tachycardia, torsades de pointes). In general, trazodone has a low potential for cardiotoxicity.

## Drug Interactions

Pharmacokinetic drug interactions are uncommon with trazodone. Elderly patients have a predisposition for developing elevated plasma trazodone levels at any given therapeutic dose. The antihypertensive effects of centrally acting α-adrenergic agents (e.g., clonidine) are inhibited by trazodone. Pharmacodynamic interactions are most common with coingestants such as ethanol, central nervous system (CNS) depressants, or α-adrenergic blockers.

## Acute Overdose Toxicity

Trazodone is relatively safe in acute overdose and most deaths from trazodone overdose occur when other medications are coingested. There is no accepted toxic dose for trazodone. Serious toxicity from trazodone has been reported with ingestions of 2 to 3 g. Other case reports indicate that amounts up to 7 to 8 g are relatively well tolerated. As a general guideline, serious toxicity is unexpected with ingestions of less than 2 g in an average adult.

The most common symptom of acute trazodone poisoning is CNS depression. Other CNS-related symptoms include ataxia, dizziness, coma, and seizures. Trazodone rarely produces coma or seizures when it is the only drug ingested. Pupils are usually normal size and remain reactive to light. Infrequently, patients may complain of muscle weakness. Trazodone-induced CNS symptoms show marked improvement within 6 to 12 h after ingestion and are almost always resolved by 24 h.

Orthostatic hypotension is the most frequently reported cardiovascular abnormality noted in trazodone overdose and usually responds to fluid administration. Most patients have a normal heart rate, rhythm, and electrocardiogram (ECG), but sinus tachycardia occurs in approximately 25 percent of patients.

Gastrointestinal complaints of nausea, vomiting, dry mouth, and nonspecific abdominal pain are common following the acute overdose. Respiratory depression is most common in the presence of other CNS depressants, but respiratory arrest has been reported following 2.2 and 3.0 g trazodone. Priapism has been reported following an acute overdose of 3.5 g.

## Management

An intravenous line should be started and cardiac monitoring initiated in all patients. In pure trazodone ingestions, significant neurologic and cardiac toxicity is not expected and supportive care is usually the only treatment required. Gastrointestinal decontamination can be applied selectively in cases where the dose ingested can be accurately predicted.

An ingestion of 1000 mg or less of trazodone in an adult carries a low risk of toxicity as long as trazodone is ingested as a single agent and the patient does not have any underlying cardiac or neurologic risk factors. These patients should receive activated charcoal (1 g/kg) and gastric lavage is probably unnecessary. Ingestions of between 1000 and 2000 mg are associated with minimal to moderate toxicity. These patients should receive activated charcoal (1 g/kg) and have 6 h of monitored observation. Gastric lavage is most beneficial when performed within the first 2 h after ingestion.

Intentional ingestion of greater than 2000 mg trazodone poses the greatest risk for associated toxicity and complications. Patients with coingestant drugs or ethanol have a higher incidence of coma, seizures, and respiratory arrest. Gastric lavage followed by activated charcoal administration is recommended in all intentional overdoses of 2000 mg or more.

Hypotension should be initially treated with isotonic intravenous crystalloid solutions. If the use of a vasopressor becomes necessary then direct-acting vasopressors (e.g., norepinephrine) are recommended. Drugs with β-adrenergic receptor activity (e.g., dopamine, epinephrine) can theoretically potentiate the hypotension in the presence of trazodone-induced α-adrenergic receptor antagonism.

Patients who have remained asymptomatic for 6 h can be safely discharged from the emergency department. This assumes that any necessary psychiatric evaluation has been completed or arranged. Routine laboratory tests are not required. Trazodone blood levels are useful only to confirm the presence of trazodone because they do not correlate with observed toxicity.

Hospital admission is suggested for patients with neurologic or cardiac symptoms persisting for 6 h after ingestion, impaired respiratory status, and significant coingestants that may have delayed or prolonged toxicity. Most hospitalized patients can be safely discharged following 24 h of observation. An intensive care unit bed is warranted in most symptomatic patients. Monitored or telemetry beds are probably sufficient for 24-h observation in patients who are not symptomatic but have underlying risk factors for complications.

## BUPROPION

Bupropion (Wellbutrin) has been available in the United States since 1989 for the treatment of major depression. At doses greater than 450 mg/d bupropion is associated with a 4 percent incidence of generalized seizures. At the currently recommended maximum daily dose of 450 mg, the incidence of seizures is approximately 0.4 percent. Bupropion comes as 75- and 100-mg tablets. The recommended starting dose is 100 mg b.i.d. This can be gradually increased to up to 100 mg t.i.d.

## Pharmacology

Bupropion has a monocyclic phenylaminoketone chemical structure that resembles phenylethylamines (e.g., amphetamine). However, bupropion does not produce stimulant effects or drug addictive behavior at therapeutic doses. Its therapeutic mechanism of action is probably related to its ability to inhibit dopamine neuronal uptake, although this remains unproven. Bupropion may also have an additional undefined dopaminergic action. It does not stimulate postsynaptic dopamine receptors or indirectly release dopamine. In vitro studies show bupropion to be a weak inhibitor of norepinephrine and serotonin neuronal uptake. This action is probably clinically insignificant.

Bupropion is rapidly absorbed after oral administration and undergoes extensive first-pass hepatic metabolism. It is highly protein bound, has an extremely large volume of distribution, and readily crosses the blood-brain barrier. Peak plasma levels occur within 2 h postingestion and elimination half-life averages 14 h. It has one active metabolite, hydroxybupropion, which is half as potent as bupropion, has a half-life twice as long, and may contribute to seizure development.

## Adverse Effects

Because bupropion does not directly interact with postsynaptic receptors, the incidence of adverse effects is very low. Therapeutic doses do not produce CNS depression, orthostatic hypotension, cardiovascular changes, or impairment of sexual function. The most commonly reported adverse effects are of mild severity and include dry mouth, nausea, headache, constipation, tremor, anxiety, confusion, blurred vision, and increased motor activity. Bupropion has been reported to produce catatonia, hallucinations, psychosis, and paranoia, which are probably related to its ability to increase CNS dopamine activity. Abrupt discontinuation of bupropion has not been associated with any withdrawal symptoms but poses a slight theoretical risk of precipitating neuroleptic malignant syndrome because bupropion is considered a dopamine agonist.

## Drug Interactions

Bupropion is relatively free of significant drug interactions. It should not be used in combination with fluoxetine, lithium, phenelzine, or levodopa. In general, bupropion should not be combined with other dopaminergic drugs (e.g., levodopa), SSRIs, MAOIs, or drugs that are known to lower patient seizure threshold (e.g., phenothiazines). There should be a 2-week abstinence period between the MAOI discontinuation and initiation of bupropion therapy.

## Acute Toxicity

Bupropion differs from other new antidepressants in that it has a low toxic-to-therapeutic ratio. Toxicity can occur at doses equal to or slightly greater than the maximum therapeutic dose of 450 mg/d. As a general rule, significant toxicity is not expected in pure bupropion overdose with adult ingestions of less than 5 mg/kg. The largest case series of bupropion overdoses reported that symptomatic patients ingested a mean of 2310 mg and the lowest symptomatic dose was 200 mg. Patients who remained asymptomatic ingested a mean of 1325 mg and the largest asymptomatic dose was 4000 mg.

Approximately one quarter of bupropion overdose patients remain asymptomatic. The most commonly reported symptoms in pure bupropion overdose include sinus tachycardia (43 percent), lethargy (41 percent), tremor (24 percent), generalized seizures (21 percent), confusion (14 percent), and vomiting (14 percent). ECGs commonly show sinus tachycardia, but no other arrhythmias or conduction abnormalities have been reported. Hypotension and coma are not seen in pure bupropion overdose but have been reported in mixed-drug overdoses. Laboratory studies are usually normal except for rare cases of mild hypokalemia.

Bupropion-induced seizures are usually generalized, single and brief and have not been associated with chronic epilepsy. The actual incidence of seizures is unknown but is probably much greater than the estimated 21 percent obtained from retrospective studies. There is no correlation between the development of seizures and the presence of other symptoms such as sinus tachycardia. Therefore, seizures can develop in otherwise asymptomatic patients. Seizures usually occur within the first 1 to 4 h after ingestion. The average time of seizure onset is 3.7 h, but they may be delayed for up to 8 h.

## Management

Emergency physicians should anticipate the possible early onset of generalized seizures in all cases of bupropion ingestion. A peripheral intravenous line should be established and cardiac monitoring initiated in all patients. Rapid gastrointestinal decontamination is recommended using gastric lavage and administering activated charcoal (1 g/kg). Syrup of ipecac is contraindicated due to risk of seizures. Significant cardiotoxicity is not expected except in mixed-drug overdoses.

Hospital admission is recommended for patients with seizures, sinus tachycardia, or lethargy. All other patients should be observed for at least 6 h and ideally up to 8 h. Any asymptomatic patient after this observation period can be safely discharged home. In some cases, a psychiatric evaluation may also be necessary. Patients with sinus tachycardia should be admitted until the tachycardia resolves.

Seizures that are single, generalized, and brief in duration do not require specific anticonvulsant therapy. However, seizures that last longer than 5 min, are focal in nature, or are repetitive should be aggressively treated with benzodiazepines. Phenobarbital is considered the second anticonvulsant of choice. Diphenylhydantoin (phenytoin) is generally less effective than benzodiazepines or phenobarbital in stopping drug-induced seizures but was reportedly effective in stopping seizure activity in one case of bupropion-induced status epilepticus.

# SELECTIVE SEROTONIN REUPTAKE INHIBITORS

The SSRIs represent a chemically heterogenous group of drugs that share a high affinity to inhibit presynaptic serotonin uptake without significantly affecting norepinephrine or dopamine neuronal uptake. They essentially have no affinity for norepinephrine, dopamine, acetylcholine, GABA, or glutamate receptors. Thus, SSRIs are associated with very few unwanted pharmacologic actions. Three SSRIs are currently available in the United States. Fluoxetine (Prozac), a phenylpropylamine derivative, represents the prototypical SSRI. It was initially released in 1988 and has become the most frequently prescribed antidepressant agent in the United States. Sertraline (Zoloft), a naphthalenamine derivative, was released in 1991 and was subsequently followed in 1993 by paroxetine (Paxil), a phenylpiperidine derivative. Fluvoxamine (Luvox) is an SSRI released in early 1995 for the treatment of obsessive-compulsive disorder.

All three SSRIs have shown similar efficacy in the treatment of depression. Therefore, selection of one SSRI over another is usually based on their pharmacokinetic differences. The SSRIs have also been used to treat other psychiatric disorders such as obsessive-compulsive disorder, bulimia nervosa, personality disorders, obesity, panic attacks, cataplexy, and myoclonic disorders. The usual daily therapeutic dose for SSRIs are fluoxetine 5 to 80 mg, sertraline 50 to 200 mg, and paroxetine 10 to 50 mg. The SSRIs have rarely been associated with mild withdrawal symptoms when discontinued.

## Pharmacology

The SSRIs acutely increase synaptic serotonin levels by inhibiting serotonin neuronal uptake, but this action may not represent the actual mechanism for their therapeutic action. As with all antidepressant agents, acute alterations in biogenic amine levels do not correlate with immediate clinical response to drug therapy. Therefore, secondary receptor or cellular compensatory mechanisms are probably responsible for the therapeutic effect of SSRIs. Paroxetine is the most potent of the SSRIs. It is at least twice as potent as sertraline and up to four times more potent than fluoxetine.

The pharmacokinetic similarities between the SSRIs include rapid and complete oral absorption, peak plasma levels between 4 and 8 h after ingestion, significant first-pass hepatic metabolism, high degree of protein binding, and large volume of distribution. Fluoxetine is the only SSRI with a clinically significant active metabolite, norfluoxetine, which is equally as potent as fluoxetine. The half-lives of fluoxetine and norfluoxetine are 1 to 4 days and 7 to 14 days, respectively. The effects of fluoxetine therapy may last for up to 5 weeks because of the prolonged period of time necessary to allow for norfluoxetine metabolism. Sertraline and paroxetine both have similar half-lives of approximately 24 h. The longer duration of action of fluoxetine is potentially beneficial in patients with poor drug compliance. However, when fluoxetine-related adverse effects or drug interactions develop they are usually very slow to resolve.

## Adverse Effects

The most serious adverse effect of SSRI pharmacotherapy is the potential to develop serotonin syndrome (see discussion below). Other CNS-related adverse effects include headache, sedation, insomnia, dizziness, weakness or fatigue, tremor, and nervousness. Seizures occur in approximately 0.2 percent of all patients taking fluoxetine. Serotonin has varying effects on the dopaminergic system. In many cases, extrapyramidal-related symptoms such as akathisia, dyskinesia, hypokinesia, dystonic reactions, and parkinsonian symptoms have been reported in association with SSRI therapy. SSRIs should be used cautiously with antipsychotic agents because of their ability to potentiate antidopaminergic activity.

Gastrointestinal complaints such as nausea, diarrhea, constipation, vomiting, and anorexia are commonly reported by patients taking SSRIs. Other adverse effects less commonly reported include dry mouth, increased sweating, blurred vision, hyponatremia, and hypoglycemia. Hyponatremia is believed to be secondary inappropriate secretion of antidiuretic hormone. Sexual dysfunction is a relatively common adverse effect of SSRIs. It is especially common in men and has been reported to resolve with cyproheptadine, which is an antiserotonergic drug.

## Drug Interactions

All SSRIs predispose to serotonin syndrome, especially when combined with other serotonergic agents (Table 131-1). Fluoxetine requires a 5-week washout period before starting MAOI therapy. Sertraline and paroxetine only require a 2-week abstinence period before MAOI therapy can be started. Conversely, there should be a 2-week washout period after stopping MAOI therapy before starting any of the SSRIs.

Fluoxetine is the most potent inhibitor of hepatic (P-450) drug metabolism of all the SSRIs. Fluoxetine therapy has been reported to cause elevated levels of carbamazepine, valproic acid, clozapine, haloperidol, perphenazine, diazepam, lithium, and TCAs. Fluoxetine can increase TCA levels between two- and tenfold, which may result in TCA toxicity. Sertraline is not associated with significant impairment of hepatic drug metabolism. Paroxetine rarely affects other drug

**Table 131-1.** Drugs Associated with Serotonin Syndrome

**Monoamine Oxidase Inhibitors**
  Isocarboxazid
  Moclobemide*
  Pargyline
  Phenelzine
  Selegiline
  Tranylcypromine
**Increase Serotonin Release**
  Amphetamines
  Cocaine
  Codeine derivatives
  Fenfluramine
  Reserpine
**Nonselective Inhibitors of Amine Uptake**
  Amitriptyline
  Amphetamines
  Clomipramine
  Cocaine
  Dextromethorphan
  Imipramine
  Venlafaxine
**Selective Inhibitor of Serotonin Uptake**
  Dextromethorphan
  Fluoxetine
  Fluvoxamine
  Meperidine
  Paroxetine
  Sertraline
  Trazodone
**Serotonin Receptor Agonists**
  Buspirone
  Lysergic acid diethylamide (LSD)
  Mescaline
**Nonspecific Serotonin Agonists**
  Bromocriptine
  Bupropion
  Diphenylhydantoin
  Electroconvulsive therapy
  L-Tryptophan
  Levodopa
  Lithium

* Denotes drug not currently available in the United States.

metabolism but may increase bleeding in association with warfarin therapy.

## Acute Toxicity

In general, all of the SSRIs are characterized by a high toxic-to-therapeutic ratio. Most of the SSRI overdose toxicity data comes from analysis of large case series involving single- and mixed-drug fluoxetine overdoses. Significant toxicity is not expected in adult patients who ingest less than 1500 mg fluoxetine. Deaths have occurred following fluoxetine overdose and in most fluoxetine-related fatalities coingestant medications were believed to be primarily responsible for patient death. Currently, there is limited information on sertraline and paroxetine overdose toxicity. Most of this information is in the form of isolated case reports that suggest their toxicity closely resembles that of fluoxetine. At the present time, all SSRIs appear to produce similar toxicity in overdose and management principles can be equally applied to all SSRIs.

Pediatric patients are reportedly less likely to develop symptoms following SSRI overdose than adult patients, which may simply reflect ingestions of lower dose per kilogram in pediatric patients. Approximately 90 percent of all pediatric patients remain asymptomatic, whereas approximately 50 percent of adult patients do not develop symptoms following single-agent SSRI ingestion.

The most common symptoms seen in SSRI overdose include sinus tachycardia, drowsiness, tremor, vomiting, and nausea. These symptoms are almost identical to the adverse effect profile of SSRIs except for sinus tachycardia, which is more common in overdose and rarely reported as an adverse effect. Tachycardia, mild hypertension, and lethargy are more commonly seen when SSRIs are combined with ethanol. Mixed-drug ingestions can produce a wide variety of additional symptoms depending on the coingestant toxicity. Serotonin syndrome can occur as a consequence of acute SSRI overdose.

Ancillary studies are usually normal in SSRI overdose. Routine chemistry tests are rarely abnormal except for the previously mentioned hyponatremia seen with chronic SSRI drug therapy. ECGs are usually normal except for the presence of sinus tachycardia. There have been rare reports nonspecific ST-T wave changes but PR, QRS and QT intervals have not been prolonged.

## Management

All SSRI overdose patients require immediate emergency physician evaluation, establishment of a peripheral intravenous line, and cardiac monitoring. Overall, single-agent SSRI overdose patients have an excellent prognosis. However, these patients occasionally develop life-threatening complications such as generalized seizures and serotonin syndrome.

The best method of gastrointestinal decontamination in SSRI poisoning remains unproven. Activated charcoal (1 g/kg) is recommended for single-agent ingestions of fluoxetine of less than 1000 mg. Gastric lavage is probably unnecessary in these patients. Gastric lavage followed by activated charcoal administration is recommended for mixed-drug overdoses and ingestions of greater than 1000 mg fluoxetine. Corresponding overdose equivalents of sertraline and paroxetine in comparison to 1000 mg fluoxetine have not been currently established. Patients with paroxetine and sertraline overdoses of up to 850 mg and 2100 mg, respectively, have been reported to have survived without sequelae, but the extent of gastrointestinal decontamination performed in these cases is unclear.

All SSRI overdose patients should be observed for 6 h. Supportive care is generally all that is required during this observation period. Hospital admission is recommended for all patients who remain tachycardic or lethargic 6 h after ingestion. Other patients at higher risk for complications include those with predisposing factors for seizures, symptoms of serotonin syndrome, and patients with mixed-drug overdoses that have the potential for delayed onset of toxicity.

Asymptomatic patients can be safely discharged home after 6 h of observation. Some patients may require a psychiatric evaluation prior to discharge.

## VENLAFAXINE

The "newest" of the new antidepressants is venlafaxine (Effexor), which was released in the United States in early 1994. It is a nonselective potent inhibitor of serotonin and norepinephrine amine uptake and a weak inhibitor of dopamine uptake capable of increasing synaptic levels of serotonin, norepinephrine, and dopamine. It remains unproven whether this nonselectivity offers any advantage over SSRIs, bupropion, or trazodone. Venlafaxine has no significant effect on presynaptic or postsynaptic neurotransmitter receptors and does not inhibit MAO activity. It is available in 25-, 37.5-, 50-, 75-, and 100-mg tablets. The recommended starting dose is 75 mg/d, which can be gradually increased up to a maximum daily dose of 375 mg.

### Pharmacology

Venlafaxine is a bicyclic compound that is structurally different from other antidepressants. Peak levels occur 2 h postingestion; it is poorly protein bound (27 percent), has volume of distribution of 7.5 L/kg, and a half-life of approximately 5 h. It has one active metabolite, *O*-desmethylvenlafaxine, which has similar pharmacologic activities as its parent compound but has a longer half-life of 11 h. The majority of venlafaxine undergoes hepatic P-450 oxidation, but it is a weak inhibitor of P-450 enzyme activity. To date, no significant pharmacokinetic drug interactions have been reported.

### Adverse Effects and Drug Interactions

The adverse effect profile for venlafaxine is similar to that described for the SSRIs. The only notable exception is the occurrence of mild to moderate hypertension when doses exceed 225 mg/d, which is probably secondary to inhibition of norepinephrine uptake.

Venlafaxine has the same potential as other serotonin agonists to produce serotonin syndrome. Therefore, it should not be combined with MAOIs or other serotonin agonists. Because of its shorter half-life, venlafaxine only requires a 1-week abstinence period before initiating MAOI therapy. However, a 2-week washout period is still required after discontinuation of MAOIs before starting venlafaxine therapy.

### Toxicity

There are limited data on venlafaxine overdose toxicity. However, its clinical toxicity is expected to resemble that seen in SSRI overdose. Therefore, many patients will probably remain asymptomatic. Patients who develop symptoms will most likely demonstrate some degree of CNS depression, which can be exacerbated by coingestant medications. Coma has occurred following the ingestion of 750 to 1500 mg. Mild to moderate hypertension and sinus tachycardia have been reported but rarely require specific pharmacologic treatment. One patient developed QT interval prolongation. No fatalities have been associated with venlafaxine poisoning. Generalized seizures have been reported but as with SSRI toxicity, seizures are relatively uncommon.

### Management

At the present time, venlafaxine overdose can be managed in a similar fashion as SSRI overdose using the same necessary precautions and observation period. The role of gastric lavage and activated charcoal is unproven in venlafaxine overdose. However, it seems prudent to follow conservative guidelines until more experience with this antidepressant is obtained.

## SEROTONIN SYNDROME

Serotonin syndrome is a recently recognized drug-induced disorder characterized by alterations in cognitive-behavior ability, autonomic nervous system function, and neuromuscular activity. It can be produced by any drug combination that has the net effect of increasing serotonin activity at postsynaptic serotonin-1A brain stem receptors (see Table 131-1). Recent evidence suggests that stimulation of postsynaptic serotonin-2 receptors is also important in mediating serotonin syndrome.

Monoamine oxidase inhibitors and SSRIs are commonly involved in the production of this syndrome, especially when they are combined with other serotonergic drugs such as meperidine, dextromethorphan, venlafaxine, clomipramine, lithium, amphetamines, cocaine, bromocriptine, levodopa, and buspirone.

Serotonin syndrome usually occurs relatively soon after either increasing the dose of a potent serotonin agonist (MAOI or SSRI) or shortly after the addition of a second serotonergic agent (e.g., lithium). Emergency physicians have acutely precipitated serotonin syndrome by administering meperidine (Demerol) to patients taking serotonergic medications, especially MAOIs and SSRIs. For the same reason, dextromethorphan and codeine should also be avoided. Morphine and fentanyl are considered safe alternative intravenous analgesics to meperidine but should be used in lower doses. There are no contraindications to using acetaminophen, salicylates, or nonsteroidal anti-inflammatory agents with serotonin agonists.

The symptoms of serotonin syndrome are nonspecific and are frequently attributed to other psychiatric and medical disorders (Table 131-2). The most common symptoms seen in serotonin syndrome include agitation, anxiety, restlessness, sinus tachycardia, mild hypertension, diaphoresis, hyperreflexia, myoclonus, shivering, tremor, diarrhea, and muscular rigidity. The neuromuscular symptoms are especially prominent in the lower extremities. Less common symptoms include coma, seizures, ventricular tachycardia, hyperthermia, and hypotension. Fatalities have been reported.

The diagnosis of serotonin syndrome is based entirely on clinical suspicion and exclusion of other psychiatric and medical conditions. There are no confirmatory laboratory tests for serotonin syndrome. Serum chemistry tests, drug levels, cerebral spinal fluid analysis, and brain computed tomography scan results are usually within normal limits. Therefore, a normal drug level (e.g., lithium) does not rule out serotonin syndrome.

The treatment of serotonin syndrome includes discontinuing all

**Table 131-2.** Symptoms of Serotonin Syndrome

**Cognitive-Behavioral**
  Agitation, anxiety
  Drowsiness, coma
  Confusion, delirium
  Euphoria, hypomania
  Headache, insomnia
  Seizures
**Autonomic Nervous System**
  Nausea, salivation
  Sinus tachycardia, ventricular tachycardia
  Diaphoresis, diarrhea, abdominal cramps
  Hyperthermia, hypertension, mydriasis
  Cutaneous piloerection, flushed skin
**Neuromuscular**
  Ankle clonus, hyperreflexia
  Restlessness, rigidity
  Shivering, teeth chattering, tremor
  Dysarthria, ataxia, incoordination (clumsiness)
  Head twitching, hyperactivity
  Myoclonic jerks
  Myoclonus, jaw quivering
  Nystagmus, paresthesias
  Babinski (bilateral) sign

serotonergic drugs and providing appropriate supportive care. Patients should be admitted to the hospital until complete resolution of symptoms has occurred. Most patients will show dramatic improvement within 24 h. Complications such as rhabdomyolysis are relatively common when significant muscle rigidity is present.

At the present time, there are no accepted guidelines for the use of serotonin antagonists in the treatment of serotonin syndrome. Isolated human case reports suggest that cyproheptadine, methysergide, and propranolol have the potential to be effective antiserotonergic agents. Benzodiazepines are nonspecific serotonin antagonists and can be used to decrease patient discomfort. Cyproheptadine is the most effective antiserotonergic. The usual dose is 4–8 mg po. This dose can be repeated every 4–6 h up to a maximum of 0.5 mg/kg/day (32 mg/day).

## BIBLIOGRAPHY

Borys DJ, Setzer SC, Ling LJ, et al. Acute fluoxetine overdose: a report of 234 cases. *Am J Emerg Med* 10:115, 1992.

Mills KC. Trazodone toxicity: current concepts. *Topics in Emergency Medicine* 15:37, 1993.

Mills KC. Serotonin toxicity: a comprehensive review for emergency medicine. *Topics in Emergency Medicine* 15:54, 1993.

Rudorfer MV, Manji HK, Potter WZ. Comparative tolerability profiles of the newer versus older antidepressants. *Drug Saf* 10:18, 1994.

Spiller HA, Ramoska EA, Krenzelok EP. Bupropion overdose: a 3-year multicenter retrospective analysis. *Am J Emerg Med* 12:43, 1994.

# 132

# MONOAMINE OXIDASE INHIBITORS
## Kirk C. Mills

## INTRODUCTION

Monoamine oxidase inhibitor (MAOI) overdose represents one of the most complex pharmacologic and toxicologic challenges faced by emergency medicine physicians. During the past 20 years the traditional MAOIs have been infrequently prescribed because of their multiple side effects, cumbersome dietary restrictions, potential for fatal drug interactions, and severe toxicity in overdose. However, MAOI pharmacotherapy is currently experiencing a significant resurgence in popularity, based on broader indications for MAOI drug therapy in a greater number of psychiatric and neurologic conditions and the development of newer MAOI antidepressants that are capable of selective and reversible enzyme inhibition. These newer MAOIs reportedly do not require dietary restrictions and demonstrate decreased toxicity in overdose. Severe drug interactions have still been reported with these newer agents (e.g., serotonin syndrome).

## BIOCHEMISTRY

Monoamine oxidase (MAO) is an intracellular enzyme bound to the outer mitochondrial membrane. It has been identified in all humans cells except erythrocytes, which do not contain mitochondria. Monoamine oxidase removes amine groups from both endogenous and exogenous biogenic amines. This oxidation process is the primary mechanism by which biogenic amines such as norepinephrine (NE), dopamine (DA), and 5-hydroxytryptamine (serotonin or 5-HT) are inactivated. A second important function of MAO is to decrease the systemic availability of absorbed dietary biogenic amines (e.g., tyramine) via hepatic and intestinal metabolism. Therefore, inhibition of MAO leads to the accumulation of neurotransmitters in presynaptic nerve terminals and allows for increased systemic availability of dietary amines.

Monoamine oxidase has a negligible role in metabolizing circulating catecholamines, which are either secreted endogenously (e.g., adrenal gland) or administered intravenously (e.g., epinephrine). This function is accomplished by a different enzyme, catechol-*O*-methyl transferase (COMT), which is not affected by MAOIs.

Monoamine oxidase is actually two separate isoenzymes, designated *MAO-A* and *MAO-B*. In most tissues both isoenzymes coexist and are complementary in function. The human brain has a predominance of type MAO-B, whereas the peripheral sympathetic adrenergic presynaptic neurons demonstrate predominantly MOA-A activity. Each isoenzyme has its own relative preference for different neurotransmitters, dietary amines, and MAOIs. MAO-A prefers NE and 5-HT, and MAO-B prefers phenylethylamine as a substrate. Both enzymes metabolize dopamine and tyramine. Importantly, substrate preference is entirely dose-dependent and can be overcome at higher MAOI doses and/or substrate concentrations.

## PHARMACOLOGY

Monoamine oxidase inhibitors share structural similarities with endogenous amines (e.g., NE, 5-HT) and amphetamines, which allows them to act as potential substrates for MAO. Irreversible MAOIs form covalent bonds with the MAO enzymes and this renders the enzyme permanently inactive. Once an irreversible MAOI has been discontinued, it takes approximately 8 to 12 days before new enzyme synthesis has returned MAO activity to 50 percent of normal.

Reversible MAOIs do not form irreversible covalent bonds with MAO. Thus, new enzyme synthesis is not necessary to restore MAO activity, and MAO activity will gradually return to normal over a period of hours as the drug-enzyme complex spontaneously dissociates. Reversible MAOIs are currently not available in the United States but approval for their release in the near future is inevitable.

Phenelzine (Nardil), tranylcypromine (Parnate), and isocarboxazid (Marplan) represent the only MAOI antidepressants currently available in the United States. They share the ability to produce nonspecific (inhibit both MAO-A and MAO-B) and irreversible inhibition of MAO activity. The daily therapeutic dose ranges for individual MAOI antidepressants are commonly listed as 45 to 90 mg for phenelzine, 30 to 60 mg for tranylcypromine, and 10 to 30 mg for isocarboxazid. The majority of their antidepressant action is believed to be related to increased NE and 5-HT brain concentrations via inhibition of MAO-A. Other potential mechanisms of action include indirect release of neurotransmitters and inhibition of neurotransmitter uptake.

Selegiline (Eldepryl) is a MAOI that is used as adjunctive therapy in Parkinson's disease. It produces selective and irreversible inhibition of MAO-B, which allows for the accumulation of dopamine within brain neurons. The therapeutic dose for selegiline is 10 mg daily. At doses greater than this, selegiline loses its selectivity and behaves similar to other MAOIs.

Pargyline is a seldom-used antihypertensive agent with a relative specificity for MOA-B inhibition. Two other relatively obscure drugs with secondary abilities to inhibit MAO activity are furazolidone (Furoxone), which is an antimicrobial agent, and procarbazine (Matulane), an antineoplastic drug.

Most MAOI antidepressants are rapidly and completely absorbed from the intestinal tract. They undergo extensive first-pass metabolism by the liver and are highly protein bound. Peak drug levels usually occur 1 to 2 h after ingestion, and their volume of distribution ranges from 1 to 5 L/kg. In general, their half-life is between 2 and 3 h. It is important to recognize that clinical toxicity is usually delayed long after most of the MAOI has already been metabolized. Thus, blood MAOI levels do not correlate with clinical toxicity.

# TYRAMINE REACTION

Tyramine is an exogenous bioamine that is normally metabolized by MAO enzymes located in the intestinal mucosa (MAO-A) and liver (MAO-B). In patients taking a nonselective MAOI, a greater proportion of ingested tyramine can potentially reach the systemic circulation. Indirect-acting biogenic amines, including tyramine, enter presynaptic neurons through amine uptake pumps. Once inside the neuron these amines are capable of displacing NE and 5-HT out of the nerve terminal and into the neuronal synapse. This action produces the so-called cheese reaction since aged cheese contains a large amount of tyramine. Thus, patients on MAOI therapy must be careful to avoid foods with high tyramine content.

Tyramine is found in over 70 foods and beverages, and any of these sources may trigger such a reaction. Patient compliance to a MAOI restrictive diet has been reported to be below 30 percent. Approximately 4 to 8 percent of all patients taking MAOIs and following a prescribed diet will experience this reaction during their course of therapy.

It is estimated that 6 to 10 mg of tyramine can produce the "cheese reaction" in patients on MAOIs. Newer guidelines call for avoiding only a few high-risk food groups such as unfresh meat or fish, sauerkraut, aged meats and cheeses, alcohol (Chianti wine and vermouth), pickled fish (herring), concentrated yeast extracts, and broad beans.

The tyramine reaction can be produced by any indirect-acting sympathomimetic, whether a dietary amine or an ingested drug such as amphetamine (see Table 132-1). Many over-the-counter preparations contain potentially dangerous indirect-acting sympathomimetics.

The typical tyramine reaction occurs within 30 to 90 min after ingesting the dietary amine. The severity of this reaction is highly variable and partially related to the total amount of tyramine ingested. Symptoms include severe occipital or temporal headache, diaphoresis, mydriasis, neck stiffness, neuromuscular excitation, and increased systolic and diastolic blood pressures. Fatalities have been reported secondary to the MAOI-tyramine interaction and are usually from an intracranial hemorrhage or myocardial infarction.

Most symptoms gradually resolve over 6 to 12 h without specific therapy. In cases of severe hypertension the drug of choice remains phentolamine (Regitine), which is given intravenously in 2.5- to 5-mg doses every 5 to 15 min until the blood pressure is controlled. An alternative treatment approach in cases of moderate hypertension is to initially give 10 mg sublingual nifedipine (Procardia). Hospital admission is recommended for patients whose symptoms do not completely resolve within 6 h after onset.

# DRUG INTERACTIONS

Chronic MAOI drug therapy predisposes to many potentially significant drug interactions (see Table 132-1). Medications that are contraindicated because they can augment sympathetic nervous system activity include any indirect-acting sympathomimetic drug, reserpine, guanethidine, bretylium, and cocaine. Other medications that should be avoided, mostly based on theoretical concerns of precipitating cardiovascular complications, include β-blockers, phenothiazines, theophylline, and ketamine. Other important MAOI-drug interactions can occur with oral hypoglycemic agents, codeine, and anticholinergic drugs.

There should always be at least a 2-week abstinence period between the time the MAOI is discontinued and the time that any contraindicated drug is administered. This abstinence period allows for new MAO enzyme synthesis.

Serotonin syndrome is an important drug-related complication that is commonly associated with MAOIs, especially in combination with any of the medications listed in Table 132-2. A partial list of medications that can produce serotonin syndrome in patients on MAOI therapy include meperidine, dextromethorphan, lithium, levodopa, fluox-

**Table 132-1.** Contraindicated Drugs with MAOIs*

| Indirect sympathomimetics | Miscellaneous drugs |
| --- | --- |
| Amphetamines | Anticholinergics |
| Bretylium | Beta-blockers |
| Cocaine | Caffeine |
| Cylert | Codeine |
| Dopamine | Dextromethorphan |
| Ephedrine | Disulfiram |
| Flenfluramine | Ketamine |
| Guanethidine | Levodopa |
| Metaraminol | Meperidine |
| Methyldopa | Oral hypoglycemic agents |
| Methylphenidate | Phenothiazines |
| Phencyclidine | Serotonin reuptake inhibitors |
| Phenylephrine | Theophylline |
| Phenylpropanolamine | Tricyclic antidepressants |
| Pseudoephedrine | Tryptophan |
| Reserpine | |
| Tyramine | |

* See Table 131-2 for additional list of drugs that cause serotonin syndrome.

etine, sertraline, paroxetine, buspirone, trazodone, and L-tryptophan. Serotonin syndrome is described in detail in Chap. 131, "Newer Antidepressants."

Aspirin, acetaminophen, ibuprofen, morphine, and fentanyl are regarded as safe analgesics in patients on MAOIs. Morphine and fentanyl should be given in decreased doses. Direct-acting sympathomimetic agents are safe to use as vasopressors because they do not rely on the release of neurotransmitters for their activity and are inactivated by the enzyme COMT, which is unaffected by MAOIs (see Table 132-2).

# TOXIC DOSE

MAOIs have a dangerously low toxic to therapeutic ratio. The lowest MAOI dose considered to be life-threatening is 2 to 3 mg per kilogram of patient body weight. Doses less than 2 mg/kg may still produce mild to moderate toxicity. The lethal dose is reported to be between 4 and 6 mg/kg. Deaths have been reported in adults with between 170 and 650 mg of tranylcypromine and 375 and 1500 mg of phenelzine. Spontaneous hypertensive episodes can occur in patients on therapeutic doses of MAOIs.

# ACUTE OVERDOSE

An important aspect of MAOI overdose is the characteristic delay in onset of initial symptoms that ranges between 6 and 12 hours postingestion but can be delayed for up to 29 h. The delayed onset of toxicity is believed to be secondary to the gradual accumulation of NE and 5-HT levels in the brain and in peripheral sympathetic neurons. Therefore, symptoms of a MAOI overdose are most consistent with a hyperadrenergic state secondary to excessive α- and β-adren-

**Table 132-2.** Drugs Considered Safe with MAOIs

| Direct sympathomimetics | Miscellaneous drugs (cont.) |
| --- | --- |
| Albuterol | Barbiturates |
| Clonidine | Benzodiazepines |
| Dobutamine | Calcium channel blockers |
| Epinephrine | Corticosteroids |
| Isoproterenol | Lidocaine |
| Methoxamine | Metoclopromide |
| Norepinephrine | Morphine |
| Salbutamol | Nitroglycerin |
| Terbutaline | Nonsteroidal anti-inflammatory drugs |
| Miscellaneous drugs | Ondansetron |
| Acetaminophen | Procainamide |
| Antibiotics | |
| Aspirin | |

ergic receptor stimulation but also include symptoms related to excessive serotonin receptor activity. Patients on chronic MAOI therapy may show earlier signs of toxicity due to preexisting enzyme inhibition. In severe cases the hyperadrenergic state can be rapidly followed by hypotension and central nervous system depression.

The initial symptoms of MAOI overdose are headache, agitation, restlessness, nausea, palpitations, and tremor. The earliest signs of MAOI toxicity include sinus tachycardia, hyperreflexia, fasciculations, mydriasis, hyperventilation, nystagmus, and generalized flushing. In cases of moderate toxicity opisthotonus, muscle rigidity, diaphoresis, chest pain, hypertension, diarrhea, hallucinations, combativeness, confusion, marked hyperthermia, and trismus may become evident.

Severe toxicity is diagnosed by bradycardia, cardiac arrest, hypoxia, papilledema, hypotension, seizures, coma, and worsening hyperthermia. Hypotension is an ominous finding and it usually remains resistant to therapeutic attempts at correction. Fetal demise, cerebral edema, pulmonary edema, and intracranial hemorrhage have all been reported in association with MAOI overdoses. The most common electrocardiographic abnormality seen in MAOI toxicity is sinus tachycardia, but T-wave abnormalities are not uncommon.

## DIFFERENTIAL DIAGNOSIS

The differential diagnosis of a MAOI overdose includes all drugs and medical conditions capable of producing a hyperadrenergic state. Toxicologic possibilities include cocaine, phencyclidine, amphetamines, phenylpropanolamine, methylphenidate, theophylline, strychnine, salicylates, nicotine, and anticholinergic drugs. The abrupt withdrawal of β blockers, clonidine, sedative-hypnotics, and alcohol can produce hyperadrenergic symptoms. Neuroleptic malignant syndrome, serotonin syndrome, and malignant hyperthermia are all capable of producing muscle rigidity, hyperthermia, and autonomic nervous system dysfunction. Medical conditions that may mimic symptoms of MAOI overdose include hypoglycemia, hyperthyroidism, pheochromocytoma, heat stroke, meningitis, sepsis, tetanus, rabies, and encephalitis.

## LABORATORY STUDIES

Monoamine oxidase inhibitor poisoning is not associated with any pathognomonic laboratory tests. Plasma MAOI levels and drug screens cannot be relied upon to assist in making the diagnosis of MAOI toxicity for two reasons: (1) plasma MAOI levels are not routinely available in most hospitals nor do they correlate with observed clinical toxicity; (2) all commonly used drug screens currently are unable to detect MAOIs. Selegiline and tranylcypromine have the potential to produce amphetamine metabolites, which are occasionally identified on routine plasma or urine drug testing.

The best use of laboratory tests is to assist in the differential diagnosis of MAOI toxicity and to identify possible complications of MAOI overdose; these complications include hypoxia, rhabdomyolysis, renal failure, hyperkalemia, metabolic acidosis, hemolysis, and disseminated intravascular coagulation.

## MANAGEMENT

### General Emergency Department Care

All MAOI overdose patients require immediate emergency physician evaluation, establishment of at least one peripheral intravenous line, and cardiac monitoring. These patients are at high risk for the rapid development of seizures, coma, respiratory insufficiency, hyperadrenergic storm, and cardiovascular collapse. Patients with predisposing medical problems, chronic use of MAOIs, or at the extremes of age will manifest greater toxicity at any given MAOI dose.

Gastric lavage is most beneficial when it is performed within 4 h

after MAOI overdose and should be followed by giving 1 g/kg of activated charcoal. There is no proven benefit in giving repeat doses of activated charcoal in MAOI poisoning. Patients who present more than 4 h postingestion probably only require activated charcoal. Syrup of ipecac is contraindicated in the setting of MAOI overdose. Hemodialysis, hemoperfusion, and peritoneal dialysis have no current role in the treatment of MAOI poisoning. Urinary acidification is not recommended because it is ineffective at enhancing MAOI elimination and it predisposes to acute renal failure secondary to myoglobin precipitation within renal tubules.

### Management of Specific Conditions

#### Hypertension

Only short-acting intravenous antihypertensive agents should be used in the acutely hypertensive patient because of the potential to develop precipitous hypotension. An intraarterial catheter is recommended for accurate blood pressure monitoring. The antihypertensive agents of choice are phentolamine and nitroprusside. Phentolamine is a nonspecific α-adrenergic receptor blocker usually administered in 2.5- to 5.0-mg doses every 10 to 15 min until blood pressure elevation is controlled. It can also be given as a continuous infusion for maintenance therapy. Nitroprusside is equally effective and is only given as a continuous infusion with an initial rate of 1 μg/kg per minute and then titrated according to blood pressure response. Nitroglycerin is indicated for the relief of anginal chest pain and in patients with evidence of myocardial ischemia.

#### Hypotension

Hypotension carries a poor prognosis in MAOI overdose. Isotonic IV fluid boluses of 10 to 20 mL/kg are the initial treatment of hypotension. When vasopressors are required it is important to avoid all indirect-acting agents (see Table 132-1). Norepinephrine is the vasopressor of choice, with epinephrine as a second-line drug due to its β-agonist vasodilation activity. MAOI patients usually demonstrate an increased sensitivity to vasopressors, and lower doses are initially recommended.

#### Dysrhythmias

Sinus tachycardia rarely requires specific drug therapy unless it is producing cardiac ischemia. Lidocaine, procainamide, and phenytoin are the most effective antiarrhythmics in treating MAOI-induced dysrhythmias. Bradycardia may quickly degrade into asystole in the later stages of the overdose and require pacemaker intervention. Pharmacologic treatment of bradycardia includes atropine, isoproterenol, and dobutamine. Bretylium should be avoided due to its indirect sympathomimetic activity.

Beta-blockers pose a theoretical risk of increasing the blood pressure through unopposed vasoconstriction. Despite this fact, β blockers have been used to treat hyperadrenergic symptoms in MAOI overdose without serious complications. At best, β blockers should be used with great caution in the setting of MAOI toxicity.

#### Seizures

Benzodiazepines and barbiturates are the anticonvulsants of choice in treating MAOI-induced seizures. Barbiturates are probably equally as effective as benzodiazepines but may cause hypotension. Phenytoin is generally ineffective in stopping drug-induced seizures. General anesthesia and/or muscle paralysis may be necessary in cases of status epilepticus to prevent the metabolic acidosis, hyperthermia, and rhabdomyolysis that commonly accompany persistent seizure activity. Muscle paralysis is best accomplished using nondepolarizing neuromuscular blocking agents.

## Hyperthermia

Antipyretics are generally ineffective at lowering drug-induced fever. Benzodiazepines help reduce muscle hyperactivity, and muscle paralysis may also be needed to reduce heat production secondary to generalized muscle rigidity. Once heat production has been controlled, then increasing evaporative and conductive heat loss is indicated. This can be accomplished by using cool mist spray, evaporative fans, and ice baths. Dantrolene can be used in resistant cases of muscle rigidity. Dantrolene doses have been reported between 2.5 and 10 mg/kg IV per day in divided doses (usually every 6 h). Older reports of MAOI-induced hyperthermia cited successful treatment with phenothiazines (chlorpromazine). However, these agents are not currently recommended because of their potential to lower the seizure threshold, worsen hypotension, and produce dystonic reactions.

## ADMISSION CRITERIA

Hospital admission to an intensive care unit is recommended for all intentional MAOI overdoses and accidental ingestions of greater than 2 mg/kg. Vital signs must be obtained frequently while the patient is being monitored. Dietary and medication restrictions should be followed during the hospitalization. Consultation with a medical toxicologist through the nearest regional poison center is also recommended.

Patients who require transfer from hospitals without intensive care capabilities should be transferred as soon as possible to avoid the problems anticipated with delayed onset of toxicity. All patients being transferred should be accompanied by medical personnel capable of performing advanced cardiac life support and endotracheal intubation.

## BIBLIOGRAPHY

Jarrott B, Vajda FLE: The current status of monoamine oxidase and its inhibitors. *Med J Aust* 146:634, 1987.

Lippman SB, Nash K: Monoamine oxidase inhibitor update: Potential adverse food and drug interactions. *Drug Safety* 5(3):195, 1990.

Mills KC: Monoamine oxidase inhibitor toxicity. *Top Emerg Med* 15(3):58, 1993.

Mills KC: Serotonin toxicity: A comprehensive review for emergency medicine. *Top Emerg Med* 15(4):54, 1993.

Wells DG: Monoamine oxidase inhibitors revisited. *Can J Anaesth* 36(1):64, 1989.

# 133
# NEUROLEPTICS
## William P. Kerns II

## INTRODUCTION

The term *neuroleptic* refers to a diverse group of antipsychotics and major tranquilizers used in the treatment of schizophrenia and other psychoses. Patients for whom neuroleptics are prescribed present a risk for therapeutic misadventure and intentional ingestion because of their behavioral unpredictability. Thus, emergency physicians need a firm understanding of the pharmacology of neuroleptic agents, potential adverse reactions, and effects of acute ingestion.

## PHARMACOLOGY

Neuroleptics comprise a group of five classes of drugs (Table 133-1) that share a basic three-ring structure. While all five classes have similar general therapeutic and adverse effects, modifications of the base structure alter the potency of the drug and prevalence of the various side effects.

Neuroleptics act by blocking dopaminergic ($D_1$ and $D_2$), adrenergic ($\alpha_1$ and $\alpha_2$), muscarinic, and histaminic ($H_1$ and $H_2$) neurotransmission receptors. The $D_2$-dopaminergic receptor blockade provides the beneficial effects of behavior modification but is also responsible for the extrapyramidal symptoms that may occur. Blockade of $\alpha$-adrenergic receptors results in vasodilation with orthostatic hypotension. Muscarinic receptor antagonism results in mydriasis, tachycardia, hyperthermia, flushing, dry mouth, urinary retention, and constipation. Histamine blockade may produce either central nervous system (CNS) stimulation or sedation.

## PHARMACOKINETICS

The pharmacokinetics of haloperidol are typical of neuroleptics. Oral bioavailability is 60 percent of a given dose. Peak plasma concentrations occur 2 to 6 h after oral administration and 10 to 20 min following intramuscular use. Peak pharmacologic activity is slightly delayed compared to peak serum concentrations, occurring 30 to 45 min after intramuscular injection. Once absorbed, approximately 90 percent of the drug is bound to plasma protein. The volume of distribution is 18 to 30 L/kg. High protein binding and a large volume of distribution preclude the use of dialysis for overdoses. Metabolism occurs in the liver via oxidation and reduction, with some enterohepatic circulation. The reported elimination half-life is 14 to 91 h. Because the drug undergoes enterohepatic circulation, multiple doses of activated charcoal may be of theoretical use to enhance drug elimination. These kinetic data are obtained from individuals taking therapeutic doses under well-controlled conditions. Kinetics may be altered in overdose situations due to the effects of large amounts of ingested drug, delays in gastric emptying, coingestants, or the premorbid condition of the patient.

## THERAPEUTIC INDICATIONS

Psychiatric indications for neuroleptics include schizophrenia, schizoaffective disorders, mania, major depression with psychotic features, paranoid disorders, and atypical psychoses.

Neuroleptics are also used for nonpsychiatric conditions. The most common nonpsychiatric use is to control nausea and emesis. The antiemetic action results from dopaminergic blockade in the chemoreceptor trigger zone of the medulla, the area that controls vomiting. Recent reports have shown beneficial effects of chlorpromazine in relief of vascular and tension headaches. Other entities for which neuroleptics have been used include hiccoughs, involuntary motor movements from Gilles de la Tourette syndrome, Huntington chorea, chorea in rheumatic fever, and Meige syndrome.

Exercise caution when considering neuroleptic use in certain clinical situations. The commonly used antiemetics, prochlorperazine and promethazine, are both class C fetal risk agents and are given to pregnant patients suffering from vomiting when the potential benefit justifies the risk to the fetus. Neuroleptics are not optimal agents to control the agitated patient experiencing alcohol withdrawal, sedative withdrawal, or acute cocaine intoxication. Treatment of cocaine toxicity in animals with haloperidol has not altered mortality, and treatment with chlorpromazine has resulted in a higher incidence of seizures. Benzodiazepines are the pharmacotherapy of choice in these situations, because they are more efficacious than neuroleptics in alcohol and sedative withdrawal and they reduce mortality in experi-

**Table 133-1.** The Five Neuroleptic Classes

| Class | Dose Range, mg/day | Dopaminergic Antagonism | Muscarinic Antagonism | Adrenergic Antagonism |
|---|---|---|---|---|
| Butyrophenone | | | | |
|   Haloperidol | 1–100 | High | Low | Moderate |
|   Droperidol | 1.25–10 | High | Low | Moderate |
| Dibenzoxazepines | | | | |
|   Loxapine | 10–300 | Low | Moderate | Low |
| Dihydroindolone | | | | |
|   Molindone | 15–225 | Low | Low | Low |
| Phenothiazines | | | | |
|   Aliphatics | | | | |
|     Chlorpromazine | 25–2000 | Low | High | High |
|     Promethazine | 50–150 | Low | High | Moderate |
|   Piperidines | | | | |
|     Mesoridazine | 75–400 | Low | High | High |
|     Thioridazine | 50–800 | Low | High | Moderate |
|   Piperazines | | | | |
|     Prochlorperazine | 15–150 | Moderate | Moderate | Low |
|     Fluphenazine | 1–25 | High | Moderate | Moderate |
| Thioxanthenes | | | | |
|   Thiothixene | 6–60 | High | Low | Moderate |

mental cocaine toxicity. However, some agitated patients may require neuroleptics as adjunctive therapy if they do not respond to benzodiazepines alone.

## ADVERSE EFFECTS

The adverse effects of neuroleptic therapy are related to the type of neurotransmitter receptors each drug antagonizes. The lower-potency agents such as chlorpromazine and mesoridazine have more anticholinergic, antiadrenergic, and antihistaminic adverse reactions. The higher-potency agents such as thiothixene and haloperidol have predominantly antidopaminergic side effects. The antimuscarinic, antihistaminic, and antiadrenergic effects are common adverse reactions of many medications and will not be considered further. Dopamine antagonism results in a variety of abnormal motor movement disorders that may be classified by time of presentation during therapy. Early reactions develop in the first few days to weeks of therapy, while late complications occur after several months of treatment (Table 133-2).

*Dystonias* are idiosyncratic drug reactions that consist of acute involuntary muscle movement and spasm. Laryngeal spasm is a rare dystonic reaction that can cause respiratory compromise. Unless a medication history is sought, the dystonia may be confused with tetanus, strychnine toxicity, atypical seizures, or hysteria. Relief of symptoms is achieved with parenteral administration of 50 mg diphenhydramine or 2 mg benztropine. Resolution occurs within 5 to 15 min. Oral therapy with either agent is then maintained for 2 to 3 days because of the prolonged action of the neuroleptic medication and risk of recurrence of the dystonic reaction. Because dystonias are idiosyncratic and not dose-dependent, prophylactic therapy is not indicated when using neuroleptics unless there is a prior history of a dystonic reaction.

*Akathisia* is a condition of motor restlessness. The symptoms may be subtle and falsely ascribed to worsening psychosis. As a result, the patient is often given increased doses of medication that result in worsening symptoms. Dosage decrease or change to a less potent neuroleptic will relieve akathisia and should occur in consultation with the patient's psychiatrist. Treatment of akathisia has also included amantadine, benztropine, and propranolol.

*Drug-induced parkinsonism* occurs due to dopamine blockade in the nigrostriatal brain pathway. Parkinsonian symptoms are reversible with reduction in dosage, change to a less potent neuroleptic, or treatment with either benztropine or amantadine.

*Tardive dyskinesia* is a movement disorder in which the patient experiences repetitive, rhythmic motions of facial muscles and limbs. Unlike the other disorders, it is secondary to increased dopaminergic effects on the nigrostriatal pathway. Postulated mechanisms include the development of supersensitivity to dopamine at the receptor site or an increased number of dopamine receptors that occur in response to the dopaminergic blockade by the neuroleptic medication. Tardive dyskinesia is a disfiguring and debilitating adverse effect that is not readily reversible. One follow-up study showed no change in symp-

**Table 133-2.** Adverse Reactions to Neuroleptics

| Type of Disorder | Presentation | Incidence | Treatment |
|---|---|---|---|
| Dystonic reaction<br>  Torticollis, facial grimacing, opisthotonos,<br>    oculogyric crisis, laryngeal spasm | Early | 12%<br>>males | Diphenhydramine, 50 mg, or benztropine,<br>  2 mg, IM/IV |
| Akathisia<br>  Restlessness, jittery feeling, insomnia | Early | 20%<br>>females | Lower dose or change to less potent drug;<br>  benztropine, amantadine, or propranolol |
| Parkinsonism<br>  Resting tremor, rigidity, masked facies | Early | 13%<br>>females | Lower dose or change to less potent drug;<br>  benztropine or amantadine |
| Tardive dyskinesia<br>  Lip smacking, tongue protrusion,<br>    grimacing, chewing motion | Late | 30%<br>>females | No proven treatment |
| NMS<br>  Hyperthermia, rigidity, altered mental status,<br>    autonomic instability | Variable | <3%<br>>males | ABCs, muscle relaxation, cooling, rehydration |

toms in two thirds of the patients 2 years after diagnosis. There is no proven beneficial treatment.

## Neuroleptic Malignant Syndrome

Neuroleptic malignant syndrome (NMS) is a life-threatening reaction to neuroleptic medication that may occur at any time during therapy. The cardinal features of the syndrome include hyperthermia, muscular rigidity, altered level of consciousness, and autonomic instability. The incidence is approximately 0.02 to 3.2 percent in patients treated with neuroleptic drugs, most commonly haloperidol. Patients receiving neuroleptics and concomitant drug therapy with lithium, cyclic antidepressants, monoamine oxidase inhibitors, and antiparkinson agents are at increased risk. The differential diagnosis includes meningitis, encephalitis, tetanus, strychnine poisoning, vascular CNS events, malignant hyperthermia, heatstroke, and fatal catatonia.

There are several proposed mechanisms, but the antidopaminergic theory is favored. This theory derives support because muscular rigidity may result from dopamine antagonism in the nigrostriatal pathway and hyperthermia may occur from blockade of hypothalamic thermoregulation. NMS has also been reported following withdrawal of dopamine agonists in parkinsonian patients. Others suggest that endorphins may have a role via modulation of dopaminergic neurotransmission.

The typical presentation is a young male brought to the hospital because of high fever and altered mental status. Temperatures may be as high as 41°C (106°F). Other signs are tachycardia and labile blood pressure. The mental status ranges from confusion to coma, but coma is more common. The muscular hypertonicity has been likened to lead-pipe rigidity.

Predominant laboratory findings include leukocytosis, elevated creatine phosphokinase (CPK), elevated hepatic transaminases, acidosis, and myoglobinuria. Electrolyte and renal function tests reflect the patient's degree of acidosis and dehydration. Cerebrospinal fluid is normal. Blood, sputum, urine, and spinal fluid cultures are negative unless a secondary infection ensues.

Successful management of NMS hinges on considering the diagnosis, followed by meticulous intensive care aimed at providing adequate ventilation, rehydration, relief of muscle rigidity, reversal of hyperthermia, and anticipation of complications (Table 133-3). Neuroleptics should be discontinued.

The use of specific drug agents as antidotes in NMS is controversial, and the rarity of this disease makes controlled clinical trials of therapeutic modalities difficult. Intravenous benzodiazepines and, if necessary, neuromuscular paralytic agents are the first-line agents for muscular relaxation. Their onset of action is rapid and predictable. Large doses of diazepam may be required to achieve the desired effect. If muscular rigidity remains after 10 to 15 min of diazepam therapy, the patient then undergoes rapid-sequence intubation followed by treatment with a paralytic agent such as pancuronium. Bromocriptine, a dopamine agonist, and dantrolene, a direct skeletal muscle relaxant, have been reported effective in anecdotal case reports. However, their efficacy in retrospective reviews is conflicting. In addition, their lack of rapid effect precludes their use in the immediate therapy of NMS, and their role as adjuncts to benzodiazepines and neuromuscular paralysis has yet to be evaluated in clinical trials.

**Table 133-3.** Initial Care of Neuroleptic Malignant Syndrome

1. Airway, breathing, IV access, and cardiac monitor.
2. Immediate skeletal muscle relaxation with repeated doses of intravenous diazepam and, if necessary, rapid-sequence intubation followed by paralysis with pancuronium.
3. Reverse hyperthermia using mist and fan technique or packing in ice.
4. Rehydrate with IV crystalloid.
5. Obtain blood samples for ABG, WBC, Hgb, Hct, glucose, electrolytes, BUN, creatinine, CPK, hepatic enzymes, PT, PTT. Send urine for myoglobin.

A recent review reports a mortality rate of 10 percent. Complications of NMS occur in one third of affected patients. Pulmonary complications predominate and include aspiration pneumonia, pulmonary embolism, pulmonary edema, and acute respiratory failure secondary to restricted chest wall motion. Other reported complications include rhabdomyolysis, renal failure, cardiac dysrhythmias, disseminated intravascular coagulation, and, rarely, seizures.

## ACUTE OVERDOSE

### Clinical Findings

Central nervous system depression, from mild sedation to coma, typically occurs. Both coma and respiratory depression are less common with isolated neuroleptic ingestion; however, their incidence increases with the coingestion of other CNS depressants. Dysfunction of hypothalamic thermal regulation may result in hypothermia or, less commonly, hyperthermia. Pinpoint pupils have been associated with phenothiazine ingestion. Any of the previously described abnormal motor movement reactions may occur. Seizures have been reported.

Anticholinergic symptoms (flushing, dry mouth, hyperthermia, tachycardia, urinary retention, and constipation) are seen with ingestion of lower-potency agents such as chlorpromazine, thioridazine, or mesoridazine.

Hypotension and reflex tachycardia due to α-adrenergic blockade occur frequently. Thioridazine and mesoridazine (piperidine phenothiazines) exert a quinidine-like action on myocardial tissue and can produce prolongation of the PR or QT interval and widening of the QRS complex. Ventricular arrhythmias, including torsade de pointes, have occurred 10 to 15 h after acute ingestion of thioridazine and mesoridazine. Several recent case reports have also implicated haloperidol as a cause of torsade both in overdose and during neuroleptization of agitated intensive care patients. Supraventricular tachycardia and atrioventricular dissociation have been reported in neuroleptic overdose.

Acute pulmonary edema associated with intentional ingestion of aliphatic phenothiazines (chlorpromazine and perphenazine) has recently been reported.

### Management

Supportive care and gastrointestinal decontamination are the mainstays of successful management (Table 133-4). Focus initial attention on ensuring a patent airway and adequate ventilation. Give naloxone

**Table 133-4.** Care of Acute Ingestion

1. Airway, breathing, IV access, cardiac monitor
2. Altered mental status
   a. Naloxone
   b. Empiric dextrose (or rapid glucose determination)
3. Hypotension
   a. Crystalloid infusion
   b. Norepinephrine or phenylephrine
4. Ventricular arrhythmias
   a. Bicarbonate, 1–2 mEq/kg IV bolus
   b. Lidocaine or phenytoin
5. Torsade de pointes
   a. Magnesium
   b. Isoproterenol
   c. Overdrive pacing
6. Gastrointestinal decontamination:
   a. Activated charcoal 1 gm/kg PO
   b. If patient is intubated, orogastric lavage using > 34 Fr tube, followed by activated charcoal
7. Warming or cooling techniques for hypo- or hyperthermia
8. Seizures
   a. Benzodiazepines
   b. Phenobarbital
   c. Phenytoin

and dextrose to patients with altered mental status. Administer crystalloid to treat hypotension. If crystalloid therapy fails and hypotension persists, initiate vasopressor therapy with a predominant α-agonist agent.

Continuous cardiac monitoring and a 12-lead ECG are essential. Manage ventricular arrhythmias with class 1B antiarrhythmics or bicarbonate therapy. Bicarbonate restores the activity of fast inward sodium channels responsible for the phase 0 depolarization of myocardial conducting tissue. Avoid class 1A antiarrhythmics (disopyramide, quinidine, and procainamide) as they may exacerbate the cardiac toxicity. Ventricular tachycardia with torsade de pointes is usually amenable to magnesium, isoproterenol, or overdrive pacing.

Obtain appropriate diagnostic studies to identify reversible effects of neuroleptics and other coingestants. Helpful laboratory tests include: glucose, electrolytes, and renal function. A qualitative urine drug screen may show the presence of neuroleptics. Blood levels are not useful as levels do not correlate with symptoms and do not alter management. A radiograph of the abdomen may demonstrate radiopaque phenothiazine pills.

Gastrointestinal decontamination to prevent systemic absorption of drug is integral in the management of acute ingestion. Give all patients activated charcoal (1 g/kg PO). Multidose charcoal (0.5 g/kg q 4 h) is of theoretical benefit in removing drug from the enterohepatic circulation, thus reducing drug bioavailability and accelerating elimination. However, there are no studies confirming clinical benefit of multidose charcoal in neuroleptic overdose. Weigh the decision to employ gastric emptying on a case-by-case basis. The mildly symptomatic patient may do well with charcoal therapy alone. A large clinical study of overdoses suggests that severely obtunded patients requiring intubation benefit from gastric lavage with a large-bore orogastric tube. Activated charcoal is instilled following lavage. The abdominal radiograph may assist in determining the need for gastric lavage and to judge its efficacy. A patient found to have a large number of radiopaque pills in the stomach might benefit from lavage.

Attempts at enhancing elimination via hemodialysis are futile as neuroleptics are highly protein-bound and have large volumes of distribution. Forced diuresis will not be of benefit as most of these drugs have minimal renal clearance.

When the patient's condition stabilizes, direct therapy to other complications. Correct temperature abnormalities. Treat abnormal motor reactions as previously described. Pharmacotherapy of seizures includes intravenous benzodiazepines, phenobarbital, or phenytoin. Physostigmine has no role in acute neuroleptic ingestion because of the risk of seizures.

### Disposition

Manage symptomatic patients in the intensive care unit. Admit patients who ingest thioridazine or mesoridazine for 24 h of cardiac monitoring, even if they are asymptomatic, because of potential delayed cardiac dysrhythmias. Patients are medically safe for psychiatric disposition from the emergency department if they meet the following criteria: (1) they are asymptomatic with normal vital signs, physical examination, and ECG after several hours of observation; (2) there is no suspicion of thioridazine or mesoridazine ingestion; (3) they receive gastrointestinal decontamination; and (4) sequelae from coingestants are not anticipated.

With strong supportive care and adequate gut decontamination, the acutely intoxicated patient experiences little morbidity or mortality. The 1992 American Association of Poison Control Centers data revealed only 27 deaths in 11,379 neuroleptic exposures.

### BIBLIOGRAPHY

Black JL, Richelson E, Richardson JW: Antipsychotic agents: A clinical update. *Mayo Clin Proc* 60:777, 1985.

Caroff SN, Mann SC: Neuroleptic malignant syndrome. *Med Clin North Am* 77:185, 1993.

Cheng L, Gefter WB: Acute pulmonary edema induced by overdosage of phenothiazines. *Chest* 101:102, 1992.

Dubin WR, Feld JA: Rapid tranquilization of the violent patient. *Am J Emerg Med* 7:313, 1989.

Goldfrank LR, Bresnitz EA, Lewin NA: Antipsychotic agents, in Goldfrank LR, Flomenbaum NE, Lewin NA, et al. (eds): *Goldfranks Toxicologic Emergencies,* 4th ed. Norwalk, CT, Appleton/Lange, 1990, pp 413–419.

Le Blaye I, Donatini B, Hall M, Krupp P: Acute overdosage with thioridazine: A review of the available clinical exposure. *Vet Hum Toxicol* 35:147, 1993.

Richelson E: Neuroleptic affinities for human brain receptors and their use in predicting adverse effects. *J Clin Psychiatry* 45:331, 1984.

Wilt JL, Minnema AM, Johnson RF, Rosenblum AM: Brief report: Torsades de pointes associated with the use of intravenous haloperidol. *Ann Intern Med* 119:391, 1993.

# 134
# LITHIUM
## P. J. Ryan

Lithium carbonate is a widely used psychotropic drug, primarily for the treatment of bipolar, manic-depressive, affective disorders. Lithium has a low therapeutic index, which is the key to understanding the narrow range between adequate dosage and drug toxicity. The most serious toxic effects involve the central nervous system, which in a severe poisoning may result in a 10 to 20 percent mortality.

### PHARMACOLOGIC PROPERTIES

Lithium, a monovalent cation, in the carbonate salt form is 99 percent absorbed following an oral dose. Peak absorption is in 1 to 4 h; complete absorption occurs in 8 h. During a 12- to 18-h distribution phase, it circulates unbound to plasma proteins, with an equilibrium volume of distribution approximating total body water, 0.6 to 0.8 L/kg. Lithium moves into and out of tissues slowly due to its property of delayed cellular membrane transfer. A blood-brain equilibrium (therapeutic state) may take 8 to 10 days. The average plasma half-life of lithium is 20 to 24 h, increasing with age and renal dysfunction.

Excretion is primarily renal and occurs in two phases. Two-thirds of a single dose is cleared in the urine by 6 to 12 h. The remainder is completely cleared over 10 to 14 days. Lithium has complete glomerular filtration; the proximal tubule reabsorbs 60 to 80 percent. No absorption occurs in the distal tubule. Renal clearance of lithium is 15 to 30 mL/min. An increased clearance is found with an alkaline urine, and a decreased clearance results with hyponatremia and renal insufficiency.

Therapeutic serum levels are 0.6 to 1.2 mEq/L. Levels should be obtained 10 to 15 h post dosage to make sure absorption and distribution are complete. A 300-mg dose of lithium carbonate equals 8.1 mEq and may increase serum levels by 0.2 to 0.4 mEq/L. Both therapeutic action and toxic effects of lithium are mediated intracellularly. Thus lithium serum levels may not be a true reflection of the biologically active tissue portion. Lithium levels are considered toxic above 2.0 mEq/L.

### PATHOPHYSIOLOGY

The exact mechanism and site at which lithium exerts its therapeutic effect remains uncertain. Lithium is known to compete with other cations, sodium, potassium, and calcium, and interferes with cyclic

**Table 134-1.** Potential Side Effects of Lithium Therapy

| Initial side effects | Chronic effects (*cont.*) |
|---|---|
| Polydipsia | Endocrine |
| Polyuria | Nontoxic goiter |
| Dry mouth | Hyperparathyroidism |
| Nausea | Teratogenesis (lithium crosses |
| Fine tremor of hands | placenta and is excreted in |
| Chronic effects | breast milk) |
| Ophthalmologic | Ebstein anomaly or other heart defects |
| Tearing | Neonatal diabetes insipidus |
| Blurring of vision | Dermatologic |
| Scotomatas | Acne |
| Exophthalmos | Localized edema |
| Papilledema (pseudotumor | Cutaneous ulcers |
| cerebri) | Hematologic |
| Renal | Neutrophilia |
| Lowered urine osmolarity | Aplastic anemia (rare) |
| Nephrogenic diabetes insipidus | |
| Nephrotic syndrome | |
| Structural damage (+/−) | |

**Table 134-2.** Signs and Symptoms of Acute Lithium Toxicity

CNS/Neuromuscular
  Tremor
  Neuromuscular irritability:
    muscle twitching, hyperreflexia, clonus, fasciculations
  Ataxia
  Transient neurologic asymmetries
  Lethargy
  Dysarthria
  Confusion
  Stupor
  Convulsions
  Coma
Gastrointestinal
  Nausea and vomiting
  Diarrhea
Cardiovascular
  ST-T-wave changes
  Sinus bradycardia
  Conduction defects
  Ventricular arrhythmias
  Hypertension (rare)

adenosine $3',5'$-monophosphate (cAMP) mediated processes that are regulated by polypeptide hormones. Lithium affects many organ systems, either as tolerable side effects or as changes resulting from chronic therapy. These effects are outlined in Table 134-1.

Side effects may escalate to toxicity during chronic lithium therapy without an actual increase in the prescribed dose. Dependence on renal clearance is the basis for a pathophysiologic cycle activated by anything which impairs kidney function or depletes water or sodium. The result will be an increase in lithium reabsorption, leading to higher lithium blood levels that incite further water and sodium loss through the kidney's response to ADH. It is important to be aware that any person receiving chronic lithium therapy and who, at the same time, has diabetes mellitus, hypertension, renal failure, advanced age, or is on a low-sodium diet is at high risk for lithium toxicity. Likewise, the same danger exists with diuretics, or nonsteroidal anti inflammatory drugs.

## LITHIUM TOXICITY

### Clinical Presentation

A patient with lithium toxicity usually presents with gastrointestinal reactions of nausea, vomiting, and diarrhea, associated with neuromuscular and central nervous system symptoms. The degree of toxicity is reflected by progression from lethargy, confusion, tremor, myoclonus, ataxia, spasticity, stupor, seizures, coma, and death. Cardiovascular alterations are usually not clinically significant despite ECG conduction defects and ST-T-wave and QT-interval changes. Signs and symptoms of acute lithium toxicity are outlined in Table 134-2.

Blood lithium levels, considered toxic above 2.0 mEq/L, cannot strictly predict the severity of an acute lithium overdose. Interpretation must consider the time of ingestion, as peak levels occur 8 to 12 h after the last dose of lithium was taken. Intracellular stores of lithium, the result of chronic therapy, are not measured in a blood level but are very important in contributing to toxicity. Patients without such active tissue stores may tolerate an acute overdose even though peak lithium levels are as high as 3 mEq/L. Careful clinical correlation is required in the interpretation of lithium levels.

### Treatment

The main treatment of lithium toxicity is good supportive care, with the addition of gastrointestinal decontamination, replacement of sodium depletion, and occasionally hemodialysis. There are no effective antidotes.

**Gastric lavage.** In the overdose state, gastric lavage should be performed, as charcoal is not effective in binding lithium. If the acute ingestion was a sustained-release lithium preparation, repeated gastric lavage in 2 to 4 h may remove additional lithium, and whole-bowel irrigation has also been reported effective. Cathartics are not helpful.

**Intravenous normal saline.** Normal saline administration ensures a good supply of sodium ions, which theoretically produce an increase in renal lithium excretion.

**Alkalinization of urine and osmotic diuresis.** If renal function is adequate, some have suggested these measures to increase lithium excretion, but they should be used with caution in the absence of good clinical studies. Anecdotally used agents are sodium bicarbonate and acetazolamide for alkalinization; and aminophylline, mannitol, and urea for osmotic diuresis.

**Good supportive care.** Supportive care should include cardiac monitoring. Careful electrolyte and renal function monitoring is required. Fluid balance needs attention. Intensive care may be required for severely toxic patients.

**Hemodialysis.** Dialysis is an effective means for removing lithium ions from the serum. The goal of hemodialysis is a lithium level of 1 mEq/L 6 to 8 h after dialysis. This will allow for redistribution of lithium from tissue stores. Repeat dialysis may be necessary based on clinical response and resultant serum lithium levels. Indications for hemodialysis are as follows:

1. Clinical signs of severe poisoning
2. Deteriorating clinical condition: seizures, coma, or ventricular arrhythmias
3. Decreasing urine output, or renal failure
4. Lack of expected drop in serum lithium level (20 percent in 6 h)

### BIBLIOGRAPHY

Amdisen A: Lithium and drug interactions. *Drugs* 24:133, 1982.

Clendeninn NJ, Pond SM, Kaysen G, et al: Potential pitfalls in the evaluation of the usefulness of hemodialysis for the removal of lithium. *J Toxicol Clin Toxicol* 19:341, 1982.

El-Mallakh RS: Treatment of acute lithium toxicity. *Vet Hum Toxicol* 26:31, 1984.

Jaeger A, Kopferschmitt SJ: Toxicokinetics of lithium intoxication treated by hemodialysis. *Clin Toxicol* 23:501, 1986.

Ramchandani D, Schindler BA: The lithium toxic patient in the medical hospital: Diagnostic and management dilemmas. *Int J Psychiatry Med* 23(1):55, 1993.

Simard M, Gumbiner B, Lee A, et al: Lithium carbonate intoxication. *Arch Intern Med* 149:36, 1989.

Smith SW, Ling LJ, Halstenson CE: Whole-bowel irrigation as a treatment for acute lithium overdose. *Ann Emerg Med* 20(5):536, 1991.

# 135

# BARBITURATES
## P. J. Ryan

Barbiturates were first introduced as a sedative in 1903. Current use has increased to include treatment of seizure disorders, induction of anesthesia, and management of increased intracranial pressure. Barbiturate poisoning is not as frequently seen now that there are numerous other tranquilizers and sedatives, but it still remains a very serious, potentially lethal problem.

## PHARMACOLOGY

The basic structure common to all barbiturates, barbituric acid, has no central nervous system activity. Only when its C-5 position is substituted with an alkyl, alkenyl, or aryl group does the resulting compound have a central nervous system effect. Four categories are classified by the duration of hypnotic activity, ranging from 0.3 h for the ultrashort-acting thiobarbiturates to 6 to 12 h for long-acting phenobarbital. (Table 135-1). The duration of action of barbiturates is dependent on lipid solubility, which is determined by the side chain structure at C-2 and secondarily by pH gradients. Thiobarbiturates, which have the oxygen at C-2 replaced by sulfur, are more lipid-soluble than oxybarbiturates.

Barbiturates with lipid solubility readily diffuse into body tissues and rapidly cross the blood-brain barrier. They are mainly metabolized by the liver. The mean half-life varies from 0.3h for the ultra-short-acting drugs to up to 37 h for intermediate-acting drugs.

Long-acting barbiturates such as phenobarbital are 80 percent absorbed by oral dosage. The volume of distribution is 0.8 L/kg, and 50 percent of the drug becomes protein-bound in the serum. Hepatic metabolism occurs, but approximately 25 percent of phenobarbital is excreted unchanged in the urine. Urinary pH varies the rate of renal clearance. The elimination half-life of phenobarbital varies from 48 to 200 h. In children, the elimination half-life is 0.5 times greater than in adults, but in infants the elimination half-life is 2 to 5 times greater than in adults. The elderly and those with hepatic disease have an increased elimination half-life. Phenobarbital readily crosses the placenta to the fetus and enters breast milk. Therapeutic levels are 10 to 40 mg/L.

Repeated use of hepatic metabolized barbiturates can lead to their shortened elimination half-life by induction of metabolizing enzymes (cytochrome $P_{450}$). Chronic use of phenobarbital can accelerate metabolism of oral anticoagulants, digoxin, glucocorticoids, quinidine, phenytoin, tricyclic antidepressants, tetracycline, and phenothiazines.

The major site of action of barbiturates is in the central nervous system, where they enhance the action of the inhibitory neurotransmitter γ-aminobutyric acid (GABA). They may also inhibit noradrenergic excitation at neuronal junctions. Barbiturates are general depressants to nerve and muscle tissues. Tolerance develops after chronic use of all barbiturates; as much as six times the usual dose may be required for the same effect.

## CLINICAL PRESENTATION

Mild to moderate barbiturate intoxication closely mimics the presentation of alcohol intoxication. Lethargy, emotional lability, and impaired thinking occur. General incoordination, slurred speech, and nystagmus may be seen.

Severe acute barbiturate toxicity results in progressive central nervous system depression ranging from lethargy to profound coma. Respiratory depression develops and may progress to respiratory arrest. Cardiovascular functions are altered, resulting in hypotension, vasodilatation, and shock. Hypothermia is common. Pupillary size may vary, either constricted or dilated. Flaccid muscle tone is present, and deep tendon reflexes are depressed or absent. Gastrointestinal activity is slowed. Skin bullae occur in about 6 percent of patients, and sweat gland necrosis has been reported. A severe overdose may show a flat line EEG.

The lethal dose of barbiturates varies considerably, but as a rule of thumb, 10 times the hypnotic dose is capable of producing severe toxicity. Short-acting, lipid-soluble barbiturates induce toxicity more rapidly and at a lower dose than the longer-acting agents. Neither drug dose nor the blood levels should be exclusively relied upon to predict the severity of an overdose or to correlate it to potential mortality. Measured plasma concentrations of barbiturates may not reflect the actual level in the brain. The laboratory should report the specific type of barbiturate ingested, which is important in understanding its duration of action and its route of excretion. Chronic barbiturate use and the patient's tolerance need to be considered.

The clinical presentation, such as the depth of coma, respiratory depression, or cardiovascular depression, must be the primary consideration in determining the severity of a barbiturate overdose. Early deaths are generally cardiovascular-related (shock or arrest), while late deaths most commonly are due to secondary pulmonary complications (aspiration pneumonitis or pulmonary edema). Less often, deaths are related to cerebral edema or renal failure. Fatalities usually have developed multiple system catastrophes.

## TREATMENT

The key to eventual recovery is the careful and skillful management of multiple depressed organ systems until the patient metabolizes and

**Table 135-1.** Barbiturate Classification

### General Formula and Substituted Derivatives

| Barbiturate | Duration of Action, h | $R_1$ | $R_2$ | $R_3$ |
|---|---|---|---|---|
| Ultrashort-acting: | | | | |
| Thiopental* | 0.3 | Ethyl | 1-Methyl butyl | –H |
| Thiamylal* | 0.3 | Allyl | 1-Methyl butyl | –H |
| Methohexital | 0.3 | Allyl | 1-Methyl-2- pentynyl | –CH₃ |
| Short-acting: | | | | |
| Hexobarbital | 3 | Methyl | 1-Cyclohexen- 1-yl | –CH₃ |
| Pentobarbital | 3 | Ethyl | 1-Methyl butyl | –H |
| Secobarbital | 3 | Allyl | 1-Methyl butyl | –H |
| Intermediate-acting: | | | | |
| Amobarbital | 3–6 | Ethyl | Isopentyl | –H |
| Aprobarbital | 3–6 | Allyl | Isopropyl | –H |
| Butabarbital | 3–6 | Ethyl | sec-Butyl | –H |
| Long-acting: | | | | |
| Barbital† | 6–12 | Ethyl | Ethyl | –H |
| Mephobarbital† | 6–12 | Ethyl | Phenyl | –CH₃ |
| Phenobarbital† | 6–12 | Ethyl | Phenyl | –H |
| Primidone* | 6–12 | Ethyl | Phenyl | –H |

\* Has S substitution for O, in thiopental and thiamylal and 2H substitution in primidone.

† Only drugs responsive to alkaline diuresis.

clears the drug. Because of this type of attention to critical care, most patients with serious barbiturate overdose now survive; only a few years ago such patients were frequently fatalities.

*Airway management* in the patient with severe overdose frequently requires intubation. Blood gas levels and chest x-ray films should be obtained periodically. Protection of the airway before gastric lavage cannot be overemphasized.

*Gastric lavage* is the method most commonly used for gastric emptying. Induction of emesis is dangerous in any patient with potential central nervous system depression.

*Activated charcoal* is instilled at the completion of an adequate lavage. In the management of patients with phenobarbital overdoses, good results occur with the use of multiple doses of charcoal. Thirty-gram doses have been used every 6 h via a nasogastric tube for a total of six doses. Results have shown a decrease in the elimination half-life of phenobarbital with use of repeated doses of charcoal.

*Intravenous fluids* are necessary for supportive or maintenance balance. A fluid challenge is the first treatment which should be given if hypotension develops. Low doses of dopamine may be used if an adequate fluid load is ineffective. Total parenteral nutrition should be considered if the coma duration is greater than 2 to 3 days.

*Forced diuresis and alkalinization* of the urine are helpful for the management of long-acting phenobarbital intoxication. Sodium bicarbonate used in 1 to 2 mEq/kg doses every 4 to 6 h to maintain urine pH at 7.5 or greater may significantly (5- to 10-fold) increase the phenobarbital excretion rate. This is not effective for intermediate- or short-acting barbiturates. Care should be taken that fluid overload does not result from too vigorous attempt of diuresis.

*Hemodialysis* can remove significant amounts of phenobarbital and is six to nine times more effective than forced diuresis and alkalinization. Charcoal hemoperfusion is even more efficacious, but is not without potential complications. Hemodialysis and hemoperfusion should only be used in the most critical overdose cases, or if the patient has underlying hepatic or renal insufficiency.

## BARBITURATE WITHDRAWAL SYNDROME

If an abrupt discontinuation of barbiturates occurs after a state of physical dependence has been established by their chronic use, withdrawal symptoms occur. Minor symptoms generally develop within 24 h after cessation of the drug. These include restlessness, anxiety, insomnia, depression, nausea, vomiting, abdominal cramps, sweating, and tremor. Such symptoms subside within 3 to 7 days. Occasionally there is progression to more severe withdrawal symptoms.

Following 2 to 3 days of abstinence, major withdrawal symptoms may appear. Increased muscular tone and jerking may progress to grand mal seizures. Auditory hallucinations and delirium could result. Hyperpyrexia, cardiovascular collapse, and death are possible.

Treatment of seizures is first the administration of diazepam and then, if this is ineffective, administration of a barbiturate. Gradual withdrawal of the addicting agent is the safest way to prevent major withdrawal symptoms.

## BIBLIOGRAPHY

Baltarowich LL: Barbiturates. *Topics in Emergency Medicine.* October 1985, pp 46–54.

Costello JB, Poklis A: Treatment of massive phenobarbital overdose with dopamine diuresis. *Arch Intern Med* 141:938, 1981.

Gaudreault P: Barbiturates. *Clin Toxicol Rev* 3:1, 1981.

Goldberg MJ, Berlinger WG: Treatment of phenobarbital overdose with activated charcoal. *JAMA* 247:2400, 1982.

Ho IK: Mechanism of action of barbiturates. *Annu Rev Pharmacol Toxicol* 21:83, 1981.

McCarron MM, Schulze BW, Walbert CB, et al: Short-acting barbiturate overdosage. *JAMA* 248:55, 1982.

Pond SM, Olson KR, Osterloh JD, et al: Randomized study of the treatment of phenobarbital overdose with repeated doses of activated charcoal. *JAMA* 251:3104, 1984.

# 136
# BENZODIAZEPINES

## George M. Bosse

Benzodiazepines are commonly used pharmacologic agents for the treatment of anxiety, insomnia, seizures, and alcohol withdrawal. They also are used in conscious sedation as well as general anesthesia. Fifteen different generic benzodiazepines are approved for use in the United States as of this writing (Table 136-1).

Benzodiazepines are frequent agents of accidental and intentional overdose. In the 1992 Annual Report of the American Association of Poison Control Centers Toxic Exposure Surveillance System, benzodiazepines accounted for 33,516 exposures, both as a single agent and in combination with other drugs. Although the ingestion of benzodiazepines alone appears to result in relatively few deaths, increased morbidity and mortality does result from mixed overdose. Parenteral administration of benzodiazepines may also result in significant complications, particularly respiratory depression and hypotension.

## PHARMACOLOGY

A specific benzodiazepine receptor has been identified in the central nervous system (CNS). Specific peripheral receptor sites also have been identified; however, the predominant clinical effects of benzodiazepines are mediated through the CNS receptors. Although not fully characterized, research supports the concept of a neuronal cell-surface protein complex containing a benzodiazepine receptor, a γ-aminobutyric acid (GABA) receptor, and a chloride channel. GABA is an inhibitory neurotransmitter; effects of stimulation of GABA pathways include sedation, anxiolysis, and striated muscle relaxation. Stimulation of the benzodiazepine receptor appears to increase the sensitivity of the GABA receptor complex to stimulation by GABA. The enhancement of GABA transmission by the administration of benzodiazepines is thought to occur by either increasing the affinity of the GABA receptor for its ligand or improving coupling between the GABA receptor and its associated chloride channel. Increased GABA output leads to inhibitory effects throughout the neuroaxis and the resultant typical clinical effects of benzodiazepines.

**Table 136-1.** Benzodiazepines Approved for Use in the US

| Generic Name | Brand Name | $t^1/_2$ (h)* | Metabolite Characteristics† |
|---|---|---|---|
| Alprazolam | Xanax | 6–26 | Inactive |
| Chlordiazepoxide | Librium | 5–30 | Active |
| Clonazepam | Klonopin | 39 | Inactive |
| Chlorazepate dipotassium | Tranxene | 1.1–2.9 | Active |
| Diazepam | Valium | 20–70 | Active |
| Estazolam | Prosom | 10–24 | Inactive |
| Flurazepam | Dalmane | 2–3 | Active |
| Halazepam | Paxipam | 14 | Active |
| Lorazepam | Ativan | 9–19 | Inactive |
| Midazolam | Versed | 2–5 | Inactive |
| Oxazepam | Serax | 5.4–9.8 | Inactive |
| Prazepam | Centrax | 0.6–2.0 | Active |
| Quazepam | Doral | 25–41 | Active |
| Temazepam | Restoril | 10–16 | Inactive |
| Triazolam | Halcion | 1.6–5.4 | Inactive |

\* Elimination half-life of parent compound.

† Some of the derivatives listed as having inactive metabolites actually are converted to active compounds. However, rapid metabolism occurs, such that there is no appreciable accumulation of active intermediates.

The presence of an endogenous ligand for the benzodiazepine receptor has been proposed but not conclusively identified.

In general, benzodiazepines are well absorbed from the gastrointestinal tract. The onset of action after oral ingestion is limited more by the rate of absorption from the gastrointestinal tract than by the relatively rapid passage from the bloodstream into the brain. With the exception of lorazepam and midazolam, intramuscular injection of benzodiazepines results in unpredictable absorption.

Benzodiazepines are all relatively lipid soluble, with some variation among the different agents. Increased lipid solubility is associated with more rapid diffusion across the blood–brain barrier. After single doses, the more highly lipophilic benzodiazepines have a shorter onset of action but also a shorter duration of activity. This short duration of activity occurs because of rapid egress of drug from the brain and bloodstream into inactive tissue storage sites. For this reason, the half-life may not be a good indicator of the duration of action in an acute ingestion. As an example, diazepam is a derivative with a long elimination half-life but relatively short duration of action.

Benzodiazepine derivatives undergo metabolism by hepatic biotransformation through either oxidation or conjugation. Several derivatives are metabolized by both oxidative and conjugative processes. Oxidation often results in active metabolities, which prolong the biologic half-life of the parent compounds. Conjugation is a rapid process that results in inactive metabolites. Oxidation is more susceptible to impairment by such factors as disease states (e.g., chronic liver disease), population characteristics (old age), and concurrent treatment with drugs that impair oxidizing capacity (e.g., cimetidine, estrogen, isoniazid, ethanol, and phenytoin). Examples of agents that undergo conjugation primarily include oxazepam, lorazepam, and temazepam. Administration of benzodiazepines that undergo conjugation may be safer in susceptible groups.

Selection of a benzodiazepine for use by a physician depends on the clinical properties of the particular derivative. Although individual drugs are marketed for specific conditions, there is considerable overlap of activity. For this reason, some hospital formulary committees have limited the number of available agents.

## CLINICAL FEATURES

Pure benzodiazepine overdose is notable for the relative lack of serious morbidity and mortality. Most reported cases of serious toxicity have occurred in the setting of coingestion of other agents or with parenteral administration. However, deaths in isolated overdose have been reported and appear to be more likely with the newer short-acting derivatives such as triazolam, alprazolam, and temazepam.

The clinical presentation of benzodiazepine intoxication is nonspecific. Clinical assessment also may be difficult because of the frequent coingestion of other agents. Except for additive effects, drug interactions of benzodiazepines with other sedative-hypnotics are unusual.

The nonspecific presentation of benzodiazepine toxicity is similar to other sedative-hypnotics. However, other agents can have at least a few distinguishing features. Chloral hydrate is known to precipitate cardiac arrhythmias. Etchchlorvinol can produce prolonged coma and may be suspected by the presence of a vinyl-like odor. Glutethimide may give rise to fluctuating levels of CNS impairment and anticholinergic signs. Barbiturates are more likely than benzodiazepines to produce coma and depressant myocardial effects.

The predominant manifestations of benzodiazepines are neurologic. CNS effects include drowsiness, dizziness, slurred speech, confusion, ataxia, and impairment of intellectual function. Coma, particularly if prolonged, is atypical and should prompt suspicion of intoxication with other agents or a nontoxin-related medical condition. The elderly are more prone to manifest the CNS effects of benzodiazepines.

Paradoxical reactions, including excitement, anxiety, aggression, hostile behavior, rage, and delirium, are reported but are uncommon. Although unclear, the etiology of such effects is probably not on an idiosyncratic basis. Benzodiazepines may have a disinhibiting effect, which in the presence of various extrinsic factors, can lead to such actions as aggressive or hostile behavior. Other effects, which are reported and which have unclear etiologies, include headache, nausea, vomiting, chest pain, joint pain, diarrhea, and incontinence.

Uncommonly, respiratory depression and hypotension may occur. These generally occur with either parenteral administration or in the presence of coingestants. Intravenous administration is more likely to cause serious cardiorespiratory effects with rapid administration of large doses. In addition, the elderly and those with underlying cardiorespiratory disease are more susceptible to adverse effects of intravenous administration. The use of propylene glycol as a diluent in parenteral preparations of diazepam has also been implicated as a factor in cardiorespiratory arrest.

Extrapyramidal reactions have been associated with the use of benzodiazepines. Various allergic, hepatotoxic, and hematologic reactions also have been reported; however, these are infrequent. In general, benzodiazepines have no long-term organ system toxicity other than what can be ascribed to indirect effects from CNS or cardiorespiratory depression.

Laboratory data in benzodiazepine ingestion is of limited value. Serum benzodiazepine levels are not indicated routinely because they do not correlate well with the clinical state. Qualitative testing may be helpful, but the laboratory may not test routinely for all available derivatives. Familiarity with laboratory capabilities at the particular institution is essential.

## MANAGEMENT

Benzodiazepines often are ingested with other agents, and the history frequently is inaccurate. Therefore, administration of concentrated dextrose, thiamine, and naloxone should be considered in such patients when depressed or altered mental status is present. Induction of emesis should be avoided in benzodiazepine overdose because CNS depression may ensue. Gastric lavage is safer and is recommended if the amount ingested is large or in coingestions with toxic agents. Activated charcoal binds benzodiazepines effectively and should be administered in most situations. Elimination enhancement by forced diuresis, hemodialysis, or hemoperfusion is not effective, and most patients do not manifest toxicity serious enough to warrant consideration of such measures. The patient should be monitored closely for CNS and respiratory depression. If CNS depression persists or is profound, other agents or conditions must be considered.

Flumazenil is a unique selective antagonist of the central effects of benzodiazepines. Clinical applications include the management of benzodiazepine overdose and reversal of benzodiazepine-induced conscious sedation. It use in benzodiazepine toxicity may obviate the need for tracheal intubation and respiratory support. As a diagnostic aid in obscure alterations of mental status, flumazenil may reduce the need for expensive and invasive procedures such as computed tomography or lumbar puncture.

In the emergency department, flumazenil is useful mainly in reversing the effects of benzodiazepines administered for diagnostic and therapeutic procedures. The plasma elimination half-life of flumazenil is approximately 1 h. Its duration of action is variable and depends on the dose of flumazenil and the benzodiazepine administered. Recurrent benzodiazepine toxicity may result once its effects have worn off. This is less likely for an agent with a short duration of action such as midazolam. The dose of flumazenil is 0.2 mg IV q minute to response or to a total of 3mg.

There are several considerations that should limit the empirical administration of flumazenil in the poisoned patient. Generalized seizures have occurred in patients given flumazenil after coingestions of benzodiazepines and seizure-inducing agents, particularly cyclic antidepressants. Seizure activity after flumazenil administration has also occurred in patients physically dependent on benzodiazepines and in patients receiving benzodiazepines for control of a seizure disorder. The putative explanation for this convulsive activity is either the reversal of the cerebroprotective and anticonvulsive effects of benzodiazepines or the precipitation of a benzodiazepine withdrawal syndrome. Another reason to avoid empirical administration of flumazenil in overdose patients is that the history is often unreliable or unavailable. Flumazenil is also contraindicated in patients with a suspected elevation of intracranial pressure, such as in severe head injury. This is due to its effects on cerebral hemodynamics. In all cases of benzodiazepine toxicity, supportive care takes precedence.

## BENZODIAZEPINE ABUSE AND DEPENDENCE

Genuine physiologic addiction to benzodiazepines may occur, particularly with prolonged and high doses. However, the abuse potential of benzodiazepines appears to be low in comparison with agents such as cocaine, opiates, and barbiturates. Benzodiazepine abuse usually occurs in individuals with a history of abuse of other psychoactive drugs. Primary drug abuse with benzodiazepines is not common.

Benzodiazepine withdrawal may occur on abrupt discontinuation and is more likely in patients with prolonged use and high doses. Because of the long biologic half-life of several derivatives, withdrawal manifestations may not occur for several days to over 1 week after the benzodiazepine is discontinued. Unfortunately, it is often difficult to distinguish between withdrawal and underlying symptoms for which the drugs were prescribed initially.

Reported withdrawal manifestations include anxiety, irritability, insomnia, nausea, vomiting, tremor, sweating, and anorexia. Serious manifestations, including confusion, disorientation, psychosis, and seizures, also have been reported. For patients with an acute organic brain syndrome, a history of possible benzodiazepine withdrawal should always be pursued. Withdrawal reactions may be avoided by dose tapering. Treatment of withdrawal reactions may be accomplished by drug substitution or by reintroduction of a benzodiazepine and subsequent tapering.

## BIBLIOGRAPHY

Hojer J, Baehrendtz S, Gustafsson L. Benzodiazepine poisoning: experience of 702 admissions to an intensive care unit during a 14 year period. *J Intern Med* 226:117, 1989.

Litovitz TL, Holm KC, Clancy C, et al: 1992 Annual report of the American Association of Poison Control Centers toxic exposure surveillance system. *Am J Emer Med* 11:494, 1993.

Spivey WH. Flumazenil and seizures: analysis of 43 cases. *Clin Ther* 14:292, 1992.

Votey SR, Bosse GM, Bayer MJ, et al. Flumazenil: a new benzodiazepine antagonist. *Ann Emerg Med* 20:181, 1991.

Warneke LB: Benzodiazepines: abuse and new use. *Can J Psychiatry* 36:194, 1991.

# 137
# NONBENZODIAZEPINE SEDATIVE-HYPNOTICS
## Suzanne R. White

This chapter reviews the clinical presentation, complications, and management of nonbenzodiazepine sedative-hypnotics toxicity. Some agents, such as etchlorvynol, meprobamate, glutethimide, and metha-qualone, are no longer commonly used, but they may be encountered in the elderly or in combination with more contemporary drugs of abuse (i.e., cocaine). Newer agents such as buspirone and zolpidem have the potential for toxicity and emergency physicians should be familiar with their effects (Tables 137-1 and 137-2).

## ETHCHLORVYNOL

Even though ethchlorvynol (Placidyl) was introduced nearly 40 years ago and has been widely replaced by other safer sedative-hypnotics, the emergency physician may still occasionally encounter patients who abuse this schedule IV substance. The most common pattern of ethchlorvynol abuse is that of intentional adult overdose, and such situations are complicated with a high incidence of serious adverse effects. The available form, a liquid-filled capsule, facilitates both intravenous and oral abuse. Street names include "pickles," "jelly beans," and "Mr. Green Jeans."

Like most sedative-hypnotics, ethchlorvynol is highly lipophilic, concentrates in the central nervous system (CNS) with gradual redistribution, and is hepatically metabolized. The mechanism of its sedative action is unknown. In toxicity, elimination half-lives of greater than 100 h have been reported.

Clinical manifestations of toxicity vary according to the method and chronicity of abuse: (1) chronic abuse with mild toxicity or withdrawal symptoms, (2) acute intravenous overdosage, and (3) acute oral overdosage. In the first situation, the chronically dependent patient complains primarily of neurologic disabilities such as facial numbness, incoordination, tremors, confusion, slurred speech, muscle

**Table 137-1.** Summary of Characteristic Features in Overdose

| | |
|---|---|
| Ethchlorvynol | Acute respiratory distress syndrome |
| | Prolonged coma |
| | Vinyl-like odor on breath |
| Meprobamate | Concretions |
| | Hypotension |
| Glutethimide | Anticholinergic symptoms |
| | Prolonged coma |
| Methaqualone | Bleeding diathesis |
| | Hyperacusis & hypertonicity |
| Chloral hydrate | Pearlike odor on breath |
| | Gastrointestinal bleeding |
| | Arrhythmias |

**Table 137-2.** Reported Toxic Exposures to Sedative-Hypnotic Agents in 1993

| Substance | No. of Exposures | Deaths |
|---|---|---|
| Benzodiazepines | 32,334 | 33 |
| Chloral hydrate | 556 | 2 |
| Ethchlorvynol | 195 | 2 |
| Glutethimide | 42 | 0 |
| Meprobamate | 367 | 4 |
| Methaqualone | 62 | 0 |
| Buspirone | Unknown | 0 |
| Carisoprodol | Unknown | 4 |

weakness, diplopia, or visual disturbances resulting from macular degeneration or chiasmal optic neuritis. A second distinct clinical picture arises after acute intravenous injection, which frequently causes noncardiogenic pulmonary edema. In fact, so reproducible is this pulmonary injury that ethchlorvynol has provided an excellent animal model for the study of acute respiratory distress syndrome (ARDS). Derangements in pulmonary capillary permeability are likely induced by metabolites of arachidonic acid. The third clinical scenario involves acute oral overdose. Signs and symptoms may initially include a mintlike taste in the mouth, dyspnea, and dry cough. Nystagmus and CNS depression with extremely prolonged comatose states represented by isoelectric electroencephalographic (EEG) tracings may ensue. Hemodynamic instability develops with bradycardia, hypotension, and hypothermia. Pulmonary edema may develop in massive oral overdose. Further unique complications may include bullae, sudden painless bilateral blindness, hemolysis, cholestatic jaundice, and pancytopenia. Most situations involve multiple drugs, and ethchlorvynol combined with ethanol or other CNS depressants can cause respiratory arrest.

The diagnosis of ethchlorvynol overdose may be aided by noting a pungent vinyl or sweet odor on the patient's breath. Blood ethchorvynol levels do seem to correlate with symptoms but may not be readily available.

Successful management requires aggressive, meticulous supportive care and gastrointestinal decontamination (see General Treatment below). The successful treatment of pulmonary edema may require Swan-Ganz monitoring and the use of positive end-expiratory pressure. New data suggest that ibuprofen may reduce ethchlovynol-induced lung injury. Charcoal hemoperfusion may be effective in severe cases, and suggested indications, although controversial, are the presence of life-threatening complications despite intensive supportive therapy and serum levels greater than 10 to 15 mg/dL in the first 12 h or greater than 7 mg/dL 12 h or more after ingestion. The premature termination of life support in a patient comatose from ethchlorvynol toxicity based on EEG findings alone is a potentially disastrous pitfall.

## Meprobamate

Meprobamate (Miltown, Equanil) is a propanediol carbamate first marketed in the 1950s as an anxiolytic, sedative-hypnotic agent. Combination preparations with benactyzine hydrochloride, a mild anticholinergic antidepressant (Deprol), tridihexethyl chloride (Milpath), conjugated estrogens (Milprem), and antianginal nitrates (Miltrate) are available. Although now widely replaced by the safer benzodiazepines, meprobamate continues to be implicated in cases of acute deliberate self-poisoning. Furthermore, a recent survey of ambulatory elderly patients in Florida noted long-term abuse patterns, some patients having taken the drug for nearly 30 years. Meprobamate may induce the same tolerance, physical dependence, and withdrawal syndromes seen with other sedative-hypnotics.

Meprobamate is well absorbed but has a propensity to form gastric concretions. Metabolism is primarily hepatic, with an elimination half-life of up to 27 h in overdose. The mechanism of sedative action is by a reduction in sensory transmission to the thalamus and an increase in endogenous CNS adenosine levels. As evidenced by postmortem studies, the drug is maximally concentrated in the myocardium, and direct myocardial toxicity occurs, even in absence of profound CNS depression.

Clinical manifestations of meprobamate toxicity may include all stages of CNS depression or coma. The coma may be prolonged (> 40 h) but is generally of less duration than that seen with ethchlorvynol. Fluctuating coma should alert the clinician to the possibility of continued drug absorption from concretions. Severe hypotension, characteristic of meprobamate toxicity, may be accompanied by tachycardia, bradycardia, and pulmonary edema. Seizures and myoclonus are rare and usually occur during the recovery phase. Bullous skin lesions may be seen.

Blood levels correlate with CNS symptoms in the nontolerant patient after a single ingestion.

Treatment involves stabilization of the airway and circulation (see General Treatment below). Delayed gastric lavage and whole bowel irrigation using a polyethylene glycol solution dosed at 2 L/h until the rectal effluent is clear (40 mL/kg per hour in children) may be considered, in view of possible concretion formation. In extreme cases, both gastrotomy and gastroscopic removal of pill bezoars have been reported to be effective. Pulse dose activated charcoal may enhance elimination, as will charcoal or resin hemoperfusion. The indications for hemoperfusion include the presence of life-threatening complications despite intensive supportive therapy, serum levels greater than 100 μg/mL in adults, and the inability to tolerate prolonged coma. Children may tolerate higher serum levels of meprobamate in overdose than do adults. Although forced diuresis will enhance renal elimination, it may induce pulmonary edema and has been only anecdotally successful when used in conjunction with Swan-Ganz monitoring. In view of the potential for meprobamate to induce pulmonary edema, this approach is potentially hazardous, and it is therefore not recommended. The management of hypotension includes the early use of vasopressors and inotropic agents to avoid fluid overresuscitation.

A structurally related muscle relaxant, carisoprodol (Soma), which is metabolized to meprobamate, is emerging as a street drug of abuse. Carisoprodol is often combined with Tylenol and codeine, and this combination is known as both "Soma-Do" and "Soma-Coma."

## GLUTETHIMIDE

Marketed in the 1950s as a safe, nonaddicting sedative-hypnotic drug, Doriden was soon noted to have similar disadvantages and side effects as did the barbiturates. Furthermore, patients intoxicated with glutethimide had more significant life-threatening manifestations, and the medical use of this schedule II substance has become limited. Glutethimide has now become primarily a drug of abuse, often taken in combination with codeine ("sets," "hits," "loads," "packs," "three's and eight's," "four doors"). The glutethimide/codeine combination reportedly produces a euphoric effect that is comparable to that of intravenous heroin but which is longer lasting. This combination is highly addicting, and both tolerance and withdrawal may occur. "Sets" abuse is highly localized, and the areas reporting this phenomenon include New York City, Philadelphia, Los Angeles, New Jersey, and rural Pennsylvania.

Glutethimide is erratically absorbed and hepatically metabolized in the liver to a number of active metabolites, one of which (4-HG) has twice the potency and duration of action as the parent drug. In toxicity, the half-life may be prolonged to 40 h. Side effects with chronic use include "hangover," blurred vision, headache, rash, bone marrow suppression, hypocalcemia, and osteomalacia.

The clinical effects of acute glutethimide toxicity are not unlike those seen in barbiturate overdose with prominent CNS and myocardial depression. Unique to this drug, however, is its ability to cause pronounced anticholinergic symptoms. Profound, cyclical coma may occur and is related to a number of factors including the enterohepatic recirculation of active metabolites and the anticholinergic effects of the parent drug on gut motility. Coma may last up to 100 h. Other typical manifestations of anticholinergic toxicity are seen, including dry mucous membranes, mydriasis, tachycardia, hypertension, ileus, urinary retention, hyperpyrexia, delirium, seizures, and agitation. Hypotension, pulmonary edema, and bullous skin lesions have also been reported.

Blood levels of the active metabolite 4-HG may correlate better with clinical outcome than do those of the parent drug. Like ethchlorvynol, complete recovery has been reported from prolonged coma despite isoelectric EEG tracings.

Decontamination principles are delineated in the section on general treatment. However, patients symptomatic from glutethimide overdosage may benefit from gastric lavage as late as 12 h postingestion because the anticholinergic effects of the drug may result in delayed gastric emptying. Multidose charcoal may be effective but has not been well studied. Aggressive management of hyperthermia, agitation, and seizures is necessary to prevent rhabdomyolysis and neurologic injury. The use of physostigmine to reverse anticholinergic toxicity from glutethimide has not been studied and is not recommended. Hemoperfusion clearly enhances glutethimide elimination although its role in management remains controversial. Candidates for this modality of elimination enhancement would include patients who are not responding to intensive supportive care, those who cannot tolerate prolonged coma (elderly), and those with serum levels greater than 40 mg/L. Because of the erratic and potentially delayed absorption with resultant unpredictable effects on mental status, prolonged periods of observation (24 h) are necessary if large amounts of the drug have been ingested. Advanced age and prolonged duration of coma are indicators of a poor prognosis.

## METHAQUALONE

Methaqualone (Quaalude, Parest, Mequin, Sopor; Mandrax—a combination with diphenhydramine) was first marketed as a nonaddicting sedative-hypnotic substitute for the barbiturate class and gained maximal popularity from the 1960s to the early 1980s. Subsequent discovery of its high abuse potential prompted the termination of legal synthesis in 1984 in the United States. Clandestine manufacture and smuggling have resulted in its continued availability on the street as "quads," "ludes," "sopers," "mandies," "soapers," "the love drug," and "wallbanger." Its reported ability to induce both profound relaxation and disinhibition have led to its popularity as an aphrodisiac and "cocaine downer."

The mechanism of sedative action is not yet clear but is likely related to binding of the γ-aminobutyric acid (GABA) receptor complex in the CNS. The drug is rapidly absorbed and widely distributed to the tissues, with a half-life of 20 to 50 h or longer in overdose situations. Hepatic metabolism to several inactive metabolites occurs. Adverse effects at normal doses include confusion, gastrointestinal upset, rash, paresthesias, and peripheral neuropathy.

Signs of mild intoxication are similar to those caused by ethanol or other sedative-hypnotics: the patient's movements are slow and uncoordinated (hence the name "wallbanger"), the speech is slurred, and nystagmus is present. Higher doses of the drug lead to several unique phenomena. Along with CNS depression, a paradoxical increase in muscle tone with hyperreflexia and myoclonus occurs, and ultimately seizure activity may be observed. Painful hyperacusis may be a helpful, discriminating feature. Unlike toxicity from other sedative-hypnotic drugs, respiratory depression and cardiovascular collapse are uncommon and should lead one to suspect coingestants. Pulmonary edema has been described frequently in severe overdose. Interestingly, methaqualone induces thrombocytopenia and hypoprothrombinemia in 20 percent of patients and has led to conjunctival, retinal, gastrointestinal, and bullous skin hemorrhages.

Methaqualone plasma levels do not correlate well with clinical findings.

As with other sedative-hypnotic agents, decontamination and supportive care remain the mainstays of therapy (see General Treatment below). Additionally, benzodiazepines may be used to control hypertonicity and seizures. Severe cases of rigidity have required treatment with neuromuscular paralytic agents. The administration of platelets, vitamin K, or fresh frozen plasma may be necessary to control bleeding. Charcoal hemoperfusion is more effective than hemodialysis in clearing methaqualone, but it should be reserved for patients who are

not responding to maximal supportive therapy or whose methaqualone serum levels are greater than 10 to 15 mg/dL. As with most other sedative-hypnotics discussed here, severe withdrawal symptoms may occur.

Fatalities caused by methaqualone are commonly related to trauma because intoxicated users exhibit poor judgment, incoordination, and impulsive behavior.

## CHLORAL HYDRATE

One of the oldest hypnotic drugs, introduced in 1869, chloral hydrate (Noctec) is still medically used for sedation, particularly in children. It is also abused in combination with ethanol as the notorious "Mickey Finn." Unfavorable properties of this drug include a narrow therapeutic index, the rapid development of tolerance and dependence, and withdrawal syndromes similar to alcohol withdrawal.

Absorption is rapid from the stomach and conversion to an active metabolite, trichloroethanol, occurs in the liver via alcohol dehydrogenase. A synergistic relationship with ethanol occurring at this enzyme site explains the potency of the "Mickey Finn" preparation. Trichloroethanol actually accounts for the majority of the drug's sedative activity. The onset of action is less than 30 min with a half-life of 8 h, which may be prolonged in toxicity.

As with all other drugs in this section, mild toxicity manifests clinically with sedation and incoordination. A distinct pearlike odor noted on the patient's breath may be a clue to ingestion. Other findings include gastrointestinal bleeding because the drug is caustic to mucous membranes, hepatitis, and purpuric or bullous skin lesions. Serious cardiovascular complications may occur and account for most of the mortality associated with this drug. Myocardial contractility is depressed, the refractory period is shortened, and sensitivity of the myocardial cells to catecholamines is heightened—a characteristic of all halogenated hydrocarbons. Resistant cardiac arrhythmias are therefore the usual mode of death.

Blood levels for chloral hydrate will rarely aid clinical management. Because chloral hydrate is radiopaque, abdominal x-rays may confirm the ingestion and guide intestinal decontamination.

Following the stabilization of both airway and cardiac function, gastric decontamination should be performed and charcoal should be administered if there is no evidence of caustic injury. Cardiac monitoring is mandatory, but treatment of arrhythmias is controversial. Both lidocaine and phenytoin have been reported to be effective for the treatment of ventricular arrhythmias. Still others have noted success using propranolol. Overdrive pacing may be necessary to treat refractory ventricular tachycardia. β-Adrenergic drugs such as epinephrine, isoproterenol, and dopamine can potentiate arrhythmias because the myocardium is already sensitized to catecholamines. If pressors are needed, purely α-acting agents such as norepinephrine should be used. In severe overdose situations, both hemodialysis and hemoperfusion appear equally effective, but unfortunately have not been well studied.

## NEWER AGENTS

### Buspirone

Buspirone (BuSpar) is a novel agent that has been found to be effective for the treatment of generalized anxiety disorder. It does not affect GABA or benzodiazepine receptors and reportedly has no potential for abuse. It does effect CNS dopaminergic, noradrenergic, and serotonergic neurotransmission. Experience in overdose is limited.

The drug is very well absorbed, highly protein bound, and widely distributed to the tissues. Metabolism occurs hepatically and the half-life is 2 h at therapeutic doses.

Buspirone is less sedating than diazepam and interacts less with other sedative agents such as ethanol. In toxicity, the most common effect is drowsiness and dysphoria. Hypotension, bradycardia, seizures, paresthesias, gastrointestinal upset, abnormal liver function studies, dystonic reactions, and priapism have all been described.

Treatment is supportive (see General Treatment below). Hemodialysis does not remove buspirone from the blood and the role of hemoperfusion in elimination enhancement has not been evaluated.

## Zolpidem

Zolpidem tartrate (Ambien, Stilnox, Bikalm, Niotal) is a new agent indicated for the short-term treatment of insomnia. It is an imidazopyridine, chemically unrelated to benzodiazepines, with sedative effects mediated through binding to benzodiazepine w-1 receptor subtypes in the CNS. Metabolism is hepatic and the half-life is 2.5 h at therapeutic doses; the half-life in toxicity is unknown. Experience in overdose cases is limited.

The primary effects of toxicity include CNS and respiratory depression. Like the benzodiazepines, these effects are dose related and are exacerbated by the coingestion of other CNS-depressing agents such as ethanol. Psychotic reactions to zolpidem have occurred at therapeutic doses. The ingestion of 70 to 390 mg by adults has resulted in somnolence, dizziness, amnesia, and vomiting; all patients experienced full recovery.

Zolpidem levels are not useful in guiding management.

Treatment involves aggressive supportive care and gut decontamination. Multidose charcoal has not yet been evaluated as an adjunct to therapy. Flumazenil has been effective in reversing the CNS and respiratory actions of zolpidem. The recommended initial dose is 0.2 mg intravenously over 30 s. If adequate consciousness is not obtained within 30 s, a further dose of 0.3 mg may be administered over 30 s. Additional doses of 0.5 mg may be administered at 1-min intervals up to a maximum total dose of 3 mg. Contraindications to the use of flumazenil include (1) suspected tricyclic overdose, (2) known seizure disorder, (3) chronic benzodiazepine dependence, (4) prescribed use of benzodiazepines for a life-threatening condition, (5) overdose on unknown agents and (6) signs or symptoms that could be related to tricyclic toxicity. Clearly the role for flumazenil in the emergency department, where often the exact substance ingested is unknown, is limited.

## GENERAL TREATMENT GUIDELINES

Many of the agents discussed in detail above share similarities both in chemical and pharmacologic properties as well as in clinical effects in toxicity. Certain generalities that may be useful in guiding management are discussed here.

Most oral overdosages with the nonbenzodiazepine sedative-hypnotics involve multiple agents. Therefore, a careful search for other treatable substances (such as salicylate or acetaminophen) is mandatory. Furthermore, the expected toxidrome (i.e., anticholinergic effect with glutethimide overdose), may be obscured if multiple drugs have been ingested. All of the drugs discussed, with the possible exception of buspirone, cause physical dependence and tolerance with chronic use. Therefore, hospitalized patients who have been treated for acute toxicity may subsequently develop life-threatening withdrawal states, and this must be anticipated.

General treatment remains the same for all agents:

1. Establish a clear airway in all patients prior to gastric decontamination.
2. Use arterial blood gases to monitor the adequacy of oxygenation and ventilation.
3. Provide intravenous access and initiate crystalloid fluid resuscitation, up to 2 L in adults or to a systolic blood pressure of 100 mm Hg. The early use of vasopressors is indicated because most sedative-hypnotics have the propensity to cause pulmonary edema.
4. Administer glucose, naloxone, and thiamine intravenously to all patients with an altered mental status.

5. Ipecac should not be administered because all of these agents may cause rapid CNS depression. Gastric lavage may be performed with the administration of charcoal (1 g/kg) and sorbitol (1 g/kg) or other cathartic. Repeat doses of charcoal may be useful in profoundly comatose patients or in special cases such as glutethimide. Do not use whole bowel irrigation or multiple-dose charcoal in patients with an ileus.
6. In general, hemoperfusion is superior to hemodialysis in enhancing elimination because these drugs are both highly lipophilic and protein bound.
7. Do not use CNS stimulants or physostigmine to reverse coma. The contraindications to flumazenil use should be reviewed prior to its administration, and its efficacy in reversing sedation with most of the above agents has not been well studied.
8. Most patients will recover with meticulous supportive care. Watch for complications such as aspiration pneumonia, ARDS, rhabdomyolysis, and withdrawal states during the recovery period.

## BIBLIOGRAPHY

Annsseau M, Pticholt W, Hansenne M, et al: Psychotic reaction to zolpidem. *Lancet* 339:809, 1992.

Bender FH, Cooper JV, Dreyfus R: Fatalities associated with acute overdose of glutethimide (Doriden) and codeine. *Vet Hum Toxicol* 30:332, 1988.

Delong RE, Phillis JW, Barraco RA: A possible role of endogenous adenosine in the sedative action of meprobamate. *Eur J Pharmacol* 118:359, 1985.

Dennison J, Edwards JN, Volans GN: Meprobamate overdosage. *Human Toxicology* 4:215, 1985.

Graham SR, Day RO, Lee R, Fulde GWO: Overdose with chloral hydrate: a pharmacological and therapeutic review. *Med J Aust* 149:686, 1988.

Hale WE, May FE, Moore MT, Stewart RB: Meprobamate use in the elderly. *J Am Geriatr Soc* 96:1003, 1988.

Hansen AR, Kennedy KA, Ambre JJ, et al: Glutethimide poisoning: a metabolite contributes to morbidity and mortality. *N Engl J Med* 292:251, 1975.

Kintz P, Tracqui A, Mangin P, Lugnier AAJ: Fatal meprobamate self-poisoning. *Am J Forensic Med Pathol* 9:139, 1988.

Litovitz TL, Holm KC, Clancy C, Schmitz BF, Clark LR, Oderda GM: 1992 Annual report of the American Association of Poison Control Centers toxic exposure surveillance system. *Am J Emerg Med* 11:494, 1993.

Meram D, Descotes J: Acute poisoning with zolpidem. *Rev Med Intern* 10:466, 1989.

Newton RE, Marunycz JD, Alderdice MT: Review of the side-effect profile of buspirone. *Am J Med* 80:17, 1986.

Product information. Ambien zolpidem tartrate. GD Searle & Co., Chicago, 1993.

Skoutakis VA, Acchiardo SR: Methaqualone poisoning: diagnosis and treatment. *CTC* 5:23, 1983.

Wetli CV: Changing patterns of methaqualone abuse. *JAMA* 249:621, 1983.

Yagi K, Baudendistel LJ, Dahms TE: Ibuprofen reduces ethchlorvynol lung injury: possible role of blood flow distribution. *J Appl Physiol* 72:1156, 1992.

Yell RP: Ethchlorvynol overdose. *Am J Emerg Med* 8:246, 1990.

# 138
# ALCOHOLS
### William A. Berk
### Wilma V. Henderson

## ETHANOL

Ethanol is the most frequently used and abused intoxicant in the United States and most other societies, including those where it is proscribed. Nearly three fourths of adult Americans consume at least one alcoholic drink each year, compared to only 36 percent who smoke at least one cigarette. Beer ranks as the fourth most popular beverage in terms of volume consumed, after soft drinks, milk, and coffee. Adult consumption of beverages containing ethanol peaked in 1980–1981 at 2.77 gallons as pure ethanol, but by 1990 had declined to 2.46 gallons. In recent years wine coolers have accounted for up to 25 percent of all ethanol consumption in the United States.

Ethanol use has been blamed for 3 percent of deaths in the United States, with the cost of ethanol use and dependence estimated at $117 billion in 1983. Lost work accounted for 61 percent of the cost, while 13 percent was attributed to the cost of medical care. Three percent of all hospitalizations are for complications of ethanol use, with ethanol withdrawal comprising 68 percent of case diagnoses, followed by liver disease with 16 percent. The cost to society and to individuals and the debilitating effect of ethanol abuse on the nation's health is clear.

Distilled spirits typically contain ethanol volumes of 40 to 50 percent (80 to 100 proof), although brands with volumes of 75 percent or more exist. Wines have an ethanol volume of 10 to 20 percent, while beers range from 2 to 6 percent. Ethanol is also a constituent of mouthwashes (up to 75 percent volume), colognes (40 to 60 percent), and medicinal preparations (0.4 to 65 percent).

## Alcoholism, Alcohol Abuse, and Alcohol Dependence

Alcoholism has been defined by the National Council on Alcoholism and Drug Dependence as a "primary, chronic disease with genetic, psychosocial, and environmental factors influencing its development and manifestations . . . (and) is characterized by impaired control over drinking, preoccupation with the drug ethanol, use of ethanol despite adverse consequences, and distortions in thinking, most notably denial. Each of these symptoms may be continuous or periodic." Three of four alcoholics are men and nearly 60 percent are 25 to 44 years old. Among the homeless, estimated at 250,000 on any given night and 3 million people per year, 20 to 45 percent are alcoholics. Secondary psychiatric diagnoses, including antisocial personality, mania, and schizophrenia are more common in alcoholics than the general population. Suicide attempts and problems with drugs other than ethanol are also common among alcoholics.

The traditional perspective on alcoholism as a disease with purely social and psychiatric underpinnings has been revised in recent years as evidence has accumulated that genetic factors play a major role. Data supporting a genetic influence on causation include the finding that close relatives of alcoholics have a fourfold risk of alcoholism over controls, even when they are adopted children raised away from their genetic family from birth. Similarly, twin research has shown that the risk of alcoholism for an identical twin of an alcoholic is much greater than that of a fraternal twin.

*Ethanol dependence,* defined as regular use resulting in tolerance to the drug and the likelihood of withdrawal symptoms if intake is suspended, is experienced by 6 percent of Americans. *Ethanol abuse,* affecting another 4 percent of the population, is a separate problem marked by social or medical problems that result from inappropriate use of ethanol but without the presence of dependence. Intermittent bouts of drinking resulting in aggressive or antisocial behavior or driving while intoxicated are examples of ethanol abuse. The fact that 10 percent of the population have ethanol-related problems means that alcoholism touches most Americans' lives at some time, whether at home, on the road, or in the workplace.

## Effects on Health

Ethanol abuse and its association with trauma represent a major public health issue. Forty percent of Americans will be involved in an ethanol-related motor vehicle accident in their lifetime, and nearly half of all fatal motor vehicle accidents are associated with use of ethanol. Between 1982 and 1992 ethanol-associated highway fatalities decreased by 30 percent, whereas all traffic fatalities fell by only 4 percent, an encouraging trend that is presumably the result of public education campaigns. Those who drink are also at increased risk for accidents within the home and for injuries from assault.

Alcoholics have been estimated on average to have a life span 10 to 15 years shorter than moderate or nondrinkers. Increased mortality results chiefly from heart and liver disease, cancer, and accidents. Although the occurence of coronary artery disease is decreased among alcoholics, heavy ethanol use increases the likelihood of hypertension and thus hypertensive disease, as well as itself being a direct cause of cardiomyopathy. Ethanol is the most common cause of liver failure in the United States and worldwide. Fatty liver is present in virtually all alcoholics; 10 to 35 percent develop alcoholic hepatitis. Alcoholic women are more susceptible than men to the development of cirrhosis; the risk of cirrhosis for women increases with ethanol intake greater than 21 to 40 g/d, compared to 61 to 80 g/d for men. Why women are at increased risk and why all heavy users of ethanol do not develop liver disease is unclear. Heavy ethanol use is also associated with increased risk of cancer of the esophagus, stomach, pancreas, liver, and breast.

Chronic toxicity from ethanol abuse may affect nearly every major organ system with serious health consequences (Table 138-1). A detailed discussion of these complications is beyond the scope of this chapter.

In contrast to the case of tobacco as a substance that is legal but for which there is no safe level of consumption, there are good indications that moderate ethanol use may actually promote good health. A population based study found that patients attending a health maintenance organization who consumed more than one drink a month but less than one drink per day had a lower mortality rate than those who drank either more or less. Decreased mortality may be associated with diminished coronary risk among users of ethanol, apparently mediated through increased blood high-density lipoprotein levels. Although this effect persists at higher levels of ethanol use, it is outweighed by the other deleterious effects of chronic use of the drug.

## Pharmacology

Ethanol is a central nervous system (CNS) depressant that inhibits neuronal activity, probably through its effects on cell membranes. Behavioral stimulation is often observed at low blood concentrations. Cross-tolerance exists between ethanol and other sedative-hypnotic agents, including benzodiazepines and barbiturates. Absorption occurs from the mouth and esophagus to a small extent, from the stomach and large bowel to a moderate extent, but chiefly from the proximal portion of the small bowel.

Gender-related differences in the pharmacology of ethanol explain the considerably higher blood ethanol levels in women in comparison to men after similar dosing on a gram-per-kilogram basis. Women have a smaller volume of distribution (0.6 L/kg) for ethanol than men (0.7 L/kg) and have decreased first-pass metabolism of ethanol because their gastric walls contain less alcohol dehydrogenase than men.

**Table 138-1.** Adverse Health Effects Associated with Ethanol Abuse and Dependence

**Central Nervous System**
  Acute intoxication
  Ethanol withdrawal
    Seizures
    Hallucinations
  Wernicke's encephalopathy
  Korsakoff's psychosis
  Dementia
  Depression, antisocial personality, suicidal ideation
**Gastrointestinal**
  Esophageal varices
  Erosive gastritis
  Alcoholic hepatitis/liver failure
  Peptic ulcer disease
  Pancreatitis
  Oropharyngeal, esophageal, gastric, hepatic and pancreatic malignancies
**Cardiovascular**
  Hypertension
  Cardiomyopathy
  Stroke
  Arrhythmias associated with intoxication or withdrawal
**Musculoskeletal**
  Fractures secondary to ethanol-associated trauma
  Myopathy
**Endocrine/Metabolic**
  Testicular atrophy
  Alcoholic ketoacidosis
  Folic acid and thiamine deficiencies
**Hematopoietic**
  Thrombocytopenia secondary to marrow suppression, folate deficiency, splenic sequestration
  Anemia secondary to marrow suppression, folate deficiency, gastrointestinal bleeding, splenic sequestration
  Leukopenia secondary to marrow suppression, splenic sequestration
**Other**
  Fetal alcohol syndrome
  Breast cancer in women

In the range of 2 to 10 percent of ethanol may be excreted by the lungs or in urine or sweat, the proportion being dependent on blood concentration. The remainder is metabolized to acetaldehyde in the liver, by one of two pathways. In the cell cytosol alcohol dehydrogenase with nicotinamide adenine dinucleotide (NAD) as a cofactor produces acetaldehyde, which in turn is metabolized by aldehyde dehydrogenase. The second pathway, which is clinically significant at high blood ethanol concentrations and which has increased activity with repeated exposures to ethanol, is a microsomal alcohol oxidizing system.

## Ethanol and the Emergency Physician

The medical, psychiatric, social, legal, and public health implications of ethanol use are well known to emergency physicians. Emergency physicians manage trauma associated with ethanol use and are expected by most local law enforcement authorities to provide a safe haven for intoxicated individuals. They provide early care for complications of ethanol use and must be able to accurately diagnose ethanol-related problems and distinguish them from problems with other causes.

A considerable proportion of emergency department patients exhibit evidence of recent ethanol use. Ethanol has been detected in the blood of 15 to 40 percent of unselected emergency department patients, depending on locale. At an urban hospital 23 percent of patients questioned admitted to ethanol use within 6 h prior to emergency department arrival. Yet emergency physicians fail to recognize 50 percent of patients with ethanol dependence, a proportion that is similar to that overlooked by specialists caring for inpatients.

The formal diagnosis of alcoholism has rested on various questionnaires/scoring systems, such as CAGE or the Michigan Alcohol Screening Test. In the clinical setting, pointed questioning when appropriate about quantity of ethanol intake, medical complications that are usually caused by drinking, and whether the patient himself and others have ever felt he has a drinking problem will usually uncover drinking problems.

## Acute Intoxication

Symptoms and signs of ethanol intoxication are well known and include slurred speech, disinhibited behavior or CNS depression, and decreased motor coordination and control. A decrease from a patient's usual blood pressure—or frank hypotension—may occur; these are secondary to an ethanol-mediated decrease in total peripheral resistance. Reflex tachycardia may also be observed. When hypotension is present, causes other than ethanol intoxication must be considered. Direct toxic effects on end organs, such as hepatitis or pancreatitis, may or may not be present. Although death occurs rarely as a result of respiratory depression, morbidity and mortality occurring in association with acute intoxication are predominantly the result of accidental injuries related to ethanol-induced deficits in judgment or physical capabilities.

Because of the phenomenon of tolerance, blood alcohol levels correlate poorly with degree of intoxication. Although death from respiratory depression may occur in unhabituated individuals at concentrations of 400 to 500 mg/dL, it is not uncommon for some alcoholics to appear unintoxicated at blood concentrations as high as 400 mg/dL. A habituated individual with a blood concentration reported as 1510 mg/dL survived with supportive care only. Although most states have adapted 100 mg/dL as the legal definition of intoxication for the purposes of driving a motor vehicle, evidence suggests that impairment may be seen with levels as low as 5 mg/dL, especially in unhabituated individuals.

**Ethanol intoxication and hypothermia.** Most cases of hypothermia during winter months in urban settings are associated with ethanol use. Many homeless persons are heavy users of ethanol and on cold nights may use ethanol to inure themselves to the effects of low temperature. Although the sedative effects of ethanol may result in exposure predisposing to hypothermia, ethanol also directly contributes to body cooling. It depresses central thermoregulatory mechanisms, decreases shivering, and enhances heat loss through vasodilatation. Management of the hypothermic intoxicated patient is similar to that of hypothermia in other patients. Prognosis is related to severity of hypothermia and the presence of underlying diseases, but it does not appear to be adversely affected by ethanol intoxication.

**Ethanol intoxication and trauma.** The injured intoxicated patient presents particular problems for the clinician. Not only are intoxicated patients prone to incidents of trauma, but the effect of ethanol on the sensorium complicates efforts at cost-effective diagnosis and treatment. Obtaining studies that require patient cooperation can be difficult, with the physician sometimes facing with the contradictory necessity of administering a second CNS depressant to satisfactorily evaluate injuries.

Ethanol intoxication may also complicate recognition of serious injuries. Patients with abdominal injuries may present without suggestive clinical findings, and the depressed mental status of patients with head injuries may be mistakenly ascribed to intoxication. Because clinicians are aware of these considerations, injured patients who have recently ingested ethanol are more likely to undergo procedures and studies such as intubation, diagnostic peritoneal lavage, head computed tomography (CT), and intracranial pressure monitoring. These may not be necessary in all intoxicated patients. As the results of one small study suggested, trauma victims with a Glasgow Coma Scale of 15 and no abdominal complaints or physical findings suggestive of abdominal injury are candidates for careful observation.

Evaluation of head-injured patients—intoxicated or not—remains a controversial area. Serious head injuries are easily overlooked in intoxicated patients, some of whom, especially in inner-city locales, may arrive at the emergency department with no definite history of trauma and no external signs of head trauma. In the authors' experience, the most common serious error made in management of intoxicated patients is to assume for too long that a depressed or abnormal mental status is secondary to intoxication. Intoxicated patients should undergo CT evaluation if there is a history of head injury and Glasgow Coma Scale is less than 15; for any worsening of mental status while under observation; or if there is no improvement of mental status by 3 h after admission. Once the decision to perform CT has been made, no delay should be allowed due to lack of cooperation by the patient, which may be due to ethanol or concomitant drug use, or the effects of head injury. Sedation may be required with careful attention to airway protection and paralysis and intubation if necessary.

It is uncertain whether ethanol intoxication itself worsens the prognosis of injured patients. Animal model studies of CNS trauma have suggested that this may be the case, whereas clinical studies have had contradictory results. A study of over a million motor vehicle accidents, which attempted to control for safety belt use, vehicle deformation, vehicle speed, and other factors, found that drivers who drank were more likely to suffer a serious injury or death. Hospital-based studies have not shown any tendency for ethanol intoxication to worsen the outcome of injured patients.

**Management.** Management of acute ethanol intoxication consists primarily of observing patients until clinical sobriety is attained, as well as attending to associated injuries or medical illness. A careful examination should be performed to evaluate for complicating injuries or medical conditions. Hypoglycemia should be excluded by a bedside glucose determination or approximation method. Any alcoholic with mental status changes, even if attributable to intoxication, should receive thiamine. Patients with mild to moderate intoxication do not require intravenous line placement, treatment with vitamin supplements other than thiamine, or intravenous fluid administration unless clinical signs of dehydration are present. Careful and serial observation of such patients is crucial because any deterioration in mental status should be considered secondary to causes other than ethanol and managed accordingly. Unhabituated patients eliminate ethanol from the bloodstream at a rate of 15 to 20 mg/dL per hour, whereas alcoholics average 25 to 35 mg/dL per hour. Most patients with CNS depression secondary to ethanol improve within a few hours of emergency department arrival.

Concomitant drug use by alcoholics should be considered and tested for when clinically relevant. In the past, ethylene glycol or methanol were occasionally substituted for or used in combination with ethanol by inner-city alcoholics. Today cocaine has clearly become the most commonly abused second drug by alcoholics. The attraction of abusing these drugs together may relate to the formation of a metabolite, cocaethylene, which has 40 times the affinity for cocaine receptors of cocaine itself and is thus an extremely potent intoxicant. The risk of sudden death by users of both drugs simultaneously may as high as 20 times that with cocaine alone. Ethanol is the most common cause of an osmolal gap (see below), which also characterizes isopropanol, methanol, and ethylene glycol poisoning (Table 138-2).

**Disposition.** Patients with acute ethanol intoxication rarely require hospital admission for treatment of this problem alone. However, questions frequently arise over alcoholics who appear clinically sober while still having considerable blood ethanol concentrations. Patients who will drive motor vehicles from the emergency department should have blood ethanol concentrations approaching zero. Patients whose intoxication has resolved to the extent that they do not constitute a danger to themselves or others and who will not be responsible for their own transport may be discharged on their own cognizance or

**Table 138-2.** Molecular Weight and Contribution of Alcohols to Serum Osmolality

| Substance | Molecular Weight | mOsm/L at 100 mg/dL | Correction Factor |
|---|---|---|---|
| Ethanol | 46 | 22 | 4.6 |
| Isopropanol | 60 | 17 | 6.0 |
| Methanol | 32 | 31 | 3.2 |
| Ethylene glycol | 62 | 16 | 6.2 |

To estimate concentration of an alcohol in mg/dL, use the following formula: (osmolal gap−10) × correction factor. This estimation is valid only if the alcohol is the only unmeasured abnormal contributor to osmolality.

preferably in the company of friends or relatives who can assist them and take some role in their care.

## Ethanol Withdrawal

Some alcoholics exhibit one or more symptoms of withdrawal on discontinuation of ethanol intake. Symptoms and signs include tremor, anxiety, agitation, and signs of autonomic hyperactivity. Cardiac dysrhythmias, most frequently sinus tachycardia or atrial fibrillation, may be observed. Seizures may occur, while hallucinations, usually visual, are a sign of moderate to severe withdrawal. Signs and symptoms of withdrawal are most likely to reach peak intensity at 48 h after patients' last drinks. The wide variation observed in timing of onset and peak severity of alcohol withdrawal reflects differences in patterns of ethanol intake, individual susceptibility to withdrawal, and concomitant illness. For example, significant withdrawal may be observed while alcoholics still have detectable blood ethanol or within a short time after the last drink. These situations may reflect a recent pattern of continued but decreased intake of ethanol, or the common practice of alcoholics self-treating themselves with ethanol when symptoms first appear, and then seeking medical care if those symptoms fail to resolve.

Because ethanol withdrawal is a syndrome complex, more than one sign should be present in most cases. When alcoholic patients present with a single sign compatible with ethanol withdrawal, other causes should be considered. Seizures in alcoholic patients are frequently secondary to other causes, most notably recent or remote head trauma, whether the history is recounted by the patient or not. Hallucinations may be secondary to a psychiatric disorder (although these are more likely to be auditory, whereas alcoholic hallucinosis is more likely to produce visual hallucinations) or concomitant drug use.

**Management.** After the diagnosis of alcohol withdrawal is established, an examination for complicating medical conditions or injury should be performed. Patients with alcohol withdrawal are frequently volume depleted and may require crystalloid infusion. If possible, patients should be placed in a quiet area with a minimum of stimulation. For patients who have experienced seizures, CT examination is indicated if focal seizures have occurred, when a focal neurologic finding is elicited, or when the patient has a persistent postictal defect in consciousness.

Benzodiazepines or phenobarbital are mainstays in the treatment of withdrawal. We favor the use of phenobarbital, beginning with a dose of 260 mg administered intravenously over 15 min. Subsequent doses of 130 mg are given every 30 to 45 min as needed to induce light sedation. At the same time 1 L of 5% dextrose/normal saline with 100 mg thiamine and 4 g magnesium sulfate is given over 1 to 2 h. Although magnesium has not been shown to effective against ethanol withdrawal in general, hypomagnesemia has been closely associated with tremor in alcoholics and may play a role in the genesis of seizures. Lorazepam may be substituted for phenobarbital in an initial dose of 4 mg, followed by subsequent 2-mg doses on a schedule similar to that for phenobarbital. It is important to approach ethanol withdrawal with the knowledge that repeated and cumulatively large doses of sedative agents may be required. There is no evidence that ethanol withdrawal seizures are prevented by anticonvulsant agents (e.g., phenytoin) which have no effect on the withdrawal state itself.

**Disposition.** Patients with alcohol withdrawal and complicating medical problems, such as infections or congestive heart failure, should be admitted to the hospital. Patients who fail to respond to one or two doses of sedative medications should also be admitted. Administration of more than 500 mg phenobarbital or 8 mg lorazepam is in most cases an indication for admission to a nursing unit where the patient can receive close observation by both nursing and physician staff, in many hospitals, an intensive care unit. Patients with mild alcohol withdrawal who respond to treatment may be discharged. If they have received phenobarbital, no outpatient prescription is necessary because of the drug's prolonged half-life, 24 to 96 h. In any case, the benefit of prescribing outpatient benzodiazepines is doubtful if a patient is likely to resume drinking after discharge from the emergency department.

### Long-term Outlook for Alcoholics

Alcoholic patients should be referred for counseling when possible. A fifth or more may achieve permanent abstinence with the aid of Alcoholics Anonymous or other self-help groups. Unfortunately, the rate of recidivism is related to socioeconomic status and availability of family and social support systems. Thus, although 60 percent of middle-class alcoholics will remain ethanol free for at least 1 year after completing a rehabilitation program, the outlook is considerably more bleak for those who are less advantaged.

## ISOPROPANOL

Isopropanol ($CH_3CHOHCH_3$), also known as isopropyl alcohol and 2-propanol, is commonly found in the home as rubbing alcohol. It is also used widely in industry as a solvent and disinfectant and is a component of a variety of skin and hair products, jewelry cleaners, detergents, paint thinners, and antifreeze. Poisoning usually results from ingestion but may also occur after inhalation in poorly ventilated areas, for example, during alcohol sponge bathing. Toxicity occurring after administration of an isopropanol enema has also been reported. Its principal metabolite, acetone, does not cause the eye, kidney, cardiac, or metabolic toxicity caused by the metabolites of methanol and ethylene glycol.

Isopropanol is approximately twice as potent as ethanol in causing CNS depression and has a duration of two to four times that of ethanol intoxication. As a result it is on occasion used as a substitute intoxicant by alcoholics, as well as in suicide attempts. After ethanol, it is the second most commonly ingested alcohol. It is more toxic than ethanol, although considerably less so than methanol or ethylene glycol.

### Pharmacology/Pathophysiology

Isopropanol is a clear, volatile liquid with a bitter, burning taste and an aromatic odor. It is rapidly absorbed after being ingested, with 80 percent of an oral dose being absorbed after 30 min and complete absorption within 2 h. The substance has a volume of distribution of 0.6 to 0.7 L/kg. Small and clinically insignificant amounts are resecreted by the salivary glands and stomach.

The kidneys excrete 20 to 50 percent of an absorbed dose unchanged. However, the major pathway for metabolism of isopropanol is in the liver, where it is oxidized to acetone by alcohol dehydrogenase (Fig. 138-1). Acetone is further metabolized to acetate, to formate, and then finally to carbon dioxide. Mild acidosis may result from the conversion of acetone to acetic acid and formic acid. A hallmark of isopropanol toxicity is ketonemia and ketonuria, without an elevated blood glucose level or glycosuria.

Isopropanol most closely follows concentration-dependent (first-order) kinetics. The half-life of isopropanol in the absence of ethanol

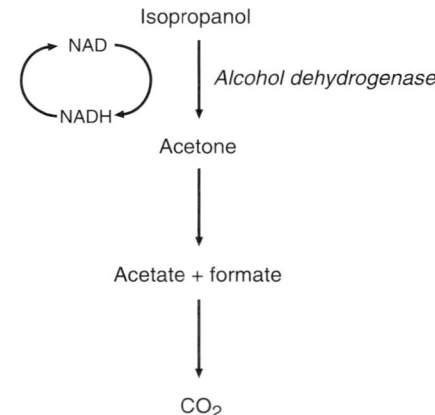

**Fig. 138-1.** Metabolic pathway of isopropanol in the liver.

is 6 to 7 h, whereas the half-life of acetone is 22 to 28 h. The long half-life of acetone may be the cause of the prolonged symptomatology often associated with isopropanol poisoning. Ethanol administration has not been used clinically to inhibit isopropanol metabolism to acetone.

The toxic dose of 70% isopropanol is approximately 1 mL/kg, with the lethal dose in an adult approximately 2 to 4 mL/kg. As little as 0.5 mL/kg may cause symptoms, but survival has been reported following ingestions of up to 1 L. Children are especially susceptible to toxic effects and may develop symptoms with as little as three swallows of 70% isopropanol.

### Clinical Presentation

The clinical features of isopropanol intoxication are similar to those seen with ethanol intoxication except that the duration of symptoms and signs are longer, and CNS depression may be more profound, due to the formation of acetone. The early phase of elation commonly seen in ethanol intoxication is absent. Onset of symptoms occurs within 30 to 60 min, with peak effects in a few hours. Nystagmus is usually present. Severe poisoning is marked by early onset of coma, respiratory depression, and hypotension.

Cardiovascular compromise is seen with massive ingestion and may be manifested by hypotension, which is secondary to peripheral vasodilatation, with contributions possible from hemorrhagic gastritis, or cardiomyopathy. Serious arrhythmias are rare.

Hemorrhagic gastritis secondary to gastric irritation appears early and is a striking feature of isopropanol ingestions, often resulting in nausea, vomiting, abdominal pain, and at times, upper gastrointestinal hemorrhage.

Hypoglycemia may occur secondary to depressed gluconeogenesis. Less common complications include hepatic dysfunction, acute tubular necrosis, myoglobinuria, hemolytic anemia, rhabdomyolysis, and myopathy.

### Diagnosis

In addition to its characteristic clinical presentation, isopropanol poisoning should be suspected when the smell of rubbing alcohol is present on the breath, when there is acidosis associated with ketonuria and ketonemia without glycosuria or hyperglycemia, and in the presence of an elevated osmolal gap. Minimal acidosis in combination with elevated serum ketones is particularly characteristic of isopropanol intoxication.

As previously mentioned, isopropanol has approximately twice the intoxicating effect of ethanol at the same blood concentration. Although isopropanol levels of 50 mg/dL are associated with mild intoxication in individuals who are not habituated to ethanol, alcoholic patients may be considerably more resistant to the CNS effects of isopropanol. Survival has been reported at concentrations up to 560 mg/dL.

The osmolal gap is the difference between measured and calculated osmolality and is normally made up of unmeasured small molecular weight substances. Calculated serum osmolality is derived from the following formula:

serum osmolality (mOsm/kg) = 2(Na$^+$)
$$+ \text{Blood urea nitrogen}/2.8 + \text{Glucose}/18$$

The result is subtracted from the serum osmolality as determined by the clinical laboratory (preferably by freezing point depression), to determine the osmolal gap, which is normally 10 mOsm or less. An elevated osmolal gap suggests the presence of abnormal low molecular weight substances; in addition to isopropanol these could include toxic agents such as methanol, ethylene glycol, or ethanol; or therapeutic agents such as glycerol or mannitol.

## Management

If suspicion of isopropanol poisoning exists, intravenous access should be established with immediate bedside testing for blood glucose and administration of thiamine and naloxone if indicated. Because of the rapid absorption of isopropanol, the utility of gastric lavage more than 2 h after ingestion is doubtful. Activated charcoal has been shown to bind isopropanol poorly, and therefore is not indicated in the absence of ingestion of other, adsorbable, substances. Patients with isopropanol ingestions should be carefully monitored for CNS or respiratory depression. In addition to serum osmolality, serum electrolytes, blood urea nitrogen, creatinine, blood glucose, acetone, arterial blood gases, and hepatic aminotransferases should be determined. Although an isopropanol level does not, in most cases, influence management, it may be helpful in cases of severe toxicity when hemodialysis is being considered to enhance elimination.

In severely obtunded patients, airway management may require intubation and ventilatory support. Hypotension usually responds to intravenous fluids; in severe cases support with pressors may be indicated. Patients with severe hemorrhagic gastritis may require blood transfusion. Although the acidosis associated with isopropanol poisoning is usually mild, it may be exacerbated by hypotension and necessitate administration of sodium bicarbonate. Hemodialysis is indicated when hypotension is refractory to conventional therapy, resulting in hemodynamic instability, or when predicted peak isopropanol level is greater than 400 mg/dL. Hemodialysis is effective in eliminating both isopropanol and acetone. Although peritoneal dialysis may be performed when hemodialysis is unavailable, it is not as effective as hemodialysis.

Patients with lethargy or prolonged CNS depression should be admitted to the hospital. Those who remain asymptomatic for 6 to 8 h may be discharged or referred for psychiatric evaluation if indicated.

## METHANOL

Methanol (CH$_3$OH), also referred to as methyl alcohol, wood spirits, or wood alcohol, is used widely in commercial, industrial, and marine solvents. It is a component of many paint removers, varnishes, shellacs, windshield washing fluids, and antifreeze formulations. A product of wood distillation, methanol poisoning has resulted from the consumption of contaminated whiskey, accidental ingestion by alcoholics, or intentional ingestion during suicide attempts. Methanol's toxicity is the result of the formation of two toxic metabolites, formaldehyde and formic acid. Therapeutic strategies are therefore based on prevention of the formation of these metabolites or their removal from the body.

### Pharmacology/Pathophysiology

Methanol is a colorless, volatile liquid with a distinctive odor. It is well absorbed from the gastrointestinal tract with peak levels attained

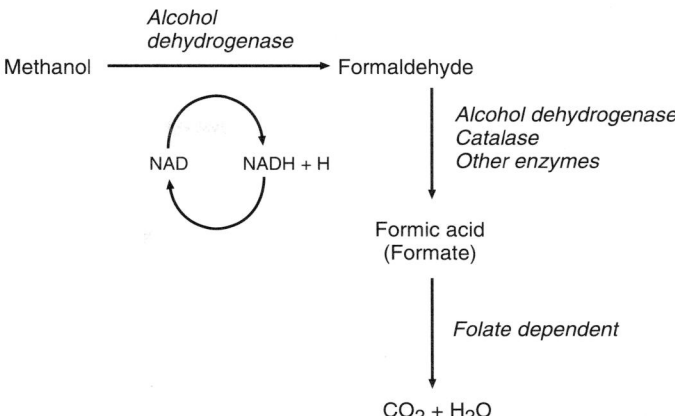

**Fig. 138-2.** Metabolism of methanol in the liver.

30 to 90 min after ingestion. Most incidents of toxicity occur after oral ingestion, but significant absorption may also occur through the lungs or skin. The serum half-life after mild toxicity is 14 to 20 h; with severe toxicity this increases to 24 to 30 h. Methanol has a volume of distribution of 0.6 to 0.7 L/kg.

Following ingestion, highest concentrations are found in the kidney, liver, and gastrointestinal tract, but high levels are also found in the vitreous humor and optic nerve. Most methanol—90 to 95 percent—is eliminated by the liver; renal excretion accounts for 2 to 5 percent, and pulmonary excretion is minimal. In overdoses, elimination follows saturation (zero-order) kinetics.

Toxicity from methanol poisoning results from the metabolism by hepatic alcohol dehydrogenase of methanol to formaldehyde and formic acid (Fig. 138-2). The accumulation of formic acid is associated with the onset of clinical symptoms. Lactate is produced from formate-induced inhibition of mitochondrial respiration, as a result of tissue hypoxia, and to a lesser extent as a result of oxidation of methanol decreasing the intracellular NAD/NADH ratio and thus stimulating anaerobic glycolysis and lactate production. Formaldehyde production in the retina causes optic papillitis and retinal edema, resulting in severe cases in blindness.

Ethanol has a 10 to 20 times greater affinity for alcohol dehydrogenase than methanol and is preferentially metabolized by the enzyme, thereby reducing the rate of oxidation of methanol to its toxic metabolites. Ethanol saturation of this enzyme may increase the serum half-life of methanol up to 30 to 35 h. Because folate is a cofactor in the breakdown of formic acid to carbon dioxide and water, alcoholics who are folate deficient may be especially susceptible to methanol toxicity.

The amount of methanol required to cause toxicity varies; death has been reported after ingestion of as small a dose as 15 mL of a 40% solution. Although 30 mL of a 40% solution is considered the minimal lethal dose, amounts as large as 500 to 600 mL have been ingested with survival reported.

### Clinical Presentation

The symptoms of methanol poisoning may not appear for up to 12 to 18 h after ingestion because of the time it takes for methanol to be metabolized to its toxic metabolites. The delay in symptoms may be even longer if ethanol has been ingested. The cardinal clinical manifestations of methanol poisoning are CNS depression similar to that of ethanol; visual disturbances; abdominal pain, nausea, and vomiting; and high anion gap metabolic acidosis. As with isopropanol, the early phase of elation commonly seen in ethanol intoxication is absent.

On arrival at the hospital, the victim may be confused, or in severe cases, comatose. There may be complaints of headache or vertigo, and seizures may occur. Visual disturbances are seen in approximately 50 percent of patients. These include diplopia, blurred vision, decreased visual acuity, photophobia, descriptions of "looking into a snow field," constricted visual fields, and blindness. The clinician may find nystagmus, fixed and dilated pupils, retinal edema, and optic atrophy or hyperemia of the optic disk. Brain CT may reveal basal ganglia infarcts consistent with the parkinsonian syndrome, which has been reported after methanol poisoning. Methanol is a potent mucosal irritant and causes severe abdominal pain, nausea, and vomiting in over one half of cases; pancreatitis has also been commonly reported. Serious ingestions may occur, however, in the absence of gastrointestinal symptoms. Although an increased osmolal gap is usually present with serious methanol ingestion, methanol poisoning with a normal osmolal gap has been reported.

Hypotension and bradycardia are late findings and suggest a poor prognosis. Outcome is best correlated with the severity of the acidosis rather than with serum methanol concentration.

## Diagnosis

Diagnosis of methanol poisoning rests on history, the presence of the characteristic clinical features outlined above, and the presence of a high anion gap metabolic acidosis and osmolal gap. Detection of an osmolal gap precedes detection of the anion gap. Although confirmation of a tentative diagnosis depends on identification of the substance in the bloodstream, treatment should be initiated based on compatible clinical presentation to avoid morbidity resulting from delay. In any case, serum methanol determinations at many institutions depend on outside laboratories and may not be available for several hours.

Normal methanol blood concentration from endogenous sources is 0.05 mg/dL. Asymptomatic individuals usually have peak levels less than 20 mg/dL; levels greater than 50 mg/dL indicate serious poisoning. CNS symptoms usually appear when levels rise above 20 mg/dL, eye problems are associated with levels greater than 50 mg/dL, and the risk of fatality rises with levels greater than 150 to 200 mg/dL.

The differential diagnosis should include other potential causes of an elevated anion gap metabolic acidosis, such as ethylene glycol, diabetic ketoacidosis, paraldehyde, isoniazid, salicylates, iron, lactic acidosis, phenformin, and uremia.

## Management

Intravenous access should be established with immediate bedside testing for blood glucose and administration of thiamine and naloxone if indicated. The general measures involved in treatment are supportive care, correction of acidosis, administration of ethanol to decrease conversion to toxic metabolites, and dialysis to eliminate the methanol. If the patient presents within 2 h of the ingestion, gastric lavage should be performed to remove any remaining methanol from the stomach. Activated charcoal has been shown to bind methanol poorly, and therefore is not indicated in the absence of ingestion of other, adsorbable, substances. Care should be taken to maintain an adequate airway with intubation if necessary for proper ventilatory support. Sodium bicarbonate should be administered with the goal of maintaining a near normal pH, because correction of metabolic acidosis moderates some of the toxic effects of methanol poisoning, including visual impairment.

Ethanol competitively inhibits the metabolism of methanol by alcohol dehydrogenase. Ethanol's affinity for the enzyme is 10 to 20 times that of methanol and its presence largely inhibits the formation of the toxic metabolites. Ethanol should be administered when methanol poisoning is suspected, in cases of high anion gap metabolic acidosis with an osmolal gap, if methanol concentration is found to be greater than 20 mg/dL, when the quantity of methanol ingested is calculated to be 0.4 mL/kg or more, or when symptoms consistent with methanol poisoning are present. Any patient considered

for dialysis should also receive ethanol. The blood ethanol level should be maintained between 100 and 150 mg/dL to completely inhibit formation of toxic metabolites. Blood concentrations less than 100 mg/dL are considerably less effective, and therefore increase the risk of severe toxicity.

Ethanol may be administered intravenously or orally or by nasogastric tube. Intravenous administration is preferred although it may result in superficial thrombophlebitis. The intravenous solution should contain 10% ethanol and 5% dextrose in water. A 20% to 30% ethanol concentration can be used for oral dosing; although higher concentrations have been used, these can cause gastritis. To maintain an ethanol level of 100 to 150 mg/dL, a loading dose of 0.6 to 0.8 g/kg should be given intravenously or orally, with maintenance doses at approximately 0.11 g/kg per hour. If the recommended solution of 10% ethanol and 5% dextrose in water is used, the loading dose is 10 mL/kg and maintenance is 1.6 mL/kg per hour. If the patient is a regular consumer of ethanol with enhanced hepatic elimination, the maintenance infusion should be started at 0.15 g/kg per hour. When intravenous ethanol is not immediately available, oral therapy can be initiated with commercial distilled spirits. To calculate the ethanol content of distilled spirits, the following formula may be used:

$$\text{Ethanol in g} = \text{Volume of beverage in mL} \times 0.9 \times (\text{proof}/200)$$

Ethanol levels should be assayed on a frequent basis, with the dose adjusted to maintain a concentration of 100 to 150 mg/dL. Administration should continue until the methanol level is zero. If dialysis is initiated, a higher maintenance infusion will be necessary because ethanol is dialyzable; starting at 0.24 g/kg per hour has been recommended. Hypoglycemia may occur with ethanol administration, especially in children, so blood glucose levels should be monitored closely.

Dialysis should be performed for methanol poisoning if there are signs of visual or CNS dysfunction, peak methanol levels are greater than 50 mg/dL, if severe metabolic acidosis develops *regardless of levels,* and if there is a history of greater than 30 mL ingestion. Hemodialysis is considerably more effective than peritoneal dialysis, but peritoneal dialysis may be used if hemodialysis is not unavailable. Dialysis eliminates both the parent compound and its toxic metabolites.

Folate is a cofactor for the conversion of formic acid to carbon dioxide. It is especially important to provide supplements to alcoholic patients who may be folate deficient. Administration of folic acid 50 mg intravenously q4h for several days to all patients is recommended.

4-Methylpyrazole has been used experimentally as an antidote for methanol and ethylene glycol poisoning. It is a competitive inhibitor of alcohol dehydrogenase and blocks the metabolism of these agents to their toxic metabolites; it does not cause CNS depression like ethanol. It has not yet been approved for clinical use in the United States.

Disposition decisions are based on criteria identical to those used for ethylene glycol poisoning (see below).

## ETHYLENE GLYCOL

Ethylene glycol has many commercial uses as a coolant, preservative, and glycerine substitute and has also been used in lacquers, cosmetics, polishes, and detergents. It may be ingested as an alcohol substitute by alcoholics, in suicide attempts, and accidentally by children. Ethylene glycol's toxicity is the result of the formation of two toxic metabolites, formaldehyde and formic acid. As with methanol, therapeutic strategies are based on prevention of formation of these metabolites or their removal from the body.

## Pharmacology/Pathophysiology

Ethylene glycol (Fig. 138-3) is a colorless, odorless, sweet-tasting substance. It is highly water soluble and rapidly absorbed when in-

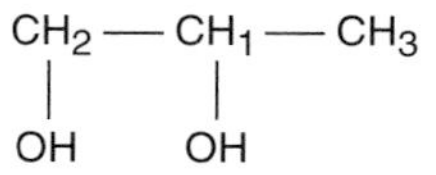

$$CH_2 - CH_1 - CH_3$$
$$\quad | \qquad\quad |$$
$$\ \ OH \qquad OH$$

**Fig. 138-3.** Chemical structure of ethylene glycol.

gested orally but not by the lungs or skin. Peak blood levels occur within 1 to 4 h of an ingestion. The volume of distribution is 0.83 L/kg and the plasma half-life is 3 to 5 h. Ethanol at a concentration of 100 to 200 mg/dL increases half-life to 17 h. Ethylene glycol is metabolized in the liver and kidneys to toxic metabolites—aldehydes, glycolate, oxalate, and lactate—which in turn cause toxicity to the lungs, heart, and kidneys. These metabolites also cause the metabolic acidosis that is associated with ethylene glycol poisoning.

Ethylene glycol is metabolized to glycoaldehyde by the alcohol dehydrogenase (Fig. 138-4). This conversion involves the reduction of $NAD^+$ to NADH, which causes inhibition of the citric acid cycle and formation of lactic acid. Glycoaldehyde is further metabolized to glycolic acid and to glyoxylic acid, which is in turn converted to several new compounds. Pyridoxal phosphate is a cofactor in the conversion of glyoxylic acid to glycine, which is nontoxic; thiamine pyrophosphate is the cofactor in the conversion of glyoxylic acid to another nontoxic compound called α-hydroxy-β-ketoadipate. A deficiency of either pyridoxal phosphate or thiamine may shift the metabolism of ethylene glycol to the production of toxic metabolites.

Glyoxylic acid is also metabolized to formic acid and oxalic acid. Glycolic acid contributes to the metabolic acidosis observed in ethylene glycol poisoning. Oxalate crystalluria is a striking feature caused by calcium oxalate salt deposition.

The potentially lethal dose in adults is 2 mL/kg although survival has been reported after ingestions ranging from 240 to 970 mL.

## Clinical Presentation

Ethylene glycol poisoning often exhibits three distinct clinical phases. The severity and progression of these phases depends on the amount ingested. The initial phase is characterized by CNS depression, usually within 1 to 12 h after ingestion. Patients may appear inebriated, with slurred speech and ataxia present, but without the odor of ethanol on their breath. Hallucinations, coma, seizures, and death may also occur during this initial phase. These CNS symptoms correlate with peak glycoaldehyde production. The optic fundus is usually normal, differentiating the syndrome from methanol poisoning, although nystagmus and ophthalmoplegia may be observed.

The second or cardiopulmonary phase develops 12 to 24 h after ingestion. Tachycardia, mild hypertension, and tachypnea are the most common symptoms, with congestive heart failure, acute respiratory distress syndrome, cardiomegaly, and circulatory collapse also observed. Myositis has also been reported less commonly during this phase.

The third phase, marked by nephrotoxicity, occurs 24 to 72 h after ingestion. Early symptoms consist of flank pain and costovertebral angle tenderness. Oliguric renal failure and acute tubular necrosis ensue. Complete anuria may occur, but most patients recover without renal damage if they receive appropriate therapy. Nephrotoxicity is caused by aldehyde metabolites and oxalic acid. Two forms of urinary calcium oxalate crystals may be identified on microscopic evaluation of the urine. The dihydrate form (octahedral crystals) is tent shaped and the monohydrate form (monclinic crystals) is dumbbell or prism shaped. The monohydrate form was at one time felt to represent a salt of hippurate, explaining previous reports of hippurate crystals in the urine.

Hypocalcemia may develop secondary to precipitation of calcium as calcium oxalate and may be severe enough to cause tetany and prolongation of the QT interval. Elevated serum creatine phosphokinase levels may accompany and explain the generalized myalgias experienced by some patients.

## Diagnosis

Ethylene glycol intoxication should be considered when a patient presents with inebriation and no ethanol scent on the breath, a high anion gap metabolic acidosis with osmolal gap, and calcium oxalate crystalluria. The mechanisms of anion gap metabolic acidosis and osmolal gap are similar to those observed with methanol.

Tentative diagnosis and initiation of treatment should be based on history and characteristic clinical presentation. As with methanol poisoning, confirmation of a tentative diagnosis depends on identification of the substance in the bloodstream, but treatment should be initiated based on compatible clinical presentation to avoid morbidity resulting from delay. Serum levels greater than 20 mg/dL are likely to result in toxicity. Survival has been reported with levels up to 650 mg/dL; fatality has been associated with levels between 98 and 775 mg/dL.

Leukocytosis is common and should not be considered a manifestation of infection unless clinical signs are present. One third of patients may have hypocalcemia, with QT interval shortening present on the electrocardiogram. Serious intoxication has been reported in the absence of an osmolal gap or calcium oxalate crystalluria.

As with methanol, the differential diagnosis should include other potential causes of an elevated anion gap metabolic acidosis.

## Management

The management of ethylene glycol poisoning is similar to that for methanol poisoning. For indications for gastric lavage, and guidelines for administration of sodium bicarbonate, refer to those given for methanol above. If the patient is hypocalcemic, 10 mL of 10% calcium gluconate should be given intravenously. Pyridoxine 100 mg and thiamine 100 mg intramuscularly or intravenously should be administered daily to facilitate metabolism of ethylene glycol by nontoxic pathways. Magnesium has also been shown to be a cofactor in the metabolism of toxic metabolites and should be given if patients are hypomagnesemic, as alcoholics are commonly observed to be. Laboratory tests that may be useful in evaluating patients suspected of ethylene glycol ingestion include complete blood count, serum electrolytes, acetone, alcohol toxicology panel (with ethanol, isopropanol, and methanol determinations), blood urea nitrogen, creatinine, salicylate level, arterial blood gases, urinalysis, serum ethylene glycol level, and calcium, creatine kinase, and magnesium levels.

Ethanol should be administered as soon as the diagnosis is suspected because the half-life of ethylene glycol is brief—only 3 h. Ethanol's affinity for alcohol dehydrogenase is 100 times that of eth-

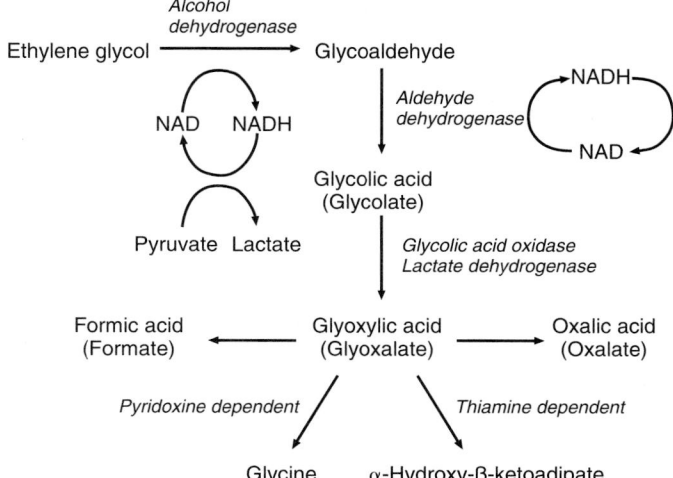

**Fig. 138-4.** Metabolic pathway of ethylene glycol.

ylene glycol, resulting in a prolongation of the half-life of ethylene glycol to 17 h. Ethanol should be administered if there is strong suspicion of ethylene glycol intoxication based on clinical presentation, if ethylene glycol level is more than 20 mg/dL, or if acidosis is present. Oral and intravenous dosing guidelines of ethanol are identical to those outlined for methanol. Dialysis should be initiated if a history, clinical presentation, or laboratory results consistent with ethylene glycol or poisoning are present, when serum concentration of ethylene glycol is greater than 20 to 25 mg/dL, for signs of nephrotoxicity, or when metabolic acidosis is present. As with methanol, hemodialysis has been shown to be considerably more effective, but peritoneal dialysis can be used if hemodialysis is unavailable. 4-Methylpyrazole is an experimental agent that inhibits alcohol dehydrogenase and may eventually prove beneficial in the treatment of ethylene glycol poisoning.

## Disposition

Any patient with the serious signs and symptoms associated with ethylene glycol or methanol intoxication should be admitted to an intensive care unit. Ethanol administration and dialysis should be continued until serum blood levels are zero and acidosis has resolved. Suicidal patients should receive a psychiatric evaluation when their condition improves and prior to discharge from any facility.

Patients seen at facilities unable to provide hemodialysis or an intensive care setting should be transferred to institutions capable of providing such care. Because the toxic symptoms of ethylene glycol and methanol may be delayed, patients with ingestions of these substances should be admitted to the hospital for observation and laboratory testing even if initially asymptomatic. Early recognition of methanol and ethylene glycol and poisoning is critical because ethanol administration, dialysis, and reversal of metabolic acidosis are potentially lifesaving measures.

## BIBLIOGRAPHY

Becker C: Acute methanol poisoning. The "blind drunk." *West J Med* 135:122, 1983.

Burkhart KK, Kulig KW: The other alcohols: methanol, ethylene glycol and isopropanol. *Emerg Med Clin North Am* 8:913, 1990.

Cadnapaphornchai P, Taher S, Bhathena D, MacDonald FD: Ethylene glycol poisoning: diagnosis based on high osmolal and anion gaps and crystalluria. *Ann Emerg Med* 10:94, 1981.

Earnest MP, Yarnell PR: Seizure admissions to a city hospital: the role of alcohol. *Epilepsia* 17:387, 1976.

Isbell H, Fraser HF, Wikler A, Belleville RE, Eisenman AJ: An experimental study of the etiology of "rum fits" and delirium tremens. *Q J Stud Alcohol* 16:1, 1955.

Jurkovich GJ, Rivara FP, Gurney JG, et al: The effect of acute alcohol intoxication and chronic alcohol abuse on outcome from trauma. *JAMA* 270:51, 1993.

Jurkovich GJ, Rivara FP, Gurney JG, Seguin D, Fligner CL, Copass M: Effects of alcohol intoxication on the initial assessment of trauma patients. *Ann Emerg Med* 21:704, 1992.

Klatsky AL, Armstrong MA, Friedman GD: Alcohol and mortality. *Ann Intern Med* 117:646, 1992.

Sullivan JB, Hauptman M, Bronstein AC: Lack of observable intoxication in humans with high blood alcohol concentrations. *J Forensic Sci* 32:1660, 1987.

Turk J, Morrell L, Avioli L: Ethylene glycol intoxication. *Arch Intern Med* 146:1601, 1986.

Waller PF, Stewart JR, Hansen AR, Stutts JC, Lederhaus C, Rodgman EA: The potentiating effects of alcohol on driver injury. *JAMA* 256:1461, 1986.

# 139
# NARCOTICS
## James A. Smith
## George L. Sternbach

The narcotic of most frequent illicit use is heroin, which is produced by the acetylation of morphine. Other narcotics include methadone, morphine, codeine, meperidine, hydromorphone (Dilaudid) and oxycodone (Percodan). Street heroin is adulterated, usually in a 20 to 200:1 ratio, with a number of agents such as quinine, lactose, sucrose, mannitol, magnesium silicate (talc), procaine, or baking soda. Quinine is most commonly used, and in itself can produce auditory, ophthalmic, muscular, gastrointestinal, and renal toxicity.

## CLINICAL FEATURES OF NARCOTIC USE

### Intoxication

Acute narcotic intoxication is characterized by drowsiness, euphoria, miosis, conjunctival injection, and slowed respirations. Decreased sensitivity of the CNS respiratory center to carbon dioxide causes a decrease in minute and tidal volume. Nausea, vomiting, and pruritus can also occur.

### Withdrawal

The classic picture of narcotic withdrawal includes piloerection, lacrimation, yawning, rhinorrhea, sweating, nasal stuffiness, myalgia, vomiting, abdominal cramping, and diarrhea. The patient may be irritable, hyperactive, or confused.

Heroin withdrawal symptoms are generally seen 12 to 14 h after the last dose, whereas symptoms of methadone withdrawal occur in 24 to 36 h. On occasion, the treatment of an overdose patient with naloxone may precipitate a withdrawal syndrome. Though discomforting, acute narcotic withdrawal in the adult is in itself not life-threatening. Many of the symptoms resemble those of a febrile illness, however, and the physician must be alert to the possibility of sepsis in a patient who appears to be undergoing withdrawal. Treatment of withdrawal is symptomatic.

The most common long-term treatment of narcotic withdrawal syndrome is through the substitution and gradual withdrawal of methadone. The antihypertensive agent clonidine has also been utilized to effect narcotic detoxification. Clonidine has been shown to alleviate the symptoms of withdrawal, especially chills, lacrimation, rhinorrhea, abdominal cramping, sweating, myalgia, and arthralgia. Although the severity of symptoms is ameliorated, their presence is not entirely eliminated by clonidine. The mechanism by which the drug acts to reduce the symptoms of opiate withdrawal appears to be by inhibiting adrenergic activity at $\alpha_2$-adrenergic receptors. Side effects of clonidine include hypotension, dizziness, drowsiness, and dry mouth. Dosage must be adjusted to individual reaction.

### Narcotic Overdose

The cardinal physical findings of narcotic overdose are pinpoint pupils and hypoventilation. However, the pupils may be midrange or dilated if CNS hypoxia has occurred. Hypertension may be present secondary to hypoxia. An injection site may be visible or absent, depending on whether the patient injected, inhaled, or ingested the drug.

Street methods of overdose "resuscitation" include packing the victim in ice, pouring milk down the throat, and injecting milk or saline intramuscularly or intravenously. Complications of such actions include hypothermia, aspiration pneumonia, and cellulitis.

## TREATMENT

The treatment of coma due to narcotic overdose is the administration of naloxone, 2.0 mg in an adult, 0.1 mg/kg in a child or neonate. The drug may be given subcutaneously, intratracheally, intramuscularly, or intravenously. When administered intravenously, it is effective in 1 to 2 min. The dose may be repeated as needed. Naloxone can also be given as a continuous intravenous infusion, with the dose titrated to clinical response; 2 mg of naloxone in 500 mL of normal saline or 5% dextrose produces a concentration of 0.004 mg/mL, or 0.4 mg/100 mL. The usual dose is 400 µg (0.4 mg) per hour.

Through antagonism at opiate receptor sites in the CNS, naloxone rapidly reverses coma and respiratory depression caused by narcotics. Pentazocine (Talwin) has been shown to occupy receptor sites other than those of the opiates, and although naloxone can reverse the CNS depressant effects of this drug, larger doses are generally required. High-dose administration of naloxone has also been shown to reverse respiratory depression produced by propoxyphene.

Zoological parks use powerful, opiate-based drugs for rapid sedation of large animals, and accidental exposure in humans has been reported. One of the most common of these compounds is carfentanil (Wildnil), which is 10,000 times as potent as morphine sulfate. A second drug, etorphine (M-99, Immobilon), has been used in the past but is no longer available in the United States. In the event of accidental human exposure, massive doses of naloxone may be required to antagonize the effects of these drugs.

Many heroin addicts also use other drugs or alcohol, so that overdose may be of a mixed type. Coma due to the action of other drugs may not be antagonized by naloxone.

The serum half-life of naloxone is about 1 h, with a duration of action of 2 to 3 h. Close observation and repeated injection or continuous intravenous infusion may be necessary, since the action of the narcotic is likely to be significantly longer than that of the antagonist. This is especially true of methadone, whose duration of action may be as long as 72 h.

Naloxone is virtually without adverse effect, even when given chronically and in large doses. Its action is purely narcotic-antagonistic, and the drug displays no intrinsic agonistic effects. In the truly addicted patient, however, its administration may precipitate a withdrawal syndrome of sudden and alarming proportions.

## COMPLICATIONS OF NARCOTIC ABUSE

### Skin

The tracks of repeated venous injection may be accompanied by the hallmark of subcutaneous use: small, oval, punctate, or depressed ulcers, or hyperpigmented atrophic lesions. Nonpitting edema of the extremities is often seen in addicts of long standing. This is the result of occlusive thrombophlebitis, lymphatic obstruction, and lymphedema.

### Infections

Among the most common sequelae of heroin addiction are infections. Narcotics cause inhibition of leukocyte motility and phagocytosis, and both humoral and cellular immune function abnormalities have been described in heroin addicts. Intravenous drug use is a known risk factor for acquired immunodeficiency syndrome (AIDS). In addition, the notorious lack of sterile technique among users contributes to the high incidence of infection.

### Abscesses, Cellulitis, Thrombophlebitis

Abscesses and cellulitis, especially of the hands and forearms, are common to subcutaneous injectors. These abscesses most often contain staphylococci, but may harbor other flora, including anaerobic bacteria. Small abscesses with no surrounding cellulitis can be treated with drainage and soaks. More extensive lesions require antibiotic therapy, usually with an agent effective against penicillinase-producing staphylococci. Since septicemia and endocarditis cannot be ruled out with certainty in most patients with a history of intravenous drug use and fever, hospitalization is often necessary. Blood cultures should be obtained before antibiotic therapy is begun.

Infections of the hand or fingers often require surgical drainage, as progression to gangrene can be rapid. Abscesses in the neck or groin are generally drained in the surgical suite because of their proximity to major vessels. Mycotic aneurysm should be considered in differential diagnosis of abscesses in these areas.

Septic thrombophlebitis, most often involving the legs or thighs, is a common result of intravenous heroin use. It is characterized by painful swelling and warmth of the affected extremity. Unlike uncomplicated deep venous thrombosis, septic thrombophlebitis requires treatment with antibiotics, not heparin alone.

Mycotic aneurysm of the brain, neck, or groin can result in life-threatening hemorrhage. Masses in the neck or groin of a drug user should be carefully evaluated for pulsation or bruits, to rule out the presence of mycotic aneurysm. Ultrasonography or angiography may be necessary to establish the diagnosis.

### Endocarditis

Endocarditis is a serious complication among addicts, with a high mortality reported in some series. The left or right side of the heart may be affected; the relative incidence varies widely in different reports.

Right-sided infections are the most common in addicts. These usually spare the pulmonic valve, attacking a previously normal tricuspid valve in almost all cases. Murmurs may be absent, faintly heard, or audible in atypical locations. Indeed, there may be no physical findings of tricuspid valvular disease per se, the diagnosis being made on the basis of multiple or repeated septic pulmonary emboli. The infecting organism is most often *Staphylococcus aureus*. The clinical picture of septic pulmonary emboli in these cases is often that of pneumonia with staphylococcal septicemia. The radiologic appearance may be one of pulmonary consolidation. Alternatively, round or wedge-shaped lesions may appear successively in the periphery of the lungs. On the other hand, initial chest roentgenograms may be unremarkable or display only minor abnormality, with typical findings appearing only as the disease progresses. Pulmonary infarcts may progress to cavitation, abscess, or empyema formation. Following treatment, the chest film may revert to normal or may display residual atelectasis or pleural thickening.

Left-sided cardiac valves may be affected in the presence or absence of previous aortic or mitral abnormality. The aortic valve in particular is susceptible even without preexisting disease. Classic physical findings of bacterial endocarditis are frequently present in left-sided disease. Organisms may be cultured from sites of extravascular embolization, such as Osler's nodes and Janeway lesions. *Escherichia coli, Streptococcus, Klebsiella,* and *Pseudomonas* species, as well as *Candida albicans* are the most frequent pathogens involved in left-sided heroin-related endocarditis. *C. albicans* never affects previously normal valves.

Complications of infective endocarditis include systemic embolization to the viscera, extremities, and brain; and acute valvular insufficiency. Focal CNS signs and progressive renal failure may develop. Embolization to a coronary vessel can result in acute myocardial infarction. Acute aortic insufficiency can lead to death within hours, and may be difficult to diagnose because the classic hallmarks of chronic aortic insufficiency (such as widened pulse pressure and prominent diastolic murmur) are often absent. The clinical picture is most often one of unexplained dyspnea, tachycardia, and hypotension, followed by cardiovascular collapse. Acute mitral valve rupture is characterized by sudden, severe pulmonary edema. A loud mitral insufficiency murmur is usually present.

## Malaria

Malaria was first described as a complication of narcotic use in 1929. During the following decade, the disease was considered endemic among addicts in New York City. Although the incidence has greatly diminished since that time, sporadic cases of syringe-transmitted malaria continue to be reported in the addict. Due to the rarity of the disease in this country, it is seldom considered in the differential diagnosis of the febrile addict, and patients experiencing the symptoms of chills, fever, and malaise may be mistakenly diagnosed as undergoing withdrawal.

## Tetanus

Tetanus was first described in addicts in 1876 and has been a relatively frequent observation among them ever since. An inordinately high mortality follows tetanus infection in the heroin user. It is a disease predominantly of the older, long-standing addict, especially the female. Some have speculated that adolescents and males are more likely to be protected by childhood or military immunization. Tetanus is more frequently seen in subcutaneous injectors, and many of these tend to be women, perhaps because the less prominent veins in many females preclude regular intravenous use. Emergency patients should be routinely questioned on the status of tetanus immunizations.

## Pulmonary Complications

The occurrence of pulmonary complications in addicts is related to the duration of heroin use, but not to the amount used or to overdose. Pneumonia is frequently seen. The bacterial agent is usually *Streptococcus pneumoniae, Haemophilus, Klebsiella,* or *Staphylococcus aureus.* Factors predisposing the drug user to pneumonia include direct drug effects: slowing of the epiglottic, cough, and sighing reflexes; alveolar hypoventilation; aspiration of gastric contents; and alterations of humoral and cellular immunity.

Lung abscess may complicate bacterial pneumonia, aspiration pneumonitis, or pulmonary infarction. Pathogens may be either aerobic or anaerobic. Heroin addicts also contract tuberculosis more frequently than nonusers. Pneumothorax may result from attempted subclavian or internal jugular vein injection.

Pulmonary edema following use of heroin is a serious complication. Although the onset of symptoms usually immediately follows injection, it may also be delayed 24 to 48 h. The mechanism is unclear, but heroin-induced pulmonary edema is characterized by an increase in capillary permeability with exudation of fluid into the alveoli. Whether the edema is due to hypoxia, allergic reaction, or the direct toxic effects of heroin is unclear. Pulmonary edema is usually bilateral, though it may appear in one or only a part of one lung.

Physical signs include cyanosis, diffuse rales, tachypnea, tachycardia, and the presence of foamy sputum. Extensive rales may be absent if pulmonary edema is perihilar or localized. Arterial blood gases reveal a profound hypoxemia and there may be hypercarbia as well.

The chest roentgenogram displays unilateral or bilateral fluffy, ill-defined densities in an alveolar pattern, radiating centrally to peripherally. The heart is usually normal in size, but may be slightly enlarged. The differential diagnosis should include head trauma, subarachnoid hemorrhage, near-drowning, noxious gas inhalation, and allergic reaction.

The treatment of heroin-induced pulmonary edema consists of ventilatory support and the administration of naloxone. Other components of cardiogenic pulmonary edema therapy—digitalis, diuretics, and rotating tourniquets—are neither effective nor necessary. Response is usually dramatic, with physical findings clearing within 1 day and radiologic changes reverting to normal within 72 to 96 h.

Angiothrombotic pulmonary hypertension, a syndrome of pulmonary hypertension and cor pulmonale, results from recurrent embolization of injected material to the pulmonary vasculature. This is most frequently seen in those injecting oral preparations intravenously, but also affects heroin users because of the talc and starch adulterants of street heroin and the cotton through which the narcotic may be filtered prior to its use. Clinical presentation of the syndrome includes dyspnea, a pulmonic ejection murmur, and signs of right ventricular hypertrophy. Roentgenographic findings include a nodular, irregular perihilar shadow pattern that is symmetrical.

Pulmonary function studies in chronic intravenous narcotic users have shown that diffusing capacity and vital capacity are decreased. It is uncertain whether these effects are due to a direct toxic action of heroin or represent sequelae of repeated episodes of the pulmonary diseases to which these patients are prone. Pulmonary infarction has been previously mentioned as a complication of right-sided endocarditis.

## Hepatic Complications

The most common side effect of parenteral drug use is acute or chronic hepatic dysfunction. Liver function tests consistent with acute hepatitis may be seen in 10 to 15 percent of addicts sampled, and approximately another 60 percent display less dramatic abnormalities. The latter are usually attributed to chronic hepatitis and, indeed, chronic hepatitis has been found in a substantial number of addicts who died suddenly and came to autopsy. This has commonly been assumed to represent type B, or serum hepatitis. However, a significant proportion of drug users with acute hepatitis test negative for hepatitis B surface antigen.

Experimental morphine addiction in animals has not been found to induce hepatitis or to exacerbate preexisting liver disease, so a toxic or allergic narcotic effect cannot be invoked to explain this extremely common association. Some heroin addicts are heavy alcohol users as well, so liver disease in addicts may in actuality be alcohol-induced. Treatment of addicts with hepatitis is essentially the same as treatment for liver impairment of any other origin. Progression from acute to chronic disease or a fatal outcome is best correlated with greatly elevated transaminase levels in the acute state.

## Gastrointestinal Complications

Intestinal hypomotility, a direct narcotic effect, may give rise to ileus. Abdominal distension and dilated loops of bowel seen on radiologic examination can be associated with this condition and may mimic intestinal obstruction. Termed "intestinal pseudoobstruction," this must be differentiated from a surgical abdomen.

Because of constipation due to hypomotility, there is a significantly increased incidence of symptomatic hemorrhoids and fecal impaction in narcotic addicts.

## CNS Complications

The neurologic complications of heroin injection are many and varied. Some have clear etiologies and others are less readily explained. Traumatic mononeuritis is easily diagnosed because there is immediate postinjection pain and paresthesia in a definite nerve distribution. The loss of function sustained in this manner is usually permanent.

Heroin and meperidine overdose have been reported to cause seizures, although this is uncommon. These are usually grand mal and of short duration. The result may be a typical postictal stupor. Seizures induced by narcotis may also be focal, even in the absence of focal lesions. However, focal CNS lesions resulting in altered states of consciousness may have grave implications in view of the addict's increased propensity for meningitis and intracerebral abscess. Focal neurologic signs are not a feature of uncomplicated addiction per se. Subarachnoid hemorrhage is a less common, though well-recognized complication of heroin addiction. This is thought to be due to vascular weakness caused by necrotizing angiitis or mycotic aneurysm.

The most frequent neurologic complication of narcotic abuse is nontraumatic mononeuropathy. This appears as a painless weakness 2 to 3 h after injection, with no history suggestive of pressure neuropathy. An entire brachial or lumbosacral plexitis may be seen, unrelated either to direct injection or pressure effect. This often occurs in association with other neurologic complications.

The narcotic user is susceptible to the development of spinal epidural abscess, most commonly on the basis of hematogenous dissemination of bacteria to the epidural space, but occasionally via direct extension of infection from vertebral osteomyelitis. *Staphylococcus aureus* is the most common infecting organism, though gram-negative bacilli may also be the cause.

The progression of signs and symptoms proceeds through phases involving spinal ache, nerve root pain, muscular weakness and, ultimately, paralysis. Fever, leukocytosis, and focal lumbar or thoracic spinal tenderness may be present in the early stage of the process, but the diagnosis may be difficult to make on early clinical grounds. Plain spinal radiographs may reveal vertebral osteomyelitis, compression fracture, or evidence of a paravertebral mass, but radiographs are often negative. Contrast-enhanced computed tomography or magnetic resonance imaging are required to make the diagnosis.

Transverse myelitis involving thoracic segments of the spinal cord is seen particularly in patients reinstituting heroin injections after a 1 to 6 month abstinence. The cause is unclear, but it has been speculated to involve a toxic or hypersensitive mechanism or vascular insufficiency to a portion of the thoracic cord. Horner's syndrome can occur as a result of neck injection.

Polyneuritis indistinguishable from Guillain-Barré syndrome has been reported. This may progress to respiratory failure.

The heroin user who presents with pain in an extremity may be the victim of a number of phenomena. Intraarterial injection, like neural trauma, results in immediate pain—in this instance in the distribution of the affected artery. Initial physical signs may be subtle and easily overlooked. The eventual outcome may include ischemic necrosis of the extremity. This is more likely if the lower extremities are involved, less so if there is involvement of the arms.

The pathophysiology of this ischemic necrosis has been postulated to include several factors. Certainly, distal embolization of particulate matter poses a threat to the circulation via occlusion. Damage caused by the needle to the intimal layer of the vessel may also result in occlusion. Arteries may release catecholamines upon such an insult, and although vasospasm has long been assumed to be a major factor in this process, recent work casts doubt upon this particular theory. Various therapeutic modalities have been employed, including sympathectomy and infusion of heparin or dextran, but the eventual outcome may not be greatly affected by such actions.

## Muscular Complications

Fascial compartment syndrome may be produced by compression of the limbs during drug-induced stupor. A vicious cycle is established in which ischemic injury produces edema, raising the pressure in fascial compartments, and aggravating ischemia. This "crush" syndrome creates a situation in which open fasciotomy may be necessary to save the involved extremity. The patient complains of increasing pain and progressive weakness as intrafascial pressure mounts, but external signs may be few. The physician may be forced to exercise clinical judgment upon hearing this history, with no more than a firm, wooden feeling to the extremity as a guide.

Signs of generalized sepsis along with raised pressure in the fascial compartment pose an even more ominous situation, these being the hallmarks of necrotizing fasciitis. This constitutes a spreading septic necrosis resulting from subfascial injection. The extremity is frequently dusky, edematous, and tender, and systemic signs of fever, tachycardia, chills, and leukocytosis are present. The bacterial agent is most likely to be streptococcal, staphylococcal or a gram-negative

organism. The entity produces a mortality rate as high as 30 percent. Treatment includes antibiotic therapy and surgical debridement.

Generalized necrosis of skeletal muscle unrelated to muscle compression sometimes occurs acutely in addicts. The rhabdomyolysis syndrome may occur in a variety of clinical situations, but if there is a mechanism peculiar to narcotic use, this is unknown. Muscles over much of the body may be tender and edematous, and the extremities weak. The hallmark of this syndrome is myoglobin in the urine. Prompt treatment is in order to prevent renal damage.

A syndrome of fever, paraspinal myalgia, and periarthritis has been reported in association with the use of brown heroin. Although this clinical picture frequently mimics an acute febrile illness, no infectious organism has been implicated, and antibiotics do not affect the outcome of this self-limited illness.

## Bone and Joint Pain

Bone or joint pain in the addict must call to mind at least two potential complications: septic arthritis and osteomyelitis. When injecting veins in the antecubital fossa or in the hand, the addict may inadvertently enter joint spaces at the elbow or wrist introducing foreign material and bacteria. More frequently, however, organisms are spread hematogenously to infect parts of the body distant from their site of introduction. There is a curious predilection for the axial skeleton in such hematogenous metastases, particulary the sternoclavicular joint. Organisms infrequently seen in septic arthritis of nonaddicts, including *Pseudomonas aeruginosa* and *Serratia marcescens,* are frequently the cause.

Hematogenous osteomyelitis, although rare, is a recognized complication of heroin addiction. There is a predilection for the spine, but other bones may be involved. *Pseudomonas* is a frequent pathogen. Osteomyelitis should come to mind whenever back pain is a presenting symptom in a patient with evidence of self-injection. Indeed, the presentation of osteomyelitis may include little more than acute localized pain, as fever is rarely present, and the white blood count and x-ray films are normal early in the course. Spinal epidural abscess should also be considered in the differential diagnosis.

## Abnormalities of Pregnancy and Menstruation

Secondary amenorrhea is common in female heroin users. In several studies, one-third of adolescent girls using narcotics ceased menstruating. An additional group displayed oligomenorrhea and hypomenorrhea. Normal menses resumed after discontinuation of the drug, but amenorrhea sometimes persisted for several months to a year.

Complications of pregnancy are frequent, and include a high incidence of toxemia, as well as delivery of premature or growth-retarded babies. Up to 70 percent of babies born to drug-using mothers experience neonatal withdrawal, a potentially fatal condition.

## Transdermal Fentanyl Patches

Transdermal fentanyl patches are becoming increasingly common in the treatment of chronic pain syndromes, especially cancer pain. This is a safe and practical alternative to short-acting analgesics. The transdermal delivery system produces a prolonged time to peak analgesic effect as well as a long elimination half-life. The side effects and complications of fentanyl use, as well as their management, are similar to those of other narcotic analgesics.

## BIBLIOGRAPHY

Ford M, Hoffman RS, Goldfrank LR: Opioids and designer drugs. *Emerg Med Clin North Am* 8:495, 1990.

Frand UI, Shim CS, Williams MH Jr: Heroin-induced pulmonary edema. *Ann Intern Med* 77:29, 1972.

Gifford DB, Patzakis M, Ivler D, et al: Septic arthritis due to *Pseudomonas* in heroin addicts. *J Bone Joint Surg* 57A:631, 1975.

Mosser KH: Transdermal fentanyl in cancer pain. *Am Fam Physician* 45(5):2289, 1992.

# 140
# COCAINE

## Jeanmarie Perrone
## Robert S. Hoffman

The recent resurgence of cocaine abuse coupled with new cocaine derivatives such as "free base" and "crack" has made cocaine a veritable challenge to the urban emergency physician. The acute and chronic manifestations on each organ system can be diverse and catastrophic, and cocaine abuse must be considered in the differential diagnosis of patients presenting with altered mental status, chest pain, seizures, intracranial hemorrhage, pneumothorax, and hyperthermia. These well-known complications of cocaine abuse are but a few of the devastating events that have been reported. The astute emergency physician must be knowledgeable about the broad scope of toxicity that may be incurred from cocaine use and the required therapeutic interventions.

## EPIDEMIOLOGY

Cocaine abuse is widespread, and few data sources can provide an accurate estimation of involved individuals. The National Institute of Drug Abuse reported 30 million people used cocaine in 1990 and cocaine was the most common illicit drug implicated in emergency department visits. Cocaine-related fatalities have paralleled this increase in abuse and many emergency physicians can comment on the trauma associated with cocaine trafficking. Although cocaine use was previously predominant in the higher socioeconomic classes due to cost, the widespread availability of the less expensive alkaloidal crack cocaine has made cocaine abuse prevalent in all socioeconomic spheres.

## PHARMACOLOGY

Cocaine is the hydrochloride salt of a naturally occurring alkaloidal extract of the *Erythroxylon coca* plant indigenous to South America. Cocaine is absorbed across all mucosal surfaces including the oral, nasal, gastrointestinal, pulmonary, and vaginal epithelium and thus can be applied topically, smoked, swallowed, or injected intravenously. Although the hydrochloride form is most often insufflated (snorted) or injected intravenously, ether extraction yields crack cocaine, a form that is heat stable and can be smoked, producing the popping sound that characterizes its name.

As with all toxins, the onset and duration of effect vary with route of administration. When insufflated nasally, the peak effect occurs within 30 min and duration of effect is 1 to 3 h. The delayed and prolonged effect is due to vasoconstrictive properties that limit mucosal absorption. A fraction of insufflated cocaine is swallowed and thus absorbed from the stomach as well. Gastrointestinal absorption is also slowed by vasoconstriction, producing a peak effect at 90 min and a duration of effect as long as 3 h. Both the intravenous and the inhalational routes produce a rapid peak effect (within 30 s to 2 min) with a duration of effect of 15 to 30 min. Cocaine is primarily metabolized to ecgonine methyl ester by plasma cholinesterase. Relative deficiency of this enzyme may predispose affected patients to life-threatening toxicity. Benzoylecgonine is the other major metabolite excreted in the urine and is the one routinely assayed for by most urine toxicology screens. It may be present for 24 to 72 h following use but has been detected in chronic users by more sensitive techniques for up to 2 weeks after discontinuation. A smaller amount is N-demethylated in the liver to form norcocaine. Knowledge of the kinetics of cocaine pharmacology and metabolism is important to guide therapy of the acutely intoxicated patient.

## PATHOPHYSIOLOGY

Cocaine is both a local anesthetic and a central nervous system (CNS) stimulant. Like other local anesthetics, cocaine inhibits conduction of nerve impulses by sodium channel blockade. Additionally, cocaine has been demonstrated to have quinidine-like effects on conduction causing QRS widening and $QT_c$ prolongation. Thus in large doses, cocaine may exert a direct toxic effect on the myocardium resulting in negative inotropy, bradycardia, and hypotension.

Central effects are mediated through activation of the sympathetic nervous system via blockade of presynaptic reuptake of norepinephrine, dopamine, and serotonin. The resultant excess of neurotransmitters at postsynaptic receptor sites leads to sympathetic activation producing the characteristic physical findings of mydriasis, tachycardia, hypertension and diaphoresis and predisposes to arrhythmias, seizures, and hyperthermia. Cocaine use produces a euphoria associated with enhanced alertness and a general sense of well being. It is thought that the psychological addiction, drug craving, and withdrawal effects are mediated through interference with dopamine and serotonin balance in the CNS.

Subsequent dopamine depletion at the nerve terminals may account for the dysphoria and depression associated with long-term abuse. Many of the emergency department visits attributed to cocaine include the vast numbers of patients seeking psychiatric help for the depression or suicidal ideation induced by chronic abuse.

## CLINICAL FEATURES
### Cardiac

Although the most vivid examples of the cardiotoxicity of cocaine abuse have been demonstrated by the publicized deaths of several famous young people, this has done little to discourage the use of cocaine. Cocaine has been reported to induce arrhythmias, myocarditis, and cardiomyopathy as well as myocardial ischemia and infarction. Other vascular complications have included aortic rupture and aortic, coronary artery dissection. Evidence in both animal and human experimental trials has shown that even at relatively low doses cocaine induces vasoconstriction in coronary arteries. Vasoconstriction is one of the proposed mechanisms of cocaine-induced myocardial ischemia and infarction. Coronary vasoconstriction is exacerbated by propanolol and antagonized by phentolamine, suggesting that it is mediated through α-adrenergic receptor stimulation. This effect is further potentiated by cigarette smoking.

Other properties of cocaine contribute to its cardiovascular toxicity. Animal data reveal increased platelet aggregation and thrombogenesis, accelerated atherosclerosis, direct myocardial toxicity, and increased myocardial oxygen demand. Myocardial ischemia has also been demonstrated in chronic abusers undergoing withdrawal from cocaine. It has been postulated that patients in cocaine withdrawal manifest a dopamine-depleted state, which results in intermittent coronary spasm.

A profile of the patient at risk can be elucidated from a compilation of 91 case reports of patients with cocaine-induced myocardial infarction. The average patient was a young man (mean age 32.8, range 18 to 52; male-to-female, 7:1), and 89 percent were cigarette smokers. Two thirds of patients presented within 3 h of cocaine use and all routes of cocaine administration were reported. Of the patients with follow-up cardiac catheterization, coronary artery disease was present in only 31 percent. Electrocardiographic (ECG) abnormalities were variably present and both q wave and non-q wave infarcts occurred. Many studies have reported myocardial infarction in patients with atypical histories and unremarkable ECGs.

### Central Nervous System

A host of neurologic syndromes have been described in association with cocaine abuse, most commonly seizures, intracranial infarctions, and hemorrhages. Pathology results from the hyperadrenergic tone inducing transient severe hypertension, focal vasospasm, and sometimes, exacerbation of underlying abnormalities of cerebral blood vessels. In a dog model, Catravas and Waters demonstrated that lethal doses of intravenous cocaine initially induced seizures, lactic acidosis, hyperthermia, and death. The increased lethality of cocaine-induced seizures is also attributed to hyperadrenergic excess. Progression of toxicity could be prevented by sedation and cooling. Catravas and Waters demonstrated that diazepam was an optimal sedative because it prevented hyperthermia and seizures in the cocaine-poisoned dog and thereby improved survival.

Other CNS manifestations reported include spinal cord infarctions, cerebral vasculitis, and intracranial abscess in an intravenous cocaine user. Acute dystonic reactions following cocaine use and withdrawal have been described. Unilateral blindness has been reported secondary to central retinal artery occlusion and bilateral blindness from diffuse vasospasm. A syndrome of corneal abrasions and ulcerations secondary to smoke and irritation has been termed "crack eye."

## Pulmonary

Complications of cocaine use on the respiratory system have become more prevalent with the epidemic of smoking crack cocaine. Pulmonary hemorrhage, barotrauma, pneumonitis, asthma, and pulmonary edema have all been reported. Pneumomediastinum, pneumothorax, and pneumopericardium result from barotrauma secondary to the Valsalva maneuvers performed following inhalation or insufflation in an attempt to enhance drug effect. Pneumonitis, asthma, and bronchiolitis may be immunologic phenomena or the results of the numerous adulterants known to be present in cocaine. Pulmonary edema may be catecholamine mediated because a similar syndrome has been described in patients with adrenergic excess from pheochromocytoma. An unusual case of pulmonary thromboembolism following crack use has also been reported.

## Gastrointestinal

Patients thought to have swallowed cocaine following police pursuit are considered "body stuffers" and often hastily ingest poorly packaged drug in an effort to avoid arrest. Such patients are often brought to the hospital by police and may or may not have signs of cocaine intoxication. In contrast, the body packer swallows a large number of well-sealed packages of cocaine to smuggle drugs into this country. Toxicity and death can occur if even a single bag ruptures. Intestinal ischemia and bowel necrosis was discovered during laparotomy for abdominal pain in two patients with a history of recent cocaine abuse. Gastrointestinal perforation in association with crack cocaine use has also been described.

## Obstetric

It is not surprising that this potent vasoconstrictor has been shown to alter uteroplacental blood flow. An increased incidence of spontaneous abortions, abruptio placentae, fetal prematurity, and intrauterine growth retardation has been attributed to cocaine abuse in pregnancy. Both spontaneous abortions and abruptio placentae appear to result from placental vasoconstriction and increased uterine contractility with concomitant maternal hypertension. Intoxication of a breast-fed infant secondary to maternal cocaine use has been reported as well.

## Renal

Multiple cases of traumatic and nontraumatic cocaine-induced rhabdomyolysis have been reported: in one series, a third of patients developed acute renal failure and half of those died. In addition to the well-known mechanism of rhabdomyolysis-induced renal failure, cocaine may further exacerbate renal susceptibility via hyperthermia,

vasoconstriction, hypotension, and hypovolemia. The emergency physician must be aware of this potential late complication and augment fluid resuscitation to maintain vigorous urine output of 1 to 3 mL/kg per hour. Renal infarction has been described in a young man following intravenous cocaine use.

## DIAGNOSIS

The cocaine-intoxicated patient can often be identified initially by vital signs. Adrenergic stimulation may produce tachycardia, tachypnea, hypertension, and possibly hyperthermia. The mental status can range from normal to paranoid or severely agitated to coma. Organ system involvement may be suspected from symptoms such as headache, chest pain, palpitations, dyspnea, or focal neurologic complaints. The patient may be postictal or present with seizures. Other physical findings may include mydriasis and diaphoresis. In the absence of adequate history it may be difficult to distinguish this presentation from other conditions of catecholamine excess such as alcohol or sedative withdrawal. Metabolic acidosis may be present following seizures or as a result of vasoconstriction and hypoperfusion. As with all intoxicated patients, occult trauma must be excluded. Concomitant use of alcohol and other drugs frequently alters the clinical presentation. Qualitative drug screens will be positive for cocaine in the presence of the drug but may be misleading in the chronic cocaine abuser who used the drug in the past several days, but now presents with a nontoxicologic condition.

## TREATMENT

The cornerstone of therapy is adequate sedation and close assessment of vital signs. The patient with hypertension and tachycardia will likely respond to treatment with benzodiazepines, which decrease central sympathetic outflow. Hyperthermia is a potentially lethal complication and patients must be aggressively cooled with mist and fan or ice baths to prevent severe metabolic consequences. Aggressive fluid resuscitation is critical to maintain urine output. Seizures may be treated with benzodiazepines as well; however, in status epilepticus phenobarbital loading or neuromuscular blockade may be necessary to control motor activity and prevent hyperthermia, acidosis, and rhabdomyolysis. Computed tomography is recommended in all cases of cocaine-induced seizures because the finding of intracranial pathology creating a seizure focus is common.

The patient complaining of chest pain should be evaluated for possible myocardial ischemia as well as the common pulmonary etiologies mentioned in this population. Suspected myocardial ischemia should be managed with nitrates, morphine, sedation, and aspirin. β-Blocker therapy is absolutely contraindicated because unopposed α-adrenergic receptor stimulation may worsen coronary and peripheral vasoconstriction, hypertension, and possibly ischemia. The successful use of thrombolytic therapy in cocaine-associated myocardial infarction has been described, but appropriate caution must be used in the hypertensive patient. Wide complex tachyarrhythmias and QRS prolongation secondary to the quinidine-like effects of cocaine may be treated with sodium bicarbonate infusion. Severe hypertension not responding to sedation may require treatment with nitroprusside or phentolamine. Although the use of labetalol (a mixed α and β blocker) has been recommended in this situation, we do not recommend it because it still has predominant β-blocking effects and again may lead to unopposed α activity worsening peripheral vasoconstriction and hypertension. Blood pressure may be lowered aggressively provided that the patient does not have chronic hypertensive disease.

The situation of an asymptomatic cocaine body packer brought in by police or customs officials constitutes a new dilemma for the emergency physician. If the patient shows no signs of toxicity, we recommend a dose of activated charcoal followed by whole bowel irrigation with polyethylene glycol electrolyte lavage solution (GoLYTELY or Colyte) to gently hasten elimination of the potentially lethal packets. If the patient begins to show signs of intoxication such as agitation, hypertension, or tachycardia, benzodiazepines should be administered while arrangements for immediate surgical intervention are made. Neither upper nor lower endoscopy should be routinely attempted because both routes have been associated with packet rupture. Following passage of the "last" packet, a radiologic imaging procedure (such as a Gastrograffin upper gastrointestinal series with small bowel follow-through) should be performed to ensure that the gut has been purged of all containers. In contrast to body packers, the body stuffers are more common in the emergency department. These patients can be given a dose of activated charcoal, sedated (if indicated), and given supportive care if intoxicated knowing that the toxicity should be shorter lived and often involves much smaller amounts of drug.

## DISPOSITION

Patient disposition depends on initial patient presentation, response to therapy, and knowledge of the kinetics of cocaine metabolism. Patients who present with adrenergic excess following recent cocaine use and who respond to sedation may be expected to improve completely during a period of observation in the emergency department secondary to the relatively limited duration of cocaine effect. In the absence of focal complaints and with a clear sensorium, patients must be advised of the life-threatening nature of their drug abuse and referred to appropriate detoxification, counseling and, social support services. In general, patients with increased creatine phosphokinase levels, hyperthermia, myoglobinuria, ECG changes, or suspected myocardial ischemia should be hospitalized in an intensive care setting where rigorous patient monitoring and directed therapy can occur.

## BIBLIOGRAPHY

Beckman KJ, Parker RB, Hariman RJ, Gallastegui JL, Javaid JI, Bauman JL. Hemodynamic and electrophysiological actions of cocaine: effects of sodium bicarbonate as an antidote in dogs. *Circulation* 83:1799, 1991.

Catravas JD, Waters IW. Acute cocaine intoxication in the conscious dog: studies on the mechanism of lethality. *J Pharmacol Exp Ther* 217:350, 1981.

Chasnoff IJ, Burns WJ, Schnoll SH, Burns KA. Cocaine use in pregnancy. *N Engl J Med* 313:666, 1985.

Ettinger NA, Albin RJ. A review of the respiratory effects of smoking cocaine. *Am J Med* 87:664, 1989.

Goldfrank LR, Hoffman RS. The cardiovascular effects of cocaine—update 1992. National Institute on Drug Abuse Research Monograph Series. Acute cocaine intoxication: current methods of treatment. 123:70, 1993.

Hollander JE, Hoffman RS. Cocaine induced myocardial infarction: an analysis and review of the literature. *J Emerg Med* 10:169, 1992.

Lange RA, Cigarroa RG, Flores ED, et al. Potentiation of cocaine-induced coronary vasoconstriction by beta-adrenergic blockade. *Ann Intern Med* 112:897, 1990.

Lange RA, Cigarroa RG, Yancy CW, et al. Cocaine-induced coronary artery vasoconstriction. *N Engl J Med* 321:1557, 1989.

# 141

# AMPHETAMINES AND AMPHETAMINE-LIKE DRUGS
## George Braitberg
## Donald B. Kunkel

Amphetamine is a generic term used to correctly describe a specific drug (β-phenylisopropylamine) and to loosely refer to a wide variety of chemical entities that may be controlled substances, legal over-the-counter (OTC) preparations, or illicit street drugs.

Historically, amphetamine was synthesized in 1887, but the first commercially available preparation did not appear until 1932, with the introduction of Benzedrine nasal inhalers. With the observation that amphetamine had powerful central nervous system (CNS) arousal effects, amphetamine began to be touted for a variety of medical disorders, including availability in tablet form for narcolepsy in 1937. Shortly thereafter, oral amphetamine was placed under Food and Drug Administration control as a prescription drug, but this move failed to curb its growing use during World War II, when military troops and home-front workers were allowed access to almost limitless supplies of the drug. Following a postwar binge of amphetamine use and with the increased use of amphetamines and other drugs during the 1960s, a number of amphetamines were moved to Class II schedule in 1970. Three factors have tended to thwart this move: (1) continued availability of potent amphetamines via prescription abuse and foreign trafficking, (2) exclusion of certain "amphetamines" (e.g., phenylpropanolamine) from control, and (3) street manufacture of a variety of these drugs.

## PHARMACOLOGY

Structurally, the amphetamines are similar to the endogenous catecholamines (epinephrine, norepinephrine) but differ in their usually marked effects on the CNS.

The clinical effects of amphetamines can be explained by their indirect sympathomimetic, dopaminergic, and serotonergic actions.

Amphetamines are taken up by the synaptic transport pump, located in the presynaptic terminal nerve ending, competitively inhibiting the uptake of neurotransmitters. In addition to this competitive displacement of synaptic neurotransmitter, amphetamines inhibit the intracellular enzyme, monoamine oxidase, leading to a decrease in the breakdown of catecholamines. Thirdly, amphetamines enter the transport vesicles located in the nerve ending and by so doing, alter intravesicular pH and cause leakage of catecholamines out of the vesicle into the cytoplasm. Eventually, the increase in cytoplasmic concentration of catecholamines from inhibited monoamine oxidase activity and displacement from terminal vesicles causes the neurotransmitter uptake pump to reverse direction and pump neurotransmitter amines into the synapse. Therefore, the net result of amphetamines is to cause an increase in synaptic neurotransmitter concentrations and hence potentiate the effects of these neurotransmitters.

Central effects are mediated by numerous pathways and receptors. Dopamine accounts for about one half of all the catecholamines in the brain and is present in greater quantities than norepinephrine and serotonin. In contrast to the diffuse distribution of noradrenergic neurons, dopaminergic neurons and receptors are highly organized and concentrated in several areas, especially in the basal ganglia, limbic system, and archicerebellum. Recent data suggest that the $D_3$ receptor is the most important subtype regulating limbic activity; $D_2$ receptors are more active in the basal ganglia. $D_4$ receptors have been identified and appear to be specifically antagonised by the antipsychotic agent clozapine. Increased dopamine receptor activity after amphetamine administration results in restlessness, hyperactivity, repetitive or stereotyped behavior, anorexia, and sleep reduction. Excessive dopaminergic activity in the striatum can cause acute choreoathetosis. Excessive dopaminergic activity in the limbic system may produce paranoid psychosis indistinguishable from paranoid schizophrenia and is thought to be responsible for the drug craving and addictive behavior in patients abusing amphetamines. Elevated synaptic serotonin levels contribute to the amphetamine-induced psychosis. The general increase in arousal observed with acute amphetamine usage may be from norepinephrine stimulation of the reticular activating system.

Peripheral effects of amphetamines reflect a largely indirect action via release of endogenous catecholamines, notably norepinephrine. Mixed α- and β-receptor effects are noted, producing pupillary dilation, peripheral vasoconstriction, increased metabolism, tachycardia, and bronchodilation, among other effects. Metabolic effects often seen are increased glycogenolysis, gluconeogenesis, and lipolysis from $\beta_3$ stimulation.

Potentially the patient on a selective serotonin uptake inhibitor who acutely uses amphetamines may be predisposed to the development of serotonin syndrome.

Amphetamines are rapidly absorbed from the gastrointestinal tract and peak plasma levels occur within 1 to 2 h following ingestion. Cerebrospinal fluid levels are 80 percent those of plasma. Approximately 30 to 40 percent of amphetamine is metabolized in the liver, and elimination of parent drug and metabolites is renal. Metabolites tend not to be active.

Amphetamines may be detected in urine for several days. Because of the high pKa of amphetamine, an acid urine will hasten the excretion of both parent drug and metabolites. However, as rhabdomyolysis occurs commonly with amphetamine toxicity, acidification of the urine is not recommended as treatment. In addition to ingestion of amphetamine, injection, inhalation, and even vaginal routes have been used. Volume of distribution of amphetamine is 3 to 6 L/kg.

## TOXICITY

Tolerance to amphetamines may dictate to a large degree the severity of reaction to otherwise toxic doses of amphetamine. Blood levels are generally of little value in determining individual prognosis. Following exposure to toxic doses, the findings outlined in Table 141-1 may occur.

## WITHDRAWAL

In the adult user, abrupt cessation of amphetamine results in abstinence symptoms, which are generally mild and rarely life-threatening, peaking within 2 to 3 days following discontinuation of drug. Depression and increased appetite are common, along with cramps, nausea, diarrhea, and headache. Withdrawal can coincide with psychosis.

Neonatal withdrawal may result in diaphoresis, restlessness, hypoglycemia, and seizures.

## MANAGEMENT OF TOXICITY

Following an acute oral exposure, avoid emesis because of the potential for seizures due to the CNS effects of amphetamine. Gastric lavage may be indicated, followed by tube instillation of activated charcoal. Cardiac monitoring is indicated due to the potential for arrhythmias and myocardial infarction.

Hyperactivity is best managed in a quiet area with decreased sensory input. Diazepam is the drug of first choice, but when this fails, haloperidol for cases of extreme hyperactivity or psychosis is recom-

**Table 141-1.** Effects of Toxic Doses of Amphetamines

**Neurologic**
Mydriasis, piloerection, diaphoresis
Extreme restlessness with repetive and bizarre behavior
Choreoathetosis
Psychosis and delirium
Coma
Extrapyramidal syndrome (rare)
Cerebral vasculitis
Intracranial hemorrhage

**Cardiovascular**
Flushing
Hypertension
Tachycardia (although rarely one may see a reflex bradycardia secondary to hypertension)
Arrhythmias
Myocardial infarction
Circulatory collapse (via catecholamine depletion from continued uptake pump inhibition)
Acute and chronic cardiomyopathy
Polyarteritis nodosa

**Gastrointestinal**
Nausea, vomiting, diarrhea (secondary to smooth muscle hyperactivity)

**Genitourinary**
Increased urinary sphincter tone may cause dysuria, hesitancy and acute urinary retention

**Other**
Hyperpyrexia
Rhabdomyolysis
Coagulopathies
Leukocytosis
Elevated thyroxine level
Acute pulmonary edema (from smoking methamphetamine)

mended. Haloperidol is a specific dopamine $D_2$ receptor antagonist and will therefore mitigate the choreoathetosis and behavioral features of acute toxicity.

Seizures may be treated with intravenous diazepam. Uncontrollable seizures may require phenobarbital or even a paralyzing agent (the use of succinylcholine may exacerbate the potential problems encountered with rhabdomyolysis).

Aggressive cooling measures may be necessary with hyperthermic states, and paralysis may be appropriate. Consider the use of dantrolene early to avert the development of malignant hyperthermia.

Severe hypertension may require the use of a nitroprusside drip. β-Blocker agents should be avoided due to the possible precipitation of unopposed α effects (hypertension). An alternative therapy for mild hypertension is the use of an α antagonist (e.g., phentolamine).

Theoretically, urinary acidification may hasten excretion of amphetamine, but the clinical effectiveness of this maneuver has not been demonstrated. In addition, urinary acidification is contraindicated in myoglobinuria, where urinary alkalinization is recommended. The best advice regarding fluid balance is to maintain good hydration and a high urine output.

## SPECIAL CONSIDERATION

Apart from Vicks nasal inhalers, no OTC preparations contain "true" amphetamines. Vicks nasal inhaler contains *l*-methamphetamine. This can only be distinguished from the *d*-isomer found in illicit "street" preparations by sophisticated isomerization techniques that are not performed in standard urine drug screens.

Phenylpropanolamine is an amphetamine-like substance that was not scheduled as a class II drug by the Controlled Substances Act of 1970. It is commonly available as an OTC agent in many diet and decongestant preparations and in the past was frequently encountered as a component of "look-alike" street drugs in combination with

**Table 141-2.** Common Chemicals Used in Illicit Manufacture of Methamphetamine

**Reagents**
Aluminum
Lead acetate
Mercuric chloride
Potassium cyanide
Phosphorous
Thionyl chloride
Hydrochloric acid
Hydroiodic acid
Sodium hydroxide

**Solvents**
Acetone
Ethyl ether
Ethanol
Isopropanol
Methanol
Pyridine
Toluene

**Precursors**
Benzyl cyanide
Benzylchloride
Dimethylformamide
Ephedrine
Formic acid
Hydrogen gas
Methylamine
N-methylformamide
Phenol-2-propanone
Phenylacetic acid

**Table 141-4.** Over-the-Counter Agents

| | |
|---|---|
| Desoxyephedrine, (L-methamphetamine) | Vicks inhaler |
| Ephedrine | Bronkaid (tablets), Marax, Tedral |
| Phenylpropanolamine | Contac, Dexatrim (tablet), Dimetapp (tablet), Triaminic |
| Propylhexedrine | Benzedrex inhaler |
| Pseudoephedrine | Actifed, Comtrex, Drixoral, Extra-Strength Sinutab, Fedahist, Novahistine, Rondec, Sudafed, Sine-Aid |

Note: Formulations may vary.

ephedrine, pseudoephedrine, and caffeine. It has been known to cause hypertension, seizures, intracerebral hemorrhage, and arrhythmias.

Propylhexedrine was introduced in the Benzedrex inhaler in 1949 as an alternative to the then-abused Benzedrine inhaler containing amphetamine. Propylhexedrine itself became the object of abuse via injection of the contents of the Benzedrex inhaler. A 1979 report listed 12 deaths following intravenous abuse of Benzedrex inhalers in Dallas. Pulmonary edema, foreign body granulomas, fibrosis, and evidence of pulmonary hypertension were frequently noted at autopsy.

Leaves of the khat shrub (*Catha edulis*) are widely used as a stimulant in eastern Africa and the Arabian peninsula. The toxic principle involved is an alkaloid called cathinone, a naturally occurring amphetamine-like substance. Khat may induce a toxic psychosis, usually of a paranoid or persecutory form.

## Designer Drugs

Designer drugs are derivatives of legal pharmaceuticals or chemicals that are illicitly developed to produce psychoactive effects and avoid legal restrictions.

Recently the first published cases of intoxication involving methcathinone, a new designer drug derivative of khat, have been reported

in the United States. In the former Soviet Union, however, methcathinone first surfaced a number of years ago in St. Petersburg and is known as "Jeff" or "Mulka." Scientific literature refers to it as ephidrone. Methcathinone is synthesized by the oxidation of ephedrine, whereas reduction of ephedrine forms methamphetamine.

Other designer drugs in the amphetamine group include 3,4-methylenedioxyamphetamine (MDA or "love drug"), 4-bromo-2,5-dimethoxyamphetamine (DOB), 3,4-methylenedioxyethamphetamine, (MDEA, "Eve") and 3,4-methylenedioxymethamphetamine (MDMA, "ecstasy," or "Adam"). All these drugs are structurally related to amphetamine and mescaline. Deaths attributable to use of MDMA and MDEA have been reported. DOB has been reported to cause diffuse vascular spasm following oral use.

Of growing concern in recent years has been the spectacular rise of methamphetamine as a street drug, with use surpassing that of cocaine in some geographical areas of the United States. Known popularly as "crank" or "ice" (smokable crystalline form), street-origin methamphetamine is commonly manufactured in clandestine laboratories, and the laboratory itself may present explosive and toxic hazards due to the storage and handling of chemicals (Table 141-2) used in the manufacture of methamphetamine.

Methamphetamine's effect is almost immediate following intravenous or intranasal use or when smoked. As compared to cocaine, users report similar effects with methamphetamine when injected or smoked, but the effects of methamphetamine are much longer (4 to 6 h) compared to cocaine's duration of action (an hour or less). In addition to the usual amphetamine effects, smoked methamphetamine has been reported to cause acute pulmonary edema, and chronic methamphetamine use seems highly prone to causing psychotic reactions. Lead poisoning has been reported due to abuse of contaminated methamphetamine.

Some common amphetamines are listed in Tables 141-3 and 141-4.

## BIBLIOGRAPHY

Baselt RC, Cravey RH (eds): *Disposition of Toxic Chemicals and Drugs in Man*, 3d ed. Chicago, Yearbook, pp 49–52, 1989.
Burton BT. Methamphetamine: drug of the 90s. *Poison Press* 1:1, 1990.
Curry SC, Agnone FA, Mills KC. Neurotransmitter principles. In: *Goldfrank's Toxicologic Emergencies*, 5th ed. Norwalk, CT: Appleton & Lange, 1994.
Emerson TS, Cisek JE. Methcathinone: a Russian designer amphetamine infiltrates the rural Midwest. *Ann Emerg Med* 22:1897, 1993.

**Table 141-3.** Common Amphetamines: Schedule II or III Agents

| Generic Name | Common Trade Name(s) |
|---|---|
| Amphetamine (racemic) | Benzedrine, Biphetamine |
| Dextroamphetamine | Dexampex, Dexedrine |
| Diethylpropion | Tenuate, Tepanil |
| Fenfluramine | Pondimin |
| Methamphetamine | Desoxyn |
| Methylphenidate | Ritalin |
| Phendimetrazine | Bontril, Dyrexan-OD, Melfiat, Prelu-2, Statobex, Weh-less |
| Phentermine | Fastin, Ionamin, Phentrol, Unifast |

# 142
# HALLUCINOGENS
## James E. Cisek

## INTRODUCTION

Hallucination is defined as *a sensory experience that does not exist outside of the mind.* Hallucinations may occur due to psychiatric illness, organic disease, withdrawal syndromes, therapeutically administered drugs, and illicit drugs. This chapter will focus on the most common agents in the last group, illicit drugs.

For centuries humans have attempted to induce altered perceptions through many different practices. Hallucinogens have traditionally been a part of many cultural and religious practices. The oracle of Delphi is said to have inhaled carbon dioxide released from a rock fissure to produce an altered state of consciousness. The 1988 National Institute on Drug Abuse Household Survey estimated that over 14.5 million Americans have used a hallucinogen at some time in their lives. Marijuana is the most commonly used drug in this class.

All of the substances discussed in this chapter can either be grown or easily synthesized in the home from readily available chemicals. Complicating the assessment, these drugs are rarely supplied in pure form. Common additives include ephedrine, pseudoephedrine, phenylpropanolamine, caffeine, lidocaine, tetracaine, benzocaine, cocaine, ketamine, strychnine, and heavy metals. In general, hallucinogens have clinical similarities, which allow for consistent management strategies. Agents discussed in this chapter are phencyclidine, lysergic acid diethylamide, mescaline, hallucinogenic amphetamines, anticholinergics, mushrooms, nutmeg, and marijuana. Their clinical features and complications are summarized in Table 142-1. Cocaine is discussed in a separate chapter.

**Table 142-1.** Hallucinogens

| Drug | Clinical Features | Complications |
|---|---|---|
| PCP | Nystagmus, agitation, ataxia, hallucinations | Muscle rigidity, seizures, coma, rhabdomyolysis, hyperpyrexia |
| LSD | Paranoia, anxiety, psychosis, hallucinations | Flashbacks |
| Peyote | Nausea, vomiting, abdominal pain, diaphoresis, headache, anxiety, paranoia | Rare |
| Hallucinogenic amphetamines | Excitement, agitation, hallucinations, confusion, anorexia | Muscle rigidity, seizures, coma, intracranial hemorrhage, hyperthermia, rhabdomyolysis, vasculitis |
| Anticholinergics | Agitation, hallucinations | Anticholinergic toxidrome |
| Marijuana | Euphoria, relaxation, impaired motor performance | Rare |
| Mushrooms | Psilocybin—nausea, vomiting, LSD-like | Rare |
| | Ibotenic acid—CNS only | Rare |
| Nutmeg | Nausea, vomiting, abdominal pain, hallucinations, delirium, stupor | Rare |

## CLINICAL FEATURES
### Phencyclidine (PCP)

PCP is a dissociative anesthetic agent that has excellent analgesic properties with preservation of brainstem function. Postoperative dysphoria, delirium, and psychosis led to its withdrawal from the market. Ketamine is a related compound still in clinical use and is also used illicitly. Many different analogues of PCP have been synthesized by clandestine chemists.

PCP is usually smoked or nasally insufflated. Inhalation is associated with the onset of symptoms in 3 min and a peak effect in 15 min. Gastrointestinal and nasal application allow for delayed onset of action. Duration of intoxication varies with the dose and route of administration. The drug is highly protein-bound and has a large volume of distribution of 6.2 L/kg. The majority of PCP is metabolized in the liver (90 percent), with subsequent urinary elimination of metabolites.

The exact cellular mechanisms of action have not been clearly defined. Multiple neurotransmitters at various locations in the brain are involved. The behavioral effects of PCP are somewhat dose-related. Low doses of PCP can cause mild agitation, confusion, bizarre behavior, hallucinations, delusions, ataxia, and nystagmus. Nystagmus is characteristic and may be vertical, horizontal, and rotatory in the same patient. Higher doses are associated with hypertension and tachycardia. Severe central nervous system (CNS) effects include combativeness, muscle rigidity, seizures, coma, and CNS hemorrhage. Hyperthermia and rhabdomyolysis are very common in significant intoxications. Young children often present with lethargy, staring episodes, apnea, and miotic pupils. Trauma is a common complication due to violent behavior and altered mentation.

### Lysergic Acid Diethylamide (LSD)

LSD is one of the most potent hallucinogens causing psychomimetic activity in microgram dosages. It can be synthesized or obtained from the fungus *Claviceps purpurea* and the seed of the morning glory family of plants.

LSD is well absorbed from the gut and all mucous membranes. After ingestion, onset of activity is within 15 to 60 min. The volume of distribution is 0.27 L/kg with over 80 percent protein bound. LSD is extensively metabolized (99 percent), with elimination of metabolites in the urine and bile.

LSD primarily affects serotonergic and dopaminergic pathways at various levels in the CNS. The drug is most commonly ingested from a sugar cube or blotting paper ("microdots," "blotter acid," "postage stamps"). The majority of patients retain insight while intoxicated and will often admit to ingesting the drug. Persons presenting to the emergency department have usually experienced a panic reaction ("bad trip") or have taken an overdose. Hallucinations, paranoia, anxiety, and psychosis occur. Synesthesias are common and are illustrated by the hearing of colors and the seeing of sounds. Flashbacks are brief and spontaneous recurrences of psychomimetic drug effect that appear during a period of abstinence. Seizures, muscle weakness, ataxia, cerebral vasospasm, and the neuroleptic malignant syndrome are rare. Sympathomimetic findings are uncommon and include mydriasis, tachycardia, hypertension, diaphoresis, and hyperthermia. Rhabdomyolysis is rare. The short half-life and lack of active metabolites allow for clinical improvement by 4 h and normalization by 12 h.

### Peyote/Mescaline

Mescaline is available in both synthetic and natural (peyote cactus) forms. Peyote is available as whole dried cactus tops ("buttons"), chopped buttons, ground powder, capsules, or a liquid extract. Peyote contains 1 to 6 percent mescaline. The usual hallucinogenic dose is 6 to 12 buttons.

Mescaline is structurally similar to amphetamine. Intoxication usually begins with nausea, vomiting, abdominal pain, diaphoresis, and headache. Rarely, a hyperadrenergic state is seen. Psychic effects begin at 2 h postingestion after the resolution of the physiologic effects. Psychiatric findings include anxiety, paranoia, flashbacks, and hallucinations. Psychic effects rarely last more than 6 to 12 h.

## Hallucinogenic Amphetamines

Phenylethylamine is the core to which various side groups are added. The addition of methoxy groups and halogens increases lipid solubility and CNS penetration. This serves to increase the psychic effects while minimizing the sympathomimetic effects. Psychic effects include enhanced mood and self-esteem, euphoria, and hallucinations. More than 50 different compounds have been developed. Many legal sympathomimetics are used for their mood-altering properties (e.g., ephedrine, caffeine, phenylpropanolamine).

The hallucinogenic amphetamines are well absorbed from all mucous membranes. Maximal effects occur within minutes after intravenous administration or smoking, within 1 h after snorting, and within several hours after oral ingestion. The duration is drug- and dose-related and can extend up to 48 h. The volume of distribution is large, with low protein binding. Over one-half of the dose is eliminated unchanged in the urine.

The mechanism of action involves sympathetic receptor stimulation, stimulation of the release of endogenous neurotransmitters, inhibition of monoamine oxidase, and inhibition of catecholamine reuptake by presynaptic neurons. If the dose is carefully titrated, desired psychic effects will predominate with a paucity of unwanted sympathomimetic symptoms. All the severe complications associated with PCP can occur, including seizures, coma, intracranial hemorrhage, hyperthermia, muscle rigidity, and rhabdomyolysis. The chronic use of amphetamines can lead to myocardial and CNS vasculitis.

## Anticholinergics

Many plants are cultivated for their hallucinogenic properties. Active ingredients include atropine, scopolamine, hyoscyamine, and hyoscine. These compounds are competitive antagonists at muscarinic receptors. Jimsonweed (*Datura stramonium*) is one of the most well known of the anticholinergic plants. The alkaloid content varies with the part of the plant ingested and with climatic conditions. Many over-the-counter antihistamines are also abused for their mind-altering properties.

Central anticholinergic findings include hypertension, altered mentation, agitation, hallucinations, seizures, and hyperthermia. Peripheral manifestations are supraventricular tachycardia, dry and flushed skin, ileus, urinary retention, mydriasis, and hyperthermia. A patient may not have all the above signs and symptoms, and rarely, the central anticholinergic toxidrome is present without peripheral effects.

## Mushrooms

Hallucinogenic mushrooms are found in many different genera. In the United States, these mushrooms grow naturally in both rural and urban locations. They can be illegally found in "clandestine mushroom farms" or grown from kits sold via the drug-oriented literature. Identification of mushrooms based on physical characteristics is very difficult and best left to individuals with significant experience.

Mushrooms purchased on the street are often commercial mushrooms that are adulterated with LSD and other hallucinogenic agents. "Magic mushrooms" are members of the genera *Psilocybe, Paneolus,* and *Gymnophilus.* Psilocybin and psilocin are the most important active ingredients, with an LSD-like effect through alteration of serotoninergic neurotransmission. The mushrooms are eaten raw, brewed in a soup or tea, or dried for future use. Extracts for intravenous use are rarely prepared. There is great variation between the history of quantity ingested and clinical effects. Psilocybin concentration will vary between genera and even in different collections of the same species from the same mycelium. Symptom onset is usually within 45 min and usually consists of nausea and vomiting. The hallucinations and other perceptual distortions are similar to those induced by LSD. Sympathomimetic effects, seizures, and coma occur mainly with large doses or in pediatric patients.

Ibotenic acid and its metabolite muscimol are hallucinogenic compounds associated with *Amanita muscaria* and *Amanita pantherina.* These toxins work through either γ-amino butyric acid, glutamate, or serotonin pathways. These mushrooms act much like the psilocybin group with the exception being a lack of significant gastrointestinal effects. Symptom onset is within 1 h and peaks at 2 to 3 h. CNS symptoms consist of agitation and altered perceptions fluctuating with somnolence and coma. Symptoms usually resolve within 8 h.

## Nutmeg/Mace

Nutmeg is the seed of *Myristica fragrans,* and mace is the fleshy, scarlet outer seed coat. The plant is most commonly grown in Grenada, the South Pacific, and East Indies. Myristicin, elemicin, and safrole make up 80 percent of the volatile oils that account for the clinical manifestations. Hallucinogenic amphetamine metabolites of the volatile oils also contribute to the intoxication. Individuals involved in the drug culture, students, and prison inmates commonly abuse this agent. One to three nutmegs, or 5 to 30 g of the ground nut, will induce psychological effects. Grinding the nut may reduce toxicity as the active ingredients are volatile. Nausea, vomiting, and abdominal pain occur within 6 h of the ingestion. This is then followed by a period of delirium and stupor that usually resolves within 24 h. Other clinical finding are very rare.

## Marijuana

Marijuana is the most commonly used illegal drug in the United States. It represents the dried leaves, stems, and flowers of the plant *Cannabis sativa.* Hashish is the dried resin of the plant, and hashish oil is a concentrated liquid extract. Delta-9-tetrahydrocannabinol (THC) is the main active ingredient of the several hundred compounds present.

THC is well absorbed through inhalation, with peak levels occurring in 7 to 8 minutes and 45 min after oral ingestion. Clinical effects are delayed, with maximal inhalation intoxication occurring after 20 min. The volume of distribution is large, with high protein binding. Extensive metabolism occurs with the majority of active and inactive metabolites eliminated through the feces.

THC-containing preparations have a high therapeutic index, with no deaths having been reported from the drug itself. Common neurologic findings include euphoria, relaxation, decreased short-term memory, and impaired performance of complex motor tasks. Less common findings include lethargy, panic, hallucinations, and paranoia. Respiratory symptoms include cough and upper-airway irritation. Marijuana contains 10 times the respiratory irritants and more carcinogens than tobacco. THC itself is a bronchodilator. Cardiovascular findings include a mild sinus tachycardia, increased cardiac output, and peripheral vasodilation.

## DIAGNOSIS

Drug-induced hallucinations are difficult to distinguish from all other causes of altered perceptual awareness. While cocaine and THC can be detected by inexpensive methods, most other hallucinogens are undetected on routine drug screens. Research, legal, and forensic interests require the application of sophisticated analytical techniques such as gas chromatography with mass spectroscopy. Absolute identification of the ingested drug does not alter the acute care management. Management of drug-induced hallucinations and other psychic effects is similar regardless of the agent, but metabolic or end-organ complications require specific treatment.

The history, physical examination, and appropriate use of laboratory and imaging techniques must be employed to quickly rule out nontoxic causes. The past medical history must be carefully evaluated, as many diseases and therapeutic drugs are associated with hallucinations. Sedative-hypnotic and alcohol withdrawal are diagnosed by history. If a history is not available, then the diagnosis of hallucinogen intoxication is one of exclusion. Physical examination should be directed to look for evidence of a specific toxidrome and evidence of trauma, especially head trauma.

## TREATMENT

Initial management must focus on stabilizing the airway, breathing, and circulation. The patient's altered mentation allows for a challenging search for associated medical and traumatic illnesses. The intoxicated patient should have continuous monitoring of cardiac rhythm and pulse oximetry. Intravenous access is required, and the patient should have an assessment of the blood sugar and receive intravenous thiamine. Early intubation is required to secure or protect an airway, provide ventilation, or for bronchial hygiene.

Gastrointestinal decontamination has little role, as the majority of the hallucinogens are rapidly absorbed. Gastric lavage may be indicated in recent large ingestions. Oral activated charcoal is sufficient for the majority of patients.

Patients with mild psychomotor stimulation may be conservatively managed with a quiet environment, reassurance, and gentle sedation with benzodiazepines. Significant intoxications will present with violent behavior, and the patient will require the immediate application of physical restraints. After the patient is physically secured, an intravenous catheter must be established for hydration and the administration of medications.

Profoundly agitated patients require pharmacologic sedation so they can be medically evaluated, and to prevent them from harming themselves and health care workers. Physician-titrated parenteral sedation is essential. Controversy exists as to the optimal drug therapy for sedation. Benzodiazepines offer definite advantages over the butyrophenones. The benzodiazepines are effective in controlling behavior, increase the seizure threshold, are safe in the management of mixed ingestions, and are optimal therapy for sedative-hypnotic and alcohol withdrawal. Lorazepam offers the advantage of a longer duration of CNS activity (3 to 6 h) and absence of active metabolites. The initial intravenous lorazepam dose is 0.05 mg/kg up to 3 mg, followed by 2 mg every 10 min. The optimal benzodiazepine dose is based on an endpoint of mild sedation and will differ for each patient. Significant intoxications will often require very large doses. Continuous infusions are commonly required after the initial bolus therapy provides sedation.

Benzodiazepines occasionally fail or require such large doses that respiratory depression occurs. Haloperidol is the second drug of choice if benzodiazepines fail in sedation. Haloperidol has the potential for lowering the seizure threshold, worsening hyperthermia through anticholinergic mechanisms, and causing dystonic reactions or the neuroleptic malignant syndrome. Haloperidol should not be used in known cocaine or anticholinergic intoxications. Haloperidol is effective within minutes and may be administered intravenously at a dose of 5 mg every 15 min until gentle sedation is achieved.

Sedation of the agitated patient will assist greatly in controlling hyperthermia. Evaporation will allow for further rapid cooling by the application of a mist of water and a high-velocity fan. Brief neuromuscular paralysis may be required in patients not responding quickly to sedation and evaporation.

There is no role for extracorporeal elimination or pH manipulation of the urine to hasten drug elimination. Multiple-dose activated charcoal is indicated in significant PCP intoxications. PCP can be trapped in the stomach and bound to charcoal as a charged weak base, regardless of the route of administration.

Hypertension that does not respond to sedation should be treated with a rapidly acting titratable agent such as nitroprusside. Supraventricular arrhythmias can be managed with a β blocker such as labetolol or esmolol. Ventricular arrhythmias in a hyperadrenergic state can be managed with β blockers. Seizures are best treated with benzodiazepines and barbiturates. Rhabdomyolysis is treated with an optimal urine output (2 mL/kg per hour), and urinary alkalinization using intravenous sodium bicarbonate. The sodium bicarbonate should be administered to achieve a urine pH of 7 to 8.

## PATIENT DISPOSITION

The decision to admit a patient will be based on clinical parameters and the resources of the emergency department. Patients require admission if they present with cardiovascular instability, seizures, hyperthermia, rhabdomyolysis, metabolic abnormalities, or other organ toxicity. Concomitant trauma associated with the intoxication may also guide admission decisions.

Mild to moderate psychomotor stimulation will usually resolve with time and mild sedation. If the emergency department cannot provide this observation period, then hospital admission is required. Patients must not be discharged until they are asymptomatic. Asymptomatic patients do not require admission as delayed toxicity does not occur.

Acute psychiatric intervention is often required after the patient is medically stable, as associated mental illness is very common. Involvement of child protective services is essential for all pediatric intoxications. Substance abuse counseling must be offered to every patient seen in the emergency department.

## BIBLIOGRAPHY

Aaron CK: Sympathomimetics. *Emerg Med Clin North Am* 8:513, 1990.

Baldridge EB, Bessen HA: Phencyclidine. *Emerg Med Clin North Am* 8:541, 1990.

Leikin J: Intoxication due to hallucinogenic drugs. *Med Toxicol Adverse Drug Exp* 4:324, 1989.

Spoerke DG, Hall AH: Plants and mushrooms of abuse. *Emerg Med Clin North Am* 8:579, 1990.

Tharratt RS, Albertson TE: Hallucinogens, in Hall JB, Schmidt GA, Wood LD (eds): *Principals of Critical Care.* New York, McGraw-Hill, 1992, pp 2141–2147.

# 143
# SALICYLATES
## Steven C. Curry

Salicylates are available in both prescription and over-the-counter preparations in many forms, usually as acetylsalicylic acid (aspirin). Oil of wintergreen (methyl salicylate) is an extremely toxic form of salicylate. Sodium salicylate is used as a kerotolytic agent. Many combination analgesics such as Darvon Compound, Percodan, and Fiorinal also contain significant amounts of salicylates.

## PATHOPHYSIOLOGY AND CLINICAL FEATURES

### General and Metabolic

Acute ingestions of salicylates are frequently accompanied by gastroenteritis from direct irritation to the gastrointestinal (GI) tract. Rare reports of gastric perforation continue to appear. Upper GI bleeding is frequent, and severe and persistent vomiting can be difficult to control. Renal failure has been rarely reported as a consequence of acute poisoning.

A mixed respiratory alkalosis and metabolic acidosis is usually seen in salicylate poisoning. Salicylate directly stimulates respiratory centers in the brain stem, resulting in respiratory alkalosis. Very high levels of salicylate depress respirations.

Salicylate enhances lipolysis, uncouples oxidative phosphorylation, and inhibits various enzymes involved in energy production and amino acid metabolism. Because oxidative phosphorylation is a major buffer of hydrogen ions, impairment of oxidative phosphorylation by salicylate results in metabolic acidosis. Ketoacids are frequently elevated due to enhanced lypolysis. Elevated circulating lactate concentrations in a minority of patients reflect increased glycolytic activity. The accumulation of other intermediate acids involved in energy metabolism has been suggested to contribute to metabolic acidosis.

Salicylate causes mobilization of glycogen stores, resulting in hyperglycemia. However, salicylate is also a potent inhibitor of gluconeogenesis. Therefore, normoglycemia, hyperglycemia, or hypoglycemia may be noted in salicylate poisoning. Children are more likely than adults to develop hypoglycemia.

### Central Nervous System

Confusion, lethargy, convulsions, respiratory arrest, coma, and brain death can all be seen in severe poisoning. Decreased adenosine triphosphate (ATP) production from uncoupling of oxidative phosphorylation and other metabolic effects result in acute brain failure and cerebral edema. Cerebrospinal fluid (CSF) glucose concentrations can be very low compared with serum glucose levels and can mimic those of bacterial meningitis. Patients who die from salicylate poisoning despite intensive supportive care frequently die a cerebral death. Even patients who die in refractory shock have developed serious neurotoxicity prior to the onset of shock.

### Cardiovascular

Cardiac toxicity is due to impaired ATP production, acidosis, electrolyte abnormalities, and, rarely, significant hyperthermia. Heart failure can occur but is usually not a major problem, except in those near death or in those with preexistent heart disease. Cardiac arrhythmias, including ventricular premature beats, ventricular tachycardia, and ventricular fibrillation, are possible.

### Pulmonary

Pulmonary edema can be a major cause of morbidity. Most pulmonary edema is noncardiogenic (acute respiratory distress syndrome [ARDS]), and ARDS complicating acute overdoses is more common in adults than in children. However, overaggressive attempts at a forced diuresis in the treatment of salicylate poisoning can result in hydrostatic pulmonary edema from fluid overload, especially in the elderly with marginal cardiac reserve. Children with inappropriate secretion of antidiuretic hormone are also predisposed to fluid overload and pulmonary edema. In contrast to acute poisoning, in which pulmonary edema is not frequent, chronic salicylate poisoning often results in ARDS.

## TOXIC DOSES AND SALICYLATE LEVELS

Some understanding of the absorption, distribution, metabolism, and excretion of salicylate is needed in order to interpret serum salicylate levels appropriately and hence provide optimum care of the patient.

Within a few minutes after absorption, acetylsalicylic acid is converted to salicylate. After ingestion of large amounts of nonenteric-coated aspirin, peak serum salicylate levels may not be reached for 18 to 24 h, although toxic levels are usually seen within 6 h. A concretion of salicylate that allows continued absorption may form in the stomach. Methyl salicylate, being a liquid, produces peak levels earlier. On the other hand, toxic levels may not be reached for hours after the ingestion of enteric-coated aspirin.

At therapeutic levels, salicylate is mainly cleared by hepatic metabolism. Even at upper therapeutic levels, hepatic enzymes are saturated, leading to zero-order elimination kinetics. In zero-order kinetics, a set amount of the drug is metabolized per unit time, regardless of plasma levels of the drug. This allows accumulation of salicylate and a prolonged elimination of salicylate from the body.

At toxic levels, renal excretion becomes a major route of elimination. Un-ionized salicylate is reabsorbed by the renal tubules, prolonging elimination. Alkaline urine favors the formation of ionized salicylate, which cannot be reabsorbed and is excreted in the urine. Because of zero-order kinetics, dehydration, and acidic urine, days may be required for salicylate levels to decrease by half in untreated patients suffering from salicylate poisoning.

After absorption, salicylate distributes throughout body tissues. At higher salicylate concentrations, a lesser percentage of the drug is protein bound. As a metabolic acidosis develops, a greater percentage of the free drug is un-ionized and is able to move into tissue. In fact, a drop in pH from 7.4 to 7.2 almost *doubles* the amount of un-ionized drug which is able to diffuse out of the plasma. The decreased protein binding and increased un-ionized fraction of the drug at lower pHs cause a change in the volume of distribution ($V_d$) of salicylate. Depending on various factors, the $V_d$ can vary over twofold from 0.15 to 0.35 L/kg. Those suffering from chronic salicylate toxicity have large $V_d$'s.

It is this changing $V_d$ that makes it difficult to interpret serum salicylate levels. Because patients can have different $V_d$'s, patients can have tremendous differences in total body burdens (and tissue levels) of salicylate while having the same serum salicylate concentrations. When elevated serum salicylate levels are decreasing in a patient, they can be decreasing not only from metabolism and renal excretion, but also because salicylate is leaving blood, moving into tissue, and causing more toxicity as the $V_d$ increases. It is for these reasons that it is more important to treat the patient than the serum salicylate level. This is especially important in chronic salicylate toxicity, in which severe toxicity may be demonstrated at serum levels that would produce minimal symptoms in acute poisoning.

The acute aspirin ingestion of 150 mg/kg or less is not expected to produce significant toxicity other than, perhaps, vomiting from a gastrointestinal irritation. Acute aspirin ingestions of 150 to 300 mg/kg produce mild to moderate toxicity with hyperpnea, vomiting, diaphoresis, tinnitus, and acid-base disturbances. The ingestion of greater than 300 mg/kg can produce moderate to severe toxicity. If aspirin has been taken within the last 24 h, potential toxicity of an acutely ingested dose is worse.

The Done nomogram can be used to *assist* in predicting the degree of toxicity after an *acute, single* ingestion of aspirin in a patient who has not been taking salicylate recently (Fig. 143-1). A serum level should not be plotted on the nomogram unless it was drawn at least 6 h after ingestion. Nontoxic levels drawn before 6 h do not rule out impending toxicity. Symptomatic patienld be treated regardless of where they fall on the Done nomogram. The Done nomogram *cannot* be used in the following instances:

1. In acute ingestions when salicylate has been taken previously within the last 24 h
2. In acute overdoses when salicylate was ingested over several hours

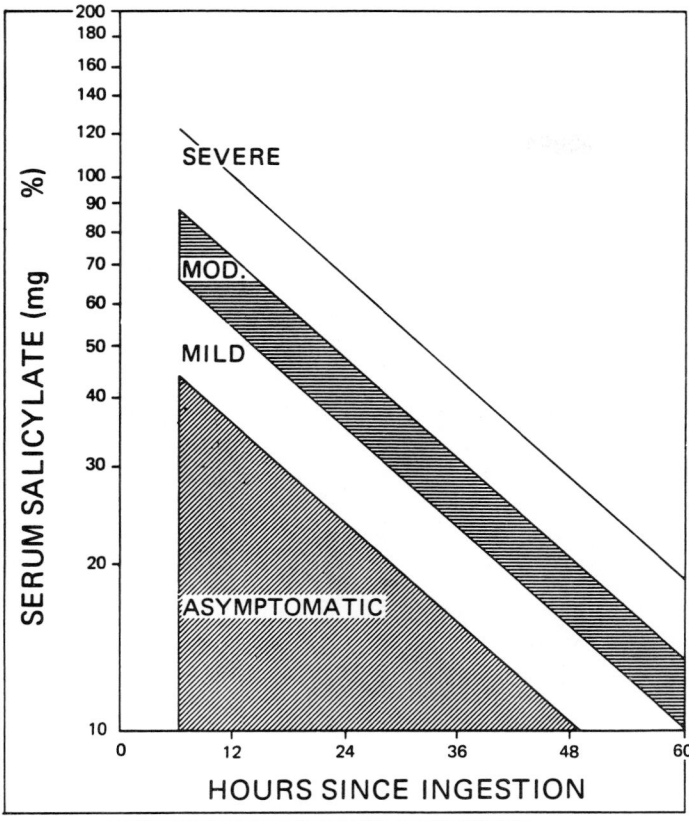

**DONE NOMOGRAM FOR SALICYLATE POISONING**

**Fig. 143-1.** The Done nomogram can be used to assist in determining the likelihood of toxicity. It can only be used after a single, acute ingestion of aspirin in which no salicylate has been taken previously in the last 24 h. Nontoxic levels drawn before 6 h cannot be used to determine degree of toxicity. This nomogram cannot be used in chronic salicylate poisoning or after the ingestion of enteric-coated aspirin. (From Done AK: Salicylate intoxication: Significance of salicylate in blood in cases of acute ingestion. *Pediatrics* 26:800, 1960. Used by permission.)

3. In chronic salicylate poisoning
4. After ingestion of enteric-coated aspirin tablets

Chronic salicylate toxicity is the result of excessive therapeutic administration over a period of 12 h or longer. Defining doses that lead to chronic toxicity is difficult. For example, if a patient is dehydrated from an illness and renal excretion of salicylate has decreased, the drug may accumulate and cause chronic toxicity in doses that otherwise would not cause problems. On the other hand, the chronic ingestion of excessive salicylate doses will cause toxicity in any otherwise healthy person. As discussed below, chronic salicylate poisoning is better described as a syndrome than as a particular dose over a particular period of time.

## ACUTE VERSUS CHRONIC POISONING

Acute and chronic salicylate poisoning have several distinct characteristics. The adult patient with acute salicylate toxicity usually presents with vomiting (sometimes hematemesis), abdominal pain, hyperventilation, diaphoresis, dehydration, alkalemia, ketonuria, and a respiratory alkalosis with metabolic acidosis. As the poisoning progresses, acidemia, lethargy, cardiovascular abnormalities, coagulation disorders, hyperthermia, and serious neurotoxicity develop. Pulmonary edema can occur but is not common. As noted earlier, children frequently present with acidemia. In acute poisoning, serum sa-

licylate levels correlate fairly well with the degree of toxicity, which is the basis for the Done nomogram described above.

In contrast to acute poisoning, patients with chronic salicylate toxicity usually do not have significant gastroenteritis, although dehydration can be severe. They are usually brought in by family members because of changes in mentation, including lethargy, disorientation, and hallucinations. Even adults are frequently, but not always, acidemic on presentation. ARDS is common in chronic toxicity. Because patients with chronic toxicity have a large $V_d$, they present with more serious toxicity at a given serum salicylate concentration compared with an acutely poisoned patient. An elevated prothrombin time is frequently present. Elevated levels of liver enzymes are present in some patients chronically using salicylates, even if chronic toxicity is not present.

Chronic salicylate toxicity must be considered in any patient with unexplained central nervous system (CNS) dysfunction, especially in the presence of a mixed acid-base disturbance. Studies have shown that about 50 percent of patients with chronic salicylate toxicity are incorrectly diagnosed at the time of hospital admission. Patients taking carbonic anhydrase inhibitors can develop chronic toxicity while using relatively low doses of salicylates because the carbonic anhydrase inhibitor alkalinizes CSF and acidifies blood, raising the $V_d$ of salicylate and concentrating salicylate in the CNS. The most important point to remember is that, because of a large $V_d$, *a patient suffering from chronic salicylate toxicity can have a therapeutic serum salicylate concentration.*

The contrast between chronic and acute poisoning is not always clear. The longer one waits after an acute ingestion, the more a patient behaves like a chronically intoxicated one. In a severely, acutely poisoned patient many hours after aspirin ingestion, CNS changes, acidemia, elevated prothrombin time, and significant toxicity in the face of decreasing or normal salicylate levels are signs that are exactly the same as those in a chronically poisoned patient. In these patients it is important to remember to treat the patient and not the serum salicylate level or degree of toxicity as determined by the nomogram.

## TREATMENT

### Gastrointestinal Decontamination

The administration of activated charcoal alone appears to be superior to induction of vomiting with ipecac. Activated charcoal (1 g/kg body weight) should be administered to patients who have ingested potentially toxic amounts of salicylate. Cathartics have not been beneficial in animal models of nonenteric-coated salicylate poisoning. There is controversy as to whether repeat doses of activated charcoal enhance salicylate elimination. Persistent and severe vomiting is common in the acutely poisoned patient and frequently limits the use of activated charcoal.

If the serum salicylate level drawn 6 h after ingestion falls in the asymptomatic portion of the Done nomogram, the patient has minimal or no symptoms, and a repeat serum salicylate determination shows that levels are falling, then the patient can be discharged. Patients whose serum salicylate levels are in the mild range can be discharged if they have minimal symptoms, if nausea and vomiting have resolved, if salicylate levels are falling, and if adequate follow-up can be provided. If nausea and vomiting persist, dehydration may prevent adequate elimination of salicylate and result in worsening toxicity. All other patients should be admitted to the hospital.

The acute ingestion of enteric-coated salicylate deserves special mention. Enteric coating allows a delayed and slower absorption of aspirin. There have been several reports of patients who have ingested toxic amounts of enteric-coated aspirin tablets and have been asymptomatic with nontoxic salicylate levels 6 h after ingestion. These patients then returned hours later with severe toxicity and elevated salicylate levels. Considering the inaccurate histories that frequently accompany overdose victims, anyone who has ingested over 150 mg of enteric-coated aspirin per kilogram should be admitted for observation and serial serum salicylate levels. Adequate follow-up should be ensured for all those who are discharged from the emergency department.

## Laboratory Studies

In symptomatic patients, blood should immediately be drawn for determination of serum levels of electrolytes, glucose, blood urea nitrogen, creatinine, and salicylate; prothrombin time; and hemoglobin and hematocrit. Arterial blood gases should be measured to determine the type and degree of acid-base imbalance. The differential diagnosis of salicylate poisoning includes theophylline toxicity, caffeine overdose, acute iron poisoning, Reye's syndrome, diabetic ketoacidosis, sepsis, and meningitis. Phenistix, a urine dipstick, used to test for phenylketonuria, detects moderate to large concentrations of salicylate in the urine.

## Intravenous Fluids and Urine Alkalinization

Almost all symptomatic patients with salicylate poisoning are dehydrated. Appropriate fluid challenges using saline or colloids should be given rapidly to replenish intravascular volume and produce adequate urine flow. All patients with CNS depression or seizures should be presumed to be hypoglycemic and should receive concentrated glucose intravenously if bedside determination of serum glucose is not readily available. After adequate hydration, intravenous fluids should include adequate amounts of sodium and potassium to replenish depleted body stores. Children should never receive plain 5% dextrose in water as an intravenous fluid.

All efforts should be made to keep arterial pH 7.4 or greater. Even the slightest fall in arterial pH results in a greater concentration of unionized salicylate, which can move into tissues to produce worsening of toxicity. The alkalinization of urine is performed to enhance urinary excretion of salicylate.

Prescott and colleagues have shown that an alkaline urine is more important than a diuresis in enhancing salicylate excretion. However, in the patient who appears to be able to handle a fluid load well, a urine output above normal is desirable. If only maintenance intravenous rates will be used, then 10% glucose should be present in the infusions.

Both bicarbonate *and* potassium are needed to produce an alkaline urine. Even if arterial pH is 7.5, alkaline urine will not be produced if, when reabsorbing sodium, the kidney is preferentially secreting hydrogen ions into the tubular lumen rather than potassium ions. Arterial blood gases, serum electrolytes, and urine pH should be monitored at least every 2 to 4 h in the severely ill patient. This is especially important in preventing hyperkalemia from the administration of large amounts of potassium, and in preventing a fall in arterial pH.

The method I use in producing an alkaline diuresis is to hydrate the patient with normal saline until a good urine output is obtained. Sodium bicarbonate as 1 mEq/kg is given intravenously in boluses until arterial pH is at least 7.5. A continuous intravenous infusion of 1 L 5% dextrose in water to which is added 50 to 100 mmol sodium bicarbonate and 40 mmol potassium chloride is started at two to three times the maintenance rate. Monitoring of urine pH, serum electrolyte levels, and arterial blood gases at least every 2 to 4 h is performed to fine-tune the infusion, to detect hyperkalemia or hypokalemia, and to detect hyponatremia. Tremendous doses of potassium may be required along with bicarbonate to produce an alkaline urine. If the blood is alkaline, if the serum potassium level is normal, and if the urine is acidic, more potassium is needed. In my experience, it may be necessary to administer as much as 110 mEq potassium every 4 h to an adult to maintain an alkaline urine. Boluses of sodium bicarbonate are given to keep arterial pH above 7.4.

Furosemide can be given if evidence of fluid overload develops, or if urine output does not approach the rate of intravenous infusion despite adequate hydration. Serum salicylate levels should be determined every few hours until they are known to be consistently falling.

The use of carbonic anhydrase inhibitors (e.g., acetazolamide) is mentioned only to be condemned. Although acetazolamide alkalinizes urine, it also alkalinizes CSF, trapping salicylate in the CNS. Acetazolamide dramatically increases mortality in animal models of salicylate toxicity.

## Dialysis

Hemodialysis greatly enhances the clearance of salicylate from the body. It also has the advantage of correcting fluid and electrolyte abnormalities at the same time. Hemodialysis is indicated in the following cases:

1. In the patient who is deteriorating despite supportive care and an alkaline diuresis
2. In the patient who is deteriorating and in whom an alkaline urine cannot be successfully produced (e.g., acidic urine despite alkalemic blood and hyperkalemia)
3. In the patient with renal failure
4. In the encephalopathic or comatose patient or in one with severe cardiac toxicity
5. In the patient with ARDS in whom the salicylate levels are not rapidly falling

Peritoneal dialysis is not nearly as effective as hemodialysis and should not be used if hemodialysis is available. If peritoneal dialysis is used, the dialysate should contain 5% albumin to enhance salicylate clearance through protein binding.

## Neurotoxicity

Except in severe cases, coma usually does not develop after acute ingestions. CNS depression is common in those with chronic toxicity. Seizures should be treated with benzodiazepines and phenobarbital. Patients receiving intensive support care who die from acute salicylate poisoning frequently die a cerebral death. Shock is usually preceded by serious neurotoxicity. Animal studies indicate that there is a critical CNS salicylate concentration responsible for malignant cerebral edema and mortality. Therefore, *the continued deterioration in level of consciousness despite supportive care is an ominous sign and is an indication for immediate dialysis and treatment for cerebral edema.* This is especially true if serum salicylate levels are not rapidly falling. Intravenous mannitol can be effective in controlling severe cerebral edema until salicylate levels have fallen.

## General

Parenteral vitamin $K_1$ can be given for a prolonged prothrombin time. Antacids may be required in the treatment of upper GI bleeding following overdose. Standard antiarrhythmic drugs can be used in treating ventricular arrhythmias. I have seen a case in which ventricular bigeminy was secondary to severe respiratory alkalosis (pH 7.68). Mild sedation and increasing dead space ventilation produced a fall in pH and a resolution of ventricular arrhythmias.

The frequent monitoring of arterial blood gases, serum electrolytes, and urine pH cannot be overemphasized. The acid-base and electrolyte status of the patient suffering from serious salicylate poisoning is constantly changing. Small changes in serum potassium levels or arterial pH can have dramatic effects on the degree of toxicity and on salicylate clearance. With close monitoring of the patient, aggressive support care, and hemodialysis when indicated, death from salicylate poisoning should be a rare occurrence.

## BIBLIOGRAPHY

Curtis RA, Barone J, Giacona N: Efficacy of ipecac and activated charcoal/cathartic: prevention of salicylate absorption in a simulated overdose. *Arch Intern Med* 144:48, 1984.

Danel V, Henry JA, Glucksman E: Activated charcoal, emesis, and gastric lavage in aspirin overdose. *Br Med J* 296:1507, 1988.

Gaudreault P, Temple AR, Lovejoy F: The relative severity of acute versus chronic salicylate poisoning in children: a clinical comparison. *Pediatrics* 70:566, 1982.

Heffner JE, Sahn SA: Salicylate-induced pulmonary edema: clinical features and prognosis. *Ann Intern Med* 95:405, 1981.

Kwong TC, Laczin J, Baum J: Self-poisoning with enteric-coated aspirin. *Am J Clin Pathol* 80:888, 1983.

Prescott LF, Balali-Mood M, Critchley JH, et al: Diuresis or urinary alkalinization for salicylate poisoning? *Br Med J* 285:1383, 1982.

Snodgrass W, Rumack BH, Petereson RG, et al: Salicylate toxicity following therapeutic doses in young children. *Clin Toxicol* 18:247, 1981.

Sweeney KR, Chapron DJ, Brandt JL, et al: Toxic interaction between acetazolamide and salicylate: case reports and a pharmacokinetic explanation. *Clin Pharmacol Ther* 40:518, 1986.

Thisted B, Krantz T, Strom J, et al: Acute salicylate self-poisoning in 177 consecutive patients treated in ICU. *Acta Anaesthesiol Scand* 31:312, 1987.

# 144
# ACETAMINOPHEN

## Christopher H. Linden

Acetaminophen, also known as paracetamol, is found in hundreds of prescription and nonprescription cough, cold, and pain-relief preparations, either alone or in combination with other drugs such as anticholinergics, antihistamines, barbiturates, caffeine, muscle relaxants, narcotics, phenothiazines, and sympathomimetics. Its widespread availability accounts for the high incidence of both intentional and accidental overdoses. Acetaminophen poisoning may result in potentially fatal hepatic necrosis. The risk of hepatotoxicity can be predicted by a nomogram that relates the serum acetaminophen concentration to the time of ingestion. Antidotal treatment with *N*-acetalycysteine can prevent or limit hepatic injury in patients with potentially toxic acetaminophen levels if therapy is started within 24 h of an overdose.

Early signs and symptoms of acetaminophen poisoning are nonspecific. They may be subtle and can easily be overlooked or masked by the more dramatic effects of other agents in patients with polydrug poisoning. In addition, biochemical evidence of hepatic injury may not become apparent until 24 to 36 h following acetaminophen overdose. Hence, unless an acetaminophen level is routinely checked in all overdose patients, acetaminophen overdose may not be discovered until signs of hepatotoxicity develop and it is too late for antidotal therapy to be effective.

## PHARMACOLOGY

Acetaminophen (*N*-acetyl-*para*-aminophenol, or APAP) is a nonnarcotic analgesic and antipyretic agent. Its antipyretic activity appears to involve the inhibition of hypothalamic prostaglandin synthetase and be effected by cutaneous vasodilation. The inhibition of central

nervous system and perhaps peripheral prostaglandin synthesis may also be responsible for APAP's analgesic activity.

APAP is available in liquid, tablet, caplet, and suppository formulations. Capsule formulations are no longer marketed. There is no commercially available intravenous formulation, but sustained-release oral preparations have recently become available (e.g., Tylenol ER). The bioavailability of APAP from suppositories is only 80 percent of that from oral formulations. The therapeutic dose is 15 to 30 mg/kg every 4 to 8 h in children and 325 to 1000 mg every 4 to 6 h in adults. The maximum recommended daily dose is 80 mg/kg in children and 4 g in adults.

Most APAP preparations are rapidly and completely absorbed from the gastrointestinal tract. Peak serum concentrations occur 1/2 to 2 h following a therapeutic oral dose. Therapeutic levels are 10 to 20 µg/mL. Pharmacologic effects are generally observed within 30 min and last about 4 h. Sustained-release formulations are designed to maintain therapeutic drug levels for 6 to 8 h. The apparent volume of distribution of APAP is 0.9 to 1 L/kg, but tissue concentrations are variable. Rapid uptake by hepatocytes results in relatively high liver concentrations. Since plasma protein binding of APAP, primarily to albumin, is low (5 to 10 percent), APAP does not significantly displace other drugs from such binding sites.

APAP is eliminated primarily by hepatic metabolism. Small amounts are also metabolized by the kidney and during absorption from the gastrointestinal tract. About 90 percent of a therapeutic dose is converted to the inactive glucuronide and sulfate conjugates, which are then excreted (Fig. 144-1). The predominant metabolite in adults is APAP-glucuronide, whereas APAP-sulfate is the major metabolite in neonates. Paralleling maturation of the glucuronidation pathway, there appears to be a gradual transition of APAP metabolism with increasing age. The adult pattern is reached between ages 9 and 12 years. Less than 4 percent of a therapeutic dose is excreted as unchanged APAP, and a similar fraction is conjugated with glutathione by hepatic cytochrome $P_{450}$-dependent mixed-function oxidases ($P_{450}$-MFOs) and excreted as mercapturic acid and cysteine conjugates. In adults, the plasma half-life of APAP is approximately 2 h after a therapeutic dose. It is slightly shorter in children and perhaps with repeated administration, and is somewhat longer in neonates, the elderly, and those with underlying liver disease.

APAP is a metabolite of two other analgesics, phenacetin and phenazopyridine (Pyridium). Although methemoglobinemia, sulfhemoglobinemia, and hemolytic anemia may occur following the ingestion of these agents, APAP itself does not produce such effects in humans. Other species (e.g., cats and dogs), however, are susceptible to this toxicity, and relatively small doses of APAP may be rapidly fatal if ingested by these common house pets.

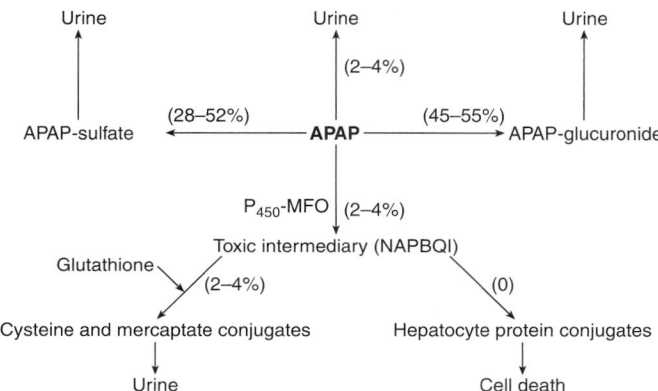

**Fig. 144-1.** Disposition of acetaminophen and metabolites. Numbers in parentheses refer to disposition following therapeutic doses. (NAPBQI, *N*-acetyl-*para*-benzoquinoneimine.)

## PATHOPHYSIOLOGY

A highly reactive metabolite of APAP, *N*-acetyl-*para*-benzo-quinoneimine (NAPBQI), formed during its metabolism by the $P_{450}$-MFO pathway, is thought to cause hepatic necrosis by covalently binding to hepatocyte protein macromolecules (Fig. 144-1). Free radical formation does not appear to be involved in the initiation of hepatotoxicity but it may be involved in its secondary propagation. Although the amount of NAPBQI formed during the metabolism of therapeutic doses of APAP can be rapidly detoxified by conjugation with hepatic glutathione, the metabolism of toxic doses of APAP eventually depletes glutathione. It also saturates the glucuronide and sulfate conjugation pathways and depletes sulfate stores, effects which may contribute to glutathione depletion by shunting more APAP into the $P_{450}$-MFO pathway. When glutathione is depleted by more than 70 percent, the capacity of the liver to detoxify NAPBQI is exceeded, and hepatic necrosis ensues. Corresponding to the region of greatest $P_{450}$-MFO activity, a centrilobular distribution pattern of hepatic necrosis is observed on histologic examination.

The minimal dose of APAP capable of causing liver toxicity following acute ingestion is estimated to be 140 mg/kg in children and 7.5 g in adults. Significant toxicity is likely after acute overdoses of 250 mg/kg. However, because of inaccuracies in overdose history; individual differences in hepatic glutathione stores, the capacity for glutathione regeneration, and $P_{450}$-MFO activity; and the variable occurrence of spontaneous emesis, only a rough correlation exists between the amount of APAP reportedly ingested and the likelihood of toxicity. In addition, the chronic use of certain drugs, such as antihistamines, phenytoin, barbiturates, and other sedatives that stimulate the $P_{450}$-MFO system, may enhance APAP toxicity. Conversely, the use of drugs such as cimetidine may inhibit this system and protect against APAP toxicity. Children appear to be less susceptible to hepatotoxicity than adults, perhaps because of differences in APAP metabolism.

The effect of ethanol consumption on APAP toxicity is variable. Since ethanol is also metabolized by $P_{450}$-MFO enzymes (the microsomal ethanol-oxidizing system, or MEOS), it may competitively inhibit the metabolism of APAP by this pathway and decrease the likelihood of hepatotoxicity following the acute ingestion of both agents. Chronic ethanol consumption may induce $P_{450}$-MFO enzymes and increase the likelihood of hepatotoxicity. Coexistent malnutrition and short-term fasting may result in decreased glutathione stores and decreased glutathione regenerative capacity and also increase susceptibility to hepatotoxicity. This may explain the observation that chronic alcoholics and patients with illnesses associated with anorexia can develop toxicity following chronic therapeutic or only slightly excessive dosing of APAP.

Very rarely, significant renal failure occurs in the presence of only mild hepatotoxicity after an acute overdose, and, also very rarely, coma and metabolic acidosis are noted in patients with massive acute ingestions. Pancreatitis and diffuse myocardial necrosis have also been reported in isolated cases. The generation of reactive APAP metabolites in the renal medulla is the postulated mechanism of nephrotoxicity. The etiology of other atypical manifestations is unknown.

Moderate but sustained elevations of serum APAP concentrations also appear to be capable of causing hepatotoxicity. However, the dose (i.e., amount, frequency, and duration) of APAP necessary to cause toxicity following chronic overdose is unknown.

## CLINICAL FEATURES

### Acute Poisoning

The clinical course of patients who became poisoned as a result of a single large overdose can be divided into four stages (Table 144-1). During stage I, nausea and vomiting are frequently present, particularly in children and those with very large overdoses. However, gas-

**Table 144-1.** Stages of Acetaminophen Poisoning

| Stage | Time Following Ingestion | Characteristics |
|---|---|---|
| I | 1/2–24 h | Anorexia, nausea, vomiting, malaise, pallor, diaphoresis |
| II | 24–48 h | Abdominal pain, liver tenderness, elevated hepatic enzymes, oliguria |
| III | 72–96 h | Peak hepatic enzyme abnormalities, increased bilirubin level and prothrombin time |
| IV | 4 days–2 weeks | Resolution of hepatotoxicity or progressive hepatic failure |

trointestinal symptoms may be mild, and some patients are entirely asymptomatic. Since APAP does not cause direct cardiovascular or respiratory abnormalities, and since it very rarely, and only after massive overdose, causes central nervous system depression, the ingestion of other drugs should be suspected if such findings are present. An increased anion gap metabolic acidosis associated with high serum lactate levels may also be noted soon after massive overdose, but this finding is also extremely rare, and, if present, should prompt a search for other causes.

During stage II, signs, symptoms, and laboratory evidence of hepatic toxicity become apparent. Transient clinical improvement with resolution of gastrointestinal symptoms may be noted despite the appearance of biochemical abnormalities indicative of hepatitis (i.e., elevated serum aminotransferase levels). The patient may then develop right upper quadrant abdominal pain with liver enlargement and tenderness. In some patients, evidence of pancreatitis may also be noted. Oliguria may develop as a result of dehydration or direct APAP-induced renal toxicity (i.e., acute tubular necrosis). Evidence of renal dysfunction occurs in about 25 percent of patients with significant hepatotoxicity. Patients with renal toxicity may complain of flank pain.

During stage III, the time of peak liver function abnormalities, nausea and vomiting may reappear, persist, or worsen. Jaundice may become evident. It is not uncommon for the ALT (SGPT) and AST (SGOT) to rise to over 10,000 IU/mL, more than 100 times the normal level. Lesser elevations in serum alkaline phosphatase and glutathione-*S*-transferase (GST) are often noted. The serum bilirubin level (primarily the indirect fraction) may also increase, and the prothrombin time (PT) may become prolonged. Elevation of the serum creatinine and BUN levels along with proteinuria, glucosuria, hematuria, pyuria, and granular casts on urinalysis are seen in patients with renal toxicity. Fetal death and spontaneous abortion have been reported following acute APAP overdose during pregnancy.

Stage IV is characterized by either recovery or progressive deterioration with death from fulminant hepatic failure. In patients who recover, hepatic function returns to normal, and liver biopsies show normal histology (unless underlying liver disease is present). In those who deteriorate, encephalopathy (ranging from confusion to coma), with worsening jaundice, elevated serum ammonia levels, coagulopathy, hypoglycemia, renal failure (i.e., hepatorenal syndrome), and ECG changes suggestive of myocardial injury may be noted.

### Chronic Poisoning

A unique syndrome of severe, combined hepatic and renal toxicity can occur in alcoholics following the ingestion of therapeutic or slightly greater doses of APAP. The etiology of this syndrome has been questioned, however, since APAP levels have not been measured to confirm drug exposure. Susceptible patients typically present with dehydration, jaundice, markedly elevated serum transaminases, coagulopathy, and hypoglycemia. Acute tubular necrosis is also present in up to 50 percent of these patients.

Nonalcoholic patients, particularly children and those with acute starvation or chronic malnutrition, can also become poisoned following the therapeutic ingestion of multiple excessive doses (small over-doses) of APAP over a period of several days. Their clinical course appears to be similar to that of patients with acute poisoning.

## PROGNOSTIC FACTORS AND RATIONALE FOR ANTIDOTAL THERAPY

In the setting of APAP poisoning, hepatotoxicity has traditionally been defined as a serum aminotransferase (AST or ALT) level above 1000 IU/L. Lesser elevations of serum transaminases are not considered clinically significant. The serum APAP concentration, measured 4 to 24 h after a single large overdose of an immediate-release preparation and related to the time of ingestion, is the best predictor of the risk of hepatotoxicity. The Rumack-Matthew nomogram (Fig. 144-2) depicts this relationship. With supportive care alone, patients with APAP levels in the "probably hepatic toxicity" area of the nomogram had a 14 to 89 percent incidence of hepatotoxicity and a mortality rate of 5 to 24 percent.

At any given time after ingestion, the risk of hepatotoxicity and death increases as the APAP concentration increases. Patients considered to be at high risk are those with APAP levels above a line parallel to that showing the lower limit of probable toxicity and connecting a 4-h APAP level of 300 μg/mL with a 24-h level of 9.4 μg/mL. As originally reported, patients with APAP levels below the lower limit of probable toxicity were not found to be at risk for clinically significant hepatotoxicity. However, because of potential errors in the reported time of ingestion and in the laboratory measurement of plasma APAP concentrations, a safety zone (the area of "possible he-

patic toxicity") was created by lowering the probable toxicity line by 25 percent. If a serum APAP concentration is not readily available, patients should be considered at risk for hepatotoxicity if they have ingested more than 140 mg/kg or 7.5 g.

Predictors of significant hepatotoxicity include early elevation of ALT, AST, or GST levels (levels greater than twice normal on presentation or within 24 h of overdose); an APAP elimination half-life of more than 4 h; and possibly the presence of severe or persistent phase I gastrointestinal symptoms. Since elevated aminotransferase levels have been noted at the time of initiation of antidotal therapy in all antidote-treated patients who have died from APAP poisoning, the absence of this finding is predictive of survival. In patients with hepatotoxicity, a serum bilirubin level greater than 4 mg/dL and a prothrombin time of more than twice normal during phase III have been associated with the subsequent occurrence of severe hepatic failure. In contrast, aminotransferase concentrations do not appear to correlate with outcome (i.e., higher enzyme levels during phase III are not associated with a poorer prognosis).

The risk of hepatotoxicity in alcoholics who ingest multiple therapeutic or slightly greater doses of APAP is unknown but appears to be low. APAP levels in these patients are not known to correlate with toxicity. Nonalcoholic patients who take multiple small overdoses of APAP and others who ingest single overdoses of sustained-release preparations and have a potentially toxic APAP level on the nomogram (timed with respect to the last dose) are clearly at risk for hepatotoxicity. Patients with ingestions of more than 140 mg/kg or 7.5 g over a period of 24 h or less and those with single ingestions of sustained-release APAP who have an elevated but nontoxic APAP level are probably also at risk, but the degree of risk is unknown. Patients with relatively smaller or larger ingestions, over relatively shorter or longer periods of time, respectively, may also be at risk.

Following the observation that APAP-induced hepatotoxicity coincided with depletion of glutathione, a number of compounds were administered to experimental animals and overdose patients in an attempt to prevent glutathione depletion and the associated liver toxicity. Since glutathione, a three-amino acid protein, does not readily enter cells, a variety of related sulfhydryl-containing compounds were studied. Cysteamine and methionine were the first compounds to be used with success, but *N*-acetylcysteine (NAC) has emerged as the treatment of choice. After entering cells, NAC is metabolized to cysteine, a glutathione precursor. However, the mechanism by which NAC prevents hepatotoxicity is unclear. It may act by increasing the supply of glutathione, combining directly with NAPBQI, or by inhibiting its formation. It may also act as a sulfate precursor and prevent saturation of the sulfate conjugation pathway.

Recent studies indicate that NAC also has a beneficial effect when given after the onset of hepatotoxicity, at a time when APAP and metabolite levels are undetectable. The mechanism(s) underlying these late effects are unclear but may involve antioxidant activity, anti-inflammatory effects, altered hepatic enzyme function, and changes in microvascular hemodynamics.

The efficacy of NAC in preventing hepatotoxicity and death decreases as the time interval between APAP overdose and the initiation of antidotal treatment increases. It also decreases as the risk of toxicity (possible, probable, or high), as identified by plotting the plasma APAP concentration on the Rumack-Matthew nomogram, increases. In patients with APAP levels in the probable risk area of the nomogram, the incidence of hepatotoxicity is 2 to 8 percent if treatment is begun within 8 to 10 h of ingestion, and death is extremely rare. The incidence of hepatotoxicity is 10 to 23 percent if NAC is started 8 to 16 h after ingestion and 24 to 40 percent if NAC is started 16 h or more after ingestion, and the mortality rate in both instances is less than 1 percent. In high-risk patients, the incidence of hepatotoxicity is 5 to 13 percent and the mortality rate is about 1 percent if treatment is begun within 10 h of ingestion. Hepatotoxicity occurs in about 34 percent of high-risk patients initially treated 10 to 24 h after

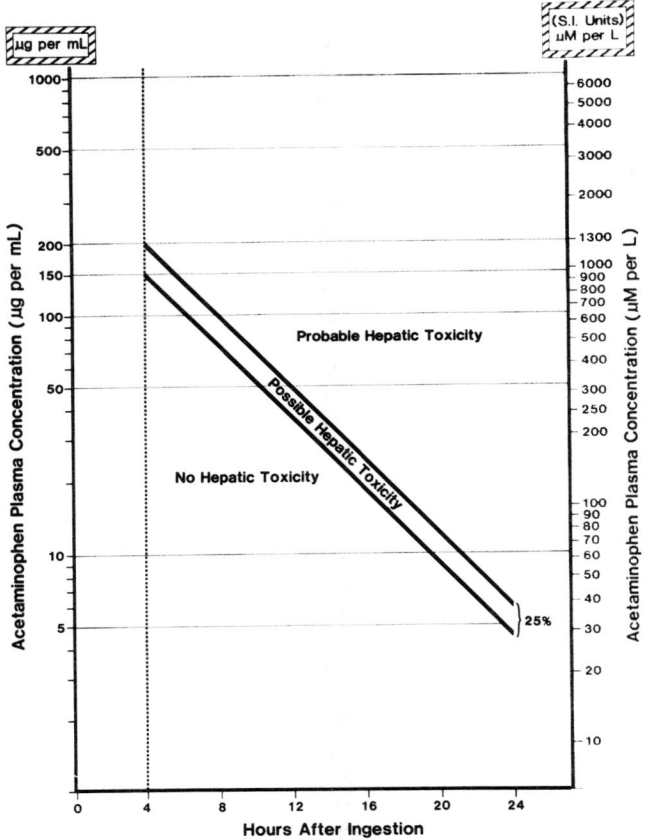

**RUMACK - MATTHEW NOMOGRAM FOR ACETAMINOPHEN POISONING**

**Fig. 144-2.** Semilogarithmic plot of plasma acetaminophen levels versus time. (Adapted from Rumack BH, Matthews H: Acetaminophen poisoning and toxicity. *Pediatrics* 55:873, 1975.)

ingestion and in 35 to 82 percent of those in whom treatment is started 16 to 24 h after ingestion. High-risk patients have a mortality of 2 to 3 percent when treatment is initiated more than 10 h after overdosage. In pregnant overdose patients, delayed treatment is associated with an increased incidence of spontaneous abortion and fetal death.

The efficacy of NAC may also be influenced by its dose. Animal studies have shown that the efficacy of NAC increases as the dose of NAC increases. When NAC is given in a dose equal to the amount of APAP administered, it is virtually 100-percent effective in preventing hepatotoxicity as long as treatment is started immediately after the overdose. Such a dose-response effect may explain why oral NAC in a dose of 1330 mg/kg over 72 h and intravenous NAC in a dose of 980 mg/kg over 48 h appear to be more effective than intravenous NAC in a dose of 300 mg/kg over 20 h in late-treated overdose patients. In addition, with shorter treatment in patients with large overdoses, significant amounts of unmetabolized APAP may still be present at the time therapy is terminated.

The efficacy of NAC does not appear to be influenced by the route of NAC administration. Intravenous therapy results in higher serum NAC concentrations than does oral therapy, whereas the oral route would be expected to produce higher hepatic concentrations (since NAC is delivered directly to the liver following absorption into the portal venous circulation). Animal studies indicate comparable potency with intravenous and oral routes of administration.

## DIFFERENTIAL DIAGNOSIS

The differential diagnosis of APAP poisoning includes viral hepatitis, alcoholic hepatitis, hepatobiliary disease, and other drug- or toxin-induced hepatitis. Acute APAP poisoning can often be distinguished from other causes of hepatitis by the presence of very high aminotransferase levels, its acute onset, and its rapid progression. Except for idiosyncratic reactions to inhalational anesthetics, other etiologies of hepatitis rarely cause aminotransferase elevations of more than 500 IU/L, and rarely begin and progress as quickly. Acute APAP poisoning may be distinguished from alcoholic hepatitis and chronic APAP poisoning in alcoholics by the AST/ALT ratio. In the former instance, this ratio is typically less than 2, whereas it is usually greater than 2 in the latter two instances. The differential diagnosis of hepatitis is discussed in further detail in Chap. 86, "Acute Jaundice and Hepatitis."

## GENERAL EVALUATION AND MANAGEMENT

Children who accidentally ingest less than 140 mg/kg of APAP and adults who accidentally ingest less than 7.5 g may be managed at home if the history is assuredly accurate. No treatment is necessary if less than 100 mg/kg has been ingested. For those ingesting 100 to 140 mg/kg, ipecac-induced emesis or activated charcoal (AC) is recommended if fewer than 4 h have passed since the time of ingestion. Intermittent follow-up (i.e., telephone contact) for 12 to 24 h is essential. Persistent gastrointestinal symptoms following induced emesis suggest the possibility of an inaccurate history, and patients who develop these findings should be evaluated in person and managed as outlined below.

Children who have accidentally ingested more than 140 mg/kg, adults who have accidentally ingested more than 7.5 g, and all patients who have taken an intentional overdose should be evaluated at a health care facility. Gastrointestinal decontamination is recommended for patients presenting within 4 h of overdose. Since food, anticholinergics, and narcotics may decrease gastric motility and delay APAP absorption, decontamination procedures may be useful after a longer interval if these substances have also been ingested.

In contrast to past recommendations, AC is now considered the preferred method of decontamination. AC effectively adsorbs APAP in vitro and prevents the absorption of APAP in vivo. AC has been shown to be equally, or more, effective than either syrup of ipecac or gastric lavage in preventing the absorption of APAP in overdose patients as well as after therapeutic doses and simulated overdose in human volunteers. When increasing, but subtoxic, doses of both AC and APAP (at a constant AC-to-APAP ratio) are given to human volunteers, the efficacy of AC in preventing APAP absorption increases, suggesting that AC may be more effective in the overdose setting than it is in volunteer studies (provided a high AC-to-APAP ratio can be achieved).

Although AC also absorbs NAC and can prevent its absorption, there are many reasons why this effect is unlikely to be clinically important. Animal studies indicate that the effective dose of NAC is equal to the amount of APAP ingested. However, patients are routinely treated with 18 doses of NAC totaling 1330 mg/kg, despite the fact that most of them have ingested far less than this amount of APAP. It follows that most patients are overtreated with NAC to begin with. Unless multiple doses of charcoal are given, the 8 to 39 percent decrease in NAC absorption reported following the near simultaneous administration of AC and NAC in human volunteers would be applicable only to the first of many doses of NAC. The potential effect on overall NAC absorption would, at worst, be a 4 percent reduction in the absorbed dose, an insignificant effect unless a very large (more than 1275 mg/kg) dose of APAP were ingested. Even if multiple doses of AC were given, this effect would potentially be significant only for patients ingesting substantial amounts (more than 821 mg/kg) of APAP.

In addition, in actual practice, the need for the near-simultaneous administration of AC and NAC almost never arises. AC is likely to decrease APAP absorption only if given within 4 h of overdose, at a time when the results of drug levels and the need for NAC therapy are not yet known and antidotal therapy is not urgently needed, since NAC is virtually 100 percent effective in preventing fatalities when given up to 8 to 10 h after overdose. Even if AC and NAC are administered together, the effect is likely to be minimal and possibly beneficial. AC has a higher affinity for APAP than NAC in vitro, and the concomitant presence of APAP has been shown to decrease the binding of NAC to AC. And, finally, and most importantly, data from controlled studies of experimental APAP poisoning in animals as well as from the retrospective analysis of cases of human poisoning indicate that treatment with a combination of AC and NAC is equally, or more, effective than treatment with NAC alone.

Syrup of ipecac not only delays the administration of the more effective AC, but its emetic effect, when combined with that caused by toxic doses of APAP and by therapeutic doses of NAC (see below), may make oral antidotal therapy difficult, if not impossible. Hence, syrup of ipecac is best reserved for patients with small overdoses who are unlikely to require antidotal therapy. The combined use of gastric lavage and AC may be optimal for the decontamination of comatose patients with mixed ingestions. However, the forcible insertion of a large-bore tube in an awake but uncooperative patient has the potential for serious complications and is not recommended. In such patients, it is easier and safer to insert a small-bore nasogastric tube, perform aspiration or lavage, and give a dose of AC.

The value of cathartics in the treatment of APAP overdose is uncertain. Although sorbitol is the most effective agent, it has not been shown to prevent drug absorption in simulated APAP overdoses, and it is associated with a higher incidence of adverse effects (i.e., nausea, cramping, and diarrhea) than other cathartics. Since these gastrointestinal side effects are similar, and potentially additive, to those caused by NAC, sorbitol is not recommended. Although the same adverse effects are also caused by other cathartics, sulfate salts can be absorbed and can theoretically prevent APAP-induced sulfate depletion. Sodium sulfate is better absorbed than magnesium sulfate, and its absorption is not inhibited by AC. Hence, if a cathartic is used at all, sodium sulfate is suggested as the agent of choice.

The serum APAP concentration should be measured as soon as

possible beginning 4 h after an acute overdose. Since colorimetric assays may be unreliable, high-pressure liquid chromatography, gas chromatography, or enzymatic immunoassay are the preferred methods of measuring APAP. An APAP level falling above the lower line of the nomogram (i.e., falling in either the possible or probable toxicity areas) indicates the need for NAC therapy. If the time of ingestion is uncertain, the earliest possible time should be used when plotting the APAP level on the nomogram. In cases where it may have been less than 4 h since the time of ingestion, APAP levels can be repeated every 30 min until the peak level is noted. If this level is greater than 150 $\mu$g/mL, the potentially toxic 4-h level, NAC therapy should be administered.

It now appears that NAC is effective in both preventing and treating hepatotoxicity if administered more than 24 h following APAP overdose. Hence, NAC therapy is recommended for patients who present more than 24 h after overdose if any APAP is detectable in the serum or if there is any biochemical evidence of hepatic dysfunction.

The serum APAP should also be measured in alcoholics with hepatotoxicity and a history of ingesting multiple therapeutic or excessive doses of APAP, in other patients with chronic overdose (i.e., more than 140 mg/kg in children or 7.5 g in adults over a period of up to 24 h or the equivalent), and in patients with single ingestions of sustained-release APAP. Since the nomogram applies only to single acute overdosage of immediate-release preparations, APAP levels in these patients are used mainly to confirm exposure. However, if the APAP level, with respect to the time of the last dose, is potentially toxic by the nomogram, NAC therapy is clearly indicated. If the APAP level is undetectable and liver function tests are normal, NAC therapy is not necessary. Although the efficacy of NAC therapy in other situations is unknown, it is potentially beneficial and therefore recommended for alcoholics with toxicity from therapeutic or excessive doses and for others with chronic overdose who have a supratherapeutic APAP level (above 20 $\mu$g/mL) or biochemical evidence of hepatotoxicity.

Routine laboratory evaluation of patients with predicted or actual toxicity should include measurement of the serum amylase, electrolytes, liver function tests (ALT, AST, bilirubin, and PT), and renal function tests (BUN, creatinine, and urinalysis). Patients with recent massive ingestions who are clinically ill should also have arterial blood gas measurements. In those with vague or unreliable histories and those with intentional ingestions, toxicology screening tests are advisable. At a minimum, because patients often confuse aspirin with acetaminophen and because salicylate poisoning may require treatment, the presence of salicylate should be excluded.

Candidates for NAC therapy require admission. Admission to a floor bed is acceptable provided that other factors (e.g., toxicity from coingestants, availability of one-to-one monitoring of suicidal patients, local customs, and hospital policy) do not necessitate a higher level of care. Therapy can even be accomplished in a psychiatric ward provided that the patient is clinically well and medical supervision is available.

Liver and renal function tests and others that are abnormal should be repeated daily for 3 days or until values begin to return to normal. Follow-up may be on an outpatient basis once antidotal therapy is complete, liver function is improving, and the patient is clinically well. Patients with intentional overdoses should have psychiatric evaluation prior to discharge.

Hepatic or renal failure should be treated by standard measures. NAC has also been shown to be beneficial in the treatment of hepatic failure. Vitamin K is effective in treating patients with a prolonged PT. However, since the PT is useful in determining the need for liver transplantation (see below), vitamin K should be reserved for patients with a prolonged PT and active bleeding. Although hemodialysis and hemoperfusion are capable of removing APAP from the plasma, they have not been shown to prevent poisoning and are not indicated for this purpose. These procedures may, however, be useful for the cor-

rection of metabolic abnormalities in patients who develop hepatic or renal dysfunction. Liver transplantation should be considered in those with advanced hepatic failure unresponsive to supportive therapy. It should not be performed prematurely (i.e., within the first week following overdose), since patients often recover despite marked aminotransferase elevations early in the course of poisoning. Recurrent hypoglycemia, lactic acidosis (pH < 7.3), a PT that continues to rise 4 days after overdose or is greater than 100 s, a serum creatinine greater than 3.4 mg/dL, and high-grade encephalopathy have been associated with a poor outcome and the need for liver transplantation. Patients with these findings should be transferred to a facility capable of performing such surgery.

## ANTIDOTAL TREATMENT

In the United States, NAC is given orally in an initial (i.e., loading) dose of 140 mg/kg followed by 17 more (i.e., maintenance) doses of 70 mg/kg every 4 h. This protocol was approved by the U.S. Food and Drug Administration (FDA) in 1985, and informed consent is no longer necessary. NAC is commercially available in a 20% (20 g/100 mL or 200 mg/mL) or 10% (10 g/100 mL or 100 mg/mL) solution (Mucomyst, Mead Johnson & Company). Since Mucomyst has a foul smell and tastes like rotten eggs, it should be diluted to a 5% solution with one or three parts of a soft drink or fruit juice to increase its palatability. Nausea and vomiting are frequent side effects. Diarrhea may also occur. The dose should be repeated if vomiting occurs within 1 h of administration. Changing the diluent, chilling the solution with ice, further diluting it, administering it slowly or in small aliquots (rather than as a bolus), having the patient sip it through a straw from a covered cup, or giving it by nasogastric or duodenal tube may be tried if repeated vomiting occurs. Metoclopramide (Reglan), 0.1 to 1.0 mg/kg IV, droperidol (Inapsine), 2.5 to 5 mg IV or IM in adults and 0.05 to 0.1 mg/kg in children, and ondansetron (Zofran), 0.15 mg/kg, or granisetron (Kytril), 0.01 mg/kg, IV over 5 min, with further doses as necessary, can also be used to prevent or treat vomiting. If multiple doses of activated charcoal are given for the treatment of coingestant poisoning, alternating doses of charcoal and NAC at 2-h intervals is recommended. Should delivery occur during the course of treatment of a pregnant patient, a complete course of NAC should be given to the newborn as well as to the mother.

Higher than usual doses of NAC may be beneficial in some patients. Since the effective dose of NAC is equal to the dose of APAP ingested in experimental animals, patients with very large APAP overdoses (e.g., those with acute ingestions of more than 1330 mg/kg or APAP levels indicating a high risk of hepatotoxicity) might benefit from higher than usual doses of NAC. This can be accomplished by increasing the NAC loading dose or increasing the first few maintenance doses. Conversely, smaller doses of NAC may be effective in patients with small overdoses. However, until further data become available, it is recommended that all patients at risk for toxicity by the nomogram receive at least a full course of therapy.

The dose of NAC used in the treatment of hepatic failure has been the same as that used for the prevention of hepatotoxicity. However, the optimal dose and duration of therapy in patients who develop hepatotoxicity is unknown. Some authorities recommend continuing therapy until liver function tests or predictors of a poor outcome begin to improve.

Intravenous NAC (300 mg/kg over 20 h) has been used with success in Europe and Canada for a number of years, and intravenous NAC (980 mg/kg over 48 h), using a dosage schedule identical to the oral protocol but stopping after a total of 12 doses, has been studied in the United States. If it is impossible to administer oral NAC (e.g., if there is active upper gastrointestinal bleeding, concomitant corrosive ingestion, or intractable vomiting), NAC should be given intravenously. Since Mucomyst is not certified as pyrogen-free, not recommended for intravenous use by the manufacturer, and not approved for intravenous administration in the United States, and since the intravenous use of NAC has resulted in anaphylactoid reactions, informed consent is essential.

The above recommendations are based on the interpretation of current data. Since definitive studies are often lacking, it is prudent to consult a toxicologist, gastroenterologist, or regional poison center for the latest treatment recommendations, especially in cases of late presentation, massive overdose, chronic exposure or poisoning, contemplated intravenous NAC therapy, and liver failure.

## BIBLIOGRAPHY

Brent J: Are activated charcoal–N-acetylcysteine interactions of clinical significance? *Ann Emerg Med* 22:1860, 1993.

Riggs BS, Brunstein AC, Kulig K, et al: Acute acetaminophen overdose during pregnancy. *Obstet Gynecol* 74:247, 1989.

Rumack DH: Acetaminophen overdose in children and adolescents. *Pediatr Clin North Am* 33:691, 1986.

Smilkstein MJ, Knapp GL, Kulig KW, et al: Efficacy of oral N-acetylcysteine in the treatment of acetaminophen overdose: Analysis of the national multicenter study (1976–1985). *N Engl J Med* 319:1557, 1988.

Whitcomb DC, Block GD: Association of acetaminophen hepatotoxicity with fasting and ethanol use. *JAMA* 272:1845, 1994.

# 145
# NONSTEROIDAL ANTI-INFLAMMATORY AGENTS

## Gregory Almond
## Richard F. Clark

## INTRODUCTION

Poisonings involving nonsteroidal anti-inflammatory agents (NSAIDs) are becoming more common as a result of their increasing availability over the counter as well as by prescription for their analgesic, anti-inflammatory, and antipyretic properties. Acute overdoses of these substances in healthy adults are rarely fatal, usually requiring only supportive care. However, when taken by patients with preexisting medical conditions or in combination with other substances, life-threatening conditions do develop. Certain categories of NSAIDs have not been adequately studied secondary to lack of documented exposure in humans.

The 1993 report from the American Association of Poison Control Centers indicates that there were 33,013 exposures to ibuprofen, with three deaths; 752 exposures to indomethacin, with one death; 12,010 exposures to other NSAID agents (including colchicine), with two deaths (one death related to piroxicam in an adult and one death related to phenylbutazone in a 9-year-old child).

NSAIDs include both salicylates and nonsalicylates (Table 145-1). In this chapter we will focus on only the nonsalicylate group, of which there are five major classes: acetic acids, fenamic (anthranilic) acids, oxicams, pyrazolones, and propionic acids. Colchicine has anti-inflammatory effects but is not related to these drugs. Diflunisal is a difluorophenyl derivative of salicylic acid that in overdose produces toxicity similar to that of members of the nonsalicylate group; it is included in this chapter. Colchicine and other forms of salicylate are discussed elsewhere in this book.

**Table 145-1.** Trade Names and Classification of Common NSAIDs

| Chemical Class | Compound | Trade Name |
|---|---|---|
| **CARBOXYLIC ACIDS** | | |
| Acetic acids | Nabumetone | Relafen |
| | Ketorolac | Toradol |
| | Diclofenac | Voltaren |
| | Indomethacin | Indocin |
| | Sulindac | Clinoril |
| | Tolmetin | Tolectin |
| Propionic acids | Flurbiprofen | Ansaid |
| | Carprofen | Rimadyl |
| | Fenoprofen | Nalfon |
| | Ibuprofen | Motrin, Advil, Medipren |
| | Ketoprofen | Orudis |
| | Naproxen | Naprosyn, Anaprox |
| Fenamic acids (anthranilic acids) | Mefenamic acids | Ponstel |
| | Meclofenamate sodium | Meclomen |
| Salicylic acid derivatives | Diflunisal | Dolobid |
| **ENOLIC ACIDS** | | |
| Pyrazolones | Phenylbutazone | Butazolidin |
| | Oxyphenbutazone | Tandearil |
| Oxicams | Piroxicam | Feldene |

## PHARMACOKINETICS

### Absorption and Distribution

Oral nonenteric-coated NSAIDs are rapidly absorbed from the gastrointestinal (GI) tract, with maximum concentrations appearing in the blood within 1 to 2 h. Enteric-coated diclofenac, sulindac, and nabumetone as well as sustained-released indomethacin peak in 2 to 5 h.

Injectable NSAIDs [ketorolac (Toradal)] are also available. Diclofenac is being evaluated in a transdermal delivery system. No reports of overdose from these formulations have been reported.

Almost all NSAIDs are greater than 90 percent protein-bound and are distributed to about 10 percent of body weight. Only free fractions of NSAIDs (normally less than 1 percent) are available for pharmacologic activity and metabolism. Elderly patients and patients with renal and hepatic disease or congestive heart failure have less circulating protein to bind free drug. These patients often have elevated levels of free NSAIDs in their circulation and develop adverse reactions at lower doses.

### Metabolism and Elimination

NSAIDs can undergo hydroxylation and oxidation but are metabolized predominantly through conjugation with glucuronic acid. Renal excretion of unchanged drug is only from 1 to 5 percent. Renal clearance and elimination half-life vary among NSAIDs, producing serum half-lives ranging from 1.5 h for tolmetin to 50 h for piroxicam. The significant difference in half-life is related to clearance rather than volume of distribution. The duration of symptoms after toxic ingestion of NSAIDs with long half-lives, such as piroxicam and phenylbutazone, is prolonged. In renal failure, certain drugs (ketoprofen, fenoprofen, naproxen, diflunisal) may be transformed to the parent compound.

Enterohepatic recirculation occurs with indomethacin and sulindac.

### Mechanism of Toxicity

The conversion of arachidonic acid to prostaglandins by the enzyme cyclooxygenase is reversibly blocked by NSAIDs. Interference with the physiologic actions of the prostaglandins results in an adverse drug reaction profile of the NSAIDs. Dilation of renal blood vessels, inhibition of gastric acid production, stimulation of gastric bicarbonate and mucin secretion, and promotion of sodium and water excretion are decreased.

## CLINICAL FEATURES

All NSAIDs can cause gastrointestinal (GI) intolerance, nephrotoxicity, headache, tinnitus, peripheral edema, and platelet dysfunction in therapeutic doses. Toxic ingestions most often manifest as mild drowsiness and GI upset. No toxic syndrome is characteristic of all NSAIDs.

### Gastrointestinal

Since prostacyclin appears to have cytoprotective effects on gastric mucosa, inhibition of prostacyclin synthesis with NSAIDs may impair this protective mucosal barrier. All available NSAIDs can produce or aggravate peptic ulcer disease and cause nausea, vomiting, and epigastric pain both in therapeutic use and overdose. Elderly patients appear to be more susceptible to these GI effects. The relative risk of GI hemorrhage in patients taking NSAIDs therapeutically may be twice as much as that of the general population.

Indomethacin is suggested to cause GI side effects most frequently among all NSAIDs and has been shown to produce ileal and jejunal ulcers in addition to gastric lesions. The fenamic acids and diclofenac also can induce small bowel erosions, which may be responsible for the high incidence (10 to 25 percent) of diarrhea reported. Acute pancreatitis has been reported in therapeutic use of sulindac, although its mechanism is uncertain.

### Renal, Acid-base and Electrolyte Abnormalities

Renal prostaglandins are necessary to maintain the glomerular filtration rate (GFR) in patients with congestive heart failure or cirrhosis and in volume-contracted patients taking diuretics. These patients, usually elderly, have less than optimal cardiac output. Since NSAIDs inhibit production of these prostaglandins, renal vasoconstriction occurs. Any NSAID can produce fluid retention and nephrotoxicity in these individuals. Indomethacin has been suggested to cause renal insufficiency and hypertension more often at therapeutic doses than other agents.

Renal vasoconstriction may be responsible for nephrotoxicity following acute NSAID poisonings. Acute renal failure has developed after massive overdoses of fenoprofen and ibuprofen. With inhibition of prostaglandin synthesis, blood flow in the kidney is redistributed; this results in increased perfusion of the juxtamedullary glomeruli, which thus have a greater capacity to absorb sodium, resulting in hypernatremia. Indomethacin impairs free water clearance by blocking the prostaglandin antagonism of antidiuretic hormone, resulting in water retention.

Acute interstitial nephritis with papillary necrosis secondary to a nephrogenic hypersensitivity reaction (analgesic abuse nephropathy) has been described with chronic therapeutic doses of some NSAIDs. The mechanism is thought to be related to glutathione depletion and metabolism of NSAIDs to toxic metabolites. Most cases of analgesic abuse nephropathy have been attributed to the propionic and acetic acids. These patients often present with hematuria and flank pain with or without rash, eosinophilia, eosinophiliuria, or fever.

Severe metabolic acidosis has occurred in NSAID overdose, most frequently with mefenamic acid and phenylbutazone. Hyperkalemia can occur, most frequently with indomethacin, ibuprofen, and piroxicam.

Hyperkalemia with a hyperchloremic metabolic acidosis can develop secondary to probable inhibition of prostaglandin-dependent secretion of renin and aldosterone, leading to a hyporenin-hypoaldosterone state. These effects may be noted in the absence of alterations in BUN or creatinine. Again, indomethacin is cited most commonly in generating this type of nephrotoxicity.

### Pulmonary

Susceptible individuals may develop a spectrum of respiratory toxicity, ranging from rhinitis to bronchospasm, that is secondary to NSAID inhibition of pulmonary prostaglandins. Aspirin-sensitive asthmatics are prone to bronchospasm when administered NSAIDs.

Overdoses of NSAIDs rarely lead to serious pulmonary toxicity. Apnea has been reported in a child after ingesting as few as 10 ibuprofen tablets. Noncardiogenic pulmonary edema, common in salicylate poisoning, has not been reported after toxic ingestions of NSAIDs.

### Hematologic

All NSAIDs reversibly inhibit platelet aggregation by altering the balance between thromboxane $A_2$ and prostacyclin, prolonging template bleeding times.

Aplastic anemia has occurred with the therapeutic use of piroxicam. Hemolytic anemia has been described with long-term use of sulindac and mefenamic acid. Thrombocytopenia has been reported.

### Hepatic

Therapeutic use of many NSAIDs may produce a transient rise in liver enzymes through a hypersensitivity response. The acetic and propionic acid species have demonstrated the highest incidence of hepatotoxicity. Sulindac has been found to cause direct hepatocellular injury and cholestatic jaundice in susceptible individuals. A similar idiosyncratic reaction led to the withdrawal of benoxaprofen from the market.

### Dermatologic

Generalized exanthems and pruritus are the most common cutaneous reactions described by patients receiving NSAIDs. Stevens-Johnson syndrome (SJS), toxic epidermal necrolysis (TEN), bullous eruptions, photosensitivity, fixed drug eruptions, urticaria, and pustular psoriasis have been reported. TEN and SJS are most frequently associated with sulindac. Photosensitivity is most common in piroxicam and other NSAIDs with extended half-lives.

### Anaphylactic Reactions

Anaphylactic shock has been reported with sulindac, zomepirac, and tolmetin. Patients allergic to any NSAID including aspirin must be considered allergic to all other NSAIDs and should not be given agents from another class.

### Central Nervous System

Subtle central nervous system (CNS) symptoms such as headache, drowsiness, and tinnitus are noted by patients taking NSAIDs in therapeutic doses. Psychological effects are seen with chronic use of most NSAIDs but appear to be described more frequently with indomethacin. Behavioral changes such as depression, confusion, and psychosis have been associated with therapeutic doses of indomethacin. The mechanism of interaction with the CNS is unclear, but it has been suggested that prostaglandins may modulate neurotransmitter release in the brain.

Aseptic meningitis has been described with sulindac, ibuprofen, and tolmetin, most often in patients suffering from connective tissue diseases such as systemic lupus erythematosus. Prostaglandin inhibition may not be the cause of the meningeal leukocytosis since patients have experienced meningitic symptoms related to one NSAID and not others.

Symptoms common in acute toxic ingestions of NSAIDs include drowsiness, dizziness, and lethargy.

Although coma and convulsions are rare in most uncomplicated NSAID overdoses, mefenamic acid poisonings are characterized by a relatively high incidence of seizures. Convulsions have occurred following acute mefenamic acid exposures as small as 7.5 g and, in one series, were present in up to 40 percent of acute ingestions where the serum mefenamic acid concentration exceeded the maximum therapeutic concentration. Mefenamic acid–induced seizures are usually self-limited, occur between 2 and 8 h after overdose, and appear unrelated to hypoxia. Propionic and acetic acid derivatives also can produce seizures after massive ingestions.

### Obstetric

Delays in onset of labor, prolongation of labor, increased bleeding in the mother and fetus, and premature closure of the ductus arteriosus in the fetus have been reported with therapeutic doses.

### Cardiac

There are no common direct cardiac effects of the NSAIDs. Sodium and water retention causes worsening of congestive heart failure in predisposed patients.

### Adverse Drug Interactions

The most serious potential drug interaction involves the concomitant use of oral anticoagulants. NSAIDs alter the effects of certain medications by displacing them from their protein-binding sites. Gastritis, peptic ulceration, and inhibition of platelet aggregation caused by NSAIDs increase the risk of GI hemorrhage in these patients.

Through effects on renal prostaglandins, the NSAIDs may cause increased toxicity when given with oral anticoagulants, oral hypoglycemics, phenytoin, sulfonamides, methotrexate, digitoxin, and lithium.

The action of NSAIDs that promotes water and sodium retention antagonizes the action of antihypertensive agents. Ibuprofen and piroxicam are well documented to act in this regard. Indomethacin has been shown to elevate the arterial pressure in hypertensive patients treated with angiotensin-converting enzyme inhibitors, diuretics, and β blockers. Indomethacin, ibuprofen, and piroxicam have also been reported to increase serum lithium concentrations by decreasing tubular lithium secretions.

A summary of the acute toxic effects reported in poisonings with each class of NSAID is presented in Table 145-2.

## DIFFERENTIAL DIAGNOSIS

There is no toxidrome associated with NSAID poisoning. The most common symptoms of NSAID poisoning are consistent with other diseases and poisonings. A mild metabolic acidosis is not uncommon with NSAID poisoning and is probably related to the weak acidity of NSAIDs and their oxidized metabolites. The standard etiologies of metabolic acidosis, including methanol, ethylene glycol, aspirin, and iron, must be considered in any patient after an unknown ingestion. A severe metabolic acidosis may also suggest a recent seizure.

Abbott TDx™ Diflunisal can cross-react with the Abbott TDx™ and colorimetric salicylate assays yielding false-positive salicylate levels. GI and CNS toxicities associated with diflunisal overdose also can resemble salicylate poisoning. However, classic symptoms of salicylism such as respiratory alkalosis and an elevated anion-gap acidosis are not observed in acute toxic ingestions of diflunisal.

## TREATMENT

### Who To Treat

Any patient who develops symptoms after an NSAID ingestion needs evaluation and observation for at least 24 h. All asymptomatic patients ingesting potentially toxic doses of NSAIDs (several times the therapeutic dose of mefenamic acid or phenylbutazone, five times the therapeutic dose of other agents in pediatric ingestions, or 10 times the therapeutic dose of other agents in adult ingestions) should be observed in the emergency department for at least 4 to 6 h.

The suspicion of phenylbutazone ingestions should be managed aggressively, especially in children. The anthranilic acids predispose to seizures (not dose-related), which can occur more than 4 h post-ingestion. Significant ingestions of agents in the phenylpropionic acid category (especially fenoprofen) are potentially lethal.

Asymptomatic patients with possible ingestions of other substances should be worked up on an individualized basis, always considering acetaminophen, salicylate, isoniazid, methanol, ethylene glycol, or iron ingestions; child abuse; and suicide attempt. All ingestions should be reported to a regional Poison Control Center.

Since ibuprofen is commonly prescribed and available over the counter, a large database of overdose information exists for this drug. Large reviews have demonstrated that patients rarely develop symptoms with acute *uncomplicated* ibuprofen ingestions of less than 100 mg/kg. Asymptomatic children fitting this description (ingesting less than 100 mg/kg) may be observed at home with specific instructions to seek medical care if symptoms occur. Patients with mixed ingestions, symptomatic or suicidal patients ingesting any type of NSAID, and those ingesting potentially toxic doses of any NSAID or more than 100 mg/kg of ibuprofen should be evaluated medically. Pediatric ingestions of greater than 400 mg/kg require immediate gastric lavage, aggressive observation and treatment, with close monitoring for development of seizures.

### Initial Stabilization

Initial stabilization should follow the standard ABC protocol. Airway management and volume replacement are most important. Altered mental status should be treated with standard measures. Hypotension should be treated with boluses of normal saline or Ringer's lactate and positioning. Symptomatic bradycardia should respond to atropine. Severe metabolic acidosis should be treated with sodium bicarbonate. Hypotension unresponsive to fluids can be treated with dopamine or norepinephrine.

Patients with evidence of severe toxicity including hyperkalemia and hypovolemia should have continuous cardiac monitoring.

There are no specific antidotes for NSAID poisoning. Decontamination with gastric lavage and charcoal, or charcoal alone, should be instituted when indicated in patients presenting after acute ingestions of NSAIDs. One dose of a cathartic can be administered with the charcoal but there is no proven benefit. Syrup of ipecac is contraindicated as NSAIDs predispose the patient to seizures, which could then be complicated by aspiration.

Patients should receive activated charcoal. Multiple doses of activated charcoal may be of benefit after ingestion of certain NSAIDs such as piroxicam, but the benefits must be weighed against the side effect of constipation.

Hemodialysis and charcoal hemoperfusion are of no benefit in removal of NSAIDs because they are highly protein-bound. However, hemodialysis may be indicated in patients who develop acute renal failure as a complication of their ingestion. Renal function usually returns to normal after a few days. Urine alkalinization or forced diuresis is unlikely to affect the clinical outcome in poisonings with NSAIDs since the kidney excretes only a small portion of the absorbed dose unchanged.

Gastrointestinal distress is common in patients with moderate to severe NSAID poisoning. GI bleeding with hematemesis or guaiac-positive stools may occur. Antacids or $H_2$ blockers may be employed for treatment or prophylaxis, but their usefulness in this situation is unproven.

Cardiac arrhythmias are not common in pure NSAID ingestions. Arrhythmias may be observed in mixed ingestions and should be treated by standard measures. Severe electrolyte abnormalities, acid-

**Table 145-2.** Clinical Findings Reported Following Toxic Ingestions of NSAIDs

| Findings | Acetic Acids | Propionic Acids | Fenamic Acids | Oxicams | Diflunisal |
|---|---|---|---|---|---|
| **Gastrointestinal** | | | | | |
| Nausea | ‡ | ‡ | † | † | † |
| Vomiting | ‡ | ‡ | † | † | † |
| Diarrhea | † | * | † | | † |
| Bloody diarrhea | | | † | † | † |
| Abdominal pain | ‡ | ‡ | | * | |
| Gastritis | * | | | | † |
| Hematemesis | * | † | | * | |
| **Neurologic** | | | | | |
| Miosis | | † | | | |
| Headache | † | † | | | |
| Blurred vision | | † | * | * | * |
| Tinnitus | † | † | | | |
| Irritability | | | ‡ | * | |
| Drowsiness | ‡ | ‡ | † | †‡ | |
| Nystagmus | * | † | | | |
| Ataxia | | † | | | |
| Diplopia | * | † | | | |
| Tremor | | | | * | |
| Agitation | † | | ‡ | * | |
| Muscle twitching | | | † | * | |
| Confusion | † | † | | * | |
| Dizziness | † | † | | * | † |
| Hallucinations | | | * | | |
| Auditory hallucinations | * | | | | |
| Respiratory depression | † | † | † | | * |
| Apnea | † | † | † | | * |
| Seizures | † | † | ‡ | * | |
| Coma | † | † | † | * | * |
| **Renal** | | | | | |
| Hematuria | * | † | | * | |
| Proteinuria | * | | | * | |
| Acute renal failure | * | † | * | | |
| **Cardiovascular** | | | | | |
| Sinus tachycardia | † | † | † | * | † |
| Bradycardia | | * | | | |
| Hypotension | * | † | * | * | † |
| **Hematologic** | | | | | |
| Abnormal coagulation studies | * | † | * | * | |
| Leukocytosis | * | | * | | |
| Bone marrow aplasia | | | | * | |
| **Laboratory** | | | | | |
| Metabolic acidosis | * | ‡ | | * | |
| Hyperkalemia | | * | | | |
| Hypokalemia | * | * | | | |
| Hypophosphatemia | | * | | | |
| Hyponatremia | | | | * | |
| Hypocalcemia | | | | * | |
| Cross-reacts with salicylate assays | | | | | ‡ |
| Elevated hepatic enzymes | | | | † | * |

\* Isolated case report.

† Several case reports.

‡ Frequently reported.

§*Source:* Adapted from Smolinske SC, Hall AH, Vandenberg SA, et al: Toxic effects of nonsteroidal anti-inflammatory drugs in overdose. *Drug Safety* 5:252, 1990.

base disturbances, hypotension, hypoxia, and preexisting cardiac disease will predispose patients with mixed ingestions to arrhythmias.

Seizures are usually brief and self-limited. NSAID-associated seizures respond to benzodiazepines. Patients with repetitive seizures or status epilepticus can be treated with phenytoin or phenobarbital.

## Laboratory Studies

Baseline laboratory studies in the symptomatic patient include arterial blood gas, complete blood count, coagulation studies, electrolytes, glucose, BUN, creatinine, aspirin level, acetaminophen level, and hepatic enzymes. Diflunisal can cross-react with the Abbott TDx™ and colorimetric salicylate assays, yielding false-positive salicylate levels. Renal and hepatic function should be monitored in ingestions of those NSAIDs associated with toxicity to those organs. Blood levels of the specific NSAIDs should not be routinely requested because the levels do not correlate with outcome. A nomogram using serum concentrations of ibuprofen in acute ibuprofen ingestions was developed, but serum concentrations of ibuprofen correlate poorly with the development of toxicity. Electrolytes should be monitored, with attention to acid-base and potassium abnormalities. Patients with GI bleeding, hematemesis, or guaiac-positive stools may require endoscopic evaluation.

## BIBLIOGRAPHY

Aaron TH, Murritt ELC: Reactions to acetylsalicylic acid. *Can Med Assoc J* 126:609, 1982.

Abramson SB, Weissmann G: The mechanisms of action of nonsteroidal anti-inflammatory drugs. *Arthritis Rheum* 32:1, 1989.

Antal EJ, Wright CE, Brown BL, et al: The influence of hemodialysis on the pharmacokinetics of ibuprofen and its major metabolites. *J Clin Pharmacol* 26:184, 1986.

Balali-Mood M, Critchley JAJH, Proudfoot AT, et al: Mefenamic acid overdose. *Lancet* 1:1354, 1981.

Bigby M, Stern R: Cutaneous reactions to nonsteroidal anti-inflammatory drugs. *J Am Acad Dermatol* 12:866, 1985.

Borda I: The spectrum of adverse gastrointestinal effects associated with nonsteroidal antiinflammatory drugs, in Borda I, Koff R (eds): *Nonsteroidal Antiinflammatory Drugs: A Profile of Adverse Effects.* Philadelphia, Hanley & Belfus, 1992, pp 25–80.

Brater DC: Clinical pharmacology of NSAIDs. *J Clin Pharmacol* 28:518, 1988.

Clive DM, Stoff JS: Renal syndromes associated with nonsteroidal antiinflammatory drugs. *N Engl J Med* 310:563, 1984.

Coles LS, Fries JF, Kraines RG: From experiment to experience: Side effects of nonsteroidal anti-inflammatory drugs. *Am J Med* 74:820, 1983.

Court H, Volens GN: Poisoning after overdose with nonsteroidal antiinflammatory drugs. *Adverse Drug React Acute Poisoning* Rev 3:1, 1984.

Fox DA, Jick H: Nonsteroidal anti-inflammatory drugs and renal disease. *JAMA* 251:1299, 1984.

Fredell BW, Strand LJ: Naproxen overdose. *JAMA* 238:938, 1977.

Hall AH, Smolinske SC, Conrad FL, et al: Ibuprofen overdose: 126 cases. *Ann Emerg Med* 15:1308, 1986.

Hall AH, Smolinske SC, Kulig KW, et al: Ibuprofen overdose—a prospective study. *West J Med* 148:653, 1988.

Harchelroad F, Evans TC, Hobbs E: Ibuprofen blood levels vary. *Ann Emerg Med* 17:186, 1988.

Ivey KJ: Mechanisms of nonsteroidal anti-inflammatory drug–induced gastric damage. *Am J Med* 84(suppl 2A):41, 1988.

Kertesz A: Neurological complications of nonsteroidal antiinflammatory agents, in Borda I, Koff R (eds): *Nonsteroidal Antiinflammatory Drugs: A Profile of Adverse Effects.* Philadelphia, Hanley & Belfus, 1992, pp 147–156.

Kwan KC, Breault GO, Umbenhauer ER, et al: Kinetics of indomethacin absorption, elimination and enterohepatic circulation in man. *J Pharmacokinet Biopharm* 4:255, 1975.

Levy RA, Smith DL: Clinical differences among nonsteroidal antiinflammatory drugs: Implications for therapeutic substitution in ambulatory patients. *Drug Intell Clin Pharmacol* 23:76, 1989.

Lewis JH: Hepatic toxicity of non-steroidal anti-inflammatory drugs. *Clin Pharmacol* 3:128, 1984.

Linden CH, Townsend PL: Metabolic acidosis after acute ibuprofen overdosage. *J Pediatrics* 111:922, 1987.

Litovitz TL, Schmitz BF, Holms KC: 1988 Annual Report of the American Association of Poison Control Centers National Data Collection System. *Am J Emerg Med* 6:495, 1989.

Litovitz TL, Clark LR, Soloway RA: 1993 Annual Report of the American Association of Poison Control Centers Toxic Exposure Surveillance System. *Am J Emerg Med* 12:546, 1994.

McElwee NE, Veltri JC, Bradford DC, et al: A prospective, population-based study of acute ibuprofen overdose: Complications are rare and routine serum levels not warranted. *Ann Emerg Med* 19:657, 1990.

Moise KJ, Huhta JC, Sharif DS, et al: Indomethacin in the treatment of premature labor: Effects on the fetal ductus arteriosus. *N Engl J Med* 319L:327, 1988.

Oates JA, FitzGerald GA, Branch RA, et al: Clinical implications of prostaglandin and thromboxane A2 formation (part 1). *N Engl J Med* 319:689, 1988.

Ragheb M, Ban TA, Buchanan D, et al: Interaction of indomethacin and ibuprofen with lithium in manic patients under a steady state lithium level. *J Clin Psychiatry* 41:397, 1980.

Reeves WB, Foley RJ, Weinman EJ: Renal dysfunction from nonsteroidal anti-inflammatory drugs. *Arch Intern Med* 144:1943, 1984.

Roth SH: Nonsteroidal anti-inflammatory drugs: Gastropathy, deaths, and medical practice. *Ann Intern Med* 109:353, 1988.

Smolinski SC, Hall AH, Vandenberg SA, et al: Toxic effects of nonsteroidal anti-inflammatory drugs in overdose. *Drug Safety* 5:252, 1990.

Somerville K, Faulkner G, Langman M: Non-steroidal anti-inflammatory drugs and bleeding peptic ulcer. *Lancet* 1:462, 1986.

Szczekik A, Gryglewski RJ, Czerniawska-Mysik G: Clinical patterns of hypersensitivity to non-steroidal anti-inflammatory drugs and their pathogenesis. *J Allergy Clin Immunol* 60:276, 1977.

Tan SY, Shapiro R, Franco R, et al: Indomethacin-induced prostaglandin inhibition with hyperkalemia. *Ann Intern Med* 90:783, 1979.

Vale JA, Meredith TJ: Acute poisoning due to non-steroidal antiinflammatory drugs. *Med Toxicol* 1:12, 1986.

Verbeeck RK, Blackburn JL, Loewen GR: Clinical pharmacokinetics of nonsteroidal anti-inflammatory drugs. *Clin Pharmacokinet* 8:302, 1983.

Webster J: Interactions of NSAIDs with diuretics and β-blockers: Mechanisms and clinical implications. *Drugs* 30:32, 1985.

Wilson T, Carruthers S: Renal and cardiovascular adverse effects of nonsteroidal antiinflammatory drugs, in Borda I, Koff R (eds): *Nonsteroidal Antiinflammatory Drugs: A Profile of Adverse Effects.* Philadelphia, Hanley & Belfus, 1992, pp 81–112.

# 146
# XANTHINES

## Charles L. Emerman

Theophylline use is complicated by its narrow therapeutic window, with a metabolism that depends on the patient's coincident medical problems and use of other medications. The 1992 Annual Report of the American Association of Poison Control Centers reported 5735 exposures to aminophylline resulting in major toxicity in 113 patients and death in 35, along with 5606 exposures to caffeine resulting in major toxicity in 6 patients with no deaths. Most consider a theophylline level greater than 20 µg/mL (110 µmol/L) as toxic although side effects may be seen at lower levels. Toxic levels are common in emergency patients with asthma or chronic obstructive pulmonary disease. Fortunately, most have a benign course, requiring little specific therapy. Life-threatening toxicity from theophylline poisoning can result in significant cardiac, neurologic, and metabolic abnormalities. Toxic side effects of caffeine share many similarities with theophylline although serious side effects are rare. Several modalities are available for treating theophylline toxicity, but indications for use in patients without life-threatening symptoms is controversial.

## PHARMACOLOGY

Theophylline and related products (Table 146-1) have a complex mechanism of action that has not been entirely elucidated. Although traditional teaching is that theophylline acts by inhibiting the action

**Table 146-1.** Theophylline Content of Related Drugs

| Drug | Theophylline Content, % |
|---|---|
| Aminophylline | 80–85 |
| Oxytriphylline | 65 |
| Dyphylline | 50 |

of phosphodiesterase, the concentration required for effective in vivo inhibition far exceeds the concentration usually produced by clinical dosages. Others have suggested that theophylline may act by affecting the binding of cyclic adenosine monophosphate, cyclic glucose monophosphate phosphodiesterase inhibition, prostaglandin antagonism, modification of intracellular calcium, stimulation of catecholamine release, or adenosine antagonism.

Theophylline is readily absorbed after oral administration, with peak levels occurring 90 to 120 min after ingestion. Oral absorption is enhanced by fasting or ingestion of large volumes of fluid and is decreased following certain foods. Enteric-coated tablets and sustained-released preparations reach peak plasma levels between 6 and 8 h. The newer "once-daily" preparations have an erratic absorption rate, particularly after eating, which may lead to drug "dumping" and elevated theophylline levels. Peak levels are reached within 30 min after intravenous administration of aminophylline. The absorption of intramuscular and rectally administered drug is erratic and unpredictable. Consequently, these routes should not be used.

Theophylline is approximately 60 percent protein bound, with less binding in neonates and patients with cirrhosis. The volume of distribution ranges from 0.3 to 0.7 L/kg with an average of 0.5 L/kg. Theophylline is primarily (85 to 90 percent) eliminated by the hepatic P-450 cytochrome system with the remaining 10 to 15 percent eliminated by urinary excretion. Metabolism generally follows first-order elimination. The half-life is 4 to 8 h in young, healthy, nonsmoking adults; children and smokers have a shorter half-life. A number of factors affect theophylline's half-life, including cigarette use, diet, cardiac or liver disease, and certain medications that interfere with the cytochrome P-450 pathway (Table 146-2). Theophylline acts as an adenosine antagonist. It has been reported to reverse adenosine-induced bronchoconstriction. Few studies have examined the effects of theophylline on the therapeutic use of adenosine to reverse supraventricular tachycardia. One study reported on the successful conversion from supraventricular tachycardia in two patients with therapeutic theophylline levels. At present, there are no established guidelines for altering the therapeutic dose of adenosine in the presence of theophylline.

Caffeine is readily absorbed after oral administration with an onset of action of 30 min and peak effect at 60 to 120 min. Caffeine is also metaboized by methylation in the liver, forming L-methyluric acid and L-methyl xanthine. Again, about 10 percent of the drug is eliminated by urinary excretion. Many of the factors that affect the half-life of theophylline, such as severe liver disease, also affect caffeine.

## TOXIC EFFECTS

### Cardiovascular

Even at therapeutic levels (10 to 20 μg/mL), theophylline can cause cardiac side effects. Sinus tachycardia may occur after administration and increased atrial automaticity with premature atrial contractions, atrial tachycardia, multifocal atrial tachycardia, atrial fibrillation, and atrial flutter is seen with increasing frequency with levels above 20 μg/mL. Ventricular arrhythmias with premature ventricular contractions and self-limited runs of ventricular tachycardia may also occur. Sustained ventricular tachycardia may occur in the older patient with chronic overdose with levels of around 40 to 60 μg/mL. Younger patients with acute intentional overdose may tolerate levels above 100 μg/mL without developing life-threatening cardiac effects. Patients with a prior history of arrhythmias may experience a recurrence of arrhythmias with levels less than 40 μg/mL. Hypotension has also been associated with acute ingestion but may also occur with chronic overmedication.

### Neurologic

Even with therapeutic levels, theophylline use can be associated with agitation, headache, irritability, sleeplessness, tremors, and muscular twitching. Seizures, including both generalized tonic-clonic and focal motor, have been reported in patients with therapeutic levels. Patients with a history of epilepsy are particularly susceptible to aminophylline-induced seizures. The incidence of seizures increases with toxic levels. Status epilepticus resistant to treatment can occur as the level rises above 25 μg/mL. When seizures occur at only mildly elevated levels there are usually underlying neurologic deficits. The occurrence of seizures does not appear to correlate with prognosis. Theophylline toxicity has also been associated with hallucinations and psychosis.

### Metabolic

Theophylline produces a dose-dependent increase in circulating catecholamines. There is a concomitant increase in glucose, free fatty acids, insulin levels, and white blood cell count. Hypokalemia may occur, with the fall in serum potassium inversely related to the theophylline concentration. Hypokalemia appears to be a particular problem in patients with acute overdose or an acute overdose superimposed on chronic use. Administration of a β agonist may also be associated with hypokalemia and, with the hypokalemia produced by theophylline overdose, may lead to cardiac arrhythmias. Lactic acidosis and ketosis also occur.

### Gastrointestinal

Theophylline has a direct central nervous system (CNS) effect leading to nausea and vomiting. In addition, theophylline increases gastric acid secretion. Nausea and vomiting can be seen with therapeutic levels, although the incidence of nausea and vomiting increases markedly with levels above 15 μg/mL. Approximately 25% of patients with levels greater than 20 μg/mL have nausea or vomiting. Gastrointestinal bleeding may also occur, with epigastric pain. Esophageal reflux has also been reported.

Caffeine shares many of the effects of theophylline. Gastrointestinal symptoms generally occur with overdose and include abdominal pain, vomiting, and occasional hematemesis. CNS effects include agitation, seizures, and coma. Ventricular arrhythmias other than premature ventricular contractions are rare, but paroxysonal atrial tachycardia may occur. Rhabdomyolysis, hyperglycemia, leukocytosis, and metabolic acidosis have been reported. Toxicity is seen after 1-g

**Table 146-2.** Factors Affecting Theophylline Half-Life

| Decreased Half-life | Increased Half-life |
|---|---|
| **Drugs** | **Drugs** |
| Carbamazepine | Cimetidine |
| Phenobarbital | Allopurinol |
| Phenytoin | ? Oral contraceptives |
| Rifampin | **Antibiotics** |
| | Erythromycin |
| | Clarithromycin |
| | Quinolones |
| | **Antiarrhythmics** |
| | Mexilitine |
| | Tocainide |
| | Propafenone |
| | **Conditions** |
| | Cirrhosis |
| | Congestive heart failure |
| | Pulmonary edema |
| | Pneumonia |
| **Conditions** | Severe acute obstructive airway disease |
| Smoking | Viral illness in children |
| Charcoal broiled foods | Obesity |
| Children | Neonates |
| Hyperthyroidism | |

doses in adults. Doses of around 80 mg/kg may lead to symptoms in children.

## TREATMENT

### Gastric Elimination

Following acute ingestion of potentially toxic doses of aminophylline or theophylline, gastric emptying should be initiated with gastric lavage. This is probably not indicated for patients whose dose is calculated to raise their levels to less than 30 μg/mL (approximately 15 mg/kg), unless coingestion of other medications is suspected. Administration of ipecac may complicate the use of other therapies for enhancing the elimination of theophylline. In addition, vomiting is usually a prominent symptom in theophylline toxicity. Therefore, the use of ipepac is limited in this syndrome

### Cathartics

Cathartics should be administered to enhance the passage of ingested theophylline through the gastrointestinal tract. Some investigators have found magnesium citrate not to be effective in lowering the theophylline level. Further, there have been reports of magnesium toxicity after magnesium cathartics.

Sorbitol may be a better choice. A 70% sorbitol solution (100 mL) can be used either alone or in combination with activated charcoal for patients with potentially toxic ingestions. There have been reports of successful use of whole bowel irrigation with polyethylene glycol although this treatment is controversial.

### Activated Charcoal

Theophylline undergoes hepatobiliary enteric circulation. Administration of repeated doses of activated charcoal at 2- to 4-h intervals significantly decreases theophylline's half-life. Doses of 30 to 60 g should be used in adults. Charcoal may also be administered as a continuous nasogastric infusion at rates of 0.25 to 0.5 g/kg per hour. In patients with markedly elevated theophylline levels, the administration of charcoal is complicated by repeated episodes of emesis. In one study, patients with levels greater than 50 μg/mL could not tolerate any of their charcoal doses because of repeated episodes of emesis. Patients who cannot tolerate oral administration of activated charcoal should be pretreated with ranitidine.

### Ranitidine

Treatment of theophylline toxicity is hindered by the recurrent nausea and vomiting producted by toxic levels. Administration of ranitidine, 50 mg intravenously, is useful when nausea and vomiting are present. This will permit the use of repeated doses of activated charcoal to enhance drug elimination.

### Antiepileptics

Diazepam, phenobarbital, and phenytoin have been used in the treatment of theophylline-induced seizures. Unfortunately, status epilepticus may be resistant to these modes of therapy. The airway should be protected in patients with theophylline-induced status epilepticus, particularly after administration of oral activated charcoal. Patients with status epilepticus resistant to traditional modes of therapy may require the induction of general anesthesia pending more aggressive measures to lower the serum theophylline level.

### Hemoperfusion/Hemodialysis

Although it is less effective than hemoperfusion, hemodialysis may be used for patients with toxicity. The clearance rate induced by hemodialysis is approximately 25 mL/kg per hour. Charcoal hemoperfusion with resin or charcoal filters is more effective than hemodialy-

**Table 146-3.** Indications for Hemoperfusion

| Clinical Conditions | Recommendation |
| --- | --- |
| Life-threatening toxicity (i.e., seizures, tachyarrhythmias) not responsible to other therapy | Hemoperfusion clearly indicated |
| Acute overdose with level > 100 μg/mL | Hemoperfusion possibly indicated |
| Chronic overdose with level > 60 μg/mL | Hemoperfusion possibly indicated |
| Elderly patient with prolonged half-life, severe liver or severe cardiac disease, or level > 30 μg/mL | Hemoperfusion controversial |
| Theophylline level < 30 μg/mL | Hemoperfusion not indicated |

sis, producing extraction ratios above 0.85 with clearance rates of 120 to 300 mL/kg per hour. The indications for hemoperfusion are controversial (Table 146-3). In the view of some investigators, hemoperfusion is not absolutely indicated at any theophylline level in the absence of life-threatening symptoms such as status epilepticus or resistant ventricular arrhythmias. Others have felt that patients with increased half-lives, advanced age, or theophylline levels above 40 μg/mL may be candidates for hemoperfusion. Young, healthy patients with an acute ingestion may be able to tolerate levels over 100 μg/mL without adverse incident. The decision to use hemoperfusion should be made considering the potential for life-threatening toxicity.

### β Blockade

Hypotension or life-threatening cardiac arrhythmias may be an indication for β-blocker therapy when symptoms do not respond to other therapy. The use of β blockers may be complicated by further cardiac depression or exacerbation of airway obstruction. They should be administered cautiously, in low doses, monitoring for adverse effect. Propanolol may be used, given in 1 mg doses, up to a total of 10 mg. Alternatively, one of the newer, β-blocker agents such as labetalol or the short-acting esmolol may be used.

### Antiarrhythmics

In addition to β blockade, cardiac arrhythmias may also be treated with other antiarrhythmics. Verapamil has been effective in animal studies. The use of digoxin, lidocaine, and phenytoin has been reported for treatment of venticular arrhythmias. Adenosine may be considered for supraventricular arrhythmias although it may induce bronchospasm. The contributory effect of hypokalemia should be considered in treating the patient with resistant ventricular arrhythmias and correction of serum electrolyte abnormalities may be effective in terminating recurrent arrhythmias.

## INDICATIONS FOR TREATMENT AND ADMISSION

Although theophylline toxicity can lead to life-threatening side effects, toxic theophylline levels are common, and most patients tolerate these with only minor toxic manifestations. No good studies have demonstrated that prophylactic use of antiarrhythmics or antiepileptics decreases morbidity or mortality. Similarly, while hemodialysis, hemoperfusion, and oral activated charcoal therapy will enhance theophylline clearance, there is no compelling evidence that their use prevents morbidity or mortality in patients with only mild toxic symptoms or minimally elevated levels.

On the other hand, ventricular arrhythmias or seizures may occur in patients before the manifestation of other minor toxic effects leading some authors to advocate aggressive therapy. Older patients with concomitant medical problems are more susceptible to life-threatening theophylline toxicity following chronic over medication than are younger patients with an acute overdose. Prophylactic use of hemoperfusion has been reported to decrease major morbidity in elderly patients.

As a general guideline, patients with a prior history of seizures or ventricular arrhythmias should be monitored until their theophylline level returns to normal. Patients with levels below 25 µg/mL do not require specific therapy other than discontinuation or modification of theophylline administration. Patients with levels above 30 µg/mL should be treated with oral activated charcoal (repeated) and monitored for toxic side effects. Hemoperfusion use is controversial, but may be indicated in older patients with levels above 30 µg/mL or in the younger patient with acute intentional overdose with levels above 100 µg/mL.

## PREVENTION

Theophylline toxicity is only rarely a result of intentional overdose. Physician prescribing errors, patient self-overmedication, and variations in plasma clearance due to deteriorating cardiac or hepatic status, smoking cessation, or concomitant administration of drugs that affect theophylline clearance all may lead to elevated levels. Aminophylline infusions should be started using standard guidelines with close monitoring of serum levels. Because the history of outpatient theophylline use has been found to be a poor guide to the serum concentration, loading doses of aminophylline should be calculated using the initial theophylline level. As a rough approximation, each milligram per kilogram of aminophylline will raise the theophylline level by 2 µg/mL. The initial dose of oral theophylline should not exceed 900 mg/d. Patients should be started at a much lower dose (400 mg/d) to avoid the nausea and vomiting frequently accompanying initial theophylline use. Levels should be obtained to monitor therapy. Patients should be cautioned not to alter their medication regimen without physician guidance. Patients being started on erythromycin or cimetidine should have their theophylline dose decreased by approximately 25 percent, with monitoring of the effect on levels.

## BIBLIOGRAPHY

Baker MD. Theophylline toxicity in children. *J Pediatr* 109:538, 1986.

Bertino JS, Walker JW. Reassessment of theophylline toxicity: serum concentrations, clinical cords, and treatment. *Arch Intern Med* 147:757, 1987.

Emerman CL, Devlin C, Connors AF. Risk of toxocity in patients with elevated theophylline levels. *Ann Emerg Med* 19:643, 1990.

Goldberg MJ, Park GD, Berlinger WG. Treatment of theophylline intoxication. *J Allergy Clin Immunol* 78:811, 1986.

Greenberg A, Piraino BH, Kroboth PD, et al. Severe theophylline toxicity: Role of conservative measures, anti-arrhythmic agents, and charcoal hemoperfusion. *Am J Med* 76:854, 1984.

Hendeles L, Weinberger M, Szefler S, et al. Safety and efficacy of theophylline in children with asthma. *J Pediatr* 120:177, 1992.

McGuigan MA: Toxicology of drug abuse. *Emerg Med Clin North Am* 2:87, 1984.

Olson KR, Benowitz NL, Woo OF, et al. Theophylline overdose: acute single ingestion vs. chronic repeated over-medication. *Ann Emerg Med* 3:386, 1985.

Sessler CN: Theophylline toxicity: clinical features of 116 consecutive cases. *Am J Med* 88:567, 1990.

Shannon M: Predictors of major toxicity after theophylline overdose. *Ann Inter Med* 119:1161,

# 147
# DIGITALIS GLYCOSIDES
## Mark A. Kirk

For centuries, digitalis glycosides have been recognized for their medicinal benefits and potential toxicity. Digitalis preparations are used most commonly in the treatment of supraventricular tachydysrhythmias and congestive heart failure. In addition to their availability as pharmaceuticals, cardiac glycosides are also found in plants such as foxglove, oleander, and lily of the valley. It is important that physicians recognize digitalis toxicity because potentially fatal cardiac dysrhythmias can develop. Prompt administration of a highly specific antidote, digoxin-specific Fab fragments, can reverse otherwise fatal toxicity.

## PHARMACOLOGY AND PATHOPHYSIOLOGY

Digoxin is currently the most widely used digitalis preparation. It is rapidly absorbed from the gastrointestinal tract and is primarily eliminated through renal excretion. It has a volume of distribution of 6 to 7 L/kg. The half-life of a therapeutic dose is 36 to 48 h.

Digitalis has a narrow margin between therapeutic and toxic effects. Toxicity results from an exaggeration of its therapeutic actions. Digitalis binds to a specific receptor site on the cardiac cell membrane, inactivating the sodium-potassium adenosine triphosphate ($Na^+,K^+ - ATPase$) pump. This pump concentrates sodium extracellularly and potassium intracellularly to maintain the electrochemical membrane potential so vital to conduction tissues. When $Na^+,K^+ - ATPase$ is inhibited, the sodium-calcium exchanger removes accumulated intracellular sodium in exchange for calcium. This exchange increases sarcoplasmic calcium and is the mechanism responsible for the positive inotropic effect of digitalis. Inhibition of the $Na^+, K^+ - ATPase$ pump also results in an increase in extracellular potassium. Digitalis increases vagal tone and decreases conduction through the atrioventricular (AV) node. In toxic doses, these effects result in various bradydysrhythmias. Slowing of the conduction tissue, along with a decreased refractory period of the myocardium, increases automaticity. Intracellular calcium overload creates transient depolarizations, giving rise to triggered dysrhythmias.

## CLINICAL FEATURES

Digitalis glycoside toxicity is determined by evaluating the entire clinical picture. The history, physical examination, and laboratory studies provide important clues, with no single element to exclude or confirm the diagnosis.

When a poisoned patient presents to the emergency department, the clinician should determine if toxicity is due to an accidental ingestion, massive intentional ingestion, or chronic toxicity from therapeutic use of digitalis. If the ingestion is intentional, historic information may be inaccurate or incomplete, and coingestants should be suspected. The time of ingestion is extremely helpful in interpreting laboratory information. Since various plants contain digitalis glycosides and cause similar toxicity to medicinal forms, attempt to accurately identify any ingested plants.

Preexisting medical conditions and current medications may identify risk factors that potentiate digitalis toxicity. Increased susceptibility is seen in patients who are elderly and in those who have coexisting diseases (heart disease, renal dysfunction, hepatic dysfunction, hypothyroidism, and chronic obstructive pulmonary disease), electrolyte disturbances (hypokalemia, hypomagnesemia, and hypercalcemia), and hypoxia. Drug interactions, most notably quinidine and calcium channel blockers, potentiate digitalis toxicity. Carefully evaluate the cardiac, neurologic, and gastrointestinal systems for clues of developing toxicity.

Cardiac dysrhythmias in digitalis toxicity are nonspecific and may be life-threatening. Suspect digitalis toxicity in patients with tachydysrhythmias or junctional escape rhythms and AV block. The most common dysrhythmia is frequent premature ventricular beats, especially in a diseased heart. Bidirectional ventricular tachycardia, a narrow complex tachycardia with right bundle branch morphology, is specific for digitalis toxicity, but is rare.

In addition to cardiac manifestations, gastrointestinal distress, dizziness, headache, weakness, syncope, and seizures may occur. Reported psychiatric symptoms include confusion, disorientation, delirium, and hallucinations. Patients with toxicity have complained of seeing yellow-green halos around objects.

## Laboratory Evaluation

Serum potassium and serum digoxin levels will assist in providing information necessary to make adequate therapeutic decisions. Acute poisoning of the $Na^+$, $K^+$ – ATPase pump may result in markedly elevated serum potassium levels. A high incidence of hyperkalemia has been noted in patients with severe acute poisoning. In fact, the serum potassium may be a better indicator of end-organ toxicity and a better prognostic indicator than the serum digoxin level in the acutely poisoned patient. Hyperkalemia is uncommon in chronically poisoned patients.

Accepted therapeutic digoxin levels are 0.5 to 2.0 ng/mL. In most laboratories, the serum digoxin level is not part of the routine toxicologic screen and must be specifically requested.

Serum digoxin levels in both acute and chronic toxicity should be interpreted in the overall clinical context and not relied upon as the sole indicator of the presence or absence of toxicity. In acute exposures, digoxin is absorbed into the plasma compartment and then redistributed slowly into the tissue compartment. Hence, high digoxin levels are not always associated with clinical signs and symptoms of poisoning. Serum levels are most reliable when obtained after 6 h, when distribution is complete. In patients with clinical evidence of chronic digitalis toxicity, a "therapeutic" level does not exclude toxicity, especially when predisposing factors are present. Conversely, levels above the upper limits of normal do not always cause symptoms. Given the above limitations, it is still most common that the higher the serum level, the greater the likelihood of toxicity.

A positive serum assay is diagnostic of acute ingestion if the patient has not received digitalis glycosides therapeutically. The rare exception is in the presence of a digoxin-like immunoreactive substance that has been detected in neonates and patients with renal insufficiency or hepatic dysfunction. In addition, naturally occurring digitalis glycosides from plants and animals can cross-react with the digoxin assay. The degree of cross-reactivity is unknown, and no correlation has been established between serum levels of these glycosides and toxicity.

Additional laboratory evaluation includes the determination of adequate oxygenation, renal and hepatic function, and electrolyte levels in addition to potassium. Continuous electrocardiographic monitoring is essential to detect dysrhythmias and evidence of hyperkalemia.

## Differences in the Presentation of Acute and Chronic Toxicity

A distinct clinical presentation exists for both acute and chronic digitalis glycoside toxicity (see Table 147-1). Acute poisoning most often results from accidental or intentional ingestion. There may be an asymptomatic period of several hours prior to development of symptoms. Gastrointestinal symptoms are often the earliest manifestation of toxicity. In the early period of toxicity, increased vagal tone produces cardiac dysrhythmias that are typically bradydysrhythmias

**Table 147-1.** Clinical Presentation of Digitalis Toxicity

Acute toxicity
  Clinical history: Intentional or accidental ingestion
    GI effects: Nausea and vomiting
    CNS effects: Headache, dizziness, confusion, coma
    Cardiac effects: Predominantly supraventricular tachydysrhythmias with AV block; Bradydysrhythmias
    Electrolyte abnormalities: Hyperkalemia
    Digoxin level: Marked elevation
Chronic toxicity
  Clinical history: Typically an elderly cardiac patient taking diuretics. May have renal insufficiency
    GI effects: Nausea, vomiting, diarrhea, abdominal pain
    CNS effects: Fatigue, weakness, confusion, delirium, coma
    Cardiac effects: Ventricular dysrhythmias are common; almost any ventricular or supraventricular dysrhythmia can occur
    Electrolyte abnormalities: Hypokalemia or normal serum potassium, hypomagnesemia
    Digoxin level: Minimally elevated or "therapeutic" range

or supraventricular dysrhythmias with AV block; however, life-threatening ventricular dysrhythmias may develop at any stage in an acute massive ingestion. Acute toxicity most closely correlates with hyperkalemia and correlates poorly with the serum digoxin level.

Chronic toxicity occurs most typically in the elderly cardiac patient on digoxin and diuretics. Signs and symptoms may mimic more common illnesses such as influenza and gastroenteritis. An altered mental status or psychiatric symptoms may not be recognized as signs of digitalis toxicity. Almost any cardiac dysrhythmia may be seen, but ventricular dysrhythmias occur more frequently in chronic than in acute poisonings. The serum digoxin level is not an accurate predictor of toxicity, and the serum potassium is usually decreased or normal.

## Differential Diagnosis

Other toxins and medical illnesses may present with a similar clinical picture to digitalis toxicity. Other toxic causes of bradydysrhythmias include calcium and β-blocker overdoses, class 1A antidysrhythmic (procainamide and quinidine) overdoses, clonidine overdoses, organophosphate insecticide poisoning, and cardiotoxic plants (e.g., aconitine- and grayanotoxin-containing plants). Sinus node disease can also mimic digitalis toxicity.

## EMERGENCY DEPARTMENT CARE

The basic emergency department management of any poisoned patient includes general supportive care, treatment of specific complications of toxicity, prevention of further drug absorption, enhanced drug elimination, antidote administration, and safe disposition (Table 147-2). Patients with intentional or accidental ingestions may present with no symptoms. Assume the worst and anticipate life-threatening complications of toxicity. Focus the management of the asymptomatic patient on preventing drug absorption and closely monitoring for development of toxicity. Provide continuous cardiac monitoring, intravenous access, and frequent reevaluations for any patient with a potentially toxic ingestion of digitalis. Toxicity may not develop for several hours after an acute ingestion; therefore, extended observation (12 h) is required for anyone with a confirmed ingestion. Admission to the intensive care unit and frequent reassessment is required for any patient developing signs of toxicity.

## Treatment of Life-Threatening Conditions

Approach the symptomatic patient methodically. Ensure a patent airway, adequate ventilation, and effective circulation. Rapidly correct conditions such as hypoxia, hypoglycemia, hypovolemia, and electrolyte abnormalities.

**Table 147-2.** Treatment of Digitalis Glycoside Poisoning

**Asymptomatic patients**
  Obtain accurate history
  Continuous cardiac monitoring
  Intravenous access
  Gastrointestinal decontamination
    Activated charcoal (1 g/kg)
    ±Gastric lavage
  Frequent reevaluation
  Fab fragments at bedside (calculate dose required for emergent use)
**Symptomatic patients**
  *ABCs*
    Intravenous access
    Continuous cardiac monitoring
  *Treat altered mental status*
    Oxygen
    Dextrose (thiamine)
    Naloxone
  *Dysrhythmias*
    Bradydysrhythmias
      Atropine (0.5–2.0 mg IV)
      Pacemaker (external or transvenous)
      Fab fragments (IV infusion)
    Ventricular dysrhythmias
      Fab fragments (IV infusion or bolus)
      Phenytoin (15 mg/kg: infuse no faster than 25 mg/min) or
        lidocaine (1 mg/kg)
      Magnesium sulfate (2–4 g IV)
      Electrocardioversion (10–25 W·s; last resort)
    Cardiac arrest
      CPR
      ACLS protocols
      Fab fragments (IV bolus; give 5–10 vials if amount ingested is
        unknown)
  *Electrolyte abnormalities*
    Hyperkalemia
      Fab fragments (IV infusion or bolus)
      Glucose–insulin
      Sodium bicarbonate
      Potassium resin binder
      Hemodialysis
      Avoid calcium chloride
    Hypomagnesemia
      Evaluate renal status prior replacement
      Magnesium sulfate (2–4 g IV)
  *Gastrointestinal decontamination*
    Activated charcoal (1 g/kg then 0.5 g/kg every 4–6 h)
    ±Gastric lavage

Conventional and antidote therapy are available to treat digitalis-induced dysrhythmias. Atropine and cardiac pacing (external and transvenous) have been used successfully in treating bradydysrhythmias. Both phenytoin and lidocaine depress ventricular automaticity and increase the fibrillation threshold. Because of phenytoin's ability to accelerate conduction at the AV node, it has been considered the antidysrhythmic of choice by some for digitalis-induced ventricular dysrhythmias. Bretylium has effectively suppressed dysrhythmias. Class 1A antidysrhythmics, such as quinidine and procainamide, are contraindicated because they depress AV nodal conduction, which in turn may enhance digitalis-induced cardiac toxicity. Intravenous magnesium has been reported to counteract ventricular irritability in digitalis toxicity. Electrocardioversion may induce intractable ventricular fibrillation and should be considered only as a last resort. If necessary, use a low setting (10 to 25 W·s) and prepare to treat resulting ventricular fibrillation. In severe toxicity, conventional treatment may be unsuccessful. When available, digoxin-specific Fab fragments are the treatment of choice for those dysrhythmias that are life-threatening and do not respond immediately to conventional therapy.

Hyperkalemia may be life-threatening and needs immediate treatment. Treatment includes intravenous administration of dextrose, insulin and sodium bicarbonate and enteral administration of a potassium-binding resin. Calcium chloride administration in the face of digitalis-induced hyperkalemia may enhance cardiac toxicity and should be avoided. If digitalis-induced hyperkalemia is not rapidly corrected by conventional therapy, then Fab fragments are indicated for reversal.

## Gastrointestinal Decontamination and Enhanced Elimination

After initial stabilization, administer activated charcoal to prevent further drug absorption and consider performing gastric lavage. Ipecac has no role in the emergency department management of digitalis glycoside poisoning. Evacuate the stomach with gastric lavage in patients presenting with massive intentional ingestions. When cardiac toxicity is evident, vagal stimulation may worsen bradydysrhythmias or produce asystole, but the presence of cardiac toxicity is not a contraindication to gastric lavage. Activated charcoal effectively adsorbs digitalis glycosides and should be administered to any patient with a potentially toxic ingestion. Forced diuresis, hemodialysis, or hemoperfusion have no role in enhancing elimination of digitalis.

## Antidote Therapy

A unique aspect in the management of digitalis poisoning is the availability of drug-specific antibodies. Digoxin-specific Fab (Digibind, Burroughs-Wellcome) is derived from the IgG fragment of sheep antidigoxin antibodies. Fab fragments distribute widely throughout tissues and remove digitalis from tissue-binding sites. In a series of 150 severely poisoned patients, 90 percent showed reversal or significant improvement in life-threatening dysrhythmias and hyperkalemia after Fab fragment administration. In most cases, clinical improvement in cardiac rhythm occurs within 1 h of antidote administration. Those patients developing cardiac arrest prior to Fab administration had a 50 percent survival, which is significantly improved from survival by treatment with conventional therapies.

Indications for digitalis-specific Fab fragments are: (1) ventricular dysrhythmias, (2) hemodynamically significant bradydysrhythmias unresponsive to standard therapy, and (3) hyperkalemia in excess of 5.5 mEq/L.

Fab fragment therapy should be immediately accessible at the bedside to all patients presenting with acute massive ingestions or with risk factors for enhanced toxicity, such as old age and preexisting cardiac disease. Elevated serum digoxin levels should not be the sole indication for Fab fragment administration. Fab fragments have also been reported to be beneficial in treating digitoxin and oleander poisonings.

Fab fragment administration has resulted in few adverse effects. Cardiogenic shock has been reported in patients dependent upon digoxin for inotropic support. In addition, ventricular response to atrial fibrillation may be increased. Hypokalemia may develop rapidly as digitalis toxicity is reversed. Only mild, acute hypersensitivity reactions including rash, flushing, and facial swelling have been reported. No incidences of serum sickness or anaphylaxis have been observed, even in patients with repeated administration. Since Fab is derived from sheep protein, skin testing should be considered in patients with a strong history of allergies, especially to antibiotics, or those with asthma. If cardiac arrest is imminent, Fab fragment infusion should not be delayed for skin testing. Failures of Fab fragment therapy have been attributed to inadequate dosing, moribund state prior to administration, and incorrect diagnosis of digitalis toxicity.

The Fab fragment dosage is based on an estimation of total body load of digoxin. This can be determined from the serum digoxin level or based on the estimated dose ingested (Table 147-3). Clinical series have reported that an average of 200 to 480 mg (5 to 12 vials) were required to effectively treat severely digitalis toxic patients. When the

**Table 147-3.** Calculating Digoxin-Specific Fab Fragment Dosage

1. Calculate total body load
   Based on history of amount ingested:

   Total body load = amount ingested (mg) × 0.80 (bioavailability)

   Based on serum digoxin concentration:

   $$\text{Total body load} = \frac{\text{serum digoxin level} \times 5.6 \text{ L/kg} \times \text{patient's wt(kg)}}{1000}$$

2. Calculate number of vials of digoxin-specific Fab fragments needed to neutralize the calculated total body load:
   It is assumed that an equimolar dose of Fab fragments is required for neutralization. One vial (40 mg) of Fab fragments binds 0.6 mg of digoxin.

   $$\text{Number of vials required} = \frac{\text{total body load}}{0.6}$$

   A simple and accurate variation of the above calculations:

   $$\text{Number of vials of Fab} = \frac{\text{serum digoxin level} \times \text{patient's weight (kg)}}{100}$$

ingested dose is unknown, 5 to 10 vials are recommended as initial treatment in life-threatening situations. Fab fragments are administered intravenously through a 0.22-μm filter over 30 min, except in a cardiac arrest, where it may be given as a bolus.

The serum level has no correlation with clinical toxicity following Fab administration because the assay measures both bound and unbound digoxin. Minutes after Fab fragment administration, the free digoxin level falls to zero, but the total serum digoxin level (bound to Fab fragments) increases 10- to 20-fold. The Fab-digoxin complex is eliminated by renal excretion. In the case of renal failure, the complex may persist in the circulation for prolonged periods. Recurrent toxicity can occur up to 10 days after Fab fragment administration in patients with renal failure. Hemodialysis does not enhance the elimination of the digoxin-Fab complex.

## DISPOSITION

Patients who present with signs of toxicity or who develop toxicity in the emergency department should be admitted to the intensive care unit. Consider admitting any patient with a history of a large ingested dose, especially if coexisting risk factors increase susceptibility to digitalis toxicity. Any patient receiving Fab fragments requires observation in the intensive care unit for at least 24 h. All suspected suicidal patients should have a psychiatric evaluation prior to discharge. Patients with accidental exposures with no signs of toxicity after 12 h can be discharged home.

## BIBLIOGRAPHY

Antman EM, Wenger TL, Butler VP, et al: Treatment of 150 cases of life-threatening digitalis intoxication with digoxin-specific Fab antibody fragments. *Circulation* 81:1744, 1990.

Kelly RA, Smith TW: Recognition and management of digitalis toxicity. *Am J Cardiol* 69:108G, 1992.

Kirkpatrick CH: Allergic histories and reactions of patients treated with digoxin immune Fab (Ovine) antibody. *Am J Emerg Med* 9:7, 1991.

Springer M, Olsen KR, Feaster W: Acute massive digoxin overdose: Survival without use of digitalis-specific antibodies. *Am J Emerg Med* 4:364, 1986.

Woolf AD, Wenger TL, Smith TW, Lovejoy FH: The use of digoxin-specific Fab fragments for severe digitalis intoxication in children. *N Engl J Med* 326:1739, 1992.

# 148
# BETA BLOCKERS
## Peter Viccellio
## Mark Henry

## PHARMACOLOGY AND PROPERTIES OF AGENTS

β-blockers frequently are prescribed for hypertension, ischemic heart disease, cardiac arrhythmias, obstructive heart disease, prevention of migraines, control of glaucoma, and other conditions. Within the adrenergic nervous system, α- and β-receptor sites are activated by catecholamines. Stimulation of $\beta_1$-receptors increases the force and rate of myocardial contraction, AV node conduction velocity, and increased renin secretion. Stimulation of $\beta_2$-receptors promotes relaxation of smooth muscle in blood vessels, bronchi, and the gastrointestinal and genitourinary tract. In addition, $\beta_2$ stimulation promotes glycogenolysis from skeletal muscle and glycogenolysis and gluconeogenesis from liver. The β-blockers act as competitive antagonists to catecholamines at β-receptor sites.

Propranolol was the first β-blocker in widespread use, and much of the clinical and overdose experience was gained from case reports and clinical studies of this drug. Propranolol is a nonselective β-blocker, showing equal affinity for both $\beta_1$- and $\beta_2$-receptors. Other nonselective β-blockers include nadolol, timolol, and pindolol. Selective β-blockers ($\beta_1$-antagonists) show a greater relative affinity for $\beta_1$ over $\beta_2$ sites and are less likely to cause bronchospasm or interfere with glucose and glycogen metabolism when administered in low doses. Selective $\beta_1$-blockers include metroprolol, atenolol, esmolol, and acebutolol. Labetalol blocks $\alpha_1$ receptors as well as both $\beta_1$ and $\beta_2$.

Some β-blockers, such as pindolol and acebutolol, also have β-agonist properties. While their agonist property is weaker than the catecholamines, they are capable of stimulating β-receptors, especially when catecholamine levels are low. These agents are said to have intrinsic sympathomimetic activity.

Other properties of importance in interpreting findings and planning therapy in overdose are membrane stabilizing activity and lipid solubility. Propranolol, labetalol, and pindolol are examples of agents which show membrane stabilizing activity or quinidine-like effects in high doses. Lipid solubility, higher in agents like propranolol and low in agents like atenolol and nadolol, may influence the degree of central nervous system effects and utility of hemodialysis in removing the agent in the overdosed patient.

β-blockers can be administered intravenously, orally, and as ophthalmic preparations. Timolol eye drops have caused systemic toxicity and side effects including respiratory arrest, asthma, congestive heart failure, and depression.

## CLINICAL PRESENTATION

β-blockers are absorbed rapidly from the stomach, and the onset of toxicity after oral overdose can occur from 20 min to 1 to 2 h following ingestion. Long-acting preparations may have delayed manifestations.

A patient presenting with bradycardia, AV block, and hypotension should raise consideration of β-blocker toxicity in the differential diagnosis. Sinus bradycardia, first-degree block, widening of the QRS complex, peaked T waves, and ST changes have been reported. Bradycardia, by itself, is not necessarily helpful as a warning sign since slowing of the heart rate and damping of tachycardia in response to stress is seen with therapeutic levels. Tachycardia, while unusual, has been reported with practolol, pindolol, and sotalol. Cardiac output falls, and hypotension results, from both bradycardia and negative inotropy, which in turn jeopardizes myocardial perfusion, creating a downward spiral.

Changes in mental status are common, ranging from delirium to coma. Coma occurs often in the setting of cardiovascular collapse. It may be less pronounced in overdoses of drugs with smaller volumes of distribution (atenolol) or cardioselective agents. Grand mal seizures have been commonly reported.

Bronchospasm is not a common manifestation of overdose, although it can occur. Respiratory arrest has been described. Congestive heart failure and pulmonary edema are more apt to occur in the patient with underlying heart disease.

Hypoglycemic reactions in unstable diabetics are problematic. Nonselective β-blockers can impair the recovery from hypoglycemia, and all β-blockers can prevent tachycardia, an important warning sign of hypoglycemia. In overdose, hypoglycemia is reported in children but rare in adults.

## LABORATORY

An electrocardiogram, cardiac monitoring, blood levels of electrolytes, glucose, and tests for renal and liver function are routine. While it is possible to obtain both qualitative and quantitative levels of β-blocker agents, the turnaround time and the variability of response in individual patients require the clinician to rely on clinical judgment in most cases.

## TREATMENT

### General

Following general toxicologic principles and providing supportive care with careful monitoring is the mainstay of treatment. To remove drugs in the stomach, gastric lavage is preferred over emesis because of the rapid absorption and occasionally precipitous onset of toxicity with these agents. Some recommend that gastric lavage be undertaken after pretreatment with atropine to avoid the potential for increased vagal tone, which may compound the clinical picture. Charcoal administration is recommended, and repeat doses may be of value in management of some agents such as atenolol and nadolol.

### Specific/Antidotal

Therapy is directed at countering the effects of β-blockade. Agents used include atropine, catecholamines, and glucagon. Isoproterenol, a pure β-receptor stimulant, may aggravate hypotension by its vasodilatory effects. Agents with $\beta_1$-selective properties (dobutamine) or combined α- and β-agonist properties (epinephrine, norepinephrine, and dopamine) may be necessary to maintain blood pressure. The optimal doses of these pressors are unknown, but it may be necessary to exceed usual clinical doses in the treatment of overdoses with these agents.

Intravenous glucagon, which enhances myocardial contractility, heart rate, and AV conduction, may be most useful to counteract the bradycardia, conduction defects, and hypotension. It is considered by many to be the drug of choice in the management of these overdoses. The production of intracellular cyclic AMP is reduced with β-blockade. Glucagon stimulates the production of cyclic AMP through nonadrenergic pathways, which probably explains its efficacy. Success has been noted with a bolus dose of 3 to 10 mg or 50 to 150 μg per kg over 1 min, followed by an infusion of 2 to 5 mg/h. An upper dose limit has not been established.

In a recent survey, a total dose of 30 mg of glucagon (an amount possibly needed in the first hour of treatment of a serious beta blocker overdose) was available in 0% of emergency departments surveyed, and in only 26% of hospitals. Obviously, a patient's life may be lost if appropriate intervention cannot be realized.

A pacemaker may be necessary if there is no response to pharmacologic therapy. Fluid replacement to combat hypotension should be administered carefully with arterial pressure and Swan-Ganz monitoring as indicated to help guide therapy. In extremis, prolonged cardiopulmonary resuscitation, balloon pump, and even bypass may be indicated. Resuscitation with discharge from the hospital has followed prolonged efforts at resuscitation.

Seizures can be treated with diazepam and, if necessary, phenytoin and/or phenobarbital. Hypoglycemia should be treated with an infusion of glucose and possibly glucagon. Bronchospasm can be treated with a $\beta_2$-agonist and aminophylline.

Charcoal hemoperfusion and dialysis may be indicated for agents with a small volume of distribution, low protein binding, and high level of urinary excretion. Agents such as atenolol, nadolol, and acebutolol are reported to be dialyzable.

## RANGE OF TOXICITY

The minimum range of toxicity has not been established clearly and depends upon the particular drug, coingestions, and the underlying host.

## DISPOSITION/FOLLOW-UP

Patients with significant ingestions should be admitted to an intensive care unit and observed until all symptoms have resolved completely.

## BIBLIOGRAPHY

Gilman AG, Rall TR, Nies AS, et al: *Goodman and Gilman's The Pharmacological Basis of Therapeutics,* 8th ed. New York, Pergamon, 1990.

Henry M, Kay MM, Viccellio P: Cardiogenic shock associated with calcium-channel and beta blockers: Reversal with intravenous calcium chloride. *Am J Emerg Med* 3:334, 1985.

Lane AS, Woodwad AC, Goldman MR: Massive propranolol overdose poorly responsive to pharmacologic therapy: Use of the intra-aortic balloon pump. *Ann Emerg Med* 16:103, 1987.

Litovitz TL, Holm KC, et al: 1992 Annual Report of the American Association of Poison Control Centers Toxic Exposures Surveillance System. *Am J Emerg Med* 11:494, 1993.

Loove JN, Tandy TK: Beta-adrenoreceptor antagonist toxicity: a survey of glucagon availability.

McVey FK, Corke CF: Extracorporeal circulation in the management of massive propranolol overdose. *Anesthesia* 46:744, 1991.

Viccellio, P: *Handbook of Medical Toxicology.* Little, Brown and Company, 1993.

Weinstein RS: Recognition and management of poisoning with beta-adrenergic blocking agents. *Ann Emerg Med* 13:79, 1984.

# 149
# CALCIUM CHANNEL BLOCKERS
## Louis J. Ling

The three most common calcium channel blockers are verapamil, diltiazem, and nifedipine. In recent years new drugs, such as nicardipine, nimodipine, isradipine, felodipine, and others, have been approved. As the use of this class of drugs has increased therapeutically, the incidence of overdose has also increased. In 1992, the Toxic Exposure Surveillance System of the American Association of Poison Control Centers reported 6683 exposures with 38 deaths,

**Table 149-1.** Calcium Antagonist Pharmacokinetics

| Drug Name | Peak Levels (h) | Protein Binding | Half-life | Chemical Class | Contractility |
|---|---|---|---|---|---|
| Amlodipine | 6–9 | 93 | 30–50 | A | 60–65 |
| Bepridil | 2 | 99 | 24 | E | 60 |
| Diltiazem | 2–4, 6–11(SR) | 70–80 | 3–6, 5–7(SR) | B | 30–60 |
| Felodipine | 2.5–5 | 99 | 11–16 | A | 10–25 |
| Flunarizine | 2–4 | 99 | 18–19 d | C | ? |
| Isradipine | 1.5 | 95 | 8 | A | 15–20 |
| Nicardipine | 0.3–2 | 98–99 | 2–4 | A | 15–43 |
| Nifedipine | 0.3–0.75, 6(XL) | >90 | 2–5 | A | 30–60 |
| Nimodipine | <1 | >95 | 1–2 | A | 13 |
| Nisoldipine | 1–1.5 | >90 | 7–10 | A | 4–8 |
| Nitrendipine | 1–2 | 98 | 12 | A | 10–30 |
| Verapamil | 1–2 | 83–92 | 3–7 | D | 10–22 |

A, dihydropyridine; B, benzothiapine; C, piperazine; D, phenylalkylamine; E, other

SOURCE: (c)1974–95 Micromedex, Inc. All rights reserved. Vol. 85 expires 8/31/95. Revised from Rumack BH, Spoerkle DG (eds): Poisindex Information System. Englewood, CO, Micromedex Inc., edition expires 8/31/95.

making calcium antagonists the leading cause of death from overdose of cardiovascular drugs.

## PHARMACOLOGY

Calcium channel blockers are readily absorbed; however, they are susceptible to a first-pass effect, where the liver metabolizes a large amount of the absorbed drug before releasing it to the systemic circulation. This results in a relatively low bioavailability. There is a large volume of distribution and the amount of the drug in the serum is highly protein bound (Tables 149-1 and 149-2). Because renal excretion is not important for drug elimination, patients with renal failure are not expected to have a decrease in clearance.

## CLINICAL FEATURES

The greatest experience comes in the form of case reports, mostly related to verapamil (Table 149-3). Case reports of nifedipine and diltiazem overdose are relatively rare and there are no reports of overdose with the newer drugs. The toxicity is primarily an extension of the therapeutic effects of decreased calcium influx in myocardium and vascular smooth muscle, which includes decreased conduction through the atrioventricular (AV) node, decreased sinus node discharge, decreased cardiac contractility, and vasodilation with hypotension. The conduction delay is most frequently seen with verapamil and diltiazem, resulting in bradycardia and conduction delay. Bradycardia is the most common finding in verapamil overdose, but first-degree and second-degree intraventricular conduction delay and asystole have all been reported. Conduction delays have been re-

ported to persist up to 36 h after ingestion. Nifedipine as well as many of the newer chemically similar calcium channel blockers are more potent vasodilators and cause concomitant hypotension but have less effect on conduction. Although bradycardia occurs, the hypotension usually results in a reflex tachycardia. Hypotension is often resistant to treatment and can last up to 24 h. Coma and lactic acidosis can result from hypoperfusion and have resulted in anoxic injury. Both improve with correction of hypotension.

Other nonspecific symptoms during overdose include lethargy, slurred speech, nausea, vomiting, coma, and respiratory depression. Nausea and vomiting occur frequently and paralytic ileus has also been reported. Hyperglycemia has been reported after verapamil overdose, but only occasionally requires treatment.

## TOXIC DOSES

In one series of verapamil overdose, ingestions less than 960 mg were always asymptomatic, whereas overdoses of greater than 2 g typically caused major symptoms. The lowest dose of nifedipine was 200 mg before cardiovascular effects were present.

## TREATMENT

Gastric decontamination and general support would be similar as for other overdoses. These treatments include activated charcoal with a cathartic, possibly gastric lavage for serious ingestions soon after ingestion, whole bowel irrigation for sustained-release preparations, and observation. Symptomatic patients should be admitted with cardiac telemetry. With sustained-release verapamil, there have been

**Table 149-2.** Calcium Antagonist Pharmacology

| Drug Name | Refractory Period AV Node | Automaticity SA Node | AV Node Conduction | Heart Rate | Contractility | Cardiac Output | Peripheral Vascular Resistance |
|---|---|---|---|---|---|---|---|
| Amlodipine | 0 | 0 | 0 | +1 | 0 | +2 | −3 |
| Bepridil | +3 | −3 | −2 | −2 | −2 | 0 | 0 |
| Diltiazem | 0 | −2 | −2 | −1 | −1 | +1 | 0 |
| Felodipine | 0 | 0 | 0 | +1 | 0 | +2 | −3 |
| Flunarizine | 0 | 0 | 0 | −1 | −1 | 0 | 0 |
| Isradipine | 0 | 0 | 0 | +1 | 0 | +2 | −3 |
| Nicardipine | +/− | 0/− | 0 | +1 | 0 | +2 | −3 |
| Nifedipine | 0 | 0 | 0 | +1 | 0 | +2 | −3 |
| Nimodipine | 0 | 0/− | 0 | 0 | 0 | 0 | 0 |
| Nisoldipine | 0 | 0 | 0 | +1 | 0 | +2 | −3 |
| Nitrendipine | 0 | 0 | 0 | +1 | 0 | +2 | −3 |
| Verapamil | +2 | −3 | −3 | 0 | −3 | 0 | −3 |

0, no effect; +, positive effect; −, negative effect

SOURCE: (c)1974–94 Micromedex, Inc. All rights reserved. Vol. 80 expires 5/31/94. From Rumack BH, Spoerke DG (eds): Poisindex Information System. Englewood, CO, Micromedex Inc. Vol. 80 expires 5/31/94.

**Table 149-3.** Summary of Toxic Effects

| Effect | No. of Patients | | |
|--------|:---:|:---:|:---:|
| | **Verapamil** | **Nifedipine** | **Diltiazem** |
| **Hypotension** | | | |
| Blood pressure <100 mm Hg | 20 | 9 | 11 |
| Blood pressure <60 mm Hg | 7 | 0 | 2 |
| Blood pressure subtotal (%) | 27 (53) | 9 (32) | 13 (38) |
| **Sinoatrial Node Depression** | | | |
| Heart rate <60 | 9 | 4 | 7 |
| Heart rate <40 | 6 | 0 | 3 |
| Sinoatrial node subtotal (%) | 15 (29) | 4 (14) | 10 (29) |
| **Atrioventricular Node Depression** | | | |
| One atrioventricular block | 14 | 1 | 4 |
| Two atrioventricular blocks | 7 | 1 | 2 |
| Three atrioventricular blocks | 5 | 0 | 0 |
| Unspecified | 2 | 3 | 4 |
| Atrioventricular node subtotal (%) | 28 (55) | 5 (18) | 10 (29) |
| **Dysrhythmias** | | | |
| Sinus tachycardia | 12 | 16 | 9 |
| Atrial arrhythmia | 2 | 0 | 1 |
| Junctional rhythm | 9 | 0 | 3 |
| Premature ventricular contractions | 6 | 0 | 2 |
| Dysrhythmia subtotal (%) | 29 (57) | 16 (57) | 15 (44) |
| **Total** | 51 | 28 | 34 |

SOURCE: Ramoska EA, Spiller HA, Winter M, Borys D. *Ann Emerg Med* 22:196, 1993. Used with permission.

cases of second-degree and even third-degree AV block which occurred more than 15 h after ingestion. Therefore, asymptomatic patients after overdose of sustained-release preparations may also need to be admitted for cardiac telemetry. Although there is no accepted protocol, calcium chloride is typically given as 10 to 20 mL of 10% calcium gluconate (4.6 mEq Ca or 93 mg Ca) or 10% calcium chloride (272 mg Ca or 13.6 mEq Ca) in 100 mL 5% dextrose in water over 15 min. In many cases, calcium infusion has not resulted in clinical improvement. A therapeutic trial of intravenous calcium is probably worthwhile. Although calcium chloride contains three times more calcium than calcium gluconate, the calcium chloride may be a disadvantage in prolonging acidosis in patients with metabolic acidosis.

Sinus bradycardia and AV block should be treated if the patient is symptomatic. There has been widespread use of many treatments, including atropine, isoproterenol, and transvenous and transcutaneous pacing. Although each of these has variable success, larger than usual drug doses may be necessary for a response. Intravenous calcium administration would not be expected to improve the rate, but clinical response has been reported in some patients. Junctional, idioventricular, and third-degree block have all been treated with ventricular pacing.

Hypotension should be treated with fluid administration and pressors. Dopamine and norepinephrine have been used and a case of successful treatment with amrinone with isoproterenol has been reported. Again, higher than usual doses may be necessary. Intravenous calcium chloride may reverse myocardia depression and correct hypotension. Although hypotension may be resistant, intravenous calcium chloride should be given and repeated as necessary. Glucagon increases cyclic adenosine monophosphate levels and has been reported to reverse myocardial depression in animals and in isolated case reports in human beings. It should be tried if there is no response to calcium. The dose is 2 to 10 mg intravenously. A pulmonary artery catheter has been used in many patients to guide therapy, especially when the hypotension is resistant to therapy and requires high doses of medications and large volumes of fluid.

Verapamil has been shown to inhibit the release of insulin, and hyperglycemia is common after verapamil overdose. Serum glucose has been reported as high as 832 mg/dL, but increased extracellular calcium decreases this effect. Therefore, blood glucose becomes normal in most patients with calcium only or without other specific treatment within 24 h. Occasionally, intravenous insulin infusion has been used.

Aminopyridine is not yet available in the United States, but it shows promise as an antidote by increasing calcium flux and has been reported to be beneficial when other treatment options have failed.

Because of the hepatic metabolism, high protein binding, and large volume of distribution, hemodialysis and hemoperfusion would not be expected to be beneficial. In one case, hemoperfusion resulted in clinical improvement after an overdose of diltiazem.

## BIBLIOGRAPHY

Clark RF, Hanna TC. Calcium channel blocker toxicity. *Topics in Emergency Medicine* 15:15, 1993.

Erickson FC, Ling LJ, Grande QA, Anderson DL. Diltiazem overdose: case report and review. *J Emerg Med* 9:357, 1991.

Goenen M, Col J, Compere A, Bonte J. Treatment of severe verapamil poisoning with combined amrinone-isoproterenol therapy. *Am J Cardiol* 58:1142, 1986.

Pearigen PD, Benowitz NL. Poisoning due to calcium antagonists. *Drug Saf* 6:408, 1991.

Ramoska EA, Spiller HA, Meyers A. Calcium channel blocker toxicity. *Ann Emerg Med* 19:649, 1990.

Ramoska EA, Spiller HA, Winter M, Borys D. A one-year evaluation of calcium channel blocker overdoses: toxicity and treatment. *Ann Emerg Med* 22:196, 1993.

Spiller HA, Meyers A, Ziemba T, Riley M. Delayed onset of cardiac arrhythmias from sustained release verapamil. *Ann Emerg Med* 20:201, 1991.

Walter FG, Frye G, Mullen JT, Ekins BR, Khaasigian PA. Amelioration of nifedipine poisoning associated with glucagon therapy. *Ann Emerg Med* 22:1234, 1993.

Young GP. Calcium channel blockers in emergency medicine. *Ann Emerg Med* 13:712, 1984.

# 150
# CLONIDINE

## E. Martin Caravati

## INTRODUCTION

Clonidine hydrochloride, a synthetic imidazoline derivative, was initially investigated as an α-adrenergic agonist for use as a nasal decongestant. It was discovered to have a potent blood pressure lowering effect and is now commonly used as an antihypertensive agent. Clonidine has also been used to ameliorate withdrawal symptoms from opiates, nicotine, and alcohol. It is of particular interest because of a recent increase in therapeutic usage; the manifestations of toxicity, which resemble those in cases of opiate overdose; and controversy regarding an antidote for clonidine poisoning.

## PHARMACOLOGY AND PATHOPHYSIOLOGY

### Formulations

Clonidine is available in 0.1-, 0.2-, and 0.3-mg tablets, alone (Catapres) or in combination with chlorthalidone (Combipres). Also available are transdermal patches (Catapres-TTS), which supply 0.1-, 0.2-, or 0.3-mg/day for 7 days. These patches contain 2.5, 5.0, and 7.5 mg total drug, respectively, and the amount of active drug remaining in a patch after 7 days of use has been reported as high as 75 percent of the total content. Therefore, the patch designed to deliver only 0.1 mg/day of clonidine may still contain up to 1.9 mg of active drug after it has been used and discarded.

## Pharmacokinetics

Clonidine is rapidly and almost completely absorbed from the gastrointestinal tract. Antihypertensive effects are noted within 30 to 60 min and peak between 2 and 4 h after ingestion. It is lipid-soluble and 20 to 40 percent protein-bound in the plasma. It has a large volume of distribution (3 to 6 L/kg). The serum half-life is approximately 12 h, with a range of 6 to 24 h. Approximately 50 percent of a therapeutic dose is excreted unchanged in the urine while the remainder is metabolized in the liver; none of the metabolites are pharmacologically active.

## Mechanism of Action

The mechanism by which clonidine lowers blood pressure is not fully understood. The primary site of action appears to be in the medulla oblongata where it is a presynaptic $\alpha_2$-adrenergic agonist. This results in decreased sympathetic outflow from the central nervous system with a subsequent decrease in heart rate, cardiac output, and peripheral vascular resistance. At high doses, it may act as a peripheral $\alpha$ adrenoreceptor agonist at vascular smooth-muscle sites and cause vasoconstriction.

Clonidine also depresses the central nervous system as reflected by decreased levels of norepinephrine and metabolites in the cerebrospinal fluid after a therapeutic dose.

## Toxic Dose

The minimum toxic dose of clonidine has not been established. Significant toxicity has been reported in a 24-month-old child (11 kg) who ingested a single 0.1-mg tablet, and in a 9-month-old boy (11 kg) found sucking on a used transdermal patch. Adults have survived ingestions of up to 100 mg. The amount ingested does not always correlate with the severity of symptoms. There has been only one reported fatality from clonidine overdose: a 37-year-old who ingested an unknown amount and suffered a cardiac arrest shortly after administration of tolazoline.

Clonidine does not appear to be teratogenic in animals, and no human congenital defects have been associated with its use. It has been administered therapeutically in the second and third trimesters of pregnancy without adverse fetal effects.

## CLINICAL FEATURES

Manifestations of acute toxicity vary and reflect both the central and peripheral effects of the drug. Symptoms are usually present within 2 h of ingestion and recovery is generally complete within 72 h.

Infants and children are particularly sensitive to the drug and may manifest toxicity after ingestion of a single tablet. In a report of 42 pediatric ingestions by Wiley, 76 percent of patients had symptoms within 1 h and 100 percent within 4 h. None of these patients demonstrated clinical deterioration more than 4 h after presentation. Therefore, if a patient is asymptomatic 4 h after ingestion, it is unlikely that significant toxicity will occur. Renal insufficiency may predispose a patient to delayed or prolonged toxic effects, however.

The common signs and symptoms of clonidine poisoning are illustrated in Table 150-1. After clonidine poisoning, children tend to have a higher incidence of hypothermia and respiratory depression, particularly recurrent apnea, than adults. Hypertension may be present initially due to the peripheral $\alpha$-adrenergic agonist effect of clonidine in high doses. It is usually transient and may be followed by significant hypotension. The effects of clonidine are additive with the CNS depressant effects of other sedative-hypnotics. Irritability, pallor, my-driasis, seizures, atrioventricular block (first-, second-, and third degree), extensor plantar reflex, and diarrhea have also been reported.

**Table 150-1.** Common Signs and Symptoms of Clonidine Poisoning

| Central nervous system | Cardiovascular |
|---|---|
| Lethargy or coma | Sinus bradycardia |
| Respiratory depression | Hypotension |
| Apnea | Hypertension |
| Miosis | Other |
| Hyporeflexia | Hypothermia |
| Hypotonia | Pallor |

Toxicity may mimic narcotic overdose with the classic triad of coma, miosis, and respiratory depression. Other agents which may cause a clinical presentation similar to clonidine include β-blocking drugs (bradycardia, hypotension, coma), phenobarbital and chloral hydrate (miosis, coma, respiratory depression), phenothiazines (miosis, coma, hypotension), and pesticides (miosis, coma, bradycardia).

## LABORATORY

No laboratory tests are specific for clonidine poisoning. It can be measured in the plasma by high-pressure liquid chromatography (HPLC). Clonidine is not detected by usual hospital toxicology screening methods, but toxicology screening may help by detecting coingestants or excluding other possible agents responsible for the clinical presentation.

An ECG may reveal sinus bradycardia or heart block. An arterial blood gas can help in assessing the patient's oxygenation and ventilatory status.

## TREATMENT

**Stabilization.** All patients suspected of clonidine overdose should have intravenous access established and continuous respiratory and cardiac monitoring for at least 4 h. Symptomatic patients should be admitted and observed for at least 12 h. The patient's vital signs, mental status, and pupil size should be checked frequently. An adequate airway and ventilation must be maintained.

**Decontamination.** After the patient has been stabilized, measures to decontaminate the gut should be initiated. Gastric emptying may be of benefit in cases of recent ingestion (within 1 h) consisting of more than one or two tablets. Gastric lavage with a large-bore orogastric tube is the procedure of choice. Because of the possibility of rapid deterioration in the patient's mental status and subsequent inability to protect the airway when vomiting, it is inadvisable to use ipecac to induce emesis. Activated charcoal probably binds clonidine and should be administered to all patients after gastric lavage.

**Elimination Enhancement.** Forced diuresis is not recommended. It does not hasten renal elimination of clonidine and may complicate management of the patient's hemodynamic status. Urinary pH manipulation, dialysis, and hemoperfusion are unlikely to add any benefit to supportive care.

**Supportive Care.** The mainstay of treatment for clonidine toxicity is supportive care. Respiratory compromise may require endotrantubation and assisted ventilation. Apnea in the child should be closely monitored. It usually responds to tactile stimulation, but if it is recurrent, elective intubation should be considered. Hypothermia is generally mild and resolves with passive rewarming. Bradycardia should be treated only in association with hemodynamic compromise and is responsive to standard doses of atropine. Hypertension is usually transient, and aggressive treatment should be undertaken only when end-organ damage is evident. An appropriate agent is sodium nitroprusside, which is short-acting and easily titratable. The hypotensive patient often responds to being placed in the Trendelenburg position and given a bolus of intravenous fluids. Dopamine is indicated for hypotension not alleviated by volume expansion. Seizures, a rare complication, respond to diazepam and phenytoin, but potential underlying causes such as hypoxia or hypoglycemia must be excluded.

**Antidotes.** Although there are no proven antidotes for clonidine poisoning, agents purported to have antagonistic effects on clonidine toxicity include naloxone, tolazoline, yohimbine, and idazoxan.

Since clonidine overdose has manifestations similar to opiate intoxication, naloxone has been recommended as a potential antidote. There are conflicting reports as to its efficacy in reversing the cardiovascular and opioid effects of clonidine. There is no evidence for a consistent or predictable clinical response and naloxone cannot be relied upon to replace supportive care. It is possible, however, that there exists a subset of patients in whom naloxone is beneficial. Naloxone should be administered to patients with significant symptoms in order to reverse potential narcotic toxicity and possibly alleviate some signs of clonidine toxicity. The dose is that used for narcotic overdose, 2–4 mg IV in adults and 0.01 mg/kg IV in children. No complications of naloxone therapy for adult clonidine toxicity have been reported, but hypertension has been reported as a complication of naloxone treatment in a few children.

Tolazoline is a relatively nonselective $\alpha$-adrenoreceptor blocker. Two case reports have suggested that it reverses the cardiovascular toxicity of clonidine, but in the majority of reported cases it had no effect. Significant complications such as seizures, hypotension, gastrointestinal hemorrhage, and death have been reported with its use in other settings. In addition, the only reported fatality from clonidine overdose occurred shortly after the administration of tolazoline. It is not recommended as an antidote for clonidine toxicity.

Yohimbine, a selective $\alpha$-adrenoreceptor blocker, readily penetrates the CNS and causes an increase in blood pressure, heart rate, and motor activity. It is available in tablet form only and has not been specifically studied as an antidote. Idazoxan, also a specific $\alpha_2$-adrenoreceptor antagonist, has been shown to reverse clonidine-induced miosis in healthy adults. It is currently an investigational drug.

## CLONIDINE WITHDRAWAL SYNDROME

Abrupt cessation of chronic clonidine therapy may result in symptoms of adrenergic hyperactivity as early as 12 h after the last dose. The symptoms last approximately 5 to 7 days and consist of anxiety, diaphoresis, headache, nausea and abdominal pain, tachycardia, and hypertension. Ventricular arrhythmias, hypertensive encephalopathy, and death have been reported. Tapering the dose of clonidine over 3 to 5 days usually prevents development of withdrawal symptoms. The syndrome is most effectively treated by restarting the clonidine. Severe hypertension may require nitroprusside therapy. Theoretically, treatment with $\beta$ blockers alone may exacerbate rebound hypertension due to unopposed $\alpha$-adrenergic stimulation. Clonidine withdrawal has not been reported after an acute overdose.

## BIBLIOGRAPHY

Bamshad MJ, Wasserman GS: Pediatric clonidine intoxications. *Vet Hum Toxicol* 30:220, 1990.

Banner W Jr, Lund ME, Clawson L: Failure of naloxone to reverse clonidine toxic effect. *Am J Dis Child* 137:1170, 1983.

Caravati EM, Bennett DL: Clonidine transdermal patch poisoning. *Ann Emerg Med* 17:175, 1988.

Gremse DA, Artman M, Boerth RC: Hypertension associated with naloxone treatment for clonidine poisoning. *J Pediatr* 108: 776, 1986.

Wiley JF, Wiley CC, Torrey SB, et al: Clonidine poisoning in young children. *J Pediatr* 116:654, 1990.

# 151
# PHENYTOIN TOXICITY
## Harold H. Osborn

## INTRODUCTION

It is estimated that over 2 million Americans suffer from epilepsy, while as many as 10 percent of the population may suffer at least one seizure in their lifetime. Phenytoin is a primary anticonvulsant for all types of epilepsy except absence. It is useful in the treatment of status epilepticus in conjunction with other more rapidly acting anticonvulsants. Phenytoin has been used prophylactically in a variety of settings (head trauma, alcohol withdrawal, drug overdose), but has so far only proven useful in the setting of head trauma. Phenytoin is probably the most widely used anticonvulsant in the world and has been more thoroughly studied and evaluated than any other.

Phenytoin has been employed in the management of chronic pain syndromes. Historically, it has also been used as an antidysrhythmic agent, especially in the setting of digoxin toxicity, but it is no longer considered a first-line agent.

Death or severe morbidity is unusual following intentional phenytoin overdose, and an intact outcome is typical if good supportive care is provided. Most phenytoin-related deaths have been caused by rapid intravenous administration or hypersensitivity reactions. The acute life- and limb-threatening manifestations of phenytoin intoxication may be readily treated using conventional therapies immediately available to any acute care facility and can be prevented by adhering to the correct methods of administration.

## MECHANISM OF ACTION

Phenytoin exerts its anticonvulsant effect by blocking voltage-sensitive sodium channels in the neurons. Phenytoin stabilizes sodium channels in an inactive state, and this inhibitory effect, similar to the action of local anesthetics, is dependent on the voltage and frequency of firing of the neuron. Phenytoin has no effect on the amplitude or duration of the action potential. Rather, it limits the ability of the neuron to fire trains of action potentials at high frequency by delaying recovery. In this fashion it suppresses repetitive neuronal activity and prevents the spread of a seizure focus. At higher concentrations, phenytoin delays activation of outward potassium currents in nerves and prolongs the neuronal refractory period. It may also exert its anticonvulsant effect by influencing calcium channels or $\gamma$-aminobutyric acid (GABA) receptors, although this is not yet fully established.

## PATHOPHYSIOLOGY

The toxic effects of phenytoin depend on the route of administration, the duration of exposure, and the dosage used. Of these determinants of toxicity, the most important is the route of administration. The intravenous administration of phenytoin carries the greatest risk, primarily due to the other constituents of the parenteral vehicle (see "Effects of Propylene Glycol and Ethanol Dilvents," below). The most serious reactions following intravenous administration are cardiovascular (bradycardia, hypotension, asystole), although tissue necrosis and sloughing following extravasation have been described. Major cardiac toxicity only occurs following parenteral administration. It is more common in the elderly and those with underlying cardiac disease, but has been described in young healthy patients as well.

Many of the side effects of the oral preparation are dose-related and are predictable at higher plasma concentrations. Early toxicity is manifested by vestibular/ocular/cerebellar signs: nystagmus, dysdiadochokinesia, and ataxia. At higher levels, central nervous system (CNS) depression and other cognitive effects (confusion, dizziness, loss of concentration and memory) are seen. Only two areas of the brain normally exhibit spontaneous neuronal burst discharge: the hippocampus and the cerebellum. Phenytoin's ability to suppress these areas may result in impaired memory and balance, respectively. Paradoxically, very high levels of phenytoin may be associated with seizures. Acute oral overdose is usually manifested by nystagmus, nausea and vomiting, ataxia, and CNS depression. Deaths from oral ingestion of phenytoin are extremely rare.

The chronic administration of phenytoin is associated with numerous side effects that involve a variety of organ systems. Many of these are dose- and duration-dependent but some are idiosyncratic. Hypersensitivity reactions to phenytoin usually occur early (in the first few months of therapy) and include fever, skin rashes, blood dyscrasias, and, rarely, hepatitis. Deaths due to Stevens-Johnson syndrome have occurred and anyone exhibiting this syndrome should never receive phenytoin again.

## PHARMACOKINETICS

Phenytoin is a weak acid with a $pK_a$ of 8.3. Thus, in the acid milieu of the stomach, and even at physiologic pH, its aqueous solubility is limited. The parenteral form is adjusted to a pH of 12 to keep the drug in solution, but it is very irritating to the tissues. Intramuscular injection results in local precipitation of phenytoin with erratic absorption and is, therefore, not recommended. Absorption after oral ingestion is slow, variable, and often incomplete, especially following an overdose. Significant differences in bioavailability exist among different phenytoin preparations. Peak levels typically occur anywhere from 3 to 12 h after a single dose. Despite these limitations, single-dose oral loading with phenytoin has proven to be a safe and effective alternative to parenteral loading for many patients.

Following absorption, phenytoin is distributed throughout the body with a volume of distribution of 0.6 L/kg. Brain tissue concentrations equal those in plasma within about 10 min of intravenous infusion and correlate with therapeutic effects, while cerebrospinal fluid and myocardium equilibrate within 30 to 60 min. This slower distribution into tissue is further evidence that hypotension and arrhythmias occurring during phenytoin infusion are due to toxicity from propylene glycol, the most widely used diluent. At steady state, concentrations are higher in neural tissue than in the serum. Within the CNS, concentrations are higher in the brainstem and cerebellum that the cerebral cortex.

### Protein Binding and Free Phenytoin Fractions

Phenytoin is extensively (90 percent) bound to plasma proteins, especially albumin. The free, unbound form is the biologically active moiety responsible for the drug's clinical effect and toxicity. The free phenytoin fraction normally constitutes 10 percent of the plasma level. The unbound fraction of the drug is greater in the following groups of patients: neonates; the elderly; pregnant women; patients with uremia, hypoalbuminemia (cirrhosis, nephrosis, malnutrition, burns, trauma, cystic fibrosis), and hyperbilirubinemia; and in those taking drugs that displace phenytoin from binding sites (salicylates, valproate, phenylbutazone, tolbutamide, and sulfisoxazole).

Although patients with decreased protein binding may have higher levels of free phenytoin and a greater biological effect, they may have lower levels of total phenytoin since more of the drug is available for metabolism. These patients may become toxic with total phenytoin levels in the therapeutic range. Patients who exhibit toxic signs in the therapeutic range and those with decreased protein binding should have their free phenytoin levels measured. Recently, salivary levels of anticonvulsants have been found to correlate with the free fraction of drug in the plasma.

### Metabolism

Following absorption and distribution, only 4 to 5 percent of phenytoin is excreted unchanged in the urine. The remainder is metabolized by hepatic microsomal enzymes. The drug is primarily hydroxylated to a series of inactive compounds.

The major (60 to 70 percent) metabolite is the parahydroxyphenyl derivative. It is glucuronidated, secreted in the bile, reabsorbed, and subsequently excreted in the urine. Phenytoin removal from the body is not appreciably influenced by hemodialysis or hemoperfusion.

Unlike the other anticonvulsant agents, the metabolism of phenytoin is "capacity-limited" (dose-dependent). At plasma concentrations below 10 µg/mL, elimination is first order (a fixed percentage of drug metabolized per unit of time). However, at higher concentrations of phenytoin, including those in the therapeutic range (10 to 20 µg/mL), the metabolic pathways may become saturated, and the elimination may change to zero-order kinetics (a fixed amount metabolized per unit of time). This change in kinetics can markedly prolong the half-life of phenytoin, which is normally 6 to 24 h. An understanding of capacity-limited kinetics is essential to the proper dosing of phenytoin, the avoidance of side effects with chronic therapy, and the management of overdoses. At higher levels in the therapeutic range, any increase in the daily dose will result in a disproportionate increase in the plasma level. Thus, at phenytoin doses above 300 mg (~5 mg/kg) per day, incremental doses should be limited to 30 mg. After each increase in dose, the patient should be maintained on the new dose for at least 2 weeks and the plasma level should be reassessed before any further increase.

Because phenytoin's half-life is 24 h or less, once-a-day regimens may result in erratic levels and become problematic for patients requiring tight control. However, one phenytoin preparation (Phenytoin Kapseals) has a delayed absorption and is the only preparation approved by the Food and Drug Administration (FDA) for once-a-day use. A once-a-day regimen is advisable since this facilitates compliance. Concomitant use of drugs that either inhibit or enhance hepatic microsomal activity may result in an increase or decrease of phenytoin level respectively. Phenytoin also affects the metabolism of various other agents (see Table 151-1).

**Table 151-1.** Phenytoin-Drug Interactions

| | |
|---|---|
| Phenytoin *increases* serum level of: | |
| Acetaminophen | |
| Oral anticoagulants | |
| Primidone | |
| Phenytoin *decreases* serum level of | |
| Amiodarone | Disopyramide |
| Carbamazepine | Mexiletine |
| Levodopa | Doxycycline |
| Methadone | Furosemide |
| Contraceptives | Quinidine |
| Glucocorticoids | Theophylline |
| Cyclosporine | Valproic acid |
| Phenytoin levels are *increased* by: | |
| Amiodarone | Fluconazole |
| Oral anticoagulants | Phenylbutazone* |
| Chloramphenicol | Sulfonamides* |
| Isoniazid | Valproic acid* |
| Cimetidine | High-dose salicylate* |
| Disulfiram | Tolbutamide* |
| Trimethoprim | |
| Phenytoin levels are *decreased* by: | |
| Antineoplastic drugs | Theophylline |
| Diazoxide | Phenobarbital |
| Folic acid | Diazepam |
| Rifampin | Ethanol |
| Sucralfate | Calcium |

* These drugs displace phenytoin from its protein-binding sites, thus increasing the free phenytoin fraction, although the total phenytoin level may *decrease.*

**Table 151-2.** Correlation of Plasma Phenytoin Level and Side Effects

| Plasma level, µg/mL | Side Effects |
| --- | --- |
| <10 | Usually none |
| 10–20 | Occasional mild nystagmus |
| 20–30 | Nystagmus |
| 30–40 | Ataxia, slurred speech, nausea and vomiting |
| 40–50 | Lethargy, confusion, |
| >50 | coma, seizures |

## Effects of Propylene Glycol and Ethanol Diluents

The acute cardiovascular toxicity seen with intravenous phenytoin infusion has frequently been ascribed to its diluent. The vehicle for the most widely used parenteral formulation of phenytoin (Dilantin) is 40% propylene glycol and 10% ethanol, adjusted to a pH of 12 with sodium hydroxide. The glycol component has been shown to cause coma, seizures, circulatory collapse, ventricular arrhythmias, cardiac nodal depression, and hypotension in humans and animals. Propylene glycol is a strong myocardial depressant and vasodilator and increases vagal tone. Other toxic effects of propylene glycol include hyperosmolality, hemolysis, and lactate-associated metabolic acidosis. Louis et al. compared the acute toxicities of intravenous phenytoin and propylene glycol both alone and in combination. In a feline model, phenytoin alone did not cause significant cardiovascular effects, and instead partially reversed the toxic effects that occurred when propylene glycol was given. Acute toxic effects of propylene glycol are also strongly related to rate of infusion. This is further evidence for its etiologic role in intravenous phenytoin toxicity, a phenomenon which is almost always related to infusion rate. The ethanol intravenous diluent fraction may precipitate a reaction in patients taking disulfiram.

The limitations of the parenteral form of phenytoin (incomplete aqueous solubility, irritating nature of the vehicle, and tendency to precipitate in intravenous solutions) have prompted a search for a more suitable preparation. Recently, prodrugs of phenytoin have been synthesized that are more soluble and less irritating to the tissues. These agents are presently being field tested and may become standard in the future.

## SERUM LEVELS AND RANGE OF TOXICITY

Therapeutic phenytoin levels are described as being 10 to 20 µg/mL (40 to 80 µmol/L)[1] with a free phenytoin level of 1 to 2 µg/mL. Although 50 percent of seizure patients achieve reduction of seizure frequency with amounts below these levels, some patients require levels above 20 µg/mL for adequate seizure control.

The therapeutic range for phenytoin is rather narrow. However, some patients have a greater propensity to side effects than others. Individual variation in toxicity is a function of baseline neurologic status, individual response to the drug, and free drug fraction. Patients with underlying brain disease are predisposed to toxicity and may become toxic at much lower levels than usual. Long-term therapy must be individualized and based on the following parameters: clinical response, drug levels, and signs of toxicity. In general, toxicity correlates fairly well with increasing plasma levels (see Table 151-2). Nystagmus usually appears first at phenytoin levels of 20 µg/mL but may occur at lower levels or not appear until much higher levels are attained. Ataxia usually begins at about 30 µg/mL, and lethargy at 40 µg/mL. Altered mental status and other motor signs may occur at levels below 20 µg/mL and are not necessarily preceded by nystagmus. Conversely, some patients may tolerate levels above 40 µg/mL and only demonstrate mild impairment on neuropsychologic testing. Al-

most all patients with phenytoin-induced seizures will have levels well above 30 µg/mL. Signs of toxicity occur at free phenytoin levels of 2.0 µg/mL and are consistently severe above 5.0 µg/mL.

## CLINICAL PRESENTATIONS

### Central Nervous System Toxicity

As toxic phenytoin levels are reached, both inhibitory cortical and excitatory cerebellar-vestibular effects begin to occur. The usual initial sign of toxicity is nystagmus, which is seen first on forced lateral gaze and then becomes spontaneous. Vertical, bidirectional, or alternating nystagmus may occur with severe intoxication.

Decreased level of consciousness is routine, with initial sedation, lethargy, ataxic gait, and dysarthria progressing to confusion, coma, and even apnea in large overdose. Chronically impaired cognitive function or acute encephalopathy may occur without other common signs of ataxia and nystagmus. This is usually seen at toxic levels but again may occur in the therapeutic range. Nystagmus will commonly disappear at levels sufficient to cause coma (above 35 to 55 µg/mL), and complete ophthalmoplegia and loss of corneal reflexes may occur. Therefore, absence of nystagmus does not exclude severe phenytoin toxicity. Nystagmus then returns as serum drug levels decrease and coma lightens.

Phenytoin-induced seizures are usually brief, and are usually generalized. They are quite rare and almost always preceded by other signs of toxicity, especially in acute overdose.

Cerebellar stimulation and alteration in dopaminergic and serotonergic activity may be responsible for acute dystonias and movement disorders seen in overdose, including opisthotonos and choreoathetosis. Either depressed or hyperactive deep tendon reflexes, clonus, and extensor toe responses may also be elicited. Some signs of neurologic toxicity may outlast the presence of drug by months, especially mild peripheral neuropathy or acute reversible cerebellar degeneration with ataxia.

Psychosis, toxic delirium, visual and auditory hallucinations, euphoria, irritability, agitation, and combativeness have all been reported with toxicity.

### Cardiovascular Toxicity

Significant cardiac toxicity after oral phenytoin overdose in an otherwise healthy patient has never been reported and, if observed, should mandate a rapid assessment for other causes (e.g., hypoxia, other drugs). Cardiovascular complications have been almost entirely limited to cases of intravenous administration. These include hypotension with decreased peripheral vascular resistance, bradycardia, conduction delays progressing to complete AV nodal block, ventricular tachycardia, primary ventricular fibrillation, and asystole. Electrocardiographic changes include increased PR interval, widened QRS interval, and altered S-T and T-wave segments. Bradycardia, hypotension, and syncope in healthy volunteers have been reported even after small intravenous doses. Slowly administered (<25 mg/min) intravenous phenytoin has also been reported to cause precipitous, refractory hypotension and cardiac arrest in critically ill patients receiving dopamine infusions to support blood pressure. Most of these complications can be attributed to rapid intravenous administration of the propylene glycol diluent fraction and are avoidable with cautious administration (see Table 151-3).

### Vascular, Extravasation, and Soft Tissue Toxicity

An important but infrequently considered toxic effect is local vascular and tissue injury after injection. Although still recommended by the manufacturer, intramuscular injection results in localized crystallization of the drug, with erratic and unpredictable absorption, hematomas, sterile abscess, and myonecrosis at the injection site. Complications after intravenous infusion have included skin and soft tissue

[1] Multiply traditional units of µg/mL or mg/L by 3.964 to convert to SI units µmol/L.

**Table 151-3.** Guidelines for Safe Phenytoin Loading

Intravenous
  Loading dose is 18 mg/kg
  Mix total dose in 75–100 mL of normal saline
  Administer through a milipore filter using an infusion pump
  Rate of administration should not exceed 30 mg/min (less in patients with
    cardiovascular disease)
  Monitor the blood pressure and cardiac rhythm continually during the
    infusion
  In the event of complications, immediately stop the infusion and administer
    isotonic crystalloid and other treatment as indicated
Oral*
  Loading dose is 20 mg/kg
  Phenytoin tablets or suspension may be used
  Patient must be conscious with an intact gag reflex and not actively seizing
    or vomiting
  Administer the total amount in one dose
  Check phenytoin level 6–8 h after administration

* Unlike IV loading, not all patients orally loaded will reach a therapeutic
level.

necrosis requiring skin grafting, compartment syndrome, gangrene, amputation, and death (at a fatality rate exceeding that from oral overdose). A syndrome of delayed bluish discoloration of the affected extremity, followed by erythema, edema, vesicles, bullae, and local tissue ischemia, has also been described. This has been reported after intravenous push administration of undiluted phenytoin *even in the absence of extravasation,* and has eventually necessitated amputation in some cases. The propylene glycol diluent, strong alkalinity of the intravenous solution, and crystallization of the drug contribute.

### Hypersensitivity Reactions

Hypersensitivity reactions usually occur within 1 to 6 weeks of beginning phenytoin therapy and can include fever, systemic lupus erythematosus, erythma multiforme, toxic epidermal necrolysis, Stevens-Johnson syndrome, hepatitis, rhabdomyolysis, acute interstitial pneumonitis, lymphadenopathy, leukopenia, disseminated intravascular coagulation, and renal failure. An erythematous morbilliform rash is common after initiation of phenytoin, occurring more frequently in the summer. One should always ask about a history of previous hypersensitivity reactions before making the decision to restart phenytoin in the emergency department setting.

### MISCELLANEOUS EFFECTS

Other side effects from phenytoin include gingival hyperplasia, hirsutism, hypocalcemia, osteomalacia, megaloblastic anemia responsive to folate administration, lymphoma, and hemorrhagic disease of the newborn responsive to vitamin K (see Table 151-4). Gingival hyperplasia is so common that its absence should suggest poor compliance.

Another clinically significant effect in some is hyperglycemia, felt to be secondary to inhibition of insulin release. This can lead to diabetic ketoacidosis or nonketotic hyperosmolar coma. The teratogenic fetal hydantoin syndrome is well described, so oral phenytoin therapy in a pregnant patient should never be initiated or continued by the emergency physician without consultation and close follow-up from the attending neurologist and obstetrician.

### DIFFERENTIAL DIAGNOSIS

Intoxication with almost any CNS-active or sedative-hypnotic drug may mimic early phenytoin intoxication, especially ethanol, carbamazepine, benzodiazepines, barbiturates, and lithium. Disease states resembling phenytoin toxicity include hypoglycemia, Wernicke encephalopathy, and posterior fossa hemorrhage or tumor. Although seizures may be caused by phenytoin at toxic levels, other epileptogenic drug overdoses and seizures due to withdrawal from ethanol or other sedative-hypnotics must be considered in adults.

## LABORATORY DIAGNOSIS AND ANCILLARY STUDIES

In oral overdose, the prolonged absorption phase mandates serial assessment to determine peak serum phenytoin levels. Phenytoin concentrations are most commonly measured by an enzyme-mediated immunoassay (EMIT) technique, which is specific and sensitive to $\leq 1$ $\mu g/mL$. If available, free phenytoin concentrations are more useful to predict toxicity. Corrected serum phenytoin levels can be calculated in hypoproteinemia patients with a known serum albumin level. To calculate the phenytoin concentration ($C_{normal}$) that would be present if the patient's serum albumin were normal, the following equation is used:

$$C_{normal} = \frac{C_{measured} \times 4.4}{\text{albumin concentration}}$$

where phenytoin concentrations are in micrograms per milliliter and albumin concentration is in grams per deciliter.

Similarly, the free phenytoin fraction (FPF) may be corrected for hypoalbuminemia with this equation:

$$FPF = \frac{1}{1 + (2.1 \times \text{albumin})}$$

## TREATMENT

Initial treatment of oral phenytoin overdose, including airway management, is similar to that for other ingested drugs. Respiratory acidosis due to ventilatory insufficiency or metabolic acidosis should be corrected to decrease the active free phenytoin fraction. Multiple doses of oral activated charcoal (1 g/kg) in the first 24 h may be of benefit, given the known poor solubility and resultant extended absorptive phase of oral phenytoin in overdose. Hemodialysis and hemoperfusion are of no clinical benefit in phenytoin poisoning.

Seizures may be treated with intravenous benzodiazepines or phenobarbital, again with the caution that seizures are not common in

**Table 151-4.** Toxicity of Phenytoin

**Central nervous system**
  Dizziness, tremor (intention), visual disturbance (horizontal and vertical
    nystagmus), diplopia, miosis or mydriasis, ophthalmoplegia, abnormal gait
    (bradykinesia, truncal ataxia), choreoathetoid movements, vomiting,
    dysphagia, respiratory distress, irritability, agitation, confusion,
    hallucinations, fatigue, coma, death (rare), encephalopathy,
    pseudodegenerative disease, dysarthria, meningeal irritation with
    pleocytosis, rarely seizures
**Peripheral nervous system**
  Peripheral neuropathy, urinary incontinence
**Hypersensitivity reactions**
  Eosinophilia, rash, pseudolymphoma (diffuse lymphadenopathy), systemic
    lupus erythematosus, pancytopenia
**Metabolic**
  Osteomalacia (rickets-like metaphyseal abnormality in children), increased
    thyroid uptake, interference with folic acid metabolism, insulin secretion
    inhibition (hyperglycemia), pyridoxine deficiency
**Hematologic**
  Megaloblastic anemia, aplastic anemia, thrombocytopenia, hemorrhagic
    disease of the newborn
**Gastrointestinal**
  Nausea and vomiting, hepatotoxicity
**Skin**
  Hirsutism, acne, rashes (including Stevens-Johnson syndrome)
**Other**
  Fetal hydantoin syndrome, gingival hyperplasia, coarsening of facial
    features
**Parenteral preparations**
  May cause hypotension, bradycardia, conduction disturbances, myocardial
    depression, ventricular fibrillation, asystole, and sloughing of tissues

phenytoin overdose and other causes must be ruled out. Cardiovascular toxicity is extremely rare in oral overdose and should suggest other etiologies. Prolonged cardiac monitoring after oral ingestion is unnecessary. Atropine and temporary cardiac pacing may be used for symptomatic bradyarrhythmias associated with intravenous phenytoin. Hypotension that occurs during intravenous administration usually responds to discontinuation of the infusion and the administration of isotonic crystalloid. Hospital admission and appropriate orthopedic or plastic surgery consultation should be obtained for patients with any significant extravasation of intravenous phenytoin or other signs of local vascular or tissue toxicity after infusion.

To minimize complications due to infusion, intravenous phenytoin should be administered only under close observation with constant cardiac and blood pressure monitoring. The infused solution should be given slowly (< 25 mg/min) through a large, well-positioned catheter.

## ADMISSION INDICATIONS

Patients with serious complications following an oral ingestion (seizures, coma, altered mental status, ataxia, etc.) should be admitted for further evaluation and treatment. Others with only mild symptoms may be treated with charcoal in the emergency department and if an observation unit is available, discharged after their levels have returned to normal, provided they are not actively suicidal. Given the long and erratic absorption phase of phenytoin after oral overdose, the decision to discharge or medically clear a patient for psychiatric evaluation cannot be based on a single serum level. Patients with symptomatic chronic intoxication should be admitted for observation unless signs are minimal, adequate care can be obtained at home, and they are 8 to 12 h from their last therapeutic dose. Phenytoin therapy should be stopped in all cases, and if toxicity continues to resolve, a serum level may be reassessed in 2 to 3 days to guide resumption of therapy.

Patients with significant or persistent complications following the intravenous administration of phenytoin should be admitted. Those with transient effects need not be although, in practice, patients receiving intravenous phenytoin loading are admitted if the underlying condition warrants.

## BIBLIOGRAPHY

Cranford RE, Leppik JE, Patrick B, et al: Intravenous phenytoin: Clinical and pharmacokinetic aspects. *Neurology.* 28:874, 1978.

Howard CE, Roberts S, Ely DS, et al: Use of multiple-dose activated charcoal in phenytoin toxicity. *Ann Pharmacother* 28:201, 1994.

Louis S, Kutt H, McDowell F: The cardiocirculatory changes caused by intravenous dilantin and its solvent. *Am Heart J* 74:523, 1967.

MacDonald RL, Kelly KM: Mechanisms of action of currently prescribed and newly developed anti-epileptic drugs. *Epilepsia* 35(suppl 4):541, 1994.

Mellick LB, Morgan JA, Mellick GA: Presentations of acute phenytoin overdose. *Am J Emerg Med* 7:61, 1989.

Murphy JM, Motiwala R, Devinsky O: Phenytoin intoxication. *So Med J* 84:1199, 1991.

Osorio I, Burnstine TH, Pemler B, et al: Phenytoin-induced seizures: A paradoxical effect at toxic concentrations in epileptic patients. *Epilepsia* 30(2):230, 1989.

Wyte CD, Berk WA: Severe oral phenytoin overdose does not cause cardiovascular morbidity. *Ann Emerg Med* 20:508, 1991.

York RC, Coleridge ST: Cardiopulmonary arrest following intravenous phenytoin loading. *Am J Emerg Med* 6:255, 1988.

# 152
# IRON

## Steven C. Curry

The accidental or intentional ingestion of iron preparations continues to be a common poisoning. Prompt and aggressive management of these patients is needed to prevent mortality and serious morbidity.

## PATHOPHYSIOLOGY

About 10 percent of ingested iron, mainly in the ferrous ($Fe^{2+}$) state, is absorbed each day from the small intestine. Free unbound iron is very toxic to living tissue. Therefore, the body has many mechanisms to keep iron bound to proteins or other macromolecules at all times.

After absorption, iron changes to the ferric ($Fe^{3+}$) state and is stored in intestinal mucosa complexed to the iron storage protein, ferritin. From the intestinal mucosa, iron is transported to the liver, spleen, and bone marrow for further storage as ferritin, or to the bone marrow and other tissues for incorporation into heme molecules.

Whenever iron is transported in the blood, it is complexed with the protein, transferrin. The total amount of iron with which transferrin can bind is termed the total iron binding capacity (TIBC). Normal serum iron concentrations vary from 50 to 150 µg/dL, while normal TIBCs can range from 300 to 435 µg/dL. Because the TIBC is far in excess of the total serum iron concentration, there normally is no "free" iron circulating in blood.

Excessive iron is directly caustic to the gastrointestinal (GI) tract, resulting in hemorrhagic gastroenteritis with hypovolemia and blood loss. If enough iron is absorbed, systemic and metabolic consequences of iron poisoning develop. Iron mainly accumulates in the liver after overdose, but can have toxic effects in almost any organ, including the kidneys, brain, lungs, and heart. Iron is concentrated in mitochondria, where it disrupts oxidative phosphorylation and catalyzes the formation of oxygen-free radicals, leading to lipid peroxidation and cell death. Iron, possibly in the form of the ferritin complex, also is able to cause dilation of venules, resulting in venous pooling. Iron increases capillary membrane permeability and causes significant third spacing of fluids. The lactic acidosis seen in iron poisoning is due to various factors, including hypovolemia and tissue hypoperfusion; the hydration of the ferric ion, resulting in the generation of hydrogen ions; and the shift of cells to anaerobic metabolism as oxidative phosphorylation is impaired. An elevated serum iron level is able directly to inhibit serine proteases such as thrombin and cause a coagulopathy, even before the onset of hepatic dysfunction. While isolated hepatic dysfunction can be seen after a significant overdose, multiple organ system failure and death can be seen in severe poisonings.

## TOXIC DOSE

When determining the amount of iron ingested, *elemental* iron must be used in calculations. For example, only 20 percent of a 300-mg ferrous sulfate tablet is iron. Ferrous fumarate contains about 33 percent elemental iron, and ferrous gluconate contains about 12 percent elemental iron.

Opinions vary as to what constitutes a toxic dose of iron. Some patients become symptomatic following the ingestion of only 20 mg of elemental iron per kilogram. Serious poisoning can often be seen after the ingestion of greater than 40 mg of iron per kilogram. The unreliability of parents in estimating how many pills their child may have ingested cannot be overemphasized. Obviously, a symptomatic patient requires evaluation and possible treatment regardless of history.

## CLINICAL FEATURES

Clinical findings can help predict the degree of toxicity. Of all children who vomit or have diarrhea, the majority have serum iron concentrations greater than 300 μg/dL. Most children with a white blood-cell count > 15,000/mm³, or a serum glucose level > 150 mg/dL, have a serum iron level greater than 300 μg/dL. *Severely poisoned children can still have a normal white blood cell count and a normal serum glucose level.* The appearance of a rosé wine color to the urine after an injection or infusion of deferoxamine is due to ferrioxamine in the urine. The absence of this color is an *unreliable* indicator of lack of significant iron poisoning, and an *unreliable* indicator of lack of need for deferoxamine.

Based on clinical findings, iron poisoning can be divided into various stages. I use four stages for purposes of discussion. *Patients can die in any stage of iron poisoning. They just die for different reasons!*

The first stage of iron poisoning develops within the first few hours after ingestion. It is due to the direct corrosive effects of iron on the GI tract and is characterized by abdominal pain, vomiting, and diarrhea. Hematemesis is not unusual. In this stage, lethargy, shock, and a metabolic acidosis are due to hypovolemia, anemia (GI bleeding), and tissue hypoperfusion.

The second stage, not always seen, may continue for up to 12 h following ingestion. During this stage, toxic amounts of iron are being absorbed into the body. GI symptoms may resolve, and the patient is frequently quiet. The apparent improvement in the patient's condition can be falsely reassuring.

The third stage may appear early in severe poisonings, or may develop hours following the second stage. Toxic amounts of iron have moved from blood into tissues, disrupting cellular metabolism, causing third spacing of fluids, and producing venous pooling of blood. Shock and a metabolic acidosis in this stage of iron poisoning can be due to persistent hypovolemia; anemia; hepatic dysfunction (including hypoglycemia); impaired oxidative phosphorylation; heart failure; and renal failure. Hepatic injury is unusual when serum peak iron levels remain under 500 μg/dL.

The fourth stage develops days to weeks after recovery from iron poisoning. It is characterized by gastric outlet or small bowel obstruction secondary to scarring from the original corrosive injury produced by iron.

## TREATMENT

**Decontamination and Supportive Care.** Patients arriving in the emergency department who have remained asymptomatic for 6 h after ingestion of iron and who have a completely normal physical examination do not need medical treatment for iron poisoning.

Patients who have a significant ingestion of iron (about 20 mg/kg or greater) should receive gastric lavage. Since ipecac-induced vomiting is confused with signs of serious iron poisoning, and since there are no studies demonstrating that ipecac changes the outcome in iron poisoning, we do not use it. There are no data supporting lavage with sodium bicarbonate solutions or supporting administration of phosphates to prevent iron absorption. Cathartics should not be administered to those who already have diarrhea. A plain film of the kidneys, ureters, and bladder (KUB) may reveal iron in the GI tract; however, 50 percent of children who develop serum iron levels in excess of 300 μg/dL have a negative KUB.

Patients who have only minimal symptoms after ingestion do well with supportive care. If the patient remains well after several hours of observation, and a serum iron level drawn 3 to 5 h after ingestion is well below 350 μg/dL, the patient can be discharged. A repeat serum iron determination during observation helps to ensure that iron levels are not rising. A KUB demonstrating iron remaining in the GI tract obviously indicates that serum iron levels may continue to increase. Again, a negative KUB does not preclude a continued rise in serum iron concentration.

Intravenous hydration should be initiated in patients with significant symptoms. A fluid challenge should be given intravenously to those patients with hypotension. Laboratory work should include measurements of serum electrolytes, blood urea nitrogen, serum glucose, coagulation parameters, a complete blood cell count, and serum iron level. Blood gases should be determined in any severely symptomatic patient.

**Deferoxamine.** Deferoxamine mesylate is a chelating agent that can remove iron from tissues and free iron from plasma. It combines with iron to form water-soluble ferrioxamine, which is excreted in the urine. The preferred route of administration is as an intravenous infusion at a rate of 15 mg/kg per hour. Higher rates of infusion are recommended in severe cases by some authorities. Hypotension is occasionally seen when deferoxamine is used in acute iron poisoning. Hypotension is thought to be due to vasodilation, possibly from histamine release. This is usually not a problem if infusion rates are kept below 45 mg/kg per hour.

Deferoxamine can be given intramuscularly, but studies in patients with chronic iron overload show that intravenous administration of deferoxamine removes much more iron than intramuscular administration. Furthermore, an intramuscular injection would be expected to produce a higher peak level, making hypotension more likely. Adequate hydration should always be given before deferoxamine is administered intramuscularly. A commonly recommended dose for intramuscular deferoxamine mesylate is 90 mg/kg, up to 1 g, every 8 h. There are no human data to support a recommendation that the total daily dose of deferoxamine not exceed 6 g in the treatment of acute iron poisoning. In fact, much larger doses have been given without complications. The use of deferoxamine in patients with chronic renal failure and/or chronic iron overload has produced neurotoxicity consisting of hearing loss, decreased visual acuity, and changes in color vision. Such changes have not been reported after the short-term use of deferoxamine in patients suffering from acute iron poisoning. Deferoxamine causes a fall in glomerular filtration rate and renal blood flow in dogs, and case reports suggest the existence of deferoxamine-induced renal failure. A canine study demonstrates the importance of adequate hydration in preventing renal dysfunction from deferoxamine. The use of deferoxamine infusions for several days has been associated with rapidly progressive and fatal pneumonitis/adult respiratory distress syndrome. Again, this has not been reported after short-term use (12 to 24 h) of deferoxamine for the treatment of acute iron poisoning.

Gastric lavage with deferoxamine mesylate is not recommended because tremendous amounts of deferoxamine mesylate would be required to complex with ingested, but yet unabsorbed, iron. Fortunately, most iron is not absorbed following overdose, which is why lesser amounts of deferoxamine can be given parenterally.

To use deferoxamine wisely, one needs to understand the limitations of using serum iron levels as a basis for therapy. Serum iron levels usually peak anywhere from 2 to 6 h after ingestion. Many patients have normal serum iron levels by the time they die from iron poisoning because it is iron that has moved from blood into *tissues* that causes systemic toxicity. Although deferoxamine can remove free iron from plasma, an important reason for giving deferoxamine is to remove iron from *tissues*.

A serum iron concentration below the TIBC, then, does not mean that deferoxamine would be of no benefit. The determination of a single iron level may not reflect what iron levels have been previously, or what direction iron levels are going. For example, suppose you have just received laboratory results reporting a serum iron concentration of 310 μg/dL and a TIBC of 365 μg/dL. The serum iron concentration may have been above the TIBC earlier, resulting in significant tissue levels of iron. On the other hand, the serum iron concentration may have been rising at the time blood was drawn, and exceeds the TIBC by the time laboratory results return. Furthermore, a recent study demonstrated that commonly used methods to measure

**Table 152-1.** Errors Treating Iron Poisoning

- Waiting until results of serum iron levels are returned before administering deferoxamine to moderately or severely symptomatic patients
- Withholding deferoxamine from severely symptomatic patients only because serum iron levels are below the TIBC
- Sending a stage-2 iron poisoning victim home
- Relying only on a negative KUB, a normal WBC, and/or a normal serum glucose level to rule out significant iron ingestion
- Using radioimmunoassays when measuring serum iron
- Not recognizing that deferoxamine causes a falsely low determination of serum iron levels by most laboratory methods

TIBC result in a falsely elevated TIBC at toxic iron concentrations. Therefore, elevated serum iron concentrations are accompanied by falsely elevated TIBCs, making interpretation of the relationship between TIBC and serum iron difficult or impossible. Therefore, *one should never wait for results of a serum iron level or TIBC to decide whether to give deferoxamine to a significantly symptomatic patient.* If a patient is severely symptomatic, deferoxamine is probably indicated regardless of the serum iron concentration or TIBC.

The following patients should receive deferoxamine after adequate hydration:

1. Any moderately or severely symptomatic patient (e.g., one with hypotension, severe gastroenteritis, lethargy), even if iron levels are below the TIBC, have not yet returned, or are not available.
2. Any patient whose serum iron level is greater than the TIBC.
3. Any patient with a serum iron level greater than 350 to 400 μg/dL.

Our center recommends that deferoxamine be continued until the patient is free of any evidence of systemic iron toxicity *and* serum iron levels are normal or low.

**Dialysis and renal failure.** Dialysis and charcoal hemoperfusion can remove some ferrioxamine as well as deferoxamine. It has been recommended that deferoxamine should be continued and dialysis instituted in the face of acute renal failure during acute iron poisoning. It appears that increasing urinary elimination of ferrioxamine is not deferoxamine's main mechanism in counteracting iron poisoning. Data suggest that deferoxamine's main protective mechanism is to combine with and inactivate iron by forming ferrioxamine, regardless of how quickly ferrioxamine may be excreted in urine. While it makes sense that deferoxamine should be continued in the face of renal failure, it is not established that dialysis or hemoperfusion should be instituted only to enhance ferrioxamine clearance. When deferoxamine is used in patients with renal failure, the elimination half-life is prolonged markedly (mean value of 25.6 h versus 1 to 4 h in normal patients), and the infusion rate should be decreased appropriately.

## ERRORS IN TREATING IRON POISONING

Several common mistakes are made by those who treat iron poisoning, and these pitfalls are summarized in Table 152-1. Attention has been drawn to several of these in the previous sections, but two others deserve special mention.

Some laboratories use radioimmunoassays to measure serum iron levels. These assays *cannot* measure serum iron concentrations greater than the TIBC. Therefore, if the serum iron level is reported to be close to the TIBC, it is possible that it is really much greater than the TIBC. A colorimetric method is probably the most reliable for measuring serum iron levels after overdose, unless methods using atomic absorption are readily available.

The second important point is that deferoxamine interferes with the determination of serum iron levels, even by colorimetric methods. Once deferoxamine has been given, serum iron level measurements may be falsely depressed by as much as 30 to 50 percent, and possibly more. This must be considered when interpreting reports of serum iron concentrations. At our center we correct for the presence of

deferoxamine by adding sodium hydrosulfite. However, this is rarely done at other institutions. This is the main reason why our center recommends that serum iron level measurements be low before stopping deferoxamine therapy.

## BIBLIOGRAPHY

Chang TMS, Barre P: Effect of desferrioxamine on removal of aluminum and iron by coated charcoal haemoperfusion and haemodialysis. *Lancet* 2:1051, 1983.

Dean BS, Krenzelok EP: In vivo effectiveness of oral complexation agents in the management of iron poisoning. *Clin Toxicol* 25:221, 1987.

Evensen SA, Forde R, Opedal I, et al: Acute iron intoxication with abruptly reduced levels of vitamin K-dependent coagulation factors. *Scand J Haematol* 29:25, 1982.

Freedman MH, Grisaru D, Olivieri N, et al: Pulmonary syndrome in patients with thalassemia major receiving intravenous deferoxamine infusions. *Am J Dis Child* 144:565, 1990.

Koren G, Bentur Y, Strong D, et al: Acute changes in renal function associated with deferoxamine therapy. *Am J Dis Child* 143:1077, 1989.

Lacouture PG, Wason S, Temple AR, et al: Emergency assessment of severity in iron overdose by clinical and laboratory methods. *J Pediatr* 99:89, 1981.

Lovejoy FH: Chelation therapy in iron poisoning. *J Toxicol Clin Toxicol* 19:871, 1983.

Peck MG, Rogers JF, Rivenbark JF: Use of high doses of deferoxamine (Desferal) in an adult patient with acute iron overdosage. *J Toxicol Clin Toxicol* 19:875, 1983.

Proudfoot AT, Simpson D, Dyson EH: Management of acute iron poisoning. *Med Toxicol* 1:83, 1986.

Robotham JL, Lietman PS: Acute iron poisoning. *Am J Dis Child* 134:875, 1980.

Stivelman J, Schulman G, Fosburg M, et al: Kinetics and efficacy of deferoxamine in iron-overloaded hemodialysis patients. *Kidney Int* 36:1125, 1989.

Tenenbein M, Kowalskis, Roberts D: Pulmonary toxicity in iron poisoning: Deferoxamine induced? *Vet Hum Toxicol* 32:349, 1990 (abstract).

Tenenbein M, Yatscoff R: Total iron binding capacity (TIBC) in iron poisoning: Who needs it? *Vet Hum Toxicol* 31:343, 1989 (abstract).

# 153
# HYDROCARBONS
## Paul M. Wax

## INTRODUCTION

Hydrocarbons are a diverse group of organic compounds consisting primarily of carbon and hydrogen atoms arranged in various aliphatic and aromatic configurations. Products containing hydrocarbons are found in many households and occupational settings. Examples include fuels, lighter fluids, paints, paint removers, glues, cleaning and polishing agents, spot removers, degreasers, lubricants, solvents, and pesticides. Exposure may cause life-threatening toxicity.

### Classification

Most hydrocarbons are produced from petroleum distillation, which results in predominantly aliphatic (open-chain) mixtures of hydrocarbons of different chain lengths. Gasoline, for instance, consists of approximately 80% saturated and unsaturated aliphatic hydrocarbons of chain length C4 to C10 and 20% aromatic hydrocarbons. Chain length determines the phase of the hydrocarbon at room temperature. Short-chain aliphatic compounds, such as methane or butane, are

**Table 153-1.** Substances That Predominantly Contain Aliphatics

| Substance | Commercial Use |
| --- | --- |
| Gasoline | Motor fuel |
| Kerosene | Stove and lamp fuel |
| Mineral seal oil | Furniture polish |
| Naphtha | Lighter fluid |
| Diesel oil | Lubricant |
| N–Hexane | Plastic cement, rubber cement |

gases; long-chain aliphatic compounds, such as tar, are solids. Intermediate-chain (C5 to 15) aliphatic compounds are in liquid form and account for most hydrocarbon exposures seen in the emergency department (Table 153-1). Pulmonary toxicity secondary to aspiration is the most common complication from ingesting liquid aliphatic hydrocarbons.

The wood distillates (e.g., turpentine and pine oil) consist mainly of cyclic terpene derivatives and make up another class of hydrocarbons. Gastrointestinal (GI) absorption of wood distillates tends to be greater than that of aliphatic petroleum distillates, increasing the risk for central nervous system (CNS) depression.

Aromatic hydrocarbons (containing a benzene ring, Table 153-2) and halogenated hydrocarbons (aliphatics with a substituted halogen group, Table 153-3) are widely used industrial solvents. Exposure, usually from inhalation, is most often found in substance abusers and in certain occupational settings and may result in significant systemic toxicity. Specific cardiovascular, hepatic, renal, and hematologic effects are attributed to aromatic and halogenated hydrocarbons.

## Epidemiology

Hydrocarbon ingestions account for approximately 3 to 10 percent of all accidental childhood poisonings in the United States. Ingestions of gasoline, kerosene, lighter fluid, mineral seal oil, and turpentine are most frequent. In less developed countries, kerosene ingestions alone account for 33 to 59 percent of accidental childhood poisonings. The 1992 American Association of Poison Control Centers National Data Collection Systems revealed that of the 63,985 hydrocarbon exposures reported to poison control centers, 1846 developed moderate to severe toxicity, and 16 died. These data imply that most hydrocarbon ingestions have a benign clinical course.

## PATHOPHYSIOLOGY AND CLINICAL FEATURES

### Determinants of Toxicity

The toxic potential of hydrocarbons depends on physical characteristics (volatility, viscosity, and surface tension), chemical characteristics (aliphatic, aromatic, or halogenated), presence of toxic additives such as pesticides or heavy metals, route of exposure, concentration, and dose. Viscosity, defined as the resistance to flow, and surface tension, denoting "creeping" ability, both play a major role in determining the aspiration potential. Viscosity is measured in Saybolt Seconds Universal (SSU). Patients ingesting substances with viscosities less than 60 SSU are at greater risk for aspiration than those ingesting substances with viscosities greater than 100 SSU (Table 153-4). Volatility denotes the ability of a substance to vaporize. Inhalation of a highly volatile agent, such as the aromatic hydrocarbons, halogenated hydrocarbons, or gasoline results in systemic absorption and the potential for significant toxicity.

**Table 153-2.** Common Aromatic Hydrocarbons

| Substance | Commercial Use |
| --- | --- |
| Benzene | Chemical intermediate, gasoline (small amount; average, 0.8%) |
| Toluene | Airplane glue, plastic cement, acrylic paint |
| Xylene | Solvent, cleaning agent, degreaser |

**Table 153-3.** Common Halogenated Hydrocarbons

| Substance | Commercial Use |
| --- | --- |
| Carbon tetrachloride | Solvent, refrigerant, aerosol propellant |
| Chloroform | Solvent, chemical intermediate |
| Methylene chloride | Paint stripper, varnish remover, aerosol paint, degreaser |
| Trichloroethylene (TCE) | Spot remover, degreaser, typewriter correction fluid |
| Trichloroethane (TCA) | Spot remover, degreaser, typewriter correction fluid |
| Tetrachloroethylene (Perchloroethylene) | Dry cleaning agent, degreaser |

Dermal exposure to hydrocarbons causes local toxicity, and occasionally leads to systemic absorption. Dermal toxicity secondary to intravenous administration of hydrocarbons has also been reported. When used intravenously, hydrocarbons may cause pulmonary toxicity by their first-pass exposure to the lungs.

Toxicity from hydrocarbon exposure can be divided into different clinical syndromes based on the organ system(s) predominately affected. Characteristic presentations usually affect one or more of the following systems: pulmonary, neurologic (central and peripheral), GI, cardiac, hepatic, renal, hematologic, or dermal.

## Pulmonary Toxicity

Pulmonary complications, especially aspiration, are the most frequent adverse effects of hydrocarbon exposure. Typically, this involves the accidental childhood ingestion of small amounts of aliphatic hydrocarbon mixtures commonly stored in the household. Aliphatic hydrocarbons have a limited GI absorption; toxicity usually results from aspiration of the low-viscosity hydrocarbons or inadvertent inhalation of the high-volatility hydrocarbons. Although ingestion of aromatic or halogenated hydrocarbons may also result in aspiration, CNS and other systemic toxicity secondary to GI absorption often predominate.

Aspiration is not dependent on volume ingested. Experimentally in rats, as little as 0.2 mL instilled intratracheally has caused pneumonitis. Pulmonary toxicity does not result from GI absorption but occurs from direct aspiration of the hydrocarbon into the pulmonary tree. This occurs at the time of ingestion when the hydrocarbon migrates from the hypopharynx into the airway. There is no evidence that hydrocarbons reflux from the stomach into the airway. Spontaneous vomiting, however, does increase the risk of aspiration. Pulmonary toxicity manifested as acute bilateral pneumonitis has also been reported from the inhalation of an aerosolized aliphatic hydrocarbon such as gasoline or kerosene.

Hydrocarbon aspiration causes chemical pneumonitis by direct toxic injury to the pulmonary parenchyma. Destruction of alveolar and capillary membranes results in increased vascular permeability and edema. Altered surfactant function may also contribute. Early distal airway closure and alveolar collapse produces clinical broncho-

**Table 153-4.** Hydrocarbon Viscosities

| < 60 SSU | > 100 SSU |
| --- | --- |
| Aromatic hydrocarbons | Diesel oil |
| Gasoline | Grease |
| Halogenated hydrocarbons | Mineral oil |
| Kerosene | Paraffin wax |
| Mineral seal oil | Petroleum jelly |
| Naphtha | Tar |
| N–Hexane | |
| Turpentine | |

SOURCE: Ellenhorn MJ, Barceloux DG: *Medical Toxicology*. New York: Elsevier, 1988. Used with permission.

spasm and ventilation/perfusion mismatch. The CNS manifestations seen after ingestion of a poorly GI-absorbed aliphatic hydrocarbon are thought to be from hypoxia secondary to the hydrocarbon-induced pneumonitis and/or direct CNS toxicity following the pulmonary absorption of a volatile hydrocarbon. Studies performed in animals in which hydrocarbons were instilled into the stomach after ligation of the esophagus demonstrate negligible absorption of aliphatic compounds from the GI tract with no evidence of subsequent pneumonitis. Pneumatoceles, pneumothoraces, and/or pneumomediastinum are also associated with hydrocarbon aspiration. Other complications include bacterial superinfection, acute respiratory distress syndrome, and death. Long-term pulmonary dysfunction may occur.

Twelve to 71 percent of pediatric hydrocarbon ingestions develop clinical or radiographic evidence of pulmonary toxicity. The clinical manifestations of pulmonary aspiration are usually apparent almost immediately on ingestion. The early effects result from irritation of the oral mucosa and tracheobronchial tree. Symptoms include coughing, choking, gasping, dyspnea, and burning of the mouth. Patients with these symptoms should be assumed to have aspirated until proven otherwise. Physical examination may reveal grunting respirations, retractions, tachypnea, tachycardia, and cyanosis. An odor of the hydrocarbon may be noted on the patient's breath. An elevated temperature of 39° (102.2°F) or greater is common and may occur on admission or be delayed for 6 to 8 h.

Auscultation may be normal, or reveal wheezing, and decreased, or absent breath sounds. Arterial blood gas analysis may demonstrate a widened alveolar–arterial oxygen gradient or frank hypoxemia. The development of a necrotizing pneumonitis and hemorrhagic pulmonary edema usually occurs within hours in severe aspiration.

Most fatalities from these complications occur within 24 to 48 h. With less severe damage, symptoms usually subside within 2 to 5 days except with pneumatoceles and lipoid pneumonias where symptoms may persist for weeks to months.

Although most patients with clinically significant aspiration have abnormal chest x-rays, the time course of radiographic changes varies and correlation with physical examination may be poor. Changes may be seen as early as 30 min after aspiration, but the initial radiograph in the symptomatic patient may be deceptively clear. Radiographic changes usually appear by 2 to 6 h and are almost always present by 18 to 24 h if they are to occur. The infiltrates range in appearance from streaking to flocculent to homogeneous and are usually located in the dependent lobes. Multilobar involvement is more common than single-lobe involvement. Radiographic changes limited to bilateral perihilar involvement with clear lung bases are also common.

High-viscosity compounds such as lubricants, mineral oil, or tar are not aspirated readily and tend to be less toxic when ingested. Occasionally, however, aspiration will occur resulting in the development of lipoid pneumonia. Deaths from hydrocarbon lipoid pneumonia have been reported.

## Central Nervous System Toxicity

Central nervous system toxicity may result from either a direct toxic response to the systemic absorption of the hydrocarbon, as an indirect result of severe hypoxia secondary to aspiration, or as a result of simple asphyxiation. Systemic absorption usually occurs through the inhalation of highly volatile petroleum distillates, which may be absorbed inadvertently, for example as an occupational risk, or deliberately associated with solvent abuse.

Solvent abuse most often occurs in teenagers and younger adults, especially from lower socioeconomic backgrounds and in particular cultures (Native Americans). These patients are described as "huffers" or "baggers" depending on whether they inhale through a rag soaked with the hydrocarbon held to the mouth or rebreathe into a plastic bag containing the hydrocarbon. The act of rebreathing to facilitate inhalation may also contribute to toxicity by producing significant hypercarbia and hypoxia. Commonly abused agents include aromatic hydrocarbons such as toluene (contained in glue and acrylic spray paints), halogenated hydrocarbons such as trichloroethylene (found in typewriter correction fluid), or highly volatile aliphatics such as gasoline.

Many hydrocarbons which affect the CNS are organic solvents and have a natural affinity for the lipid-rich neural tissue. They behave similarly to the inhalational anesthetic agents. Hydrocarbon intoxication may be confused with ethanol inebriation. CNS depression ranges in severity from dizziness, slurred speech, ataxia, and lethargy to obtundation and coma. Depression of the central ventilatory drive may also occur. These effects are usually dose dependent. Although hydrocarbons are CNS depressants, they often have an initial excitatory effect manifested as euphoria, exhilaration, and giddiness, effects sought by those who abuse them. More severe excitatory features include tremor, agitation, and convulsions. Perceptual changes such as confusion, hallucinations, and psychosis may occur.

Chronic CNS sequelae may result from recurrent inhalational exposure to hydrocarbons in the work place or with solvent abuse. These sequelae are seen among house painters and solvent abusers exposed to toluene-containing substances. The syndrome is characterized by recurrent headaches, cerebellar ataxia, and a chronic encephalopathy consisting of tremors, emotional lability, mental status changes, cognitive impairment, and psychomotor impairment. These effects may be transitory or permanent. The development of encephalopathy, ataxia, tremor, chorea, and myoclonus also is associated with the habitual sniffing of leaded gasoline. In this case, symptoms are thought to be secondary to the effects of tetraethyl lead and its toxic metabolites.

## Peripheral Nervous System Toxicity

Exposure to *n*–hexane, methyl *n*–butyl ketone, and other six-carbon aliphatic hydrocarbons is associated with the development of a characteristic peripheral polyneuropathy caused by demyelinization and retrograde axonal degeneration resembling a dying-back neuropathy. Onset of symptoms may be delayed for months to years after initial exposure. Toxicity is attributed to a metabolite, 2,5-hexanedione, produced by the cytochrome P–450-mediated biotransformation of the parent compounds. This neurotoxic metabolite is thought to inhibit glutaraldehyde-3-phosphate dehydrogenase, which supplies energy for axonal transport. Long, distal nerves seem to be most vulnerable, characteristically producing foot and wrist drop with numbness and paresthesias. The electromyelogram typically shows a decrease in nerve conduction velocity.

## Gastrointestinal Toxicity

Local GI toxicity may occur after hydrocarbon ingestion. Most hydrocarbons act as intestinal irritants, resulting in burning in the mouth and throat, abdominal pain, belching, nausea, vomiting, and diarrhea. Vomiting, which occurs in about one third of the patients with aliphatic hydrocarbon ingestions, is particularly troublesome because of the increased risk of pulmonary aspiration.

## Cardiac Toxicity

Life-threatening arrhythmias, such as ventricular tachycardia and ventricular fibrillation, may be present with systemic absorption of a variety of hydrocarbon compounds. Most commonly, arrhythmias occur after exposure to halogenated hydrocarbons and aromatic hydrocarbons. Exposures to predominantly aliphatic mixtures such as gasoline or mineral spirits have also been reported to cause arrhythmias. In these cases, the aromatic fraction of the mixture may still act as the precipitant. The mechanism of toxicity is believed to be secondary to a sensitization of the heart to catecholamines. The term "sudden sniffing death" describes solvent abusers who die suddenly after exertion, panic, or fright. The sudden release of catecholamines in these situations is thought to induce these fatal arrhythmias. Cardiac arrhythmias as a consequence of industrial exposure to volatile hydrocarbons have also been described. Other mechanisms for sudden death include asphyxia, respiratory depression, and vagal inhibition. The use of exogenous catecholamines, such as epinephrine, may precipitate sudden arrhythmias and should be avoided except if required for cardiac resuscitation. A causal relationship may exist between halogenated hydrocarbon exposure and a decrease in myocardial contractility.

## Hepatic Toxicity

Hydrocarbon-induced hepatic damage resulting from halogenated hydrocarbons is well described. Carbon tetrachloride toxicity has been used as a model for toxin-induced hepatic dysfunction. As little as 3 mL carbon tetrachloride has been associated with the development of fatal liver injury. Other halogenated hydrocarbons, such as chloroform, are also associated with liver dysfunction. Free-radical metabolites of these agents that cause lipid peroxidation are apparently responsible for hepatocellular destruction.

Pathologic examination reveals acute fatty degeneration of the liver with areas of centrilobular necrosis. Phenobarbital, ethanol, and other agents that induce cytochrome P-450 enzymes are contraindicated because of the propensity to increase the production of the toxic metabolites. Liver function tests may be elevated in 24 h after ingestion with the development of liver tenderness and jaundice in 48 to 96 h. Chronic exposure to carbon tetrachloride may be associated with the development of cirrhosis and hepatomas.

## Renal and Metabolic Toxicity

Solvent abuse and occupational exposure to hydrocarbons may result in renal dysfunction. Exposure to hepatotoxic halogenerated hydrocarbons such as carbon tetrachloride and trichlorethylene has caused centrilobular hepatic necrosis and acute renal failure. Occupational hydrocarbon exposures have been associated with a variety of glomerulonephritides including Goodpasture's syndrome.

Renal tubular acidosis may occur in patients who abuse toluene-containing substances. Patients present with a nonanion gap metabolic acidosis, hypokalemia, and hypophosphatemia. The serum potassium may be so low (< 2 mEq/L) that severe muscle weakness develops, occasionally resulting in quadriparesis. Significant rhabdomyolysis may also result. Toluene toxicity may also cause a high anion gap metabolic acidosis as a result of the accumulation of hippuric acid and benzoic acid metabolites. Proteinuria and renal insufficiency can occur in patients who abuse toluene.

## Hematologic Toxicity

Chronic exposure to benzene, the prototypical aromatic hydrocarbon, is associated with an increased incidence of hematologic disorders including aplastic anemia, acute myelogenous leukemia, and multiple myeloma. This association has received much attention because of the extensive use of benzene in the workplace. The etiology of these blood dyscrasias is probably not benzene itself but rather a toxic metabolite. Although aplastic anemia is associated with glue sniffing, this is most likely due to the benzene fraction of the glue and not the toluene. Hydrocarbon-induced hemolysis has occurred following the acute ingestion of gasoline, kerosene, and tetrachloroethylene. Consumptive coagulopathy has also been reported.

A peculiar complication of methylene chloride exposure is the endogenous production of carbon monoxide. This is unlike ordinary carbon monoxide exposure from exogenous sources where maximum carboxyhemoglobin level occurs at the time of exposure. With methylene chloride exposure, carbon monoxide formation may continue after cessation of exposure due to slow release of methylene chloride from the tissues prior to its metabolism to carbon monoxide. When patients exposed to methylene chloride present with CNS and cardiac symptoms, impairment due to significant carbon monoxide production must be considered.

## Dermal Toxicity

Dermal exposure may also result in toxicity. Cutaneous injury is associated most often with the short-chain aliphatic, aromatic, and halogenated hydrocarbons. These agents act as primary irritants and as sensitizers. Clinically, skin findings can range from local erythema, papules, and vesicles to a generalized scarlatiniform eruption and an exfoliative dermatitis. A "huffer's rash" may be noted over the face of patients who chronically abuse the volatile hydrocarbons. Pruritus may also be present. A defatting dermatitis, similar to a chronic eczematoid dermatitis, may occur. Cellulitis and sterile abscesses have been associated with the injection of hydrocarbons. Extensive partial-thickness and full-thickness burns following immersion in hydrocarbons may also occur.

Exposure to heated high-viscosity, long-chain aliphatics, such as tar, asphalt, or bitumen present a particularly challenging problem because of their association with burns and hyperthermia, and difficulty with decontamination.

## TREATMENT
### Prehospital

Not all patients who have ingested hydrocarbons require emergency department evaluation. In a recent retrospective study of 211 patients with hydrocarbon ingestions called to a poison center, less than 1 percent required physician intervention. This suggests that patients who are asymptomatic or quickly become asymptomatic after ingestion can be watched safely at home. This approach of home observation for asymptomatic patients can be supported when the ingestion is accidental, the ingredients are known and do not require GI decontamination, and reliable follow-up can be ensured. All symptomatic patients should be referred to the hospital for further evaluation.

GI decontamination is indicated for hydrocarbon ingestions where the hydrocarbon or a toxic additive has good GI absorption and significant systemic toxicity. The CHAMP mnemonic (camphor, halogenated hydrocarbons, aromatic hydrocarbons, metals, pesticides) is helpful in remembering most situations that require GI decontamination. Ingestion of these substances, whether or not symptomatic, should be referred to the hospital. The use of ipecac in the home is not recommended because of the increased risk of aspiration. An exception is the ingestion of benzene where the patient's risk of delayed toxicity following absorption may be higher than the risk of aspiration.

### Emergency Department

General principles of poison management apply to the initial approach to patients exposed to hydrocarbons once they reach the hospital. Establishing the airway and maintaining ventilation is the critical first maneuver. A sweet odor associated with hydrocarbon exposure (especially chloroform and trichloroethylene) may be detected. Glucose, thiamine, and naloxone should be administered in cases of altered mental status. Hypotension should be treated with aggressive fluid resuscitation. Catecholamines, such as dopamine, norephinephrine, or epinephrine, are avoided to prevent precipitating arrhythmias, especially following exposure to halogenated hydrocarbons and aromatic hydrocarbons. Obtaining an electrocardiogram and continued cardiac monitoring are especially important in these situations. The patient needs to be fully undressed to prevent ongoing contamination from hydrocarbon-soaked clothes. Dermal decontamination with soap and water and eye decontamination with saline irrigation should be performed. Protective gloves and aprons should be worn by the staff to prevent possible secondary exposure. Specific antidotal treatment directed at the complications of toxic additives such as organophosphates or heavy metals may also be needed.

Useful diagnostic tests include the chest x-ray and arterial blood gas to detect pulmonary aspiration and hypoxemia. Abdominal x-ray examination may show evidence of chlorinated hydrocarbon ingestions, such as carbon tetrachloride, because of the radiopaque nature of these substances. Tests of liver and renal function should be obtained in all aromatic and halogenated hydrocarbon exposures to check for the development of hepatic and renal injury. A serum lead level may be helpful when evaluating patients with chronic gasoline exposure. A carboxyhemoglobin level is useful to evaluate the extent of endogenous carbon monoxide production following methylene chloride exposure. Routine drug screens are not useful for the detection of hydrocarbons, but as in all intentional ingestions, an acetaminophen level, ethanol level, anion gap, and osmolality may be helpful in assessing for the presence of other coingestants.

## Gastrointestinal Decontamination

For most hydrocarbon ingestions, ipecac and gastric lavage are of no benefit; supportive care and appropriate treatment of coexisting ingestions are all that is required. The necessity for GI decontamination depends on the type of hydrocarbon and route of exposure. The risk of systemic toxicity by intestinal absorption has to be weighed against the risks of aspiration associated with gastric emptying. The majority of hydrocarbon ingestions, which consist of aliphatic hydrocarbons mixtures (see Table 153-1), do not require GI decontamination. These agents have poor GI absorption and their toxicity is limited primarily to pulmonary aspiration. In the typical childhood accidental ingestion, the actual amount ingested is usually about one swallow or about 5 mL. Suicidal ingestions, which involve larger amounts of hydrocarbons, frequently are associated with spontaneous emesis, and further decontamination is usually not required. Some recommend GI decontamination if emesis has not occurred and the dose is greater than 1 to 2 mL/kg, although this strategy has not been studied.

The preferred method of gastric emptying for ingestions of CHAMP-type hydrocarbons, significant amounts of wood distillates, or coingestants is controversial. Some recommend ipecac in the alert patient who has an intact gag reflex. Ipecac should never be used in patients with altered mental status or potential for sudden deterioration, such as following a camphor or organophosphate ingestion. Lavage is recommended for significant wood distillate ingestions because of their GI absorption and tendency to cause CNS depression. If the ingestion is limited to liquid preparations only, lavage with a small nasogastric tube should suffice, but if there is a concern about a concomitant solid ingestion, a large-bore orogastric tube is used. In patients with altered mental status, it is preferable to protect the airway with a cuffed endotracheal tube, although in smaller children under 8 years of age, the cuff should be kept inflated only during the period of lavage because of cuff-related injury from prolonged inflation.

Activated charcoal has not been shown to be efficacious in adsorbing hydrocarbon compounds. Charcoal instillation may distend the stomach increasing the risk for vomiting and aspiration. The use of charcoal is not recommended unless a dangerous hydrocarbon (such as benzene or toluene), toxic additive, or coingested absorbable toxin has been ingested.

The use of cathartics to hasten GI transit and facilitate decontamination has no proven efficacy in hydrocarbon ingestions. Many patients will already have diarrhea from the hydrocarbon, and further catharsis is not required. Oil-based cathartics, which had been used in the past to thicken the ingested hydrocarbon in order to increase its viscosity and decrease subsequent risk of aspiration, are contraindicated. They may actually increase GI absorption and are associated with an increased risk of lipoid pneumonia when aspirated.

## Pulmonary Treatment

Nebulized oxygen is helpful in the treatment of pulmonary aspiration. Positive end-expiratory pressure (PEEP) or continuous positive-airway pressure (CPAP) may sometimes be required, but because of the additional barotrauma this creates, one should observe for the development of pneumatoceles or pneumothoraces. In cases of severe pulmonary aspiration resulting in refractory hypoxemia, treatment with extracorporeal membrane oxygenation (EMCO) has proved successful. Corticosteroids are contraindicated because they impair the cellular immune response and increase the chance of bacterial superinfection. Antibiotics have no proven role in prophylaxis and are usually not required except in cases of continued pulmonary deterioration because of the risk of a superimposed bacterial pneumonitis.

## Other

There are few antidotes to counteract the actions of hydrocarbons. N-Acetyl cysteine and hyperbaric oxygen may have a role in preventing hepatic toxicity after carbon tetrachloride (and possibly chloroform) exposure, but more studies are needed. Hyperbaric oxygen therapy is indicated for patients who develop significant carbon monoxide toxicity after exposure to methylene chloride. β-Blocking drugs may be useful in the treatment of hydrocarbon-induced malignant arrhythmias. Although extracorporeal removal with hemodialysis, hemoperfusion, or peritoneal dialysis has been attempted for severe intoxications, clinically controlled evidence of efficacy is lacking.

Undoubtedly, the best therapy begins with preventive measures to reduce accessibility of these compounds to young children. Proper labeling of containers that store hydrocarbons, mandatory use of safety closures, and public education on the risks of hydrocarbons also limit the potential for inadvertent hydrocarbon toxicity.

The treatment of tar and asphalt injuries is a particular problem because of the difficulty in removing these substances without causing further tissue injury. Immediate cooling with cold water for at least 30 min is critical. Debridement of blistered skin can aid in the removal of adherent substances. De-Solv-It, a surface-active petroeumbased solvent, has proven both nonirritating and effective in removing these agents. Polyoxyethylene sorbitan containing ointments such as Polysorbate 80 or Tween 80 have also proven useful. Petrolatumcontaining preparations such as Neosporin (although occasionally sensitizing) or Polysporin may also work and are readily available. In some instances, early excision and skin grafting will be required to treat the more significant hot tar burns.

## DISPOSITION

Hospitalization is required for patients who have ingested aliphatic hydrocarbons who are symptomatic at the time of evaluation. After a 6-h observation period, asymptomatic patients with a normal chest x-ray may be discharged home. Similar disposition of asymptomatic patients with abnormal chest x-rays has also been suggested if reliable follow-up can be ensured. However some physicians prefer to watch these patients for 24 h in the hospital. Hospitalization is advisable for those who ingest hydrocarbons capable of producing delayed complications (e.g., halogenated hydrocarbons causing hepatic toxicity) and those with toxic additives (organophosphates). All patients taking ingestions with suicidal intent or presenting with complications of solvent abuse should have psychiatric evaluation following medical clearance.

## BIBLIOGRAPHY

Algren JT, Rodgers GC: Intravascular hemolysis associated with hydrocarbon poisoning. *Pediatr Emerg Care* 8:34, 1992.

Anas N, Namasonthi V, Ginsburg CM: Criteria for hospitalizing children who have ingested products containing hydrocarbons. *JAMA* 246:840, 1981.

Bombassei GJ, Kaplan AA: The association between hydrocarbon exposure and anti-glomerular basement membrane antibody-mediated disease (Goodpasture's syndrome). *Am J Indust Med* 21:141, 1992.

Dice WH, Ward G, Kelly J, et al: Pulmonary toxicity following gastrointestinal ingestion of kerosene. *Ann Emerg Med* 11:138, 1982.

Gupta P, Singh RP, Murali MV, et al: Kerosene oil poisoning—a childhood menace. *Indian Pediatr* 29:979, 1992.

James NK, Moss AL: Review of burns caused by bitumen and the problems of its removal. *Burns* 16:214, 1990.

Leikin JB, Kaufman D, Lipscomb JW, Burda AM, Hryhorczuk DO: Methylene chloride: report of five exposures and two deaths. *Am J Emerg Med* 8:534, 1990.

Machado B, Cross K, Snodgrass WR: Accidental hydrocarbon ingestion cases telephoned to a regional poison center. *Ann Emerg Med* 17:804, 1988.

Nierenberg DW, Horowitz MB, Harris KM, James DH: Mineral spirits inhalation associated with hemolysis, pulmonary edema, and ventricular fibrillation. *Arch Intern Med* 151:1437, 1991.

Ruprah M, Mant TGK, Flanagan RJ: Acute carbon tetrachloride poisoning in 19 patients: implications for diagnosis and treatment. *Lancet* 1:1027, 1985.

Scalzo AJ, Weber TR, Jaeger RW, Connors RH, Thompson MW: Extracorporeal membrane oxygenation for hydrocarbon aspiration. *Am J Dis Child* 144:867, 1990.

Shepherd RT: Mechanism of death associated with volatile substance abuse. *Human Toxicology* 8:289, 1989.

Steele RW, Conklin RH, Mark HM: Corticosteroids and antibiotics for the treatment of fulminant hydrocarbon aspiration. *JAMA* 219:1434, 1972.

Streicher HZ, Gabow PA, Moss AT, et al: Syndromes of toluene sniffing in adults. *Ann Intern Med* 94:758, 1981.

# 154
# CAUSTIC INGESTIONS
## Monica Parraga
## Diane Sauter

Accidental and intentional exposure to caustic agents represents a significant source of morbidity and mortality. The most recent report from the American Association of Poison Control Centers Toxic Exposure Surveillance System documented approximately 10,000 exposures in 1993, with 136 major complications or deaths. Strong acids and bases can be found in both household and industrial settings. In the home, caustics represent a particularly serious danger for children who may sustain serious perioral, gastrointestinal, or cutaneous burns as a result of an accidental exposure. When ingested or spilled on the skin, caustic acids or bases may produce extensive tissue destruction and possibly death. Effective management requires aggressive but careful diagnostic and therapeutic intervention to minimize morbidity and maximize the probability of survival.

## PATHOPHYSIOLOGY OF ALKALINE BURNS

When ingested, alkaline agents, such as sodium hydroxide and potassium hydroxide, may result in severe injury to the gastrointestinal tract. With a pH of 12.5 or greater, they produce an injury described histologically as liquefaction necrosis. Solid alkali, when swallowed, tends to adhere to the mucous membranes of the oropharynx and esophagus, producing severe proximal burns. In contrast, liquid lye, a strong alkali found in household drain cleaners such as Drano, Liquid Plumr and Plunge is easier to swallow, tasteless, and odorless. It causes less damage to the oropharynx and greater damage to the esophagus. In addition, liquids, because of their high specific gravity,

can pass rapidly through the esophagus and reach the stomach, injuring tissue on contact.

Acutely, direct cellular destruction results from the saponification of fats and proteins. Blood vessels thrombose, resulting in further tissue necrosis and cellular death. This is followed in 2 to 3 days by the sloughing of a thin layer of necrotic tissue. If the acute injury is survived, a healing phase occurs between days 5 and 14 in which granulation tissue develops and collagen is deposited. During this period there is maximal softening of the injured tissue and, therefore, an increased risk of perforation. By day 21 following severe injuries, stricture formation begins, when the collagen contracts circumferentially and longitudinally.

Esophageal injury may result in a nonulcerative, mild or severe ulcerative esophagitis. Nonulcerative esophagitis is characterized by erythema, edema, and an intact mucous membrane. Mild ulcerative esophagitis is characterized by the presence of isolated areas of superficial ulceration with areas of vesiculation. Injuries that result in severe ulcerative esophagitis are characterized by total denudation of the esophageal epithelium and necrosis that may involve the entire esophageal wall and extend into underlying structures. Alkaline products do not directly produce systemic effects, apart from the systemic consequences of extensive tissue destruction.

Household bleaches are probably the most common caustic ingestant. Although perceived as moderately dangerous, household bleach (5% sodium hypochlorite) is not a strong caustic. When ingested, it may produce emesis, a burning sensation, and superficial mucosal erythema. Occasionally, following the ingestion of very large quantities of household bleach or following the ingestion of more highly concentrated industrial bleach, significant injury with strictures has resulted. In general, nothing more than symptomatic treatment is required, and most result in a favorable outcome. Ammonia or ammonium hydroxide and nonphosphate detergents, on the other hand, may produce serious injury with mucosal burns, ulceration, and sometimes full-thickness burns.

## PATHOPHYSIOLOGY OF ACID BURNS

Strong or corrosive acids are characterized by a pH of less than 2. Commonly ingested acids include sulfuric and hydrochloric acid, which may be found in household products such as toilet bowl cleaners and drain openers. The ingestion of acids occurs less frequently but results in a higher rate of complications and mortality. Acids produce coagulation necrosis and eschar formation, which allegedly protects underlying tissue from further caustic damage. On ingestion, acids have their major effect on the columnar epithelium of the stomach. The esophagus tends to be spared. This effect has been attributed to a rapid transit time through the esophagus and to the resistance of esophageal squamous epithelium to acid injury. Once the acid reaches the gastroesophageal junction it tends to follow the lesser curvature of the stomach, pooling in the antrum and eventually inducing pylorospasm and extensive antral damage. Destruction of the gastric mucosa and musculature results in edema, inflammation, the loss of glandular tissue and sometimes immediate or delayed hemorrhage. Eventually, if the initial injury is survived, fibrosis develops and may result in gastric outlet obstruction. Serious ingestions may result in complete gastric necrosis, hemorrhage, early perforation, and the destruction of adjacent structures. In addition, acids are well absorbed and may produce a profound systemic acidemia as well as massive hemolysis.

### Clinical Presentation

Acutely, patients who have ingested a strong acid or base may present with burns of the face, oropharyngeal pain, dysphagia, drooling, dyspnea, retching, or emesis. Hoarseness, stridor, and dyspnea are strong indicators of laryngeal and epiglottic edema. Esophageal injury is suggested by complaints of dysphagia and odynophagia. Intravascular volume depletion, resulting from the third spacing of fluids, vomiting or hemorrhage may result in hypotension or shock.

Acids cause immediate, severe pain in the oropharynx and are usually expelled rapidly following an accidental ingestion. Epigastric pain and retching develop initially, followed by intractable ulcer-type pain that is associated with vomiting. Hematemesis and melena are common sequelae. Acidemia and hemolysis are frequent accompaniments of large acid ingestions. Gastric perforation and the subsequent development of peritoneal involvement may become evident and must be watched for vigilantly.

The ingestion of solid alkaline agents will result in severe oropharyngeal pain. The mouth and pharynx may have a soapy white film over the mucosa that eventually becomes brown and edematous. Perforation of the esophagus can produce severe chest pain from subsequent chemical and later bacterial mediastinitis.

It is important to note that no constellation of signs and symptoms will accurately predict the presence or severity of esophageal injury. Recently, it has been demonstrated that the occurrence of two or more of the symptoms of stridor, drooling, or vomiting accurately predicts the presence of significant esophageal injury 50 percent of the time. The absence of visible lesions in the oropharynx cannot exclude visceral burns. The ingestion of strong acids has resulted in complete gastric necrosis and death in the absence of any demonstrable proximal injury. Although patients with significant injuries are very likely to be symptomatic, children and patients who are suicidal may inaccurately report the presence or absence of symptoms.

## Stabilization

Following a caustic ingestion, the initial management of the patient begins with stabilization. Health care workers must take precautions to ensure their own protection from exposure to the caustic agents on the patient's skin or in emesis or gastric aspirate. Airway obstruction secondary to oropharyngeal or laryngeal edema is the most life-threatening immediate sequela. Endotracheal intubation may be necessary for airway protection or for the prevention or treatment of upper airway obstruction. Ideally, intubation should be done under direct visualization, with the patient sedated or paralyzed to prevent additional soft tissue damage that inevitably results from the intubation of an agitated, uncooperative patient. If the treating physician is skilled in the use of fiberoptic laryngoscopy, intubation may be most safely accomplished over the laryngoscope. When the extent of soft tissue edema prevents the passage of an endotracheal tube, the patient may require a cricothyrotomy. Blind nasotracheal intubation is contraindicated because the tube may be passed through an area of necrotic tissue.

Following (or simultaneously with) airway management, two large-bore intravenous catheters need to be placed and an infusion of crystalloid begun. Blood specimens should be sent to the laboratory for an analysis of serum electrolytes and a complete blood count, type, and crossmatching. Profound hypovolemia may develop (as in the setting of a significant thermal burn) and should be treated with crystalloid, colloid, or blood products when indicated. Acid-base disorders, when clinically significant, need to be corrected. Most often, metabolic acidosis results from the ingestion of a strong acid. Following the ingestion of sulfuric, phosphoric, or acetic acid, the disorder will be an anion gap metabolic acidosis due to the absorption of hydrogen and the respective anions. Following the ingestion of hydrochloric acid, and in the absence of a significant lactic acidosis, a nonanion gap metabolioc acidosis will result from the systemic absorption of hydrogen and chloride ions. Difference of opinion exists regarding the indication for the treatment of a metabolic acidosis. Although some practitioners would treat a pH of 7.2, most physicians would agree that a pH of less than 7.1 is an indication for the judicious intravenous administration of sodium bicarbonate. An in-depth discussion of this issue may be found elsewhere.

## Gastric Decontamination

Dilution with water or milk is controversial. The administration of a diluent may cause vomiting, leading to repeated exposure of esophageal and oropharyngeal tissues to the caustic, thus exacerbating damage. Dilution is contraindicated prior to airway interventions in patients with acute or impending airway obstruction. In addition, dilution should not be attempted in patients with clinical signs of esophageal or gastric perforation. Dilution with milk will make it impossible to visualize tissues by endoscopy. Neutralization of an acid or a base is not recommended because the heat of neutralization may result in additional thermal injury to already damaged tissues. Ipecac is absolutely contraindicated because emesis will expose the oropharyngeal and esophageal tissues to a repeated caustic insult. The blind passage of a nasogastric tube is not recommended and in the setting of an alkaline injury is contraindicated. The risk of perforating an area of compromised and fragile tissue is great. Because alkaline ingestions are not associated with systemic effects (in contrast to acid ingestions), the benefits of gastric evacuation do not clearly outweigh this risk. Some authors advocate the blind passage of a small soft feeding tube for gastric aspiration in patients who have ingested large amounts of acid. These authors argue that the eschar formation that accompanies acid ingestions protects the underlying tissues so the risk of iatrogenic perforation is small. In addition, the elimination of the acid from the stomach may prevent or ameliorate the systemic consequences of acid ingestion and minimize tissue damage. This recommendation is controversial, however, and no good clinical data exist to support this practice. Under direct visualization, however, insertion of a nasogastric tube may serve several purposes such as the removal of caustic materials, the measurement of gastric pH and maintenance of esophageal lumen patency. Patients with clinical evidence of perforation (peritoneal findings on physical examination) are best managed by surgical intervention. Caustics will not be bound by activated charcoal, and it, therefore, has no utility in this setting.

An upright chest radiograph is essential because it may provide evidence of the presence of a gastric or esophageal perforation. In addition, a chest radiograph may provide the findings of an aspiration pneumonitis. Ocular, cutaneous, and oral burns must not be overlooked. All require irrigation with copious amounts of normal saline until a physiologic pH is achieved.

Prior to further evaluation or diagnostic testing, a directed history and physical examination should be completed. Product identification, when possible, is extremely helpful and allows health care workers to form judgments about the likely quality and extent of damage and will help in the anticipation of potential complications.

## DIAGNOSTICS

### Endoscopy

It is well recognized that the presence or absence of oropharyngeal lesions cannot be used to accurately predict the pattern or extent of esophageal pathology. Ten to 30 percent of patients with esophageal burns have no identifiable oropharyngeal lesions. Endoscopy is the most reliable and accurate method for the evaluation of esophageal injury. It has value in the identification of injuries that require pharmacologic intervention (such as the administration of steroids and antibiotics), as well as esophageal or gastric perforations that require immediate surgical intervention. The procedure should be performed on all patients with a history of caustic ingestion. Endoscopy should be accomplished as early as possible following stabilization, and certainly within the first 12 to 24 h. Caustic burns may be classified by their gross endoscopic appearance in terms of depth and extent. First-degree burns are characterized by superficial hyperemia, mucosal edema, and areas of superficial mucosal epithelial sloughing. Second-degree burns involve damage to deeper layers. Typically, transmucosal injury with white exudative ulcerations is evident. Third-degree burns involve the entire esophageal wall and possibly penetrate to involve adjacent structures. The pattern of caustic burns may be linear and streaky or patchy and circumferential. Gross perforation may be apparent.

The standard recommendation has been to advance the endoscope only as far as the first circumferential second-degree burn or any third-degree burn because the risk of iatrogenic perforation is felt to be high. Some authors advocate the complete evaluation of the esophagus and stomach using a flexible endoscope until an area of obvious necrosis is identified. If frank necrosis is identified, many authors advocate surgical intervention to evaluate the extent of injury and to remove dead tissue. The presence of esophageal or gastric burns is an indication for hospitalization. Patients should have nothing by mouth. Repeated endoscopy during the first 2 to 3 days is helpful in the identification of progressive injury requiring surgical intervention. In addition, it also allows for the insertion of stents, strings, and feeding tubes that may help maintain esophageal lumen patency while healing occurs. Endoscopy should be avoided from the fifth day until one and one half weeks following ingestion. At this time the risk of perforation increases due to wound softening that occurs as healing progresses. Endoscopy is contraindicated in patients with necrosis of the pharynx or in patients in respiratory distress who have not undergone airway management.

### Radiographic Contrast Imaging

Contrast-enhanced visualization of the esophagus is not recommended in the initial evaluation of esophageal or gastric burns. Most authors agree that these studies are rarely sensitive enough for the detection of mucosal injuries. Some features of injury evident from esophagrams are the intramucosal retention of contrast material and gaseous dilatation of esophagus due to air trapping. The blurring of mucosal margins, linear streaking of contrast material and abnormal displacement of the pleural reflection may be seen. Following the third week postingestion, serial barium swallows will identify the development of strictures.

## MANAGEMENT
### Steroids and Antibiotics

Evidence in support of the use of steroids for the prevention of stricture formation following significant caustic ingestions is somewhat controversial. Steroids are believed to prevent stricture formation by inhibiting the degree of fibroplasia. Adequately controlled clinical trials to prove the efficacy of steroids have not been performed. However, animal studies support their use. In general, first-degree burns of the esophagus will heal completely without stricture formation and, therefore, steroid use is not indicated. Third-degree burns are felt to consistently result in stricture formation. However, the additional risk of immune supression, wound softening with perforation, and bacterial invasion that occurs secondary to steroid use is very significant and probably not justified. Steroid use is recommended by many authors for patients with circumferential second-degree burns because it is felt that the risk of perforation is lower in these patients but the benefits of reduced scar formation are greater. The use of steroids may increase the risk of bacterial invasion and mask infection, so antibiotics are always recommended in conjunction with steroids. Contraindications for the use of steroids include signs of infection, perforation, or gastrointestinal bleeding. Treatment will only have benefit when initiated within 48 h of ingestion. The dosage of methyl prednisolone is 40 mg q8h for 2 to 3 weeks followed by a 6-week taper. The antibiotics of choice include penicillin 12 million units or ampicillin 8 to 12 g intravenously over 24 h in divided doses. Other antibiotics may include clindamycin, vanomycin, or tetracycline. If steroids are not used, antibiotics are recommended only if signs of infection develop.

Additional treatment for esophageal strictures is undergoing further study. Substances with lathyrogenic properties have been reported to prevent stricture formation in animals. β-Aminopropionitrile inhibits intermolecular covalent cross-linking in newly formed collagen and decreases the tensile strength of scar tissue. Penicillamine has also been used experimentally in animal studies. It inhibits lysine-derived aldehyde groups and prevents the cross-bonding of collagen. Currently, these treatments are not available or recommended for human use.

### Delayed Complications

The most common delayed complication secondary to lye ingestions is stricture formation. Strictures are usually the result of second- and third-degree burns. Patients may become symptomatic with signs of gradual esophageal obstruction between 3 weeks and 1 year postingestion. Acid burns may result in gastric outlet obstruction. Symptoms of early satiety and weight loss occur and may develop any time after the first 6 weeks or several years following ingestion. Esophageal carcinoma has been reported to be a late complication of lye ingestion with an average latency period of 40 years. The incidence of esophageal carcinoma is reported to be 1,000 times that of the general population.

### Dilatation

The use of bougienage to treat stricture formation in the esophagus following caustic ingestion is controversial. Prophylactic bougienage has been started as early as the week following ingestion. However, many authors believe that dilatation prior to the third week following ingestion is contraindicated because the risk of trauma and perforation is high. If stricture formation is apparent, steroid administration may be reduced and dilatation begun cautiously. Strictures of moderate degree may be dilated successfully by antegrade bougienage. In patients with more severe stricture formation, retrograde dilatation using an indwelling string is considered by some the safest and most successful method, but it requires a gastrostomy. Strictures that do not respond to dilatation may require surgical reconstruction and colonic interposition. Surgical management at this point is controversial. Many authors advocate esophagectomy and colonic interposition as prophylaxis against the later development of esophageal carcinoma. Some believe that the risk of thoracotomy and resection of the esophagus is greater than that of the development of esophageal carcinoma.

## OTHER CAUSTIC AGENTS
### Clinitest Tablets

Clinitest tablets, which are used by some diabetic patients to test urine for ketones, contain caustic chemicals including copper sulfate 20 mg, citric acid 300 mg, sodium hydroxide 232.5 mg, and sodium bicarbonate 80 mg. The sodium hydroxide in each tablet provides the strongly basic pH required for its reducing action. The tablets are approximately the same size and shape as a tablet of acetaminophen or salicylate. Patients often keep bottles of Clinitest tablets in the medicine cabinet alongside other over-the-counter products. Occasionally an error results in the accidental ingestion of Clinitest tablets, most frequently by children, but adults have also made this error. Full-thickness burns of the esophagus and esophageal strictures have resulted. The preferred treatment is dilution with cold milk or water to decrease the causticity and to absorb the heats of solution and neutralization. Management recommendations include stabilization as described above, esophagoscopy, with further management decisions based on the results.

## Button Batteries

Button batteries are an occasional source of foreign body ingestion, most frequently by children, but occasionally by adults. The chemical composition of the batteries is variable, but they may contain potassium or sodium hydroxide, and salts of mercury, zinc, or other metals. A knowledge of the diameter of the battery and the identification of the chemical system is helpful in patient management. Batteries with a diameter of greater than 15 mm usually contain mercuric oxide. Following ingestion, most batteries pass uneventfully through the gastrointestinal (GI) tract. However, if the battery becomes impacted in the esophagus, at some other site, or aspirated into a bronchus, it must be removed. The impacted battery can produce a local pressure necrosis. Furthermore, if the battery opens, the leakage of alkali can result in an area of liquefaction necrosis with subsequent perforation. In addition, the systemic absorption of heavy metal salts can occur and is of concern.

On presentation, radiographs should be done to identify the position of the ingested battery. Batteries that have passed beyond the esophagus need not be removed unless the patient develops signs of necrosis, obstruction, or hemorrhage. Patients with batteries lodged in the esophagus may develop dysphagia, vomiting, anorexia, or fever. Batteries lodged in the GI tract, and batteries that have split open, need to be removed emergently, either surgically or endoscopically. Recently, the use of endoscopes with magnetized probes and drugs that decrease esophageal tone have been used to dislodge these batteries. Syrup of ipecac has not been shown to be effective and may encourage aspiration of the battery. Follow-up radiographs are necessary only to confirm passage of the button battery. Confirmation by inspection of the stools is preferred, however, because it eliminates the need to perform additional abdominal radiography. Mercury levels in blood and urine need only be followed if the battery splits open. Although elevated blood mercury levels have been found in this setting, no case has been reported in which chelation has been necessary.

## Hydrofluoric Acid

Hydrofluoric (HF) acid is an inorganic compound used widely in industry and in some household products. Fluorine compounds are found in plastics, germicides, dyes, fire-proofing materials, and resins. In addition, HF acid is used in the pickling of stainless steel; the polishing of metal; the polishing, etching, and frosting of glass; in making rust removers; and in manufacturing semiconductors. It is found in solutions of various concentrations ranging from 20% to 70%. It is highly toxic, producing severe injury to exposed tissues as well as significant and potentially lethal systemic effects. Exposure to the skin, eyes, or respiratory system may result in extensive burns and death from tissue destruction or the systemic effects of hypocalcemia, hypomagnesemia, and other electrolyte abnormalities.

## Pathophysiology

Hydrofluoric acid is a weak acid when compared with other mineral acids. It is poorly dissociated in solution and produces less free hydrogen ion than other acids of equimolar solutions. HF acid exposure results in the desiccation of skin and severe local tissue injury. Because it is relatively nonpolar, it is highly lipophilic. It therefore readily crosses cell membranes and penetrates deeply. The fluoride ion dissociates slowly and is responsible for much of the tissue destruction. It has a strong affinity for positively charged ions and is not neutralized until contact with calcium or other cations occurs. Insoluble calcium fluoride and magnesium fluoride salts are formed. The removal of these essential ions from biologic systems interferes with the electrical activity of cellular membranes and disrupts cellular metabolism. As fluoride ion penetrates more deeply, bony destruction occurs through the interaction of fluoride ion with the calcium of bone. In addition, the absorption of fluoride ion can have significant systemic effects. Death from profound hypocalcemia has been reported following the exposure of a relatively small skin area (< 2.5 percent total body surface area) to a highly concentrated solution.

Because HF exposure most frequently occurs in an occupational setting, patients frequently present with complaints of burns to the hand and nail bed. HF acid will penetrate pin holes in rubber gloves. Exposure of the nail plate will result in the penetration of subungual tissue. The patient may complain of excruciating pain, throbbing and burning in character. Early following exposure to relatively dilute solutions, there may be pain but no gross evidence of injury to the tissues. Pallor of the exposed skin or sometimes mild erythema may be evident on presentation. Typically, the physical findings are so unimpressive that the significance of the injury is missed initially. Unless the physician is careful to elicit the source of the exposure, the patient may be discharged without appropriate treatment only to return with necrosis of the involved tissue. The intensity and rapidity of onset of the signs and symptoms varies with the concentration of the acid and the duration of contact. Solutions of 50% to 70% concentration will produce immediate signs and symptoms, whereas solutions with concentrations of 20% or less will produce signs and symptoms up to 12 h later.

Burns secondary to exposure to highly concentrated HF acid will progress to complete necrosis of the involved area unless treated correctly. The affected skin will become firmly edematous and pasty white with vesiculation. The vesicles may appear cloudy and usually contain caseous material which is necrotic tissue. The burns may progress to ulceration with full thickness tissue loss.

## Management

Prior to arrival in the emergency department, initial management of a cutaneous exposure involves the removal of saturated clothing and copious irrigation of the affected area with water. This should be followed by immersion of the affected part in an iced solution of magnesium sulfate, calcium salts, or a high molecular weight quarternary ammonium compound (benzethonium chloride). The cold constricts lymph and blood vessels, retarding the diffusion of fluoride ions. The cations bind with fluoride to produce a nonionized complex preventing further tissue penetration. Care must be taken not to produce a superimposed thermal injury.

Initial emergency department management includes stabilization as described previously. Cardiac monitoring and routine laboratory studies and are essential. A 12-lead electrocardiogram (ECG) will be valuable initially. In particular, the QT interval should be inspected for evidence of the lengthening that occurs with various electrolyte disturbances. In addition, the physician should look carefully for ECG evidence of hyperkalemia. Systemic acidosis, hypocalcemia, hypomagnesemia, and hyperkalemia are common potentially lethal complications of exposure to highly concentrated HF.

Successful therapy for mild HF acid burns may be accomplished with the topical application of a 2.5% calcium gluconate gel. The gel can be made by mixing 3.5 g calcium gluconate with 5 oz of water-soluble lubricant. The gel may be placed in a surgical glove and used to cover the affected part. If the patient experiences relief from pain, remains pain free, and the burn does not appear to progress, no more aggressive treatment is required. If involvement of the nail bed is suspected, the nail must be removed and the nail bed treated as the rest of the skin. Burns not responding to topical treatment and severe burns may require intradermal injection with 10% calcium gluconate. A 30-gauge needle should be used for intradermal injections. No more than 5 mL of 10% calcium gluconate per square centimeter of tissue should be injected into the affected area. Pain relief is the end point of treatment. Recurrence of pain is an indication for additional treatment. Intradermal injections of the hand and fingers requires the infiltration of limited amounts of volume as vascular compromise may occur and result in further necrosis. Calcium chloride should never be used intradermally because it causes tissue necrosis.

An alternative to intradermal calcium gluconate or magnesium sulfate injection is the intra-arterial perfusion of calcium gluconate. This type of therapy is effective if the area of exposure is an area with a discreet vascular supply, such as a digit. Placement of an intra-arterial catheter proximal to the site of injury (radial, ulnar, or brachial arteries) is performed. Proper placement of the catheter is confirmed by blood flow and pressure tracing or by angiography. An infusion of 10 mL of 10% calcium gluconate diluted in 40 to 50 mL of 5% dextrose is given over 4 h. Calcium chloride solutions have also been used effectively; however, they are not recommended by most authors because extravasation of solution will result in tissue necrosis at the site. Patients may require multiple treatments. This mode of treatment has significant advantages over intradermal injections. Selective arterial perfusion avoids the need to remove the fingernail and avoids the pressure necrosis that may result from the injection of liquid into a closed space. In addition, it provides a greater concentration of calcium to the affected area. The disadvantages of intra-arterial infusion include the requirement for hospitalization and the risk of arterial spasm or thrombosis. Following either mode of treatment, the serum calcium must be carefully monitored.

Ocular exposure to HF acid results in the rapid onset of pain, tearing, conjunctival inflammation, corneal opacification, and erosion. An immediate single irrigation with normal saline or water for 15 min is thought to be appropriate intervention. Injections of calcium gluconate or magnesium sulfate are very toxic to the eye and increase the risk for corneal ulceration. There is now evidence that repeated instillation of 1% calcium gluconate drops may be efficacious in the treatment of ocular burns. All patients with an ocular exposure to HF acid require a consultation with an ophthalmologist.

Patients who ingest HF acid will develop gastrointestinal symptoms, nausea, vomiting, and sometimes hemorrhage. Oral ingestions of HF acid require the administration of calcium or magnesium salts. Ideally, the magnesium or calcium should be given on a milliequivalent-for-milliequivalent basis. Although it is usually impossible to know the amount of ingested HF acid, an attempt must be made to get a reasonable estimate from the historical data. Otherwise, 300 mL magnesium citrate or calcium salts can be given empirically. Ipecac is contraindicated in this setting. Therapy should be initiated quickly because the ingestion of HF acid often results in death.

Inhalation burns with very concentrated or anhydrous fluoride may result in a compromised airway, systemic fluorosis, delayed pulmonary edema, electrolyte abnormalities, and arrhythmias. Following the inhalation of HF acid, the patient must be moved to an uncontaminated area, the airway must be protected, 100% oxygen administered, and treatment begun with bronchodilators and systemic steroids as indicated. Nebulized 2.5% calcium gluconate has been recommended; however, insufficient studies exist in support of its use. The prognosis following fluoride inhalation is poor.

## BIBLIOGRAPHY

Anderson, KD, Rause T, Randolph JG. A controlled trial of corticosteroids in children with corrosive injury of esophagus. *N Engl J Med* 323:637, 1990.

Gorman RL, Khin-Maung-Gyi MT, Klein-Schwartz W, et al. Initial symptoms as predictors of esophageal injury in alkaline corrosive injections. *Am J Med* 10:189, 1992.

Hoffman RS. Caustics and batteries. In: Goldfrank LR, Flomenbaum NE, Lewin NA, Weisman RS, Howland MA, Hoffman RS (eds). *Goldfrank's Toxicologic Emergencies*, 5th ed. Norwalk, CT: Appleton & Lange, pp. 1245–1260, 1994.

Homan CS, Maitra SR, Lane BP, Geller ER. Effective treatment of acute alkali injury of the rat esophagus with early saline dilution therapy. *Ann Emerg Med* 22:178, 1993.

Homan CS, Maitra SR, Lane BP, Thode HC, Sable M. Therapeutic effects of water and milk for acute alkali injury of the esophagus: *Ann Emerg Med* 24:14, 1994.

Howell JM, Daisey WC, Hartsell TW, Butzin CA. Steroids for the treatment of corrosive esophageal injury: a statistical analysis of past studies. *Am J Emerg Med* 10:421, 1992.

Litovitz TL, Clark LR, Soloway RA. 1993 Annual Report of the American Association of Poison Control Centers toxic exposure surveillance system. *Am J Emerg Med* 12:546, 1994.

Previtera C, Guisti F, Guglielmi M. Predictive value of visible lesions (cheeks, lips, oropharynx) in suspected caustic ingestion: may endoscopy reasonably be omitted in completely negative pediatric patients? *Pediatr Emerg Care* 6:176, 1990.

Zargar SA, Kochhar R, Mehta SK. The role of fiberoptic endoscopy in the management of corrosive ingestion and modified endoscopic classification of burns. *Gastrointest Endosc* 37:165, 1991.

### Button Batteries

Kulig K, Rumack C, Rumack B, Duff XJ. Disk battery ingestion: elevated urine mercury levels and enema removal of battery fragments. *JAMA* 249:2502, 1983.

Litovitz T, Schmitz BF: Ingestion of cylindrical and button batteries: an analysis of 2382 cases. *Pediatrics* 89:747, 1992.

### Hydrofluoric Acid

Bentur Y, Tannebaum S, Yaffe Y, Halpert M. The role of calcium gluconate in the treatment of hydrofluoric acid eye burn. *Ann Emerg Med* 22:161, 1993.

Burkhart KK, Brent J, Kirk MA, Baker DC, Kulig KN. Comparison of topical magnesium and calcium treatment for dermal hydrofluoric acid burns. *Ann Emerg Med* 24:9, 1994.

Caravati EM. Acute hydrofluoric acid exposure. *Ann J Emerg Med* 6:143, 1988.

Konok, Yoshida Y, Watanabe M, et al. An experimental study on the treatment of hydrofluoric acid burns. *Arch Environ Contam Toxicol* 22:414, 1992.

Seigal DC, Heard JM. Intra-arterial calcium infusion for hydrofluoric acid burns. *Aviat Space Environ Med* 63:206, 1992.

Vance MV, Curry SC, Kunkel DB, Ryan PS, Ruggeri SB. Digital hydrofluoric acid burns: treatment with intra-arterial calcium infusion. *Ann Emerg Med* 15:890, 1986.

## 155
# ORGANOPHOSPHATE AND CARBAMATE POISONING
### James Roberts
### John Tafuri

There are two major classes of insecticides—the organophosphates and the carbamates. The organophosphate compounds are most commonly associated with serious human toxicity, accounting for over 80 percent of pesticide-related hospitalizations. The more toxic chlorinated hydrocarbon compounds, such as DDT, heptachlor, chlordane, and Kepone, were commonly used in the past but these compounds have been banned from private or commercial use. Organophosphate and carbamate insecticides have become increasingly popular for both agricultural and home use because their unstable chemical structure leads to rapid hydrolysis into harmless compounds with little long-term accumulation in the environment. This widespread use, however, has resulted in increased numbers of human poisonings.

Potent organophosphates are the principal toxins found in some nerve gases used in chemical warfare (soman, VX, and others).

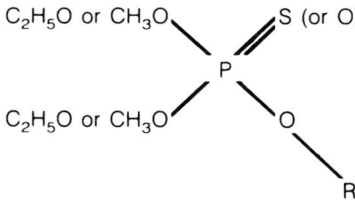

**Fig. 155-1.** The general chemical structure of organophosphates. (From Tafuri J, Roberts J: Organophosphate poisoning. *Ann Emerg Med* 16:193, 1987, with permission.)

## PATHOPHYSIOLOGY

Organophosphate insecticides are a class of compounds that avidly and permanently bind to cholinesterase molecules and share a similar chemical structure (Fig. 155-1). Carbamates exhibit similar pathophysiology except that they form a reversible bond with cholinesterase. A list of common commercial organophosphate insecticides is included in Table 155-1, and common carbamate insecticides are given in Table 155-2. Unless otherwise specified, all comments in the following discussion about organophosphates apply to carbamates as well.

Acetylcholine is present throughout the autonomic and central nervous systems, functioning as a chemical neurotransmitter at pre- and postganglionic parasympathetic synapses, preganglionic sympathetic synapses, and at the neuromuscular junction (Fig. 155-2). Normally, cholinesterases rapidly hydrolyze acetylcholine into inactive fragments of choline and acetic acid after the completion of neurochemical transmission. The two principal cholinesterases are erythrocyte (RBC) or true cholinesterase (acetylcholinesterase), and serum cholinesterase (pseudocholinesterase), which is present in plasma, liver, heart, pancreas, and brain tissue. The major toxicity of organophosphates is related to the covalent binding of the insecticide's phosphate radicals to the active sites of the cholinesterases, transforming the cholinesterases into enzymatically inert proteins. Organophosphates act as irreversible cholinesterase inhibitors. The organophosphate–cholinesterase bond is not spontaneously reversible without pharmacologic intervention and after 24 to 48 h of continuous binding, cholinesterase is irreversibly destroyed. The carbamate–cholinesterase bond reverses spontaneously in 4 to 8 h, yielding a normal cholinesterase molecule.

The inhibition of cholinesterase activity leads to the excess accumulation of acetylcholine at synapses. This causes initial overstimulation (cholinergic crisis) and subsequently paralysis of neurotransmission in both the central and peripheral nervous systems where acetylcholine serves as a neurotransmitter, leading to a variety of physiologic and metabolic derangements. Exposure to cholinesterase inhibitors will, therefore, interfere with synaptic transmission in the central nervous system and peripherally at both the muscarinic neuroeffector junctions (postganglionic parasympathetic nerve endings) and nicotinic receptors (autonomic ganglia and skeletal myoneural junctions).

Organophosphates and carbamates produce a similar clinical spectrum of poisoning and have identical pathophysiologic mechanisms. However, the carbamates are considered less toxic and have poor CNS penetration. Generally, the carbamates produce a similar but shorter and more benign clinical course.

## EXPOSURE

The mode of contact in organophosphate and carbamate poisoning may be quite variable, as these compounds are absorbed efficiently by oral, dermal, conjunctival, gastrointestinal, and respiratory routes. Poisoning commonly occurs as a result of agricultural use, accidental exposure, suicide, and, rarely, homicide. There have been numerous

**Table 155-1.** Common Commercial Organophosphate Insecticides*

| Highly Toxic | Moderately Toxic |
|---|---|
| TEPP | Bromophos-ethyl (Nexagan) |
| Phorate (Thimet) | Leptophos (Phosvel) |
| Disulfoton (Di-Syston) | Dichlorvos (DDVP, Vapona) |
| Fensulfothion (Dasanit) | Coumaphos (Co-Ral) |
| Demeton (Systox) | Ethoprop (Mocap) |
| Terbufos (Counter) | Quinalphos (Bayrusil) |
| Mevinphos (Phosdrin) | Triazophos (Hostathion) |
| Methidathion (Supracide) | Demeton-methyl (Metasystox) |
| Chlormephos (Dotan) | Propetamphos (Safrotin) |
| Sulfotepp (Bladafum) | Chlorpyrifos (Lorsban) |
| Chlorthiophos (Celathion) | Dioxanthion (Delnav) |
| Monocrotophos (Azodrin) | Isoxathion (Karphos) |
| Fonofos (Dyfonate) | Phosalone (Zolone) |
| Prothoate (Fac) | Thiometon (Ekatin) |
| Fenamiphos (Nemacur) | Heptenophos (Hostaquick) |
| Phosfolan (Cyolane) | Crotoxyphos (Ciodrin) |
| Methyl parathion (Dalf) | Cythioate (Proban) |
| Schradan (OMPA) | Phencapton (G28029) |
| Chlorfenvinphos (Birlane) | DEF (De-Green, E-Z-off D) |
| Ethyl parathion (Parathion) | Ethion |
| Azinphos-methyl (Guthion) | Dimethoate (Cygon, De-Fend) |
| Phosphamidon (Dimecron) | Fenthion (Baytex, Entex) |
| Methamidophos (Monitor) | Dichlorfenthion (Mobilawn) |
| Dicrotophos (Bidrin) | EPBP (S-Seven) |
| Isofenphos (Amaze, Oftanol) | Diazinon (Spectacide) |
| Bomyl (Swat) | Phosmet (Imidan, Prolate) |
| Carbophenothion (Trithion) | Formothion (Anthio) |
| EPN | Profenfos (Curacron) |
| Famphur (Warbex, Bo-Ana) | Naled (Dibrom) |
| Fenophosphon (Agritox) | Phenthoate |
| Dialifor (Torak) | Trichlorfon (Dylox, Dipterex) |
| Cyanofenphos (Surecide) | Pyrazophos (Afugan, Curamil) |
| | Fenitrothion (Agrothion) |
| | Cyanphos (Cyanox) |
| | Pyridaphenthion (Ofunack) |
| | Propylthiopyrophosphate (Aspon) |
| | Acephate (Orthene) |
| | Merphos (Folex) |
| | Malathion (Cythion) |
| | Etrimfox (Ekamet) |
| | Phoxim (Baython) |
| | Pirimiphosmethyl (Actellic) |
| | Iodofenphos (Nuvanol-N) |
| | Bromophos (Nexion) |
| | Tetrachlorvinphos (Gardona, Rabon) |
| | Temephos (Abate, Abathion) |

* Compounds are listed in order of decreasing toxicity. "Highly toxic" compounds have listed LD50 values of less than 50 mg/kg in the rat.
*Source:* Modified from Morgan DP: *Recognition and management of pesticide poisonings.* U.S. Government Printing Office, Washington, D.C., 1982.

reports of agricultural worker contamination after application on crops, and less frequently among industrial workers who are involved in the manufacture or transport of these chemicals. Nonagricultural workers also have been poisoned after working in areas recently treated for insect control. Low-grade chronic organophosphate poisoning has been reported in pet groomers who are exposed to flea-dip products and in workers who wear clothing contaminated with the insecticide. Children are frequently poisoned while playing in areas re-

**Table 155-2.** Carbamate Insecticides

| | |
|---|---|
| Aldicarb (Temik) | Mexacarbate (Zectran) |
| Aminocarb (Matacil) | Methiocarb (Mesurol) |
| Oxamyl (Vydate) | Dimetilan (Snip, Snipfly) |
| Isolan (Isolan) | Propoxur (Baygon) |
| Carbofuran (Furadan) | Carbaryl (Sevin) |
| Methomyl (Lannate) | |

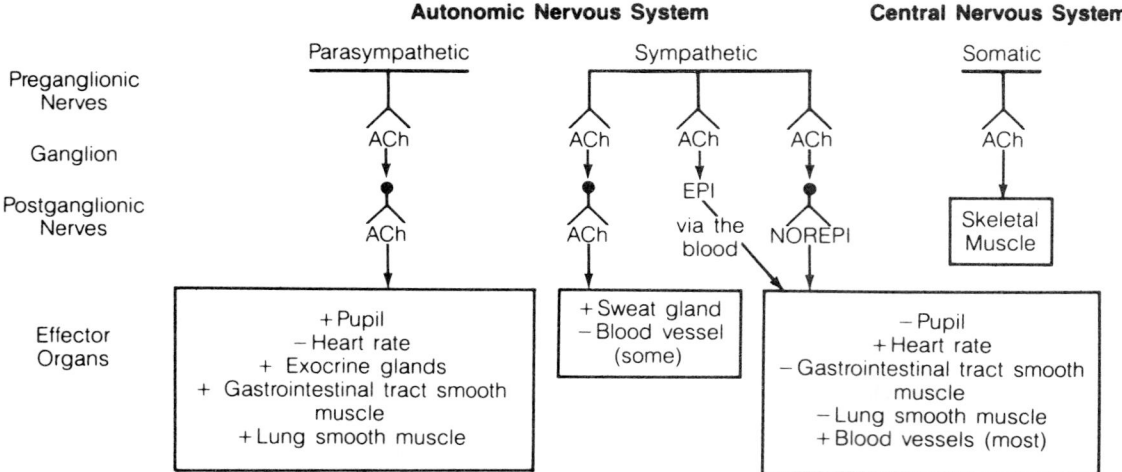

**Fig. 155-2.** Schematic representation of the human peripheral nervous system. Hyperstimulation of peripheral nerves during organophosphate intoxication will occur at *all* synapses where the neurotransmitter acetylcholine (ACh) is present, including the parasympathetic and somatic divisions. Parasympathetic stimulation will cause miosis, bradycardia, secretion of the exocrine glands (lacrimal, salivary, bronchial, and pancreatic), hyperactivity of GI smooth muscle, and bronchoconstriction. Sympathetic cholinergic stimulation will cause diaphoresis and perhaps vasodilation within skeletal muscle. Sympathetic adrenergic stimulation, mediated by cholinergic sympathetic ganglia, produces mydriasis, tachycardia, vasoconstriction of blood vessels, slowing of GI motor activity, and bronchodilation. The degree to which either the sympathetic or parasympathetic system will predominate during organophosphate intoxication depends on the type and dose of organophosphate, rate of absorption, and individual physiologic factors. (EPI, epinephrine; NOREPI, norepinephrine.) (From Tafuri J, Roberts J: Organophosphate poisoning. *Ann Emerg Med* 16:193, 1987, with permission.)

cently treated with organophosphates. Suicide is the most common mode of serious contamination, followed by accidental agricultural and industrial contacts and accidental poisoning of children within the home. Mass poisoning secondary to widespread food contamination also has been observed in India, Colombia, Egypt, Singapore, and Mexico. The organophosphates in nerve gases are effectively absorbed through the skin and respiratory tract.

The onset of the signs and symptoms of poisoning will vary with the route and degree of exposure; however, the time interval between exposure and symptoms generally is less than 12 to 24 h. Nerve gases may produce symptoms within seconds of inhalation. It should be noted, however, that certain newer, more lipid-soluble organophosphates, such as dichlorfenthion and fenthion, may not produce cholinergic crisis for up to several days, and symptoms may persist for up to several weeks to months with periodic relapses despite adequate therapy, probably because of initial lipid storage and subsequent redistribution. Low-grade chronic exposure is associated with the insidious onset of many vague and ill-defined symptoms (headache, fatigue, GI upset).

## CLINICAL PRESENTATION

In mild to moderate poisoning with a cholinesterase-inhibiting agent, the patient will initially be alert and oriented and will complain of a variety of symptoms including headache, dizziness, blurred vision, weakness, incoordination, muscle fasciculation, tremor, diarrhea, abdominal cramping, and occasionally chest tightness, wheezing, and a productive cough (Tables 155-3 and 155-5). Any episodes of incontinence, convulsions, or altered mental status are indicative of severe poisoning. Symptoms from a single moderate dose exposure may persist for weeks after initial contact. Chronic intermediate dose exposure may be manifested as nonspecific symptoms including weakness, fatigue, malaise, anorexia, and neurobehavioral abnormalities.

Signs and symptoms may be more conveniently understood by differentiating them into the effect of cholinergic excess as it relates to overstimulation of muscarinic, nicotinic, and CNS receptors (Table 155-4). *Muscarinic* overstimulation is manifested as hyperactivity of the parasympathetic system, including miosis; hypersecretion of the

salivary, lacrimal, and bronchial glands; bronchoconstriction; nausea; vomiting; diarrhea; urinary and fecal incontinence; and bradycardia. This syndrome is often referred to as SLUDGE (*s*alivation, *l*acrimation, *u*rination, *d*iarrhea, *g*astrointestinal, *e*mesis). The *nicotinic* effects include muscle fasciculations, cramping, and muscle weakness. In addition, overstimulation of the nicotinic receptors in the sympathetic ganglia may overwhelm parasympathetic stimulation and produce tachycardia, hypertension, and stimulation of the adrenal medulla. Many authors consider miosis and muscle fasciculations to be the most reliable clinical signs of organophosphate toxicity. Cholinergic excess in the *central nervous system* (CNS) produces varying degrees of delirium, confusion, coma, and seizure activity. The usual cause of death is respiratory failure, which is due to a combination of depression of the CNS respiratory center, weakness of the respiratory muscles, and increased bronchial secretions.

## LABORATORY FINDINGS

Routine laboratory studies are nondiagnostic of organophosphate or carbamate poisoning and are typically unremarkable with several occasional exceptions: Nonketotic hyperglycemia, hypokalemia, leukocytosis (both with and without a left shift), elevated serum amylase, glycosuria, and proteinuria are not uncommon findings (Table 155-3). A chest radiograph is usually unremarkable but may reveal evidence of pulmonary edema in severe cases.

From a pathophysiologic standpoint, one might expect bradycardia to be a universal finding due to vagal (parasympathetic) stimulation by excess acetylcholine. However, since the nicotinic receptors (autonomic ganglia) are also stimulated, there may be a combination of both parasympathetic and sympathetic responses, and some patients (especially children) may exhibit tachycardia. The ECG may display a variety of abnormalities in acute organophosphate poisoning. Idioventricular rhythms, multiform ventricular extrasystoles, ventricular tachycardia, torsade de pointes, ventricular fibrillation, complete heart block, and asystole have been reported. Classically, cardiac arrhythmias in organophosphate poisoning consist of two phases: first, a transient phase of intense sympathetic tone causing sinus tachycardia, followed by a second phase of extreme parasympathetic tone

**Table 155-3.** Incidence of Clinical and Laboratory Features in Acute Organophosphate Poisoning

| Symptom | Whorton, % | MMWR, % |
|---|---|---|
| Weakness | 100 | 28 |
| Blurred vision | 100 | 48 |
| Nausea | 100 | 38 |
| Headache | 79 | 48 |
| Vomiting | 63 | — |
| Abdominal pain | 58 | — |
| Dizziness | 58 | 41 |
| Night sweats | 37 | 7 |
| Collapse | 11 | — |
| Eye irritation | — | 76 |
| Chest pain/SOB | — | 21 |
| Skin irritation | — | 17 |
| Diarrhea | — | 7 |

| Sign | Hayes, % |
|---|---|
| Constricted pupils | 85 |
| Vomiting | 59 |
| Salivation excess | 58 |
| Respiratory distress | 48 |
| Abdominal pain | 42 |
| Depressed level of consciousness | 42 |
| Muscle fasciculation | 40 |
| Diarrhea | 37 |
| Diaphoresis | 26 |
| Pyrexia | 24 |
| Muscle weakness | 23 |
| Tachypnea | 22 |
| Tachycardia | 21 |
| Hypertension | 18 |
| Pulmonary edema | 16 |
| Smell of poison | 11 |
| Bradycardia | 10 |
| Restlessness | 9 |
| Cyanosis | 8 |
| Hypothermia | 7 |
| Hypotension | 7 |
| Lacrimation | 7 |
| Seizures | 6 |
| Urinary incontinence | 6 |
| Fecal incontinence | 5 |
| Conjunctival injection | 3 |
| Dilated pupils | 2 |

| Laboratory | Hayes, % |
|---|---|
| Serum cholinesterase (markedly depleted) | 97 |
| Neutrophil leukocytosis | 46 |
| Proteinuria | 19 |
| Glycosuria | 14 |
| Hyperglycemia | 7 |
| Abnormal ECG (other than bradycardia/tachycardia) | 5 |

*Source:* From Tafuri J, Robert J: Organophosphate poisoning. *Ann Emerg Med* 16:193, 1987. Published with permission.

causing sinus bradycardia, atrioventricular block, and ST- and T-wave abnormalities. Prolongation of the Q-T interval is commonly noted.

## DIAGNOSIS

The classic clinical presentation of serious organophosphate or carbamate poisoning includes an agitated or comatose patient with diaphoresis, pinpoint pupils, muscle fasciculations, bradycardia, and varying degrees of respiratory distress. There are often increased oral and bronchial secretions with urinary and bowel incontinence. Occasionally the patient will manifest a petroleum or garliclike odor associated with organophosphates.

The definitive diagnosis of organophosphate insecticide poisoning

**Table 155-4.** Classification of the Signs and Symptoms of Acute Organophosphate or Carbamate Poisoning According to Receptor Site and Type

| Muscarinic | Nicotinic | Central† |
|---|---|---|
| Miosis* | Muscle fasciculations* | Unconsciousness |
| Blurred vision | (striated muscle) | Confusion |
| Nausea | Paralysis | Toxic psychosis |
| Vomiting | Muscle weakness | Seizures |
| Diarrhea | Hypertension | Fatigue |
| Salivation | Tachycardia | Respiratory depression |
| Lacrimation | Pallor | Dysarthria |
| Bradycardia | Mydriasis (rare) | Ataxia |
| Abdominal pain | | Anxiety |
| (cramping) | | |
| Diaphoresis | | |
| Wheezing | | |
| Urinary incontinence | | |
| Fecal incontinence | | |

\* Most specific clinical findings.
† Less prominent with carbamate exposure.
*Source:* From Tafuri J, Roberts J: Organophosphate poisoning. *Ann Emerg Med* 16:193, 1987. Published with permission.

is established by demonstrating decreased cholinesterase activity in the blood. Both serum cholinesterase and RBC cholinesterase can and should be measured, although the laboratory results will not be readily available to the emergency physician. RBC cholinesterase is theoretically a more accurate test and is believed to more closely reflect the degree of synaptic cholinesterase activity. The serum (pseudocholinesterase) level is a more sensitive test and is more readily measured by most laboratories, but it may be a less specific indicator of organophosphate poisoning than is the RBC cholinesterase level. Low pseudocholinesterase activity can be seen as a genetic variant and in a number of disease states, such as malnutrition, acute infections, or liver disease. The pseudocholinesterase level will gradually return to normal in days to weeks after exposure without treatment, but regeneration of RBC cholinesterase occurs at a rate of only 1 percent per day or less and can require 3 to 4 months to normalize in severe cases. In mild cases the cholinesterase levels are decreased by 20 to 50 percent of normal, and less than 10 percent cholinesterase activity produces severe clinical manifestations. It should be noted that the quoted normal ranges of cholinesterase levels are variable and quite broad, and individuals may manifest some organophosphate toxicity with "normal" (but significantly decreased from baseline) cholinesterase levels. In some cases, especially low-grade chronic exposures, serial levels must be measured to demonstrate a trend rather than relying on a single determination of enzyme activity. Cholinesterase levels are diagnostic aids only and have no specific value in management of the clinical symptoms. Some laboratories can identify the organophosphates in containers, gastric washings, or urine. The laboratory is less useful in the diagnosis of carbamate poisoning, since cholinesterase levels may return to normal in 4 to 8 h after exposure has been terminated.

## MANAGEMENT

A history or suspicion of organophosphate or carbamate exposure, coupled with the appropriate findings on physical examination, will direct the specific treatment. Asymptomatic patients require 6 to 8 h observation only. The aim of treatment of seriously poisoned patients consists of vigorous decontamination and respiratory support and the use of specific antidotes. A classification of the degree of poisoning and a guide to treatment are given outlined in Table 155-5.

### Establishment of Airway

The initial objective of treatment should be the establishment of an airway and adequate ventilation. The patient with serious organo-

**Table 155-5.** Classification and Treatment of Organophosphate
Poisoning

**Latent Poisoning**

Clinical manifestations: None.
Serum cholinesterase: Greater than 50% of normal value.
Treatment: None. Observation for 6 h to monitor for progression of
symptoms.

**Mild Poisoning**

Clinical manifestations: Fatigue, headache, dizziness, numbness of
extremities, nausea and vomiting, diaphoresis, excessive salivation,
wheezing, abdominal pain, diarrhea. The patient is able to ambulate.
Serum cholinesterase: 20 to 50% of normal value.
Treatment: Atropine 1 mg intravenously and pralidoxime 1 g intravenously.

**Moderate Poisoning**

Clinical manifestations: Generalized weakness, dysarthria, muscle
fasciculations, miosis, and symptoms described in mild poisoning. The
patient is unable to ambulate.
Serum cholinesterase: 10 to 20% of normal value.
Treatment: Atropine 1 to 2 mg intravenously every 15 to 30 min until signs of
atropinization appear, and pralidoxime 1 g intravenously.

**Severe Poisoning**

Clinical manifestations: Marked miosis and loss of pupillary reflex to light,
muscle fasciculations, flaccid paralysis, pulmonary rales, respiratory distress,
cyanosis. The patient is unconscious.
Serum cholinesterase: Less than 10% of normal value.
Treatment: Atropine 5 mg every 15 to 30 min until signs of atropinization
appear. Pralidoxime 1 to 2 g intravenously. If therapy is not followed by
improvement, intravenous infusion of pralidoxime at 0.5 g per hour.

*Source:* Modified from Namba T. Nolte C, Jackrel J, et al: Poisoning due to
organophosphate insecticides. *Am J Med* 50:475, 1971.

phosphate poisoning commonly presents with respiratory distress
secondary to excessive oropharyngeal secretions, bronchospasm, and
respiratory muscle paralysis. Acute management in these cases consists of suctioning the copious oropharyngeal secretions and any
vomitus. Tracheal intubation and mechanical ventilation are often required in serious poisoning. If the depolarizing neuromuscular blocking agent succinylcholine is used as an aid to intubation, it should be
noted that its effect may be quite prolonged due to the inhibition of
pseudocholinesterase. It is essential to improve tissue oxygenation as
much as possible prior to the administration of atropine in order to
minimize the risk of ventricular fibrillation.

## Atropine

All patients poisoned with organophosphates/carbamates are candidates for atropine therapy. Atropine acts as a physiologic antidote in
the state of acetylcholine excess by competitively blocking the action
of acetylcholine at muscarinic (but not nicotinic) receptors, thereby
ameliorating the excessive parasympathetic stimulation caused by
acetylcholinesterase inactivation. Atropine sulfate should be administered intravenously. Repeated doses of atropine should be administered until signs of atropinization (mydriasis, tachycardia, flushing,
xerostomia, anhydrosis, etc.) appear. Pupils frequently dilate with atropine therapy but it is difficult to use only pupil size as a clinical
guide to adequate atropine therapy. Drying of secretions can be used
as an endpoint of therapy. In moderately severe poisoning, adults
should receive 2 mg intravenously every 5 to 15 min until adequate
atropinization is established. The pediatric dosage is 0.05 mg/kg, repeated every 15 min as necessary. A continuous infusion of atropine
(50 mg in 500 mL normal saline solution) titrated for effect may be
used.

It is essential to recognize that a severely poisoned individual will
exhibit marked atropine refractoriness and may require massive
doses, occasionally depleting the hospital's entire supply of the drug.
Atropine refractoriness is a semidiagnostic parameter that can aid di-

agnosis in confusing cases. Aggressive therapy is mandatory, as the
most common cause of treatment failure is probably *inadequate atropinization.* Tachycardia, usually due to hypoxia or ganglionic stimulation, is not a contraindication to atropine, and it frequently (paradoxically) produces a slowing of the heart rate. It should be noted
that atropine will have no effect on the nicotinic receptors at skeletal
myoneural junctions or within the sympathetic ganglia, although it
may be therapeutic for CNS symptoms (especially in children). Atropine does not hasten the regeneration of the inhibited or destroyed
cholinesterases. Glycopyrrolate (Robinul) administered intravenously
in doses approximately half those of atropine may be equally effective with fewer CNS side effects.

## Decontamination

After initial stabilization, the patient should be decontaminated. This
involves the removal of all exposed clothing and vigorous washing of
the skin with soap and water. Some suggest a second washing with
ethanol and water. It is essential that all personnel who have contact
with the patient wear protective clothing and gloves to prevent accidental dermal absorption.

## Ipecac, Charcoal, Cathartic

If the patient has ingested a significant amount of organophosphate or
carbamate, gastric emptying is indicated. A small taste or sip may not
require gastric emptying, but oral activated charcoal should be given.
Gastric lavage is preferred over ipecac-induced emesis because of the
potential for seizures and the delayed onset of ipecac. Ideally, activated charcoal should be added to the lavage fluid and administered
again with a cathartic following lavage. The value of multiple doses
of oral activated charcoal is unknown, but the regimen is recommended by the authors. An intestinal ileus caused by atropine can
make repeated doses of charcoal problematic. Whole bowel irrigation
and cathartics are of theoretical (but unproven) benefit. Hemodialysis
and/or hemoperfusion are of no known value in treating organophosphate or carbamate poisoning.

## Pralidoxime

After blood samples have been obtained for basic laboratory studies
and serum and RBC cholinesterase levels, pralidoxime may be administered. Pralidoxime (Protopam, 2-PAM chloride) is a biochemical antidote for primarily organophosphate intoxication but probably
not for pure carbamate poisoning. Pralidoxime reverses the cholinergic nicotinic effects that are unaffected by the use of atropine alone.
These nicotinic effects include muscle weakness and fasciculations
and stimulation of the sympathetic ganglia. Pralidoxime has also been
demonstrated to reactivate the cholinesterase that has been phosphorylated by an organophosphate if it is given with 24 to 36 h of acute
exposure. If it is not administered within this period, a change in the
organophosphate-enzyme complex may occur, irreversibly destroying
the cholinesterase. After this has occurred, restoration of normal
function requires the total regeneration of the destroyed cholinesterase molecules, a process which requires weeks.

The beneficial effects of pralidoxime include (1) reactivation of
cholinesterase by cleavage of phosphorylated active sites, (2) direct
reaction and detoxification of unbounded organophosphate molecules, and (3) an endogenous anticholinergic effect in normal doses.
Although pralidoxime is not equally effective against all cholinesterase inhibitors, it has been documented to be efficacious in numerous organophosphate insecticide intoxications. Pralidoxime
should be administered, however, regardless of the type of organophosphate involved. Pralidoxime should not be given routinely to
asymptomatic patients or in cases of known carbamate exposure with
minimal symptoms. Pralidoxime probably does not help a patient
with carbamate toxicity but it is not harmful. In instances of symptomatic mixed carbamate/organophosphate exposure or in cases of

unknown exposure with significant symptoms, the use of pralidoxime is warranted.

The initial dose of pralidoxime is 1 g given intravenously over 15 to 30 min. The pediatric dose is 20 to 50 mg/kg given over 15 to 30 min. Subsequent doses may be repeated 1 to 2 h after the initial dose and every 10 to 12 h thereafter as needed. A continuous intravenous infusion of pralidoxime (0.5 g/h in adults and 10 to 20 mg/kg per hour in children) has also been recommended. Reversal of muscle weakness and fasciculations usually begins within 10 to 40 min after administration. Treatment is usually continued for 24 to 48 h.

Pralidoxime possesses little inherent toxicity. In normal doses of 1 to 2 g, pralidoxime has been shown to produce no significant side effects in normal subjects when given intravenously, but it has been noted to produce hypertension, headache, electrocardiographic changes, dizziness, and gastrointestinal upset at high doses. Although pralidoxime is usually considered routine therapy, its value in reducing morbidity and mortality has never been unequivocally demonstrated and has been questioned by some.

## ORGANOPHOSPHATE/CARBAMATE POISONING IN CHILDREN

Infants and children may be poisoned with these insecticides through a variety of routes. Inhalation exposures and dermal absorption may be more common than in adults. Infants are often mistakenly fed toxic solutions resembling formula that have been stored in unmarked soda or juice containers. Young children can present a confusing and unrecognized clinical picture if one extrapolates to them the data and typical descriptions obtained from reports on poisoned adults. Importantly, the clinical scenario in young children is quite different from that classically seen in adults. In children, CNS symptoms (especially lethargy, stupor, coma, and seizures) and hypotonia/weakness predominate, while the more characteristic muscarinic symptoms (SLUDGE) may be mild or absent. Miosis, muscle fasciculations, bradycardia, diaphoresis, excessive salivation, and severe gastrointestinal symptoms occur decidedly less frequently in infants and children. Curiously, atropine readily reverses CNS toxicity in children, and this antidote may be used in a therapeutic (or diagnostic) trial in confusing cases. Pralidoxime may also be used. Pseudocholinesterase activity may be in the normal range in the face of serious toxicity.

## COMPLICATIONS

Acute complications of organophosphate insecticide poisoning that may require urgent treatment include seizure activity and complex ventricular arrhythmias. Seizures may be easily treated with intravenous diazepam or lorazepam until the acute poisoning has resolved. Significant ventricular arrhythmias that are not responsive to lidocaine, bretylium, and/or cardioversion have been shown to be best treated with intravenous isoproterenol and overdrive pacing and continuous cardiac monitoring.

Nonspecific symptoms such as headache, memory impairment, depression, confusion, and peripheral neuropathies may persist for some time following significant exposure, but the exact biochemical nature of these impairments is unknown.

### Delayed/Long-Term Sequelae

Some patients will experience a variety of neurologic sequelae following recovery from the acute phase of organophosphate toxicity. For weeks to months following exposures of varying intensity, patients report symptoms such as peripheral neuropathies, fatigue, irritability, memory impairment, personality changes, headache, mood swings, trouble concentrating, and depression, but these abnormalities are difficult to quantify or document clinically. Neuropsychiatric testing may be abnormal. The cause of these abnormalities is unknown, and there is no specific treatment.

From a few days to weeks following clinical recovery from the

acute cholinergic phase of organophosphate poisoning (due to diazinon, fenthion, parathion, and others), some patients develop what has been termed the *intermediate syndrome*. It is characterized by a predominantly motor polyneuropathy consisting of generalized weakness, hyporeflexia, and cranial nerve abnormalities and may progress to acute respiratory paresis requiring mechanical ventilation. Muscarinic symptoms are lacking during this apparent relapse, and patients do not respond to atropine or pralidoxime. The syndrome is probably due to prolonged cholinesterase inhibition. Treatment of this potentially lethal syndrome, which can last for up to 3 weeks, is supportive.

## BIBLIOGRAPHY

Bardin PG, Van Eeden SF: Organophosphate poisoning: Grading the severity and comparing treatment between atropine and glycopyrrolate *Crit Care Med* 18:956, 1990.

Bardin P, van Eeden S, Moolman J, et al: Organophosphate and carbamate poisoning. *Arch Intern Med* 154:1433, 1994.

De Bleecker J, Van Den Neuker K, Colardyn F: Intermediate syndrome in organophosphate poisoning: A prospective study. *Crit Care Med* 21:1706, 1993.

Tafuri J, Roberts J: Organophosphate poisoning. *Ann Emerg Med* 16:193, 1987.

# 156
# CYANIDE
## Kathleen Delaney

## INTRODUCTION

Cyanide is a potent cellular toxin with an infamous history. The ability of extracts of bitter almonds and cherry laurel leaves to cause rapid death has been known for centuries, although the causative agent was not identified as cyanide until the end of the eighteenth century. Cyanide was used in state executions by the ancient Greeks and Romans and, until recently, by the state of California. The first chemist to synthesize hydrogen cyanide gas succumbed dramatically in 1786 when a vial of the gas broke on his laboratory floor. In 1978 hundreds of people died in Jonestown, British Guiana, following a mass suicidal cyanide ingestion.

Cyanide is a simple, highly reactive compound of carbon and nitrogen that has many uses in industry and the chemical laboratory. Its wide availability was emphasized by the experience of investigators who found 65 legitimate sources of cyanide in the Chicago area during attempts to trace the source of cyanide used in the infamous Tylenol-substitution poisonings. In nature, it is found in large amounts in certain nuts, plants, and fruit pits in the form of cyanogenic glycosides. Tobacco smoke has been estimated to contain from 100 to 1600 parts per million (ppm) of cyanide, and smokers have been shown to have higher levels of cyanide and thiocyanate, a "detoxified" form of cyanide. Since it is so ubiquitous in nature, animals have evolved biochemical means of detoxifying cyanide. In humans and many other mammals, the enzyme rhodanese detoxifies cyanide by binding it to sulfate to form the less toxic thiocyanate, which is excreted by the kidneys.

## SOURCES OF EXPOSURE

Acute cyanide poisoning occurs in a number of settings: (1) accidental occupational poisonings; (2) nonoccupational accidental or suicical ingestion of cyanide or chemicals metabolized to cyanide, such as acetonitrile-containing solvents; (3) iatrogenic toxicity due to prolonged exposure to intravenous nitroprusside; and (4) ingestion of plants or foods containing naturally occurring cyanogenic glycosides.

Cyanide is produced in industry by combining ammonia ($NH_3$) and methane ($CH_4$) to form hydrogen cyanide gas (HCN). Commercial quantities of water-soluble salts such as sodium cyanide (NaCN) and potassium cyanide (KCN) are synthesized from hydrogen cyanide gas. HCN is readily liberated when cyanide salts are exposed to acid. Cyanide compounds are both precursors and incidental by-products in the production of plastics, solvents, enamels, high-strength paper, paints, glues, wrinkle-resistant fabrics, herbicides, pesticides, and fertilizers. Hydrogen cyanide gas is produced in large quantities during the manufacture of acrylonitrile, a precursor of many plastic compounds. The affinity of cyanide for metals makes it useful in the extraction of ores, in metal polishing, and in the electroplating industry. It is also used to strip hair from hides in the leather industry. The recent widespread use of cyanide as a fumigant resulted in many poisonings. Industrial exposures most commonly occur through inhalation, but skin exposure to solutions of cyanide salts has also resulted in poisoning. Inadvertent ingestion of cyanide salts while eating in a contaminated work setting has also been proposed as a cause of accidental subacute poisoning in the workplace.

Large amounts of hydrogen cyanide may be released when natural and synthetic nitrogen-containing polymers such as wool, silk, polyurethane, or vinyl are burned. Elevated cyanide levels have been frequently reported in victims of smoke inhalation, often in association with elevated carbon monoxide levels, and have been implicated in fire-related fatalities.

Adverse physiologic effects due to chronic subacute cyanide exposure have been proposed but are poorly defined. Studies of workers chronically exposed to cyanide have demonstrated a higher incidence of thyroid disease and vitamin $B_{12}$ deficiency. Linamarin is a cyanogenic glycoside found in the cassava plant, a significant source of carbohydrate to many peoples in developing countries. In areas of the world where cassava ingestion is high, goiter and tropical ataxic neuropathy are endemic and plasma and urinary levels of cyanide are elevated.

## BIOCHEMICAL TOXICOLOGY

The avidity with which cyanide binds to metals accounts for most of its serious physiologic effects in poisoning. Cyanide disrupts metabolism by binding and inhibiting the function of important metal-containing enzymes, particularly those that contain trivalent ferric (+3) iron. Although cyanide has been shown to inhibit a substantial number of biochemically important enzymes, the most dramatic physiologic effects are produced by its disruption of mitochondrial oxidative phosphorylation through the inhibition of cytochrome $A_3$, also called cytochrome oxidase. This binding is labile and readily reversible. Cytochrome $A_3$ catalyzes the final step in electron transport, in which molecular oxygen is reduced to water. Without this enzyme, the body tissues cannot utilize oxygen and only anaerobic metabolism occurs.

## CLINICAL TIME COURSE OF POISONING: ROUTES OF EXPOSURE

The time course and severity of the clinical effects of cyanide are a function of the nature of the cyanide-containing compound, the route of exposure, and the concentration of cyanide to which the patient is exposed. The absorption of cyanide following inhalational exposures to hydrogen cyanide gas is virtually immediate. Symptoms depend on the concentration of inspired gas. Toxicity occurs when the rate of accumulation of cyanide is greater than the rate of detoxification. Several hours of exposure to low concentrations of gas (<50 ppm) cause restlessness, anxiety, palpitations, dyspnea, and headache. Death may

occur following prolonged exposure at these levels. Exposure to 100 ppm may be fatal within 30 min. Higher levels lead to severe dyspnea, loss of consciousness, seizures, and cardiac dysrhythmia. Coma and cardiovascular collapse can occur immediately upon exposure to levels of hydrogen cyanide greater than 270 ppm. Survival with aggressive resuscitation has been reported following a 3-min industrial exposure to 500 ppm. Although in most industrial accidents it has been difficult to separate the effects of inhalational absorption from percutaneous absorption, animal studies and studies of human skin have clearly shown that absorption of both cyanide ion ($CN^-$) and HCN vapor occur through intact skin. In one industrial case reported in the 1950s, a fully protected worker was poisoned when he removed a glove and allowed his hand to contact aqueous HCN.

The onset of symptoms following ingestion of a cyanide salt may occur within minutes, depending on the amount of cyanide ingested and the rate of absorption. Deaths have occurred in adults following the ingestion of as little as 50 mg, and survival has been reported in much larger ingestions with aggressive resuscitation and use of antidotes.

Certain cyanide-containing compounds, such as nitrile or cyanogenic glycosides, require enzymatic breakdown and release of free cyanide before the symptoms of poisoning occur. Acetonitrile is a solvent sold commercially as a nail polish remover. It undergoes hepatic oxidative metabolism, which results in the release of hydrogen cyanide. Severe poisoning and death attributed to cyanide poisoning have been reported following latency periods as long as 12 h after ingestion. Amygdalin is a cyanogenic glycoside that is found in particularly high concentrations in apricot pits and bitter almonds. It is the principal constituent of Laetrile, a compound popular for nontraditional cancer therapies in the late 1970s. Because the release of cyanide requires hydrolysis of the glycoside by enzymes in the alkaline environment of the small intestine, the progression of symptoms following ingestion is characteristically slow, with a latency of onset of several hours. Amygdalin does not produce cyanide poisoning when given intravenously.

## CLINICAL PRESENTATION OF CYANIDE POISONING

Cyanide-poisoned patients frequently present to emergency departments without any history of exposure. Although isolated individual poisonings with cyanide are relatively rare, it is important that emergency physicians recognize signs of serious poisoning, as specific antidotal treatment is available and effective. A deeply comatose, bradycardic, acidotic patient without evidence of cyanosis or hypoxia on arterial blood gas examination should cause the clinician to think of cyanide. The finding of bright-red retinal vessels, an abnormally elevated venous oxygen pressure, oral burns, or the smell of bitter almonds supports the diagnosis, although clues of this nature are frequently absent. It is estimated that only 60 to 80 percent of the population can detect the characteristic almond odor of cyanide.

The clinical signs and symptoms of cyanide poisoning mimic those of hypoxia, with one exception: unless respiratory arrest has occurred, patients are not cyanotic. These clinical effects are readily understood based on the effect of cyanide on cytochrome oxidase activity. Blockade of the ability of mitochondria to utilize oxygen produces a state of severe hypoxia despite the presence of oxygen. Anaerobic metabolism is switched on, generating large amounts of lactic acid. Severe, unexplained acidosis is an important clinical clue to the timely diagnosis of cyanide poisoning in case of an "unknown" exposure.

At the onset of poisoning, there is an inspiratory gasp followed by hyperventilation. Patients complain of breathlessness and anxiety. Symptoms related to anxiety about the exposure may also mimic these initial symptoms of toxicity. During inhalational exposure, these symptoms will resolve following removal from the toxic exposure. Cerebral function is rapidly affected in significant exposures.

**Table 156-1.** Signs and Symptoms of Acute Cyanide Toxicity

| Central nervous system effects | Local effects |
|---|---|
| Headache | Oropharyngeal burns |
| Obtundation | Nausea |
| Seizures | Gastrointestinal irritation |
| Coma | Odor of almonds |
| Arterialization of retinal veins | |
| Cardiopulmonary effects | |
| Early stage | |
| Dyspnea | |
| Hypertension | |
| Tachycardia | |
| Dysrhythmias | |
| Late stage | |
| Apnea | |
| Hypotension | |
| Bradycardia | |
| Asystole | |

Loss of consciousness occurs, often associated with seizures. Even such severely poisoned patients may recover rapidly and spontaneously when removed from an inhalational exposure.

Early cardiac effects include sinus tachycardia, atrial dysrhythmia, and premature ventricular contractions. When exposure continues, bradycardia and apnea occur, followed by asystolic arrest. As with severe hypoxia, ventricular tachycardia and fibrillation are uncommon (see Table 156-1).

Although small amounts of cyanide bind to the ferrous (+2) form of hemoglobin, there is no significant interference with the ability of hemoglobin to bind oxygen. As noted above, cyanosis does not occur except as a terminal event. The inability to use oxygen leads to decreased oxygen extraction from hemoglobin and a concomitant increase in the oxygen content of venous blood. This may be clinically detectable as a decrease in the normal arteriolar-venous oxygen difference $[(A - V)_{O_2}]$, a measure of the amount of oxygen extracted by the tissues. It may also be demonstrated on funduscopic examination as "arterialized" retinal veins. Accurate determination of the $(A - V)_{O_2}$ requires pulmonary artery sampling and a time-consuming calculation. Although peripheral venous samples do not reflect whole-body oxygen extraction, it is clinically useful to recall that the venous pressure of oxygen in forearm blood is around 40 mmHg in patients on room air under normal circumstances. A high forearm venous oxygen pressure would support the diagnosis of cyanide poisoning. The necessity of administering oxygen to these patients affects this finding in an unpredictable way (see Table 156-2).

A brief occupational history may provide a clue to the diagnosis of cyanide poisoning in an acutely ill adult. In patients with work-related industrial poisoning, the exposure is usually accidental and

**Table 156-2.** Anticipated Laboratory Abnormalities in Cyanide Poisoning

| Test | Result | Cause |
|---|---|---|
| Serum electrolytes | Elevated anion gap | Lactic acidosis from increased anaerobic metabolism |
| Arterial blood gas | Metabolic acidosis Normal $P_{O_2}$ | As above |
| Calculated % $O_2$ saturation | Normal | |
| Measured % $O_2$ saturation | May be slightly decreased | Small amount of binding of $CN^-$ to hemoglobin |
| Arterial-central venous $P_{O_2}$ difference | Increased (normal is 5 mL $O_2$/100 mL blood) | Decreased tissue $O_2$ utilization |

*Source:* Adapted with permission from Hall and Rumack.

the diagnosis suggested by the patient's job and circumstances. Frequently multiple exposures result from the same incident. Suicidal ingestion of cyanide often occurs in patients whose occupations provide access to cyanide salts, such as industrial and research chemists, laboratory technicians, science students, or jewelers. Cyanide salts are caustic and may cause oral burns when concentrated solutions or undiluted salts are ingested. Accidental or suicidal ingestion of cyanide-containing commercial products, such as metal polishes or acetonitrile-containing solvents, has been associated with severe cyanide toxicity. A history of use of nontraditional cancer therapies would provide a clue to the ingestion of Laetrile or other cyanogen-containing preparations. Careful identification of ingestants in asymptomatic patients will prevent the mistaken discharge of a patient who has ingested a compound with delayed toxicity.

## DIFFERENTIAL DIAGNOSIS OF CYANIDE POISONING

Cyanide poisoning should always be considered in the poisoned patient with metabolic acidosis. The differential diagnosis of acidosis in the setting of inhalational exposure includes other cellular toxins, such as hydrogen sulfide and carbon monoxide, and simple asphyxiants. Hydrogen sulfide is a product of organic decomposition, encountered in septic tanks and sewers, petroleum production, and a number of other occupational settings. The characteristic odor of "rotten eggs" is frequently detectable. Carbon monoxide poisoning is readily confirmed by measurement of a carboxyhemoglobin level. The differential diagnosis of acidosis in patients with suspected ingestions includes methanol, ethylene glycol, salicylates, and iron. The slower time course of deterioration and the variable depth of mental status depression frequently help to distinguish the effects of these agents from those of cyanide. Severe isoniazid and cocaine poisoning are also associated with significant acidosis that occurs in the setting of seizures. The initial manifestations of severe intoxication with these agents may be clinically indistinguishable from cyanide intoxication.

## PHARMACOLOGIC PRINCIPLES OF TREATMENT

Standard accepted therapy for cyanide poisoning in the United States is based on experimental and chemical principles developed in 1933. It is provided by the Lilly Cyanide Antidote Kit. The kit contains nitrites in two forms, an ampule of amyl nitrite for inhalation and 10 mL of a 3% solution of sodium nitrite for intravenous infusion. It also contains 50 mL of a 25% solution of sodium thiosulfate. The usual adult dose of sodium nitrite is 300 mg, followed by 12.5 g of sodium thiosulfate. The pediatric dose is 0.33 mL/kg of 10% sodium nitrite and 1.65 mL/kg of 25% sodium thiosulfate. Pediatric dosages of sodium nitrite should be adjusted if anemia is known to be present (see Table 156-3). The amyl nitrite is used to temporize in the prehospital setting or until intravenous access can be obtained and does not need to be administered when sodium nitrite is readily available. Nitrites act quickly and therefore are the first antidote to be used when the diagnosis of cyanide poisoning is clear.

The initial rationale for using nitrites was based on their capacity to form methemoglobin. Methemoglobin binds avidly to cyanide and prevents its binding to cytochrome oxidase. Although the antidotal efficacy of nitrites is not disputed, their actual mechanism of action has recently been questioned. The formation of methemoglobin is a slow process relative to the rapidity of the therapeutic response to nitrites. In addition, the reversal of cyanide toxicity in animals by nitrites has been demonstrated to occur in the presence of methylene blue, which prevents the formation of methemoglobin. Rapid methemoglobin formers, such as dimethyl-4-aminophenol, which is now used in Germany to treat cyanide poisoning, do not appear to work any faster than sodium nitrite. Many papers imply that a level of methemoglobin of at least 25% should be a goal of therapy. This is

**Table 156-3.** Treatment of Cyanide Poisoning

**CHILDREN**

1. Amyl nitrite inhaler: crack vial and inhale 30 s/min.*
2. Administration of IV sodium nitrite and sodium thiosulfate:

| Hb, g/100mL | 3% $NaNO_2$, mL/kg | 25% $Na_2S_2O_3$, mL/kg |
| --- | --- | --- |
| 7 | 0.19 | 0.95 |
| 8 | 0.22 | 1.10 |
| 9 | 0.25 | 1.25 |
| 10 | 0.27 | 1.35 |
| 11 | 0.30 | 1.50 |
| 12 | 0.33* | 1.65 |
| 13 | 0.36 | 1.80 |
| 14 | 0.39 | 1.95 |

3. May repeat once at one-half dose.
4. Monitor methemoglobin to keep level less than 30%.

**ADULTS**

1. Amyl nitrite: crack and inhale 30 s/min.*
2. Sodium nitrite: 10 mL IV (10-mL ampule, 3% $NaNO_2$ = 300 mg).
3. Sodium thiosulfate: 50 mL IV (50-mL ampule, 25% $Na_2S_2O_3$ = 12.5 g).
4. May repeat once at one-half dose.

* Administration of amyl nitrite is only necessary if venous access has not been obtained.
*Source:* Adapted with permission from Hall and Rumack.

based on work in dogs, who are much more sensitive to the methemoglobin-forming effects of nitrites than humans. It has been repeatedly demonstrated that the rapid clinical reversal of cyanide toxicity occurs despite the demonstration of only very small amounts of methemoglobin. Rapid detoxification of cyanide has been reported using solutions of methemoglobin stripped of the red cell walls, so-called stroma-free methemoglobin. Nitrites have a potential to cause serious side effects. Their vasodilatory properties can exacerbate hypotension. A single death has been reported secondary to massive methemoglobinemia in an asymptomatic child with an inconsequential cyanide ingestion.

Following the administration of sodium nitrite, sodium thiosulfate is given. Studies of the cyanide $LD_{50}$ in animals demonstrate that the therapeutic effect of the combination of sodium nitrite and sodium thiosulfate is greater than the additive effects of either agent alone. Sodium thiosulfate enhances the activity of the body's own detoxification enzyme, rhodanese, by acting as a sulfur donor. Rhodanese removes the cyanide molecule from methemoglobin and transfers it to sulfur, forming thiocyanate, which is renally excreted. The rate of this detoxification reaction in humans is limited by the availability of sulfur. The speed of the antidotal effect of sodium thiosulfate administration has been noted to be species-dependent: very slow in rabbits, intermediate in dogs, and very rapid in sheep. There are limited data on the efficacy of sodium thiosulfate as sole therapy for cyanide poisoning in humans, although anecdotal reports suggest that it may be very effective as a sole therapy. This is an important question because sodium thiosulfate has very limited toxicity in comparison with the nitrites and is a safer empirical therapy in cases where the diagnosis is not clear. Administration of 100% oxygen has been clearly shown in animal studies to significantly enhance the therapeutic efficacy of sodium thiosulfate alone and of the nitrite-thiosulfate combination. If the only mechanism of toxicity of cyanide were its binding to cytochrome $A_3$, then rationally oxygen would not be expected to have any therapeutic effect. It has been proposed that oxygen may affect the binding of cyanide to cytochrome oxidase or the ability to form methemoglobin. Hyperbaric oxygen has not been shown to offer any benefit over 100% oxygen in animal studies of cyanide poisoning. Hyperbaric oxygen is very useful in the management of the patient with suspected cyanide poisoning who has concomitant carbon monoxide poisoning.

Because of the potential side effects of the nitrites, a great deal of effort has been made to develop equally efficacious but less toxic therapies. Many agents bind cyanide and render it nontoxic. Hydroxocobalamin (vitamin $B_{12a}$) has been shown to reverse cyanide toxicity in animal models and used to protect patients on prolonged nitroprusside infusions from cyanide toxicity. The large amounts of the agent needed to neutralize cyanide require large volume infusions in the concentrations currently available. Studies are currently being conducted using hydroxocobalamin alone or in combination with sodium thiosulfate, an intervention widely used in France. The concurrent use of sodium thiosulfate is thought to "recycle" the hydroxocobalamin binding sites, allowing administration of a smaller dose. Recent studies support this concept. It appears that when only hydroxocobalamin is administered, cyanide is held in the form of cyanocobalamin. When the combination is used, cyanide appears in the form of thiocyanate. This effect has been termed "antidotal synergy." Anaphylactoid reactions have been reported with the use of hydroxocobalamin alone, and this toxicity may be increased by the addition of sodium thiosulfate.

Dicobalt edetate (Kelocyanor) is the therapeutic agent used as first-line treatment of cyanide poisoning in the United Kingdom. It is highly effective as a cyanide antidote but is not devoid of toxicity. Metabolic acidosis and hypotension have occurred in animals, and massive edema and ventricular tachycardia have been attributed to its administration to humans. The toxicity of dicobalt edetate is greater when cyanide is not present, limiting its use as an empirical therapy or in minimally symptomatic patients with cyanide exposure.

4-Dimethylaminophenol (DMAP) is an agent developed in Germany for the treatment of cyanide poisoning. It rapidly produces methemoglobinemia but has not been demonstrated to be more clinically efficacious than sodium nitrite. It does not cause the same degree of hypotension but has been associated with renal failure in experimental animals. Unlike dicobalt edetate, it does not have greater side effects in the absence of cyanide. In practice, most of these agents are used in combination with sodium thiosulfate.

## MANAGEMENT DECISIONS: USE OF SPECIFIC ANTIDOTES

Severely poisoned patients have survived with supportive therapy alone, although survival in many cases of massive exposure has undoubtedly been facilitated by specific antidotal therapy. The largest reported ingestion where survival occurred with supportive care alone was 600 mg. Much larger ingestions have resulted in survival when specific antidotes were used. All patients should receive 100% oxygen and be put on a cardiac monitor with an intravenous line in place. Patients with a history of cyanide ingestion should have careful gastric lavage. Ipecac is absolutely contraindicated due to the expected rapid onset of symptoms. Gastric decontamination should never take priority over resuscitation of the symptomatic patient. Superactivated charcoal has been shown to bind small amounts of cyanide and may be useful in decreasing the significance of an ingestion.

Patients with inhalational exposures do not require gastric decontamination. Extensive decontamination of the skin should be accomplished in patients with cutaneous exposure, with adequate precautions to protect the staff from skin contamination. Patients with inhalational exposures often evidence recovery following their rescue from the toxic environment. They do not require specific antidotal therapy if significant recovery has occurred prior to reaching medical attention.

The decision regarding the administration of the sodium nitrite-thiosulfate antidote is straightforward when faced with a comatose, bradycardic patient with a clear history of cyanide exposure. Hypotension is not a contraindication to sodium nitrite therapy in this setting. At the other end of the spectrum, because of the potential toxicity of the nitrites, it is never appropriate to treat an asymptomatic patient. A patient with mild to moderate symptoms may be closely observed for more serious signs prior to the initiation of treatment. More difficult management decisions arise in (1) patients with smoke inhalation who have, or may have, carbon monoxide exposure as well as suspected cyanide exposure; and (2) patients who are critically ill and acidotic without any history of cyanide exposure. In these cases, an antidote that is effective and has no toxicity would obviously be useful. Empirical administration of nitrites to victims of smoke inhalation who have, or may have, elevated carboxyhemoglobin levels has been considered to be contraindicated because of the decreased oxygen-carrying capacity caused by simultaneous induction of methemoglobinemia. A recent study of seven patients with smoke inhalation and elevated cyanide and carboxyhemoglobin levels who were treated empirically with both sodium nitrite and sodium thiosulfate demonstrated that the measured decrease in oxygen-carrying capacity accounted for by carboxyhemoglobin and methemoglobin ranged from 10 to 21 percent and was not clinically significant in those patients. The safety of administering both agents in this setting remains unclear. Lactic acidosis in a victim of smoke inhalation may be caused by cyanide, carbon monoxide, hypoxia from airway injuries, severe burns, or shock. The safest immediate empirical therapy that avoids the hypotensive effects of nitrites and the concerns about decreased oxygen-carrying capacity due to methemoglobin formation is the administration of 100% oxygen and sodium thiosulfate. Sodium thiosulfate is safe, and its efficacy as a sole therapy has been demonstrated in anecdotal case reports.

The institution of hyperbaric oxygen therapy for patients with carbon monoxide poisoning in addition to suspected cyanide poisoning obviates the concerns about induction of methemoglobinemia. If lactic acidosis persists following hemodynamic resuscitation, oxygenation, and the administration of thiosulfate, sodium nitrite may then be cautiously administered.

The differential diagnosis of the comatose patient with metabolic acidosis is extensive. Empirical therapy in the unknown patient with possible toxic ingestion who is critically ill and acidotic should include 100% oxygen, thiamine, 50% dextrose in water, and naloxone, in addition to aggressive supportive care. When cyanide poisoning is considered, empirical administration of sodium thiosulfate is indicated. Significant hypotension is a contraindication to empirical administration of sodium nitrite. Following the demonstration of adequate blood pressure, adequate oxygenation, and the absence of an elevated carboxyhemoglobin level, sodium nitrite may be administered after the sodium thiosulfate if the diagnosis is strongly entertained.

## LABORATORY EVALUATION

In order to be effective, treatment of cyanide poisoning must be instituted long before confirmatory laboratory studies can be accomplished. Cyanide levels are useful to confirm a clinical diagnosis in retrospect; they cannot be obtained in time to make the diagnosis at the bedside. Because cyanide is sequestered in erythrocytes, red blood cell levels should be obtained. Cyanide levels do not correlate well with toxicity but will support a diagnosis. Whole blood levels greater than 40 μmol/L have been associated with fatal poisoning. Arterial blood gas measurement is a rapid and useful test as noted above, as is the determination of carboxyhemoglobin, oxyhemoglobin, and methemoglobin levels on a cooximeter. Whenever a patient is poisoned with an agent that alters hemoglobin so that it cannot bind oxygen, a "saturation gap" can be noted between the oxygen saturation measured by a cooximeter and the calculated oxygen saturation reported from the blood gas measurement. Patients with carbon monoxide poisoning and methemoglobinemia have large saturation gaps. Patients with hydrogen sulfide poisoning and cyanide poisoning rarely have small gaps related to the less common effects of direct interactions of these substances with hemoglobin. The absence of a

metabolic acidosis is inconsistent with the diagnosis of acute cyanide poisoning in a symptomatic patient. Recently, the demonstration of a serum lactate level greater than 10 mmol/L was shown to have a significant correlation with toxic cyanide levels in victims of smoke inhalation from residential fires.

## PROGNOSIS

Full recovery is anticipated in many cases of severe poisoning where treatment is initiated rapidly and cardiac arrest has not yet occurred. Recovery despite cardiac arrest has also been reported. Most patients who survive do not suffer neurologic injury, although anoxic encephalopathy may ensue.

## BIBLIOGRAPHY

Ballantyne B: Toxicology of cyanides, in Ballantyne B, Marrs TC (eds): *Clinical and Experimental Toxicology of Cyanide.* Bristol, Wright, 1987, pp 40–125.

Baud FJ, Barriot P, Torris V, et al: Elevated blood cyanide concentrations in victims of smoke inhalation. *N Engl J Med* 325:1761, 1991.

Chen K, Rose CL: Nitrite and thiosulfate therapy in cyanide poisoning. *JAMA* 149:113, 1952.

Hall AH, Rumack BH: Clinical toxicology of cyanide. *Ann Emerg Med* 15:1067, 1986.

Kirk MA, Gerace R, Kulig KW: Cyanide and methemoglobin kinetics in smoke inhalation victims treated with the cyanide antidote kit. *Ann Emerg Med* 22:1413, 1993.

Kulig K: Cyanide antidotes and fire toxicology (editorial). *N Engl J Med* 325:1801, 1991.

Marrs TC: The choice of cyanide antidotes, in Ballantyne B, Marrs TC (eds): *Clinical and Experimental Toxicology of Cyanide.* Bristol, Wright, 1987, pp 382–400.

Way JL: Cyanide intoxication and its mechanism of antagonism. *Annu Rev Toxicol* 24:451, 1984.

# 157
# ANTICHOLINERGIC TOXICITY
## Leslie R. Wolf

Because of the frequent use of tricyclic antidepressants, phenothiazines, antihistamines, and antiparkinsonian drugs, anticholinergic toxicity is commonly seen in the emergency department. Anticholinergic medications are commonly prescribed for elderly patients, often resulting in drug-induced delirium. Many drugs have anticholinergic properties (Table 157-1) that may be mild at therapeutic doses but are life-threatening in overdose. The use and abuse of some plants and mushrooms may also result in anticholinergic toxicity.

## PHARMACOLOGIC PROPERTIES

Drug absorption can occur after ingestion, smoking, or ocular use. The rate of absorption varies depending on the drug and the route of exposure. Because cholinergic blockade delays gastric emptying and decreases intestinal motility, absorption and peak clinical effects are often delayed.

The signs and symptoms of anticholinergic toxicity are a result of both central and peripheral cholinergic blockade. Muscarinic acetylcholine receptors predominate in the brain, while nicotinic receptors predominate in the spinal cord. Depending on the drug involved, an-

**Table 157-1.** Anticholinergic Substances

| | |
|---|---|
| **Antihistamines**<br>  Ethanolamines<br>    Dimenhydrinate (Dramamine)<br>    Diphenhydramine (Benadryl)<br>  Ethylenediamines<br>    Tripelennamine (Pyribenzamine)<br>  Alkylamines<br>    Chlorpheniramine (Teldrin)<br>  Piperazines<br>    Astemizole (Hismanal)<br>    Terfenadine (Seldane)<br>    Loratadine (Claritin)<br>    Cyclizine (Marezine)<br>    Meclizine (Antivert)<br>  Phenothiazines<br>    Promethazine (Phenergan)<br>**Antiparkinsonian drugs**<br>  Benztropine mesylate (Cogentin)<br>  Biperiden (Akineton)<br>  Ethopropazine (Parsidol)<br>  Trihexyphenidyl (Artane)<br>  Procyclidine (Kemadrin)<br>**Antipsychotics**<br>  Phenothiazines<br>    Chlorpromazine (Thorazine)<br>    Thioridazine (Mellaril)<br>    Perphenazine (Trilafon)<br>  Nonphenothiazines<br>    Molindone (Moban)<br>    Loxapine (Loxitane)<br>**Antispasmodics**<br>  Clidinium bromide (Quarzan, Librax)<br>  Dicyclomine (Bentyl)<br>  Methantheline bromide (Banthine)<br>  Propantheline bromide (Pro-Banthine)<br>  Tridihexethyl chloride (Pathilon)<br>**Plants**<br>  Deadly nightshade<br>  Mandrake<br>  Jimsonweed | **Belladonna alkaloids, synthetic cogeners**<br>  Atropine (Hyoscyamine)<br>  Belladonna alkaloid mixtures<br>  Glycopyrrolate (Robinul)<br>  Homatropine (Dia-Quel, Malcotran)<br>  Methscopolamine bromide (Pamine)<br>  Scopolamine hydrobromide (Hyoscine)<br>**Cyclic antidepressants**<br>  Amitryptyline hydrochloride (Elavil, Amitril, Endep)<br>  Desipramine hydrochloride (Norpramin, Pertofrane)<br>  Doxepin hydrochloride (Sinequan, Adapin)<br>  Imipramine hydrochloride (Tofranil, Pramine)<br>  Nortriptyline hydrochloride (Aventyl, Pamelor)<br>  Protriptyline hydrochloride (Vivactil)<br>  Trimipramine (Surmontil)<br>  Maprotiline hydrochloride (Ludiomil)<br>  Zimelidine hydrochloride<br>  Fluoxetine (Prozac)<br>  Amoxapine (Asendin)<br>**Ophthalmic products**<br>  Atropine and scopolamine solutions<br>  Cyclopentolate hydrochloride (Cyclogyl)<br>  Tropicamide (Mydriacyl)<br>**OTC medications** (including antihistamines and belladonna alkaloids)<br>  Analgesics: Excedrin PM, Percogesic<br>  Cold remedies: Actifed, Allerest, Coricidin, Dristan, Flavihist, Romex, Sine-Off<br>  Hypnotics: Compoz, Sleep-Eze, Sominex<br>  Menstrual products: Pamprin, Premesyn PMS<br>**Skeletal muscle relaxants**<br>  Orphenadrine citrate (Norflex)<br>  Cyclobenzaprine hydrochloride (Flexeril)<br>**Mushrooms**<br>  *Amanita muscaria*<br>  *Amanita pantherina* |

*Source:* Adapted from LR Goldfrank, et al, 1990.

tagonism of muscarinic, nicotinic, or both receptors may occur. The central effects of cholinergic blockade include agitation, amnesia, anxiety, ataxia, coma, confusion, delirium, disorientation, dysarthria, hallucinations, hyperactivity, lethargy, somnolence, seizures, circulatory collapse, mydriasis, and respiratory failure. The peripheral effects include arrhythmias, tachycardia, decreased bronchial secretions, dysphagia, decreased gastrointestinal motility, hyperthermia, hypo- or hypertension, decreased salivation, decreased sweating, urinary retention, and vasodilation.

## CLINICAL PRESENTATION

The classic presentation of patients with anticholinergic toxicity can be remembered as:

> **Hot as Hades**
> **Blind as a Bat**
> **Dry as a Bone**
> **Red as a Beet**
> **Mad as a Hatter**

Clinical characteristics include unreactive mydriasis, hypo- or hypertension, absent bowel sounds, tachycardia, flushed skin, disorientation, urinary retention, hyperthermia, dry skin and mucous mem-

branes, and auditory and visual hallucinations. Patients can also present with seizures or coma. Cardiogenic pulmonary edema may occur secondary to depression of myocardial contraction.

The diagnosis of anticholinergic toxicity must be based on clinical presentation. The diagnosis may be confused with delirium tremens or an acute psychiatric disorder. Anticholinergic toxicity can be differentiated from delirium tremens and sympathomimetic toxicity by the presence of dry skin and the absence of bowel sounds. Acute psychiatric disorders may have associated tachycardia and tachypnea, but usually the physical examination is normal. Complications from anticholinergic toxicity occur secondary to hyperthermia, arrhythmias, seizures, and circulatory collapse.

Electrocardiographic abnormalities may include QRS prolongation, abnormal conduction, bundle branch block, AV dissociation, and atrial and ventricular tachycardias. Sinus tachycardia is the most common abnormality. Routine laboratory evaluations, including measurement of electrolytes, glucose, and arterial blood gases, should be checked in the presence of abnormal mental status but should be normal in isolated anticholinergic toxicity. Comprehensive toxicologic screens are of little value in the acute setting, and some anticholinergic agents (e.g., scopolamine) may not be detected. The screen can be used for confirmation, but the diagnosis should be based on clinical findings.

## TREATMENT

Conservative, supportive therapy is the mainstay of treatment of anticholinergic toxicity. Evaluation of the airway, breathing, and circulation is a priority. An intravenous line should be established and an ECG monitor placed in any patient with significant symptoms. Because gastrointestinal motility is delayed, gastric emptying may be effective after several hours. Activated charcoal may be useful to decrease drug absorption, particularly with agents that undergo enterohepatic circulation or when the agents ingested are unknown. A cathartic should also be administered.

Hyperthermia should be controlled with conventional therapy. Seizures can be treated with benzodiazepines and barbiturates. Hypertension usually does not require treatment, but conventional therapy should be used if necessary. The treatment of arrhythmias depends on the type and on the causative agent. Standard antiarrhythmics are usually effective, but class Ia agents should be avoided due to the quinidine-like effect of many anticholinergic drugs. Agitation can be treated with benzodiazepines. Because of their anticholinergic effects, phenothiazines should be avoided.

The most controversial topic surrounding anticholinergic toxicity is the use of physostigmine. Physostigmine is a tertiary ammonium compound which is a reversible acetylcholinesterase inhibitor that crosses the blood-brain barrier and reverses both central and peripheral anticholinergic effects. Physostigmine may aggravate arrhythmias and seizures and must be used with extreme caution. The indications for its use include the presence of peripheral anticholinergic signs and seizures unresponsive to conventional therapy, uncontrollable agitation, hemodynamically unstable arrhythmias unresponsive to conventional therapy, coma with respiratory depression, malignant hypertension, or refractory hypotension. Physostigmine should be avoided in cyclic antidepressant overdose as it may potentiate toxicity and increase mortality. The initial dose of physostigmine is 0.5 to 2.0 mg IV over 5 min. Improvement of central signs usually occurs within 5 to 15 min. The minimal effective dose should be used. Due to rapid elimination, repeat doses may be necessary every 30 to 60 min. Physostigmine use is contraindicated in patients with cardiovascular disease, bronchospasm, intestinal obstruction, heart block, peripheral vascular disease, and bladder obstruction. Patients receiving physostigmine should be on a monitor and observed for cholinergic symptoms (salivation, lacrimation, urination, and defecation).

Patients with mild symptoms of anticholinergic toxicity can be discharged after 6 h of observation, if their symptoms are improving. Patients receiving physostigmine usually require admission for at least 24 h.

## JIMSONWEED

Many plants have anticholinergic effects, including deadly nightshade, henbane, mandrake, burdock root, Jimsonweed, and others. They are often used for medicinal purposes or brewed in teas. *Datura stramonium,* also known as Jimsonweed, is a member of the Solanaceae family. It is a common weed that grows to be 3 to 6 ft high and can be found throughout the United States. Its leaves are large, jagged, and have a bitter taste and foul odor. The plant has large white or purple trumpet-shaped flowers that bloom in the late spring and become thorny quadripartite capsules in the fall, filled with black seeds. The entire plant is toxic and contains atropine, hyoscyamine, and scopolamine in various amounts. In the past, Jimsonweed was marketed and sold in health food stores in a preparation for the treatment of asthma. Many accidental childhood poisonings from Jimsonweed have been reported. Over the past 20 to 30 years, Jimsonweed has been involved in inadvertent overdoses in persons experimenting with mind-altering drugs. The plant can be smoked or ingested. Fifty to one hundred seeds contain the equivalent of 3 to 6 mg atropine.

Symptoms of anticholinergic toxicity occur within 2 to 6 h after the ingestion of Jimsonweed. As with other agents causing anticholinergic toxicity, patients present with fever, erythema, mydriasis, delirium, hallucinations, tachycardia, and amnesia. The treatment is the same as that described above. Because the seeds may remain in the stomach for prolonged periods, gastric emptying is recommended up to 12 to 24 h after the ingestion of seeds. The most persistent symptom of Jimsonweed toxicity is blurred vision, as mydriasis can persist for up to 1 week. Mydriasis can also occur from isolated local contact of Jimsonweed with the eye ("cornpicker's pupil").

## BIBLIOGRAPHY

Ellenhorn MJ, Barceloux DG: *Medical Toxicology, Diagnosis and Treatment of Human Poisoning.* New York, Elsevier, 1988.

Goldfrank LR, Flomenbaum NE, Lewin NA, et al (eds): *Goldfrank's Toxicologic Emergencies,* 4th ed. Norwalk, Appleton & Lange, 1990.

Goldfrank L, Flomenbaum N, Lewin N: Anticholinergic poisoning. *J Toxicol Clin Toxicol* 19:17, 1982.

Goodman LS, Gilman A: *The Pharmacologic Basis of Therapeutics,* 8th ed. Elmsford, NY, Pergamon, 1990.

Savitt DL, Roberts JR, Siegel EG: Anisocoria from Jimsonweed. *JAMA* 255:1439, 1986.

# 158
# HEAVY METALS
## Marsha D. Ford

Acute heavy metal toxicity is an uncommon clinical entity that can be a cause of significant morbidity and mortality if unrecognized and inappropriately treated. Because of their effects on numerous enzymatic systems in the body, the heavy metals often present with protean manifestations primarily affecting four systems: neurologic, gastro-intestinal, hematologic, and renal. Emergency physicians should be familiar with the common toxic manifestations of the most common metals—lead, arsenic, and mercury—in order to appropriately diagnose poisoned patients and to recognize an initial "index case" in order to prevent others from being poisoned when the metal source is environmental or industrial (see Table 158-1).

## LEAD

Lead is the most common cause of chronic heavy metal poisoning and remains a major environmental contaminant. The National Health and Nutrition Examination Survey II (NHANES II), conducted from 1976 to 1980, found that 1.9 percent of persons aged 6 months to 74 years had blood lead levels $\geq$ 30 $\mu$g/dL, with significantly higher levels being found in blacks and in children from lower socioeconomic groups. More recently phase 1 of NHANES III, 1988 to 1991, found that 0.4 percent of persons aged 1 year and older had blood lead levels $\geq$ 25 $\mu$g/dL, representing an overall improvement. However, the data for children aged 1 to 5 years indicate that an estimated 1.7 million children have blood lead levels $\geq$ 10 $\mu$g/dL. These elevated levels may have detrimental effects on development, and, thus, lead tox-icity remains a significant public health problem. Both inorganic and organic forms of lead produce clinical toxicity. Inorganic lead affects the central and peripheral nervous systems, hematopoietic system, kidney, gastrointestinal tract, liver, myocardium, and reproductive capacity. With organic lead intoxication, central nervous system effects predominate.

**Table 158-1.** Sources of Heavy Metals

| Heavy Metal | Source |
| --- | --- |
| **Lead** | |
| Inorganic | Soldering; battery burning/reclamation; bronzing; brassmaking; glassmaking; ingesting ceramic lead glaze; stripping old paint, "deleading" homes; "moonshine" whiskey; liquids in improperly glazed pottery; contaminated herbal medications; indoor shooting ranges; ingestion of paint chips, lead-laden floor dust, lead foreign bodies; lead bullets in abdomen or joint spaces. Workers at risk: jewelers, painters, lead burners and smelters, pipe cutters, pigment makers, printers, welders, pottery makers, radiator repair personnel, battery reclamation workers, construction workers. |
| Organic | Leaded gasoline |
| **Arsenic** | |
| Inorganic [arsenite ($As^{3+}$), arsenate ($As^{5+}$), elemental] | Insecticides, rodenticides, herbicides; mining smelting/refining; homeopathic medicines; kelp. |
| Organic | Parasitical medicines (veterinary) |
| Gas (arsine) | Mining smelting/refining; semiconductor industry; made by mixing acids with arsenic-containing insecticides. |
| **Mercury** | |
| Elemental | Battery and thermometer manufacture; sphygmomanometer repair; dentistry; jewelry and lamp manufacture; photography; mercury mining; manufacture of scientific instruments. |
| Salts | Taxidermy; fur processing; tannery work; chemical laboratories; manufacture of explosives, fireworks, disinfectants, button batteries, inks, and vinyl chloride. |
| Organic (methylmercury, ethylmercury, phenylmercury) | Contaminated seafood; embalming; manufacture of drugs, fungicides, bactericides; handling of insecticides; pesticides, coated seeds; manufacture of chloralkali; working with wood perservatives. |

## Inorganic Lead

### Pharmacology

Absorption is by the respiratory and gastrointestinal tracts, while skin absorption is negligible. In the body, lead distributes into the blood, soft tissues, and bone. Greater than 90 percent of the total body lead is stored in bone, where it easily exchanges with the blood. Excretion of lead occurs slowly; the biologic half-life of lead in bone has been estimated to be 30 years.

### Toxicopathology

Like all the heavy metals, lead combines with sulfhydryl groups in proteins, thereby interfering with enzymatic activity. In the hematopoietic system lead interferes with porphyrin metabolism, which may contribute to lead-induced anemia (see Fig. 158-1). The two enzymes chiefly affected are Δ-aminolevulinic acid dehydratase and ferrochelatase, the latter being the enzyme that catalyzes the transfer of iron from ferritin to protoporphyrin to form hemoglobin. Coexistent iron deficiency may act synergistically with lead toxicity to produce a more profound anemia and, in children, may be more important than lead as the cause of a microcytic anemia. Hemolytic anemia also occurs due to inhibition of red blood cell (RBC) pyrimidine 5′-nucleotidase, an enzyme responsible for clearing cellular RNA degradation products. On a blood peripheral smear, these prod-

ucts produce the RBC basophilic stippling sometimes seen in lead-poisoned patients.

Interference with enzymatic activity and neurotransmitters in the central nervous system (CNS) produces acute cytotoxicity, cerebral edema, hyperactivity, and seizures. In the peripheral nervous system (PNS), nerves undergo primary segmental demyelination followed by secondary axonal degeneration, primarily of the motor nerves. In the kidney acute lead toxicity affects the proximal tubule, producing a Fanconi-like syndrome with aminoaciduria, glucosuria, phosphaturia, and renal tubular acidosis. Chronic effects include interstitial nephritis and increased uric acid levels due to increased tubular reabsorption of urate. The relationship between chronic lead toxicity, gout, hypertension, and chronic renal failure remains controversial.

Toxic hepatitis with mildly elevated transaminases, normal bilirubin, and normal alkaline phosphatase can occur. Lead-induced adverse effects on the reproductive system include increased fetal wastage, premature membrane rupture, depressed sperm counts, abnormal/nonmotile sperm, and sterility. Chronic lead toxicity can depress free thyroxine levels without producing clinical hypothyroidism.

### Clinical Effects

The common signs and symptoms of acute, chronic, and delayed toxicity are listed in Table 158-2. A few points bear emphasis. Young children are more susceptible than adults to the effects of lead. Encephalopathy, a major cause of morbidity and mortality, may begin dramatically with seizures and coma or develop indolently over weeks to months with decreased alertness and memory progressing to mania, delirium, and cerebral edema. Gastrointestinal and hematologic manifestations occur more frequently with acute than with chronic poisoning, and the colicky abdominal pains may be associated with concurrent hemolysis. Patients may complain of a metallic taste and have bluish gingival lead lines. Delayed cognitive development can occur in infants and children whose cord and blood lead (PbB) levels are $\geq 10$ μg/dL. Finally, patients may be asymptomatic in the face of significantly elevated PbB levels.

### Diagnosis

History of an exposure—occupational, hobby, environmental, or alcohol-related—is the most important clue to making the diagnosis. The combination of abdominal or neurologic dysfunctions with a hemolytic anemia should raise the suspicion of lead toxicity. Emergency physicians should consider the diagnosis in all children presenting with encephalopathy.

Laboratory studies in the emergency department should focus on evaluation for anemia and examination of bone radiographs in chil-

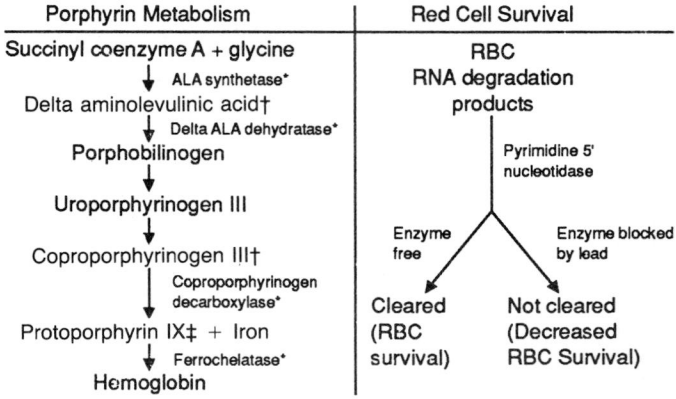

**Fig. 158-1.** Effects of lead on the hematopoietic system. * Enzymes affected by lead; † levels elevated in urine; and ‡ level elevated in RBCs.

**Table 158-2.** Clinical Effects of Inorganic Lead Toxicity

| System | Acute | Chronic | Late |
|---|---|---|---|
| Central nervous system | Encephalopathy (more common in children); seizures (focal or generalized); confusion, obtundation, coma; papilledema; optic neuritis; vomiting; ataxia. May have complaints listed under Chronic. Normal cerebellar and cranial nerve function. | Headache; irritability; depression, fatigue, behavioral change; memory deficit; apathy; sleep disturbances. | |
| Peripheral nervous system | Paresthesias. May have some or all findings listed under Chronic | Motor weakness, including classic wrist drop (peripheral neuropathy rare in children); depressed/absent DTRs; normal sensory function. | |
| Hematologic | Hypoproliferative and/or hemolytic anemias. Basophilic stippling (uncommon). | Same as in Acute. | |
| Gastrointestinal | Abdominal pain (colicky). | Abdominal pain (usually not severe, often absent); constipation; diarrhea. | |
| Renal | Fanconi-like syndrome: aminoaciduria, glucosuria, phosphaturia, renal tubular acidosis. | Interstitial nephritis. | Chronic renal failure; ? hypertension; gout. |
| Reproductive | | Decreased libido; impotence; sterility; abortions; premature births; insufficient and abnormal sperm production. | |
| Other | Bone pain. | Arthralgias; weakness; weight loss. | |

dren for "lead bands." The anemia can be normocytic or microcytic, possibly with evidence of hemolysis, including an elevated reticulocyte count and increased serum free hemoglobin. The peripheral smear may show basophilic stippling of the RBCs. Both anemia and basophilic stippling occur variably, and their absence does not rule out lead toxicity. Basophilic stippling of RBCs is nonspecific for lead toxicity, as it is also found in arsenic toxicity, sideroblastic anemia, and the thalassemias. In children radiographs of long bones, especially of the knee, may reveal horizontal, metaphyseal "lead bands," which represent failure of bone remodeling rather than deposition of lead.

The definitive diagnosis rests upon finding an elevated PbB level, with or without symptoms. The PbB level is the best single test for evaluating lead toxicity, and levels $\geq 10$ µg/dL are considered toxic. Screening levels may be performed on fingerstick capillary blood but, due to the potential for environmental Pb contamination, elevated levels should always be confirmed on a venous blood sample. Previously, a Calcium Disodium Versenate (CaNa$_2$-EDTA) provocation test was utilized to evaluate total-body lead stores and the need for chelation therapy when PbB levels were between 25 and 55 µg/dL. However, animal data demonstrating that one dose of CaNa$_2$-EDTA redistributes lead to the brain, the technical difficulties in performing the test, the lowering of the toxic PbB level to $\geq 10$ µg/dL, and the advent of dimercaptosuccinic acid (DMSA) as a safe and effective oral chelator raise concerns about the utility of the provocation test. Some major lead treatment centers have abandoned its use. Also with the lowering of the toxic PbB level to $\geq 10$ µg/dL, the erythrocyte protoporphyrin (EP) test can no longer be used to screen for lead toxicity, due to its unacceptably low sensitivity at these lower PbB levels.

## Differential Diagnosis

The differential diagnosis of lead toxicity includes causes of encephalopathy such as Wernicke's encephalopathy; withdrawal from ethanol and other sedative-hypnotic drugs; meningitis; encephalitis; human immunodeficiency virus (HIV) infection; intracerebral hemorrhage; hypoglycemia; severe fluid and electrolyte imbalances; hy-poxia; arsenic, thallium, and mercury toxicity; and poisoning with cyclic antidepressants, and anticholinergic drugs, ethylene glycol, or carbon monoxide. The abdominal pains can mimic sickle cell crisis or the hepatic porphyrias. Chronic lead toxicity can masquerade as depression, neurosis, hypothyroidism, polyneuritis, gout, iron deficiency anemia, and learning disability.

## Management

All patients with appropriate symptoms and an elevated PbB level are classified as lead toxic and should be treated. Fortunately, lead-induced encephalopathy rarely occurs now, but, unfortunately, it remains a major cause of serious morbidity and mortality in lead-toxic patients. In severely toxic patients, standard life support measures should be instituted and seizures treated with benzodiazepines, phenobarbital, phenytoin, and general anesthesia, if necessary. If abdominal films demonstrate radiopaque flecks consistent with lead, whole-bowel irrigation with a polyethylene glycol electrolyte solution (Colyte, Golytely) should be instituted. The solution should be administered continuously at a rate of 1000 to 2000 mL/h for adults and 100 to 500 mL/h for children until the abdominal radiograph is clear. It will not alter fluid or electrolyte balance in the patient. Fluid administration should be carefully controlled to avoid worsening the cerebral edema. Lumbar puncture may precipitate cerebral herniation and should be performed carefully, if at all, with the removal of a small amount of cerebrospinal fluid only.

Chelation therapy should be instituted immediately, prior to obtaining laboratory verification of the diagnosis. All chelating agents supply sulfhydryl groups to which the lead attaches. Dimercaprol (British anti-Lewisite, or BAL), 75 mg/m$^2$, should be administered IM first, followed 4 h later by CaNa$_2$-EDTA, 1500 mg/m$^2$ per 24 h, in a continuous IV infusion. The BAL administration is continued every 4 h. BAL chelates intracellular as well as extracellular lead and may be administered to patients in renal failure since it is also excreted in the bile. It is mixed in peanut oil and must be given IM. CaNa$_2$-EDTA chelates extracellular lead only and may exacerbate lead-induced CNS toxicity in patients with high PbB levels unless preceded by BAL therapy. Continuous IV infusion is the preferred method of delivery. CaNa$_2$-EDTA can cause renal toxicity, and patients should be adequately hydrated to promote diuresis and minimize the risk of this complication. It should not be used in patients with renal failure. Adverse effects of the chelating agents are listed in Table 158-3.

For symptomatic patients without encephalopathy and for asymptomatic patients with elevated PbB levels requiring chelation, the use of BAL and/or CaNa$_2$-EDTA and the dosing schedules are determined by the PbB levels and the presence or absence of symptoms. Children who are symptomatic but not encephalopathic should be treated as above except with doses of BAL, 50 mg/m$^2$, and CaNa$_2$-EDTA, 1000 mg/m$^2$ per 24 h. Symptomatic, nonencephalopathic

**Table 158-3.** Adverse Effects of Chelating Agents

| Chelating Agent | Adverse Effects |
| --- | --- |
| BAL (dimercaprol) | Hypertension<br>Febrile reaction, diaphoresis<br>Painful injection<br>Nausea/vomiting, salivation<br>Headache<br>Lacrimation, rhinorrhea<br>Hemolysis in G-6-PD-deficient patients<br>BAL-iron complex very toxic |
| CaNa$_2$-EDTA | Renal toxicity (especially if dehydrated)<br>Can increase CNS levels of lead if given prior to BAL<br>Chelates essential metals (e.g., copper, zinc, iron)<br>Dermatitis<br>Minor: Headache, chills, fever, myalgias, fatigue |
| D-Penicillamine | Nausea/vomiting<br>Fever<br>Rash<br>Leukopenia, thrombocytopenia<br>Eosinophilia<br>Hemolytic anemia<br>Stevens-Johnson syndrome<br>(Probably safe in penicillin-allergic patients) |
| DMSA | Nausea, vomiting, diarrhea<br>Abdominal gas, pain<br>Transient elevated AST, alkaline phosphatase<br>Rash, pruritus<br>Sore throat, rhinorrhea<br>Drowsiness, paresthesia<br>Thrombocytosis, esinophilia |

adults may be treated with BAL and CaNa$_2$-EDTA or with CaNa$_2$-EDTA alone. In asymptomatic patients, the standards for determining lead toxicity and the necessity for treatment differ for children and adults. In asymptomatic children, chelation therapy should be performed if the PbB level is $\geq$ 45 µg/dL. If the PbB level is 20 to 44 µg/dL, treatment strategies include environmental and nutritional evaluation, medical examination, and possibly chelation therapy, either with DMSA or CaNa$_2$-EDTA. For children with PbB levels between 10 and 19 µg/dL, interventions include nutritional and medical evaluation, repeat screening PbB levels, and environmental investigation for persistently high levels. In asymptomatic adults, the guidelines are less rigorous. In asymptomatic workers, a PbB of < 40 µg/dL is accepted as normal, levels of 40 to 50 µg/dL require increased job surveillance, and levels > 50 µg/dL require temporary removal from the job until the PbB drops below 40 µg/dL. Details on therapy for these various groups can be found in standard toxicology references.

Two oral chelating agents are being used in lead toxicity. DMSA, an analogue of dimercaprol, effectively chelates lead in adults and children. Its advantages include oral administration without increasing lead absorption from the gastrointestinal tract, no serious adverse effects, and minimal chelation of essential metals. High cost is its main disadvantage. The dose is 10 mg/kg every 8 h for 5 days, followed by the same dose every 12 h for 14 days. Repeat treatment may be necessary after a 2-week drug-free period. D-Penicillamine is a less effective chelating agent but has the advantage of being inexpensive It has been used for outpatient therapy in both asymptomatic children and adults with mild PbB elevations.

Removal of the source of lead is mandatory for all patients. Patients should not be discharged to their former environments until appropriate deleading and decontamination measures have been accomplished. Family members and coworkers should be evaluated for occult lead toxicity.

A guide for hospitalization would be to hospitalize:

1. All children with symptoms or with a PbB $\geq$ 70 µg/dL.
2. All adults with CNS symptoms.
3. All patients with suspected toxicity, when returning to the environment is considered dangerous.

## Prognosis

Approximately 85 percent of patients who suffer encephalopathy develop permanent CNS damage including seizures, mental retardation in children, and cognitive deficits in adults. Abdominal colic usually subsides within days after beginning chelation therapy, and other acute manifestations clear within 1 to 16 weeks with therapy. Lead-induced nephropathy may be partially reversible with chelation therapy.

## Organic Lead Intoxication

Exposure to tetraethyl lead (TEL), found in leaded gasoline, can occur with gasoline sniffing or in the occupational setting. Tetraethyl lead is metabolized to inorganic lead and triethyl lead. Triethyl lead is the primary toxic product which produces predominantly CNS toxicity. Symptoms range from behavioral changes with irritability, insomnia, restlessness, and nausea/vomiting to tremor, chorea, convulsions, and mania. Muscle, hepatic, and renal damage can occur. Anemia and elevated EP levels are usually not found. PbB levels may be normal or elevated. Therapy consists of removal from the source, symptomatic treatment, and chelation only if the PbB is elevated.

## ARSENIC

Arsenic is a nearly tasteless, odorless metal; it is the most common cause of acute heavy metal poisoning and the second leading source of chronic heavy metal toxicity. Arsenicals are found in a variety of compounds and industries (see Table 158-1) and continue to be used as tools for homicides and suicides. Elemental, inorganic and, organic salts, and gaseous forms exist. Elemental and organic forms have little to no toxicity and will not be discussed further. Inorganic compounds include arsenite (As$^{3+}$) and arsenate (As$^{5+}$). These compounds are the most toxic forms, and the discussion below will focus on inorganic arsenic toxicity. Arsine, a gaseous form, has toxicopathologic mechanisms and treatment that differ from those of other arsenical compounds. It will be discussed under a separate heading.

## Pharmacology

Arsenic is well absorbed via the gastrointestinal (GI), respiratory, and parenteral routes, and may be absorbed through damaged skin. Due to its water solubility, pentavalent arsenic (arsenate) is more readily absorbed through mucous membranes, for example, the GI tract, than trivalent arsenic (arsenite). Arsenite penetrates the skin more readily due to its increased lipid solubility. After absorption, arsenic localizes in erythrocytes and leukocytes or binds to serum proteins. Within 24 h redistribution into the liver, kidney, spleen, lung, GI tract, muscle, and nervous tissues occurs with subsequent integration into hair, nails, and bone. Metabolism of inorganic arsenic occurs via methylation. Elimination from the blood is rapid, and excretion is predominantly renal. Toxicity of the various forms is partially determined by excretory rates, with the more toxic arsenite being excreted at a slower rate than arsenate or the organic arsenical compounds. Arsenic crosses the placenta and has produced teratogenicity in both animals and humans.

## Toxicopathology

Arsenic reversibly binds with sulfhydryl groups found in many tissues and enzyme systems. The mechanisms of toxicity for inorganic arsenic are as follows:

1. For arsenite, inhibition of the pyruvate dehydrogenase complex is the primary biochemical lesion. This inhibition results in diminished adenosine triphosphate (ATP) production and, indirectly, in decreased gluconeogenesis possibly leading to hypoglycemia.
2. For arsenate, uncoupling of oxidative phosphorylation and loss of ATP occurs when $As^{5+}$ substitutes for inorganic phosphate in one step of the glycolysis reaction.

Pathologically, acute exposure produces dilation and increased permeability of small blood vessels, resulting in GI mucosal and submucosal inflammation and necrosis, cerebral edema and hemorrhage, myocardial tissue destruction, and fatty degeneration of the liver and kidneys. Subacute or chronic exposure can cause a primary peripheral axonal neuropathy with secondary demyelination.

## Clinical Effects

The signs and symptoms of toxicity vary with the form, amount, and concentration ingested and the rates of absorption and excretion of the various arsenical compounds. Arsenite (trivalent) is more toxic than arsenate (pentavalent). Symptoms usually occur within 30 min to several hours of ingestion. Severe gastroenteritis with nausea, vomiting, and cholera-like diarrhea is the hallmark of acute poisoning and may last several days to weeks, frequently necessitating hospitalization. Patients may complain of a metallic taste. Hypotension and tachycardia secondary to volume depletion, capillary leak, and myocardial dysfunction occur in moderate to severe cases. The ECG may demonstrate nonspecific ST- and T-wave changes with a prolonged $QT_c$, although these findings are more common in chronic intoxication. Ventricular tachycardia with a torsade de pointes morphology has been reported. Secondary myocardial ischemia may occur, leading to an erroneous diagnosis of primary myocardial infarction. Acute encephalopathy with delirium, seizures, and coma; pulmonary edema; acute renal failure; rhabdomyolysis; and death may ensue.

Patients with subacute or chronic toxicity typically present with complaints of a peripheral neuropathy, skin rash, or a nonspecific malaise and weakness, often with a history of gastroenteritis occurring 1 to 6 weeks earlier. Survivors of acute poisonings can develop the same problems. The peripheral neuropathy develops in a stocking-glove distribution and is initially sensory, with later motor symptoms. Severe cases can develop an ascending paralysis mimicking Guillain-Barré syndrome. The dermatologic manifestations vary. Hyperpigmentation, hyperkeratosis of the palms and soles, morbilliform rash, and epidermoid cancer have been reported. Mee lines (1- to 2-mm-wide transverse white lines in the nails) may be seen 4 to 6 weeks after an acute ingestion, while nasal septal perforation has been found in workers exposed occupationally to arsenic. Patients may complain of weakness, muscular aching, abdominal pain, memory loss, personality changes, periorbital and extremity edema, or decreased hearing secondary to sensorineural damage. Chronic encephalopathy with delirium, hallucinations, disorientation, agitation, and confabulation resembling Korsakoff syndrome has been reported. Chronic exposure to arsenic has been linked with the development of squamous cell and basal skin carcinomas, respiratory tract cancer, hepatic angiosarcoma, and possibly with leukemia (see Table 158-4).

## Diagnosis

Without a history of known exposure to arsenic, the diagnosis must be based on the presenting signs and symptoms and a strong index of clinical suspicion. Physicians rarely encounter arsenic toxicity, and, unfortunately, criminal poisonings often go undetected. The diagnosis of acute arsenic poisoning should be considered in any patient with hypotension of unknown etiology that was preceded by a severe gastroenteritis. The diagnosis of chronic arsenic toxicity should be considered in a patient with a peripheral neuropathy, typical skin manifestations, or recurrent bouts of unexplained gastroenteritis.

An abdominal radiograph may demonstrate intestinal radiopaque metallic flecks in cases of arsenic ingestions. The complete blood count may reveal either a normocytic, normochromic, or megaloblastic anemia and/or a thrombocytopenia. The white blood cell (WBC) count may be elevated in acute toxicity and decreased in chronic cases. A relative eosinophilia, up to 21 percent, and basophilic stippling of the RBCs have been reported. Elevated reticulocyte counts are found in cases with a component of hemolytic anemia. The electrocardiogram often reveals a prolonged $QT_c$ interval, especially in cases of chronic poisoning.

Definitive diagnosis of acute poisoning depends upon finding elevated arsenic levels in a 24-h urine collection. All urinary measurements of heavy metals should be collected in metal-free containers. Normal urinary arsenic is < 0.05 mg/L, and total urinary arsenic excretion in an unexposed patient should not exceed 0.1 mg/24 h. If the baseline urinary level is within normal limits and arsenic intoxication is still suspected, hair and nail clippings should be harvested for laboratory analysis. Due to the rapid distribution of arsenic in tissues, blood arsenic levels are unreliable. The reader is referred to *Goldfrank's Toxicologic Emergencies,* 5th edition, for a detailed discussion of laboratory testing and interpretation of results in arsenic toxicity.

## Differential Diagnosis

Arsenic toxicity should be included in the differential diagnosis for septic shock; peripheral neuropathy, including Guillain-Barré syndrome; Addison disease; hypo- and hyperthyroidism; patients with the previously mentioned dermatologic manifestations; Korsakoff syndrome; persistent gastroenteritis and/or cholera-like diarrhea; porphyria; other heavy metal toxicities such as thallium; and unexplained, prolonged malaise and weakness.

## Management

Acute arsenical toxicity is a life-threatening illness requiring aggressive management. The first task is to ensure adequate respiratory and circulatory function. Hypotension and arrhythmias are the chief causes of death. Hypotension, usually due to volume depletion, should be managed initially with crystalloid volume replacement. Invasive hemodynamic monitoring followed by further crystalloid and pressor therapy with dopamine or norepinephrine (levarterenol) may be required. Overhydration should be avoided since pulmonary and cerebral edema can occur. Cardiac monitoring should be instituted. Ventricular tachycardia and fibrillation may be treated with lidocaine, bretylium, and electrical defibrillation as necessary. Isoproterenol, magnesium, and overdrive pacing therapies should be considered for torsade de pointes arrhythmias. Drugs that prolong the $QT_c$, including classes IA (procainamide, quinidine, disopyramide), IC, and III antidysrhythmics should be avoided. Potassium, calcium, and magnesium levels should be monitored and corrected as necessary to prevent further prolongation of the $QT_c$ with possible exacerbation of torsade de pointes arrhythmias.

Gastric lavage with a large-bore orogastric tube should be performed in all cases of acute ingestion, and activated charcoal (1 g/kg body weight) and a cathartic should be instilled. Activated charcoal poorly adsorbs arsenic but may be effective if coingestants were taken. Whole-bowel irrigation should be considered if abdominal radiographs reveal intestinal radiopaque materials consistent with arsenic.

Seizures can be treated with benzodiazepines, phenobarbital, phenytoin, and general anesthesia as necessary.

Initial management of chronic toxicity should be directed toward

**Table 158-4.** Signs and Symptoms of Arsenic Toxicity

| System | Toxicity | | |
| --- | --- | --- | --- |
| | Acute | Subacute | Chronic |
| CNS | Encephalopathy<br>Delirium<br>Seizures<br>Coma | Encephalopathy develops/<br>persists<br>Irritableness<br>Confusion<br>Decreased memory<br>Hallucinations<br>VI cranial nerve palsy | Encephalopathy develops/<br>persists |
| PNS | Subacute symptoms can<br>develop early | Sensory symptoms early<br>Diminished/absent<br>vibration, DTRs,<br>pinprick, light touch<br>Motor weakness<br>ascending paralysis<br>Severe extremity pain with<br>light touch | Sensorimotor neuropathy<br>develops/persists |
| Cardiovascular | Arrhythmias<br>Prolonged $QT_c$<br>Torsade de pointes<br>Pulmonary edema<br>Myocarditis<br>Hypotension | Arrhythmias<br>Prolonged $QT_c$<br>Torsade de pointes | |
| Gastrointestinal | Nausea, vomiting<br>Diarrhea<br>Abdominal pain<br>Toxic hepatitis | Persistence of<br>acute symptoms<br>Anorexia<br>Weight loss | May be absent<br>Nausea, diarrhea<br>Colicky abdominal pain |
| Pulmonary | Pulmonary edema<br>Respiratory failure | Cough, rales, hemoptysis<br>Chest pain<br>Interstitial lung infiltrates | Cough |
| Hematologic | Hemolytic anemia | Pancytopenia | Anemia<br>Aplastic anemia<br>Agranulocytosis |
| Renal | Acute tubular<br>necrosis<br>Cortical necrosis | | |
| ENT | Metallic taste<br>Mucous membrane<br>irritation | | |
| Dermatologic | | Alopecia<br>Macular pruritic rash<br>Brawny desquamation<br>Mee's lines<br>Facial/peripheral edema | Hypopigmentation/hyperpigmentation<br>Palmoplantar keratoses<br>Papular keratoses<br>Ulcerative lesions<br>Facial/peripheral edema<br>Skin carcinomas—basal cell,<br>squamous, Bowen's |
| Other | Fever<br>Rhabdomyolysis,<br>acute myopathy | Fever<br>Diaphoresis<br>Fatigue | Fatigue<br>Cancer<br>Lung, hemangiosarcoma<br>Cirrhosis<br>Noncirrhotic portal hypertension<br>Blackfoot's disease |

*Source:* Reprinted with permission from Ford M: Arsenic, in Goldfrank LR, Flomenbaum NE, Lewin NA, et al (eds): *Goldfrank's Toxicologic Emergencies,* 5th ed. Norwalk, Appleton/Lange, 1994, pp 1011–1025.

prevention of further arsenic absorption and gastrointestinal decontamination, if appropriate. In cases of suspected homicidal intent, patients should be advised to avoid food and drinks prepared by others, and visitor contact with hospitalized patients should be carefully monitored.

Chelation therapy with BAL should be instituted immediately in all cases of known or suspected acute arsenical poisoning and in proven cases of chronic toxicity. In cases of suspected chronic toxicity with stable symptoms, therapy may be withheld pending diagnosis. BAL doses range 3 to 5 mg/kg IM every 4 h for 2 days followed by 3 to 5 mg/kg every 6 to 12 h. In severe, life-threatening toxicity

BAL therapy should be continued until the clinical condition stabilizes and a less toxic oral chelating agent can be substituted. Two oral chelating agents discussed in the section on lead toxicity, DMSA and D-penicillamine, can also be used to enhance arsenic excretion. DMSA is preferred and is given according to the dosing regimen for lead, but therapy may be required beyond the initial 19-day regimen. D-Penicillamine (100 mg/kg per day with a maximum dose of 2 g for adults and 1 g for children) should be given in four divided doses per day for 5 days. During chelation intermittent 24-h urinary arsenic levels should be measured and therapy continued until the urine level falls below 0.05 mg/L per 24 h.

Hemodialysis can remove small amounts of arsenic (2 to 4.5 mg) in patients with acute renal failure but is not indicated otherwise.

Hospitalize:

1. All patients with acute or life-threatening known or suspected arsenic poisoning.
2. All chronically poisoned patients requiring BAL therapy.
3. All patients in whom suicidal or homicidal intent is suspected.

## Prognosis and Sequelae

In acute toxicity, prognosis may be influenced favorably by the rapid institution of BAL therapy. Recovery from arsenical neuropathy appears to be related more to initial severity of symptoms than to institution of chelation therapy, although in those patients who do recover, BAL appears to significantly shorten the duration of illness. Often, neurologic recovery occurs slowly over months to years. Normalization of hematologic values can occur in the absence of any specific therapy. BAL has a variable effect on the dermatologic manifestations; hyperpigmentation is unresponsive to this therapy.

## Arsine

Arsine is a colorless, nonirritating gas encountered in the semiconductor industry, ore smelting, and refining processes and is also produced when arsenic-containing insecticides are mixed with acids. Arsine attaches to sulfhydryl groups of hemoglobin, producing an acute hemolytic anemia with resultant jaundice, abdominal pain, and hemoglobinuria-induced acute renal failure. Acute poisonings are managed with blood transfusions, exchange transfusion to remove the nondialyzable arsine, and hemodialysis for the acute renal failure. BAL therapy has no role in the management of arsine toxicity.

## MERCURY

Mercury occurs in both inorganic and organic forms. Inorganic compounds are divided further into elemental mercury and mercurous and mercuric salts. Organic mercurials exist as short- and long-chained alkyl and aryl compounds. The short-chained alkyls, such as methyl mercury and ethyl mercury, are more toxic to humans. All forms of mercury are toxic but differ in the routes of absorption, constellations of clinical findings, and responses to therapy.

## Pharmacology

Elemental mercury is primarily absorbed via inhalation of its vapor but may also be absorbed dermally. Absorption by the gastrointestinal tract is usually negligible. Intramuscular injections of mercury can induce abscess and granuloma formation; delayed systemic toxicity can occur. Intravenous injections have produced mercury pulmonary and systemic emboli. Both mercuric salts and organic mercury are primarily absorbed through the GI tract, with the short-chained alkyl organic compounds being better absorbed than the aryl organic compounds.

Elemental mercury crosses the blood-brain barrier where it is ionized and trapped in the CNS. Mercuric salts are deposited in the ionized form primarily in the kidney and also in the liver and spleen. The salts do not enter the CNS in consequential amounts. With organic mercury compounds, the highly lipid-soluble short-chained alkyls easily cross membranes, accumulating in RBCs, the CNS, liver, kidney, and the fetus. Longer-chained alkyl and the aryl compounds are biotransformed into inorganic mercuric ions in the body. Therefore, toxicity with these compounds more closely resembles inorganic mercury toxicity.

Inorganic and the aryl organic mercurials are eliminated in the urine and feces. The short-chained alkyl compounds are primarily excreted in the bile where they undergo significant enterohepatic circulation.

## Toxicopathology

Mercury binds with sulfhydryl groups, affecting a diverse number of enzyme and protein systems. Methylmercury also inhibits choline acetyl transferase, which catalyzes the final step in the production of acetylcholine, and may produce an acetylcholine deficiency.

## Clinical Effects

The clinical effects of mercury poisoning depend upon the form and, in some cases, the route of administration. In general, the neurologic, gastrointestinal, and renal systems are predominantly affected. The short-chained alkyl compounds, methyl- and ethylmercury, have the most devastating effects on the CNS, followed by elemental mercury, whose primary toxicity is neurologic. Both forms of mercury produce erethism, a constellation of neuropsychiatric abnormalities including anxiety, depression, irritability, mania, sleep disturbances, excessive shyness, and memory loss. Tremor, either intention or nonintention, is a common physical finding. The short-chained alkyls produce paresthesias (early sign), ataxia, muscular rigidity or spasticity, and visual and hearing impairment and induce CNS teratogenic effects. Gastrointestinal effects of both elemental and short-chained alkyl compounds are mild. In cases of severe, chronic poisoning with elemental mercury, stomatitis, gingivitis, and excessive salivation are seen. Chronic toxicity of elemental and organic forms may cause renal glomerular and tubular damage.

In contrast, the mercury salts have little to no effect on the CNS but produce a severe corrosive gastroenteritis with abdominal pain which may be followed rapidly by cardiovascular collapse. Renal effects are typical, including acute tubular necrosis within 24 h. Children exposed to all forms of mercury except the short-chained alkyls can develop acrodynia, a condition characterized by a generalized rash, fever, irritability, splenomegaly, and generalized hypotonia with particular weakness of the pelvic and pectoral muscles. Further details of clinical findings are listed in Table 158-5. Swallowing mercury contained in a glass thermometer usually does not produce adverse effects because the mercury is not absorbed from the gastrointestinal tract unless the GI tract is damaged or contains fistulas.

## Diagnosis

A thorough history, including occupational exposures, and typical physical findings, especially tremor or a constellation of signs and symptoms suggesting erethism or acrodynia, may alert the emergency physician to mercury toxicity. Ingestion of mercuric chloride can produce a rapidly fatal course and should be considered in any patient presenting with a corrosive gastroenteritis. Often, however, the diagnosis of mercury toxicity is subtle, arrived at only after many other diagnoses have been investigated.

For all forms of mercury except short-chained alkyls, a 24-h urinary measurement of mercury should be performed. Most unexposed individuals will have levels ≤ 10 to 15 µg/L. A level of > 20 µg/dL either before or after therapy indicates meaningful exposure. In cases of chronic toxicity this measurement may be falsely low. Whole-blood mercury levels are less reliable diagnostically. A seafood meal can temporarily elevate the blood level to the toxic range.

Short-chained alkyl mercury compounds are predominantly excreted via the bile, rendering urinary measurements invalid. Laboratory diagnosis rests on finding elevated whole-blood mercury levels, since these compounds concentrate in erythrocytes. Whole-blood mercury levels are normally < 1.5 µg/dL.

## Differential Diagnosis

The differential diagnosis of mercury toxicity depends upon the form ingested. Hypothyroidism, apathetic hyperthryroidism, metabolic encephalopathy, senile dementia, adverse effects of therapeutic drugs

**Table 158-5.** Clinical Effects of Mercury Toxicity

| | Inorganic | | Organic | |
| System | Elemental | Salts | Short-Chained Alkyls* | Long-Chained Alkyls, Aryls |
|---|---|---|---|---|
| Neurologic | Tremor (intention and nonintention), peripheral neuropathy (sensorimotor). Seizures (vapor inhalation). | (−) | Paresthesias (early sign); ataxia; sensory and hearing impairment; constricted visual fields; dysarthria; muscular rigidity or spasticity; seizures (rare); muscle tenderness; and optic atrophy (EM only). MM: Sensorimotor neuropathy. | |
| Erethism** | + | − | + | |
| GI | Stomatitis, gingivitis, excessive salivation (severe chronic poisoning). Blue gum line. | Severe gastroenteritis, may be hemorrhagic; abdominal pain, stomatitis, proctitis, colitis. | MM: Rarely symptoms. EM: Nausea/vomiting, abdominal cramps. | Similar to elemental. |
| Renal | Glomerular and tubular damage (chronic). | Acute tubular necrosis (severe poisoning); proteinuria, hematuria and casts (mild poisoning). Nephrotic syndrome. | MM: − EM: Polyuria, proteinuria. | Similar to elemental. |
| Pulmonary (inhaled) | Pneumonitis, pulmonary edema, pneumothorax, pneumomediastinum. | − | Same as elemental. | Same as elemental. |
| Skin | Slate-gray pigmentation. Brownish-yellow discoloration of anterior capsule of eye. Allergic dermatitis. | Urticaria, vesication, allergic dermatitis. | Erythroderma, pruritus. | |
| Teratogenicity | − | − | Cerebral palsy, mental retardation, micrognathia, microcephaly, cleft palate, blindness, chorea, ataxia. | |
| Acrodynia† | + | + | − | + |
| Other | | Rapid cardiovascular collapse with mercuric chloride. | EM: Severe musculoskeletal pain. | |

* MM, methylmercury; EM, ethylmercury.

† Generalized rash with erythema and desquamation of hands, feet, and nose; fever, diaphoresis, splenomegaly; hypotonia, irritability, weakness of pelvic/pectoral muscles. Does not occur in newborns or adults.

** Systemic or organ specific irritability.

(such as lithium, theophylline, phenytoin), Parkinson disease, delayed neuropsychiatric sequelae of carbon monoxide poisoning, lacunar infarction, cerebellar degenerative disease or tumor, and ethanol or sedative-hypnotic drug withdrawal may produce behavioral changes or tremor similar to those caused by elemental mercury. Causes of corrosive gastroenteritis such as iron, arsenic, phosphorus, acids, or alkalis should be considered in the differential diagnosis for mercury salts. Many of the differential diagnoses for elemental mercury also apply to the organic mercury compounds. Cerebral palsy, intrauterine hypoxia, and teratogenic effects of therapeutic and illicit drugs and environmental contaminants should be considered when evaluating an infant thought to be affected in utero by the short-chained alkyl mercury compounds.

## Treatment

General therapeutic measures include removal from exposure and supportive therapy. Ingestion of mercury salts should be treated with aggressive gastrointestinal decontamination including instillation of milk or egg whites to bind the mercury, lavage, and activated charcoal. Given the profuse diarrhea that may ensue, a cathartic may not be indicated. A polythiolated resin (commercially unavailable) has been used to bind intestinal methylmercury and interrupt the enterohepatic circulation. Neostigmine may improve motor function in methylmercury-poisoned patients by improving acetylcholine levels.

Both BAL and D-penicillamine may be used for chelation therapy. BAL is the preferred chelator for mercury salts and is administered in a regimen of 3 to 5 mg/kg per dose IM every 4 h for 2 days, then every 6 h for 2 days, followed by every 12 h for 7 days. BAL is contraindicated in methylmercury poisoning due to exacerbation of CNS

symptoms. The BAL-mercury complex is dialyzable, and hemodialysis may be helpful in patients receiving BAL who have diminished renal function. D-Penicillamine is used in elemental mercury and less severe cases of mercury salt toxicities. The dose is 100 mg/kg per day, to a maximum of 1 g in four divided doses for 3 to 10 days. D-Penicillamine has been used with variable results in organic mercury poisoning. DMSA has demonstrated efficacy in binding mercury, including organic forms, and may become the treatment of choice for the short-chained alkyl compounds.

Hospitalize:

1. All patients known or suspected of ingesting mercury salts.
2. All patients known to have or suspected to have inhaled elemental mercury vapor with pulmonary injury.
3. All patients requiring BAL therapy.

## Prognosis and Sequelae

Outcome depends upon the form of mercury and the severity of toxicity. Mild cases of elemental and mercury salt poisoning and very mild cases of organic mercury toxicity may result in complete recovery. Death can occur in severe cases of mercuric chloride poisoning. Most cases of organic mercury poisoning are left with residual neurologic deficits.

## BIBLIOGRAPHY

### General

Goldfrank LR, Flomenbaum NE, Lewin NA, et al (eds): *Goldfrank's Toxicologic Emergencies,* 5th ed. Norwalk, Appleton/Lange, 1994.

Graziano JH: Role of 2,3-dimercaptosuccinic acid in the treatment of heavy metal poisoning. *Med Toxicol* 1:155, 1986.

## Lead

Baghurst PA, McMichael AJ, Wigg NR, et al: Environmental exposure to lead and children's intelligence at the age of seven years. The Port Pirie Cohort Study. *N Engl J Med* 327:1279, 1992.

Brody DJ, Pirkle JL, Kramer RA, et al: Blood lead levels in the US population: Phase 1 of the Third National Health and Nutrition Examination Survey (NHANES III, 1988 to 1991). *JAMA* 272:277, 1994.

Centers for Disease Control: *Preventing Lead Poisoning in Young Children,* US Dept of Health and Human Services, October, 1991.

Cory-Slechta D, Weiss B, Cox C: Mobilization and redistribution of lead over the course of calcium disodium ethylenediamine tetraacetate chelation therapy. *J Pharmacol Exp Ther* 243:804, 1987.

Glotzer DE, Bauchner H: Management of childhood lead poisoning: A survey. *Pediatrics* 89:614, 1992.

Graziano JH, Lolacono NJ, Moulton T: Controlled study of meso 2,3-dimercaptosuccinic acid for the management of childhood lead intoxication. *J Pediatr* 120:133, 1992.

Kapoor SC, Wielopolski L, Graziano JH, et al: Influence of 2,3-dimercaptosuccinic acid on gastrointestinal lead absorption and whole-body lead retention. *Toxicol Appl Pharmacol* 97:525, 1989.

Kobayashi H, Suzuki T, Sato I, et al: Neurotoxicological aspects of organotoxin and lead compounds on cellular and molecular mechanisms. *TEN* 1:23, 1994.

McElvaine MD, Orbach HG, Binder S, et al: Evaluation of the erythrocyte protoporphyrin test as a screen for elevated blood lead levels. *J Pediatr* 119:548, 1991.

## Arsenic

Beckman KJ, Bauman JL, Pimental PA, et al: Arsenic-induced torsades de pointes. *Crit Care Med* 19:290, 1991.

Fowler BA, Weissberg JB: Arsine poisoning. *N Engl J Med* 291:1171, 1974.

Graziano JH, Cuccia D, Friedheim E: The pharmacology of 2,3-dimercaptosuccininc acid and its potential use in arsenic poisoning. *J Pharmacol Exp Ther* 20:1051, 1978.

Hilfer RJ, Mandel A: Acute arsenic intoxication diagnosed by roentgenograms. *N Engl J Med* 266:663, 1962.

Kyle RA, Pease GL: Hematologic aspects of arsenic intoxication. *N Engl J Med* 273:18, 1965.

Mahieu P, Buchet JP, Roels HA, et al: The metabolism of arsenic in humans acutely intoxicated by $As_2O_3$: Its significance for the duration of BAL therapy. *J Toxicol Clin Toxicol* 18:1067, 1981.

McKinney JD: Metabolism and disposition of inorganic arsenic in laboratory animals and humans. *Environ Geochem Health* 14:43, 1992.

Park MJ, Currier M: Arsenic exposures in Mississippi: A review of cases *South Med J* 84: 461, 1991.

Schoolmeester WL, White DR: Arsenic poisoning. *South Med J* 73:198, 1980.

## Mercury

Agocs MM, Etzel RA, Parrish RG, et al: Mercury exposure from interior latex paint. *N Engl J Med* 323:1096, 1990.

Ambre JJ, Welsh MJ, Svare CW, et al: Intravenous elemental mercury injection: Blood levels and excretion of mercury. *Ann Intern Med* 87:451, 1977.

Elhassani SA: The many faces of methylmercury poisoning. *Clin Toxicol* 19:875, 1982–83.

Laundy T, Adam AE, Kershaw JB, et al: Deaths after peritoneal lavage with mercuric chloride solutions: Case report and review of the literature. *Br Med J* 289:96, 1984.

Levin SP, Cavender GD, Langoff GD, et al: Elemental mercury exposure: Peripheral neurotoxicity. *Br J Indust Med* 39:136, 1982.

Lilis R, Miller A, Lerman Y: Acute mercury poisoning with severe chronic pulmonary manifestations. *Chest* 88:306, 1985.

Roels HA, Boeckx M, Ceulemans E, et al: Urinary excretion of mercury after occupational exposure to mercury vapour and influence of the chelating agent meso-2,3-dimercaptosuccinic acid (DMSA) *Br J Ind Med* 48:247, 1991.

Schwartz JG, Snider TE, Montiel MM: Toxicity of a family from vacuumed mercury. *Am J Emerg Med* 10:258, 1992.

Sketris IS, Gray JD: Mercury poisoning. *Clin Toxicol Consult* 5:10, 1983.

Takeuchi T: Pathology of Minamata disease. *Acta Pathol Jpn* 32:73, 1982.

Winek CL, Fochtman FW, Bricker JD, et al: Fatal mercuric chloride ingestion. *Clin Toxicol* 18:261, 1981.

## 159

# FROSTBITE AND OTHER LOCALIZED COLD-RELATED INJURIES

### Mark Rabold*

Throughout history the most celebrated and extreme reports of cold-related injuries have been in the field of military endeavor. From Hannibal losing half his 46,000 man army crossing the Pyrenean Alps to frostbite and hypothermia, to the tens of thousands of cases of trench foot during World War I, we have learned much. But perhaps the most famous cold injury mass casualty incident was Napoleon's retreat from Moscow during the dreadful winter of 1812–1813. This first authoritative account as described by Napoleon's Surgeon-in-Chief, Baron de Larrey, described how each evening thousands of French soldiers thawed, and often inadvertently burned, their frozen extremities over campfires, only to refreeze them again on the next day's march. Combined heat and cold injury coupled with refreezing and forced ambulation resulted in abysmal outcomes. Additionally, thousands died from the tetanus sustained from their frostbite wounds. It was from this experience that Larrey recommended rubbing frostbitten extremities with snow. This destructive therapy was the standard of care until the 1950s and is still used occasionally by the lay public. It was not until 1956 that rapid rewarming of frozen extremities was studied by a Public Health Service medical officer in Tanana, Alaska, which laid the foundation of modern therapy.

## PATHOPHYSIOLOGY

It is man's inability to physiologically compensate and protect himself from the cold that produces injury. However, cold itself is not the only factor in determining whether injury will occur. Duration of contact, humidity, wind, altitude, clothing, medical conditions, behavior, and individual variability all contribute to the picture.

Cold-induced injury may be instantaneous, as with contact frostbite after touching a cold metal bottle of fuel or more chronic as in chilblains. The humidity also is important because this contributes to evaporative heat loss. Wet skin is more conducive to both ice crystal formation subcutaneously and to trench foot as well. Wind velocity and cold, the wind-chill factor, have a synergistic affect on heat loss. For example, an ambient temperature of −7°C (19.4°F) when combined with a wind of 72.5 kph (45 mph) will feel equivalent to −40°C (−40°F) on a windless day. The rigors of travel at high altitude may also predispose to cold injury. Although the lower barometric pressure has not been shown to directly influence susceptibility to cold injury, a variety of factors associated with high altitude travel have. The fatigue, dehydration, and hypoxia seen so often in climbers or trekkers, coupled with the sometimes extreme weather conditions and remote locations, all contribute to the incidence and severity of cold-related injuries at altitude.

Inadequate clothing is probably the most avoidable cause of cold-related injuries. Constrictive clothing and boots can reduce circulation to extremities and predispose to frostbite. An exposed head and

neck can account for 80% of body heat loss. Natural fiber clothing, such as wool and cotton, when compared to modern synthetics such as polypropylene, have poorer wicking ability and greater thermal conductance and moisture retention. Simply changing out of cold, wet clothes into dry ones can also be preventive. During World War I, the British decreased the number of trench foot cases from 29,172 in 1915 to a total of only 443 in 1916–1918 by frequent foot drying and sock changing.

Certain disease states such as atherosclerosis, arteritis, hypovolemia, diabetes, vascular injury secondary to trauma or infection, and previous cold-related injuries may predispose to subsequent injury.

Individual behavior is extremely important as well. In fact, alcohol- or drug-intoxicated persons, as well as psychiatric patients, account for the majority of frostbite cases in the United States. The impaired judgment and lack of self-preservation instincts prevent this population from dressing adequately and making rational decisions about exposure to the cold. Alcohol consumption also increases peripheral vasodilatation and heat loss, which increases the risk for hypothermia. In addition, many of these patients smoke, which results in peripheral vasoconstriction and increases the risk of frostbite.

Military studies suggest that dark-skinned soldiers and those from warmer climatic regions are more susceptible to frostbite. Conversely, peoples indigenous to frigid climates, such as Eskimos, Tibetans, and Laplanders are often "acclimated" to the cold and are less prone to injury.

Local cold-related injuries are classified into nonfreezing and freezing injuries.

## NONFREEZING COLD INJURIES: CHILBLAINS AND TRENCH FOOT

### Clinical Features

Chilblains or pernio is characterized by painful, inflammatory lesions of the skin of bared extremities caused by chronic, intermittent exposure to damp, nonfreezing ambient temperatures; it is acutely precipitated by acute exposure to cold. The hands, ears, lower legs, and feet are most commonly involved. The cutaneous manifestations, which appear up to 12 h after acute exposure, are characterized by localized edema, erythema, cyanosis, plaques, nodules, and in rare cases, ulcerations, vesicles, and bullae. The patient may complain of pruritus and burning paresthesias. Rewarming may result in the formation of tender, blue nodules, which may persist for several days. This is primarily a disease of women, and although rare in the United States, chilblains is common in the United Kingdom. Also, it appears that young females with Raynaud phenomenon are at greatest risk.

Trench foot was given its current name after it was frequently found among World War I troops who had been confined for long periods in trenches filled with standing cold water. Significant numbers of cases were also seen in the Falkland and Vietnam wars. Immersion foot describes a more severe variant of trench foot seen in downed pilots and shipwrecked sailors exposed for extended periods in life rafts in the North Atlantic Ocean. Although they are a significant problem in military operations, trench foot and immersion foot are rarely seen in the civilian population.

The pathophysiology is multifactorial but involves direct injury to soft tissue sustained from prolonged cooling, and is accelerated by wet conditions. The peripheral nerves seem to be the most sensitive

---

* Dr. Rabold reached the summit of Mt. Everest in May, 1993.

to this form of injury. Trench foot develops slowly over hours to days and is initially reversible, but if allowed to progress will become irreversible. Early symptoms progress from tingling to numbness of the affected tissues. On initial examination, the foot is pale, mottled, anesthetic, pulseless, and immobile, which initially does not change after rewarming. A hyperemic phase begins within hours and is associated with severe burning pain and reappearance of proximal sensation. As perfusion returns to the foot over 2 to 3 days, edema and bullae form and the hyperemia may worsen. Anesthesia frequently persists for weeks but may be permanent. In more severe cases, tissue sloughing and gangrene may develop. Hyperhidrosis and cold sensitivity are common late features and may persist for months to years. Severe cases may be associated with prolonged convalescence and permanent disability.

## Treatment

Management of chilblains is supportive. The affected skin should be rewarmed, gently bandaged, and elevated. Some European studies support the use of nifedipine (Procardia), at a dose of 20 mg t.i.d, as both prophylactic and therapeutic. Topical corticosteroids (.025% fluocinolone cream), or even a brief burst of oral corticosteroids, such as prednisone, have been shown to be useful. Affected areas are more prone to reinjury.

Effective prophylaxis for trench foot includes keeping warm, ensuring good boot fit, changing out of wet socks several times a day, never sleeping in wet socks and boots, and once early symptoms are identified, maximizing efforts to warm, dry, and elevate the feet. Once injury has occurred, treatment is supportive. Currently there is no specific therapy. Feet should be kept clean, warm, dryly bandaged, and elevated. Signs of early infection should be monitored.

## FREEZING COLD INJURIES (FCI): FROSTNIP AND FROSTBITE

### Pathophysiology

Cutaneous vascular tone can be altered by direct heating (warming hands over a fire) and indirect heating (putting on a hat to increase core temperature), and is modulated by sympathetic adrenergic vasoconstrictive fibers. In a euthermic 70-kg male, the total basal cutaneous blood flow is 200 to 500 mL/min. However, as the skin temperature drops to 14°C (57°F), the flow falls to 20 to 50 mL/min. As cooling continues to 10°C (50°F), cutaneous blood flow becomes negligible, and 5- to 10-min cycles of vasodilatation and vasoconstriction, known as the hunter's response or cold-induced vasoconstriction occurs. For individuals who are well "acclimated" to the cold, such as Eskimos, the intervals between cycles are often much shorter. As the vasodilatory phases carry cooled blood back from the extremities, the core temperature begins to fall. These cycles continue until the core temperature is threatened. The body attempts to maintain thermal integrity by completely shutting down flow to the coldest extremities. This begins phase I of frostbite and irreversible tissue damage commences. As skin temperatures fall well below 0°C (32°F), ice crystals form in the extracellular space. Crystals exert an osmotic force and pull fluid from the intracellular space, resulting in cellular dehydration and hyperosmolarity. The intracellular NaCl concentration may rise 10-fold. As the damage continues, proteins are denatured, enzymes are destroyed, and the cellular membranes are altered. Theoretically, intracellular ice crystals then form, especially in rapid freeze and refreeze injuries, and may be even more lethal to the cell. Actual structural damage from the ice crystals may result.

Phase II is characterized by reperfusion injury as the involved extremity is rewarmed and some initial blood flow returns. Over a period of several hours to days, the damaged endothelium-lined capillaries allow leakage of fluid into the interstitium, intracellular swelling occurs, and oxygen free radicals are generated, which furthers endothelial damage. An arachidonic acid cascade forms, which liberates prostaglandin and thromboxane. This cascade promotes vasoconstriction, platelet aggregation, and leukocyte sludging, which results in venule and arterial thrombosis and subsequent ischemia, necrosis, and dry gangrene. Profound vasoconstriction and arteriovenous shunting occurs at the margin between injured and noninjured tissue. Phase II is remarkably similar to the dynamics of a burn injury.

Frostbite injury can be divided into three zones. The *zone of coagulation* is the most severe, distal region of damage and is irreversible. The *zone of hyperemia* is the more superficial, proximal region with the least cellular damage and generally recovers without treatment in less than 10 days. The *zone of stasis* is the middle ground and is characterized by severe, but possibly reversible, cell damage. It is here that treatment is directed.

## Clinical Features

Frostbite can occur on any skin surface but is generally limited to the nose, ears, face, hands, and feet. Frostbite has been reported in the penis and scrotum of joggers and in burn patients after prolonged treatment with ice. Also, a freezing keratitis of the cornea has been reported in snowmobilers and skiers who did not wear protective goggles.

*Frostnip* is on a continuum with frostbite and is a superficial freeze injury characterized by lack of extracellular ice crystal formation and absence of progressive tissue loss. The involved extremity appears pale from intense vasoconstriction and is associated with some discomfort. Symptoms resolve on rewarming, and tissue loss does not occur.

There has been much debate over the proper classification of the severity of frostbite. One may classify frostbite into degrees of injury or into superficial and deep groups (Table 159-1). First- and second-degree injuries are classified as superficial, whereas third- and fourth-degree injuries are classified as deep. The initial clinical appearance

**Table 159-1.** Classification of Cold Injury According to Severity

| | **Symptoms** |
|---|---|
| SUPERFICIAL | |
| **First degree:** partial skin freezing<br>Erythema, edema, hyperemia<br>No blisters or necrosis<br>Occasional skin desquamation (5–10 d later) | Transient stinging and burning<br>Throbbing and aching possible<br>May have hyperhidrosis |
| **Second degree:** full-thickness injury<br>Erythema, substantial edema<br>vesicles with clear fluid<br>Blisters that desquamate and form<br>blackened eschar | Numbness; vasomotor disturbances<br>in severe cases |
| DEEP | |
| **Third degree:** full-thickness skin<br>and subcutaneous freezing<br>Violaceous/hemorrhagic blisters<br>Skin necrosis<br>Blue-gray discoloration | Initially no sensation<br>Tissue feels like "block of wood"<br>Later, shooting pains, burning,<br>throbbing, aching |
| **Fourth degree:** full-thickness skin,<br>subcutaneous tissue, muscle,<br>tendon, and bone freezing<br>Little edema<br>Initially mottled, deep red, or<br>cyanotic<br>Eventually dry, black, mummified | Possible joint discomfort |

SOURCE: Britt LD, Dascombe W, Rodriquez A: *Surg Clin North Am* 71:359, 1991, with permission.

is often deceiving, especially if some warming has not occurred. Most patients present after some warming has occurred and are in phase II of the injury. Frostbite classification is based on this time of presentation.

*First-degree injury* is characterized by partial skin freezing, erythema, mild edema, lack of blisters, and occasional skin desquamation several days later. The patient may complain of transient stinging and burning, followed by throbbing. Prognosis is excellent.

*Second-degree injury* is characterized by full-thickness skin freezing, formation of substantial edema over 3 to 4 h, erythema, and formation of clear blisters rich in thromboxane and prostaglandins. The blisters form within 6 to 24 h, extend to the end of the digit and usually desquamate and form black, hard eschars over several days. The patient complains of numbness, followed later by aching and throbbing. Prognosis is good.

*Third-degree injury* is characterized by damage that extends into the subdermal plexus. Hemorrhagic blisters form and are associated with skin necrosis and a blue-gray discoloration to the skin. The patient may complain of the involved extremity feeling like a "block of wood," followed later by burning, throbbing, and shooting pains. Prognosis is often poor.

*Fourth-degree injury* is characterized by extension into subcutaneous tissues, muscle, bone, and tendon. There is little edema. The skin is mottled, with nonblanching cyanosis, and will eventually form a deep, dry, black, mummified eschar. Vesicles often present late, if at all, and may be small, bloody blebs that do not extend to the digit tips. The patient may complain of a deep, aching joint pain. Prognosis is extremely poor.

## Treatment

### Field Management

Field management of frostbite by emergency medical service personnel is simple. The hypothermia and dehydration associated with frostbite should be addressed. Wet and constrictive clothing should be removed. The involved extremities should be elevated and carefully wrapped in dry sterile gauze, remembering to separate affected fingers and toes. Further cold injury should be avoided. In most cases, more aggressive wound management should be avoided and the patient transported to the emergency department. However, in some cases the patient may be several days away from evacuation and medical services and more complex management might be indicated before arrival to the hospital.

There is a correlation between the length of time tissue is frozen and the degree of cellular damage. Rapid rewarming is the single most effective therapy for frostbite. However, rewarming in the field is often impractical and is sometimes dangerous. In fact, in some unusual circumstances, it is best to endeavor to keep the affected part frozen until definitive care can be administered. For instance, if the victim has frozen feet and the only avenue to evacuation is prolonged ambulation, then rewarming can significantly complicate matters. The risk of refreezing the feet and causing even more severe damage is a real concern. Also, if adequate analgesia is not available, the rewarming process itself can be excessively painful. Ambulation on edematous and blistered feet may not be possible secondary to pain. In extreme situations such as this, it may be wise to keep the feet frozen and ambulate the patient to a location where more advanced evacuation can occur. If rewarming is attempted in the field, only clean water warmed to 40° to 42°C (104° to 108°F), as measured by thermometer, should be used. Avoid the use of hot, untested tap water because the 50° to 60°C (122° to 140°F) temperatures will cause a destructive thermal injury and worsen the prognosis. Attempts to directly warm with dry air, such as camp fires and heaters, should be avoided. Dry heat tends to desiccate damaged tissue and temperature cannot be adequately measured. Adding a thermal injury on top of frostbite will worsen outcome. Rubbing snow on frostbitten tissue to stimulate circulation is ineffective, destructive, and absolutely contraindicated.

Controversy surrounds management of the blisters associated with frostbite. Clear blisters are rich in tissue-injurious thromboxane and prostaglandins. Common sense would suggest that blister debridement or aspiration would limit contact with these chemicals and allow direct contact of aloe vera (Dermaide Aloe Cream) to counteract their injurious effects. Also tense blisters, which tend to only worsen when immobilization is not possible, are painful. Debridement or aspiration can bring some pain relief. When the patient is ambulating on rewarmed, frostbitten feet the associated blisters often rupture anyway. Field debridement of clear blisters is controversial, but adequate research is lacking to support or condemn this practice. Hemorrhagic blisters should not be drained in the field.

One possible complication of field aspiration or debridement is the theoretical increased risk of infection. Prophylactic use of penicillin might be wise in the field setting to combat any potential wound infection. Wounds should be cleansed daily and if feet are involved, socks should be clean and changed at least once or twice per day. Affected digits should be covered with aloe vera and separated by dry, sterile cotton and dressings should be changed daily. Pain management should begin with nonsteroidal anti-inflammatory drugs, such as ibuprofen, 12 mg/kg per day in divided doses, to counteract the arachidonic acid cascade, and should be continued even if narcotic analgesics are required as well. The victim should be discouraged from smoking because this will exacerbate vasoconstriction and tissue damage.

### Emergency Department Management

In taking the patient's history it is important to determine as many prognostic factors as possible. What was the temperature and wind velocity? How long was the extremity frozen and if thawed, did any refreezing occur? Was there any self-treatment, such as rubbing with snow or use of aloe vera or ibuprofen? Were recreational drugs, alcohol, or tobacco involved? Are there any predisposing medical conditions?

Frostbite is often associated with systemic hypothermia and dehydration, both of which can have a negative impact on the prognosis for tissue salvage. Rehydration and general warming are important adjuncts to therapy when indicated.

All too often the frostbitten patient presents to the emergency department subacutely (> 24 h after injury) and with the involved extremity in a partially thawed state. This more prolonged injury and slow, partial thaw usually translates to significantly longer hospital stays and greater tissue loss. However, this should not mean the patient is treated any less aggressively than the acute patient. The target of treatment remains minimizing tissue loss by focusing on the zone of stasis where damaged but potentially salvageable tissue exists.

Rapid rewarming is the core of frostbite therapy and should be initiated as soon as possible. The injured extremity should be placed in gently circulating water at a temperature of 40° to 42°C (104° to 108°F) for approximately 10 to 30 min, until the distal extremity is pliable and erythematous. Anticipate severe pain during rewarming and titrate with parenteral narcotics. The patient will probably require daily hydrotherapy and physical therapy during the inpatient phase.

Blister management is somewhat controversial, as is the use of prophylactic antibiotics. The current consensus is that clear blisters should be debrided or at least aspirated. The blister fluid is rich in destructive thromboxane and prostaglandins. Removal limits damage from these chemicals and enables access to the underlying tissue for topical therapy. Hemorrhagic blisters should not be debrided because this often results in tissue desiccation and worsened outcome. However, there is some controversy as to whether or not aspiration is helpful. Both blister types should be treated with topical aloe vera (Dermaide Aloe Cream) q6h, which helps to combat the arachidonic acid cascade. Affected digits should be separated with cotton and wrapped with sterile dry gauze. Elevation of the involved extremities will help decrease edema and pain.

The role of prophylactic antibiotics is unclear. The edema associated with the first several days after injury does appear to predispose to infection. *Staphylococcus aureus, Staphylococcus epidermidis,* and β-hemolytic streptococci account for nearly half of infections, but anaerobes, *Pseudomonas,* and *Enterococcus* are important pathogens as well. Therapy with penicillin G 500,000 units intravenously q6h, for 48 to 72 h, is recommended in several successful protocols and seems to be beneficial. One study, however, demonstrated better infection prophylaxis using topical bacitracin. Silver sulfadiazine (Silvadene) cream has also been advocated by some, but it has not been shown to be consistently beneficial. One disadvantage of using topical antibiotics is that it complicates the concurrent use of aloe vera (Dermaide Aloe Cream). It is important to address tetanus status and administer appropriate vaccination, if needed, because frostbite is considered to be a tetanus-prone wound.

Several agents beyond aloe vera (Dermaid Aloe Cream) have been advocated to battle the arachidonic acid cascade and thereby limit tissue damage. The most commonly advocated oral medication is ibuprofen (Motrin) at a daily dose of 12 mg/kg. Animal studies suggest possible future roles for oral methimazole, a thromboxane synthetase inhibitor, and topical 1% methylprednisolone acetate, which acts as a phospholipase A inhibitor preventing the formation of arachidonic acid.

Another controversial area is the use of sympathectomy to relieve vasospasm and edema. The treatment may be medical, as in the use of intra-arterial reserpine, or surgical. There is no role for early sympathectomy and the controversy is beyond the scope of emergency department management.

Heparin, low molecular weight dextran, and hyperbaric oxygen therapy have been studied and appear to be of little value. However, some preliminary data from a study using intra-arterial recombinant tissue plasminogen activator in patients with third-degree frostbite suggests that it may hold some promise in decreasing the rate of amputation.

Early surgical intervention is not indicated in the management of frostbite. Premature surgery has been an important contributor to unnecessary tissue loss and poor results in the past. This is primarily due to the inability to assess the depth of frostbite at early stages, and the fact that the blackened, mummified carapace is protective to the underlying regenerating tissue. Limited, early escharotomy may be indicated if the eschar is preventing adequate range of motion or circulation. Fasciotomy is rarely, if ever, indicated. Amputation may be unavoidable, however, if wet gangrene or infection complicate recovery. It usually takes 3 to 4 weeks for full demarcation to occur. Most amputations and grafts occur during this third week. The mean length of hospital stay for all degrees of frostbite is reported to be 8.5 days to 33.2 days. To minimize these extended hospital stays some have advocated the early use of radionuclide angiography with bone scan, at 7 to 14 days, to assess tissue viability and possible early surgical debridement.

### Admission Criteria

It is difficult to determine the extent of frostbite on initial examination and so it is best to be conservative when contemplating admission. It has been the standard of care in the past to admit all but the most isolated and superficial frostbite cases. It is important to consider the associated social factors as well. The homeless or elderly, especially when unable to care for themselves adequately, should never be discharged into subfreezing temperatures. If the frostbite is extensive and the hospital and staff are not equipped to treat this degree of severity, then transfer to a tertiary hospital should be considered after initial rewarming and treatment has been accomplished. Pa-

tients who are discharged from the emergency department should be treated with topical aloe vera (Dermaid Aloe Cream) and oral ibuprofen and encouraged not to smoke. Close surgical follow-up should be arranged.

### Sequelae

The sequelae of frostbite can be significant and prolonged. Permanent cold sensitivity, pain, tingling, and hyperhidrosis are common. Skin color changes may occur. When deep frostbite involves bone or joint, arthritis may result. In pediatric patients growth plate damage may result in digit shortening and radial deviation. Infection is a possible complication and often results in poor outcome. Deep frostbite often results in amputation.

### BIBLIOGRAPHY

Burr RE: Trench foot. *Journal of Wilderness Medicine* 4:348, 1993.

Carruthers R: Chilblains (perniosis). *Aust Fam Physician* 17:968, 1988.

Heggers JP, Phillips LG, McCauley RL, Robson MC: Frostbite: experimental and clinical evaluations of treatment. *Journal of Wilderness Medicine* 1:27, 1990.

Heggers JP, Robson MC, Manaualen K, et al: Experimental and clinical observations on frostbite. *Ann Emerg Med* 16:1956(191), 1987.

McCauley RL, Heggers JP, Robson MC: Frostbite: methods to minimize tissue loss. *Postgrad Med* 88:8, 1990.

McCauley RL, et al: Frostbite injuries: a rational approach based on the pathophysiology. *J Trauma* 23:143, 1983.

Mehta RC, Wilson MA: Frostbite injury: prediction of tissue viability with triple-phase bone scanning. *Radiology* 170:511, 1989.

Salini Z, Vas W, Tang-Barton P, et al: Assessment of tissue viability in frostbite by 99m-Tc pertechnetate scintigraphy. AJR Am J Roentgenol 42:415, 1984.

Skolnick AA: Early data suggest clot-dissolving drug may help save frostbitten limbs from amputation. *JAMA* 267:2008, 1992.

Smith DJ, Robson MC, Heggers JP: Frostbite and other cold related injuries. In: Auerbach PS, Geehr EC (eds). *Management of Wilderness and Environmental Injuries,* 2d ed. St. Louis: CV Mosby, pp. 101–118, 1989.

Tek DT, Mackey S: Non-freezing injury in a Marine infantry battalion. *Journal of Wilderness Medicine* 4:353, 1993.

Valnicek SM, Chasmar LR, Clapson JB: Frostbite in the Prairies: a 12 year review. *Plast Reconstr Surg* 92:4, 1993.

Vogel EJ, Dellon AL: Frostbite injuries of the hand. *Clin Plast Surg* 16:565, 1989.

# 160
# HYPOTHERMIA
### Howard A. Bessen

Hypothermia is defined as a core temperature less than 35°C (95°F). While most commonly seen in cold climates, it may develop without exposure to extreme environmental conditions. Indeed, hypothermia is not uncommon in temperate regions and may develop indoors during the summer.

## PHYSIOLOGY OF TEMPERATURE HOMEOSTASIS

Body temperature may fall as a result of heat loss by conduction, convection, radiation, or evaporation. Conduction is the transfer of heat by direct contact, down a temperature gradient, e.g., from a warm body to the cold environment. Since the thermal conductivity of water is approximately 30 times that of air, the body loses heat rapidly when immersed in water, producing a rapid decline in body temperature.

Convection is the transfer of heat by the actual movement of heated material, for example, wind disrupting the layer of warm air surrounding the body. Convective heat loss increases in windy conditions, a particular hazard for outdoors enthusiasts.

Heat may also be lost by radiation to the environment (primarily from noninsulated body areas) and by evaporation of water. Evaporation of the water contained in exhaled, water-saturated air occurs over a wide range of ambient temperatures and may be prevented by inhalation of warmed humidified air.

Opposing the loss of body heat are the mechanisms of heat conservation and gain. In general, these are controlled by the hypothalamus; thus, hypothalamic dysfunction may cause an impairment in temperature homeostasis. Heat is conserved by peripheral vasoconstriction and, importantly, by behavioral responses. If behavioral responses such as putting on clothing or coming indoors from a cold environment are impaired for any reason (e.g., drug intoxication or trauma), the risk of hypothermia is increased.

Heat gain is effected by shivering, and by "nonshivering thermogenesis." The nonshivering component of heat production consists of an increase in metabolic rate brought about by increased output from the thyroid and adrenal glands.

## HIGH-RISK PATIENTS

Individuals at the extremes of age, and those with an altered sensorium for any reason, are particularly susceptible to developing hypothermia.

The elderly may lose their ability to sense cold; neonates easily become hypothermic because of their large surface area to volume ratio. Both groups have a limited ability to increase heat production and to conserve body heat. Individuals with an altered sensorium, if unable to carry out the appropriate behavioral responses to cold stress, may develop hypothermia despite otherwise intact thermoregulatory mechanisms.

## ETIOLOGY OF HYPOTHERMIA: CLINICAL SETTINGS

Table 160-1 lists the common causes of hypothermia. Although there are other, more unusual etiologies of hypothermia, nearly all patients seen in the emergency department will have hypothermia due to one or more of these causes.

"Accidental" hypothermia may be divided into immersion and nonimmersion cold exposure. Exposure to cold environmental conditions may lead to hypothermia even in healthy subjects, especially in wind and rain. Inadequate clothing and physical exhaustion contribute to the loss of body heat. The high thermal conductivity of water leads to the rapid development of immersion hypothermia. Though the rate of heat loss is determined by water temperature, immersion in any water less than 16 to 21°C (61 to 70°F) may lead to hypothermia.

Metabolic causes of hypothermia include various hypoendocrine states (hypothyroidism, hypoadrenalism, hypopituitarism), which lead to a decrease in metabolic rate. Hypoglycemia may also lead to

**Table 160-1.** Causes of Hypothermia: Clinical Settings

"Accidental" (environmental)
Metabolic
Hypothalamic and CNS dysfunction
Drug-induced
Sepsis
Dermal disease
Acute incapacitating illness

hypothermia; the probable mechanism is hypothalamic dysfunction secondary to glucopenia.

Other causes of hypothalamic and CNS dysfunction (e.g., head trauma, tumor, stroke) may interfere with mechanisms of temperature regulation. Wernicke's disease may involve the hypothalamus; this is a rare but important cause of hypothermia, since it is potentially reversible with parenteral thiamine.

In the United States, the vast majority of hypothermic patients are intoxicated with ethanol or other drugs. Ethanol is a vasodilator, and, because of its anesthetic and CNS-depressant effects, intoxicated subjects neither feel the cold nor respond to it appropriately. Other drugs commonly implicated in the development of hypothermia include barbiturates and other sedative-hypnotics, phenothiazines, and occasionally insulin.

Sepsis may alter the hypothalamic temperature set point and is a well-known cause of hypothermia. Subnormal body temperature is a poor prognostic factor in patients with bacteremia.

Severe dermal disease may impair the skin's thermoregulatory functions. Significant burns or severe exfoliative dermatitis may prevent cutaneous vasoconstriction and increase transcutaneous water loss, predisposing to the development of hypothermia.

Finally, hypothermia may develop in anyone with an acute incapacitating illness. Thus, patients with severe infections, diabetic ketoacidosis, immobilizing injuries, and various other conditions may have impaired thermoregulatory function, including altered behavioral responses.

## PATHOPHYSIOLOGY AND CLINICAL FEATURES

In general, body temperatures from 32 to 35°C (90 to 95°F) constitute "mild" hypothermia. In this temperature range, the patient is in an excitation (responsive) stage, in which physiologic adjustments attempt to retain and generate heat.

When temperature drops below 32°C, (90°F), general excitation gives way to the slowing (adynamic) stage, in which there is a progressive slowdown of bodily functions. Metabolism slows, causing a decrease in both oxygen utilization and $CO_2$ production. Shivering ceases when body temperature falls below 30 to 32°C (86 to 90°F).

In the initial excitation phase, heart rate, cardiac output, and blood pressure all rise. With decreasing temperature, these all decline. Cardiac output and blood pressure may be markedly depressed by the negative inotropic and chronotropic effects of hypothermia and further depressed by concomitant hypovolemia.

Hypothermia causes characteristic ECG changes and may induce life-threatening arrhythmias (Table 160-2). The Osborn (J) wave, a slow, positive deflection at the end of the QRS complex (Fig. 160-1), is characteristic, though not pathognomic, of hypothermia.

Patients are at risk for arrhythmias at body temperatures below 30°C (86°F); the risk increases as body temperature decreases. Although various arrhythmias may occur at any time, the typical sequence is a progression from sinus bradycardia to atrial fibrillation with a slow ventricular response, to ventricular fibrillation, and, ultimately, to asystole. The hypothermic myocardium is extremely irrita-

**Table 160-2.** ECG Changes in Hypothermia

T-wave inversions
PR, QRS, QT prolongation
Muscle tremor artifact
Osborn (J) wave
Arrhythmias:
  Sinus bradycardia
  Atrial fibrillation or flutter
  Nodal rhythms
  AV block
  PVCs
  Ventricular fibrillation
  Asystole

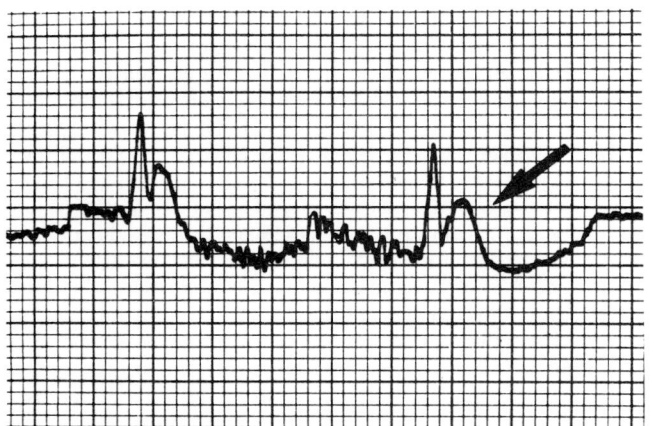

**Fig. 160-1.** Rhythm strip from patient with temperature of 25°C (77°F), showing atrial fibrillation with a slow ventricular response, muscle tremor artifact, and Osborn (J) wave (arrow).

ble, and ventricular fibrillation may be induced by a variety of manipulations and interventions that stimulate the heart, including rough handling of the patient.

Pulmonary effects include initial tachypnea, followed by a progressive decrease in respiratory rate and tidal volume. Cold-induced bronchorrhea, along with a depression of cough and gag reflexes, makes aspiration pneumonia a common complication.

Much attention has been paid to the temperature correction of arterial blood gases in the hypothermic patient. Since the blood gas analyzer warms the blood to 37°C, (99°F), thus increasing the partial pressure of dissolved gases, the machine will report a higher $P_{O_2}$ and $P_{CO_2}$, and lower pH than the actual values at the patient's body temperature. Correction factors and nomograms are available to determine the actual values in the patient's body; however, the optimal or "normal" values in hypothermia are not known. The simplest solution is to use the uncorrected values as if the patient were normothermic; studies suggest that this approach is the most physiologically sound. $P_{CO_2}$ is often quite low secondary to depressed metabolism and decreased $CO_2$ production, and iatrogenic hyperventilation may lead to marked respiratory alkalosis.

Hypothermia causes a leftward shift of the oxyhemoglobin dissociation curve, potentially impairing oxygen release to tissues. Patients may have minimal oxygen reserves despite diminished oxygen requirements, warranting the administration of supplemental oxygen.

The central nervous system is affected by hypothermia, with a progressive depression of consciousness with decreasing temperature. Mild incoordination is followed by confusion, lethargy, and coma; pupils may be dilated and unreactive. These changes are associated with a decrease in cerebral blood flow. An even greater decrease in cerebral oxygen requirements may protect the brain against anoxic or ischemic damage.

Hypothermia impairs renal concentrating abilities and induces a "cold diuresis," leading to significant volume losses. Because of this concentrating defect, urine flow and specific gravity are unreliable indicators of intravascular volume and circulatory status. The immobile hypothermic patient is prone to rhabdomyolysis, and acute tubular necrosis may occur because of myoglobinuria and renal hypoperfusion.

Intravascular volume is also lost due to a plasma shift to the extravascular space. The combination of hemoconcentration, cold-induced increase in blood viscosity, and poor circulation may lead to intravascular thrombosis and subsequent embolic complications. Disseminated intravascular coagulation may occur because of release of tissue thromboplastins into the bloodstream, especially when circulation is restored during rewarming.

Endocrine function is fairly well preserved at low body temperatures. Plasma cortisol and thyroid hormone levels are usually normal or elevated unless the patient has a preexisting deficiency. Glucose levels may be normal, low, or elevated. Though hyperglycemia is common due to decreased insulin release as well as decreased glucose utilization, hypoglycemia may occur in up to 40 percent of patients.

Acid-base disturbances are common in hypothermia but follow no uniform pattern. Acidosis may occur due to severe respiratory depression and $CO_2$ retention and to lactic acid production from shivering and poor tissue perfusion. Alkalosis may result from diminished $CO_2$ production with low metabolic rates, or from iatrogenic hyperventilation or sodium bicarbonate administration.

Pancreatitis (not only hyperamylasemia but true pancreatic necrosis) may occur in hypothermia. Hepatic function is depressed by cold, so drugs normally metabolized, conjugated, or detoxified by the liver (e.g., lidocaine) may rapidly accumulate to toxic levels.

Finally, local cold injury and frostbite need special attention.

## DIAGNOSIS

The diagnosis of hypothermia is often not obvious; exposure to profound cold is *not* necessary to produce hypothermia. Since many standard clinical thermometers record only to 34.4°C (94°F), low-reading glass or electronic thermometers are required to accurately measure the temperature of hypothermic patients. Electronic thermometers with flexible probes can be used to continuously monitor rectal or esophageal temperatures; tympanic thermometers may also be useful.

## MANAGEMENT

Treatment includes both general supportive measures and specific rewarming techniques. Therapy begins with careful, gentle handling, since manipulation can precipitate ventricular fibrillation in the irritable hypothermic myocardium.

Controversy has arisen regarding the performance of CPR on an unmonitored patient who appears to be profoundly hypothermic and in cardiopulmonary arrest. Opponents of CPR argue that pulses may be difficult to detect in this setting, and that chest compressions may precipitate ventricular fibrillation. They recommend withholding CPR until the presence of an arrested rhythm (ventricular fibrillation or asystole) is confirmed. Alternatively, withholding CPR in the patient who is truly in cardiac arrest may unnecessarily subject the brain and other organs to prolonged ischemia. This CPR controversy applies only to patients with severe hypothermia, with core temperatures less than 28°C (82°F); practically, it may be difficult to confirm this diagnosis in the field. To avoid inappropriate chest compressions, prehospital care personnel should examine the patient for 30 to 60 s before diagnosing pulselessness. If no pulses are detected, most recommend initiating CPR. The optimal rate of chest compressions and ventilations has not been determined.

Similar considerations apply to monitored patients. Some authors recommend avoiding chest compressions in severely hypothermic patients with "nonarrested rhythms" (sinus bradycardia, atrial fibrillation with slow ventricular response, junctional rhythms), even without a palpable pulse. Most, however, recommend full CPR in patients with pulseless electrical activity, even with profound hypothermia.

Oxygen and intravenous fluids should be warmed, and patients should have constant monitoring of their core temperature and cardiac rhythm. If central venous lines are placed, care should be taken to avoid entering and irritating the heart. In general, indications for endotracheal intubation are the same as in the normothermic patient. Concern has been raised regarding induction of arrhythmias during intubation; however, there is a very low complication rate with gentle intubation after oxygenation.

Although arrhythmias in the hypothermic patient may represent an immediate threat to life, most rhythm disturbances (e.g., sinus brady-cardia, atrial fibrillation or flutter) require no therapy and revert spontaneously with rewarming. In addition, the activity of antiarrhythmic and cardioactive drugs is unpredictable in hypothermia, and the hypothermic heart is relatively resistant to atropine, pacing, and countershock.

Ventricular fibrillation is often refractory to therapy until the patient is rewarmed. The American Heart Association's 1992 guidelines suggest initial defibrillation attempts with up to three shocks. If this is unsuccessful, CPR should be instituted and rapid rewarming begun. Defibrillation should be reattempted when the core temperature rises above 30°C (86°F). Bretylium has been suggested as the drug of choice for the prophylaxis or treatment of ventricular fibrillation in hypothermic patients, although data concerning its efficacy are conflicting.

## Drug Therapy

Because many hypothermic patients are thiamine-depleted alcoholics (and because Wernicke's disease may cause hypothermia), patients should be given intravenous thiamine. Fifty to 100 mL of 50% dextrose should be administered if a dipstick serum glucose measurement is low or if a rapid test is unavailable.

Administration of antibiotics, steroids, and thyroid hormone must be individualized. Serious, often occult, infections may either precipitate or complicate hypothermia, and a thorough search for infection is indicated. Routine steroid therapy is generally not indicated, but hydrocortisone (100 mg) should be given to the patient with a history of adrenal suppression or insufficiency preceding the hypothermic episode, as well as to the patient with myxedema coma.

Hypothermia and hypothyroidism share many clinical features. While the majority of patients with myxedema coma are hypothermic, only a small minority of hypothermic patients are hypothyroid; thyroid hormone levels are most often normal or elevated. Thyroxine in large doses is necessary for the patient in myxedema coma, but could potentially cause arrhythmias or cardiac ischemia in other hypothermic patients. Therefore, thyroid hormone replacement is indicated only in patients with a known history of hypothyroidism, a thyroidectomy scar, or other strong clinical evidence of myxedema coma.

## Rewarming Techniques

Modalities available for rewarming are listed in Table 160-3. The choice of method is a matter of controversy. There are no prospective, controlled studies comparing rewarming methods in humans, and each method has advantages and disadvantages.

Passive rewarming allows patients to rewarm on their own, using endogenous heat produced by metabolism. Since patients often become hypothermic over a period of hours to days, slow, passive

**Table 160-3.** Rewarming Techniques

Passive rewarming:
  Removal from cold environment
  Insulation
Active external rewarming:
  Warm water immersion
  Heating blankets
  Heated objects (water bottles, etc.)
  Radiant heat
Active core rewarming:
  Inhalation rewarming
  Heated IV fluids
  GI tract lavage
  Bladder lavage
  Peritoneal lavage
  Pleural lavage
  Extracorporeal rewarming
  Mediastinal lavage via thoracotomy

rewarming is physiologically sound, avoiding rapid changes in cardiovascular status and the complications associated with active rewarming methods.

Patients must have intact thermoregulatory mechanisms and be capable of metabolic heat production for successful passive rewarming. With severe hypothermia or hypothermia secondary to an underlying illness (see Table 160-1), patients may fail to rewarm passively; active rewarming is then indicated. In addition, since temperature rises slowly with passive rewarming, it is inappropriate for patients with cardiovascular compromise.

Active external rewarming (application of exogenous heat to the body) is often rapidly effective in raising body temperature and has been used successfully in many patients. However, this method has several potential disadvantages. Application of external heat may cause peripheral vasodilation, returning cold blood to the core. While warming the periphery, this may paradoxically cause central cooling ("core temperature afterdrop"), potentially leading to arrhythmias. Although the mechanism and significance of this afterdrop phenomenon have been questioned, its occurrence with external rewarming has been well documented. The peripheral vasodilation and venous pooling can also lead to relative hypovolemia and hypotension (rewarming shock). Washout of lactic acid from the peripheral tissues may lead to "rewarming acidosis," and an increase in metabolic demands of the periphery before the hypothermic heart can provide adequate tissue perfusion may lead to further tissue hypoxia and acidosis. Finally, resuscitation and monitoring of a patient immersed in warm water are technically difficult.

Active core rewarming has several theoretical advantages. Internal organs including the heart are preferentially rewarmed, decreasing myocardial irritability and returning cardiac function. Peripheral vasodilation is avoided, decreasing the incidence and magnitude of core temperature afterdrop, rewarming shock, and acidosis. However, some internal rewarming techniques are invasive and may be difficult to institute.

Inhalation rewarming—administration of warmed, humidified oxygen via mask or endotracheal tube—provides a fairly small heat gain, and is not effective for rapid rewarming. This is an important modality, however, as it minimizes heat loss from the lungs, a potential loss of up to 30 percent of the total metabolic heat production. Similarly, IV fluids should be warmed to avoid further cooling by the administration of fluids at room temperature. IV bags may be warmed in a microwave oven, although commercial fluid warmers allow the temperature of infused fluids to be more precisely controlled. Inhalation rewarming and warm IV fluids should be used in all but mild cases of hypothermia, as these are simple, noninvasive techniques with minimal risk of complications.

GI tract (gastric or colonic) lavage with warmed saline is technically simple, and patients can be lavaged with large volumes of fluid in a short time period. The obtunded hypothermic patient may develop pulmonary aspiration if lavaged with an unprotected airway. In a manner similar to GI tract lavage, the bladder can be lavaged with warm saline solution using a Foley catheter.

Peritoneal lavage affords relatively rapid rewarming. It is widely available, may be instituted rapidly and with little technical difficulty, and has been shown to be effective in both animal studies and human applications. Potassium-free dialysis solution is warmed to 40 to 45°C (104 to 113°F), instilled, and then removed; the use of two catheters (one for fluid instillation and one for removal) may increase the rewarming rate.

Pleural lavage using thoracostomy tubes has provided effective rewarming in animal studies and a few human cases. Lavaging the left thoracic cavity delivers heated fluid in close proximity to the heart, potentially allowing rapid cardiac warming. Two thoracostomy tubes (for fluid inflow and outflow) have generally been employed. If this technique is chosen, care must be taken to monitor the net fluid infusion, as increased intrathoracic pressure and tension hydrothorax may complicate the procedure. The risk of precipitating arrhythmias during chest tube insertion is unknown.

Rapid internal rewarming can also be accomplished through an extracorporeal circuit. This consists of an arteriovenous shunt in which blood is routed to a warming device and then returned to the patient. The femoral vessels are usually used for vascular access. Pump-assisted cardiopulmonary bypass and heated hemodialysis are the most commonly used extracorporeal techniques. Recently, continuous arteriovenous rewarming using a countercurrent heat exchanger (a modified commercial fluid warmer) interposed between catheters placed in the femoral vessels, with flow driven by the patient's blood pressure, has been reported. This technique obviates the need for pump support and systemic heparinization but is ineffective in hypotensive patients. Full cardiopulmonary bypass using a median sternotomy has also been employed.

Profoundly hypothermic patients may be rewarmed in a very short time period with these methods. In addition to allowing rapid rewarming, pump-driven partial (femoral-femoral) or complete cardiopulmonary bypass provides circulatory support and oxygenation of blood, a great advantage in the management of patients in cardiac arrest or with severe cardiovascular compromise. Specialized equipment and personnel are required, however, and lack of immediate availability often precludes the use of this technique. In addition, the heparinization required for some extracorporeal techniques may cause complications in hypothermic trauma patients.

Various diathermy and radiowave techniques, although promising, have had limited use in hypothermic humans.

Finally, mediastinal irrigation using open thoracotomy has been used successfully as a rewarming technique in a few patients. It is possible that these patients could have been resuscitated using less invasive modalities. Thoracotomy has many potential complications and should only be considered in arrested patients. Even then, indications for this procedure are unclear.

### Approach to Rewarming

No prospective controlled studies comparing the various rewarming modalities have been done in humans. Therefore, firm guidelines for therapy cannot be given.

Patients with mild hypothermia, who are still in the "excitation" stage, generally improve spontaneously, as long as endogenous heat production mechanisms are functional. In addition, at temperatures above 30°C (86°F) the incidence of arrhythmias is low, and rapid rewarming is rarely necessary.

By far the most important consideration is the patient's cardiovascular status; a secondary consideration is the presenting temperature. Some feel that patients with a stable cardiac rhythm (including sinus bradycardia and atrial fibrillation) and stable vital signs do not need rapid rewarming, even if the temperature is very low. They recommend passive rewarming and noninvasive internal modalities (e.g., warm moist oxygen and warm IV fluids) in this setting. Others argue that profoundly hypothermic patients, even if currently "stable," are at risk of developing life-threatening arrhythmias. They recommend rapid rewarming until the temperature has reached 30 to 32°C (86 to 90°F) to minimize the time period during which arrhythmias may develop. The relative merits of each approach have not been studied.

Patients with cardiovascular insufficiency or instability, including persistent hypotension and life-threatening arrhythmias, need to be rewarmed rapidly. The best method remains to be definitively determined. Extracorporeal techniques offer many advantages but are often unavailable. If extracorporeal rewarming is not available, multiple other rewarming modalities can be used simultaneously.

### PROGNOSIS

Many hypothermic patients have severe infections or other threatening illnesses. Patients with "uncomplicated" hypothermia (often purely due to cold exposure) have a fairly low mortality rate; patients with significant associated diseases have a much worse prognosis. In terms of ultimate outcome, the underlying disease process is far more important than the initial temperature or the rewarming method chosen. Therefore, evaluation and treatment of these patients must include a search for associated diseases as well as treatment of the hypothermia itself.

The protective effect of hypothermia may have an important influence on prognosis; decreased oxygen requirements can protect the brain and other organs against anoxic and ischemic damage. This means that the usual criteria indicating death or irreversibility of disease are not valid in the hypothermic patient, who may even survive prolonged cardiac arrest without neurologic sequelae.

Hypothermic patients may recover completely after presenting in a rigid, apneic state with fixed and dilated pupils. Recovery has been documented with core temperatures as low as 15°C (59°F), and with cardiac arrest for 4.5 h. Death in hypothermia must be defined as a failure to revive with rewarming; unless there is strong evidence that the patient is not viable, resuscitative efforts should be continued until core temperature is at least 30 to 32°C (86 to 90°F).

### DISPOSITION

Patients with mild accidental hypothermia caused purely by environmental exposure may be discharged after rewarming in the emergency department, provided that they are asymptomatic and can return to a warm environment. Most other hypothermic patients require hospital admission, both for the management of hypothermia and for the evaluation and management of underlying diseases.

### BIBLIOGRAPHY

Bolgiano E, Sykes L, Barish RA, et al: Accidental hypothermia with cardiac arrest: Recovery following rewarming by cardiopulmonary bypass. *J Emerg Med* 10:427, 1992.

Corneli HM: Accidental hypothermia. *J Pediatr* 120:671, 1992.

Danzl DF, Pozos RS: Multicenter hypothermia survey. *Ann Emerg Med* 16:1042, 1987.

Gentilello LM, Cobean RA, Offner PJ, et al: Continuous arteriovenous rewarming: Rapid reversal of hypothermia in critically ill patients. *J Trauma* 32:316, 1992.

Reuler JB: Hypothermia: Pathophysiology, clinical settings and management. *Ann Intern Med* 89:519, 1978.

Weinberg AD: Hypothermia. *Ann Emerg Med* 22 (part 2):370, 1993.

Zell SC, Kurtz KJ: Severe exposure hypothermia: A resuscitation protocol. *Ann Emerg Med* 14:339, 1985.

# 161
# HEAT EMERGENCIES
## James S. Walker
## Michael V. Vance

Since the days of earliest recorded history, people have recognized that prolonged exposure to the sun or heat can be deleterious to their health. Steel mill workers, foundry workers, miners, firefighters, military recruits, soldiers, amateur and professional athletes, and farm workers are examples of those whose employment requires them to work or exercise under sweltering conditions. Furthermore, the elderly, those who are chronically ill, alcoholics, and patients taking antipsychotic, anticholinergic, or cardiovascular medications are at risk for developing heat-related illnesses even with only a moderate exposure to ambient heat. Heatstroke remains a frequent cause of death, with mortality rates ranging from 10 to 75 percent. In the United States alone, more than 4000 people die of heatstroke annually, and it is the second leading cause of death in young athletes. Additionally, many authorities speculate that numerous heat-related illnesses go unreported or unrecognized.

In this chapter we will discuss the physiology of thermoregulation, the pathophysiology of heat illness, and the features and treatment of the heat syndromes. The minor heat illnesses are disorders that develop in response to a heat load but in which thermoregulation is preserved. Heatstroke develops when thermoregulation fails.

## CONCEPTS OF THERMOREGULATION

Body temperature is dependent on the balance between heat production and heat loss; it is normally maintained within narrow limits through a variety of mechanisms.

### Heat Production

Under normal circumstances, heat production results from exothermic intracellular metabolic processes and absorption of heat from external sources. The normal heat production of the body (basal metabolic activity) is 60 to 70 kcal/h and would result in a temperature rise of 1.1°C/h if there were no cooling mechanisms. Strenuous physical activity increases body heat production up to 900 kcal/h for short periods of time. Furthermore, a large radiant heat load from the sun will contribute to even greater levels of heat gain. Solar irradiation under summer conditions may add up to 300 kcal/h of heat production. Black skin absorbs approximately 20 percent more heat than does white skin but adds protection from ultraviolet sunlight. As the ambient temperature rises above 33°C (91.4°F), the incidence of heat stroke increases significantly.

### Heat Loss

Regulation of body temperature is contingent not only on heat production but also on heat loss. Heat loss, or dissipation, is accomplished by radiation, convection, conduction, and evaporation. *Radiation* is heat transfer by electromagnetic waves. When the air temperature is lower than body temperature, radiant heat loss accounts for 65 percent of cooling. However, when the air temperature is greater than body temperature, radiation can be a source of major heat gain. To facilitate heat loss by radiation in a hot environment, the peripheral blood flow to the skin can increase by a factor of 20. *Convection* is heat loss to air and to water vapor molecules circulating around the body. As the ambient temperature rises, the amount of heat dispersed by convection decreases, and once air temperature exceeds skin temperature, heat is gained by the body. Convection accounts for about 10 to 15 percent of heat loss of the body and is greatly affected by wind velocity. As the wind speed increases so does the rate of convection and heat loss. Loose-fitting clothing maximizes convective heat loss. *Conduction* is the transfer of heat energy from warmer to cooler objects by direct physical contact. This accounts for 2 percent of body heat loss under normal conditions, but immersion in cool water can enhance heat loss through this mechanism by a factor of 32. *Evaporation* is the conversion of a liquid to a gaseous phase at the expense of energy. This is accomplished by the loss of 0.58 kcal/mL of water evaporated. Evaporation of water from the body as sweat and insensible water losses accounts for 25 percent of total heat loss of a nude individual at rest. Surprisingly, the respiratory evaporative heat loss component is not significant in humans but only in panting mammals. In humans, the primary means of evaporative heat loss is sweat from the skin.

Under ordinary circumstances, radiation and evaporation are the major mechanisms by which the body can eliminate heat. When the ambient temperature approaches or exceeds body temperature, heat loss by radiation stops and the body may begin to take on heat by radiation. High humidity renders the evaporative heat loss mechanism ineffective. Accordingly, conditions of high humidity and high ambient temperature block both of the body's defenses against heat loss and can lead to heatstroke.

### Physiologic Coordination

The body's temperature-regulating system generally functions well in the face of diverse metabolic and environmental conditions. Responses to core temperature changes are directed by the anterior hypothalamus and are mediated by the autonomic nervous system, neuromuscular activity, and the endocrine system. The primary response to increased core temperature is cutaneous vasodilation, resulting in greater heat transfer from the skin to the atmosphere. However, as ambient temperature approaches body temperature, heat loss becomes increasingly dependent on evaporation of sweat produced by the activity of cholinergic sympathetic nerve fibers. The efficiency of evaporative heat loss is in turn influenced greatly by ambient temperature.

### Physiologic Adaptation

The human body is remarkably capable of adapting to dramatic changes through the process of acclimatization. Acclimatization occurs gradually over days to weeks and primarily involves alterations of sodium and water balance mediated by aldosterone. When a human is initially exposed to a hot and humid environment, sodium and water are lost through sweating. In addition, blood is shunted to the skin to aid in heat dissipation. The net result is contraction of the extracellular fluid volume, decreased renal plasma flow, and, consequently, an increase in aldosterone secretion. The concentration of sodium in urine and sweat then decreases markedly. Sodium retention results in expansion of extracellular fluid volume, and, at some point, acclimatization to the new environment is completed.

## PATHOGENESIS OF HEAT-RELATED ILLNESSES

After reviewing these basic concepts of thermoregulation, it becomes evident that the three most important variables that affect temperature regulation are: (1) exogenous heat gain, (2) increased endogenous heat production, and (3) decreased heat dispersion. Any factor that increases the amount of heat produced or diminishes the amount of heat dissipated can potentially exceed the capacity of the body to adjust to these heat stressors and produce a heat illness. A reevaluation of these three variables of thermoregulation is now in order, especially when one takes into consideration the numerous agents that can alter these respective variables and the ability to respond to heat stress.

### Exogenous Heat Gain

High ambient temperature and high ambient humidity result in an environmental heat load. Heat waves predispose to heatstroke epidemics, and direct exposure to sunlight or heat increases the heat burden. The best indicator of environmental heat stress is the wet-bulb globe temperature, which factors the effect of humidity upon the temperature. Many agencies, including the military, utilize the wet-bulb globe temperature as a guide for recommended activity levels (see Table 161-1). At wet-bulb temperatures of 33°C or more the incidence of heatstroke increases.

Working close to furnaces or boilers or in mines has been associated with heat-related injuries. Amateur athletes and military recruits who start training in the summer are also at high risk for developing heat emergencies. The ability of people to remove themselves from the hot environment can reduce the frequency of heat-related illness. During the heat wave of 1980 in Kansas City, the risk of heatstroke was 49 times greater for people without home air-conditioning than

**Table 161-1.** Wet-Bulb Globe Temperature and Recommended Activity Restrictions

| Temperature | | |
| --- | --- | --- |
| C° | F° | **Activity Level Restrictions** |
| 15.6 | 60 | No precautions |
| 19–21 | 66–70 | No precautions provided water, salt, and food intake are adequate |
| 22–24 | 71–75 | Postpone sports practice, avoid hiking |
| 24 | 76 | Lighter practice and work with rest breaks |
| 27 | 80 | No hiking or sports |
| 28 | 82 | Heavy exertion with caution |
| 30 | 85 | Cancel all exertion for unacclimatized persons; avoid sun exposure |
| 31.5 | 88 | Limited brief activity for acclimatized fit personnel only |

*Source:* From Callaham M: *Emergency Management of Heat Illness.* ACEP: Emergency Physicians Monograph Series, Chicago, Abbott Laboratories, 1979, with permission.

those with continuous air-conditioning. It was also reported that spending 2 h/day in an air-conditioned shopping mall decreased the risk of heatstroke for those without air-conditioning.

### Increased Endogenous Heat Production

The three main elements that are responsible for an increase in endogenous heat production are febrile illnesses, physical activity, and pharmacologic agents. Patients with febrile illnesses have an increased metabolic rate that increases the heat burden. Diseases such as hyperthyroidism may predispose to heat illness. Vigorous physical activity increases endogenous heat production. If the environment impedes heat loss, exercise can increase core temperature by 1°C (1.8°F) every 5 min. Any condition causing skeletal muscle contraction increases endogenous heat production. Seizures, drug withdrawal states, neuroleptic malignant syndrome, malignant hyperthermia, and combative behavior are examples.

A number of pharmacologic agents are associated with hyperthermia. Cocaine, amphetamines, and tricyclic antidepressants can increase endogenous heat production by directly stimulating the hypothalamus and by increasing muscle contractions. In cocaine poisoning, hyperthermia can result from convulsions. Lysergic acid diethylamide (LSD) and phencyclidine act on the central nervous system to induce a hypermetabolic state. Monoamine-oxidase inhibitors can cause muscular hyperactivity and hyperthermia.

Salicylates and parachlorophenol increase metabolic heat production by enhancing the uncoupling of oxidative phosphyloration. This means that the cellular energy generated by the oxidation of fats and glucose is released as heat rather than being stored in adenosine triphosphate molecules. Sympathomimetics generate heat by stimulating hepatic metabolism.

### Decreased Heat Dispersion

There are seven primary factors that impair the body's ability to disperse or dissipate heat: (1) dehydration, (2) cardiovascular disease, (3) extremes of age, (4) obesity, (5) improper clothing, (6) skin diseases, and (7) drugs.

Dehydration is an important risk factor for heat illness and results in hyperthermia through a number of mechanisms. Dehydration increases the body temperature even at rest by increasing the work of the cellular sodium-potassium pump, which accounts for 20 to 45 percent of the basic metabolic rate. Volume depletion also limits sweating and predisposes to cardiovascular impairment by the effects of hypovolemia on the Starling curve. Additionally, core body temperature has been found to increase as a function of dehydration, especially when dehydration was greater than 3 percent.

A second important risk factor is cardiovascular disease. An intact cardiovascular system is necessary for dispersing or losing heat. Ninety-seven percent of cooling takes place at the vascular beds supplying the skin. As the body's heat load increases, the cutaneous vessels dilate to maximize the cooling surface. This, in turn, increases blood flow to the skin up to 20-fold and greatly decreases peripheral vascular resistance. This physiologic response adequately dissipates heat but taxes the heart by decreasing the venous return and requiring an increase in cardiac output by two- to four-fold to maintain a normal blood pressure. Heat stress in patients with cardiovascular disease may precipitate cardiac dysrhythmias, myocardial infarction, congestive heart failure, cerebral vascular accident, or heatstroke. Diuretics, vasodilators, β blockers, calcium channel blockers, and other cardiovascular drugs blunt the ability to increase cardiac output in response to a heat load.

The very young and the very old are most susceptible to heat illness. Neonates lack mature thermoregulatory and sweating responses. Children produce more metabolic heat per kilogram of body weight and sweat proportionally less than adults. Furthermore, children have a larger surface area to mass ratio than adults. In contrast, the elderly are less able to increase and maintain cardiac output in response to a heat load because of the presence of cardiovascular disease, use of multiple drugs, reduced sweat production, and poor physical conditioning.

Obese people are less heat tolerant than people of normal weight. Obese individuals have more insulation and a larger surface area to mass ratio. The obese person may also be unable to attain the necessary cardiac output for effective cooling due to a lack of physical conditioning.

Clothing can prevent evaporation of sweat and thus retain heat. Garments which tend to be thick, have less thermal conductance, have a low evaporative ability as well as resistance to wind can significantly impair heat loss. Multilayer occlusive garments can cause heatstroke with just short heat exposures, as can result when a child is bundled in blankets in the summer.

Skin diseases that diminish sweating can decrease the body's ability to disperse a heat load. Scleroderma, cystic fibrosis, eczema, psoriasis, heat rash, and even sunburn (>30 percent of body surface area) interfere with heat dissipation.

Many drugs contribute to the development of heat disorders by decreasing the body's ability to disperse heat, especially anticholinergic agents, diuretics, phenothiazines, cardiovascular drugs, and sympathomimetic agents. These five groups and their respective mechanisms can be easily remembered by the mnemonic: *a*ll *d*esert *p*eople *c*apitulate *s*weat. Anticholinergic agents or medications with anticholinergic properties impair the sweating response. Diuretics may cause relative volume depletion, decrease cardiac output, and diminish sweating. Phenothiazines (and butyrophenones) result in the blockade or depletion of the central stores of dopamine and interfere with the thermoregulatory center of the anterior hypothalamus. Phenothiazines also have anticholinergic properties. Cardiovascular medications such as β blockers or calcium channel blockers can diminish the body's cardiovascular response to heat stress. Sympathomimetics decrease the body's ability to lose heat by causing cutaneous vasoconstriction.

Many investigators have observed and reported that alcoholics have an increased susceptibility to heat-related illnesses. In one study by the Centers for Disease Control and Prevention, the relative risk for heatstroke death was 15 times greater in alcoholic patients than in nonalcoholic patients. Alcohol's primary effect is to impair or interfere with normal behavioral responses to a heat stressor. The recognition of the need to move to a cooler place, turn on the air conditioner, or remove heavy clothing is altered by alcohol. Physiologically, moderate alcohol consumption may result in peripheral vasodilation and blunt the cardiovascular response to a heat load. Also, alcohol ingestion leads to a relative dehydration by the inhibition of ADH.

# MINOR HEAT ILLNESSES

## Heat Edema

Heat edema is a self-limited process manifested by mild swelling and tightening of the hands and feet; it appears in the first few days of exposure to a hot environment. It is found most commonly in elderly nonacclimatized individuals who are physically active after a prolonged period of sitting in a car, bus, or plane. To a lesser extent, it is seen in healthy travelers just arriving from a colder climate. Edema is usually mild and does not restrict normal activities. Rarely, pitting edema of the ankles may develop, but heat edema does not progress to the pretibial region. A typical history and thorough physical examination are sufficient to exclude systemic causes of edema. Heat edema is due to cutaneous vasodilatation and orthostatic pooling of interstitial fluid in the extremities. Some authorities feel increased secretion of aldosterone and antidiuretic hormone (ADH) also plays a role.

Heat edema usually resolves spontaneously in a few days but may take up to 6 weeks. No special treatment is necessary. If the patient is insistent upon treatment, elevation of the legs and the use of support hose will facilitate the removal of the interstitial fluid. Diuretics are not effective and can predispose to electrolyte abnormalities, volume depletion, or a more serious heat illness.

## Prickly Heat

Prickly heat is a pruritic, maculopapular, erythematous rash found over clothed areas of the body. Also known as lichen tropicus, miliaria rubra, or "heat rash," it is an acute inflammation of the sweat ducts caused by blockage of the sweat pores by macerated stratum corneum. The ducts become dilated under pressure and ultimately rupture, producing superficial vesicles in the malpighian layer of the skin on a red base. Itching is the predominant clinical feature during this phase and is treated successfully with antihistamines. Prevention can be accomplished by wearing clean, light, and loose-fitting clothing and avoiding sweat-generating situations. The use of talc or babypowder is of no benefit. Sometimes ducts become secondarily infected with *Staphylococcus aureus*. Chlorhexidine in a light cream or lotion is the treatment of choice in the acute phase.

With prolonged heat exposure, a keratin plug fills the duct, causing obstruction in the stratum malpighian layer. When the duct ruptures a second time, the resultant vesicle will be driven deeper into the dermis. This rash simulates the white papules of piloerection and is not pruritic. This is known as the profunda stage of prickly heat and it can readily advance into a chronic dermatitis. Infection with *S. aureus* is a common complication and requires the use of dicloxacillin or erythromycin. Desquamation of the skin can be accomplished by applying 1% salicylic acid to the affected area three times a day. Caution should be utilized to avoid salicylate toxicity.

## Heat Syncope

Heat syncope is a variant of postural hypotension resulting from the cumulative effect of peripheral vasodilation, decreased vasomotor tone, and relative volume depletion. It occurs most commonly in unacclimatized individuals during the early stages of heat exposure. It does not necessarily represent a state of significant volume depletion.

Evaluation of patients with heat syncope requires the usual exclusion of serious neurologic, metabolic, and cardiovascular disorders. The patient should also be examined for any injuries acquired as a result of the syncopal episode and subsequent fall. Treatment consists of removal from the heat source, oral or intravenous rehydration, and rest. Hospitalization is usually not necessary. Most patients with heat syncope recover promptly with fluids.

## Heat Cramps

Heat cramps are painful, involuntary, spasmodic contractions of skeletal muscles, usually those of the calves, thighs, and shoulders.

Heat cramps usually occur in individuals who are sweating liberally and replace fluid loss with water or other hypotonic solutions. Cramps may occur during exercise or after a latent period of several hours. Unconditioned or nonacclimated individuals who are just starting manual labor in a hot environment are at high risk for developing heat cramps. Although heat cramps do not cause significant morbidity and are considered to be self-limiting, the pain associated with them can readily result in an emergency department visit.

The exact pathogenesis of heat cramps is not known. However, a relative deficiency of sodium, potassium, and fluid at the muscle level is generally accepted. The production of large amounts of sweat, which has a high sodium content, coupled with inadequate sodium replacement results in hyponatremia. This in turn produces muscle cramps by interfering with calcium-dependent muscle relaxation. Hypokalemia from hyperventilation and dehydration may also play a contributing role.

Treatment consists of rest in a cool environment and fluid and salt replacement. Salt and fluid repletion can be accomplished either orally or intravenously. For mild cases, or if an overwhelming number of patients require treatment, a 0.1 to 0.2% saline solution can be given orally. Many electrolyte drinks are commercially available. More severe cases of heat cramps will respond to intravenous rehydration with normal saline.

Heat cramps can be prevented by maintaining adequate dietary salt intake or by drinking commercial electrolyte beverages. Salt tablets by themselves should not be used for the following reasons: (1) the tablets are a gastric irritant and often result in nausea and vomiting, and (2) they do not replace volume.

## Heat Tetany

Heat tetany is characterized by hyperventilation resulting in respiratory alkalosis, paraesthesias, and carpopedal spasm. Heat tetany is usually associated with short periods of intense heat stress. Treatment consists of removal from heat and decreasing the respiratory rate. Generally concomitant heat cramps are not present.

## Heat Exhaustion

Heat exhaustion is an obscure syndrome characterized by nonspecific symptoms such as dizziness, weakness, malaise, lightheadedness, fatigue, nausea, vomiting, headache, and myalgias. Clinical manifestations include syncope, orthostatic hypotension, sinus tachycardia, tachypnea, diaphoresis, and hyperthermia. However, the core temperature is variable and can range from normal to 40°C (104°F). Mental status remains normal. Because of the ill-defined and nonspecific symptoms, heat exhaustion is a diagnosis of exclusion. Physiologically, heat exhaustion is characterized by a combination of salt and water depletion.

Laboratory studies will almost universally demonstrate hemoconcentration, although specific electrolyte abnormalities depend on the ratio of fluid and electrolyte losses to intake. Patients who have virtually no fluid intake of any kind will usually develop hypernatremia, while those who partially rehydrate with salt-containing fluids may develop isotonic dehydration with normal sodium and chloride levels. Serum potassium and magnesium levels are variable.

The treatment of heat exhaustion is rest and volume and electrolyte replacement. Rapid administration of moderate amounts of intravenous fluids (1 to 2 L of saline solution) may be necessary in occasional patients who demonstrate significant tissue hypoperfusion. The choice of solution is guided by laboratory determinations, but balanced salt solutions may be utilized until specific electrolyte abnormalities are determined to be present. Generally these patients do not require hospitalization.

The signs and symptoms of early heatstroke may be difficult to differentiate from heat exhaustion. Patients with heat exhaustion will have a normal neurologic examination and normal mental status, although they may complain of headache, dizziness, weakness, or blurring of vision. Any patient with altered mental status has the diagnosis of heatstroke.

## HEATSTROKE

Classically, heatstroke was defined as the triad of hyperpyrexia [usually core temperature > 40.5°C (105°F)], central nervous system (CNS) dysfunction, and anhidrosis. However, anhidrosis, or a lack of sweating, is not an absolute diagnostic criterion. Heatstroke is a true medical emergency that may result in widespread organ system injury. It requires immediate intervention due to its high potential for mortality.

The CNS is particularly vulnerable in heatstroke. Heatstroke should be suspected in anyone with heat exposure, hyperthermia, and CNS dysfunction, such as syncope, irritability, bizarre behavior, combativeness, hallucinations, or coma. The cerebellum is highly sensitive to heat, and ataxia is an early finding. Virtually any neurologic abnormality may be present in heatstroke, including plantar responses, decorticate and decerebrate posturing, hemiplegia, status epilepticus, and coma. Cerebral edema is a common finding. CNS dysfunction is universal at core temperatures greater than 42°C (108°F). However, there is no arbitrary core temperature at which heatstroke begins. Cellular injury is a function of both the maximum temperature reached and the time of exposure. Patients with lower temperatures for longer periods of time can do worse than patients with higher temperatures for shorter periods of time.

The presence or absence of sweating has classically been one of the important distinctions between true heatstroke and other heat emergencies. However, the presence of sweating does not exclude the diagnosis of heatstroke. Patients with early heatstroke typically demonstrate marked sweating but eventually develop anhidrosis due to profound volume depletion or sweat gland dysfunction. However, anticholinergic agents are the most common cause of impaired sweating.

Heatstroke is a total breakdown of thermoregulation. Historically, two forms of heatstroke have been described: nonexertional and exertional. Classic, or nonexertional, heatstroke usually occurs during summer heat waves. The poor, the elderly, and the chronically ill are at greatest risk. The pathophysiology is increased exogenous heat gain and diminished heat dispersion. The specific stressors are lack of air-conditioning, presence of cardiovascular disease, older age, and cardiovascular or anticholinergic drugs.

Exertional heatstroke usually strikes a younger segment of the population as a consequence of vigorous physical activity. The primary cause is increased endogenous heat production. Individuals who perform physical labor or exercise in a hot, humid climate are especially prone to develop heatstroke. The distinction between exertional and nonexertional heatstroke is moot because signs, symptoms, and management are the same.

The definitive diagnosis of environmental heatstroke is a diagnosis of exclusion. The differential diagnosis for fever and altered mental status is varied and lengthy (Table 161-2). However, once heatstroke is suspected, efforts to lower the body temperature must be initiated immediately by whatever means available, whether in the prehospital or emergency department setting.

**Table 161-2.** Differential Diagnosis of Heat Stroke

| | |
|---|---|
| Alcohol withdrawal syndrome | Meningitis |
| Neuroleptic malignant syndrome | Brain abscess |
| Malignant hyperthermia | Malaria (cerebral falciparum) |
| Anticholinergic toxicity | Typhoid fever |
| Salicylate toxicity | Status epilepticus |
| PCP, cocaine, or amphetamine toxicity | Cerebral hemorrhage |
| Tetanus | Diabetic ketoacidosis |
| Sepsis | Thyroid storm |
| Encephalitis | |

## TREATMENT OF HEAT STROKE

### Initial Resuscitation Measures

Initial attention must be paid to the airway, breathing, circulation, debilitation, etc. High-flow supplemental oxygen is indicated. Continuous pulse oximetry and cardiac monitoring are necessary. Intravenous access should be obtained quickly, but fluid administration should be cautious. We recommend the initial infusion of normal saline or lactated Ringer's solution at 250 mL/h. If the patient is elderly or has cardiovascular disease, it is wise to monitor pulmonary wedge pressure to guide fluid therapy. A Foley catheter should be inserted. Of paramount importance is the serial monitoring of the patient's core temperature. This is best accomplished by inserting an electronic rectal thermistor probe. Glass thermometers are dangerous in patients with seizures or altered mental status.

Diagnostic studies necessary to detect the end-organ sequelae of heat stroke include a complete blood cell count, electrolytes, liver chemistries, blood urea nitrogen, creatinine, calcium, magnesium, coagulation profile (prothrombin time, partial thromboplastin time) arterial blood gases, urinalysis, urinary myoglobin, and a toxicology screen. An electrocardiogram and chest x-ray are also necessary. A CT scan of the head and lumbar puncture may also be indicated as part of the evaluation of altered mental status.

### Cooling Techniques

Rapid reduction of core temperature to 40°C (104°F) is the primary goal of treatment and is accomplished by physical cooling techniques. Antipyretics are not effective in heatstroke. The fastest cooling techniques reported in the literature are usually implemented in a structured research laboratory environment, utilizing animal models and equipment and techniques that are not universally available. In clinical practice, a technique that allows easy patient access and is readily available is preferable to a technique that may be faster, but is difficult to perform or does not permit easy access to the patient.

A comparison of the cooling rates achieved in several animal and human models with various cooling techniques is shown in Table 161-3. The advantages and disadvantages are summarized in Table 161-4. Immersion cooling is relatively contraindicated if the patient may require defibrillation or cardiac monitoring. Iced gastric lavage

**Table 161-3.** Cooling Rates Achieved with Various Cooling Techniques

| Technique | Author/Year | Species | Rate, °C/min |
|---|---|---|---|
| Evaporative | Weiner/1980 | Human | 0.31 |
| | Barner/1984 | Human | 0.04 |
| | Al-Aska/1987 | Human | 0.09 |
| | Kielblock/1986 | Human | 0.034 |
| | Wyndam/1959 | Human | 0.23 |
| | White/1987 | Dog | 0.14 |
| | Daily/1948 | Rat | 0.93 |
| Immersion (ice water) | Weiner/1980 | Human | 0.14 |
| | Wyndam/1959 | Human | 0.14 |
| | Magazanik/1980 | Dog | 0.27 |
| | Daily/1948 | Rat | 1.86 |
| Icepacking (whole body) | Kielblock/1986 | Human | 0.034 |
| | Bynum/1978 | Dog | 0.11 |
| Strategic ice packs | Kielblock/1986 | Human | 0.028 |
| Evaporative and strategic ice packs | Kielblock/1986 | Human | 0.036 |
| Cold gastric lavage | Syverud/1985 | Dog | 0.15 |
| | White/1987 | Dog | 0.06 |
| Cold peritoneal lavage | Bynum/1978 | Dog | 0.56 |

*Source:* Helmrich DE, Syverud SA: Procedures pertaining to hyperthermia, in Roberts JR, Hedges JR (eds): *Clinical Procedures in Emergency Medicine,* 2d ed. Philadelphia, Saunders, 1991, with permission.

**Table 161-4.** Various Cooling Techniques

| Technique | Advantages | Disadvantages |
|---|---|---|
| Evaporative | Simple, readily available | Constant moistening of skin |
| | Noninvasive | surface required to maximize |
| | Easy monitoring and patient | heat loss |
| | access | |
| | Relatively more rapid | |
| Immersion | Noninvasive | Cumbersome |
| | Relatively more rapid | Patient monitoring and access |
| | | difficult |
| | | Shivering |
| | | Poorly tolerated by conscious |
| | | patients |
| Ice packing | Noninvasive | Shivering |
| | Readily available | Poorly tolerated by conscious |
| | | patients |
| Strategic ice packs | Noninvasive | Relatively slower |
| | Readily available | Shivering |
| | Can be combined with other | Poorly tolerated by conscious |
| | techniques | patients |
| Cold gastric lavage | Can be combined with other | Relatively slower |
| | techniques | Invasive |
| | | May require airway protection |
| | | Human experience limited |
| Cold peritoneal lavage | Very rapid | Invasive |
| | | Human experience limited |

*Source:* Helmrich DE, Syverud SA: Procedures pertaining to hyperthermia, in: Roberts JR, Hedges JR (eds): *Clinical Procedures in Emergency Medicine,* 2d ed. Philadelphia, Saunders, 1991, with permission.

should not be utilized unless the airway is protected. Iced lavage is relatively contraindicated if the patient is pregnant or has had previous abdominal surgery.

We favor evaporative cooling as the technique of choice. It is the fastest noninvasive cooling technique in humans. Evaporative cooling combines the advantages of simplicity and noninvasiveness with the most rapid cooling rates that can be achieved with any external techniques. Ice packs can be placed at the groin and axillae. Gastric lavage is safe if the patient is intubated. Cooling with peritoneal lavage is an effective and rapid central cooling technique. Immersion cooling should be limited to situations where evaporative cooling is not possible.

Evaporative cooling is performed by positioning fan(s) close to the completely undressed patient and then sponging the skin or spraying tepid water on the patient. Inexpensive plastic spray bottles work the best. We avoid covering the patient with sheets and then wetting the sheets because this impairs evaporation of heat from the skin. Only one person is needed to monitor and continue cooling the patient.

There are only two complications of evaporative cooling: (1) shivering, and (2) inability of cardiac electrodes to adhere to the skin. Shivering is treated primarily with intravenous benzodiazepines and secondarily with phenothiazines. Cardiac electrodes can be applied to the patient's back.

In comparison, immersion cooling is performed by placing the undressed patient into a tub of water deep enough to cover the trunk and extremities. The head must be kept out of the water. Cardiac monitoring electrodes and rectal temperature probes must be secured to the patient. The complications of immersion cooling include shivering, displacement of monitoring leads, and inability to perform defibrillation or rescuscitative procedures.

Regardless of the cooling technique that is chosen, cooling efforts should be discontinued when the rectal temperature reaches 40°C (104°F). Continued cooling below this temperature will lead to "overshoot hypothermia."

## Complications of Heatstroke

In the patient with a relatively intact cardiovascular system, heat stress causes an increase in heart rate and cardiac index. Most heat-stroke victims have a high cardiac index, elevated central venous pressure, and a low peripheral resistance. However, heart failure, pulmonary edema, and cardiovascular collapse can occur even in young healthy individuals. In any age group, the presence of hypotension, decreased cardiac output, and a falling cardiac index indicates a particularly poor prognosis. A Swan-Ganz catheter may be necessary in the assessment of appropriate volume replacement.

Hepatic and renal abnormalities may be found in patients with heatstroke. Centrilobular necrosis due to direct thermal injury results in abnormal liver function studies, although recovery is to be expected. Jaundice is unusual. Microscopic hematuria, proteinuria, and hyaline and granular casts rapidly become evident on urinalysis. Patients with hypovolemic complications and decreased renal blood flow may develop acute tubular necrosis (ATN). Exercise-induced heatstroke is often complicated by rhabdomyolysis, sometimes with massive myoglobinuria and renal failure. This complication may not develop until several days after the initial injury, so that careful monitoring of creatine phosphokinase levels and renal function is necessary. Occasionally, a patient may present to the emergency department with the dark urine of myoglobinuria, and historical considerations should include recent heat exposure or heavy exertion.

Widespread hematologic disorders may be apparent both clinically and on laboratory evaluation. Purpura, conjunctival hemorrhages, petechiae, and pulmonary, gastrointestinal, and renal hemorrhages may be present. Coagulation studies may show thrombocytopenia, hypoprothrombinemia, and hypofibrinogenemia. Thermal injury to the vascular endothelium causes increased platelet aggregation, changes in capillary permeability, thermal deactivation of plasma proteins resulting in a decreased level of clotting factors, and, rarely, disseminated intravascular coagulation or fibrinolysis.

As expected, the fluid and electrolyte abnormalities vary with the onset and duration of the disorder, underlying disease (especially cardiovascular disease), and prior use of medications such as diuretics. The most important consideration with respect to fluid and electrolyte abnormalities in heatstroke is that dehydration and volume depletion may not occur in classic heatstroke, whereas they are common signs of heat exhaustion. Vigorous fluid administration may produce pulmonary edema, especially in the elderly. A myriad of blood gas abnormalities may be encountered, from respiratory alkalosis to severe metabolic acidosis.

## BIBLIOGRAPHY

Al-Aska AK, Abu-Aisha H, Yaqub B, et al: Simplified cooling bed for heatstroke (letter). *Lancet* Feb 14, 381, 1987.

Bynum G, Patton J, Bowers W, et al: Peritoneal lavage cooling in an anesthetized dog heatstroke model. *Aviat Space Environ* Med 49:779, 1978.

Callaham ML: *Emergency Management of Heat Illness.* Emergency Physician Series. Chicago, Abbott Laboratories, 1979, pp 1–23.

Daily WM, Harrison TR: A study of the mechanism and treatment of experimental heat pyrexia. *Am J Med Sci* 215:42, 1948.

Helmrich DE, Syverud SA: Procedures pertaining to hyperthermia, in Roberts JR, Hedges JR (eds): *Clinical Procedures in Emergency Medicine,* 2d ed. Philadelphia, Saunders, 1991, pp 1109–1116.

Jones TS, Liang AP, Kibourne EM, et al: Morbidity and mortality associated with the July 1980 heat wave in St. Louis and Kansas City, MO. *JAMA* 247:3327, 1982.

Kielblock AJ, Van Renshurg JP, Franz RM: Body cooling as a method for reducing hyperthermia. *S Afr Med* J 69:378, 1986.

Magazanik A, Epstein Y, Udassin R, et al: Tap water, an efficient method for cooling heatstroke victims—a model in dogs. *Aviat Space Environ Med* 51:864, 1980.

Stewart CE: Acute hyperthermia: The spectrum of heat emergencies. *Emerg Med Rep* 13:134, 1993.

Syverud SA, Barker WJ, Amsterdam J, et al: Iced gastric lavage for treatment of heat stroke: Efficacy in a canine model. *Ann Emerg Med* 14:424, 1985.

Tek D, Olshaker JS: Heat illness. *Emerg Med Clin North Am* 10:299, 1992.

Vassalo SU, Delaney KA: Pharmacologic effects on thermoregulation: Mechanism of drug-related heat stroke. *Clin Toxicol* 27:199, 1989.

Weiner JS, Khogali M: A physiological body-cooling unit for treatment of heatstroke. *Lancet* Mar 8, 507, 1980.

White JD, Riccobene E, Nucci R, et al: Evaporation versus iced gastric lavage treatment of heatstroke: Comparative efficacy in a canine model. *Crit Care Med* 15:748, 1987.

Wyndham CH, Strydom NB, Cooke HM, et al: Methods of cooling subjects with hyperpyrexia. *J Appl Physiol* 14:771, 1959.

# 162
# INSECT AND SPIDER BITES
## Richard F. Salluzzo

## INTRODUCTION

Insects that sting are members of the order Hymenoptera of the class Insecta. Toxic reactions to multiple stings by members of the order of Hymenoptera and severe systemic reactions to one or two stings or to bites of some other insects such as deerflies, blackflies, horseflies, and kissing bugs can both present an emergency, life-threatening situation. (See Table 162-1 for a listing of harmful arthropods of the United States.) However, fatalities due to biting insects are far rarer than those caused by the venom of Hymenoptera.

## HYMENOPTERA (WASPS, BEES, AND ANTS)

The Hymenoptera are the most important venomous insects known to humans. There are two major subgroups; *vespids* include the yellow jackets, hornet, and wasp, and *apids* include the honeybee and bumblebee (Fig. 162-1). Generally speaking, the yellow jackets cause most of the allergic reactions to insect stings. These organisms are

**Table 162-1.** Harmful Arthropods of the United States

| Class and Order | Common Name | Bite | Sting |
|---|---|---|---|
| Hexapoda (Insecta) | | | |
| Hymenoptera | Bees: | | |
| | Bumblebees | | x |
| | Sweat bees | | x |
| | Honeybees | | x |
| | Wasps: | | |
| | Hornets | | x |
| | Yellow jackets | | x |
| | Ants: | | |
| | Fire ants | | x |
| | Harvester ants | | x |
| Diptera | Mosquitoes | x | |
| | Deerflies | x | |
| | Horseflies | x | |
| | Stable flies | x | |
| | Blackflies | x | |
| | Biting midges | x | |
| Hemiptera | Bedbugs | x | |
| | Wheel bugs | | |
| | Kissing bugs | x | |
| Coleoptera | Blister beetles | | x |
| Lepidoptera | Puss caterpillars | | x |
| | Browntail caterpillars | | x |
| | Buck mouth caterpillars | | x |
| Siphonaptera | Fleas (human, cat, dog) | x | |
| Anoplura | Lice, (body, head, pubic) | x | |
| Arachnida | | | |
| Araneida | Black widow spiders | x | |
| | Brown recluse spiders | x | |
| Acarina | Mites | x | |
| | Ticks | x | |
| Scorpionida | Scorpions | | x |

*Source:* Frazier CA: *Insect Allergy.* St. Louis, WH Green, revised edition, 1987, p 421. Used by permission.

found nesting in the ground or in walls and may be disturbed by work around the yard, including mowing, gardening, and outdoor sports.

Honeybees and bumblebees are docile and tend to sting only when provoked. In general, the honeybee stings only once since its stinger has multiple barbs that causes the sting apparatus to detach from the insect. The African honeybees, or "killer bees," are now found in Texas, Arizona, and California. Their venom is no more toxic than that of the American counterpart, but African honeybees are very aggressive and can cause massive stinging leading to death from severe venom toxicity.

The normal response to Hymenoptera venom consists of pain, slight erythema, edema, and pruritus at the sting site. In addition to this response, there are several more significant reactions that may occur.

**Local reaction.** A local reaction consists of marked and prolonged edema contiguous with the sting site (Fig. 162-2). Although there are no systemic signs or symptoms, a severe local reaction may involve one or more neighboring joints. A local reaction occurring in the mouth or throat can produce airway obstruction. Stings around the eye or on the lid may result in the development of an anterior capsule cataract, atrophy of the iris, lens abscess, perforation of the globe, glaucoma, or refractive changes. When local reactions become increasingly severe, the likelihood of future systemic reactions appears to increase and, if skin tests are positive, may warrant immunotherapy.

**Toxic reactions.** When there is a history of multiple stings, often more than 10, a toxic reaction may occur. Symptoms of a toxic reaction may resemble those of a systemic reaction, but there is generally a greater frequency of gastrointestinal disturbance. Vomiting, diarrhea, light-headedness, and syncope are common signs. There also may be headache, fever, drowsiness, involuntary muscle spasms,

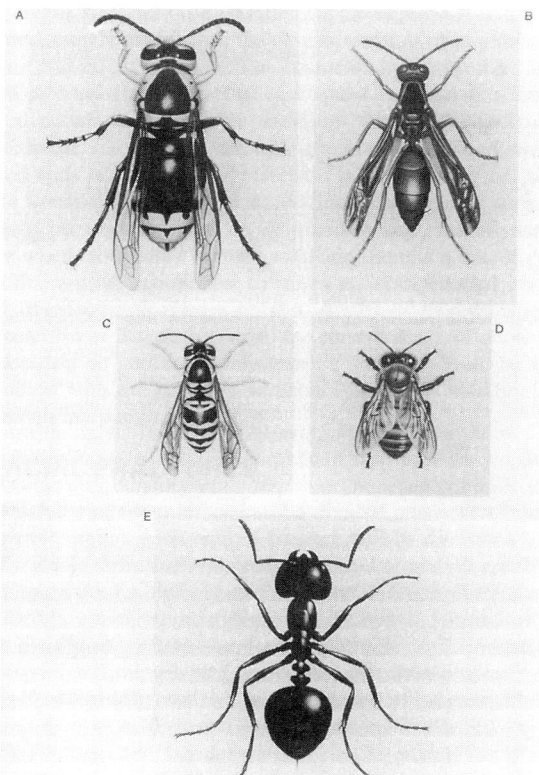

**Fig. 162-1.** Representative venomous hymenoptera. **A.** Hornet (*Vespula maculata*); **B.** wasp (*Chlorion ichneumerea*); **C.** yellow jacket (*Vespula maculiforma*); **D.** honey bee (*Apis mellifera*), and **E.** fire ant (*Solenopsis invicta*). (Reproduced by permission of Merck Sharp & Dohme, Division of Merck & Co., Inc.)

edema without urticaria, and occasionally seizures. Urticaria and bronchospasm are not present. Symptoms usual subside within 48 h. Toxic reactions are believed to be a response to the nonantigenic properties of Hymenoptera venom.

**Systemic or anaphylactic reactions.** A generalized systemic reaction, whether in response to a single sting or multiple stings, may range from mild to fatal, and death can occur within minutes. The majority of such reactions occur within the first 15 min, and nearly all occur within 6 h. There is no correlation between systemic reactions and the number of stings. In general, the shorter the interval between the sting and the onset of symptoms, the more severe the reaction. Fatalities that occur within the first hour of the sting usually result from airway obstruction or hypotension. Initial symptoms usually consist of itching eyes, facial flushing, generalized urticaria, and dry cough. Symptoms may intensify rapidly with chest or throat constriction, wheezing, dyspnea, cyanosis, abdominal cramps, diarrhea, nausea, vomiting, vertigo, chills and fever, laryngeal stridor, shock, loss of consciousness, involuntary bowel or bladder action, and bloody, frothy sputum. Initial mild symptoms may progress swiftly to anaphylactic shock. Patients can deteriorate rapidly and undergo respiratory failure or cardiovascular collapse.

**Delayed reaction.** A delayed reaction, appearing 10 to 14 days after a sting, consists of serum sickness–like signs and symptoms of fever, malaise, headache, urticaria, lymphadenopathy, and polyarthritis. Frequently, the patient has forgotten about the encounter and is puzzled by the sudden appearance of symptoms.

**Unusual reactions.** Infrequently, a reaction to Hymenoptera venom produces neurologic, cardiovascular, and urologic symptoms, with signs of encephalopathy, neuritis, vasculitis, and nephrosis. A case of Guillain-Barré syndrome has been reported as a possible con-

sequence of a Hymenoptera sting. Another unusual reaction is intense apprehension following a sting, with symptoms of faintness, excessive sweating, and an increased heart rate.

## Pathophysiology of Systemic Reaction

A generalized systemic reaction to Hymenoptera venom is thought to be IgE-mediated. When an individual predisposed to allergy to bees is stung, there is usually an increase in the production of IgE antibodies, which become attached to the mast cells and basophils. This sensitizes the individual so that a subsequent sting may result in an antigen-antibody interaction that releases pharmacologically active mediators, histamine, the slow-reacting substance of anaphylaxis (SRS-A), and eosinophil chemotactic factors of anaphylaxis (ECF-A). It is these mediators that actually cause tissue damage and systemic symptoms.

The pharmacologic effects of histamine are vasodilation, urticaria or angioedema, either an increased or decreased respiratory rate, fall in blood pressure, vomiting, and tenesmus. Histamine is believed responsible for symptoms of bronchoconstriction in a systemic reaction. SRS-A is also believed to be a constrictor of bronchial smooth muscle and may potentiate the effect of histamine. In addition to producing the eosinophil cell increase, ECF-A may serve to counteract the activity of SRS-A and histamine, which may diminish the acuteness of the reaction. Platelet-activating factors may contribute to the reaction by platelet aggregation and degranulation.

Electrophoretic, chromatographic, and fractionating techniques have recently increased our knowledge of the chemical and immunologic characteristics of Hymenoptera venoms. These venoms are similar in some substances but differ in others. Honeybee venom contains histamine; wasp venom contains histamine and serotonin; hornet venom contains both histamine and serotonin, as well as acetylcholine. Pharmacologically active amines in the venoms have

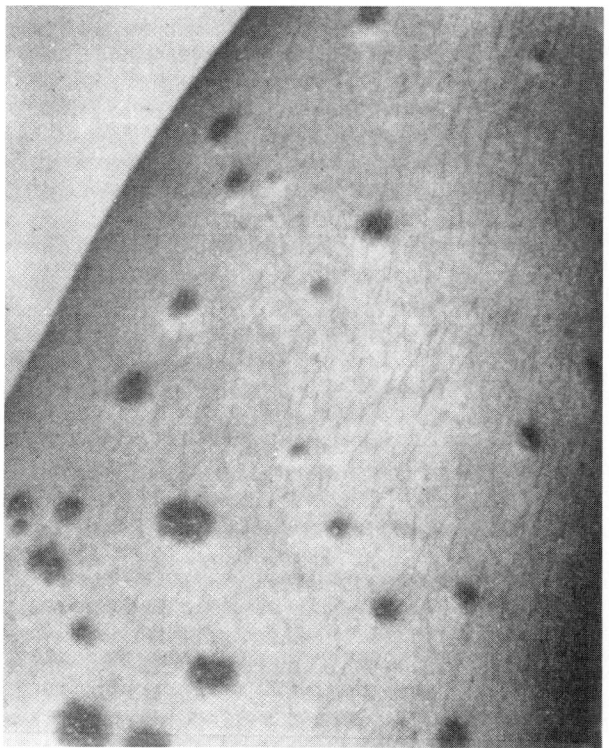

**Fig. 162-2.** Inflamed nodular reaction to insect bites. (From Moschella SL, Hurley HJ, eds: *Dermatology*, 2d ed. Philadelphia, Saunders, 1985, with permission.)

been identified as histamine, serotonin, acetylcholine, adrenaline, noradrenaline, and dopamine. Melittin and apamin are among the polypeptides, while phospholipase A and hyaluronidase are the major enzymes. The five important allergens in honeybee venom are phospholipase A, hyaluronidase, melittin, acid phosphatase, and diphenylpyraline (Allergen C). There is some controversy as to whether phospholipase A or hyaluronidase is the main allergen.

The venom of other members of Hymenoptera differs from honeybee venom in several respects. Wasp venom contains histamine, 5-hydroxytryptamine, and kinins, while hornet venom contains these fractions plus acetylcholine. This allergenic specificity resides in the fact that bees belong to the superfamily Apoidea, while wasps, hornets, and yellow jackets belong to Vespoidea. A common antigen occurs in the body of a wasp and a honeybee, but it is not common to their respective venoms. There is also a common antigen in the body of a bee and a yellow jacket. Cross-reactivity appears to be the greatest between the wasp and yellow jacket, for they share a common body antigen as well as a common antigen in their venom sacs.

## Diagnosis

Identification of the offending insect can be difficult, except for the honeybee, which almost invariably leaves its stinger with venom sac attached in the lesion. A careful history is often necessary to distinguish members of Vespoidea from each other, and slides or pictures of the various species can aid the patient in recall. Some questions that can be asked in an effort to identify the offending insect are: Where did the encounter occur? Was a nest noted, and, if so, was it in the ground (yellow jackets), under leaves or windowsills (wasps), in bushes or low-hanging tree limbs (hornets)? Skin tests are not always reliable in identification since most individuals allergic to insects are sensitive to two or three species. This high incidence of cross-reactivity underlines the importance of mixed species extracts in immunotherapy.

If edema persists at the sting site, secondary infection, such as cellulitis, must be considered. Severe local reactions on the foot or ankle can be misdiagnosed as gout if the insect bite is not visible.

If the bee sting is present in the wound, try to remove it without squeezing since this will force more venom from the attached sac into the wound. In case of the honeybee, remove the stinger as quickly as possible as it continues to pulse even after the bee has flown away. As a general rule, the sting site should be thoroughly washed with soap and water to minimize the possibility of infection. For local reactions, ice packs at the site will diminish swelling and delay the absorption of the venom while limiting edema. Oral antihistamines and analgesics may limit discomfort and pruritus. NSAIDs are effective if given immediately. A dose of 800 mg ibuprofen or equivalent can be

given orally to adults or 20 mg/kg PO in children. If edema is significant, elevation and rest of the affected limb should limit swelling unless secondary infection develops, in which case antibiotics will be necessary. In local tissue reactions, there is often significant erythema and swelling, making it difficult to distinguish from infection; as a general rule infection is only present in a minority of cases.

While the initial symptoms of a systemic reaction may be mild, symptoms can intensify rapidly to become life-threatening in a matter of minutes. It is vital to administer epinephrine hydrochloride; 1:1000, 0.3 to 0.5 mL for an adult, and 0.01 mL/kg for a child (never more than 0.3 mL). It should be injected subcutaneously and the injection site massaged to hasten absorption of the drug. The patient should then be observed for several hours to ensure that symptoms do not intensify.

More severe symptoms of a systemic reaction, such as chest constriction, nausea, faintness, and pronounced uneasiness, may require a second injection of epinephrine in 10 to 15 min. Antihistamines, such as diphenhydramine, 25 to 50 mg, should be administered parenterally.

If bronchospasm develops, a secure intravenous line should be established and an infusion of aminophylline administered IV over 20 to 30 min. Beta agonists by nebulizer may also be effective in treating the bronchospasm. Maintain an open airway and administer oxygen as needed. If laryngeal edema is present with impending airway obstruction, insert an endotracheal tube. Hypotension may require massive crystalloid infusion, and central venous pressure monitoring may be helpful in some cases. Persistent hypotension after massive volume replacement may call for an initial infusion of dopamine, 200 mg in 250 mL of normal saline, at 5 µg/kg per minute, which may be increased gradually to 20 to 50 µg/kg per minute. While steroids are of little help in combating the immediate problem, their administration tends to limit urticaria and edema and may potentiate the effects of other measures.

The patient who suffers a severe systemic reaction should be kept under observation for 24 to 48 h and examined for evidence of cardiac problems, bleeding, proteinuria, or neurologic complications.

## Long-Term Management and Preventive Care

If skin tests are positive, immunotherapy should be initiated and the patient maintained thereafter on an optimum dose (see Table 162-2). There is controversy over the relative effectiveness and safety of whole body and venom extracts. Nor has the question of which patients should undergo immunotherapy been totally resolved. Generally speaking, a rise in IgE levels indicates sensitivity, and an increase in IgG levels may indicate protection, but unfortunately this is not always the case. Nor are skin tests and radioallergosorbent tests

**Table 162-2.**

| Type of Past Reaction | Risk of Systemic Reaction to Subsequent Stings | Should Skin Testing be Performed? | Results of Skin Testing | Recommended Treatment |
|---|---|---|---|---|
| Never stung | Minimal | No | | None |
| Minor local reaction (immediate pain, swelling, and itching at sting site; subsides in 1 day) | Minimal | No | | None |
| Extensive local reaction (swelling contiguous to sting site; develops 24–48 h after the sting and resolves in a few days to a week) | Less than 10% | No | | Epinephrine syringe (ANA-Kit, Epi-Pen) |
| Systemic reaction: | | | | |
| Adult (urticaria, angioedema, or anaphylaxis) | High | Yes | + | Venom immunotherapy |
| | | | − | Epinephrine syringe |
| Child (urticaria and mild angioedema only) | Low | Yes | + | Venom immunotherapy or epinephrine syringe |
| | | | − | Epinephrine syringe |
| Child (anaphylaxis) | Moderate | Yes | + | Venom immunotherapy |
| | | | − | Epinephrine syringe |

**Table 162-3.** Prevention of Insect Stings

1. Seek and destroy Hymenoptera nests that may be in the vicinity of the home, outbuildings, and yard. Begin with the advent of warm weather and conduct the searches periodically until the first hard frost. This task, however, should not be undertaken by the insect-allergic individual, but rather by a nonallergic person or by a professional exterminator.
2. Avoid going barefoot or wearing sandals outdoors.
3. When outdoors, wear light colors such as white, tan, khaki, or light green. Do not wear bright colors or flowery prints.
4. Do not use perfumed lotions, aftershaves, or shampoos during the warm months.
5. Cover up with long sleeves and long pants and wear gloves when working outdoors; refrain from wearing floppy clothing that could entangle an irate stinging insect and from wearing bright jewelry that could attract one. Suede and leather articles may also not only attract but irritate Hymenoptera.
6. Anyone severely allergic to insects should not mow lawns, pick flowers, or clip hedges. Such an individual should be wary when eating outdoors, especially sugary food or drinks, and should avoid areas near garbage cans, littered picnic grounds, or fruit trees where fruit lies rotting on the ground.
7. If confronted by a member or members of Hymenoptera, remain calm, never swat or move hastily, but rather retreat as slowly and calmly as possible. If retreat seems impossible, lie on the ground and cover your head with your arms.

*Source:* Fraizer CA: *Insect Allergy.* St. Louis, WH Green, 1969.

(RAST) fully reliable in determining the need for patient protection, for patients with negative results may have been sensitized by the skin tests themselves. Every patient who has had a systemic reaction must be provided with an insect sting kit containing premeasured epinephrine and be carefully instructed in its use.

There are several insect sting kits available. Probably the simplest to use is the Ana-Kit, which contains a sterile syringe preloaded with two doses of epinephrine 1:1000, 0.5 mL in each dose with a stop between. The kit also contains a tourniquet, sterile alcohol pads, several antihistamine tablets, and instructions for self-injection. When prescribing this kit, the physician should stress that the patient must not rely on simply taking the antihistamine tablets, since these would not mitigate intensifying symptoms, but should inject the epinephrine subcutaneously at the first sign of a systemic reaction.

A second kit, the Epi-Pen, contains a single self-injecting, spring-loaded syringe of epinephrine 1:1000. Its advantage is the ease of injection; its disadvantages are that to be on the safe side the patient should carry two kits, and there is no way to measure proper dosage for children.

Physicians should, as a matter of course, advise their patients who are allergic to insects to wear Medic-alert tags, and they should provide those patients with a list of avoidance measures to prevent being stung (Table 162-3).

Armed with these preventive measures—a medical warning tag and three insect sting kits, one for the home, one for the car, and one to carry in the field—the individual allergic to insects has taken every possible precautionary measure.

When immunotherapy with venom extracts is decided upon, the injection schedule may be rapid, with weekly visits until the optimum (for most patients) maintenance dose of 100 µg is reached. A slower schedule may be used, with the advantage of fewer systemic reactions during the process, but the goal should remain 100 µg. There are no absolute contraindications to immunotherapy, although pregnancy may require extra caution against the possibility of systemic reactions during treatment.

Proposed guidelines for the safe cessation of venom immunotherapy are evolving. In general, conversion from a previously positive venom skin test to a negative test is a criterion for stopping therapy. Some studies suggest that 3 to 5 years of treatment even with the persistence of positive venom skin tests provides effective long-term protection.

## FIRE ANTS

There are five known species of fire ant (*Solenopsis*) in the United States; *S. aurea, S. geminata, S. xyloni,* and the two imported species, *S. invicta* and *S. richteri.* The two imported species entered the United States through Mobile, Alabama, in the 1930s and have now spread to all the Gulf Coast states and South Carolina. The fire ant inhabits a loose amount of dirt and breeds nine to ten months of the year. One mature nest can produce 200,000 ants during a 3-year period, which accounts for the rapid spread of this insect. The venom of the fire ant is almost entirely an insoluble alkaloid. There is no significant cross-reactivity between the fire ant and Hymenoptera, and individual stings produce limited toxicity.

**Fig. 162-3.** External anatomy of a spider. **A.** Dorsal; **B.** ventral; **C.** frontal. (Reproduced with permission from *Management of Wilderness and Environmental Emergencies,* St. Louis, Mosby, 1989.)

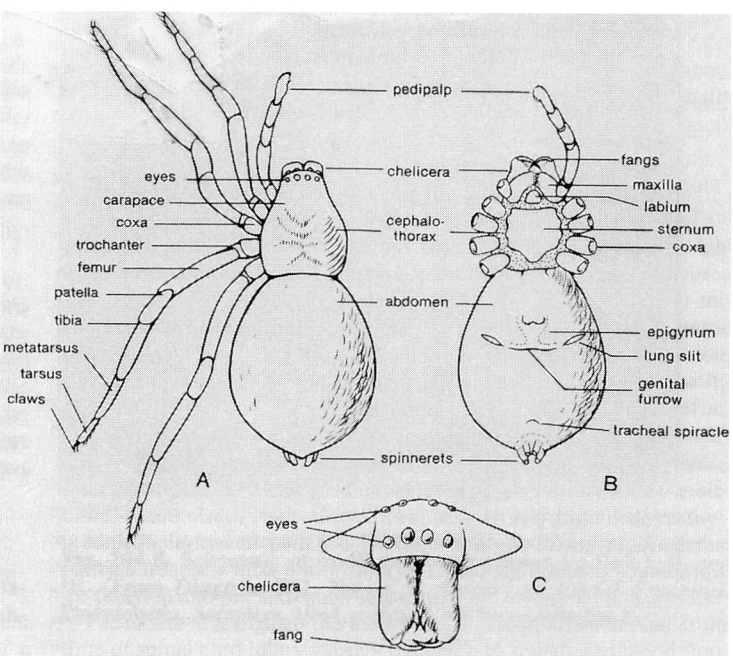

## Clinical Presentation

Fire ants are characterized by their tendency to swarm if provoked and may attack in great numbers. Each sting usually results in a papule, which becomes a sterile postule in 6 to 24 h. Localized necrosis, scarring, and secondary infection can result. There may be a systemic reaction manifested by urticaria and angioedema.

One study has estimated a hypersensitivity rate to the fire ant of 16 percent in the general population. Treatment of individual stings consists of local wound care. If there is evidence of systemic reaction, the usual treatment for anaphylaxis should be undertaken. Desensitization should be directed to any person exhibiting a potentially life-threatening reaction to the fire ant.

## SPIDER BITES

There are over 30,000 species of spiders worldwide, of which approximately 50 species in the United States have been implicated in medically significant envenomations. Spiders belong to the class Arachnida, one of the major divisions of the Arthropoda, the insects being a second major class. All spiders are carnivores utilizing venom to paralyze their prey prior to ingestion. Figure 162-3 shows the external anatomy of the spider. The *Loxosceles* have a worldwide distribution. There are 18 species in the genus *Loxosceles* in North America, with 13 of these found in the United States. Five of these, *L. reclusa, L. laeta, L. refuscens, L. arizona,* and *L. unicolor,* have been associated with ulcers and necrotic skin lesions. *Loxosceles reclusa* (the brown recluse spider) is one of the most common species found in the United States and has been reported in over 20 states, particularly those in the region of the Missouri, Ohio, and Mississippi river basins, but also in several southwestern, southern, and midwestern states. *Loxosceles reclusa* prefers warm dry areas such as abandoned buildings, wood piles, and cellars and is generally nocturnal in activity. It is difficult to find the exact incidence of these spider bites, though one U.S. study of 460 deaths from venomous bites attributed 63, or 14 percent, to *L. reclusa.* Loxoscelism is the reaction to the envenomation by species of the brown spider. Given their innocent appearance, indoor habitat, and relatively large numbers in endemic areas, the brown spider represents a greater public health hazard than that of the much-feared black widow spider.

The most frequent manifestation of an *L. reclusa* bite consists of a mild erythematous lesion that may become firm and heal over several days to weeks. Occasionally, a more severe reaction occurs, with mild to severe pain several hours after the bite. There may be erythema and blister formation and bluish discoloration within the first 24 h (Fig. 162-4). This lesion may become necrotic over the next 3 to 4 days (Fig. 162-5) with eschar formation by the end of the first week. These lesions may vary in size from 1 to 30 cm and may require 6 weeks to 4 months to heal.

The necrosis is caused by aggregation of leukocytes and platelets forming a hemostatic plug in venules and arterioles. The bite of the brown recluse spider may also cause systemic involvement, which generally occurs 24 to 48 h after the bite. The patient may experience fever, chills, nausea, vomiting, myalgias, arthralgias, petechiae, hemolysis, and even seizures. Hemolysis is apparently mediated by direct effect of the spider venom on red cell membranes and may be severe, causing hemoglobinuria, renal failure, disseminated intravascular coagulation, and, ultimately, death.

Though the systemic symptoms are proportional to the amount of envenomation, the severity of the skin lesions is not; relatively minor-appearing skin lesions may be accompanied by severe systemic symptoms.

The venom of *L. reclusa* consists of multiple proteases, alkaline phosphatase, lipase, anaronadase, and other substances that involve the complement system. It is still unclear which of these substances is the major factor related to the necrosis-producing activity of the spider.

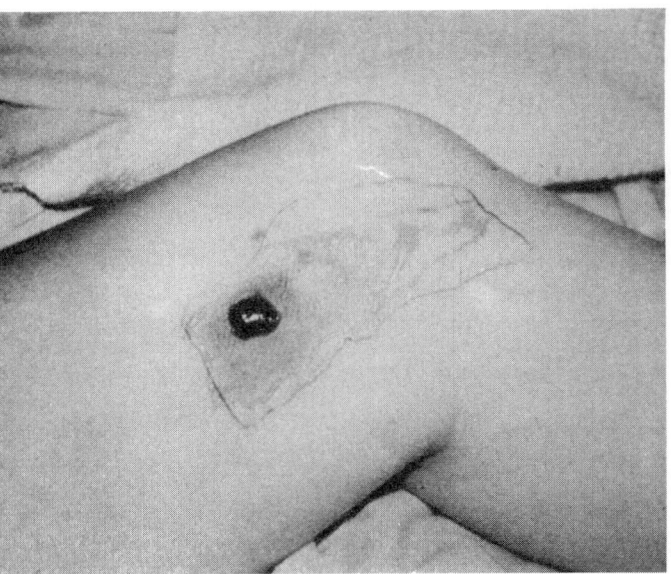

**Fig. 162-4.** Brown recluse spider bite approximately 12 hours old. Note central hemorrhagic vesicle with surrounding spread of toxin. (Reproduced by permission of author from *Management of Wilderness and Environmental Emergencies,* St. Louis, Mosby, 1989.)

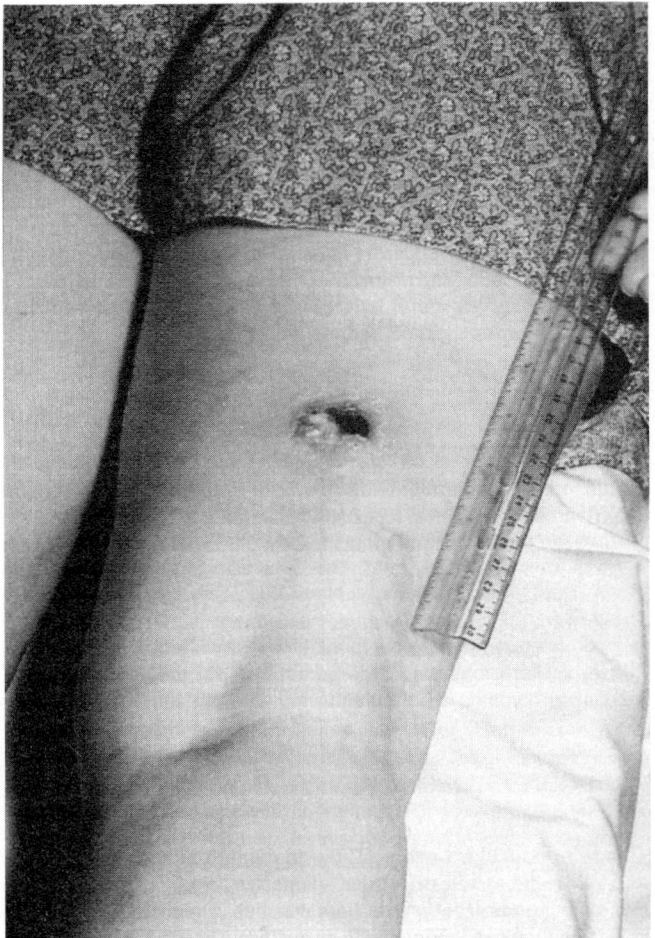

**Fig. 162-5.** Brown spider bite four days after injury. (Reproduced with permission from *Emergency Medicine,* June 1988.)

## Diagnosis

Since many spiders can produce skin lesions that are similar to those of the brown recluse bite, diagnosis of a bite from *L. reclusa* is sometimes very difficult. In the United States *L. argiope, L. atrax, L. chiracanthium, L. lycosa,* and *L. phidippus* can all cause similar bites to *L. reclusa.* In the absence of the actual spider for examination, the diagnosis is usually based upon clinical presentation and known presence of *L. reclusa* in the area.

In patients suspected of having a bite from *L. reclusa,* a CBC, BUN, electrolytes, blood sugar, creatinine, and coagulation profile should be ordered, as well as an urinalysis for hemoglobinuria.

## Treatment

Treatment of the brown recluse spider bite should include the usual supportive measures. Currently no antivenom is commercially available. For those bites with cytotoxic reactions and necrosis, tetanus prophylaxis and daily wound care should be given. Antibiotics should be utilized if evidence of infection exists. In some cases, analgesic therapy will be required. In general, surgery should not be done until the necrotic ulcers are greater than 2 cm in diameter and the borders of the ulcers are well established, usually 2 to 3 weeks after the bite.

Some recent studies have evaluated the use of dapsone in patients with *L. reclusa* bites. Dapsone may inhibit local infiltration by polymorphonuclear leukocytes, and although there is some suggestion that it may prevent ongoing necrosis, there are as yet no controlled data to substantiate this claim.

Adults and children with evidence of significant systemic reaction warrant hospitalization and close observation. If hemolysis occurs, appropriate hydration, red cell transfusion, and monitoring of renal function are important to avoid complications such as acute renal failure.

## Black Widow Spider Bites

The black widow spider is found throughout the United States, though predominantly in the southern states. Of the estimated 30,000 species of spiders, the black widow is probably the most feared. There are five species found commonly in the United States, only three of which, *L. mactans, L. variolus,* and *L. hesperus,* are actually black.

The classic orange-red hourglass-shaped marking is noted in only one species, *L. mactans.* Female spiders are relatively large, with a body size ranging up to 1.5 cm in length and leg spans of 4 to 5 cm. The male spider is approximately one-third the size of the female, and his bite can not penetrate human skin. Black widow spiders are relatively aggressive and most often found in wood piles, basements, garages, and other outdoor structures. The black widow will aggressively defend her turf, particularly when guarding her eggs. Most black widow bites occur between April and October and usually occur on the hands and forearms.

## Pathophysiology

The black widow spider injures its victim by secretion of one of the most potent venoms secreted by any animal. The venom is a neurotoxic protein that causes release of acetylcholine and norepinephrine at the neurosynoptic junction. The result of continued release of these neurotransmitters is protracted muscle contractions and, ultimately, muscle fatigue due to neurotransmitter depletion.

## Clinical Presentation

Initially the bite of the female black widow spider is generally mildly to moderately painful. Approximately 20 min to 1 h after the bite, erythema and swelling occur with muscle cramps that begin at the site and gradually spread. The pain progressively increases and can become very severe. Large muscle groups such as the thighs, shoulders, and back are often involved. Classically involvement of the abdominal wall musculature causes severe pain and a boardlike abdomen that can mimic peritonitis.

Severe muscle pain generally subsides after a few hours but may recur over 2 to 3 days. Muscle weakness and spasms may persist for weeks to months. The most serious complications include hypertension, which is reported in 10 to 30 percent of envenomations and remains of unclear etiology. In addition, severe envenomation may also cause shock, coma, and respiratory failure secondary to muscle paralysis.

## Diagnosis

If the spider bite goes unnoticed by the patient, a number of other diseases may be considered in the differential diagnosis as the cause of pain, muscle spasms, and the generally toxic appearance of the patient. There is no specific laboratory study that can confirm the diagnosis, and consequently it should be considered in the differential diagnosis in patients with the clinical presentation described above.

## Treatment

The initial therapy for black widow spider bites is basic supportive care of airway, breathing, and circulation. In addition, local wound care should consist of routine cleansing of the bite site and tetanus prophylaxis.

### Pain Relief and Muscle Relaxation

Patients should be given appropriate narcotic analgesics and benzodiazepines for pain relief and muscle relaxation. Intravenous calcium gluconate has been advocated to relieve pain and muscle spasms from the black widow bite, although controlled data are lacking. In a recent review of 163 patients treated with calcium, very few had effective relief of muscle spasm and pain.

### Antivenom

Antivenom is very effective for relieving symptoms caused by severe envenomation by the black widow spider bite. The usual dose is one to two vials of antivenom over 20 to 30 min. Since the antivenom is a horse serum preparation, skin testing should be done prior to administration as major complications including anaphylaxis have occurred with this therapy.

## Other Spider Bites

Although the black widow spider and the brown recluse spider are the best known, the most common biting spider in the United States is the so-called jumping spider, one of the *Phidippus* species. These small, furry, and relatively aggressive spiders are sometimes confused with the black widow spider because of their black and red markings.

Though jumping spiders bite and tend to hang on to the victim, they generally only produce a local reaction, which may take hours to days to subside. Treatment should include local wound care, analgesia, and occasionally antihistamine for pruritus.

## Tarantula

The term *tarantula* is used for several species of large spiders such as the desert tarantula, which is found in the southwest region of the United States and is a member of the family Theraphosidae. Despite their large size (up to 7 cm), the venom is very mild and does not produce systemic reactions. The typical tarantula bite causes local swelling and pain at the bite site; this may last for a few hours and is treated successfully with local wound care.

The South American tarantula, also known as "banana spider," does have potent venom and its bite may cause systemic reactions.

For these reasons, an antitoxin has been developed for the bite of the South American tarantula.

## CHIGGERS

Chigger infestations are caused by mite larvae that feed on the host skin cells. The combination of the effect of digestive enzymes secreted by the mite and the immune response of the host produces the typical chigger bite. The usual response is intense pruritus at the bite site, but more severe reactions and chigger-borne disease may also occur. Mites live comfortably in warm and cold climates. There are approximately 50,000 known species, making mites the most numerous form of arthropods on the planet. There are approximately 2500 species of chigger mites, with *Trombicula alfreddugesi* the most common. Mites are quite small, 0.3 to 1.0 mm in length, and attach themselves to the host skin with their mandibular structures, known as the chelicerae. They then release their digestive enzymes that lead to the host immune response and subsequent symptomotology. In general, itching begins a few hours after the chigger bite, with a papule developing initially that ultimately enlarges over 24 to 48 h to form a nodule. Pruritus is usually at its peak on the second day, and the nodules persist for up to 14 days. Children who play or sit on the grass are prone to chigger bites in the genital area. Bites are characterized by impressive soft tissue edema, which is pathognomic of chigger bites (Fig. 162-6). Mite infestations may be associated with fever and an erythema multiforme–like rash. The diagnosis of chigger infestation can usually be made on the basis of known outdoor exposure and typical skin lesions.

The treatment of chigger bites consists largely of symptomatic measures to control the itching. Chiggers may also be killed with lindane (Kwell, Scabene) or crotamiton (Eurax). For moderate to severe cases, topical steroid creams and oral antihistamines may provide some relief. Occasionally, there have been reports of systemic steroids providing relief for severe pruritus. If secondary infection occurs, antibiotic therapy is indicated.

The main approach to preventing chigger infestation is a preventive one. For outdoor activities, field clothing should be laundered in hot water to kill any chiggers that may be present. In addition, clothing should fit snugly at the neck, wrists, and ankles to prevent chigger infestation. Insect repellents are very effective in preventing chigger bites and should be utilized in areas of likely chigger habitation.

## MOSQUITO AND FLY BITES

### Mosquito Bites

From available evidence, it is apparent that a characteristic sequence of events takes place in all subjects exposed to mosquito bites over a period of time. Human reaction to bites of the mosquito may be classified as follows:

1. Immediate and delayed reactions, both negative
2. Immediate reaction negative; delayed reaction positive
3. Immediate and delayed reactions, both positive
4. Immediate reaction positive and delayed reaction negative

An immediate skin reaction to mosquito bites includes redness, wheal, and itching. A delayed reaction usually consists of edema and a burning pruritus. The immediate reaction tends to be of short duration, whereas a delayed reaction may persist for hours, days, and even weeks.

Hypersensitivity reactions are of three types: tuberculin, urticarial, and eczemoid. Arthus' phenomenon with skin necrosis occurs occasionally. The history of an allergy to mosquito saliva constituents consists of an increasing reaction to seasonal exposures with more and more pronounced edematous and pruritic lesions, accompanied sometimes by complications such as fever, malaise, generalized edema, severe nausea and vomiting, and necrosis with resulting scarring.

### Fly Bites

Bloodsucking flies that stab and pierce the skin can cause some degree of pain and, commonly, subsequent pruritus. Several species, such as deerflies, blackflies, horseflies, and sand flies, can produce allergic reactions, although rarely as severe as those produced by Hymenoptera venom. There is also the possibility of myiasis with fly bites, but this, too, is rare in the United States.

The diagnosis of fly bites depends chiefly on the patient's history and a knowledge of the insects that frequent the area of the encounter.

Treatment for the more severe normal reactions to insect bites is symptomatic while treatment of systemic reactions is the same as it is for Hymenoptera venom. Prevention of secondary infection, especially in the case of fly bites, is important, although antibiotics should not be given prophylactically. Oral antihistamines and cyproheptadine or hydroxyzine hyrochloride are helpful in relieving pruritus; trimeprazine tartrate is particularly effective in relieving pruritus of mosquito bites. Use of topical antihistamines runs the risk of contact dermatitis. However, topical steroid ointments are helpful when local reactions are severe or if scarring occurs.

Cold compresses may alleviate localized edema. For severe systemic reactions oral or parenteral steroids may be indicated. While immunotherapy has not proved as successful for mosquito or fly bite allergies as for Hymenoptera allergies, it is well worth the attempt for patients who suffer severe systemic reactions.

## FLEA, LICE, AND SCABIES BITES

### Flea Bites

Bites of fleas, lice, and scabies produce lesions so similar that diagnosis is often difficult. Flea bites are frequently found in zigzag lines, especially on the legs and in the waist area. The lesions have hemorrhagic puncta surrounded by erythematous and urticarial patches. Pruritus is intense, and often, even after the lesions clear, dull red spots persist. Children may develop impetigo as a complication.

The main concern in the treatment of flea bites is the possibility of secondary infection. The lesions should be washed thoroughly with soap and water. For children, keep the fingernails cut short to prevent scratching. To relieve discomfort and itching, starch baths at bedtime (about 1 kg starch to a tubful of water), local application of calamine, cool soaks, and an oral antihistamine such as trimeprazine may be helpful. For severe discomfort, application of a topical steroid cream or spray may be necessary.

If secondary infection develops, a topical antibiotic such as neomycin or polymyxin may be needed.

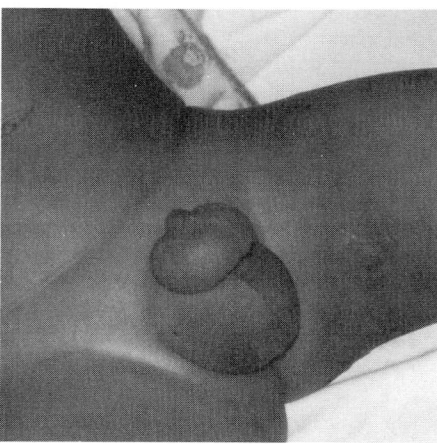

**Fig. 162-6.** Chigger bites. Edema of the foreskin, scrotum, and penis is dramatic. There is no meatal obstruction.

## Lice

Body lice concentrate about the waist, shoulders, axillae, and neck. The lice and their eggs can often be found in the seams of clothing. The lesions begin as small, noninflammatory red spots that quickly become papular wheals. They are so intensely pruritic that their linear scratch marks are diagnostically suggestive of infestation.

The white ova of head lice can be mistaken for dandruff, but unlike dandruff, they cannot be brushed out, for they are glued to the hair itself.

Pubic lice leave bluish spots in the abdomen and thighs, and ova are evident on the shafts of pubic hairs. If sensitization to lice saliva and feces components takes place, delayed reactions may develop. Fever and malaise are possible, and secondary infection may produce enlarged lymph glands. Long periods of infestation may bring a decrease in pruritus and often impart a thick, dry, scaly appearance to the skin. A brownish pigmentation characteristic of vagabond's disease can occur on the neck, shoulders, and back, or can become generalized and include even the mucuous membranes.

Treatment for body lice infestation consists of a thorough application of lindane or crotamiton (or permethrin), plus sterilization of clothing, bedding, and personal articles. Lindane, however, must be employed with caution for infants and children since it can be absorbed more readily by their skin. It can be toxic to the central nervous system. Crotamiton should not be employed on raw or weeping areas. Head lice are treated with either of the above medications, daily shampoos, and fine combing the hair. Personal articles should be sterilized.

## Scabies

While scabies infestation resemblies that of lice, scabies bites are generally concentrated around the hands and feet, especially in the webs between the fingers and toes. In children, however, the face and scalp may be infested as well. In adults, scabies frequently affects the nipples in females, the penis in males.

The scabies mite, an arachnid like the spider, is a universal pest that appear to follow a 30-year cycle of waxing and waning. During the past several years, there has been an epidemic of scabies infestation in the United States. In general, scabies infestation is more likely to occur by direct contact between the infested individual and the non-infested individual than by indirect contact with clothing and personal articles.

Diagnostically, pruritus is the dominant symptom, although it takes about a month for sensitization to develop and itching to begin. However, a patient who becomes infested, and who is already sensitized, develops inflammation and pruritus within a few hours of contact.

The distinctive feature of scabies infestation is the burrow that the female mite digs into the skin to lay her eggs. Vesicles and papules form at the surface of these zigzag, whitish, threadlike channels that contain small gray spots at the closed ends where the parasite rests. Burrows tend to enlarge and be more visible in children. The burrows can be traced with the hand lens and the female mite scraped out with a needle or razor blade. A thin shaving of skin containing both burrow and mite can be examined under a microscope to establish diagnosis clearly. Unfortunately, the burrows are often disguised by the results of fierce scratching. These distinctive physical findings are then obscured by crusting, eczematization, and secondary infection.

Treatment for scabies infestation consists of a thorough application of permethrin (Elemite) or lindane (cream or lotion) from the neck down, following a warm bath with liberal use of soap. The patient should be cautioned to keep the substance from eyes and mucous membranes and to avoid inhaling the vapors. Again, since lindane is toxic, it probably should not be employed for young children or pregnant women. A 5% sulfur ointment can be substituted if necessary, although it is apt to be somewhat odoriferous and messy. It should be applied twice from the neck down, with a 24-h interval between ap-

plications, followed each time by a soap and water bath. A third application following the second by 12 h should be effective.

Crotamiton, which is also antipruritic in action, can be applied from the neck down in two applications 24 h apart and followed 24 to 48 h later by a bath. The safety of its use, too, is somewhat in doubt, and it should be employed with caution.

Even after the scabies mites have been destroyed, lesions and pruritus can persist. No further use of scabicide is needed, but calamine lotion, oral antipruritic agents, and analgesics will help alleviate discomfort. Antibiotics are only necessary where secondary infection is a problem.

## KISSING BUG BITES

*Triatoma* species, commonly known as conenose or kissing bugs, are found mainly in the southeastern and Pacific coast regions of the United States. They feed on the blood of vertebrate animals, including humans. Their common name derives from their habit of feeding at night on any exposed surface of a sleeping victim, which commonly is the face. Since their bite is relatively painless, the victim is rarely aware of the attack.

Kissing bugs, like bedbugs, live in baseboards, between cracks in walls and floors, and in furniture.

Bites are usually multiple and consist of hemorrhagic papules or bullae if the bites occur on the hands or feet, and large wheals if they are on the trunk.

Diagnostically, kissing bug bites can be differentiated from bedbug bites in that they do not appear to form a linear formation nor do they leave the telltale brown or black patterns of excrement on the bed linen. They can be distinguished from spider bites, since the latter tend to be single lesions, and they usually can be distinguished from erythema multiforme by their unilateral, local distribution.

Generally, treatment is symptomatic with cool local applications and mild analgesics to relieve pruritus. Some individuals become highly sensitive to the kissing bug and react with systemic symptoms, which should be treated as previously outlined for Hymenoptera venom. There are enough recorded cases of successful results with immunotherapy for allergy to kissing bugs to make it well worth the attempt for the hypersensitive individual.

## CATERPILLAR STINGS

Some caterpillars possess hollow spines among their hairs that contain urticating poison that can cause symptoms ranging from local dermatitis to generalized systemic reactions. The puss caterpillar, larval stage of the flannel moth *Megalopyge opercularis,* is perhaps the most toxic in the United States and is especially hazardous for children who tend to find it intriguing and thus handle it.

Found primarily in the southeastern states and especially in Texas and Florida, the venom of the puss caterpillar has demonstrated hemolytic action in laboratory studies and an ability to increase vascular permeability. It is believed to be proteinaceous in nature.

The dominant feature of the puss caterpillar's sting is intense immediate pain, often rhythmic. Local edema and pruritus follow quickly, and a rash of red blotches and ridges develops. The lesions consist of white or red papules and vesicles, and frequently they form a perfect gridlike mark where the caterpillar made contact. The patient may be notably restless and frightened. In addition, generalized symptoms commonly occur with fever and muscle cramps. Shocklike symptoms have also been reported. Within several hours or days, local desquamation may develop. Lymphadenopathy has been described.

Treatment should begin with immediate removal of broken-off spines by placing cellophane tape over the sting site. Calcium gluconate, 10 mL of a 10% solution, intravenously, is effective in relieving pain in severe cases, while tripelennamine usually brings relief in milder cases. Generalized symptoms are treated symptomatically.

## BLISTER BEETLE STINGS

Blister beetles are found most frequently in the western section of the United States. When disturbed, they exude a vesicating agent, cantharidin, which can penetrate the epidermis to produce irritation and blistering within a few hours of contact. If ingested, cantharidin can produce intense gastrointestinal disturbances with symptoms of nausea, vomiting, diarrhea, and abdominal cramps. Initial contact with the beetle produces a burning, tingling sensation and a mild rash. Within a few hours, flaccid, elongated vesicles and bullae develop.

## Treatment

Treatment consists of protecting the bullae from trauma by an occlusive dressing. Large bullae should be drained and an antibiotic ointment applied. If bullae occur on the feet, the patient should be advised to stay off the feet and wet dressings should be applied for 24 to 48 h.

## BIBLIOGRAPHY

Clark RF, Wethern-Kestner S, Vance MV, Gerkin R: Clinical presentation and treatment of black widow spider envenomation: A review of 163 cases. *Ann Emerg Med* 21(7):782, 1992.

DeShazo RD, Butcher BT, Banks WA: Reactions to the stings of the imported fire ant. *N Engl J Med* 323(7):462, 1990.

Grendron BP: *Loxosceles reclusa* envenomation. *Am J Emerg Med* 8(1):51, 1990.

Rees RS, Campbell DS: Spider bites, in Auerbach P, Geehr EC (eds): *Management of Wilderness and Environmental Emergencies.* Chicago, Year Book, 1988, pp 543–547.

Reisman RE: Current concepts: Insect stings. *N Engl J Med* 331(8):523, 1994.

Reisman RE: Natural history of insect sting allergy: Relationship of severity of symptoms of initial sting anaphylaxis to re-sting reactions. *J Allergy Clin Immunol* 90:335, 1992.

Sinkinson CA, Graft DF, McLean D: Individualizing therapy for Hymenoptera stings. *American Health Consultants,* ER Reports, July 1990, vol 11, no 14.

Valentine MD, Lichtenstein LM: Anaphylaxis and stinging insect hypersensitivity. *JAMA* 258:2881, 1987.

Valentine MD, Schuberth KC, Kagey-Sobotka A, et al: The value of immunotherapy with venom in children with allergy to insect stings. *N Engl J Med* 323:1601, 1991.

# 163
# REPTILE BITES AND SCORPION STINGS

### Richard C. Dart
### Hernan F. Gomez

## RATTLESNAKE BITES

Approximately 19 of the 115 snake species in the United States are venomous. Snakes inflict about 45,000 bites each year in the United States, of which 8000 are inflicted by venomous snakes. Most bites occur in the warm summer months, when snakes and victims are most active. In the past, it was estimated that mortality from venomous snakebite approached 25 percent. Due to the availability of antivenin and advances in emergency and critical care, mortality rates today are below 0.5 percent. Approximately 10 deaths occur per year.

Except for bites by imported species, North American venomous snakebite involves the pit vipers (Crotalidae family) or coral snakes (Elapidae family). The crotalids are represented by the rattlesnakes (*Crotalus* species), pygmy rattlesnakes and massasauga (*Sistrurus* species), and the copperheads and water moccasins (*Agkistrodon* species).

Poisonous snakebites from imported exotic species are infrequent but may occur in zoo personnel as well as in amateur herpetologists. A regional poison center may be able to provide information on snake identification, expected toxicity, and antivenin location. The Antivenin Index, a list of exotic snake antivenins available in the United States, can be accessed by calling (602) 626-6016.

The crotalid snakes are called pit vipers because of bilateral depressions or pits located midway between and below the level of the eye and the nostril (Fig. 163-1). The pit is a heat receptor that guides strikes against warm-blooded prey or predators. Crotalid snakes are also distinguished by two fangs, which can be folded against the roof of the mouth, in contrast to the coral snakes, which have shorter, fixed, and erect fangs. Within the pit vipers, the rattle distinguishes the rattlesnake from other crotalids. The mistaken belief that rattlesnakes always rattle before striking has persisted for centuries. In truth, many strikes occur without a warning rattle.

## Pathophysiology

Crotalid venom is a complex enzyme mixture that causes local tissue injury, systemic vascular damage, hemolysis, fibrinolysis, and neuromuscular dysfunction, resulting in a combination of local and systemic effects. Venom proteins range in molecular weight from less than 6000 to over 100,000. Crotalid venom quickly alters blood vessel permeability, leading to loss of plasma and blood into the surrounding tissue. It also consumes fibrinogen and platelets, causing a coagulopathy. In some species, specific venom fractions block neuromuscular transmission leading to ptosis, respiratory failure, and other neurologic effects.

## Clinical Features

Up to 25 percent of crotalid snakebites are termed dry: venom effects do not develop. The manifestations of crotalid venom poisoning are a complex interaction of the venom and the prey. The species and size of the snake, the age and size of the victim, the time elapsed since the bite, and characteristics of the bite (location, depth, and number, the amount of venom injected) all affect the clinical appearance. The severity of poisoning following a crotalid bite is therefore variable. Crotalid bites are generally classified as *minimal, moderate,* or *severe* depending on the degree of local and systemic injury (Table 163-1). An initially minimal bite may evolve into a moderate or severe bite and require large amounts of antivenin.

The cardinal manifestations of crotalid venom poisoning are the presence of one or more fang marks, localized pain, and progressive edema extending from the bite site. Other early symptoms and signs of rattlesnake venom poisoning are nausea and vomiting, weakness, oral numbness or tingling of tongue and mouth, tachycardia, dizziness, hematemesis, hematuria, thrombocytopenia, and fasciculation. In general, swelling becomes apparent within 15 to 30 min, but in some cases may not start for several hours. In severe cases edema may progress to involve an entire limb within an hour. In less severe cases, edema may progress over a 1- to 2-day period. Edema near an airway or in a muscle compartment may threaten life or limb without the presence of systemic effects.

Progressive ecchymosis may also occur because of leakage of blood into subcutaneous tissue. Ecchymoses may appear within minutes or hours in the area of the snakebite. Hemorrhagic blebs may occur within several hours for similar reasons. Hemoconcentration may initially be present as a result of fluid loss into subcutaneous tissue, followed by a decrease in hemoglobin over several days from blood loss secondary to coagulopathy.

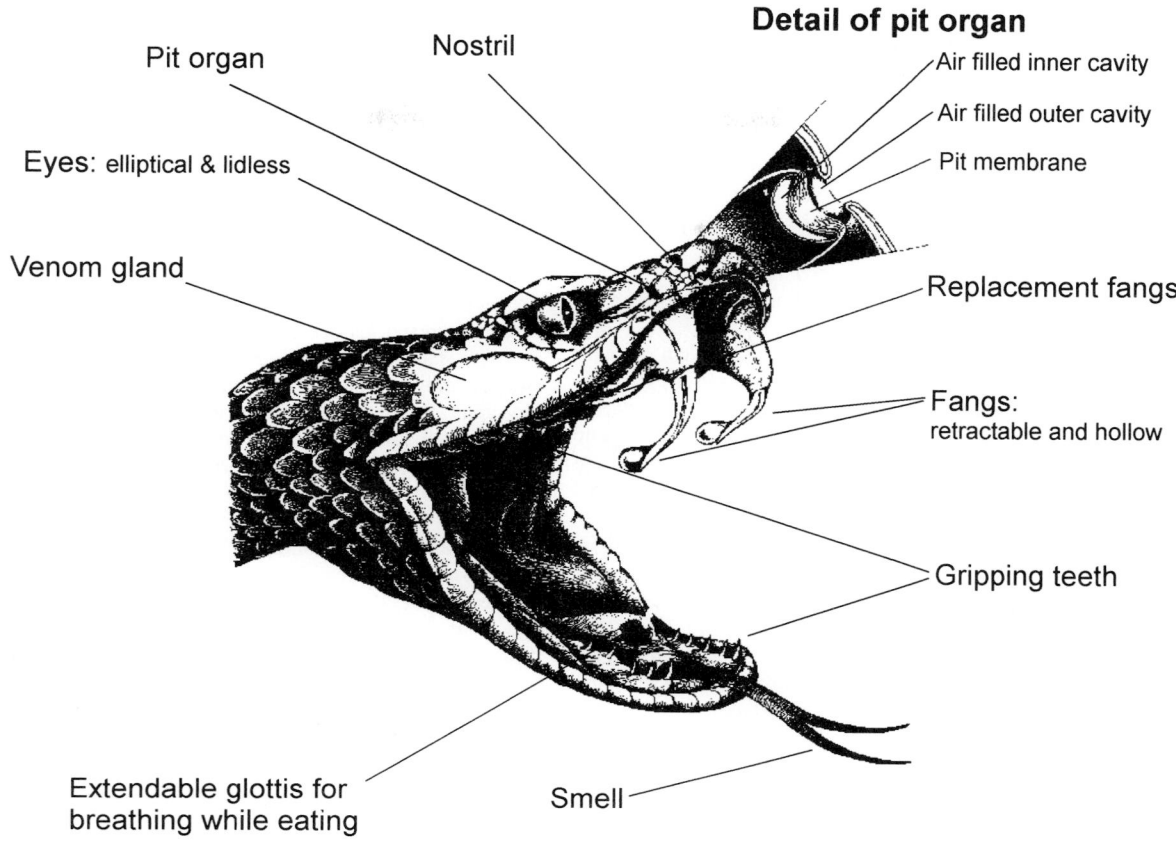

**Detail of pit organ**

Air filled inner cavity

Air filled outer cavity

Pit membrane

Pit organ

Nostril

Eyes: elliptical & lidless

Venom gland

Replacement fangs

Fangs:
retractable and hollow

Gripping teeth

Extendable glottis for
breathing while eating

Smell

**Fig. 163-1.** Anatomy of a rattlesnake.

**Table 163-1.** Grading of Envenomation by Crotalid Snakes

**Minimal Envenomation**

*Swelling, erythema, or ecchymosis* limited to immediate area of the bite site.

*Systemic signs and symptoms* not present or minimal.

*Coagulation parameters* all normal. No other significant laboratory abnormalities.

**Moderate Envenomation**

*Swelling, erythema, or ecchymosis* present, may involve most of an extremity, and may be spreading slowly.

*Systemic signs and symptoms* present, but not life-threatening. These may include nausea, vomiting, oral paresthesia or unusual tastes, mild hypotension (systolic blood pressure > 80 mm Hg), mild tachycardia, and tachypnea.

*Coagulation parameters* may be abnormal, but no clinically significant bleeding is present. Severe abnormalities of other laboratory tests are not present.

**Severe Envenomation**

*Swelling or ecchymosis* involve the entire extremity and are spreading rapidly.

*Systemic signs and symptoms* are markedly abnormal, including severe alteration of mental status, nausea and vomiting, hypotension (systemic blood pressure < 80 mm Hg), severe tachycardia, tachypnea, or other respiratory compromise.

*Coagulation parameters* abnormal with serious bleeding present or threat of spontaneous bleeding, including prothrombin time unmeasurable, partial thromboplastin time unmeasurable, platelets < 20,000/μL, or fibrinogen undetectable. Severe abnormalities of other laboratory values should also be considered severe envenomations.

## Diagnosis

Diagnosis is based on the presence of a clinical syndrome consistent with envenomation combined with corroborating laboratory studies. Laboratory evaluation should include a complete blood count and platelet count, coagulation tests (including prothrombin time and fibrinogen level), electrolytes, renal function tests, and urinalysis. In patients with severe or rapidly worsening envenomation, type and crossmatch, arterial blood gas, and an electrocardiogram should be added and all studies performed serially until the patient is improving.

## Treatment

### First Aid

First aid measures should never substitute for definitive medical care nor delay the administration of antivenin. All patients bitten by a pit viper should be taken to a health care facility. Table 163-2 lists one prudent approach to first aid. Several first aid products are marketed. The Cutter Snakebite Kit should not be used because it contains cups that produce little suction and seal poorly on digits. The blade in the kit or any method of incision can injure digital nerves, arteries, and tendons; incision is not recommended. The Sawyer Extractor Vacuum Pump, removes venom without incision, producing up to 750 mm Hg of suction over a puncture site. The usefulness of this device is unknown although it has been shown to remove some venom in one animal study. Other useless or dangerous techniques are electric shock and ice. Electric shock treatment of the bite site is mentioned

**Table 163-2.** Recommended First Aid Measures

| |
|---|
| Retreat well beyond striking range. Many victims are bitten repeatedly while trying to capture the snake. |
| Remain calm. Movement will increase venom absorption. |
| Immobilize the extremity in a neutral position below the level of the heart. |
| Keep physical activity minimal. |
| Promptly transport victim to medical facility regardless of whether overt signs of envenomation are quickly apparent. Signs and symptoms of snakebite may be delayed. |

only to be condemned. This dangerous procedure is not effective and has resulted in electrical injuries. Ice water immersion worsens the injury.

Constriction bands may be of some use, especially when immediate medical care is not available. In theory, a constriction band retards venom absorption. This should increase local tissue injury, but reduce the severity of systemic effects. Anecdotal human reports and animal studies suggest that constriction band use delays venom absorption without causing increased swelling. Additional controlled studies are needed to better define the clinical indications for constriction band use. If used, the band should restrict only superficial venous and lymphatic flow.

## Emergency

In the prehospital phase, personnel should be directed to immobilize the limb, establish intravenous access in another limb, administer oxygen, and transport the victim to a medical facility. Previously placed tourniquets and constriction bands should not be removed until intravenous access is established.

As in any emergency, initial snakebite management should include advanced cardiac life support. If the patient is hypotensive, initial treatment should include rapid intravenous isotonic fluid infusion. Other supportive care measures should include limb immobilization to reduce further venom absorption. Consultation with a physician or poison center familiar with the management of snake envenomation is recommended for all but the simplest of cases.

Antivenin (Crotalidae) Polyvalent is the mainstay of therapy for poisonous snakebite. All crotalid bites that show evidence of progressive signs and symptoms should immediately receive the antivenin. Progression is defined as worsening of local injury (e.g., pain, ecchymosis, or swelling), laboratory abnormalities (e.g., worsening platelet count, clotting times, or other tests), or systemic manifestations (e.g., unstable vital signs or abnormal mental status).

Because Antivenin (Crotalidae) Polyvalent is derived from horse serum, it is common for patients to develop an allergic reaction during infusion. An intradermal skin test should be applied before antivenin is given, but only when a definite decision to administer the antivenin has been made. This is to prevent unnecessary sensitization. A positive test (wheal or erythema > 10 mm in diameter) indicates that the patient may develop an allergic reaction, whereas a negative result usually indicates that the patient will tolerate the infusion. Some patients with negative skin tests will develop acute allergic reactions, and likewise, some patients with positive skin tests tolerate antivenin infusion without difficulty. The skin test is a guide and antivenin decisions should be based on a risk-benefit analysis of the patient's condition. To prevent a delay while waiting for the skin test results, the antivenin should be mixed simultaneously with placement of the skin test. Because the antivenin takes 20 to 30 min to enter solution, it will be ready when the skin test is interpreted.

The recommended dose of antivenin has increased over the years. The use of at least 10 vials is recommended as the initial dose in rattlesnake bites. In rapidly progressive envenomations or hemodynamically unstable cases, an initial dose of at least 20 vials of antivenin is recommended in addition to aggressive supportive care. Poisoning by water moccasins usually requires lesser doses, whereas in copperhead bites, antivenin is often not required, except for children and the el-

derly. Under no circumstances should antivenin be injected directly into finger or toes. Intramuscular injection is also not recommended because venom-induced hypovolemia may retard absorption of antivenin. Hospital pharmacies in those regions of the United States where poisonous snakes are prevalent should maintain adequate stocks of antivenin. Unfortunately, many hospitals stock insufficient amounts of antivenin, even in endemic areas.

The package insert may be used as a guide for antivenin preparation. Antivenin should only administered in a critical care facility such as the emergency department or intensive care unit. After reconstitution, the antivenin should be diluted in 250 to 500 mL of crystalloid and infused slowly, until it is evident that anaphylaxis will not occur. If a reaction does not develop, the rate should be increased in a stepwise manner until the infusion is complete, usually in 1 h. Infusion of antivenin should be done under the direct supervision of a physician. If an acute allergic reaction occurs, the infusion should be stopped immediately and antihistamines administered (both $H_1$- and $H_2$-receptor blockade). Epinephrine should be added depending on the severity of the reaction.

The end point of antivenin therapy is arrest of progression or improvement of clinical findings. One infusion of 10 to 20 vials is often sufficient. It is extremely important, however, that observation for progression of edema and systemic signs of envenomation be continued even after antivenin infusion. Limb circumference should be measured at several sites above and below the bite, and the advancing border of edema should be outlined with a pen every 30 to 60 min. This serves as an index of the progression as well as a guide for antivenin administration. Laboratory determinations are repeated q4h or after each course of antivenin therapy, whichever is more frequent. Additional antivenin therapy may be warranted if the patient's condition worsens.

The value of aggressive supportive care cannot be overemphasized. Isotonic fluid resuscitation followed by pressor agents is appropriate for hypotension. Antivenin is the best treatment for coagulopathy, but if active bleeding occurs, blood component replacement may be necessary. Another complication of snakebite is compartment syndrome. Increased compartment pressure may occur when venom is injected into a compartment during a bite. This is usually manifested by severe pain, localized to a compartment, that is resistant to narcotics. The use of fasciotomy is controversial. Recommended management is shown in Table 163-3.

The wound area should be cleaned and the need for tetanus booster determined. Cultures and antibiotic therapy should be initiated only if signs of infection are present. Although recommended by some authors, no objective evidence supports the use of prophylactic antibi-

**Table 163-3.** Management of Compartment Syndrome

1. Determine intracompartmental pressure.
2. If not elevated, continue standard management.
3. If signs of compartment syndrome are present and compartment pressure is > 30 mm Hg:
   Elevate limb.
   Administer mannitol 1–2 g/kg IV over 30 min.
   Simultaneously administer *additional* Antivenin (Crotalidae) Polyvalent, 10 to 15 vials IV over 60 min.
   if elevated compartment pressure persists another 60 min, consider fasciotomy.

*Notes:*

1. Elevated compartment pressure is caused by the action of the venom on the tissues, and thus, the most effective treatment is to neutralize the venom, which may reduce the compartment pressure.

2. This protocol delivers a high osmotic load and should not be used when contraindicated. The protocol must be completed promptly so that, if ever needed, fasciotomy may be performed as early as possible.

otics. The use of steroids is also controversial. Several studies suggest lack of efficacy or even deleterious effects. Without evidence of efficacy, steroids should be reserved for the treatment of allergic reactions or the treatment of serum sickness.

Patients are ready for discharge when swelling begins to resolve, the coagulopathy has been reversed, and the patient is ambulatory. During recovery, the bitten part (particularly the hand) should be regularly exercised to preserve as much function and strength as possible. Outpatient follow-up is necessary to monitor for infection and serum sickness.

### Admission

It cannot be overemphasized that one can easily be deceived by a bite that initially appears innocuous. An unremarkable physical and laboratory examination at presentation does not reliably indicate an insignificant envenomation. We recommended that physicians observe patients for at least 8 h. Patients with severe or life-threatening bites and patients receiving antivenin should be admitted to an intensive care unit. The general ward is appropriate for patients with mild or moderate envenomations who have completed or do not require further antivenin therapy.

### Outpatient

Patients with dry bites that have been observed for at least 8 h may be discharged. They should return if pain, swelling, or bleeding develops.

## CORAL SNAKE BITE

North American coral snakes include the eastern coral snake (*Micrurus fulvius fulvius*), the Texas coral snake (*Micrurus fulvius tenere*), and the Arizona (Sonoran) coral snake (*Micruroides euryxanthus*). The eastern coral snake is found primarily in the southeast United States. The Texas and Arizona coral snakes are found primarily in the states that bear their names. Coral snakes account for 20 to 25 bites a year.

All coral snakes are brightly colored with black, red, and yellow rings. The red and yellow rings touch in coral snakes, but they are separated by black rings in nonpoisonous snakes, creating the well known rhyme: "Red on yellow, kill a fellow; red on black, venom lack." This rule is *not* true outside of the United States.

Coral snake venom is primarily composed of neurotoxic components that do not cause marked local injury. Elapid bites produce primarily neurologic effects: tremors, salivation, dysarthria, diplopia, bulbar paralysis with ptosis, fixed and contracted pupils, dysphagia, dyspnea, and seizures. The immediate cause of death is paralysis of respiratory muscles. Signs and symptoms may be delayed up to 12 h.

The potential coral snake victim should be admitted to the hospital for 24 to 48 h of observation. Coral snake venom effects may develop hours after a bite and are not easily reversed. It is suggested that 3 vials of the Antivenin (*Micrurus fulvius*) be administered to patients who have definitely been bitten because it may not be possible to prevent further effects or reverse effects that have already developed. Additional coral snake antivenin is reserved for the appearance of symptoms or signs of coral snake envenomation. However, because respiratory failure may result from clinical effects of the neurotoxin, baseline and serial pulmonary function parameters (such as inspiratory pressure and vital capacity) in addition to intensive care observation may be useful. Prolonged ventilatory support may be required in severe cases. The patient must be observed closely for signs of respiratory muscle weakness and hypoventilation. Bites by the Sonoran coral snake are mild. Medical care is not usually needed.

## GILA MONSTER BITE

Gila monsters are slow-moving lizards that inhabit the desert in the southwestern United States. They possess a venom as potent as rat-tlesnake venom but lack the apparatus to effectively inject it. Instead of fangs, they simply have short, grooved teeth down which their venom flows. Therefore, envenomation requires a prolonged bite. Gila monsters bite tenaciously and may be difficult to remove from the bitten extremity.

Most bites result in local pain and swelling only, which worsens over several hours and then subsides over several more hours. Dislodged teeth often contaminate the wound. Occasionally, a more severe syndrome of systemic toxicity develops, including weakness, light-headedness, paresthesia, and diaphoresis. Severe hypertension may occur, which also resolves over several hours. There are few, if any, documented deaths from gila monster bite.

First aid involves removal of the reptile from the bite site without sustaining another bite. This may require force. It helps to place the animal on a solid surface; like other animals, it will often loosen its grip when it is no longer suspended in midair. Otherwise, standard local wound care is sufficient, taking care to remove any teeth in the wound. The usefulness of prophylactic antibiotics is unknown and tetanus status should be determined.

## SCORPION STING

Although there are several species of scorpions in the United States, only the bark scorpion (*Centruroides exilicauda*) produces effects other than local pain. *C. exilicauda* is found in Arizona and adjacent regions of California, Nevada, and Texas. Children are common victims while playing outside or sleeping.

Scorpion venom contains components that activate sodium channels. These components produce sympathetic, parasympathetic, and somatic nerve discharge. This is manifested by immediate burning and tingling at the site although no local injury is apparent. The local effect may persist or it may subside briefly to be replaced over minutes to hours by generalized pain and paresthesia. Autonomic effects include tachycardia and excessive secretions. Motor nerve effects include the pathognomonic roving eye movements, opisthotonus, fasciculation, and difficulty swallowing. Death is rare. When it occurs, it is probably due to the combination of secretions, difficulty swallowing, and respiratory compromise.

Diagnosis is clinical. Initially it can be confused with anything that causes local pain, especially in children. As the syndrome progresses the diagnosis becomes apparent. Airway management is the mainstay of therapy. Patients with minimal to moderate effects can be treated symptomatically with oral or parenteral analgesics or sedation. Severe cases should receive the antivenin produced by Arizona State University. It is an unlicensed, goat serum-derived antivenin available within Arizona only. Like all partially purified animal serum products, allergic reactions occur regularly and therefore it should be used only in severe cases. The patient should be skin tested first, while the antivenin is reconstituted. One to 2 vials is sufficient to reverse effects.

## BIBLIOGRAPHY

Banner WB Jr. Scorpion envenomation. In: Auerbach PS, Geehr EC (eds). *Management of Wilderness and Environmental Emergencies,* 2nd ed. St. Louis: CV Mosby, pp. 603–616, 1989.

Dart RC, McNally DW, Spaite DW, Gustafson R. The sequelae of pitviper poisoning in the United States. In: Campbell JA, Brodie, ED Jr (eds). *Biology of the Pitvipers.* Arlington, TX: Selva Publishing, pp. 395–403, 1992.

Kitchens CS, Van Mierop LHS. Envenomation by the eastern coral snake (*Micrurus fulvius fulvius*): a study of 39 victims. *JAMA* 258:1615, 1987.

Klauber LM. *Rattlesnakes: Their Habits, Life, Histories and Influence on Mankind,* 2nd ed. San Diego: University of California Press, Zoological Society of San Diego, vol. 2, 1972.

Russell FE. *Snake Venom Poisoning,* 3rd ed. Great Neck, NY: Scholium International, 1983.

# 164

# TRAUMA AND ENVENOMATIONS FROM MARINE FAUNA

## Daniel G. Guenin
## Paul S. Auerbach

Although noxious marine organisms are concentrated predominantly in warm temperatures and tropical seas, particularly in the Indo-Pacific region, dangerous marine animals may be found as far north as 50° N latitude. Because of increasing numbers of recreational divers and private salt water aquariums, as well as the ease of international travel, emergency physicians everywhere should be familiar with the hazards of the marine environment. Included among these dangers are injuries from traumatizing and envenoming animals. Exposure to these creatures may occur while walking on the beach, wading in tidal pools, deep-water diving, or simply changing the water in a home aquarium. The infections that may occur after marine trauma are also important.

## MARINE TRAUMA

The notoriety of the shark attack seems undeserved when the statistics are examined. Fewer than 100 attacks occur annually worldwide, with 10 or fewer fatalities. Of approximately 370 shark species, only 32 have been definitely implicated in human attacks—the majority by the tiger, great white, blue, mako, hammerhead, bull, and reef sharks. The shark attack zone includes the temperate and tropical waters between 42° N and 42° S latitudes with seasonal variations.

Two general attack behaviors have been described: feeding and agonistic. Feeding attacks appear to be the result of mistaking a human for a pinniped or more typical prey. These attacks often terminate as soon as the shark realizes the mistake. Agonistic attacks seem to be defensive or territorial-protective.

Shark attack wounds range from severe dermal abrasions (due to shark skin denticles) following a "bumping" to massive tissue loss with fractures and hemorrhage. This occurs from the razor sharp teeth on jaws brought together with an estimated force that approaches 18 tons per square inch. "Hit and run" attacks occur in the majority of instances, and 70 percent of victims are bitten only once or twice. The lower extremity is most frequently injured, followed by the upper extremity. Death is usually the result of hemorrhagic shock and drowning.

As with other resuscitative endeavors, the ABCs are fundamental, with special attention to hemorrhage control, volume resuscitation, and rewarming as needed. Tetanus toxoid and tetanus immune globulin should be administered. Prophylactic intravenous antibiotics are empirically recommended. Third-generation cephalosporins, trimethoprim-sulfamethoxazole, chloramphenicol, ciprofloxacin, or an aminoglycoside may be given. Meticulous wound care is most appropriately performed in the operating room for adequate surgical exploration, irrigation, and debridement of wounds. Wounds should be packed open for delayed primary closure or closed around drainage systems.

It has been suggested that most shark attacks could be prevented if a few precautionary measures were taken: (1) avoid swimming in river mouths, low-visibility waters, or shark-infested waters; (2) avoid wearing bright or shiny clothing, jewelry, or equipment; (3) avoid swimming with an open wound; and (4) obey beach authorities.

The great barracuda (*Sphyraena barracuda*) is the only barracuda species to be implicated in human attacks. Attacks are generally by solitary fish and occur only in tropical climes. Moray eels, found in tropical to temperate waters, can inflict severe puncture wounds, commonly to the hands of inquisitive divers. Other marine vertebrates known to cause traumatic injuries to humans include giant groupers, sea lions, seals, crocodiles, alligators, needlefish, wahoos, piranas, and triggerfish. Wounds resulting from interactions with these creatures are a combination of crush injury, abrasion, puncture, and laceration. Treatment of these injuries is analogous to that of shark bites, with an emphasis on irrigation, removal of foreign bodies (e.g., teeth), and leaving puncture wounds open.

Coral cuts are probably the most common injuries sustained underwater. The initial reaction to a coral cut is stinging pain, erythema, and pruritus, most commonly on the hands, forearms, elbows, and knees. A break in the skin may be surrounded by an erythematous wheal within minutes, which fades over 1 to 2 h. The local reaction of red, raised welts and local pruritus is called *coral poisoning*. With or without prompt treatment, this may progress to cellulitis with ulceration and tissue sloughing. The wounds heal slowly over 3 to 6 weeks. In extreme cases, the victim develops cellulitis with lymphangitis, reactive bursitis, local ulceration, and wound necrosis.

Coral cuts should be promptly and vigorously irrigated to remove all foreign matter. Any fragments that remain can become embedded and increase the risk for infection or foreign body granuloma. If stinging is a major symptom, there may be an element of envenomation by nematocysts. A brief rinse with dilute acetic acid (vinegar) may diminish the discomfort. If a coral-induced laceration is severe, it should be closed with adhesive strips rather than sutures if possible. Sharp debridement each day for 3 to 4 days is preferable.

## Bacteriology of the Marine Environment and Antibiotic Therapy

Ocean water provides a rich saline milieu for microbes. Although the greatest number and variety of bacteria are found near the ocean surface, diverse bacteria and fungi are found in marine silts, sediments, and sand. Microbes, including bacteria, microalgae, protozoa, yeasts, and viruses, are most abundant in areas with the greatest number of life forms. Marine bacteria are generally gram-negative rods. Bacteria isolated from the marine environment or from marine-acquired wounds of greatest concern to humans include: *Aeromonas hydrophila, Bacteroides fragilis, Chromobacterium violaceum, Clostridium perfringens, Erysipelothrix rhusopathiae, Escherichia coli, Mycobacterium marinum, Pseudomonas aeruginosa, Salmonella enteritidis, Staphylococcus aureus, Streptococcus* species, and *Vibrio* species.

There is no substitute for meticulous wound care, including irrigation and debridement of devitalized tissue with particular attention to retained foreign bodies such as teeth, vegetable matter, and spines. Quantitative wound culture prior to the appearance of clincially evident wound infection has not been shown to be useful. The issue of prophylactic antibiotics in the treatment of marine wounds has not been well studied. Pending a prospective study of prophylactic antibiotics in this setting, the following recommendations are generally advised and are based on the morbidity of soft tissue infections caused by *Vibrio* species:

1. Minor abrasions and lacerations of the normal, immunocompetent patient do not require prophylactic antibiotics.
2. Minor abrasions and lacerations of the immunocompromised or chronically ill patient require initiation of therapy with trimethoprim-sulfamethoxasole, tetracycline, cefuroxime axetil, or ciprofloxacin.
3. High-risk wounds (e.g., extensive lacerations or burns; deep puncture wounds, particularly involving the joint space; or grossly contaminated wounds) require initiation of parenteral trimetho-

prim-sulfamethoxasole, a third-generation cephalosporin, an aminoglycoside, or chloramphenicol, or one of the oral agents mentioned above.

The objectives for the management of infections from marine microorganisms are to recognize the clinical condition, culture the organism, and provide antimicrobial therapy. The appearance of an infection indicates the need for prompt debridement and search for a retained foreign body. Infected wounds should be cultured for aerobes and anaerobes. Since special media may be necessary for culture and sensitivity testing, the clinician should alert the microbiology laboratory that a marine-acquired organism may be present. Empirical antibiotic therapy should be initiated based on the clinical condition.

Management of marine-acquired infections must include coverage against *Vibrio* species with a third-generation cephalosporin, trimethoprim-sulfamethoxasole, tetracycline, ciprofloxacin, or cefuroxime. Fresh-water infections may be treated with the above agents, in addition to imipenem or an aminoglycoside, to cover *Aeromonas* species. Appropriate antibiotic coverage against staphylococcal and streptococcal species is mandatory since they remain the most common infecting organisms. Imipenem-cilastatin is reserved for established wound infections and/or sepsis.

Several special clinical conditions are of note. A patient with a rapidly progressive cellulitis, myositis, or necrotizing fasciitis warrants consideration of *V. parahaemolyticus* or *V. vulnificus* infection. *V. vulnificus* can also cause a primary septicemia in chronically ill individuals, particularly those with hepatic disease. Mortality in these patients approaches 60 percent. *E. rhusopathiae* is the infectious agent in "fish-handler's disease" and causes sharply marginated, painful, expanding plaques on the fingers or hands following cutaneous inoculation. It responds to penicillin, cephalexin, or erythromycin. *M. marinum* is an acid-fast bacillus that causes "swimming pool granuloma" or "aquarium granuloma." Some 3 to 4 weeks following an abrasion or puncture wound, the patient develops a red papule, which progresses to a cutaneous granuloma. Excision or antibiotics (minocycline, trimethoprim-sulfamethoxasole, rifampin, or ethambutol) are the treatments of choice, although spontaneous resolution typically occurs over 2 to 3 years. *A. hydrophila* is a gram-negative bacteria found in marine and fresh-water environments; it causes wound infections that can rapidly become cellulitic and progress to necrotizing myositis.

## MARINE ENVENOMATIONS

Marine venoms are large-molecular-weight compounds of vasoactive and proteolytic enzymes with diffuse effects on the circulatory, neurologic, immunologic, and respiratory systems. They require a specialized delivery system, are commonly heat and gastric acid labile, show nonseasonal toxicity, and can be released in varying amounts. Conversely, poisons are usually metabolic byproducts of lower molecular weight. They are ingested (thereby requiring no delivery system), are usually heat and gastric acid stable, and carry some seasonal toxicity.

Venoms are produced in specialized glands and are broadly classified as parenteral toxins, which are injected mechanically, or crinotoxins, which are delivered topically as slimes—mucous or gastric secretions. Practically, venoms are used offensively or defensively. An offensive venom is employed to kill prey and is typically located near the mouth or on the tentacles. Defensive venoms are used to protect the animal and are usually located near the tail. A human's reaction to an envenomation can be allergic or toxic.

## INVERTEBRATE ENVENOMATIONS

Envenoming invertebrates are found in five phyla: Cnidaria (Coelenterates), Porifera, Echinodermata, Mollusca, and Annelida.

## Cnidaria (Coelenterates)

The phylum Cnidaria is an enormous group of approximately 9000 species, at least 100 of which are dangerous to humans. The phylum contains three classes: Hydrozoa, Scyphozoa, and Anthozoa. Cnidariae, from *cnid,* the stem of the Greek word "nettle," are known for their specialized venom-containing stinging cells called cnidocytes. The cnidocytes are located near the mouth or on the outer surfaces of tentacles. A physical or chemical stimulus causes the release of a hollow, sharply pointed threadlike tube from the contained nematocyst. This tube penetrates the victim's skin, allowing injection of the viscous venom with diffusion into the general circulation. Detached, moistened tentacles carry live nematocysts capable of discharging for months. Air-dried nematocysts may retain considerable potency for weeks.

The class Hydrozoa includes the hydroids, milleporina (fire corals), and siphonophores (Portuguese man-of-war and bluebottle jellyfish). Hydroids are the most numerous of the hydrozoans. The feather hydroids are plumelike animals that sting the victim who brushes against or handles them. Coastal storms can break off feather hydroid branches and infest a local swimming area.

Contact with the nematocysts of a feather hydroid induces a mild reaction, which consists of instantaneous burning, itching, and urticaria. If the exposure is brief, the skin rash may not be noticeable or may consist of a faintly erythematous morbilliform eruption. A second variety of envenomation consists of a delayed papular, hemorrhagic, or zosteriform reaction occurring 4 to 12 h after contact. Rarely, erythema multiforme or a desquamative eruption may develop. Systemic manifestations are rarely reported.

The *Millepora* species, or fire corals, are not true corals. The fire coral *M. alcicornis* probably accounts for the majority of coelenterate envenomations. They are widely distributed in shallow tropical waters and often mistaken for seaweed. Tiny nematocyst-bearing tentacles protrude from numerous minute surface gastropores. Immediately following contact with fire coral, the victim notices burning or stinging pain, with rare proximal radiation. Over the course of 5 to 30 min, pruritic urticarial lesions develop. The pain generally resolves without treatment in 30 to 90 min. In the case of multiple stings, regional lymph nodes may become inflamed. Skin lesions resolve over 3 to 7 days, occasionally resulting in postinflammatory hyperpigmentation, which may take months to disappear.

The Atlantic Portuguese man-of-war (*Physalia physalis*) inhabits the surface of the ocean. It is constructed of a floating sail (pneumatophore) from which are suspended multiple nematocyst-bearing tentacles, measuring up to 30 m in length. The smaller Pacific bluebottle (*Physalia utriculus*) usually has a single fishing tentacle that attains lengths of up to 15 m. Each tentacle in a larger specimen may carry more than 750,000 nematocysts. Nematocysts from fractured tentacles may remain active for months. The most common reaction from contact is an immediate, toxic, dermal reaction with linearly arranged urticarial lesions. Respiratory distress and death have been reported following *P. physalis* envenomation.

The class Scyphozoa, or jellyfish, includes the Indo-Pacific box jellyfish (*Chironex fleckeri*), the sea nettle (*Chrysaora quinquecirrha*), and the thimble jellyfish (*Linuche unguiculata*). The Indo-Pacific chirodropids are armed with some of the most potent venoms in existence. The extreme example of envenomation occurs with the Indo-Pacific box jellyfish. Found along the northern coast of Australia, *C. fleckeri* has killed at least 65 people in the past century. Death is attributed to hypotension, profound muscle spasm, muscular and respiratory paralysis, and subsequent cardiac arrest. The overall mortality following box jellyfish stings approaches 15 to 20 percent. Most stings are minor, although severe reactions or death can follow skin contact with tentacles in excess of 6 to 7 m. The sting is instantly and intensely painful, and the victim may struggle purposefully for only a minute or two prior to collapse. The toxic skin reaction may be quite intense, with rapid formation of wheals, vesicles, and a darkened reddish-brown or purple whiplike flare pattern with stripes of 8 to 10 mm in width. Major stings show skin blistering within 6 h, with superficial necrosis in 12 to 18 h. On occasion, a pathognomonic "frosted" appearance with a transverse cross-hatched pattern may be present.

Sea nettles (*Chrysaora* and *Cyanea* species) are found in tropical and temperate waters, particularly the Chesapeake Bay, and are far less dangerous. Sea nettle envenomation presents similarly to that from *Physalia* species.

Seabather's eruption, commonly misnomered "sea lice," refers to a pruritic dermatitis that is vesicular or morbilliform. It occurs a few minutes to 12 h after salt water exposure. The eruption primarily involves skin surfaces covered by bathing suits, swim caps, or fins. Dermatitis persists for 2 to 14 days and resolves spontaneously. Other symptoms include headache, chills, pronounced nocturnal pruritus, malaise, conjunctivitis, and urethritis. The 0.5-mm larval form of the thimble jellyfish *Linuche unguiculata* has been recently identified as the cause of outbreaks in southern Florida and the Caribbean. The planula form of the sea anemone *Edwardsiella lineata* has been implicated in outbreaks off the coast of Long Island, New York.

The class Anthozoa includes the sea anemones, stony (true) corals, and the soft corals. Anemones are attractive creatures often found in tidal pools, where the unwary may brush up against them or inquisitively touch them. Like other coelenterates, they possess tentacles loaded with nematocysts. The dermatitis resulting from contact is identical to that produced by fire coral. If the envenomation is severe, hemorrhagic bullae with necrosis and ulceration may occur.

Due to considerable phylogenetic resemblance among Cnidaria species, the clinical features of Cnidaria envenomation are similar across a wide spectrum of severity. The toxicity of envenomation depends on the venom dose, the marine species, and the victim. Mild envenomation results in bothersome dermatitides that resolve spontaneously over 1 to 2 weeks, with occasional postinflammatory hyperpigmentation. Anemones, *Physalia* species, and scyphozoans may cause moderate to severe envenomations compounded by systemic symptoms. These symptoms may appear immediately or within several hours.

Therapy is directed at securing the ABCs, detoxifying the venom, and providing symptomatic and pain relief. Nematocysts still attached to the patient need to be deactivated and removed to prevent continued envenomation. All victims with systemic signs or symptoms should be observed for at least 8 h, as rebound of symptoms can occur. *Chironex fleckeri* produces the only venom for which there is a specific antidote. While the venoms are heat labile, this does not appear to be of clinical significance, and hot water immersion is not recommended.

Deactivation of attached nematocysts is important but controversial, due to locale-dependent variations in therapy. A generally accepted method is to start with salt (not fresh) water rinsing and removing obvious tentacles with forceps or a protected hand. Acetic acid 5% (vinegar) is the treatment of choice to inactivate most venoms. An alternative therapy is isopropyl alcohol (40 to 70%). For *Chrysaora* or *Cyanea,* a slurry of baking soda (sodium bicarbonate) is effective. The detoxicant should be applied continuously for at least 30 min or until there is no further pain. Once the nematocysts have been inactivated, the easiest way to remove them is to apply shaving cream or a paste of baking soda, flour, or talc and then shave the area with a razor or similar instrument. Topical anesthetics, antihistamines, or steroids may be of benefit. Corneal envenomations can be irrigated with an isotonic solution and treated judiciously with topical steroids. Prophylactic antibiotics are not needed, but standard antitetanus prophylaxis and diligent wound care should be carried out.

In general, only severe *Physalia* and box jellyfish stings will result in rapid decompensation. Other than the usual resuscitative measures and the *Chironex* antivenin, only systemic steroids and verapamil

have been suggested to have any therapeutic promise. Pain can be excruciating and requires narcotic analgesia.

## Porifera

The phylum *Porifera* contains approximately 4000 species of sponges which are composed of horny but elastic skeletons. Embedded in the connective tissue matrices are spicules of silicon dioxide or calcium carbonate. Secondary coelenterate inhabitants are responsible for the dermatitis and local necrotic skin reaction termed *sponge diver's disease.* A number of sponges produce crinotoxins that may be direct dermal irritants.

Two general syndromes are induced by contact with sponges. The first is a pruritic dermatitis similar to plant-induced allergic dermatitis. Within a few hours after skin contact, itching and burning develop, which may then progress to local joint swelling and stiffness, soft tissue edema, and vesiculation, particularly if small pieces of broken sponge are retained in the skin near the interphalangeal or metacarpophalangeal joints. The skin may become mottled or purpuric. Untreated mild reactions will subside within 3 to 7 days. With large surface area exposure, the victim may complain of fever, chills, malaise, dizziness, nausea, and muscle cramps. Bullae may become purulent. Erythema multiforme or an anaphylactoid reaction may develop 1 to 2 weeks after a severe exposure.

The second syndrome is an irritant dermatitis and follows the penetration of small spicules of silica or calcium carbonate into the skin. Crinotoxins enter microtraumatic lesions caused by the spicules. In severe cases, superficial desquamation of the skin may follow in 10 days to 2 months. There is no medical intervention that can prevent this process. Recurrent eczema and persistent arthralgias are rare complications.

Because it is usually impossible to distinguish clinically between the allergic and spicule-induced reactions, it is safest to treat for both. The skin should be gently dried. Spicules should be removed, if possible, using adhesive tape or a facial peel. Beginning as soon as possible, acetic acid 5% (vinegar) soaks should be applied for 10 to 30 min three to four times daily to affected areas. Isopropyl alcohol (40 to 70%) is a reasonable second choice. Although topical steroids may help to relieve the secondary inflammation, they are of no initial value. If steroids are applied before the vinegar soaks, they appear to worsen the primary reaction. Delayed primary therapy or inadequate decontamination may result in the persistence of bullae. Erythema multiforme may require supportive care including intravenous hydration, particularly if mucosal surfaces are involved, and topical steroids for symptomatic relief. The use of systemic steroids for erythema multiforme is controversial. If the allergic component is severe, systemic glucocorticoids (prednisone, 40 to 80 mg, tapered over 2 weeks) may be beneficial. Severe itching may be controlled with an antihistamine.

## Echinodermata

The phylum Echinodermata has five classes: sea lilies, brittle stars, starfish, sea urchins, and sea cucumbers. Only the last three are of emergency medical interest. The venom apparatuses of sea urchins consist of the sharp, brittle, and venom-filled spines and the triple-jawed globiferous pedicellariae. Venomous spines cause immediate and intense pain. Burning pain rapidly evolves into severe local muscle aching with erythema and swelling of the skin surrounding the puncture sites. Frequently, spines break off and lodge in the victim. If a spine enters a joint, it may rapidly induce severe synovitis. If multiple spines have penetrated the skin, particularly if deeply embedded, the victim may rapidly develop systemic symptoms, including nausea, vomiting, paresthesias, muscular paralysis, abdominal pain, syncope, hypotension, and respiratory distress. Pedicellariae can cause more severe symptoms, which are predominantly neurologic.

Starfish (Asteroidea) are covered with thorny spines that deliver a slimy venom produced in special glandular tissue. The crown-of-thorns sea star, *Acanthaster planci,* is a particularly venomous species. The sharp, rigid, and venomous aboral spines of this animal may grow to 4 to 6 cm. As the spines enter the skin, they carry venom into the wound, causing immediate pain, copious bleeding, and mild edema. The wound may become dusky or discolored. Multiple puncture wounds may result in acute systemic reactions, including paresthesias, nausea, vomiting, lymphadenopathy, and muscular paralysis.

Sea cucumbers (Holothuroidea) produce a toxin that is concentrated in the tentacular organs. Direct contact may induce a contact dermatitis, which is usually mild since the venom is diluted in sea water. The greater risk is to the corneae and conjunctivae, which may become intensely inflamed.

Treatment of echinoderm wounds consists of immediate immersion in hot water to tolerance [45°C (113° F)] for 30 to 90 min or until there is significant pain relief. Prompt removal of pedicellariae and spines, especially those in intraarticular areas, is necessary. Soft tissue radiographs or magnetic resonance imaging are helpful in locating retained spines. Treatment of systemic symptoms is supportive, and analgesia may be needed. Granuloma formation does occur and may require excision. Sea cucumbers dine on coelenterates and secrete the nematocyst venom; therefore, topical vinegar may provide some symptomatic relief.

## Annelida

The phylum Annelida contains the fireworms, or bristleworms, which are segmented worms covered with cactuslike bristles that can penetrate the skin. These bristles easily detach in the skin and can be difficult to remove. Envenomation causes intense inflammation with a burning sensation and erythema. Untreated, the pain generally resolves within a few hours, but erythema may last for 2 to 3 days. Bristles should be removed with forceps or adhesive tape, and topical vinegar or isopropyl alcohol may be applied.

## Mollusca

The phylum Mollusca contains two potentially envenoming classes: the gastropods (cone shells, nudibranchs) and the cephalopods (octopuses). Cone shells are beautiful, univalve creatures found in shallow Indo-Pacific waters. They are predators that feed by injecting a potent neurotoxin via detachable, dartlike, and radular teeth. Mild stings resemble Hymenoptera envenomations. More severe reactions include local, then generalized, paresthesias and muscular paralysis with ventilatory failure.

The Australian blue-ringed octopus also produces the neurotoxin tetrodotoxin. Octopus bites typically occur on the upper extremity and consist of two small puncture wounds. Local reactions are often absent, and generalized paresthesias may be the first indication of an envenomation. Further neurologic symptoms may develop, with flaccid paralysis and ensuing ventilatory failure. Treatment is supportive, with mechanical ventilation as needed, and full recovery is expected. No antivenin is available. Wide excision of the bite wound has been done to remove sequestered venom; however, there is no scientific evidence of speedier recovery to support this practice.

## VERTEBRATE ENVENOMATIONS

The stingrays are the most commonly incriminated group of fishes involved in human envenomations. The venom organ of stingrays consists of one to four venomous spines on the dorsum of a whiplike tail. When an unwary human handles, corners, or steps on a ray, the tail reflexively whips upward and accurately thrusts the spines into the victim, producing a puncture wound or jagged laceration in addition to an envenomation. On occasion, the entire spine tip is broken off and remains in the wound. Envenomation causes immediate local intense pain, edema, and variable bleeding. The pain, which may radiate centrally, peaks at 30 to 60 min and may last for up to 48 h. The wound is initially dusky or cyanotic and rapidly progresses to become erythematous and hemorrhagic, with fat and muscle involvement and possible necrosis. Systemic manifestations include weakness, nausea, vomiting, diarrhea, diaphoresis, vertigo, headache, syncope, seizures, muscle cramps, fasciculations, generalized edema (with truncal wounds), paralysis, hypotension, arrhythmias, and death.

Scorpionfish are distributed in tropical and, less commonly, temperate oceans and, unfortunately, in private aquariums. They can be grouped according to the severity of their envenomation in ascending order from the beautifully ornate lionfish (mild) to the camouflaged scorpionfish (moderate to severe) to the motionless stonefish (severe to life-threatening). The venom organs consist of 12 to 13 dorsal, 2 pelvic, and 3 anal spines, with associated venom glands. Although they are frequently large, plumelike, and ornate, the pectoral spines are not associated with venom glands.

Scorpionfish venom has been likened in potency to cobra venom. Its principal action appears to be direct muscle toxicity, resulting in paralysis of cardiac, involuntary, and skeletal muscles. The presentation of injury is similar to stingray envenomation. Pain is immediate and intense with radiation centrally. Untreated, the pain peaks at 60 to 90 min and persists for 6 to 12 h. In the case of the stonefish, the pain may be severe enough to cause delirium and may persist at high levels for days. The wound and surrounding area are initally ischemic and then cyanotic, with surrounding areas of erythema, edema, and warmth. Vesicles may form, and rapid tissue sloughing with surrounding areas of cellulitis may develop within 48 h. Systemic effects are similar to those of coelenterate envenomation.

Other venomous fish that sting in a manner similar to scorpionfish include catfish, weeverfish, surgeonfish, horned sharks, toadfish, ratfish, rabbitfish, stargazers, and leatherbacks. Approximately 1000 species of catfish inhabit both fresh and salt waters. Catfish venom apparatus consists of the single dorsal and two pectoral fin spines and the axillary venom glands. Catfish also produce a crinotoxin which can be introduced into the wound during envenomation. The sting of the marine catfish is usually more severe than that of its freshwater counterpart. The weeverfish, the most venomous fish in the temperate zone, is found in the Mediterranean and European coastal areas. Weeverfish are bottom dwellers that sting when stepped upon. The five to seven envenoming dorsal spines can penetrate a leather boot and create a substantial puncture wound.

The success of therapy for stings from marine animal spines is dependent upon rapid initiation. Treatment is directed at combating the effects of the venom, alleviating pain, and preventing infection. The wound should be irrigated immediately, and any visible pieces of the spine or integumentary sheath should be removed. As soon as possible, the wound should be immersed in hot water to tolerance [45°C (113°F)] for 30 to 90 min or until there is pain relief. During the hot water soak, the wound should be explored and foreign material removed.

Narcotics may be necessary for pain control. Local infiltration of the wound with lidocaine without epinephrine or a regional nerve block may be very useful.

After the soaking procedure, the wound should be prepared in an aseptic fashion, reexplored, and thoroughly debrided. Soft tissue radiography should be employed to visualize calcified matter. Wounds should remain open for delayed primary closure or sutured loosely with adequate drainage. Prophylactic antibiotics are recommended because of the high incidence of ulceration and necrosis with subsequent secondary infection. If a victim is to be treated and released, he or she should be observed for at least 4 h for systemic side effects. A stonefish antivenin (Commonwealth Serum Laboratories, Melbourne, Australia) is available for severe systemic reactions to stonefish or other scorpionfish.

Sea snakes (family Hydrophidae) are the most abundant venomous

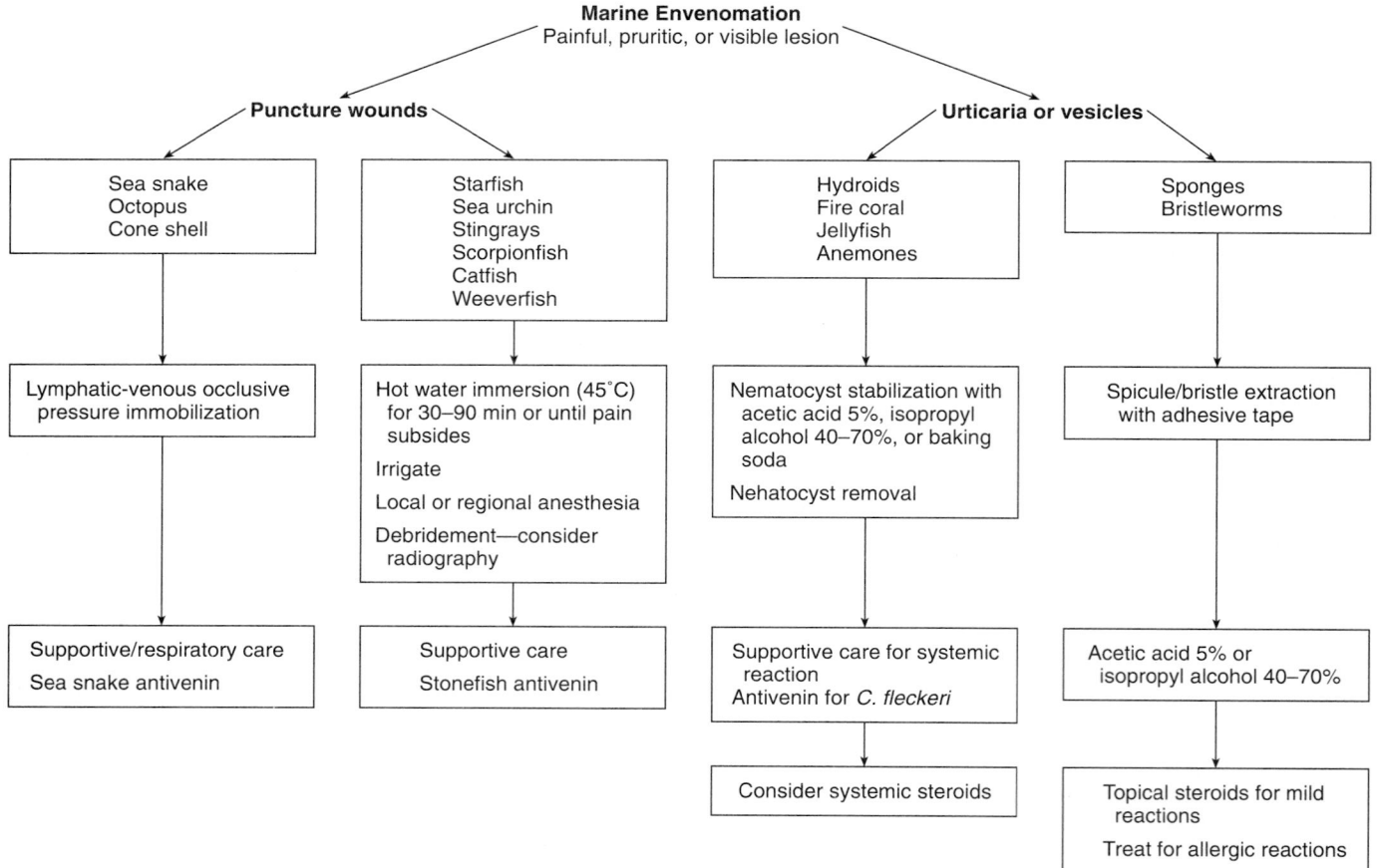

**Fig. 164-1.** Algorithmic approach to marine envenomation. (Adapted from Auerbach PS: Marine envenomations. *N Engl J Med* 325:490, 1991, with permission.)

reptiles. There are 52 species of sea snakes, all of which are venomous. The snakes are distributed in the tropical and warm temperate Pacific and Indian Oceans. None are found in the Atlantic Ocean, the Caribbean, or in North American coastal waters. Hawaii is the only U.S. state that has sea snakes.

Most sea snakes are 3 to 4 ft (about 1 m) long, although some attain lengths of up to 9 ft (3 m). They can be distinguished from land snakes by their flat tails and valvelike nostril flaps and from eels by the presence of scales and absence of gills and fins. Sea snakes swim in an undulating fashion and can move backward or forward in the water with equal speed. The venom apparatus consists of two to four hollow maxillary fangs and a pair of associated venom glands. The fangs are short and easily detached. Approximately 80 percent of bites do not result in significant envenomations.

The sea snake venom contains a peripherally acting neurotoxin that causes paralysis and a myotoxin that causes muscle necrosis. Due to the lack of an immediate local reaction, the bite often goes unnoticed. Symptoms typically become apparent 2 h after the bite but may begin as soon as 5 min or as late as 8 h afterward. The first complaint may be one of euphoria, malaise, or anxiety. Classic muscle aches then develop, along with a "thick tongue" and sialorrhea. Ascending flaccid or spastic paralysis follows shortly and is accompanied by other neurologic signs and symptoms such as ophthalmoplegia, ptosis, facial paralysis, and pupillary changes. Death is most commonly due to ventilatory failure.

Diagnosis of a sea snake bite is based on the combination of snake identification and the presence of a multiple-puncture bite wound, which was initially painless and occurred in the water. Envenomation should be suspected if the characteristic symptoms develop, primarily

myalgias. The presence of myoglobinuria and elevated SGOT levels are also typical. Neurotoxic symptoms are rapid in onset and usually appear within 2 to 3 h. If no symptoms develop by 6 to 8 h, envenomation did not occur.

Treatment of a sea snake bite involves pressure-immobilization of the dependent limb to provide venom sequestration. Incision and suction therapy is not recommended. Supportive measures are necessary but are not an adequate substitute for sea snake antivenin, which is absolutely indicated. With any clinical evidence of envenomation, polyvalent sea snake antivenin (Commonwealth Serum Laboratories, Melbourne, Australia) should be administered after skin testing. Tiger snake (*Notechis scutatus*) antivenin is also available as a second choice. If neither of these is available, polyvalent *Elapidae* antivenin can be used.

The administration of antivenin should begin as soon as possible but remains useful up to 36 h after envenomation. Intensive supportive care and monitoring of renal, metabolic, and respiratory function are critical. The relatively small molecular weight of sea snake neurotoxin makes it dialyzable; therefore, hemodialysis may be of benefit. An algorithmic approach to the unidentified marine envenomation is provided (Fig. 164-1).

## BIBLIOGRAPHY

Auerbach PS: Clinical therapy of marine envenomation and poisoning, in Tu At (ed): *Handbook of Natural Toxins,* vol 3, *Marine Toxins and Venoms.* New York, Dekker, 1988, pp 493–565.

Auerbach PS: Marine envenomation, in Auerbach PS (ed): *Wilderness Medicine. Magement of Wilderness and Environmental Emergencies,* 3d ed. St. Louis, Mosby, 1995, p. 1327.

Auerbach PS, Halstead BW: Injuries from nonvenomous aquatic animals, in Auerbach PS, (ed): *Wilderness Medicine. Management of Wilderness and Environmental Emergencies,* 3d ed. St. Louis, Mosby, 1995, p 1303.

Auerbach PS, Yaijko DM, Nassos PS, et al: Bacteriology of the marine environment: Implications for clinical therapy. *Ann Emerg Med* 16:643, 1987.

Burnett JW, Calton CJ: Jellyfish envenomation syndromes updated. *Ann Emerg Med* 16:1000, 1987.

Halstead BW: *Poisonous and Venomous Marine Animals.* Princeton, NJ, Darwin, 1988.

Halstead BW, Auerbach PS: *Dangerous Aquatic Animals of the World: A Color Atlas.* Princeton, NJ, Darwin, 1992.

Hessinger DA, Lenhoff HM (eds): *The Biology of Nematocysts.* San Diego, Academic, 1989.

Kizer KW, McKinney HE, Auerbach PS: Scorpaenidae envenomation: A five-year poison center experience. *JAMA* 253:807, 1985.

Rifkin JF, Fenner PJ, Williamson JAH: First aid treatment of the sting from the hydroid *Lytocarpus philippinus:* The structure of and in vitro discharge experiments with its nematocysts. *J Wild Med* 4:252, 1993.

Tomchik RS, Russell MT, Szmant AM, Black NA: Clinical perspectives—seabather's eruption, also known as "sea lice." *JAMA* 269:1669, 1993.

Tu AT: Biotoxicology of sea snake venoms. *Ann Emerg Med* 16:1023, 1987.

Williamson J: Current challenges in marine envenomation: An overview. *J Wild Med* 3:422, 1992.

# 165

# HIGH ALTITUDE MEDICAL PROBLEMS

### Peter H. Hackett
### Mark Rabold

Over 40 million visitors to the western United States went to altitudes over 2400 m (8000 ft) in 1989, and tens of thousands traveled to other high altitude locations in Alaska, Europe, Asia, South America, and Africa. Physicians working or traveling in or near these locations therefore are increasingly likely to encounter persons ill with a high altitude illness or suffering an untoward effect of altitude on a preexisting condition. Although the focus of this chapter is hypoxia-related problems, patients in the mountain environment also may require care for associated illnesses such as hypothermia, frostbite, trauma, ultraviolet keratitis, dehydration, and lightning injury, which are covered elsewhere in this text.

High altitude is a hypoxic environment. Since the concentration of oxygen in the troposphere remains constant at 21 percent, the partial pressure of oxygen decreases as a function of the barometric pressure (Fig. 165-1). In Denver (1610 m), air pressure is 17 percent less than at sea level and therefore contains 17 percent less oxygen. The air of Aspen, Colorado (2438 m) has 26 percent less oxygen, and the barometric pressure on top of Mt. Everest is merely one-third that of sea level. Paul Bert, in his classic experiments of the late 19th century, showed that supplemental oxygen prevented symptoms of altitude illness during hypobaric exposure and concluded that hypoxia, not hypobaria, was responsible for illness.

For purposes of discussion, the range of high altitude may be divided based on physiological effects. From 1500 to 3500 m above sea level (4900 ft to 11,500 ft) is considered *high altitude;* decreased exercise performance and increased ventilation (lower arterial $P_{CO_2}$) occur, without a major impairment in arterial oxygen transport, even though altitude illness is common with abrupt ascent to over 2500 m

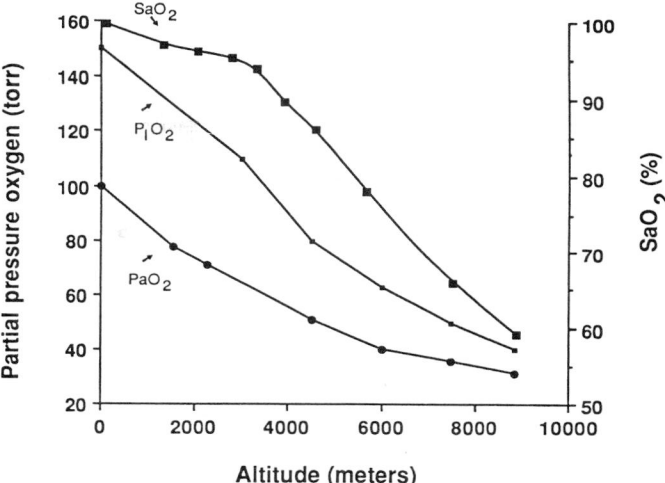

**Fig. 165-1.** Increasing altitude results in a fall of inspired $P_{O_2}$ ($PI_{O_2}$), arterial $P_{O_2}$ ($Pa_{O_2}$), and arterial oxygen saturation ($Sa_{O_2}$). *Note:* (1) the difference between inspired and arterial $P_{O_2}$ narrows at high altitude and (2) $Sa_{O_2}$% is well maintained while awake until nearly 4000 m. (From Auerbach PS, Geehr EC (eds): *Management of Wilderness and Environmental Emergencies.* St. Louis, Mosby, 1989. Used by permission.)

(8200 ft). *Very high altitude* encompasses the range of 3500 to 5500 m (11,500 to 18,000 ft), where maximum arterial oxygen saturation falls to less than 90 percent ($Pa_{O_2}$ < 60 mmHg), and extreme hypoxemia may occur during exercise, sleep, and altitude illness. Abrupt ascent to these altitudes may be dangerous; a period of acclimatization is required. *Extreme altitude,* over 5500 m (18,000 ft), is accompanied by severe hypoxemia and hypocapnia, and abrupt ascent precipitates illness in nearly all individuals. At this altitude, progressive physiologic deterioration eventually outstrips acclimatization; no human habitations are higher.

## ACCLIMATIZATION TO HIGH ALTITUDE

Persons rendered acutely hypoxic become dizzy, faint, and rapidly unconscious if hypoxic stress is sufficient. These same individuals, given days to weeks to develop the exact same degree of hypoxia, are able to function quite well. While the fundamental process of this acclimatization takes place in the metabolic machinery of cells and mitochondria, acute "struggle" responses are critical while allowing the cells time to adjust.

### Ventilation

Defense of alveolar $P_{O_2}$ through increased ventilation is the primary initial adaptation. The hypoxic ventilatory response (HVR) is effected by the carotid body, which senses a decrease in arterial oxygenation and inputs to the central respiratory center in the medulla to increase ventilation. The vigor of this inborn response is related to successful acclimatization and increased performance. Respiratory depressants or stimulants may affect HVR, as does chronic hypoxia, which eventually blunts the response. A low hypoxic drive may allow extreme hypoxemia to develop during sleep. The initial hyperventilation is quickly attenuated by respiratory alkalosis, which acts as a brake on the respiratory center. As renal excretion of bicarbonate compensates for the respiratory alkalosis, pH returns toward normal, and ventilation continues to increase. This process of maximizing ventilation, termed ventilatory acclimatization, culminates after 4 to 7 days at a given altitude. With continuing ascent to higher altitudes, the central chemoreceptors reset to progressively lower $P_{CO_2}$ values, and the completeness of acclimatization can be gauged by the arterial

**Table 165-1.** Blood Gases and Altitude

| Altitude (meters) | $Pa_{O_2}$ (mmHg) | $Sa_{O_2}\%$ | $Pa_{CO_2}$ (mmHg) |
|---|---|---|---|
| Sea level | 90–95 | 96 | 40 |
| 1524(5000 ft) | 75–81 | 95 | 32–33 |
| 2286(7500 ft) | 69–74 | 92–93 | 31–33 |
| 4572(15,000 ft) | 48–53 | 86 | 25 |
| 6096(20,000 ft) | 37–45 | 76 | 20 |
| 7620(25,000 ft) | 32–39 | 68 | 13 |
| 8848(29,029 ft) | 26–33 | 58 | 9.5–13.8 |

*Source:* Auerbach PS, Geehr EC (eds): *Management of Wilderness and Environmental Emergencies.* St. Louis, Mosby, 1989. Used by permission.

$P_{CO_2}$. Acetazolamide, which forces a bicarbonate diuresis, greatly facilitates this process. An appreciation of the normal values for blood gases and acid-base status with acclimatization at various altitudes is necessary in order to distinguish abnormalities (Table 165-1).

## Blood

The hematopoietic response to altitude was first observed in 1890 by Viault. We now know that within 2 h of ascent to altitude, erythropoietin is increased in plasma and, over days to weeks, results in increased red cell mass. This adaptation has no importance during initial acclimatization when altitude illness develops and, when excessive, results in chronic mountain polycythemia. Shifts in the oxyhemoglobin dissociation curve are thought to be minimal *in vivo* at altitude, since the increase in 2,3-diphosphoglyceric acid, which is proportional to the severity of hypoxia and shifts the curve to the right, is offset by the alkalosis, which shifts the curve to the left. Naturally occurring left-shifted hemoglobin is an advantage at high altitude.

## Fluid Balance

Peripheral venous constriction on ascent to altitude causes an increase in central blood volume, which triggers baroreceptors to suppress antidiuretic hormone (ADH) and aldosterone and induce a diuresis. Combined with the bicarbonate diuresis from the respiratory alkalosis, this can result in decreased plasma volume and hyperosmolality (serum osmolality of 290 to 300), which the body appears to permit by a reset of the osmol center of the brain. Clinically, diuresis and hemoconcentration is considered a healthy response.

## Cardiovascular

Stroke volume is decreased initially, and an increased heart rate maintains cardiac output. Maximum exercising heart rate declines at altitude proportional to the decrease in $V_{O_2}$ max. Cardiac muscle in healthy persons is able to withstand extreme levels of hypoxemia ($Pa_{O_2} < 30$ mmHg) without evidence of ST segment changes or ischemic events. Blood pressure is mildly elevated on ascent secondary to increased sympathetic tone.

The pulmonary circulation constricts with exposure to hypoxia. This is an advantage during regional alveolar hypoxia, such as pneumonia, but is a disadvantage during the global hypoxia of altitude exposure. As a result, pulmonary pressure increases. This degree of hypertension is quite variable, with those having a hyperreactive response much more susceptible to high altitude pulmonary edema.

Cerebral blood flow transiently increases on ascent to altitude (despite the hypocapnic alkalosis), which increases oxygen delivery to the brain. This response, however, is limited by the increase in cerebral blood volume, which may increase intracranial pressure and produce and/or aggravate symptoms of altitude illness.

## Effects on Exercise

Exercise capacity, as measured by maximum oxygen consumption, drops dramatically on ascent to altitude, approximately 10 percent for each 1000-m altitude gain above 1500 m. During acclimatization, submaximal endurance increases appreciably after 10 days, but $V_{O_2}$ max does not. The mechanism of the decrement is probably lack of adequate oxygen supply to the muscle cells due to the low driving pressure for diffusion of oxygen from the capillary.

## Limitations

There are limits to acclimatization. Even those who are by nature good acclimatizers cannot tolerate the hypoxia of extreme altitude for long. Miners from South America report that they cannot live at altitudes above 5800 m because of weight loss, increasing lethargy, poor quality sleep, weakness, and headache. High altitude mountaineers cannot survive for more than a few days above 8000 m without supplemental oxygen because of more acute deterioration in physiologic functioning. Considerable weight loss, both of fat and lean body mass, are unavoidable at extreme altitude, and help contribute to demise. Other factors limiting ability to acclimatize to extreme altitude include right ventricular strain from excessive pulmonary hypertension, intestinal malabsorption, impaired renal function, polycythemia and microcirculatory sludging, and prolonged cerebral hypoxia. Even at more modest altitudes, some individuals are very slow or poor acclimatizers for reasons not entirely known but, at least in part, due to poor carotid body function and inadequate ventilation.

## Sleep at High Altitude

Sleep stages III and IV are reduced at altitude while sleep stage I is increased. More time is spent awake, with a significant increase in arousals, but only slightly less rapid eye movement (REM) time. The frequent arousals are a common source of bitter complaints from skiers and others, but they are innocuous and improve with time at altitude. The typical periodic breathing (Cheyne-Stokes) in those sleeping above 2700 m (9000 ft) consists of 6- to 12-s apneic pauses interspersed with cycles of vigorous ventilation. Interestingly, the frequent awakenings are not necessarily related to the sleep periodic breathing, and neither are they related to acute mountain sickness. Presumably, the mechanism of the lighter sleep is related to cerebral hypoxia. Quality of sleep and also arterial oxygenation during sleep improves with acclimatization and with acetazolamide.

## HIGH ALTITUDE SYNDROMES

High altitude syndromes of primary concern are those problems attributed directly to the hypoxia: acute hypoxia, acute mountain sickness, pulmonary edema, cerebral edema, retinopathy, peripheral edema, sleeping problems, and a group of neurologic syndromes. The other syndromes, not necessarily related to hypoxia, include thromboembolic events (which may be attributable to dehydration, prolonged incapacitation, polycythemia, and cold), high altitude pharyngitis and bronchitis, and ultraviolet keratitis. Although the different hypoxic clinical syndromes overlap, all share a fundamental mechanism, all are seen in the same setting of rapid ascent in unacclimatized persons, and all respond to the same essential therapy: descent and oxygen.

## Acute Hypoxia

The syndrome of acute hypoxia occurs in the setting of sudden and severe hypoxic insult, such as accidental decompression of a pressurized aircraft cabin or a failed oxygen system in a pilot or high altitude mountaineer. Sudden overexertion precipitating arterial desaturation, acute onset of pulmonary edema, carbon monoxide poisoning, and sleep apnea may result in relatively acute hypoxia as well. Unacclimatized persons become unconscious at an arterial oxygen saturation of 50 to 60 percent, an arterial $P_{O_2}$ of less than about 30 mmHg, or a jugular venous $P_{O_2}$ less than 15 mmHg. Acute hypoxia is reversed by immediate administration of oxygen, rapid descent, and correction of the underlying cause such as removal of the carbon monoxide source or repair of the oxygen delivery system. Symptoms of acute hypoxia reflect the sensitivity of the central nervous system (CNS) to this insult: dizziness, light-headedness, and dimmed vision progressing to loss of consciousness. Hyperventilation has been shown to increase the time of useful consciousness during acute alveolar hypoxia.

## Acute Mountain Sickness (AMS)

### Incidence

AMS occurs in the setting of more gradual and less severe hypoxic insult than with acute hypoxic syndrome. Its incidence varies by location, depending on ease of access, rate of ascent, and sleeping altitude reached. A recent study at 2100 m (6900 ft) found a 25 percent incidence of AMS in physicians attending a continuing-education meeting in Colorado. Other studies at resorts between 2220 and 2700 m (7200 and 9000 ft, respectively) claimed an incidence between 17 and 40 percent, and a sleeping altitude of 2750 m (9000 ft) seemed to be a threshold for increased attack rate. Approximately 40 percent of trekkers in Nepal on the path to Mt. Everest suffer AMS, while climbers on Mt. Rainier have the very high incidence of 70 percent because of the rapidity of ascent.

### Susceptibility

In addition to rate of ascent and sleeping altitude, inherent factors determine individual susceptibility to acute mountain sickness. Factors identified so far are low hypoxic ventilatory response and low vital capacity. Age has a small influence on incidence, with children being somewhat more susceptible. Women are just as likely, if not more so, to develop mountain sickness but appear to have less pulmonary edema. Susceptibility to AMS is generally reproducible in an individual or repeated exposures. Persons living at intermediate altitudes of 1000 to 2000 m already are acclimatized partially and do much better than lowlanders upon ascent to higher altitudes. There is no relationship of susceptibility to AMS and physical fitness.

### Clinical Presentation

The diagnosis of AMS is based on the setting, symptoms, and physical findings. The setting is rapid ascent of an unacclimatized person to 2000 m (6600 ft) or higher. Typically, the person on arrival feels lightheaded and slightly breathless, especially with exercise. One to six h later, but sometimes delayed for 1 day or more (and especially after a night's sleep), the typical symptoms of mild AMS develop; they are similar to an alcohol hangover. The headache usually is described as bifrontal and worsened with bending over and the valsalva maneuver. Gastrointestinal symptoms include anorexia, nausea, and sometimes vomiting, and the chief constitutional symptoms are lassitude and weakness. The person with AMS is often irritable and wants to be left alone. Sleepiness and a deep inner chill, especially in a cold environment, also are common. If the illness progresses, the headache becomes more severe, and vomiting, oliguria, and increased dyspnea develop. Lassitude may progress to the victim requiring assistance for eating and dressing. The most severe form of AMS, high altitude cerebral edema (HACE), is heralded by onset of ataxia and altered level of consciousness; coma may ensue within 12 h if treatment is delayed.

Physical findings in mild AMS are nonspecific. Heart rate and blood pressure are variable, and usually in the normal range, although postural hypotension may be present. Localized rales are detectable in up to 20 percent of persons with AMS. Fever is unusual except in the presence of pulmonary edema. Funduscopy reveals venous tortuosity and dilatation, and retinal hemorrhages are common over 5000 m or in those with pulmonary and cerebral edema. Fluid retention is a hallmark of AMS, in contrast to the usual diuresis of acclimatization, and may result in peripheral edema, especially of the face. Differential diagnosis in this setting includes hypothermia, carbon monoxide

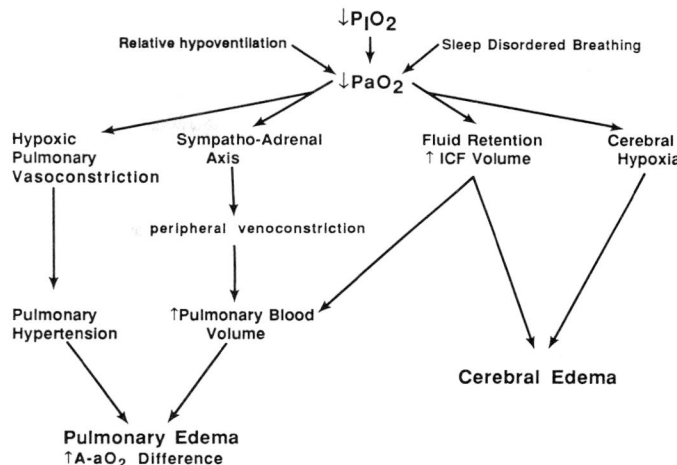

**Fig. 165-2.** A schema of pathophysiology for high altitude illness. (From Hackett and Roach, *Ann Emerg Med* 16:980, 1987. Used by permission.)

poisoning, pulmonary or CNS infection, dehydration, and exhaustion.

The natural history of AMS at a Colorado resort (3000 m or 10,000 ft) recently was documented. Mean duration of symptoms was 15 h, with a range to 94 h, despite the fact that one-half of those with symptoms self-medicated. At higher sleeping altitudes, the illness may last much longer, even weeks if untreated, and is more likely to progress to pulmonary or cerebral edema. Eight percent of those with AMS at 4243 m (14,000 ft) in Nepal developed cerebral or pulmonary edema, or both.

### Pathophysiology

AMS is due to hypobaric hypoxia, but the exact sequence of events leading to illness is unclear. Figure 165-2 offers a schema for the pathophysiology. The symptoms indicate a neurologic etiology and elevated cerebrospinal fluid pressure; scans confirming cerebral edema have been obtained in persons severely ill. Whether the more common mild illness of headache, anorexia, and malaise is due to mild cerebral edema has yet to be confirmed, but seems likely. Two types of cerebral edema have been proposed. One is cytotoxic edema, due to failure of the sodium-potassium pump with subsequent intracellular accumulation of sodium and water. The other is a vasogenic edema, due to a leaky blood-brain barrier.

No direct evidence for cytotoxic edema in humans at altitude has been reported, but a large shift of fluid into the total intracellular space, presumably including the brain, was demonstrated to take place over the first 3 days at altitude, when AMS occurs. The time required for fluid shift and overhydration of the brain may explain the time lag in onset of symptoms, which distinguishes AMS from acute hypoxia. In support of the vasogenic theory, white-matter brain edema on magnetic resonance imaging (MRI) recently was demonstrated in persons with high altitude cerebral edema, and it may also occur in AMS. The leaky blood-brain barrier is due either to loss of autoregulation and overperfusion or to hypoxia-induced increased permeability. The fact that corticosteroids so effectively treat AMS also supports the notion of vasogenic edema, since this is the only type of cerebral edema responsive to steroids. Further research is likely to reveal that brain swelling is due to both cytotoxic and vasogenic mechanisms.

The cerebral edema, interstitial pulmonary edema, peripheral edema, and the antidiuresis observed in AMS all point to an abnormality of water handling by the body. The mechanism is thought to be increased renin-angiotensin, aldosterone, and ADH in contrast to the normal ADH and aldosterone suppression at high altitude and usual diuresis. A decrease in glomerular filtration also has been observed. The effectiveness of diuretics in prevention and treatment of AMS reinforces the importance of fluid retention in the pathophysiology.

Relative hypoventilation due to a sluggish hypoxic ventilatory response is a characteristic of AMS-susceptible individuals and has been linked to fluid retention. Hypoventilation, of course, results in greater hypoxic stress and is equivalent to being at a higher altitude. Higher $P_{CO_2}$ and lower $P_{O_2}$ also increase cerebral blood flow and aggravate brain swelling. Less hypocapnia also may reduce the stimulus for bicarbonate diuresis and aggravate fluid retention.

## Treatment (Table 165-2)

### Descent and Oxygen

The goals of treatment are to prevent progression, abort the illness, and improve acclimatization; early diagnosis is essential. Initial clinical presentation does not predict eventual severity, and all persons with AMS must be observed carefully for progression. The three principles of treatment are (1) to not proceed to a higher sleeping altitude in the presence of symptoms, (2) to descend if symptoms do not abate or become worse despite treatment, and (3) to descend and treat immediately in the presence of a change in consciousness, ataxia, or pulmonary edema. Mild AMS is self-limited and generally improves with an extra 12 to 36 h of acclimatization if ascent is halted. Descent is the definitive treatment for all forms of altitude illness, although it is not always an option, nor always necessary. Remarkably, a drop in altitude of only 500 to 1000 m usually is effective promptly. Evacuation to a hospital or to sea level is unnecessary except in the most severe cases. To simulate descent, portable hyperbaric bags are being used in various locations to treat AMS. The patient is inserted into the fabric chamber, and a pressure of 2 psi is achieved by means of a manual or automated pump; the pressure is equivalent to a drop in altitude of 1500 m (5000 ft). A valve system creates sufficient ventilation to avoid $CO_2$ accumulation or $O_2$ depletion.

Oxygen effectively relieves symptoms, but it often is unavailable in the field and generally reserved for moderate to severe AMS in order to conserve supplies. Oxygen promptly relieves headache, dizziness, and most other symptoms, although ataxia may resolve more slowly. Nocturnal low flow oxygen (0.5 to 1 L/min) is particularly helpful and efficient. The combination of oxygen and descent provides optimal therapy, especially in more severe cases.

**Table 165-2.** Suggested Treatment of High Altitude Illness

| | |
|---|---|
| Mild AMS | Stop ascent |
| | Descend to lower altitude or acclimatize at same altitude |
| | Acetazolamide 125–250 mg b.i.d. to speed acclimatization |
| | Symptomatic treatment as necessary with analgesics and antiemetics |
| Moderate AMS | Immediate descent for worsening symptoms |
| | Low flow oxygen if available |
| | Acetazolamide 250 mg b.i.d. and/or dexamethasone 4 mg q 6 h |
| | Hyperbaric therapy |
| HACE | Immediate descent or evacuation |
| | Oxygen 2–4 L/min |
| | Dexamethasone 8 mg PO, IM, or IV, then 4 mg q 6 h |
| | Hyperbaric therapy if cannot descend |
| HAPE | Immediate descent or evacuation |
| | Oxygen 4 L/min |
| | Nifedipine 10 mg PO or 30 mg q 4–6 h extended-release q 6 h if no oxygen or descent |
| | Hyperbaric therapy if cannot descend |
| | Continuous positive airway pressure |
| | Minimize exertion and keep warm |
| Periodic Breathing | Acetazolamide 125 mg at bedtime as needed |

### Medical Therapy

Pharmacologic treatment offers an alternative to descent or oxygen in mild to moderately severe AMS. Acetazolamide is very helpful in speeding acclimatization and aborting illness, especially when used early. The drug acts by inhibiting the enzyme carbonic anhydrase, slowing the hydration of carbon dioxide to hydrogen and bicarbonate ions. In the kidney, acetazolamide reduces reabsorption of bicarbonate, causing a bicarbonate diuresis and metabolic acidosis, which stimulates ventilation. The drug essentially mimics the process of ventilatory acclimatization. As a result, arterial $P_{O_2}$ is higher, and sleep oxygenation remains high and stable, without periods of apnea (Fig. 165-3). The drug also maintains cerebral blood flow despite greater hypocapnia, and because of its diuretic action, it counteracts the fluid retention of AMS. Many trials have shown its value for prevention; although widely used empirically for treatment, controlled studies have been hindered by the reluctance of ill persons to enroll in placebo trials. Current indications for acetazolamide are (1) a history of altitude illness, (2) abrupt ascent to over 3000 m (10,000 ft), (3) for treatment of AMS, and (4) bothersome sleep periodic breathing. The dosage regimen varies; 5 mg/kg per day in two or three divided doses is sufficient, whether for prevention or treatment. An extended-release formulation of acetazolamide, 500 mg 24 h, is a convenient regimen. Treatment should be continued until symptoms of AMS resolve, and then the drug should be restarted if symptoms return. Since the drug acts by improving acclimatization, fear of masking serious illness is unwarranted. Common side effects of acetazolamide include peripheral paresthesias and sometimes nausea or drowsiness, and the usual precautions of sulfa drugs apply to acetazolamide because of the sulfhydryl moiety. Since the drug inhibits the instant hydration of $CO_2$ on the tongue, the carbon dioxide in carbonated beverages can be tasted, ruining the flavor of beer and other drinks.

Symptomatic treatment of AMS is sometimes sufficient. Aspirin 650 mg or acetaminophen 650 to 1000 mg (with or without codeine) can be given for headache. Prochlorperazine 5 to 10 mg intramuscularly is useful for nausea and vomiting and has the advantage of augmenting the hypoxic ventilatory response. The short-acting benzodiazepines such as triazolam 0.25 mg and temazepam 15 mg also can be used to treat the complaint of frequent wakening, but they are potentially dangerous in ill persons because of respiratory depression and may decrease oxygenation even in persons acclimatizing well. A combination of acetazolamide and benzodiazepine may work very well.

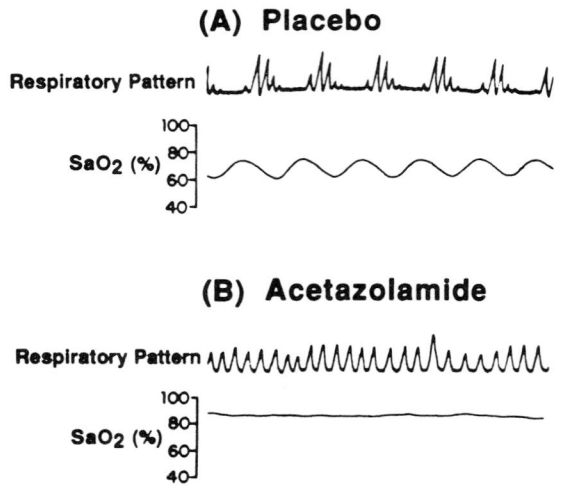

**Fig. 165-3.** Respiratory patterns and arterial oxygen saturation ($S_{O_2}\%$) with placebo and acetazolamide in two sleep studies of a subject at 4400 m. (From Hackett and Roach, *Ann Emerg Med* 16:980, 1987. Used by permission.)

Dexamethasone 4 mg PO, IM, or IV every six h is quite effective therapy for mountain sickness, but it is best reserved for moderate to severe AMS, since it may be associated with significant side effects and does not aid acclimatization, sometimes resulting in rebound symptoms when discontinued. A short taper period may prevent this rebound phenomenon. The mechanism of action of dexamethasone may be to reduce vasogenic edema, to lower intracranial pressure, or to act as an antiemetic and mood elevator. The use of acetazolamide to speed acclimatization and a brief course of dexamethasone to treat illness can be a useful combination. The use of diuretics is reasonable because of the fluid retention associated with mountain sickness. Furosemide 20 to 40 mg every 12 h until improved was reported effective by the Indian army, although other investigators have not been enthusiastic about its use because of concerns for avoiding hypovolemia, hypotension, and incapacitation.

## Prevention

Graded ascent with adequate time for acclimatization is the best prevention. A recommendation for those visiting medium altitude resorts in the western United States is to spend a night at an intermediate altitude of 1500 to 2000 m (Denver or Salt Lake City) before sleeping at altitudes above 2500 m (8200 ft). Mountaineers and trekkers should avoid abrupt ascent to sleeping altitudes over 3000 m and then allow two nights for each 1000-m altitude gain in camp altitude, starting at 3000 m. Other preventative measures include avoiding overexertion, alcohol, and respiratory depressants, and eating a high carbohydrate diet. Acetazolamide is a useful prophylactic agent for those with a history of AMS or for forced abrupt ascent without acclimatization stages. The drug should be started 24 h before the ascent and continued for the first 2 days at altitude. The medication then can be discontinued and started again if illness develops. Acetazolamide can be expected to reduce the symptoms of AMS by approximately 75 percent in persons ascending rapidly to sleeping altitudes of over 2500 m. An alternative for those allergic to sulfa is dexamethasone 4 mg every 12 h starting the day of ascent and continuing for the first 2 days at altitude.

## Neurologic Syndromes of High Altitude

Until recently, most neurologic events at high altitude were attributed to HACE or AMS. Clearly, this has been a diagnostic oversimplification. Other syndromes now recognized as related to high altitude include altitude syncope, cerebrovascular spasm (migraine equivalent), cerebral arterial or venous thrombosis (infarct), transient ischemic attack, and cerebral hemorrhage. These syndromes are characterized by more focal neurologic findings than in cerebral edema, though differentiation in the field may be impossible.

Other problems may be due to exacerbation or unmasking of underlying disease, such as previously asymptomatic brain tumors and epilepsy. Presumably, space-occupying lesions become symptomatic because of increased brain volume at altitude. Hyperventilation (hypocapnic alkalosis), which is commonly used to induce seizure activity on electroencephalography, may explain unmasking of a seizure disorder at altitude, while changes in cerebral blood flow may exacerbate vascular lesions. Even generalized encephalopathy or coma, considered the hallmark of HACE, may be due to factors other than edema. Indeed, unconsciousness from acute hypoxia at sea level clearly is not due to edema, but rather to neurotransmitter failure, similar to the neuroglycopenia of insulin reactions.

## High Altitude Cerebral Edema (HACE)

HACE is defined clinically as the presence of progressive neurologic deterioration in someone with AMS or high altitude pulmonary edema (HAPE). It is characterized by altered mental status, ataxia, stupor, and progression to coma if untreated. Headache, nausea, and vomiting are not always present. Because of raised intracranial pressure, focal neurologic signs such as third and sixth cranial nerve palsies may result from distortion of brain structures or by extraxial compression.

HACE is usually associated with pulmonary edema. Pathologically, necropsies have described severe, diffuse cerebral edema with multiple small hemorrhages and sometimes thrombosis.

The treatment of HACE is the same as for severe AMS: oxygen, descent, and steroids (Table 165-2). Descent is the highest priority. Acetazolamide may be an adjunct, but immediate reversal of the illness is the goal; improving acclimatization comes later. In acutely ill patients who cannot descend, the combination of steroids, supplemental oxygen, and a hyperbaric bag is optimal therapy, but rarely available. Comatose patients require additional airway management, bladder drainage, and other coma care. For coma, the use of hyperventilation to decrease intracranial pressure is a reasonable approach, keeping in mind that the $P_{CO_2}$ is already low and pH high in these individuals. Additional acute hyperventilation could produce cerebral ischemia; monitoring of arterial blood gases and, if available, cerebral blood velocities by transcranial Doppler ultrasonography may be advisable. Loop diuretics such as furosemide 40 to 80 mg or bumetanide 1 to 2 mg may help reduce brain overhydration, but hypoperfusion must be avoided. Hypertonic solutions of saline, mannitol, or urea have been used too infrequently to establish clinical guidelines. In the hospital setting, mannitol in a patient who does not respond immediately is worth considering. Coma may persist for days, even for weeks after evacuation to lower altitude, and the patient may still recover, sometimes with permanent sequelae. Persistent coma is unusual, however, and mandates exclusion of other possible etiologies.

## Cerebrovascular Syndromes of Altitude

Strokes, due both to infarct and hemorrhage in the arterial circulation, as well as venous thrombosis have been reported in young healthy persons at altitude who otherwise would not be considered at risk for such conditions. Transient ischemic attack, cortical blindness, and various focal neurologic signs such as hemiparesis or hemiplegia of a transient nature also occur. Since these latter events are reversible, they suggest etiologies such as vasospasm, watershed hypoxia between arterial zones, or transient ischemia attack.

Differentiation of the various neurologic syndromes may be impossible in the field, and treating as if cerebral edema were present may be reasonable, with a rapid descent to lower altitude, oxygen, and steroids, and evacuation to a hospital if symptoms persist despite treatment. Fortunately, focal neurologic signs usually resolve spontaneously and do not recur upon reascent. However, a thorough cerebrovascular evaluation before advising reascent may be prudent.

## High Altitude Pulmonary Edema (HAPE)

HAPE is the most lethal of the altitude illnesses. Since the condition is easily reversible with descent and oxygen, the cause of death is usually lack of early recognition, misdiagnosis, or inability to descend to a lower altitude.

## Epidemiology

The incidence of HAPE varies from less than one in 10,000 skiers in Colorado to 2 to 3 percent of climbers on Mt. McKinley and was reported as high as 15 percent in some regiments in the Indian army who were airlifted to high altitude during the Indian/Chinese war. Children appear more susceptible; women appear less susceptible than men. Risk factors include heavy exertion, rapid ascent, cold, excessive salt ingestion, use of sleeping medication, and a previous history indicating inherent individual susceptibility.

## Clinical Presentation (Table 165-3)

Early in the course of illness, when the edema is still interstitial or localized, the victim develops a dry cough, decreased exercise performance, dyspnea on exertion, increased recovery time from exercise, and localized rales, usually in the right midlung field. Late in the course of the illness, there develops tachycardia, tachypnea, and dyspnea at rest, marked weakness, productive cough, cyanosis, and more generalized rales. As hypoxemia worsens, consciousness becomes impaired. Victims usually become comatose and then die. Early diagnosis is critical, and decreased exercise performance and dry cough is enough to raise the suspicion of early HAPE. The typical victim is strong and fit and may or may not have symptoms of AMS before onset of HAPE. The condition typically worsens at night and is noticed most commonly on the second night at a new altitude. Unfortunately, rales may not be audible in 30 percent of persons with HAPE at rest but can be elicited immediately after a short bout of exercise. Fever up to 38.5°C is common, and tachycardia and tachypnea generally correlate with the severity of illness. On cardiac auscultation, a prominent P2 and right ventricular heave may be appreciated. ECG generally reveals right axis deviation and a right ventricular strain pattern consistent with acute pulmonary hypertension. Chest x-ray findings progress from interstitial to localized alveolar to generalized alveolar infiltrates as the illness progresses from mild to severe.

## Pathophysiology

The pioneering work of Hultgren established HAPE as a noncardiogenic edema. Left ventricular function is normal. Left ventricular end diastolic pressure, wedge pressures, and left atrial pressures are low to normal, cardiac output is low, and pulmonary vascular resistance and pulmonary artery pressure are markedly elevated. The exact cause of the edema is still unclear. Pulmonary hypertension is an essential component, and persons with a history of HAPE have been shown to have exaggerated pulmonary pressor responses to hypoxia. Whether this represents one end of a normal distribution or a pathologic subpopulation is unknown. However, not all persons with pulmonary hypertension develop HAPE; another factor must also be present, which induces a change in capillary membrane permeability. Pulmonary venous constriction, fibrin and platelet thrombi, and uneven arterial vasoconstriction leading to overperfusion of some areas of the vasculature have all been proposed. Predisposed individuals have a low hypoxic ventilatory response, an abnormal pulmonary circulation, and tend to suffer HAPE on repeated exposures.

## Treatment

The key to successful treatment of HAPE (Table 165-2) is early recognition, since the condition in its early stage is easily reversible. The optimal therapy depends upon the environmental setting, evacuation options, availability of oxygen or hyperbaric units, and ease of descent. Immediate descent is the treatment of choice, but this is not always possible. During descent, exertion by the victim must be mini-

mized. Reports of victims dying during descent probably are related to overexertion offsetting the benefit of lower altitude. With descent, oxygen is unnecessary except in severe cases. Oxygen provides excellent results and can completely resolve pulmonary edema without descent to a lower altitude, but may require 36 to 72 h to do so. Such quantities of oxygen rarely are available to trekking, mountaineering, and skiing groups, but they may be available at ski resorts or medical facilities. Oxygen immediately lowers pulmonary artery pressure and improves arterial oxygenation. Its use is life saving when descent is not an option; in such cases, rescue groups should make delivery of oxygen to the victim the highest priority. As in the treatment of AMS and HACE, the portable hyperbaric bag is a very useful adjunct to therapy when immediate descent is not possible.

Bed rest may be adequate for very mild cases, and bed rest with supplemental oxygen may suffice for moderate illness, as long as the safety of the patient can be assured by the presence of a medical facility, adequate oxygen, or immediate descent capability should the patient's condition deteriorate. Since cold stress elevates pulmonary artery pressure, the patient should be kept warm. The use of an expiratory positive airway pressure (EPAP) mask has been shown to increase arterial oxygen saturation by 10–20% in HAPE patients by enhancing alveolar recruitment. The mask is lightweight, well tolerated, and may be a useful adjunct to descent.

Since oxygen and descent are so effective, experience with drugs has been limited. Morphine and furosemide were used with good results by the Indian army, and both seem physiologically reasonable since they augment venous pooling, reduce pulmonary blood flow, and therefore reduce hydrostatic force for fluid extravasation in the lung. However, patients with HAPE often are dehydrated intravascularly, and caution must be exercised to avoid hypotension. Several studies have demonstrated that nifedipine, either 10 mg capsule or 30 mg extended-release formulation orally was reported to be of clinical benefit, to reduce pulmonary artery pressure by 30 to 50 percent, and to increase arterial oxygen saturation. Nifedipine, at a dose of 20 mg slow release preparation every 8 hours while ascending, has also been shown to be an effective prophylactic agent in those who have had previous episodes of HAPE. Other vasodilators, such as hydralazine and phentolamine, show promise, as well, in the treatment of HAPE. The mechanism presumably is by lowering pulmonary pressure and, therefore, the pressure gradient for flux of fluid across the membrane. Hypotension is a potential problem with nifedipine, and the results are not nearly as dramatic as with oxygen or descent, which still remain the treatments of choice.

Hospitalization may be warranted for severe cases that do not respond immediately to descent, especially if cerebral edema is present. Intubation, high F$_{IO_2}$, and positive end-expiratory pressure ventilation are rarely required. Antibiotics are indicated for coexisting infection when present. Occasionally pulmonary artery catheterization is useful to exclude a cardiac component to the edema in persons with heart disease. The patient with HAPE who does not make the usual rapid improvement should be evaluated for pulmonary emboli, mediastinal pulmonary artery obstruction, or other pulmonary circulatory abnor-

**Table 165-3.** Severity Classification of HAPE

| Grade | Symptoms | Signs | Chest Film |
|---|---|---|---|
| 1 Mild | Dyspnea on exertion, dry cough fatigue while moving uphill | Heart rate (HR) (rest) < 90–100, respiratory rate (RR) (rest) < 20, Dusky nailbeds, Localized rales, if any | Minor exudate involving less than one-fourth of one lung field |
| 2 Moderate | Dyspnea, weakness, fatigue on level walking, raspy cough, headache, anorexia | HR 90–100, RR 16–30, cyanotic nailbeds, rales present, ataxia may be present | Some infiltrate involving 50% of one lung or smaller area of both lungs |
| 3 Severe | Dyspnea at rest, productive cough, orthopnea, extreme weakness stupor, coma, blood-tinged sputum | Bilateral rales, HR > 110, RR > 30, Facial and nailbed cyanosis, ataxia, | Bilateral infiltrates > 50% each lung |

*Source:* Hultgren HN: High altitude pulmonary edema, in Staub NC (ed): *Lung Water and Solute Exchange.* New York, Marcel Dekker, 1978, pp 437–469.

malities, such as congenital absence of a pulmonary artery. Adequate discharge criteria are progressive clinical and radiographic improvement, and an arterial $P_{O_2}$ of 60 mmHg or arterial oxygen saturation greater than 90 percent. Residua such as fibrosis and impaired pulmonary function tests have not been reported. Patients are advised to resume activities gradually and are warned that they may feel weak for 1 to 2 weeks. An episode of HAPE is not a contraindication to subsequent ascent, but patients should be advised on staged ascent, acetazolamide and/or nifedipine prophylaxis, and recognition of early signs and symptoms.

## Reentry Pulmonary Edema

A rather high incidence of HAPE, especially in children, has been reported in residents of high altitude who sojourn to a lower altitude and then suffer HAPE when returning home. In Peru, Hultgren found a prevalence of 6.4 per 100 exposures in the 1 to 20-year-old age group, and 0.4 per 100 exposures in persons over 21. Reports have also been published from Leadville, Colorado. The mechanism is thought to be more vigorous pulmonary vasoconstriction and pulmonary hypertension upon reexposure to hypoxia because of increased muscularization of pulmonary arterioles.

## Peripheral Edema

Swelling of the face and distal extremities is common at high altitude. Peripheral edema was reported in 18 percent of trekkers at 4200 m in Nepal and was twice as likely in women. It was often associated with AMS, but not necessarily. The presence of peripheral edema should raise suspicion of altitude illness and prompt a thorough examination for pulmonary and cerebral edema. The problem can be treated with diuretics, but if left untreated, it will resolve spontaneously with descent. The mechanism is presumably similar to that of the fluid retention of AMS but with edema formation peripherally rather than in the brain and lung.

## High Altitude Retinopathy

Retinal abnormalities described at high altitude include retinal edema, tortuosity and dilatation of retinal veins, disc hyperemia, retinal hemorrhages, and, rarely, cotton-wool exudates. Retinal hemorrhages are asymptomatic, except for rarely occurring macular hemorrhages, and are not considered an indication for descent unless visual changes are present. They resolve spontaneously in 10 to 14 days. Hemorrhages are common above a sleeping altitude of 5000 m and occur at lower altitudes in persons with altitude illness.

## High Altitude Pharyngitis and Bronchitis

Most unacclimatized persons exercising at altitudes over 2500 m develop a dry, hacking cough. With exposure to extreme altitudes for prolonged periods of time, a purulent bronchitis and a painful pharyngitis become nearly universal. These problems may not be of an infectious nature; high volumes of dry, cold air through the lungs may induce respiratory heat loss and cause purulent secretions on that basis alone. Bronchospasm may also be triggered by respiratory heat loss. Severe coughing spasms can result in cough fracture of the ribs.

Pharyngeal membranes become dry, painful, and cracked because of the dehydration and high ventilation. Mucosal cracks may be an entry for pathogens, or the erythema and dryness may cause discomfort strictly on a mechanical basis. Antibiotics generally are not helpful, supporting the concept of a noninfectious etiology. Breathing of steam, ingesting hard candies or lozenges to increase salivation, and forcing hydration may provide some benefit with systemic analgesics as necessary. A silk Balaclava or similar material across the nose and mouth that is sufficiently porous to allow large volume ventilation but trap some moisture and heat helps ameliorate these bothersome high altitude conditions.

## Chronic Mountain Polycythemia (CMP)

Monge's disease, also called chronic mountain sickness or CMP, has now been recognized in all high altitude locations of the world. Both long-term high altitude residents and lowlanders who relocate to high altitude may develop this condition after variable length of residence. The incidence is much higher in males and increases with age. The disease is characterized by excessive polycythemia for a given altitude, which causes symptoms such as headache, muddled thinking, difficulty sleeping, impaired peripheral circulation, drowsiness, and chest congestion. The diagnosis is made by the characteristic symptoms and a hemoglobin value greater than expected for the altitude, generally over 20 to 22 g/dL. Any problem causing hypoxemia at sea level causes greater hypoxemia at altitude, and the etiology of CMP can be traced to problems such as chronic obstructive pulmonary disease (COPD) and sleep apnea in 50 percent of patients. The etiology of pure CMP is attributed to idiopathic hypoventilation on the basis of diminished respiratory drive.

Therapy includes phlebotomy, relocation to lower altitude, or home oxygen use. Respiratory stimulants such as acetazolamide (250 mg twice a day) and medroxyprogesterone acetate (20 to 60 mg/day) have also been employed successfully. The response to respiratory stimulants supports the role of hypoventilation in this disorder.

## Ultraviolet Keratitis (Snow Blindness)

Ultraviolet light (UVA and UVB) penetrates the atmosphere to a greater degree at high altitude because of less cloud cover, less water vapor, and less particulate matter in the air. Radiation increases roughly 5 percent for every 300 m (1000 ft) gained, and it is exacerbated by reflection back from snow. UV radiation below 300 nm (UVB) is absorbed by the cornea, and high exposure levels can cause corneal burns in 1 h, although symptoms do not become apparent for 6 to 12 h. The typical symptoms of photokeratitis are severe pain, a foreign body or gritty sensation, photophobia, tearing, marked conjunctival erythema, chemosis, and eyelid swelling. UV keratitis generally is self-limited and heals within 24 h, but the condition is sufficiently painful to warrant systemic analgesics. Cold compresses may also provide some relief, and eye patches may be necessary for comfort. Prevention is obviously of great importance, since this condition can be disabling, especially in hazardous terrain. Adequate sunglasses should transmit less than 10 percent of UVB light. Side shields are necessary if traveling on snow, and polarizing lenses help by absorbing glare. Makeshift protection can be fashioned by cutting narrow horizontal slits in cardboard, foam, or any available material (Eskimo sunglasses).

# ILLNESSES AGGRAVATED BY HIGH ALTITUDE

## Chronic Lung Disease

COPD patients ascending to altitude often report increased dyspnea and reduced exercise ability. Obviously, those with hypoxemia, pulmonary hypertension, disordered control of ventilation, and sleep disordered breathing at sea level will have greater problems at altitude because of the greater alveolar hypoxia. Such patients may require supplemental oxygen at altitude when they do not at sea level (and avoid having to descend), and oxygen-dependent patients at sea level may need to increase the $F_{I_{O_2}}$. The required $F_{I_{O_2}}$ can be calculated by multiplying low-altitude $F_{I_{O_2}}$ by the ratio of low altitude barometric pressure divided by high altitude barometric pressure. This will ensure the delivery of the same partial pressure of oxygen as at low altitude. There are no data to suggest that persons with COPD are more likely to develop AMS or HAPE, although such persons may be self-selected to avoid travel to high altitude locations. In fact, persons with mild to moderate COPD already are partially acclimatized and may do well at modest altitude, as suggested by Graham and Houston. High altitude per se does not exacerbate asthma, and persons with chronic bronchospasm often report easier breathing at high altitude, due to lower air density and/or cleaner air.

## Arteriosclerotic Heart Disease (ASHD)

The healthy heart and cardiovascular system tolerates even extreme hypoxia very well. Numerous ECG studies, echocardiograms, heart catheterizations and exercise tests do not demonstrate cardiac ischemia or cardiac dysfunction in healthy persons at high altitude, even when arterial $P_{O_2}$ was less than 30 mmHg. Those with arteriosclerotic disease may not have the same adaptive capabilities and intuitively seem more likely to suffer from acute cardiac events. Epidemiologic data, however, do not support this supposition. Morbidity and mortality from arteriosclerotic heart disease is reduced in persons with long-term residence at high altitude, and visitors apparently do not have increased risk of acute myocardial infarction. Recent work, however, suggested earlier onset of angina at high altitude compared with sea level. Congestive heart failure (CHF) may worsen in tourists arriving at the medium altitude of ski resorts, and it is related apparently to fluid retention rather than depressed ventricular function from hypoxia. Patients with CHF should therefore maintain or increase their diuretic regimen during travel to high altitude, and clinicians may want to consider low flow oxygen during sleep for CHF patients, at least for the first few nights. Patients' status postcoronary artery bypass grafting have trekked to altitudes over 5000 m without problems, the issue of safety having generated much debate. Overall, high altitude does not impose as much stress on the heart as would seem intuitively obvious. Further study will more clearly define subcategories of cardiac patients at risk.

Ascent to altitude produces a mild increase in blood pressure in normotensive persons, secondary to increased sympathetic tone; the matter has not been studied in hypertensives. Patients should continue hypertensive medications at altitude. No data suggest that hypertensives are more likely to succumb to any of the altitude illnesses, and in general, hypertension would not seem to be a contraindication to altitude exposure.

## Sickle Cell Disease

Even the modest simulated altitude of a pressurized aircraft (1500 to 2000 m) may cause persons with hemoglobin SC and sickle-thalassemia to have a vasoocclusive crisis. High altitude exposure without supplemental oxygen is considered a contraindication in these persons. Sickle cell trait is not considered an increased risk, although splenic infarction syndrome during heavy exercise at altitude has been reported in those with trait.

## Pregnancy

Pregnant residents of high altitude have an increased prevalence of hypertension, low-birth-weight infants, and neonatal hyperbilirubinemia. However, an increased incidence of pregnancy complications in lowlanders who visit high altitude has not been reported. The normal $P_{O_2}$ of the fetus is 29 to 33 mmHg, and the mild maternal hypoxia induced by traveling to resort-type altitudes does not generate significantly more hypoxic stress. Until more data become available, pregnant patients should not be advised to curtail reasonable activities they wish to undertake. Perhaps of more concern than mild hypoxia is the fact that high altitude locations are often remote from medical facilities, and patients need to be aware that without access to sophisticated medical care, complications could have more serious consequences than at home.

## BIBLIOGRAPHY

Bartsch P, Maggioini M, Ritter M, et al: Prevention of high-altitude pulmonary edema by nefedipine. *N Engl J Med* 325(18): 1284, 1991.

Bert P: *Barometric Pressure.* Bethesda, MD, Undersea Medical Society, 1978.

Blume FD, Boyer SJ, Braverman LE, et al: Impaired osmoregulation at high altitude. *JAMA* 252:524, 1984.

Dean AG, Yip R, Hoffmann RE: High incidence of mild acute mountain sickness in conference attendees at 10000 foot altitude. *J Wilderness Med* 1:86, 1990.

Fasules JW, Wiggins JW, Wolfe RR: Increased lung vasoreactivity in children from Leadville, Colorado after recovery from high altitude pulmonary edema. *Circulation* 72:957, 1985.

Hackett PH, Rennie ID: Rales, peripheral edema, retinal hemorrhage and acute mountain sickness. *Am J Med* 67:214, 1979.

Hackett PH, Rennie ID, Hofmeister SE, et al: Fluid retention and relative hypoventilation in acute mountain sickness. *Respiration* 43:321, 1982.

Hackett PH, Rennie ID, Levine HD: The incidence, importance, and prophylaxis of acute mountain sickness. *Lancet* 2:1149, 1976.

Hackett PH, Roach RC: Medical therapy of altitude illness. *Ann Emerg Med* 16:980, 1987.

Hackett PH, Roach RC: High altitude pulmonary edema. *J Wilderness Med* 1:3, 1990.

Hultgren HN, Marticorena E: High altitude pulmonary edema: Epidemiologic observations in Peru. *Chest* 74:372, 1978.

Johnson TS, Rock PB: Acute mountain sickness. *N Engl J Med* 319:841, 1988.

Karliner JS, Sarnquist FH, Graber DJ, et al: The electrocardiogram at extreme altitude: Experience on Mt. Everest. *Am Heart J* 109:505, 1985.

Kasic JF, Yaron M, Nicholas RA, et al: Treatment of acute mountain sickness: hyperbaric versus oxygen therapy. *Ann Emerg Med* 20(10):1109, 1991.

King SJ, Greenlee R, Goldings HJ: Acute mountain sickness (Letter). *N Engl J Med* 320:1492, 1989.

Levine BD, Yoshimura K, Kobayashi T, et al: Dexamethasone in the treatment of acute mountain sickness. *N Engl J Med* 321:1707, 1989.

Mairbaurl H, Schobersberger W, Oelz O, et al: Unchanged in vivo P50 at high altitude despite decreased erythrocyte age and elevated 2, 3 diphosphoglycerate. *J Appl Physiol* 68:1186, 1990.

Montgomery AB, Mills J, Luce JM: Incidence of acute mountain sickness at intermediate altitude. *JAMA* 261:732, 1989.

Mortimer EA, Monson RR, MacMahon B: Reduction in mortality from coronary heart disease in men residing at high altitude. *N Engl J Med* 296:581, 1977.

Oelz O, Maggiorini M, Ritter M, et al: Nifedipine for high altitude pulmonary edema. *Lancet* 2:1241, 1989.

Schoene RB, Roach RC, Hackett PH, et al: High altitude pulmonary edema and exercise at 4400 meters on Mt McKinley: Effect of expiratory positive airway pressure. *Chest* 87:330, 1985.

Sophocles AM: High-altitude pulmonary edema in Vail, Colorado, 1975–1982. *West J Med* 144:569, 1986.

Viault F: On the large increase in the number of red cells in the blood of the inhabitants of the high plateaus of South America, in West JB (ed): *High Altitude Physiology.* Stroudsberg, PA, Hutchinson Ross, 1981, pp 333–334.

Vock P, Fretz C, Franciolli M, et al: High-altitude pulmonary edema: Findings at high-altitude chest radiography and physical examination. *Radiology* 170:661, 1989.

Wohns RN: High altitude cerebral edema: A pathophysiological review. *Crit Care Med* 9:880, 1981.

# 166
# DYSBARISM
## Kenneth W. Kizer

## DYSBARIC DIVING CASUALTIES

There are now over 4 million recreational scuba[1] divers in the United States, and over 400,000 new sport divers are certified each year. In addition, diving is an integral part of many commercial and scientific activities (Table 166-1).

The health problems associated with diving are due to the hazards of the aquatic environment and the breathing of compressed gases at higher than normal atmospheric pressure. Table 166-2 categorizes a number of diving-related medical problems.

### Physical Principles

#### Pressure

Many adverse physical conditions are encountered in the underwater environment. These include cold, wetness, changes in light and sound conduction, increased density of the surrounding environment, and increased atmospheric pressure. Of these, the indirect or direct effects of pressure account for the majority of serious diving medical problems.

Pressure is force per unit area and is measured in a number of different units (Table 166-3). The weight of air at sea level is equal to 14.7 lb/in$^2$ (psi) or 1 atm absolute (ATA). Under water, pressure increases because of the weight of the water. Because water is much denser than air, large changes in pressure will accompany small fluctuations in depth. Thus (Table 166-4), at a depth of 33 ft of seawater (fsw) the pressure is 2 ATA, and at 165 fsw it is 6 ATA.[2] The proportionate change in pressure per unit depth is greatest near the surface and progressively diminishes with increasing depth. Because fresh water is less dense than saltwater, it takes a depth change of 34 ft of fresh water (ffw) to change the pressure 1 ATA. Scuba diving is generally done at pressure of less than 6 ATA, with the overwhelming majority in the 2- to 4-ATA range.

Because body tissues are composed mostly of water, which is not compressible, they are not directly affected by pressure changes. However, gases are compressible, and, consequently, gas-filled organs of the body are directly affected by pressure changes.

**Table 166-1.** Types of Commercial Diving

| | |
|---|---|
| Recovery of natural resources | Construction |
| Oil and natural gas | Piers and harbors |
| Minerals | Bridges and tunnels |
| Fish and shellfish | Dams |
| Pearls, corals, and shells | Underwater photography and motion |
| Algae | picture production |
| Wood (logging) | Marine studies |
| Aquaculture | Biology |
| Salvage and recovery operations | Geology |
| Maintenance and repair work | Archeology |
| Ship hulls | Other sciences |
| Nuclear power plants | Rescue and recovery operations |
| Bridges and tunnels | Sport diving instructors and tour guides |
| Piers and harbors | |
| Aquariums | |
| Water treatment plants | |

[1] *Scuba* is an acronym for *self-contained underwater breathing apparatus.*
[2] In diving and hyperbaric medicine the most commonly used units of pressure and depth are ATA and fsw.

**Table 166-2.** Medical Problems of Scuba Divers

Environmental exposure problems
  Motion sickness
  Near drowning
  Hypothermia
  Heat illness
  Sunburn
  Phototoxic and photoallergic reactions
  Irritant dermatitides
  Infectious diseases
  Mechanical trauma
Dysbarism
  Barotrauma
  Dysbaric air embolism
  Decompression sickness
  Dysbaric osteonecrosis
  Dysbaric retinopathy
  Hyperbaric cephalgia
Breathing gas-related problems
  Nitrogen narcosis
  Hypoxia
  Oxygen toxicity
  Hypo- or hypercarbia
  Carbon monoxide poisoning
  Nitrogen oxide toxicity
  Lipoid pneumonitis
Hazardous marine life
  Envenomations
  Animals that inflict trauma
  Toxic ingestions
Miscellaneous
  Hearing loss
  Carotogenic blackout
  Panic and other psychological problems

SOURCE: Adapted from Kizer KW: Management of dysbaric diving casualties. *Emerg Med Clin North Am* 1:659, 1983. Used by permission.

### Gas Laws

Diving physiology is largely explained by three gas laws.

The first is *Boyle's law,* which states that the volume of a gas is inversely proportional to its pressure at a constant temperature. This is expressed by the equation.

$$PV = K$$

where $P$ is pressure, $V$ is volume, and $K$ is a constant. Thus, as shown (see Table 166-4), when the pressure is doubled the volume of a unit of gas is halved, and conversely. Boyle's law explains the basic mechanism of all types of barotrauma.

The second is *Dalton's law,* which states that the pressure exerted by each gas in a mixture of gases is the same as it would exert if it alone occupied the same volume, or, alternatively, the total pressure of mixture of gases is equal to the sum of the partial pressures of the

**Table 166-3.** Pressure Equivalents

| 1 atmosphere absolute (ATA) | = 33 ft seawater (fsw)* |
|---|---|
| | = 5.5 fathoms seawater |
| | = 34 ft fresh water (ffw) |
| | = 14.7 psi |
| | = 760 mm Hg |
| | = 29.9 in Hg |
| | = 1.033 kg/cm$^2$ |
| | = 1.013 bar |
| | = 10.06 m |
| | = 0 atm gauge |

* 1 fsw = 0.445 psi = 0.0303 atm.
SOURCE: From Kizer KW: Management of dysbaric diving casualties. *Emerg Med Clin North Am* 1:659, 1983. Used by permission.

**Table 166-4.** Pressure-Volume Relationships According to Boyle's Law

|  | Depth, fsw | Gauge Pressure, atm* | Absolute Pressure, atm | Gas Volume, % | Bubble Diameter,† % |
|---|---|---|---|---|---|
| Air | 0 | 0 | 1 | 100 | 100 |
| Seawater | 33 | 1 | 2 | 50 | 79 |
|  | 66 | 2 | 3 | 33 | 69 |
|  | 99 | 3 | 4 | 25 | 63 |
|  | . | . | . | . | . |
|  | . | . | . | . | . |
|  | . | . | . | . | . |
|  | 165 | 5 | 6 | 17 | 54 |

\* Gauge pressure is always 1 atm less than absolute pressure.

† Bubble diameter is probably more important than volume in consideration of the ability of recompression to restore circulation to a gas-embolized blood vessel.

SOURCE: Adapted from Kizer KW: Management of dysbaric diving casualties. *Emerg Med Clin North Am* 1:659, 1983. Used by permission.

component gases. This is mathematically stated as

$$P_t = P_{O_2} + P_{N_2} + P_x$$

where $P_t$ is the total pressure, $P_{O_2}$ is the partial pressure of oxygen, $P_{N_2}$ is the partial pressure of nitrogen, and $P_x$ is the partial pressure of the remaining gases in the mixture. This law explains why the partial pressures of component gases in a mixture change proportionately to changes in ambient pressure even though their absolute concentrations remain constant. This law is fundamental to the understanding of decompression sickness and other breathing gas-related problems.

*Henry's law* states that the amount of gas dissolved in a given volume of fluid is proportional to the pressure of the gas with which it is in equilibrium. The formula is

$$\%X = P_X P_t \times 100$$

where $\%X$ is the amount of gas dissolved in a liquid, $P_X$ is the partial pressure of gas $X$ and $P_t$ is the total atmospheric pressure. This law explains why more inert gas (e.g., nitrogen) dissolves in the diver's body as ambient pressure is increased with descent and, conversely, is released from tissue with ascent.

### Direct Effects of Pressure—Barotrauma

The pressure-related diving syndromes can be divided into problems caused by the mechanical effects of pressure (i.e., barotrauma) and problems caused by breathing gases at elevated partial pressures (i.e., gas toxicities and decompression sickness [DCS]).

*Barotrauma* is the most common affliction of divers. It is defined as tissue damage resulting from contraction or expansion of gas spaces that occurs when the gas pressure in the body, or its compartments, is not equal to ambient pressure. For purposes of discussion, barotrauma can be viewed according to whether it occurs during descent or ascent.

### Barotrauma of Descent

Barotrauma of descent, or "squeeze," as it is known in common diving parlance, results from the compression of gas in enclosed spaces as ambient pressure increases with underwater descent. Gas pressure in the various air-filled spaces of the body is normally in equilibrium with the environment; however, if something obstructs the portals of gas exchange, pressure equalization is precluded. If the air-filled space is not collapsible, the resulting pressure imbalance will cause tissue distortion, vascular engorgement and muscosal edema, hemorrhage, and other tissue damage. The ears and paranasal sinuses are most likely to be affected by such a process.

Aural barotrauma is the most common type of barotrauma and is a major cause of morbidity among divers, experienced by essentially all divers at one time or another. There are three main types of aural barotrauma, depending on which part of the ear is affected, and they may occur singly or in combination.

The first type involves the external auditory canal and is generally referred to as *external ear squeeze,* or *barotitis externa.* The external ear canal normally communicates with the environment and, consequently, the air in the canal is replaced by water when a diver is submerged. However, if the external ear canal is occluded (e.g., by cerumen, foreign bodies, exostoses, or earplugs), water entry is prevented, and compression of the enclosed air with descent will have to be compensated for by tissue collapse, outward bulging of the tympanic membrane, or hemorrhage. This is typically manifested by pain or bloody otorrhea. Physical examination may reveal petechiae or blood-filled cutaneous blebs along the canal, along with erythema or rupture of the tympanic membrane. Treatment involves keeping the canal dry, prohibiting of swimming or diving until healed, and, in special cases, taking antibiotics and analgesics.

The next and by far the most common type of aural barotrauma is *middle ear squeeze,* or *barotitis media.* This results from a failure to equalize the middle ear and environmental pressures because of occlusion or dysfunction of the eustachian tube.

The eustachian tubes normally open and allow equalization of middle ear pressure when the pressure difference between the middle ear and pharynx reaches about 20 mm Hg. This can be facilitated by yawning, swallowing, or using various autoinflation techniques (e.g., the Valsalva or Frenzel maneuvers). If middle ear pressure equalization is not achieved, the diver will notice discomfort or pain when the pressure differential reaches 100 to 150 mm Hg or, roughly, when there has been a 20 percent reduction in middle ear gas volume. As the pressure differential is increased, mucosal engorgement and edema, hemorrhage, and inward bulging of the tympanic membrane develop. Eventually, these will be inadequate to compensate for the gas volume contraction, and the tympanic membrane ruptures. Fortunately, this is uncommon.

A number of factors may cause eustachian tube blockage or dysfunction—mucosal congestion secondary to upper respiratory infection, allergies, or smoking; mucosal polyps; excessively vigorous autoinflation maneuvers; and previous maxillofacial trauma. Persons with such conditions are at increased risk of middle ear barotrauma.

Divers having a middle ear squeeze usually complain of ear fullness or pain. As would be expected from the way that pressure changes with depth (see Table 166-4), most problems occur near the surface. The pain is substantial and usually causes the diver to abort the dive. If not, it will continue to worsen until the eardrum ruptures, at which time the diver may feel air bubbles escaping from the ear and experience disorientation, nausea, and vertigo secondary to the caloric stimulation of cold water entering the middle ear. This sequence has been responsible for cases of panic and near drowning.

The otoscopic appearance of the tympanic membrane in cases of middle ear squeeze varies according to the severity of the injury and can be graded according to the amount of hemorrhage in the eardrum, with grades running from 0 (symptoms only) to 5 (gross hemorrhage and rupture). Physical examination may also disclose blood around the nose or mouth and a mild conductive hearing loss, which is usually only temporary.

Treatment of middle ear squeeze involves abstinence from diving until the condition has resolved and use of decongestants, which may be combined with antihistamines if there is an allergic component to the eustachian tube dysfunction. A combination of oral and long-acting spray decongestants is usually most efficacious. Antibiotics should be used when there is a tympanic membrane rupture or a pre-existing infection, or after diving in polluted waters. No diving should be done until a perforated eardrum has healed. Oral analgesics or topical aural anesthetics may be needed for a couple of days. In general, eardrops should not be used when there is a tympanic membrane perforation. Ideally, an audiogram should be obtained in anyone having more than a trivial middle ear squeeze, and serial audiograms should be obtained in patients having hearing loss. Most middle ear squeezes will resolve without complication in 3 to 7 days. Prevention is preferable; a diver should refrain from diving when unable to easily equalize pressure in the ears and should always heed warning signs of ear pain.

Although less common, the third type of aural barotrauma, *inner ear barotrauma,* is much more serious than middle ear barotrauma because of possible permanently disabling injury to the cochleovestibular system. Inner ear barotrauma typically results from the sudden or rapid development of markedly different pressures between the middle and inner ear, such as may occur as a result of an overly forceful Valsalva maneuver intended to equalize the pressure in the middle ear or an exceptionally rapid descent during which the middle ear pressure is not equalized.

Patients with inner ear barotrauma typically are quite symptomatic, having a feeling of fullness or "blockage" of the affected ear, nausea, vomiting, nystagmus, diaphoresis, disorientation, or ataxia. The classic triad of symptoms indicating inner ear barotrauma is roaring tinnitus, vertigo, and deafness. The onset of these symptoms may occur soon after the injury or may be delayed many hours, depending on the specific type of inner ear injury and the diver's activities during and after the dive. Findings on physical examination may be normal or may reveal signs of middle ear barotrauma or vestibular dysfunction, and audiometry may demonstrate a mild to severe sensorineural hearing loss. Any scuba diver with a hearing loss or vestibular symptoms following a nondecompression dive should be considered to have inner ear barotrauma until shown otherwise.

Clinically, there appear to be four categories or mechanisms for these injuries: (1) hemorrhage within the inner ear (especially in the basal turn of the cochlea); (2) rupture of the Reissner's membrane, resulting in mixing of endolymph and perilymph; (3) fistulation of the round or oval window; and (4) a mixed injury involving a combination of any or all of the other three. Injury to the membranous labyrinth may be either implosive or explosive.

Hemorrhage within the inner ear usually is associated with findings of middle ear barotrauma, no or transient vestibular symptoms, and a diffuse mild to severe sensorineural hearing loss (SNHL). Treatment of these patients should consist of bed rest with head elevated, avoidance of strain or strenuous activities, and symptomatic measures, as needed. The potential for full recovery is excellent, with the hearing loss usually completely resolved in 3 weeks to 3 months.

Manifestations of a tear in Reissner's membrane are similar to those of inner ear hemorrhage, although a persistent localized SNHL remains commensurate with the area of membrane tear. Treatment is similar to that of inner ear hemorrhage.

Inner ear fistulas typically present with a mild high-frequency SNHL or a marked cochleovestibular deficit and no or little evidence of middle ear barotrauma. Initially, these should be treated with bed rest, avoidance of strain, and other symptomatic measures, as needed. Worsening of hearing or vestibular symptoms or persistence of significant vestibular symptoms after a few days indicates the need for surgical exploration and repair. Some authorities, however, recommend immediate tympanotomy if severe symptoms are present initially. Importantly, recompression is contraindicated unless DCS or air embolism is also suspected to be present.

Any of the paranasal sinuses may fail to equalize pressure during descent. Manifestations of sinus squeeze include a sensation of fullness or pressure in the affected sinus, pain, or hemorrhage. Predisposing conditions for barosinusitis include upper respiratory infections, sinusitis, nasal polyps, or anything else that impairs the free flow of air from sinus cavity to nose. The maxillary and frontal sinuses are most often affected (Fig. 166-1). Treatment for sinus squeeze is much the same as for middle ear squeeze although antibiotics are usually indicated in cases involving the frontal sinuses.

Squeeze can also affect any other gas space that does not equilibrate with ambient pressure. For example, conjunctival, scleral, and

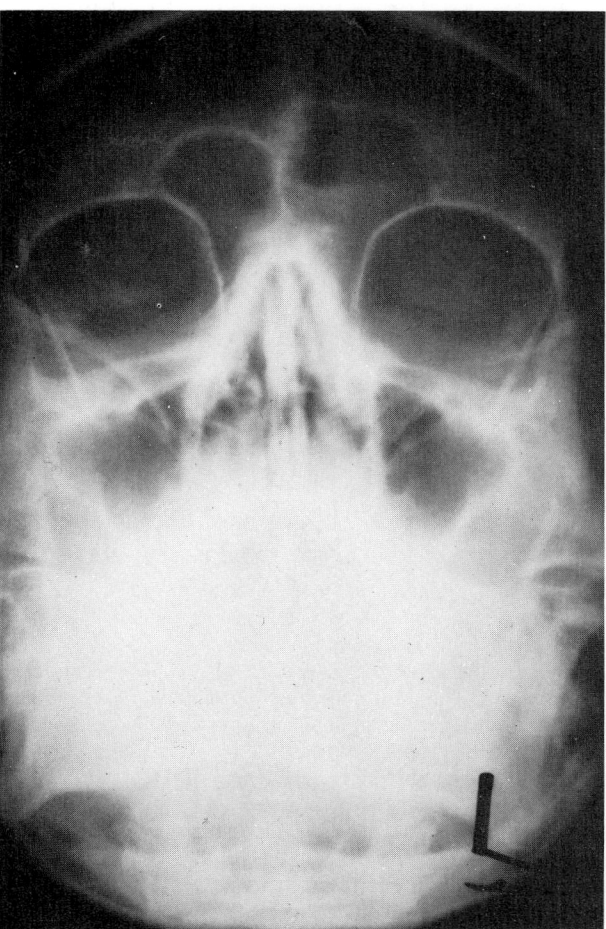

**Fig. 166-1.** Radiograph showing an air-fluid level in the left frontal sinus from a sinus squeeze. (Photograph by KW Kizer.)

periorbital hemorrhage may result if the diver fails to exhale into the mask during descent, resulting in telltale erythema, ecchymosis, and petechiae of the part of the face enclosed by the face mask—"face mask squeeze." If an area of skin is tightly enclosed by a dry diving suit a "suit squeeze" may occur. Although the appearance of these injuries may be spectacular, no special treatment is required, and they usually resolve in a few days.

Another special kind of squeeze may occur in divers who, while holding their breath, descend below the depth at which their total lung volume is reduced to less than residual volume. As occurs in other types of barotrauma of descent, the underventilated lung air spaces fill with tissue fluids and blood in an attempt to relieve the negative pressure. Clinical manifestations include chest pain, cough, hemoptysis, dyspnea, and pulmonary edema. Treatment includes administration of 100% oxygen, fluid replacement, and other supportive measures as clinically indicated. Because of the intrinsic lung injury and consequent potential for gas embolism, positive-pressure breathing (e.g., positive end-expiratory pressure or continuous positive airway pressure) should be avoided if possible. Very few divers attempt to free dive to depths likely to cause lung squeeze, and it is rare.

## Barotrauma of Ascent

If there has been adequate equilibration of the pressure in the body's air-filled spaces during descent, the gas in those spaces will expand according to Boyle's law as ambient pressure decreases with ascent. The resulting excess gas is normally vented to the atmosphere. However, if this is prevented by obstruction of the air passages, the expanding gases will distend the tissues surrounding them; the resulting damage is known as *barotrauma of ascent* and is the reverse process of squeeze.

Although the ears and sinuses may be affected by barotrauma of ascent, this is unusual, because impediment of air egress is highly unlikely if pressure equalization is achieved with descent. However, middle ear and sinus barotrauma of ascent, or *reverse squeeze,* can occur, especially in divers having upper respiratory congestion treated with a short-acting nasal spray whose vasoconstrictive effect wears off while the diver is submerged. Similarly, *alternobaric vertigo* (ABV) resulting from unequal vestibular stimulation due to asymmetric middle ear pressure may occur during ascent. Although usually only transient, ABV may be severe enough to cause panic. Rarely, it may last for several hours, or even a day or two, after a dive.

Three other types of barotrauma of ascent should be discussed. The first of these may occur with either ascent or descent, although more commonly with ascent, and is known as *barodontalgia,* or, less accurately, "tooth squeeze." Several specific conditions are associated with this problem (e.g., pulp decay, peridontal infections, or recent extraction sockets or fillings), but it may be due to anything that causes a pressure disequilibrium in an air-filled space in or about a tooth. Although rare and usually self-limited, anyone presenting with a toothache after diving should be referred for dental evaluation after maxillary sinus squeeze has been excluded.

Another unusual type of barotrauma of ascent is gastrointestinal barotrauma, which is also known as *aerogastralgia,* or "gas in the gut." This occurs most commonly in novice scuba divers, who are more prone to aerophagia, and is caused by expansion of intraluminal bowel gas as ambient pressure is decreased during ascent. Other predisposing conditions include repeated performance of the Valsalva maneuver in the head-down position (which forces air into the stomach), drinking carbonated beverages or eating a heavy meal before diving (especially one containing legumes or other flatogenic substances), or chewing gum while diving. Symptoms of gastrointestinal barotrauma include abdominal fullness, colicky abdominal pain, belching, and flatulence. It is rarely severe because most divers will readily vent any excess bowel gas during ascent; however, it has been know to cause syncope and shocklike states. Actual gastric rupture from GI barotrauma has occurred, but this is exceedingly rare.

The last and most serious type of barotrauma of ascent is pulmonary barotrauma (PBT). Several different injuries can result from PBT of ascent, and these are collectively referred to as the pulmonary overpressurization syndrome (POPS) or "burst lung" (Table 166-5).

Diving equipment is designed to deliver compressed gas to the diver at the same pressure as the surrounding environment (e.g., at 33 fsw the diver breathes gas at a pressure of 2 ATA). Consequently, the compressed gas will expand during ascent according to Boyle's law, and the diver must allow the expanding gas to escape from the lungs, or it will rupture and dissect into the surrounding tissue. The resultant injury will depend on the location and amount of escaped gas. Overt symptoms may appear immediately on surfacing or may be delayed for several hours.

Mediastinal and subcutaneous emphysema are the most common

**Table 166-5.** Manifestations of Pulmonary Barotrauma

Pneumomediastinum
Subcutaneous emphysema
Pneumopericardium
Pneumothorax
Pulmonary interstitial emphysema
Pneumoperitoneum
Diffuse alveolar hemorrhage
Arterial gas embolisma.
   Brain
   Heart
   Visceral

forms of the POPS. The patient usually presents with gradually increasing hoarseness, neck fullness, and substernal chest pain several hours after diving. Dyspnea, dysphagia, syncope, and other symptoms may be present as well. The history is usually diagnostic, although radiographs are indicated to verify the location of gas and exclude the presence of a pneumothorax (Fig. 166-2).

The development of a pneumothorax as a result of PBT is uncommon but especially serious, for intrapleural gas cannot be released to the environment and is likely to progress to tension pneumothorax during ascent, leading to syncope, shock, or unconsciousness on surfacing.

Except for pneumothorax, which may require needle aspiration or tube thoracostomy, treatment of uncomplicated POPS typically requires only observation, rest, and, sometimes, supplemental oxygen. Recompression is necessary only in extremely severe cases.

## Air Embolism

The most feared complication of PBT is air embolism. Indeed, dysbaric air embolism (DAE), or arterial gas embolism (AGE), is one of the most dramatic and serious injuries associated with diving and is a major cause of death and disability among sport divers.

DAE results from the entry of gas bubbles into the systemic circulation through ruptured pulmonary veins. This usually occurs at the alveolar or terminal bronchiole level. After passing through the heart, bubbles lodge in small arteries, occluding the more distal circulation. The resulting manifestations will depend on the location of the occlusion. Depending on the site, even minute quantities of gas can have disastrous consequences.

DAE usually presents immediately after a diver surfaces, at which time the high intrapulmonic pressure resulting from lung overexpansion is relieved, which allows air bubble-laden blood to return to the heart. Although the classic history is that the diver ascends rapidly because of running out of air, panic, or some similar circumstance, this is not always the case. Localized overinflation also may result from focally increased elastic recoil of the lungs in some divers. It is axiomatic that symptoms of DAE develop within 10 min of surfacing from a dive, although most often they are clearly evident within the first 2 min.

The presenting manifestations of DAE are sudden, dramatic, and often life-threatening. Coronary occlusion and cardiac arrest or arrhythmias may occur, although the brain is by far the most often affected organ. The neurologic manifestations are typical of an acute stroke, such as mono- or multiplegia, focal paralysis, sensory disturbance, blindness, deafness, vertigo, dizziness, confusion, convulsions, or aphasia. Asymmetric multiplegias are the most common presentation, and the differentiation of DAE from severe neurologic DCS is sometimes impossible. *Sudden loss of consciousness on surfacing should always be assumed to be due to gas embolism until proved otherwise.* Other reported clinical findings such as visualization of bubbles in the retinal arteries or Liebermeister's sign (a sharply circumscribed area of glossal pallor) are exceedingly rare.

All cases of suspected DAE must be referred for recompression treatment—hyperbolic oxygen treatment—as quickly as possible. This is the primary and essential treatment for this condition, as is discussed later.

Some patients with very severe initial neurologic symptoms may improve spontaneously. The mechanism of spontaneous recovery is not clear. Nonetheless, such patients should still be referred for recompression because even subtle dysbaric injuries may become irreversible without definitive care. Before recompression, pneumothorax should be ruled out.

## Indirect Effects of Pressure

Nitrogen narcosis and DCS sickness may develop as a result of breathing gases at higher-than-normal atmospheric pressure.

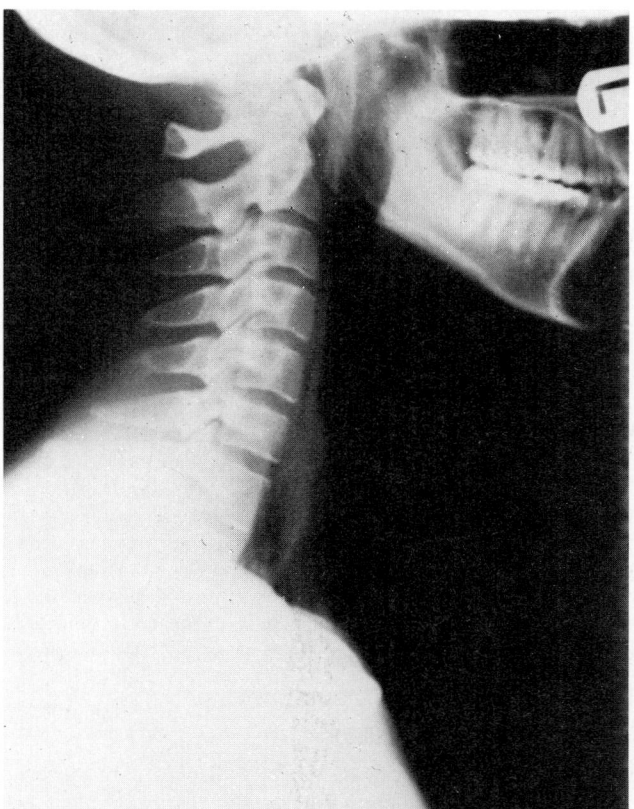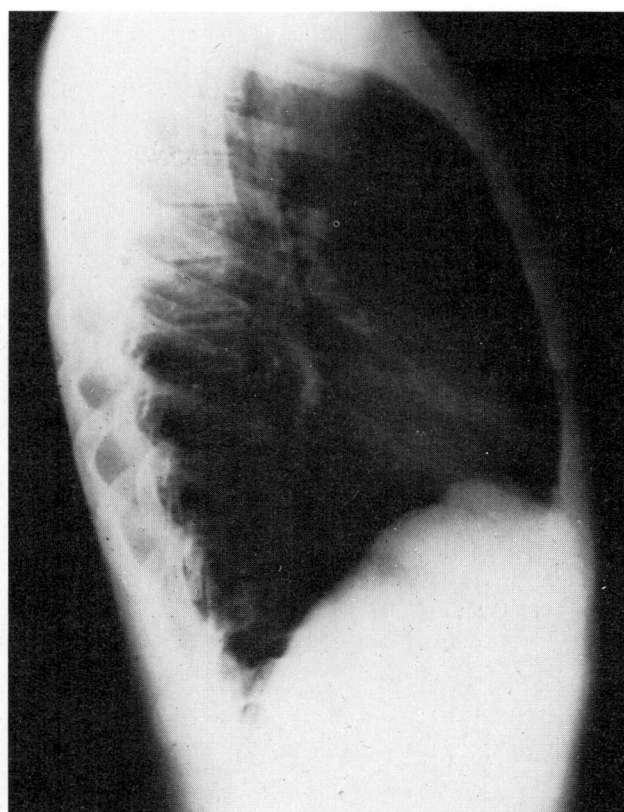

**Fig. 166-2.** Radiographs showing air dissection through the mediastinum and into the neck from pulmonary barotrauma. (Photograph by KW Kizer.)

## Nitrogen Narcosis

Nitrogen and other lipid-soluble inert gases have an anesthetic effect at elevated partial pressures. The narcotic effects are similar to those of alcohol and become evident in most divers between 70 and 100 fsw. Many divers are so markedly impaired at 200 fsw that they can do no useful work, and at depths over 300 to 350fsw unconsciousness ensues. Although narcotic effects are reversed as the $P_{N_2}$ decreases with ascent, nitrogen narcosis is not an uncommon precipitating factor in diving accidents and may impair a diver's memory of the circumstances leading up to the accident.

## Decompression Sickness

Decompression sickness is a multisystem disorder resulting from the liberation of inert gas from solution with the formation of gas bubbles in blood and body tissues when ambient pressure is decreased. The critical factor in its pathogenesis is increased tissue absorption of inert gas, which in most diving situations is nitrogen.

As an air-breathing diver descends, ambient pressure increases, giving rise to a positive pressure gradient of nitrogen from alveoli to blood to tissue. After a time at depth this gradient will diminish, eventually becoming zero as a new equilibrium is reached. The time that it takes for the new equilibrium to be achieved will depend on the alveolar-to-tissue inert gas gradient, the tissue blood flow, and the ratio of blood-to-tissue inert gas solubility. Consequently, the rate at which a diver reaches a new inert gas equilibrium will be an exponential function of the diffusion and perfusion characteristics of the different tissues.

The tissue absorption of increased gas is the first step toward DCS, but it is only when ambient pressure is, in turn, decreased too rapidly to allow the diffusion of inert gas from tissues that DCS occurs.

The pathophysiology of decompression sickness results from both the mechanical and biophysical effects of bubbles (Fig. 166-3). The major mechanical effect of bubbles in DCS is vascular occlusion. Of note, the bubbles in DCS form primarily in the venous circulation and thus impair venous return, in contrast to the more usual arterial occlusion that occurs in most other conditions. However, the bubbles in DCS can form anywhere, such as in lymphatics, or intracellularly or extravascularly. Lymphedema, cellular distention and rupture, and intercellular dislocation can all compound the effects of vascular occlusion. Also, venous gas emboli may cause paradoxical arterial embolization via intrapulmonic and intracardiac shunts. Indeed, it is now clear that some dysbaric cerebral injuries are due to paradoxical embolization through previously unrecognized right-to-left intracardiac shunts that may only be open during abnormal pressure conditions found during diving. For example, in two series, 60 to 80 percent of serious neurologic DCS patients had paradoxical shunting. Such paradoxical embolization may explain the high frequency of apparent combined DCS/air embolism noted in some series.

Bubbles also exert a variety of biophysical effects due to blood-bubble surface interaction. In essence, bubbles are viewed by the immune system as foreign matter, and they incite an inflammatory reaction. The key step in the process is activation of Hageman factor, which, in turn, activates the intrinsic clotting mechanisms and kinin and complement systems, which results in platelet activation, cellular clumping, lipid embolization, increased vascular permeability, interstitial edema, and microvascular sludging. The net effect of all these processes is decreased tissue perfusion and ischemic injury.

The clinical manifestations of DCS are protean (Table 166-6), but the joints and spinal cord are most often affected. Technically, the term *bends* refers only to the musculoskeletal form of DCS, but it is commonly used in a generic sense to mean any type of DCS. The various forms of DCS have also been arbitrarily categorized as either types I or II, with type I referring to the mild forms of DCS (skin,

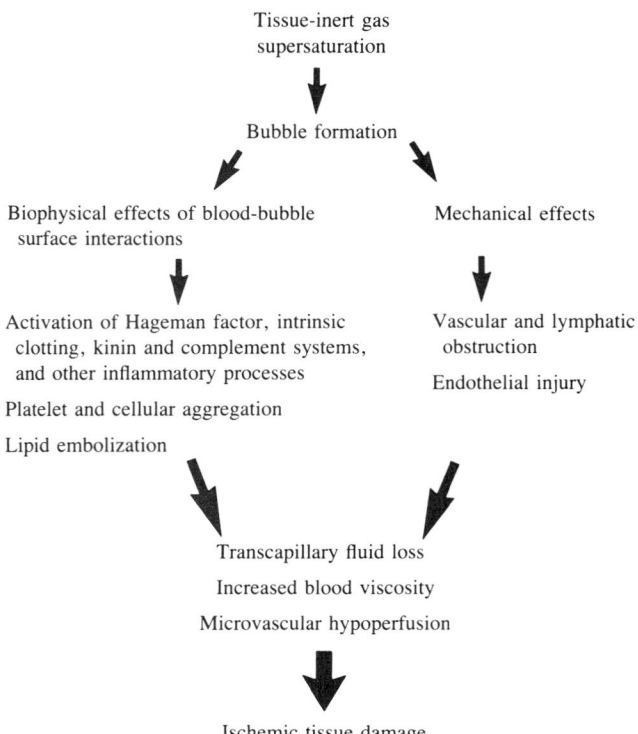

**Fig. 166-3.** Schematic representation of the pathogenesis of decompression sickness. (Adapted from Kizer KW: Management of dysbaric diving casualties. *Emerg Med Clin North Am* 1:659, 1983. Used by permission.)

lymphatic, and musculoskeletal systems) and type II including the neurologic and other serious types. Although this latter categorization is firmly entrenched in the literature, it is clinically more meaningful to refer to the systems affected when discussing patients with DCS.

Cutaneous manifestations of DCS include pruritus, subcutaneous emphysema, and scarlatiniform, erysipeloid, or mottled rashes. Localized swelling or peau d'orange may result from lymphatic obstruction.

Periarticular joint pain is typically described as a deep, dull ache, although it may be throbbing or sharp. There may be a vague area of numbness or dysesthesia around the affected joint. Movement of the affected extremity usually aggravates the pain, but inflation of a blood pressure cuff around the involved joint may relieve the pain for as long as the cuff is inflated. The shoulders and elbows are the joints most often affected in scuba divers, although essentially any joint may be involved.

Neurologic DCS may be manifested by a vast array of symptoms and signs. In fact, essentially any symptom is compatible with neurologic DCS. Classically, however, neurologic DCS involves the lower thoracic, lumbar, and sacral portions of the spinal cord and produces

**Table 166-6.** Forms of Decompression Sickness

Cutaneous ("skin bends")
Lymphatic
Musculoskeletal (the "bends" or pain-only bends)
Neurologic
    Spinal cord
    Cerebral
    Cerebellar (the "staggers")
    Inner ear
    Peripheral nerves
Pulmonary (the "chokes")
Cardiovascular (decompression shock)
Visceral

paraplegia or paraparesis, lower extremity paresthesias, and bladder dysfunction. Historically, urinary retention was such a frequent manifestation of spinal cord DCS that a urethral catheter used to be part of the diver's standard equipment. Hallenbeck and colleagues have convincingly demonstrated that at least some cases of spinal cord DCS result from venous infarction of the cord due to obstruction of venous drainage in the epidural vertebral venous plexus.

Pulmonary DCS results from massive venous air embolization and usually does not become symptomatic until at least 10 percent of the pulmonary vascular bed is obstructed. Signs and symptoms include chest pain, cough, dyspnea, shock, and pulmonary edema. The clinical course is often fulminant and downhill.

Many divers develop intravascular bubbles but no apparent illness; these have been called "silent bubbles" and their clinical significance is unclear.

A variety of laboratory abnormalities may be demonstrated in DCS, but most of them have little clinical relevance to acute care. Two tests that may be useful, though, are the urine specific gravity and hematocrit, because intravascular volume depletion and hemoconcentration are common in serious DCS. These two tests can help guide fluid replacement, which is an integral part of therapy.

Dysbaric casualties should be rapidly referred for hyperbaric treatment. However, the patient should also be evaluated for life-threatening nondysbaric injuries and, if present, resuscitation commenced.

## Treatment of Diving Casualties

### The Diving Accident History

Most diving problems can be properly diagnosed by history and physical examination alone. The specific diving accident history should encompass the following key points.

1. The type of diving engaged in and the equipment used. Some kinds of diving or certain types of equipment are associated with specific problems (e.g., hypercarbia or oxygen toxicity with re-breathing apparatus). And always make sure that the patient was actually breathing compressed air before sending him or her for recompression treatment.
2. The number, depth, bottom time, and surface interval between repetitive dives for all dives in the 72 h preceding symptom onset. Even though this information may not be especially meaningful to you, having it available will facilitate communication with the diving medicine consultant, who will want to ascertain whether required decompression steps were omitted.
3. In-water decompression. Again, this is relevant to the determination of the likelihood of the diver having DCS.
4. In-water recompression. Except in very unusual situations using 100% oxygen, full face mask, and other specialized support, in-water recompression should never be attempted. Recompression with compressed air should not be done, for it almost always leaves the diver in worse condition than originally and is fraught with other hazards.
5. Site of diving (e.g., ocean, lake, or quarry) and environmental conditions (e.g., water temperature, amount of current) associated with the dive. Other things being equal, DCS is more likely to occur after diving in cold water, but nondysbaric problems related to the environment (e.g., motion sickness) must be excluded.
6. Primary diving activity (e.g., spearfishing, photography). DCS is more likely after an arduous dive.
7. Presence of predisposing factors. A number of factors have been anecdotally related to the development of DCS. These include advanced age (decreased tissue perfusion), obesity (increased absorption of inert gas), dehydration, recent alcohol intoxication, cold water (decreased peripheral perfusion), vigorous underwater exercise (increased gas uptake), local physical injury (decreased local perfusion), and multiple repetitive dives in unacclimatized individuals (gradual buildup of inert gas).

8. Dive complications. These include running out of air, marine animal envenomation, mechanical trauma, or some other unexpected event. Musculoskeletal pain may be due to overexertion or muscle strain, and numbness in an extremity may be from a jellyfish sting rather than DCS.

9. Predive and postdive activities. Activities such as jogging and unpressurized airplane travel after diving may precipitate DCS. Likewise, trivial dysbaric symptoms may become severe after similar activities.

10. Onset of symptoms. Certain conditions are more likely to occur at given times in the dive profile, and a differential scheme can be derived on the basis of time of symptom onset.

## Differential Diagnosis of Diving Accidents

In general, a scuba dive can be divided into five stages, each of which is associated with characteristic problems.

### The Predive Surface Phase

The predive surface phase includes all activities prior to going underwater and beginning to breathe compressed air. This often involves considerable surface swimming to the dive site. The most often encountered problems during this phase of the dive are motion sickness, hyperventilation, mechanical trauma, near drowning, and untoward marine animal encounters.

### Descent Phase

The primary problems associated with descent are the squeeze syndromes, especially aural barotrauma, although inner ear barotrauma and ABV may also occur. Similarly, carbon monoxide poisoning, hypoxia, or other breathing gas problems may develop early in the dive.

### At-Depth or Bottom Phase

Overall, few problems occur "on the bottom," and the most likely ones are mechanical trauma or encounters with dangerous marine life. Nitrogen narcosis may contribute to an underwater accident. Inner ear barotrauma or gas mixture problems may first become symptomatic at this time even though they occurred earlier.

### Ascent Phase

Again, barotrauma is the problem most often encountered with ascent although much less frequently than during descent. The relationship of POPS, ABV, and inner ear barotrauma with ascent have already been discussed. Gas mixture problems may become manifest at this time, and hypercarbia can be experienced toward the end of a dive. DCS may occasionally occur while a diver is still submerged; if this happens it usually implies a very serious problem.

### Postdive Surface Phase

The postdive surface phase is divided into immediate (within 10 min of surfacing) and delayed (after 10 min). Any symptom occurring in the immediate postdive phase should be considered an air embolism until shown otherwise. Any symptom that begins more than 10 min after the dive should be viewed as DCS until otherwise explained. More than half of all DCS patients will become symptomatic in the first hour after surfacing, with most of the rest experiencing symptoms within 6 h. A very few patients (1 to 2 percent) may first note their symptoms 24 to 48 h after diving. Other problems that may be first noted in the delayed postdive phase include mild forms of the POPS, sequelae of barotrauma, inner ear barotrauma, motion sickness, exhaustion, irritant or venomous dermatoses, and nondysbaric conditions related to physical activity.

## Immediate Management

The victim should be rescued from the water and life support measures begun as needed. Hypothermia should be considered an aggravating factor in every aquatic accident victim.

If DAE is suspected, it is recommended that the patient be maintained supine in the field and during transport. Placement in the Trendelenburg or Durant positions is no longer recommended because of the uncertain benefit of such maneuvers and concerns about causing or aggravating cerebral edema (especially if left in the head-down position for longer than 30 to 60 min) and the increased respiratory difficulty attendant to being in such positions.

Supplemental 100% oxygen should always be given as soon as possible, being best administered by mask at 6 to 8 L/min. This facilitates offgassing of the nitrogen bubbles and improves oxygenation of damaged tissues.

Depending on local circumstances, patients with suspected DAE or DCS may be taken directly to the recompression chamber (Fig. 166-4) or may need emergency department intervention. Whichever the case, transportation should be as expeditious as possible. If air transportation is used, the patient should be subjected to the least possible pressure reduction so as not to cause any further gas expansion. Either a low-flying helicopter or light airplane, capable of flight at 1000 ft (300 m) or less, should be used. Alternatively, aircraft that can be pressurized to 1 ATA (e.g., Lear jet, Cessna Citation, or C-130 Hercules) can be used.

Advanced life support drugs should be administered according to the victim's condition and standard protocols. In general, most DCS victims will be at least mildly volume depleted, so parenteral and oral (if the patient is alert) fluids should be given at a brisk rate unless they are contraindicated for other reasons.

Although high-dose parenteral corticosteroids have been widely recommended and used in the past two decades as an adjunct to recompression treatment of both neurologic DCS and DAE, little evidence supports their use. The use of glucocorticoids became prevalent based on the belief that they were beneficial in the treatment of cerebral edema, shock, and other conditions pertinent to DCS, but their benefit in many of these other conditions is now questioned. A few anecdotal cases suggesting that steroids are beneficial, either alone or with other pharmacologic interventions combined with standard recompression therapy, have been reported, but there have been no published clinical series or controlled trials demonstrating their efficacy. In contrast, recent controlled studies of high-dose parenteral dexamethasone or methyl prednisolone in DCS-affected dogs showed that the use of glucocorticoids as an adjunct to conventional hyperbaric oxygen treatment produced no benefit and even suggested that the steroid-treated animals did less well.

If the need for recompression or the location of the nearest hyperbaric treatment facility is uncertain, assistance is available 24 h a day through the National Diving Alert Network at Duke University, (919) 684-8111.

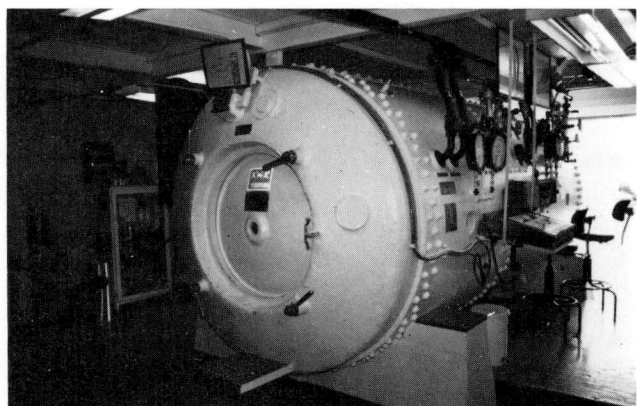

**Fig. 166-4.** Typical multiplace recompression chamber. The two compartments can be pressurized independently of each other up to at least 6 ATA, and as many as 12 persons can be seated in the chamber. (Photograph by KW Kizer.)

## Hyperbaric Treatment

Pressure and oxygen are the keystones of treatment for DCS and DAE and are administered according to well-established protocols. Various types of hyperbaric chambers may be used for treatment, and the relative merits of one type or another need not be recounted here.

The outcome of recompression treatment will, of course, depend on the severity of the disease, the delay in commencing hyperbaric treatment, and the victim's health prior to the accident. Overall, 80 to 90 percent success rates have been reported from a variety of sources, and even though recompression is generally believed to be more likely to be beneficial the sooner that it is commenced after the onset of symptoms, it should not be refused to someone who presents 2, 3, or more days after an accident, for dramatic recoveries have been reported after treatment delays of 10 days or longer. It is not possible to determine in advance what the effect of a delay in recompression will be for any individual patient.

## Postrecompression Evaluation

Because recompression treatment does not always result in complete resolution of dysbaric neurologic injury and because occasional situations arise when the differential diagnosis of acute diving-related neurologic dysfunction includes intracranial hemorrhage, trauma, or other nondysbaric injury, it is sometimes important to be able to characterize the site, extent, and origin of central nervous system (CNS) lesions beyond what can be achieved by the traditional means of history and physical examination.

Both computed tomography (CT) and magnetic resonance imaging (MRI) have been used in this regard. Regrettably, conventional CT has not been found to be an efficient investigative tool for the posttreatment evaluation of DCS, and CT imaging of spinal cord lesions (which constitute the majority of neurologic DCS) is not feasible. In contrast, limited clinical data support the feasibility and efficacy of MRI of these conditions, especially when intracranial injury is present.

## BLAST INJURY

The phenomenon of blast injury has been recognized for as long as human beings have used explosives although it has been mainly a wartime concern. However, in the past few decades there has been a dramatic increase in the incidence of peacetime civilian explosive blast injuries because of the popularity of the homemade bomb as a vehicle of social protest and the continued hazard of explosions in mining, grain storage, and other industries. In addition, blast injuries remain a prominent cause of fire-related morbidity.

### Blast Physics and Terminology

*Explosives* are materials that are rapidly converted into gases when detonated. *Blast* and *blast injury* are, respectively, general terms used to describe this gaseous decomposition and the damage occurring in an organism subjected to the pressure field produced by an explosion.

Blasts are characterized by the release of large quantities of energy in the form of pressure and heat, with the exact amount depending on the type and amount of explosive. If the explosion in confined within some sort of casing (e.g., a bomb), the pressure will rupture the housing and eject the resulting fragments at high velocity. The remaining energy is transmitted to the surrounding environment in the form of a blast wave, blast winds, ground shock, and fire.

The *blast wave* begins as a single pulse of increased pressure that rises to peak levels within a few milliseconds and then rapidly falls to a minimum pressure that is lower than the original atmospheric pressure (Fig. 166-5). It is propagated outward radially from the explosion, with the sharply marginated periphery of the sphere becoming the blast, overpressure, or shock wave, as it has been variously called. The duration and level of the high-pressure peak depends on the na-

**Table 166-7.** Selected Pressure Effects

| Pressure, psi* | Effect |
|---|---|
| 5 | Possible tympanic membrane rupture |
| 15 | 50% incidence of tympanic membrane rupture |
| 30 | Possible lung injury |
| 75 | 50% incidence of lung injury |
| 100 | Possible fatal injuries |
| 200 | Death more likely than not |

* 1 psi = 51.7 mm Hg.

ture of the explosive, the conducting medium, and the distance from the detonation point. This blast wave pressure peak determines the *overpressure* that an object in its path is subjected to and is the main determinant of primary blast injury. Conversely, the negative pressure wave, or suction of the blast wave, lasts several times longer than the high-pressure wave but can never be greater than −700 mm Hg (−14.7 psi). Representative pressure effects are listed in Table 166-7.

The rapidly expanding gases from an explosion also displace air, causing it to move away at very high velocity and produce transient *blast winds* that travel immediately behind the shock front of the blast wave. The blast wave may also accelerate loose objects (e.g., people) through the air, causing acceleration-deceleration injuries. In the immediate vicinity of an explosion this *windage* can cause atomization, or total disintegration, of a body, evisceration, or traumatic amputations, depending on the force of the explosion. Illustrative of the force of such winds, an overpressure of about 5200 mm Hg (100 psi) produces a blast wind having a velocity of about 2400 kph (1500 mph).

In addition to the amount and duration of overpressure caused by an explosion, the overall effect of the blast wave will also depend on the exact waveform of the overpressure (i.e., its rise time), the victim's body mass and orientation to the explosion, the presence of deflecting and reflecting surfaces in the environment, and the medium through which the shock wave is conducted. For example, because of the greater density of water and its relative incompressibility, blast waves produced by underwater explosions travel much faster and farther than those produced by terrestrial explosions. Consequently,

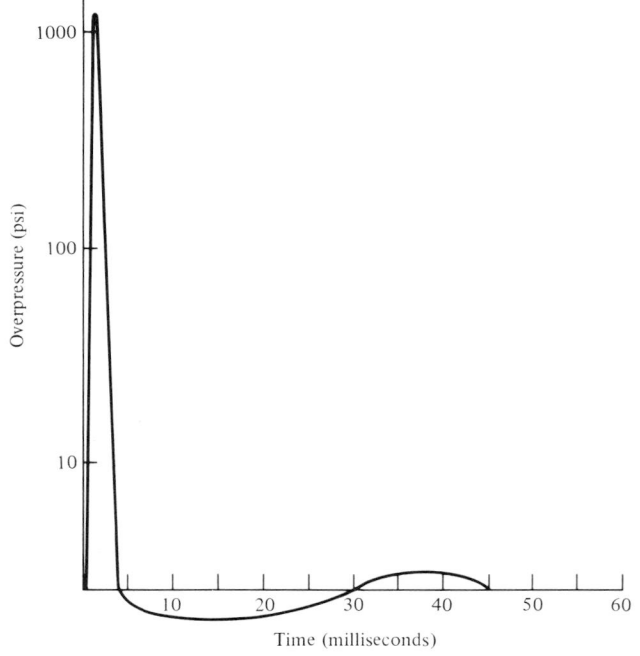

**Fig. 166-5.** The general form of a blast wave − 700 mmHg (− 14.7 psi).

blast injuries in water occur at greater distances from the detonation point and tend to be more severe. Underwater blast injury has other peculiarities, too, but these are beyond the scope of this discussion.

## Categories and Manifestations of Blast Injury

Explosive blast injuries can be divided into four categories (Table 166-8).

### Primary Blast Injury

*Type I,* or *primary, blast injury* results directly from the sudden changes in environmental pressure caused by the blast wave. Tissues vary in their susceptibility to primary blast injury, with homogeneous or solid tissues being at least risk because they are essentially noncompressible and merely vibrate as a whole when subjected to a blast wave. Conversely, gas-filled organs are compressible and have tissue-gas interfaces, which means that displacement occurs wherever tissues of different densities interface, resulting in tissue distortion and tearing. Thus, primary blast injury mainly affects organs containing air and causes the most severe damage at the junctions between tissues, where loose, poorly supported tissue is displaced beyond its elastic limit.

There are three general mechanisms whereby a blast shock wave can damage living tissue. The first of these is known as *spalling* and occurs when a shock wave traveling through a medium of higher density (e.g., liquid) passes into a medium of lower density (e.g., gas), creating a negative reflection at the interface and, thus, fragmenting the surface of the heavier medium. This is analogous to hitting the outside of a rusty bucket with a hammer, which causes flakes to come off inside the bucket.

The second mechanism is implosion of gas-filled spaces as the high pressure in the surrounding fluid or solid compresses these spaces. Similarly, because there is a pressure differential between the air-filled and vascular spaces, blood and fluid are forced into the air-filled spaces. This mechanism is of particular importance in the lungs, where it contributes to pulmonary hemorrhage. In addition, as the negative pressure wave follows the initial positive pressure, smaller internal secondary explosions occur as the compressed gas reexpands.

Third, tissues of different densities will be accelerated and decelerated at different rates relative to each other, producing shearing forces that can tear or otherwise damage the tissue.

The organs most vulnerable to primary blast injuries are the ears, lungs, CNS, and gastrointestinal tract. Abdominal visceral injury is relatively rare in air blast casualties but is of considerable concern in persons exposed to underwater blasts.

#### Otolaryngologic Manifestations

The ears are most often affected by explosive blasts, with hearing loss being the primary manifestation. Hearing can be damaged by one of three ways. First, the tympanic membranes may rupture. This usually occurs in adults at a pressure differential between the middle and external ears of around 360 mm Hg (7 psi), and most often presents as a linear perforation of the pars tensa. The second way is dislocation of the ossicles, which may accompany tympanic membrane rupture or occur as the sole injury. Finally, deafness may result from blast effects on the inner ear, causing perilymph fistula and other damage. In addition to hearing loss, primary symptoms of inner ear damage include vertigo and tinnitus.

The paranasal sinuses are also susceptible to blast injury, usually manifesting barotraumatic damage similar to the squeeze syndromes that occur with compressed air diving.

#### Pulmonary Manifestations

The lungs are generally the organs most severely affected by blast injury, and these injuries are likely to present a threat to life. (Of course, the severe injuries resulting from windage in the immediate vicinity of the explosion are also life-threatening.) The blast wave causes widespread alveolar damage because of its effects on tissue-gas interfaces, producing interstitial and intra-alveolar hemorrhage and edema, parenchymal and pleural lacerations, and alveolar-venous fistulas. Because of the widespread nature of this damage a variety of specific injuries may be found, including pulmonary edema, pneumothorax and other extra-alveolar air syndromes, and air embolism. Similarly, pulmonary contusions result from compression of the lung between the spine, thoracic wall, and rising diaphragm, as well as from being thrown against solid objects in the environment.

The actual symptoms experienced by victims of blast lung injury will vary with the severity and nature of their specific injuries, but, in general, they will present with dyspnea, shortness of breath, chest pain, hemoptysis, rales, rhonchi and signs of pulmonary edema or hemorrhage, as well as symptoms of the POPS.

#### Gastrointestinal Manifestations

Blast injuries to the stomach and bowels are due to damage at tissue-gas interfaces, producing hemorrhage into the wall and lumen along with perforations, which tend to be multifocal. Because the large bowel usually contains more gas than the small bowel, it tends to be more severely affected. Common clinical manifestations include abdominal pain, melena, signs of peritonitis, and free air in the abdomen. Evisceration and other gross damage may be found in victims who were very close to the detonation site, but these types of injury are nearly always fatal.

#### Neurologic Manifestations

Blast injuries of the CNS are of two main types. First are the direct shock wave effects, which produce a concussion syndrome and various types of intra- and extra-axial hemorrhage, and second are the effects of cerebral air embolism. As with dysbaric diving casualties, the specific neurologic manifestations of air embolism are myriad.

### Other Categories of Blast Injury

*Type II,* or *secondary, blast injuries* are due largely to the blast wind and result from the victim being struck by flying debris. Conversely, *type III,* or *tertiary, blast injuries* are those that result from the victim being displaced through space by the blast wind and impacting a stationary object; this sudden deceleration usually causes more harm than the acceleration through space. *Type IV blast injuries* include a wide variety of injuries resulting from inhalation of dust and toxic gases, exposure to radiation, thermal burns, and so on.

The myriad number of bodily insults that can result from these latter types of blast injury are far too numerous to list here. Of particular concern, though, are the traumatic amputations, occurring in about 25 percent of severely wounded victims, and liver, spleen, or other visceral injury produced from the acceleration-deceleration forces of the blast wind. Likewise, bomb casing fragments or missiles such

**Table 166-8.** Categories of Blast Injury

| Category | Injury Caused by | Primary Target Organs |
|---|---|---|
| I. Primary blast injury | Blast wave | Ears, lungs, GI tract, CNS |
| II. Secondary blast injury | Victim struck by flying debris | Integument, CNS, eyes, musculoskeletal system |
| III. Tertiary blast injury | Bodily displacement, i.e., victim impact with stationary objects | Abdominal viscera, CNS, lungs, integument, musculoskeletal system |
| IV. Miscellaneous | Inhalation of dust or toxic gases, thermal burns, radiation, other | Lungs, integument, eyes |

as nails, nuts and bolts, screws, ball bearings, etc., can cause high-velocity missile injuries.

## Management of Blast Casualties

Blast injury victims should be managed in the same manner as any multiple trauma victim, except that particular attention should be directed to the respiratory system. This includes giving special attention to maintenance of a patent airway (especially when maxillofacial, cervical spine, or other head and neck injuries are present), administering supplemental oxygen, judiciously using intravenous fluids and analgesics, evacuating pneumo- and hemothoraxes, and promptly implementing mechanical ventilation if signs of respiratory failure or inadequate oxygenation are present. Although positive pressure ventilation may be necessary to maintain adequate oxygenation, its use is fraught with hazard because the diffuse alveolar-capillary damage present in blast lung greatly increases the risk of causing extraalveolar extravasation of air, including air embolism.

Systemic air embolization presents particular problems in the management of blast casualties, since the effects on the brain, heart, and viscera caused by air emboli may be indistinguishable from other types of injury. Yet, the preferred therapy for air embolism is hyperbaric oxygen treatment, which may not be readily available or may be impractical because of coexistent injuries or other logistical problems. Whenever possible, though, hyperbaric oxygen treatment should be implemented as expeditiously as possible, being given in a manner similar to the treatment of dysbaric diving casualties, because it is usually very effective in reversing cerebral or coronary injuries.

Tympanic membrane rupture and other otolaryngologic trauma, as well as most other types of blast injury, should be treated essentially the same as they are treated when due to other causes. Closed abdominal injuries are always of particular concern and should be treated according to the patient's signs and symptoms, with prompt surgical exploration being undertaken whenever there are signs of peritonitis or peritoneal free air. Abdominal visceral injuries should be especially looked for in victims of underwater explosion. Lacerations, fractures, amputations, and missile wounds should be treated in the usual manner, except for delayed primary closure being the generally preferred method of wound management.

Explosions in confined spaces typically produce worse injuries than those occurring in the open because of the greater likelihood of inhalation injury from dust, smoke, and toxic gases. Again, though, the inhalation injury is treated essentially the same as that resulting from other circumstances.

Because primary blast injuries may not always be present when the victim is first evaluated, all blast-injured patients should be closely observed for at least 6 to 12 h after the accident. This is particularly true if there is perforation of the eardrums, which is generally an indication of significant exposure to high pressure.

## BIBLIOGRAPHY

### Dysbaric Diving Casualties

Bove AA: The basis for drug therapy in decompression sickness. *Undersea Biomed Res* 9:91, 1982.
Colebatch HJM, Smith MM, Ng CKY: Increased elastic recoil as a determinant of pulmonary barotrauma in divers. *Respir Physiol* 26:55, 1976.
Cramer FS, Heimbach RD: Stomach rupture as as result of gastrointestinal barotrauma in a scuba diver. *J Trauma* 22:238, 1982.
Gillen HW: Symptomatology of cerebral gas embolism. *Neurology* 18:507, 1968.
Hallenbeck JM, Bove AA, Elliott DH: Mechanisms underlying spinal cord damage in decompression sickness. *Neurology* 25:308, 1975.
Kizer KW: Delayed treatment of dysbarism; a retrospective review of 50 cases. *JAMA* 247:2555, 1982.
Kizer KW: Dysbaric cerebral air embolism in Hawaii. *Ann Emerg Med* 16:535, 1987.

Kizer KW, Goodman PG: Radiographic manifestations of venous air embolism. *Radiology* 144:35, 1982.
Lundgren CEG, Tjernstrom O, Ornhagen H: Alternobaric vertigo and hearing disturbances in connection with diving: an epidemiologic study. *Undersea Biomed Res* 1:251, 1974.
Parell GJ, Becker GD: Conservative management of inner ear barotrauma resulting from scuba diving. *Otolaryngol Head Neck Surg* 93:393, 1985.

### Blast Injury

Benzinger T: Physiological effects of blast in air and water. In *German Aviation Medicine, World War II*. Washington, DC: US Government Printing Office, vol. II, pp. 1225–1259, 1950.
Caseby NG, Porter MF: Blast injuries to the lungs: Clinical presentation, management and course. *Injury* 8:1, 1976.
Clemedson CJ: Blast injury. *Physiol Rev* 36:336, 1956.
Hadden WA, Rutherford WH, Merrett JD: The injuries of terrorist bombing: a study of 1532 consecutive patients. *Br J Surg* 65:525, 1978.
Huller T, Bazini Y: Blast injuries of the chest and abdomen. *Arch Surg* 100:24, 1970.
Kerr AG: Trauma and the temporal bone—the effects of blast on the ear. *J Laryngol Otol* 94:107, 1980.
Pahor AL: Blast injuries to the ear: an historical and literary review. *J Laryngol Otol* 93:225, 1979.
Pahor AL: The ENT problems following the Birmingham bombings. *J Laryngol Otol* 95:399, 1981.
Rawlings JSP: Physical and pathophysiological effects of blast. *Injury* 9:313, 1977.
Roy D: Gunshot and bomb blast injuries: a review of experience in Belfast. *J Roy Soc Med* 75:542, 1982.

# 167
# NEAR DROWNING
## Bruce E. Haynes

Drowning, like other causes of accidental death, often strikes young, otherwise healthy individuals, and prevention is the most important way to reduce these unnecessary deaths. The patient's prognosis after near drowning depends on the speed of rescue and resuscitation, emphasizing the role of emergency medical care.

## DEFINITIONS

Almost as many definitions of drowning exist as authors in the field. One approach is to define drowning as death from suffocation after submersion, while those who suffer near drowning survive, at least temporarily, after suffocation by submersion. A few use the more generic term *immersion syndrome* to highlight the blurred margins between the two entities, although this term has also been used to refer to sudden death after immersion in cold water. Postimmersion syndrome, or secondary drowning, refers to the deterioration of a seemingly well patient after immersion.

## EPIDEMIOLOGY

About 4500 people die of submersion in the United States each year, making drowning the third leading cause of accidental death. Many more—the exact number is uncertain—experience serious submersion episodes.

Fresh water drowning, especially in pools, is more common than saltwater drowning, even in coastal areas. There is a bimodal age distribution, with large numbers of deaths among children under age 4 and then later among teenagers, although risk climbs again in the elderly from bathtub drowning. Young children are also at risk for drowning in a bathtub, even in the presence of siblings, and abuse or neglect should be considered in such cases. Caretakers should ensure constant attention by an individual of appropriate age.

Alcohol or drug use by victims or by supervising adults often plays a role in drowning and boating accidents; trauma, especially to the lower cervical spine, results in some cases. Children may be oblivious to potentially dangerous situations especially in rivers and lakes. Once a person is in trouble poor swimming skills cause numerous drownings; swimming lessons can be targeted at those, including ethnic groups, who need them. Hypothermia, hyperventilation before underwater swimming, or seizure disorders are also factors. Patients with seizure disorders must receive careful supervision if swimming and should, depending on seizure control, probably bathe in showers or tubs with open drains and plastic stalls. This patient education is important when first-time seizure patients are discharged from emergency departments.

Drowning deaths should be prevented by adequate, well-maintained fencing with self-locking gates that surrounds pools themselves, rather than simply isolating the backyard, leaving access to the pool from the house and yard. Drowning occurs extraordinarily rapidly, and caretakers must be taught that attention to children must not be diverted by chores, socializing, telephone calls, or other seemingly momentary distractions. Cardiopulmonary resuscitation (CPR) is frequently not started by rescuers, and pool owners should be encouraged to learn CPR and have telephones in the pool area.

## CLINICAL COURSE

Respiratory failure and ischemic neurologic injury are the threats to life after submersion although associated injuries are occasionally present. Childhood drowning happens quickly and silently. Older victims who are not immediately unconscious may panic, struggle in the water, hold their breath, or hyperventilate. Once under water, involuntary breathing resumes at a break point determined by the $P_{O_2}$ or $P_{CO_2}$. This soon leads to vomiting and aspiration of water and emesis. "Dry drowning" without aspiration results from laryngospasm and glottal closure. Whatever the mechanism, the final common pathway is profound hypoxemia.

Initial hypoxemia results from flooding of alveoli and impairment of gas exchange. Although both seawater and fresh water wash surfactant out of alveoli, fresh water also changes the surface tension properties of surfactant. Surfactant loss leads to atelectasis, ventilation perfusion mismatch, and breakdown of the alveolar capillary membrane. Hypoxemia follows aspiration of small amounts of water and is seen experimentally with aspiration of 2.2 mL/kg of either fresh water or saltwater. Contributing to pulmonary injury may be aspiration of bacteria, algae, sand, particulate matter, emesis, and chemical irritants. Noncardiogenic pulmonary edema results from direct pulmonary injury, surfactant loss, inflammatory contaminants, and cerebral hypoxia.

Poor perfusion and hypoxemia lead to metabolic acidosis in a majority of patients; yet perhaps as a result of the young age of most victims, the cardiovascular status is remarkably stable. Blood volume shifts depend on the nature and quantity of the fluid aspirated, although life-threatening changes are unusual, because most human drowning victims aspirate quantities of water far below those that produce significant disturbances. Electrolyte abnormalities in near-drowning patients are seldom significant, and hematologic values are usually normal, although the clinician will occasionally see hemoconcentration or hemolysis that results in anemia. Rarely, disseminated intravascular coagulation will occur.

Renal function is usually adequate although proteinuria may occur and hemoglobinuria can follow hemolysis. Acute tubular necrosis can result from hypoxia or myoglobinuria.

**Table 167-1.** Prehospital Care of Near-Drowning Victims

Rapid, cautious rescue
Spinal precautions
Cardiopulmonary resuscitation
Supplemental oxygen on all patients
Transport all patients

## THERAPY

### Prehospital Care

Treatment of near drowning begins at the scene with rapid, cautious removal of the victim from the water (Table 167-1). Spinal precautions should be observed if the mechanism of injury, such as diving or surfing, raises suspicion of such injury. The vast majority of spinal injuries are to the lower cervical spine after diving. Clues to spinal injury may be paradoxical respiration (abdominal breathing without movement of intercostal muscles), flaccidity, priapism, or unexplained hypotension or bradycardia. Lifeguards and emergency medical technicians should maintain spinal precautions during rescue if possible. Initial history may be unreliable, and the physician should have a low threshold for obtaining cervical spine x-rays.

A patent airway must be maintained and ventilation assisted as needed; patients should receive supplemental oxygen. CPR should be started on any arrested patient with even a remote possibility of success. Sodium bicarbonate may be considered in unstable patients, and any patient with a significant episode, including those asymptomatic at the scene, should be transported to the hospital for evaluation.

In-water CPR is generally ineffective and dangerous for the rescuer, and should not be attempted unless a firm, stable surface is available. Human near-drowning victims aspirate small quantities of water; postural drainage or the abdominal thrust (Heimlich maneuver) is of unproven efficacy in removing water from the lungs or improving oxygenation. No drainage procedure appears to significantly affect oxygenation in experimental preparations. Field limitations to postural drainage include the danger of aspiration from an uncontrolled airway, interruption of ventilation or CPR, the danger of spinal injury, and the possibility of aggravating other undiagnosed injuries. An appropriate maneuver for airway obstruction should be used only if ventilation is obstructed.

### Hospital Care

Hospital evaluation and care of drowning victims emphasizes initial resuscitation, treatment of respiratory failure, and evaluation of associated injuries (Table 167-2).

Although patient survival in a persistent vegetative state is a con-

**Table 167-2.** Hospital Care of Near-Drowning Victims

Clear spine
Laboratory studies:
    CBC, electrolytes, glucose, clotting studies, urinalysis
    Arterial blood gases, pulse oximetry
    Chest x-ray
    Electrocardiogram
Pulmonary support:
    Supplemental oxygen on all patients
    High-flow $O_2$ as needed
    Intubation and positive pressure (PEEP, CPAP)
Nasogastric tube
Foley catheter
Monitor:
    Oxygenation
    Acid-base balance
    Temperature
    Volume status
Evaluate and treat:
    Associated injuries
    Specific conditions: hypoglycemia, hypothermia, etc.

cern, substantial numbers of patients, predominantly children, requiring CPR on emergency department arrival have survived with good outcomes, and physicians should err on the side of providing resuscitation. The physician should gather sufficient history to allow an estimate of prognosis and gauge the patient's response to resuscitative efforts.

On the victim's arrival in the emergency department adequate oxygenation should be ensured, the integrity of the patient's spine should be confirmed if necessary, and associated injuries should be sought. Pulmonary insufficiency may be indicated by dyspnea, tachypnea, or use of accessory muscles of respiration. Physical examination may reveal wheezing, rales, or rhonchi, although the chest may be completely normal to auscultation after aspiration.

All patients should receive supplemental oxygen during evaluation, and those with more than mild symptoms should be on 100% oxygen until adequate oxygenation is documented. If high-flow oxygen (40% to 50%) cannot maintain the arterial $P_{O_2}$ greater than 60 mm Hg in adults or 80 mm Hg in children, the patient should be intubated and mechanical ventilation used.

Intubated patients generally require positive end-expiratory pressure or continuous positive airway pressure (CPAP). Muscular paralysis will be needed in some patients, and moderate fluid restriction and hyperventilation to a $P_{CO_2}$ of 30 may help control cerebral edema.

Occasionally, a patient may require only increased oxygenation and CPAP without mechanical ventilation. Only patients who are alert and unlikely to vomit are candidates for mask CPAP ventilation.

Those patients whose temperatures register at the low end of standard thermometers need further investigation. A hypothermia thermometer is best, but emergency departments can usually obtain low-reading thermometers from their clinical laboratory or operating room. Hypothermia can immobilize a swimmer, resulting in drowning, may cause primary ventricular fibrillation, or may be responsible for a variety of adverse metabolic effects. Severe hypothermia often indicates prolonged submersion and is a bad prognostic sign. Despite this, individuals have survived after prolonged submersion (up to 40 min) in cold water. These patients have body temperatures less than 30°C (86°F) after submersion in water less than 20°C (68°F). The nature of the protective effect of hypothermia is unclear. It may be general slowing of metabolism or preferential shunting of blood to the brain, heart, and lungs (diving reflex). Hypothermic near-drowning victims who are resuscitated should be warmed to at least 30° to 32.5°C (86° to 90°F) before resuscitation efforts are abandoned.

Appropriate laboratory data should be obtained (see Table 167-2). Direct measurement of oxygenation and acid-base status by arterial blood gas analysis and on-line pulse oximetry guide pulmonary therapy and the need for sodium bicarbonate.

Roentgenograms of the chest may be normal after a significant near-drowning incident or may show generalized pulmonary edema (Fig. 167-1), perihilar infiltrates, or other patterns. Chest films do not necessarily correlate with arterial $P_{O_2}$, making direct measurement of oxygen saturation important, although many patients with significantly abnormal films will require intubation.

Standard treatment of bronchospasm, electrolyte imbalance (especially hypoglycemia), seizures, hypothermia, arrhythmias, and hypotension should be undertaken as needed. Some patients may need fluid resuscitation in the face of noncardiogenic pulmonary edema. To avoid inducing arrhythmias, central venous catheters, if used, should not enter the heart in hypothermic patients. A nasogastric tube will empty the stomach and help prevent vomiting, and a Foley catheter will help to monitor urine output. Neither antibiotics nor steroids alter the course of aspiration pneumonia or pulmonary edema in drowning, and they should not be given prophylactically.

## PROGNOSIS AND CEREBRAL RESUSCITATION

Statistics on survival and the incidence of severe neurologic deficits after near drowning are difficult to interpret. They vary with regard to

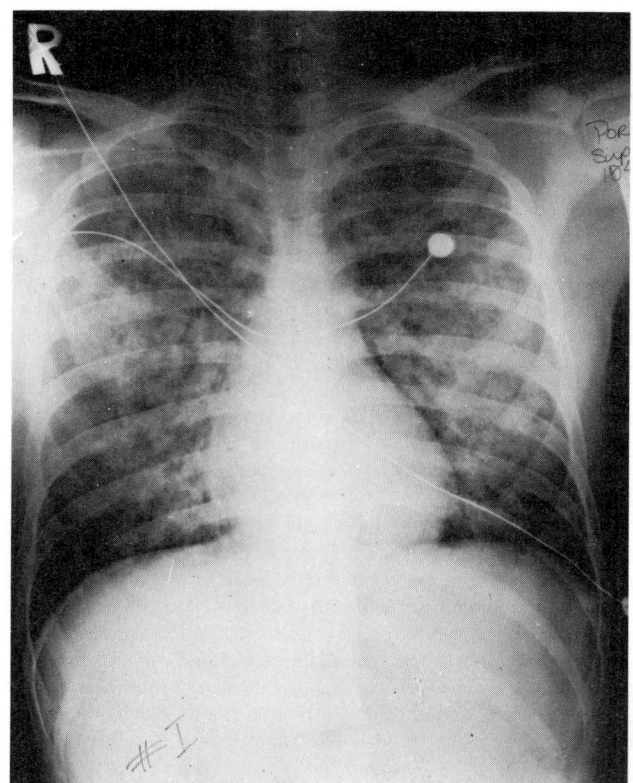

**Fig. 167-1.** Chest roentgenogram of near-drowning patient demonstrating diffuse noncardiogenic pulmonary edema.

definitions, patient age, water temperature, treatment regimens, and many other variables. Almost all patients who are alert and fully conscious will survive without sequelae, as will the vast majority of victims who are obtunded but have a purposeful response to pain. As many as 24 percent of children admitted to intensive care units who required full CPR and had an initial Glasgow Coma Scale of 3 in the referring emergency department have survived with intact neurologic function. CPR, requiring cardiotonic medications, or unreactive pupils all indicate a poor prognosis, but no one indicator or scoring system fully differentiates survivors with acceptable neurologic outcome from children who die. Quan and Kinder have suggested resuscitation is indicated if the time of submersion is likely to be 10 min or less, and that patients not responding to advanced life support measures within 25 min will not live.

Life support can be withdrawn in the intensive care unit once the patient's condition is stable, the likely outcome more clear, and the family has had time to consider treatment options.

Outcome depends primarily on the duration of submersion but also on the amount of time until resuscitative efforts begin.

## DISPOSITION

Most older reports on drowning recommend admission and monitoring of all near-drowning victims. This recommendation arose from descriptions of "secondary drowning" in which 2 to 25 percent of near-drowning patients deteriorated significantly or died after a seemingly successful rescue or resuscitation. Most of the patients in these reports, however, simply had pulmonary insufficiency that progressed and symptoms or signs that today would be discovered easily by an adequate evaluation. The decision of whom to admit must focus on those at risk for pulmonary insufficiency or other complications.

Patients at risk have undergone a "significant" episode and display symptoms such as coughing, dyspnea tachypnea, or have historical factors such as unconsciousness in the water. Occasionally, patients who suffered transient severe hypoxia or who have underlying cardiovascular disease will fall into the same group.

The physician's approach should depend on the patient's symptoms and the results of screening examinations. For convenience, patients may be separated into four groups, although one should take particular care in evaluating young children. One group will have no evidence of significant submersion and may be discharged quickly. Chest roentgenograms and arterial blood gas determinations are unnecessary in the face of a benign history, but the studies or pulse oximetry may lend weight to the decision to discharge.

A second group will be asymptomatic or have mild symptoms after a significant episode. They can frequently be observed in the emergency department for several hours and then discharged if their social situation allows adequate follow-up. The third group will have mild to moderate hypoxemia corrected by oxygen therapy. These patients are admitted and then discharged when the hypoxemia resolves if no complications ensue.

The final group is composed of patients who require intubation and mechanical ventilation whose prognosis usually depends more on their neurologic status than on pulmonary injury, unless they develop serious aspiration pneumonia or progressive, irreversible lung injury.

## BIBLIOGRAPHY

Lavelle JM et al: Ten-year review of pediatric bathtub near drowings: evaluation for child abuse and neglect. *Ann Emerg Med* 25:344, 1995.

Lavelle JM, Shaw KN: Near drowning: is emergency department cardiopulmonary resuscitation or intensive care unit cerebral resuscitation indicated? *Crit Care Med* 21:368, 1993.

Modell JH: Drowning. *N Engl J Med* 328:253, 1993.

Quan L, Kinder D: Pediatric submersions: prehospital predictors of outcome. *Pediatrics* 90:909, 1992.

# 168
# THERMAL BURNS

## Lawrence R. Schwartz

## INTRODUCTION

Of the approximately 2 million patients who present to emergency departments with burn injuries in the United States each year, about 100,000 are hospitalized and 12,000 die. The remainder sustain minor injuries and are treated as outpatients. There is a high incidence in children 1 to 5 years of age, most of whom are scalded by hot liquids. The risk of burns is highest in the 18- to 35-year-old age group, with a male:female ratio of 2:1 for both injury and death. Burns are the second most common cause of accidental death in this country. The death rate in children less than 4 years of age is twice that of the overall burn population. The death rate in patients over 65 years of age is three times greater than that of the overall burn population.

## PATHOPHYSIOLOGY OF THE BURN WOUND

A burn is defined by its size and depth. The size and depth are a function of the burning agent, its temperature, and the duration of exposure. Cell damage occurs at temperatures greater than 45°C (113°F) due to denaturation of cellular protein.

The burn wound is described as having three zones. The most damaged area, the zone of coagulation, is that which came in contact with the heat source. The tissue is destroyed, and the blood vessels thrombosed. The next adjacent zone is the zone of stasis, described as hav-

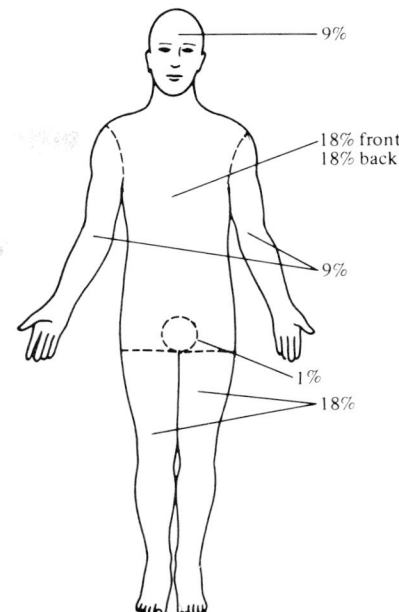

**Fig. 168-1.** Rule of nines.

ing stagnant but not clotted blood in the microcirculation. As the stasis persists the tissue in that zone can get progressively more hypoxic and ischemic. The next adjacent zone is the zone of hyperemia or inflammation. This zone has increased blood flow. It has sustained minimal damage and will recover.

## Burn Size

The size of a burn is quantified as the percentage of total body surface area (TBSA). One method of approximating the percentage of TBSA burned is to use the *rule of nines* (Fig. 168-1). This method divides the adult body into segments that are approximately 9 percent TBSA each or multiples of 9 percent (Table 168-1). In infants and children, the head has a larger percentage of TBSA and the legs a smaller one.

Another method is that the area of the back of a patient's hand is approximately 1 percent of the TBSA. The percentage of TBSA burned can be approximated by estimating the number of "hands" that are equal to the burn.

A more precise estimation of the percentage of TBSA burned is obtained by using a Lund and Browder burn diagram (Fig. 168-2). This allows the burn to be diagrammed by size and depth, and the area of each depth of burn to be calculated. These charts are age-adjusted, allowing for the changing percentages of TBSA for children aged 0, 1, 5, 10, and 15 years.

## Burn Depth

The depth of a burn is described either in degree: first, second, or third; or by the depth of the skin injured. The latter describes burns in terms of partial thickness or full thickness.

First-degree burns involve the epidermis layer of the skin only. They are most commonly caused by ultraviolet light. Sunburn is the

**Table 168-1.** Body Segments for the Rule of Nines

| | |
|---|---|
| Head and neck, anterior and posterior | 9% |
| Each arm, including the hand | 9% |
| Each thigh | 9% |
| Each lower leg, including foot | 9% |
| Anterior trunk, clavicles to pubis | 18% |
| Posterior trunk, root of neck to and including buttocks | 18% |
| Perineum | 1% |

most common example. The burned skin is painful and red, and there is no blister formation. It heals without scarring in 7 days.

Partial-thickness burns, or second-degree burns, are subdivided into *superficial* and *deep.* In superficial partial-thickness, or superficial second-degree burns, the epidermis and part of the dermis are involved. The deeper layers of the dermis are spared, as are the hair follicles and sweat and sebaceous glands. These burns are usually caused by hot liquids. There is blister formation, under which the skin is red and moist, and the burns are very painful to touch. If the blisters are broken, the wound is moist. Wounds heal in 14 to 21 days and may or may not leave a scar, depending on the extent of the burn.

Deep second-degree burns, or deep partial-thickness burns, involve the deeper layers of the dermis. There is damage to the hair follicles and sweat glands, but their deeper portions survive. Causes of deep second-degree burns are hot liquids, steam, oil, or flame. They may be difficult to distinguish from full-thickness burns. The skin appears blistered to charred and is tender. Healing takes 3 to 4 weeks. There will be some scarring, which will be related to the amount and depth of the dermal injury. Surgical repair or grafting may be necessary.

Third-degree, or full-thickness, burns involve the entire thickness of the skin, epidermis through dermis, down to the subcutaneous fat. All epidermal and dermal structures are destroyed. Common causes of full-thickness burns are flame, steam, and hot oil. The skin is charred, pale, *painless,* and leathery. This burn will not heal spontaneously. Surgical repair and/or skin grafts are necessary, and there is significant scarring (Fig. 168-3).

Fourth-degree burns are those described as going through the skin, involving the underlying fat, muscle, and bone. These are devastating, life-threatening injuries.

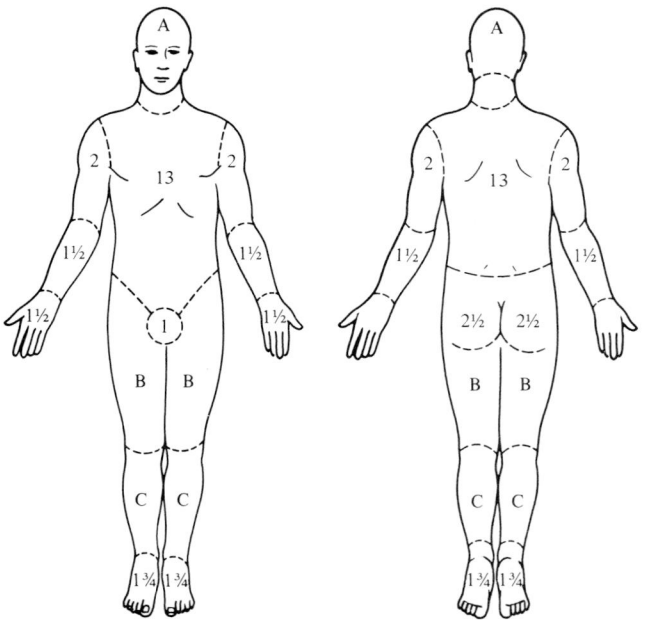

Relative Percentages of Areas Affected by Growth (Age in Years)

|  | 0 | 1 | 5 | 10 | 15 | Adult |
| --- | --- | --- | --- | --- | --- | --- |
| A: half of head | $9\frac{1}{2}$ | $8\frac{1}{2}$ | $6\frac{1}{2}$ | $5\frac{1}{2}$ | $4\frac{1}{2}$ | $3\frac{1}{2}$ |
| B: half of thigh | $2\frac{3}{4}$ | $3\frac{1}{4}$ | 4 | $4\frac{1}{4}$ | $4\frac{1}{2}$ | $4\frac{3}{4}$ |
| C: half of leg | $2\frac{1}{2}$ | $2\frac{1}{2}$ | $2\frac{3}{4}$ | 3 | $3\frac{1}{4}$ | $3\frac{1}{2}$ |

Second degree _____ and

Third degree _____ =

Total percent burned ___

**Fig. 168-2.** Classic Lund and Browder chart.

## American Burn Association Classification of Burns

The American Burn Association has devised a classification of burns, dividing them into major, moderate, and minor burns. Low-risk adults are patients between the ages of 10 and 50 years. Higher-risk patients are less than 10 and greater than 50 years old. Other patients considered "poor risk" are those with underlying medical illnesses such as heart disease, diabetes, or chronic pulmonary problems.

### Major Burns

Major burns are defined as partial-thickness burns greater than 25 percent TBSA in the 10- to 50-year-old age group, or greater than 20 percent TBSA in children under 10 years or adults over 50; full-thickness burns of greater than 10 percent TBSA in anyone; burns involving the hands, face, feet, or perineum; burns crossing major joints; circumferential limb burns; burns complicated by inhalation injury; electrical burns; burns complicated by fractures or other trauma; burns in infants and the elderly; and burns in poor-risk patients.

### Moderate Burns

Moderate burns are partial-thickness burns of 15 to 25 percent TBSA in the 10- to 50-year-old age group, 10 to 20 percent TBSA in children under 10 years or adults over 50; full-thickness burns of ≤ 10 percent TBSA in anyone; burns *not* involving the hands, face, feet, or perineum, or circumferential limb burns.

### Minor Burns

Minor burns, which imply outpatient treatment, involve a TBSA of less than 15 percent in the 10- to 50-year-old age group or 10 percent in children less than 10 years or adults over 50; full-thickness burns that are less than 2 percent TBSA in anyone; and no other injuries.

## SYSTEMIC RESPONSE OF THE BURN PATIENT

Burns wounds that cover 20 to 25 percent TBSA cause a systemic inflammatory reaction and edema. The tissue injury results in complement activation and the release of mediators. Cytokines such as tumor necrosis factor and interleukins 1 and 6 are released. The arachidonic acid metabolites prostaglandin $I_2$ ($PGI_2$), a vasodilator, and thromboxane $A_2$ ($TxA_2$), a vasoconstrictor, and leukotrienes are also released.

Prostaglandin inhibitors, such as ibuprofen, have been used to suppress or reduce the systemic inflammatory response that occurs with a major burn injury. The use of nonsteroidal antiinflammatory agents (NSAIDs) varies with different burn centers. Many centers use NSAIDs initially on burns of all severity. Others do not use them at all. Oxidants such as superoxide and hydrogen peroxide are produced. These compromise the fatty acid portion of the cell membrane, disrupting its function, and cause it to leak fluid and proteins, resulting in edema.

The mediators along with oxidants are immunosuppressive. They cause a hypermetabolic state and muscle catabolism. Endotoxin, produced by burn wound colonization and/or an early gut leak, is a potent macrophage and neutrophil stimulator that prompts the release of more mediators.

There are large endothelial cell gaps formed in the microvasculature, allowing leaks of proteins and fluid. The leaky membrane allows a large flux of fluid and protein from the vascular space into the interstitial space. This increases the oncotic pressure of the interstitial space. Simultaneously there is a decrease in the oncotic pressure in the vascular space due to the large loss of plasma proteins and fluids both through the burn wound itself and into the nonburned tissue through leaky cell membranes. Increased interstitial oncotic pressure coupled with decreased vascular oncotic pressure and a leaky cell membrane cause more edema. The edema reaches its maximum at 12 to 24 h postburn.

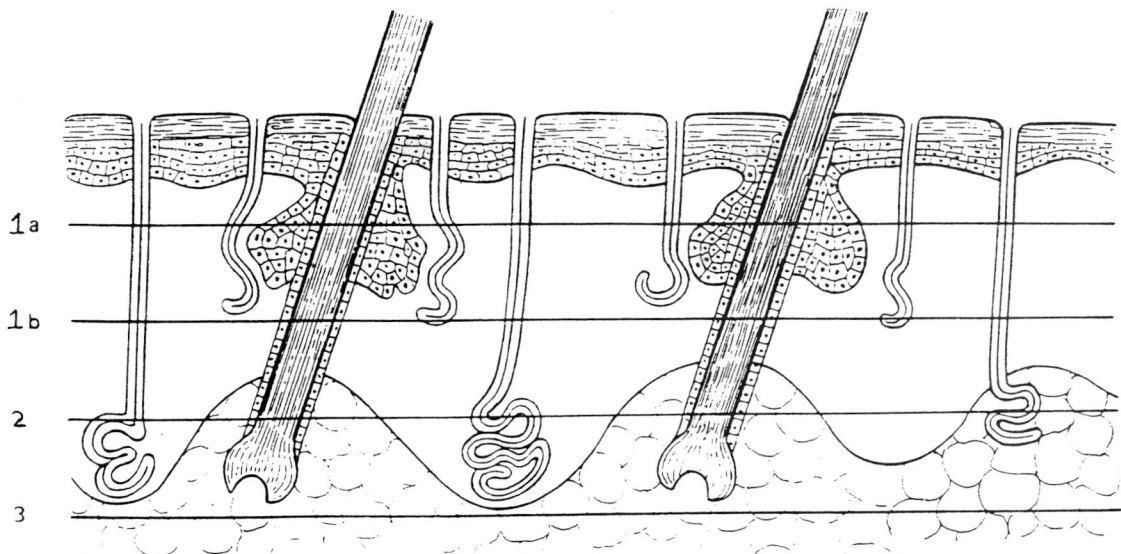

**Fig. 168-3.** Diagram showing the microstructure of the skin and its relationship to the different depths of burning. Level 1a: superficial partial-thickness burn passes through hair follicles, sebaceous glands, and sweat glands. Level 1b: also superficial partial-thickness burn, but deep to the sebaceous glands. It passes through hair roots and sweat glands. The dermis-fat interface is not breached. Level 2: deep partial-thickness burn passes through hair roots and sweat glands but breaches the dermis-fat interface and cuts across the fat domes. Level 3: full-thickness burn passes deep to all epithelial structures. (From Muir I et al. (eds): *Burns and Their Treatment.* London, Butterworth-Heinemann, 1987, with permission.)

Other organ systems are affected by the burn injury. The lungs are affected by interstitial edema, which is compounded by smoke inhalation.

Decreased cardiac output occurs. There is thought to be a "myocardial depressant factor" that decreases the contractility of the heart. This may be the result of carbon monoxide combined with cardiac myoglobin. Another etiology may be the diminished vascular volume that exists.

There is decreased renal blood flow and a decreased glomerular filtration rate. This may likewise be due to the decreased intravascular volume.

There is impaired humoral and cell-mediated immunity. IgG and IgA concentrations are depressed. T lymphocytes do not respond normally, and their cytotoxicity is diminished. There is an increase in the number of suppressor T cells. This makes the patient susceptible to infection, which so often is the cause of death.

## SMOKE INHALATION

Half of all fire-related deaths are due to smoke inhalation. Smoke inhalation injury doubles the mortality rate for a burn of any size.

*Smoke inhalation injury* is a general term that comprises several types of injury. Carbon monoxide poisoning is a well-known consequence of smoke inhalation. Carbon monoxide has an affinity for the hemoglobin molecule that is 200 times that of oxygen. Therefore carbon monoxide displaces oxygen, and the patient suffers tissue hypoxia. Oxygen cannot get transported to the tissue.

Carboxyhemoglobin levels are measured as the percentage of hemoglobin bound to carbon monoxide. The following carboxyhemoglobin levels correlate with the following clinical symptoms:

| | |
|---|---|
| < 10 percent | no symptoms |
| 20 percent | headache, nausea, vomiting, loss of dexterity |
| 30 percent | confusion, lethargy, ECG ST depression |
| 40 to 60 percent | coma |
| > 60 percent | death |

The half-life of carboxyhemoglobin is 4 to 5 h at room air, 90 min with 100% oxygen, and 20 to 25 min at 3 atm in a hyperbaric chamber. Treatment consists of 100% oxygen if the carboxyhemoglobin level is <40 percent. The hyperbaric chamber should be considered in patients with a carboxyhemoglobin level of 40 percent or greater; in any patient displaying neurologic symptoms, regardless of the measured carboxyhemoglobin level; and in pregnant patients.

Asphyxiation is another cause of injury or death associated with smoke inhalation. Victims may lose consciousness due to hypoxia or hypercarbia in a fire.

Thermal injury is an unusual injury due to smoke inhalation. The injury is usually a burn to the upper airway. The laryngeal and/or pharyngeal tissues get burned. Edema then follows, jeopardizing the airway. Early endotracheal intubation is advised.

*Smoke poisoning* is the inhalation of noxious gases that are the products of combustion. Cyanide poisoning is known to occur in victims of smoke inhalation. Other toxic gases released are sulfur dioxide, hydrogen chloride, phosgene, and ammonia. These gases cause injury to the respiratory endothelium, similar to a chemical burn.

The inhalation injury causes injury to the endothelial cells with a loss of function of the bronchial epithelial cilia. Mucosal edema of the small airways causes obstruction and wheezing. Decreased alveolar surfactant activity leads to atelectasis. Tracheal and bronchial epithelial sloughing causes hemorrhagic tracheobronchitis. This can progress to a necrotizing bronchiolitis. Hyaline membranes then form. Intraalveolar hemorrhage leads to fibrinothrombus formation. The injured lung is very susceptible to pulmonary edema and the adult respiratory distress syndrome (ARDS). Careful fluid management is essential in these patients.

The pulmonary macrophages are injured. If patients survive lung injury, they are susceptible to bacterial pneumonia, which is a later complication of inhalation injury.

The diagnosis of smoke inhalation is made by the history of a fire in an enclosed space. Physical signs include facial burns, intraoral or pharyngeal burns, singed nasal hairs, soot in the mouth or nose, hoarseness, carbonaceous sputum, and expiratory wheezing. Bronchoscopy may be helpful in determining the extent of the injury. Signs of pulmonary injury can be delayed for 12 to 24 h after the exposure to noxious gases. Chest x-ray may likewise be normal initially.

Treatment of suspected inhalation injury includes humidified oxygen, early intubation and ventilation, vigorous pulmonary toilet, and bronchodilators.

## MANAGEMENT OF PATIENTS WITH MODERATE TO MAJOR BURNS

### Prehospital Care

Before any attempt at resuscitation is made the patient must be removed from the burning environment. The ABCs of trauma resuscitation must be initiated. Any burning clothing should be removed immediately, and the remainder of the clothing removed after airway, breathing, and circulation are secured. The airway needs to be assessed and protected if necessary. Thought must be given to an airway that has the potential of rapid swelling, even though initial assessment may be acceptable. If not breathing adequately, the patient must be intubated and ventilated. Blood pressure and pulse must be assessed and supported with intravenous (IV) fluids. Cool soaks can be applied to the burned area if it is not large; otherwise, the patient should be covered in clean sheets. The patient should not be allowed to become chilled or hypothermic. Routine stabilization procedures should be instituted. The patient should be placed on a 100% oxygen mask, assuming carbon monoxide poisoning. IV fluid rates should be calculated as discussed subsequently and titrated to support the patient's vital signs. Analgesia, most commonly IV morphine sulfate, should be administered in doses of 2- to 5-mg aliquots at the discretion of the physician assuming medical direction. The patient should be transported to the nearest hospital capable of caring for a burn patient or, if none is available, the nearest hospital, for stabilization.

### Emergency Department Management

Once in the emergency department a rapid assessment needs to be made. The history of the mechanism of injury needs to be obtained. What was the burning agent? Was it flame, hot liquid, grease, oil, steam, chemical, or electrical? What was the duration of exposure to the burning substance? Was the fire in an open or enclosed space? Was there an explosion causing the patient to suffer a blast injury? If the fire was in an enclosed area, what substances burned? What toxins could have been released by the combustion of the materials in the fire? How much smoke inhalation was there? Was there any other trauma sustained? A general medical history must be obtained. The patient's age and past history of chronic medical illnesses should be determined. Medications currently being taken as well as any allergies need to be known. The patient's tetanus immunization history needs to be ascertained. Regardless of status, all patients should get a 0.5-mL tetanus toxoid booster intramuscularly (IM). If there is any doubt as to the adequacy of previous immunizations, then 250 units of tetanus immune globulin should be given IM in another extremity.

A general physical examination needs to be performed, starting with a reassessment of airway, breathing, and circulation. If the patient is not already intubated, the airway needs to be reassessed. Carbonaceous sputum, singed nasal hairs, soot in the patient's mouth or pharynx, and wheezing are signs of smoke inhalation and/or an airway burn. If there is any compromise of the airway, early intubation is recommended. If the breathing is labored or if there is tachypnea or hypoxia, the patient should be intubated and given assisted ventilation with 100% oxygen.

The adequacy of circulation is assessed by the patient's blood pressure and pulse. If an IV line was not established in the field, it needs to be done as soon as possible.

The patient then needs a head-to-toe examination to look for evidence of trauma other than the burn. Attention should be paid to the head and neurologic status (Glasgow coma score), neck, chest (heart and lungs), abdomen, spine, pelvis, extremities, and perineum.

Lastly, the burn needs to be assessed. The size of the burn should be estimated either with the rule of nines or using a Lund and Browder chart, and the depth estimated by the initial appearance of the burn and the presence or absence of sensation. The depth and size take about 24 h to be more precisely defined. A complete blood count, electrolyte, BUN, creatinine, and glucose levels are baseline laboratory investigations that should be obtained. Measurement of arterial blood gases and carboxyhemoglobin levels and a chest x-ray must be obtained as a baseline of the patient's respiratory status and to assess for smoke inhalation. Fiberoptic bronchoscopy is indicated when there is a suspicion that smoke inhalation occurred. A urinalysis, urine myoglobin and CPK levels should be obtained to assess the patient for rhabdomyolysis. Other x-rays should be taken as indicated by the trauma sustained.

### Emergency Department Treatment/Resuscitation

Airway, breathing, and circulation are the first things that must be stabilized. All patients need supplemental oxygen, even if they do not need intubation and ventilation. Patients need a nasogastric tube because an ileus frequently accompanies the burn; a Foley catheter is necessary so that fluid resuscitation can be monitored.

Fluid resuscitation of burn patients remains a subject of investigation. The generally accepted initial resuscitation fluid of choice is lactated Ringer's solution. Other solutions used in burn units are hypertonic saline, protein solutions such as albumin or plasma, and heat-fixed protein solutions like Plasmanate. Nonprotein colloids or high-molecular-weight polysaccharides such as dextran are also used. The purpose of the various other solutions is to maintain vascular volume and renal perfusion with a minimum of edema. Since the cell membranes leak even large molecules for the first 24 h after a burn, the initial fluid of choice remains Ringer's lactate.

Ringer's lactate should be infused through two large-bore peripheral IV lines placed through uninjured nonburned skin, if at all possible. Central lines are to be avoided as they tend to become infected. However, in major burns, a cutdown or femoral venous catheter insertion may be very difficult to perform once edema develops.

There are many burn formulae in use to estimate fluid administration rates. All are calculated in mL/kg per percentage of TBSA burned per 24 h. The formulae are *suggested* rates of infusion. The rate can be modified depending on the patient's age, cardiac status, and parameters of vascular volume. Half of the calculated 24-h fluid total is given over the first 8 h from the time the burn occurred. The second half is infused over the remaining 16 h. It is important to infuse one-half the calculated amount within 8 h of the onset of the *burn,* not the insertion of the IV. The Parkland formula uses 4 mL/kg per %TBSA per 24 h. The modified Brooke Army formula uses 2 mL/kg per %TBSA per 24 h. Initial fluid resuscitation is therefore 2 to 4 mL/kg per %TBSA per 24 h. The resuscitation is monitored closely by frequent assessment of the patient's vital signs, signs of cerebral and skin perfusion, and urinary output. In adults urinary output should be 0.5 to 1.0 mL/kg per h.

There are several methods of calculating fluid resuscitation for infants and children. One method is to use the Parkland formula of 4 mL of Ringers lactate/kg per %TBSA per 24 h and modify it to maintain a urine output of 1 mL/kg per h. Alternatively, a pediatric maintenance rate for 24 h can be calculated, and anywhere from 2 to 4 mL/kg per %TBSA per 24 h can be added for the burn injury, monitoring vital signs and mentation, and maintaining a urine output of 1 mL/kg per h.

It is common for patients with major burns to receive excessive IV fluids both prehospital and in the emergency department. Total fluids infused in these settings should be carefully monitored and titrated to the patient's response, determined by vital signs, mentation, skin perfusion, and urinary output. Pulmonary edema and hypoxia are exacerbated by overvigorous fluid administration. This is especially true in patients who have sustained a pulmonary injury due to smoke inhalation.

## Burn Care

After the patient is evaluated and resuscitation begun, the burn wound needs to be addressed. The patient may need intravenous narcotic analgesia. The burns should be washed gently with a mild soap and water or saline. There should be sharp debridement of blisters. The blister fluid contains vasoactive peptides that promote ischemia to the underlying tissue.

If the patient is *not* going to be transferred, cover the burns with moist saline-soaked dressings while awaiting the consulting/admitting service. Be careful to avoid chilling the patient. Do not apply antibiotic ointment and a dressing. The admitting team will need to undress the burn and wash off the ointment to assess it. Always consult the admitting service early. They should have an active role in care of the patient.

If the patient *is* going to be transferred, the accepting burn unit should be contacted for specific instructions for burn care. The transferring facility should have access to the regional burn center treatment protocols. Intravenous antibiotics are not to be started by the emergency physician in the emergency department. They are not part of the initial resuscitation and treatment of burns.

Patients with circumferential burns of the limbs may develop compromise to distal circulation. Distal pulses need to be monitored closely. A Doppler flow probe may be very helpful. If circulation is compromised, an escharotomy will be needed. The eschar needs to be incised on the side of the limb, allowing the fat to bulge through. This relieves pressure, restoring circulation. If necessary, the incision can be continued onto the dorsal hand or foot. If there is a need for escharotomy of a finger, it likewise is incised on the lateral surface (Figs. 168-4 and 168-5).

If there is a circumferential burn to the chest, there may be mechanical restriction to ventilation by the eschar. An escharotomy of the chest wall needs to be done to allow adequate ventilation. A square needs to be cut through the eschar on the anterior chest wall, letting fat bulge out and releasing the restriction. Incisions need to be made at the anterior axillary lines from the level of the second rib down to the level of the twelfth rib. These two incisions need to be joined by parallel perpendicular incisions creating a floating box on the anterior chest wall (Fig. 168-6).

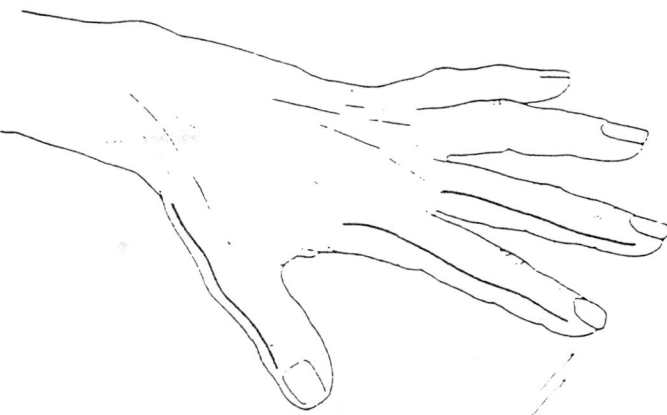

**Fig. 168-5.** Escharotomy of the hand. (From Robertson C, Fenton O: Management of severe burns. *BMJ* 301:285, 1990, with permission.)

## Admission

Burn patients with the following circumstances require inpatient care:

1. Those between 10 and 50 years of age with partial-thickness burns of greater than 15 percent TBSA or deep partial-thickness burns or full-thickness burns of greater than 5 percent TBSA
2. Those less than 10 years or greater than 50 years of age with partial-thickness burns greater than 10 percent TBSA or deep partial-thickness or full-thickness burns greater than 3 percent TBSA
3. Any patient with partial-thickness to full-thickness burns of the face, hands, feet, or perineum or burns across major joints or circumferential limb burns
4. Electrical burns
5. Chemical burns
6. Burns with inhalation injury
7. Burns in patients who have underlying medical problems or who are immunocompromised
8. Burns associated with other trauma

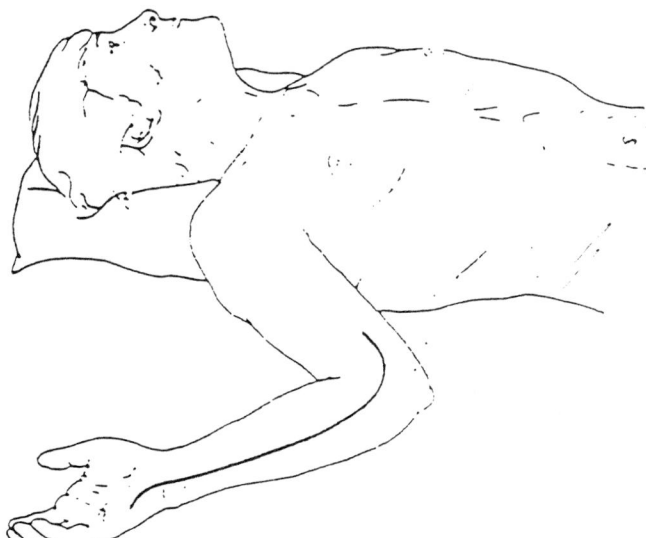

**Fig. 168-4.** Escharotomy of the arm. The incision is made on the side of the limb. (From Robertson C, Fenton O: Management of severe burns. *BMJ* 301:285, 1990, with permission.)

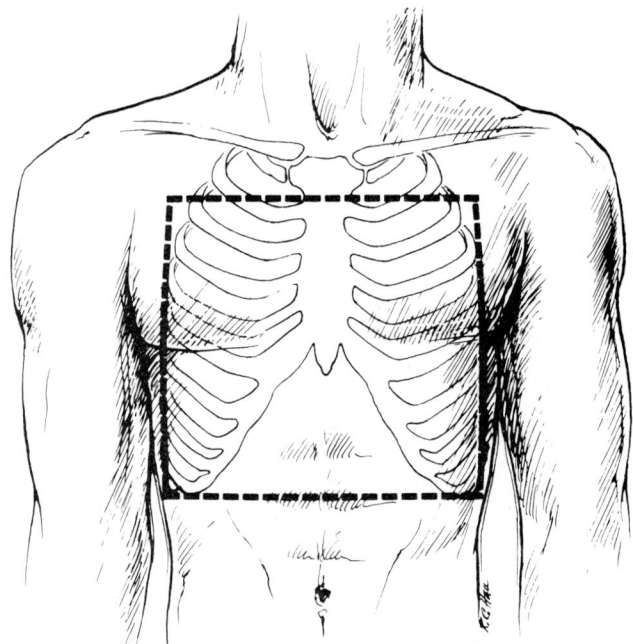

**Fig. 168-6.** In escharotomy of the chest wall, the constricting eschar that may impair ventilation is cut and a floating square of tissue is defined.

The American Burn Association recommends that patients with any of the above circumstances be admitted to a burn unit. This is a decision to be made by the emergency physician and the consultant who manages burns in each hospital setting. There are patients who may be managed well in a large general hospital and may not need transfer. In small hospitals with minimal physician coverage, any of the above criteria would warrant transfer.

There are conditions where patients should be transferred from even large general hospitals to specialized burn units. These include:

1. Major partial-thickness burns with a TBSA of greater than 25 percent in the 10- to 50-year-old age group or greater than 20 percent in children less than 10 years and adults older than 50 years
2. Any full-thickness burn greater than 10 percent TBSA
3. Burns involving the hands, face, feet, or perineum; circumferential limb burns; or burns across major joints
4. Major or moderate burns associated with inhalation injury
5. Major or moderate burns complicated by fractures or other trauma
6. Electrical burns
7. Burns in infants or the elderly
8. Major or moderate burns in patients who are poor risk due to underlying conditions

Transfer to a burn unit should be considered for any patient where long-term social or emotional support is needed or where there is going to be a long, difficult rehabilitation and/or recovery period.

## MINOR BURNS

Minor burns are defined by the American Burn Association as partial-thickness burns less than 15 percent TBSA in people aged 10 to 50 years, and less than 10 percent TBSA in people less than 10 years or greater than 50 years of age. Full-thickness burns are defined as minor if they are less than 2 percent of TBSA.

To qualify as minor, the burn must be an isolated injury and *not* involve the hands, face, feet, or perineum; cross major joints; or be a circumferential limb burn. Not every patient with burns to the above areas needs to be admitted. However, only the smallest and most superficial of hand, face, feet, or perineum burns can be considered for outpatient management.

The patient's medical and social situation needs to be considered when the admission decision is being made. An elderly patient or a patient with medical problems may be admitted for a burn that is less than 10 percent TBSA. The same size and depth of burn may be comfortably treated in the outpatient setting in a young, healthy, compliant patient. The patient's reliability is also a factor in outpatient care. The patient who seems unable or unwilling to follow burn care instructions and make and keep follow-up appointments may need admission.

### Care of the Minor Burn in the Emergency Department

Minor burns are painful. There is no reason to withhold analgesia. Children especially need analgesia as soon as possible. Ibuprofen is a good analgesic and its antiinflammatory properties may speed up healing. After giving the patient an appropriate analgesic, the burn needs to be cleansed with mild soap and water or saline, and the blisters debrided. Tetanus toxoid and tetanus immune globulin should be administered as needed, and then a dressing should be applied.

There are several ways to dress minor burns. Classically the burn is covered by a thin layer of antibiotic ointment, most commonly silver sulfadiazine, then covered with a gauze dressing. Although Silvadene is used most commonly, it cannot be used in patients with sulfa allergies or on the face, because of silver staining. Alternative topical agents are ophthalmic gentamicin ointment, Neosporin, or bacitracin. The dressing is removed once or twice a day, the burn washed, more

antibiotic ointment applied, and then it is redressed. This regimen goes on for 7 to 10 days, after which the burn should be healed.

This method of therapy may dry out the wound, impeding healing. Another dressing approach for the superficial partial-thickness burn is to cover the burn with a fine-mesh gauze, such as Owen's Gauze or Xeroform Gauze, without a topical antibiotic. The fine-mesh gauze is covered with 4 × 4s, and a bulky absorbent dressing like Kerlex is then wrapped around the burn. The burn is reevaluated in 5 to 7 days, and the bulky dressing removed. If the fine-mesh gauze is still in place adherent to the burn without any fluid collection, it is left in place and the burn rewrapped. The patient then is seen in another 5 to 7 days, and by then the burn should be healed. The fine-mesh gauze impregnated with the crust from the burn will separate from the epithelium below, revealing healed epithelium. If there is a fluid collection beneath the fine-mesh gauze it needs to be removed, the wound cleansed, and new fine-mesh gauze applied.

Another method of managing partial-thickness burns is with the use of the semisynthetic occlusive dressings. There are several commercially available. Examples include Biobrane, Duoderm, and Tegaderm. These have been used successfully on flat surface partial-thickness burns of the trunk and extremities. The burn wounds are cleansed and debrided. The occlusive dressing is placed on the wound. The goal is for the dressing to adhere to the wound surface and for there to be no fluid or exudate between the dressing and the burn. The dressing is removed at 7 to 10 days, as usually the wound is healed by then. If there is nonadherence or leaking at any time, the dressing must be changed. The superficial partial-thickness burns healed faster with this method. The patients found it more comfortable and were more compliant.

Although dressing changes may be advised at 5- to 7-day intervals, *all burn patients must be seen in 24 h* for a burn check to reassess the depth and extent of the burn.

Patients must be given discharge instructions that explain burn care and symptoms and signs of infection. They should be advised to elevate the burned area, especially if it is an extremity, and return to the emergency department at once if there are any symptoms or signs of an infection. The follow-up visit schedule should be clearly explained. Patients should also be given a prescription for analgesic medication.

## BIBLIOGRAPHY

American Burn Association: Hospital and prehospital resources for optimal care of patients with burn injury: Guidelines for development and operation of burn centers. *J Burn Care Rehab* 11:98, 1990.

Clark WR Jr, Nieman GF: Smoke inhalation. *Burns* 14(6):473, 1988.

Dziewulski P: Burn wound healing: James Ellsworth Laing Memorial Essay for 1991. *Burns* 18(6):466, 1992.

Griglak MJ: Thermal injury. *Emerg Med Clin North Am* 10(2):369, 1992.

Hermans MHE: Treatment of burns with occlusive dressings: Some pathophysiological and quality of life aspects. *Burns* 18(suppl 2):S15, 1992.

Robson MC, Burns BF, Smith DJ Jr: Acute management of the burned patient. *Plastic Recon Surg* 89(6):1155, 1992.

Warden GD: Burn shock resuscitation. *World J Surg* 16:16, 1992.

Wong L, Munster AM: New techniques in burn wound management. *Surg Clin North Am* 73(2):363, 1993.

Youn YK, LaLonde C, Demling R: The role of mediators in the response to thermal injury. *World J Surg* 16:30, 1992.

# 169
# CHEMICAL BURNS

### Marcus L. Martin
### Fred P. Harchelroad, Jr.

Chemical burns occur in the home, industrial, agriculture, and military settings, school and research laboratories, and as a result of civilian assaults, hobby accidents, and other accidents. Chemical burns also occur as a result of innocent application of products for medical purposes and for hair and skin care.

More than 25,000 products are capable of producing chemical burns. Both occupational exposure and contact with numerous chemicals during daily life contribute to the large number of chemical injuries to the skin. There are no good epidemiologic data on the incidence of toxic cutaneous exposure in the nonoccupational setting. However, about 40 percent of all occupationally related diseases reported concern the skin, and about 25 percent of these are due to chemical burns.

Common household chemical burns are caused by lye (drain cleaners, paint removers, urine sugar reagent test tablets), phenols (deodorizers, sanitizers, disinfectants), sodium hypochlorite (disinfectants, bleaches), and sulfuric acid (toilet bowl cleaners). In industries, chemicals are used for cleaning, tanning, curing, extracting, preserving, soldering, and other functions. The most commonly used industrial acids are tungstic, picric, sulfosalicylic, tannic, formic, sulfuric, acetic, cresylic, trichloroacetic, chromic, hydrochloric, and hydrofluoric. Widely used alkalis are the hydroxide salts of sodium, potassium, ammonium, lithium, barium, and calcium. White phosphorus used in munitions was the most common cause for chemical burns to military personnel during times of armed conflict in the 1960s. White phosphorus is also found in rodenticides and pesticides.

The body sites most often burned by chemicals are the face, eyes, and extremities. Less than 5 percent of patients admitted to major burn centers suffer from chemical burns. In general, chemical burn average sizes are small, and the mortality rate is lower than for thermal burns, but wound healing and hospital stay times are higher.

## PATHOPHYSIOLOGY

The skin interfaces with the external environment and constitutes a barrier and transition zone between the internal and external milieus. The outer stratum corneum layer of the skin functions as an excellent barrier against certain chemical agents, whereas others may penetrate readily. The skin contains three main layers: an outer layer of epithelial tissue (epidermis), a loose connective tissue layer (dermis), and a variable-thickness inner layer containing adipose and connective tissue (hypodermis or panniculus adiposus).

Chemicals can produce burns, dermatitis, allergic reaction, thermal injury, or systemic toxicity. Pathophysiologically, burns produced by all chemicals are similar. The skin has a limited variety of toxic responses, corresponding to the major patterns of possible structural or functional changes. Toxic reactions are described mainly on the basis of morphologic rather than functional responses. There are morphologic, physiologic, and biochemical protective mechanisms and elements in the skin which include the epidermal barrier, eccrine sweating, phagocytic cells, metabolic detoxification, immunologic processes, and melanin pigmentation. However, these vary on a phenotypic basis and may be affected by systemic or local disease.

Skin damage by chemicals may demonstrate the classic manifestations of thermal injury (erythema, blistering, or full-thickness loss); however, the acute injury may be deceptively mild, only to be followed by extensive skin damage and systemic toxicity. A superficial (first-degree) burn causes capillary and arterial dilatation. Initially, this involves only the superficial vessels, but then extends to the deeper subcutaneous vessels by both direct and reflex action. Tissue hyperemia and congestion results in symptoms of itching, burning, or pain. More extensive inflammatory reactions result in an outpouring of fluid into the extracellular space causing edema and vesicle or bulla formation characteristic of partial-thickness (second-degree) burns. Continued chemical damage through the dermis or into the hypodermis results in a full-thickness (third-degree) burn.

Tissue damage is determined by:

- Strength/concentration of the agent
- Manner of contact
- Quantity of agent
- Duration of contact
- Mechanism of action
- Extent of penetration

Factors enhancing percutaneous absorption of chemical are: body site (areas of thin skin, i.e., genitalia, face; chemical contact between skin folds; amount of surface area exposed); integrity of skin (traumatized skin; elderly skin; decreased lipid; dehydration; inflammation); nature of the chemical (lipid solubility; pH; concentration) and occlusion (garments; occlusive dressings).

The majority of chemical burns are caused by acids or alkalis. At similar volumes and manner of contact, alkalis usually produce far more tissue damage than acids. Acids in general cause coagulation necrosis with protein precipitation. Tough leathery eschar may form with development of underlying ulcers. The eschar limits spread of the agent. Heat may be released during reaction of acid with skin. Alkalis produce liquefaction necrosis with loosening of material which allows deeper penetration of the unattached chemical into tissue. Since not all chemicals causing burns can be considered as acid or alkali, a useful classification by C. Jelenko groups chemicals by the manner in which they damage protein:

1. Oxidizing agents: Damage is produced when a chemical becomes oxidized in contact with tissue. Often a toxic moiety is released during this reaction.
2. Corrosives: Extensive protein denaturation is produced, resulting in soft eschar and shallow, indolent ulcers.
3. Reducing agents: Protein denaturation is produced by binding of free electrons in tissue protein.
4. Desiccants: Severe cellular dehydration is produced, and thermal injury occurs due to exothermic reaction.
5. Vesicant: Blisters are produced, tissue amines are liberated, local ischemia and anoxic tissue damage and pandermic inflammation occurs.
6. Protoplasmic poisons: Protein is denatured by salt formation or by metabolic competition/inhibition (i.e., binding calcium or other inorganic ions necessary for tissue viability and function).

## GENERAL APPROACH

The goal of treatment is to minimize any area of irreversible injury and maximize salvage of the zone of reversible damage. Hydrotherapy is the cornerstone of initial treatment for chemical burns with few exceptions. Chemical agents may continue to damage tissue until they are removed or inactivated. The first priority is to stop the burning process. Immediate removal from the offending chemical, removal of garments, and counteraction of the chemical remaining on the body by dilution, debridement, or neutralization are important measures. Dry chemical particles such as lime should be brushed away before irrigation. Initially sodium metal and related compounds should be covered with mineral oil or excised, since water can cause a severe exothermic reaction. Dilution of phenol (carbolic acid) with water may enhance penetration. For the most part, however, use of water or saline to irrigate a chemical burn should not be delayed while searching for a neutralizing agent and should begin at the scene of the accident. In general, the earlier the irrigation, the better the prognosis.

The amount of elapsed time to initiate dilution or removal of chemical agents relates to the depth and degree of injury. Wounds irrigated 3 min after contact with some chemicals have a twofold greater chance of becoming full-thickness burns than wounds irrigated within 1 min of chemical contact. When using agents to neutralize a chemical burn, additional tissue injury may occur through heat production. In some cases, heat of dilution may be produced using water irrigation, but copious amounts will decrease the rate and amount of chemical reaction and dissipate the heat. Irrigation should be maintained at a gentle flow to avoid driving the chemical deeper into tissue or splashing chemical into the victim's or rescuer's eyes. The time required for irrigation varies; irrigation may need to be continued for hours in the case of alkali burns. Use of pH litmus paper may help determine continued presence of alkali or acid in burn wounds.

After irrigation and debridement of remaining particles and devitalized tissue, antimicrobial agents should be used and tetanus immunization should be updated as needed. Other than measures specific for a particular chemical burn, treatment following initial therapy is basically the same as for thermal burns. Patients sustaining chemical burns require the same aggressive fluid replacement as those with thermal burns. Analgesics may be needed, and, in the case of allergic responses to chemicals, antihistamines, steroids, and epinephrine may be required. Hemodialysis may be required in cases of severe systemic toxicity and renal failure. Autografts, heterografts, homografts, or synthetic material may be necessary for full-thickness burns. Hyperbaric oxygen may be utilized to assist healing of resistant burn wounds.

## SPECIFIC CHEMICALS

### Acids

With the exception of hydrofluoric acid, strong acids produce coagulation necrosis as a result of the desiccating action of the acid on proteins in the superficial tissue. Injury severity is related to certain physical characteristics of the acid. Most substances with a pH less than 2 are strong corrosives. Other important factors increasing the tissue-damaging properties of acids include concentration, molarity, and complexing affinity for hydroxy ions. The higher each of these factors is, the greater the tissue damage. Contact time with the skin is the most important feature of chemical burns which health care professionals may alter. Instantaneous skin decontamination of 18 $M$ sulfuric acid will cause no burn; however, a 1-min exposure can cause full-thickness skin damage. Examination of the patient with a significant chemical burn from these acids should not be limited to observation of the skin because several of these acids are respiratory and mucous membrane irritants as well. Furthermore, skin absorption of some compounds may occur and result in systemic signs and symptoms. The most commonly used chemicals that cause burns are listed in Table 169-1.

### Acetic Acid

The dilute (< 40%) acetic acid solution found in hair wave neutralizer solutions is perhaps the most common cause of chemical burns to the scalp in women. Prolonged contact, especially with an already damaged scalp, may cause a partial thickness burn which heals slowly because of the constant bacterial flora on the hair. Initial treatment is copious water irrigation. As trimming the hair is not a viable option in these patients, oral antibiotics are often given if the entire scalp is involved.

### Phenol

Phenol (carbolic acid), a corrosive organic acid used widely in industry and medicine, denatures proteins and causes chemical burns characterized by a white- or brown-colored coagulum that is relatively painless. Its unpleasant, acrid odor, detectable in air at 0.047 parts per million, and its low volatility help prevent airborne exposure. Though commercially available in concentrations of 1 to 90%, even dilute solutions of 1 to 2% phenol may cause a burn if contact is prolonged. Hexylresorcinol is a bactericidal phenol derivative. Chemically related phenolic compounds that induce skin damage include cresol, creosote, and cresylic acid.

Coagulation necrosis of the involved area is common. Necrotic tissue may delay absorption temporarily, but phenol may become entrapped under the eschar. Contaminated clothing should be removed and water lavage begun immediately. Water lavage alone may be ineffective, presumably because the necrotic coagulum inhibits water penetration to the deeper layers. Paradoxically, dilute phenol penetrates tissue more readily than when concentrated.

More effective decontamination has been demonstrated with a 5- to 10-min swab with a combination of polyethylene glycol 300 (PEG 300) and industrial methylated spirits (IMS) in a 2:1 mixture. This should not only reduce the extent of cutaneous corrosion but also decrease systemic toxicity. The PEG 300 is mixed with the IMS to form a more liquid (and therefore easier to use formulation). However, the viscous PEG 300 or PEG 400 may be used alone, and, indeed, glycerol is an acceptable substitute if the PEG 300/IMS mixture is not available. The use of an isopropyl alcohol rinse may be superior to PEG/IMS or water alone in removing phenol. The advantage of isopropyl alcohol is its easy availability.

### Chromic Acid

The toxicity of chromium compounds is related to the powerful oxidizing action of the hexavalent compounds ($Cr^{6+}$). The chromate ion in chromic acid will produce a chronic penetrating ulcerating lesion of the skin. Associated signs and symptoms are conjunctivitis, lacrimation, ulceration of the nasal septum, and systemic chromium toxicity. A 10 percent total body surface area cutaneous burn caused by chromic acid was fatal due to systemic toxicity. Any acute skin exposure to chromic acid should be treated with copious water irrigation and observation for systemic effects.

### Formic Acid

Formic acid in 60% solution is used by airplane-glue makers, cellulose formate workers, and tanning workers. Formic acid produces coagulation necrosis of the skin. Treatment includes immediate decontamination and irrigation with water. Open lesions should be treated like any damaged skin: with debridement of devitalized tissue, prevention of further damage and infection, and skin grafting if the defect is full thickness and of a size requiring closure.

### Hydrochloric and Sulfuric Acids

The dermal toxicity of hydrochloric and sulfuric acid is so well recognized that early decontamination and water irrigation usually prevent severe burns to the skin. These acids can turn the skin dark-brown or black when burned. Toilet bowl cleaners may contain 80% solutions of sulfuric acid. Some drain cleaners may be 95 to 99% sulfuric acid solutions. Munitions, chemical, and fertilizer manufacturers commonly use 95 to 98% sulfuric acid solutions in their industrial processes. Automobile battery fluid is 25% sulfuric acid. Most household bleaches are only 3 to 6% hypochlorite solutions, which, though acidic, cause little damage unless they are in contact with skin for a prolonged time. Treatment is the same as for formic acid burns.

**Table 169-1.** Chemicals That Cause Burns

| Agent | Use | Initial Treatment |
|---|---|---|
| Acetic acid | Permanent wave neutralizers, printing, dyeing, hat making | Water irrigation |
| Alkyl mercury compounds | Disinfectants, fungicides, wood preservatives | Water irrigation & prompt removal of blister fluid and overlying skin to prevent intoxication |
| Cantharides ("Spanish fly") | Veterinary aphrodisiac | Water irrigation |
| Chromic acid | Microelectronics/microinstruments, photography, metal cleaning and plating, leather tanning, cement manufacture | Water irrigation |
| Cresol (Lysol) | Disinfectant | Water irrigation |
| Creosote | Fungicides, wood preservative | Water irrigation |
| Cresylic acid | Industry | Water irrigation |
| Dimethyl sulfoxide (DMSO) | Topical treatment for sprains, arthritis | Water irrigation |
| Diquat dibromide | Herbicides | Water irrigation |
| Formic acid | Airplane-glue making | Water irrigation |
| Hydrocarbons | Industry, commerce | Water irrigation |
| Hydrochloric acid (muriatic acid) | Bleaching agents, metal cleaning, chemistry laboratories, fire proofing material, semiconductor industry | Water irrigation |
| Hydrofluoric acid | Microelectronics/microinstruments, petroleum refining, glass etching/frosting, metal etching, rust removal, dyes, plastics, germicides, leather tanning | Water irrigation Calcium gluconate |
| Lime | Agriculture Cement | Brush off, water irrigation |
| Lyes (alkalis) KOH, NaOH, | Industrial cleansers, washing powders, drain cleaners, $NH_4OH$, $LiOH$, $Ba_2(OH)_3$, $Ca(OH)_3$ | Water irrigation paint removers, urine sugar reagent tablets, portland cement |
| Metals | Industry | Cover with mineral oil, excision |
| Mustard gas | Chemical warfare | Water irrigation/mineral oil/adsorbent powders/ M258A1 Kit |
| Nitric acid | Electroplating, engraving, fertilizer manufacturing, casting iron/steel | Water irrigation |
| Oxalic acid | Leather tanning, blueprint paper | Water irrigation, IV calcium gluconate |
| Phenols (carbolic acid) | Dyes, deodorizers, sanitizers, disinfectants, cosmetics, plastics manufacture, agriculture | Water irrigation, PEG/IMS or glycerol, or isopropyl alcohol |
| Phosphoric acid | Metal cleaning, disinfectants, rust proofing | Water irrigation |
| Picric acid | Industry | Water irrigation |
| Potassium permanganate | Disinfectants, bleach, deodorizers, medical | Water irrigation |
| Sodium hypochlorite (Clorox) | Cleanser | Water irrigation |
| Sulfosalicylic acid | Industry | Water irrigation |
| Sulfuric acid | Casting iron/steel, chemistry laboratories | Water irrigation |
| Tannic acid | Industry | Water irrigation |
| Trichloracetic acid | Industry | Water irrigation |
| Tungstic acid | Industry | Water irrigation |
| White phosphorus | Warfare incendiary, insecticides, rodent poison, fertilizers | Water irrigation, 1% copper sulfate irrigation |

## Hydrofluoric Acid

Hydrofluoric acid (HF) is unique among the corrosives in its mechanism of action and degree of toxicity. HF acts like alkalis and will cause progressive tissue loss, including bony destruction. Hydrofluoric acid, considered a protoplasmic poison, penetrates the skin, dissociates, and releases fluoride ions. Fluoride ions immobilize intracellular calcium and magnesium and poison cellular enzymatic reactions. Potassium permeability is increased and results in spontaneous depolarization of nerve tissue and pain.

Industrial applications include use in production of high-octane fuel; etching and frosting glass; semiconductors; microelectronics/ microinstruments; germicides; dyes; plastics; tanning; and fireproofing material and use in cleaning stone and brick buildings. It is also a very effective rust remover.

HF rapidly penetrates the skin and causes both local and systemic toxicity. Its systemic effects include hypocalcemia, hypomagnesemia, and hyperkalemia. The dermal effects may not be immediately noted and appear to be more related to the concentration of HF than to the duration of exposure. Solutions greater than 50% produce immediate pain and tissue destruction; solutions less than 20% may not produce signs and symptoms until 12 to 24 h after exposure. The skin may develop a blue-gray appearance with a surrounding region of erythema.

Unlike the treatment of dermal injury caused by other acids, the treatment of HF burns consists of two phases. The first, which should be immediate, is copious water irrigation of the affected skin for 15 to 30 min. This may be the only treatment that is needed if the HF solution is less than 20% concentrated, the duration of exposure was very brief, and decontamination is begun immediately. Unfortunately, this is rarely the case. Severe, persistent pain denotes a more serious injury requiring the second phase of treatment.

The second phase of treatment is aimed at detoxifying the enzyme-poisoning fluoride ion. Two ions, calcium ($Ca^{2+}$) and magnesium ($Mg^{2+}$) have been shown to be beneficial in binding the fluoride and curtailing its toxic effects. However, the overwhelming clinical experience to date has been with the use of calcium gluconate, and it should be considered the agent of choice at present. Several therapeutic modalities are available for using calcium gluconate: topical, subcutaneous/intradermal injection, or intraarterial infusion. An intravenous regional perfusion technique based on Bier's method has been described and reported effective in one case report.

A calcium gluconate gel made of either Surgilube or dimethylsulfoxide (DMSO) in a 2.5 to 10% concentration may be applied directly to the affected area. The main limitation of topical therapy is the impermeability of the skin to calcium. Penetration into the dermis and subcutaneous tissues may be enhanced if the formulation with DMSO is used. The topical therapy can be utilized in the outpatient setting, and industries utilizing HF should keep this topical formulation on hand for emergency use.

Subcutaneous and intradermal injection of a 5 to 10% calcium gluconate solution through a 30-gauge needle into the HF-burned skin is the most widely used treatment. A maximum dose of 0.5 mL of 10% calcium gluconate per square centimeter of burned skin is recommended. Pain relief is near immediate, and indeed, the elimination of pain may be used as a guide for further therapy. Recurrence of pain indicates the need for further therapy. Unfortunately, injection therapy has several disadvantages: (1) only limited amounts of calcium are delivered to the tissue, (2) hyperosmolarity and inherent toxicity of free calcium ions cause more pain initially, and more tissue damage is possible if calcium is not bound to fluoride; (3) vascular compromise can result if too much fluid is injected, especially into digits; and (4) rapid penetration of HF beneath the nail requires nail removal to administer the calcium gluconate into the nail bed adequately.

Intraarterial infusion of calcium gluconate may be used to prevent tissue necrosis and stop the pain associated with HF burns. This should be performed as soon as possible after the initial burn, preferably within 6 h of insult. An intraarterial catheter should be placed in the appropriate vascular supply (the brachial artery if the entire hand is affected) and connected to a three-way stopcock to which is attached an arterial pressure monitoring device and the infusion syringe of calcium gluconate. A 50-mL syringe may be filled with 10 mL of a 10% calcium gluconate solution and 40 mL of 5% dextrose. This should be infused over 2 to 4 h. The arterial pressure monitoring device ensures that the catheter has not dislodged from the lumen of the cannulated artery. Infusion of the calcium solution into the deep tissues may cause further tissue damage. Repeat infusion may be needed if pain recurs within 4 h. This intraarterial infusion avoids the disadvantages of local infiltration therapy; however, it has its own disadvantages: an invasive vascular procedure (1) may result in arterial spasm or thrombosis and (2) requires more time and resources, including hospital admission.

Nebulized calcium gluconate is a recognized treatment for inhalational exposures to HF. Ocular exposure to HF requires water irrigation for at least 30 min. Treatment with calcium chloride or magnesium chloride by subconjunctival injection or irrigation may increase corneal damage. There is a reported case, however, of complete and quick recovery utilizing 1% calcium carbonate eye drops in a patient who had sustained a large corneal erosion due to a 49% HF burn.

Systemic toxicity related to dermal HF exposure has resulted in death. This appears to be related to myocardial irritability and subsequent ventricular fibrillation as a result of systemic acidosis, hyperkalemia, hypomagnesemia, and hypocalcemia. Cardiac monitoring, intravenous access, and electrolyte monitoring should be performed in all significant HF dermal burns.

## Nitric Acid

Nitric acid is used in industry for casting iron and steel, electroplating, engraving, and fertilizer manufacturing. Upon contact with skin, nitric acid can produce tissue damage by oxidation and may turn the skin a yellowish color as it is burned.

## Oxalic Acid

Oxalic acid is used for leather tanning and blueprint paper. Like hydrofluoric acid, it poisons enzymatic processes. Oxalic acid binds calcium and prevents muscle contraction. The burn wounds should be irrigated with water, intravenous calcium may be required. Serum electrolytes and renal function should be checked, and cardiac monitoring should be performed after serious dermal exposure.

## ALKALIS

Alkalis penetrate skin much more deeply and longer than acids, causing liquefaction necrosis of tissue with danger of toxicity from systemic absorption. Wounds may look superficial and in 2 to 3 days become full-thickness burns. Alkalis combine with protein and lipids in tissue to form soluble protein complexes and soaps which permit passage of hydroxyl ions deep into tissue. Soft, gelatinous, friable, brownish eschars are often produced. Strong alkalis have a pH ≥ 12.

### Lyes

Strong, corrosive alkalis ("lyes") include ammonium, barium, calcium, lithium, potassium (caustic potash), and sodium (caustic soda) hydroxides. Lyes are widely used in industry and found in home products (drain and toilet cleaners, washing powders, and paint removers). The urine sugar reagent tablet Clinitest contains anhydrous sodium hydroxide. As a mode of assault, lyes cause lower mortality than gunshot wounds or stabbings, but victims often suffer long-term pain, scarring and blindness. Lyes are extremely corrosive and penetrating, and burns require copious irrigation for long periods. Suicidal ingestion of lye requires aggressive airway management. Early death results from uppper airway occlusion. Late morbidity related to esophageal and gastric necrosis may be minimized by early surgical intervention with esophago-gastrectomy.

### Lime

Lime (calcium oxide) is found in agriculture products and cements. It is converted by water to the alkali calcium hydroxide. Contact with lime draws water out of the skin. All dry particles should be brushed away prior to irrigation. Paradoxically, a small amount of water may generate an exothermic reaction with tissue injury secondary to calcium hyroxide formation. A large amount and strong stream of water taking care to avoid splashing in eyes should be used and will permit dissipation of heat. There is considerable variability of lime content in different grades of cement, with fine to textured masonry cement having more than concrete.

### Portland Cement

Portland cement, which accounts for a major proportion of the cement used in the United States, is a mixture of sand, lime, and other metal oxides. In the presence of water, calcium hydroxide, sodium hydroxide, and potassium hydroxide may all be formed. Workers who kneel in wet cement or get cement in their boots may discover burns hours after initial contact. In addition, skin may become irritated from gritty material, and a contact dermatitis may develop in individuals sensitive to the chromate contained in the material.

### Metals

Burns due to molten metal occur in foundry workers. Molten metal may spill or splash on body parts and may run down into the boots of workers. Elemental metals, sodium, lithium, potassium, magnesium, aluminum, and calcium may all cause burns. When exposed to air, some elemental metals spontaneously ignite. Water is generally contraindicated in extinguishing burning metal fragments embedded in the skin because the explosive exothermic reaction that may result can lead to significant tissue injury. Burning metal may be extinguished with a class D fire extinguisher or smothered with sand. Covering metal fragments with mineral oil, however, appears to be the favored treatment method. Wound debridement should include excision of metal fragments which cannot be wiped away. Metal fragments should be placed in mineral oil to prevent further accidents.

## OTHERS

### Hydrocarbons

Hydrocarbons will cause a fat-dissolving corrosive injury to the skin. In our present petroleum-dependent society, gasoline is a common agent of burns. Patients sustaining gasoline immersion burns usually have undergone some other traumatic insult (i.e., a motor vehicle accident). Gasoline is a complex mixture of alkanes, cycloalkanes, and aromatic hydrocarbons. The hydrocarbon chemical burn resembles either a thermal scald or a partial-thickness burn. Full-thickness burns secondary to prolonged contact with gasoline have been reported. Topical gasoline exposure in cold weather can result in frostbite of the digits due to rapid evaporation of gasoline resulting in heat loss from the skin. Any potential for systemic effects of the involved hydrocarbon (or what it was a solvent for) must be recognized, as this may expose the patient to greater morbidity than the skin damage. Dehydration of the skin associated with solvent contact contributes to injury. Treatment involves decontamination and otherwise management is as for a thermal burn.

Hot tar is derived from long-chain petroleum and coal hydrocarbons. Roofing tars and asphalt are heated to temperatures in excess of 500°F and the burns sustained are usually thought of more as thermal than chemical. Liquefaction injury to tissue can occur. Though the surface area size of the burn is usually small, solidified material, stuck to skin and hair is hard to remove. The tar should be cooled to prevent continued thermal injury. Manual mechanical debridement can be painful and destructive to skin structures. Polyoxylene sorbitan (polysorbate) contained in neosporin is an emulsifying agent that can be used to remove tar. De-solv-it, a citrus and petroleum distillate, is also reported effective in tar removal. The use of mayonnaise topically has been reported as a home remedy utilized in a similar fashion.

## DMSO, Cantharides, and Mustard Gas

DMSO, cantharides, and mustard gas are considered to be vesicant agents. Skin burns with edema and blister formation can occur due to production of ischemia and anoxic necrosis at the site of contact. DMSO is a water-soluble organic solvent that has been used industrially since the 1940s. General therapeutic interest in DMSO began in the 1960s, when it was used by thousands of patients topically for sprains, bruises, minor burns, and arthritis. Its use has declined substantially because of eye toxicity, although it is still used for research and some clinical problems. Cantharides, "Spanish fly," is used as a veterinary aphrodisiac and occasionally by human beings as well for its supposed aphrodisiac effects. Mustard gas is a war gas that is unlikely to be seen in civilian practice. Historically, the most important of these agents, and still used in battle most often, is sulfur mustard. Burns resulting from vesicants should be irrigated copiously with water or saline. Skin decontamination can be accomplished using adsorbent powders (flour, talcum powder, (Fuller's earth) if water is limited in supply. The powder adsorbs the mustard from the skin and should be wiped away with a moist towel. The military uses M258A1 kits for skin decontamination. These kits contain 3 sets of towelettes, one of each containing phenol, hydroxide and chloramine. Chloramine produces "free" chlorine which inactivates sulfur mustard. Mineral oil is also recommended for mustard gas burns.

## Potassium Permanganate

Potassium permanganate is an oxidizing agent which is mildly irritating in dilute solution but in concentrated solution can produce dermal burns with a thick, brownish-purple eschar of coagulated protein. Burns should be copiously irrigated.

## Alkyl Mercury Compounds

Alkyl mercury compounds are reducing agents used in disinfectants, fungicides, and wood preservatives. Alkyl mercury can produce dermatitis or burn lesions. Lesions typically are erythematous with blister formation. The blister fluid is high in metallic mercury content. The burning process continues as long as the agent remains in contact with skin. Partial-thickness burns deepen if the blister fluid is allowed

to remain. The treatment is to debride, and remove blister fluid, and irrigate copiously.

## Diquat Dibromide

Full-thickness skin burns have been reported to occur after prolonged exposure to the herbicide diquat dibromide. These burns were treated with skin grafting. It is unknown if earlier therapy would have prevented the chain of events.

## Lacrimators (Chloroacetophenone, Chlorobenzylidenemalonitrile and Dibenzoxapine)

Lacrimators (tear gas) such as chloroacetophenone (CN), chlorobenzylidenemalonitrile (CS) and dibenzoxazepine (CR) cause skin and mucosal irritation and contact dermatitis. The epidermal injury is limited, in contrast to the possible pulmonary parenchymal damage. Burns to the skin are treated with standard water irrigation. Ocular irritation is treated with copious water irrigation, followed by slit-lamp exam for corneal damage. Structural damage to the cornea occurs at high concentrations of these lacrimators. Pepper gas (trichloronitromethane), so named because of its pepper-like odor and propensity to induce sneezing, is used in some areas by law enforcement agencies. As with the other lacrimators, it will cause mucous membrane, ocular and upper airway irritation (as well as bronchospasm in susceptible patients). Treatment is copious irrigation with saline and removal of the patient from the offending agent.

## White Phosphorus

White phosphorus is a chemical used as an incendiary and in insecticides, rodenticides, and fertilizers. It can ignite spontaneously when exposed to air and is rapidly oxidized to phosphorus pentoxide. White phosphorus is commonly found in hand grenades and other warfare munitions and thus is implicated in wartime and accidental burns to military personnel. In munitions, white phosphorus is solid in form, but some of it may liquefy with detonation. Burns may be caused by liquid or solid forms. White phosphorus burns may be complicated by multiple traumatic injuries as a result of shell fragments and the force of weapon explosions. Because of its many uses, white phosphorus burns also occur in civilians.

Flaming droplets of inorganic phosphorus may embed beneath the skin. The heat of reaction can be directly destructive to tissue. Particles continue to oxidize slowly until either debrided, neutralized, or completely oxidized. Contaminated clothing should be removed. Debride visible particles and irrigate the burns copiously with normal saline or water. A brief rinse with 1% copper sulfate solution may be helpful. Copper sulfate combines with phosphorus to form a dark-copper phosphide coating on the particles which make them easier to see and debride and also impedes further oxidation. After copper sulfate use, the burn should be irrigated again to remove copper and prevent systemic copper toxicity. Some investigators have found copper sulfate ineffective in preventing death and also toxic in animal studies.

## OCULAR BURNS

Chemical burns to the eyes are common and considered true ocular emergencies requiring immediate treatment. Typically, chemical burns to the eye occur in the industrial setting, in laboratories, or as a result of accidents such as battery explosion and intentional assaults. Rupture of automobile airbags with spillage of chemicals onto the face represents a new potential for ocular as well as skin burns. Early signs and symptoms of eye burns include tearing, rubbing, redness, pain, and blepharospasm. Conjunctivas, if severely injured, may appear pale due to ischemia. Swelling of the corneal epithelium, clouding of the anterior chamber, pupillary dilatation, and corneal ulceration may all occur.

If the nature of the chemical is not known, pH paper should be used to determine the presence of acid or alkali. Acid quickly precipitates the superficial tissue proteins of the eye, but penetration is generally limited by local buffering and barrier effects. The damage sustained secondary to acid burns in most cases is immediate and limited to the area of contact. The posterior segment of the eye rarely suffers injury, and there are usually no late effects such as cell disruption or tissue softening.

Alkali burns are much more serious, and results are frequently unsightly and disastrous. In general, the higher the pH of the alkali, the more damage occurs. In a short period of time, strong alkali can penetrate the cornea, anterior chamber, and the retina with destruction of all sensory elements, thus causing complete blindness. Alkali combines with cellular membrane lipids, resulting in cell disruption and tissue softening. Severe disruption of stromal mucopolysaccharides of the cornea occurs. The penetration of alkali can continue for hours to days. An opaque, marbled appearance of the cornea and even perforation may occur with deep injury. Conjunctival and scleral blood vessels and collecting veins of the anterior chamber may be destroyed, leading to secondary glaucoma.

Chronic inflammation of the iris and ciliary body (iridocyclitis) and adhesions between lens and iris (posterior synechiae) are complications. Other complications of eye burns include ectropion (lid deformity), cataract formation, scarring and marked revascularization of the cornea, and scarring of both palpebral and bulbar conjunctiva with resulting adhesions between the lids and globe (symblepharon).

Treatment of eye burns should begin immediately with the rare exception of burns from chemicals that react violently with water. Immediate treatment is copious and continuous irrigation at the scene, in transport, and at the hospital. Time should not be wasted in search for a neutralizing substance. Special eye-irrigating kits may be used, but in general IV tubing set up using 1 to 2 L of normal saline for 1-h continuous irrigation is the minimum treatment, particularly for alkali burns.

Acid burns may not require as much volume or treatment time. Twenty-four hours or more of continuous irrigation for alkali burns has been recommended by some. Checking the pH in the conjunctival sac to see if it has returned to normal may be helpful in determining need for further irrigation (tears have a pH between 7.3 to 7.7). The eyelid may have to be held open manually or with retractors due to severe orbicularis spasm. The eyelids should be everted if they are not too edematous. All particulate matter should be removed using a moistened cotton applicator or forceps.

Pain control with topical anesthetics initially and subsequent systemic analgesics may be necessary. Cycloplegics, mydriatics, and antibiotics should be used and the use of an eye patch may encourage corneal reepithelialization. The patient should be hospitalized and ophthalmology consultation obtained for severe burns.

Another treatment modality is the use of collagenase inhibitors such as cysteine and acetylcysteine (Mucomyst) to prevent loss of corneal stroma which occurs with liberation of collagenase from injured corneal and conjunctival epithelium. Topical steroids may reduce iridocyclitis but may also exacerbate collagenase-induced corneal ulceration. Use of scleral contact lens may reduce adhesions and scarring. Agents to reduce intraocular pressure should be used if glaucoma develops. Paracentesis may be required in severe alkali burns to introduce sterile phosphate buffer solution into the anterior chamber in attempt to reduce the pH of the inner eye. Surgery to the eye is usually not indicated during the early phase of burn management unless for corneal grafting following corneal perforation. Blepharoplasty, keratoplasty, or keratoprosthesis may be eventually required.

## IATROGENIC CHEMICAL BURNS

Iatrogenic chemical burns have been caused by the use of potassium permanganate for dermatologic problems at an inappropriately high concentration. DMSO used as a transcutaneous vehicle for minor sprains has caused burns. Patients in the operating room may develop burns from skin prep solutions. Thimerosal, which has a high mercury content, is the most common agent implicated. Mechanical abrasion of the skin from scrubbing and from pooling of the skin prep agent under the torso or tourniquet predisposes to burns. Blister formation, skin sloughing, and eschar development has been reported in neonates when isopropyl alcohol pledgets were substituted for conducting paste beneath limb ECG electrodes. Silver nitrate utilized to cauterize umbilical granulomas in infants reportedly has caused periumbilical burns.

## SYSTEMIC TOXICITY

Death early after severe chemical burns is usually related to hypotension, acute tubular necrosis, and shock as a result of fluid loss. However, systemic toxicity and subsequent morbidity and mortality may also occur with some chemicals which are absorbed through denuded dermis. Acidosis, hypotension, and shock can occur with significant absorption of acids. Hypocalcemia has been reported with both oxalic acid and hydrofluoric acid burns. Profound hypocalcemia and hypomagnesemia may be accompanied by hyperkalemia, cardiac arrhythmias, and sudden death. Tannic acid, chromic acid, formic acid, picric acid, and phosphorus may cause hepatic necrosis and nephrotoxicity. Cresol can cause methemoglobinemia, massive hemolysis, and multiple organ failure. Gasoline immersion with large surface area exposure and absorption of hydrocarbon aromatic components may result in severe pulmonary, cardiovascular, neurologic, renal, and hepatic complications. The gasoline lead additives such as tetraethyl and tetramethyl can cause lead encephalopathy. Carburetor cleaning solvent containing phenol and methylene chloride may cause renal and hepatic failure. Phenol (carbolic acid) when absorbed can lead to intravascular hemolysis, cardiovascular, pulmonary, and central nervous system toxicity. The use of phenolkin disinfectant by medical personnel in the 1800s caused chronic toxicity (carbolic marasmus) characterized by weight loss, vertigo, salivation, and increased skin and scleral pigmentation.

Sodium nitrate and potassium nitrate can cause a severe toxic methemoglobinemia from absorption with refractory cyanosis. Significant absorption of dichromate solution can result in liver failure and acute tubular necrosis and death despite hemodialysis.

Just as with thermal burns, overwhelming sepsis can be a systemic complication with chemical burns.

## BIBLIOGRAPHY

Benda B: Chemical Injuries, in Rosen P, Barkin R, et al: *Emergency Medicine: Concepts and Clinical Practice.* St. Louis, Mosby, 1992, pp. 965–968.

Bertolini JC: Hydroflouric acid: a review of toxicity. *Emerg Med* 10:163, 1992.

Borak J, Sidell FR: Agents of chemical warfare: sulfur mustard. *Ann Emerg Med* 21:303, 1992.

Caravati EM: Acute hydrofluoric acid exposure. *Am J Emerg Med* 6:143, 1988.

Emmett EA: Toxic responses of the skin, in Klaassen CD, Amdur MO, Doull J (eds): *Cassaret and Doull's Toxicology: The Basic Science of Poisons.* New York, Macmillan, 1986, pp 412–423.

Estrera A, Taylor W, Mills L. Platt M: Corrosive burns of the esophagus and stomach: a recommendation for an aggressive surgical approach. *Ann Thorac Surg* 41:276, 1986.

Goldberg MF, Paton D: Ocular emergencies, In Peyman GA, Sanders DR, Goldberg MF (eds): *Principles and Practice of Ophthalmology.* Philadelphia, Saunders, 1980, pp. 2425–2512.

Hansbrough JF, Zapata-Sirvent R, Dominic W, et al: Hydrocarbon contact injuries. *J Trauma* 25:250, 1985.

Hunter DM, Timerding BL, Leonard RB, et al: Effects of isopropyl alcohol, ethanol, and polyethylene glycol/industrial methylated spirits in the treatment of acute phenol burns. *Ann Emerg Med* 21:1303, 1992.

Jelenko C: Chemicals that "burn." *J Trauma* 14:65, 1974.

Konjoyan TR: White phosphorus burns: Case report and literature review. *Military Med* 148:881, 1983.

Leonard LG, Scheulen JJ, Munster AM: Chemical burns: Effect of prompt first aid. *J Trauma* 22:420, 1982.

Luterman A, Curreri PW: Chemical burn injury in Boswick JA (ed): *The Art and Science of Burn Care*. Rockville, MD, Aspen, 1987, pp 233–239.

Vance MV, Curry SC, Kunkel DB, et al: Digital hydrofluoric acid burns: Treatment with intraarterial calcium infusion. *Ann Emerg Med* 15:890, 1986.

Williams JM, Hammad A, Cottington EC, Harchelroad FP: Intravenous magnesium in the treatment of hydrofluoric acid burns in rats. *Ann Emerg Med* 23:464, 1994.

# 170
# ELECTRICAL AND LIGHTNING INJURIES

## Phil B. Fontanarosa

## ELECTRICAL INJURIES

Electrical injuries frequently are associated with multisystem involvement and can result in significant morbidity and mortality. Electrical injuries account for approximately 1000 deaths annually in the United States and comprise 3 to 5 percent of burn center admissions. Electrocution is the fifth leading cause of fatal occupational injuries and is the second leading cause of death in the construction industry, with the highest death rates occurring among electrical power linesmen and electricians.

Approximately 60 to 70 percent of reported electrical injuries are due to low-voltage current sources, which account for nearly half of deaths from electrical shock and cause 1 percent of accidental deaths in the home. The majority of household electrocutions involve 110- or 220-V current and most commonly result from failure to ground tools or appliances properly or from using electrical devices (e.g., hair driers) near water. More than 20 percent of all electrical injuries occur in adolescents and children. Risk-taking behavior among adolescent boys (e.g., climbing utility poles) can cause them to become exposed to high-tension electrical sources. Among children younger than 6 years of age, the most frequent causes of electrical injury are oral contact with electrical cords or wall sockets and placement of conductive foreign bodies in wall sockets.

## Pathophysiology

### Factors Related to Injury Severity

Electrical injuries result from the direct effects of current and from the conversion of electrical energy into thermal energy as current passes through body tissues. Systemic effects and tissue damage resulting from electrical shock are proportional to the magnitude and intensity of current delivered to the victim. In general, the greater the voltage, the more severe the injury, although fatal electrocutions can occur secondary to contact with low-voltage current sources (e.g., 110-V household current). Other factors that determine the severity of electrical injury include current flow, type of current, duration of contact, and current pathway (Table 170-1).

Current flow (amperage) is directly related to voltage in the system and is inversely related to resistance in the current path (according to Ohm's law, amperage = voltage/resistance). The amount of heat produced by an electrical shock and the concomitant degree of thermal injury is primarily dependent on amperage and, to a lesser degree, on tissue resistance and duration of contact (as governed by Joule's law: heat = amperage$^2$ × resistance × time). However, the exact amperage seldom is known in cases of electrical shock. The voltage of the power source usually can be determined and therefore is used to gauge the potential magnitude of current exposure and to classify electrical shock into high-voltage or low-voltage injuries. The National Electric Code defines high voltage as greater than 600 V, whereas in the medical literature, high voltage generally refers to current levels greater than 1000 V.

Body tissues differ in their resistance to the passage of electricity. In general, tissues with high fluid and electrolyte content conduct electrical current better than others. Bone is most resistant to the passage of electrical energy, followed in decreasing order of resistance by fat, tendon, skin, muscle, blood vessels, and nerves. Skin resistance is the most important factor impeding current flow. High skin resistance and a small area of contact usually concentrate electrical energy in a relatively small area and produce a severe local skin wound, limiting internal current flow. Once the skin becomes damaged, the external barrier to flow is removed, allowing the current internal access. Skin resistance also can be reduced substantially by moisture, sweat, or skin contaminants, which decrease the impediment to current flow and convert what ordinarily may be a minor low-voltage injury into a life-threatening shock. In cases of low skin resistance, current with a low-voltage electrical source may cause fatal electrocution but leave no cutaneous evidence of current contact.

Alternating current at 60 cycles per second (Hertz, or Hz)—the frequency used in most household and commercial sources of electricity—is more dangerous than direct current of the same magnitude. Low-voltage alternating current (60 Hz) has a narrow margin of safety between its amperage and amperage levels that are dangerous to humans (Table 170-2). Low-intensity current at 1 to 5 milliamps (mA) is perceived as an unpleasant tingling sensation. Contact with alternating current at 10 to 20 mA may cause repetitive stimulation of muscle fibers, produce tetanic skeletal muscle contractions, and prevent the victim from releasing hold (the hand is the most common current contact point) from the energized source. The result is increased duration of contact with the electrical source and thus increased current delivery to the victim. In contrast, direct current and high-voltage alternating current commonly cause a single powerful, involuntary contraction of skeletal muscle and often will thrust the victim away from the current source.

Tissues and organs in the current pathway are at increased risk for injury and secondary complications, although structures at sites distant from the apparent current path also can be involved. Electrical current passing through the head or crossing the thorax is more likely to cause respiratory arrest or ventricular fibrillation (VF) than current

**Table 170-1.** Factors Associated with Severity of Electrical Injuries

Current power (high voltage vs. low voltage)
Current intensity (amperage delivered)
Type of current (alternating vs. direct)
Resistance of tissues (skin resistance, internal tissue resistance)
Duration of contact (instantaneous vs. prolonged)
Contact surface area involved (localized vs. diffuse)
Current pathway (horizontal—"hand-to-hand"; vertical—"hand-to-foot" or "head-to-toe"; straddle—"foot-to-foot")
Extent of multisystem involvement (e.g., cardiac, neurologic, traumatic)
Circumstances surrounding the injury (e.g., water immersion, contact with metallic conductor)

**Table 170-2.** Effects of Electrical Current

| Current Intensity | Effect |
| --- | --- |
| 1–5 mA | Tingling sensation |
| 5–10 mA | Painful sensation |
| 10–20 mA | If contacted by hand, induces tetanic muscle contraction and prevents voluntary release of grip from current source |
| 30–50 mA | Respiratory arrest secondary to diaphragmatic and thoracic muscle tetany |
| 30–90 mA | Respiratory arrest if current directed through medulla |
| 50–100 mA | Ventricular fibrillation |
| 2–5 A | Cutaneous burns |
| 5–10 A | Asystole |

passing through the legs. The passage of current through the thorax increases the likelihood of cardiac complications, such as dysrhythmias and myocardial damage. Sudden death from VF is more likely with horizontal (hand-to-hand) current flow than with vertical (hand-to-foot) current passage, although one study found that patients with a vertical current pathway had an increased incidence of cardiac muscle damage compared to patients with a horizontal current pathway.

## Cellular Injury

Although Joule heating is thought to mediate tissue destruction in electrical injuries, particularly at skin contact points, it does not explain the extensiveness of tissue injury observed. Nonthermal mechanisms that occur secondary to the direct effects of current produce primary cellular injury and are important components of tissue injury in electrical shock. Cellular damage induced by large transmembrane electrical potentials contributes significantly to the tissue destruction associated with electrical injury and may help to explain the occurrence of tissue injury at sites distant from the apparent current pathway based on skin contact points. Cellular disruption appears to be mediated by electroporation, the process by which electrical current creates defects in the cell membrane, and probably occurs before Joule heating becomes significant. Although these processes may cause tissue damage independently, some evidence suggests that they are synergistic and that heating appears to increase the probability of membrane rupture by electroporation.

Cell membrane permeability changes and cellular rupture have been demonstrated in skeletal muscle cells and nerve cells, although a similar mechanism may occur in myocardial cells. The morphologic and functional changes in the myocardial cell membrane may result in leakage of potassium and cardiac enzymes from the cell and increased intracellular calcium. These processes, along with direct electrical depolarization of myocardial cell membranes and alterations of myocardial cell transmembrane potentials, may be contributing factors for the development of ventricular dysrhythmias and cardiac dysfunction.

## Tissue Damage

Electrical current may cause tissue damage by conductive electrothermal injury and nonconductive thermal trauma. Electrical energy density is greatest at the current contact points, and the greatest observable degree of tissue damage generally involves the skin. As current passes into the subcutaneous tissues, the electric field strength distributes throughout the tissues, with the current density and amount of tissue damage inversely proportional to the cross-sectional diameter of the contact area. Thus, current flow through a small cross-sectional area, such as a digit, may result in more local tissue destruction than current flow through a larger cross-sectional area, such as the thorax or trunk.

As current flows from the contact points, tissues with the least electrical resistance (i.e., nerves, blood vessels, and muscle) sustain the greatest current density and destructive heating. Muscle and neural tissue damage occurs secondary to cell membrane disruption, edema, coagulation necrosis, and ischemia. Vascular damage results from thrombosis, disruption of the intima and media layers, and coagulation necrosis. The net effects of these processes—neurovascular compromise, ischemia, and local tissue necrosis—coupled with electrothermal damage to muscle tissue and the corresponding release of myoglobin and hemoglobin pigments result in an injury pattern that resembles a crush injury rather than a thermal burn. Moreover, the extent of the underlying tissue destruction does not correlate with the observable skin damage. Relatively small, unimpressive cutaneous burns may be evident, but with extensive amounts of damage to underlying tissues, vascular structures, and internal organs, and thereby may result in underestimation of the severity of the electrical injury.

Nonconductive cutaneous injuries may result from exposure to electrical current arcs and are similar to conventional thermal burns. Radiant heat from electrical current arcs, which can have temperatures of 5000°C or greater, can cause burns even when the victim is not in direct contact with the electrical current. Thermal injuries also may result from hot debris from faulty electrical equipment, ignition of the victim's clothing, or from heating of metallic objects, such as rings or belt buckles.

## Cardiopulmonary Arrest

Several mechanisms may be involved in precipitating sudden death from electrical shock. Fatal accidental electrocution may be the consequence of a brief, powerful positive inotropic stimulus, perhaps tetanic in nature, resulting from the current itself. Other factors implicated in immediate cardiopulmonary arrest from electrical shock include malignant dysrhythmias resulting from myocardial cell damage, electrically induced alterations in myocardial transmembrane potentials, release of adrenomedullary and neuronal catecholamines, and asphyxia with tissue hypoxia secondary to central respiratory arrest or sustained thoracic muscle contraction.

Ventricular fibrillation may occur with exposure to as little as 50 to 100 mA. The repetitive frequency of alternating current increases the likelihood of current delivery to the myocardium during the vulnerable recovery period of the cardiac cycle and can precipitate VF, analogous to the "R-on-T" phenomenon. A single stimulus of alternating current ranging from 1 to 10 msec in duration is capable of inducing VF. The likelihood of VF increases if the electrical shock continues for a complete cardiac cycle.

Respiratory arrest may occur immediately following electrical shock and may result from one or a combination of the following mechanisms: electrical current passing through the brain may cause inhibition of medullary respiratory center function; tetanic contraction of the diaphragm and chest wall musculature may occur during current exposure; prolonged paralysis of respiratory muscles may continue after contact with the electrical current has terminated; and respiratory arrest accompanies cardiac arrest in patients with VF or asystole. Thoracic muscle tetany involving the diaphragm and intercostal muscles occurs at 30 to 50 mA and can result in respiratory arrest. Prolonged contact with the current source leads to sustained apnea with hypoxemia and secondary cardiac arrest.

In addition to the direct effects of current on myocardial tissue, coronary artery spasm appears to be an important mechanism in the development of myocardial injury and ischemia. An electrogenic mechanism of smooth muscle activation may exist in human coronary artery, and, theoretically, electrical shock could produce direct coronary artery spasm and myocardial ischemia. Prolonged electrical stimulation may generate free oxygen radicals that inhibit coronary artery smooth muscle relaxation. On the other hand, transmural myocardial infarction due to acute coronary artery occlusion following electrical shock is rare.

## Neurologic Involvement

Neural tissue is highly susceptible to the effects of electrical current. Central nervous system (CNS) involvement affecting the brain, spinal cord, or both is common following electrical shock and may occur whether or not the head or spine is the point of direct current contact or is in the current pathway traversed. Neurologic damage and brain dysfunction may result from the direct effects of electrical current on neuronal tissue or from secondary mechanisms. Direct effects include coagulation necrosis, reactive gliosis, demyelination, and cerebral edema. Secondary mechanisms include primary intracerebral or spinal injury; cerebral anoxia from prolonged seizures, aspiration, or respiratory arrest; or spinal cord ischemia resulting from vascular insufficiency or thrombosis.

Peripheral nerves in electrically injured extremities are highly sensitive to damage. Mechanisms of injury include direct electrothermal damage to neural tissue along the current pathway, ischemia secondary to swelling of injured tissues, and compromise of the local blood supply from vascular thrombosis, tissue edema, and development of compartment syndrome.

## Renal Failure

Renal failure is a significant potential complication following electrical current exposure. Although renal damage caused by the direct effects of current on the kidneys is uncommon, acute tubular necrosis from hemochromogen deposition and hypovolemia may occur and represents a serious complication. Myoglobin is released into the circulation from electrically damaged skeletal muscle, and free hemoglobin is released secondary to intravascular hemolysis. Fluid losses from damaged tissues can be profound and lead to hypovolemia, decreased glomerular filtration, and renal cortical ischemia.

## Clinical Features

Victims of electrical shock may experience a wide spectrum of injury, ranging from a transient unpleasant sensation from brief exposure to low-intensity current to instantaneous sudden death from accidental electrocution. Following significant current exposure, multisystem involvement is common (Table 170-3) and may manifest immediately after current contact or may become apparent several hours after the injury.

### Cardiopulmonary

Cardiopulmonary arrest is the primary cause of immediate death due to electrical injury. The initial dysrhythmia producing sudden death is a function of the magnitude of the current. Low-tension alternating current (50 to 100 mA) generally causes ventricular fibrillation, whereas higher intensity current (greater than 10 A) may cause either VF or asystole. Exposure to either low- or high-voltage current may produce other life-threatening cardiac dysrhythmias, such as ventricular tachycardia or ventricular ectopy, which may progress to VF. Respiratory arrest may last minutes to hours after the electrical shock terminates and may persist following restoration of spontaneous circulation. In some patients, cardiac activity may be maintained in the absence of spontaneous ventilations. However, if respiratory arrest is not corrected promptly by artificial ventilation and oxygenation, secondary hypoxic cardiac arrest may occur.

Dysrhythmias are common following electrical shock, with an incidence up to 30 percent. The most frequent dysrhythmias are sinus tachycardia and premature ventricular contractions. Ventricular tachycardia, atrial fibrillation, atrial tachycardia, atrial ectopic beats, sinus bradycardia, first- and second-degree heart block, bundle branch block, and ST-T-wave changes have been documented. Although the majority of significant dysrhythmias occur immediately following electrical shock, cases of life-threatening ventricular dysrhythmias occurring up to 12 h after electrical current exposure have

**Table 170-3.** Complications Associated With Electrical Shock

| Type of Involvement | Complications |
| --- | --- |
| Cardiovascular | Sudden death (ventricular fibrillation, asystole), chest pain, dysrhythmias, ST-T-segment abnormalities, bundle branch block, myocardial damage, ventricular dysfunction, myocardial infarction (rare), hypotension (secondary to volume depletion), hypertension (secondary to endogenous catecholamine release) |
| Neurologic | Altered level of consciousness, confusion, agitation, amnesia, coma, seizures, cerebral edema, hypoxic encephalopathy, headache, aphasia, quadriplegia, paraplegic, focal motor weakness, spinal cord dysfunction (may be delayed), peripheral neuropathy, cognitive impairment, insomnia, emotional lability |
| Cutaneous | Electrothermal contact injuries; noncontact arc burns and "flash" burns, secondary thermal burns (clothing ignition, heating of metal objects, e.g., rings or belt buckles) |
| Vascular | Vascular thrombosis, coagulation necrosis, intravascular hemolysis, delayed vessel rupture, compartment syndrome |
| Pulmonary | Respiratory arrest, aspiration pneumonia, pulmonary edema, pulmonary contusion (rare) |
| Renal/metabolic | Acute renal failure (secondary to heme pigment deposition and hypovolemia), myoglobinuria, metabolic (lactic) acidosis, hypokalemia, hypocalcemia, hyperglycemia |
| Gastrointestinal | Paralytic ileus ("electroileus"), intestinal perforation, intramural esophageal hemorrhage, hepatic necrosis, pancreatic necrosis, stress ulceration (Curling ulcers), GI bleeding, GI tract dysfunction |
| Muscular | Myonecrosis, compartment syndrome, clostridial myositis, muscle fibrosis |
| Skeletal | Vertebral compression fractures, long bone fractures, shoulder dislocations (anterior and posterior), scapular fractures, aseptic necrosis, periosteal burns, bony matrix destruction, osteomyelitis |
| Infectious | Sepsis, local wound infection, clostridial myonecrosis, cellulitis, pneumonia, osteomyelitis |
| Ophthalmologic | Corneal burns, delayed cataract formation, intraocular hemorrhage or thrombosis, uveitis, retinal detachment, orbital fracture |
| Auditory | Hearing loss, tinnitus, tympanic membrane perforation (rare) |
| Oral burns | Delayed labial artery hemorrhage, scarring and facial deformity, delayed speech development, hypoplastic mandible growth, impaired dentition development |
| Fetal | Spontaneous abortion, fetal death, oligohydramnios, intrauterine growth retardation, hyperbilirubinemia |

been reported. Functional cardiac impairment following electrical injury also has been documented, including global left ventricular hypokinesis, biventricular dysfunction, and reduced cardiac ejection fraction.

Myocardial damage after electrical accidents is an uncommon but potentially life-threatening complication. Patients at highest risk for myocardial damage after high-voltage electrical injuries are those with extensive body surface burns or with transthoracic current flow. Electrically induced myocardial injury tends to be diffuse and nonfocal, and most cases involve subepicardial injury, with only rare cases of transmural involvement.

Clinical information and available diagnostic studies have limitations for confirming the presence of myocardial damage. Consequently, the diagnosis is easily missed. The clinical presentation varies, and most patients lack the characteristic chest discomfort indicative of myocardial ischemia. Electrocardiographic (ECG) abnormalities usually are transient and most commonly include nonspecific ST-T-wave changes; ST-segment elevation seldom occurs. Although creatine kinase MB (CK-MB) enzyme levels usually are increased in patients with myocardial damage, the sensitivity of these levels in electrical shock is controversial. Electrical injuries involving skeletal muscle damage may cause significant elevations of CK-MB isoenzymes in the absence of cardiac damage and may lead to false-positive diagnoses of myocardial infarction.

## Neurologic

Neurologic involvement occurs in the majority of patients with significant electrical injuries and both acute and delayed neurologic complications have been reported. Temporary loss of consciousness is frequent following current exposure, although alterations of consciousness can range from acute confusion or agitation to deep coma. Other CNS manifestations include seizures, amnesia, headache, quadriplegia, focal motor weakness, aphasia, tinnitus or deafness, and visual disturbances. Diverse neuropsychiatric sequelae, including cognitive, behavioral, and emotional disturbances, have been reported and may persist for years following electrical injury.

Peripheral nerve injury may be apparent immediately following current exposure or may manifest days to months after electrical trauma. Peripheral neuropathies range from transient, mild paresthesias to complete and irreversible impairment of sensory or motor function or both. In cases in which the current contact point includes the hand, the median nerve is injured most commonly, although a combination of mixed motor and sensory deficits involving more than one peripheral nerve occurs frequently. Recovery from significant peripheral nerve injury generally is poor, and a high incidence of delayed causalgia has been reported.

## Cutaneous

Contact with electrical current frequently produces cutaneous burns, with entrance wounds at the point of current contact and one or more exit wounds as the current leaves the body. The vast majority of entry wounds are on the upper extremities, usually the hand, whereas exit wounds are most common on the lower extremities, typically the heels. Electrical skin wounds consist of a charred central area, surrounded by an adjacent firm middle zone that appears white to grayish white, and an outer region of brighter red, swollen, damaged tissue. Entry wounds characteristically are relatively small and well localized, whereas exit wounds may be larger with an explosive appearance. Contact with current having energy levels sufficient to generate a significant amount of heat will produce blistering, charring, and destruction of the dermis and, at times, evidence of thermal injury to subcutaneous tissues. Partial-thickness nonconductive thermal burns also may occur.

## Vascullar

Acute vascular complications may result from direct damage to the vessel wall from the electrical current, from secondary arterial spasm, or from arterial or venous thrombosis. Clinical findings may include absence of pulses, decreased peripheral perfusion, and impaired neurologic function. Electrically injured extremities often develop rapid swelling of the muscles and soft tissues, thereby setting the stage for the development of a compartment syndrome, which further endangers the vascular supply to the limb. Thrombosis of peripheral veins may occur and precludes using them for establishing intravenous access. Delayed rupture of injured vessels may result in significant hemorrhage.

## Blunt Trauma

Victims of electrical shock may sustain injuries by being thrown from the energized current source, from forceful tetanic muscle contraction associated with alternating current, or from falls after losing consciousness and muscle control. Consequently, blunt trauma secondary to electrical injuries is relatively common and encompasses a wide range of potential injuries, including head and spinal cord, intrathoracic, and intraabdominal injuries.

Fractures occur in 5 to 15 percent of patients with electrical shock, with vertebral compression fractures and long bone fractures from falls among the most common musculoskeletal injuries. Anterior and posterior shoulder dislocations and bilateral scapular fractures caused by severe tetanic muscle contractions also have been reported.

## Oral Burns

Oral and perioral burns are the most common electrical injury in young children. The injury results when a curious toddler sucks or chews on a live electrical wire, extension cord, plug, or outlet. Saliva on the lips and mouth conducts current flow and may lead to arcing, which can produce temperatures approaching 2500°C. The child displays an obvious burn near the corner of the mouth, typically consisting of an oval ulcer with surrounding erythema and usually involving the upper and lower lips and oral commissure. Occasionally, injuries to the teeth and tongue or further facial burns are noted. The majority of children with oral burns have no systemic involvement and, except for being frightened from the burn, appear normal and alert. Nonetheless, a thorough search for associated problems is indicated.

Delayed hemorrhage from the labial artery is a major concern following oral electrical burns and occurs in 10 to 15 percent of patients. Several days to 2 weeks after the initial injury, the local tissues begin to separate (or the child can dislodge the healing tissues) and the damaged labial artery may be exposed, resulting in brisk hemorrhage. Children with perioral electrical burns also are at risk for scarring and deformation of the lips and mouth, impaired jaw growth, and abnormal speech development.

## Electric Shock during Pregnancy

Electrical shock in pregnant women is associated with significant fetal morbidity and mortality. Amniotic fluid effectively transmits current flow to the fetus and thereby increases the risk of spontaneous abortion and fetal demise. Surviving infants have an increased risk of postnatal complications, including growth retardation.

## Other Complications

The gastrointestinal tract is susceptible to injury when electrical current contacts the abdominal wall or traverses the abdominal contents. Perforation of a hollow viscus or necrosis of intraabdominal organs may occur secondary to the effects of current. Paralytic ileus, stress ulcerations of the stomach and duodenum, and hepatic and pancreatic dysfunction have been reported.

Ophthalmologic complications are associated with electrical current flow near the head or eyes and include corneal burns, intraocular thrombosis and hemorrhage, and retinal detachment. Cataract formation is a well-recognized delayed complication and usually occurs several months after the acute electrical injury.

Local and systemic infections are common complications following significant electrical trauma. Local wound infections in burned surface tissues or in areas with occult deep necrotic tissues may be caused by aerobic or anaerobic pathogens, including *Pseudomonas* or *Clostridium*. Overwhelming systemic infection, such as sepsis from wound infection or pneumonia, is among the leading causes of death among patients hospitalized following serious electrical injuries.

Despite improvements in initial resuscitation, advances in critical care, and refinements of surgical techniques, electrical injuries remain a devastating form of trauma. Patients with serious electrical injuries frequently require multiple operations for sequential debridement and coverage of skin defects and commonly undergo major amputations. Despite aggressive treatment and prolonged rehabilitation, permanent sequelae and long-term disability occur in a significant proportion of survivors.

## Diagnosis

The diagnosis of electrical injury usually is based on the history surrounding the event. If the patient's clinical status permits, a thorough history should be obtained to attempt to determine the magnitude of voltage involved, the type of current, the duration of current contact, the likely current pathway, and symptoms suggestive of multisystem complications. Circumstances surrounding the electrical injuries (e.g., faulty equipment, wet flooring) should be sought to determine the possible mechanism for current exposure and to identify future efforts at prevention. Precipitating factors, such as intoxication, suicidal intention, or foul play, also should be considered. The presence of underlying medical conditions, such as cardiovascular disease, diabetes mellitus, and neurologic disease should be determined. Occasionally, the diagnosis of electrical injury may be unclear, such as in unwitnessed cases in which the victim is confused, amnestic, or unconscious or in instances when external signs of electric injury are absent, such as with electrocution occurring in swimming pools or bathtubs.

A thorough physical examination should be performed to evaluate apparent tissue damage and to identify associated complications. Assessment of airway, respirations, and hemodynamic status is essential, along with careful evaluation for evidence of cutaneous burns and secondary trauma. Detailed neurologic and vascular examinations should be performed, with particular attention to mental status and neurovascular function of electrically injured extremities. Despite the importance of a thorough initial assessment, clinical findings alone may not be sensitive or specific enough to identify precisely the extent of electrical injuries. Clinicians must be aware that the absence of physical findings does not necessarily rule out potentially serious underlying involvement.

All patients with electrical injury should have a 12-lead electrocardiogram performed and should be placed on continuous cardiac monitoring. Patients with high-voltage current exposure, high- or low-voltage conductive injury, extensive cutaneous burns, or evidence of associated complications require laboratory evaluation. Initial studies should include complete blood count, electrolytes and calcium, urea nitrogen and creatinine, coagulation studies, arterial blood gases, creatine kinase (CK) levels and CK-MB fraction, and myoglobin level. Urinalysis and urine myoglobin level should be obtained, and a rapid examination of urine should be performed to screen for myoglobinuria. Liver function studies and amylase level should be obtained for patients with suspected intraabdominal involvement. Blood type and cross match are indicated for patients with severe electrical injury and for those in whom surgical intervention or extensive debridement is anticipated.

Cervical spine radiographs should be obtained in patients with suspected spinal injuries, evidence of head or facial trauma secondary to falls, or in obtunded patients in whom a history of trauma is uncertain. Cranial computed tomography should be considered in patients with altered level of consciousness following electrical shock who have evidence of associated head trauma and in those without apparent head injury who fail to show improvement in CNS function. Indications for additional radiographic studies should be based on patient complaints or clinical findings. Consideration of other diagnostic studies, such as arteriography to evaluate suspected vascular compromise or radionuclide scanning to evaluate underlying muscle damage, should be coordinated with the consulting surgeon.

## Management

Principles of management for electrically injured victims include providing aggressive and sustained resuscitation measures and using a combination of basic and advanced cardiac and trauma life-support techniques to achieve initial stabilization and to manage associated acute complications. Recovery from electrical shock is not readily predictable because the magnitude of current delivered, the nature of the underlying injuries, and the degree of cardiac or cerebral ischemia may not be apparent. However, given that most victims of electrical trauma are young, healthy, and lack significant underlying cardiac disease, aggressive and vigorous resuscitation measures are indicated and may be effective even for those who appear unlikely to survive based on initial evaluation.

Immediate priorities for patients with severe electrical injuries include securing the airway, supporting respiration and ensuring adequate oxygenation, and stabilization of circulation. Establishing an artificial airway may be difficult in patients with electrical burns of the face, mouth, or anterior neck. Extensive soft tissue swelling may develop rapidly and complicate airway management. During airway control measures and initial resuscitation, spinal protection and immobilization should be maintained if there is any likelihood of head or neck trauma.

Ventricular fibrillation, ventricular asystole, and other serious dysrhythmias should be treated with standard advanced life-support (ALS) techniques and cardiac drug therapy. If defibrillation or cardioversion is necessary, energy levels recommended by standard ALS protocols should be used. Most dysrhythmias are transient and, except for those causing circulatory compromise, treatment with antiarrhythmic agents usually is unnecessary.

Patients with significant underlying tissue destruction or hypovolemic shock require rapid intravenous fluid administration to correct ongoing fluid losses, counteract shock, and maintain urine output to facilitate clearance of myoglobin and avoid renal shutdown. Ringer's lactate solution or normal saline is the preferred resuscitation fluid. Because fluid requirements generally are substantially greater for electrically injured patients than for victims of thermal burns, standard burn formulas for calculating fluid needs based on cutaneous injury markedly underestimate the amount of fluid necessary to maintain perfusion and counteract rhabdomyolysis. An initial fluid bolus of 10 to 20 mL/kg should be administered to hypotensive patients, with subsequent fluid administration sufficient to maintain urinary output at approximately 1.0 mL/kg per hour. Central venous or pulmonary artery pressure monitoring may be necessary to help guide fluid replacement and prevent circulatory overload in patients at risk for congestive heart failure.

Evidence of heme pigments in the urine requires additional measures to treat myoglobinuria. Urinary alkalinization, which increases the solubility of myoglobin and facilitates its excretion, is accomplished by adding sodium bicarbonate to the IV fluids (i.e., 44 to 50 mEq of bicarbonate to each liter of normal or half-normal saline). Blood pH should be monitored and maintained at 7.45 or greater, and urine output should be maintained at 1.5 to 2.0 mL/kg per hour. Administration of mannitol also may be useful to maintain and enhance urinary flow. The initial dose is 25 g IV, followed by 12.5 g IV per hour until the urine is cleared of heme pigment. If thermal burns are present in addition to electrical injury, mannitol should not be given.

Wound care depends on the extent of cutaneous involvement and the likelihood of underlying tissue injury. Because relatively innocuous-appearing surface wounds may exist with significant underlying tissue destruction, consultation with a surgeon experienced in the treatment of electrical injuries should be considered to evaluate the need for formal wound exploration and for cases in which debridement may be necessary. Care for minor, localized wounds involving only cutaneous structures includes cleansing the wound thoroughly and covering it with a topical antimicrobial preparation. Silver sulfadiazine is appropriate for superficial wounds. Mafenide acetate has better eschar penetration and is preferred for localized full-thickness electrothermal burns.

For minor cutaneous burns, tetanus prophylaxis should be administered based on the patient's tetanus immunization status. The use of tetanus immune globulin should be considered for electrical burns with increased risk of tetanus, including those that are greater than 6 h old, are contaminated (especially by soil), or have devitalized subcutaneous tissue or muscle tissue. The administration of prophylactic antibiotics varies with the extent of the electrical injury and with the policies of the institution. Most centers do not routinely administer antimicrobial agents if only cutaneous injury is present. However, prophylaxis with parenteral antibiotics (e.g., high-dose penicillin) effective against anaerobic organisms to prevent clostridial myonecrosis should be considered in patients with apparent or suspected devitalized muscle tissue.

Management of other complications resulting from electrical trauma generally follows standard emergency therapy. Seizures should be treated with usual anticonvulsant agents. Fractures and dislocations should be reduced and immobilized in the usual fashion, with careful monitoring of neurovascular status of the involved extremity. Patients with multisystem involvement or severe electrical injuries should have nasogastric tube insertion because of the attendant risks of ileus and gastric dilatation.

## Patient Disposition

### Admission

After resuscitation and stabilization, all patients with significant electrical injuries require admission to a center with appropriate capabilities for providing specialized, comprehensive care for electrical trauma victims. Given the devastating nature of serious electrical trauma and the potential benefits of a multidisciplinary approach to management of the associated acute and long-term complications, most patients with serious electrical injury should be admitted to regional burn centers or trauma intensive care units staffed by surgeons, critical care specialist physicians and nurses, and support personnel (e.g., physical therapists, occupational therapists, psychological counselors) experienced in the management of electrical trauma.

Admission is indicated for all patients with high-tension (>1000 V) current exposure. Patients with low-tension (<1000 V) current exposure and any evidence of complications (Table 170-4) also should be admitted, either to a critical care setting or, for less severe electrical shock injuries, to a setting with capabilities for careful clinical monitoring and electrocardiographic monitoring for at least 24 h.

### Discharge

The management of asymptomatic patients with brief exposure to low-intensity current (i.e., up to 110 or 220 V) is controversial. Although prospective studies evaluating the safety and cost-effectiveness of optimal management strategies for these patients are lacking, it appears that selected asymptomatic patients may be safely discharged home after appropriate evaluation and observation in the emergency department.

To be considered for discharge from the emergency department after electrical shock, the patient should have no evidence of significant electrothermal burns, the physical examination and ECG should be normal, and the urine should be negative for any evidence of heme pigment. The patient should have remained asymptomatic and should have had no evidence of dysrhythmias during a 6- to 8-h period of observation and cardiac monitoring in the emergency department. All discharged patients should have reliable home support, should be advised to return immediately if any symptoms occur, and should have specific follow-up arranged with a physician familiar with electrical

**Table 170-4.** Indications for Admission

High-tension (>1000 V) current exposure
Low-tension (<1000 V) current exposure and any of the following:
  Any suspected conductive current flow, especially involving current through the chest, trunk, or head
  Any symptoms suggestive of systemic involvement or involvement of the cardiovascular (e.g., chest pain, palpitations), gastrointestinal (e.g., abdominal pain, vomiting), neurologic (e.g., headache, loss of consciousness, confusion, weakness, paresthesias), or respiratory (e.g., dyspnea) system
  Electrical injury involving an extremity or a digit with suspected or potential neurovascular compromise
  Electrothermal burns with evidence of or suspected involvement of subcutaneous tissues
  Abnormal findings on physical examination
  Abnormal findings on laboratory studies or urinalysis
  Abnormal findings on electrocardiogram
  Documented or suspected dysrhythmia
  History of cardiac disease, renal disease, or other underlying medical problems
  Electrical injuries associated with suspected foul play, abuse, or suicidal intent
  Associated injuries necessitating admission

injures. If the emergency physician has any doubt concerning the extent of current exposure, the degree of injury, associated complications, or the patient's reliability, admission is advisable.

### Consultation

In addition to liberal involvement of surgical specialists for evaluation and management of electrothermal burns, several other types of patients with electrical injuries require prompt specialty consultation. Patients with hemodynamic compromise and multisystem involvement may benefit from early involvement of an intensive care specialist, whereas those with renal involvement should have a nephrologist consulted. Patients with isolated involvement of the hand or significant involvement of a digit should be evaluated by a hand surgeon or plastic surgeon. Children with isolated burns involving the oral commissure should be seen promptly by a plastic surgeon or oral surgeon to evaluate the injury, plan for treatment (such as splinting or debridement), and, depending on the philosophy of the center, aid in decision-making regarding admission. Pregnant women who sustain electric shock should be evaluated by an obstetrician. Abdominal ultrasound and fetal monitoring are indicated for patients in their second and third trimesters, along with close follow-up during the remainder of the pregnancy.

### Documentation

Clear, complete, detailed documentation of the emergency department assessment and management is essential in all cases of electrical injuries, both for issues related to patient care and for legal reasons. Given the significant mortality and morbidity associated with electrical trauma, the emergency management of victims of electrical trauma carries the potential for claims of malpractice against treating physicians. In addition, significant electrical injuries virtually always result in tort claims, either as charges of negligence against a power company, litigation against a private corporation or manufacturer, or claims involving workman's compensation. It is therefore necessary not only to deliver timely, appropriate care for patients with electrical injuries but also to have a carefully documented record that contains the reported circumstances surrounding the electrical shock, the clinical evaluation and findings, and the treatment provided.

## LIGHTNING INJURIES

Lightning strike is an unusual form of trauma yet represents one of the leading causes of death from environmental phenomenon. Lightning accounts for approximately 150 to 300 fatalities per year in the United States and causes serious injuries to an additional 1000 to 1500 persons. Victims of lightning strike have a 20 to 30 percent fatality rate, with the majority of deaths due to immediate cardiac arrest. Among survivors of lightning injuries, approximately 75 percent sustain significant permanent sequelae. Although lightning is an electrical phenomenon that follows many of the same laws of physics that govern manmade electricity, lightning injuries differ substantially from high-voltage electrical injuries, not only in terms of the types and severity of injuries that occur but also with respect to emergency management.

## Pathophysiology

Compared with manmade electricity, lightning has a much greater magnitude of energy, a substantially shorter duration of exposure, and a different current pathway. The lightning current may have an energy level that exceeds 100 million V and 100,000 A. However, because of the instantaneous duration of current flow, the amount of energy delivered internally to the victim may be less than with high-voltage electrical shock (Table 170-5).

Victims of lightning may be injured by one of several mechanisms. Direct strike occurs when lightning current contacts the victim and energy passes through or over the victim. Direct strike most commonly occurs when the victim is in contact with an object, such as a tree or metal pole, that becomes part of the current path. Direct strike also may occur when the victim is the tallest structure in the vicinity, such as when caught in a thunderstorm on a hilltop or on an open flat area. Direct strike is considered to be the most serious type of lightning exposure and generally results in the most severe injuries, although it is not uniformly fatal.

Side flash or splash injury occurs when lightning strikes a primary site, such as a tree, light pole, or building, but then splashes from the structure to involve a nearby victim in its pathway. Side flash occurs when the primary strike site has a relatively greater resistance to the lightning current than the air between the object and the victim. Side flash also may occur when lightning splashes off one victim and strikes another nearby person, thereby contributing to the occurrence of simultaneous injury of several individuals from a single lightning strike.

Ground current or step voltage occurs when lightning strikes the earth and spreads through the ground toward the victim. The victim may have one leg in contact with the ground closer to the strike point than the other leg, producing a potential difference (orstride potential) between the legs. The result is passage of current through the legs and into the trunk.

Lightning also may cause injury by thermal mechanisms or blunt trauma. Thermal burns may occur when clothing is ignited by lightning strike or when metal objects worn by the victim become superheated by the lightning current. If the victim's skin is wet from rainwater or sweat, the high temperatures from the lightning current (estimated between 8000° and 30,000°C) may cause first- and second-degree burns as the moisture is converted to steam. Lightning causes rapid expansion of the surrounding air through which it passes and creates an implosive force. As the sudden force from the lightning passes near the victim, it may cause blunt injury from the shock waves it produces or may cause the victim to be thrown from the strike current, leading to secondary blunt trauma.

Except for lightning strike in which the victim absorbs a substantial amount of charge, the short duration of lightning usually limits internal current flow and prevents significant tissue damage from occurring. Instead, in many cases, the majority of the lightning current instantaneously passes over the outside of the victim. This so-called flashover phenomenon, which is analogous to current flow over the outside of a metal conductor, may account for the relatively high survival rate considering the magnitude of current involved in lightning injuries. However, some of the lightning current may enter the victim and produce sudden disruption of cardiac, respiratory, or neurologic function.

Immediate cardiac arrest is the primary cause of death following lightning strike. Lightning may act as a sudden direct-current countershock that depolarizes the entire myocardium, produces a sustained cardiac contraction, and results in cardiac standstill. Although asystole has been considered the primary rhythm in lightning-induced sudden death, VF also has been reported and may be more common than traditionally acknowledged.

Following asystole, cardiac automaticity may restore organized electrical activity in the heart, which may lead to the development of bradycardia accompanied by return of spontaneous circulation. However, concomitant respiratory arrest due to paralysis of the medullary respiratory center frequently is prolonged and may outlast cardiac arrest. The duration of apnea, rather than the duration of asystole, appears to be a critical factor in mortality. If timely ventilatory assistance is not provided, hypoxic cardiac arrest with VF eventually ensues.

## Clinical Features

The nature and severity of lightning injuries depends on the magnitude of energy delivered to the victim, the type of lightning exposure, the body systems involved, acute secondary complications, and un-

**Table 170-5.** Comparison of Lightning Injuries and High Voltage Electrical Injuries

| Factor | Lightning | High Voltage |
|---|---|---|
| Current exposure duration | Instantaneous | May be prolonged |
| Energy level | | |
|   Voltage | 3000–30,000,000 V | 1000–70000 V |
|   Amperage | 50,000 A | 10–10,000 A |
| Current characteristics | Unidirectional (direct) | Alternating |
| Current pathway | Flashover | Horizontal (hand-to-hand) Vertical (hand-to-foot) |
| Burn characteristics | Superficial, minor | Deep, destruction of underlying tissues |
| Initial rhythm in cardiac arrest | Asystole more common | Ventricular fibrillation more common |
| Renal involvement | Myoglobinuria or hemoglobinuria rare | Myoglobinuria and renal failure common |
| Fasciotomy and amputation | Rarely necessary | Relatively common and extensive |
| Blunt injury | Explosive effect with "shock wave" | Falls, being thrown from current source |

*Source:* Modified from: Cooper MA, Lightning injuries, in Auerbach PS, Geehr EC (eds): *Wilderness Medicine: Management of Wilderness and Environmental Emergencies,* 3rd ed. St Louis, Mosby, 1995.

derlying medical disorders. In most instances, cardiac and neurologic findings predominate (Table 170-6).

Lightning injuries encompass a wide spectrum ranging from minor to severe injuries, with prognosis correlating roughly with the initial severity of the injury. For example, patients with minor lightning injuries typically appear "stunned," i.e., they are awake but somewhat confused, amnestic for the event, and have problems with short-term memory. Common complaints include headache, muscle pain, paresthesias, and temporary vision loss or hearing loss. Except for mild tachycardia and hypertension, vital signs usually are stable. For most patients with mild injury, gradual recovery occurs. In contrast, patients with severe lightning injury may present in refractory cardiac arrest, may have associated central nervous system damage, and generally have a poor prognosis.

In addition to cardiac arrest, other cardiovascular complications are common in victims of lightning strike. Cardiac damage may result from direct myocardial damage, coronary artery spasm, and blunt cardiac injury. ECG evidence of acute ischemia and injury, elevation of creatine phosphokinase cardiac (MB) fraction, and myocardial necrosis on autopsy have been documented. Atrial and ventricular dysrhythmias occur frequently, and a variety of ECG changes, including ST-segment and T-wave changes and Q-T interval prolonga-

**Table 170-6.** Complications Associated With Lightning Strike

| Type of Involvement | Complications |
| --- | --- |
| Cardiovascular | Sudden death (asystole, ventricular fibrillation), dysrhythmias (premature ventricular contractions, ventricular tachycardia, atrial dysrhythmias), ST-segment abnormalities, cardiac necrosis, myocardial infarction, cardiac dysfunction, pericardial effusion, hypertension |
| Pulmonary | Respiratory arrest, pulmonary edema, pulmonary contusion, pulmonary hemorrhage |
| Neurologic (acute) | Confusion, amnesia, loss of consciousness, seizures, intracranial hemorrhage (epidural, subdural, intraventricular) respiratory center paralysis, cerebral edema, cerebral infarction or hemorrhage, extremity paralysis, paresthesias, dyscoordination, ataxia, hemiplegia, aphasia, vision loss |
| Neurologic (long term) | Paraplegia, hemiplegia, paresis, paeresthesias, neuralgia, difficulty with balance, insommia, panic attacks, aphasia, post-traumatic stress disorder symptoms, difficulty with fine motor function, cognitive dysfunction, headaches, depression, mood disturbances, emotional lability, storm phobia |
| Cutaneous | Linear burns, punctate burns, arborescent feathering burns (keraunographic markings, Lichtenberg figures), full-thickness burns, thermal burns |
| Extremities | Mottling, intense vasomotor spasm, keraunoparalysis (severe vascular spasm, motor paralysis, sensory loss) |
| Ophthalmologic | Cataracts, corneal lesions, hyphema, uveitis, iridocyclitis, vitreous hemorrhage, diplopia, chorioretinitis, retinal detachment, macular degeneration, optic atrophy, ocular autonomic disturbances |
| Auditory | Tympanic membrane rupture, cerebrospinal fluid otorrhea, hemotympanum, temporaty or chronic deafness |
| Renal | Myoglobinuria, hemoglobinuria, renal failure (rare) |
| Miscellaneous | Secondary blunt trauma (head, spine, chest, abdomen, extremity), muscle compartment syndrome, disseminated intravascular coagulation |

tion, have been observed. Acute global cardiac dysfunction, life-threatening acute pericardial effusion, and both immediate and delayed pulmonary edema have been reported. Transient hypertension and tachycardia are common in the acute phase of lightning strike and have been attributed to excess catecholamine release leading to a relative hyperadrenergic state.

Neurologic injuries are among the most common and most serious complications of lightning strike. Neurologic findings may be immediate and transient or delayed and progressive. Temporary loss of consciousness is the most common neurologic event, occurs in 72 percent of victims, and almost invariably is accompanied by confusion and amnesia for the lightning strike event. Patients who remain unresponsive following lightning strike have a relatively poor prognosis. Coma may result from brain injury from the lightning current; prolonged cerebral anoxia prior to resuscitation; acute cerebral edema; closed head injury; or cerebral infarction, ischemia, or hemorrhage. The usual causes of altered level of consciousness also should be considered, including hypoglycemia, drug ingestion, or, in some cases, hypothermia. Acute neurologic complications also may include seizures, vision loss, and cognitive disturbances. Long-term neurologic sequelae occur frequently and include paralysis, paresthesias, neuralgias, cognitive dysfunction, and psychological disturbances such as depression, anxiety, posttraumatic stress disorder, and storm phobias.

Keraunoparalysis, which is transient flaccid paralysis that usually involves the lower extremities, is common following lightning strike. Paralysis occurs in combination with complete or partial sensory loss and is accompanied by marked vasomotor changes. The victim typically awakens on the ground but is unable to move the extremities, which appear cold and mottled and are insensitive and pulseless. This phenomenon usually is due to vascular spasm and sympathetic instability. In most patients with keraunoparalysis, motor and sensory deficits and circulatory disturbances begin to resolve within several hours and usually resolve completely within 24 h, although some patients develop permanent paralysis and paresthesias. However, acute spinal cord injury must be considered in the differential diagnosis.

Cutaneous injuries from lightning generally are superficial and relatively minor. Unless the patient has sustained significant thermal burns from the ignition of clothing, discrete entry and exit wounds as well as burns involving underlying soft tissues or muscle are uncommon. Superficial cutaneous burns from lightning have several common patterns, including discrete, multiple, clustered punctate burns or linear burns that typically involve areas of sweat and moisture collection, such as the axilla or groin. Another type of superficial burn unique to lightning injury is the keraunographic skin marking. These markings are thought to result from the superficial pathway of the lightning current as it "flashes over" the skin; they appear as arborescent, fernlike erythematous steaks and are pathognomonic for lightning injury. The lesions appear within several hours after the lightning strike, usually begin to fade within 12 h, and disappear within 48 h.

Otologic complications frequently accompany lightning injury. More than 50 percent of lightning victims sustain bilateral or unilateral tympanic membrane rupture. This complication most commonly occurs secondary to the concussive force of the lightning strike but also may be caused by basilar skull fracture, local trauma to the ear canal, or direct lightning burns.

Ophthalmologic disorders are commonly associated with lightning and may result from direct effects of current or forces transmitted to the orbit from the lightning shock wave. Cataract development is a frequent occurrence and may manifest within the first several days after the injury or may develop up to 2 years after the incident. A number of additional ocular complications have been reported, including vision loss, diplopia, corneal lesions, hyphema, uveitis, iritis, retinal detachment, and optic nerve injury. Because ocular autonomic disturbances may occur after lightning strike, dilated unresponsive pupils should not be used as a sign of brain death.

Lightning victims may sustain blunt trauma from the force generated by the lightning strike or from falls. A variety of fractures may occur, including those involving the skull, spine, and long bones. Blunt abdominal trauma, chest trauma, and head injury also may occur, depending on the circumstances and mechanism of injury.

Compared with electrical injuries, renal involvement is unusual in victims of lightning strike. Lightning seldom causes extensive tissue damage, deep burns, muscle injury, or significant fluid losses. Consequently, renal failure secondary to hemoglobinuria or myoglobinuria is uncommon.

## Diagnosis

The diagnosis of lightning injuries is usually based on the history surrounding the event. If the patient's clinical status permits, a thorough history should be obtained to attempt to determine the circumstances surrounding the strike, the possible mechanism of exposure, and the immediate effects on the victim, particularly regarding loss of consciousness. The presence of underlying medical conditions, such as cardiovascular disease, diabetes mellitus, and neurologic disease, should be identified. At times, the diagnosis of lightning strike injury may be difficult, particularly for unwitnessed events following which the victim is rendered unconscious or is confused or amnestic.

A careful physical examination should be performed. Assessment of airway, respirations, and hemodynamic status is essential, along with careful neurologic evaluation for mental status abnormalities, motor weakness, and neurovascular deficits in the extremities. An accurate temperature reading should be obtained to rule out hypothermia, particularly in rain-soaked victims. The skin should be examined carefully for evidence of cutaneous burns. Baseline ophthalmologic examination should be performed, along with visual acuity testing if the patient can cooperate. The tympanic membranes should be inspected for evidence of rupture, and simple hearing tests should be performed. In an unconscious victim found outdoors, but for whom the history is unknown, the presence of arborescent burns coupled with ruptured tympanic membranes should suggest the diagnosis of lightning injury.

All patients with lightning injury should have a 12-lead electrocardiogram performed and should be placed on continuous cardiac monitoring. Complete blood count and CK levels and CK-MB fraction should be obtained for most patients, along with a urinalysis and test for urinary myoglobin. Additional laboratory studies in patients with moderate to severe injuries should include electrolytes with calcium and magnesium, urea nitrogen and creatinine, coagulation studies, arterial blood gases, and myoglobin level.

Cervical spine radiographs should be obtained in patients with suspected spinal injuries, evidence of head or facial trauma secondary to falls, or in obtunded patients in whom a history of trauma is uncertain. Cranial CT should be considered in patients with altered or deteriorating level of consciousness, confusion that fails to clear, or evidence of head injury. A chest radiograph should be obtained to look for evidence of aspiration, pulmonary edema, or trauma. Additional diagnostic studies should be based on clinical findings. Intracranial pressure monitoring may be necessary to guide therapy but should be coordinated with the consulting neurosurgeon.

## Management

Approximately 70 percent of lightning fatalities involve single victims, and the remainder involve deaths in groups of two or more victims struck at once. Given the cardiac effects of lightning and considering that a single lightning strike frequently injuries several victims simultaneously, triage principles for multiple lightning victims differ from standard triage. Because virtually all victims of lightning strike who do not experience cardiac or respiratory arrest survive, the usual prehospital triage priorities should be reversed when several victims are struck by lightning. Victims who appear clinically dead following the strike should be treated before other victims showing signs of life.

For patients in cardiac arrest, basic resuscitation and ALS measures should be instituted immediately. Because many victims of lightning strike are young and healthy and are unlikely to have serious underlying cardiac disease, aggressive resuscitation measures are indicated, including prompt airway control, adequate ventilatory assistance, and circulatory support as indicated by the clinical status. Some victims with respiratory arrest may require only ventilation and oxygenation to avoid secondary hypoxic cardiac arrest.

Resuscitation efforts, including indications and energy levels for defibrillation, and administration schedules and dosages for cardiac medications are the same as for victims of cardiac arrest from other causes. Spinal protection and immobilization are indicated for unconscious patients and those who may have trauma. Unlike electrical shock victims, patients with lightning strike seldom have significant underlying tissue destruction, and fluid loading is unnecessary. If signs of shock due to blood loss or blunt trauma are evident, vigorous fluid resuscitation is indicated. Otherwise, as soon as spontaneous circulation and adequate blood pressure are established, fluid administration should be restricted, especially for patients with cardiac arrest or head trauma, to prevent cerebral edema that may accompany these complications.

Resuscitation attempts may have higher success rates in lightning victims than in patients with other etiologies for cardiac arrest, and efforts may be effective even when the interval before resuscitation begins is prolonged. Several anecdotal case reports have documented successful recovery after prolonged anoxia in victims of lightning strike. Other reports suggest that patients with initial postarrest rhythms traditionally associated with poor outcomes, such as asystole, may recover with prompt institution of cardiac and respiratory support.

Management of lightning strike victims without cardiac arrest generally follows standard emergency therapy. Dysrhythmias are treated with usual ALS agents, and seizures are treated with usual anticonvulsant agents. Care for superficial lightning burns involves cleansing the wound thoroughly, covering it with a topical antimicrobial preparation, and administering tetanus prophylaxis based on the patient's tetanus immunization status. Because lightning burns are superficial, aggressive fluid loading, the use of osmotic agents, and urinary alkalinization are seldom used. Likewise, repeated wound debridement, fasciotomies, and escharotomies are rarely required.

## Patient Disposition

The vast majority of patients with lightning strike injuries require admission to a center with appropriate capabilities for providing specialized, comprehensive care. Patients who survive severe or moderately severe lightning injury require admission to a critical care setting that has capabilities for invasive monitoring and for management of complications. Consultation with the critical care specialist physician, the neurosurgeon, and perhaps the cardiologist and trauma surgeon may be helpful.

Patients with minor lightning injuries generally demonstrate progressive improvement during the first several hours following the lightning strike event. Nonetheless, these patients require careful monitoring of neurologic and cardiovascular status, and most patients should be admitted to a hospital unit that has capabilities for clinical and electrocardiographic monitoring.

## BIBLIOGRAPHY

### Electrical Injuries

Chandra NC, Siu CO, Munster AM: Clinical predictors of myocardial damage after high voltage electrical injury. *Crit Care Med* 18:293, 1990.

Fish R: Electric shock, parts I–III. *J Emerg Med* 11:309, 457, 599, 1993.

Fontanarosa PB: Electrical shock and lightning strike. *Ann Emerg Med* 22 (pt 2):378, 1993.

Lee RC, Capelli-Schellpfeffer M, Kelley KM (eds): *Electrical Injury: A Multidisciplinary Approach to Therapy, Prevention, and Rehabilitation.* New York, New York Academy of Sciences, 1994.

McBride JW, Labrosse KR, McCoy HG, et al: Is serum creatine kinase-MB in electrically injured patients predictive of myocardial injury? *JAMA* 255:764, 1986.

## Lightning Injuries

Andrews CJ, Cooper MA, Darveniza M, Mackerras D: *Lightning Injuries: Electrical, Medical, and Legal Aspects.* Boca Raton, FL, CRC Press, 1992.

Cherington M, Yarnell P, Lammereste D: Lightning strikes: Nature of neurological damage in patients evaluated in hospital emergency departments. *Ann Emerg Med* 21:575, 1992.

Cooper MA: Lightning injuries, in Rosen P, Barkin R, Braen GR, et al (eds): *Emergency Medicine—Concepts and Clinical Practice,* 3d ed. St Louis, Mosby, 1992, pp 979–985.

Cooper MA: Lightning injuries, in Auerbach PS, Geehr EC (eds): *Management of Wilderness and Environmental Emergencies,* 2d ed. St Louis, Mosby, 1989, pp 173–193.

Lichtenberg R, Dries D, Ward K, et al: Cardiovascular effects of lightning strike. *J Am Coll Cardiol* 21:531, 1993.

# 171
# CARBON MONOXIDE POISONING
## Earl J. Reisdorff
## John G. Wiegenstein

Carbon monoxide (CO) is the single leading cause of toxin-related death in the United States. From 1979 to 1988, 56,133 death certificates filed in the United States contained codes implicating CO as a contributing cause of death. The incidence of nonlethal CO poisoning is not established. CO is a colorless, odorless, nonirritating gas. Its specific gravity is 0.97 relative to air, so it does not stratify. CO has a high affinity for hemoglobin. It reversibly displaces oxygen from hemoglobin to produce carboxyhemoglobin (COHb), resulting in tissue hypoxia.

The symptoms of CO poisoning are protean and vague, resulting in a high rate of misdiagnosis. Correct treatment requires aggressive oxygen therapy and the select use of hyperbaric oxygen (HBO).

## SOURCES

Carbon monoxide is endogenously produced during the metabolism of heme pigments. When protoporphyrin is converted into bilirubin, CO is released. This generates 75 percent of the endogenous production of CO, producing a serum COHb level of 0.4 to 0.7 percent. This level increases slightly during the menstrual cycle and pregnancy. Higher levels (4 to 6 percent) are seen with acute hemolytic anemia due to the accelerated metabolism of hemoglobin. CO is eliminated primarily unchanged during pulmonary respiration, though a small amount is metabolized to $CO_2$.

Exogenous CO is produced by the incomplete combustion of organic fuels. Gas-powered engines produce significant amounts of CO. Other sources include furnaces, home water heaters, gas heaters, pool heaters, wood stoves, kerosene heaters, indoor charcoal fires, and Sterno fuel. Industrial sources include steel foundries, pulp paper mills, and plants producing formaldehyde and coke. Exposures have resulted from wildland firefighting, airplane crashes, military ship explosions, propane-fueled forklifts, smoke-filled bingo halls, self-immolation, ice skating rink zambonis, and indoor tractor pulls. Fire fighters are at high risk, and most immediate deaths from building fires are due to CO poisoning. All patients from a fire scene must, therefore, be evaluated for CO toxicity.

Tobacco smoke is a significant source of CO. Serum COHb levels in smokers often approach 9 percent but may reach 20 percent. These levels can compromise patients with preexisting cardiopulmonary disease. Furthermore, CO toxicity from cigarette smoking has been implicated as a major factor in atherogenesis. It is also known to be a precipitating factor in angina, myocardial infarction, and cardiac arrhythmias. Smoke released from the tip of the cigarette contains 2.5 times more CO than the inhaled smoke. Cigarette smoking in poorly ventilated rooms can cause CO toxicity in the exposed nonsmoker.

Methylene chloride is found in many paint removers and its vapors are readily absorbed through the lungs. In the liver it is converted into CO. Since methylene chloride is stored in tissues and gradually released, the CO elimination half-life in patients exposed to this substance is about twice that of inhaled CO.

## PATHOPHYSIOLOGY

The pathophysiology of CO poisoning is not completely understood. Nevertheless, five mechanisms explaining the toxic effects of CO have been proposed: (1) direct binding of CO to hemoglobin; (2) shifting of the oxygen-hemoglobin dissociation curve; (3) CO binding to myoglobin; (4) inhibition of cellular respiration; and (5) brain lipid peroxidation.

### Tissue Hypoxia

Carbon monoxide readily crosses the pulmonary alveolar membrane. It acts as a competitive inhibitor of oxygen binding by reversibly coupling with hemoglobin. The affinity of CO for hemoglobin is 210 to 270 times greater than the affinity of oxygen for hemoglobin. This results in high serum COHb levels from exposures to environments with relatively low partial pressures of CO. When inhaled air contains 0.01% CO, the resulting serum COHb level is 10 percent. The net effect of COHb production is a reduction of the oxygen-carrying capacity in the blood. This produces tissue hypoxia, the predominant toxicologic property of CO.

### Shifting the Oxygen-Hemoglobin Curve

The tissue hypoxia caused by the formation of COHb does not adequately explain the toxic effects of CO. Hemoglobin has four binding sites for oxygen. When CO binds to one of these sites, the hemoglobin molecule is altered in such a way that the remaining three oxygen molecules are held more tightly. This shifts the oxygen-hemoglobin curve to the left, further reducing the amount of oxygen available at the cellular level (see Fig. 171-1).

### Myoglobin Binding

Carbon monoxide has a high affinity for myoglobin, especially cardiac myoglobin. Carbon monoxide impairs cardiac performance because cardiac carboxymyoglobin reduces the oxygen available to myocardial tissue. Cardiac ischemia and arrhythmias can also be caused by CO. Since carboxymyoglobin dissociates more slowly than COHb, a rebound increase of the serum COHb level may occur after treatment. After oxygen therapy causes the serum COHb to decrease, the myoglobin releases its bound CO, causing an increase in the serum COHb concentration.

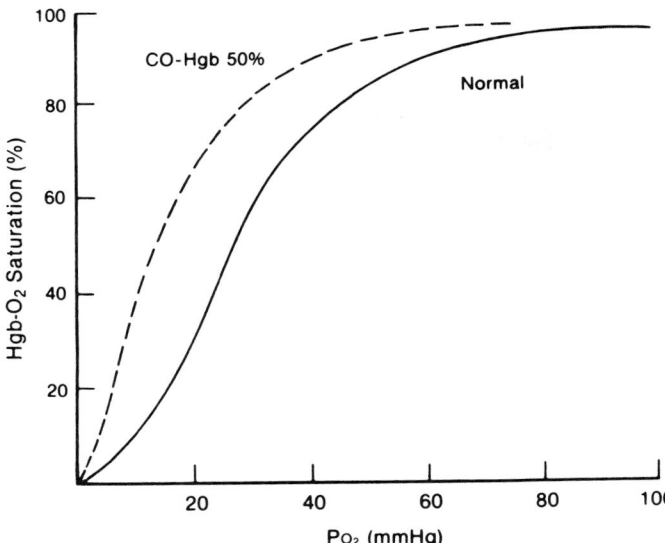

Fig. 171-1. Normal oxygen-hemoglobin dissociation curve compared with oxygen-hemoglobin dissociation curve of 50% carboxyhemoglobin. (Used with permission from Auerbach PS, Geehr EC: *Management of Wilderness and Environmental Emergencies,* 2d ed. St. Louis, Mosby, 1989, p 161.)

## Inhibition of Cellular Respiration

Carbon monoxide also binds to cytochromes $A_3$ and P-450. By reversibly binding to the cytochrome oxidase system, CO may cause inhibition of cellular (mitochondrial) respiration. The affinity of cytochrome oxidase for oxygen is much greater than the affinity of cytochrome for CO. Therefore, an environment with a low oxygen tension (hypoxia) is required for significant CO-cytochrome binding to occur. The exact impact that the inhibition of cellular respiration produces in CO poisoning remains unclear.

## Brain Lipid Peroxidation

A recent theory suggests that the neurologic findings associated with CO poisoning may result from brain lipid peroxidation. Carbon monoxide converts xanthine dehydrogenase into xanthine oxidase. Xanthine oxidase reacts with hypoxanthine, eventually producing superoxide, a free-radical reduction product of oxygen. Superoxide reacts with the body's iron stores and ultimately causes cell membrane lipid peroxidation, which results in neuronal damage. This strongly suggests that CO-mediated brain injury is similar to postischemic reperfusion phenomena.

## CLINICAL PRESENTATION

The manifestations of CO poisoning are often vague, leading to frequent misdiagnoses with subsequent delays in therapy. Initial symptoms commonly include headache, dizziness, weakness, and nausea. Other symptoms include difficulty in thinking, chest pain, palpitations, visual disturbances, and abdominal pain. CO poisoning is often misdiagnosed as "flu," gastroenteritis, and psychiatric disorders.

Routine CO screening of emergency patients during the winter months revealed a 2.8 percent incidence of elevated CO levels. With patients complaining of headache during colder months, a similar incidence was found. In addition, physicians were unable to predict elevated COHb levels in patients.

At the scene of the exposure, COHb levels correlate fairly well to symptoms (see Table 171-1). When patients are removed from CO or have been breathing 100% oxygen, there is a poor correlation between COHb levels and the clinical manifestations. Despite "nontoxic" COHb levels after treatment, patients may still demonstrate

**Table 171-1.** Signs and Symptoms at Various Carboxyhemoglobin Concentrations

| COHb Level, % | Signs and Symptoms |
|---|---|
| 0 | Usually none |
| 10 | Frontal headache |
| 20 | Throbbing headache, dyspnea with exertion |
| 30 | Impaired judgment, nausea, dizziness, visual disturbance, fatigue |
| 40 | Confusion, syncope |
| 50 | Coma, seizures |
| 60 | Hypotension, respiratory failure |
| 70 | Death |

signs of severe poisoning. Patients may lapse into coma and die without intermediary symptoms when exposed to high levels of CO. Low-level exposures over a long period of time may be more harmful than high-level exposures over a brief time, though COHb levels may be similar. It is therefore important that a serum sample be drawn by emergency medical personnel at the scene. The field specimen COHb level will correlate best with the clinical presentation.

## SYSTEMIC MANIFESTATIONS

### Cardiac

Although CO poisoning affects every organ system (see Table 171-2), the brain and heart, having the highest metabolic require-

**Table 171-2.** Reported Complications of Carbon Monoxide Poisoning

| System Involved | Complication |
|---|---|
| Neuropsychiatric | Coma, seizures, agitation, leukoencephalopathy, cerebral edema, behavioral disorders, decreased cognitive ability, Tourette-like syndrome, mutism, fecal and urinary incontinence, parietal lobe dysfunction, ataxia, muscular rigidity, parkinsonism, peripheral neuropathy, psychosis, memory impairment, gait disturbance, abnormal EEG, personality changes |
| Cardiovascular | Angina, tachycardia, ST-segment changes, hypotension, arrhythmias, myocardial infarction, heart block |
| Pulmonary | Pulmonary edema and hemorrhage, unilateral diaphragmatic paralysis |
| Ophthalmologic | Flame-shaped retinal hemorrhages, decreased light sensitivity, decreased visual acuity, cortical blindness, retrobulbar neuritis, papilledema, paracentral scotomas |
| Vestibular and auditory | Central hearing loss, tinnitus, vertigo, nystagmus |
| Gastrointestinal | Vomiting, diarrhea, hepatic necrosis, hematochezia, melena |
| Dermatologic | Bullae, alopecia, sweat gland necrosis, "cherry-red" skin color (rare), edema, cyanosis, pallor, erythematous patches |
| Hematologic | Disseminated intravascular coagulation, thrombotic thrombocytopenic purpura, leukocytosis |
| Musculoskeletal | Rhabdomyolysis, myonecrosis, compartment syndrome |
| Renal | Acute renal failure secondary to myoglobinuria, proteinuria |
| Metabolic | Lactic acidosis, nonpancreatic hyperamylasemia, diabetes insipidus, hyperglycemia, hypocalcemia |
| Fetal | Death, cerebral atrophy, microcephalus, low birth weight, psychomotor retardation, seizures, spasticity |

ments, are most susceptible to CO toxicity. When coronary artery disease is present, a low serum COHb level can produce myocardial ischemia and infarction. In fact, ischemia and infarction can occur in the absence of coronary artery disease. In a study of burn victims, 5 of 18 patients (28 percent) with COHb levels greater than 10 percent sustained myocardial infarctions. Decreased exercise tolerance also results from CO poisoning.

Myocardial ischemia is most prominent in the subendocardial and subepicardial regions of the ventricles. This may produce papillary muscle dysfunction, abnormal ventricular wall motion, and mitral valve prolapse. The electrocardiogram often reflects ischemia, showing ST-segment and T-wave abnormalities. Atrial flutter, atrial fibrillation, premature ventricular tachycardia, and conduction system disturbances are also seen. The ventricular fibrillation threshold is lowered in cases of severe CO poisoning. However, in patients with existing cardiac arrhythmias, mild elevations of COHb (up to 5 percent) are not reported to increase the frequency of single or multiple ventricular ectopic beats during rest or exercise.

## Ophthalmologic

Visual disturbances are frequent and correlate with the duration of exposure. Funduscopic examination may reveal flame-shaped retinal hemorrhages. They are caused by hypoxia and may be unilateral. The hemorrhages often resolve without visual deficit. A sensitive indicator of CO toxicity is the presence of bright red retinal veins. These may be seen before the mucous membranes become erythematous and appear at lower COHb levels. Blindness is infrequent and is usually temporary.

## Dermatologic

The classic "cherry-red" skin of CO poisoning is rarely seen; more often, victims are pale or cyanotic. Dermal necrosis with bullae formation may occur anywhere but especially at pressure point areas in the comatose patient and over areas of myonecrosis. Myonecrosis from pressure or prolonged tissue hypoxia may cause rhabdomyolysis, a potential cause of renal failure. Other dermal changes include sweat gland necrosis, alopecia, edema, and erythematous patches.

## Other

Other physiologic effects of CO poisoning include noncardiogenic pulmonary edema, bowel ischemia, hepatic failure, vestibular dysfunction, hearing loss, disseminated intravascular coagulation, and thrombotic thrombocytopenic purpura. Even low COHb levels can significantly diminish exercise tolerance in patients with chronic destructive pulmonary disease.

## Fetal

Up to 10 percent of patients receiving HBO are pregnant. In pregnancy, the fetus is particularly susceptible, as CO readily crosses the placenta. During exposure, fetal COHb levels lag behind the maternal level, achieving equilibration after 14 to 24 h. After equilibration with maternal blood, fetal COHb levels are 10 to 15 percent higher than maternal levels. In addition, because the fetal oxygen-hemoglobin dissociation curve is shifted to the left (see Fig. 171-2), small amounts of COHb can markedly decrease the fetal oxygen tension and content. Fetal elimination of CO is prolonged, resulting in a fetal CO elimination half-life that is three and a half times longer than that of the mother. Pregnant women should receive more aggressive and prolonged oxygen therapy. Longo suggests that the mother should receive oxygen for a period five times longer than the time period needed to complete just the maternal course of therapy (see Fig. 171-2). For example, if 4 h is required to completely treat the mother, an additional 20 h of oxygen treatment is required. Fetal heart tones

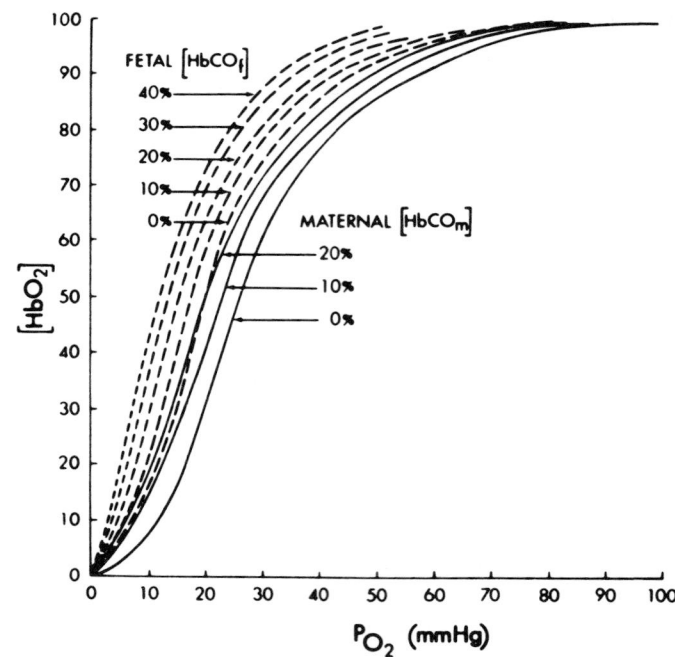

**Fig. 171-2.** Human maternal and fetal oxyhemoglobin saturation curves showing carbon monoxide effect. The oxyhemoglobin saturation (HbO$_2$) is that percentage of hemoglobin not bound as carboxyhemoglobin. (Used with permission from Longo LD. The biological effects of carbon monoxide on the pregnant woman, fetus, and newborn infant. *Am J Obstet Gynecol* 129:75, 1977.)

should be obtained, and cardiotachodynomanometry instituted at 20 weeks' gestation or greater. Up to 60 percent of children born to women surviving CO poisoning have neurologic sequelae. In addition, CO is teratogenic and causes lower-birth-weight infants. Fetal death has occurred in cases of nonlethal maternal poisoning. Fetal demise may be seen immediately or be delayed. Fetal outcome roughly correlates to maternal symptoms at the time of CO exposure; however, there may be no relationship between fetal death and maternal COHb levels.

## Pediatric

Children make up 37 percent of patients receiving HBO therapy; children less than 5 years old account for 25 percent of victims receiving HBO. Among acutely exposed children, as many as 17 percent die and 48 percent require cardiopulmonary resuscitation (CPR). Most childhood deaths from CO poisoning are fire-related. Newborns are more susceptible to the effects of CO poisoning due to a higher fetal hemoglobin concentration which shifts the oxygen-hemoglobin curve to the left.

In children, in whom nausea is a common complaint, CO toxicity is frequently misdiagnosed as acute gastroenteritis; in young infants it can be confused with colic. Carbon monoxide toxicity has been implicated as a cause for some cases of sudden infant death syndrome.

Children are frequently affected by riding in vehicles with faulty exhaust systems, especially in the back seats of cars or in the enclosed backs of pickup trucks. In one study of 68 children requiring HBO therapy, 20 (29 percent) were exposed from riding in pickup trucks. Children riding in the same vehicle can have different symptoms with the same COHb levels or have markedly different COHb levels from the same exposure.

The treatment of CO toxicity for children is similar to that for adults; however, myringotomy is more commonly performed in children undergoing HBO therapy.

## Neurologic

Since the brain has a high oxygen requirement, most acute symptoms are related to the central nervous system (CNS). In a mass exposure of 184 victims, the most common complaints were headache (90 percent) dizziness (82 percent), and weakness (53 percent). Carbon monoxide poisoning has been suggested as an occult cause of syncope. Of CO-poisoned patients, 35 percent complained of "spells" which mimicked near-syncope. The prevalence of CO poisoning among patients presenting with seizures may be 5 to 7 percent.

The most significant pathologic changes of the brain seen with CO poisoning are white matter lesions. These include white matter demyelination, edema, focal and laminar necrosis, and petechiae. Lesions of the hippocampus are reported in half of the cases. Gray matter lesions also occur in the watershed area between the anterior and middle cerebral arteries. The characteristic pathologic injury of CO poisoning is bilateral lesions of the globus pallidus. These lesions are seen with other hypoxic-ischemic insults and may be unilateral or asymmetric. The globus pallidus lesions are most likely the result of hypoxia with concomitant ischemia. This area has relatively low oxygen requirements, protecting it from pure hypoxia, but it has a poor blood supply, making it vulnerable to hypoperfusion. Low-density lesions of the globus pallidus demonstrated on CT scan or magnetic resonance imaging (MRI) are associated with a high incidence of neurologic sequelae.

Neurologic abnormalities are frequent in acute poisoning (Table 171-2). The most common neurologic complaints are headache, dizziness, agitation, stupor, seizures, and coma. Other aberrations include behavioral disorders, decreased cognitive ability, gait disturbance, memory deficits, emotional lability, parkinsonism, mutism, tic disorders, and impairment of parietal lobe functions. Long-term psychiatric and neurologic sequelae are grossly apparent in 11 percent of survivors. Memory impairment occurs in up to 43 percent. The most common personality change, "affective incontinence," is characterized by emotional lability and may be a consequence of damage to the hippocampus. Resolution of the neurologic sequelae, when it occurs, may take 2 years. These deficits may be permanent.

A syndrome of delayed neurologic sequelae has been described. Delayed sequelae usually occur after coma from a prolonged exposure. The patient recovers, has a symptom-free interval, then undergoes rapid neurologic deterioration. In 10 to 30 percent of poisonings, neuropsychiatric symptoms will appear within 2 to 3 weeks after exposure. The common symptoms are mental deterioration, urinary and fecal incontinence, and gait disturbance. Complete recovery occurs in two-thirds. Older patients are at greater risk for developing delayed sequelae. Diffuse demyelinization of white matter is associated with delayed deterioration. More aggressive oxygen therapy may reduce the incidence of sequelae.

## CLINICAL EVALUATION AND LABORATORY STUDIES

### History

The diagnosis of CO poisoning is most often suggested by the circumstances in which the patient is found. Victims of a house fire who are comatose pose little diagnostic difficulty. In patients with vague symptoms who have been chronically exposed to low CO levels (e.g., smokers), reaching the diagnosis may be difficult. In the absence of a reliable history of CO exposure, alternative diagnoses include viral illness, food poisoning, depression, functional illness, encephalitis, and toxin-induced encephalopathy.

The physician should continually suspect CO poisoning during the colder months. Common complaints associated with CO poisoning include headache, nausea, weakness, fatigue, difficulty in thinking, dizziness, paresthesias, chest pain, palpitations, visual disturbances, diarrhea, and abdominal pain. In addition, CO poisoning has been confused with psychogenic hyperventilation and polycythemia.

One feature in the medical history which is suggestive of CO poisoning is when another person in the same dwelling also experiences similar symptoms. The appropriate agency should then be notified to measure ambient CO levels at the suspected site. The physician should further ask about the source of home heating and the condition of the exhaust system on the patient's car.

### Physical Examination

The physical examination is of limited use in establishing the diagnosis of CO poisoning. Nevertheless, once the diagnosis is established, the physical examination does help define the severity of the poisoning. Vital sign abnormalities reflect the severity of the intoxication. The presence of singed nasal hairs, carbonaceous sputum, and thermal injury to the oral mucosa suggests thermal airway injury and severe CO poisoning. Auscultation may reveal wheezing from the exacerbation of preexisting pulmonary disease or from bronchospasm that results from irritation due to inhalation injury. Rales can be heard from the development of noncardiogenic pulmonary edema.

### Laboratory Evaluation

The diagnostic evaluation of the CO poisoning victim must be guided by the situation. For example, the fire victim should be evaluated for cyanide toxicity. When evaluating those attempting suicide, a routine drug screen and measurement of ethanol, phenobarbital, salicylate, and acetaminophen levels may be required. Asymptomatic individuals with minor exposure do not require extensive evaluations.

A COHb level should be obtained in all cases. This should not delay the administration of 100% oxygen. Levels should be obtained by a modified spectrophotometric blood gas analyzer or, less accurately, by measuring expired CO concentration with a hand-held breath analyzer. A high expired CO concentration or serum COHb level confirms CO poisoning, but a low level does not exclude the diagnosis. If a patient has been removed from the CO-containing environment and has been given 100% oxygen, the COHb level may be deceptively normal.

An arterial blood gas measurement calculates the reported oxygen tension from the amount of oxygen that is dissolved in the blood, not from the amount of oxygen that is bound to hemoglobin. The amount of oxygen that is dissolved in the blood is essentially unaffected by CO. In addition, pulse oximetry units mistakenly measure COHb as oxyhemoglobin. Therefore, the oxygen saturation as reported by most arterial blood gas measurements and pulse oximeters will be falsely elevated. The difference between the oxygen saturation that is accurately measured and the false elevated oximetry reading is called the *saturation gap*. This saturation gap is characteristic of CO poisoning and correlates with the COHb level. For example, if the oximeter reads 93 percent and the arterial blood gas directly measures (not calculates) the saturation to be 88 percent, the COHb is about 5 percent. Likewise, if the pulse oximeter is 95 percent and the measured COHb is 5 percent, the true oxygen saturation is only 90 percent.

An ECG should be performed on patients with cardiac symptoms, coronary artery disease, altered mental status, or a COHb level greater than 10 percent. The ECG is often abnormal. Sinus tachycardia and ST-segment changes are the most frequently seen aberrations, although almost any abnormality may be present.

Fire victims must have a chest radiograph taken. Though frequently normal acutely, it serves as a valuable baseline study. Cyanide levels can be obtained but are of limited value. Assays for other toxic inhalants, such as acrolein, phosgene, or gaseous hydrogen chloride, are unavailable. Spirometry and fiberoptic bronchoscopy may be required.

Serial creatine phosphokinase (CPK) and lactic dehydrogenase (LDH) levels assist in determining myocardial damage. The CPK is frequently elevated. Isoenzymes, especially of the CPK, differentiate rhabdomyolysis from cardiac necrosis or infarction. In addition, a urinalysis may reveal myoglobinuria.

Alcohol is frequently consumed with both suicidal and accidental CO poisoning, sometimes making a rapid diagnosis difficult. Therefore, a blood alcohol level should be measured. If a suicide attempt is suspected, a drug screen may be sent for analysis. In addition, quantitative aspirin, phenobarbital, and acetaminophen levels should be obtained.

Other laboratory tests assist in confirming CO poisoning. A routine complete blood count (CBC) may show a leukocytosis. Determination of arterial blood gas and electrolyte levels may demonstrate an anion gap acidosis. The acidosis results from lactic acid production. Abnormalities are commonly seen with measurements of the blood glucose, amylase, and transaminases. These findings, however, are of limited clinical significance.

Brain CT is used to define focal or otherwise unexplainable neurologic symptoms as well as to assess for cerebral edema. MRI is a more sensitive neuroimaging modality for detecting CO-induced CNS lesions. MRI can demonstrate cerebral findings associated with CO poisoning, which include necrosis of the globus pallidus, demyelinated lesions of the white matter, and necrotic lesions of the hippocampus. MRI has also defined lesions in the anterior thalami in a CO-poisoned child.

Psychometric testing is performed on CO-poisoned patients at some hospitals. The Carbon Monoxide Screening Battery has been developed to detect patients with subtle cognitive deficit resulting from CO exposure. The battery includes: the general orientation, digit spans, trail-making, digit symbols, aphasia screening, and block design. This battery is used to assess the need for HBO treatment. After HBO treatment, the patient is tested again to determine the effectiveness of therapy.

## TREATMENT

### Initial Approach

In treating CO-poisoned patients, one should remove the victims from the CO-containing atmosphere, keep them at rest to minimize oxygen requirements, immediately administer 100% oxygen, and institute cardiac monitoring. Pulse oximetry will not adequately measure oxygen status. A simple mask which allows for mixture with room air is inadequate. A tight-fitting mask with a bag reservoir is required to deliver a high $F_{IO_2}$. The serum elimination half-life of COHb when breathing room air is 240 to 320 min, compared to 50 to 80 min when breathing 100% oxygen. Oxygen therapy should not be discontinued until the patient is asymptomatic and the COHb level is less than 10 percent. In patients with angina, 100% oxygen should be applied until the COHb is below 2 percent or the patient is pain free.

### Hyperbaric Oxygen Therapy

HBO use is empiric but is recommended for severe cases of CO toxicity. HBO is delivered in monoplace or multiplace chambers. The multiplace chamber permits treatment of multiple patients simultaneously and provides room for staff and accessory equipment, e.g., ventilators. Most treatment regimens have been empirically developed; they usually involve 100% oxygen at pressures of 2 to 3 atm for 46 to 120 min. A second treatment is given in 6 to 8 h if symptoms persist. With HBO therapy, the elimination half-life of CO is reduced to 23 min. When HBO is used to treat methylene chloride–induced CO toxicity, the CO half-life changes from 13.0 h at room air to 5.8 h.

With HBO therapy at 3 atm pressure, the amount of oxygen dissolved in the blood is increased to 6.6 vol percent. This amount is sufficient to meet the demands of cerebral metabolism independent of the COHb concentration. HBO therapy may also reduce the amount of cerebral edema. HBO therapy has been shown to prevent CO-mediated lipid peroxidation in the brain.

HBO use remains somewhat empiric since no well-designed prospective study has adequately defined the benefits of HBO. Nevertheless, the growing weight of scientific evidence suggests an advantage of HBO in severe poisoning or in cases with protracted symptoms. The prompt application of HBO may reduce mortality. In one study, patients treated within 6 h of CO exposure had a mortality rate of 13.5 percent; of those treated after 6 h, 30.1 percent died. Reports have demonstrated a dramatic reduction in the incidence of neuropsychiatric sequelae when HBO is used.

As many as 10 percent of patients requiring HBO therapy are pregnant. Animal studies have raised concerns regarding the potential adverse effects of high partial pressures of oxygen on the fetus, but the pressures and durations used were greater than those used in humans. The Russians have the largest experience with HBO in pregnancy. They found a decrease in perinatal complications and mortality. A Canadian study involving pregnant women exposed to CO had five cases of severe poisoning. Of the three patients treated with high-flow (non-HBO) oxygen, two had stillbirths; the child of the third patient had cerebral palsy. The two patients treated with HBO had normal outcomes. The greatest advantage of HBO over 100% normobaric oxygen is that it reduces the time required to decrease fetal COHb. Given the safety of HBO and the danger of CO toxicity to the fetus, many recommend liberal use of HBO in pregnant women.

When HBO therapy is required, it should be started promptly. Nevertheless, delays of 7 to 20 h have still resulted in favorable outcomes. Treatment guidelines have been developed to assist in defining those patients needing HBO therapy (Table 171-3). How-

**Table 171-3.** Treatment Guidelines Based on Severity of CO Poisoning

**Mild poisoning**
  Criteria
    COHb levels < 30%
    No signs or symptoms of impaired cardiovascular or neurologic function
    May complain of headache, nausea, or vomiting
  Treatment
    Admission of patients with COHb levels > 25%
    Symptomatic medication
    100% oxygen by non-rebreathing mask until COHb remains < 5%
    Patients with underlying heart disease should be admitted and cardiac function appropriately monitored regardless of COHb level.
**Moderate poisoning**
  Criteria
    COHB levels from 30–40%
    No signs or symptoms of impaired cardiovascular or neurologic function
  Treatment
    Admission
    Cardiovascular status should be followed closely even in the absence of clear cardiac effects, especially in those patients with underlying heart disease
    Determination of acid-base status (will be corrected by high-flow oxgyen)
    100% oxygen by non-rebreathing mask until COHb remains < 5%
**Severe poisoning**
  Criteria
    COHb levels > 40%
         or
    Cardiovascular or neurologic functional impairment at any COHb level
  Treatment
    Admission
    Cardiovascular function monitoring
    Acid-base status monitoring
    100% oxygen by non-rebreathing mask
    Transport to a hyperbaric oxygen facility immediately if available, or if no improvement in cardiovascular or neurologic function is seen within 4 h

*Source:* Used with permission from Ilano AL, Raffin TA; Management of CO poisoning. *Chest* 97:169, 1990.

ever, assigning patients into different treatment plans based on the clinical presentation and the COHb level is imprecise. In addition, HBO should be used more readily in cases of pregnancy, age extremes, cardiovascular or neurologic impairment, and metabolic acidosis.

The potential benefits of HBO are based upon sound physiologic principles; the risks of treatment are minimal. During HBO treatment patients may develop otalgia and sinus discomfort. Myringotomy can be performed to ease otic pressure. Tympanic membrane rupture and epistaxis are rare. Of patients with severe CO poisoning who undergo HBO, 5 percent will have a seizure and 6 percent will vomit. The cause of these adverse reactions (CO toxicity versus HBO treatment) is unclear.

Patients with significant neurologic abnormalities, cardiovascular abnormalities, or symptomatic pregnant patients require prompt HBO treatment. Such patients should be stabilized and prepared for transfer to the nearest HBO chamber. The indications for transfer and HBO therapy may be unclear, or the patient's condition may remain unstable. Therefore, the patient's transfer and interim treatment should be discussed with the HBO chamber physician. To locate the nearest hyperbaric chamber, one should call Diver's Alert Network (DAN) at Duke University at (919) 684-2948.

The role of nitrites with mixed cyanide and CO exposures is not clearly defined and is theoretically harmful. The nitrites given to treat cyanide toxicity cause methemoglobinemia. This shifts the oxygen-hemoglobin dissociation curve further to the left, exacerbating tissue hypoxia. If the patient has been removed from the source and presents to the emergency department alive, sodium thiosulfate, 12.5 g intravenously, should detoxify the cyanide.

Cerebral edema should be treated with mannitol and by elevation of the head of the bed. Hyperventilation should be used in severe cases. The efficacy of glucocorticoids is debated.

Correcting the metabolic acidosis may be harmful; a mild acidosis is often a normal compensatory response. A low pH shifts the oxygen-hemoglobin dissociation curve to the right, increasing oxygen unloading to the tissue. Alkalinization will shift the oxygen-hemoglobin curve to the left, further reducing tissue availability of oxygen and exacerbating the toxic effect of CO. Nevertheless, if the pH is less than 7.20, cardiovascular performance is compromised, and judicious alkalinization is required.

## PROGNOSIS

Many variables, such as age, smoking habit, existing cardiopulmonary disease, severity of exposure, prior state of health, and form of therapy, influence outcome. Coma, cardiac arrest, metabolic acidosis, and high COHb levels have been associated with poor neurologic outcome. These factors, however, are inconsistent predictors of outcome and therefore are of limited value. Abnormal CT findings are associated with neurologic sequelae, which will often persist.

## BIBLIOGRAPHY

Binder JW, Roberts RJ: Carbon monoxide intoxication in children. *Clin Toxicol* 16:287, 1980.

Burney RE, Wu SC, Nemiroff MJ: Mass carbon monoxide poisoning: Clinical effects and results of treatment in 184 victims. *Ann Emerg Med* 11:394, 1982.

Cobb N, Etzel RA: Unintentional carbon monoxide-related deaths in the United States, 1979 through 1988. *JAMA* 266:659, 1991.

Hyperbaric Center Advisory Committee Emergency Medical Service, City of New York: A registry for carbon monoxide poisoning in New York City. *Clin Toxicol* 26:419, 1988.

Koren G, Sharav T, Pastuszak A, et al: A multicenter, prospective study of fetal outcome following accidental carbon monoxide in pregnancy. *Reprod Toxicol* 5:397, 1991.

Peirce EC, Kaufmann H, Bensky WH, et al: A registry for carbon monoxide poisoning in New York City. *Clin Toxicol* 26:419, 1988.

Reisdorff EJ, Shah SM: Carbon monoxide poisoning: From crib death to pickup trucks. *Emerg Med Rep* 14:181, 1993.

Thom SR: Carbon monoxide–mediated lipid peroxidation in the rat. *J Appl Physiol* 68:997, 1990.

# 172
# ACUTE EXPOSURE TO TOXIC AGENTS
## Constance J. Doyle

Acute exposure to hazardous materials is a very probable event in today's society. Workplace accidents and transportation accidents can result in acute exposure to the worker, surrounding workers, and even emergency medical services and emergency department personnel. Health morbidity can occur from both acute accidental exposure and chronic long-term exposure.

The U.S. Department of Transportation list seven major classes of hazardous materials, with 2750 subcategories. These involve only transportation. There were 9294 hazardous materials incidents reported to the Department of Transportation in 1992. The majority of these occurred on the highway, rather than on the railroads or in the air. More than 65,000 substances are produced, with an average of 600 new chemicals being developed each year. There is no estimate of additional hazardous materials that may result from combinations of chemicals, products of combustion, and combinations in abandoned waste dumps that may result in exposure. In 1990 to 1992, data pertaining to health and hazardous materials collected by the Agency for Toxic Substances and Disease Registry showed 3125 incidents, of which 77 percent were at fixed facilities. In 15 percent of all of the events there were 1446 persons injured and 11 deaths. These statistics were only from five states. Respiratory injuries were the most frequently reported. More than 10,000 people in surrounding areas of incidents were evacuated.

Transportation accidents result in additional traumatic injuries from explosion, burns, and smoke inhalation, which must be treated along with the chemical exposure and/or contamination. All emergency personnel may be at risk of exposure. If the patient is improperly handled, the emergency department may become contaminated and may need decontamination and/or evacuation until decontamination is complete. The emergency physician and poison control centers may be called upon to access data to help emergency personnel care for patients and to aid in evacuation decisions. CHEMTREC has logged over 189,000 calls in the past year for emergency assistance. Most of these voluntary calls were transportation related, and only 5 percent involved medical emergencies. CHEMTREC has thousands of Materials Safety Data Sheets available to give immediate first-aid information. Each year one-third of them are updated. They are also a resource for shipping and manufacturing information and have links with poison control centers.

## PLANNING

Every emergency department should have a hazardous materials plan. It should include: on-site prehospital decontamination, decontamination at the hospital, types of protective equipment available, decontamination equipment, decontamination location, and personnel responsible for the decontamination and treatment process. Responsibilities for decontamination, triage, and treatment should be written into the plan.

Medical control should be involved early to access toxicity data and to ensure that proper safety equipment is used and that decontamination begins on site if necessary. Compliance in protection of rescuers and scene evaluation from a safe distance are most often ignored and may result in rescuer exposure and morbidity. Continuing education and practice in prehospital procedures are both necessary. Hazardous materials patient-care protocols should be clearly outlined. Guidebooks and resource lists of telephone numbers for information and equipment should be available to medical control and rescue personnel at the scene of a hazardous materials emergency.

Hospital planning should be more than a written addendum to a disaster plan. It should cover the following: (1) the entrance by which casualties are to enter the emergency department; (2) a plan for an "unknown chemical contamination" protocol for when a patient arrives at the triage desk unannounced; (3) a list of available protective equipment and its location, location of the decontamination area, and identification of personnel who will be involved in the decontamination/treatment process; and (4) a list of resources for chemical information and help. For this last item there are multiple sources of information from multiple agencies through toll-free hot lines and computer-based information, such as the Poisindex and Tomes systems from Micromedex and TOXNET. General toxicology texts and occupational medicine tests are also helpful.

## DECONTAMINATION

If possible, decontamination should occur at the site of the chemical incident, and the contaminated material should not leave the site until environmental cleanup personnel arrive. The more toxic the substance, the more immediate the need for decontamination. With injuries necessitating medical treatment, one must simultaneously treat the injury, effect rapid decontamination, and avoid exposing others to the contaminated material. Rescue personnel should wear protective clothing and/or respiratory protection as dictated by the toxicity of the chemical involved. If such protection is unavailable, local "hazmat" team members from the fire service may be used. If none are available, then firefighters in "full turnout gear" may be the best available solution. With attention to airway and cervical spine precautions if indicated, the patient should be stripped of all apparel and washed rapidly with water from a nearby hose or from buckets of water. Only life-saving treatment with personnel in protective gear should be carried out in the immediate "hot" area of the spill. The patient may need further decontamination and treatment in an intermediate area. Other advanced life support (ALS) measures are started in this area. Some protective gear may still be necessary for the rescuers. After the patient is washed and wrapped in clean blankets, further therapy and transport to a hospital for further care should be carried out in the most basic vehicle possible.

Decontamination of an ALS vehicle can be expensive and may result in a long time out of service. If the hospital emergency department is contaminated, the entire department or part of the department may be closed for a period of time. There is additional liability if other patients or personnel are exposed to a toxic material.

The ideal decontamination facility has a separate entrance from the outside and contains a shower, separate wastewater collection, and separate venting. No consensus exists for the minimum level of protection for the hospital decontamination suite or for the minimum amount of respiratory protection. Outside decontamination protocols should include a source of warm water and some ability to contain wash water, such as a wading pool or a cart with a top that permits collection of all wash water in a barrel. A major source of contamination is clothing and shoes, which should be removed as soon as possible. Attention to privacy during this step is a must. Additional essential supplies are clean sheets and/or blankets for the patient,

protective clothing and eye wear for staff, irrigation supplies for eye contamination, pH paper for strong alkali or acid exposures to ensure that the toxin has been neutralized, and ALS supplies.

## PATTERNS OF INJURY

Most industrial and transportation exposures are either by inhalation or dermal exposure with or without systemic effects. Some chemicals on the skin can vaporize and result in a simultaneous inhalation injury. Cutaneous injury results from materials contacting the skin. A contact dermatitis, a chemical burn, or an allergic reaction may result. Some chemicals penetrate the superficial skin layers, such as the deep burns that occur from hydrofluoric acid. Hydrofluoric acid can also bind calcium systemically and lead to arrhythmias, seizures, and death. Other strong acids can cause coagulation necrosis of the skin. Alkali can saponify the upper layers of the skin and destroy the deeper layers of tissue. Other chemicals may be absorbed systemically or volatilize and be inhaled, causing systemic symptoms. Decontamination of the skin and/or eye with copious amounts of water prevents further exposure. There are rare agents that react violently with water, such as chlorosulfonic acid, titanium tetrachloride, and calcium oxide, or that are insoluble in water, such as phosphorus. Metals such as lithium, calcium, magnesium, and sodium will burn in contact with water. These should be wiped off with a dry cloth, and all clothing removed. If there is burning metal on the skin, it should be wiped off and covered with sand, blankets, or cooking oil to prevent its contact with air. References should be consulted for specific decontamination procedures for these agents.

Inhalation injuries from volatile chemicals or their products of combustion can result in asphyxiation, irritation, systemic absorption, or a combination of these (see Table 172-1). Asphyxiants cause toxicity by replacing oxygen in the lungs. Biologically inert substances such as nitrogen, methane, and carbon dioxide are examples.

Chemical asphyxiants interfere with tissue oxygenation by preventing delivery of oxygen to the cell or by inhibiting the use of oxygen at the cellular level. Examples include carbon monoxide and cyanide. Both types of asphyxiant gases cause little direct lung damage but can have a profound effect on the neurologic, metabolic, and cardiovascular systems secondary to the hypoxia they cause. Treatment is aimed at restoring cellular oxygenation.

Irritant gases act directly on the mucosa of the respiratory tree. The location of the pulmonary damage depends on their water solubility. Ammonia, very water soluble, is absorbed in the upper airway and produces such signs of upper airway irritation as cough, laryngeal edema, and pharyngitis. Phosgene, which has little water solubility, reaches the lower airways and causes pneumonitis and pulmonary edema. Gases with intermediate solubility cause upper airway symptoms if exposure is brief. If exposure is prolonged, lower respiratory systems predominate.

A fourth class of gases such as hydrogen sulfide, methylated halogens, and metal fumes act both as irritants and asphyxiants. Smoke includes multiple products of combustion. Carbon monoxide, toluene diisocyanate, hydrocyanic acid, acrolein, ammonia, acetic acid, and

**Table 172-1.** Classification of Noxious Gases

Asphyxiants, simple:
  Carbon dioxide, nitrogen, hydrocarbons, helium, argon, neon, hydrogen, ethane, acetylene, silo gas
Asphyxiants, chemical:
  Carbon monoxide, cyanide, hydrogen sulfide, acetonitrile, acrylonitrile
Irritant gases:
  Ammonia, phosgene, nitrogen dioxide, hydrogen halides, acrolein, methyl bromide, ethylene oxide, fluorine nitric acid, sulfur dioxide
Combined asphyxiants and irritants:
  Hydrogen sulfide, metal fumes, metallic oxides, aromatic hydrocarbons ozone, paraquat, methylated halogens

formic acid are common products produced by burning nylon and plastics. Thermal injury from heat and irritation from inhaled soot add to the injury. Immediate application of 100% oxygen must be done until carbon monoxide inhalation and respiratory impairment are ruled out and complete respiratory evaluation has been done.

Additional injury may come from trauma, including blast injuries if there is an explosion, heat from fire or a hot atmosphere, and cold exposure from cold liquids or gases, which can freeze tissues, or from a cold environment.

## TOXIDROMES

Hemoglobinopathies, such as carboxyhemoglobinemia, sulfhemoglobinemia, and methemoglobinemia, result from exposures to chemicals that impair oxygen transport by hemoglobin. Symptoms of cellular hypoxia from these agents include dizziness, headache, nausea and vomiting, disorientation, seizures, and coma as well as cardiac toxicity, including tachycardia, arrhythmias, myocardial infarction, and cardiovascular collapse. Methemoglobinemia, sulfhemoglobinemia, and cyanide poisoning present with cyanosis unresponsive to oxygen therapy. Organophosphate and carbamate poisoning present with a syndrome of salivation, lacrimation, urination, and defecation (SLUD); sweating, bronchospasm, and pulmonary edema; and CNS symptoms such as restlessness, ataxia, convulsions, and respiratory and circulatory depression. Metal fume fever occurs when volatilized metals are inhaled and produces chills, fever, severe muscle aching, headache, fatigue, and dry throat. The symptoms may be delayed by hours, and the worker may not connect the symptoms with an on-the-job toxin. It is found in metal workers, welders, foundry workers, and shipyard workers.

## INITIAL STABILIZATION

Treatment of chemical injuries begins with initial hazard assessment and protection of rescuers with proper protective clothing and respiratory protection. Early decontamination not only mitigates some effects of some toxic substances but also contains environmental hazards to prevent further exposure.

Immediate attention to airway is paramount, along with stabilization of the cervical spine if there is concern about trauma. If there are highly toxic fumes, an open bag-valve-mask respirator should not be used. A demand valve or a closed system with 100% oxygen ensures that no additional fumes are ventilated into the patient's airway. After the airway and breathing are established, exsanguinating hemorrhage is controlled, any sucking chest injury is sealed, and tension pneumothorax is relieved. When the patient has been exposed to fumes and/or has CNS alteration, 100% oxygen should be administered pending full respiratory and systemic investigation.

In the absence of a specific antidote, all medical treatment is supportive. This includes a meticulous history of the exposure, including agent, length of exposure, route, interval since the exposure, and associated trauma. Was the exposure in an enclosed space? Were any unusual odors noted? Long-term and delayed effects should be checked in available references to counsel the patient in long-term surveillance and to anticipate delayed medical consequences that may mean that close medical supervision is needed. The patient's prior health status and any previous similar injuries or episodes must be documented since some cases may involve compensation claims. Ensure that decontamination is complete or whether further decontamination is necessary and treatment needs to begin during decontamination.

A physical examination with careful attention to signs of covert trauma must be done. Intravenous lines with crystalloid are started, and blood is drawn for definitive testing. Pulse oximetry can give an immediate estimate of oxygen saturation while other tests are completed. Arterial blood gas, for saturation levels, and carboxyhemoglobin measurements must be done for anyone with an inhalation injury due to fire, smoke, and/or explosion and any unknown inhalation. Blood and/or urine specimens for specific toxicologic agents should be sent. However, supportive treatment of the specific injury should proceed without waiting for definitive laboratory test results to return. Confirmation from a reference laboratory may take weeks and may be helpful only for long-term surveillance and compensation issues. Bear in mind that some toxic illnesses are "contagious," with other persons developing respiratory and systemic symptoms without real exposure.

## CUTANEOUS INJURY

Cutaneous injury is treated with copious washing and treatment of the specific injury present. Wounds are decontaminated first to prevent further internal exposure. Then the wound is sealed with dressings, and the surrounding skin, including skinfolds, irrigated and washed with detergent to remove any material remaining. The hair is cleansed in a similar manner. Burns are treated by stopping the burning process with removal of the agent and any burning clothing and debris. Strong alkali burns are irrigated under running water for prolonged periods. Burns are then cleaned, debrided, and dressed. Consultation with a burn surgeon should be considered in all but the most minor chemical burns. Contact dermatitis and local allergic reactions should be treated with standard agents to reduce swelling, itching, and irritation. Systemic toxicity from injury to the skin is related to the lipid solubility of the material and to inhalation of vapors from volatile substances.

Strong alkali burns of the eye require immediate, on-site irrigation with normal saline solution or running water, and irrigation should be continued en route and in the emergency department. Irrigation may need to continue until consultation with an ophthalmologist is obtained. Other eye exposures should be irrigated copiously with the goal of bringing the pH of the lacrimal fluid to about 7.0. Topical anesthetic may be used but should not delay copious irrigation. Surface testing in alkali exposure is inadequate since residual alkali may persist in the tissues and act as a reservoir. Repeated pH testing and consultation may be necessary. A thorough eye examination should follow to check for abrasions, embedded foreign bodies, visual acuity, and fundal integrity. Consultation with an ophthalmologist and close follow-up ensure that complications and problems are addressed.

## INHALATION INJURY

Examination of the patient with inhalation injury should include examination of the entire respiratory tree. Singed nasal vibrissae and soot in the posterior pharynx indicate inhaled smoke and hot gases. Cough and change in voice may indicate upper airway irritation. The presence of stridor and the use of accessory muscles should be noted. Tachypnea, respiratory rate, and dyspnea as well as wheezing, rales, and rhonchi should be noted. Patients with inhalation injuries receive supportive treatment dependent on signs and symptoms uncovered during the physical and laboratory examinations. Unless symptoms are very mild and involve only the nose and pharynx, oxygen should be started while a history and physical examination are completed. If CNS signs or respiratory distress are present, 100% oxygen is started until the causative entity can be further defined. If hypotension is present, it is treated with isotonic fluids and vasopressors if needed. Consult poisoning references to ensure that the vasopressor is not contraindicated by the exposure. If upper airway edema is present, early prompt intubation must be considered. Humidification aids in tracheobronchitis, and bronchospasm is treated with nebulized β agonists and subcutaneous terbutaline or epinephrine. Aminophylline can be added if needed.

If pulmonary edema develops, the judicious use of diuretics (only if fluid overload is suspected) and vasodilators is indicated. If severe or if respiratory failure ensues, intubation, mechanical ventilation, and positive end-expiratory pressure are indicated.

Baseline ECG, chest x-ray, and arterial blood gas and carboxyhemoglobin levels are baseline studies. Other studies depend on the patient's signs and symptoms, references on the inhaled toxin, and previous medical history. Patients with thermal injury to the airway may need laryngoscopy, bronchoscopy, or intubation and then bronchoscopy if severe laryngeal or tracheal injury is present. Pulmonary function tests may add information about parenchymal involvement and will provide baseline values if long-term follow-up is necessary. Use of prophylactic antibiotics and steroids is controversial.

**Admission criteria.** Criteria for admission to the hospital include anticipated delayed effects from a particular chemical, hypoxia, a carboxyhemoglobin level above 15 to 20 percent or lower with systemic symptoms, dyspnea in room air, thermal injury, evidence of lower airway injury, tracheobronchitis, pulmonary edema, severe bronchospasm, pneumonia, and severe upper airway irritation that may progress to obstruction. Systemic signs may be due to hypoxia or systemic toxicity and should be treated supportively.

## ENTITIES WITH SPECIFIC ANTIDOTES

### Carbon Monoxide (See Chap. 171)

### Cyanide

Cyanide is used in industry in electroplating, silver recovery from x-ray film, ore extraction, in fumigation, and as a fertilizer. It is one of the products of combustion from burning nylon, polyurethane, wool, silk, and cellulose.

Cyanide is absorbed through the lung and interferes with the cytochrome oxidase system. It is a rapidly acting toxin, and a high index of suspicion must be maintained. Symptoms include weakness, dizziness that may be mistaken for anxiety, headache, palpitations, rapidly progressing dyspnea without cyanosis, rapid unconsciousness, and seizures. There may be an odor of bitter almonds on the breath or on the body, but 20 to 40 percent of the population is unable to detect this odor. Bright-red venous blood may be present in early stages and may not be present in later stages. Blood should be drawn for measurement of arterial blood gases, electrolytes, lactate, and carbon monoxide. Specimens should be sent to the laboratory for testing for cyanide levels. Results are not available on an emergency basis but may be useful for forensic or compensation purposes. There may be a lactic acidosis with a high anion gap with no other source. There will be a gap greater than 5 percentage points between the measured and calculated oxygen saturation. Because this gap may also occur with carbon monoxide poisoning and with both entities in smoke inhalation, 100% oxygen should be started immediately. Fluids and vasopressors are used for hypotension.

Treatment of symptomatic patients uses the specific antidotes contained in the Lily Cyanide Poison Kit (amyl nitrite, sodium nitrite,

**Table 172-2.** Therapy for Hydrofluoric Acid Burns

**Topical treatment:** 2.5% calcium gluconate gel:
  Surgical lubricant 120 g and 30 mL of 10% calcium gluconate
  Surgical lubricant 5 oz tube and 3.5 g calcium gluconate powder
**Zephiran solution (0.13%)**
  1.3 g of benzalkonium chloride in 1 L of ice water
  H-F antidote gel, Pharmascience, Inc., Quebec, Canada
  Magnesium sulfate 25% solution
**Subcutaneous injection treatment:** 10% calcium gluconate solution
**Intraarterial infusion:** 10 mL of 10% calcium gluconate diluted with 40 to
  50 ml of dextrose and water infused over 4 h
**Inhalation treatment:** 2.5% calcium gluconate nebulization solution:
  0.15 g of calcium gluconate powder mixed with 6 mL of sterile water or
   saline
1.5 mL of 10% calcium gluconate solution of 4.5 mL of sterile water or saline

*Source:* From Upfal M, Doyle CJ: *J Occup Med* 32(8):726, 1990.

and sodium thiosulfate). The objective of treatment is to induce methemoglobinemia with the nitrites. Methemoglobin combines with cyanide and thus unbinds the cytochrome oxidase system. Thiosulfate then combines with the cyanide to form sodium thiocyanate, which is excreted by the kidneys.

Rapid decontamination with protection of rescuers from contact with the chemical is paramount. Gastric emptying in cases of ingestion should not delay the use of the antidote.

A pearl of amyl nitrite is crushed and held under the patient's nose or may be placed in the Ambubag or face mask for 15 to 30 s out of each minute. As soon as possible, 10 mL of a 3% solution of sodium nitrite is injected over a 3- to 5-min period. The dosage for children is 0.15 to 0.33 mL/kg and varies with hemoglobin level. Blood pressure is carefully monitored and treated with fluids and vasopressors if necessary. Sodium thiosulfate is then given in a dose of 50 mL of 25% solution intravenously. The pediatric dose is 1.6 mL/kg. Additional doses of sodium nitrite and sodium thiosulfate at half the original amount are given in 1/2 to 1 h if there is no clinical response. Hyperbaric oxygen has been reported as useful for those not responding to antidotes. Its use is controversial, and there is a problem with safe transport of patients who are not located in a center with a chamber. Hospitalization for 24 to 48 h for careful monitoring and close follow-up are recommended.

### Hydrogen Sulfide

Hydrogen sulfide is a very rapidly acting cellular poison that is also an irritant gas. Hydrogen sulfide is found in sewers and septic tanks, decaying organic matter, and in some industrial settings. There are multiple descriptions of rescuer and bystander morbidity and mortality with this material. Its odor is of rotten eggs and causes olfactory fatigue, so rescuers may not be aware of continued exposure.

Hydrogen sulfide poisoning is similar to cyanide poisoning, and hydrogen sulfide binding of the cytochrome oxidase system can be displaced by sodium nitrite induction of methemoglobin. Amyl nitrite and sodium nitrite are used, but sodium thiosulfate is not. Unfortunately, few reach medical facilities in time for treatment to be of help. Supportive care should be begun immediately, and nitrites may be tried. Hyperbaric oxygen has been tried for those who have not responded to nitrite.

### Organophosphates and Carbamate Insecticides

Organophosphate and carbamate insecticides are prevalent in farming and are present in weaker strengths in household insecticide preparations. These compounds inhibit acetylcholine in the nervous system, and acetylcholine accumulates at the myoneural junction and synapses. Carbamates are reversible inhibitors.

These agents produce the SLUD syndrome and bronchorrhea, sweating, wheezing, bradycardia, muscular weakness, cramping, and respiratory and circulatory collapse.

Treatment is begun with respiratory support, decontamination of the patient by rescuers with respiratory and skin protection, and removal of all of the patient's clothing. Clothing should be isolated and discarded. Fumes from clothing are a hazard to emergency personnel. The patient should be washed at least three times with soap and water. An ethyl alcohol washing is also recommended. Respiratory status should be monitored and adequate oxygenation ensured since the patient will have excessive secretions and severe bronchospasm. With cardiac monitoring, atropine is given intravenously in large doses. A trial dose of 2 mg may be given. A repeat dose of 2 mg is given in 15 min and is increased in increments to 5 mg every 15 min until the patient demonstrates signs of atropinization: dry mouth, drying of bronchial secretions, flushing, and dilated pupils. Tachycardia may not always appear. The initial dose for children is 0.05 mg/kg IV, with maintainance doses of 0.02 to 0.05 mg/kg.

Atropine needs to be continued for at least 24 h and may be needed for several days. Adrenergic amines, aminophylline, physostigmine, phenothiazines, morphine, succinylcholine, or reserpine should not be used.

Treatment for organophosphates also includes the antidote pralidoxime. Treatment for carbamate insecticides is with atropine alone. Pralidoxime (2-PAM) reverses the neuromuscular blockade by reactivating the acetylcholinesterase. Its use may reduce the need for large doses of atropine. It is given in doses of 1 g diluted in dextrose and water, over 15 to 30 min. If there are severe symptoms, the dosage may be repeated in 1 to 2 h and may continue at 1 g every 6 to 8 h for 48 h if symptoms persist.

## Methemoglobinemia

Methemoglobinemia is caused by abnormal hemoglobin or exposure to various nitrates, including nitroglycerin, explosives, aniline dye derivatives, and some sulfonamides. Brown color of arterial blood, and cyanosis that does not clear with oxygenation are clues to the diagnosis. There may be marked cyanosis with little respiratory distress.

Treatment is supportive with oxygen administration, and decontamination with soap and water if the exposure was dermal. A 1% solution of methylene blue is used for symptomatic patients who have cardiac symptoms such as angina, arrhythmias, hypotension, seizures, or coma. Levels as low as 15 percent in patients with underlying cardiac disease or anemia may be treated. The dose is 1 to 2 mg/kg or 0.1 to 0.2 mL/kg given intravenously over 5 min. Methemoglobin levels are then remeasured 1 h after infusion. The dose may be repeated if the patient is still symptomatic and still has significant levels. Exchange transfusions and hyperbaric oxygen have been used in very severe cases.

## Hydrofluoric Acid

Hydrofluoric acid is a strong inorganic acid that can penetrate intact skin and cause coagulation necrosis of subcutaneous tissues. It causes severe pain that may be out of proportion to the visible injury. The onset of pain is delayed with household and weaker strengths, and the patient may present with severe burning 8 to 12 h after the exposure. Sometimes it takes a detailed history to ascertain that an exposure has occurred hours earlier. Severe damage can occur to subcutaneous structures including muscle and bone. Systemic hypocalcemia and hypomagnesemia are due to complexing of cations by fluoride. Hyperkalemia due to extracellular efflux of potassium can occur with resulting arrhythmias and death. A third-degree burn with concentrated hydrofluoric acid as small as 2.5 percent of the body surface area can cause death.

Calcium will precipitate the fluoride ion. A 2.5% solution of calcium gluconate gel or other available treatment (Table 172-2) should be massaged into the skin, using pain relief as an endpoint. Subcutaneous injection of 10% calcium gluconate may be used, with a maximum of 0.5 mL per digit. This treatment is painful, and nail bed removal may be needed if the distal dorsal digit is involved. If regional anesthesia is used, the endpoint of pain relief is obscured. Alternative treatment of interarterial calcium gluconate will obviate the need for nail removal and painful local injection. Pain is often so severe that narcotic analgesia may be needed. Consultation with a burn surgeon is necessary for severe burns, circumferential burns, burns of nail plates, and burns that do not respond to simple treatment. If systemic hypocalcemia occurs, intravenous calcium replacement will be necessary.

## Phenol

Phenol, or carbolic acid, and its derivatives are used as deodorizers, disinfectants, and sanitizers. It is absorbed through the skin and causes liver and kidney end-organ damage, as well as CNS depression. On contact with the skin it denatures protein and causes intense pain and burning and may form an eschar that traps the phenol in the subcutaneous tissues. Gangrene may develop. Dinitrophenol and hydroquinolone can cause methemoglobinemia. Management includes immediate washing with soap and water. Olive oil and polyethylene glycol have been recommended.

## Additional Antidotes

Additional antidotes are available to chelate heavy metals, such as deferoxamine for iron; British anti-lewisite (BAL, Dimercaprol) for arsenic; D-penicillamine for chronic arsenic exposure; BAL and EDTA for lead; and BAL and D-penicillamine for mercury.

## BIBLIOGRAPHY

Agency for Toxic Substances and Disease Registry: *Managing Hazardous Materials Incidents,* vol 1: *Emergency Medical Systems.* Washington, DC, US Department of Health and Human Services, 1993.

Agency for Toxic Substances and Disease Registry: *Managing Hazardous Materials Incidents,* vol 2: *Hospital Emergency Departments.* Washington, DC, US Department of Health and Human Services, 1993.

Agency for Toxic Substances and Disease Registry: *Managing Hazardous Materials Incidents,* vol 3: *Medical Management Guidelines for Acute Chemical Exposures.* Washington, DC, US Department of Health and Human Services, 1994.

Binder S: Deaths, injuries, and evacuations from acute hazardous materials releases. *Am J Public Health* 79:1042, 1989.

Borak J, Callan M, Abbott W: *Hazardous Materials Exposure.* Englewood Cliffs, NJ, Brady, 1991.

Burgess WA: *Recognition of Health Hazards in Industry: A Review of Materials and Processes.* New York, Wiley, 1981.

CHEMTREC data, personal communication, Mr Hank Sauer, Oct 1994.

Doyle CJ: Hazardous chemicals. *Emerg Med Clin North Am* 1:653, 1983.

Doyle CJ: Resources for toxicology (appendix), in Little NE (ed.): *Critical Decisions in Emergency Medicine,* vol 6. Dallas, TX, ACEP Publishing, 1993.

Goldberg MJ, Spector R, Park GD: et al: An approach to the management of the poisoned patient. *Arch Intern Med,* July, 1986.

Goldfrank LR, Flomenbaum NE, Lewin NA: *Toxicologic Emergencies.* Norwalk, CT, Appleton/Lange, 1990.

Guzzardi L: Toxic products of combustion. *Top Emerg Med* 7:45, 1985.

Haddad LM, Winchester JF (eds): *Clinical Management of Poisoning and Overdose, 2d ed.* Philadelphia, Saunders, 1990.

Hall IH, Dara VR, Price-Green PA, et al: Surveillance for emergency events involving hazardous substances—United States, 1990–1992 *MMWR* 43: ss-2, July 22, 1994.

Hedges JR: Acute noxious gas exposure. *Curr Top Emerg Med* 2:59, 1978.

Kirk MA, Cisek J, Rose SR: Emergency department response to hazardous materials incidents. *Emerg Med Clin North Am* 12: 461, 1994.

Kizer KW: Toxic inhalations. *Emerg Med Clin North Am* 2:649, 1984.

Klaassen CD, Amdur MO, Doull J: *Casarett and Doull's Toxicology,* 3d ed, New York, Macmillan, 1986.

Leonard RB: Hazardous materials accidents: Initial scene assessment and patient care. *Aviat Space Environ Med* 64:(6) 546, 1993.

Maibach HI: *Occupational and Industrial Dermatology,* 2d ed. Chicago, Year Book, 1987.

Marrs TC: Organophosphate poisoning. *Pharmacol Ther* 58:51, 1993.

Noji EK, Kelen GD (eds): *Manual of Toxicologic Emergencies.* Chicago, Year Book, 1989.

Proctor NH, Hughes JP: *Chemical Hazards of the Workplace* 2d ed. Philadelphia, Lippincott, 1988.

Reiffenstein RJ, Hulbert WC, Roth SH: Toxicology of hydrogen sulfide. *Annu Rev Pharmacol Toxicol* 32:109, 1992.

Rorison DG, McPherson SJ: Acute toxic inhalations. *Emerg Med Clin North Am* 10:2, 1992.

Rumack BH et al: *Poisindex.* Micromedex, Denver, CO, 11/1994.

Student FJ: *Emergency Handling of Hazardous Materials in Surface Transportation.* Washington, DC, Bureau of Explosives, 1981.

Stutz DR, Ricks RC, Olsen MF: *Hazardous Materials Injuries: A Handbook for Pre-Hospital Care.* Greenbelt, MD, Bradford Communications, 1982.

Upfal M, Doyle CJ: Medical management of hydrofluoric acid exposure. *J Occup Med* 32(8):726, 1990.

US Department of Transportation: *National Transportation Statistics,* annual report. Washington, DC, US Department of Transportation, Sept. 1993.

US Department of Transportation: *Hazardous Material—Emergency Response Guidebook.* Washington, DC, US Department of Transportation, 1994.

# 173

# RADIATION INJURIES

## H. Arnold Muller

We cannot see, smell, feel, or hear radiation, yet it captured our attention during the 1979 Three Mile Island accident. And on April 26, 1986, the worst commercial nuclear power plant disaster in history occurred with the explosion and fire at the Chernobyl No. 4 nuclear power plant in the Soviet Union. In terms of the amount of radioactivity released into the environment, the size of the affected area, long-term consequences, the numerous acute injuries, and 29 known deaths, the Chernobyl accident was the most significant nuclear event since the bombing of Hiroshima and Nagasaki.

Some elements of radiation physics, common sources of radiation (Table 173-1), the tissue effects of radiation, the signs and symptoms of radiation injury, and the evaluation and therapy of radiation injuries and exposure will be briefly covered in this chapter.

## PATHOPHYSIOLOGY

Radiation may be classified as *ionizing* or *nonionizing.* Ionizing radiation is produced by nuclear weapons and reactors, radioactive material, and x-ray machines. The term *ionizing* is derived from the effect that such radiation produces when it interacts with matter, that is, it causes atoms to convert to ions as a result of the atoms' loss or gain of electrons. Biological function may be affected if such ionized atoms are in the human body. On the other hand, light, radio waves, and microwaves are examples of *nonionizing radiation.*

Radiation is either *particulate* or *electromagnetic.* Electromagnetic

**Table 173-1.** Common Sources of Radiation

| Source | Whole Body, mrem/yr | Dose Rate |
|---|---|---|
| Natural sources: | | |
| Radon | 200 | |
| Natural background radiation | 35 | |
| Air | 5 | |
| Building materials | 34 | |
| Food | 25 | |
| Ground | 11 | |
| Medical | 50 | |
| Total | 360 | |
| Technological sources: | | |
| Coast-to-coast jet flight | | 5 mrem/round trip |
| Color television | | 1 mrem/yr |
| AP chest film | | 10 mrem/film |

*Source:* Linnemann RE: *Background Information on Radiation.* April 4, 1979. San Jose, California, General Electric Nuclear Energy Group. Used by permission. Above table has been altered with permission of Dr. Linnemann to reflect more recent information regarding common sources of radiation.

radiation occurs in waveform and has no mass or charge. It belongs to a family of radiant energies that is described by wavelengths. Electromagnetic radiations, in order of decreasing energy content are γ rays, x-rays (photons), ultraviolet rays, visible rays, infrared rays, microwaves, and radio waves. Gamma waves and x-rays are electromagnetic radiations that can cause ionization. The electrons lost from atoms act as secondary particles and produce additional ionizations. X-rays differ from γ rays only in that x-rays are produced outside the nucleus of an atom; γ rays are emitted from the nucleus. Both travel great distances and readily penetrate body cells. X-rays and γ rays can easily be detected by Geiger-Müller (GM) counters.

Although α and β particles are not electromagnetic, they do cause ionization. The α particle consists of two protons and two neutrons (identical to a helium atom without electrons) emitted from the nucleus of a high atomic number (≥82) radioactive atom. The α particles travel only a few centimeters in air and are completely stopped by paper or the keratin layer of the skin. The β particle is an electron emitted from the nucleus of a radioactive atom. Beta particles travel up to a few meters in air but barely penetrate the skin. Both α and β particles are harmful, however, if they contaminate wounds or are ingested or inhaled. Contamination of the body surfaces by α and β particles can be detected by counters.

Energy deposited by radiation per unit of mass is referred to as the *dose.* A *rad* (radiation *a*bsorbed *d*ose) is 100 ergs of energy deposited in 1 g of material. The Système International (SI) unit for dose is the Gray (Gy): 1 Gy = 100 rad; 1 cGy = 1 rad. The rem (roentgen *e*quivalent *m*an) is a calculated radiation unit of dose equivalent in which the absorbed dose in rad (or Gy) is multiplied by a quality factor to account for the biological effectiveness of different types of radiation. The SI unit for dose equivalent is the Sievert (Sv). 1 Sv = 100 rem; 1 cSv = 1 rem. We generally use the term *rem* or *millirem* (mrem) when referring to the exposure of biological systems. For x-rays, γ rays, and β particles, the rad and the rem and the Gray and the Sievert are equivalent. A given rad dose from neutrons of α particles produces up to 20 times as much biological damage as the same dose in rad from x-rays or γ rays. The whole body dose of ionizing radiation that will kill half of those who are exposed is approximately 400 rem (4 Sv). At about 600 rem (6 Sv) the mortality has been nearly 100 percent. Mental retardation has been associated with radiation doses as low as 5 rem to the fetus during the eighth to fifteenth week of gestation. The human average annual "normal" exposure to radiation in the United States from all sources, including radon, is approximately 360 mrem (3.6 mSv). A person or object exposed to radiation, other than high-dose neutron radiation, does not become radioactive. However, a person may be a risk to caregivers if contaminated with radioactive dirt or imbedded radioactive shrapnel, etc.

Equivalent doses received over a long time are less harmful than those received over a short period of time. For example, 100 rem (1 Sv) delivered over 1 year is much less harmful than 100 rem delivered in 1 s. The radiation dose from a point source of radiation decreases inversely as the square of the distance from the source.

The biological effects of radiation are a consequence of ionization. Free radicals are formed from water and can cause DNA and RNA strands to be broken. The most susceptible cells are those whose nucleic acids turn over most rapidly, i.e., cells of developing gametes, embryo, bone marrow, and the epithelium of the gastrointestinal tract. Cell and chromosomal changes may be minor and not pose a hazard to the organism. They may result in aberrations that are passed on to subsequent generations, or they may result in cell death, or the inability to replicate.

## CLINICAL FEATURES

The most prominent systemic signs and symptoms of high [>100 rem (1 Sv)] whole body radiation exposure are malaise, nausea, vomiting, and diarrhea; seizures; erythema of the skin; and later, bleeding, anemia, and infection. Nausea and vomiting occasionally occur at about 100-rem exposure (Table 173-2). If they develop within 2 h of exposure, it suggests a dose of more than 400 rem (4 Sv); after 2 h from exposure, less than 200 rem (2 Sv); if none after 6 h from exposure, less than 50 rem (0.5 Sv). Erythema, local or generalized, indicates skin exposure greater than 300 rem (3 Sv); diarrhea indicates exposure of the gastrointestinal tract to greater than 400 rem (4 Sv); and seizures indicate central nervous system exposure greater than 2000 rem (20 Sv). Lymphocyte counts are useful prognostically. If after 48 h the lymphocyte count is >1200/μL, the prognosis is good; 300 to 1200, fair; less than 300/μL, poor. Bleeding, anemia, and infection may occur after a latent period of 20 to 30 days.

Erythema and brawniness of the skin, indicating exposure of 300 or more rem (3 Sv), develop in a few hours and progress over days, just as with a thermal burn. While radiation burns are initially less painful than thermal burns, when pain does develop, and it often starts quickly, it may rapidly dominate the clinical picture. During circumstances in which fire as well as radioactive contamination may have occurred, ask the patient if he or she recalls exposure to fire or hot objects or caustic chemicals. Loss of hair, vesiculation, and ulceration may eventually develop if the radiation dose is high enough.

Following radiation exposure the likelihood of significant systemic effects can be estimated based on time of onset of nausea, vomiting, and diarrhea; changes in lymphocyte count; and knowledge of the accident, the radiation source, the dose readings at the site of the accident, and the duration of exposure.

Often a health physicist at the scene of an industrial accident is able to provide some indication of dose. Severity of symptoms varies and does not correlate with dose, but onset following exposure does. The earlier signs and symptoms develop, the higher the dose and the worse the prognosis. Initial symptoms (nausea, vomiting, and general malaise) generally subside within a few hours to several days and are followed by a latent period of 1 or more weeks. In general, if exposure is less than 125 rem (1.25 Sv), prognosis is good. For patients with doses less than 200 rem (2 Sv), probably nothing more than symptomatic treatment is needed, and recovery should occur. Those with exposure of 200 to 1000 rem should be promptly placed into a reverse isolation atmosphere. Further treatment need is probable to certain, and aggressive treatment can make a great difference in pa-

**Table 173-2.** Dose-Effect Relations Following Acute Whole Body Irradiation (X- or γ-Ray)

| Whole Body Dose, rad | Clinical and Laboratory Findings |
|---|---|
| 5–25 | Asymptomatic. Conventional blood studies are normal. Chromosome aberrations detectable. |
| 50–75 | Asymptomatic. Minor depressions of white cells and platelets detectable in a few persons, especially if baseline values established. |
| 75–125 | Minimal acute doses that produce prodromal symptoms (anorexia, nausea, vomiting, fatigue) in about 10–20% of persons within 2 days. Mild depressions of white cells and platelets in some persons. |
| 125–200 | Symptomatic course with transient disability and clear hematologic changes in a majority of exposed persons. Lymphocyte depression of about 50% within 48 h. |
| 240–340 | Serious, disabling illness in most persons with about 50% mortality if untreated. Lymphocyte depression of about ≥75% within 48 h. |
| 500+ | Accelerated version of acute radiation syndrome with GI complications within 2 weeks, bleeding, and death in most exposed persons. |
| 5000+ | Fulminating course with cardiovascular, GI, and CNS complications resulting in death within 24–72 h. |

*Source:* Mettler FD: Emergency management of radiation accidents. *JACEP* 7:302, 1978. Used by permission.

tient survival. Other than prompt external and internal body decontamination of radioactive material, and fluid replacement, when indicated, there is no *emergency* treatment specific to radiation exposure that will make any difference in long-term survival. Whatever symptoms occur should be treated symptomatically.

Following exposure to radiation, the exposed population is at risk for delayed complications such as leukemia and thyroid carcinoma. Contraception should be practiced for several months to avoid congenital defects in offspring.

## TREATMENT

Initial treatment of radiation-exposed patients must first involve management of life-threatening injuries: airway impairment, bleeding, and circulation impairment. Patients who have been irradiated, that is, subjected to a high flux of γ rays or x-rays, are not radioactive. As such, no radiation is detected on the patient's body or clothes. Any tissue damage occurs instantaneously and will manifest itself in time. An irradiated person may sustain local or total body exposure. Following immediate management of life-threatening injuries, the patient should be checked with a GM counter for surface contamination, and it should be determined whether radioactive material has been ingested or inhaled. The GM counter is very useful for detecting β and γ radiation. If used to detect α radiation, it must contain a special window because of the low penetrating power of α particles. In 1987, following the radiation accident in Goiania, Brazil, it was discovered that the axilla was the most representative point for measurement of dose rate using GM monitors in relation to internal cesium 137 body burden. Such an approach might be applicable when internal contamination with other whole body critical organ radionuclides is suspected. The health physicist at the site should be contacted so that data regarding dose, nature of exposure, type of radiation, and duration of exposure can be obtained.

Treatment protocol is as follows: Cover open wounds, remove the patient's clothing, and deposit contaminated material in closed receptacles. Protect open wounds to avoid contamination while washing or disrobing the patient. Next, wash the patient with soap and water. If the patient is on a drainage table, contaminated water can be collected in containers. If radioactive material in the form of solid particles, liquid, or dust is inhaled or ingested or contaminates an open wound, then incorporation has occurred. Since such material will irradiate internal tissues and may well cause extensive cellular damage, and since some radioactive elements may become permanently incorporated in the body's molecules, immediate treatment (decorporation) is indicated. Decorporation emphasis is directed at the gastrointestinal tract since even inhaled radioactive particulates tend to be coughed up and swallowed. Chelating agents provide an ion-exchange matrix that results in formation of an excretable stable complex containing the radioactivity. Radioactive actinide isotopes can be chelated effectively and subsequently excreted when diethylenetriaminepentaacetic acid (DTPA) is administered. Such action should be taken within 1 h of internal contamination. Chelating agents are useful only for transuranics and certain heavy metals. They would probably only be needed for accidents near a fuel-processing or military weapons facility. Although nuclear medicine departments may have stock DTPA solutions, they are too dilute to be useful as chelating agents for the removal of internal radioactive contamination. DTPA may be ordered from the Radiation Emergency Assistance Center/Training Site (REAC/TS) at Oak Ridge, Tennessee. If one anticipates the possible future need for DTPA, a request for current acquisition of it should be made to REAC/TS. DTPA is itself dangerous to use.

Primary wound closure is acceptable if successful decontamination is possible; however, if, in spite of irrigation and cleansing, a significant amount of contamination is retained in a wound, the wound should be left open for 24 h. Much of the remaining contamination will be freed up by bleeding and exudate and can then be removed by debridement. If an extremity is severely contaminated and adequate decontamination is not possible, the question of amputation may be raised. In general, unless the extremity is so severely traumatized that functional recovery is unlikely or unless contamination by radionuclides is so severe that extensive and severe radiation-induced necrosis can be expected, amputation is rarely indicated. The dictum is, decontaminate, but do not mutilate.

Though amputation is rarely required, one should aggressively debride and surgically decontaminate. Such procedures can usually be done without endangering a functional recovery. As surgical instruments become contaminated, they should be removed from the surgical field in order to prevent extension of contamination.

For contamination by plutonium or another long-lived $\alpha$ emitter for which DTPA is an effective chelating agent, prompt treatment locally and intravenously is indicated, preferably prior to surgical decontamination.

Potassium iodide, a blocking agent, effectively prevents the uptake of radioactive iodine by the thyroid if it is given within a few hours of exposure. The National Council on Radiation Protection and Measurements recommends treatment to protect the thyroid when the dose is, or is expected to be, 10 to 30 rem. Persons 13 years of age or older should receive 130 mg of potassium iodide (100 mg stable iodine) by mouth daily for 14 days. However, pregnant women and children from 3 to 12 years of age should receive 65 mg potassium iodide (50 mg potassium iodine), and children under a year old, 32.5 mg potassium iodide (25 mg stable iodine) to minimize risk of side effects. Following the Chernobyl accident, 0.37 percent of Polish newborns who received potassium iodide prophylaxis on the second day of life showed transient increases in serum thyroid-stimulating hormone (TSH) levels and concomitant decreases in the serum free $T_4$ levels. The transient thyroid inhibition had no sequelae. However, the findings indicate the need for careful observation in the event that more prolonged periods of treatment are indicated for infants. Antacids in the stomach precipitate many metals in the form of insoluble hydroxides, and can shorten the internal transit time of such material. Aluminum phosphate gel (100 mL) reduces the intestinal absorption of radioactive strontium by 85 percent, and barium sulfate precipitates radium.

A baseline complete blood cell count, differential blood cell count, and platelet count should be done during this initial treatment phase. For patients who have received >200 rem, protective isolation is indicated, and blood transfusions may be necessary later. Bone marrow depression is usually evident 20 to 30 days after exposure. Appropriate cultures, antibiotic therapy as soon as there is evidence of infection, prophylaxis against fungal infections, and HLA typing of the patient and family members are all indicated in serious cases. Such supportive measures help to permit autologous bone marrow recovery, as does use of hemopoietic growth factors, when indicated. Bone marrow transplant may be considered if there is no recovery or if the stem cell pool is sufficiently damaged. Such damage would be evidenced by severe granulocytopenia, severe lymphopenia, and beginning thrymbocytopenia around day 5 to 7. These findings are evident when only 6 to 8 of every 10,000 stem cells have survived, i.e., irreversible stem cell damage.

Radiation burns are like electrical burns in that physical findings may be minimal initially. For $\beta$-particle burns, excision followed by full-thickness grafting may be necessary.

Patients from a radiation accident scene may also have been exposed to chemical hazards. Thus, beryllium, which is present in many nuclear weapons, may be released as fumes and smoke, which in turn may cause respiratory distress, nervousness, and fever. Contamination of open wounds with beryllium results in greatly delayed wound healing. Treatment of the pulmonary problem includes, in addition to oxygen, ethylenediaminetetraacetic acid (EDTA) or another effective chelating agent.

When lead, used in nuclear weapon devices for shielding, burns it releases toxic fumes that can cause pneumonitis and dermatitis. Dermatitis and delayed-onset pneumonitis may also occur as a result of the inhalation of fumes from the combustion of plastics, which are used in most nuclear devices.

Finally, if a U.S. nuclear weapon were to accidentally detonate, such detonation would in all probability be incomplete. It would, however, be associated with blast effects, fires, and the spread of radioactive material. Unexploded pieces of the explosive might be scattered around an accident site. Such pieces frequently look like natural rock and should not be touched or moved unless absolutely necessary for evacuation of casualties.

## DECONTAMINATION IN THE EMERGENCY DEPARTMENT

Advance notice of the arrival of a radiation-injured patient is important so that the emergency department can be prepared. Given such notice, emergency personnel can also advise on prior decontamination in the field.

Every nuclear facility must have identified primary and tertiary referral facilities. It is necessary to develop and maintain open channels of communication between the nuclear facility and the emergency department so that each will be prepared in times of individual injury or major accident. One should not rely on telephone communication being available within the hospital or between the hospital and other facilities in the event of a major nuclear accident or disaster. A predetermined plan involving backup radio communication is advised. Periodic exercises in which the facility is suddenly faced with the hypothetical need to treat a few or hundreds of irradiated and/or radioactive-contaminated patients is the best means to ensure the capability of dealing with such problems.

In the emergency department, a designated area, the radiation emergency area, isolated and preferably with a separate entryway, should be available for the management of patients with radiation exposure. Contamination should be prevented by covering the floor with plastic or paper sheets. Patients and personnel should be monitored for evidence of contamination. Personnel treating or attending the patient must be gowned and wear caps, masks, foot covers, double gloves, and personnel monitoring devices (i.e., film badge, thermoluminescent dosimeter badge, and/or pocket dosimeters). All personnel caring for patients suspected of contamination with radioiodine should, if possible, take potassium iodide prior to the arrival of the patient(s).

In rare cases it may also be necessary to provide a lead shield to protect personnel, especially in cases in which there are highly contaminated foreign bodies. Exposure can also be minimized by decreasing exposure time (several people would share care of a patient) and maintaining a distance from the patient whenever possible. Those providing care should not be exposed to more than 5 rem (0.05 Sv) except to save a life. The National Council on Radiation Protection has established that a once-in-a-lifetime exposure to 100 rem (1.0 Sv) for purposes of saving a life is acceptable and will result in no undue morbidity. Individuals not involved in the treatment should be kept away from the roped-off area. All attendant personnel should be monitored and decontaminated and their garments appropriately disposed of following completion of their involvement in the treatment process. Everyone working in the radiation emergency area must remain there, and traffic should never move in the reverse direction without first being appropriately monitored. Ambulance personnel and their vehicle(s) should also be checked for the presence of contamination before leaving the facility.

## PREHOSPITAL DECONTAMINATION

R. E. Linnemann suggests an order of priority for treating a number of individuals involved in radiation accidents:

1. Injured and contaminated patients
2. Patients with certain types of internal contamination
3. Patients exposed only to external total body radiation
4. Patients exposed only to external local body radiation

If treatment of great numbers of radiation-exposed and contaminated patients is necessary, different modes may be indicated. Home treatment with showers or garden hoses should be considered, as should treatment at nearby facilities such as schools. An alternative decontamination facility within the hospital should be such that ready access and shelter available from fallout may be provided for a large number of contaminated patients. Triage should be performed to identify those who may require immediate medical care and/or decontamination. Those found to be contaminated should pass through a disrobing area and a shower, and ultimately be garbed with hospital gowns and reassessed for residual contamination. Again, resuscitation and stabilization always take precedence over decontamination.

Under these circumstances all available GM counters and dosimeters would be commandeered. Provision should be made for initial and follow-up treatment of any injuries. One should also consider establishing a large holding area, with subsequent transfer, if necessary, to other institutions where there is no area-wide radiation risk.

## THE EVACUATION DILEMMA

Emergency physicians should be aware of the burden carried by local and state government officials who must make evacuation decisions. A population should be evacuated if the estimated per capita whole body radiation dose will be 50 rem (0.5 Sv) or more and seek shelter if the dose is expected to be 5 rem (0.05 Sv) or more. Emphasis is placed on predetermined actions for predetermined conditions. Thus, in a nuclear power plant accident if significant core damage has occurred, evacuation of the public from within a 2-mile radius is indicated. If the operator of the plant cannot assure the situation is under control, evacuation is indicated from within a 5-mile radius. If control is assured, all persons beyond 2 miles would be instructed to remain in available shelter. However, the present methods of dose assessment have a great range of uncertainty. The timing of a decision to evacuate may be crucial. Thus, officials fail if they wait too long, that is, until dangerous levels of radiation are present in populated areas, and they fail, too, if an unnecessary evacuation is ordered, for there are many risks inherent in an evacuation including adverse effects on moving hospitalized patients, panic reactions, and injuries and death from automobile crashes.

## HOSPITAL EVACUATION

It is conceivable that internal hospital evacuation may be necessary in the event of radiation threat. Emergency radiation disaster plans should include designation of preselected sites within the hospital which afford the most protection for patients and health care personnel. Such sites are usually at ground level or below. Indeed, the dose can be increased by a factor of 10 or more if basement level is used. As much "concrete" as possible should be placed between personnel and the environment. Provision should be made for ensuring appropriate medical equipment, food, medications, and electric power and heat at the new care site (Table 173-3). Consideration should be given to shutting off fans and air conditioning during the critical exposure period (plume phase) and turning them back on following the plume phase in order to reduce exposure to radionuclides which have entered the building. The duration of such an internal evacuation would be related to the type of radiation and its half-life, atmospheric conditions, availability of supplies, and the condition of the patients.

External evacuation in the event of a radiation threat can be even more chaotic if not properly planned. One central source must provide for the evacuation needs of the hospitals in the area and determine the availability of off-site hospitals. Such an external evacuation

**Table 173-3.** Emergency Supplies for Use in Radiation Emergencies

Radiation detection instruments including Geiger-Müller counters, spare batteries, film badges, ring badges, self-reading dosimeters
Surgical scrub suits
Surgical gowns
Surgical caps
Surgical masks
Surgical gloves
Plastic shoe covers
Adhesive tape
Plastic sheets and bags
Step-off pads
Plastic containers for collection of decontamination fluids
Decontamination stretcher
Roll of plastic floor covering for use in the hallway
Radiation "mark off" rope
Radioactive signs and labels
Filter paper for smears
Clipboard, paper, and pens
Assorted containers for sample collection

would entail the need to categorize patients, effect discharge of ambulatory patients if possible, and provide clinical summaries plus radiographs and reports, a listing of medications and treatments needed, and a 24-h supply of food, water, and medications. Categorized patients would be taken to different and appropriate facility staging areas within the facility to await their external evacuation.

## LESSONS LEARNED FROM CHERNOBYL

In the Three Mile Island incident, two workers received 3 to 4 (0.03 to 0.04 Sv) total body dose and several received $\beta$ radiation skin exposure of about 300 rem (3 Sv). No acute injury resulted in any of these cases. By contrast, 203 people were hospitalized and 29 died of radiation exposure as a result of the Chernobyl accident.

The lesson: build safe nuclear power plants. The Chernobyl No. 4 reactor, unlike U.S. nuclear power plants, contained a large mass of combustible material (2700 tons of graphite) and had much less contamination protection than do U.S. reactors.

A radiation disaster plan should include provision for (1) on-site triage; (2) a nearby hospital prepared for secondary triage, further decontamination, and treatment of life-threatening injuries; and (3) identified tertiary care radiation injury treatment centers to deal with contaminated injuries, including those of burn patients and patients in the advanced hematologic and immune system-suppressed states.

Based on the Chernobyl experience, most patients receiving less than 400 rem (4 Sv) whole body radiation can be expected to recover, if provided with optimal supportive care. Indeed, survival following a dose of 600 rem now appears possible.

The human immune system is vulnerable between 150 and 200 rem (1.5 and 2.0 Sv). At total body radiation exposures between 200 and 1500 rem (2 and 15 Sv), marrow damage is a major cause of death. And at higher doses, survival is limited by damage to skin, liver, lung, and gastrointestinal tract. At 5000 rem (50 Sv), death occurs in less than 2 days from central nervous system vasculitis.

Inhalation of particulate radioactivity can be significantly reduced (by a factor of 3 to 5) by breathing through several layers of moistened handkerchiefs, although the method is almost ineffective against gaseous radioiodines.

Emergency physicians might be faced with evaluating patients at times other than after acute exposure. In that context, the following points are important: granulocytopenic patients who develop fever require treatment with antibiotics, generally with those that cover enteric bacteria. Acyclovir is helpful in treating oral herpes simplex infection, which is apt to recrudesce following radiation exposure. If fever persists in a patient being treated with antibiotics, one should think of the possibility of systemic fungal infections and consider treating with amphotericin B.

Thermal burns and significant musculoskeletal and visceral injuries, if present, contribute significantly to radiation-related deaths. Physical radiation monitoring devices may prove inadequate, as they did at Chernobyl, in a nuclear accident. The devices may be destroyed, or they may not have been designed for the high levels of radiation encountered.

At Chernobyl biological dosimetry was used for dose assessment. Thus, serial measurements of granulocyte and lymphocyte levels as well as analyses of blood and bone marrow cell chromosomes for dicentrics, tricentrics, and rings were performed. In the case of cell chromosome analyses, the number of changes per cell is linearly related to exposures between 15 and 600 rem (0.15 and 6.0 Sv). The time elapsed between exposure and the onset of nausea and/or vomiting was also used for dose assessment purposes.

The world's ongoing need for nonfossil energy sources is borne out by the choices of other nations. The Japanese and Russians are adding significantly to their nuclear plant numbers, and the great majority of France's power generation is by nuclear plant.

## SPECIAL ASPECTS OF RADIATION ACCIDENTS AND DISASTERS

In the absence of nuclear war or nuclear power plant disaster, such as occurred at Chernobyl, it is unlikely that most hospitals will receive any patients who have been involved in life-threatening radiation accidents. It is more likely that a given hospital's emergency department personnel will be called upon to handle a patient with routine injuries complicated by inadvertent radiation exposure or the presence of low-level radioactive contamination. Such a circumstance might result from an accident involving transportation of radioactive materials or a contaminating incident in a hospital's nuclear medicine department. Since radiation accidents are so uncommon, it is wise for emergency physicians to include in their planning discussions personnel from operating rooms, ICUs, and any other disciplines likely to be involved in the care of patients who have been exposed to and are contaminated with radioactive material.

Despite the Chernobyl accident, radiation injuries are an infrequent medical event, even though there are ever-increasing production and use of radiation-producing machines, radioactive products, nuclear plants, and nuclear weapons. Thus, as of 1988, worldwide there had been 69 peacetime deaths secondary to radiation exposure. And of these 69, nine were in the United States. No significant injuries or deaths due to radiation overexposure have occurred in the U.S. commercial nuclear power industry since its inception in 1957. The majority of industrial radiation accidents involve personnel radiated from high-activity sealed sources used in radiography. Nevertheless, as we plan for the more likely minor radiation accident, we must recognize that it is possible that the United States might sustain a terrorist attack with a nuclear weapon or suffer the accidental discharge and detonation of a nuclear weapon by another nation. An all-out exchange of thermonuclear weapons would not likely leave enough medical facilities and staff to provide an effective response, nor would any medical response under such conditions be apt to be sustainable.

Whatever the basis for a radiation accident or disaster, prior communication, instruction, and staff exercises are the best preparation for any eventuality. As a corollary, ongoing communication with staff during an exercise or "real life" accident or disaster is a must. The role of the public relations department is very important, for it is such personnel who, under such circumstances, deal with the media and the public.

In addition to your own staff and others who are experienced and knowledgeable about radiation, there are other individuals and organizations, private, state, and federal, willing and able to promptly respond to your call for aid. REAC/TS can be contacted 24 hours a day for radiation accident assistance at (615) 576-1004, and Radiation Management Consultants (RMC) may be contacted at (215) 537-0672.

Finally, nuclear facilities do not "blow up" like nuclear bombs. It is physically impossible. Instead, a nuclear plant accident is more apt to be associated with a potentially large number of people being slightly exposed, slightly contaminated, and very anxious.

## BIBLIOGRAPHY

Linnemann RE: Medical experience and preparedness for handling radiation injuries. *J Med Assoc Georgia* 78:95, 1989.

Nauman J, Wolff J: Iodide prophylaxis in Poland after the Chernobyl reactor accident: Benefits and risks. *Am J Med* 94:524, 1993.

Oliveira A, Hunt J, Valverde N, et al: Medical and related aspects of the Goiania accident: An overview. *Health Phys* 60:17, 1991.

Perry AR, Iglar AF: The accident at Chernobyl: Radiation doses and effects. *Radiotechnol* 61:290, 1990.

Task Group of Committee 4 of the International Commission on Radiological Protection: Principles for intervention for protection of the public in a radiological emergency. *Ann ICRP* 22:1, 1991.

Weinsheimer W, Szepesi T, Fliedner TM: Early indicators of response to accidental radiation exposure and relevance for clinical management strategies. *Prog Clin Biol Res* 372:155, 1991.

# 174
# MUSHROOM POISONING
**Christopher H. Linden**
**Robert P. Dowsett**

Mushrooms, also known as toadstools, are the visible fruit of certain fungi. Of the thousands of species known to exist, only about 100 can cause serious illness, and only about 10 are responsible for fatal poisoning. Parallel with the increased popularity of foraging for edible wild mushrooms, the incidence of mushroom poisoning has risen in recent years. Of the thousands of ingestions of potentially toxic mushrooms reported annually in the United States, however, only a few hundred result in significant morbidity or death.

Poisoning is most common during the late summer and early fall, since wild mushrooms are most abundant during these seasons. It most often occurs when amateur foragers (and their friends and relatives) mistake poisonous species for edible ones. *Amanita phalloides* (the "death cap") and *A. virosa* (the "destroying angel") are the species responsible for most fatalities. Young children who accidentally ingest a wild mushroom rarely become seriously ill (unless they partake of a mushroom meal served to them by adults), probably because uncooked wild mushrooms are generally not very palatable. Recreational drug users may experience untoward effects after intentionally ingesting hallucinogenic mushrooms. They may also become poisoned by phencyclidine (PCP) or lysergic acid diethylamide (LSD), since edible mushrooms laced with these chemicals are frequently sold on the street as psychoactive species. Although hallucinogenic mushrooms are usually ingested as dried or fresh mushroom pieces or occasionally after brewing as a tea, they are sometimes snorted, smoked, or injected intravenously. The inhalation of vapors evolved during the boiling (i.e., attempted detoxification) of some species of wild mushrooms can also cause poisoning.

Under certain circumstances, or in susceptible persons, poisoning can occur after the ingestion of normally edible mushrooms. Some species cause an adverse reaction only if ingested with ethanol. Edible mushrooms contaminated with bacteria or chemicals (e.g., insecticides) can result in poisoning unrelated to mushroom toxins. The common grocery store mushroom, *Agaricus bisporus,* can cause unpleasant gastrointestinal effects in individuals who are inherently intolerant to this species. And finally, immunologic reactions (e.g., food allergy, hemolytic anemia) may sometimes occur following mushroom ingestion.

There are no easy rules for differentiating poisonous from edible species. That boiling, drying, or salting a poisonous mushroom will detoxify it are common misconceptions. Correctly identifying a mushroom as edible or poisonous requires careful analysis of its morphologic features by an experienced mycologist. Even when the mushroom thought to be responsible for poisoning is available, toxic and nontoxic species may be found growing side by side and gathered and eaten together, and the mushroom available for identification may not be the one (or the only one) ingested. In addition, the appearance and toxicity of a given species of mushroom may vary depending on such factors as mushroom maturity, geographic location, and growing conditions; poisonous strains of reportedly edible mushrooms may exist; and the treatment of poisoning by one species of mushroom may be harmful if another species or condition is the true source. For all these reasons, the diagnosis and the appropriate treatment should ultimately be determined by the clinical presentation (rather than by mushroom identification).

## PHARMACOLOGY

Poisonous mushrooms can be divided into eight different groups based on their principal toxins and the nature and time of onset of clinical toxicity (Table 174-1). *Amatoxins* are bicyclic octapeptides that act by inhibiting RNA polymerase II and thus interfere with DNA and RNA transcription. The resultant disintegration of nucleoli and disruption of protein synthesis ultimately causes potentially fatal intestinal, hepatic, and renal tubular necrosis. Intestinal effects may be mediated or enhanced by cyclic heptapeptides (phallotoxins) also present in species containing amatoxins. Amatoxins are rapidly absorbed, metabolized, and excreted in bile and urine. They are not significantly bound to plasma proteins and do not cross the placental barrier. Metabolic activation of amatoxins by hepatic cytochrome $P_{450}$ microsomal enzymes may be involved in the pathogenesis of poisoning. Amatoxins are heat stable and nonvolatile; boiling, cooking, or drying mushrooms containing these toxins does not affect their potency.

*Gyromitrins* are hydrazones whose hydrazine metabolites (e.g., *N*-methyl-*N*-formylhydrazine and *N*-monomethyl-hydrazine) can oxidize hemoglobin, inhibit glutamic acid decarboxylase, and cause fatal hepatitis and, possibly, interstitial nephritis. The oxidization of hemoglobin could potentially cause methemoglobinemia and Heinz body hemolytic anemia. Inhibition of glutamic acid decarboxylase results in decreased γ-aminobutyric acid (GABA) synthesis. Low central nervous system (CNS) levels of this inhibitory neurotransmitter may be responsible for the neurologic toxicity of gyromitrins. Hepatic damage may result from a direct interaction between gyromitrins and mixed function oxidase enzymes.

These toxins are eliminated primarily by hepatic metabolism, with lesser amounts excreted unchanged in the urine. Small amounts also undergo pulmonary excretion. Since gyromitrins are volatile, boiling or drying reduces the toxicity of gyromitrin-containing mushrooms. Such processing does not, however, necessarily render them harmless.

*Orellanine* and *orelline* are bipyridine cyclopeptides that can inhibit renal alkaline phosphatase, decrease adenosine triphosphate production, and cause a tubulointerstitial nephritis. Orelline is a metabolite of orellanine. Their biological disposition is unclear. The concomitant presence of other polypeptides (e.g., cortinarin A and B) may contribute to nephrotoxicity. Heating or drying mushrooms containing these toxins does not reduce their toxicity.

*Coprine* is a glutamine derivative whose metabolite(s) appear to act by inhibiting aldehyde dehydrogenase and dopamine decarboxylase. If ingested with ethanol, mushrooms containing coprine can cause β-adrenergic stimulation similar to that which results from disulfiram-ethanol reactions. Coprine and its metabolites are metabolized by the liver and excreted in urine. These toxins are not destroyed by heat.

*Ibotenic acid* and *muscimol* are isoxazole derivatives that are similar to GABA in structure. They interact with multiple central and peripheral neurotransmitters and neuroreceptors causing hallucinations and manifestations of inhibited cholinergic activity. Mushrooms containing ibotenic acid and muscimol may also contain small amounts of muscarine. Ibotenic acid and its metabolite, muscimol, are eliminated primarily by hepatic metabolism. These toxins and their inactive metabolites are excreted in the urine. Boiling or cooking does not affect the toxicity of mushrooms containing these chemicals, but drying may reduce their potency.

*Muscarine,* an aminofuran alkaloid, acts by stimulating peripheral parasympathetic (cholinergic) neurons. It also may have histamine-releasing or receptor-stimulating activity. Muscarine is eliminated primarily by hepatic metabolism. The parent chemical and its metabolites are excreted in the urine. Muscarine is heat stable and nonvolatile.

*Psilocybin* and *psilocin* are dimethyltryptamines, similar in structure to serotonin. Interactions with CNS neuroreceptors appear to be responsible for their hallucinogenic and sympathomimetic activity. Psilocybin undergoes hepatic metabolism to the more active psilocin. Psilocin is eliminated primarily by metabolism, with small amounts excreted unchanged in the urine. Cooking or drying mushrooms containing these chemicals does not detoxify them.

*Miscellaneous/unidentified* toxins probably act locally on the gastrointestinal tract as mucosal irritants or motility stimulants. Some of these toxins may be inactivated by freezing or cooking.

For most toxins and mushrooms, the minimal dose that will result in human poisoning is unknown. Hence, it is prudent to assume that all intentional ingestions (i.e., mushroom consumption for food or hallucinogenic effects) and all accidental ingestions of more than one mushroom are capable of causing poisoning.

## CLINICAL TOXICITY

Except for mushrooms containing hallucinogens, initial symptoms of poisoning consist of nausea, vomiting, diarrhea, and abdominal cramps regardless of the species ingested. The time of onset and severity of these symptoms and the nature and severity of subsequent toxicity differ from group to group. The severity of poisoning may also reflect differences in the amount of toxin ingested or absorbed, in individual susceptibility, or in toxin metabolism.

*Amatoxin* poisoning has a delayed onset. Nausea, vomiting, thirst, colicky abdominal pain, and profuse diarrhea typically begin abruptly 6 to 24 h (up to 48 h) after the ingestion of mushrooms containing these toxins (Table 174-1). The emesis and diarrhea may be bloody. Gastrointestinal effects tend to be more severe and prolonged than those caused by other groups. Severe dehydration with hypotension, tachycardia, and oliguria can occur. Laboratory findings may include acidosis, hyperamylasemia, hypoglycemia, leukocytosis, increased BUN and creatinine, and abnormalities of serum sodium and potassium due to fluid and electrolyte losses. The hematocrit may decrease as a result of blood loss or increase as a result of hemoconcentration.

Gastrointestinal symptoms may last 12 to 24 h and end with a period of apparent improvement, or they may continue unabated. Adynamic ileus can occur as a consequence of gut mucosal necrosis. One

**Table 174-1.** Classification of Poisonous Mushrooms

| Principal Toxin | Genus (Species)* | Clinical Toxicity† | Onset‡ |
|---|---|---|---|
| Amatoxins | *Amanita* (*bisporigia, ocreata, phalloides, suballiacae, tennifolia, verna, virosa*); *Conocybe* (*filaris*); *Galerina* (*autumnalis, marginata, vererata*); *Lepiota* (*helveola, brunneoincarnata*) | Hepatitis<br>Renal tubular necrosis | Late |
| Gyromitrins | *Gyromitra* (*brunnea, caroliniana, fastigiate, infula, umbigna*); *Paxina* (*involutus*); *Sarcosphaera* (*coronaria*) | Hepatitis<br>CNS depression/stimulation<br>Hemolysis<br>?Methemoglobinemia | Late |
| Orellanine/orelline | *Cortinarius* (*calisteus, cinnamomeus, gentilis, orellanus, rainierensis, semisanguineus, speciosissimus*) | Tubulointerstitial nephritis | Late |
| Coprine | *Clitocybe* (*calvipes*); *Coprinus* (*atramentarius*) | Disulfiram-ethanol-like reaction | Variable |
| Ibotenic acid/muscimol | *Amanita* (*cokeri, cothurna, gemmata, musaria, pantherina*) | Hallucinations<br>Anticholinergic and cholinergic effects | Early |
| Muscarine | *Boletus* (*calopus, luridus, pulcherrimus, satanas*); *Clitocybe* (*cerbissata, dealbata, illudens, and rivulosa*); *Inocybe* (*fatigata, geophylla, lilacina, patuoillardi, purica, rimosus*); *phalotus* (*olearius*) | Cholinergic effects | Early |
| Psilocybin/psilocin | *Conocybe* (*cyanopus*); *Gymmopilus* (*auruginosa, spetabilis, validipes*); *Psilocybe* (*balocystis, caerulescens, cubensis, cyanescens, fimentaria, mexicana, semilanceata, silvatica*); *Strophans* (*coronilla*) | Hallucinations<br>Sympathomimetic effects | Early |
| Miscellaneous/unidentified | *Boletus, Chorophyllum, Entoloma, Gomphius, Hebeloma, Lacterius, Omphalotus, Paxillus, Pholiota, Ramaria, Russula, Tricholoma*, and *Verpa* species | Gastroenteritis | Early |

\* Partial listing (other toxic species may exist).
† Includes gastroenteritis in virtually all cases of mushroom poisoning.
‡ Late indicates effects begin more than 6 h after ingestion, whereas early indicates onset within 3 h of ingestion.

to three days following ingestion, serum aminotransferase levels, bilirubin, and the PT and PTT may begin to rise. Right upper quadrant pain, liver enlargement and tenderness, jaundice, hypoglycemia, metabolic acidosis, hyperammonemia, coagulopathy, cardiomyopathy, asterixis, encephalopathy, seizures, coma, and other features of hepatic failure may ensue. Concomitant renal failure with increasing levels of BUN and creatinine, oliguria, hematuria, and proteinuria may be noted. Kidney dysfunction can occasionally occur without significant hepatotoxicity.

Most patients with amatoxin poisoning recover slowly over a period of 1 or more weeks. Some patients who recover clinically have biochemical evidence of persistent hepatic dysfunction. In severe cases, progressive hepatic failure may end in death (most commonly about 7 days after mushroom ingestion).

*Gyromitrin* poisoning also has a delayed onset. Gastrointestinal symptoms typically begin 6 to 8 h (sometimes as long as 24 h) after the ingestion of certain species (Table 174-1). They tend to be mild to moderate in severity and duration and are often accompanied by agitation, ataxia, hyperreflexia, muscle cramps, vertigo, and weakness. A severe headache is typically present. Gyromitrin poisoning can also occur following the inhalation of vapors during the cooking of mushrooms containing these toxins.

In severe cases, dehydration and biochemical evidence of hepatitis, sometimes progressing to hepatic failure, may ensue. Laboratory findings are similar to those seen in amatoxin poisoning but are usually less pronounced. Additional complications may include hemolysis with anemia and hemoglobinuria, and renal failure. Hypoglycemia and methemoglobinemia have been observed in experimental animal poisoning. In severe cases, recovery often takes several weeks. Fatalities are rare.

*Orellanine* and *orelline* poisoning is even more slow and insidious in onset. Gastrointestinal symptoms are typically mild, transient, and do not occur until 1 to 3 days after the ingestion of mushrooms containing these toxins (Table 174-1). Constipation, rather than diarrhea, is often present. Patients frequently do not seek medical attention until 3 days to 3 weeks after ingestion, when they develop renal toxicity. Anorexia, chills, headache, paresthesias, malaise, night sweats, back pain, polyuria or oliguria, and thirst (often intense and burning)

are the usual presenting complaints. Examination may reveal flank tenderness. Typical laboratory findings include increased BUN and creatinine, albuminuria (sometimes massive), hematuria, leukocyturia, and red cell casts in the urine. Hematuria and leukocyturia can occur without renal failure, and some patients have laboratory evidence of concomitant hepatotoxicity. Renal failure may be permanent and is potentially fatal. In most cases, renal function returns to normal, or near normal, over a period of several weeks to several months.

*Coprine* poisoning occurs only if ethanol is consumed within several hours to several days of the ingestion of certain normally edible mushroom species (Table 174-1). If the interval between mushroom and ethanol ingestion is longer than a few hours, patients may not relate the two events and the cause of symptoms may not be appreciated. Symptoms typically begin within a half hour of ethanol ingestion and last 3 to 6 h. The severity of poisoning appears to correlate directly with the quantity of mushrooms ingested and inversely with the time interval between mushroom and ethanol ingestion.

Gastrointestinal symptoms can occur abruptly and be severe. Other manifestations of the coprine-ethanol reaction include agitation, confusion, diaphoresis, dyspnea, flushed skin, headache, hypotension (supine or orthostatic), chest tightness, palpitations, tachycardia, paresthesias, vertigo, and weakness. Arrhythmias (atrial fibrillation and premature atrial and ventricular beats) have been reported.

*Ibotenic acid* and *muscimol* poisoning is typically associated with the recreational use of certain species of mushrooms (Table 174-1) for their mind-altering effects. Symptoms usually begin 20 min to 2 h following mushroom ingestion. Although vomiting can occur, gastrointestinal effects are often absent. Drowsiness, dizziness, and lethargy may be followed by agitation, ataxia, confusion, delirium, euphoria, hallucinations, and psychosis. Children may present with crying, screaming, or incoherent babbling. Muscle fasciculations, twitching, myoclonic jerking, and hyperreflexia may also be seen. The level of consciousness often fluctuates. Coma and tonic-clonic seizures can occur in severe cases. Hallucinations are characteristically visual (e.g., misperceptions of color and shape) and tend to be illusionary. In addition to neuromuscular findings, anticholinergic effects such as dry skin, fever, mydriasis, myoclonus, hypertension, and tachycardia or cholinergic effects such as miosis, salivation, and bradycardia may present. Except for a headache, which may last several days following acute intoxication, symptoms rarely last more than 12 h.

*Muscarine* poisoning typically begins 15 min to 2 h after the ingestion of mushrooms containing this toxin (Table 174-1). Gastrointestinal symptoms are usually mild to moderate in severity. They are often associated with manifestations of cholinergic hyperactivity such as blurred vision, diaphoresis, headache, lacrimation, miosis, salivation, and urinary frequency. Skin flushing may sometimes be noted. Bradycardia, hypotension, seizures, and wheezing can occur in severe cases. Transient increases in hepatic enzymes have also been reported. Symptoms usually last from 2 to 10 h.

*Psilocin* and *psilocybin* poisoning occur primarily in the setting of the recreational use of certain psychoactive mushroom species (Table 174-1). Symptoms begin 30 to 60 min after ingestion and include ataxia, blurred vision, headache, confusion, dysphoria, hallucinations, incoordination, paresthesias, and weakness. If present, nausea and vomiting are usually mild and transient. Hallucinations are most often visual, but they can also be auditory or tactile. Although psychic effects are usually perceived as pleasant, "bad trips" with aggressive, irrational, and suicidal behavior can occur. Physical manifestations, usually mild, may include hyperreflexia, hypertension or hypotension, mydriasis, and tachycardia or bradycardia. Symptoms rarely last longer than 4 to 6 h following ingestion, but "flashbacks" may occur for months following acute intoxication.

Severe poisoning can result in coma, hyperthermia, seizures, and death. It occurs primarily in children and follows ingestion. Severe poisoning may also occur in adults following the intravenous injection of mushroom extracts. Manifestations of poisoning by this route may include arthralgias, cyanosis, chills, fever, and myalgias. Laboratory findings may include hypoxia, mild methemoglobinemia, and biochemical evidence of hepatorenal dysfunction.

*Miscellaneous/unidentified toxins* are present in a variety of mushrooms (Table 174-1). They cause poisoning of variable duration and severity. Gastrointestinal symptoms may begin 30 min to 6 h after mushroom ingestion and last 4 to 48 h. They are usually mild, but gastrointestinal fluid losses can sometimes lead to dehydration. Bloody diarrhea may occasionally be present. Infrequent complaints include chills, diaphoresis, dyspnea, headache, myalgias, light-headedness, carpopedal spasm, paresthesias, and weakness.

## DIAGNOSTIC EVALUATION

Unless a history of mushroom ingestion is volunteered, there may be nothing to suggest that what first appears to be a self-limited gastrointestinal process such as viral gastroenteritis or food poisoning may progress to a more serious or even fatal illness. Only by routinely asking about mushroom ingestion and including it in the differential diagnosis of "gastroenteritis" can subsequent morbidity and mortality be averted.

If a history of mushroom ingestion is elicited, the time of ingestion, the number of mushrooms and mushroom species that were consumed, who else ate them, and the nature, severity, and time of onset of symptoms should be determined. The clinical course and manifestations of poisoning can be used to presumptively identify the offending toxin. Although gastrointestinal symptoms are nonspecific, the time between mushroom ingestion and their onset depends on the toxin involved and is useful in the differential diagnosis.

An interval of more than 6 h between mushroom ingestion and the onset of symptoms suggests amatoxin, gyromitrin, or orellanine/orelline poisoning; an interval of less than 3 h suggests ibotenic acid/muscimol, muscarine, psilocin/psilocybin, or miscellaneous/unidentified toxin poisoning. A temporal association between the onset of symptoms and ethanol ingestion suggests coprine poisoning. The distinction between early and late onset of symptoms is important because it differentiates mushrooms which are cytotoxic and can cause permanent organ damage with serious or fatal consequences from those which are physiotoxic and cause only transient autonomic and central nervous system dysfunction.

Both the very young and the elderly appear to be more susceptible to fluid and electrolyte disturbances secondary to vomiting and diarrhea than those of intermediate age. Small children also appear to be more sensitive to other effects of ingested toxins, and the elderly are more likely to have underlying health problems which could adversely effect the outcome of poisoning. The method of mushroom preparation sometimes influences the severity of poisoning. Cooking can decrease the toxicity of mushrooms containing gyromitrins, but it can also generate toxic vapors.

The physical exam should initially be directed toward assessing the patient for potential dehydration. Orthostatic vital signs should be routinely measured. The pulse, blood pressure, temperature, pupil size, neuromuscular function, and skin characteristics should also be evaluated for signs of cholinergic, anticholinergic, or sympathetic stimulation. The level of consciousness and mental status should be documented with particular attention to the presence or absence of hallucinations. A general cardiopulmonary exam should be performed. The abdomen should be examined for tenderness and bowel sounds. The presence or absence of jaundice and flank pain should be noted. If signs of peritoneal irritation are present, a diagnosis other than mushroom poisoning should be considered. Any available stool or vomitus should be tested for the presence of occult blood.

In patients with moderate or severe gastrointestinal symptoms or signs of dehydration, routine laboratory tests should include a complete blood count, electrolytes, BUN, creatinine, glucose, and urinalysis. If symptoms began more than 6 h after mushroom ingestion or if ingestion of a cytotoxic species is suspected or confirmed by mushroom identification, a serum amylase level and liver function tests [i.e., alkaline phosphatase, AST(SGOT), ALT(SGPT), bilirubin, PT] should also be obtained. Toxicology screening may be useful to rule out other etiologies of poisoning. Except for psilocin, however, mushroom toxins cannot be identified by routine urine testing. Specific assays can detect other toxins but they are not routinely available. Abdominal x-rays can confirm the diagnosis of an ileus but are not otherwise helpful. Cardiac rhythm analysis by monitor or ECG should be performed in patients with chest pain, hypotension, palpitations, respiratory symptoms, or an abnormal cardiopulmonary finding.

If a sample of the ingested mushroom can be obtained, analysis of the shape, texture, and color of the pileus (cap), gills, stipe (stem), base, and spores can be used to identify its genus and species and hence the offending toxin. The odor, food substrate (e.g., soil, wood, dung, or another mushroom), habitat, geographic location, and the season of harvest are also helpful. It is best to have the mushroom examined by a competent mycologist. Prior arrangements will prevent confusion and costly or even fatal delays when an emergency arises. Mycologists may be located through university biology departments, botanical gardens, mycological societies and clubs, and poison centers. A listing of state mycological societies and color photographs of common poisonous mushrooms (and their spores) may be found in *Poisindex.*

If a mycologist is not physically available to examine the mushroom, the mushroom can be sent to one. When shipping a mushroom, it should first be dried in air, by hot light, hairdryer, or in an oven (microwaves excluded) at 95°C (200°F). It should be shipped in a paper container rather than a plastic one to avoid decomposition. Alternatively, the physician may describe the mushroom to the mycologist or attempt to identify the mushroom utilizing one of the many available field guides.

When a sample of the mushroom is not available, a mycologist may still be be able to identify the species ingested by microscopic examination of spores recovered from the patient's vomitus, gastric aspirate, or stool. Spores may also be found on the gills of a partially eaten mushroom or on the dish from which the mushroom was served. Techniques used for the isolation and staining of spore samples can be found in reference texts. Spores are oval or popcorn-kernel-shaped and are similar in size to red blood cells (8 to 20 μm). The parent mushroom may be identified by its characteristic spore features (e.g., color, size, shape, surface texture, wall thickness, presence or absence of an apical pore).

## GENERAL MANAGEMENT

Treatment begins with supportive care. Airway management, ventilatory support, oxygenation, anticonvulsant therapy for seizures, and correction of hemodynamic instability should be instituted as necessary. Treatment of dehydration should begin with the intravenous administration of isotonic saline. A bolus of glucose should be given to patients with altered mental status, and acid-base and electrolyte abnormalities should be corrected. Except when using atropine for cholinergic poisoning, antiemetics and antispasmodics should be avoided, since such therapy may delay spontaneous evacuation of stool or vomitus and lead to increased toxin absorption.

Attention should then be focused on gastrointestinal decontamination. Activated charcoal (0.5 to 1 g/kg orally or by nasogastric tube) is recommended for all patients. In the absence of spontaneous diarrhea, a cathartic such as sorbitol should be administered along with activated charcoal. Syrup of ipecac can be used for the home treatment of children with accidental ingestions. In addition to a dose of charcoal, whole bowel irrigation (e.g., 0.5 to 2 L/h of a Colyte or Golightly bowel prep solution orally or by nasogastric tube) should also be considered if the ingestion of a cytotoxic species is suspected and treatment can be accomplished within 24 h of ingestion. Multiple-dose activated charcoal therapy (i.e., repeated dosing every 2 to 4 h during the first 48 h after ingestion) may enhance the elimination of these toxins and is also recommended.

Patients with potential amatoxin, gyromitrin, or orellanine/orelline poisoning and those with moderate to severe poisoning caused by other mushroom toxins should be admitted for observation and/or treatment. Other patients can be discharged from the emergency department if they remain or become asymptomatic after a 4- to 6-h period of observation and treatment. Those who are discharged should be instructed to return promptly if symptoms recur. Patients who intentionally ingest hallucinogenic mushrooms should be referred for drug abuse counseling.

## TOXIN-SPECIFIC TREATMENT

A number of toxin elimination measures, metabolic antidotes, and physiologic antagonists have been used in the treatment of specific types of mushroom poisoning. Unfortunately, there are few if any controlled trials documenting the efficacy of these measures. Consultation with a toxicologist or poison center is therefore recommended.

Specific interventions that may be helpful in the treatment of *amatoxin* poisoning include forced diuresis, charcoal hemoperfusion, high-dose penicillin, high-dose cimetidine, liver transplantation, and possibly hyperbaric oxygen therapy, high-dose ascorbic acid, and N-acetylcysteine. Silibinin, aucubin, and kutkin may also be effective. Glucocorticoids and thioctic acid are of no benefit and are no longer recommended.

Forced diuresis and charcoal hemoperfusion may enhance amatoxin elimination. Diuresis (i.e., maintaining a urine output of 2 to 4 mL/kg per hour) using normal saline is likely to be effective only if employed during the first 10 h following ingestion. Hemoperfusion is likely to be effective only if undertaken within 24 h (or possibly 48 h) of ingestion. Whether it offers any advantage over multiple doses of oral charcoal is unknown. Hemoperfusion may also be used supportively (i.e., for the correction of metabolic and neurologic abnormalities associated with severe liver failure). Hemodialysis does not enhance amatoxin elimination, but it can be used as a supportive procedure in patients with renal failure.

Penicillin is thought to act by inhibiting the uptake of amatoxin by hepatocytes. It may also act by sterilizing the gut and inhibiting the bacterial production of GABA, a neurotransmitter thought to be involved in the pathogenesis of hepatic encephalopathy. Recommended doses of penicillin G (benzyl penicillin) range from 0.3 to 1 million units/kg per day (in divided doses) for 2 to 3 days following mushroom ingestion. Seizures are a potential complication of high-dose penicillin therapy. In addition, the commonly available potassium salt contains 1.5 mEq of potassium per million units and high doses may result in hyperkalemia, particularly in patients with renal failure. Hyperbaric oxygen therapy may enhance the efficacy of penicillin and is reasonable to employ as an adjunctive measure if it is readily available.

Large doses of cimetidine prevent amatoxin-induced hepatic damage in experimental animals. Cimetidine appears to act by inhibiting hepatic cytochrome $P_{450}$ enzymes, since other $H_2$ blockers are not as effective. It might be beneficial in humans if given during the first 2 to 3 days after mushroom ingestion. Doses of up to 2 g intravenously every 4 h have been used. High-dose ascorbic acid enhances the efficacy of cimetidine in experimental amatoxin poisoning. Hence, adjunctive therapy with maximal human doses of this vitamin (i.e., 10 to 40 mg/kg per day orally or intravenously in divided doses) might also be helpful.

*N*-Acetylcysteine (Mucomyst) might also be effective in amatoxin poisoning since amatoxin metabolites generated by cytochrome $P_{450}$ enzymes appear to be involved in the pathogenesis of hepatoxicity. Although it is not effective in experimental animals when given in a single dose, a regimen similar to that used in the treatment of human acetaminophen poisoning might be beneficial.

Silibinin, the active component of silymarin, a milk thistle extract, appears to be effective in preventing hepatotoxicity when given intravenously in doses of 20 to 50 mg/kg per day for 2 to 4 days. It is thought to inhibit the uptake of amatoxins by hepatocytes. Silibinin is currently being studied in clinical trials in Europe. In an uncontrolled study, silibinin therapy (along with other modalities) was associated with a three- to fourfold reduction in mortality. Silibinin is not yet available for use in the United States. Dietary preparations of silymarin (sold in health food stores) may also be effective, but the therapeutic oral dose is unknown. Doses of 1.4 to 4.2 g/day have been suggested. Aucubin and kutkin, iridoid glycosides obtained from the plants aucuba japonica and picrorhiza kurroa, may also be effective antidotes, but they have thus far only been studied in animals.

In addition to standard treatments of hepatic failure, liver transplantation has been used with success in patients with severe amatoxin poisoning. It should not be performed prematurely, however, as some patients spontaneously recover despite having marked hepatic dysfunction during the first week after mushroom ingestion.

Specific treatments that may be helpful in patients with *gyromitrin* poisoning include pyridoxine, benzodiazepines, diuresis, blood transfusions, and possibly methylene blue. As in isoniazid poisoning, pyridoxine may reverse the inhibition of glutamic acid decarboxylase by substituting for pyridoxal phosphate, the enzyme's cofactor. It may be effective in reversing neurologic toxicity. The recommended dose is 25 mg/kg, given intravenously over 15 to 30 min. The dose can be repeated up to four times in 24 h if symptoms persist or recur. Higher doses are unlikely to be of additional benefit and may result in pyridoxine toxicity. Benzodiazepines may also be used to control agitation and neuromuscular hyperactivity.

Maintenance of a normal or brisk urine output may enhance hemoglobin excretion and prevent associated renal dysfunction in patients with hemolysis. Red blood cell transfusions might also be necessary. Although probably only a theoretical concern, significant methemoglobinemia (i.e., levels above 30 percent or lower levels associated with hypoxic or ischemic manifestations) could require treatment with intravenous methylene blue (0.1 to 0.2 mL/kg of a 1% solution).

The treatment of *orellanine/orelline* poisoning consists primarily of maintaining fluid and electrolyte homeostasis and temporary or chronic support of renal function using dialysis. Furosemide and other loop diuretics should be avoided as they enhance nephrotoxicity in experimental animals. Steroids have not been shown to be effective in treating nephrotoxicity. Charcoal hemoperfusion may enhance toxin elimination. It is probably most effective if started within 2 days of mushroom ingestion but may be of some benefit up to 1 week after ingestion. Whether hemoperfusion is superior to repeated oral doses of charcoal is unknown.

In patients with *coprine-ethanol reactions,* dopamine or norepinephrine may be required for the treatment of hypotension unresponsive to fluid administration. Pharmacologic therapy may also be required for tachyarrhythmias. Beta blockers are the most theoretically attractive choice, but any antiarrhythmic drug that is appropriate may be used. Myocardial ischemia and infarction should be treated with standard measures.

Patients with *ibotenic acid/muscimol* poisoning may require control of neuromuscular hyperactivity. Benzodiazepines and barbiturates are the preferred agents for treating seizures. Reassurance and a quiet atmosphere may be effective in calming agitated patients. If necessary, restraint should be accomplished by pharmacologic rather than physical measures. Benzodiazepines are preferable to neuroleptic agents since the latter may lower the seizure threshold. Physostigmine may also be used for the management of severe or refractory agitation, but only if ECG analysis reveals sinus tachycardia with normal PR, QRS, and QT intervals and peripheral anticholinergic findings are also present. It is given as a slow intravenous bolus over several minutes in an initial dose of 1 to 2 mg in adults and 0.5 mg in children. The dose may be repeated if the response is incomplete or transient.

Specific treatments that may be helpful in patients with *muscarine* poisoning include atropine, inhaled bronchodilators (i.e., $\beta_2$ agonists), and possibly antihistamines. Atropine is effective in decreasing excessive pharyngeal or pulmonary secretions. It may also be used to treat hypotension unresponsive to fluid administration when it is accompanied by bradycardia. Atropine is also effective in treating gastrointestinal cramps, vomiting, diarrhea, and diaphoresis. However, it should not be used solely for this purpose unless there is a clear history of ingestion of mushrooms containing muscarine, since ibotenic acid/muscimol poisoning may be exacerbated by atropine. The usual dose of atropine is 0.5 to 1.0 mg in adults and 0.01 mg/kg in children, given intravenously. Similar or smaller doses may be repeated as necessary until secretions are controlled or tachycardia develops.

Inhaled bronchodilators (e.g., albuterol, isoetharine, or metaproterenol) may be useful as an adjunctive therapy in patients with wheezing. Antihistamines (both $H_1$ and $H_2$ receptor antagonists) are also of theoretical value in the treatment of effects possibly mediated by histamine (e.g., wheezing, hypotension, and flushing).

The treatment of *psilocin/psilocybin* poisoning includes reassurance, avoidance of unnecessary stimulation, and pharmacologic control of behavioral, physiological, and CNS hyperactivity as described for ibotenic acid/muscimol poisoning. Sedation and therapeutic paralysis as well as physical cooling measures may be necessary for the treatment of hyperthermia.

Supportive therapy is all that is necessary for the treatment of patients poisoned by *miscellaneous/unidentified* mushroom toxins.

## BIBLIOGRAPHY

Bouget J, Bousser J, Pats B, et al: Acute renal failure following collective intoxication by *cortinarius orellanus. Intensive Care Med* 16:506, 1990.

Koppel C: Clinical symptomatology and management of mushroom poisoning. *Toxicon* 31:1513, 1993.

Lampe KF: Differential diagnosis of poisoning by North American mushrooms, with emphasis on *Amanita phalloides*-like intoxication. *Ann Emerg Med* 16:956, 1987.

Lincoff G, Mitchell DH: *Toxic and Hallucinogenic Mushroom Poisoning: A Handbook for Physicians and Mushroom Hunters.* New York, Van Nostrand Reinhold, 1977.

Pinson CW, Daya MR, Benner KG, et al: Liver transplantation for severe *Amanita phalloides* mushroom poisoniing. *Am J Surg* 159:493, 1990.

Rumack BH, Spoerke DG (eds); *Handbook of Mushroom Poisoning; Diagnosis and Treatment,* 2d ed. Boca Raton, FL, CRC Press, 1994.

# 175
# POISONOUS PLANTS

## David C. Michener
## Rodger Keller
## Robert F. Kowalski

Plants have evolved an extraordinarily complex and diverse array of secondary metabolites that are toxic to the animals (especially insects) that feed on them. That some of these compounds are toxic to humans is inconsequential from an evolutionary perspective. The presence and distribution of pyrrolizidine alkaloids, nonprotein amino acids, cyanogenic and cardiac glycosides, glucosinolates, iridoids, sesquiterpene lactones, saponins, sterols (including estrogens and other vertebrate sex hormones; insect moulting hormones), and tannins vary by plant division (phylum), family, genus, and even within an individual plant both by season and by tissue. As a result, reports from the chemical and ecological literature on the presence or distribution of such compounds in roots, foliage, or fruits may be difficult to place in a clinical context. Since toxic compounds are ubiquitous in noncrop plants (an aspect of domestication is selection for palatability), we focus only on those plants that are reported ingestions with emphasis on the subset that are generally considered to be dangerous to humans.

The tables (Tables 175-1 and 175-2) and descriptions are intended only to allow an initial decision whether the plant involved (determined either by samples or from rough narratives) is the plant featured and whether the toxic parts have been encountered. Good color photographs, although no substitute for a knowledgeable consultant, can be found in the books by Graf, Lampe and McCann, and Westbrooks and Preacher cited in the bibliography of this chapter and may help nonbotanists eliminate candidate plants. Scientific names, family names, and toxins are listed to facilitate cross referencing.

A complex array of herbicides, insecticides, fertilizers, fungicides, and phytohormones are often applied to cultivated plants, especially to their leaves. These organics or their "inert" carriers may be the cause of or may confound symptoms.

Table 175-1 lists the "little red berries" most likely to be ingested by children or, from our experience, to be encountered in North America. The most toxic plants are marked (!). Since brightly colored fruits have coevolved with their seed dispersers (primarily birds, occasionally other vertebrates such as turtles), it is noteworthy how few are truly dangerous rather than just unpleasant to humans. *Note that fleshy pulp may be essentially harmless while the seeds, if chewed, may be severely toxic.* This is especially true in *Taxus* and to a lesser extent for many cultivated members of the Rosaceae including apples, apricots, cherries, and pears.

**Table 175-1.** "Little Red Berries" of North America Likely to Be Ingested by Children

| Scientific Name | Common Names | Family | Key* |
|---|---|---|---|
| !*Abrus precatorius* | Rosary pea | Fabaceae | v |
| !*Actaea rubra* | Red baneberry | Ranunculaceae | h |
| *Amelanchier* spp. | Shad. rowan | Rosaceae | s/t |
| *Arisaema triphyllum* | Jack-in-the-pulpit | Araceae | h |
| *Berberis* spp. | Barberries | Berberidaceae | s |
| *Capsicum* spp. | Ornamental peppers | Solanaceae | h |
| *Celastrus scandens* | Bittersweet | Celastraceae | v |
| !*Convallaria majalis* | Lily-of-the-valley | Liliaceae | h |
| *Cornus* spp.† | Dogwoods | Cornaceae | s/t |
| *Cotoneaster* spp.† | Cotoneasters | Rosaceae | s |
| *Crataegus* spp. | Hawthorns | Rosaceae | t |
| !*Daphne mezereum* | Daphne | Thymeliaceae | s |
| *Elaeagnus* spp. | Autumn and Russian olives | Elaeagnaceae | s |
| !*Ilex* spp.† | Hollies | Aquifoliaceae | s/t |
| *Lonicera* spp.† | Honeysuckles | Caprifoliaceae | s/v |
| *Magnolia* spp. | Magnolias | Magnoliaceae | s/t |
| *Malus* spp. | Apples and crabapples | Rosaceae | t |
| *Prunus* spp.† | Bird and wild cherries | Rosaceae | s/t |
| *Pyracantha* | Firethorns | Rosaceae | s |
| *Rhamnus* spp.† | Buckthorns | Rhamnaceae | s/t |
| *Schinus* spp.† | Pepper trees | Anacardiaceae | s/t |
| *Smilacina racemosa* | False Solomon's seal | Liliaceae | h |
| !*Solanum* spp.† | Nightshades | Solanaceae | h/v |
| *Sorbus* spp. | Mountain ashes | Rosaceae | s/t |
| !*Taxus* spp. | Yews | Taxaceae | s/t |
| *Viburnum* spp.† | Viburnums | Caprifoliaceae | s/t |

\* h , herb; s, shrub; t, tree; v, vine; combinations allowed.

† Fruits may also be black, blue, or purple, especially with age.

! Generally considered to be dangerous; see text.

## SPECIFIC TOXIC PLANTS AND MANAGEMENT

Approximately 10 percent of calls to poison control centers concern plants. Fortunately, in most cases, patients are asymptomatic or have a mild gastrointestinal irritation. However, in some cases, plants and plant products can be extremely toxic. When treating patients with plant ingestions, one must remember to treat the patient and not the plant.

The effects seen may be those of pesticides, fertilizers, or adjacent plants, as stated above. The following recommendations for general management of plant ingestions do not include mushroom ingestion or contact dermatitis, which are covered elsewhere in this study guide.

**Table 175-2.** Seasonally Common Houseplants and Decorative Materials

| Scientific Name | Common Names | Family |
|---|---|---|
| THANKSGIVING–NEW YEARS | | |
| *Capsicum annuum* | Ornamental pepper | Solanaceae |
| *Celastrus scandens* | Bittersweet | Celastraceae |
| *Chrysanthemum* spp. | Chrysanthemums | Asteraceae |
| *Euphorbia pulcherrima* | Poinsettia | Euphorbiaceae |
| !*Ilex* spp. | Hollies | Aquifoliaceae |
| *Phoradendron* | Mistletoes | Loranthaceae |
| *Solanum pseudocapsicum* | Jerusalem cherry | Solanaceae |
| EASTER–PASSOVER | | |
| *Crocus* spp. | Crocus | Iridaceae |
| !*Convallaria* spp. | Lily-of-the-valley | Liliaceae |
| *Cyclamen* spp. | Florists' cyclamen | Primulaceae |
| *Hyacinthus* spp. | Hyacinths | Liliaceae |
| *Lilium* spp. | Lilies | Liliaceae |
| *Narcissus* spp. | Daffodils | Liliaceae |
| *Tulipa* spp. | Tulips | Liliaceae |

! Generally considered to be dangerous; see text.

## Initial Management

Initial management of plant ingestions is similar to that of other poisonings. However, emergency physicians should be aware that there are a few specific plant ingestions in which standard detoxification procedures are not indicated.

Forced emesis has been questioned, in the recent literature, as effective in the management of poisonings. This may also be true for plant ingestions because the volume of the plant material ingested is almost always small and there is usually a delay in seeking medical attention. In two specific plant ingestions, use of ipecac is contraindicated:

1. The jequirity bean (*Abrus precatorius*), which is strongly alkaline and may cause esophageal and pharyngeal burns similar to caustics
2. The poison hemlocks (*Conium* or *Circuta* species), which may cause seizures

Gastric lavage has little benefit except possibly for large ingestions, and most plant ingestions are of small quantities. The use of lavage depends on clinical judgment. Activated charcoal with a cathartic in standard doses may be the safest detoxificant, especially if the plant cannot be identified.

Hypotension should be treated with intravenous fluids and the patient placed in the Trendelenburg position. In severe cases, vasopressors may be needed.

If seizures ensue, standard management with diazepam is indicated. If seizures are not controlled, phenytoin or phenobarbital may be used.

Hallucinations may be caused by ingestion of certain plant parts (i.e., morning glory seeds, Convolvulus, and Ipomea). Patients may also exhibit nicotinic, cholinergic, or anticholinergic symptoms for which treatment is specific. In most cases, a calm, quiet environment with friends or family is helpful.

If the patient is uncontrollable and dangerous to himself or herself or others, the use of diazepam for sedation is indicated.

Prolonged vomiting and diarrhea secondary to plant ingestions may require intravenous fluids and monitoring of electrolytes.

Based on the patient's symptoms in most cases, a period of observation in the emergency department is the best diagnostic procedure. The use of the laboratory for identification in plant ingestions is usually not helpful. However, if an emergency department has access to consultation with botanical experts, macro- and microscopic examination of plant products from gastric contents may be helpful in identification. Specific management for every plant ingestion is beyond the scope of this chapter. There are several references available that every emergency department should have access to.

## COMMONLY INGESTED PLANTS, EFFECTS, AND MANAGEMENT

### Abrus precatorius

There is usually a delay in symptoms from hours to a few days, depending on the amount ingested or chewed. There may be nausea, vomiting, diarrhea, and occasionally ulcerations in the pharynx, esophagus, stomach, and ileum. An ileus may develop. There also may be massive fluid with electrolyte loss.

### Management

Treatment is mainly supportive with fluid and electrolyte replacement. However, ingestion of one chewed seed may be fatal even with intensive care.

### Actaea

There is hypersalivation with blisters and ulcers to the oropharynx. Bloody vomiting and diarrhea occur with abdominal pain secondary to cramping. Renal injury occurs, starting with polyuria, dysuria, and hematuria, and followed by oliguria. Central nervous system symptoms such as dizziness, confusion, and syncope with seizures may occur 30 min after ingestion. Hallucinations were reported in one case.

### Management

Lavage should be instituted if a large amount has been ingested, followed by the use of a demulcent (egg white in milk), and monitoring of fluids, electrolytes, and renal function with appropriate replacement.

### Aloe

A marked catharsis occurs 6 to 12 h after ingestion. Alkaline urine may turn red. Large doses may cause nephritis.

### Management

Fluids may be necessary. Otherwise, no therapy is usually required. Symptomatic treatment of pain may be instituted.

### Capsicum

Children may experience painful, but harmless, irritation to the oropharynx. Exposure to skin may cause erythema, but not blistering.

### Management

No therapy is usually required. Symptomatic treatment of pain may be instituted.

### Conium

This is similar to nicotine poisoning. There is an onset of irritation to the oropharynx with nausea, salivation, and vomiting. Headache, thirst, diaphoresis, mydriasis and light-headedness may occur. Severe cases may have seizures, coma, and death, secondary to pulmonary failure.

### Management

Treatment is symptomatic with administration of activated charcoal slurry after vomiting ceases.

### Lily of the Valley (*Convallaria*)

Oropharyngeal pain, nausea, vomiting, diarrhea, abdominal pain, and cramping may develop. Digitalis-type toxicity depends upon the amount ingested and may take hours to express itself. Toxic effects are usually conduction defects, sinus bradycardia, and hyperkalemia. Arrhythmias are uncommon, except for escape beats.

### Management

Standard detoxification procedures may be performed. One should monitor electrocardiogram and serum potassium. Atropine or cardiac pacing may be required for conduction defects. If rhythm disturbances ensue, phenytoin is the drug of choice. Hemodialysis and forced diuresis are not helpful.

### Daphne

Ingestion produces blistering and swelling of the entire oropharynx with salivation and dysphagia. Other later symptoms include thirst, vomiting, bloody diarrhea, and abdominal pain. Renal damage, hypovolemia, and electrolyte imbalance may occur.

### Management

This ingestion is potentially lethal. Airway must be maintained along with monitoring fluid and electrolytes. Symptoms may last for days.

### Datura

Ingestion may cause anticholinergic symptoms, including dry mouth, mydriasis, erythema, tachycardia, delirium, hallucinations, fever, hypertension, decrease in peristalsis, and urinary retention.

### Management

As for anticholinergic poisoning.

### Dieffenbachia

Mastication causes sudden, severe pain. It is occasionally followed by swelling of the oropharynx and bullae formation. The name "dumbcane" came about because in severe cases, speech is affected. Swallowing of the plant causes laryngeal edema, but this is not common because severe pain usually prevents swallowing. The swelling and pain may last for days and cause necrosis of the oral mucosa.

### Management

The swelling and pain in the oropharynx resolve over time without intervention. Cool oral fluids may give some symptomatic relief. Judicious use of analgesics may be indicated. Systemic poisoning is not produced by the insoluble oxalates in these plants.

### Euphorbia

Contact dermatitis may occur and may be corrosive. Conjunctivitis may occur with contamination to the eyes. Vomiting may follow after ingestion.

### Management

If vomiting is present, patients should have electrolytes monitored and appropriate intravenous fluids given.

### *Ilex*

Nausea, protracted vomiting, and occasional diarrhea occur after ingestion of berries.

### Management

This includes monitoring of electrolytes and use of intravenous fluids to prevent dehydration. This is especially important in children.

### *Laportea* and *Urtica*

These nettles rapidly cause an intensive burning sensation when contacted; they are unlikely to be held long enough to be eaten.

### Management

Standard treatment with antihistamines is usually helpful.

### *Lonicera*

The old European literature reports of deaths and toxicity due to *Lonicera* may be in error; the fruits are generally considered innocuous in the United States.

### *Nerium oleander*

See *Convallaria.*

### *Philodendron*

See *Dieffenbachia.*

### *Phytolacca*

Two to 3 h after ingestion, nausea, abdominal cramping, vomiting, diaphoresis, and diarrhea develop. These symptoms may last for 48 h.

### Management

This includes monitoring of electrolytes with appropriate replacement. Paint may also be treated.

### *Rhododendron*

Severe intoxications have occurred from chewing leaves and from eating honey made from rhododendron nectar. Upon ingestion, there is an initial burning sensation in the oropharynx. This is followed hours later by salivation, vomiting, diarrhea, and paresthesias. Other complaints include cephalgia, weakness, and decreased vision. In severe cases, bradycardia may develop followed by hypotension, coma, and seizures, leading to an increase in morbidity and mortality.

### Management

Respiratory and fluid therapy are essential. If bradycardia ensues, atropine may be indicated. Hypotension is treated by intravenous fluids, Trendelenburg positioning, and ephedrine, if necessary. Cardiac telemetry is required. Complete recovery can be expected in 24 h.

### *Ricinus*

Nausea, vomiting, and diarrhea ensue several hours after ingestion. Other symptoms are the result of fluid and electrolyte loss and bowel dysfunction.

### Management

Fluid and electrolyte replacement are indicated. Parenteral alimentation may be necessary in severe cases. Fatalities have been recorded with the ingestion of two to six seeds.

### *Solanum*

This is rarely toxic in adults. However, fatal ingestions have occurred in children. Gastrointestinal upset, oropharyngeal irritation, fever, and diarrhea occur after ingestion. The clinical picture is similar to bacterial gastroenteritis. After ingestion, there is a latent period of several hours, and the symptoms may last for days.

### Management

Supportive care with monitoring of fluids and electrolytes is indicated.

### *Taxus*

Within 1 h after ingestion, light-headedness, dry oropharynx, mydriasis, abdominal cramping, salivation, and vomiting may occur. Facial pallor, circumoral cyanosis, and a rash may appear. Generalized weakness followed by coma is seen in severe intoxications. Cardiopulmonary symptoms include bradycardia, hypotension, dysrhythmias, and dyspnea. Death is secondary to cardiac or respiratory failure. Anaphylaxis may occur from chewing the needles.

### Management

Oral administration of activated charcoal is indicated. Cardiac monitoring is necessary. A cardiac pacemaker and appropriate respiratory therapy may be indicated. Standard treatment for anaphylaxis, if present, with epinephrine fluids and respiratory support is indicated.

## DISCHARGE INSTRUCTIONS

Discharge instructions for general plant ingestions should include returning to seek medical care for:

1. Delayed vomiting 8 to 24 h after ingestion
2. Abdominal pain
3. Diarrhea
4. Hallucinations or bizarre behavior

## DESCRIPTIONS OF COMMONLY INGESTED PLANTS

*Abrus precatorius* **L.** Common names: Coral-bead, crabs'-eye, jequerity, licorice vine, love bean, prayer bean, precatory bean, rosary pea, weather vine. Family: Leguminosae (Fabaceae). Note: Dangerous with known fatalities; ingestion and chewing of one of these brightly colored beans exceeds lethal dose for adults; toxin soluble in saliva has killed children. Seeds resemble small sugar candies and are used in native American necklaces and rosaries purchased by unsuspecting tourists. Toxins: Abrin, one of the most lethal toxins known. Presence: Seeds; fatality in children known from chewing seeds without swallowing seeds. Grows: Outdoors in tropical United States (including Hawaii). Description: Vine to 6 m spread, leaves small, alternate, pinnate; flowers pealike, rose, purple, or white; seeds rather uniform in size, about 7 mm (5 to 10 mm) long, shiny, two-thirds orange-red and one-third black, seed attachment scar in the black zone (colors fade with age); seeds produced in papery, hairy pods.

*Actaea rubra* **(Ait.) Willd.,** *Actaea pachypoda* **Ell.** Common names: baneberry, doll's eyes, necklaceweed, red baneberry. Family: Ranunculaceae. Note: Generally considered dangerous. Toxins: Protoanemonin; destroyed by drying or cooking. Presence: In berries and roots; berries only likely to be ingested by children. Grows: Forested, temperate North America, unusual but present in wildflower gardens, otherwise rarely grown. Description: Perennial from stout root; leaves compound through multiple divisions; leaflets cleft and toothed; fruits berry-like, red (white with black spot in *Actaea pachypoda*) usually with 5 to 15 seeds.

*Aloe barbadensis* **Mill.** Common names: aloe vera, Barbados aloe, burn plant, curacoe, medicinal aloe. Family: Liliaceae. Toxins: Some of the more than 200 species of *Aloe* contain unspecified cathartic and irritating compounds. Presence: leaves. Grows: Common houseplant in northern regions, grown outdoors in subtropical and desert regions. Description: Clump-forming succulent; leaves yellow-green, may be speckled when young, to 30 to 50 cm long at maturity; flowers yellowish on stalks to 1 m long.

***Capsicum annuum* L.** Common names: pepper (banana, bell, green, hot, ornamental, red, sweet, etc.). Family: Solanaceae. Note: Generally considered nontoxic (common green peppers of grocery stores), but some ornamental and "hot" cultivars may cause severe irritation if ingested or contacted. Toxins: Capsicine. Presence: fruits and seeds. Grows: Common vegetable and house plants cultivated for both edible and ornamental fruits. Description: perennial herb (treated as an annual in cold climates) with alternate, simple leaves; fruits inflated, green, red, yellow, purple, or white.

***Chlorophytum comosum* (Thunb.) Jacques.** Common names: Ribbon plant, spider plant, walking plant. Family: Liliaceae. Note: Generally considered nontoxic but is among the 25 most frequently ingested houseplants. Grows: Common houseplant in north, used as a ground cover in shade in tropics. Description: Clump-forming perennial with broad grassy leaves (these often variegated with a white to yellow-green stripe); in pot culture often with pendant young plants on the ends of flexible stems; flowers small, white to yellow on long scapes.

***Conium maculatum* L.** Common names: fool's parsley, poison hemlock, poison parsley, spotted hemlock, spotted parsley, winter fern. Family: Apiaceae (Umbelliferae). Note: Dangerous with known fatalities. Toxins: Alkaloids, especially coniine and derivatives. Presence: Whole plant; roots and seeds most likely ingested by adults mistaking it for edible wild carrots or anise seed. Grows: An escaped weed of waste and moist places throughout temperate North America. Description: Large, branching biennial herb to more than 2 m tall from solid taproot; stems hollow; leaves pinnately and repeatedly compound; flowers small, white, in clusters.

***Convallaria majalis* L.** Common names: Lily-of-the-valley. Family: Liliaceae. Note: Generally considered dangerous. Toxins: Cardiac glycosides. Presence: Throughout plant; also water in vases when these are used as cut flowers. Outdoors the berries and indoors the vase water have been ingested by children. Grows: Cultivated garden perennial throughout temperate North America; often forced in pots indoors for flowers. Description: Low perennial herb from creeping underground rootstock, leaves usually two or three, oblong, entire; flowers white, bell-like, fragrant, pendant from scape; fruits orange to red pulpy berries with few seeds.

***Crassula argentea* (Thunb.).** Common names: Chinese rubber plant, dollar plant, jade plant, jade tree. Family: Crassulaceae. Note: Generally considered nontoxic; leaves commonly ingested by children. Grows: Common houseplant, used outdoors in subtropics. Description: Sturdy succulent-stemmed perennial, ultimately a shrub, with thick, oval, succulent leaves that may be striped with red or white; flowers small, white, star-shaped, in many-flowered clusters.

***Daphne mezerium* L.** Common names: Daphne. Family: Thymeliaceae. Note: Dangerous; 10 to 12 fruits can be lethal for children; 30 percent mortality reported for ingestions. Toxins: Daphnetoxin and mezerein. Presence: All parts; ingestion of fruits is the rare but expected exposure. Grows: Uncommon ornamental shrub of temperate North America; grown for its intensely fragrant flowers. Description: Small shrubs often less than 1 m tall with relatively thick stems; leaves alternate and simple, elliptical; flowers white to purple, flowering before leaves are present; fruits bright red to yellow.

***Datura* species (including *Brugmansia* sp.).** Common names: angel's trumpet, horn-of-plenty, Indian apple, Jimson weed, thorn apple. Family: Solanaceae. Note: Dangerous, potentially lethal; cultivated for millenia for ornament and hallucinogens. Toxins: Alkaloids; atropine, hyoscyamine. Presence: All parts including nectar; leaves smoked or seeds eaten by adults seeking a "high." Grows:

These are occasionally garden plants of temperate zone, also as escaped weeds of subtropical and tropical states. Description: Rank, short-lived perennials and annuals with coarse, soft, alternate leaves foul-smelling when crushed; flowers medium to large funnels, white to yellow usually extremely fragrant lasting one to a few days; fruits a spiny (sometimes smooth) pepper-like pod.

***Dieffenbachia* species (over 30).** Common names: dumbcane, dumb plant, mother-in-law's tongue. Family: Araceae. Note: Members of the Araceae possess raphides: numerous needle-shaped crystals of calcium oxalate that are physically ejected by turgor pressure when the cell containing them is disturbed. The immediate and intense reaction is due to this physical assault. If leaves are chewed, the swelling may become so intense the individual cannot speak and is rendered "dumb." Toxins: Calcium oxalate crystals; proteolytic enzymes also reported to be present. Presence: Primarily leaves, ingested by both children and adults; stems equally noxious if chewed. Grows: One of the most common house and office plants; common outdoors in tropical climates. Description: Long-lived erect perennial herbs to shrubs over 1 m tall with large entire leaves; numerous cultivars with variegated leaves; flowers and fruits uncommon in indoor culture.

***Euphorbia pulcherrima* Willd.** Common names: Christmas flower, poinsettia. Family: Euphorbiaceae. Notes: Foliage and latex of this species evidently harmless but cause for numerous inquiries; other species (2000 are known) can cause dermatitis. Grows: Common houseplant forced for Christmas displays; used outdoors in tropical states. Description: Shrub to 3 m tall with alternate, toothed leaves; floral bracts red, pink, orange, or white (commonly mistaken for petals); flowers insignificant, in a complex structure.

***Ficus* species (over 800 species).** Common names: banyan, botree, climbing figs, figs, rubber tree, weeping fig. Family: Moraceae. Notes: One of the top 25 causes of ingestion inquiries; most generally considered to be nontoxic. Grows: Common house and office shrubs and trees; very common outdoors in tropical regions. Description: Trees and shrubs with often thick, evergreen leaves; leaf size and lobing quite variable between species.

***Ilex* species (400 species).** Common names: American holly, cassena, dahoon, English holly, holly, inkberry, possum haw, winterberry, yaupon. Family: Aquifoliaceae. Note: Dangerous: 20 to 30 berries can be fatal to children; native American Indians used infusions of *Ilex vomitoria* berries to promote vomiting. Toxins: Uncertain; saponins in some cases. Presence: Berries only; leaves are used as a tea substitute. Grows: Native or cultivated plants throughout North America except in very arid or northern climates. Description: Trees and shrubs with often prickly evergreen leaves (some species with simple deciduous or evergreen leaves); fruits bright red, yellow, or black. Common Christmas decoration.

***Laportea* and *Urtica* species.** Common names: bull nettle, stinging nettle, wood nettle. Family: Urticaceae. Toxins: histamines(?). Presence: Leaves and stems. Grows: Moist woods and fields in temperate North America. Description: Short to tall perennial herbs; leaves alternate, somewhat heart-shaped (*Laportea*) or elongate (*Urtica*), covered with short, stiff, stinging glandular hairs; flowers minute, clustered near leaf bases.

***Lonicera* species (200 species).** Common names: honeysuckle, woodbine. Family: Caprifoliaceae. Generally considered nontoxic. Grows: Common ornamental and native shrubs and vines found throughout temperate North America; shrubs especially common in colder regions. Description: Shrubs and vines with opposite and usually entire leaves; flowers white, cream, yellow, or red; fruits paired, red (rarely yellow or blue), often translucent.

***Nerium oleander* L.** Common names: oleander, rose bay. Family: Apocynaceae. Note: Dangerous with known fatalities; all plant parts, smoke from plants, vase water from cut flowers. Notorious for poisoning food if stems used to roast hot dogs, marshmallows, etc. Toxins: Cardioactive glycosides. Presence: Entire plant. Grows: Subtropical to tropical states; grown as a tub or garden room plant in colder climates. Very common highway planting in central and southern California. Description: Large shrub to over 5 m; leaves narrow, opposite (or often in threes), evergreen; flowers in terminal clusters, white, yellow, red, or purple.

***Philodendron* species (275 species).** Common names: Philodendron. Family: Araceae. Note: The most common houseplant and leading cause of infant exposures due to leaf ingestion; see *Dieffenbachia*. Description: Perennial tropical vines tolerant of low light levels (as homes and offices); leaves heart-shaped to oval, thick, evergreen; flowers and fruits uncommon in cultivation.

***Phytolacca americana* L.** Common names: inkberry, phytolacca, pigeonberry, poke, pokeweed, salat. Family: Phytolaccaceae. Toxins: Triterpenes. Presence: Roots, leaves, and berries; however, cooked roots, greens, and berries (for pies) are featured in some Appalachian and Southern recipes; commercially canned greens are marketed as "salat"; adult poisonings result from improper cooking of fresh roots or use of raw greens. Grows: Common weed of disturbed places and fencerows in eastern North America. Description: Rank perennial from fleshy rootstock growing to over 3 m tall (often mistaken for a shrub); leaves alternate, elliptical, often with purplish tinge; berries succulent, bright purplish-black with intense purplish-red stain.

***Pyracantha* species (10 species).** Common names: firethorn, pyracantha. Family: Rosaceae. Note: Generally considered nontoxic but one of 25 most commonly ingested berries. Grows: Ornamental shrub throughout temperate North America. Description: Multiple trunked thorny shrub to over 3 m tall, leaves alternate, linear to elliptical, deciduous to semievergreen (depending on climate); fruits orange to red, shaped like miniature apples.

***Rhododendron* species (over 500 species).** Common names: azalea, rhododendron. Family: Ericaceae. Toxins: Andromedotoxins. Presence: Leaves, flowers, and their honey; children known to chew leaves; adults may experiment with flowers in foods. Grows: Common ornamental and native shrubs in temperate North America except for the Great Plains and arid Southwest. Common houseplants. Description: Evergreen to deciduous shrubs with simple, alternate and often glossy leaves; flowers bellshaped to flaring, in most colors but blue.

*Rhus.* See *Toxicodendron.*

***Ricinus communis* L.** Common names: castor bean, castor-oil plant. Family: Euphorbiaceae. Note: Dangerous with known fatalities. Toxins: Ricin, one of the most toxic compounds known. Seeds used in necklaces in tropical America and purchased by unsuspecting tourists. Presence: Concentrated in seeds but present in most of plant. Grows: Cultivated throughout North America. Description: Rank annual to 4 m, widely grown both as an ornamental and for the oil extracted from the seeds; variable in size and coloration (dull green to bronze/red), colors brightest in new growth; leaves large, star-shaped; flowers in upper leaf axils, small; seed pods usually brightly colored, densely hairy to prickly, borne in tight clusters; seeds quite variable, oval with a white to gray nodule at the smaller end; seed coloration intricately marbled or striped, silver, gold, brown, and black.

***Schefflera* species (including *Brassaia*).** Common names: Australian umbrella tree, dwarf schefflera, umbrella tree. Family: Araliaceae. Notes: Generally considered nontoxic but a leading cause of ingestion inquiries. Grows: Common house and office plant; used outdoors in subtropics. Description: Shrubs to trees with shiny, dull to dark green, alternate, palmately compound leaves (leaflets arranged in a circle on a common leaf stalk).

***Solanum* species.** Common names: deadly nightshade, eggplant, Jerusalem cherry, nightshade, potato, woody nightshade. Family: Solanaceae. Note: Some species dangerous and potentially lethal; over 2000 species of mostly tropical herbs, shrubs, small trees, and vines and thus extremely variable. Includes the potato and eggplant as well as attractive houseplants and toxic weeds; the foliage is often malodorous when crushed; the fruits of some species are frequently ingested by children. Toxins: Solanine, glycoalkaloids. Presence: Foliage, fruits (especially immature), green skins of potatoes. Grows: Common in gardens and as weeds. Descriptions: (1) *S. dulcamara* L., deadly nightshade. Perennial weedy vine to 5 m; leaves alternate, lobed or divided, hairy; flowers star-shaped, purple; fruits red, produced in clusters, egg-shaped, about 1 cm long. (2) *S. nigrum* L., black nightshade. Low spreading annual; leaves glossy, shallowly lobed to entire; flowers white, star-shaped arising from leaf axils; fruits green becoming black. Cultivated forms as "garden huckleberry" leaves are edible when cooked and fruits when ripe; wild types reportedly toxic. (3) *S. pseudocapsicum* L., Jerusalem cherry. Unlike the previous two species, this is most commonly encountered as a winter houseplant and grown outdoors in subtropics. Shrub to 1.5 m, pot plant often less than 50 cm; leaves small, oblong, dull green; flowers small, star-shaped, white; fruits orange-red about 1.5 cm long, spherical.

***Taxus* species (10 species).** Common names: Yew. Family: Taxaceae. Note: Dangerous with known fatalities especially if ingestion of "berries" (actually a modified cone structure) is accompanied by chewing of seeds. Toxins: Taxine alkaloids. Presence: Foliage and seeds (but not the fleshy red aril = "berry" pulp). Grows: Common ornamentals and one uncommon native in temperate North America often clipped for hedges, foundation plantings, etc. Description: Shrubs to small trees with flat dark-green evergreen needles; cones highly modified and commonly called "berries" but technically a fleshy red aril surrounding the naked seed.

## BIBLIOGRAPHY

Andrews J: *Peppers. The Domesticated Capsicums.* Austin, TX: University of Texas Press, 1984.

Bailey Hortorium staff: *Hortus Third.* New York: Macmillan, 1976.

Graf AB: *Exotica,* series 4 (2 vols). East Rutherford, NJ: Roehrs, 1982.

Harborne JB: *Introduction to Ecological Biochemistry,* 2d ed. London, Academic, 1982.

Keeler RF, Tu AT (eds): *Handbook of Natural Toxins, Plant and Fungal Toxins.* New York, Dekker, vol 1, 1983.

Kingsbury JM: The evolutionary and ecological significance of plant toxins. In Keeler RF, Tu AT: *Handbook of Natural Toxins, Plant and Fungal Toxins.* New York, Dekker, vol 1, pp 675–706, 1983.

Lampe KF, McCann MA: *AMA Handbook of Poisonous and Injurious Plants.* Chicago: American Medical Association, 1985.

Levey CK, Primack PB: *A Field Guide to Poisonous Plants and Mushrooms of North America.* Brattleboro, VT: Stephen Green, 1984.

Litovitz TL, Schmitz BF, Holm KC: 1988 Annual Report of the American Association of Poison Control Centers National Data Collections System. *Am J Emerg Med* 7:495, 1988.

Rumack BH (ed): *Poisonindex.* Micromedex, Inc., vol 67, 1991.

Smith PM: *The Chemotaxonomy of Plants.* New York: Elsevier, 1976.

Westbrooks RG, Preacher JW: *Poisonous Plants of Eastern North America.* Columbia, SC: University of South Carolina Press, 1986.

Willis JC, Shaw HKA: *A Dictionary of the Flowering Plants and Ferns,* 8th ed. Cambridge: Cambridge University Press, 1973.

# Endocrine Emergencies

## 176
# HYPOGLYCEMIA
### Gene Ragland

Glucose is the main energy source of the brain, and prolonged, severe hypoglycemia has been reported to cause brain damage and death. The blood glucose level at which hypoglycemia occurs is variable but has been generally accepted as <50 mg/dL. Hypoglycemia occurs most often in insulin-dependent diabetics as a complication of insulin therapy and accounts for 3 to 7 percent of deaths in patients with insulin-dependent diabetes mellitus. Treatment includes the administration of glucose, in most instances, and the outcome is usually favorable. Hypoglycemia in childhood is discussed in Chap. 39.

## CNS GLUCOSE DEPRIVATION

The central nervous system (CNS) depends upon glucose as its sole source of energy, except under conditions of prolonged starvation, when it can utilize ketones to meet energy needs. Hypoglycemia can be defined as a fall in blood glucose concentration to a level that elicits symptoms due to glucose deprivation in the CNS. The symptoms of hypoglycemia are therefore due to CNS dysfunction. It has been hypothesized that glucopenia within the CNS is sensed by a glucoregulatory center located in the hypothalamus. When CNS glucose concentration falls below a critical level, the autonomic centers in the hypothalamus are triggered producing stimulation of various end organs supplied by the peripheral autonomic innervation and resulting in the secretion of epinephrine.

A subset of hypoglycemia symptoms is therefore due to release of the counterregulatory hormone epinephrine via this mechanism and are termed *autonomic* or sympathomimetic symptoms. The most common autonomic symptoms are sweating, trembling, warmness, anxiety and nausea.

CNS glucose deprivation also produces certain symptoms through a direct effect on the brain. This subset of symptoms is termed *neuroglycopenic* and consists of dizziness, confusion, tiredness, difficulty speaking, headache and inability to concentrate. Coma is the end expression of neuroglycopenic symptoms.

Additional hypoglycemia symptoms do occur that overlap these two categories and cannot be attributed to autonomic or neuroglycopenic mechanisms per se. These include drowsiness, weakness, hunger and blurred vision.

The actual level of blood glucose that causes CNS deprivation and produces symptoms is highly individual. The glucose level may be influenced by factors such as age, sex, weight, dietary history, physical activity, emotion, and coexisting disease. Many reports exist of asymptomatic individuals with plasma glucose levels of 35 mg/dL or lower and of individuals who are symptomatic with glucose levels in the "normal" range. The actual value of plasma glucose that defines hypoglycemia is somewhat arbitrary. The clinical state of the patient must be correlated with the glucose determination.

## GLUCOSE HOMEOSTASIS

Glucose homeostasis in humans involves a complex, dynamic synchronized interaction of neural and hormonal factors. The primary glucoregulatory organs are the liver, the pancreas, the adrenal glands, and the pituitary gland, and glucose homeostasis is maintained by the interaction of insulin, glucagon, catecholamines, glucocorticoids, and growth hormone from these organs.

Recent experimental studies have demonstrated that among the counterregulatory hormones, glucagon and epinephrine are of special importance. They are the only counterregulatory hormones capable of stimulating hepatic glucose production within minutes. Their long-term action, beyond 1–2 h, is predominately through their effect on gluconeogenesis. In contrast to glucagon and epinephrine, catecholamine and growth hormone responses to hypoglycemia are thought to be of minor importance.

This hormonal interaction is largely determined by glucose intake and varies in the fed and the fasting state. During the fed state, glucose intake stimulates the release of insulin, which initiates tissue uptake and storage of fuels. During fasting, low insulin levels initiate the mobilization of stored fuels from tissue sources.

The fed state begins with the ingestion of food and extends for 2 to 3 h. The fasting state begins 3 to 4 h after eating. Because of the human's continuous energy needs but intermittent food intake, fuel for use between feedings and during fasting must be stored. The major forms of stored fuel are glycogen in the liver, triglycerides in adipose tissue, and protein in muscle.

Following food intake and absorption from the gut, glucose stimulates the release of insulin from pancreatic β cells. Insulin promotes the uptake of glucose by the liver; the glucose is converted to glycogen and stored in that form. Insulin also acts on the liver to decrease glucose output by inhibiting glycogenolysis (breakdown of glycogen to glucose) and gluconeogenesis (formation of glucose from precursors). Insulin promotes the storage of other energy sources by restraining lipolysis and enhancing lipogenesis in adipose cells and by promoting the uptake of amino acids into muscle protein and inhibiting proteolysis.

In the fasting state, the most readily available source of glucose is hepatic glycogen, which is utilized first. Hepatic glycogenolysis is enzyme-mediated and is stimulated by glucagon and catecholamines. This glycogen reserve is depleted in 24 to 48 h, and other fuel stores must be mobilized if fasting is prolonged. As hepatic glycogen stores are exhausted, blood glucose and plasma insulin levels decrease. The inhibitory action of insulin on lipolysis and proteolysis is removed, and alternative fuel stores can be mobilized and utilized.

During fasting, after several hours' worth of liver glycogen has been utilized, gluconeogenesis becomes the primary source of blood glucose needed for brain metabolism. Gluconeogenesis occurs primarily in the liver. Amino acids, principally alanine, are mobilized from the muscles via proteolysis. This process is facilitated by low insulin levels and mediated by glucocorticoids from the adrenal glands. Glucagon aids the conversion of amino acids to glucose in the liver. Lactate, from recycled glucose, and glycerol, from fat breakdown, can also be transformed to glucose but are minor sources of energy. During nonprolonged overnight fasting, 90 percent of gluconeogenesis occurs via proteolysis and conversion of amino acids to glucose. In starvation states, the kidneys play an important role in gluconeogenesis.

Fat stores are a major source of energy. Fat is stored as triglycerides (free fatty acids plus glycerol), and this process is promoted by insulin. Lipolysis can occur with low insulin levels and is enhanced by epinephrine and growth hormone. When triglycerides are broken down, free fatty acids (FFA) and glycerol are released. Most tissues, except brain and formed blood elements, can utilize FFA as a source of energy. This mechanism allows the body to conserve glucose for use in the CNS and to spare protein from breakdown for conversion to glucose. Additionally, the released glycerol can be converted to glucose in the liver.

In brief summary, glucose homeostasis involves a complex interaction between insulin and the counterregulatory hormones glucagon, catecholamines, glucocorticoids, and growth hormone. The action of insulin depends upon its concentration, which is determined by the level of blood glucose through a sensitive feedback loop. In the fed state, insulin acts to convert glucose to stored energy and inhibits the release of other fuel stores. The glucose concentration during the transition from a fed to a fasting state depends upon the relative balance between glucose use and glucose production. The CNS is the primary consumer of glucose. The production of glucose during a brief fast occurs through glycogenolysis. When the fast is more than a few hours, such as overnight, gluconeogenesis is the primary mechanism responsible for glucose production. Hypoglycemia may result from disease of any of the glucoregulatory organs or as a breakdown of normal glucose homeostasis.

## PATHOPHYSIOLOGY

Hypoglycemia has been classified in a variety of ways. Table 176-1 lists the common causes of hypoglycemia seen in the emergency department and divides these into spontaneous and induced causes. This classification is arbitrary, and overlap occurs.

### Spontaneous Hypoglycemia

#### Fed Hypoglycemia

Hypoglycemia occurring during the fed state has also been termed *reactive* and *postprandial hypoglycemia*. Fed hypoglycemias are characterized by normal fasting serum glucose levels with a decline to hypoglycemic levels within 6 h of a glucose load. Most commonly fed hypoglycemia occurs several hours after eating, usually in the late

**Table 176-1.** Causes of Hypoglycemia

| Spontaneous | Induced |
| --- | --- |
| Fed—reactive—postprandial | Insulin |
|   Alimentary | Factitious |
|   Early diabetes mellitus | Sulfonylureas |
|   Idiopathic | Alcohol |
| Fasting | Miscellaneous drugs |
|   Islet-cell tumor of pancreas | Posthyperalimentation or |
|     (insulinoma) |   -hemodialysis |
|   Extrapancreatic neoplasms | |
|   Endocrine-related | |
|     Pituitary insufficiency | |
|     Adrenal insufficiency | |
|     Glucagon deficiency | |
|     Thyroid insufficiency | |
| Hepatic disease | |
| Miscellaneous | |
|   Sepsis | |
|   Chronic renal failure | |
|   Starvation | |
|   Autoimmune | |
|   Exercise | |
|   Artifactual | |

morning or the late afternoon. The critical period in which hypoglycemia may develop is during the transition from the fed to the fasting state, between 2 and 4 h after the ingestion of glucose. The glucose tolerance test (GTT) no longer has a role in confirmation of this diagnosis.

#### Alimentary

The major causes of fed hypoglycemia are alimentary causes, early diabetes mellitus, and idiopathic. Following partial or total gastrectomy, gastrojejunostomy, or pyloroplasty, 5 to 10 percent of the patients may develop symptomatic hypoglycemia $1\frac{1}{2}$ to 3 h after a meal. The cause appears to be rapid gastric emptying and an exaggerated insulin response. A correlation of hypoglycemia with peak insulin levels has been shown.

Postgastrectomy hypoglycemia is not the same as dumping syndrome, which is due to rapid dilution of a hyperosmolar load in the jejunum and produces symptoms of weakness, pallor, nausea, epigastric discomfort, palpitations, dizziness, and diarrhea. These symptoms occur within 10 min after a meal, subside within 1 h, and are not due to hypoglycemia. Alimentary hypoglycemia in the absence of gastrointestinal (GI) surgery has been described. Patients with this entity may have a gut defect with rapid glucose absorption, or release of gut factors that stimulate insulin secretion. Treatment of alimentary hypoglycemia is aimed at minimizing insulin release by decreasing the amount of ingested carbohydrate.

#### Early Diabetes

Spontaneous hypoglycemia occurring 3 to 5 h after a meal may be seen as an early manifestation of non-insulin dependent diabetes (NIDDM). It is postulated that there is a delay in the early release of insulin with subsequent excessive insulin secretion in response to the initial hyperglycemia. The symptoms are usually brief and mild, lasting 15 to 20 min. A family history of diabetes is usual.

#### Idiopathic

Idiopathic hypoglycemia is probably rare and may simply reflect the transition in intermediary metabolism between the fed and fasting state. It is diagnosed far more often than justified. It is usually described as occurring 2 to 4 h after meals or with minor deprivation of food such as a missed meal. The patient is often a healthy young adult with no known underlying cause of hypoglycemia. Symptoms of sweating, shakiness, weakness, light-headedness, numbness, confusion, and anxiety are commonly reported and may lead the physician to obtain a 6-h GTT. If the blood glucose level goes below 50 mg/dL, the patient is diagnosed as having hypoglycemia and placed on a high-protein, low-carbohydrate diet. The GTT no longer has a role in the evaluation of hypoglycemia.

Many question the diagnosis. Several investigations of patients with idiopathic hypoglycemia have shown a poor correlation between symptoms and the blood glucose levels. If the serum glucose level is less than 50 mg/dL and is associated with spontaneous symptoms, the diagnosis should be considered and the patient referred for further evaluation.

According to the American Diabetes Association, the following are criteria for the diagnosis of idiopathic hypoglycemia: the occurrence of documented low blood sugar; the particular symptoms of which the patient complains must be shown to be due to low blood sugar; the symptoms must be relieved by the ingestion of food or sugar; and the particular kind of hypoglycemia causing symptoms must be established.

#### Fasting Hypoglycemia

Fasting hypoglycemia is by far the most important hypoglycemic state for the emergency physician to recognize. Fasting hypoglycemia often reflects serious underlying organic disease. Hypoglycemia may develop slowly so that the signs of hyperepinephrinemia may not be seen, and the patient may simply lapse into coma.

By definition, fasting hypoglycemia begins 5 to 6 h after a meal. Most patients with a disorder that causes fasting hypoglycemia develop low glucose levels during a 24-h fast. Occasionally a 72-h fast is required to establish or rule out this diagnosis. Not uncommonly, the patient is difficult to arouse in the morning following an overnight fast. Evaluation of the cause of this type of hypoglycemia may require hospitalization.

## Insulinoma

Hypoglycemia due to insulinoma may occur in the fasting or the fed state. In 80 percent of the cases, the tumor is small, single, and nonmalignant and is located anywhere within the pancreas. About 10 percent of the patients have multiple tumors and also a high association with multiple endocrine neoplasia (MEN), type I. The remaining 10 percent have metastatic malignant insulinoma.

Insulinoma occurs somewhat more often in women in the later decades of life (40 to 70 years). Most of the patients have symptoms consisting of various combinations of sweating, palpitations, weakness, diplopia, and blurred vision. Confusion or abnormal behavior is seen in 80 percent of the cases. Coma or amnesia for the hypoglycemic episode occurs in about half the patients and seizures in 12 percent. Symptoms occur at irregular intervals, more often in the late afternoon or early morning before breakfast and may be induced by exercise. The symptoms are of varying duration and are alleviated by food in the majority of instances. The interval between the appearance of the first hypoglycemic symptoms and the diagnosis of insulinoma is usually months (19 months) and may be years. Many of these patients are diagnosed to have a neurologic abnormality such as a convulsive disorder, a cerebrovascular accident, a brain tumor, or narcolepsy, or they may be thought to have a psychiatric problem such as psychosis or hysteria. Some patients have been diagnosed to have Adams-Stokes attacks.

In one series of 78 patients with insulinoma, 38 (49 percent) were evaluated in an emergency department because of CNS symptoms. Twenty patients were identified as hypoglycemic, and eight of those were immediately admitted to rule out hyperinsulinism. Eight patients did not have a blood glucose determination, and the remaining ten patients had various neurologic or psychiatric diagnoses. For 15 of these patients (39 percent) their presentation to the emergency department was for their first symptomatic episode.

The hypoglycemia of insulinoma is thought to be due to excess insulin secreted by the tumor. The diagnosis is made by the demonstration of hypoglycemia and hyperinsulinemia at the time of spontaneous symptoms. A prolonged fast (72 h) may be required to provoke hypoglycemia, but most patients (75 to 90 percent) develop it before 24 h of fasting. A variety of provocative tests based upon the administration of insulin secretagogues, and several suppression tests utilizing insulin inhibitors, can be used as diagnostic aids. The ratio of immunoreactive insulin to glucose (IRI/G) can be determined to see if the insulin level is inappropriate to the concomitant level of blood glucose.

The differential diagnosis of insulinoma includes surreptitious self-administration of insulin. In someone taking exogenous insulin, factitious hypoglycemia from excess insulin administration can be diagnosed by the determination of immunoreactive C-peptide levels. Proinsulin is converted to insulin and C peptide in the pancreatic β cells, and these two peptides are secreted in equimolar concentrations. If insulin is endogenously produced, the insulin and the C-peptide levels are proportionately elevated. If insulin is exogenously administered, the insulin level is elevated but the C-peptide level is low. In patients who are not known to be taking insulin, the presence of insulin antibodies in the serum suggests the self-

administration of insulin. These antibodies may not be detectable before 6 weeks to 2 months of exogenous insulin administration.

The treatment of insulinoma is surgical excision of the tumor, and this is curative in most cases. In those patients in whom surgical therapy is not feasible or curative or in whom surgery must be delayed, drug treatment and diet can be used. More frequent feedings using slowly absorbable forms of carbohydrate are indicated. Benign tumors can be treated with diazoxide and thiazide. Diazoxide acts to directly inhibit the release of insulin by the β cells and has an extrapancreatic hyperglycemic effect. The diuretic prevents edema caused by diazoxide-induced sodium retention. With malignant insulinoma, streptozotocin is the most effective antitumor agent to date.

## Extrapancreatic Neoplasms

Hypoglycemia may be associated with, and caused by, neoplasms of virtually every histopathologic type. Hypoglycemia-causing tumors may be unsuspected and discovered during systemic evaluation of a patient with fasting hypoglycemia; or hypoglycemia may occur as a late or preterminal event in a patient with known neoplasia.

Mesenchymal tumors are the most common tumors of nonpancreatic origin associated with tumor hypoglycemia. Thoracic and retroperitoneal tumors, especially fibrosarcomas and mesotheliomas, are most common. Mesenchymal tumors are slow-growing and large and may be massive (20 kg or more). Other endocrinopathies may be present because of the ectopic production of a variety of hormones by these tumors. The presenting signs and symptoms may include profound hypoglycemia, depressed cerebral function, weight loss, and a large intrathoracic or intraabdominal mass.

Epithelial and endothelial tumors involving the lung, breast, kidney, ovary, and GI tract can cause hypoglycemia. The epithelial tumors most often associated with hypoglycemia are hepatic carcinomas, adrenocortical neoplasms, and carcinoid tumors. Hepatic carcinomas are invariably large, occur more commonly in men than women (4 to 1), and usually have a rapid clinical course with a fatal outcome in 1 to 6 months. Hypoglycemia occurs as a terminal or a preterminal event. Adrenocortical neoplasms are usually malignant and large. Carcinoid tumors develop from cells of the amine precursor uptake and decarboxylation (APUD) series and may occur in a variety of locations. These tumors are slow-growing and elaborate a variety of biologically active substances. They are capable of producing hypoglycemia as well as the carcinoid syndrome. Diagnosis is made by the demonstration of increased 5-hydroxyindoleacetic acids (5-HIAA) in a 24-h urine collection.

Tumor hypoglycemia is a heterogeneous disorder that no single mechanism can satisfactorily explain. Some tumors secrete substances with insulinlike biological activity. Other causes of tumor hypoglycemia include increased utilization of glucose by the tumor, decreased gluconeogenesis from cachexia and depletion of substrates, liver impairment due to metastasis or tumor products, or depression of glucagon secretion and activity. Regardless of the mechanism, the treatment is intravenous or oral glucose replacement.

## Endocrine-Related

The crucial role of the counterregulatory hormones in the maintenance of glucose homeostasis has been reviewed. Deficiency of any of these hormones could result in hypoglycemia. Catecholamine deficiency has not been documented to cause hypoglycemia, but deficiency of glucagon, glucocorticoids, and growth hormone has. Glucagon or pancreatic α-cell deficiency is a rare cause of hypoglycemia. Glucocorticoid deficiency as a cause of fasting hypoglycemia is seen with primary or secondary adrenal insufficiency. Hypoglycemia is more pronounced with secondary adrenal insufficiency (hypopituitarism) because of concomitant growth hormone and glucocorticoid deficiencies. Patients with growth hormone deficiency may have fasting or fed hypoglycemia even when growth hormone deficiency is not accompanied by deficits in other pituitary hormones. Hypothyroidism can also cause hypoglycemia, especially when severe enough to cause myxedema coma.

## Hepatic Disease

Diffuse, severe liver disease, in which 80 to 85 percent of the liver is functionally impaired or destroyed, may result in hypoglycemia due to impaired glycogenolysis and gluconeogenesis. Diseases such as acute hepatic necrosis, acute viral hepatitis, Reye's syndrome, and severe passive congestion have been implicated. Metastatic or primary liver neoplasia may cause hypoglycemia if a large portion of the liver is involved, but liver metastases usually do not produce hypoglycemia. Hypoglycemia has been described as part of the syndrome of fatty liver of pregnancy. An association between hypoglycemia and the HELLP syndrome (hemolysis, elevated liver enzyme levels, and low platelet count) has also been reported. A spectrum of hepatic damage ranging from preeclampsia to HELLP syndrome to acute fatty liver may occur in pregnancy. All ill women in the third trimester should have glucose level determinations. Chronic liver disease only rarely is a cause of hypoglycemia. Patients with hepatic failure severe enough to cause hypoglycemia are often in a coma. Hypoglycemia as a cause of coma may be missed if it is assumed that coma is due to hepatic encephalopathy.

## Miscellaneous

Hypoglycemia has been described in a wide variety of other clinical situations. Sepsis can cause hypoglycemia, more often in elderly patients with underlying liver and renal disease. It has also been described in a 6-month-old patient with *Neisseria* meningitis and in other patients in whom no cause for hypoglycemia other than sepsis was present. Spontaneous, fasting hypoglycemia with chronic renal failure in diabetic and non-diabetic patients is well-documented. The pathogenesis is poorly understood, but is often accompanied by severe lactic acidosis.

Starvation-related hypoglycemia is occasionally seen. The majority of the case reports on starvation hypoglycemia involve children with kwashiorkor, but adult cases, especially associated with anorexia nervosa, have been described. Hypoglycemia can be severe and refractory to therapy. The mechanisms are obscure, but include the failure of gluconeogenesis due to the depletion of fat and protein stores, or abnormally increased cellular glucose consumption. An infusion of 20% dextrose and lactated Ringer's solution containing hydrocortisone is used to treat this condition.

Fasting and fed autoimmune hypoglycemia has been described. The presence of anti-insulin antibodies in patients not known to have received insulin injections has been confirmed in several reports. This syndrome has both hypoglycemia and hyperglycemia which is the hallmark for its discovery. The autoantibodies tie up insulin resulting in hyperglycemia. Hypoglycemia occurs later when they dissociate giving a dramatic rise to free insulin. Saturation of the insulin-binding capacity with the continued release of insulin from the pancreas has also been suggested. Additionally, hypoglycemia associated with antibodies to the insulin receptor has been identified. These autoantibodies may mimic the bioactivity of insulin on target tissues, causing hypoglycemia.

Prolonged exercise may result in hypoglycemia. With intense, continued exercise (longer than 90 min), liver glycogen stores are depleted, and the rate of glucose production may fail to keep pace with the rate of glucose use, resulting in a fall in the blood glucose concentration. With the current popularity of endurance training, a patient with exercise-induced hypoglycemia could present to the emergency department.

Artifactual hypoglycemia may occur in conditions in which either the leukocyte or lymphocyte count is markedly increased (>60,000 mm³, regardless of the underlying disease). This is thought to be due to continued glycolysis by the large number of leukocytes or lymphocytes between the time the blood is drawn and the time the glucose determination is made. Artifactual hypoglycemia has been reported in various leukemias, with nucleated red blood cells during a hemolytic crisis, and in polycythemia rubra vera. True hypoglycemia has been reported in terminal leukemia and must be distinguished from artifactual hypoglycemia, which is asymptomatic. The refrigeration of blood samples and the addition of an antiglycolytic agent, such as sodium fluoride, decreases glucose consumption by the white blood cells.

## Induced Hypoglycemia

Induced hypoglycemia is almost always due to drugs, commonly insulin, sulfonylureas, alcohol, and salicylates. During the first 2 years of life, salicylates account for most cases of drug-induced hypoglycemia. During the next 8 years, alcohol is the most likely cause. In patients 11 to 30 years of age, two-thirds of all comas have been caused by sulfonylureas or insulin, with half of these occurring in nondiabetic young women attempting suicide. Alcohol alone or in combination with insulin is a common cause of hypoglycemic coma in patients between 30 and 50 years of age who have drug-related hypoglycemia. Hypoglycemia caused by sulfonylurea agents is more likely after 60 years of age.

Factors predisposing to drug-induced hypoglycemia include restricted carbohydrate intake and renal or hepatic disease.

## Insulin-Induced

Insulin reaction in the diabetic patient is by far the most common cause of hypoglycemia seen in the emergency department.

Multiple factors affect the severity and the frequency of insulin reactions. The severity of the diabetes is directly related to the incidence of insulin reactions. Those with the least endogenous insulin have the widest variation in blood glucose levels. It is well-documented that the counterregulatory hormones increase in response to insulin-induced hypoglycemia.

Recent investigations concerning the role of the counterregulatory hormones in the prevention or correction of hypoglycemic reactions in insulin-dependent diabetic patients have shown that glucagon is the primary hormone protecting against hypoglycemia. Epinephrine is not normally critical but becomes so when glucagon is deficient. The effects of cortisol and growth hormone require several hours to occur, and thus they are not factors in rapid counterregulation of hypoglycemia but are more important in recovery from prolonged hypoglycemia.

Patients who have been diabetic for less than 2 years generally have an intact defense against hypoglycemia with a normal glucagon and epinephrine response. Eventually, most patients with insulin-dependent diabetes acquire a deficiency in glucagon secretory response during hypoglycemia. This defect is almost universally present after 5 years of diabetes. These patients are dependent upon epinephrine to promote recovery from hypoglycemia. However, after 5 to 10 years of IDDM, glucose counterregulation becomes further impaired when epinephrine secretion also becomes deficient. One study of patients with long-standing IDDM reported a 40% incidence. Additionally, diabetic autonomic neuropathy or blockade with the use of a non-selective β adrenergic antagonist places these patients at increased risk of prolonged, severe hypoglycemic reactions.

Some other factors that may precipitate hypoglycemia in an insulin-dependent diabetic patient include exercise, emotions, late meals, gastroparesis, undereating of carbohydrates, alcohol ingestion, errors of insulin dosage, erratic absorption of insulin from subcutaneous sites, and overtreatment with insulin. Of these factors, overtreatment with insulin deserves further discussion. Hypoglycemia commonly occurs during intensive insulin treatment for near euglycemia glucose control. Following the classic report by Somogyi, excess insulin as a cause of hypoglycemia, nocturnal hypoglycemia, and rebound hyperglycemia has been well-documented and is fairly common in adults and children.

Nocturnal hypoglycemia is often difficult to recognize clinically. It is most likely to be associated with the use of long-acting insulin preparations taken once daily. Suggestive features include lethargy, depression, night sweats, nightmares, morning headaches, seizures, hepatomegaly due to glycogen accumulation, and acquired tolerance to high doses of insulin. Polyuria, nocturia, or enuresis despite increasing insulin dosage, excessive appetite, weight gain, mood swings, and frequent bouts of rapidly developing ketoacidosis are additional clues to the recognition of insulin overdosage (see Table 176-2). Fasting early-morning blood glucose levels may be normal in spite of nocturnal hypoglycemia. They may also be elevated and lead to an increase in the insulin dose and a worsening of the symptoms. When insulin-dependent diabetic patients are brought to the emergency department with early morning hyperglycemia or with symptoms of undetermined cause, follow-up arrangements should be made with their physicians through personal communication.

Another cause of early morning hyperglycemia is the dawn phenomenon. This condition has been described in insulin-dependent and non-insulin-dependent diabetic patients and in nondiabetics. It is characterized by an abrupt increase in fasting levels of plasma glucose between 5 and 9 A.M. in the absence of antecedent hypoglycemia. This phenomenon is extremely common, occurring in the vast majority of those patients who have been studied. The mechanism is unknown. Elevated glucose levels occur irrespective of insulin levels and may reflect a circadian variation in glucose tolerance.

Clinically, it is important to distinguish among the Somogyi phenomenon, the dawn phenomenon, and simple waning of previously injected insulin as a cause of early morning hyperglycemia, as treatments differ. Management of the Somogyi phenomenon consists of reducing insulin doses and providing late-evening carbohydrate to avoid hypoglycemia. Treatment of the dawn phenomenon and insulin waning generally consists of adjusting the evening dose of intermediate- or long-acting insulin to provide additional coverage in the early morning hours. Attribution of early-morning hyperglycemia to an incorrect cause could result in inappropriate treatment. A coordinated management effort between the emergency physician and the patient's personal physician is important in such cases.

The question of rigid or tight control of diabetes is even more vital following a policy statement from the American Diabetes Association in 1976 calling for "a serious effort to achieve levels of blood glucose as close to those in the nondiabetic state as feasible." This therapeutic goal is based upon the belief that the long-term vascular complications of diabetes, particularly retinopathy and nephropathy, are decreased by reduction of the blood glucose concentration. To this end, newer methods for tight diabetic control have been introduced. These include home blood glucose monitoring with multiple insulin injections (two or three times a day) based upon glucose levels, continuous subcutaneous insulin infusion using a portable pump, and the development of an artificial pancreas.

Several authors have cautioned against too-rigid control. In spite of

the efficacy of home blood glucose monitoring and the apparent effectiveness of the infusion pump, complications have been reported. Results from the Diabetes Control and Complications Trial, a large, multicenter study comparing intensive insulin therapy with standard treatment regimens for insulin-dependent patients, indicate that the incidence of severe hypoglycemia or coma is approximately three times higher in patients receiving intensive therapy.

Recent reports have affirmed the benefits of intensive diabetes therapy in delaying the onset and slowing the progression of retinopathy and neuropathy in patients with IDDM. However, several studies have demonstrated reduced counterregulatory response to hypoglycemia in those patients who have achieved tight glycemia control. Strict control itself may produce physiologic adaptations that impair glucose counterregulation and place this patient population at increased risk for repeated episodes of severe hypoglycemia.

Several authors have stressed that the glycemic goals for insulin-dependent diabetic patients must be individualized. Intensive insulin therapy should be utilized only in those patients who are apt to benefit from such regimens and who are at relatively low risk of sustained hypoglycemia. Individuals whose life expectancy is reduced by advanced age, life-shortening disorders, and end-stage diabetic complications are unlikely to obtain long-term benefits from rigorous glucose control. Additionally, those patients with defective glucose counterregulation from deficient glucagon and epinephrine responses are not candidates for meticulous control.

It is important to prevent hypoglycemic reactions in the insulin-dependent diabetic patient. Studies with continuous blood glucose sampling in IDDM have suggested that less than a third of all hypoglycemic episodes are symptomatic.

The best defense against hypoglycemia is the ability of the patient to recognize its symptoms and to abort a full-blown episode by the oral ingestion of carbohydrates. Hepburn found that in diabetic and non-diabetic subjects, the most common initial symptoms of hypoglycemia were neuroglycopenia, inability to concentrate, weakness and drowsiness. When analyzing the diabetic group alone, autonomic symptoms were experienced more frequently among the initial symptoms. Many diabetic subjects miss or fail to recognize the early warning cues provided by neuroglycopenic symptoms and therefore have to rely on the autonomic symptoms of sweating, trembling, warmness, pounding heart and anxiety as indicators of hypoglycemia. Patients with long-standing IDDM and those treated by strict glycemic control are less likely to experience autonomic symptoms of hypoglycemia and are more likely to quietly slip into a coma in response to CNS glucose deprivation.

The emergency physician must be prepared to identify and advise the diabetic patient who drives a motor vehicle and is prone to hypoglycemic reactions, especially neuroglycopenic ones. One survey of 250 insulin-dependent diabetic patient drivers identified 34 percent with severe or frequent hypoglycemia in the preceding 6 months, during which they had been driving regularly. Thirty-four patients (13.6 percent) had been involved in a driving accident since commencing treatment with insulin, and 13 of those patients were aware that hypoglycemia had been an important causal factor. Another survey of 85 young diabetic patients identified 5 percent who experienced unexpected hypoglycemic reactions while driving or operating machinery.

The emergency physicians must directly question the insulin-dependent diabetic driver about unexpected hypoglycemic reactions. If any have occurred, the patient should be instructed to self-monitor the blood glucose level just before driving and at 1- to 2-h intervals on long trips. The blood glucose level should be maintained at about 200 mg/dL, and the patient should take supplemental feedings whenever the glucose falls below that level. Patients subject to unexpected hypoglycemia should have sugar and glucagon available in the vehicle and should drive accompanied by an informed person who can administer them. Finally, the hypoglycemia-prone patient must avoid

**Table 176-2.** Clinical Clues of Nocturnal Hypoglycemia

| |
|---|
| Lassitude, depression, difficulty with waking in morning |
| Early morning headaches or irritability |
| Night sweats, nightmares |
| Polyuria, nocturia, enuresis in children |
| Convulsions |
| Increased appetite and weight gain |
| Hepatomegaly |
| Morning ketonuria without glucosuria or disproportionate to glucosuria |
| Worsening of symptoms with increased insulin dose |
| Insulin dose greater than 1.0 unit/kg of body weight per day |

**Table 176-3.** Differentiation between Hypoglycemia and Ketoacidosis

| | **Hypoglycemia** | **Ketoacidosis** |
|---|---|---|
| History | Insufficient food, excess insulin, excess exercise | Insufficient insulin, infection, gastrointestinal upset |
| Onset | Following *short-acting insulin:* Sudden, a few hours after injection<br><br>Following *long-acting insulin:* Relatively slower, many hours after injection | Gradual over many hours |
| Course | Anxiety, sweating, hunger, headache, diplopia, incoordination, twitching, convulsions, coma (headache, nausea, and haziness especially following long-acting insulin) | Polyuria, polydipsia, anorexia, nausea, vomiting, labored deep breathing, weakness, drowsiness, possible fever and abdominal pain, coma |
| Physical findings | Pale moist skin, full rapid pulse, dilated pupils, normal breathing, blood pressure normal or elevated, overactive reflexes, positive Babinski sign | Florid, dry skin. Kussmaul breathing with acetone odor, decreased blood pressure, weak rapid pulse, soft eyeballs |
| Laboratory findings | Second urine specimen sugar- and ketone-free, low blood sugar, normal serum $CO_2$ | Urine contains sugar and ketone bodies; high blood sugar, low serum $CO_2$ |

*Source:* Ensinck JW, Williams RH: Disorders causing hypoglycemia, in Williams RH (ed): *Textbook of Endocrinology,* 6th ed, Philadelphia, Saunders, 1981, p 873.

alcohol and all medications that may cause or potentiate hypoglycemic reactions.

A cooperative effort between the patient, the patient's primary physician, and the emergency physician is essential for the appropriate follow-up of a diabetic patient presenting to the emergency department.

When a diabetic patient is brought to the emergency department with depressed cerebral function or in coma, rapid differentiation between hypoglycemia and ketoacidosis must be made (see Table 176-3). Testing a drop of blood with a glucose reagent strip reliably allows differentiation between high and low blood glucose levels within minutes. If there is still uncertainty about the cause, 50 mL of a 50% glucose solution should be given intravenously after blood has been obtained for appropriate studies. The hypoglycemic patient benefits, and the patient in ketoacidosis is not unduly harmed.

## Factitious Hypoglycemia

An occasional emotionally unstable patient surreptitiously administers insulin or an oral hypoglycemic drug to induce hypoglycemia and simulate organic disease. These patients may be medical personnel or diabetic, or they may be related to someone who is diabetic or in the medical profession. These patients often exhibit erratic patterns of hypoglycemia and usually deny drug misuse even when confronted directly. The use of insulin or oral hypoglycemic agents causes hyperinsulinemia, which may be mistaken for an insulinoma. Factitious hypoglycemia resulting from oral hypoglycemics can be diagnosed by detecting sulfonylurea agents in the blood. Proinsulin and C-peptide determinations are not useful for ruling out factitious hypoglycemia due to ingestion of sulfonylurea agents. Those drugs stimulate the pancreas to secrete insulin, and equivalent amounts of C-peptide and insulin are present. Additionally, no insulin antibodies are present. Because the second-generation sulfonylurea agents are more potent, smaller doses are used and the plasma levels are not very high. Differentiating between surreptitious ingestion of these agents and insulinoma may be difficult.

Insulin antibodies may be detected in the serum of patients who claim to have never used insulin if the insulin has been administered for 6 to 8 weeks. The measurement of C-peptide levels is indicated if insulin antibodies are not detected or if a diabetic patient is suspected of factitious hypoglycemia. The C-peptide levels are low if the source of the insulin is exogenous and high in cases of endogenous hyperinsulinemia.

## Sulfonylureas

The sulfonylureas are commonly used as oral hypoglycemic agents and include the first-generation agents chlorpropamide, tolbutamide, acetohexamide, and tolazamide. Second-generation sulfonylurea

drugs are glyburide and glipizide. These newer drugs have a greater hypoglycemic effect per milligram than older agents. All sulfonylurea drugs stimulate the release of insulin from the pancreas with a subsequent decrease in hepatic glucose output. These agents are commonly used to treat NIDDM. Hypoglycemic reactions may be profound, prolonged, and life-threatening. Sulfonylurea overdose and surreptitious self-administration may also produce hypoglycemia. Encephalopathy from recurrent hypoglycemic reactions induced by oral hypoglycemic drugs has been reported.

Other drugs may potentiate the hypoglycemic effect of sulfonylurea agents. Alcohol, salicylates, sulfonamides, bis-hydroxycoumarin, and phenylbutazone should be avoided in patients on sulfonylureas. All the sulfonylurea compounds have caused hypoglycemia, but chlorpropamide is responsible for most cases. Hypoglycemia due to chlorpropamide has occurred during normal food intake, with intact renal function, and at ordinary dosages. Chlorpropamide causes the most prolonged hypoglycemia of all sulfonylurea drugs. Its half-life in the serum is 36 h, and 3 to 5 days are required for complete elimination from the body. Severe and prolonged hypoglycemia due to glyburide has also been described.

Sulfonylurea-induced hypoglycemia may be refractory to treatment by intravenous glucose alone. This is particularly true in nondiabetic patients in whom insulin-release mechanisms are intact. Infused glucose stimulates insulin release, which may further lower the blood glucose level. Diazoxide, 300 mg by slow intravenous infusion over a 30-min period, repeated every 4 h, has been successful in raising the blood glucose to supranormal levels without causing hypotension. All patients with sulfonylurea-induced hypoglycemia require hospitalization, observation, and treatment.

## Alcohol

Alcohol-induced hypoglycemia is usually seen in malnourished chronic alcoholics. It may also occur in spree drinkers, in occasional drinkers who have missed a meal or two, and in children and adolescents. Severe alcoholic intoxication and hypoglycemic coma has also been reported from continuous sponging of a febrile child with rubbing alcohol.

Patients with alcohol-induced hypoglycemia usually present in coma or semicoma 2 to 10 h after alcohol ingestion. The presenting physical findings may include hypothermia, tachypnea, and the smell of alcohol on the breath. The absence of alcohol fetor does not rule out alcohol as a cause of hypoglycemia or coma. Most patients are unresponsive except to deep pain stimulation. Convulsions are a particularly frequent occurrence in children with alcoholic hypoglycemia. Laboratory findings, in addition to hypoglycemia, usually include an elevated blood alcohol level, ketonuria without glucosuria, and mild acidosis.

Alcohol-induced hypoglycemia is attributed primarily to the inhibition of gluconeogenesis during alcohol metabolism. Ethyl alcohol is metabolized primarily in the cytoplasm of the liver cells, utilizing nicotinamide adenine dinucleotide (NAD) as the hydrogen acceptor. During this process the rate of NAD reduction exceeds the rate of NADH oxidation, and the NADH/NAD ratio increases severalfold. The NAD available for those oxidation-reduction reactions necessary to sustain gluconeogenesis is thus decreased, and the level of plasma glucose subsequently falls. The chronic alcoholic with reduced caloric intake and depleted liver glycogen stores has no glucogenic reserve, and hypoglycemic coma results. The mechanism by which alcohol induces hypoglycemia in the well-fed person is less well defined.

Treatment with intravenous glucose is usually sufficient to correct alcohol-induced hypoglycemia. Thiamine should be given before glucose in chronic or suspected alcoholics. Glucagon is not recommended in the chronic alcoholic, as liver glycogen stores are usually exhausted.

## Miscellaneous Drugs

Several other drugs should be mentioned in relation to drug-induced hypoglycemia. Salicylate-induced hypoglycemic coma in children can occur with overtreatment of febrile illnesses with aspirin, and from accidental overdose. Salicylate toxicity and hypoglycemia should be considered in any child with coma, convulsions, or cardiovascular collapse. Salicylate-related hypoglycemia in adults most often occurs when aspirin is used in conjunction with other compounds that lower the levels of glucose. Propranolol has been reported to precipitate hypoglycemia, and several authors have expressed concern over the use of β-adrenergic blockers in diabetic patients. They believe that β blockers may mask the adrenergic symptoms of hypoglycemia and increase the risk and the severity of hypoglycemic reactions. Experimental and clinical evidence is contradictory. Some researchers find that β blockers potentiate insulin-induced hypoglycemia and delay the blood glucose recovery after hypoglycemic reactions, while others have disputed these findings. The β blockers are widely used among diabetic patients for the treatment of angina and hypertension. Cardioselective β blockers have been recommended when diabetic patients require β-blocking drugs. The possible induction, potentiation, or masking of hypoglycemia by β-blocking drugs in diabetics should be considered.

A wide variety of drugs have been found to cause hypoglycemia in isolated instances (Table 176-4). Disopyramide-induced hypoglycemia has been reported increasingly since 1978 and usually occurs in elderly patients who are poorly nourished and have mild abnormalities in glucose homeostasis.

A final cause of induced hypoglycemia is the sudden cessation of a high-concentration glucose infusion. Hypoglycemia from this cause may occur in patients receiving hyperalimentation or hemodialysis. An occasional patient undergoing outpatient hemodialysis may be brought to the emergency department with hypoglycemia due to this reason.

## CLINICAL PRESENTATION

The clinical manifestations of hypoglycemia vary widely. Some patients are asymptomatic even though the hypoglycemia is significant. As glucose is the main source of energy for the brain, it is not surprising that most symptomatic hypoglycemia produces neurologic and mental dysfunction. The autonomic symptoms of hypoglycemia and the neuroglycopenic symptoms were described earlier.

Hypoglycemia can cause other neurologic manifestations such as cranial nerve palsies, paresthesias, and transient hemiplegia. Hemiplegia may be due to spontaneous or induced hypoglycemia. The paralysis is usually abrupt in onset, is associated with extensor plantar responses, and may last a few hours to a few days. This phenomenon is thought to be due to decreased glucose perfusion of a selected area of the brain because of arteriosclerotic narrowing of a blood vessel. Hypoglycemic hemiplegia has also been described in children and adolescents, however. Additional neurologic abnormalities due to hypoglycemia include diplopia, clonus, and decerebrate posturing. In the absence of neuronal damage, these neurologic deficits should reverse with the administration of glucose.

Moderate hypothermia may occur with hypoglycemia and can be a useful clue in cases of unsuspected hypoglycemia. Sweating, peripheral vasodilatation, hyperventilation, and reduced heat production contribute to hypoglycemic-induced hypothermia. When hypoglycemia is accompanied by elevated temperature, infection, dehydration, or cerebral edema may be the cause.

Unsuspected hypoglycemia may masquerade as neurologic, psychiatric, or cardiovascular disorders. Hypoglycemia has been misdiagnosed as a cerebrovascular accident, a transient ischemic attack, a seizure disorder, a brain tumor, narcolepsy, multiple sclerosis, psychosis, hysteria, depression, and Adams-Stokes attacks. Particular care should be exercised when dealing with these entities so that hypoglycemia is not missed.

### Evaluation of Hypoglycemia

The ability to detect and evaluate hypoglycemia in the emergency department is limited. A history, a physical examination, selected x-ray studies, and laboratory studies, such as random glucose, are the main investigative tools available to the emergency physician. One test that could assist in the diagnosis of suspected transient hypoglycemia is the cerebrospinal fluid glucose analysis. Gruber has reported that the CSF glucose level lags behind the blood glucose level during the return to the normal range. The delay in the return to a baseline level may be as much as 4 to 6 h. Transient hypoglycemia could be reflected in a low CSF glucose level at a time when the blood glucose concentration is normal. Other laboratory studies, such as measurement of the levels of insulin, insulin antibodies, and C peptides, should be obtained in conjunction with the patient's primary physician.

Fed hypoglycemic reactions are suspected based upon the proximity of the symptoms to eating, especially when a repetitive pattern is evident. A history of gastric surgery or relatives with diabetes may be obtained. If idiopathic hypoglycemia is suspected, home blood glucose monitoring or random blood glucose levels obtained at the time of the symptoms are indicated. Fasting hypoglycemia may occasionally be detected in the emergency department if the patient presents in a fasting state or if a random blood glucose level is low. Patients suspected of having fasting hypoglycemia should be admitted to the hospital for evaluation.

**Table 176-4.** Potentially Hypoglycemic Agents

| | |
|---|---|
| Acetaminophen | Lithium |
| Amphetamine | Manganese |
| Aspirin | Monoamine oxidase inhibitors |
| Chloramphenicol | Onion extract |
| Dextropropoxyphene | Orphenadrine |
| Dicumarol | Oxytetracycline |
| Disopyramide | Pentamidine |
| Ethylenediaminetetraacetate | Phenothiazines |
| Halofenate | Phenylbutazone |
| Haloperidol | Propranolol |
| Hypoglycin (akee nut) | Quinine |
| Kerola (herb) | Sulfa drugs |

*Source:* Malouf R, Brust JCM: Hypoglycemia: Causes, neurological manifestations, and outcome. *Ann Neurol* 17:421, 1985.

The plasma glucose levels should be determined in all patients who are comatose, have a seizure, have a disturbance of sensorium, have taken a drug overdose, smell of alcohol, or have "funny spells" that are undefined. Random glucose levels should be determined in all diabetic patients with clinically significant complaints.

## TREATMENT

Many aspects of treating hypoglycemia have been discussed in conjunction with specific disorders. The armamentarium of the emergency physician in combating hypoglycemia consists of intravenous or oral glucose solutions, glucagon, and hydrocortisone.

Outpatient treatment of insulin reactions can often be self-administered by the ingestion of glucose. One study recommends 20 g of D-glucose as most efficacious, correcting moderate to severe hypoglycemia in 20 min without causing prolonged hyperglycemia. See Table 176-5 for a list of common sources of D-glucose.

Diabetic adults in coma, or other patients who have coma of uncertain cause, should be given 50 mL of a 50% glucose solution by intravenous bolus, after blood has been obtained for appropriate studies. In confirmed hypoglycemia, a follow-up infusion of a 5, 10, or 20% glucose solution should be started. Continuous intravenous glucose for 4 to 6 h is needed for most hypoglycemic reactions. Prolonged therapy may be indicated in some cases, and knowledge of the cause of the hypoglycemia should guide the duration of treatment. Care must be taken not to discontinue the glucose infusion too soon, as the hypoglycemia may recur. Fructose should not be used to correct hypoglycemia in diabetics. This low caloric sugar does not cross the blood–brain barrier effectively.

The glucose level with the infusion running should be 100 mg/dL or greater. The blood glucose level should be monitored every 2 to 3 h. If the first liter of glucose solution fails to establish and maintain elevated glucose levels, 100 mg of hydrocortisone and 1 mg of glucagon should be added to each liter of infusate for as long as necessary. Persistent hyperglycemia, maintained by slow administration of 5% glucose, is a sign that the glucose infusion may be withdrawn. After intravenous therapy has been discontinued, the blood glucose level should be determined in every patient discharged from the emergency department. Patients should be instructed to continue oral carbohydrate intake and to return if any symptoms of hypoglycemia recur.

The required duration of continuous glucose infusion is unpredictable. Most diabetic patients with insulin reactions respond fairly rapidly to intravenous glucose. Similarly, alcohol-induced hypoglycemia usually responds quickly to glucose administration. Sulfonylurea-induced hypoglycemia can be prolonged and may not respond to intravenous glucose alone. Diazoxide as adjunctive therapy may be required. All patients with sulfonylurea hypoglycemia should be admitted to the hospital.

Glucagon is effective adjunctive therapy in selected cases. Glucagon increases glucose production by the liver providing that glycogen stores are adequate. Glucagon can be administered intramuscularly, subcutaneously, or intravenously in 0.5- to 2.0-mg doses. It is effective in 10 to 20 min and may be repeated twice. If glucagon is given intravenously, continuous infusion should be used because of glucagon's short half-life in the circulation. Glucagon is not effective in the treatment of alcohol-induced hypoglycemia in chronic alcoholics because of the depletion of liver glycogen stores.

If a patient does not respond clinically to intravenous glucose, glucagon or hydrocortisone should be considered and other causes of coma should be investigated.

## BIBLIOGRAPHY

Campbell PJ, Gerich JE: Mechanisms for prevention, development, and reversal of hypoglycemia. *Adv Intern Med* 33:205, 1988.

Field JB: Hypoglycemia. *Endocrinol Metab Clin North Am* 18:March 1989.

Gerich JE: Oral hypoglycemic agents. *N Engl J Med* 321:1231, 1989.

Hepburn DA, Deary IJ, Frier BM, et al: Symptoms of acute insulin-induced hypoglycemia in humans with and without IDDM. A factor-analysis approach. *Diabetes Care* 14:949, 1991.

Hoeldtke RD, Boden G: Epinephrine secretion, hypoglycemia unawareness, and diabetic autonomic neuropathy. *Ann Intern Med* 120:512, 1994.

Malouf R, Brust JCM: Hypoglycemia: Causes, neurological manifestations, and outcome. *Ann Neurol* 17:421, 1985.

Service FJ, Dale AJD, Elveback LR, et al: Insulinoma: Clinical and diagnostic features of 60 consecutive cases. *Mayo Clin Proc* 51:417, 1976.

**Table 176-5.** Common Sources of 20 g of D-GLUCOSE

| Food | Amount |
| --- | --- |
| Kool-Aid with sugar | 13.4 fl oz* |
| Coke | 13.3 fl oz† |
| Orange soda (Fanta) | 10.0 fl oz† |
| Ginger ale (Fanta) | 15.5 fl oz† |
| Tang (orange with sugar) | 12.0 fl oz* |
| Hershey milk chocolate bar | 2.5 fl oz‡ |
| Gelatin sweetened with sugar | 6.4 oz |
| Orange juice | 12.0 fl oz* |
| Apple juice | 12.0 fl oz* |
| Banana (flecked) | 6.4 oz§ |

* One cup equals 8 oz.

† One can equals 12 oz.

‡ One bar equals 1.45 oz.

§ One large or two small bananas equal 7 oz.

*Source:* Brodows RG, Williams C, Amatruda JM: Treatment of insulin reactions in diabetics. *JAMA* 252:3378, 1984.

# 177
# DIABETIC KETOACIDOSIS
## Gene Ragland

Diabetic ketoacidosis occurs exclusively in the diabetic population. It is characterized by hyperglycemia and ketonemia. A relative deficiency of insulin and a concurrent excess of stress hormones are responsible for the metabolic derangement. Therapy includes the replacement of fluids and insulin using low doses administered with various techniques.

## PATHOPHYSIOLOGY

The major metabolic abnormalities that occur during diabetic ketoacidosis are hyperglycemia and ketonemia. The metabolic derangements can be explained by relative insulin insufficiency and counterregulatory hormone excess. Insulin is the prime anabolic hormone and is responsible for the metabolism and storage of carbohydrates, fats, and proteins. The counterregulatory hormones are glucagon, catecholamines, cortisol, and growth hormone.

### Insulin

Ingested glucose is the primary stimulant of insulin release from the β cells of the pancreas. Insulin acts on the liver to facilitate the uptake of glucose and its conversion to glycogen. Insulin inhibits glycogen breakdown (glycogenolysis) and suppresses gluconeogenesis. The net effect of these actions is to promote the storage of glucose in the form of glycogen.

Insulin's effect on lipid metabolism is to increase lipogenesis in the liver and adipose cells and simultaneously to prevent lipolysis. Insulin promotes the production of triglycerides from free fatty acids and facilitates the storage of fat. The breakdown of triglycerides to free fatty acids and glycerol is inhibited by insulin. The overall result is the conversion of glucose to stored energy as triglycerides.

Insulin's action in protein metabolism is to stimulate the uptake of amino acids into muscle cells and to mediate the incorporation of amino acids into muscle protein. It prevents the release of amino acids from muscle protein and from hepatic protein sources.

Deficiency in the insulin-secretory mechanism of the β cells of the pancreas is the predominant lesion in diabetes mellitus. This defect results in insulin lack that may be partial or total.

Absolute insulin lack is rare but may be found in insulin-dependent diabetes (IDDM) patients. In the typical non-insulin dependent diabetes (NIDDM) patient, secretory failure involves primarily the initial rapid-release phase of insulin secretion. Minimal insulin inadequacy causes a decrease in the storage of body fuels, and β-cell failure is evident only by the abnormal response to a glucose load—abnormal glucose tolerance test. With more severe failure of insulin secretion, not only is fuel storage impaired, but fuel stores are mobilized during fasting, resulting in hyperglycemia. The increase in the blood glucose level is due to increased glycogenolysis and may elicit an increase in insulin secretion if β-cell reserve is present. The glucose metabolism and concentration may then return to normal.

When there is an absolute or relative failure in insulin secretion, hyperglycemia does not produce increased insulin activity. Loss of the normal physiologic effects of insulin results in catabolism, and hyperglycemia and ketonemia occur.

### Counterregulatory Hormones

During insulin insufficiency, glucose transport into the cells is inhibited. The physiologic response to cellular starvation and other stresses is to increase the hormones glucagon, catecholamines, cortisol, and growth hormone. These hormones are grouped as counterregulatory hormones because of their anti-insulin effects. The relative roles of each and their mechanisms of action in diabetic ketoacidosis have not been completely elucidated. However, glucagon in excess has been implicated as the main hormone contributing to hyperglycemia and ketonemia. Excess counterregulatory hormone secretion, in conjunction with relative insulin deficiency, is essential to the development of diabetic ketoacidosis. This is shown by the failure of diabetic animals to develop ketoacidosis in the absence of counterregulatory hormones, the elevation of at least one hormone in every case of diabetic ketoacidosis, a delay or reduction of ketoacidosis with pharmacologic blockade of individual stress hormones, and an increase in ketogenic activity when each of the counterregulatory hormones is infused in high physiologic concentrations. No correlation has been reported between the plasma level of insulin during diabetic ketoacidosis and the severity of the ketoacidosis. Finally, the association between antecedent stress and diabetic ketoacidosis has long been recognized. Secretion of the counterregulatory hormones characterizes all major forms of stress.

The counterregulatory hormones are catabolic and, in general, reverse the physiologic processes promoted by insulin. They affect carbohydrate metabolism by increasing glycogenolysis and gluconeogenesis, thereby raising the blood glucose level. Lipolysis is stimulated by glucagon and catecholamines, and this results in increased free fatty acids for conversion to ketones. Protein breakdown is accelerated and provides amino acids for gluconeogenesis. The net effect of relative insulin insufficiency and excess counterregulatory hormones is hyperglycemia and ketonemia (Figure 177-1).

Hyperglycemia occurs earlier than ketonemia during diabetic ketoacidosis. Glucose is underutilized because of insulin lack and overproduced because of enhanced glycogenolysis and gluconeogenesis. Gluconeogenesis is faciliated by increased levels of glucogenic precursors such as glycerol and amino acids resulting from unopposed lipolysis and proteolysis.

Ketonemia occurs because of increased lipolysis and ketogenesis. Insulin deficiency and excess stress hormones lead to the breakdown of triglycerides and the release of large amounts of fatty acids into the circulation. These fatty acids are assimilated in the liver, where they are converted to ketone bodies. The peripheral utilization of ketones is decreased during insulin insufficiency, and they accumulate in the usual 3:1 ratio (β-hydroxybutyrate to acetoacetate).

Factors known to precipitate diabetic ketoacidosis include omission of daily insulin injections and a variety of stressful events, such as infections, stroke, myocardial infarction, trauma, pregnancy, hyperthyroidism, and pancreatitis. However, in some patients, there is no clear precipitating cause.

## CLINICAL PRESENTATION

Most of the clinical manifestations of diabetic ketoacidosis are related to the biochemical derangements. Hyperglycemia causes an increased osmotic load, and intracellular water is lost because cellular membranes are not freely permeable to glucose. Osmotic diuresis produces total body fluid depletion. Dehydration, hypotension, and reflex tachycardia are consequences. Osmotic diuresis also causes loss of sodium, chloride, potassium, phosphorus, calcium, and magnesium. The serum sodium level may be further decreased by a dilution effect of hyperglycemia. The dilutional effect is a serum sodium decrease of about 5 mEq/L for every 180 mg/dL increase of blood glucose. Electrolyte loss may be worsened by repeated bouts of vomiting.

Dissociation of hydrogen ions from circulating ketone bodies is responsible for the development of acidosis and the fall in the serum bicarbonate level. Some of the ketone bodies are oxidized to acetone, a neutral, soluble, volatile substance that causes the characteristic fruity

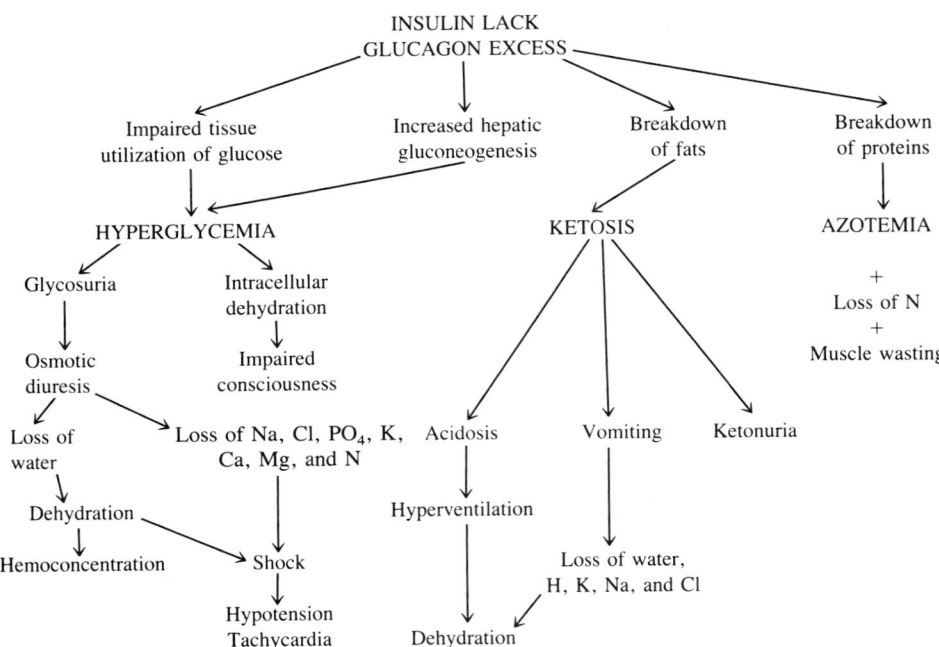

**Fig. 177-1.** Metabolic consequences of insulin lack, accelerated by glucagon excess. (From Baruh S, Sherman L, Markowitz S: Diabetic ketoacidosis and coma. *Med Clin North Am* 65:117, 1981. Used by permission.)

odor on the breath of a patient with ketoacidosis. Hepatomegaly due to accumulation of fat within the liver may occur and should resolve with reversal of ketogenesis.

Acidosis produces other clinical consequences. Compensatory hyperventilation is commonly seen. Exchange of H⁺ ions for K⁺ across the intracellular membrane is partially responsible for the elevated serum potassium level seen in patients in diabetic ketoacidosis. Peripheral vasodilatation and vascular collapse can result from acidosis.

There is no apparent correlation between the state of consciousness of the patient and the degree of ketonemia, hyperglycemia, electrolyte imbalance, or acidosis. The most direct correlation is with serum osmolality. Some degree of mental confusion or coma is more likely with serum osmolality levels above 340 mOsm/kg. In addition, if the serum osmolality is <340 mOsm/kg in a patient with diabetic ketoacidosis, some other cause of coma should be sought.

Nausea, vomiting, and abdominal pain are common presenting complaints. The cause of these disturbances is not clear. Gastric dilatation, paralytic ileus, and abdominal tenderness may be present. Although pancreatitis may develop as a result of ketoacidosis, the diagnosis is difficult since the serum amylase level and the amylase clearance can be elevated in both conditions. Of course, the reverse can occur, so that acute inflammatory or hemorrhagic pancreatitis can result in ketoacidosis. In general, abdominal signs and symptoms should disappear with the resolution of ketoacidosis, and carefully repeated evaluation is necessary to rule out a serious intraabdominal disorder.

Inappropriate normothermia can occur, so that infection must be presumed even in the absence of fever.

Diabetic ketoacidosis may develop rapidly or over a few days. If the patient is able to maintain an adequate fluid and salt intake, a state of compensated ketosis may develop. During the early stages of ketoacidosis or when nausea and vomiting occur, the patient may decrease or omit insulin, thus hastening full-blown diabetic ketoacidosis. The typical patient has nausea, vomiting, abdominal pain, weight loss, dehydration, hypotension, tachycardia, hyperventilation or Kussmaul's respirations, and the odor of acetone on the breath.

## LABORATORY

Laboratory abnormalities that are always present during diabetic ketoacidosis include elevated levels of blood glucose, β-hydroxybutyrate, and acetoacetate. Similarly, glucosuria and ketonuria are con-

sistent findings. A decreased pH, low serum bicarbonate level, and decreased $P_{CO_2}$ are present because of metabolic acidosis with respiratory compensation.

The serum sodium level is variable. More water is lost than solutes, and even if the serum sodium level is low, the patient is hypertonic. Initially, the serum potassium level is usually elevated or normal, but it falls as the acidosis is corrected and potassium shifts intracellularly. The serum chloride level may be low if excessive vomiting has occurred. An increased anion-gap acidosis is present because of ketonemia.

The diagnosis of diabetic ketoacidosis should be suspected based upon the clinical presentation previously described. Confirmatory laboratory findings include a blood glucose level greater than 300 mg/dL, a bicarbonate level less than 15 mEq/L, a serum acetone level greater than 2:1 dilution, and a pH less than 7.3. Venous blood should be drawn for a complete blood cell count and determinations of serum glucose, electrolytes, blood urea nitrogen (BUN), creatinine, phosphorus, calcium, magnesium, and acetone. Arterial blood gases are essential. Urinalysis and a chest roentgenogram to search for infection, and an ECG to identify acute myocardial infarction and hyperkalemia, are necessary.

## Differential Diagnosis

The differential diagnosis of metabolic coma in a diabetic patient includes hypoglycemia, nonketotic hyperosmolar coma, alcoholic ketoacidosis, and lactic acidosis. A rapid differentiation can be made in the emergency department (Figure 177-2). The result of the analysis of blood gases should be available in a few minutes, and acidosis, if present, will be confirmed. While the physician is awaiting other laboratory results, a drop of blood can be tested for blood glucose and serum ketones.

Reagent strips that measure blood glucose levels can be interpreted visually, or can be read in a reflectance meter. Visual interpretation identifies a range but not a precise number, and this method reliably distinguishes between hyperglycemic and hypoglycemic levels. Semiquantitative estimation of serum ketones can be made by testing a drop of blood with a nitroprusside-impregnated tablet. The nitroprusside reaction measures acetoacetate but not β-hydroxybutyrate. This test can be misleading if most of the serum ketones are in the form of β-hydroxybutyrate. Additionally, lactic acidosis may occur simultaneously with diabetic ketoacidosis. Measurement of serum

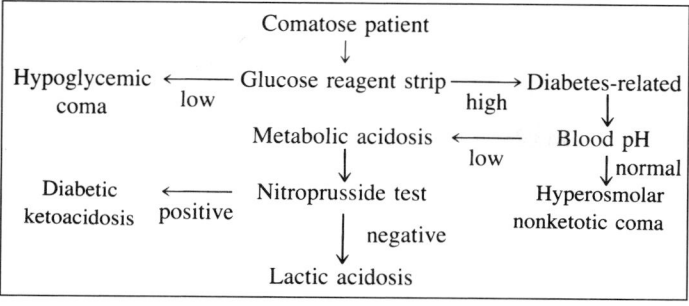

**Fig. 177-2.** Differential diagnosis of metabolic causes of coma in a diabetic patient. (Adapted from Skillman TG: Diabetic ketoacidosis. *Heart Lung* 7:598, 1978. Used by permission.)

lactate levels may be indicated to determine the contribution of lactic acid to the metabolic acidosis. Finally, in mixed acid-base disturbance, the pH may not accurately reflect the degree of acidosis. The anion gap can assist in identifying unmeasured acids.

## TREATMENT

Once the diagnosis of diabetic ketoacidosis has been established, therapy must be started immediately. Specific therapeutic goals include rehydration, correction of electrolyte and acid-base imbalance, reversal of the metabolic consequences of insulin insufficiency, treatment of precipitating causes, and avoidance of complications.

A variety of therapeutic approaches are advocated. Regardless of the approach used, frequent monitoring of the effects is essential. The levels of blood glucose, the anion gap, potassium, and carbon dioxide should be determined every 1 to 2 h until recovery is well-established. A flow sheet to record vital signs, level of consciousness, intake and output, therapeutic measures, and blood chemistry determinations is recommended. Complete clearing of hyperglycemia and ketonemia usually requires 8 to 16 h.

### Fluid Administration

Rapid fluid administration is the most important initial step in the treatment of diabetic ketoacidosis. The average patient in diabetic ketoacidosis has a water deficit of 5 to 10 L and a sodium deficit of 450 to 500 mEq. Normal saline is the most frequently recommended fluid for initial rehydration even though the extracellular fluid of the patient is hypertonic. The normal saline does not provide "free water" to correct intracellular dehydration, but it does prevent a too-rapid fall in extracellular osmolality and excessive transfer of water into the central nervous system (CNS). Most authors favor alternating the administration of normal saline with the administration of half-normal saline.

The first liter of fluid should be administered rapidly, usually over $^1/_2$ to 1 h. During the first 3 to 4 h, 3 to 5 L of fluid may be required. The blood glucose level and ketone body concentration fall after fluid administration and before implementation of any other therapeutic modality. With rehydration, tissue perfusion is restored, improving the effectiveness of insulin, and renal blood flow increases, allowing the excretion of ketone bodies.

The fluid should be changed to a hypotonic solution after the initial replacement of intravascular volume or if the serum sodium level is 155 mEq/L. Central venous pressure or pulmonary artery wedge pressure should be monitored during fluid replacement in the elderly patients or those with heart disease.

### Bicarbonate

Sodium bicarbonate is given to correct the negative effects of acidosis. At a pH of 7, peripheral vasodilatation, decreased cardiac output, and hypotension can occur. Respiratory and CNS depression can occur with severe acidosis (pH less than 6.8).

The hazards of excessive alkali replacement can outweigh the potential benefits. These include paradoxical spinal fluid acidosis, hypokalemia, impaired oxyhemoglobin dissociation, rebound alkalosis, and sodium overload.

It has been established that cerebrospinal fluid (CSF) acidosis is deleterious to brain function. Systemic acidosis per se does not cause mental aberration as long as the CSF is protected against large pH changes. When sodium bicarbonate is administered in large doses, the carbon dioxide loss is diminished, and extracellular fluid and levels of carbon dioxide and bicarbonate increase. Carbon dioxide diffuses freely across the blood-brain barrier, but bicarbonate diffuses into the CSF much more slowly. The difference in the rates of movement into the spinal fluid results in an increase in CSF carbonic acid, a fall in CSF pH, and paradoxical spinal fluid acidosis.

Alkali administration causes a shift of potassium intracellularly. In a patient who already has total body potassium depletion, severe hypokalemia could result. During acidosis, the oxyhemoglobin dissociation curve shifts to the right, facilitating the off-loading of oxygen at the tissue level. This beneficial effect of acidosis could be lost with sudden restoration of the pH toward normal. Final complications of excessive sodium bicarbonate administration include overcompensated rebound alkalosis and sodium overload.

Current recommendations are to administer sodium bicarbonate in modest amounts, i.e., 44 to 100 mEq, when the pH is less than 6.9 for adults. Some studies have shown that use of bicarbonate therapy in patients with diabetic ketoacidosis has provided no beneficial effects in terms of clinical recovery or biochemical variables, even with a pH as low as 6.9. Hydrogen ion production ceases when ketogenesis stops; excessive hydrogen ions are eliminated through the urine and through the respiratory tract, and ketone body metabolism results in the endogenous production of alkali.

### Potassium

The deficiency of total body potassium is created by insulin deficit, acidosis, diuresis, and frequent vomiting. The potassium deficit is about 3 to 5 mEq/kg. The initial serum potassium level is usually normal or high because of a deficit of body fluid, diminished renal function, and intracellular exchange of potassium for hydrogen ions during acidosis. Initial hypokalemia indicates severe total body potassium depletion, and massive amounts of potassium for replacement are required during the next 24 h.

The goals of potassium replacement are to maintain a normal extracellular potassium concentration during the acute phases of therapy and to replace the intracellular deficit over a period of days or weeks. With initiation of therapy for diabetic ketoacidosis, the serum potassium concentration falls. This is due to dilution of extracellular fluid, correction of acidosis, increased urinary loss of potassium, and the action of insulin in promoting reentry of potassium into the cells. If these changes occur too rapidly, precipitous hypokalemia may result in fatal cardiac arrhythmias, respiratory paralysis, and paralytic ileus. These complications are avoidable if the pathophysiology is understood and the effects of therapy are frequently monitored.

The ability of insulin to drive potassium into the cells is directly proportional to the insulin concentration. Low-dose insulin therapy provides greater stabilization of the extracellular potassium concentration during the early stages of therapy.

Early potassium replacement is now a standard modality of care. Some authors recommend that small doses of potassium (20 mEq) be added to the intravenous fluid given initially. Others favor administering potassium within the first 2 to 3 h, when insulin therapy is initiated, or after volume expansion has been accomplished. If oliguria is present, renal function must be evaluated and potassium replacement must be decreased. Potassium determinations every 1 to 2 h and continuous ECG monitoring for changes reflecting the potassium concentration should be employed. From 100 to 200 mEq of potassium during the first 12 to 24 h is usually required. Occasionally, as much as 500 mEq of potassium may be necessary.

## Insulin

Familiarity with a particular insulin replacement regimen, continuous monitoring, and attention to detail are the most important factors in successfully treating a patient in diabetic ketoacidosis. The amount and route of insulin administration are of secondary importance.

Large doses of insulin are not required to reverse the metabolic derangements of diabetic ketoacidosis and hypoglycemia, osmotic disequilibrium, and hypokalemia are more frequent with large-dose insulin therapy.

Low-dose insulin techniques for treatment of diabetic ketoacidosis are simple, safe, and effective. Techniques for continuous intravenous infusion and intramuscular, subcutaneous, and intravenous bolus therapy have been developed. Blood insulin concentrations of 20 to 200 μ units/mL inhibit gluconeogenesis and lipogenesis, stimulate the uptake of potassium by peripheral tissues, and achieve maximum rates of fall of blood glucose concentrations. A continuous insulin infusion of 1 units/h raises the plasma insulin concentration by 20 μ units/mL. Similarly, 5 units/h produces a therapeutic level of 100 μ units/mL. This level is generally sufficient to achieve normal metabolic homeostasis. The half-life of insulin given intravenously is 4 to 5 min, with an effective biological half-life at the tissue level of approximately 20 to 30 min.

Hypoglycemia using low-dose insulin techniques is almost nonexistent as long as monitoring is done carefully. With low-dose insulin therapies and proper potassium replacement, the occurrence of hypokalemia is less than 5 percent. The more gradual, even insulin effect achieved by low-dose therapy avoids rapid osmotic fluid shifts and the development of cerebral edema.

All low-dose insulin techniques are effective in reversing the metabolic consequences of insulin insufficiency (Figure 177-3). In continuous intravenous infusion of low doses of insulin, 5 to 10 units of regular insulin are administered per hour. The effect of insulin begins almost immediately after the initiation of the infusion, and a "priming" intravenous bolus is not required. Continuous insulin administration ensures that a steady blood concentration is maintained in an effective range, and this technique allows flexibility in adjusting the insulin dose. When the infusion is stopped, the insulin already in the blood is quickly degraded, providing greater control of the amount of insulin given in comparison with the intramuscular or subcutaneous routes.

Serious complications with continuous intravenous low-dose insulin infusion are minimal. The main disadvantage is that it requires an infusion pump and frequent monitoring to ensure that insulin is being administered in the desired amount. A separate intravenous site for the insulin infusion is desirable but not required.

The technique of low-dose intramuscular or subcutaneous insulin therapy is better suited to a hospital environment in which constant nursing supervision is not always possible. The main disadvantage to this approach, more marked with the subcutaneous route, is that insulin absorption may be erratic in a hypotensive, peripherally vasoconstricted patient. Erratic absorption may result in a delay in achieving adequate insulin levels. Further, delayed absorption can produce deposits of insulin that may later be absorbed, causing hypoglycemia. These problems can largely be eliminated by ensuring adequate hydration of the patient and by using small enough doses of insulin to preclude accumulation of large insulin deposits.

The onset of action of insulin given intramuscularly is delayed in comparison with that of insulin given intravenously. The most current protocols recommend an initial dose of 20 units of insulin intramuscularly, intravenously, or divided between these routes, followed by 5 to 10 units/h intramuscularly. The half-life of insulin given intramuscularly is 2 h. Hourly injections produce a continuous, effective blood concentration of insulin.

There are common problems with insulin therapy regardless of the technique used. The incidence of nonresponders to low-dose therapies is 1 to 2 percent. Infection is the main reason for failure to respond to low-dose insulin therapy. If the patient fails to respond to low-dose insulin therapy in the first hour, most protocols recommend doubling the infusion rate or administering an intravenous bolus of insulin. The insulin dose is increased in a similar fashion each hour until a satisfactory response is achieved.

Glucose should be added to the intravenous fluid when the blood glucose concentration falls to 250 mg/dL. Insulin therapy should not be stopped just because the blood glucose level declines but should be continued until the ketonemia and acidosis have cleared. Intravenous insulin should not be abruptly discontinued. An overlap period in which subcutaneous insulin is given should precede discontinuation of the insulin infusion.

## Phosphate Replacement

The role of phosphate replacement during the treatment of diabetic ketoacidosis remains controversial. Hyperphosphatemia is the initial finding in most cases of diabetic ketoacidosis. However, one author estimates that up to 90 percent of patients have acute hypophosphatemia within 6 to 12 h after initiation of therapy for diabetic ketoacidosis. The decrease is primarily due to a sudden shift of phosphate from the extracellular to the intracellular compartment following insulin administration and accelerated glucose storage. Phosphate is found in all body tissues, and this sudden shift deprives them of this essential constituent. Hypophosphatemia is usually most severe 24 to 48 h after the start of insulin therapy.

Phosphate plays an integral part in the conversion of energy from adenosine triphosphate (ATP) and in the delivery of oxygen at the tissue level through 2,3-diphosphoglyceric acid (2,3-DPG). In addition, many important enzymes, cofactors, and biochemical intermediates depend upon phosphate. Acute phosphate deficiency has been associated with a variety of clinical disorders including neuromuscular paralysis leading to respiratory failure and possibly myocardial dysfunction.

Acute hypophosphatemia can be corrected by intravenous or oral administration of phosphorus. Several oral forms are available but may cause diarrhea and be erratically absorbed. A commercial intravenous preparation ($KH_2PO_4$ plus $K_2HPO_4$) containing $K^+$ at a con-

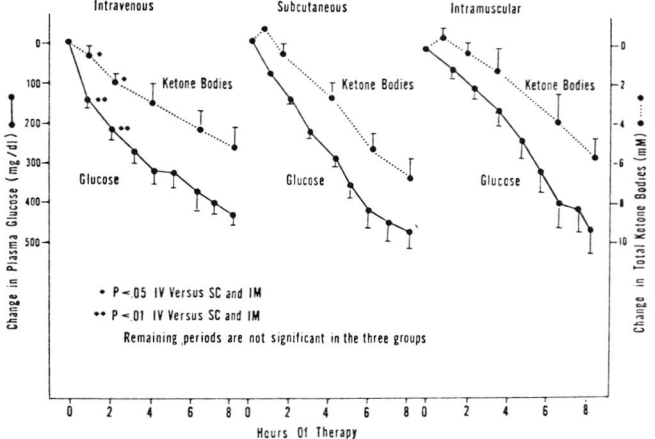

**Fig. 177-3.** Change in levels of plasma glucose and total ketone bodies (β-hydroxybutyrate plus acetoacetate) after intravenous, subcutaneous, or intramuscular low-dose insulin therapy (15 patients in each group). (From Fisher JN, Shahshahani MN, Kitabchi AE: Diabetic ketoacidosis: Low-dose insulin therapy by various routes. *N Engl J Med* 297:238, 1977. Used by permission.)

centration of 4 mEq/mL and phosphorus at a concentration of 96 mg/mL can be used. Five milliliters of this commercial potassium phosphate preparation added to 1 L of intravenous fluid provides approximately 20 mEq of $K^+$ and 480 mg of $PO_4^{2+}$.

Hypophosphatemia is not associated with untoward consequences until a serum concentration of less than 1.0 mg/dL is reached. Phosphorus supplementation is not indicated and should not be given as long as the level remains above this concentration. Some authors have recommended the use of potassium phosphate salts instead of potassium chloride as a means of potassium replacement during therapy for diabetic ketoacidosis. Early routine use of potassium phosphate solutions to replace potassium should be discouraged. The need for phosphorus replacement, if at all, occurs several hours after therapy for diabetic ketoacidosis has begun, and potassium is usually required much sooner.

Several undesirable side effects from phosphate administration have been reported. These include hyperphosphatemia, hypocalcemia, hypomagnesemia, metastatic soft tissue calcifications, and hypernatremia and dehydration from osmotic diuresis. The serum phosphate level should be monitored during treatment of diabetic ketoacidosis, but the case for routine phosphate replacement has not been made.

## COMPLICATIONS AND MORTALITY

Complications related to the disease state include aspiration of gastric contents by an unconscious patient, vascular stasis and deep vein thrombosis, and disseminated intravascular coagulation (DIC). Rhabdomyolysis during diabetic ketoacidosis has also been recently reported. Protection of the airway and evacuation of gastric contents are indicated in an unconscious patient. Prophylactic heparin therapy may help to prevent thrombotic complications.

Major complications related to the therapy of diabetic ketoacidosis include hypoglycemia, hypokalemia, paradoxical spinal fluid acidosis, and cerebral edema. The goal of therapy of diabetic ketoacidosis is to produce a gradual, even return to normal metabolic balance. Rapids shifts of the levels of water, electrolytes, and other solutes can be avoided by using isotonic saline as the initial intravenous fluid, refraining from excessive bicarbonate administration, replacing potassium early in the course of treatment, and using low-dose insulin techniques. Above all, a basic understanding of the pathophysiology of diabetic ketoacidosis, constant monitoring of the patient, and attention to detail are essential to prevent complications of treatment.

The development of cerebral edema during the treatment of diabetic ketoacidosis, especially in young patients, is a continuing problem. An extensive review found no specific treatment variables that contributed to the development of cerebral edema. Variables included overhydration, rapid osmolar changes, hemodynamic compromise and hypoxia. Young age and new-onset diabetes were the only identified contributing risk factors.

Approximately one-half of the patients who developed cerebral edema had premonitory symptoms of severe headache, incontinence, change in arousal or behavior, pupillary changes, blood pressure changes, seizures, bradycardia, or disturbed temperature regulation. Early recognition of neurologic deterioration and treatment of cerebral edema by hyperventilation and mannitol is the best hope for survival of this disastrous complication.

In general, the greater the presenting serum osmolality, blood urea nitrogen (BUN), and blood glucose concentration, the greater the mortality. There is also increased mortality for patients presenting with a serum bicarbonate level of less than 10 mEq/L.

Of the factors responsibile for precipitating diabetic ketoacidosis, infection and myocardial infarction are the main contributors to high mortality. Half the patients in diabetic ketoacidosis die when myocardial infarction is the precipitating event. Additional factors that reduce the chances of survival include old age, severe hypotension, prolonged and severe coma, and underlying renal and cardiovascular disease.

## BIBLIOGRAPHY

Fisher JN, Kitabchi AE: A randomized study of phosphate therapy in the treatment of diabetic ketoacidosis. *J Clin Endocrinol Metab* 57:177, 1983.

Fisher JN, Shahshahani MN, Kitabchi AE: Diabetic ketoacidosis: Low-dose insulin therapy by various routes. *N Engl J Med* 297:238, 1977.

Foster DW, McGarry JD: The metabolic derangements and treatment of diabetic ketoacidosis. *N Engl J Med* 309:159, 1983.

Kitabchi AE: Low-dose insulin therapy in diabetic ketoacidosis: Fact or fiction? *Diabetes Metab Rev* 5:337, 1989.

Page MM, Alberti KGMM, Greenwood R, et al: Treatment of diabetic coma with continuous low-dose infusion of insulin. *Br Med J* 2:687, 1974.

Rosenbloom AL: Intracerebral crises during treatment of diabetic ketoacidosis. *Diabetes Care* 13:22, 1990.

# 178
# ALCOHOLIC KETOACIDOSIS
## Gene Ragland

Alcoholic ketoacidosis is characterized by an anion gap acidosis due to high levels of ketoacids. It occurs exclusively in relation to alcohol abuse but not just in chronic alcoholics. It has been reported in first-time drinkers whose food intake is minimal.

The true incidence is unknown, and the frequency is probably directly related to the incidence of alcoholism in a population.

## PATHOPHYSIOLOGY

Several mechanisms have been postulated. In one explanation, ketosis results from increased mobilization of free fatty acids from adipose tissue coupled with simultaneous enhancement of the liver's capacity to convert these substrates into acetoacetate and β-hydroxybutyrate.

During the metabolism of alcohol in the liver the rate of nicotinamide adenine dinucleotide (NAD) reduction exceeds the rate of mitochondrial NADH oxidation, causing a decrease in available NAD. This state persists for a few days in spite of no further alcohol consumption. An NAD-dependent step in the oxidation of fatty acids in the mitochondria of the hepatocyte is displaced in favor of ketone body formation.

During alcoholic ketoacidosis insulin levels are low, whereas levels of cortisol, growth hormone, glucagon, and epinephrine are increased, possibly as a result of alcohol-induced hypoglycemia. This hormonal milieu promotes lipolysis, which increases the levels of free fatty acids available for conversion to ketones.

Additional mechanisms that may contribute to ketosis include the conversion of acetate, an alcohol breakdown product, to ketones; alcohol-induced mitochondrial structural changes which enhance the rate of ketosis; and mitochondrial phosphorus depletion, which inhibits the utilization for NADH and increases ketone body formation. Finally, vomiting and starvation superimposed on chronic malnutrition also contribute to ketoacidosis.

## CLINICAL PRESENTATION

The usual history is one of heavy alcohol consumption or binge drinking with decreased or absent food intake for several days. Food and alcohol intake are usually terminated by nausea, protracted vomiting, and abdominal pain occurring 24 to 72 h before presentation. It is during this period that ketoacidosis develops.

Clinically the patient appears acutely ill with dehydration, tachypnea, tachycardia, and diffuse abdominal pain. Most patients are alert, but they may be mildly disoriented or occasionally comatose.

There are no specific physical findings. Evidence of dehydration such as hypotension, orthostatic changes in blood pressure, tachycardia, and decreased urine output may be present. The temperature varies from hypothermia to mildly elevated. Abdominal pain due to non-specific causes or due to gastritis, pancreatitis, or hepatitis is common. Sepsis, meningitis, pyelonephritis, or pneumonia may be present, and delirium tremens may develop.

## LABORATORY

Alcohol levels are usually low or undetectable, as the alcohol intake is decreased or discontinued during the period of anorexia and vomiting. Essential to the diagnosis of alcoholic ketoacidosis is a large anion gap due to high levels of serum ketones. Most patients have a blood pH reflective of the underlying metabolic acidosis, but many may present with normal or alkalemic pH values.

### Acid-Base Balance

Fulop and Hoberman compared typical laboratory data from patients with diabetic ketoacidosis with data from patients with alcoholic ketoacidosis (Table 178-1). The alcoholic patients tended to have a higher blood pH, lower levels of serum $K^+$ and $Cl^-$, and a higher level of plasma $HCO_3^-$ than the diabetic patients. This difference is attributed to the severe recurrent vomiting experienced by the alcoholic patients. Vomiting causes chloride depletion and metabolic alkalosis. In addition, respiratory alkalosis may occur secondary to fever, sepsis, or alcohol withdrawal and further increases the blood pH.

### Ketones

The anion gap $[Na^+ - (Cl^- + HCO_3^-) = 12 \pm 4$ mEq/L] in the patient groups is very similar and is due primarily to high levels of β-hydroxybutyrate and to a lesser extent to lactic acid accumulation. The principal ketones are acetoacetate and β-hydroxybutyrate. These ketones are intermediates in the oxidation of fatty acids; they are normally produced in equal amounts and are not normally detectable in the serum. Acetoacetate and β-hydroxybutyrate are a redox pair and are interconverted by an oxidation-reduction reaction with NAD and NADH as cofactors. In alcoholic ketoacidosis, perhaps because of lack of NAD, β-hydroxybutyrate accumulates to levels several times higher than the levels of acetoacetate. Acetone is a volatile, neutral ketone that is formed from acetoacetate by irreversible spontaneous decarboxylation. Its presence reflects the level and duration of acetoacetate elevation and is indicative of a sustained, severe acidosis.

### Nitroprusside Test

The nitroprusside test is used to detect the presence of ketones in serum and urine. This is a semiquantitative test that gives a reaction with acetoacetate, is less sensitive to acetone, and does not detect β-hydroxybutyrate at all. There is no practical test that measures β-hydroxybutyrate levels. In most series on alcoholic ketoacidosis, the nitroprusside test has shown moderate or large ketonemia or ketonuria. But in a significant minority of patients, the reaction may be weakly positive or negative even though ketoacidosis, because of high levels of β-hydroxybutyrate, is pronounced. Reliance on this test alone as a measure of ketoacidosis may lead to failure to recognize the presence of ketoacidosis or to an underestimation of the severity of the ketoacidosis.

### Glucose

The blood glucose level in alcoholic ketoacidosis varies from hypoglycemia to mild elevation. In most series it is normal or slightly increased. Glucosuria is usually mild or absent. A subset of alcoholic patients in whom hypoglycemia and ketoacidosis are coexistent has been described.

The pathogenesis of alcohol-induced hypoglycemia includes acute starvation, depletion of liver glycogen stores because of chronic malnutrition, and inhibition of gluconeogenesis because of alcohol-induced alteration of the NAD/NADH ratio. Alcohol also causes decreased peripheral utilization of glucose, and this acts to balance the glucose-depleting processes. Devenyi asks if alcoholic hypoglycemia and alcoholic ketoacidosis are sequential events of the same process. He theorizes that alcohol-induced hypoglycemia occurs first, causing increased levels of cortisol, growth hormone, glucagon, and epinephrine; this may correct the hypoglycemia and mobilize free fatty acids,

**Table 178-1.** Comparison of Admission Laboratory Data in Patients with Diabetic Ketoacidosis and Alcoholic Ketosis*

| Variable† | Diabetic Ketoacidosis | | Alcoholic Ketoacidosis ($N = 18$) |
|---|---|---|---|
| | Oh and Co-workers ($N = 35$) | Our Series ($N = 27$) | |
| Blood pH | $7.07 \pm 0$ | $7.17 \pm 0.02$ | $7.35 \pm 0.05$ |
| Serum $Na^-$ | $135.5 \pm 1.6$ | $133.0 \pm 1.2$ | $135.2 \pm 1.6$ |
| Serum $K^+$ | | $4.9 \pm 0.2$ | $4.1 \pm 0.3$ |
| Serum $Cl^-$ | $101.0 \pm 1.4$ | $97.3 \pm 1.1$ | $90.9 \pm 3.9$ |
| Plasma $HCO_3^-$ | $9.4‡$ | $6.7 \pm 0.6$ | $16.5 \pm 2.4$ |
| $\Delta HCO_3^-$ | $14.6$ | $17.3 \pm 0.6$ | $7.5 \pm 2.4$ |
| Anion gap§ | $26.1$ | $28.9 \pm 1.1$ | $27.8 \pm 2.5$ |
| Plasma lactate | $2.7 \pm 0.3$ | $2.1 \pm 0.1$ | $3.9 \pm 1.2$ |
| Plasma β-hydroxybutyrate | $10.3 \pm 0.3$ | $10.8 \pm 0.6$ | $9.3 \pm 1.1$ |
| Plasma lactate + β-hydroxybutyrate | $13.0$ | $12.9 \pm 0.6$ | $13.2 \pm 1.6$ |
| Excess anion gap¶ | $14.1$ | $17.0 \pm 1.1$ | $15.8 \pm 2.5$ |

* Data given as mean $\pm$ SEM.

† All units except blood pH are in mEq/L.

‡ This and all succeeding values in this column refer to 15 patients.

§ Calculated as serum $Na^+ - (Cl^- + HCO_3^-)$.

¶ Calculated as anion gap $- 12$ mEq/L.

*Source:* Fulop M, Hoberman HD: Diabetic ketoacidosis and alcoholic ketoacidosis. *Ann Intern Med* 91:796, 1979.

which are converted to ketones. If this theory is correct, the diagnosis of alcoholic hypoglycemia or alcoholic ketoacidosis may depend upon the point in this process at which the disorder is detected.

## DIAGNOSIS

The diagnosis of alcoholic ketoacidosis is easily established in those patients with an antecedent history of alcohol intake, decreased food intake, vomiting, and abdominal pain, and laboratory findings of metabolic acidosis, a positive nitroprusside test, and a low or mildly elevated glucose level.

Several factors may contribute to the failure to recognize this metabolic disorder. The blood alcohol level may be zero, and, in the absence of a history of alcohol intake, this diagnosis may not be considered. The nitroprusside test may be weakly positive or negative in spite of significant ketoacidosis. The pH may be mildly acidotic, normal, or even alkalemic in the face of pronounced metabolic acidosis. There are no specific physical findings which suggest the diagnosis of alcoholic ketoacidosis. Alcoholic patients may have a variety of alcohol-induced associated illnesses which may obscure or distract from this diagnosis. Mental confusion or coma may be incorrectly attributed to alcoholic intoxication or other causes if the appropriate laboratory studies are not performed or if they are incorrectly interpreted.

Soffer and Hamburger's criteria to define alcoholic ketoacidosis are a serum glucose level less than 300 mg/dL, a recent history of alcohol intake with a relative or absolute decline in ethanol consumption 24 to 72 h before hospitalization, a history of vomiting, and a metabolic acidosis for which other causes, such as diabetic ketoacidosis, lactic acidosis, renal failure, or drug ingestion, are excluded by clinical observations or laboratory studies. A positive serum nitroprusside test, because of its limitations, is not a criterion for diagnosis.

### Differential Diagnosis

A positive nitroprusside test and a very low plasma bicarbonate concentration suggest ketosis with a high level of β-hydroxybutyrate. The combination of a barely positive nitroprusside test and a low plasma bicarbonate concentration signifies either a very reduced state with high concentrations of β-hydroxybutyrate or else a coincidental lactic acidosis. The measurement of serum lactate levels aids in this differential diagnosis.

The entity with which alcoholic ketoacidosis is most often confused is diabetic ketoacidosis. The magnitude of ketoacidosis is equal in these two disorders. It is important to make the proper distinction, as the treatment of each entity is different. In diabetic ketoacidosis, hyperglycemia and glucosuria are present. The serum glucose level in alcoholic ketoacidosis varies from hypoglycemia to mild elevation, and glucosuria is usually mild or absent. This differential diagnosis can be made in the emergency department.

## TREATMENT

Therapy of alcoholic ketoacidosis is simple and effective and consists of the intravenous administration of a glucose and saline solution. Patients given only saline improve, but not as rapidly as those who are also given glucose. Thiamine, 50 to 100 mg intravenously, should be given before the glucose to prevent precipitation of Wernicke's disease. Reversal of ketoacidosis usually occurs in 12 to 18 h.

Restoration of intravascular volume is best accomplished by alternating infusions of glucose-containing normal and half-normal saline. Volume repletion is necessary to correct insulin-release inhibition by adrenergic nerve endings in the islets of Langerhans as well as by circulating catecholamines. Glucose infusion stimulates insulin release, and insulin inhibits lipolysis and terminates ketoacid production. Glucose may inhibit further ketoacid production by increasing oxidation

of accumulated NADH via glucose-induced uptake of phosphorus by the hepatic mitochondria.

Exogenous administration of insulin is not indicated in treatment of alcoholic ketoacidosis; this aspect of therapy differs from therapy of diabetic ketoacidosis. Inappropriate administration of insulin to a patient with a normal or low glucose level could be dangerous.

Administration of sodium bicarbonate is usually not required. As ketoacid levels fall, plasma bicarbonate levels increase, and the pH returns to normal. A small amount of bicarbonate may be indicated if the pH is less than 7.1 or if the patient is clinically deteriorating as evidenced by a weak, rapid pulse, hypotension, or inability to compensate by hyperventilation because of weakness. The role of phosphorus replenishment in therapy of alcoholic ketoacidosis is not clear.

With recovery and reversal of the acidosis, β-hydroxybutyrate is converted to acetoacetate. As this process occurs, the nitroprusside test becomes more positive because of higher levels of acetoacetate. This factitious hyperketonemia may cause the uninformed clinician unnecessary concern, as it appears that the ketoacidosis is worsening. Clinical improvement of the patient and increasing blood pH values are more reliable parameters of recovery than the nitroprusside test.

The survival rates of patients with alcoholic ketoacidosis are good. Those patients that die usually do so because of other complications of chronic alcoholism. A thorough search for and treatment of associated alcoholic disorders is essential. Recurrent episodes of alcoholic ketoacidosis after subsequent alcoholic debauch are not uncommon.

## BIBLIOGRAPHY

Fulop M, Ben-Ezra J, Bock J: Alcoholic ketosis. *Alcoholism: Clin Exp Res* 10:610, 1986.
Fulop M, Hoberman HD: Alcoholic ketosis. *Diabetes* 24:785, 1975.
Levy LJ, Duga J, Girgis M, et al: Ketoacidosis associated with alcoholism in nondiabetic subjects. *Ann Intern Med* 78:213, 1973.
Miller PD, Heinig RE, Waterhouse C: Treatment of alcoholic acidosis—The role of dextrose and phosphorus. *Arch Intern Med* 138:67, 1978.
Soffer A, Hamburger S: Alcoholic ketoacidosis: A review of 30 cases. *J Am Med Wom Assoc* 37:106, 1982.

# 179
# NONKETOTIC HYPEROSMOLAR COMA
## Gene Ragland

Nonketotic hyperosmolar coma is characterized by severe hyperglycemia, hyperosmolality, and dehydration, but no ketoacidosis. This metabolic derangement occurs primarily in diabetics but may occur in nondiabetics under certain circumstances. Many names have been used to identify this entity, but the term *nonketotic hyperosmolar coma* is used in this chapter.

This syndrome shares many features with diabetic ketoacidosis, including hyperglycemia and hyperosmolality, but the lack of ketoacidosis is its main distinguishing feature. Nonketotic hyperosmolar coma is much less common than diabetic ketoacidosis. Nonketotic hyperosmolar coma and diabetic ketoacidosis are part of a continuum, and when present in pure form, they represent the opposite ends of a spectrum with regard to lipid mobilization. In general, a patient with nonketotic hyperosmolar coma has a blood glucose concentration greater than 800 mg/dL, usually 1000 mg/dL or more, a serum osmolality greater than 350 mOsm/kg, and a negative test for serum ketones. By comparison, the average blood glucose level of a patient in diabetic ketoacidosis is usually less than 600 mg/dL, the serum osmolality is rarely above 350 mOsm/kg, and the test for serum ketones is strongly positive.

Nonketotic hyperosmolar coma occurs most commonly as the initial manifestation of non-insulin dependent diabetes (NIDDM). Most known diabetics who develop this syndrome have mild, NIDDM controlled by diet or oral hypoglycemic agents. A small minority of insulin-dependent patients on parenteral therapy develop nonketotic hyperosmolar coma. Both extremes—nonketotic hyperosmolar coma and diabetic ketoacidosis—have been reported to occur in the same patient.

## PATHOPHYSIOLOGY

Any explanation of the pathogenesis of nonketotic hyperosmolar coma must explain why extreme hyperglycemia develops and why ketoacidosis does not. Neither of these questions has been answered with certainty. Simply put, extreme hyperglycemia develops because ketoacidosis does not. The failure of ketoacidosis to occur allows the underlying process to continue unrecognized and much higher levels of glucose to result. In addition, glucose enters the extracellular space more rapidly than it is excreted, leading to profound hyperglycemia.

When a patient with NIDDM is subjected to stress, the β cells of the pancreas respond to the increased glucose concentration by increasing the secretion of insulin. Continued diabetogenic stress eventually exhausts the insulinogenic reserve of the β cells, and plasma insulin levels fall. Because of the increased insulinogenic capacity of the patient with mild diabetes, higher levels of blood glucose occur before this reserve is depleted. If the patient is receiving insulin therapy, supplemental insulin allows additional time for β-cell recovery and further prolongs the time required for exhaustion of the insulin reserve. In addition, elevated levels of glucagon may promote gluconeogenesis in the liver, resulting in massive hyperglycemia.

The reason ketoacidosis does not occur is not well understood, and explanations conflict. Some have found low levels of free fatty acids (FFAs), with normal insulin, glucocorticoid, and growth hormone levels. They believe that inhibition of lipolysis occurs because of relatively higher circulating insulin levels or lower lipolytic hormone levels than are present with diabetic ketoacidosis. When lipolysis is inhibited, the precursors required for ketone body formation are not released and ketoacidosis does not develop. It is known that the quantity of insulin required to inhibit lipolysis in adipose tissue is less than the quantity required to promote the utilization of glucose by peripheral tissues. Ketoacidosis may not develop because there is enough circulating insulin to inhibit lipolysis but an insufficient amount to protect against the development of hyperglycemia.

Others have reported similar high FFA levels and low circulating insulin levels in both nonketotic hyperosmolar coma and diabetic ketoacidosis. Additionally, glucagon and glucocorticoids (cortisol) have been found to be increased to the same extent in both conditions. These authors conclude that in nonketotic hyperosmolar coma the FFAs are mobilized to the same extent as in diabetic ketoacidosis, but that the intrahepatic oxidation of the incoming FFAs is directed along nonketogenic metabolic pathways, such as triglyceride synthesis, because of relatively low but adequate insulin action in the liver. Prehepatic and posthepatic insulin levels have been measured. In diabetic ketoacidosis, both pre- and posthepatic insulin levels are low, but in nonketotic hyperosmolar coma, prehepatic insulin levels twice the posthepatic ones have been found. Subscribers to this theory conclude that the liver is selectively bathed in insulin while the periphery is in a "diabetic" state. They conclude that the available insulin exerts its antiketogenic effect at the hepatic and not the adipocyte level.

Regardless of the pathogenesis of nonketotic hyperosmolar coma, the effect of hyperglycemia in producing osmotic diuresis and fluid and electrolyte imbalance is understood. When relative insulin insufficiency develops in the diabetic patient, osmotically active glucose is located in the extracellular fluid compartment. During insulin insufficiency the cell membrane is not freely permeable to glucose, and water is drawn from the intracellular compartment into the extracellular compartment in an attempt to achieve equal osmolality. The presence of large amounts of glucose in the extracellular compartment tends to preserve that compartment at the expense of cellular volume. Relative expansion of the extracellular fluid volume may protect against hypotension until late in the course of nonketotic hyperosmolar coma.

In addition to the internal shifts in body fluids, an osmotic diuresis also occurs. Normally, antidiuretic hormone (ADH) from the posterior pituitary gland acts to maintain water balance. With severe hyperglycemia, glucosuria produces an increased volume and rate of urine flow through the kidneys. Despite maximum levels of ADH, water can no longer be maximally reabsorbed, and an increased volume of urine results. Total body water is decreased and serum osmolality is increased. Fluid losses during nonketotic hyperosmolar coma range from 8 to 12 L.

Sodium balance is also upset by osmotic diuresis. Sodium reabsorption normally occurs in the distal tubules, mediated by the renin-aldosterone system. The concentration gradient against which sodium must be actively transported into the distal tubules is increased as water reabsorption diminishes. Thus a large proportion of the filtered sodium remains unabsorbed and passes into the urine. Nevertheless, the water loss during osmotic diuresis is greater than the sodium loss, and the patient becomes hypertonic relative to sodium. Prolonged diuresis results in hypovolemia and hypertonic dehydration.

Total body potassium depletion is also a consequence of osmotic diuresis. The distal tubules are under maximal stimulation by aldosterone, and some sodium is reabsorbed in exchange for potassium. Because of the longer duration of osmotic diuresis with nonketotic hyperosmolar coma, potassium depletion is greater than that which occurs with diabetic ketoacidosis and may reach 400 to 1000 mEq. Potassium depletion may not become evident until the patient is rehydrated. Other solutes such as magnesium and phosphate are also lost during osmotic diuresis (see Fig. 179-1).

## CLINICAL PRESENTATION

Nonketotic hyperosmolar coma is most common in the middle-aged or elderly and occurs most commonly in diabetics, although the majority are undiagnosed at the time of presentation. Patients who depend upon others to meet their needs, such as infants, nursing home patients, and the mentally retarded, are particularly vulnerable to its insidious onset. Inaccessibility to water coupled with an inability to communicate masks the early signs and symptoms.

### Precipitating Factors

Minor upper respiratory infection or gastroenteritis is capable of precipitating diabetic ketoacidosis, but an illness of greater magnitude is usually required before nonketotic hyperosmolar coma results. Infection is a common precipitating cause, especially gram-negative pneumonias. Other precipitating illnesses include myocardial infarction, cerebrovascular accidents, gastrointestinal (GI) hemorrhage, acute pyelonephritis, acute pancreatitis, uremia, subdural hematomas, and peripheral vascular occlusion. Chronic renal and cardiovascular disease is common.

Various drugs have been linked to the onset of nonketotic hyperosmolar coma (Table 179-1). Most are dehydrating agents or have side effects of impairing insulin release from the pancreas or of interfering with the peripheral action of insulin. Thiazide diuretics and diazoxide possess both characteristics and are well-recognized causes of nonketotic hyperosmolar coma. Other drugs causally related to this syndrome include corticosteroids, phenytoin, mannitol, cimetidine, propranolol, calcium channel blockers, and immunosuppressive agents.

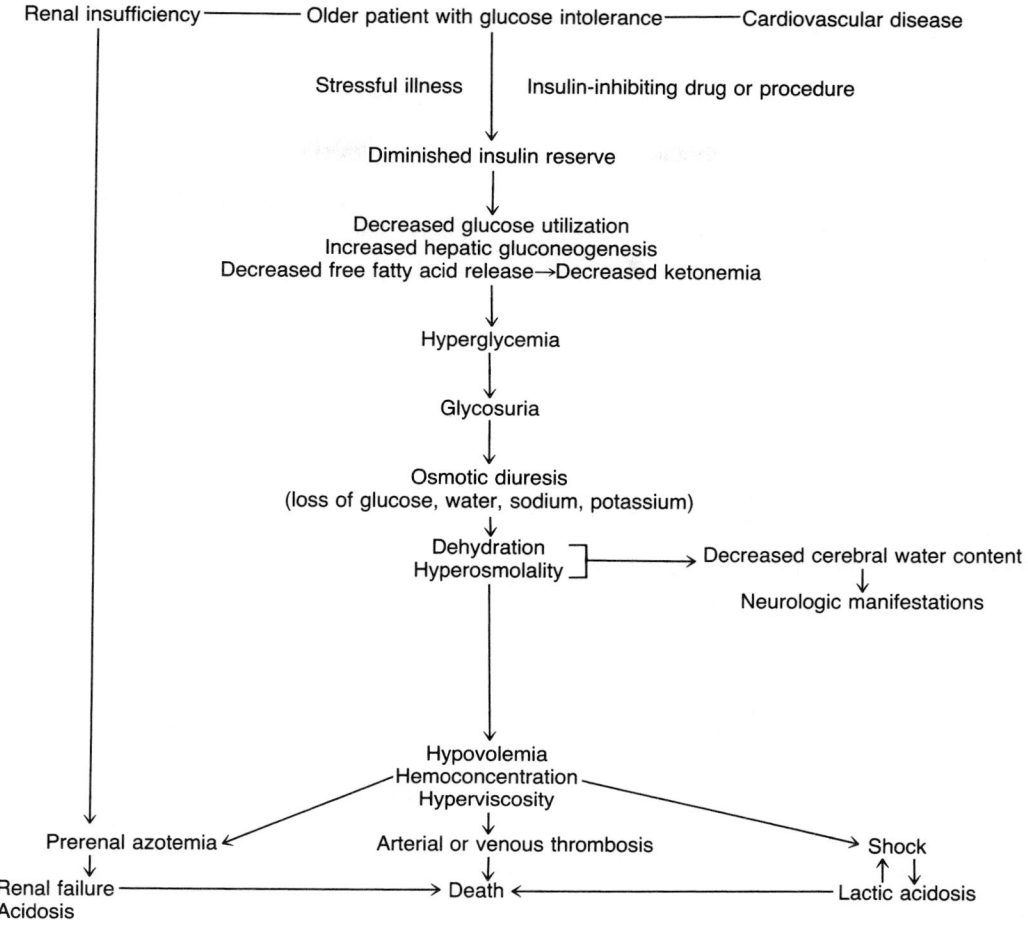

**Fig. 179-1.** Pathophysiology of nonketotic hyperosmolar coma. (From Grace TW: Hyperosmolar non-ketotic diabetic coma. *Am Fam Physician* 32:119, 1985. Used by permission.)

Clinical situations that can result in severe dehydration or an excessive glucose load or both may produce this syndrome in nondiabetic patients. These include extensive burns, heatstroke, hypothermia, peritoneal or hemodialysis with a hypertonic glucose solution, and hyperalimentation; these causes are most commonly seen in hospitalized patients.

An occasional patient may have a history of ingesting enormous quantities of sugar-containing fluids. This patient is usually alert and has a lesser degree of dehydration than the usual patient with nonketotic hyperosmolar coma.

The prodromal period during the development of nonketotic hyperosmolar coma is longer than that for diabetic ketoacidosis. Metabolic changes occur over many days to several weeks. Symptoms of polyuria, polydipsia, and increasing lethargy are almost always present but may not be appreciated. Failure to develop ketoacidosis and its clinical manifestations may allow the underlying process to go unrecognized until stupor or coma develops. Decreased responsiveness is the main reason patients receive medical attention.

## Physical Findings

There are no specific physical findings. Virtually all are significantly dehydrated. Fever, hypotension, and tachycardia may be present. Shock is especially common if gram-negative pneumonia is present. Respirations are variable. Kussmaul's breathing is not a feature of uncomplicated nonketotic hyperosmolar coma, but hyperventilation may be present if the patient is acidotic for other reasons. Shallow respirations with hyperpnea and tachypnea are usual. The smell of acetone on the breath is absent.

The most prominent physical findings are neurologic (Table 179-2). Almost all patients exhibit some disturbance in mentation, ranging from inappropriate response to confusion, drowsiness, stupor, or coma. The higher the osmolality, the greater the obtundation. The average osmolality for a comatose patient with nonketotic hyperosmolar coma is 380 mOsm/kg. Depression of the sensorium does not correlate with the glucose concentration or with the pH of the plasma or cerebrospinal fluid.

The most common focal signs are hemisensory deficits or hemiparesis or both. Approximately 15 percent of the patients exhibit seizure activity, usually of the focal motor type (85 percent). Grand mal seizures can occur. Tremors, fasciculations, and a variety of other neurologic abnormalities including aphasia, hyperreflexia, flac-

**Table 179-1.** Drugs and Procedures that May Cause Hyperosmolar Coma

| | |
|---|---|
| Hydrochlorothiazide and other thiazide diuretics | Cimetidine (Tagamet) |
| Chlorthalidone (Hygroton, Thalitone) | Propranolol (Inderal) |
| Furosemide (Lasix) | Asparaginase (Elspar) |
| Ethacrynic acid (Edecrin) | Immunosuppressive agents |
| Diazoxide (Hyperstat, Proglycem) | Mannitol |
| Calcium channel blockers | Peritoneal dialysis |
| Glucocorticoids | Hemodialysis |
| Phenytoin (Dilantin) | Intravenous hyperosmolar alimentation |
| Chlorpromazine (Thorazine) | |

*Source:* Grace TW: Hyperosmolar non-ketotic diabetic coma. *Am Fam Physician* 32:119, 1985.

**Table 179-2.** Neurologic Manifestations of Nonketotic Hyperosmolar Coma

| Diffuse | Focal |
|---|---|
| Seizures | Focal seizures |
| Lethargy | Todd's paralysis |
| Confusion | Hemisensory loss |
| Delirium and hallucinations | Hemiparesis |
| Stupor | Babinski's reflex |
| Coma | Aphasia |
| | Hemianopsia |
| | Tonic eye deviation |
| | Nystagmus |
| | Hyperreflexia |
| | Choreoathetosis |

*Source:* Grace TW: Hyperosmolar non-ketotic diabetic coma. *Am Fam Physician* 32:119, 1985, with permission.

cidity, depressed deep tendon reflexes, positive plantar response, and nuchal rigidity may be seen. In one series by Arieff and Carroll, 12 of 33 patients with nonketotic hyperosmolar coma were initially diagnosed as "probably acute stroke." This diagnosis was not confirmed in any of the patients.

Considering the age of the patient population and the frequency of neurologic findings, it is not surprising that the misdiagnosis of stroke or organic brain syndrome is common. Nonketotic hyperosmolar coma must be suspected in every elderly, dehydrated patient with glucosuria or hyperglycemia, especially if they are mild diabetics and receiving diuretic drugs or glucocorticoids.

### Laboratory

Confirmation of the diagnosis is with laboratory findings. The essential tests are blood glucose levels, calculated and measured serum osmolality, and serum ketone levels. A reasonable approximation of the blood glucose and serum ketone levels can be made promptly at the bedside by use of the nitroprusside test and glucose reagent strips. Additional tests should include a complete blood cell count and levels of electrolytes, blood urea nitrogen (BUN), creatinine, and arterial blood gases.

Serum electrolytes display a variable pattern. Serum sodium values usually range from 120 to 160 mEq/L, but because water is lost in excess of sodium through osmotic diuresis, the patient is almost always hypertonic. There is a sodium decrement of 1.6 mEq/L for every 100 mg/dL increase in blood glucose. Total body potassium depletion is usually severe. Potassium loss in nonketotic hyperosmolar coma is greater than that with diabetic ketoacidosis because of the longer duration of osmotic diuresis, GI loss, and prior diuretic use.

The BUN level is almost always elevated because of extracellular volume depletion and underlying renal disease. The initial BUN level is elevated out of proportion to the creatinine level. Ratios of BUN to creatinine may be 30:1. Prerenal azotemia resolves with volume replacement, but most patients have underlying chronic renal impairment.

Metabolic acidosis due to the accumulation of ketone bodies is not a feature of nonketotic hyperosmolar coma, but metabolic acidosis due to other causes can occur. In most series, 30 to 40 percent of the patients have a mild metabolic acidosis attributed to accumulation of lactic acid or due to uremia. However, in a significant number of these cases, no cause of the acidosis can be identified. Striking elevations of creatine phosphokinase (CPK) in patients with nonketotic hyperosmolar coma have been reported and are attributed to the complication of rhabdomyolysis. This condition as a complication of severe hyperosmolality has been reported.

Because of the frequency of underlying chronic disease and precipitating illnesses, a search for a precipitating cause must be made. Urinalysis, chest roentgenogram, ECG, and cultures of the blood, urine, and sputum should be performed. Because of the frequency of fever and neurologic signs, including nuchal rigidity, a CT scan and lumbar puncture may be necessary. Typical findings in the spinal fluid include a normal opening pressure, a markedly elevated glucose level (usually 50 percent of the serum value), a normal or slightly elevated protein level, and an osmolality identical to that of the serum.

## TREATMENT

Attention to detail and constant monitoring are necessary. Serial measurements of glucose, electrolyte, and serum osmolality levels are essential. A flow sheet to record therapeutic measures and patient response is recommended. The specific goals of therapy of nonketotic hyperosmolar coma include correction of hypovolemia and dehydration, restoration of electrolyte balance, and reduction of serum glucose and hyperosmolality levels. Reasonable end points that can usually be achieved within 36 h are a blood glucose level of 250 mg/dL, a serum osmolality of 320 mOsm/kg, and a urine output of at least 50 mL/h.

### Crystalloid

No agreement exists on the composition of the initial replacement fluid. Some authors advocate the use of isotonic saline (0.9% NaCl), and others recommend the use of half-normal saline (0.45% NaCl). Those who advocate isotonic saline believe that the most immediate threat to life is hypovolemic shock. Even though the patient has lost water in excess of solute and is hypertonic, normal saline is still hypotonic to the patient with nonketotic hyperosmolar coma. Normal saline corrects the extracellular volume deficit, stabilizes the blood pressure, and maintains adequate urinary flow. Once this has been achieved, hypotonic saline can be administered to provide free water for correction of intracellular volume deficits.

Those who recommend half-normal or hypotonic saline as initial fluid therapy argue that any osmotically active solute in the replacement fluid prolongs and enhances the hyperosmotic state. Further, since the patient has lost water in excess of solute, a hypotonic solution is the logical replacement.

All authors agree that if the patient is in hypovolemic shock, isotonic saline should be given until volume has been restored. Most agree that if the patient has significant hypernatremia (155 mEq/L) or hypertension, hypotonic saline should be the initial fluid of choice.

Rarely a patient has hyperglycemia, hyponatremia, and a low or normal osmolality. This indicates a significant excess of water, probably due to the ingestion of enormous quantities. The use of hypotonic saline in this setting can precipitate water intoxication.

There are no controlled studies that compare the advantages of isotonic solutions with those of hypotonic solutions in the initial management of nonketotic hyperosmolar coma. Regardless of the fluid used, there are guidelines to determine the rate and amount of fluid administration.

The average fluid deficit in nonketotic hyperosmolar coma is usually between 20 and 25 percent of total body water (TBW), or 8 to 12 L. In elderly subjects, it is assumed that 50 percent of the body weight is due to TBW. By using the patient's usual weight in kilograms, normal TBW and water deficit (20 to 25 percent of TBW) can be calculated. One-half of the estimated water deficit should be replaced during the first 12 h and the balance during the next 24 h. Ongoing insensible and urinary losses should also be replaced.

Renal cardiac and cerebral function must be monitored. Too rapid correction of glucose and osmolality can result in cerebral edema.

### Electrolytes

Electrolyte replacement is an essential part of therapy for nonketotic hyperosmolar coma. In the average patient, for every liter of body water lost, 70 mEq of monovalent ions is concomitantly lost. That translates into 300 to 800 mEq of sodium and potassium that usually needs to be replaced.

The sodium deficit is replenished by the administration of normal saline (154 mEq of sodium per liter) or half-normal saline (77 mEq of sodium per liter). Potassium replacement, as with diabetic ketoacidosis, should be started early in the course of treatment. Potassium supplement should be started within 2 h of the institution of fluid and insulin therapy or as soon as adequate renal function has been confirmed. Most authors recommend the infusion of KCl at a rate of 10 to 20 mEq/h during the acute phase of therapy (24 to 36 h). Potassium should be added to the initial intravenous fluid if the patient presents with hypokalemia. Magnesium levels should be obtained and replacement given if the level is low. Caution is necessary in the presence of renal dysfunction.

## Insulin

Traditionally it has been taught that the insulin requirement of a patient with nonketotic hyperosmolar coma is less than that of a patient with diabetic ketoacidosis. The difference in insulin requirement was attributed to decreased insulin resistance in the patient with nonketotic hyperosmolar coma because of the absence of acidosis.

Changing concepts have led to a reappraisal of insulin therapy, and continuous intravenous infusion of low doses of insulin and intermittent intramuscular injections of low doses of insulin are effective therapy.

The usual insulin dose is 0.1 units/kg/h, given by continuous intravenous infusion or by intramuscular injection. If the intramuscular route is chosen, 20 units of regular insulin can initially be administered intramuscularly or by intravenous bolus. Often no additional insulin is required after the initial dose. No insulin should be given after the blood glucose level reaches approximately 300 mg/dL.

The reasons for not using large doses of insulin when treating nonketotic hyperosmolar coma are even more compelling than those stated for diabetic ketoacidosis. In addition to producing a more gradual reduction of the glucose concentration, thus avoiding hypoglycemia, hypokalemia, and cerebral edema, low-dose insulin techniques may help to avoid vascular collapse and renal shutdown in the patient with nonketotic hyperosmolar coma.

Cerebral edema in nonketoic hyperosmolar coma is far less common than in patients with diabetic ketoacidosis. It usually occurs when the metabolic abnormalities have largely been corrected. As the patients' clinical condition is improving, there is an abrupt decrease in the sensorium, increased lethargy, elevated blood pressure and decreasing heart rate. The pediatric population may be more prone to this complication than adults. One study suggests that rapid lowering of the blood glucose below 300 mg/dl during the first 24 h of insulin therapy may contribute to the genesis of cerebral edema. Treatment of this complication is usually ineffectual and the mortality rate is 75%.

A high glucose concentration in the extracellular fluid compartment protects that compartment against hypovolemia at the expense of intracellular water. If the concentration of glucose is rapidly lowered by the administration of large doses of insulin, insufficient extracellular osmotic solute may result in a net intracellular shift of large volumes of water, producing hypovolemia and vascular collapse. Similarly, osmotic diuresis induced by hyperglycemia acts to protect the kidney against acute tubular necrosis (ATN) in the presence of reduced renal perfusion. If the blood glucose concentration is rapidly reduced, the osmotic diuresis decreases, and ATN may result. Acute tubular necrosis after institution of large-dose insulin therapy was reported in 5 of 30 patients in the series studied by Arieff and Carroll.

## Glucose

Glucose should be added to the intravenous solution when the blood glucose level declines to 250 mg/dL. It is at this level that further rapid lowering of the blood glucose concentration may result in cerebral edema. Cerebral edema can be recognized clinically by the sudden onset of hyperpyrexia, hypotension, and deepening of coma in spite of biochemical improvement. Though cerebral edema during treatment of nonhyperosmolar coma is rare, it is usually fatal and can be prevented.

## Additional Treatment

The role of phosphate replacement during treatment of nonketotic hyperosmolar coma is controversial. The plasma phosphorus level should be monitored during therapy, but a case for routine phosphate infusion has not been made convincingly.

Patients with nonketotic hyperosmolar coma are at risk for the development of arterial and venous thrombosis. Low-dose prophylactic heparin therapy should be considered.

Seizures are usually due to hyperosmolality and electrolyte abnormalities, but CNS mass lesions and meningitis or encephalitis should be considered. Unless the patient has an underlying seizure disorder or has status epilepticus, specific treatment for single seizures is not necessary. Phenytoin may precipitate nonketotic hyperosmolar coma and should be given with caution.

## BIBLIOGRAPHY

Arieff AI: Cerebral edema complicating nonketotic hyperosmolar coma. *Mineral Electrolyte Metab* 12:383, 1986.

Arieff AI, Carroll HJ: Nonketotic hyperosmolar coma with hyperglycemia: Clinical features, pathophysiology, renal function, acid-base balance, plasma-cerebrospinal fluid equilibria and the effects of therapy in 37 cases. *Medicine* 51:73, 1972.

Bendezu R, Wieland RH, Furst BH, et al: Experience with low-dose insulin infusion in diabetic ketoacidosis and diabetic hyperosmolarity. *Arch Intern Med* 138:60, 1978.

Gerich JE, Martin MM, Recant L: Clinical and metabolic characteristics of hyperosmolar nonketotic coma. *Diabetes* 20:228, 1971.

Podolsky S: Hyperosmolar nonketotic coma in the elderly diabetic. *Med Clin North Am* 62:815, 1978.

# 180
# LACTIC ACIDOSIS
## Gene Ragland

Lactic acidosis is the most common metabolic acidosis. It occurs in association with a wide variety of underlying processes and may represent a well-tolerated, physiologic event or a life-threatening, pathologic condition. Lactic acidosis is classified based upon oxygen supply to the tissues. Type A is that clearly associated with clinically evident hypoperfusion or hypoxia, and type B includes all other forms, those in which there is no evidence of tissue anoxia. Lactic acidosis is often diagnosed during the evaluation of an anion gap acidosis. Treatment is directed toward identification and correction of the underlying disorder and restitution of normal acid-base equilibrium.

## PATHOPHYSIOLOGY

### Lactate

Lactate is a metabolic product of anaerobic glycolysis and under normal conditions is in equilibrium with its immediate precursor, pyruvate. The basal production of lactate in a 70-kg person is approximately 1300 mEq/day, and the normal lactate concentration in extracellular fluid is about 1 mEq/L. The maintenance of lactate homeostasis is a complex, dynamic process involving interorgan balance between lactate production and utilization. Virtually all body tissues are capable of producing lactate, but skeletal muscle, erythrocytes, brain, skin, and intestinal mucosa are the most active. The utilization of lactate takes place in the liver and kidneys and to a lesser extent in the heart and skeletal muscle. Lactate is primarily disposed of in the liver and kidneys via gluconeogenesis, a process that requires the conversion of lactate back to pyruvate.

Lactate is formed from pyruvate as an end product of anaerobic glycolysis. This oxidation-reduction reaction requires reduced nicotinamide adenine dinucleotide (NADH) and hydrogen ion (H+) and is catalyzed by lactate dehydrogenase (LDH). This reaction is expressed by the equation

$$\text{Pyruvate} + \text{NADH} + \text{H}^+ \overset{\text{LDH}}{\rightleftharpoons} \text{Lactate} + \text{NAD}$$

The equilibrium of this reaction strongly favors the formation of lactate. The normal ratio of lactate to pyruvate is 10:1. Lactate is a metabolic blind end; it cannot be utilized in any other intracellular reactions and must be converted back to pyruvate for gluconeogenesis or oxidation to $CO_2$ and $H_2O$ via the Krebs cycle. The result of this biochemical reaction is to produce energy in the form of adenosine triphosphate (ATP) and to oxidize NADH to NAD. A small amount of lactic acid is produced even at rest and under aerobic conditions. In the presence of oxygen and essential cofactors, lactate is converted back to pyruvate; it does not accumulate and maintains equilibrium with pyruvate.

A variety of factors may alter this normal process. The concentration of lactate in the cytosol depends primarily upon the concentration of pyruvate, the intracellular redox state (NADH/NAD), and the intracellular pH. The net effect of these multiple factors determines the intracellular concentration of lactate.

## Pyruvate

Since lactate can be eliminated only by conversion back to pyruvate, lactate concentration is intimately interrelated to the fate of pyruvate. Pyruvate is a key intermediary at the junction of several important pathways. The major sources of pyruvate are glycolysis, in which pyruvate is formed from the oxidation of glucose, and transamination, a process by which pyruvate can be derived from amino acids, especially alanine. Pyruvate may be utilized via gluconeogenesis in which pyruvate is a substrate in the formation of glucose, and mitochondrial oxidation, in which pyruvate enters the mitochondria for oxidation to $CO_2$ and $H_2O$. A variety of factors may alter these normal pathways. For example, rapid glycolysis can be induced by alkalosis, protein catabolic states may increase transamination, metabolic poisons may impair mitochondrial function, or key enzymes and cofactors may be inactivated or unavailable. The concentration of pyruvate, and thus the concentration of lactate, depends upon the net production and consumption of pyruvate by these various routes.

## Redox State

The intracellular redox state is a critical factor in determining the concentration of lactate. The availability of oxygen at the tissue level is an important determinant of the cellular redox. During prolonged anaerobic conditions, lactate cannot be reoxidized back to pyruvate because of a lack of NAD. Normally, NADH can be reoxidized to NAD within the mitochondria via the electron transport chain coupled with oxidative phosphorylation. Electron transport abruptly ceases during anoxia. NAD is not available for lactate conversion, and lactate accumulates. This mechanism is thought to be operative during type A lactic acidosis. Other factors may alter the cellular re-

dox, and consequently, alterations in the NADH/NAD ratio do not solely reflect tissue oxygenation.

## Intracellular pH

A third major determinant of lactate concentration within the cytosol is the intracellular hydrogen ion concentration. Changes in the intracellular pH affect enzymatic reactions, lactate transport, and the lactate/pyruvate ratio. Some of these effects may counterbalance each other. In general, a fall in pH causes decreased lactate production, whereas an increase in pH causes increased lactate concentration. One important aspect of a change in intracellular pH is its effect on the liver. As the pH declines, lactate uptake by the liver decreases. Additionally, when the pH is 7.0 or less, the liver becomes an organ of lactate production instead of lactate clearance.

## Lactate Utilization

The liver and kidneys are the major organs that consume lactate. Gluconeogenesis is the main pathway utilized by these organs in lactate removal. This process utilizes the hydrogen ions produced during the formation of lactic acid and this acts to maintain acid-base balance. The liver normally clears more than half the total daily lactate load, and the kidneys remove approximately 30 percent. Some researchers believe that the kidneys have a negligible role in lactate clearance and that other extrahepatic sites are more important. Of the approximately 1300 mEq of lactate produced each day, 60 to 70 mEq of lactate is extracted by the liver every 2 h. The hydrogen ion that is consumed by the liver during this period is roughly equivalent to the total amount of hydrogen ion excreted daily by the kidneys. By virtue of the liver's ability to clear lactate, the role of the liver in the maintenance of the overall acid-base balance is very important. In addition, the liver has a large reserve capacity to extract lactate; this has been estimated to be as high as 3400 to 4000 mEq/day. Obviously, any situation which converts the liver from a lactate-consuming to a lactate-producing organ results in serious acid-base disturbance. Lactic acid clearance by the liver may be reduced with decreased hepatic blood flow or parenchymal hypoxia.

The kidneys carry out their role in lactate clearance primarily through gluconeogenesis, not excretion. The renal threshold for lactate is about 7 to 10 mEq/L, so the amount of lactate excreted by the kidneys at normal plasma levels is negligible. The kidneys may also dispose of lactate through oxidation, but this is not the preferred pathway. At a pH of less than 7.1, lactate uptake by the kidneys may be decreased, and at a pH of 7.0 or below, the kidneys—like the liver—may produce lactic acid.

Skeletal and cardiac muscle is capable of extracting some lactate from the circulation. The relative role of these sites of lactate clearance is not clear. Lactate utilization by skeletal muscle may depend on the concentration of lactate and whether the muscle is active or at rest.

## Lactic Acidosis

Lactic acidosis can be thought of as an imbalance between the rate of production of lactate by tissues active in glycolysis and the rate of utilization by tissues active in gluconeogenesis. Disagreement exists over whether the primary mechanism responsible for lactic acidosis is overproduction or underutilization.

Lactic acid is a strong organic acid that is almost completely dissociated at physiologic pH. The ratio of lactate ion to undissociated lactic acid at a pH of 7.4 is more than 3000:1. For each milliequivalent of lactic acid produced, equal amounts of hydrogen ion and lactate are liberated. Hydrogen ions are initially buffered by bicarbonate and other buffers and then consumed during the utilization of lactate via gluconeogenesis or oxidation. Acid-base balance is therefore maintained. Under circumstances of increased lactic acid production and/or decreased lactic acid utilization, body buffers are saturated by the excess hydrogen ions. When this is of sufficient magnitude, acidosis results. Whether the resultant lactic acidosis is clinically significant depends upon the underlying process responsible for the lactic acid accumulation and the preexistent acid-base status.

## Diagnosis

Lactic acidosis is a metabolic acidosis caused by the accumulation of lactate and hydrogen ion. It is accompanied by an elevated blood lactate concentration, but there is no consensus on what level of lactate defines lactic acidosis. The normal plasma lactate level is 0.5 to 1.5 mEq/L. In general, a lactate concentration of 5 to 6 mEq/L is considered indicative of significant acid-base disturbance. Some authors have included demonstration of a reduced arterial pH, $\leq 7.35$, as a criterion for diagnosis. However, if there is a coexistent alkalosis, the pH could be normal or even alkalemic in the face of significant lactic acidosis.

The presence of hyperlactemia per se does not mean that the patient has clinically significant lactic acidosis. Many situations encountered clinically may result in elevation of blood lactate levels but not produce significant clinical consequences. Exercise; hyperventilation; infusions of glucose, saline, or bicarbonate; or injections of insulin or epinephrine may all cause elevation of lactate levels without clinical manifestations. Plasma lactate concentrations after vigorous exercise or maximum work have been reported to reach 14 to 30 mEq/L. In patients with grand mal seizures, levels of 12.7 mEq/L have been recorded. In spite of these high levels, the lactate production is self-limited, and the lactate is rapidly cleared from the circulation without untoward consequences. Persistent elevation of lactate levels may occur with chronic disorders such as severe congestive heart failure, pulmonary disease, liver disease, and diabetes mellitus. These levels are generally well-tolerated. To identify the patient in whom an increased lactate level is significant, the physician must assess the clinical state and correlate it with the extent to which increased lactate and hydrogen ion levels contribute to clinical abnormalities.

A presumptive diagnosis of lactic acidosis can be made in many instances. This diagnosis is based upon the recognition of an anion gap acidosis in a patient with a clinical disorder in which lactic acidosis is known to occur. For this impression to be confirmed, other causes of an increased anion gap metabolic acidosis must be excluded, and the plasma lactate concentration must be shown to be elevated.

### Anion Gap Acidosis

The anion gap is generally determined by subtracting the concentration of chloride plus bicarbonate ions from the concentration of sodium ion: $Na^+ - (Cl^- + HCO_3^-)$. The normal value is 12 mEq/L $\pm 4$. Any value greater than 16 mEq/L suggests the presence of an "unmeasured ion," usually an accumulation of organic anions. Most patients with lactic acidosis have an anion gap that averages 25 to 30 mEq/L. The major causes of anion gap acidosis in addition to lactic acidosis include diabetic ketoacidosis, uremic acidosis, alcoholic ketoacidosis, and ingestion of the toxins salicylate, methanol, ethylene glycol, paraldehyde, or cyanide (Table 180-1). Laboratory determinations of the levels of arterial blood gases, electrolytes, glucose, blood urea nitrogen, creatinine, and lactate, and liver function studies and appropriate drug screens, should help establish the correct cause of acidosis.

Particular caution should be used with diabetic and alcoholic patients to ensure that the unmeasured anion is correctly identified. The major organic anion in diabetic and alcoholic ketoacidosis is β-hydroxybutyrate, which is not measured by the serum nitroprusside test. Lactic acidosis and ketoacidosis may occur simultaneously. If lactate levels do not account for the entire increase in the anion gap, ketoacidosis should be suspected, even with a weakly positive acetone test. The bicarbonate level may provide additional help with this differential point. In uncomplicated diabetic ketoacidosis, the increase in the anion gap is identical to the decrease in the bicarbonate concentration, whereas in lactic acidosis, the increase in the anion gap is usually greater than the decrease in the bicarbonate concentration.

## Clinical Presentation

The clinical findings in lactic acidosis are nonspecific. The onset may be abrupt, often occurring over several hours. Generally the patient appears ill. Hyperventilation or Kussmaul's respiration is the most constant feature. The level of consciousness may vary from lethargy to coma. Vomiting and abdominal pain sometimes occur. Hypotension and evidence of hypoxia occur with type A lactic acidosis but not with type B.

Laboratory abnormalities that occur during lactic acidosis include elevated lactate levels, increased anion gap, hyperkalemia, decreased bicarbonate levels, and decreased pH unless altered by compensatory alkalosis. Serum potassium concentrations are most likely to be elevated in those patients with underlying renal insufficiency or tissue destruction. Marked hyperphosphatemia and hyperuricemia may be seen. The white blood cell count is usually elevated and may reach leukemoid proportions. Hypoglycemia has also been reported, especially in conjunction with liver disease.

## Classification of Lactic Acidosis

Lactic acidosis is classified on clinical grounds and occurs in two principal clinical settings. According to Cohen and Woods' classification, type A lactic acidosis occurs with clinically evident tissue anoxia, such as during shock or severe hypoxia. Type B lactic acidosis includes all other forms, those in which there is no evidence of tissue anoxia (Table 180-2). Spontaneous or idiopathic lactic acidosis

**Table 180-1.** Causes of Increased Anion Gap Metabolic Acidosis

| | |
|---|---|
| Increased endogenous organic acids: | Ingestion of toxins: |
| Diabetic ketoacidosis | Salicylates |
| Alcoholic ketoacidosis | Methanol |
| Lactic acidosis | Ethylene glycol |
| Decreased excretion of organic and inorganic acids: | Paraldehyde |
| Renal failure (uremia) | Cyanide |

**Table 180-2.** Classification of Lactic Acidosis

Type A:
  Clinically evident tissue anoxia (e.g., shock, hypoxia)
Type B:
  Various common disorders
    Diabetes mellitus
    Renal failure
    Liver disease
    Infection
    Leukemia and certain other malignant conditions
    Convulsions
  Drugs, toxins
    Biguanides (phenformin)
    Ethanol
    Fructose and other saccharides
    Methanol
    Various other drugs
  Hereditary forms
    Type I glycogen storage disease
    Fructose-biphosphatase deficiency
    Subacute necrotizing encephalomyelopathy (Leigh's syndrome)
    Methylmalonic aciduria
    Others

*Source:* Adapted from Cohen RD, Woods HF: *Clinical and Biochemical Aspects of Lactic Acidosis.* Oxford, Blackwell, 1976.

has been described but is now felt to be nonexistent. Recognition of an increasing array of disorders in which lactic acidosis can occur without evident tissue anoxia has virtually eliminated this category. A new metabolic disorder, D-lactic acidosis, has been described. It occurs in patients with anatomically or functionally shortened small bowel. Bacterial fermentation produces D-lactic acid, which can be absorbed and cause an increased anion gap acidosis and stupor or coma. The plasma levels of L-lactate are normal. Treatment with neomycin or vancomycin results in correction of the metabolic abnormalities.

## Type A Lactic Acidosis

This is the most common form of lactic acidosis seen in the emergency department and is most often due to shock. Hemorrhagic, hypovolemic, cardiogenic, or septic shock have been shown to cause lactic acidosis. The pathogenesis of lactic acidosis during shock is inadequate tissue perfusion with subsequent anoxia and lactate and hydrogen ion accumulation. Clearance of lactate by the liver is reduced because of decreased splanchnic and hepatic artery perfusion, and hepatocellular ischemia. At a pH of around 7.0 or less, the liver and kidneys may become organs of lactate production.

The association between shock and lactic acidosis is so common that a presumptive diagnosis can be made in a critically ill patient in shock who suddenly develops severe hyperventilation and an increased anion gap acidosis. Treatment should be directed toward correction of the cause of shock. In general, the higher the lactate level, the higher the mortality.

Hypoxia may also cause type A lactic acidosis. The hypoxia must be acute and severe. Adaptations such as polycythemia, diminished hemoglobin affinity for oxygen, and increased tissue extraction of oxygen protect patients with chronic, stable lung disease from developing lactic acidosis.

These patients may not develop significant lactic acidosis until an arterial $P_{O_2}$ of 30 to 35 mmHg is reached. In patients with a diminished ability to compensate for a respiratory insult, lactic acidosis may arise at considerably higher arterial oxygen tensions. Acute asphyxiation, pulmonary edema, status asthmaticus, acute exacerbation of chronic obstructive pulmonary disease, and displacement of oxygen by carboxyhemoglobin, sulfhemoglobin, or methemoglobin have been associated with lactic acidosis.

## Type B Lactic Acidosis

Type B lactic acidosis includes all forms in which there is no clinical evidence of tissue anoxia. This form may occur abruptly, over a few hours. The diagnosis may be missed or delayed because of no clear antecedent event, or because of lack of familiarity with the disorders associated with type B lactic acidosis. The mechanisms by which these disorders predispose to lactic acidosis are not well understood. By definition, the cardiovascular function is not impaired and the blood pressure is not decreased. Subclinical, regional underperfusion of tissue has been suggested as a possible cause. In many cases of severe type B lactic acidosis, circulatory insufficiency may occur after a few hours, making this condition clinically indistinguishable from type A lactic acidosis. Type B lactic acidosis is divided into three subgroups.

### Type B₁

Type $B_1$ lactic acidosis comprises those cases that occur in association with other medical disorders such as diabetes, renal and hepatic disease, infection, neoplasia, and convulsions. There is no clear causal relation between diabetes and lactic acidosis, but the association between them has been noted by many authors. Massive hepatic necrosis and cirrhosis are associated with lactic acidosis. Decreased lactate clearance by the liver because of insufficient liver tissue for gluconeogenesis may be the cause. Acute and chronic renal insuffi-

ciency is commonly associated with lactic acidosis but is probably not a cause in its own right. Some patients with severe infections, especially bacteremia, develop lactic acidosis for unknown reasons. Myeloproliferative disorders such as leukemia, multiple myeloma, generalized lymphoma, and Hodgkin's disease are associated with lactic acidosis. Grand mal seizures may result in lactic acidosis because of muscular hyperactivity and probably hypoxia. Lactic acidosis in Reye's syndrome has been reported. A close correspondence between the stage of coma and lactate levels has been noted.

### Type B₂

This subgroup includes cases of lactic acidosis due to drugs, chemicals, and toxins. This category was formerly dominated by the oral hypoglycemic agent phenformin, which has been withdrawn from U.S. markets. Ethanol is currently the most common drug associated with lactic acidosis. During the oxidation of alcohol, NADH levels increase, causing utilization of the pyruvate-lactate pathway for the reoxidation of NADH. This reaction produces a moderate increase in the lactate level. In the presence of other causes of lactic acidosis, ethanol ingestion may cause increased acidosis. Other drugs associated with lactic acidosis include fructose; sorbitol; excess amounts of epinephrine and other catecholamines; methanol; and possibly salicylates. Many other drugs have also been implicated as causally related to lactic acidosis.

### Type B₃

This form of lactic acidosis is rare and is due to inborn errors of metabolism such as type I glycogen storage disease (glucose-6 phosphatase deficiency) and hepatic fructose-biphosphatase deficiency. These congenital lactic acidoses include defects in gluconeogenesis, the pyruvate dehydrogenase complex, the krebs cycle, and cellular respiratory mechanisms.

## Treatment

The basic therapeutic goals in treatment of lactic acidosis are to identify and correct the underlying cause of the lactic acid accumulation and to counteract the deleterious effects of the acidosis.

The specifics of therapy depend upon the cause. Shock and hypoxia must be corrected as soon as possible. Adequate ventilation is imperative. Restoration of blood pressure, cardiac output, and tissue perfusion with well-oxygenated blood is essential. Volume replacement with fluids, plasma expanders, or blood, as indicated, should be instituted. Vasopressors should probably be avoided as they may decrease tissue perfusion and worsen the acidosis. Low cardiac output states should be treated with inotropic compounds along with afterload-reducing agents. Catecholamines are glycogenolytic and may enhance lactic acid production. In type B lactic acidosis, the underlying disorder may not be readily identifiable or amenable to therapy. Drugs known to be associated with lactic acidosis should be discontinued, and infection must be aggressively treated.

### Sodium bicarbonate

Treatment of acidosis with intravenous sodium bicarbonate ($NaHCO_3$) has been a mainstay of therapy for lactic acidosis. The purpose of this therapy is to reverse the untoward effects of acidosis and allow time for other therapeutic modalities to correct the cause of the acidosis. If the cause of lactic acidosis can be quickly corrected, such as with respiratory failure or pulmonary edema, alkali therapy may not be needed. The undesirable effects of acidosis include depression of myocardal contractility and decreased cardiac output at a pH below 7.1. Arteriolar dilatation and hypotension may occur when the blood pH falls below 7.0. Additionally, a pH below 7.0 impairs hepatic utilization of lactate and may induce production of lactate by the liver and kidneys. These effects may be the cause of the cardiovascular collapse that occurs during the course of type B lactic acidosis.

Several authors have suggested that alkali administration may not only lack benefit but actually be deleterious in the treatment of lactic acidosis. This position is based upon experimental animal studies and the reevaluation of the use of sodium bicarbonate in the treatment of such conditions as diabetic ketoacidosis and cardiopulmonary arrest. This question will most likely remain unresolved for some time. Until an efficacious alternative is identified, sodium bicarbonate will continue to be used in conjunction with cause-specific measures.

In general, sodium bicarbonate should be given when the pH is 7.1 or less. The smallest possible amount of bicarbonate that will return the systemic pH to hemodynamically safe levels (e.g., pH of 7.2) should be used. Frequent monitoring of the acid-base status during bicarbonate therapy is essential for appraisal of additional bicarbonate requirements. Some undesirable effects of sodium bicarbonate include fluid and sodium overload, hyperosmolarity, alkaline overshoot which could increase lactate production, displacement of the oxyhemoglobin dissociation curve to the left, and paradoxical cerebrospinal fluid acidosis.

The approximate dose of bicarbonate required to correct the acidosis can be calculated from the following formula:

$$HCO_3 \text{ deficit} = (25 \text{ mEq/L } HCO_3 - \text{measured } HCO_3) \times 0.5(\text{body weight in kg})$$

This equation is based upon the assumption that bicarbonate distributes in a space equal to 50 percent of the body weight in kilograms. The apparent space of distribution for bicarbonate is enlarged in hypobicarbonatemic states; thus, using 50 percent body weight to calculate the space for distribution of bicarbonate may underestimate the bicarbonate requirements.

Some patients may require massive amounts of sodium bicarbonate to correct acidemia. Those unable to tolerate fluid and sodium overload can be treated with a bicarbonate infusion, potent loop diuretic, or tris(hydroxymethyl)aminomethane (THAM). Hyperosmolarity can be reduced by adding 3 to 4 ampoules of $NaHCO_3$ (44 mEq/L) to 1 L of 5% dextrose and water. This solution provides 132 to 176 mEq/L, respectively. Use of a potent loop diuretic creates intravascular space for fluid and sodium. A diuretic should be given in whatever dose is required to maintain a brisk diuresis (300 to 500 mL/h). Urinary sodium and potassium losses can be measured and replaced along with the urinary volume loss on an equal basis.

Oliguric patients require hemodialysis to permit administration of large amounts of sodium bicarbonate. Standard dialysis baths can be replaced by a bicarbonate bath so that the fluid and sodium chloride removed by the hypertonic solution can be replaced as the bicarbonate salt. Hemodialysis and peritoneal dialysis remove lactate. As there is no evidence that lactate ion per se is harmful, this approach is unnecessary. Removal of lactate, however, can minimize the rebound alkalosis that often occurs after correction of the acidosis.

There is often a delay of many hours between the return of the pH to the normal range and a fall in the blood lactate level. The bicarbonate infusion can be decreased after several hours of a normal pH. If the pH begins to drop, the bicarbonate infusion can be increased. When the pH stabilizes in an acceptable range, the infusion can be discontinued. As always, the clinical status of the patient is the best parameter to follow during recovery.

## Additional Treatment

A variety of other therapies have been advocated in treatment of lactic acidosis. These include insulin, glucose, thiamine, methylene blue, vasodilator drugs such as sodium nitroprusside, carbicarb, and the experimental drug dichloroacetate. Most authors do not favor the use of insulin, or insulin in conjunction with glucose, in treatment of lactic acidosis. Insulin may be indicated in a diabetic patient with concomitant lactic acidosis or in a diabetic with an unexplained increased anion gap acidosis. Insulin therapy in these instances should be based upon individual need. Glucose infusion in the setting of hypoglycemia and lactic acidosis has been reported to correct the lactic acidosis.

Thiamine is a necessary cofactor for the enzyme that catalyzes the first step in the oxidation of pyruvate. This vitamin should be given to alcoholic patients with lactic acidosis, but a role for thiamine therapy in other patients has not been established. Methylene blue is a redox dye that is capable of accepting $H^+$ and thereby oxidizing $NADH_2$ to $NAD^+$ and theoretically limiting the conversion of pyruvate to lactate. Clinical trials have not supported the benefit of this drug. Vasodilator therapy is based upon the premise that tissue perfusion improves with reduced peripheral vascular resistance and increased cardiac output. The value of vasodilator agents in treatment of lactic acidosis remains to be proved.

Carbicarb is an equimolar solution of sodium bicarbonate and sodium carbonate. This mixture buffers hydrogen ion without the net generation of $CO_2$. Carbicarb also consumes excess $CO_2$ to yield more bicarbonate buffer. The deleterious effect of an increase in tissue $P_{CO_2}$ is avoided. Experimentation with carbicarb is ongoing and no clear clinical benefit has been demonstrated.

Dichloroacetate (DCA) is an experimental drug that increases the activity of pyruvate dehydrogenase, and this promotes the oxidation of glucose, pyruvate, and lactate and thus reduces blood lactate levels. Since oxygen is required for this metabolic process, DCA has no role in treatment of type A lactic acidosis. Its role in therapy for type B lactic acidosis may be limited by the increased ketosis and neurologic complications that occur with its use.

The fact that so many experimental therapies have been tried in lactic acidosis reflects the poor outcome of this disorder with the use of current treatment. The mortality of patients with type A lactic acidosis is approximately 80 percent; with type B it is 50 to 80 percent. Earlier recognition and correction of the underlying disorder responsible for the lactic acidosis is the best hope for reduction of this high mortality.

## BIBLIOGRAPHY

Kreisberg RA: Pathogenesis and management of lactic acidosis. *Annu Rev Med* 35:181, 1984.

Narins RG, Cohen JJ: Bicarbonate therapy for organic acidosis: The case for its continued use. *Ann Intern Med* 106:615, 1987.

Oliva PB: Lactic acidosis. *Am J Med* 48:209, 1970.

Park R, Arieff AI: Lactic acidosis: Current concepts. *Clin Endocrinol Metab* 12:339, 1983.

Stacpoole PW, Wright EC, Baumgartner TG, et al: A controlled clinical trial of dichloroacetate for treatment of lactic acidosis in adults. *N Engl J Med* 327:1564, 1992.

# 181

# THYROID STORM

## Gene Ragland

Thyroid storm is a rare complication of hyperthyroidism in which the manifestations of thyrotoxicosis are exaggerated to life-threatening proportions. Thyroid storm is most often seen in a patient with moderate to severe antecedent Graves' disease and is usually precipitated by a stressful event. It must be suspected and treated based upon a clinical impression, as there are no pathognomonic findings or confirmatory tests.

Hyperthyroid patients who are undiagnosed or undertreated are at risk for this complication. The duration of uncomplicated thyrotoxicosis preceding the onset of storm varies from months to years. A majority of the patients have had symptoms of hyperthyroidism for fewer than 24 months. It is not possible to predict accurately which thyrotoxic patient will develop storm as there is no predisposition by age, sex, or race.

## PRECIPITATING FACTORS

A wide variety of factors have been reported as precipitating events. Thyroid surgery for treatment of hyperthyroidism used to be the most common cause of storm. Medically identified causes of thyroid storm are numerous and now predominate over surgical ones. Infection, especially pulmonary infection, is the most common precipitating event. In diabetic patients, ketoacidosis, hyperosmolar coma, and insulin-induced hypoglycemia have provoked storm. Events known to increase the levels of circulating thyroid hormones and initiate storm in susceptible persons, include premature withdrawal of antithyroid drugs, administration of radioactive iodide, use of an iodinated contrast medium during x-ray study, thyroid hormone overdose, administration of a saturated solution of potassium iodide to patients with nontoxic goiters, and vigorous palpation of the thyroid gland in thyrotoxic patients. Additional events implicated as causes of storm include vascular accidents, pulmonary emboli, toxemia of pregnancy, and emotional stress. Finally, hospitalization may lead to storm because of the rigors of diagnostic procedures.

## PATHOPHYSIOLOGY

The exact pathogenesis of thyroid storm has not been defined. It is attractive to attribute storm to excess thyroid hormone production or secretion. The results of thyroid function studies are elevated in the vast majority of patients during storm, but the values are not significantly different from those found in uncomplicated thyrotoxicosis. An increase in free triiodothyronine ($T_3$) or free thyroxine ($T_4$) levels has been suggested as causative of storm. But storm has occurred in the absence of elevated free $T_3$ or $T_4$ levels. Something in addition to excess amounts or forms of thyroid hormones must occur during storm.

Adrenergic hyperreactivity due to either patient sensitization by thyroid hormones or altered interaction between thyroid hormones and catecholamines has been suggested. Plasma levels of epinephrine and norepinephrine are not increased during thyroid storm. The exact role of catecholamines in storm awaits further study.

Altered peripheral response to thyroid hormone, causing increased lipolysis and overproduction of heat, is another theory. This theory maintains that excessive lipolysis due to catecholamine-thyroid hormone interaction results in excessive thermal energy and fever. Finally, exhaustion of the body's tolerance to the action of thyroid hormones, leading to "decompensated thyrotoxicosis," is a long-standing viewpoint. This implies an altered response to thyroid hormones rather than a sudden increase in their concentration.

## CLINICAL PRESENTATION

Thyroid storm is a clinical diagnosis as there are no laboratory studies that distinguish it from thyrotoxicosis. Although the clinical presentation is extremely variable, there are clues to diagnosis. A history of hyperthyroidism, eye signs of Graves' disease, widened pulse pressure, and a palpable goiter are present in most patients who develop thyroid storm. However, the history may be unobtainable and the usual features of Graves' disease absent, including no obvious goiter in up to 9 percent of patients with Graves' disease.

### Diagnostic Criteria

The generally accepted diagnostic criteria for thyroid storm are a temperature higher than 37.8°C (100°F); marked tachycardia out of proportion to the fever; dysfunction of the CNS, cardiovascular system or gastrointestinal (GI) system; and exaggerated peripheral manifestations of thyrotoxicosis.

The signs and symptoms of storm usually occur suddenly, but there may be a prodromal period with subtle increases in the manifestations of thyrotoxicosis.

### Signs and Symptoms

The earliest signs are fever, tachycardia, diaphoresis, increased CNS activity, and emotional lability. If the condition is untreated, a hyperkinetic toxic state ensues in which the symptoms are intensified. Progression to congestive heart failure, refractory pulmonary edema, circulatory collapse, coma, and death may occur within 72 h.

Fever ranges from 38°C (100.4°F) to 41°C (105.8°F). The pulse rate may range between 120 and 200 beats per minute but has been reported as high as 300 beats per minute. Sweating may be profuse, leading to dehydration from insensible fluid loss.

Central nervous system disturbance occurs in 90 percent of patients with thyroid storm. Symptoms vary from restlessness, anxiety, and emotional lability, manic behavior, agitation, and psychosis, to mental confusion, obtundation, and coma. Extreme muscle weakness can occur. Thyrotoxic myopathy can occur and usually involves the proximal muscles. In severe forms, muscles of the more distal extremities and muscles of the trunk and face may be involved. About 1 percent of patients with Graves' disease develop myasthenia gravis, producing an occasional confusing clinical situation. The response of thyrotoxic myopathy to edrophonium (Tensilon test) is incomplete, unlike the complete response that occurs with myasthenia gravis. Hypokalemic periodic paralysis may also occur in patients with thyrotoxicosis.

Cardiovascular abnormalities are present in 50 percent of the patients regardless of underlying heart disease. Sinus tachycardia is usual. Arrhythmias, especially atrial fibrillation, but also including premature ventricular contractions and, rarely, complete heart block, may be present. In addition to increased heart rate, there is increased stroke volume, cardiac output, and myocardial oxygen consumption. Pulse pressure is characteristically widened. Congestive heart failure, pulmonary edema, and circulatory collapse may be terminal events.

Gastrointestinal symptoms develop in most patients in storm. Before the onset of storm, a history of severe weight loss is usual. Diarrhea and hyperdefecation seem to herald impending storm and can be severe, contributing to dehydration. During storm, anorexia, nausea, vomiting, and crampy abdominal pain may occur. Jaundice and tender hepatomegaly due to passive congestion of the liver, or even hepatic necrosis, have been reported. Jaundice is a poor prognostic sign.

## LABORATORY

There are no laboratory tests that confirm thyroid storm. The combination of free $T_4$ assay and a sensitive TSH assay are the primary means of assessing thyroid status in all patients. Some authors feel a single TSH assay is an appropriate screening tool. Both tests are needed in an emergency setting. When the clinical impression is thyrotoxicosis, an elevated free $T_4$ and a suppressed unmeasurable TSH confirms the diagnosis.

In an emergency setting rarely would additional thyroid tests be necessary to establish a diagnosis of thyrotoxicosis. The uncommon $T_3$ thyrotoxicosis would present with a suppressed TSH and a normal or low free $T_4$. With this entity, the total $T_3$ or free $T_3$ would be required to accurately make the diagnosis.

Routine laboratory data during thyroid storm show wide variation. Nonspecific abnormalities in the complete blood cell count, electrolyte levels, and liver function studies may be found. Bacterial infection may be reflected only by a leftward shift in the differential white count without elevation in the total white cell count. Hyperglycemia (>120 mg/dL) is common, and hypercalcemia is occasionally present. One series reported all patients to have low cholesterol levels with a mean value of 117 mg/dL. Plasma cortisol levels have been observed to be inappropriately low for the degree of stress, suggesting a lack of adrenal reserve.

## APATHETIC THYROTOXICOSIS

Apathetic thyrotoxicosis is a rare, distinct form that usually occurs in the elderly and is frequently misdiagnosed. These patients may develop thyroid storm without the usual hyperkinetic manifestations and may quietly lapse into coma and die. There are some salient clinical characteristics which are helpful in establishing this diagnosis. The patient is generally in the seventh decade or older, with lethargy, slowed mentation, and placid apathetic facies. Goiter is usually present but may be small and multinodular. The usual eye signs of exophthalmos, stare, and lid lag are absent, but blepharoptosis (drooping upper eye lid) is common. Excessive weight loss and proximal muscle weakness are usual. These patients generally have had symptoms longer than nonapathetic thyrotoxic patients.

"Masked" thyrotoxicosis occurs when signs and symptoms referable to dysfunction of one organ system dominate and obscure the underlying thyrotoxicosis. Signs and symptoms referable to the cardiovascular system tend to mask thyrotoxicosis in apathetic patients. These patients frequently present with atrial fibrillation and congestive heart failure. In one series of nine patients, the diagnosis of hyperthyroidism was unsuspected in each case because of the predominance of cardiovascular symptoms. Congestive heart failure in this setting may be refractory to the usual therapy unless the underlying hyperthyroidism is diagnosed and treated.

The pathogenesis of an apathetic response to thyrotoxicosis is not understood. Age alone is not the determining factor, as apathetic thyrotoxicosis has been described in the pediatric age group. A high index of suspicion must be maintained for this diagnosis.

## TREATMENT

The importance of early treatment of thyroid storm based upon the clinical impression cannot be overemphasized. Before the therapy is begun, blood should be drawn for sensitive TSH assay, free $T_4$ index or free $T_4$ assay and free $T_3$ and cortisol levels, a complete blood cell count, and routine chemistries. Appropriate cultures in search of infection are indicated.

Specific therapeutic goals can be divided into five areas; general supportive care, inhibition of thyroid hormone synthesis, retardation of thyroid hormone release, blockade of peripheral thyroid hormone effects, and identification and treatment of precipitating events. Each of these goals must be pursued concurrently.

### General Supportive Care

Adequate hydration with intravenous fluids and electrolytes to replace insensible and GI losses is indicated. Supplemental oxygen is needed because of increased oxygen consumption. Hyperglycemia

and hypercalcemia usually improve with fluid administration but occasionally require specific therapy. Fever should be controlled through the use of antipyretics and a cooling blanket. Aspirin should be used with caution or not at all during storm because salicylates increase free $T_3$ and $T_4$ levels because of decreased protein binding. This objection to the use of aspirin is theoretical, as no untoward clinical effect from aspirin use has been demonstrated. Caution should also be exercised in the use of sedatives during thyroid storm. Sedation depresses the level of consciousness and reduces the value of this parameter as an indicator of clinical improvement. Sedation may also cause hypoventilation.

Congestive heart failure should be treated with digitalis and diuretics even though congestive failure due to hyperthyroidism may be refractory to digitalis. Cardiac arrhythmias are treated with the usual antiarrhythmic agents. Atropine should be avoided, as its parasympatholytic effect may accelerate the heart rate. Atropine also may counteract the effect of propranolol.

Intravenous glucocorticoids equivalent to 300 mg of hydrocortisone per day should be given. The role of the adrenal glands in the pathogenesis of thyroid storm is uncertain, but the use of hydrocortisone has been reported to increase the rate of survival. Dexamethasone offers an advantage over other glucocorticoids as it decreases the peripheral conversion of $T_4$ to $T_3$.

### Inhibition of Thyroid Hormone Synthesis

The antithyroid drugs propylthiouracil (PTU) and methimazole act to block the synthesis of thyroid hormone by inhibiting the organification of tyrosine residues. This action begins within 1 h after administration, but a full therapeutic effect is not achieved for weeks. An initial loading dose of PTU, 900 to 1200 mg, should be given, followed by 300 to 600 mg daily for 3 to 6 weeks or until the thyrotoxicosis comes under control. Methimazole, 90 to 120 mg initially followed by 30 to 60 mg daily, is an acceptable alternative. Both preparations must be given orally or via a nasogastric tube, as no parenteral form is available. The PTU has an advantage over methimazole because it inhibits the peripheral conversion of $T_4$ to $T_3$ and produces a more rapid clinical response. Although these drugs inhibit the synthesis of new thyroid hormone, they do not affect the release of stored hormone.

### Retardation of Thyroid Hormone Release

Iodide administration promptly retards thyroidal release of stored hormones. Iodide can be provided by various preparations. It can be given as strong iodine solution, 1 mL 3 times daily, as potassium iodide, 10 drops of a solution containing 1 g/mL every 4 to 6 h, or as sodium iodide, 1 g every 8 to 12 h by slow intravenous infusion. Caution should be used in those patients taking potassium-sparing diuretics or potassium-containing drugs as potassium iodide preparations will add to the potassium load. Concomitant use of iodides and lithium salts may result in an additive hypothyroid effect. Iodide should be administered 1 h after the loading dose of antithyroid medication to prevent utilization of the iodide by the thyroid in the synthesis of new hormone.

### Blockade of Peripheral Thyroid Hormone Effects

Adrenergic blockade is a mainstay of therapy for thyroid storm. Currently, the β-adrenergic blocking agent propranolol is the drug of choice. In addition to reducing sympathetic hyperactivity, propranolol also partially blocks the peripheral conversion of $T_4$ to $T_3$.

Propranolol can be given intravenously at a rate of 1 mg/min with cautious incremental increases of 1 mg every 10 to 15 min to a total dose of 10 mg. The effects of the drug in controlling cardiac and psychomotor manifestations of storm should be seen in 10 min. The lowest possible dose required to control thyrotoxic symptoms should be used, and this dose can be repeated every 3 to 4 h as needed. The oral dose of propranolol is 20 to 120 mg every 4 to 6 h. When given by mouth, propranolol is effective in about 1 h. Propranolol has been used successfully in treatment of thyroid storm in childhood. Younger patients may require a dosage as high as 240 to 320 mg/day orally.

The usual precaution of avoiding propranolol in patients with bronchospastic disease and heart block should be observed. Electrocardiographic evaluation for conduction disturbance should occur before the administration of propranolol. In patients with congestive heart failure, the benefit of slowing the heart rate and controlling certain arrhythmias must be weighed against the risk of depressing myocardial contractility with β-adrenergic blockade. Urbanic believes the benefit outweighs the risk in this situation but recommends administration of digitalis before propranolol.

Guanethidine and reserpine also provide effective autonomic blockade and are alternatives to propranolol. Guanethidine depletes catecholamine stores and blocks their release. When given 1 to 2 mg/kg per day orally (50 to 150 mg), it is effective in 24 h, but it may not have its maximum effect for several days. Toxic reactions are cumulative and include postural hypotension, myocardial decompensation and diarrhea. It has an advantage over reserpine because it does not cause the pronounced sedation observed with that drug.

Reserpine acts to deplete catecholamine stores. As the initial dose, 1 to 5 mg is given intramuscularly, followed by 1 to 2.5 mg every 4 to 6 h. Improvement may be seen within 4 to 8 h. Side effects include sedation; psychic depression, which can be severe; abdominal cramping; and diarrhea.

Finally, a thorough evaluation for a precipitating cause of thyroid storm should be made. The treatment of thyroid storm should not be delayed by this evaluation, which may have to wait until the patient is at least partially stabilized.

Following the initiation of therapy, symptomatic improvement should occur within a few hours, primarily due to adrenergic blockade. Resolution of thyroid storm requires degradation of the already-circulating thyroid hormones, whose biological half-life is 6 days for $T_4$ and 22 h for $T_3$. Storm may last from 1 to 8 days, with an average duration of 3 days. If conventional therapy is not successful in controlling storm, alternative therapeutic modalities include peritoneal dialysis, plasmapheresis, and charcoal hemoperfusion to remove circulating thyroid hormone. Following recovery from thyroid storm, radioactive iodine therapy is the treatment of choice for hyperthyroidism. The mortality in untreated thyroid storm approaches 100 percent. Decreased mortality has occurred with the use of antithyroid drugs. Underlying illness is the cause of death in many cases. Prevention of thyroid storm is the ultimate solution to reduce mortality.

## BIBLIOGRAPHY

Cooper DS: Antithyroid drugs. *N Engl J Med* 311:1353, 1984.

Davis PJ, Davis FB: Hyperthyroidism in patients over the age of 60 years: Clinical features in 85 patients. *Medicine* 53:161, 1974.

Hay ID, Bayer MF, Kaplan MM, et al: American thyroid association assessment of current free thyroid hormone and thyrotropin measurements and guidelines for future clinical assays. *Clin Chem* 37:2002, 1991.

Mazzaferri EL, Reynolds JC, Young RL, et al: Propranolol as primary therapy for thyrotoxicosis: Results of a long-term prospective study. *Arch Intern Med* 136:50, 1976.

Thomas FB, Mazzaferri EL, Skillman TG: Apathetic thyrotoxicosis: A distinctive clinical and laboratory entity. *Ann Intern Med* 72:679, 1970.

Woeber KA: Thyrotoxicosis and the heart. *N Engl J Med* 327:94, 1992.

# 182
# HYPOTHYROIDISM AND MYXEDEMA COMA
## Gene Ragland

Myxedema coma is a life-threatening expression of hypothyroidism in its most severe form. It occurs most often during the winter months in elderly women with long-standing, undiagnosed, or undertreated hypothyroidism. It may be precipitated by infection or other stresses, and the diagnosis must be suspected based upon the clinical presentation. Treatment should be prompt and requires the administration of thyroid hormone in large doses. The mortality is greater than 50 percent in spite of optimum therapy.

## CAUSES OF HYPOTHYROIDISM

Hypothyroidism is a chronic systemic disorder characterized by progressive slowing of all bodily functions because of thyroid hormone deficiency. The prevalence of hypothyroidism is about 1 percent in women and 0.1 percent in men. After age 60, the prevalence may be as high as 6 to 7 percent in women. Thyroid hormone is secreted in response to stimulation of the thyroid gland by thyroid-stimulating hormone (TSH) from the anterior pituitary gland. The TSH release is promoted by thyrotropin releasing hormone (TRH) from the hypothalamus. Therefore, thyroid failure may be primary, due to intrinsic failure of the thyroid gland, or secondary, due to disease or destruction of the hypothalamus or pituitary gland (Table 182-1).

### Primary Hypothyroidism

Primary thyroid failure is by far the most common cause, accounting for 95 percent of the cases of hypothyroidism. The most common cause of hypothyroidism in the adult is treatment of Graves' disease by radioactive iodine or subtotal thyroidectomy. Postoperative hypothyroidism is usually evident within 12 to 15 months after surgery. The incidence of hypothyroidism following destruction of thyroid tissue with radioiodine increases progressively with time. The develop-

**Table 182-1.** Differentiation of Primary and Secondary Myxedema*

| Primary (Thyroid) | Secondary (Pituitary) |
| --- | --- |
| Previous thyroid operation | No previous thyroid operation |
| Obese | Less obese |
| Goiter present | No goiter present |
| Hypothermia more common | Hypothermia less common |
| Increased serum cholesterol | Normal serum cholesterol |
| Voice coarse | Voice less coarse |
| Pubic hair present | Pubic hair absent |
| Sella turcica normal | Sella turcica may be increased in size |
| Plasma cortisol level normal | Plasma cortisol level decreased |
| Skin dry and coarse | Skin fine and soft |
| Heart increased in size | Heart usually small |
| Normal menses and lactation | Traumatic delivery, no lactation; amenorrhea |
| No response to TSH | Good response to TSH |
| Good response to levothyroxine without steroids | Poor response to levothyroxine without steroids |
| PBI < 2 µg/dL | PBI > 2µg/dL |
| Serum TSH increased | Serum TSH decreased |

* TSH signifies thyroid-stimulating hormone; PBI, protein-bound iodine.

*Source:* Senior RM, Birge SJ: The recognition and management of myxedema coma. *JAMA* 217:61, 1971.

ment of hypothyroidism as a consequence of surgical or radioiodine therapy may take years or decades. If hypothyroidism develops, these patients are committed to replacement thyroid hormone therapy for life.

Autoimmune thyroid disorders are the next most common cause of hypothyroidism. These include primary hypothyroidism and Hashimoto's thyroiditis. Primary hypothyroidism is thought to be the end result of an autoimmune destruction of the thyroid gland and produces thyroid failure because of glandular atrophy. Hashimoto's thyroiditis is the most common cause of goitrous hypothyroidism in areas with adequate iodine and may cause hypothyroidism because of defective hormone synthesis. There is clinical and immunologic overlap of these entities. Other causes of primary thyroid failure are rare and include iodine deficiency, antithyroid drugs such as lithium and phenylbutazone, spontaneous hypothyroidism from Graves' disease, and congenital causes.

## Secondary Hypothyroidism

Secondary thyroid failure accounts for 5 percent of the cases of hypothyroidism. Pituitary tumors, postpartum hemorrhage, or infiltrative disorders, such as sarcoidosis, may result in secondary thyroid failure. There are clinical and historical differences that distinguish primary thyroid insufficiency from pituitary failure (see Table 182-1.) This differential diagnosis is difficult on clinical grounds and requires laboratory evaluation. In general, the TSH level is high in primary hypothyroidism and low or normal in secondary hypothyroidism. Disease of the hypothalamus may cause failure to secrete TRH and may result in thyroid failure. This condition has been termed *tertiary hypothyroidism.* A few hypothyroid patients have been identified who have presumed hypothalamic disease and respond to TRH administration by increasing TSH above baseline levels.

## Clinical Presentation

All patients who develop myxedema are hypothyroid, but not all hypothyroid patients have myxedema. Hypothyroidism is a graded phenomenon with various signs and symptoms along the clinical spectrum. With moderate to severe hypothyroidism, a nonpitting, dry, waxy swelling of the skin and subcutaneous tissue may occur, resulting in a puffy face and extremities. The term *myxedema* refers to this particular presentation of hypothyroidism.

The signs and symptoms of mild hypothyroidism may be subtle and the diagnosis difficult. With advanced hypothyroidism, the patients present with characteristic features. Typically, they complain of fatigue, weakness, cold intolerance, constipation, and weight gain without an increase in appetite. Muscle cramps, decreased hearing, mental disturbances, and menstrual irregularities are additional symptoms. Cutaneous features noted on physical examination include dry, scaly, yellow skin, puffy eyes, thinning of the eyebrows, and scant body hair. The voice may be deep and coarse and the tongue thickened. Paresthesia, ataxia, and prolongation of the deep tendon reflexes are characteristic neurologic manifestations. Bell's palsy due to hypothyroidism has been reported. In advanced cases, delusions, hallucinations, and psychosis (myxedema madness) may occur. Abdominal distension and fecal impaction may be present. Cardiac findings include bradycardia, enlarged heart, and low voltage on ECG. Mild hypertension rather than hypotension is the rule. Hypertension in conjunction with hypercholesterolemia may contribute to coronary artery disease and angina pectoris. A surgical scar on the neck may be present, but a palpable goiter is uncommon.

Diagnosis of hypothyroidism in a patient with these signs and symptoms can be made essentially on clinical grounds. Abnormally low levels of thyroid hormones confirm the diagnosis. Serum TSH levels should also be measured, and elevated levels are virtually diagnostic of primary hypothyroidism. If the disease is not treated, death follows a progressive intensification of these signs and symptoms.

The time from onset to death varies between 10 and 15 years. Appropriate therapy is L-thyroxine in an average maintenance dosage of 0.1 to 0.3 mg once daily. The dosage must be individualized and may be higher or lower. Other thyroid preparations are available and acceptable as replacement thyroid hormone therapy.

## MYXEDEMA COMA

Myxedema coma is a rare complication of hypothyroidism. The incidence is greater in women than men, and approximately half the patients are between 60 and 70 years old. A patient with undiagnosed hypothyroidism may develop coma as the initial manifestation. More commonly, the disease progresses insidiously, and coma develops when the patient is subjected to stress.

## Precipitating Factors

A precipitating factor can be found in most cases of myxedema coma. Exposure to a cold environment is a significant antecedent occurrence with pulmonary infection and heart failure the most frequent precipitating events. Other stresses reported to initiate coma include hemorrhage, cerebrovascular accident, hypoxia, hypercapnia, hyponatremia, hypoglycemia, and trauma.

Significantly, it has been observed that more than 50 percent of the patients whose cases were reported in the literature lapsed into coma after admission to the hospital. In this setting, the stress of diagnostic and therapeutic procedures, acquisition of nosocomial infections, and the administration of certain drugs have been implicated as causative factors. Hypothyroid patients metabolize drugs more slowly than normal persons, and narcotics, anesthetics, phenothiazines, and other tranquilizers or sedatives have been reported to induce coma. Disastrous results may occur in a patient with advanced hypothyroidism and myxedema madness whose psychosis is treated with phenothiazines. The β-blocking drugs may cause myxedema coma by reducing thyroid hormone levels through peripheral conversion of thyroxine to triiodothyronine. Amiodarone-induced hypothyroidism leading to myxedema coma has been reported. Caution must be used when administering drugs, even in normal amounts, to hypothyroid patients. A final drug-related cause of myxedema coma is the failure to take necessary replacement thyroid hormone medication.

## Clinical Presentation

The diagnosis of myxedema coma may easily be made in a patient who presents with the previously described general appearance and physical findings and with a history of previous thyroid hormone medication, radioactive iodine therapy, or subtotal thyroidectomy. Unfortunately, the diagnosis is not always that easy. A wide variety of clinical and laboratory abnormalities occur and may tend to occupy the physician's attention. Coma may be attributed to hypothermia, respiratory failure, and $CO_2$ narcosis; electrolye imbalance and hyponatremia; hypoglycemia; congestive heart failure; stroke; drug overdose; and other causes. Indeed, any of these disorders may lead to or worsen coma in the hypothyroid patient, but unless the underlying thyroid failure is diagnosed and treated, therapeutic efforts are unsuccessful. The overall clinical picture must be correlated and the diagnosis of myxedema coma considered.

### Hypothermia

Hypothermia, unaccompanied by sweating or shivering, is typical of patients in myxedema coma and occurs in 80 percent of the cases. Approximately 15 percent have a temperature of 29.5°C (85°F) or less. A normal or elevated temperature suggests underlying infection. It is not coincidental that most patients develop myxedema coma during the winter, as normal thermogenesis is impaired in hypothyroidism.

This important diagnostic sign may be missed if a low-reading thermometer is not used or if the mercury in the thermometer is not shaken down. Hypothermia should be treated by gradual rewarming at room temperature. Too-rapid rewarming may cause peripheral vasodilation and circulatory collapse.

## Respiratory Failure

Hypoventilation, hypercapnia, and hypoxia are common in patients with myxedema coma and may be the cause of death in many instances. Multiple factors have been implicated as causes of respiratory failure. Impaired respiratory mechanics due to dysfunction of the muscles of the respiratory system may lead to alveolar hypoventilation, hypercapnia, and hypoxia, and loss of responsiveness of the respiratory center to these stimuli. With thyroid hormone replacement hypoxic ventilatory drive is increased but hypercapnic ventilatory drive is not.

Additional factors that may further impair pulmonary function include obesity, congestive heart failure, pleural effusions, ascites, parenchymal lung involvement by myxedematous infiltrate, enlarged tongue, and changes in the airway, which may occur over its entire length. Airway obstruction due to myxedematous infiltration of the laryngeal mucosa has been reported. Patients should be evaluated by chest roentgenography and arterial blood gas levels, and require close monitoring. Drugs that may further depress respirations should be avoided. Mechanical ventilation may be required, and initial tracheostomy has been recommended because of the long recovery time for normal ventilatory function.

## Hyponatremia

Water retention with hyponatremia and hypochloremia is another common finding in myxedema coma. Hyponatremia is dilutional, due to extracellular volume expansion and impaired ability to excrete a water load. Several mechanisms to account for the hyponatremia have been proposed. These range from deficiency of adrenal cortical hormones to decreased water delivery to the distal nephron to inappropriate secretion of antidiuretic hormone. Regardless of the etiology, hyponatremia is a potentially grave complication that can lead to water intoxication, brain edema, and death.

Conventional therapy is fluid restriction, but hypertonic saline is recommended if the serum sodium level is less than 115 mEq/L. A convincing case for a different therapeutic approach utilizing hypertonic saline, furosemide, and thyroid hormone has been presented. A review of the 24 hyponatremic-hypothyroid patients described in the literature since 1953 showed the serum sodium levels to range from 120 to 129 mEq/L in 8 patients and from 110 to 119 mEq/L in 10 patients, and to be less than 110 mEq/L in 6 others. All 6 patients treated with hypertonic saline survived, while 13 out of 18 who did not receive this treatment died. Intravenous furosemide induces negative water balance, while hypertonic saline replaces urinary sodium losses. Extreme caution must be used to avoid heart failure during the administration of hypertonic saline.

## Cardiovascular System

The cardiovascular system is altered in structure and function with advanced hypothyroidism. Hypotension, cardiac enlargement detectable on x-ray films, and bradycardia are the most significant abnormalities to occur during myxedema coma. Thyroid hormones and sympathomimetic amines act synergistically to maintain left ventricular performance and vascular tone. Hypotension may result from a decreased synergistic effect due to thyroid hormone deficiency. Left ventricular dysfunction and hypotension are usually corrected by thyroid hormone replacement. Vasopressors do not work well in the absence of thyroid hormone and should be used, with caution, only in cases of severe hypotension unresponsive to other therapy. Ventricular arrhythmias may occur because of the synergistic actions of simultaneously administered thyroid hormone and vasopressors on a myxedematous myocardium.

Cardiomegaly is common, and is thought to be due to either pericardial effusion or underlying heart disease and not to ventricular dilation induced by hypothyroidism. The presence or absence of cardiomegaly on x-ray film is not a reliable indicator of a pericardial effusion, and echocardiography is the best way to identify a pericardial effusion. In spite of the frequency of pericardial effusions, cardiac tamponade in myxedema coma is rare because of the slow formation of the effusion and the ability of the pericardium to distend. Most pericardial effusions resolve with thyroid hormone replacement, but some may require pericardiocentesis or pericardial fenestration.

Sinus bradycardia is the most common electrocardiographic abnormality during myxedema coma. Other findings include low voltage, flattening or inversion of the T waves, and prolongation of the PR interval. In spite of impaired cardiac contractility, pericardial effusions, and conduction disturbances, congestive heart failure is unusual in myxedema coma and probably reflects underlying heart disease.

## Nervous System

Coma is the terminal expression of neurologic dysfunction in myxedema and may be directly due to a lack of thyroid hormone in the brain. A variety of neurologic symptoms premonitory of myxedema coma do occur. Psychiatric disorders include slowed mentation, memory loss, personality changes, hallucinations, delusions, and psychosis. Cerebellar ataxia, intention tremor, nystagmus, and difficulty with coordinated movements may occur. Twenty-five percent of those who develop myxedema coma initially present with grand mal seizure. Many of the neuropsychiatric abnormalities improve with thyroid hormone replacement, but permanent dementia may remain after treatment. The role of hypothermia, $CO_2$ narcosis, cerebral edema, and other metabolic disturbances in the genesis of coma must not be overlooked.

## Gastrointestinal System

Patients with myxedema may have abdominal distension due to ascites, paralytic ileus, or fecal impaction. Acquired megacolon is almost uniformly observed and has been the cause of unnecessary abdominal surgery. Urinary retention may occur, causing lower abdominal discomfort from a distended bladder. The weight gain that occurs with hypothyroidism is due to accumulation of some adipose tissue and retention of fluid. Patients with myxedema coma may be emaciated because of long-standing illness and decreased food intake. The treatment of abdominal complications consists of thyroid replacement and conservative measures such as nasogastric aspiration and enemas.

## Laboratory

Although some laboratory findings are characteristic of myxedema coma, only thyroid function tests can confirm hypothyroidism. The combination of free $T_4$ assay and a sensitive TSH assay are the primary means of assessing thyroid status in all patients. The patient with hypothyroidism has a low free $T_4$. TSH is elevated in primary hypothyroidism, whereas when pituitary or hypothalamic disease is the cause of hypothyroidism, TSH is low. The results of these tests will not be available for use in the emergent situation but can later be used to support the clinical impression.

Characteristic laboratory abnormalities of myxedema coma already mentioned include hypoxemia, hypercapnia, hyponatremia, and hypochloremia. Serum potassium levels are extremely variable. Blood glucose levels are generally in the normal range, but severe hypoglycemia can occur. Hypercalcemia is rare, but hypocalcemia can occur in thyroidectomized patients in whom the parathyroids have been removed.

Bacterial infection may be reflected only by a leftward shift in the differential white blood cell count without appreciable elevation of the total white cell count.

Elevated serum cholesterol levels occur in approximately two-thirds of myxedematous patients. Malnutrition may lower the serum cholesterol level in some cases. Carotenemia has also been reported and may be the cause of the yellowish skin discoloration. Occasionally, striking elevations of the levels of muscle enzymes such as creatine kinase (CPK), serum glutamic-oxaloacetic transaminase (SGOT), lactate dehydrogenase (LDH), and fructose-biphosphate aldolase may be present. The elevations are thought to be due to changes in membrane permeability in skeletal muscle rather than to muscle destruction. The concentrations of these enzymes fall quickly when thyroid hormone is replaced. Finally, in most hypothyroid patients the CSF protein level is elevated to 100 mg/dL or more. The CSF pressure may occasionally be increased to over 400 mmH$_2$O. The significance of these CSF abnormalities remains obscure.

## TREATMENT

Patients with myxedema coma are critically ill with a multiplicity of precarious and complex management problems. Specific therapy requires the administration of large doses of thyroid hormone. This decision must be based upon clinical judgment and made with extreme caution. The recommended dose of thyroid hormone could be fatal to the euthyroid comatose patient and harmful to the patient with ordinary myxedema. Every attempt to rule out causes of coma unrelated to hypothyroidism must be made first.

### Supportive Therapy

Coma in myxedema may be primary, from a cerebral lack of thyroid hormone, or secondary, due to complications or precipitating causes. Treatment of the secondary causes of coma already mentioned includes oxygen administration and ventilatory support for respiratory failure, avoidance of drugs that may further depress respiratory or metabolic function, gradual rewarming of hypothermic patients, correction of hyponatremia by fluid restriction or hypertonic saline and furosemide, correction of hypoglycemia by glucose infusion, and treatment of hypotension with thyroid hormone and vasopressors, as needed. A thorough search for precipitating causes of coma should be made. Antibiotics are indicated for underlying infection. Additional adjunctive therapy is hydrocortisone, 300 mg/day, to protect against adrenal insufficiency.

### Thyroid Hormome

Thyroid hormone replacement is the most critical and specific aspect of therapy for myxedema coma. The treatment already mentioned is largely supportive and is not fully effective until adequate thyroid hormone is given. Disagreement exists over the type, doses, and route of thyroid hormone administration.

Intravenous thyroxine is the drug of choice of most authors. It has been shown to be fully effective within 24 h with an onset of action in 6 h. The initial intravenous dose is 400 to 500 µg infused slowly; this is followed by 50 to 100 µg IV daily. Following the initial dose, some authors recommend no further thyroxine therapy until 3 to 7 days later. Once-daily therapy allows a smooth rise in hormone levels, as the turnover rate for L-thyroxine is about 10 percent per day. An oral dosage of thyroxine, 100 to 200 µg/day, can be started when possible. Cardiac arrest following the intravenous administration of L-thyroxine has been reported. The dose of thyroxine should be reduced in the face of cardiac ischemia or arrhythmias.

Triiodothyronine is an effective drug for treatment of myxedema coma. Triiodothyronine is four times more pharmacologically active than thyroxine. It has previously been available only in tablet form but intravenous L-triiodothyronine is now available. An initial IV dose of 25 to 50 µg is recommended for the emergent treatment of myxedema coma or precoma in adults. The dose should be lowered to 10 to 20 µg is patients with known or suspected cardiovascular disease. Subsequent dosage is 65 to 100 µg per 24 h in 3 to 4 divided doses and half of this amount in patients with cardiovascular disease. There is no difference in the contraindications or drug interactions between IV T$_3$ or T$_4$. With either replacement medication, overall clinical improvement should be seen in 24 to 36 h.

## BIBLIOGRAPHY

Holvey, DN, Goodner CJ, Nicoloff JT, et al: Treatment of myxedema coma with intravenous thyroxine. *Arch Intern Med* 113:89, 1964.

Ladenson PW, Goldenheim PD, Ridgway C: Rapid pituitary and peripheral tissue responses to intravenous L-triiodothyronine in hypothyroidism. *J Clin Endocrinol Metab* 56:1252, 1983.

Mitchell JM: Thyroid disease in the emergency department: Thyroid function tests and hypothyroidism and myxedema coma. *Emerg Med Clin North Am* 7:885, 1989.

# 183
# ADRENAL INSUFFICIENCY AND ADRENAL CRISIS
## Gene Ragland

Adrenal insufficiency consists of decreased levels of or absent hormones produced by the adrenal glands and results from structural or functional lesions of the adrenal cortex, the anterior pituitary gland, or the hypothalamus. Deficit of adrenal hormones may manifest clinically as a chronic, insidious disorder, or as an acute, life-threatening emergency. Therapy of adrenal insufficiency is specific and includes replacement of the deficient hormones.

Chronic adrenal insufficiency is due to a variety of causes. It may be primary (Addison's disease), due to failure of the adrenal glands. It may also occur secondarily because of failure of the pituitary gland (hypopituitarism) or as a tertiary insufficiency due to hypothalamic dysfunction. Iatrogenic adrenal suppression from chronic steroid use is termed iatrogenic tertiary adrenal insufficiency. Acute adrenal insufficiency (adrenal crisis) may result from certain acute events, or when a person with chronic adrenal insufficiency is subjected to stress and exhausts reserve adrenal hormones, or when replacement hormone medication is discontinued.

## PATHOPHYSIOLOGY OF THE ADRENAL GLANDS

The adrenal glands are divisible into the cortex and medulla. The adrenal cortex is essential for life and produces glucocorticoid, mineralocorticoid, and androgenic steroid hormones. The medulla secretes the catecholamines epinephrine and norepinephrine, largely under neural control. No definite clinical condition has been ascribed to hypofunction of the adrenal medulla. Most of the manifestations of adrenal insufficiency occur when the physiologic requirement for glucocorticoid and mineralocorticoid hormones exceeds the capacity of the adrenal glands to produce them.

### Cortisol

The major glucocorticoid is cortisol, which is secreted in response to direct stimulation by adrenocorticotropic hormone (ACTH) from the anterior pituitary gland. Secretion of ACTH is governed by the hormone corticotropin-releasing factor (CRF) from the hypothalamus. This normally occurs with a diurnal rhythm, with the highest levels in the morning and the lowest levels in the late evening. Upon stimulation by ACTH, the adrenal glands respond in minutes to secrete cortisol in direct proportion to the ACTH concentration. Cortisol is normally secreted at the rate of 20 to 25 mg/day. Through negative feedback inhibition, the plasma cortisol level acts to suppress ACTH release.

By an undefined mechanism, stress factors such as anoxia, trauma, infections, and hypoglycemia can also trigger CRF and ACTH release and produce cortisol levels several times normal. The release of CRF in response to stress is resistant to suppression through negative feedback inhibition.

Cortisol is a potent hormone and affects the metabolism of most body tissues. In general, cortisol acts to maintain blood glucose levels by decreasing glucose uptake at extrahepatic sites and by providing precursors for gluconeogenesis via protein and fat breakdown. Cortisol governs the distribution of water between extracellular and intracellular compartments and possesses a minor sodium-retaining effect. It also acts to enhance the pressor effects of catecholamines on heart muscle and arterioles. In supraphysiologic amounts, cortisol inhibits inflammatory and allergic reactions. Finally, through negative feedback inhibition, cortisol suppresses the secretion of ACTH and melanocyte-stimulating hormone (MSH) from the anterior pituitary gland.

## Aldosterone

The major mineralocorticoid is aldosterone. The renin-angiotensin system and plasma potassium concentration regulate aldosterone through negative feedback loops. These mechanisms are probably of equal importance and far more important than the minor aldosterone-stimulating effect of ACTH.

Aldosterone acts to increase sodium reabsorption and potassium excretion, primarily in the distal tubules of the kidneys. Other tissue effects of aldosterone are minor in comparison with its regulation of sodium and potassium levels.

## Androgens

Androgenic hormone production by the adrenal glands is regulated by ACTH and is trivial in men in comparison with the production of these hormones by the gonads. In women, however, androgens from the adrenal glands *do* contribute a significant proportion to androgen metabolism.

## PRIMARY ADRENAL INSUFFICIENCY

### Idiopathic

Primary adrenal insufficiency, or Addison's disease, is due to disease or destruction of the adrenal cortex and has a wide variety of causes (see Table 183-1). Approximately 90 percent of the adrenal cortex must be involved before clinical manifestations of adrenal failure result. Idiopathic atrophy of the adrenal glands is the leading cause of chronic adrenal insufficiency. Idiopathic adrenal insufficiency has been further divided into autoimmune (70 to 75 percent) and truly idiopathic (25 to 30 percent).

There is an overwhelming association between idiopathic adrenal insufficiency and other autoimmune diseases. Associated diseases include diabetes mellitus, Hashimoto's thyroiditis, pernicious anemia, and primary ovarian failure. Other investigators have reported frequent association with hypoparathyroidism, chronic active hepatitis, malabsorption, chronic mucocutaneous candidiasis, alopecia, and vitiligo.

**Table 183-1.** Pathogenesis of Primary Adrenal Insufficiency

Primary, chronic
    Idiopathic (autoimmune)
    Infiltrative or infectious
        Tuberculosis
        Fungal infections
        Sarcoidosis
        Amyloidosis
        Hemochromatosis
        Acquired immunodeficiency syndrome (AIDS)
        Neoplastic (metastatic) disease
        Adrenoleukodystrophy
    Hemorrhage or infarction
    Bilateral adrenalectomy
    Drugs
    Congenital adrenal hyperplasia
    Congenital unresponsiveness to ACTH
Primary, acute
    Hemorrhage (adrenal apoplexy)
        Fulminant septicemia
        Newborn
        Anticoagulants
    Discontinuation of replacement steroids

### Infiltrative or Infectious

Adrenal tuberculosis has declined in frequency as a cause of Addison's disease but is still reported to be a cause in 17 to 21 percent of the cases. Fungal infections and other infiltrative processes are infrequent causes of adrenal insufficiency during active, disseminated disease. Adrenal insufficiency as a complication of the acquired immunodeficiency syndrome (AIDS) has been reported. Infectious infiltration of the adrenal glands with *Mycobacterium avium* or *M. intracellulare* or with cytomegalovirus may have caused the adrenal failure. Metastatic carcinoma in the adrenal glands is a relatively frequent finding at autopsy in patients with certain carcinomas, but it only rarely causes adrenal insufficiency.

### Bilateral Adrenal Hemorrhage

Bilateral adrenal gland hemorrhage (adrenal apoplexy) is rare. In general, patients with a serious underlying condition whose adrenal glands are stressed are at risk for this complication. Stress-stimulated adrenal glands are hemorrhage prone. The association between adrenal hemorrhage and anticoagulant therapy with heparin and dicumarol is well established. Adrenal hemorrhage in this setting is most likely to occur between the third and eighteenth day of anticoagulation. Sudden deterioration with hypotension and pain in the flank, costovertebral angle, or epigastrium should suggest this disastrous event. Associated findings may include fever, nausea, vomiting, and disturbed sensorium. Computed tomography and ultrasound can assist in establishing this diagnosis. Other stressful events that have been associated with adrenal hemorrhage include surgery, trauma, burns, convulsions, pregnancy, and adrenal vein thrombosis.

Adrenal crisis as a consequence of adrenal hemorrhage also occurs with overwhelming septicemia and in the newborn. Fulminant septicemia with meningococcus, pneumococcus, staphylococcus, streptococcus, *Haemophilus influenzae,* and gram-negative organisms has been reported to cause adrenal hemorrhage. The Waterhouse-Friderichsen syndrome is a life-threatening disorder resulting from overwhelming septicemia due to meningococcemia. The patient is acutely ill and has shaking chills, severe headache, and a petechial rash that may progress to extensive purpura. Bilateral adrenal gland hemorrhage frequently occurs with this disorder. Vascular collapse and death may result unless the patient is promptly treated.

## Miscellaneous

Another cause of primary adrenal failure is bilateral adrenalectomy for metastatic breast or prostate cancer or for Cushing's syndrome. Following such a procedure the patient is totally dependent upon replacement corticosteroids for life. Chemotherapeutic agents such as mitotane (*o,p'*-DDD) used in treatment of Cushing's disease can produce adrenal failure. Other drugs such as methadone, rifampin, and ketoconazole have been reported to cause adrenal insufficiency. Finally, rare congenital and inherited disorders can cause adrenal insufficiency.

In children, adrenal insufficiency is due to rare congenital causes or to acquired lesions of the hypothalamus, pituitary or adrenal cortex. By far, the most common cause of acquired chronic adrenal insufficiency is autoimmune destruction of the adrenal glands. Type I autoimmune polyendocrinopathy manifests with chronic mucocutaneous candidiasis, hypoparathyroidism and Addison's disease. Type II autoimmune disease presents with adrenal failure in association with thyroid disorder or insulin dependent diabetes mellitus.

Infections account for approximately 20 percent of the cases of pediatric adrenal insufficiency. Among those are infiltrative destruction of the gland by fungal infections and tuberculosis. Hemorrhage into the adrenal glands may occur in the neonatal period as a consequence of a complicated labor or asphyxia. Another cause of adrenal gland hemorrhage is the Waterhouse-Friderichsen syndrome resulting from meningococcemia and producting shock. Finally, about one-third of patients with adrenoleukodystrophy will develop adrenal insufficiency, usually after 4 years of age.

## Clinical Presentation

The clinical manifestations of chronic adrenal insufficiency develop gradually with subtle signs and symptoms that provide a diagnostic challenge. The clinical presentation of Addison's disease can be explained on the basis of a deficiency of cortisol and aldosterone and a lack of feedback suppression of ACTH and MSH.

Cortisol deficiency manifests clinically with anorexia, nausea, vomiting, lethargy, hypoglycemia with fasting, and inability to withstand even minor stresses without shock. The ability to excrete a free water load is also impaired and can lead to water intoxication. Lack of aldosterone results in impaired ability to conserve sodium and excrete potassium. The patient with aldosterone deficiency presents with sodium depletion, dehydration, hypotension, postural syncope, and decreased cardiac size and output. Renal blood flow is decreased, and azotemia may develop. Hyperkalemia is commonly seen but rarely is severe. Lack of suppression of ACTH and MSH secretion occurs because of deficient cortisol levels and results in increased pigmentation.

The overall clinical picture of a patient with Addison's disease is that of one who is weak and lethargic, with loss of vigor, and fatigue on exertion. The patient may have a feeble tachycardic pulse. Postural hypotension and syncope are common. In spite of hypotension, the extremities usually remain warm. Heart sounds may be soft or almost inaudible on auscultation.

Gastrointestinal (GI) symptoms are a prominent feature of chronic adrenal insufficiency and include anorexia, nausea, vomiting, weight loss, abdominal pain, and sometimes diarrhea.

Cutaneous manifestations of Addison's disease include increased brownish pigmentation over exposed body areas such as the face, neck, arms, and dorsum of the hands, and over friction or pressure points such as the elbows, knees, fingers, toes, and nipples. Pigmentation of mucous membranes, darkening of nevi and hair, and longitudinal pigmented bands in the nails may be seen. Vitiligo, mucocutaneous candidiasis, and alopecia may occur with Addison's disease that has an autoimmune cause. Women with Addison's disease may exhibit decreased growth of axillary and pubic hair because of

adrenal androgen deficiency. This is not seen in men because of adequate testicular androgen.

Mentally these patients vary from alert to confused. Unconsciousness is rare unless the condition is preterminal. The sensory modalities of taste, olfaction, and hearing may be increased. Hyperkalemic paralysis is a rare, emergent complication of adrenal insufficiency; the patient presents with a rapidly ascending muscular weakness which leads to flaccid quadriplegia. Treatment of this complication consists of the intravenous administration of glucose and insulin or bicarbonate.

## Laboratory

The usual laboratory findings in patients with primary adrenal insufficiency include hyponatremia, hyperkalemia, hypoglycemia, and azotemia. Hyponatremia is usually mild to moderate, and severe hyponatremia (<120 mEq/L) is rare. Hyperkalemia is usually mild, and the potassium level rarely exceeds 7 mEq/L. Initial potassium levels may be normal or low if protracted vomiting has occurred. Rarely, hyperkalemia may be severe and cause cardiac arrhythmia or paralysis.

Hypoglycemia is infrequent in adults with chronic adrenal insufficiency in the absence of infection, fever or alcohol ingestion. Moderate elevation of the blood urea nitrogen (BUN) level may occur because of dehydration secondary to aldosterone deficiency. Azotemia is usually reversible with rehydration.

Electrocardiographic changes include flat or inverted T waves, a prolonged QT interval, low voltage, a prolonged PR or QRS interval, and a depressed ST segment. The ECG changes reflective of hyperkalemia may also be present. The chest x-ray film may show a small, narrow cardiac silhouette due to decreased intravascular volume. A flat plate film of the abdomen may show adrenal calcification, which is most commonly due to tuberculosis but may occur with infection or hemorrhage.

## SECONDARY AND TERTIARY ADRENAL INSUFFICIENCY

Secondary adrenal insufficiency may be due to disease or destruction of the pituitary gland, and tertiary insufficiency due to hypothalamic dysfunction, resulting in impaired capacity of the pituitary to secrete ACTH. Those disorders responsible for secondary or tertiary adrenal failure are listed in Table 183-2.

The most common cause of tertiary adrenal insufficiency and adrenal crisis is iatrogenic adrenal suppression from prolonged steroid use. Rapid withdrawal of steroids from patients with adrenal

**Table 183-2.** Pathogenesis of Secondary or Tertiary Adrenal
Insuffciency

| |
|---|
| Secondary |
|     Pituitary tumor (chromophobe adenoma, craniopharyngioma, hamartoma, meningioma, glioma) |
|     Pituitary hemorrhage or vascular accident |
|     Postpartum pituitary infarction (Sheehan's syndrome) |
|     Infiltrative and granulomatous disease |
|         Sarcoidosis |
|         Hemochromatosis |
|         Histiocytosis X |
|     Internal carotid artery aneurysm |
|     Head trauma (basilar skull fracture) |
|     Infection (meningitis, cavernous sinus thrombosis) |
|     Hypophysectomy |
|     Pituitary gland irradiation |
|     Isolated ACTH deficiency |
| Tertiary |
|     Iatrogenic HPA suppression due to steroid therapy |
|     Discontinuation of replacement steroids. |

atrophy secondary to chronic steroid use may result in collapse and death, especially under circumstances of increased stress. Exogenous administration of glucocorticoids may cause hypothalamic-pituitary-adrenal (HPA) suppression and subsequent adrenal atrophy. This complication has been reported to occur not only with oral steroids but also with those given by the intrathecal, topical, and inhalant routes.

The mechanism of continued adrenal atrophy following discontinuation of exogenous steroids may be a failure of normal diurnal release of CRF. Stress-induced release of ACTH may remain intact, but the atrophic adrenal glands are unable to secrete sufficient cortisol to meet the physiologic requirements in response to stress. The shortest time interval or the smallest dose at which HPA suppression occurs is unknown. As a general rule, there is no suppression regardless of the dose if its duration of use is less than three weeks. In addition, there is no suppression if the dose is <10 mg of prednisone regardless of the duration unless it is given on an h.s. timetable. Any patient who is on more than 20 mg of prednisone for greater than three weeks is suppressed and should have the necessary precautions taken.

Following prolonged supraphysiologic dosages of steroids, it may take up to 6 to 12 months for recovery of HPA function when steroids are withdrawn completely. Until complete recovery has occurred, it is wise to assume the patient will need basal steroid therapy and supplementary therapy during intercurrent illness or stress. Adrenal suppression must be suspected based upon the history of prior steroid use. When in doubt about the HPA status of a seriously ill or deteriorating patient, steroids should be given.

## Clinical Presentation

Significant clinical and laboratory differences exist between patients with primary and those with secondary adrenal insufficiency. With secondary adrenal failure, the capacity of the pituitary to secrete ACTH is impaired. The level of aldosterone is largely unaffected because of its regulation by the renin-angiotensin system and the plasma potassium concentration. The clinical manifestations of secondary adrenal failure are due to insufficiency of cortisol and adrenal androgens. In addition, insufficiency of other anterior pituitary hormones such as growth hormone, thyroid hormone, and gonadotropic hormone may cause clinical abnormalities.

Patients with secondary adrenal insufficiency are better able to tolerate sodium deprivation without developing shock. This is true because of intact aldosterone secretion. Hyponatremia, hyperkalemia, and azotemia are not prominent features of secondary failure. Hypoglycemia, however, may be more common in patients with hypopituitarism because of concomitant growth hormone deficiency. Hyperpigmentation does not occur with secondary failure because ACTH and MSH are eliminated at their source, the pituitary gland. Finally, with secondary failure, men as well as women may exhibit signs of androgen deficiency because of insufficient gonadotopic hormone from the pituitary.

## DIAGNOSIS

Primary adrenal insufficiency is diagnosed by demonstrating a low baseline plasma cortisol level and failure to increase this level in response to exogenous administration of ACTH. Any patient who has cortisol level of >20 μg/dl does not have adrenal insufficiency of any type. Failure to respond to ACTH stimulation occurs because the adrenal cortex is damaged or destroyed and has no functional capacity to respond. Secondary adrenal insufficiency is diagnosed by demonstrating low plasma cortisol and urinary metabolite levels that increase in a stepwise fashion with repetitive ACTH stimulation over a period of days. A variety of tests to assess the integrity of the HPA axis are available.

A rapid screening test can reliably distinguish patients with normal adrenal function from those with adrenal insufficiency. This test is based on the fact that adrenal response to a single injection of ACTH is maximal within 1 h. Plasma for measurement of baseline cortisol level is drawn, and then 25 units of corticotropin (synthetic ACTH) is administered subcutaneously, intramuscularly, or intravenously. Another plasma cortisol level is obtained 30 to 60 min later. Normal persons should respond with a doubling of the baseline cortisol level, unless the patient has an already existing high basal level due to stress or some other factor. In this instance, the cortisol level would not double but the patient could still have normal physiology. Patients with primary adrenal insufficiency show no increase in plasma cortisol levels, whereas those with secondary adrenal failure may show no, or a slight, response to corticotropin. A normal response is defined by a peak cortisol value of greater than or equal to 20 μg/dL. However, both falsely normal and abnormal rapid ACTH test results have been reported. This test should be used as a screening test, or to assess adrenal reserve in patients previously receiving steroids, but not as a diagnostic test for adrenocortical failure. A more prolonged period of ACTH stimulation is necessary to confirm adrenal failure and to reliably distinguish primary from secondary adrenal insufficiency. However, measurement of ACTH will also help clarify this differential and will be less labor-intensive.

## TREATMENT

### Glucocorticoid

Therapy of primary adrenal insufficiency consists of replacement of cortisol and aldosterone, and, on occasion, supplemental androgen therapy in the female patient. The usual maintenance dosage for glucocorticoid replacement varies from 20 to 37.5 mg of cortisol per day. Various preparations may be used (see Table 183-3 for steroid equivalents). A generally accepted dosage schedule is 5 mg of prednisone in the morning followed by 2.5 mg of prednisone in the afternoon. This simulates the normal diurnal variation of cortisol secretion. A few patients, especially large active men, may require a total daily dose of 10 mg of prednisone for optimum response.

Another treatment alternative is 5 mg of prednisone h.s. or 15 to 20 mg of hydrocortisone on awakening and 5 to 10 mg in the early afternoon. Finally, once a day dosing for prednisone is sufficient.

### Mineralocorticoid

Mineralocorticoid replacement in patients with primary adrenal insufficiency can be achieved by administration of the synthetic mineralocorticoid fludrocortisone acetate (Florinef), 0.05 to 0.2 mg/day orally. This dosage should be appropriately reduced in patients in whom hypertension develops. It is also important for the patient with Addison's disease to maintain an adequate dietary salt intake.

### Androgen

The woman with primary adrenal insufficiency may show signs of androgen deficiency such as decreased growth of axillary and pubic

**Table 183-3.** Steroid Equivalents

| Drug | Equivalent Dose, mg | Na⁺ Retention |
|---|---|---|
| Short-acting | | |
| Cortisone | 25 | 2+ |
| Hydrocortisone (cortisol) | 20 | 2+ |
| Prednisone | 5 | 1+ |
| Prednisolone | 5 | 1+ |
| Methylprednisolone | 4 | 0 |
| Intermediate-acting | | |
| Triamcinolone | 4 | 0 |
| Long-acting | | |
| Dexamethasone | 0.75 | 0 |
| Betamethasone | 0.6 | 0 |

hair. Supplemental androgen therapy can be achieved with 2 to 5 mg of fluoxymesterone (Halotestin) orally per day.

## Secondary Insufficiency

Treatment of secondary adrenal insufficiency differs from that of primary adrenal insufficiency with regard to mineralocorticoid and androgen replacement. Patients with secondary adrenal failure usually do not require mineralocorticoid therapy and can maintain salt and fluid balance with a diet generous in sodium chloride. In the presence of hypotension, however, supplementary fludrocortisone acetate, 0.05 to 0.1 mg/day, is indicated. Evidence of androgen insufficiency may occur with male and female patients with hypopituitarism. Sufficient androgen in the female patient can be achieved with 2 to 5 mg of fluoxymesterone orally per day. Larger dosages of this preparation or long-acting testosterone (Depo-Testosterone) can be used in the male patient. Patients with secondary insufficiency will also require thyroid hormone replacement.

## ADRENAL CRISIS

Adrenal crisis is an acute, life-threatening emergency that must be suspected and treated based upon clinical impression. It is due primarily to cortisol insufficiency and to a lesser extent, aldosterone insufficiency, and occurs when the physiologic demand for these hormones exceeds the capacity of the adrenal glands to produce them.

Adrenal reserve may be exhausted in patients with chronic adrenal insufficiency when they are subjected to intercurrent illness or stress. These patients should be taught to respond to minor febrile illness or stress by increasing their glucocorticoid dose by 2 to 3 times the usual dose for a few days during the illness. Mineralocorticoid dose does not need to be changed. During an emergency from severe trauma or stress, dexamethasone 4 mg IM can be self-administered. A variety of conditions may precipitate crisis; these include major or minor infections, trauma, surgery, burns, pregnancy, hypermetabolic states such as hyperthyroidism, and drugs, especially hypnotics or general anesthetics. Adrenal crisis may also occur in patients with chronic adrenal failure if the patient fails to or is unable to take replacement steroid medication. The most common cause of adrenal crisis is abrupt withdrawal of steroids from a patient with iatrogenic adrenal suppression due to prolonged steroid use. Finally, bilateral adrenal gland hemorrhage from fulminant septicemia or other causes can produce adrenal crisis.

## Clinical Presentation

The clinical manifestations of adrenal crisis are due primarily to insufficiency of cortisol and to a lesser extent, insufficiency of aldosterone. Patients appear acutely ill. They are profoundly weak and may be confused. Hypotension, especially postural hypotension, is usual. Circulatory collapse may be profound. The pulse is feeble and rapid, and heart sounds may be soft. Temperature elevation is common but may be due to underlying infection. Anorexia, nausea, vomiting, and abdominal pain are almost universal. The abdominal pain may be severe, simulating an acute abdomen. Patients in crisis may exhibit increased motor activity which can progress to delirium or seizures.

Laboratory findings vary. The serum sodium level is usually moderately decreased but may be normal. Potassium levels may be normal or slightly increased. Rarely the potassium concentration may be markedly increased, and this can cause cardiac arrhythmias or hyperkalemic paralysis. Hypoglycemia is characteristic and can be severe.

## Treatment

Treatment must be instituted promptly based upon clinical impression and should not be delayed for confirmatory testing of adrenal function. Therapeutic measures in treatment of adrenal crisis include re-placement of fluids and sodium, administration of glucocorticoid, correction of hypotension and hypoglycemia, reduction of hyperkalemia, and identification and treatment of a precipitating cause of the crisis.

## Fluids

A rapid infusion of 5% dextrose and isotonic saline should be started immediately. This acts to correct dehydration, hypotension, hyponatremia, and hypoglycemia. The extracellular volume deficit in the average adult in adrenal crisis is approximately 20 percent, or 3 L. The first liter should be given over 1 h, and 2 or 3 L may be required during the first 8 h of therapy. The functional capacity of the cardiovascular system is reduced with adrenal insufficiency, and the usual precautions with the rapid administration of saline should be observed.

## Steroids

A water-soluable glucocorticoid should be administered promptly. As soon as the diagnosis of adrenal crisis is entertained, 100 mg of hydrocortisone sodium succinate (Solu-Cortef) or phosphate should be given in an intravenous bolus. In addition, 100 mg of hydrocortisone should be added to the intravenous solution. Usually, 200 mg of hydrocortisone is given every 6 h during the first 24 h of therapy. Glucocorticoid therapy acts to correct hypotension, hyponatremia, hyperkalemia, and hypoglycemia.

Mineralcorticoid therapy is not required during initial treatment of adrenal crisis. High dosages of hydrocortisone provide sufficient mineralocorticoid effect. As the total dosage of glucocorticoid is reduced below 100 mg/24 h, many patients need supplementary mineralocorticoid, which can be provided as desoxycorticosterone acetate (Percorten), 2.5 to 5.0 mg intramuscularly one or twice daily. If hypotension persists despite adequate volume and corticosteroid replacement, additional corticosteroid can be given and other causes of hypotension should be investigated. Vasopressors may be needed to correct hypotension. Adrenal hemorrhage should be considered, especially if the patient is receiving anticoagulants.

## Simultaneous Treatment and Testing

It is possible to treat adrenal crisis and to perform simultaneous, confirmatory diagnostic testing for adrenal insufficiency. Physiologic saline is administered, but instead of hydrocortisone, 4 mg of dexamethasone is added to the infusion. Additionally, 25 units of corticotropin is added to the solution and this liter is infused in the first hour. Blood for plasma cortisol assay is obtained before and at the completion of the infusion. A 24-h urine collection for measurement of 17-hydroxycorticosteroid (17-OHCS) is collected. Additional corticotropin is added to subsequent intravenous solutions so that at least 3 units is infused each hour for 8 h. A third blood specimen for cortisol assay is obtained between the sixth and eighth hours of intravenous therapy.

If the patient has primary adrenal insufficiency, all plasma cortisol levels are low (<15 µg/dL), and the urinary 17-OHCS is also low, confirming the inability of the adrenals to respond to ACTH stimulation. An adequate rise in the plasma cortisol level excludes the diagnosis of adrenal insufficiency. A response indicative of partially intact adrenocortical reserve excludes the diagnosis of primary adrenal failure in favor of secondary adrenal insufficiency, but further testing is required to confirm this diagnosis. Other methods for simultaneous diagnosis and treatment have been described.

The adrenal crisis should begin to resolve favorably within a few hours after initiation of appropriate therapy. Intensive treatment and monitoring should continue for 24 to 48 h. Once the patient's condition has stabilized, the transition to an oral maintenance program can begin. Usually, 7 to 10 days are required for this transition.

The main causes of death during adrenal crisis are circulatory collapse and hyperkalemia-induced arrhythmias. Hypoglycemia may contribute to demise in some cases. With prompt recognition and appropriate treatment, most patients in adrenal crisis should do well.

## BIBLIOGRAPHY

Addison T: On the constitutional and local effects of disease of the supra-renal capsules. *Med Classics* 2:244, 1937.

Axelrod L: Glucocorticoid therapy. *Medicine* 55:39, 1976.

Nerup J: Addison's disease—clinical studies. A report of 108 cases. *Acta Endocrinol* 76:127, 1974.

Tapper ML, Rotterdam HZ, Lerner CW, et al: Adrenal necrosis in the acquired immunodeficiency syndrome. *Ann Intern Med* 100:239, 1984.

Thorn GW, Lauler DP: Clinical therapeutics of adrenal disorders. *Am J Med* 53:673, 1972.

Xarli VP, Steele AA, David PJ, et al: Adrenal hemorrhage in the adult. *Medicine* 57:211, 1978.

# Hematologic and Oncologic Emergencies

## 184
## EVALUATION OF THE BLEEDING PATIENT

**Mary E. Eberst**

Most bleeding that is seen in the emergency department is normal—the result of local wounds, lacerations, or other structural lesions. The majority occurs in patients with normal hemostasis. With careful attention to the history and physical findings, patients with pathologic bleeding can often be readily identified. Generally speaking, patients who manifest spontaneous bleeding from multiple sites, bleeding from untraumatized sites, delayed bleeding several hours after trauma, and bleeding into deep tissues or joints should be considered to possibly have a bleeding disorder.

Important historical data for the presence of a congenital bleeding disorder include the presence or absence of unusual or abnormal bleeding in the patient and other family members and the possible occurrence of excessive bleeding after dental extractions, surgical procedures, or trauma. Many patients with abnormal bleeding have an acquired disorder. Questioning about liver disease and drug use (particularly ethanol, aspirin, nonsteroidal anti-inflammatory drugs, coumadin, antibiotics, and other aspirin-containing products) may be helpful.

The site(s) of bleeding may provide an indication of the hemostatic abnormality. Mucocutaneous bleeding, including petechiae, ecchymoses, epistaxis, gastrointestinal, genitourinary, or heavy menstrual bleeding is characteristic of qualitative or quantitative platelet disorders. Purpura often are associated with thrombocytopenia and commonly indicate systemic illness. Bleeding into joints and potential spaces, such as between fascial planes and into the retroperitoneum, as well as delayed bleeding, is most commonly associated with coagulation factor deficiencies. Patients who demonstrate both mucocutaneous bleeding and bleeding in deep spaces often have disorders such as disseminated intravascular coagulation, where both platelet abnormalities and coagulation factor abnormalities are present.

### REVIEW OF NORMAL COAGULATION

The normal hemostatic system consists of a complex process that limits blood loss by the formation of a platelet plug (primary hemostasis) and the production of cross-linked fibrin (secondary hemostasis), which strengthens the platelet plug. These reactions are counter-regulated by the fibrinolytic system, which limits the size of fibrin clot that is formed, thereby preventing excessive clot formation. Congenital and acquired abnormalities occur in all of these systems. The affected patients may have excessive hemorrhage, excessive thrombus formation, or both.

### Primary Hemostasis

*Primary hemostasis* is the platelet interaction with the vascular subendothelium that results in the formation of a platelet plug at the site of injury. Required components for this to occur are: normal vascular subendothelium (collagen); functional platelets; normal von Willebrand factor (connects the platelet to the endothelium via glycoprotein Ib); and normal fibrinogen (connects the platelets to each other via glycoprotein IIb-IIIa). Figure 184-1 depicts primary hemostasis.

### Secondary Hemostasis

*Secondary hemostasis* describes the reactions of the plasma coagulation proteins by a tightly regulated mechanism. The final product is cross-linked fibrin, which is insoluble and strengthens the platelet plug formed in primary hemostasis. Figure 184-2 diagrams the reactions of secondary hemostasis.

### The Fibrinolytic System

This complex system regulates the hemostatic mechanism by limiting the size of fibrin clots that are formed. A simplified schema is depicted in Figure 184-3. The principle physiologic activator is tissue plasminogen activator (tPA) which is released from endothelial cells. tPA converts plasminogen, which is synthesized in the liver and adsorbed in the fibrin clot, to plasmin. Plasmin degrades fibrinogen and fibrin monomer into low molecular weight fragments known as fibrin degradation products (FDPs) and cross-linked fibrin into D-dimers.

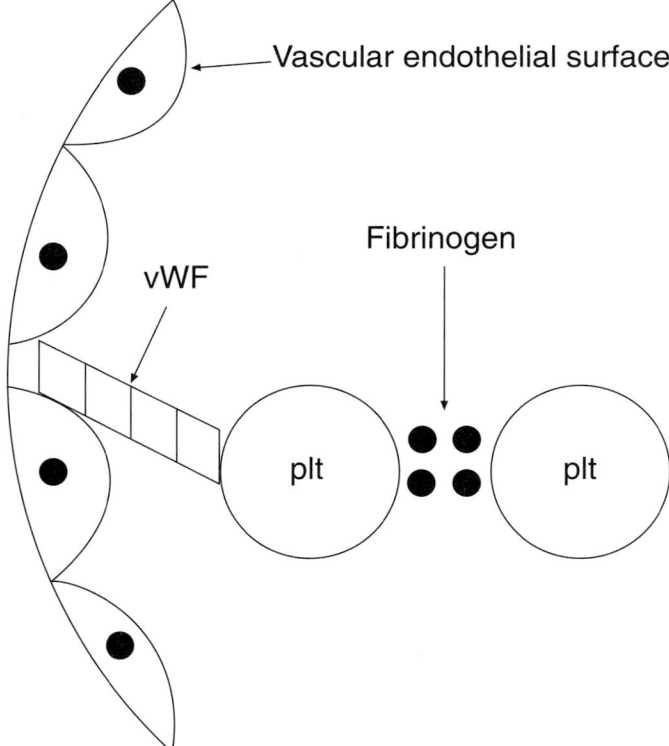

**Fig. 184-1.** Primary hemostasis. See text for details. vWF, von Willebrand factor; plt, platelet.

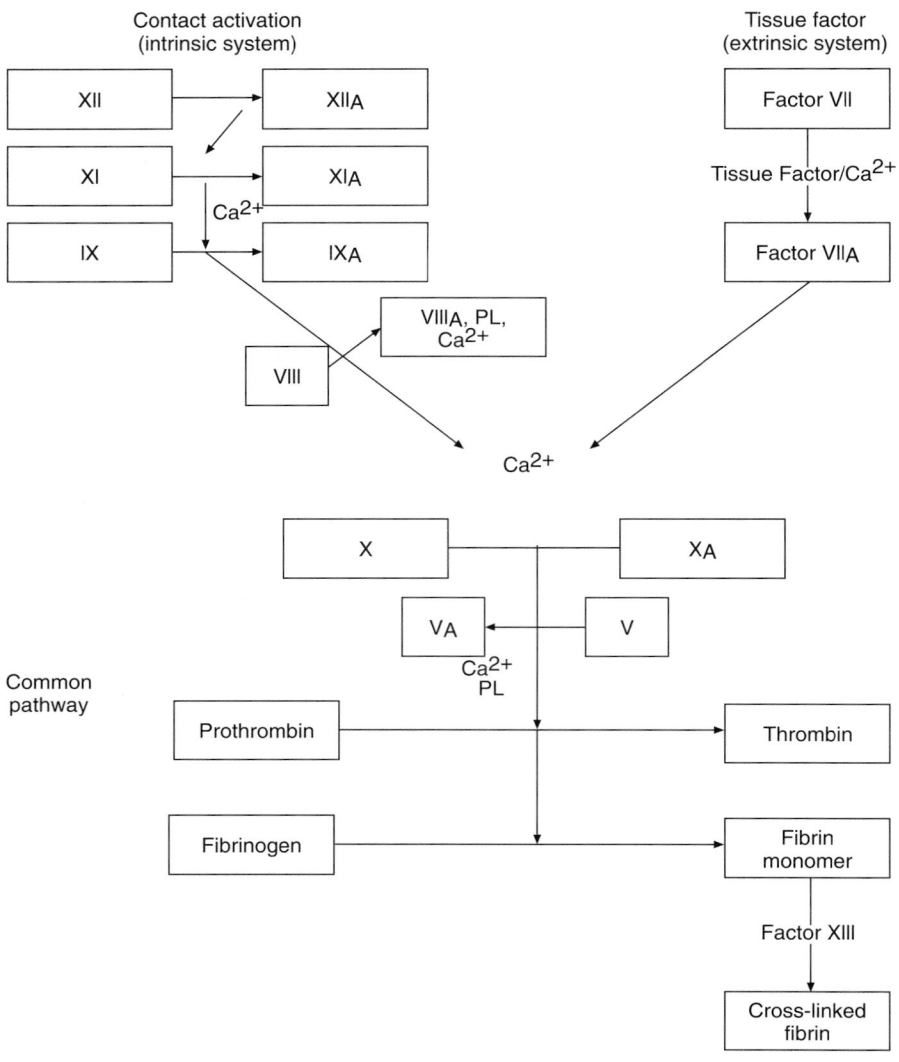

**Fig. 184-2.** Secondary hemostasis, also known as the coagulation cascade. The unactivated coagulation proteins (factors) are indicated by roman numerals; after the reaction occurs, the factor is activated and designated by subscript A. There are two independent activation pathways. The contact system is known as the intrinsic pathway, and the tissue factor system is known as the extrinsic pathway. The pathways merge at the point of activation of factor X. This begins the common pathway that generates the final product, cross-linked fibrin. $Ca^{2+}$, calcium; fibrinogen is factor I; PL, phospholipid surface (often platelets); prothrombin is factor II.

Other physiologic inhibitors of hemostasis with prevalent clinical applicability include antithrombin III and the protein C–protein S system. Antithrombin III is a protein that forms complexes with all the serine protease coagulation factors (factors XII, XI, X, IX, VII, and prothrombin) thereby inhibiting their function. Heparin potentiates this interaction and this is the basis for its use as an anticoagulant. Protein C, which requires the presence of protein S for activation, is capable of inactivating the two plasma cofactors, factors V and VIII, and inhibiting their participation in the coagulation cascade.

## TESTS OF HEMOSTASIS

Table 184-1 outlines the screening tests of primary and secondary hemostasis as well as other commonly used coagulation tests. Table

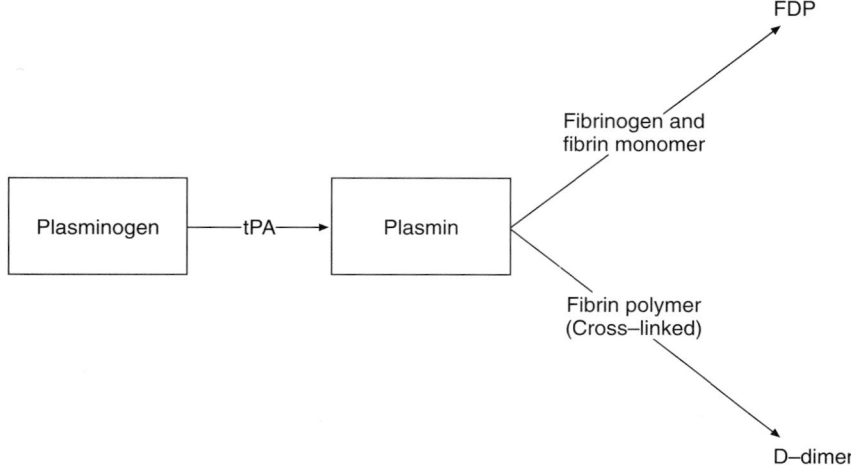

**Fig. 184-3.** The fibrinolytic pathway. See text for details. FDP, fibrin degradation product; tPA, tissue plasminogen activator.

**Table 184-1.** Tests of Hemostasis

| Screening Tests | Normal Value | Measures | Clinical Correlations |
|---|---|---|---|
| Platelet count | 150,000–300,000/mm³ | Number of platelets per mm³ | Decreased platelet count (thrombocytopenia)<br>Bleeding usually not a problem until platelet count < 50,000; high risk of spontaneous bleeding including CNS with count < 10,000/mm³.<br>Causes<br>　Decreased production—viral infections (measles); marrow infiltration; drugs (thiazides, ETOH, estrogens, interferon-α) (see Table 184-2)<br>　Increased destruction—viral infections (mumps, varicella, EBV, HIV); ITP, TTP, DIC, HUS; drugs heparin, protamine (see Table 184-2)<br>　Splenic sequestration (hypersplenism, hypothermia)<br>　Loss of platelets (hemorrhage, hemodialysis, extracorporeal circulation)<br>　Pseudothrombocytopenia—platelets are clumped but not truly decreased in number; examine blood smear to recognize this<br>Elevated platelet count (thrombocytosis)—commonly reactive to inflammation or malignancy, or in polycythemia vera; can be associated with hemorrhage or thrombosis |
| Bleeding time (BT) | 2.5–10 min (template BT) | Interaction between platelets and the subendothelium | Prolonged BT caused by:<br>　Thrombocytopenia (platelet count < 50,000/mm³)<br>　Abnormal platelet function (vWD, ASA, NSAIDs, uremia, liver disease)<br>　Collagen abnormalities (congenital abnormality or prolonged use of steroids) |

Secondary Hemostasis

| Screening Tests | Normal Value | Measures | Clinical Correlations |
|---|---|---|---|
| Prothrombin time (PT) | 10–12 s, but laboratory variation | Extrinsic system and common pathway—factors VII, X, V, prothrombin, and fibrinogen | *Prolonged PT*—most commonly caused by:<br>　Use of coumadin/warfarin (inhibits vitamin K dependent factors II, VII, IX and X)<br>　Liver disease with decreased factor synthesis<br>　Antibiotics, some cephalosporins, (moxalactam, cefamandole, cefotaxime, cefoperazone) that inhibit vitamin K-dependent factors |
| Activated partial thromboplastin time (aPTT) | Depends on type of thromboplastin used; "activated" with Kaolin | Intrinsic system and common pathway including factors XII, XI, IX, VIII, X, V, prothrombin, and fibrinogen | *Prolongation of aPTT* most commonly caused by:<br>　Heparin therapy<br>　Factor deficiencies; factor levels have to be < 30% of normal to cause prolongation<br>　**Note:** high doses of heparin or warfarin can cause prolongation of both the PT and aPTT due to their activity in the common pathway. |
| Thrombin clotting time (TCT) | 10–12 s | Conversion of fibrinogen to fibrin monomer | *Prolonged TCT* caused by:<br>　Low fibrinogen level (DIC)<br>　Abnormal fibrinogen molecule (liver disease)<br>　Presence of heparin, FDPs or a paraprotein (multiple myeloma); these interfere with the conversion<br>　Very high fibrinogen level (acute phase reactant) |
| "Mixes" | Variable | Performed when one or more of the above screening tests is prolonged; the patients plasma ("abnormal") is mixed with "normal" plasma and the screening test is repeated | *If the "mix" corrects* the screening test, one or more factor deficiencies are present.<br>*If the "mix" does not correct the screening test,* an inhibitor is present. |

Other Hemostatic Tests

| Screening Tests | Normal Value | Measures | Clinical Correlations |
|---|---|---|---|
| Fibrin degradation products and D-dimer (evaluate fibrinolysis) | Variable | *FDPs* measure breakdown products from fibrinogen and fibrin monomer;<br>*D-dimer* measures breakdown products of cross-linked fibrin | Levels of these are elevated in DIC, thrombosis, pulmonary embolus, liver disease. |
| Factor level assays | 60–130% (0.60–1.30 units/mL) | Measures the % activity of a specified factor compared to normal | Used to identify specific factor deficiencies and in therapeutic management of patients with deficiencies |
| Inhibitor screens | Variable | Verifies the presence or absence of antibodies directed against one or more of the coagulation factors | *Specific inhibitors*—directed against one coagulation factor, most commonly against factor VIII; can be in patients with congenital or acquired deficiency.<br>*Nonspecific inhibitors*—directed against more than one of the coagulation factors; example is lupus-type anticoagulant |

ASA, aspirin; CNS, central nervous system; DIC, disseminated intravascular coagulation; EBV, Epstein-Barr virus; ETOH, ethanol; FDPs, fibrin degradation products; HIV, human immunodeficiency virus; HUS, hemolytic uremic syndrome; ITP, idiopathic thrombocytopenic purpura; NSAIDs, nonsteroidal anti-inflammatory drugs; TTP, thrombotic thrombocytopenic purpura; vWD, von Willebrand disease.

**Table 184-2.** Drugs Associated with Thrombocytopenia

| | Relative Incidence | | Relative Incidence |
|---|---|---|---|
| Heparin | 4+ | Thiazides | 2+ |
| Gold salts | 4+ | Furosemide | 2+ |
| Sulfa-containing antibiotics | 4+ | Procainamide | 2+ |
| Quinine/Quinidine | 4+ | Digoxin/Digitoxin | 2+ |
| Amrinone | 3+ | Cimetidine/Ranitidine | 2+ |
| Ethanol (chronic use) | 3+ | Phenytoin | 1+ |
| Aspirin | 3+ | Penicillins/Cephalosporins | 1+ |
| Indomethacin | 3+ | Estrogens | 1+ |
| Valproic acid | 3+ | Protamine sulfate | 1+ |
| Heroin | 3+ | Interferon-$\alpha$ | 1+ |

Relative incidence based on number of case reports: 4+ equivalent to at least 50–100 reports; 3+ is 20 or more reports; 2+ is 10–20 reports; 1+ is 10 or less case reports.

184-2 lists many commonly used drugs that are associated with thrombocytopenia.

## Laboratory Investigation

The basic laboratory parameters that should be obtained in a patient with a suspected bleeding disorder are a complete blood count and platelet count, prothrombin time, and activated partial thromboplastin time. The results of these tests coupled with clinical evaluation should enable one to formulate a differential diagnosis. Further hematologic evaluation, using the tables provided in the chapter, can then follow. Hematologic consultation should be sought if the differential diagnosis or the laboratory approach is unclear.

## BIBLIOGRAPHY

Kitchens CS: Approach to the bleeding patient. In: Penner VA, Hassouna HI (eds). *Hematology/Oncology Clinics of North America, Coagulation Disorders I.* Philadelphia: WB Saunders, pp. 983–989, 1992.

Goldhaber SZ, Simons GR, Elliott CG, et al: Quantitative plasma D-dimer levels among patients undergoing pulmonary angiography for suspected pulmonary embolism. *JAMA* 270:2819, 1993.

Goebel RA: Thrombocytopenia. In: Moore GP, Jorden RC (eds). *Emergency Medicine Clinics of North America, Hematologic/Oncologic Emergencies,* pp. 445–464, 1993.

Hansson PO, Eriksson H, Ericksson E, et al: Can laboratory testing improve screening strategies for deep vein thrombosis at an emergency unit? *J Intern Med* 235:143, 1994.

# 185
# ACQUIRED BLEEDING DISORDERS
## Mary E. Eberst

## PLATELET ABNORMALITIES

Acquired platelet abnormalities include both quantitative and qualitative defects. Quantitative problems are usually associated with bleeding complications at a platelet level of less than 50,000/mm³ with spontaneous bleeding, including central nervous system (CNS) hemorrhage, likely at a level below 10,000/mm³. Table 185-1 depicts the causes of acquired thrombocytopenia; Table 184-2 displays the drugs most commonly associated with thrombocytopenia. Platelet counts above 400,000/mm³ are encountered most commonly in inflamma-

**Table 185-1.** Pathophysiologic Mechanisms of Acquired Thrombocytopenia

| Mechanism | Associated Clinical Conditions |
|---|---|
| Decreased platelet production | Marrow infiltration (tumor or infection) |
| | Aplastic anemia |
| | Viral infections (measles, tuberculosis) |
| | Drugs (thiazides, estrogens, ethanol, interferon-$\alpha$, chemotherapeutic agents) |
| | Radiation |
| | Vitamin $B_{12}$ and/or folate deficiency |
| Increased platelet destruction | Idiopathic thrombocytopenic purpura |
| | Thrombotic thrombocytopenic purpura |
| | Hemolytic uremic syndrome |
| | Disseminated intravascular coagulation |
| | Viral infections (HIV, mumps, varicella, EBV) |
| | Drugs (heparin, protamine) |
| Splenic sequestration | Hypersplenism |
| | Hypothermia |
| Platelet loss | Excessive hemorrhage |
| | Hemodialysis |
| | Extracorporeal circulation |
| Pseudothrombocytopenia | Not a disease state, laboratory phenonemon |

EBV, Epstein-Barr virus; HIV, human immunodeficiency virus

tory reactions, patients with malignancy, splenectomized patients, and those with polycythemia vera. Thrombocytosis can be associated with bleeding or thrombosis and is considered an emergency when platelet levels exceed 1 million/mm³ or are associated with evidence of CNS dysfunction or acute thrombosis or hemorrhage.

Acquired qualitative platelet abnormalities, characterized by abnormal platelet function, occur in many disease states (Table 185-2). When present, functional abnormalities can be associated with excessive bleeding regardless of the platelet count. Table 185-3 outlines some commonly used drugs that can cause platelet dysfunction.

The emergency management of patients with thrombocytopenia is based on the control of acute hemorrhage and maintenance of an adequate intravascular volume to maintain normal hemodynamics. Most patients with active bleeding and platelet counts less than 50,000/mm³ should receive platelet transfusion. Each unit of platelets infused should raise the platelet count by 10,000/mm³. Patients with platelet antibodies, such as those with idiopathic thrombocytopenic purpura (ITP) or hypersplenism are unlikely to respond to platelet transfusions. Some disease states, such as disseminated intravascular coagulation (DIC) and thrombotic thrombocytopenic purpura (TTP), may actually be exacerbated by platelet transfusion; hematologic consultation should be obtained. All patients with platelet counts less than 10,000/mm³ should receive immediate platelet transfusion, regardless of the underlying etiology, because of the high risk of spontaneous hemorrhage. Nonemergency therapies for thrombocytopenia with which the emergency physician should be familiar include antithymocyte globulin (ATG) for aplastic anemia; prednisone, intra-

**Table 185-2.** Clinical Conditions Associated with Qualitative Platelet Abnormalities

Uremia
Liver disease
Disseminated intravascular coagulation
Drugs (see Table 185-3)
Antiplatelet antibodies (ITP, SLE)
Cardiopulmonary bypass
Myeloproliferative disorders (PCV, CML)
Dysproteinemias (multiple myeloma, Waldenstrom macroglobulinemia)
Preleukemias, AML, ALL
von Willebrand disease (congenital or acquired)

ALL, acute lymphocytic leukemia; AML, acute myelogenous leukemia; CML, chronic myelogenous leukemia; ITP, idiopathic thrombocytopenic purpura; PCV, polycythemia vera; SLE, systemic lupus erythematosus

**Table 185-3.** Commonly Used Drugs Associated with Platelet Dysfunction

| | |
|---|---|
| Aspirin, NSAIDs | Calcium channel blockers |
| Heparin and thrombolytics | Propranolol |
| Penicillins and cephalosporins | Nitroprusside |
| Nitrofurantoin | Nitroglycerin |
| Prostaglandins | Tricyclic antidepressants |
| Dextran | Phenothiazines |
| Chemotherapeutics | Antihistamines |

NSAIDs, nonsteroidal anti-inflammatory drugs

venous gamma globulin, and splenectomy for ITP; prednisone, aspirin (ASA), plasma infusion, and plasma exchange for TTP and hemolytic uremic syndrome (HUS); as well as other immunosuppressive and chemotherapeutic agents with direct effect on the bone marrow or peripheral antibody production.

The long-term management of qualitative platelet abnormalities that result from underlying disease is directed at treatment of the underlying problem. Acute hemorrhage in these patients can sometimes be controlled with platelet transfusion, but often this is only a temporary solution because the transfused platelets soon acquire the same functional defect. Other management options in patients with the more common acquired types of platelet dysfunction, such as liver disease, uremia, and DIC, are discussed below.

## WARFARIN AND VITAMIN K DEFICIENCY

Prothrombin (factor II) is a vitamin K-dependent coagulation factor as are factors VII, IX, and X, protein C, and protein S. In the liver, reduced vitamin K is required as a cofactor for the carboxylation of glutamic acid residues in the precursors of these coagulation proteins. Deficiency of vitamin K or inhibition of this process by an antagonist such as warfarin results in decreased levels of these factors in the plasma. In the United States, all hospital-born infants are prophylactically treated with intramuscular vitamin K. Nutritional deficiency of vitamin K is rare in adults; however, it does occur as a result of poor nutrition and malabsorption in patients with liver disease.

Sodium warfarin (Coumadin), a vitamin K antagonist, is widely used as an oral anticoagulant. Even in those who are closely monitored, as many as 25 percent of patients taking warfarin develop hemorrhagic complications due to severe coagulation factor deficiencies. Routinely monitored by the prothrombin time (PT), large doses of warfarin can also cause prolongation of the activated partial thromboplastin time (aPTT). The treatment of overdosage of warfarin depends on the severity of clinical manifestations, not the degree of prolongation of the PT. If there is no evidence of bleeding, temporary discontinuation of the warfarin may be all that is needed. Warfarin has a half-life of 2.5 days in patients with normal hepatic function. Patients who manifest bleeding complications can be treated with fresh frozen plasma (FFP) or vitamin K (intravenous, intramuscular, or subcutaneous)—each has advantages and disadvantages. Infusion of FFP can result in the rapid repletion of coagulation factors and control of hemorrhage. FFP, however, carries some risk of viral transmission and the risk of volume overload. Parenteral administration of vitamin K will reverse the warfarin effect in 12 to 24 h. Some do not advise intravenous administration of vitamin K because of the risk of hypersensitive anaphylactic reactions, although usually 1 mg can be given intravenously safely. Intramuscular or subcutaneous vitamin K is typically given in doses of 5 to 10 mg daily in states of coagulation factor deficiency. In addition to the risk of intravenous administration of vitamin K, the major disadvantage to its use is that its effect may last up to 2 weeks, making it difficult or impossible to anticoagulate the patient using warfarin during that time.

Drug-induced deficiency of the vitamin K-dependent factors can also be seen in patients receiving some antibiotics, particularly the third-generation cephalosporins that contain the *N*-methylthiotetra-zole side chain (moxalactam, cefamandole, cefotaxime, cefoperazone).

Warfarin has long been used as a rodenticide; however, resistance has developed in the animals and new products known as "superwarfarins" are now used. Brodifacoum is the most widely available of these agents. Many case reports now in the literature describe intentional and accidental ingestion of these products. Such patients present with a severe coagulopathy: major mucosal bleeding and internal bleeding are common and can be fatal. Treatment with high doses of vitamin K, up to 50 to 100 mg/day for several weeks is often required to correct this coagulopathy because of the long half-life of these products.

## LIVER DISEASE

Acute and chronic diseases of the liver can be associated with many hemostatic abnormalities of clinical significance. Parenchymal diseases such as cirrhosis and hepatitis, and infiltrative diseases, such as metastatic neoplasms, cause a variety of coagulation problems (Table 185-4).

**Decreased protein synthesis.** The hepatocytes are the site of synthesis of all the coagulation factors except factor VIII. Diseases affecting the hepatic parenchyma result in decreased synthesis of coagulation factors.

**Vitamin K deficiency.** The synthesis of factors II (prothrombin), VII, IX, and X depends on vitamin K carboxylation. Vitamin K deficiency in patients with liver disease results from nutritional deficiency, malabsorption, and cholestasis, which prevents the absorption of this fat-soluble vitamin.

**Thrombocytopenia.** This is most often due to portal hypertension, which leads to hypersplenism and splenic sequestration. Ethanol causes direct bone marrow suppression and reduced production of all hematopoietic cells including platelets.

**Increased fibrinolysis.** Several findings indicate that patients with significant liver disease have increased fibrinolysis, and according to some, a compensated, low-grade DIC. Fibrinogen levels are often low and abnormal fibrinogen molecules are synthesized (dysfibrinogenemia). Fibrin and fibrinogen degradation products (FDPs and D-dimers) are often elevated due to poor hepatic clearance. The inactivator of plasmin, $\alpha_2$-plasmin inhibitor, is synthesized in the liver. Decreased synthetic capability reduces the amount of this enzyme that is present and can lead to unregulated plasmin activity and increased fibrinolysis.

**Anemia.** Although not directly a result of the liver disease, anemia is common in patients with liver disease, particularly those whose hepatic dysfunction results from the use of ethanol. Ethanol causes direct bone marrow suppression and is commonly associated with folate and iron deficiency.

Patients with mild or moderate hepatic dysfunction most often have subclinical hemostatic abnormalities. Those with severe liver disease may have life-threatening bleeding. Laboratory studies that should be obtained include hemoglobin/hematocrit, PT, aPTT, thrombin clotting time (TCT), and platelet count. Fibrinogen levels and measurement of FDPs or D-dimers may not be readily available. In general, prolongation of the PT is a poor prognostic sign in patients with liver disease.

The management of patients with liver disease and a coagulopathy depends on the presence or absence of active bleeding and the need to

**Table 185-4.** Hemostatic Abnormalities in Patients with Liver Disease

Coagulation factor deficiency due to decreased protein synthesis
Vitamin K deficiency
Thrombocytopenia
Increased fibrinolysis
Anemia

**Table 185-5.** Treatment Options for Patients with Liver Disease and Bleeding

Packed red blood cells to maintain hemodynamic stability
Vitamin K
Fresh frozen plasma
Platelet transfusions
Desmopressin (DDAVP)

do invasive procedures (Table 185-5). If there is no evidence of bleeding and no need for invasive procedures, treatment is not mandatory. When treatment is indicated, the following should be used. *Packed red blood cells* should be transfused if there is significant bleeding or blood loss to maintain hemodynamic stability. *Vitamin K* should be given to all patients with liver disease and bleeding. A trial dose of 10 to 15 mg given subcutaneously or intramuscularly may take up to 24 h to have an effect. In most patients with significant liver disease, vitamin K alone will not totally correct the prolonged PT. *FFP* can be given to temporarily replace coagulation factors. Its use is limited by the potential for volume overload; often the patient cannot tolerate the volume that would be required to completely replete the coagulation factors. Each unit is 200 to 250 mL and contains 200 to 250 units of each coagulation factor. *Platelet transfusions* may be used in severe bleeding situations, but, in general, this will have a transient effect before the transfused platelets are sequestered in the spleen. *Desmopressin (DDAVP),* a synthetic analog of vasopressin, shortens the prolonged bleeding time in some patients with liver disease. There are no controlled trials to support its use, but generally its side effects are mild and there are few adverse effects from a trial administration. The dose is 0.3 μg/kg subcutaneously or intravenously q 12 h up to three doses.

## RENAL DISEASE

Hemostatic abnormalities are commonly encountered in patients with renal disease. Bleeding can be a complication of acute or chronic renal failure. Spontaneous bleeding commonly occurs involving the skin (purpura), mucous membranes (epistaxis and menorrhagia), and gastrointestinal and urinary systems. Less common is bleeding involving the central nervous system, retroperitoneum, pericardium, and other internal bleeding. Surgery or trauma can lead to fatal hemorrhage, even with aggressive management.

The bleeding tendency in patients with renal disease is related to the degree and duration of uremia. The bleeding time is the clinical test most often prolonged in uremia, although it cannot be directly used to predict hemorrhage. In patients with uremia, a number of factors contribute to the bleeding diathesis: uremic retention products, chronic anemia, platelet dysfunction, deficiency of coagulation factors, and thrombocytopenia. Anemia contributes to the bleeding by making it difficult for the platelets to adhere to the subendothelium at sites of damage. Platelet function is optimized when the hematocrit is maintained between 26 and 30 percent. Acquired deficiencies of clotting factors are common in patients with the nephrotic syndrome. Mild thrombocytopenia is common in patients with renal failure; the

**Table 185-6.** Treatment Options for Patients with Uremia and Excessive Bleeding

Dialysis
Optimize hematocrit (recombinant human erythropoietin or transfusion of PRBCs)
Desmopressin (DDAVP)
Conjugated estrogens
Cryoprecipitate infusion*
Platelet transfusion*

* Only in life-threatening bleeding situation

PRBCs, packed red blood cells

etiology is multifactorial, but the platelet count is generally above 100,000/mm³.

Management of these hemostatic defects is both preventive and directed at acute bleeding episodes (Table 185-6). *Dialysis* improves platelet function transiently, lasting for 1 to 2 days. Optimally, patients are well dialyzed three times per week. *Partial correction of the anemia* of chronic renal disease also improves platelet function. This can be accomplished by the use of recombinant human erythro-

**Table 185-7.** Common Causes of Disseminated Intravascular Coagulation

| Clinical Setting | Comments |
|---|---|
| **INFECTION**<br>Bacterial<br>Viral<br>Fungal | Probably the most common cause of DIC; 10–20% of patients with gram-negative sepsis have DIC; endotoxins stimulate monocytes and endothelial cells to express tissue factor; Rocky Mountain spotted fever causes direct endothelial damage; DIC more likely to develop in asplenic patients or those with cirrhosis; septic patients are more likely to have thrombosis than bleeding. |
| **CARCINOMA**<br>Adenocarcinoma<br>Lymphoma | Malignant cells may cause endothelial damage and allow the expression of tissue factor as well as other procoagulant materials; most adenocarcinomas tend to have thrombosis (Trousseau syndrome), except prostate cancer tends to have more bleeding; DIC is often chronic and compensated. |
| **ACUTE LEUKEMIA** | DIC most common with promyelocytic leukemia (M₃); blast cells release procoagulant enzymes, there is excessive release at time of cell lysis (chemotherapy); more likely to have bleeding than thrombosis. |
| **TRAUMA** | DIC especially with brain injury, crush injury, burns, hypothermia, hyperthermia, rhabdomyolysis, fat embolism, hypoxia. |
| **SHOCK** | |
| **LIVER DISEASE** | May have chronic compensated DIC; have acute DIC in the setting of acute hepatic failure, tissue factor is released from the injured hepatocytes. |
| **PREGNANCY** | Placental abruption, amniotic fluid embolus, septic abortion, intrauterine fetal death (can be chronic DIC); can get DIC in HELLP syndrome (hemolysis, elevated liver enzymes, low platelets). |
| **VASCULAR DISEASE** | Large aortic aneurysms (chronic DIC can become acute at time of surgery), giant hemangiomas, vasculitis, multiple telangiectasias. |
| **ENVENOMATION** | DIC can develop with bites of rattlesnakes and other vipers; the venom damages the endothelial cells; bleeding is not as bad as expected from laboratory values. |
| **ARDS** | Microthrombi are deposited in the small pulmonary vessels, the pulmonary capillary endothelium is damaged; 20% of patients with ARDS develop DIC and 20% of patients with DIC develop ARDS. |
| **TRANSFUSION REACTIONS**<br>Acute hemolytic reaction<br>Massive transfusion | DIC with severe bleeding, shock and acute renal failure. |
| **SURGICAL PROCEDURES**<br>Liver transplantation<br>Vascular surgery | |

Note: M₃ in the table is rendered with subscript 3, i.e., $M_3$.

**Fig. 185-1.** Pathophysiology of disseminated intravascular coagulation. Refer to text for details. FDPs: fibrin/fibrinogen degradation products

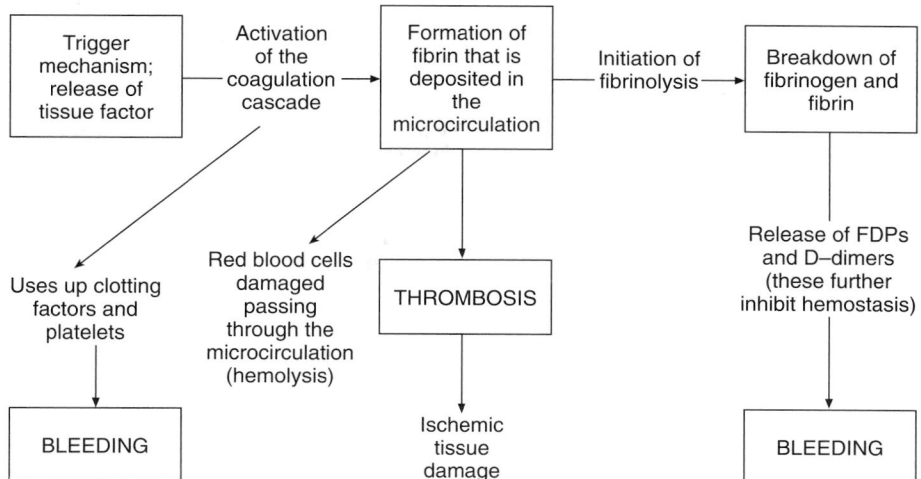

poietin on a chronic basis or transfusion of packed red blood cells in the acute setting. *Desmopressin* (DDAVP) is a synthetic analog of vasopressin. In uremic patients with prolonged bleeding times, 50 to 75 percent will have shortening or normalization of the bleeding time when treated with DDAVP. The usual dose is 0.3 μg/kg body weight given subcutaneously or intravenously. This dose is given q 12h up to three or four doses before transient tachyphylaxis develops. Side effects associated with DDAVP are generally mild and include headache, flushing, minor hypotension, tachycardia, nausea, abdominal cramps, and local site reaction. Severe complications—hyponatremia and thrombosis—rarely occur. Although the mechanism is unknown, *conjugated estrogens* also improve the bleeding time and clinical bleeding in more than 80 percent of uremic patients treated. *Cryoprecipitate infusion* is one of the older treatments for bleeding associated with renal failure. Its use has largely been replaced by the use of DDAVP, which has no risk of viral transmission because it is not a blood product. *Platelet transfusions* are not routinely used in this setting and are not effective because the infused platelets quickly acquire the uremic defect. Infusions of cryoprecipitate and platelets are only indicated for life-threatening bleeding used in combination with packed red blood cells, DDAVP, and conjugated estrogens.

## DISSEMINATED INTRAVASCULAR COAGULATION

Disseminated intravascular coagulation is a loosely defined syndrome that is reflective of serious underlying disease. Patients who have severe DIC have a mortality rate of up to 85 percent. DIC can be triggered by a wide variety of disorders (Table 185-7) and can be acute and life-threatening or chronic and compensated. The most common trigger of DIC is the liberation of tissue factor. Tissue factor is usually confined within the extravascular space; when it is released, the coagulation system is activated (Fig. 185-1). Small fibrin clots are formed and deposited as thrombi or emboli in the microcirculation. Fibrinolysis then occurs and can be massive. FDPs are released and further inhibit hemostasis. The usually tightly regulated system of coagulation and fibrinolysis becomes unbalanced. Because of clot formation, coagulation factors and platelets are consumed. Microthrombi in the circulation can lead to tissue hypoxia, and the red blood cells are damaged trying to pass through the microcirculation. The severity of DIC that develops depends on the synthetic function of the liver, the integrity of the vascular endothelium, and the capacity of the bone marrow to replace platelets. Chronic, compensated DIC occurs when the rate of consumption of clotting factors and platelets does not exceed their rate of production.

Table 185-7 lists the more common causes of DIC, particularly as

encountered in the emergency setting. The reader is referred to a standard text for a complete list of causes. DIC occurs in its most extreme form in *Neisseria meningitidis* sepsis and acute myelogenous leukemia, promyelocytic (M3) type.

The clinical complications of DIC are bleeding, thrombosis, and purpura fulminans. Although hemorrhage and thrombosis may occur simultaneously, in an individual patient, one may predominate. Bleeding occurs in up to 75 percent of patients with DIC. Bleeding from the skin and mucous membranes is most common; usually there is bleeding from several sites including venipuncture sites, surgical wounds, epistaxis, petechiae, and ecchymoses. Hematuria and gastrointestinal bleeding are seen; intracerebral bleeding carries a very poor prognosis. Thromboses (usually microthrombi) predominate in some patients. Clinical signs of this include mental status changes, focal ischemia or gangrene, oliguria, renal cortical necrosis, and adult respiratory distress syndrome (ARDS). Purpura fulminans occurs when there are widespread arterial and venous thromboses. Gangrene develops in the digits or extremities and there is hemorrhagic infarction of the skin. Purpura fulminans is most commonly seen with high-grade bacteremia (*Streptococcus pneumoniae* or *N. meningitidis*).

The diagnosis of DIC is based on the clinical setting and characteristic laboratory abnormalities. The typical laboratory results in DIC are outlined in Table 185-8. Patients with chronic DIC have laboratory evidence of the disorder but no clinical evidence of hemorrhage or thrombosis.

The management of acute DIC is based on the symptoms demonstrated by the patient and the underlying disease state. Many patients with DIC require no specific therapy if there is no evidence of bleeding or thrombosis and laboratory studies are not deteriorating. The first principle of management is to stabilize the patient hemodynamically, providing oxygen, fluids, and life support as needed. If possible, the primary cause of the DIC needs to be treated. The high mortality rate in severe DIC is primarily due to the underlying disorder. Antibiotics can be given and the fetus or retained uterine products removed; however, in many circumstances, little can be done rapidly. Further management depends on the predominant symptoms of the patient—bleeding or thrombosis. Bleeding requires replacement therapy based on the amount of bleeding, risk of bleeding (i.e., postoperative), and the extent of depletion of coagulation factors and platelets. The PT is the best indicator of clotting factor depletion. If the PT is prolonged by more than 2 to 3 s and there is bleeding, replacement is indicated. Factor levels can also be used to guide therapy if they are readily available. The fibrinogen level should be maintained above 100 to 150 mg/dL and the other factor levels at or above 50 percent of normal. FFP is used to replace clotting factors; each unit contains 200 to 250 units of each factor. Usually given 2 units at a time, there

**Table 185-8.** Laboratory Abnormalities Characteristic of Disseminated Intravascular Coagulation

| Studies | Result |
|---|---|
| Most Useful | |
| Prothrombin time | Prolonged |
| Platelet count* | Usually low |
| Fibrinogen level[†] | Low |
| Helpful | |
| Activated partial thromboplastin time | Usually prolonged |
| Thrombin clot time[‡] | Prolonged |
| Fragmented red blood cells[§] | Should be present |
| FDPs and D-dimers[¶] | Elevated |
| *Specific Factor Assays*** | |
| Factor II | Low |
| Factor V | Low |
| Factor VII[††] | Low |
| Factor VIII[‡‡] | Low, normal, high |
| Factor IX | Low (decreases later than other factors) |
| Factor X | Low |

* Platelet count usually low, most important that it is falling if it started at an elevated level.

[†] Fibrinogen level correlates best with bleeding complications; it is an acute phase reactant so it may actually start out at an elevated level; fibrinogen level < 100 mg/dL correlates with severe DIC.

[‡] Not a sensitive test, prolonged by many abnormalities.

[§] Fragmented red blood cells and schistocytes are not specific for DIC.

[¶] Levels may be chronically elevated in patients with liver or renal disease.
** The factors in the extrinsic pathway are most affected (VII, X, V, and II).

[††] Factor VII is usually low early because it has the shortest half-life.

[‡‡] Factor VIII is an acute phase reactant so its level may be normal, low, or elevated in DIC.

FDP, fibrin degradation products

are 200 to 250 mL of fluid per unit, making volume overload a potential problem. Cryoprecipitate is used to replace fibrinogen. There are 100 to 250 mg fibrinogen per bag of cryoprecipitate; 10 bags are typically given at one time. Platelet replacement is indicated if the count is less than 50,000/mm³ and there is bleeding, or if it is less than 20,000/mm³ regardless of bleeding. Each unit of platelets transfused should raise the platelet count 10,000/mm³; typically 6 units of random donor platelets (or one apheresis unit) are given at a time. As with the use of any blood products, there is a small risk of viral transmission. Patients with DIC should also be given vitamin K and folate. The treatment of microthromboses in DIC with systemic heparinization is controversial. Its use has not been conclusively shown to improve survival and may make the overall clinical situation worse. Heparin should be considered and may be beneficial for some patients with DIC if the underlying condition is carcinoma, acute promyelocytic leukemia, or retained uterine products. Patients with purpura fulminans may also benefit from anticoagulation. In this setting, the continuous infusion of low-dose heparin (5 to 10 units/kg per hour) is recommended. Patient's with large thromboses, such as seen with Trousseau syndrome, should receive full-dose heparinization. Antifibrinolytic agents such as Amicar (ε-aminocaproic acid, EACA) and Cyklokapron (tranexamic acid) are used in DIC with great caution. Although these drugs may reduce bleeding and fibrinogen consumption, they may convert a bleeding disorder into a thrombotic disorder. When used, these antifibrinolytic agents are usually given in conjunction with low-dose heparin infusion to minimize the potential for thrombosis. They are occasionally used in DIC patients with acute promyelocytic leukemia or prostate cancer.

# HEPARIN AND THROMBOLYTIC THERAPY

## Heparin

Heparin is an anticoagulant widely used for the treatment and prevention of venous thrombotic and thromboembolic disease. Administered intravenously or subcutaneously, heparin prevents thrombus formation and the extension and propagation of the preformed thrombus. Heparin reduces the ability of blood to clot by enhancing the ability of antithrombin III to form complexes with the activated serene protease coagulation factors (XIIa, XIa, IXa, and prothrombin), thereby inhibiting their activity in the coagulation cascade. Heparin may also have an anti-inflammatory effect. Because it does not cross the placenta, heparin is the drug of choice when anticoagulation is needed during pregnancy. The dosing of heparin depends on the clinical setting, with standard regimens available in most medicine and hematology texts. Heparin therapy is generally monitored by the aPTT, with variable goals dependent on the clinical setting and laboratory standards. As with any drug, there are risks when heparin is used; these risks need to be weighed against the risk of not using heparin. The fatality rate is up to 15 percent for untreated venous thromboses.

Bleeding is the major complication of heparin therapy, occurring in up to 33 percent of all treated patients with 1 to 7 percent of these episodes considered serious or life-threatening (requiring transfusion of blood). Some patients are at higher risk of developing bleeding complications, particularly those with a history of renal failure, gastrointestinal bleeding, head injury, heavy alcohol use, malignancy, recent surgery or trauma, or hemorrhagic disorders. Concomitant use of medications such as aspirin, warfarin, steroids, or nonsteroidal anti-inflammatory drugs (NSAIDs) also places patients at higher risk of bleeding complications. If significant bleeding complications develop, the heparin is stopped immediately. The half-life of heparin is 60 to 90 min, but can be longer if high levels are present. Protamine sulfate can be used to neutralize heparin; 1 mg protamine sulfate neutralizes 100 units of standard molecular weight heparin.

Thrombocytopenia is the other major complication of heparin therapy. Two types of thrombocytopenia can occur. The more common type of thrombocytopenia develops in up to 25 percent of patients treated with heparin. This is a benign, transient decrease in platelets; the platelet count usually remains greater than 100,000/mm³, and is thought to be due to platelet aggregation and sequestration in the spleen. Heparin therapy generally does not have to be discontinued and the platelet count rises spontaneously. The second type of thrombocytopenia, known as heparin-associated thrombocytopenia, occurs in 1 to 5 percent of patients treated with heparin and can be life-threatening. Heparin-associated thrombocytopenia occurs when antibodies are formed against the platelets. This can occur immediately in patients who have received heparin previously, but it takes 6 to 10 days for the antibodies to form in previously untreated patients. Severe thrombocytopenia results; platelet counts less than 50,000/mm³ and arterial thromboses can occur. In this setting, the heparin must be completely eliminated, and other anticoagulants can be used if necessary (warfarin, dextran). The platelet count will usually return to normal 4 to 6 days after the heparin is stopped. It is controversial whether these patients should ever be treated with heparin again. Long-term use of heparin, for greater than 1 month, is associated with accelerated osteoporosis.

Lower molecular weight heparin compounds are now becoming available. They are said to be as effective as the high molecular weight heparins with the advantages of once or twice a day dosing and less incidence of heparin-associated thrombocytopenia. Their use, however, is difficult because they cannot be monitored by the aPTT.

## Thrombolytics

Thrombolytic agents are able to dissolve preformed arterial and venous thrombi and emboli and restore blood flow to anoxic tissue.

**Table 185-9.** Currently Available Thrombolytic Agents

| Agent | Abbreviation |
|---|---|
| Streptokinase | SK |
| Urokinase | UK |
| Recombinant tissue plasminogen activator | r-tPA |
| Anisoylated plasminogen streptokinase activator complex | APSAC |

Currently available thrombolytics are listed in Table 185-9. These products work by inducing a systemic fibrinolytic state. This fibrinolytic state is not limited to the thrombus; it occurs throughout the circulation. This results in the potential for major hemorrhagic complications, which occur in about 9 percent of patients treated with thrombolytics compared to an average of 4 percent significant bleeding complications in patients treated with heparin. Because of this risk, the diagnosis of thrombus or embolus should be firmly established before treatment begins. Although theoretically more thrombus specific, major and minor bleeding complications are as common with recombinant tissue plasminogen activator (r-tPA) as with streptokinase.

Clinical indications for the use of thrombolytic therapy are as follows:

*Deep venous thrombosis*—Streptokinase is the most common thrombolytic agent used in this setting. Lytic therapy should be considered for acute thromboses (less than 5 to 7 days old) that are large. Lytic therapy allows for lysis of the thrombus and decreases the risk of postphlebitic syndrome. In carefully selected patients, major bleeding complications are no more common than with heparin.

*Acute myocardial infarction*—Vascular reperfusion is the major determinant of improved clinical outcome and mortality reduction. The best results are found in patients with recent onset of chest pain (less than 6 h) and those with thrombosis involving the left anterior descending artery.

*Pulmonary embolism*—The role of thrombolytic therapy in patients with pulmonary embolism is not clearly defined; however, it should be considered in patients with acute onset of symptoms (less than 48 h), evidence of hemodynamic compromise, presence of massive emboli, or the presence of submassive emboli superimposed on chronic cardiopulmonary disease. Patients with pulmonary embolism who receive thrombolytic therapy have greater reperfusion, earlier normalization of the perfusion scan, and decreased pulmonary artery pressures.

*Peripheral arterial occlusion*—Acute peripheral arterial occlusions as well as those in some central sites are commonly treated with systemic or intra-arterial infusion of thrombolytic agents. In this setting, urokinase may be superior to streptokinase.

Specific recommendations for the use of thrombolytic agents in various clinical settings are available in many standard texts. Many institutions have protocols for the use of thrombolytic agents.

Contraindications to use the thrombolytic therapy are outlined in Table 185-10.

**Table 185-10.** Contraindications to Thrombolytic Therapy

**Absolute Contraindications**
   Active bleeding from any site
   Central nervous system pathology within 1–2 mo: surgery, infarction, hemorrhage, trauma, neoplasms

**Relative Contraindications**
   Surgical procedures or other invasive procedures within 10 d
   History of gastrointestinal bleeding
   Baseline hemostatic defects including thrombocytopenia
   Severe arterial hypertension, diastolic blood pressure > 120 mm Hg
   Pregnancy or first 10 d postpartum
   Known allergy to agent
   Known active cavitary lung disease

Bleeding is the major complication of thrombolytic therapy. Less common complications include fever, embolization of thrombi, and allergic reactions. Bleeding complications are primarily due to the dissolution of hemostatic plugs at sites of recent vascular injury. Superficial bleeding is usually not a major problem and can be controlled with local measures. Thrombolytic agents are discontinued at the first indication of major bleeding. Although the half-life of the thrombolytics is short, the systemic fibrinolytic state remains for 12 to 36 h after the infusion is stopped because it takes that long for fibrinogen to replenish itself. Cryoprecipitate can be given to replete fibrinogen and reverse the lytic state. Amicar (EACA) can also be given to inhibit the fibrinolytic state.

## INFECTION WITH HUMAN IMMUNODEFICIENCY VIRUS

The most common hemostatic abnormalities observed in patients infected with the human immunodeficiency virus (HIV) are thrombocytopenia and acquired circulating anticoagulants—lupus-type anticoagulants and anticardiolipin antibodies.

Thrombocytopenia is one of the earliest findings in asymptomatic HIV-infected individuals. Three to 60 percent of all HIV-infected patients will have thrombocytopenia at some time during the course of their illness. Both increased peripheral platelet destruction and decreased platelet production occur. Patients infected with HIV have an increased incidence of immune platelet destruction, such as ITP. HIV also can directly infect bone marrow megakaryocytes, resulting in decreased thrombopoiesis. The use of zidovudine (AZT) may result in improved platelet counts and rarely causes thrombocytopenia.

After thrombocytopenia, the most common hemostatic abnormality in HIV-infected patients is prolongation of the aPTT. This is usually due to the presence of a lupus-type anticoagulant. Often a transient defect, the lupus-type anticoagulant may appear with an acute opportunistic infection and disappear when the infection is treated. Anticardiolipin antibodies, which are detected by enzyme-linked immunosorbent assay (ELISA) and do not affect the basic hemostatic screening tests, are also more common in HIV-infected patients. One or both of these antibodies occur in 22 to 82 percent of patients with HIV. These antibodies themselves do not predispose to clinical bleeding, but they result in an increased risk of thrombosis. However, concomitant hemostatic abnormalities such as platelet dysfunction or hypoprothrombinemia (associated with lupus-type anticoagulant) may lead to bleeding manifestations.

Another hemostatic complication of HIV-infection is anemia, which occurs in the majority of patients at some time in the course of their disease. Etiologies include ineffective erythropoiesis, the effect of HIV and opportunistic infections on the bone marrow, and the use of AZT, which causes significant anemia in at least one third of patients. TTP is an uncommon but well-described complication of HIV infection. TTP may be the initial manifestation of the infection and is characterized by the pentad of fever, thrombocytopenia, neurologic symptoms, renal insufficiency, and microangiopathic hemolytic anemia (see Chapter 188). Many patients infected with HIV are also infected with the hepatitis viruses and have significant liver disease and resultant coagulation abnormalities.

## USE OF ASPIRIN AND NONSTEROIDAL ANTI-INFLAMMATORY DRUGS

Table 185-3 depicts many of the commonly used drugs that can affect platelet function. Of these, the most commonly used are ASA and the NSAIDs, which will be discussed in more detail.

Aspirin inhibits platelet function by acetylating and irreversibly inactivating platelet cyclooxygenase. Normally, platelet cyclooxygenase allows the formation of endoperoxides and thromboxanes, which stimulate platelet aggregation. This effect can be seen with as little as 80 mg ASA per day and can continue for as long as 7 to 10 days after the ASA is stopped, until the affected platelets are replaced by new platelets. The clinical significance of ASA ingestion and bleeding is usually minimal except in some surgeries, cardiothoracic, plastic, and neurosurgery, where small amounts of blood loss are crucial, and in patients with underlying bleeding disorders (congenital or acquired) such as von Willebrand disease, hemophilia, liver disease, uremia, or heavy ethanol ingestion. Chronic ASA ingestion can lead to gastrointestinal blood loss; however, this is primarily from the direct affect of ASA on the gastric mucosa. Platelet transfusion is the only acute treatment to overcome the platelet dysfunction induced by ASA, but this is rarely required.

The NSAIDs such as ibuprofen, indomethacin, and naproxen reversibly inhibit platelet cyclooxygenase. Inhibition of platelet cyclooxygenase occurs only as long as there is active drug in the circulation. The transient defect in platelet aggregation usually lasts less than 24 h. An exception is the drug piroxicam, which has a 2-day half-life; the resultant platelet dysfunction may be present for days. NSAIDs can be safely used in patients with hemophilia.

## CIRCULATING ANTICOAGULANTS

Acquired inhibitors of blood coagulation, also known as circulating anticoagulants, can have serious clinical consequences or only be laboratory phenomena that have little clinical impact. These inhibitors are antibodies directed against one or more of the coagulation factors. Although inhibitors have been described against most of the coagulation factors the two most common are discussed here. Factor VIII inhibitors are a type of "specific" inhibitor, directed only against factor VIII. The lupus anticoagulant is a "nonspecific" inhibitor that is directed against several of the coagulation factors.

### Factor VIII Inhibitors

Factor VIII inhibitors most commonly occur in patients with congenital factor VIII deficiency, hemophilia A (see Chapter 186). Factor VIII inhibitors can also develop in patients with previously normal hemostasis; the incidence is estimated at 0.2 to 1.0 per million persons per year. Although uncommon, this is an important clinical entity to recognize because the mortality rate approaches 50 percent. About one half of the affected patients are otherwise healthy individuals, usually older than 65. The other patients have underlying associated conditions such as autoimmune disorders (systemic lupus erythematosus [SLE], rheumatoid arthritis, ulcerative colitis), lymphoproliferative disorders (multiple myeloma, Waldenstrom macroglobulinemia, benign monoclonal gammopathy of uncertain significance), women in pregnancy and the postpartum period, and patients with allergic drug reactions (penicillins, sulfonamides, phenytoin). Clinically, these patients without a prior bleeding history present with massive spontaneous bruises, ecchymoses, and hematomas. Laboratory studies classically show a normal PT, normal TCT, and greatly prolonged aPTT that does not correct with "mixing." A factor VIII-specific assay will show that the factor VIII activity is very low or absent. The other specific factor assays should be normal or only slightly decreased. Quantitative measurement of the inhibitor by the Bethesda inhibitor assay is important for the emergency management of bleeding episodes. Long-term management is directed at the suppression of antibody production by steroids, intravenous gamma globulin or cytotoxic agents. The management of acute, often life-threatening bleeding episodes should be directed by a hematologist or coagulation specialist. Treatment options include high doses of factor VIII concentrates, the use of unactivated or activated prothrombin complex concentrates, porcine factor VIII, and potentially recombinant factor VIIa.

### Lupus Anticoagulant

The lupus anticoagulant is an antiphospholipid antibody that interferes in vitro with many of the coagulation reactions. Its name is a misnomer because the majority of affected patients do not have lupus and very few have a clinical bleeding disorder. The lupus anticoagulant is identified in 5 to 15 percent of patients with SLE. Associated conditions include other autoimmune disorders, drug reactions (procainamide and phenothiazines), malignancies, and patients with HIV in the setting of acute opportunistic infections. Many affected patients have no underlying disease state. Clinically, many patients are asymptomatic, with the abnormality discovered on routine coagulation screening tests. Arterial or venous thromboses occur in 23 to 58 percent of patients. Recurrent fetal loss, thought to be due to thrombosis of placental vessels and placental infarction, is also common. Some patients have thrombocytopenia, but they may also have ITP. Bleeding abnormalities are uncommon in patients with the lupus anticoagulant unless they have associated hypoprothrombinemia (usually patients with SLE), significant thrombocytopenia, or other underlying abnormality predisposing them to hemorrhage, such as uremia.

Laboratory studies of patients with the lupus anticoagulant typically show a normal or slightly prolonged PT, mild to moderate prolongation of the aPTT, (not usually more than 10 to 15 s prolonged) and a normal TCT. The prolonged aPTT will not correct with "mixing." If the PT is prolonged by more than 3 s, the patient should be evaluated for concomitant hypoprothrombinemia (factor II). Factor-specific assays done in this setting will show a decrease in all the factor levels, although none are extremely low. Various tests can be done to verify the presence of the lupus anticoagulant. These are the dilute Russell viper venom time, kaolin clot time, platelet neutralization procedure, and tissue thromboplastin inhibition test. Asymptomatic patients found to have the lupus anticoagulant require no treatment. If there is an associated underlying disorder, it should be treated, and with resolution, the lupus anticoagulant may disappear. Patients who suffer thrombotic events are managed with long-term anticoagulation (those with venous thrombosis) or low-dose ASA (those with arterial thrombosis). Patients with the lupus anticoagulant can often be managed through a successful pregnancy when treated with prednisone and ASA.

## BIBLIOGRAPHY

Burgess JL, Dart RC: Snake venom coagulopathy: use and abuse of blood products in the treatment of pit viper envenomation. *Ann Emerg Med* 20:795, 1991.

Cappell MS, Simon T, Tiku M: Splenic infarction associated with anticardiolipin antibodies in a patient with acquired immunodeficiency syndrome. *Dig Dis Sci* 37:1152, 1993.

Clark J, Rubin RN: A practical approach to managing disseminated intravascular coagulation. *J Crit Ill* 9:265, 1994.

Eberst ME, Berkowitz LR: Hemostasis in renal disease: pathophysiology and management. *Am J Med* 96:168, 1994.

Gando S, Tedo I, Kubota M: Posttrauma coagulation and fibrinolysis. *Crit Care Med* 20:594, 1992.

George JN, Shattil SJ: The clinical importance of acquired abnormalities of platelet function. *N Engl J Med* 324:27, 1991.

Goldhaber SZ: What role for thrombolysis in patients with pulmonary embolism? *J Crit Ill* 7:192, 1992.

Kruse JA, Carlson RW: Fatal rodenticide poisoning with brodifacoum. *Ann Emerg Med* 21:331, 1992.

Levine JD, Groopman JE: Hemostatic complication of HIV infection, in Loscalzo J, Schafer AI (eds): *Thrombosis and Hemorrhage.* Cambridge, MA, Blackwell Science, pp. 1027–1037, 1994.

O'Meara JJ III, McNutt RA, Evans AT, et al: A decision analysis of streptokinase plus heparin as compared with heparin alone for deep-vein thrombosis. *N Engl J Med* 330:1864, 1994.

Rogers LQ, Lutcher CL: Streptokinase therapy for deep vein thrombosis: a comprehensive review of the English literature. *Am J Med* 88:389, 1990.

Williams EC: Disseminated intravascular coagulation. In: Loscalzo J, Schafer AI (eds): *Thrombosis and Hemorrhage.* Cambridge, MA: Blackwell Science, pp. 921–943, 1994.

# 186

# HEMOPHILIAS AND VON WILLEBRAND DISEASE

## Mary E. Eberst

Hemophilias are hereditary bleeding disorders due to deficiency of factor VIII (hemophilia A, classic hemophilia) or factor IX (hemophilia B, Christmas disease). Von Willebrand disease is a related hereditary deficiency of a portion of the factor VIII complex. These disorders are discussed below.

## HEMOPHILIA

Patients with hemophilia A, factor VIII deficiency, account for 85 percent of patients with hemophilia. This X-linked, recessive disorder occurs in 1 in 10,000 live male births. Hemophilia B, factor IX deficiency, is also an X-linked recessive disorder and occurs in 1 in 25,000 to 30,000 live male births. Thirty percent of affected patients have no family history of hemophilia; spontaneous mutations are believed to be responsible. Females are generally carriers of hemophilia A or B, have 50 percent of normal factor VIII or factor IX activity, and are asymptomatic. On occasion, due to extreme lyonization, a female carrier can have lower factor VIII or factor IX levels and have clinical manifestations of the disease.

The clinical classification of the hemophilias is based on the severity of deficiency. Patients classified as mildly deficient have 6 to 60 percent of normal factor VIII or factor IX activity; moderate disease is 1 to 5 percent of normal; severe hemophilia describes patients with less than 1 percent of normal factor activity and accounts for 60 percent of all patients. The most common bleeding manifestations are outlined in Table 186-1. Unless there is other underlying disease, patients with hemophilia do not have problems with minor cuts and abrasions. Bleeding in hemophiliacs is characterized by deep hematomas and hematroses that occur spontaneously or with minimal trauma; the bleeding is often delayed several hours after minor injury. Unfortunately, bleeding is not the only problem facing patients with hemophilia. Many hemophiliacs also have chronic hepatitis and are infected with the human immunodeficiency virus (HIV) as a result of their exposure to blood products. In hemophilic patients who received plasma products prior to the mid-1980s, 90 percent have serologic evidence of hepatitis B, 85 to 100 percent have hepatitis C antibodies, and 60 to 90 percent have HIV infection. Those most likely to be infected with HIV are patients with severe hemophilia A

without an inhibitor. Hemophilia B patients are less likely to be infected with HIV as a result of the products they receive for treatment—about 50 percent are infected. Since 1985, acquired immunodeficiency syndrome (AIDS) has become the leading cause of death in patients with hemophilia. Hemophilic patients with AIDS account for 1 percent of the total U.S. AIDS population. Since 1986, as a result of new viral inactivation procedures, there have been few seroconversions resulting from the use of currently available factor replacement products.

Patients with hemophilia are usually identified in childhood or adolescence; however, those with a mild deficiency may go undetected until there is a major hemostatic challenge. Coagulation screening tests in patients with hemophilia typically show a normal prothrombin time (PT), normal thrombin clot time (TCT), and prolonged activated partial thromboplastin time (aPTT), reflective of the abnormality in the intrinsic pathway. However, if the factor VIII level in hemophilia A or factor IX level in hemophilia B is greater than 30 percent of normal activity (mild hemophilia), the aPTT can be normal. The only way to distinguish hemophilia A and hemophilia B is by specific factor assays of factors VIII and IX. Inhibitors are circulating antibodies, usually IgG, that are directed against factor VIII or factor IX, whichever factor the patient is lacking. Inhibitors occur in 10 to 15 percent of patients with severe hemophilia A and in about 10 percent of patients with severe hemophilia B. Inhibitors develop in response to exposure to the "missing factor" through replacement therapy. Most of these develop early in life. The quantity of inhibitor that is present is measured most commonly by the Bethesda inhibitor assay (BIA) and is reported in BIA units. This quantitation is important in determining what type of factor replacement therapy the patient will require.

The emergency physician needs to be aware of major bleeding emergencies that can develop in patients with hemophilia. These patients require emergent factor replacement therapy and management by hemophilia specialists. Air transport should be considered, if available. Bleeding into the *central nervous system* (CNS) can occur spontaneously as well as with trauma. Any patient with hemophilia who complains of a new headache or any neurologic symptoms requires immediate factor replacement therapy followed by computed tomography (CT) scanning of the head. Spontaneous or traumatic bleeding into *the neck, retropharynx, or pharynx* has a high potential for airway compromise. Such bleeding can be spontaneous or precipitated by successful or unsuccessful placement of external jugular lines or other trauma. These patients require immediate factor replacement and CT scanning to define the bleeding area. Airway management, including oral intubation, takes priority. If not preceded by factor replacement therapy, intubation must be followed immediately by factor replacement. Hemophilic patients with complaints of back, thigh, groin, or abdominal pain may have bleeding into the *retroperitoneum*. Bleeding into this potential space can be life-threatening because of the large potential area and the ability of the bleeding to dissect along fascial planes. Immediate factor replacement and CT scanning are indicated. *Compartment syndromes* result from muscle bleeds within the fascial compartments of the extremities. Complaints of pain and paresthesias and the findings of sensory, motor, or vascular deficits raise this possibility. After factor replacement therapy is initiated, the compartment pressure can be measured. Surgical fasciotomy may be required and needs to be done within 8 h after the onset of symptoms for best chance of full neurovascular recovery. Patients with hemophilia should never receive intramuscular injections unless factor replacement is given and maintained for several days. Central lines, including femoral lines and external jugular lines, should not be placed in patients with hemophilia prior to factor replacement therapy. Life-threatening bleeding can result. Arterial blood gases should not be performed on patients with hemophilia without coverage of factor replacement therapy. A compartment syndrome can result.

**Table 186-1.** Common Bleeding Manifestations in Patients with Hemophilia

| Site | Comments |
|------|----------|
| Hemarthroses | Lead to joint destruction and chronic arthropathy if not treated aggressively |
| Hematomas | Bleeding into soft tissues or muscle; this bleeding can dissect along fascial planes; most dangerous near in the neck (airway compromise), limbs (compartment syndromes) and retroperitoneum (massive blood loss) |
| Mucocutaneous bleeding | Bleeding in the oropharynx, gastrointestinal tract, epistaxis, hemoptysis, bleeding after dental extractions |
| Central nervous system | Intracranial bleeding is the most common cause of bleeding death in hemophiliacs, has a 34% mortality; also get subdural hematomas—occur spontaneously or with minimal trauma |
| Hematuria | Common, usually not serious, and the source is rarely found |
| Pseudotumor | Bone cysts that result from unresolved hematomas; usually have to be removed surgically |

The management of hemophilic bleeding is dependent on the type of hemophilia that is present, the severity of deficiency, the presence or absence of an inhibitor, and the location of the bleeding. Each of these will be discussed separately.

## Management of Factor VIII Deficiency (Hemophilia A) without an Inhibitor

Patients with mild or moderate hemophilia A may respond to treatment with desmopressin (1-desamino-8-D-arginine vasopressin, DDAVP). It is helpful to know if the patient has been previously treated with DDAVP successfully. In patients who respond, DDAVP can raise the factor VIII activity level up to threefold. Its mechanism of action is not entirely understood, but DDAVP is believed to cause release of von Willebrand factor (vWF) from storage sites in the endothelial cells; the increased amount of vWF is then capable of carrying additional amounts of factor VIII in the plasma. The usual dose of DDAVP is 0.3 µg/kg of body weight administered intravenously or subcutaneously every 12 h. Some authors suggest 30 µg as a maximum dose. A response in the factor VIII level should be seen in 1 h. This dose can be repeated three or four times before temporary tachyphylaxis develops. The advantages of DDAVP are that it is not a blood product, and therefore carries no risk of viral transmission, and it is easily administered in the hospital or home setting. Serious side effects are uncommon. Common reactions include facial flushing and headache, and mild hyponatremia can develop, especially in pediatric patients.

Patients with moderate or severe hemophilia A and significant bleeding will require treatment with factor VIII concentrates. In settings where virally safe factor VIII concentrates are not available and life-threatening bleeding requires treatment, cryoprecipitate or fresh-frozen plasma (FFP) can be used temporarily; however, these products carry a risk of viral transmission so they should be administered for this purpose only in true emergencies. Each bag of cryoprecipitate contains about 100 units of factor VIII. FFP contains 1 unit of factor VIII per milliliter of FFP. The most commonly used factor VIII concentrates in 1994 are those that are monoclonal antibody–purified (Monoclate-P, Hemophil-M, Factor VIII-M) or the new recombinant products (Recombinate, Kogenate). Other products of lesser purity, which carry some small risk of hepatitis transmission (but not HIV), are still available and electively used by some patients who are already infected, because of their lower price. These products should not be given to patients with negative or uncertain infection status un-

less it is a true emergency. Factor VIII concentrates are dosed by units; 1 unit is the amount of factor VIII activity in 1 milliliter of normal plasma. One unit of factor VIII concentrate should raise the circulating factor VIII level by 2 percent. Table 186-2 outlines specific treatment recommendations for factor VIII replacement therapy in patients with hemophilia A. After the loading dose, subsequent doses of factor VIII should be adjusted based on factor VIII level assays.

Ancillary therapies in the management of bleeding episodes include rest, potential immobilization, analgesia, and the use of antifibrinolytic agents, which are most commonly used in patients undergoing dental or oral surgery. Amicar (ε-aminocaproic acid, EACA) and tranexamic acid (Cyklokapron) are examples. These can be used alone in some cases or in conjunction with factor VIII concentrates. These agents are contraindicated in patients with hematuria.

## Management of Factor VIII Deficiency (Hemophilia A) with Inhibitor Present

The use of factor replacement therapy in hemophilic patients with inhibitors is guided by the inhibitor titer (number of BIA units) and the type of response the patient has to factor VIII concentrates. This anamnestic response is usually either a rapid increase in the inhibitor titer within 2 to 3 days (high responders) or a low response where the inhibitor increases little or none (low responders). Table 186-3 outlines the treatment options available for treatment of hemophilia A patients with inhibitors.

## Management of Factor IX Deficiency (Hemophilia B) without an Inhibitor

Table 186-4 outlines the goals of replacement therapy for patients with hemophilia B. The products that are available for replacement therapy are listed in Table 186-5. The highly purified factor IX concentrates are the treatment of choice if available. If it is necessary to raise the factor IX level to 75 to 100 percent (life-threatening situations), this should be done with the highly purified concentrates because they carry essentially no risk of thrombogenicity. In settings where factor IX concentrates are not available, FFP can be used to raise the factor IX level. The use of FFP in this setting should be limited to emergency treatment because of the small risk of viral transmission and the inability to raise the factor IX levels adequately because of volume constraints. One unit of FFP will raise the factor IX level by 3 percent in an average-size person.

**Table 186-2.** Factor VIII Replacement Therapy for Patients with Hemophilia A (No Inhibitor)

| Type of Hemorrhage | Factor VIII Level Required for Hemostasis, % of normal | Factor VIII Dose in Units/kg (Initial Dose) | Dosing Interval, h* | Duration of Therapy, days |
|---|---|---|---|---|
| Minor | | | | |
| Hemarthroses | 30–50 | 15–25 | 24 | 1–2 |
| Superficial muscular or soft tissue | 30–50 | 15–25 | 24 | 1–2 |
| Moderate | | | | |
| Epistaxis | 30–50 | 15–25 | 12 | Until resolved |
| Dental extractions | 50 | 25 | 12–24 | 1–2 |
| Muscular or soft tissue with dissection | 50–100 | 25–50 | 12 | Variable |
| GI bleeding | 50–100 | 25–50 | 12 | 7–10 |
| Hematuria | 50–100 | 25–50 | 12 | Until resolved |
| Life threatening | | | | |
| Central nervous system | 75–100 | 50 | 12 | 10–14 |
| Retropharynx/pharnyx | 75–100 | 50 | 12 | 10–14 |
| Retroperitoneum | 75–100 | 50 | 12 | 10–14 |
| Surgery | 75–100 | 50 | 12 | Variable |

* Continuous infusion of factor VIII concentrate may be used in hospitalized patients; a typical dose after the loading dose is 150 units/h; this is adjusted based on factor VIII levels.

*Note:* GI, gastrointestinal.

**Table 186-3.** Replacement Therapy for Hemophilia A Patients with Inhibitors

| Type of Product (Trade Names) | Used for | Dose | Frequency, h | Comments |
|---|---|---|---|---|
| *Factor VIII concentrates* | Inhibitor titer less than 5–10 BIA units | 5,000–10,000 unit bolus | Continuous infusion at about 1000 units/h | If patient is a "high responder," in about 3 days the inhibitor titer will rise |
| *Prothrombin complex concentrates* (PCCs) PCCs contain factors II, VII, IX, X (Bebulin VH, Proplex T, Profilnine HT, and Konyne-80) | Inhibitor titer >10 units; known good response to these products | 75–100 units/kg of bodyweight | Repeat dose every 8–12 h | Complications of use include development of thromboembolic disease, DIC, very low risk of hepatitis transmission |
| *Activated prothrombin complex concentrates* aPCCs contain factors II, VII, IX, and X with variable amounts of activated factors $VII_a$, $IX_a$, and $X_a$ (Autoplex, FEIBA) | Patients who do not respond to PCCs | Same as with PCCs | Repeat dose every 12–24 h | Same as with PCCs |
| *Porcine factor VIII* | Patients with high inhibitor titers not responsive to the above products | Variable | Variable | Patients will often develop an inhibitor to the procine product |
| *Recombinant factor $VII_a$* | Not yet commercially available | Variable | Variable | Less thrombogenic risk than PCCs and no risk of viral transmission |

**Table 186-4.** Factor IX Replacement Therapy for Patients with Hemophilia B

| Type of Hemorrhage | Factor IX level Required for Hemostasis, % of Normal | Initial Factor IX dose in Units/kg | Duration of Therapy, days |
|---|---|---|---|
| Minor | | | |
| Hemarthroses | 20–30 | 20–30 | 1–2 |
| Superficial muscular or soft tissue | 20–30 | 20–30 | 1–2 |
| Moderate | | | |
| Epistaxis | 25–50 | 25–50 | Until resolved |
| Dental extractions | 25–50 | 25–50 | 2–7 |
| Muscular or soft tissue bleeds with dissection | 25–50 | 25–50 | Until resolved |
| Hematuria | 25–50 | 25–50 | Until resolved |
| GI bleeding | 50 | 50 | 5–10 |
| Life-threatening* | | | |
| Central nervous system | 50 | 50 | 7–10 |
| Retropharynx/pharynx | 50 | 50 | 7–10 |
| Retroperitoneum | 50 | 50 | 7–10 |
| Surgery | 50 | 50 | 7–10 |

* Factor IX levels higher than 50% may be necessary and are safely obtained using the highly purified factor IX concentrates.

**Table 186-5.** Products Used for Replacement Therapy in Patients with Hemophilia B

| Type of Product | Typical Dose |
|---|---|
| Highly purified factor IX concentrates Alpha Nine Alpha Nine-SD Mononine | One unit/kg raises the factor IX level by 1 percent; these products require dosing every 18–30 h |
| Prothrombin complex concentrates Bebulin VH Proplex T Profilnine HT Konyne-80 | One unit/kg raises the factor IX level by 1 percent; subsequent doses every 12 h |

## Management of Factor IX Deficiency (Hemophilia B) with Inhibitor Present

The products available for the treatment of hemophilia B patients with inhibitors are outlined in Table 186-6, along with treatment guidelines. The treatment of each patient must be individualized based on the clinical response.

## Indications for Hospital Admission

Hemophilic patients with bleeding episodes will require hospital admission in these situations:

- The patient has potentially life-threatening bleeding involving the CNS, neck, pharynx, retropharynx or retroperitoneum, or potential compartment syndrome.
- The patient is not capable of administering factor replacement therapy at home.
- The patient requires treatment for several days.
- The patient needs close monitoring.
- The patient requires parenteral pain control.

## VON WILLEBRAND DISEASE

Von Willebrand disease, which is caused by a deficiency or abnormality of vWF, is the most common inherited bleeding disorder. The vWF is a glycoprotein that is synthesized, stored, and secreted by vascular endothelial cells; it is also found in plasma and platelets. vWF has two functions: (1) in primary hemostasis, vWF allows platelets to adhere to the damaged endothelium; and (2) vWF carries factor VIII in the plasma.

It is estimated that 1 in 100 persons has a gene defective for vWF, which is inherited in an autosomal dominant pattern. However, only 1 in 10,000 manifests a clinically significant bleeding disorder. The most severe type of von Willebrand disease (vWD), known as type III, is very rare, occurring in 1 in 1 million persons; it results from an autosomal recessive defect.

A variety of tests are used to establish the diagnosis of vWD. Co-

**Table 186-6.** Products Used for Replacement Therapy in Patients with Hemophilia B with Inhibitors

| Type of Product | Used for | Initial Dose |
|---|---|---|
| Highly purified factor IX concentrates | Bethesda inhibitor titer <10 units | Variable |
| Prothrombin complex concentrates | Bethesda inhibitor titer <10 units | 75 units/kg |
| Activated prothrombin complex concentrates | Bethesda inhibitor titers > 10 units or unresponsive to the above | Variable, about 75 units/kg |
| Recombinant factor VII$_a$ | Not yet commercially available | Variable |

agulation screening tests will show a normal PT, normal TCT, and usually normal aPTT, although it may be prolonged in moderate or severe vWD due to the decreased factor VIII activity. The other tests used in the evaluation of vWD are outlined in Table 186-7. The diagnosis of vWD can be difficult to establish because of variability in test results. Oftentimes, patients have to be tested repeatedly when there is a high index of suspicion in order to establish the diagnosis. The tests can be affected by estrogens, progesterones, oral contraceptive agents, thyroid disease, infections, and exercise.

Based on the results of testing, patients with vWD can be classified into three main types, outlined in Table 186-8. There are many subtypes that are clinically unimportant.

Von Willebrand disease can be difficult to distinguish from mild hemophilia A. The bleeding time should be normal in hemophilia, although it is also often normal in patients with vWD. The von Willebrand antigen and activity should be normal or elevated in patients with hemophilia. The factor VIII activity level will be low in patients with hemophilia and may be normal or slightly low in patients with vWD. In some cases, it is nearly impossible to distinguish type I vWD and mild hemophilia A.

The hemorrhagic tendency in patients with vWD is highly variable among patients with the same type of vWD, even among patients from the same family who have an identical genetic defect. Most characteristic are mild bleeding symptoms from mucocutaneous surfaces (such as epistaxis), easy bruising, bleeding after dental extractions, menorrhagia, and gastrointestinal bleeding. Patients with type III vWD have a severe bleeding diathesis with spontaneous hematomas and hemarthroses similar to patients with severe hemophilia.

The treatment of vWD depends on the type of disease that is pre-

**Table 186-7.** Laboratory Evaluation of Patients with von Willebrand Disease*

| Test | Typical Result in vWD | Comments |
|---|---|---|
| Bleeding time | Prolonged | Measures platelet and vessel wall interaction (primary hemostasis); this test has high variability—if prolonged, it is important data; if normal, does not rule out vWD |
| vWF antigen | Low or normal | Is an acute phase reactant, increased in stress and pregnancy |
| vWF activity | Low | Evaluates the function of vWF by measuring the ability of vWF to agglutinate platelets in the presence of the antibiotic ristocetin |
| Factor VIII activity | Low or normal | May be normal or slightly decreased in vWD, except very low or absent in type III vWD |
| Multimeric analysis | Variable | Separates the vWF molecule into its subunits (multimers) based on molecular weight; needed to distinguish types of vWD |

*Note:* vWF, von Willebrand factor; vWD, von Willebrand disease.

**Table 186-8.** Classification of von Willebrand Disease

| Type | Occurrence | Defect |
|---|---|---|
| I | 70–80% of patients with vWD | All multimeric forms are present but their quantity is diminished |
| II | 10–15% | The vWF molecule is abnormal, missing some of the multimers |
| III | <10% | Essentially no vWF is present |

*Note:* vWD, von Willebrand disease; vWF, von Willebrand factor.

**Table 186-9.** Suggested Treatment for Patients with von Willebrand Disease

| Type I | DDAVP (desmopressin) |
|---|---|
| Type II | Humate-P or Koate-HS (factor VIII concentrates) or cryoprecipitate |
| Type III | Humate-P or Koate-HS (factor VIII concentrates) or cryoprecipitate |

sent and the severity of bleeding. Table 186-9 shows the recommended therapy for patients with vWD. DDAVP is the mainstay of therapy for patients with type I vWD; plasma products that contain vWF are used for types II and III. DDAVP can be administered subcutaneously or intravenously at a dose of 0.3 μg/kg of body weight. This dose is given every 12 h to a total of three or four doses before temporary tachyphylaxis develops. In a setting where treatment is essential and DDAVP or the specifically recommended factor VIII concentrates are not available, cryoprecipitate can be used to replace the vWF that is needed for hemostasis. Each bag of cryoprecipitate contains about 100 units of vWF activity. Cryoprecipitate should only be used in emergencies because there is a small risk of viral transmission. Women with vWD are often treated with hormonal agents (estrogens and/or progesterones), which cause an increase in the vWF activity. Bleeding associated with dental procedures can often be managed with fibrinolytic inhibitor agents such as EACA and tranexamic acid.

## BIBLIOGRAPHY

Chorba TL, Holman RC, Strine TW, et al: Changes in longevity and causes of death among persons with hemophilia A. *Am J Hematol* 45:112, 1994.

Coyne MA: Avoiding indecision and hesitation with hemophilia-related emergencies. *Emerg Med Rep* 13:165, 1992.

Dietrich AM, James CD, King DR, et al: Head trauma in children with congenital coagulation disorders. *J Pediatr Surg* 29:28, 1994.

Hanna WT, Bona RD, Zimmerman CE, et al: The use of intermediate and high purity factor VIII products in the treatment of von Willebrand disease. *Thromb Hemost* 71:173, 1994.

Mannucci PM, Cattaneo M: Desmopressin: A nontransfusional treatment of hemophilia and von Willebrand disease. *Haemostasis* 22:276, 1992.

Morgan LM, Kissoon N, de Vebber BL: Experience with the hemophiliac child in a pediatric emergency department. *J Emerg Med* 11:519, 1993.

Pfaff JA, Geninatti M: Hemophilia. *Emerg Med Clin North Am* 11:337, 1993.

Roberts HR, Eberst ME: Current Management of Hemophilia B, in Penner JA, Hassouna HI (eds): *Hematol Oncol Clin North Am* 7:1269, 1993.

Roberts HR, Eberst ME: The molecular biology of classic hemophilia and a review of factor VIII concentrates, in Spivak JV, Bell WR, et al (eds): *The Yearbook of Hematology*. St. Louis, Mosby, 1992, pp 121–144.

# 187
# HEREDITARY HEMOLYTIC ANEMIAS
## Mary E. Eberst

In this chapter, we will discuss the most common inherited hemolytic anemias including the hemoglobinopathies; sickle cell anemia and its variants; glucose-6-phosphate dehydrogenase deficiency, which is a red blood cell enzymatic defect; and hereditary spherocytosis, a defect in the red blood cell membrane.

## SICKLE CELL ANEMIA
### Pathophysiology

A hemoglobinopathy is an inherited disease resulting from the presence of one or more abnormal hemoglobins. More than 400 hemoglobin variants have been described. Normal human hemoglobin consists of four polypeptide chains and four heme groups. The four polypeptide chains consist of two $\alpha$ (alpha) chains and two nonalpha chains, which are most commonly $\beta$ (beta). The majority of hemoglobin in a normal adult consists of two alpha chains and two beta chains and is called hemoglobin A (HbA, $\alpha_2\beta_2$). Other normal nonalpha chains are gamma (hemoglobin F) and delta (hemoglobin $A_2$) (see Table 187-1).

The most common hemoglobin variant, known as hemoglobin S (Hb S), results from a single point mutation on the beta chain: valine is substituted for glutamic acid in the sixth position. Hemoglobin S is little problem when it is carrying oxygen (oxyhemoglobin form), but when it is deoxygenated, Hb S polymerizes within the red blood cell causing the sickle shape. Sickled red blood cells increase the viscosity of the blood, leading to sludging or obstruction in the microcirculation. Eventually, the cells may become irreversibly sickled. Conditions that increase the amount of sickling include acidosis and increased 2, 3-diphosphoglycerate (both cause the oxygen dissociation curve to shift to the right, which favors the formation of the deoxyhemoglobin form); vascular stasis; dehydration; the presence of higher levels of Hb S in the cells; and low oxygen tension. The presence of hemoglobin F (Hb F) has a protective role; higher Hb F levels are associated with less sickling phenomena. Sickled red blood cells are rapidly hemolyzed resulting in a red blood cell survival of 10 to 20 days, compared with the normal red blood cell lifespan of 120 days.

In the U.S. African-American population, about 8 percent carry the sickle cell gene; these persons have Hb AS ($\alpha_2\beta S$, sickle cell trait). Inherited in an autosomal codominant pattern, sickle cell disease (SCD) results when the patient inherits the sickle gene from both parents. This is hemoglobin SS ($\alpha_2 S_2$) and occurs in 0.14 to 0.20 percent of the U.S. African-American population, resulting in about 50,000

patients with SCD. When the sickle gene is inherited from one parent and another abnormal beta-chain gene is inherited from the other parent, heterozygous hemoglobinopathies result, such as hemoglobin SC disease and sickle–$\beta$ thalassemia (see below).

### Clinical Features

The clinical manifestations of SCD are variable between patients but all are related to chronic hemolytic anemia, and virtually every organ system can be affected by recurrent vasoocclusive events. First we will review the common clinical findings in patients with SCD, then we will discuss the problems that are likely to bring the patient to the emergency department (Table 187-2).

Patients with SCD have a chronic hemolytic anemia with a baseline hemoglobin of 6 to 9 g/dL and a reticulocyte count of 5 to 15 percent. These patients commonly have cardiopulmonary disease, including decreased pulmonary function and reserve, decreased resting arterial oxygen tension, systolic and diastolic flow murmurs, congestive heart failure, cardiomegaly, and cor pulmonale. Myocardial infarction is rare in patients with sickle cell disease. Icterus is the rule as a result of chronic hemolysis. Bilirubin gallstones are found in up to 75 percent of patients with SCD. Hepatomegaly and liver function test abnormalities are common. Splenomegaly is seen in children with SCD; however, by adulthood, the spleen is usually small as a result of recurrent infarction. Renal abnormalities including isosthenuria (inability to concentrate urine) and papillary necrosis occur commonly because of sickling phenomena in the hypertonic, acidic renal medulla. Bony abnormalities, resulting from expansion of the marrow space, and bony infarcts are typical. Radiographs of the bones show thinning of the cortices and sparseness of the trabecular pattern; the biconcave "fishmouth" changes in the vertebrae are pathognomonic of SCD. Skin ulcerations occur over the distal lower extremities. Ophthalmologic problems primarily involving the retinae are common. Chronic disabilities resulting from central nervous system vasoocclusive events are seen.

Table 187-2 outlines the types of crises that occur in patients with SCD. Frequently, a patient will have more than one type of crisis at a time.

### Vasoocclusive Crises

Painful vasoocclusive crises are the most common reason for visits to the emergency department by patients with SCD. These crises account for the greatest morbidity and mortality among these patients. The average adult sickle cell patient has four severe attacks per year; however, some patients experience crises daily. Vasoocclusive events are more common in adult patients with higher hemoglobin levels and lower amounts of Hb F. The underlying pathophysiology is sludging of sickled red blood cells in the microcirculation with infarction. This event can be precipitated by infection, exposure to cold, dehydration, and high altitude. In children, up to 80 percent of the vasoocclusive events are infection-related. In adults, up to one-third of vasoocclusive crises are related to bacterial or viral infections, but the majority of crises are unexplained. Patients can have

**Table 187-1.** Composition of Normal Human Hemoglobin and the Sickle Hemoglobin Variants.

| Phenotype | Types of Hemoglobin Present | Percent | Genotype |
|---|---|---|---|
| Normal adult | Hb A | 96–98 | 2 alpha 2 beta |
|  | Hb F | 0.5–0.8 | 2 alpha 2 gamma |
|  | Hb $A_2$ | 1.5–3.2 | 2 alpha 2 delta |
| Sickle cell trait (heterozygons) | Hb AS | A 60–65 | 2 alpha 1 beta 1 sickle |
|  |  | S 35–40 |  |
| Sickle cell disease (homozygous) | Hb SS | S 80–90 | 2 alpha 2 sickle |
|  | Hb F | F 2–20 | 2 alpha 2 gamma |
|  | Hb $A_2$ | $A_2$ 2–4 | 2 alpha 2 delta |

**Table 187-2.** Clinical Emergencies in Patients with Sickle Cell Anemia.

| Vasoocclusive Crises | Hematologic Crises | Infectious Crises |
|---|---|---|
| Musculoskeletal pain | Splenic sequestration | Pneumonia |
| Abdominal pain | Aplastic crisis | Meningitis |
| Pulmonary crisis |  | Osteomyelitis |
| Central nervous system crisis |  | Urinary tract infection |
| Priapism |  | Sepsis |
| Hand and foot syndrome |  |  |
| Renal crisis |  |  |

"typical" crises with pain in the same location recurrently, but the pain can be anywhere.

**Musculoskeletal pain.** Vasoocclusive crisis with pain involving the bones, joints, and muscles is the most prominent manifestation of SCD. This pain can be anywhere but most often involves the humerus, tibia, femur, and low back area. Examination may reveal local tenderness, but often there are no physical findings. The differential diagnosis includes osteomyelitis and acute arthritides such as gout and rheumatoid arthritis. Pain in the hip with difficulty walking raises the possibility of avascular necrosis (AVN) of the femoral head. If there is local tenderness or an effusion, an aspirate should be obtained for culture or the joint fluid evaluated for signs of infection. Plain radiographs may show changes of osteomyelitis or AVN but are of little value in detecting bony infarction. Magnetic resonance imaging (MRI) can be used to document infarction. Bone scans and gallium scans can differentiate infarction from osteomyelitis and may show osteomyelitis in the early stages before plain radiographs will show abnormalities.

**Abdominal pain.** This is the second most common type of vasoocclusive crisis experienced by patients with SCD. Abdominal pain due to vasoocclusive crisis typically is of relatively acute onset, diffuse, poorly localized, and often recurrent. These patients have diffuse pain without peritoneal signs; bowel sounds should be present. Pain in the right upper quadrant (RUQ) raises the possibility of cholecystitis and the RUQ syndrome. At least 75 percent of patients with SCD have bilirubin gallstones; however, only 10 percent are ever symptomatic. The RUQ syndrome involves the sudden onset of RUQ pain, progressive hepatomegaly, and extreme hyperbilirubinemia (>50 mg/dL). Resulting from intrahepatic cholestasis, the outcome of the RUQ syndrome is usually benign in pediatric patients, but some adult patients progress to liver failure. The remainder of the differential diagnosis of sickle cell patients with abdominal pain suspected of having vasoocclusive crisis includes pancreatitis, mesenteric infarction, hepatitis, hepatic infarction, appendicitis, perforated viscus, and pelvic inflammatory disease. Ultrasound examination and computed tomographic (CT) scanning of the abdomen and pelvis may be helpful. Surgical consultation is indicated if the diagnosis remains uncertain.

**Pulmonary crisis.** This problem occurs in up to 30 percent of patients with SCD and accounts for 15 percent of adult deaths. The presentation of pleuritic chest pain, fever, leukocytosis, and possible pulmonary infiltrate raises the differential diagnosis of pulmonary infarction, acute chest syndrome, bacterial or viral pneumonia, and pulmonary thromboembolus. The acute chest syndrome occurs when a pulmonary infarct becomes secondarily infected. This is a major cause of death in patients with SCD above age 10. Such patients often have a precipitous decrease in pulmonary function and severe hypoxia. The chest radiograph may not show an infiltrate for up to 2 days. Arterial blood gas analysis, complete blood count (CBC), and the presence of sputum may be helpful. Ventilation-perfusion (V/Q) scan of the lung may be helpful, especially if a baseline study for comparison is available. Pulmonary angiography should be avoided, if possible, as the contrast material can induce more pulmonary sickling. Sickle cell patients with significant pulmonary signs or symptoms should be admitted to the hospital. Empiric antibiotics are often given until the diagnosis becomes clear.

**Central nervous system crisis.** This is the only type of vasoocclusive crisis that is painless. Overall, neurologic complications occur in 15 to 25 percent of patients with SCD. The most common problems are cerebral infarction in children and cerebral hemorrhage in adults. Other complications of central nervous system (CNS) vasoocclusive events are transient ischemic attacks, seizures, headache, dizziness, cranial nerve palsies, unexplained coma, paresthesias, meningitis, vestibular dysfunction, and sensory hearing loss. There is an increased incidence of subarachnoid hemorrhage (SAH) in patients with SCD. Evaluation of patients with CNS complaints should include a CT scan of the head and a lumbar puncture to rule out SAH

and meningitis. MRI is better than CT scanning for demonstrating the CNS effects of vasoocclusive phenomena.

**Priapism.** This complication occurs in up to 30 percent of males with SCD. The persistent, painful erection results from the sickling of cells in the corpus cavernosum, which prevents the emptying of blood from the penis. Surgical decompression may be required, and permanent impotence may result.

**Hand and foot syndrome (dactylitis).** This complication of SCD usually occurs in the first 2 years of life and may be the first sign that a child has SCD. The patient presents with swelling of the hands and/or feet (one to four extremities involved) that is the result of vasoocclusion of the nutrient arteries to the metacarpals and/or metatarsals. Avascular necrosis of the bone marrow in the involved bones occurs.

**Renal crisis.** Vasoocclusive events involving the kidneys are very common but often asymptomatic. Infarction in the renal medulla may cause flank pain, renal colic-type pain, and costovertebral angle tenderness. Patients may have gross or microscopic hematuria and may pass tissue resulting from papillary necrosis. Pyelonephritis and urinary tract infection must be excluded, and adequate/stable renal function should be documented.

## Hematologic Crises

Heralded by an acute drop in the hemoglobin level, patients with hematologic crisis will present with weakness, shortness of breath, fatigue, worsening of congestive heart failure, or shock. There are two types of hematologic crisis.

**Acute splenic sequestration.** This occurs primarily in children and is the second most common cause of death in children with SCD under the age of 5. Often preceded by viral infections, sickled cells block the splenic outflow, causing pooling of peripheral blood and sickled cells in the spleen. Such patients present in hypovolemic shock with an enlarged spleen. These crises are divided into major and minor. In a major sequestration crisis, the spleen enlarges rapidly and the hemoglobin drops to less than 6 g/dL or by 3 g/dL from baseline. A minor sequestration crisis is specified by an enlarging spleen and a hemoglobin greater than 6 g/dL. These patients will have a higher-than-usual reticulocyte count reflective of normal compensatory bone marrow activity. Such patients are managed with transfusion of red blood cells and exchange transfusions; splenectomy may be considered.

**Aplastic crisis.** This life-threatening complication of SCD occurs when bone marrow erythropoiesis is slowed or stopped. The hematocrit falls to as low as 10 percent, and the reticulocyte count falls to as low as 0.5 percent. The white blood cell count and platelet counts usually remain stable. Aplastic crises can be precipitated by viral infections (particularly parvovirus $B_{19}$), folic acid deficiency, or the ingestion of bone marrow toxins such as phenylbutazone. This is usually a self-limited problem, but red blood cell transfusions may be required for severe anemia or cardiopulmonary compromise.

## Infectious Crises

Infection is a common contributor to death in patients of all ages with SCD, especially children under the age of 5. Functionally asplenic after early childhood and with impaired phagocyte functioning, patients with SCD are and should be treated as immunocompromised hosts. Sickle cell patients who present with an unexplained fever of $\geq 38°C$ (101°F) require evaluation for a source of bacterial infection and consideration for early treatment with broad-spectrum antibiotics. Sickle cell patients can be rapidly overwhelmed by bacterial sepsis, particularly with encapsulated organisms, such as *Haemophilus influenzae* and *Streptococcus pneumoniae*. Other common diseases are pneumonia, caused by these organisms as well as *Mycoplasma pneumoniae;* meningitis; and osteomyelitis due to *Salmonella typhimurium, Staphylococcus aureus,* and *Escherichia coli.* Patients with iron overload from frequent transfusions who are treated with the chelating agent deferoxamine are at risk for infection with *Yersinia enterocolitica.*

## Diagnosis—Laboratory and Radiologic Evaluation

The diagnosis of sickle cell disease is usually established in early life based on the family history, ideally before the child begins to develop complications. The diagnosis is made by documenting the presence of sickle hemoglobin. Sickled red blood cells should be seen on the peripheral smear. Quick tests to determine the presence of sickle hemoglobin are the Metabisulfite test and the Sickledex test. Hemoglobin electrophoresis is required to distinguish homozygous SS disease from sickle cell trait and the other heterozygous sickle syndromes.

### Laboratory Studies

The laboratory evaluation required for an individual patient who presents to the emergency department can be tailored to the symptoms of the patient and the physical findings. Commonly obtained studies include

**Complete blood count.** A complete blood count (CBC) should be obtained in most sickle cell patients with severe crisis. The "normal" white blood cell count in patients with SCD ranges from 12,000/μL (mm³) to 18,000/μL (mm³) but usually has a normal differential. Elevations higher than the patient's baseline or the presence of a left shift are notable. The baseline hemoglobin in sickle cell patients is typically 6 to 9 g/dL. A fall in the hemoglobin by 2 g/dL or a fall in the hematocrit by 4 to 6 percent may reflect hematologic crisis or blood loss. The platelet count is often elevated at baseline. The peripheral smear should show sickled cells and Howell-Jolly bodies, which indicate the loss of splenic function.

**Reticulocyte count.** A reticulocyte count should be obtained if the hemoglobin has fallen by 2 g/dL or more. The baseline reticulocyte count is typically 5 to 15 percent; lower values may reflect aplastic crisis.

**Electrolytes.** Electrolytes should be obtained in any patient who appears significantly dehydrated, because imbalances occur readily because of isosthenuria.

**Liver function tests.** Liver function tests should be obtained in sickle cell patients who present with abdominal pain. These patients often have baseline abnormalities and a chronically elevated indirect bilirubin due to chronic hemolysis.

**Erythrocyte sedimentation rate.** The erythrocyte sedimentation rate (ESR) is not a reliable indicator of inflammation or infection in patients with SCD because sickled cells cannot form rouleaux, which is the basis for the test. The ESR is helpful only if it is elevated, since a normal value does not rule out infection or inflammation.

**Arterial blood gas.** An arterial blood gas should be obtained in any patient with sickle cell disease who presents with respiratory complaints. It is very helpful to know a baseline value because adults may have chronic mild to moderate hypoxia. A $P_{O_2} < 60$ mmHg in adults or < 70 mmHg in children usually indicates an acute problem.

**Urinalysis.** A urinalysis should be obtained in any sickle cell patient with urinary symptoms or fever.

### Radiologic Studies

**Chest x-ray.** A chest x-ray should be obtained in any patient with pulmonary signs or symptoms. In the acute chest syndrome, the chest x-ray may be normal for 2 days, so a normal radiograph does not exclude a problem.

**Bone films.** Bone films should be considered for the patient who presents with localized bone tenderness. Plain radiographs will not show infarction and will only show osteomyelitis after about 10 days. A bone scan or MRI can show changes of osteomyelitis within 24 h.

**Abdominal ultrasound or CT scan.** An abdominal ultrasound or CT scan may be helpful in patients with abdominal pain. The pres-

ence of vasoocclusive crisis will not alter these studies; however, they may show changes of cholecystitis, pancreatitis, bowel infarction, abscesses, or appendicitis.

**Computed tomography of head or MRI scan.** Computed tomography of the head (head CT) or an MRI scan should be obtained in any sickle cell patient who presents with neurologic symptoms or signs. MRI is a more sensitive study in this setting.

## General Management

General recommendations will be reviewed here as well as some specific guidelines for the initial treatment of complications. Additional suggestions are included above under the types of crises and laboratory and radiologic evaluation.

The general management of patients with sickle cell disease who present to the emergency department is primarily supportive. Patients with unstable vital signs or neurologic compromise need emergency care. The basic care of patients who present with "crisis" include the following:

*Hydration:* Any type of crisis may be precipitated or exacerbated by dehydration. Oral rehydration can be attempted if the patient can tolerate fluids and the episode is relatively mild. Intravenous rehydration will be needed for patients who are orthostatic or in severe pain. Fluid overload needs to be avoided in light of potential underlying cardiopulmonary disease. One-half normal saline at a rate of one to one and a half times maintenance dose is a reasonable fluid choice.

*Analgesia:* Sickle cell patients need prompt pain relief with adequate analgesia. The presence of narcotic addiction or the potential for its development should not alter what is prescribed in the emergency department. Sickle cell patients who frequently seek help in the emergency department will benefit from a protocol treatment plan so they know what to expect and manipulative behavior is minimized. The emergency staff should have a consistent approach to the use of narcotics in these patients. It is reasonable to administer up to two doses of narcotics in the emergency department over a 4- to 6-h period; if patients still have significant pain, they should be admitted to the hospital. Nonnarcotic analgesics such as Tylenol or ibuprofen can be used for mild pain, although most sickle cell patients do not come to the emergency department for mild pain. Oral narcotics such as Tylenol #3 or Percocet may be adequate for moderate pain. Parenteral narcotics are necessary for severe pain. A combination of meperidine and promethazine is commonly used. A typical dose would be 100 mg of meperidine and 25 mg of promethazine intravenously or intramuscularly. Some patients will have developed tolerance to narcotics and require larger doses.

*Supplemental oxygen:* Supplemental oxygen is only beneficial if the patient is hypoxic.

*Cardiac monitoring:* Cardiac monitoring should be considered if the patient has a history of cardiopulmonary compromise or any acute complaints referable to those systems.

## Specific Recommendations for Complications

### Infections

Sickle cell patients with infectious symptoms or a temperature greater than 38°C (101°F) should be presumed to have a bacterial infection. Basic laboratory studies should be obtained as well as cultures of blood, sputum, and urine as indicated. Radiographs should be obtained. There should be a low threshold for lumbar puncture. In most patients, parenteral antibiotics should be administered for 48 h or until the cultures are finalized. Intravenous cephalosporins such as cefuroxime or ceftriaxone are generally used. Suggested oral or outpatient regimens would be Ceclor or Augmentin.

Sickle cell patients need to be vaccinated in childhood against *Strep. pneumoniae, H. influenzae,* and hepatitis B. Children with

SCD generally receive prophylactic daily oral penicillin up to age 6; this practice is not known to be helpful in adults.

## Pulmonary Crisis

Sickle cell patients with pulmonary crisis need aggressive management including hospitalization until the diagnosis becomes apparent. Since the differential diagnosis includes pneumonia, empiric antibiotics such as cefuroxime and erythromycin are often given. Oxygen is administered for hypoxia, and close monitoring is needed for possible decompensation. Pulmonary thromboembolism is also in this differential diagnosis. If significant V/Q mismatch is demonstrated on V/Q scan, or large vessel occlusion on pulmonary angiography, heparinization is indicated. Patients with significant cardiopulmonary decompensation may be treated with exchange transfusion.

## Central Nervous System Crisis

Sickle cell patients with signs or symptoms of neurologic compromise need emergent care and close monitoring. After the patient is stabilized, a head CT or MRI should be obtained. If there is no contraindication, a lumbar puncture should be performed to rule out SAH and meningitis. Seizures and cerebral edema are managed conventionally. These patients require admission to an intensive care unit. When there is an acute CNS event, exchange transfusion is used to lower the Hb S concentration to less than 30 percent.

## Localized Bone Pain

This finding, especially when accompanied by fever and leukocytosis, raises the possibility of osteomyelitis. Radiographs, bone scan, or MRI may not be immediately helpful or available. The site should be directly aspirated for culture, and the patient started on parenteral antibiotics to cover *Staph. aureus* and *S. typhimurium.*

## Priapism

When a patient with sickle cell disease presents with priapism, urologic consultation should be obtained. The patient should receive analgesia and hydration, and the bladder should be emptied by catheterization, if possible. Exchange transfusions may be instituted, but if not successful, surgical intervention will be necessary.

## Disposition and Follow-up

After evaluation in the emergency department (including physical examination and laboratory and radiographic studies as indicated), conservative supportive therapy, and observation, a diagnosis can usually be established that will dictate the disposition of the patient.

The following are some guidelines for hospital admission for sickle cell patients:

1. Patients with pulmonary, neurologic, or infectious crisis
2. Patients with splenic sequestration or aplastic crisis
3. Patients with other types of vasoocclusive crises who do not have adequate pain control after analgesics in the emergency department, the determination to be made after 4 to 6 h and no more than 2 doses of narcotic analgesics
4. Patients who are unable to maintain adequate hydration
5. Patients in whom the diagnosis is uncertain.

Patients with SCD who are discharged from the emergency department need to have the following:

1. The ability to maintain adequate oral hydration
2. A 2- or 3-day supply of oral analgesics that provide adequate pain relief
3. Instructions to return to the emergency department for increased pain, fever >38°C (100.4°F), or a change in their symptoms
4. Follow-up, preferably with their primary care physician, in 12 to 24 h for children or 24 to 48 h for adults.

## VARIANTS OF SICKLE CELL DISEASE

### Sickle Cell Trait

This carrier state for SCD is the most frequently encountered sickle hemoglobin variant; it is *not* a mild form of sickle cell disease. Approximately 8 percent of the U.S. African-American population, or 2.5 million people, carry the gene for sickle hemoglobin. This heterozygous state is a result of autosomal dominant inheritance and results in Hb AS. Each red blood cell contains both normal Hb A (60 percent) and Hb S (40 percent). The abundance of normal Hb A prevents sickling under most physiologic circumstances. Hematologically, these patients are normal. Their red blood cells have a normal life span, so they are not anemic. Sickled red blood cells should not be seen on peripheral blood smear except under extreme hypoxia; if seen under normal circumstances, the diagnosis is incorrect.

Clinically, patients with sickle cell trait have minimal complications. The kidney is the most frequently affected organ. Microinfarcts occur in the medulla, leading to papillary necrosis and impaired concentrating ability. Hematuria can be found in 1 percent of patients with sickle cell trait. Exposure to high altitude has been associated with splenic infarction and cerebrovascular complications. Women with sickle cell trait have an increased incidence of urinary tract infections and hematuria during pregnancy. Persons with sickle cell trait have an increased incidence of sudden death during physical training, presumably due to increased sickling with extreme exertion. However, the majority of patients with sickle cell trait are asymptomatic, lead normal lives, and overall have a normal life expectancy.

### Sickle Cell–Hemoglobin C Disease (Hb SC Disease)

This heterozygous sickle cell variant results when the gene for Hb S is inherited from one parent and the gene for Hb C is inherited from the other parent. Hemoglobin C results from a single point mutation in the beta-chain gene. Lysine is substituted for glutamic acid at the sixth position. Some 2.4 percent of U.S. African-Americans carry the gene for Hb C. This gene frequency is one-fourth that for Hb S, but the prevalence among adults of SC and SS disease is almost the same because those with Hb C have a near-normal life expectancy. The red blood cells of these patients contain 50 percent Hb S and 50 percent Hb C. Because Hb C does not polymerize as readily as Hb S, the disease generally has less severe clinical consequences. These patients have a mild to moderate hemolytic anemia and mild reticulocytosis. The peripheral smear shows abundant target cells and a few sickle cells, and Hb C may be seen precipitated as a rhomboid crystal in the red blood cells. Splenomegaly is a feature of Hb SC disease and persists into adulthood in 60 percent of patients. Overall, patients with Hb SC disease have few clinical complications, although some have profound medical problems as complex as those seen in patients with SCD. Patients with Hb SC disease can have painful crises and organ infarcts. They are at higher-than-normal risk for bacterial infections. Ocular complications and visual loss occur, as well as infarcts in the renal medulla and avascular necrosis of the femoral heads. Women with Hb SC disease have an increased incidence of complications in pregnancy.

### Sickle Cell–Beta (β) Thalassemia Disease

This heterozygous sickle cell variant occurs when the gene for sickle hemoglobin is inherited from one parent and the gene for β thalassemia is inherited from the other parent. In U.S. African-Americans, the gene frequency for β thalassemia is 0.8 to 1.0 percent. The frequency of sickle cell–β thalassemia disease is 1 per 3200 births. The severity of the disease that results, including the degree of anemia and frequency of clinical complications, depends on the type of β-thalassemia gene that is inherited. Between 80 and 90 percent of affected individuals have a β-thalassemia gene that results in the production of some normal beta chains; thus some normal Hb A is made. These patients have a mild hemolytic anemia with near-normal hemoglobin levels, few crises, and minimal organ damage. Those 10 to 20 percent of patients who inherit a β-thalassemia gene that produces no beta chains, and therefore no normal hemoglobin, have severe hemolytic anemia and vasoocclusive symptoms comparable to patients with SCD. Splenomegaly is found in 70 percent of patients with sickle cell–β thalassemia disease.

## DEFICIENCY OF GLUCOSE-6-PHOSPHATE DEHYDROGENASE

Deficiency of the red blood cell (RBC) enzyme glucose-6-phosphate dehydrogenase (G-6-PD) is the most common human enzyme defect, affecting nearly one-tenth of the world's population. In this inherited abnormality, the activity of this enzyme is markedly diminished. As a result, the RBC is unable to protect itself against oxidant stress. Normally, reduced glutathione is generated to protect the sulfhydryl groups of hemoglobin and the red cell membrane from oxidation. When the enzyme is deficient, the hemoglobin sulfhydryl groups become oxidized and the hemoglobin precipitates within the RBC, forming Heinz bodies that are readily removed from the circulation.

Clinically, the resultant hemolytic anemia varies greatly in severity. It is an X-linked disorder, and clinical manifestations are seen in male heterozygotes and female homozygotes. In the United States, 15 percent of African-American males have a mild form of this deficiency. Acute hemolytic crises occur that are incited by bacterial and viral infections, exposure to oxidant drugs, metabolic acidosis (such as diabetic ketoacidosis), and ingestion of fava beans in some patients. Within 1 to 3 days following oxidant stress, the patient can develop hemoglobinuria and the potential for vascular collapse. These hemolytic crises are generally well tolerated and self-limited because only the older RBCs will hemolyze. In more severe but less common variants of this disease, the patient can have severe chronic hemolytic anemia. The diagnosis of G-6-PD deficiency can be established by the demonstration of decreased enzyme activity through quantitative assay. There is no specific treatment for this disease. Prevention of hemolytic episodes is crucial, with prompt treatment of infections and the avoidance of oxidant drugs. The drugs most commonly associated with oxidant stress are sulfa drugs, antimalarials, pyridium, and nitrofurantoin. HIV-positive patients are commonly screened for this defect because of the common use of the sulfa drugs for the treatment and prophylaxis of *Pneumocystis carinii* pneumonia.

## HEREDITARY SPHEROCYTOSIS

Hereditary spherocytosis (HS) is the most prevalent hereditary hemolytic anemia among people of northern European descent. An estimated 1 in 4500 persons is affected. The disease is typically inherited in an autosomal dominant pattern, but in up to 20 percent of patients it is the result of an apparent spontaneous mutation. The abnormal shape of the RBCs results from molecular abnormalities in the cytoskeleton of the RBC membrane, most commonly with the proteins spectrin and ankyrin. Because of their abnormal shape, the RBCs are caught in the spleen and destroyed. As a result of the typically mild symptoms, the diagnosis may not be established until adulthood. Clinically, HS is characterized by a hemolytic anemia that is usually mild (a small minority of patients have severe anemia), splenomegaly, and intermittent jaundice from indirect bilirubin (due to hemolysis). Pigment gallstones are common.

Patients with HS have a mild anemia, and the peripheral blood smear shows spherocytes with a normal mean corpuscular volume and increased mean corpuscular hemoglobin concentration (>36 percent). The diagnosis of HS is established by the osmotic fragility test. Splenectomy is the treatment for patients with HS. This cures the anemia, although the spherocytes are still present.

## BIBLIOGRAPHY

Kark JA, Posey DM, Schumacher HR, Ruehle CV: Sickle cell trait as a risk factor for sudden death in physical training. *N Engl J Med* 317:781, 1987.

Krachman SL, Lodato RF, D'Alonzo GE: Managing the acute chest syndrome in sickle cell patients. *J Crit Illness* 9:375, 1994.

Losek JD, Hellmich TR, Hoffman GM: Diagnostic value of anemia, red blood cell morphology, and reticulocyte count for sickle cell disease. *Ann Emerg Med* 21:915, 1992.

Platt OS, Brambilla DJ, Rosse WF, et al: Mortality in sickle cell disease, life expectancy and risk factors for early death. *N Engl J Med* 330:1639, 1994.

Platt OS, Thorington BD, Brambilla DJ, et al: Pain in sickle cell disease—rates and risk factors. *N Engl J Med* 335:11, 1991.

Pollack CV Jr: Emergencies in sickle cell disease. *Emerg Med Clin North Am* 11:365, 1993.

Pollack CV Jr: Usefulness in empiric chest radiography and urinalysis testing in adults with acute sickle cell pain crisis. *Ann Emerg Med* 20:1210, 1991.

Schiffman MA: Preventable sudden death in children with sickle hemoglobinopathies and fever: The need for a protocolized approach (editorial). *Ann Emerg Med* 20:1043, 1991.

# 188
# ACQUIRED HEMOLYTIC ANEMIAS
## Mary E. Eberst

In this chapter we will review some of the anemias that result from hemolysis that is precipitated by an acquired or extrinsic abnormality. Table 188-1 outlines these conditions, which include antibody-mediated (immune) hemolytic anemias; fragmentation hemolysis, either microvascular or macrovascular; anemias resulting from direct toxic effects; anemias resulting from mechanical injury; and anemia that is the result of abnormal splenic function (hypersplenism).

The general laboratory evaluation of patients with suspected he-

**Table 188-1.** Classification of Acquired Hemolytic Anemias

I. Autoimmune hemolytic anemia (antibody-mediated)
  A. Warm antibodies
  B. Cold antibodies
    1. Cold agglutin disease
    2. Paroxysmal cold hemoglobinuria
  C. Drug-induced
II. Fragmentation hemolysis
  A. Microangiopathic hemolytic anemia (MAHA)
    1. Thrombotic thrombocytopenic purpura (TTP)/hemolytic uremic syndrome (HUS)
    2. Pregnancy-associated hemolysis (HELLP)
    3. Disseminated intravascular coagulation (DIC)
    4. Malignancy-associated hemolysis
    5. Hemolysis in vasculitis
    6. Hemolysis in malignant hypertension
  B. Macrovascular hemolysis
    1. Due to abnormal cardiac valves
III. Direct toxic effects causing hemolysis
  A. Infections
  B. Other toxins—bites, copper
  C. Drug-induced oxidative hemolysis—methemoglobinemia
IV. Mechanical damage causing hemolysis
  A. Heat denaturation
  B. March hemoglobinuria
  C. Cardiopulmonary bypass
V. Anemia due to abnormal splenic function (hypersplenism)

molysis is reviewed here; the characteristic results for each type of anemia will be discussed below.

## LABORATORY EVALUATION OF HEMOLYTIC ANEMIA

1. *Complete blood count* (CBC): The anemia that occurs may be mild or severe; verify normal/abnormal white blood cell count and platelet count.
2. *Reticulocyte count:* This is the single most useful test in ascertaining the presence of hemolysis and a normal bone marrow response; this should be elevated and can be as high as 30 to 40 percent.
3. *Review of the peripheral blood smear:* Most hemolytic disorders are associated with changes in the morphology of the red blood cells (RBCs); typical changes may include:
   a. *Spherocytes:* These are the most common morphologic abnormality in hemolytic diseases; they will be most abundant in patients with warm antibody immune hemolysis and those with hereditary spherocytosis (Chap. 187).
   b. *Schistocytes:* These are fragmented RBCs that result from direct trauma within the vasculature, most often in the microvasculature (known as microangiopathic hemolytic anemia, MAHA), but can also occur in the macrovasculature; schistocytes are markers of nonimmune hemolysis.
4. *Unconjugated (indirect) bilirubin:* This should be elevated in the presence of hemolysis as a result of heme catabolism; the direct (conjugated) bilirubin should be normal unless there is concomitant hepatic or biliary dysfunction.
5. *Haptoglobin:* This binds to the protein globin that is released when hemoglobin is catabolized, so this should be low or absent in the presence of hemolysis; it is an acute-phase reactant so it may be deceptively elevated.
6. *Plasma free hemoglobin:* This should be elevated in hemolysis.
7. *Lactic dehydrogenase* (LDH): This should be elevated in hemolysis; it can be a relatively sensitive marker used to follow the course of a hemolytic disease.

## AUTOIMMUNE HEMOLYTIC ANEMIAS

There are three types of antibody-mediated, so-called immune, hemolytic anemias:

1. Warm antibody hemolytic anemia. These antibodies are reactive at body temperature.
2. Cold antibody hemolytic anemia. These antibodies react with the patient's RBCs at temperatures below normal body temperature.
3. Drug-induced immune hemolytic anemia. Certain drugs can cause an immune reaction in some patients that results in destruction of their RBCs.

Immune hemolytic anemias are characterized in the laboratory by the Coombs antiglobulin test, also known as the direct Coombs test, or direct antiglobulin test (DAT). This test demonstrates the presence of immunoglobulin (IgG) or complement (C3) on the surface of the RBC. It is only positive in immune-mediated hemolytic anemias. The indirect Coombs test is primarily used for pretransfusion screening for antibodies; it demonstrates the presence of free antibodies in the patient's serum. Immune hemolysis is typified by abundant spherocytes on the peripheral blood smear.

### Warm Antibody Hemolytic Anemia

This disease is characterized by the presence of antibodies directed against IgG and/or C3 that are deposited on the surface of the RBC. It comprises 70 percent of all cases of immune hemolytic anemia. These antibodies react with the RBCs at 37°C. After the antibody-RBC interaction, the RBCs are trapped and destroyed in the spleen.

Patients of any age may be affected, but warm antibody hemolytic anemia is most likely to occur in older adults, women more often than men. Most often it is idiopathic; however, up to 25 percent of affected patients have an underlying disease that affects the immune system such as chronic lymphocytic leukemia, Hodgkin or non-Hodgkin lymphoma, or systemic lupus erythematosus (SLE). In adults, the disease is typically relapsing. In young children, it often follows an acute infection or immunizations and is unlikely to recur.

The clinical presentation and course of disease are highly variable depending on the severity of the anemia and how rapidly it develops. Many patients will have a mild anemia with splenomegaly. In this setting, the Coombs test will be positive for IgG but not C3, and the indirect Coombs test will be negative. Life-threatening anemia can also occur with hemoglobin levels less than 7 g/dL and a reticulocyte count greater than 30 percent. These patients may have marked splenomegaly, pulmonary edema, and mental status changes. Venous thrombosis can also occur. Patients with severe hemolysis generally have a Coombs test that is positive for both IgG and C3, and the indirect Coombs test is also often positive. Rare patients have Evans syndrome, where there is coexistent immune destruction both of RBCs and platelets by different antibodies.

The treatment of warm antibody hemolytic anemia depends on the degree of anemia that develops and the ability of the patient to hemodynamically tolerate anemia. When there is only mild anemia, no treatment is necessary. When significant hemolysis is present, the first-line treatment is prednisone, 1.0 mg/kg per day. About 75 percent of patients will respond to steroid therapy, but up to one-half of these will relapse after the steroids are tapered. Transfusion of red blood cells is difficult in these patients because they will be impossible to crossmatch. Transfusion is indicated for symptoms of angina, congestive heart failure, mental status changes, orthostasis, or hypoxia. In this setting, the patient is slowly transfused with the best match available; acute transfusion reactions can occur. Splenectomy is the second-choice treatment for patients who fail or cannot tolerate steroids. Immunosuppressive drugs such as azathioprine and cyclophosphamide are occasionally used. Treatment of any underlying immunologic disease may also help control the hemolytic anemia. Death in these patients results from severe anemia that cannot be corrected, immunosuppression, venous thrombosis, or underlying immunologic disease.

### Cold Antibody Hemolytic Anemia

Cold-reactive antibodies, those that react maximally at temperatures between 4° and 20°C and not usually above 32°C, account for 10 to 20 percent of patients with immune hemolytic anemia. There are two types of diseases where this occurs: cold agglutinin disease and paroxysmal cold hemoglobinuria. These antibodies react with the RBCs in the superficial microcirculation where it is cool, then the hemolysis occurs when the red blood cells reenter the central circulation and are warmed.

### Cold Agglutin Disease

This can be an acute, transient disease mostly seen in younger people or a chronic disease primarily in older patients. It is typically caused by an IgM antibody, and the Coombs test will only be positive for C3, because the IgM will not be attached to the RBCs at warmer temperatures. The acute form of this disease is mostly seen in patients with *Mycoplasma* pneumonia or infectious mononucleosis. The IgM antibodies are directed against the "I" antigen or "i" antigen on the RBC surface, respectively. Only rare patients develop significant hemolysis, but severe anemia and renal failure can occur. The acute form of this disease is self-limited. Chronic cold agglutin disease is more common than the acute form and primarily occurs in patients with underlying lymphoid neoplasms. These patients typically have a mild to moderate anemia that results from hemolysis occurring in portions of the body exposed to lower temperatures (acrocyanosis).

These patients should be kept in a warm environment, and treatment is directed against the underlying disease. Some of the hemolysis may respond to treatment with prednisone.

## Paroxysmal Cold Hemoglobinemia

This disease is characterized by acute episodes of hemolysis following exposure to cold. Two groups of patients can be affected by this disease: (1) those with congenital or tertiary syphilis that is untreated, or (2) patients with viral illnesses such as mumps or measles. In this disease, the immune hemolysis is caused by an IgG antibody called the Donath-Landsteiner antibody, which is directed against the P-antigen complex on the RBC surface. Clinically, after exposure to cold, affected patients will have hemoglobinuria, chills, fever, and pain involving the back, legs, and abdomen. The direct Coombs test is only positive during an acute attack. When associated with syphilis, this disease goes away after appropriate antibiotic therapy. Now most commonly seen in patients with viral infections, the hemolysis is self-limited but can cause transient severe anemia.

## Drug-Induced Hemolytic Anemia

Many drugs have been directly linked to immune hemolytic anemia. There are three types of reactions that can occur and result in hemolysis:

**Autoantibody induction.** Alpha-methyldopa is the prototype drug of this reaction, and 10 to 20 percent of patients taking moderate-to-high doses will develop a positive direct Coombs test. In this drug reaction, the RBCs become coated with an IgG that is directed against the Rh complex. Other drugs that can cause this are L-dopa, procainamide, ibuprofen, diclofenac, and thioridazine. Generally, it takes an extended period of drug exposure to develop the positive Coombs test, and only a small number of those patients will develop severe hemolysis. The hemolysis ceases after the drug is stopped, but the Coombs test may remain positive for a year or more.

**Hapten-induced immune hemolysis.** Penicillin is the classic drug associated with this reaction. Immune hemolysis can develop in patients receiving large intravenous doses of penicillin or penicillin-type antibiotics and usually starts 1 to 2 weeks after the therapy begins. The patient forms an antibody against the offending drug, then the antibody combines with the drug-RBC complex and causes hemolysis. Other drugs that can cause hemolysis by this mechanism include oxacillin, ampicillin, methicillin, carbenicillin, and some cephalosporins. The hemolysis stops when the drug is discontinued.

**Innocent bystander immune hemolysis.** Quinidine is the prototype drug for this reaction. Antibodies (IgG or IgM) are formed against the drug, then the drug-antibody complex binds to the RBC and hemolyzes it. Other drugs linked to this mechanism include quinine, isoniazid, sulfonamides, hydrochlorothiazide, antihistamines, insulin, chlorpromazine, tetracycline, acetaminophen, hydralazine, probenecid, cephalosporins, fenoprofen, and sulindac. Even a small dose of the drug can cause hemolysis; however, these drugs are very commonly prescribed and the associated hemolysis is very rare.

# FRAGMENTATION HEMOLYSIS

## Microangiopathic Hemolytic Anemia (MAHA)

This type of hemolytic anemia is associated with a variety of disorders; however, the mechanism leading to hemolysis is consistent. The fragmentation of RBCs results from their passage through abnormal arterioles: usually there is damage to the vessel wall or endothelial surface or fibrin has been deposited in the arteriole. Schistocytes are characteristically found on the peripheral blood smear.

## Thrombotic Thrombocytopenic Purpura (TTP) and Hemolytic Uremic Syndrome (HUS)

Those diseases will be discussed separately; however, TTP and HUS may well represent variant clinical presentations of a single disease. In selected patients, the specific diagnosis may be impossible to establish.

### Thrombotic Thrombocytopenic Purpura

TTP is a heterogeneous clinical syndrome characterized by this pentad of symptoms and signs:

1. Microangiopathic hemolytic anemia (MAHA) with characteristic schistocytes on the peripheral blood smear and a reticulocytosis
2. Thrombocytopenia with platelet counts ranging from 5000 to 100,000/μL (mm³)
3. Renal abnormalities including renal insufficiency, azotemia, proteinuria, or hematuria
4. Fever
5. Neurologic abnormalities including headache, confusion, cranial nerve palsies, seizures, or coma

TTP has been diagnosed in patients of all ages but occurs most commonly in ages 10 to 60. Women are affected more commonly than men. The course of the disease is typically acute and fulminant, lasting days to months, but it can be chronic and relapsing in 10 percent of patients. The overall survival rate is 80 percent, but the course is rapidly fatal in some patients. The majority of patients diagnosed with TTP have no apparent predisposing condition. In a small number of patients, TTP has been linked to genetic predisposition, pregnancy, immunologic diseases (SLE, rheumatoid arthritis, Sjögren syndrome), or infections (viral, *Mycoplasma* pneumonia, subacute bacterial endocarditis, human immunodeficiency virus).

The pathogenesis of TTP is uncertain, but the presence of one or more platelet aggregating agents is likely responsible. Several abnormalities of the vascular endothelium and endothelial cell function have been implicated, including the release and presence of large von Willebrand multimers, decreased production of prostacyclin, inadequate fibrinolysis as a result of deficient tissue plasminogen activator (tPA) production, the presence of a platelet agglutinating protein, and deficient production of IgG molecules. Whatever the etiology, the result is the deposition of hyaline material within the lumina of capillaries and arterioles. These microthrombi are made of platelets and a small amount of fibrinlike material. These deposits may be found in any tissue but occur most frequently in the heart, brain, kidneys, pancreas, and adrenal glands.

The diagnosis of TTP is established clinically by the presence of the signs and symptoms listed above. Treatment should begin immediately based on these clinical and laboratory features. Biopsies are sometimes done of the gingiva, kidney, or bone marrow but are not essential to establish the diagnosis and should not delay therapy.

Clinically, the neurologic abnormalities are the most common presenting complaint, but hemorrhagic signs and symptoms and those referable to anemia are also common presentations. Laboratory studies will reflect the presence of MAHA with an anemia of variable degree (the hemoglobin will be less than 6 g/dL in one out of three patients), reticulocytosis, elevated indirect bilirubin, elevated LDH, negative Coombs test, and the presence of schistocytes on the peripheral smear (the diagnosis of TTP is doubtful without schistocytes). Thrombocytopenia, reflective of the intravascular microthrombi, is often severe with the count less than 20,000/μL (mm³) in 50 percent of patients. A mild leukocytosis with a left shift is common. The blood urea nitrogen (BUN) and creatinine are typically elevated to a mild to moderate degree. Urinalysis usually shows some degree of proteinuria and may show microscopic hematuria. Coagulation screening tests should be normal.

The salient features in the differential diagnosis of TTP are outlined in Table 188-2.

The diagnosis of TTP represents a medical emergency. Patients should be treated by experienced specialists. Rapid transport to a tertiary care center is indicated. Some centers have a policy of initially admitting all TTP patients to an intensive care unit. The foundation of

**Table 188-2.** Characteristics of Acquired Hemolytic Anemias*

| | Evans' Syndrome | TTP | HUS | DIC | HELLP |
|---|---|---|---|---|---|
| Autoimmune hemolytic anemia | Present | No | No | No | No |
| Microangiopathic hemolytic anemia (MAHA) | No | Prominent | Prominent | Often present | Present |
| Coombs test | Positive | Negative | Negative | Negative | Negative |
| Thrombocytopenia | Present | Prominent | Present | Present | Present |
| Renal abnormalities | No | Mild | Prominent | No | No |
| Neurologic abnormalities | No | Prominent | No or mild | No | No |
| Hepatic dysfunction | No | May have | May have | May have | Prominent |
| Fever | No | Present | Present | May have | No |
| Coagulation studies | Normal | Normal | Normal | Abnormal | Normal |
| Pregnancy-associated | No | Can be | Can be | Can be | Always |

* Disease descriptions here are based on presence of isolated disease without complications; individual patients often have other problems that make syndromes less readily identified.

*Note:* TTP, thrombotic thrombocytopenic purpura; HUS, hemolytic uremic syndrome; DIC, disseminated intravascular coagulation; HELLP, hemolysis, elevated liver functions, low platelets.

therapy for TTP is plasma exchange transfusion (PLEX). Some patients will respond favorably to plasma infusions alone, and these can be given until the exchanges can be initiated. The plasma exchange uses fresh-frozen plasma (FFP) or fresh unfrozen plasma (FUP). The plasma is thought to provide a substance that the patient is lacking or remove an unknown toxic substance. These exchanges may be required daily for a period of several months. TTP patients are also treated with prednisone (or methylprednisolone), 1 mg/kg per day, and antiplatelet therapy consisting of aspirin or dipyridamole. Refractory patients may receive immunosuppressive therapy such as vincristine, azathioprine, or cyclophosphamide. Splenectomy is sometimes done but has little correlation with clinical improvement. Supportive care includes the transfusion of packed red blood cells as needed and hemodialysis if indicated. Platelet transfusions should be avoided, unless there is uncontrolled hemorrhage, because they can aggravate the thrombotic process. Clinical and hematologic progress in patients with TTP is assessed by improvement in neurologic and renal function, decrease in the reticulocyte count, decrease in the LDH, and increase in the platelet count.

### Hemolytic Uremic Syndrome

HUS is a disease mainly of infancy and early childhood, with a peak incidence between 6 months and 4 years of age. An adult form also exists (see below). The overall mortality rate is 5 to 15 percent, and the prognosis is worse in older children and adults. HUS is one of the most common causes of acute renal failure in childhood. HUS is characterized by acute renal failure, microangiopathic hemolytic anemia, fever, and thrombocytopenia.

In children, the development of HUS often follows a prodromal infectious disease, usually diarrhea or an upper respiratory infection. Diarrhea, particularly that associated with *Escherichia coli* serotype 0157:H7, as well as with *Shigella, Yersinia, Campylobacter,* and *Salmonella,* may be antecedent. Other implicated bacteria and viruses include *Streptococcus pneumoniae,* varicella, echovirus, and coxsackie A and B. Some cases of HUS are familial, with a genetic or HLA-type predisposition.

As noted above, HUS and TTP may actually be clinical variations of the same disease. Like TTP, HUS is pathologically identified by microthrombi, consisting of platelet aggregates, that occlude the arterioles and capillaries. In HUS, the microthrombi are confined mostly to the kidneys; in TTP, they occur throughout the microcirculation. The platelet-fibrin hyaline material is found in the afferent arterioles and glomerular capillaries. A defect in the vascular endothelium is thought to cause these platelet aggregates. It is not precisely known how the endothelial damage occurs, but the toxins released from bacteria or viruses have been implicated. The damaged endothelial cells are then thought to release large and ultralarge vonWillebrand factor multimers that lead to platelet aggregation.

Like TTP, HUS is primarily a clinical and laboratory diagnosis. The signs and symptoms of acute renal failure predominate. Although neurologic dysfunction is not a key feature of HUS, it does occur in up to one-third of HUS patients at some point in the course of their disease. Laboratory studies reflect the presence of MAHA. Thrombocytopenia is present but generally not to the degree seen in TTP. The BUN and creatinine will be markedly elevated, and urine, if present, will contain protein and red blood cells. Coagulation studies are usually normal.

The treatment of HUS primarily consists of early dialysis for management of renal failure and general supportive care. Up to 90 percent of HUS patients with acute renal failure will eventually regain normal renal function. Plasma exchange or infusion is not usually used in the treatment of childhood HUS. HUS is rarely a recurrent disease, but it has been known to recur in patients who have undergone renal transplantation.

**Adult HUS.** When HUS occurs in adult patients, it can be difficult or impossible to differentiate between HUS and TTP. HUS is diagnosed when there is prominent renal failure and minimal neurologic dysfunction. Of adults diagnosed with HUS, two-thirds are women. Associated factors are the use of oral contraceptive agents, preeclampsia, eclampsia, other obstetric complications, and the postpartum period. HUS also rarely occurs in association with the chemotherapeutic drug mitomycin C and in other cancer patients who may or may not have received chemotherapy. The renal failure in adults with HUS may be reversible, even after as long as 1 year.

### Pregnancy-Associated Hemolysis

Microangiopathic hemolytic anemia (MAHA) can occur in pregnancy as a complication of preeclampsia, eclampsia, or placental abruption. The presence of preeclampsia, hemolysis, elevated liver enzymes, and low platelet counts is known as the *HELLP syndrome.* The HELLP syndrome can occur with minimal signs or symptoms of preeclampsia. The pathogenesis is not entirely known, but preeclampsia can be associated with microvesicular fatty infiltration of the liver and with localized or systemic endothelial damage that can lead to MAHA. Untreated, HELLP can result in hepatic failure or rupture, disseminated intravascular coagulation (DIC), or congestive heart failure. Treatment begins with prompt delivery of the infant followed by supportive care.

### Disseminated Intravascular Coagulation (DIC)

DIC is discussed in Chap. 185. MAHA occurs in about 25 percent of patients with DIC. The degree of hemolysis that occurs in DIC is much less than that seen in TTP or HUS. The basic pathology in DIC is the deposition of fibrin in the microvasculature. Fragmentation and hemolysis of the RBCs occur as they pass through the microcirculation. Schistocytes, reflective of MAHA, are often found on the peripheral smear of patients with DIC, but their absence does not rule out DIC. Along with the factor replacement therapy required in DIC, patients with significant hemolysis and anemia will require transfusion of packed red blood cells to maintain adequate circulation and oxygenation.

## Malignancy-Associated Hemolysis

MAHA can be seen in patients with widely disseminated cancer. Gastric adenocarcinoma is the malignancy most frequently associated with MAHA, although it also occurs with adenocarcinomas of the lung, breast, and of unknown primary. The pathogenesis is uncertain, but hypotheses include the following: vessels that supply malignant tumors may be structurally abnormal; circulating tumor cells may damage the endothelial surface; or tumor cells may give off factors that promote platelet aggregation and microvascular changes. Patients with MAHA due to widespread malignancy have a very poor prognosis.

## Hemolysis in Vasculitis

MAHA can be seen in vascular diseases such as SLE, polyarteritis nodosa, Wegener granulomatosis, and scleroderma. In this setting, damage to the endothelial surface is thought to result from deposition of immune complexes and fibrin in the microcirculation.

## Hemolysis in Malignant Hypertension

Patients with malignant or accelerated hypertension can develop MAHA as a result of narrowing and hardening of the afferent arterioles and swelling of the endothelial cells. This hemolysis subsides after normalization of the blood pressure.

## Macrovascular Hemolysis

Traumatic hemolysis can occur in patients with artificial heart valves or severe calcific aortic stenosis. Some degree of hemolysis occurs in up to 10 percent of patients with aortic prostheses; mechanical valves are more likely to cause hemolysis than porcine valves. Mitral valve replacements cause less hemolysis because of the lower pressure gradient. Hemolysis can also occur in patients with prosthetic patches in the heart and, rarely, in patients who have undergone aortofemoral bypass. The hemolysis that occurs in this setting is generally mild and well tolerated. These patients should receive supplemental iron and folate. If the hemolysis is severe, the defective valve may have to be replaced.

## DIRECT TOXIC EFFECTS CAUSING HEMOLYSIS

### Infections

Destruction of red blood cells occurs commonly in the course of many infectious diseases. Those disease with the most profound effect on RBCs will be reviewed here.

Transmitted by mosquitoes, *malaria* is the world's most common cause of hemolytic anemia. Red cell hemolysis results from direct parasitization of the RBCs. Hemolysis also results from direct parasitization of RBCs in *babesiosis,* which is transmitted by ticks or blood transfusions. Infection with *Bartonella* is also associated with direct parasitization of RBCs and resultant hemolysis.

*Haemophilus influenzae type B* infection can produce hemolysis by altering the RBC surface. The capsular polysaccharide of the bacterium binds to the RBC surface, then antibodies destroy the bacterium as well as the RBC. Those with *H. influenzae* meningitis have the greatest potential to develop severe hemolysis.

*Clostridium perfringens (welchii)* infection can result in severe hemolysis by direct lysis of red blood cells. The organism releases enzymes that acutely degrade the phospholipids of the RBC membrane bilayer and the proteins in the structural membrane. This infection is seen most commonly in patients with acute cholecystitis, after surgery involving the biliary tree, after abortions, and in uterine infections. Clinically, the patient may have acute hemodynamic collapse and profound intravascular hemolysis. *Clostridium* septicemia has a mortality rate over 50 percent.

*M. pneumoniae* and *infectious mononucleosis* are associated with cold agglutin disease, as described above.

Many viral infections can be accompanied by hemolytic anemia, including measles, cytomegalovirus, varicella, herpes simplex, coxsackie, and human immunodeficiency virus.

## Other Toxins that Cause Hemolysis

**Insect, spider, and snake bites.** Acute intravascular hemolysis can occur following bites/stings of bees, wasps, the southern black widow spider, and the brown recluse spider. The bites of American snakes, pit vipers and coral snakes, are known to cause coagulation abnormalities but rarely cause hemolysis. The bite of the cobra snake does cause intravascular hemolysis.

**Copper.** Copper has a direct hemolytic effect on red blood cells. Copper sulfate contamination from copper pipes can taint hemodialysis fluid, and copper sulfate is sometimes used in suicide attempts. Patients with Wilson disease experience transient episodes of hemolysis as a result of their elevated copper levels.

## Drug-Induced Oxidative Hemolysis

Oxidative hemolysis of RBCs can result from exposure to a number of drugs that cause the formation of methemoglobin. These drugs oxidize ferrous hemoglobin (+2) to ferric hemoglobin (+3), which is methemoglobin. Methemoglobin cannot bind oxygen, so the oxygen-carrying capacity of the blood is decreased. A large number of commonly used drugs can cause methemoglobinemia, but not at therapeutic doses (Table 188-3). Toxic methemoglobinemia occurs when more than 1 percent of the hemoglobin has been oxidized to the ferric form. Clinically, methemoglobinemia should be suspected in patients who are cyanotic without cardiopulmonary disease. This cyanosis is not relieved by oxygen. The venous blood appears chocolate brown. The arterial blood gas will reflect a normal $P_{O_2}$, but decreased oxygen saturation. Table 188-4 shows the clinical effects of acute methemoglobinemia. Levels of methemoglobin greater than 20 to 30 percent of the total hemoglobin should be treated. Methylene blue is given intravenously at a dose of 1 to 2 mg/kg in a 1% solution over 5 min. Methylene blue reduces methemoglobin back to oxygen-carrying hemoglobin through a series of reactions.

**Table 188-3.** Drugs that Cause Oxidative Hemolysis

| |
|---|
| Benzocaine, lidocaine |
| Nitrates, nitrites |
| Sulfonamides |
| Sulfonamides |
| Phenacetin |
| Azulfidine |
| Pyridium |
| Dapsone and other antimalarials |

**Table 188-4.** Clinical Effect of Acute Methemoglobinemia

| % of Total Hemoglobin that is Methemoglobin | Clinical Effects |
|---|---|
| 10–15 | Peripheral cyanosis |
| 30–35 | Headache, weakness, breathlessness |
| 55 | Dyspnea, bradycardia, seizures, arrhythmias |
| 60–70 | Vascular collapse, coma |
| 80 or more | Incompatible with life |

**Table 188-5.** Disease States Associated with Hypersplenism and Hemolysis

| Cause of Splenic Enlargement | Disease Example(s) |
|---|---|
| Splenic congestion due to elevated portal pressure | Cirrhosis, portal vein thrombosis, splenic vein obstruction, congestive heart failure, Budd-Chiari syndrome |
| Infiltrative disease | Leukemia, lymphoma, amyloidosis, polycythemia vera |
| Inflammatory states | Rheumatoid arthritis, SLE, sarcoidosis |
| Infections | Bacterial endocarditis, infectious mononucleosis, military tuberculosis, malaria, schistosomiasis |
| Hereditary hemolytic anemias | Sickle cell anemia |
| Acquired hemolytic anemias | Autoimmune hemolytic anemia |

*Note:* SLE, systemic lupus erythematosus.

## MECHANICAL DAMAGE CAUSING HEMOLYSIS

**Heat denaturation.** Temperatures above 47°C cause direct damage to erythrocytes by denaturation of the cytoskeletal protein, spectrin. This can occur in patients with extensive burns. Within 24 h of the burns, acute hemolytic anemia can develop with gross hemoglobinuria and spherocytes and schistocytes on the peripheral blood smear.

**March hemoglobinuria.** This type of hemolysis can occur in soldiers and joggers and in karate and conga-drumming enthusiasts. Red blood cell destruction is the result of direct trauma to the cells in the vessels of the feet or hands. These patients rarely become anemic but do have hemoglobinuria after strenuous exercise or activity.

**Cardiopulmonary bypass.** Patients who have been on cardiopulmonary bypass can develop a "postperfusion syndrome" that consists of acute intravascular hemolysis, leukopenia, and fever. This hemolysis is thought to result from the activation of complement as blood passes through the oxygenator.

## ANEMIA DUE TO ABNORMAL SPLENIC FUNCTION

There are many disease states that result in splenic enlargement (Table 188-5). The main function of the normal spleen is to filter defective red blood cells and foreign particles and to participate in antigen processing and antibody synthesis. When the spleen is enlarged, its activity is increased, a condition known as hypersplenism. Hypersplenism results in the sequestration of red blood cells as well as platelets and white blood cells. Unlike the platelets and white blood cells, which can survive within the spleen and be released back into the circulation, the sequestered red blood cells are not metabolically self-sufficient and are prematurely destroyed within the spleen. Hemolysis within the spleen is greatest when the splenomegaly is caused by inflammatory states or splenic congestion due to elevated portal pressure.

## BIBLIOGRAPHY

Leo PL, Cooper C, Songco C: Hemolytic uremic syndrome: Just another case of gastroenteritis? *Am J Emerg Med* 12:358, 1994.

Moake JL: Thrombotic microangiopathies: Thrombotic thrombocytopenic purpura and the hemolytic-uremic syndrome, in Loscalzo J, Schafer AI (eds): *Thrombosis and Hemorrhage.* Cambridge, MA, Blackwell Scientific, 1994, pp 517–527.

Neild GH: Haemolytic-uremic syndrome in practice. *Lancet* 343:398, 1994.

Reubinoff BE, Sohenker JG: HELLP syndrome—a syndrome of hemolysis, elevated liver enzymes and low platelet count—complicating preeclampsia-eclampsia. *Int J Gynaecol Obstet* 36:95, 1991.

Schwartz RS, Berkman EM, Silberstein LE: The autoimmune hemolytic anemias, in Hoffman R, Benz EJ, Shattil SJ, et al (eds): *Hematology: Basic Principles and Practice.* New York, Churchill Livingstone, 1991, pp 422–441.

White CD, Weiss LD: Varying presentations of methemoglobinemia: Two cases. *J Emerg Med* 9:45, 1991.

# 189
# BLOOD TRANSFUSIONS AND COMPONENT THERAPY
## Mary E. Eberst

Since the time of the first blood transfusions in the late 1600s and the recognition of the ABO blood grouping system by Landsteiner in 1900, transfusion medicine has become a complex medical specialty. It is not important that all practitioners be familiar with the intricacies of blood banking, but any physician who is responsible for the transfusion of blood products to patients needs to have a basic understanding of what products are available, what product is appropriate in a given clinical situation, and what are the potential complications of the transfusion.

In this chapter, we will review the different types of blood products that are available, with an emphasis on component therapy. The potential complications of transfusions, immediate and delayed, are reviewed. Two topics of particular importance in emergency medicine, emergency transfusion and massive transfusion, are briefly discussed.

## AVAILABLE BLOOD PRODUCTS

### Whole Blood

Modern transfusion medicine recommends that it is preferable to give patients only the specific portions of blood that they require. This is achieved by the use of component therapy. Therefore, whole blood is rarely used in current practice, except for exchange transfusions for neonates. A unit of whole blood contains 435 to 500 mL of blood plus a preservative/anticoagulant solution. CPDA-1 (citrate phosphate dextrose adenine) is the additive in current use. With proper collection and storage of the blood at 2° to 6°C, in the presence of this additive, whole blood has a shelf life of 35 days. The shelf life is defined as viability of at least 70 percent of the red blood cells 24 h after infusion. Whole blood is not entirely "whole" at the time of administration because during storage, beginning 24 h after collection, there is a loss of platelets and some coagulation factors. By 72 h after collection, there are virtually no viable platelets and negligible factor VIII activity in "whole" blood. Experts suggest that fewer than 10 percent of all patients requiring transfusions actually require all the components of whole blood. Whole blood has the advantage of simultaneously providing volume and oxygen-carrying capacity. This is also accomplished by the use of packed red blood cells (PRBCs) and crystalloid solution, and this is the preferred procedure. Disadvantages to the use of whole blood transfusion are: it is a rarely available in the United States; clotting factors are present in low levels; whole blood often contains elevated levels of potassium, hydrogen ion, and ammonia; the patient is exposed to a large number of antigens; and volume overload can occur before the needed components are replenished.

### Component Therapy

A unit of donated blood contains about 450 mL of whole blood. In current practice, shortly after collection this blood is separated into its components: red blood cells, platelets, plasma, and cryoprecipitate. This method allows for the widest usage of available blood and optimal storage for each component.

### Packed Red Blood Cells

Packed red blood cells (PRBCs) are prepared from whole blood by centrifugation followed by the removal of 80 to 90 percent of the plasma. A preservative solution, such as Adsol (dextrose, adenine, and mannitol), is added, resulting in a storage time of up to 42 days. PRBCs are stored at 4°C. Each unit of PRBCs transfused should raise the hemoglobin by 1 g/dL or the hematocrit by 3 percent. The advantages to the use of PRBCs compared to whole blood include reduced risk of volume overload; decreased infusion of citrate, ammonia, and organic acids; and the decreased risk of alloimmunization because the patient is exposed to fewer antigens. PRBCs provide rapid restoration of oxygen-carrying capacity in patients with acute or chronic blood loss.

It is impossible to set specific criteria for the transfusion of PRBCs, although general guidelines can be used and adapted to each clinical setting. The impact of blood loss is variable among patients, depending on the underlying cause, the rate of blood loss, the patient's underlying health status, the cardiopulmonary reserve, and the activity level of the patient. There are three common settings where the transfusion of PRBCs should be considered:

1. *Acute hemorrhage:* Acute hemorrhage, as seen in patients with trauma, bleeding from the gastrointestinal (GI) tract, or from a ruptured aortic aneurysm, often requires emergency transfusion of PRBCs. In otherwise healthy patients, the loss of up to about 1500 mL of blood (about 25 to 30 percent of the blood volume in a 70-kg person) can be replaced entirely with crystalloid solutions. Blood losses greater than this usually require the transfusion of PCRBs to replace oxygen-carrying capacity and crystalloid solution to replace volume.
2. *Surgical blood loss:* Otherwise healthy surgical patients usually do not require preoperative transfusion of PRBCs unless the hemoglobin is less than 7 g/dL or large amounts of blood loss are expected. Intraoperative blood loss of 1500 to 2000 mL can often be replaced with just crystalloid if the patient initially had a normal hemogram. Most patients will require transfusion of PRCBs and crystalloid when blood loss exceeds 2 L.
3. *Chronic anemia:* Patients with chronic stable anemia probably only require transfusion of PRBCs if the hemoglobin falls to less than 7 g/dL or if they are symptomatic or have underlying cardiopulmonary disease.

Patients in the emergency department whose blood should be typed and crossmatched for potential transfusion include those with: (1) evidence of shock from whatever cause; (2) known blood loss of more than 100 mL; (3) gross GI bleeding; (4) those with a hemoglobin less than 10 g/dL or hematocrit less than 30 percent; or (5) patients who are potentially going for surgery where blood may be lost (laparotomy after trauma or for ectopic pregnancy).

Other patients who may need blood products but do not meet these criteria should have blood sent to the blood bank for typing and antibody screening. Many institutions have criteria for the number of units to be crossmatched in a particular clinical setting.

In addition to PRBCs, red blood cells are available as leukocyte-poor, frozen, or washed, when required for certain patients. *Leukocyte-poor RBCs* have 70 to 85 percent of the leukocytes removed by centrifugation, filters, or ultraviolet irradiation. This preparation is indicated for patients who are transplant recipients or transplant candidates (bone marrow or solid organ), in order to prevent immunization against leukocytes, and in patients who have a history of previous febrile nonhemolytic transfusion reactions. *Frozen RBCs* are prepared by adding a cryoprotective agent, then storing the cells for as long as several years at below freezing temperatures. The freezing process destroys the other blood constituents except for a small number of immunocompetent lymphocytes. Prior to transfusion, the cells are thawed and washed with a solution that removes 99.9 percent of the plasma and cellular debris. This process is expensive but can provide a supply of rare blood types, provides metabolically superior RBCs, and results in reduced antigen exposure for transplant candidates. *Washed RBCs* are prepared from whole blood or PRBCs. Isotonic saline is used to wash the RBCs, resulting in the removal of plasma proteins, some leukocytes, and some platelets. Washed RBCs must be infused within 24 h because of the risk of bacterial contamination during processing. Washed RBCs are used for patients who have hypersensitive reactions to plasma (usually IgA-deficient patients), neonatal transfusions, and in patients with paroxysmal nocturnal hemoglobinuria in order to avoid the precipitation of hemolytic episodes.

## Platelets

Platelets for transfusion are obtained through whole blood donations or by plateletpheresis of a single donor. Platelets can be stored for up to 5 days at 20° to 24°C with agitation, although platelet recovery and survival is sometimes better with shorter storage periods. Generally, random donor units are given six at a time (6-pack) or the patient is given one plateletpheresis pack. Each of these totals 250 to 350 mL and contains about $4 \times 10^{11}$ platelets. Six random donor packs or one plateletpheresis pack should raise the platelet count by 50,000 to 60,000/$\mu$L (mm$^3$) in an average-size adult. The posttransfusion platelet count should be checked 1 h and 24 h after platelet infusion. Transfused platelets should survive 3 to 5 days unless there is platelet consumption or refractoriness. Patients with fever, certain infections, disseminated intravascular coagulation (DIC), excessive bleeding, splenomegaly, or antibodies against the transfused platelets may be refractory to platelet transfusion. It is preferable to use ABO-compatible platelets whenever possible to avoid the passive administration of ABO-incompatible plasma. This is particularly true in patients weighing less than 40 kg and patients who receive numerous transfusions. A small amount of RBCs contaminate the platelets, so Rh-negative women of childbearing age should receive Rh-negative platelets.

The clinical indications for the transfusion of platelets depend on the underlying etiology of the thrombocytopenia, the presence or absence of active bleeding, the presence of other disease states that may cause platelet dysfunction, and the need for surgical or invasive procedures. When the patient has thrombocytopenia due to the presence of antiplatelet antibodies, platelet transfusion is generally futile. General guidelines for platelet transfusion in adults include the following:

1. When the platelet count is above 50,000/$\mu$L (mm$^3$), excessive bleeding due to thrombocytopenia is unlikely unless there is platelet dysfunction present.
2. The platelet count should be maintained at 50,000/$\mu$L (mm$^3$) or greater in patients undergoing major surgery or in those with ongoing significant bleeding.
3. When the platelet count is between 10,000 and 50,000/$\mu$L (mm$^3$), there is an increased risk of bleeding with trauma or invasive procedures; bleeding that develops spontaneously or as a result of invasion should be treated with platelet transfusions; patients with concurrent disease (renal or liver) causing platelet dysfunction can bleed spontaneously with these counts.
4. When the platelet count is below 10,000/$\mu$L (mm$^3$), there is a high risk of spontaneous hemorrhage and platelets should be transfused prophylactically.

Special platelet preparations are indicated for some patients. Those who become refractory after multiple transfusions may need HLA-matched platelets. Immunosuppressed patients should receive irradiated platelets to prevent the alloimmunization that can occur as a result of leukocyte contamination.

## Fresh-Frozen Plasma (FFP)

FFP is plasma that is obtained after the separation of whole blood donations into its plasma and cellular (RBCs and platelets) components. Frozen within 6 h of the collection, FFP is stored at −18°C for up to 1 year. Each bag of FFP contains 200 to 250 mL and, by definition, contains 1 unit of each coagulation factor per milliliter of FFP and 1 to 2 mg of fibrinogen per milliliter of FFP. Transfused FFP should be ABO-compatible. The desired dose to be transfused can be estimated from the plasma volume and the desired incremental increase in factor activity. A typical starting dose is 8 to 10 mL/kg, or approximately two bags of FFP. After infusion, the patient should be reevaluated for clinical bleeding and posttransfusion coagulation studies obtained.

The indications for transfusion of FFP are as follows:

1. The presence of a coagulopathy due to acquired factor(s) deficiency with active bleeding or prior to invasive procedures; the patient should have significant (1.5×) prolongation of the prothrombin time (PT) and/or activated partial thromboplastin time (aPTT), or a specific coagulation factor assay less than 25 percent of normal; patients in this category include those with liver disease, DIC, and those taking warfarin.
2. Patients with congenital isolated factor deficiencies when specific virally safe replacement products are not available (see below); those with isolated deficiencies of fibrinogen, factor VIII, or factor XIII are probably better treated with cryoprecipitate.
3. Patients with thrombotic thrombocytopenic purpura (TTP) in the process of plasma exchange (see Chap. 185).
4. Some patients who receive massive transfusion and have evidence of a coagulopathy and active bleeding (see below).
5. Patients with antithrombin III deficiency when antithrombin III concentrates are not available.

FFP is *not* indicated for patients who require volume expansion.

## Cryoprecipitate

Cryoprecipitate is the cold precipitable protein fraction derived from FFP thawed at 1° to 6°C; it can be stored frozen for up to 1 year. The contents of a bag of cryoprecipitate are outlined in Table 189-1. The typical dose of cryoprecipitate given is two to four bags per 10 kg—usually 10 to 20 bags at a time. Each bag of cryoprecipitate exposes the recipient to 10 donors. When given in large volumes, it is preferable to use ABO-compatible cryoprecipitate.

The indications for transfusion of cryoprecipitate are as follows:

1. For patients with hypofibrinogenemia. In patients with congenital deficiency of fibrinogen or those with consumptive coagulopathy such as DIC, transfusion is indicated when the fibrinogen level is less than 100 mg/dL.
2. For patients with von Willebrand disease and active bleeding, cryoprecipitate should only be used when desmopressin (DDAVP) is not available or does not work and factor VIII concentrates containing von Willebrand factor are not available.
3. For patients with hemophilia A, only when virally inactivated factor VIII concentrates are not available.
4. For use as fibrin glue surgical adhesives.
5. For fibronectin replacement, which may be beneficial to promote healing in patients with trauma, severe burns, or sepsis.

## Albumin

Albumin accounts for about 50 percent of the circulating protein and accounts for 75 percent of the plasma oncotic pressure. Albumin replacement products are available as 5 or 25% solutions in saline. Plasma protein fraction (PPF) is a similar product; it is a 5% solution

**Table 189-1.** The Contents of Cryoprecipitate (per Bag)

| | |
|---|---|
| Factor VIIIC | 80–120 units |
| von Willebrand Factor | 80 units |
| Fibrinogen | 200–300 mg |
| Factor XIII | 40–60 units |
| Fibronectin | Variable |

containing 88 percent albumin and 12 percent globulins. These products undergo heat inactivation for 10 h at 60°C and are not known to transmit viral diseases.

The clinical indications for albumin infusion are controversial but may include the following:

1. As colloid replacement to replace or maintain oncotic pressure. Most clinical experimental studies suggest that there is no advantage to colloid solutions over crystalloid in the acute management of hemorrhagic shock. Infused albumin solutions rapidly distribute to the extravascular space and are expensive.
2. In conjunction with large volume paracentesis in patients with refractory ascites.
3. In patients with severe burns. Most centers are moving away from this practice.

## Immunoglobulins

Intravenous immunoglobulins, commonly referred to as *IVIg,* are being increasingly used for a variety of medical conditions. There are six preparations currently available in the United States. They have never been shown to transmit viral infections. The current indications for use are as follows:

1. Primary and secondary immunodeficiency, such as in patients with congenital immunodeficiency or chronic lymphocytic leukemia, bone marrow transplant patients, pediatric patients infected with the human immunodeficiency virus (HIV), and for the prevention of sepsis in premature infants and of infection in patients in intensive care settings.
2. Patients with immune or inflammatory disorders such as immune thrombocytopenic purpura or Kawasaki disease.

Two notable and interesting complications that may occur with the infusion of immunoglobulins are: (1) anaphylaxis, which can occur in patients with IgA deficiency; these patients need to be given the IgA-depleted product; and (2) development of transient positive serologies in some patients due to the passive transfer of antibodies against hepatitis C and cytomegalovirus (CMV).

## Antithrombin III (ATIII)

Antithrombin III is a serum protein that has inhibitory effects on coagulation factors, activated factor II (thrombin), as well as activated factors IX, X, XI, and XII. Deficiency of ATIII can be congenital or acquired. Replacement ATIII is available in two preparations obtained by heparin-affinity chromatography. The products undergo viral inactivation for 10 h at 60°C, which inactivates HIV. There are ever-expanding uses for ATIII replacement, but currently its main use is for patients with hereditary deficiency of ATIII with acute thromboembolism or the prophylaxis of thrombosis in these patients. It is also being used experimentally for the prevention of thrombosis in surgical patients, for obstetric emergencies, and for shock and DIC.

## Specific Factor Replacement Therapy

The most common congenital factor deficiencies, hemophilia A and hemophilia B, are discussed in Chap. 186. Other congenital factor deficiencies are rare and unlikely to be encountered, but the emergency physician needs to be aware of their existence and have a basic knowledge of what products are used for the management of acute bleeding episodes. Table 189-2 outlines the recommended therapy for congenital factor deficiencies.

## COMPLICATIONS OF TRANSFUSIONS

Up to 20 percent of all transfusions may lead to some type of adverse reaction. Fortunately, most of these reactions are mild and not of long-term consequence to the patient. Transfusion reactions can oc-

**Table 189-2.** Replacement Therapy for Congenital Factor Deficiencies

| Coagulation Factor | Incidence* | Replacement Therapy |
|---|---|---|
| Factor I (fibrinogen) | 150 cases | Cryoprecipitate |
| Factor II (prothrombin) | 30 cases | FFP for minor bleeding episodes<br>Prothrombin complex concentrate† for major bleeding |
| Factor V | 150 cases | FFP |
| Factor VII | 150 cases | FFP for minor bleeding episodes<br>Prothrombin complex concentrates for major bleeding<br>Recombinant factor VII$_A$ (experimental) |
| Factor VIII‡ | 1 in 10,000 males | Factor VIII concentrates<br>DDAVP for those with mild hemophilia |
| Factor IX‡ | 1 in 30,000 males | Factor IX concentrates |
| Factor X | 1 in 500,000 | FFP for minor bleeding episodes<br>Prothrombin complex concentrates for major bleeding |
| Factor XI§ | 3 in 10,000 Ashkenazi Jews<br>1 in 1,000,000 in general | FFP |
| Factor XII | Several hundred cases | Replacement not required |
| Factor XIII | 100 cases | FFP or cryoprecipitate |

* Incidence as of 1992.

† See Chap. 186 for details concerning prothrombin complex concentrates.

‡ See Chap. 186 for detailed management recommendations for patients with hemophilia A and hemophilia B.

§ Factor XI levels correlate poorly with bleeding complications; many patients have low levels, but no bleeding complications.

cur while the transfusion is in process (immediate reactions) or the adverse result may not become apparent for hours to years (delayed reactions).

## Immediate Transfusion Reactions

### Acute Hemolytic Transfusion Reaction

This is a medical emergency that occurs when incompatible RBCs are transfused. Most often this is an intravascular event resulting from incompatibility in the ABO blood group system. Table 189-3 reviews compatibility in the ABO blood group system. An acute hemolytic reaction occurs when the incompatible transfused cells are immediately destroyed by antibodies. The overall incidence of acute hemolytic transfusion reactions is unknown, but the outcome is fatal in 1 in 100,000 transfusions.

Clinically, a transfusion reaction should be suspected when the patient complains of fever, chills, low back pain, breathlessness, or a burning sensation at the site of infusion. If the reaction progresses, the patient may develop hypotension, bleeding, respiratory failure, and acute tubular necrosis. More severe reactions occur in anesthetized or unconscious patients because of their inability to alert the staff that something is amiss. The management of a patient with a possible transfusion reaction begins with the immediate discontinuation of the transfusion. While the transfusion work-up is in progress, the patient should be aggressively hydrated in order to maintain a brisk diuresis (at least 100 mL/h) for at least 24 h. Furosemide may be required to maintain the diuresis. Cardiorespiratory support may be needed. The laboratory evaluation of a possible hemolytic transfusion reaction includes the finding of hemoglobinemia (elevated plasma free hemoglobin) and hemoglobinuria. Other tests for hemolysis should be performed including haptoglobin and bilirubin. Direct and indirect Coombs test should be performed on pre- and posttrans-

fusion blood samples. A complete blood count, creatinine, and coagulation tests will also be helpful.

A less common and less serious type of acute hemolytic transfusion reaction is extravascular hemolysis (in the spleen), usually caused by transfusion of incompatible Rh cells. These patients may be asymptomatic and only rarely have hemoglobinemia and hemoglobinuria. Laboratory studies in this situation will show a positive Coombs test, elevated level of indirect bilirubin, and a poor response to the transfusion—the hemoglobin and hematocrit do not rise as expected. This type of hemolytic reaction usually does not require any treatment.

### Febrile Nonhemolytic Transfusion Reaction

This reaction is estimated to occur once for every 200 units transfused. During the transfusion or within a few hours after its completion, the patient has a temperature elevation of at least 1°C and usually has chills. The usual cause of this febrile reaction is an antigen-antibody reaction involving the plasma, platelets, or white blood cells that are passively transfused to the recipient along with the RBCs. Such a reaction occurs most commonly in patients who have been multiply transfused or in multiparous women. Febrile reactions not involving hemolysis are usually mild but can be life-threatening in patients with tenuous cardiopulmonary status or in those who are already critically ill. As in the acute hemolytic transfusion reaction, the first step in management is to stop the transfusion. Clinically, it is impossible to distinguish initially between a febrile nonhemolytic reaction and the more serious acute hemolytic transfusion reaction. The hemolytic transfusion reaction must be ruled out by repeat crossmatching of the blood and repeat Coombs testing. Infections that could potentially be responsible for the fever and chills should be considered. Patients with a known history of febrile reactions to transfusions can be pretreated with acetaminophen or aspirin and meperidine or be given leukocyte-depleted blood components.

### Allergic Transfusion Reaction

Allergic reactions to the transfused products occur in about 1 percent of all transfusions. The reaction is thought to be due to exposure to plasma proteins. Such reactions most commonly occur in IgA-deficient patients. Typical allergic symptoms such as skin erythema, urticaria, pruritus, bronchospasm, vasomotor instability, and, rarely, anaphylaxis occur. True anaphylaxis occurs only once in 20,000 transfusions. Such reactions are rarely serious and often do not recur with subsequent transfusions. The severity of the reaction is not dose related—the transfusion often can be completed. When an apparent allergic transfusion reaction occurs, the infusion should be discontinued while the patient is evaluated and treated with diphenhydramine. If the patient improves with this therapy, the transfusion can be restarted. Some clinicians routinely premedicate patients who have a history of allergic transfusion reactions.

## Delayed Reactions

### Infections

Since HIV was identified in the U.S. blood supply in the mid-1980s, several screening methods have been instituted to ensure the safety of

**Table 189-3.** ABO Blood Group System Compatibility

| Phenotype | Antigens on RBCs | Antibodies in Serum | Can Receive Blood Type |
|---|---|---|---|
| A | A | anti-B | A, O |
| B | B | anti-A | B, O |
| AB | A and B | None | A, B, O |
| O | None | anti-A; anti-B | O |

**Table 189-4.** Tests Performed on Donated Blood

| | |
|---|---|
| ABO, Rh determination | Hepatitis B surface antigen |
| Antibody to HIV-1 | Hepatitis B core antibody |
| Antibody to HIV-2 | Antibody to hepatitis C |
| Antibody to HTLV-1 | ALT/SGPT |
| Serology for syphilis | |

*Note:* HIV, human immunodeficiency virus; HTLV, human T-cell leukemia virus; ALT/SGPT, alanine transaminase/serum glutamic–pyruvic transaminase.

the blood products in current use. The majority of blood products available in the United States today are collected from volunteer donors who reliably provide a safer product than that obtained from paid donors. There are two levels of screening of the donors and blood: (1) donor prescreening by a questionnaire that excludes persons with a high risk of viral exposure; and (2) serologic testing of the donor blood. The tests typically performed on donor blood are outlined in Table 189-4. Some component products, factor replacement products in particular, undergo further treatment to ensure viral inactivation. The risks of transmission of various infections by transfused blood products are listed in Table 189-5. These risks are averages; the actual risk may be higher or lower depending on the incidence of infection in the area the blood is collected. Rarely, blood products become contaminated with bacteria during preparation or bacterial infection can come from an infected donor. This should be considered when a patient develops fever during or shortly after the transfusion of blood products.

## Delayed Hemolytic Reaction

This reaction occurs 7 to 10 days after transfusion as a result of an antigen-antibody reaction that develops after the transfusion. Laboratory studies reflect a slowly falling hemoglobin, and a previously negative Coombs test becomes positive. The patient is generally asymptomatic. Further blood bank work-up is needed to detect the causative antibody.

## Hypervolemia

The transfusion of PRBCs or plasma results in the rapid expansion of intravascular volume. Such expansion may not be well tolerated by patients with limited cardiovascular reserve, particularly infants and elderly patients. Patients may complain of headaches and shortness of breath; on examination, they will have signs of congestive heart failure. Treatment consists of slowing the rate of infusion and diuresis of the patient.

**Table 189-5.** Estimated Risk of Infection Transmission via Blood Products—1994

| Virus | Risk per Units Transfused | Infection | Risk |
|---|---|---|---|
| HIV* | 1 in 150,000 units | Epstein-Barr virus (EBV) | Rare |
| Hepatitis C | 3 in 10,000 units | Syphilis | Rare |
| Hepatitis B | 1 in 50,000 units | Malaria | Rare |
| HTLV I/II† | 1 in 70,000–100,000 units | Babesiosis | Rare |
| CMV‡ | Positive or negative | Toxoplasmosis | Rare |
| | | Trypanosomiasis§ | Rare |

* These data are for the HIV-1 virus; HIV-2 is very rarely found in the United States; 60–90% of HIV-2 antibodies are detected by the currently used test.
† HTLV I and II cause adult T-cell leukemia and myelopathy.
‡ CMV is not transmitted by plasma or cryoprecipitate; CMV-negative blood products should be considered for immunosuppressed patients, bone marrow or solid organ transplant candidates or recipients.
§ Trypanosomiasis is a parasite that causes Chagas disease.
*Note:* HIV, human immunodeficiency virus; HTLV, human T-cell leukemia virus; CMV, cytomegalovirus.

## Hypothermia

Hypothermia may develop in patients who receive rapid infusion of large quantities of refrigerated blood. This is generally only a problem if three or more units are given rapidly. PRBCs are stored at 4°C, platelets at 20° to 24°C, and FFP at −18°C. Electric blood warmers may be used but should not raise the temperature to more than 40°C or hemolysis can occur. The easiest method for warming blood is to infuse it along with warmed (39° to 43°C) normal saline, which will warm and dilute the blood.

## Noncardiogenic Pulmonary Edema

Noncardiogenic pulmonary edema occurs in approximately 1 in 5000 transfusions. Believed to be due to incompatibility of passively transferred leukocyte antibodies, the problem usually develops within 4 h of the transfusion. Clinically, the patient has respiratory distress, fever, chills, and tachycardia, and a chest radiograph shows diffuse patchy infiltrates without cardiomegaly. There is no evidence of fluid overload or congestive heart failure. In the majority of cases, the pulmonary infiltrates resolve over a few days and only supportive care is needed. This reaction can, however, be fatal in patients who are already critically ill.

## Electrolyte Imbalance

Citrate is a component of the preservative solution used in blood storage; it functions as an anticoagulant by chelating calcium. Significant hypocalcemia rarely occurs as a result of transfusion-related citrate exposure because patients with normal hepatic function readily metabolize citrate to bicarbonate. Even with massive transfusion, calcium replacement is rarely needed.

Hypokalemia can be a problem when large amounts of blood are transfused. When the citrate is metabolized to bicarbonate, the blood becomes alkalotic and potassium is driven to the intracellular compartment.

Hyperkalemia rarely is a problem after blood transfusions even though the potassium content increases in stored blood. This may be a problem for patients with renal failure or neonates.

## Graft-Versus-Host Disease

This unfortunate reaction, which is fatal in more than 90 percent of cases, can occur after the transfusion of nonirradiated cellular blood components into an immunocompromised host. Graft-versus-host disease occurs when immunologically competent lymphocytes are passively transferred to an immunoincompetent host who is unable to destroy the donor lymphocytes. The donor lymphocytes engraft, recognize the host as foreign, then attack the host tissues. Bone marrow aplasia commonly results.

## EMERGENCY TRANSFUSIONS

In the emergency department, the administration of type O blood or type-specific incompletely crossmatched blood may be lifesaving; however, it carries the risk of severe, life-threatening transfusion reactions. Many experts now believe that there are virtually no indications for the use of uncrossmatched type O blood. Certainly its use is limited to the early resuscitative phase of patients with shock from exsanguinating hemorrhage and insufficient response to infused crystalloid solutions. Patients with trauma, massive GI bleeding, ruptured aortic aneurysm, or unexpected intraoperative hemorrhage may be candidates to receive emergency transfusions. Current practice is moving away from the use of type O negative uncrossmatched blood to the use of ABO group– and RH type–specific blood, which can usually be obtained from the blood bank within 10 to 15 min after the sample is received. Fully crossmatched blood can typically be obtained in 30 to 60 min. Most hospitals use Rh-negative blood when it has not been fully crossmatched. PRBCs are the only blood product that can be given for emergency transfusion. Plasma products contain too many antibodies and should not have a role in the early phase of treatment of massive hemorrhage. As soon as type-specific cross-matched PRBCs are available, they should be given. Subsequent crossmatching will become more difficult as increasing amounts of uncrossmatched blood are transfused.

## MASSIVE TRANSFUSION

Massive transfusion is defined as the replacement of a volume equivalent to the patient's normal blood volume within a 24-h period. Potential complications of this procedure are bleeding, citrate toxicity, and hypothermia. Bleeding is the most frequent complication and is related to platelet and factor deficiencies. Actual thrombocytopenia does not regularly occur in this setting because even after the replacement of one blood volume, most patients still have about 35 to 40 percent of their original platelet count, about 100,000/µL. Bleeding is the result of mild thrombocytopenia combined with platelet dysfunction from renal or liver disease or DIC, and coagulation factor deficiencies. Coagulation factor deficiencies can develop in the setting of massive transfusion because stored blood has low levels of coagulation factors, especially factors V and VIII. The coagulopathy may be worsened by hypothermia, shock, sepsis, underlying liver disease, or DIC. In current practice, the routine use of platelet transfusions and FFP in massive transfusion is unwarranted, costly, and dangerous. Platelet transfusions should be given only if there is thrombocytopenia with oozing or excess bleeding. FFP should be given only when there is a documented coagulopathy and bleeding.

In modern blood banking, citrate toxicity is rarely a problem unless whole blood is being transfused. Patients receiving more than five units of whole blood, neonates, or patients with liver disease are at risk of hypocalcemia. An ionized calcium level should be obtained. The QT interval is not a reliable indicator of hypocalcemia in this setting. If calcium needs to be repleted, 5 to 10 mL of calcium gluconate given slowly IV is recommended.

Hypothermia is a potential risk when the patient receives three or more units of blood rapidly. When giving large quantities of blood rapidly, the blood itself needs to be warmed or it can be administered with warm saline (see above) in order to prevent iatrogenic hypothermia.

## BLOOD ADMINISTRATION

The administration of blood products begins with the absolute identification of the patient and the unit to be transfused. Blood products are generally infused through large bore intravenous tubing (16 gauge or greater) to prevent hemolysis and permit rapid infusion if needed. Normal saline is the only crystalloid fluid compatible with PRBCs. Saline is usually given with the blood to dilute it and facilitate infusion. If multiple units of blood are to be given or are being given rapidly, warmed saline can be given concurrently (warmed to 39° to 43°C) or the blood itself can be warmed in an electric blood warmer. Blood will hemolyze if warmed to more than 40°C. Except in emergency settings, the infusion of blood is started slowly over the first 30 min, when reactions are most likely to occur. Patients without cardiovascular disease can be given a unit of PRBCs over 1 to 2 h. Those with a risk of hypervolemia should receive each unit over 3 to 4 h. Micropore filters should be used when giving any blood product in order to filter microaggregates of platelets, fibrin, and leukocytes. Rapid infusion of blood in the emergency setting may be facilitated by the use of pressure infusion devices that apply pneumatic pressure (up to 300 mmHg) to the blood unit.

## BIBLIOGRAPHY

Buetler E: Platelet transfusions: The 20,000/ml trigger. *Blood* 81:1411, 1993.
Falk JL, O'Brien JF, Kerr R: Fluid resuscitation in traumatic hemorrhagic shock. *Crit Care Clin* 8:323, 1992.
Labadie LL: Transfusion therapy in the emergency department. *Emerg Med Clin North Am* 11:379, 1993.
Leslie SD, Toy PTCY: Laboratory hemostatic abnormalities in massively transfused patients given red blood cells and crystalloid. *Am J Clin Pathol* 96:770, 1991.
Lundberg GD: Practice parameter for the use of fresh frozen plasma, cryoprecipitate, and platelets. *JAMA* 271:777, 1994.
Morris JA, Wilcox TR, Reed GW, et al: Safety of the blood supply. *Ann Surg* 219:517, 1994.
Rasmussen GE, Grande CM: Blood, fluids and electrolytes in the pediatric trauma patient. *Int Anesthesiol Clin* 32:79, 1994.
Wilson RF, Binkley LE, Sabo FM, et al: Electrolyte and acid-base changes with massive blood transfusions. *Am Surg* 58:535, 1992.

# 190
# EMERGENCY COMPLICATIONS OF MALIGNANCY
## Judith E. Tintinalli

The increasing prevalence of malignant disease, longer patient survival, and complications of treatment demand the ability to recognize and treat a wide spectrum of oncologic emergencies. Myelosuppression from chemotherapy and radiotherapy can result in coagulopathies and infection. Tumor growth can produce signs and symptoms of local compression on the spinal cord or airway, and certain tumors are associated with unique complications, such as hyperviscosity syndromes from tumor-related gammopathies. Table 190-1 lists the most important life-threatening oncologic emergencies.

## ACUTE SPINAL CORD COMPRESSION

> Multiple myeloma
> Non-Hodgkin and Hodgkin lymphomas
> Carcinoma of lung
> Carcinoma of prostate
> Carcinoma of breast

Spinal cord compression can result from bleeding, infection, or fracture. It may be the first sign of a neoplasm, or can complicate pre-existing metastatic disease. The incidence is estimated at > 5 percent, and repeated occurrences in the same patient have been reported.

**Table 190-1.** Emergency Complications of Malignancy

Related to local tumor compression
  Acute spinal cord compression
  Upper airway obstruction
  Malignant pericardial effusion with tamponade
  Superior vena cava syndrome
Related to biochemical derangement and systemic collapse
  Hypercalcemia of malignancy
  Syndrome of inappropriate ADH (SIADH)
  Hyperviscosity syndrome
  Adrenocortical insufficiency with shock
Related to myelosuppression and infection
  Granulocytopenia and sepsis
  Immunosuppression and opportunistic infections
  Thrombocytopenia and hemorrhage
  Anaphylaxis and transfusion reactions

Spinal cord compression occurs most commonly with multiple myeloma and lymphoma. It is generally suspected in individuals with previously documented malignancy who develop paraparesis, paraplegia, sensory deficits, or urinary incontinence. Spinal cord compression may also present as acute urinary retention. All patients with acute urinary retention should have a careful neurologic examination, including assessment of reflexes, motor and sensory function, rectal sphincter tone, and gait, to rule out spinal cord compression. Pain localized to involved vertebrae may be present and intensified by local percussion during the physical examination. However, as is often the case in lymphomas, if lytic bony lesions are not present, local pain is absent and the patient may have only a sensory level or distal flaccid paralysis. Hypoesthesia, lower extremity weakness, or gait disturbance are early symptoms and should alert the emergency physician to the possibility of spinal cord compression. Early treatment may avert progression to paraplegia and prevent sphincter loss.

The emergency physician's role includes not only suspicion and recognition of cord compression but also institution of measures to prepare the patient for potential emergency surgery. This includes assessment of fluid status, hematologic parameters and cardiorespiratory functions. CT scanning of the thoracolumbar spine may demonstrate the level of compression. Myelography is definitive. Decadron, 10 mg IV, or Solumedrol, 30 mg/kg IV, as recommended for acute traumatic spinal cord injury, should be given. Emergency surgical decompression or emergency radiotherapy is necessary to prevent irreversible neural damage.

## UPPER AIRWAY OBSTRUCTION

> Carcinoma of larynx
> Thyroid carcinoma
> Lymphoma
> Metastatic lung carcinoma

Acute upper airway obstruction is generally associated with aspiration of foreign bodies or food, with epiglottitis, or with other oropharyngeal infections. Malignancy-related obstruction to airflow is more insidious and often attended by voice change. This is generally a late manifestation of tumors arising in the oropharynx, neck, and superior mediastinum. Acute compromise is uncommon unless infection, hemorrhage, or inspissated secretions supervene. Rapidly growing tumors such as Burkitt's lymphoma and anaplastic carcinoma of the thyroid are capable of compromising airflow within weeks and should be suspected in afebrile individuals with stridor and palpable anterior neck masses.

Fiberoptic laryngoscopy is usually necessary to evaluate airway lumen size, because local anatomy is generally greatly distorted. Lateral soft-tissue x-rays are of value in assessing laryngotracheal patency. Establishment of an effective airway is primary and surgical tracheostomy may be required prior to the intitiation of radiotherapy.

## CARDIAC EMERGENCIES
### Malignant Pericardial Effusion with Tamponade

> Malignant melanoma
> Hodgkin lymphoma
> Acute leukemia
> Carcinoma of lung
> Carcinoma of breast
> Carcinoma of ovary
> Radiation pericarditis

Malignant melanoma has special predilection for the heart, but the commonest cause of malignant pericardial effusion is carcinoma of the lung and breast. Pericardial disease can also result from media-stinal irradiation, infection, or drugs such as cyclophosphamide, granulocyte-macrophage colony-stimulating factor (GM-CSF), and cytarabine.

The hemodynamic consequences of malignant pericardial effusions are a function of the volume and speed of accumulation. Even collections greater than 500 mL may be well tolerated if development is slow. Sudden intrapericardial bleeding is associated with dyspnea, chest pain, and hypotension. If the myocardium is also involved with metastatic disease, cardiac dysfunction will result in a decrease in cardiac output as well.

The classical clinical features of cardiac tamponade are (1) hypotension and a narrowed pulse pressure; (2) jugular venous distension; (3) diminished heart sounds; (4) pulsus paradoxus greater than 10 mmHg; (5) low QRS voltage; and (6) cardiomegaly without evidence of congestive heart failure on chest x-ray. Diagnosis is confirmed by echocardiography. Emergency percutaneous pericardiocentesis may be life-saving. It can be done blindly, if extreme haste is needed, or under fluoroscopic guidance. Definitive treatment consists of pericardiectomy, establishment of a pericardial window, radiation, or intrapericardial chemotherapy.

## Coronary Artery Disease

Many cancer patients also have coronary artery disease. Anemia from bone marrow suppression or malignant infiltration can result in decreased myocardial oxygen supply. Interferon and interleukin 2 (IL-2) can increase cardiac output, resulting in an increased myocardial oxygen demand. Several chemotherapeutic agents have been associated with cardiac ischemia, including 5-fluorouracil, vinblastine, and IL-2. Sternal pain mimicking angina has been associated with GM-CSF.

Many agents have been associated with tachyarrhythmias, bradyarrhythmias, and blocks. These include the anthracyclines, 5-fluorouracil, interferon, IL-2, GM-CSF, and taxol. Myocarditis has been reported in association with anthracyclines and cyclophosphamide. Anthracyclines are directly toxic to myocardial cells, while cyclophosphamide toxicity appears to be vascular. Anthracycline-induced cardiomyopathy may occur months to years after cessation of treatment and is thought to be related to both the total cumulative dose and mode of administration.

## Superior Vena Cava Syndrome

> Small-cell (oat-cell) carcinoma of lung
> Squamous cell carcinoma of lung
> Lymphoma

The superior vena cava syndrome is frequently a de novo diagnosis first established in the emergency department. A history of previously documented malignancy is often lacking, and patients may seek medical attention because of the insidious and progressive nature of their symptoms. Obstruction to blood flow in the superior vena cava elevates venous pressure in the arms, neck, face, and cerebrum. Patients with moderate obstruction complain of headache, edema of the face and arms, or a nondescript feeling of head congestion and fullness in the neck and face. As venous pressure rises, intracranial pressure also rises and syncope may ensue. Critical intracranial pressure elevations are a true medical emergency and are usually associated with bilateral papilledema.

On physical examination, neck vein and upper chest vein distension may be apparent. Facial plethora and telangiectasia often are prominent, but edema of the face and arms is generally subtle. Papilledema on fundoscopic examination indicates critical intracranial pressure and justifies early diuretic therapy. A palpable supraclavicular mass due to direct tumor extension can occasionally be noted with tumors of the superior mediastinum. Chest x-ray will demonstrate an enlarged mediastinum and possibly an isolated primary lesion in the lung parenchyma.

Prompt administration of diuretics and glucocorticoids may help reduce venous pressure prior to initiation of mediastinal irradiation. Furosemide (Lasix), 40 mg intravenously, and methylprednisolone (Solumedrol), 120 mg intravenously, are frequently used to reduce intracerebral edema. In advanced disease, radiotherapy to improve cardiodynamics is frequently necessary before tissue diagnosis can be obtained.

## HYPERCALCEMIA OF MALIGNANCY

> Renal cell carcinoma
> Multiple myeloma
> Bone metastases from carcinoma of breast, prostate, or lung
> Humoral-induced non-Hodgkin lymphoma and adult T-cell lymphoma-leukemia

Mild elevations of serum calcium are well tolerated and produce little in the way of symptoms. However, when serum calcium levels rise rapidly or exceed ionic thresholds, cardiac, neural, and muscular electrophysiology may be greatly altered. A number of mechanisms have been identified that promote release of bony calcium into the circulation. Bony involvement with myeloma or carcinoma of the breast, prostate, or lung will release calcium by local matrix destruction. Squamous cell carcinoma of the lung may produce a parathormone-like substance, and an osteoclast-activating factor has been associated with non-Hodgkin lymphoma (diffuse histiocytic) and retrovirus adult T-cell lymphoma-leukemia.

Approximately 40 percent of patients with multiple myeloma will have hypercalcemia. An often encountered clinical triad includes back pain, constipation, and depression in the level of consciousness. Hypercalcemia from any cause may induce hypertension, constipation, and an altered sensorium. Elevated ionized calcium is responsible for neuromuscular dysfunction and therefore serum calcium levels should be interpreted with phosphorus, serum albumin, and blood pH determinations. The QT interval of the electrocardiogram may shorten as the serum calcium rises.

The majority of patients with malignancy-induced hypercalcemia will improve with saline infusion and intravenous furosemide (1 to 2 L saline load and 80 mg of IV furosemide). This will promote renal calcium excretion but depends upon adequate renal function and glomerular filtration. Because renal insufficiency is a common accompaniment in myeloma, assessment of blood urea nitrogen and creatinine levels is important to ensure both adequacy of response and avoidance of iatrogenic fluid overload. Hemoconcentration and dehydration may additionally aggravate elevating calcium. For severe hypercalcemia, hemodialysis or peritoneal dialysis against a low- or no-calcium dialysate may be necessary. The IV administration of inorganic phosphate is a rapid and effective method for decreasing blood calcium, but its use is controversial because of the associated adverse effects. Phosphate administration can initiate and accelerate metastatic soft tissue calcification and can cause hypocalcemia, hypotension, renal failure, and death. The dose of intravenous phosphate is 1 g infused over 8 h. Serum calcium may fall within minutes, and decline in calcium levels may continue for several days. Oral phosphate, given as 1 g of sodium acid phosphate daily, produces maximum effect after several days. Glucocorticoids can be given empirically in comatose or obtunded patients with serum calcium levels greater than 13 mg/dL. The dose is 100 mg of prednisone or equivalent, but the hypocalcemic effect takes several days to develop. The effect of glucocorticoids is greatest in the hematologic malignancies and breast cancer and is unpredictable in solid tumors. Mithramycin acts by inhibiting bone resorption. The dose is 25 μg/kg delivered as an IV infusion. Its effect is usually evident in 24 to 48 h.

## SYNDROME OF INAPPROPRIATE ADH

> Malignancy of the brain, lung, pancreas, duodenum, thymus, prostate
> Lymphosarcoma

Ectopic secretion of antidiuretic hormone (ADH) may come from a variety of malignancies, but in any case the end result is the syndrome of inappropriate ADH (SIADH), which consists of serum hyponatremia, less than maximally dilute urine, excessive urine Na excretion (>30 mEq/L), and normal renal, adrenal, and thyroid functions. Treatment is aimed at removing the source of ADH secretion. Water restriction usually raises the serum sodium over a period of several days. The intravenous infusion of 100 to 250 mL of hypertonic saline solution (3 percent) may be necessary in the face of hyponatremic-induced seizures or cardiac arrhythmias.

## HYPERVISCOSITY SYNDROME

> Multiple myeloma
> Waldenström macroglobulinemia
> Chronic myelocytic leukemia

Viscosity is the flow-resisting characteristic of fluids. Marked elevations in certain serum proteins will produce sludging and a reduction in microcirculatory perfusion. IgA myeloma components and IgG subtype 3 proteins have a tendency to polymerize, leading to symptomatic hyperviscosity. Macroglobulinemia is the most common cause for hyperviscosity by virtue of the high molecular weight and high intrinsic viscosity of IgM proteins. Serum viscosity relative to water is normally 1.4 to 1.8, and symptoms develop at viscosities greater than five times that of water.

Fatigue, headache, anorexia, and somnolence are early nonspecific symptoms. As blood flow slows, microthromboses may occur, with the advent of local symptoms such as deafness, visual disturbances, and jacksonian or generalized seizures. The diagnosis of hyperviscosity must be considered in the emergency department when patients with unexplained stupor or coma are found to have anemia, with rouleau formation on the peripheral blood smear. The most readily appreciated physical findings are in the ocular fundi and include "sausage-linked" retinal vessels, hemorrhages, and exudates. Laboratory evaluation should include coagulation, renal, and electrolyte profiles. Hypercalcemia can coincide, and when M-component protein concentrations are high, "factitious" hyponatremia may also be present. A clue to the presence of hyperviscosity may be the laboratory's inability to perform chemical tests because of the serum stasis in the analyzers, undoubtedly due to "too thick" blood. Serum viscosity and protein electrophoresis determinations are diagnostic.

The emergency physician's role is predominantly suspicion and recognition of the syndrome in patients with unexplained stupor and coma. Hyperviscosity is generally a presenting manifestation of certain plasma cell dyscrasias, and a history of previously documented disease is often lacking. Initial therapy is rehydration followed by emergency plasmapheresis. When coma is present and the diagnosis rapidly established, a temporizing measure may be a two-unit phlebotomy with saline infusion and replacement of the patient's red cells.

## ADRENAL INSUFFICIENCY AND SHOCK

> Carcinoma of the lung
> Carcinoma of the breast
> Malignant melanoma
> Retroperitoneal malignancies
> Withdrawal of chronic steroid therapy

Adrenal insufficiency may be related to adrenal gland replacement by metastatic tumors or to adrenocortical suppression by therapeutic glucocorticoid administration. In either case, maximal adrenal function may be inadequate to support the individual when stressed by infection, dehydration, surgery, or trauma. Adrenal crisis and shock with vasomotor collapse may be sudden and fatal. The differential diagnosis of cancer patients with fever, dehydration, hypotension, and shock would more frequently include sepsis and hemorrhagic shock. Adrenal crisis is less common than bleeding and sepsis but the steroid-dependent patient should be empirically given intravenous glucocorticoids.

Laboratory clues to the possible concomitant presence of adrenal insufficiency may be mild hypoglycemia, hyponatremia, hyperkalemia, and eosinophilia. Azotemia is, however, nonspecific and is often present in dehydration from any cause. In suspected cases, a serum cortisol should be drawn prior to steroid treatment.

Normal adrenal glands maximally produce approximately 300 mg per day of hydrocortisone when stressed. This has served as a guideline for replacement therapy. Adrenalectomized individuals are maintained on average doses of 35 to 40 mg of hydrocortisone per day and this is increased during potential stress. Appropriate emergency doses of hydrocortisone (Solucortef) would be 250 to 500 mg intravenously. Somewhat larger doses have been employed in septic shock.

## GRANULOCYTOPENIA, IMMUNOSUPPRESSION, AND INFECTION

Overwhelming infection is a common cause of death in the immuno-compromised host. A variety of factors may contribute to increased susceptibility to infection in cancer patients. Important factors include

1. Malnutrition and cachexia
2. Granulocytopenia
3. Impaired humoral immunity and antibody production, as in chronic lymphocytic leukemia or multiple myeloma
4. Altered cellular immunity, as in Hodgkin and other lymphomas
5. Postsplenectomy susceptibility to serious pneumococcal infections
6. Reactivation tuberculosis with concurrent glucocorticoid therapy
7. Polymicrobial enteric sepsis from bowel organism entry; carcinoma of colon or mucosal damage from chemotherapy
8. Nosocomial infections transmitted through blood transfusion and blood products
9. Immunosuppression and myelosuppression of chemotherapy

Both the frequency of infection and the mortality rate increase significantly when the circulating granulocyte pool is below 1000 to 1500 per cubic millimeter. Cancer patients are at risk for a variety of bacterial, viral, and fungal infections. Frequently encountered infections include pneumococcal sepsis and pneumonia; *Staphylococcus aureus* infection; enteric gram-negative pneumonia or sepsis, including *Pseudomonas* infections; and localized or disseminated varicella zoster viral and cytomegaloviral infections. Immunosuppression predisposes to invasion by organisms that are normally held at bay by host defenses and biocompetition from normal body flora. Such opportunistic infections include *Pneumocystis carinii* pneumonia (protozoal), disseminated candidiasis, aspergillosis, cryptococcal meningitis, pulmonary nocardiosis, and histoplasmosis.

For fever in the presence of malignancy or a history of chills and rigor, the emergency physician should assume an infectious etiology and initiate appropriate laboratory studies and cultures. Life-threatening gram-negative sepsis with hypotension should be aggressively treated after appropriate cultures. Fluids, broad-spectrum antibiotics, and intravenous glucocorticoids are advised. Few bacterial organisms would be missed with regimens containing a second- or third-generation cephalosporin (cefazolin, cefoxitin, cefoperazone, cefotaxime) and an aminoglycoside (gentamicin, tobramycin, amikacin). Anaerobic coverage may be added (clindamycin) if peritonitis or abdominal

symptomatology exists. Other choices include piperacillin/lazobactam, 3.375 g IV q6h, or ampicillin/sulbactam, 3.0 g IV q6h, or ticarcillin clavulanate, 3.1 g IV q6h.

## HEMATOLOGIC SYNDROMES

Thromboembolism is not uncommon in cancer patients and is due to a number of factors such as a hypercoagulable state; decreased proteins C, S, and antithrombin III; and the effect of metastases on activation of the coagulation pathway. Cancer patients are at increased risk for both deep venous thrombosis and pulmonary embolism. However, anticoagulation may result in bleeding at sites of metastatic disease, so that treatment options are more complex and may include placement of a filter in the inferior vena cava.

Polycythemia is enhanced production of red cells due to increases in sensitivity of erythropoietin. Any organ system can be affected by resultant thrombosis, bleeding, or hyperviscosity, but CNS affects are the most devastating. Celiac or mesenteric vessel ischemia, or Budd-Chiari syndrome, is seen when GI vessels are involved. If the hematocrit is >60 percent and symptoms are present, emergency phlebotomy is necessary.

Either acute or chronic leukemias can result in white blood cell counts >100,000 per μL. A leukocrit of > 10 percent is often associated with clinically significant hyperviscosity, and CNS dysfunction and respiratory distress can occur from capillary leukostasis. Diuretics worsen symptoms because they will increase the leukocrit. Treatment is directed at the underlying malignancy, and allopurinol should also be administered in anticipation of massive tumor lysis, to prevent acute gouty arthropathy and renal failure.

## GASTROINTESTINAL SYNDROMES

Acute gastrointestinal complications may or may not be related to the underlying malignancy. In patients with cancer, even gastric cancer, the major causes of GI bleeding are still hemorrhagic gastritis and peptic ulcer disease. Intraarterial hepatic chemotherapy infusions have been associated with GI bleeding, especially from the duodenum. Chemotherapy or radiotherapy can cause vomiting, resulting in Mallory-Weiss tears or reflux esophagitis.

Cancer patients with acute abdominal processes present with typical signs and symptoms unless they are receiving exogenous steroids. Acute appendicitis has been reported to occur in up to 4 percent of patients with leukemia.

## ACUTE RENAL FAILURE

Prerenal azotemia can be a result of dehydration from vomiting and disease, from chemotherapy, anorexia, or diuretics. Hepatic and peritoneal disease may cause sequestration of fluid in the peritoneal cavity, leading to intravascular volume depletion. Interleukin 2 and cyclosporine can also cause prerenal azotemia.

Multiple myeloma and lymphoma can cause amyloid deposition in the glomeruli, resulting in rapidly progressive renal failure. Interstitial nephritis can also result from renal infiltration by lymphoma. Intratubular obstruction can result from tumor lysis syndrome, hypercalcemia, and gammopathies and has also been reported with high-dose methotrexate and acyclovir.

## BIBLIOGRAPHY

Gibbs HR, Swafford J: Cardiac emergencies in the cancer patient. *Oncology* 6:25, 1992.

Thomas CR, Edmondson EA: Common emergencies in cancer medicine: Cardiovascular and neurologic syndromes. *J Natl Med Assoc* 83:1001, 1991.

Thomas CR, Imhotep KAC, Leslie WT, et al: Common emergencies in cancer medicine: Hematologic and gastrointestinal syndromes. *J Natl Med Assoc* 84:165, 1992.

Weinman EJ, Patak RV: Acute renal failure in cancer patients. *Oncology* 6:47, 1992.

## 191
# THE NEUROLOGIC EXAMINATION
### Gregory L. Henry

The individual components of the nervous system can be easily tested and analyzed in a simple but structured fashion. It is common for the less organized examiner to spend a vast amount of time and yet obtain little information. The objective of this chapter is to set the foundation for the emergency department diagnosis of neurologic disorders and complaints.

A systematic approach for performing the neurologic examination must be accompanied by an equally effective method for recording the examination findings. It is not adequate to write "Neuro within normal limits" when dealing with a complex neurologic problem. The pertinent positive and negative findings should be recorded on the chart, with degree of elaboration depending on the patient's chief complaint.

The basic areas of the neurologic examination should be approached quickly and directly. Further tests in any specific area should be prompted only by positive findings.

The object of the neurologic examination is to answer the questions: "What is it?" and "Where is it?" The question "What is it?" is asked to determine the mechanism by which the nervous system is being compromised. As a general rule, this question is best answered by history. The second question usually refers to the level of the nervous system involvement: peripheral nerve, spinal cord, cerebellum, brainstem, or cerebral hemisphere. This question is best answered by the physical examination. A disease can involve a number of these areas, and a patient can have more than one disease, so that all data must be synthesized before any conclusions are reached.

## HISTORY

Entities with rapid onset in seconds to minutes and with distinct neurological signs and symptoms are almost invariably vascular in nature. Vascular events may be large, with huge deficits at the onset, or may represent multiple small infarcts with accumulation of deficits which lead to more and more progressive neurologic decline.

The transient ischemic attack is a warning signal of an imminent vascular catastrophe. Transient ischemic attacks should be viewed as prestroke lesions and treated aggressively.

A history obtained from family and friends is essential to determine the patient's premorbid level of function. It is not adequate to ask the family if the patient was "all right" prior to presentation to the emergency department. Many families have an unusual perception of what normal mental status and function is, and these perceptions must be carefully determined. It is helpful to have a family member in the room with the patient to assist in monitoring the veracity of the patient's statements. Most patients with a history of progressive downhill function over weeks to years are affected with degenerative disease or some chronic dementing process. If the patient has had a slow downhill course with little change in mental status, it is unlikely that a definitive diagnosis will be made in the emergency department. The emergency physician should always beware of the patient with

mild to moderate CNS impairment, or dementia who presents with sudden deterioration over 2 or 3 days. Such a patient is a prime candidate for a subdural hematoma, CNS infection, overmedication, dehydration, or another toxic metabolic condition. Patients with rapidly fluctuating, nonfocal neurologic signs should be considered to have a primarily metabolic insult until proved otherwise.

Multiple sclerosis is, as always, nebulous and difficult to diagnose. There is no definitive test for this disease, but it may be suspected in patients who have rapidly changing multiple focal neurologic findings that are unrelated to a specific anatomic site.

## SCREENING EXAMINATION

The basic neurologic screening examination evaluates six areas: (1) mental status, (2) cranial nerves, (3) motor response, (4) sensory response, (5) coordination (cerebellar function and gait), and (6) reflexes. Each area is described below, and the areas evaluated and tests employed are summarized in Table 191-1.

### Mental Status

Examination of mental status is performed simply by speaking with the patient. In the emergency department detailed tests for hemispheric function are not necessary in a patient who is conversing normally, is making reasonable responses to questions, and is well oriented. Observation of simple speech, reasoning power, and communications skills are the elements of the screening examination of mental status. If subtle mental status changes are suspected, more involved testing is required. In the vast majority of human beings, the left-sided brain is dominant. Dominant functions include speech, mathematical ability, and certain other communications skills. It is more difficult to test nondominant hemisphere functions. The nondominant hemisphere is involved with spatial orientation, sound localization, and body self-image. Specific tests for these areas need be performed if initial screening evaluation reveals difficulties.

### Cranial Nerves

Tests for intact brainstem function are concerned chiefly with the second through seventh cranial nerves.

Mass lesions that cause pressure either directly or indirectly on the diencephalon can alter the visual fields and pupillary response to light. Insidious tumors of the cerebral hemispheres, which may have very few gross neurologic findings, can cause early changes in the vi-

**Table 191-1.** Neurologic Screening Examination

| Area | Test |
| --- | --- |
| Mental status | Normal orientation, speech, global affect |
| Cranial nerves | Funduscopic, extraocular movements and pupillary response, visual fields, corneal reflexes, and facial muscular strength |
| Motor | Basic muscle groups, tone, drift, heel-and-toe walking |
| Sensory | Cold and vibration on areas indicated by patient or on distal extremities |
| Coordination (gait) | Observation of gait, and finger-to-nose testing |
| Reflexes | Deep tendons—knees, ankles, elbows, and wrists; degenerative reflexes—Babinski's signs, snout, grasp, and root |

sual fields. An intact pupillary response to light requires both reception by the second cranial nerve and motor outflow from the third cranial nerve. Visual fields can be tested simply by having the patient look at the examiner's nose from an arm's length distance. With both arms extended and the elbows at right angles, the examiner quickly flicks both index fingers at the same time. The patient is then asked which finger moved. If the patient responds that both fingers moved, gross bitemporal lesions can be eliminated. This test should be performed to evaluate all four quadrants of vision.

Midbrain and pontine dysfunction can be detected by observing extraocular movements. The extraocular muscles are innervated by the third, fourth, and sixth cranial nerves. The nuclei for these nerves cover a large area in the pons and midbrain, making them good indications of brainstem function. The patient is asked to follow the examiner's light into the six cardinal positions of gaze, making sure that the eyes are put through the full range of motion. The patient can also be observed simultaneously for nystagmus. Any abnormal findings should prompt a more detailed examination.

The fifth cranial nerve has extensive motor and sensory functions. The corneal reflex is often affected in hemispheric disease long before general facial sensation or the muscles of mastication are involved. Corneal sensation is tested by lightly touching the cornea with a small wisp of cotton. To do this, the patient must look opposite to the direction from which the examiner approaches. Scleral or lid response does not count, and only by touching the cornea can this sensation be tested. Unilateral depression of the corneal reflex is objective evidence of intracranial disease.

Seventh nerve function is commonly tested by having a patient smile or show the teeth. While considerable emphasis has been placed on the significance of asymmetry of the nasolabial folds, many people have slight asymmetry. A better test for facial strength is to ask the patient to squeeze the eyes tightly, and observe the degree to which the eyelashes are buried. Then, try to open the patient's eyes against such resistance. Another test is to have the patient purse the lips as in a whistle. Upper motor neuron lesions are characterized by unilateral weakness of the lower half of the face, while peripheral lesions involve the entire half of the face.

The eighth cranial nerve rarely requires testing in the emergency department unless there are specific complaints related to vertigo or hearing difficulties. Whenever questions with regard to the eighth cranial nerve function are raised, tests of both the vestibular and cochlear portions of the nerve are necessary. Speech reception testing by whispering numbers and words, as well as tuning fork evaluation for both the standard Weber and Rinne responses, is usually sufficient to separate out gross hearing abnormalities.

Tests for the ninth, tenth, eleventh, and twelfth cranial nerves are generally not important in the emergency department. There are no acute diseases that will manifest themselves with findings only in these areas, and in a rapid neurologic screening examination they are of little value. Lower cranial nerve testing is important, however, if screening examination findings are referable to other cranial nerves or posterior fossa structures.

## Motor Response

Evaluation of general muscle strength, tone, and symmetry is the objective of the screening examination. The patient should lie on the back so that the legs and arms can be observed. To check tone, quickly lift the knee off the cot and observe the actions of the foot. The normal response is to drag the heel along the bed as the knee is quickly jerked upward. If the leg comes up as a single unit, tone is probably increased. Tone in the upper extremities is best appreciated by moving the joints passively through a range of motion. Increased tone is often readily apparent with this technique. Gross bulk is estimated by observing the muscles of the calf and upper arm for mass, asymmetry, or fasciculations.

As a general rule, muscle groups essential in maintaining the body's normal posture have bilateral innervation and are less useful for determining lateralized weakness. In the upper extremities, the dorsiflexors of the wrist and the extensors of the forearm at the elbow have sufficiently uncrossed fibers to be useful in examination. In the lower extremities, evaluation of the dorsiflexors of the great toe and the flexors of the lower leg at the knee is all that is required to get a general idea of focal weakness.

An extremely sensitive indicator of focal weakness is testing for drift. In this examination, the patient is asked to extend both arms in front of the body, with the palms up and eyes closed. The patient is then carefully observed to see if there is any movement of one arm downward while the eyes remain closed. This test can be especially helpful in the minimally cooperative patient who is exhibiting give-way weakness on specific muscle testing. Another exceptionally good test for gross strength is to have the patient walk on the heels and then on the toes. This requires intact muscular strength. Simple resistance testing using the examiner's arm strength against the patient's leg strength is not sufficiently reliable. It requires considerably greater strength for the patient to walk distances on the toes and heels than to overcome the resistance of the examiner's hand.

## Sensory Response

Testing sensation is the least exacting and least informative part of the neurologic screening examination. If the patient has an area of decreased sensation, it is probably best to have the patient outline that area before attempting to isolate the lesion. If a definitive nerve root or peripheral nerve is outlined, direct testing for sensation should confirm the diagnosis.

A much more useful system in the emergency department is to think of sensory and motor loss in terms of patterns. Whenever sensation is found to be lacking in the "stocking/glove" distribution, peripheral nerve lesions should be considered. Loss of either motor or sensory response in the upper extremities and across the chest in a cloak or capelike distribution is often associated with lesions in the spinal column. Syringomyelia, a degenerative disease process, may present in such a fashion. More important to the emergency physician is that traumatic central cord syndrome of the cervical cord may likewise present with a capelike distribution. Loss of all sensation below a specific vertebral level defines a spinal cord injury. A mixed picture may be seen with only partial cord involvement, as in the Brown-Séquard syndrome. Loss of sensation on one entire side of the body denotes a lesion high in the central nervous system before entering into brainstem structures. Areas of alternating hemianesthesia or hemiplegia, that is, facial findings on one side and trunk and extremity findings on the opposite side, always indicate a lesion in the brainstem itself.

In the patient who does not have a specific sensory complaint, testing with a cold stethoscope, reflex hammer, or tuning fork is probably as accurate as any other method. Remember that sensory loss confined to one-half of the body usually involves a CNS lesion and most often is a hemispheric problem. If there is some decrease in response to vibratory sensation or hot and cold in either the hands or the feet, compare the lower extremities with each other, and against the upper extremities. Peripheral neuropathies tend to be symmetrical and show increasing sensation as one moves proximally along the limb. In symmetrical metabolic peripheral neuropathies there should be approximately the same level of nerve loss in both lower and upper extremities, and the legs tend to be involved earlier than the hands and arms.

The Romberg test requires explanation. A properly performed Romberg examination should be done with the patient standing and unsupported by any aids. With the feet together and arms at the side, the patient is asked to stand with the eyes open. If a patient cannot stand with the eyes open, the problem is usually related to one of

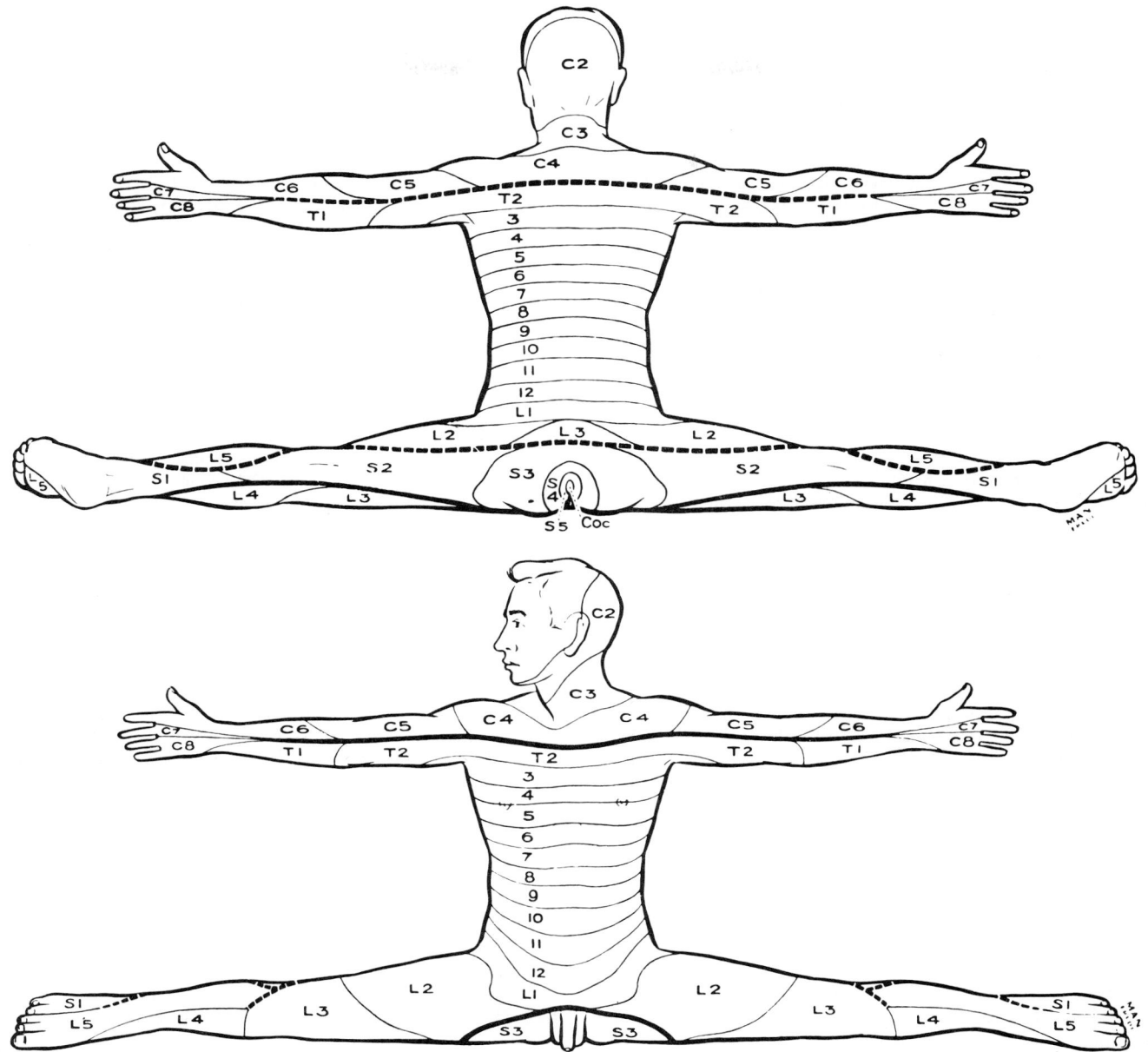

**Fig. 191-1.** Nerve root origin of various reflexes. (From Haymaker W, Woodhall B: *Peripheral Nerve Injuries: Principles of Diagnosis,* 1st ed. Philadelphia, Saunders, 1945, p. 16. Used by permission.)

cerebellar coordination. If the patient is able to stand with the eyes open but has difficulty in holding this position with the eyes closed, the problem is not one of coordination but one of sensation, with abnormality in position sense. This usually indicates involvement of posterior column function or may be seen as an isolated finding or as part of a general peripheral neuropathy.

## Coordination (Gait)

This part of the neurologic examination is frequently referred to as *cerebellar testing.* In truth, it is difficult to isolate the cerebellum because many areas are responsible for coordinating motor activity. Observing the patient's stance and gait is useful for testing both motor function and coordination. A broad-based, unsteady gait suggests cerebellar dysfunction. Patients with midline cerebellar lesions may have difficulty sitting up in bed without help. One good test for peripheral cerebellar lesions is finger-to-nose testing. Ask the patient to be precise, and to touch the tip of your finger to the tip of his or her

nose in rapid sequence. Development of oscillation the last few inches before touching the target is abnormal. Hysterical patients commonly produce wide oscillations from the moment they begin the motor task, or always touch precisely off the target. Romberg testing, as previously mentioned, has a cerebellar component. If the patient is unable to stand with the feet together, despite the input of vision, cerebellar lesions can be suspected.

## Reflexes

Both deep tendon and regressive reflexes can be rapidly tested. Asymmetry of response is the significant finding. The patient with brisk reflexes in all extremities, and no other signs of neurologic disease, probably has a normal variant. Likewise, the patient who essentially has no deep tendon reflexes without other neurologic findings is probably exhibiting a baseline state. A change, however, in the threshold required to elicit a reflex or clonus on one side of the body suggests a lateralizing lesion high in the CNS. A difference in

**Table 191-2.** Diagnostic Neurologic Tests Correlated with Specific Abnormal Neurologic Complaints

| Presenting Signs, Symptoms | Accessory Tests | Presenting Signs, Symptoms | Accessory Tests |
|---|---|---|---|
| Confusion, delirium, paucity of affect | Basic neurologic examination plus: Formal mental status testing Aphasia testing Psychological assessment Thought process and content evaluation (remember that the patient with decreased affect may be psychologically depressed, so try to obtain a measure of thought content) Snout, grasp, root, Babinski's reflexes Physical examination of head, supple neck | Dizziness | Basic neurologic examination plus: Orthostatic vital signs taken on both arms Enough history should be taken to divide the patient into those with: Vertigo—positional and cold water caloric testing Syncope—cardiac examination, ECG, perhaps in-house monitoring |
| Blurred, dim, absent, or double vision | Basic neurologic examination plus: Visual acuity and light perception Optokinetic nystagmus—in blindness Red glass testing—diplopia Careful fundoscopic examination | Coma | Completely separate examination: Level of consciousness Respirations Doll's-eye movements or caloric testing Pupillary responses Motor responses and general physical examination |
| Headache | Basic neurologic examination plus: Careful palpation of the head and neck, particularly the temporal arteries, sinuses, teeth, scalp | Trauma | Coma: go directly to coma protocol Awake: do limited examination Fine-motor movements Drift Do not put patients through major testing until cervical spine x-ray films are reviewed; the ABCs (airway, breathing, and circulation) precede all else in traumatized patients |
| Focal weakness | Basic neurologic examination plus: Systematic testing of each nerve root or peripheral nerve involved in both motor and sensory function Hemispheric testing | Back pain without history of direct trauma | Basic neurologic examination plus: Straight-leg raising Anal wink or tone Expanded motor, sensory, reflex examinations Gait |
| Nonfocal weakness | Basic neurological examination plus: Test for muscle fatigue, including lid lag and drift (suspect myasthenia gravis, Lambert-Eaton syndrome, alcoholic myopathy) | | |

reflexes between the arms and the legs suggests a lesion involving the spinal cord. Depression of reflexes in only one limb, while the others are symmetrical, is consistent with a root or peripheral nerve lesion. The various reflexes and their nerve roots of innervation are listed in Fig. 191-1.

Pathologic reflexes, such as Babinski's reflex and snout, root, and grasp reflexes, indicate a lack of inhibition from higher cortical centers to primitive stereotypic behavior. Babinski's reflex, which is elicited by stroking the lateral aspect of the foot, is the most commonly used, and is a good lateralizing sign. The presence of snout, root, and grasp reflexes indicates diffuse, bilateral frontal hemispheric disease.

Depending on the chief complaint of the patient and positive findings in the neurologic examination, a more thorough examination may be necessary. Some aspects of such an examination require special training, but frequently you can further delineate the patient's problems by just a few simple testing procedures. Listed in Table 191-2 are various presenting complaints and the accessory tests that can aid the emergency physician in making a diagnosis.

## BIBLIOGRAPHY

Henry G, Little N: *Acute Neurologic Emergencies: A Symptom Oriented Approach.* New York, McGraw-Hill, 1985.

Plum F, Posner JB: *The Diagnosis of Stupor and Coma,* 3d ed. Philadelphia, Davis, 1982.

# 192
# HEADACHE AND FACIAL PAIN
## Gwendolyn L. Hoffman

## HEADACHE

Approximately 40 percent of all Americans have a significant headache at some time, with 10 percent of the population seeing a physician episodically for headaches. Migraine headache alone affects 23 million Americans. Headache pain can originate extracranially from the skin, fat, muscle, blood vessels, periosteum, and fascial planes of the neck. It can also originate intracranially, from the great venous sinuses, their tributaries, the dura at the base of the skull, the dural arteries, the falx cerebri, and the large arteries at the base of the brain, all of which have pain fibers. Actual brain parenchyma, most of the dura, the arachnoid, and the pia mater are incapable of producing painful stimuli. The fifth cranial nerve is responsible for pain arising from above the tentorium and serves most of the facial areas. The ninth, tenth, and eleventh cranial nerves and upper cervical spinal nerves serve the region below the tentorium; pain is often referred to the neck and back of the head.

The pain-sensitive structures of the head and neck are affected by the following pain-producing mechanisms: distention, dilation, inflammation, tension, and traction. Approximately 1 percent of all headaches are symptoms of significant underlying pathology. The emergency physician must distinguish serious and life-threatening presentations from those that are less serious. This is best accomplished by a directed history and physical examination supported by ancillary testing.

## Pathophysiology

Recent biochemical and pharmacologic advances suggest that neither Wolff's vascular theory of migraine nor the muscle contraction theory of tension headache is any longer viable. Evidence now suggests that migraine may not be due to vasoconstriction followed by vasodilatation and that tension-type headache may not be due to excessive muscle contraction. Headache was thought to be caused by displacement, inflammation, or tension of the pain-sensitive structures; by increased intracranial pressure secondary to obstruction of cerebrospinal fluid (CSF) pathways; or by dilation of intracranial arteries.

Current pathophysiologic theories focus on central serotonergic transmission abnormalities, trigeminovascular neuronal transmission abnormalities, vascular structures, and neurogenic inflammation. Platelet aggregation with subsequent release of vasoactive substances as well as prostaglandin synthesis have been implicated. Moskowitz and colleagues suggest that trigeminovascular system activation induces vasodilatation and neurogenic plasma development of neurogenic inflammation. Vascular studies and electromyographic studies indicate that primary headache may be a continuum between tension-type headache and migraine. The basic pathophysiology of cluster headache remains undetermined, but there is clearly a neuronal component with implication of the trigeminal nerve. At this time, no one theory can explain all headache phenomena but most likely when one unified theory is developed, it will include aspects of all the current theories.

Postlumbar puncture headache, on the other hand, is caused by leakage of fluid through the dural puncture site. This causes a reduction of CSF volume below the cisterna magna with downward movement resulting in pain.

## Clinical Features

The International Headache Society (IHS) developed and published new classification and diagnostic criteria in 1988. Previously, the only classification was from 1962 and had been developed by the Ad Hoc Committee on Classification of Headache. The new system is felt to be an improvement over the prior one. The new criteria are more specific and ensure a better homogeneity in diagnosis by different physicians.

Approximately 12 percent of the population is affected by migraine with approximately 70 percent of these having a positive family history for similar headaches. Social history may document important drinking and smoking habits as well as contact with other toxins. Mood and anxiety disorders can be associated with migraine with depression more common than anxiety. Migraine occurs three or four times more commonly in women than it does in men and usually begins in adolescence or young adulthood.

### Migraine without Aura

The vast majority of people with migraine do not have an aura. Previously, this headache was called common migraine. Its duration is 4 to 72 h. At least two of the following characteristics should be present: (1) unilateral position, (2) pulsating quality, (3) moderate or severe intensity (inhibits or prohibits daily activities), (4) aggravation by walking stairs or similar routine physical activity. At least one of the following should be present during the headache: (1) nausea or vomiting or both, (2) photophobia and phonophobia. The patient must have at least five attacks fulfilling the above criteria before the diagnosis can be made. Migraine is a recurrent phenomenon, and the diagnosis should not be applied to the first headache experienced by the patient. In addition, history, physical examination, and, where appropriate, diagnostic tests should exclude a secondary cause. The most common markers of the migraine syndrome are the gastrointestinal symptoms of nausea and vomiting combined with photophobia and phonophobia along with increased intensity with physical activity.

### Migraine with Aura

Approximately 15 percent of people who have migraine will experience an aura prior to some of their attacks. This was previously called classic migraine. At least three of the following four characteristics should be present: (1) one or more fully reversible aura symptoms indicating brain dysfunction, (2) at least one aura symptom develops gradually over more than 4 min or two or more symptoms occur in succession, (3) no single aura symptom lasts more than 60 min, (4) headache follows aura with a free interval of less than 60 min (it may also begin before or simultaneously with the aura). There should be at least two attacks before the diagnosis is made. In addition, history, physical examination, and, where appropriate, diagnostic tests should exclude a secondary cause.

The most common auras are visual. The positive scotoma in the form of an arc of scintillating lights in a herringbone-like pattern is almost pathognomonic. Virtually any symptom or sign of brain dysfunction may be a feature of the aura. Some other examples are homonymous visual disturbance, unilateral paresthesias or numbness, unilateral weakness, and aphasia or unclassifiable speech difficulty. In some instances, one type of aura follows the other: sensory phenomena may occur as visual phenomena fade and motor phenomena develop as sensory phenomena dissipate. Previously used terms were *ophthalmoplegic migraine* and *hemiplegic migraine*.

## Factors Common to Migraine with or without Aura

A migrainous attack can be provoked or intensified by changes in the body's internal milieu and by environmental factors. Menstruation is the most common bodily change, but changes in body rhythm such as too little sleep, too much sleep, or fasting may provoke an attack. Physical activity makes the pain worse; minor head trauma may precipitate a headache. Often relaxation following stress such as after a strenuous day, on vacations, or weekends will result in a headache. Hot, humid weather or changes in weather may trigger an attack.

Foods may precipitate an attack in about 15 to 20 percent of migraine sufferers. Because of their tyramine content (especially red wines) and vasodilation properties, alcoholic beverages may cause a headache. Phenylethylamine in chocolate-containing foods as well as hard cheeses and herring containing tyramine and citrus fruits containing 1-octopamine may precipitate an attack. Consuming foods containing nitrites in processed meats and foods containing the additive monosodium glutamate may result in headache. Caffeine withdrawal and excessive caffeine intake may also trigger an attack.

Medications such as contraceptive estrogens may cause an increase in frequency or severity of headaches. If this occurs, the medication should be discontinued. Coronary artery disease and hypertension medications may provoke migraines in part by their vasodilating effects such as is seen with nitroglycerin.

## Cluster Headache

This is probably one of the most severe forms of head pain known to man and is relatively uncommon. It predominantly affects men with a 4:1 to 9:1 male/female ratio. The onset is usually in the late 20s with periodicity as the main feature. Episodes seem to occur more frequently in spring and autumn. The period during which a series of headaches occurs lasts about 2 to 3 months and occurs every year or two. Remissions do occur and range from 2 months to 20 years but the average is 2 years.

There is no associated aura and the peak pain is 10 to 15 min after onset, generally lasting 45 to 60 min. Attacks may occur one to three times per day. The pain is always unilateral, excruciating, penetrating, usually nonthrobbing, and located in the distribution of the trigeminal nerve. Maximum pain is usually felt behind the eye in the region of the supraorbital nerve and the temples. A component of the pain virtually always affects the orbit itself. The pain may also be above or to the side of the orbit or below the orbit in a so-called lower-half distribution. Certain autonomic features are attributable to sympathetic system paresis and parasympathetic overaction. These features include ipsilateral lacrimation, conjunctival injection, and nasal stuffiness or rhinorrhea. Ptosis and myosis may also occur. In more than 50 percent of patients, the attacks tend to be nocturnal and are characterized by a circadian regularity with attacks occurring at a particular time. There is often a history of excessive alcohol intake and heavy smoking. Alcohol, nitroglycerin, and histamine may actually trigger an attack.

## Tension-type Headache

This is the new term used to describe what was previously called tension headache, muscle contraction headache, stress headache, ordinary headache, idiopathic headache, or psychogenic headache. This is the most common type of headache and affects people of all ages. It can last from 30 min to 7 days. At least two of the following pain characteristics should be present: (1) pressing/tightness (nonpulsating) quality; (2) mild or moderate intensity (may inhibit but does not prohibit activities); (3) bilateral location; (4) no aggravation by walking, climbing stairs, or performing similar routine physical activity. Associated symptoms may include anorexia, photophobia, or phonophobia but not nausea and vomiting. The pain may worsen as the day progresses. In addition, history and physical, and, where appropriate, diagnostic tests must exclude a secondary cause.

A distinction is made by the IHS between patients with episodic tension-type headaches and chronic tension-type headaches (formerly chronic daily headaches). It is based on frequency with the episodic type occurring less than 15 times per month and the chronic occurring more than 15 times per month.

## Postlumbar Puncture Headache

This can occur in 5 to 30 percent of patients following lumbar puncture usually occurring within hours of the procedure and lasting 1 to 2 days. It is bicranial, pulsatile, and exacerbated by the upright position. The pain can involve the entire cranium but is usually cervical and suboccipital in location.

## Differential Diagnosis

Because many headache patients have normal physical and neurologic examinations, the most important tool for making a correct diagnosis is a detailed and relevant history.

### History

#### Age at Onset

Migraine headaches usually start in childhood, adolescence, or young adulthood. Tension-type headaches can occur at all ages. Organic etiologies such as temporal arteritis, cerebrovascular disease, or tumor may be the cause of headaches that start later in life.

#### Frequency and Pattern

Cluster headaches typically occur in brief attacks lasting 45 to 60 min and may occur several times a day. Migraine and tension-type headaches last longer.

#### Location

Unilateral headaches that alternate sides suggest migraine. Bilateral headaches suggest tension type. Cluster headache is suggested by strictly unilateral, orbital pain of brief duration.

#### Onset, Duration, Character, and Severity

Beware of the acute-onset, "thunderclap" headache. The cause may be a subarachnoid hemorrhage. A sudden onset of severe headache, especially associated with other symptoms, suggests a serious condition such as subarachnoid hemorrhage. The pain of migraine may be pulsating or throbbing. Tension-type headache is dull, nagging, and persistent. It is often described as though a band were wrapped around the head. A deep, piercing, intense unilateral pain is often seen with cluster headaches. A transient shocklike pain in the distribution of the fifth cranial nerve is seen with trigeminal neuralgia.

#### Course

The headache that progressively worsens may have an organic cause such as tumor. The longer the headache has existed in its present form, the more likely it is to be benign. Periodicity is the main feature of cluster headache.

#### Prodromes and Auras

This is usually seen with migraine headaches.

#### Associated Signs and Symptoms

Nausea and vomiting are commonly seen in migraine headaches but not in tension-type headaches. Unilateral nasal congestion, tearing, and conjunctival injection are seen with cluster headaches.

#### Signs of Neurologic Dysfunction

Neurologic symptoms of weakness, aphasia, diplopia, visual loss, and paresthesias may be seen in migraine with aura. Usually the patient will have a prior history of migraines. These symptoms along with vertigo and faintness may suggest a possible space-occupying lesion or aneurysm. If this is suspected, further workup must be done.

#### Precipitating Factors

Certain foods, drugs, and alcohol can trigger migraine headaches. Menstruation, bright lights, and loss of sleep can also precipitate an attack. Exercise or orgasm can trigger a migraine or result in the rupture of an aneurysm. With the rupture of an aneurysm, neurologic findings are usually seen on physical examination.

#### Family History

A positive family history is present in 70 percent of patients with migraine. There is no family history in cluster headaches.

### Physical Examination

A thorough examination can rule out many systemic causes of headache. This must include the vital signs. Hypertension may be seen with subarachnoid hemorrhage. Tachycardia may be seen with severe pain. Tachypnea is possible with headaches associated with anoxia, such as carbon monoxide poisoning. Fever may indicate meningitis, brain abscess, or encephalitis.

In funduscopic examination, spontaneous venous pulsations as viewed in the upright patient indicate normal intracranial pressure. This is an important finding, especially if later lost. Papilledema indicates increased intracranial pressure. Subhyaloid or preretinal hemorrhages are diagnostic of subarachnoid hemorrhage. Acute hemorrhages and exudates may be seen with hypertensive encephalopathy.

Palpation of the head conveys a sense of thoroughness to the patient. In addition, the finding of tenderness may be related to trauma or muscle spasm. Tenderness in the temporal arteries is important in the elderly because it may indicate temporal arteritis. Tenderness in the areas of sinuses, teeth, and fifth cranial nerve may also be helpful in making a diagnosis.

Stiffness indicates irritation of the meninges. To check for it the patient should be relaxed and in the supine position. With the patient relaxed, the examiner flexes the neck to determine whether there is involuntary resistance.

A sensitive sign of unilateral weakness is "drift" in one of the outstretched, palm-up arms of the patient. Abnormal gait, inability to touch finger to nose, and tandem walk may be the only clues to a posterior fossa mass.

## Ancillary Tests

When the diagnosis of migraine, tension-type, cluster, or postlumbar puncture headache can be made from a thorough history and physical examination, no other tests are needed. If the diagnosis is unclear, computed tomography (CT) scanning is indicated. It has replaced the skull x-ray for diagnostic evaluation. It can discover, define, and locate any causative lesion and is approximately 90 percent accurate in locating subarachnoid blood.

Lumbar puncture is necessary to identify intracranial infection or to detect subarachnoid blood not evident on CT scanning. Magnetic resonance imaging (MRI), visually evoked potential, and noninvasive transcranial Doppler ultrasound are not emergency department tests but may be required for elective evaluation.

The laboratory studies ordered will depend on the clinical differential diagnosis. For example, a complete blood count may be ordered if meningitis is suspected or an erythrocyte sedimentation rate (ESR) if temporal artery dysfunction is suspected.

## Emergency Presentation of Headache Patients

Basically, three categories of headache patients will present to the emergency department.

1. The chronic headache patient who has been thoroughly evaluated presents for pain control with no change in the headache pattern
2. The person who has never been evaluated presents with the first severe headache
3. The patient with prior history of evaluated headaches who now presents with a change in the quality and intensity or character of the headache

The emergency physician should be especially concerned if any of the following are present:

1. The first or worst headache of the patient's life, especially if the onset is acute and associated neurologic symptoms are present
2. A headache that gets progressively worse over days or weeks and was subacute in onset
3. A headache without a systemic illness but associated with fever, nausea, and vomiting
4. A headache associated with a stiff neck, focal neurologic findings, papilledema, and changes in consciousness or cognition
5. No obvious identifiable headache etiology

### Subarachnoid Hemorrhage

In North America, 28,000 people per year have a subarachnoid hemorrhage from a ruptured aneurysm. In a younger person, bleeding is more likely to be from an arteriovenous malformation. The onset is sudden and the pain is intense. It is often described as "the worst headache" of the patient's life. Loss of consciousness may occur. Meningismus develops as well as signs of increasing intracranial pressure such as vomiting. If CT scanning does not locate the source of bleeding, a lumbar puncture must be performed. Cerebral edema can be controlled by the usual means of hyperventilation and hypocapnia. Nimodipine can be used to reduce spasm. Urgent neurosurgical consultation is required.

### Hypertensive Headache

These throbbing occipital headaches do not generally occur until the diastolic pressure exceeds 130 mm Hg. Hypertension is an overdiagnosed cause of headaches, but if the headache is due to hypertension, control of the blood pressure with appropriate antihypertensive agents will alleviate the headache.

### Meningitis

Headache due to meningitis usually involves the entire head with associated fever and evidence of meningismus.

### Mass Lesions

Mass lesions can be in the subdural and epidural spaces or in the brain parenchyma itself.

*Subdural hematoma* is characterized by depression of mental status out of proportion to focal findings with a headache of variable quality. A chronic subdural hematoma is often seen in the elderly after previously forgotten minor injuries; it may also be atraumatic. Patients with an acute subdural hematoma are often too obtunded to complain of headache. Diagnosis is by CT scanning followed by neurosurgical consultation.

*Epidural hematoma* may progress to uncal herniation. There is usually a history of trauma and a brief episode of unconsciousness, followed by consciousness with headache. There is usually a fracture line through the middle meningeal groove. Diagnosis is by CT scan with an urgent neurosurgical consultation.

*Brain tumors* above the tentorium produce pain referred to the frontal region or vertex. Subtentorial lesions cause pain in the occipital region. An index of suspicion is raised if there is pain on awakening, if the pain is worse with the Valsalva maneuver, and if there is a new or unfamiliar headache associated with nausea and vomiting. The initial examination may be without focal findings. Follow-up must be arranged and diagnosis can be made by CT scan with contrast.

### Brain Abscess

The findings in cases of headache due to brain abscess will be similar to those for other space-occupying lesions, but the patient will also have a history of fever and possible sinusitis. Diagnosis is made by CT scanning. Neurosurgical consultation is necessary.

### Sinusitis

Acute infections of the nasal, paranasal, and mastoid sinuses may be associated with severe headaches, along with other symptoms. The pain is either stabbing or aching. It is made worse by bending or coughing and lessens when the patient is supine.

### Toxic Metabolic Headaches

Toxic metabolic headaches are bicranial and are caused by vasodilatation of the pain-sensitive arteries often combined with a lowering of the pain threshold by the toxic metabolic substance itself.

Fever greater than 38.8°C (102°F) is the most common cause. Hypoxia and hypercapnia are both potent cerebral vasodilators. Carbon monoxide produces cellular hypoxia with headache presenting when carboxyhemoglobin levels are greater than 20 percent. High altitude headaches may occur in nonacclimated mountain climbers at 3000 to 3600 m (10,000 to 12,000 ft) above sea level.

After a generalized seizure, postictal distention of vasculature with resultant headache may occur. The patient may identify this as a part of the usual postictal state, but if the pain is described as being different from what is usually experienced, further investigation is needed.

Acute anemia secondary to blood loss may result in headache due to vasodilatation and a relative oxygen deficiency.

Definitive treatment of most toxic metabolic headaches is removal of the cause with analgesic supplementation as needed. Additional definitive treatment such as blood transfusion with anemia may be indicated.

## Postconcussion Headache

Postconcussive headaches may follow trauma within hours to days. There can be associated vertigo, nausea and vomiting, difficulty with concentration, and mood alterations. The physical examination and CT scan are normal. These headaches are usually self-limiting, but nonsteroidal anti-inflammatory drugs (NSAIDs) may be beneficial. The prognosis is excellent.

## Pseudotumor Cerebri (Benign Intracranial Hypertension)

The usual patient with benign intracranial hypertension is a young, obese female with irregular menstrual cycles or amenorrhea. She presents with visual complaints and a nonspecific, often severe, headache. On physical examination, papilledema is found. CT scanning reveals slitlike ventricles and no mass effect. Treatment consists of repeated lumbar puncture to relieve the pressure, which can be above 500 mm water, and steroids.

## Acute Glaucoma

Nausea, vomiting, and orbital pain are present. The cornea may be edematous and the pupil midposition. The conjunctiva will be injected and visual acuity is decreased. Elevated intraoccular pressure as determined by tonometry is diagnostic.

# Treatment

For the treatment of migraine one must consider acute or abortive medications, general comfort measures, and prophylactic therapy.

## Emergency Department Management

Acute or abortive treatment measures are generally used because the patient already has the headache and may have accompanying nausea and vomiting. Antiemetics, rehydration, and pain control may be indicated.

Ergotamine constricts the external carotid artery and its branches with stabilization of serotonergic neurotransmission. It is thus contraindicated in patients with focal neurologic signs, peripheral vascular disease, hypertension, coronary artery disease, and pregnancy. The best absorbed route of administration is by inhalation or rectally. Blood levels following rectal administration are 20 to 30 times higher than those with the same oral dose.

Phenothiazines have antiemetic and antimigraine properties. Intravenous chlorpromazine (0.1 mg/kg) and prochlorperazine (10 mg) can provide complete or partial relief of migraine. Increased sedation and orthostatic hypotension may be seen with chlorpromazine. Metoclopramide (Reglan) is available in tablets, syrups, and injectable form (dose 10 to 20 mg). Besides being an antiemetic, it decreases gastric atony and enhances the absorption of any coadministered medications. It has been shown to be efficacious by itself as well as when coadministered with an analgesic. Any of these phenothiazines may cause extrapyramidal effects.

Specific serotonin or 5-hydroxytryptamine (5-HT) agonists have become popular in the treatment of migraine. Dihydroergotamine mesylate (DHE) is a weak vasoconstrictor but a strong venoconstrictor. It has a half-life of 18 h. The risk of headache recurrence is small, and there is no risk of addition or rebound. Pretreatment with an antiemetic is required. After this, a 0.75- to 1-mg dose is given intravenously over 2 min. If necessary, the process can be repeated in 30 min. Sumatriptan, a 5-HT agonist, has intrinsic antiemetic properties as well as intrinsic antimigraine properties. It is effective even late in an attack and is given as a 6-mg dose subcutaneously with a rapid onset of action. Within 60 min, 70 percent of patients have no headache and within 2 h, 80 percent are headache free. About one third of those treated have a recurrence of their headache within 24 h. This can be easily retreated, even by patients (using an "autoinjector" device) at home. Because pretreatment with an antiemetic is unnecessary, sedation and hypotension are avoided.

The NSAID, ketorolac 60 mg intramuscularly, has been moderately effective. The advantage over narcotic analgesics is that it causes no respiratory depression, has no addictive potential, and has no significant effect on mental or physical performance. Oral NSAIDs especially naproxen may also be helpful. For an acute attack, an oral dose of no less than 750 mg of naproxen should be considered.

Narcotic analgesics are the most common agents used in treating migraines in the emergency department. Their disadvantages are that they increase nausea and vomiting, cause respiratory depression, and may attract those patients with drug-seeking behavior. About 40 percent of emergency physicians use meperidine as their treatment for migraine, despite the availability of other effective drugs.

General comfort measures in the emergency department may include a darkened, quiet room and a cool, damp cloth for the forehead.

Prophylactic medications should not be used when attacks occur no more than two or three times per month, unless the attacks are incapacitating, associated with focal neurologic signs, or of prolonged duration. The patient's primary physician will need to monitor the effectiveness of the treatment. The emergency physician will probably not be ordering these but will certainly care for patients taking them. Several different types of drugs are used. β-Blockers, in particular, atenolol, propranolol, nadolol, and timolol, are useful. The effective benefit of calcium channel blockers such as verapamil, nifedipine, and nimodipine may lag 3 to 4 weeks, making them less popular. Serotonin antagonist such as cyproheptadine and methysergide are effective. However, methysergide is not a drug of choice due to its potential idiosyncratic reaction of retroperitoneal, pulmonary, or endocardial fibrosis (1 of 5000). Tricyclic antidepressants, especially nortriptyline, amitriptyline, and doxepin, are effective for headache treatment independent of antidepressant effect. The antiepileptic valproic acid has been used but has a lag time of 1 week and the possibility of hepatotoxicity. The monoamine oxidase inhibitor, phenelzine, can be effective but the patient must adhere to a tyramine-free diet. Nonpharmacologic therapies such as biofeedback, behavioral counseling, and transcutaneous electrical nerve stimulation, alone or with drugs, have had varied success.

The treatment for cluster headaches is similar to that for other migraines, although β blockers are not used. Additionally, oxygen inhalation of 5 to 8 L/min for 10 min at the onset is effective in aborting the headache in about 70 percent of the patients. Instillation of 4% intranasal lidocaine into the ipsilateral nostril is also useful. Effective prophylactic medications include ergotamine, methysergide, corticosteroids, calcium channel blockers, lithium, indomethacin, and valproate. In selected cases, surgical procedures for chronic cluster headaches, such as radiofrequency trigeminal gangliolysis, are available.

Treatment of tension-type headaches consists of mild analgesics such as aspirin and acetaminophen. NSAIDs are also useful. Relaxation techniques, stress management, biofeedback, and hypnosis may be helpful. If the headache becomes chronic in nature, amitriptyline is useful.

It is best to decrease the risk of postlumbar headache from occurring in the first place. Using a small needle, removing the least amount of fluid possible and being successful on the first puncture may prevent a headache. Bed rest versus early immobilization has been studied with contradicting results. However, patients should avoid lifting, bending, or squatting for 3 days to allow the dural puncture site to heal. Intravenous fluids are helpful to avoid dehydration because the lumbar puncture lowers CSF pressure with possible aggravation of the headache. Many medications have been used: simple analgesics, narcotic analgesics, ergots, barbiturates, and caffeine. If medications and rehydration are not successful, an epidural blood patch can be placed by an experienced anesthesiologist. This has proven to be highly successful.

## Admission

Admission criteria to the hospital for headache may vary with locale, insurance status, and ability to provide close follow-up care. Some reasonable indications for admission are:

1. Continuous migraine lasting for days and associated with nausea, vomiting and dehydration.
2. Headache complicated by overuse of analgesics, narcotics, caffeine, barbiturates, or ergots.
3. Chronic daily refractory headache that does not respond to outpatient treatment.
4. Headache secondary to suspected organic CNS disease (subarachnoid hemorrhage, tumor, meningitis, pseudotumor cerebri).
5. Headache accompanied by significant medical or surgical problem.
6. Intractable cluster headache.
7. Headache causing interruption and compromise of the ability to carry out activities of daily living.

## Outpatient

**Discharge instructions.** If patients have received medications that may alter mentation, the instructions must be given to a responsible adult. Patients should be assigned a primary care physician if they do not already have one. If the headache recurs, patients should call in the primary physician. At times, patients may return to the emergency department if the primary care physician is not available. For patients on prophylactic medications who present with a headache, they should be instructed to see their own doctor within 3 to 4 days for possible medication adjustment. Anytime that patients have a change in symptoms such as the development of fever, they should be instructed to call their own physician or return to the emergency department for further evaluation.

**Time course of disease symptoms.** By the time patients leave the emergency department, they should be greatly improved. The recurrence of symptoms will depend on how successful prescribed treatment is and if precipitating causes are avoided.

**Ambulatory treatment.** Patients can be sent home with a limited supply of combination analgesics. The advantages of combination analgesics are several: (1) combining two analgesics with different mechanisms of action can enhance analgesia; (2) combining lower doses of different drugs reduces side effects; (3) caffeine enhances analgesia and is analgesic itself; (4) barbiturates or benzodiazepines can alleviate anxiety; and (5) analgesic combination drugs offer dosing convenience. Commonly used combinations include acetaminophen or aspirin plus butalbital, a short-acting barbiturate. They are available without caffeine (Phrenilin) or with caffeine (Fiorinal, Fioricet, Esgic). If needed these are also available with codeine. Midrin, an analgesic, combines acetaminophen, isometheptene (a sympathomimetic agent), and dichloralphenazone (a chloral hydrate derivative) and is effective. Ergotamine tartrate, if not contraindicated, is available sublingually (Ergostat) or in combination with caffeine as an oral tablet or suppository (Cafergot, Wigraine). An NSAID may be all that is needed.

## FACIAL PAIN

## Temporal Arteritis

### Pathophysiology

Temporal vasculitis is a vasculitis in which a branch of the external carotid artery, most frequently the temporal artery, becomes infiltrated with lymphocytes, plasma cells, and multinucleate giant cells.

### Clinical Features

Women are affected up to four times more frequently than men, and it is usually a disease of people over 50 years of age. Average age of onset is 70 years, with a range of 50 to 85. Frequently it is associated with polymyalgia rheumatica. The pain is usually unilateral but can be bilateral and has a piercing or burning quality. Frequent jabs, often excruciating, are experienced at night. The inflamed artery is tender and pulseless and can sometimes be rolled between the fingers and the skull. Numerous signs and symptoms of systemic involvement may be present, including fever, malaise, weight loss, anorexia, visual defects (diplopia, blurred vision), and polymyalgia.

### Differential Diagnosis

The systemic signs and symptoms will distinguish it from other conditions. In addition an ESR of over 50 mm/h (Westergren) with the other clinical features is essentially pathognomonic. There also is a mild anemia and a leukocytosis. Biopsy of the artery (not an emergency department procedure) will yield a definitive diagnosis.

### Treatment

**Emergency.** Treatment should not be withheld while waiting diagnosis because blindness is the most common sequela and can develop rapidly secondary to ischemic papillitis. Prednisone 60 to 80 mg/d can be started in an attempt to prevent progression of the visual loss. NSAIDs may be beneficial for managing the initial pain. Emergent rheumatology consultation is necessary.

**Admission.** This will depend on the degree of the patient's systemic signs and symptoms and ability to care for his or her own needs or to have someone else do so.

**Outpatient.** If the patient is able to go home, close follow-up must be arranged before discharge from the department. If blindness occurs unilaterally, the patient will lose sight in the other eye within 1 to 20 days in 75 percent of cases. By starting prednisone immediately, the second eye can be saved and total symptomatic relief is evident within a few days. Within 4 weeks total remission of the disease is possible. A maintenance dose of prednisone is often recommended for a year or more. Progress can also be followed by periodic ESR determinations.

## Trigeminal Neuralgia

### Pathophysiology

Trigeminal neuralgia is considered a form of "deafferentation" pain involving peripheral and central components of trigeminal nerve fibers. Partial segmental demyelinization of the trigeminal root secondary to vascular compression may induce changes within the trigeminal nuclei in the brain stem. This may be responsible for intermittent bursts of the typical neuronal hyperactivity.

### Clinical Features

Each year in the United States, about 15,000 new patients will become affected with trigeminal neuralgia or tic douloureux. It rarely occurs before the fifth decade and women are slightly more prone to develop it than men. The right side of the face is more commonly involved than the left. In less than 4 percent of the patients is it bilateral and both sides are never involved simultaneously. The attacks of pain are brief, intermittent, lancinating and often have an "electric-like" quality. The midface (V2) or the lower face (V3) are involved exclusively or in combination with each other. Pain confined only to the eyebrow and forehead (V1) is not common, but a combination of V1 and V2 may be seen. Most often the attacks are "triggered" by a variety of maneuvers such as eating, talking, washing the face, or applying cosmetics. The most sensitive areas are the medial or lateral portion of the eyebrow (V1), the ala nasi (V2), the lower lip or one of the molar or premolar teeth (V3). The tendency is to refrain from any maneuver that might trigger an attack. Eating is often drastically reduced and weight loss is not uncommon. The neurologic examination is normal.

## Differential Diagnosis

Several conditions are associated with unilateral facial pain, which must be considered and excluded. These include postherpetic neuralgia, dental and maxillary sinus problems, cluster headaches, and atypical facial pain. The key to the diagnosis of trigeminal neuralgia is the history. It is not associated with any abnormalities on physical examination. If neurologic defects (hearing loss, facial sensory deficits, facial weakness, etc.) do occur with intermittent unilateral facial pain, a possible structural lesion could exist. The lesion would usually be in the cerebellopontine angle associated with irritability and distortion of the trigeminal nerve. Also, if symptoms develop before the fifth decade, multiple sclerosis as well as a cerebellopontine angle abnormality must be ruled out. MRI has become the gold standard diagnosis.

**Emergency.** Treatment in the emergency department may require parenteral analgesics such as morphine or meperidine. Most likely the patient is already taking carbamazepine and may need a dosage adjustment.

**Admission.** An initial painful episode may require admission, but most patients can be treated as outpatients.

**Outpatient.** At the time of discharge the patient should be advised to call his or her physician for follow-up. Medical therapy may need to be changed. Carbamazepine 200 mg orally tid is the medication of choice. Phenytoin can also be used. Baclofen is often added to both of them for its synergistic effect. If medical management fails, surgery can be done. Minor operative procedures include: (1) percutaneous injection of ethanol into the affected peripheral trigeminal branch, (2) neurectomy of the affected peripheral branch, (3) gangliolysis by either injection of alcohol or glycerol, and (4) radiofrequency gangliolysis. These are all neurodestructive and neuroablative. Major operative procedures are limited to microvascular decompression, rhizotomy, and medullary tractotomy.

## Temporomandibular Joint Syndrome

### Pathophysiology

Temporomandibular joint syndrome (TMJ; Kostin's syndrome) is usually secondary to periarticular spasm of muscles used in mastication. It may be secondary to an overbite, recent dental work, dentures, nocturnal grinding of teeth, or chewing. Physical derangement of the joint is possible with a history of prior trauma. A psychological component may also be present.

### Clinical Features

Presentation is with unilateral or bilateral pain in the TMJ and its associated craniofacial musculature. The area may be tender to palpation. Additional symptoms may include clicking and sticking of the joint and limitation of opening of the mandible with deviation to the affected side. A sense of fullness, popping, or tinnitus in the ear may be present.

### Differential Diagnosis

Temporal arteritis, trigeminal neuralgia, and cluster headache may be considered but should be able to be excluded on history and physical examination. A possible dental abnormality should be considered. Impaired sensation, paresthesia of any kind, or facial weakness necessitates a CT scan or MRI to exclude the rare possibility of a nasal, pharyngeal, or cerebral tumor.

### Treatment

**Emergency.** Anti-inflammatory medications should be sufficient.
**Admission.** This is not indicated.
**Outpatient.** The patient will need referral to a dentist or oral surgeon at the time of discharge from the emergency department for

more definitive treatment. This often consists of an occlusal splint or bite guard. If this is not sufficient, a tricyclic antidepressant such as nortriptyline can be added.

## BIBLIOGRAPHY

Duarte C, Dunaway F, Turner L, et al. Ketorolac versus meperidine and hydroryzine in the treatment of acute migraine headache: randomized prospective, double-blind trial. *Ann Emerg Med* 21:9, 1992.

Ellis GL, Delaney J, DeHart DA, Owens A. The efficacy of metoclopramide in the treatment of migraine headache. *Ann Emerg Med* 22:2, 1993.

Ferrari MD. Sumatriptan in the treatment of migraine. *Neurology* 43(suppl 3):543, 1993.

Fromm GH. Clinical pharmacology of drugs used to treat head and face pain: *Neurol Clin* 8:143, 1990.

Harris M, Feenman C, Wise M, Treasure F. Temporomandibular joint and orofacial pain: clinical and medicolegal management problems. *Br Dent J* 174:129, 1993.

Kooiker JC. Spinal puncture and cerebrospinal fluid examination. In: Roberts JR, Hedges JR (eds). *Clinical Procedures in Emergency Medicine*, 2nd ed. Philadelphia: WB Saunders, pp. 974–975, 1991.

Lance JW. Current concepts of migraine pathogenesis. *Neurology* 43(suppl 3):511, 1993.

Mathew NT. Cluster headache. *Neurology* 42(suppl 2):22, 1992.

Moskowitz MA, Cutrer FM. Sumatriptan: a receptor-targeted treatment for migraine. *Annu Rev Med* 44:145, 1993.

Rapoport AM. The diagnosis of migraine and tension-type headache, then and now. *Neurology* 42(suppl 2):11, 1992.

Raskin NH. Acute and prophylactic treatment of migraine: practical approaches and pharmacologic rationale. *Neurology* 43(suppl 3):539, 1993.

Schulman EA, Silberstein SD. Symptomatic and prophylactic treatment of migraine and tension-type headache. *Neurology* 42(suppl 2):16, 1992.

Silberstein SD. Advances in understanding the pathophysiology of headache. *Neurology* 42(suppl 2):6, 1992.

Silberstein SD. Evaluation and emergency treatment of headache, review article. *Headache* 32:396, 1992.

Solomon S, Lipton RB, Newman LC. Migraine: clinical features and diagnosis. *Neuropsychiatry* 18:25, 1992.

# 193
# MANAGEMENT OF STROKE

**Rashmi U. Kothari**
**William Barsan**

## INTRODUCTION

Stroke is the third leading cause of death and the leading cause of disability in the United States. Nearly 500,000 Americans are afflicted yearly; of these, almost 20 percent will die within the first year. Those who survive are often socially and financially devastated, losing their ability to walk, speak, or care for themselves. Stroke-related costs, including physician and nursing services, hospital and nursing home care, and lost wages amount to almost $20 billion a year. Research suggests that early accurate diagnosis and management of patients presenting to the emergency department with stroke may lessen the impact of this disease.

Unfortunately, when patients present to the emergency department with unilateral weakness they are often given a cursory evaluation, quickly diagnosed with a "stroke," and admitted to a general medical bed. Emergency department treatment may involve an intravenous line and oxygen. Little thought is put into the cause of the stroke and how it may affect management. The etiology of strokes is diverse, ranging from cardiac emboli to rupture of a congenital berry aneurysm. Effective treatment for one stroke type may be disastrous when applied to another stroke type. The anatomic location of the lesion and the mechanism of the stroke must be known before effective treatment can be given.

## STROKE TYPE

A stroke can be defined as any disease process that disrupts vascular blood flow to a distinct region of the brain. Brain damage due to stroke occurs via two major mechanisms: (1) ischemia due to vessel occlusion, which deprives neurons of needed oxygen and fuel; or (2) hemorrhage due to vessel rupture, which causes brain injury by direct cell trauma, mass effect, elevated intracranial pressure, and/or the release of deleterious biochemical substances. From 80 to 85 percent of all strokes are ischemic in nature; 15 to 20 percent are hemorrhagic.

### Ischemic Stroke

Ischemic stroke can be subdivided into three major categories: thrombotic, embolic, and hypoperfusion. The majority of all strokes are caused by vessel thrombosis, which occurs when clot formation is superimposed upon gradual vessel narrowing or alterations in the luminal lining of the vessel. Atherosclerotic disease is the most common cause of thrombotic stroke in the United States. Atherosclerosis primarily affects the larger intra- and extracranial arteries and causes hyperplasia and fibrous disposition in the subintimal area with plaque formation. Plaques cause luminal narrowing and platelet adhesion, which lead to vessel thrombosis. Other causes of thrombosis include vasculitis, dissection, polycythemia, and hypercoagulable states. Less common causes are infectious diseases, such as syphilis and trichinosis, that lead to vessel wall injury. The signs and symptoms of a thrombotic stroke usually develop gradually over minutes to hours and may wax and wane in severity. Upon questioning, patients often give a history of similar but transient symptoms that have occurred in the past, suggesting a transient ischemic attack (TIA) in the same vascular distribution.

One-fifth of all strokes are embolic in nature. In embolism, intravascular material from a proximal source is released and then occludes a distal vessel. In contrast to thrombotic stroke, there is no intrinsic vascular disease in the occluded vessel. Thus, emboli are less adherent to the vessel walls and are more likely to fragment and move distally than clots due to thrombosis. The most common sources of emboli are the heart and major vessels (aorta, carotid arteries, and vertebral arteries). Cardiac sources of emboli include valvular vegetations, mural thrombi (due to atrial fibrillation, myocardial infarction, or arrhythmia), paradoxical emboli (due to an atrial or ventricular septal defect), or cardiac tumor. Artery-to-artery emboli usually occur when a platelet-fibrin clump is dislodged from a tight stenotic lesion or from a large-vessel atherosclerotic plaque. Rarer causes of embolic stroke include fat emboli, particulate emboli from intravenous drug injection, or septic emboli.

Systemic hypoperfusion is a less common mechanism of ischemic stroke than thrombosis or embolism. It is most commonly due to cardiac pump failure (myocardial infarction or arrhythmias). Hypoperfusion leads to a more generalized or diffuse injury pattern than thrombosis or emboli. It is most evident in border zones or so-called watershed regions at the periphery of the major vascular-supply territories. Patients often present with diffuse findings that wax and wane according to their hemodynamic status.

### Hemorrhagic Stroke

Although hemorrhagic strokes comprise only one of every five strokes, they have a 30-day mortality of 30 to 50 percent and occur in a younger population of patients. Hemorrhagic strokes can be divided into two subtypes: intracerebral and subarachnoid hemorrhage.

The majority of hemorrhagic strokes are intracerebral hemorrhages. In intracerebral hemorrhage (ICH), bleeding occurs directly into the brain parenchyma. Increasing age and history of prior stroke are the leading risk factors for developing an ICH. The majority of ICH are associated with chronic hypertension. In hypertensive ICH, blood is thought to leak from small intracerebral arterioles damaged by chronically elevated blood pressure. Amyloidosis is another major cause of intracerebral hemorrhage, especially among elderly patients with lobar or multiple hemorrhages. Other causes of ICH include bleeding diathesis due to iatrogenic anticoagulation, vascular malformations, and cocaine use.

Subarachnoid hemorrhage (SAH) is half as common as intracerebral hemorrhage. In SAH, blood leaks from a cerebral vessel into the subarachnoid space. Blood from a ruptured artery is released at near systemic arterial pressure, in contrast to ICH in which arteriolar rupture occurs more gradually at lower pressures. The sudden release of blood under high pressure leads to direct cellular trauma as well as a rapid increase in intracranial pressure. Half of all subarachnoid hemorrhages are due to berry aneurysm rupture, most commonly occurring at arterial bifurcations or branchings. Arteriovenous malformations make up another 6 percent of all subarachnoid hemorrhages.

## PATHOPHYSIOLOGY

Basic knowledge of the anatomy and pathophysiology of the brain can assist the physician in identifying the location of the lesion and in understanding the rationale behind various therapeutic interventions.

### Ischemic Stroke

Neurons are very sensitive to changes in cerebral blood flow. Brain cells die within a few minutes of complete cessation of blood flow. However, despite complete occlusion of a cerebral vessel during an acute ischemic stroke, some perfusion remains even in the center of the ischemic brain region due to collateral flow and variations in local tissue pressure gradients. Cells vary from irreversibly injured neurons in the center of the ischemic region to reversibly injured neurons in the periphery (the penumbra). The degree and duration of occlusion determine the viability of the cells in the penumbra. Theoretically, the sooner reperfusion occurs the greater the chance of cell survival. Recent investigational use of intravenous and intraarterial thrombolytic therapy for ischemic stroke is based on this rationale.

### Hemorrhagic Stroke

In intracerebral and subarachnoid hemorrhage, a cerebral blood vessel ruptures, with a dramatic increase in intracranial pressure and a decrease in global cerebral perfusion that can last for minutes. After these immediate changes, intracranial pressure and perfusion pressure gradually improve, although not back to baseline. A marked reduction in cerebral perfusion occurs near the hematoma and is probably due to local compression. Areas of the brain remote from the bleed also have alterations in perfusion. These alterations in perfusion are thought to be due to vasoconstriction, caused either by chemical release from blood breakdown products or by neuronal mediation (diaschisis).

## ANATOMY

The vascular supply to the brain is derived from two sources: the anterior and posterior circulations, which supply blood to different regions of the brain. Hypoperfusion of specific areas of the brain leads to typical neurologic findings that can help clinically differentiate the location of the lesion and the vessels that may be involved.

The anterior circulation originates from the carotid system. It supplies blood to four-fifths of the brain. The common carotid arteries divide into the right and left internal and external carotid arteries at the level of the angle of the mandible. The internal carotid arteries then course intracranially along the sella turcica within the cavernous sinus. The first branch off the internal carotid artery is the ophthalmic artery, which supplies the optic nerve and retina. Sudden onset of painless monocular blindness (amaurosis fugax) identifies the stroke as involving the anterior circulation (specifically the carotid artery) at or below the level of the ophthalmic artery. The internal carotid arteries terminate by branching into the anterior and middle cerebral arteries at the circle of Willis. The anterior circulation supplies blood to the optic nerve, retina, and frontoparietal and anterotemporal lobes of the brain.

Although the posterior circulation is smaller (supplying blood to only one-fifth of the brain), it supplies the brainstem, which is critical for normal consciousness, movement, and sensation. The posterior circulation is derived from the two vertebral arteries that ascend through the transverse processes of the cervical vertebrae. The vertebral arteries enter the cranium through the foramen magnum, supplying the cerebellum via the posteroinferior cerebellar arteries. They join to form the basilar artery, which branches to form the posterior cerebral arteries. The posterior circulation supplies the brainstem, cerebellum, thalamus, auditory and vestibular functions of the ear, medial temporal lobe, and the visual occipital cortex.

The extent of stroke is also dependent on the presence of collateral blood flow distal to the vessel occlusion. A patient with excellent collateral blood flow from the contralateral hemisphere may have minimal clinical deficits despite a complete carotid occlusion. In contrast, a patient with poor collateral flow may be hemiplegic with the same lesion.

## CLINICAL FEATURES

The clinical presentation of stroke is often subtle and varied. The physician must approach the patient in a systematic and logical manner. Armed with the basic knowledge of the various stroke types and anatomy, the history and physical examination should be aimed at determining the underlying cause of the stroke and the location of the lesion.

### History

A review of the patient's demographics and past medical history can often suggest the etiology of the stroke. A 40-year-old patient presenting with a strokelike syndrome is more likely to have a hemorrhagic stroke (rather than a thrombotic stroke) than a 65-year-old patient. A history of hypertension, coronary artery disease, and diabetes mellitus are all suggestive of underlying atherosclerotic disease and vessel thrombosis. In contrast, atrial fibrillation, valvular replacement, or recent myocardial infarction suggest a cardioembolic source of infarction.

The patient should be thoroughly questioned regarding a recent history of TIA-like symptoms since this can help differentiate stroke types. A transient neurologic deficit in the same vascular distribution is suggestive of underlying vascular disease consistent with a thrombotic stroke, in contrast to multiple TIAs involving different vascular distributions, which suggest emboli.

An accurate and detailed history of the presenting illness can further direct the physician to the cause of the stroke. Initial onset of symptoms and any fluctuations in symptoms should be documented, since diagnostic studies and emergency management may differ depending on this history. Sudden onset of symptoms suggests an embolic or hemorrhagic stroke, whereas a stuttering or waxing and waning deficit suggests a thrombotic stroke or a stroke due to hypoperfusion. Concomitant complaints such as headache, vomiting, or recent trauma should be recorded. Headache occurs in the majority of patients with hemorrhage but in only 10 to 20 percent of those with ischemic stroke. A recent history of neck injury, such as a motor vehicle accident or a sports-related injury, suggests a carotid dissection.

## Physical Examination

Prior to initiating a neurologic examination, a general physical examination should be completed. If the patient is febrile, the source of infection should be identified. An infection may be the cause of the patient's deterioration or may be a complication of the stroke (e.g., aspiration pneumonia). A skin examination for signs of emboli (e.g., Janeway lesions and Osler nodes) or bleeding dyscrasia (e.g., ecchymosis or petechiae) should be done. A funduscopic examination to identify signs of papilledema (suggesting a mass lesion or hypertensive crisis), preretinal hemorrhage (consistent with a subarachnoid hemorrhage), or evidence of extensive hypertensive retinopathy should be completed. A history of physical findings suggestive of possible cardiac disease such as myocardial infarction, angina, arrhythmias, palpitation, or worsening of congestive heart failure should be investigated. Physical findings such as rales, an $S_3$ gallop, or carotid bruit should be recorded.

## Neurologic Examination

The goal of the neurologic examination is to localize the brain lesion and rule out other neurologic disease processes. The NIH Stroke Scale is a 15-item neurologic evaluation that is reproducible, correlates to infarct volume, and can be performed in less than 7 min (see Fig. 193-1). This allows a serial, standardized neurologic evaluation of a patient over time by either a nurse or a physician. The neurologic examination can be broken down into six major areas: (1) level of consciousness, (2) visual assessment, (3) motor function, (4) sensation and neglect, (5) cerebellar function, and (6) cranial nerves.

### Level of Consciousness

The patient's level of alertness should be evaluated by asking simple questions (birth date or month of the year) and by having the patient follow simple commands (close their eyes, make a fist). The patient may be alert, drowsy (requiring minor stimulation to answer or obey), lethargic (requiring repeated or painful stimulation to respond), or obtunded (postures or is totally unresponsive).

### Visual Assessment

Evaluation of visual fields and extraocular movements can give information regarding occipital lobe or brainstem lesions. Visual fields can be tested by confrontation, using finger counting, or visual threat as appropriate. Gaze palsy can be assessed by evaluating both voluntary and reflex (by turning the patient's head) horizontal eye movements.

### Motor Function

Upper extremity motor weakness is best determined by testing for pronator drift. Patients close their eyes and extend their arms with palms facing the ceiling. The test is positive if one arm pronates or drifts lower than the other within 10 s. Lower extremity strength can be similarly evaluated by the patient's ability to individually elevate each leg 45° for 5 s while lying in bed. For subtle signs of lower extremity weakness, observe the patients' gait or have them walk on their toes and then on their heels. Facial motor weakness (facial droop) due to a central nervous system lesion can be distinguished from a peripheral seventh nerve palsy (e.g., Bell's palsy) by the patient's ability to wrinkle the forehead on the affected side.

### Cerebellar Function

Cerebellar function can be tested by observing the patient's gait, finger-nose testing, heel-to-shin testing, and by having the patient stand with eyes closed and arms outstretched (Romberg test).

**Fig. 193-1.** National Institute of Health Stroke Scale. A rapid, reproducible neurologic evaluation of patients with stroke.

| | | | | |
|---|---|---|---|---|
| 1a. | Level of Consciousness (LOC) | Alert<br>Drowsy<br>Stuporous<br>Coma | 0<br>1<br>2<br>3 | |
| 1b. | LOC Questions | Answers both correctly<br>Answers one correctly<br>Incorrect | 0<br>1<br>2 | |
| 1c. | LOC Commands | Obeys both correctly<br>Obeys one correctly<br>Incorrect | 0<br>1<br>2 | |
| 2. | Pupillary Response | Both reactive<br>One reactive<br>Neither reactive | 0<br>1<br>2 | |
| 3. | Best Gaze | Normal<br>Partial gaze palsy<br>Forced deviation | 0<br>1<br>2 | |
| 4. | Best Visual | No visual loss<br>Partial hemianopsia<br>Complete hemianopsia | 0<br>1<br>2 | |
| 5. | Facial Palsy | Normal<br>Minor<br>Partial<br>Complete | 0<br>1<br>2<br>3 | |
| 6. | Best Motor Arm | No drift<br>Drift<br>Can't resist gravity<br>No effort against gravity | 0<br>1<br>2<br>3 | |
| 7. | Best Motor Leg | No drift<br>Drift<br>Can't resist gravity<br>No effort against gravity | 0<br>1<br>2<br>3 | |
| 8. | Plantar Reflex | Normal<br>Equivocal<br>Extensor<br>Bilateral extensor | 0<br>1<br>2<br>3 | |
| 9. | Limb Ataxia | Absent<br>Present in upper or lower<br>Present in both | 0<br>1<br>2 | |
| 10. | Sensory | Normal<br>Partial loss<br>Dense loss | 0<br>1<br>2 | |
| 11. | Neglect | No neglect<br>Partial neglect<br>Complete neglect | 0<br>1<br>2 | |
| 12. | Dysarthria | Normal articulation<br>Mild to moderate dysarthria<br>Near unintelligible or worse | 0<br>1<br>2 | |
| 13. | Best Language | No aphasia<br>Mild to moderate aphasia<br>Severe aphasia<br>Mute | 0<br>1<br>2<br>3 | |
| 14. | Change form Previous Exam | Same<br>Better<br>Worse | S<br>B<br>W | |
| 15. | Change from Baseline | Same<br>Better<br>Worse | S<br>B<br>W | |

## Sensation and Neglect

Sensory deficits and neglect should be evaluated by pin-prick testing, having the patient identify numbers gently written on the palm (graphesthesia), and by double-simultaneous extinction (the physician touches the patient's right and left limbs individually and then simultaneously). The double-simultaneous extinction test is positive if the patient feels the sensation in either limb individually but only on one side when touched simultaneously, and it suggests neglect. Neglect can be further confirmed by having the patient draw a box or house. Patients with neglect will often omit figures on one side of the drawing.

## Language

The terms *dysarthria* and *aphasia* are often erroneously interchanged. Dysarthria is a disturbance in articulation due to paralysis or incoordination of muscles used for speech. Dysarthric speech is often slurred. Subtle cases can be identified by having the patient repeat simple nursery rhymes. In contrast, aphasia is due to a disturbance in processing language (either written or spoken). Aphasia can be receptive (difficulty in comprehension), expressive (difficulty in communicating thoughts), or both. Receptive aphasia can be tested by having the patient follow simple commands (either vocal or written). An expressive aphasia is assessed by having the patient identify simple objects or describe what is happening in a magazine picture. A patient with expressive aphasia will use inappropriate words or use nonfluent sentences, whereas the words of a patient with dysarthria will be slurred.

### Cranial Nerves

Cranial nerves should be individually tested in all patients to identify possible brainstem involvement. Unlike anterior circulation strokes, which cause contralateral motor deficits, brainstem involvement causes ipsilateral cranial nerve deficits with contralateral motor weakness.

## STROKE SYNDROMES

After a complete history and physical examination the physician must integrate physical findings with brain anatomy and function to determine the anatomic location of the lesion and the possible vessels that may be involved. Physical findings often follow classical patterns that can assist the physician in localizing the lesion.

### Ischemic Stroke Syndromes

#### Dominant Hemispheric Infarction

In all right-handed patients and up to 80 percent of left-handed patients, the left hemisphere is the dominant hemisphere. A stroke involving the dominant hemisphere often presents with contralateral weakness and numbness, contralateral visual field cut, a gaze preference, dysarthria, and aphasia.

#### Nondominant Hemispheric Infarction

Strokes involving the nondominant hemisphere can similarly cause contralateral weakness, numbness, and visual field cuts. Patients with such strokes often neglect the contralateral extremities and fail to sense double-simultaneous stimulation on the contralateral side. Constructional apraxia can be demonstrated by the inability to draw a clock and fill in the appropriate numbers. Patients may be dysarthric but typically are not aphasic.

#### Middle Cerebral Artery Infarcts

Lesions of the middle cerebral artery are associated with contralateral sensory deficit and motor weakness, with the arm and face weaker than the leg. Patients often have an associated receptive and/or expressive aphasia if the dominant hemisphere is involved.

#### Anterior Cerebral Artery Infarct

In contrast to middle cerebral infarctions, lesions of the anterior cerebral artery cause leg weakness greater than arm weakness, mild contralateral cortical sensory deficit, and dyspraxia.

#### Vertebrobasilar Syndrome

The posterior circulation supplies blood to the brainstem, cerebellum, and visual cortex. Signs and symptoms attributable to a stroke in this distribution may be subtle. They include findings such as dizziness, vertigo, diplopia, dysphagia, ataxia, cranial nerve palsies, and bilateral limb weakness. The hallmark of posterior circulation stroke is crossed neurologic deficits (i.e., ipsilateral cranial nerve deficits with contralateral motor weakness).

### Basilar Artery Occlusion

Occlusion of the basilar artery causes severe quadriplegia, coma, and the locked-in syndrome. The locked-in syndrome occurs with lesions in the pontine tectum, causing complete muscle paralysis except for upward gaze.

### Transient Ischemic Attack

A TIA is a neurologic deficit that resolves within 24 h (although most resolve within 30 min) and is most commonly associated with thrombotic strokes. The incidence of prior TIAs is 50 to 75 percent in patients with subsequent thrombotic, extracranial carotid artery strokes but only 10 percent in all other stroke types. TIAs have been thought to cause reversible brain injury; however, recent studies indicate that over 60 percent may be associated with computed tomography (CT) findings of infarction. The true significance of TIAs is that they are associated with a 5 to 6 percent risk of stroke per year.

### Lacunar Infarct

Lacunar infarcts are pure motor or sensory deficits that are due to infarction of small penetrating arteries and are commonly associated with chronic hypertension. Lesions are primarily located in the pons and the basal ganglia.

### Arterial Dissection

Dissections are often associated with severe trauma but can occur from such mild events as turning the head sharply. Patients may complain of severe neck pain or headache hours to days prior to onset of neurologic deficits. Dissections may occur in the carotid or vertebral circulation.

### Hemorrhagic Syndromes

#### Intracerebral Hemorrhage

Intracerebral hemorrhage may be clinically indistinguishable from cerebral infarction. Intracerebral hemorrhage also presents with contralateral hemiplegia, hemianesthesia, hemianopsia, and aphasia or neglect (depending on the hemisphere involved). The presentation may differ from infarction in that the patients are more commonly lethargic and have marked hypertension. Headache, nausea, and vomiting often precede the neurologic deficit. Patients can quickly deteriorate and require emergent intubation. Bleeding is usually localized to the putamen, thalamus, pons, or cerebellum (in decreasing frequency) in patients with hypertensive intracerebral hemorrhage. Lobar hemorrhages are suggestive of amyloid angiopathy and are associated with a better prognosis than are deep hypertensive bleeds.

#### Cerebellar Hemorrhage

A patient presenting with sudden onset of dizziness, vomiting, marked truncal ataxia, and inability to walk must be immediately suspected of having a cerebellar infarction or hemorrhage. These findings may be associated with gaze palsies and increasing stupor. Patients may rapidly progress to coma and herniation unless surgical decompression and/or hematoma evacuation are quickly initiated.

#### Subarachnoid Hemorrhage

SAH occurs more commonly in women, but men dominate in the age group below 40 years. Patients present with sudden onset of a severe constant headache that is often occipital or nuchal in location. A recent history of a "sentinel hemorrhage" with a severe headache lasting for days can be obtained in 15 to 31 percent of cases. Vomiting often presents with the onset of headache, and the patient may be noted to have a decreased level of consciousness. Neurologic deficits may be present due to the aneurysm compressing adjacent brain tis-

**Table 193-1.** Hunt and Hess Classification of Subarachnoid
Hemorrhage

| Classification | Symptoms |
|---|---|
| Grade I | Asymptomatic or minimal headache and mild nuchal rigidity |
| Grade II | Moderate to severe headache, nuchal rigidity, no neurologic deficit other than cranial-nerve palsy |
| Grade III | Drowsiness, confusion, or mild focal deficit |
| Grade IV | Stupor, moderate to severe hemiparesis, possible early decerebrate rigidity, and vegetative disturbance |
| Grade V | Deep coma, decerebrate rigidity, moribund appearance |

sue or cranial nerves. A grading classification based on neurologic
condition can aid in determining eligibility for surgery and prognosis
(see Table 193-1).

## DIFFERENTIAL DIAGNOSIS

Although strokes are the most common cause of unilateral weakness,
other causes must be considered (see Table 193-2). All patients with
neurologic deficits should have their blood sugar checked to rule out
hypoglycemia. Bell's palsy (peripheral seventh cranial nerve palsy)
usually occurs in younger patients, is associated with upper and lower
facial paralysis, and does not involve the extremities. Evidence of
trauma should be sought since an epidural or subdural hematoma can
mimic an acute stroke. Although stroke can present with marked hypertension, one can usually differentiate stroke from hypertensive encephalopathy by history and physical examination. Unlike stroke, the
onset of hypertensive encephalopathy is more gradual, and focal neurologic deficits, if present, are superimposed upon global cerebral
dysfunction (e.g., decreased level of consciousness), rather than isolated to one brain region. Papilledema, flame-shaped retinal hemorrhages, and acute renal failure are all indicative of hypertensive encephalopathy. Other diseases that may mimic the mental status
changes of stroke include diabetic ketoacidosis, hyperosmotic coma,
and meningoencephalitis.

## DIAGNOSTIC TESTS

Although clinical data can direct the physician toward the diagnosis
of stroke, including the cause and location of the lesion, diagnostic
tests are often required to confirm these suspicions and to rule out
other causes of the deficits. Tests that may require immediate emergency department interventions include a blood sugar determination,
CT, and an ECG. A blood sugar determination should be obtained
early (by prehospital providers if possible) to rule out hypoglycemia
as the cause of the neurologic deficit. 50% dextrose should be given
immediately in any patient with neurologic deficit and hypoglycemia.

An emergent noncontrast CT of the head is essential since it can
quickly differentiate ischemic from hemorrhagic infarction. This information is crucial for subsequent therapeutic decisions. CT can
identify almost all parenchymal bleeds greater than 1 cm and up to 95
percent of all subarachnoid hemorrhages. A lumbar puncture is required in all patients suspected of having SAH when the CT scan is
normal. Most ischemic strokes will not be visualized by routine CT

**Table 193-2.** Differential Diagnosis of Acute Stroke

Hypoglycemia
Postictal paralysis (Todd's paralysis)
Bell's palsy
Hypertensive encephalopathy
Epidural/subdural hematoma
Brain tumor/abscess
Complicated migraine
Encephalitis
Diabetic ketoacidosis
Hyperosmotic coma
Meningoencephalitis

for at least 6 h and often considerably longer, depending on the size
of the infarct. In addition to distinguishing ischemia from hemorrhage, CT can also rule out other life-threatening processes such as
abscess, tumor, and subdural or epidural hematoma.

An ECG should be obtained to rule out an associated cardiac cause
of the stroke. Atrial fibrillation and acute myocardial infarction are
associated with up to 60 percent of all cardioembolic strokes. Untreated chronic atrial fibrillation may increase the risk of stroke up to
6 percent yearly. In addition, stroke occurrence is 2.5 percent in patients with acute myocardial infarction within the first 4 weeks of
their cardiac event.

Blood tests that may be helpful include a complete blood count
with platelet count, coagulation studies, toxic screen, and cardiac enzymes. A hematocrit can identify abnormalities in blood viscosity.
Elevated blood viscosity, even when hematocrit levels are not frankly
polycythemic, can affect blood flow and prognosis. A platelet count
can identify thrombocytosis or thrombocytopenia that may precipitate
thrombosis or hemorrhage. Coagulation studies are especially helpful
in patients with hemorrhagic stroke to rule out coagulopathy or excessive anticoagulation with warfarin. A toxic screen to rule out cocaine or amphetamine use should be obtained in patients with either
ischemic or hemorrhagic stroke in which substance abuse is suspected. Although of minimal use in the emergency department, cardiac enzymes will assist inpatient evaluation for a possible myocardial infarction.

Other diagnostic tests that may be of assistance, depending upon
the circumstances, include an echocardiogram, carotid duplex scanning, angiogram, and a magnetic resonance imaging (MRI) or magnetic resonance imaging angiography (MRA). An echocardiogram
can identify a mural thrombus, tumor, or valvular vegetation in patients with a suspected cardioembolic stroke. Carotid duplex scanning
may be helpful in patients with worsening neurologic deficit or
crescendo TIAs with known or suspected high-grade carotid stenosis.
Such patients may be candidates for emergent carotid endarterectomy
or heparinization. Carotid duplex scanning can accurately identify
carotid stenosis of greater than 60 percent, but an angiogram is required to distinguish 95 percent stenosis from complete occlusion.

Angiography is the definitive test to demonstrate stenosis or occlusion of both large and small blood vessels of the head and neck. It
can detect subtle arterial abnormalities, such as dissection, which
may be missed with other imaging techniques. Angiography is the
"gold standard" for demonstrating the cause of subarachnoid hemorrhage and for defining the anatomical relationships of aneurysms.
The use of angiography has been limited by its cost, availability, and
invasiveness.

MRI currently has a marginal role in the emergency department
evaluation of stroke. MRI will visualize ischemic infarcts earlier than
CT and is more effective than CT at identifying acute posterior circulation strokes. However, it is less accurate at differentiating ischemia
from hemorrhage. MRA allows demonstration of large vessel occlusions at the base of the skull, but small intracranial vascular occlusion
may not be readily apparent. Improvement in MRA speed and resolution may allow greater use of this technology, and MRAs may replace the need for angiograms in the future.

## TREATMENT

Few therapeutic interventions have proven to be beneficial in stroke.
Until large randomized studies are completed, treatment must be
based on personal experience and published reports. In the following
section, management guidelines are given based on the current stroke
literature.

### General Approach to Treatment of Ischemic Stroke

Priority should be given to airway and oxygenation in patients with
ischemic stroke. Patients should be placed on oxygen, the head of the

bed should be slightly elevated, and a monitor and intravenous line should be established. Fluids should be administered judiciously to prevent cerebral edema unless there is hypotension. Dehydration in the patient with ischemic stroke should be treated promptly as it may contribute to decreased cerebral blood flow in the ischemic region. Dextrose-containing solutions should be avoided in patients suspected of having a stroke except in those with proven hypoglycemia. Hyperglycemia has been associated with an increase in infarct volume and poor long-term outcome.

Emergency physicians should take a cautious approach to the management of elevated blood pressure in patients with acute ischemic stroke. Only severe hypertension (≥220 mm Hg systolic or ≥120 mm Hg diastolic) should be treated. Pharmacologic lowering of systemic blood pressure may reduce perfusion to the penumbra, converting an area with reversible injury to an area of infarction. Numerous clinical case series have reported neurologic deterioration immediately following iatrogenic reduction of blood pressure. In contrast, elevating blood pressure by means of vasopressors may be indicated in patients with ischemic stroke and relative hypotension.

The use of anticonvulsants for seizure prophylaxis in ischemic stroke is not recommended. If seizures occur, the patient should be treated acutely with benzodiazepines and then given a loading dose of phenytoin, 20 mg/kg IV at 25 mg/min.

### Transient Ischemic Attacks

Though the effectiveness of heparin is unproven in the management of acute stroke, it should considered in patients with recent TIAs who are at high risk for recurrence. These include patients with: (1) known high-grade stenosis in the appropriate vascular distribution for the symptoms, (2) a cardioembolic source, (3) TIAs of increasing frequency (crescendo TIAs), and (4) TIAs despite antiplatelet therapy.

Urgent carotid endarterectomy should be considered for TIAs that resolve within the first 6 h but that are associated with 70 to 99 percent stenosis of the appropriate carotid artery. Endarterectomy has been shown to significantly reduce the risk of future strokes in these patients with anterior circulation TIAs.

### Embolic Stroke

Patients with embolic stroke who have minor deficits should be anticoagulated. About 10 to 15 percent of recurrent emboli occur within 2 weeks of the initial event, some within 24 h. Anticoagulation with heparin should be withheld for 3 to 4 days following large cardioembolic stroke, due to the increased risk of spontaneous hemorrhagic changes associated with heparin in these types of strokes.

### Thrombotic Stroke

Treatment for stable completed thrombotic stroke is largely supportive. Anticoagulation has not proved beneficial and should not be used in patients with completed strokes. Large randomized stroke trials studying the efficacy of thrombolytic therapy within 3 to 6 h of symptom onset are currently underway and appear promising. Immediate heparinization should be considered in patients with stuttering or progressively worsening symptoms.

Emergency thrombectomy or endarterectomy in patients with persistent neurologic deficit due to cerebral ischemia is controversial and unproven. Some authors suggest that emergency surgery should be considered for progressive stroke in the extracranial anterior circulation where there are favorable angiographic findings such as stenosis greater than 90 percent, carotid dissection or aortic aneurysm, or intraluminal clot attached to a plaque.

Use of agents that prevent platelet aggregation, such as aspirin and ticlopidine, has been suggested for acute treatment of recent stroke. It is unlikely that these agents would be effective if given in the first few hours after a stroke, but they may be useful in preventing strokes in patients with TIAs and small strokes when given chronically.

### Vertebrobasilar Infarction

Unfortunately, no study definitively establishes the advantages or disadvantages of a specific therapy for patients with acute, well-defined, occlusive vascular disease within the posterior circulation. Published studies are either small or not randomized. Most authors suggest the use of heparin in patients with posterior circulation TIAs or progressive vertebrobasilar strokes.

### Cerebellar Infarction

Early neurosurgical consultation is needed in all patients with cerebellar infarction. Cerebellar swelling can lead to rapid deterioration with herniation. Neurosurgical consultation is required to determine the need for emergency posterior fossa decompression in these patients.

## General Approach to Hemorrhagic Stroke

After appropriate attention to the ABCs, early management of hemorrhagic stroke should focus on regulation of blood pressure, control of brain edema, and prompt neurosurgical evaluation.

### Intracerebral Hemorrhage

To date there are no large randomized studies evaluating the appropriate management of blood pressure in intracerebral hemorrhage. Current published recommendations are that only severe hypertension (i.e., ≥200 mm Hg systolic or >120 mm Hg diastolic) be treated. When treated, blood pressure should be lowered gradually to prehemorrhage levels using either labetalol or nitroprusside. The exceptions to this rule are cases of intracerebral hemorrhage associated with cardiac failure or arterial dissection, in which more rapid reduction is required. If a patient is known to have chronic hypertension, the blood pressure should not be lowered to normotensive levels but rather to an approximation of the patient's usual hypertensive blood pressure.

The use of hyperventilation, mannitol, and furosemide is recommended in patients with evidence of increased intracranial pressure with features such as mass effect, midline shift, or herniation.

The role of acute surgical intervention remains controversial and is dependent on the neurologic status of the patient as well as the size and location of the hemorrhage. Surgical decompression and hematoma evacuation are strongly recommended in patients with cerebellar hematomas greater than 3 cm diameter or those near the brainstem.

### Subarachnoid Hemorrhage

Rebleeding and vasospasm are the major morbid complications in SAH. Risk of rebleeding is greatest in the first 24 h. Lowering systolic blood pressure to 160 mm Hg and/or maintaining a mean arterial pressure of 110 mm Hg has been associated with lower risk of rebleeding and decreased mortality. Current recommendations are that blood pressure should be maintained at prehemorrhage levels.

Cerebral ischemia due to vasospasm occurs from 2 days to 3 weeks after aneurysm rupture. Nimodipine, given orally 60 mg every 6 h, has been found to reduce the incidence and severity of vasospasm and should be given to all patients with SAH who are in good neurologic condition (grades I to III). Preliminary studies indicate that trilazad mesylate may also be beneficial in patients with SAH.

Seizures and persistent vomiting can cause elevations in systemic and intracranial pressure. Phenytoin loading is recommended as prophylaxis against seizures. Nausea and vomiting should be promptly treated with antiemetics.

Usually, candidates for early angiography and surgical intervention are stable patients with good neurologic condition (Hunt and Hess grades 1 to 3). However, there is little published evidence that this regimen reduces long-term morbidity or mortality.

## ADMISSION GUIDELINES

All patients with new onset strokes should be admitted for further evaluation, education, and early rehabilitation. Patients with anterior circulation strokes should be evaluated for surgically correctable lesions and observed for any progression in their symptoms that may require anticoagulation. Patients with vertebrobasilar strokes should be admitted for heparinization and observation.

Patients with new onset TIAs should be admitted for evaluation of possible cardiac source of TIAs or high-grade stenosis in the carotid arteries. The incidence of stroke after TIA may be as high as 20 to 25 percent in the first year, with the highest incidence in the first month. Because of the proven efficacy of carotid endarterectomy, patients should be admitted unless high-grade stenosis of the carotid artery can be ruled out.

Patients with a prior history of an anterior circulation stroke who have been previously studied, who present with a minor, completed (>24-h old), recurrent stroke or TIA, and who have a reliable support system may be discharged home after an appropriate emergency department workup. The use of aspirin or ticlopidine should be discussed with the family physician or neurologist, and follow-up within 48 h should be arranged. The patient and family members should be given clear instructions to return for further medical treatment if the patient experiences worsening of symptoms.

## BIBLIOGRAPHY

American Heart Association: *Heart and Stroke Facts:* 1994 Statistical Supplement.

Barnett HJM: *Stroke: Pathophysiology, Diagnosis, and Management,* 2d ed. New York, Churchill Livingston, 1992.

Bogousslausky J, Van Melle G, Regli F: The Lausanne Stroke Registry of 1000 consecutive patients with first stroke. *Stroke* 15:249, 1984.

Broderick JP: Population-based natural history of primary intracerebral hemorrhage, in Whisnant JP (ed): *Stroke: Populations, Cohorts and Clinical Trials.* Oxford, Butterworth-Heinemann, 1993.

Brott T, Adams HP, Olinger CP, et al: Measurements of acute cerebral infarction: A clinical examination scale. *Stroke* 20:864, 1989.

Brott T, Broderick JP: Intracerebral hemorrhage. *Heart Dis Stroke* 2:59, 1993.

Caplan LR: *Stroke: A Clinical Approach,* 2d ed. Stoneham, MA, Butterworth-Heinemann, 1993.

Caplan LR, Hier D, D'Cruz I: Cerebral embolism in the Michael Registry. *Stroke* 14:530, 1983.

Duke RJ, Bloch RF, Turpia AG, et al: Intravenous heparin for the prevention of stroke progression in acute partial stable stroke. *Ann Intern Med* 105:825, 1986.

European Carotid Surgery Trialists' Collaborative Group: MRC European carotid surgery trial: Interim results for symptomatic patients with severe (70–99%) or with mild (0–29%) carotid stenosis. *Lancet* 337:1235, 1991.

Fieschi C, Argentino C, Lenzi GL, et al: Clinical and instrumental evaluation of patients with ischemic stroke within the first six hours. *J Neurol Sci* 91:311, 1989.

Hier DB, Babcock DJ, Foulkes MA, et al: Influence of site on course of intracerebral hemorrhage. *Stroke Cerebrovasc Dis* 3:65, 1993.

Kase CS: Diagnosis and management of intracerebral hemorrhage in elderly patients. *Clin Geriatric Med* 7:549, 1991.

Kassell NJ, Torner J, Haley EC Jr, et al: The international cooperative study on the timing of aneurysm surgery. Part I: Overall management results. *J Neurosurg* 73:18, 1990.

Matsumoto N, Whisnant J, Kurland L, et al: Natural history of stroke in Rochester, Minnesota, 1955–1969. *Stroke* 4:20, 1973.

Mohr J, Caplan LR, Melski J, et al: The Harvard Cooperative Stroke Registry: A prospective registry of patients hospitalized with stroke. *Neurology* 28:754, 1978.

National Stroke Association: Early treatment of acute ischemic stroke. *Stroke Clinical Updates* 1:5, 1990.

National Stroke Association Consensus Statement: Stroke: The first six hours. *Stroke Clinical Updates* 4:1, 1993.

National Stroke Association: Acute stroke management: Part III. *Stroke Clinical Updates* 4:13, 1993.

National Stroke Association: Acute stroke management: Diagnosis (part I.) *Stroke Clinical Updates* 3:17, 1993.

National Stroke Association: Acute stroke management: Part II. *Stroke Clinical Updates* 3:21, 1993.

Powers WJ: Acute hypertension after stroke: The scientific basis for treatment decisions. *Neurology* 43:461, 1993.

Sacco R, Wolf PA, Bharncho NF: Subarachnoid and intracerebral hemorrhage: Natural history, prognosis, and precursive factors in the Framingham Study. *Neurology* 34:847, 1984.

Whisnant J, Fitzgibbons J, Kurland L, et al: Natural history of stroke in Rochester, Minnesota, 1945–1954. *Stroke* 2:11, 1971.

# 194
# VERTIGO AND DIZZINESS
## Neal Little

Complaints of dizziness and light-headedness are among the most common in emergency medicine, and their evaluation can test the problem-solving ability of the physician. Dizziness itself may not be life-threatening, but it is usually bothersome and potentially disabling. The primary challenge to the emergency physician is establishing what a given patient means by "dizziness," which is an ambiguous, nonmedical, subjective term that derives from the old English word *dysig,* meaning *foolish* or *stupid.* It may be used to articulate a sensation of weakness, unsteadiness, giddiness, malaise, instability, swimming in the head, faintness or near faintness, or a disturbance of mentation. A variety of disorders affecting the central nervous system, ears, cardiovascular system, eyes, and psyche may all produce dizziness, and thus a systematic approach is imperative.

*Vertigo* is used to refer to an illusion of motion where no motion exists and derives from the Latin *vertere,* meaning *to turn.* Either the patient or the environment seems to be moving. Movement is classically described as spinning or whirling, but may also be described as rocking, staggering, or swaying, or as a sensation of "impulsion," where the person feels as though he or she is being pulled to one side or to the ground as if by a magnet. The distinction between a feeling that the patient is moving versus a feeling that the environment is moving (subjective versus objective vertigo) is not useful. Oscillopsia, a visual illusion that objects in the environment are moving, may occur.

*Syncope* means a transient loss of consciousness, with rapid return to normal, on the basis of diminished cerebral blood flow, oxygen, or glucose. *Near syncope* is an impending loss of consciousness, or a "gray-out" feeling.

*Disequilibrium* refers to a feeling of imbalance or unsteadiness while walking. When the subjective complaint of dizziness is not well defined and cannot be classified as vertigo or near syncope, the term ill-defined dizziness is often used.

## PATHOPHYSIOLOGY

Spatial orientation is determined by the interaction between the visual, labyrinthine, and proprioceptive systems and the integration of impulses by the central nervous system. Dysfunction in either the pathways that integrate those systems or the sensors themselves may be the cause of disordered sensations of spatial orientation, position, and motion.

The visual system, consisting of the eyes, the optic pathways, and the visual cortex create for the person a visual-spatial orientation. The labyrinthine system consists of the otoliths, which primarily produce an orientation to gravity, and the semicircular canals, which produce an orientation to movement or the tilt of the head. The semicircular canals are filled with fluid and lined by hair cells. Movement of the fluid causes movement of the hair cells, which results in a change in afferent vestibular nerve impulses. There is a balanced vestibular neuronal input to the brain stem from both vestibular nerves. Alteration of input from one is perceived as motion. The proprioceptors in the joints and muscles of limbs and neck relate movement and the tilt of the head to that of the body and also sense body position when lying, walking, or sitting.

The integrative structures involved in mediating the sensory input from the receptor systems are the cerebellum, the brain stem (primarily the vestibular nuclei and the medial longitudinal fasciculus), the basal ganglia (red nuclei), and the cerebral cortex (superior temporal gyrus and parietal lobes). Dizziness can occur as a result of dysfunction in one or all of the receptor systems or the mediating structures.

The pathophysiologic mechanisms that can affect these structures include all of the processes which affect the nervous system in general, including vascular, metabolic-nutritional, toxic, neuronal, and psychogenic.

Age-related changes that can contribute to dizziness or vertigo include diminished labyrinthine hair cells, diminished labyrinthine nerve fibers, diminished visual, auditory, and proprioceptive sensations, and diminished integrative abilities.

Nystagmus due to injury to the vestibular system is a to-and-fro movement of the eyes that has a slow component (due to vestibular-ocular reflex) and a fast component. It is named for the fast component. Excitation of one semicircular canal produces eye movement away from that canal (vestibular-ocular reflex). The cortex exerts a quick corrective movement in the opposite direction, resulting in nystagmus. Ocular fixation tends to suppress nystagmus of peripheral vestibular origin. The normally balanced input from the semicircular canals of both ears results in no net eye movement. Most peripheral (vestibular) disorders result in inhibition of one more semicircular canals, and thus nystagmus beating with the quick phase away from the affected ear. Patients with peripheral vertigo feel that the environment is spinning in the direction of the fast component, or that their bodies are spinning in the direction of the slow component. Vestibular nystagmus occurs in the plane of the affected semicircular canal and may be either horizontal or torsional-vertical. Strictly vertical nystagmus is rarely the result of vestibular involvement and usually points to a brain stem origin. It is normal to have a few beats of nystagmus on extreme lateral gaze.

## ETIOLOGY AND CLINICAL MANIFESTATIONS

The major characteristics of central and peripheral vertigo are given in Table 194-1. The etiologies of vertigo are classically separated into

**Table 194-1.** Characteristics of Vertigo

Peripheral origin
  Intense spinning, swaying or impulsion
  Nausea, vomiting, possibly diarrhea
  Diaphoresis
  Aggravated by change of position, movement
  Possible tinnitus, hearing loss
  Acute onset
  Fatiguable, unidirectional nystagmus
  Nystagmus inhibited by ocular fixation
Central origin
  Ill-defined, less intense vertigo
  Not positionally related, concomitant brain stem or cerebellar signs and
    symptoms (diplopia, dysphagia, facial numbness or weakness, ataxia,
    hemiparesis)
  Nystagmus not inhibited by ocular fixation
  Nonfatiguable, multidirectional nystagmus

*peripheral vertigo,* which is caused by disease processes affecting structures peripheral to the brain stem (eighth nerve, vestibular apparatus), and *central vertigo,* which is caused by processes affecting structures central to the brain stem (cerebellum).

Associated symptoms leading away from a vestibular disturbance include headache, loss of consciousness and neurologic symptons including seizures.

## Disorders Causing Peripheral Vertigo

The vast majority of patients with vertigo seen in emergency practice have peripheral vertigo. Peripheral vertigo is characterized by an intense vertiginous or whirling feeling, often accompanied by profound associated symptoms such as nausea, vomiting, sweating, pallor, diarrhea, and alteration of blood pressure and pulse. Impulsion is very strongly suggestive of peripheral vertigo. These symptoms may be of abrupt onset. Peripheral vertigo may be dramatically influenced by position change, greatly worsened by movement or by the assumption of certain positions of the head, and is extremely distressing to the patient. The symptoms of patients with peripheral vertigo resemble those of classic motion sickness.

## Vestibular Neuronitis

Vestibular neuronitis is characterized by peripheral vertigo without hearing loss. If tests of cochlear function are done, they show no abnormality. Patients may complain of fullness in the ear or tinnitus. Positional nystagmus occurs in one-third of cases. Caloric vestibular testing is usually abnormal on one side. This illness is of suspected viral origin and may occur in epidemics. It may be a mild viral encephalitis affecting the brain stem or a neuronitis affecting the vestibular nerve. The exact site of the lesion is not known. Patients typically complain of acute onset and severe symptoms and may have had an upper respiratory infection in the preceeding two to three weeks. The vertigo is worsened by any movement of the head. It may last for days, and residual symptoms may persist for weeks. Most cases of casually diagnosed labyrinthitis probably fall into this category.

## Labyrinthitis

Labyrinthitis is characterized by peripheral vertigo associated with hearing loss. While the etiology of many cases of labyrinthitis is a presumed viral infection, there is no proof of this. Occasional cases occur in association with mumps and measles. Bacterial labyrinthitis is an extremely rare condition usually associated with long-standing otitis media with fistula, meningitis, mastoid disease, dermoid tumor, or postsurgical infection. Bacterial labyrinthitis is potentially devastating and requires appropriate antibiotic therapy.

If there is a perilympathic leak from a fistula at the round or oval window, pneumatic changes in the middle ear may be transmitted to the labyrinthine apparatus and cause subjective vertigo. This may occur as a result of trauma. Patients with perilymphatic fistula complain of intermittent or positional vertigo exacerbated by straining, sneezing, and coughing, which may also cause such a fistula. Fluctuating hearing loss occurs. Hennebert's sign, which is subjective vertigo and nystagmus induced by pneumatic otoscopy, is diagnostic.

Menière's disease is a condition characterized by recurrent attacks of severe vertigo, vomiting, and prostration, and usually associated with progressive deafness and tinnitus. It tends to run a recurrent and protracted course over time associated with less severe attacks of vertigo and progressively more severe deafness. It occurs in middle age, and in men and women equally. While little is known about the underlying etiology, there is a gross dilatation of the endolymphatic system of the internal ear.

The typical history in Menière's disease is that of a patient over the age of 50 with slowly progressive tinnitus and deafness in one or rarely both ears over months to years who suddenly develops severe vertigo. It may occur so suddenly that the patient falls. More commonly, it worsens over several minutes. There is an intense sensation of rotation, more commonly of the surroundings than of the patient. nausea and vomiting are common and may be severe. The pulse may be rapid or slow, and the blood pressure raised or lowered. Occasionally patients may develop diarrhea. There may be profound diaphoresis. Preexisting deafness and tinnitus, usually unilateral, may become intensified. The attack may last from half an hour to many hours with gradual offset. The patient is frequently unable to stand or walk and may be unsteady and staggering on attempted ambulation. Between attacks, deafness, usually unilateral, is found. The attacks often occur at regular intervals separated by weeks to years. The severity of the attacks tends to diminish and finally cease as deafness increases. A similar picture may be produced by tertiary syphilis. Tumors at the cerebellopontine angle, such as acoustic schwannoma, may produce progressive unilateral hearing loss and vertigo and simulate Menière's disease.

### Drug Effects

A variety of drugs affect the inner ear. Most affect both vestibular and cochlear mechanisms, but the degree to which they affect them is variable. Aspirin in toxic doses affects predominantly cochlear function and produces tinnitus and hearing loss, but little vertigo. Aminoglycosides may produce vestibular neuroepithelial damage before any cochlear damage is evident. Anticonvulsants such as phenytoin may produce exclusively vestibular symptoms. Drugs which affect the inner ear are listed in Table 194-2.

### Benign Positional Vertigo

Benign positional vertigo is a syndrome in which patients have repeated attacks of vertigo precipitated by changes in posture, typically a sudden turning of the head as in rolling over in bed. There is no acute hearing loss or tinnitus. It is a very common cause of vertigo, and the most common cause in the elderly. The attacks usually last a few seconds to minutes, and usually subside within a few weeks. Nylen-Barany (Hallpike) testing is diagnostic, and distinguishes between peripheral and central vertigo (Table 194-3). Some patients with positional vertigo may not have nystagmus elicited on exam. Benign positional vertigo is also known as Barany's vertigo, and is thought to result from calcium carbonate crystals which have detached from the otoconia of the utricle and fallen against the cupula of the posterior semicircular canal.

### Eighth-Nerve Lesions

Eighth-nerve lesions, such as acoustic schwannomas or meningiomas, may affect the eighth nerve and produce vertigo. Typically,

**Table 194-2.** Drugs and Chemicals Affecting the Inner Ear

| Antibiotics | Cytotoxic agents |
|---|---|
| Aminoglycosides | Vinblastine |
| Erythromycin | Cisplatin |
| Minocycline | Nitrogen mustard |
| Diuretics | Anticonvulsants |
| Ethacrinic acid | Phenytoin |
| Furosemide | Barbiturates |
| Bumetanide | Carbamazepine |
| Nonsteroidal anti-inflamma- | Ethosuccimide |
| tory agents | Others |
| Salicylates | Quinine |
| Ibuprofen | Chloroquine |
| Naproxen | Propylene glycol |
| Indomethacin | Ethanol |
| | Methanol |
| | Mercury |

**Table 194-3.** Nylen-Barany (Hallpike) Maneuver

*Test:* Patient is in sitting position on stretcher. Clinician supports head and has patient rapidly assume supine position, first with head straight, then with head turned 45 degrees left, then 45 degrees right.
Findings with peripheral vertigo:
  Vertigo and nystagmus produced, latency 2–20 s
  Duration less than 1 min
  Unidirectional nystagmus
  Nystagmus and vertigo fatigue with repeated testing
  Even straight head position may elicit vertigo (Barany's)
Findings with central vertigo
  Latency of nystagmus, none
  Nystagmus nonfatiguing, multidirectional
  Duration greater than 1 min

this gradual-onset vertigo is preceded by hearing loss, and there may be other symptoms to suggest involvement of the cerebellopontine (CP) angle, such as a constant unsteadiness or ataxia and a chronically progressive course. Patients typically complain more of unsteadiness than vertigo. Patients with unilateral sensorineural hearing loss, including those who seem to have Menière's disease, should be evaluated for cerebellopontine angle tumor.

### Cerebellopontine Angle Tumor

Many patients with tumors at the CP angle, such as meningiomas and dermoids, exhibit chronic deafness and disequilibrium, and occasionally vertigo. They may demonstrate ipsilateral impairment of the corneal reflex, facial weakness, and cerebellar signs on the involved side.

### Posttraumatic Vertigo

The delicate labyrinthine membranes are susceptible to accelerational forces, and head trauma may result in unilateral contusion or concussion to the labyrinth. After cerebral concussion, up to 20 percent of people develop vertigo. *Acute posttraumatic vertigo* caused by labyrinthine concussion begins immediately after head injury and results in continuous vertigo, nausea, and vomiting. Symptoms usually improve over the first few days, with gradual resolution over a few weeks. *Posttraumatic positional vertigo* may develop days to weeks after injury, and may replace the constant vertigo of acute posttraumatic vertigo. Symptoms are precipitated by changes in head position, as with benign positional vertigo. Symptoms tend to resolve over months, and most are gone by 2 years post injury.

### Benign Paroxysmal Vertigo of Childhood

A condition of severe brief attacks of vertigo in children, usually under the age of 3 years, benign paroxysmal vertigo of childhood, is generally self-limited, resolving spontaneously within months to a few years. It is felt to be labyrinthine in origin and of unknown etiology. Because vertigo may represent the aura of a seizure, EEG might be considered in very selected cases of childhood vertigo.

## Disorders Causing Central Vertigo

Central vertigo is characterized symptomatically by a much less dramatic vertiginous feeling than peripheral vertigo and is not exacerbated by motion or by assuming specific positions. Typically, central vertigo is not an intense feeling, and has little or no associated nausea, vomiting, pallor, or diaphoresis. The onset is gradual. The nystagmus characteristic of central vertigo may be present in the absence of the subjective sensation of vertigo. Central vertigo is produced by conditions that affect the cerebellum and brain stem. All conditions that affect the brain stem and cause vertigo typically have other brain stem signs associated with them, such as dysphagia, dysarthria, ataxia, diplopia, facial numbness, bilateral limb weakness, or bilateral visual blurring. Oscillopsia may occur.

Conditions producing central vertigo affect the brain stem and cerebellum. Hearing is characteristically unimpaired, and tinnitus is rare. Cerebellar infarction and hemorrhage may result in central vertigo. The typical history of cerebellar hemorrhage is acute vertigo and ataxia, with or without nausea and vomiting, and with or without acute headache. Less typically there may be conjugate eye deviation to the side opposite the hemorrhage, or a sixth-nerve palsy. The patient with cerebellar hemorrhage may not be able to sit without support, although casual neurologic testing done only in the supine position or a supported position may not be abnormal. Cerebellar infarction may present in a similar fashion. Vertigo from cerebellar disease may be described as recurrent front-to-back or side-to-side movement, which may be evoked by position change.

Conditions affecting the brain stem can produce vertigo as part of their clinical symptomatology, particularly lateral medullary infarction (Wallenberg's syndrome), which consists of vertigo; ipsilateral paralysis of the soft palate, pharynx, and larynx with dysphagia and dysphonia; ipsilateral facial numbness with loss of corneal reflex; ipsilateral Horner's syndrome; and ipsilateral cerebellar asynergia and hypotonia. Sixth-, seventh-, and eighth-nerve lesions have been reported with vertigo, nausea and vomiting, nystagmus, and hiccups. There is contralateral loss of pain and temperature on the limbs and trunk.

Transient ischemic attacks affecting the brain stem may produce similar short-lasting symptoms and positional nystagmus, but by definition must include more than simply vertigo. Other structures in the brain stem must be affected in order to render the diagnosis.

Neoplasms of the fourth ventricle, typically ependymomas in young patients and metastases in elderly patients, can likewise affect the brain stem.

Multiple sclerosis, with its myriad manifestations, may produce isolated lesions in the brain stem, producing vertigo and other brain stem findings. Marked nystagmus with little no vertigo should suggest a brain stem origin.

## Miscellaneous Causes of Vertigo

Physiologic vertigo, as in motion sickness, results from mismatched vestibular, visual, and somatosensory input. Similar mismatch may occur when the visual sensation of motion, as in watching a movie of an automobile chase, is not accompanied by matching vestibular input.

Vertigo may occur on a psychogenic basis, typically as a longstanding vertiginous feeling unaffected by motion and position and without associated nausea or vomiting. As a prodrome to seizure, a cortical focus may produce transient vertigo prior to the seizure. This is very rare. Rare ocular causes of vertigo include watching a rapidly moving series of objects, such as the car or train from a stationary position or telephone poles from a moving car, inducing a sensation of vertigo and motion sickness. Recent ophthalmoplegia may cause brief vertigo. Serous labyrinthitis due to otitis media may produce vertigo.

The blood supply to the inner ear is not supported by a collateral circulation, and is tenuous. However, direct evidence for reduced blood flow to the inner ear as a cause of vertigo is lacking. While it is postulated that vertigo may occur as a result of imbalanced proprioceptive input due to cervical muscle lesions, its clinical occurrence is doubtful. Basilar migraine may cause throbbing occipital headache, visual hallucinations, vertigo, tinnitus, dysarthria, and drop attacks. Patients with herpetic vesicles of the auditory canal and fascial palsy ("Ramsay Hunt" syndrome) may have deafness and vertigo.

## Disequilibrium Syndrome

Disequilibrium syndrome consists of an ill-defined dizziness as a result of multiple sensory abnormalities. There is a chronic mismatch of input from the body systems providing spatial orientation. The patient, typically elderly, may have diminished vision, diminished hearing, and diminished proprioceptive, cerebellar, or peripheral neurologic function. The disequilibrium may be exaggerated or precipitated by sudden worsening in one or more of these sensory modalities, and typically worsens at night when diminished ambient lighting reduces visual input. Unfamiliar situations and surroundings may exacerbate the symptoms. Sedative medications can exaggerate or precipitate the problem. Typically these patients have multiple etiologies for near syncope as well; at times it is difficult to establish a precise diagnosis.

## Ill-Defined Light-Headedness

Patients with ill-defined light-headedness frequently cannot characterize their symptomatology in any way that is useful for the physician. They may have concomitant complaints of generalized fatigue or aching and nonfocal weakness. It is very difficult to ascribe a specific etiology to these subjective complaints.

## Hyperventilation Syndrome

Some patients with dizziness or light-headedness may suffer from a primary hyperventilation syndrome. Reproduction of their symptoms with directed hyperventilation aids in the diagnosis. Primary hyperventilation must be distinguished from hyperventilation secondary to a variety of medical disorders or insufficient oxygenation.

## Anxiety

Anxiety itself may produce dizziness characterized by disequilibrium. Many times the dizziness has been present for very long periods of time, there is no clear relationship to any exacerbating or precipitating factors, and the history and physical and neurologic examinations do not reveal any recognizable pattern. It is sometimes difficult to isolate other possible causes of dizziness when the patient presents with a host of symptoms seemingly precipitated by anxiety.

## Near Syncope

Patients with near syncope may complain of dizziness. On detailed questioning, it can usually be elicited that patients have a feeling that they would pass out if the symptomatology became worse. The causes of syncope and near syncope are essentially identical and only differ in magnitude. Near syncope may be produced by orthostatic, autonomic, reflex, and cardiac mechanisms, or by hypoglycemia. Possible orthostatic causes include volume depletion, poor conditioning, venous insufficiency, peripheral neuropathy including that produced by diabetes mellitus, and the effects of antihypertensive, vasodilating, and anti-Parkinson drugs. Preganglionic autonomic dysfunction, such as that presenting with Shy-Drager syndrome, may produce a near syncopal feeling. Reflex causes include a hyperactive carotid sinus, micturition, cough, and swallow syncope. Vasovagal syncope is actually less common in elderly patients and may be associated with multiple causes for stress or prolonged bed rest. Cardiac mechanisms for syncope include mechanical causes, such as valvular disease or subaortic stenosis, and arrhythmias.

## Unknown Causes

Despite thorough history, physical, and neurological exam, extensive neurological and cardiac testing and specialty follow-up, many patients will not have a cause for their dizziness found.

## Multiple Causes

In intensive studies of patients with persistent dizziness, only about one-half have a single cause.

# DIAGNOSIS

## History

Most causes of vertigo are benign, but potentially disabling. Some forms of dizziness may represent life-threatening emergencies, e.g., arrhythmia. Since the primary problem in the diagnosis of a patient with dizziness is establishing a precise definition of the patient's symptomatology, the history is of paramount importance. There is nowhere that the classic neurologic approach to the patient (defining the nature of the disturbance first and its localization second) is more important.

Even though the symptoms may be very difficult for the patient to describe, it is important not to ask leading questions or to suggest to the patient what the symptoms might mean because patients may incorporate the words used by the examiner into the description of their symptoms, whether they fit or not. In general, patients must be given time to elaborate exactly what the subjective feeling of dizziness means to them. At some point it must be established whether or not they have a vertiginous feeling. Whether the feeling is that of syncope should be determined, as well as the relationship to movement, head position, and particular postures.

The temporal profile at onset, such as the rate of development of symptoms and the duration of symptoms, should be elicited. The time of day of any worsening of symptoms should be elicited. All associated symptoms, such as nausea, vomiting, blurriness or double vision, tinnitus, focal or generalized weakness, numbness, visual loss, palpitations, and loss of consciousness should be noted. Past medical facts of most importance are the use of medications, both prescribed and over the counter, any history of trauma, and a history of similar episodes.

## Physical Examination

The physical examination should focus on several areas. Bedside tests of hearing and physical examination of the ears should be done. Eye movements, with particular emphasis on nystagmus, both direction and fatigue, should be evaluated. The details of cranial nerve testing are important, particularly eighth-nerve function; the cranial nerves most closely associated with the eighth nerve, specifically fifth-nerve function, including corneal reflex; seventh-nerve function; and ninth- and tenth-nerve function (gag reflex, swallowing). Of particular importance on the motor examination is testing of coordination, such as finger-to-nose testing or rapid alternating movements. Gait testing and an evaluation of the patient's ability to sit without support, as a test for truncal ataxia, may be necessary. Orthostatic vital signs are not reliable unless there are marked changes and reproduce identically the clinical symptomatology. The range of pulse and blood pressure changes in normal patients is wide and encompasses many recommended parameters for the diagnosis of orthostasis.

Perhaps the best bedside test of hearing is that of the soft whispered voice. One masks the ear not being tested with light pressure on the external canal or by rubbing the fingers in front of it and whispers names or letters in the unmasked ear that the patient must repeat. If there is a decrease in hearing, then Webber's and Rinne's test may be done to help distinguish between conductive and neurosensory loss.

Of particular importance in the evaluation of the potentially vertiginous patient is the Nylen-Barany maneuver outlined in Table 194-3. The type and duration of nystagmus are noted. In addition to the findings noted in the table, peripheral vertigo is more likely than central vertigo to be associated with nausea and vomiting and relatively severe symptoms (Table 194-1).

Other tests can be done as indicated by the initial history and physical examination. Drachman's dizziness stimulation battery is given in Table 194-4.

Of particular importance on the cardiac exam is to note the rate and

**Table 194-4.** Drachman's Dizziness Battery

Blood pressure lying and standing
Valsalva maneuver
Head turn—standing with eyes open
Sudden turn when walking
3 min hyperventilation
Nylen-Barany testing

rhythm of the heart and to evaluate for evidence of valvular heart disease.

History and physical examination alone may provide the diagnosis in the vast majority of patients.

## Laboratory Evaluation

Laboratory testing is selected based on the history and physical examination. Glucose testing in particular may be a productive test in patients with disequilibrium syndrome. Diabetes is one major cause of diminished peripheral neurologic function. In patients with typical peripheral vertigo and little else to suggest other medical problems, laboratory testing is not needed. In patients with presyncopal feeling, cardiac rhythm monitoring may be in order. Depending upon the physical examination, other testing to detect cardiac etiology may be indicated, such as echocardiography, ambulatory cardiac rhythm monitoring, etc. In the evaluation of long-term hearing loss with vestibular dysfunction, serologic testing for syphilis is commonly done.

When cerebellar hemorrhage or infarction is suspected, CT scanning should be considered. If tumor at the CP angle is a possibility, CT scanning may be done, although MRI is more sensitive. Patients with suspected central vertigo will require an imaging study and neurologic consultation. Most patients with peripheral vertigo and no suspicion of eighth-nerve lesion or CP angle tumor do not require an urgent imaging study.

## TREATMENT

*The principle of most importance in emergency department management is to firmly establish the nature of the patient's dizziness.* Virtually all of the medications that are useful for peripheral vertigo will result in worsening symptoms of patients with disequilibrium syndromes or ill-defined light-headedness.

There are multiple medications used in the emergency department and outpatient management of peripheral vertigo. Antihistamines have been known to be effective for the treatment of peripheral vertigo for 40 years. Not all antihistamines are useful, and their peripheral potency as antihistamines does not correlate with suppression of vertigo. The most useful ones have anticholinergic properties. Antihistamines may act both centrally, at the brain stem level, and peripherally, within the labyrinthine apparatus. Anticholinergics such as atropine and scopolamine are also quite effective. The efferent nerves of the vestibular sensory cells are cholinergic, and thus affected by anticholinergics. The central effects of anticholinergics may also mediate their action. Diazepam acts centrally on the lateral vestibular nucleus and is useful in acute peripheral vertigo. More recently the calcium channel blocker flunarizine has been found useful in the management of vertigo. Other commonly used antiemetics, such as prochlorperazine and chlorpromazine, are of little use in relieving patients with vertigo. Hydroxyzine and promethazine, however, with their antihistaminic activity, are. Effective agents for the management of peripheral vertigo are listed in Table 194-5.

Most patients need reassurance that the symptoms, while overpowering, are self-limiting, are not a reflection of serious pathology, and are not a serious threat to their health. An explanation that symptoms are caused by an imbalanced input from the two ears, and that the nervous system will accommodate to it, is helpful. The component of management that usually requires little explanation for the vertigi-

**Table 194-5.** Drugs used for Vertigo of Peripheral Origin

| | |
|---|---|
| Antihistamines | |
| Diphenhydramine | 25–50 mg PO q6h |
| Dimenhydrinate | 50 mg PO q4h |
| Cyclizine | 50 mg PO q4h* |
| Meclizine | 25 mg PO q6h |
| Promethazine | 25–50 mg PO q4–6h |
| Anticholinergics | |
| Atropine | 1 mg IM or IV |
| Scopolamine | 0.5 mg patch behind ear q3d |
| Antiemetics | |
| Hydroxyzine | 0.5 mg/kg up to 25–50 mg PO q4–6h |
| Promethazine | 25–50 mg PO q4–6h |
| Sedatives | |
| Diazepam | 2–10 mg PO q6–8h |
| Chlordiazepoxide | 5–25 mg PO Q6–8h |

* *Not* to exceed 200 mg in 24 h.

nous patient is that of either bed rest or resting in a position of comfort and a slowing of all movements so as to not precipitate the vertiginous feeling. Visual fixation on a nearby object may inhibit vertigo of peripheral origin and is preferable to lying with closed eyes.

The efficacy of the many regimens used in the chronic treatment of Menière's disease (low salt diet, ammonium chloride, diuretics, glycerol) has not been proved. Acute management is the same as for other forms of peripheral vertigo. Surgical destruction of the labyrinth or endolymphatic shunt can be done in the long-term management of Menière's disease.

Benign positional vertigo (Barany's) is treated with the same medications as other peripheral disorders, but is seldom very responsive. Some advocate repeated head movement to provoke attacks, fatiguing the response and or dispersion of the otolithic fragments.

In cases of disequilibrium syndrome, if no specific causes are found, one might consider withdrawal of any sedative or hypnotic medications. If the problem appears to be one of multiple sensory deficit syndrome, consideration of changes in ambient light, especially later in the day, and changing some factors in the surroundings may be indicated.

Emergency department management of patients with near syncope is similar to that for those with syncope (see Chap. 30).

For ill-defined light-headedness, when it is impossible to place the patient in a better-defined category of dizziness and when preliminary emergency department testing does not indicate any specific pathology, it is best to avoid medications used for vertigo.

### SUMMARY

The evaluation of the dizzy patient is a challenge to the skills of the physician. An initial open-ended history is important to define the clinical symptomatology precisely, without suggesting a particular entity. Precision in history taking will be rewarded by narrowing the field of potential insults causing symptoms. A thorough neurologic examination, with particular emphasis upon nystagmus, must be done. If vertigo is indeed the problem, one must separate peripheral (benign) causes from more ominous central causes. Recognition that symptoms may be quite disabling yet reflect benign processes may be reassuring to the patient. Careful selection of medications for vertigo can only be done when the syndrome is precisely defined and should be avoided unless the diagnosis of peripheral vertigo is established.

### BIBLIOGRAPHY

Adams RD, Victor M: *Principles of Neurology,* 4th ed. New York, McGraw Hill, 1989, p 238.

Baloh RW: Dizziness in older people. *J Am Geriatr Soc* 40.0, 1992.

Bannister R: *Brain's Clinical Neurology,* 6th ed. New York, Oxford, 1985, p 75.

Brandt T, Daroff RB: The multisensory physiological and pathological vertigo syndromes. *Ann Neurol* 7:195, 1980.

Cohen NL: The dizzy patient: update on vestibular disorders. *Med Clin North Am* 75:6, 1991.

Drachman DA, Apfelbaum RI, Posner JB: Dizziness and disorders of equilibrium, panel 8. *Arch Neurol* 36:806, 1979.

Drachman DA, Hart CW: An approach to the dizzy patient. *Neurology* 22:323, 1972.

Froehling DA, Silverstein MD, Mohr DN, Beatty CW: Does this dizzy patient have a serious form of vertigo? *JAMA* 271:5, 1994.

Herr RD, Zun L, Mathews JJ: A directed approach to the dizzy patient. *Ann Emerg Med* 18:664, 1989.

Linstrom CJ: Office management of the dizzy patient. *Otolaryngol Clin North Am* 25:4, 1992.

Mohr DN: The syndrome of paroxysmal positional vertigo, a review. *West J Med* 145:645, 1986.

Norris CH: Drugs affecting the inner ear: A review of their clinical efficacy, mechanisms of action, toxicity, and place in therapy. *Drugs* 36:754, 1988.

Olsky M, Murray J: Dizziness and fainting in the elderly. *Emerg Med Clin North Am* 8:295, 1990.

Olsson JE, Atkins JS: Vestibular disorders, *Otolaryngol Clin North Am* 20:83, 1987.

Scheinberg P: *An Introduction to Diagnosis and Management of Common Neurologic Disorders,* 3d ed. New York, Raven, 1986, p 99.

Slater R: Vertigo: How serious are recurrent and single attacks? *Postgrad Med.* 84:58, 1988.

Todd PA, Benfield P: Flunarizine: A reappraisal of its pharmacological properties and therapeutic use in neurological disorders. *Drugs* 38:481, 1989.

Warner EA, Wallach PM, Adelman HM, Sahlin-Hughes K: Dizziness in primary care patients. *J Gen Intern Med 7, 1992.*

## 195
# SEIZURES AND STATUS EPILEPTICUS IN ADULTS
### Thomas R. Pellegrino

A seizure is defined as an episode of abnormal neurologic function caused by an abnormal electrical discharge of brain neurons. Note that the seizure is the clinical attack experienced by the patient; some patients with "epileptic" electroencephalographic (EEG) discharges may not experience any clinical symptoms. Conversely, some seizure-like clinical episodes may be due to causes other than abnormal brain electrical activity; such attacks, however impressive, are not true seizures.

The term *epilepsy* denotes a clinical condition in which an individual is subject to recurrent seizures; it implies a more or less fixed condition of the brain responsible for the seizures. Ordinarily, the term *epileptic* is not used to refer to an individual with recurrent seizures caused by reversible conditions such as alcohol withdrawal, hypoglycemia, or other metabolic derangements.

The occurrence of one or more seizures indicates abnormal function of cerebral neurons. When this occurs in patients who are otherwise normal and in whom no evident cause for the attacks can be discerned, the seizures are referred to as primary or idiopathic. Seizures which occur as a consequence of some other identifiable neurologic condition are referred to as secondary or symptomatic.

Seizures are very common; approximately 1 to 2 percent of persons are subject to recurrent seizures. About 10 percent of individuals will experience at least one seizure during their lives. It is important to note that any individual can be caused to have a seizure under appropriate conditions. Electrical stimulation of the brain, convulsant drugs, profound metabolic disturbances, or a sharp blow to the head may induce seizures in otherwise normal individuals. Such attacks are generally self-limited, and such persons are not considered to have a seizure disorder or epilepsy. From such otherwise normal persons, there extends a continuum which includes, at its other extreme, persons who have frequent recurrent seizures without discernible cause.

The precise mechanisms involved in generating clinical seizures remain unknown, despite intense investigation. The process appears to require both intense and prolonged neuronal electrical discharges and failure or inhibition of normal protective mechanisms, but the molecular mechanisms underlying the events remain unclear. Once the seizure discharge begins, it may remain localized, it may spread to involve nearby populations of neurons, or it may spread rapidly to involve the entire cerebral cortex. The mechanisms by which these electrical discharges cause clinical seizures remain unknown. As mentioned earlier, EEG tracings frequently demonstrate electrical seizure discharges without any associated clinical signs.

## SEIZURE CLASSIFICATION

Over the years, many attempts have been made to provide a clinically useful classification of seizure types, both to facilitate communication among physicians and provide a basis for treatment decisions. Seizures may be classified based on the observed clinical features of the attacks, on their presumed etiologies, on EEG findings, on their clinical context, or on some combination of these.

The simplest scheme is to identify seizures as "big ones, little ones, and funny ones," a tradition maintained in the terms "grand mal, petit mal, and psychomotor." Unfortunately, these common terms are neither precise nor very informative. While commonly used informally, they have been largely replaced for most purposes by more formal terminology proposed by the International League Against Epilepsy. In this scheme, seizures are divided into two major groups; generalized seizures and focal seizures. (Table 195-1).

*Generalized seizures* are thought to be caused by nearly simultaneous activation of the entire cerebral cortex, perhaps caused by an electrical discharge originating deep in the brain and spreading outward. The attacks begin with abrupt loss of consciousness. This may be the only clinical manifestation of the seizures (as in absence attacks), or there may be a variety of motor manifestations (myoclonic jerks, drop attacks, tonic posturing, clonic jerking of the body and extremities, etc.) Motor activity, when present, typically involves all four extremities and is symmetrical (from side to side). Although generalized seizures may be preceded by several hours or days of prodromal symptoms (irritability, tension, isolated myoclonic jerks, etc.), true sensory auras do not occur in generalized seizures. The

**Table 195-1.** Classification of Seizures

Generalized seizures (consciousness always lost)
   Absence seizures (petit mal)
   Myoclonic seizures
   Tonic seizures
   Clonic seizures
   Tonic-clonic seizures
   Atonic seizures
Partial (focal) seizures
   Simple (elementary), no alteration of consciousness
      Motor seizures
      Sensory seizures
      Autonomic seizures
   Complex (psychomotor or temporal lobe seizures) consciousness
     impaired
     With psychic, cognitive, or affective symptoms
     With automatisms
Partial seizures (elementary or complex) with secondary generaization
Unclassified (due to inadequate information)

most familiar varieties of generalized seizures are absence (petit mal) and tonic-clonic (grand mal) attacks.

*Petit mal* attacks are very brief, generally lasting only a few seconds. The patients abruptly lose consciousness and seem "out of contact." Current activity ceases. They may stare and may have twitching of their eyelids; they do not respond to voice or to other stimulation. They do not fall or exhibit involuntary movements, and they do not lose continence. The attacks cease abruptly, and the patients are able to resume their previous activity with no postictal symptoms. Both patients and witnesses may be unaware that anything has happened. Classic petit mal attacks are virtually limited to school-age children and are often attributed by parents and teachers to daydreaming or not paying attention. The attacks may be very frequent, sometimes occurring 100 or more times daily, and may result in poor school performance. Petit mal attacks may occur alone or be associated with other kinds of seizures, especially as the children enter their adolescent or teenage years. Petit mal attacks usually resolve as the child matures, and true absence attacks are unusual in adults. It is usually incorrect to refer to minor seizures in adults as petit mal. Similar attacks in adults are more likely to be minor complex partial seizures. The distinction is important, since the causes and treatment of the two types of seizures are quite different.

*Grand mal* attacks are among the most dramatic of medical events. The true generalized grand mal attack begins with an abrupt loss of consciousness; there is usually no warning, and true auras do not occur. In a typical attack, the patient suddenly becomes rigid, with trunk and extremities extended, and falls to the ground. Patients are often apneic during this period and may be deeply cyanotic; they often urinate or defecate and may vomit. As the rigid (tonic) phase of the attack subsides, there is increasing coarse trembling which evolves into rhythmic (clonic) jerking of the trunk and extremities. As the attack ends, the patient is left flaccid and unconscious, often with deep rapid breathing. Typical attacks last from 60 to 90 s (occasionally longer). Bystanders generally grossly overestimate the duration of the attack. Consciousness returns gradually, and postictal confusion and fatigue may last several hours or longer.

*Partial (focal) seizures* are due to electrical discharges which begin in a localized region of the cerebral cortex; the discharge may remain localized or may spread to involve nearby cortical regions or to the entire cortex. Focal seizures are generally thought to be secondary or symptomatic seizures; their occurrence often implies a focal structural lesion of the brain. It is often possible to deduce the likely location of the initial cortical discharge from the clinical features at the onset of the attack. Unilateral tonic or clonic movements (often limited to one extremity) suggest a focus in the motor cortex. Tonic deviation of the head and eyes (usually to the side *away* from the discharge) suggests a frontal lobe focus. Sensory hallucinations (e.g., paresthesias or numbness) suggest a discharge in the sensory cortex. Visual symptoms, especially flashing lights or distortions of vision, suggest an occipital focus. Bizarre olfactory or gustatory hallucinations suggest a focus in the medial temporal lobe. Such sensory phenomena are often the initial symptoms of attacks which then become more widespread. The auras which may precede other kinds of seizures are examples of such focal sensory seizures; the presence of an aura implies that the attack is a focal seizure. In simple or elementary focal seizures, the seizure remains localized, and consciousness and mentation are not affected.

*Complex partial seizures* are focal seizures in which consciousness and/or mentation are affected. They are often caused by a focal discharge originating in the temporal lobe and are sometimes referred to as temporal lobe seizures. Because of their alterations of thinking and behavior, they are sometimes referred to as psychomotor seizures. Because such seizures may originate from brain regions other than the temporal lobes, and to avoid any confusion with psychiatric illness, the term *complex partial seizures* is preferred. Often thought to be rare, they are in fact quite common.

Because of their frequently bizarre symptoms and psychic features, complex partial seizures are commonly misdiagnosed as psychiatric problems. Their symptoms may include visceral symptoms, hallucinations, memory disturbances, dream-like states, automatisms, and affective disorders. Visceral symptoms often consist of a sensation of "butterflies" beginning in the stomach or epigastrium, rising up through the chest to the face. Other visceral auras include nausea or abdominal pains. Hallucinations may involve any sensory modality including smell, taste, hearing, or vision. There may be complex distortions of perception such that objects may appear to change color, shapes may be distorted, or objects may appear larger, smaller, closer, or more distant than they really are. The perception of time is commonly distorted; patients cannot usually estimate the length of the attack and may describe time as passing very slowly or standing still. Rarely, the passage of time seems accelerated. Memory disturbances may include *déjà vu,* a sense of familiarity in an unfamiliar environment, or *jamais vu,* a sense of unfamiliarity or strangeness in familiar surroundings. Patients may experience brief "reruns" of past experiences or may describe a sensation that they are seeing themselves in a movie. Automatisms are typically simple, repetitive, purposeless movements such as lip smacking, fiddling with clothing or buttons, or repeating short phrases. More complex behaviors may occur, but well-organized, purposeful activity is very rare. Affective disorders may include intense sensations of fear, paranoia, depression, or rarely, elation or ecstasy.

A focal seizure discharge may spread to involve both hemispheres, mimicking a typical generalized seizure. For purposes of classification, diagnosis, and treatment, such attacks are regarded as focal seizures. In some patients, the discharge may spread so rapidly that no focal symptoms are evident, and the correct diagnosis may depend on demonstration of the focal discharge on an EEG recording. In many cases, however, a very careful history will reveal focal symptoms at the onset of the attack and allow a correct diagnosis. The distinction is very important since, as noted previously, the diagnosis of the focal seizure disorder should prompt a search for an underlying structural lesion.

## CLINICAL EVALUATION OF SEIZURE PATIENTS

### History

The first and most important step in evaluating a seizure patient is to determine if the attack was truly a seizure. Unfortunately, it is common practice to use a diagnosis of "rule out seizure" in patients who have had any transient spells for which no more specific diagnosis is available. This practice is to be condemned, not only for being intellectually and diagnostically sloppy, but also because of the consequences to the individual of being erroneously labeled a seizure patient. There may be serious adverse effects on employability, driving privileges, insurability, etc. Also, it should be remembered that all anticonvulsant drugs are more or less toxic. An erroneous or hasty diagnosis of epilepsy may expose the patient to substantial harm with no prospect of benefit, not to mention delaying appropriate treatment for the correct diagnosis. A basic rule is that "everything which falls down and shakes is not a seizure." There are many episodic disturbances of neurologic function which may be mistaken for seizures by the unwary physician (Table 195-2). A complete review of these conditions would be too lengthy for inclusion here, but several of the more important possibilities should be mentioned.

Syncope usually is attended by premonitory symptoms such as pallor, diaphoresis, and a "graying out" of vision. Patients often are aware that they are going to pass out and can clearly describe the onset of the attacks. Syncope may be attended by injury or incontinence; in addition, some patients may experience some myoclonic jerks, especially if they are prevented from falling. Recovery is usually rapid, with few or no postictal symptoms.

Narcolepsy is characterized by brief attacks of uncontrollable day-

**Table 195-2.** Paroxysmal Disorders: Differential Diagnosis

Seizures
Syncope
Narcolepsy/cataplexy
Movement disorders
Hyperventilation syndrome
Psychogenic seizures
Paroxysmal vertigo
Rage attacks, fugue states
Transient ischemic attacks
Migraine

time sleepiness. Patients are able to feel their attacks coming on and can sometimes control them with judiciously timed naps. An associated symptom is cataplexy, characterized by a sudden brief loss of postural muscle tone. The patient collapses but remains fully conscious; there are no involuntary movements. The attacks are often triggered by emotional upset, laughter, crying, etc. Other symptoms of narcolepsy include vivid dreams, often at the onset of sleep or immediately upon awakening, and attacks of sleep paralysis.

Movement disorders such as myoclonic jerks, tremors, or tics may occur in a variety of neurologic disorders. Consciousness is always preserved during these movements; the movements, though involuntary, often can be suppressed temporarily by the patient.

Hyperventilation syndrome is very common and is often misdiagnosed as a seizure disorder. A careful history normally will reveal the gradual onset of the attacks with shortness of breath, anxiety, and perioral numbness. Such attacks may progress to involuntary spasm of the extremities and even loss of consciousness. The attacks often are reproduced easily in the emergency room or office by asking the patient to overbreathe.

Psychogenic seizures are common and may be extremely difficult to distinguish from true seizures. This diagnosis should be suspected when seizures occur regularly in response to emotional upset or when seizures only occur with witnesses present. The attacks are often very bizarre and highly variable. Patients often are able to protect themselves from noxious stimuli during the attack. Incontinence and injury are very rare, and there is often no postictal confusion. In some cases, accurate diagnosis may require prolonged EEG monitoring to demonstrate the presence of normal EEG activity during an attack.

A careful history of the details of the attack usually will allow a diagnosis to be made with a high degree of certainty. The history should be obtained from the patient, if possible, and from any bystanders who actually witnessed the attack. Be very wary of accepting a diagnosis of seizure from witnesses, including other physicians. Also, do not assume that a given episode was a seizure, even if the patient has a history of seizures. The original diagnosis may be incorrect, or the patient may have experienced another kind of attack. In each case, try to get a detailed description of the attack, and draw your own conclusions.

Try to determine how the attack began. Was there any aura? Did the attack begin abruptly or gradually? Ask about staring, lip smacking, blinking, breath holding, etc. Ask about motor activity as the attack progressed. Determine if motor activity was local or generalized, symmetrical or not. Did the motor activity begin in one part of the body and then spread? Finally, ask about the duration of the attack and about any postictal confusion or lethargy. Ask the patient if he or she has any recollection of the attack. Clinical features that help to distinguish seizures from other kinds of attacks include:

1. Abrupt onset and termination. Although some focal seizures are preceded by auras which last 20 to 30 s (or more), most attacks begin abruptly. Attacks which develop over several minutes, or longer, should be regarded with suspicion. Most seizures last only 1 or 2 min, occasionally more. Be wary of an attack which lasts 30 min or several hours or longer.

2. A true sensory or other aura, if present, is helpful in recognizing focal (especially complex partial) seizures. Absence of an aura is not helpful.

3. True seizures are generally stereotyped. Attacks may vary in intensity or duration, of course, but the basic features will be consistent. There are patients who have more than one type of seizure, but each type will maintain its own pattern. Be very wary if the attacks are highly variable and inconsistent.

4. Lack of recall. Except for simple partial seizures, patients usually cannot recall the details of an attack, the responses and acts of bystanders, etc. Be wary of attacks in which the patient "could hear everyone talking but could not respond."

5. True seizures are not generally provoked by environmental cues or stimuli. There are rare cases of true reflex epilepsy, and seizures may be provoked by sleep deprivation, drugs, or alcohol withdrawal. True seizures, however, are usually not provoked by emotional distress, being yelled at by parents, etc.

6. Movements or behavior during the attack generally are purposeless or inappropriate. Occasional rare exceptions have been described, but popular literature to the contrary, persons do not rob banks, engage in direct violence, or carry out other coherent, purposeful activity during seizures.

7. Most seizures, except for simple absence attacks (petit mal) or simple partial seizures, will be followed by a period of postictal confusion and lethargy. Be very wary of a dramatic convulsion followed immediately by normal mental function.

Although a clinical diagnosis of seizures often can be made with a high degree of certainty, there are some occasions when the diagnosis is not convincing. In such cases, it is better to admit uncertainty and not use the term *seizure* or begin inappropriate and potentially hazardous treatment. In some cases, multiple EEG recordings, prolonged EEG monitoring, and evaluation by a neurologist all may be necessary to establish a diagnosis.

Once it is decided that the patient actually has had a seizure, the next step is to determine the clinical context in which the attack occurred. In the case of a patient with a previously documented and evaluated seizure disorder who has had a typical attack, little further evaluation is required. If the patient is receiving anticonvulsant medication, ask about any recent changes in medication, missed doses, etc. Even a single missed dose may result in a marked drop in blood levels of medication and result in a seizure. Ask about a recent change from brand-name to generic medication or from one generic formulation to another. Other possible factors which might provoke a seizure include sleep deprivation, alcohol withdrawal, and use of other drugs.

If there is no previous history of seizures, a much more detailed history is needed. Ask about any symptoms that might suggest previous unwitnessed or unrecognized seizures: blank spells or staring spells in school, involuntary movement, unexplained injuries, nocturnal tongue biting, and enuresis. Ask about any other neurologic symptoms, such as mental retardation, delayed development, progressive headache, head trauma, and focal symptoms. Inquire into any systemic illness: cancer, hypo- or hyperglycemia, electrolyte abnormalities, drug ingestion (licit and illicit), and alcohol use. Finally, ask about any family history of seizures or other neurologic illness (Table 195-3).

## Physical Examination

The general physical examination should be directed toward discovering any injuries that might have resulted from the seizure and any systemic illness which might have caused the attack. Seizures may cause injuries such as fractures, sprains, and bruises; posterior dislocations of the shoulder are common and often overlooked. Look for tongue lacerations and broken teeth or any suggestion of aspiration. Look also for any dysmorphic features or birthmarks.

**Table 195-3.** Some Causes of Secondary Seizures

Intracranial etiologies
   Trauma (recent or remote)
   Infection (meningitis, encephalitis, abscess)
   Vascular lesion (stroke, arteriovenous malformation, vasculitis)
   Mass lesions (neoplasms, subdural hematoma)
   Degenerative disease
Extracranial etiologies
   Anoxic-ischemic injury (e.g., cardiac arrest, severe hypoxemia)
   Endocrine/electrolyte disorders
      Hypoglycemia
      Hyperosmolar states
      Hyponatremia
      Hypocalcemia, hypomagnesemia (rare)
   Toxins and drugs
      Cocaine, lidocaine
      Antidepressants
      Theophylline
      Alcohol withdrawal
      Barbiturate withdrawal
      Benzodiazepine withdrawal
      Anticonvulsant withdrawal
        and *many* others
   Eclampsia of pregnancy (may occur postpartum)
   Hypertensive encephalopathy

The neurologic examination should evaluate the patient's level of consciousness and mentation. Mental status should be followed closely with serial examinations. Profound obtundation which improves steadily is probably benign, while progressive deterioration should cause great concern. Search for any signs of increased intracranial pressure and any signs of focal weakness or reflex changes. Focal signs following a seizure, even if transient, strongly suggest a focal seizure.

## Laboratory Examination

### Blood Chemistry

There are no standard or routine laboratory studies to be obtained in seizure patients; the need for such studies must be assessed on an individual basis. In a patient with a well-documented seizure disorder who has had a single unprovoked seizure, no laboratory studies may be needed. Anticonvulsant drug levels may be helpful but should be interpreted with caution.

In the case of a patient with a first seizure or when the history is unclear, more extensive studies may be helpful. Arterial blood gas studies may demonstrate a metabolic acidemia following a major convulsion; similarly, muscle enzyme levels (e.g., creatine kinase) may be elevated. Serum electrolytes, glucose, blood urea nitrogen (BUN) and creatinine, calcium and magnesium, and a toxicology screen may be indicated depending on the clinical context. Blood prolactin levels may be elevated for a brief period (30 to 60 min) immediately after a true seizure (but not after pseudoseizures) and are sometimes helpful in confirming that an attack was a true seizure. A normal prolactin level is not helpful. The presence of anticonvulsant drugs in the blood of a patient from whom no history is available suggests (but does not prove) the presence of a seizure disorder.

Anticonvulsant drug levels must be interpreted with caution. The usual therapeutic and toxic levels indicated in laboratory reports are helpful only as very rough guides. The therapeutic level of a drug is that level which provides adequate seizure control without unacceptable side effects; a phenytoin level of only 8 µg/mL may be therapeutic if a patient is having only occasional seizures and if higher levels cause symptoms of toxicity. Similarly a toxic level is one which causes symptoms of intoxication. A phenytoin level of 15 µg/mL (or less) may be toxic in a given patient. Conversely, a phenytoin level of 24 µg/mL may result in excellent seizure control and be well tolerated. A marked change in previously stable drug levels may indicate noncompliance, a change in medication (e.g., from one brand to another), malabsorption of a drug (as in severe diarrhea or vomiting), or ingestion of a competing drug.

## Radiographic Studies

In the case of a patient with a known seizure disorder, radiographic studies usually are not needed. There is no rational basis for the common practice of obtaining routine CT scans on each patient who presents to the emergency department after a seizure.

In the case of a patient with a first seizure, CT scanning may be appropriate to look for evidence of a structural lesion responsible for the attack. Whenever possible, such scans should be done both without and with contrast enhancement, since many important processes, such as metastatic or primary tumors or vascular anomalies, may be missed on noncontrast studies. In most cases, the scan may be delayed until the patient has recovered and the results of BUN and creatinine levels are available, and the patient has been asked about any relevant allergies. Emergency scanning is only necessary in a patient whose condition is deteriorating or in whom there is evidence of a structural lesion.

Magnetic resonance (MR) scanning is substantially more sensitive than CT in detecting subtle alterations of brain structure, and it is often the study of choice in the evaluation of patients with seizures. Especially in patients with uncomplicated first seizures, it is reasonable to omit the CT scan and obtain an MR scan instead. Consultation with a radiologist may be helpful in choosing the best approach and avoiding unnecessary examinations.

Other radiographic studies may be indicated in some cases. Chest x-rays may reveal primary or metastatic tumors or evidence of aspiration. Skull x-rays may reveal fractures or other bony lesions (though CT scanning is often superior). Special examinations such as angiography may be helpful in some cases but are rarely included in an emergency department evaluation.

## EEG

The EEG may be very helpful in the evaluation of patients with seizures. It is sometimes said that the only way to be certain of the diagnosis of epilepsy is to record an attack and demonstrate the characteristic electrical discharge. More commonly, the EEG provides support for the diagnosis of seizures by recording interictal EEG discharges without clinical accompaniment; the EEG can help distinguish focal from generalized seizures and may indicate an underlying disturbance of cerebral function. However, a normal interictal EEG does not exclude the diagnosis of epilepsy. An EEG obtained shortly (within hours) after a clinical attack may demonstrate postictal slowing of EEG rhythms and support the clinical impression that the attack was a true seizure. Finally, the EEG findings may be very helpful in identifying specific epileptic syndromes.

The diagnostic yield of EEG recordings can be increased by appropriate patient preparation (especially sleep deprivation) or by activation techniques such as hyperventilation, photic stimulation, and sleep recordings. More elaborate examinations such as 24-h recordings or video-EEG recordings also may be used. Consultation with a neurologist can help ensure that the appropriate studies are chosen and inappropriate and unnecessary studies avoided.

## TREATMENT

Appropriate emergency treatment of a patient with seizures will vary depending on the specific clinical situation. It should be stressed that the first step in providing appropriate treatment is to make an accurate diagnosis; only in patients with status epilepticus is it sometimes necessary to initiate treatment before diagnostic evaluation has been completed. Certain general measures should be taken for any seizure patient. Vital functions should stabilized; in unconscious patients, it may be necessary to secure the airway. Emptying the stomach will reduce the risk of aspiration and remove any unabsorbed drugs or toxins in the case of ingestion. Standard measures for management of any unconscious patient should be employed.

Definitive management of the patient with seizures should begin, if possible, with treatment of any underlying condition causing the attacks. Seizures caused by hypoglycemia, hyperosmolar states, or hyponatremia, for example, should be treated by managing the metabolic derangement. Anticonvulsant drugs are not indicated and usually are ineffective. In most patients, of course, no such specific cause is present, or if present, may not be amenable to immediate direct treatment. In these patients, anticonvulsant drug therapy is appropriate.

With regard to the specific management of seizures, four clinical scenarios will be reviewed: the patient who is actually having a seizure, the patient with previous epilepsy who has had a recent seizure, the patient with a first seizure, and the patient in status epilepticus.

## The Acute Seizure

There is little to be done during the course of an actual seizure other than to protect the patient from injury. Gentle but firm restraint should be used to prevent falls. If possible the patient should be turned to one side to reduce the risk of aspiration should vomiting occur. It is usually not possible to get a bite block between the teeth without using considerable force; there is little point in risking damage to teeth in order to prevent tongue biting. If a bite block is used, be certain that it cannot be aspirated or swallowed. It is usually not necessary or even possible to ventilate a patient effectively during a seizure, but once the attack subsides, it is appropriate to make sure the airway is clear. There is no indication for intravenous anticonvulsant medications during the course of an uncomplicated seizure.

## Patients with Previous Seizures

Proper management of a patient with a well-documented seizure disorder who presents after one or more seizures depends on the particular circumstance of the case. Ask about any changes in routine or regimen which might have caused the seizure, such as sleep deprivation, excessive alcohol intake (or alcohol withdrawal), or medication changes. Many such seizures occur because of failure to take anticonvulsant medication as prescribed. Review of the pharmacologic properties of commonly used anticonvulsant drugs (Table 195-4) shows that several of them have very short serum half-lives. This means that missing even a single dose may result in a sharp drop in serum levels and recurrence of seizures. If anticonvulsant levels are very low, supplemental doses may be given and the patient restarted on their regular regimen. If no supplemental medication is given, several days may be required for steady-state blood levels to be reestablished. During that time the patient will be at increased risk for further seizures.

If anticonvulsant levels are adequate and the patient has had a single attack, treatment usually is not needed since even well-controlled patients may have occasional breakthrough seizures. If there has been a recent increase in the frequency of breakthrough seizures, a change in medication may be needed. This decision usually does not need to be made in the emergency department, and the patient can be referred to their regular physician for definitive management. If it is decided to increase the patient's maintenance dose of medication, only very small increments should be made, and close follow-up should be provided since even small dose changes may result in dramatic increases in serum levels of drugs.

## The Patient with a First Seizure

There has been considerable controversy about the appropriate management of a patient who has experienced an apparent first seizure.

**Table 195-4.** Properties of Commonly Used Anticonvulsant Drugs

| Drug | Oral Dose, mg/day* | Therapeutic Level, μg/mL† | Days to Reach Steady State‡ | Serum Half-life, h |
|------|------|------|------|------|
| Phenytoin | 300–400 | 10–20 | 5–10 | 24 ± 12 |
| Carbamazepine | 800–1200 | 8–12 | 2–4 | 12 ± 3 |
| Phenobarbital | 90–120 | 15–40 | 15–20 | 96 ± 12 |
| Primidone | 150–1000 | 8–12 | 2–4 | 12 ± 3 |
| Valproic acid | 1500–3000 | 50–150 | 2–4 | 12–18 |
| Ethosuximide | 750–1000 | 40–100 | 5–7 | 24–36 |

\* Daily dose must be individualized for each patient. Drug-drug interactions may dramatically change daily doses in patients receiving multiple drugs.
† See text for definition of therapeutic and toxic levels. Serum levels are for rough guidance *only*.
‡ Indicates times required to establish stable serum level after any change in dose.

The goal of treatment is to reduce the risk of recurrent seizures; rational treatment decisions depend on the likelihood of a recurrence and on the effectiveness of treatment in preventing further seizures. Until recently, reliable data on these questions have been unavailable. Previous studies have suggested rates of recurrence ranging from 23 to 71 percent. Some studies have found no benefit from treatment while others have reported a 50 percent reduction in the risk of recurrence. Clearly, those patients with active medical or neurologic illnesses causing seizures should have those illnesses treated if possible. Some of these patients will require treatment with anticonvulsant drugs, and the effectiveness of such treatment depends on the nature of the underlying illness. More problematic are patients who have no apparent cause for their seizures or those who have evidence of a previous neurologic illness or injury but no evidence of any active process.

A very careful analysis by Berg and Shinnar (1991) found that in patients with an apparent first seizure, the most important predictors of the risk of recurrence were the etiology of the seizure and the results of the EEG. Seizures were considered to be *idiopathic* if there was no neurologic history and a normal neurologic examination. The term *remote symptomatic* was used to describe seizures thought to be caused by a previous neurologic illness or injury as evidenced by the history or by an abnormal examination. In patients with idiopathic seizures (as defined above) the risk of a recurrent seizure within two years was 24 percent if the EEG was normal and 48 percent if the EEG was abnormal. In patients with remove symptomatic seizures, the risk was 48 percent if the EEG was normal and 65 percent if the EEG was abnormal. Family history, age, sex, and even the presence of status epilepticus at the time of the first seizure were not strong predictors of the risk of recurrence. Unfortunately EEG results are often not available to the emergency physician who must make a treatment decision. Concerning the effectiveness of treatment, two recent studies have found that treatment appears to reduce the risk of recurrent seizures by about 50 percent during two years of follow-up, but some 30 percent of patients experience potentially significant side effects from the drugs (Camfield, et al, 1989; First Seizure Trial Group, 1993).

Given these data, some general recommendations can be made. Patients with remote symptomatic seizures (as defined above) should generally be treated. Their risk of recurrence is quite high (50 to 65 percent) and their absolute risk reduction (25 to 30 percent) is substantial. In patients with idiopathic seizures, the decision is less clear. Their risk of recurrence may be as low as 24 percent (10 to 12 percent with treatment) if the EEG is normal. Given the expense, inconvenience, and potential side effects of treatment, some patients may wish to defer a decision about treatment until an EEG is obtained. In these patients, the only realistic approach is a full discussion of the risks and benefits of treatment. Often, a decision need not be made in the emergency department and patients can be referred to their regular physicians for further care.

If treatment is started, either phenytoin or carbamazepine would be an appropriate choice for most adults. The two drugs are about equally effective and have similar risks of side effects. The choice can be based on cost, convenience, and physician preference (Table 195-5). There is no need to give intravenous or oral loading doses of phenytoin; either drug may be given in regular maintenance doses which will provide adequate blood levels within a few days. Hospitalization is not necessary if the patient has made a full recovery. Diagnostic studies can be completed on an outpatient basis.

Patients should be instructed to take precautions to minimize the risks from further seizures. Swimming should be avoided unless a competent lifeguard is present. Working with hazardous tools or machines or on ladders or scaffolds should be avoided. The emergency physician should be familiar with state driving regulations, including any reporting requirements. The emergency department record should document the precise instructions given to the patient.

## Alcohol Withdrawal Seizures

The management of seizures in alcoholic patients remains controversial. It is important to distinguish between patients who experience seizures only in the setting of alcohol withdrawal and patients with epilepsy whose seizures are exacerbated by alcohol withdrawal. Most authorities agree that patients whose seizures occur only in the setting of alcohol withdrawal usually do not require specific anticonvulsant therapy. Use of benzodiazepines in doses adequate to manage withdrawal will usually afford adequate protection. Exceptions would be patients with a history of severe or prolonged alcohol withdrawal seizures or patients with status epilepticus. Patients with epilepsy exacerbated by alcohol withdrawal should be managed as any other seizure patient with recurrent seizures.

## STATUS EPILEPTICUS

Status epilepticus is defined as either continuous seizure activity for 30 minutes or more, or two or more seizures which occur without full recovery of consciousness between the attacks. In the emergency department, a presumptive diagnosis should be made and treatment initiated in all patients with continuous seizure activity without regard to the 30 minute criterion.

The diagnosis of status epilepticus is usually obvious in patients with continuous convulsions, but it must be remembered that patients

**Table 195-5.** Anticonvulsant Drugs: Indications

| | |
|------|------|
| Generalized seizures | |
|   Absence seizures: | Ethosuximide (1st) |
| | Valproic acid (2nd) |
|   Myoclonic seizures: | Valproic acid |
|   Tonic-clonic seizures: | Carbamazepine or phenytoin (1st) |
| | Phenobarbital or primidone (2nd) |
| | Valproic acid (3rd) |
| Partial seizures: (simple or complex, with or without generalization) | Carbamazepine or phenytoin (1st) |
| | Phenobarbital or primidone (2nd) |
| | Valproic acid (3rd) |

with pseudoseizures may also present with apparent "status epilepticus." This is not rare in patients with psychogenic seizures, some of whom may have had previous episodes of aggressive treatment for their non-epileptic seizures. In addition, seizures other than tonic-clonic seizures may occur continuously or in rapid succession, fulfilling the criteria for status epilepticus. Patients may present with continuous or repeated simple partial or complex partial seizures (epilepsia partialis continua). In patients with simple partial seizures, status epilepticus may present with continuous twitching or jerking movements of an extremity or persistant sensory or autonomic symptoms; consciousness may be preserved. Patients with complex partial status epilepticus may have persistent bizarre behaviors, automatisms, or hallucinations and may be erroneously thought to have a psychiatric disorder. Finally, patients may have continuous or repeated absence seizures; their clinical symptoms may include altered mentation, diminished responsiveness, confusion, amnesia, dream-like states, etc., without motor symptoms. Such instances of "nonconvulsive status" may occur in up to 25 percent of patients with status epilepticus (Cascino, 1993; Celesia, 1976). In some patients with convulsive status epilepticus, convulsions may gradually lessen over time or with partial treatment, giving the impression that the seizures have been controlled; such patients may continue to have non-convulsive seizures misdiagnosed as a postictal state. Correct diagnosis requires a high index of suspicion, a perceptive physician, and often an EEG.

Convulsive status epilepticus and epilepsia partialis continua demand urgent treatment. Patients are at risk for serious injury, hypoxemia, circulatory collapse, and other complications. In addition, uncontrolled seizure discharges may cause permanent neuronal injury within 30 to 60 minutes even in the absence of convulsions. Finally, the longer seizures are allowed to continue the more difficult it will be to control the seizures. The overall prognosis depends in large part on the underlying cause of the seizures. Convulsive status epilepticus has an overall mortality of up to 30 percent. The mortality of status epilepticus *per se* is about 10 percent. Status epilepticus may result from a wide variety of causes including changes in anticonvulsant therapy (including noncompliance), CNS infections, trauma, anoxia, stroke, metabolic encephalopathies, etc. In addition, about 10 percent of epileptic patients will present with status epilepticus as their initial seizure event; about 50 percent of patients with status will have no previous seizure history (Hauser, 1990).

Management of patients with status epilepticus requires rapid diagnostic evaluation, general supportive care, and specific anticonvulsant therapy, all of which should be carried out nearly simultaneously.

## Initial Evaluation and Treatment

The history and physical examination should be directed toward discovery of the cause of the seizures and to any injury which may have resulted from the seizures. Any of the causes of seizures previously noted (see Table 195-3) may result in status epilepticus; in many patients, no specific cause will be found.

The patients should be protected from injury; mechanical restraints should be used only with great caution. A large-bore intravenous (IV) line should be established. Use of an IV fluid without glucose will facilitate administration of anticonvulsant drugs. Endotracheal intubation should be done if there is any concern about the adequacy of ventilation or safety of the airway. A nasogastric tube may be used to empty the stomach. Initial blood work should include blood glucose and electrolytes and, where indicated, toxicology screens and anticonvulsant levels. In patients with prolonged seizures, serum creatine kinase (CK) levels and urine myoglobin should be done. Blood-gas studies are rarely helpful; when in doubt, intubate the patient. Emergency lumbar puncture is rarely indicated and is likely to be very difficult. If bacterial meningitis is suspected, empiric antibiotic therapy

should be started. Radiographic studies (such as a CT scan) will usually need to be delayed until the seizures are controlled.

Thiamine (100 mg) and glucose (25 to 50 g) should be given IV if hypoglycemia is suspected or confirmed; there is no benefit to giving additional glucose to normoglycemic patients.

## Anticonvulsant Drugs

The choice of an appropriate drug regimen depends on the frequency and intensity of the seizures. The drugs most often used in the therapy of status epilepticus are the benzodiazepines (diazepam or lorazepam), phenytoin, and phenobarbital (Table 195-6).

Benzodiazepines are used in patients with continuous or very frequent seizures to temporarily control the seizures until more specific agents can be given. Either diazepam or lorazepam may be used (lorazepam is not FDA approved for this indication). Diazepam 5 to 20 mg is given by slow (not more than 5 mg/min) IV infusion. Lorazepam is given by slow IV infusion (not more than 2 mg/min) up to a total of 0.1 mg/kg. Both drugs are equally effective but lorazepam has a longer duration of action and is considered the agent of choice by some authorities. Midazolam is also effective but not as well studied or as widely used as diazepam and lorazepam. Respiratory depression and hypotension may occur when benzodiazepines are used and are especially likely in patients who have taken alcohol, barbiturates, narcotics, or other sedatives. Because of their short duration of action, benzodiazepines should be followed immediately by a major anticonvulsant drug (usually phenytoin).

Phenytoin is the most important drug used in the management of status epilepticus. It may be given immediately after a benzodiazepine or may be used as primary therapy in patients whose seizures are less frequent. It is usually given as an IV loading dose of 20 mg/kg. Doses well in excess of the usual 1000 mg may be required; a smaller loading dose (15 mg/kg) may be used in the elderly but the loading dose is not reduced in patients with renal failure or other illnesses. The drug should be infused at a rate not greater than 50 mg/min; a rate of 25 mg/min is safer in elderly patients. Dilantin

**Table 195-6.** Management of Status Epilepticus

General measures
   Establish/maintain airway
   Thiamine 100 mg IV
   Dextrose 25–50 g IV
Standard regimen
   Diazepam 5 mg IV (repeat as necessary q 5 min to total of 20 mg) or
     lorazepam up to 0.1 mg/kg) and
   Phenytoin 18 mg/kg IV at 25 mg/min
   *If not effective, then:*
   Phenobarbital IV 100 mg/min to total of 10 mg/kg or seizures are
     controlled.
   *If not effective, then:*
   Phenobarbital 50 mg/min to total (including previous doses) of 20 mg/kg
     or seizures are controlled.
   *If not effective, then:*
   Phenobarbital 50 mg/min to total (including previous doses) of 30 mg/kg
     or seizures are controlled.
   *If not effective, then:*
   Consider barbiturate coma, general anesthesia, or diazepam drip.
Alternative regimen
   Phenobarbital 100 mg/min IV to total of 10 mg/kg or seizures are
     controlled.
   *If not effective, then:*
   Phenytoin 18 mg/kg IV (at dose of 25–50 mg/min) and phenobarbital 50
     mg/min to total dose of 20 mg/kg or seizures are controlled.
   *If not effective, then:*
   Phenobarbital 50 mg/kg to total dose (including previous doses) of 30 mg/
     kg or seizures are controlled.
   *If not effective, then:*
   Consider barbiturate coma or general anesthesia

should not be mixed with any glucose-containing IV fluid and should *never* be given intramuscularly due to erratic absorption. Adverse effects of IV dilantin include hypotension, decreased myocardial contractility, and increased atrioventricular (AV) block (these may be related to the propylene glycol used as a diluent). The drug is contraindicated in the presence of second- or third-degree AV block. Patients should be monitored closely during phenytoin infusions; if side effects develop, the infusion should be stopped. The drug may be restarted at a lower rate when the side effects have resolved; in some cases, patients are unable to tolerate the drug.

Phenobarbital is usually used as a second-line drug in patients unable to tolerate phenytoin or in patients whose seizures are not controlled despite full loading doses of dilantin. An initial loading dose of 10 mg/kg is given IV at a rate of 100 mg/min. If necessary, an additional 10 mg/kg can be given at a rate of 50 mg/min. Additional doses of 5 to 10 mg/kg may be given; total doses of 30 mg/kg or more may be required. Respiratory depression is common, especially at higher doses or when diazepam or lorazepam was used previously. Ventilator support is often required. Hypotension may also occur. Because of very slow elimination, large doses of phenobarbital may result in prolonged obtundation or coma.

Phenobarbital may also be used as initial therapy. Shaner et al. (1988) found that initial treatment was more effective and easier to use than regimens using benzodiazepines and phenytoin. They suggest an initial dose of 10 mg/kg infused at 100 mg/min. If necessary, this is followed by phenytoin 18 mg/kg infused at 40 mg/min or by additional doses of phenobarbital to a total dose of 20 to 30 mg/kg.

In a few patients, seizure control is not obtained with these regimens and further treatment is needed.

### Refractory Status Epilepticus

The standard regimens of benzodiazepines, phenytoin, and phenobarbital will suffice to control status epilepticus in most patients. In a few cases (generally patients with structural lesions or CNS infections), seizures will continue even after such treatment. Various approaches have been advocated, including IV infusions of lidocaine (2 to 4 mg/min) or diazepam (up to 8 to 10 mg/h). Intravenous infusions of paraldehyde have also been used. The easiest and most direct approach is to obtain general anesthesia with IV barbiturates. Pentobarbital 5 to 15 mg/kg is given initially, followed by a constant infusion of 1 to 3 mg/h. Continuous EEG monitoring is needed to assess response and guide dosage, and consultation from an anesthesiologist and neurologist should be obtained.

Neuromuscular blocking agents (usually pancuronium or vecuronium) are sometimes helpful. These drugs will abolish tonic-clonic movements and may facilitate ventilation and other measures; they have no effect on abnormal neuronal activity. EEG monitoring is necessary to assess the effectiveness of anticonvulsant therapy when neuromuscular blockers are utilized.

### BIBLIOGRAPHY

Aggarwal P, Wali JP: Lidocaine in refractory status epilepticus: a forgotten drug in the emergency department. *Am J Emerg Med* 11:243, 1993.

Berg AT, Shinnar S: The risk of seizure recurrence following a first unprovoked seizure: a quantitative review. *Neurology* 41:965, 1991.

Camfield P, Camfield C, Dooley J, et al: A randomized study of carbamazepine versus no medication after a first unprovoked seizure in childhood. *Neurology* 30:851, 1989.

Cascino G: Non-convulsive status epilepticus in adults and children. *Epilepsia* 34;Suppl 1:S21, 1993.

Celesia G: Modern concepts of status epilepticus. *JAMA* 235:1571, 1976.

Commission on Classification and Terminology of the International League Against Epilepsy: Proposal for revised clinical and electroencephalographic classification of epileptic seizures. *Epilepsia* 22:489, 1981.

DeLorenzo RJ: The Epilepsies, in Bradley WG, Daroff RB, Fenichel GM, et al (eds): *Neurology in Clinical Practice: Principles of Diagnosis and Management.* Boston, Butterworth-Heinemann, 1991, pp 1443–1477.

First Seizure Trial Group: A randomized clinical trial on the efficacy of antiepileptic drugs in reducing the risk of relapse after a first unprovoked tonic-clonic seizure. *Neurology* 43:478, 1993.

Hauser WA: Status epilepticus: epidemiologic considerations. *Neurology* 40;Suppl 2:9, 1990.

McMicken DB, Freedland ES: Alcohol-related seizures. *Emerg Med Clin North Am* 12:1057, 1994.

Pascual J, Sedano MJ, Polo JM, et al: Intravenous lidocaine for status epilepticus. *Epilepsia* 29:584, 1988.

Shaner DM, McCurdy SA, Herring MO, et al: Treatment of status epilepticus: a prospective comparison of diazepam and phenytoin versus phenobarbital and optional phenytoin. *Neurology* 38:202, 1988.

Shepherd SM: Management of status epilepticus. *Emerg Med Clin North Am* 12:941, 1994.

Working Group on Status Epilepticus: Treatment of convulsive status epilepticus. *JAMA* 270:854, 1993.

# 196
# ACUTE PERIPHERAL NEUROLOGIC LESIONS
### Gregory L. Henry

A systematic approach to the evaluation of neurologic symptoms of the extremities consists of (1) differentiation between acute and chronic symptoms, (2) separation of central and peripheral origin, (3) reflex assessment, and (4) close follow-up (Fig. 196-1).

First, most peripheral neuropathies and myopathies are slowly developing processes with an often confusing history of downhill progression. Family members and the patient should be carefully questioned to determine if the process is acute or chronic. Diffuse, bilateral nerve-muscle lesions are those that evolve over a few hours to days (or at least worsen acutely) and that do not involve severe changes in mental status, at least as their predominant symptomatology.

Second, peripheral nerve lesions must be separated from central nervous system disease. For example, patients with numbness and aching in the right hand may be so occupied with this symptom that they fail to realize they are also having trouble with word finding and facial numbness. It is absolutely essential that by history and physical examination a search is made that will exclude lesions of the central nervous system (see Table 196-1).

Third, reflexes are notoriously difficult to evaluate in the amount of time generally available in the emergency department. A few general statements, however, can be made.

*Hyperreflexia in the face of down-going toes and no other pathological reflexes is probably a normal variant.* Lesions such as previous stroke, multiple sclerosis, cerebral palsy, and amyotrophic lateral sclerosis may all give hyperreflexia, but these lesions are usually quickly separated out by history and physical examination.

In the hyporeflexic patient the situation is more difficult. *The patient who is truly areflexic—that is, no reflexes—usually has a neuropathic as opposed to a myopathic disorder.* However, hyporeflexia may be a normal variant, a sign of spinal shock, a sign of acute cerebral vascular accident, or may accompany a variety of myopathies and neuropathies, and is therefore a nonspecific finding.

Fourth, of all examinations done in medicine, motor and sensory examinations are often the most imprecise. When unsure as to the cause of specific symptom, it is prudent to advise the patient to return

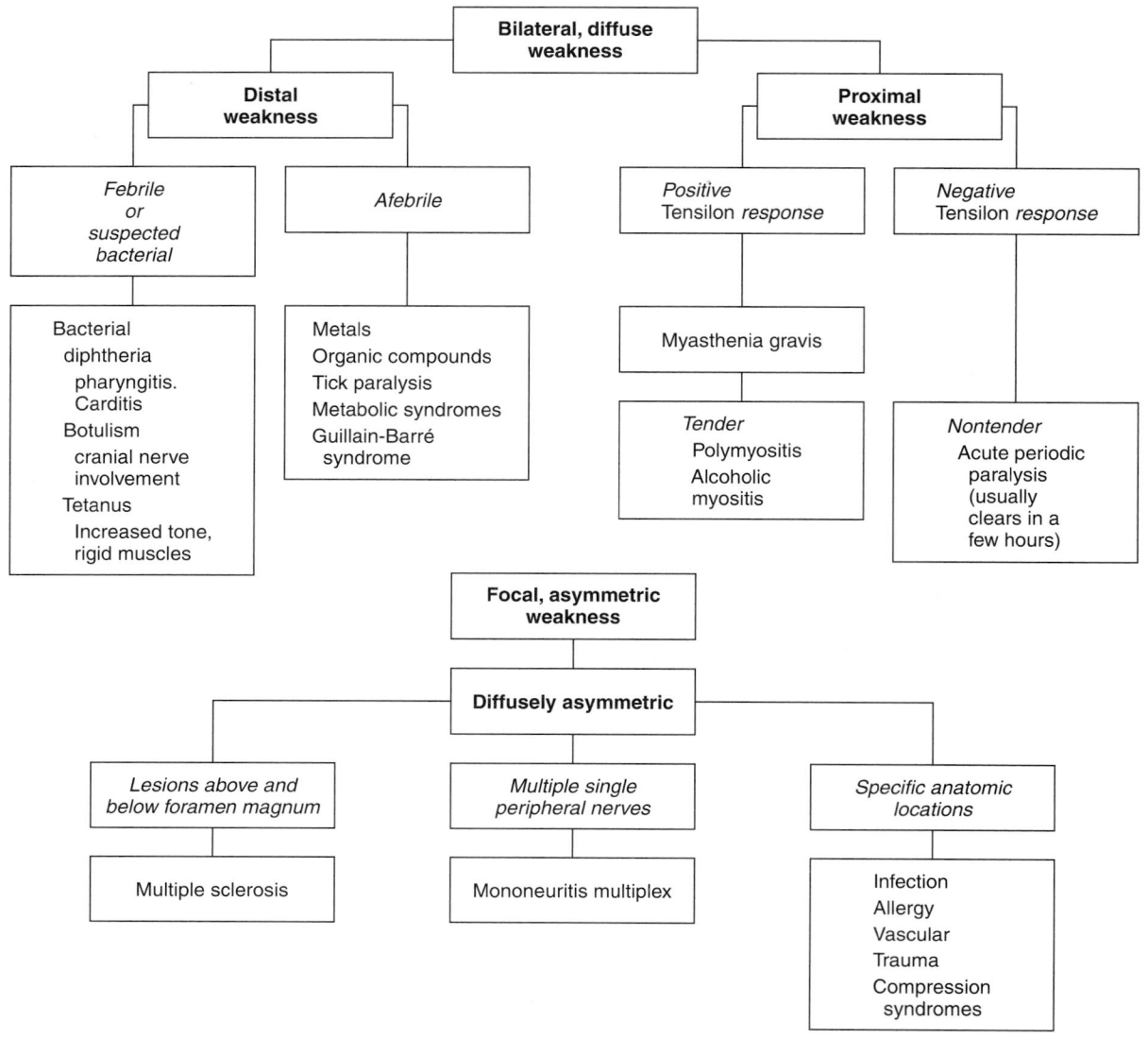

**Fig. 196-1.** Differential diagnosis of weakness. (From Henry G: The patient complaining of weakness. *Emerg Med* Jan 15, 1984, with permission.)

should the symptoms worsen and insure proper outpatient follow-up. A brief emergency department evaluation is not the basis for diagnosis of hysteria or functional disorder.

Keeping in mind the order and extent of the physical examination described in Chap. 191, "The Neurologic Examination," and with the above basic guidelines, we are ready to construct the working differential diagnosis of acute peripheral problems.

It is beyond the scope of this chapter to discuss the myriad diseases that produce myopathies and neuropathies. We will concentrate on those entities that are both common and acute. No attempt will be made to describe the chronic disease processes that can usually be segregated out by history, but the main causes of both acute and chronic peripheral neuropathy are summarized in Table 196-2.

## ACUTE GENERALIZED WEAKNESS

A listing of the major causes of acute generalized weakness is shown in Table 196-3.

## ACUTE TOXIC NEUROPATHIES

### Bacterial Illnesses

Overwhelming bacterial sepsis may cause generalized weakness and lack of motor coordination, but only a limited number of bacterial ill-

**Table 196-1.** Focal Weakness

| Area of Weakness | Location |
|---|---|
| Contralateral face, arm, leg (hemiplegia) | Cortex, internal capsule, rarely brainstem |
| Ipsilateral face, contralateral arm and leg | Brainstem |
| Bilateral arm and leg without neck and head (quadriplegia) | Cervical spinal cord, rarely medulla or pons |
| Arms bilaterally without involvement of the head, neck, or legs (diplegia) | Central cord syndrome or syringomyelia of the cervical spinal cord |
| Legs bilaterally without involvement of upper body or head (paraplegia) | Thoracic or lumbar spinal cord |
| Ipsilateral weakness one leg, with contralateral leg decreased pin and temperature sensation | Hemisection spinal cord (Brown-Séquard syndrome) |
| Unilateral or bilateral single dermatome weakness with associated sensory changes | Spinal-nerve-root lesion |
| Specific peripheral nerve, with associated sensory findings | Isolated peripheral nerve |
| Isolated arm or leg (monoplegia) | Pons, occasionally central cortex, spinal cord; small lesion, extremely rare |

*Source:* Henry G, Little N: *Neurologic Emergencies: A Symptom Oriented Approach.* New York, McGraw-Hill, 1985. Used by permission.

**Table 196-2.** Causes of Acute and Chronic Peripheral Neuropathy

| Diseases | | Vitamin Deficiencies | Intoxications | Commonly Used Drugs |
|---|---|---|---|---|
| Multiple myeloma | Renal failure | Thiamine | Arsenic | Chloroquine |
| Carcinoma | Diabetes mellitus | Pyridoxine | Lead | Clioquinol |
| Myxedema | Porphyria | Pantothenic acid | Mercury | Dapsone |
| Systemic lupus erythematosus | Refsum disease | Riboflavin | Thallium | Phenytoin |
| Cryoglobulinemia | Tangier disease | Vitamin $B_{12}$ | Acrylamide | Disulfiram |
| Rheumatoid arthritis | Metachromatic leukodystrophy | Folic acid | Carbon tetrachloride | Glutethimide |
| Scleroderma | Polyarteritis nodosa | | Chlorinated hydrocarbons | Gold |
| Diphtheria | Sarcoidosis | | Methyl butyl ketone | Hydralazine |
| Hepatic failure | Tuberculosis | | Triorthocresyl phosphate | Isoniazid |
| Vasculitis | Waldenström disease | | Hexachlorophene | Nitrofurantoin |
| | Acromegaly | | Plastic model glue | Stilbamidine |
| | Amyloidosis | | | Vincristine |
| | | | | Immunization |

nesses will present early with severe peripheral neurologic findings. These are diphtheria, botulism, and tetanus.

## Diphtheria

Infections with *Corynebacterium diphtheriae* are usually characterized by an acute onset, exudative pharyngitis, high fever, and malaise. The organism gives off a powerful exotoxin that acts directly on the heart, kidneys, and the nervous system. The most common presenting neurologic problem with diphtheria is mononeuritis or a mononeuritis multiplex. For example, neurologic involvement of the palate with difficulty in speaking and changing quality of voice can occur. The most commonly observed paralyses, however, involve the intrinsic and extrinsic muscles of the eye, producing ptosis, strabismus, and problems in accommodation. When the limbs are involved, the patient is critically ill and has bilateral flaccid weakness or paralysis accompanied by absent deep tendon reflexes and, in longstanding cases, atrophy. Sensory involvement is rare. However, bladder and rectal sphincter muscles may be involved, producing urinary retention, overflowing incontinence, and incompetent anal sphincter tone. The ascending transverse myelitis of the Guillain-Barré type has been recorded with cases of diphtheria. Although diphtheria has been considered a rare disease in North America over the past 40 years, pockets of nonimmunized and poorly immunized patients do exist. Recent immigrants, the poor, and religious sects that do not have children immunized should all be considered at risk.

## Botulism

Botulism toxin is a preformed toxin, elaborated by *Clostridium botulinum,* an anaerobic gram-positive bacillus that affects both striated and smooth muscle. The toxin exerts its effect principally at the myoneural junction, without direct toxicity to the muscle fibers or the peripheral nerve itself. The principal mode of action is in prevention of the release of acetylcholine. There are at least seven major toxins,

but toxins A, B, and E are the ones primarily causing disease in humans.

The principal source of botulism in the United States is food that has been improperly prepared. There are no definitive telltale signs or smells of the organism so that it may exist in food which is normal on inspection. The neurologic symptoms usually appear in 24 to 48 h after ingestion of contaminated foods and may or may not be preceded by nausea, vomiting, and diarrhea. The most common early presenting neurologic complaints are related to the eyes and bulbar musculature. Symptoms spread very rapidly, however, to involve all the muscles of the trunk and extremities. The smooth muscle of the intestine and the bladder may occasionally be involved, resulting in ileus and acute urinary retention. Good mental status is maintained until the patient is terminal.

It is important to differentiate botulism from diphtheria or Guillain-Barré syndrome. Guillain-Barré syndrome is usually an ascending process and does not usually begin with involvement of bulbar musculature. Diphtheria is an acute febrile illness, with pseudomembranous oropharyngitis and cardiac involvement. With rapid deterioration, botulism may occasionally be confused with undiagnosed myasthenia gravis. The two are easily differentiated with the edrophonium chloride (Tensilon) test. Botulism should not improve with the administration of cholinesterase inhibitors.

A variant form of botulism, infant botulism, has recently had a resurgence. In almost 40 percent of affected infants, the source of the botulism can be traced to raw honey containing botulinum spores. Children affected with this disease may exhibit lethargy and failure to thrive, eventually leading to paralysis and death. It is almost always insidious in infants because of the extremely small amounts of botulinum toxin ingested along with the honey.

After diagnosis and respiratory support, further treatment of botulism patients is usually carried out in the intensive care unit. As with all ingested toxins, removal of the remaining offending agent by gastric lavage, activated charcoal, and instillation of cathartics may be needed. The decision to use botulinum antitoxin is usually made following consultation with infectious disease specialists.

## Tetanus

Tetanus is described more fully in Chap. 123. The symptoms of tetanus are due to the toxin elaborated by *Clostridium tetani.* Tetanus may cause local tetany where it diffuses through the perineural tissues at the site of innoculation. More commonly, however, the patient will have generalized tetanus 5 to 10 days after inoculation. The most common presenting symptom is trismus, but it is usually rapidly followed by neck stiffness, rigidity of the back muscles to the point of opisthotonos, and a characteristic tight rigid facial expression that is referred to as *risus sardonicus.*

There are no specific blood, urine, or cerebral spinal fluid (CSF) abnormalities that will confirm the diagnosis. The combination of

**Table 196-3.** Acute Generalized Weakness

| Neuropathies | Myopathies | Motor End Plate | Cancer Syndromes |
|---|---|---|---|
| Infection | Polymyositis | Myasthenia gravis | Eaton-Lambert |
| Idiopathic | Alcohol myositis | | Chemotherapy |
| Toxins | Acute periodic paralysis | Botulism | Radiation therapy |
| Organic compounds | Metabolic | Tick paralysis | Cerebellar degeneration |
| Metals | Infection | Drugs | Polymyositis |
| | | | Metabolic |
| | | | Affective (frontal lobe) weakness |
| | Psychiatric | | |

rapidly progressive trismus, persistent truncal and extremity tetany, risus sardonicus, and intermittent convulsions give little problem in formulating a differential diagnosis. Strychnine can produce tetany and convulsions, but pronounced muscle relaxation between convulsions is characteristic of strychnine poisoning.

## Metallic Poisons

Poisoning by metallic compounds usually results in prominent central nervous system as well as peripheral nervous system findings. It is impossible to mention all the various types of metallic poisoning syndromes, but arsenic and lead poisoning are worth reviewing. Arsenic is still found in insecticides, rat poisons, and herbicides, and in certain medicinal compounds. Acute gastrointestinal irritation with vomiting and diarrhea are usually presenting signs following ingestions of large amounts of arsenic. In patients receiving lower doses, however, polyneuritis may be one of the presenting complaints. In such cases, a history of occupational exposure is usually found.

Lead poisoning usually results from accidental or industrial toxic exposure. Lead may be absorbed through the skin or the lungs, or ingested through the gastrointestinal tract. In severe acute lead poisoning the principal symptoms are acute weakness, prostration, and abdominal pain. In those patients who have received chronic smaller doses of lead, a peripheral motor neuropathy is common. These patients will have minor sensory findings but may have pronounced distal weakness.

## Organic Compounds

Neuromuscular toxic effects can result from a wide variety of organic compounds. The alcohols, phenothiazines, and aminoglycoside antibiotics are discussed here.

Ethanol, methanol, and other alcohols may produce long-standing, slowly progressive peripheral neuropathies, predominantly sensory. Myopathies can be present as well. Acute intoxication with these agents usually causes pronounced central nervous system effects.

The phenothiazines may produce local dystonias even though the mechanism is central. Buccolingual dyskinesias caused by phenothiazine derivatives should be well known to emergency physicians. Often these are not seen in persons taking chronic psychiatric medication, but in those receiving small amounts of phenothiazines for symptoms such as nausea and vomiting, or in those who abuse street drugs.

Neuromuscular blockade, causing profound weakness, can be enhanced by aminoglycoside antibiotics. This is usually encountered in hospitalized patients, especially postoperatively.

## Tick Paralysis

Tick paralysis is also discussed in Chap. 127. Tick paralysis is a reversible, rapidly progressive ascending paralysis in which neuromuscular end-plate conduction is affected without morphologic changes. The symptoms of tick paralysis are almost identical to those of Guillain-Barré syndrome. Flaccid paralysis begins at the extremities and trunk and moves up to involve the bulbar musculature. There are no specific blood, urine, or CSF changes to aid in the diagnosis. The diagnosis of tick paralysis is made by finding the tick after a thorough examination of the body, including the hairy areas. Formerly, acute poliomyelitis would also be considered in the differential diagnosis of tick paralysis and Guillain-Barré syndrome. However, polio can usually be differentiated from the other two types of paralysis by their lack of fever or neck stiffness, or of cellular and protein changes in the cerebrospinal fluid.

## Metabolic Neuropathy

The majority of nutritional and metabolic neuropathies have a slow onset, are progressive, and are clearly beyond the scope of the emergency physician. There are, however, several variants that may occur in a rapid fashion and are thus worth considering in a differential diagnosis: hyperinsulinism, gout, and acute intermittent porphyria. In contrast to diabetic neuropathy, which is symmetric and slow in onset, hyperinsulinism associated with pancreatic tumors may produce acute paresthesia, impaired sensation, muscle weakness, and hyporeflexia. It is virtually always seen in conjunction with symptomatic hypoglycemia.

During gouty attacks there may be a sudden onset of generalized extremity neuropathy or neuropathies, particularly of the lumbar plexus. The neuropathies seem to disappear when symptoms of gout are controlled. The pathophysiology of this form of paralysis is unknown.

Acute intermittent porphyria is characterized by psychosis, abdominal pains, and polyneuropathy of the Guillain-Barré type.

## Neuropathy of Guillain-Barré

Today, the neuropathy of the Landry-Guillain-Barré disease is thought to be not a disease but a symptom complex that may follow many infectious diseases, exposure to toxins, and collagen vascular diseases. This syndrome usually follows an acute febrile episode or an acute metabolic problem by days or weeks and may be rapidly progressive. Persons in the third to fourth decades are most frequently affected, but it may occur in young children and in older adults.

The usual pattern of presentation is that of an ascending motor neuron involvement. The lower extremities are usually involved first and are more severely affected than the upper extremities. The bulbar musculature, however, may be involved partially or totally. Although paralysis usually reaches the maximum within a week, in some patients maximum paralysis is reached within hours. This is considered to be a motor neuron disease, but sensory symptoms are not uncommon and radicular pain is often noted. Although paralysis is rapid in onset, recovery may take months to years but is usually complete.

In the emergency department differential diagnosis is difficult. Frequently the patient gives a vague history of weakness in the lower extremities without any other antecedent history. Since this is a motor neuron disease, reflex arcs are often affected early. A patient who has weakness and loss of lower extremity reflexes should be considered to have Guillain-Barré disease until proven otherwise. Acute exacerbations of lead poisoning, porphyria, botulism, and diphtheria may all enter into the differential diagnosis and must be separated out by history and other pertinent clinical findings.

## ACUTE MYOPATHIES

Like neuropathies, most myopathies, particularly in young people, progress slowly. The rapidly progressive acquired myopathies are relatively few in number, and a reasonable differential diagnosis can be made in the emergency department.

The first task is to differentiate neuropathies from myopathies. Neuropathies tend to give distal symptoms, with pronounced distal weakness progressing proximally. With myopathies, large muscle and central muscle groups are frequently affected at the same time as distal muscle groups, so diffuse or predominantly proximal weakness is a striking finding. A second important clue in differentiating neuropathies and myopathies is that myopathies rarely include sensory symptoms. There may be aching in the involved musculature, but paresthesias and decreased sensation are not noted. A third differentiating feature is the fact that in myopathies, despite rather pronounced weakness, the patient will maintain deep-tendon reflexes until the disease process is extremely advanced. Neuropathies usually affect reflexes early in the disease process.

Laboratory testing is usually more fruitful for the emergency physician in myopathies as opposed to neuropathies. Elevated leukocyte count, sedimentation rate, and elevated muscle enzymes along with normal spinal fluid parameters characterize myopathies.

## Polymyositis Syndrome

It is of little value for the emergency physician to subclassify acute polymyositis into its multiple causes. Polymyositis is more a syndrome than a specific disease. This form of myopathy, however, usually evolves rapidly, and, within weeks of onset, the patient has pronounced symptoms. In severe cases, however, severe weakness may develop over several days. Most patients have muscular pain and tenderness. A significant number also have dysphasia. Accompanying signs and symptoms, such as arthralgia, fever, and Raynaud phenomenon, all lend support to the diagnosis of polymyositis. After the polymyositis syndrome is suspected, investigation is necessary to isolate the various treatable causes. Such a complex workup is beyond the scope of emergency diagnosis.

Many infections, including trichinosis and toxoplasmosis, and many viral entities have been associated with polymyositis. All the collagen vascular diseases except periarteritis nodosa have also been implicated. Endocrinopathies, including both hyperthyroidism and hypothyroidism as well as adrenal-cortical and parathyroid lesions, are part of the differential diagnosis. Steroids, which are used in treating many forms of polymyositis, can actually exacerbate the problem. Several of the drugs used to treat malaria and other protozoan infection have been associated with polymyositis. This can be confusing, as malaria itself can cause polymyositis. In approximately 10 percent of adults, polymyositis is a remote manifestation of carcinoma. There is no specific emergency department therapy for polymyositis, and use of steroids should await correct diagnosis.

## Alcoholic Myopathy

Along with the well-known alcoholic peripheral neuropathy and the propensity to develop other skeletal disorders, alcoholics are prone to at least one type of unique myopathic syndrome. During prolonged periods of heavy alcohol intake, an alcoholic may have severe muscle tenderness and swelling, muscle cramps, and severe weakness. Signs and symptoms may be generalized or focal. This syndrome represents the acute diffuse necrosis of skeletal muscle fibers all in one stage of degeneration, or acute rhabdomyolysis. Muscle degeneration can lead to life-threatening hyperkalemia or hypocalcemia and secondary binding without released intracellular $PO_4$, and myoglobinuria can cause renal failure. In the alcoholic with acute muscle pain and weakness, serum electrolyte levels, muscle enzymes, and urinalysis for myoglobin are necessary. Although most patients recover within several weeks, return to normal motor functions may take many months.

## Myasthenia Gravis

Myasthenia gravis is not a true myopathy, but the presenting symptoms and examination features closely resemble those of the other myopathic diseases. It is discussed in detail in Chap. 198.

## Acute Periodic Paralysis

The most bizarre of the acute weakness syndromes is acute periodic paralysis. There are three basic types or primary forms: hyperkalemic, hypokalemic, and normokalemic. The exact mechanisms of these types have not been fully delineated, but an abnormal number of mitochondria and abnormalities in the sarcoplasmic reticulum have been noted by electron microscopy.

This disease complex is rarely suspected before the ninth or tenth attack. Periodic paralysis occurs predominantly in males (by 4:1 or 5:1 ratio), and generally the onset is between the seventh and twenty-first years of life.

Interestingly, the patient may often be awakened from sleep by the weakness. A history of extreme physical exertion on that day is important in establishing the diagnosis. Cold weather, large meals, trauma, and surgery may provoke an attack. Some patients will have the attacks on a regular basis, almost daily; others will have only a limited number throughout their lifetime. But the usual story is one of sudden extreme weakness without associated pain. Patients will give a history of being normal before and after the episodes, which usually last 1 or 2 h. Episodes may be so severe that patients will fall while walking or gag while eating.

An in-depth discussion of the various forms of periodic paralysis and paramyotonia congenita is beyond the scope of this basic review, but an understanding of these attacks should alert the emergency physician to consider the diagnosis, obtain a serum potassium level, and provide referral to a neurologist in suspected cases.

## NONMYASTHENIC SYNDROMES OF MALIGNANCY

As the average age of the population increases, there will by sheer weight of numbers be more interaction between emergency physicians and patients suffering from or being treated for various forms of cancer. Many acute side effects of cancer or its treatment are due to local disease extension or metastases. The following entities, however, are unrelated to the tumor mass itself but represent the remote effects of the tumor or its treatment: Lambert-Eaton syndrome, effects of drugs and radiation, cerebellar degeneration, polymyositis, and acute dementia.

## Lambert-Eaton Syndrome

For a number of years it has been recognized that there is abnormal neuromuscular transmission associated with certain malignancies, particularly oat-cell carcinoma of the lung. This syndrome, when first described by Eaton and Lambert, was thought to be a mild variant form of myasthenia gravis. However, as the syndrome became more fully delineated, it was clear that the differences between the two were multiple. In the Lambert-Eaton syndrome the patient will occasionally have aching muscle pain and will rarely be as weak as the patient with myasthenia gravis. There is less fluctuation of weakness and strength than found in myasthenia gravis. The cranial nerves are almost always spared in the Lambert-Eaton syndrome.

A rather remarkable finding is the fact that unlike myasthenia gravis, which gets worse with repeated activity, with the Lambert-Eaton syndrome grip strength actually improves with repeated activity. There is no response to edrophonium.

## Drugs and Radiation Therapy

For cancer patients currently under treatment, medications and dosage schedules must be carefully reviewed to determine the cause of weakness. Many chemotherapeutic agents are metabolic poisons and this may be the reason for the patient's weakness. *Steroids may produce a polymyositis syndrome.* Many tumors are treated with radiation. If the spinal column is involved, transverse myelitis may develop very suddenly, months to even years later. This is a true medical emergency. The differential diagnosis is radiation myelitis, or a compressive lesion due to metastasis. Emergency neurosurgical consultation and myelography or magnetic resonance imaging (MRI) are often necessary.

## Cerebellar Degeneration

Another and yet unexplained remote effect of cancer is acute weakness and cerebellar degeneration. Patients may have a rapid history of deterioration with inability to walk and control the upper extremities, and there is evidence of pancerebellar involvement.

## Polymyositis

Polymyositis may be a remote effect of carcinoma. Occult malignancy will be discovered in about 10 percent of adults with polymyositis.

## MONONEURITIS AND MONONEURITIS MULTIPLEX

Acute temporal arteritis is probably the prototype for this disorder. The principle lesion is infarction of peripheral nerves due to arteritis in the vasa nervorum of the peripheral nerves. It occurs in diabetic patients and those with collagen vascular disease. The patient may complain of a specific peripheral nerve lesion in the right arm, another one in the left leg, and still another in the region of the cervical plexus. On specific testing, perfectly anatomic localizations can be delineated and usually the underlying disease has already been diagnosed. Treatment with high dose steroids may be indicated.

## SPECIFIC ISOLATED PERIPHERAL NERVE LESIONS

### Herpes Zoster

Herpes zoster represents the most important infection that clinically presents as an isolated peripheral nerve lesion. Herpes as a whole tends to present as an independent condition, but it may be associated with surgical procedures, diabetes, and occasionally trauma. Elderly and immunocompromised patients are at the greatest risk of developing herpes zoster. Younger adults who develop the disease should be considered at high risk for having an underlying illness involving the immune system. Extreme pain, which is generally in a dermatomal distribution, usually precedes the skin lesions by several days. The dermatomes most often affected are the thoracic, followed by the trigeminal nerve, lumbar plexus, and finally the cervical plexus. Although herpes produces principally sensory involvement, motor dysfunction may be seen in up to 25 percent of patients. Although the sensory disturbances and skin lesions usually abate with time, the motor disturbances seen with herpes do not usually completely resolve. Herpes zoster may involve the cranial nerves. Skin lesions in the various divisions of the fifth and seventh cranial nerves are frequently seen. Tympanic membrane and corneal involvement may be seen as part of the Ramsay Hunt syndrome. Whenever corneal lesions are suspected, ophthalmologic consultation for consideration of antiviral medications is appropriate. The role of steroids following the initial phase of the lesions is controversial. Current treatment consists of oral acyclovir, 200 mg 5 times a day, for 10 days. Patients do not require admission unless the disease is disseminated, or unless patients are immunocompromised or receiving steroids or chemotherapy. As acyclovir can cause interstitial nephritis, creatinine and BUN should be obtained before beginning the medication.

### Allergic Neuropathy

An unusual phenomenon that is seen approximately nine times more in males than in females is an allergic neuropathy following the injection of immunologic materials, usually tetanus toxoid. The neurologic complications usually develop about 2 days after signs of generalized serum sickness. Although central nervous system signs are reported, the most common neurologic complication is a motor peripheral neuropathy involving the brachial plexus. It may or may not be bilateral. A single nerve such as the radial or optic nerve may be involved.

### Vascular Peripheral Nerve Lesions

#### Volkmann Paralysis

Volkmann ischemic paralysis is the prototype for vascular peripheral nerve lesions. The paralysis is due primarily to injury to the nutrient vessels of a peripheral nerve, and it can be iatrogenically induced by a tight-fitting cast. During the first few hours, severe pain is the principal symptom. As the disease process progresses, nerves and muscles undergo extensive fibrosis with resultant contractures and impairment of both motor and sensory functions.

### Tic Douloureux

Tic douloureux, or trigeminal neuralgia, should be mentioned. There is probably no one explanation for the source of pain in trigeminal neuralgia. It is believed by many that pulsations from a branch of the basilar artery serve as irritants and decrease the trigeminal nerve's threshold for pain. The principal symptom is severe lancinating pain usually confined to the area of distribution of the third portion of the trigeminal nerve. Often multiple portions of the trigeminal nerve will be involved, but bilaterality is unusual. Such pain usually presents little problem in differential diagnosis, but treatment may be difficult. During acute attacks opiates are helpful. It is inappropriate for the emergency physician to initiate chronic therapy without consulting a physician who will follow the patient.

Ninth-nerve neuralgia, or glossopharyngeal tic, is less common. Although rare, this disorder is characterized by intense pain localized to the area of the ear and throat on the affected side. Pain may radiate to the posterior third of the tongue, tonsillar pillars, and the oropharynx and larynx. The most common irritants that initiate this unusual pain are swallowing, talking, or chewing. Unlike tic douloureux, the pain of glossopharyngeal neuralgia may last for longer periods of time and usually tends to come in waves or clusters at a particular time of the year. There is no single theory as to the cause of glossopharyngeal neuralgia, but a vascular etiology is hypothesized.

### Cranial Nerve Neuropathies

The cranial nerve neuropathies represent a separate subcategory of specific isolated nerve lesions. The general maxim from neurology and ear, nose, and throat surgery is that any cranial nerve neuropathy may represent a tumor until proven otherwise. In all practicality, however, most cranial nerve neuropathies seen by the emergency physician are more likely to be vascular or idiopathic lesions of sudden onset. It is beyond the scope of this discussion to detail each cranial neuropathy, but because the seventh nerve is frequently involved in both traumatic and infectious conditions and is the most commonly involved with idiopathic dysfunction, it will be discussed here.

The seventh cranial nerve, or facial nerve, has two principal divisions as it leaves the brainstem. These are a motor root and the nervus intermedius, which functions to supply taste to the anterior two thirds of the tongue and automatic fibers to the salivary and lacrimal glands. Above the brainstem, the seventh nerve has both crossed and uncrossed fibers, while below the seventh nerve nucleus fibers are uncrossed. If a patient retains muscular strength in the forehead and upper face but not the lower face, the lesion is probably central, i.e., in the brainstem or above. If the patient has weakness of the forehead, around the eyes, and lower face, this probably represents a lower motor neuron involvement of the type usually seen with Bell palsy. Taste may be affected by involvement of the chorda tympani nerve but is of little clinical value since taste is very difficult to test in the outpatient setting.

### Bell's Palsy

Bell's palsy is not a specific disease but represents a constellation of symptoms of multiple etiologies. Idiopathic Bell palsy is a diagnosis of exclusion. Disease processes such as Lyme disease, parotid tumors, lesions of the middle ear, cerebellopontine angle tumors, eighth-nerve lesions, and vascular disease can all present as Bell's palsy (Table 196-4). The exact location of the disorder along the seventh nerve or in the brainstem can often be ascertained by careful physical examination. It is important to localize the level of involvement to determine if a structural lesion or idiopathic Bell's palsy is present. It is essential to check for otitis media, mastoiditis, or chcolesteatoma, since Bell's palsy in association with these disorders is an ear, nose, and throat emergency. In endemic areas, Lyme disease should always be considered in patients with Bell's palsy. Le-

**Table 196-4.** Common Causes of Peripheral Seventh-Nerve Palsy

Middle ear disorders
    Otitis media
    Mastoiditis
    Cholesteatoma
Viral diseases
    Herpes zoster (Ramsay Hunt syndrome)
    Mumps
    Echovirus
    Herpes simplex
    Human immunodeficiency virus
    Rubella
Systemic disorders
    Lyme disease
    Lymphoma
    Kawasaki disease

**Table 196-5.** Nerve Entrapment Syndromes

| Nerve Entrapment Syndromes | Signs and Symptoms |
| --- | --- |
| Carpal tunnel syndrome (median nerve) | Tingling in the hand—first, second, third, and one-half of fourth digit; late muscular wasting, thenar area |
| Pronator syndrome (median nerve at the muscle) | Pain from the elbow to the wrist; weakness of the thenar muscles |
| Ulnar nerve–wrist | Paresthesia, fourth and fifth fingers; atrophy, intrinsic muscles of the hand |
| Ulnar nerve–elbow | Same as ulnar nerve–wrist, plus decreased strength in ulnar deviation also of the hand at the wrist |
| Radial nerve | Weakness of the finger extension and wrist extension |
| Lateral cutaneous of the thigh | Numbness in the lateral part of the thigh |
| Posterior tibial (tarsal tunnel) | Numbness of the sole of the foot; decreased sensation |
| Bell facial-nerve palsy | Weakness of facial musculature all divisions of the seventh cranial nerve ipsilateral to the lesion |

*Source:* Henry G, Little N: *Neurologic Emergencies: A Symptom Oriented Approach.* New York, McGraw-Hill, 1985. Used by permission.

sions in the tegmentum of the brainstem involve the nucleus of the seventh nerve and almost invariably have an accompanying sixth-nerve palsy. Lesions of the seventh nerve at the point of emergence from the brainstem frequently have associated auditory components due to involvement of the eighth nerve as well. If the lesion is peripheral to the lateral geniculate ganglion, lacrimal fibers are spared and there is usually an excess collection of tears in the conjunctival sac on that side. Beyond the point where the chorda tympani nerve arises, autonomic functions are no longer involved, and a lesion beyond the stylomastoid foramen results in motor weakness and is characteristic of Bell's palsy. Jaw pain or external ear pain is also a common complaint.

If idiopathic Bell's palsy is suspected, the next problem is treatment. There is a considerable growing body of evidence that high-dose steroid therapy in short bursts may be of benefit in treatment of Bell's palsy. If steroids are given, they should be prescribed in consultation with an otolaryngologist or neurologist who can also initiate electro-stimulatory therapy for the patient's muscles while waiting for recovery of the seventh nerve. There is a small but firm group who advocate unroofing the canal of the seventh nerve if recovery has not occurred after approximately 6 weeks. However, 98 percent of patients with Bell's palsy recover at least partial function, and operative intervention should be reserved for those patients with prolonged or severe difficulty.

## TRAUMA AND NERVE COMPRESSION SYNDROMES

### Spinal Cord Compression

Lesions along the cord may produce distinct isolated neurological syndromes. One of the emergency problems is compression of the spinal cord. This may occur as a result of trauma, herniation of intervertebral disks, primary or metastatic tumors, AV malformations, radiation myelitis, or cysts. It is important to remember that acute spinal cord compression is often associated with areflexia. Cremasteric reflexes, anal sphincter tone, and motor activity in the extremities all help to localize the lesion. Emergency neurosurgical consultation and emergent imaging studies are indicated.

### Root and Trunk Syndromes

The peripheral nerve is the endpoint in a long process of combinations and divisions of nervous tissues. After exiting the cord in the cervical, upper thoracic, and lumbosacral regions, nerve roots at each particular level combine with other nerves to form plexuses. Plexuses then form major and minor trunks which divide to form specific peripheral nerves. Therefore, depending on the lesion along the nerve, different symptoms can result. The patient with a C6 root lesion will have a different distribution in the hand than a patient with a median nerve injury. When evaluating isolated complaints, do not overlook the possible multiple levels at which a nerve might be involved.

### Common Nerve Entrapments

There is not adequate room to list all the various nerve root compression syndromes that the emergency physician might encounter. Two texts are useful: *Aids to the Investigation of Peripheral Nerve Injuries,* which was first published in 1942 as an aid to British trauma surgeons and has stood the test of time as an excellent reference for acute neuromuscular problems, and *Peripheral Entrapment Neuropathies,* by H. P. Kopel and W. A. Thompson, which carefully reviews the physical findings in entrapment disorders and lists possible locations on the nerve where they are involved. Table 196-5 gives a brief overview to the common nerve entrapments and their symptomatology.

The most common causes of acute mononeuropathies are usually traumatic, following fractures, dislocations, or acute soft tissue swelling. A mononeuropathy can be a result of repetitive motor activity that causes increased connective tissue in small spaces. It should be remembered that with high-velocity missile injuries, direct contact with a nerve is not necessary to produce a palsy. Besides trauma, causes of entrapment neuropathies include any inflammation or degeneration in and around tight canals where nerves must pass. This is frequently seen in patients with rheumatoid arthritis, myxedema of thyroid disease, amyloidosis, and pregnancy.

## BIBLIOGRAPHY

Henry G, Little N: *Neurologic Emergencies: A Symptom Oriented Approach* New York, McGraw-Hill, 1985.

Long Island Neuroborreliosis Collaborative Study Group: Lyme borreliosis in Bell's Palsy. *Neurology* 42(7): 1268, 1992.

## 197

# MULTIPLE SCLEROSIS

### Richard F. Edlich
### Marie-Louise Hammarskjöld

## INTRODUCTION

The demyelinating diseases consist of a group of diseases that cause central nervous system dysfunction by damaging the myelin sheaths covering axons. There are two basic types of such disorders. In the first, myelin loss occurs in the absence of an inflammatory reaction and this group includes genetic defects in myelin metabolism, toxin-induced injury (e.g., carbon monoxide), and opportunistic viral infection of oligodendrocytes (e.g., progressive multifocal leukoencephalopathy).

In the second, the demyelinating diseases exhibit focal or patchy destruction of the myelin sheaths in the central nervous system in the presence of inflammation. Of the latter group, we will review here only multiple sclerosis (MS).

MS is the leading cause of neurologic morbidity and mortality among young adults. The average age of onset is in the third and fourth decades, and females are affected more commonly than males. The female-to-male incidence ratio may be as high as 2.5:1. The prevalence rate in the white population is 62 per 100,000 people, compared to 31 per 100,000 people in the nonwhite population. This disease is uncommon in Orientals. Generally, MS is more common in people who live in the northern and southern temperate latitudes. There is a familial incidence, and approximately 10 percent of MS patients have an affected relative.

## PATHOPHYSIOLOGY

MS is an inflammatory disease of the central nervous system that has its primary effect in the oligodendroglia cells, which are responsible for the production and maintenance of the myelin sheaths covering the axons. The initial event in multiple sclerosis appears to be functional interference with or injury to the myelinating capacity of the oligodendrocytes. There is subsequent degeneration of the myelin lamellae, which antedates complete destruction of the myelin sheaths. As a consequence of injury, antigens are presented by microglial cells, which result in the infiltration of inflammatory cells, including T and B lymphocytes as well as macrophages.

The key pathologic lesion in MS is the plaque, which is a more or less circumscribed lesion, varying in size from a few to many cubic centimeters, oriented around venules. The characteristic findings in the plaque are primary destruction of myelin with relative preservation of axons and gliosis. Conduction of nerve impulses along axons without myelin is slowed; this defect in nerve conduction is made worse by hyperthermia. The plaques are present in scattered areas of the white matter of the central nervous system, with a predilection for the periventricular areas of the cerebrum and subpially, and within the brainstem, spinal cord, and optic nerves. The acute lesions usually contain inflammatory infiltrates with lymphocytes at the site of subsequent demyelination.

## CLINICAL FEATURES

This disease presents as recurrent attacks of a focal neurologic disease. The presence of clinical remissions remains the clinical rule. In addition, the disease should be disseminated over time and location within the nervous system. MS can be viewed as the "great imitator" in neurologic disease. The first episode of MS presents as more than one symptom or sign in the majority (55 percent) of cases; the remaining cases become evident as a single sign or symptom.

Symptoms and signs of neurologic dysfunction in MS arise from lesions in the optic nerve, posterior visual pathways (optic chiasm, tracts, and radiations), brainstem, cerebellum, and spinal cord. More than one-third of patients with MS present with sensory or motor visual symptoms, and they occur at some stage of the disease in nearly all patients with MS.

The first symptom of MS in 10 to 30 percent of patients in the United States is optic neuritis. It often begins with pain around the eye, which is increased by eye movement. Blurring of vision usually follows within days. This blurring of vision may precede the pain. Visual loss evolves over a week, reaching a maximum level of severity that ranges from minimal loss of vision to no light perception. Color vision is altered early, with the colors being broken in a pointillist manner.

Examination reveals a variable loss of visual acuity. The classical field loss is a central scotoma, but a range of defects may be found. Color vision is almost invariably impaired. Fundal examination is normal in approximately 50 percent of the patients. In the remainder, there is swelling of the disk (papillitis) that may be indistinguishable from papilledema. After approximately 1 month, pallor of the optic disk frequently develops.

Three transient phenomena are encountered in patients with optic neuritis. Phosphenes (flashes of light), frequently precipitated by eye movements, are noted in one-third of patients. Deterioration of vision induced by exercise, a hot meal, or hot bath (Uhthoff's phenomenon) is usually not encountered in the acute stage of optic neuritis, though it can rarely be the presenting feature of MS. This variability in vision is attributed to the extreme sensitivity of conduction in partially demyelinated fibers to small changes in temperature. The third phenomenon is a sense of disorientation in moving traffic experienced by some patients and is probably due to the Pulfrich effect, a phenomenon attributable to unequal latencies between the two eyes.

Between 85 and 95 percent of patients with optic neuritis make an excellent recovery over 1 to 3 months. Even if the final visual acuity is normal, residual symptoms may persist. Impairment of contrast sensitivity and color vision are common, and abnormal depth perception may interfere with recreational activities. Recurrence of optic neuritis in either eye occurs in 20 to 35 percent of patients.

Practically all known types of abnormalities in eye movements have been described in patients with MS. Diplopia is encountered in one-third of patients, and nystagmus is noted in two-thirds. The most common eye movement disorders are bilateral internuclear ophthalmoplegia (INO) and pendular nystagmus. While these disorders must alert the emergency physician to the diagnosis of MS, neither are specific to MS or any other disease.

The best known clinical eye movement disorder in MS is INO. This disorder is due specifically to a lesion of the medial longitudinal fasciculus (MLF), which is an important pathway for both horizontal and vertical eye movements. The cardinal feature of INO is slow or, less commonly, incomplete abduction of the eye ipsilateral to the affected MLF. Bilateral INO causes bilateral adduction weakness, bilateral abduction nystagmus, and impaired vestibular and pursuit eye movements. Despite loss of adduction on lateral gaze, convergence is preserved. Consequently, patients with acute bilateral INO have horizontal double vision on lateral gaze in either direction, with minimal or no diplopia on primary gaze.

Unilateral INO is a less common manifestation of MS than bilateral INO. Unilateral lesions of the MLF cause weakness of the ipsilateral medial rectus and a dissociated nystagmus of the abducting eye. When a patient with a right-sided INO attempts to look to the left, the adducting right eye moves slowly. In addition, the abducting left eye gives the appearance of a dissociated nystagmus.

In a young adult, acute bilateral INO due to lesions of the MLF bilaterally is considered by some to be diagnostic of MS. However, there are other possible causes of this disorder, including systemic lupus erythematosus, metastatic cancer, or an arteriovenous malformation. While MS is a common cause of unilateral INO, other possible disorders, such as vascular disease or tumor, must be considered in the differential diagnosis.

Lesions of the cerebellum and its connections occur frequently in MS and produce characteristic eye movement disorders that are frequently associated with other symptoms and signs of cerebellar dysfunction. Saccadic dysmetria is one of the most common cerebellar eye movement disorders. It is most easily recognized by asking patients to center their eyes quickly from a position of lateral deviation. Truncal or limb ataxia frequently coexist.

Acquired pendular nystagmus occurs frequently in MS and is characterized by sinusoidal involuntary oscillations of one or both eyes. Oscillations may occur in any plane and result in linear elliptical or torsional movements of the globe.

Isolated ocular motor palsies not associated with other defects, such as nystagmus on upward gaze, are uncommon in MS. When they do occur, the sixth and third nerves are most commonly involved. While isolated ocular palsies are uncommon in MS, the diagnosis should be considered in a young patient with no other obvious cause.

Lesions in the brainstem, affecting the fifth, seventh, and eighth cranial nerves, can occur in MS. When the seventh nerve is involved, there may be a unilateral peripheral facial nerve palsy that almost never causes changes in taste. The descending root of the fifth cranial nerve may be involved, producing unilateral facial numbness, paresthesia, or pain. Paroxysmal unilateral facial pain, indistinguishable from trigeminal neuralgia (tic douloureux) without concomitant sensory loss, occurs in approximately 2 percent of MS patients. Vertigo, vomiting, and nystagmus due to lesions near the vestibular complex are noted in nearly 30 percent of patients at some time during their illness. Clinical experience suggests that deafness is quite rare. Lesions in the cerebellum result in ataxia, scanning monotonous speech, and intention tremor.

Spinal cord lesions in MS may involve the lateral corticospinal tracts, lateral spinothalamic tracts, and dorsal columns. Most MS patients will have abnormalities in the motor systems, largely in the corticospinal tracts, which result in features of upper motoneuron dysfunction characterized by paresis, spasticity, hyperflexia, clonus, Babinski response, and loss of abdominal reflexes. Posterior column lesions produce a decrease in joint-position and vibration sense. Spinothalamic tract involvement, as evidenced by diminution of pain and temperature sensation, is occasionally encountered. A few develop painful tonic spasms in all muscles of the limb due to spinal cord lesions. Patients with MS frequently complain of a symptom of tingling down the back and into the leg that has an electric shock–like quality produced by flexion of the neck (Lhermitt's sign).

Beyond the well-recognized abnormalities of the somatic neural component of the spinal cord in MS, the spinal cord involvement can produce dysautonomias that can be as devastating as their somatic counterparts. These dysautonomias involve primarily the vesicourethra, gastrointestinal tract, and sexual function. The severity of dysautonomias in MS is clearly related to the severity of disease, and this is particularly evident in relation to spastic weakness due to damage to the corticospinal tracts. From a practical point of view, vesicourethral dysfunction in MS can be categorized as failure to store urine, failure to empty urine, or a combination of these with detrusor–external sphincter dyssynergia (DESD). Three major risk factors that predispose patients with MS to grave urologic complications are the presence of an indwelling catheter, the presence of DESD in men, and the presence of poor bladder compliance with associated high detrusor pressures (greater than 40 cmH$_2$O). These urologic abnormalities have been associated with considerable morbidity and mortality. In 55 percent of MS patients who had undergone autopsy, death could be directly attributed to hydronephrosis, pyelonephritis, or septicemia arising from the upper urinary tract. Severe constipation and sexual dysfunction frequently accompany urinary bladder dysfunction in patients with advanced MS. Dysautonomias involving the cardiorespiratory systems are rarely encountered in MS patients with severe neurologic dysfunction.

On rare occasions, severe spinal cord lesions herald the advent of MS. They can result in either complete or incomplete loss of function and are called *transverse myelitis.* Much more frequent causes of acute transverse myelitis are postinfectious vasculomyelopathy and complications from various vaccinations. When there is evidence of a fairly circumscribed level of neurologic deficit, mechanical compression of the spinal cord must always be considered. The association of acute transverse myelitis with concomitant acute bilateral optic neuritis is sometimes referred to as Devic's syndrome. This ill-defined symptom complex is considered by some to be an entity distinct from MS.

Even though cerebral MS is seen in fewer than 5 percent of patients, it is the most disabling and tragic form of MS, with serious deterioration of intellect. The most frequent subtle cerebral symptom is depression. Euphoria is associated with widespread cerebral disease, dementia, and pseudobulbar palsy. Up to 5 percent of patients with MS have seizures. Some of these seizures are focal, caused by subcortical lesions.

The adverse effects of elevated core temperature on the neurologic signs and symptoms of MS have been well known for more than 50 years. Many patients experience worsening of their neurologic deficits with exercise and other states of induced hyperthermia. The physiologic basis for the adverse effects of increased core temperature on the neurologic symptoms in MS involves a blocking of impulse conduction in a demyelinated nerve. There is growing evidence that significant elevation in core body temperature is not without risk in these patients, either precipitating permanent neurologic deficits or exposing the patients to circumstances that predispose to serious injury.

Symptomatic fatigue is the most common symptom of persons with MS, occurring in approximately 70 percent. Fatigue manifests itself by extreme tiredness and the need to rest. Simple tasks, such as dressing, are exhausting to some patients, occasionally even when the individual has normal or near-normal strength. This symptomatic fatigue usually takes place over a day's activity. It can be exacerbated by exercise and increased environmental temperature, probably secondary to the conduction blocks in demyelinated fibers.

Patients with MS have a high incidence of psychological disorders. More than half experience serious depression. Bipolar disorder occurs more frequently among people with MS.

The signs and symptoms of MS are often mistaken for a psychiatric disorder, and a substantial proportion of patients with MS are initially referred to psychiatrists. Psychiatrists in turn may mistake symptoms of MS for those of psychiatric disorder.

## CLINICAL COURSE

The clinical course of the disease is variable. At onset, approximately 65 percent of patients have a *relapsing and remitting* form of the disease. These patients have exacerbations with symptoms associated with central nervous system lesions or plaques. The exacerbations usually resolve over weeks to months. About 15 percent of patients have exacerbations similar to the relapsing and remitting form of the disease but exhibit less recovery, developing significant residual disability. This latter form is referred to as the *relapsing and progressive* form of the disease. In addition, there is a *chronic progressive form* dominated by spinal cord and cerebellar dysfunction. In nearly 20 percent of these patients, the chronic progressive form starts with the initial symptoms. More commonly, it develops from the relapsing and remitting form of the disease over time. A progressive course from disease onset in the younger patient should make one doubt the diagnosis of MS, suggesting the presence of a degenerative disease or tumor. Long-term follow-up studies frequently report that 20 to 35 percent of patients have a very benign disorder, with minimal or no disability. They exhibit a normal lifespan of relatively unencumbered physical activities. Fewer than 5 to 10 percent of patients have a very malignant course, with severe disability within months to a few years and, in a rare subset, within days. In general, symptoms that appear acutely and those involving the sensory pathways and/or cranial nerves have a more favorable prognosis than those developing insidiously with either motor deficits or cerebellar dysfunction.

Pregnancy and infection are factors that influence the course of the disease. The MS relapse rate during pregnancy is half that expected. However, after delivery, the relapse rate increases two- to sixfold. Upper viral respiratory and urinary tract infections appear to exacerbate MS. Immunization, overexertion, and stress do not enhance the relapse rate.

The majority of deaths occur in advanced disease and in patients with high disability scores and of advanced age. Nearly half die due to complications of MS (e.g., pneumonia, renal failure). Of the remaining deaths, malignancy (30 percent), acute myocardial infarction (27 percent), and stroke (11 percent) occur at the same rate as in the age-matched general population. Suicides account for 30 percent of the deaths, a rate that is seven and one-half times that for the age-matched general population.

## DIAGNOSIS

Clinical diagnostic criteria remain the standard method of diagnosis of MS and require the demonstration that a patient of an appropriate age has had at least two episodes of neurologic disturbances that must implicate two distinct sites in the white matter. In the latter circumstance, the diagnosis can be made with greater than 95 percent certainty. In recent years, clinical assessment has been supplemented by a number of tests, but none are specific for MS and the data they provide must be interpreted in light of the clinical picture. Magnetic resonance imaging (MRI) is the recommended imaging technique for supporting the diagnosis (Fig. 197-1). The typical abnormalities of MS are multiple discrete lesions located in the supratentorial white matter, especially in periventricular areas. Lesions are less commonly detected in the cerebellum and brainstem. The MRI detects abnormalities consistent with MS in 70 to 95 percent of MS patients. Gadolinium-enhanced MRI may demonstrate breakdown of the blood-brain barrier and can distinguish acute and chronic lesions. While computed tomography (CT) is not as sensitive as MRI in the detection of MS lesions, it does reveal a wide variety of findings. It provides a reliable assessment of cerebral atrophy and ventricular enlargement and detects low-density focal lesions in the cerebrum, brainstem, or optic nerves.

Evoked-response testing measures the electric response to stimulation of a sensory pathway, recorded through surface electrodes, amplified and subjected to signal averaging. It is a sensitive method to detect slowed conduction of visual, auditory, or somatosensory impulses. One or more evoked-response tests will reveal a slowing of conduction in approximately 80 percent of MS patients.

In addition, cerebrospinal fluid (CSF) examination in MS patients is used to support the diagnosis. The CSF has a normal cell number in most patients. While slight increases in cell counts have been reported, cell counts greater than 50 cells/µL are rare. The cells in the CSF are usually T lymphocytes. Immunocytochemical analysis of the CSF can differentiate benign from malignant lymphoproliferation. The protein concentration is increased in approximately 25 percent of patients. The most characteristic CSF finding in MS is an increase in immunoglobulin (IgG) caused by synthesis of IgG in the central nervous system. An unenhanced CT scan should be obtained before lumbar puncture, searching for evidence of increased intracranial pressure and/or a mass lesion.

## DIFFERENTIAL DIAGNOSIS

A list of the clinical features that cast doubt on the diagnosis of MS includes the following: (1) absence of eye findings (optic nerve involvement or extraocular movement abnormalities); (2) absence of clinical remissions, especially in young patients; (3) localized disease (posterior fossa, craniocervical junction, spinal cord); (4) absence of CSF abnormalities; and (5) atypical clinical features (absence of sensory findings and bladder involvement). The frequency of misdiagnosis, even in MS specialty clinics, has been estimated to be at least 10 percent.

Clinical features common in MS patients may be seen in patients with systemic lupus erythematosus (SLE). Clinically, SLE and MS have several features characteristic of diseases with HLA gene products, including a chronic and/or relapsing course, an inflammatory component, and a weak familial propensity. Based on the American Rheumatism Association's criteria, a diagnosis of SLE rests on serologic findings (elevated ANA, positive anti-DNA antibodies) and a specific pattern of organ involvement.

Lyme disease, neurosyphilis and HIV disease may mimic some aspects of MS. The best clinical marker of acute Lyme disease is erythema chronicum migrans. In many patients, infection progresses to chronic Lyme disease, a spectrum of clinical signs and symptoms characterized by neurologic dysfunction and persistent musculoskeletal and cardiac disease.

The differential diagnosis of neurosyphilis is extensive and beyond the scope of this chapter. Diagnostic criteria include reactive CSF VDRL, reactive serum nontreponemal test results, five or more lymphocytes per µl of CSF, and CSF total protein ≥ 45 mg/dL.

Human immunodeficiency virus (HIV) infections can also present with relapsing and remitting symptoms that are similar to MS. Recent studies suggest that human T-lymphotrophic virus (HTLV-I) may also play an important role in certain disorders of the CNS whose clinical manifestations may mimic MS. The progressive spastic para-

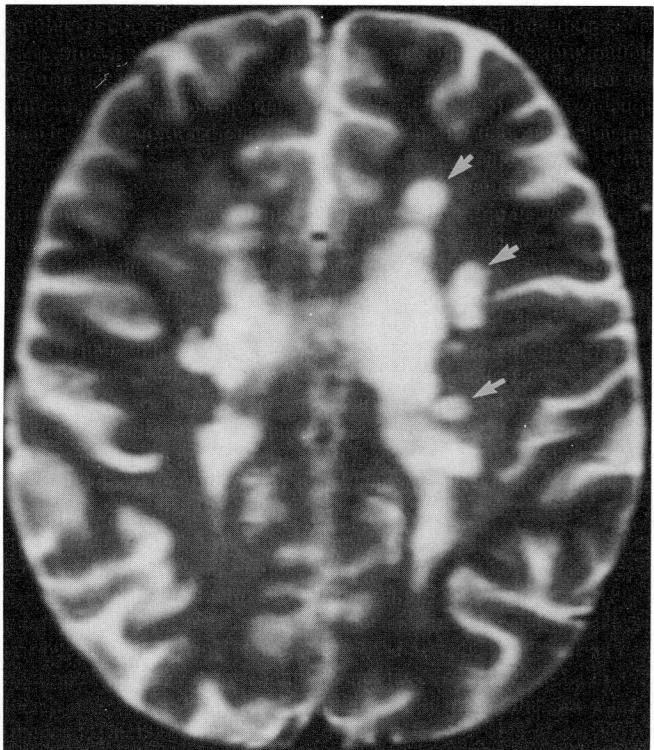

**Fig. 197-1.** A magnetic resonance image from a patient with MS. Multiple lesions of the white matter (arrows) in the periventricular areas support the diagnosis of MS in a patient with an appropriate history and physical findings.

paretic form of MS seen in Caucasian males is virtually identical to tropical spastic paraparesis of HTLV-1-associated myelopathy, which is widely distributed in Africa, the Caribbean, and southern Japan. This disease is associated with HTLV-1.

## EMERGENCY DEPARTMENT CARE

In spite of the fact that there is no single diagnostic test, an emergency physician can suspect the diagnosis through a careful history and examination. Because support from paraclinical data, such as MRI, evoked-potential, and CSF studies, is necessary to confirm the diagnosis, referral to a neurologist who will complete these studies in an ambulatory care setting is necessary. Because the diagnosis is difficult, the neurologist is the best health professional to convey the diagnosis to the patient.

## TREATMENT

Treatment of multiple sclerosis has focused on four aspects of management: delaying the onset of MS, amelioration of an acute exacerbation, slowing the progression of the disease, and relief of symptoms. Optic neuritis is frequently the first manifestation of MS. Even when optic neuritis occurs without any clinical signs of multiple sclerosis (isolated optic neuritis), MRI of the brain often detects signal abnormalities of white matter and analysis of the CSF often shows oligoclonal bands. In patients with acute optic neuritis with signal abnormalities detected on MRI of the brain, treatment with a 3-day course of high-dose intravenous methylprednisolone reduces the rate of development of MS over a 2-year period. Methylprednisolone (250 mg) is administered every 6 h for 3 days followed by 1 mg of oral prednisone per kilogram of body weight per day for 11 days. The beneficial effects of the intravenous steroid appear to lessen after the first 2 years of follow-up. Prednisone given orally is ineffective in reducing the rate of developing MS in patients with acute optic neuritis.

Exacerbations often develop over hours to days, after which the clinical symptoms stabilize and then begin to resolve over weeks to months. If the exacerbation is severe with significant motor and/or cerebellar dysfunction, the patient may be treated with steroids. A short-term (5 days) high-dose (500 mg) course of pulsed intravenous methylprednisolone, followed by an oral tapering course of prednisone for 3 weeks, has been recently reported to be beneficial in acute exacerbation of MS. It is not known if the long-term recovery of function is any different whether or not the patient is given steroids, except in patients with isolated optic neuritis. Long-term daily or alternate-day steroids are not recommended.

Preservation of the integrity of the upper urinary tract is of primary importance in the management of MS urinary dysfunction. Consequently, the initial steps in the detection of urologic dysfunction in these patients is a careful history and physical examination, followed by a microscopic analysis of the Gram stain of unspun urine. When bacteria are detected, cultures of the urine are indicated. Symptomatic patients usually complain of either irritative bladder symptoms with urgency, frequency, and incontinence or obstructive bladder symptoms with hesitancy, flow decrease, and retention, or of a combination of both. Because the likelihood of infection is associated with excessive postvoiding residual (PVR) urine, all MS patients should have serial PVR urine determinations during the course of their disease. The history alone is inadequate in identifying those patients with incomplete bladder emptying. The PVR urine can be determined accurately either by catheterization using aseptic technique or by ultrasonography after the patient has voided.

The treatment of the urologic dysfunction will depend on the magnitude of PVR urine as well as the patient's symptoms. If the MS patient presenting to the emergency department has symptomatic voiding or evidence of bacteriuria, a PVR urine determination is indicated. When the amount of residual urine is either greater than 100 mL or more than 20 percent of the voided volume, the treatment of choice is intermittent catheterization by the clean technique. When the bladder does not empty completely with a PVR urine volume of less than 100 mL, the treatment will depend on the patient's symptoms. In the symptomatic patient, appropriate and effective pharmacologic therapy can be instituted based on specific findings from the urodynamic evaluation by the urologist.

Acute urinary tract infections may be asymptomatic, may produce nonspecific symptoms, or may produce specific symptoms. Patients with dysuria, frequency, urgency, and suprapubic pain usually have cystitis without systemic manifestations. Prominent systemic signs and symptoms, such as fever over 39.2°C (103°F), nausea, vomiting, and costovertebral angle tenderness, usually indicate renal infection. However, some patients with significant bacteriuria from either cystitis or renal infection are asymptomatic. In addition, urinary tract infections may aggravate seemingly unrelated neurologic symptoms, such as lower extremity weakness or spasticity, in MS patients. Consequently, any change in neurologic symptoms in an MS patient should lead to the consideration of urinary tract infection. Although recurrent urinary tract infection may reflect an inadequately treated infection, chronic infection may indicate significant structural pathology (e.g., calculi, abscess) that warrants further diagnostic study.

In the febrile MS patient, it is vitally important to lower the body temperature. Small increases in the body temperature of MS patients can worsen existing signs and symptoms as well as produce additional neurologic manifestations.

Many other symptoms of MS, which can be ameliorated by appropriate therapy, include gait dysfunction, fatigue, tremors, constipation, seizures, and bowel symptoms. Management of these symptoms is optimal in an MS comprehensive care center with its multidisciplinary staff, rather than in the emergency department. An MS comprehensive care center will be able to coordinate delivery of a uniform standard of care in keeping with modern management guidelines.

When MS patients are subjected to diseases or injuries that warrant surgical intervention, special considerations in the management of these patients are warranted. Before surgery, the patient's respiratory function must be assessed. Failure of spontaneous ventilation may occur in MS patients. Some will have a labile autonomic nervous system that may precipitate hypotension during anesthesia and surgery. Because the autonomic nervous system of the gastrointestinal tract may be affected, MS patients may have gastric and intestinal atony with constipation, bloating, and fecal incontinence. This delayed emptying of the stomach is an invitation to aspiration and subsequent pneumonia during intubation. The use of preoperative medications to enhance gastric motility, followed by rapid-sequence intubation, minimizes the chance for aspiration pneumonia.

Newer agents used in the treatment of MS include interferons (IFN) and immunosuppressive therapy. Interferons, proteins secreted by virus-infected cells that act on other cells to prevent them from becoming infected, have been considered as drugs to treat MS because viral infections have been found to trigger new attacks of MS. On the basis of the results of 2-year multicenter, randomized, double-blind, placebo-controlled clinical trial, the Food and Drug Administration approved INF-β for relapsing-remitting MS.

Immunosuppressive therapy with several drugs (methotrexate, azathioprine, cyclophosphamide, etc.) in patients with the chronic progressive form of the disease is encouraging in that some statistically significant results have been obtained, but disappointing by immediate or late adverse effects. When indicated, the patient with MS should be treated in a medical center that is experienced in the use of immunosuppressive agents and involved in well-designed clinical trials.

## Acknowledgment

This Chapter is dedicated to Charles H. Ross, who died on May 27, 1994 leaving a legacy of integrity, compassion and love that has inspired his friends and family.

## BIBLIOGRAPHY

Bellian KT, Devlin PM, Zimmer CA, et al: Concurrence of multiple sclerosis and Hodgkin's disease. *J Emerg Med* 10:13, 1992.

Edlich RF, Muir A, Persing JA, et al: Special considerations in the management of a patient with multiple sclerosis and a burn injury. *J Burn Care Rehab* 12:162, 1991.

Edlich RF, Westwater JJ, Lombardi SA, et al: Multiple sclerosis and asymptomatic urinary tract infection. *J Emerg Med* 8:25, 1990.

IFNB Multiple Sclerosis Study Group: Interferon beta-1b is effective in relapsing-remitting multiple sclerosis. I. Clinical results of a multicenter, randomized, double-blind, placebo-controlled trial. *Neurology* 43:665, 1993.

Optic Neuritis Study: Effect of corticosteroids for acute optic neuritis on the subsequent development of multiple sclerosis. *N Engl J Med* 32:1764, 1993.

Ransohoff RM: Multiple sclerosis: New concepts of pathogenesis, diagnosis, and treatment. *Comp Therapy* 15:39, 1989.

Rodriguez M: Multiple sclerosis: Basic concepts and hypothesis. *Mayo Clin Proc* 64:570, 1989.

Rodriguez M, Scheithauer BW, Forbes G, Kelly PJ: Oligodendrocyte injury is an early event in lesions of multiple sclerosis. *Mayo Clin Proc* 68:627, 1993.

Rudick RA, Schiffer RB, Schwetz KM, Herndon RM: Multiple sclerosis. The problem of incorrect diagnosis. *Arch Neurol* 43:578, 1986.

Weinshenker BG, Bass B, Rice GPA, et al: The natural history of multiple sclerosis: A geographically based study. 2. Predictive value of early clinical course. *Brain* 112:1419, 1989.

# 198
# DISORDERS OF NEUROMUSCULAR TRANSMISSION*

## Lawrence H. Phillips
## Richard F. Edlich

## INTRODUCTION

Disorders of neuromuscular transmission are characterized by fatigable weakness in a child or adult. The pathophysiology of these disorders relates to a disturbance of neuromuscular transmission at the myoneural junction (motor end plate) of skeletal muscle. A classification of these disorders divides them into autoimmune (myasthenia gravis, Lambert-Eaton myasthenic syndrome), genetic, toxic (botulism), and drug-induced forms. The onset of symptoms of the genetic form occurs in the newborn period or infancy and they are caused by either presynaptic defects (abnormal acetylcholine (Ach) resynthesis or mobilization, abnormal Ach release), or postsynaptic defects [endplate acetylcholinesterase (AChE) deficiency, reduced number of acetylcholine receptors (AchR), inpaired function of AchR, and slow channel syndrome]. These genetic forms are not caused by antibodies to AchR.

## MYASTHENIA GRAVIS (MG)

While MG is an uncommon disease, it remains the most common disorder of neuromuscular transmission, which produces varying degrees of muscle weakness. It is an autoimmune disease that is classified as a disorder of neuromuscular transmission because the cause

* This research was supported by a grant from the Charles Edison Fund, East Orange, NJ.

for weakness is an antibody-mediated depletion of AchR at the muscle end plate. This depletion results in faulty transmission at the neuromuscular junction by preventing Ach from stimulating the muscle to contract. Because patients with this disorder may develop acute changes in their condition that may be life-threatening, the emergency physician must be prepared to act quickly when patients present with symptoms suggestive of an exacerbation.

The disease is relatively rare. The average annual incidence is approximately two to five cases per million population. The estimated patient prevalence is 5 to 10 cases per 100,000 population. The disease occurs in all ages, with a greater incidence in females than males (2:1 female to male ratio). The peak prevalence is in the third decade of life for females and in the fifth or sixth decade for males, thus producing a bimodal distribution.

## Pathophysiology

There is a circulating antibody against the AchR in the sera of myasthenic patients that binds with the AchR at the motor end plate. The bound antibody mobilizes complement and produces a cascade of destructive events, ending in a marked reduction in the number of AchR.

In the normal motor end plate, there is a large redundancy of AchR. This produces a safety margin for neuromuscular transmission that can only be exceeded under extraordinary conditions, such as repetitive activation of the motor nerve terminal at sustained high rates. In the case of the myasthenic end plate, the safety margin is markedly reduced. The result is that repeated activation of an affected muscle fiber at even low rates will exceed the safety margin, and that fiber will become refractory to additional nerve impulses. This phenomenon is the basis for the clinical hallmark of MG, fatigable weakness. In muscles that are affected, the reduced safety margin will result in a certain number of muscle fibers being refractory to nerve impulses after an initial period of activation. Thus, an initially strong muscle contraction will rapidly become weaker with repeated contractions.

The association of MG with other recognized autoimmune diseases, such as rheumatoid arthritis, pernicious anemia, systemic lupus erythematosus, sarcoidosis, and thyroiditis, provides further support for the belief of its autoimmune etiology. The interaction of MG with some of the other autoimmune disorders can become clinically important. For example, the hyperthyroid phase of autoimmune thyroiditis can be associated with an increase of muscle weakness due to MG.

Approximately 10 to 25 percent of patients with MG have an associated thymoma, and 30 to 59 percent of patients with thymoma will develop clinical MG. Although thymomas are most commonly benign tumors, they are associated with a more severe form of MG. Frequently, control of the disease can only be attained after removal of the thymic tumor.

## Clinical Features

As noted above, the clinical hallmark of MG is muscle weakness, usually with some component of fatigability. Most patients will have demonstrable weakness present throughout the day. They typically observe that their strength improves after a period of resting and that weakness of a particular muscle group will increase after sustained or repetitive use.

There is a typical pattern of evolution of muscle weakness that affects the majority of patients. Most frequently the first muscles to become weak are the extraocular muscles, although weakness in other muscle groups, such as the bulbar muscles, may be the presenting symptom. The initial symptoms of the disease are usually either diplopia or eyelid ptosis, frequently fluctuating from side to side over the course of the day or from day to day. In approximately 20 percent of patients, the disease remains confined to the extraocular muscles throughout its course. The typical course is for weakness of other muscle groups to develop within months of the ocular symptoms.

Symptoms of the disease are frequently influenced by environmental, emotional, and physical factors. Bright light will often exacerbate ptosis and diplopia, and heat may increase muscle weakness. Emotional stress, viral illness, surgery, menses, pregnancy, immunization, and other physical factors all may precipitate a change in the expression of MG, although not in a predictable direction. Changes in strength associated with these factors are usually transient, lasting only as long as the precipitating cause.

When limb muscles become symptomatic, proximal muscles are typically weakest. The most severe manifestation of the disease produces weakness of respiratory muscles, precipitating a life-threatening situation, the *myasthenic crisis*. Myasthenic crisis occurs in a severe MG patient who is either not being treated or who is being undertreated because of insufficient medication or drug resistance. Improved treatment of myasthenic crisis has resulted in a dramatic decrease in the mortality of the disease, but this still remains the most likely cause of death. Disease progression is most rapid within the first 3 years, and more than one half of the deaths occur within this period. Spontaneous remissions lasting from weeks to years have been noted.

## Diagnosis

In the generalized form of MG, the diagnosis is generally not difficult. The combination of ocular, bulbar, and limb weakness, which fluctuates during the day and decreases with resting, is so typical of the disease that few other disorders need to be considered in the differential diagnosis. The patients who present with disease limited to ocular muscles, particularly when it is mild, sometimes present a diagnostic challenge. The patients who have minimal ocular signs and symptoms and more severe weakness in other muscle groups are particularly difficult to diagnose with certainty. A variety of laboratory and bedside tests have been devised to supplement the clinical examination and provide more certainty about the diagnosis.

### Anticholinesterase Tests

The diagnosis can be confirmed at the bedside, often very dramatically, through the use of the edrophonium test. Edrophonium bromide is administered as an intravenous bolus while the patient's muscle strength is tested. Edrophonium chloride is an AchE inhibitor, which prevents rapid breakdown of Ach at the myoneural junction. It acts within a few seconds and its effects last 5 to 10 min. Its pharmacologic effect of improving muscle strength is dramatic but transient. A positive result is a definite increase in strength of a previously weak muscle which lasts for several minutes. Muscle weakness then slowly returns. In adults, 1 to 2 mg of the drug is injected intravenously to identify the occasional patient who is hypersensitive to the drug. This would be manifested by the appearance of muscular fasiculations and respiratory depression. This drug must be given cautiously to patients with cardiac disease because it may cause sinus bradycardia, AV block, and, rarely, cardiac arrest. Atropine is an effective antidote for the muscarinic effects of edrophonium chloride but is of no value in counteracting the nicotinic effects on the motor end plate that might result in secondary partial paralysis of skeletal muscles. If there are no untoward cholinergic effects in 30 s, a larger dose of 5 to 8 mg is administered. The usual intravenous dose in children is 0.15 mg/kg body weight, not to exceed 10 mg per dose; a test dose of one tenth of the total dose is administered first to test for hypersensitivity. Intramuscular neostigmine in adults, 0.5 to 1.0 mg, acts maximally in about 30 min, allowing a more prolonged evaluation of changes in the clinical status.

Special considerations are in order for the use of edrophonium chloride in the emergency department. Only patients with ocular myasthenia or those with mild generalized disease should be tested in the emergency department. Patients with bronchial asthma or cardiac arrhythmia should not be evaluated in the emergency department but rather in a hospital setting that can appropriately treat increased tracheobronchial secretions and cardiac arrhythmia.

The value of edrophonium chloride testing may be negated if the test is not performed carefully. Particular care must be taken to select weak muscles for evaluation prior to administration of the drug. While some suggest that reversal of eyelid ptosis is the only reliable indicator of a positive test, other muscles can be monitored. The performance of the test in a double-blinded fashion is the most reliable strategy to follow. The examiner must have an assistant draw up the edrophonium chloride and an inactive solution, such as normal saline, in identical, coded syringes. The contents of the two syringes are administered sequentially, and the examiner and the patient independently rate the effect on the two agents, prior to breaking the code. Caution must be used in interpreting the results of even a clearly positive test, because other diseases (e.g., amyotrophic lateral sclerosis, Guillain-Barré syndrome, lesions in the cavernous sinus, and Lambert-Eaton myasthenic syndrome) may, at times, produce a response to edrophonium chloride. Additionally, patients with neurasthenia may have a temporary improvement in strength.

### Electromyography (EMG)

Electromyographic testing has two roles in the diagnosis of MG. The first is to confirm the diagnosis through demonstration of the typical findings of abnormal neuromuscular transmission. The second is to exclude the presence of other diseases, which may form part of the differential diagnosis. The typical electrophysiologic hallmark of a defect of neuromuscular transmission is a decrement in the amplitude of the compound muscle action potential in response to repetitive nerve stimulation. It is recognized that abnormal neuromuscular transmission can be found in a number of disorders, and a complete electromyographic study is necessary to exclude such disorders as amyotrophic lateral sclerosis, Lambert-Eaton syndrome, various neuropathies, and myotonic muscular dystrophy.

At times specialized techniques, such as single-fiber EMG, are necessary to demonstrate the defect of neuromuscular transmission in patients with mild MG. In ocular MG, in particular, all electrophysiologic tests may be normal, and other diagnostic modalities are necessary to confirm the diagnosis.

### Serologic Tests

The most specific test for MG is the demonstration of AchR antibodies in the serum. The assay is relatively insensitive in milder forms of the disease. In ocular MG, fully one third of patients will not have demonstrable AchR antibodies. Striated muscle antibodies also occur in MG patients, but their role is not known. Because there is no single test that is absolutely reliable in the diagnosis of the disease, a battery of tests is usually used.

## Differential Diagnosis

### Mitochondrial Myopathy

An increasingly large number of disorders of mitochondrial metabolism are being recognized. One of the most typical manifestations of a mitochondrial disease is progressive external ophthalmoplegia. This disorder may resemble MG in that there is often a severe degree of weakness of extraocular muscles. Other cranial muscles as well as trunk and extremity muscles may also be weak, but the weakness is not variable through the day. A variety of laboratory abnormalities have been encountered in this heterogeneous group of disorders, including lactic acidosis and varying degrees of heart block.

### Oculopharyngeal Muscular Dystrophy

This rare form of muscular dystrophy is inherited in an autosomal dominant pattern. The muscles most commonly found to be weak in this disorder are reflected in its name. Virtually all cases described to date are in individuals who can trace their ancestry to French Canada.

## Inflammatory Myopathies

Occasional patients with polymyositis will have a pattern of weakness that includes cranial and facial muscles. The demonstration of elevated muscle enzyme levels in the blood usually provides a clue to the correct diagnosis. A rare form of inflammatory myopathy, inclusion body myositis, may provide more of a diagnostic challenge. In this disorder, an atypical distribution of weakness may include facial muscles, but muscle enzyme levels may not be elevated. The disease is otherwise typical of inflammatory myopathy, and muscle biopsy may be necessary for accurate diagnosis.

## Amyotrophic Lateral Sclerosis (ALS)

The distinction between ALS and MG is generally not difficult to make. Occasional patients with ALS respond to acetylcholinesterase inhibitors, which can make the distinction from MG less clear. Two facts can help in distinguishing ALS from MG. The first is that ALS rarely, or never, causes weakness of extraocular muscles. The second is that patients with limb muscle weakness due to MG will almost always have a positive AchR antibody titer in their serum.

## Periodic Paralysis Syndromes

The various forms of periodic paralysis associated with hypo- or hyperkalemia, paramyotonia congenita, or hyperthyroidism present with distinct episodes of muscle weakness. If the episodes are frequent, they may be mistaken for the fatigable weakness of MG. Clinical distinction can be made from MG in that muscle strength is generally normal between episodes in all of the periodic paralysis syndromes.

## Neurasthenia

There are patients with a syndrome, which is a form of somatization disorder, that may be misdiagnosed as MG. The presenting symptoms are usually expressed as complaints of excessive fatigue, especially later in the day. Mild degrees of muscle weakness may apparently be present, but it is often difficult to be certain that patients cooperate fully with manual muscle testing. When such patients are given drugs such as pyridostigmine, they are often able to tolerate enormous daily dosage without experiencing drug side effects. That MG is not the cause for the symptoms can be inferred from negative findings on the more objective diagnostic studies.

## Emergency Department Care

Because the spectrum of the disease can vary from mild ocular weakness to severe, life-threatening generalized weakness, a variety of treatment strategies are used.

## Acetylcholinesterase Inhibitors

The most commonly used preparation is pyridostigmine bromide. A standard 60-mg dose typically has onset of effect within 30 min to 1 h of administration. The peak drug effect is at 1 1/2 to 2 h, and the effect of the dose disappears within 4 h. Various dosage strategies are used, but the typical patient will take 60 mg three to four times per day, often taking each dose prior to a meal. Other preparations have shorter (neostigmine bromide) or longer (ambenonium chloride) durations of therapeutic effect.

Side effects of anticholinesterase therapy are generally related to peripheral cholinergic excess because the drugs do not penetrate the blood-brain barrier well. The drugs work at muscarinic as well as nicotinic synapses, producing symptoms of abdominal cramping, excessive sweating, lacrimation, and, infrequently, cardiac arrhythmia. Most patients tolerate or adapt to the muscarinic side effects after a period of adjustment. When side effects are intolerable, supplemental doses of anticholinergic drugs, such as atropine sulfate, can be given concurrently with each dose of cholinesterase inhibitor.

The major complication of the use of cholinesterase inhibitors is the development of muscle weakness as a consequence of depolarization block of neuromuscular transmission. This typically occurs in the setting of overdosage of the drug, and is particularly likely to occur in patients with more severe degrees of weakness and larger dosage requirements. Distinction of "cholinergic crisis" from "myasthenic crisis" is sometimes difficult. An edrophonium test performed at the time of expected peak effect of a dose of pyridostigmine may help to distinguish between the two. If the patient becomes stronger after intravenous edrophonium, the patient is undermedicated. If, on the other hand, the patient becomes weaker, a condition of cholinergic blockade of neuromuscular transmission can be inferred. In the latter case, treatment consists of withdrawal of drug until a clear response to edrophonium returns. A return of response may not occur for several days, and many patients require monitoring in hospital during this time. Patients who have increasing difficulty in breathing, feeding, and handling tracheobronchial secretions and are refractory to relatively high doses of AChE are best treated by drug withdrawal, respiratory support, and intravenous fluids in an intensive care setting.

## Hospital Care

### Admission Indications

Patients with MG who come to the emergency department complaining of increasing weakness should be admitted to the hospital. The patient with MG can quickly develop ventilatory insufficiency or bulbar dysfunction with an inability to handle secretions. This progressive weakness may be due to a variety of causes, including acute exacerbation of disease precipitated by an underlying infection, administration of a neuromuscular blocking agent, thyroid disease, or hypokalemia. It can also be mimicked by cholinergic crisis, overtreatment by anticholinesterase drugs.

### Thymectomy

The thymus is normal or involuted in 20 percent of patients with MG; the remaining 80 percent have either hyperplasia (65 percent) or thymoma (15 percent). Thymomas tend to occur from the fourth decade onward. Approximately 60 percent are well encapsulated and benign; the other 40 percent are locally invasive and typically spread in a subpleural distribution. Distant metastases are rare. Plain radiography is the simplest technique to identify thymoma. Computed tomography (CT) and magnetic resonance imaging (MRI) may diagnose small tumors in a few additional patients and successfully negate the possibility in others. Additionally, CT or MRI scan can identify discontinuous or aberrant thymic tissue and help guide surgical resection in patients undergoing thymectomy.

The presence of a thymoma is an absolute indication for thymectomy because the disease may not be controlled otherwise. The practice in most centers today is to advocate thymectomy for all MG patients as early in the course of the disease as possible. Exceptions would be patients with mild disease whose symptoms are controlled adequately with anticholinesterase medication, patients with a contraindication to surgery, and elderly patients. The last situation reflects the fact that the therapeutic effect of thymectomy may take 5 to 7 years to be realized fully. Patients with a limited projected life span should not be subjected to the major surgery necessary for thymectomy.

### Anesthetic Management

The anesthetic management of a patient with MG must be individualized according to the type of surgery and the severity of the disease.

Whenever possible, the use of local anesthesia or regional anesthesia is recommended. When local or regional anesthesia is used, the dose of the anesthetic agents should be reduced to decrease their possible effects on neuromuscular transmission.

General anesthesia can be performed safely, providing that the patient is optimally prepared and neuromuscular transmission is carefully monitored during and after surgery. A balanced technique of general anesthesia, which includes the use of muscle relaxants, can be safely used. Patients with MG are sensitive to nondepolarizing relaxants, but intermediate-acting nondepolarizing relaxants such as atracurium and vecuronium are eliminated rapidly and can be titrated to achieve the required neuromuscular blockade, which can be reversed completely after surgery. The dose necessary to produce adequate surgical relaxation is often as little as 10 percent of the standard dose. In high-risk patients, postoperative ventilatory support is often required.

## Immunosuppressive Drug Treatment

Patients with the more severe manifestations of the disease generally require some form of immunosuppression. The drug that has been used most frequently in the United States for initial immunosuppression is prednisone. Various dosing strategies are used but most call for high doses tapered slowly over periods of 2 or more years. Initiation of steroid therapy should be done cautiously, because approximately 10 percent of patients will experience a pronounced increase of weakness within the first 21 days after first exposure to high doses of the drug. However, the usual response to prednisone is rapid and sustained improvement in strength shortly after beginning the drug.

In the United States other immunosuppressive drugs, mainly azathioprine, have been used to supplement the therapeutic effect of prednisone and to allow lowering its dose. In some American centers and in Europe, however, azathioprine has been used as the primary modality of therapy. The usual effective dose is in the range of 2 to 3.5 mg/kg of body weight. The onset of therapeutic effect of the drug is often several months, therefore supplementary therapy, such as plasma exchange, is often necessary. Drug toxicity is primarily on the bone marrow and liver. Initial treatment requires frequent monitoring of blood counts and liver function because some patients may have idiosyncratic reactions at even very low dosage levels. An additional drug now available in the United States is cyclosporine. Its primary use appears to be for supplementation of prednisone therapy.

## Plasmapheresis

Plasma exchange involves the removal of the antibody-rich plasma from the blood and replacing it with an inactive protein substitute. In MG, a course of plasma exchange, usually four to six sessions, is marked by dramatic, rapid improvement in strength. Unfortunately, if therapy is not supplemented by immunosuppressive drugs, weakness returns within days to several weeks after the plasma exchange is ended. In some centers, particularly difficult-to-control cases are sometimes treated with a regimen of a weekly session of plasma exchange in addition to immunosuppressive drug therapy. In most centers, however, the use of plasma exchange is reserved for treatment of acute myasthenic crisis. A secondary indication is to use plasma exchange to improve strength rapidly in preparation for thymectomy.

## Drug Interaction

A number of medications have the potential to increase weakness in patients with MG. Although no drug is absolutely contraindicated, several are known to be particularly hazardous and should be used with proper precautions. A partial listing of drugs known to produce increased weakness or to have an exaggerated effect is given in Table 198-1. When it is necessary to use any of the drugs listed in a patient with MG, one should be prepared to deal with increased muscle weakness that may result.

Various antibiotics are known to produce neuromuscular blockade. The aminoglycosides are particularly likely to produce increased weakness in MG. The clinical situation will arise, nevertheless, where the choice of antibiotic to use takes precedence over concern about neuromuscular blockade. In this situation, special care should be taken to monitor the strength of the patient with MG. The increased weakness produced by systemically administered antibiotics is usually not marked, and strength reverts to baseline after discontinuation of the drug.

The neuromuscular blocking agents must be used with great caution. Patients with MG are already suffering from partial neuromuscular blockade and may not need any neuromuscular blockers to achieve adequate levels of surgical muscle relaxation. If a patient does not achieve adequate relaxation with general anesthesia alone, very small doses of neuromuscular blockers should be given. If normal doses are used, the effect is usually markedly prolonged, and the patient will likely require prolonged intubation postoperatively.

**Table 198-1.** Drugs That Should Be Used With Caution in Myasthenia Gravis

| | | | | |
|---|---|---|---|---|
| **Steroids** | Kanamycin* | Amitriptyline | Lidocaine | **Others** |
| ACTH* | Gentamicin | Droperidol | Dilantin | Amantadine |
| Methylprednisolone* | Tobramycin | Haloperidol | Trimethaphan | Diphenhydramine |
| Prednisone* | Dihydrostreptomycin* | Imipramine | | Emetine |
| **Anticonvulsants** | Amikacin | Paraldehyde | **Local Anesthetic** | Diuretics |
| Dilantin | Polymyxin A | Trichlorethanol | Lidocaine* | Muscle relaxants |
| Ethosuximide | Polymyxin B | | Procaine* | CNS depressants |
| Trimethadione | Bacitracin | **Antirheumatics** | | Respiratory depressants |
| Paraldehyde | Sulfonamides | D-Penicillamine | **Analgesics** | Sedatives |
| Magnesium sulfate | Viomycin | Colchicine | Narcotics | Procaine* |
| Barbiturates | Colistin | Chloroquine | Morphine | Tranquilizers |
| **Antimalarials** | Colistimethate* | | Dilaudid | |
| Chloroquine* | Lincomycin | **Cardiovascular** | Codeine | **Neuromuscular blocking** |
| Quinine* | Clindamycin | Quinidine* | Pantopon | **agents** |
| **IV Fluids** | Tetracycline | Procainamide* | Meperidine | Tubocurarine |
| Na lactate solution | Oxytetracycline | Beta blockers | | Pancuronium |
| **Antibiotics** | Rolitetracycline | Propranolol | **Endocrine** | Gallamine |
| Aminoglycosides | **Psychotropics** | Oxprenolol | Thyroid* replacement | Dimethyl tubocurarine |
| Neomycin* | Chlorpromazine* | Practolol | **Eyedrops** | Succinylcholine |
| Streptomycin* | Lithium carbonate* | Pindolol | Timolol* | Decamethonium |
| | | Sotalol | Ecothiopate | |

* Case reports implicate drugs in exacerbations of MG.

*Source:* This table is a modified version of the table from Adams SL, Matthews J. Drugs that may exacerbate myasthenia gravis. *Ann Emerg Med* 13:532, 1984. Used by permission.

## TRANSITORY MYASTHENIA GRAVIS (TMG)

TMG is noted in 10 to 15 percent of offspring of MG mothers. It is of interest that the affected and unaffected infants exhibit the same high titer of AchR antibodies as their mothers. However, infants are affected only when they produce antibodies independently, either because of adoptive transfer of immunocytes from the mother or perhaps because fetal AchR damaged by maternal antibodies trigger a transient immune response in infants. Difficulty feeding and generalized hypotonia are the major clinical features of TMG. Symptoms frequently begin within hours after birth but can be delayed until the third postnatal day. Respiratory insufficiency is uncommon. Recovery is complete, and infants with TMG do not develop MG later in life. The diagnosis of TMG is made by demonstrating high serum concentrations of AchR antibodies in the newborn and temporary reversal of weakness after a subcutaneous injection of edrophonium chloride.

Newborns with severe generalized weakness and respiratory distress may require exchange transfusions. For those who are less impaired, intermittent intramuscular injections of anticholinesterase prior to feeding may provide sufficient improvement.

## LAMBERT-EATON MYASTHENIC SYNDROME (LEMS)

LEMS is another disorder of neuromuscular transmission. The defect is an antibody-mediated decrease in the number of Ach release sites on motor nerve terminals. The clinical hallmark is proximal muscle weakness, particularly of the lower extremities, which may decrease with repetitive activation of the muscle. Patients rarely have weakness of extraocular or respiratory muscles. In addition to the pattern of weakness, which differs from MG, tendon stretch reflexes are markedly diminished or absent. Patients also have autonomic symptoms, principally dry mouth, as a consequence of decreased cholinergic transmission at peripheral autonomic synapses.

The syndrome is slightly more common in men than women. Approximately 30 to 50 percent of the patients have a malignant neoplasm, more commonly oat-cell carcinoma of the lung. The disease may precede or follow the discovery of the tumor.

On electromyography, the compound muscle action potential evoked by a single nerve stimulus in a resting muscle is abnormally small. Repetitive stimulation at 2 Hz results in a further fall in the amplitude of successive motor responses. Brief exercise of the muscles or stimulation at frequencies higher than 10 Hz for a brief period markedly facilitates the amplitude of the response to normal levels.

There is ample evidence that LEMS is an autoimmune disease. This evidence is based, in part, on its responsiveness to glucocorticoids as well as to other immunosuppressants and plasmapheresis. Furthermore, nonneoplastic LEMS is associated with autoimmune diseases and organ-specific antibodies. The most compelling evidence for an autoimmune cause of both neoplastic and nonneoplastic LEMS is the passive transfer of the main electrophysiologic features of the disease from humans to mice.

The most effective treatment of nonneoplastic cases of LEMS is combined therapy with prednisone and azathioprine. Acetylcholinesterases have limited effectiveness.

## BOTULISM

Botulism is a rare neuroparalytic disease caused by a potent polypeptide toxin elaborated by the organism *Clostridium botulinum*. The disease occurs in three forms: food-borne, wound, and infantile. In the food-borne disease, symptoms arise when food containing the toxin is eaten without proper cooking necessary to denature the toxin. Most commonly, the food-borne disease is produced by consumption of improperly canned food. Typically, more than one case of the disease occurs because the contaminated food is usually consumed as part of a common meal shared by several individuals. In infantile botulism, organisms in the gut, arising from ingested spores, produce toxin that is systemically absorbed. Spores in dust, vacuum cleaner dust, honey, and corn syrup have been implicated. Wound botulism should be considered in any patient with a wound and/or a chronic history of drug abuse associated with a progressive descending symmetric paralysis. The organisms contaminating the wound produce a toxin that is systemically absorbed.

The clinical manifestations of botulism resemble LEMS more than MG because the toxin impairs release of Ach from motor terminals. Symptoms of infantile botulism are poor suck, constipation, listlessness, regurgitation, and generalized weakness. Cranial nerve deficits appear, manifested by a flaccid facial expression, ptosis, and ophthalmoplegia. Adults present with complaints of nausea, vomiting, blurred vision, and dysphagia, which is followed by a descending symmetric muscle weakness and respiratory insufficiency. Impairment of cholinergic function is encountered and may result in constipation, urinary retention, and reduced salivation and lacrimation.

Diagnosis depends on epidemiologic, clinical, and electrophysiologic findings and may be confirmed by the finding of the toxin and/or organism in the food, stool, or wound. Diminished amplitude of the evoked muscle action potential with facilitation reaching normal amplitude after exercise or repetitive stimuli is a classic electromyographic finding in botulism.

Precipitous respiratory failure is the most serious threat to the patient. Early elective intubation and the use of ventilatory assistance can be life-saving. Although the effectiveness of antitoxin therapy remains uncertain, its use is recommended. Because most infants are no longer acutely ill when the diagnosis is established, antitoxin is rarely administered. If ileus is profound, nasogastric suction and parenteral nutrition may be necessary. The use of antitoxin, respiratory support, and parenteral nutrition has reduced fatality rates from 60 to 25 percent over the past 30 years. In addition to the above therapies, wound excision is mandatory for wound botulism.

## DRUG-INDUCED DISTURBANCES IN NEUROMUSCULAR TRANSMISSION

Drugs resulting in neuromuscular transmission disturbances affect either pre- or postsynaptic mechanisms or both. These drugs, given parenterally or in cathartics, limit the safety margin of neuromuscular transmission (Table 198-1). Such drug-induced disturbances in neuromuscular transmission cause symptoms that resemble MG, with prominent extraocular muscle weakness and ptosis and variable degrees of facial, bulbar, and generalized muscular weakness. Respiratory paralysis may occur early and be severe. However, overt MG symptoms do not appear unless an overdose of the drug has been administered or hepatic or renal elimination of the drug is impaired. These same drugs also can enhance the activity of neuromuscular blocking agents used during surgical procedures and thereby delay recovery of strength.

## BIBLIOGRAPHY

### Myasthenia Gravis

Baraka A: Anaesthesia and myasthenia gravis. *Can J Anaesth* 39:476, 1992.
Engel AG: Myasthenia gravis and myasthenic syndromes. *Ann Neurol* 16:519, 1984.
Keesey JC: Electrodiagnostic approaches to defects of neuromuscular transmission. *Muscle Nerve* 12:613, 1989.
Moore DR: Imaging in myasthenia gravis. *Clin Radiol* 40:115, 1989.
Phillips LH II, Melnick PA: Diagnosis of myasthenia gravis in the 1990's. *Semin Neurol* 10:62, 1990.
Seybold ME: The office Tensilon test for ocular myasthenia gravis. *Arch Neurol* 43:842, 1986.
Shah A, Lisak RP: Immunopharmacologic therapy in myasthenia gravis. *Clin Neuropharmacol* 16:97, 1993.

## Genetic Forms of Myasthenia Gravis

Misulis KE, Feichel GM: Genetic forms of myasthenia gravis. *Pediatr Neurol* 5:205, 1989.

## Lambert-Eaton Myasthenia Syndrome

Newsome-Davis J, Murray NMF: Plasma exchange and immunosuppressive drug treatment in Lambert-Eaton myasthenia gravis. *Neurology* 34:480, 1984.

## Botulism

Arnon SS: Infant botulism. *Annu Rev Med* 31:541, 1980.

Dowell VR Jr: Botulism and tetanus. Selected epidemiologic and microbiologic aspects. *Rev Infect Dis* 6(suppl 1):S202, 1984.

## Drug-Induced Disorders of Neuromuscular Transmission

Adams SL, Matthews J, Grammer LC: Drugs that may exacerbate myasthenia gravis. *Ann Emerg Med* 13:532, 1984.

Howard JF Jr: Adverse drug effects on neuromuscular transmission. *Semin Neurol* 10:89, 1990.

Swift TR: Disorders of neuromuscular transmission other than myasthenia gravis. *Muscle Nerve* 4:334, 1981.

# 199

# MENINGITIS, ENCEPHALITIS, AND BRAIN ABSCESS

## David C. Anderson
## Alan J. Kozak

## BACTERIAL MENINGITIS

In cases of bacterial meningitis, the primary goal in the emergency department is to recognize it and begin empirical treatment promptly. It is often not possible to distinguish with certainty meningitides due to viruses, fungi, and other organisms or those due to neoplastic, toxic, and autoimmune processes from bacterial meningitis on the basis of clinical findings and even lumbar puncture (LP) results. Obtaining appropriate studies, particularly cultures, early on in the emergency department is enormously helpful in eventually arriving at an appropriate diagnosis. Hence, while initiating therapy for the most imminently dangerous possibility, the emergency physician must also lay the diagnostic groundwork for establishing alternative diagnoses.

Approximately 25,000 cases of bacterial meningitis occur yearly in the United States. Attack rates are age-specific, ranging from almost 400 per 100,000 in neonates to 1 to 2 per 100,000 in adults. Two thirds of cases are in children. Mortality is about 5 percent in children beyond infancy, 25 percent in neonates, and 25 percent in adults. Long-term complications such as cognitive deficits, epilepsy, hydrocephalus, and hearing loss affect about a quarter of survivors. The discussion that follows will focus on bacterial meningitis, touching on other processes in the differential diagnosis.

## Pathophysiology

Bacterial meningitis begins with the entry of organisms into the well-defended subarachnoid space. The ability to infect the subarachnoid space is not shared equally by all bacteria. The dominance of three organisms, *Streptococcus pneumoniae, Haemophilus influenzae* type b, and *Neisseria meningitidis,* the organisms causing over two thirds of bacterial meningitis cases, is no accident. These encapsulated organisms share the ability to invade the host through the upper airway, survive dissemination through the bloodstream, and from there gain access to the subarachnoid space. Also important in the pathogenesis of disease caused by these organisms are their subcapsular constituents, which trigger inflammatory cascades in the host. The resulting processes attack the enemy invader and, as a byproduct, initiate and amplify the meningeal and parenchymal inflammation responsible for the clinical picture.

Neural structures are innocent bystanders and secondary victims in the battle taking place around them. Stimulation of pain-sensitive structures in meninges and posterior spinal roots leads to headache and meningeal signs. The brain, meanwhile, is put at risk for serious ischemia by a constellation of events. Encased in its fixed-volume container, it is squeezed by its own swelling as well as by the expanding sizes of other intracranial compartments. These include the swollen and inflamed meninges themselves. Cerebrospinal fluid (CSF) drainage is reduced by interference with its flow in the subarachnoid pathways as well as its absorption by the arachnoid granulations. Hence, the quantity of CSF increases, causing communicating or noncommunicating hydrocephalus. Intracranial blood vessels initially expand, increasing the volume occupied by that compartment. The brain itself swells by several mechanisms. Disruption of the blood-brain barrier allows entry of protein and ultimately water (vasogenic edema), while hydrocephalus forces CSF into the periventricular parenchyma (interstitial edema). Eventually, cell membrane homeostasis may be compromised, leading to increased intracellular water (cytotoxic edema).

The sum of these expanded volumes overwhelms the compensatory displacement of CSF into the more compliant spinal compartment, and intracranial pressure rises as a result. Since brain perfusion depends on arterial pressure exceeding tissue pressure (in this case intracranial pressure), ischemia may develop. This is all the more likely since the vascular supply is bathed in inflammatory infiltrate with additional functional and structural consequences. These include faulty autoregulation, inflammatory narrowing, and a prothrombotic situation.

There are some variations on the pathophysiologic themes described above. For example, organisms sometimes gain entry to the CSF not by hematogenous seeding but through direct contiguity. Such direct spread may be from infected parameningeal structures (e.g., brain abscess, otitis media, sinusitis), traumatic or congenital communications with the exterior, or neurosurgery. The bacteriology of these infections may be different, since the organisms that inhabit these contiguous sources are selected by different determinants. Finally, immunologic deficiency states are increasingly common and predispose to yet other organisms. The meningitis picture produced by organisms other than *S. pneumoniae, H. influenzae* type b, and *N. meningitidis* will depend on their capacity to stimulate the host's immune processes as well as the host's capacity to respond.

## Clinical Features

### Symptoms and Signs

Definitive diagnosis is based on demonstrating bacterial organisms in the subarachnoid space along with an appropriate inflammatory response. The possibility of meningitis must be considered if the diagnosis is to be made. In classic and fulminant cases, about 25 percent of adult cases, there is little diagnostic challenge; the patient presents with rapidly developing fever, headache, stiff neck, photophobia, and disordered cognition. Seizures occur in 25 percent of adults and at least that many children. In some patients, typically the very young and the elderly, the presenting picture may be incomplete and nonspecific. The challenge to consider meningitis is accordingly greater.

In the newborn, irritability and poor feeding may be the sole manifestations. In the elderly, confusion and fever may be signs of meningeal infection or more mundane processes.

Historic data may increase the likelihood of meningitis and suggest specific pathogens. Several areas deserve special attention: living conditions, trauma, immunocompetence, immunization history, and antibiotic use. Army barracks and college dormitories are typical environments in which clusters of cases due to *N. meningitidis* occur. Day-care centers may become a source for multiple cases due to *H. influenzae* type b. A history of head trauma (*S. pneumoniae*) or neurosurgery (staphylococcal species, gram-negative rods) may be significant. Conditions that affect immune competence (e.g., history of surgical or functional splenectomy, glucocorticoid therapy, HIV) should be sought. On the other hand, a history of immunization to *H. influenzae* type b in the past will make meningitis due to this organism unlikely. It is important to inquire about recent exposure to antibiotics, which may have influenced the clinical course in a less than florid case. If so, CSF findings will also likely be modified. A history of antibiotic allergy is of obvious relevance.

Examination must include assessment for meningeal irritation with resistance to passive neck flexion, Brudzinski sign (flexion of hips and knees in response to passive neck flexion), and Kernig sign (contraction of hamstrings in response to knee extension while hip is flexed). One or more of these will be present in 80 percent of cases. Also crucial is an examination of the skin seeking the purpuric rash characteristic of meningococcemia and, less commonly, other pathogens. Cutaneous stigmata suggesting microembolization (petechiae, splinter hemorrhages, pustular lesions) should be aspirated for Gram stain and culture. Paranasal sinuses should be percussed, and ears examined for evidence of primary infection in those sites. Fundi must be assessed, and in infants, the fontanel should be palpated; evidence of increased intracranial pressure will influence the diagnostic priorities. Neurologic examination should seek evidence for focal neurologic dysfunction, present in 25 percent of cases. Disordered eye movements, homonymous visual field deficits, facial asymmetry, and hemiparesis are typical findings in such cases.

## Laboratory Studies

Germane laboratory studies when bacterial meningitis is a leading diagnostic concern include, at a minimum, white blood cell and platelet counts, partial thromboplastin and prothrombin times, blood glucose, as well as serum sodium and creatinine. Blood cultures (two specimens drawn 15 min apart) yield the responsible organism in about 50 percent of bacterial meningitis cases. Obviously, however, CSF analysis is paramount. Appropriate sequencing of LP, cranial imaging studies, and initiation of empirical antibiotics will be further discussed below. However, LP should be carried out as quickly as possible. Proper technique and thoughtful planning maximize the diagnostic yield and avoid later questions and uncertainties.

## Lumbar Puncture

Lumbar puncture should be performed if intracranial mass lesions and florid coagulopathy are unlikely on clinical grounds. When clinical suspicion of meningitis is high, informed consent should be waived if obtaining it would delay the procedure unduly. Local anesthetic is optional but will improve likelihood that the patient will be relaxed and cooperative. The L3–L4 interspace should be punctured (L4–L5 in newborn infants) while the patient is coiled as tightly as possible in a fetal position. In adults a line drawn between the iliac crests crosses the spine at the L3–L4 interspace. Alternatively, the patient may be seated on the edge of a bed or cart leaning over a tray stand. This latter technique is particularly useful when landmarks are uncertain as they may be in an obese patient. After puncture, using a two and one half inch 22-gauge needle in children and a three and one half inch 20-gauge needle in adults, the opening pressure should be measured manometrically. To obtain meaningful results the pressure must be measured with the patient lying extended on his or her side. Pressures measured with the patient still coiled or while sitting will be artifactually elevated. Normal pressure is less than 170 mm $H_2O$. Repositioning (uncoiling the coiled patient, helping the seated patient to a lying position on his or her side) is performed with the needle in situ. Modifying these procedures in cases with evidence of increased intracranial pressure or coagulopathy is of doubtful value. Tapping at the level of the foramen magnum will not protect against transtentorial herniation, and using a smaller needle is no guarantee against herniation or bleeding complications.

Four tubes, each containing several milliliters of CSF, are typically obtained. Red and white cell counts with differential are requested for tubes 1 and 4. The two-tube assessment is carried out to detect a traumatic tap, in which case the rate of bleeding will likely be inconstant causing a difference in red cell count between the two tubes. Tube 4 may also be used for culture and Gram stain. Tube 2 is sent for protein and glucose. Tube 3 should be saved for other studies discussed below, should they be necessary. Closing pressure is not necessary.

## Differential Diagnosis

The differential diagnoses may be categorized into parenchymal or meningeal disorders. When fever and focal neurologic symptoms and signs predominate, parenchymal central nervous system infections are concerns (brain abscess, viral encephalitis, cerebral toxoplasmosis, other parenchymal processes). When meningeal signs predominate, other infectious meningitides, meningeal neoplasm, and subarachnoid hemorrhage are possible.

For evaluation of parenchymal brain infections, LP is unhelpful and potentially dangerous as it can lead to transtentorial or tonsillar herniation. Cranial CT scan should be done first if there is papilledema or focal neurologic signs. Cranial CT scan is also the preferred mode in diagnosing subarachnoid hemorrhage.

For meningeal disorders other than subarachnoid hemorrhage, CSF examination is most helpful. Typical CSF formulae for bacterial, viral, fungal, and neoplastic meningitides are displayed in Table 199-1, but there is considerable overlap in findings. Some bacteria (e.g., *Mycoplasma* and *Listeria* and spirochetes, syphilis, leptospira, Lyme) produce spinal fluid alterations that resemble the viral profile, while CSF findings in tuberculous meningitis resemble the fungal profile of the table. An "aseptic" profile suggesting viral infection is typical of partially treated bacterial infections (one-third or more of pediatric

**Table 199-1.** Typical Spinal Fluid Results for Meningeal Processes

| Parameter (Normal) | Bacterial | Viral | Neoplastic | Fungal |
|---|---|---|---|---|
| O.P. (<170 mm CSF) | >300 mm | 200 mm | 200 mm | 300 mm |
| WBC (<5 mononuclear) | >1000/μL | <1000/μL | <500/μL | <500/μL |
| % pmns (0) | ≥80% | 1–50% | 1–50% | 1–50% |
| Glucose (>40 mg/dL) | <40 mg/dL | >40 mg/dL | <40 mg/dL | <40 mg/dL |
| Protein (<50 mg/dL) | >200 mg/dL | <200 mg/dL | >200 mg/dL | >200 mg/dL |
| Gram stain (−) | + | − | − | − |
| Cytology (−) | − | − | + | + |

*Note:* O.P., opening pressure; WBC, white blood cells; pmns, polymorphonuclear cells.

cases have received antimicrobial treatment before presenting with meningitis). The same is true of untreated bacterial infections adjacent to but not communicating with the subarachnoid space, such as abscesses of the brain and subdural or epidural spaces. The percentage of polymorphonuclear cells may be higher in early viral meningitis, and glucose may be reduced in some viral cases.

Additional tests that may be helpful include viral cultures in suspected viral meningitis, *Borrelia* antibodies in patients with possible Lyme disease, india ink and latex agglutination assay for fungal antigen in cryptococcal meningitis, acid-fast stain and culture for mycobacteria in tuberculous meningitis, and latex agglutination or counterimmune electrophoresis for bacterial antigens in potentially partially treated bacterial cases. Assays are most widely available for *S. pneumoniae*, other group B streptococci, *H. influenzae* type b, and *N. meningitidis*. Rarely, CSF may be normal or nearly so in very early bacterial meningitis, especially during meningococcemia. Empirical antibiotic treatment, admission, and repeat LP are appropriate if clinical suspicion is great despite negative initial CSF results.

## Treatment

Ideal management has several goals. First priority is the rapid administration of a bactericidal antibiotic that gains rapid entry to the subarachnoid space. A secondary priority in some cases is use of an antiinflammatory agent to suppress the normal inflammatory processes, which are amplified by antibiotic-induced bacteriolysis. A tertiary concern is to counter the adverse effects of unchecked inflammation, especially brain ischemia related to increased intracranial pressure and vasculopathy. Finally, when several options that accomplish these goals are available, those with the lowest expense and treatment morbidity are chosen.

Agents to which local bacterial resistance has developed should be avoided. Currently, for example, about 30 percent of *H. influenzae* type b isolates are resistant to ampicillin. Bacteriostatic agents should not be used alone or in combination with a bactericidal agent, since the action of the latter may be interfered with. Agents of current choice for given bacterial meningitides are indicated in Table 199-2. Empirical therapy in cases warranting antibiotics before LP or when the Gram stain is negative (about 30 percent of untreated cases, 50 percent of those receiving antibiotics before LP) is based on the patient's age and should also take risk factors into consideration. Once culture results are available, antibiotic choice should be reassessed, considering both efficacy and cost.

A variety of inflammation suppressants have been shown to improve outcome in experimental bacterial meningitis. Only glucocorticoids, and specifically dexamethasone, have been tested in clinical trials. Evidence is persuasive that dexamethasone given before or at the time of the first antibiotic dose reduces the morbidity of bacterial meningitis. Most data have been collected in children infected with *H. influenzae* type b, and many authorities now recommend dexa-

**Table 199-2.** Bacterial Meningitis

| | Potential Pathogens | Initial Empirical Therapy |
|---|---|---|
| **AGE** | | |
| Neonate (0–7 days) | Group B Streptococcus, *Listeria monocytogenes*, aerobic Gram-negative bacilli | Cefotaxime 50 mg/kg IV q 12 h **plus** Ampicillin 50 mg/kg IV q 12 h *or* Ampicillin 50 mg/kg IV q 12 h **plus** Gentamicin 2.5 mg/kg IV q 12 h **or** Amikacin 7.5 mg/kg IV q 12 h |
| Neonate (8–28 days) | **As above** | Cefotaxime 50 mg/kg IV q 8 h **plus** Ampicillin 50 mg/kg IV q 8 h |
| Infants (1–3 months) | Group B Streptococcus, *Listeria monocytogenes*, *Haemophilus influenzae*, *Streptococcus pneumoniae*, *Neisseria meningitidis* | Cefotaxime 50 mg/kg IV q 6 h **plus** Ampicillin 50–75 mg/kg IV q 6 h |
| 3 months–18 years | *Haemophilus influenzae*, *Streptococcus pneumoniae*, *Neisseria meningitidis* | Ceftriaxone 50 mg/kg IV, q 12 h (not to exceed 4 g/24 h) *or* Cefotaxime 50 mg/kg IV q 6 h (not to exceed 8 g/24 h) |
| 18–50 years | *Streptococcus pneumoniae*, *Neisseria meningitidis* | Ceftriaxone 2 g IV q 12 h |
| Older than 50 years | *Streptococcus pneumoniae*, *Neisseria meningitidis*, *Listeria monocytogenes*, aerobic Gram-negative bacilli | Ceftriaxone 2 g IV q 12 h **plus** Ampicillin 2 g IV q 4 h |
| **SPECIAL CIRCUMSTANCES** | | |
| CSF leak with history of closed head trauma | *Streptococcus pneumoniae*, *Haemophilus influenzae*, group B-hemolytic streptococcus | Ceftriaxone 2 g IV q 12 h |
| History of recent penetrating head injury, neurosurgery, or CSF shunt | *Staphylococcus aureus*, *Staphylococcus epidermidis*, diphtheroids, aerobic Gram-negative bacilli | Vancomycin 25 mg/kg IV load (not more than 500 mg infused per hour) followed by 19 mg/kg at intervals dictated by Matzke nomogram* **plus** Ceftazidime 2 g IV q 8 h |
| Immunocompromised host | *Streptococcus pneumoniae*, *Neisseria meningitidis*, *Listeria monocytogenes*, aerobic Gram-negative bacilli | Vancomycin 25 mg/kg IV load (not more than 500 mg infused per hour) followed by 19 mg/kg at intervals dictated by Matzke nomogram* **plus** Ampicillin 2 g IV q 4 h **plus** Ceftazidime 2 g IV q 8 h |

* See Matzke GR et al: Evaluation of the vancomycin-clearance: creatinine-clearance relationship for predicting vancomycin dosage. *Clin Pharm* 4:311, 1985.

methasone, 0.15 mg/kg IV, as adjunctive therapy in children. Some would extrapolate the favorable results noted in children to adults, especially those with a heavy burden of organisms (reflected by a positive CSF Gram stain) or evidence of increased intracranial pressure. Dexamethasone would be the glucocorticoid of choice for these patients as well, at the same dosage.

Additionally important in management is surveillance for and correction of complications. These include seizures, hyponatremia, hydrocephalus, and cerebrovascular accidents.

Management of tuberculous, fungal, and neoplastic meningitis is beyond the scope of this discussion. Viral meningitis without encephalitis is generally self-limiting and can probably be managed at home. Practically speaking, however, it is a diagnosis by exclusion; unless the diagnosis is obvious (for example, with classic symptoms and CSF findings and typical maculopapular enteroviral rash during late summer), admission is warranted.

### Emergency Department Care

The most crucial management of community-acquired bacterial meningitis occurs in the emergency department. Triage must be accurate and rapid. Protocols should be in place to facilitate speedy progress through a series of decisions. Protocols should address the sequencing of LP and initial dose of antibiotic, the need for a pre-LP imaging study, and the use of preantibiotic dexamethasone.

An acceptable approach would be to give antibiotics first to all in whom bacterial meningitis is seriously considered on clinical grounds. In fact, there is no argument that some meningitis suspects should receive antibiotics immediately after blood cultures. Such patients include those with clinical features suggesting meningococcemia, e.g., purpuric skin rash or hypotension. Antibiotics should also be given before LP to meningitis suspects for whom the procedure must be delayed, e.g., those for whom an imaging study is warranted beforehand.

In other bacterial meningitis suspects, a strong argument can be made for expeditious LP in the emergency department before or during initiation of empirical antibiotics. Obtaining CSF before antibiotics are started or within the first few hours after the first dose enhances the likelihood that a specific bacteriologic diagnosis will be established or can be confidently ruled out. Although the rate at which Gram stain and culture become negative is uncertain, delay beyond a few hours after starting empirical antibiotics reduces the likelihood of positive cultures by 20 to 30 percent. When a meningitis suspect leaves the emergency department on antibiotics, the tempo of management frequently slackens. If LP has not been accomplished already, the opportunity for a very early and definitive study may be lost. The best solution is for LP to be done in the emergency department while awaiting arrival of antibiotics from the pharmacy. Antibiotics may be started during the procedure or immediately thereafter. Patients in whom the leading diagnostic concern is bacterial meningitis should have antibiotics started before they leave the emergency department. Shock or hypotension and hypoxemia should be corrected before LP. For critically ill patients, antibiotics should be given simultaneously with resuscitation and before LP.

Antibiotics may be withheld in patients whose clinical presentation suggests viral meningitis if close observation is possible, pending results of CSF examination.

Cranial imaging may play several roles in a meningitis suspect. In some patients the clinical presentation may be ambiguous. Focal findings and signs of increased intracranial pressure (coma or papilledema) may add parenchymal brain lesions to the differential diagnosis, or the clinical story may be compatible with subarachnoid hemorrhage. Emergent unenhanced CT scan is needed to avoid an inappropriate LP. Evidence of very severe cerebral edema in the CT of a stuporous or comatose patient with presumed meningitis may be grounds for treating empirically and avoiding LP altogether, although

risk of herniation after LP is probably lower if pressure is generalized rather than from a focal mass. Marked cerebral edema may be grounds for administering dexamethasone as an inflammation suppressant in adult cases. Imaging may show an opacified sinus compatible with an unsuspected sinusitis or CSF leak or may detect complications that alter treatment, such as hydrocephalus, arterial or venous infarction, and subdural effusions or empyema.

Because glucocorticoids counter the cytokine-mediated adverse neurologic effects of bacteriolysis, they will have the greatest effect if they can be given before the first dose of antibiotics, if practical. Hence, use of dexamethasone is an emergency decision. Dexamethasone should be given to all children with meningitis and considered in adults, particularly those with clinical evidence of brain involvement manifested by reduced level of consciousness or edema on imaging.

General treatment measures include maintenance of normal blood volume. Hypotonic fluids should be avoided. Serum sodium should be monitored serially to detect a syndrome of inappropriate antidiuretic hormone or cerebral salt-wasting. Hyperpyrexia should be treated. Coagulopathies should be corrected using specific replacement therapies. Phenytoin loading is indicated in patients who develop seizures. For marked cerebral edema on clinical or CT grounds, the following are indicated: head elevation, hyperventilation to a $P_{CO_2}$ of 25 to 30 mmHg, and use of mannitol. Measurement of intracranial and systemic arterial pressure is useful in severe cases to enable monitoring of cerebral perfusion pressure.

Finally, intimate contacts of patients with documented *N. meningitidis* or *H. influenzae* type b meningitis may be carriers of these organisms. They should be treated with rifampin and instructed to return at once if they develop symptoms.

## VIRAL ENCEPHALITIS

Viral encephalitis is a viral infection of brain parenchyma producing an inflammatory response. It is distinct from, although often coexists with, viral meningitis, in which the infectious agent and inflammatory response are in the subarachnoid space. Clinically the distinction is made by the presence of neurologic abnormality in encephalitis, whereas only meningeal symptoms and signs (photophobia, headache, stiff neck) occur in meningitis. The true incidence of viral encephalitis is difficult to estimate because of the variability of clinical expression, ranging from profound neurologic involvement to inapparent cases, as well as in reporting policies. Several thousand cases are reported yearly in the United States.

### Pathophysiology

A number of viruses may cause either meningitis or encephalitis; however, certain ones predominate in encephalitis. In North America, these include the arboviruses, herpes simplex (HSV) type I, herpes zoster, Epstein-Barr virus (EBV), and rabies. On the other hand, enteroviruses, mumps, cytomegalovirus (CMV), HSV type II, lymphocytic choriomeningitis, adenoviruses, and acute HIV infection are typically responsible for the aseptic meningitis syndrome and rarely cause encephalitis.

Entry portals are highly virus-specific for the encephalitis-producing viruses. The arboviruses are inoculated by mosquitos, and rabies is transferred by the bite of an infected animal, whereas the others are common human viruses that accidentally cause encephalitis. Impaired immune status may play a role in herpes zoster and cytomegalovirus encephalitis. Common to all is preliminary viral invasion of the host at a non-CNS site where replication takes place. Most viruses then reach the nervous system hematogenously during viremia. However, at least three important viruses—rabies, herpes simplex, and herpes zoster—reach the spinal cord and eventually the brain by travelling backwards within axons from a distal site where they have gained access to nerve endings.

Once in the brain, the virus enters neural cells. Neurologic dysfunction and damage are caused by the disruption of neural cell functions by the virus and by the effects of the host's inflammatory responses. Gray matter is predominantly affected, resulting in cognitive and psychiatric signs, lethargy, and seizures. By contrast, postinfectious encephalomyelitis causes multifocal white matter damage. Sensorimotor deficits referable to one hemisphere or to the spinal cord would be more typical of this immune-mediated pathologic process, which may follow viral infection at any site.

## Clinical Features

Encephalitis should be considered in patients presenting with the following clinical features singly or in combination: new psychiatric symptoms, cognitive deficits (aphasia, amnestic syndrome, acute confusional state), seizures, and movement disorders. Features of meningeal involvement, such as headache and photophobia, are usually, but not invariably, present. The same is true for fever.

Patients with herpes zoster (shingles or chicken pox), EBV, or CMV encephalitis (lymphadenopathy and hepatosplenomegaly) may have a history and signs typical of the non-CNS clinical syndromes caused by these viruses. Other circumstances of the case may suggest the diagnosis as well as the offending agent (Table 199-3). For example, a late summer encephalopathy should suggest the possibility of an arbovirus encephalitis. An animal bite for which no antirabies treatment was obtained would be of obvious relevance.

Signs of meningeal irritation and increased intracranial pressure should be sought. Neurologic findings reflect the areas of involvement. A careful assessment of cognition is crucial. Sensorimotor deficits are not typical. Encephalitides may show special regional tropism. HSV involves limbic structures of the temporal and frontal lobes, with prominent psychiatric features, memory disturbance, and aphasia. Some arboviruses predominantly affect the basal ganglia, causing chorea-athetosis and parkinsonism. Involvement of brainstem nuclei involved in swallowing is responsible for the choking response to water characteristic of rabies encephalitis.

## Differential Diagnosis

Diagnosis rests on imaging using MRI, electroencephalography (EEG), and LP. Imaging not only excludes other potential lesions, such as brain abscess, but may display findings that are highly suggestive of HSV encephalitis, a treatable infection, with involvement of medial temporal and inferior frontal gray matter. MRI is more sensitive than CT in this regard. The EEG is quite useful in establishing the diagnosis. Almost by definition it is abnormal in encephalitis, in contrast to isolated viral meningitis, which may be a differential concern in some cases, or to a primary psychiatric disorder, which will be a consideration in others. Furthermore, HSV produces an almost pathognomonic picture in the setting of acute febrile encephalopathy with periodic, usually asymmetric sharp waves. The EEG may detect abnormalities before the MRI. Lumbar puncture is the next step. Findings of aseptic meningitis are typical. It is at least theoretically possible to have encephalitis without meningitis; however, this situation must be quite unusual.

Differential diagnosis will depend on the nature of the presentation. When fever and meningeal symptoms predominate, bacterial meningitis will be a concern. In less fulminant meningeal cases, Lyme disease, subacute subarachnoid hemorrhage, and tuberculous, fungal, and neoplastic meningitis will be concerns. In cases in which parenchymal features are prominent, brain abscess, bacterial endocarditis, postinfectious encephalomyelitis, and toxic or metabolic encephalopathies will be considered. Finally, primary psychiatric disease will be mimicked by some cases.

The clear diagnostic imperative is to exclude alternative processes requiring specific treatment. Once that is satisfactorily accomplished, the mandate is less definite. Of the viruses causing encephalitis, only HSV has been shown by clinical trial to be responsive to antiviral therapy. The diagnosis of HSV encephalitis cannot currently be reliably established in most centers without brain biopsy. Because current antiviral treatment is relatively risk- and side effect–free, empirical therapy is advocated for cases of clinical encephalitis. Use of the polymerase chain reaction may allow specific diagnosis of HSV infection from a CSF sample in the near future.

## Treatment

The agent of choice for HSV is acyclovir. Based on anecdotal data, cases of herpes zoster and CMV encephalitis may also benefit from antiviral therapy: acyclovir for herpes zoster and gancyclovir for CMV encephalitis.

Complications of encephalitis include seizures, disorders of sodium metabolism, occasional increased intracranial pressure, and the systemic consequences of a comatose state. These should be dealt with in the standard ways.

Prognosis depends on the virus and host. Rabies encephalitis, while rare, continues to be neurologically devastating and usually fatal. Eastern equine encephalitis and HSV also carry high mortality and frequently produce residual deficits. For the others, adverse outcome is seen mainly in elderly patients or in those with compromising preexisting systemic or neurologic conditions.

## Emergency Department Care

Patients with encephalitis should in general be admitted. The outcome in cases of HSV encephalitis is related to the neurologic condition at the time that antiviral therapy is initiated. Patients who are already in coma do very poorly, making timely diagnosis and therapy a priority for this form of encephalitis. At this point, however, empirical initiation of acyclovir, 10 mg/kg, in the emergency department in encephalitis suspects has not become standard.

## BRAIN ABSCESS

A brain abscess is a focal pyogenic infection. When fully developed, it is composed of a central pus-filled cavity, ringed by a layer of granulation tissue and an outer fibrous capsule. Surrounding this is edematous brain tissue infiltrated with inflammatory cells. It is a pathologic response typical of a relatively competent immune system against a bacterial invader. Focal brain infections due to other organisms, such as granulomas due to tuberculosis, the necrotic lesions of toxoplasmosis in the immunocompromised patient, or the cystic lesions of cysticercosis, are not abscesses in the pathologic sense. These nonpurulent focal lesions will not be considered here.

**Table 199-3.** Viral Pathogens Causing Encephalitis in North America

|  | Clinical Clues | Diagnosis | Prognosis |
|---|---|---|---|
| Herpes simplex type I | "Psychiatric" presentation | MRI, EEG, PCR* of CSF, biopsy | 30% die; 30% have deficits |
| Herpes zoster | Shingles, chicken pox, immuno-suppressed state | Skin vesicle/CSF culture, serology | Mortality 10–20% |
| E-B virus | Mononucleosis | Serology | 5–10% die |
| Rabies | Animal bite | Saliva/CSF culture, biopsy, serology | 90% die |
| Arboviruses | Seasonal |  |  |
| California | Midwest, children | CSF/blood culture, serology | Good |
| W. Equine | West, outside workers | As above | 5–10% die |
| E. Equine | Southeast, outside workers | As above | 50% die |
| St. Louis | Midwest, older urban dwellers | As above | 5–10% die |

* PCR, polymerase chain reaction.

Compared with bacterial meningitis, brain abscess is uncommon, with an incidence of 3 to 5 per 100,000, a rate that has gradually fallen over the past century, probably reflecting the effect of antibiotics on predisposing conditions such as otitis media. Mortality of diagnosed cases has also fallen, from about 50 percent early in the 20th century to a current level of 10 to 20 percent. Long-term sequelae are seen in about a third of survivors.

## Pathophysiology

Organisms reach the brain by one of three known routes: hematogenously (one-third of cases); from contiguous infections of middle ear, sinus, or teeth (one-third of cases); or by direct implantation by neurosurgery or penetrating trauma (about 10 percent of cases). The route is unknown in about 20 percent. Circumstances that reduce oxygenation of brain parenchyma are important predisposing factors for bacterial invasion. For example, spread from a contiguous infection usually involves intervening cerebral thrombophlebitis with congestive ischemic hypoxemia of tissue destined to become infected. Hematogenous seeding is facilitated by systemic hypoxemia, as in congenital heart diseases with right-to-left shunt and chronic pulmonary suppuration. This is demonstrated by the prominent role of anaerobic bacteria in brain abscesses.

Identification of the mechanism of abscess formation is important in management not only because the underlying cause deserves attention but because the bacteriology of the abscess, often polymicrobial, will be influenced by its source. For examples, gram-negative rods, especially *Bacteroides,* are the usual pathogens in otogenic brain abscesses, which are generally single and located in the adjacent temporal lobe or cerebellum. Anaerobic and microaerophilic streptococci are the most common pathogens in sinogenic and odontogenic abscesses, which are more typically located in the frontal lobes. Abscesses formed from hematogenous spread are often multiple and polymicrobial, with anaerobic and microaerophilic streptococci commonly represented. Staphylococci are typical pathogens in abscesses due to direct implantation. Gram-negative rods would also be concerns in cases related to a neurosurgical procedure.

## Clinical Features

Presenting features of brain abscess are unfortunately nonspecific. Patients are typically not acutely ill. For these reasons, diagnosis is often delayed. Symptoms reflect the infectious and neurologic (focal and mass effect–producing) aspects of the disease. Fever is present in about half, and neck stiffness in fewer than that. Focal neurologic symptoms, such as hemiparesis or seizures, are present in about a third. The most common symptom is headache, which is a complaint in almost all cases. Other symptoms of increased intracranial pressure such as vomiting, confusion, or obtundation are present in about half. The presentation may be dominated by the origin of the infection, e.g., ear or sinus pain.

Meningeal signs are present less than half the time on examination. Papilledema is noted on funduscopy in about a third of patients. Focal neurologic signs reflecting the site of the lesion (frontal lobes—hemiparesis; temporal lobes—homonymous superior quadrant visual field deficits, aphasia; cerebellum—limb incoordination, nystagmus) are present in about 60 percent of patients on careful examination. Discovery of potential sites of origin may raise suspicion about the presence of brain abscess when presentation is otherwise nonspecific, e.g., otitis media, sinus tenderness, evidence of pulmonary suppuration, or right-to-left shunting in a patient with subacute headache and lethargy.

## Differential Diagnosis

Brain abscess is diagnosed by imaging. CT with contrast infusion classically demonstrates one or several thin, smoothly contoured rings of enhancement surrounding a low-density center and in turn surrounded by white matter edema. Early in the course a ring may be thicker and less well defined. MRI usually demonstrates a ring, even without gadolinium enhancement. Both are highly sensitive and there is no practical advantage of one imaging modality over the other. Other studies, such as blood work, EEG, and CSF examination, are too nonspecific to be of help, and LP is contraindicated. Cultures of blood or other sites of infection may provide guidance in management later.

Differential diagnosis of the clinical presentation is broad because of its nonspecificity and variability. A sudden onset with focal features may suggest cerebrovascular disease. Prominent fever, stiff neck, and confusion may suggest meningitis. A protracted course with features of increased intracranial pressure may bring neoplasm to mind. Imaging features may be mimicked by brain neoplasm, subacute brain hemorrhage, and other focal lesions, as well as other focal brain infections such as toxoplasmosis. Biopsy or aspiration for confirmation of diagnosis as well as for bacteriology will be necessary in most cases.

## Treatment

The cornerstone of treatment of brain abscess is antibiotics. The susceptibility of the likely pathogen and the penetration of the agent into the lesion should be considered when choosing an antibiotic. The bacteriology of the lesion may be inferred if the origin is obvious, and initial empirical antibiotic choice should take advantage of such information. Initial treatment in a suspected otogenic case would be a third-generation cephalosporin, such as cefotaxime, or trimethoprin-sulfamethoxazole with metronidazole or chloramphenicol. For presumed abscess of sinogenic or odontogenic origin, high-dose penicillin would be a good choice. Penicillin would also be a good choice for an abscess of hematogenous origin. Chloramphenicol or metronidazole, which by virtue of their lipophilic natures penetrate abscesses very well, are usually added to these penicillin regimes. When communication with the exterior is suspected, as in penetrating trauma or after neurosurgery, nafcillin or vancomycin would be a reasonable empirical choice. Addition of ceftazidime may be required if gram-negative aerobes are suspected. Finally, for patients in whom no mechanism is apparent or suspected, the combination of a third-generation cephalosporin, such as cefotaxime, and metronidazole would provide good coverage.

Most cases will require neurosurgery for diagnosis and bacteriology, if not for definitive treatment. Total excision has become necessary less often with the availability of imaging to follow the course of abscesses treated medically after surgical aspiration. In cases in which intracranial pressure is high, excision is still carried out. The role of glucocorticoids is controversial. Steroids may produce temporary improvement of increased intracranial pressure.

## Emergency Department Care

The challenge in the emergency department is recognition of the possibility of brain abscess. This relatively rare problem presents nonspecifically. Avoidance of LP and admission for definitive treatment are priorities. In cases presenting with impending herniation or with coexisting meningitis, emergency management of these complications will be appropriate.

## BIBLIOGRAPHY

Anderson DC, Kozak AJ: Brain abscess, in Joynt RJ (ed): *Clinical Neurology,* vol 2. Philadelphia, Lippincott, 1989.

Ashwal S, Tomasi L, Schneider S, et al: Bacterial meningitis in children: Pathophysiology and treatment. *Neurology* 42:739, 1992.

Bale JF Jr: Viral encephalitis. *Med Clin North Am* 77:25, 1993.

Durand ML, Calderwood SB, Weber DJ, et al: Acute bacterial meningitis in adults: A review of 493 episodes. *N Engl J Med* 328:21, 1993.

Feigin RD, McCracken GH Jr, Klein JO: Diagnosis and management of meningitis. *Pediatr Infect Dis J* 11:785, 1992.

Geiman BJ, Smith AL: Dexamethasone and bacterial meningitis: A meta-analysis of randomized controlled trials. *West J Med* 157:27, 1992.

Greenlee JE: Approach to diagnosis of meningitis: Cerebrospinal fluid evaluation. *Infect Dis Clin North Am* 4:583, 1990.

Kaplan SL: New aspects of prevention and therapy of meningitis. *Infect Dis Clin North Am* 6:197, 1992.

Kaufman BA, Tunkel AR, Pryor JC, Dacey RG Jr: Meningitis in the neurosurgical patient. *Infect Dis Clin North Am* 4:677, 1990.

Lebel MH: Dexamethasone therapy of bacterial meningitis. *Antibiot Chemother* 45:169, 1992.

Quagliarello VJ, Scheld WM: Bacterial meningitis: Pathogenesis, pathophysiology, and progress. *N Engl J Med* 327:864, 1992.

Rowley AH, Whitley RJ, Lakeman FD, et al: Rapid detection of herpes simplex-virus DNA in cerebrospinal fluid of patients with herpes simplex encephalitis. *Lancet* 335:440, 1990.

Schaad UB, Lips U, Gnehm HE, et al: Dexamethasone therapy for bacterial meningitis in children. *Lancet* 342:457, 1993.

Talan DA, Hoffman JR, Yoshikawa TT, Overturf GD: Role of empiric parenteral antibiotics prior to lumbar puncture in suspected bacterial meningitis: State of the art. *Rev Infect Dis* 10:365, 1988.

Tauber MG, Sande MA: General principles of therapy of pyogenic meningitis. *Infect Dis Clin North Am* 4:661, 1990.

# 200
# NEUROLEPTIC MALIGNANT SYNDROME

## Philip L. Henneman

Neuroleptic malignant syndrome (NMS) is a rare syndrome that is associated with the use of neuroleptic medications; it is characterized by hyperthermia, muscular rigidity, altered mental status, and autonomic dysfunction. Neuroleptic medications were introduced in 1954, and NMS was first described in 1968 by Delay and Deniker. Although diagnosed much less frequently, NMS occurs in 0.07 to 0.15 percent of patients treated with neuroleptics. In a pooled review of 16 studies, the incidence of NMS was 0.2 percent.

NMS is found primarily in young and middle-aged adults, paralleling the use of neuroleptics, but it can occur in patients of any age and is equally common in men and women. NMS occurs independently of ambient conditions and climate, but high temperatures and humidity may augment the risk of NMS.

## PATHOPHYSIOLOGY

NMS may occur in any patient taking any of the neuroleptic medications, regardless of the duration of use. The frequency of NMS caused by each of the neuroleptic agents depends on the frequency of their use and their antidopaminergic potency. The most common medication associated with NMS is haloperidol (Haldol) but NMS may occur with many medications, including fluphenazine (Prolixin), prochlorperazine (Compazine), promethazine (Phenergan), metoclopramide (Reglan), hydroxyzine (Vistaril), or amoxapine (Asendin). NMS has also been reported in patients being withdrawn from dopaminergic agonists (anti-Parkinson drugs), in patients abusing cocaine, and in one patient taking amphetamines.

NMS is believed to be related to dopaminergic blockade or depletion in the central nervous system. Neuroleptic agents block dopamine receptors in the hypothalamus, corpus striatum, and spinal areas. This blockage or depletion of dopamine may lead to hyperthermia, muscular contractions, sympathetic discharge, and vasomotor abnormalities. In animals, acute dopaminergic depletion leads to extrapyramidal symptoms including dysarthria, dysphagia, involuntary movements, and muscular rigidity. Parkinson disease is treated with dopaminergic agonists such as levodopa or carbidopa. When patients are abruptly withdrawn from these medications, they may develop hyperthermia and muscular rigidity. Cocaine and amphetamine release dopamine, and it has been postulated that abusers may deplete dopamine stores, resulting in agitation, delirium, hyperthermia, and muscular rigidity.

## CLINICAL FEATURES

A history of psychiatric illness is common. Phenothiazine use is almost always present in patients with NMS. A small percentage of patients will be withdrawing from anti-Parkinson medication, and even fewer patients may admit recreational drug use. As many as 17 percent of patients may have experienced a similar episode during prior treatment with neuroleptics.

Patients with NMS almost uniformly have hyperthermia, muscular rigidity, mental status changes, and autonomic instability. Hyperthermia, associated with profuse sweating, occurs in 98 percent of reported cases; 40 percent have a temperature above 40°C. Generalized rigidity, often described as feeling like a "lead pipe," is reported in 97 percent of patients. Muscular rigidity is usually associated with various degrees of myonecrosis. Increased muscular activity is the primary cause of fever. Other symptoms of muscular rigidity include akinesia, tremor, dysarthria, and dysphagia. Changes in mental status are reported in 97 percent of cases. These changes may range from confusion to stupor or coma. Fluctuating levels of consciousness are common. Classically, the NMS patient is alert but appears dazed and mute. Finally, autonomic instability is seen in 95 percent of patients; most commonly this is manifested as tachycardia, fluctuations in blood pressure, or cardiac dysrhythmias.

Symptoms usually develop between 1 and 7 days after treatment with a neuroleptic. One-third of patients, however, will develop signs of NMS between 1 and 4 weeks after initiating neuroleptics. Once neuroleptics are stopped, untreated NMS lasts approximately 10 days. Patients receiving long-acting depot neuroleptics may have NMS for twice as long. Symptoms may also not be so dramatic; it is often suggested that milder cases of NMS are never diagnosed.

No laboratory results are diagnostic of NMS, but laboratory evaluation is important to exclude other causes of the patient's symptoms. A lumbar puncture and chest radiograph are appropriate to exclude meningitis and pneumonia. Elevation of creatine phosphokinase (CK) from skeletal muscle occurs in 95 percent of patients, and myoglobinuria has been reported in two-thirds of patients. It is, therefore, important to evaluate the urine of all patients with NMS for myoglobinuria (dipstick is positive for heme but without red blood cells) and, if present, to measure CK to determine the risk of acute renal failure.

Other nonspecific findings include leukocytosis (98 percent), metabolic acidosis or hypoxemia on arterial blood gas analysis (75 percent), and hypocalcemia (50 percent). Less common findings include hyponatremia, hypernatremia, azotemia, and coagulopathies.

Death may occur from respiratory failure or cardiac arrest. Respiratory failure is most often due to chest wall rigidity and hypoventilation or from aspiration pneumonia. Other causes of death include myocardial infarction, pulmonary embolus, renal failure, and disseminated intravascular coagulation. Between 1980 and 1987, 10 percent of the reported patients with NMS died. In a more recent, prospective study of 24 patients with NMS there were no deaths, but 2 required hemodialysis and 5 required intubation.

**Table 200-1.** Differential Diagnosis of Neuroleptic Malignant Syndrome

| | |
|---|---|
| Endocrine | Psychiatric |
|   Hyperthyroidism |   Lethal catatonia |
| Environmental | Rhabdomyolysis |
|   Heat stroke | Toxic |
| Infectious |   Cocaine |
|   Meningitis |   Amphetamines |
|   Encephalitis |   Strychnine |
|   Sepsis |   Anticholinergics |
|   Tetanus |   Monoamine oxidase inhibitors |
|   Rabies | |
| Neuromuscular | |
|   Malignant hyperthermia | |
|   Parkinson disease | |
|   Severe dystonia | |

## DIAGNOSIS

The diagnosis of NMS is made after excluding other causes of the patient's signs and symptoms. Levenson has suggested diagnostic criteria for NMS involving major and minor manifestations. Major criteria include fever, rigidity, and elevated CK; minor criteria include tachycardia, abnormal blood pressure, tachypnea, altered mental status, diaphoresis, and leukocytosis. To make the diagnosis of NMS, Levenson suggests that three major or two major and four minor manifestations must be present, as well as a suggestive clinical history (e.g., history of neuroleptic use). Similar diagnostic criteria have been proposed by others.

The differential diagnosis of NMS is listed in Table 200-1. After excluding infection (predominantly meningitis), heat stroke, and hyperthyroidism, there are few diagnoses to consider. Lethal catatonia and malignant hyperthermia are two rare syndromes that are similar but distinct from NMS. Lethal catatonia is a condition first described in the 1800s as a hyperthermic episode with decreased muscle activity, often followed by severe excitability. It is not associated with autonomic dysfunction or neuroleptic use and is presently felt to represent a form of heat exhaustion brought on by uncontrolled manic type hyperactivity. Malignant hyperthermia is an autosomal dominant syndrome that results in abnormal muscular contractions in the presence of certain anesthetics. As with NMS, this syndrome has fever, muscle rigidity, and some autonomic dysfunction but is not associated with neuroleptic use and is associated with anesthetic use. Toxins are also possible diagnoses.

## TREATMENT

The basis of treatment for NMS is early recognition, cessation of neuroleptic medications, institution of rapid cooling, fluid replacement, support of cardiovascular and pulmonary systems, and prevention of complications (Table 200-2). All patients should be undressed and placed on a cardiac and oxygen saturation monitor. The patient's airway and breathing should be quickly assessed. Respiratory failure should be treated with intubation, ventilation, and oxygenation. An intravenous line should be placed, and hypotension should initially be treated with fluid resuscitation, most often with normal saline. Fluid replacement should be continued to maintain good urine output (e.g., greater than 30 mL/h). A Foley catheter will aid in determining accurate urine output. After initial stabilization of the patient, rapid cooling should be instituted. This is best accomplished with evaporation (mist and fan), cooling blankets, ice, and antipyretics (e.g., acetaminophen). Rhabdomyolysis should be promptly diagnosed and treated. Steps should be taken to exclude other diagnoses and complications of NMS, such as aspiration pneumonia, dysrhythmias, and thromboembolism.

The value of pharmacology in the treatment of NMS is less clear. There are no controlled trials evaluating drug treatment of NMS. Per-

**Table 200-2.** Treatment of Neuroleptic Malignant Syndrome

Remove stimulus
Airway/breathing
  Oxygen
  Pulse oximetry
  Consider intubation
Circulation
  Cardiac monitor
  Intravenous access
  Fluid resuscitation
  Consider nitroprusside if severe vasoconstriction
Cooling measures
  Evaporation
    Mist and fan
  Cooling blanket
  Ice
  Antipyretics
Bromocriptine
  Consider for hyperthermia
  Dose: 5 mg initially then 2.5–10 mg PO or nasogastric tube t.i.d.
Dantrolene
  Consider for muscular rigidity and hyperthermia
  Intravenous dose: 0.8–3.0 mg/kg q 6 h (maximum dose 10 mg/kg per 24 h)
  Oral dose: 50–100 mg PO bid
Benzodiazepines
  Consider for muscular rigidity

haps the best approach is to tailor therapy to the patient's presenting symptomatology (Table 200-2). Fever unresponsive to cooling measures may benefit from bromocryptine. Bromocriptine (Parlodel) is a direct dopamine agonist. The usual first dose is 5 mg, then 2.5 to 10 mg orally or via nasogastric tube t.i.d. Patients with severe vasoconstriction contributing to the hyperthermia may benefit from vasodilators such as nitroprusside. Muscular rigidity and hyperthermia may benefit from the nonspecific muscle relaxant, dantrolene (Dantrium). The dose of dantrolene is 0.8 to 3 mg/kg intravenously every 6 h (maximum dose 10 mg/kg per 24 h). Oral dosing of dantrolene is 50 to 100 mg b.i.d. Many authors recommend benzodiazepine for muscular rigidity, but its use has not been studied. Finally, patients who are dopamine-depleted, such as those on holiday from their Parkinson medications, would benefit from a combination of levodopa and carbidopa (Sinemet), with or without amantadine (Symmetrel).

Patients with the diagnosis of NMS should be admitted to the hospital, most often to an intensive care unit. Patients with very mild symptoms or unclear diagnosis may be considered for close outpatient management after exclusion of serious diagnoses and treatment of their symptoms. Patients discharged home should be instructed to discontinue their neuroleptics (or restart their Parkinson medications) and closely monitor their temperature. They should be instructed to return to the emergency department if they develop a fever, difficulty breathing, dysphagia, dysarthria, or muscle stiffness. A short course of bromocriptine (2.5 mg PO tid) and dantrolene (50 mg PO bid) may be given, and frequent follow-up is needed until symptoms have resolved.

## BIBLIOGRAPHY

Caroff SN, Mann SC: Neuroleptic malignant syndrome. *Med Clin North Am* 77:185, 1993.

Caroff SN, Mann SC, Lazarus A, et al: Neuroleptic malignant syndrome: Diagnostic issues. *Psychiatr Ann* 21:130, 1991.

Delay J, Deniker P: Drug-induced extra pyramidal syndromes, in Vinken PJ, Bruyn GW (eds): *Diseases of the Basal Ganglia: Handbook of Clinical Neurology* (vol 6). Amsterdam, North-Holland, 1968, p 248.

Granner MA, Wooten GF: Neuroleptic malignant syndrome or Parkinsonism hyperpyrexia syndrome. *Semin Neurol* 11:228, 1991.

Gurrera RJ, Chang SS, Romero JA: A comparison of diagnostic criteria for neuroleptic malignant syndrome. *J Clin Psychiatr* 53:56, 1992.

Keck PE, Pope HG, Cohen BM, et al: Risk factors for neuroleptic malignant syndrome. *Arch Gen Psychiatr* 46:914, 1989.

Levenson JL: Neuroleptic malignant syndrome. *Am J Psychiatr* 142:1137, 1985.

Nierenberg D, Disch M, Manheimer E, et al: Facilitating prompt diagnosis and treatment of the neuroleptic malignant syndrome. *Clin Pharmacol Ther* 50:580, 1991.

Rosebush P, Stewart T: A prospective analysis of 24 episodes of neuroleptic malignant syndrome. *Am J Psychiatr* 146:717, 1989.

Rosebush PI, Stewart TD, Mazurek MF: The treatment of neuroleptic malignant syndrome. Are dantrolene and bromocriptine useful adjuncts to supportive care? *Br J Psychiatr* 159:709, 1991.

Schneider SM: Neuroleptic malignant syndrome: Controversies in treatment. *Am J Emerg Med* 9:360, 1991.

# Eye, Ear, Nose, Throat, and Oral Surgery

## 201
## OCULAR EMERGENCIES
### Alvina M. Janda

The spectrum of ocular trauma is broad and varies from minor corneal abrasions with no long-term visual impairment to permanently blinding injuries such as extensive ruptures of the globe. Nontraumatic ocular emergencies span an equally broad spectrum of visual consequences from the relatively benign "pink eye" to the ominous central retinal artery occlusion (CRAO). The only two true *urgent* ocular emergencies consist of chemical burns (need for immediate irrigation) and an acute CRAO (need to stimulate perfusion within the first 90 min of obstruction). Appropriate evaluation and triage of the patient with an ocular emergency cannot be overemphasized. Life-threatening injuries (e.g., respiratory distress, hemorrhaging, etc.) obviously require stabilization prior to assessment of ocular status. Once stabilized, history taking can commence, followed by the examination, at times doing them concurrently.

### EYE EXAMINATION

#### History

Obtain any information on past ocular trauma, ocular/periocular surgery, or other eye-related problems. Ask specifically if there was any preexisting visual impairment. Inquire as to the use of glasses or contact lenses, and, if so, what kind (i.e., soft, gas permeable, or hard contacts; if soft, ask if daily or extended wear usage: extended wear lenses carry an increased risk of corneal ulcers). Obtain a detailed description of the current eye problem or injury regarding time of onset and associated symptoms such as change in vision, redness, pain, or discharge. If this is a trauma-induced ocular emergency, inquire as to the use of safety glasses and document this as well as time/place/activity when injury occurred. Of particular significance is hammering metal on metal or working with or near equipment that could fracture off tiny, high-speed fragments. With trauma always ask about flashes of light because this can suggest a retinal detachment. Ask if any "treatment" has been used such as drops, ointments, or irrigating solutions, and if so, for how long. Obtain a thorough general medical history because the eye can be affected by systemic disease.

#### Physical Examination

The examination of the eye/ocular adnexa can then proceed. It is helpful to break down the examination as follows, streamlining your approach appropriate to each patient's presenting signs and symptoms.

**Visual acuity.** *Always* evaluate and document the visual acuity in *both* eyes. Typically, this is done as the initial part of the examination, the exception being chemical burns to the eyes, where irrigation takes priority. Have patients use their glasses if they wear them and note this on the chart. Test each eye separately, making sure to occlude the opposite eye well. If glasses are not available, vision should be tested through a pinhole. A distance visual acuity chart is preferable to the near card. If the patient is unable to see the largest print, continue to assess the vision by determining if there is no light perception, light perception, hand motions (move your hand 1 to 2 ft in front of the eye), or counting fingers (hold up several fingers at various distances from the eye). Document clearly, as, e.g., count fingers at 1 ft.

**Lids/ocular adnexa.** Evaluate the position, contour, and color of the lids and periocular areas. Check for swelling or evidence of discharge.

**Pupils.** Evaluating the pupillary light response as well as checking for afferent pupillary defects (the consensual light response) should be done routinely. Patients with previous intraocular surgery or trauma or those taking either miotics (e.g., pilocarpine) or mydriatrics (e.g., atropine) or cyclopentolate (e.g., Cyclogyl) may have poorly reactive or nonreactive pupils. An accurate history can help sort this out. A positive test for an afferent pupillary defect is indicative of an optic nerve abnormality.

**Motility.** Range of motion of the eyes can be evaluated by having the patient look in all fields of gaze. Diplopia is generally caused by restriction or paresis of an extraocular muscle in a previously binocular individual. Cranial nerves III, IV, and VI are responsible for ocular motility. Partial or complete paresis of the cranial nerves can be isolated or multiple. It can be seen in diabetes, intracranial aneurysms/tumors, intraorbital masses, myasthenia gravis, demyelinating diseases, intracranial inflammatory disease, sphenoid sinusitis, and trauma.

**Anterior segment.** This includes the cornea, conjunctiva, anterior chamber, iris, and lens. It is best evaluated by using a slit lamp. The slit lamp functions as a biomicroscope with specialized optics to allow for high resolution and detail of structures of the anterior segment.

Most slit lamps have two levels of magnification to allow increased anterior segment detail. The patient must be able to sit up and place the chin on a rest and forehead against a bar to allow the examiner to focus on the eye. Focusing is manual and done by moving the slit lamp with a joy stick located on the base. Because the slit lamp is binocular, excellent depth of focus is possible. A broad beam as well as a "slit" beam can be created of variable lengths. An "optical section" can be cut across the cornea to evaluate all the layers by using a slit beam. A fine point of light focused in the anterior chamber will determine the presence of cells (white blood cells are indications of inflammation in the aqueous and red blood cells indicate a hyphema) or flare (so-called headlights in fog phenomenon) that indicates increased protein content of the aqueous. Several filters are also available on most slit lamps to change the color of the light beam to blue (used to look for corneal or conjunctival epithelial defects after instillation of fluorescein) or green (helps delineate vasculature and iron lines). The detail available with a slit lamp is far superior to loupes or other magnifying devices and, if available, its use is encouraged in evaluating anterior segment problems.

**Intraocular pressure.** When concerned about possible glaucoma or situations in which pressures may be elevated (e.g., hyphema, iritis) or very low (ruptured globe, wound leak after surgery), the intraocular pressure (IOP) should be measured. Among the several methods available to measure IOP, those most commonly used in the emergency department are Goldmann applanation, Schiötz tonometry, or the Tono-pen. Normal IOP ranges from 10 to 21 mm Hg. Measuring IOP accurately requires a cooperative patient as well as an experienced physician or assistant. All methods mentioned require an anesthetized cornea. The Goldmann applanation tonometer is attached to the slit lamp and is the standard to which other methods of measurement are compared. With applanation, pressure is measured in terms of the force needed to flatten a small area of the cornea. The Tono-pen is a hand-held, battery-operated applanator that has gained increasing popularity because of its size and ease of use. Proper use and calibration are critical to obtain meaningful results. The Tono-pen can momentarily increase the IOP by up to 12 mm Hg by indenting the cornea. For a potential ruptured globe, care should be exercised in using it: the preferred method to measure the IOP would be the Goldmann tonometer. In addition, the Tono-pen tends to underestimate IOPs in the higher range of greater than 16 mm Hg. The Schiötz tonometer is transportable and available. It is based on indentation tonometry (IOP measured by the response of the cornea to an externally applied force). It can be misleading in situations of altered ocular rigidity. If the ocular rigidity is high, the pressure measurement will be high. With the 5.5-g weight on this instrument, a scale rating of less than 4 is abnormal (greater than 20 mm Hg). Always use the scale ratings supplied with the Schiötz tonometer, and make sure you use the scale that corresponds to the weight on the tonometer.

**Fundus.** The optic nerve, retina, and retinal vessels can be examined through an undilated pupil, but it is easier with dilation. Certainly not all patients with eye problems need dilating drops. There are a few contraindications for dilation. Do not dilate any eye with an iris-supported intraocular lens or untreated narrow angle glaucoma (i.e., patient has not received a laser peripheral iridectomy). Readily available and relatively short-acting (4 h) dilating drops are 1% tropicamide (Mydriacyl) and 2.5% phenylephrine (Neo-Synephrine). One drop of each can be instilled into the eyes and repeated in 15 min if dilation is not occurring. A good posterior and peripheral retinal examination can then be done with the indirect ophthalmoscope.

**Orbit.** Evaluation of orbital symmetry and proptosis can be easily done by simply looking at the patient face on. Orbital floor or wall fractures occur most commonly in the setting of blunt trauma. Palpation of the orbital rim to feel for step-offs can be helpful, as well as evaluation of ocular motility (checking for entrapments). Plain x-ray films (skull anteroposterior and Water's view) are useful. A computed tomography (CT) scan with coronal cuts will show the full extent of the fracture as well as the amount of entrapped tissue in severe cases. Orbital hemorrhage, emphysema (air), edema, and tumor are all potential etiologies for proptosis.

Table 201-1 lists the ocular emergencies that are described in this chapter.

## TRAUMATIC OCULAR EMERGENCIES

### Blunt Trauma

#### Subconjunctival Hemorrhage

This is caused by disruption of a blood vessel within the normally clear conjunctiva. Although commonly seen in blunt trauma, rarely is it a harbinger of any serious injury, but if extensive enough may obstruct visualization of a ruptured globe. A circumferential elevated dense subconjunctival hemorrhage is highly suspicious for a ruptured globe and requires close evaluation and possible exploration of the globe to rule out an occult rupture. Assuming an intact globe, there is no treatment and the hemorrhage will spontaneously resolve. If it is a recurrent spontaneous (nontraumatic) subconjunctival hemorrhage, consider a coagulopathy or hypertension.

#### Corneal Abrasions

Traumatic abrasions will cause partial or complete removal of the corneal epithelium. Symptoms are severe pain, tearing, and blepharospasm. A topical anesthetic (tetracaine, proparacaine [Ophthetic]) will facilitate the examination. Fluorescein strips or drops are then used to dye the tear film. Uptake of fluorescein is seen whenever corneal epithelial cells are damaged or lost. *Always* evaluate for a retained foreign body, everting the upper lid as well. Assess if it is a "clean" abrasion or "dirty" (e.g., dog scratch).

Treatment of "clean" abrasion:

1. Cycloplegic drop (dilates pupils and relaxes any ciliary body spasm that can cause a deep ache)
   1% cyclopentolate or 5% homatropine (useful in dark-eyed patients), instill one drop
2. Antibiotic ointment—several choices
   tobramycin
   gentamicin
   bacitracin/polymixin (Polysporin)
3. Tape lid closed
4. Light pressure dressing (two eye pads)
5. Reexamine in 24 to 36 h or refer to an ophthalmologist
6. *Never* prescribe topical anesthetic—repeated use leads to corneal epithelial breakdown, ulceration, and potential blindness.
7. Oral analgesic if needed

Treatment of "dirty" abrasion:

1. Cycloplegic
2. Frequent broad-spectrum antibiotic drops (every 1 to 2 h while awake), such as ciprofloxacin (Ciloxan), tobramycin, norfloxacin (Chibroxin), gentamicin
3. No patching
4. Reexamine in 24 to 36 h or refer to an ophthalmologist
5. Oral analgesic if needed

#### Contact Lens-Related Abrasions

These may be caused by several different factors, including a foreign body between the lens and cornea, poorly fitting lens, damage to the corneal epithelium on insertion or removal of the contact lens, or

**Table 201-1.** Ocular Emergencies

| Trauma Induced | Nontraumatic |
|---|---|
| BLUNT OCULAR TRAUMA | RED EYE |
| Subconjunctival hemorrhage | Conjunctivitis |
| Corneal abrasions | Keratitis |
| External foreign bodies | Episcleritis |
| Trauma to the iris | Iritis |
| Blowout fractures | Scleritis |
| Hyphema | Acute angle closure glaucoma |
| Traumatic retinopathies | "WHITE" EYES WITH SUDDEN |
| Ruptured globe from blunt trauma | VISUAL LOSS |
| Optic nerve trauma | Uveitis |
| SHARP OCULAR TRAUMA | Ectopia lentis |
| Lid lacerations | Acute cataract formation |
| Corneal/scleral lacerations | Amaurosis fugax |
| Severed extraocular muscles | Central retinal artery occlusion |
| Retained intraocular foreign body | Central retinal vein occlusion |
| | Retinal detachment |
| CHEMICAL BURNS | Retinal hemorrhage |
| Acid | Optic neuritis |
| Alkali | Ischemic optic neuropathy |
| Others | Migraine headaches |
| LIGHT-INDUCED TRAUMA | Hypertensive crisis |
| Ultraviolet keratitis | Cerebral blindness |
| Laser-induced scotomas | Functional disease |
| Solar retinopathy | |

overwear of the lens with secondary corneal edema. Always maintain suspicion of a potential corneal ulcer in a contact lens-related problem. The ulcer will stain with fluorescein, but in addition, will have an underlying or surrounding corneal infiltrate (white spot/haze). Obtain an emergency ophthalmology consult for a suspected corneal ulcer. *Pseudomonas* is the leading organism in contact lens-related bacterial ulcers and can devastate a cornea in 24 to 48 h. Corneal ulcers should not be patched, and cultures and frequent topical antibiotics (every 1 to 2 h) will be prescribed by the ophthalmologist.

## External Foreign Bodies

### Foreign Bodies of the Conjunctiva

Foreign bodies of the conjunctiva can be removed under topical anesthetic using a sterile cotton-tip applicator moistened with saline. The superior tarsal plate is a common lodging spot for foreign bodies and requires upper lid eversion for removal. Topical antibiotic drops can be instilled on completion of foreign body removal but are generally not mandatory.

### Foreign Bodies of the Cornea

Foreign bodies of the cornea are best removed under slit lamp control to assess the depth of the foreign body. A topical anesthetic must be used and a foreign body spud is helpful. Typically a small corneal abrasion will result after removal of the foreign body, and the eye can then be treated similarly to a corneal abrasion. If a metallic foreign body containing iron was removed, an underlying rust ring likely will be noted in the superficial corneal layers. The rust ring can be removed immediately by careful use of a spud or burr but is best left alone for 18 to 36 h because it will "soften" and be considerably easier to remove at that time. Treat the eye with a residual rust ring after foreign body removal as a corneal abrasion and refer the patient for rust ring removal the next day. Lastly, discussion of usage of safety glasses is certainly appropriate for any patient presenting with an ocular foreign body.

### Cyanoacrylate (Super-Glue, Krazy-Glue) Removal

Adhesives containing cyanoacrylate are prevalent and extremely efficient at forming strong bonds between dissimilar surfaces in seconds. Although many of these products are packaged in tubes, some are in bottles that have marked similarity to eyedrop containers. Inadvertent instillations into the eye or accidental splashes of cyanoacrylate adhesives occur regularly. Acetone or water/ethanol mixtures will soften the bond but *neither* of these is an acceptable treatment for the eye and lids. A definitive therapy for removal from the lids or ocular surface does not exist, but immediate copious irrigation (within 15 min of the splash) of the lids and eye with warm water for a minimum of 15 min can decrease the frequency of corneal abrasions. Mineral oil can be applied to eyelid adhesions after irrigation to soften the glue. Surgical separation of the eyelids has been done but must be done with extreme caution to prevent laceration of the lid margins or underlying globe. Although cyanoacrylate adhesives will cause a corneal abrasion when removed from the cornea, the deeper layers sustain no permanent damage that would cause a corneal scar. The abrasion can be treated as such and should heal readily. An ophthalmologist should be consulted for almost all cases.

## Trauma to the Iris

### Traumatic Iritis/Iridocyclitis

Commonly seen after blunt trauma, this is usually a mild inflammatory reaction of the iris or ciliary body. Symptoms include pain (usually described as a deep ache), headache above the eyebrow, photophobia, and occasionally epiphora (excessive tearing). Signs are seen best with the slit lamp and consist of ciliary injection and flare and cells in the anterior chamber. Treatment includes topical cycloplegics (1% cyclopentolate or 5% homatropine 1 drop to affected eye up to t.i.d.). Avoid long-lasting cycloplegic agents such as scopolamine and atropine. Use of steroids should be left to the ophthalmologist.

### Traumatic Miosis/Mydriasis

The iris and ciliary body may respond to some forms of blunt trauma with a constricted pupil (miosis) and spasm of accommodation *or* with dilation (mydriasis) and cycloplegia. Treatment is not required.

### Iris Sphincter Ruptures

Ruptures can cause small triangular defects in the pupillary margin, leaving a permanent "notch" in the border of the pupil. No treatment is available for this injury.

### Iridodialysis

This is a much more serious and permanent injury to the iris, usually associated with a hyphema. The base of the iris separates from the ciliary body and scleral spur creating an "accessory pupil" at the limbus. Pupillary light testing for afferent defects may be confusing secondary to irregular constriction of the pupil. The resulting hyphema should be treated, but no intervention is required for the iridodialysis itself.

## Blowout Fractures

The thinnest part of the orbital wall is in the floor of the orbit (maxillary bone) with the next thinnest being the ethmoid bones along the medial orbital wall. Fractures of the orbital floor occur from transmission of forces through the orbital soft tissues by a nonpenetrating object (e.g., fist, ball). They often occur with fractures of the orbital rim and adjacent facial bones. Medial wall fractures into the ethmoid sinuses may result in orbital emphysema. Medial and floor fractures may be complicated by entrapment of orbital contents (fat, extraocular muscles) such that significant restriction of gaze (with diplopia) or enophthalmos occurs. If this occurs or persists, repair can be undertaken. Although fractures can often be seen on a Water's view, CT scan is best (coronal) to delineate the extent of herniated tissue into the sinuses. Medial wall fractures are typically "covered" with an oral antibiotic for 7 days (using a first-generation cephalosporin) because the mucosal lining of the ethmoid is usually torn, thus allowing sinus-to-orbital connection and potential contamination.

All patients with blowout fractures deserve a complete eye examination in the emergency department. If there is extraocular muscle entrapment, obtain an ophthalmology consult. If there is no entrapment, and the ocular examination is normal, ophthalmology follow-up should be provided in a few days.

## Hyphema

Hyphema is blood in the anterior chamber resulting from rupture of one or more iris stromal vessels. The extent of a hyphema varies from microscopic (detectable with slit lamp only) to "8-ball" hyphemas in which the anterior chamber is filled with blood or clot. Anywhere from 8 to 33 percent of hyphemas rebleed between 2 and 5 days postinjury. Rebleeds are almost invariably worse than the original bleed and are associated with reduced vision, secondary glaucoma, and potential corneal blood staining.

Treatment includes topical atropine drops (1% atropine, 1 gtt bid), usually topical steroids (prednisolone 1 gtt, q.i.d.), and a Fox metallic eye shield. Bed rest for 5 days (to prevent clot dislodgment and a rebleed) remains controversial. Oral prednisone at a dose of 20 mg b.i.d. for 5 days has been shown to decrease the incidence of rebleeds. The patient is checked regularly during this period. Patients with sickle cell disease or trait require special consideration because sickle cells can sludge, raising IOP. The eyes of sickle cell patients tolerate elevated IOP poorly and medications that promote sickling (e.g., Diamox, epinephrine, and hyperosmotics) need to be avoided.

Surgical washout of the hyphema may need to be considered. Major complications of hyphemas include acute glaucoma (32 percent), chronic late glaucoma (7 percent), optic atrophy (7 to 10 percent), and angle recession (71 to 86 percent). Ophthalmologic consultation and close follow-up should be obtained.

## Traumatic Retinopathies

### Commotio Retinae

This is a common result of blunt trauma and is transient retinal edema that on ophthalmoscopy appears as white patchy areas of retina. It is of long-term significance only if it involves the macula because after resolution it may be associated with impaired vision consequent to retinal pigmentary disturbances, macular holes, or cysts. Ophthalmologic consultation should be obtained.

### Macular Cysts and Holes

Microcystoid degeneration of the retina is seen occasionally after blunt trauma. A macular cyst may occur a few days to years after the injury. Most macular holes are thought to develop from cysts that have deteriorated. Full-thickness macular holes render a patient legally blind (20/200). An ophthalmologic referral should be obtained.

### Choroidal Rupture

This is a break in Bruch's membrane (outer retinal layer) frequently concentric with the disk. If it involves the macular area, it will cause significant loss of vision. The choroidal rupture disrupts all the overlying retinal layers. No treatment is available unless secondary neovascular membranes develop, which could cause extensive hemorrhaging. These new vessels can be ablated by laser treatment. Refer patients to an ophthalmologist for evaluation and follow-up.

### Traumatic Retinal Detachments

In acute injury, if the patient reports seeing flashes of light, consider detachment. Typically there will be a latent period between injury and detachment (50 percent develop by 8 months; 80 percent develop by 2 years). Dialysis (tear at ora serrata) is the most common type of tear and occurs in the inferotemporal quadrant most often followed in frequency by the superonasal quadrant. A scleral buckling procedure is indicated for the detachment. Visual outcome depends on the extent of involvement of the macula. Refer these patients to an ophthalmologist.

### Retinal Pigmentary Changes

Retinal pigmentary changes occur secondary to damage to the retinal pigment epithelium from concussive injury. These changes are more commonly seen in the periphery and cause no symptoms, but if involvement of the macula occurs, permanent decrease in vision may occur. They are not seen in the acute injury period.

### Retinal/Vitreous Hemorrhages

These can occur if a severe enough force is applied or transmitted to the globe. If the hemorrhages are small, they self-absorb with usually no sequellae. If located in the macula (center of vision) they will cause significant visual impairment until they are absorbed. Refer these patients to an ophthalmologist.

The victim of "shaken baby syndrome" may also present with multiple retinal and vitreous hemorrhages, as well as intracranial bleeds. There may be severe visual as well as developmental impairment. Evaluation of suspected child abuse (3 years old and under) should include a dilated funduscopic examination by an ophthalmologist.

## Ruptured Globe from Blunt Trauma

Prognosis for visual recovery is poor due to the potentially significant disruption of all intraocular structures from the force required to rupture the sclera/cornea. Careful evaluation/manipulation of the globe must be done to prevent further prolapse of intraocular contents. Notify an ophthalmologist immediately.

Management of ruptured globe:

1. Assess vision and do as much of the ocular evaluation that can be safely performed.
2. Do not instill any drops or ointment.
3. Keep patient NPO.
4. Initiate intravenous antibiotics. Cover for both gram-negative and gram-positive organisms. Vancomycin is an excellent gram-positive choice.
5. Place a Fox metallic shield over the eye; *no* underlying pressure patch
6. Tetanus update and immune globulin if indicated
7. Sedation/analgesia
8. Radiographic studies (CT or magnetic resonance imaging [MRI])
9. Repair of globe by an ophthalmologist (under general anesthesia)

## Optic Nerve Trauma

Trauma to the optic nerve may be isolated and present with visual loss and an intact globe (or decreased vision out of proportion to the ocular injury). Patients will present with an afferent pupillary defect on the involved side.

Orbital pressure elevation may occur with large hematomas or significant orbital emphysema. If orbital pressure exceeds the profusion pressure of the optic nerve or retina, profound ischemia will occur. Treatment consists of a lateral canthotomy or lateral orbital window to decompress the orbit. Orbital emphysema occurs with fractures of the orbit walls/floor, but most commonly is seen with medial wall blowout fractures. If the air is in a "pocket" and there is optic nerve compromise, careful placement into the orbit of a needle on a syringe without a plunger will allow evacuation of the air. These procedures should be done by an ophthalmologist.

### Traumatic Optic Neuropathies

**Avulsion or laceration of the nerve.** This will lead to immediate, irreversible visual loss. Optic nerve disruption may be visible on CT scan, or even funduscopically if it was avulsed at the entry into the globe. Le Fort III fractures can rarely cause blindness due to disruption of the optic nerves. No treatment is available.

**Optic nerve contusion.** This is felt to represent capillary disruption and results in immediate, irreversible visual loss. The CT scan is normal. The optic nerve will become pale within several weeks. No treatment is available.

**Optic nerve compression.** This is potentially reversible and may be associated with delayed visual loss. There are two main areas for compression to occur:

1. Within the optic canal. There may or may not be an associated fracture in the canal. If obvious canal narrowing is *not* evident on high-resolution CT scanning, megadose corticosteroids can be initiated (methylprednisolone 30 mg/kg loading dose then 15 mg/kg in 2 h and repeat q6h). Strongly consider antibiotic coverage. Treat any underlying peptic ulcer disease. Discontinue intravenous steroids in 3 days if no improvement is seen.

Optic canal decompression is indicated if the canal is narrowed or if deterioration occurs on steroid withdrawal.

2. Within the optic nerve sheath. Typically occurs with a large intrasheath hematoma. Optic nerve sheath decompression is indicated. Immediate ophthalmologic consultation should be obtained.

## Sharp Ocular Trauma

### Lid Lacerations

Always evaluate the globe for potential trauma as well.

Lid margin lacerations require a specific three-stitch closure under magnification to prevent development of a lid notch and can be done in the emergency department with a cooperative patient by an ophthalmologist.

Medial eyelid lacerations must be scrutinized for potential trauma to the nasolacrimal system (i.e., evaluate patency and integrity of canaliculus and punctum). Canalicular patency can be evaluated by irrigating fluorescein-stained saline through the punctum (use a 22- or 25-gauge blunt-tip cannula on a syringe) and looking for any appearance of fluorescein in the laceration site. If a canalicular laceration exists, this should be stented and closed in the operating room by an ophthalmologist.

Upper lid lacerations parallel to the lid margin may involve damage to the levator muscle/aponeurosis in which case muscle reattachment should be done primarily to prevent ptosis. This is best accomplished in the operating room.

## Corneal/Scleral Lacerations

The spectrum of severity of these injuries varies from partial-thickness corneal lacerations to irreparable penetrating injuries with extensive loss of retinal tissue. Principles for evaluation/preparation for repair of sharp penetrating trauma is the same as for blunt trauma, but prognosis is generally better. Evaluation of the partial-thickness versus full-thickness corneal laceration is done by "painting" the area of laceration with fluorescein (instill 1 gtt anesthetic first) and look for "streaming" of the fluorescein from the site using a slit lamp. Partial-thickness lacerations can often be managed with a bandage soft contact lens as can an occasional self-sealing, small, full-thickness laceration. An ophthalmologist needs to evaluate and make these treatment decisions. Repair should be performed as soon as possible to avoid wound edema, prolapse of ocular contents, hemorrhage, or late infection. General anesthesia is best. This avoids unnecessary pressure on the globe from the manipulation required with, as well as the volume from, a retrobulbar injection. For general anesthesia, depolarizing muscle relaxants are to be avoided as is excessive manipulation during intubation. Potential sequelae of corneoscleral lacerations include irregular corneal astigmatism and scarring, cataract, glaucoma, and formation of fibromembranous vitreous bands with subsequent retinal detachment.

## Severed Extraocular Muscles

Severance of extraocular muscles is a rare occurrence but a difficult problem. If the muscle is completely severed, it retracts along the fascial planes posteriorly and may be unrecoverable. If identified, it is reattached to its usual insertion site. If not recoverable, significant strabismus will develop with overaction in the direction of the unapposed antagonist muscle. A transposition procedure can be performed at a later date. Botulinum toxin can be used against the antagonist muscle in selected cases. Evaluation by an ophthalmologist is required.

## Retained Intraocular Foreign Body

Maintain a high level of suspicion whenever periorbital ocular tissue damage or wounds are apparent. Foreign bodies can enter the globe, leaving little evidence of penetration. Inquire as to composition of the foreign body and velocity with which it struck. Consider potential intracranial extension of the injury.

Identification/localization of foreign body includes the following methods:

1. Direct visualization (slit lamp, ophthalmoscopy)
2. Water's view and lateral skull x-rays
3. CT scan
4. Ultrasound
5. MRI (avoid if foreign body is magnetic)

The presence of more than one foreign body must always be considered. Table 201-2 lists common foreign bodies.

**Table 201-2.** Most Commonly Seen Intraocular Metallic and Nonmetallic Foreign Bodies

| Metallic | | Nonmetallic | |
|----------|----------|-------------|----------|
| Toxic | Nontoxic | Toxic | Nontoxic |
| Lead | Gold | Wood, other | Stone |
| Zinc | Silver | plant matter | Glass |
| Nickel | Platinum | Cloth particles | Porcelain |
| Aluminum | | Cilia | Carbon |
| Copper | | Eyelid particle | Some plastics |
| Iron | | | |

If the foreign body is magnetic, it indicates the presence of a toxic iron content and also indicates that the foreign body is amenable to removal from the eye using magnetic devices.

Techniques of foreign body extraction depend on the location and type of foreign body and include limbal or clear corneal extraction, magnet extraction, vitrectomy instrumentation, and scleral cutdown.

Final visual acuity correlates best with the extent of damage at the time of initial injury. Immediate ophthalmologic consultation should be obtained.

## Chemical Burns

Acid burns (e.g., battery acid, glacial acetic acid) precipitate tissue proteins that set up barriers against deeper penetration. Damage is usually localized to the area of contact with exception of hydrofluoric acid and acids containing heavy metals, which tend to penetrate the cornea and anterior chamber.

Alkali burns (e.g., lye, fresh lime, ammonia) penetrate the cornea rapidly due to their ability to lyse cell membranes. Damage is related to the alkalinity (pH) and permanent injury is determined by the nature and concentration of the chemical burn, as well as the time lapsed before irrigation. Table 201-3 lists the prognosis of these burns according to initial findings.

Other chemicals include burns from tear gas and Mace. These result in an injury similar to an alkali burn and should be managed as such. Injury from sparklers and flares that contain magnesium hydroxide should be managed as chemical burns rather than thermal burns.

Treatment of chemical burns:

1. Immediate lavage at site of injury
2. Subsequent lavage with normal saline in the emergency department with a minimum of 1 to 2 L. Instill topical anesthetic q20min. Evaluate palpebral conjunctiva and conjunctival fornices for any retained foreign material and remove it. Continue lavage until pH is 7.4 to 7.6. Once this pH is achieved, wait 10 min and recheck to ascertain that more chemical is not leaching out of the ocular tissue. This is particularly a concern in alkali injuries.
3. During irrigation, evaluate for any aspirated or swallowed chemicals and be aware of the potential of acute airway obstruction if the former occurred.

**Table 201-3.** Hughes Classification of Alkali Burns to the Eye

| | |
|---|---|
| Grade I | Good prognosis |
| | Corneal epithelial damage |
| | No ischemia |
| Grade II | Good prognosis |
| | Cornea hazy but iris details seen |
| | Ischemia of less than one third limbus |
| Grade III | Guarded prognosis |
| | Total corneal epithelial loss |
| | Stromal haze blurring iris details |
| | Ischemia of one third to one half of limbus |
| Grade IV | Poor prognosis |
| | Cornea opaque, obscuring view of iris or pupil |
| | Ischemia of more than one half limbus |

4. Dilate the eye with 1% cyclopentolate or 5% homatropine.
5. Check IOP (important in alkali burns). If 22 mm Hg or greater, contact an ophthalmologist.
6. Apply an ophthalmic antibiotic ointment (needs to be used until reepithelialization is completed). Bacitracin/polymyxin ointment is a good choice.
7. Pain medications. These patients have severe pain—be generous with analgesics.
8. Follow-up the next day. If the burn is severe (grade III or IV) or you are uncertain about the grade, notify an ophthalmologist immediately. Aggressive treatment is necessary in severe burns to minimize scarring and to prevent perforation. Topical steroids and citrate drops are used. Bandage contact lenses and oral ascorbate may be considered.

### Light-Induced Ocular Trauma

#### Ultraviolet Keratitis

Ultraviolet keratitis represents a "sunburn" of the anterior surface of the globe. Potential exposure sources include arc welding, tanning booths, and prolonged time outdoors in sunny, snow-covered areas, typically at high altitude. Severe pain and photophobia occur 4 to 8 h after the exposure. Examination reveals an injected conjunctiva with diffuse punctate staining of the cornea. Treatment includes cycloplegic drops (1% cyclopentolate or 5% homatropine instilled × 1 in the emergency department) and consider antibiotic ointment. Patching is optional. Pain medication is mandatory. No visual deficit will persist beyond 24 to 48 h after the pain has resolved.

#### Laser-Induced Scotomas

Lasers are increasingly being used as a therapeutic modality in many specialties. Reflected or scattered laser beams have potential for causing ocular (retinal) burns in bystanders. Treatment lies in prevention with appropriate eye shields, because once a thermal or nonthermal retinal burn occurs, a scotoma (blind spot) will develop for which there is no treatment.

#### Solar Retinopathy

Sungazing can cause permanent visual loss by virtue of retinal damage to the photoreceptors in the area of the fovea (center of vision). Initially, on examination, a small gray zone is seen that, in time, changes to pigmentary scarring. Treatment lies in prevention because once the damage has occurred, no medical or surgical treatment is available to reverse or decrease the scotoma.

### NONTRAUMATIC OCULAR EMERGENCIES

#### Red Eye

#### Conjunctivitis

Conjunctivitis is inflammation of the conjunctiva, which normally appears as a relatively clear mucous membrane on the surface of the eye. Multiple etiologic factors can cause swelling (chemosis) or dilation of the blood vessels in the conjunctiva. Not all conjunctivitis is infectious, and an accurate history and examination will identify cases that require appropriate precautions to prevent spread (particularly an issue in day care centers and other large group facilities where hygiene is not optimal). Differential diagnosis includes other more serious forms of "red eye": keratitis, episcleritis, uveitis, scleritis, and narrow angle glaucoma.

*Viral conjunctivitis* accounts for the large majority of "pink eye" and frequently occurs in conjunction with an upper respiratory infection. Redness and epiphora (tearing) are common. Preauricular adenopathy is frequently found and a mild palpebral (lid) conjunctival follicular response can be seen. Treatment is supportive. A particularly contagious form of viral conjunctivitis known as epidemic keratoconjunctivitis (EKC) can cause significant signs and symptoms. EKC is caused by several subtypes of adenovirus and causes marked hyperemia of the conjunctiva, chemosis, epiphora, and occasionally, superficial viral corneal infiltrates that can drop vision by several lines. The time course of EKC varies from 2 to 8 weeks and there is no specific treatment. The exception is when corneal infiltrates cause reduction in visual acuity at which time topical steroids can be used cautiously with frequent monitoring by an ophthalmologist. Physicians should use gloves when examining patients with an acute red eye to minimize the possibility of cross-infection. The examining chair and slit lamp table and bars should be cleansed with an antiseptic solution after use by a patient with EKC, to minimize spread to the next patient.

*Bacterial conjunctivitis* presents with a mucopurulent discharge of varying colors (gray, yellow, green). Typically there is matting of the lashes in the morning, but minimal, if any, pain. The conjunctival injection is variable, and there is no preauricular adenopathy. Treatment consists of topical antibiotic drops (trimethoprim/polymyxin, tobramycin, gentamicin, norfloxacin) q.i.d. for 1 week. Warm soaks should be used to keep the lids/lashes free of debris. A review of good hygiene and points for cross-contamination in the home (towels, pillows, makeup) should be reviewed. An eye that is "pouring out pus" must be cultured for gonorrhea and Gram stained as well. Urgent treatment is needed to prevent corneal ulceration with *Neisseria gonorrhea* and consists of intramuscular ceftriaxone plus frequent ocular irrigation with saline. Topical tetracycline or bacitracin ointment or penicillin G drops can be initiated q2h decreasing to q.i.d. dosing after 2 to 3 days. Inquiry as to personal contacts and their treatment must also be done. Refer to an ophthalmologist.

*Chlamydial conjunctivitis* in an adult presents with a mucopurulent discharge and redness. Examination shows a follicular conjunctival response that becomes more pronounced with chronicity. This has been typically described in sexually active adults so inquiry as to contacts may be warranted. Treatment consists of topical tetracycline or sulfonamide drops q.i.d. for 3 weeks but, most importantly, systemic treatment with doxycyline 100 mg orally bid or erythromycin base, 250 to 500 mg orally qid or sulfasoxazole, 500 to 1000 mg orally qid, all for 3 weeks.

*Allergic conjunctivitis* is noninfectious and often has a seasonal occurrence. Symptoms include mild to severe itching, a stringy white discharge, and redness. Signs often show a conjunctival papillary response and relatively pale swelling (chemosis) of the conjunctiva. Treatment includes levocobastine (Livostin), a histamine receptor site blocker. Dosage is q.i.d. as needed for itching and cold compresses as needed. Less effective is the topical decongestant and antihistamine combination drop, naphazoline HCl-antizoline phosphate (Naphcon A), that can be used up to four times daily. It is contraindicated in patients with narrow angles. Contact lens wear should be eliminated during periods of active allergic conjunctivitis. For chronic allergic conjunctivitis, lodoxamide tromethamine (Alomide) is recommended q.i.d. to minimize symptoms. Alomide stabilizes mast cells and inhibits eosinophil migration.

*Toxic conjunctivitis* occurs with either airborne irritants (e.g., smoke, particulate matter) or a direct splash of liquid or powder to the eye. Irrigation *must* be done immediately when direct substance contact occurs. Subsequent treatment of residual redness and irritation consists primarily of lubrication with artificial tears/ointment. (See Chemical Burns for further details.)

### Keratitis

Keratitis is a generic term used to refer to inflammation/irritation of the cornea from any number of etiologies.

## Corneal Ulcer or Bacterial/Fungal Keratitis

Bacterial or fungal keratitis typically presents with a "white spot" or infiltrate on the cornea, often with an overlying epithelial defect, hence the name, "corneal ulcer." This is a serious ocular problem and requires referral to an ophthalmologist for culturing and evaluation. Frequent topical broad spectrum antibiotics and possibly antifungal drops are started around the clock as well as cycloplegic with 5% homatropine t.i.d. or 1% atropine b.i.d. Most corneal ulcers are painful and generally have an associated iritis that can be severe enough to cause a hypopyon (layering out of white blood cells in the anterior chamber). There is an increased incidence of corneal ulcers with extended overnight wear soft contact lenses, notably caused by *Pseudomonas,* which can devastate a cornea in 24 to 48 h. Corneal ulcers need emergent ophthalmologic evaluation and management.

## Viral Keratitis

***Herpes simplex keratoconjunctivitis*** usually presents primarily with one or more dendriform corneal ulcers (no infiltrate). They can be well demonstrated with rose bengal dye, applied with strips analogous to fluorescein strips. Rarely, there can be associated skin/periocular lesions. Treatment of the dendriform ulcers consist of topical 0.3% trifluridine (Viroptic) nine times per day for 2 to 3 weeks. The herpes simplex virus is capable of establishing a latent state in the trigeminal ganglion and reactivating under situations of increased patient stress. Recurrent disease presents multiple ways and includes iridocyclitis, disciform keratitis, infectious ulcers, trophic ulcers, or interstitial keratitis. The initial dendriform ulcer is unique but can easily be confused with the herpes zoster dendrite. Generally concomitant dermatomal lesions in zoster aid in the differentiation. Refer to an ophthalmologist for initiation of treatment.

***Herpes zoster dermatitis,*** when involving the $V_I$ branch of the trigeminal nerve, has a 70% incidence of ocular involvement. Virtually any part of the eye as well as the lids and extraocular muscles can be affected. Lid lesions, conjunctivitis, iritis, and dendriform corneal ulcers are most often seen in ophthalmic zoster. Oral acyclovir (800 mg orally five times a day for 10 days) decreases the incidence and severity of the ocular complications but must be initiated early in the course of the disease (best if within 72 h of onset). Topical steroids are used to treat any associated iritis. Topical antibiotic ointment or drops can be used prophylactically against secondary bacterial infection of the epithelial ulcers. The typical antiviral therapy used in treating herpes simplex is not effective for herpes zoster. The iritis and stromal keratitis that can occur in zoster may last months to years after the initial dermatomal outbreak. It is important to inform all patients with active herpes zoster ophthalmicus to be alert for any ocular problems and seek immediate attention if ocular redness, pain, or blurred vision occur. Refer to an ophthalmologist any patient with herpes zoster virus-1 who has any ocular complaint.

## Episcleritis

Episcleritis is a generally benign, self-limiting inflammation of the episclera (tissue between the conjunctiva and sclera). It is characterized by localized or diffuse vascular dilation as well as edema. Patients report discomfort but no change in vision. A subtype known as "nodular" episcleritis can occur with collagen vascular disease, gout, rheumatoid arthritis, or herpes zoster virus-1.

Treatment may not be necessary in mild cases. Topical decongestants (naphazoline HCl or Vasocon [Naphcon]) can be used up to t.i.d. for relief. With more pain, oral nonsteroidal anti-inflammatory drugs (NSAIDs)—indomethacin (Indocin) 25 mg b.i.d., naproxen (Naprosyn) 250 mg b.i.d., or diflunisal (Dolobid) 500 mg b.i.d.—can be instituted along with topical steroids (1% prednisolone t.i.d. to q.i.d.). Topical NSAIDs such as diclofenac sodium (Voltaren) can be considered as well, although their efficacy as compared to topical steroids has not been adequately studied in episcleritis. Differential diagnosis includes conjunctivitis, uveitis, and scleritis. Refer these patients to an ophthalmologist.

## Iritis

See Uveitis below.

## Scleritis

This refers to inflammation of the sclera and can cause severe deep pain and potentially visual loss. The majority of cases occur in the anterior sclera (visible by slit lamp) and present with deep violaceous injection and potential corneal involvement (infiltration or peripheral thinning). Three subtypes are described: diffuse, nodular, or necrotizing (least frequent but most ominous). There is a high incidence of associated systemic or collagen vascular diseases and full medical evaluation is appropriate. Treatment is best managed by an ophthalmologist and can include topical steroids or NSAIDs, systemic steroids, or immunosuppressive agents.

## Acute Angle Closure Glaucoma

Smaller eyes with "crowded" anterior segments may be seen at the slit lamp to have very shallow (or narrow) anterior chambers. Such eyes may experience a sudden increase in IOP when the pupil is mid-dilated owing to pupillary block. This causes the aqueous humor to remain and accumulate in the posterior chamber, pushing the peripheral iris against the trabecular meshwork and obstructing outflow, hence increasing the IOP.

Subclinical attacks of narrow angle glaucoma are perhaps more frequent than we realize. The acute, full-blown narrow angle glaucoma attack presents with a very injected eye, a "steamy" (hazy) cornea, and iritis. The pupil is typically mid-dilated and minimally, or not at all, reactive. IOP ranges from 40 to 70 mm Hg. The patient not only experiences severe pain and blurring, but often nausea and vomiting. Treatment acutely is directed at decreasing the IOP with topical medications (β blockers such as timolol maleate [Timoptic] and apraclonidine [Iopidine]; oral agents if possible, (e.g., acetazolamide [Diamox] or methazolamide [Neptazane]); miotics to constrict the pupil (pilocarpine drops); and, possibly, intravenous agents (e.g., acetazolamide or mannitol). Once the pressure has been lowered and the cornea cleared, a peripheral iridectomy (full-thickness opening in the iris) is made with the yttrium-aluminum-garnet +/– argon laser to prevent subsequent attacks. The fellow eye is evaluated for its potential for narrow angle glaucoma and a prophylactic peripheral iridectomy is done, if indicated. Management requires an ophthalmologist.

## White Eyes

### Uveitis

Inflammation of one or all parts of the uveal tract is termed uveitis. The uveal tract consists of the iris, ciliary body, and choroid. The majority of uveal tract inflammation affects the anterior aspect of the uveal tract and is categorized more specifically as iritis. If the inflammation is severe enough, it can substantially impair vision, down to 20/200 or worse. Evaluating nontraumatic uveitis requires a systemic evaluation to eliminate conditions such as sarcoid, collagen vascular disorders, ankylosing spondylitis, Reiter syndrome, tuberculosis, syphilis, toxoplasmosis and toxocariasis, juvenile rheumatoid arthritis, and Lyme disease.

Symptoms typically are blurred vision, deep aching, photophobia, and varying degrees of redness. The more posterior in the eye the inflammation, the less the redness. Signs are best seen at the slit lamp and include cells in the anterior or posterior chamber, "flare" (headlights in fog) in the aqueous humor, and variable conjunctival injection. Cells and fibrin may be seen in varying degrees in the vitreous gel in posterior uveitis.

Treatment consists of topical corticosteroids initially with possible topical cycloplegic agents. More refractory posterior or severe cases may require periocular or oral steroids. An ophthalmologist needs to diagnose and treat this disorder.

## Lenticular Etiologies

It is rare for "acute" cataract formation to occur in a nontraumatic setting; however, rapid progression of a posterior subcapsular cataract can, in fact, drop vision rapidly over the course of a few days to weeks. The so-called "osmotic" cataract that occurs with rapid blood sugar changes is rare. "Ectopia lentis" refers to a subluxated lens and may occur in homocystinuria, Weill-Marchesani syndrome, and Marfan syndrome. Once the lens has become displaced enough, it is no longer able to focus light and monocular diplopia or blurred vision occurs. Dislocation into the vitreous can occur in these conditions as well as in trauma. If increased IOP occurs in the setting of a dislocated lens, a vitrectomy and lens removal is necessary to save the eye. Acutely, medication to lower the IOP can be used (topical β blockers, apraclonidine, oral carbonic anhydrase inhibitors, or intravenous hyperosmotics) until surgery can be done to remove the lens. An ophthalmologist needs to manage these cases.

## Amaurosis Fugax

This refers to the ocular transient ischemic attack and is typically a painless, monocular, transient (5 to 30 min) loss of vision. It is often described as a "graying" or "blurring" of part or all of the visual field. It occurs due to transient obstruction of a retinal artery/arteriole from cholesterol emboli ("Hollenhorst" plaque) or fibrin-platelet emboli. It is completely reversible, but systemic evaluation to identify etiology is necessary. Collagen vascular disease, syphilis, sickle cell disease, and temporal arteritis should be considered. Both cardiac and carotid ultrasound examinations are appropriate. Hollenhorst plaques in the retina typically have their origin from a carotid plaque, and depending on the extent of the carotid blockage, may be surgically treatable. An ophthalmologist should perform a complete eye examination and an internal medicine physician should be consulted to evaluate sources of plaque.

## Central Retinal Artery Occlusion (CRAO)

Central retinal artery occlusion is an event requiring *emergency* intervention. With a CRAO, the blood supply to the retina is obstructed, producing a painless, total, or near total "black-out" of vision. Reestablishment of retinal circulation must be accomplished within 90 min to regain useful vision. Initially, examination may show an afferent pupillary defect and extreme narrowing of the retinal arterioles. A very sluggish flow can occasionally be seen and is termed "boxcarring" owing to the appearance of segmentation of blood in the arterioles. A distal obstruction affecting a branch of a retinal arteriole (branch retinal artery obstruction) will affect the visual field only in that area supplied by the obstructed vessel. After the first few hours, a gray appearance develops across the area of infarcted retina. The macular area in CRAO develops a "cherry-red" spot owing to the thinness of the retina here and the clearer view of the underlying choroidal vasculature. Treatment of a CRAO is generally futile if the obstruction has been present for over 2 h. Nonetheless, given the extreme hopelessness (outcome varies from counting fingers to no light perception vision), an attempt to regain perfusion should be done at least up to 48 h. Off and on pressure on the globe (known as ballotment) should be initiated immediately and done for 5 to 30 min. Paracentesis of the anterior chamber rapidly decompresses the eye and may dislodge a clot. If an orbital compressive lesion is responsible for the CRAO, (e.g., retrobulbar hemorrhage), urgent orbital decompression is needed. Refer all cases of suspected CRAO to an ophthalmologist immediately.

## Central Retinal Vein Occlusion

Obstruction of the retinal vein behind the optic nerve head results in a painless loss of vision of varying severity, depending on the extent of the obstruction. Examination of a severe central retinal vein occlusion (CRVO) reveals deep and superficial retinal hemorrhages, cotton wool spots (localized nerve fiber layer infarcts), and macular edema. The retinal venous system can appear markedly dilated. If the venous obstruction occurs anterior to the optic nerve head, a branch retinal vein obstruction (BRVO) will occur. Retinal hemorrhages will be seen in the hemisphere or quadrant drained by the obstructed vein and, depending on the location, macular edema may occur. Conditions associated with CRVO and BRVO include systemic hypertension, diabetes, and hyperviscosity syndromes. CRVO has been divided into ischemic and nonischemic subtypes, identifiable by retinal perfusion on fluorescein angiography. Acutely, no treatment is necessary. Ischemic CRVOs are treated with panretinal photocoagulation to prevent retinal and iris neovascularization (with subsequent rubeotic glaucoma). Persistent, significant macular edema can also be treated with laser photocoagulation. Refer the patient to an ophthalmologist.

## Retinal Detachment

A retinal detachment refers to the separation of the inner layers of the retina from the outermost retinal pigment epithelial layer. Patients may experience one or all of the typical triad of symptoms characteristic of a retinal detachment: sudden increase in floaters, photopsia (flashing lights), and a gray cloud or film over part of the visual field. Visual acuity can be quite good until the detachment affects the macula. Timely treatment by an ophthalmologist is required and consists of laser or cryopexy if the detached area is localized or a scleral buckling procedure for larger detachments. Risk factors for detachment include high degrees of myopia (nearsightedness), peripheral retinal thinning, prior cataract surgery, trauma, and a positive family history.

## Vitreo/Retinal Hemorrhages (Atraumatic)

Many retinal hemorrhages are "quiet," causing no symptoms unless they affect the macula, thereby decreasing visual acuity. Vitreous hemorrhages often will cause symptoms of floaters, as the blood in the gel of the eye tends to disperse. Both retinal and vitreous hemorrhages are painless events and are most commonly seen in diabetics with retinopathy. Numerous other causes for retinal and vitreous hemorrhage exist, including posterior vitreous detachments, CRVO, BRVO, submacular neovascularization (seen with histoplasmosis and age-related macular degeneration), and retinal hole or tear. Evaluation of vitreo/retinal hemorrhages needs to be done by an ophthalmologist and treatment rendered appropriate to the etiology.

## Optic Neuritis

Optic neuritis is inflammation or demyelination at any point along the optic nerve. Patients present with mild to profound levels of visual loss that typically occur over hours to a few days. Pain occurs in over 60 percent of cases, varying from dull to sharp and often exacerbated by extraocular movement. "Desaturation" or dimness of vision has been described as well as poor color vision. Examination will reveal an afferent pupillary defect on the affected side. The disk may appear swollen and hyperemic; however, in "retrobulbar optic neuritis" the disk is normal. Visual field defects are common and varied. A central scotoma is most common, but other defects including peripheral and midperipheral scotomas can occur. A general neurologic history and examination is warranted. Causes include multiple sclerosis, toxin exposure, drug abuse, alcoholism, lupus, sarcoid, Lyme disease, neurosyphilis, and idiopathic. Evaluation, treatment and follow-up are best directed by an ophthalmologist or neurologist. Treatment of optic neuritis is evolving as ongoing data from the National Optic Neuritis Treatment Trial is being evaluated. Primary treatment with oral steroids is *contraindicated* owing to the increased recurrence rate of optic neuritis over the subsequent 2 years. Intravenous steroids for 3 days followed by oral steroids can shorten the period of visual impairment and appears to have additional benefit in decreasing the number of patients progressing to symptomatic multiple sclerosis.

## Ischemic Optic Neuropathy

Obstruction of the main posterior ciliary arteries (blood supply to optic nerve and choroid) will cause an infarction of the anterior optic nerve. Up to 90 percent are caused by "nonarteritic" atherosclerosis. In the past, no treatment was available for this subgroup, but optic nerve sheath decompression may be of some benefit in selected patients. The remaining 10 percent comprise the granulomatous form of ischemic optic neuropathy, known as temporal arteritis. Patients typically are over 55 years of age and will have several systemic symptoms (e.g., anorexia, fever, fatigue, weight loss, and jaw claudication or pain over the temporal artery). Examination acutely may show pale disk swelling with nerve fiber layer hemorrhages on and near the disk. A palpably tender temporal artery or one that is nodular or nonpulsable is suspicious. A Westergren sedimentation rate is abnormally high in the majority of cases. Diagnosis is based on careful histopathology of a temporal artery biopsy. Treatment of temporal arteritis consists of high-dose oral steroids that are started even prior to the temporal artery biopsy to prevent further visual loss and protect the fellow eye (up to 10 percent of these patients will have a CRVO). Typically both an ophthalmologist and rheumatologist will follow these patients.

## Migraine Headaches

This broad grouping of headaches varies from the "common" migraine to the classical migraine with the visual aura, to the more disconcerting complicated migraine.

Migraine headaches will have at least several, if not all, of the following characteristics: aura, throbbing pain, unilateral location, nausea/vomiting, relief after sleep, and a positive family history. Patients who experience the visual aura for the first time often seek evaluation because it is frightening for many. The scotomas and scintillations may be monocular or binocular, in color or black and white, depending on their origin in the visual system. A number of patients experience a "march" of the scintillation and scotomas across their visual field. Sharp angles or zigzags are commonly described along the leading edge of a scotoma. The duration is typically 15 to 20 min and generally is followed by a headache. If no headache occurs, the phenomenon is known as an acephalgic (no pain) migraine. When a headache does not occur, the diagnosis may not be immediately evident and retinal tears or detachment may be suspected. These patients should be encouraged to have a thorough dilated examination by an ophthalmologist.

Complicated migraines have neurologic symptoms beyond the aura and headache. An ophthalmoplegic migraine involves paresis typically of cranial nerve III; however, cranial nerve IV or VI can be involved. These generally occur in early childhood (under 5 years old) and recovery takes 1 to 4 weeks. If it is a recurrent attack, permanent damage may occur. Differential diagnosis needs to include evaluation for possible causes of increased intracranial pressure, intracranial aneurysm, and diabetes. Basilar artery migraines are rare and present with scotomas and then complete loss of vision. This is followed by severe headache, vertigo, dysarthria, tinnitus, and altered consciousness. Young females are most prone to this and permanent damage is rare. Permanent visual field defects rarely occur with migraines. This results secondary to severe ischemia and essentially is a migraine-induced cerebrovascular accident. A neurologist needs to evaluate the patient and recommend prophylactic treatment.

## Hypertensive Crisis

Chronic hypertension will cause the well-known arteriolar attenuation visible on funduscopic examination. With increased blood pressure, over time, arteriolar-venous crossing changes occur (so-called AV nicking). Fluid transudation across the vessels results in hard exudates (yellow deposits in the retina) as well as small hemorrhages. As the degree of ischemia and hypertension increases, cotton wool spots (nerve fiber layer infarcts) will be seen in the posterior pole and with extreme levels of hypertension, disk edema occurs. Because this is a systemic condition, the findings of disk edema, retinal hemorrhages, hard exudates, cotton wool spots, and arteriolar narrowing should occur bilaterally. Visual loss as a result of the hypertensive crisis varies and is generally reversible with appropriate control of the blood pressure. The exception is if venous occlusion occurs, which could chronically decrease visual acuity. These patients need a primary care physician for blood pressure control with follow-up by an ophthalmologist.

## Cerebral Blindness

A number of central nervous system conditions that may have an impact on the optic tract, chiasm, optic radiations, or occipital lobe can all potentially affect central or peripheral vision profoundly. Patients will have unremarkable anterior segment and fundus examinations; pupillary involvement may occur with anterior lesions, but frequently there is no afferent pupillary defect. Etiologies include tumor, cerebrovascular accident, hydrocephalus, encephalitis, meningitis, and anoxia. Systemic symptoms such as headache, confusion, seizures, or paralysis may be seen. An MRI of the head/anterior visual pathways is indicated. Visual field testing should be attempted in patients who are cooperative. Typically both an ophthalmologist and neurologist are involved in patient management.

## Functional Disease

In patients with profound visual loss, either monocular or binocular, for which no organic reason can be found after doing a thorough examination, one needs to consider functional loss. Distinction between those patients with hysteria versus the malingerer can be difficult, although often the hysterical patient is far more cooperative. A number of tests can be performed in the ophthalmologist's office to better assess the visual function and thereby level the claims of "blindness" by the malingerer or allow one to reassure the hysterical patient that return of vision would be expected.

## BIBLIOGRAPHY

Buys, YM, Levin AV, Enzenauer RW. Retinal findings after head trauma in infants and young children. *Ophthalmology* 99:1718, 1992.

Corbet JJ. Neuro-ophthalmic complications of migraine and cluster headaches. *Neurol Clin* 1:973, 1983.

Dean BS, Krenzelok EP. Cyanoacrylates and corneal abrasion. *J Toxicol Clin Toxicol* 27:169, 1989.

Faber AS. Preventing eye injuries: what to tell patients. *Postgrad Med* 89:121, 1991.

Farber MD, Fiscella R, Goldberg MF. Aminocaproic acid versus prednisone for the treatment of traumatic hyphema. *Ophthalmology* 98:279, 1991.

Hayreh SS. The role of optic nerve sheath fenestration in management of anterior ischemic optic neuropathy. *Arch Ophthalmol* 108:1063, 1990.

Janda AM. Ophthalmic disorders in primary care. *Hosp Physician* 29:44, 1993.

Janda AM. Sudden nontraumatic visual loss. *Postgrad Med* 91:111, 1992.

Janda AM. Ocular trauma: triage and treatment. *Postgrad Med* 90:51, 1991.

Joseph MP, Simmons L, Rizzo J, et al. Extracranial optic nerve decompression for traumatic optic neuropathy. *Arch Ophthalmol* 108:1091, 1990.

Kelman SE, Elman MJ. Optic nerve sheath decompression for nonarteritic ischemic optic neuropathy improves multiple visual function measurements. *Arch Ophthalmol* 109:667, 1991.

Keltner JL. Giant-cell arteritis: signs and symptoms. *Ophthalmology* 89:1101, 1982.

Kooner KS, Cooksey JC, Barron JB, et al. Tonometry comparison: Goldmann versus Tono-Pen. *Ann Ophthalmol* 24:29, 1992.

Liesegang TJ. Diagnosis and therapy of herpes zoster ophthalmicus. *Ophthalmology* 98:1216, 1991.

Linberg JV. Orbital compartment syndromes following trauma. *Adv Ophthalmic Plastic Reconstruct Surg* 6:51, 1987.

Miller NR. The management of traumatic optic neuropathy. *Arch Ophthalmol* 108:1086, 1990.

Nichols B. Continuing education in ophthalmology. Section 4. Ophthalmology Basic and Clinical Science Course. American Academy of Ophthalmology, 1985.

Pavan-Langston D. *Manual of Ocular Diagnosis and Therapy,* 2d ed. Boston: Little, Brown, 1985.

Pederson J. Glaucoma: a primer for primary care physicians. *Postgrad Med* 90:41, 1991.

Rosenwasser GO, Holland S, Pflugfelder SC, et al. Topical anesthetic abuse. *Ophthalmology* 97:967, 1990.

Shingleton BJ, Hersh PS, Kenyon KR. *Eye Trauma.* St. Louis: Mosby-Year Book, 1991.

Shingleton BJ. Eye injuries. *N Engl J Med* 325:408, 1991.

Slamovits TL, Macklin R, Beck RW, et al. What to tell the patient with optic neuritis about multiple sclerosis. *Surv Ophthalmol* 36:47, 1991.

Smith CH, Beck RW, Mills RP. Functional disease in neuro-ophthalmology. *Neurol Clin* 1:955, 1983.

Spalding SC, Sternberg P. Controversies in the management of posterior segment ocular trauma. *Retina* 10:S76, 1990.

Spoor TC, Hartel WC, Lensink DB, et al. Treatment of traumatic optic neuropathy with corticosteroids. *Am J Ophthalmol* 110:665, 1990.

Thompson HS. Functional visual loss. *Am J Ophthalmol* 100:209, 1985.

Weinstein JM. Pupillary disorders. *Curr Opin Ophthalmol* 1:453, 1990.

Whiteacre MM, Emig M, Hassanein K. The effect of Perkins, Tono-Pen and Schiötz tonometry on intraocular pressure. *Am J Ophthalmol* 111:59, 1991.

# 202
# OTOLARYNGOLOGIC EMERGENCIES
## W. F. Peacock IV

## OTOLOGIC EMERGENCIES

### Otalgia

Ear pain is a common complaint with many causes. The approach should focus on the diagnosis and treatment of acute events, while excluding serious underlying pathology. A careful history and physical examination will usually identify the appropriate management course.

Auricular sensation is supplied by branches of cranial nerves V, VII, IX, and X as well as by the cervical plexus. Pathologic processes affecting these nerves may manifest as ear discomfort. Therefore, pain from the high cervical region, temporomandibular joint, mandible, teeth, tongue, tonsil, larynx, and cervical esophagus may be referred to the ear. An otologic examination should include these areas as potential causes of discomfort.

Treatment consists of analgesics and specific therapy directed at the underlying disease. A nondiagnostic examination should prompt outpatient follow-up with an otolaryngologist [ear-nose-throat (ENT) specialist].

### Infections

**External otitis and malignant external otitis (necrotizing external otitis).** These entities represent a spectrum of disease that begins with dermatitis of the external auditory canal (EAC). It may progress to cellulitis, chondritis, or osteomyelitis of the temporal bone and skull base. The advanced stages of this illness are termed *malignant external otitis* or, more appropriately, *necrotizing external otitis* (NEO). The necrotizing variety occurs primarily in elderly diabetics (80 to 90 percent of cases) but may occur in immunosuppressed or debilitated patients. The limited form of otitis externa is common to swimmers.

In otitis externa, patients present with pain in the affected ear exacerbated by movement of the pinna or tragus. Physical findings may be limited to erythema of the EAC. With progression, there is swelling and exudate from the EAC, and there may be an associated otitis media. If the lumen of the EAC is completely obstructed by edema or debris, examination of the tympanic membrane may be impossible. With canal occlusion, there will be an associated conductive hearing loss.

In NEO, there is erythema and edema of the pinna and periauricular tissues, the patient may be febrile or demonstrate other signs of sepsis, and there may be trismus. The EAC may have evidence of granulation tissue. In severe cases cranial nerve palsies, most frequently involving the ipsilateral seventh nerve, can be seen. Untreated, NEO can result in septic cerebral thromboembolism, meningitis, or brain abscess.

The diagnosis of these infections is made strictly by history and physical examination. In long-standing cases of NEO, radiographs or nuclear scan may demonstrate osteomyelitis but are usually not needed in the emergency department. In diabetics with NEO, serum glucose should be tightly controlled.

Culture of EAC exudate is unnecessary unless the patient has systemic illness or increased susceptibility to NEO. The most frequently demonstrated organism is *Pseudomonas.* Less frequently described pathogens are *Proteus, Staphylococcus,* and *Streptococcus.*

Treatment is based upon clinical findings. When symptoms are limited to erythema of the EAC, with pain on movement of the pinna, therapy should be analgesics and topical antibiotics directed at the suspected pathogens. Therapy is usually a combination of polymyxin B and neomycin, or colistin sulfate with hydrocortisone, placed in the EAC four times per day. The use of these antibiotics in solution commonly results in much more discomfort than when the suspension formulation is used. If possible, debris within the EAC should be removed by gentle irrigation and suctioning to ensure antibiotic contact with the skin. The patient should be instructed to keep all water out of the ear for 2 to 3 weeks.

If EAC edema is sufficient to obstruct the lumen, a "wick" must be placed to facilitate topical antibiotic penetration. These can be purchased specifically manufactured for otitis externa, or a gauze strip may be used. The patient is instructed to keep the wick moist with antibiotic solution. When the tympanic membrane (TM) cannot be visualized, oral antibiotics for a presumptive concurrent otitis media should be considered.

Patients with only mild erythema of the auricle who are not septic and not at risk for NEO can be closely followed as outpatients. In patients at risk for NEO, inpatient parenteral antibiotics should be considered if there is significant involvement of the pinna or if there are signs of systemic illness. Recommended antibiotics in NEO are antipseudomonal β lactams in combination with an aminoglycoside. Successful treatment with cephalosporins active against *Pseudomonas* has been reported. In severe cases, or those associated with facial nerve palsy, urgent ENT consultation should be arranged.

**Furuncles.** Furuncles of the external auditory canal are a painful condition until spontaneous rupture. Examination reveals a local area of tenderness and erythema. Treatment is as for external otitis, along with incision and drainage.

**Bullous myringitis.** This is a variant of acute otitis media, with similar presentation. On examination, bullae or vesicles are noted on the TM. The implicated etiologic organisms may be similar to those causing acute otitis media. The role of *Mycoplasma* has been questioned. Therapy consists of analgesics, antipyretics, and antibiotics covering the common otitis media organisms and *Mycoplasma*. Since TM blebs resolve spontaneously, they require no specific therapy.

**Otitis media.** Otitis media represents a spectrum of disease that includes the initial acute infection, otitis media with effusion, and chronic otitis media.

The most frequent pediatric bacterial infection, and a common complaint of adults, acute otitis media (AOM) is frequently heralded by the rapid onset of ear discomfort. While pain and fever occur, there may be neither. In the infant, nonspecific findings of fever, irritability, poor sleep, poor feeding, vomiting, otorrhea, or ear pulling may indicate AOM.

The diagnosis requires visualization of the TM. At onset, the normally clear to pearly white and freely mobile TM develops erythema and opacification. This may progress to a poorly mobile, bulging TM. In otitis media with effusion, bubbles or air-fluid levels may be visualized through the TM. While bilateral AOM occurs, erythema of both TMs may be the result of fever or crying in children. There are no laboratory tests that are diagnostically helpful.

*Pneumatic otoscopy* may aid diagnosis. The normal TM is a freely mobile structure that should move as a result of positive and negative pressure fluxes. Middle ear pathology is reflected in mobility changes. Absent TM motion in response to pressure changes suggests perforation. A bulging TM with poor movement to positive pressure indicates middle ear fluid or TM thickening. A TM that moves only to negative pressure indicates TM retraction.

*Tympanometry and acoustic otoscopy* may assist in the diagnosis of middle ear abnormality. In tympanometry, a probe placed in the EAC measures reflected sound. There must be a hermetic seal between the probe and the canal. The resulting data curve (tympanograph) indicates alterations within the acoustic system. When coupled with clinical information, this may be used to predict accurately middle ear pathology such as acute otitis media, serous otitis, otosclerosis, etc. Acoustic otoscopy is a newer, less widely accepted technique. This tool emits a variable frequency tone while recording reflected sound amplitude. It produces similar data to tympanometry but does not require an EAC seal.

In the pediatric cohort, AOM is most commonly the result of *Strep. pneumoniae* (26 percent), nontypable *Haemophilus influenzae* (21 percent), and *Moraxella catarrhalis* (3 percent). Less often, *Strep. pyogenes* (3 percent), *Staph. aureus* (3 percent), and others (26 percent) occur. Importantly, up to 25 percent of cases may be sterile. Chronic otitis media may be due to *Pseudomonas*.

Adult bacteriology yields *Strep. pneumoniae* more frequently (63 percent), with *H. influenzae* (10 percent), *Staph. aureus* (11 percent), *Strep. pyogenes* (7 percent), and others (9 percent) completing the spectrum.

Adult treatment consists of analgesics, antipyretics, and antibiotics. Amoxicillin is a reasonable first choice, with trimethoprim-sulfamethoxazole or erythromycin-sulfisoxazole in the penicillin-allergic patient. A significant response should be noted in 2 to 3 days. Failing this, antibiotic therapy should be changed to address β-lactamase species. Cefaclor or amoxicillin–clavulanic acid should be considered. Antibiotics should be continued for 10 days, with follow-up after completion to evaluate for possible persistent effusion. Patients with frequent infections or persistent effusion should also be referred for outpatient follow-up. Refer to Chap. 107, "Otitis and Pharyngitis," for details of pediatric treatment.

Complications include treatment failure, TM perforation, cholesteatoma, hearing changes, facial nerve injury, lateral sinus thrombophlebitis, or the suppurative complications of mastoiditis, intracranial abscess, and meningitis.

*Myringotomy* is the incision or excision of a portion of the TM for the purpose of allowing middle ear drainage. *Tympanocentesis* involves removal of middle ear fluid and is the definitive procedure for diagnosis and culture. While rarely indicated, tympanocentesis may be considered for patients with otitis media if any of the following occur:

1. Severe otalgia, serious illness, or toxicity
2. Unsatisfactory response to antimicrobial therapy
3. A confirmed or potential suppurative complication
4. Development of AOM while already on antibiotics
5. Occurrence in the newborn infant, a sick neonate, or in the immunocompromised patient where unusual organisms may be present

This procedure should be performed by an otolaryngologist or other personnel specifically trained in the technique.

## Mastoiditis

An uncommon disorder since the advent of antibiotics, mastoiditis is most frequently a complication of inadequately treated otitis media. Predictably it occurs with greatest frequency in the pediatric age group. There is no sex predilection. Clinical deterioration in a patient with otitis media should prompt concern for the possibility of acute mastoiditis.

Mastoiditis presents as a spectrum of diseases. Because of the communication between the middle ear and mastoid sinus, all cases of otitis media are accompanied by mastoiditis. The majority of subclinical cases resolve with appropriate antibiotic therapy. However, treatment failure results in clearing of the middle ear process while allowing persistent infection of the mastoid. This state has been referred to as *masked mastoiditis*. Untreated, progression results in clinically apparent mastoiditis.

Acute mastoiditis is usually secondary to obstruction of the middle ear and mastoid sinus communication by pus or engorged mucosa. Blockage causes the accumulation of mucopurulent material and results in inflammatory changes within the mastoid. *Coalescent mastoiditis* occurs with the resorption of the mastoid's bony trabeculae from long-standing inflammation. Finally, erosion through the mastoid's bony cortex leads to a *subperiosteal abscess*. Chronic mastoiditis is defined as infection lasting longer than 3 months.

The complications of mastoiditis occur frequently and include osteitis, subperiosteal abscess, facial palsies, and extension of the abscess into the neck (Bezold abscess) or cranial structures. Meningitis, intracranial abscesses, and intracerebral septic thrombophlebitis can occur.

While there is frequently a recent history of otitis media, antibiotic use, persistent otalgia, or possibly otorrhea, this "prodrome" may be absent. The symptoms of mastoiditis may include otalgia, otorrhea, headache, and hearing loss. In the very young infant, presentation may be limited to be fever, irritability, and diarrhea. Fever can be a variable finding.

Physical examination may demonstrate mastoid tenderness and erythema, loss of the postauricular crease, outward or inferior displacement of the pinna, or postaural fluctuance. While common, postauricular swelling is not always present. The TM usually demonstrates some abnormality of erythema, opacity, gross edema, loss of landmarks, or perforation with pus in the EAC. Visualization of the TM can be prevented by sagging of the posterior canal wall. As many as 10 percent of cases will have a normal TM examination.

The diagnosis of mastoiditis is based on clinical findings. Laboratory evaluation may identify leukocytosis. In patients with acute mastoiditis, cultures obtained at the time of surgical drainage may grow *Strep. pyogenes, Strep. pneumoniae, Staph. aureus, H. influenzae, Pseudomonas* species, anaerobes, or may be sterile. Tuberculosis of the mastoid occurs rarely. In chronic mastoiditis, anaerobes, most frequently *Bacteroides* species, are seen more often.

Plain radiographs can demonstrate mastoid opacity or cloudiness, although these findings may be absent. In all patients suspected of having mastoiditis, a computed tomography (CT) scan is indicated. This not only distinguishes soft tissue swelling from mastoiditis, but also evaluates the intracranial structures.

The mainstay of treatment is emergent surgical drainage by an otolaryngologist. While antibiotics will have little effect until the abscess is drained, they should be started in the emergency department. Appropriate choices include ampicillin/sulbactam, ceftriaxone (possibly in combination with metronidazole), imipenem, or chloramphenicol with vancomycin or nafcillin. When chronic mastoiditis is suspected, antibiotic selection should ensure anaerobic coverage.

## Sudden Hearing Loss

Sudden hearing loss is defined as occurring within a 72-h period. Although distressing to the patient, it is most frequently the result of benign cerumen impaction. While cerumen impaction is easily remedied, the entire differential diagnosis must be considered in cases where there is no EAC foreign body responsible for the hearing deficit.

Historical considerations to address are if one or both ears are involved, recent viral illness, trauma (including Q-tip usage), swimming, diving, flying, a forceful Valsalva maneuver (as in weight lifting), or associated neurologic symptoms. An in-depth past medical history is indicated to evaluate specifically the presence of collagen vascular disease, previous cerebrovascular events, diabetes, hyperlipidemia, hypertension, a history of syphilis, or ototoxin exposure, all of which have been reported to cause acute sensory hearing loss.

The physical examination consists of visualization of the EAC and TM. If the canal is impacted with cerumen, the cerumen may be removed by curettage. If TM perforation is unlikely, irrigation with warmed water may be attempted. Cerumenolytics, such as 10% triethanolamine polypeptide oleate, may be used as an adjunct with irrigation to soften earwax prior to removal. A clear canal should prompt the performance of a thorough otologic and neurologic examination.

In acute deafness, hearing loss is categorized to be either conductive or sensorineural by the Rinne and Weber tests, respectively. The Rinne test is performed by placing a tuning fork vibrating at 512 Hz on the mastoid. When the patient can no longer hear vibrations, the fork is moved over the EAC. The normal patient will hear the vibrating fork over the EAC after it becomes inaudible at the mastoid. In conductive hearing loss, vibrations are not heard at the EAC despite still hearing them at the mastoid.

In Weber's test, the vibrating fork is placed on the forehead while the patient reports in which ear sound is loudest. It should be equal in both ears. With sensorineural loss, lateralization occurs to the normal ear. In conductive hearing loss, vibrations are heard in the abnormal ear.

Conductive hearing losses occur on the basis of EAC obstruction (e.g., foreign body, cerumen, or external otitis) or interference with sound conduction via the TM-ossicle complex (e.g., TM perforation, sclerosis of TM or ossicles, or middle ear fluid).

The diagnosis of sensory hearing loss may be suggested based on whether one or both ears are involved. Unilateral sensory loss (normal Rinne test; Weber test lateralizes to normal ear) results most frequently from viral neuronitis. In the pediatric age group this is most commonly the result of mumps. Vesicles of the outer ear or tympanic membrane suggest herpes zoster oticus. An acoustic neuroma may give similar findings and is often associated with cranial nerve deficits. The most common neuropathy with an acoustic neuroma is loss of the corneal reflex via trigeminal nucleus involvement. Ménière's disease is characterized by fluctuating sensorineural hearing loss, vertigo, tinnitus, and a sensation of aural fullness. Autoimmune disorders, blood dyscrasias, and idiopathic causes may also present as sensory hearing loss.

Bilateral sensory hearing loss (normal Weber and Rinne tests, with decreased hearing) suggests noise or ototoxin exposure. Ototoxicity

has been reported after the use of certain antibiotics (aminoglycosides, erythromycin, vancomycin), nonsteroidal anti-inflammatory drugs (NSAIDs), antimalarials, antineoplastics (cisplatin, nitrogen mustards), and loop diuretics (ethacrynic acid, furosemide).

Except for cerumen impaction, specific treatment is based upon the underlying disease. Unfortunately, the long and complicated differential diagnosis of sudden sensory hearing loss is frequently dependent upon results of investigations not available to the emergency physician. It is essential that life-threatening illnesses are excluded, after which outpatient ENT referral should be arranged within 1 to 2 days. Although controversial, steroids may be prescribed for sensorineural hearing loss when there is a completely negative examination. This may be done after discussion with the otolaryngologist who will be following the patient.

## Trauma

Trauma to the ear should be managed only after more critical injuries have been addressed. Blunt auricular trauma results in three categories of injury: ecchymosis, seroma, and hematoma. Ecchymosis requires little therapy other than analgesics and cold compresses. Lacerations of the auricle are reviewed in Chap. 47.

**Seromas and hematomas.** Each of these presents as a firm painful swelling of the auricle. Once organized, this may result in an unacceptable cosmetic outcome. Initial treatment is by large-gauge needle aspiration using aseptic technique, followed by the placement of periauricular packing and a firm fitting mastoid dressing (see Fig. 202-1). Follow-up, to evaluate recurrence of fluid, should occur in 24 h. Reaccumulation of fluid requires repeat drainage and mastoid dressing replacement. In the absence of fluid, the dressing may be discontinued.

**Thermal injuries.** Thermal injuries of the auricle are injuries caused by both extremes of temperature. Superficial injury usually requires minimal therapy. Partial-thickness injury is treated with a topical antimicrobial ointment and gentle cleansing several times per day. Full-thickness injury may require debridement. If outpatient management is selected, there should be close follow-up, and antibiotics to cover *Pseudomonas* and *Staph. aureus* may be given. Auricular full-thickness burns, involving cartilage, should be debrided, with immediate skin closure or grafting of the resected edges. Local anesthesia may be obtained in Chap. 43.

In frostbite, rapid rewarming with saline-soaked gauze at 38° to 42°C (100.4° to 107.6°F) should be performed. Debridement should be deferred, but other measures are the same as described above. See Chap. 159 for further discussion on the care of frostbite.

**Chemical injuries.** Chemical injuries to the auricle may result in damage to the pinna or its canal. It is unusual for inner or middle ear damage to result from such trauma. The primary symptom is pain. Associated injuries, such as airway or ocular exposure, may take precedence.

The most important predictor of injury is the offending agent itself; therefore its identification is critical. Strong acid or alkali produces immediate burning on contact. Either may be removed initially by copious water irrigation, making sure that external particles are not washed into the EAC. The canal should be irrigated by syringe. Further specific therapies are guided by the involved caustic. After decontamination and any toxin-specific therapy, disposition is as for thermal burns of the auricle, described above.

**Perichondritis and chondritis.** These represent true otologic emergencies. Usually following trauma, the patient complains of pain, fever, swelling, and tenderness of the ear. Erythema and warmth are localized to the perichondral region of the auricle. Initially the cartilage maintains its firm consistency; however, as the disease advances it is destroyed. Diagnosis, with treatment initiated early in the course, is necessary to avoid permanent deformity. Parenteral antibiotics active against *Pseudomonas, Proteus,* and *Staphylococcus,* as

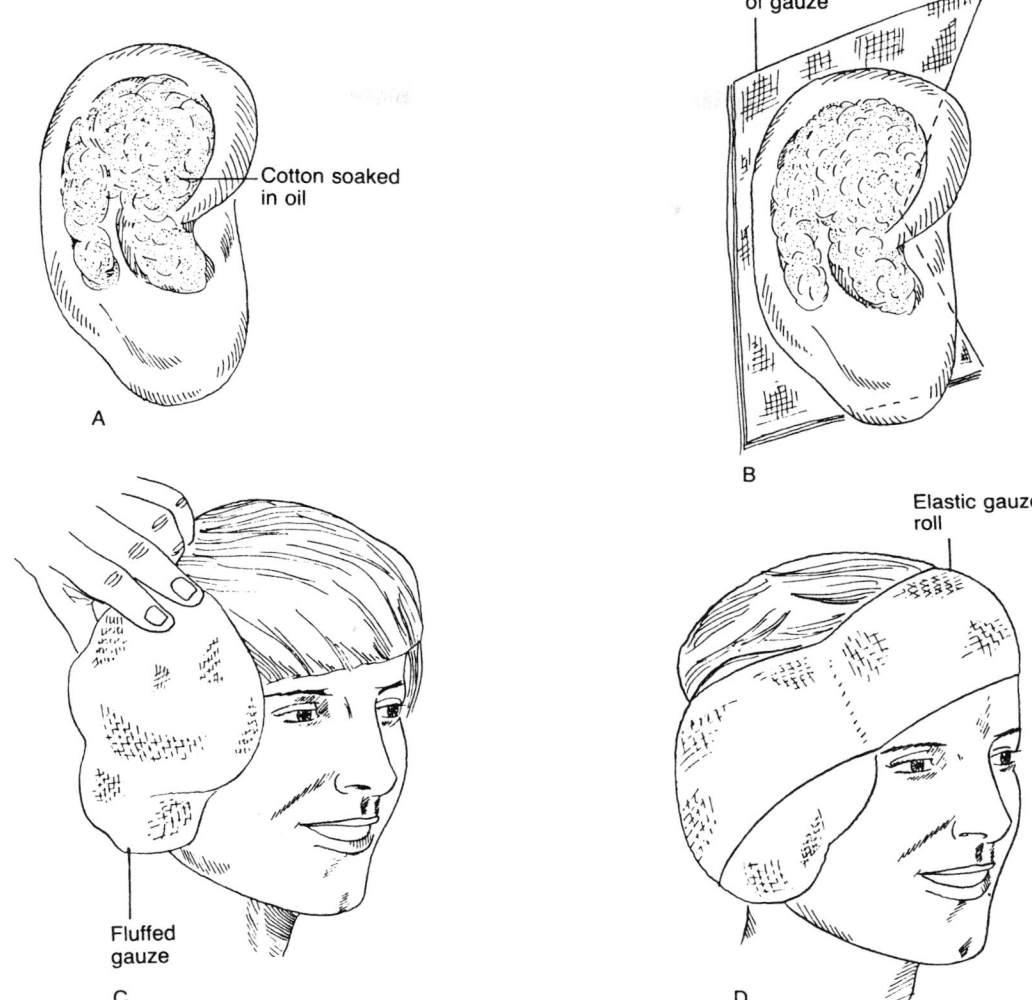

**Fig. 202-1.** Compression dressing of the ear. Following successful aspiration of an auricular hematoma a compression dressing is used to prevent reaccumulation of the hematoma or fluid. *A.* Dry cotton is first placed into the ear canal. A conforming material is then carefully molded into all the convolutions of the auricle. One may use Vaseline gauze or cotton soaked in mineral oil or saline. *B.* When the convolutions are fully packed, a posterior gauze pack is placed behind the ear. A V-shaped section has been cut from the gauze to allow it to easily fit behind the ear. *C.* Multiple layers of fluffed gauze are placed over the packed ear, and the entire dressing is held in place with Kling or an elastic gauze roll (*D*). The ear is thus compressed between two layers of gauze, and the packing assures even distribution of pressure to all parts of the auricle. (From Abelson TI, Witt WJ in Roberts JR, Hedges JR (eds): *Clinical Procedures in Emergency Medicine*, 2d ed. Philadelphia, Saunders 1991, p 1042, with permission).

well as consultation with an ENT specialist for surgical drainage, are recommended.

## Foreign Body of the Ear

Foreign bodies (FB) of the ear occur most often in children and may present in a delayed fashion. Insects and other animate objects are seen in all ages, usually promptly after the occurrence. Adults will present when there is accidental loss of materials used in self-instrumentation of the EAC, such as Q-tips or earplugs. Always attempt to identify the FB.

Inanimate objects in the EAC of children rarely cause extreme discomfort unless there is associated infection or injury. If the object has been in the canal chronically, there may be malodorous discharge with signs of infection. In the cooperative adult patient, inaminate FBs may present with pain, fullness, and hearing loss.

On examination, the FB should be visualized. Ensure that there is no TM perforation or evidence of infection. A conductive hearing loss may be present.

A live object trapped in the EAC will cause acute distress to the patient. Movement of a trapped insect against the TM will result in impressive agitation of the patient. There may be ipsilateral tearing and nausea. The initial therapy is to immobilize the offending creature. This should be done with an agent that will not complicate later attempts at carcass removal. Two percent lidocaine, placed in the EAC, will result in prompt termination of all movement. Foreign body removal may then proceed as for inanimate material.

There are many descriptions on how to remove EAC foreign bodies, but most important is patient cooperation. In difficult cases, this may require conscious sedation or restraints. To attempt removal in an agitated patient risks pushing the object further into the canal or damaging the TM and ossicles. ENT consultation and general anesthesia may be required.

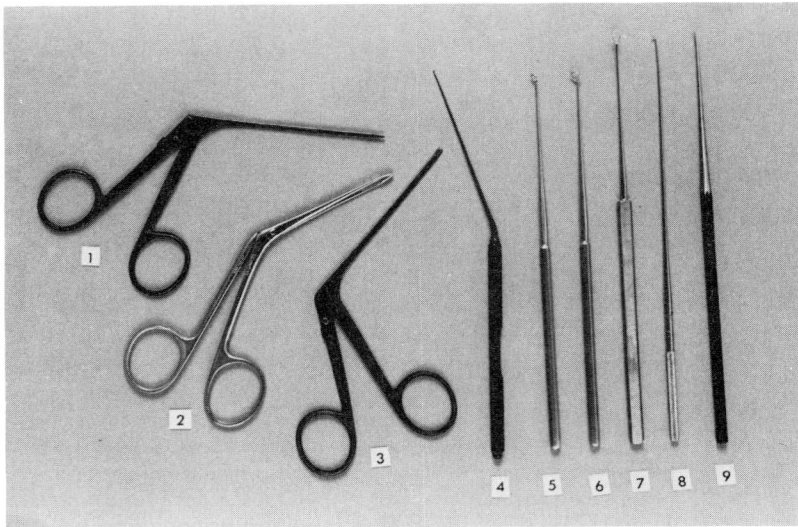

**Fig. 202-2.** Useful ear foreign body tools. *1.* Alligator forceps; *2.* Hartman ear forceps; *3.* cupped forceps; *4.* Schuknecht pick; *5.* small Buck curette; *6.* large Buck curette; *7.* Sharpleigh curette; *8.* Day hook; *9.* Turner needle. (From Peterson LJ in Cummings CW (ed): *Otolaryngology—Head and Neck Surgery*, 2d ed. Vol. 2. St. Louis, Mosby Year Book, 1993, p.1207, with permission.)

Options for removal include the use of microforceps for small-diameter objects. Larger objects may be removed with forceps or by placing a hook behind the foreign body and applying gentle traction. See Fig. 202-2 for tools useful in EAC foreign body management. These techniques should be performed only under direct visualization. Suctioning of the foreign body may assist in its removal. More exotic is the reported use of cyanoacrylate glue to attach a probe to the foreign body.

Irrigation, possibly the safest method of foreign body extraction, may be attempted unless there is a known TM perforation. Butterfly syringe tubing or an intravenous catheter can be used to direct a stream of warm saline around the periphery of the object so that back pressure pushes the material out of the canal. Caution should be exercised if the foreign object is plant material, as it may swell with the introduction of water.

If removal is successful and there is no infection or TM perforation, the patient may be discharged. Antibiotics are needed only if there is associated infection. EAC lacerations usually require only observation. In TM perforation, ENT follow-up is needed. Ossicular damage requires emergent ENT consultation.

If an impacted EAC foreign body cannot be removed, ENT follow-up can be provided the next day as long as the object is not alive. Emergent ENT consultation is needed if there is severe pain or the foreign body is a caustic substance.

## Tympanic Membrane Perforations

Perforations of the TM result from acute changes in air or water pressure (blast injury), direct trauma (foreign body, Q-tips), molten metal, caustics, lightening strike, otitis media, or associated temporal bone fractures. Associated injuries should be excluded.

The patient may complain of slight hearing loss or pain. Physical examination usually identifies the violation of the TM. Bulb insufflation will demonstrate absent movement of the TM.

The presence of concurrent vertigo or acute deafness suggests associated injuries to the ossicles, labyrinth, or temporal bone. Immediate ENT consultation is indicated. In the absence of these findings, nonemergent ENT follow-up is recommended for all perforations, regardless of size.

The majority of TM perforations heal without specific therapy. The patient should be counseled to put nothing in the ear. Water should be kept out of the ear by a cotton ball, with petroleum jelly on the exterior surface, placed in the EAC prior to bathing.

Antibiotics have no demonstrated value in uncomplicated TM perforations unless there is a coexistent otitis media. In the presence of otitis media, standard antibiotics are appropriate. In external otitis

with concomitant TM perforation, antibiotic otic suspension should be utilized. Some authors suggest prophylactic antibiotics for TM perforations when there has been contamination with potentially polluted water.

## Otic Barotrauma

*Squeeze* is the scuba diver's term for the various syndromes resulting from changes in ambient pressure. Boyle's law states that the volume of gas at constant temperature varies indirectly with pressure. Descent, either underwater or in a plane, results in increasing ambient pressure and a decreasing volume of gas in a closed space. The converse occurs with ascent. Because of the greater density of water, there is larger clinical impact during diving than during flying. Pressure differentials between various closed spaces result in the syndromes, which occur independently, discussed below.

**Ear canal barotrauma (canal squeeze).** This occurs when pressures in the EAC cannot equalize externally because of cerumen or ear plugs. With descent, increasing ambient pressure causes decreasing EAC volume. This creates suction forces that result in outward bulging of the TM and the surrounding soft tissue. The diver may experience otalgia and bloody discharge from the affected ear. Petechiae, hemorrhagic blebs, and TM rupture may be seen. Therapy is as for routine TM ruptures.

**Barotitis media (middle ear squeeze).** This is the most common form of barotrauma in recreational scuba divers. On descent, middle ear gas volume decreases. With normal eustachian tube function, pressure is equalized with the nasopharynx. Eustachian dysfunction, due to anatomic abnormality or respiratory infection, may impair equalization with the rigid cavity of the middle ear. Continued decrease in middle ear volume results in retraction of the TM and engorgement of the mucosa. Further descent results in mucosal hemorrhage and possible TM rupture.

The patient may complain of acute pain with diminished hearing. Vertigo, nausea, and vomiting may result from cold water vestibular stimulation following TM rupture. Physical examination may demonstrate a conductive hearing loss, hemotympanum, or TM rupture.

Less commonly, TM perforation is reported to result during underwater ascent, or in airplane travel, when gas expands in the middle ear concurrently with an obstructed eustachian tube.

Treatment is abstention from diving or flying until the patient is asymptomatic. Antihistamine and/or decongestants have been recommended and may be used prophylactically. Therapy is as for routine TM rupture.

**Inner ear barotrauma.** This may be seen when there is a large pressure differential between the middle and inner ear. With rapid descent, the TM and stapes may move inward enough to implode the oval window. Alternatively, an explosive injury can occur during a forceful Valsalva maneuver, as when attempting to equalize the middle ear and nasopharyngeal pressures. When there is a sufficient increase in CSF pressure from the Valsalva maneuver, oval or round window protrusion and rupture may result.

Clinically, the presentations of implosive or explosive injury are similar. The patient complains of severe vertigo unrelieved by ascent, with usually unilateral loud tinnitus and a fullness in the ear. Nystagmus and ipsilateral sensorineural hearing loss are found on physical examination. Emergent ENT consultation is needed.

## SALIVARY GLAND PROBLEMS

The diagnosis of salivary gland dysfunction is based on clinical features. Important aspects include which glands are involved; whether single or multiple glands are affected; the presence of pain, tenderness, or mass; acuity and precipitants of symptoms; whether the symptoms are persistent rather than recurrent; and whether associated systemic symptoms are present (e.g., dry mouth or eyes, joint symptoms, diabetes).

## Sialoadenitis

Sialoadenitis may occur secondary to viral or bacterial etiology. While many viruses may involve the salivary glands, the paramyxovirus, causing mumps, is most common.

**Mumps.** Mumps is the most common cause of painful parotid swelling in the pediatric age group. It is spread by fomites, with an incubation period of 12 to 21 days. The greatest incidence occurs in the 5- to 15-year-old age group. Patients are infective from 3 days before until 7 days after salivary gland swelling. Repeat episodes of mumps occur but are rare.

Symptoms progress from initial fever and malaise to increasing pain and stiffness with chewing. Parotid swelling, bilateral in 70 percent, follows. There may be edema of the surrounding area, but there is no discharge from Stensen's duct. In 10 percent, the submandibular glands are involved. The diagnosis of mumps is made on clinical grounds. Laboratory evaluation is nonspecific, and treatment is symptomatic.

Usually benign in children, mumps can be severe in adults. Although 25 percent of men suffer orchitis, only 5 percent of women manifest oophoritis. Complications consist of mastitis, pancreatitis, myocarditis, meningoencephalitis, encephalomyelitis, and sensorineural deafness.

**Bacterial parotitis.** This can occur in any debilitated or dehydrated patient, with 30 percent of cases occurring postoperatively. Drugs or therapies decreasing the flow of saliva predispose to infection; examples include irradiation, phenothiazines, antihistamines, and parasympathetic inhibitors.

Bilateral in 20 percent of cases, suppurative parotitis clinically presents as a red, tender, and swollen parotid. With progression, swelling extends over the face and neck, fever and trismus are present, and pus (which should be cultured) may be expressed from Stensen's duct.

Treatment consists of hydration, massage, local heat, and sialogogues. The patient should receive antibiotics selected for penicillinase-resistant *Staph. aureus,* until culture results are known. If there is an abscess or failure to improve, ENT consultation and surgical drainage may be necessary.

**Miscellaneous causes of sialoadenitis.** Severe uremia, irradiation, or the result of certain medications can cause sialoadenitis. Other than drug withdrawal and symptomatic therapy, no specific treatment is indicated.

**Chronic relapsing sialoadenitis.** This occurs in patients with ductal abnormalities or obstructions or can occur idiopathically. Emergency department treatment centers on therapy for acute exacerbations and ENT referral.

**Systemic diseases.** Sarcoidosis, cat-scratch disease, tuberculosis, atypical mycobacterial infections, and actinomycoses may present as a chronic form of sialoadenitis. When primary, tuberculosis occurs most frequently in the parotid. Such patients present with slow painless enlargement of the major salivary glands. Additionally, lymphoma and squamous carcinomas may arise within the salivary glands. Treatment is specific for the underlying disorder.

## Salivary Calculi

Salivary calculi are seen at any age but peak in the third to sixth decades, with a male predilection. More than 80 percent of stones occur in the submandibular gland, with 5 to 20 percent occurring in the parotid. The sublingual glands are rarely involved.

Symptoms are exacerbated by meals, when salivary secretion is stimulated. Sialolithiasis usually presents with unilateral swelling and pain in the affected gland. The stone may be palpated along the course of the salivary duct. If there is superimposed infection, the diagnosis may be difficult.

Stones are composed mainly of calcium phosphate and organic matrix, and more than 90 percent of calculi can be visualized by intraoral radiographs. Extraoral radiographs demonstrate only approximately 50 percent of calculi. Sialography, diagnostically limited in the detection of small stones and extrinsic masses, is being replaced by ultrasound, CT, or MRI. However, these diagnostic procedures are rarely emergently indicated. Diagnosis and therapy may be initiated based upon clinical findings.

Initial treatment consists of analgesics, antibiotics (if there is concurrent infection), and sialogogues (e.g., lemon drops). Easily located distal calculi may be digitally "milked" from the duct. Alternatively, they may be removed by either dilation or incision of the ductal orifice. Patients with proximal or intraglandular sialoliths should be referred to ENT on an outpatient basis.

Complications of salivary duct obstruction are recurrent or persistent obstruction, sialectasia (irregular dilations of the ductal system resulting in stasis and further stone formation), and superimposed infection.

**Salivary gland enlargement.** This may result from a large number of conditions. Metabolic causes include malnutrition, alcoholism, celiac disease, and heavy metal poisoning. It may be seen in the pathologic conditions of uremia, cirrhosis, diabetes, cystic fibrosis, hypothyroidism, and hyperlipidemia. Hormonal causes, such as testicular atrophy, pregnancy, lactation, and menopause, have been reported. Finally, drugs such as thiourea, methimazole, isoproterenol, phenothiazines, and thiocyanate may result in salivary gland enlargement. No acute intervention is required, and these patients should be referred to an internist for evaluation.

## POSTADENOTONSILLECTOMY BLEEDING

Bleeding is a rare, but potentially fatal, complication of tonsillectomy. With treatment, fewer than 1 percent of patients will require transfusion or reoperation. Presentation usually results from secondary bleeding, defined as greater than 8 h postsurgery. Management consists of ensuring an adequate airway and suctioning for clot removal. If active bleeding from the tonsillar fossa is identified, direct pressure should be applied. This is performed by using ring forceps and oxidized cellulose, thrombin packs, or gauze moistened with an equivolume solution of 1:1000 epinephrine and 4% lidocaine. Active bleeding requires emergent ENT consultation.

In massive bleeding, standard therapy for hemorrhagic shock should be instituted. Airway control is paramount, as well as volume resuscitation and preparation for emergent reoperation. Significant adenoidal bleeding is treated by the placement of a posterior nasal pack (see Chap. 203, "Nasal Emergencies and Sinusitis.")

Direct pressure or silver nitrate cautery sticks may be helpful in controlling less significant oozing of blood. If direct pressure fails, local infiltration of 1 to 3 mL lidocaine with 1:1000 epinephrine may be attempted. If bleeding is controlled, and after a period of observation, the patient may be discharged home with close follow-up. The patient should avoid salicylate use during the postoperative period.

## FACIAL CELLULITIS

Facial cellulitis represents a group of diseases requiring individualized diagnosis and treatment. Specific diagnoses, such as orbital cellulitis, are covered in other chapters of this text. Cellulitis is classically defined by pain, erythema, edema, increased tactile temperature, and dysfunction of the involved structure. The diagnosis is usually based on clinical findings.

The history should examine recent prodromal events, such as insect bites, trauma, allergen exposure, chronic dental caries, or painful mastication. The presence of dental appliances, nasal discharge, or vision changes should be ascertained. Systemic signs of infection, e.g., fever and vomiting, should be excluded.

A thorough head and neck examination, specifically addressing periorbital and intraoral regions, is required. Occult infection, with extension to facial structures, should be excluded.

Laboratory evaluation may demonstrate a leukocytosis. Cultures are rarely useful in the outpatient population but should be obtained if hospital admission is anticipated. There are no reliable methods for obtaining cultures of the offending organism in routine cellulitis. When there is a focus with purulent drainage, such as an abscess, cultures may yield the organism.

Antibiotics are the mainstay of therapy. They should be directed at the most likely underlying etiology if the cause is identified. When the source of the cellulitis is unknown, broad-spectrum antibiotic therapy, ensuring coverage of staphylococcal and streptococcal species, is indicated. In adults, a penicillinase-resistant synthetic penicillin, first-generation cephalosporin, or vancomycin is appropriate. However, in children, *H. influenzae* should be covered with cefuroxime, amoxicillin/clavulanate, or trimethoprim/sulfamethoxazole.

The differential diagnosis includes insect envenomation or other traumatic event, dental caries with abscess formation, occult head and neck infection, orbital or periorbital cellulitis, sinusitis with erosion of the bony cortex, otitis externa, erysipelas, viral exanthems (e.g., erythema infectiosum), parotitis, impetigo, systemic lupus erythematosus, herpes zoster, dermatitides, angioneurotic edema, and allergy.

Hospitalization, with antibiotic therapy initiated in the emergency department, is required in patients with facial cellulitis and the following associated conditions:

1. Systemic signs of sepsis
2. Antibiotic intolerance for any reason (e.g., emesis)
3. Immunosuppressive therapies or illness
4. Extensive areas of erythema or induration
5. Unremovable head/neck appliances or foreign bodies
6. Inability to comply with outpatient therapy

Patients at the extremes of age should have a lower admission threshold.

Outpatient therapy is appropriate in selected cases. Patients should be instructed to return to the emergency department for fever, difficulty swallowing or breathing, inability to take their antibiotics for any reason, or if there is worsening of their condition. Patients should be seen the following day for evaluation. If there is continued progression, admission for inpatient antibiotics is warranted.

## ACUTE UPPER AIRWAY OBSTRUCTION

### History

Management of airway obstruction always takes precedence over any other event. History and physical examination are of secondary importance in patients who are apneic or in severe respiratory distress. If the patient is able to communicate, the history will frequently provide the etiology of upper airway obstruction. Establish acuity of symptoms; prodromal complaints of fever, pain, or cough; and review the events surrounding the onset, such as trauma, eating, choking, holding something in the mouth, etc. The past medical history may suggest a progression of chronic disease. Specifically discern if the patient has dental or oropharyngeal appliances.

### Physical Examination

A complete, but necessarily brief, examination focusing on the head, neck, and chest should be performed. The pharynx should be examined for evidence of infection, swelling, tenderness, or lymphadenopathy. Dentition should be inspected. The neck should be examined for mobility, meningismus, laryngeal tenderness, and crepitance. The chest examination should ensure equal and clear breath sounds and that the trachea is midline at the sternal notch.

Upper airway obstruction is usually manifest by stridor. Stridor is difficulty during the inspiratory phase of respiration. If there is accompanying wheezing, it should be differentiated from that of asthma or chronic obstructive pulmonary disease. Wheezing from bronchospasm is usually worse during the expiratory phase of respiration. Stridor is a critical point in the diagnostic algorithm. With worsening airway obstruction, stridor may become biphasic, occurring in both inspiration and expiration.

### Differential Diagnosis

#### Foreign Bodies

The majority of aspirated foreign bodies occur in young children and represent a significant mortality risk. These aspirations are frequently food products; however, toy parts, coins, and any small object may be found in the upper airway of children. Older patients with a history of stroke, altered mental status, or neuromuscular disease and those with intraoral or nasopharyngeal appliances are also at risk for aspiration.

The patient may report a precise description of foreign body aspiration with an antecedent history of fish or fowl consumption. Conversely, symptoms may be subtle, with insidious onset of progressive stridor or recurrent pneumonia secondary to a retained bronchial foreign body.

Symptoms of aspiration are predicted by the location of the foreign body. When it is in the upper airway, there may be marked acute stridor, odynophagia, or respiratory distress. With total obstruction, there is profound asphyxia, apnea, and cyanosis.

Bronchial obstruction, most frequently the right mainstem, may present with a range of symptoms from cough, dyspnea, and wheezing to respiratory distress and hypoxia. Wheezing may be unilateral but is often referred to the entire chest. New-onset wheezing should prompt investigation for a foreign body.

In the stable patient, simple inspection of the pharynx may demonstrate the foreign body. With mild symptoms, care should be taken to prevent converting a partial blockage to a complete obstruction. Attempts at removal should be accompanied by the necessary materials for definitive airway control and for prevention of aspiration in the case of emesis. Soft tissue radiographs are useful if the foreign body is radiopaque. Indirect and flexible fiberoptic laryngoscopy can be helpful for visualization of laryngeal structures and foreign bodies but is of limited use for removal of impacted material. Direct laryngoscopy, with topical anesthesia, can be used in the cooperative patient for both visualization and removal of foreign objects. Failing these techniques, patients with persistently impacted foreign bodies should receive emergent ENT consultation.

In the prehospital environment, an unstable patient suffering asphyxia should have a Heimlich maneuver performed. In the emergency department, a quick attempt at removal by direct laryngoscopy is indicated. If this fails, a surgical airway is the only option. For very distal foreign bodies in unstable patients, a deeply placed double-lumen endotracheal tube may allow ventilation of one lung while preparations are made for rigid bronchoscopic removal of the foreign body.

## Epiglottitis

Epiglottitis is an acute life-threatening upper respiratory infection, primarily in children 2 to 7 years old but occurring in all ages. Anatomically, it is an infection of the supraglottic structures (also called supraglottitis) and involves the lingual tonsillar area, epiglottic folds, false vocal cords, and the epiglottis. Children deteriorate more rapidly and suffer airway obstruction more frequently than adults. This is felt to be due to a more flaccid mucosa and smaller airway. Epiglottitis may be rapidly fatal in all ages. The fatal event is thought to result from an edematous epiglottis obstructing the airway.

In adults and children, epiglottitis is most commonly due to *H. influenzae* type B. Other pathogens occur, more often in adults, and are usually *Streptococcus* or *Staphylococcus* species. It is expected that with wide use of the *H. influenzae* vaccine will result in a decline in epiglottitis in children. Epiglottitis is principally a primary infection but may arise secondarily. Concurrent bacteremia is seen in approximately 75 percent of pediatric cases but in only about 30 percent of adults.

Pediatric epiglottitis is an acute febrile illness associated with respiratory distress. Symptoms generally present over 12 to 24 h. Other findings include stridor, toxic appearance, anxiety, dysphagia, drooling, sore throat, level of consciousness changes, and cyanosis. The child may assume a characteristic tripod position, sitting upright and leaning forward, and refuse to lie down. Although rare, a crouplike cough and wheezing have been reported in pediatric epiglottitis. Many of the "classic" symptoms may be absent in the very young patient.

Details of diagnosis and management of pediatric epiglottitis are discussed in Chapter 37, "Upper Respiratory Emergencies."

In adults, the most common initial symptoms are sore throat and dysphagia, which may have been present for hours to days. The sore throat is out of proportion to physical findings. Less consistently the voice is muffled, and there may be tenderness to palpation of the larynx. With progression, drooling and stridor appear. Respiratory difficulty is not a prominent symptom in the early stages of adult epiglottitis.

Emergent laboratory evaluation is minimally helpful. Blood cultures should be obtained, although they are often negative. Laryngeal swabs are more frequently helpful but should be performed only if the airway has been controlled. Leukocytosis is a usual finding.

Soft tissue x-rays of the neck (see Fig. 202-3) may show edema of the epiglottis, aryepiglottic folds, arytenoids, uvula, and retropharyngeal soft tissues. There may be ballooning of the hypopharynx and obliteration of the vallecula. The enlarged epiglottis may appear as a thumbprint on the lateral soft tissue neck x-ray. Radiographs should not delay appropriate airway management or prevent adequate observation of the patient.

With stridor or respiratory distress present, the value of any diagnostic procedure must be carefully weighed against the need for immediate airway control. In the obvious or unstable case, it is appropriate to diagnose epiglottitis at the time of direct laryngoscopy. This should be done in the operating room, with an ENT specialist in attendance to perform an emergency tracheostomy, if needed.

The role of intubation in the management of the stable adult is unclear. There are many reports of successful management with only observation, antibiotics, and supportive care. The decision to place an airway depends on the acuity of the patient's presentation and the immediate availability of personnel skilled in difficult airway management. Early controlled intubation, performed in the operating room

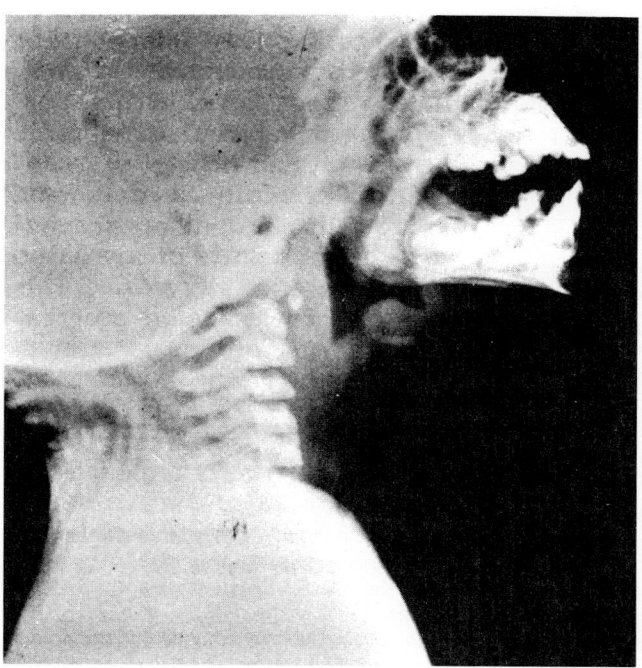

**Fig. 202-3.** The diagnosis of epiglottitis is confirmed by lateral neck film that shows an enlarged epiglottis obstructing the airway. (Courtesy of the Children's Hospital Center of Akron, Ohio.)

by an otolaryngologist, is the safest route. All patients with epiglottitis should be admitted to an intensive care unit, with ENT consultation.

Parenteral antibiotics, directed at the suspected pathogens, should be administered. Cefuroxime, cefotaxime, ceftriaxone, ampicillin/sulbactam, or trimethoprim/sulfamethoxazole are generally accepted choices. Aztreonam or chloramphenicol can be used in patients allergic to first-line agents. Steroids, still controversial, may be of benefit in treating airway edema.

Complications include airway obstruction, respiratory arrest, asphyxia, hypoxic brain damage, and death.

In instances of invasive *H. influenzae* infection, chemoprophylaxis is recommended in certain situations. If there is a contact in the household under 4 years of age, rifampin, at a daily dose of 20 mg/kg (maximum 600 mg), is given for 4 days to all nonpregnant household members. Prophylaxis is unnecessary if there are no contacts under the age of 4. The index case should also receive rifampin after primary infection treatment.

## Laryngeal Trauma

Blunt trauma secondary to motor vehicle accidents is the most common etiology of laryngeal damage, although penetrating trauma is increasing in frequency. Laryngeal damage ranges from hematomas and mucosal lacerations to thyroid cartilage fractures and complete avulsion of the laryngotracheal junction. Recurrent laryngeal nerve injury may present as airway obstruction with what appears to be minimal laryngeal symptoms. Associated trauma, including occult cervical fracture, must always be considered.

Symptoms vary with severity of injury. There may be hoarseness, hemoptysis, dyspnea, dysphagia, aphonia, stridor, or severe respiratory distress. Physical examination may demonstrate any of the following: laryngeal swelling, tenderness, anterior neck contusion, abnormality of the laryngeal contour, tracheal deviation, or subcutaneous emphysema.

It is important to identify and repair laryngeal injuries early, thereby preventing the long-term sequelae of voice and airway compromise. These injuries are rare, with significant morbidity and possible mortality. Indirect and flexible laryngoscopy are excellent investigative modalities. CT is a useful diagnostic adjunct.

Stable patients with limited manifestations may be placed on humidified oxygen while awaiting ENT consultation for laryngoscopy. Initially minor laryngeal injuries may rapidly progress due to expanding hematoma or edema, and close observation is essential.

Unstable patients with laryngeal trauma requiring airway control represent the most difficult of emergency airway problems. Because of blood, distorted anatomy, and cervical spine precautions, endotracheal, retrograde, or fiberoptic intubation techniques may be unsuccessful. Furthermore, exacerbation of laryngeal injuries may occur with endotracheal manipulation. A tracheotomy, performed under local anesthesia, is the preferred method of airway management. However, this may be precluded by airway instability or lack of readily available personnel with expertise in the performance of this procedure. Gentle endotracheal intubation, emergency cricothyrotomy, or needle cricothyrotomy may be required.

The management of complete laryngotracheal transection is different than for other laryngeal injuries. There is usually a significant space, 6 to 8 cm, between the parts of the divided trachea and larynx. The soft tissue and prevertebral fascia may retain their shape around the area the trachea occupied before its separation. If a cricothyrotomy is performed, it will be above the level of the division and may fail in controlling the airway. Obviously, immediate emergent operative intervention is desirable. However, if the patient is too unstable or operative support is not available, endotracheal intubation and ventilation may be possible, depending on the ability of the soft tissues to retain their shape. This may temporize long enough to arrange definitive operative repair.

Patients should receive antibiotics active against oral and respiratory flora when there is suspicion of mucosal violation, or if there is subcutaneous emphysema. Ampicillin/sulbactam or amoxicillin/clavulanate are good choices. Emergent ENT consultation is warranted for all patients with signs or findings suggestive of laryngeal injury.

## Irritants and Corrosives

Damage to the airway may occur as the result of inhalation injury from toxic and irritant gases, steam, heat, or from the ingestion of materials such as caustics and corrosives.

Irritant gases (e.g., chlorine) exert their effects from direct mucosal damage, while toxic gases (e.g., cyanide, carbon monoxide) manifest systemic symptoms specific to the toxin. Both mechanisms may occur simultaneously, as in a closed-space fire, where there may be inhaled irritant particulate matter, direct airway burns, and systemic effects from toxic gases.

Heat injury is primarily restricted to the upper airway, although steam, with a much higher specific heat, may impart lower airway damage.

Ingested corrosives predominantly result in oropharyngeal and esophageal injury; however, laryngeal involvement can occur with devastating consequences. These injuries are usually accidental in children or the result of a suicide attempt in the adult. Nonairway management of corrosive and/or caustic ingestions is reviewed in Chap. 154.

Patients may present demonstrating a spectrum of symptoms, from asymptomatic to acute severe respiratory distress. Oropharyngeal pain, drooling, dysphagia, coughing, vomiting, stridor, or dyspnea suggests airway involvement. Nasal and oropharyngeal injury should be viewed as a high-risk marker for airway damage.

In the asymptomatic patient with a history suggesting risk for airway injury, humidified oxygen, supportive care, and observation may suffice. The absence of respiratory distress does not exclude airway damage. Indirect laryngoscopy is useful in the evaluation of potential upper airway burns in stable victims.

In the mildly symptomatic patient, rapid progression to complete airway obstruction should be anticipated. Close observation, with treatment as in the asymptomatic patient, should occur. If there is progression of symptoms, emergent consultation for fiberoptic bronchoscopy should take place. If airway edema is suspected, aerosolized racemic epinephrine may be given. Lower airway symptoms of wheezing, chest tightness, and dyspnea may be treated with the addition of aerosolized bronchodilators.

In symptomatic patients demonstrating stridor, croupy cough, or hoarseness, upper airway injury has occurred and preparations for early endotracheal intubation are needed. Emergent consultation for fiberoptic bronchoscopy should be arranged. Progressive airway edema may make delayed airway management extremely difficult. In the awake patient who has suffered inhalation injury, routine endotracheal, blind nasotracheal, or fiberoptic intubation may be attempted. Failing this, lighted stylet, retrograde intubation, or a surgial airway is required. Airway placement by blind technique is not recommended following a caustic ingestion. Blind techniques may result in iatrogenic injury from the endotracheal tube perforating injured oropharyngeal or tracheoesophageal tissue.

Steroid therapy is controversial. The role of broad-spectrum systemic antibiotics is unclear. Tetanus status should be addressed.

Disposition of patients with these injuries is frequently predicated on associated symptoms. Those demonstrating any symptoms or potential for airway involvement should be admitted for observation.

## Angioneurotic Edema

Angioneurotic edema is a well-demarcated, nonpitting edema occurring in large areas of the face, lips, tongue, and mucous membranes. It may be accompanied by erythema. Progression leads to laryngeal edema, airway compromise, asphyxia, and possibly death.

In the majority of patients, no certain antigenic exposure can be identified. Immediate hypersensitivity allergic reactions to a large number of drugs, food products, or insect venoms are frequently implicated. Angiotensin-converting enzyme inhibitors can cause angioedema that may present at any time, but usually within a month of starting the drug. Other etiologies include medications resulting in histamine release (morphine, radiocontrast dye), circulating immune complexes (lupus), and physical stimuli.

Symptoms are throat tightness, hoarseness, drooling, lip or face swelling, dyspnea, and stridor. If untreated, it may lead to respiratory arrest. The onset can be rapid, on the scale of minutes, following antigen exposure. All cases must be urgently evaluated for impending airway compromise.

Physical findings reveal edema of the tongue, lips, or palate, and there may be massive uvular swelling. Wheezing, vital sign abnormalities, and associated urticaria may be noted.

Treatment is based on airway manifestations. If only subjective or mild symptoms are present, antihistamines, oxygen, and observation may be sufficient.

With respiratory distress or wheezing, inhalational β agonists and parenteral steroids are indicated. Epinephrine should be considered if there is hypotension or respiratory manifestations. The benefit of epinephrine should be weighed carefully in the elderly and those with known coronary disease. Although controversial, $H_2$ antagonists, such as cimetidine, may be used in those failing standard therapy. In the patient with significant airway compromise or in those who worsen despite appropriate therapy, early airway control should be considered before laryngeal edema makes endotracheal intubation technically difficult. Flexible bronchoscopy, cricothyrotomy, or tracheostomy may be required in the unstable patient if an airway cannot be obtained endotracheally.

Patients with any significant airway symptoms should be admitted, for observation and continued therapy, to an area with personnel capable of managing the unstable airway. Discharge on antihistamines and steroids is appropriate in the asymptomatic patient. Patients should be observed for a significant period in the emergency department to ensure that there is no further deterioration. Follow-up with an allergist, or private physician, is recommended. Patients may be prescribed anaphylaxis kits containing epinephrine autoinjectors and antihistamines.

**Hereditary angioneurotic edema (HAE).** HAE is a rare congenital cause of this disorder. It results from insufficient synthesis of C1 esterase inhibitor, with inappropriate activation of the complement cascade.

In patients with HAE and severe symptoms, danazol should be considered in addition to standard therapy. Danazol increases the hepatic synthesis of C1 esterase inhibitor. It is administered orally at an initial daily dose of 400 to 600 mg, in two to three divided doses. If an attack occurs while the patient is on danazol, the dosage may be increased by up to 200 mg daily. Since the androgenic effects of danazol may be harmful to children and pregnant women, ε-aminocaproic acid (E-ACA) may be substituted. E-ACA reduces plasmin-induced complement activation and is administered either orally or intravenously. Dose requirements are variable; however, most patients will require at least 8 to 10 g/day. Doses as high as 30 g/day have been reported. In intravenous use, 4 to 5 g are administered over 1 h, followed by a 1-g/h infusion. Treatment is continued for approximately 8 h or until improvement is noted.

## Peritonsillar Abscess

Peritonsillar abscess is the most frequent abscess of the head and neck in adults and occurs predominantly in teenagers and young adults. It may be prefaced by throat infection in the weeks before presentation.

The classic symptoms are fever, sore throat, drooling, muffled voice, and trismus. There may be accompanying dysphagia, odynophagia, otalgia, pain with lateral movement of the head, and foul-smelling breath. Later presentations may be complicated by respiratory compromise. Physical findings are a unilaterally enlarged and edematous tonsil, deviation and edema of the uvula, coexistent swelling of the anterior tonsillar pillar, and soft palate edema (see Fig. 202-4). Cervical adenopathy is frequently present. Complications from a peritonsillar abscess include airway obstruction, aspiration, and mediastinal extension.

Laboratory evaluation may demonstrate leukocytosis. There are no reliable criteria differentiating peritonsillar abscess from adenitis.

Therapy and diagnosis in the cooperative nontoxic patient without airway compromise may be performed by needle aspiration. Abscess aspiration should result in prompt resolution of trismus and odynophagia, allowing discharge on oral antibiotics with close ENT follow-up. Commonly used oral antibiotics are broad-spectrum antistaphylococcals, such as the newer cephalosporins, clindamycin, or amoxicillin/clavulanate.

Patients with nondiagnostic aspirations, inadequate symptom relief, intolerance of oral fluids, toxic appearance, or airway concerns require inpatient treatment with IV fluids, parenteral antibiotics, and ENT consultation. Unreliable patients and those in whom close follow-up will be difficult should have a lower threshold for admission.

In patients unable to undergo aspiration because they are too young, uncooperative, or have excessive trismus, admission for general anesthesia incision and drainage, parenteral antibiotics, and IV fluids is indicated.

**Peritonsillar abscess aspiration.** This should be performed only by individuals trained in the technique and by those with the ability to manage the complications of the procedure. Aspiration is performed with the patient seated, as for a routine head and neck examination. The examiner requires adequate lighting, and oral suction must be immediately available. Topical anesthesia is obtained with Xylocaine or Cetacaine. A 10-mL syringe, with an 18- to 20-gauge needle, is introduced into the most fluctuant portion of the tonsil at the soft palate, while withdrawing the plunger. The needle should penetrate no deeper than 1 cm. A needle guard, to prevent deep penetration, may be used. The guard is made by amputating the distal tip of a plastic needle cover and replacing it over the needle so that only 0.5 cm of needle protrudes. The operator should keep the needle medially oriented to avoid the carotid artery lying lateral to the tonsil. A positive aspiration should obtain at least 1 mL of pus. Complications of this procedure include aspiration of pus, uncontrolled bleeding, and carotid artery laceration.

Antibiotics are selected to cover suspected bacteria. A wide range of pathogens have been reported including group A *Streptococcus,* other streptococci, oral flora, *H. influenzae* type B, *Bacteroides* species, staphylococci, and mixed flora. Penicillin, amoxicillin, ampicillin/sulbactam, clindamycin, and erythromycin are all appropriate outpatient antibiotic selections. Inpatient antibiotics should address β lactamase–producing species.

## Retropharyngeal Abscess

Retropharyngeal abscess is predominantly a disease of young children. Prior to age 5, when retropharyngeal lymph nodes atrophy,

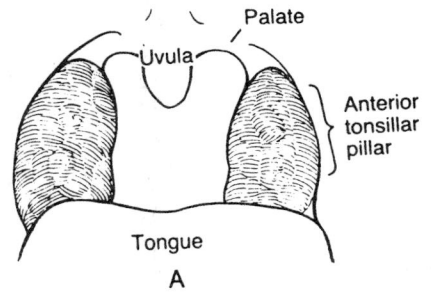
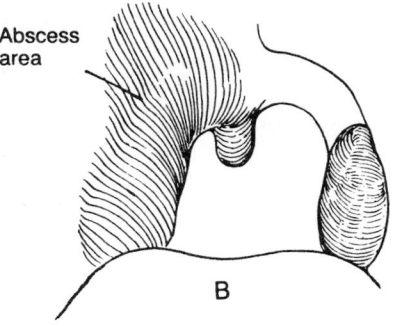

**Fig. 202-4.** *A.* In tonsillitis, the tonsils are enlarged. They may be covered by white exudate. The margin between the tonsil and the anterior tonsillar pillar and palate is well defined. *B.* In peritonsillar abscess, the tonsil, palate, and anterior tonsillar pillar may be bulging medially in one unit. The margin between the tonsil, palate, and anterior tonsillar pillar is somewhat effaced. The uvula is usually edematous and may be pointing toward the opposite tonsil. The safest area to aspirate a peritonsillar abscess is usually just above the tonsil in the soft palate. This location will serve to guard the deep vessels of the neck from inadvertent injury. (From Abelson TI, Witt WJ in Roberts JR, Hedges JR (eds): *Clinical Procedures in Emergency Medicine,* 2d ed. Philadelphia, Saunders, 1991, p.1044, with permission.)

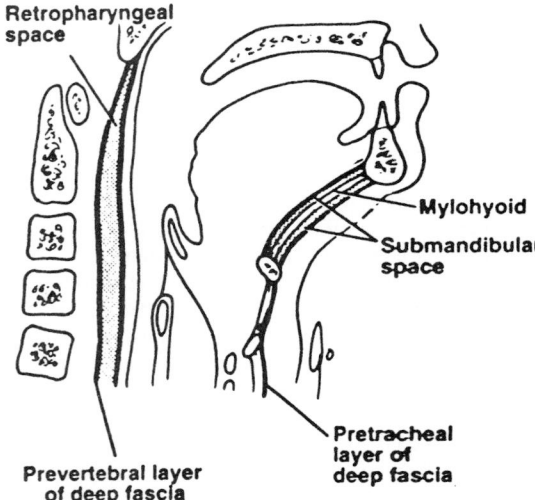

**Fig. 202-5.** Sagittal section of the neck showing the positions of the retropharyngeal space and the submandibular space. (From Snell RS, Smith MS: *Clinical Anatomy for Emergency Medicine.* St Louis, Mosby, 1993, with permission.)

head and neck infection can result in lymphangitis, suppuration, and abscess formation. In older patients, foreign bodies or trauma may predispose to this condition.

Because of the contiguous nature of the fascial planes of the retropharyngeal space with the mediastinum, infectious spread is a significant risk (see Fig. 202-5). Retropharyngeal abscesses can result

in acute airway obstruction, sepsis, mediastinitis, aspiration pneumonia, empyema, thrombosis of the jugular vein, or erosion into the carotid artery.

Signs and symptoms include fever, odynophagia, neck swelling, drooling, torticollis, meningismus, cervical adenopathy, and stridor in younger children.

Clinical suspicion and radiographic imaging procedures are the mainstay of diagnosis. The lateral neck radiograph has a diagnostic sensitivity of 88 percent. The prevertebral soft tissues should not exceed half the width of the vertebral bodies. This finding may be mimicked by neck flexion. CT scan may aid in differentiating abscess from cellulitis. The role of ultrasound is not completely evaluated for this diagnosis.

Patients with retropharyngeal abscess should be admitted for parenteral antibiotics and urgent ENT consultation. Treatment consists of incision and drainage, usually under general anesthesia.

Intravenous antibiotics should be administered in the emergency department. They are selected for activity against mixed gram-negative and anaerobic bacteria, *Staph. aureus, Klebsiella* sp., *Neisseria* sp., and streptococci. A penicillinase-resistant penicillin, combined with a third-generation cephalosporin and metronidazole, or clindamycin and an aminoglycoside are appropriate.

## Parapharyngeal Abscess

Also known as the lateral pharyngeal space, or the pharyngomaxillary space, the parapharyngeal space is an inverted cone extending from the base of the skull to the hyoid; it is in contact with the carotid sheath (see Fig. 202-6).

Abscess in the parapharyngeal space usually presents with fever,

**Fig. 202-6.** Oblique section through neck. (From Echerarria J in Schlossber D (ed): *Infections of the Head and Neck.* New York, Springer-Verlag, 1993, with permission.)

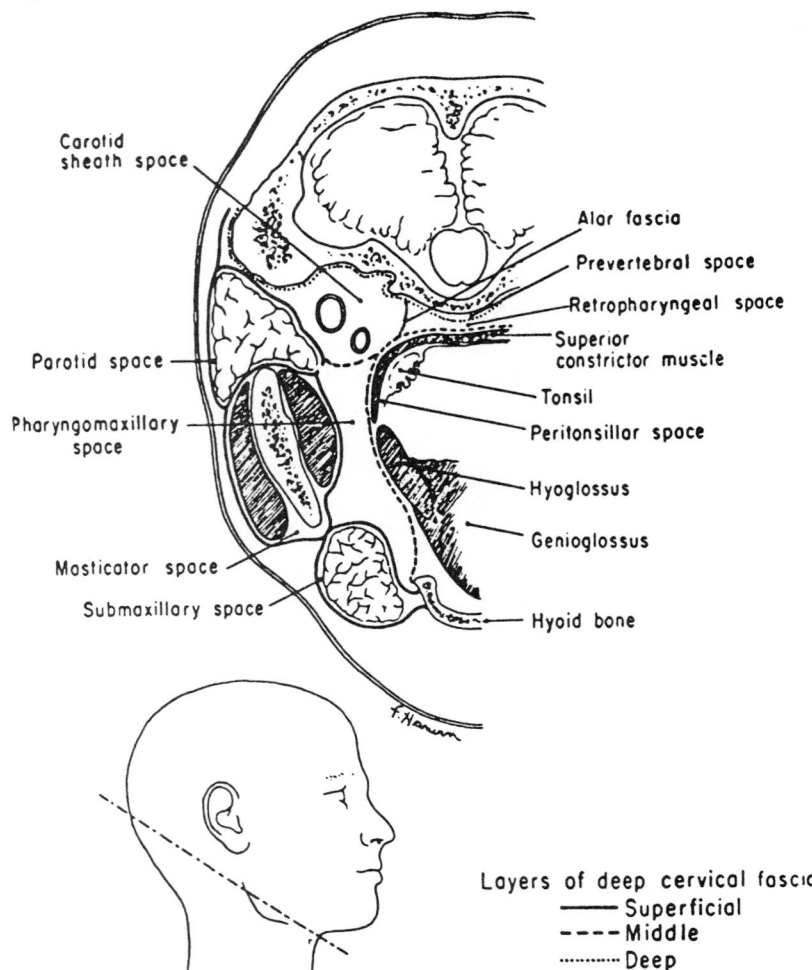

limitation of neck movement, poor oral intake, sore throat, dysphagia, and drooling. There may be a recent history of head and neck infection, trauma, or dental procedure. Physical findings include cervical adenopathy, pharyngitis, torticollis, and bulging of the pharyngeal wall.

Complications from abscess in this space include respiratory obstruction, internal jugular vein thrombosis, or erosion of the carotid artery.

Diagnostically there may be leukocytosis. A lateral neck x-ray may demonstrate retropharyngeal swelling. CT scan localizes soft tissue swelling to the parapharyngeal region. There may be air-fluid levels or a cystic lesion.

Treatment is admission for IV antibiotics. Patients with respiratory distress should ideally have an emergency surgical airway established in the operating room, prior to incision and drainage of the abscess. If intubation must be performed, it should be done carefully so as to prevent possible abscess rupture and aspiration of pus. Patients with a stable airway require emergent ENT consultation. Successful treatment of cellulitis (without abscess) by antibiotics alone has been reported.

Intravenous antibiotics should be started in the emergency department. Selection should be directed against the often mixed infections of aerobes and anaerobes. This includes group A β-hemolytic *Streptococcus, Staph. aureus, Neisseria, Moraxella catarrhalis, Haemophilus* sp., Enterobacteriaceae, *Bacteroides, Peptostreptococcus,* and *Fusobacterium.* Ampicillin/sulbactam is an appropriate selection. Clindamycin is an acceptable alternative if gram-negative aerobes are unlikely.

## Masticator Space Abscess

The masticator space consists of four spaces bounded by the muscles of mastication (see Fig. 202-7). This space comprises the masseteric, superficial temporal, deep temporal, and the pterygomandibular spaces. Since these spaces are contiguous, it is rare for only one to be infected. Infection is considered secondary, as it usually occurs by extension from one of the anterior spaces (the buccal, sublingual, or submandibular spaces).

Infection in the masseteric space usually results from extension of buccal space infection or from soft tissue infection around the third molar. There will be posterior inferior facial swelling and mild to moderate trismus.

The temporal spaces are rarely involved. When this occurs, it is usually the result of serious overwhelming infection. There is soft tissue swelling over the temporalis, with significant trismus.

The pterygomandibular space is usually infected secondarily by extension from the sublingual or submandibular spaces or from infection around the third molar. There is minimal swelling on examination; however, there is significant trismus. Trismus without swelling suggests pterygomandibular space abscess.

Other nonspecific signs of infection occur. The patient may complain of fever and malaise. Dehydration (secondary to poor oral intake), dysphagia, nausea, or vomiting may complicate the clinical course. In more advanced cases, systemic signs of sepsis may be present.

The diagnosis of masticator space infection is clinical. Leukocytosis is a variable finding. Radiographs occasionally demonstrate osteomyelitis of the mandible. CT scan may define the extent of an abscess but is not required in the management of those well enough to be treated as outpatients. However, CT scan is needed in patients who appear more ill. Abscess culture usually yields streptococci and oral anaerobes but is unnecessary in uncomplicated immunocompetent patients.

Treatment is determined by the patient's condition. In unilateral masticator space infections, airway compromise is rare, but the possibility should always be considered. Emergent ENT consultation is re-

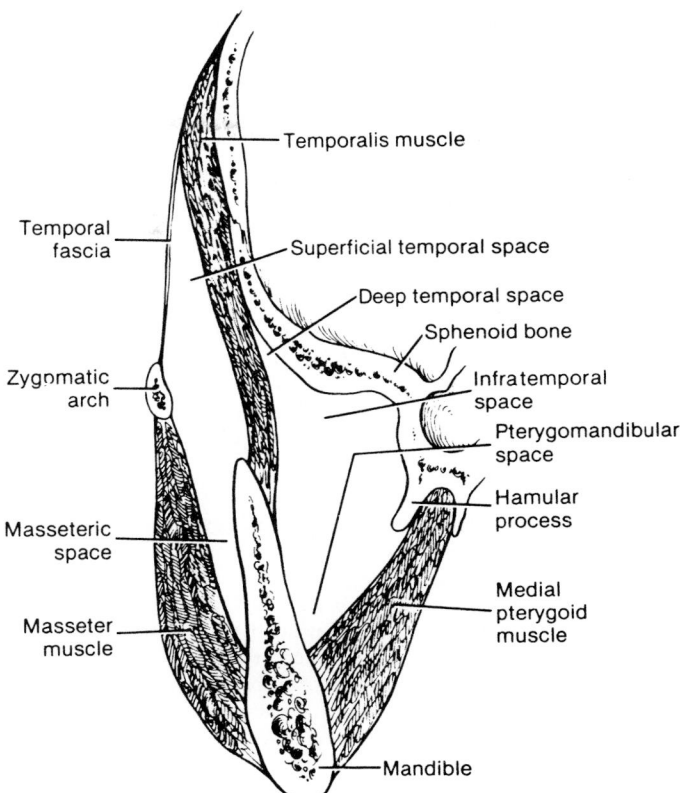

**Fig. 202-7.** Spaces of ramus of mandible are bounded by masseter muscle, medial pterygoid muscle, temporal fascia, and skull. Temporal space is divided into two portions, deep and superficial, by temporalis muscle. (From Peterson LJ in Cummings CW (ed): *Otolaryngology—Head and Neck Surgery,* 2d ed. Vol. 2 St. Louis Mosby Year Book, 1993, p.1207, with permission.)

quired in patients with airway compromise, trismus, vomiting, palpable abscess, large or diffuse areas of cellulitis, large areas of induration, or systemic signs of sepsis. Intravenous antibiotics should be started in the emergency department. Large doses of penicillin, 20 million units daily, are appropriate. In penicillin-allergic patients, clindamycin is a good alternative. Analgesics should be administered as needed.

Stable afebrile patients with minimal symptoms, only slight trismus, no palpable abscess or induration, and without vomiting or systemic signs of infection are candidates for discharge on oral antibiotics and analgesics. Penicillin as a first choice, erythromycin, or clindamycin may be selected. Patients should have follow-up within 24 h. They should also receive precise discharge instructions to return for difficulty in swallowing or breathing, fever, vomiting, or inability to take their medication for any reason.

## Ludwig's Angina

Ludwig's angina is defined as bilateral cellulitis of the submandibular space, involving connective tissue, fascia, and muscles but excluding the glandular structures. It is frequently odontogenic in origin, from the posterior mandibular molars, either as a result of abscess or recent trauma. Patients are predominantly healthy males age 20 to 60, although Ludwig's angina may complicate lupus, diabetes, chronic alcoholism, and immunodeficient states.

This is a febrile illness manifest clinically by brawny painful edema of the submandibular area. Progression of soft tissue swelling results in restricted neck motion, trismus, dysphonia, odynophagia, dysphagia, drooling, and displacement of the tongue posteriorly and cephalad. Generally there is no palpable fluctuance.

Stridor with respiratory compromise, progression to acute airway obstruction, and asphyxia can occur. The infection may dissect along head and neck fascial planes, resulting in mediastinitis with its attendant complications. Other complications include aspiration, thrombophlebitis of the jugular vein, carotid artery rupture, metastatic abscesses, and tongue necrosis.

Frequently there is a leukocytosis. Since attempts at direct visualization of the laryngeal structures may result in laryngospasm, radiographs have been the diagnostic modality of choice. A lateral soft tissue neck radiograph, performed with the patient sitting, may demonstrate airway narrowing, soft tissue swelling, or air in the soft tissues. CT scan has been reported a useful diagnostic adjunct. Since it is difficult for the anxious stridorous patient to assume the supine position, it should be performed only if adequate airway control is ensured. A panorex radiograph of the jaw may reveal an odontogenic source of infection.

Frequently, mixed anaerobic and aerobic oral flora are the etiologic agents of this disease. *Streptococcus, Staphylococcus,* and *Bacteroides* species are the most common pathogens.

Treatment requires analgesics, antibiotics, and possibly surgical drainage. Appropriate antibiotics, usually high-dose penicillin, should be started in the emergency department. If the patient is penicillin-allergic, clindamycin or chloramphenicol may be used. Aminoglycosides can be added for the treatment of suspected resistant organisms. The role of steroids in the treatment of airway edema is undefined. Equipment for airway control should be readily available. Acute laryngospasm is a constant concern until a definitive airway control is ensured. Since as many as one-third of patients with Ludwig's angina ultimately require tracheostomy or intubation, these patients should be admitted to an intensive care unit.

## Miscellaneous Causes

Mononucleosis, in young adults or teenagers, may rarely present with tonsillar hypertrophy of such extent as to compromise the airway. While there is no specific therapy except supportive care, inpatient observation is sometimes required for intravenous hydration, humidified oxygen, and intravenous steroids.

## BIBLIOGRAPHY

### Otologic Emergencies

#### External Otitis and Necrotizing External Otitis

Blake GB, Gianoli GJ: Necrotizing external otitis. *J La State Med Soc* 145:43, 1993.

Johnson MP, Ramphal R: Malignant external otitis: Report on therapy with ceftazidime and review of therapy and prognosis. *Rev Infect Dis* 12:173, 1990.

Strauss M: Current therapy of malignant external otitis. *Otolaryngol Head Neck Surg* 102:174, 1990.

Timon CI, O'Dwyer T: Diagnosis, complications, and treatment of malignant otitis externa. *Irish Med J* 82:30, 1989.

#### Furuncles and Bullous Myringitis

Reich JJ: Ear infections. *Emerg Med Clin North Am* 5:227, 1987.

#### Otitis Media

Celin ES, Bluestone CD, Stephenson J, et al: Bacteriology of acute otitis media in adults. *JAMA* 266:2249, 1991.

Jung TT, Rhee CK: Otolaryngologic approach to the diagnosis and management of otitis media. *Otolaryngol Clin North Am* 24:931, 1991.

Kemp ED: Otitis media. *Prim Care* 17:267, 1990.

Kempthorne J, Giebink GS: Pediatric approach to the diagnosis and management of otitis media. *Otolaryngol Clin North Am* 24:905, 1991.

Sugita R, Fujimaki Y, Deguchi K: Bacteriological features and chemotherapy of adult acute purulent otitis media. *J Laryngol Otol* 99:629, 1985.

#### Tympanometry and Acoustic Otoscopy

Dietrich J, Cottington E: Acoustic otoscopy in the diagnosis of otitis media. *Ann Emerg Med* 18:396, 1989.

Margolis RH, Hunter LL: Audiologic evaluation of the otitis media patient. *Otolaryngol Clin North Am* 24:877, 1991.

Shanks J, Shelton C: Basic principles and clinical applications of tympanometry. *Otolaryngol Clin North Am* 24:299, 1991.

Sutherland JE, Campbell K: Immitance audiometry. *Prim Care* 17(2):233, 1990.

#### Myringotomy/Tympanocentesis

Bluestone CD: Modern management of otitis media. *Pediatr Clin North Am* 36:1371, 1989.

#### Mastoiditis

Gaffney RJ, O'Dwyer TP, Maguire AJ: Bezold's abscess. *J Laryngol Otol* 105:765, 1991.

Matthews TJ, Oliver SP: Bacteriology of mastoiditis (a five year experience at Groote Schuur Hospital). *J Laryngol Otol* 102:397, 1988.

Neely JG: Complications of temporal bone infection, in Cummings CW (ed): *Otolaryngology—Head and Neck Surgery,* 2d ed. St. Louis, Mosby Year Book, 1993, pp 2840–2864.

Palva T, Virtanen H, Makinen J: Acute and latent mastoiditis in children. *J Laryngol Otol* 99:127, 1985.

Samuel J, Fernandes CM: Otogenic complications with an intact tympanic membrane. *Laryngoscope* 95:1387, 1985.

#### Sudden Hearing Loss

Lawrence LJ, Brown CG: Approach to decreased hearing. *Emerg Med Clin North Am* 5:193, 1987.

Shikowitz MJ: Sudden sensorineural hearing loss. *Med Clin North Am* 75:1239, 1991.

#### Auricular Trauma

Kirsch JP, Amedee RG: Management of external ear trauma. *J La State Med Soc* 143:13, 1991.

Turbiak TW: Ear trauma. *Emerg Med Clin North Am* 5:243, 1987.

#### Foreign Body of the Ear

Fritz S, Kelen GD, Sivertson KT: Foreign bodies of the external auditory canal. *Emerg Med Clin North Am* 5:183, 1987.

#### Traumatic Tympanic Membrane Perforations

Kristensen S, Juul A, Gammelgaard NP, Rasmussen OR: Traumatic tympanic membrane perforations: Complications and management. *Ear Nose Throat J* 68:503, 1989.

Kristensen S: Spontaneous healing of traumatic tympanic membrane perforations in man: A century of experience. *J Laryngol Otol* 106:1037, 1992.

#### Otic Barotrauma

Jerrard DA: Diving medicine. *Emerg Med Clin North Am* 10:329, 1992.

Melamed Y, Shupak A, Bitterman H: Medical problems associated with underwater diving. *N Engl J Med* 326:30, 1992.

Talmi YP, Finkelstein Y, Yuval Z: Barotrauma-induced hearing loss. *Scand Audiol* 20:1, 1991.

### Salivary Gland Problems

Bodner L: Salivary gland calculi: Diagnostic imaging and surgical management. *Compend Contin Educ Dent* 14:572, 1990.

Johnson A: Inflammatory conditions of the major salivary glands. *Ear Nose Throat J* 68:94, 1989.

Langlais RP, Benson BW, Barnett DA: Salivary gland dysfunction: Infections, sialoliths, and tumors. *Ear Nose Throat J* 68:758, 1989.

Lustman J, Regev E, Melamed Y: Sialolithiasis. A survey on 245 patients and a review of the literature. *Int J Oral Maxillofac Surg* 19:135, 1990.

White AK: Salivary gland disease in infancy and childhood. *J Otolaryngol* 21:422, 1992.

## Postadenotonsillectomy Bleeding

Chowdhury K, Tewfik TL, Schloss MD: Post-tonsillectomy and adenoidectomy hemorrhage. *J Otolaryngol* 17:46, 1988.

Kendrick D, Gibbin K: An audit of the complications of paediatric tonsillectomy, adenoidectomy and adenotonsillectomy. *Clin Otolaryngol* 18:115, 1993.

Wiatrak BJ, Myer CM 3rd, Andrews TM: Complications of adenotonsillectomy in children under 3 years of age. *Am J Otolaryngol* 12:170, 1991.

## Facial Cellulitis

Middleton DB, Ferrante JA: Periorbital and facial cellulitis, *Am Fam Physician* 21:98, 1980.

Waldman LA: Facial cellulitis caused by an unrecognized foreign body. *Oral Surg Oral Med Oral Pathol* 48:408, 1979.

## Acute Upper Airway Obstruction

### Epiglottitis

Andreassen UK, Baer S, Nielsen TG, et al: Acute epiglottitis—25 years experience with nasotracheal intubation, current management policy and future trends. *J Laryngol Otol* 106:1072, 1992.

Barrow HN, Vastola AP, Wang RC: Adult supraglottitis. *Otolaryngol Head Neck Surg* 109(3 pt 1):474, 1993.

Crosby E, Reid D: Acute epiglottitis in the adult: Is intubation mandatory? *Can J Anesth* 38:914, 1991.

Mayo-Smith M: Fatal respiratory arrest in adult epiglottitis in the intensive care unit. Implications for airway management. *Chest* 104:964, 1993.

Ziad ED: Approach to supraglottitis. *Emerg Med Clin North Am* 5:353, 1987.

### Laryngeal Trauma

Bent JP, Silver JR, Porubsky ES: Acute laryngeal trauma: A review of 77 patients. *Otolaryngol Head Neck Surg* 109:441, 1993.

Fuhrman GM, Steif FH 3rd, Buerk CA: Blunt laryngeal trauma: Classification and management protocol. *J Trauma* 30:87, 1990.

Minard G: Laryngotracheal transection. *J Tenn Med Assoc* 83:402, 1990.

Schafer SD: Use of CT scanning in the management of the acutely injured larynx. *Otolaryngol Clin North Am* 24:31, 1991.

Schafer SD: The acute management of external laryngeal trauma. *Arch Otolaryngol Head Neck Surg* 118:598, 1992.

### Irritants and Corrosives

Goldberg RM, Lee S, Line WS: Laryngeal burns secondary to the ingestion of microwave-heated food. *J Emerg Med* 8:281, 1990.

Gough D, Young G: Airway burns and toxic gases, in Dailey RH, Simon B, Young G, Stewart RD (eds): *The Airway: Emergency Management.* St. Louis, Mosby Year Book, 1992, pp 297–308.

Scott JC, Bronwyn J, Eisele DW, Ravich WJ: Caustic ingestion injuries of the upper aerodigestive tract. *Laryngoscope* 102:1, 1992.

Snyderman C, Weissmann J, Tabor E, Curtin H: Crack cocaine burns of the larynx. *Arch Otolaryngol Head Neck Surg.* 117:792, 1991.

Vergauwen P, Moulin D, Buts JP, et al: Caustic burns of the upper digestive and respiratory tracts. *Eur J Pediatr* 150:700, 1991.

### Angioneurotic Edema

Davidson AE, Miller SD, Settipane G, Klein D: Urticaria and angioedema. *Clev Clin J Med* 59:529, 1992.

Frank MM, Gelfand JA, Atkinson JP: Hereditary angioneurotic edema: The clinical syndrome and its management. *Ann Intern Med* 84:580, 1976.

Lundh B, Laurell A, Wetterqvist H, et al: A case of hereditary angioneurotic oedema successfully treated with epsilon-aminocaproic acid. *Clin Exp Immunol* 3:733, 1968.

Megerian CA, Arnold JE, Berger M: Angioedema: 5 years' experience, with a review of the disorder's presentation and treatment. *Laryngoscope* 102:256, 1992.

## Peritonsillar Abscess

Epperly TD, Wood TC: New trends in the management of peritonsillar abscess. *Am Fam Physician* 42:102, 1990.

Ophir D, Bawnik J, Poria Y, et al: Peritonsillar abscess: A prospective evaluation of outpatient management by needle aspiration. *Arch Otolaryngol Head Neck Surg* 114:661, 1988.

Shoemaker M, Lampe RM, Weir MR: Peritonsillitis: Abscess or cellulitis? *Pediatr Infect Dis* 5:435, 1986.

Weinberg E, Brodsky L, Stanievich J: Needle aspiration of peritonsillar abscess in children. *Arch Otolaryngol Head Neck Surg* 119:169, 1993.

## Peritonsillar Abscess Aspiration

Abelson TI, Witt WJ: Otolaryngologic procedures, in Roberts JR, Hedges JR (eds): *Clinical Procedures in Emergency Medicine,* 2d ed. Philadelphia, Saunders, 1991, pp 1041–45.

Schechter GL: Peritonsillar abscess, in Gates GA (ed): *Current Therapy in Otolaryngology—Head and Neck Surgery,* 2d ed. Philadelphia, Decker, 1984, pp 371–372.

## Retropharyngeal Abscess

Coulthard M, Isaacs D: Retropharyngeal abscess. *Arch Dis Child* 66:1227, 1991.

Hartman RW: Recognition of retropharyngeal abscess in children. *Am Fam Physician* 46:193, 1992.

Robinson MH, Young JD, Burge PD: Retropharyngeal abscess, airway obstruction, and tetraplegia after hyperextension injury of the cervical spine: A case report. *J Trauma* 32:107, 1992.

## Parapharyngeal Abscess

Broughton RA: Nonsurgical management of deep neck infections in children. *Pediatr Infect Dis* 11:14, 1992.

Ortiz JA, Hudkins C, Kornblut A: Adenitis, adenopathy, and abscesses of the head and neck. *Emerg Med Clin North Am* 5:359, 1987.

Sethi DS, Stanley RE: Parapharyngeal abscesses. *J Laryngol Otol* 105:1025, 1991.

## Masticator Space Abscess

Chow AW: Odontogenic infections, in Schlossberg D (ed): *Infections of the Head and Neck.* New York, Springer, 1987, pp 153–60.

Peterson LJ: Odontogenic infections, in Cummings CW (ed): *Otolaryngology—Head and Neck Surgery,* 2d ed. St. Louis, Mosby Year Book, 1993, pp 1199–1215.

## Ludwig's Angina

Fritsch DE, Klein DG: Ludwig's angina. *Heart Lung* 21:39, 1992.

Juang YC, Cheng DL, Wang LS: Ludwig's angina: An analysis of 14 cases. *Scand J Infect Dis* 21:121, 1989.

Nguyen VD, Potter JL, Hersh-Schick MR: Ludwig's angina: An uncommon and potentially lethal neck infection. *Am J Neuroradiol* 13:215, 1992.

Steinberg DG, Stollerman GH: Dangerous pyogenic skin infections. *Hosp Pract* 24:101, 1989.

# 203

# NASAL EMERGENCIES AND SINUSITIS

## James A. Smith

## EPISTAXIS

### Introduction

The blood supply to the nasal cavity ultimately originates from the internal and external carotid arteries and thus epistaxis may result in serious bleeding. The initial priority is to secure the patient's airway, breathing, and circulation. Never underestimate the amount of blood that can be lost from a "simple nosebleed," either acute or chronic.

After the patient's ABCs have been evaluated, the emergency physician should then determine if the bleeding originates in the anterior or posterior part of the nasal cavity. This will determine how best to achieve control of the hemorrhage. The site of blood loss should be identified in *all* patients, even those in whom the bleeding has stopped.

The origin of epistaxis may be either anterior or posterior. The causes are many, involving both local and systemic disorders, and some of the more common etiologies are listed in Table 203-1. Important questions that should be asked of all patients presenting with

**Table 203-1.** Common Etiologies of Epistaxis

Infection
  Rhinitis
  Nasopharyngitis
  Sinusitis
Trauma
  Self-induced (i.e., nose-picking)
  Facial bone fractures
  Nasal foreign body
  Iatrogenic
  Nasal surgery
  Local irritants
    OTC nasal sprays
    Cocaine abuse
    Other chemical irritants
    Dry nasal mucosa
Allergic rhinitis
Atrophic rhinitis
Hypertension and atherosclerotic cardiovascular disease
Tumors (benign or malignant)
  Primary
  Secondary
Congenital or acquired nasal defects
Predisposing factors
  Congenital
    Hemophilia A
    Hemophilia B
    von Willebrand Disease
    Osler-Weber-Rendu syndrome
  Disease-mediated
    Thrombocytopenia
    Hypoprothrombinemia
    Hypofibrinogenemia
    Liver disease
    Renal failure/uremia
    Disseminated intravascular coagulation
  Drug-induced
    Salicylates and other NSAIDS
    Heparin
    Coumadin
    Thrombolytics
    Heavy metals

**Table 203-2.** Important Historical Considerations in Epistaxis

How long has the patient been bleeding?
How severe has the bleeding been?
What has the patient done to try to stop the bleeding?
What medications is the patient on that may contribute to or exacerbate the bleeding (e.g., coumadin, aspirin, NSAIDS, over-the-counter nasal sprays)?
Is the patient using any illicit drugs (e.g., cocaine) that might contribute to or exacerbate the bleeding?
Does the patient have any preexisting medical problem, such as hemophilia or thrombocytopenia, that may contribute to or exacerbate the bleeding?
Has the patient seen a physician or come to the emergency department for epistaxis within the past several days (evidence of continued bleeding despite prior attempts at control)?
Is bleeding associated with recent nasal surgery?

epistaxis can be found in Table 203-2. Postoperative bleeding requires notification of the responsibe otolaryngologist.

### Anterior Epistaxis

#### Pathophysiology

Most cases of epistaxis originate from the anterior aspect of the nasal septum at a site called *Little's area.* This is a superficial region of the nasal mucosa where a complex anastomosis of arterioles, referred to as *Kisselbach's plexus* (also known as *Woodruff's plexus*) can be found. This collection of vessels is fed by the septal branches of the anterior ethmoidal, sphenopalatine, and superior labial arteries as well as the greater palatine artery (Fig. 203-1).

#### Clinical Features

It may be difficult to determine clinically if the source of bleeding is anterior or posterior. It may also be difficult to tell which side of the nasal cavity is involved because blood can reflux into the unaffected side through the posterior choanae. Proper lighting and suction are essential for a good physical examination. Such lighting is best accomplished by the use of a head mirror or specialized ENT (ear-nose-

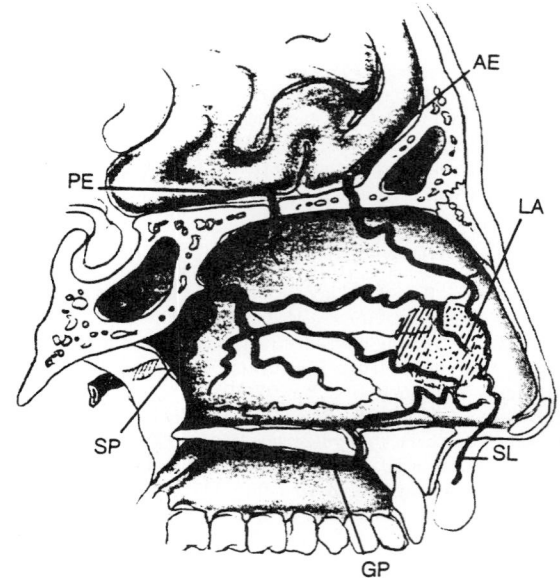

**Fig. 203-1.** Arterial blood supply to the nasal cavity. The most common site of nasal hemorrhage is at Little's area, located on the nasal septum. The most common site of posterior epistaxis is at the lateral nasal branch of the sphenopalatine artery, which enters the nasal cavity behind the middle turbinate. AE, anterior ethmoid; GP, greater palatine; LA, Little's area; PE, posterior ethmoid; SL, superior labial; SP, sphenopalatine (lateral nasal branch).

**Table 203-3.** Steps in the Initial Evaluation and Treatment of Epistaxis

It is often difficult to determine if epistaxis is anterior or posterior in origin. In general, the following sequence of events should be followed:

1. A quick history is obtained to determine the duration and severity of bleeding as well as the presence of any contributing factors such as anticoagulant use, history of bleeding diathesis, etc. If these conditions are present, IV access and laboratory studies (CBC, PT/PTT, type and screen) are obtained.

2. The patient is told to blow his or her nose to dislodge clots.

3. A quick inspection of the nasal cavity is made to determine if the bleeding site is anterior. Suction with an 8 or 10 French Fraizer suction tip catheter may help enormously. If an anterior site is visualized, this does not rule out an additional posterior bleed.

4. A cotton or gauze pledget is moistened with vasoconstrictive and anesthetic agents and inserted into the nasal cavity with a bayonet forceps. A pledget is preferred over nasal spray as it provides greater contact with the nasal mucosa and provides a tamponade effect.

5. The patient is shown the correct method to apply firm pressure to the nose for 10 min (Fig. 203-2). If blood flows down the back of the throat, either compression is inadequate, a clot is still present in the posterior nasal cavity, or there is posterior bleeding.

6. During the application of nasal compression, orthostatic vital signs may be obtained.

7. After 10 min of compression, remove the pledgets and inspect the nasal cavity with a speculum. If there is no evidence of continued bleeding, no further treatment may be necessary. If anterior bleeding continues after three attempts at vasoconstriction and direct pressure, an anterior nasal pack should be inserted using strips of petrolatum-impregnated gauze or an appropriate commercial device. If nasal packing does not control isolated anterior bleeding, the anterior pack should be re-inserted to insure proper placement.

8. If the patient continues to note blood flowing down the back of his/her throat, then posterior epistaxis should be considered. A combined anterior and posterior pack should be placed. The patient is then closely monitored for continued blood loss and an otolaryngologist consulted.

9. After the combined anterior and posterior packs are placed, an intravenous line should be started and laboratory studies such as a CBC, PT/PTT, type and hold clot are obtained, if not done previously. The patient is closely monitored for continued blood loss.

*Note:* CBC, complete blood count; PT, prothrombin time; PTT, partial thromboplastin time.

throat) head lamp. Having an assistant hold a flashlight does not provide adequate illumination. The physical examination must include the determination of vital signs, including orthostatic blood pressure measurements, as well as a thorough inspection of the oral cavity and nasopharynx.

The fact that Kisselbach's plexus is readily accessible to objects inserted past the nasal vestibule explains why this is the most common site of epistaxis. Specific features of the history that suggest an anterior site of bleeding include the following:

The presence of a specific inciting event (e.g., nasal trauma)
The recent use of agents that irritate or promote vasoconstriction of the nasal mucosa (such as cocaine or over-the-counter nasal sprays)
The insertion or presence of a foreign body in the nasal cavity
Symptoms of a recent cold, flu, or allergy
Bleeding from the anterior nares with no sensation of blood flowing down the back of the throat

## Treatment

The treatment of anterior epistaxis includes direct pressure, use of vasoconstrictors, cautery, and packing. The initial approach to a patient with epistaxis is listed in Table 203-3. Additional details regarding these steps can be found in the discussion below and in the sections detailing the treatment of posterior epistaxis.

**Direct pressure**

The most effective way to apply pressure is to use the closed hand technique (Fig. 203-2). This method provides firm compression of the entire elastic area of the nose and makes it less likely that the patient will loosen his or her grip. The duration of compression (5 to 10 min) should be confirmed by a watch or clock since patients invariably underestimate the amount of time that has elapsed.

**Vasoconstrictive and Anesthetic Agents**

There are many vasoconstrictive agents that are useful in the control of epistaxis. These compounds may be instilled into the nasal cavity by using a spray bottle, atomizer, or pledget. Moistening a pledget is the preferred route since this provides for better contact with the nasal mucosa and also provides an excellent tamponade effect.

The use of a vasoconstrictor alone is not sufficient, however. The nasal mucosa is exquisitely sensitive, and an appropriate anesthetic should also be used. Table 203-4 lists common topical agents. Cocaine provides excellent vasoconstriction and anesthesia but should be used with extreme caution in patients who are elderly, have a history of cocaine abuse, or have significant cardiovascular disease. It should not be used in children.

**Cautery**

*Chemical Cautery*

Silver nitrate sticks have long been used as an aid in the management of well-visualized, minor sources of anterior nasal bleeding. After the bleeding from an anterior site has been stopped, the mucosa is cauterized by touching the area with the tip of a silver nitrate stick for 10 to 15 s. Some authors also recommend application to the surrounding area to cauterize the arterioles that feed the disrupted mucosa. Care should be exercised during application as septal perforations have been reported with overzealous use. Bleeding should be stopped by vasoconstrictors or direct pressure *before* silver nitrate is applied because it is extremely difficult, if not impossible, to cauterize an actively bleeding area by chemical means alone.

**Electrical and Thermal Cautery**

Few emergency departments have access to the specialized equipment necessary for the electrical cautery of epistaxis. A recent study by Toner et al. has demonstrated that there appears to be no signifi-

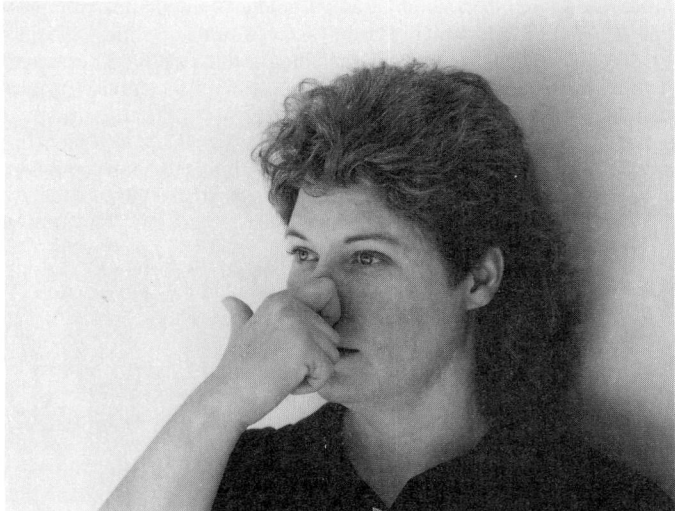

**A**

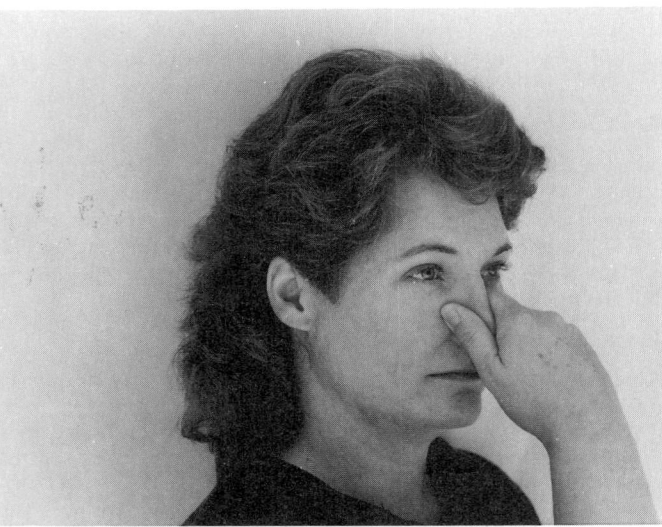

**B**

**Fig. 203-2.** The closed hand technique for complete compression of the nasal septum. With this technique, the radial aspect of the second digit between the proximal and distal interphalangeal joints rests against the side of the nose and the thumb applies pressure from the opposite side. The arm and elbow can rest against the chest to help maintain good hand position.

cant difference in the control of hemorrhage when electrocautery is compared to chemical cautery. This is best left to an otolaryngologist.

Battery-powered, disposable heat cautery devices are now standard in many emergency departments. Unfortunately, it is difficult to control or estimate the depth of cautery achieved with these devices, and significant injury can occur to the nasal mucosa or septal perichondrium. For these reasons, heat cautery of intractable epistaxis should not be attempted by the emergency physician.

### Anterior Nasal Packing

Anterior nasal packing should be inserted in any patient who has anterior epistaxis that cannot be controlled with vasoconstrictors and direct pressure.

### Standard Gauze Packing

Correct technique is important since inadequate packing is probably the most common cause of treatment failure. The procedure is as follows (see also Fig. 203-3):

**Table 203-4.** Vasoconstrictive and Anesthetic Agents Used in Epistaxis

Phenylephrine (Neo-Synephrine) 0.5–1.0% concentration mixed with 4% lidocaine*
Oxymetozaline (Afrin) 0.05% concentration mixed with 4% lidocaine*
Epinephrine 0.25 mL of 1:1000 concentration mixed with 20 mL of 4% lidocaine*
Cocaine (4%)†; total dosage of 2 to 3 mg/kg in adults

* The maximum dose of lidocaine applied to the nasal mucosa should not exceed 4 mg/kg.
† Please note that 4% cocaine = 40 mg/mL.

1. The nasal cavity is adequately prepared with combined vasoconstrictor and anesthetic agents as noted above.
2. A speculum is used to visualize the nasal cavity and ensure that the gauze is placed correctly. Blind packing or loose placement of gauze results in inadequate compression.
3. Using a bayonet forceps, one end of a long strip of petrolatum-impregnated gauze or iodoform gauze saturated with antibiotic ointment is inserted all the way to the posterior limit of the cavity, and the forceps is removed.
4. The speculum is then removed and reinserted so that the packing material is gently pushed toward the floor of the cavity. The bayonet forceps is reinserted and used to gently push the posterior end of the strip downward.
5. Another strip of gauze is inserted on top of the first using an "accordion" technique. The speculum is again removed and reinserted, and the forceps used to gently push the pack downward.
6. This procedure is continued until the entire nasal cavity is filled with layers of packing material. The folded end of each layer of gauze should be visible anteriorly.
7. The patient should be observed for 30 min after packing is complete to make sure that adequate hemostasis has been achieved.

### Commercial Devices

There are many commercial products that have been specifically designed to make the insertion of an anterior nasal pack faster, more convenient, and more comfortable for the patient. One such device is the Merocel nasal sponge (Merocel Corp., Mystic, CT). This is a dehydrated, synthetic spongelike material that expands upon contact with moisture (see Fig. 203-4). When inserted, the sponge absorbs the blood and secretions present in the nasal cavity and quickly expands to provide a good tamponade effect. Insertion should be accomplished rapidly, as the sponge will start to expand almost immediately on contact with any blood or secretions. Expansion can be delayed slightly by coating the desiccated sponge with a water-soluble antibiotic ointment. If there is inadequate expansion after insertion, the sponge can be rehydrated by injecting sterile water, using an intravenous catheter attached to a syringe, into the sponge. Parents report that the Merocel sponge is more comfortable than balloon or gauze packing. It has been reported that the efficacy of this device is comparable to other methods. Gelfoam packs can also be used.

If you should decide to use a commercial device as an isolated anterior nasal pack, it is important not to use one that is designed for both anterior and posterior tamponade. Devices designed for the control of posterior epistaxis have been associated with significant morbidity and should not be used for the control of isolated anterior nasal bleeding.

### Complications

Anterior nasal packing is a relatively benign procedure, but some problems have been reported. Complications include dislodgement of the packing, recurrent bleeding, sinusitis, and, although rare, toxic shock syndrome. Any patient who presents to the emergency department following nasal packing or recent nasal surgery and the complaint of fever, nausea, or vomiting should be thought to have early

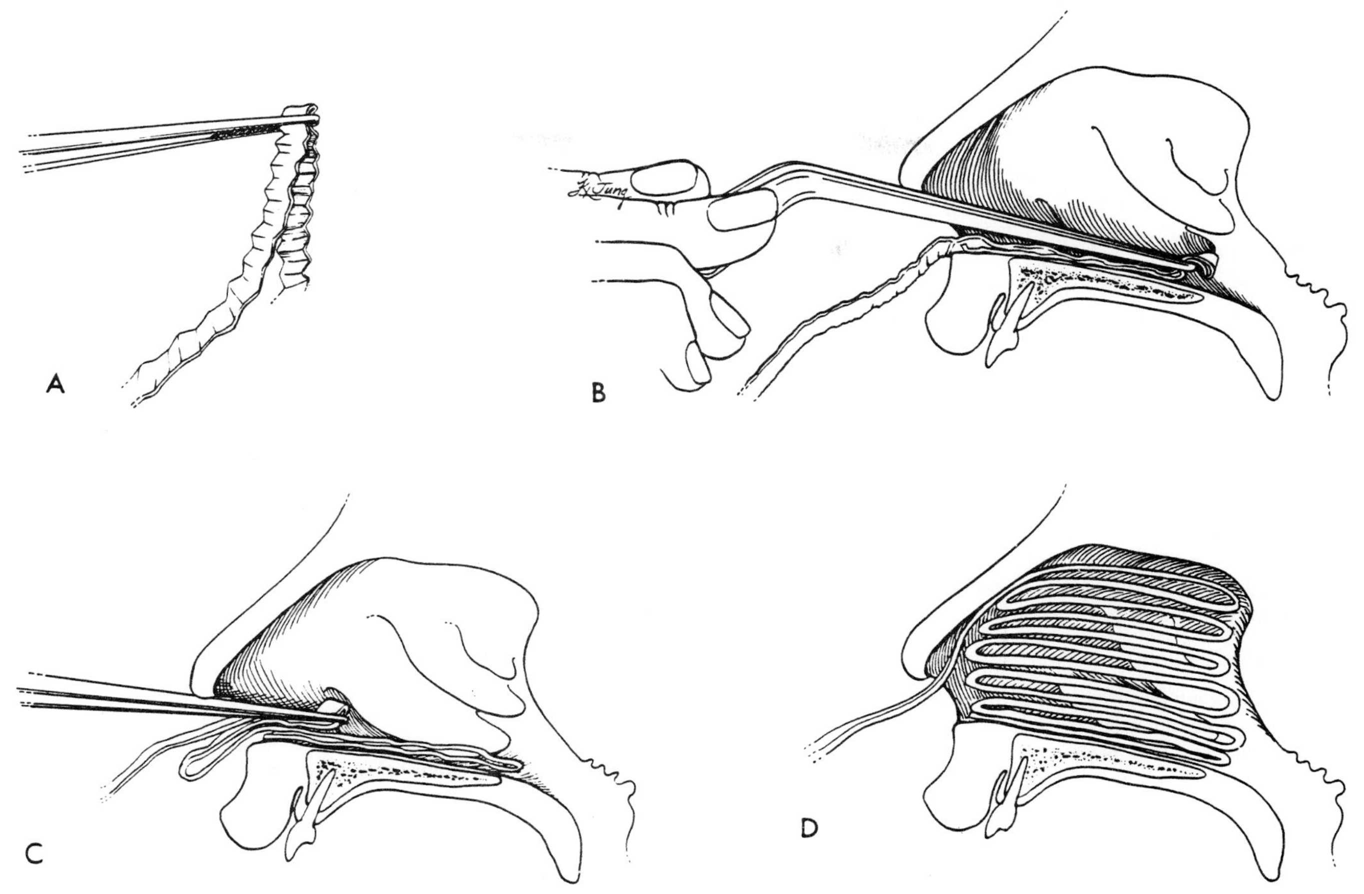

**Fig. 203-3.** The key to placement of an anterior nasal pack that will control epistaxis adequately and stay in place is to lay the packing into the nasal cavity in an "accordion" manner, so that part of each layer of packing lies anteriorly, preventing the gauze from falling posteriorly into the nasopharynx. **A.** The first layer of ¼-inch petrolatum-impregnated gauze strip is grasped approximately 2 to 3 cm from its end. **B.** The first layer is then placed on the floor of the nose through the nasal speculum (not pictured here). The bayonet forceps and nasal speculum are then withdrawn. **C.** The nasal speculum is reintroduced on top of the first layer of packing, and a second layer is placed in an identical manner. After several layers have been placed, it is often useful to reintroduce the bayonet forceps to push the previously placed packing down onto the floor of the nose, making it tighter and more secure. **D.** A complete anterior nasal pack can tamponade a bleeding point anywhere in the anterior nasal cavities and will stay in place until removed by the physician or patient.

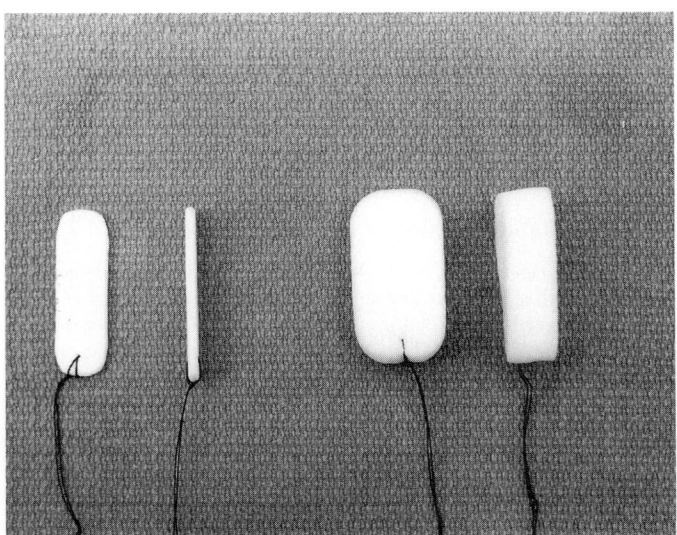

**Fig. 203-4.** The Merocel nasal sponge in its desiccated (left) and hydrated (right) forms.

toxic shock syndrome until proven otherwise. The effectiveness of antistaphylococcal anti-biotics in the prevention of this syndrome has not yet been proven. Nevertheless, it is still recommended that all patients with nasal packing be given appropriate antibiotics. A good choice is cephalexin (250 to 500 mg four times a day) or amoxicillin/clavulanate (250 to 500 mg three times a day). In the patient who cannot tolerate cephalexin or amoxicillin/clavulanate, clindamycin (150 to 300 mg four times a day) or trimethoprim/sulfamethoxazole DS (twice a day) are good second choices. Regardless of the antibiotic chosen, the patient should follow-up with an otolaryngologist in 2 to 3 days.

Another complication occurs if the layers of an anterior nasal pack fall backward into the nasopharynx. The patient usually complains of choking or the sensation of a foreign body in the back of the throat. If this occurs, the existing gauze needs to be removed and the packing replaced. If repacking results in the same problem, a posterior pack may need to be placed to act as a buttress. Because of the morbidity and mortality associated with its placement, all patients with posterior nasal packing should have immediate otolaryngologic evaluation for possible hospital admission.

Continued bleeding may also occur after an anterior nasal pack has been inserted. Although improper technique is the most common cause, Montgomery and Reardon have reported that even properly placed gauze packing can be associated with a 25 percent failure rate. Patient discomfort, secondary to the blockage of normal sinus drainage from the ostia, and reflux of blood through the ocular puncta may also occur. Finally, significant injury to the nasal mucosa can occur if blind packing is attempted. If the emergency physician is unable to visualize the packing process or is uncomfortable with performing this procedure, a commercial device such as the Merocel sponge should be used instead.

### *Placement of Anterior Packs in Children*

Nosebleeds in children are common, are usually anterior, and almost always subside with direct pressure. In the rare case of a patient with intractable bleeding, the placement of gauze strips is identical to the procedure used in adults. Care must be taken, however, because children tend to be less cooperative and packing may be extremely difficult. If there is any problem with patient cooperation, an otolaryngologist should be consulted.

### *Removal of Anterior Nasal Packing*

Gelfoam is biodegradable and, if used for nasal packing, is left to be absorbed by the body. Removal of the other types of packing materials is best left to an otolaryngologist at the time of follow-up. This generally takes place 2 to 3 days after the initial insertion.

### *Admission Indications*

Hospital admission is not necessary for patients who have had good control of simple, anterior epistaxis or epistaxis where the bleeding has been stopped by the placement of an anterior nasal pack. If there is evidence of continued bleeding after the insertion of an anterior pack, the possibility of inadequate packing technique or a posterior bleeding site should be considered. If attempts to control the bleeding fail, immediate consultation with an otolaryngologist is advised.

### Discharge Instructions

At the time of discharge, patients who have had adequate control of their anterior epistaxis should be given the following instructions:

1. Patients should not manipulate the external nares or insert any foreign object into the nasal cavity. As an exception, the patient may apply petrolatum or triple antibiotic ointment to dry mucosa *gently* with a sterile Q-tip once or twice a day for 3 to 4 days.
2. Patients should not use aspirin or nonsteroidal anti-inflammatory agents for 3 or 4 days.
3. If bleeding should recur in a patient with simple, anterior epistaxis where no packing has been inserted, home measures should be tried before returning to the emergency department. Patients may be advised to use an over-the-counter nasal spray (such as phenylephrine or oxymetozaline) and pinch their nose, using proper technique, for 5 to 10 min. If bleeding continues, compression may be repeated twice more. If bleeding continues after three attempts, the patient should return to the emergency department immediately. These instructions should be given only to patients in whom a well-visualized site of anterior mucosal disruption is thought to be the cause of bleeding, in patients without medical problems that might exacerbate bleeding, and in patients not taking medications that may affect hemostasis.
4. Patients who have had an anterior pack inserted should return *immediately* if bleeding occurs around the packing or if there is a sensation of blood trickling down the back of the throat. Also, these patients should be advised to leave the pack in place and not attempt to remove it themselves.
5. Antibiotics such as cephalexin, amoxicillin/clavulanate, trimethoprim/sulfamethoxazole, or clindamycin are necessary if an anterior nasal pack has been inserted to prevent sinusitis and possibly reduce the risk of toxic shock syndrome. The patient should be advised to return immediately if he or she has any problems with fever, nausea, or vomiting as these symptoms may represent early toxic shock syndrome.
6. The patient should follow-up with an otolaryngologic in 2 to 3 days.

## Posterior Epistaxis

### Pathophysiology

Although less common than anterior epistaxis, posterior epistaxis can result in more blood loss for several reasons. The posterior nature of the bleeding means that it cannot be controlled by direct pressure, and compression by packing may be difficult. The usual source of bleeding in these patients is from the lateral nasal branch of the sphenopalatine artery, which enters the nasal cavity behind the middle turbinate (Fig. 203-1).

### Physical Examination

With posterior epistaxis, blood can usually be seen flowing down the oropharynx when the patient opens the mouth. Direct visualization of the posterior bleeding site may be impossible without the aid of a fiberoptic nasopharyngoscope. Posterior epistaxis is suspected in the following circumstances:

The physician is unable to identify an anterior site of bleeding or the disrupted mucosa cannot be visualized if bleeding has been stopped.

Bleeding occurs from both nares. This is thought to be more common with posterior epistaxis because the site of hemorrhage is closer to the choanae and blood is more likely to reflex to the unaffected side.

The patient reports a sensation of blood trickling down the back of the throat, especially after an anterior pack has been placed.

### Initial Treatment

The initial approach to epistaxis is outlined in Table 203-3. Additional details regarding these steps can be found in the discussion below and in the section on the treatment of anterior epistaxis. The emergency department treatment for posterior epistaxis is posterior nasal packing. Direct pressure is ineffective. The use of vasoconstrictive and anesthetic agents in the initial treatment of posterior epistaxis is the same as for anterior bleeding.

The use of chemical, thermal, or electrocautery by an emergency physician in cases of posterior epistaxis should be discouraged. First, posterior bleeding tends to be more severe than that from an anterior source, and cautery is difficult, if not impossible, in an actively bleeding patient. Second, attempts to cauterize a posterior vessel are likely to lead to more severe bleeding. Finally, it is often difficult to visualize the bleeding site in posterior epistaxis. The use of blind chemical, heat, or electrocautery is dangerous and can result in severe damage to the posterior nasal structures.

### Posterior Nasal Packing

A posterior nasal pack should be inserted in anyone who has suspected posterior nasal hemorrhage. This includes patients in whom a bleeding site cannot be identified, patients who continue to bleed after an anterior source has been ruled out by direct visualization, and patients who continue to bleed after an anterior pack has been inserted. Another indication for posterior packing occurs when it is needed to act as a buttress for an anterior pack, to prevent the posterior displacement of gauze.

#### Procedure

In the past, many physicians were taught to construct a posterior nasal pack using a gauze roll and silk ties as detailed in Fig. 203-5. In actual practice, however, this can be a time-consuming, complicated, and frustrating venture. In addition, the availability of many commercial products has made this exercise largely unnecessary. Most commercial devices, such as the Nasostat epistaxis balloon (Sparta Surgical Corp., Hayward, CA) or the Storz epistaxis catheter (Storz Instrument Co., St. Louis, MO), provide both anterior and posterior tamponade by using two independently inflatable balloons (Fig. 203-6). These devices allow for the rapid control of refractory epistaxis with a minimum of preparation. The procedure for their insertion is as follows:

1. The nasal cavity is adequately prepared with vasoconstrictors and anesthetic agents as previously described.
2. A test is made for leakage by filling the anterior balloon with 25 mL of water and the posterior balloon with 8 mL of water. If no leak is detected, the water is removed from the balloons.
3. The device is lubricated and inserted into the nasopharynx. The patient opens his or her mouth, and the device is advanced until the distal balloon tip is visible in the posterior pharynx.
4. The posterior balloon is slowly filled with 4 to 8 mL of water, and the device is pulled forward to wedge it in the posterior nasopharynx.
5. While gentle tension is maintained, the anterior balloon is slowly inflated with 10 to 25 mL of water to provide anterior tamponade. Inflation should be stopped immediately if the patient complains of significant pain. Be aware, however, that some discomfort is usually present.
6. Bilateral packing may be necessary to stop the bleeding in some patients.

The Merocel nasal sponge is also effective in the treatment of posterior epistaxis. See the discussion on anterior epistaxis for more information on its use.

If a commercial device is not available, an excellent posterior pack can be constructed using a simple Foley catheter. The procedure is as follows:

1. The nasal cavity is adequately prepared with vasoconstrictors and anesthetic agents as previously described.
2. The distal tip of a standard 12F or 16F Foley catheter with a 30-mL balloon is cut off to minimize stimulation of the posterior pharynx and minimize gagging after insertion.
3. The balloon is tested for leakage by filling it with 15 mL of water. If no leak is present the water is removed.
4. The catheter is lubricated and inserted into the nasopharynx. The patient opens his or her mouth, and the catheter is advanced until the balloon is visible in the posterior pharynx.
5. The balloon is slowly filled with between 4 and 8 mL of water, and the catheter is pulled forward to wedge it in the posterior nasopharynx.
6. While gentle tension is maintained on the catheter, standard petrolatum-impregnated gauze is used for anterior packing as previously described.
7. Gauze padding is placed over the nasal alae and columella, and a plastic umbilical clamp (commonly referred to as a Hollister clamp) is placed to prevent deflation of the balloon. If such a clamp is not available, then several knots can be tied and the remaining end is cut off. It is necessary for slight tension to be maintained to ensure good placement of the posterior balloon.

**Complications**

There have been serious complications associated with the use of posterior nasal packs. Among the problems reported are patient hypoventilation with resultant hypoxia and/or hypercarbia, cardiac arrhythmias, cardiac arrest, infection, severe patient discomfort, dysphagia, accidental dislodgment into the airway, and aseptic necrosis of the nasal alae, columella, palate, or nasal mucosa.

**Removal of Posterior Nasal Packing**

In general, posterior nasal packs should not be left in place for more than 2 to 3 days. The task of removal is usually left to the consulting otolaryngologist.

## Specialized Techniques

If epistaxis is refractory to all of the above attempts at control, more extensive and specialized techniques may be called for. Surgical arterial ligation of the vessels that supply the nasal cavity is regarded as the last resort for the control of nasal hemorrhage. The anterior and posterior ethmoidal arteries may be ligated in cases of uncontrollable anterior epistaxis. In posterior epistaxis, one of three techniques may be used: (1) external carotid artery ligation, (2) transantral ligation of the maxillary artery, or (3) intraoral ligation of the maxillary artery. If the site of bleeding cannot be determined, the ethmoidal arteries are ligated in conjunction with the maxillary artery.

With modern advances in digital subtraction angiography, a less drastic option has recently become available for the treatment of recalcitrant posterior epistaxis. Transarterial embolization of the vessels that supply the bleeding site can be performed under local anesthesia and has a complication rate as low as 0.1 percent in experienced hands. Embolization cannot be used for the treatment of anterior epistaxis, since the blood supply to the anterior septum arises from the anterior and posterior ethmoidal arteries. These vessels receive their blood from the internal carotid system via the ophthalmic artery, and the potential complications associated with catheterization preclude this approach.

## Admission Indications

All patients with posterior epistaxis should have immediate consultation with an otolaryngologist. Although relatively uncomplicated, the placement of posterior nasal packing is not a benign procedure and complications may be serious. This is especially true in patients with preexisting chronic obstructive pulmonary disease. Although postulated, the presence of a "nasopulmonary reflex" has yet to be confirmed.

Because of the significant morbidity and mortality associated with this procedure, patients who have had a posterior nasal pack inserted may be admitted to the hospital for close observation. In addition, patients with nasal packing of any kind should receive antibiotics as prophylaxis against sinusitis.

## NASAL FRACTURE

### Pathophysiology

The trauma that produces a fracture of the nasal bones may come from a frontal, superior to inferior, or lateral direction. Of these mechanisms, laterally directed trauma is most likely to cause a fracture since there is no cartilage to absorb or dissipate the impact energy. The pattern and extent of a resulting break vary according to the site, direction, and intensity of the impact as well as the characteristics of the bone that is struck. This latter consideration is a function of age, in which a younger patient's bones have greater density and elasticity and an older patient's bones have less.

### Clinical Features

#### History

Nasal fractures should be suspected in all patients with significant facial trauma. In adults, a broken nose is most likely to result from an interpersonal altercation or sports injury, while motor vehicle accidents, falls, and other mechanisms are less common. In children, play and sports injuries predominate. Trauma inflicted on a child may also be the result of physical abuse.

## Physical Examination

Findings suggestive of a nasal fracture include swelling, tenderness, crepitance, ecchymosis, or deformity of the nose. There may also be indirect evidence of nasal trauma such as periorbital ecchymosis, epistaxis, rhinorrhea, or other associated injuries to the face. Al-though many systems have been proposed to classify the severity of nasal fractures and predict treatment outcome, all require complex criteria and are not practical for the emergency physician. The complications of a nasal fracture include the development of a septal hematoma, cribriform plate fracture, and associated facial or spinal injuries.

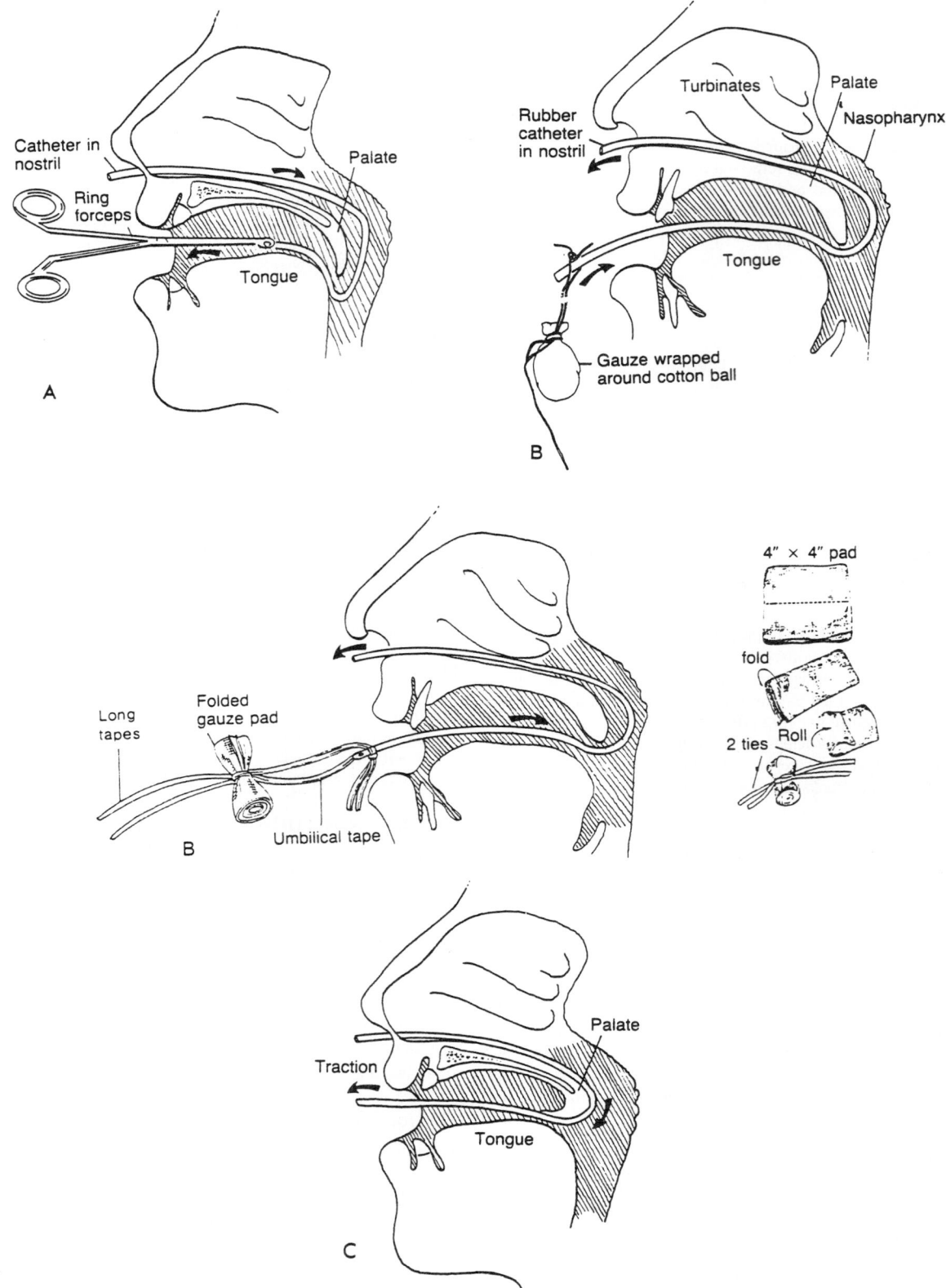

**Fig. 203-5.**

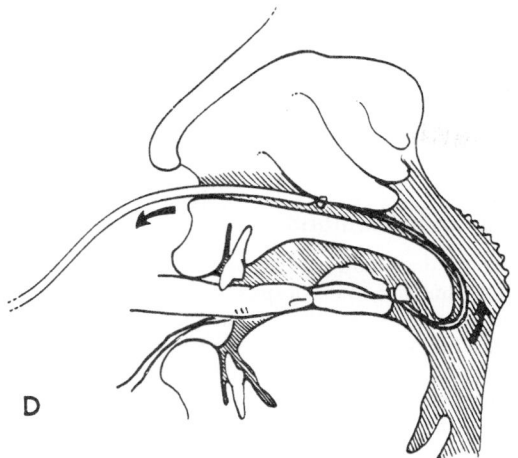

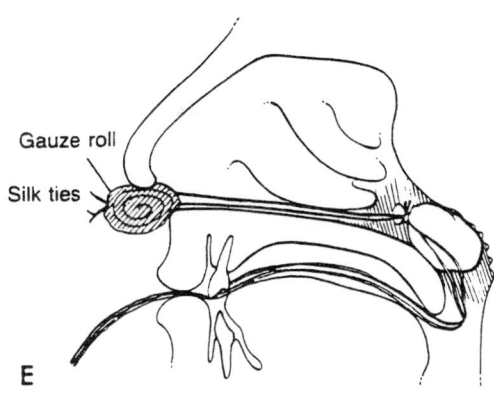

**Fig. 203-5.** Posterior nasal pack. **A.** Following topical anesthesia, a red rubber catheter is passed through the nose and carefully grasped in the oral pharynx with ringed forceps and brought out through the mouth. **B, Upper.** A posterior nasal pack made by wrapping a cotton ball in a 4-in by 4-in gauze pad and tying two long silk sutures or umbilical tapes around the neck of the pack. **Lower.** Alternatively, a gauze pad can be folded and rolled into a cylinder and tied with two strings. Two of the strings are used to tie the pack to the tip of the catheter. **C.** As an option, a second catheter, which has been passed through the nonbleeding side and brought out the mouth, can be used to retract the palate forward to aid in the placement of the pack (not shown). The optional catheter is removed after the pack is in the proper position. **D.** The finger is used to guide the pack through the

mouth and into the proper position as traction on the catheter pulls the pack from above. This uncomfortable step is the most difficult of the procedure and must be performed deliberately and smoothly. If the patient has teeth, a dental roll or bite block is placed to prevent the patient from biting the physician's finger. **E.** Proper position of the posterior pack, wedged in the posterior portion of the nose. A long strand attached to the pack exits from the mouth and is taped to the cheek. If the pack slips posteriorly, the mouth string is pulled to prevent suffocation. A large gauze pad or roll is used to keep slight tension on the pack (after the anterior pack has been placed). A large roll is used to prevent pressure necrosis on the nasal ala and columella.

## Complications

### Septal Hematoma

Development of a septal hematoma is a rare but serious complication of nasal trauma. This is a collection of blood beneath the perichondrium and is easily identified on physical examination by the presence of a bluish, fluid-filled sac overlying the nasal septum. Such a hematoma is easily managed by making an incision to allow adequate drainage, followed by packing of the anterior nasal cavity to prevent the reaccumulation of blood (Fig. 203-7). If untreated, a septal hematoma may progress to form an abscess or result in avascular necrosis of the nasal septum in as little as 3 to 4 days. This latter complication is associated with a saddlenose deformity, retraction of the columella, and changes in phonation.

### Fracture of the Cribriform Plate

Another significant injury associated with nasal trauma involves a fracture through the cribriform plate of the ethmoid bone. In this fracture, cerebrospinal fluid (CSF) may leak through torn meninges, and this represents a violation in the integrity of the subarachnoid space. Cerebrospinal fluid rhinorrhea should be suspected in any patient who presents with a clear nasal discharge following facial injury. Although it may start days or weeks following the traumatic event, CSF rhinorrhea usually manifests itself within the first week as cerebral edema resolves. If left untreated, possible sequelae include the development of meningoencephalitis or a brain abscess. Fortunately, this injury is rare.

The identification of CSF rhinorrhea can be a problem in nasal injuries because it is not unusual for there to be a clear transudate from the traumatized nasal mucosa. Medical tradition has taught that one method of detecting CSF is to put a drop of the suspected liquid on a piece of filter paper and see if a clear area surrounds a central blood stain. This so-called ring test is unreliable and should not be used to

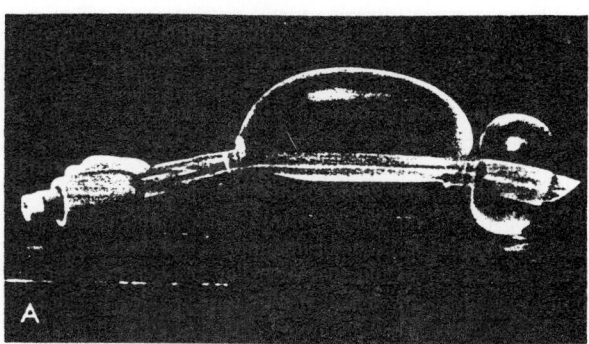

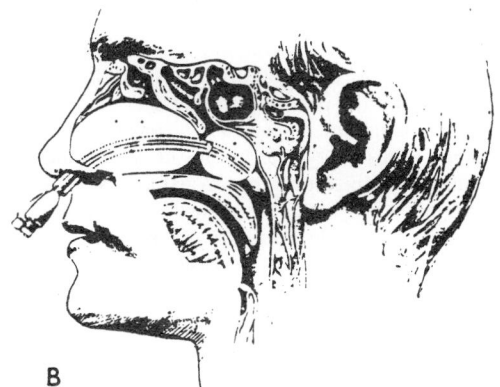

**Fig. 203-6. A.** and **B.** The balloon tamponade device serves as both an anterior and posterior pack. It is easily inserted and is often successful for the temporary control of posterior epistaxis in the emergency department. The balloon shown here is the Epistat balloon. (*Courtesy of Exomed Inc., Jacksonville, FL.*)

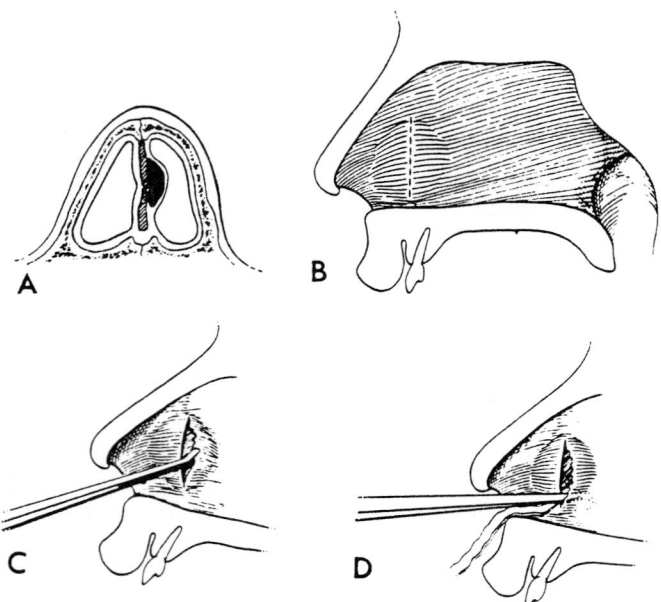

**Fig. 203-7. A.** A small left-sided septal hematoma. **B.** After applying appropriate topical anesthesia, supplemented with local infiltrative anesthesia if necessary, an incision is made through the mucosa and the perichondrium covering the hematoma. **C.** A small cup forceps or scissor is used to remove enough mucosa to help prevent premature closure of the wound and reaccumulation of hematoma. **D.** A sterile rubber band is then placed as a drain, and the nares is packed as described in the section "Anterior Epistaxis."

confirm or exclude the diagnosis. Another part of medical folklore states that CSF can be detected by using a glucose reagent strip. If the glucose content of suspected fluid is greater than 30 mg/dL, then the presence of CSF is confirmed. This test also has its limitations and should not be used to exclude the diagnosis either.

The most accurate way to diagnose CSF rhinorrhea is through the use of metrizamide computed tomography cisternography (MCTC), a highly specialized procedure involving the injection of contrast dye into the subarachnoid space. The diagnosis is confirmed if there is radiographic demonstration of extracranial CSF extravasation. If a fracture of the cribriform plate is clinically suspected, the patient should be placed in an upright position, intranasal packing avoided, and immediate neurosurgical consultation obtained. Coughing, sneezing, nose blowing, and straining by the patient should be avoided.

## Other Complications

Other injuries associated with nasal trauma include blowout fractures of the orbital floor, isolated orbital floor fractures, tripod fractures of the zygomatic bone, and open nasal fractures. The emergency physician should also be suspicious of a cervical spine or closed head injury in any patient who has received significant facial trauma.

## Treatment/Emergency Department Care

A simple, nondisplaced fracture of the nasal bones does not require any treatment other than mild analgesia, protection from further injury, and possibly over-the-counter nasal decongestants. If significant bleeding is present, then an anterior nasal pack, as for uncomplicated epistaxis, should be inserted.

If the patient has a displaced nasal fracture, there may be so much soft tissue swelling that it is impossible to provide definitive treatment in the emergency department. Such swelling tends to prohibit a good evaluation of the amount of displacement and makes the assessment of any subsequent reduction extremely difficult. In these cases,

the patient may be given oral analgesics, advised to avoid further injury, and have an over-the-counter nasal decongestant prescribed. The patient is then advised to follow up with an appropriate specialist once the swelling has subsided, usually in 2 to 5 days. Reduction of displaced nasal fractures should be performed by a plastic surgeon, otolaryngologist, or oral and maxillofacial surgeon.

## Admission Indications

A fracture of the nasal bones, even with displacement, is not an indication for admission to the hospital. Of concern, however, is the presence of some coexisting injury such as a cribriform plate fracture, closed head injury, or cervical spine fracture. One of the emergency physician's primary tasks in treating nasal fractures is to rule out these other causes of significant morbidity.

## Discharge Instructions

The patient is advised to begin measures to reduce the swelling as soon as possible. These modalities include the application of ice packs to the face and elevation of the head. In addition, the patient should be given standard head injury instructions and advised to watch for the onset of CSF rhinorrhea.

## Ambulatory Treatment

A summary of the ambulatory treatment for nasal fractures is as follows:

Ice to the area of swelling for 24 to 48 h
Head elevation, including when asleep
Over-the-counter nasal decongestants as necessary. The patient should be advised not use these agents for more than 3 days to reduce the possibility of a rebound phenomenon).

## Follow-up Care

The patient should follow up with a plastic surgeon, otolaryngologist, or oral and maxillofacial surgeon once the swelling has subsided, usually in 3 to 5 days. Although nondisplaced fractures rarely need further treatment, follow-up should be provided due to the cosmetic importance of the injury.

## FOREIGN BODIES

### Pathophysiology

A nasal foreign body is the most common cause of nasal obstruction in children. Items that may be found in the nose are limited only by a child's imagination and the persistence necessary to insert an object where it does not belong. Dried beans and vegetable matter are especially worrisome because they tend to absorb water and swell, enhancing discomfort and making removal extremely difficult. Common nasal foreign bodies include buttons, button batteries, beads, fabric scraps, beans, vegetable matter, toys, toy parts, and any other object small enough to fit past the nasal vestibule.

### Clinical Features

#### History

When obtaining the history, interact with the child in a nonjudgmental manner. Many children are hesitant to admit placing an object in the nose for fear they will elicit displeasure from their parents or the physician. The following aspects of a patient's history should make an emergency physician suspicious of the diagnosis:

The sensation of a nasal obstruction, especially if unilateral

Persistent, foul-smelling rhinorrhea that recurs despite the use of antibiotics

Persistent unilateral epistaxis

## Physical Examination

The nasal mucosa is prepared with vasoconstrictors and anesthetics by nasal spray or atomizer (see below). Following this, visualization of the nasopharynx with an appropriately sized speculum is attempted.

## Diagnosis/Differential Diagnosis

The diagnosis of a nasal foreign body is best made by direct visualization of the offending object. If a child is especially young or uncooperative, a plain radiograph of the skull may demonstrate the presence of a radiopaque object. If the radiograph is negative but strong clinical suspicion exists, the patient should follow up with an otolaryngologist to further explore the possibility of a radiolucent foreign body.

In a child with nasal obstruction and persistent rhinorrhea, the differential diagnosis includes tumors (both benign and malignant), abscess of the nasal septum, and chronic sinusitis.

## Treatment/Emergency Department Care

If the child is cooperative and the foreign body visible, it may be possible to remove it in the emergency department. The procedure for this is as follows:

1. The mucosa is prepared and anesthetized by spraying the nasal cavity with a children's nasal decongestant [0.25% phenylephrine mixed with a *small amount* of 4% xylocaine is a good choice (see Table 203-4)]. Pledget insertion should not be attempted as this may push the object further back or dislodge it posteriorly, resulting in aspiration.
2. Using an appropriately sized speculum, the foreign body is visualized within the nasal cavity.
3. If the object appears to be loose after vasoconstriction, the tip of a suction catheter may be used to try and remove it.
4. If the object is small and irregularly shaped, it may be possible to grasp it with a bayonet or alligator forceps. Care must be taken not to push the object further back into the nasopharynx.
5. If the object is round and/or smooth and is difficult to remove using the above two methods, a small hooked instrument may be used to facilitate removal (Fig. 203-8).
6. If necessary, a number 4 Fogarty vascular catheter can be inserted past the foreign body, the balloon inflated, and traction applied to loosen or remove it. Alternatively, the balloon may be inflated and used as a buttress to prevent pushing the object further back as other techniques are tried.
7. If the child is uncooperative, conscious sedation may be administered (see Chap. 43).
8. If the above measures are unsuccessful, the patient should be referred to an otolaryngologist.

## Admission Indications

Despite the anxiety generated in the mind of the parent, a nasal foreign body is relatively benign and can await referral to an otolaryngologist the next day if removal has been unsuccessful. If there is any concern that the foreign body might prolapse into the oropharynx and be aspirated, or if the child should exhibit any constitutional symptoms (such as fever, malaise, lethargy, etc.), immediate consultation with an otolaryngologist for evaluation and possible admission is mandatory.

## Discharge Instructions

After removal of the foreign body, the child should be cautioned not to insert further objects into his or her nose. The parents should be advised to keep all items small enough to be swallowed, aspirated, or inserted into body orifices away from the child and in a safe place.

## Ambulatory Treatment

No further treatment is needed after a foreign body has been removed. Antibiotics are not required because the persistent rhinorrhea usually resolves in a few days. Nasal decongestants are also not necessary.

## Follow-up Care

Following the successful removal of a foreign body from the nose, no follow-up is required. If the emergency physician has been unsuccessful in his attempts to remove the object and there is no evidence of constitutional symptoms or concern that the foreign body might be aspirated, the patient may follow up with an otolaryngologist in 1 or 2 days.

## SINUSITIS

### Pathophysiology

Sinusitis occurs when there is an acute obstruction of the normal drainage mechanism of the paranasal sinuses. This mechanism consists of three elements: the patency of the ostia, the function of the ciliary apparatus, and the quality of the nasal secretions. Although problems may occur following a malfunction in any one of these components, obstruction is most common and is frequently produced by a viral rhinitis. Edema from the rhinitis produces a dysfunction of the osteomeatal complex, a confluence of the drainage openings from the frontal, ethmoidal, and maxillary sinuses.

Following obstruction, the air in the sinus is reabsorbed and the resulting negative pressure produces a collection of transudate. The sinuses are usually sterile, but bacteria may be present and multiply, resulting in suppuration. Acute sinusitis is said to occur in patients who have had typical signs and symptoms of infection for less than 3 weeks and is usually caused by *Haemophilus influenzae, Streptococ-*

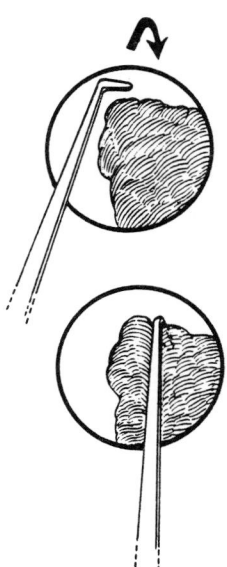

**Fig. 203-8.** Hook technique for foreign body removal. Under direct vision a small, blunt, right-angle hook is passed between the foreign body and the nasal mucosa. After the tip is past the foreign body, it is rotated 90° and withdrawn.

cus pneumoniae, Strep. pyogenes, Staphylococcus aureus, or Branhamella catarrhalis. Chronic sinusitis is said to occur if signs and symptoms persist for longer than 3 weeks and is more likely to involve infection with an anaerobic organism such as Corynebacterium, Bacteroides, and Veillonnella species.

## Clinical Features

### History

Classically, patients with acute sinusitis complain of pain overlying the affected area, with maxillary sinusitis causing discomfort beneath the eyes and frontal sinusitis resulting in pain along the supraorbital ridge and lower forehead. Surprisingly, most of the classic signs and symptoms thought to indicate sinusitis have been found to be poor indicators of infection. The best predictors are maxillary toothache, poor response to nasal decongestants, a history of colored nasal discharge, and abnormal transillumination. There is a poor correlation between the presence of bacterial infection and the quality, intensity, or radiation of facial pain.

Ethmoid sinusitis, which is especially serious in children because of its tendency to extend toward the retroorbital area and central nervous system, tends to produce a "dull and aching" sensation behind the eyes. The presence of fever and chills suggests the extension of infection. Isolated sphenoidal sinusitis is extremely uncommon and is accompanied by vague signs and symptoms. Chronic sinusitus is usually associated with nonspecific symptoms, although a chronic, purulent exudate is usually a prominent feature.

### Physical Examination

The physical examination usually demonstrates evidence of an underlying infection. Specifically, the emergency physician may find erythema, warmth, and tenderness to palpation/percussion over the involved sinus. Direct visualization of the nasal cavity often reveals a swollen, erythematous mucosa with purulent exudate draining from the ostia. There is also diminished transillumination of the affected sinus.

## Diagnosis/Differential Diagnosis

In most cases, the diagnosis of acute sinusitis is made by the history and physical examination. A recent study by Williams and Simel has demonstrated that the findings of sinusitus on x-ray are extremely variable and accurately predict infection only 72 to 96 percent of the time. The radiographic findings that are most reliable include sinus opacity, an air-fluid level, or at least 6 mm of mucosal thickening.

The absence of radiographic evidence does not exclude the diagnosis. It has also been shown that a single Water view is almost as good at detecting sinusitus as a full sinus series. In children less than 6 years of age, the sinuses are not fully developed and radiographs commonly appear abnormal regardless of the presence or absence of disease.

The differential diagnosis in a patient who presents with signs and symptoms of acute sinusitis includes:

Uncomplicated viral rhinitis
Uncomplicated allergic rhinitis
Chemical rhinitis (from inhalation of irritants)
Traumatic rhinitis
Tension headache
Nasal foreign bodies
Tumors
Nasal polyps
Brain abscess
Fungal infection (especially in the immunocompromised patient)

## Treatment/Emergency Department Care

The initial insufflation of a common, over-the-counter nasal decongestant such as oxymetazoline (Afrin), 0.05%, or phenylephrine (Neo-Synephrine), 0.5% to 1.0%, can provide significant and immediate relief while the patient is still in the emergency department.

## Admission Indications

Any patient who shows evidence that an infection has spread beyond the sinus cavity should be admitted to the hospital. These patients usually present with a toxic appearance and may appear to have an orbital/periorbital cellulitis or facial abscess. Frontal sinusitus can lead to osteomyelitis of the posterior table of the frontal bone and produce a meningitis, epidural abscess, subdural empyema, or brain abscess. Finally, there may be destruction of the anterior table of the skull with the formation of a large forehead abscess, sometimes referred to as Pott puffy tumor.

## Discharge Instructions

The following instructions should be given to patients with acute sinusitis:

1. The patient should use a cool-mist vaporizer or humidifier to add moisture to the ambient air. With proper use, fabrics in the room should feel slightly damp.
2. Warm compresses to the face may be applied as necessary to provide relief from pain or discomfort. Nonnarcotic analgesics may also be used as directed on the package.
3. The patient should be advised to blow the nose gently. For infants and children, a nasal bulb aspirator and saline may be used to clear thick secretions.
4. Over-the-counter nasal sprays such as oxymetazoline (Afrin) or phenylephrine (Neo-Synephrine) may provide significant relief, especially if used just prior to bedtime. The patient should be advised not to use these preparations for more than 3 days to avoid the occurrence of a rebound phenomenon.
5. The patient should drink plenty of fluids.
6. An immediate return to the emergency department is necessary if it appears the infection has extended beyond the sinus cavity. Such signs and symptoms include high fever, blurred vision, lethargy, and vomiting. Worsening of the erythema, warmth, and swelling of the face despite antibiotics also necessitates a return visit to the emergency department.

## Ambulatory Treatment

Antibiotics have been shown to be effective in patients with bacterial sinusitus. A common choice is ampicillin (250 to 500 mg orally, every 6 h for 10 days) or amoxicillin/clavulanate (250 to 500 mg three times a day for 10 days). In patients who are allergic to penicillin, the emergency physician may prescribe erythromycin (250 to 500 mg, four times a day for 10 days), cephalexin (250 to 500 mg four times a day for 10 days), or trimethoprim/sulfamethoxazole DS (one tablet twice a day for 10 days).

## Follow-up Care

Patients should be advised to follow up with their regular physician or an otolaryngologist if their symptoms persist for longer than 5 to 7 days despite the use of antibiotics. Patients who have evidence of chronic sinusitis (i.e., symptoms for longer than 3 weeks) and who do not appear toxic should follow up with an otolaryngologist within 2 to 3 days.

# BIBLIOGRAPHY

Bailey BJ, Johnson JT, Kohut RI, et al: *Head and Neck Surgery—Otolaryngology.* Philadelphia, Lippincott, 1993.

Cummings CW, Fredrickson JM, Harker LA, et al: *Otolaryngology—Head and Neck Surgery.* St. Louis, Mosby Year Book, 1993.

Montogmery WW, Reardon EJ: Early vessel ligations for control of severe epistaxis, in Snow JB (ed): *Controversy in Otolaryngology.* Philadelphia, Saunders, 1980.

Roberts JR, Hedges JR: *Clinical Procedures in Emergency Medicine,* 2d ed. Philadelphia, Saunders, 1991.

Toner JG, et al: Comparison of electro and chemical cautery in the treatment of anterior epistaxis. *J Laryngol Otol* 104(8):616, 1990.

Wald ER: Sinusitis in children. *N Engl J Med* 326:5, 319, 1992.

Williams JW, Simel DL: Does this patient have sinusitis? Diagnosing acute sinusitis by history and physical examination. *JAMA* 270(10):1242, 1993.

# 204
# MAXILLOFACIAL TRAUMA
## Barry H. Hendler

## GENERAL PRINCIPLES

The patient's general medical condition must always be the primary concern in the immediate posttraumatic phase of facial injury. It is rare for a patient to die as a direct result of maxillofacial injuries, yet because of the alarming nature, grotesqueness, and apparent severity of facial injuries, personnel may give these injuries priority over more critical problems.

In the absence of gross soft tissue injury, facial fractures are most often treated several days after initial assessment when the soft tissue swelling resolves and an accurate plan for reduction can be developed through definitive radiological evaluation and patient assessment. Three basic principles of treatment are (1) preservation of life; (2) maintenance of function, specifically the masticatory apparatus; and (3) restoration of appearance.

## SOFT TISSUE INJURIES

After initial stabilization, attention may be directed to the specific sites of the maxillofacial injury, with assessment of any associated bony injuries or damage to vital structures such as the facial nerve and the parotid and submandibular ducts. The adequate assessment of specific soft tissue injuries may require local anesthesia prior to inspection. Soft tissue contusions usually heal well with conservative management. Abrasions should be thoroughly irrigated with normal saline, 1% betadine, or 50% hydrogen peroxide diluted in normal saline in a pulsatile fashion. After debridement of the wound, it should be covered with a triple antibiotic ointment. Reepithelialization usually occurs within 7 to 10 days.

All injured and lacerated tissues should be retained until the final plan for definitive surgical repair has been formulated. Foreign bodies within the wound should be removed, followed by copious irrigation to the depth of the wound margins. This is followed by debridement of necrotic or severely avulsed tissue, while smaller avulsive defects may be retained by local undermining and advancement of adjacent tissue (local flaps). Stellate or contused tissue margins often require debridement or "freshening of the edges" in order to obtain a clean edge-to-edge primary closure. Areas of hemorrhage should be controlled with local pressure, the use of cautery, or suture ligatures. See Chaps. 44 and 45 for details of wound management.

## Antibiotic Prophylaxis

Antibiotics may not be necessary for clean wounds or for those that have occured within 24 h of presentation to the emergency room. For those injuries considered clean-contaminated, contaminated, or dirty or for those more than 24-h old, antibiotics should be given, since the incidence of infection is directly proportional to the classification of the wound and the time elapsed since injury.

Oral soft tissue injuries may require the administration of adjunctive antibiotics because of potential for contamination of the wound by the multibacterial oral secretions. Penicillin remains the antibiotic of choice for prophylaxis against this flora. Overlying skin lacerations are better treated with a first-generation cephalosporin to cover staphyloccocus.

## Regional Anesthesia

Simple lacerations may be amenable to the use of local anesthesia, usually lidocaine 1% to 2%, injected through the edges of the laceration. A vasoconstrictor (epinephrine 1:100,000) may be used for hemostasis in certain instances but should be avoided at wound margins in areas with a questionable blood supply. Care must be taken to avoid distortion of the wound margins with local anesthetic solution, which may result in a poor cosmetic result.

When more complicated primary repair under local anesthesia is performed, the use of regional nerve blocks should be considered. The advantages include a decrease in the total anesthetic dosage, avoidance of tissue distortion at the site of injury, and a decrease in wound edge edema, resulting in better healing.

The various regions of the oral cavity may be anesthetized with infiltration or via the use of regional techniques including inferior alveolar, mental, and lingual nerve blocks. The use of infiltration anesthesia is usually reserved for the maxilla, where the solution is injected in a supraperiosteal location, and the thin porous cortex and highly vascular bone permits diffusion and uptake of the anesthetic to the root apices of the maxillary teeth.

The inferior alveolar nerve block, (mandibular block), is performed to anesthetize the teeth and gingiva on the side of the block. The needle is directed just lateral to the pterygomandibular raphe at approximately 1 cm above the occlusal surfaces of the mandibular teeth and advanced until bone is contacted (Fig. 204-1). The syringe is aspirated to rule out intravascular placement, and then the solution is injected.

The lingual nerve can be anesthetized during the administration of the inferior alveolar block by injecting anesthetic as the needle is withdrawn. Alternatively, the lingual nerve can be blocked by injecting anesthetic in the posterolateral floor of the mouth, or the region just lingual to the premolar teeth.

The mental nerve block will anesthetize the anterior mandibular teeth and gingiva in front of the mental foramen, which usually lies between the root apices of the first and second premolar teeth, (Fig. 204-2). Therefore, the needle is directed to a point in the mandibular mucobuccal fold inferior to the premolar teeth in the region of the mental foramen. A spray of benzocaine aerosol (Cetacaine) on the oral mucosa will make these injections almost painless.

## Lip Lacerations

Lacerations of the lip can result in signficant cosmetic deformity, especially since secondary revision is often difficult after primary healing is complete. Despite aggressive irrigation and debridement, a lip laceration will not remain clean during repair because of oral contamination, and antibiotic prophylaxis is uaually considered. Regional

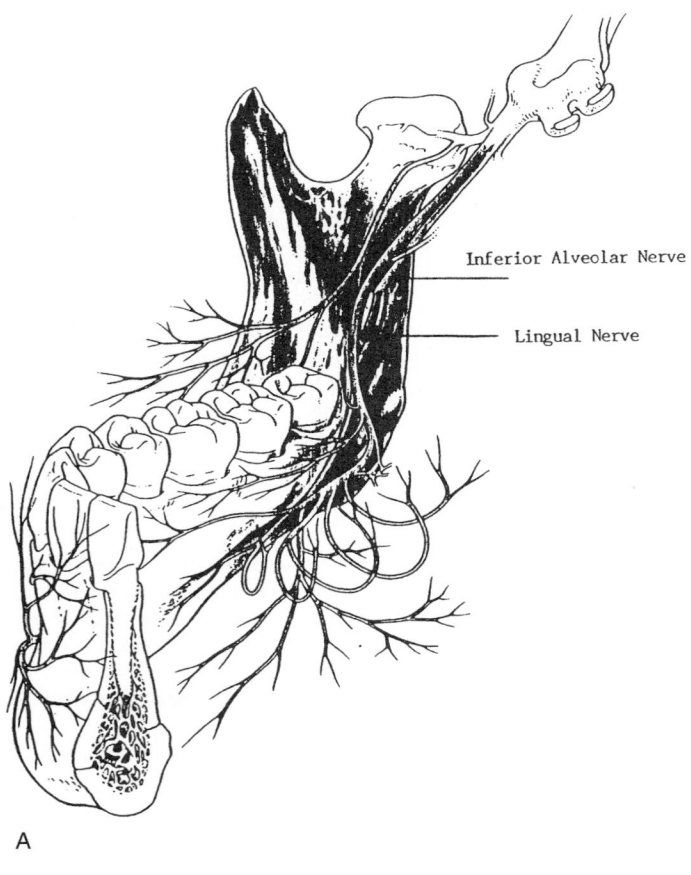

Inferior Alveolar Nerve

Lingual Nerve

A

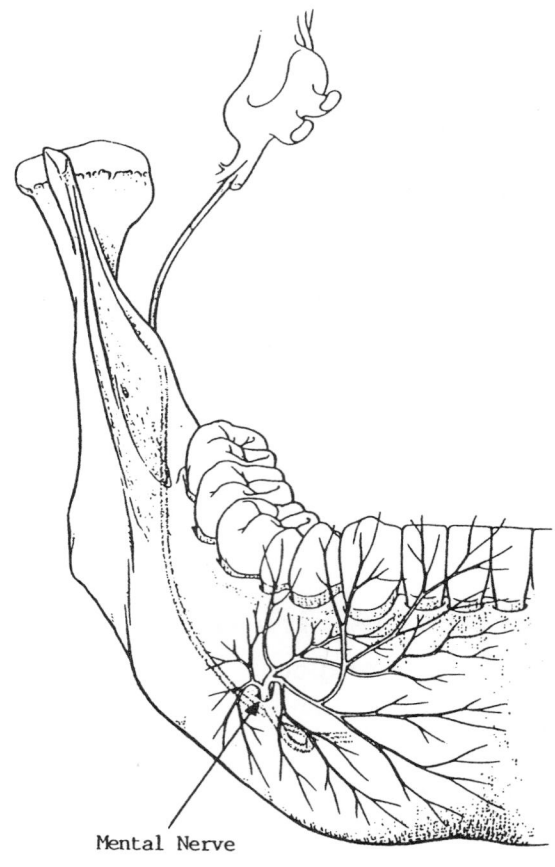

Mental Nerve

A

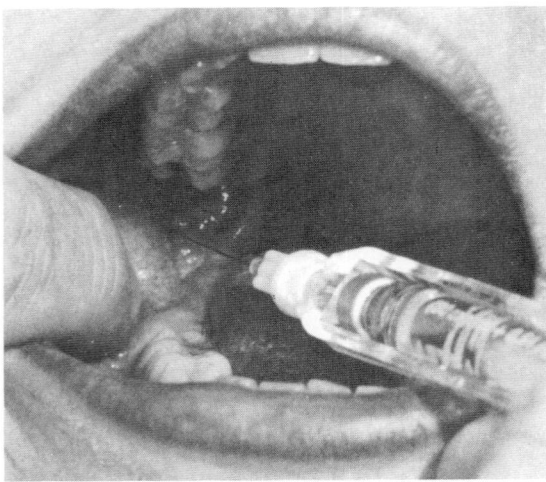

B

**Fig. 204-1. A.** This drawing shows the anatomic position of the inferior alveolar nerve and the lingual nerve as they course along the inner aspect of the ramus of the mandible. The alveolar nerve divides into branches that enter the mandibular foramen and course along the mylohyoid groove of the mandible. The lingual nerve curves inward to course along the floor of the mouth. The buttressing ridge of the coronoid process serves as a landmark for these nerves. **B.** A regional block is being obtained by injecting local anesthetic just behind the buttressing ridge of the coronoid process about 1 cm above the molars of the mandible.

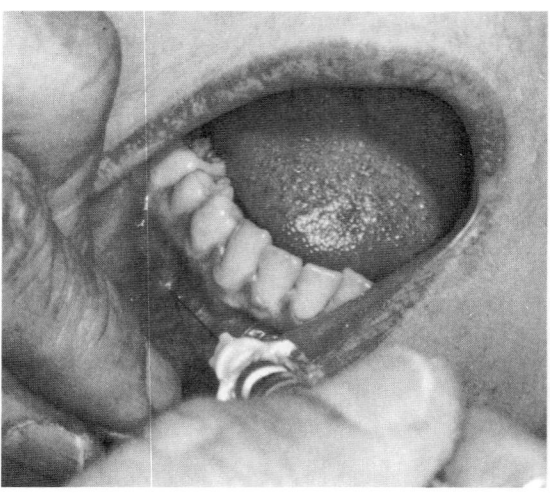

B

**Fig. 204-2. A.** Branches of the alveolar nerve are shown exiting the mental foramen of the right mandible. A regional block of these branches will provide anesthesia of the lower lip as well as dental anesthesia. **B.** An injection of local anesthetic is being directed towards the root apex of the first premolar tooth through the mucobuccal fold.

anesthesia for repair of upper lip lacerations may be accomplished with infiltration nerve blocks in the mucolabial fold. When the avoidance of tissue distortion is critical for lower lip injury, bilateral mental nerve blocks are indicated. Since lip lacerations can occur secondary to blunt trauma where teeth are responsible for cutting the lip, devitalized and contaminated tissue should be carefully debrided, while associated damage to teeth or alveolar bone should be assessed and tooth fragments or other foreign bodies removed.

In general, up to one-third of the lower lip can be removed during debridement, or as a result of an avulsive injury, and closed primarily without cosmetic deformity. The upper lip, due to its intimate association with the philtrum, columella, and alar bases, is less amenable to even minimal tissue loss. Upper lip defects may be secondarily reconstructed using local tissue flaps or skin grafts.

After debridement, closure is performed in layers. The first, and most critical, suture is placed to reapproximate the vermilion border (junction of skin and lip mucosa) using a nonresorbable suture of 5–0 monofilament nylon. The importance of this step cannot be overemphasized since misalignment of even 1 to 2 mm will be easily noticed and cosmetically unacceptable. The next important suture is placed at the wet-dry line (junction of lip and intraoral mucosa). Lacerations of the orbicularis oris muscle require layered closure with reapproximation using deep 4–0 or 5–0 absorbable gut or polyglycolic acid suture to restore function. Through-and-through laccerations are closed from the inside out. After placement of the two key sutures, the intraoral mucosa is closed with 4–0 resorbable sutures, the entire wound is thoroughly irrigated once again, and the remainder of the lip laceration is closed extraorally with 4–0 or 5–0 monofilament nylon. Antibiotic ointment is placed on the lip post repair for 1 to 2 weeks. The nonresorable sutures are usually removed in approximately 5 days.

## Oral Mucosal Lacerations

Almost any injury within the oral cavity poses the potential threat of airway obstruction. Inspection of the oral cavity requires assessment of associated injuries to other structures, including both hard and soft tissues. If teeth are fractured, all fragments must be accounted for; if doubt exists regarding the presence of tooth or bone fragments or foreign bodies (e.g., amalgam silver fillings) in the oral soft tissues, radiological examination may be performed for localization.

In general, small intraoral mucosal lacerations between 1 and 2 cm will heal without primary repair if the wound edges are not significantly separated. Larger lacerations may be repaired using 4–0 resorable sutures to approximate the wound edges. Copious irrigation is initially performed, but extensive debridement is usually not necessary. Gingival lacerations are repaired easily with the use of the remaining teeth as guides for proper repositioning. Intraoral trauma mandates evaluation of submandibular duct patency in the anterior floor of the mouth, as well as the parotid (Stensen) duct orifice in the posterior buccal mucosa. If injury is suspected, cannulation and sialography using water-soluble nonionic contrast dye may be performed. Salivary duct lacerations may be repaired primarily over a stent (e.g., a plastic angiocath) which is removed in 7 to 10 days as long as adequate salivary flow is demonstrated. When a salivary duct injury is suspected, consultation with an oral and maxillofacial surgeon would be prudent.

Anesthesia for oral mucosal lacerations depends on the site of the injury and may be performed through infiltration in the area of the laceration, since the mucosa is generally mobile and distortion of tissue usually does not pose a problem. In specific areas, regional nerve blocks may be performed using inferior alveolar or mental nerve blocks.

Oral mucosal lacerations heal well despite the multibacterial flora of the oral cavity. Penicillin prophylaxis is usually prescribed. Patients should be instructed to rinse their mouths frequently with a mouthwash solution such as chlorhexidine gluconate (Peridex).

## Tongue Lacerations

Tongue lacerations smaller than 1 cm will heal without primary repair. Larger lacerations require repair performed in layers, while maintaining forward traction of the tongue out of the mouth with a dry gauze or the use of two 2–0 silk sutures passed through the anterior portion of the tongue on each side of the midline. Since the tongue is highly vascular, hemostasis may be obtained with pressure, a cautery unit, or suture ligatures as needed. Injury to structures in the floor of the mouth must also be ruled out. The tongue heals well with placement of deep interrupted absorbable sutures of 4–0 gut or polyglycolic acid. Anesthesia for tongue repair may be performed locally or with the use of regional lingual nerve blocks. In small children, sedation with ketamine, 2 mg/kg, atropine, 0.02 mg/kg, and midazolam, 0.1 mg/kg IM, will provide adequate control.

## MANDIBULAR FRACTURES

The classic signs and symptoms of fracture of the mandible are (1) history of trauma; (2) malocclusion; (3) pain; (4) abnormal mobility or crepitus of the fracture segments; (5) interference with function and decreased range of motion; (6) deformity, either facial deformity or deformity of the dental arches; (7) deviation on opening; (8) swelling and ecchymosis; (9) mental nerve anesthesia; and (10) radiological confirmation.

As with any facial fracture, the primary consideration in the treatment of fractures of the mandible is the assessment and treatment of the general condition of the patient. Mandibular fractures are rarely treated at the time of injury in the absence of gross soft tissue wounds.

There are several approaches to the examination of a patient to make the diagnosis of mandibular fracture. Extra- and intraoral examinations, as well as a radiological survey, are required to complete the assessment of mandibular trauma.

### Extraoral Examination

This will usually reveal unilateral or bilateral swelling, deformity, and ecchymosis associated with the ascending ramus or body of the mandible or both. The mandible should be palpated beginning at the mandibular condyle and proceeding along the entire length of the mandibular border, and any tenderness or break in contour of the posterior or inferior border should be noted. Point tenderness is pathognomonic of fracture and frequently a step deformity may be noted at the inferior border. Bilateral inferior alveolar nerves run through the inferior alveolar canal of the mandible and terminate as the mental nerves that supply sensation to the lower lip. Numbness of the lower lip on one or both sides is a strong indication of mandibular fracture.

### Intraoral Examination

Bloodstained saliva will be evident in the mouth shortly after injury and if sufficient time has elapsed prior to examination, a marked fetor oris may be noted. If there is a mucosal laceration of the alveolar ridge, the fracture should be considered an open fracture. The lower dental arch should be examined for disruption of arch continuity, gross malalignment of the teeth should be noted, and the teeth inspected for looseness. Malocclusion may indicate mandibular fracture. In cases where abnormal occlusion is suspected to have existed prior to the fracture, careful inspection of the wear facets on the teeth should be made. More simply, the patient should be asked to bite on the back teeth as if chewing, and tell the examiner if the bite has changed. Biting down on a tongue blade will usually cause pain at the fracture site.

Movement of the mandible is also important. The patient should place the mouth through a full range of motion, with protrusion, lateral excursion, opening and closing, and any limitation of motion or associated pain should be noted. Unilateral subcondylar fractures will cause the mouth to deviate toward the side of fracture on maximum opening. The buccolingual sulcus of the mandible and the mucobuccal and labial gutters should be palpated and these areas examined for tenderness or alteration in contour, break in continuity of the mucosa, or existence of ecchymoses or a sublingual hematoma. A large sublingual hematoma can compromise the airway.

## X-Ray Evaluation

A routine x-ray film series of the mandible involves three views: a posteroanterior (PA) view of the face and skull, and right and left lateral oblique views. The whole outline of the mandible is visible in the PA view, but owing to the superimposition of the zygomatic bone and the mastoid process, it may be impossible to accurately interpret the region of the condylar head. In the lateral oblique views, the outline of the mandible may be visualized from the first premolar to the condyle. In all cases, films of both sides of the mandible should be obtained to rule out bilateral or multiple fractures.

Perhaps the best roentgenogram for suspected fracture of the mandible is the panoramic view of the maxilla and mandible. This view is essentially a clear curved surface tomogram at the level of the facial bones taken by an x-ray beam moving around the head. The problem areas that frequently occur in interpretation with the PA and lateral oblique views are virtually eliminated.

## Classification of Mandibular Fractures by Region

By site, the most common area of fracture is the angle of the mandible, followed closely by the condyle, molar, and mental regions. The symphysis is least frequently fractured due to the thickness of this area.

### Alveolar Fractures

The most common type of mandibular fracture is a fracture of the alveolus, or tooth-bearing segment of the mandible. Alveolar fractures are most frequently observed in the anterior or incisor region, since this area is more directly exposed to trauma. Viable teeth should be preserved even if they have been avulsed, and no segments of alveolus should be removed if they are firmly attached to mucoperiosteum (Fig. 204-3). Injudicious debridement of the oral cavity will leave the patient with large defects in the alveolus that cannot be corrected prosthetically. Direct pressure should be applied with gauze sponges to the attached dental segments and they should then be covered with a saline-soaked sponge. Most alveolar fractures can then be stabilized with wires or arch bar fixation.

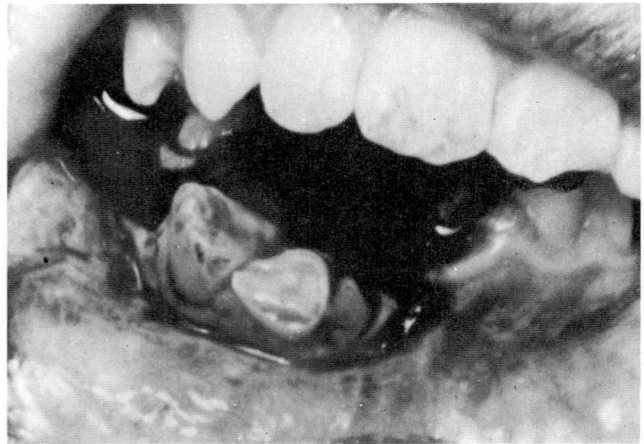

**Fig. 204-3.** Alveolar fracture with avulsed teeth. Preservation of supporting bone and viable teeth is an important early consideration.

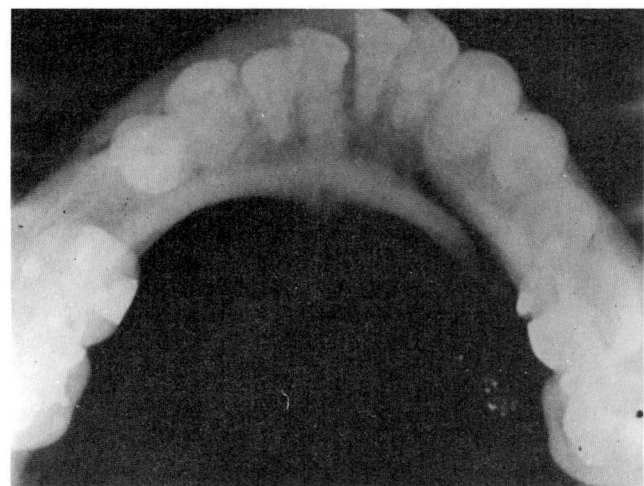

**Fig. 204-4.** Occlusal view of the mandible showing symphysis fracture with telescoping fragments.

### Condyle Fractures

Unilateral fractures of the condyle will cause the jaw to deviate toward the side of fracture on maximum opening. In a bilateral subcondylar fracture the patient usually has an anterior bite, occlusion on the posterior molars, and no contact of the incisor teeth.

### Symphysis Fractures

Fractures of the mandibular symphysis are easily noted by observation of displacement of the lower incisor teeth, disruption of arch continuity, and the ease with which segments can be moved on bimanual palpation. Bilateral fracture in the mental region can result in loss of anterior tongue support with possible acute airway obstruction (Fig. 204-4).

### Angle and Body Fractures

Unfavorable angle fractures are usually acted upon by muscle pull of the pterygomasseteric sling causing the proximal fragment to ride superiorly. This is best found by roentgenographic examination.

### Edentulous Fractures

Since many teeth may be missing in one or more of the fragments and the occlusion may be difficult to evaluate, the only way to accurately diagnose edentulous or partially edentulous mandibular fractures is by roentgenography. Always salvage dentures from the edentulous patient who has sustained facial fractures. The dentures can not only be used to splint bony fragments, but they may also help maintain occlusal vertical dimension.

## Treatment

Most mandibular fractures can be reduced and fixed in position by wiring upper and lower teeth in occlusion (intermaxillary fixation). Nonviable, loose teeth in the fracture site should be removed unless essential for splinting and alignment of the fractures. When many teeth are missing in any or all of the fragments, the problem is more complex but still lends itself to surgical management.

All dental appliances (bridges, etc.) may be utilized in intraoral fixation of fractures and should be preserved for the oral and maxillofacial surgeon.

When there are teeth on either side of the fracture site that can be brought into satisfactory occlusion with opposing maxillary teeth, a closed reduction is indicated. When the fracture line is unfavorable and posterior to the last tooth in the dental arch, or in a large edentulous segment, open reduction is most often required.

The use of rigid internal fixation for mandibular fixation has become increasingly useful with the development of mini-plates that are both safe and effective, as well as cosmetically acceptable. The goal of rigid internal fixation is the early pain-free mobilization of the fractured mandible without jeopardizing healing. Rigid fixation affords absolute stabilization through absence of motion between the fractured ends or between the plate and bone enabling the patient to eat with intermaxillary fixation almost immediately after surgery.

Tetanus prophylaxis must be instituted in any case of mandibular fracture where soft tissue injuries exist and there is a risk of contamination. Since most mandibular fractures are compounded intraorally, the risk of infection is always present. Antibiotic therapy is indicated with penicillin or a cephalosporin, the current drugs of choice. However, decision on antibiotic maintenance therapy should be made in consultation with the patient's surgeon. Almost all mandibular fracture patients are admitted acute.

## MIDFACIAL FRACTURES

Since fractures of the midface can be divided into several categories by anatomic region, each type of fracture will be discussed individually. Obviously these fractures can occur in any and all combinations depending on the multiplicity and direction of force. Once the patient is stabilized, immediate treatment of midfacial and mandibular fractures is mainly supportive. Avulsed or partially avulsed teeth should be preserved and reimplanted as soon as possible, preferably within an hour if completely avulsed. In the balance of gross overlying soft tissue injuries, most fractures can be reduced in several days when swelling resolves and facial incisions can be placed more aesthetically.

### Zygomatic Arch

Isolated fractures of the zygomatic arch are uncommon, because the force must be directly over the midlateral position of the arch to break it.

### Clinical Features

A facial dimpling or depression over the affected region of the zygomatic arch may be evident. This depression may be palpated to elicit point tenderness. In addition, owing to mechanical impingement of the coronoid process of the mandible by the inwardly fractured arch, the patient may not be able to open the mouth or, rarely, may have a partially open mouth and be unable to close it or move it in lateral excursion.

### X-Ray Evaluation

The zygomatic arches are best visualized by a modified basal view of the skull. Other names for the survey include submentaloccipital, submental-vertical, or jug-handle view of the skull (Fig. 204-5).

### Treatment

Treatment of zygomatic arch fractures is usually delayed. Criteria for surgical intervention are residual cosmetic deformity or restriction of mandibular motion. Frequently several days elapse for resolution of facial swelling before surgery is contemplated.

### Zygoma or Zygomatic-Maxillary Complex

The zygoma has major articulations with the frontal bone, maxilla, zygomatic process of the temporal bone, and lateral wall of the sinus, and it is usually subjected to multiple fractures at or near these articulations. A blow to the zygomatic prominence is unlikely to shatter the bone, but probably will result in a line of fracture at the frontal zygomatic suture line; the zygomaticomaxillary suture line or infraorbital rim; the lateral wall of the maxillary sinus at the buttress of the zy-

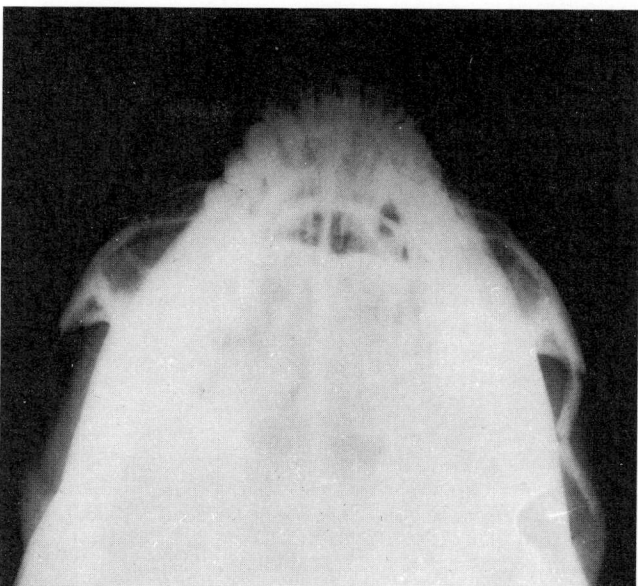

**Fig. 204-5.** Basal view of skull demonstrating unilateral fracture of the zygomatic arch.

goma; or at the zygomatic arch slightly behind the suture, between the short temporal process of the zygomatic bone and the longer zygomatic process of the temporal bone.

Frequently the central portion of the orbital floor will also fracture as part of the zygomaticomaxillary complex. A comminuted depressed fracture may lead to serious complications with entrapment of extraocular muscles. This type of orbital floor fracture should not be confused with the blowout type of orbital fracture.

A pure blowout is caused by direct intraocular trauma, forcing the eye posteriorly, at which time a plunger effect takes place upon the surrounding structures, particularly the relatively incompressible periorbital fat. The dense, strong, laterally angled outer wall of the orbit resists this force that is reflected downward on the thin bone of the floor of the orbit. The bone is forced into the underlying cavity of the maxillary antrum, thus the term *orbital blowout*. Extraocular muscle entrapment may occur with this type of fracture.

### Clinical Features

The major clinical signs of a fracture of the zygomatic bone or zygomaticomaxillary complex are (1) edema of the cheek and periorbita; (2) facial flattening shortly after injury or after initial edema subsides; (3) circumorbital or subconjunctival ecchymosis; (4) unilateral epistaxis; (5) anesthesia of the cheek, upper lip, teeth, and gum; (6) step deformity and tenderness over the inferior orbital margin, the frontal zygomatic suture line area, the zygomatic arch, and the lateral wall of the maxillary sinus (intraorally in the region of the zygomatic buttress); (7) diplopia with possible asymmetry of the ocular levels; (8) limitation of mandibular movement; and (9) emphysema of the overlying tissues.

Within 2 or 3 h of injury, the underlying skeletal deformity will be masked by edema. Therefore a great number of these injuries remain undiagnosed until swelling subsides so that resultant disfigurement can be evaluated.

A characteristic flattening of the upper part of the cheek can be seen, either immediately following injury or after the acute phase of edema has subsided, usually in 3 to 5 days (Fig. 204-6).

Palpation, beginning at the medial aspect of the superior orbital margin, will often elicit step deformities at the infraorbital rim and at the frontal zygomatic suture area. The tip of the index finger should

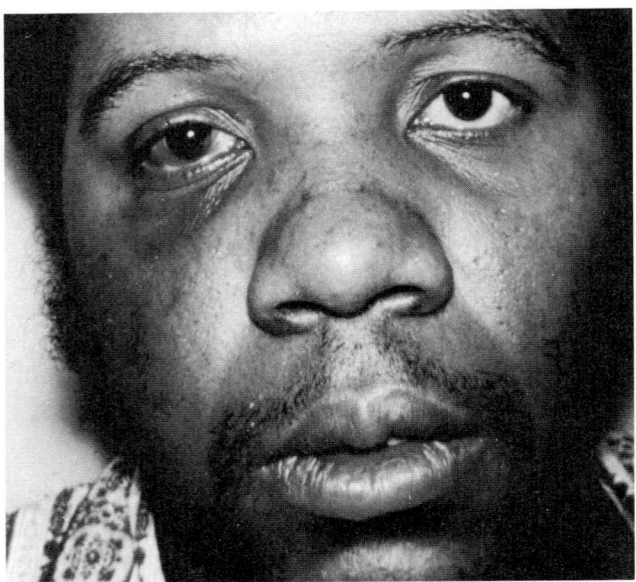

**Fig. 204-6.** Clinical presentation of fractured zygoma. Note facial flattening and lateral subconjunctival hemorrhage.

be carefully passed around the entire orbital rim. Owing to the thinness of the overlying tissue, step defects are usually easily palpated. Then palpation should proceed along the prominence of the zygoma and along the zygomatic arch. Point tenderness at the fracture sites is usually elicited.

Circumorbital ecchymosis and severe lateral subconjunctival hemorrhage are often present. Carefully examine the pupillary level on both sides to detect unilateral depression of the ocular level. Visual acuity and the range of ocular movement should be tested. Complaints of diplopia or blurring of vision should be noted.

Limitation of mandibular movement may be a result of mechanical obstruction by the depressed zygomatic bone or arch. Intraorally, ecchymosis of the upper buccal sulcus is often evident. Anesthesia of the teeth, gum, cheek, upper lip, and lateral ala nasi on the affected side is caused by injury to the infraorbital nerve at the zygomaticomaxillary fracture site. Subcutaneous emphysema may be caused by fracture of the lateral antral wall at the zygomatic buttress. Unilatertaxis may occur, but this usually ceases spontaneously.

## X-Ray Evaluation

The Waters' projection and a basal view of the skull are most important in the initial evaluation of fractures of the zygomatic bone. The Waters' or occipitomental projection, commonly used to visualize the maxillary sinus, offers complete visualization of three of the four areas that commonly fracture and displace in zygomaticomaxillary complex injuries: the frontozygomatic suture area; the zygomaticomaxillary or infraorbital area; and the lateral wall of the maxillary sinus. The presence of opacity or an air-fluid level in the sinus may signify antral hemorrhage secondary to trauma.

A basal view of the skull demonstrates the fourth point of fracture at the zygomatic arch. This view can also demonstrate inward displacement of the prominence of the zygoma and confirm intrusion or rotation of that bone in relation to the undisplaced zygoma on the opposite side. Further evaluation can be obtained through orbital tomograms that confirm fractures at the aforementioned articulations, as well as suspected fractures of the floor of the orbit. Frequently, herniation of orbital contents through the roof of the maxillary antrum can be seen on tomography (see "Computed Tomography in Maxillofacial Trauma").

## Treatment

The treatment is surgical through a number of approaches, the most common of which is open reduction and wire fixation or antral packing. The surgeon should be consulted regarding antibiotic choices and the timing of the procedure.

Again, rigid fixation can be used, especially when the surgeon's goals are to promote stabilization after anatomic reduction or to avoid intermaxillary fixation. Absolute stabilization is helpful after reduction of midface fracture in that it permits undisturbed healing. Rigid internal fixation applies forces that will exceed the functioning forces at all times with direct bone contact.

## Orbital Floor Fractures

Fracture of the orbital floor may occur as a component of a massive zygomaticomaxillary complex fracture, which usually causes comminution of the thin orbital floor, or as an isolated fracture—the less common orbital blowout fracture—caused by a very rapid increase in intraorbital pressure. This form of orbital floor fracture is described and discussed in chap. 201.

## Clinical Features

The two most common presenting ocular problems from orbital floor injury are diplopia and lowering of the globe. Diplopia occurs particularly in zygomaticomaxillary fractures when the thin orbital floor is fractured and comminuted as the stronger zygomatic complex is depressed downward and medially.

Evaluation of the eye is best performed before periorbital swelling has occurred, if possible. Corneal abrasions or scleral tears must be sought and foreign bodies on the ocular surface carefully removed. Having determined that there is no penetrating injury to the globe, evert the upper lid and check the conjunctival cul-de-sac for foreign material. Retinal function should be assessed by visual acuity testing, reactivity to light and accommodation, and ophthalmoscopy. Also evaluate extraocular muscle function. Diplopia may follow soft tissue entrapment of the inferior rectus or oblique muscles, disruption of muscular attachments, interruption of muscle innervation, orbital hemorrhage, or edema. Carefully inspect the anterior chamber of the eye for presence of a hyphema. Such hemorrhage, secondary to torn blood vessels in the peripheral iris, can cause blindness if not treated.

## X-Ray Evaluation

Diagnostic studies should include Waters' view x-rays and tomograms. On x-ray, the orbital floor may appear fragmented and displaced bony fragments may be seen in the maxillary sinus. In orbital floor fractures, orbital soft tissue may be seen protruding into the upper portion of the maxillary sinus (Fig. 204-7). In either fracture there may be emphysema of the soft tissues of the orbit. The soft tissue shadow on the x-ray usually appears as a semilunar mass protruding into the upper half of the maxillary sinus.

## Treatment

The goal of treatment of orbital floor fractures is to relieve restricted extraocular muscle function and elevate the lowered globe. This can be accomplished through an infraorbital approach, which permits direct inspection of the floor, removal of the small pieces of comminuted bone, and reconstruction of the orbital floor with an implant of alloplastic material or autogenous bone or cartilage. An ophthalmologist should be consulted regarding any injury to the eye. Consider antibiotics if there is significant ocular emphysema. Generally, surgery for the fracture itself is delayed.

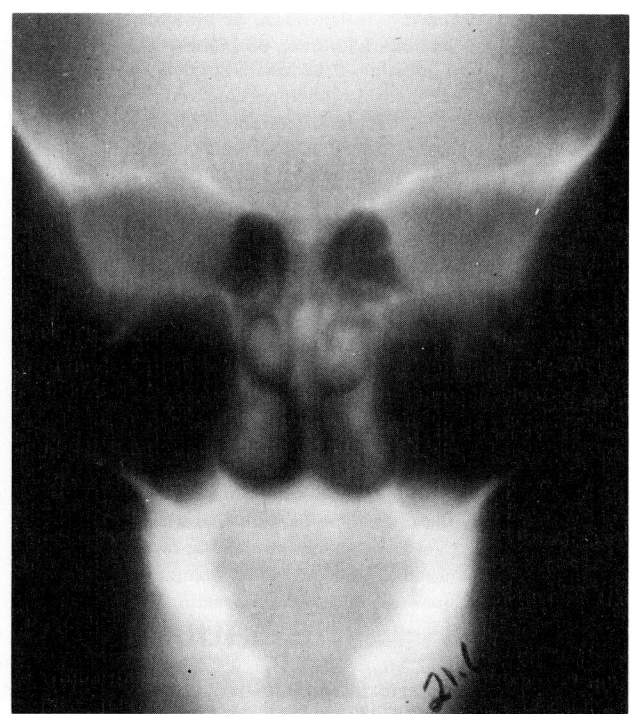

**Fig. 204-7.** Orbital tomogram showing classical "teardrop" herniation of orbital tissue into the maxillary sinus.

# MAXILLARY FRACTURES

Fractures of the alveolar process alone are the most common form of maxillary fracture and have been previously discussed.

## Le Fort Fractures

The characteristic of most maxillary fractures is a separation of attachments to the bony framework of the face or the skull. Studies by the French scientist, René Le Fort, at the turn of the century, produced the Le Fort classification of midfacial maxillary fractures (Fig. 204-8).

## Le Fort I or Horizontal Maxillary Fracture

As in all the Le Fort-type fractures, a free-floating jaw is encountered. The horizontal fracture is one in which the body of the maxilla is separated from the base of the skull above the level of the palate, and below the attachment of the zygomatic process. The fracture line runs from the lateral nasal apertures, along the lateral wall of the maxillary sinuses bilaterally, and across the pterygomaxillary tissue to the lateral pterygoid plates.

### Clinical Features

Many horizontal maxillary fractures are not significantly displaced and their diagnosis may be missed. Displacement is dependent upon the force of the blow and the muscular pull. Diagnosis is most easily made by grasping the alveolar process and anterior teeth between the thumb and forefinger and causing a forward-backward motion. The visualization of movement of the entire upper dental arch means that the patient has, at the very least, a Le Fort I fracture. An x-ray often does not establish the diagnosis.

## Le Fort II or Pyramidal Fracture

The pyramidal fracture consists of vertical fractures through the facial aspects of the maxilla extending upwards to the nasal and eth-moid bones. The fractures extend through the maxillary sinuses and the infraorbital rims bilaterally across the bridge of the nose.

### Clinical Features

The entire midface, nose, lips, and eyes are swollen. Bilateral subconjunctival hemorrhage is present and there is often blood in the nares. If clear fluid is seen in the nose, cerebrospinal rhinorrhea must be suspected (see chap. 203), and the neurosurgical service should be consulted prior to consultation with the oral and maxillofacial surgery service. Cerebrospinal rhinorrhea is a result of fracture of the cribriform plate of the ethmoid bone. It is for this reason that a clinical examination for suspected Le Fort II fracture must be done gently with as little movement as possible. However, the diagnosis of Le Fort II fracture can usually be confirmed by grasping the premaxilla, as with the Le Fort I fracture, in conjunction with palpation of the base of the nose (Fig. 204-9).

### X-Ray Evaluation

The diagnosis of Le Fort II fracture is usually confirmed by a Water view roentgenogram for evaluation of the infraorbital rims bilaterally, together with bilateral orbital tomograms. Films of the nasal bones may be desired by the consultant.

## Le Fort III Fracture or Craniofacial Dysjunction

The Le Fort III fracture extends through the frontozygomatic suture lines bilaterally, across the orbits, and through the base of the nose and the ethmoid region (Fig. 204-10). The lateral rim of the orbit is separated and the infraorbital rim may be fractured, along with associated fractures of the zygoma. A pyramidal or horizontal fracture may also be present.

### Clinical Features

A characteristic "dishface" may be evident because of retroposition of the entire midface at a 45° angle, along the base of the skull. On profile, the face appears spooned-out in the nasal area and the patient

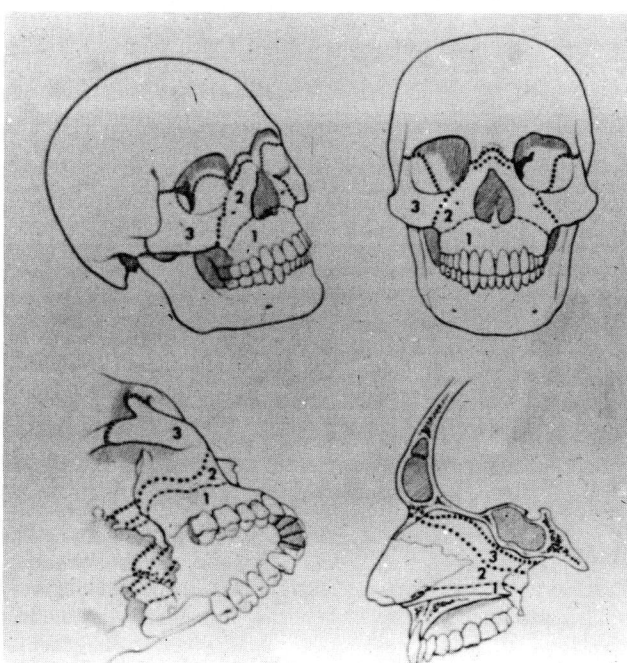

**Fig. 204-8.** Schematic of midfacial fracture lines: Le Fort I, II, and III. (From Dingman RO, Natvig P: *Surgery of Facial Fractures.* Philadelphia, Saunders, 1964, p. 248. Used by permission.)

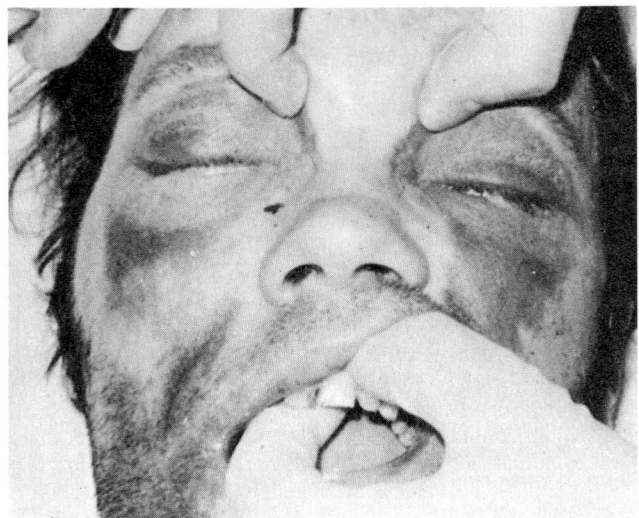

**Fig. 204-9.** Method of examination for Le Fort II fractures of maxilla.

often has an anterior open bite. As the face is repositioned by the force of impact, the teeth in contact on occlusion are the posterior molars while there is no contact of the anterior or incisor teeth. Cerebrospinal rhinorrhea is more common than with the Le Fort II fracture. Palpation should be done gently (Fig. 204-11). If movement of the midface and zygoma occur concurrently, LeFort III fracture is confirmed.

### X-Ray Evaluation

A Water view roentgenogram and bilateral orbital tomograms confirm the diagnosis.

### Treatment

The usual treatment of midfacial fractures is surgical. The objective is to reduce the fracture accurately and fix it internally to support the sagging face and restore normal occlusion. The bones of the face must be mobilized and displacements of the zygoma, lacrimal, and

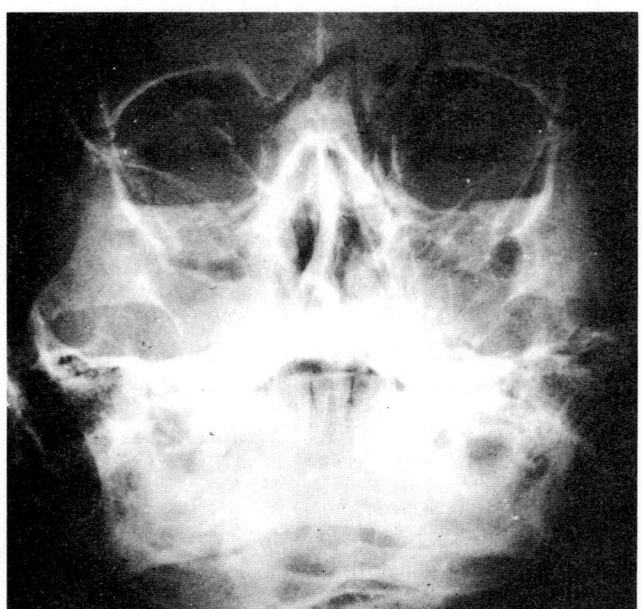

**Fig. 204-10.** Waters' view roentgenogram of Le Fort III fracture. Note bilateral fracture at the frontozygomatic area and the craniofacial dysjunction.

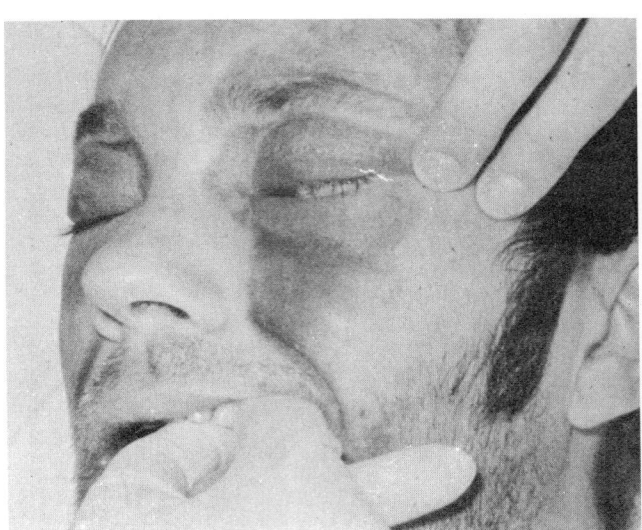

**Fig. 204-11.** Movement of zygomas on examination indicates probable Le Fort III fracture.

other facial bones corrected. Fractures of the nasal bones are usually treated by closed reduction with intranasal reduction and manual molding. Tetanus toxoid and antibiotic prophylaxis should be administered.

## NASO-ORBITAL INJURY

Blunt trauma to the naso-orbital area may cause disruption and detachment of the medial canthal ligaments. Because of the resilience of the lateral canthal ligament, increased intercanthal distance, or telecanthus, will result. It is not uncommon to see an intercanthal distance of 40 or 45 mm in naso-orbital injuries in the white adult, as opposed to the usual intercanthal distance of approximately 35 mm. The medial canthal ligament is normally attached to the anterior and posterior lacrimal crests of the lacrimal bone; the majority of the attachments are to the anterior lacrimal crest. Between these two leaves of the medial canthal ligament the nasolacrimal duct passes through in the nasolacrimal fossa. In naso-orbital injury the medial portion of the palpebral fissure assumes an almond configuration, in contrast to its normal elliptical shape.

### Clinical Signs

The triad of a widened bridge of the nose, telecanthus, and an almond-shaped palpebral fissure following trauma to the midface area should lead the clinician to suspect a nasal skeleton fracture along with disruption of the medial canthal ligaments.

### X-Ray Evaluation

Radiographic examination should include Waters' projection, x-ray of the paranasal sinuses, and tomograms when indicated. A maxillofacial and/or ophthalmologic consult should be obtained for acute or delayed management.

## COMPUTED TOMOGRAPHY IN MAXILLOFACIAL TRAUMA

The use of computed tomography (CT) in the evaluation of maxillofacial injuries has been extremely helpful in assessing orbital fractures, midfacial trauma, and potential airway obstruction. This technique not only can be used when conventional techniques fail but actually offers some distinct advantages as a primary assessment tool.

The advantages are

1. Soft tissues are clearly displayed and related to the bony framework so that exact margins of lesions can be defined.
2. Both axial and coronal views are available as well as sagittal reconstruction.
3. Blurring does not occur as with conventional tomograms.
4. There is approximately 40 percent less radiation exposure than with the latter.
5. Density determination and identification (e.g., blood, pus, muscle) of tissues are possible by measuring their absorption values.
6. It is the diagnostic modality of choice in the assessment of intracranial lesions.

### Orbital and Midfacial Fractures

Fractures of this region are often complicated by edema, making initial clinical assessment of bony injury difficult. Since the bones are thin and lie in various planes, superimposition often occurs and may be further obscured by the dense cranial base.

Fractures of the cribriform plate of the ethmoid can be identified, which is especially important in the diagnosis of cerebrospinal fluid leakage. In addition, persistent leaks can be evaluated by the intrathecal placement of metrizamide (Fig. 204-12).

CT is the only technique that clearly shows the complete skeletal distortion often occurring in middle third fractures. The amount of comminution and degree of displacement, especially at the posterior aspects of the maxilla, are often unobtainable by a routine radiographic study.

## DISTURBANCES OF THE TEMPOROMANDIBULAR JOINT (TMJ)

### Dislocation of the Mandible

Acute dislocation causes considerable pain, discomfort, and swelling. The anatomic structure of the TMJ fossa and anterior articular eminence of that fossa may predispose to dislocation. The weakness of the connective tissue capsule forming the temporomandibular ligaments also may be a predisposing factor. The capsule may have loose attachments, may be excessively stretched, and more rarely, may be torn. Dislocation is generally caused by trauma to the chin while the mouth is in the open position, but it may occur while yawning, laughing excessively, or opening the mouth widely to chew food. Dislocation can also occur by overstretching the mouth while the patient is under general anesthesia. In addition, hysterical dislocations have been recorded.

### Clinical Features

In an acute dislocation, the condyle becomes locked anterior to the articular eminence and is prevented from sliding back by muscular

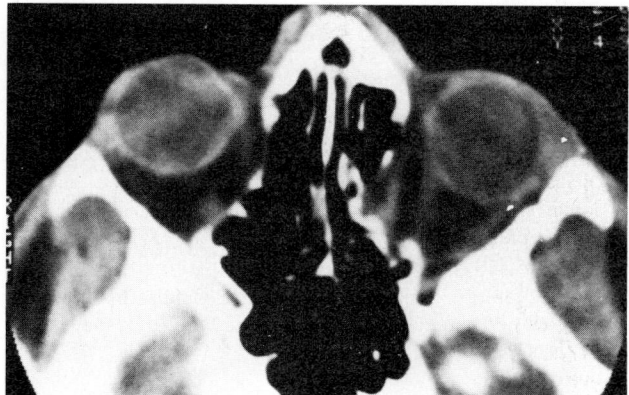

**Fig. 204-12.** orbital CT scan showing enophthalmos and fracture of the medial wall of the orbit. Note that the extraocular muscles can also be visualized.

trismus. The external pterygoid, masseter, and internal pterygoid muscles then go into spasm. Characteristically the patient has the mouth open, and is unable to close the anterior teeth. Bilateral dislocation will thus present with an anterior open bite, but if the dislocation is unilateral, the jaw is displaced toward the unaffected side. The head of the condyle may produce swelling in front of the ear below the zygomatic arch. Since the jaw is locked in an open position, talking and swallowing are difficult. Examination of the TMJs will demonstrate the condyle in front of the anterior articular eminence of the joint fossa.

### X-Ray Evaluation

The roentgenogram may be an important aid in differentiating dislocation from fracture of the condyle, since these conditions may produce similar occlusal disturbances. It should beed prior to reduction to assure that no fracture is present.

### Treatment

Temporomandibular joint dislocation can usually be successfully treated by manual manipulation. Occasionally, owing to the intensity of the muscle spasms, the muscles of mastication may have to be injected with a local anesthetic solution to enable them to relax. More frequently, 10 mg of diazepam is injected slowly intravenously to aid in muscle relaxation and to allay some of the anxiety of the patient during the relocation procedure.

The patient should be in a sitting position with the physician standing on the side of the dislocation. The thumb is then wrapped in gauze and placed on the occlusal surfaces of the posterior teeth with the fingertips placed around the inferior border of the mandible in the region of the mandibular angles. Downward pressure is then exerted while the jaw is opened wide to free the condyle from the stuck position anterior to the eminence. A great deal of patience is needed rather than great force. The masseter muscles eventually relax, allowing reduction. The chin is then pressed back after it has been forced down so that the mouth is closed while the condyle returns to the fossa. Since the jaw may snap back quickly, the gauze protects the physician's thumb from injury. The procedure is then repeated on the opposite side if the dislocation is bilateral.

After reduction of an acute dislocation, the patient is cautioned against further wide excursions of the mandible, and placed on a soft diet for 1 week. Analgesics and muscle relaxants help override the acute phase of trauma.

In chronic dislocations, or in acute recurrences, a Barton bandage is applied for 1 week to prevent the patient from opening the jaw widely. In severe cases, intermaxillary wiring and fixation may be applied to restrict and control jaw motion during healing. Chronic dislocation may occasionally require surgical intervention, with most procedures aimed at recontour of the articular eminence to prevent dislocation or eliminate locking.

### Temporomandibular Joint Dysfunction

The TMJ dysfunction syndrome, usually referred to as myofascial pain dysfunction, is a form of fibrositis that accounts for the majority of patients who seek treatment for TMJ pain. The diagnosis is suspected when an adult patient, usually female, presents with pain in the region of the jaw, earache, "popping" or crepitus, and difficulty with chewing or opening the mouth. Other symptoms include burning sensation in the tongue or roof of the mouth, bruxism, tinnitus, and vertigo. Clinical evidence suggests that pain in the neck, shoulders, arms, and fingers may be related to disorders in the cervical spine that may be associated with temporomandibular disorders. Muscle pain often affects the temporalis, the masseter, and muscles of the occipital areas and the neck.

Physical examination of the TMJ may elicit tenderness on palpation of the joint capsule and of the muscles of mastication. Patients with TMJ disorders fall into three diagnostic categories:

1. Those with joint abnormalities resulting from trauma or from conditions such as ankylosis, synovitis, arthritis, and neoplasm;
2. Those with structural defects of the articular disc (meniscus), ligaments of the disc, condyles, glenoid fossae, or articular tubercles;
3. Those who present with pain or restricted jaw motion but do not have evidence of organic disease or structural defects.

No clear etiology has been established. It is believed that the disease is a neuromuscular disturbance and that occlusal factors are contributory in nature. In addition to irregularities of the teeth and occlusion, factors such as trauma, psychic tension, and neuromuscular habits, such as bruxism and clenching of teeth, are all considered to play a major role in the development of this syndrome.

## Clinical Features

Typically, the patient with the TMJ syndrome will have unilateral facial pain, mainly around the immediate region of the joint. The pain is of a dull, aching character that intensifies toward evening because of the use of the jaw during the day. Pain may be referred to the temporal, supraorbital, occipital, and cervical regions.

Commonly, the patient will have acute otalgia mimicking external otitis or otitis media, yet the otologic examination is negative. Inability to open the mouth widely is another complaint. The mouth may deviate on opening toward the side of the mandibular dysfunction or facial pain. Stiffness of the jaw generally worsens with use. Myofascial spasm or trismus may also be associated with clicking of the affected joint.

Clinical examination will usually reveal acute tenderness over the lateral capsular ligament of the TMJ, anterior to the external auditory canal. Placing the fingers on the joint and having the patient open and close the mouth will elicit this tenderness. The masseter and the internal pterygoid muscles may also be tender.

## X-Ray Evaluation

Radiological diagnosis is usually unrewarding. TMJ films are taken in the open and closed position. It is uncommon to find irregularities of the joint unless the patient has temporomandibular degenerative joint disease. In that case, osteophyte proliferation and flattening out or erosions of the head of the condyle are characteristic changes.

## Treatment

The TMJ syndrome is treated by physiotherapy, dietary restrictions, analgesics, muscle relaxants, and occlusive therapy. Warm, moist compresses should be applied to the affected side of the face for 15 min four times a day for 7 to 10 days. A pureed diet should be followed for 1 to 2 weeks. Analgesics and muscle relaxants help disrupt the pain-muscle spasm-pain cycle.

It is surprising how often relief can be obtained by placing the upper and lower jaws in their proper occlusal relationship and maintaining the joint in its maximum rest position. When the acute phase has subsided, or as an adjunct to the treatment of the acute phase, the patient should be referred for a dental consultation for equilibration of occlusion, and for possible construction of bite splints to disarticulate the posterior teeth and help relieve muscle spasm.

Direct intraarticular injection of steroids is beneficial in many patients who do not respond to conservative therapy, if they show signs of synovitis.

## Internal Derangements of the TMJ

In internal derangements and dislocation of the TMJ the menisci become displaced because of tears, perforation, or stretching of the posterior attachments. The term *internal derangements of the TMJ* refers to any disturbance between the articular components in the joint proper. It implies a localized structural derangement that interferes with the smooth function of the joint. It has been adopted in the last few years mainly for changes in the disc-condyle relationship. The disc is most commonly displaced in an anteromedial direction. It often produces pain and/or functional disturbances in the masticatory system. It is most common in young adults, particularly women. The patient often hears a click in the ear with each mouth opening. The joint may lock in the closed position, severe pain inhibiting opening of the mouth. Range of motion of the jaw is limited and with opening of the mouth there may be deviation to the affected side.

Determine whether the click is accompanied by pain. Patients with internal derangements frequently experience an increase in pain before the click followed by a decrease in pain afterward. It is important to notice whether the noise changes, whether it occurs more or less frequently or later during opening, or whether it gets louder or changes otherwise. Changing joint noise may indicate the presence of an active etiologic factor and progression of the disorder. Crepitus is generally considered to represent advanced disease and occurs as a result of movement across irregular surfaces. Internal-derangement patients typically report having previously had a clicking TMJ followed by a period of no joint noise (associated with locking) and then a grating or grinding noise. Frequent crepitus indicates a perforation of the disc or its attachments. This is especially true when degenerative changes are observed in the radiographs. Limited range of movement presents in three forms that usually occur together: opening, protrusive, and lateral movements. Normal opening is 35–50 mm when measured from the tip of the upper to lower incisors. When the disc is anteriorly displaced and does not reduce to a normal position during opening, the patient has limited opening (closed lock). The closed lock condition may be either intermittent or persistent. With intermittent closed lock, the patient usually reports that their jaw suddenly catches or gets stuck. If pain is present, it generally is reported to be worse during the closed lock condition. Disc position is most easily determined with an MRI. Treatment may be surgical via arthroscopy or open arthroplasty.

## Osteoarthritis (OA or DJD)

Middle-aged to elderly patients with TMJ osteoarthritis complain of pain and crepitus in the jaw. The latter is evident on movement of the jaw and is worse at the end of the day. Tenderness and spurs may be noted. Conventional roentgenographs show thinning and loss of cortical bone, flattening of the joint contour and spurs in established disease. The roentgenograph is usually sufficient for diagnosis, but a CT scan may be required.

## Rheumatoid Arthritis (RA)

Rheumatoid arthritis of the TMJ is almost always part of a generalized arthritic process but it may be the chief complaint, overshadowing other joints. The joint is limited in motion, tender and perhaps swollen. Roentgenographs show erosion of the head and neck of the condyle, flattening of the joint surface, and joint space narrowing. CT scans are particularly useful in the evaluation of RA.

## Treatment

TMJ dysfunction and pain tend to be a chronic and difficult problem. Referral to an oral surgeon should be arranged. NSAIDs may be helpful short term.

## ACKNOWLEDGMENT

The author would like to acknowledge the assistance of Michael Miloro, M.D., D.M.D., in the updating of this chapter.

## BIBLIOGRAPHY

Helms CA, Katzberg RW, Morrish R, et al: Computed tomography of the temporomandibular joint meniscus. *J Oral Maxillofacial Surg* 41:512, 1983.

Hendler BH: Maxillofacial trauma in the emergency unit. *Current Topics Emerg Med* 2:00, 1985.

Le Fort R: Étude experimentale sur les fractures de la machoire supérieure. *Rev Chir* (Paris) 23:360, 479, 1901.

Rowe NL, Williams JL: *Maxillofacial Injuries,* 2d ed. New York, Churchill Livingstone, 1985, vols I, II.

# 205
# GENERAL DENTAL EMERGENCIES
## James T. Amsterdam

There are four categories of general dental emergencies of importance to the emergency physician: (1) oral-facial pain, primarily of odontogenic origin; (2) dentoalveolar trauma; (3) hemorrhage; and (4) oral medicine emergencies including oral manifestations of systemic disease. An understanding of the anatomy of the tooth and attachment apparatus is essential for the recognition and management of these emergencies.

## ANATOMY OF THE TEETH

A tooth is a homogeneous body of dentin, a microporous structure which surrounds a central pulp—the neurovascular supply—from which it is nourished and was initially derived. The pulp continuously lays down additional dentin throughout life. The coronal portion of the tooth is that part which is normally seen in the mouth and is covered by enamel; the root portion serves to anchor the tooth and is covered with cementum, a substance which is much softer than enamel.

Thirty-two teeth are generally found in the permanent dentition, consisting of four types of teeth—incisors, canines, premolars, and molars. Beginning from the midline and counting backward, the normal dental anatomy will consist of one central incisor, one lateral incisor, one canine, two premolars, and three permanent molars. The third molar is commonly referred to as the *wisdom tooth. Agenesis* or absence of any of these teeth or additional (*supernumerary*) teeth can occur. It is best for the emergency physician simply to describe the type of tooth and location involved in a particular emergency, e.g., an upper right second premolar or a lower left canine. Useful dental nomenclature consists of the following:

Facial: Referring to that part of a tooth that faces the oral vestibule
Incisors to canines: Labial
Premolars to molars: Buccal
Oral: Referring to that part of a tooth that faces the tongue (lingual) or palate (palatal)
Approximal: Referring to the contacting areas of adjacent teeth; those closest to the midline are mesial, those toward the posterior aspect of the mouth are distal
Occlusal: Referring to the biting surfaces of the premolars and molars
Incisal: Referring to the biting surface of the incisors and canines
Apical: Referring to the tip of the root
Coronal: Toward the biting surface of the tooth

## THE NORMAL PERIODONTIUM

The normal periodontium is divided into two major components, the gingival unit and the attachment apparatus.

The *gingival unit* is composed of the soft tissues investing the teeth and the alveolar bone. The *gingiva* is covered by a stratified squamous keratinized epithelium. It extends from the free gingival margin to the mucogingival junction. Apical to the mucogingival junction is the *alveolar mucosa,* which is covered by nonkeratinized, stratified squamous epithelium and is continuous with the mucosa of the lip and cheek.

In healthy individuals, the gingiva is attached tightly to the tooth, except for a 2- to 3-mm cuff of tissue surrounding the neck of the tooth (*gingival sulcus*), bounded on one side by enamel and on the other by a continuation of the gingival epithelium. The *attachment apparatus* or anchoring mechanism consists of the cementum covering the root, the alveolar bone surrounding the root, and the periodontal ligament. The periodontal ligament is composed of collagen fibers that insert on one end in the alveolar bone and on the other end in the cementum forming a fibrous attachment, not a calcific union. The periodontal ligament as a double periosteum laying down cementum on the root and bone on the alveolus. The anatomy of the dental unit (crown and root) and the periodontium are illustrated in cross section in Fig. 205-1.

## ORAL AND FACIAL PAIN

If pain is of odontogenic (tooth) origin, patients usually will be able to localize the pain. The emergency physician should also recognize nonodontogenic causes for facial and oral pain (e.g., temporomandibular joint disturbances, Bell's palsy) and consider ischemic heart disease in the adult presenting with mandibular pain of unclear etiology.

## Odontogenic Pain

### Tooth Eruption

The earliest pain of odontogenic origin is associated with eruption of the primary teeth in the infant. Although there is some controversy over whether diarrhea and low-grade fever are associated with tooth eruption, an infant with dental pain may refuse to eat or drink and become dehydrated. The associated symptoms of diarrhea may be due to increased salivary gland production which also leads to drooling. The low grade fever 37.9°C (100.6°F) is most likely associated with some degree of dehydration similar to the post-operative pediatric patient. This same age group is also subject to various viral upper respiratory and gastrointestinal infections which confuse most studies. Care must be taken not to attribute significant fevers 37.9°C (100.6°F) to this relatively benign process. Management is directed

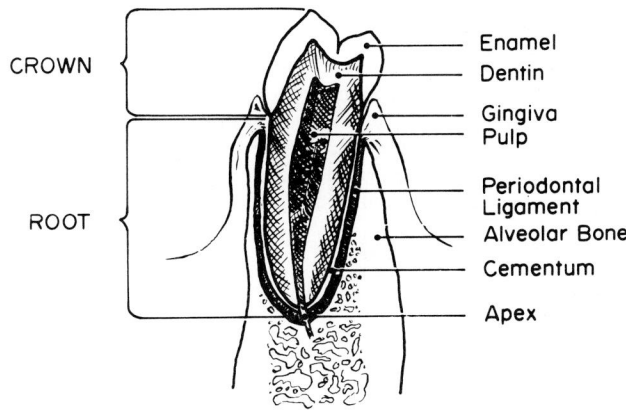

**Fig. 205-1.** The dental anatomic unit and attachment apparatus.

toward (1) pain control and (2) adequate hydration. Topical application every 15 to 30 min of an oral topical anesthetic (benzocaine) agent may be a useful method of analgesia. On rare occasions, the infant may be dehydrated enough to warrant bolus intravenous fluids or admission for observation. Adult patients may suffer from pain associated with erupting teeth, most commonly third molars. The gingiva surrounding crowded, malerupted or impacted third molar teeth has a tendency for food impaction and subsequent inflammation, termed *pericoronitis.* Local therapy consists of saline irrigation and mouth rinses; if fluctuance and pus are present, a conservative and superficial incision and drainage may be useful. If local infection, fever, or malaise are evident, phenoxymethyl penicillin or erythromycin, 250 to 500 mg qid, are prescribed. Once local inflammation has resolved, definitive treatment involves the surgical removal of these teeth. Therefore, referral to an oral and maxillofacial surgeon in 24 to 48 h is important.

## Dental Caries

The most common odontogenic pain, *odontalgia* or *toothache,* is associated with a carious tooth. A history of sudden or gradual onset of sharp to dull throbbing pain localized to a specific area of the mouth, aggravated by changes in temperature or possibly relieved by cool temperature, is consistent with caries. Such a history is consistent with pulp involvement and may indicate that the tooth is abscessed (periapical abscess). The pain may be generalized or referred to other areas such as the ear, temple, eye, neck, or even opposite jaw. Physical examination frequently will reveal a grossly decayed tooth (or teeth), or there may be no apparent pathology. Localization is most easily accomplished by percussing individual teeth with a tongue blade; if abscessed, sharp pain is elicited when the tooth is tapped. Treatment is with analgesics such as codeine, acetaminophen-codeine combinations, or even, on occasion, parenteral narcotic analgesics. Patients who have undergone endodontic treatment may experience exquisite pain secondary to instrumentation during therapy and/or the build-up of gas in the tooth after it has been sealed (pericementitis) which may be unrelieved by any analgesic; a general dentist or endodontist should be notified so that the tooth can be reopened.

Any associated oral or facial swelling secondary to abscessed teeth may produce pain. Swelling may range from a parulis (a small swelling in the gingiva opposite an abscessed tooth) to subperiosteal extension or a facial cellulitis. Fluctuant swellings require incision and drainage, antibiotics, and warm saline rinses every 2 h until seen the following day for definitive treatment.

## Postextraction Pain

Pain experienced within 24 h of an extraction, termed *periosteitis,* responds well to analgesics. Severe pain associated with a foul odor and taste in the mouth 2 to 3 days after an extraction is termed *alveolar osteitis* ("dry socket"). This pain is often excruciating and not relieved by oral analgesics. The pathophysiology is due to a combination of loss of the healing blood clot and a localized infection (localized osteomyelitis). Treatment consists of irrigation of the socket and the application of a medicated dental packing, or simply 1 in. of iodoform gauze slightly dampened with eugenol or Campho-Phenique which may be performed by the emergency physician. The patient should be seen by a dentist in 12 to 24 h.

## Periodontal Emergencies

### Periodontal Abscess

A swelling of the gingiva secondary to entrapment of plaque and debris in a so-called *pocket* (space between the tooth and the gingiva) is termed a *periodontal abscess* and may result in severe pain. Abscesses of this nature usually respond to local therapy consisting of warm saline irrigation and antibiotics (phenoxymethyl penicillin, 250 mg po qid; if allergic to penicillin and not pregnant, tetracycline 250 mg po qid). Larger abscesses may require a conservative and superficial ("stab incision") incision and drainage.

## Acute Necrotizing Ulcerative Gingivitis

Acute necrotizing ulcerative gingivitis (ANUG) is an acute destructive disease of the periodontium found most often in adolescents and young adults. ANUG is the only periodontal lesion in which bacteria (*Fusobacteria,* spirochetes) actually invade nonnecrotic tissue. Patients complain of generalized gingival pain associated with a foul taste and odor. Signs that may be present are fever, malaise, and regional lymphadenopathy. On physical examination the gingiva appears edematous and fiery red; the interdental papillae (tissue between the teeth) are edematous, ulcerated, and covered with a grayish pseudomembrane.

ANUG is initially managed with antibiotics (tetracycline 250 mg po qid, preferred; or phenoxymethyl penicillin, 250 mg po qid), warm saline rinses, as well as the application of topical local anesthetic agents such as viscous lidocaine or 10% carbamide peroxide in a specially prepared anhydrous glycerol. Symptomatic improvement is impressive; however, the potential complication of destruction of underlying alveolar bone requires dental follow-up.

## Oral Medicine Emergencies

Although it is beyond the scope of this chapter to discuss the myriad of oral medicine emergencies which may result in pain, there are several important classes that represent common problems.

### Oral Lesions

Patients frequently present because of pain from oral lesions. It is often difficult to distinguish a primary herpetic gingivostomatitis from recurrent infection, herpangina, or herpes zoster. Such ulcerations when recognized are often best treated palliatively in the emergency department with topical anesthetic agents, e.g., viscous xylocaine and the application of warm saline rinses. Some are now advocating the use of oral acyclovir for primary herpetic infections in the adult. Its use should certainly be considered in the immune-compromised patient. These lesions are usually secondarily infected and since much of the pain is due to the secondary infection itself, the prescription of antibiotics (erythromycin 250 mg qid or phenoxymethyl penicillin 250 mg qid) is often appropriate. In most circumstances, the prescription of topical or systemic corticosteroid preparations should be avoided. Although steroids have been useful in treatment of erythema multiforme, their use with viral oral infection is not indicated. Owing to the complexity of the differential diagnosis of oral vesicular lesions, definitive treatment is best managed by a dentist or oral and maxillofacial surgeon.

### Paroxysmal Pain of Neuropathic Origin

Tic douloureux, or trigeminal neuralgia, is the most common cause for paroxysmal pain of neuropathic origin involving the trigeminal (fifth) cranial nerve. The diagnosis is made primarily on history. Patients report a paroxysmal pain, i.e., an episode of sudden pain separated by pain-free periods, which is recurrent, excruciating, normally of short duration, and resembling the pain due to a severe electric shock. The key to the diagnosis is the fact that the pain follows the anatomical distribution of the cranial nerve involved. Often, a similar pain can be initiated by minor sensory stimuli to areas called *trigger zones* that consistently reproduce the pain. Tic douloureux may respond well to the administration of carbamazepine (100 mg bid initially and gradually increased if needed to a maximum dose of 1200 mg daily). The pain of tic douloureux may not necessarily be idiopathic, as it may be the result of a tumor, such as a cerebellopontine angle tumor (e.g., acoustic neuroma); a nasopharyngeal carcinoma; or a manifestation of multiple sclerosis. Any patient in whom the diagnosis of tic douloureux is made requires a careful neurologic examination, a referral to a dentist to rule out oral pathology, and a referral to a neurologist to rule out intracranial pathology.

Nonparoxysmal pain of neuropathic origin may develop (1) in patients who have suffered for a long time from tic douloureux; (2) secondary to surgical trauma along the distribution of the fifth cranial nerve, most frequently the mandibular branch; or (3) in association with viral infections, drugs, or heavy metal intoxication. Other neuropathies, such as alcoholic and diabetic sensory neuropathies, may affect the oral cavity as well.

### Other

The differential diagnosis of oral facial pain includes cluster headache, temporal arteritis, and polymyalgia rheumatica. Referred pain from an ischemic myocardium must be considered in the differential diagnosis of jaw pain.

## Oral Manifestations of Systemic Disease

Several systemic diseases are associated with important oral manifestations, often as the first manifestation.

### Diabetes Mellitus

Acute gingival abscesses and sessile or pedunculated gingival proliferations (granulation tissue that protrudes from under the gingiva, producing a red-gingival hypertrophy) occur frequently in diabetics. Dry burning mouth, gingival tenderness, lip dryness, spontaneous gingival bleeding, and tooth mobility may be seen. Chronic oral disease, particularly periodontal disease, may contribute to out-of-control diabetes.

### Collagen Vascular Disease

Systemic lupus erythematosus (SLE) may be associated with large intraoral necrotic ulcerations which may become secondarily infected.

Scleroderma may present with a characteristic facies or thickening of the periodontal ligament on x-ray. Midline lethal granuloma or Wegener's granulomatosis may present with large palatal ulcerations. All ulcerations of the oral cavity which do not respond to palliative treatment warrant biopsy within 7 to 10 days.

### Granulomatous Disease

Rarely, tuberculosis may manifest itself orally as granulomatous ulcerations. Other infections such as actinomycosis must be ruled out. These lesions may frequently be confused with syphilitic ulcerations in the oral cavity, with the tongue and tonsil areas being common locations.

A more benign and common entity is a pedunculated or sessile mass, termed *pyogenic granuloma*. This is a proliferation of highly vascularized connective tissue in response to nonspecific infection seen on the gingiva. A specific pyogenic granuloma, occurring primarily during pregnancy, is referred to as a *pregnancy tumor* (Fig. 205-2). The tumor is benign and frequently recurs if removed during pregnancy. If the tumor does not regress 2 to 3 months postpartum, definitive removal is indicated.

### Blood Dyscrasias

Acute leukemia, particularly the acute granulocytic form, causes massive infiltration of leukemic cells into the gingival tissues, resulting in a hyperplastic gingivitis so marked as to almost cover the teeth; it is edematous and bluish in color. Chronic leukemia rarely causes oral disorders.

Oral complications that occur during the disease include gingival

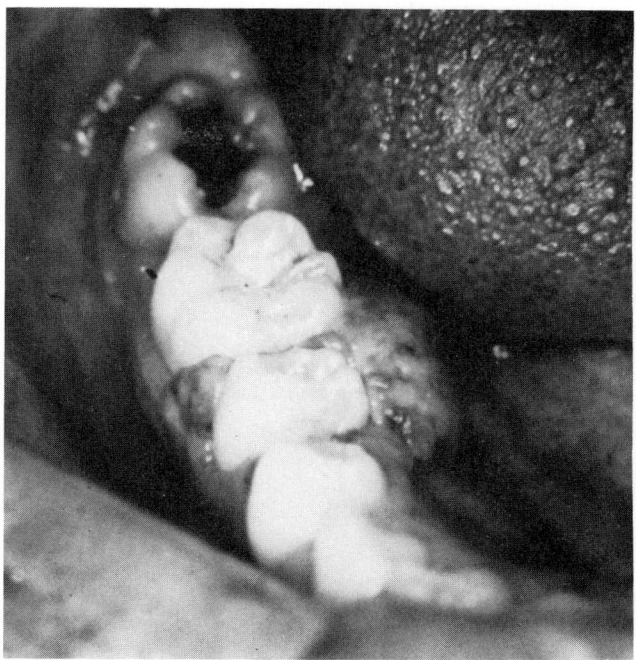

**Fig. 205-2.** Pyogenic granuloma

hemorrhage, local infection, marked discomfort, and loss of appetite. During the acute phase of the disease, only those procedures necessary to alleviate the discomfort and hemorrhaging should be performed (Fig. 205-3).

Intraoral signs and symptoms of thrombocytopenic purpura consist of gingival bleeding, intramucosal hemorrhages, and prolonged bleeding from trauma. In addition, gingival hypertrophy has been reported.

### Phenytoin Hyperplasia

Phenytoin hyperplasia of the gingiva occurs in approximately 40 percent of patients and is more prevalent in younger patients. Its severity may be unrelated to either dosage or blood levels. The initial appearance of hyperplasia is an enlargement of the interdental papillae, which encroaches on the crowns of the teeth with the marginal gingival tissue lobulated, firm, and pale pink in color. Inflammation secondary to local irritants alters the appearance of the hyperplastic gingiva and responds to improved oral hygiene. Surgical removal of tissue is effective, but hyperplasia recurs if the drug is continued. A similar reaction can be associated with nifedipine.

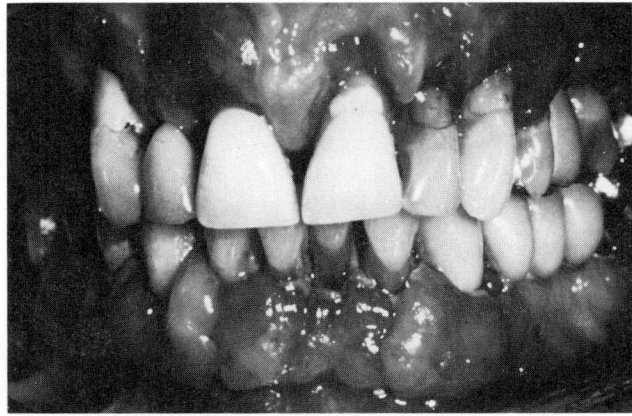

**Fig. 205-3.** Oral manifestations of leukemia.

## Acquired Immunodeficiency Syndrome

There are numerous intraoral manifestations of acquired immunodeficiency syndrome (AIDS). Many of these are exaggerated responses to the viral conditions described above. Viral conditions that are potentially life-threatening may respond to intravenous acyclovir. A host of other opportunistic infections may be present in addition to the AIDS-related malignancies, such as Kaposi's sarcoma and non-Hodgkin's lymphoma, or conditions such as hairy leukoplakia (white lesions on the side of the tongue possibly associated with Epstein-Barr virus). Oropharyngeal thrush is perhaps one of the most common and perhaps earliest manifestations of AIDS, and this diagnosis should be suspected in any adult patient who presents with this condition. Periodontal conditions that are seen in the AIDS patient include a variety of advanced periodontitis very similar to the clinical picture of the patient with leukemia in Fig. 205-3 as well as isolated areas of gingival recession (a relatively nonspecific finding) or unusual gingival pigmentation. Premature onset of periodontitis without excessive local etiologic factors includes in its differential diagnosis: juvenile periodontitis, diabetes, and AIDS (17% of HIV-infected homosexual males).

## DENTOALVEOLAR TRAUMA

The simplest type of dental trauma involves the fracture of anterior teeth. The management of dental fractures is based on (1) the extent of the fracture in relation to the pulp of the tooth, and (2) the age of the patient. A classification, the Ellis system, has been developed to describe the fracture anatomy of teeth. However, the emergency physician may also use a descriptive classification of traumatic injuries to teeth and supporting structures as advocated by Johnson (Fig. 205-4).

### Fractures

The Ellis class I fracture involves only the enamel portion of the tooth. This is generally a minor problem and requires immediate intervention only if a sharp piece of tooth is causing trauma to soft tissues. In such situations, the rough edge may be smoothed with something as simple as an emery board and/or referred to a general dentist for cosmetic restoration.

The Ellis class II fracture is a more complicated fracture involving not only the enamel but also exposure of dentin. The patient may complain of sensitivity to heat, cold, or even air. Immediate treatment of the Ellis class II fracture is dictated by the age of the patient, since less dentin is present in younger patients (under 12 years). Passage of

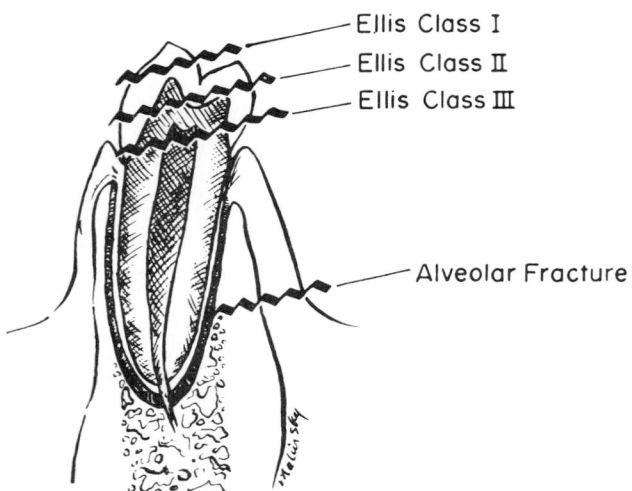

**Fig. 205-4.** Ellis classification for fractures of anterior teeth.

microorganisms through the microtubules of exposed dentin can contaminate the pulp.

The management of Ellis class II fractures in younger patients requires the immediate placement of a calcium hydroxide dressing on the exposed dentin which is then covered with dry gauze, aluminum foil or dental dry foil with an adhesive backing. The patient requires dental referral within 24 h. Older patients (12 to 14 years) who have a greater dentin to pulp ratio may be advised to avoid extremes in temperature and to seek dental care the following day. Patients with severe Ellis class II fractures (which may be recognized by a pinkish tinge to the dentin) should be treated as younger patients. Analgesics may also be required. The correct management of Ellis class II fractures may obviate the need for root canal therapy. The emergency physician should warn any patient who has sustained trauma to the anterior teeth, no matter how minor, that disruption of the tooth's neurovascular supply may have occurred; long-term complications may be pulpal necrosis or resorption (dissolving) of the tooth.

Ellis class III fractures of the teeth involve, in addition to fracture of enamel and the exposure of dentin, the actual exposure of the pulp. These fractures may be differentiated from Ellis class II fractures by gently wiping a tooth clean with a piece of gauze to eliminate the possibility of blood from soft tissue trauma. The tooth is then examined for any red blush of dentin or frank drop of blood. A patient may complain of exquisite pain or no pain if the neurovascular supply is disrupted. Ellis class III fractures are true dental emergencies and require immediate attention from a general dentist or endodontist since delay in treatment may result in significant pain and probably abscess formation. If a dentist is not immediately available, the tooth may be temporarily covered with aluminum foil or sealed with "cavet," a temporary root canal sealer, so as to minimize pulpal irritation and pain. Analgesics should be prescribed and the patient should see a dentist as soon as possible. The emergency physician would be ill-advised to introduce any instrument into the tooth for the removal of pulpal tissue since instrument breakage or tooth fracture may result, making endodontic treatment difficult or impossible. Over-the-counter topical dental analgesic preparations should neither be prescribed nor applied in the adult. Although these agents may give the patient temporary relief from pulpal pain, they often cause severe soft tissue irritation and sterile abscesses. In all cases of tooth fracture, lacerated soft tissue should be palpated for tooth fragments and radiographed if swelling limits the examination.

### Subluxated and Avulsed Teeth

The same force which may have resulted in the fracture of anterior teeth may also result in actual loosening of the tooth, termed subluxation. A traumatized tooth should always be examined for subluxation with use of finger pressure or the application of gentle rocking pressure with two tongue blades on each side of the tooth. A more subtle indication that teeth have been traumatized is the appearance of blood in the gingival crevice of the tooth. Minimally mobile teeth heal well with a soft diet for 1 to 2 weeks. Grossly mobile teeth require prompt stabilization. As a temporizing procedure for teeth which are very loose, it is often useful to have the patient bite gently on a piece of gauze to keep the tooth in place pending examination by a dentist or oral-maxillofacial surgeon.

A tooth that has been completely avulsed from the socket is a true dental emergency. If the patient is unaware of the location of the missing tooth, x-rays should be taken to determine if the missing tooth has been forced beneath the gingiva. Intruded primary ("baby") teeth are allowed to erupt for 6 weeks. Permanent teeth are surgically repositioned with a forceps and stabilized. Failure to diagnose intruded teeth may result in cosmetic deformity or infection. The management of an avulsed tooth depends upon the age of the patient and the length of time that the tooth has been absent from the oral cavity. Avulsed primary anterior teeth in the pediatric patient (ages 6 months to 5 years) are not replaced into their sockets. Replanted primary teeth have a high tendency to ankylose or fuse to the bone itself, resulting in facial deformity.

Traditional teaching is that a permanent tooth should be replaced in its socket as soon as possible if avulsion is less than 2 to 3 h. A percentage point for successful replantation is lost each minute that the tooth is absent from the oral cavity. When a call is received about an avulsed tooth, determine the age of the patient. If it appears that the tooth is permanent, the parent or patient should be instructed to quickly rinse the tooth under running tap water, holding it by the crown portion *only,* and to replant it immediately back in its socket. If actual replantation is not possible, the patient should be advised to bring the tooth to the emergency department as quickly as possible in a tooth transport container, "Save-A-Tooth," or if not available, in moist gauze or, preferably, a glass of milk. The patient may also be allowed to place the tooth in his or her own mouth to bathe in saliva, with care taken not to swallow the tooth.

New advances have been made in the development of a more ideal storage and transport media for avulsed teeth. When a tooth is avulsed from its socket, periodontal ligament fibers remain attached to both the tooth and the socket. Key to successful replantation is the survival of the remaining periodontal ligament fibers on the root. Milk is an acceptable storage media due to its osmolarity and essential ion concentration of $Ca^{2+}$ and $Mg^{2+}$. However, it is now known that the best storage and transport medium is Hank's solution, which is a pH-balanced cell culture medium. This solution is commercially available in a kit called "Save-A-Tooth." (TPS, Biological Rescue Products, Inc.). It has also been found that Hank's solution can maintain the viability of the periodontal ligament cells for 4 to 6 h or longer. Finally, if the tooth has been avulsed for longer than 30 min, placement of the tooth in the Hank's solution for 20 to 30 min helps restore cell viability. The use of the TPS system is illustrated in Fig. 205-5. The tooth is dropped in a basket and immersed in the Hank's solution; at the time of removal, the basket is lifted out of the solution and tipped over on the padded lid for retrieval.

If the tooth has not been replanted by the time the patient reaches the emergency department, it should be held by the crown at all times, rinsed under saline or running water, or preferably in the TPS system but *not* scrubbed (so as to conserve as many of the remaining periodontal ligament fibers as possible for reattachment) and re-

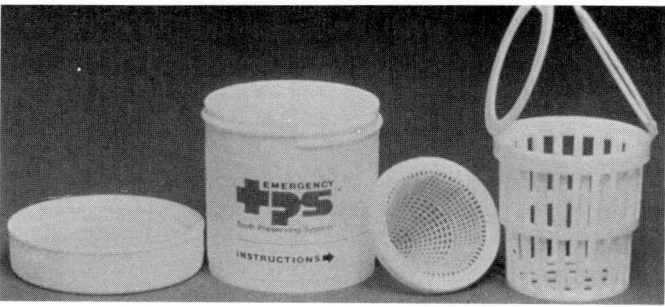

A

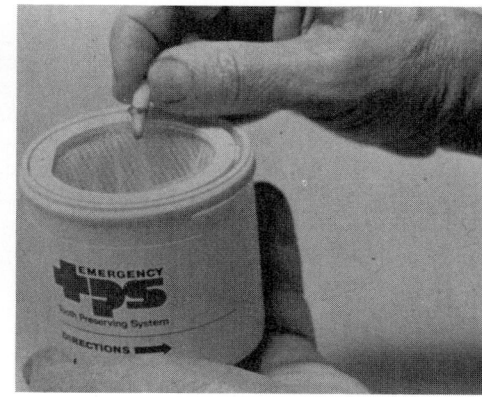

B

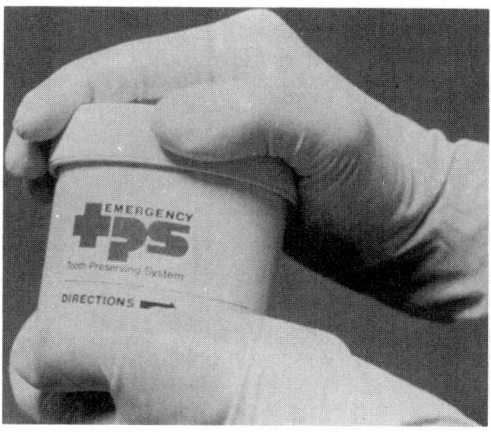

C

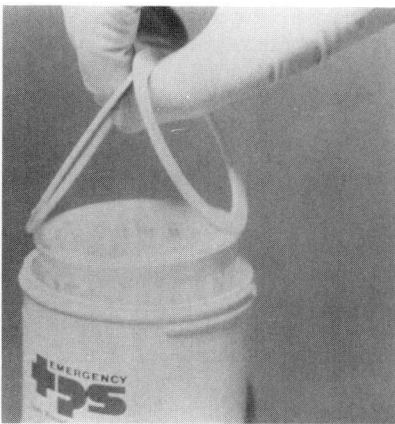

D

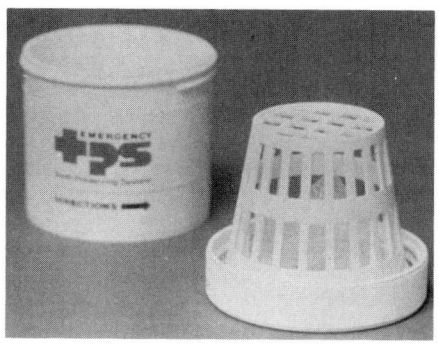

E

**Fig. 205-5. A.** The Tooth Preserving System (TPS). **B.** Each avulsed tooth is dropped into a separate TPS container of Hank"s solution. **C.** The lid is tightly secured. The container can be gently swirled to clean the tooth. **D.** The tooth is removed from the container by lifting up the basket. **E.** The tooth is retrieved by turning the basket over onto the cushioned interior lining of the lid. (Courtesy of Paul Krasner, D.D.S., Biological Rescue Products, Inc., 566 High Street, Pottstown, PA., 19464.)

planted into the socket. If absent longer than 30 min, placement in the TPS system should be considered prior to replantation. If a blood clot prevents replantation, or in the case of long time intervals since avulsion, the clot should be quickly suctioned or debrided under local anesthesia and then the tooth should be replanted.

Both maxillary central incisors may be avulsed at the same time. In order to determine which tooth is right or left, hold the tooth with the convex portion facing you. The side of the tooth which faces the midline comes to more of a sharp right angle at the incisal corner; the side which goes posteriorly is usually more curved. Extreme wear of the tooth can make this differentiation quite difficult. If the teeth are inadvertently placed in the wrong socket, the dentist can correct this at the time of definitive stabilization (Fig. 205-6).

Avulsed teeth require immediate stabilization or they will exfoliate; biting on gauze is a temporizing measure. Though stabilization is normally performed by the general dentist or oral-maxillofacial surgeon, there are situations where stabilization may be performed by the emergency physician. Indications would be a single avulsed tooth which has been placed back into the socket with satisfactory alignment, e.g., no prematurity of occlusion on jaw closure. Any tooth stabilized by the emergency physician should be evaluated by the general dentist or oral-maxillofacial surgeon within 24 h.

Several techniques are at the disposal of the emergency physician for stabilization of subluxated or avulsed teeth. A simple method described by Medford involves the application of a periodontal dressing ("Coe-Pak") which consists of zinc oxide and a catalyst that set when mixed to a semihard consistency. When molded over the reimplanted tooth and adjacent teeth, 24 h of stabilization can be achieved (Fig. 205-7).

## Alveolar Fractures

Avulsed teeth are stabilized for approximately 10 days to 2 weeks and then placed back into function to avoid ankylosis. When there are concomitant alveolar fractures, the stabilization of avulsed or subluxated teeth serves to stabilize the alveolar bone; stabilization is then left for a minimum of 6 weeks. Indiscriminate loss of alveolar bone will lead to more difficult prosthetic restoration of this area than the removal of any ankylosed tooth. Generally, prophylactic antibiotics, e.g., phenoxymethyl penicillin, 250 to 500 mg qid, are used when avulsed teeth are reimplanted in the oral cavity and appropriate tetanus prophylaxis should also be instituted.

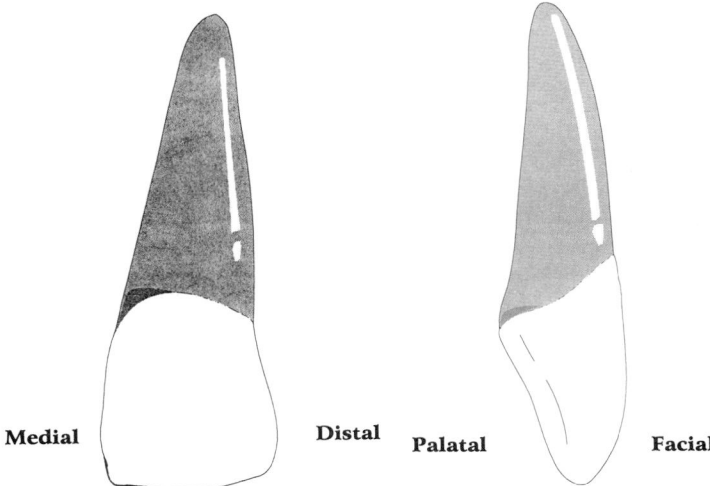

**Fig. 205-6.** Illustration of an upper (maxillary) left central incisor. Note that the part of the tooth facing medially comes to more of a right angle at the incisal edge than occurs distally. The facial portion of the tooth is more convex.

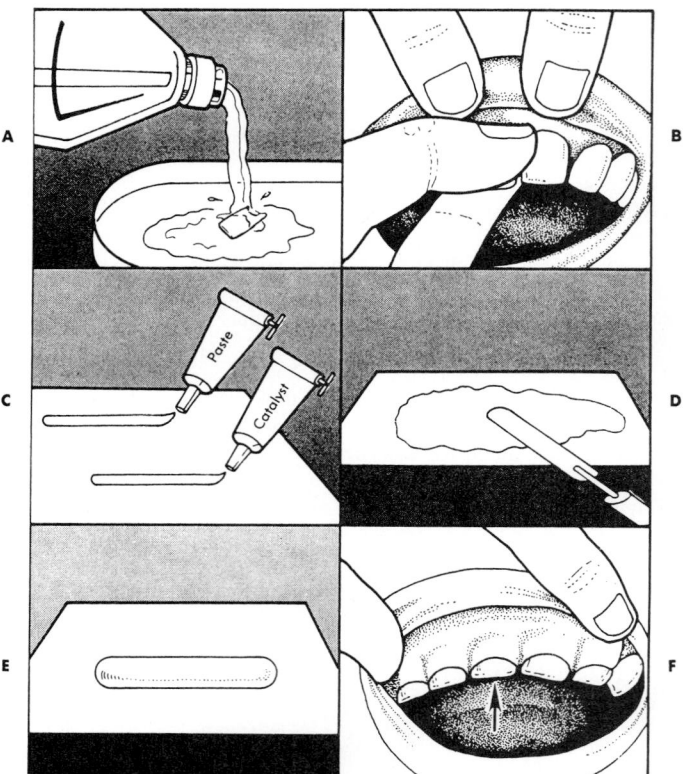

**Fig. 205-7.** Reimplantation and stabilization of an avulsed tooth. **A.** Tooth is rinsed. **B.** Tooth is placed back into socket. **C, D.** Periodontal pack is mixed. **E.** Splint Material is ready for application. **F.** Packing is molded over reimplanted tooth and two adjacent teeth to each side. (From Rosen P, Barkin R, Braen G, et. al. (eds): *Emergency Medicine: Concept and Clinical Practice,* 3rd ed. St. Louis, Mosby, 1992, p. 2393. Used by permission.)

## Soft Tissue Injury

Closure of associated laceration of the gingiva, mucosa, lips, and other facial soft tissues is performed after the teeth have been stabilized in the oral cavity. Stabilization of these teeth involves various methods of wiring or application of plastic materials or both, all of which require stretching of soft tissues, especially the lips and oral mucosa. Thus, carefully placed sutures will simply be torn and increase the soft tissue injury. The emergency physician should await final stabilization of the dentoalveolar component before instituting soft tissue closure and plastic repair.

### Oral Lacerations

Oral lacerations can involve either the lips, mucosa, gingiva, hard palate, tongue, or combinations of each. If lip lacerations are associated with intraoral injuries, the intraoral injuries should be managed first and a new sterile instrument tray used for the skin closure.

Gaping intraoral mucosal lacerations (greater than 1.5 cm) tend to become ulcerated, secondarily infected, and heal in a fibrotic manner resulting in a lump of tissue that is subject to repeated trauma unless sutured. Mucosal lacerations should be inspected carefully for debris (including tooth structure), crushed and nonviable tissue should be removed, the wound copiously irrigated, and closed with 4–0 chromic suture material. Black silk suture (4–0) is an acceptable alternative and easier to use but will require removal in 7 to 10 days. Good tissue approximation is preferred to a watertight seal so that drainage can occur should the wound become infected. Extensive mucosal lacerations or those involving large amounts of crushed tissue are best covered with antibiotics (phenoxymethyl penicillin or erythromycin 250 mg po qid) based on clinical experience although there are not much data to support the practice. Laceration of the frenulum alone does not usually require repair.

### Tongue Lacerations

Tongue lacerations greater than 1 cm should be closed with either 4–0 black silk suture or 4–0 chromic. If one finds a laceration of the dorsum of the tongue, the ventral surface should be carefully inspected for additional lacerations from the teeth. Careful attention must be paid to detail in approximating the edges of the wound in a laceration of the dorsum of the tongue. Reepithelialization across the wound margin is desired; if the wound edges are not well approximated, the epithelium will marginate downward to the base of the wound on each side and result in a "bifid" tongue appearance. A bifid tongue results in cosmetic as well as functional deformity and will require revision. Even in the best of hands, this is a potential complication of a tongue laceration, and the patient should be so advised. Extensive lacerations of the mucosal surface of the tongue warrant antibiotic treatment similar to other intraoral mucosal lacerations.

### Palate Lacerations

Palatal lacerations may involve either the hard or the soft palate. Soft palate injuries occur commonly in children who fall with a pointed object in their mouth. These lacerations should be treated as puncture wounds. Gaping skin edges can be loosely approximated with 5–0 chromic, but for the most part the wound should be allowed to drain. Injury to the retropharynx and vascular structures should be considered. Lacerations of the hard palate are difficult to close since this tissue is not very mobile. Closure can be performed with a 4–0 or 5–0 silk or chromic suture using a fine needle. Abrasions of the palate can heal by granulation; a dental emollient paste such as Orabase can be prescribed for comfort. Palatal lacerations tend not to become infected. Prophylactic antibiotic coverage is recommended with the same rationale as that for other intraoral mucosal injuries.

Good patient control is necessary for management of these wounds. An intraoral bite block is a very useful adjunct and makes the procedure more comfortable for the patient. Very young and uncooperative patients who require closure of the wound need sedation and may even require repair in the operating room.

### Lip Lacerations

Lacerations of the lip require meticulous closure, especially if the vermilion border is involved. As with any facial skin closure, suture removal should occur within 4 to 5 days to avoid suture marks. However, due to the musculature of the lips, premature wound separation can occur with deep lacerations. Therefore, when lip lacerations involve deep subcutaneous tissue and muscle, these structures should be approximated with a resorbable material (5–0 polyvicryl). The skin is then closed with a 6–0 nylon monofilament material. If the vermilion border of the lip is involved, the first step is to approximate the border as precisely as possible. The remainder of the closure is then accomplished. If possible, the suture through the vermilion border itself should be removed (making sure that the wound remains approximated) so that no suture mark will appear on the vermillion border. The patient should keep the wound clean with hydrogen peroxide wipes and maintain a layer of triple antibiotic ointment on the wound. Caution should be exercised not to distend the lips with such activity as laughing, yawning, or trying to examine the injury at home.

Controversy surrounds the management of the through-and-through laceration involving communication between the skin and the oral cavity. Some advocate not closing the intraoral component. It is this author's recommendation that if the mucosal laceration meets the criteria specified above, then it should be approximated. Through-and-through wounds should be irrigated well. The patient should be instructed in the use of saline rinses at home. Some well-controlled studies support the practice of prescribing antibiotics (phenoxymethyl penicillin or erythromycin 250 mg qid) as a prophylactic measure. These patients should have the wound checked in 48 to 72 h for infection. Care must be taken not to misinterpret normal mucosal edema associated with initial wound healing for infection. The need for tetanus prophylaxis should be considered with all oral and intraoral lacerations.

## HEMORRHAGE

### Spontaneous Hemorrhage

Oral hemorrhage may be spontaneous from gingiva. The history should include inquiry as to recent dental scaling or prophylaxis. If this history exists, bleeding usually responds to peroxide mouth rinse and local pressure with gauze compresses. Spontaneous gingival hemorrhage may also be the initial presentaton of a systemic process, such as leukemia or coagulopathy. Extent of the hemorrhage, age of the patient, and results of general examination determine the need for laboratory testing.

### Hemorrhage Secondary to Extraction

Bleeding secondary to dental extraction is usually controlled by having the patient apply sustained pressure by biting gauze. Spitting, smoking cigarettes, and the use of straws create a negative pressure intraorally that exudes blood clots from sockets and aggravates postextraction bleeding.

If the bleeding fails to respond to gauze pressure and there are large clots present, the clots should be wiped from the oral cavity, the socket suctioned, and gauze pressure attempted once again. If this is unsuccessful, local anesthesia consisting of 2% lidocaine with 1:100,000 or 1:50,000 epinephrine may be infiltrated in the area of the socket and gingiva, and gauze pressure reapplied for 20 min. If oozing persists, a small piece of absorbable gelatin sponge can be placed in the socket and secured with one or two 3–0 black silk sutures.

If there is sustained, vigorous oozing after all of the above procedures, a screening coagulation profile consisting of a CBC, platelet count, PT, and PTT should be drawn, since postextraction hemorrhage is often the initial manifestation of a coagulopathy. In some instances, postextraction bleeding is due to improper surgical technique or flap design, and lack of a sufficient number of sutures for hemostasis. Flaps may be sutured together and gauze pressure applied.

### Postoperative Hemorrhage

In case of bleeding after periodontal surgery, the emergency physician should contact the periodontist, for periodontal packs placed during surgery are extremely important to wound healing and incorrect placement can result in treatment failure.

## BIBLIOGRAPHY

Amsterdam J. Dental disorders, in Rosen P, Barkin R, Braen G, et al (eds): *Emergency Medicine: Concepts and Clinical Practice,* 3d ed. St. Louis, Mosby, 1992, pp 2381–2398.

Amsterdam J. Emergency Dental Procedures, in Roberts J, Hedges J (eds): *Clinical Procedures in Emergency Medicine,* 2nd ed. Philadelphia, Saunders, 1991, pp 1045–1064.

Amsterdam J, Hendler B, Rose L: Dental emergencies, in Schwartz G, Safer P, Stone J, et al (eds): *Principles and Practice of Emergency Medicine,* 2d ed. Philadelphia, Saunders, 1986, pp 1557–1585.

Blomlof L: Milk and saliva as possible storage media for traumatically exarticulated teeth prior to replantation, *Swed Dent J* 8 (suppl):1, 1981.

Jaber L, Cohen I, Mor A: Fever associated with teething, *Arch Disease Child* 67:234, 1992.

Johnson R: Descriptive classification of trauma: The injuries to the teeth and supporting structures. *J Am Dent Assoc* 102:195, 1981.

Kristerson L, Soder PO, and Otteskog P: Transport and storage of human teeth in vitro for autotransplantation and replantation, *J Oral Surg* 34:13, 1976.

Kruger GO: *Textbook of Oral and Maxillofacial Surgery,* 6th ed. St. Louis, Mosby, 1984.

Leung A: Teething. *AFP* 39(2): 131, 1989.

Lindskog S, Blomlof L: Influence of osmolality and composition of some storage media on human periodontal ligament cells, *Acta Odontol Scand* 40:435, 1982.

Lynch M (ed): *Burket's Oral Medicine,* 8th ed. Philadelphia, Lippincott, 1984.

Masci J. Primary and ambulatory care of the HIV-infected adult, in Rosen P, Barkin R, Braen G, et al (eds): *Emergency Medicine: Concepts and Clinical Practice,* 3rd ed. St. Louis, Mosby, 1992, pp 93–94.

Medford HM: Temporary stabilization of avulsed teeth. *Ann Emergy Med* 11:490, 1982.

# Skin and Soft Tissue Emergencies

## 206

# TOXICODENDRON DERMATITIS

**Thomas A. Chapel**
**Johanna Chapel**

Kligman states that the *Toxicodendron* species—poison ivy, poison oak, and poison sumac—are responsible for more cases of allergic contact dermatitis in the United States than all other allergens combined. Fisher estimates that at least 70 percent of the population of the United States if casually exposed to the plants would develop allergic contact sensitivity to the *Toxicodendron* species, and the percentage would be even greater if contact were more prolonged. Dark-skinned individuals seem less susceptible than others to *Toxicodendron* dermatitis, and elderly persons are not as susceptible to poison ivy as younger people are.

## CHARACTERISTICS OF *Toxicodendron spp.*

Poison ivy and poison oak are the principal causes of plant dermatitis in North America. Poison ivy occurs throughout the United States, while poison oak is more common on the west coast. In the United States there are two species of poison oak, *Toxicodendron diversilobum* (western poison oak) and *T. toxicarium* (eastern poison oak). There also are two species of poison ivy, *T. rydbergii,* a nonclimbing subshrub, and *T. radicans,* which may be either a shrub or a climbing vine. One species of poison sumac, *T. vernix,* occurs in the United States. It grows as a coarse, woody shrub or as a tree and is found in wooded, swampy areas.

All species of poison oak and poison ivy have leaves with three leaflets, and poison sumac has 7 to 13 leaflets per leaf. The *Toxicodendron* species can also be recognized by their U- or V-shaped leaf scars, typical lenticels, and flowers and fruit that arise in the angle between the leaf and the branch. Off-white mature fruit is borne on a doubly branched structure called a *panicle.*

The leaves, stems, seeds, flowers, berries, and roots of the *Toxicodendron* species contain a milky sap which darkens to the appearance of black lacquer on exposure to the air. The black deposit is present where plants have been injured, and its presence proves that a suspicious plant is a toxicodendron. This characteristic can be used by novices or persons working with unfamiliar vegetation to identify these plants. Guin suggests that several leaves from the plant in question be crushed on a sheet of white paper. The sap stain from poison ivy, poison oak, and poison sumac darkens markedly within a few minutes. This black spot test is used only to augment classic methods of plant identification, and care must be taken to avoid contamination of fingers and clothing with sap.

## THE DERMATITIS-PRODUCING FACTORS OF THE *Toxicodendron* SPECIES

The antigenic oleoresin of *Toxicodendron* species is easily extracted from plant sap with alcohol and other solvents. The residue left after evaporation of the solvent is called *urushiol,* and its dermatitis-producing principle is pentadecylcatechol. The *Toxicodendron* species share similar antigens, and therefore cross-sensitivity exists between poison ivy, poison oak, and poison sumac.

Urushiol oxidizes and with complete oxidation is rendered nonallergenic. The speed of the breakdown is promoted by moisture and heat. The antigenic film on clothing or other objects may become inactive within 1 week in a hot, humid environment, while the substance remains allergenic for much longer periods in a dry atmosphere. Washing with soap and water rapidly destroys the antigen. The allergenicity of the oleoresin is maximal in fresh plants and diminishes as the plant ages. However, sensitive individuals must avoid handling plants of any age, for even withered leaves produce contact dermatitis.

The persistence of the allergen permits its spread by contaminated fingers, clothing, tools, animals, and sports equipment. Smoke carrying particles of the plant can, and often does, disseminate the disease. However, complete incineration of the plant destroys the allergen.

Toxicodendron antigen may remain under a person's fingernails for several days unless deliberately removed by thorough cleansing. Scratching with antigen-contaminated fingers disseminates the dermatitis to the face, genitals, and covered areas. The dermatitigenic effect of minute amounts of allergen in highly sensitized individuals is astonishing. Kligman contaminated the thumb of a nonsensitized subject with the juice from crushed leaves. The thumb was then pressed onto the back of a nonsensitized subject 99 times, then once onto the back of a highly sensitive individual. This sequence was repeated four more times. The fifth contact on the highly sensitive individual caused a slight dermatitis, even after 500 impressions.

## PRESENTATION AND DIAGNOSIS

### Clinical Features

*Toxicodendron* antigen enters the skin rapidly, and in order to prevent a reaction the sap must be totally removed within 30 min after exposure. Under ordinary circumstances such prophylaxis is impossible. Contact dermatitis in susceptible people generally develops within 2 days following exposure. However, Fisher reports that in a few cases the eruption appears 8 h after exposure, and, rarely, the interval may exceed 10 days.

The temporal difference in onset of the eruption and variations in the clinical expression of toxicodendron dermatitis depend upon the patient's degree of sensitivity, the amount of contact with the allergen, and the regional variations in cutaneous reactivity. Mildly sensitive persons can probably withstand casual exposure to the plant without difficulty. Some individuals develop simple erythema, others erythema and papules, and yet others erythema, papules, vesicles, and bullae. The dermatitis usually begins with pruritus and redness. Streaks of erythema or papulovesicles in linear arrangement soon appear (Figs. 206-1 and 206-2). The linear configuration of some lesions is highly suggestive of toxicodendron dermatitis; it is produced by portions of the plant rubbing across the skin or by dissemination of the allergen by scratching with contaminated fingernails. A common myth is that the disorder is spread by rupturing vesicles. However, blister fluid contains no antigen, and therefore it cannot transmit the dermatitis.

The eruption usually disappears without a trace, but leukodermia or hyperpigmentation are occasional sequelae. Urticaria and erythema multiforme infrequently occur as a result of systemic absorption of toxicodendron antigen.

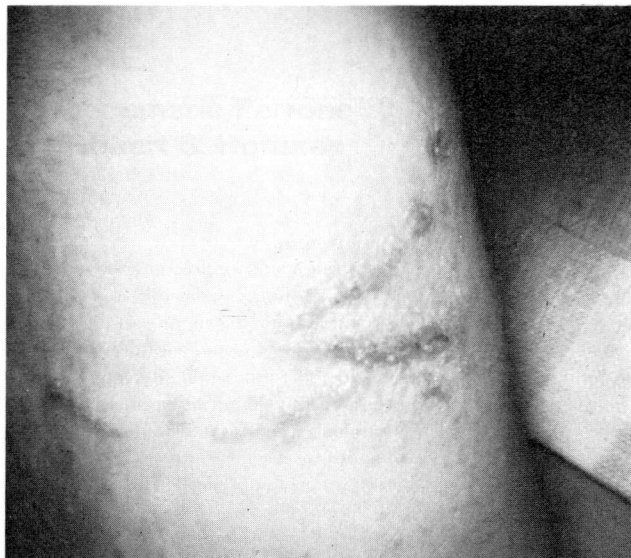

**Fig. 206-1.** Erythematous, edematous papules and vesicles of the poison ivy in typical linear arrangement.

Laboratory findings in patients with poison ivy dermatitis are minimal. Leukocytosis and eosinophils of 5 to 10 percent occur in a small percentage of patients with severe dermatitis.

### Differential Diagnosis

Toxicodendron dermatitis is quite distinctive, but occasionally it may be confused with contact dermatitis of other origin. A mimic is phytophotodermatitis caused by lime, parsley, celery, figs, and buttercups. Juices from these plants contain psoralens, which are activated by long-wave ultraviolet light and produce a phototoxic eruption. The eruption consists of striate lesions and irregularly liner bullae in sun-exposed areas. The blisters usually heal with pigmentation that lasts for months. Poison ivy dermatitis is not photoactivated, and it can be distinguished from phytophotodermatitis by lesions that occur on both covered and uncovered areas of the body.

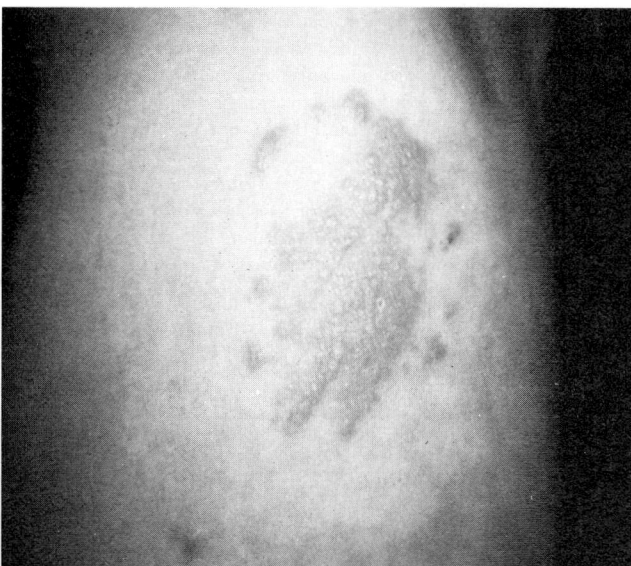

**Fig. 206-2.** Plaque of poison ivy dermatitis with streaks of erythema and papulovesicles.

## TREATMENT

Treatment of toxicodendron dermatitis is determined by the severity of the eruption. Mild dermatitis consisting of erythema, edema, and papules limited to a few anatomic regions can be managed with shake lotions such as calamine or steroid sprays, creams, or lotions. Compresses or soaks with cold or moderately hot water bring temporary relief from pruritus, and antihistaminics by mouth effectively control persistent itch.

More aggressive treatment is required for moderate and severe dermatitis with vesicles and bullae distributed over large areas of the body's surface. Compresses with cool aluminum sulfate diluted 1:10 (Domeboro) help dry lesions and minimize itch. Compresses are applied for 30 to 60 min two to three times each day until blisters dry. Large bullae can be aseptically aspirated with roofs left intact. Potassium permanganate baths aid in drying ruptured blisters. The patient dissolves one-half tablespoon of potassium permanganate crystals in a tub of lukewarm water and soaks for 15 to 20 min each day. Baths with colloidal oatmeal (Aveeno), mixed 1 cupful per tub of water, are also soothing. The pruritus accompanying severe dermatitis should be treated with antihistaminics in full therapeutic doses.

Systemic corticosteroids are effective in bringing relief and are often used if there are no contraindications. If corticosteroids are used, they should be initiated at a level equivalent to 40 to 60 mg of prednisone daily, gradually tapered over a 2- to 3-week period, and then discontinued. Shorter courses of corticosteroids should be avoided as they are frequently associated with a rebound exacerbation of the dermatitis.

The speed with which the eruption heals depends upon the severity and the extent of the cutaneous injury. Mild dermatitis often disappears within 7 to 10 days, while severe eruptions often require 3 or more weeks for normalization.

## PROPHYLAXIS

The salient points of toxicodendron dermatitis must be explained carefully to patients, and common myths should be dispelled. The best prophylaxis against recurrent dermatitis is avoidance of the *Toxicodendron* species. This requires that patients recognize poison ivy and related species. Display posters and illustrated pamphlets are helpful teaching aids in educating patients. Persons allergic to the *Toxicodendron* species may have cross reactions to Japanese lacquer and cashew nut trees, the mango, and the marking nut tree of India. Contact with these items also should be avoided.

Individuals exposed to toxicodendrons should wash the entire body with soap and water and carefully clean their fingernails. Clean clothing should be worn, and contaminated clothing laundered. Poison ivy, poison oak, and poison sumac growing in areas of unavoidable contact should be destroyed with herbicides or removed physically to prevent future reexposure.

Epstein and associates advise highly sensitive individuals at increased risk of reexposure because of work or hobbies to try hyposensitization. Hyposensitization requires oral administration of very large doses of urushiol over a 4- to 8-month interval. Unfortunately, hyposensitization lasts no more than several months after the last dose of oil.

## BIBLIOGRAPHY

Baer R: Poison ivy dermatitis. *Cutis* 46:34, 1990.
Epstein WL: The poison ivy picker of pennypack park: the continuing saga of poison ivy. *J Invest Dermatol* 88:7, 1987.
Epstein WL: Topical prevention of poison ivy/oak dermatitis. *Arch Dermatol* 125:499, 1989.
Epstein WL, Byers VS, Baer H: Induction of persistent tolerance to urushiol in humans. *J Allergy Clin Immunol* 68:20, 1981.
Guin JD: The black spot test for recognizing poison ivy and related species. *J Am Acad Dermatol* 2:332, 1980.

Guin JD, Gillis WT, Beaman JH: Recognizing the *Toxicodendron* (poison ivy, poison oak, poison sumac). *J Am Acad Dermatol* 4:99, 1981.

Resnick SD: Poison-ivy and poison-oak dermatitis. *Clin Dermatol* 4:208, 1986.

# 207
# EXFOLIATIVE DERMATITIS

## Thomas A. Chapel
## Johanna Chapel

*Exfoliative dermatitis* refers to a condition in which most or all of the skin surface is involved with a scaly erythematous dermatitis. Males are afflicted with the condition twice as often as females, and at least 75 percent of the patients are over the age of 40. The widespread inflammatory exfoliation often is accompanied by immediate or delayed effects in other organ systems.

## ETIOLOGY AND PATHOGENESIS

Exfoliative dermatitis is a cutaneous reaction produced in response to a drug or chemical agent or to an underlying cutaneous or systemic disease. The etiologic classification and relative incidence of the more common underlying conditions are listed in Table 207-1. Aside from acute exacerbation of a preexisting dermatosis or generalized exposure to a contact allergen, the mechanisms responsible for exfoliative dermatitis are not known. However, it has been postulated that drug-induced exfoliative dermatitis may be mediated by an excessive number of drug-sensitized suppressor-cytotoxic T lymphocytes and may represent a disorder of immunoregulatory T cells.

Exfoliative dermatitis can have an abrupt onset when related to a drug or contact allergen or to malignancy. Outbreaks arising from an underlying cutaneous disorder usually evolve more slowly, and the identifiable features of the underlying disease may be lost. However, careful observation and a thorough physical examination can sometimes uncover changes characteristic of the primary disease.

In a study of 101 cases, Abrahams et al. found that exfoliative dermatitis tends to be a chronic condition, with a mean duration of 5 years and a median duration of 10 months. A shorter course often follows suppression of the underlying dermatosis, discontinuation of inciting drugs, or avoidance of the inciting allergen. Exfoliative dermatitis with no associated discernible cause can continue for 20 or

**Table 207-1.** Causes of Dermatitis

| Disease | Range of Reported Incidence, % |
| --- | --- |
| Generalized flares of preexisting cutaneous disease: | 25–40 |
| Psoriasis | |
| Atopic dermatitis | |
| Seborrheic dermatitis | |
| Lichen planus | |
| Pemphigus foliaceus | |
| Pityriasis rubra pilaris | |
| Contact dermatitis | |
| Drugs | 3–10 |
| Lymphoma, leukemia, solid tumors | 10–40 |
| Idiopathic | 15–45 |

more years. Death may occur and in general is attributable to hepatocellular damage from severe drug reactions or to underlying malignancies.

There is generalized erythema and warmth of the skin, accompanied by scaling or flaking of the epidermis. The patient usually has a low-grade fever and often complains of pruritus, a chilly sensation, and tightness of the skin. Chronic inflammatory exfoliation produces many changes, such as dystrophic nails, thinning of scalp and body hair, and patchy or diffuse postinflammatory hyperpigmentation or, less commonly, hypopigmentation. Gynecomastia and generalized lymphadenopathy are common in longstanding cases.

Active erythroderma is complicated by excessive heat loss, impairment of temperature regulation, and sometimes hypothermia. The widespread cutaneous vasodilation can cause increased cardiac output. In marginally compensated patients the hemodynamic changes may produce a high-output cardiac failure with dyspnea and dependent edema. Splenomegaly occurred in 3 to 14 percent of the 236 cases reported by Abrahams et al. and Nicolis and Helwig. When associated with exfoliative dermatitis, splenomegaly suggests an underlying leukemia or lymphoma.

The disruption of the epidermis results in increased transepidermal water loss, and continued exfoliation can result in significant protein loss and negative nitrogen balance. Steatorrhea sometimes results from the widespread inflammatory exfoliation, but the enteropathy resolves with improvement of the exfoliative dermatitis. The serum albumin level is lowered because of steatorrhea, cutaneous scaling, and plasma dilution arising from cardiovascular alterations.

## DIAGNOSIS AND TREATMENT
### Differential Diagnosis

The various ichthyoses may mimic exfoliative dermatitis; however, the presence of ichthyosis in other family members, the lifelong presence of disease, and the morphologic detail in scale and anatomic distribution make differentiation easy.

### Clinical Evaluation and Treatment

A patient with a newly diagnosed case of exfoliative dermatitis or one who is experiencing an acute exacerbation should be hospitalized for dermatologic nursing care, supportive treatment, and investigative studies. Considerable effort must be made to determine the underlying etiology by a careful history of previous cutaneous disease and of recent drug use, and laboratory tests to establish whether there is possible association with leukemia, lymphoma, or solid tumor. A cutaneous biopsy is indicated, and if there is significant lymphadenopathy, lymph nodes should likewise be biopsied. The patient should also be evaluated for cardiac failure and intestinal dysfunction.

Some patients respond to topical application of corticosteroid cream or ointment and oral antihistamines to control pruritus. However, many require systemic corticosteroids beginning with 40 to 60 mg of prednisone each day. If no response is observed, the dose may be increased by 20 mg. With a favorable response the dose is gradually tapered over weeks or months and eventually discontinued. When systemic steroids are used, the patient can apply bland lotions or creams rather than topical corticosteroid preparations. Tepid colloidal baths, such as cornstarch or oatmeal powder suspension, are of some benefit.

### SUMMARY

Exfoliative dermatitis is a cutaneous reaction produced in response to a drug or chemical agent or to an underlying cutaneous or systemic disease. It can be abrupt or insidious in onset. Clinically, it is characterized by generalized erythroderma and flaking or scaling of the epidermis.

Treatment includes control of the underlying cutaneous disorder, avoidance of the inciting drugs or allergen, or treatment of the underlying malignancy. Topical steroids and antipruritic agents may provide relief in many cases, but for more serious disorders systemic corticosteroids may be necessary.

## BIBLIOGRAPHY

Abrahams I, McCarthy J, Sanders S: 101 Cases of exfoliative dermatitis. *Arch Dermatol* 87:96, 1963.

Nicolis GD, Helwig EB: Exfoliative dermatitis: A clinicopathologic study of 135 cases. *Arch Dermatol* 108:788, 1973.

Wong KS, Wong SM, Tham SM, et al: Generalized exfoliative dermatitis—a clinical study of 108 patients. *Ann Acad Med* 17:520, 1988.

# 208
# ERYTHEMA MULTIFORME

### Thomas A. Chapel
### Johanna Chapel

## PATHOLOGY AND CLINICAL CHARACTERISTICS

*Erythema multiforme* represents a spectrum of disease that ranges from trivial cutaneous lesions to severe, sometimes fatal, multisystem illness. Tissue reaction is of variable expression, yet the histologic features are sufficiently characteristic to differentiate this disorder from other erythematous and vesiculobullous eruptions. The histo-

**Table 208-1.** Common Causes of Erythema Multiforme

Associated infectious diseases
  Adenovirus
  Coxsackie B5
  Echoviruses
  Enteroviruses
  Hepatitis A
  Hepatitis B
  Measles
  Vaccinia
  Herpes simplex infection, types I and II
  *Mycoplasma* pneumonia
  Influenza
  Mumps
  Psittacosis
  Cat-scratch disease
  Typhoid fever
  Diphtheria
  Lymphogranuloma venereum
  Histoplasmosis
  Cholera
Drugs commonly implicated
  Antituberculous drugs
  Sulfonamides
  Oral hypoglycemic agent: chlorpropamide
  Pyrazolone derivatives: phenylbutazone, oxyphenbutazone, phenazone
  Phenytoin and related anticonvulsants
  Barbiturates
  Tetracyclines
  Penicillins
  Carbamazepine
Malignancy with or without radiation therapy
  Carcinoma
  Lymphoma

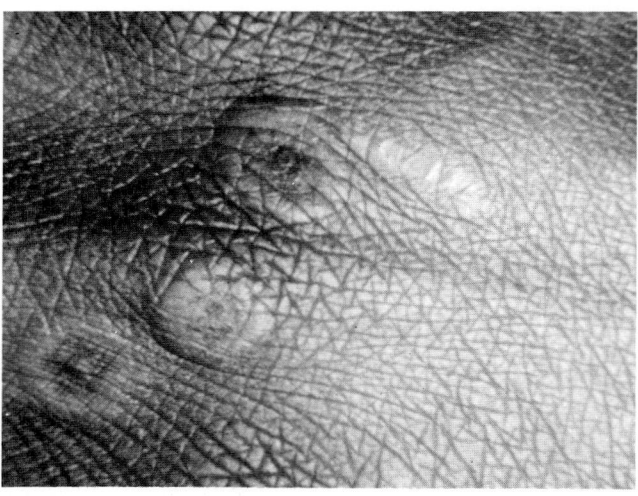

**Fig. 208-1.** Erythema multiforme secondary to heroin snuff.

pathologic spectrum of erythema multiforme has been described by Bedi and Pinkus. Bullae are subepidermal, and epidermal cell necrosis is often noted. The dermis is usually edematous, and a lymphocytic infiltrate is often present about the capillaries and venules of the upper dermis. The disorder is a hypersensitivity reaction precipitated by many agents and conditions (Table 208-1).

Recent data suggest an important role for circulating immune complexes. Direct immunofluorescence studies of erythema multiforme skin lesions have shown deposits of complement components and immunoglobulin in the superficial dermal blood vessels or at the dermal-epidermal junction, and immune complexes have been detected in serum samples of patients with erythema multiforme.

Infections are generally more important as the cause in children, while drugs (Fig. 208-1) and malignancies (Fig. 208-2) are more often implicated in adult cases. About half the cases lack an identifiable cause. Many cases of erythema multiforme occur during epidemics of atypical pneumonia, adenovirus infection, and histoplasmosis.

The disorder occurs at any age, affects males twice as often as females, and is most common in the spring and the fall. The morphology of the cutaneous lesions is variable; they can be macular, urticarial, or vesiculobullous. The skin lesions typically begin as erythematous macules or urticarial-like plaques, and they often contain

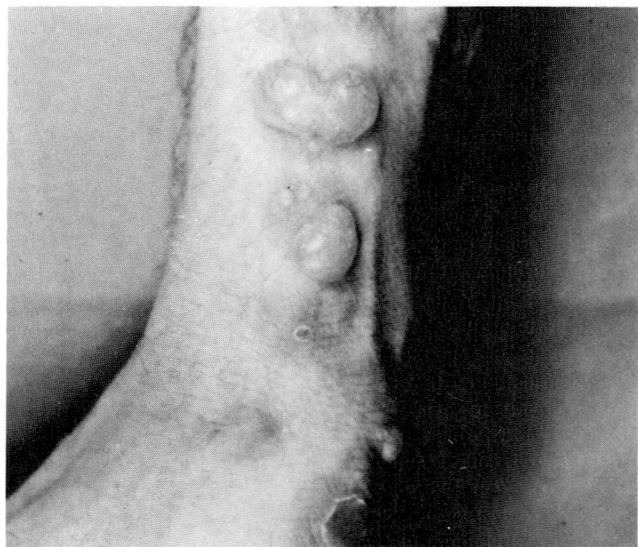

**Fig. 208-2.** Erythema multiforme bullosum secondary to cancer of the stomach.

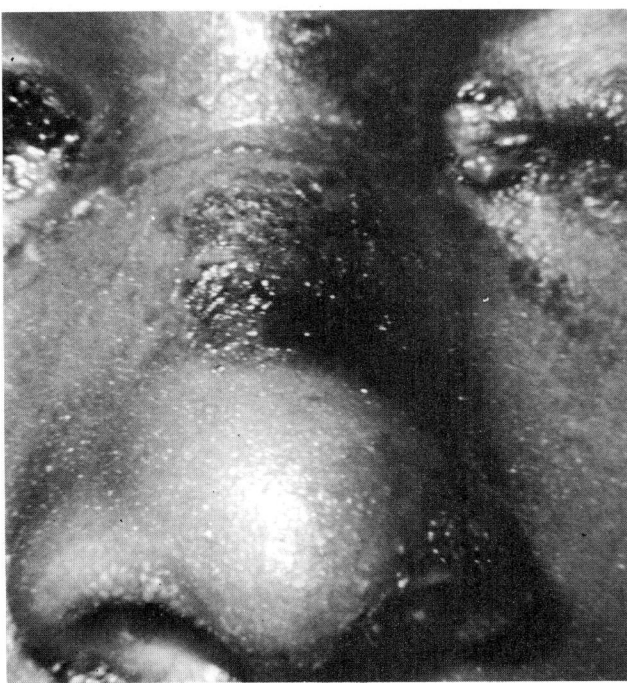

**Fig. 208-3.** Bullous erythema multiforme of the face.

scattered petechiae. Unlike true hives, the urticarial lesions of erythema multiforme are not usually pruritic. Vesiculobullous lesions develop centrally within preexisting macules, papules, or wheals (Figs. 208-3 and 208-4). Blistering of the mucous membranes occurs in about a quarter of cases, and at times it represents the sole expression of the disease. The characteristic iris lesions of erythema multiforme are erythematous plaques with dusky centers and bright red borders, resembling the bull's-eye of a target (Fig. 208-5).

The eruption has a predilection for dorsum of the hands, palms, soles, and extensor surfaces of the extremities. Lesions tend to appear in crops over a period of 2 to 4 weeks, and, rarely, over many

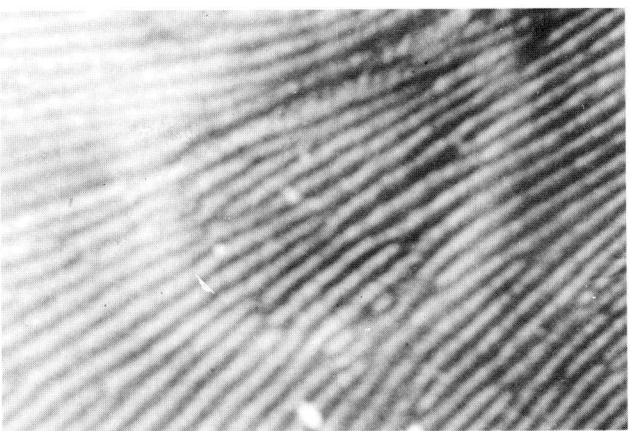

**Fig. 208-5.** Erythema multiforme lesions tend to appear in crops over a period of 2 to 4 weeks.

months. The individual lesions heal in 7 to 10 days without scarring unless the site is secondarily infected. However, in dark-skinned patients postinflammatory hyperpigmentation or hypopigmentation is common. When associated with herpes simplex virus, erythema multiforme can recur 5 to 7 days after each viral relapse and with drug incitant can recur upon repeat exposure.

The Stevens-Johnson eponym is reserved for the most severe bullous form of erythema multiforme. It is frequently preceded by a prodrome of variable symptoms, such as fever, malaise, myalgias, and arthralgias, which probably stem from an underlying infectious disease. The mucocutaneous lesions have abrupt onset and are associated with marked constitutional symptoms and multisystem pathology. The mucosal surfaces of the lips, cheeks, palate, eyes, urethra, vagina, nose, and anus are involved (Fig. 208-6). In severe cases the linings of the pharynx, tracheobronchial tree, and esophagus are also affected. The lesions begin as blisters, which rupture to leave shreds of necrotic grayish-white epithelium and blood-crusted denuded bases. Patients are often unable to eat because of the painful stomatitis. The eyes have a catarrhal or purulent conjunctivitis, and vesicles are sometimes observed on the conjunctivae. Rarely, widespread de-

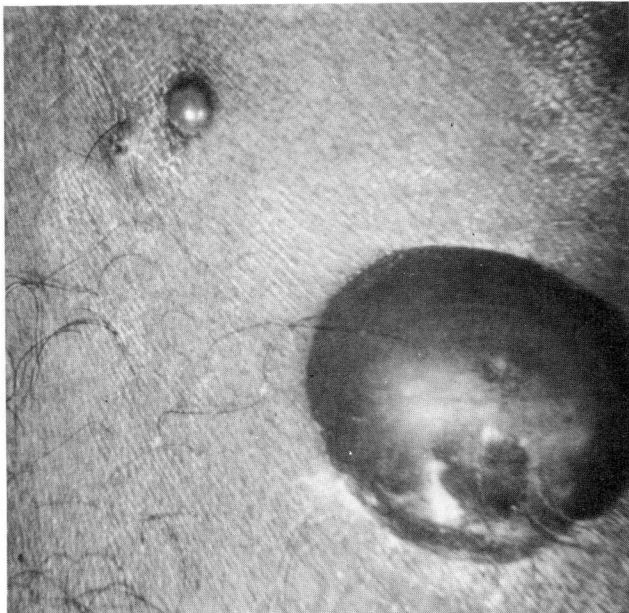

**Fig. 208-4.** Erythema multiforme bullosum lesions are usually annular and sharply demarcated from normal skin.

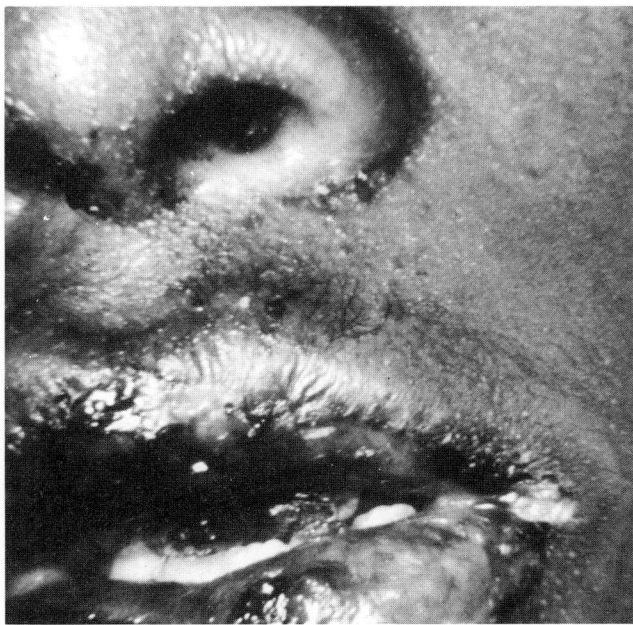

**Fig. 208-6.** Bullous erythema multiforme of the mouth, a commonly involved orifice.

nudation of skin typical of toxic epidermal necrolysis has been reported in patients with lesions of erythema multiforme, suggesting that toxic epidermal necrolysis is the most severe expression of erythema multiforme.

The Stevens-Johnson syndrome has substantial morbidity and a mortality of 5 to 10 percent. Denuded surfaces are susceptible to secondary bacterial infection, and, when untreated, these can lead to scar formation. Nails may occasionally be shed, balanitis can lead to scarred attachment of the foreskin to the glans, and vulvovaginitis can lead to stenosis of the vagina. Hematuria, renal tubular necrosis, and progressive renal failure can occur but are rare. More common are significant ocular sequelae, including corneal ulceration, anterior uveitis, panophthalmitis, corneal opacities, and blindness.

### Differential Diagnosis

Conditions to be differentiated include the migratory annular erythemas such as erythema annulare centrifugum; toxic erythemas of infectious or drug origin; blistering disorders such as bullous pemphigoid, pemphigus vulgaris, herpes gestationis; and the cutaneous and systemic vasculitides. Erythema multiforme has also been seen in association with erythema nodosum and toxic epidermal necrolysis.

### DIAGNOSIS AND TREATMENT

The clinical features are usually distinctive enough to permit a diagnosis, but a skin biopsy should be obtained in equivocal cases. Because erythema multiforme is a pattern reaction, appropriate investigative studies should be undertaken to determine the underlying cause, and all drugs of potential etiologic significance must be stopped. Respiratory failure can develop secondary to mucosal sloughing. While renal complications are uncommon, kidney function should be monitored.

Patients with limited disease can be treated on an outpatient basis with topical corticosteroids. However, those with severe mucous membrane involvement require hospitalization, preferably in a burn unit, where fluids and electrolytes can be managed and frequent secondary bacterial infections controlled. Ophthalmologic consultation is necessary if there is eye involvement. Relief from painful stomatitis can sometimes be achieved with diphenhydramine hydrochloride elixir or viscous lidocaine held in the mouth for 3 to 5 min before expectorating. Systemic corticosteroids give symptomatic relief but are of unproven value in influencing the duration and outcome of the disease. Indeed, many authorities believe that systemic corticosteroid therapy is contraindicated in the treatment of Stevens-Johnson syndrome.

### BIBLIOGRAPHY

Bedi TR, Pinkus H: Histopathological spectrum of erythema multiforme. *Br J Dermatol* 95:243, 1976.

Chan H-L, Stern R, Arndt K, et al: The incidence of erythema multiforme, Stevens–Johnson syndrome, and toxic epidermal necrolysis. *Arch Dermatol* 126:43, 1990.

Hurwitz A: Erythema multiforme: A review of its characteristics, diagnostic criteria, and management. *Pediatr Rev* 11:217, 1990.

## 209
## TOXIC EPIDERMAL NECROLYSIS AND THE STAPHYLOCOCCAL SCALDED SKIN SYNDROME

**Thomas A. Chapel**
**Johanna Chapel**

Toxic epidermal necrolysis and the staphylococcal scalded skin syndrome present with skin findings suggesting scalded skin. However, despite this morphologic similarity, staphylococcal scalded skin syndrome and toxic epidermal necrolysis are clinically, histologically, and etiologically distinct.

Toxic epidermal necrolysis is due to a drug or chemical agent or graft-versus-host reaction. It occurs most often but not exclusively in adults, and it is characterized by the sudden appearance of patches of intense, tender erythema that is followed by widespread loosening of skin and denudation to a glistening base. The skin separates at the dermal-epidermal junction. Some researchers consider toxic epidermal necrolysis a separate disease, while others feel that it is a severe form of erythema multiforme.

Staphylococcal scalded skin syndrome usually afflicts children under the age of 5 years, but rarely has been reported in adults (Fig. 209-1). The disorder is associated with an underlying staphylococcal infection and is due to the production of a toxin that cleaves the epidermis beneath the stratum granulosum. The exact mode of action of the toxin is unknown, although studies suggest an intercellular target, probably desmosomes.

### CLINICAL FEATURES

Toxic epidermal necrolysis occurs chiefly in adults and is characterized by separation of the skin at the dermal-epidermal junction (Fig. 209-2). The involved epidermis is necrotic, but little infiltrate is seen in the dermis. Lesions are widespread, the skin tender, and the mucous membranes are commonly involved (Figs. 209-3 and 209-4). Lateral pressure on the skin causes separation of the epidermis from the dermis (positive Nikolsky sign). At times, the skin lesions may resemble those of erythema multiforme. The complete loss of the epidermis is associated with slow healing, and reepithelialization takes 1 to 3 weeks.

Systemic signs include high fever, leukocytosis, elevation of transaminases, albuminuria, and water and electrolyte imbalance that may proceed to hemodynamic shock, pulmonary edema, and renal

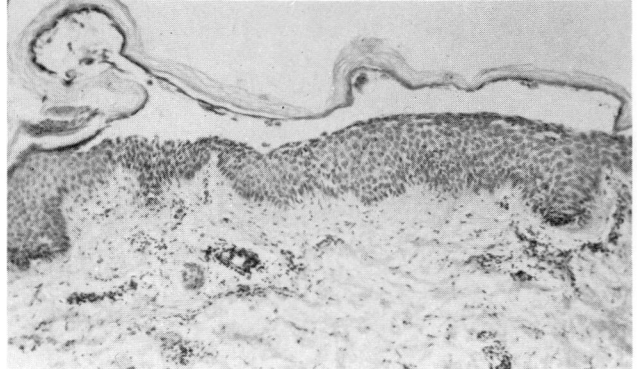

**Fig. 209-1.** Staphylococcal scalded skin syndrome.

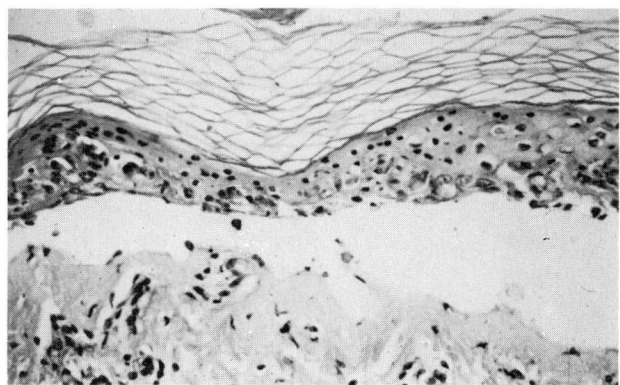

**Fig. 209-2.** Drug-induced toxic epidermal necrolysis.

failure. Toxic epidermal necrolysis carries a 5 to 50 percent mortality due to fluid loss and secondary infection (Table 209-1).

Staphylococcal scalded skin syndrome comprises a spectrum of skin lesions ranging from localized bullous impetigo to generalized exfoliation. The disease begins as tender, erythematous patches of scarlatiniform lesions that often follow an upper respiratory tract infection or purulent conjunctivitis. The initiated lesions are characteristically distributed on the periorificial areas of the face, the neck, the axillae, and the groin. At this stage, lateral pressure on the skin produces a positive Nikolsky sign. Large flaccid bullae sometimes develop, and within 24 to 48 h the epidermis spontaneously separates in rumpled sheets, revealing a moist, erythematous base. Despite widespread exfoliation of the skin, the mucous membranes are not involved. The denuded bases dry rapidly, leading to a postinflammatory desquamation that resolves in 5 to 7 days. Because the cleavage plane is intraepidermal, fluid loss may not be extreme, and the mortality is less than 5 percent.

### Differential Diagnosis

Clinically, toxic epidermal necrolysis and staphylococcal scalded skin syndrome may be confused with pemphigus vulgaris or thermal or chemical burns.

### DIAGNOSIS

The distinctive morphology of toxic epidermal necrolysis and staphylococcal scalded skin syndrome suggests the clinical diagnosis. However, the age of the patient is not an absolute indication of the underlying cause. A history of drug usage or chemical exposure, maternal-fetal transfusion, or administration of blood products or bone marrow transplants leading to graft-versus-host reaction and the

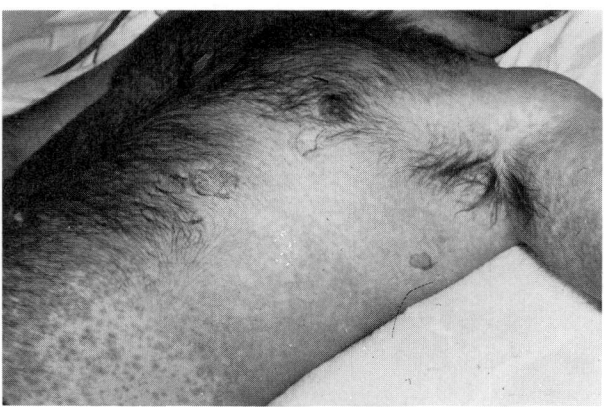

**Fig. 209-3.** Toxic epidermal necrolysis secondary to a sulfone.

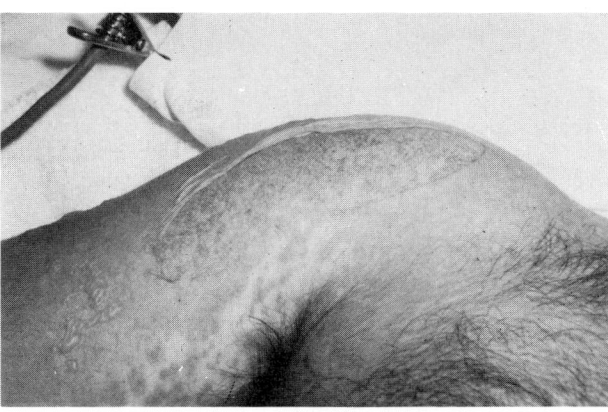

**Fig. 209-4.** Closeup view of toxic epidermal necrolysis secondary to a sulfone.

results of bacterial culture and skin biopsy allow differentiation of the two diseases. Amon and Dimond have suggested methods for more rapid differentiation. The level of separation in the cutaneum can be determined by examining the cells from denuded areas or by examining frozen sections of bullae roofs.

The first technique involves scraping the denuded bases with a no. 15 surgical blade. The material collected is smeared on a clean glass slide and examined. In the staphylococcal scalded skin syndrome, a few acantholytic keratinocytes will be evident; in toxic epidermal necrolysis, inflammatory cells, cellular debris, and basal cell keratinocytes will be present.

The second technique involves histologic examination of a frozen section of skin peeled from a fresh lesion. In toxic epidermal necrolysis, the split is at the dermal-epidermal junction and a full thickness of epidermis is present; in the staphylococcal scalded skin syndrome, only stratum corneum and a few granular cells are seen.

The growth of *Staphylococcus aureus* on cultures obtained from the conjuctiva, nose, throat, perineum, and skin strongly suggests an infectious cause. Definitive diagnosis is made by excisional or punch biopsy specimen of involved skin.

### TREATMENT

A patient with toxic epidermal necrolysis has temporarily lost his or her skin barrier against percutaneous water loss. Adults with toxic necrolysis lose an average of 2 to 4 L/day by evaporation for the first 9 days. In general, greater losses of plasma occur within the first few days, whereas water loss predominates later in the course. At any rate, volume and electrolyte replacement should be done in the emergency department if there are signs of hypovolemia. The possibility of septic shock should also be considered in the differential diagnosis of hypotension.

Staphylococcal scalded skin syndrome should be treated with an oral or intravenous penicillinase-resistant penicillin, even though antibiotic therapy does not seem to alter the course of the cutaneous disease. Glucocorticoids are contraindicated in staphylococcal scalded skin syndrome. Their value has not been proven in drug-related toxic epidermal necrolysis.

Until barrier function is restored, the lesions of toxic epidermal

**Table 209-1.** Drugs Most Commonly Implicated in Toxic Epidermal Necrolysis

Sulfonamides and sulfones
Pyrazolone derivatives: phenylbutazone, oxyphenbutazone, phenazone
Barbiturates
Antiepileptics
Antibiotics

necrolysis are treated as second-degree burns. Patients with less than 10 percent loss of skin usually can be treated successfully with tub baths of potassium permanganate or dressings soaked in 0.5% silver nitrate. Silver sulfadiazine and mafenide acetate creams should be avoided because sulfonamide drugs are often the cause of toxic epidermal necrolysis and because these drugs delay epithelialization. Antibiotics in toxic necrolysis are reserved for treating disease caused by identified pathogens. If the eyes are involved, an ophthalmologist should be consulted.

Patients with more than 10 percent loss of skin should be admitted to the burn unit. Intensive supportive care available in burn units coupled with newer grafting techniques using cadaver allografts, porcine xenografts, and hydrocolloid dressings have reduced morbidity and mortality.

## SUMMARY

Toxic epidermal necrolysis and staphylococcal scalded skin syndrome are morphologically similar but different diseases.

The staphylococcal scalded skin syndrome generally occurs in children and, if appropriately treated, carries a favorable prognosis. Toxic epidermal necrolysis is caused by a drug or chemical agent or graft-versus-host reaction and carries a 5 to 50 percent mortality due to fluid loss and secondary infection. The age of the patient is not an absolute indicator of the cause. The two diseases are differentiated by a history of drug usage or chemical exposure and by the results of bacterial culture and skin biopsy.

The lesions are treated as second-degree burns. The form associated with staphylococcal infection is treated with antibiotics, and steroids are contraindicated. Patients with the toxic epidermal reactions are most appropriately cared for in the burn unit.

## BIBLIOGRAPHY

Amon RB, Dimond RL: Toxic epidermal necrolysis: Rapid differentiation between staphylococcal-induced disease and drug-induced disease. *Arch Dermatol* 111:1433, 1975.

Birke G, Liljedahl S, Rajka G: Lyell's syndrome: Metabolic and clinical results of a new form of treatment. *Acta Dermatol Venereol* (Stockh) 51:199, 1971.

Elias PM, Fritsch P, Dahl MV, et al: Staphylococcal toxic epidermal necrolysis: Pathogenesis and studies on the subcellular site of action of exfoliation. *J Invest Dermatol* 65:501, 1975.

Elias PM, Fritsch P, Epstein EH Jr: Staphylococcal scalded skin syndrome: Clinical features, pathogenesis, and recent microbiological and biochemical developments. *Arch Dermatol* 113:207, 1977.

Lillibridge CB, Melish ME, Glasgow LA: Site of action of exfoliative toxin in the staphylococcal scalded skin syndrome. *Pediatrics* 50:728, 1972.

Lyell A: Toxic epidermal necrolysis: The scalded skin syndrome. *J Contin Ed Dermatol* 16:15, 1978.

Rudolph RI, Schwartz W, Leyden JJ: Treatment of staphylococcal toxic epidermal necrolysis. *Arch Dermatol* 110:559, 1974.

Schöpf E, Stühmer A, Rzany B, et al: Toxic epidermal necrolysis and Stevens-Johnson syndrome. *Arch Dermatol* 127:839, 1991.

Villada G, Roujeau J-C, Clerici T: Immunopathology of toxic epidermal necrolysis. *Arch Dermatol* 128:50, 1992.

# 210
# CUTANEOUS ABSCESSES
## E. Jackson Allison, Jr.
## John E. Gough

Generally, intact healthy skin provides significant protection from the development of skin infections and cutaneous abscess formation. The outer keratinous layer serves as a mechanical barrier against invasion of pathogenic organisms. In addition, the continuous desquamation of the epidermis contributes protection by constantly shedding bacteria present on the skin. Chemical factors, such as the normally low pH (3.0 to 5.0) of the skin, help diminish bacterial growth. Host factors, such as cellular defense (phagocytosis) and humoral components (antibodies and complement), also contribute to protect the body from invasion of pathogens and subsequent infections.

Since the skin provides the body with a formidable barrier against invasion by pathogenic organisms, skin infections and abscesses generally arise in an area of skin that has been injured. The damage may be traumatic (mechanical, chemical, thermal), infectious, or inflammatory. More recently immunosuppression, either congenital or acquired, has been increasingly implicated in the development of cutaneous abscesses.

All individuals possess resident bacteria, or "normal flora," on their skin. The number and type of these organisms vary with relation to the anatomic area of the body, environmental factors (humidity, pH), hygienic factors, and the underlying health of the individual.

While the normal flora inhabiting a given anatomic site may give a clue as to the bacteriologic etiology of the abscess, many abscesses are composed of organisms not normally part of the resident flora. For example, *Staphylococcus aureus*, a common resident bacteria of the nose and perineum, is found on less than 10 percent of normal skin. However, *S. aureus* is the most common aerobic pathogen present in cutaneous infections, abscesses, and around foreign bodies, particularly on the extremities and trunk. Other staphylococcal species, particularly *S. epidermis* and *S. hominis,* are commonly isolated on the axilla, head, and extremities.

Streptococci are not frequently isolated on normal skin. They are common residents of the oropharynx and are sometimes found in abscesses in adjoining skin.

Gram-negative aerobic pathogens of note are *Escherichia coli, Klebsiella,* and *Proteus.* All of these organisms form a very small portion of normal flora in healthy individuals. They are most often seen in the moist intertriginous and perineal areas. For unknown reasons, *Proteus* is sometimes found in abscesses of the upper torso.

Abscesses involving the perirectal, genitalia, buttock, inguinal, and cervical areas are predominantly caused by anaerobic bacteria. Most commonly they are found in abscesses involving mixed flora of both aerobes and anaerobes. *Bacteroides fragilis* is the most common gram-negative anaerobe in human feces and is often found in abscesses on the perineum. Abscesses in the perineal area occurring in diabetic patients require special attention and aggressive treatment to prevent evolution of a disseminated necrotizing infection (Fournier's gangrene).

*Propionibacteria acne* is the predominant aerobe associated with areas rich in sebaceous glands. *P. acne* is the organism mainly responsible for acne vulgaris.

*Pityrosporum* species are the only yeasts found in significant numbers on healthy skin. In immunocompromised patients (particularly those with AIDS), *Cryptococcus neoformans,* coccidioidomycosis, and aspergillosis have been reported as etiologies of cutaneous abscesses. Other opportunistic organisms that may present as cutaneous abscesses in the immunocompromised patient are *Mycobacterium kansasii, M. tuberculosis,* and *Yersinia enterocolitica.*

Patients who abuse injectable drugs, either intravenously or intradermally ("skin poppers"), are at significant risk of developing skin abscesses. This may be a result of the direct trauma to the skin as well as a generally decreased state of health (nutritionally, immunocompromised). Further, chemical irritation from both the drug and diluents may form a sterile abscess.

## LABORATORY STUDIES

The most common laboratory test utilized in the treatment of cutaneous abscesses is the Gram stain of the aspirate. Often, this is usually followed by culture and sensitivities. While not necessary in all cases (e.g., a simple abscess in a healthy individual), the Gram stain remains a useful test. If the stain does not demonstrate any organisms, it is most likely a sterile abscess. If many different organisms are seen, a mixed infection of both aerobic and anaerobic organisms should be suspected. A Gram stain demonstrating gram-positive cocci in clusters is suggestive of an *S. aureus* infection, which commonly presents as a pure culture.

Cultures are useful in differentiating aerobic from anaerobic organisms as well as assisting in the identification of the organism(s) present. Sensitivities will assess the appropriateness of antibiotic choice, if one is given. These tests are usually reserved for the compromised host or if evidence of systemic involvement is present. They may be useful in cases where empirical antibiotic therapy has been started, as may be the case with abscesses involving the head, neck, or hand.

Since diabetes mellitus (DM) is a common disease and abscesses are common in the diabetic patient, patients presenting with abscesses should be screened for DM with a fingerstick or venous glucose determination. Other tests such as a complete blood count, blood cultures, and radiography may be employed on an individual basis. These tests may be useful in determining systemic involvement as well as in helping to identify the source of the infection. They are often utilized if there is suspicion that the abscess is secondary to extension of an infection from an adjacent site or through hematogenous spread.

## CLINICAL PRESENTATION

Most patients present with a complaint of a localized area of pain and swelling. It is not unusual for the patient to have attempted self-treatment prior to presentation. This treatment may range from squeezing the abscess to application of salves and/or lotions. Some patients may have attempted more innovative "home remedies" such as placing salt, bacon, or turpentine on the abscess. Frequently, the result is an abscess that has been extensively traumatized and incompletely drained.

Often the abscess is fluctuant, indurated, and erythematous. Lymphadenitis, cellulitis, and regional lymphadenopathy may be clues to dissemination of the infection. Cutaneous abscesses in the otherwise healthy host are generally localized and do not show signs of systemic involvement. Fever should not be present. If the patient is febrile, a search for signs of systemic involvement (or a source of the fever unrelated to the cutaneous abscess) should be undertaken.

Since cutaneous abscesses often form secondary to traumatic impairment of the natural defenses of the skin, a thorough examination of the skin should be performed. If there is a history consistent with the possibility of a foreign body, a careful search utilizing radiography or ultrasonography should be undertaken. Ultrasonography has been shown to be very useful in the detection of nonradiopaque foreign bodies.

A complete medical history must be obtained. Identification of chronic conditions such as DM, collagen vascular disease, neoplasm, or inflammatory bowel disease may give clues to the etiology of the abscess. Identification of HIV risk factors may also prove helpful. Furthermore, a history of organ transplantation and any drug use (steroid, chemotherapeutic agents, illicit drugs) should be procured. An occupational history may identify patients at risk for specific infections (e.g., truck driving is a risk factor for pilonidal abscesses).

The following are specific abscesses commonly encountered in the emergency department:

**Furuncle.** A furuncle arises from an infected hair follicle (folliculitis). The result is an inflammatory node with a purulent center often containing necrotic tissue. Staphylococcal species are the most common etiology. DM may be a predisposing factor. Furuncles most often occur on the back, axilla, and lower extremities.

**Carbuncle.** A carbuncle is a staphylococcal infection most commonly occurring on the back of the neck. A carbuncle is much larger than a furuncle and often contains a "honeycomb" system of abscesses that do not adequately drain spontaneously. Carbuncles are most commonly seen in diabetic patients, and if one occurs in a patient not known to be diabetic, screening for DM is indicated.

**Pilonidal abscess.** Pilonidal abscesses occur in the gluteal fold over the coccyx. Pilonidal abscesses are felt to arise from a disruption of the epithelium, which leads to a formation of a pit. The pit is lined with epithelial cells and may become plugged with hair and keratin, leading to an abscess. The patient typically presents with a painful, fluctuant nodule in the gluteal fold. Acute treatment of a pilonidal abscess involves incision and drainage (I&D). Recurrent or deep abscesses should receive surgical referral for a more extensive excision of the cyst, sinuses, and granulation tissue. The organisms present within the abscess generally represent cutaneous flora, with staphylococcal species being the most common; however, a mixed infection containing perineal flora is not uncommon.

**Bartholin abscess.** Bartholin cyst abscess occurs with obstruction of a Bartholin duct. The abscess is usually composed of a mixed infection of vaginal flora and may contain *Neisseria gonorrhoeae, Chlamydia trachomatis,* and *E. coli.* The patient presents with unilateral swelling of the labia. Acute treatment of the abscess includes I&D, with the incision made on the mucosal surface. Placement of iodoform gauze or a Word catheter and the use of sitz baths will help promote drainage. Marsupialization of the cyst may help prevent recurrence.

**Hidradenitis suppurativa.** Hidradenitis suppurativa is characterized by chronic suppurative abscesses of the apocrine sweat glands, particularly in the groin and axilla. Risk factors include female gender (3:1 versus males), young age, obesity, black race, shaving, and poor hygiene. The patient typically presents with a tender subcutaneous nodule that may or may not drain spontaneously. *S. aureus, Streptococcus viridans,* and *Proteus* are common pathogens. Incision and drainage is the preferred treatment of an acute presentation. Chronic or extensive involvement often requires surgical referral for removal of the apocrine glands.

**Paronychia.** A paronychia is a superficial abscess over the lateral nail fold. The abscess may result from nail biting. Common organisms include *S. aureus, Candida,* and anaerobes. Treatment consists of I&D. Care must be taken to avoid damage to the germinal matrix.

**Perirectal abscess.** Perirectal abscesses originate in the anal crypts and extend through the ischiorectal space. The patient often complains of pain in the rectal area with sitting and defecation. Pregnancy, DM, immunodeficiency, and inflammatory bowel disease are predisposing factors. Abscesses are named by the position where the purulence accumulates (perianal, perirectal, ischiorectal, pelvirectal/supralevator). *B. fragilis* is the predominant anaerobe, and most abscesses contain a mixed culture. Fistula formation is not uncommon. Simple abscesses may be drained in the emergency department; however, the abscess is often very extensive, necessitating drainage in the surgical suite under general anesthesia.

**Infected sebaceous cyst.** Sebaceous cysts are very common and may occur in any location on the body. The cysts result from obstruction of the ducts of the sebaceous gland. The cysts may be present for extended periods without signs of infection. Once infection occurs, abscess formation is common. The patient presents with a tender, fluctuant, erythematous mass. The treatment consists of I&D. The cyst capsule should be excised to prevent recurrence; however, it is often best to perform the I&D initially and excise the capsule on a follow-up visit.

## TREATMENT

### Incision and Drainage

Incision and drainage of the cutaneous abscess remain the cornerstone of definitive therapy. In cases of a localized abscess in an immunocompetent patient, I&D is all that is necessary for proper treatment. Often the patient presents with a localized area of tenderness and fluctuance, and the need for I&D is obvious. At times, fluctuance may be difficult to determine, and a needle aspiration of the site will help to distinguish an abscess from an area of cellulitis. If no pus is aspirated, a period of treatment with warm soaks and antibiotics is indicated. If any amount of pus is aspirated, I&D is needed.

The decision on where to perform the I&D (emergency department versus operating room) is based on several factors. Simple abscesses that are localized can often be easily drained in the emergency department. Deep abscesses, those in proximity to major neurovascular structures, and those involving the palm are usually best handled in the surgical suite. The ability to provide sufficient anesthesia is another determining factor as to whether to perform the I&D in the emergency department or in the operating room. It is often difficult to obtain sufficient anesthesia with local infiltration. In some cases, a field block may be sufficient. Parenteral sedation and/or analgesia with narcotics, benzodiazepines, or nitrous oxide can all aid in making the procedure easier for both the patient and the physician. Agents such as midazolam and fentanyl possess several advantages as adjuncts in the performance of I&Ds in the emergency department; they have a quick onset of action, short duration, are titratable, and can be reversed easily. While these agents are not without potential adverse effects (e.g., respiratory depression, particularly if they are used in combination), with careful monitoring (pulse oximetry, cardiac monitoring, frequent assessment of vital signs) by personnel skilled in airway management, they can be safely given in the emergency department.

Informed consent should be obtained from the patient. The patient should then be placed in a comfortable position that also provides the physician with complete visualization and access to the abscess. The area should be properly prepped and draped. An incision is made through the entire length of the abscess cavity. An incision that is too small will not allow for adequate drainage. When possible, the incision should conform with the natural skin folds and creases to prevent excessive scar formation. The abscess is then probed bluntly with a finger or hemostat. Care should be taken not to damage adjacent neurovascular structures. However, the cavity should be sufficiently explored to determine its extent as well as to break up any loculated areas of pus to allow adequate drainage. If anaerobic cultures are to be obtained, it is best to do this by needle aspiration prior to the incision or immediately after the incision to avoid prolonged exposure to air by the organisms. The cavity should then be irrigated to remove any remaining debris. Once the abscess is drained, the cav-

**Table 210-1.** Treatment of Cutaneous Abscesses

Normal host defenses
    Incision and drainage
High-risk patients
    Incision and drainage
    Gram stain and culture
    Antibiotics

**Table 210-2.** Oral Therapy of Superficial Soft Tissue Infections

| | |
|---|---|
| Streptococcus, group A: | |
| Penicillin V (phenoxymethyl penicillin) | 250–500 mg q 6 h |
| Erythromycin | 500 mg–1 g q 6 h |
| *Staphylococcus aureus:* | |
| Cloxacillin | 250–500 mg q 8 h |
| Dicloxacillin | 125–500 mg q 6 h |
| Erythromycin | 500 mg–1 g q 6 h |
| Clindamycin | 150–450 mg q 6 h |
| Cephradine | 250–500 mg q 6 h |
| Cephalexin | 250–500 mg q 6 h |
| Amoxicillin/clavulanate | 250–500 mg q 8 h |
| *Haemophilus influenzae:* | |
| Cefaclor | 250–500 mg q 8 h |
| Cephradine | 250–500 mg q 6 h |
| Cephalexin | 250–500 mg q 6 h |
| Amoxicillin/clavulanate | 250–500 mg q 8 h |
| Trimethoprim/sulfamethoxazole | 160 mg TMP/800 mg SMX q 12 h |

**Table 210-3.** Conditions at Risk for Endocarditis

Prosthetic heart valves
Valvular dysfunction
Mitral valve prolapse with insufficiency
History of endocarditis
Idiopathic hypertrophic subaortic stenosis
Congenital cardiac malformation

ity should be loosely packed with gauze to provide continued drainage and to prevent the wound edges from closing prematurely.

Follow-up care should be individualized to the specific patient and infection. Patients with abscesses involving the face or hands or who have impaired health (immunocompromised or with DM) may need hospital admission. If not admitted, they should be seen back in the emergency department within 24 h. Most other abscesses may be followed up in 48 h. Patients who will require long-term follow-up are best referred to a local physician, as this increases the likelihood that a single physician is monitoring the progress.

### Antibiotics

The use of antibiotics in the treatment of cutaneous abscesses remains controversial. Most physicians agree that if the abscess is localized and the patient possesses normal host defenses, I&D is all that is needed and no antibiotics are indicated (see Table 210-1). Patients at high risk for infections (immunocompromised or with DM or collagen vascular diseases), those with facial abscesses in areas drained into the cavernous sinus, or those demonstrating signs of systemic toxicity are often treated empirically with antibiotics.

The choice of antibiotic therapy is directed by knowledge of probable pathogen (based on the area of the body involved) and the Gram stain. Definitive treatment may be altered by results of cultures, sensitivities, and patient response. A table of common antibiotic regimens is given in Table 210-2.

Another group of patients who require special attention are those at risk for endocarditis (Table 210-3). Since tissue manipulation from even simple I&Ds can cause a transient bacteremia, it is recommended that patients at risk for endocarditis receive a parenteral antibiotic prophylactically prior to I&D.

### BIBLIOGRAPHY

Aly R: Cutaneous microbiology, in Orkin M, Maibach HI, Dahl MV (eds): *Dermatology.* Norwalk, CT, Appleton/Lange, 1991.

Bailey PL, Pace NL, Ashburn MA, et al: Frequent hypoxemia and apnea after sedation with midazolam and fentanyl. *Anesthesiology* 73(5):826, 1990.

Brook I, Frazier EH: Aerobic and anaerobic bacteriology of wounds and cutaneous abscesses. *Arch Surg* 125(11):1445, 1990.

Ghosh AK, Verma PP, Jha V, et al: Disseminated tuberculosis in a renal transplant recipient presenting as a non healing ulcer. *Int J Artif Organs* 16(3):132, 1993.

Ginsberg MJ, Ellis GL, Flom LL: Detection of soft-tissue foreign bodies by plain radiography, xerography, computed tomography, and ultrasonography. *Ann Emerg Med* 19(6):701, 1990.

Helm TN, Mazanec D: Disseminated aspergillosis presenting as a skin abscess. *Cleveland J Med* 57(1):92, 1990.

Hirshmann JV: Bacterial infections of the skin, in Sams WM, Lynch PJ (eds): *Principles and Practice of Dermatology.* New York, Churchill Livingstone, 1990.

Krogstad P, Mendelman PM, Miller VL: Clinical and microbiologic characteristics of cutaneous infection with *Yersinia enterocolitica. J Infect Dis* 165(4):740, 1992.

Quimby SR, Connolly SM, Winkelmann RK, et al: Clinicopathic spectrum of specific cutaneous lesions of disseminated coccidioidomycosis. *J Am Acad Dermatol* 26(1):79, 1992.

Salvino C, Harford FJ, Dobrin PB: Necrotizing infections of the perineum. *South Med J* 86(8):908, 1993.

Stellbrink HJ, Koperski K, Albrecht H, et al: *Mycobacterium kansaii* infection limited to skin and lymph node in a patient with AIDS. *Clin Exper Dermatol* 15(6):457, 1990.

Warden TM, Fourre MW: Incision and drainage of cutaneous abscesses and soft tissue infections, in Roberts JR, Hedges JR (eds): *Clinical Procedures in Emergency Medicine,* 6th ed. Philadelphia, Saunders, 1991.

# 211
# SOFT TISSUE INFECTIONS
## Steven G. Folstad

## TETANUS

Tetanus is a life-threatening disease characterized by muscular rigidity, reflex spasm, and autonomic instability. Its prevalence is greatest in underdeveloped countries without immunization programs, but in the United States it is primarily a disease of the elderly who lack adequate immunization. The overall case fatality rate in the United States is 24 percent, but it increases to 50 percent in patients over the age of 80.

## Pathophysiology

Tetanus is caused by local wound contamination with the anaerobic, gram-positive bacillus *Clostridium tetani,* a spore-forming organism that is commonly found in soil, manure, dust, clothing, and in up to 25 percent of human intestinal tracts. This ubiquitous organism produces the exotoxin tetanospasmin that is responsible for the clinical features of the disease. Clinical tetanus is most commonly associated with an open skin wound but can also be a complication of otitis media, thermal burns, chronic wounds, intranasal foreign bodies, corneal injuries, injections, childbirth, abortions, and gastrointestinal and gynecologic surgery.

Tetanospasmin is a neurotoxic protoplasmic protein synthesized within the bacteria and released by spontaneous bacterial autolysis. Once released the toxin travels by retrograde axonal transport via the peripheral nerves to the central nervous system (CNS), where it binds to presynaptic membranes blocking the release of the inhibitory neurotransmitters γ-aminobutyric acid (GABA) and glycine. This produces unopposed excitation of the alpha motor neurons in the spinal cord and brainstem as well as sympathetic overactivity by blocking the inhibitory synapses in the preganglionic neurons of the thoracic spinal cord.

Initially the toxin is spread to the peripheral nerves local to the infection. As the amount of toxin increases it is picked up by the adjacent capillary circulation and disseminated throughout the body. Clinical presentation and progression of the disease are dependent on the length of the nerves involved. Typically the first signs of muscular rigidity are seen in the facial muscles because of their short axons, and the rigidity tends to progress in a descending pattern toward the lower extremities. It appears that the blood-brain barrier blocks toxin from crossing into the CNS via the bloodstream, and all toxin reaching the CNS arrives via retrograde axonal transport.

## Clinical Features

Clinically tetanus is divided into four types: generalized, local, cephalic, and neonatal.

*Generalized tetanus* occurs in 50 to 75 percent of cases, with patients typically presenting with trismus secondary to masseter spasm, nuchal rigidity, or dysphagia. Early in the course of the disease, facial muscle rigidity may cause a sneering grin known as *risus sardonicus* (the ironic smile). As the disease progresses, generalized muscular rigidity worsens, often progressing to reflex spasms, a sudden tonic contraction causing opisthotonus-flexion, adduction of the arms with clenching of the fists over the thorax, and extension of the lower extremities. They are precipitated by external stimuli such as noise and touch and may last from seconds to minutes. The patient, having an intact sensorium, experiences extreme pain. Severe reflex spasms may cause fractures of vertebrae and long bones and may avulse tendons from their insertions. Prior to the advent of neuromuscular blockade and mechanical ventilation, asphyxiation from recurrent spasms was the most common cause of death. Autonomic instability presents as labile hypertension, tachycardia, arrhythmias, diaphoresis, hyperpyrexia, and peripheral vasoconstriction alternating with sudden episodes of bradycardia, hypotension, and cardiac standstill. Sudden cardiac death secondary to autonomic instability is now the leading cause of death in tetanus.

The incubation period varies from a few days to a few months, with the majority of patients developing symptoms within 2 weeks. In general, the shorter the incubation period the more severe the disease. In more severe cases the generalized muscular rigidity progresses over several days to reflex spasms. This interval is termed the *period of onset,* and as with the incubation period, the shorter the interval the more severe the disease.

The clinical course of generalized tetanus varies, but typically the spasms resolve after the second week, with residual muscular rigidity possibly lasting for a period of months. The toxin itself does not cause permanent neurologic damage, and with uncomplicated tetanus recovery may be complete. Complications primarily related to autonomic instability, prolonged ventilator dependence, and infection still maintain a case mortality rate from 17 to 50 percent, depending on age.

*Local tetanus* is the clinical form in which symptoms are limited to a group of muscles closely related to a wound; it often progresses to intermittent, intensely painful spasms. Local tetanus may remain localized, with a gradual resolution of symptoms over weeks to months, but often progresses to the generalized form of the disease.

*Cephalic tetanus* is uncommon, occurring in fewer than 1 percent of cases. It typically follows a head injury or otitis media and involves the muscles innervated by one or more of the cranial nerves. The facial nerve is the most commonly involved, producing furrowing of the forehead, blepharospasm, and retraction of the corner of the mouth. Like local tetanus, cephalic tetanus often progresses to a generalized form.

*Neonatal tetanus* is a significant problem in underdeveloped countries where tetanus prophylaxis is lacking and obstetric conditions are poor. It typically occurs near the end of the first week of life and is characterized by irritability and poor feeding, later developing into generalized rigidity with spasms and opisthotonos. The prognosis is very poor.

In the United States tetanus is now primarily a disease of the elderly. From 1989 to 1990 there were 117 cases of tetanus reported to the Centers for Disease Control and Prevention (CDC), with 58 percent involving patients over the age of 60. This is mainly due to absent or inadequate immunizations including appropriate booster injections. A 1990 study found that only 55 percent of patients greater than age 65 presenting to an emergency department with an open wound had adequate protective serum antitoxin levels. Furthermore, when the inadequately protected patients were immunized, 44 percent of them failed to seroconvert after 2 weeks.

## Diagnosis

The diagnosis of tetanus is based on history and physical findings. *C. tetani* is isolated from wounds in fewer than 30 percent of cases. Serum antitoxin levels greater than or equal to 0.01 IU/mL are considered protective and make the diagnosis unlikely. Appropriately immunized patients are very unlikely to have the disease.

The differential diagnosis of trismus includes parotitis, peritonsillar abscess, mandible fracture, temporomandibular joint pathology, dystonic reaction, and hysterical reaction. For muscle spasms, strychnine poisoning, dystonic reaction, hyperventilation syndrome, and hypocalcemia should be considered.

## Treatment

The goals of treatment are neutralization of circulating toxin, halting production of the toxin, and supportive care.

1. Human tetanus immune globulin (HTIG) neutralizes circulating tetanospasmin, preventing further uptake by motor neurons. It has no effect on already absorbed toxin. It should be administered in a single intramuscular dose of 3000 to 5000 units as soon as the disease is diagnosed. Since the half life is 25 days, subsequent doses are not needed. Earlier reports suggesting a benefit from intrathecal HTIG therapy have not been confirmed by further study. Infection with tetanus does not impart immunity to the host against subsequent infections, so tetanus toxoid should be administered intramuscularly, at a separate site, at the same time.
2. Antibiotic therapy and surgical wound management are used to stop further production of toxin by eradicating the *C. tetani* organism from the wound site. High-dose penicillin is the most commonly used antibiotic, but recent studies have shown metronidazole to be equally or possibly more effective. Other antibiotic options include cephalosporins, imipenem, tetracycline, and erythromycin. Aggressive surgical cleansing and debridement, to a 2-cm margin of normal-appearing tissue around the wound edges, should follow antitoxin and antibiotic therapy.
3. All patients should be admitted to an intensive care unit with continuous hemodynamic monitoring and a minimal stimulus environment to reduce reflex spasms. Muscular rigidity and mild spasms are best treated with intravenous benzodiazepines, but dantrolene has been used in less severe cases. In cases where laryngospasm threatens the airway, neuromuscular blockade and mechanical ventilation are necessary. Vecuronium is the recommended neuromuscular blocking agent due to its minimal cardiovascular effects. Intrathecal baclofen has been shown to shorten the length of ventilation dependence in a few patients.

The correct treatment of autonomic instability is not well established. Long-acting medications are undesirable because of the rapid swings in hemodynamics. One study used a combination infusion of esmolol and norepinephrine for a total of 44 days and showed improved hemodynamic stability. Morphine sulfate may be useful in re-

**Table 211-1.** Summary Guide to Tetanus Prophylaxis in Routine Wound Management, 1991

| | Clean, Minor Wounds | | All Other Wounds | |
|---|---|---|---|---|
| | Td | TIG | Td | TIG |
| Uncertain or <3 doses | Yes | No | Yes | Yes |
| 3 or more doses and <5 years since last dose | No | No | No | No |
| 3 or more doses and 5–10 years since last dose | No | No | Yes | No |
| 3 or more doses and >10 years since last dose | Yes | No | Yes | No |

*Source:* Adapted from: Summary of recommendations of ACIP for tetanus prophylaxis in routine wound management—United States, 1991. *MMWR,* vol. 41, No. SS-8, 1–9, December 11, 1992.

ducing peripheral vasoconstriction via histamine release, and intravenous magnesium sulfate suppresses catecholamine release. Continuous epidural or spinal anesthesia has been beneficial in very severe cases.

## Emergency Department Care

Proper wound management with passive and active immunization are the fundamentals of emergency department care in the prevention of tetanus. Wounds that are prone to tetanus infection are those that are greater than 6 h old; have necrotic, crushed, or ischemic edges; are contaminated with dirt or other debris; or are infected. Wounds must be well cleansed and irrigated and debrided aggressively, and antibiotics used when indicated. Early follow-up for a wound check is recommended.

Careful questioning regarding immunization history is very important. Attempts must be made to determine if all or part of a primary series of vaccinations has been given and when the last booster was received. Table 211-1 outlines the steps recommended by the 1991 CDC Advisory Committee on Immunization Practices for tetanus prophylaxis. Children less than 7 years old should receive DPT instead of Td (DT, when pertussis is contraindicated). Boosters are given at 10-year intervals but given at 5 years in the case of a dirty wound. Those patients in whom previous primary immunization cannot be established should be assumed to have not been primarily immunized.

At discharge, patients should be given written wound care instructions as well as instructions for follow-up for wound checks and further vaccinations as needed.

## GAS GANGRENE

Gas gangrene, or clostridial myonecrosis, is a rapidly progressive and life- and limb-threatening soft tissue infection caused by one of the spore-forming clostridial species of organism. Severe myonecrosis with gas production and sepsis are the hallmarks of this disease, and early diagnosis and aggressive management are needed to prevent mortality.

## Pathophysiology

There have been seven clostridium species identified as causing gas gangrene. Between 80 and 95 percent of cases are attributed to *C. perfringens,* with *C. septicum* being the second most common etiology. The clostridial organisms are large, gram-positive, spore-forming anaerobic bacilli normally found in the soil, gastrointestinal tract, and female genitourinary tract. They produce several exotoxins that are responsible for the cellular destruction as well as the rapid progression and systemic toxicity of the disease. Bacteremia is rare. Secondary toxic effects may be caused by the release of myoglobin, CPK, and potassium from tissue breakdown.

There are two potential mechanisms for infection with clostridial organisms. The first and most common is through direct inoculation from an open wound. Similar to tetanus, clostridial species thrive best in contaminated wounds with crushed or ischemic edges that tend to offer a favorable anaerobic environment. The second mechanism for infection is by hematogenous spread, usually in immunocompromised patients with diabetes mellitus, peripheral vascular disease, alcoholism, drug abuse, or hematologic or gastrointestinal malignancies. Almost a third of cases of "spontaneous gas gangrene" are caused by *C. septicum*, with an even higher association to malignancies.

## Clinical Features

The incubation period is usually less than 3 days. The most common presenting complaints in early gas gangrene are pain out of proportion to physical findings as well as a sensation of "heaviness" of the affected part. On examination the area may demonstrate a brawny, woody edema with crepitance and may be cool to the touch. The skin will develop a bronze or brownish discoloration with a malodorous serosanguinous discharge, and bullae may be present. Systemic manifestations include a low-grade fever with tachycardia out of proportion to the fever. The patient may be confused or irritable and have a rapid deterioration of the sensorium. Laboratory evaluation may reveal any or all of the following: metabolic acidosis, leukocytosis, anemia, thrombocytopenia, coagulopathy, myoglobinemia and myoglobinuria, or liver or kidney dysfunction. Gram stain of the bullae often shows pleomorphic gram-positive bacilli with or without spores, red blood cells, but very few white blood cells. Radiologic studies may demonstrate gas within soft tissue fascial planes and possibly gas within the peritoneal or retroperitoneal space.

## Diagnosis

Early diagnosis and treatment are essential. Familiarity with the disease and its clinical features is important to avoid overlooking the subtle early signs of its presentation. Any patient presenting with pain out of proportion to physical findings, low-grade fever, and significant tachycardia, with or without a cutaneous injury, should be carefully evaluated for possible clostridial infection. Crepitus detectable on physical examination may be a later finding, and its absence does not rule out the diagnosis. A Gram stain of exudate or tissue showing gram-positive rods with a relative lack of leukocytes is considered diagnostic. Surgical exploration is also helpful in the diagnosis. In the early stages the muscles are edematous and pale but still bleed when cut; in later stages the muscle looses its contractility and upon dissection appears beefy red without bleeding, and gas bubbles may be evident between the tissues.

The differential diagnosis of clostridial myonecrosis must include other forms of gas-forming infections, including necrotizing fasciitis, streptococcal myositis, acute streptococcal hemolytic gangrene, crepitant cellulitis, and synergistic necrotizing cellulitis. The crepitance should be differentiated from other causes of subcutaneous emphysema such as pneumothorax, pneumomediastinum, and fractured larynx or trachea. The edema and pallor with loss of distal pulses seen in an affected extremity should be differentiated from vascular thrombosis conditions such as phlegmasia cerulea dolens.

## Treatment

Treatment consists of four main phases.

1. *Resuscitation* should begin in the emergency department immediately upon making a presumptive diagnosis. Aggressive fluid resuscitation using crystalloid, plasma, and packed red blood cells is usually needed to replace red blood cells lost to hemolysis and to correct shock. Volume status should be closely monitored using urine output and central venous pressure readings. Vasoconstrictors should be avoided since they may decrease perfusion to an already ischemic area.
2. *Antibiotic therapy* using penicillin G, 10 to 40 million units per day in divided doses is recommended. Clindamycin, metronidazole, and chloramphenicol are alternative choices for the penicillin-allergic patient. Sodium penicillin is recommended over potassium penicillin to avoid hyperkalemia in patients with hemolysis and tissue necrosis. Mixed infections with other anaerobes, gram-negative rods, and staphylococci are common, so multiple antibiotic therapy using aminoglycosides, penicillinase-resistant penicillins, or vancomycin is recommended. Tetanus prophylaxis should be given as indicated.
3. *Surgical debridement* is a mainstay of therapy and may include fasciotomy, debridement, or amputation. The borders for debridement are guided by the appearance of the muscle.
4. *Hyperbaric oxygen therapy* (HBO) has been widely used since the early 1960s. Its use in relation to surgical debridement remains somewhat controversial. Standard therapy has consisted of surgical debridement prior to HBO, partly for confirmation of the diagnosis based on muscle appearance. Some argue that since elevated partial pressures of oxygen are bactericidal in tissues, as well as inhibitory to toxin production, early HBO may allow for sharper demarcation of necrotic tissue at debridement, lead to less loss of tissue to amputation, and decrease systemic toxicity. Certainly fasciotomy for cases of compartment syndrome must precede HBO, but in cases where it is readily available a trial of HBO prior to surgery may be beneficial. Typical HBO therapy consists of 100% oxygen at 3 atmospheres of pressure for 90 min, with two to three dives in the first 24 h followed by two to three dives a day for a total of seven to ten dives.

## Prevention

Wound care at the time of initial evaluation and treatment and providing proper immunization are the most important factors in preventing clostridial infections. Debridement of crushed or dead tissue and copious irrigation prior to wound closure will help prevent the development of an environment favorable to clostridial growth. Prophylactic antibiotics may prevent subsequent infection.

# CELLULITIS

Cellulitis is a local soft tissue inflammatory reaction secondary to bacterial invasion of the skin. The classic symptoms of cellulitis have previously been attributed to the bacterial invasion and subsequent proliferation within the local tissues; however, new evidence suggests that the majority of symptoms may instead be secondary to a complex set of immune and inflammatory reactions triggered by cells within the skin itself.

## Pathophysiology

Cellulitis is a local inflammation of the skin characterized by pain, induration, warmth, and erythema. It is caused by invasion of the tissues with bacteria, most commonly staphylococci or streptococci in adults, and *Haemophilus influenzae* in children. Lymphangitis and lymphadenopathy are occasionally seen in previously healthy patients, but purely local inflammation is much more common. Systemic involvement with fever, leukocytosis, and bacteremia is most typically seen in patients with underlying immunosuppressive diseases. Traditional thought has been that the symptoms of cellulitis are related to the effects of the bacteria and its proliferation on the local tissues. However, efforts to isolate organisms from infected tissue are often unsuccessful. Needle aspiration of the leading edge of an area of cellulitis produces organisms in fewer than 10 percent of cultures, and even punch biopsy from the same area yields organisms in only around 20 percent. Only areas with suppuration or abscess formation have significantly higher yield. Recent studies now suggest that although bacterial invasion is what triggers the inflammation, the organisms are largely cleared from the site within the first 12 h and the infiltration of lymphoid and reticular cells and their products is what produces the majority of symptoms. Cells such as Langerhans cells and keratinocytes release the cytokines interleukin-1 and tumor necrosis factor, which enhance the infiltration of the skin by circulating lymphocytes and macrophages. The net effect of this is much more rapid clearing of bacteria but at the price of a significantly larger inflammatory response. Theoretically, the addition of anti-inflammatory agents to the treatment regimen of cellulitis would be beneficial. Further study needs to be done to identify what specific role, if any, they should play.

## Clinical Features

Patients with cellulitis typically present with local tenderness, warmth, induration, and erythema. Specific note should be made on physical examination of evidence of lymphangitis or lymphadenitis as this may suggest more serious infection. The presence of high fever and chills suggests bacteremia, especially in patients with underlying medical disorders.

## Diagnosis

In otherwise healthy patients, the clinical presentation is sufficient for diagnosing cellulitis. The high likelihood of typical organisms and the low yield of isolation techniques makes further efforts unwarranted. In patients with underlying disease or signs of bacteremia, blood cultures and leukocyte counts are indicated. Local means of isolating the organism are controversial but in the case of a toxic-appearing patient may be worth the effort.

Differentiating deep venous thrombosis from cellulitis in the lower extremities is often difficult and may require Doppler studies or a venogram. Other forms of local soft tissue infections should also be ruled out.

## Treatment

Simple cellulitis in otherwise healthy adult patients can be treated in the ambulatory setting with an oral cephalosporin, erythromycin, trimethoprim/sulfamethoxazole, or amoxicillin/clavulanate. The exception to this is the patient with cellulitis involving the head or neck, who in most cases should be admitted for intravenous antibiotics. Appropriate antibiotics for the latter include cephalosporins, penicillinase-resistant penicillins, vancomycin, ampicillin/sulbactam, or ticarcillin/clavulanate. Anti-inflammatory agents for the treatment of cellulitis are experimental at this time, and until further research identifies a specific role they should be used with caution.

Patients with evidence of bacteremia and those with underlying diseases such as diabetes mellitus, alcoholism, or other immunosuppressive disorders should be admitted for intravenous antibiotics. Empiric therapy may be started with the antibiotics listed above and changed as indicated by culture results.

## ERYSIPELAS

### Pathophysiology

Erysipelas is a superficial cellulitis with lymphatic involvement that is usually caused primarily by group A *Streptococcus*. Atypical infections most commonly seen with other groups of streptococcus are also noted. Infection is typically achieved through a portal of entry in the skin with traumatic wounds, ulcers, and infected dermatoses of the lower extremities being the most common sites. Peripheral vascular disease, especially venous insufficiency, is a local risk factor for infection. Most often erysipelas occurs proximal to the portal of entry into the skin.

## Clinical Features

The onset of symptoms is usually abrupt, with a sudden onset of high fever, chills, malaise, and nausea. Over the next 1 to 2 days a small area of erythema with a burning sensation develops. As the infection continues a red, shiny, hot plaque forms. The plaque has a tense, painful induration that is sharply demarcated from the surrounding normal tissue. Lymphangitis and local lymphadenopathy are common. Purpura, bullae, and small areas of necrosis are also often seen. Systemic symptoms continue until antibiotic therapy is initiated. Upon resolution of the infection, desquamation of the site typically occurs. There has been a dramatic increase in the incidence in erysipelas over the past 20 years as well as a change in location on the body. Previously it most commonly involved the face but now is primarily an infection of the lower extremities.

## Diagnosis

The diagnosis is based primarily on physical findings. The differential diagnosis includes other forms of local cellulitis. Leukocytosis with an increase in the neutrophil count is common. Needle aspiration of the site is very poor at isolating an organism, but swabs of the portal of entry, when identifiable, may have a higher success rate. Blood cultures are positive in only around 5 percent of cases. Serologic testing to determine ASO and anti-DNAase B titers may be more specific but are of little use acutely.

Some believe that streptococcal necrotizing fasciitis is a complication of erysipelas infections and should be considered in all cases. Necrotizing fasciitis is most often caused by group A *Streptococcus* and, other than tending to have more severe local and systemic symptoms, shares a similar clinical course with erysipelas. Antibiotic therapy alone is insufficient, and often massive surgical debridement is needed. Epidemiologic similarities between erysipelas and streptococcal necrotizing fasciitis have not been identified.

## Treatment

Mild, well-localized cases of erysipelas can be treated on an ambulatory basis with oral penicillin. Essentially all serious cases should be admitted for intravenous antibiotics. Penicillin G, 4 to 6 million units per day, should be given in divided doses. Erythromycin, cephalosporins, or a macrolide should be used in patients with penicillin allergy.

## SPOROTRICHOSIS

Sporotrichosis is a mycotic infection caused by the fungus *Sporothrix schenckii* commonly found on plants and vegetation and in soil. Infection is caused by traumatic inoculation and usually remains within the local soft tissues and lymphatics. Disseminated forms, although more rare, do occur.

### Pathophysiology

*Sporothrix schenckii* is a thermally dimorphic fungus, changing from its mycelial form to its yeast form upon entering a body temperature environment. Inoculation into the host most commonly occurs from a spine or barb on a plant puncturing the skin during handling. It is a common disease among florists, gardeners, and agricultural workers. Transmission from infected animals, especially cats, has been documented, and veterinarians and animal handlers are also at increased risk. Extracutaneous forms including pulmonary and disseminated forms are rare.

### Clinical Features

The incubation period averages 3 weeks from the time of initial inoculation but varies from a few days to several weeks. After entering the body through a break in the skin, three types of localized infection may occur. The fixed cutaneous type is characterized by lesions restricted to the site of inoculation and may appear as a crusted ulcer or verrucous plaque. The local cutaneous type also remains local but presents as a subcutaneous nodule or pustule. The surrounding skin becomes erythematous and may ulcerate, resulting in a chancre. Local lymphadenitis is common. The lymphocutaneous type is the third and most common type. It is characterized by an initial painless nodule or papule at the site of inoculation, with the later development of subcutaneous nodules with clear skip areas along local lymphatic channels. The local reactions in all three types of infection tend to be relatively painless but show no signs of improvement without treatment.

## Diagnosis

History and physical findings are the key to the diagnosis. Histopathologic stains are of little help as the organisms are scarce in tissues. Fungal cultures are the best way to isolate the fungus, and tissue biopsy cultures are often diagnostic. Routine laboratory tests are nonspecific but an increased WBC, eosinophil count, and erythrocyte sedimentation rate may be noted.

The differential diagnosis includes tuberculosis, tularemia, cat-scratch disease, leishmaniasis, staphylococcal lymphangitis, and nocardiosis.

## Treatment

The treatment of choice for cutaneous sporotrichosis is potassium iodide (SSKI), 3 to 4 g tid, PO, to be continued for at least 1 month beyond resolution of clinical symptoms. Oral ketoconazole is an alternative in patients who do not tolerate SSKI. Intravenous amphotericin B is effective, but adverse reactions usually limit its use to disseminated forms.

Patients with the cutaneous form of sporotrichosis can be treated as outpatients. Discharge instructions should include basic wound care for open lesions, and close follow-up should be arranged.

## BIBLIOGRAPHY

### Tetanus

Gareau A, Eby R, et al: Tetanus immunization status and immunologic response to a booster in an emergency department geriatric population. *Ann Emerg Med* 19:1377, 1990.

Groleau G: Tetanus. *Emerg Med Clin North Am* 10:351, 1992.

King W, Cave D: Use of esmolol to control autonomic instability of tetanus. *Am J Med* 91:425, 1991.

Prevots R, Sutter R, et al: Tetanus surveillance—United States, 1989–1990. *MMWR* 41:1, 1992.

Roos K: Tetanus. *Semin Neurol* 11:206, 1991.

### Gas Gangrene

Corey E: Nontraumatic gas gangrene: Case report and review of emergency therapeutics. *J Emerg Med* 9:431, 1991.

Rich R, Salluzzo R: Spontaneous clostridial myonecrosis with abdominal involvement in a nonimmunocompromised patient. *Ann Emerg Med* 22:1477, 1993.

### Cellulitis and Erysipelas

Chartier C, Grosshans E: Erysipelas. *Int J Dermatol* 29:459, 1990.

Ochs M, Dolwick F: Facial erysipelas: Report of a case and review of the literature. *J Oral Maxillofac Surg* 49:1116, 1991.

Sachs M: Cutaneous cellulitis. *Arch Dermatol* 127:493, 1991.

### Sporotrichosis

Fitzpatrick T, Johnson R, et al (eds): *Color Atlas and Synopsis of Clinical Dermatology,* 2d ed. New York, McGraw-Hill, 1992, pp 330–334.

Rafal E, Rasmussen J: An unusual presentation of fixed cutaneous sporotrichosis: A case report and review of the literature. *J Am Acad Dermatol* 25:928, 1991.

Yalisove B, Berzin M, et al: Multiple pruritic purple plaques. *Arch Dermatol* 127:721, 1991.

# Trauma

## 212
## INITIAL APPROACH TO THE TRAUMA PATIENT

### Ernest Ruiz

Despite the advent of sophisticated transportation systems and the designation of regional trauma centers, community hospital emergency departments remain the critical link in the resuscitation of a large percentage of trauma victims in this country. Because of weather, distances, and geography, this will continue to be the case. All physicians covering emergency departments should be skilled in trauma resuscitation.

In this chapter we outline the process of trauma resuscitation in the prehospital phase and during the first few minutes after arrival in the emergency department. Other chapters will elaborate on the techniques and process of resuscitation when certain injuries are identified.

### THE INCIDENCE OF TRAUMA

In the United States, trauma is responsible for more deaths in the 5- to 34-year age group than all diseases combined and is the leading cause of death up to age 44.

### Motor Vehicle Accidents

Motor vehicle accidents account for the largest share of trauma deaths (Fig. 212-1). In 1988 about 48,000 people were killed in crashes. More than half were automobile occupants. About 40 percent of adult victims were legally classified as intoxicated.

Motorcylist deaths accounted for 7 percent of the highway death toll in 1988. The motorcycle death rate is more than 35 times greater than the automobile death rate.

Bicyclist fatalities in collisions with motor vehicles account for about 2 percent of traffic deaths. Two-thirds of bicyclist deaths occur in the 5- to 14-year age group, with 13-year-old males constituting the largest group.

Pedestrian deaths account for 10 to 15 percent of motor vehicle deaths, making it the second largest category, the largest group of which is the elderly.

### Other Unintentional Trauma

The leading causes of unintentional trauma fatalities are listed in Table 212-1. More than half of the fatal falls are in the elderly, who account for 4 percent of the population. Fractured hips are the most common type of injury resulting in hospital admission.

### Distribution

Unintentional injury death rates are more than 50 percent greater in rural areas than in central cities. There are many logistical explanations for this, including longer times to discovery, response, and delivery to the hospital. However, prehospital care systems and emergency department, operating room, and in-hospital management deserve positive attention.

### PREVENTION

Trauma can be prevented through public education, state and federal legislation, and modification of the physical environment. The latter includes highway improvement, passive restraints, and other measures. The seat belt issue has taught us that although education and physical changes are important, legislation is effective and legislators are receptive to the input of physicians.

### PREHOSPITAL CARE

The "load and go" method of managing trauma in the field requires skill and resourcefulness to accomplish safely and rapidly. The objec-

**Table 212-1.** Twenty Leading Causes of Unintentional Injury Death, 1988

| Rank | Cause | Number of Deaths |
|------|-------|------------------|
| 1 | Motor vehicle crashes—(traffic) | 48,024 |
| 2 | Falls | 12,096 |
| 3 | Poisoning by solids/liquids | 5353 |
| 4 | Fires and burns | 5087 |
| 5 | Drowning | 4966 |
| 6 | Aspiration—nonfood | 2230 |
| 7 | Aspiration—food | 1575 |
| 8 | Firearm | 1501 |
| 9 | Machinery | 1176 |
| 10 | Aircraft | 1012 |
| 11 | Suffocation | 956 |
| 12 | Poisoning by gas/vapor | 873 |
| 13 | Excessive cold | 846 |
| 14 | Struck by falling object | 835 |
| 15 | Electric current | 714 |
| 16 | Pedestrian—train | 470 |
| 17 | Excessive heat | 454 |
| 18 | Pedestrian—nontraffic | 380 |
| 19 | Collision with object/person | 239 |
| 20 | Exposure, neglect | 199 |

*Source:* Baker et al. Used by permission.

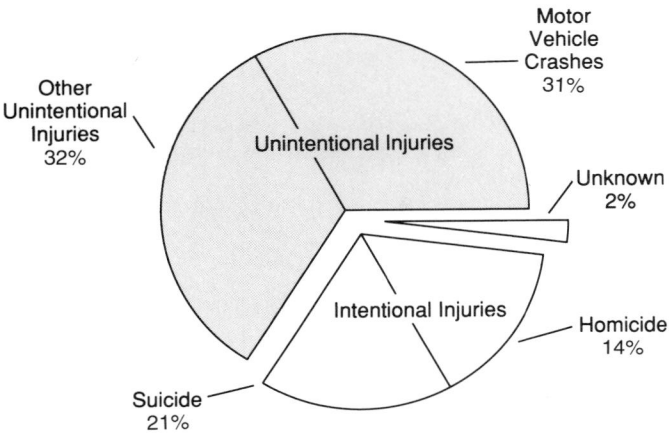

**Fig. 212-1.** Percent of injury deaths by manner of death, 1986. (From Baker et al. Used by permission.)

tive is to immobilize patients and move them to the hospital as quickly as possible, inserting IV lines while on route rather than at the scene. The receiving emergency department should be contacted early and put on notice that an injured patient is on the way.

**Table 212-2.** A Step-by-Step Procedure for Trauma Resuscitation

1. *Notification by Prehospital Personnel:* The receiving emergency department should be informed about:
   Airway patency
   Pulse and respirations
   Level of consciousness
   Immobilization
   Mechanism of injury and blood loss at the scene
   Anatomic sites of apparent injury
2. *Preparation for Receiving the Trauma Victim*
   Assign tasks to team members
   Check and prepare vital equipment
   Summon surgical consultant and other team members not present
3. *Primary Survey:* The most immediately lethal injuries are taken care of as they are identified.
   Airway
       Clear airway: chin lift, suction, finger sweep
       Protect airway
           Depressed level of consciousness or bleeding, tracheal intubation without neck movement
       Surgical airway
   Breathing
       Ventilate with 100% oxygen
       Check thorax and neck
           Deviated trachea
           Tension pneumothorax (intervention—needle decompression)
           Chest wounds and chest wall motion
           Sucking chest wound (intervention—occlusive dressing)
           Neck and chest crepitation
           Multiple broken ribs
           Fractured sternum
           Pneumothorax
       Listen for breath sounds
           Correct tracheal tube placement?
           Hemopneumothorax?
               Chest tube(s)—38 F
               Collect blood for autotransfusion
   Circulation
       Apply pressure to sites of external exsanguination
       Assure that two large-bore IVs established
           Begin with rapid infusion of warm crystalloid solution
           If arm sites unavailable, insert a large central line or perform a saphenous cutdown at the ankle
       Assess for blood volume status
           Radial and carotid pulse, BP determination
           Jugular venous filling
           Quality of heart tones
       Beck triad present?
           Pericardiocentesis or echocardiogram
           Decompress tamponade
               Pericardiocentesis
               Thoracotomy with pericardiotomy
       Hypovolemia
           After 2 L of crystalloid begin blood infusion if still hypovolemic; in children use two 20 mL/kg boluses then 10 mL/kg blood boluses if still unstable
       Near-term pregnant patient—place roll under right hip
   Disability
       Brief neurological examination
           Pupil size and reactivity
           Limb movement
           Glasgow Coma Scale
   Continuing resuscitation
       Monitor fluid administration
           Consider central line for CVP monitoring
           Use fetal heart rate as indicator in pregnant women
           Record all events

4. *Secondary Survey:* A thorough search for injuries is carried out in order to set further priorities.
   Trauma series x-rays: lateral cervical spine, supine chest, AP pelvis
   Head-to-toe examination looking and feeling; quickly bring problems under control as they are discovered
       Scalp wound bleeding controlled with Raney clips
       Hemotympanum?
       Facial stability?
       Epistaxis tamponaded with balloons if severe
       Avulsed teeth, broken jaw?
       Penetrating injuries?
       Abdominal distension and tenderness?
       Pelvic stability?
       Perineal laceration/hematoma?
       Urethral meatus blood?
       Rectal examination for tone, blood, and prostate position
       Bimanual vaginal examination
       Peripheral pulses
       Deformities, open fractures
       Reflexes, sensation
   Large gastric tube (32 F) inserted
   Foley catheter inserted
       Blood?
       Pregnancy test
   Deflate the MAST sequentially beginning with the abdominal portion if the BP is near normal; consider bicarbonate therapy
   Log-roll the patient to feel and see the back, flanks, and buttocks
   Splint unstable fractures/dislocations
   Assure that tetanus prophylaxis is given
   Consult with surgeon regarding further tests or immediate need for surgery or preferred IV medications; consider:
       Emergency thoracotomy to provide aortic compression or cross-clamping
       Aortogram or upright chest x-ray to r/o ruptured aorta
       Cystogram if pelvic fracture present or blood in urine
       IVP or enhanced CT scan of the abdomen
       Diagnostic peritoneal lavage: open or closed
       Head CT scan
       IV mannitol for neurologic decompensation
       IV steroids for possible spinal cord injury
       IV antibiotics for possible ruptured abdominal viscus
       IV antibiotics for perineal, vaginal, or rectal laceration
       Pelvic arteriogram and embolization for pelvic hemorrhage

## RESUSCITATION OF THE TRAUMA PATIENT IN THE EMERGENCY DEPARTMENT

The types of injuries trauma victims can suffer are innumerable, but the ABCs of trauma resuscitation, (airway, breathing, circulation), which are described below, apply to all cases. Table 212–2 outlines the flow of the process.

### Role of Assistants

The physician should assign tasks for assistants prior to patient arrival so that time is not wasted. Before the patient arrives, assistants should do the following:

1. Obtain two units of type O blood if it is known that the patient is hypotensive.
2. Prepare blood tubes and laboratory slips for type and crossmatching, CBC, electrolytes, BUN, glucose, coagulation, and blood alcohol studies. Ideally, a packet of tubes and laboratory slips stand ready at all times already filled out and identified by number so that the blood can be processed as soon as the number is attached to the patient.
3. Have airway and IV equipment at hand.

In hospitals where a trauma surgeon is not on staff, the surgeon on call should be summoned even before the patient arrives.

Once the patient arrives in the emergency department, the assistants should:

1. Restrain the patient's arms and legs.
2. Cut off the clothing on the torso.
3. Palpate the radial or brachial pulse.
4. Insert large-bore (16- or 14-gauge) IV catheters in each arm, and send blood specimens to the laboratory.
5. Apply ECG monitor leads to the chest, avoiding the subclavicular areas, where they would interfere with central venous line placement.

Failure to restrain the patient who appears quiet on arrival frequently results in a struggle when an airway is inserted or an IV line attempted. Personnel must hold down the patient, delaying IV access and airway management and preventing adequate cervical spine immobilization. A determination of the blood pressure is not essential during the first minutes of the resuscitation. The presence of a radial pulse indicates a blood pressure of at least 80 mmHg.

## Role of the Team Captain

The resuscitating physician should supervise the placement of the patient on the cart and listen to the report of the ambulance personnel while beginning the primary survey. The assistants should carry out their assigned tasks.

## The Primary Survey

A quick look at the patient gives a rough impression as to size, sex, age, body build, color, and alertness, but the first conscious step should be to institute the ABCs. The primary survey rapidly identifies the most immediately lethal injuries and assures that they are managed with the highest priority.

### Airway

If the patient is not able to breathe or is not making an effort to breathe, a chin lift or the insertion of an oral or nasal airway may suffice for the moment. Any movement of the neck should be avoided in the usual blunt trauma case. Obtunded or unconscious patients should be tracheally intubated to protect the airway and to provide a means of hyperventilation. Large-bore or dental suction and a transtracheal needle ventilation device should be on hand in case the patient vomits prior to intubation. Log rolling and pharyngeal suction may be necessary if the patient vomits, to prevent aspiration. If the patient is not breathing or if there is severe facial injury, cricothyrotomy or transtracheal needle ventilation may be indicated.

The very agitated trauma patient suffering from head injury, hypoxia, or drug- or alcohol-induced delirium may harbor a cervical spine fracture. A paralyzing agent such as succinylcholine or vecuronium bromide, along with a small dose of diazepam or midazolam, may be necessary to enable safe airway management. Disadvantages of immediate sedation and paralysis are interference with neurologic evaluation and the necessity of taking an emergent head CT scan to rule out intracranial bleeding or mass lesion. This is a small price to pay if the victim has been rendered so irrational as to jeopardize effective resuscitation.

### Breathing

With the patient breathing, or now intubated and being ventilated with 100% oxygen, the thorax and neck should be examined and felt to detect abnormalities such as a deviated trachea, crepitation, flail chest, sucking chest wound, fractured sternum, and the absence of breath sounds or both sides of the chest. Possible interventions here include (1) insertion of a needle in the chest to relieve a tension pneumothorax; (2) application of an occlusive dressing to a sucking chest wound; (3) withdrawal of the endotracheal tube from the right mainstem bronchus; (4) reintubation of the trachea if no breath sounds are heard; and (5) insertion of large chest tubes (38F). If blood returns, the blood can be collected in an autotransfusion device. The volume of blood that returns should immediately be noted. If 1500 to 2000 mL of blood comes from the chest tube, thoracotomy may be indicated.

### Circulation

Any exsanguinating external hemorrhage should have become apparent by now. Direct pressure should be used to control bleeding. Hemostats can cause injury to adjacent structures. If the bleeding site is on an extremity, a blood pressure cuff can be inflated to a pressure greater than the patient's systolic pressure.

By this time, assistants should have cut off the clothing from the patient's chest and reported the presence or absence of a pulse. Military antishock trousers (MAST) should not be deflated until the circulating volume has been sufficiently restored to raise the systemic blood pressure to normal or near-normal levels. Two large-bore IV lines should have been established, and blood should have been obtained for the laboratory studies already ordered. If arm veins are not available, a large-bore central line should be inserted. Alternatively, there should be a cut down of the saphenous vein at the ankle and a large cannula inserted. Warm crystalloid should be infused as rapidly as possible, using manual or pneumatic pressure on the IV bags. If there is no palpable pulse on admission, or no marked improvement after the very rapid infusion of 2 L of crystalloid, O-negative blood should be administered. All team members should be alert to the dangers of iatrogenic air embolism associated with pressure infusion. A blood and fluid warmer should be in use.

The team captain should now listen for heart sounds, observe for neck vein distension, and assess cardiac rhythm on the cardiac monitor. If the clinical findings suggest cardiac tamponade (Beck triad—low blood pressure, elevated venous pressure, and muffled heart sounds), and if tension pneumothorax has been excluded and the patient is in shock and unresponsive to rapid volume infusion, a pericardiocentesis should be attempted. If pericardiocentesis fails, a left thoracotomy should be performed to directly decompress the pericardial sac. Echocardiography, using a subcostal window, is replacing diagnostic pericardiocentesis in many emergency departments. It is noninvasive, rapid, and accurate.

### Disability

An abbreviated neurologic evaluation should now be performed, including level of consciousness, pupil size and reactivity, and motor function. The Glasgow Coma Scale (Table 212-3) should be used to

**Table 212-3.** The Glasgow Coma Scale Measure of Level of Consciousness

| Measure | Response | Score |
|---|---|---|
| Eye opening | Opens: | |
| | Spontaneously | 4 |
| | To verbal command | 3 |
| | To pain | 2 |
| | No response | 1 |
| Verbal | Oriented and converses | 5 |
| | Disoriented and converses | 4 |
| | Inappropriate words | 3 |
| | Incomprehensible sounds | 2 |
| | No response | 1 |
| Motor | Obeys verbal command | 6 |
| | To painful stimulus: | |
| | Localizes pain | 5 |
| | Flexion-withdrawal | 4 |
| | Abnormal flexion (decorticate rigidity) | 3 |
| | Extension (decerebrate rigidity) | 2 |
| | No response | 1 |

quantify the patient's level of consciousness: possible scores range from 3 (no response) to 15 (high response on all measures).

### Continuing Resuscitation

At this stage of the primary survey, the blood pressure, pulse pressure, pulse rate, and rectal temperature should be recorded. A narrow pulse pressure is common to both cardiac tamponade and hypovolemia. Ventilation should continue with 100% oxygen. If large volumes are being infused, trends in central venous pressure (CVP) should be followed. However, the central venous pressure is sometimes elevated in conditions such as tension pneumothorax and hemothorax, even in the presence of hypovolemia. For rapid fluid infusion, the guidewire technique can be used to replace a peripheral IV with an 8F or 9F sheath. If there is little or no response to the rapid infusion of 2 L of crystalloid, type O blood should be given if type-specific or fully crossmatched blood is not yet available. Documentation of resuscitative events should be entered on a flow sheet, listing the volumes and type of fluid given, blood pressure and pulse rate, CVP, urine output, gastric suction volume, and neurologic status. Recent experimental work indicates that large fluid infusions can be detrimental when hemorrhage is ongoing. When it is likely that the patient is continuing to bleed, use blood instead of electrolyte solution to avoid hemodilution. Under these circumstances it is probably best to accept a systolic blood pressure of 90 to 100 mmHg until surgical repair is underway.

## Secondary Survey

While resuscitation continues, the team captain should proceed with the secondary survey. The secondary survey is a rapid but thorough physical examination for the purpose of identifying as many injuries as possible. With this information, the resuscitating physician and his or her surgical colleague can set logical priorities for evaluation and management. Frequent assessments of the patient's blood pressure, pulse rate, and central venous pressure should continue.

The examination is conducted in a head-to-toe fashion, beginning with the scalp. Scalp lacerations can bleed profusely. This bleeding can be controlled with plastic Raney clips that grasp the full thickness of the scalp and galea. The tympanic membranes should be visualized to detect hemotympanum, and the pupil examination should be repeated. If epistaxis is a problem, a Foley catheter or a nasal balloon should be inserted to provide posterior tamponade. The examination continues over the neck and thorax. A lateral cervical spine x-ray (if not already obtained), a chest x-ray, and an anteroposterior pelvic x-ray should be obtained while the secondary survey continues. A 32F gastric tube should be inserted into the stomach and connected to suction. When there is facial trauma or basilar skull fracture, the gastric tube should be inserted through the mouth rather than the nose. The clothing at the crotch of the MAST is cut away, and the urinary meatus, scrotum, and perineum are inspected for the presence of blood, hematoma, or laceration.

A rectal examination is done, noting sphincter function and whether the prostate is boggy or displaced. Rectal blood indicates rectal laceration. If the prostate is normal and there is no blood at the urethral meatus, a Foley catheter can be placed in the bladder. If a urethral injury is suspected (meatal blood present), a urethrogram (described in Chap. 221) should be obtained prior to passing the catheter. If the prostate is displaced, it should be assumed that the urethra is disrupted. Catheterization should not be attempted if the urethra is injured. The urine should be examined for blood. If the patient is a woman of childbearing age, a pregnancy test should be obtained. A bimanual vaginal examination should be performed. If blood is present, a speculum examination will be necessary to identify a possible vaginal laceration in the presence of a pelvic fracture. Palpate all peripheral pulses. The patient should be log-rolled to either side while keeping the neck immobilized, so that every inch of the patient's body is seen and felt. The extremities should be evaluated for fracture and soft tissue injury. Peripheral pulses should be felt. A more thorough neurologic examination can now be done, carefully checking motor and sensory function.

If the blood pressure rises and stabilizes with volume replacement, the MAST can be sequentially deflated. Start with the abdominal compartment, and then proceed one leg at a time while monitoring the blood pressure. If the prfalls, the suit should be reinflated. Consider administering sodium bicarbonate solution if shock has been present for a prolonged period (5 to 10 minutes or longer). Follow arterial or mixed venous pH if possible because ischemic tissues under the trousers will release lactic acid as blood flow returns.

The three trauma series x-rays—cervical spine, chest, and pelvis—should be carefully read. Every anatomic structure should be checked. Flank stripes (radiopaque lines separating the wall of the colon from the properitoneal fat lines on either flank) signify free fluid in the peritoneal cavity. Diaphragmatic ruptures may be difficult to discern, but if the gastric tube is seen in the left chest, the diagnosis is obvious. If a pelvic fracture is present, a cystogram is useful for outlining the extent of the retroperitoneal hematoma present and for demonstrating an intraperitoneal bladder rupture. The cystogram should be obtained early because it may obviate the need for a diagnostic peritoneal lavage.

If the patient's blood pressure has not responded or stabilized with crystalloid or blood by the end of the secondary survey (which should take only about 10 min in most cases), transfer of the patient to the operating room for abdominal or thoracic exploration should be considered. Ideally, the trauma surgeon will be present during the secondary survey to observe the patient's progress.

On occasion, it will be necessary to perform emergency department thoracotomy to allow tamponade of the aorta at the diaphragm or aortic cross clamping. One indication for thoracotomy—cardiac tamponade—has already been described. Other indications are (1) persistent profound shock despite ventilation and rapid volume and blood infusion and (2) cardiac arrest. Thoracotomy has not been found to be useful when signs of life are not observed by first responders at the scene of the incident.

## PATIENT DISPOSITION FROM THE EMERGENCY DEPARTMENT

Options include moving the patient to the operating room, admission to the hospital, or transfer to another facility. The primary and secondary survey must have been completed and a gastric tube and a Foley catheter should be in place unless a urethral injury was detected. In most urban hospitals, the trauma surgeon should have been present for the secondary survey and he or she should assume direction of the diagnostic workup and disposition of the case at that time. In rural hospitals that transfer severe trauma cases, the resuscitating physician should relate all of the physical findings discovered during the primary and secondary surveys to the physician receiving the patient. Laboratory results, x-rays, and the flow sheet showing blood pressure, pulse, fluids infused, urine output, gastric output, and neurologic findings should accompany the patient. If a diagnostic peritoneal lavage was performed, a sample of the lavage fluid should accompany the patient. A patient who is being transported to another facility should be accompanied by personnel capable of administering fluids and monitoring vital signs and pupillary changes. Mannitol should be available if there is neurologic deterioration on route.

MAST, as they are commonly used in the field, are inflated to a pressure of about 100 mmHg. When a patient is left in the trousers for a period of more than 2 to 3 h, the pressure should be reduced to 20 to 30 mmHg to avoid skin necrosis and compartment syndromes. At this reduced pressure the MAST garment is still an effective splint and will tamponade venous and small arterial bleeding. Splinting of long bone fractures and especially pelvic fractures helps prevent continuing blood loss.

## FOUNDATIONS OF TRAUMA RESUSCITATION

**Time.** The primary enemy of the resuscitating physician is elapsing time. The injured patient may harbor continuing hemorrhage or other sources of shock that will kill if not quickly identified and managed. *The most skilled resuscitators make good use of every second of time starting from the moment of notification.* A definite and practiced routine such as outlined here is essential to enable decisive, timesaving leadership.

**Go back to the beginning.** If, during the course of the resuscitation, the patient reverses course and deteriorates, the resuscitation team must go back to the beginning and repeat the ABCs.

**Be thorough.** Attention to detail by all team members is critical. Do not compromise patient safety by skipping steps. A central venous line for CVP measurement is essential when large fluid volumes are administered. Do not allow dramatic wounds, such as a limb amputation, to distract you from your systematic search for lethal injuries.

**Be skilled.** Surgical and nonsurgical airway management, chest tube insertion, venous cannulation and cutdowns, Foley catheter insertion, central venous catheter insertion, and gastric intubation are the basic skills required of resuscitating physicians. The ability to perform emergency thoracotomy, diagnostic peritoneal lavage, and arterial cutdown are also desirable skills.

**Be a team player.** It is essential that resuscitating physicians and their surgical colleagues work well and closely together. Small minds dwell on who's in charge. The fact that 70 percent of fatal trauma occurs in rural America where trauma surgeons and fully trained emergency physicians are in short supply makes it essential that all physicians who cover emergency departments be well versed in the basics of resuscitation.

**Be suspicious.** If the mechanism of injury suggests aortic rupture, proceed accordingly. A bent steering wheel or a known high-speed impact should result in referral from a hospital without vascular surgery capabilities to a trauma center. Seat belts, while life-saving, can result in occult abdominal injuries such as "bucket handle" bowel devascularization. An inocuous looking laceration may, in fact, be a bullet or knife wound.

In conclusion, the ABC system of managing the resuscitation of severely injured patients during the first few minutes to 1 hour of arrival offers a safe, efficient initial approach to the trauma patient. The flow of the process identifies rapidly lethal injuries first and takes steps to reverse them as they are discovered. The process is also painstakingly thorough in order to allow good priority setting. It also saves time by providing a framework for action.

## BIBLIOGRAPHY

Asbun HJ, Irani H, Roe EJ, et al: Intra-abdominal seatbelt injury. *J Trauma* 30:189, 1990.
Baker SP, O'Neill B, Ginsburg MJ, Li G: *The Injury Fact Book,* 2d ed. New York, Oxford University Press, 1992.
Bickell WH, Bruttig SP, Millnamow GA, et al: The detrimental effects of intravenous crystalloid after aortotomy in swine. *Surgery* 110:529, 1991.
Committee on Trauma Research: *Injury in America.* Washington, D.C,, National Academy Press, 1985.
Committee on Trauma, American College of Surgeons: *Advanced Trauma Life Support Instructor Manual,* 5th ed. Chicago, American College of Surgeons, 1993.
Esposito TJ, Jurkovich GJ, Rice CL, et al: Reappraisal of emergency room thoracotomy in a changing environment. *J Trauma* 31(7):881, 1991.
Flint LM Jr, Babikian G, Anders M, et al: Definitive control of mortality from severe pelvic fracture. *Ann Surg* 211:703, 1990.
Kowalenko T, Stern S, Dronen S, et al: Improved outcome with hypotensive resuscitation of uncontrolled hemorrhagic shock in a swine model. *J Trauma* 33:349, 1992.
Niemi TA, Norton LW: Vaginal injuries in patients with pelvic fractures. *J Trauma* 25:547, 1985.
Orsay EM, Dunne M, Turnbull TL, et al: Prospective study of the effect of safety belts in motor vehicle crashes. *Ann Emerg Med* 19:258, 1990.
Stern SA, Dronen SC, Birrer P, et al: Effect of blood pressure on hemorrhagic volume and survival in a near fatal hemorrhage model incorporating a vascular injury. *Ann Emerg Med* 22:155, 1993.

# 213
# PEDIATRIC TRAUMA
## Marte E. Baro
## Gary C. Fifield

Trauma is the most common cause of death in children over 1 y of age. It accounts for approximately one half of all deaths in the pediatric age group. Some 13 to 16 million children per year visit an emergency department with trauma-related complaints and, of these, 400,000 to 600,000 children are hospitalized each year.

Although accidental trauma remains the leading cause of morbidity in the pediatric age group, nonaccidental trauma represents a higher proportion of morbidity and mortality in certain locations and age groups. Homicide is the most common cause of infant death, most often as a result of child abuse. In New York City, gunshot wounds account for the greatest mortality in adolescents. Motor vehicle accidents, bicycle accidents, drownings, and burns are the most frequent causes of accidental injury.

Even though pediatric trauma is common, most emergency departments tend to see more adult trauma patients and the staff are often more comfortable with the older trauma patient. The priorities of management of the pediatric and adult trauma patients remain the same, but some physiologic and psychological differences must be considered by emergency physicians when they are caring for an injured child.

## OVERVIEW OF MANAGEMENT

The general initial assessment and management of an injured child is the same as that of the injured adult. Airway and breathing must be evaluated and managed first, followed by assessment of circulation, then a brief neurologic examination and complete exposure of the patient. The ratio of body surface area to mass is greater in children than adults, so hypothermia occurs more rapidly in children. Warming lights, warm blankets, and warmed intravenous fluids should be used early in the resuscitation.

Children who are conscious during this rapid unexplained examination and placement of various catheters and intravenous lines are apt to be frightened and may be combative. A staff member should talk to the child directly, using the child's name, and explain briefly what is happening and why. Sedation may be needed and should not be withheld once a neurologic examination has been done.

## AIRWAY MANAGEMENT

The pediatric airway is different from that of an adult not only in the obvious smaller size, but the proportions of anatomic features and the mechanics of breathing. A baby is an obligate nose breather until about 6 months of age. The tongue is relatively larger in proportion to the mouth. The larynx is more cephalad, located at approximately C3–4 in an infant and C4–5 in an adult. The vocal cords are shorter and more concave, and their anterior attachment is relatively more cephalad. In children less than 8 years old, the narrowest portion of the trachea is subglottic and may block passage of an endotracheal tube that has passed through the vocal cords easily. The size of the cricoid ring is the pertinent measurement for assessing endotracheal tube size and can be approximated by the formula:

$$\text{Internal Diameter in mm} = \frac{16 + \text{Patient's Age in Years}}{4}$$

The mechanics of breathing differ between childhood and adulthood in that children are more dependent on diaphragmatic excursion to generate an adequate tidal volume. The compliant chest wall of the child cannot compensate for impeded excursion, which may be due to an intra-abdominal process and may result in parodoxical motion with retractions.

Signs of respiratory distress in a child include tachypnea, grunting, flaring, and use of accessory muscles. Any child exhibiting these signs should receive 100% oxygen by face mask, as should patients with decreased level of consciousness, head injury, or significant trauma.

Any airway intervention should be accompanied by cervical spine immobilization. Initial airway maintenance should consist of jaw thrust or chin lift maneuvers. If this does not clear the airway, an oral airway may be inserted using a tongue blade. The child can then be bag-valve-mask ventilated using a 15 L/min oxygen flow to the bag. Ventilation can be assessed for adequacy by watching chest rise.

Orotracheal intubation will be required in patients needing prolonged ventilatory support. The endotracheal tube also prevents aspiration, aids in pulmonary toilet, and can be used to administer positive end-expiratory pressure. The orotracheal tube should be uncuffed in children less than 8 years old. Orotracheal intubation, with in-line immobilization of the cervical spine, is the preferred route of intubation. Nasotracheal intubation can be difficult and can cause damage and swelling of the nasopharynx. Before intubation is attempted, the patient should be maximally oxygenated with a bag-valve-mask device and high-flow oxygen. A pulse oximeter should be used to assess both oxygen saturation and pulse during intubation attempts. Once an airway is secured, the endotracheal tube placement should be checked by auscultation of both axillae and abdomen, checking for a right main stem intubation or esophageal intubation. The initial ventilatory rate should be approximately 20 breaths/min and tidal volume can be assessed by chest rise.

Rapid sequence intubation, as outlined in Table 213-1, is appropriate for use in children with head injuries or combative patients. For children with facial trauma who have a compromised airway, the procedure of choice is placement of a transtracheal catheter for jet insufflation. The catheter should be placed using the Seldinger technique.

In some infants, the cricothyroid membrane is easily palpable and direct puncture with an exploring needle is worth trying. In other infants, the cricothyroid membrane is not so easily identified. The cricoid cartilage itself is easily damaged, so cricothyrotomy is not recommended in small children. A safe approach when transtracheal catheter ventilation will be difficult is to cutdown on the trachea prior to needle insertion. Make a midline skin incision caudad to the cricoid cartilage using a no. 15 scalpel. Carry this incision down to the trachea using blunt dissection with a curved mosquito clamp. A small self-retaining retractor (Alm minor surgery retractor) is helpful. When the trachea can be definitely felt or visualized, insert the exploring needle of a pediatric transtracheal needle ventilation kit (Cook Critical Care, T7.0-32-5-P-NS-O) into the trachea aspirating with a syringe to detect air. The guidewire is then inserted into the trachea through the needle. Remove the needle; then insert the 7 F cannula into the trachea over the guidewire. Aspirate with a syringe again to confirm correct placement. Attach the oxygen source (Sanders Venturi Ventilation System, Pilling-Rusch, Inc., #50-2575) at a pressure of 25 psi and attempt ventilation. The pressure can be gradually increased to achieve adequate chest rise. The transtracheal catheter can be replaced with a tracheostomy tube by replacing the guidewire through the cannula into the trachea and removing the cannula. The opening into the trachea is then carefully enlarged by spreading with an iris scissors. A tracheostomy tube with its obturator in place can then be inserted alongside the guidewire into the trachea. Figure 213-1 shows the steps of this procedure. Table 213-2 gives the sizes of tracheostomy tubes corresponding to endotracheal tube size. A shortened endotracheal tube could be used instead of a tracheostomy tube. Cricothyroidotomy is difficult in small children due to the small size and because the connecting tissues are fragile. Indeed, neck trauma commonly results in transection of the trachea at this level.

## CIRCULATION, SHOCK, ACCESS

Pediatric patients who have lost a significant amount of blood may exhibit signs of shock differently than do adults. Children are able to increase their systemic vascular resistance significantly, thereby maintaining a normal or close to normal blood pressure despite hypovolemia. They maintain an adequate cardiac output by increasing their heart rate. Therefore, tachycardia is the most sensitive indicator of shock in children. Blood pressure may not drop until 40 to 45 percent of circulating volume is lost. Other clues to alterations in volume status include narrowing of pulse pressure, decrease in mental status, prolonged capillary refill, decreased skin temperature, and decreased urine output.

Pediatric shock patients require volume expansion, but vascular access is often more difficult to obtain. Initially, venous access should be attempted using saphenous and antecubital veins. When venous access cannot be established quickly (two attempts per advanced trauma life support guidelines and three attempts per pediatric advanced life support guidelines), intraosseous cannulation is the procedure of choice. In our experience, intraosseous cannulation is the first route chosen in infants. This technique has been successful in children up to 10 y old and has a low complication rate. Any intravenous medication or blood product can be infused via an interosseous line, although a pump may be required. Femoral and subclavian lines are appropriate if they can be placed quickly.

Initial fluid resuscitation should consist of 20 mL/kg boluses of normal saline or Ringer's lactate. If there is no response to the fluid bolus or deterioration occurs after an initial improvement in vital signs, blood loss should be suspected. Further volume expansion should include 10 mL/kg boluses of whole blood or, as is more commonly available, packed red blood cells reconstituted with saline.

## NEUROLOGIC INJURY

The incidence of traumatic brain injury is approximately 200/100,000 children per year. Of these, 82 percent are mild, 14 percent are moderately severe, and 5 percent are fatal. Motor vehicle accidents, bicy-

**Table 213-1.** Procedure for Rapid Sequence Intubation in the Child

100% oxygen by mask for 3 min
Restrain
Establish reliable IV
Atropine, 0.02 mg/kg IV (minimum dose 0.1 mg and maximum dose 1.0 mg)
Midazolam HCl, 0.05–0.1 mg/kg IV
Succinylcholine Cl, 2.0 mg/kg IV
*or*
Vecuronium Br, 0.15 mg/kg IV
Selleck's maneuver (cricoid pressure)
Orotracheal intubation with in-line immobilization
Succinylcholine results in histamine release, so vecuronium is preferable in asthmatics. The onset of paralysis with succinylcholine is 50 s and 2.5 min with vecuronium. Paralysis lasts 10 min with succinylcholine and about 30 min with vecuronium.

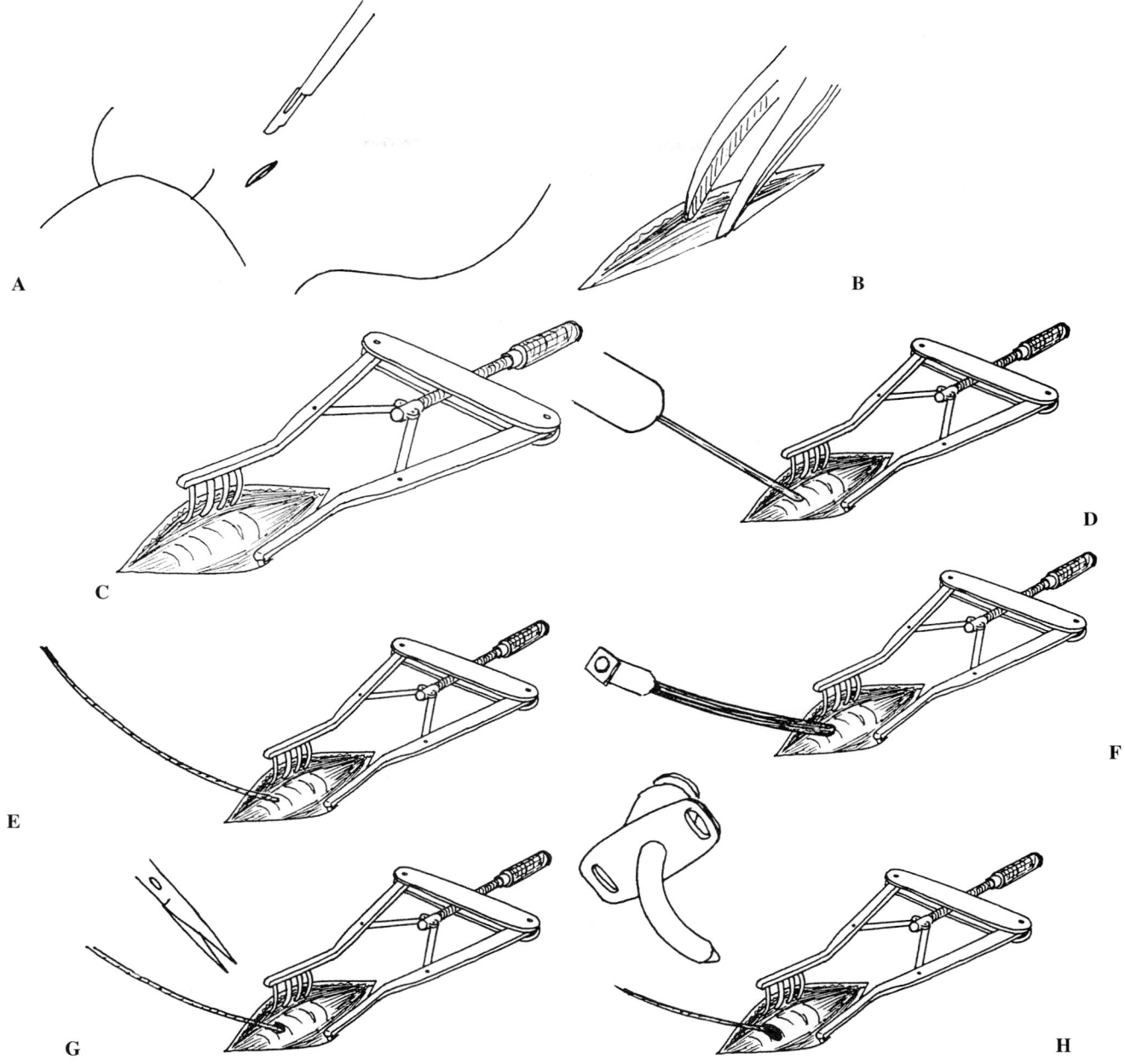

**Fig. 213-1.** The steps in performing transtracheal catheter ventilation and tracheostomy in infants. **A.** A midline incision is made over the trachea below the cricoid cartilage. A no. 15 scalpel is used. **B.** A mosquito clamp is used to spread the strap muscles. **C.** The Alm self-retaining retractor is inserted to spread the strap muscles apart. Some additional dissection may be necessary to expose the tracheal rings. **D.** Under direct vision, a needle is placed in the trachea between tracheal rings. Air is aspirated when the trachea is entered. **E.** A guidewire is inserted through the needle. **F.** A 7 F pediatric transtracheal cannula is then inserted. Aspirate again to check position, then ventilate. **G.** To convert to a tracheostomy, the guidewire is reinserted and the cannula removed. Use iris scissors to gently spread the hole. **H.** Insert the pediatric tracheostomy tube along side the guidewire into the trachea.

cle accidents, and falls account for most of head trauma in children. Isolated head injury is usually secondary to a fall.

Overall, children recover better from head injury than do adults, but younger children tend to do more poorly than children over 3 years old. Adverse prognostic features include hypoxia and, especially, hypotension. Preclinical assessment and treatment of hypotension seems to be most important in ameliorating its detrimental effects.

Neurologic assessment of the child can be difficult in the setting of a busy and scary emergency department. The physician must know appropriate developmental stages, consider the apprehensiveness of the child, and modify conventional neurologic scoring strategies (i.e., Glasgow coma score) based on age. The remainder of the examina-

tion is similar to that of adults, with attention to pupillary size and reactivity, reflexes, motor activity, and signs of cerebrospinal fluid leakage or basilar skull fracture. In an infant, the fontanelle can provide information regarding intracranial pressure (ICP). The presence of an open fontanelle does not appear to be protective of acute changes in intracranial tissue volumes.

Children who bump their heads often vomit. Emesis is rarely a sign of increased ICP. In addition, young children often are transiently pale, diaphoretic, and lethargic immediately following even mild head injury. The cause of the pediatric concussion syndrome is not known but it may be associated with posttraumatic epilepsy.

The primary method of radiographically assessing a head-injured child is computed tomography (CT) scan. Indications for CT scan in-

**Table 213-2.** Endotracheal Tube Size and Tracheostomy Tube Size in mm according to the age of the child. These are estimates only because of the variability of patient size.

| Patient Age | Endotracheal Tube | | Tracheostomy Tube | | |
| --- | --- | --- | --- | --- | --- |
| | I.D. | O.D. | Size | I.D. | O.D. |
| Premie | 2.5 | 3.4 | oo | 3.1 | 4.5 |
| Newborn | 3.0 | 4.4 | oo | 3.1 | 4.5 |
| 1 month | 4.0 | 5.4 | o | 3.4 | 5.0 |
| 6 months | 4.5 | 6.1 | 1 | 3.7 | 5.5 |
| 1 year | 5.0 | 6.9 | 2 | 4.1 | 6.0 |
| 2–3 years | 5.5 | 7.5 | 3 | 4.8 | 7.0 |
| 4–5 years | 6.0 | 8.2 | 3 | 4.8 | 7.0 |
| 6–8 years | 6.5 | 9.0 | 4 | 5.5 | 8.0 cuffed |

clude loss of consciousness, a change in the level of consciousness, headache, persistent emesis, skull fracture, or seizure. Skull x-rays may be helpful to detect foreign bodies and depressed skull fracture.

The "growing skull fracture" is a pediatric entity. It involves a skull fracture with an underlying dural tear that continues to leak. Children present up to weeks after the initial injury with a boggy mass or sunken defect at the fracture site. The dural defect needs to be repaired for definitive treatment.

Children who have sustained a severe head injury and who have evidence of, or are at risk for, increased ICP should be hyperventilated to maintain a $P_{CO2}$ of 25 to 29. The head of the bed should be elevated to 20° to 30°; and the neck should be straight, not kinked, to optimize venous drainage. Intravenous mannitol in a dose of 0.5 to 1.0 g/kg can be used to lower ICP. Lasix, at a dose of 1.0 mg/kg, may decrease edema as well. Currently no studies have shown steroids to be helpful.

Posttraumatic seizures occur more frequently in children than adults. Those occurring within minutes of the injury are not associated with subsequent epilepsy. However, seizures increase the metabolic demands of an already compromised brain. Therefore, seizure prophylaxis is often started on children with moderate to severe head injury. The drug of choice is phenytoin, with a 15 mg/kg load intravenously at a rate of 50 mg/min.

## SPINAL CORD INJURY

Spinal cord injuries are caused by motor vehicle accidents, falls, sports injuries, and gunshot wounds, in decreasing order of frequency. Young children have a higher incidence of upper cervical spine and cranioverterbral junction injuries, as well as complete spinal cord injuries and spinal cord injury without radiographic abnormalities as compared to adults. Teenagers more frequently suffer nondisplaced fractures of the vertebral bodies and posterior elements.

The upper cervical spine and cranioverterbral junction are susceptible to injury in the younger child because the relatively large head shifts the fulcrum of cervical motion from the C5–6 area to C2–3. In addition, the facet joints are horizontally oriented, allowing the vertebrae to slip in an anteroposterior direction.

Imaging of the spine should begin with conventional trauma views of the cervical spine, and anteroposterior and lateral views of the thoracic, lumbar, and sacral spine. If a fracture or dislocation is seen, then CT scan or standard tomograms should be used to further evaluate the position of the vertebrae or fragments. If a neurologic deficit is present, with or without radiographic abnormality, a magnetic resonance imaging or CT myelogram can help exclude or identify a surgically correctable lesion.

Treatment of spinal cord injuries in the prehospital and emergency department setting consists of immobilization, diagnosis of the specific injury, and steroids. Prehospital personnel must be instructed that an infant's relatively large head may cause the neck to flex in the standard supine position, so they require padding behind the shoulders to prevent this. Steroids should be started with evidence of a

neurologic deficit with a loading dose of 30 mg/kg of methylprednisolone. In the event of spinal cord injury or head injury, a neurosurgeon should be consulted.

## CHEST TRAUMA

Children, with their relatively compliant chest walls, may not show external evidence of serious intrathoracic trauma. Blunt trauma occurs more frequently than penetrating trauma and may be equally as serious. Isolated chest trauma in children carries a 4 to 12 percent mortality rate.

Evaluation of a patient who has evidence of, or who has a good mechanism for, chest injury should include a thorough physical examination looking for bony defects, crepitus, paradoxical chest movement, and unequal breath sounds. A chest x-ray should be taken. A rib fracture is a sensitive indicator of serious underlying injury. The most commonly seen injury is pulmonary contusion, which may not be visible on the original chest x-ray.

Tube thoracostomy alone is usually sufficient management for pneumothorax or hemothorax. Emergent thoracotomy is indicated in children for the same reasons as adults. As with adults, children with penetrating chest injuries benefit more from thoracotomy than those with blunt injuries. Children who have sustained blunt trauma and whose vital signs deteriorate after they are in the emergency department may benefit from emergent thoracotomy but survival is rare.

## ABDOMINAL TRAUMA

Abdominal trauma is common in children and difficult to evaluate on physical examination. Studies have found an initial abdominal examination to have a 22 to 50 percent false positive rate and a 15 percent false negative rate.

Because physical examination can be unreliable, other means of evaluation must be used. The commonly used techniques include diagnostic peritoneal lavage (DPL), CT scan, and ultrasound. Ultrasound can detect intraperitoneal fluid quite accurately, but often cannot locate the specific injury. DPL is more sensitive than CT scan, but may be too sensitive, leading to laparotomy in a patient who may have been managed conservatively. CT scans may miss significant lesions, especially in a hastily prepped patient.

Evaluation of a child who has sustained abdominal trauma can follow two paths. In a child who has a high likelihood of requiring laparotomy, the initial screening examination should be DPL. This may be followed by CT in a stable child to define the specific injury. This approach would obviate unnecessary surgery. The unstable child should be evaluated with DPL or immediate surgical intervention. The stable child who is less likely to have significant intra-abdominal trauma can be evaluated by CT scan followed by serial abdominal examinations by a surgeon in an intensive care unit setting.

Any child undergoing DPL should have a Foley catheter and, especially, a nasogastric tube in place. Children are prone to aerophagia resulting in impressive distention of the stomach. Often, the evacuation of air from the stomach results in complete relief of symptoms as well as distention.

## BURNS

Burns are the second most common cause of accidental death in children less than 5 years old. Initial evaluation of the burned child should be directed at the airway. The small diameter of the trachea places the pediatric burn patient at risk for airway compromise should even moderate swelling occur. Approximately 30 percent of patients with major burns have inhalation injuries, and all burn patients are at risk for carbon monoxide poisoning.

After an airway is secured, the depth and extent of burns should be assessed using burn charts. In children with a major burn, volume resuscitation is vital to avoid shock and renal failure. Children have a high surface area-to-mass ratio and require relatively higher fluid volumes than adults. The patient in shock should receive 20 mL/kg fluid boluses until the pressure is stable, with ongoing volume resuscitation consisting of 3 to 4 mL/kg per percent of body surface area burned, over 24 h. The crystalloid of choice in the emergency department is Ringer's lactate. Potassium should not be given with the initial fluids because the injured tissue releases large quantities of potassium.

## TRANSPORT

Children with significant trauma or burns have better survival rates when treated in trauma and burn centers. Transport to an appropriate facility should be arranged with adequate monitoring and personnel who are familiar with the care of injured children. Errors made during transport accounted for a significant proportion of all errors in management of potentially salvageable pediatric trauma patients who died in one study.

Any child who is expected to have airway difficulty should be intubated. All tubes should be secured, as should intravenous and intraosseous lines. During transport, pulse oximetry, electrocardiographic monitoring, and frequent blood pressure measurements should be used and recorded. The receiving facility should be contacted prior to transport, and a copy of all pertinent notes, laboratory results, and x-rays should accompany the child. Often, parents may need transport to a distant center and it may be appropriate for them to accompany the patient.

## BIBLIOGRAPHY

Alexander R, Proctor H. *Advanced Trauma Life Support Student Manual.* American College of Surgeons, 1993.

Chameides L (ed). *Textbook of Pediatric Advanced Life Support.* American Heart Association, 1990.

Cooper A, Barlow B, et al. Epidemiology of pediatric trauma: importance of population based statistics. *J Pediatr Surg* 27:2, 1992.

Fifield GC, Morton T, Ruiz E. Transtracheal catheter ventilation in a small animal model. *Ann Emerg Med* 17:397, 1988. Abstract.

Graneto J, Soglin D. Transport and stabilization of the pediatric trauma patient. *Pediatr Clin North Am* 40:2, 1993.

Guy J, Haley K, et al. Use of intraosseous infusion in the pediatric trauma patient. *J Pediatr Surg* 28:2, 1993.

Harris B, Barlow B, et al. American Pediatric Surgical Association principles of pediatric trauma care. *J Pediatr Surg* 27:4, 1992.

Krauss B, Harakal T, et al. General trauma in a pediatric emergency department: spectrum and consultation patterns. *Pediatr Emerg Care* 9:3, 1993.

Leschohier I, DiScala C. Blunt trauma in children: causes and outcomes of head versus intracranial injury. *Pediatrics* 91:4, 1993.

Luerssen T. Head injuries in children. *Neurosurg Clin North Am* 2:2, 1991.

Mayer T (ed). *Emergency Management of Pediatric Trauma.* Philadelphia, WB Saunders, 1985.

Meyer D, Thal E. Computed tomography in the evaluation of children with blunt abdominal trauma. *Ann Surg* 217:3, 1993.

Michaud L, Duhaime A, et al. Traumatic brain injury in children. *Ped Clin North Am* 40:3, 1993.

Nakagama D, Copes W, et al. Differences in trauma care among pediatric and nonpediatric trauma centers. *J Pediatr Surg* 27:4, 1992.

Osenbach R, Menezes A. Pediatric spinal cord and vertebral column injury. *Neurosurgery* 30:3, 1992.

Pigula F, Wald S, et al. The effect of hypotension and hypoxia on children with severe head injuries. *J Pediatr Surg* 28:3, 1993.

Reilly J, Brandt M, et al. Thoracic trauma in children. *J Trauma* 34:3, 1993.

Sheikh A, Culbertson C. Emergency department thoracotomy in children: rationale for selective application. *J Trauma* 34:3, 1993.

Stewart G, Meert K, et al. Trauma in infants less than three months of age. *Pediatr Emerg Care* 9:4, 1993.

Todres I. Pediatric airway control and ventilation. *Ann Emerg Med* 22:2, Part 2, 1993.

# 214
# GERIATRIC TRAUMA
## O. John Ma
## Daniel J. DeBehnke

With the rapid growth in the size of the elderly population, the incidence of geriatric trauma is expected to increase as well. Although the elderly experience the same type of injuries that younger individuals do, there are differences in the incidence and patterns of trauma. Emergency physicians need to stay abreast with many of these unique injury mechanisms and patterns associated with geriatric trauma. Elderly patients also respond differently to traumatic injuries because age-related changes may produce a diminished physiologic reserve. Therefore, special management principles need to be applied in caring for geriatric trauma victims.

## EPIDEMIOLOGY

Persons 65 years of age and older represent a large and growing segment of the population. According to the 1990 U.S. census, 30.9 million people, representing 12.5 percent of the total population, were 65 years of age or older. This marked a 21.3 percent increase in this segment of the population from the 1980 census figures. The U.S. Census Bureau projects that those over 65 years will increase to 52 million by the year 2020. The number of people over 85 years of age is also growing at an accelerated pace, with estimates that they will number 6.7 million by the year 2020.

While persons over 65 years of age represent 12 percent of the population, they account for 36 percent of all ambulance transports, 25 percent of hospitalizations, and 25 percent of total trauma costs. Although the elderly are less likely to be involved in trauma compared to other age groups, they are more likely to have fatal outcomes when they are injured. Approximately 28 percent of deaths due to accidental causes involve persons 65 years and older. Also, the elderly have the highest population-based mortality rate of any age group.

## DEFINITIONS

Defining the term *elderly* is a difficult task since it involves both chronologic and physiologic components. The literature has divided the elderly population into two groups: the "young old" (65 to 80 years of age) and the "old old" (80 years of age and older). Although this is a somewhat arbitrary division, it is helpful in interpreting the literature of geriatric trauma.

One of the difficulties in describing the elderly population is the potential discrepancy between chronologic age and physiologic age. *Chronologic age* is the actual number of years the individual has lived. *Physiologic age* describes the actual functional capacity of the patients' organ systems in a physiologic sense. Comorbid disease states such as diabetes mellitus, coronary artery disease, renal disease, arthritis, and pulmonary disease can decrease the physiologic reserve of certain patients, which makes it more difficult for them to recover from a traumatic injury. Physiologic reserve describes the various levels of functioning of the patients' organ systems that allows them to compensate for traumatic derangement. For example, a 65-year-old patient with diabetes, arthritis, and chronic obstructive pulmonary disease may have less physiologic reserve and, hence, an older physiologic age compared to an 80-year-old without any comorbid conditions.

## COMMON MECHANISMS OF INJURY

The elderly will experience similar types of injuries as younger individuals do. However, there are differences in the incidence and patterns of injury for elderly patients compared to younger persons.

## Falls

Falls are the most common accidental injury in patients over 75 years of age and the second most common injury in the group aged 65 to 74 years. Most individuals who fall will do so on a level surface, and most will suffer an isolated orthopaedic injury. Falls are reported as the underlying cause of 9500 deaths each year in patients over the age of 65 years. There are age-related changes in postural stability, balance, motor strength, and coordination that make the elderly more prone to tripping and falling and may explain the increased incidence of falls in this population. Also, decreased visual acuity and increased memory loss can cause the patient difficulty in recognizing and avoiding environmental hazards. Acute, preexisting, and chronic diseases also may lead to falls. Syncope has been implicated in many cases of elderly patients who fall and may be secondary to dysrhythmias, venous pooling, autonomic derangement, hypoxia, anemia, and hypoglycemia.

## Motor Vehicle Crashes

Motor vehicle–related injuries rank as the leading mechanism of injury that brings elderly patients to a trauma center in the United States. Motor vehicle crashes are the most common mechanism for fatal incidents in elderly persons through 80 years of age. Emergency physicians should anticipate an increase in motor vehicle trauma involving the elderly due to the growth in this subset of the population and the increase in elderly drivers and occupants. Although there is most likely a cause-and-effect relationship between increasing age and incidence and outcome from motor vehicle crashes, no data exist to support this hypothesis. As noted above, similar effects of acute and chronic medical conditions can influence the incidence of motor vehicle crashes. The patient may have decreased cerebral and motor skills and may have memory and judgment losses that can compound the difficulty in operating a motor vehicle. The patient also may have decreased auditory or visual acuity that makes it more difficult to recognize dangerous traffic situations. Furthermore, decreased strength and slower reaction times may hinder an individual's ability to respond to a hazardous traffic situation.

## Pedestrian-Automobile Accidents

When elderly patients are struck by automobiles, devastating injuries may result. The group aged 65 years and older accounts for 22 percent of pedestrian-automobile fatalities in the United States. Postural changes due to musculoskeletal decline may lead to kyphosis, which results in difficulty in lifting the head to see and obey traffic signals. Traffic signals, which operate at a crossing rate of 4 ft/s, may not allow for the slower walking speeds of the elderly. Thus, elderly individuals may not have enough time to safely cross an intersection. Reduced peripheral vision and decreased hearing may limit access to information needed to make rational decisions about crossing the street. Again, cognitive, memory, and judgment skills may be diminished and could play a role in pedestrians being struck by automobiles.

## Violence

The overall increase in violent crimes in the United States has not spared the elderly. Violent assaults account for 4 to 14 percent of trauma admissions in this age group. Elderly persons are seen as ideal targets for robberies because they may possess various age-related physical deficiencies. Just as in the younger population, ethanol consumption by the assailant or victim has been found to be involved in the majority of fatal assaults. While blunt trauma, to date, has been the most frequent injury mechanism, penetrating injuries are on the rise. Just as in pediatric cases, emergency physicians should have a heightened suspicion for elder or parental abuse in the geriatric trauma patient.

## ASSESSMENT

### Primary and Secondary Surveys

As in all trauma patients, the ABCDEs of the primary survey should be assessed expeditiously. Special attention should be paid to anatomical variation that may make airway management more difficult. These include the presence of dentures (which may occlude the airway), cervical arthritis (which adds danger to extending the neck), or temporomandibular joint arthritis (which may hinder mouth opening). A thorough secondary survey is essential to uncover less serious injuries. These injuries, which include various orthopaedic and "minor" head trauma, may not be severe enough to cause problems during the initial resuscitation but cumulatively may cause significant morbidity and mortality. An important point to note is that patients with no apparent life-threatening injuries can actually have potentially fatal injuries if there is some degree of limited physiologic reserve. Seemingly stable geriatric trauma patients can deteriorate rapidly and without warning.

### History

Since elderly patients may have a significant past medical history that impacts their trauma care, obtaining a precise history is vital. Often, the time frame for obtaining information about the traumatic event, past medical history, medications, and allergies is quite short. Medical records and consultation with the patient's family physician may be helpful. Family members also may be able to provide information regarding the traumatic event and the patient's previous level of function.

### Vital Signs

Early assessment and frequent monitoring of vital signs are essential in the geriatric trauma patient. However, the clinician should not be led into a false sense of security by "normal" vital signs. In a study by Scalea et al. of 15 patients initially considered to be hemodynamically "stable," 8 had cardiac outputs of less than 3.5 L/min and none had an adequate response to volume loading. Of seven patients with a normal cardiac output, five had inadequate oxygen delivery.

There is progressive stiffening of the myocardium with age that results in a decreased effectiveness of the pumping mechanism. An 80-year-old will have approximately 50 percent of the cardiac output of a 20-year-old, even without significant atherosclerotic coronary artery disease. The myocardium also becomes less sensitive to endogenous and exogenous catecholamines. Conduction defects may be exacerbated by the stress of illness or trauma. A normal tachycardic response to pain, hypovolemia, or anxiety may be absent or blunted in the elderly trauma patient. Medications such as β blockers may mask tachycardia and hinder the evaluation of the elderly patient. Emergency physicians should be wary of a "normal" heart rate in the geriatric trauma victim.

## RECOGNITION AND DIAGNOSIS OF COMMON INJURY PATTERNS

### Head Injury

With aging, the brain undergoes progressive atrophy and decreases in size by about 10 percent between the ages of 30 and 70 years. Subtle changes in cognition, memory, and data acquisition may confound the emergency physician's evaluation of the elderly patient's mental status. When evaluating the patient's mental status during the neurologic examination, it would be a grave error to assume that alterations in mental status are due solely to any underlying dementia or senility.

Elderly persons suffer a much lower incidence of epidural hematomas than the general population. This has been attributed to the relatively more dense fibrous bond between the dura mater and the inner table of the skull in older individuals. There is, however, a higher incidence of subdural hematomas in elderly patients. As the brain mass decreases with advancing age, there is greater stretching and tension of the bridging veins that pass from the brain to the dural sinuses. The increased "dead space" within the skull may delay symptoms of intracranial bleeding. More liberal indications for computed tomography (CT) scanning are justified.

## Cervical Spine Injuries

With advancing age, there is a decline in the incidence of cervical spine fractures. In one study, cervical spine injuries in patients 60 years of age and older accounted for 12 percent of the injuries. The pattern of cervical spine injuries in the elderly is very different than in younger patients. Ryan et al. found that the incidence of C1 and C2 fractures rose as the population aged. This rise in upper level fractures was due to a significant increase in the incidence of odontoid fractures in the elderly. When the elderly trauma patient presents with neck pain, emergency physicians need to place special emphasis on maintaining cervical immobilization until the cervical spine is properly assessed. Because underlying cervical arthritis may obscure fracture lines, the elderly patient with persistent neck pain and negative plain radiographs should undergo CT scanning of the neck.

## Chest Trauma

Chest trauma, both minor and severe, can compromise elderly individuals. In blunt trauma, there is an increased incidence of rib fractures due to osteoporotic changes. The pain associated with rib fractures, along with any decreased physiologic reserve, may predispose patients to respiratory complications. More severe thoracic injuries, such as hemopneumothorax, pulmonary contusion, flail chest, and cardiac contusion, can quickly lead to decompensation in elderly individuals whose baseline oxygenation status may already be diminished.

Geriatric patients are more susceptible to developing hypoxia and respiratory infections following trauma. In the elderly, diminished elasticity of the lungs along with progressive changes in the chest wall can lead to a reduction in pulmonary compliance and in the ability to cough effectively. Total lung surface area decreases as alveolar and small airway support diminishes with advancing age. There is also reduced mucociliary clearance of foreign material and bacteria and increased colonization of the oropharynx with gram-negative organisms. All of these factors result in an increased risk for elderly patients to develop nosocomial gram-negative pneumonia.

The main therapeutic goal is aggressively maintaining adequate oxygen delivery. Frequent arterial blood gas analysis may provide early insight into elderly patients' respiratory function and reserve. Prompt tracheal intubation and use of mechanical ventilation should be considered in patients with more severe injuries, respiratory rates greater than 40 breaths per minute, or when the $Pa_{O_2}$ is < 60 mmHg or $Pa_{CO_2}$ > 50 mmHg. While nonventilatory therapy helps to prevent respiratory infections and is always desirable, early mechanical ventilation may avert the disastrous results associated with hypoxia.

Emergency physicians should remember that chest trauma alone does not necessarily forecast a bleak outcome. In one series, most of the patients sustaining blunt chest injuries were discharged home to their preinjury level of independence.

## Abdominal Trauma

The abdominal examination in elderly patients is notoriously unreliable compared to younger patients. Even with an initially benign physical examination, emergency physicians must have a high index of suspicion for intraabdominal injuries in patients who have associated pelvic and lower rib cage fractures. For older patients, the adhesions associated with previous abdominal surgical procedures may increase the risk of performing diagnostic peritoneal lavage in the emergency department. Therefore, CT scanning with contrast is a valuable diagnostic test. It is important to ensure adequate hydration and baseline assessment of renal function prior to the contrast load for the CT scan. Some patients may be volume-depleted due to medications such as diuretics. This hypovolemia coupled with contrast administration may exacerbate any underlying renal pathology.

## Orthopaedic Injuries

### Hip Fractures

Many elderly patients are predisposed to orthopaedic injuries due to osteopenic and osteoporotic changes in their skeletal structure. Hip fractures occur primarily in four areas: intertrochanteric, transcervical, subcapital, and subtrochanteric. Intertrochanteric fractures are the most common, followed by transcervical fractures. Emergency physicians must be aware that pelvic and long bone fractures are not infrequently the sole etiology for hypovolemia in elderly patients. Timely orthopaedic consultation, evaluation, and treatment with open reduction and internal fixation should be coordinated with the diagnosis and management of other injuries.

### Long Bone Fractures

Long bone fractures of the femur, tibia, and humerus may produce a loss of mobility with a resulting decrease in the independent lifestyle of elderly patients. Early orthopaedic consultation for intramedullary rodding of these fractures may result in increased early mobilization.

## Upper Extremity Injuries

Falls on the outstretched hand increase the elderly's risk for Colles fractures. After the diagnosis is confirmed radiologically, these fractures can usually be treated with closed reduction and immobilization. The incidence of humeral head and surgical neck fractures in elderly patients also is increased by falls on the outstretched hand or elbow. Localized tenderness, swelling, and ecchymosis to the proximal humerus are characteristic of these injuries. Early orthopaedic consultation and treatment with a shoulder immobilizer or surgical fixation should be arranged. Social services may need to be contacted to arrange for assistance with routine daily activities for some elderly patients being discharged home after an orthopaedic injury.

## SPECIAL MANAGEMENT PRINCIPLES

Emergency physicians are often faced with the challenging task of assessing elderly trauma patients' cardiovascular status and reserve. The work by Scalea et al. demonstrated that trauma physicians frequently fail to recognize the severity of hemodynamic instability in geriatric patients. Therefore, early invasive monitoring has been advocated to help physicians assess the elderly's hemodynamic status. Scalea and coworkers showed that by reducing the time to invasive monitoring in elderly trauma patients from 5.5 to 2.2 h, and thus recognizing and appropriately treating occult shock, the survival rate of their patients increased from 7 to 53 percent. Survival was improved because of enhanced oxygen delivery through the use of adequate volume loading and inotropic support. They concluded that urgent invasive monitoring provides important hemodynamic information early, aids in identifying occult shock, limits hypoperfusion, helps prevent multiple organ failure, and improves survival.

The insertion of invasive monitoring lines seldom occurs in the emergency department because of institutional practice and availability of equipment. Thus, every effort should be made by emergency physicians to expedite emergency department care of elderly trauma patients and prevent unnecessary delays. In the emergency department evaluation of blunt trauma patients, the chest radiograph, cervical spine series, and pelvic radiographs are necessary diagnostic tests during the secondary survey. After ordering this set of plain radiographs, emergency physicians must resist the temptation of trying to appease consultants by immediately obtaining plain films of every other body region that may have sustained minor trauma. While it is vital to be thorough in the diagnosis of occult orthopaedic injuries, expending a great deal of time in the radiology suite may compromise patient care. Only a few radiologic studies, such as emergent head and abdominal CT scans, should take precedence over obtaining vital information from invasive monitoring. Elderly trauma patients will benefit most from an expeditious transfer to the intensive care unit for invasive monitoring so that their hemodynamic status can be further assessed. Invasive monitoring in the intensive care environment may provide clues to subtle hemodynamic changes that may compromise geriatric patients with limited physiologic reserve. After being assured that their hemodynamic status has been stabilized, patients can be transported back to the radiology suite for further plain radiographic studies.

In the emergency department, emergency physicians must make critical management decisions regarding volume resuscitation without the benefit of sophisticated invasive monitoring devices. Geriatric trauma patients can decompensate with overresuscitation just as quickly as they can with inadequate resuscitation. Elderly patients with underlying coronary artery disease and cerebrovascular disease are at a much greater risk of suffering the consequences of ischemia to vital organs when they become hypotensive after sustaining trauma. During the initial resuscitative phase, crystalloid, while the primary option, should be administered judiciously since elderly patients with diminished cardiac compliance are more susceptible to volume overload. Strong consideration should be made for early and more liberal use of red blood cell transfusion. This practice early in the resuscitation would enhance oxygen delivery and help minimize tissue ischemia.

## PROGNOSIS AND OUTCOME

The mortality rate of hospitalized geriatric trauma patients has been reported to be between 15 and 30 percent. These figures far exceed the mortality rate of 4 to 8 percent found in younger patients. In general, multiple organ failure and sepsis cause more deaths in elderly patients than in younger trauma victims. Geriatric patients also are more likely to die following minor traumatic events.

Several markers for poor outcome in elderly trauma victims have been determined. Age greater than 75 years, Glasgow Coma Scale score ≤ 7, presence of shock upon admission, severe head injury, and the development of sepsis are associated with worse outcome and higher mortality figures. The Injury Severity Score has been found by many investigators to have poor correlation with mortality rates.

The ultimate goal in the care of elderly trauma patients is to return them to their preinjury state of independent function. There are conflicting data on the ability of elderly patients to return to independent living. A study by Oreskovich et al. showed a mortality rate of 15 percent among their geriatric trauma patients and a dismal 12 percent of patients returning to their baseline independent state. Some authors have raised questions about the ethics and cost benefits of trauma care for the elderly. However, DeMaria et al. demonstrated that immediately after discharge one-third of trauma survivors return to independent living, one-third return to dependent status but living at home, and one-third require nursing home facilities. Altogether, at long-term follow-up, 89 percent returned home after trauma and 57 percent returned to independent living. The findings of DeMaria et al. are supported by another team of investigators, who also showed that the majority of elderly trauma patients regained an independent level of function.

Many questions regarding the ultimate outcome of geriatric trauma patients remain unanswered. In light of the investigations by DeMaria and others, showing that elderly patients can return to independent living after trauma, and the study by Scalea, demonstrating the bene-

**Table 214-1.** Geriatric Trauma Management Axioms

Assume that patients have limited physiologic reserve.
Seemingly minor injuries may actually be life-threatening in the face of limited physiologic reserve.
"Stable" patients may become unstable quickly and with little warning.
Liberal use of head and abdominal CT scanning is justified in diagnosing injuries.
Early invasive hemodynamic monitoring often will provide valuable diagnostic and resuscitation information.
Early, aggressive oxygen use and mechanical ventilation may be necessary in some patients.
Blood transfusion for volume replacement early in the resuscitation phase will improve oxygen delivery in hypovolemic patients.
Overresuscitation is as detrimental as inadequate resuscitation.

ficial effect of early invasive monitoring, it appears that aggressive resuscitation efforts for geriatric trauma patients are warranted.

In summary, the acute management principles of geriatric trauma continue to evolve. Emergency physicians must remain familiar with the various mechanisms of injury unique to the elderly trauma patient. Special management and treatment axioms, outlined in Table 214-1, should be applied early when caring for the geriatric trauma patient.

## BIBLIOGRAPHY

Allen JE, Schwab CW: Blunt chest trauma in the elderly. *Am Surg* 51:697, 1985.

DeMaria EJ, Kenney PR, Merriam MA, et al: Survival after trauma in geriatric patients. *Ann Surg* 206:738, 1987.

DeMaria EJ, Kenney PR, Merriam MA, et al: Aggressive trauma care benefits the elderly. *J Trauma* 27:1200, 1987.

Evans L: Risk of fatality from physical trauma versus sex and age. *J Trauma* 28:369, 1988.

Finelli FC, Jonsson J, Champion HR, et al: A case control study for major trauma in geriatric patients. *J Trauma* 29:541, 1989.

Horst HM, Obeid FN, Sorensen VJ, et al: Factors influencing survival of elderly trauma patients. *Crit Care Med* 14:681, 1986.

Kirkpatrick JB, Pearson J: Fatal cerebral injury in the elderly. *J Am Geriatr Soc* 26:489, 1978.

MacKenzie EJ, Morris JA, Edelstein SL: Effect of pre-existing disease on length of hospital stay in trauma patients. *J Trauma* 29:757, 1989.

Morris JA, MacKenzie EJ, Edelstein SL: The effect of pre-existing conditions on mortality in trauma patients. *JAMA* 263:1942, 1990.

Oreskovich MR, Howard JD, Copass MK, et al: Geriatric trauma: Injury patterns and outcome. *J Trauma* 24:565, 1984.

Osler T, Hales K, Baack B, et al: Trauma in the elderly. *Am J Surg* 156:537, 1988.

Ryan MD, Henderson JJ: The epidemiology of fractures and fracture-dislocations of the cervical spine. *Injury* 23:38, 1992.

Scalea TM, Simon HM, Duncan AO, et al: Geriatric blunt trauma: Improved survival with early invasive monitoring. *J Trauma* 30:129, 1990.

Schwab CW, Kauder DR: Trauma in the geriatric patient. *Arch Surg* 127:701, 1992.

Sklar DP, Demarest GB, McFeeley P: Increased pedestrian mortality among the elderly. *Am J Emerg Med* 7:387, 1989.

Smith DP, Enderson BL, Maull KI: Trauma in the elderly: Determinants of outcome. *South Med J* 83:171, 1990.

# 215
# HEAD INJURY
## Gaylan L. Rockswold

The leading cause of death in persons up to age 44 years in the United States is trauma, and head injury accounts for approximately half of the deaths related to trauma. The mortality rate from severe head injury is approximately 35 percent, and functional recovery occurs in only 40 to 50 percent of patients with severe head injury.

## ANATOMY AND PHYSIOLOGY

### Scalp

The scalp consists of five layers: (1) skin, (2) subcutaneous tissue, (3) galea, (4) areolar tissue, and (5) pericranium. The scalp has a very rich blood supply and can be the source of major blood loss. In addition, there is a loose attachment between the galea and the pericranium, allowing for large subgaleal hematomas.

### Skull

The skull is a bony container for the brain and provides considerable protection. For practical purposes it is rigid and inflexible, thus contributing to problems with increased intracranial pressure (ICP). Cerebral contusion and contrecoup injuries frequently occur against uneven surfaces of the skull such as the orbital roofs, the sphenoid wing, and the petrous apex.

### Brain

The intracranial volume is approximately 1900 mL in the average adult. The brain weighs 1300 to 1500 g and occupies approximately 80 percent of the volume of the intracranial cavity. The brain is partially compartmentalized by attachments of the dura. In the midline, the falx cerebri partially divides the right hemisphere from the left hemisphere of the brain. The tentorium cerebelli partially divides the supratentorial cerebral hemispheres from the brainstem and cerebellum. The cerebral hemispheres are connected to the posterior fossa contents by the midbrain, which occupies the tentorial hiatus. The brain consists of gray and white matter, with the latter consisting primarily of axons and myelin sheaths. Deep in the white matter are nuclei of gray matter. The gray matter also forms the surface of the brain. It consists of nerve cells, and the connecting dendrites and axons of these cells form myriad synapses. The extracellular space is considerably smaller in gray matter than in white matter. The arteries and veins run vertically through the gray and white matter, giving off capillaries at right angles.

### Cerebral Blood Flow

Under normal circumstances the blood volume of the brain is approximately 3 to 4 mL/100 g of brain tissue. In the average patient, the average cerebral blood flow (CBF) to the whole brain is about 50 mL/100 g per min, with approximately 75 mL/100 g per min going to the gray matter and 25 mL/100 g per min going to the white matter. Although the brain constitutes only 2 percent of the total body weight, it receives approximately 15 percent of cardiac output and about 20 percent of the oxygen consumed by the body. Variations in arterial $P_{CO_2}$ exert a profound effect on CBF. Hypercapnia causes cerebral vasodilatation, and hypocapnia causes vasoconstriction that can be so marked that brain hypoxia can result. Changes in oxygen tension in arterial blood also influence CBF. As the $P_{O_2}$ falls below 50 mmHg, there is a marked increase in CBF, while hyperbaric oxygen ventilation at 2 atmospheres absolute decreases CBF by 20 to 25 percent.

The brain is unique in the sense that it is autonomous in controlling blood flow within it. This intrinsic property has been labeled *autoregulation,* defined as the tendency of the brain to maintain a constant blood flow despite perfusion changes. Cerebral perfusion pressure (CPP) is defined as the difference between mean systemic arterial blood pressure (SAP) and mean intracranial pressure (ICP) (CPP = SAP − ICP). If autoregulation is intact, CBF remains constant when the CPP ranges between 45 and 160 mmHg. When it falls below 40 mmHg, CBF and cerebral metabolism are critically affected.

### Cerebrospinal Fluid

Of the approximate 1900-mL volume of the intracranial cavity, 150 mL is cerebrospinal fluid (CSF), of which 25 to 30 mL is found in the ventricles. The ventricles are ependymal lined cavities deep within the brain. Cerebrospinal fluid is formed primarily by the choroid plexuses within the ventricular system at a rate of 0.35 mL/min or 500 mL/24 h. Cerebrospinal fluid moves from the lateral ventricles through the foramen of Monro into the third ventricle and then via the aqueduct of Sylvius into the fourth ventricle and out through the foramina of Luschka and Magendi. Cerebrospinal fluid then flows through the basal cisterns and is absorbed in the arachnoid villi along the sagittal sinus and the lateral sinuses. The CSF cushions and buffers the brain and spinal cord against trauma. It also provides a fluid pathway for chemical substances to reach the intercellular spaces of the brain and for metabolites to be returned to the venous system.

## PATHOLOGY AND PATHOPHYSIOLOGY

The concept of primary and secondary brain injury due to trauma has become well established. An initial impact injury to the brain produces varying degrees of mechanical neuronal and axonal injury which, at the present state of medical science, cannot be treated. Secondary brain injury occurs from potentially treatable factors such as intracranial hemorrhage, cerebral edema, ischemia, hypoxia, hypercarbia, and increased ICP. Optimal management minimizes the secondary brain injury and decreases the overall mortality and morbidity.

### Intracranial Pressure

The craniospinal intradural space is nearly constant in volume, and its contents are relatively noncompressible. Therefore, the sum of the volumes of brain, blood, and CSF remains relatively constant. If there is an increase in volume of one of these three components, it must be offset by an equal decrease in some other component or ICP rises. If the brain were completely incompressible and the cranium unexpandable, the addition of even minimal volume to the intracranial space would lead to dramatic increase in ICP (Fig. 215-1). Initially, as a mass lesion or diffuse edema develops, CSF buffering occurs by the displacement of CSF into the spinal canal. Once CSF buffering becomes exhausted, the elastic properties of the brain tissue itself and its blood vessels play the major buffering role as the pressure begins to elevate rapidly (Fig. 215-1). *Elastance* is the increase in pressure with a given increase in intracranial volume. *Compliance* is the reciprocal of elastance. The elastic properties of the brain are not constant but will depend on the presence of pathologic processes such as cerebral edema or a mass lesion. For example, an increase in the arterial pressure stiffens the brain, producing a decreased compliance, whereas a decrease in arterial pressure will have the reverse effect. The pressure-volume curve explains why a patient can appear relatively intact neurologically and then undergo rapid deterioration because of transtentorial herniation.

Increased ICP is defined as CSF pressure greater than 15 mmHg. Following removal of a traumatic intracranial hematoma at least half

## Pressure-Volume Curves for the Cranium

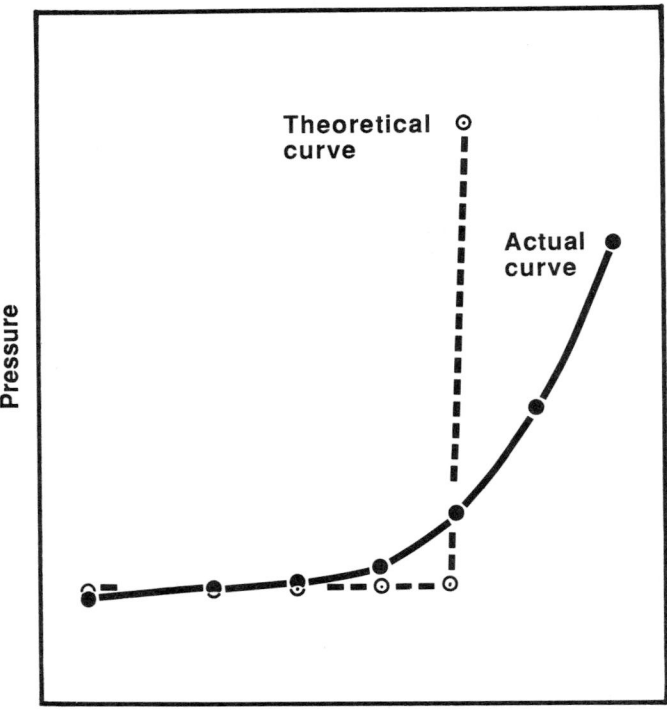

**Fig. 215-1.** Theoretical pressure-volume curve (broken line) derived if the modified Monro-Kellie hypothesis were strictly true. Actual pressure-volume curve (solid line).

of comatose patients display an elevated ICP. Approximately a third of patients with diffuse brain injury have elevated ICP. Uncontrollably elevated ICP (defined as an ICP of 20 mmHg or more refractory to treatment) is present in over half of all head-injury deaths. If ICP repeatedly elevates to the point where CPP is inadequate, vasoparalysis results, whereupon CBF passively follows systemic arterial pressure. Massive vasodilatation occurs with further elevations in ICP. Autoregulation can be lost in one area and preserved in another. For example, CBF may be markedly lowered in an area of contusion and edema while global ICP and CPP remain relatively normal. Loss of autoregulation leads to the failure of the resistant vessels to constrict normally, and systemic pressure communicated to the capillaries and veins, resulting in the outpouring of fluid from the intravascular space to the extracellular space (vasogenic edema). The production of lactic acid by anaerobic metabolism may play a role in the loss of CBF autoregulation. The ICP eventually rises to the level of SAP and there is no CPP. Brain death results.

### Herniation

Diffusely or focally increased ICP can result in herniation of the brain at several locations. The least important herniation is cingulate or subfalcial, occurring when one cerebral hemisphere is displaced underneath the falx cerebri into the opposite supratentorial space. This is rarely clinically diagnosed. A herniation of major clinical importance in head injury is transtentorial or uncal herniation (Fig. 215-2). A subdural hematoma or temporal lobe mass forces the ipsilateral uncus of the temporal lobe through the tentorial hiatus into the space between the cerebral peduncle and the tentorium. This results in compression of the oculomotor nerve and parasympathetic paralysis of the pupil on the same side, causing it to become fixed and dilated. The cerebral peduncle is simultaneously compressed, resulting in a contralateral hemiparesis. The increased ICP and brainstem com-

pression result in progressive deterioration in the level of consciousness. Occasionally the contralateral cerebral peduncle is forced against the free edge of the tentorium on the opposite side, resulting in paralysis ipsilateral to the lesion—a false localizing sign. The posterior cerebral artery can be compressed against the free edge of the tentorium, resulting in an infarction of the occipital lobe. If the herniation continues untreated, there is progressive brainstem deterioration progressing to hyperventilation and decerebration (extensor response) and then to apnea and death. Uncal herniation can occur bilaterally in cases of diffuse brain swelling or bilateral lesions. Cerebellar tonsillar herniation through the foramen magnum occurs much less frequently in head trauma. Resultant medullary compression causes bradycardia, respiratory arrest, and death.

### Diffuse Lesions

Closed-head injuries (CHI) can be divided into diffuse and focal lesions. Diffuse injuries are divided into concussion syndromes and prolonged traumatic coma. Concussion is a transient loss of consciousness that occurs immediately following a nonpenetrating blunt impact to the head. Concussion generally occurs when the head, while moving, strikes or is struck by an object. The duration of unconsciousness is usually short (from seconds to minutes), although it may last for several hours. Loss of consciousness is due to impairment of the reticular activating system, caused by rotation of the cerebral hemispheres on the brainstem. Classically, recovery from concussion was regarded as complete, without pathologic lesions of the brain or neurologic sequelae. However, persistent headache and problems with memory, anxiety, insomnia, and dizziness can persist in some patients for weeks and sometimes months.

Diffuse axonal injury is a tearing or shearing of nerve fibers occurring at the time of impact. The site and degree of axonal injury are determined by the direction, magnitude, and duration of the angular force applied to the head. It results in functional, or physiologic, rather than grossly demonstrable, anatomic abnormalities.

Although diffuse axonal injury has frequently been associated with the severely head injured, it has been demonstrated in patients with mild head injury and can occur either diffusely or focally. Prolonged traumatic coma lasting for at least 6 h appears to result from diffuse axonal injury produced by the accelerating and decelerating forces of the impact. Prolonged coma is present in about one-third of all patients who die from head injury and is associated with poor neurologic outcome in survivors.

### Focal Lesions

#### Skull Fractures

Linear nondepressed fractures with the scalp intact do not of themselves require treatment. Severe intracranial bleeding can result if the fracture also causes disruption of the middle meningeal artery or a major dural sinus. Depressed skull fractures are classified as open or closed, if the overlying skin is lacerated or intact respectively.

Basilar skull fractures can occur at any point in the base of the skull, but the typical location is in the petrous portion of the temporal bone. Longitudinal fractures occur much more frequently than do transverse fractures and typically begin with a fracture in the vault extending into the petrous bone. Hemotympanum, otorrhea, disarticulation of the ossicles, and ecchymosis in the mastoid region (Battle sign) are frequently seen. Transverse fractures of the petrous bone are associated with severe head injury and are secondary to blows to the occiput. Seventh- or eighth-nerve transection can occur.

#### Contusion

Contusion typically occurs over the crest of gyri, largest at the surface and tapering into the white matter (Fig. 215-3). The area of contusion is usually hemorrhagic and surrounded by edema, with overly-

**Fig. 215-2.** Anterior view of transtentorial uncal herniation caused by a large hematoma. Note skull fracture overlying the hematoma.

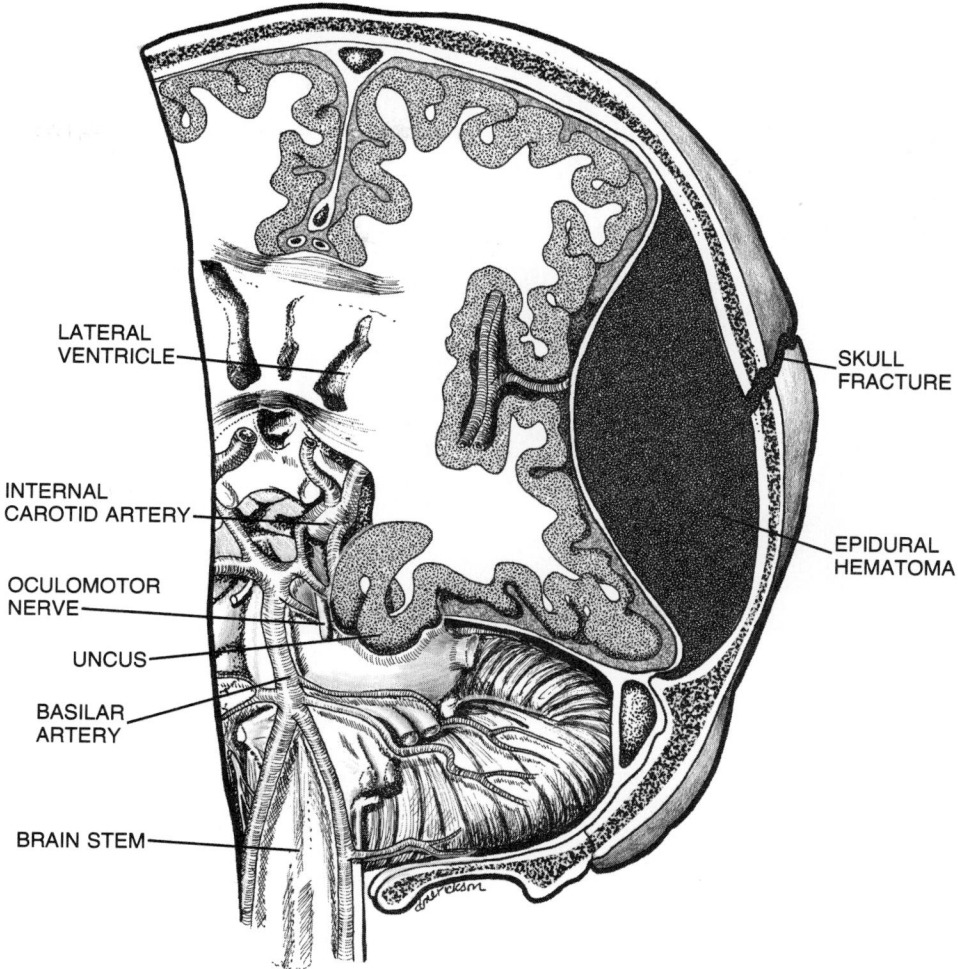

LATERAL VENTRICLE

INTERNAL CAROTID ARTERY

OCULOMOTOR NERVE

UNCUS

BASILAR ARTERY

BRAIN STEM

SKULL FRACTURE

EPIDURAL HEMATOMA

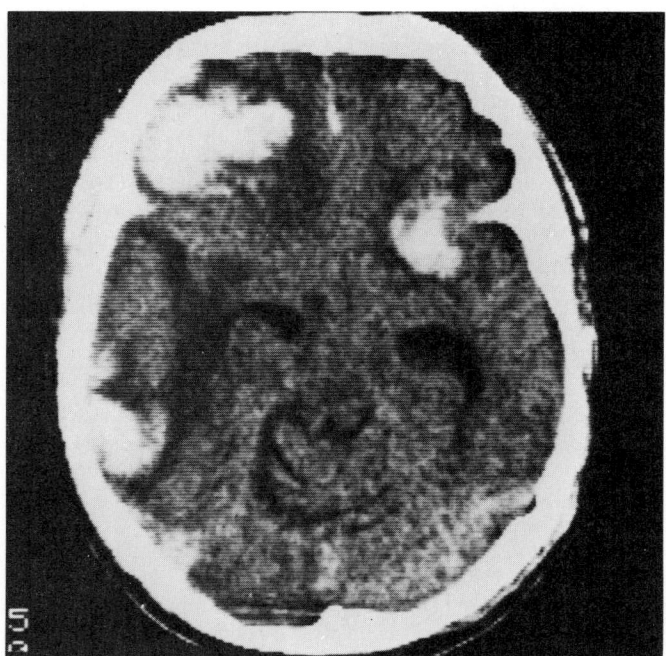

**Fig. 215-3.** Cerebral contusion with associated hemorrhage occurring subfrontally on the left, superior to the right sphenoid wing, and in the left posterior temporal region. Note the soft tissue swelling in the left frontotemporal region.

ing subarachnoid hemorrhage frequently present. Contusions may occur directly under the site of impact or on the contralateral side (a contrecoup lesion). Contusions may occur anywhere, but typical locations are the frontal poles, the subfrontal cortex, and the anterior temporal lobes. Movement of the cortical gyri over rough skull surfaces such as the orbital plates or the sphenoid ridge are conducive to contusion.

## Intracerebral Hemorrhage

Torn blood vessels can cause parenchymal hemorrhage (Fig. 215-3). Most intracerebral hemorrhages are delayed for days and only occasionally are seen on the initial computed tomography (CT) scan taken within a few hours of injury. Combined contusion and parenchymal hemorrhage can produce an expanding mass lesion which is particularly treacherous when present in the anterior temporal lobe, since uncal herniation can occur without a diffuse increase in ICP.

## Epidural Hematoma

An epidural hematoma is a collection of blood between the inner table of the skull and the dura (Fig. 215-4). Approximately 80 percent of the time, an epidural hematoma is associated with a skull fracture that tears a meningeal artery, usually the middle meningeal. Fracture through a large venous lake or through a major dural sinus can also produce an epidural hematoma. The underlying brain injury is seldom severe. Epidural hematomas are rare in the elderly, presumably because of the very close attachment of the dura to the periosteum of the inner table.

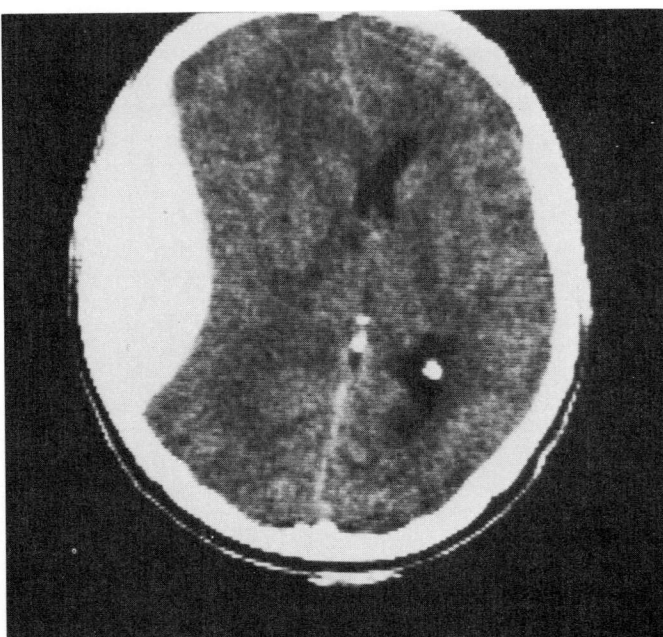

**Fig. 215-4.** A typical epidural hematoma with a lenticular-shaped configuration.

## Subdural Hematoma

A subdural hematoma is a collection of blood beneath the dura and overlying the arachnoid and brain (Fig. 215-5). It is usually located over the cerebral convexities and results from tears of bridging veins that extend from the subarachnoid space to the dural venous sinuses or from tears in pial arteries. Blood dissects over the cerebral convexities, frequently extending from the sagittal sinus to the floor of the temporal fossa or from the frontal region back to the parietal and occipital lobes. The mechanism of injury is usually acceleration-deceleration. Patients with brain atrophy due either to aging or alcoholism are particularly susceptible to the development of subdural hematomas because the bridging veins span a greater dis-

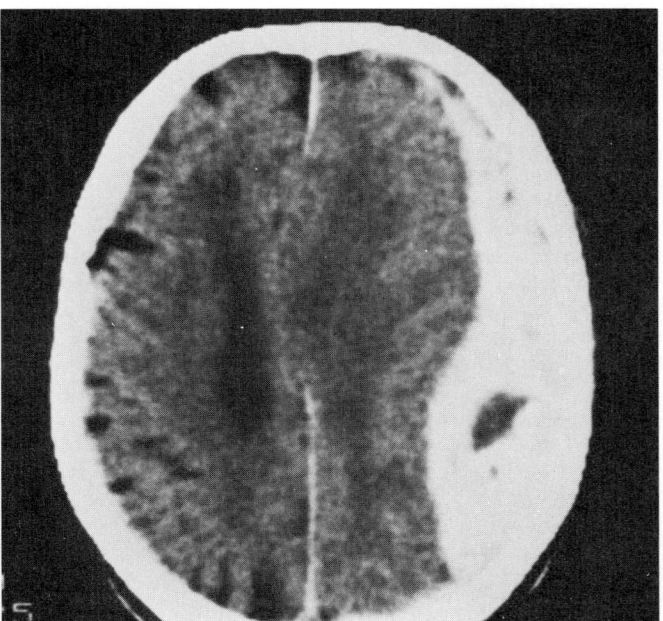

**Fig. 215-5.** A large acute subdural hematoma with marked midline shift and ipsilateral ventral ventricular collapse.

tance and are more easily torn. Acute subdural hematomas become symptomatic within 24 h of injury. These lesions are caused by acceleration-deceleration forces that cause significant primary impact injury to the brain. Contusions of areas of the brain remote from the site of primary impact also occur. Subacute subdural hematomas become symptomatic from 24 h to approximately 2 weeks after injury. Chronic subdurals become symptomatic 2 weeks or more after injury when the blood clot has liquefied. Occasionally a specific history of trauma cannot be obtained and it is difficult to date the hematoma exactly in terms of the initial trauma. It is important to distinguish this more chronic lesion from the acute subdural hematoma because *immediate surgery may not be necessary or advisable.*

### Brain Laceration

A tear in the brain parenchyma can be produced by a crude penetrating injury or depressed skull fracture. There is frequently associated hemorrhage and necrosis of the brain.

### Penetrating Injuries

Penetrating sharp objects and gunshot wounds can result in penetrating injury to the brain. Gunshot wounds inflict injury far beyond their direct penetration of the brain because of the energy exerted as shown by the formula $E = \frac{1}{2}mV^2$ (where $E$ is the energy of the missile, $m$ is its mass, and $V$ is the velocity). The degree of neurological injury will depend on the energy of the missile, whether the trajectory involves a single or multiple lobes or hemispheres of the brain, the amount of scatter of bone and metallic fragments, and whether a mass lesion is present. Hemorrhage can be profuse and life-threatening if a major artery or dural sinus is involved.

## ASSESSMENT

### History

Prehospital personnel must obtain a history from observers or family regarding the patient's condition immediately after the injury. This includes respiratory effort, duration of unconsciousness, verbalization, and movement of the extremities. In addition, the mechanism of injury, the time of the injury, the presence of a lucid interval, and prior use of drugs and alcohol should be noted. This information should be recorded on the ambulance data sheet and delivered with the patient to the emergency department. Ongoing observations by the prehospital personnel are essential.

### Vital Signs

Adequate oxygenation and ventilation are essential to the head-injured patient, since hypoxia and hypercarbia can convert reversible brain injury to irreversible injury. Moderate hypercarbia can cause profound cerebral vasodilatation, resulting in an increased ICP with further ventilatory deterioration. A vicious cycle can ensue whereby the secondary brain injury becomes more profound than the initial primary impact injury.

An elevated systolic blood pressure can reflect a rise in ICP and be part of the Cushing reflex (hypertension and bradycardia). Hypertension is the brain's attempt to maintain CPP. Hypotension is rarely due to head injury except as a terminal event with medullary collapse. Important exceptions are (1) profound blood loss from scalp lacerations and (2) the infant or small child with a relatively small circulating blood volume in whom hemorrhage into the epidural or subgaleal spaces can produce hypovolemic shock. Hypotension in the severely head-injured patient can greatly impair neurologic function. Blood pressure must be restored before an accurate neurologic assessment can be made.

**Table 215-1.** The Glasgow Coma Scale

| | EYES | |
|---|---|---|
| Open: | Spontaneously | 4 |
| | To verbal command | 3 |
| | To pain | 2 |
| No response: | | 1 |
| | BEST VERBAL RESPONSE | |
| | Oriented and converses | 5 |
| | Disoriented and converses | 4 |
| | Inappropriate words | 3 |
| | Incomprehensible sounds | 2 |
| | No response | 1 |
| | BEST MOTOR RESPONSE | |
| To verbal command: | Obeys | 6 |
| To painful stimulus: | Localizes pain | 5 |
| | Flexion-withdrawal | 4 |
| | Abnormal flexion (decorticate rigidity) | 3 |
| | Extension (decerebrate rigidity) | 2 |
| | No response | 1 |
| Total | | 3–15 |

## Neurologic Examination

The neurologic examination is essential in establishing the severity of the head injury and its clinical course. Examination must be adequate to accomplish the goals described above but rapid enough not to delay emergency management of the patient. Repeated examinations are required to determine if the patient is stable, improving, or deteriorating. The level of consciousness is the single most important factor in neurologically assessing the head-injured patient. The Glasgow Coma Scale (GCS) (Table 215-1) as devised by Teasdale and Jennett is a system of examination which can be performed by all levels of medical personnel and is highly reproducible. The scale evaluates three aspects of the patient's responsiveness: (1) eye opening, (2) best verbal response, and (3) best motor response. Each category is described according to a well-defined series of responses that indicate progressive degrees of neurological impairment.

### Eye Opening

Spontaneous eye opening suggests that the reticular activating centers are functioning. This does not imply awareness, however. If spontaneous eye opening is not present, verbal stimuli or commands should be used next. If there is no eye opening with verbal stimulation, painful stimulation, such as vigorous pinching or pressure on the nail beds, should be applied.

### Verbal Response

Speech suggests a relatively intact central nervous system. Oriented speech implies awareness of oneself and one's environment. A patient should be oriented in all three spheres of name, place, and date. To be characterized as "disoriented and converses," speech should be well articulated and organized but the patient disoriented. Inappropriate words are those which are exclamatory or random only. Incomprehensible speech consists of moaning or groaning but no recognizable words.

### Motor Responses

This is the most important and reproducible portion of the GCS. Obeying verbal commands means the ability to move one's limbs readily and without the need for painful stimulation. Localizing pain means that the patient moves a limb sequentially to the location of the painful stimulus in an effort to remove it. Flexion-withdrawal implies that the patient pulls in flexion away from a pain stimulus. Abnormal flexion means a decorticate response which is consistently apparent. An extensor response is decerebration, with abduction and internal

rotation of the shoulder and pronation of the forearm. No response is hypotonia or flaccidity, which strongly suggests loss of medullary function. In a head-injured patient who exhibits flaccidity, concomitant spinal cord injury may be present.

A maximum score of 15 can be obtained on the GCS, with a low score of 3. Severe head injury is defined as a GCS of 8 or less persisting for 6 h. Moderate head injury is defined as GCS of 9 to 12, and mild head injury, 13 to 15.

Pupil size in millimeters, and reactivity to light, should be carefully recorded. An enlarging pupil in the face of a decreasing level of consciousness is strongly suggestive of uncal herniation with associated oculomotor nerve compression.

Brainstem function can be further tested by checking corneal reflexes with a wisp of Kleenex or cotton. This reflex originates in the pons, with the afferent limb conducted by the ophthalmic branch of the fifth nerve and the efferent limb by the facial nerve. In addition, oculocephalic (doll's eyes) or oculovestibular responses (ice water calorics) are important in testing the integrity of the brainstem. Oculocephalic reflexes should not be tested until the cervical spine has been cleared for the presence of fractures. A lateral cervical spine x-ray alone does not suffice. The presence or absence of a gag reflex and spontaneous respirations will further assess the status of the lower pons and medulla.

Since the diagnosis of basilar skull fracture is primarily clinical, it is important to recognize the physical findings of this entity. They include (1) hemotympanum or bloody discharge from the ear; (2) rhinorrhea or otorrhea; (3) retroauricular ecchymosis (Battle sign); (4) periorbital ecchymosis ("raccoon's eyes"); and (5) first-, second-, seventh-, and eighth-cranial nerve deficits.

## Diagnostic Tests

Approximately 5 percent of patients suffering from severe head injury will have an associated cervical spine fracture. Cervical spine x-rays should be taken in all unconscious patients, in patients with cervical pain, in those with neurologic deficits suggesting cervical cord injury, or if the mechanism of injury can produce cervical damage.

Anteroposterior and lateral skull films should be obtained for penetrating wounds of the skull or for suspected depressed skull fracture. Skull x-rays localize the position of a foreign body within the cranium and can determine the amount of bony depression. Skull films also identify significant linear fractures, and if a fracture crosses the vascular groove of the middle meningeal artery or dural sinuses, an epidural hematoma should be anticipated. With an occipital fracture, a contrecoup frontal lobe contusion is likely. The Towne view reveals fractures of the occiput extending down to the foramen magnum. Anteroposterior and lateral views alone will not demonstrate all fractures. If a CT head scan will be obtained, bone windows can be obtained, eliminating the need for skull films. For patients who have not lost consciousness, and have no focal neurologic deficit, no evidence of depressed or basilar skull fracture, no evidence of penetration of the skull, and no indwelling shunt, skull x-rays are not necessary. Intoxicated patients are a particular problem since history is unreliable and drugs or alcohol alter the neurologic examination. When there are findings suggesting head trauma, head CT is usually indicated.

The main indications for CT scanning in the assessment of head-injured patients are (1) persistent decrease in level of consciousness, (2) clinical neurologic deterioration, (3) persistent focal neurologic or mental status deficit, and (4) skull fractures in the vicinity of the middle meningeal artery or major venous sinuses. The CT scan defines the location and extent of hemorrhage and distinguishes intraparenchymal hemorrhage from brain swelling or edema (Figs. 215-3 to 215-5). The amount of midline shift can be readily determined. CT scanning has been found to be superior to conventional skull x-rays in diagnosing basilar skull fractures but inferior in diagnosing linear skull fractures of the vault.

Laboratory work in all significant head injury should include CBC, electrolytes, blood glucose, arterial blood gases, urinalysis, ethanol level, and directed toxicologic analysis where indicated. Coagulation parameters, including partial thromboplastin time, prothrombin time, platelets, and fibrinogen level, should be obtained. Blood for type and crossmatch should be sent immediately. In addition to possible skull x-rays and cervical spine x-rays, a chest x-ray and pelvic x-ray are performed routinely in all cases of severe trauma.

## DISPOSITION AND MANAGEMENT

### Mild and Moderate Head Injury

The major question is which patient can be safely discharged to home and which patient should be admitted for observation (Fig. 215-6). The decision depends on the reliability of the patient and the patient's friends or family as well as the degree to which the examining physician is familiar with the patient. For example, a patient who could be observed at home by reliable family members and who is neurologically intact could be discharged home following a relatively minor head injury with a brief loss of consciousness. However, if there is a history of unconsciousness in an unreliable patient or in a patient about whom very little is known, admission to the hospital is advisable. Any patient with a persisting decreased level of consciousness, deterioration in neurologic function, focal neurologic deficit, seizures, penetrating injuries, or open or depressed skull fractures should be admitted. Seizures should be treated with intravenous phenytoin, 18 mg/kg, at 25 mg/min with cardiac and blood pressure monitoring. Neurologic evaluation by the nursing staff should include an assessment and documentation every 15 to 60 min of the level of consciousness, pupillary size and reactivity, movement of the extremities, and vital signs. Any deterioration should be reported immediately to the neurosurgical staff.

### Head Injury Referral

In hospitals where neurosurgical care is not available, some patients can be safely observed at the local hospital and some should be referred to a neurosurgical unit (Fig 215-7). Patients who have a per-sisting decreased level of consciousness such that they cannot follow simple commands or utter recognizable words should be referred. Patients who can follow commands or utter recognizable words but who have pupil inequality, lateralized extremity weakness, depressed skull fractures, or basilar skull fractures should be referred. Any patient with neurologic deterioration, regardless of the state of consciousness, should be quickly referred. Patients with intracranial hemorrhage of any significance are best observed where neurosurgical care is quickly available. The above categories include the vast majority of patients who sustain acute mortality or significant morbidity.

Prior to transfer, direct communication between the referring physician and the receiving physician should occur. The cardiorespiratory status, the neurologic condition, the presence and rate of any neurologic deterioration, and the presence of any multiple injuries should be presented. A plan for the best mode of transport, the need for artificial ventilation, the administration of any significant drugs, and the potential need for blood transfusion, especially in the small child or infant, should be determined before the patient leaves the referring institution.

### Severe Head Injury

Patients with severe head injuries or those with unequal pupils or focal deficits must be treated aggressively (Fig 215-7). Establishment of an adequate airway with mechanical hyperventilation is a first priority. Whenever possible, it is important during intubation to use topical nasopharyngeal and laryngotracheal anesthesia. In agitated patients a paralytic agent and sedation may be needed to prevent elevation of ICP, even though these agents will compromise neurologic assessment. Nasotracheal intubation is a preferred method for possible cervical spinal injury, unless severe facial fractures or cribriform plate fractures are present. Following intubation, if the cervical spine injury is still suspected and the patient is agitated, the cervical spine must be physically immobilized or the patient then sedated or paralyzed. Patients are artificially ventilated to maintain an arterial $P_{CO_2}$ of 28 to 32 mmHg.

Hypotension can greatly depress neurologic function because cerebral perfusion pressure falls and cerebral metabolism is adversely af-

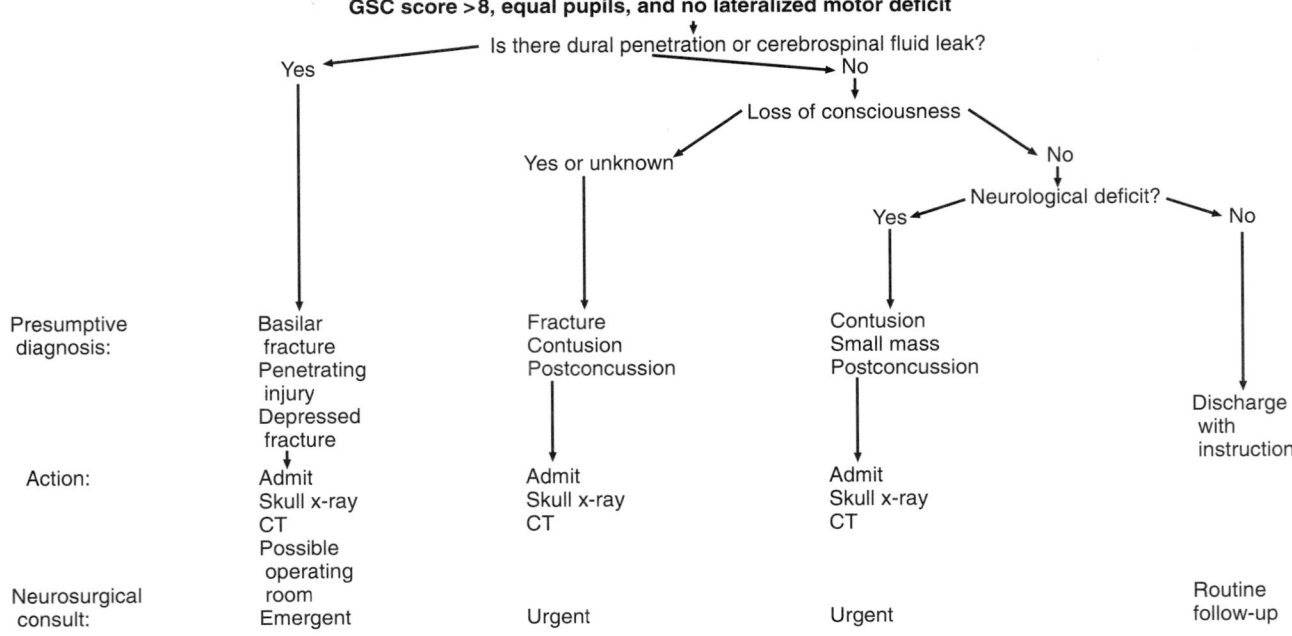

**Fig. 215-6.** Concussion-fracture patient flow.

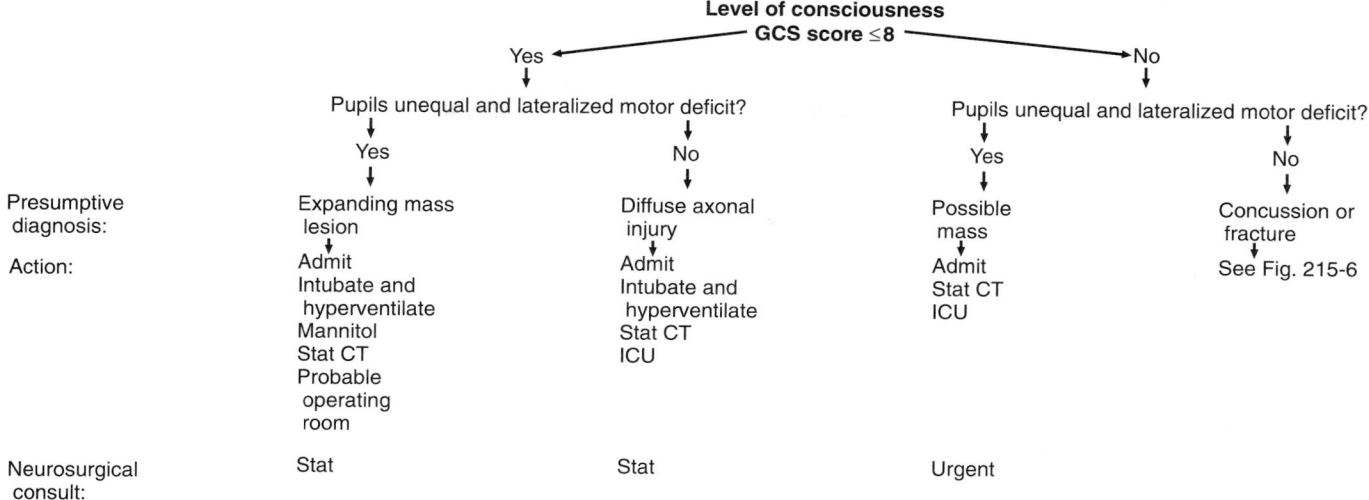

**Fig. 215-7.** Disposition of head-injured patients.

fected. Every attempt must be made to restore adequate blood pressure so that an accurate neurologic assessment can be made. Hypertension in conjunction with increased ICP must be treated with caution. Attempts at decreasing the blood pressure may result in inadequate CPP. Also, the blood pressure can be very sensitive to hypertensive medication, resulting in wide swings in the blood pressure. Treatment of hypertension is best directed initially toward reducing increased ICP.

In patients with focal deficits, pupil inequality, neurologic deterioration, or a GCS score of 6 or less, 1 g/kg of intravenous mannitol as a solution of 500 mL of 20 percent Osmitrol is infused as rapidly as possible through a large-bore intravenous catheter. An indwelling Foley catheter is essential. Mannitol acts as an osmotic diuretic, so significant hypovolemia is a relative contraindication. The agent draws water out of the normal brain by creating an osmotic gradient and can dramatically reduce ICP. An intracranial hematoma can expand somewhat as the brain shrinks, so mannitol should be given only when a definitive study or definitive surgery is to be performed. The head of the bed is elevated 30°, and any kinking of the neck is carefully avoided. All patients with focal brain lesions such as extracerebral hematomas, contusions, or intraparenchymal hematomas are given intravenous phenytoin, 18 mg/kg, at 20 mg/min and with cardiac and blood pressure monitoring.

Immediately after stabilization in the emergency department a CT scan of the head is obtained. A high-quality study is ensured by a combination of sedation with intravenous lorazepam (Ativan) 2 mg and vecuronium bromide (Norcuron) 0.15 mg/kg as needed. Patients with extracerebral or intracerebral hematomas, with 5 mm or more shift of midline structures, and with depressed skull fractures are taken directly to the operating suite. Penetrating foreign bodies should be removed from the skull and brain in the operating room. Patients sustaining gunshot wounds, unless they are moribund, are also taken to the operating room for debridement of their wounds and removal of hematomas and foreign bodies as indicated.

## "Talk and Deteriorate" Syndrome

Patients who talk and deteriorate are defined as those who utter recognizable words at some time after head injury and then deteriorate to a severe brain-injured condition within 48 h of their injuries. They represent approximately 10 to 20 percent of all patients sustaining severe head injury.

A patient's ability to talk following injury presumably indicates the initial impact was not lethal. Clinical experience, however, has demonstrated that lesions producing deterioration are very serious, and the process of deterioration is a marker of poor prognosis. Recognizing the symptoms of early deterioration, identifying the etiology of ongoing deterioration, and initiating prompt treatment represent a distinct challenge to emergency physicians.

The most frequent neurologic findings in parients who talk and deteriorate are altered mental status and focal hemispheric deficits. Progressive transtentorial herniation develops in a significant number of these patients either gradually or with frightening speed. A significant problem in managing these patients is identifying those at risk within the much larger group of patients with mild to moderate brain injuries. In contrast, patients demonstrating severe brain injury from the time of the impact are easily identified and receive immediate, aggressive care. Early and appropriate use of CT scanning is helpful in detecting significant intracranial lesions before clinical neurologic deterioration occurs or very early in the course of deterioration.

Rapid surgical evacuation of a developing mass lesion is important for improving outcome in a patient who initially talks and then deteriorates after brain injury. Rapid CT scanning followed by surgical evacuation of a hematoma has been found to be optimal in these patients. Intracranial hematomas, primarily subdural and epidural, are the cause of deterioration in approximately 70 to 80 percent of such patients. If the patients who talk and deteriorate with signs of transtentorial herniation do not respond promptly to medical management, they are taken directly to the operating room for immediate exploratory burr holes with ultrasound exploration of the intracranial contents. Outcome for patients who talk and deteriorate has improved with aggressive treatment. The challenge for emergency physicians is to distinguish the patients at risk for deterioration from the many patients presenting after traumatic brain injury.

## Intracranial Pressure

Management of ICP beginning as soon as possible, often in the emergency department, and continuing throughout the clinical course of the patient is essential to the optimal management of the severely head-injured patient. Intracranial pressure monitoring is routinely instituted in severely injured patients following removal of surgical mass lesions, or in the case of diffuse brain injuries, on admission to the intensive care unit. Patients without focal findings who have purposeful movement of the extremities, and have a normal CT scan, are not monitored. Ventriculostomies are preferred for ICP monitoring because of their accuracy and the ability to remove CSF as a treatment for increased ICP.

If ICP cannot be maintained at less than 20 mmHg with the above routine measures, the following treatments are instituted in a stepwise fashion: (1) cerebral spinal fluid drainage is instituted; (2) mannitol is administered intravenously, to reduce ICP to less than 20 mmHg; (3) vecuronium (Norcuron) is administered intravenously to prevent any movement on the part of the patient; (4) barbiturate coma is initiated if the patient's cardiac status is stable; and (5) repeat craniotomy to remove significant mass lesions is carefully considered in appropriate patients.

In addition, CPP must be maintained and adequate intravascular volume ensured. Not infrequently, barbiturate coma, osmotic dehydration, and sedation can cause hypotension. A Swan-Ganz catheter is essential in ensuring adequate vascular volume and cardiac output.

## Seizures

Seizures following trauma are classified as: immediate, early, and late. Immediate seizures are due to traumatic neuronal depolarization and have little morbidity. Early seizures occur the first week after injury, and late seizures occur any time afterward. Five percent of patients sustaining blunt head injury will have an early seizure. Early seizures suggest the presence of focal cerebral contusions, intracranial hemorrhage, hypoxia, or metabolic abnormalities. In addition, early seizures can damage the already injured brain by producing hypoxia, acidosis, and increased ICP, despite adequate controlled ventilation. They also increase the incidence of late seizures from an overall incidence of 5 percent to 25 percent in blunt head injury. The likelihood of late epilepsy is increased by acute intracranial hematomas and depressed fractures.

Early seizures should be treated aggressively. Prophylactic intravenous phenytoin loading at 18 mg/kg should be instituted in all severely head-injured patients with intracranial blood, depressed skull fractures with dural penetration, penetrating wounds, intracranial infections, or early seizures.

## PITFALLS TO AVOID IN THE ASSESSMENT AND MANAGEMENT OF THE HEAD-INJURED PATIENT

The following errors should be avoided:

- Inaccurately attributing decreased level of consciousness to alcohol or drugs. Obtain blood alcohol levels and toxicologic screens to help with difficult problems.
- Discharging a patient from the emergency department during a "lucid interval." Err on the conservative side when a period of unconsciousness is documented or if unknown.
- Failure to diagnose a cervical fracture or spinal cord injury. Persist with further views or tomograms when in doubt.
- Failure to adequately immobilize an agitated patient with a cervical fracture. When usual restraint systems are inadequate, consider paralyzing the patient.
- Failure to establish an adequate airway. All obtunded or unconscious patients should be intubated and hyperventilated.
- Failure to recognize progressive neurologic deterioration. Frequent, documented examinations are necessary.
- Failure to rapidly and correctly manage the "talk and deteriorate" patient. This is an extreme emergency.

## PROGNOSIS

Prognosis from mild to moderate severe head injury is usually regarded as good. Mortality rates of patients with head injuries and GCS scores of 10 or greater approach zero unless there has been deterioration to a severe head-injured state. However, a patient who appears to display a good or favorable recovery can exhibit subtle alterations in memory, concentration, and cognition which interfere with function.

The overall mortality rate for severe head injuries is approximately 35 percent with a favorable or functional outcome accounting for another 40 to 50 percent. Even in the functional or favorably recovered patients, formal neuropsychological tests will uncover significant deficits.

The major factors influencing outcome in the severely head-injured patient is the initial GCS score which reflects the severity of the neurologic injury and the particular type of lesion causing the neurologic deficit. The mortality rate for patients with GCS scores of 3 to 5 is approximately three times that of patients with scores of 6 to 8 (60 vs. 20 percent). Acute subdural hematoma with a GCS score of 3 to 5 will have an approximately 75 percent mortality rate and less than a 10 percent chance for a favorable recovery. On the other hand, diffuse injury without mass lesions with a GCS score of 6 to 8 will have an approximately 10 percent mortality and two-thirds will make a good recovery. Acute subdural hematomas and diffuse injuries associated with coma of longer than 24 h account for 75 percent of head-injury deaths. In addition, bilaterally absent pupillary responses or oculocephalic responses are associated with an approximately 75 percent mortality rate. This is true regardless of whether a surgical or a nonsurgical lesion is present. Increasing age appears to adversely affect the outcome of head injury in general.

Despite improvement in the ability to prognosticate based on the neurologic examination and other factors, it is difficult to ascertain the ultimate prognosis in the early phases of treatment. Aggressive stabilization and treatment is indicated in all severely head-injured patients.

## DELAYED TRAUMATIC PROBLEMS

### Postconcussion Syndromes

The term *postconcussion syndrome* evokes the image of a psychophysiologic reaction in many physicians' minds. This probably is because many of the symptoms such as insomnia, loss of memory, hearing problems, sensitivity to alcohol, depression, and visual disturbances seem, superficially at least, to have no organic basis. There is increasing documentation that the mildly and moderately head-injured patients have evidence of organic brain damage on formal neuropsychological testing. In one study of minor head injury, 34 percent of patients gainfully employed before the accident were unemployed 3 months after the injury. This was felt to be due primarily to problems with attention, concentration, memory, and judgment and also the emotional stress caused by the persistent symptoms. Litigation and compensation may obviously play a role in some cases, but the burden of proof would appear to be on the physician. These patients should be referred for appropriate evaluation if symptoms appear to be legitimately interfering with normal functioning.

### Delayed Posttraumatic Cerebral Spinal Fluid Leak

The exact incidence of recurrent posttraumatic CSF leak is difficult to ascertain but is probably as high as 10 percent. Previous head injury with loss of the integrity of the meningeal coverings of the brain is the most common cause of recurrent meningitis in adults. Not all patients having posttraumatic meningitis will necessarily have active CSF leak, although the majority will. Because of this risk of delayed bacterial meningitis, all patients with suspected CSF leak must be referred to a neurosurgeon without delay.

### Delayed Posttraumatic Seizures

Delayed posttraumatic seizures, defined as the first seizures occurring after 1 week from the time of trauma, occur in anywhere from 2 to 6 percent of the head-injured population. Eighty-five percent of these seizures occur for the first time within 1 year of the injury. Depressed fractures with tear of the dura or brain associated with intracranial hematomas have a significant increased incidence of posttraumatic seizures. Outpatients with delayed posttraumatic seizures should be loaded with phenytoin as described above and placed on a maintenance dose which should be continued until a 2-year seizure-free interval has passed.

## BIBLIOGRAPHY

Adams JH, Graham DI, Murray LS, et al: Diffuse axonal injury due to non-missile head injury in humans: An analysis of 45 cases. *Ann Neurol* 12:557, 1982.

Gennarelli TA, Spielman GM, Langfitt TW, et al: Influence of the type of intracranial lesion on outcome from severe head injury. A multicenter study using a new classification system. *J Neurosurg* 56:26, 1982.

Jeret JS, Mandel M, Anziska B, et al: Clinical predictors of abnormality disclosed by computed tomography after mild head injury. *Neurosurgery* 32:9, 1993.

Rockswold GL, Pheley PJ: Patients who talk and deteriorate. *Ann Emerg Med* 22:1004, 1993.

# 216
# SPINAL INJURIES
### Brian D. Mahoney

It is difficult to imagine an injury more devastating than acute quadriplegia. Kraus and coworkers estimated the incidence of new spinal cord injury at 50 per million U.S. population. This extrapolates to approximately 13,000 new spinal cord injury victims in 1994 in the United States. The typical patient is a man in his early twenties involved in a motor vehicle accident. Motor vehicle accidents (41 percent) are followed in frequency by falls (13 percent), firearms (9 percent), and recreation (5 percent) as sources of spinal cord injury.

## PATHOPHYSIOLOGY

### Spinal Cord Injury Syndromes

Severe injury to the spinal cord may cause spinal shock. This is a sudden transient distal areflexia that may last hours to weeks. The patient initially presents with a flaccid quadriplegia. As spinal shock passes (usually within 24 h), segmental reflexes return and the patient develops a spastic paralysis. Spinal neurogenic shock is that part of spinal shock relating to the vasomotor instability that is due to loss of sympathetic tone. The patient typically has a systolic blood pressure of 80 to 100 mmHg. Despite hypotension, the skin is warm, pink, and dry, and there is adequate urine output. In addition, despite the hypotension, there is a paradoxical bradycardia.

The patient also may have other autonomic nervous system dysfunction. Paralysis of the bowel and bladder may lead to paralytic ileus, gastric dilation, and acute urinary retention. Loss of anal sphincter tone leads to fecal incontinence. Priapism may occur and serve as a sign of cord injury. The patient may lose temperature control because of inability to vasoconstrict, vasodilate, shiver, or sweat over a large portion of his or her body. The patient may become poikilothermic and require external thermal control with a warming blanket.

### Complete and Partial Cord Syndromes

Cord injury is physiologically complete when all cord function is absent distal to the level of injury. Long-term prognosis assessment cannot be made until spinal shock has resolved. The presence of a complete versus an incomplete lesion has tremendous implications for prognosis and treatment. The prognosis of a complete lesion after spinal shock has resolved is for continued quadriplegia. In contrast, partial cord lesions often have at least some degree of recovery. Maynard and coworkers reported the neurologic prognosis after traumatic quadriplegia among 103 cognitively intact patients. None with complete injury at 72 h were walking at 1 year. Of patients with sensory incomplete function at 72 h postinjury, 47 percent were walking at 1 year, and 87 percent of patients with motor incomplete function at 72 h postinjury were walking at 1 year.

### Anterior Spinal Cord Syndrome

The anterior spinal cord syndrome has been related to compression of the anterior spinal cord itself or compression of the anterior spinal artery with resultant ischemic injury to the cord. There is complete motor paralysis and loss of pain and temperature sensation distal to the lesion. Because the posterior columns are spared, the senses of light touch, motion, vibration, and gross proprioception are preserved. After bony reduction, an emergent CT myelogram is obtained to check for a removable extrinsic mass pressing on the cord.

### Central Spinal Cord Syndrome

The central spinal cord syndrome typically occurs with hyperextension injuries in patients with a narrow spinal canal due to spondylosis or congenital stenosis. It is a partial cord syndrome characterized by weakness greater in the arms than the legs and worse in the hands than in the proximal upper extremity. There are variable bladder and scattered sensory losses. The cause is unknown, but it is often attributed to buckling of the ligamentum flavum into the cord during extension injury. Ischemic injury primarily to the center of the cord has been found at autopsy. The order of the motor fibers of the corticospinal tract explains the neurologic findings. The more-damaged motor fibers serving the arms are nearer the injured center of the cord, and those serving the legs more lateral. Treatment usually is nonoperative, and there is a relatively good prognosis.

### Brown-Séquard Syndrome

Brown-Séquard syndrome involves injury to one side of the cord. There are paralysis and loss of gross proprioception and vibratory sensation on the side of the lesion and loss of pain and temperature sensation on the contralateral side. This crossed lesion is explained by the level of decussation of motor fibers in the medulla and the decussation of pain and temperature fibers two dermatome levels about their point of nerve root entry. This partial cord syndrome is usually due to penetrating wounds, although lateral placed disk protrusion, tumor, or hematoma can cause it.

### Research

Allen's animal model for graded spinal cord injury uses a weight dropped a fixed distance through a vented tube onto the exposed spinal cord. Initial impact causes immediate paraplegia without microscopic or pathologic changes. Later, the cord develops a central hemorrhagic lesion. Animal models have shown a 4- to 8-h period in which gray and then white matter necrosis develops. Therapeutic interventions attempt to halt or limit this ongoing process. Areas of investigation have included glucocorticoids, osmotic diuretics, antiadrenergic compounds, naloxone, thyrotropic-releasing hormone, dimethylsulfoxide, hyperbaric oxygen, and hypothermia. In a double-blind, randomized, controlled clinical trial of very high dose methylprednisolone-treated patients, Bracken and coworkers reported that patients treated within 8 h of injury showed significantly greater motor function and pin and touch sensation.

Faden has investigated the theory that β endorphins released at the time of spinal cord injury cause a reduction in spinal cord blood flow, allowing secondary injury to occur. Using a cat model he reported that animals treated with naloxone or thyrotropic-releasing hormone showed less damage and significantly improved neurologic recovery than did animals receiving glucocorticoids or placebo. Unfortunately, in Bracken and coworkers' multicenter human trial, naloxone showed no evidence of efficacy.

## CLINICAL FEATURES

### Stability

Panjabi and White define stability as the ability of the spine to maintain vertebral relations when a load is applied such that there is no damage or irritation to the spinal cord or the nerve roots and no deformity or pain. Trafton has ranked cervical spine injuries according to their degree of instability (Table 216-1). Cervical sprain, that is, damage to ligaments, may lead to dangerous instability and neurologic loss with or without fracture. The atlantoaxial joint is principally maintained by the cruciform ligament. Disruption of this ligament leads to widening of the predental space.

Using CT and Denis' three-column system of categorizing spinal injuries, one can accurately assess spinal stability. The anterior column includes the anterior longitudinal ligament, the anterior two-thirds of the vertebral body, the annulus fibrosus, and the disk. The middle column includes the posterior one-third of the vertebral body, the annulus fibrosus, the disk, and the posterior longitudinal ligament. The posterior column includes all the remaining posterior elements: the pedicles, lateral masses, intertransverse ligaments, facet capsular ligaments, lamina, ligamentum flavum, spinous processes, interspinous and supraspinous ligaments, and ligamentum nuchae. To be unstable, the injury must involve two of the columns.

Some fracture dislocations are obviously unstable, but others, such as severe compression fractures, seat belt fractures, or burst fractures may or may not be unstable, depending on associated ligamentous injury. In some questionable cases, acute stability can be assessed on careful flexion-extension studies. Check for subluxation greater than 3 mm or angulation of one vertebral body over the next greater than 11°. CT avoids the risk of these dynamic studies by more accurately describing the injury.

A principal goal is to identify and protect all patients with acutely unstable spinal columns. There is, in addition, a subset of patients who on initial films, including flexion and extension views, will have what appears to be a stable column that within 3 weeks will develop subacute instability. This phenomenon is thought to be due to the prevention of subluxation by muscle tension at the initial visit and the occurrence of progressive instability as the muscles relax. It is important that patients with acute cervical strains are referred for follow-up before 3 weeks.

## Mechanisms of Injury and Common Fractures/Dislocations

Approximately 39 percent of cervical fractures have associated neurologic injury. Factors that increase the risk of neurologic injury include block vertebrae, spina bifida, os odontoideum, ankylosing spondylitis, rheumatoid arthritis, spinal stenosis, and age-related degenerative changes. Although approximately 20 percent of patients with cervical spine injuries have facial injuries, the converse is not true. People with facial injuries rarely have cervical spine injuries. In a study of 2555 patients with facial fractures severe enough for hospital admission, Davidson and Birdsell found that only 1.3 percent had associated neck injuries. The vast majority of the patients with combined face and neck injuries had multiple-system trauma from motor vehicle accidents.

Harris and coworkers have classified the various injuries of the cervical spine according to seven mechanisms of injury (Table 216-2). The *Jefferson fracture* is a burst of the ring of C1 from a vertical compression force. It is most often seen on the open-mouth odontoid view, although tomograms may be necessary. The *hangman's fracture* is a bilateral fracture through the pedicles of C2. It is often due to hyperextension in a motor vehicle accident. Fortunately, the generous size of the spinal canal at C2 and spontaneous decompression help to limit cord damage. The *flexion teardrop fracture* refers to the mechanism and shape of the large triangular fragment displaced from the anterior aspect of the involved vertebral body. There is extensive associated posterior and anterior ligamentous disruption and, with it, cord injury. The *extension teardrop fracture* also has a triangular anterior, inferior fragment, but the mechanism is extension with avulsion of the fragment, leaving the posterior ligaments intact. The *burst fracture* is a vertical compression injury in which pieces of the comminuted vertebral body are often forced posteriorly into the spinal canal. Some authors consider it a variation of the flexion teardrop fracture. The *clay-shoveler's fracture* is due to avulsion of the spin-

**Table 216-1.** The Spectrum of Acute Instability in Cervical Spine Injuries

***Most Unstable***

- Rupture of transverse atlantal ligament
- Fracture of dens
- Burst fracture with posterior ligamentous disruption ("flexion teardrop")
- Bilateral facet dislocation (or equivalent posterior disruption)
- Burst fracture of vertebral body without posterior ligamentous disruption
- Hyperextension fracture dislocation
- Hangman's fracture
- Extension teardrop fracture (stable in flexion)
- Jefferson fracture (burst of C1)
- Unilateral facet dislocation (or equivalent posterior disruption)
- Anterior subluxation
- Simple wedge compression fracture without posterior disruption
- Pillar fracture
- Fracture of posterior arch of C1
- Spinous process fracture (clay-shoveler)

***Least Unstable***

*Source:* Trafton G: Spinal cord injuries. *Surg Clin North Am* 62:61, 1982. Reprinted with permission.

**Table 216-2.** Cervical Spine Injuries: Mechanism of Injury

Flexion
    Anterior subluxation (hyperflexion sprain)
    Bilateral interfacetal dislocation
    Simple wedge (compression) fracture
    Clay-shoveler (coal-shoveler) fracture
Flexion teardrop fracture
Flexion-rotation
    Unilateral interfacetal dislocation
Extension-rotation
    Pillar fracture
Vertical compression
    Jefferson bursting fracture of atlas
    Burst (bursting, dispersion, axial loading) fracture
Hyperextension
    Hyperextension dislocation
    Avulsion fracture of anterior arch of atlas
    Extension teardrop fracture of axis
    Fracture of posterior arch of atlas
    Laminar fracture
    Traumatic spondylolisthesis (hangman's fracture)
    Hyperextension fracture-dislocation
Lateral flexion
    Uncinate process fracture
Diverse or imprecisely understood mechanisms
    Atlantooccipital disassociation
    Odontoid fractures

*Source:* Harris JH, Edeiken-Monroe B, Kopanily DR: A practical classification of acute cervical spine injuries. *Orthop Clin North Am* 17:15, 1986. Reproduced by permission.

ous process of C7, C6, or T1 (in order of frequency) from a flexion mechanism. It is also caused by direct blows to the spinous process.

*Bilateral interfacetal dislocation* occurs in flexion. The lesion is unstable, with total ligamentous disruption. On lateral x-ray views, there is anterior displacement of 50 percent or greater of one vertebral body on the next lower body. *Unilateral facet dislocation* occurs in combined flexion with rotation injuries. It is potentially unstable, depending on ligamentous disruption, and on lateral x-ray views there is anterior dislocation of 25 to 33 percent of one vertebral body on the next lower body. In addition, the vertebrae inferior to the injury appear in true lateral projection, and above the level of injury there is a sudden change to an oblique view.

## Thoracolumbar Injuries

The greatest number of thoracolumbar injuries occur at the junction of the relatively fixed upper thoracic spine (T1–T9) and the relatively mobile thoracolumbar (T10–L5) spine. Because of the buttressing provided by the rib cage, it takes great force to cause a thoracic fracture dislocation. Thoracic fracture dislocations are less common than lower thoracolumbar ones, but when they occur the spinal cord injury is typically more severe for three reasons: the diameter of the thoracic spinal canal is narrow, the thoracic spinal cord fills a larger portion of the canal, and the thoracic cord's blood supply is in a watershed area such that compression on the anterior spinal artery can cause ischemic injury much higher up in the thoracic cord. The greater radicular artery of Adamkiewicz enters the spinal canal at L1 but provides circulation as high as T4.

There are four major types of thoracolumbar fractures. The first is the *wedge,* or *compression, fracture.* It results from axial loading and flexion with failure of the anterior column. Wedge fractures are generally acutely stable. Severe wedge fractures are potentially unstable if the anterior margin of the vertebral body has lost more than 50 percent of its height and there is partial failure of the posterior ligaments. Wedge fractures are particularly common in elderly patients. The order of frequency is L1 > L2 > T12. Neurologic injury is uncommon, and treatment is symptomatic. Patients with acute wedge fracture of greater than 50 percent are often admitted for pain control and in anticipation of an ileus.

The second type of thoracolumbar fracture is the *burst fracture.* It results from axial loading, causing failure of the anterior and middle columns. The vertebral end plates fracture, forcing the nucleus pulposus into the vertebral body, resulting in explosion of the body. There is loss of vertebral height both anteriorly and posteriorly. On the anteroposterior (AP) x-ray the burst may be identified by a widening of the interpedicular distance. In severe burst fractures the posterior portion of the vertebral body explodes into the spinal canal, causing spinal cord compression. CT scan is often necessary to show clearly the true extent of these retropulsed fragments.

The third type of thoracolumbar fracture is a *distraction* or *seat belt injury.* In these injuries the seat belt serves as the axis of rotation during distraction, with failure of the spine in its posterior ligamentous and bony components. In the *Chance distraction fracture* the spine fails entirely in bone, splitting horizontally through the spinous process, laminae, pedicles, and the vertebral body. Abdominal injuries are common with seat belt spinal injuries.

*Fracture dislocations* involve failure of all three columns. The mechanism is flexion with rotation or shearing from massive blows such as from a cave in. These types of injuries are unstable and have the most associated spinal cord injury.

### Radiographic Evaluation of Thoracolumbar Injuries

The AP and lateral are the minimum views of the thoracolumbar spine. After initial AP and lateral films identify the level of injury, cone-down views will give more details, especially of the posterior elements. On the lateral radiograph, check the anterior and posterior height of the vertebral bodies, the alignment of the bodies, the posterior bony elements for fracture, and the interspinous distance for evidence of ligamentous disruption. On the AP, check the height of the vertebral bodies, the width between pedicles, and the alignment of the vertebral bodies and follow the spinous processes down the midline. Besides being checked for spinal injury, the AP film should be assessed for associated chest and abdominal injuries. Look for a paraspinal hematoma and for transverse process fractures correlated with trauma to adjacent organs, particularly the kidneys.

Do a CT scan if plain films are equivocal or suggest posterior element injury or if the patient has a neural deficit but no obvious fracture. CT scanning will frequently identify additional injuries, especially injuries of the posterior elements. Do CT myelography if initial x-rays do not explain a neurologic deficit, if the deficit progresses, or if the patient has an unexplained plateau during recovery from a deficit.

## Sacral and Coccygeal Injuries

Overlying bowel and soft tissue shadows make plain film diagnosis difficult. CT will identify fractures of the sacrum and pelvis and associated hematoma. Neurologic injury is rare in sacral injuries. When it occurs, it involves damage to sacral nerve roots, impairing bowel, bladder, and sexual functions and motor and sensory function in the posterior legs.

Coccygeal injuries occur due to direct blows and, if severe, may have associated rectal tears. X-rays are not indicated, nor are they helpful in isolated coccygeal injury. Make the diagnosis of coccygeal fracture on rectal examination. Treatment in uncomplicated fractures is symptomatic, with pain medication and a doughnut pillow. Chronic coccydynia occasionally complicates recovery.

## Penetrating Injuries

Acute bony instability is very rare in penetrating wounds of the spine. High-velocity missile wounds can cause direct injury and more remote injury due to concussive forces. Treatment includes antibiotics; tetanus prophylaxis; methylprednisolone; and surgery to remove any extrinsic mass compressing the cord, to repair dural tears, and to debride devitalized tissue.

## Sports Injuries

Bruce and coworkers reported that football caused 66 percent of organized-sports-related cervical spine injuries, diving 18 percent, and rugby 9 percent. High school football in the United States causes 20 to 30 quadriplegic injuries per year. C5–C6 is the most common level of injury. Approximately 72 percent of cervical cord injuries occur during tackling, and 50 percent of college football players have experienced a paresthesia at least once.

In rugby, cervical injuries occur primarily when the scrimmage collapses in the center and players behind keep pushing. Injuries during tackling are uncommon, since the lack of a helmet leads to different tackling techniques. Although soccer is the most widely played team sport in the world, soccer-related spinal cord injuries are uncommon. In soccer, central nervous system injuries are largely limited to closed head trauma. Wrestling, horseback riding, gymnastics, and trampoline yield an additional small number of cord injuries.

## Posttraumatic Syringomyelia

Posttraumatic syringomyelia is characterized by progression of neurologic deficits distant from the level of a preceding injury. It occurs in approximately 1 percent of spinal-cord-injured patients but does not show itself for 4 to 9 years. The most common initial complaint is pain with coughing or straining, followed by paresthesias, numbness, weakness, and hyperhidrosis. Physical examination reveals hypesthesia, weakness, and diminished reflexes cephalad from the original lesion. Incomplete cord lesions may progress to spasticity and loss of retained bowel, bladder, and sexual function. It is usually unilateral in onset and remains asymmetric over time.

## DIAGNOSIS

### Cervical X-Ray Studies

Obtain cervical spine x-ray views on all trauma patients with any of the following: (1) posttraumatic neck pain or tenderness; (2) transient or persistent numbness or paresthesia; (3) loss of consciousness; (4) impaired level of consciousness, such as from intoxication, with evidence of head or neck injury; (5) an examination consistent with cervical cord injury; and (6) other painful, distracting injuries, especially multiple injuries, resulting from high-energy accidents or falls. The minimum views needed are a lateral, AP, and open-mouth odontoid.

The lateral view shows 90 percent of the significant injuries, the open-mouth odontoid 10 percent, and the AP fewer than 1 percent. Other views may add substantial information, but the presence of an injury is usually at least suspected based upon these first three views. In reading an x-ray, it is acceptable to do an initial rapid survey, but this must be followed by an explicit sequence of evaluation, as follows:

1. On the true lateral view (Fig. 216-1), look for all seven cervical vertebrae, including the cervicothoracic junction. If all seven cervical vertebrae plus the upper margin of T1 cannot be seen, then do a repeat lateral with arm traction applied to lower the shoulders, a swimmer's view, or bilateral supine oblique projections. In managing a seriously injured patient, valuable time can be saved by automatically doing the swimmer's view immediately after the lateral view with arm traction applied.
2. Check prevertebral soft tissue; 5 mm or greater down to the C3 to C4 level suggests hematoma secondary to fracture.
3. Check each vertebra for fracture.
4. Check for alignment of the four lordotic curves, consisting of the anterior margin of the vertebral body, the posterior margin of the vertebral body, the spinolaminal line, and the tips of the

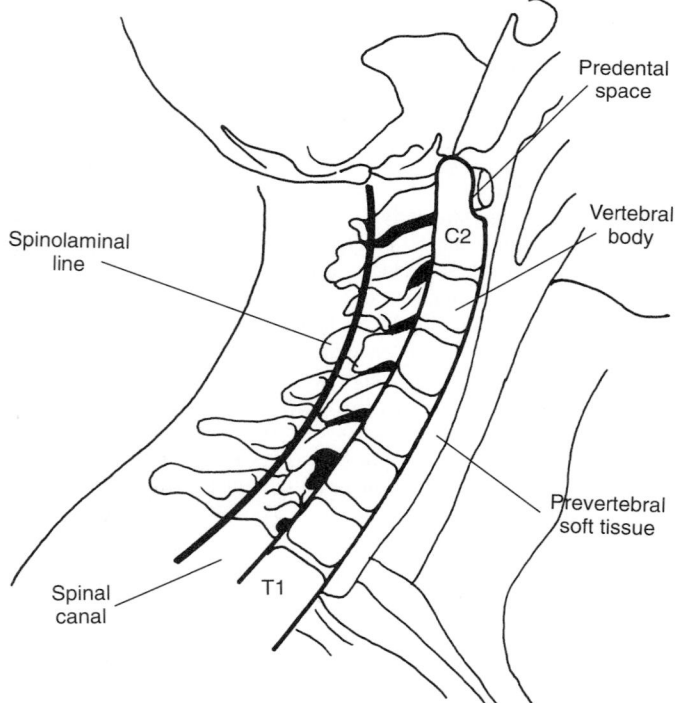

**Fig. 216-1.** Schematic of lateral cervical x-ray.

spinous processes. In an adult, up to 3.5 mm of anterior subluxation on a true lateral view taken at 6 ft (2 m) may be normal. Yet to assess ligamentous stability, careful flexion and extension views may be required.

5. Check for an abrupt change in angulation of the cervical column of greater than 11° at a single interspace.
6. Check for fanning of spinous processes, suggesting posterior ligamentous disruption.
7. Check the lateral masses for abrupt change in rotation, suggesting facet dislocation.
8. Check the AP diameter of the spinal canal for congenital stenosis or stenosis due to spondylosis. The anatomic upper limit of the normal AP diameter of the adult cord is 9.3 mm—about the size of your little finger. Yet, due to the magnification on plain films, if the canal diameter is less than 13 mm, the patient risks cord injury in otherwise minor strain injuries.
9. Check the predental space. If it is greater than 3 mm in adults or 4 mm in children, there may be disruption of the cruciform ligament holding the dens (odontoid) forward against the body of C1.
10. Check the atlantooccipital relation for dislocation.
11. On the open-mouth odontoid view, look for fracture of the odontoid or body of C2, alignment of the lateral masses of C1 with C2, and symmetry of the C1–C2 interspace.

According to a retrospective review by Shaffer and Doris, the lateral view alone failed to show 6 out of 35 cervical spine fractures or dislocations. On 3 more of the 35, the injury was very difficult to see on the lateral view and best seen on the odontoid or AP view. If the patient is unconscious or immobilized so that the patient cannot open his or her mouth, the authors recommend a modified axial supine odontoid process view instead of the open-mouth odontoid view.

If, after obtaining a quality lateral, AP, and open-mouth odontoid view, there is a question about whether a lesion is unstable, CT is the usual next step. If the lesion is most likely stable, then careful lateral views in flexion and extension can be made. Take these views with the patient still supine on a stretcher. Use extreme care, with a knowledgeable physician guiding the patient as the patient slowly flexes and later extends his or her neck. If the patient complains of pain or paresthesias, attempt no further motion. Do not do flexion-extension views if the original three views predict an unstable spinal column. In such a case, the neurosurgeon should order and conduct subsequent radiographic examinations.

If there is concern about a lamina, pedicle, facet, or foramen, then order oblique views after interpreting the first three views as stable. Pillar views are for assessing lateral masses. Tomograms add greatly to the accuracy of the diagnosis. CT is indicated in any patient with a neurologic deficit, fracture of the posterior arch, or burst fracture with vertebral fragments retropulsed into the spinal canal, and for equivocal plain films. In general the CT provides a better view of bony injuries. MRI provides information about soft tissues. Limited access to the patient and the need for prolonged immobility limit the usefulness of MRI in early patient management.

## TREATMENT

### Priorities

There are three priorities in the emergency medical management of the patient with a spinal injury. The first is to ensure patient survival by following the ABCDEs of trauma care. The second priority is to preserve residual spinal cord function by stabilizing the injured spinal column and avoiding secondary injury to the spinal cord. The third priority is to initiate treatments aimed at allowing the highest possible chance for the injured cord to recover. After the completion of emergency care, a fourth priority is to restore the bony stability of the spinal column. Even the permanently quadriplegic patient needs bony vertebral stability.

The patient suffers the primary injury at the time of impact. Emergency physicians can have the most influence on primary injury by being vocal advocates of public safety issues such as endorsing seat belt usage and penalties for those who drive while intoxicated. Once the patient has sustained primary injury, the critical role of all emergency personnel is to avoid secondary injury.

Secondary injury to the cord may occur when there is unnecessary motion of an unstable spinal column, hypoxemia, edema, continued pressure on the cord by an extrinsic mass, or shock that reduces perfusion of the injured cord.

## Prehospital Spinal Immobilization

After surveying the scene for hazard and mechanism of injury, the emergency medical technician immediately controls the patient's head and neck. Management of airway, breathing, and circulation follows. Next a semirigid collar and spinal immobilization board are applied. These devices are used to immobilize the spine and not to apply traction, since excessive traction may cause secondary injury. The degree of immobilization provided by a cervical collar varies from minimal with the soft sponge variety to substantial but not complete with semirigid varieties. Sponge collars have no role in prehospital or emergency department care except for symptomatic relief when a patient with a stable neck injury is ready for discharge. No collar can adequately immobilize the occiput, C1, and C2. The semirigid collar is an important adjunct to aid in transfer onto the long spinal immobilization board. Immobilization continues until history and physical examination or x-ray studies rule out an acutely unstable spinal column. The semirigid collar may be opened to examine the neck, trachea, and jugular veins but then should be reapplied until the indicated spinal x-rays are cleared. Patients should be immobilized for posttraumatic spinal pain or tenderness, unconsciousness, neurologic findings, paresthesias, or a suspicious mechanism and distracting painful injuries. Because a patient is walking at the accident scene does not eliminate the need for proper immobilization.

## Emergency Department Care

Maintain spinal immobilization during assessment and management of airway, breathing, circulation, and disability. Airway management is a controversial topic. The apneic patient needs rapid, definitive airway control, since gastric distension followed by regurgitation is likely during unprotected positive-pressure ventilation. Options include orotracheal intubation with in-line immobilization, transtracheal catheter ventilation while x-rays are taken and cleared, or immediate cricothyrotomy. In-line immobilization means immobilization and not traction. During in-line immobilization, pressure on the cricoid cartilage (Sellick maneuver) will usually allow direct visualization of the vocal cords. For unconscious patients with adequate spontaneous breathing, the usual approach is supplemental oxygen until completion of x-ray studies. Be prepared to logroll patients immediately and suction them. Leave patients attached to the backboard so that if they regurgitate, they can be rolled with reasonable safety. Unfortunately, log rolling with or without a spinal immobilization board does not completely prevent all spinal column motion. Patient exposure for examination requires temporarily releasing straps, but these should be reattached after cutting and removing the clothing.

Resuscitation involves intravenous access, nasogastric tube, and Foley catheter. Adequate volume resuscitation continues until occult hemorrhage is ruled out or controlled. Next, the critical trauma series of x-ray studies is performed, including lateral cervical spine, chest, and pelvic x-rays.

The secondary survey follows and includes assessment of motor function (graded 0/5 for flaccid, 3/5 for overcoming gravity, and up to 5/5 for normal), perception of pain, reflexes, flaccidity or spasticity of extremities, gross proprioception, diaphragmatic breathing, rectal tone, perirectal sensation and wink, bulbocavernosus reflex, and pri-

**Table 216-3.** Muscle Innervation

| Root Level | Muscle | Function Lost |
|---|---|---|
| C3, C4 | Trapezius | Shoulder elevation |
| C4 | Diaphragm | Respiration |
| C5, C6 | Biceps | Forearm flexion |
| C7 | Triceps | Forearm extension |
| C8 | Flexor digitorum | Finger flexion |
| T1 | Interossei | Finger abduction/adduction |
| T1 to T12 | Intercostals and abdominals | Respiration |
| L1, L2 | Iliopsoas | Hip flexion |
| L3, L4 | Quadriceps | Knee extension |
| L5 | Extensor hallucis | Great toe dorsiflexion |
| S1 | Biceps femoris | Knee flexion |
| S1, S2 | Soleus and gastrocnemius | Foot plantar flexion |
| S2 to S4 | Rectal sphincter | Sphincter tone |

apism. A common oversight is to leave out assessment of posterior column function (vibration, gross proprioception, light touch, and motion). Preserved posterior column function is significant in identifying the anterior cord syndrome. The assessment for preserved neurologic function around the anus is vital to identifying sacral sparing and therefore an incomplete lesion. The absence of reflex activity shows the presence of spinal shock. The level of spinal cord injury can be estimated using Tables 216-3 and 216-4. Information must be accurately and serially recorded. Improvement or loss will have significant impact on the patient's management by the neurosurgeon.

The patient's vital signs may indicate spinal neurogenic shock characterized by hypotension, paradoxical bradycardia, warm dry skin, and adequate urine output. Consider all causes of shock in a patient with possible multiple injuries and vital signs indicative of spinal neurogenic shock. Look for hemorrhagic; mechanical (tamponade, tension pneumothorax); cardiogenic; and, to a lesser extent, septic shock. Complete a thorough search for occult hemorrhage before attributing hypotension to spinal cord injury. Emergency evaluation after physical examination includes chest x-ray, peritoneal lavage or abdominal CT, ECG, echocardiogram, urinalysis, and further x-ray studies as appropriate.

If the patient is still hypotensive after occult blood loss and other causes of shock are controlled, support blood pressure with a dopamine infusion. Patients with otherwise healthy cardiovascular systems tolerate very well the systolic pressures of 80 to 100 mmHg common with acute quadriplegia. The optimal blood pressure to maintain is unknown. In animal experiments and theoretically in humans, a pressure nearer normal might aid in perfusing injured areas of the cord. The patient can be overhydrated, and in some cases a central venous pressure line or Swan-Ganz catheter plus Foley catheter may be needed to guide fluid therapy to avoid pulmonary edema.

After completion of the primary survey, resuscitation, trauma series of x-rays, and secondary survey, the presence of spinal column or

**Table 216-4.** Sensory Innervation

| Root | Sensory Level |
|---|---|
| C2 | Occiput |
| C4 | Shoulder tops |
| C6 | Thumb |
| C7 | Long finger |
| C8 | Little finger |
| T2 | Nipple |
| T10 | Umbilicus |
| L1 | Inguinal crease |
| L2, L3 | Medial thigh |
| L4 | Medial calf |
| L5 | Lateral calf |
| S1 | Lateral foot |
| S2 to S4 | Perianal |

cord injury should be evident. If the emergency physician is not certain whether a spinal injury is stable or unstable, the patient must remain on the backboard. Consult a neurosurgeon for significant spinal cord or column injuries.

Start very high dose methylprednisolone as soon as practical after diagnosing spinal cord injury. Bracken and coworkers reported significant improvement of motor, pin, and touch sensation when this treatment began within 8 h of injury. The patient should receive a 30-mg/kg loading dose of methylprednisolone over 15 min in the first hour. Follow this with a 5.4-mg/kg per hour continuous infusion for the next 23 h.

## Traction

A key means of preserving and regaining cord function is to remove any extrinsic source of pressure on the spinal cord. Remarkable degrees of recovery have been achieved with early reduction of displaced fracture dislocations. The first step is to reduce any displacement of the spinal column. Thoracolumbar injuries usually reduce in the supine position on a rotary bed. For cervical injuries, apply tongs such as the Gardner-Wells Traction Tong (Fig. 216-2). Skull fracture, thin and diseased skulls, and scalp infection have varying degrees of contraindication. Complications include osteomyelitis, cerebral infarction, intracerebral hemorrhage following cranial penetration, cerebral aneurysm, and scalp infection. After aseptic prep and local anesthesia, advance the needle-sharp cone-shaped points into the skull above the bony ear canal and just below the temporal ridges. Shaving is not necessary. The metal instruction plate on the tongs should be with the writing face up. Advance the points into the skull by turning the knurled handles alternately until the spring tension indicator advances 1 mm from its recess in the knurled handle. Gently

rock the tongs back and forth to further seat the points. Retighten the knurled handles until the spring tension indicator again protrudes 1 mm. Tighten the lock nuts on each side of the handle to prevent loosening. After 24 h the points will often advance approximately 1 mm into the skull and further tightening will be needed until the tension spring indicator protrudes 1 mm from its recess. Carefully move the patient to a circle or rotary bed. Immobilize the cervical spine by applying 5 lb (2 kg) of traction to the s-hook on the tongs. Use 2 lb (1 kg) for atlantooccipital injuries. Add weight in 5-lb (2 kg) increments every 15 min up to certain weight limits of approximately 5 lb (2 kg) per interspace. Traction must be applied carefully, using serial x-ray films and neurologic examinations as a guide. Excessive traction can permanently destroy cord or nerve root function. Reduction by traction continues until restoration of the AP canal diameter to at least two-thirds of normal, there is neurologic deterioration, or an intervertebral disk space exceeds 5 mm, suggesting that distraction may be occurring. Sedation and muscle relaxation may be needed. If reduction cannot be achieved or maintained, surgery follows.

## Myelography

After reduction of bony displacement, the patient has an emergent myelogram if (1) there has been a documented loss of function since the first prehospital evaluation, (2) there is an anterior cord syndrome, or (3) the patient has a partial cord syndrome that is not improving. The myelogram identifies bone, disk, or hematoma pressing on the cord. Continued unrelieved pressure on the cord will prevent optimal cord recovery and may lead to continuing deterioration. The myelogram is done via a lateral C1–C2 puncture with the stretcher angled head up. Interpretation involves searching for flattening of the cord, tissue visibly pressing on the cord, swelling of the cord, or inability to pass dye inferior to the lesion showing occlusion. Using CT metrizamide myelography, Allen and coworkers reported that approximately 24 percent of patients (11 of 46) with acute nonpenetrating cervical spinal cord injuries can be shown to have significant continuing spinal cord compression after restoration of adequate alignment.

## Disposition

The patient with significant spinal column or cord injury should be managed at a regional trauma center or spinal cord injury center. Transfer should be accomplished when the patient's other injuries allow. If the injured cord progresses in humans in a fashion analogous to that in animal experiments, reduction, decompression, and active experimental interventions must be completed within 4 to 8 h after the injury.

The indications and benefits of early surgery remain controversial. Wagner and Chehrazi recommend considering immediate surgery on patients with (1) acute spinal cord injuries with incomplete sensorimotor loss who have undergone a failed attempt at closed reduction, (2) a successful reduction but continued compression proven on myelography, (3) continued bony encroachment despite reduction, or (4) failure to maintain reduction. They do not recommend immediate surgery for patients with incomplete lesions who are improving or for patients with complete lesions despite adequate reduction.

## Admission Indications

Patients should be admitted for any unstable spinal column injury, cord injury or root injury, pain control, or ileus.

## Discharge Instructions

As with all injuries, patients should be warned they will probably have more pain on the following day and the next day after that. On the third day symptoms often plateau, and then gradual progressive recovery occurs. Instruct the patient to return for worsening pain not

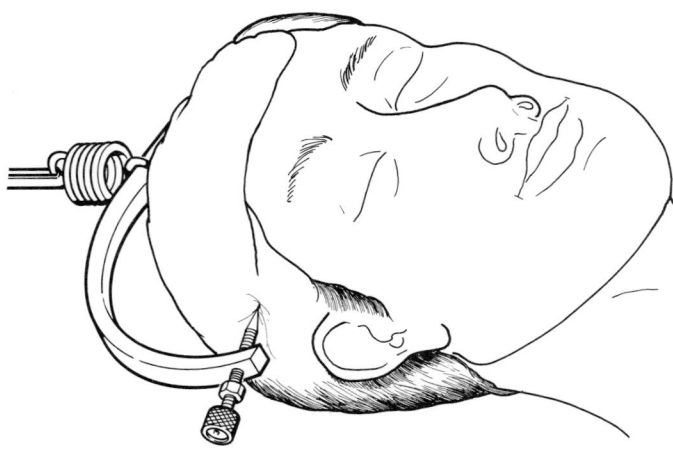

**Fig. 216-2.** Gardner-Wells Traction Tong.

relieved by medication, sudden worsening pain, paresthesias, weakness, numbness, fecal incontinence, or urinary retention.

## Ambulatory Treatment

Ease pain and promote recovery with nonsteroidal medications, physical therapy using massage—first cold, later heat, and later still flexibility and strengthening. For more painful injuries, short periods of bedrest and cervical collar immobilization will be needed.

## Follow-up Interval

The patient with acute spinal strain should have follow-up within 3 weeks of injury. This will provide opportunities to discover signs of subacute cervical instability. Worsening symptoms or pain out of proportion to the stage of recovery should lead to further radiographic studies.

## BIBLIOGRAPHY

Allen RL, Perot PL, Gudeman SK: Evaluation of acute nonpenetrating cervical spine cord injuries with CT metrizamide myelography. *J Neurosurg* 63:510, 1985.

Bracken MB, Shepard MJ, Collins WF, et al: A randomized controlled trial of methylprednisolone or naloxone in the treatment of acute spinal-cord injury. *N Engl J Med* 322:20, 1990.

Bruce DA, Schut L, Sutton LN: Brain and cervical spine injuries occurring during organized sports activities in children and adolescents. *Primary Care* 11:175, 1984.

Brunette DD, Rockswold GL: Neurologic recovery following rapid spinal realignment for complete cervical spinal cord injury. *J Trauma* 27:445, 1987.

Chilton J, Dagi TF: Acute cervical spinal cord injury. *Am J Emerg Med* 3:340, 1985.

Davidson JS, Birdsell DC: Cervical spine injury in patients with facial skeletal trauma. *Trauma* 29:9, 1989.

Denis F: Spinal instability as defined by the three-column spine concept in acute spinal trauma. *Clin Orthop* 189:65, 1984.

Faden AI: Neuropeptides and central nervous system injury. *Arch Neurol* 43:501, 1986.

Gardner WJ: The principle of spring-loaded points for cervical traction. *J Neurosurg* 39:543, 1973.

Harris JH, Edeiken-Monroe B, Kopaniky DR: A practical classification of acute cervical spine injuries. *Orthop Clin North Am* 17:15, 1986.

Kalsbeek WD, McLaurin RL, Harris BS, et al: The national head and spinal cord injury survey: Major findings. *J Neurosurg* 53:519, 1980.

Kraus JF, Franti CE, Riggins RS, et al: Incidence of traumatic spinal cord lesions. *J Chronic Dis* 28:471, 1975.

Lamont A, Zachary J, Sheldon P: Cervical cord size in metrizamide myelography. *Clin Radiol* 32:409, 1981.

Ljunggren B, al Refai M, Sharma S, et al: Functional recovery after near complete traumatic deficit of the cervical cord lasting more than 24 hours. *Br J Neurosurg* 6:375, 1992.

Maynard FM, Reynolds GG, Fountain S, et al: Neurological prognosis after traumatic quadriplegia. *J Neurosurg* 50:611, 1979.

McArdle CB et al: Surface coil MR of spinal trauma: Preliminary experience. *Am J Neuroradiol* 7:885, 1986.

Meyer GA, Berman IR, Doty DB, et al: Hemodynamic responses to acute quadriplegia with or without chest trauma. *J Neurosurg* 34:168, 1971.

Panjabi MM, White AA: Basic biomechanics of the spine. *Neurosurgery* 7:76, 1980.

Riggins RS, Kraus JF: The risk of neurologic damage with fractures of the vertebrae. *J Trauma* 17:126, 1977.

Shaffer MA, Doris PE: Limitation of the cross table lateral in detecting cervical spine injuries: A retrospective analysis. *Ann Emerg Med* 10:508, 1981.

Trafton G: Spinal cord injuries. *Surg Clin North Am* 62:61, 1982.

Wagner FC, Chehrazi B: Spinal cord injury: Indications for operative intervention. *Surg Clin North Am* 60:1049, 1980.

Weir DC: Roentgenographic signs of cervical injury. *Clin Orthoped* 109:9, 1975.

Wilkins RH, Rengachary SS (eds): *Neurosurgery,* 2/e. New York, McGraw-Hill, 1996.

# 217
# PENETRATING AND BLUNT NECK TRAUMA
## Robert A. Swor

The management of the patient with a direct injury to the neck is a difficult problem in the emergency department. The physician must be concerned with airway patency, control of major hemorrhage, and stability of osseous structures and must also evaluate for other, less apparent but potentially lethal injuries.

The neck is unique in the body in that it has many important visceral structures that are not well protected by bone. It is in part protected by both the face and the chest but is still a region vulnerable to both penetrating injury and, less commonly, blunt trauma.

## ANATOMY

The platysma is a major landmark in the discussion of *penetrating neck injury,* which is defined as any wound that violates the platysma. Along its entire length, this muscle is invested in fascia originating on the clavicle. It inserts on the mandible and extends over the proximal half of the sternocleidomastoid. It tamponades bleeding from neck injury and makes direct clinical evaluation difficult.

The sternocleidomastoid muscle (SCM) extends diagonally from the mastoid process of the skull to the superior sternum and clavicle. It divides the neck into the anterior triangle, bounded by the SCM, the midline, and the mandible. This triangle contains most of the major vascular and visceral structures and the airway. The posterior triangle is bounded by the SCM, the trapezius, and the clavicle. It has relatively few structures except at its base. The posterior triangle is further divided by the spinal accessory nerve into a so-called careful region at the base and a carefree region that has a paucity of vital structures (Fig. 217-1).

Major vessels that are frequently injured by both blunt and penetrating injury lie in the anterior triangle. These include carotid arteries, jugular veins, and the thyrocervical trunk. The vertebral arteries are well protected by bone and infrequently injured. The subclavian vessels lie at the base of the posterior triangle and may be injured by a vertical blow to that region. In penetrating injury, and less commonly in blunt injury, contiguous neurologic structures can be involved. Understanding their location is important in predicting injury to contiguous structures. The sympathetic chain ganglia lie posteriorly to the carotid sheath and are protected by it (Fig. 217-2). The spinal accessory nerve courses through the midportion of the posterior triangle and is used as an anatomic boundary between areas with vital structures and less worrisome areas.

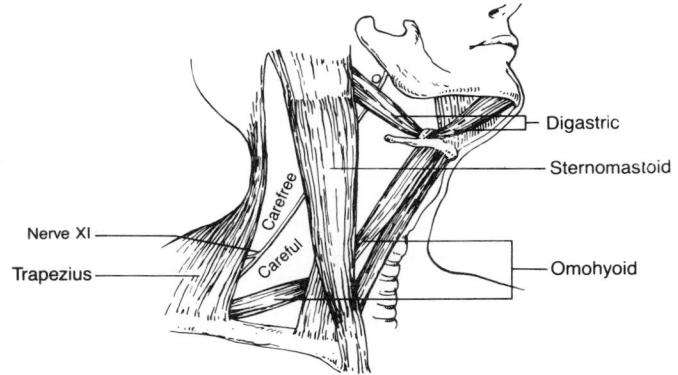

**Fig. 217-1.** Triangles of the neck.

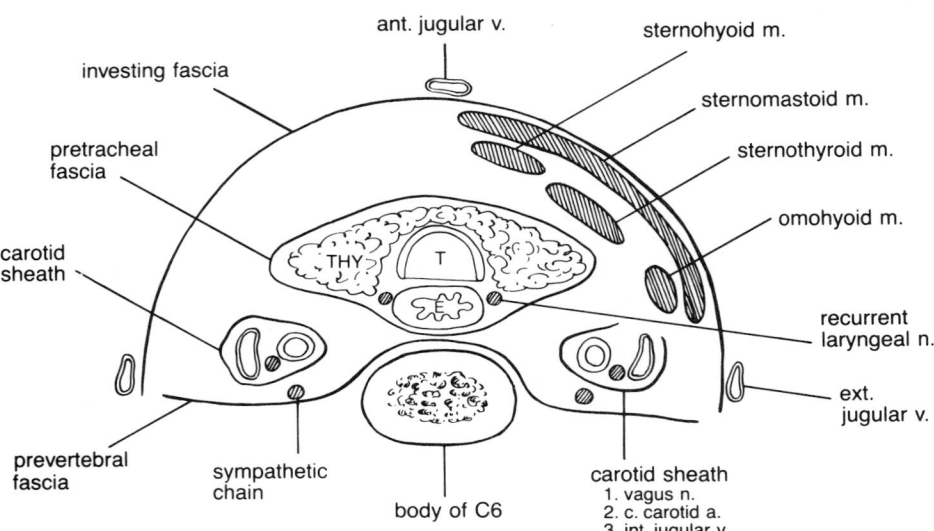

**Fig. 217-2.** Fascial planes of the neck.

Fascial planes play a major role in the management of neck trauma. The fascia that invests the platysma tamponades bleeding. The carotid sheath is tough enough to deflect low-velocity missiles such as knives and small-caliber bullets. The cervical visceral fascia envelopes the esophagus and thyroid (Fig. 217-2). It is continuous with the mediastinum and can be a conduit for mediastinal soilage with esophageal injury.

## TYPES OF INJURY

Most early experience with penetrating neck injuries was related to high-velocity missile injury encountered in warfare. Increasing numbers of civilian injuries occur secondary to stab wounds and low-velocity gunshot wounds from handguns.

The majority of injuries caused by penetrating injury are vascular. These injuries may present with massive or occult hemorrhage. Both central nervous system (CNS) and peripheral nerve injury are frequent in most series, and brachial plexus injury can occur with low neck injury. Neurologic injuries are difficult to assess in patients who are intoxicated or in shock. CNS deficits secondary to vascular injury are important injuries to diagnose before surgical intervention. Air embolus secondary to venous injury is a rare but lethal complication. Arteriovenous fistulas are also reported in most series. Cervical spine injuries are often overlooked and must be suspected in all neck injuries. Pharyngeal and esophageal injuries are frequently not apparent on initial presentation.

In blunt injury, the force is commonly a direct blow. Common mechanisms for such injury are steering wheel injury to a restrained driver of a car, direct blows during sports, "clothesline"-type injuries to drivers of recreational vehicles (motorcycles, all-terrain vehicles, snowmobiles), and strangulation. Such injuries may cause laryngeal edema or fracture resulting in upper airway obstruction. Laryngotracheal separation has also been reported.

Airway injury is common in blunt trauma secondary to the anterior and fixed position of the larynx and trachea in the neck. Blunt injury to the vasculature and viscera also occurs. Avulsion of the carotid arteries has been reported after hangings. Cerebrovascular infarcts have also been reported after blunt injury, due to carotid dissection, formation of an intimal flap or plaque embolization. Perforation of the pharynx and the esophagus, though rare, may result from the transient increase in intraluminal pressure that occurs during blunt injury.

## MAJOR CAUSES OF DEATH

Early death after neck injury occurs by one of three mechanisms: CNS injury, exsanguination, or airway compromise. Most CNS in-

jury occurs at the time of neck injury and is thus not preventable. Exsanguination and airway compromise should be treatable if recognition and appropriate emergency care are available. Late deaths occur secondary to sepsis, which may be the result of missed injury.

## RESUSCITATION

### Airway

The first priority in the management of a patient with a neck injury is the maintenance of the airway and control of the cervical spine. With both penetrating and blunt neck injuries cervical spine injury must be assumed until ruled out by examination or cervical radiography. Management of the airway is most difficult because there may be direct damage to the airway itself. For patients in respiratory distress, emergent airway management via endotracheal or nasotracheal intubation may be lifesaving. Several caveats, however, are necessary. The neck must be maintained in a neutral position. The patient must not be made to gag or cough because this could dislodge a clot and produce massive bleeding. The airway itself must be evaluated for possible false passages secondary to the injury. An endotracheal tube, or a blind nasotracheal tube introduced into a false channel, could be a fatal error. Blunt injury may result in acute respiratory distress or may produce respiratory embarrassment over a period of hours secondary to increasing edema. For patients with direct airway injury or patients with airway compromise secondary to extrinsic compression from an expanding hematoma, a secure airway is crucial.

For many patients with traumatic neck injury, control of the airway from above may not be possible. Intubation without movement of the cervical spine is a difficult procedure and may not be technically possible. If the patient has associated maxillofacial injury, profuse emesis, or uncontrolled upper airway bleeding, endotracheal or nasotracheal intubation will not be accomplished and the patient will require a surgical airway. Cricothyrotomy is the procedure of choice in these cases, with formal tracheotomy being performed as soon as practical. Although emergency cricothyrotomy is a procedure with a relatively high complication rate, the superficial location of the cricothyroid membrane and the relative paucity of vascular structures overlying the membrane make cricothyrotomy preferable to tracheostomy as an emergency airway. Tracheotomy, however, is indicated in the setting of a complete laryngotracheal separation, which may occur as a consequence of blunt trauma to the larynx.

An alternative airway advocated by some is transtracheal jet ventilation. This procedure is performed by introducing a large-gauge intravenous catheter into the cricothyroid membrane and ventilating the patient with high-pressure oxygen. Complete upper airway obstruction is a contraindication because increased intratracheal pressure from continued inhalation without adequate exhalation, results in barotrauma and tension pneumothorax.

## Breathing

Because of the proximity of the apex of the lung to the base of the neck, pneumothorax is frequently associated with neck trauma. Most commonly it occurs with penetrating injury, but it may occur secondary to disruption of the airway from blunt trauma. In both instances, needle decompression and tube thoracostomy may be lifesaving. Subclavian injury with subsequent hemothorax must also be suspected in low neck injury and, if found, must be drained.

## Circulation

Priorities that must be simultaneously addressed are control of external hemorrhage, assessment of degree of hemorrhage, and establishment of vascular access. Control of external hemorrhage may be established by direct pressure at the bleeding site without fear of compromising cerebral blood flow. One of the lessons learned during the Vietnam war was that young healthy brains could tolerate up to 100 min of no flow through a carotid artery without neurologic sequelae. One must not, of course, compromise the airway with direct pressure or circumferential bandages. Attempts to control bleeding by blindly clamping vessels are inappropriate in the emergency department. Dissection of a wound to a bleeding site should only be done in the surgical suite, where proximal and distal control of vessels can be obtained.

Vascular access may be done as for any trauma resuscitation with a few notable differences. Central venous access should not be attempted in the region of an injury because the resuscitation fluid may leak into the surrounding tissues. Similarly, if one suspects injury to the subclavian vessels, at least one intravenous line should be established in a lower extremity.

Air embolus is a potentially fatal complication of central venous injury. If such injury is suspected, the patient should be kept in Trendelenberg's position to minimize this risk.

## EVALUATION

The most important part of evaluation is a careful history and physical examination. Injury to the neck produces many incipient injuries and may produce only subtle clues to diagnosis (Table 217-1).

The history is focused on complaints related to the aerodigestive systems. Initial complaints of respiratory distress or hoarseness may indicate upper airway injury. Other symptoms suggestive of upper airway injury include neck pain, hemoptysis, or pain with speaking. Pharyngeal or esophageal injury may be indicated by dysphagia, odynophagia, or hematemesis. Complaints regarding neurologic function should also be elicited.

Physical examination must be careful and complete despite the lo-

**Table 217-1.** Indications for Neck Exploration

Vascular
   Continued hemorrhage
   Unstable vital signs
   Diminished or absent pulses
   Large or expanding hematoma
Airway
   Difficulty breathing
   Voice change
Visceral
   Difficulty swallowing
   Subcutaneous emphysema
   Coughing, spitting, or vomiting of blood
Neurologic

cal nature of the injury. One must look carefully for evidence of pneumothorax or hemothorax. A thorough neurologic examination is important (although often difficult in the shocky or intoxicated patient) to establish whether there is peripheral nervous system injury or more importantly CNS injury. The presence of a CNS deficit may be the result of direct CNS trauma or secondary to carotid or vertebral artery injury. The presence or absence of a deficit dictates whether or not revascularization is attempted.

Examination of the neck itself requires a search for evidence of significant injury. One must look for active bleeding or hematoma, drooling, stridor, or tracheal deviation. Normal anatomic landmarks are often lost, especially in a man if there is laryngeal injury. The neck should be palpated for tenderness or crepitance. The neck and upper extremities must be assessed for pulse deficits, thrill, or bruit.

Evaluation of the wound itself after a penetrating injury should be limited. The purpose is only to establish whether or not the platysma has been violated. Further probing of a wound in the emergency department is an invitation to disaster. Full wound evaluation must be reserved for the operating room, where adequate proximal and distal control of vessels can be obtained. Early surgical consultation is mandatory if the platysma is violated.

## Radiographic Evaluation

Fundamental studies in the patient with a cervical injury include a complete cervical spine series for blunt and penetrating injury. This is to assess not only the bony structures but also to evaluate for air in the soft tissues or soft tissue swelling. If airway injury is suspected, as with blunt injury, soft tissue technique should be requested for better airway evaluation. A good quality chest x-ray must also be obtained to evaluate for the presence of pneumothorax, hemothorax, or air in the mediastinum. This finding mandates further evaluation for possible esophageal or tracheal injury.

Esophageal injury may be evaluated by the use of barium or Gastrograffin esophagrams. Most authorities prefer the use of Gastrograffin, even though it is not as good diagnostically, because it is less irritating to surrounding tissues if extravasated. Regardless of contrast media used, this technique has a high false negative rate (up to 25 percent) and is therefore only helpful if positive.

## Interventional Studies

Fiberoptic endoscopy of both the gastrointestinal tract and the respiratory tract have been used in many series to evaluate for acute injury. Esophagoscopy is a helpful adjunct, but many authors question its accuracy. Bronchoscopy is difficult in a patient in acute respiratory distress secondary to airway injury and may increase edema in an already traumatized airway. If attempted, both techniques should be performed under sedation to minimize trauma.

## Arteriography

Early studies of penetrating trauma rarely used arteriography as a diagnostic modality. In their review of 20 years' experience in penetrating trauma, Mattox and coworkers report using three arteriograms.

Roon and Christianson used arteriography based on the level of injury to the neck. Dividing the neck into three zones: (1) below the cricoid cartilage (zone I); (2) between the mandible and the cricoid (zone II), and (3) above the angle of the mandible (zone III, Fig. 217-3), they performed arteriography on all patients with penetrating injury to both high and low zones. The information obtained by arteriogram changed the operative strategy in 29% of patients with such injuries. Other authors have suggested that clinical findings of vascular injury are not sensitive enough to identify major vascular injuries in all cases. Therefore, angiography, particularly for zone I and III injuries, has become a standard diagnostic approach in the evaluation of penetrating injuries in most large centers.

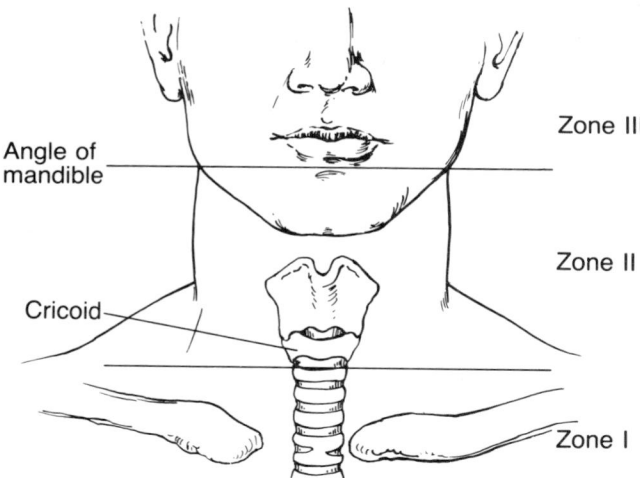

**Fig. 217-3.** Regions of the neck.

## Computed Tomography

Computed tomography (CT) has proved to be a valuable adjunct in the evaluation of the airway after blunt trauma, serving to delineate the type and degree of injury. It is time consuming and should not be attempted in a patient with respiratory distress who may require emergency airway management. For stable patients with symptoms of laryngeal injury (e.g., hoarseness, hemoptysis, odynophagia) or a suspicious mechanism of injury (e.g., direct blow to the larynx), CT is invaluable for identifying injuries to the glottis and supporting cartilaginous structures. A high index of suspicion must be maintained because these injuries may have few symptoms. The need for operative intervention or more conservative care may be identified by this modality.

## MANAGEMENT OF PENETRATING INJURY

Management of penetrating neck injury is an area of controversy that continues to be debated in the surgical literature. Some authors argue that all wounds that penetrate the platysma should have surgical exploration in the operating suite. Others argue that such a radical approach is unnecessary, and these wounds can be evaluated using ancillary modalities, and exploration can be reserved for unstable patients or those with specific indications.

Penetrating injuries are difficult to evaluate and the hazards of missed injury are considerable. Therefore, for the emergency physician, surgical consultation is mandatory for all penetrating wounds that penetrate the platysma, regardless of whether operative intervention is required.

## MANAGEMENT OF BLUNT INJURY

Blunt injury to the neck often poses a diagnostic challenge to the clinician, who should maintain a high index of suspicion with minimal signs of injury. Most cases will be due to motor vehicle accidents, sports injuries, or strangulation. Forces that result in injury are a direct blow to the airway, hyperextension of the neck, or increase of intraluminal pressure due thoracic injury or Valsalva maneuvers at the time of injury.

External signs of injury may be limited to soft tissue injury to the anterior portion of the neck, and patient complaints may be minimal. Hoarseness, dysphonia, and dyspnea demand a more complete evaluation of the neck. Focal neurologic signs may be the result of carotid artery dissection, or intimal flap formation, or injury to the cervical cord. Initial evaluation should include indirect laryngoscopy in the emergency department. Radiographic evaluation may show the presence of soft tissue air or displacement or fracture of the hyoid bone.

Early signs of airway instability require control of the airway be-

cause progression to complete compromise may be rapid. Control of the airway by intubation may not be definitive and may exacerbate injury because of the risk (albeit rare) of laryngotracheal separation. Close observation of the patient after airway measures will ascertain whether a partial airway injury has been worsened by treatment. Some authors argue that laryngotracheal injury is a contraindication to cricothyrotomy and emergent tracheostomy is the airway procedure of choice.

If laryngeal injury is suspected due to mechanism of injury or nature of complaints, the stable airway should be evaluated by CT scanning of the larynx, which is extremely sensitive in identifying subtle injury.

Blunt trauma with symptoms of airway, vascular, or other soft tissue injury should receive aggressive evaluation and consultation until the airway is found to be stable and the full extent of injury is delineated.

## BIBLIOGRAPHY

Camnitz S, et al. Acute blunt laryngeal and tracheal trauma. *Am J Emerg Med* 5:157, 1987.
Carducci B, et al. Collective review—penetrating neck trauma: consensus and controversies. *Ann Emerg Med* 15:208, 1986.
Fogelman MJ, Stewart RD. Penetrating wounds of the neck. *Am J Surg* 91:581, 1956.
Gussack GS, Jurkovich GJ. Treatment dilemmas in laryngotracheal trauma. *J Trauma* 28:1439, 1988.
Line WS, Stanley RB, Choi JH. Strangulation: a full spectrum of blunt neck trauma. *Ann Otol Rhinol Laryngol* 94:542, 1985.
Mansour MA, Moore EE, Moore FA, Whitehall TA. Validating the selective management of penetrating neck wounds. *Am J Surg* 162:517, 1991.
Roon AJ, Christianson. Evaluation and treatment of penetrating cervical injuries. *J Trauma* 19:391, 1979.
Schaider JJ, Dunne P. Head and neck trauma. In: Rosen P (ed). *Diagnostic Radiology in Emergency Medicine.* St. Louis: Mosby-Year Book, 1992.

# 218
# THORACIC TRAUMA
### Robert F. Wilson

## INTRODUCTION

Thoracic trauma directly causes at least 25 percent of trauma deaths and is a contributing factor in another 25 percent. About 80 percent of patients with chest trauma do not have hypotension or severe respiratory distress when first seen in the emergency department. Such patients will generally do very well, and if no other injuries are present, will have a mortality rate of less than 1 percent. However, if the patient with chest trauma has a systolic blood pressure less than 80 mmHg on admission and/or requires urgent endotracheal intubation, the mortality rate will generally exceed 10 to 20 percent. Most of these patients can be treated adequately by ensuring adequate ventilation and oxygenation, providing rapid fluid resuscitation, and inserting one or more chest tubes as needed. Only 5 to 15 percent of patients with chest trauma admitted to a hospital require an emergency thoracotomy.

## CHEST WALL, BRONCHI, LUNG, AND DIAPHRAGM

Patients with chest trauma who develop acute severe respiratory distress have a high mortality rate. In the series reported by Wilson et al., 11 percent of patients admitted with chest trauma required endotracheal intubation almost immediately upon entrance to the emer-

**Table 218-1.** Injuries in Patients with Respiratory Failure After Blunt Chest Trauma

| Injury | Incidence, % | Mortality Rate, % |
|---|---|---|
| Flail chest/multiple rib fracture | 75 | 52 |
| Hemopneumothorax | 55 | 39 |
| Lung contusion | 39 | 45 |
| Extremity fracture | 30 | 53 |
| Intraabdominal | 23 | 46 |
| Intracranial | 23 | 46 |
| Myocardial contusion | 13 | 57 |
| Diaphragm | 9 | 20 |
| Paraplegia | 4 | 100 |
| Other | 7 | 100 |

*Note:* 56 (16.4%) of 340 patients admitted with blunt chest trauma had respiratory failure in the ED.

gency department. Of these, 58 percent died. If shock accompanied the respiratory distress, the mortality rate rose to 73 percent. In patients with blunt chest trauma, the most frequent factors associated with acute respiratory distress included shock, coma, multiple rib fractures, and hemopneumothorax (Table 218-1). In patients with penetrating trauma, respiratory distress was usually due to severe shock or hemopneumothorax (Table 218-2).

## Initial Resuscitation, Airway Control, and Ventilation

Diagnosis of the cause of respiratory distress must be made promptly. If the patient is making little or no effort to breathe, central nervous system dysfunction due to head trauma, drugs, or spinal cord injury is the most likely problem. If the patient is attempting to breathe but is moving little or no air, upper airway obstruction should be suspected.

The most common cause of upper airway obstruction in comatose patients is prolapse of the tongue into the pharynx. Other causes of upper airway obstruction include dentures; vomitus; or blood clots in the pharynx, larynx, or upper trachea. Occasionally, direct trauma may cause fracture of the larynx or cricotracheal separation. Inspiratory stridor does not usually occur unless there is at least a 70 percent occlusion of the larynx or upper trachea. With any suspected laryngeal injury, cautious endoscopy should be performed in the operating room as soon as possible, but one must also be prepared to perform an emergency tracheostomy immediately if the airway occludes.

If the patient is attempting to breathe and the upper airway appears to be intact but the breath sounds are poor, thoracic problems such as flail chest, hemopneumothorax, diaphragmatic injury, or parenchymal lung damage should be considered. In all cases of respiratory distress, the airway must be secured. Following airway control, optimal oxygenation and ventilation should be provided.

### Cardiac Arrest During or Just After Endotracheal Intubation

Although Rotondo et al. have pointed out that urgent paralysis and intubation of trauma patients who are combative or have complex in-

**Table 218-2.** Injuries in Patients with Respiratory Failure After Penetrating Chest Trauma

| Injury | Incidence, % | Mortality Rate, % |
|---|---|---|
| Lung | 55 | 69 |
| Intraabdominal | 36 | 83 |
| Heart | 29 | 63 |
| Hemopneumothorax | 18 | 42 |
| Diaphragm | 17 | 64 |
| Chest wall | 8 | 60 |
| Extremity vessels | 8 | 20 |
| Other | 41 | 63 |

*Note:* 66 (8.3%) of 796 patients admitted with penetrating chest trauma had acute respiratory failure in the ED.

**Table 218-3.** Causes of Cardiac Arrest with Endotracheal Intubation

Inadequate preintubation oxygenation and ventilation
Esophageal intubation
Intubation of the right (or left) main bronchus
Excess ventilation, further reducing venous return
Development of a tension pneumothorax
Systemic air embolism
Vasovagal response (rare)
Sudden development of severe alkalosis

juries is safe, with only 12 percent intubation mishaps (multiple attempts: 7 percent; aspiration: 3.5 percent; esophageal intubation: 1.5 percent) one of the most frequent times for an emergency department patient to have a cardiac arrest is during or right after endotracheal intubation. Table 218-3 lists common causes for cardiac arrest during intubation. If the patient has poor venous return because of hypovolemia, ventilation with excessive pressures can further reduce venous return and cause cardiac arrest. Hypovolemic patients should probably be ventilated with tidal volumes of only 5 to 8 mL/kg at 10 to 14 times per minute until venous return is improved.

If there is a lung injury or if there are fragile subpleural blebs, bagging the patient vigorously can also cause a tension pneumothorax to develop rapidly, further reducing venous return. Even if the lungs are normal, ventilatory pressure exceeding 70 to 80 cmH$_2$O can cause pulmonary damage. Excessive hyperventilation can also cause severe alkalosis, reducing ionized calcium levels and producing serious arrhythmias.

Any patient with a lung injury, especially with hemoptysis, should be considered at risk for developing a systemic air embolus, particularly if high ventilatory pressures are used. Intrabronchial bleeding may also flood normal alveoli, causing severe hypoxemia.

Vasovagal responses are rare in injured patients, but they can occur during insertion of endotracheal, nasogastric, or chest tubes. One should be alert for the development of this problem in patients with nausea or inappropriate bradycardia that worsens as a procedure is being performed.

### Relief of Hemopneumothorax

If a tension pneumothorax is suspected, a large needle or intravenous (IV) catheter with an attached stopcock and syringe to provide an immediate decompression of the pleural cavity should be inserted in the second intercostal space (Fig. 218-1). A chest tube should be inserted as soon as possible.

If a large hemothorax or nontension pneumothorax is suspected in a patient with acute severe respiratory distress, a "blind" chest tube (a chest tube inserted without waiting for a chest roentgenogram) should be inserted through the fourth or fifth intercostal space in the anterior axillary line on the affected side. Digital examination of the pleural cavity before the chest tube is inserted should reduce the chances of inserting the chest tube into the lung parenchyma (if the lung is adherent to the chest wall), through a high diaphragm, or into herniated abdominal viscera. Once a properly functioning chest tube is in place, it is usually connected to 20 to 30 cmH$_2$O suction. The amount of bloody drainage should be monitored closely.

### Intercostal Nerve Blocks

The severe pain caused by multiple fractured ribs can greatly impair ventilation. In such circumstances, blocking the intercostal nerves of the fractured ribs plus two ribs above and two ribs below with a long-acting local anesthetic, such as 0.5% bupivacaine hydrochloride (Marcaine) mixed with an equal quantity of 1% lidocaine with epinephrine, may dramatically relieve pain and improve ventilation for 6 to 8 h or longer. If there are any residual tender spots after the intercostal block, they should also be injected with the local anesthetic.

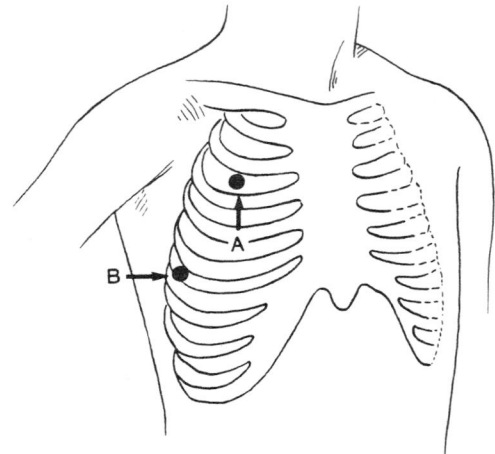

**Fig. 218-1.** Standard sites for tube thoracostomy. A, second intercostal space, midclavicular line, for relief of tension pneumothorax; B, fifth intercostal space, anterior axillary line, for standard tube thoracostomy. (From Roberts JR, Hedges JR: *Clinical Procedures in Emergency Medicine,* 2d ed. Philadelphia, Saunders, 1991, with permission.)

## Ventilatory Support

In patients with chest trauma, impaired ventilation in spite of an open airway, relief of chest wall pain, and drainage of hemopneumothorax is an indication for ventilatory support. Respiratory failure associated with a flail chest is best treated by early endotracheal intubation and ventilatory assistance, particularly if there are associated injuries. Even if the patient's breathing initially seems adequate, ventilatory assistance should be strongly considered in patients with a flail chest if the patient is in shock, has had multiple injuries, is comatose, requires multiple transfusions, is elderly, or has preexisting pulmonary disease. A respiratory rate greater than 30 to 35 breaths per minute, a vital capacity less than 10 to 15 mL/kg, and/or a negative inspiratory force (NIF) less than 25 to 30 cmH$_2$O can also be considered early indications for ventilatory support.

In patients with severe chest trauma, an arterial blood gas should be drawn soon after admission and at frequent intervals thereafter. If arterial P$_{O_2}$ is less than 50mm Hg while the patient is breathing room air or less than 80 mmHg while the patient is breathing supplemental oxygen (equivalent to an F$_{IO_2}$ of 0.4 or more), the patient should generally be given ventilatory assistance. Metabolic acidosis with an arterial P$_{CO_2}$ above 40 mmHg is also evidence of a significant reduction in pulmonary function and is another indication for ventilatory support. If the ventilatory response is adequate, the P$_{CO_2}$ will be less than 35 mmHg if the pH < 7.30, less than 30 mmHg if the pH < 7.20, and less than 25 mmHg if the pH < 7.10.

Continuous pulse oximetry should be part of the initial and continuing evaluation of anyone with moderate to severe chest trauma. Pulse oximetry may allow one to detect pulmonary deterioration much earlier than might be apparent clinically. When used properly, pulse oximetry can also reduce the need for arterial blood gas (ABG) determinations; however, since the Sa$_{O_2}$ indicated by the pulse oximeter is often 2 to 3 percent higher than that seen with ABG, one should try to keep the saturation more than 92 to 93 percent.

## Shock

At the same time that one is ensuring an adequate ventilation, efforts should be directed toward rapidly restoring a more than adequate tissue perfusion. Diebel et al. have shown that after hemorrhagic shock, the cardiac output and oxygen delivery must be 25 to 50 percent

**Table 218-4.** Injuries Present in Patients with Shock After Blunt Chest Trauma

| Injury | Incidence, % | Mortality Rate, % |
|---|---|---|
| Flail chest/multiple rib fracture | 78 | 67 |
| Pelvic/extremity fracture | 59 | 50 |
| Cranial | 48 | 85 |
| Intraabdominal | 41 | 55 |
| Hemothorax | 30 | 38 |
| Lung contusion | 26 | 71 |
| Myocardial contusion | 15 | 75 |
| Diaphragm | 7 | 50 |
| Paraplegia | 7 | 100 |
| Other | 19 | 80 |

*Note:* 27 (7.9%) of 390 patients admitted with blunt chest trauma were in shock in ED.

greater than normal to adequately perfuse and oxygenate the intestinal mucosa and liver.

Other preliminary studies indicate that capnometry [to determine the end tidal P$_{CO_2}$ (PET$_{CO_2}$), particularly if combined with arterial P$_{CO_2}$ determinations so that one can determine the arterial–end tidal CO$_2$ difference [P (a − ET)$_{CO_2}$], can also help monitor the adequacy of tissue perfusion ventilation. In general, a persistent PET$_{CO_2}$ < 28 mmHg or P (a − ET)$_{CO_2}$ > 10 mmHg is an indication of a poor prognosis.

Wilson et al. found that if hypotension is present in patients with blunt chest trauma, it is most likely due to pelvic or extremity fractures (59 percent), intraabdominal injuries (41 percent), and/or intrathoracic bleeding (30 percent). They also noted that 15 percent of these patients had ECG evidence of myocardial contusion (Table 218-4).

In patients with penetrating chest trauma, Wilson et al. found the cause of shock to be intrathoracic injury in 74 percent. The most frequent sources of intrathoracic bleeding were lung (36 percent), heart (25 percent), great vessels (14 percent), and intercostal or internal mammary arteries (10 percent) (Table 218-5). In addition, 40 percent of the patients with penetrating chest trauma had extrathoracic injuries contributing to the shock. These included intraabdominal bleeding (34 percent), bleeding from extremity vessels (6 percent), and spinal cord injuries (5 percent).

## Treatment

### Fluid

Failure to correct hypotension within 15 to 30 min greatly increases the mortality rate. In previously healthy patients requiring massive transfusions but having hypotension for less than 30 min, the mortal-

**Table 218-5.** Injuries in Patients with Shock After Penetrating Chest Trauma

| Injury | Incidence, % | Mortality Rate, % |
|---|---|---|
| Lung | 36 | 52 |
| Intraabdominal | 34 | 51 |
| Heart | 25 | 36 |
| Hemothorax | 14 | 19 |
| Diaphragm | 10 | 40 |
| Chest wall | 7 | 20 |
| Superficial extensive lacerations | 6 | 10 |
| Extremity vessels | 6 | 11 |
| Paraplegia | 5 | 14 |
| Subclavian/innominate artery | 4 | 33 |
| Pulmonary artery or vein | 3 | 80 |
| Aorta | 3 | 80 |
| Superior/inferior vena cava | 3 | 50 |

*Note:* 147 (18.5%) of 796 patients admitted with penetrating chest trauma were in shock in the ED.

ity rate has averaged about 10 percent. However, if the hypotension is present for more than 30 min, the mortality rises to almost 50 percent. If the patient has preexisting disease or is over 65 years of age, the mortality with massive transfusions plus prolonged hypotension exceeds 90 percent.

To provide fluids rapidly in hypotensive patients, one usually needs at least two large IV catheters. If peripheral veins are not readily available, one may be forced to cannulate the subclavian or internal jugular veins. If a subclavian vein line is required, it should be inserted on the side of the injury. If one side of a chest is injured and the other lung is collapsed during insertion of a central IV line, the impaired function of both lungs could be rapidly fatal.

**Chest Tube and Thoracotomy**

A large hemothorax or pneumothorax can seriously interfere with ventilation and venous return; consequently, it should be evacuated as rapidly as possible. If blood is being removed rapidly through the chest tube, the vital signs should be followed very closely. If the vital signs are improving, one can continue to evacuate the blood. However, if the vital signs deteriorate as the blood is being evacuated, in spite of the rapid infusion of IV fluids, the patient may be exsanguinating via the chest tube because the tamponading effect of the hemothorax has been removed. In such circumstances, the chest tube should be clamped and the patient taken directly to the operating room for an emergency thoracotomy.

If it is thought that the bleeding is from an internal mammary or intercostal artery, one can insert a 30-mL balloon Foley catheter into the chest at the injured site, inflate the balloon, and pull it back tightly against the inside of the chest wall. The Foley catheter can also be used to drain blood or air from the pleural cavity, and if adequate pressure is applied with the inflated balloon against the chest wall for 12 to 24 h by taping the stretched tube to the chest wall, the bleeding will usually remain controlled.

## Cardiac Arrest

### External Massage

In patients with cardiac arrest due to chest trauma, external cardiac massage is generally of no value and is in fact likely to be harmful. Since the trauma patient suffering cardiac arrest is generally hypovolemic, external massage is usually ineffective and may actually cause severe additional injury to the heart, liver, lungs, or great vessels. In one series, major cardiovascular disruption was found in all patients receiving external cardiac compressions after truncal trauma. In addition, of the patients receiving forced ventilation and prehospital external cardiac compression, 12 percent died with air emboli in their coronary arteries.

Open cardiac massage is usually performed through an anterolateral incision in the fifth intercostal space on the side of the injury. The pericardium is opened vertically 1 to 2 cm anterior to the phrenic nerve. The thoracic incision allows direct inspection of the heart, control of bleeding sites in the chest, and complete evacuation of any pericardial tamponade or hemopneumothorax. In addition, a left thoracotomy allows the physician to compress or clamp the descending thoracic aorta.

Since about 60 percent of the cardiac output normally goes to the tissues below the diaphragm, clamping the descending thoracic aorta can increase coronary and carotid blood flow almost threefold. If the arterial systolic blood pressure does not rise to 90 mmHg within 5 to 10 min of aortic cross-clamping, further resuscitation will probably be of no avail. On the other hand, if the proximal aortic pressure rises above 160 to 180 mmHg in a previously normotensive individual, it can damage the brain and/or left ventricle.

It is becoming increasingly clear that an emergency department resuscitative thoracotomy can be helpful in selected patients with signs of life within 5 min of arrival in the emergency department and pene-

trating wounds of the chest, neck, or extremities. However, a resuscitative thoracotomy is seldom of benefit in (1) patients with blunt trauma, (2) patients with penetrating abdominal or head injuries, and (3) patients "dead at the scene."

## Diagnosis

### Symptoms

The most frequent symptoms of thoracic trauma are chest pain and shortness of breath. The pain is usually well localized to the involved area of the chest wall, but not infrequently it is referred to the abdomen, neck, shoulder, or arms. Dyspnea and tachypnea are nonspecific and may also be caused by anxiety or pain from other injuries.

### Physical Examination

The most frequent symptoms of thoracic trauma are chest pain and shortness of breath. The pain is usually well localized to the involved area of the chest wall, but not infrequently it is referred to the abdomen, neck, shoulder, or arms. Dyspnea and tachypnea are nonspecific and may also be caused by anxiety or pain from other injuries.

### Physical Examination

Excessive reliance on chest x-rays may lead to delay in performing life-saving procedures. A rather thorough physical examination can be performed rapidly and may provide valuable information to help confirm or rule out any equivocal findings on the x-ray. Tension pneumothorax, in particular, should be diagnosed and treated before obtaining a chest x-ray.

#### Inspection

*Chest Wall*

Without careful inspection of the chest wall, one can easily overlook contusions, flail chest, intrathoracic bleeding, and open ("sucking") chest wounds. The paradoxical motion of a flail chest may be minimal when the patient is first seen, especially if it involves the lateral or posterior thorax.

Although external bleeding is easily recognized, it may be difficult to determine whether the source is intrathoracic or from the chest wall itself. Most chest wounds that communicate with the pleural cavity are readily apparent because of the noise air makes as it passes through the tissue of the chest wall during ventilatory efforts. However, some wounds are open only intermittently and may not be discovered until or unless the patient makes increased ventilatory efforts.

*Neck*

Distended neck veins, especially when the patient is sitting upright, may indicate the presence of pericardial tamponade, tension pneumothorax, cardiac failure, or air embolism. However, distended neck veins may not appear until hypovolemia has been at least partially corrected. If the face and neck are cyanotic and swollen, severe damage to the superior mediastinum, with occlusion or compression of the superior vena cava, should be suspected. Subcutaneous emphysema from a torn bronchus or laceration of the lung can cause severe swelling of the neck and face.

*Abdomen*

A scaphoid abdomen may indicate a diaphragmatic injury with herniation of abdominal contents into the chest. Excessive abdominal movement during breathing may indicate chest wall damage that might not otherwise be apparent. A rocking-horse type of ventilation may indicate a high spinal cord injury with paralysis of intercostal muscles.

*Palpation*

Palpation of the chest should begin with determining whether the trachea is in its normal position, which is in the midline or slightly to the right. Palpation of the chest wall may reveal areas of localized tenderness or crepitation from fractured ribs or subcutaneous emphysema. Well-localized and consistent tenderness over ribs should be considered to be due to rib fractures, even if the initial x-rays appear to be normal.

Motion of a portion of the sternum or severe localized tenderness may be the only objective evidence of a fractured sternum. When a patient is coughing or straining, palpation can sometimes detect abnormal motion of an unstable portion of the chest wall better than visual inspection.

### Percussion

Percussion of the chest wall can be of some help in differentiating between a hemothorax and pneumothorax. Dullness to percussion over one side of the chest following trauma may be the first evidence that a hemothorax is present; hyperresonance, on the other hand, may indicate the presence of a pneumothorax. A fairly large hemothorax can be missed if the chest x-ray is taken while the patient is lying supine.

If the pericardial cavity is greatly distended by an effusion or tamponade, the area of cardiac dullness may extend beyond the midclavicular line on the left or the sternal border on the right. This sign is especially helpful if the point of maximal impulse is located more than an inch inside the left border of cardiac dullness.

### Auscultation

Whenever possible, the chest should be auscultated systematically and thoroughly, anteriorly, laterally, and posteriorly, and at both the bases and apices. If the breath sounds are equal bilaterally, the major bronchi are probably intact.

The presence of bowel sounds high in the chest may be the first indication of a diaphragmatic injury. Decreased breath sounds on one side usually indicate the presence of hemothorax or pneumothorax, but this may also occur if the endotracheal tube is in too far and only one lung is being ventilated. Before inserting a chest tube into a patient with an endotracheal tube and acute respiratory distress, with decreased breath sounds on one side, one should check the position of the endotracheal tube. Occasionally, persistently decreased breath sounds on one side are due to a bronchial foreign body or ruptured bronchus.

## Injury to the Chest Wall

### Soft Tissue Injuries

#### Bleeding

Probing of a penetrating chest wound to determine its depth or direction can be dangerous because it can damage underlying structures and can cause severe recurrent bleeding or a pneumothorax or air leak. Bleeding from chest wall muscles can be rather brisk at times and is best controlled initially by local pressure. Later, one can inspect the depths of the wound in the operating room and use ligatures to control the bleeding and carefully close the wound.

#### Open (Sucking) Chest Wounds

Small open chest wounds can act as one-way valves, allowing air to enter during inspiration but none to leave during expiration, thereby causing an increasing pneumothorax. This not only reduces tidal volume but can also interfere with venous return. If the open chest wound exceeds two-thirds the area of the trachea, air will preferentially enter the pleural cavity through the chest wall opening rather than through the tracheobronchial tree into the lungs.

Sucking wounds of the chest should be covered immediately by a sterile airtight dressing, such as a petrolatum gauze, and a chest tube should be inserted almost simultaneously at a separate site to relieve the pneumothorax. The chest tube is not inserted through the trauma wound because it is then likely to follow the missile or knife tract into the lung or diaphragm.

### Tissue Loss

Injuries caused by close-range shotgun blasts or high-powered rifles may destroy such large quantities of chest wall that it may be impossible to close the chest wall in the usual manner. It is important, however, to cover the lungs and heart and close the diaphragm. For small defects, resection of adjacent ribs and a thoracoplasty may be adequate. With large defects, rotated muscle flaps and/or Marlex mesh may be required.

### Subcutaneous Emphysema

Subcutaneous emphysema usually develops because air from lung parenchyma or the tracheobronchial tree gains access to the chest wall through an opening in the parietal pleura. The air may also reach the chest wall from an interstitial lung injury by dissecting back along the bronchi into the hilum and mediastinum and then into the extrapleural spaces. Extensive subcutaneous emphysema should make one suspect an injury to the pharynx, larynx, or esophagus.

Patients with subcutaneous emphysema should be presumed to have an underlying pneumothorax, even if it is not visible on the chest x-ray. If the patient requires a general anesthetic or is to be placed on a ventilator, a chest tube should be inserted on the involved side(s), after inserting a finger to ensure that a pleural space is present. If subcutaneous emphysema is severe, a major bronchial injury should be suspected and sought by bronchoscopy.

If there appears to be any respiratory difficulty that may be due to mediastinal emphysema, a tracheostomy around which the skin and fascia are closed only loosely may serve to maintain adequate ventilation and also allow a route for air to escape from the mediastinum and subcutaneous tissue. Very rarely, linear incisions into the subcutaneous space of the chest wall may be required to relieve massive subcutaneous emphysema. Once the initiating cause is controlled, subcutaneous emphysema usually disappears gradually over a period of several days.

## Bony Injuries

### Clavicular Fractures

Isolated clavicular fractures due to blunt trauma are usually relatively harmless. Occasionally, however, direct trauma produces sharp fragments that may injure the subclavian vein and produce a moderately large hematoma or venous thrombosis. Rarely, excess callus forming later at the site of a clavicular fracture may press against the subclavian artery or brachial plexus, producing a thoracic outlet syndrome.

### Rib Fractures

#### Simple Fractures

Rib fractures should be assumed to be present in any patient who has localized pain and tenderness over one or more ribs after chest trauma. Up to 50 percent of rib fractures (especially those involving the anterior and lateral portions of the first five ribs) may not be apparent on x-ray, particularly for the first few days after injury. Furthermore, injuries to the cartilaginous portions of the ribs may never be seen on x-ray.

The principal diagnostic goal with clinically suspected rib fractures is the detection of significant complications, especially hemopneumothorax, pulmonary contusion, or major vascular injury. If there is a suspicion of a pneumothorax that is not seen on the initial chest x-ray, the patient should also have inspiratory and expiratory films taken. As a general rule, a pneumothorax is seen better on expiratory chest films where the pneumothorax space takes up a larger percentage of the hemithorax. If the patient has severe trauma, if the rib fractures have sharp fragments, or if the patient has other injuries, serial chest roentgenograms (every 6 to 12 h for 24 to 48 h) should be obtained.

The pain of rib fractures can greatly interfere with ventilation. Strapping the chest with adhesive tape or a rib belt to relieve the pain may be effective in young athletic individuals with only a few rib fractures; however, in less vigorous patients, strapping may significantly reduce ventilation and cause progressive atelectasis. Probably the best analgesic for mild to moderate chest wall pain is acetaminophen with codeine (Tylenol no. 3) or ibuprofen, 600 to 800 mg every 6 to 8 h as needed.

If the patient is admitted, an intercostal nerve block with bupivacaine (Marcaine) may dramatically relieve pain, muscle spasm, and ventilation for 6 to 12 h. Intrapleural catheters for administration of local anesthetics can also relieve chest wall pain quite well. Luchette et al. have shown that epidural analgesia usually works even better, but in many hospitals this requires admission to a step-down intensive care unit (ICU) for apnea monitoring.

### First and Second Rib Fractures

Except with direct trauma, such as with a hammer, it takes great force to fracture the first and second ribs. In one series, 40 percent of patients with fractures of the first and second ribs had myocardial contusion, bronchial tears, or a major vascular injury.

First rib fractures are usually associated with higher mortalities (15 to 36 percent) than any other rib fractures because of the frequent severe associated injuries. However, in the series of Richardson et al., patients with second rib fractures had a higher mortality (27 percent) than those with first rib fractures (15 percent). Two-thirds of the deaths were due to head injury or rupture of major vessels.

### Multiple Rib Fractures

If a patient with fractured ribs, especially ribs 9, 10, and 11, becomes hypotensive and does not have a large hemothorax or tension pneumothorax, intraabdominal bleeding from the liver or spleen should be suspected. In one series of 783 patients with blunt chest trauma, Wilson et al. showed that 71 percent of the patients admitted in shock had a ruptured intraabdominal viscus.

In general, it is wise to hospitalize patients with fractured ribs for at least 24 to 48 h if they cannot cough and clear their secretions adequately, especially if they are elderly or have preexisting pulmonary disease. Admitting the patient also provides time to observe the patient for associated injuries that might not be apparent initially. Aspiration pneumonitis and fat embolism often do not become apparent clinically or on chest x-ray for at least 24 to 48 h.

## Flail Chest

### Pathophysiology

Segmental fractures (i.e., fractures in two or more locations on the same rib) of three or more adjacent ribs anteriorly or laterally often result in an unstable chest wall and the phenomenon known as flail chest. This injury is characterized by a paradoxical inward movement of the involved portion of the chest wall during spontaneous inspiration and outward movement during expiration.

Although the paradoxical motion of the involved chest wall can greatly increase the work of breathing, the main cause of the hypoxemia of flail chest is the underlying lung contusion. In the past, pendelluft (a ventilatory phenomenon referring to movement of air back and forth between the injured and uninjured lungs with each breath) was considered to be an important cause of the hypoxemia seen with flail chest. However, pendulluft is probably significant only when the upper airway is partially obstructed.

Immediately after the injury, little flail may be apparent. Later, as fluid moves into the area of the pulmonary contusion, lung compliance falls, and more pressure is needed to inflate the lungs. The increasing pressure differential between intrathoracic and atmospheric pressure may then overcome the resistance of the muscles attached to the fractured ribs, thereby allowing the involved chest wall to de-velop increasing paradox. In addition, the patient may fatigue rapidly because of the decreased efficiency of ventilation and increased muscle effort. Thus, a vicious cycle of decreasing efficiency of ventilation, increasing fatigue, and hypoxemia may develop. In some instances, the increasing ventilatory fatigue can result in a sudden respiratory arrest.

### Treatment

**Initial therapy.** A severe flail chest can most quickly be managed initially by applying a sandbag or direct pressure over the unstable portion of the chest wall. Although this reduces vital capacity, it can relieve some of the pain, and it increases the efficiency of ventilation.

**Nonventilatory therapy.** Patients with mild to moderate flail chest and little or no underlying pulmonary contusion or associated injuries can often be managed without a ventilator. Trinkle et al. noted that mechanical ventilation is not necessary in many patients with a flail chest and might even be deleterious. Important aspects of their nonventilatory therapy included: (1) relief of pain by analgesics or intercostal nerve block, (2) frequent coughing and chest physiotherapy, and (3) restriction of intravenous fluids to prevent fluid overload. However, ventilatory support was provided if, in spite of this regimen, the arterial $P_{O_2}$ remained less than 80 mmHg on supplemental oxygen.

**Ventilatory support.** Our usual indications for early ventilatory support of patients with flail chest include shock, three or more associated injuries, severe head injury, previous severe pulmonary disease, fracture of eight or more ribs, or age greater than 65 years. In our experience, early (prophylactic) ventilatory assistance in patients with flail chest and one or two additional injuries is associated with a mortality of only 7 percent. This is in sharp contrast to a mortality rate of 69 percent in similar patients in whom ventilatory assistance is delayed until there is clinical evidence of respiratory failure. Ventilated patients seem to do better if intermittent mandatory ventilation (IMV), rather than controlled mandatory ventilation (CMV), is used.

One of the most controversial areas in flail chest management is the role of surgical fixation of the fractured ribs or the sternum. The aim of surgical fixation of the chest is to reduce the need for ventilatory assistance; however, this same objective can often be achieved with improved pain relief and ventilatory support. Although some European surgeons have claimed significant reductions in mortality and morbidity with surgical fixation of the flail chest, it is performed only infrequently in the United States. Galan et al. have pointed out that up to a third of the patients with severe flail chest have severe brain damage and about two-thirds have significant lung contusions. Both of these injuries are considered by some to be contraindications to surgical fixation of the chest wall. Thus, the ideal candidate for surgical fixation of the chest wall is a young patient without lung contusion or brain damage who has a severe and persistent anterolateral flail.

## Sternal Fractures

Fracture of the sternum has long been considered a serious and life-threatening injury. Some authors have reported the mortality rates in patients with sternal fractures to be as high as 45 percent. Sternal fractures occur most often in motor vehicle accidents and have been thought to be associated frequently with cardiovascular injury, particularly myocardial contusions, especially in older women wearing seat belts. Because one study noted a 91 percent (10/11) incidence of impaired motion of the anterior heart wall in patients with a fractured sternum, it was felt that the serial ECGs and creatine phosphokinase isoenzyme (CPK-MB) studies should be done on all these patients every 8 h for the first 24 to 32 h. In clinically suspicious cases, a two-dimensional echocardiogram or radionuclide angiogram is also recommended.

In a large recent study of patients with sternal fractures collected over 6 1/2 years by Brookes et al., it was found that the incidence of sternal fracture as a result of motor vehicle collisions was 3 percent. Contrary to many other studies, the patients with sternal fracture in this series had a very low incidence of cardiac arrhythmias requiring treatment [1.5 percent (4/272)], and the mortality rate was only 0.7 percent. Nevertheless, one should look for underlying injuries, and unstable sternal fractures may produce a significant flail requiring ventilatory support.

## Traumatic Asphyxia

Sudden, severe crushing of the chest may cause subconjunctival hemorrhage or petechiae together with vascular engorgement; edema; and cyanosis of the head, neck, and upper extremities. This clinical picture appears to be due to an abrupt sustained rise in superior vena caval pressure and concurrent closure of the airway after deep inspiration. Although these patients often look moribund initially, Jongewaard et al. have shown that neurologic impairment is usually only temporary, and long-term morbidity is due primarily to associated injuries.

## Injury to the Lungs

### Pulmonary Contusions

#### Pathophysiology

The pathologic changes in pulmonary contusion include interstitial edema with capillary damage, resulting in interstitial and intraalveolar accumulations of fluid. The increasing interstitial edema plus varied amounts of peribronchial extravasation of red blood cells tend to cause a progressive decrease in compliance and an increasing physiologic shunt and hypoxemia for at least 24 to 48 h. If atelectasis and pneumonia can be prevented, the lungs usually improve rapidly over the next 2 to 6 days.

#### Diagnosis

Areas of opacification of the lung seen on the chest x-ray within 6 h of blunt trauma are usually considered to be pulmonary contusions. The lung changes with aspiration pneumonia and fat embolism are not usually seen on chest x-rays for at least 12 to 24 h. The extent of the lung injury seen at thoracotomy or autopsy or on CT scan is usually much greater than suspected from chest x-rays.

#### Treatment

Treatment of pulmonary contusions primarily involves maintenance of adequate ventilation. Chest physiotherapy, intercostal nerve blocks, epidural analgesia, and nasotracheal suction are used as needed to ensure that the patient takes deep breaths and coughs adequately. If ventilatory assistance is required, ventilation with IMV and positive end-expiratory pressure (PEEP) usually provides much better ventilation-perfusion matching, better venous return, and quicker weaning than does standard controlled ventilation.

Patients who have a severe unilateral lung injury and are responding poorly to conventional mechanical ventilation may benefit from synchronous independent lung ventilation (SILV) provided through a double-lumen endobronchial catheter. This technique helps prevent overinflation of the normal lung and underinflation of the damaged, poorly compliant lung.

## Pulmonary Hematomas

Pulmonary hematomas are parenchymal tears filled with blood. These generally resolve spontaneously over a few weeks; however, if they become infected, they can form lung abscesses that may be very difficult to manage. These hematomas are more likely to become infected if a thoracotomy is performed, if there is prolonged chest tube drainage of the pleural cavity, and/or if prolonged ventilatory assistance is required.

## Pulmonary Lacerations with Hemopneumothorax

Major hemorrhage from lacerations of the lung following blunt trauma are usually caused by the sharp ends of fractured ribs. Occasionally, they may be caused by tearing of the lung at pleural adhesions during rapid deceleration injuries. Rarely, the adhesions themselves are quite vascular, and a torn adhesion will bleed enough to cause shock.

## Systemic Air Embolism

In patients with penetrating chest wounds, and particularly those with hemoptysis, positive-pressure ventilation must be used with great care. High ventilatory pressures, especially over 50 cmH$_2$O, may force air from an injured bronchus into an adjacent injured vessel, producing systemic air emboli. This probably accounts for many of the severe arrhythmias or central nervous system (CNS) changes that occur when patients with penetrating chest wounds are intubated and ventilated. One should be particularly concerned about causing systemic air emboli if the patient has hemoptysis.

If systemic air embolism occurs, the head should be lowered, and an immediate thoracotomy should be performed to clamp the injured area of lung and then aspirate air from the heart and ascending aorta. Open cardiac massage with clamping of the ascending aorta may help push air through the coronary arteries. Cardiopulmonary bypass should be instituted promptly if available.

## Intrabronchial Bleeding

Intrabronchial bleeding is poorly tolerated and can rapidly cause death from severe hypoxemia by flooding dependent alveoli. Patients with intrabronchial blood tend to die from "drowning" rather than from hypovolemia. Relatively small amounts of blood infused into a dog trachea over 30 to 60 min cause severe rapid reductions in the P$_{O_2}$ with minimal changes in the Pa$_{CO_2}$ or airway resistance.

In patients with hemoptysis due to trauma, the noninvolved lung should be kept as free of blood as possible, and nasotracheal suction and bronchoscopy should be used as often as necessary. If the bleeding is severe, a double-lumen endotracheal (Carlen) tube can sometimes be used to confine the bleeding to one lung. If a Carlen or similar split-function tube is not available or cannot be inserted, one may insert an endotracheal tube over a flexible bronchoscope into the bleeding main-stem bronchus. The balloon on the endotracheal tube can then be inflated as needed. If the bleeding is from the intubated lung, the endotracheal tube prevents blood from passing into the other lung, and ventilation of the other lung may then be maintained either spontaneously or via a mask or another endotracheal tube.

In some instances, the bleeding can only be controlled by occluding the involved bronchus with a Fogarty balloon catheter or by packing it with gauze until the bleeding site can be controlled surgically.

## Pulmonary Arteriovenous Fistulas

Posttraumatic pulmonary arteriovenous (AV) fistula is rare. Patients with this condition have a history of chest trauma, symptoms and signs of hypoxemia, and may have a bruit on auscultation of the chest. They frequently have an abnormal density on chest roentgenograms. The fistula is treated by surgery or transcatheter embolization.

## Aspiration

Aspiration of gastric contents is quite common after severe trauma, especially if the patient is unconscious. If it is recognized promptly, immediate bronchoscopy should be performed to remove any residual food particles. Immediate irrigation of the tracheobronchial tree with buffered saline or a bicarbonate solution may also help reduce the severity of the chemical pneumonitis, but the value of such irrigation is controversial.

Radiologic changes are usually delayed for more than 12 to 24 h. If an opaque foreign body is aspirated into the tracheobronchial tree, it is usually readily diagnosed on x-ray. However, radiolucent foreign bodies are easily missed. Inspiratory and expiratory chest films may help diagnosis of a one-way valve effect due to a foreign body by demonstrating failure of one lung to empty properly during expiration. Occasionally, a foreign body can remain lodged in various bronchi, causing repeated pulmonary infections or hemoptysis for years before being discovered. Persistent or recurrent cough, atelectasis, or pneumonia after trauma should be indications for bronchoscopy and/or bronchography.

## Hemothorax

### Etiology

Hemothorax requiring a thoracotomy is most frequently caused by bleeding from lung injuries. However, the compressing effect of the shed blood, the high concentration of thromboplastin in the lungs, and the low pulmonary arterial pressure combine to help reduce bleeding from torn lung parenchyma, so that a thoracotomy is needed only in about 5 to 15 percent of patients admitted with chest trauma. The other causes of severe and/or continuing intrathoracic bleeding include damage to the great vessels of the chest or intercostal or internal mammary arteries.

### Pathophysiology

If there is more than 300 to 500 mL of blood in the pleural cavity, it should be removed as completely and rapidly as possible. Large clots can act as a local anticoagulant by releasing fibrinolysins and fibrinogenolysins from their surface. A large hemothorax also restricts ventilation and venous return. Bleeding from multiple small intrathoracic vessels often stops fairly rapidly after the hemothorax is completely evacuated.

### Diagnosis

A hemothorax should be suspected following trauma if the breath sounds are reduced and the chest is dull to percussion on the involved side. Fluid collections greater than 200 to 300 mL can usually be seen on good upright or decubitus roentgenograms of the chest. However, if the patient is supine, more than 1000 mL of blood may easily be missed because it may only produce a mild to moderate diffuse haziness on that side.

Ultrasound diagnostic imaging is a valuable tool in the evaluation of trauma patients. Rozycki et al. feel that ultrasound is a rapid, sensitive, and specific diagnostic modality for detecting abnormal intraabdominal, pleural, and pericardial fluid collections. Of 90 patients with clinically significant injuries, ultrasound imaging successfully detected injury in 71, with a sensitivity of 79 percent and specificity of 96 percent.

### Treatment

#### Thoracentesis

A very small stable hemothorax does not always have to be removed, but it should be carefully observed. If the hemothorax seems large enough to drain, we have avoided needle aspiration and have relied on chest tubes. Needle aspiration of a hemothorax is usually incomplete and may cause a pneumothorax or infection of the hemothorax.

#### Chest Tubes

**Technique.** Chest tubes for treatment of traumatic pneumothorax or hemothorax are usually inserted in the anterior axillary line just behind the lateral edge of the pectoralis major muscle. For a pneumothorax we tend to direct the tube as high and anteriorly as possible without the tip pressing on the mediastinum. For a hemothorax, the tube is usually inserted at the level of the nipple and directed posteriorly and laterally.

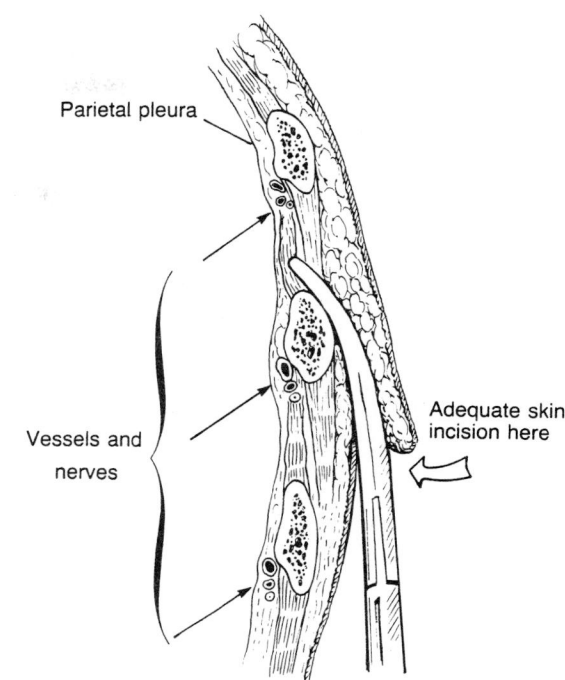

**Fig. 218-2.** The clamp is inserted through the incision and is tunneled up to the next intercostal space. (From Roberts JR, Hedges JR: *Clinical Procedures in Emergency Medicine,* 2d ed. Philadelphia, Saunders, 1991, with permission.)

Once the insertion site is selected, the area around it is painted liberally with an iodophor preparation and then widely draped with a fenestrated sheet. A 22-gauge needle is used to liberally infiltrate the skin, subcutaneous tissue, and intercostal muscles down to the parietal pleura with 1% lidocaine (Xylocaine) with adrenalin, keeping the total amount of lidocaine used below 0.5 mL/kg (5 mg/kg).

A transverse incision 2 to 3 cm in length is then made and extended down to the intercostal muscles. The skin incision for the chest tube should be at least 1 to 2 cm below the interspace through which the tube will be placed. A large clamp is then inserted through the intercostal muscles in the next higher intercostal space, with care taken to prevent the tip of the clamp from penetrating the lung (Fig. 218-2). The resulting oblique tunnel through the subcutaneous tissue and intercostal muscles usually closes promptly after the chest tube is removed, thereby reducing the chances of recurrent pneumothorax.

Once the clamp is pushed through the internal intercostal fascia, it is opened to enlarge the hole to approximately 1.5 to 2 cm. A finger is inserted along the top of the clamp through the hole to verify the position within the thorax and to make sure the lung is not stuck to the chest wall (Fig. 218-3). This is particularly important if a chest x-ray has not been taken or if the x-ray does not clearly show that the lung is away from the chest wall.

For a simple pneumothorax, a 24F or 28F chest tube can be inserted. For a hemothorax, a 32F to 40F chest tube is preferred. The chest tube is grasped at its tip with the clamp and directed through the hole into the pleural space and advanced in the appropriate direction (Fig. 218-4). The tube is advanced until the last side hole is 2.5 to 5 cm (1 to 2 in) inside the chest wall. The tube is secured in place with a long, heavy suture (2–0 or 1–0) of nonabsorbable material placed in a U fashion around the tube. The suture is tied so as to pull the soft tissues snugly around the tube and provide an airtight seal. The tails of the suture can be wrapped around the tube in opposite directions approximately half a dozen times and then tied to secure the tube to the chest wall.

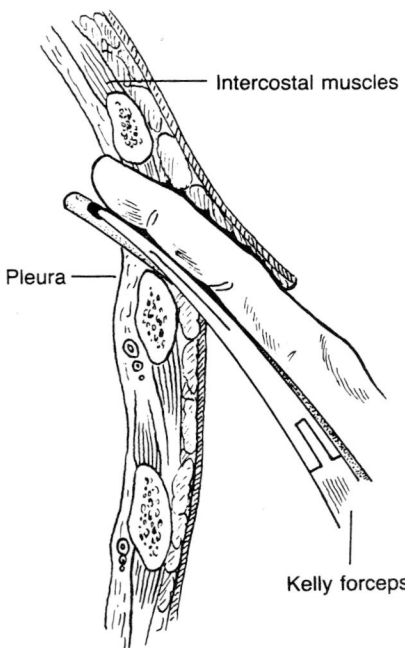

**Fig. 218-3.** Using the finger as a guide, one places the tip into the pleural cavity. The pleura is punctured just above the rib to avoid intercostal vessels and nerves. (From Roberts JR, Hedges JR: *Clinical Procedures in Emergency Medicine,* 2d ed. Philadelphia, Saunders, 1991, with permission.)

The open end of the tube is attached to a combination fluid-collection water-seal suction device, such as the Pleur-evac, with 20- to 30-cmH$_2$O suction (Fig. 218-5). If a significant hemothorax is known to be present or if a large amount of blood starts to drain immediately, consideration should be given to collection of blood in a heparinized autotransfusion device so that it can be returned to the patient either directly or after washing the red blood cells in saline.

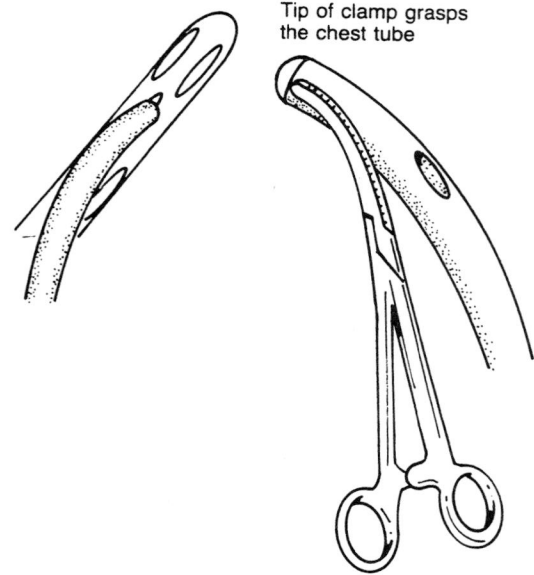

**Fig. 218-4.** The tube is grasped with the curved clamp, with the tube tip protruding from the jaws. (From Roberts JR, Hedges JR: *Clinical Procedures in Emergency Medicine,* 2d ed. Philadelphia, Saunders, 1991, with permission.)

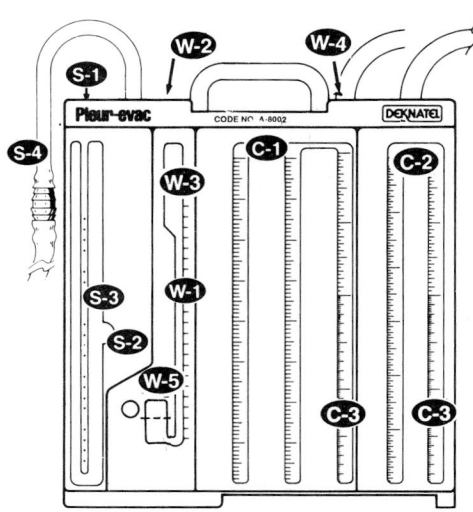

**Fig. 218-5.** Chest drainage. A. Suction control. S-1, atmospheric vent. Use this opening for filling the suction control chamber. This is also the vent to atmosphere. S-2, self-sealing diaphragm on face of unit. Use an 18- or higher-gauge needle, attached to a syringe, to remove fluid from this chamber. S-3, suction control pressure scale. When suction is applied and bubbling occurs, the approximate level of suction imposed is determined by the original fluid level. S-4, suction tubing for connection to suction source. If suction is not required, tubing should remain uncapped and unclamped, to allow air to exit and minimize possibility of tension pneumothorax. B. Water-seal chamber. The water-seal chamber serves three purposes: (1) acts as a one-way valve to allow air to exit from the pleural space; (2) serves as a manometer, measuring the amount of negativity in the patient's chest cavity; (3) allows for observation of the degree of air leak. W-1, water-seal pressure scale (to determine negativity in patient's chest cavity). Without suction, the pressure in the chest cavity is read directly by the fluid level in the calibrated water-seal pressure scale. With suction, add the reading from the suction control chamber setting to the reading of the water-seal pressure scale (e.g., −20 suction plus −10 water seal = −30 cmH$_2$O patient negativity). Patency of the patient's thoracic catheter can be observed as oscillation in the water-seal chamber. The water level rises and falls as the patient breathes. Oscillations may not be present when suction is operative, the lung is fully expanded, or the tubing is blocked or kinked. W-2, positive-pressure relief valve opens with increases in positive pressure, preventing pressure accumulation. W-3, high-negativity float valve preserves the water seal in the presence of high negativity. W-4, filtered high-negativity relief valve is provided to vent excessive negativity. W-5, self-sealing diaphragm is provided in the front of the unit to adjust the water level in the water-seal chamber. C. The major collection chamber is calibrated in 2-mL increments up to 200 mL. Over 200 mL, calibrations are in 5-mL increments. Fluids overflow from one section to the next. The capacity of the major collection chamber is 2000 mL. C-2, the minor collection chamber. Its collection capacity is 1000 mL. C-3, self-sealing diaphragms are provided on the back of the unit for taking laboratory samples of patient drainage. (Adapted from instructions for use of the Pleur-evac, Deknatel, Inc., Fall River, MA.)

After it appears that the chest tube is correctly situated and working properly, a sterile occlusive dressing is placed over the incision, and additional layers of tape are used to secure the tube to the chest wall so that it will not be accidentally pulled out.

The intrathoracic position of the chest tube and its last hole and the amount of air or fluid remaining in the pleural cavity should be checked with a chest x-ray as soon as possible after the tube is inserted. If there is a significant air leak, the chest films are best done as portables at the patient's bedside so as not to risk the development of a tension pneumothorax while the patient is off suction en route to the x-ray department.

If the patient is sent to the radiology department for x-rays, the chest tube should not be clamped because any continuing air leakage can rapidly collapse the lung and/or cause a tension pneumothorax. While the tube is unclamped, the water-seal bottle should be kept 1 to 2 feet lower than the patient's chest.

Serial chest auscultation, chest x-rays, and careful recording of the volume of blood loss and the amount of air leakage are important guides to the functioning of chest tubes. If a chest tube becomes blocked and a significant pneumothorax or hemothorax is still present, the tube should be replaced. This can often be done easily through the same incision. Irrigating an occluded chest tube or passing a Fogarty catheter through it in an effort to reestablish its patency seldom works well and almost certainly increases the risk of infection. If the chest tube is functional and well placed but a decubitus film shows a shift of some of the pleural fluid, the hemothorax is partially clotted; another chest tube placed with ultrasound guidance may be helpful. If a significant hemothorax persists, Mancini et al. report that early evacuation of the clotted blood via thoracoscopy can prevent atelectasis.

If a chest tube is inserted because of a pneumothorax, it is left in place on suction for at least 24 h after all air leaks have stopped. If inserted for bleeding, it is left in place until the drainage is serous and less than 100 mL/24 h. However, if the patient is on a ventilator, many physicians would prefer to keep the chest tubes in to act as a safety valve in case a new pneumothorax suddenly develops.

When the tube is to be removed, the patient is asked to take a deep breath and bear down, as in a Valsalva maneuver. While intrathoracic pressure and lung volume are at their maximum, the tube is quickly pulled out and petrolatum or vaseline gauze is immediately applied as an airtight dressing over the chest tube site. It is important that the patient be in full inspiration when the tube is pulled. The involuntary reflex while the tube is being pulled is a quick inspiratory effort because of the pleural pain. This may rapidly suck in several hundred milliliters of air just as the tube is being removed, necessitating reinsertion of another tube. Some surgeons put only one throw in their initial chest tube suture so that the ends can be unwound from the chest tube and then tied down to provide an airtight seal of the chest tube hole.

Following removal of the chest tube, a chest x-ray should be obtained to rule out a recurrent pneumothorax. Another chest x-ray should be obtained 12 to 24 h later to confirm continued complete expansion of the lungs.

Although there continues to be controversy about the need for prophylactic antibiotics in patients requiring a chest tube for a traumatic hemothorax and/or pneumothorax, a recent review by Wilson of the six available double-blind prospective studies showed a clear reduction in the incidence of pneumonia and/or empyema [18 percent (41/234) versus 3 percent (7/238)] when antibiotics were given until the chest tubes were removed. Studies by Cant et al. suggest that giving antibiotics for just 24 h is adequate, and a study by Demetriades et al. suggests that only one dose of antibiotic need be given.

### Autotransfusion

In patients with massive bleeding into a body cavity, proper collection and autotransfusion of the shed blood may reduce the need for bank blood and its associated risks. Intrathoracic bleeding is generally ideal for this technique because there is usually no contamination of the blood by bile or intestinal contents.

To use shed blood for autotransfusion, one adds citrate or heparin to it as it is removed (to keep it from clotting) and collects it in a special sterile container. The red blood cells are then usually washed with saline. Autotransfused blood can greatly reduce many of the risks of blood transfusion, but in emergency situations, attempts at autotransfusion can be time-consuming and difficult. The suction used for collecting blood for autotransfusion is also not as efficient as the regular suction for keeping the operative field clear. As a consequence, if adequate type-specific blood is readily available, there is little effort to use autotransfusions in many centers. Furthermore, using more than five units of autotransfused blood may contribute to a tendency to a coagulopathy. If the cells are washed in a cell-saver, more autotransfused blood can be given safely, but there is still some concern about the patient developing a coagulopathy. In our own hospital it is generally easier and much faster to use bank blood unless: (1) the bleeding is massive and not rapidly controllable by surgery, (2) the blood type is rare, and (3) there is difficulty with the cross-matching.

### Thoracotomy

Most patients with intrathoracic bleeding can be treated adequately by intravenous administration of fluids and evacuation of the hemothorax with a chest tube. Only 9 percent of our patients with penetrating chest wounds have required a thoracotomy for continuing hemorrhage. Thoracotomy for intrathoracic bleeding is generally indicated if (1) the patient's vital signs remain or become unstable, (2) more than 1500 mL of blood is lost from the chest tube in the first 12 to 24 h and there is continued bleeding, (3) the drainage of blood from the chest tubes exceeds 300 mL/h for 3 to 4 h, or (4) the chest remains more than half full of blood on x-ray.

Occasionally, when the chest tube is initially inserted, blood emerges at an alarmingly rapid rate. If the patient's condition improves as the blood is being removed, continuing drainage of the blood and observation of the patient are in order. However, if the patient's vital signs deteriorate as the blood is being removed, loss of the tamponading effect of the hemothorax has probably allowed serious bleeding from the lung to recur. Consequently, the chest tube should be clamped, and the patient taken directly to surgery.

## Pneumothorax

### Pathophysiology

Collections of air or blood within the pleural cavity reduce vital capacity and increase intrathoracic pressure, thereby decreasing minute ventilation and venous return to the heart. During inspiration, the negative intrapleural pressure increases the tendency for air or blood to leak into the pleural cavity through any wound in the lung or chest wall. If there is any obstruction of the upper airway or if the patient has chronic obstructive lung disease, additional air may be forced into the pleural cavity during expiration, increasing the likelihood of tension pneumothorax with intrapleural pressures exceeding atmospheric pressure.

### Diagnosis

Failure to obtain a chest x-ray soon after admission and again in 4 to 8 h may result in missing significant intrathoracic injuries. The presence of a chest injury is usually readily apparent from the history and physical examination; however, accurate assessment of the damage, especially to intrathoracic organs, often requires serial chest x-rays and/or a CT scan.

A pneumothorax is not likely to cause severe symptoms unless it (1) is a tension pneumothorax, (2) occupies more than 40 percent of one hemithorax, or (3) occurs in a patient with shock or preexisting cardiopulmonary disease. If there is a suspicion of a pneumothorax but it is not clearly seen on the first chest roentgenogram, repeat films during expiration may be helpful. Apical-lordotic films may allow better visualization of an apical pneumothorax. Occasionally, a pneumothorax after a stab wound is delayed for more than 12 h. Consequently, serial chest x-rays every 6 h for 12 to 24 h are indicated in selected patients. In a recent study of 4106 patients with initially asymptomatic stab wounds of the chest, Ordog et al. found that 12 percent of the patients required a tube thoracostomy for a delayed hemothorax or pneumothorax.

One should assume that a tension pneumothorax is present and begin treatment without waiting for a chest x-ray if the patient has: (1) severe respiratory distress, (2) decreased breath sounds and hyperresonance on one side of the chest, (3) distended neck veins, and (4) deviation of the trachea away from the involved side. Insertion of a large needle into the involved side through the second intercostal space in the midclavicular line may help confirm the diagnosis and provide temporary relief while a chest tube is inserted.

A small pneumothorax (less than 1.0 cm wide and confined to the upper one-third of the chest) that is unchanged on two chest roentgenograms taken 4 to 6 h apart in an otherwise healthy individual can usually be treated by observation alone. However, in most instances after trauma, a chest tube or small catheter should be inserted as a precautionary measure, especially if the patient cannot continue to be observed closely.

Occasionally a small pneumothorax is not apparent on chest x-rays but is seen on a CT scan of the chest or abdomen. This is referred to as an "occult pneumothorax." Collins et al. have found that chest tube drainage of an occult pneumothorax is not required unless the patient is going to be on a ventilator. Enderson et al. noted that 38 percent (8/21) of occult pneumothoraces had progression in patients who were on positive pressure ventilation.

If only a pneumothorax is present, a small- to moderate-sized (24F to 28F) chest tube may be inserted anteriorly in the second intercostal space in the midclavicular line. However, a high midaxillary tube is generally preferable. Although some physicians insert chest tubes over trocars because it is less painful, especially if the lung is well away from the chest wall, we believe it is safer to avoid the trocar and insert chest tubes using a large hemostat. Catheter aspiration of a simple pneumothorax (CASP) is most suitable for the treatment of pneumothoraces caused by needles or catheters.

### Complications

In general, a small- or moderate-sized pneumothorax does not cause problems unless there is a continuing air leak or the patient has other trauma or preexisting cardiopulmonary disease. Also, a continuing air leak does not usually result in complications if the lung is completely expanded. However, if a combination of a pneumothorax and continued air leak is allowed to exist for more than 24 to 48 h, the incidence of empyema and bronchopleural fistula is greatly increased.

The most frequent reasons for failure to evacuate a pneumothorax rapidly and to completely expand the lungs are: (1) improper connections or leaks in the external tubing or water-seal collection apparatus, (2) improper position of the chest tube(s), (3) occlusion of bronchi by secretions or a foreign body, (4) a tear of one of the large bronchi, or (5) a large tear of the lung parenchyma. If a pneumothorax persists in spite of one or two well-placed chest tubes and there is a large leak, emergency bronchoscopy should be performed to clear the bronchi and identify any damage to the tracheobronchial tree that may need repair. Continued large air leakage and failure of the lung to expand adequately in spite of these measures is an indication for early thoracotomy to control the air leak.

## Pneumomediastinum

Subcutaneous emphysema in the neck should make one look closely for a pneumomediastinum. The diagnosis of pneumomediastinum should also be suspected from the presence of a crunching sound (Hamman sign) over the heart during systole. The diagnosis is usually readily apparent on CT scans, but it can easily be missed on chest x-rays. Traumatic pneumomediastinum is of itself usually asymptomatic, but one must look closely for an injury to the larynx, trachea, major bronchi, pharynx, or esophagus.

## Tracheobronchial Injury

### Lower Trachea and Major Bronchi

Most injuries to major bronchi are due to rapid deceleration and shearing of more mobile bronchi from relatively fixed proximal structures. However, forced expiration against a closed glottis and/or compression against the vertebral column may cause bursting of these structures.

Numerous reports have emphasized that the most common presenting signs and symptoms are dyspnea, hemoptysis, subcutaneous emphysema, Hamman sign, and sternal tenderness. A large pneumothorax, pneumomediastinum, deep cervical emphysema, and an endotracheal tube balloon with a round appearance on chest roentgenograms may suggest tracheobronchial injury; however, approximately 10 percent are almost completely asymptomatic.

Most tracheobronchial injuries occur within 2 cm of the carina or at the origin of lobar bronchi. On bronchoscopy the usual bronchial injury seen is a transverse tear in a main bronchus or a disruption at the origin of an upper lobe bronchus. The characteristic injury in the trachea is a vertical tear in the membranous portion near its attachment to the tracheal cartilages.

Even if the lung expands and the air leak stops, lacerations of the bronchi involving more than a third of the circumference should be repaired because they tend to eventually cause severe bronchial stenosis with repeated pulmonary infections or complete atelectasis. Untreated tracheal tears may result in severe mediastinitis.

The majority of airway injuries can be corrected using standard techniques. With complex ruptures, cardiopulmonary bypass can provide safety during correction of the lesion and may encourage repair of the involved lung rather than its resection.

The only patients who survive a tracheal transection generally have their injury in the cervical trachea and have no associated injuries. Intrathoracic tracheal transection is usually associated with two or more major injuries and is almost invariably fatal. Concurrent esophageal injuries occur in almost 25 percent of penetrating tracheobronchial injuries and are easily missed unless esophagoscopy or contrast studies are also performed.

### Cervical Tracheal Injuries

Injuries to the cervical trachea from blunt trauma usually occur at the junction of the trachea and cricoid cartilage. This is most frequently caused by striking the anterior neck against the dashboard in an automobile accident. Evidence of trauma to the neck with subcutaneous emphysema should arouse suspicion of this injury. Inspiratory stridor usually indicates a 70 to 80 percent upper airway obstruction. However, cricotracheal separation is often only suspected when an endotracheal tube or bronchoscope cannot be inserted past the cricoid cartilage.

If the patient has a laceration of the trachea that is small and high, it may be managed simply by performing a tracheostomy below the injury. All lacerations of the trachea should be repaired.

## Diaphragmatic Injury

### Etiology

In urban centers, diaphragmatic injuries are caused most frequently by penetrating trauma, particularly gunshot wounds of the lower chest or upper abdomen. Rupture due to blunt trauma is much less frequent and occurs in only 4 to 5 percent of patients hospitalized with chest trauma. If there is a fracture of the pelvis, the incidence increases to about 8 to 10 percent.

Because of the protective effect of the liver on the right and the possible increased weakness of the left posterolateral diaphragm, most series report that 80 to 90 percent of the diaphragmatic injuries following blunt trauma occur in that area. However, in the series of

Brown and Richardson, the incidence of right- and left-sided diaphragmatic rupture was almost equal.

## Natural History

Since 60 to 70 percent of normal ventilation depends on proper function of the diaphragm, trauma to this structure can cause serious ventilatory problems. However, the initial signs and symptoms are often masked by other injuries. Unless the diaphragmatic lesion is large, symptoms due to abdominal viscera in the thoracic cavity usually occur rather late. Over time, sometimes even years, a large amount of viscera can gradually work up into the chest through small diaphragmatic tears. The intrathoracic bowel may then become obstructed or strangulated or cause severe compression of the adjacent lung, a phenomenon we have referred to as "tension enterothorax."

## Diagnosis

With penetrating trauma, the diagnosis of diaphragmatic injury is often made only intraoperatively. However, if the entrance wound is in the abdomen and there is evidence of an intrathoracic injury or foreign body, one can assume that the missile or knife has transgressed the diaphragm. In the series just mentioned, 59 percent of the patients with diaphragmatic injuries had diagnostic chest x-rays. However, eight of nine peritoneal lavages done in these patients were negative. In the only positive lavage, the lavage fluid drained out through a previously placed chest tube.

With blunt trauma, any abnormality of the diaphragm or lower lung fields on chest x-ray should arouse suspicion of a diaphragmatic tear. Occasionally a nasogastric tube is seen to go into the abdomen and then back up into the chest because the stomach has passed through a diaphragmatic tear.

Techniques for diagnosing the less obvious diaphragmatic injuries include: (1) peritoneal lavage with a chest tube in place; (2) upper gastrointestinal (GI) series, looking for displacement of viscera into the chest; (3) pneumoperitoneum with carbon dioxide; (4) CT scan with contrast; and (5) intraperitoneal technetium sulfur colloid. However, up to 50 percent of diaphragmatic injuries are only diagnosed during a thoracotomy or laparotomy. Blunt injury of the right diaphragm may be particularly difficult to diagnose.

## Therapy

Laparotomy is necessary to repair the diaphragm. Thoracotomy may be necessary for associated chest injury, for resuscitation, for delayed repair of the diaphragm, or for management of thoracic complications.

## HEART

## Penetrating Injury to the Heart

The many factors affecting survival from penetrating injury to the heart include the weapon used, the size of the myocardial injury, the injured cardiac chamber, coronary artery damage, the presence of tamponade, associated injuries, and the time taken to reach the hospital. Every patient with penetrating chest injury anywhere near the heart and shock on admission should be considered as having a cardiac injury until proven otherwise.

With early aggressive resuscitation and surgery, up to one-third of patients arriving in a trauma center "in extremis" with a cardiac injury can be saved. In patients brought to the operating room with signs of life and a recordable blood pressure, the survival rate should exceed 70 percent for gunshot wounds and 85 percent for stab wounds. In one series, 23 consecutive patients with isolated penetrating injuries of the heart reaching the operating room alive survived.

Prognosis with penetrating cardiac injuries is closely related to the cardiovascular-respiratory component of the Trauma Score (CVRS).

The CVRS reflects individual elements of blood pressure (0–4), respiratory rate (0–4), respiratory effort (0–1), and capillary refill (0–2). A highest possible CVRS of 11 indicates a systolic blood pressure greater than 90 mmHg, a respiratory rate between 10 and 24/min with normal effort, and normal capillary refill. A lowest possible CVRS of 0 indicates no blood pressure, no carotid pulse, no respiratory effort, and no capillary refill.

## Pathophysiology

Penetrating wounds of the heart are usually rapidly fatal, generally because of massive hemorrhage; fewer than one-fourth of the patients with this injury reach the hospital alive. Patients surviving more than 15 to 30 min usually have either a small wound or some component of pericardial tamponade. In a sense, pericardial tamponade is a two-edged sword; although it may prolong life by reducing the initial blood loss, the tamponade itself can be fatal by interfering with diastolic filling of the heart.

## Diagnosis

### Clinical Features

All patients in shock with a penetrating wound of the chest between the midclavicular line on the right and the anterior axillary line on the left should be considered to have a cardiac injury until proven otherwise. If the only problem is tamponade and the patient is not hypovolemic, the Beck I triad may be present. This consists of distended neck veins, hypotension, and muffled heart tones. The last is the least reliable sign; even with a large acute pericardial tamponade, which seldom is more than 200 mL, the heart tones are usually fairly clear.

Since patients with penetrating heart wounds are usually hypotensive, the neck veins will generally not distend until the blood volume is at least partially restored. On the other hand, chest injuries can cause the patient to breathe abnormally or strain, thereby causing neck vein distension, even in the absence of tamponade. Other causes of Beck's triad include tension pneumothorax, myocardial contusion, acute myocardial infarction, and systemic air embolism.

Tamponade may also cause two Kussmaul signs. One is increased distension of neck veins during inspiration, and the other is pulsus paradoxus. Paradoxical pulse is characterized by a drop in systolic blood pressure of more than 10 to 15 mmHg during normal spontaneous inspiration. The amount of paradox may be increased by hypovolemia, and bronchospasm is the most frequent cause of pulsus paradoxus.

### Invasive Monitoring

As the volume of blood in the pericardial cavity increases, this will produce an equalization of the diastolic pressures in all chambers, which should make one suspicious of tamponade. At the same time, stroke volume will tend to fall.

Central venous catheters that are inserted past the superior vena cava–right atrial junction can perforate the heart and cause tamponade.

### X-Rays

Chest films are generally of little help in diagnosing acute cardiac injury, except in the unusual patient with intrapericardial air. Since the average acute tamponade has only 150 to 200 mL of blood and clots, significant early enlargement of the cardiac shadow is unusual. The x-ray may, however, reveal a hemopneumothorax or mediastinal pathology that might not otherwise be noted.

### ECG

Electrocardiography changes following cardiac injury are usually nonspecific. ST-T wave changes may indicate pericardial irritation or may reflect associated ischemia or hypoxia.

### Echocardiography

Echocardiography can identify pericardial fluid and may help localize missile fragments in the pericardium.

### Pericardiocentesis

#### *Accuracy*

There is an increasing tendency to avoid the use of pericardiocentesis as a diagnostic procedure in acutely injured patients with possible tamponade. In Demetriades' series, the incidence of false-negative pericardiocentesis was 80%, and the incidence of false-positives was 33%. In addition to its inaccuracy, attempts at pericardiocentesis may injure the heart or cause dangerous delays in needed surgery.

#### *Technique*

The paraxiphoid approach is commonly used. An 18-gauge, 10-cm spinal needle is attached to a stopcock and then to a 20-mL syringe. The pericardiocentesis should be done with continuous ECG monitoring if possible. The ECG monitoring is more sensitive if one attaches the V lead of the ECG to the metal pericardiocentesis needle using an insulated wire with alligator clips on both ends.

The needle is passed upward and backward at an angle of 45° for 4 to 5 cm and advanced slowly until the point seems to enter a cavity (Fig. 218-6). Most authors direct the needle toward the left scapula tip; however, directing the needle toward the right scapula is more likely to parallel the right border of the heart and is less likely to penetrate the right ventricle.

One should aspirate every 1 to 2 mm as the needle is advanced. One can insert a stylet or inject 0.5 to 1.0 mL of saline solution at intervals to be certain that the needle is not plugged. The needle is then carefully advanced until blood is obtained, cardiac pulsations are felt, or the ECG shows an abrupt change.

Generally, a large portion of the blood in the pericardial cavity is clotted. Consequently, one can usually remove only a few milliliters of blood without manipulating the needle. If 20 mL of blood can be drawn out easily and rapidly, it usually indicates that the blood is being aspirated from the right ventricle.

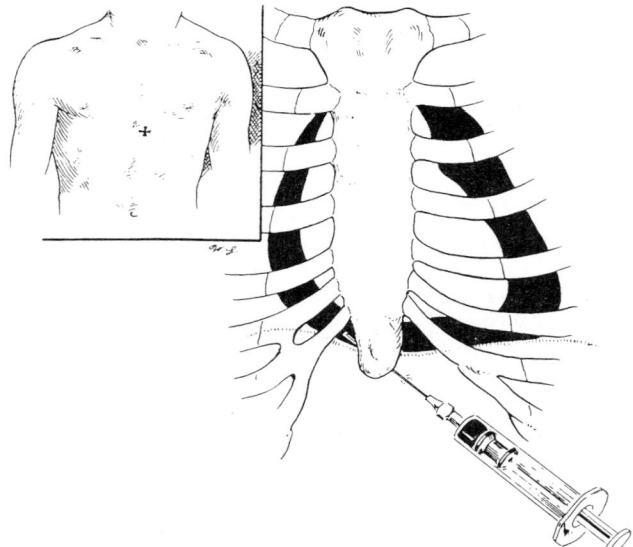

**Fig. 218-6.** The paraxiphoid technique for pericardiocentesis is usually performed with the needle directed toward the left shoulder or left scapula tip. *However,* if one aims toward the tip of the right scapula, the needle tends to go parallel to the lateral border of the right heart and is less apt to penetrate the coronary artery or myocardium. [From Wilson RF: Injury to the heart and great vessels, in Henning RS (ed): *Critical Care Cardiology.* NY, Churchill, 1989.]

If an immediate thoracotomy is not possible in a patient with a positive pericardiocentesis, a plastic catheter (inserted over a needle or Seldinger wire) can be left in place for continuous drainage of intrapericardial blood until the cardiac wound can be surgically repaired.

#### *Complications*

The pericardiocentesis needle can perforate the right ventricle or a coronary artery and cause tamponade. Arrhythmias may also occur. A falsely negative pericardiocentesis may delay needed surgery.

### Subxiphoid Pericardial Windows

If the patient has been hemodynamically stable and echocardiography is either not available or is equivocal, an alternative method for diagnosing pericardial tamponade is a subxiphoid pericardial window. Although this can occasionally be performed under local anesthesia in the emergency department in a cooperative patient, it is best done in the operating room under general anesthesia. If blood is found in the pericardium, the incision can be extended up as a midsternotomy to repair the cardiac wound.

In a recent study by Ordog et al. of 4106 patients who were initially asymptomatic after a stab of the chest, four patients had initially unsuspected cardiac wounds and two of these patients died in the operating room. A subxiphoid pericardial window or thoracoscopy might have provided an earlier diagnosis in these patients. In hemodynamically stable patients with precordial stab wounds, a subxiphoid window will reveal intrapericardial blood in about 14 percent.

## Treatment

### Fluid Replacement

It is essential that patients with penetrating wounds of the chest have two or more large IV lines in place, with at least one line in a leg vein in the event that the superior vena cava or one of its major branches is injured. It is particularly important to have an adequate or increased blood volume if hypovolemia or tamponade is present. If tamponade is present with an elevated central venous pressure, one should generally not be reluctant to administer further fluid and blood to improve venous return to the heart while moving the patient to an operating room. Gyhra has shown that rapid infusions of saline can restart bleeding from wounds in the heart in spite of the tamponade.

### Pericardiocentesis

Patients who are in shock and may have a cardiac injury should have an emergency thoracotomy as soon as possible. If it is not possible to perform an emergency thoracotomy promptly, continuing pericardiocentesis to relieve the suspected tamponade should be attempted.

Pericardiocentesis is primarily a diagnostic procedure, but removal of as little as 5 to 10 mL of blood from the pericardial sac may increase stroke volume by 25 to 50 percent, with a dramatic improvement in cardiac output and blood pressure. In patients who have small puncture wounds of the heart, pericardiocentesis may be curative, and the patient may not require a thoracotomy as long as the vital signs remain stable for at least 24 to 48 h after the procedure.

### Thoracotomy

Occasionally, a highly selected stable patient with a small penetrating cardiac injury, such as by a needle or ice pick, may be successfully treated without surgery. However, virtually all patients with shock and a suspected injury to the heart should have emergency thoracotomy to completely relieve the tamponade and to repair any injuries found.

#### *Incision*

For penetrating wounds over the precordium thought to involve the heart, an anterolateral thoracotomy is performed in the left fifth intercostal space, which is one interspace below the male nipple (Fig. 218-7). The incision should be as long as possible, extending from just lateral to the sternum to a point high in the axilla. In females, the

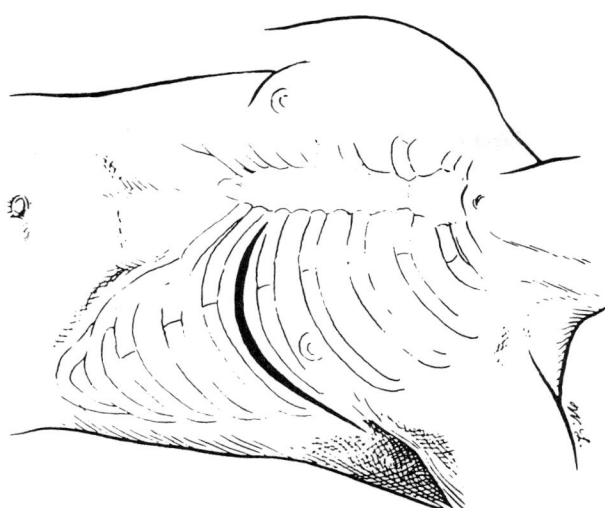

**Fig. 218-7.** Emergency thoracotomy to treat a stab wound of the heart or to perform open cardiac massage is usually done through an anterolateral thoracotomy approach. The incision extends along the fifth intercostal space with the skin incision placed in the inframammary crease. It extends from just lateral to the sternum to the midaxillary line. (From Geller ER: *Shock and Resuscitation.* New York, McGraw-Hill, 1993.)

breast is displaced upward, and the incision is made through the breast crease. The incision is extended through the intercostal muscle into the pleural cavity, with care taken not to injure the underlying lung or heart. A rib spreader is then inserted and opened widely so that two hands can fit inside the chest (Fig. 218-8). Cutting the intercostal cartilages above and below the incision may help increase the exposure. Not infrequently the internal mammary vessels, which lie about 0.5 to 1.0 cm lateral to the sternum, are cut, and, if so, they must be clamped and tied or suture-ligated.

When the injury is to the right of the sternum, a right thoracotomy

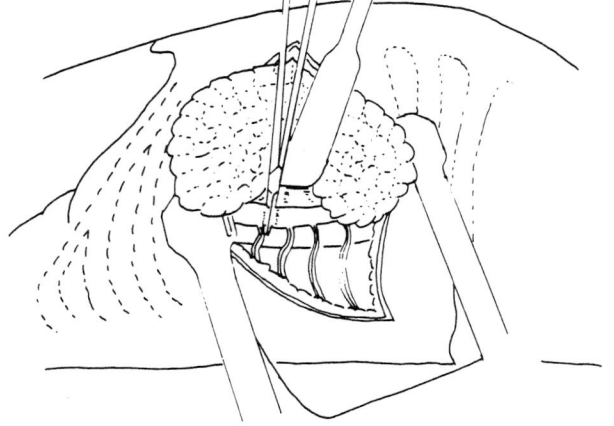

**Fig. 218-8.** If the descending thoracic aorta is to be cross-clamped, it is best done under direct vision. To accomplish this, the anterior thoracotomy must be large and the incision opened as widely as possible. The left lung is pulled up anteriorly as far as possible by an assistant standing at the right side of the table. The pleura and fascia anterior to the aorta is thin, but the tissue between the aorta and the vertebral column is often rather tough and must be incised for the surgeon to get around the aorta properly. A straight clamp is often easier to put around the aorta than a curved clamp and is less likely to rupture the intercostal vessels. (From Geller ER: *Shock and Resuscitation.* New York, McGraw-Hill, 1993.)

is initially performed to control any bleeding sites, but strong consideration should be given to extending the incision across the sternum as a bilateral thoracotomy so as to be able to also control the descending aorta and, if needed, massage the heart more effectively. The sternum can be divided with a rib cutter. A bilateral anterolateral thoracotomy allows wide exposure of both sides of the heart and the proximal great vessels. In patients with a cardiac arrest, there is usually minimal bleeding from the thoracotomy incision until the circulation is restored. However, once circulation is restored, incisional bleeding may become quite severe, especially from the internal mammary arteries, which should be suture-ligated.

In hemodynamically stable patients with penetrating anterior chest trauma, Mitchell et al. have pointed out that a midsternotomy provides superior exposure for the organs most apt to be injured. They feel that an anterolateral or lateral thoracotomy should be reserved for hemodynamically unstable patients, particularly if posterior mediastinal injury is suspected or aortic cross-clamping is apt to be needed.

### Pericardiotomy

Even when the pericardial sac is not distended with blood, it can be difficult to grasp the pericardium with a forceps. It may be necessary at times to "hook" the pericardium with one blade of a scissors and then grab it with a forceps or clamp. Another technique is to very carefully incise the pericardium near the apex of the heart with a small-bladed knife to produce a hole just big enough to allow the tip of one blade of a scissors. If a scalpel is used to open the pericardial sac, inadvertent injury to the underlying myocardium or left anterior descending coronary artery can easily occur.

The pericardial sac should then be opened from the diaphragm below to the great vessels above with a scissors in a longitudinal direction 1 to 2 cm anterior to the left (or right) phrenic nerve. If the pericardial sac is still tight around the heart, a transverse cut of the anterior pericardium just above the central diaphragm may greatly help with exposure. The surgeon should then manually evacuate the liquid blood and clots in the pericardial sac and begin cardiac massage if it is needed.

### Clamping the Descending Aorta

The second maneuver in the patient with severe hypotension or a cardiac arrest is compression or clamping of the descending thoracic aorta to help improve coronary and cerebral arterial flow. Since more than 60 percent of the cardiac output goes through the descending thoracic aorta, cross-clamping this vessel can increase blood flow to the coronary and cerebral arteries two- to threefold.

To expose the descending aorta, an assistant on the right side of the patient lifts the left lung anteriorly, almost out of the hemithorax, so that the aorta can be seen from the left side of the table. The pleura and fascia in front of the aorta are easily opened, but the tougher posterior tissue between the aorta and the vertebral bodies often has to be incised sharply.

After the aorta has been exposed, a finger or a vascular clamp can be hooked around it. In this way, clamping is performed under direct vision, and the chances of intercostal or esophageal injuries are reduced. To be sure that the clamp is applied properly, one should feel pulsations from the spontaneous heart beat or cardiac massage above the clamp but none below. If a nasogastric tube is not in place and there is little or no blood pressure, one can sometimes mistake the esophagus for the aorta. After the clamp is applied, the time is noted, and the left lung is allowed to drop back into the thorax.

### Clamping Injured Lung

If there is an obvious associated lung injury, it should be controlled with a vascular clamp or a lung clamp to prevent systemic air embolism and to stop the bleeding and air leak until more definitive control can be accomplished. If there is a large central lung injury, one should put a clamp across the hilum. If the hilar clamp does not control the bleeding because the injury is too close to the heart, one may have to clamp the pulmonary vessels inside the pericardium.

### Examining the Heart

If the bleeding site(s) is (are) not obvious, one should first carefully examine the right ventricle and right atrium, which are the chambers most apt to be injured. If an injury is still not seen, the heart can be swung out laterally and anteriorly into the left hemithorax to allow better examination of the remainder of the heart. When examining the posterior heart, one should be very careful because lifting the heart straight up increases the possibility of entry of air into a left-sided or posterior cardiac perforation, and this could result in sudden fatal coronary or cerebral air embolism.

### Controlling Cardiac Wounds

Most atrial wounds can be controlled by the application of a Satinsky vascular clamp and then sewn with a running 3–0 or 4–0 polypropylene suture. Wounds of the ventricles can generally be tamponaded by the operator's finger while pledgeted horizontal mattress sutures of 2–0 silk or Prolene are passed under the finger and tied by an assistant. When a wound lies next to a major coronary artery, mattress sutures are placed beneath the artery so as to avoid ligation or compression of the vessel. Cardiac stapling can also be highly effective in the initial management of simple penetrating cardiac wounds.

For handling more difficult cardiac wounds, several other techniques are available. The insertion of a 5- or 30-mL balloon Foley catheter into a large or inaccessible (posterior) defect may allow for control of hemorrhage until a purse-string suture can be applied around the hole. Use of such a catheter also allows one to infuse fluids very rapidly, directly into the heart.

Wide horizontal mattress sutures placed on either side of a large defect and pulled together can also be used to control hemorrhage until cardiopulmonary bypass can be instituted. If cardiopulmonary bypass is not readily available, occlusion of the superior vena cava and inferior vena cava by vascular tapes or clamps can allow quick repair of large defects without causing exsanguinating hemorrhage. Before restarting the heart, if the caval occlusion technique is used, all air is evacuated from the various cardiac chambers by allowing bleeding through the injury prior to tying the final suture and then inserting large needles into the apex of the right and left ventricles while the heart is cautiously massaged.

### Cardiac Massage

Once cardiorrhaphy had been completed, internal cardiac massage can be performed as needed by compressing the heart between the palms of two hands or between one palm and the sternum. Warm— preferably 40 to 42.2°C (104 to 108°F)—saline solution poured over the heart may help prevent ventricular fibrillation. If ventricular fibrillation occurs, defibrillation with internal paddles, starting at 20 to 40 W·s should be performed. Lidocaine, correction of severe acidosis or alkalosis, and IV infusions of 1 to 2 g of $MgSO_4$ may help prevent recurrent ventricular fibrillation.

### Air Embolism

If severe arrhythmias or cardiac arrest develops during endotracheal intubation or while the chest is being opened, aspiration of the cardiac chambers for air should be performed immediately. Systemic air embolism is most frequently diagnosed by seeing air bubbles in the coronary arteries. This serious complication is seldom mentioned in the literature, but we see it in at least 20 percent of our patients with penetrating truncal trauma who have a cardiac arrest in the emergency department after endotracheal intubation.

### Continued Care

Once the heart develops a satisfactory rhythm, the descending thoracic aorta is gradually declamped as infusions of fluid and blood are administered, with care taken to keep the systolic blood pressure

above 90 to 100 mmHg. One should also avoid systolic blood pressures greater than 160 to 180 mmHg because it may tear open cardiac repairs, excessively dilate the left ventricle, and/or cause intracerebral bleeding. The use of vigorous inotropes, such as epinephrine, should be particularly avoided at this point, as they may cause sudden, severe hypertension and can also increase the risk of recurrent ventricular fibrillation.

After the cardiac wounds and all bleeding vessels are controlled and an adequate cardiac output has been obtained, all clot is washed out of the pericardial and pleural cavities. One must look closely to make sure that the internal mammary arteries are intact or carefully suture-ligated. If the heart is edematous or dilated, the pericardium can be left open. Occasionally, the sternum cannot even be closed. In such instances, the skin can usually be stapled. The sternum can then be closed after several days when the cardiac edema and dilatation have resolved.

### Coronary Artery Injuries

Ligation of the cut ends is the treatment of choice for lacerations of small coronary vessels. Torn proximal coronary arteries may also be ligated if there is no evidence of cardiovascular dysfunction. However, such patients must be observed closely. If a large proximal coronary artery laceration results in arrhythmias, myocardial infarction, or impaired hemodynamic function, an aortocoronary revascularization with a saphenous vein graft should be performed under cardiopulmonary bypass.

### Ventricular Septal Defects

Up to 5 percent of patients with penetrating cardiac trauma will be found to have a ventricular septal defect postoperatively. Cross-sectional echocardiography is ideally suited for such assessment. If the patient is in heart failure, emergency cardiac catheterization and surgery may be required; however, in most instances, one can wait 2 to 3 months to correct the defect.

### Valve Injuries

Most valvular injuries that are detected postoperatively can be corrected 3 to 6 months later on an elective basis after cardiac catheterization. Occasionally, however, severe cardiac failure or dysfunction at the initial procedure will require an emergency valve repair or replacement.

## Blunt Injury to the Heart

### Etiology and Mechanisms of Injury

The most common cause of blunt cardiac trauma is a high-speed motor vehicle accident. However, myocardial injury has been documented in accidents involving vehicles going less than 20 mph. Other causes include direct blows to the chest, industrial crush injuries, falls from heights, blast injuries, and athletic trauma.

The heart is suspended relatively freely within the chest cavity from the great vessels, and this mobility plus its location between the sternum and the thoracic vertebrae make it susceptible to injury as a result of several mechanisms: (1) sudden horizontal acceleration and/or deceleration, causing the heart to impact against the sternum and vertebrae; (2) a compression between the sternum and vertebrae following a direct forceful blow to the chest; (3) a sudden increase in intrathoracic and intracardiac pressures, causing disruption of the myocardium or cardiac valves; (4) a "hydraulic ram effect," with compression of the abdomen forcibly displacing abdominal viscera against the heart with sudden great force; and (5) strenuous or prolonged cardiac massage, particularly if done through the intact chest wall.

### Types of Injuries

Blunt trauma to the heart can cause a wide spectrum of injuries, including (1) rupture of an outer chamber wall, with resulting death

**Table 218-6.** Predominant Injury in 546 Cases of Fatal Nonpenetrating Cardiac Trauma

| Predominant Injury | Number |
| --- | --- |
| Myocardial rupture, including septum | 353 |
| Myocardial contusion or surface laceration | 129 |
| Pericardial laceration | 36 |
| Hemopericardium | 25 |
| Papillary muscle rupture or lacerations | 1 (23)* |
| Coronary artery injury | 1 (9) |
| Laceration of valve | 1 (6) |
| Coronary artery thrombosis | 0 |

*The number in parentheses is the number combined with other more serious cardiac injury.

*Source:* Modified from Parmley LF, Manion WC, Mattingly TW: Nonpenetrating traumatic injury to the heart. *Circulation* 18:371, 1958, with permission.

from tamponade or bleeding; (2) septal rupture; (3) valvular injuries, of which injury to the aortic valve is the most common; (4) direct myocardial injury (contusion); (5) laceration or thrombosis of coronary arteries; and (6) pericardial injury (Table 218-6).

Some authors have stressed the differences between myocardial concussion and myocardial contusion. With myocardial concussion, there is no anatomic cellular injury, but there is some dysfunction, as demonstrated by abnormal wall motion studies. With contusion, there is an anatomic injury, as demonstrated either by elevated CPK-MB isoenzymes or by direct visualization at surgery or autopsy.

## Diagnostic Problems

Blunt cardiac trauma can be very difficult to detect at times. The victim may have experienced severe multiple-system trauma, and the presence of a cardiac injury may be overshadowed by other, more obvious injuries. In addition, the forces that produce blunt cardiac trauma may cause little or no external evidence of injury. Therefore, a history of moderate to severe chest or upper abdominal injury, even without abnormalities on physical examination, should make one suspect cardiac injury (Table 218-7).

## Cardiac Rupture

Cardiac rupture due to blunt chest trauma is the lesion most frequently found at autopsy in patients dying at the scene of an accident.

**Table 218-7.** Clues to Diagnosis of Blunt Cardiac Injury

History
  High-speed motor vehicle accident
  Crushed steering wheel
  Angina-like chest pain
Physical examination
  Tachycardia out of proportion to other findings
  Any dysrhythmia
  Any part of Beck triad
  Evidence of severe anterior chest injury
  Any evidence of heart failure
Radiography
  Fractured sternum or first two ribs
  Widened pericardial silhouette
Laboratory
  Elevated CPK-MB levels
ECG
  Dysrythmias or conduction disturbance
  Elevated ST segments
Other studies
  Impaired motion of anterior heart on two-dimensional echocardiogram or radionuclide angiography
  PA catheter monitoring showing elevated PAWP, low cardiac output, and/or poor response to fluid

As with myocardial contusion, the anterior right ventricle is the area most apt to be involved.

About 80 to 90 percent of patients with cardiac rupture die almost immediately at the scene of the accident. The most common site of cardiac rupture in patients who reach the hospital alive is a tear of the right atrium at its junction with the superior or inferior vena cava. With today's rapid transport systems, some patients, especially those with small tears of the right atrium, may arrive in the emergency department with little or no evidence of hemorrhagic shock or tamponade. Unfortunately, most of these patients suddenly deteriorate a short time later and die before appropriate surgery can be performed.

The diagnosis of cardiac rupture and/or tamponade should be suspected when shock exists out of proportion to the degree of recognized injury or when shock persists despite control of hemorrhage elsewhere and rapid volume replacement. An immediate left anterior thoracotomy or median sternotomy, preferably with cardiopulmonary bypass on standby, is required to repair these devastating injuries successfully.

## Septal Defects

Septal defects after blunt chest trauma are rare but should be looked for carefully if there is a murmur plus evidence of myocardial damage. The muscular interventricular septum near the apex is particularly susceptible to perforation after blunt trauma. The triad of chest trauma, systolic murmur, and an infarct pattern on ECG should suggest a ventricular septal defect (VSD). It is also important to suspect septal injury in patients with severe early hypoxemia and a relatively normal chest x-ray following chest trauma. Any right-to-left shunt will increase hypoxemia, and high-pressure mechanical ventilation will tend to increase such shunting.

If there is severe heart failure, prompt cardiac catheterization with rapid surgical repair may be required to restore adequate oxygen delivery to the tissues. Although small traumatic VSDs in the muscular septum may close spontaneously, surgical repair, preferably 6 to 8 weeks after the trauma, is the treatment of choice for persistent defects.

Isolated atrial septal defects (ASD) due to blunt trauma are extremely rare, and most patients with this defect die within minutes of the injury. Nevertheless, if an ASD is suspected, cardiac catheterization and subsequent repair are appropriate.

## Valve Injury

Rupture of the aortic valve is the most common valvular lesion found in patients who survive nonpenetrating cardiac injury. Patients with bioprosthetic heart valves are particularly likely to have traumatic valve injury. The next most frequent blunt valvular injury is laceration of a papillary muscle or chordae tendineae of the mitral valve. The prognosis for rupture of a mitral papillary muscle or a mitral valve leaflet is grave, and death usually occurs within a few days after injury.

The tricuspid valve is rarely involved in blunt trauma, and tricuspid insufficiency does not usually cause a significant hemodynamic problem unless the patient has pulmonary hypertension.

## Myocardial Contusion

### Pathologic Changes

The pathologic changes seen with an acute myocardial contusion typically include subendocardial hemorrhage and a much larger area of focal myocardial edema, interstitial hemorrhage, and myocytolysis with infiltrates of polymorphonuclear leukocytes. The areas most frequently involved are: (1) the anterior right ventricular wall, (2) the anterior interventricular septum, and (3) the anterior-apical left ventricle.

Additional myocardial injury may occur if there are concomitant coronary arterial problems such as spasm, intimal tears, or compression from adjacent hemorrhage and edema. Indeed, some feel that much of the myocardial injury seen is due to coronary blood flow redistribution. Very occasionally, transient hypotension may cause complete occlusion of a previously diseased coronary artery.

Usually there is complete clinical recovery with minimal residual scarring within 3 to 6 weeks of a myocardial contusion. However, in rare cases with severe transmural injury, a ventricular aneurysm may develop.

**Physiologic Changes**

In addition to rhythm and conduction disturbances, myocardial contusion can significantly impair myocardial function. In an otherwise normal individual without severe associated injuries, the hemodynamic impairment may not even be noticed. However, in patients who have preexisting cardiac disease or multiple other injuries or require a prolonged general anesthetic, the incidence of arrhythmias and/or hypotension is greatly increased.

Some reduction in cardiac output can be found in most victims studied. The degree of cardiac depression is directly related to the mass of contused myocardium. This has been confirmed in experimental animal studies and has been shown to persist for 2 to 3 weeks or longer. Abnormal wall motion and a decreased ejection fraction are also commonly seen. Although screening tests, such as the ECG and CPK-MB isoenzymes, can help diagnose myocardial contusions, they usually do not accurately indicate the severity of the injury, nor are they predictive of major morbidity or mortality.

Although there seems to be a great concern about making the diagnosis, most patients with myocardial contusions have relatively little problem. However, occasionally there is a problem with an arrhythmia, especially premature ventricular contractions (PVCs), atrial fibrillation, or a conduction defect, or there is clinical evidence of heart failure. Such problems are most apt to occur in patients with: (1) preexisting cardiac disease, (2) prolonged general anesthetics, or (3) hypotension because of other injuries.

**Diagnosis (See Table 218-6)**

There continues to be much debate about how to diagnose myocardial contusion. The value of various diagnostic tests varies greatly in the large number of papers written on the subject.

*Clinical Features*

Any patient involved in a motor vehicle accident involving speeds exceeding 35 mph and having any chest symptoms or signs should be suspected of having a myocardial contusion. Rarely, a patient with a myocardial contusion will have angina-like pain that is not relieved by nitroglycerin. Differentiation from an acute myocardial infarction in older individuals may be difficult under such circumstances.

A tachycardia that is out of proportion to the degree of trauma or blood loss may be the first sign of a myocardial contusion. Aside from evidence of significant chest wall injury, the only other helpful physical signs are an occasional friction rub or abnormality in the heart sounds. Occasionally, an irregular rhythm due to atrial fibrillation or multiple premature atrial or ventricular contractions may be noted.

*Radiologic Examination*

The chest x-ray has its greatest value in the recognition of associated injuries. The closest x-ray correlates of myocardial contusion are pulmonary contusion or fractures of the first two ribs, the clavicles, or the sternum. Sternal fractures are particularly important. In many series, the presence of a fractured sternum is the clinical finding most significantly associated with myocardial contusion. In the series reported by Harley and Mena of 11 patients with sternal fractures studied with radionuclide angiography (RNA), 10 (91 percent) had functional defects involving the anterior heart. Only four of these patients had an ECG abnormality, and none had elevated CPK-MB isoenzymes.

Acute cardiac decompensation may be diagnosed by x-ray evidence of acute pulmonary edema associated with a normal-sized heart. Cardiac tamponade usually does not cause an enlarged cardiac silhouette, but a widened azygous vein is suggestive of this diagnosis.

*ECG*

Some authors feel that the ECG is the best screening test for an acute myocardial contusion, but this is extremely controversial. Nevertheless, an ECG should be obtained initially and at 24 and 48 h postinjury in anyone suspected of having a myocardial injury. ST-T wave abnormalities may be present on admission or may develop only after 12 or 24 h, but such changes are very nonspecific. New atrial fibrillation, multiple PVCs, or conduction disturbances are much more important and are almost diagnostic.

ECG changes have been noted in 33 to 88 percent of patients with myocardial contusions. In one series of 108 patients with clinically diagnosed myocardial contusions, 12 percent had normal ECGs, 22 percent had ventricular rhythm disorders, 32 percent had other arrhythmias or disturbances of conduction, 61 percent had disturbances of repolarization, and 3 percent had ECG evidence of a myocardial infarction.

In a report by Fabian et al. continuous Holter monitoring for 3 to 5 days revealed "significant arrhythmias" (SARRs), usually short runs of ventricular tachycardia, in up to 78 percent of patients with such monitoring; however, the effect, if any, of SARRs on outcome was not clear.

It must be emphasized that a normal ECG does not exclude a significant myocardial lesion at autopsy. The initial ECG may be normal, and significant changes may develop only 24 to 72 h later, as occurred in 12 of 52 patients in one series. However, in most series the incidence of new ECG changes developing after 24 h is extremely low.

Although physicians often rely heavily on the ECG to help diagnose acute myocardial contusion, many patients with otherwise proven contusions will have normal ECG patterns. In particular, Sutherland et al. (1983) found that almost two-thirds of their patients with anterior myocardial dysfunction had a normal ECG. This is partly because the ECG tends to reflect changes in the left ventricle, while contusion tends to primarily involve the right ventricle.

*Enzymes*

SGOT, LDH, and CPK levels are often elevated in patients with severe blunt chest trauma because of associated injuries to the liver, lung, bone, brain, or skeletal muscle. Consequently, they are of little value in diagnosing cardiac injuries. However, myocardial (CPK-MB) isoenzymes should be more accurate. These should be drawn initially when the patient is first seen in the emergency department and at 8, 16, and 24 h postinjury. With myocardial contusions, the CPK-MB should peak at about 18 to 24 h.

Most authors consider a ratio of CPK-MB to total CPK of 5 percent or more to be indicative of myocardial damage. Since CPK-MB isoenzymes usually comprise less than 1 percent of the CPK in young normal hearts, this isoenzyme is of relatively little help if such hearts are injured. Even when CPK-MB isoenzymes are released by a contused heart, they can be diluted out to very low levels if the total CPK release from other injuries is very high. Consequently, there often appears to be no correlation between the severity of cardiac injury and the level of CPK-MB isoenzymes. Likewise, normal CPK-MB levels do not entirely rule out blunt myocardial injury. In the Sutherland et al. study, up to two-thirds of patients with impaired ventricular motion on gated radionuclide angiography had normal CPK-MB levels.

*Technetium Pyrophosphate (PYP) Scan*

PYP scans lack sensitivity in patients with myocardial contusions because a transmural injury is necessary to bind enough scintigraphic tracer to distinguish the lesion from background noise. The sensitivity of the scan is further hampered because it cannot differentiate a contusion of the right ventricle from an overlying sternal fracture or chest wall contusion.

### Radionuclide Angiography

First-pass biventricular RNA, including left ventricular segmental wall motion (LVSWM) analysis, can now be performed at the bedside as well as in the radiology department. The acquisitions are processed for both right and left ventricular ejection fractions (RVEF and LVEF) and for right and left ventricular segmental wall motion analysis. The normal LVEF is 62 ± 5 percent (mean ± SD), and the normal RVEF is 50 ± 4 percent. An LVEF less than 50 percent (>2.5 SD below the mean) and an RVEF less than 40 percent are considered as abnormal. Using this technique, Harley and Mena found that 11 of 12 patients with sternal fractures had abnormalities of ventricular contraction and motion; however, only 4 had ECG changes, and none had abnormal CPK-MB levels.

As a result of recent studies of emergency department patients with first-pass RNA, some authors have recommended the use of RNA on all trauma patients with no other problems except suspected cardiac injury. They feel that patients with a normal RNA can be observed in the emergency department for 4 to 6 h and then safely discharged home to be followed as outpatients.

### Single Photon Emission Computed Tomography

Thallous chloride $^{201}$Tl imaging of the heart has been used effectively for the investigation of a number of myocardial conditions such as ischemia and myocardial infarction. Unfortunately, conventional thallous chloride $^{201}$Tl imaging is unreliable for detecting small, partial-thickness lesions. However, if the thallous chloride $^{201}$Tl images of the heart are displayed by computer in the form of tomographic slides in different planes of the heart, a process referred to as single photon emission computed tomography (SPECT), the accuracy of the imaging is greatly increased. In the series of Waxman et al. of 48 patients with blunt chest trauma, 23 had normal SPECT studies, and none of these 23 developed any serious arrhythmias; in contrast, 5 of 25 patients with abnormal or ambiguous SPECT studies developed arrhythmias requiring treatment. In some other studies, however, SPECT scanning has predictive values inferior to the initial ECG.

### Echocardiography

Two-dimensional echocardiography has many advantages in the diagnosis and subsequent management of acute myocardial contusion. Quantitative and qualitative information can be obtained noninvasively on the status of the cardiac chambers, wall motion abnormalities, functional integrity of the valves, cardiac tamponade, and intracardiac thrombus or shunts. In addition, two-dimensional echocardiography can differentiate right and left ventricular contusions both from each other and from pericardial tamponade. Contused myocardium can be identified on two-dimensional echocardiogram by (1) increased echo brightness, (2) increased end-diastolic wall thickness, and (3) impaired regional systolic function.

The most common abnormality seen with myocardial contusion is right ventricular free wall dyskinesia, often with some dilation, of the involved chamber. Frazee et al. have noted that if patients with myocardial dysfunction demonstrated by abnormal anterior heart wall motion are given a general anesthetic, they have a significantly increased incidence of hypotension and arrhythmias for up to a month after the injury.

Many authors currently advocate obtaining a two-dimensional echocardiogram on all patients with suspected cardiac injuries, particularly if they have an abnormal ECG or elevated cardiac isoenzymes. Karalis et al., using both transthoracic and transesophageal echocardiography, diagnosed a myocardial contusion by cardiac wall motion abnormalities in 31 of 105 patients with severe blunt chest trauma; however, only 10 patients developed any cardiac problem requiring treatment.

### Monitoring of Pulmonary Artery Wedge Pressure and Cardiac Output

A pulmonary artery catheter should be inserted to monitor pulmonary artery pressures and cardiac output in patients with suspected myocardial contusion if there is any hemodynamic impairment, preexisting cardiac disease, or need for a major operative procedure under general anesthesia. Determinations of ventricular function curves with fluid loading have revealed a high incidence of subclinical biventricular dysfunction in patients with myocardial contusion. Baseline cardiac output may be relatively normal, but there is often a poor response to fluid loading.

### Summary of Diagnostic Approach

Patients with known or clinically suspected cardiac injury should have continuous cardioscopic monitoring. If the CPK-MB levels and ECGs are all negative for 24 h, it is unlikely that a significant cardiac injury exists. Nevertheless, two-dimensional echocardiography or RNA are more accurate tests and should probably be performed in individuals who have other significant injuries or may require a general anesthetic.

## Treatment

Although Glinz's series of 108 patients with myocardial contusions had 37 patients who required treatment of heart failure or rhythm or conduction disturbances, specific treatment interventions are seldom required. It has been suggested that cardiac monitoring is only necessary in patients with preexisting cardiac disease, severe associated injuries, or ECG evidence of ischemia or arrhythmias. In general, blunt cardiac injuries cause death very rarely, and the incidence of clinically significant dysrhythmias or other cardiac complications is generally greatly overestimated.

Supplemental oxygen should be administered as needed to maintain the arterial $P_{O_2}$ above 80 mmHg, and analgesics should be given as needed to reduce excessive pain. Coronary vasodilators should not be used unless the patient has suspected preexisting coronary artery disease. Cardiac arrhythmias should be diagnosed early and treated appropriately. Prophylactic treatment of arrhythmias is not indicated. Low cardiac output or hypotension should be treated with fluids or inotropic agents as indicated.

Patients with myocardial contusion can safely undergo surgical procedures if the pulmonary artery wedge pressure and cardiac output are closely monitored. In one series (Snow et al.), no significant problems or operative deaths were recorded in 27 patients. In another series (Flancbaum et al.), of 19 patients with myocardial contusion proven by RNA who had surgery for associated injuries, 11 required perioperative inotropic support and 1 needed intraaortic balloon pumping (IABP). However, no patient died or had complications directly due to the myocardial contusion. Thus, important surgery should not be delayed because of a suspected myocardial contusion unless the patient has arrhythmias or is hemodynamically unstable.

If the patient remains in a low-output state despite adequate fluid resuscitation, inotropic support, and correction of any mechanical problems, such as tamponade, use of an intraaortic balloon counterpulsation device should be considered.

There is some question as to whether patients with a myocardial contusion and an intramural thrombus seen on two-dimensional echocardiography should have prophylactic anticoagulation if not otherwise contraindicated. Although five of seven patients with chest trauma in the series reported by Miller et al. had echocardiographically proven right ventricular thrombi, none of the patients had subsequent systemic or pulmonary embolization. Furthermore, anticoagulation is contraindicated in most cases of multiple trauma because of the potential for severe hemorrhage.

## Coronary Artery Injury

Direct injury to the coronary arteries from blunt chest trauma occurs very rarely, but if it causes pericardial tamponade or intrathoracic bleeding, immediate operation is required. Coronary artery thrombosis is also rare but has been reported.

Several investigators have studied postmortem angiograms of myocardial trauma in dogs. Almost immediately following the impact, transmural redistribution of small vessel perfusion to the myocardium could be demonstrated distal to the site of injury. The researchers found no associated coronary artery spasm; in fact, a significant decrease in distal small vessel resistance was noted.

## Pericardial Injury and Effusion

The incidence of major cardiac injury from blunt trauma resulting in cardiac tamponade or acute hemopericardium at autopsy has been reported to be about 6 percent. Hemopericardium or pericardial effusion with or without frank tamponade can occur without any evidence of blunt cardiac injury. This may develop acutely or may be delayed for more than a week. As with other causes of pericardial effusion, the rate of fluid accumulation is the main determinant of its hemodynamic consequences.

Pericardial injury from blunt trauma should be suspected if there is ECG or other evidence of myocardial damage. However, a normal ECG does not rule out traumatic pericarditis. In some instances, only echocardiography or autopsy may provide the diagnosis.

Small posttraumatic pericardial effusions can be seen with many cardiac injuries following blunt chest trauma but are usually of little or no consequence. They generally remain asymptomatic and resolve without any therapy. In rare instances, a patient may develop late constrictive pericarditis, occasionally with extensive calcification of the pericardium.

Occasionally, severe blunt chest trauma may tear the parietal pericardium. If the hole is large enough and near the apex, the heart may actually herniate out through the defect, causing sudden severe shock or cardiac arrest.

## Follow-up

It is important that patients with proven or suspected cardiac injury be closely observed, not only throughout their hospital stay but also later, for undiagnosed injuries or complications. One should look particularly for posttraumatic pericarditis, ventricular septal defect, valvular defects, and ventricular aneurysms.

## Postpericardiotomy Syndrome

### Etiology and Pathogenesis

The cause of the postpericardiotomy syndrome (PPCS) is still largely unknown, but it may be a delayed hypersensitivity reaction to the presence of damaged myocardium in the pericardial cavity. This damaged tissue can act as a foreign protein, inducing the production of autoantibodies against similar tissues. In fact, antimyocardial antibodies can be measured, and their serum concentration varies with the severity of the symptoms. Autogenous blood and lipids in the pericardium can also set up an inflammatory response that may be a contributing factor.

### Diagnosis

PPCS should be suspected in individuals who develop chest pain, fever, and pleural or pericardial effusions 2 to 4 weeks after heart surgery or trauma. Patients may also have friction rubs, arthralgia, and pulmonary infiltrates. The blood count often shows a leukocytosis, and the ECG will often show ST-T wave changes consistent with pericarditis.

### Treatment

Treatment is primarily symptomatic. Salicylates and rest can often reduce symptoms dramatically within 12 to 24 h, but glucocorticoids are occasionally required. Rarely, drainage of pleural or pericardial fluid may be required to relieve symptoms or rule out other problems.

# GREAT VESSELS OF THE CHEST

## Penetrating Trauma

Of the patients who reach the hospital with penetrating chest wounds and require admission, only 5 to 15 percent require a thoracotomy, but up to 25 percent of the patients having such surgery have an injury to a great vessel. The survival rate with stab wounds is generally much higher than with gunshot wounds. Small knife wounds are often rapidly sealed off by surrounding tissue, especially vascular adventitia. This limits the amount of blood loss, particularly after hypotension develops. If the knife stays in place, it may temporarily seal the involved vessel.

The amount of tissue destruction caused by a bullet is determined largely by the kinetic energy (KE) lost after the missile enters the tissue. This can be calculated as $KE = \frac{1}{2} m(V_1^2 - V_2^2)$. Thus, the tissue destruction is proportional to the mass ($m$) of the missile and the entering velocity squared ($V_2^2$) minus the exiting velocity squared ($V_2^2$) as the bullet leaves the tissue. If the bullet remains in the patient, $V_2^2$ is zero. Thus, a rifle bullet with a velocity of 3000 ft/s can impart 25 times as much damage to tissue as a pistol bullet of similar mass going at 600 ft/s. A close-range shotgun blast, particularly by 12-gauge shotgun pellets, can be even more destructive.

## Types of Vascular Injuries

Simple lacerations of the great arteries of the chest can cause exsanguination, tamponade, hemothorax, or air embolism. Other vascular injuries include AV fistulas and false aneurysms, which may not be apparent for days or even months. As time goes on, AV fistulas tend to increase in size. Eventually, if more than 25 percent of the cardiac output goes through an AV fistula, high-output cardiac failure is likely to develop.

Pulmonary AV fistulas after penetrating chest trauma are said to be extremely rare because of the small pressure differential that usually exists between the pulmonary arteries and veins. However, if the patient develops hypoxemia out of proportion to the apparent lung injury and has a persisting pulmonary density, one should suspect this problem.

## Diagnosis

### History

Most penetrating wounds of the chest are quite obvious. However, certain historical facts can be helpful. For example, the amount of time the patient spent at the scene and in transit may be extremely important in considering whether to perform an emergency department thoracotomy on a patient who arrives in cardiac arrest. A "down time" exceeding 5 min rarely allows one to perform a successful resuscitation with satisfactory neurologic outcome.

The size of a knife, its depth, and the angle of penetration may indicate the vessels or organs most likely to be injured. If there are two skin wounds, it is helpful to know whether they represent two entrance wounds or an exit and an entrance wound. In some instances, a bullet that entered the chest without exiting is not evident on chest or abdominal x-rays because it is in lateral subcutaneous tissues or has entered a major vessel and has embolized. It is also extremely important to know, if possible, the caliber of the bullet and whether it was a high-velocity missile (>1000 ft/s).

## Physical Examination

Small wounds, especially in the axilla or in heavy chest hair, may easily be missed. Although one does not usually probe chest wounds because this may start severe external or internal bleeding, careful superficial instrumentation may provide important information on the direction of the tract.

A large upper mediastinal hematoma may cause an acute superior vena caval syndrome, tracheal compression, and/or respiratory distress. Occasionally, a decreased upper extremity pulse may be noted. However, Flint et al. found that 45 (32 percent) of 146 patients with 206 injuries to major vessels at the thoracic inlet had none of the usual diagnostic signs of significant vascular injury.

One should auscultate the entire chest for bruits after a penetrating injury. A systolic bruit, particularly over the back or upper chest, should make one suspect a false aneurysm involving one of the great vessels. A continuous bruit suggests an AV fistula. A millwheel murmur, thought to be due to the churning of air in the heart, may be diagnostic of air embolism. Loss of a peripheral pulse caused by an embolization of a bullet from a thoracic vascular injury is occasionally seen.

## Radiography

### Plain Radiographs

Evidence of cervical or supraclavicular swelling or widening of the upper mediastinal silhouette on chest x-ray is often present in patients with injury to brachiocephalic vessels. A "fuzzy" foreign body (bullet) can be an important radiologic sign, and one should not assume that it is due to poor radiologic technique. Because foreign bodies tend to pulsate when they lie next to major vessels, their margins may appear indistinct on chest films. Therefore, a fuzzy foreign body contiguous with clear mediastinal structures on chest films can be an important x-ray clue to a vascular injury. Even if an angiogram is normal, a fuzzy foreign body should still be considered an indication for surgery.

### Computed Tomography Scan

CT scans are rarely performed immediately for penetrating wounds of the chest because of the usually precarious condition of the patient. However, in a stable patient, a CT scan can identify localized hematomas or collections of blood that may not be apparent on routine x-rays. If a persistent "mass" is adjacent to a great vessel and does not move with position changes by the patient, one should assume a contained hematoma is present. IV contrast provides additional help for demonstrating a vascular defect or false aneurysm on the CT scan. CT scans can be particularly helpful for suspecting thoracic aorta trauma or dissection, and false-negative studies without an adjacent hematoma are very unusual if the CT scan has been performed and interpreted properly. Nevertheless, CT scans should be used primarily for screening for great vessel injuries rather than for definitive diagnosis.

### Arteriogram

Arteriograms may be particularly helpful in identifying major intrathoracic vascular injuries within contained hematomas, especially those resulting from penetrating wounds of the lower neck. Indeed, before exploring penetrating injuries of the thoracic inlet in hemodynamically stable patients, one should obtain a preoperative arteriogram to visualize the arch of the aorta and its major branches.

### Venograms

Venograms to identify major vascular injuries in the chest are seldom performed. A patient who is actively bleeding from a major venous injury is usually explored emergently because of unstable vital signs or continued blood loss through chest tubes. However, once a venous injury stops bleeding, the hemorrhage generally does not recur and does not require a thoracotomy.

### Contrast Swallows

A contrast swallow may be performed on a stable patient if there is concern about an associated esophageal injury. Gastrographin is used first but may miss up to half of esophageal leaks. Barium swallows have fewer false-negatives but can cause a worse mediastinitis if a perforation is present.

### Endoscopy

With penetrating wounds of the chest or lower neck in hemodynamically stable patients, it may be prudent to perform bronchoscopy and esophagoscopy to rule out an injury to the aerodigestive tract. In some patients with "hemoptysis," the source may not be clear, and such bleeding may result from injury to lung parenchyma, trachea, or a major bronchus. In other instances, it may be unclear as to whether mediastinal air is caused by an esophageal, pulmonary, or tracheobronchial injury.

### Ultrasound

There is much controversy on how to evaluate hemodynamically stable patients with transmediastinal gunshot wounds. Such injuries often result in either prompt surgical exploration or an extensive evaluation to rule out injury to the heart, great vessels, esophagus, or tracheobronchial tree. Recently, however, transesophageal echocardiography has been noted to be of great diagnostic help, particularly if the aortogram demonstrates an equivocal injury.

## Treatment

### Initial Resuscitation

The standard ABCs of initial resuscitation should be followed aggressively if the patient is in shock. One of the problems occasionally seen with injuries to vessels in the thoracic outlet is massive mediastinal hematoma formation with resulting tracheal compression. Consequently, early endotracheal intubation should be performed. Tracheostomy should be avoided in patients with injuries at the thoracic inlet, at least initially, because of the possibility of precipitating massive bleeding from an otherwise controlled hematoma.

If the patient is in severe shock (systolic blood pressure < 60 mmHg), surgery should be performed promptly and aggressive fluid replacement should not be employed until the major bleeding sites are controlled. With mild to moderate shock (systolic blood pressure = 60 to 88 mmHg), one should infuse 2000 to 3000 mL of balanced electrolyte solution in 10 to 15 min. If the shock is persistent, the patient is rushed to the operating room. If the patient is about to have a cardiac arrest in the emergency department, an immediate resuscitative thoracotomy should be performed there to control bleeding, provide internal cardiac massage, and cross-clamp the descending thoracic aorta as needed.

If rapid control of the bleeding sites and cross-clamping of the descending thoracic aortic arch do not raise the systolic blood pressure to at least 90 mmHg within 5 min, terminal cardiovascular failure is present; almost all of these patients will die in the operating room. Even if large doses of epinephrine or dopamine combined with aortic cross-clamping can raise the systolic blood pressure over 90 mmHg, death is still almost invariably the outcome.

Even if the patient's vital signs are relatively stable, one should probably perform a thoracotomy for continued bleeding if (1) a total of more than 1500 mL of blood is lost from the chest within the first 4 to 8 h and the patient is still bleeding, (2) the drainage of blood from the chest tubes continues to exceed 200 to 300 mL/h, or (3) the chest continues to be more than half full of blood on x-ray after the chest tubes are inserted and functioning well.

Bullets entering large systemic veins or the right heart can embolize to the lungs, whereas bullets entering the pulmonary veins or left heart can embolize to major systemic arteries. Some of these emboli cause no symptoms or signs and cannot be found except with multiple x-rays. Fluoroscopy in the operating room can be important in tracing these bullets, especially in the central veins or heart, because they can change position rapidly during the surgery itself.

## Blunt Trauma to the Great Vessels of the Chest

### Incidence

Approximately 80 to 90 percent of patients with blunt trauma to thoracic great vessels, particularly the aorta, die at the scene, and up to 50 percent of the remaining patients die within 24 h if not promptly treated. The frequency of these injuries appears to be increasing and is primarily related to the use of high-speed automobiles. Each year at least 5000 to 8000 individuals in the United States suffer traumatic rupture of the thoracic aorta or one of the other great arteries in the chest.

### Mechanism of Injury

The mechanical factors responsible for traumatic rupture of the thoracic aorta and its major branches are probably somewhat different for each anatomic area. For the descending aorta at the level of the isthmus, three mechanical factors thought to contribute to rupture are shearing stress, bending stress, and torsion stress. The difference in deceleration between the mobile aortic arch and the relatively immobile descending aorta puts the aortic isthmus under tension, and the resultant shearing stress can lead to rupture or tears opposite the site of fixation. Bending stress is produced as the heart exerts downward traction on the aortic arch, resulting in the hyperflexion of the blood-filled aortic arch on a transverse fulcrum created by the hilar structures of the left lung. Torsion stress occurs when anteroposterior compression of the chest with resultant displacement of the heart to the left is combined with an intravascular pressure wave transmitted to the aorta. These three forces can combine to produce maximum stress to the inner surface of the aorta at the ligamentum arteriosum, which is its point of greatest fixation.

The aortic injury tends to progress from the intima out toward the adventitia. The adventitia, which has the lowest elastic limit, seems to withstand these stresses better than the intima or media.

Ben-Menachem has noted an increased incidence of partial shearing of the distal aortic arch from broadside motor vehicle impacts. With vertical deceleration injuries, the ascending aorta may be involved, particularly in those who die immediately. Vertical deceleration produces acute lengthening of the aorta, with resultant development of a pressure wave in the aortic blood column. This water-hammer effect, which is greatest in the ascending aorta, is believed to contribute greatly to rupture in that location.

Rupture of the innominate or left subclavian artery at their origins probably results primarily from the interaction of two forces. One is a compression force that displaces the heart into the left chest and places the brachiocephalic vessels under tension at their attachment to the aortic arch. The other force occurs when hyperextension of the neck with rotation of the head to one side places the contralateral subclavian arteries under tension. Subclavian artery injuries can also occur just over the first rib, and injuries at that site are usually caused by direct trauma and/or excessive stretching.

### Pathologic Changes

Blunt aortic tears usually extend partially or completely around the vessel in a transverse or spiral direction. Preexisting disease, such as atherosclerosis or medial necrosis, does not appear to predispose to traumatic rupture. When the aortic tear involves all layers of the aortic wall, death by exsanguination is usually almost instantaneous. If the aortic tear does not involve the adventitia, and the parietal pleura and the surrounding mediastinal tissues remain intact, a false aneurysm often forms. The false aneurysm tends to expand, particularly if the patient is hypertensive, and about 50 percent of these, if untreated, will rupture within 24 h. However, some posttraumatic aortic false aneurysm remain intact and may not be detected for 20 years or longer. Although a lacerated subclavian artery occasionally forms a false aneurysm, it usually just occludes and does not require surgery.

It should be emphasized that the small hemothorax that is often present with blunt trauma to the aorta does not result from the aortic injury itself but rather from tears to adjacent small mediastinal vessels or other structures. In the same manner, although the widened mediastinum may be partly due to the aortic pseudoaneurysm, much of it is actually caused by bleeding from small mediastinal vessels.

### Natural History

Parmley et al. found that, of the patients who reach a hospital and survive for 1 h, 20 to 30 percent die within 6 h, 40 to 50 percent die within 24 h, and 60 to 80 percent die within 7 days. Of the remainder, most die within the next 1 to 3 months.

Many of the early deaths are caused by associated injuries, but even when the aortic injury is an isolated problem, diagnosis and repair should usually be accomplished on an urgent basis. All too often the patient dies of exsanguination before a definitive repair can be effected. Keeping the systolic blood pressure <120 mmHg and prevention of Valsalva maneuvers probably would have prevented virtually all of these early deaths.

### Location

At least 90 percent of blunt aortic injuries in patients who reach the hospital alive occur in the isthmus of the aorta, between the left subclavian artery and the ligamentum arteriosum. The next most common sites involved are the innominate or left subclavian artery at their origin or a subclavian artery over the first rib. Patients do not usually survive injury to the ascending aorta, but this injury may be seen in up to one-third of the individuals who die at the scene of an accident, especially with vertical deceleration from falls from great heights or plane crashes. Tears in the lower aorta below the ligamentum arteriosum are quite uncommon but tend to occur adjacent to severely comminuted fractures of vertebral bodies.

### Diagnosis

#### History

The single most important factor in establishing the diagnosis of acute traumatic rupture of the aorta (TRA) is a high index of suspicion because of the nature of the trauma (Table 218-8). Even if there is no external evidence of chest injury, one should still be acutely aware of the possibility of this injury in anyone who has sustained an accident characterized by sudden severe deceleration or a high-speed impact from the side.

Patients with TRA usually complain primarily of their associated injuries and generally have no symptoms related to the aortic injury itself. The most common complaint that may be due to the aortic injury itself is retrosternal or interscapular pain from "stretching" or

**Table 218-8.** Clinical Factors Suggesting Possible Traumatic Rupture of the Aorta

High-speed deceleration injury or side impact
Multiple rib fractures or flail chest
Pulse deficits
Hypertension
Systolic murmur over back
Hoarseness without laryngeal injury
Superior vena caval syndrome

dissection of the adventitia of the aorta. Recurrence or exacerbation of the pain, particularly if associated with a rise in blood pressure (which may be due to excess fluid administration or inadequate pain control), may herald an impending rupture of the pseudoaneurysm. Less frequent symptoms, due primarily to pressure from the associated hematoma, include dysphagia, stridor, dyspnea, or hoarseness.

## Physical Examination

In many reports, at least one-third of the patients with blunt trauma to the aorta have no external evidence of thoracic injury at the time of the initial physical examination. In fact, Kirsch and Sloan reported that only 15 (27 percent) of 55 patients with TRA sustained identifiable chest wall contusion or rib fractures.

Physical findings that suggest aortic injury include (1) an acute onset of upper extremity hypertension, (2) difference in pulse amplitude between the upper and lower extremities, and (3) the presence of a harsh systolic murmur over the precordium or posterior interscapular area. Upper extremity hypertension has occurred in 31 to 43 percent of the patients reported in the literature and has been attributed to compression of the aortic lumen by a periaortic hematoma. However, the hypertension may also be secondary to stretching or stimulation of special receptors located in the vicinity of the aortic isthmus. This mechanism could account for the upper extremity hypertension that occurs without aortic narrowing after trauma to the aortic isthmus and for the slowly resolving postoperative hypertension that is seen in up to one-third of patients who have a TRA successfully repaired.

If the torn intima and media form a flap that acts as a "ball valve," partial or complete aortic obstruction can occur. With partial obstruction, an "acute coarctation syndrome" can develop, with hypertension in the upper extremities and weak pulses or hypotension in the lower extremities. A systolic murmur, thought to be caused by turbulent blood flow across the area of transection, is found in fewer than 30 percent of the patients with acute aortic rupture. If complete aortic obstruction occurs, anuria and paraplegia can develop almost immediately. Other, less frequently encountered physical findings include hoarseness, voice change, superior vena cava syndrome, swelling at the base of the neck, and paraplegia.

## Plain Chest X-ray

Although the circumstances of the accident and the physical examination may be helpful, the diagnosis of TRA is usually suspected from findings on the routine chest x-ray (Table 218-9). The most frequent radiologic finding noted is widening of the superior mediastinum, usually to more than 8.0 to 8.5 cm, caused primarily by subadventitial and periadventitial hematoma (Fig. 218-9). The ratio of the mediastinal width to the width of the chest may provide more objective measurements, but it does not seem to be as accurate as the subjective impression of mediastinal widening on a good upright chest film.

One of the main reasons that many unnecessary aortograms are preformed is a technically poor chest x-ray. The upper mediastinum tends to appear wider than normal if the chest x-ray is taken (1) anteroposteriorly (AP) rather than posteroanteriorly (PA), (2) with the patient less than 3 1/4 ft (100 cm) from the origin of the x-ray beam, (3) with the patient lying flat, or (4) with poor inspiration. The opti-

**Table 218-9.** Chest Radiographic Findings Associated With
Traumatic Rupture of the Aorta

Superior mediastinal widening
Deviation of esophagus and/or trachea at T4
Obscuration of aortic knob and/or descending aorta
Obliteration of the aortopulmonary window
Obscuration of medial aspects of left upper lobe
Widening of the paravertebral stripe
Fracture of first or second rib
Apical cap

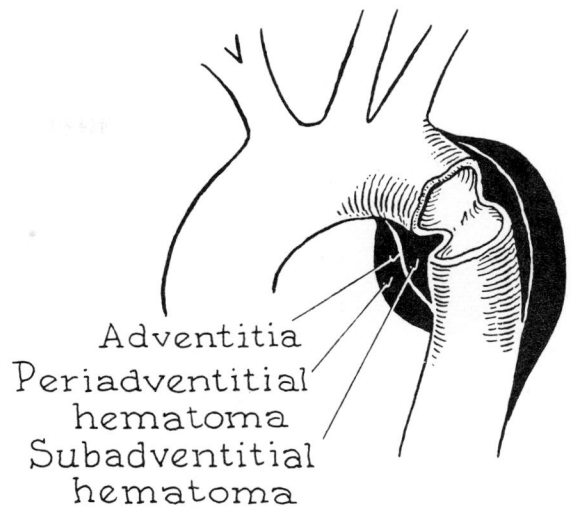

**Fig. 218-9.** The widening of the mediastinum around a traumatic rupture of the aorta usually results from hematoma in the subadventitial and periadventitial spaces. The periadventitial hematoma may be very large and is due primarily to bleeding from small mediastinal vessels.

mal chest x-ray is an upright PA chest x-ray taken at a distance of 6 ft (about 2 m) with the patient leaning forward about 10 to 15°.

The most accurate radiographic sign of TRA is usually deviation of the esophagus more than 1 to 2 cm to the right of the spinous process of T4 (Fig. 218-10). In Ayella's large series, none of the patients with the esophagus less than 1.0 cm from the midline had a TRA. In a series of 45 patients, Gerlock and associates also noted that none of the patients with a nasogastric tube in a normal position had TRA.

Blurring or obscuration of the aortic knob or descending aorta is almost as accurate an indication of TRA. In a study of 86 patients

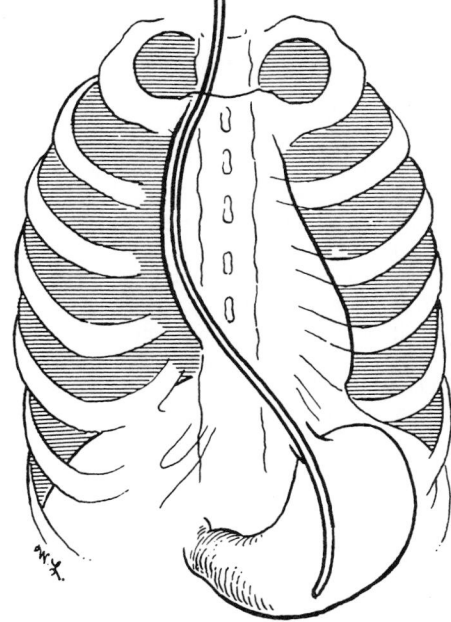

**Fig. 218-10.** Deviation of the esophagus (nasogastric tube) to the right is generally a very accurate sign of traumatic rupture of the aorta. If the distance from the nasogastric tube to the spinous process of the fourth thoracic vertebra is greater than 2.0 cm, it is almost 100 percent indicative of a torn descending thoracic aorta.

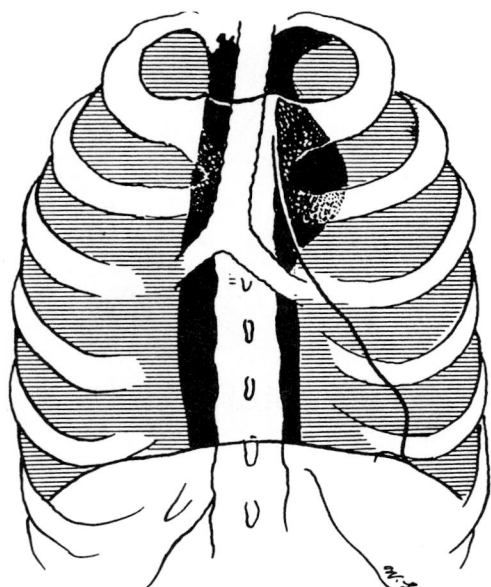

**Fig. 218-11.** Mediastinal hematomas, indicated by the blackened areas, may widen and displace the paratracheal stripe separating the right side of the tracheal air column from the medial border of the right lung by more than 5 mm. Mediastinal hematomas may also displace the right and left paraspinal lines in the lower thorax rather widely from the lateral edges of the thoracic spine. The paraspinal lines are not readily seen on most x-rays because of overlying structures.

with blunt chest trauma, 13 patients had TRA and 73 did not. No patient with a normal aortic contour and no evidence of deviation of the trachea or nasogastric tube to the right on the chest x-ray had TRA.

Other chest x-ray signs include displacement of the left main-stem bronchus more than 40° below the horizontal, obliteration of the usual clear space between the aortic knob and the left pulmonary artery (apical cap), widening of the right paratracheal stripe, and displacement of the right paraspinous interface (Fig. 218-11).

The paratracheal stripe is a linear structure just to the right of the tracheal air column (Fig. 218-11). It extends from the thoracic inlet to the proximal right bronchus and normally measures less than 5 mm in thickness at a level 2 cm above the azygous vein. If the paratracheal stripe is more than 5 mm wide and/or is deviated to the right, this may be another sign of mediastinal hemorrhage.

The paraspinal lines lie between the pleura and the lung, projected away from the lateral margin of the thoracic spine. The right paraspinal line is usually not visible on routine chest x-rays, but if it is seen and if it is displaced to the right in the absence of spinal or sternal fractures, it may be of some diagnostic value.

The left paraspinal line may be distinguished from the image of the descending aorta by the fact that it is not continuous with the aortic knob. When displaced more than one-half the distance from the spine to the left margin of the descending aorta without spinal or sternal fractures, it is highly specific.

It often takes great force to fracture the first or second ribs or sternum, especially in young patients. Consequently, such fractures tend to be associated with an increased incidence of major intrathoracic injuries; however, it is now very controversial whether fractures of the first or second ribs are associated with a significantly increased incidence of TRA.

One should not assume that a TRA has been ruled out if the initial chest x-ray is normal. In up to one-third of patients with TRA, widening of the mediastinum and other characteristic changes may not be apparent on the chest x-ray for several hours after the injury. Simi-

larly, Gundry et al. reported that up to two-thirds of patients older than 65 years with TRA may not show mediastinal widening. Consequently, serial chest films should be taken in any patient with severe chest trauma at 6- to 12-h intervals during the first day and then daily for at least the next 3 days. Indeed, the circumstances of the accident in such individuals should be the main indication for ordering an aortogram.

### Transesophageal Ultrasound

If transesophageal ultrasound (TEUS) is available and it can be performed without excessive gagging or vomiting, it can be a great help in the early diagnosis of intrathoracic problems after severe chest trauma. Indeed, it increasingly appears to be more sensitive than aortography for diagnosing TRA.

TEUS can offer a quick assessment of the thoracic aorta at the patient's bedside with almost negligible disruption of the continuous resuscitative measures. It can also be performed during an urgent laparotomy required for massive intraabdominal blood loss. TEUS visualizes the aortic isthmus and descending aorta very well and allows assessment of the pericardial cavity (hemopericardium, tamponade), valve function, (traumatic rupture of valves), pulmonary veins (avulsion), and regional wall motion abnormalities (myocardial contusion).

It is not known how well ascending aortic ruptures are seen with TEUS, but with practice, they may be visualized as readily as type A dissections. Avulsions of the great vessels, particularly the innominate artery, are unlikely to be seen clearly and, if suspected, would warrant angiography.

### CT Scans

Although aortography has been considered the ideal method of diagnosing TRA, there has been some enthusiasm for performing contrast-enhanced CT scans to screen for these lesions. Heiberg et al. reported in their study of 10 trauma patients, of whom 4 had TRA, that CT examination provided no false-positives or -negatives, whereas 1 of 13 "positive" aortograms was falsely positive.

Miller et al. studied 104 chest trauma patients with both CT scans and thoracic aortograms looking for great vessel injuries. Of 67 with "negative" CT scans, 2 had an aortic injury. However, one CT scan was misread and one was performed without contrast. Durham et al. also had a series with two false-negative aortograms, but the films may have been suboptimal.

The presence of a mediastinal hematoma on CT scan after severe blunt chest trauma is an indication for aortography. Subtle changes in the aortic contour indicating transection or a thin filling defect caused by torn intima and media may be missed between the various CT scanning planes, which are usually 10 mm apart. Consequently, the newer spiral CT scans should be much more accurate.

We have used the CT scan primarily as a screening tool, and if there is a mediastinal hematoma adjacent to a great vessel, we order an aortogram. Indeed, although we are not aware of a TRA requiring surgery that did not have a mediastinal hematoma on a properly done and properly read CT scan, more than a few have been reported in the literature.

Poole et al. have noted that chest x-rays are superior to CT for identifying rib fractures; however, CT was more sensitive than chest x-ray for diagnosing pneumothorax, pulmonary infiltrates, and effusions. Nevertheless, the lesions detected on CT, but not on chest x-ray, usually resolved without any therapeutic intervention.

### Magnetic Resonance Imaging

The newer generations of MRI may be particularly good for diagnosing dissecting aneurysms and therefore should be ideal for posttraumatic studies of the thoracic vessels if the patient is stable and can lie still long enough.

## Aortography

If an aortic rupture is suspected on clinical or radiologic grounds, an aortogram should be performed. While waiting for the aortogram or surgery, it is important to ensure that the systolic blood pressure is kept below 120 mmHg. It is also important to protect the patient from excessive gagging or straining.

The most common finding on aortogram is a pseudoaneurysm of the isthmus of the aorta. A slight pouching out of the inferior or inner border of isthmus, sometimes referred to as a pseudodiverticulum, is normal but may be confused with a traumatic pseudoaneurysm. Bulging of the aorta laterally is a more reliable indicator of TRA. A linear filling defect caused by torn intima and media is the best evidence that a TRA is present.

The left anterior oblique (LAO) x-ray appears to be optimal for examining the aortic arch and proximal descending aorta. In addition, the entire aorta and its branches, particularly those coming off the arch, should be visualized to rule out the less common or multiple ruptures that might otherwise be missed. A patient who is in shock from a suspected TRA or who has a rapidly expanding mediastinal hematoma should be taken directly to the operating room without undergoing aortography. It should be remembered that occasional false-negatives occur with aortography. Indeed, this author has had two such cases personally and knows of two others.

Although it is often thought that there is relatively little risk to angiography, Waugh and Sacharias noted that local complications with conventional angiography may occur in up to 23 percent of cases, and systemic complications may occur in up to 9 percent. Although the rates of amputation (0.1 percent) or death (0.3 percent) resulting from transfemoral studies is relatively low, if they occur in an individual with a negative study, the indications for the aortogram are apt to be questioned. Death has also occurred in at least two instances when the angiographic catheter was manipulated through the aorta at the level of a tear. If angiography is done in a hospital where relatively few cases are done each year, the incidence of complications can be increased up to 32-fold.

### Intraarterial Digital Subtraction Angiography

In an effort to improve the speed and accuracy of angiography and reduce the dose of contrast material, Mirvis et al. studied 61 consecutive patients with blunt thoracic trauma and obscuration of the aortic knob or mediastinal widening on the chest x-ray using intraarterial digital subtraction angiography (IA-DSA). Ten of these patients had aortic ruptures diagnosed by IA-DSA. Digital subtraction aortography proved 100 percent accurate, as indicated by the results of surgery, conventional arteriography, serial chest x-rays, and clinical follow-up. The method was 50 percent faster than conventional aortography, and it significantly reduced x-ray film costs. The use of smaller-caliber catheters for the intraaortic injection and a decrease in radiographic contrast media requirements also make this method safer than conventional arteriography.

## Treatment

Although it is essential to resuscitate severely injured patients aggressively and to rapidly correct hypotension and hypoxemia, the patient with a TRA should not be allowed to develop a systolic blood pressure over 120 mmHg or to perform a Valsalva maneuver. Fluid administration should be watched carefully, and administration of sedatives, analgesics, vasodilators, or even beta-adrenergic blockers may be required to keep the patient's systolic blood pressure at safe levels.

It is often important to insert a nasogastric tube in patients with multiple injuries, but it is essential that the patient with a suspected TRA not perform a vigorous Valsalva maneuver. Sudden gagging or bearing down can cause intraaortic pressure to rise abruptly to well over 200 mmHg and complete the rupture of a partially torn aorta.

Similar precautions must be undertaken when inserting an endotracheal tube.

Since the initial report of a successful repair of an acute traumatic thoracic aortic disruption in 1958, emergency operation has become the accepted standard for treatment. However, in selected cases, delays in surgical intervention may be warranted and safe. Such delay should be considered if (1) the patient is stable but the conditions for surgery are not ideal, or (2) the patient represents an extremely high operative risk because of associated injuries or preexisting medical conditions.

In a few centers with extensive experience with thoracic aortic surgery, the aortic repair may be preferentially performed by a rapid "clamp and sew" technique without an external shunt or cardiopulmonary bypass. Under these circumstances, an IV infusion of an $\alpha$ and a $\beta$ blocker may be used to keep the systolic blood pressure in the upper portion of the body less than 150 mmHg to diminish the chances of intracerebral hemorrhage or left heart failure while the aorta is clamped. The operation must be rapid and precise, because clamping of the descending aorta for more than 30 min without perfusion of the distal aorta greatly increases the risk of damage to the spinal cord and abdominal viscera.

Because it allows increased time for a meticulous, unhurried repair, and because it reduces the risk of ischemic damage to the spinal cord and abdominal viscera, repair of traumatic rupture of the thoracic aorta is often performed under partial cardiopulmonary bypass. If the patient's condition is stable, transfer to a hospital where cardiopulmonary bypass is available is wise, just in case problems develop during the repair. The usual cardiopulmonary bypass circuit, from the femoral vein to the femoral artery, requires an oxygenator and heparin, which increases the risk of dangerous bleeding, particularly into injuries of the brain, eyes, or retroperitoneum.

Recent use of a special vortex (Biomedicus) bypass pump with catheters in the left atrium and femoral artery may be particularly helpful and safe because no oxygenator and no heparin are required. In the four published series using this technique, there have been only two (7 percent) deaths and no paraplegia.

An alternative to cardiopulmonary bypass is a shunt to divert blood around the involved aorta. The proximal end of the tubing (filled with heparinized saline) can be inserted into the ascending aorta, the aortic arch, or the apex of the heart. The distal end can be inserted into the mid or lower descending thoracic aorta or the femoral artery. If special heparin-coated polyvinyl tubing is used, the patient may not have to be exposed to the risk of systemic heparinization.

## Special Considerations in Less Frequent Great Vessel Injuries

### Ascending Aorta

#### Incidence

Very few patients with ascending aortic injury survive long enough for the diagnosis to be established and repair to be carried out. These injuries are frequently associated with cardiac rupture or severe myocardial contusion, and the aortic tears are multiple in up to 15 to 20 percent. Most victims have been hit by or thrown from moving vehicles or have fallen from great heights.

#### Diagnosis

Since most ascending aortic tears occur within the pericardium, if there is a small complete tear, there is often evidence of both shock and pericardial tamponade. The chest x-ray findings often show a widened superior mediastinum with or without obscuration of the aortic knob. Aortography is generally required for the diagnosis to be established. The aortogram usually shows a pseudoaneurysm with an intimal tear seen as an irregular filling defect within the lumen. If there is an associated valvular injury, aortic insufficiency of varying severity will usually also be seen.

## Lower Thoracic Aorta

Thoracic aortic injuries distal to the isthmus should be suspected with severe chest trauma in which a lower thoracic vertebra is severely crushed.

## Other Great Vessel Injuries

### Innominate Artery

#### Incidence

In patients reaching the hospital alive, blunt injuries of the innominate artery are second in frequency only to rupture of the aorta at the isthmus. Associated injuries, such as rib fractures, flail chest, hemopneumothorax, fractured extremities, head injuries, facial fractures, and abdominal injuries, are found in more than 75 percent of these patients.

#### Diagnosis

Making a diagnosis of blunt injury to the innominate artery can be very difficult because there are no characteristic physical findings except for some diminution of the right radial or brachial pulse, which occurs in about 50 percent of the patients. Signs and symptoms of distal ischemia are uncommon. Occasionally, a systolic murmur may draw attention to a possible lesion in this area.

The chest x-ray findings are somewhat similar to those seen with TRA, but the mediastinal hematoma tends to be higher and the trachea and esophagus may be pushed to the left. Aortography must generally be performed for the diagnosis to be established. Tears of the innominate artery typically show bulbous dilation of the vessel just distal to its origin, associated with a crescentic line across its base, representing retraction of the torn intima into the lumen of the vessel. Associated injuries in other brachycephalic vessels or the aorta are found in about 10 percent of patients.

### Subclavian Artery

#### Etiology

Although a subclavian artery is occasionally avulsed at its origin because of sudden deceleration, direct trauma to the distal artery with intimal damage and occlusion associated with fractures of the first rib or clavicle are more likely. Shoulder restraints that are loose may be a major factor in causing this injury.

#### Diagnosis

The most important sign of a subclavian occlusion is absence of a radial pulse. In the patient with only a partial laceration and no occlusion, the radial pulse may be preserved. Other physical findings that are highly suggestive of subclavian artery rupture are a pulsatile mass or a bruit in the root of the neck. Occasionally a patient may develop an acute subclavian steal syndrome if the subclavian artery occludes proximal to the origin of the vertebral artery.

Up to 60 percent of patients with blunt injury to the subclavian artery, especially from motor vehicle accidents, will also have some damage to the brachial plexus. Consequently, a complete neurologic examination preoperatively is important in these patients. A Horner's syndrome often indicates avulsion of nerve roots from the spinal cord.

The chest x-ray with subclavian artery injuries may show the presence of a widened superior mediastinum without obscuration of the aortic knob. The angiogram usually shows occlusion, but a pseudoaneurysm is occasionally found. Blunt subclavian artery injuries are associated with other major vascular injuries in about 10 percent of patients.

#### Treatment

The treatment of acute subclavian artery injury is usually immediate repair. However, in certain high-risk patients who are doing poorly, occlusion by an interventional radiologist may be the treatment of choice. If the artery is already occluded, observation may be all that is required. The collateral circulation to the distal portions of the vessel is usually very good; however, if there has been severe blunt trauma to the shoulder girdle, many of the collateral vessels may be damaged, resulting in critical ischemia of the hand or upper extremity gangrene in 29 percent of cases.

## ESOPHAGEAL AND THORACIC DUCT INJURIES

### Esophageal Injuries

#### Mechanical Trauma

Lacerations of the esophagus occur most frequently during endoscopic biopsy or dilatation of a narrowed or obstructed esophagus. The esophagus can also be injured by swallowed foreign bodies. Injury to the thoracic esophagus is seen only rarely in patients who reach the hospital alive.

If esophageal injury is suspected, an esophagogram should be performed. Many physicians prefer a water-soluble radiopaque material, such as Gastrografin, because it causes less reaction than barium if it leaks into surrounding tissues. However, with such contrast material, there is at least a 25 percent incidence of false-negatives. Contrast swallows with barium are less likely to be falsely negative. In addition, if the Gastrografin is aspirated into the lungs, it can cause a more severe pneumonitis than barium would.

Flexible esophagoscopy is being performed increasingly for diagnosis but may miss more than 20 percent of injuries, even if combined with an esophagogram. Some prefer rigid esophagoscopy in combination with bronchoscopy to rule out associated tracheobronchial injuries.

If treatment is delayed beyond 24 h, primary closure of a torn esophagus is usually not advisable because local edema, tissue necrosis, and infection make secure suturing and primary healing unlikely. If mediastinitis develops, it may be rapidly fatal unless the site is drained early and completely. Even if an esophageal repair is not attempted, continuous complete drainage of the stomach (preferably with a gastrostomy tube) and the adjacent mediastinum (with chest tubes) is important and may be necessary for up to several weeks.

In spite of all our technical and nutritional advances in recent years, the mortality rate for esophageal injuries ranges from 5 to 25 percent for those treated definitively within 12 h, and 25 to 66 percent for those treated after 24 h.

## Thoracic Duct Injuries

Most injuries to the thoracic duct in the chest result in a chylothorax. Because the thoracic duct in the chest tends to be slightly to the right of the midline, injuries to it usually cause a chylothorax on the right. Initially, the chyle may just accumulate in the mediastinum as a chyloma, but eventually, usually within 7 to 13 days, it will cause an increasing pleural effusion, especially after the patient begins to eat. Thoracic duct leakage in the chest can result in the loss of 1500 to 2500 mL/day of fluid with fat globules (demonstrated by Sudan III) and/or chylomicrons (demonstrated by lipoprotein electrophoresis) with minimal cholesterol.

Keeping the patient from eating and providing adequate drainage of the pleural cavity with a chest tube for several days usually results in spontaneous closure of the fistula. If the fistula persists and is large, nasogastric suction can help reduce the amount of chyle draining, and intravenous hyperalimentation can help prevent the protein malnutrition that can rapidly develop in these patients. If the patient is allowed to eat, a strict no-fat diet or a diet in which fat is given only as medium-chain triglycerides is preferred. If the drainage is greater than 1500 mL/day and leads to metabolic and nutritional problems or persists for more than 14 days, surgery to ligate the duct is generally indicated.

## BIBLIOGRAPHY

### Chest Wall, Bronchi, Lung, and Diaphragm

Bassett JS, Gibson RD, Wilson RF: Blunt injuries to the chest. *J Trauma* 8:418. 1968.

Brookes JG, Dunn RJ, Rogers IR: Sternal fractures: A retrospective analysis of 272 cases. *J Trauma* 35:46, 1993.

Brown GL, Richardson JD: Traumatic diaphragmatic hernia. *Ann Thorac Surg* 39:172, 1985.

Cant PJ, Smyth S, Smart DO: Antibiotic prophylaxis is indicated for chest stab wounds requiring closed tube thoracostomy. *Br J Surg* 80:464, 1993.

Collins JC, Levine G, Waxman K: Occult traumatic pneumothorax: Immediate tube thoracostomy versus expectant management. *Am Surg* 58:743, 1992.

Demetriades D, Breckon V, Breckon C, et al: Antibiotic prophylaxis in penetrating injuries of the chest. *Ann R Coll Surg Engl* 73:348, 1991.

Diebel LN, Robinson RL, Wilson RF, Dulchavsky SA: Splanchnic mucosal perfusion effects of hypertonic versus isotonic resuscitation of hemorrhagic shock. *Am Surg* 59:495, 1993.

Enderson BL, Abdalla R, Frame SB, et al: Tube thoracostomy for occult pneumothorax: A prospective randomized study of its use. *J Trauma* 35:726, 1993.

Galan G, Penalver JC, Paris E, et al: Blunt chest injuries in 1696 patients. *Eur J Cardiothorac Surg* 6:284, 1992.

Inoue H, Suzuki I, Iwasaki M, et al: Selective exclusion of the injured lung. *J Trauma* 34:496, 1993.

Jongewaard WR, Cogbill TH, Landercasper J: Neurologic consequences of traumatic asphyxia. *J Trauma* 32:28, 1992.

Luchette FA, Radfshar MR, Kaiser R, et al: Prospective evaluation of epidural versus intrapleural catheters for analgesia in chest wall trauma. *J Trauma* 35:165, 1993.

Mancini M, Smith LM, Nein A, Buechter KJ: Early evacuation of clotted blood in hemothorax using thoracoscopy: Case reports. *J Trauma* 34:144, 1993.

Ordog GJ, Wasserberger J, Balasubramanium S, Shoemaker W: Asymptomatic stab wounds of the chest. *J Trauma* 36:680, 1994.

Pagliarelo G, Carter J: Traumatic injury to the diaphragm: Timely diagnosis and treatment. *J Trauma* 33:194, 1992.

Richardson JD, McElvein RB, Trinkle JK: First rib fracture: A hallmark of severe trauma. *Ann Surg* 181:251, 1975.

Rotondo MF, McGonigal MD, Schwab CW, et al: Urgent paralysis and intubation of trauma patients: Is it safe? *J Trauma* 34:242, 1993.

Rozycki GS, Ochsner MG, Jaffin JH, Champion HR: Prospective evaluation of surgeons' use of ultrasound in the evaluation of trauma patients. *J Trauma* 34:516, 1993.

Trinkle JK, Richardson JD, Franz JL, et al: Management of flail chest without mechanical ventilation. *Ann Thorac Surg* 19:355, 1975.

Washington B, Wilson RF, Steiger Z, et al: Emergency thoracotomy: A four-year review. *Ann Thorac Surg* 40:188, 1985.

Wilson RF, Antonenko D, Gibson DB: Shock and acute respiratory failure after chest trauma. *J Trauma* 17:697, 1977.

Wilson RF: *Handbook of Antibiotic Therapy for Surgery Related Infections.* Philadelphia, Scientific Therapeutic Information, 1994, pp 29–31.

### Heart

Baker CC, Thomas ANM, Trunkey DD: The role of emergency room thoracotomy in trauma. *J Trauma* 20:848, 1980.

Buckman RF, Badellino MM, Mauro LH, et al: Penetrating cardiac wounds: Prospective study of factors influencing initial resuscitation. *J Trauma* 34:717, 1993.

Cogbill MH, Moore EE, Millikan JS, et al: Rationale for selective application of emergency department thoracotomy in trauma. *J Trauma* 23:453, 1983.

Demetriades D: Cardiac wounds. *Ann Surg* 203:315, 1985.

Fabian TC, Cicala RS, Croce MA, et al: A prospective evaluation of myocardial contusion: Correlation of significant arrhythmias and cardiac output with CPK-MB measurements. *J Trauma* 31:653, 1991.

Flancbaum L, Wright J, Siegel JH: Emergency surgery in patients with post-traumatic myocardial contusion. *J Trauma* 26:795, 1986.

Frazee RC, Mucha P, Farnell MB, et al: Objective evaluation of blunt cardiac trauma. *J Trauma* 26:510, 1986.

Gyhra A, Pierart J, Torres P, Prieto L: Experimental cardiac tamponade with a myocardial wound: The effect of rapid intravenous infusion of saline. *J Trauma* 33:25, 1992.

Glinz W: Problems caused by the unstable thoracic wall and by cardiac injury due to blunt injury. *Injury* 17:322, 1986.

Harley DP, Mena I: Cardiac and vascular sequelae of sternal fractures. *J Trauma* 26:553, 1986.

Karalis DG, Victor MF, Davis GA, et al: The role of echocardiography in blunt chest trauma: A transthoracic and transesophageal echocardiographic study. *J Trauma* 36:53, 1994.

Mattox KL, Flint LM, Carrico CJ: Blunt cardiac injury (formerly termed "Myocardial Contusion"), editorial. *J Trauma* 33:649, 1992.

Miller FA, Seward JB, Gersh BJ, et al: Two-dimensional echocardiographic findings in cardiac trauma. *Am J Cardiol* 50:1022, 1982.

Mitchell ME, Muakkassa FF, Poole GV, et al: Surgical approach of choice for penetrating cardiac wounds. *J Trauma* 34:17, 1993.

Ordog GJ, Wasserberger J, Balasubramanium S, Shoemaker W: Asymptomatic stab wounds of the chest. *J Trauma* 36:680, 1994.

Rozycki GS, Ochsner MG, Jaffin JH, Champion HR: Prospective evaluation of surgeons' use of ultrasound in the evaluation of trauma patients. *J Trauma* 34:516, 1993.

Snow N, Richardson JD, Flint IM: Myocardial contusion: Implications for patients with multiple traumatic injuries. *Surgery* 92:744, 1982.

Sutherland GR, Cheung HW, Holliday RL, et al: Hemodynamic adaptation to acute myocardial contusion complicating blunt chest injury. *Am J Cardiol* 57:291, 1986.

Sutherland GR, Driedger AA, Holliday RL, et al: Frequency of myocardial injury after blunt chest treatment as evaluated by radionuclide angiography. *Am J Cardiol* 52:1099, 1983.

Waxman K, Soliman MH, Braunstein P, et al: Diagnosis of traumatic cardiac contusion. *Arch Surg* 121:689, 1986.

### Great Vessels

Ayella RJ: *Radiologic Management of the Massively Traumatic Patient.* Baltimore, Williams & Wilkins, 1978.

Ben-Menachem Y: Rupture of the thoracic aorta by broadside impacts in road traffic and other collisions: Further angiographic observations and preliminary autopsy findings. *J Trauma* 35:363, 1993.

Durham RM, Zuckerman D, Wolverson M, et al: Computed tomography as a screening exam in patients with suspected blunt aortic injury. *J Trauma* 35:161, 1993.

Flint IM, Snyder WH, Perry MD, et al: Management of major vascular injuries in the base of the neck. *Arch Surg* 106:407, 1973.

Gerlock AJ, Muhletaler CA, Coulam CM, et al: Traumatic aortic aneurysm: Validity of esophageal tube displacement sign. *Am J Radiol* 135:713, 1980.

Gundry SR, Williams S, Burney RE: Indications for aortography in blunt thoracic trauma. A reassessment. *J Trauma* 22:664, 1982.

Heiberg E, Wolveson MK, Sundaram M, et al: CT in aortic trauma. *Am J Radiol* 140:1119, 1983.

Hilgenberg AD, Logan DL, Akins CW, et al: Blunt injuries of the thoracic aorta. *Ann Thorac Surg* 53:233, 1992.

Jones WG, Ginsberg RJ: Esophageal perforation: A continuing challenge. *Ann Thorac Surg* 53:534, 1992.

Kearney PA, Smith W, Johnson SB, et al: Use of transesophageal echocardiography in the evaluation of traumatic aortic injury. *J Trauma* 34:696, 1993.

Kirsch MM, Sloan H: *Blunt Chest Trauma.* Boston, Little Brown, 1977.

Miller FB, Richardson JD, Thomas HA, et al: Role of CT in diagnosis of major arterial injury after blunt thoracic trauma. *Surgery* 106:596, 1989.

Mirvis SE, Pais OS, Gens DR: Thoracic aortic rupture: Advantages of intra-arterial digital subtraction angiography. *Am J Radiol* 146:987, 1986.

Parmley LF, Mattingly TW, Manion WC: Nonpenetrating traumatic injury of the aorta. *Circulation* 17:1086, 1958.

Poole GV, Morgan DB, Cranston PE, et al: Computed tomography in the management of blunt thoracic trauma. *J Trauma* 35:296, 1993.

Van Normal GA, Pavlin EG, Eddy AC, Pavlin DJ: Hemodynamic and metabolic effects of aortic unclamping following emergency surgery for traumatic thoracic aortic tears in shunted and unshunted patients. *J Trauma* 31:1007, 1991.

Waugh JR, Sacharias N: Arteriographic complications in the DSA eras. *Radiology* 182:243, 1992.

### Esophagus and Thoracic Duct

Wilson RF, Steiger Z: Oesophageal injuries, in Champion HR, Robbs JV, Trunkey DD (eds): *Trauma Surgery,* 4th ed. London, Butterworths, 1989, pp 327–340.

# 219
# ABDOMINAL TRAUMA

### Arthur L. Ney
### Jeremy Hollerman
### Robert C. Andersen

Abdominal trauma is difficult to evaluate because of the many possible injuries and their varied presentations. The thrust of the abdominal examination and resuscitation should be to recognize surgical lesions, not to diagnose specific injuries. The findings at surgery will dictate management, and a prolonged examination to pinpoint the exact injury is potentially detrimental. The most serious mistake is to delay surgical intervention when it is needed. Most preventable deaths are a result of uncontrolled hemorrhage during that delay.

The evaluation of the patient with abdominal trauma must be done in the context of the entire patient, and all potential and actual injuries must be prioritized. This means that a head, cardiac, great vessel, or respiratory injury may take precedence over an abdominal injury. In an unstable patient, the diagnostic peritoneal lavage (DPL) remains the gold standard in the evaluation of abdominal injury. Retroperitoneal injuries are, however, rarely diagnosed with this test. Computed tomography (CT) scanning is extremely valuable and in some centers has replaced DPL in specific clinical circumstances. The choice of examination will depend on local resources. Neither test will eliminate the need for careful clinical evaluation and follow-up to monitor for progression or development of findings suggesting injury. The role of thoracoscopy and laparoscopy in the evaluation and treatment of abdominal trauma is yet to be defined, as is the role of ultrasound.

## PATHOPHYSIOLOGY

Abdominal injuries are frequently divided into two main types on the basis of the wounding mechanism: blunt and penetrating. A fundamental point to be remembered is that combined injuries often occur. For example, a patient who has been stabbed may also have been kicked or beaten. Likewise, a patient in a motor vehicle accident will be expected to have significant blunt injury, but penetration from sharp objects can also occur. This concept of evaluating injuries focuses attention on the more likely injuries and directs further diagnostic maneuvers.

## Blunt Trauma

With blunt trauma there are three common mechanisms of injury: (1) the direct blow, (2) crush, and (3) the deceleration injury. The first two cause injury by direct compression and the latter by organ trac-

tion beyond a point of internal fixation (i.e., renal pedicle, aorta at ligamentum arterosum, trachea at the carina).

The main divisions within the abdomen are the peritoneal cavity and the extraperitoneal potential space. The extraperitoneal area includes the retroperitoneum and the extraperitoneal pelvis. The retro-peritoneum and extraperitoneal pelvis are difficult to examine, often with minimal findings on clinical examination. Peritoneal lavage is unreliable for injuries in this area and negative lavage can actually give a false sense of security. Ancillary tests are of the most help in evaluating the retroperitoneum and pelvis. Intravenous pyelography, upper gastrointestinal contrast studies, cystography, angiography, and CT scanning will all be helpful in selected cases. CT scanning with oral and intravenous contrast appears to be the most helpful single test in evaluating injury to retroperitoneal organs. Serum amylase is a helpful indicator of potential injury; however, significant pancreatic injury may be present in the presence of a normal serum amylase level. A digital rectal examination with testing of stool for occult blood is essential. Because of the insidious nature of these injuries, it is essential to maintain a high index of suspicion.

Injuries in the peritoneal cavity usually result in findings on examination of the anterior abdomen. Guarding, rigidity, rebound tenderness, or the presence of a palpable mass all suggest injury. In the absence of these signs, significant injury is unlikely but can occasionally occur, even in the presence of normal neurologic function. When there is doubt, a CT or DPL will help identify a surgical lesion in this portion of the abdomen.

## Penetrating Injuries

Penetrating injuries can result from gunshot and stab wounds. Gunshot wounds have three main injury-causing mechanisms: (1) direct missile penetration of tissues by the projectile, (2) missile fragmentation after the original impact, and (3) "shock waves" transmitted to neighboring organs. Injuries from gunshot wounds should be routinely explored. The only somewhat controversial area is the management of injuries close to the abdominal cavity where it is felt that peritoneal penetration is unlikely but remotely possible. In this situation, DPL can help differentiate patients with and without peritoneal penetration. Use of DPL in these cases will need to be done in conjunction with the surgeon caring for the patient. An example is a low chest gunshot wound with hemopneumothorax where there remains a remote possibility that the bullet traversed the diaphragm. Some surgeons favor lavage followed by exploration if any red blood cells are present. Many would, however, routinely explore any patient with a gunshot injury when it is even remotely possible that the abdomen has been entered. High-velocity gunshot wounds may cause intra-abdominal injury without peritoneal penetration through shock wave generation. A false-negative DPL may occur with these injuries, and lesions that require surgery will not be identified.

Stab wounds cause injury primarily by direct laceration of the tissue traversed. Penetrating injuries from stab wounds are associated with a high incidence of negative laparotomy if routinely explored. For this reason, patients are managed in a more selective manner in trauma centers where experienced clinical monitoring and operating rooms are immediately available. Celiotomy is clearly indicated in patients with evisceration, peritoneal irritation, or persistent hypotension. We evaluate the remainder by wound exploration under local anesthesia. A *positive wound exploration* is the finding of penetration of the superficial fascia. It is difficult, and as a result unreliable, to explore deeper wounds to detect peritoneal penetration in most patients. Sinograms are generally of no value. The next maneuver for evaluating peritoneal penetration is peritoneal lavage with an aliquot of the lavage fluid sent for evaluation. The accepted value for a positive count is still controversial, with trauma surgeons advocating celiotomy for a red blood cell count as low as 1000 cells/mm$^3$ to a high of 100,000 cells/mm$^3$. At our institution the positive value is 10,000 cells/mm³ when the diaphragm may be involved, and 100,000/mm³ when the lower abdomen is involved. In patients with fewer or no red blood cells per cubic millimeter, an observation period of at least 24 h is indicated. These patients *must* have a normal neurologic examination before they are discharged. Drug intoxication and head or spinal cord injuries limit the sensitivity of physical examination for the identification of injuries.

## CLINICAL FEATURES OF SPECIFIC ORGAN INJURY

In the evaluation of patients with abdominal injury, it is important to keep in mind the management techniques that will be used for different injuries. A concept of the surgical management of different injuries gives perspective to adequate preoperative evaluation and preparation. A prime example would be the case of a low rectal injury in the face of other abdominal injuries. This is easily missed at exploratory laparotomy, and an appropriate colostomy will not be done if that injury is not detected preoperatively. What follows is a brief discussion of specific injuries and the diagnostic and therapeutic techniques in their management.

### Hollow Organs

Injury to these organs is insidious and has the potential for significant morbidity and mortality. Sudden compression by a seat belt may result in a hollow viscus rupture as a result of "submarining" when only a lap belt is used. A high index of suspicion should be present when lap belt bruises or abrasions are seen. Bacterial flora that represent a significant risk when organ contents spill into the peritoneal cavity. Injuries to these organs usually result in symptoms of peritonitis.

Most of these injuries will be detected with DPL, but water-soluble contrast studies may be necessary to document organ disruption.

### Stomach

The stomach is resistant to blunt injury. In addition, when injury does occur its excellent blood supply makes primary repair the most common technique used, with generally excellent results. In trauma patients, a distended stomach will increase the chances of injury. Heme-positive nasogastric return is usually present with injury. Confusion occurs when there has been nasopharyngeal trauma either from the original injury or iatrogenically with tube insertion. Contrast studies may occasionally be necessary to confirm the diagnosis.

### Duodenum

The retroperitoneal position of the duodenum makes the diagnosis of injury difficult. Signs and symptoms are often slow to develop and, when present, indicate significant injury. Specific clues as to the presence of duodenal injury include retroperitoneal air or elevation of the serum amylase level. The definitive test for evaluating duodenal injury is a contrast study showing extravasation (Fig. 219-1). On CT scan the contrast may not adequately distend the duodenum, and formal fluoroscopic examination may be necessary. Duodenal injuries may range in severity from an intramural hematoma to an extensive crush or laceration too severe for simple closure. Hematoma is best managed nonoperatively if the diagnosis can be ensured without exploration. If the lesion is found incidentally at surgery, it is difficult to decide how to manage it. The hematoma is usually drained at that point, which carries somewhat higher morbidity.

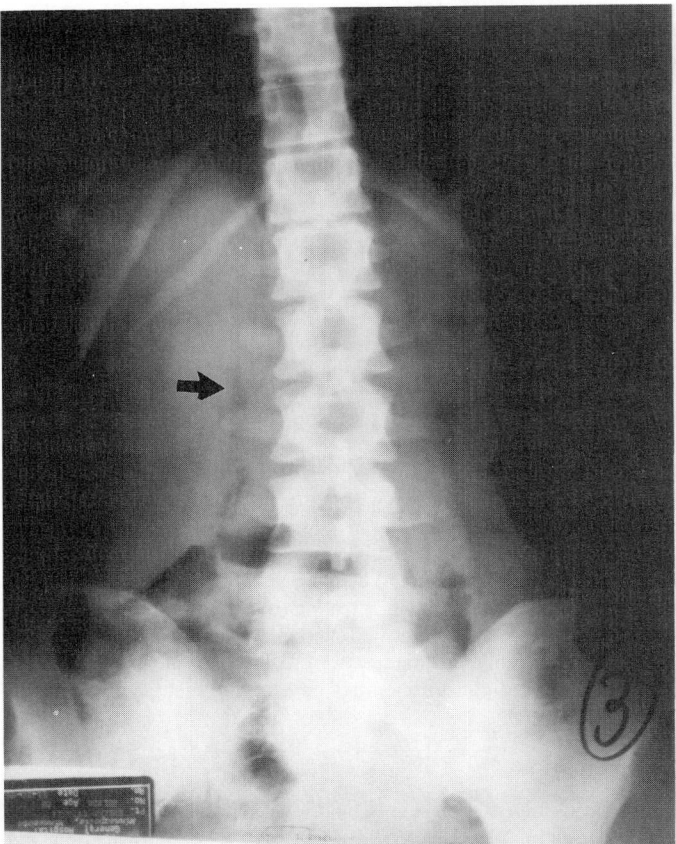

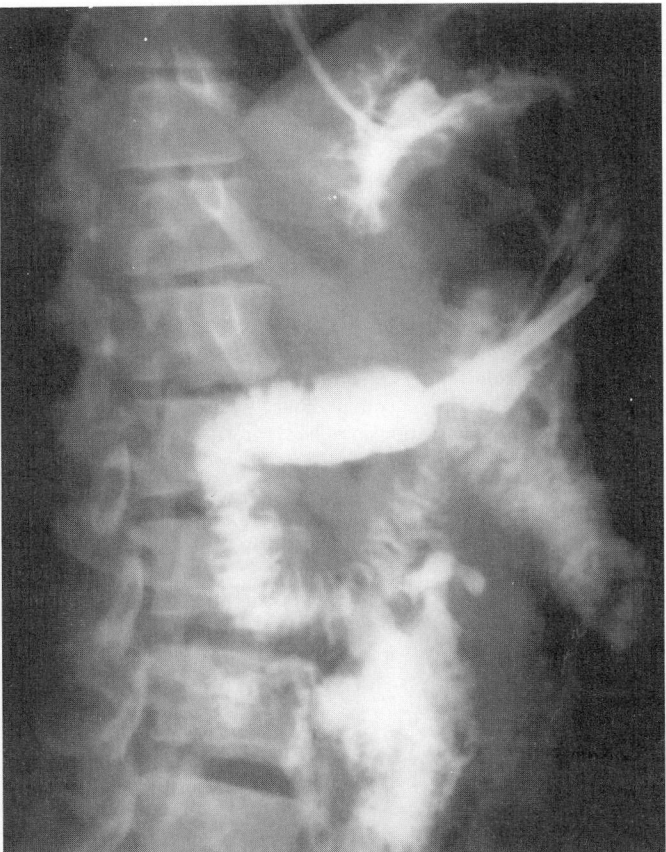

**A**

**B**

**Fig. 219-1. A.** A flat plate radiograph of the abdomen revealing vertically oriented air bubbles (arrow) over the upper psoas shadow. About 20 percent of patients with duodenal rupture will have this finding.

**B.** Gastrograffin study of the same patient showing leakage of duodenal contents into the retroperitoneal space.

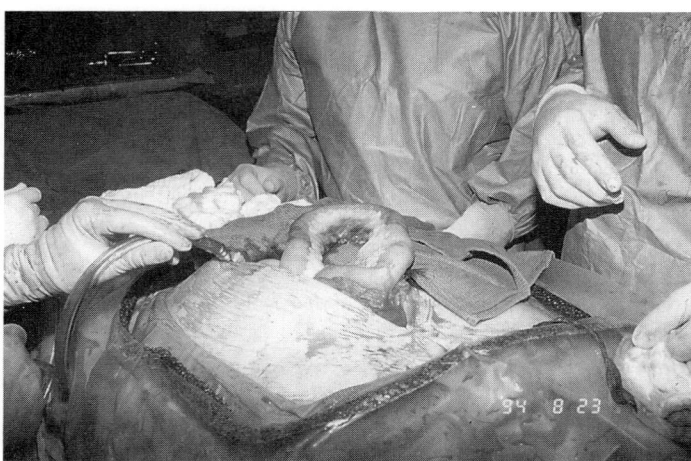

**Fig. 219-2.** "Bucket handle" tear of the mesentery of the bowel resulting in ischemia of the affected segment.

## Small Bowel

Small bowel injuries are similar to stomach injuries in that they are most frequently the result of penetrating injury and generally carry a good prognosis. In most cases, injury to the small bowel will result in early peritoneal irritation from spillage of bowel contents causing significant symptoms. A deceleration injury can cause a bucket-handle tear of the mesentery (Fig. 219-2) or a blow-out injury of the antimesenteric border (Fig. 219-3). The bowel can lose its viability over a period of time. Such injuries are often diagnosed late, especially in head-injured patients. DPL is usually positive, and CT scan is also a good modality for diagnosis. The majority of small bowel injuries can be repaired primarily after local debridement. In more extensive injuries or those with compromise to the blood supply, resection and anastomosis will be necessary.

## Colon

The management of injury to the large bowel is controversial. The number of lesions felt to be amenable to management without stoma (colostomy) is considerable, and some surgeons feel that most lesions may be repaired primarily. This practice is certainly well accepted for right-sided lesions and left-sided lesions found early with minimal contamination. Colostomy is frequently used in any left-sided lesion with extensive injury or any colonic injury with extensive contamination. Excessive contamination may be the result of delayed surgical treatment. To avoid this situation, colonic lesions must be suspected and specifically searched for early. The use of CT scanning with rectal contrast is the best way to detect injury. If there is any doubt, a Gastrograffin enema with fluoroscopy remains the optimal test for evaluating colonic perforation. Barium, though giving superior contrast studies, is extremely irritating to the peritoneal cavity and causes an intense inflammatory response. When perforation is suspected, water-soluble contrast should be used. If doubt persists exploration may be prudent.

## Rectum

Injuries to the rectum are especially important to diagnose preoperatively because diagnosis at surgery is difficult. The rectum is an extraperitoneal organ, and physical findings may be minimal. Careful rectal palpation should be done to search for evidence of bony penetration with a pelvic fracture, and stool should be tested for blood. Undetected, an open pelvic fracture (exposed to a rectal injury) will rapidly develop into overwhelming sepsis. Surgical management of these patients involves both an abdominal and a perineal approach. If the diagnosis is not made before exploratory laparotomy, reoperation for colostomy will be necessary. Management includes preoperative broad-spectrum antibiotics, repair of associated injuries, drainage, and fecal diversion. This usually includes a diverting end-on sigmoid colostomy proximal to the rectal injury, washout of the distal rectum with saline solution, and placement of presacral drains through the perineum. This combination of complete diversion and rectal washout has markedly reduced the morbidity and mortality of this injury. Clearly, early accurate diagnosis is essential because the rectum is below the peritoneal reflection making it difficult to detect at celiotomy.

## Gallbladder and Biliary Ducts

Injuries to the gallbladder and biliary ducts are rare. Gallbladder injury occurs most frequently as a result of penetrating trauma but may occur after blunt injury and frequently involves transection near the papilla. This injury is extremely difficult to diagnose preoperatively. It is suspected when peritoneal lavage fluid is positive for bile. It should, however, be found during exploration. An intraoperative cholangiogram can provide the definitive diagnosis.

## Genitourinary Tract

Lesions of the genitourinary tract are addressed more fully elsewhere (see Chapter 221). In the presence of persistent microscopic or gross hematuria, contrast studies are necessary for diagnosis. The contrast CT scan provides an excellent study when time allows. In situations where this is not possible, a rapid cystogram and intravenous pyelogram (IVP) in the resuscitation area are helpful. When time allows, oblique and lateral films as well as postvoid films improve visualization of subtle injuries. In the hypotensive patient, nonvisualization of IVPs is common, and so should be obtained after patient stabilization. Intraoperative studies, although technially inferior, frequently identify extravasation or absence of function, which are the major concerns. At operation, dyes that are excreted in the urine, such as methylene blue and indigo carmine, may be useful to identify the location of extravasation.

## Solid Organs

Injury to the solid organs causes morbidity and mortality primarily as a result of blood loss. The products of secretion are potential sources of morbidity but are generally sterile and, as such, are less of an infection risk. Blood loss is usually more of a problem and may be life-threatening. Immediate surgery to control the bleeding will be critical. Presentation will be with tachycardia and hypotension in addition to the abdominal findings. When the hemorrhage is contained within

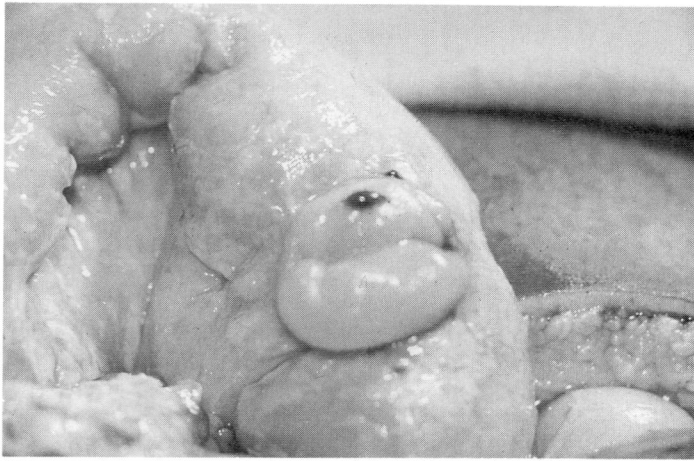

**Fig. 219-3.** "Blow-out" injury to the jejunum.

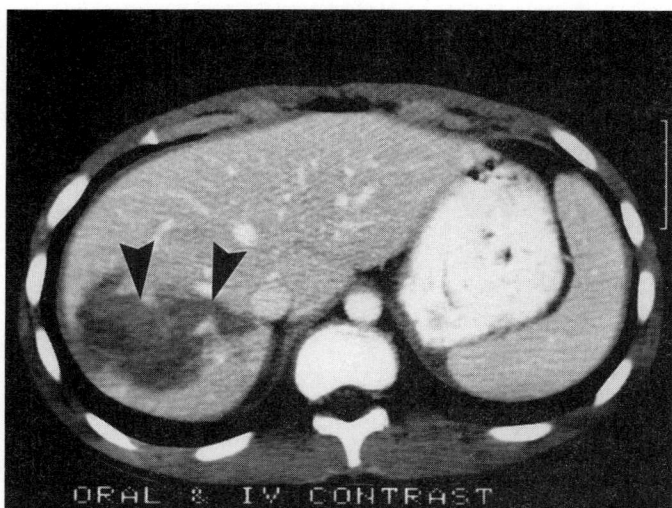

**Fig. 219-4.** Computed tomogram showing an intra-hepatic hematoma.

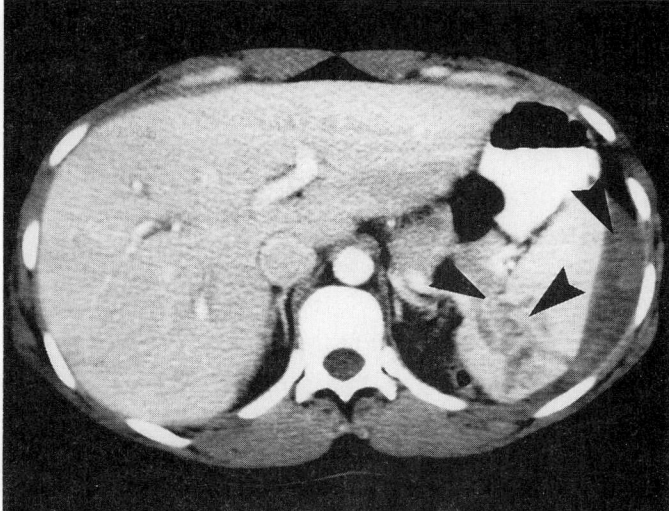

**Fig. 219-5.** Computed tomogram showing an intrasplenic, hilar, and perisplenic hematoma.

a fixed space, a mass may develop that may be clinically palpated or found on radiologic examinations. In isolated injuries to the spleen or the liver, autotransfusion at the time of surgery is often of benefit.

## Liver

The liver is commonly injured in both blunt and penetrating trauma to the abdomen. Most injuries are self-limited, with the bleeding stopped at the time of laparotomy. With CT scanning, some lesions are now being identified that can be managed nonoperatively (Fig. 219-4). In massive liver injury with caval or hepatic vein injury, total vascular isolation of the liver may be necessary. The mortality from this injury is high (50 to 100 percent), with rapid control of bleeding the key to survival. Control is with a shunt from the lower cava to above the liver. A Pringle maneuver (occlusion of the vessels at the hilum of the liver) will complete the vascular isolation of the liver. In some cases, vascular control (aortic) by thoracotomy before abdominal exploration will prevent the excessive blood loss related to the removal of tamponade before control can be achieved. Liver packing has gained prominence in situations where control cannot be obtained by other techniques or resection is inadvisable because of the time required and associated blood loss with major resection. This is often most appropriate when hypothermia and coagulopathy have developed. Late potential complications of liver injury include bile fistula, sepsis (intrahepatic or abdominal), and vascular injury with pseudoaneurysm and hematobilia. Septic foci are usually diagnosed with CT scanning and are treated with drainage. This can be done either surgically or with CT or ultrasound guidance. Hematobilia often presents weeks to months after injury, and the trauma history may need to be specifically sought. Findings in this syndrome include gastrointestinal bleeding, jaundice, and colicky abdominal pain relieved by hematemesis. Selective angiography is used to make the diagnosis and has been used in reported cases to embolize the fistula. Bile fistulas usually are noted early postoperatively and will often close spontaneously if drainage is adequate and there is no distal obstruction.

## Spleen

The spleen is the most frequently injured organ in blunt abdominal trauma and is commonly associated with other intra-abdominal injuries. The traditional treatment for splenic injuries had been splenectomy, but multiple reports have highlighted the risks of postsplenectomy sepsis, and currently a selective approach is optimal. In some cases, splenectomy is still the treatment of choice, but splenorrhaphy and nonoperative observation are also indicated in some cases. Symp-

toms of injury to the spleen include those of blood loss with tachycardia, hypotension, and syncope as a late sign. Kehr's sign, or left shoulder-strap pain, is a classic finding in rupture of the spleen. Abdominal pain and tenderness in the left upper quadrant are usually attendant. Lower rib fractures on the left should suggest injury to the spleen and warrant further evaluation. Diagnosis of splenic injury is confirmed with surgical exploration in patients who require laparotomy or by CT scanning with contrast in those managed nonoperatively. Liver and spleen scanning may be helpful but are generally not as useful as CT scanning (Fig. 219-5). Management after diagnosis depends on associated injuries, hemodynamic stability, and transfusion requirements.

Delayed splenic rupture is a rare injury, which is reported to occur in 1 to 2 percent of cases of abdominal trauma. The rupture may occur at a remote time from the original trauma and not be readily associated with injury by the patient. Symptoms are similar to those in the acute injury, with diagnosis frequently made by scanning techniques. Late complications associated with splenic injury are related to the treatment modality. With splenorrhaphy or nonoperative management, secondary bleeding episodes or abscess formation may occur. With splenectomy, the late development of overwhelming bacterial sepsis is seen in children, and recent reports indicate a definite risk in adults even after polyvalent pneumococcal vaccine prophylaxis. Studies are not conclusive as to the role of prophylactic antibiotics. Patients who require splenectomy should be immunized and appraised of the risk of infection because close monitoring of infections can have a significant positive effect on the outcome of septic episodes. Antibiotic prophylaxis is controversial in this situation. Immunization should include coverage for pneumococcus, *Haemophilus influenzae,* and meningococcus.

## Pancreas

Pancreatic injury is most common with penetrating trauma. It may also occur as a result of a crushing injury, dividing the pancreas over the vertebral column. The classic case is a blow to the midepigastrium such as that from a steering wheel or the handlebar of a bicycle. CT scanning has been helpful in the diagnosis of these injuries (Fig. 219-6). Unrecognized, this injury has considerable morbidity and mortality. The exocrine products from the pancreas have an irritative effect on the peritoneum. A form of autodigestion occurs, resulting in an ideal medium for bacterial proliferation. In some situations it is clear that there is a possibility of this injury preoperatively, although most cases are discovered at exploration. If ductal injury is suspected

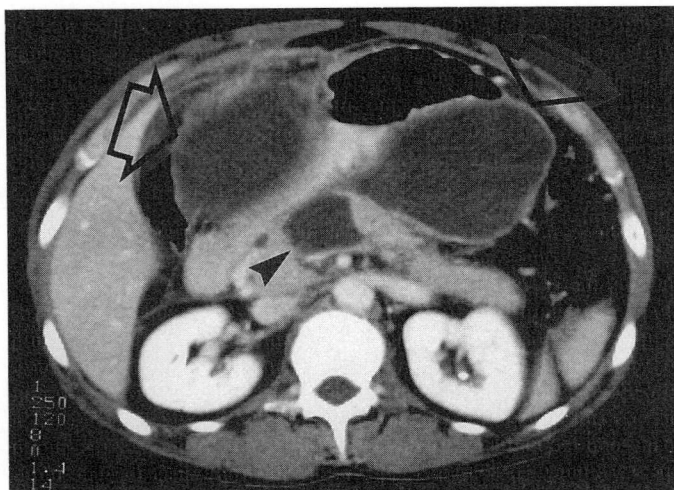

**Fig. 219-6.** Computed tomogram showing fracture of the pancreas and early formation of multiple pseudocysts.

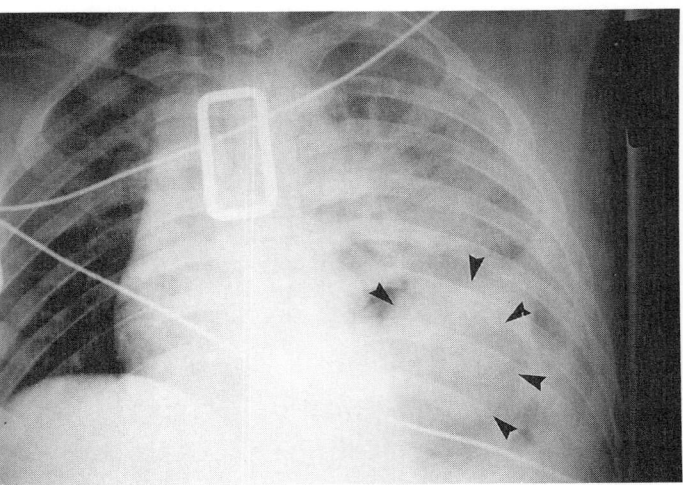

**Fig. 219-8.** Chest X-ray showing an indistinct left diaphragm and "hazy" left lower lung field with a suggestion of a mass in the area. This is suspicious for a left diaphragm rupture.

and if the patient is stable, an endoscopic retrograde cholangiopancreatography (ERCP) study will help identify the anatomy. The surgical management of these lesions is difficult because the ducts are small and hard to identify. The "road map" provided by ERCP can be helpful. Its greatest value is in documenting the absence of major ductal injury because these lesions can be managed by drainage alone, without resection.

Diagnosis at surgery is usually difficult without opening the duodenum for a contrast study via the papilla. Because this adds risk to the procedure, it is rarely done. Isolated pancreas injury is rare in blunt trauma. When associated with duodenal or biliary tract injury, management includes many options, and specific treatment will depend on the combination of injuries. Pseudocyst is a late complication possible with any type of pancreatic injury.

## Kidney

Renal parenchymal injury usually results in hematuria. Most renal injuries can be managed nonoperatively, but accurate diagnosis is essential (Fig. 219-7). Prior to laparotomy or at surgery, an IVP will

identify major lesions. Most contusions and some lacerations can be managed nonoperatively. Renal vascular lesions can be diagnosed with selective angiography or, in many cases, with contrast and CT scanning. Indications for surgery include evidence of continuing blood loss, laceration through Gerota's fascia, or loss of function.

## Diaphragm

Diaphragm injuries are often insidious, with the diagnosis made late. In many cases there is no herniation, and the only finding is blurring of the diaphragm or an effusion (Fig. 219-8). With herniation of the abdominal viscera into the chest, the diagnosis is usually clear (Fig. 219-9). Inability to pass a nasogastric tube should suggest this possibility. Diagnosis frequently is made or alluded to with contrast studies, CT scans, or DPL. This injury is diagnosed most often on the left, although it can occur on the right. Treatment is surgical, with the abdominal approach usually used in acute cases to manage the frequently associated intra-abdominal injuries. In chronic cases, presentation may be with symptoms of obstruction or bowel strangulation.

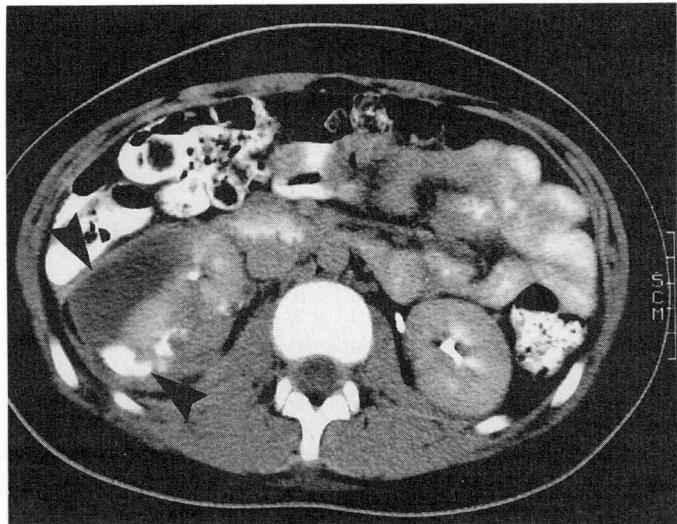

**Fig. 219-7.** Computed tomogram showing renal disruption and extrarenal urine accumulation.

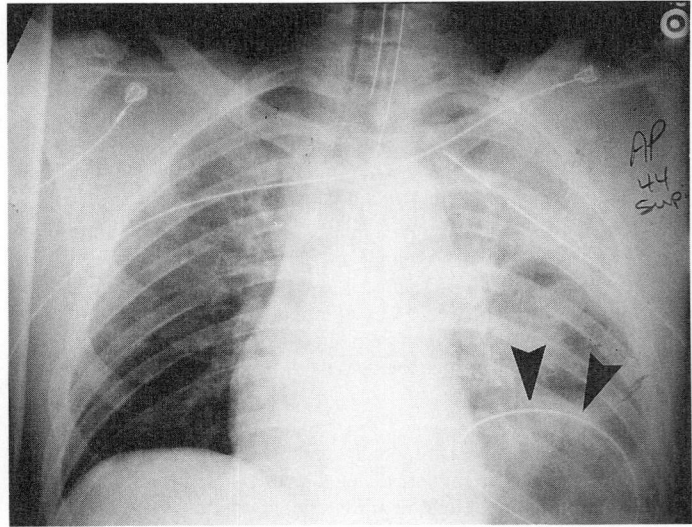

**Fig. 219-9.** Chest X-ray with a gastric tube in the left chest and obliterated left lower lung field indicating a rupture of the left diaphragm.

## Abdominal Wall

With abdominal wall penetrating injuries, there is the potential for evisceration. These patients have a high incidence of associated intra-abdominal visceral injuries, necessitating a complete abdominal exploration, making a DPL unnecessary. Repair of the associated lesions is followed by repair of the abdominal wall defect. If necessary, polypropylene mesh is used to cover the defect. In cases where the only organ eviscerated is omentum, confusion may occur, because the appearance is similar to that of subcutaneous fat. It is important to make the correct diagnosis because laparotomy is necessary. Any eviscerated organ should be covered with moist sterile dressings and replaced when examined at surgery. Replacement of organs that appear to have vascular compromise is rarely necessary and should be done in consultation with the surgeon who will be caring for the patient. Such replacement is usually done in patients who are being transferred and a delay in exploration is unavoidable.

## Vascular Structures

Both abdominal arterial and venous injuries are potentially life-threatening as a result of hemorrhage. As in solid viscera injury, lesions present with the signs of hypovolemia and occasionally an abdominal mass. Management is directed at early control of hemorrhage. Military antishock trousers (MAST) may be particularly helpful with these lesions. Prior to abdominal exploration, thoracotomy for control of the proximal aorta or use of the intra-aortic Fogarty balloon can help minimize blood loss with release of the tamponade of the MAST. The key to the surgical management of all vascular injuries is proximal and distal control of the vessels. In all cases the chest as well as the upper thighs must be prepared. This will give exposure for control of thoracic vessels and open cardiac massage should it be necessary and the saphenous vein if grafting is necessary. In isolated injuries to the abdominal vasculature the use of autotransfusion should be considered, and appropriate personnel for the use of that device should be arranged prior to exploration.

## COMPLICATIONS AND IATROGENIC INJURIES

The major problems that result from abdominal injuries are related to either missed injuries or overtreatment of suspected injuries; preventable deaths are those of patients with surgically correctable in whom the diagnosis was missed or delayed. In missed solid organ and vascular injuries, hemorrhage and the complications of organ secretion predominate. In hollow viscus injury, local or systemic sepsis, the result of leaking, is the major risk. Negative laparotomy has minimal associated morbidity and is often necessary to be certain that a life-threatening injury is not present. Finding no correctable lesion at surgery does not make that surgery inappropriate if the indications were appropriate. Hypothermia is a major risk to the traumatized patient. Trauma patients often present to the emergency department cold, and the use of blood without use of warmers and room temperature crystalloid solution intravenously and in DPL solutions contributes to the problem. In addition, these patients need to be undressed for complete examination, also contributing to heat loss. Patient temperature needs to be monitored carefully preferably with a central thermometer. Fluid warmers, warming blankets, warm lavage, and warm examination rooms help to avoid this problem.

## EMERGENCY DEPARTMENT EVALUATION

### History and Physical Examination

A directed history and physical examination are essential. The history should include a brief past medical history in addition to that relative to the wounding mechanism. Paramedical personnel are important sources of information, particularly for neurologically impaired pa-

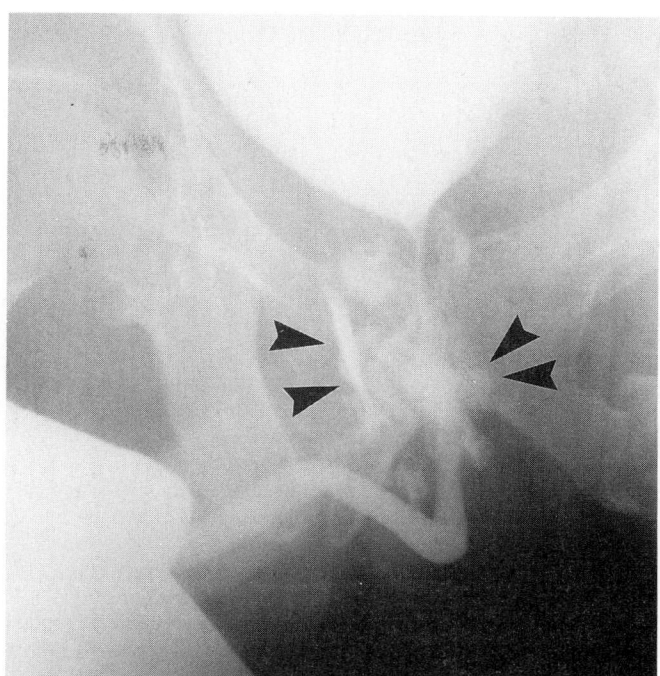

**Fig. 219-10.** Urethrogram showing extravasation of contrast from a ureteral disruption.

tients. The condition of the vehicle and the status of other passengers in a motor vehicle accident are helpful indicators of the severity of the injuring mechanism. Preexisting conditions, medications, and allergies must be considered because all can affect the diagnosis, management, and outcome.

Physical examination of the abdomen includes evaluation of the back, lower chest, and perineum, with rectal and vaginal examinations. Such an examination is especially important in patients who require emergent exploratory celiotomy. An injury to the back or perineum is difficult to diagnose (evaluate) at celiotomy, and appropriate intraoperative management depends on accurate preoperative evaluation.

### Resuscitation Room Radiographs

A pelvic x-ray is important in all multiply injured patients but has particular importance in patients with abdominal trauma. Pelvic injuries can result in significant blood loss and are often associated with intra-abdominal visceral injury. In the presence of a fracture, DPL should be done through a supraumbilical incision to avoid entering the pelvic hematoma with a resultant false positive examination. When urethral tear is suspected, a urethrogram should be done before Foley catheter placement (Fig. 219-10). An IVP and a cystogram are helpful in the presence of hematuria and may negate the need for DPL if intraperitoneal bladder rupture is identified (Fig. 219-11). Any x-ray revealing free air, suggesting hollow visceral injury, would also negate the DPL.

### Adjunctive Tests

#### Diagnostic Peritoneal Lavage

Diagnostic peritoneal lavage remains an excellent test for quickly evaluating the abdomen. Advantages of the test include its sensitivity (98 percent in many reports), its availability, and the relative speed with which it can be performed. Problems with the test are related to the potential for iatrogenic injury and its misapplication to the evaluation of retroperitoneal injuries. The fairly high incidence of false pos-

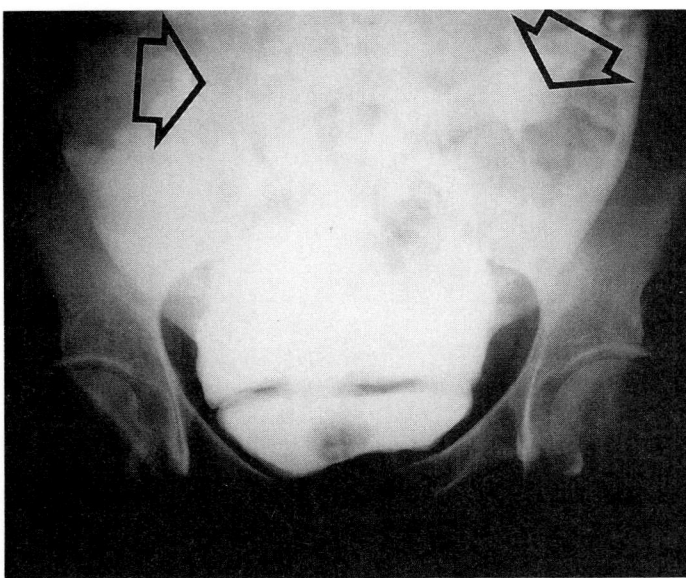

**Fig. 219-11.** Cystogram showing intraperitoneal bladder rupture demonstrated by contrast flowing freely intraperitoneally.

itive examinations has been used as an argument for the superiority of the CT scan. The relative lack of specificity has also been pointed out. When one considers the question of the need for emergency exploratory celiotomy, and not whether a particular abdominal injury exists, the examination has a high level of sensitivity and specificity.

Indications for DPL in blunt trauma include a history of significant abdominal trauma when the physical examination is equivocal. DPL is especially useful in patients in whom the examination is unreliable, as in patients with a head or spinal cord injury or with drug intoxication. Unexplained hypotension when intra-abdominal hemorrhage is a possibility is another indication. Patients who will be unavailable for monitoring by abdominal examination, such as those who will require general anesthesia for other injuries, may also benefit from a preoperative DPL.

In penetrating injury, lavage should be used when it is not clear that celiotomy is necessary. In stab wounds, this is when clinical signs of peritoneal irritation are absent and local wound exploration indicates that the superficial muscle fascia has been violated. In low-velocity gunshot wounds, there may be some value when peritoneal penetration is unclear and the clinical examination is negative. DPL in tangential wounds or wounds of the low chest may be helpful in confirming a negative examination. In high-velocity gunshot wounds, most surgeons feel exploratory celiotomy should be done when any question of penetration exists.

There are no absolute contraindications to peritoneal lavage, only relative contraindications. It is clearly *not necessary* in patients in whom indications for surgery are present because it will delay surgery and does have potential complications. The relative contraindications are in patients for whom the procedure carries a greater risk, such as advanced hepatic dysfunction with portal hypertension, severe coagulopathies, among others. In patients with previous abdominal surgery or gravid uterus, DPL may be performed with a modified or open technique. By making the incision away from previous incisions or the uterus and using the open technique, the examination can be done safely. Extensive adhesions may result in loculation and prevent distribution of fluid throughout the entire abdomen. This can result in a false negative examination. Marked gaseous distention, which may result from external ventilation with a mask, increases the risk of bowel injury. Open lavage should be used if DPL is felt to be necessary.

Three techniques can be used: closed, semiclosed, or open. In all

three, the patient should have a Foley catheter and nasogastric tube placed first for drainage and for decompression of those organs. The area should be prepared, draped, and anesthetized with local anesthetic with epinephrine in a concentration of 1:100,000. In the closed technique, a skin nick is made, followed by needle placement in the peritoneum. Using the Seldinger technique, a lavage catheter is placed. In the semiclosed technique, the incision is carried down to the fascia, which is visualized prior to peritoneal puncture. In the open technique, the incision is carried down to the peritoneum, which is opened under direct visualization, and a catheter is placed in the peritoneal cavity. The incision is usually made in the midline below the umbilicus, but it can be made paramedianly or supraumbilically, depending on the location of previous incisions or the presence of a pelvic fracture.

After catheter placement, fluid is aspirated, and if more than 5 mL of blood is returned the test is positive. If no blood is aspirated, then 20 mL/kg of lactated Ringer's solution up to 1000 mL is instilled into the peritoneum. The patient's position may be changed or the abdomen massaged to ensure complete distribution and sampling throughout the abdomen. Fluid is returned by placing the intravenous bag below the level of the abdomen to siphon the fluid out of the abdomen. Slight reverse Trendelenburg's position may facilitate return. Inadequate return of the lavage fluid is a common problem. Usually this is a result of catheter positioning, but translocation of the fluid into the thorax can occur with diaphragm rupture. An aliquot of the lavage fluid is then examined. The examination is positive if the red blood cell count is greater than 100,000 cells/$\mu$L, the white blood cell count is greater than 500 cells/$\mu$L, the amylase level is above 200 units/100 mL, or bile is present or if, on microscopic examination, bacteria or vegetable material is seen.

In penetrating injury, the criteria for a positive examination are controversial. Many centers reduce the red blood cell count considered to be a positive test. In gunshot wounds, the use of lavage remains controversial.

In situations where the initial appearance of the fluid is slightly pink, suggesting an equivocal test, or when the patient will be transferred, the catheter may be left in place for a repeat examination later. If the patient is to be transferred, a sample of the lavage fluid should accompany the patient.

## Computed Tomography

The CT scan is an excellent test and complements the DPL. When performed under optimal conditions, the scan has a much greater specificity than DPL. A useful examination requires a cooperative patient and personnel skilled in the examination of trauma patients. For optimal resolution, oral and intravenous contrast material should be given. The oral contrast should be in two boluses. This is generally given by nasogastric tube. The first bolus is 900 mL of 3.67% water-soluble contrast given as soon as possible before the examination. A second bolus of 250 mL is given in the CT unit. The intravenous contrast is given as a bolus at the time of the study; iodinated contrast material, 150 mL of a 60% solution, is used in adults. Studies are now being done to determine the value of contrast by enema to increase the sensitivity in evaluation of colon perforation.

The main advantage of CT scanning is to better evaluate the retroperitoneum and to more precisely locate an intra-abdominal injury preoperatively. In addition, the study may be able to clearly identify injuries that are best managed nonoperatively, for example, liver hematoma. There are conflicting reports as to the sensitivity of the test, and there are multiple reports of missed surgical lesions. Jejunal perforations appear to be the most difficult to diagnose. It should be emphasized that both DPL and CT scanning should be evaluated in the context of the clinical status. Neither test is perfect, and each should be used in conjunction with the clinical findings over time.

## Ultrasound

Up to four views are obtained in the abdominal ultrasound examination. The right lateral subcostal position gives visualization of the kidney-liver junction and is the easiest area to identify fluid, making this site the most frequently used. The relative role of ultrasound in evaluation of trauma patients has not yet been defined. Most use the study in patients who need quick evaluation and are too unstable for transfer to the scan area. Serial examination is possible using portable machines and may eliminate many of the false negative examinations that were identified when this test was first used. The interpretation of ultrasound findings is operator dependent. However, the ability to identify blood in Morrison's pouch is learned quickly.

## Arteriography

The evaluation of major vessel injuries may best be accomplished by arteriography. The CT scan with contrast does, however, appear to be replacing the arteriogram as a screening test for renal arterial lesion. However, in pelvic fractures, for example, bleeding sites can be located, and there is the potential for control of these bleeding sites through embolization. An aortogram remains the diagnostic test of choice to rule out the possibility of thoracic aortic injury although transosophageal echo and high-speed computerized scanning are being evaluated in this context.

## MANAGEMENT

The approach to the patient with abdominal trauma is not unique. All traumatized patients should have a similar approach. The airways, breathing, and circulation are assessed and managed first. The airway is managed with cervical spine control. Breathing is with ventilatory assistance, if necessary, followed by evaluation and resuscitation of circulation. Fluid resuscitation is managed by several large-bore intravenous lines. The rate at which fluid can be delivered depends on the caliber of the catheter inserted. When massive fluid replacement is necessary, a 9 F catheter can be placed either peripherally or centrally using the Seldinger technique. At the time of line placement, blood can be drawn for laboratory studies. A routine trauma laboratory series should be obtained, including at least a complete blood count, electrolytes, blood sugar, amylase, type and crossmatch, pregnancy test, urinalysis, and toxicology as indicated. Additional evaluation as a baseline in the severely injured patient should include renal, hepatic, and clotting function tests.

A nasogastric tube may be useful for both diagnostic and therapeutic reasons. The presence of bloody gastric aspirate suggests nasopharyngeal or gastrointestinal injury. Patients with trauma frequently have gastric distention and nasogastric tube placement will help to prevent aspiration. Nasal placement of the tube is contraindicated in the presence of facial injury with suspected cribriform plate fracture. Foley catheter placement should follow a urethrogram when there is an injury or findings suggestive of urethral tear. Blood at the urethral meatus or a large perineal hematoma suggests urethral tear.

When there is a suspected pelvic fracture, a rectal examination should be done before Foley catheter placement to determine the position of the prostate gland. If the position of the gland is abnormal, a urethrogram should be done. With hematuria, an IVP and cystogram should be considered. In the evaluation of more stable patients, CT scanning with contrast gives better resolution in renal parenchymal injuries. Subsequent management depends on the findings of the above-mentioned examinations. DPL, CT scanning, and exploratory laparotomy may all be indicated under certain circumstances (Table 219-1). In cases where there is a suspicion of bowel injury, antibiotics active against both aerobes and anaerobes should be given preoperatively. Most commonly a single broad-spectrum antibiotic is given intravenously.

## BIBLIOGRAPHY

American College of Surgeons Committee on Trauma. *Advanced Trauma Life Support Course* (manual). Chicago: 1984.

Anderson PA, Rivera FP, Maier RV, et al. The epidemiology of seatbelt associated injuries. *J Trauma* 31:60, 1991.

Ang JGP, Hanslits ML, Clark RA, et al. Computed tomography of abdominal and pelvic trauma. *J Emerg Med* 3:311, 1985.

Cue JL, Miller FB, Cryer HM, et al. A prospective, randomized comparison between open and closed peritoneal lavage techniques. *J Trauma* 30:880, 1990.

Marx JA, Moore EE, Jorden RC, et al. Limitations of computed tomography in the evaluation of acute abdominal trauma: a prospective comparison with diagnostic peritoneal lavage. *J Trauma* 25:933, 1985.

McAnena OL, Moore EE, Marx JA. Initial evaluation of the patient with blunt abdominal trauma. *Abdom Trauma* 70:495, 515, 1990.

Moore EE, Marx JA. Penetrating abdominal wounds: rationale for exploratory laparotomy. *JAMA* 253:2705, 1985.

Rothlin MA, Naf R, Amgwerd M, et al. Ultrasound in blunt abdominal and thoracic trauma. *J Trauma* 34(4), 1993.

Thal ER, May RA, Bessinger OD. Peritoneal lavage: its unreliability in gunshot wounds of the lower chest and abdomen. *Arch Surg* 115:430, 1980.

Wisner DH, Wold RL, Frey CF. Diagnosis and treatment of pancreatic injuries: an analysis of management principles. *Arch Surg* 125:1109, 1990.

**Table 219-1.** Indications for Exploratory Celiotomy

Abdominal trauma and hemodynamic instability
Abdominal wall disruption with evisceration
Clinical findings of peritoneal irritation
Free air in abdomen on x-ray
Retroperitoneal air on x-ray
Ruptured urinary bladder (intraperitoneal)
Positive peritoneal tap or lavage
Rectal perforation
Surgically correctable lesions suggested by CT scan

# 220

# PENETRATING TRAUMA TO THE POSTERIOR ABDOMEN AND BUTTOCK

**Mark D. Odland**
**Arthur L. Ney**

Penetrating trauma to the back, flank, and buttock is most likely to occur from gunshot and stab wounds. The extent of injury can be difficult to assess when extraperitoneal injury occurs and there is a desire to avoid nontherapeutic or diagnostic celiotomy. Due to the increasing sophistication of diagnostic testing, selective management is now possible, at least in some cases. This chapter outlines the evaluation of patients with penetrating trauma to the posterior abdomen and buttock and the rationale for safer selective management.

## PENETRATING TRAUMA TO THE POSTERIOR ABDOMEN

### Pathophysiology

Penetrating trauma to the posterior abdomen is a distinct subcategory of penetrating torso trauma. Because of the protection afforded by the pelvis, spine, and thick musculature of the back, intraperitoneal and retroperitoneal contents are less likely to be injured. However, extraperitoneal visceral injury can occur without associated intraperitoneal injury, with minimal physical findings seen on examination. This apparent absence of physical findings will delay the diagnosis of duodenal, renal, colonic, rectal, and pancreatic injuries. Given the morbidity and mortality of such injuries when left untreated, diagnostic accuracy is of the utmost importance. Suspicion of injury and frequent reevaluation are paramount to successful outcome.

The posterior abdomen, namely the flank and back, is the area posterior to the anterior axillary line, extending from the tip of the scapula to the iliac crest. The organs most commonly injured by penetrating trauma to this area are the liver, kidney, and colon. With any thoracic injury below the tip of the scapula, diaphragmatic injury and subsequent intraperitoneal injury may occur. Consequently, both the abdomen and chest must be evaluated in all cases of penetrating injury to the posterior abdomen or thorax. The treatment of specific organ injuries is covered in the chapters on abdominal trauma (Chapter 219) and genitourinary tract trauma (Chapter 221).

## Clinical Features

All patients with penetrating trauma to the posterior abdomen should be evaluated according to a routine regimen. Initial resuscitation should follow the ABCs, as outlined in Chapter 212. The importance of obtaining a complete history and performing a thorough physical examination cannot be overemphasized. Mechanism of injury, description of the wounding object, and time elapsed since wounding are all important to the evaluation of these patients. Baseline hemogram, chest radiograph, urinalysis, and rectal examination are performed on all patients. Physical examination followed by observation was highly accurate in identifying significant injuries in Los Angeles County–USC Medical Center emergency department admissions for injuries of this type. Diagnostic accuracy can be further improved by the use of other diagnostic modalities. False-negative examinations result from the absence of physical findings in cases of hidden retroperitoneal injury. Unrecognized, such injuries can lead to significant morbidity and mortality.

## Diagnosis

### Exploratory Celiotomy

If any of the following signs or symptoms exist, immediate celiotomy should be performed:

Shock
Hemodynamic instability
Evisceration
Peritonitis
Transabdominal missile path
Intraperitoneal free air
Ongoing blood loss

All intraperitoneal and retroperitoneal organs should be visualized using appropriate operative maneuvers.

### Adjunctive Diagnostic Measures

If immediate celiotomy is not indicated, adjunctive diagnostic measures can be used. These measures include wound exploration, diagnostic peritoneal lavage (DPL), and computed tomography (CT).

#### Local Wound Exploration

In the patient with a history and physical examination consistent with a low probability of visceral injury, wound exploration may be performed. Only on rare occasions should a missile wound be explored. Local wound exploration using sterile technique, adequate anesthesia, good exposure, and hemostasis has been used to decide whether further evaluation or hospitalization is necessary. If the injury does not extend through fascia or muscle, the patient may be treated as an outpatient. With deeper penetrating injuries, exploration can be terminated and other diagnostic studies performed. Wound exploration through deep tissue planes may lead to hemorrhage, further tissue damage, and a false sense of security. More information is obtained from DPL or CT scanning. Wound exploration has a very limited role in evaluating the patient with penetrating trauma to the posterior abdomen.

#### Diagnostic Peritoneal Lavage

Diagnostic peritoneal lavage is highly accurate in determining whether intraperitoneal injury exists, but poorly detects the presence of retroperitoneal injury. If, on DPL, blood is obtained on aspiration or a red blood cell (RBC) count of $10,000/mm^3$ or greater is obtained, it is the authors' custom to perform a celiotomy. Other trauma surgeons use different RBC criteria, ranging from $1000/mm^3$ to $100,000/mm^3$. Controversy exists over whether to perform DPL before CT scanning, which more accurately examines the retroperitoneal contents. In the stable patient in whom there is a low suspicion of intraperitoneal injury, the authors perform a CT scan before DPL, to avoid confusion caused by the infused fluid. The unstable patient is taken to the operating room for definitive therapy, without any adjunctive diagnostic testing. DPL is performed after CT scan in hemodynamically stable patients with no indications for immediate celiotomy, but in whom injury to the diaphragm or hollow viscus is suspected.

#### Computed Tomography

CT scanning has become a valuable adjunct in the evaluation of patients with posterior abdominal penetrating trauma. A diagnostic accuracy of nearly 97 percent has been achieved in some series. Oral and intravenous contrast are necessary for an optimal study, and some centers include rectal contrast. Organ injuries can be visualized and management based on the findings and the type of injury. More commonly, a retroperitoneal hematoma without associated organ injury is found. Angiography is necessary if the hematoma is located near the great vessels or in a perinephric location. If a hematoma is located near a hollow organ, fluoroscopic contrast studies or celiotomy may be required. Free peritoneal fluid suggests intraperitoneal penetration and the need for celiotomy.

## Treatment

Treatment of penetrating trauma to the posterior abdomen remains controversial. Some have advocated mandatory celiotomy to detect insidious injuries early. With the increasing availability and accuracy of computed tomography, many surgeons now favor close observation of the patient and selective management. Mandatory celiotomy is indicated in gunshot wounds or other missile injuries, since missile wounding results in visceral injury in 80 to 90 percent of cases. If history and physical examination indicate a low likelihood of intraperitoneal injury, as with superficial tangential wounds, then selective management may be entertained. However, cases suitable for selective management are rare. Blast effect does occur, making possible a visceral injury from a missile on an extraperitoneal course; this must be taken into account when evaluating and treating these superficial missile injuries. Selective management is more appropriately applied in cases of stab wounding.

It is the authors' practice to manage penetrating trauma to the posterior abdomen as follows.

1. When the diagnosis of intraperitoneal or vascular injury can be made on the basis of history and physical examination alone, immediate celiotomy is performed.
2. Gross hematuria without other signs and symptoms that warrant immediate celiotomy is further clarified through CT scanning and/or angiography.

3. When there are no signs or symptoms of significant organ injury, other adjunctive diagnostic measures are used to identify hidden injuries. CT scanning with oral contrast, rectally administered contrast, and intravenous contrast is done to identify duodenal, pancreatic, colonic, and renal injuries or hematomas.
4. Further diagnostic workup, such as DPL, angiography, or ERCP is then performed as indicated.

Patient management is directed by the findings. All patients are hospitalized and examined frequently for any changes in their condition. In the authors' experience, this regimen identifies nearly all significant injuries.

## PENETRATING BUTTOCK INJURIES

### Pathophysiology

Penetrating trauma to the buttock has the potential to injure multiple organ systems, including the gastrointestinal (GI), genitourinary (GU), and neurologic systems, and evaluation must assess each of these systems. In addition, intraperitoneal injury may be present, necessitating celiotomy. Indications for mandatory celiotomy include shock, intraperitoneal penetration as evidenced by missile trajectory, peritonitis, free air, or evidence of vascular, GU, or bowel injury.

### Clinical Features and Diagnosis

After initial resuscitation, evaluation begins with a thorough history and physical examination and an assessment of the likelihood of visceral injury. Abdominal examination results consistent with peritonitis, hemodynamic instability, or blood within the GI tract all indicate the need for operative therapy. Routine radiologic examination of the pelvis may reveal bony injury, suggesting penetration of the pelvis and possibly the intraperitoneal cavity. Routine proctosigmoidoscopy will accurately identify rectal injuries. If there is blood within the GI tract, contrast enemas may identify colon injury. Hematuria, scrotal hematoma, or penile hematoma could signify lower GU tract injuries, prompting further investigation with retrograde urethrograms, cystograms, and intravenous pyelography. Signs of vascular injury, such as pulselessness, pain, pallor, paresthesias, or paralysis, should prompt operation or further investigation. Hypotension, evidence of ongoing blood loss, and nerve injuries are suggestive of significant vascular injury. CT scanning of the pelvis can determine the presence or absence of a hematoma and indicate any need for further investigation.

The mechanisms of nerve injury include transection, concussion, and stretch injury secondary to hematoma or false aneurysm. With sciatic nerve or femoral nerve injuries, early operative intervention is necessary to assess the nature of the injury and repair the nerve.

### Treatment

When a patient has sustained a penetrating injury to the buttock and presents with signs or symptoms of organ injury, such as shock, peritonitis, hematuria, or gastrointestinal bleeding, the authors recommend proctosigmoidoscopy to identify rectal injury, followed by celiotomy. In the stable patient without evidence of intraperitoneal or retroperitoneal organ injury, further evaluation is done by proctosigmoidoscopy and cystourethrogram. CT scanning with rectal and intravenous contrast may be done to look for colon, urinary tract, or vascular injury. When the CT scan reveals the presence of a pelvic hematoma, angiography and venography may detect significant vascular injury. If femoral or sciatic nerve deficit exists, nerve exploration is performed.

Operative therapy for penetrating buttock injuries should follow standard surgical principles for the injured organ system. Debridement and closure of bowel injuries, or colostomy if indicated, are standard operative therapies for small or large bowel injury. Proximal sigmoid colostomy, distal washout, and presacral drainage continue to be the treatment of choice for rectal injuries. Lower GU tract injuries are safely treated with suprapubic cystostomy, debridement, and drainage, as indicated. Vascular injuries are best treated with primary repair or autogenous grafts.

## SUMMARY

Penetrating trauma to the posterior abdomen is a distinct subcategory of penetrating abdominal and thoracic trauma. Insidious injuries may occur; therefore a systematic approach to the evaluation of these injuries is necessary. Because significant retroperitoneal injury can occur without intraperitoneal injury, there may be an absence of physical findings. Left untreated, these injuries can cause significant morbidity and mortality.

Penetrating injuries to the buttock can injure several different organ systems and result in significant morbidity and mortality. The associated visceral injuries are often extraperitoneal and have subtle or minimal physical findings. Successful management requires a thorough, systematic evaluation to identify these injuries early. With appropriate surgical mangement, morbidity and mortality should be kept to a minimum.

## BIBLIOGRAPHY

Berne TV: Management of penetrating back trauma. *Surg Clin North Am* 70:671, 1990.

Demetriades D, Rabinowitz B, Sofianos C, et al: The management of penetrating injuries to the back. *Ann Surg* 207:72, 1988.

Fallon WF, Reyna TM, Brunner RG, Cromms C, Alexander RH: Penetrating trauma to the buttock. *South Med J* 81:1237, 1988.

Ferraro FJ, Livingston DH, Odom J, et al: The role of sigmoidoscopy in the management of gunshot wounds to the buttocks. *Am Surgeon* 59:350, 1993.

Henneman PL: Abdominal CT in the evaluation of patients with stab wounds of the back [letter; comment]. *J Trauma* 30:754, 1990.

Henneman PL, Marx JA, Moore EE, et al: Diagnostic peritoneal lavage: Accuracy in predicting necessary laparotomy following blunt and penetrating trauma. *J Trauma* 30:1345, 1990.

Himmelman RG, Martin M, Gilkey S, et al: Triple-contrast CT scans in penetrating back and flank trauma. *J Trauma* 31:852, 1991.

Meyer DM, Thal ER, Weigelt JA, et al: The role of abdominal CT in the evaluation of stab wounds to the back. *J Trauma* 29:1226, 1989.

Phillips T, Scalafani JA, Goldstein A, et al: The use of contrast-enhanced CT enema in the management of penetrating trauma to the flank and back. *J Trauma* 26:1226, 1989.

# 221
# TRAUMA TO THE GENITOURINARY TRACT

Joe Y. Lee
Alexander S. Cass

In the multiply injured patient the management of life-threatening injuries takes precedence over urologic injury, and the diagnostic evaluation of genitourinary trauma is often delayed. Early diagnosis and surgical management, however, can optimize the restoration of urinary function. The basic processes of obtaining a patient history, performing a physical examination, examining the urine, and properly using and interpreting radiographic imaging are essential for accurate diagnosis and treatment.

## PERINEAL INSPECTION DURING THE SECONDARY SURVEY

During the head-to-toe search for injury that takes place during the secondary survey, a concerted effort should be made to closely inspect the perineum. It is not necessary to deflate pneumatic antishock garments during this search. The clothing at the crotch can be cut away with scissors by slightly spreading the legs. Blood on the underwear is an important finding and should be duly noted. In both male and female patients, spread the folds of the buttocks in search of perineal lacerations. If such are found, they usually denote an open pelvic fracture. Do not insert a finger lest a clot be disrupted and exsanguinating hemorrhage result. This finding means that the patient will need a diverting colostomy. It is also an indication for antibiotics. A second-generation cephalosporin such as cefoxitin, 2 g IV, would suffice. Next, perform a rectal examination noting sphincter tone, the position and quality of the prostate gland, and whether or not blood is present in the rectum. Blood in the rectum may signify rectal perforation. Start antibiotics if this finding is present. Decreased sphincter tone may mean spinal cord injury. If the sacrum is fractured, it may signify a cauda equina syndrome and this should be tested for later. If the prostate is riding high or has a boggy feeling, there has been a disruption of the membranous urethra. Next, palpate the scrotum, checking for ecchymoses, laceration, and testicular disruption. Palpate the length of the penis while looking for blood at the meatus. In females, inspect the labia looking for lacerations. Perform a bimanual vaginal examination feeling for vaginal lacerations. If the patient is of child-bearing age and there is blood in the vagina, a speculum examination will be necessary to rule out vaginal laceration. If a vaginal laceration is present, start IV antibiotics. It is helpful to include palpation of the femoral pulses in this examination.

During the secondary survey, the trauma series x-rays are obtained, including cervical spine films, a chest x-ray, and an anteroposterior (AP) view of the pelvis. The presence of a pelvic fracture will have important implications in the workup for genitourinary injuries.

## RADIOGRAPHIC EVALUATION

The indications for radiographic evaluation of the urinary tract following trauma continue to evolve. Previously, patients with any degree of hematuria required a complete radiographic evaluation. In adult patients with blunt trauma and only microscopic hematuria, the diagnostic yield of a significant urologic injury was extremely low. Currently, adult patients with blunt trauma who have gross hematuria or microscopic hematuria that is associated with either shock or significant nongenitourinary injuries are evaluated radiographically. Adult patients with penetrating trauma require radiographic studies regardless of the degree of hematuria. In contrast, pediatric patients require radiographic studies with any degree of hematuria with either blunt or penetrating trauma. Clinical assessment may mandate further evaluation. Transverse lumbar process or bony pelvic fractures; high-velocity deceleration injuries; and flank pain, tenderness, and masses should prompt radiographic studies. The studies should follow a caudal to cephalad direction (retrograde urethrogram, cystogram, intravenous pyelogram, etc.).

### Retrograde Urethrogram

When blood is found at the urethral meatus, a retrograde urethrogram with contrast solution determines the integrity of the urethra before any urethral instrumentation, in order to prevent the conversion of a partial urethral laceration into a complete transection. If the prostate gland was grossly displaced on rectal examination, the urethra is transected and a retrograde study is not needed, at least not in the initial evaluation. Approximately 30 mL of radiocontrast solution is injected into the urethra by holding the syringe tip in the meatus with lead gloves or with a Foley catheter inserted 1 to 2 cm into the urethra into the navicular fossa of the distal urethra and the balloon inflated with 1 mL of saline. An oblique view is obtained by placing the x-ray tube at an oblique angle above the supine patient. The entire length of the urethra is seen on the plain film when the x-ray is taken as the last 10 mL of the contrast solution is injected. Occasionally a patient may be transferred from another facility with an indwelling urethral catheter in place. A retrograde urethrogram can be performed without removing the urethral catheter by injecting contrast solution into the urethra through a small feeding tube placed adjacent to the urethral catheter.

### Cystogram

In the presence of a pelvic ring fracture or gross hematuria, a cystogram is performed to evaluate the urinary bladder. Contrast solution, 400 to 500 mL in adults and 5 mL/kg in children, is instilled into the bladder under gravity from 2 ft (60 cm) above the patient. In both adults and children the instillation is halted if a bladder contraction is elicited. At a height of 2 ft the intravesical pressure generated approximates the physiologic voiding pressure. Unless adequate bladder pressure is generated, the cystogram may be falsely negative. After the AP film is obtained, the bladder is emptied of the contrast solution and washed out with saline solution; then another AP film is taken as the "washout film."

### Intravenous Pyelogram

An intravenous pyelogram (IVP) is seldom indicated in the emergency setting. It has been replaced by the enhanced computed tomography (CT) scan. However, there may be a need for an IVP in an unstable patient who is headed for the operating room. If the patient's blood pressure is 70 mmHg or less, however, the kidneys may not concentrate the contrast and are more susceptible to injury by it.

### Enhanced Abdominal CT

In the multiply injured patient in stable condition, CT may be the initial study obtained to assess associated abdominal injuries and to stage the extent of renal injury. CT of the abdomen details the retroperitoneal anatomy, hematomas, renal lacerations, and renal devascularization. In children with hematuria, CT is the radiographic study of choice in evaluating renal injuries because a significant nonrenal intraabdominal injury is more likely than a renal injury. Thus, if an IVP is the only study obtained in children, significant associated injuries will be missed. If the IVP or CT reveal nonfunction, a renal arteriogram may be required in selected cases.

The following should be considered when ordering studies in the trauma patient: (1) IV contrast agents can cause false-positive scans for blood; (2) the total quantity of contrast required may limit the number of contrast studies, especially with shock; (3) hypotensive patients are at risk for developing contrast-induced acute renal failure; (4) abdominal CT reveals more information but requires a hemodynamically stable condition; and (5) an intraoperative IVP during an emergency laparotomy is needed to determine the status of the contralateral kidney.

## RENAL INJURIES

Renal injury is the most frequent form of genitourinary trauma (Table 221-1).

Penetrating injuries to the kidneys are secondary to gunshot and stab wounds. Gunshot wounds require surgical exploration because of the high incidence of associated injuries to adjacent structures such as bowel, liver, and spleen. An intraoperative IVP should be obtained to document contralateral renal function. Patients in hemodynamically stable condition with stab wounds to the flank (posterior to the

**Table 221-1.** Incidence of Sites of Genitourinary Injuries 1959–1985,
St. Paul Ramsey Hospital and Hennepin County
Medical Center

| Site | Number | Percent |
|------|--------|---------|
| Kidney | 1667 | 67 |
| Ureter | 30 | 1 |
| Bladder | 534 | 22 |
| Urethra | 79 | 3 |
| Testis | 75 | 3 |
| Penis/scrotum | 101 | 4 |
| Total | 2486 | 100 |

anterior axillary line) are evaluated with CT. Isolated minor renal injuries may be managed conservatively. Conversely, stab wounds to the abdomen are associated with injuries to other organs and thus require exploration.

Blunt renal injuries are evaluated radiographically. The kidneys are well protected in the retroperitoneal location surrounded by bulky musculature, fascia, and lower ribs. Considerable force is generally necessary to cause significant renal injury. Fractured ribs, vertebral transverse process fractures, flank bruises or hematomas, and hematuria are indications for radiographic evaluation.

## Renal Contusion

Renal contusions are minor renal injuries with renal parenchymal ecchymosis, minor lacerations, and subcapsular hematomas with an intact renal capsule. Contusions account for 92 percent of renal injuries. Radiographically, the IVP is usually normal and the CT may reveal edema with microextravasation of contrast within the renal parenchyma. Subcapsular hematoma appears as a flattened portion of the renal cortex compressed by the hematoma under the renal capsule.

Minor renal injuries are managed conservatively with bed rest, hydration, serial hematocrits, vital signs, and serial urine specimens for the degree of gross hematuria. Patients with gross hematuria remain at bedrest until the gross hematuria resolves and remain at limited activity until the microscopic hematuria resolves. Renal contusions almost always resolve without sequelae unless there is a preexisting renal lesion such as hydronephrosis, cyst, or tumor.

## Renal Laceration

Renal lacerations are classified as either minor cortical lacerations that do not involve the medulla or collecting system or major renal lacerations that extend deep into the corticomedullary junction or collecting system. The resulting perirenal hematoma may fill the perirenal space before it is tamponaded by the Gerota fascia. Renal lacerations account for approximately 5 percent of renal injuries. Radiographic studies demonstrate disruption of the renal outline, a perirenal hematoma, and possibly extravasation of contrast adjacent to the kidney.

The management of renal lacerations remains controversial. Almost all minor lacerations heal without sequelae with conservative management. Major lacerations may develop complications despite remaining in a stable hemodynamic condition with conservative therapy. The absolute indication for surgical exploration of a renal injury is persistent retroperitoneal bleeding with hemodynamic instability. Relative indications include stable patients with extensive urinary extravasation, large devitalized renal fragments, and renal pedicle injuries. Surgical exploration consists of preliminary vascular control, debridement, and surgical repair. Early control of the renal vessels decreases the nephrectomy rate in the potentially salvageable kidney. Nephrectomy, however, may be necessary in the patient in unstable condition.

## Renal Rupture

Renal ruptures or shattered kidneys account for 1 percent of renal injuries. A large expanding perirenal hematoma accompanies renal rupture, and the patient becomes clinically unstable from the continued bleeding. Radiographic studies reveal multiple deep lacerations, devitalized kidney fragments, and extravasation of contrast. Renal exploration, with preliminary pedicle control with vascular clamps, and nephrectomy is the treatment of choice.

## Renal Pedicle Injury

Renal pedicle injuries include lacerations and thrombosis of the renal artery, vein, and their branches. Renal pedicle injuries make up 2 percent of all renal injuries. These injuries result from high-velocity deceleration injuries and penetrating trauma. In blunt trauma the most common renal pedicle injury is thrombosis of the renal artery that follows tearing of the intima with intact adventitial and medial layers. There is bruising surrounding the renal artery, but no perirenal hematoma as found in renal pedicle lacerations. When the renal artery is occluded or divided, the IVP shows nonfunction and an arteriogram reveals renal artery occlusion or bleeding. CT demonstrates a nonenhanced kidney with minimal peripheral enhancement from the renal capsular vessels ("rim sign"). Renal vein thrombosis results in delayed renal function and parenchymal swelling in the absence of ureteral obstruction.

Renal pedicle injuries are usually associated with multiple life-threatening injuries, and the safest surgical option is nephrectomy. In the patient in stable condition with an isolated renal pedicle injury, repair should be undertaken within 12 h of the injury if a viable kidney is to result. Intimal tears of the renal artery are excised with an end-to-end anastomosis. Otherwise, a saphenous vein graft is used to shunt blood from the aorta to the distal renal artery. Laceration or rupture of the renal vein is repaired by direct suture. Thrombosis of segmental arteries is treated conservatively.

## Renal Pelvis Rupture

Ruptures of the renal pelvis result in extravasation of urine into the perirenal space and along the psoas muscle. Renal pelvis ruptures are rare and are often associated with congenital renal anomalies. Radiographic studies reveal a normally functioning kidney, filling of the calyceal system, and extravasation of contrast without visualization of the ureter. Renal pelvis ruptures are often misdiagnosed as small renal lacerations. If the diagnosis is delayed, the patient develops high fever, increasing abdominal pain, and tenderness as the extravasation of urine continues into the retroperitoneal space. The diagnosis is confirmed by retrograde pyelogram. Upon surgical repair, the ureteropelvic junction should be examined for congenital obstruction.

## URETERAL INJURIES

Ureteral injuries are the rarest of all genitourinary injuries from external trauma. Blunt trauma can induce a rupture at or just below the ureteropelvic junction as a result of hyperextension of the spine with the distal ureter fixed at the trigone of the bladder. With penetrating injuries, contusion and partial or complete rupture of the ureter may result. Blast effects from gunshot wounds may cause microvascular thrombosis in the ureteral wall, delayed ureteral necrosis, and urinary fistula formation (Fig. 221-1). Ureteral injuries are surgically repaired with wide debridement and ureterouretostomy. Distal retrovesical ureteral lacerations are repaired with a neoureterocystostomy.

## BLADDER INJURIES

The bladder is an intraabdominal organ in the child but is situated deep in the bony pelvis in the adult. It is protected from all but the most severe injuries to the abdomen and pelvis. Bladder injuries are

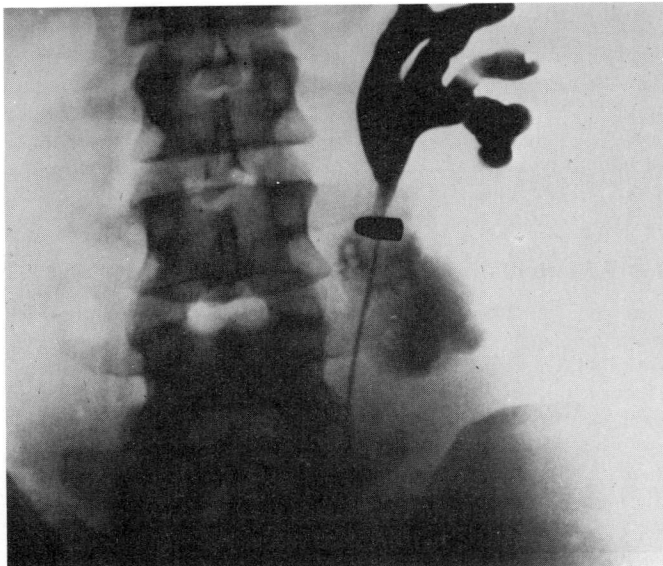

**Fig. 221-1.** Rare ureteral injury from gunshot wound, with extravasation of contrast on retrograde pyelogram.

the second most common injury to the genitourinary tract after renal injury and are usually associated with blunt trauma and pelvic fracture. Penetrating bladder injuries are often associated with injuries to other abdominal and pelvic organs.

## Bladder Contusion

Bladder contusion is bruising of the bladder wall with hematuria. The cystogram demonstrates an intact bladder outline. With a fractured pelvis, a large hematoma often results inside the bony pelvis that causes displacement of the bladder superiorly and laterally (Fig. 221-2). This bladder displacement can serve as an indicator of pelvic hemorrhage. Management is conservative, as the bruise will resolve, leaving an intact bladder wall.

## Intraperitoneal Bladder Rupture

Intraperitoneal bladder rupture is usually a burst injury of a full bladder resulting in a 1-in laceration in the dome and spillage of urine

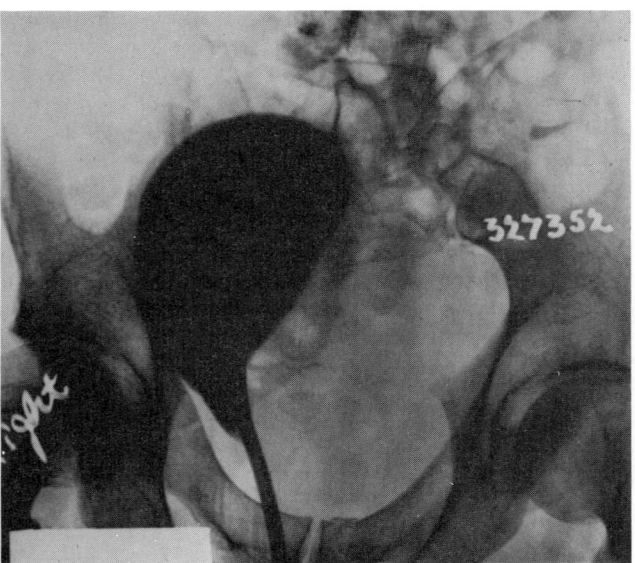

**Fig. 221-2.** Bladder contusion and displacement from pelvic hematoma.

into the peritoneal cavity. The cystogram demonstrates intraperitoneal extravasation of contrast in the cul de sac posterior to the bladder, along the paracolic gutters, and between the loops of intestine. Exploration of the abdominal cavity and repair of the rupture in the dome of the bladder are required.

## Extraperitoneal Bladder Rupture

In extraperitoneal bladder rupture, the cystogram shows extravasation of contrast streaking into the perivesical tissues. The washout film is helpful when the extravasation is predominantly behind the bladder and obscured by contrast in the full-bladder film of the cystogram. Extraperitoneal bladder ruptures are treated with urethral catheter drainage alone. The catheter remains indwelling for 10 to 14 days. The cystogram is repeated to verify healing before the urethral catheter is removed. Rarely, persistent urinary extravasation is seen, with a bony fragment remaining in the bladder wall or a pelvic fixation impinging the bladder.

## URETHRAL INJURIES

### Male Urethral Injuries

Urethral injuries in males occur in the posterior (prostatomembranous) urethra and in the anterior (bulbous and penile) urethra. Posterior urethral injuries are associated with pelvic fractures. The digital rectal and perineal examinations reveal the presence of a perineal hematoma or high-riding detached prostate that is associated with complete posterior urethral disruption. Anterior urethral injuries result from direct blows to the urethra (fall-astride injuries, straddle injury, kick), instrumentation, and in conjunction with a penile fracture. Examination reveals the classic "butterfly" perineal hematoma limited by the attachments of the fascia lata.

### Anterior Urethral Injuries

In anterior urethral contusions, there is blood at the external urinary meatus but the retrograde urethrogram is normal. The contusion heals with conservative management, with or without a urethral catheter.

In partial anterior urethral lacerations, the retrograde urethrogram reveals contrast extravasation at the site of injury and contrast outlining the urethra proximal to the site of injury (Fig. 221-3). Partial urethral lacerations are managed with an indwelling urethral catheter (placed coaxially over a guidewire under fluoroscopic control) or with a suprapubic cystostomy.

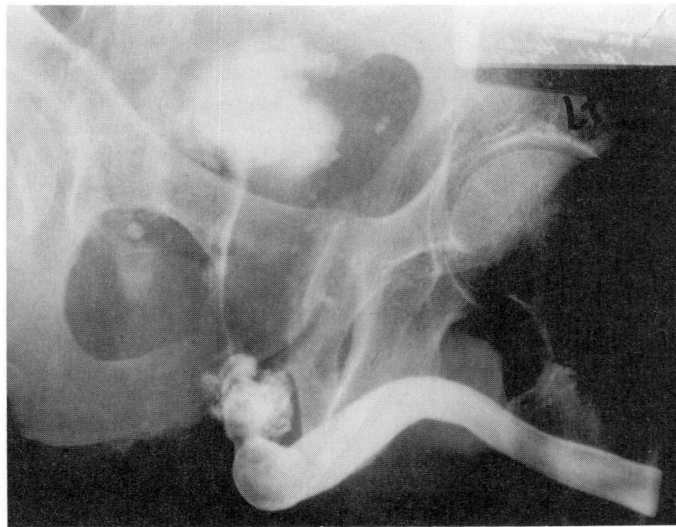

**Fig. 221-3.** Partial urethral laceration, with contrast extravasation at the site of injury and outlining the prostatic urethra and bladder.

In complete anterior urethral lacerations, the retrograde urethrogram reveals contrast extravasation at the site of injury without contrast proximal to the site of injury. Complete lacerations of the anterior urethra are repaired surgically with debridement and end-to-end anastomosis over a urethral catheter.

## Posterior Urethral Injuries

Partial posterior urethral lacerations are managed with a urethral catheter placed coaxially over a guidewire under fluoroscopic control or with a suprapubic catheter.

In complete posterior urethral lacerations, the management remains controversial. The injury is managed with primary realignment of the lacerated urethra or with suprapubic cystostomy alone. In primary realignment, a catheter realigns the bladder, prostate, and urethra as the pelvic hematoma resolves. A urethrogram is repeated to verify satisfactory healing before removing the catheter. In suprapubic cystostomy alone, the prostate returns to its normal position as the pelvic hematoma resolves. Stricture formation occurs with both techniques. However, the subsequent urethral stricture in patients with primary realignment tends to be less extensive. The advantage of suprapubic cystostomy alone, especially in the patient in an unstable condition, is its simplicity. The impotence and incontinence rates are thought to be related to the extent of injury and are the same in both techniques.

## The Full Bladder Dilemma

Emergency physicians in nontrauma centers may be faced with a patient with a urethral injury precluding bladder catheterization but with a full urinary bladder. Such a patient may have to be transferred many miles to reach a center with a urologic service. Spontaneous or conscious bladder contraction may ensure, with spillage of urine into the perivesicle space, increasing the risk of infection. Guidewire-aided placement of a temporary suprapubic catheter into the bladder can alleviate this problem. A large-bore Seldinger-technique central venous catheter or cavity drainage catheter may provide temporary relief. Insert the exploring needle perpendicularly about two finger breadths above the symphysis pubis and, when urine returns, insert the guidewire. The catheter selected should be long enough to coil within the bladder so that it remains in the lumen of the bladder when it is empty. Because the bladder may be displaced by a large hematoma or extravasated urine, it would be advisable to inject a few milliliters of contrast into the bladder while obtaining an x-ray to confirm that the catheter is actually in the bladder.

## Female Urethral Injuries

Female urethral injuries should be suspected in extensive pelvic fractures. Eighty percent of female urethral injuries present with vaginal bleeding. Careful vaginal and endoscopic examination should be undertaken, even when the patient has menstrual bleeding or an indwelling tampon. Delayed diagnosis has resulted in labial edema, necrotizing fasciitis, and sepsis. A layer repair of the urethral and associated vaginal injuries are performed over a urethral catheter. The voiding phase of the repeat cystogram is essential in confirming complete urethral healing.

## GENITAL INJURIES

## Testicular and Scrotal Injuries

The mobility of the testicle, cremaster muscle contraction, and the tough capsule of the testis (tunica albuginea) are responsible for the infrequent rate of injury to the testis. A direct blow to the testis impinging it against the symphysis pubis is the primary cause of blunt testicular injury. Blunt testicular injuries are either contusions or ruptures. The rare traumatic dislocation of the testicle to the inguinal canal has been reported. In testicular contusions or ruptures, the tunica vaginalis sac fills with blood (hematocele) and appears as a large, blue, tender scrotal mass. Penetrating injuries to the scrotum through the tunica vaginalis require exploration. Bilateral testicular injuries are often seen in penetrating trauma. Testicular ultrasound with colored Doppler studies can help delineate the extent of testicular trauma. Early exploration, evacuation of blood clots, and repair of testicular rupture tend to result in an earlier return to normal activity, decreased hematoma infection, and less testicular atrophy than conservative management.

Scrotal skin avulsion is managed by housing the testicle in the remaining scrotal skin even though the reconstruction places the skin under tension. Usually the scrotum returns to nearly normal size within a few months. In complete scrotal skin loss, the testicles are placed in pouches in the inner thighs.

## Injuries to the Penis

### Vacuum and Sharp Wounds

Self-inflicted injuries of the penis include vacuum cleaner injuries and blade injuries. Vacuum cleaners cause extensive injury to the glans penis and some loss of the urethra, requiring debridement of devitalized tissue and reconstruction. Blade injuries range from superficial lacerations to complete amputation. Amputation of the penis is managed by reimplantation or local repair. Reimplantation is preferable if the distal penis is in satisfactory condition, and the ischemia time is less than 18 h.

### Penile Rupture

Traumatic rupture of the corpus cavernosum of the penis or fracture of the penis occurs when the erect penis impacts forcibly on a hard object (sexual partner's pubis or the floor), receives a direct blow, or is subjected to abnormal bending. A cracking sound is heard, followed by penile pain, immediate detumescence, rapid swelling, discoloration, and distension. Urethral injuries may accompany penile ruptures. Penile ruptures are managed by immediate surgical evacuation of blood clot, and repair of the torn tunica albuginea of the corpus cavernosum and urethra.

### Penile Denuding

Loss of penile skin by avulsion injury or burns is managed by split thickness skin grafts after the denuded penis is clean and uninfected. The avulsed skin should not be reapplied, for it invariably becomes necrotic and infected and must be subsequently removed.

### Zipper Injury

Zipper injury to the penis is caused when the penile skin is trapped in the trouser zipper. Mineral oil and lidocaine infiltration are useful in freeing the penile skin from the zipper. Otherwise, wire-cutting or bone-cutting pliers are used to divide the median bar (or diamond) of the zipper, which causes the zipper to fall apart, freeing the penile skin.

### Contusions

Contusions of the perineum or penis, which can result from straddle or toilet seat injuries, are treated conservatively with cold packs, rest, and elevation. If the patient is unable to void, catheter drainage is elected.

## CONCLUSION

Genitourinary injuries are common; they are also easily overlooked, with drastic consequences. A careful search for injury and a high index of suspicion are necessary. Ready consultation with a urologic surgeon will help set correct priorities in the multiply injured patient.

## BIBLIOGRAPHY

Carroll PR, McAninch JW, Klosterman P, et al: Renovascular Trauma: risk assessment, surgical management and outcome. *J Trauma* 30:547, 1990.

Fournier GR, Laing FC, McAninch JW: Scrotal Ultrasonography and the Management of Testicular Trauma 16:377, 1989.

Guerriero WG: Ureteral Injury. *Urol Clin North Am* 16:237, 1989.

Lee JY, Cass AS: Evaluating lower urinary tract injuries. *Contemporary Urology* 5:75, 1993.

Lee JY, Cass AS: Pediatric genitourinary trauma. *Problems in Urology* 8:315, 1994.

Mee SL, McAninch JW, Robinson AI, et al: Radiographic assessment of renal trauma: a ten year prospective study of patient selection. *J. Urol* 141:1095, 1989.

Perry MO, Hussmann DA: Urethral injuries in female subjects following pelvic fractures. *J Urol* 147:139, 1992.

Taylor GA, Eichelberger MR, O'Donnell R, et al: Indications for computed tomography in children with blunt abdominal trauma. *Ann Surg* 213:212, 1991.

# 222

# WOUND BALLISTICS

### Jeremy J. Hollerman
### Martin L. Fackler

The medical literature is full of erroneous articles classifying gunshot wounds based on bullet velocity. It is wrong to think that one can predict the characteristics of a wound based on whether the bullet inflicting it is "high velocity" or "low velocity." Bullet velocity is certainly an important factor in wounding, but it is only one factor. Other bullet and tissue characteristics are at least as important as velocity. Bullet *mass,* which is related to diameter and length, is a major determinant of how deeply the bullet will penetrate tissue. Bullet *construction* (such as whether the bullet is solid lead with no bullet jacket, is partially jacketed, or has a full metal jacket) is a primary determinant of whether the bullet will deform or fragment. Bullet *shape* and center of mass (which determine how soon it will yaw in its path through tissue), the *thickness of the body part wounded* (determining whether the bullet has a long enough path through tissue to deform or yaw) (Fig. 222-1); *tissue type* struck (e.g., femur versus lung), and tissue elasticity, density, specific gravity, and internal cohesiveness (which determine how well the tissue will withstand tissue stretch [temporary cavitation forces]) are all extremely important, in addition to bullet *velocity,* in determining the nature of the wound produced. Wound classification systems based on bullet kinetic energy or velocity markedly overemphasize the importance of velocity in determining the wound produced and largely ignore the other factors stated above. The amount of kinetic energy "deposited" or "retained" in a victim wounded by a projectile is not a reliable predictor of wound severity. Muzzle energy is not a reliable indicator of bullet performance.

An understanding of wound ballistics allows the physician to evaluate and treat missile wounds without repeating the errors of conventional "wisdom." Many papers have suggested harmful and unnecessary treatment for gunshot wounds based on common misconceptions about wound ballistics. An example of such an unnecessary and harmful recommendation is for mandatory surgical excision of the tissue surrounding the bullet track (the path of the projectile through tissue) whenever an extremity wound is caused by a high-velocity

bullet. This is based on the belief that these tissues will become necrotic. Clinical experience and research show this to be false.

## COMMON *MISCONCEPTIONS* ABOUT WOUND BALLISTICS

1. Missile velocity and missile kinetic energy are erroneously viewed as the main factors that determine the wound produced.

2. Kinetic energy transfer is erroneously believed to be the main mechanism of wounding.

3. It is incorrectly thought that there is a constant and fundamental difference between the wound produced by a high-velocity bullet compared to that produced by a low-velocity bullet.

4. A common misconception is that the main wounding mechanism of all high-velocity bullets is the explosive effect of temporary cavity formation.

5. A common misconception is that one wound path through tissue is pretty much like another in terms of the effect a bullet will produce in tissue. The changes in the wound when the bullet contacts a large bone (versus if it had not) are often ignored.

6. Some erroneously believe that military bullets are more damaging to tissue than civilian bullets.

7. The erroneous statement that when an undeformed bullet is present in tissue, its lack of deformation is diagnostic of the bullet being jacketed, is sometimes found in medical literature.

8. A common misconception is that rounds of the same caliber (bullet diameter) have the same wounding potential.

9. Some erroneously believe that bullets usually tumble in flight.

10. Some authors have the misconception that wound ballistics research conducted with small animals and spherical projectiles can accurately predict the tissue effect of bullets in human beings. Some authors erroneously believe that when using inanimate material to "catch" the bullet, recording media such as duct-sealing compound, clay blocks, and soap blocks are as useful and accurate as properly calibrated ballistic gelatin.

To understand why these are misconceptions, one must understand the mechanisms by which missiles wound tissue. These are the *crushing* of tissue and the *stretching* of tissue.

## WOUNDING POTENTIAL

Every moving bullet has a maximum wounding *potential* determined by its mass and velocity. Bullets of equal wounding *potential* may produce wounds of very different severity, depending on bullet shape, internal and extrenal construction, and which tissues they traverse.

Bullets with equal wounding potential often do not produce similar wounds. A heavier, slower bullet crushes more tissue but induces less temporary cavitation; most of the wounding potential of a lighter, faster bullet is likely to be used up forming a larger temporary cavity, but this bullet leaves a smaller permanent cavity (crushes less tissue). The heavier, slower bullet causes a more severe wound in elastic tissue than the lighter, faster bullet, which uses up much of its wounding potential producing tissue stretch (temporary cavitation). This tissue stretch may be absorbed with little or no ill effect by elastic tissue such as lung or muscle. In less elastic tissue such as liver or brain, the temporary cavity produced by the lighter, faster bullet can produce a more severe wound. Penetration depth will be less with the lighter, faster bullet, and critical structures such as the heart may not be reached.

## MECHANISMS OF WOUNDING

Both missile and tissue characteristics determine the nature of the wound. Missile characteristics are partly inherent (mass, shape, construction) and are partly conferred by the weapon (longitudinal and rotational velocity). Tissue characteristics (elasticity, density, ana-

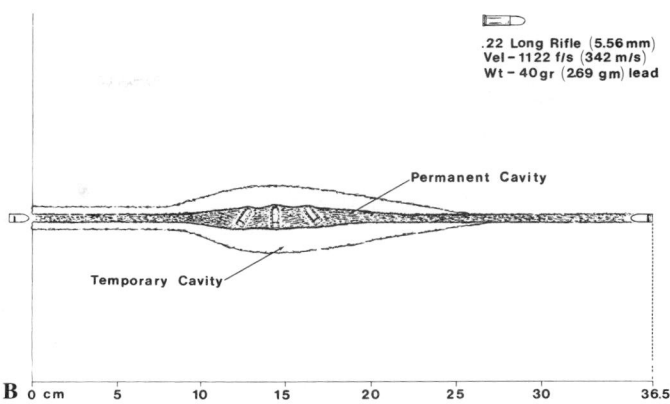

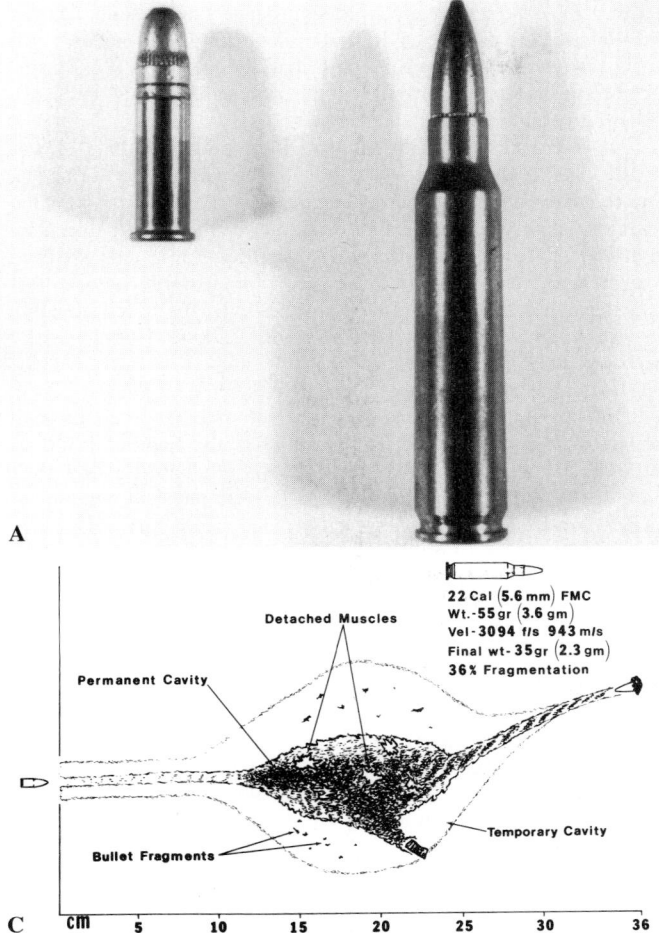

**Fig. 222-1.** (A) The photograph shows a .22 long rifle round (*left*) and an M16 round (*right*). (B) and (C) These are the wound profiles of the same .22 long rifle (B) and .224 cal M-193 round of the M16A1 rifle (C). (Full metal case (FMC) is a synonym of full metal jacket (FMJ), the type of bullet used in the military.)

This figure shows that caliber (bullet diameter in hundredths of an inch) is only one indicator of wounding potential, and not a very good one. Because of much higher velocity (943 m/s [3094 ft/s]) as opposed to 342 m/s [1122 ft/s] for the .22 long rifle bullet), because it fragments in tissue, and because of greater bullet mass, the M16 bullet has the potential to cause a much more severe wound if the anatomic part struck is sufficiently thick. Note that in the gelatin block, both the permanent cavity and the temporary cavity caused by the M16 bullet are much larger than those of the .22 long rifle bullet. As is usual for a nondeforming bullet, the temporary and permanent cavities caused by the .22 long rifle bullet are largest when the bullet is at 90° of yaw. (From Hollerman JJ, Fackler ML, Coldwell DM et al. *AJR Am J Roentgenol* 155:686, 1990. Used with permission.)

tomic relationships) also strongly affect the nature of the wound. The severity of a bullet wound is influenced by the bullet's orientation during its flight through tissue and by whether the bullet fragments or deforms (into the typical mushroom shape of the expanding hollow-point or soft-point bullet).

Two major mechanisms of wounding occur: the *crushing* of the tissue struck by the projectile (forming the permanent cavity) and the radial *stretching* of the projectile path walls (forming a temporary cavity) (see Fig. 222-1).

In addition, a sonic pressure wave precedes the projectile through tissue. The sonic pressure wave plays no part in wounding.

## Crushing of Tissue

A missile crushes the tissue it strikes, thereby creating a permanent wound channel (permanent cavity). If the bullet is traveling with its pointed end forward and its long axis parallel to the longitudinal axis of flight (0° of yaw, the angle between the long axis of the bullet and its path of flight), it crushes a tube of tissue no greater than its approximate diameter. When the bullet yaws to 90°, the entire long axis of the bullet strikes tissue. The amount of tissue crushed may be three times greater than at 0° of yaw.

When striking soft tissue with sufficient velocity, soft-point and hollow-point bullets deform into a mushroom shape. This increases surface area and the amount of tissue crushed. For most big-game hunting, such bullets are mandated by law. This is to increase the probability of prompt lethality, rather than the creation of a disabling but nonlethal wound causing the animal prolonged suffering. If the mushroomed diameter is 2.5 times greater than the initial diameter of the bullet, the area of tissue crushed by the bullet is 6.25 times greater

than the amount that would have been crushed by the undeformed bullet.

Bullet fragmentation also increases the volume of tissue crushed. After bullet fragmentation, bullet surface area is increased and much more tissue is crushed. For large handgun (e.g., .44 magnum) and rifle bullets, the striking of bone is one of the causes of early bullet fragmentation. The lighter bullet fragments often do not penetrate tissue as deeply as the intact heavier bullet would have

Comminuted fracture may be created by rifle and large handgun bullets striking bone. Bone fragments can become secondary missiles, crushing tissue. Many handgun bullets are unable to significantly fragment bone. When a large bone is struck, it is likely that the bullet will expend its wounding potential in the patient and will not exit.

Bullet fragments and secondary missiles, such as bone fragments, teeth, or coins propelled by contact with the bullet, are likely to increase the severity of the wound. Multiple perforations weaken tissue and create focal points for stress (stress risers). Tissue tears are particularly likely to occur at stress risers during temporary cavitation stretch.

Unjacketed lead bullets cannot be driven faster than about 610 m/s (2000 ft/s) without some of the lead stripping off in the barrel. This is avoided if a jacket made of a harder metal (such as copper or a copper alloy) is used to surround the lead.

The jacket of a military bullet completely covers the bullet tip (a full metal jacket). Civilians often use hollow-point or soft-point bullets. Hollow-point bullets have a hole in the jacket at the bullet tip, and soft-point bullets have some of the lead core of the bullet exposed at the bullet tip. These constructions weaken the bullet tip, causing it to flatten on impact. This flattening often greatly exceeds bullet diameter, resulting in a mushroom-shaped projectile.

The hollow-point and soft-point bullets used by civilians are often more damaging to tissue than military bullets fired from rounds otherwise configured identically. Because of this, wounds produced by civilian hunting rifles, shotguns, and large-caliber handguns are usually more severe than wounds produced by military rifle bullets of the same mass and velocity.

Hollow-point and soft-point bullets either deform into a mushroom shape or stay undeformed. Up to one third of hollow-point and soft-point handgun bullets fail to deform into a mushroom shape, usually due to insufficient bullet velocity or an excessively stiff or thick bullet jacket, preventing deformation.

When the tip of a hollow-point bullet is plugged with material such as clothing or drywall, bullet expansion into a mushroom shape in tissue is usually delayed and sometimes prevented. This causes deeper penetration of tissue, sometimes causing a perforating wound (having both an entrance and an exit). This may result in the injury of bystanders. Some recent handgun bullets have designs attempting to overcome this problem.

All projectiles penetrate more deeply as projectile velocity is increased, only up to the point where velocity gets high enough to deform the projectile; penetration depth decreases markedly from that point on. The greater the bullet diameter expansion from mushrooming, the less the depth of penetration.

There is a critical range of velocity for each handgun hollow-point and soft-point bullet, within which the bullet may perform as expected. Below this velocity range the bullet will have insufficient velocity to mushroom on impact, and at velocities above this range the bullet may fragment after impact, resulting in many light bullet pieces crushing tissue at a superficial depth.

Military full metal jacket bullets do not flatten at the bullet tip, (they do not mushroom), but sometimes they can break and fragment as a result of yawing to 90°. The stress on the bullet as its long axis strikes tissue causes flattening of the sides of the bullet as if it had been squeezed in a vise. If the bullet breaks, it will usually do so at the *cannelure,* a circular groove around the bullet where it is crimped into the cartridge case. Although the M-193 military bullet of the M16 rifle fragments in soft-tissue wounds with a characteristic pattern depending on range, most other full metal jacket military bullets, such as those fired from the AK-47, the AK-74, and the NATO 7.62 mm rifle (USA version), do not fragment unless they strike a large bone.

If a bullet is jacketed, the bullet jacket usually cannot be distinguished from the lead core on standard radiographs because the entire bullet is metallic density. Occasionally, as the bullet deforms or fragments, the bullet jacket separates from the bullet and is visible on a radiograph.

In extremity wounds, when a radiograph reveals an undeformed bullet lying in the soft tissues and no fracture is present, tissue disruption is usually minor. However, if a major vessel or nerve is divided, even a simple wound can have a severe effect.

Wounding is like real estate—location is the most important factor. A bullet of low wounding potential can cause a severe wound if it passes through a vital structure such as the spinal cord.

## Temporary Cavitation (Tissue Stretch)

Fired from an appropriate and well-designed weapon, a bullet flies in air with its nose pointed forward; it yaws only 1° to 3°. Yaw occurs around the bullet's center of mass. In pointed rifle bullets, the center of mass is behind the midpoint of the bullet's long axis. Although the bullet's most naturally stable in-flight orientation would be with its heaviest part (its base) forward, for aerodynamically efficient flight it must fly point forward.

During flight, a bullet is stabilized against yaw by the spin imparted to it by the spiral grooves (rifling) in the gun barrel. The longer (and heavier) the bullet in relation to its diameter, the more rapidly it must be rotated to avoid significant yaw in flight. A gun barrel intended to fire a heavier bullet has rifling that makes a full turn in fewer inches of barrel length than the rifling in a barrel intended for a shorter, lighter bullet of the same caliber. This will cause a faster rate of bullet spin.

A gun with a shorter barrel will generally produce a bullet of lower velocity than would a weapon with a longer barrel when firing the same round. With shorter barrel length, the expanding gases of the burning gunpowder have less time to accelerate the bullet before they are discharged into the atmosphere. When identical rounds are fired by a rifle and a handgun, bullet velocity is often significantly different because of different barrel length. A .22 long rifle round fired in a rifle will produce a bullet with up to 91.5 m/s (300 ft/s) more velocity than would the same round fired in a handgun.

Although the bullet's spin is adequate to stabilize it against yaw in its flight through air, it is not adequate to stabilize it in its path through tissue because of the higher density of the medium. If it does not deform, a pointed bullet eventually yaws to a base-forward position (180° of yaw). Expanding bullets lose the physical stimulus to yaw because after mushrooming their heaviest part is forward.

As a bullet passes through 90° of yaw or after it deforms into a mushroom shape, it is crushing its maximal amount of tissue (unless it fragments, which will crush more). It is slowed down rapidly as its wounding potential is used up. The bullet creates a splash-type force in tissue, which spreads out radially. This force creates the temporary cavity. This aspect of the wounding process is analogous to the splash of a diver entering the water.

If a diver enters the water very straight and point forward (similar to the point-forward configuration of a bullet at 0° of yaw), the splash may be minimal. If the diver does a belly-flop (similar to a bullet at 90° of yaw), a large splash is induced. In tissue, this splash, the temporary cavity, produces localized blunt trauma.

The maximal size of the temporary cavity occurs several milliseconds after the bullet has passed through the tissue. Because forces follow paths of least resistance, temporary cavitation is likely to be asymmetrical and spread out through tissue planes.

The temporary cavity caused by common handgun bullets is generally too small to be a significant wounding factor in all but the most sensitive tissues (brain and liver). Center-fire rifle bullets and large handgun bullets (e.g., .44 magnum) often induce a large temporary cavity (10 to 25 cm [4 to 10 in.] diameter) in tissue. This can be a significant wounding factor, depending on the characteristics of the tissue in which it forms.

Near-water density, less elastic tissue (such as brain, liver, or spleen), fluid-filled organs (including the heart, bladder, or gastrointestinal tract), and dense tissue (such as bone) may be damaged severely when a large temporary cavity contacts them or forms within them. More elastic tissue (such as skeletal muscle) and lower-density elastic tissue (such as lung) are less affected by the formation of a temporary cavity.

Although the formation of a large temporary cavity often has devastating effects in the brain or liver, its effect in wounds of the extremities has frequently been exaggerated. Fracture of large bones not hit by the bullet and tearing of major vessels or nerves by the temporary cavity are often mentioned in the literature, but they are rare in clinical experience. This includes a systematic review of 1400 rifle wounds sustained in the Vietnam conflict and analyzed in the Wound Data and Munitions Effectiveness Team study (RF Bellamy, personal communication). Most of the permanent damage done in wounds of the extremities is the result of structures being hit by the intact bullet, bullet fragments, or secondary missiles. As in all blunt trauma, shear forces develop and tear structures at points where one side is fixed and the other side is free to move. The temporary cavity is no exception. In the unlikely event that the blunt trauma caused by the temporary cavity tears a vessel wall, this is particularly likely to occur at the vessel origin.

## BALLISTIC PROPERTIES AND THE WOUND PRODUCED

Animal experiments using military rifle bullets have clearly disproved the assertion that all tissue exposed to temporary cavitation is destroyed. These studies also show that not only does the 14-cm diameter temporary cavity produced by the AK-74 assault rifle not destroy a great amount of muscle, but the sizable stellate exit wound it causes in the uncomplicated thigh wound ensures excellent wound drainage, which assists healing. A history that the wound was caused by a high-velocity bullet does *not* mandate radical excision of the wound path.

The characteristics of the wounded tissue, the thickness of the body part, the point in the path of the bullet at which deformation into a mushroom shape, yaw, or fragmentation occurs, and other factors strongly influence the wound produced. As discussed above, bullets of equal wounding *potential* may produce wounds of quite different severity, depending on which tissues they traverse.

Experiments with ballistic gelatin (which reproduces the projectile deformation and penetration depth of living animal muscle) have shown that most full metal jacketed rifle bullets yaw significantly only at tissue depths greater than the diameter of human extremities.

In the first 12 cm (the average thickness of an adult human thigh) of a soft tissue wound path, there is often little or no difference between the wounding effect of low- and high-velocity bullets when the high-velocity bullet is of the military full metal jacket type. This is particularly true of the relatively heavier military rifle bullets such as those fired by the AK-47 and NATO 7.62 mm (USA version) rifles. A wound of an extremity caused by an AK-47 bullet that does not hit bone is often similar to a handgun bullet wound. If a high-velocity, nondeforming, heavy bullet does not break, fragment, or hit a large bone, it may exit an extremity with much of its wounding potential unspent. These same bullets are often lethal in chest or abdominal wounds because the trunk is thicker than an extremity and allows the bullet a sufficiently long path through tissue to yaw. Maximal temporary cavitation induced by the AK-47 bullet usually occurs at a tissue depth of 28 cm, much greater than the diameter of a human extremity.

A soft- or hollow-point bullet fired from a civilian center-fire rifle deforms soon after entering tissue and produces a much more severe extremity wound than a military full metal jacket bullet that does not break and fragment.

The more recently developed, smaller caliber, AK-74 fires a bullet that is lighter than the AK-47 bullet and yaws earlier. Its maximal temporary cavity occurs at a tissue depth of 11 cm. Extremity wounds from the AK-74 can be expected to be more severe than those from the AK-47. The lighter, smaller AK-74 round allows a soldier to carry many more rounds of ammunition. This was the primary motivation for development of the M16 and the AK-74.

### Caliber

*Caliber* (bullet diameter in hundredths of an inch) is only one indicator of wounding potential and not a very good one (see Fig. 222-1). Although the .22 long rifle bullet (.22LR) and the M16 bullet (which is .224 inches in diameter) are similar in diameter (caliber), the M16 bullet is heavier (3.6 g versus 2.7 g for the .22LR bullet), mainly because the M16 bullet is longer. Caliber indicates bullet diameter but not bullet length and, therefore, does not disclose bullet mass. Caliber also is independent of bullet velocity and bullet construction (deforming or nondeforming, etc.). The M16 bullet, which is fired from a center-fire cartridge holding much more gunpowder, travels at much higher velocity than the .22LR bullet. Because the M16 bullet breaks then fragments in tissue, because of its greater bullet mass, and because of its higher velocity (943 m/s [3094 ft/s] as opposed to 342 m/s [1122 ft/s] for the .22LR bullet), the M16 bullet has the potential

to cause a much more severe wound. If it traverses only extremity muscle, does not yaw, does not fragment, and does not hit a bone, the M16 may still produce a relatively minor ice pick-type extremity wound. Usually the M16 produces a much larger permanent cavity and much larger temporary cavity than the .22LR.

The large temporary and permanent cavities formed by the M16 bullet occur mainly from 11 to 30 cm deep in tissue. Remember that the bullet has its highest velocity when it enters the tissue, but it forms a small wound channel at that point. Only when it deforms, fragments, or yaws to 90° is its severe wounding effect realized. At that point it is travelling more slowly and has less than its maximum velocity. Velocity is only one factor in wounding.

Unfortunately, commonly used weapon and bullet designations are often numerically incorrect. As an example, the .38 special and the .357 magnum use bullets that have the same diameter (9.07 mm [.357 in.]) (Table 222-1). These bullets are often exactly the same weight. The longer cartridge case of the magnum can hold more powder, giving the bullet higher velocity and greater wounding potential.

### Gunshot Fractures

Handgun wounds of the extremities yield characteristic fracture patterns. Frequently seen are divot fractures of cortical bone, drill-hole fractures, butterfly fractures, and double butterfly fractures. Nondisplaced fracture lines sometimes radiate from these defects. These usually heal well. The bullet hole itself can act as a stress riser. Spiral fractures extending proximally or distally from the bullet hole may result from the dissipation of stress forces at the bullet hole. Occasionally, remote spiral fractures at some distance proximal or distal to the bony gunshot wound also occur, probably because of the presence of stress risers such as vascular channels in the bone, and the fact that the bone was under load and often torsional stress at the time of impact.

In gunshot fractures from rifles and large handguns, a greater extent of comminution may be seen. These fractures often have complications because of the soft tissue damage these bullets cause. The vascular compromise associated with these comminuted gunshot fractures increases the likelihood of delayed union or nonunion of the fracture. Wound infections are more common in this group. Early fasciotomy to prevent compartment syndrome is important, when needed.

At some hospitals, outpatient treatment is being used successfully for extremity fractures caused by handguns, if no significant neurologic or vascular compromise has occurred.

### Trunk Wounds

Bullets are not sterilized by the heat of firing. They can carry bacteria from the body surface or body organs, such as a perforated colon, deep into the wound.

In trunk wounds, an analysis of the bullet path is mandatory to determine whether a laparotomy is needed. Two radiographs in planes separated by 90°, computed tomography (CT), clinical examination, and peritoneal lavage are all useful. Abdominal CT is more accurate if performed before peritoneal lavage. If peritoneal penetration by a bullet is suspected, laparotomy is indicated. The morbidity and mortality of an exploratory laparotomy that shows no significant intraabdominal injury is low compared with that of missed intestinal injury. CT is useful, especially when an exclusively body wall or retroperitoneal path is suspected. CT has largely replaced excretory urography as the preferred means of evaluating the urinary tract after penetrating trauma.

Any bullet wound below the nipple line should raise the question of whether the diaphragm or abdomen has been penetrated. CT or peritoneal lavage, sometimes can be used to make this determination. Laparotomy is required if peritoneal penetration cannot be excluded. As in the rest of the body, because of the skin's elastic properties, a

**Table 222-1.** Cartridge Case Name and Actual Bullet Diameter Used

| Cartridge Cases of Common Interest | Actual Bullet Diameter |
| --- | --- |
| 32 Auto (ACP) | .312″ |
| 380 Auto (ACP) | .355″ |
| 9 mm Luger (9 mm Parabellum) | .355″ |
| 38 Super | .355″ or .357″ |
| 38 Special | .357″ |
| 357 Magnum | .357″ |
| 44 Special | .4295″ |
| 44 Magnum | .4295″ |
| 444 Marlin | .4295″ |

| Others Cartridge Cases of Interest | Actual Bullet Diameter |
| --- | --- |
| 22 Hornet | .223″ and .224″ |
| 218 Bee | .224″ |
| 219 Donaldson Wasp | .224″ |
| 219 Zipper | .224″ |
| 221 Remington Fireball | .224″ |
| 222 Remington | .224″ |
| 222 Remington Magnum | .224″ |
| 223 Remington | .224″ |
| 224 Weatherby Magnum | .224″ |
| 225 Winchester | .224″ |
| 22-250 Remington | .224″ |
| 220 Swift | .224″ |
| 243 Winchester | .243″ |
| 244 Remington/6 mm Remington | .243″ |
| 240 Weatherby Magnum | .243″ |
| 256 Winchester Magnum | .257″ |
| 250/3000 Savage | .257″ |
| 257 Roberts | .257″ |
| 25/06 Remington | .257″ |
| 257 Weatherby Magnum | .257″ |
| 30-06 | .308″ |
| 30-30 Winchester | .308″ |
| 30 M1 Carbine | .308″ |
| 7.62 × 39 mm (AK-47 rifle) | .308″ |
| 30/40 Krag | .308″ |
| 7.5 × 55 mm Swiss (Schmidt-Rubin) | .308″ |
| 300 Savage | .308″ |
| 7.62 mm Russian | .308″ |
| 308 Winchester | .308″ |
| 7.62 mm NATO | .308″ |
| 30-06 Springfield | .308″ |
| 300 H & H Magnum | .308″ |
| 30-338 | .308″ |
| 300 Winchester Magnum | .308″ |
| 308 Norma Magnum | .308″ |
| 300 Weatherby Magnum | .308″ |
| 303 British | .311″ |
| 7.65 mm Mauser | .311″ |
| 7.7 mm Japanese | .311″ |

Often, both the numerical designation associated with the bullet and the cartridge case do not reflect exact measurements. As an example, the 44 Remington Magnum Pistol cartridge is .456 in. in diameter at its distal end and uses a bullet with a .43-in. diameter. Both the .38 special and the .357 magnum use bullets that have the same diameter (.357 in. [9.07 mm]). These bullets are often exactly the same weight. When trying to determine bullet type from a radiograph, in addition to correcting for magnification or deformation, one must look up actual bullet diameter rather than relying on the bullet name for its size. ACP, Automatic Colt Pistol

*Source:* Sierra Rifle and Sierra Handgun Reloading manuals (both 3rd ed., 1989). Sierra Bullets, L.P., 1400 W. Henry, Sedalia, Mo 65301

nearly spent bullet is often arrested subcutaneously at the end of the wound path.

Whenever a gunshot wound traverses the midline of the neck or the width of the mediastinum, perforation of the esophagus should be suspected. Esophageal evaluation should not be overlooked after angiographic evaluation of the neck or chest.

## Head Wounds

In skull wounds, as elsewhere in bone gunshot fractures, inward beveling of the calvarial defect at the bullet entrance and outward beveling of the skull at the exit wound are typical. This is due partly to the geometry of the skull and partly to the bullet-bone interaction. Characteristic fracture patterns of the skull can be used to identify entrance and exit wounds. When there is a cranial exit wound, skull fractures propagate across the calvarium faster than the bullet travels through the brain, producing characteristic patterns of fracture. These fracture patterns sometimes allow differentiation of entrance and exit wounds. Radial fractures often spread out in a star pattern from the entrance and to a lesser extent from the exit holes in the skull. Concentric heaving fractures may occur, connecting the arcs of the radial fractures around both the entrance and exit holes, if sufficient temporary cavitation forces are generated inside the brain to cause significant outwardly directed tissue splash forces inside the skull, pushing the calvarium out. Because a fracture will not cross a preexisting fracture line, the temporal sequence of the occurrence of the fractures can often be determined from the pattern of the fractures.

Brain, whose tissue properties include near-water density, very little elasticity, and poor tissue cohesiveness, is extremely sensitive to temporary cavitation forces. When disrupted by such forces, severe brain injury often results. In addition to the relative lack of elasticity of brain tissue, its enclosure in the rigid cranial vault magnifies brain disruption by temporary cavitation forces.

## Pellet Wounds

Compared with the pointed rifle bullet, the spherical pellet slows rapidly in its flight through air or tissue. In tissue, the entire wounding potential of the shot pellet at its entrance velocity is likely to be delivered to the target, often with no exit wound. At close range (< 3 m [10 ft]) shotgun pellets remain tightly clustered. Therefore, shot pellet size makes little difference because the entire load of the pellets functions as a unit, with a velocity virtually equal to muzzle velocity. Shotgun wounds at ranges less than 5 m (16 ft) consist of multiple parallel wound channels. This grossly disrupts the blood supply to tissue between the wound channels.

The most severe civilian firearm wounds typically seen are those inflicted by a shotgun from close range. After a close-range or contact shotgun wound to the trunk, external examination of the patient, particularly after adequate volume resuscitation, often does not disclose the severity of the internal injuries present.

Major neural injury after shotgun wounding may be more important than fracture or major vascular injury in determining the final outcome.

During surgical exploration of a close-range shotgun wound, it is important to search for wadding, casing debris, plastic shot cup, and surface materials carried into the wound (e.g., clothing, glass, or wood). Many of these are radiolucent.

Diagnosing long-range injury on the basis of the pattern of pellet spread is sometimes problematic. When shotgun pellets are tightly clustered or widely spread out, close-range or long-range injury (respectively) is usually suspected. However, in close-range injuries, the *"billiard ball" effect* may cause considerable pellet spread. When the tightly clustered group of shot at close-range contacts the skin, the pellets at the front of the group are slowed. The pellets behind them in the group strike the pellets in front with an effect like a billiard ball break. This causes much more pellet spread in tissue than would be expected at close range. On radiographs, particularly in trunk wounds, this effect can simulate the pellet spread of a longer-range injury. This pitfall can be avoided if the skin physical examination is correlated with the radiologic findings. If there is only one entrance wound hole, it is a close-range injury. If the distribution of the multiple skin entrance wounds is the same as the pellet spread on the radiograph, the injury occurred at longer range.

Recent BB guns and airguns that fire small pellets have considerably higher muzzle velocity than older guns of this type. Penetrating injuries from these weapons are sometimes fatal. These firearms should not be considered toys. It is possible to be shot with a BB pellet that has penetrated the scalp, skull, and brain and think only a scalp wound is present. Patients and doctors suspecting only a scalp abrasion have been surprised by skull radiographs showing that a BB fired by an air rifle has penetrated the forehead scalp and the anteroposterior length of the brain of an awake and alert patient with only skin puncture-type complaints.

## ASSESSMENT OF MISSILE TYPE AND LOCATION IN THE BODY

As in all of radiology, localization requires two views at 90° or a tomographic image. CT of the head and body is often useful for analysis of bullet path.

The CT digital scout radiograph can be used for missile localization. It usually can be taken in anteroposterior and lateral projections without moving the patient. The ability to manipulate the display window and level allows visualization of bullets seen through dense structures, such as the shoulders and pelvis.

### Assessment of Missile Type

On a radiograph, assessment of missile caliber is difficult because of magnification and missile deformation. If an undeformed bullet is seen in two views at 90°, and its degree of magnification is known, it is possible to determine the approximate caliber of the bullet. The focus-object distance and focus-image distance (also known as the focus-film distance) must be known. This requires knowing the position of the bullet in the patient's body and its location relative to the film. You often can distinguish an undeformed .22 from a .25, a .38 from a .44, but probably cannot distinguish a .357 or .38 from a 9 mm because they are too similar in diameter. The actual diameter of the .38 is .357 in., the .357 bullet is .357 in. in diameter, the 9 mm bullet is .355 in. in diameter and the .44 bullet is .4295 in. in diameter (see Table 222-1). Sometimes even deformed bullets can be accurately characterized radiologically for intact bullet caliber and weight.

Many radiographs show only fragments of the bullet and do not allow determination of the type of weapon and projectile causing the wound. However, certain bullets deform or fragment in a characteristic pattern (such as the M16 military bullet, the Winchester Black Talon or SXT handgun bullets, the .357 magnum 125-grain Remington semijacketed soft-point, and others). Sometimes the pattern of fragments can be used to identify the bullet. Deformation of large lead shotgun pellets (e.g., 00 buckshot) after contact with bone can cause these to be confused with deformed bullet fragments.

### Missile Embolization

It always must be ascertained that the path from the entrance wound is consistent with the bullet's current location because a bullet may have reached its present location by embolization. Arterial and venous embolization of bullets and shotgun pellets, as well as bullet movement within the subarachnoid space in the head and spine, have been reported. It is generally accepted that a missile freely floating within a cardiac chamber should be removed to prevent embolization. Missiles clearly embedded in chamber walls are relatively safe. In one case, a shotgun pellet was probably dislodged from the heart during cardiopulmonary resuscitation, and embolized to the intracranial circulation, with a fatal result. Missile size does not seem to be especially important because all sizes can produce morbidity after embolization. Two-dimensional echocardiography is useful in determining whether a missile is embedded in a chamber wall. CT (particularly high-speed CT) and magnetic resonance imaging for nonmagnetic missiles also have a role. On chest radiographs, blurring

of the margins of a pericardiac missile or fragment is a reason to suspect that the missile is in or next to the heart.

Whenever a bullet is not found on radiographs of the body part predicted to contain it based on the entrance wound, the bullet's location is not known, and there is no exit wound, additional radiography or fluoroscopy to find the bullet is mandatory. Immediately before surgery for removal of a missile, repeat radiographic confirmation of the exact location of the missile is usually indicated.

Interventional radiologic techniques are useful in bullet removal, including the removal of intravascular and intrarenal bullets. Significant deformation of an intravascular bullet is a relative contraindication to retrieval using a transarterial catheter because of potential damage to the intima. Arthroscopy sometimes can be used for removing bullets from joints, especially the knee.

Most bullets follow straight paths through the body. But sometimes, even in the absence of embolization, a bullet, particularly a handgun bullet, will not follow a straight path in the body. It may ricochet off body structures, especially bone, or may follow fascial or tissue planes. Bullets traveling less than 335 m/s (1100 ft/s) are the ones most likely to be deflected by anatomic structures or to follow tissue planes. Bullet shape also influences the tendency to be deflected.

## LEAD FRAGMENTS AND LEAD POISONING

Lead fragments in soft tissue usually become encapsulated with fibrous tissue and do not cause problems. Intra-articular, disk space, and bursal locations of bullet fragments are common for bullet-induced lead poisoning. Lead fragments in the brain are usually benign unless they are copper plated (as are many civilian .22 caliber bullets). Copper-plated lead pellets produced a sterile abscess or granuloma in the brain of cats surgically implanted with missiles of this type. This can be associated with downward migration of the missile, resorption of copper from the surface of the missile, progressive neurologic deficit, and sometimes the death of the cat. These findings were absent in cats whose brains were implanted with uncoated lead pellets.

Intra-articular fragments should be removed to avoid both the mechanical trauma and the destructive synovitis lead can cause. Fragments within a joint space may be distributed by joint mechanics creating an arthrogram-like effect on radiographs, delineating cartilage surfaces and joint capsule recesses. Significant damage to the articular cartilage visible at surgery may be present as a result of lead synovitis, when radiographs remain normal except for bullet fragments. If large fragments are present in the joint, they can cause severe mechanical trauma during motion. This motion can lead to further lead fragmentation. Lead is relatively soluble in synovial fluid.

Whether lead poisoning occurs depends largely on the surface area of the retained lead particles and their location in the body. In a few cases, a fibrotic mass containing gray fluid with a high lead content has been observed adjacent to the site of large bullet fragment(s). Sometimes the onset of clinical lead poisoning can be quite rapid, but usually it takes years.

Patients with retained lead pellets or lead bullet fragments should be advised that, on rare occasions, a fragment might erode into a bursa or joint space and cause lead poisoning. They should be assured that lead poisoning poses a threat *only if unrecognized and untreated.* They should be cautioned to inform their physician of the retained lead any time they seek treatment for problems such as headache, abdominal pain, personality change, or bizarre neurologic symptoms. Once the possibility of lead poisoning is considered, it can be easily confirmed or ruled out simply by determining the blood lead level.

## EPIDEMIOLOGY

Violence involving firearms is a significant problem in the United States. Handguns are used in the overwhelming majority of cases because they are easy to carry and conceal. Many criminals now use semiautomatic handguns that carry up to 15 cartridges in their clips. Funds produced in the lucrative illegal drug trade allow drug traffickers to switch from cheap "Saturday-night special" revolvers to expensive modern high-technology semiautomatic pistols. Law enforcement has followed suit in this "arms race." It is not surprising that multiple gunshot wounds are becoming more common. Recently, a higher percentage of patients wounded by semiautomatic pistols are dead at the scene, increasing from 5 percent in 1985 to 34 percent in 1990 in Philadelphia County. In that study, the percentage of firearm homicide victims with criminal records increased from 43 percent in 1985 to 67 percent in 1990. Among all the 1990 Philadelphia firearm homicide victims, 61 percent were intoxicated at the time they were killed; 39 percent were using cocaine at the time of death compared to 9 percent in 1985.

Between 1983 and 1992, 37 million handguns, rifles, and shotguns were produced in the United States. These were added to the pool of existing firearms in the United States. This figure does not include guns imported during the same period. In 1992, 3.0 million handguns, rifles, and shotguns were produced in the United States and 2.85 million more were imported.

Each day in the United States, 65 murders occur. At least 68 percent of these are committed with firearms. Many of these murders and much of the urban gun violence results from disputes between criminals. Criminals are often the victims. The medical literature about the epidemiology of firearm-involved trauma is often misleading and sometimes outright false.

When tracing the ownership history of a weapon for a crime investigation, the record often stops at the point of the weapon's first private sale. Except where expressly outlawed by individual states, anyone who owns a firearm is free to sell it to whomever he wishes without demanding identification and without keeping any record of the sale. The new Brady law does not apply. Like most federal gun sale laws, it regulates only transactions through federally licensed gun dealers.

## EVIDENTIARY CONCERNS

Physicians must be aware of the importance of preserving evidence in patients being resuscitated after penetrating trauma. Do not cut through bullet holes or knife holes in clothing when removing clothing. Do not incise through skin wounds unless absolutely necessary. To preserve powder marks, do not scrub wounds unless necessary. The emergency department must have a protocol for collecting clothing and other evidence so that it can be documented that it was always under surveillance or otherwise kept in such a way that tampering could not occur. Do not describe wounds as entry or exit wounds; instead describe the appearance of the wound in detail without interpretation. When a bullet or fragment is encountered, do not pick it up with a metallic clamp so that markings can be interpreted without the possibility that marks were made with an instrument. Prehospital personnel should receive similar instruction relative to preserving evidence at the scene. The history of the episode can be useful if the number of shots fired is recalled or if the position of the victim in relation to the assailant was observed.

## CONCLUSION

The common misconceptions about wound ballistics listed at the chapter beginning are discussed in order.

1. The primary determinants of wounding are: the properties of the tissue through which the missile passes (tissue elasticity, density, cohesiveness, internal architecture); the diameter, shape, mass and velocity of the projectile; whether it fragments or expands; its internal construction; the length of the wound path; and whether the path is sufficiently long to allow yaw to 90°.

A center-fire high-velocity rifle bullet usually causes a fairly minor wound if it traverses only elastic tissue such as skeletal muscle, does not yaw to 90°, does not fragment or deform, and does not hit a major blood vessel or nerve. It will exit the extremity with most of its wounding *potential* unspent. If this same bullet hits a large bone, fragments, and does not exit, it will crush a large volume of tissue, will create secondary missiles such as bone fracture fragments, which also crush tissue, and is likely to disrupt the neurovascular integrity of the area wounded, expending much or all of its wounding potential in the patient, usually producing a severe wound.

The amount of tissue crushed by a bullet depends on projectile size and shape and whether it deforms or fragments. If the tissue wounded is relatively elastic and cohesive, the amount of tissue crushed is the primary determinant of wounding because the tissue stretch of temporary cavitation may have relatively little wounding effect. If an organ is inelastic, of near-water density, and not very cohesive, tissue stretch (temporary cavitation) can cause a severe wound.

The bullet's mass and velocity, the depth of the organ in the body, whether the bullet has deformed into a mushroom shape or traveled a long enough tissue path to yaw significantly and then sometimes to break and fragment in an organ, will be the primary determinants of the wound produced. Significant temporary cavitation blunt trauma forces occur only if the bullet enters the body with sufficient velocity and then deforms, fragments, or yaws to 90°.

2. It is apparent that bullet velocity is only one factor in wounding and in some wounds may be a minor factor. Kinetic energy expended in elastic tissue may produce little damage because tissue stretch may be well tolerated. Crushed tissue is always damaged. If a rubber ball and a raw egg of equal weight are dropped on a cement floor from the same height, these two missiles of equal kinetic energy will sustain different degrees of damage. Missile mass and velocity establish an upper limit of *possible* tissue damage (the *wounding potential*). Whether or not this tissue damage occurs depends on numerous properties of the tissue, the missile, and its path. Also, collisions between bullets and tissue are not elastic, and kinetic energy is not conserved. Some, possibly most, is lost as heat.

3. Many factors determine wound severity. Some high-velocity wounds are minor, and some low-velocity wounds are devastating. A stab wound to the brain, heart, spinal cord, aorta, or other vital structure, with properties similar to a small handgun bullet wound, is often lethal. An AK-47 military assault rifle wound of an extremity often is like an ice pick stab wound and may have little effect.

Bullet mass has a great deal to do with determining the maximum penetration depth that will be achieved. A light high-velocity bullet may cause a substantial but superficial wound, sparing deep vital structures. A heavier slower bullet usually penetrates more deeply, reaching vital structures. It is important to examine each patient and "treat the wound not the weapon."

A missile with much wounding potential may cause a minor wound. A missile with little wounding potential may cause a wound with devastating consequences. Adherence to treatment guidelines including no primary closure, the administration of prophylactic antibiotics to prevent streptococcal bacteremia, and performance of fasciotomy when necessary to prevent compartment syndrome will serve the patient well. Delayed primary closure or no wound closure is recommended. Never attribute hypesthesia, pallor, or weak pulse to arterial spasm after a gunshot wound because it is more likely caused by arterial thrombus. Appropriate diagnostic evaluation and treatment are required.

4. See discussion of point 1.

5. The length of the bullet path through tissue, the sequence of tissues encountered, and each tissue's properties are critical in determining whether the wounding potential of the missile will be expended in tissue. The bullet was spinning fast enough (because of the rifling of the barrel) to be stable in air, and it takes some distance in the higher density medium of tissue for the bullet to deform or become unstable and yaw. This requires a sufficiently long tissue path.

A nondeforming bullet may yaw little or not at all in a short tissue path such as an extremity. In trunk wounds, organs deeper in the body such as in the abdomen or mediastinum are more likely to experience blunt trauma from temporary cavitation in the region where the bullet deformed or yawed to 90°.

Hard objects such as a large bone or a belt buckle are wound-modifying structures. When these are hit by a bullet with substantial wounding potential, the severity of tissue damage may increase because bullet fragmentation or deformation increases the volume of tissue crushed and decreases the likelihood of missile exit.

6. Because civilian bullets deform and fragment much more easily than their full metal jacket military analogs, they cause more tissue crush and tissue stretch at shallower penetration depth. Frequently this means that the wounding potential of a civilian rifle bullet is expended in the wounded animal, rather than the bullet exiting with wounding potential unspent. Civilian rounds have as much powder in the cartridge case and as much bullet mass as the comparable military round. The difference lies in the bullet jacket.

7. When an undeformed bullet is seen on a radiograph, it is usually not possible to state accurately whether it is fully jacketed or not. It may not have deformed because it entered the patient with insufficient velocity, it did not strike a structure causing it to deform, or it is a full metal jacket bullet. Unless the bullet jacket has separated from the bullet, the jacket, if present, is not visible on standard radiographs.

8. Caliber alone is a poor indicator of the wounding potential of a round (see Fig. 222-1). Bullet caliber does not tell you how much powder is in the cartridge case. The cartridge case may have a different diameter than the bullet and may be any length. Caliber does not disclose bullet mass. The bullet also may be any length. Caliber only specifies diameter. The bullet's composition and construction (and therefore tendency to yaw, fragment, or deform) do not relate to caliber.

9. Bullets typically yaw only 1° to 3° in flight when fired from a properly designed weapon. If the bullet strikes an intermediate target, the bullet may yaw, deform, or decelerate as a result, and its wounding properties will be altered.

10. To be useful, wound ballistics research must be conducted using appropriate materials and methods. Erroneous conclusions frequently result from poor experimental design.

In essence, bullet wounds are assessed like all other trauma. The amount, site, and type of tissue injury, assessed primarily by physical examination and radiologic studies, determine the treatment needed.

## BIBLIOGRAPHY

Bixler RP, Ahrens CR, Rossi RP, et al. Bullet identification with radiography. *Radiology* 178:563, 1991.

Bowen TE, Bellamy RF. *Emergency War Surgery: Second United States Revision of the Emergency War Surgery NATO Handbook,* 2nd ed. Washington, DC: US Department of Defense, US Government Printing Office, 1988.

Bureau of Alcohol, Tobacco and Firearms. Civilian firearms—domestic production, importation, exportation, and availability for sale 1899–1992. In: *ATF Ready Reference 1993 (with Addendum 1994).* Washington, DC: US Department of the Treasury, 1994.

Fackler ML. Wound ballistics: a review of common misconceptions. *JAMA* 259:2730, 1988.

Fackler ML. Wounding patterns of military rifle bullets. *Int Defense Rev* 22:59, 1989.

Fackler ML, Dougherty PJ. Theodor Kocher and the scientific foundation of wound ballistics. *Surg Gynecol Obstet* 172:153, 1991.

Fackler ML, Surinchak JS, Malinowski JA, et al. Bullet fragmentation: a major cause of tissue disruption. *J Trauma* 24:35, 1984.

Federal Bureau of Investigation. *Crime in the United States 1992: Uniform Crime Reports.* Washington, DC: US Department of Justice, 1993.

Feliciano DV, Burch JM, Spjut-Patrinely V, et al. Abdominal gunshot wounds: an urban trauma center's experience with 300 consecutive patients. *Ann Surg* 208:362, 1988.

Fragomeni LSM, Azambuja PC. Bullets retained within the heart: diagnosis and management in three cases. *Thorax* 42:980, 1987.

Froede RC, Pitt MJ, Bridgemon RR. Shotgun diagnosis: "it ought to be something else." *J Forensic Sci* 27:428, 1982.

Hampton OP Jr. The indications for debridement of gun shot (bullet) wounds of the extremities in civilian practice. *J Trauma* 1:368, 1961.

Harvey EN, Korr IM, Oster G, et al. Secondary damage in wounding due to pressure changes accompanying the passage of high velocity missiles. *Surgery* 21:218, 1947.

Hollerman JJ, Fackler ML. Bullets, pellets and wound ballistics. In: Hunter TB, Bragg DG (eds). *Radiologic Guide to Medical Devices and Foreign Bodies.* St. Louis: CV Mosby, pp. 524–572, 1994.

Hollerman JJ, Fackler ML, Coldwell DM, et al. Gunshot wounds: 1. Bullets, ballistics and mechanisms of injury. *AJR Am J Roentgenol* 155:685, 1990.

Hollerman JJ, Fackler ML, Coldwell DM, et al. Gunshot wounds: 2. Radiology. *AJR Am J Roentgenol* 155:691, 1990.

Hornady Manufacturing Company. *Hornady Handbook of Cartridge Reloading: Rifle-Pistol,* 3rd ed. Grand Island, NE, Hornady Manufacturing Company, 1980.

Linden MA, Manton WI, Stewart RM, et al. Lead poisoning from retained bullets: pathogenesis, diagnosis, and management. *Ann Surg* 195:305, 1982.

Lucas RM, Mitterer D. Pneumatic firearm injuries: trivial trauma or perilous pitfalls? *J Emerg Med* 8:433, 1990.

McGonigal MD, Cole J, Schwab CW, et al. Urban firearm deaths: a five-year perspective. *J Trauma* 35:532, 1993.

Messmer JM, Fierro MF. Radiologic forensic investigation of fatal gunshot wounds. *RadioGraphics* 6:457, 1986.

Miner ME, Cabrera JA, Ford E, et al. Intracranial penetration due to BB air rifle injuries, *Neurosurgery* 19:952, 1986.

Moore EE, Moore JB, VanDuzer-Moore S, et al. Mandatory laparotomy for gunshot wounds penetrating the abdomen. *Am J Surg* 140:847, 1980.

Reddick EJ, Carter PL, Bickerstaff L. Air gun injuries in children. *Ann Emerg Med* 14:1108, 1985.

Robison RJ, Brown JW, Caldwell R, et al. Management of asymptomatic intracardiac missiles using echocardiography. *J Trauma* 28:1402, 1988.

Ryan JR, Hensel RT, Salciccioli GG, et al. Fractures of the femur secondary to low-velocity gunshot wounds. *J Trauma* 21:160, 1981.

Sights WP, Bye RJ. The fate of retained intracerebral shotgun pellets: an experimental study. *J Neurosurg* 33:646, 1970.

Smith HW, Wheatley KK Jr. Biomechanics of femur fractures secondary to gunshot wounds. *J Trauma* 24:970, 1984.

Smith OC, Berryman HE, Lahren CH. Cranial fracture patterns and estimate of direction from low velocity gunshot wounds. *J Forensic Sci* 32:1416, 1987.

Wang ZG, Feng JX, Liu YQ. Pathomorphological observations of gunshot wounds. *Acta Chir Scand Suppl* 508:185, 1982.

Wolberg EJ. Performance of the Winchester 9mm 147 grain subsonic jacketed hollow point bullet in human tissue and tissue simulant. *J Int Wound Ballistics Assoc* 1:10, 1991.

Woloszyn JT, Uitvlugt GM, Castle ME. Management of civilian gunshot fractures of the extremities. *Clin Orthop* 226:247, 1988.

# SECTION 21
# Fractures and Dislocations

## 223
## EARLY MANAGEMENT OF FRACTURES AND DISLOCATIONS
### Jeffrey S. Menkes

## CLINICAL PHYSIOLOGY OF FRACTURES

The ability to properly assess and treat acutely injured patients in the emergency department depends largely on an understanding of the way fractures are created and how they heal. Practical knowledge of fracture physiology may provide the index of suspicion needed to diagnose an injury that might otherwise be missed. It may also help prevent or minimize complications and may form the basis for advising the patient regarding the outlook for ultimate recovery of function.

## How Fractures Occur

Although fractures are sometimes described in terms of the external mechanism by which they are created, they may also be thought of simply in terms of the physiologic processes involved.

### "Typical" Fractures

Most fractures are the result of significant trauma to healthy bone. The bony cortex may be disrupted by a variety of forces, including a direct blow, axial loading, angular (bending) forces, torque (twisting) stress, or a combination of these.

### Pathologic Fractures

Fractures that occur from relatively minor trauma to *diseased or otherwise abnormal* bone are termed *pathologic* fractures. This implies that a preexisting pathologic process has weakened the bone and rendered it susceptible to fracture by forces which, under normal circumstances, would not disrupt the cortex. Common examples of such injuries are fractures through metastatic lytic lesions, fractures through benign bone cysts (as in the humerus of Little League pitchers), and—perhaps most common—vertebral compression fractures in patients with advanced osteoporosis. Numerous other disease processes may render patients susceptible to pathologic fracture.

Because these injuries are often not associated with a history of significant trauma, pathologic fractures may go undetected unless there is a preexisting index of suspicion, based on the knowledge that such injuries can occur.

### Stress Fractures

In some cases, bone may undergo a "fatigue" fracture from repetitive forces, applied before the bone and its supporting tissues have had adequate time to accommodate to such forces. An example is the insidious occurrence of a metatarsal shaft fracture in unconditioned foot soldiers (the so-called march fracture). The physiologic principle of stress fracture can be easily envisioned by anyone who has "cut" an aluminum finger splint to the desired length by bending it back and forth. The pliable metal—too hard to cut with an ordinary scis-

sors—ultimately gives way in the face of repeated stresses requiring relatively little force.

The exact processes that render bone susceptible to stress fracture are controversial. The important point is that diagnosis depends on a familiarity with the entity, because *x-rays are typically negative* early in the patient's course. Early diagnosis may be purely clinical, based on the history and physical findings. Days or weeks may pass before the fracture line or new bone formation become visible on x-ray, ultimately confirming the suspicions of the physician who, having made the correct presumptive diagnosis, will have treated the patient appropriately from the outset.

## Salter (Epiphyseal) Fractures

Fractures involving the *physis*—the cartilaginous epiphyseal plate near the ends of the long bones of growing children—are called Salter fractures after Salter and Harris, the physicians who devised the most popular method for classifying these injuries. The supply of new bone material needed for the elongation of bones during growth is provided by specialized cells within the physis. When growth is completed, the physis is transformed into bone, ultimately fusing with the surrounding bone and disappearing as a distinct entity. By definition, Salter fractures cannot occur in fully grown adults.

Any damage to the epiphyseal plate during a child's growth may destroy part or all of its ability to produce new bone substance, resulting in aborted or deformed growth of the bone thereafter. The potential for growth disturbance from an epiphyseal injury is related to the number of years the child has yet to grow (the older the child, the less time remains for deformity to develop) and to the pattern of the fracture line through the epiphyseal area. Classification of Salter fractures and their clinical implications are discussed later in this chapter.

## Fracture Healing

The physiology of fracture healing constitutes the basis for many decisions in the emergency department. The judgment as to whether an angulated fracture requires reduction or can be left to heal "as is," the choice of treatment modality in relation to the patient's age, and the prognosis for regaining function or being left with residual deformity all require familiarity with the short- and long-term aspects of the healing process.

Fracture healing can be described in terms of three phases, each of which gradually blends into the next.

### Inflammatory Phase

When a fracture occurs, the microscopic vessels crossing the fracture line are severed, depriving the damaged bone ends of their blood supply. In the ensuing hours and days, the bone ends necrose, triggering a classic *inflammatory response*. This early phase is brief but creates the tissue environment for the most predominant aspect of fracture healing: the *reparative phase.*

### Reparative Phase

Soon, granulation tissue begins to infiltrate the area. Within this tissue are specialized cells capable of forming collagen, cartilage, and bone—the ingredients of *callus,* which gradually surrounds the fractured ends and stabilizes them. With time, the callus becomes more densely mineralized.

Meanwhile, the necrotic edges of the fragments are removed by osteoclasts—cells whose specific function is to *resorb* bone. That is why some "hairline" fractures do not appear on x-ray until days after injury: initially invisible, the diagnostic fracture line appears only after necrotic bone has been resorbed from the area.

### Remodeling Phase

This final phase of bone healing is the longest, often lasting *years*. Remodeling refers to the tendency of bone to gradually regain its original shape and contour. During this phase, the superfluous portions of callus are resorbed, and new bone is laid down along natural lines of stress. These internal layers, easily visible in x-rays of normal bone, are the bony *trabeculae*. Formation of trabecular bone is a physiologically efficient process, providing maximum strength relative to the amount of bone material used.

The anticipated success of remodeling is related to a number of factors. Young children have a greater capacity for remodeling than adults do. Accordingly, their potential for residual deformity is less, other circumstances being equal. Remodeling is also related to the magnitude and direction of unreduced angulation and to the fracture's location along the bone. Specific predictors of satisfactory remodeling include youth, proximity of the fracture to the end of the bone (but not involving the epiphyseal plate), and direction of angulation being in the plane of natural joint motion.

Clinical decisions regarding the aggressiveness of fracture reduction are directly linked to a knowledge of this physiology. Angulation near the end of a long bone, for example, is more acceptable than angulation near the midshaft. Dorsal or volar angulation at the wrist has a better prognosis than ulnar or radial angulation because the natural plane of wrist motion is dorsal-volar. Mild angulation in a 2-year old might be left to remodel on its own, whereas the same angulation in an adult might require correction.

## ORTHOPEDIC EMERGENCIES

Some types of musculoskeletal trauma deserve special mention because a delay in their diagnosis or treatment can increase the chance of significant complications or a negative outcome.

### Open Fracture

An *open fracture* (called "compound" in older terminology) is a fracture associated with overlying soft tissue injury, creating communication between the fracture site and the external surface of the body. Although open fracture may initially convey the image of grossly exposed bone, the term is equally applicable to a simple puncture wound extending to the depth of an underlying fracture. Such puncture wounds may be created by external forces or by a sharp bone fragment transiently protruding through the skin before receding back beneath the surface.

The most dreaded complication of open fracture is osteomyelitis. Once established, osteomyelitis may result in months or years of pain, disability, medical therapy, surgical procedures, and ultimately amputation. Although osteomyelitis may be unavoidable in some cases, it becomes less likely when treatment is prompt and meticulous.

Open fractures are sometimes classified by severity, based on the length of the overlying laceration, extent of tissue damage, kinetic energy of the injuring force, and evidence or likelihood of significant contamination. Irrespective of these factors, *any* open fracture should be promptly and carefully treated. Elements in the care of open fractures are described later in this chapter.

### Dislocation

A joint is said to be dislocated when the articular surfaces of the bones that normally meet at the joint are completely out of contact with one another. This is distinct from *subluxation,* a condition in which the articular surfaces are only partially out of contact.

The urgency of treating dislocated joints is based on several factors. One is the potential for neurologic or circulatory compromise. The neurovascular bundle passing close to the affected joint is typically "kinked" around the deformity associated with the dislocation. Persistence of this condition can result in a neurologic or vascular deficit that may be temporary if the deformity is reduced promptly but irreversible if treatment is delayed.

Another consideration is that the longer a joint has been dislocated, the more difficult it may be to reduce, and the more likely it is to be unstable after reduction. This is probably due at least in part to edema, muscle spasm, and other tissue changes that increase over time.

Dislocation of the *hip* carries its own particular urgency in addition to those mentioned above: the danger of avascular necrosis of the femoral head. Avascular necrosis occurs because much of the blood supply to the femoral head is delivered through vessels that emerge from the acetabulum. When the joint is dislocated, circulation to the femoral head is disrupted. At some point, the vascular insult becomes irreversible, and bony necrosis is the ultimate result. Although aseptic necrosis may occur despite the physician's best efforts, its likelihood increases with the time delay until reduction.

### Neurovascular Deficit

Naturally, any injury associated with neurologic or vascular compromise—as may result from a severely deformed fracture—should be addressed as soon as possible. The longer a deficit goes untreated, the longer it is likely to persist and the greater the possibility it will be irreversible. In some cases, simply reducing a deformity by means of longitudinal traction may restore circulation or nerve function, allowing the remainder of the patient's evaluation and treatment to proceed at a calmer pace.

## PREHOSPITAL CARE

With the growing sophistication of emergency medical service (EMS) programs in many areas of the country, important aspects of early care are no longer overlooked.

### Preliminary Splinting

Effective splinting of the injured extremity is crucial for several reasons. (1) It reduces the patient's pain. (2) It reduces damage to nerves and vessels by preventing them from being repeatedly ground between the fragments or being stretched by increased angulation at the fracture site. (3) It reduces the chance of inadvertently converting a closed fracture to an open one as a sharp bone fragment pokes its way through the skin (considered a mishap of severe consequence, because of the potential for the disastrous complication of osteomyelitis). (4) It facilitates patient transport and the taking of x-rays, by reducing the pain and manipulation associated with moving the patient from ground to ambulance to emergency department stretcher to x-ray table.

### Prehospital Splinting Devices

Many splinting devices are available to EMS systems. For injuries of the wrist or forearm, a foam-padded intravenous board can be wrapped in place, supplemented by a sling. The sling is important because optimal immobilization includes the "joint above and the joint below" the fracture. The sling keeps the elbow (the "joint above") at rest.

For suspected injuries to the elbow or humerus, a sling-and-swathe arrangement does nicely. This involves applying a sling, then binding the affected arm to the thorax with a gauze wrap. An *exception* to this principle is immobilization of patients with suspected anterior dislocation of the shoulder. These patients are unable to adduct the fore-arm against the thorax, and forcibly binding it there is painful and not recommended. A simple sling is adequate. (Anterior dislocation is unlikely if the patient *prefers* to keep the arm tightly bound against the thorax and abdomen.)

Injuries to the ankle can be immobilized in a pillow or well-padded cardboard splint. If fracture of the tibial shaft or knee is suspected, the device should extend well above the knee (to immobilize the joint above as well as the joint below).

Some injuries warrant specialized splints, such as winch-mechanism traction devices for femoral shaft fractures. Although such devices do not immobilize the hip (the joint above), the added element of traction makes this unnecessary. If a traction device is unavailable, then the hip does need to be immobilized. This can be accomplished with military antishock trousers (MAST) with all compartments inflated or, less elegantly, by binding the legs together, then binding the patient to a backboard from ankles to thorax.

Other types of splints exist, but their use is controversial. Inflatable plastic splints, for example, are acceptable for injuries to the ankle or wrist, but are often used inappropriately for fractures of the humerus or femur. Because these devices normally do not extend above the elbow or knee, they provide inadequate immobilization for such injuries. Also, overinflation of plastic splints can seriously impair circulation. (If the splint cannot be dented by moderate thumb pressure, it is probably overinflated.) Inflatable splints should not be applied over clothing because underlying wrinkles in the clothing may cause pressure sores in swollen and vulnerable tissue.

Also controversial are nonmalleable aluminum splints because they are based on the "one size fits all" principle, which some physicians regard as "this size fits none." If used, aluminum splints should be very well padded because their hard surface may cause pressure sores. Like any splint, they should immobilize the joint above and the joint below the fracture if they are used for long bone injuries. For example, an above-knee splint would be needed for fracture of the tibial shaft. Aluminum splints should be removed as soon as possible, once a fracture is diagnosed or ruled out. If a fracture is confirmed, the splint should be replaced with another type of immobilization dressing before the patient leaves the emergency department.

## Reducing Deformity in the Field

Many EMS programs do not recommend prehospital reduction of deformity of an injured extremity. If the deformity is near a joint (suggesting the possibility of dislocation), this is certainly good advice. Injudicious manipulation may convert a pure dislocation to a fracture-dislocation. Even if a fracture already exists, there will be no way to prove it was not *caused* by the manipulation.

A circumstance in which prehospital reduction of obvious fractures along the *shaft* of a long bone can be justified is the absence of a distal pulse. Minutes count in such cases. If reduction is attempted, it should be performed by means of longitudinal traction (rather than an "unbending" force).

In the absence of a common standard, the indications for reduction of deformity by prehospital personnel ultimately remain at the discretion of the supervising EMS program.

## EMERGENCY DEPARTMENT EVALUATION AND DIFFERENTIAL DIAGNOSIS

The importance of a careful history and physical examination cannot be overstated. Orthopedic diagnosis is sometimes thought of as being as simple as taking an x-ray where the patient says the pain is. This philosophy is probably responsible more than any other factor for significant injuries being missed.

Although x-ray is of course an important adjunct, it is not the ultimate diagnostic resource for the following reasons. The pain of a fracture, or even a dislocation, may be referred to another area. For example, patients with disruption of the sternoclavicular joint or fracture of the humeral shaft may present complaining of *shoulder* pain. If the x-ray is based solely on where the patient reports subjective discomfort, then the injury might not even be included on the film. The area x-rayed should be determined not only by the patient's chief complaint, but also by systematic *palpation,* looking for subtle deformity or significant point tenderness.

Some fractures or dislocations are apparent only on *special x-ray views,* which are not part of the standard series for that body part. Such special views will never be ordered, unless the physician has already formulated a presumptive differential diagnosis *before* x-ray, based on the history and physical findings.

Some injuries may not be radiologically apparent on the first day, regardless of what views are taken. Common examples are fracture of the carpal navicular, nondisplaced fracture of the radial head, and stress fracture of a metatarsal. The classic radiologic signs accompanying such injuries, like the fat pad sign of the elbow, are not always conveniently present. But suggestive history and findings commonly are. In such cases, the diagnosis of fracture may have to be purely clinical until 7 to 10 days after injury, when enough bony resorption has occurred at the fracture site to reveal a lucency on x-ray. A bone scan may suggest the fracture even sooner. But on the day of injury, there may be no readily available "test" capable of demonstrating the pathology. Only the physician's clinical impression—arrived at through a systematic history and physical examination—will result in proper and timely treatment of a radiologically undemonstrable fracture.

## History

The value of history-taking in the case of orthopedic injuries is often underestimated. In fact, knowing the precise mechanism of injury or listening carefully to the patient's symptoms can be the key to diagnosing fractures or dislocations. For example, a history of shoulder injury *combined with the complaint of dysphagia* may be the only clue to the existence of posterior sternoclavicular dislocation. This entity, which causes pressure on the mediastinal structures, can often be demonstrated only by computed tomography (CT) scan and is associated with severe complications if treatment is delayed. Another example is a history of landing flat on the feet from a significant height, which should prompt the physician to consider fracture of one or both calcanei, as well as lumbar vertebral compression fracture.

History is often the only means of correctly assessing and treating the young child who "just won't use the arm." These children, who present with a seemingly paralyzed arm ("pseudoparalysis") after being pulled or yanked, may be incorrectly diagnosed as having a brachial plexus injury, when in fact the history and presentation are classic for subluxed radial head—an entity *not discernible on x-ray* and easily and quickly remedied by a proper reduction maneuver.

A careful history may enable the physician to diagnose posterior dislocation of the shoulder—another entity commonly missed on routine films. If the patient has (1) experienced a direct blow to the front of the shoulder, (2) landed forward on the outstretched arm, or (3) had a seizure or undergone violent muscle contraction for any other reason (such as contact with high-voltage current), and now complains of excruciating shoulder pain and severely limited motion, the diagnosis of posterior dislocation should be entertained. If the implications of the history are not appreciated, then the specific x-ray views needed to demonstrate the injury may never be ordered.

## Physical Examination

Essential components of the examination for musculoskeletal trauma are: (1) inspection for swelling, discoloration, or deformity; (2) assessment of active and passive range of motion of the joints proximal and distal to the injury; (3) palpation for tenderness or subtle deformity; and (4) verification of neurovascular status.

## Inspection and Range of Motion

Gross deformity along the shaft of a long bone is of course pathogno-monic for fracture. The presence of most dislocations, or fractures near a joint, can be inferred by deformity at the joint, loss of range of motion, and severe pain at rest. An exception is posterior dislocation of the shoulder, which, though intensely painful, may not be accompanied by obvious deformity. Chapter 226 has a more complete discussion of this entity.

## Palpation

When gross deformity is not present, presumptive orthopedic diagnosis depends strongly on the findings noted on palpation. Palpation will disclose areas of bony step-off, as well as the precise location of point tenderness. If films are ordered before performing this phase of the examination, the wrong area may be x-rayed, because pain is commonly referred to a location distant from the injury site.

The palpation examination should be done systematically and consistently, from one patient to the next. The area palpated should extend well beyond the location of the patient's subjective pain. For example, when an injured patient complains of shoulder pain, palpation should begin at the sternoclavicular joint, then proceed along the extent of the clavicle, onto the acromioclavicular joint, then onto the humeral head and along the entire humeral shaft. In addition, the scapula should be palpated for tenderness and the posterior aspect of the shoulder palpated for any unnatural prominence that might suggest a posterior dislocation. Injury to any of these areas may be reported by the patient as pain in the shoulder. Only a meticulous palpation examination may protect the physician from being misled by referred pain and missing a crucial diagnosis.

## Neurovascular Assessment

When injury involves an extremity, as opposed to the vertebral column, sensorimotor testing should be performed on the basis of *peripheral nerve* function, rather than nerve root and dermatomal distribution. In the upper extremity, the radial, median, and ulnar nerves should be tested. When the shoulder is anteriorly dislocated, two additional nerves—the axillary (supplying sensation to the lateral aspect of the shoulder) and the musculocutaneous (supplying sensation to the extensor aspect of the forearm)—should be checked as well. In the lower extremity, examination of the saphenous (sensory only), peroneal, and tibial nerves should be performed. Neurologic deficit, although not necessarily immediately reversible, is important to document early, particularly before the patient has undergone any significant manipulation or reduction maneuvers.

Assessment of vascular status should be performed early as well. The sooner circulatory compromise is identified and addressed, the greater the chance of avoiding tissue infarction and necrosis. Injuries such as dislocation of the knee (tibiofemoral joint), fracture-dislocation of the ankle, and displaced supracondylar fracture of the elbow in children are commonly associated with vascular occlusion or disruption, with resulting circulatory impairment.

## RADIOLOGIC EVALUATION

The area x-rayed and the particular views ordered should be based on the history and physical examination rather than simply on where the patient reports subjective pain. The joint above and the joint below a fracture should be included on the films because injury at the proximal or distal joint may coexist with long bone fractures.

Injuries that may require special views to be visualized include acromioclavicular separation, fracture of the carpal navicular, posterior shoulder dislocation, and sternoclavicular dislocation. That is why formulation of a presumptive diagnosis *prior to* x-ray is crucial. The physician may never order the specialized views needed to

demonstrate a particular injury unless he or she has already anticipated the injury by virtue of the history and physical examination.

Children who have sustained trauma at or near a joint may need comparison studies of the opposite extremity, to differentiate fracture lines from normal epiphyseal plates or ossifying growth centers. This is particularly true for the pediatric elbow, which typically has six separate ossification centers appearing sequentially as the child grows.

Although the physician may be tempted to base diagnostic and treatment decisions on the radiologist's written report, this is not advisable for at least two reasons. First, a negative report does not rule out significant injury. Fractures of the radial head, carpal navicular, or metatarsal shaft, for example, may initially be undetectable on x-ray, even when special views are taken. Second, the terminology used by radiologists to describe malposition of fracture fragments or disrupted joints is often different from the terminology used by orthopedists. Because the emergency physician will often be conferring with an orthopedist regarding the initial management of a patient, and because this interaction commonly involves describing the radiologic appearance of a patient's injury, it is important that the two physicians "speak the same language." This might not be achieved by simply relaying the radiologist's written description.

## Describing Radiographs

When orthopedic consultation is indicated, proper management of the patient may rest on the emergency physician's accurate description of the x-ray. Often the narrative will influence the orthopedist's decision regarding the need for hospital admission and whether surgical versus nonsurgical management is warranted. In essence, the emergency physician should be able to transmit a virtual FAX of the x-ray by means of verbal description.

There are various ways to classify or categorize fractures. The method presented here is intended to be the most practical from the standpoint of effective communication with a consultant who is not physically present.

## Open versus Closed

Although not a radiologic finding per se, this aspect of an injury is among the most important and should be conveyed to the orthopedist before any other. The implications of open fracture are of such significant consequence that this factor alone may determine the patient's immediate care or ultimate disposition.

## Location of the Fracture

Typical reference points used by orthopedists to describe the location of a fracture along the shaft of a long bone are the midshaft, the junction of the proximal and middle thirds, and the junction of the middle and distal thirds. Any fracture more proximal or distal than this may be localized in terms of its distance, in centimeters, from the bone end.

When a proximal or distal fracture extends into the adjacent joint, it is termed intra-articular. Intra-articular fractures have special significance because disruption of the joint surface may warrant surgery to restore the joint's contour and prevent subsequent traumatic arthritis. This feature of a fracture line, if present, constitutes important information.

Anatomic bony reference points should be cited when applicable. A fracture just above the condyles of the distal humerus or femur, for example, is most precisely called a *supracondylar* fracture. A fracture running from the greater to the lesser trochanter of the proximal femur is an *intertrochanteric* hip fracture, whereas a fracture just below the trochanters is *subtrochanteric,* and a fracture just above is said to involve the femoral *neck.* The area at or proximal to the coronoid process of the ulna is the *olecranon,* and should be referred to as such, rather than simply the proximal ulna. Other bony landmarks include the radial head (proximal), radial styloid (distal), and greater tuberosity of the humerus. Numerous additional examples exist.

## Orientation of the Fracture Line

The most common orientations of fracture lines are illustrated in Fig. 223-1. Torus and greenstick fractures are seen almost exclusively in young children, whose bones are more pliable than those of adults. Note the segmental fracture, which is commonly described incor-

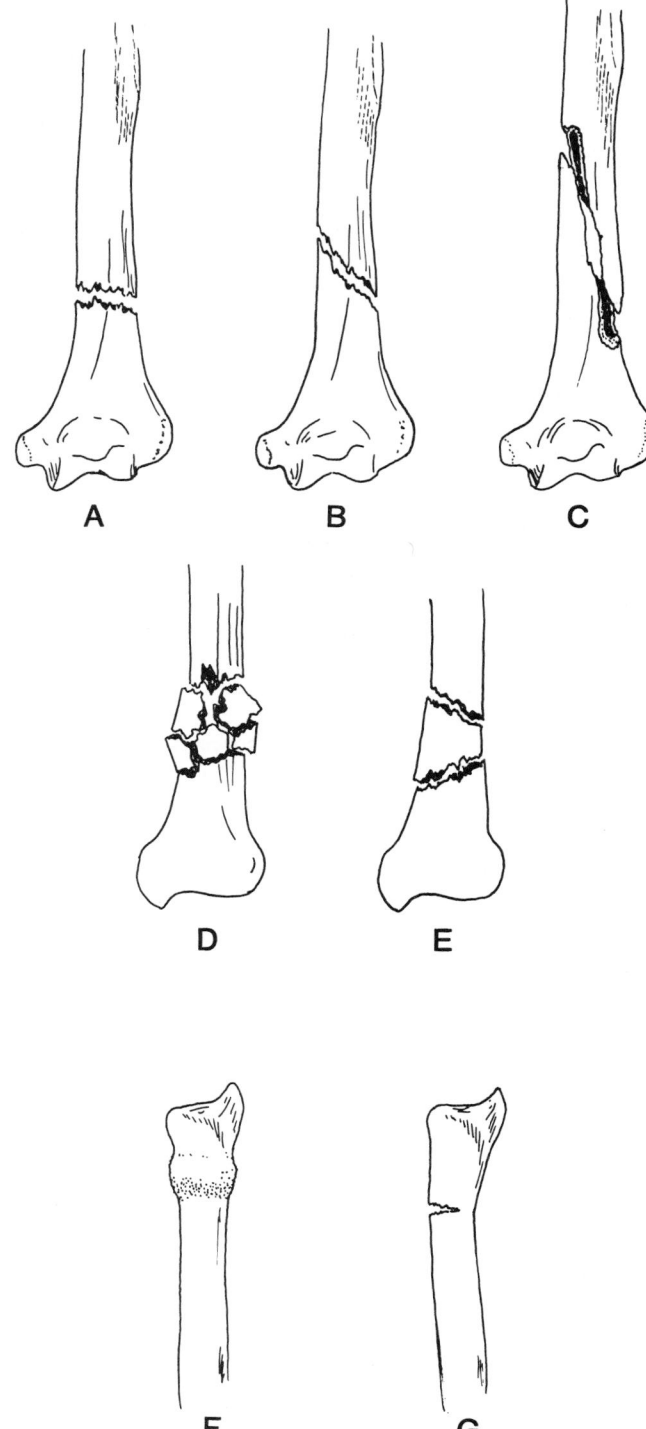

**Fig. 223-1.** Fracture line orientation. (A) Transverse. (B) Oblique. (C) Spiral. (D) Comminuted. (E) Segmental. (F) Torus. (G) Green-stick.

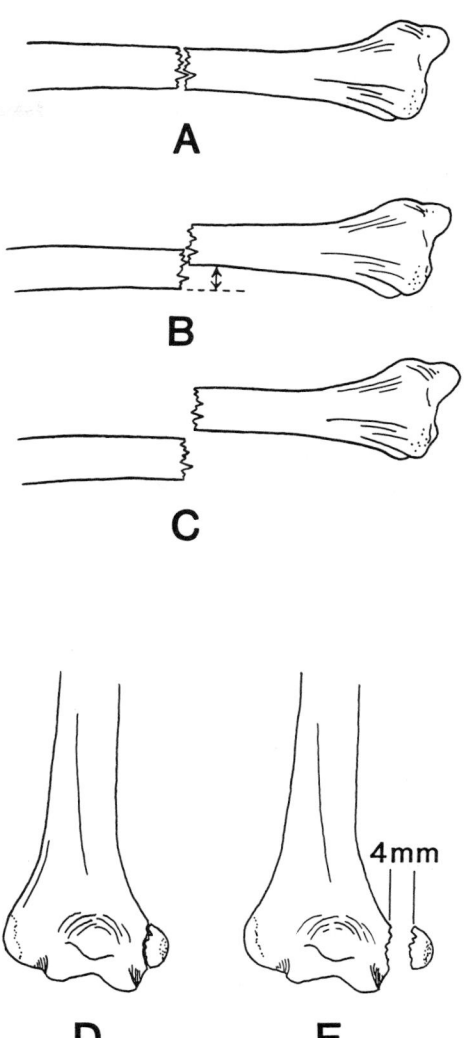

**Fig. 223-2.** Fracture displacement and separation. (A) No displacement, slight separation. (B) 50% dorsal displacement. (C) Complete dorsal displacement. (D) Nondisplaced, no separation. (E) 4 mm separation.

rectly as a comminuted fracture. To an orthopedist, the term *comminuted* implies splintering or shattering. When there is a single large free-floating segment of bone between two well-defined fracture lines, this is properly called a *segmental fracture.*

## Displacement and Separation

*Displacement* refers to the fracture fragments being *nonconcentric* or *offset* from each other. It is expressed in terms of direct measurement (4-mm displacement), or in terms of the percent of the width of the bone (50 percent displacement, complete displacement). The direction of displacement is based on the position of the distal fragment in relation to the proximal.

Displacement should not be confused with *separation,* which is the distance two fragments have been pulled apart. Figure 223-2 illustrates principles of displacement and separation.

## Shortening

Shortening is the amount by which the bone's length has been reduced and is expressed in millimeters or centimeters. This can occur by *impaction* (telescoping of the fragments into one another) or by the overlap of two completely displaced fragments (Fig. 223-3). The

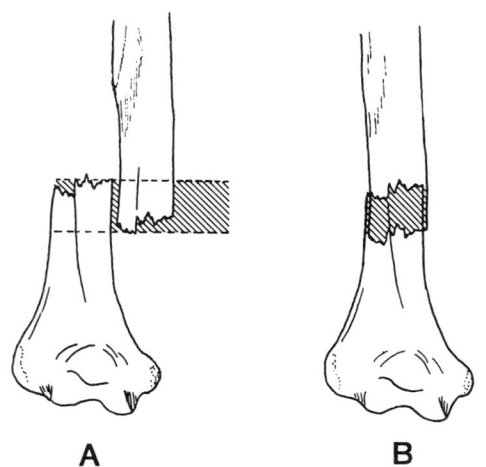

**Fig. 223-3.** Shortening at fracture site. (A) Complete displacement with overriding. (B) Impaction. In both cases, the width of the shaded area represents the amount of shortening.

latter is referred to by some orthopedists as *overriding.* Because an x-ray affords no depth perception, a fracture that appears impacted on one view must also be visualized at an angle 90° from the first, to differentiate it from a fracture whose ends are completely displaced and overriding.

Depending on the location of the fracture and the age of the patient, shortening may have long-range functional implications and may have to be corrected by closed manipulation or by surgery.

## Angulation

Angulation is expressed in terms of two parameters—direction and amount (Fig. 223-4). Quantifying the angulation is relatively simple.

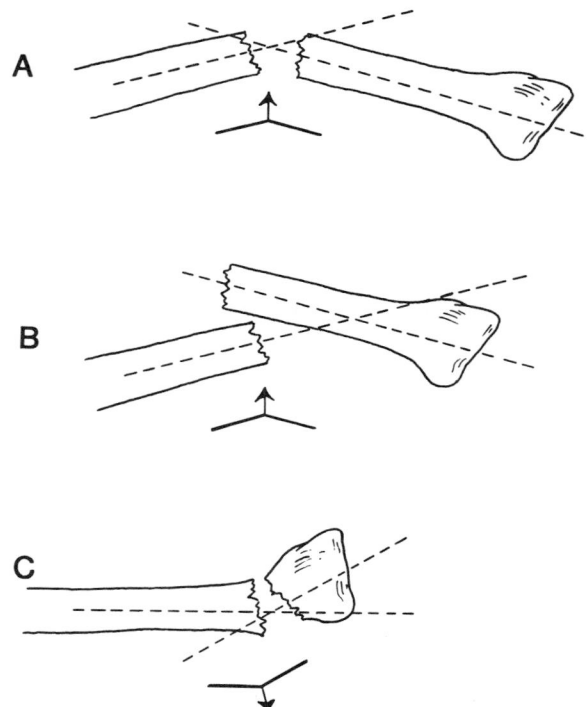

**Fig. 223-4.** Fracture angulation. All figures depict 30° dorsal angulation. (A) and (B) Direction is based on the apex of the angle drawn below the figures. (C) Direction is based on the direction of the terminal fragment.

The physician need only estimate the amount of "unbending" (expressed in degrees) that would be required to make the fragments *parallel.*

Describing the direction of angulation is more difficult because the terminology is less consistent among clinicians. Generally, when a fracture is near the midshaft of a long bone, the direction of angulation is the direction of the *apex* of the angle formed by the two fragments. Figures 223-4A and B, both represent 30° of dorsal angulation. When a fracture is located near the *end* of a bone, however, angulation is described in terms of the direction the *terminal fragment* is deviated. Figure 223-4C also represents 30° of dorsal angulation, even though the apex of the angle formed by the fragments is pointing in the opposite direction from that in the preceding figures. If there is a possibility of ambiguity in the description, specifying the *direction of deviation of the distal fragment* can usually resolve it.

Depending on the anatomic area involved, direction of angulation may be expressed as radial or ulnar, dorsal or volar, anterior or posterior, or lateral or medial.

### Rotational Deformity

Rotational deformity—the extent to which the distal fracture fragment is "twisted" on its own axis relative to the proximal fragment—is generally *not* measurable on x-ray and sometimes not even radiologically apparent. This element of fracture description depends on physical examination. Its detection is particularly important in the phalanges of the fingers where, if rotational deformity goes unrecognized and is left uncorrected, the affected finger will always be malaligned when the hand is closed.

### Fracture Combined with Dislocation or Subluxation

Injuries near a joint may involve dislocation or subluxation in combination with a proximate fracture. An example is fracture of one or more ankle malleoli, together with partial or complete displacement of the talus from beneath the tibia. Fracture-dislocations are significant injuries, often requiring surgical intervention. If, in describing the injury, the physician emphasizes the fracture component but expresses the dislocation or subluxation component as mere displacement, then the full severity may not be appreciated by the orthopedist. Such injuries should be described as fracture-dislocations or fracture-subluxations.

### Salter Fractures

The physiology of Salter fractures—fractures involving the epiphyseal plate at the end of the long bone of a growing child—has already been discussed. Salter fractures are classified into five types, based on the pattern of the fracture line. Because the type generally correlates with the potential for future growth disturbance (and, consequently, with the aggressiveness of treatment required), the ability to classify these injuries based on their x-ray appearance is important.

Perhaps the easiest way to remember the Salter classification system is to think of these injuries not in terms of where the fracture line runs, but in terms of *what has been broken off.* Figure 223-5 illus-

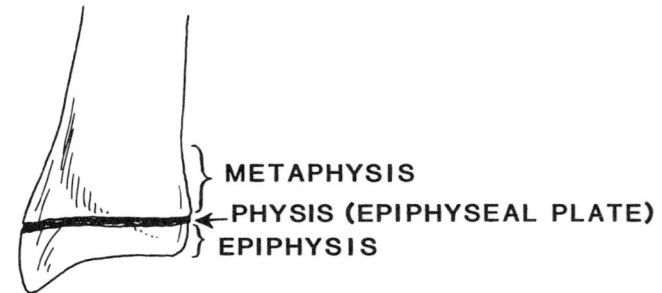

**Fig. 223-5.** Epiphyseal anatomy.

**Table 223-1.** Description of Salter Fractures

| Salter Type | What Is Broken Off |
|---|---|
| I | The entire epiphysis |
| II | The entire epiphysis *with* a portion of the metaphysis |
| III | A portion of the epiphysis |
| IV | A portion of the epiphysis *with* a portion of the metaphysis |
| V | Nothing "broken off;" compression injury of the epiphyseal plate |

trates the anatomy involved. Table 223-1 describes the five types of Salter fractures, which are illustrated in Fig. 223-6. The potential for growth disturbance is least for type I, and increases with the classification number, the worst prognosis being associated with type V injuries.

Type I and type V Salter fractures may be *radiologically undetectable*. Type I injuries usually involve little or no separation of the epiphysis from the rest of the bone, and the lucent fracture line is not visible along the equally lucent epiphyseal plate. If the epiphysis and plate "slip" transversely along the end of the shaft, the abnormal position will be seen on x-ray, but slippage does not always occur. Diagnosis of acute Salter I fractures is usually clinical, based on the presence of swelling and tenderness in the region of the physis.

Type V injuries may be evident only retrospectively, when growth disturbance first begins to appear. At time of initial presentation, however, a history of a significant axial loading force, coupled with significant tenderness in the area of the epiphyseal plate, should suggest the possibility of a type V injury. Such children should be immobilized and referred for orthopedic follow-up.

## TREATMENT IN THE EMERGENCY DEPARTMENT

### Control of Pain and Swelling

Measures to reduce swelling should be initiated early. Severe swelling not only intensifies the patient's discomfort, but may also prevent the application of a long-term definitive immobilization dressing, and may make the skin more susceptible to pressure sores. Although sometimes regarded as trivial modalities, the application of cold and elevation are both effective in keeping swelling to a minimum or at least preventing its progression. When cold is applied, the skin should be protected from direct contact with ice-cold temperatures.

Parenteral analgesics should be administered as necessary. If the patient is relatively comfortable at rest, medication may not be required. Analgesics have virtually no effect on the pain of movement or manipulation, unless combined with hypnotics or other central nervous system active agents. Jewelry, watches, or rings that can cause compression as an extremity swells, should always be removed if there is suspicion or confirmation of proximal injury.

### Keeping the Patient NPO

Any patient who might be a candidate for prompt surgical fixation, manipulation, or any other procedure under general anesthesia or conscious sedation, should be kept NPO from the moment of arrival until the need for, and timing of, such a procedure has been ascertained. This seemingly obvious point is commonly overlooked, particularly in a busy emergency department, where the process of clinical evaluation might be prolonged and hunger may develop in the interim.

### Reducing Fracture Deformity

The long-term purpose of reducing significant deformity associated with fractures is, of course, restoration of normal appearance and function of the extremity. However, there are also short-term reasons for reducing deformity early in the patient's course. These include: (1) alleviating pain, (2) relieving the tension on nerves or vessels that may be stretched as they pass over the deformity, (3) eliminating or significantly minimizing the possibility of inadvertently converting a closed fracture to an open one when the skin is tented by a sharp bony fragment, and (4) restoring circulation to a pulseless distal extremity.

After the patient has been sedated, deformity at or near the midshaft of a long bone is usually easy to reduce with gradual, steady *longitudinal traction*. Any rotational deformity should be corrected only after the angular component has been addressed and should be performed while traction is maintained. If reduction is performed as a definitive procedure prior to immobilization, attention to rotational deformity is particularly important because of its profound effect on ultimate function. As discussed earlier, rotational deformity is much easier to appreciate by examining the patient than by examining the x-ray.

The nearer the deformity is to a joint, the more difficult it may be to correct, and the more specialized the reduction maneuver may have to be. Who performs the procedure, the emergency physician or the orthopedist, is determined by a variety of circumstances, some of which may be specific for the particular practice environment. When deformity is associated with circulatory deficit, a true emergency exists, and the anticipated delay until reduction should be considered.

### Reducing Dislocations

The techniques used to reduce specific dislocations are discussed in subsequent chapters. In general, reduction should not be performed prior to x-ray, unless circulation is threatened and prompt radiologic evaluation is not available. This is because dislocations and fracture-dislocations may have the same clinical appearance on physical examination, but the techniques used to treat them may be markedly different. An example is simple anterior dislocation of the shoulder, as opposed to the same injury associated with complete fracture through the humeral neck. If the fracture is identified at the outset, the patient will be spared the pain of prolonged unsuccessful reduction attempts, and no question will arise as to exactly when the fracture might have occurred. Even "pure" dislocations may be associated with minute fracture fragments. A prereduction film will usually furnish proof of the preexistence of such fragments.

Postreduction films are equally important. Occasionally a joint may feel as though it has been reduced, when in fact it has not. Even

**Fig. 223-6.** Epiphyseal fractures based on Salter-Harris classification.

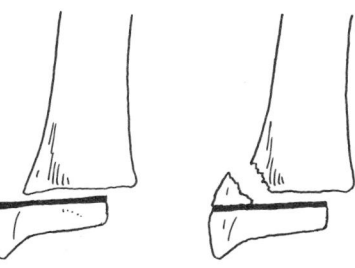
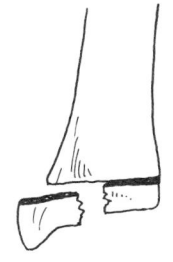
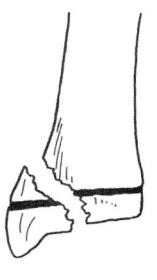
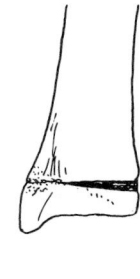

I            II            III            IV            V

when a maneuver is successful, the joint may re-dislocate after the patient leaves the emergency department. There is no way to prove the joint was in anatomic position at the time of discharge, without a postreduction film.

## Initial Management of Open Fractures

Open fractures, which may be complicated by subsequent osteomyelitis, warrant prompt and meticulous attention. The most important elements in the treatment of open fractures, aside from tetanus prophylaxis that applies generally to any wound, are irrigation, debridement, and antibiotics—each implemented as early as is practical. Although irrigation and debridement are commonly performed in the operating room, antibiotics can be administered in the emergency department.

The role of prophylactic antibiotics in preventing osteomyelitis remains a subject of study, but their early use in open fractures is common practice. The longer the interval between the time of injury and the initiation of antibiotic therapy, the less likely it becomes that such therapy will be of any benefit. Exactly what constitutes the ideal antibiotic is controversial. An accepted combination is a first-generation cephalosporin plus an aminoglycoside, although this is by no means the only regimen in use. Aerobic and anaerobic wound cultures can be obtained before antibiotics are administered.

Antibiotics by themselves are no substitute for irrigation and debridement, both of which have been well demonstrated as crucial to reducing the incidence of osteomyelitis in open fractures by reducing bacterial contamination and the potential for bacterial colonization. Irrigation should be extensive to (1) make the area more visible for inspection for foreign material, (2) float out nonviable tissue, or at least float it into the field of vision so it can be removed, and (3) float out contaminated blood clots and bits of tissue. Pulsatile pumps may increase the effectiveness of irrigation, provided the stream is not too forceful. Excessive force will simply pack debris further into the recesses of the wound.

Debridement of minor wounds that overlie a fracture may sometimes be performed in the emergency department. When tissue damage is moderate or severe, however, formal debridement and irrigation are commonly performed in the operating room.

## IMMOBILIZATION TECHNIQUES

Immobilization is indicated not only for fractures but also for dislocated joints that have been reduced. When a joint becomes dislocated, the ligaments that had provided it with stability are disrupted, and the joint is susceptible to re-dislocation until healing has occurred.

## To Cast or to Splint?

The issue of *splinting* as opposed to circumferential casting by the emergency physician is controversial. Those who advocate splinting point out that casts have a higher potential for complications, including pressure sores, circulatory compromise, and neuropraxia, than splints do, and might therefore be more appropriately applied by the same physician who will provide the patient's long-term follow-up. Furthermore, a properly and carefully fashioned splint can provide immobilization essentially equal to that of a cast during the interval between the patient's emergency department visit and initial follow-up. Yet another consideration is that during this interval, much of the initial swelling may subside, allowing excessive mobility inside the original dressing regardless of whether it is a cast or a splint and necessitating its replacement by another dressing in any case. For these reasons, this chapter will focus on splinting techniques.

## Material Used

Whether plaster or fiberglass is used in the dressing depends on a number of factors, including the emergency physician's preference, the philosophy of the orthopedic community, the needs of the patient, and the hospital's resources. Fiberglass has the advantages of being lightweight, fast setting, and resistant to damage by moisture (although most splint dressings contain additional bandaging materials that need to be kept dry). Ultimately, the physician should use the material he or she is most comfortable with and can use most skillfully with best results.

## Principles of Splinting

With the exception of the specific chemical substance involved, references to plaster in the following description are equally applicable to fiberglass.

The chemical reaction that causes plaster of Paris (calcium sulfate) to crystallize, or set, is initiated by contact with water. The higher the water temperature, the faster the hardening process. However, the setting of plaster is an *exothermic* chemical reaction, which liberates heat—and the faster plaster sets, the more heat it generates. This means the maximum temperature to which the patient's skin is exposed will be the *additive* result of the water temperature *plus* the heat released by the plaster. For this reason, severe burns can result when plaster has been immersed in hot water, even though the temperature of the water itself was not sufficient to cause such burns. Although there is no universally prescribed ideal water temperature, a safe practice is to make the water slightly warmer than room temperature. If steam is visible, the water is almost certainly too hot.

To avoid irritation and minimize the potential for pressure sores, plaster dressings need to include several layers of padding between the plaster and the skin. When longitudinal splints are used, the padding need not be circumferential. Longitudinal padding will effectively protect the skin, as long as it slightly exceeds the width and length of the splint. The best way to ensure this is to fashion the dry splint first, then measure the padding over it.

The length of a splint should be sufficient to provide ample leverage to immobilize the injured joint. To immobilize the elbow, for example, a splint should begin distal to the wrist and extend *high* up the lateral arm, to the level of the humeral neck. To effectively immobilize the ankle, a splint should extend from beneath the metatarsal heads to high calf. If the fracture is located along the midshaft of the distal extremity rather than at a joint, the splint should be long enough to immobilize the joint above and the joint below the fracture.

Splints may be fashioned from the plaster rolls normally used for casting, or from prepadded material supplied on a continuous roll, which can be cut to length. When using common plaster rolls, determine the necessary length of the splint by measuring out a single layer along the extremity. Then, on a flat surface, unroll the plaster back and forth over itself to make a multilayered splint. For an adult, the splint should be at least 12 layers thick. Even more layers should be used for children, who typically remain as active as possible and have little regard for protecting the dressing.

When the dry splint has been prepared, measure out several layers of padding over it, making the padding longer and wider than the plaster. After setting the padding aside, grip each end of the splint and immerse it in water, keeping it submerged until bubbling stops (indicating the water has been fully absorbed into the interstices of the material). Then withdraw the splint and strip out the excess water by sliding the thumb and index finger along the length of the plaster on each side. (Be sure to use a stripping motion, rather than crumpling the dressing to wring out the excess water, or much of the plaster will be wrung out as well.)

The next step, frequently overlooked, is to lay the splint on a flat surface and massage the layers into one another, so that they fuse together. This creates a strong dressing that is solid on cross-section. A splint whose separate layers are still visible on cross section is much weaker.

The padding should now be laid over the plaster and the dressing applied to the extremity, with the padded surface against the skin. An assistant can hold the splint against the extremity while it is wrapped in place with gauze bandage. Make sure the assistant uses the palms, rather than fingertips, when holding the plaster. Hardened finger dents can cause irritation or even pressure sores. If a compressive effect is desired, an elastic bandage may now be wrapped over the gauze. *Note:* If an elastic bandage is wrapped directly onto plaster without an intervening layer of gauze, it will set into the plaster and lose its compressive function.

While the plaster is setting, the physician may need to maintain the affected joint in a particular position. Again, the palms rather than the fingers should be used. Once the setting process is well underway, the position of a joint cannot be changed, or the dressing will crack and become functionally useless. If the joint has gradually migrated from the desired position, the physician must decide either to accept the current position or remove the dressing and start over. There is no need to feel self-conscious about the latter course. Patients generally appreciate perfection in their physician.

## Types of Immobilization Dressings

The more common immobilization dressings used in the emergency department are discussed below.

### Shoulder Immobilizer

This is a removable, Velcro-fastened device that keeps the arm in "sling position" but allows less mobility than a sling (Fig. 223-7). A wide band wraps around the thorax. Two cuffs are attached to the thoracic piece—one on the lateral side that grasps the upper arm, keeping it adducted against the thorax, and one anteriorly that grasps the wrist, keeping the forearm against the abdomen. This dressing is suitable for fractures about the shoulder girdle, including clavicle and well-positioned humeral neck fractures, as well as for reduced anterior shoulder dislocations.

The shoulder immobilizer is also commonly used for acromioclavicular separations, although the ideal dressing for this injury is one that exerts upward pressure on the elbow and downward pressure on the clavicle. Commercial versions of such dressings do exist, but they are cumbersome to apply and uncomfortable to wear, leading to noncompliance. A shoulder immobilizer (or sling-and-swathe) is an acceptable alternative dressing.

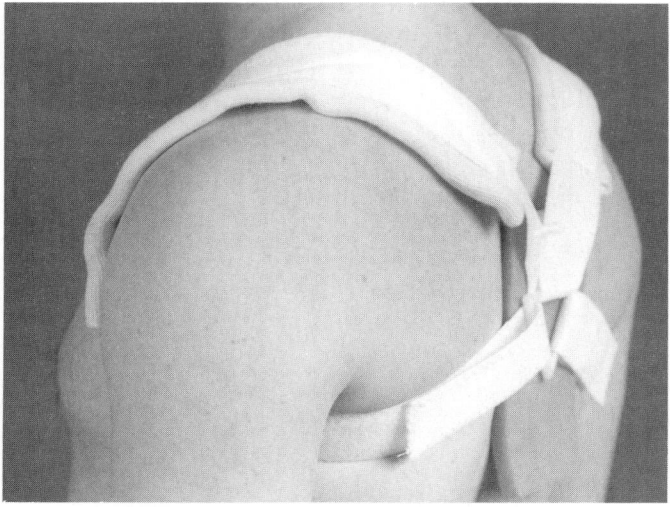

**Fig. 223-8.** Clavicle strap.

### Clavicle Strap (Figure-of-Eight Bandage)

This is a dressing used for fracture of the clavicle (Fig. 223-8). It consists of padded straps that pass down the anterior aspect of both shoulders and under the axillae. The right and left halves of the dressing meet in back, where they are attached to clips centered between the scapulae. The straps, whose tension is adjustable, exert backward pressure on each shoulder. This dressing is designed specifically for fractures of the clavicle (except for very distal fractures, which are better treated with a shoulder immobilizer). It may be combined with a sling, according to the patient's comfort.

The purpose of a clavicle strap is to reduce pain by minimizing free motion of the fracture fragments. It is not intended to maintain optimal alignment. Some patients, usually adults, are more comfortable in a simple sling, without a clavicle strap. When that is the case, the strap can be omitted.

Patients or their parents should be cautioned to watch for paresthesias or swelling in the hands or fingers. If such symptoms occur, the dressing is too tight and should be removed completely until symptoms disappear. The strap may then be reapplied more loosely.

### Long-Arm Ulnar Gutter Splint

This is a plaster splint that maintains the elbow in flexion, usually at 90° (Fig. 223-9). The upper extremity is placed in sling position (elbow flexed and palm facing the abdomen). The splint begins on the

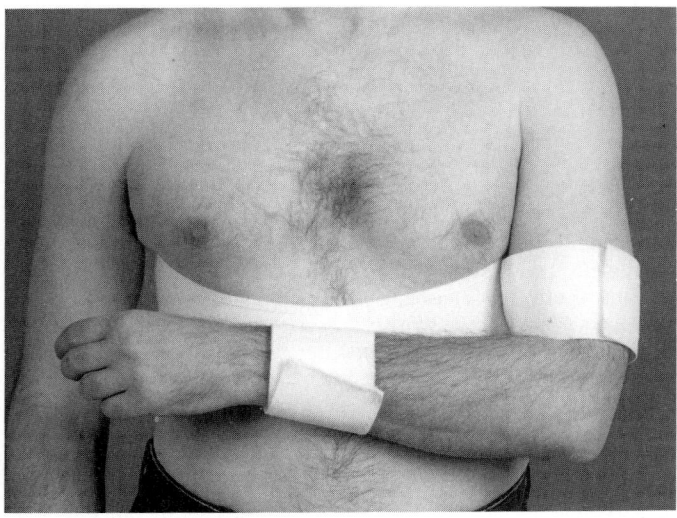

**Fig. 223-7.** Shoulder immobilizer.

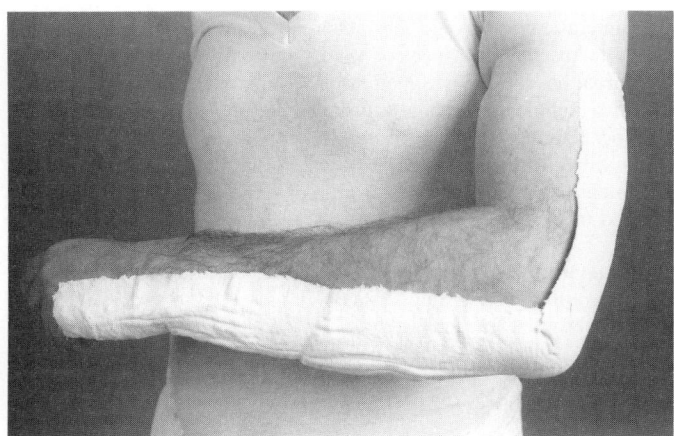

**Fig. 223-9.** Long-arm ulnar gutter splint.

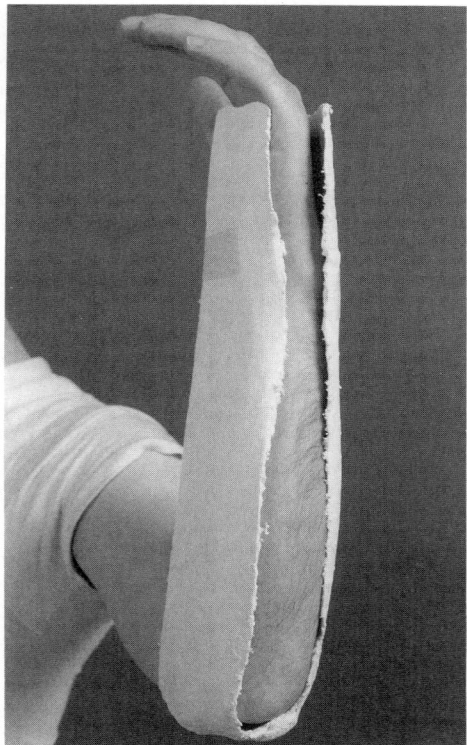

**Fig. 223-10.** Sugar tong splint.

ulnar surface of the hand at the metacarpal heads and extends along the ulnar surface of the forearm, past the apex of the elbow, to a spot *high* on the lateral surface of the upper arm just opposite and a bit below the axillary crease. It should be supplemented with a sling.

The most common error associated with fashioning this dressing is insufficient length. If the splint is not carried far enough above the elbow, it will not be able to exert enough leverage to prevent motion of the joint.

The long-arm ulnar gutter is useful for injuries about the elbow, including radial head fractures, nondisplaced supracondylar humeral fractures, and reduced dislocation of the elbow.

## Sugar Tong Splint

This is a plaster splint that prevents motion of the wrist and elbow, including pronation-supination (Fig. 223-10). The upper extremity is placed in sling position as described above. The splint begins on the extensor aspect of the hand at the level of the metacarpal heads and extends along the extensor aspect of the forearm, around the elbow and humeral condyles onto the flexor aspect of the forearm, and ultimately to the palmar aspect of the hand, ending at the level of the metacarpal heads. It is wrapped in place with gauze and often topped off with a compression bandage. It should be supplemented with a sling.

Proper length of the sugar tong dressing is important. Too short a splint will fail to immobilize the wrist. If the dressing is too long it will impair motion of the metacarpophalangeal joints, leaving them stiff and making the fingers more susceptible to swelling due to immobility.

The sugar tong splint is appropriate for fractures about the wrist or distal forearm. Some orthopedists use it as a definitive dressing after reduction of wrist fractures.

## "Cock-up" Wrist Splint (To Be Avoided)

The "cock-up" splint is a removable device that encloses the forearm and hand, maintaining the wrist in a dorsiflexed position. The splint is fastened with Velcro straps. *Cock-up splints should not be used for*

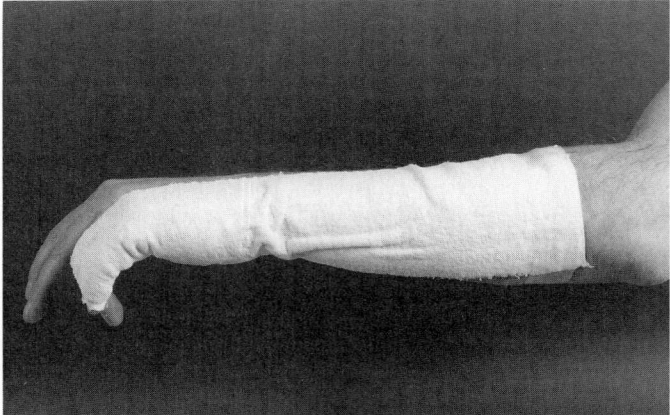

**Fig. 223-11.** Short-arm ulnar gutter splint.

*fractures of the wrist or carpals* because such injuries are usually caused by forceful dorsiflexion, and the splint only reproduces the position of injury, imposing considerable pain in the process. Fractures about the wrist are generally immobilized in neutral position with plaster dressings. Colles fractures may even be immobilized in slight palmar flexion after reduction.

"Cock-up" splints can be useful in some situations, such as to immobilize the wrist for tendinitis, or to support it in the case of wrist drop due to radial nerve palsy. In those instances, dorsiflexion of the wrist will preserve the patient's grip strength.

## Short-Arm Ulnar Gutter Splint

This plaster splint immobilizes the wrist and ulnar half of the hand (Fig. 223-11). It extends along the ulnar surface of the hand and forearm, beginning just proximal to the tip of the fifth finger and ending high onto the forearm. The splint should be wide enough to encompass the fourth and fifth rays (fingers and metacarpals) on both the extensor and palmar aspects of the hand. The splint is wrapped in place with the fourth and fifth fingers bound together, separated by a thin layer of padding to prevent maceration of the skin. The metacarpophalangeal joints and interphalangeal joints should be positioned in gentle flexion. The dressing should be supplemented with a sling.

The short-arm ulnar gutter is useful for fractures of the proximal phalanx of the ring or little finger, or for fractures of the fourth or fifth metacarpal (including the common "boxer's fracture"). The counterpart of this splint, the short-arm radial gutter, is designed in similar fashion, but extends along the radial surface of the hand and forearm, and is used for comparable injuries of the index or middle rays. It is fashioned with a hole that allows the thumb to pass through.

## Thumb Spica

This plaster dressing immobilizes the wrist and thumb (Fig. 223-12). The term spica applies to any dressing that encompasses a main trunk plus one or more of its branches—in this case, the forearm plus the thumb. It is used for fractures of the carpal navicular or for fractures of the thumb metacarpal or proximal phalanx.

A thumb spica can be fashioned from a single wide plaster splint, but a more effective and better-looking dressing can be made from two separate splints. The wrist piece runs along the extensor aspect of the hand and forearm, beginning at the metacarpal heads and ending just short of the elbow. The more narrow thumb piece, approximately 2 in. wide, extends from the tip of the thumb (which has been padded separately), along the outer aspect of the thumb metacarpal, and onto the extensor aspect of the forearm, well overlapping the first splint. Along their area of contact, the two splints are molded into each other, with no padding between them, to form a sturdy dressing. The plaster is wrapped in place with gauze, and a compression wrap may

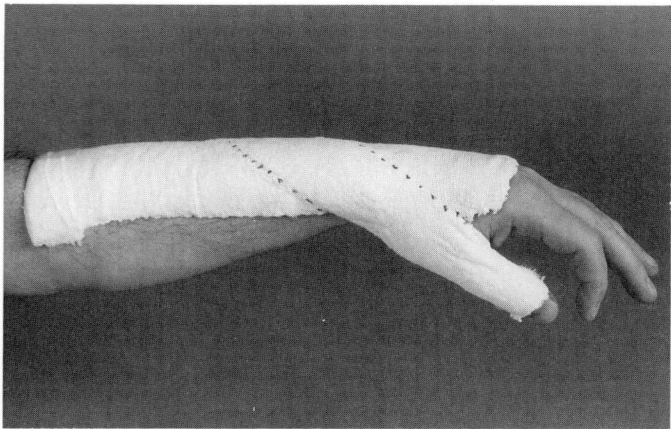

**Fig. 223-12.** Thumb spica splint.

be added at the physician's discretion. The dressing is supplemented with a sling.

While the plaster is setting, optimal position can be achieved by keeping the wrist in *neutral* position and having the patient oppose the tips of the thumb and index fingers in the form of an "OK" sign. This preserves thumb-index pinch function, minimizing the patient's incapacitation. It also avoids reproducing the position of injury in the case of navicular fractures, which are typically caused by forced dorsiflexion of the wrist.

### Knee Immobilizer

This is a removable device that wraps around the upper and lower leg and maintains the knee in a fully or almost fully extended position (Fig. 223-13). The splint contains longitudinal metal struts and is fastened with Velcro straps.

The knee immobilizer is useful for a variety of injuries, including fracture of the lateral or medial tibial plateau, fracture or subluxation of the patella, meniscal injuries (provided the patient's knee is not "locked" in partial flexion), and ligamentous strains or tears.

### Posterior Ankle Mold

This is a plaster splint that immobilizes the ankle (Fig. 223-14). It begins beneath the metatarsal heads, runs along the plantar aspect of the foot, and continues up the back of the lower leg, ending at high calf. The splint is used for severe ankle sprains or for stable ankle fractures, such as minimally displaced fractures of the distal fibula. Unstable fractures, such as those involving more than one malleolus or widening of the medial joint space (disruption of the deltoid ligament), may be supplemented by a sugar tong component running down one side of the leg, beneath the heel, and up the other side. Where the two components overlap, they are molded together. The additional component helps minimize inversion-eversion of the ankle. Even more stability is provided by continuing the posterior splint past the back of the knee to high posterior thigh, using wider plaster for this area. With the knee slightly flexed, rotational motion at the ankle will be prevented as well.

While the plaster is setting, the ankle should be maintained in a position as close as possible to neutral, that is, at 90° to the leg. This maintains the width of the ankle joint and allows the patient to regain range of motion more quickly after the dressing is removed. Because most patients with ankle injuries tend to keep the ankle plantar flexed, the physician will usually have to maintain passive dorsiflexion by exerting gentle pressure with a palm beneath the sole of the foot. An exception to the 90° principle is immobilization for rupture of the Achilles tendon. Patients with this injury should be immobilized in plantar flexion to reduce tension on the tendon.

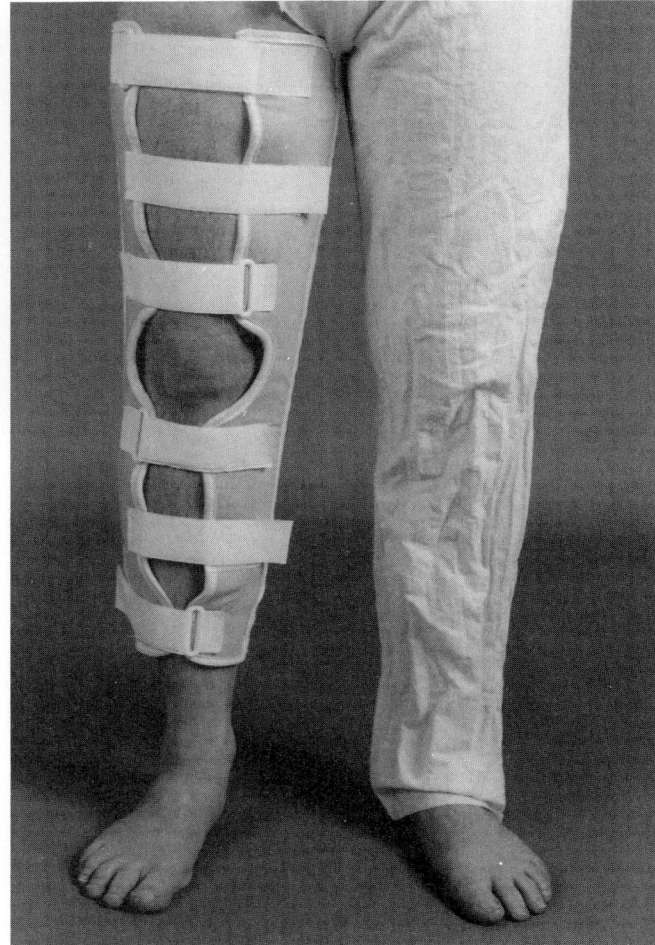

**Fig. 223-13.** Knee immobilizer.

Commercially available ankle splints (air-cast splints) are also useful for ankle sprains and minor avulsion fractures. They prevent eversion and inversion but do not limit plantar flexion or extension.

## ADJUNCTS TO AMBULATION

### Crutches

Crutches should be used by patients who can bear no weight at all on an injured lower extremity. Ideal crutch height is one hand width below the axillae. The grip bar should be adjusted to a height at which the elbows are still mildly flexed while supporting the body weight.

The patient should be instructed to bear the pressure of the pads against the sides of the thorax rather than in the axillae, or brachial plexus injury might result (crutch palsy). During ambulation, the patient should advance the crutches first, then bring the well leg up to, or just past, the crutches. Ascending stairs, the patient advances the well extremity up to the next step, followed by the crutches. Descending stairs, the crutches are lowered first. Either a two-point or three-point gait can be used with crutches, depending on whether some or no weight-bearing is allowed. The physician should specify the type of gait he or she wishes the patient to use.

### Walkers and Canes

Most elderly or infirm patients do not have the strength to use crutches safely. For them, a walker or cane is more suitable. Unfortunately, these devices are more appropriate for partial weight-bearing than for full non–weight-bearing conditions. Elderly patients who can

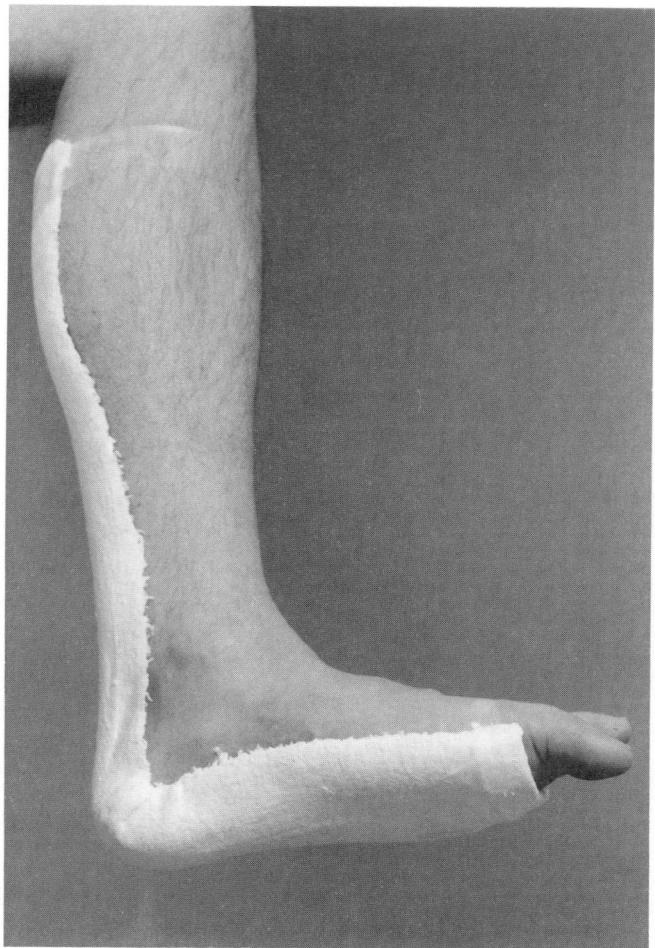

**Fig. 223-14.** Posterior ankle mold.

bear no weight at all on an injured extremity may require initial bed rest and subsequent rehabilitation.

The technique for using a walker is essentially intuitive, the patient simply lifting it and placing it a short distance ahead, then advancing up to it. By contrast, the technique for using a cane tends to be counterintuitive. Most patients instinctively hold a cane on the same side as the injured extremity. In fact, when the cane is held in the hand on the *well* side, much less strength is required to maintain balance, resulting in an easier and less awkward gait. This can be substantiated with geometric diagrams and physical equations but is much more easily appreciated by personally comparing the two methods.

## DISCHARGE INSTRUCTIONS

Continuous elevation of the injured part will usually help minimize swelling and pain. However, most individuals do not share the physician's knowledge that to be effective, elevation must be above the level of the heart. Patients with an injured lower extremity will often sit at home or at work with the leg resting on a chair, thinking they are complying with instructions. The patient should understand that the benefits of elevating a lower extremity can only be achieved in a recumbent or near-recumbent position, with the leg supported higher than the rest of the body.

Patients discharged in a lower extremity plaster dressing should be cautioned not to rest the heel on the floor or any other hard surface. Plaster takes about 24 h to fully set. During this time, prolonged pressure on the heel can gradually create an indentation that may cause significant discomfort or even a pressure sore. This is not a consideration with fiberglass, which sets immediately.

If an upper extremity sugar tong dressing has been applied, the patient should be instructed to work the fingers (wiggle or wave) as much as possible to minimize stiffness and swelling. The sugar tong splint should allow full flexion of the metacarpophalangeal joints.

Patients should be advised to watch the fingers or toes for excessive swelling, decreased sensation, or cyanosis, and to be alert for a significant increase in pain. Any of these signs or symptoms warrant a return to the emergency department or prompt evaluation by the follow-up physician.

When crutches, a cane, or a walker are supplied, instructions for their use should be provided, and the patient's ability to navigate with such aids should be verified.

## FOLLOW-UP

There is no universally prescribed follow-up interval for specific injuries. Physicians differ in their opinion as to how soon patients should be seen. Generally, unreduced fractures or injuries that may require future surgical intervention should be seen within a few days.

Sometimes the situation may be discussed with the follow-up physician and an appointment arranged while the patient is still in the emergency department. Alternatively, the emergency physician may instruct the patient to contact the follow-up physician or clinic as soon as possible. If the name of the injury is written on the discharge instruction sheet, the patient can convey it at the time of the call. Based on this information, the follow-up physician can decide when the patient should be seen.

## COMPLICATIONS

The earliest complications associated with skeletal injuries include neurovascular deficit and compartment syndrome (see Chap. 237). Neurologic injury is usually due to traction or pressure. Recovery may take hours, days, or weeks, or may sometimes be irreversible. Compartment syndrome is a true emergency, requiring expeditious diagnosis and aggressive treatment to prevent muscle necrosis and permanent disability.

A later complication is a pulmonary fat embolus, usually originating from the marrow of a large bone such as the femur. If fat embolism occurs, it usually does so within the first few days after injury, rather than in the first hours. This event may have a variable effect on pulmonary function, ranging from mild distress to severe or even fatal respiratory failure.

The most delayed complications of fractures include nonunion, malunion (healing with deformity), joint stiffness, traumatic arthritis of an involved joint, avascular necrosis of one of the bone fragments, and, in the case of open fractures, osteomyelitis.

## ACKNOWLEDGMENTS

Original art work: Eleanore Denton Rhodes, A.M.I.
Photography: Joy Miller, B.P.A.

## BIBLIOGRAPHY

Buckwalter JA, Cruess RL. Healing of the musculoskeletal tissues. In: Rockwood CA Jr, Green DP (eds). *Fractures in Adults,* 3rd ed. Philadelphia: JB Lippincott, vol. 1, pp. 181–222, 1991.

Chapman MW. Open Fractures. In: Rockwood CA Jr, Green DP (eds). *Fractures in Adults,* 3rd ed. Philadelphia: JB Lippincott, vol. 1, pp. 223–264, 1991.

Chudnofsky CR, Otten EJ, Newmeyer WL. Splinting techniques. In: Roberts JR, Hedges JR (eds). *Clinical Procedures in Emergency Medicine,* 2nd ed. Philadelphia: WB Saunders, pp. 792–810, 1991.

Salter RB, Harris WR. Injuries involving the epiphyseal plate. *J Bone Joint Surg* 45A:587, 1963.

Schultz RJ. *The Language of Fractures.* Baltimore: Williams & Wilkins, 1972.

Wallace KK. Extremities. In: Keats TE (ed). *Emergency Radiology.* St. Louis: Mosby-Year Book, pp. 403–477, 1989.

# 224

# INJURIES TO THE WRIST AND HAND

### Robert R. Simon

### David Slobodkin

## GENERAL PRINCIPLES

The hand is an immensely complex organ and evaluating and treating injuries requires a more than casual knowledge of anatomy and function.

The key concept in dealing with hand disorders is to preserve range of motion by splinting in the proper position to maintain function, followed by early mobilization. Although in injuries to joints elsewhere in the body, one attempts to preserve stability, in hand injuries the principle goal is to preserve dexterity.

The metacarpophalangeal (MCP) joints and their collateral ligaments are lax in extension and taut in flexion. Thus, during immobilization of the MCP joints, they should be positioned as close to 90° and no less than 50° of flexion to prevent ligament shortening. This can be achieved in the "safe" position or "position of function" (Fig. 224-1).

## Motions of the Hand

Figure 224-2 shows the motions of the hand. Note that flexion and extension of the thumb are demonstrated by holding the hand open horizontally and moving the thumb in the same plane. With the hand still horizontal, abduction and adduction are demonstrated by raising and lowering the thumb in the vertical plane.

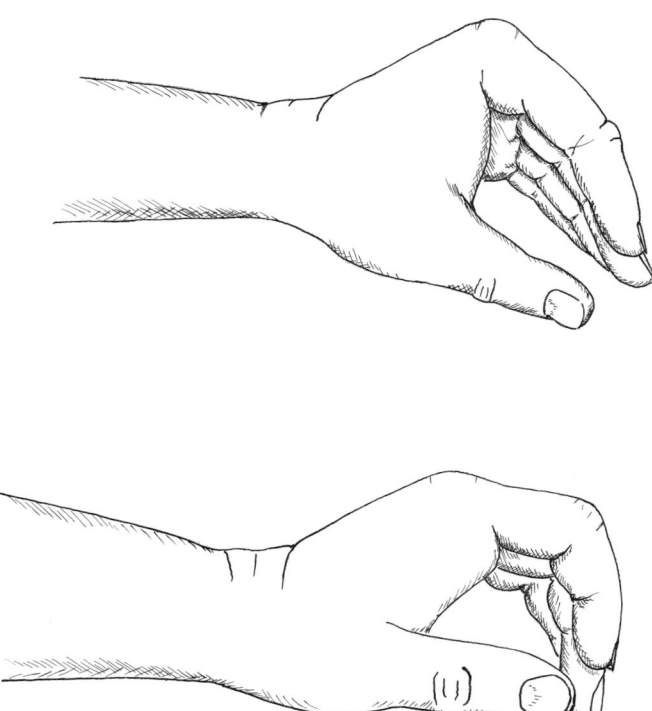

**Figure 224-1.** Positioning the hand during immobilization. (A) This position is used when splints are applied for fractures or severe sprains. (B) This is the position of function used when applying a soft tissue dressing.

## Examination

The key to hand examination is to test the *function* of each individual structure in isolation. With appropriate knowledge of anatomy, it is usually easy to demonstrate a motor or sensory deficit distal to the injury. The injured hand should be examined systematically to assess integrity of circulation, sensation, skin coverage, bones, joints, ligaments, flexor tendons, extensor tendons, and intrinsic muscle function. When in doubt, comparison of the injured and the noninjured hand may be invaluable. Complete documentation is extremely important.

### Circulation

Vascular integrity is the first determinant of viability. Radial and ulnar pulses should be assessed, by Doppler if necessary. Capillary refill, color, and temperature of each digit must be noted.

### Sensation

Sensation of the radial and ulnar aspects of each finger pad must be accurately assessed. Two-point discrimination is an objective test and can be elicited even in children. A small iris scissors or a paper clip provides two convenient points for this purpose. Proximal integrity of the radial, ulnar, and median nerves can be established by the presence of normal sensation in the first dorsal web space, the tip of the long finger, and the tip of the small finger, respectively.

Normal two-point discrimination does not rule out a partial nerve laceration. If the patient states that he or she has a subjective sensation of numbness distal to a laceration, even if the objective examination is negative, the patient has a partial nerve injury. This injury may later develop a neuroma, and the patient should be referred if any problems persist.

### Skin Coverage

Skin defects too large to heal by contracture, or in areas where contracture will result in tethering or limitation of motion, will require grafting, usually in the operating room. Bone, tendons, nerves, and vessels must be covered primarily, to avoid desiccation and secondary injury. *There is no dead space in the hand.* Subcutaneous sutures should almost never be placed in the emergency room. Closure can be achieved by approximation of skin with a minimum number of simple interrupted sutures. In cases where skin is inadequate for coverage, or in which severe contamination precludes skin closure, strictly sterile moist saline dressings (wet to wet) are appropriate, followed by a delayed closure or referral.

### Bones, Joints, and Ligaments

Bony integrity is evaluated by assessing any deformities and by palpation of each of the 14 phalangeal bones and the 5 metacarpals. Each of the interphalangeal (IP) and MCP joints and its related ligaments is assessed for range of motion and stability, both active and passive. This may require the use of anesthesia. Evaluation of the carpal bones requires a knowledge of anatomic location. The navicular bone can be individually palpated in the "anatomic snuffbox" and at the palmar navicular tubercle. The lunate can be palpated dorsally in a "hollow" just distal to Lister's tubercle, with the wrist in flexion. The triquetrum can be palpated volarly just distal to the ulnar styloid. The pisiform and the hook of the hamate are palpable on the volar surface at the base of the hypothenar eminence.

### Tendons

It is critical to check for the presence of tendon function and to assess strength against resistance. A tendon that is 90 percent lacerated can still have function. However, motion against resistance (strength) is

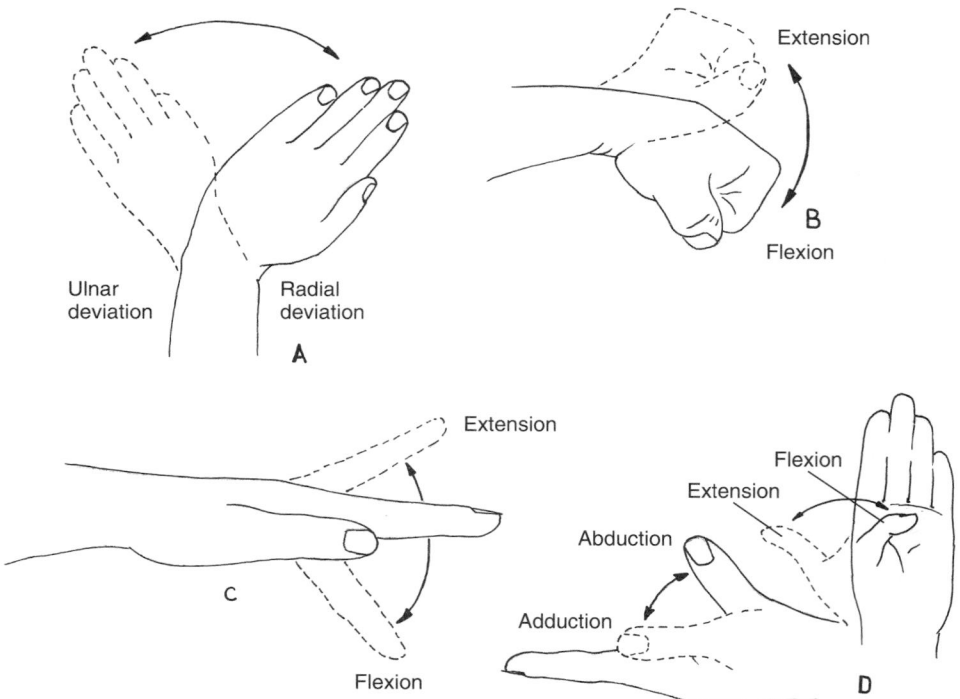

**Figure 224-2.** Describing motions of the hand, these are the common term used.

markedly reduced. It is important to determine the position of the hand at the time of injury to tell where along its course a tendon was injured.

The site of pain along the course of a tendon correlates with the site of tendon injury in patients with both blunt and penetrating tendon disruption. A negative examination in an uncooperative patient is entirely unreliable in ruling out the presence of tendon injury and must be repeated later.

Flexor carpi radialis and flexor carpi ulnaris can be individually palpated just proximal to the wrist with the wrist flexed and radially deviated and flexed and ulnarly deviated, respectively. In examination of the flexor digitorum profundus (Fig. 224-3), the digit should be held extended at the MCP and proximal interphalangeal (PIP) joints. In testing the flexor digitorum superficialis, one must hold the MCP and IP joints of adjacent digits extended, to remove the effect of the profundus, as shown in Fig. 224-4. It is important to realize that the MCP joints are flexed by the intrinsic muscles, and hence, gross finger motion may be present in the complete absence of extrinsic flexors.

The extensor tendons lie in six fibro-osseous tunnels over the dorsum of the wrist (Fig. 224-5). The extensor carpi radialis longus and extensor carpi radialis brevis are critical tendons to examine because they hold the hand in an extended position necessary for maximum grip strength. These two tendons are superficial and easily involved in a laceration on the dorsal surface of the hand. By asking the patient to make a fist and dorsiflex the wrist, they can be palpated as they enter the second extensor canal proximal and dorsal to the radial styloid. By asking the patient to flex the thumb and radially deviate the wrist, abductor pollicis longus and extensor pollicis brevis and extensor pollicis longus can be demonstrated distally. These tendons form the edges of the "anatomic snuffbox." Extensor digitorum communis and extensor indicis proprius lie in the fourth canal, extensor digiti quinti proprius in the fifth, and extensor carpi ulnaris in the sixth. The independent finger extensors of the index or small finger can be demonstrated by asking the patient to hyperextend the appropriate finger while making a fist with the other fingers. The integrity of the extensor mechanism and hood in the fingers must be assessed by extension of each finger against resistance *from a position of flexion.* Failure to do so may miss an isolated injury of the extensor hood, with severe late sequelae.

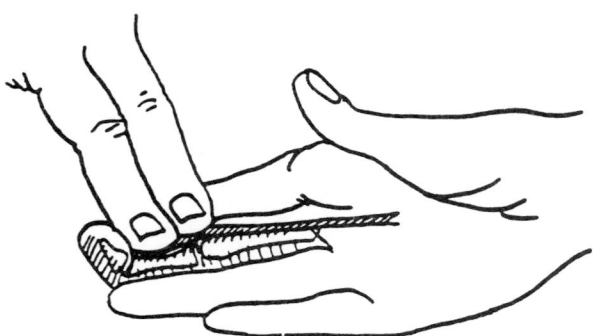

**Figure 224-3.** Testing function of flexor profundus.

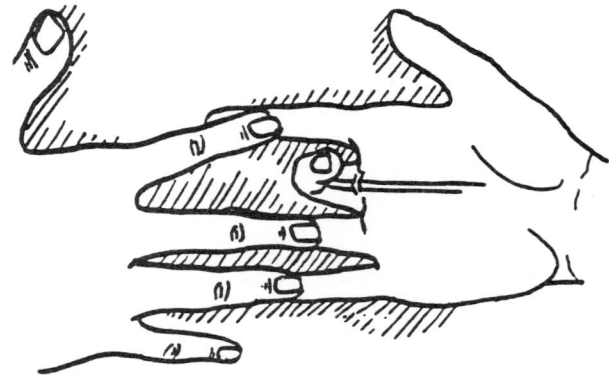

**Figure 224-4.** Testing function of flexor superficialis.

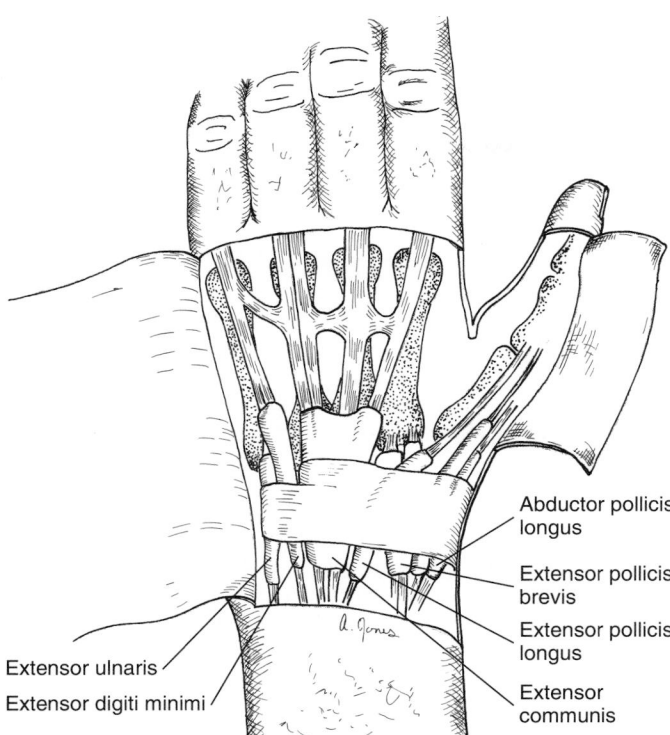

**Figure 224-5.** A fibrous canal system courses over the dorsum of the wrist through which the extensor tendons pass to insert on the hand.

### General Principles of Treatment

Many injuries of the hand can be appropriately treated, splinted, and referred to a specialist. Others require immediate definitive care to achieve optimal results.

Various splinting materials are available; however, the emergency physician will usually be using either commercial padded aluminum strips or plaster of Paris. Aluminum splints, in an appropriate width, provide excellent control of the distal interphalangeal (DIP) and PIP joints, whose normal movements are limited to flexion and extension. As a rule, aluminum splints alone provide poor control of the MCP and wrist joints because they cannot control rotatory motion. Because splints should usually be applied to control one joint distal and one joint proximal to the injury, plaster of Paris is the splint of choice for the MCP and wrist joints. If precise and complete control of the proximal phalanx and MCP is required, an aluminum splint embedded in a short arm plaster cast provides excellent immobilization (Fig. 224-6). This technique should not be used by the emergency physician if swelling of the wrist or forearm is anticipated.

Open fractures or open dislocations should be irrigated and debrided in the operating room within a few hours of injury. Any injury that has contaminated a joint space or has resulted in extensive contamination of nonviable tissue requires similarly urgent treatment. Immediate intravenous antibiotics are indicated in all of these situations but do not replace local decontamination.

Dislocations and fractures with neurovascular findings, or with deformity severe enough to place tension on neurovascular structures or that threaten intact skin, require urgent reduction. In many cases this may be accomplished by the emergency physician familiar with the specific injury. In cases where closed reduction is unsuccessful, such injuries should be reduced in the operating room.

Crush injuries of the hand or forearm in which a compartment syndrome is suspected must be assessed and treated by a hand surgeon as soon as possible to prevent irreversible tissue necrosis. Injuries to the radial or ulnar arteries should be repaired emergently, usually along with any coexisting major nerve injuries.

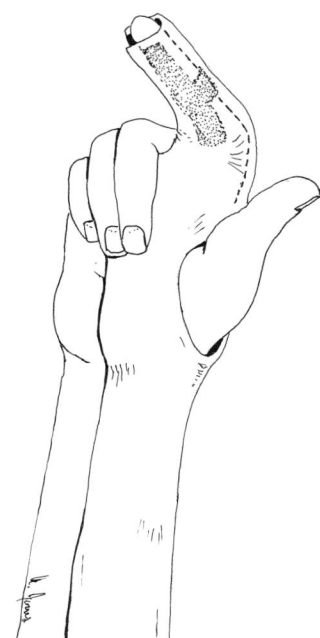

**Figure 224-6.** A gutter splint is used to maintain reduction. The proper position is shown.

## SOFT TISSUE INJURIES
### Tendon Injuries
#### General

A partial tendon injury can be treated by protective splinting and requires no repair. Complete tendon disruption can be treated by primary, delayed, or secondary repair. A primary repair is optimal when the laceration is clean and incisive. Delayed repair should be used if the wound is dirty or a proper repair cannot be done in a reasonable time limit. Secondary repair is used in wounds where there is loss of tendon tissue or when circumstances do not permit a primary or delayed repair. Although many hand surgeons find repair of some extensor tendon injuries in the emergency department acceptable, flexor tendon repair is *never* to be attempted except by a qualified hand surgeon in the operating room. Appropriate follow-up and rehabilitation of all tendon injuries are necessary.

#### Special Tendon Injuries

**Mallet finger.** A mallet finger is a disruption of the extensor tendon at its attachment at the base of the distal phalanx or an avulsion of the bone on which the tendon inserts. A tendinous avulsion, or a small bony avulsion, is easily treated with a dorsal splint that permits motion of the PIP joint but prevents motion of the DIP joint (Fig. 224-7). A bony avulsion involving more than one third of the DIP articular surface may be most appropriately treated by open reduction and internal fixation.

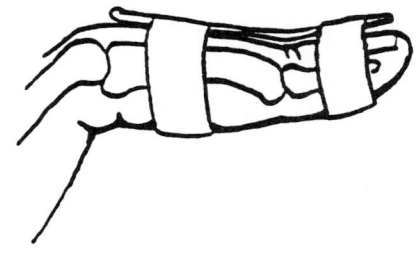

**Figure 224-7.** Dorsal splint for extensor rupture.

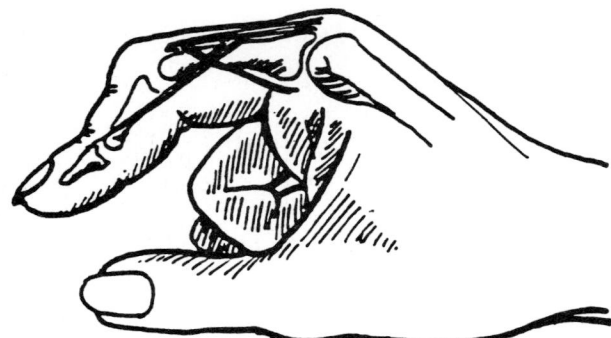

**Figure 224-8.** Boutonnière deformity secondary to rupture of extensor apparatus at PIP joint.

**Boutonnière deformity.** A boutonnière deformity results from a disruption of the extensor hood apparatus near the PIP joint. The lateral bands of the extensor mechanism sublux anterior to the axis of the PIP joint, becoming flexors of the PIP and hyperextensors of the DIP. Contraction over the course of several weeks produces the typical deformity shown in Fig. 224-8. Extensor hood injuries can be easily missed in the emergency department. Injuries over the PIP dorsum should be regarded with suspicion and reexamined after a 7- to 10-day interval.

## Injuries to the Collateral Ligaments and Volar Plate

It is critical to understand the functional anatomy of the collateral ligaments and the volar plate. The collateral ligaments and volar plate are interconnected, forming a U-shaped hood around the lateral and volar aspect of the IP and MCP joints. Because of the cam effect of the metacarpal heads, the MCP joints are taut in flexion and lax in ex-

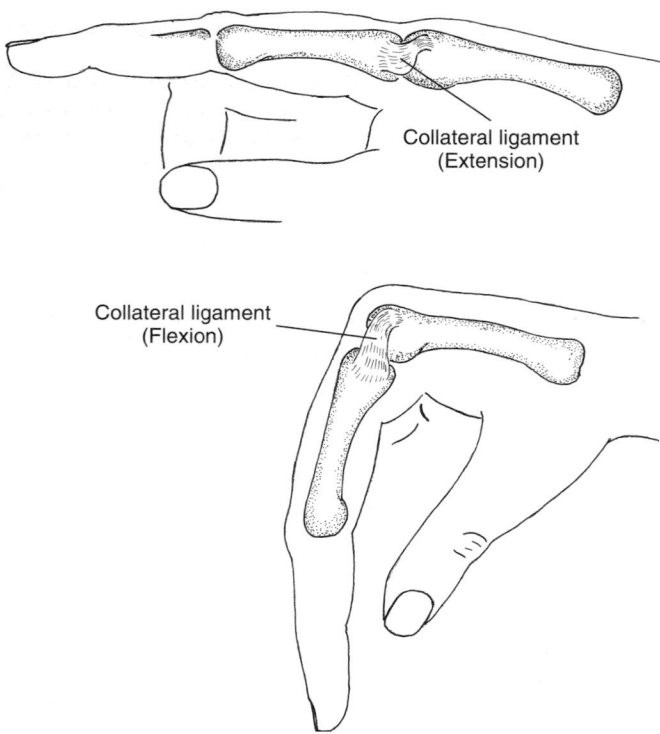

Collateral ligament
(Extension)

Collateral ligament
(Flexion)

**Figure 224-9.** Because of the condyloid shape of the metacarpal head, the collateral ligaments are taut and flexion and relaxed in extension. This is unique in that in most joints (knee, ankle, elbow) the opposite is true.

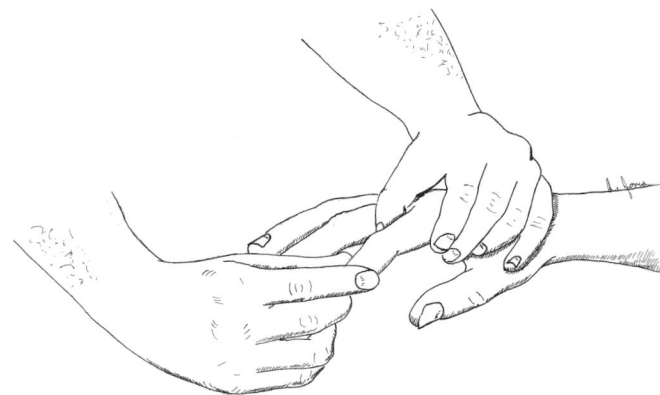

**Figure 224-10.** A stress test of the collateral ligaments of the IP joints is shown.

tension (Fig. 224-9). This is the opposite of collateral ligaments elsewhere in the body, which are taut in extension and lax in flexion. For this reason, the MCP collateral ligaments should be immobilized in flexion to preserve maximum length and dexterity.

Collateral ligament injuries should be immobilized for the shortest necessary time to prevent stiffness, which is the most common complication following these injuries.

Sprains of the collateral ligaments can be first degree, second degree, or third degree. One can determine the extent of sprain by performing a "stress test" perpendicular to the axis of motion of the involved joint (Fig. 224-10). If there is no opening, but pain and swelling are present, the patient has a first-degree injury. If there is minimal opening with a firm end point, the patient has a second-degree injury. If there is significant opening of more than 3 to 5 mm, the patient has a collateral ligament tear and a volar plate injury. If the volar plate is intact, there cannot be wide opening of the IP joint or MCP joint on stress testing. Disruption of both structures should be splinted and referred because they may need surgical repair.

## Treatment of Collateral Ligament Sprains

Never immobilize the MCP joint in extension. It should always be immobilized at 50° to 90° of flexion. A partial tear of a collateral ligament of the IP joints can be treated with dynamic splinting ("buddy-taping"), as shown in Fig. 224-11. A complete disruption of the collateral ligament with a normal volar plate should be treated in an aluminum splint in the position shown in Figs. 224-6 and 224-12.

Third-degree sprains involving disruption of collateral ligaments of the volar plate should be treated in a gutter splint or an aluminum splint, and the patient should be referred to an orthopedist. An ulnar

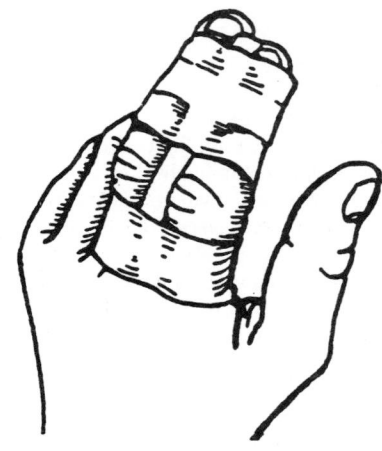

**Figure 224-11.** Dynamic splinting of the digits.

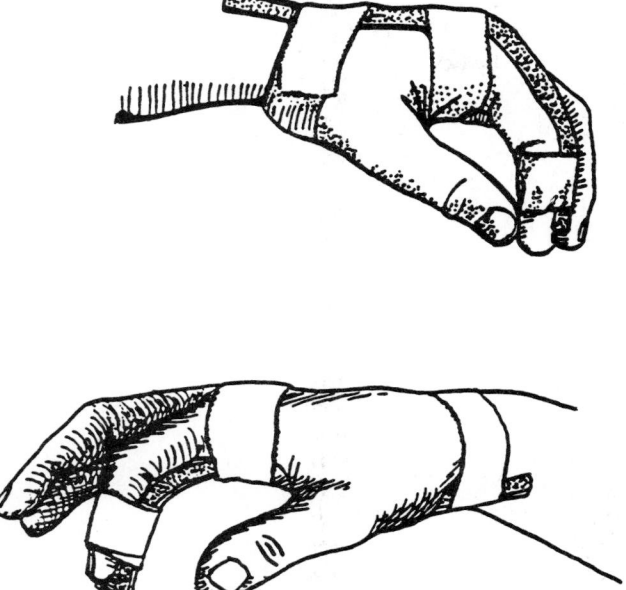

**Figure 224-12.** Splints for DIP and PIP joints. Notice that flexion of the MCP joint should be between 50° and 90°.

gutter splint is easily fashioned by moistening eight or nine layers of 5- or 6-inch plaster to make a solid slab stretching from the proximal forearm to the tip of the fingers. After placing absorbent cotton padding between the fingers to avoid maceration and a layer of cast padding or stockinette to cover the plaster, the slab is applied along the ulnar aspect of the extremity and folded to immobilize the small and ring fingers. A radial gutter is constructed analogously, but a hole for the thumb must be cut in the plaster before moistening. The plaster is held in position with an elastic bandage. As always, the MCP must be placed in at least 50° of flexion (Fig. 224-13).

Isolated injuries of the volar plate are secondary to hyperextension forces and can be partial or complete. A digital block should be performed to do a proper stress test when pain prevents the test from being done. A hyperextension stress is applied to the involved joint and compared to the normal side. In a partial volar plate injury, the joint should be immobilized in the position shown in Fig. 224-12.

A complete volar plate injury should be referred because the patient may need surgical repair.

## Interphalangeal Joint Dislocations

Interphalangeal joint dislocations are common and are usually secondary to a blow to the tip of the flexed digit. The most common dislocation is a posterior or dorsal dislocation of the PIP or DIP joint. One should always x-ray the digit involved to be certain it is not a fracture dislocation.

Proximal interphalangeal or DIP joint dislocations are easily reduced after digital block anesthesia by applying a distracting force

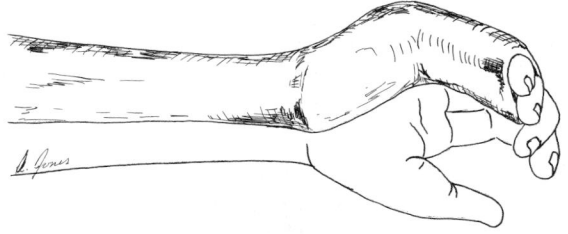

**Figure 224-13.** A gutter splint is shown. See text for discussion.

along the long axis of the digit while holding the phalanx proximal to the dislocation with the opposite hand.

After distracting the joint, slight hyperextension followed by repositioning of the distal phalanx (DIP joint dislocations) or middle phalanx (PIP joint dislocations) into its anatomic position is easily accomplished. A PIP joint dislocation may be difficult to reduce because of volar plate entrapment. When this occurs, surgical repair is needed.

Following reduction, the examiner should check for collateral ligament injury, which should be treated as indicated above. If there is no collateral ligament disruption, the digit should be splinted to the adjacent digit (dynamic splinting).

Volar dislocations of the PIP must be recognized by the emergency physician and the precise diagnosis communicated to the hand surgeon. These uncommon dislocations require treatment of the accompanying extensor mechanism injury.

## Metacarpophalangeal Joint Dislocations

These joint dislocations have a mechanism similar to that of IP joint dislocations. Involvement of the volar plate with entrapment in the joint is far more common than in PIP or DIP joint injuries. At the same time, the head of the metacarpal buttonholes volarly between the flexors and the lumbrical. The interposed proximal edge of the volar plate prevents reduction in flexion, and the flexor tendons and lumbrical tighten around the narrow MCP neck if reduction is attempted in extension. Thus, unreducible MCP joint dislocations are common. When this occurs, the MCP joint should be splinted and referred for surgical reduction and repair.

## Complications of Metacarpophalangeal and Interphalangeal Joint Injuries

The most common complication of IP and MCP joint injuries, whether they are dislocations or ligamentous sprains, is persistent thickening around the joint and stiffness. Both of these can be prevented or markedly reduced by early mobilization. It is critical that the hand be splinted in the proper position to maintain ligamentous length.

Volar plate injuries are not uncommon, and one should examine for them. If they are present and complete, the patient should be referred.

Occasionally, a small fleck of bone is avulsed with the collateral ligament in an IP or MCP joint injury. One should treat this depending on the degree of ligamentous disruption. However, if the bony avulsion involves more than a 1- to 2-mm fleck of bone, it may require pinning, and the patient should be splinted and referred.

## Gamekeeper's Thumb

The ulnar collateral ligament of the MCP joint of the thumb is of special significance. When it is completely disrupted, the patient loses the pincer ability to grasp with the thumb. Thus, this is the most critical of all the collateral ligament injuries of the hand.

Any injury in which the thumb is forcefully abducted should be viewed with suspicion, as should any injury in which an object is forcefully torn from the patient's clenched hand. Injuries involving ski poles or steering wheels are associated with this diagnosis, as is a history of a missed punch, which makes contact with the thumb rather than the knuckles. Patients with point tenderness along the medial aspect of the thumb IP joint or inability to grasp between the thumb and index finger, should be considered to have a serious injury until proven otherwise.

Complete disruption of the ulnar collateral ligament of the thumb can be determined easily by a stress test following infiltration with anesthesia. If the stress test demonstrates laxity with more than 20° of opening compared to the opposite normal side, the patient needs surgical repair. If the opening is less than 20° compared to the opposite side and there is a firm end point, the patient may be treated conservatively with a splint similar to that for a collateral ligament injury involving other digits. A thumb spica splint or cast is favored by some.

Patients in whom a gamekeeper's thumb is suspected should be referred to a hand surgeon for follow-up.

### Nerve Injuries of the Hand

The most common nerve injury of the hand involves a laceration of a digit with partial or complete transection of the digital nerve. Not uncommonly, the median nerve, branches of the radial nerve, or the ulnar nerve may be injured. Complete ulnar injuries occur proximal to the wrist as the nerve divides into a superficial and deep branch approximately 5 cm proximal to the wrist.

There are three general types of nerve injuries: neuropraxia, a blunt contusion of the nerve; axonotmesis, a more severe contusive injury of the nerve resulting in destruction of the nerve fibers but with preservation of the myelin sheaths; and neurotmesis, a complete transection of the nerve, which occurs only in penetrating trauma.

### Treatment

Complete nerve disruption should be repaired by a hand surgeon, either primarily or secondarily (contaminated wounds), when it involves one of the major nerves supplying the hand or a digital nerve proximal to the PIP joint.

The digital sensory nerves most critical to function are the ulnar digital nerve of the thumb and the radial digital nerves of the index and long fingers because these surfaces are involved in the manipulation of small objects. The radial digital nerve of the thumb and the ulnar digital nerve of the small finger are important to protect the hand from inadvertent injury.

### Volkmann's Contracture

Inadequate circulation to the forearm from any cause may result in necrosis and Volkmann's ischemic contracture of the forearm muscles. It is critical to prevent this.

Prevention involves early recognition. Whenever a patient complains of increasing pain, a dressing or cast around the arm, forearm, or hand should be removed immediately. Swelling and paresthesia are symptoms that occur later, and distal pulses may be entirely normal. If the patient has tenderness in the forearm on either the volar or dorsal aspect, a fasciotomy may be indicated because of elevated compartment pressures. This syndrome should be suspected in any patient with a fracture around the elbow (supracondylar), severe forearm fractures involving both the ulna and radius, or compressive injuries along the forearm. Early suspicion and referral are essential for preservation of hand function. Irreversible damage may occur in as little as 6 h.

## FRACTURES OF THE WRIST

### Fractures of the Carpus

Carpal trauma is complex and diagnosis may be subtle. A good rule is that significant pain or tenderness in the wrist should be taken seriously and never dismissed as "only" a soft tissue injury. Some soft tissue injuries of the wrist require surgical repair, and some fractures of the wrist are radiographically occult. Patients with significant complaints should be placed in a thumb spica splint and referred to a hand surgeon.

The three most common carpal fractures are fractures of the scaphoid, followed by dorsal chip fractures of the triquetrum, and,

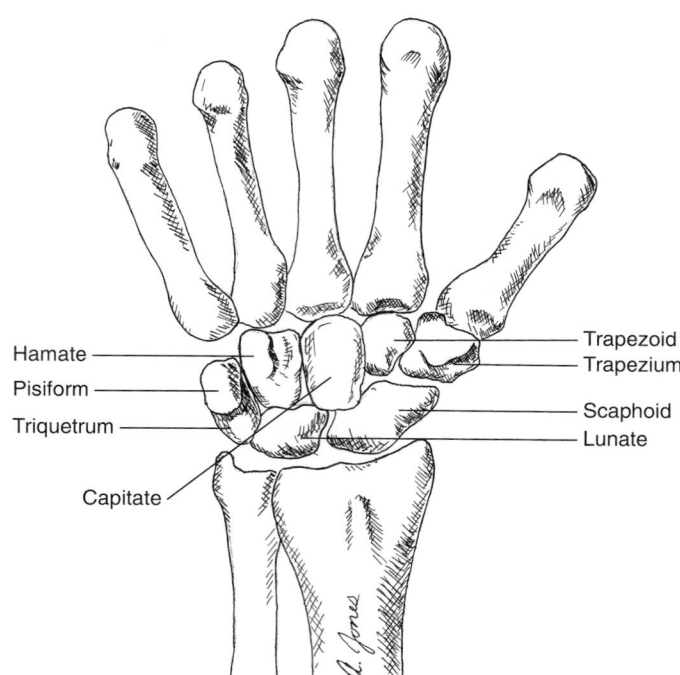

**Figure 224-14.** The carpal bones of the wrist are shown.

most importantly, fractures of the lunate (Fig. 224-14). All of these occur from falls on the outstretched hand.

### Scaphoid Fractures

Scaphoid fractures are the most common of all carpal fractures. The patient presents with tenderness in the anatomic "snuff box." The scaphoid can fracture in four locations. The more proximal the fracture site, the more common is avascular necrosis. Scaphoid views will often demonstrate a fracture that cannot be seen on routine wrist views. Nonetheless, patients with tenderness over the scaphoid should be treated as if a fracture were present, even if x-rays are normal. These patients should be placed in a thumb spica splint and referred to an orthopedist. Fractures will usually become radiographically evident within 2 weeks.

### Dorsal Chip Fractures

Dorsal chip fractures are the second most common type of carpal fracture. The most common bone involved is the triquetrum. The patient presents with tenderness dorsally over the ulnar aspect of the wrist. Lateral views of the wrist may demonstrate a small chip of bone on the dorsal aspect of the wrist. Often, the x-ray is negative. If the patient presents with tenderness over the dorsal and ulnar aspect of the wrist following an extension injury, the patient should be treated with a volar splint with the wrist in 10° extension. These fractures heal without compromise, and although most orthopedic surgeons treat them in cast immobilization, a volar splint is adequate.

### Lunate Fractures

Lunate fractures are the third most common type of carpal fracture and the most important. The lunate is the most critical and pivotal bone of all the carpals in the proximal row. Because none of the carpals articulate with the ulna and only the scaphoid and lunate articulate with the radius, the lunate occupies two thirds of the radial surface.

Patients with lunate fractures present with tenderness over the lunate fossa, which is located just distal to the rim of the radius, directly at the base of the long finger metacarpal.

When this condition is suspected, the patient should be treated with a thumb spica cast and referred. Wrist x-rays may or may not demonstrate the fracture. This fracture may be associated with avascular necrosis of the lunate, which is called Kienbock's disease. Kienbock's disease may cause complete collapse of the lunate. This must be prevented at all costs by early detection and proper immobilization. All of these patients should be referred to an orthopedic surgeon.

## Colles' and Smith's Fractures

A Colles' fracture is a fracture of the distal radius at the metaphysis, which is dorsally displaced. This occurs from a fall on the outstretched hand. Typically, this produces a "dinner fork" deformity Fig. 224-15. One should examine the radiocarpal joint to determine whether the fracture involves that joint. In addition, the radioulnar joint should be examined. Fractures involving the radiocarpal or radioulnar joint predict a much worse prognosis in terms of swelling, persistent pain, and limitation of motion.

Colles' fractures are reduced by placing the patient's hand in a finger trap traction apparatus followed by reduction of the distal radius.

A hematoma block usually provides adequate anesthesia. This is achieved using the strictest aseptic precautions, by creating a small skin weal, and then probing the fracture site with a 22-gauge needle until dark blood is aspirated and the fracture site is felt; 10 mL of 1% lidocaine is then injected.

A Smith's fracture is a reversed Colles' fracture (see Fig. 224-15). In a Smith's fracture, there is a volar displacement of the distal radius. This fracture is reduced easily in a finger trap traction apparatus, but one must be certain there is no associated median nerve or flexor tendon injury.

## DISLOCATIONS OF THE WRIST

### Lunate Dislocations

Lunate dislocations can occur dorsally or volarly, as shown in Fig. 224-16. Dorsal lunate dislocations are easily diagnosed on the lateral view of the wrist, whereby the lunate is seen dorsal to its normal position within the radial fossa. The lunate is easily palpated over the dorsum of the wrist. Volar dislocations involve displacement of the lunate in the volar direction.

The lunate should be reduced by a hand surgeon. Patients may require surgical intervention for proper reduction and ligamentous stability.

### Perilunate Dislocations

Perilunate dislocations involve dislocations of the carpal bones around the lunate. In this dislocation, the lunate remains in its normal position of alignment with the radial head. However, the remainder of the carpal bones are dislocated dorsally or volarly. This can be readily diagnosed on the anteroposterior and lateral views. Reduction of this dislocation can be accomplished by longitudinal traction using finger traps. However, the patient should be referred to an orthopedic surgeon for early repair and immobilization.

### Scapholunate Disassociation

The normal distance between the lunate and scaphoid on an anteroposterior view of the wrist is less than 3 mm. If the space between the scaphoid and lunate is greater than 3 to 5 mm, the patient has a scapholunate dissociation.

This is a very serious injury in that the ligaments connecting the scaphoid and lunate are ruptured and require surgical repair. This must be diagnosed early and referred to a hand surgeon. This condition is one of the most commonly missed diagnoses among emergency physicians.

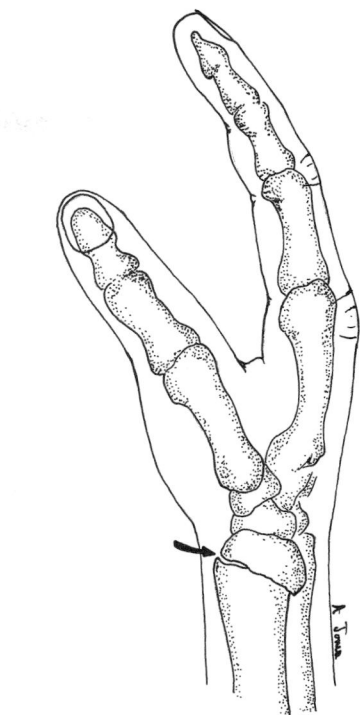

**Figure 224-15.** A Colles' fracture. A Smith's fracture is the same fracture with volar displacement rather than dorsal displacement.

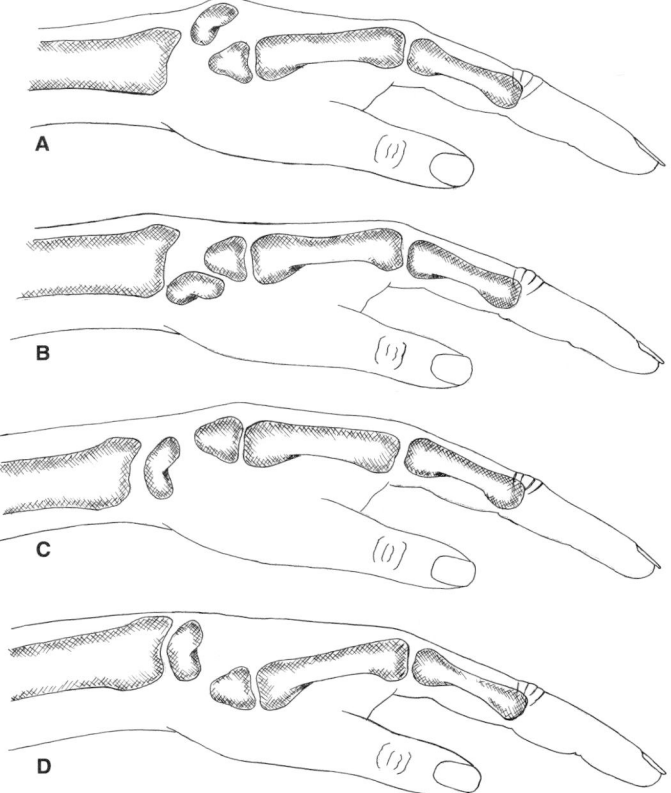

**Figure 224-16.** The four common dislocations of the wrist are shown. (A) Dorsal dislocation of the lunate. (B) Volar dislocation of the lunate. (C) Dorsal perilunate dislocation. (D) Volar perilunate dislocation.

## FRACTURES OF THE HAND

### Distal Phalanx

There are five types of fractures of the distal phalanx (Fig. 224-17). The most common distal phalanx fracture is a comminuted fracture, where the comminution involves only the distal tuft. It is often referred to as a "tuft fracture." These fractures are treated in a protective splint, leaving all joints free. If a subungual hematoma is present, this should be drained. Transverse fractures with displacement are always associated with a nail bed laceration. The nail bed laceration should be repaired.

Mallet fractures, which involve an avulsion injury at the attachment of the extensor tendon to the distal phalanx, should be treated in an extension splint. If the fragment is large, this may require surgical pinning.

### Middle and Proximal Phalanx Fractures

Many hand surgeons prefer internal fixation of these fractures to allow earlier mobilization and prevent tendon adhesion at the fracture site. Extra-articular fractures of the middle and proximal phalanx that are not displaced should be treated in an ulnar or radial gutter splint and referred (see Fig. 224-13). An ulnar splint is used in fractures involving the fourth and fifth digits. Fractures of the index and long finger phalanges should be treated in a radial gutter splint. In fractures that are oblique or spiral and in those that are grossly displaced and unstable, a gutter splint can be used temporarily, but the patient will require more definitive therapy, which may involve pinning or some other type of surgical intervention.

Fractures involving the articular surface that are nondisplaced can also be treated in an ulnar or radial gutter splint. Even minimally displaced fractures involving the articular surface should be reduced anatomically, and this may require surgical intervention. Thus, these patients should be referred.

When applying a radial or ulnar gutter splint for a middle or proximal phalanx fracture, the MCP joint should be at 50° to 90° of flexion, the IP joints should be 10° to 15° of flexion, and the wrist should be at 15° extension.

### Metacarpal Fractures

Fractures of the metacarpal neck are the most common of all metacarpal fractures. The most common of these is called a boxer's fracture and involves the fifth digit and sometimes the fourth. When fractures of the metacarpal neck involve the second or third metacarpal, the fracture needs to be reduced if the angulation is greater than 15°. The index and long finger metacarpals are relatively stationary bones in the hand, and any angulation of a neck fracture of these metacarpals is poorly tolerated.

The name delineates the mechanism, which is basically that of a clenched fist striking an unyielding object. Angulation in a boxer's fracture is usually apex dorsal, and if the fracture involves a fourth or fifth digit, one can tolerate up to 30° of angulation without reduction.

### Fractures of the Metacarpal Shafts

Fractures of the metacarpal shafts can be transverse, oblique, spiral, or comminuted. Oblique and spiral fractures are often angulated or displaced.

Rotational malalignment is a common problem in metacarpal, middle, and proximal phalanx fractures. It must be detected early because it is difficult to treat later.

Fractures of the base of the metacarpal are uncommon and often unstable. Displaced fractures of the metacarpal shaft or base should be referred early.

All fractures of the metacarpal neck, shaft, or base can be treated in a gutter splint. In many cases, when the fracture is stable, this therapy can be definitive.

## CLASS A: EXTRA-ARTICULAR FRACTURES

**Type I: Longitudinal**     **Type II: Transverse**

**Type III: Comminuted**     **Type IV: Transverse with displacement**

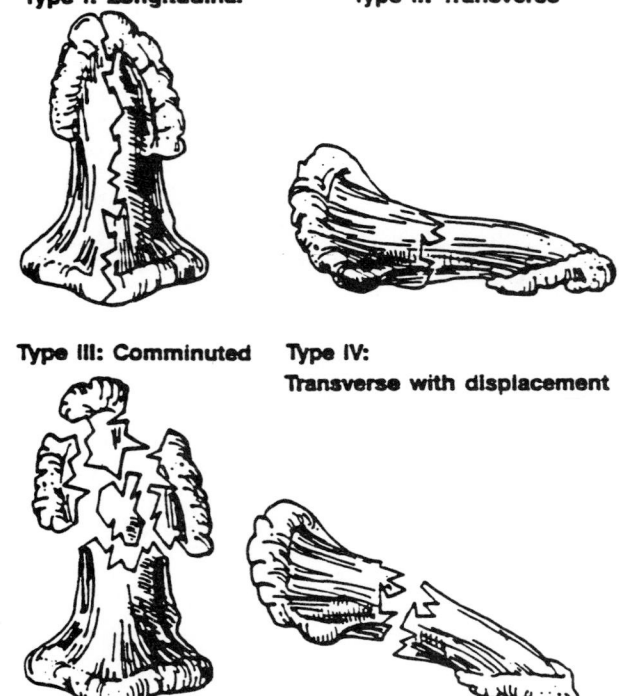

## CLASS B: INTRA-ARTICULAR AVULSION FRACTURES

**Type I: Dorsal avulsion fracture**

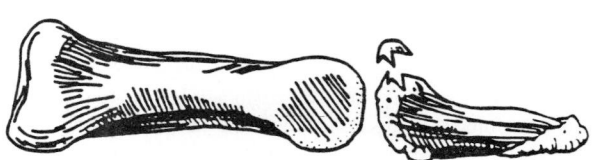

A: "Mallet" fracture (<25% of articular surface)

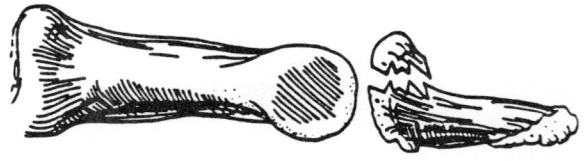

B: "Mallet" fracture (>25% of articular surface)

**Figure 224-17.** Distal phalangeal fractures.

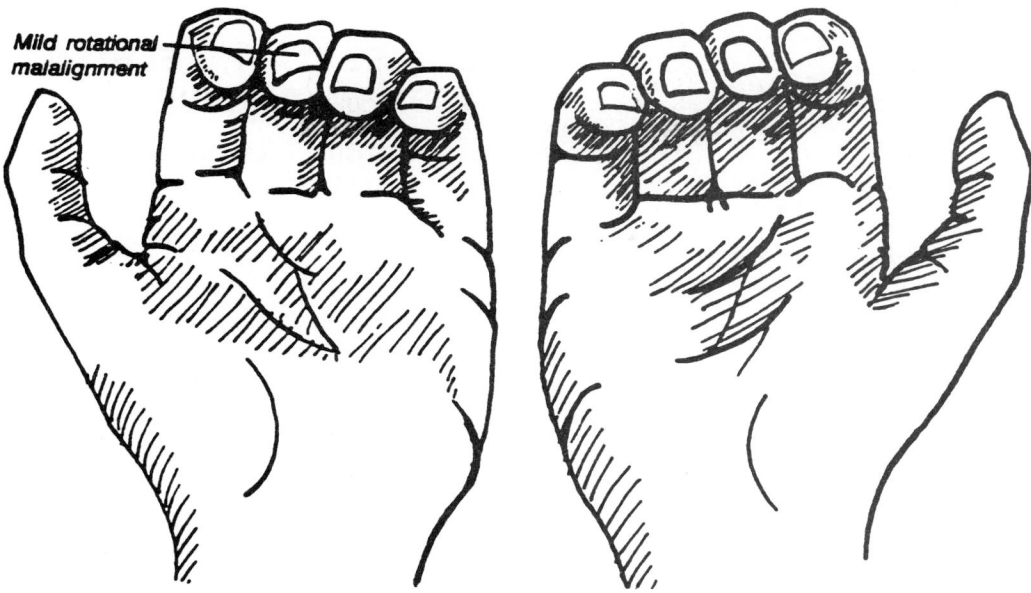

**Figure 224-18.** Checking for rotational malalignment.

## Rotational Malalignment

Rotational malalignment must be detected early and looked for in all patients with middle or proximal phalanx or metacarpal fractures. It is very difficult to detect unless one looks for it. One can diagnose rotational malalignment by comparing the planes of the fingernails of the partially closed hand to that of the involved digit, as shown in Fig. 224-18.

Malalignment of the plane of the fingernail indicates rotational malalignment. Another technique used to detect this is to close the hand as much as possible without pain, as shown in Fig. 224-19, and ascertain whether the fingernails all point to the same spot—if not there is rotational malalignment.

## Bennett's Fracture

A fracture of the base of the thumb metacarpal involving the joint is called a Bennett's fracture. It is due to an axial load applied to the thumb with the hand closed. This fracture must be anatomically reduced and requires surgical intervention.

## FINGERTIP INJURIES

Finger injuries distal to the tendon insertions are common. They may involve simple lacerations, skin loss, nail bed laceration, open or closed distal phalanx fractures, and crush injuries. The goal of treatment is to maintain sensation, avoid permanent tenderness, maintain

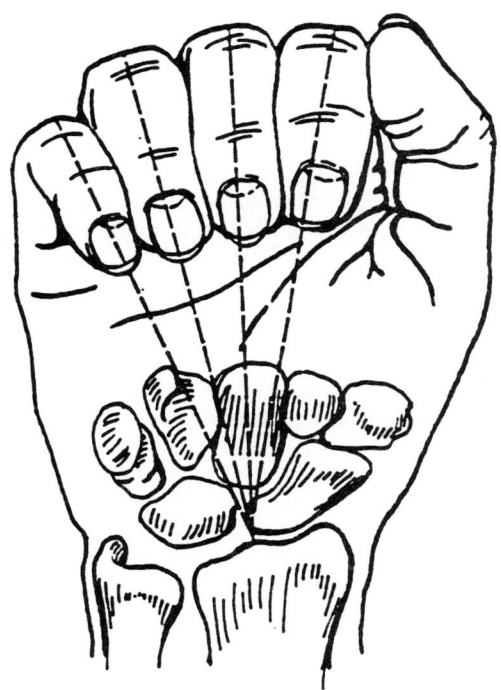
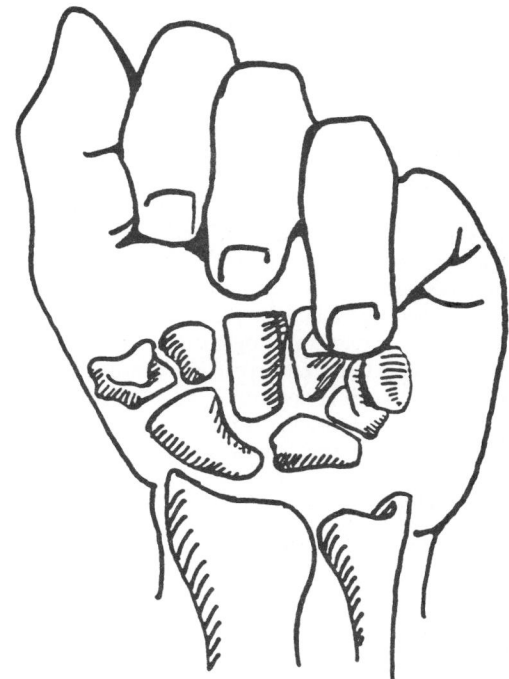

**Figure 224-19.** These drawings show another test for rotational malalignment. See text for discussion.

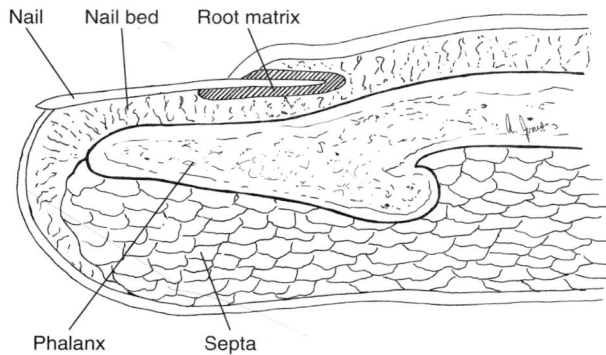

**Figure 224-20.** The nail bed anatomy is shown in a sagittal section.

length, and preserve an adherent and normally shaped nail. In injuries to the thumb, maintenance of length has special importance.

Simple lacerations that can be closed without tension pose no special problems, although the patient should be warned of the possibility of a tender scar. Closed fractures are similarly straightforward, being treated as previously described. Most surgeons consider copious irrigation and tissue coverage in the emergency department to be adequate treatment of open tuft fractures.

Treatment of injuries involving actual skin loss is more controversial and in most cases should be discussed with a hand surgeon. The emergency physician must have a clear understanding of the anatomy (Fig. 224-20). Although a variety of ingenious methods are available to provide coverage, most authors now agree that healing by secondary intention is most likely to achieve a good long-term result. Time off from work is not significantly longer using this method. If bone is exposed, the options are to preserve length and provide coverage using a graft or flap or to rongeur the bone until the stump is covered. This decision should be made in consultation with a hand surgeon, who will want to know the patient's occupation, avocations, and hand dominance.

Injuries involving the nail bed may result in splitting, clawing or nonadherence of the nail, as well as more minor cosmetic problems. Such a result is surprisingly burdensome to the patient, and these injuries should be treated meticulously. A relatively normal nail can be expected if the proximal half of the nail matrix and the nail fold can be anatomically reconstructed. Theoretically, an adherent and intact nail may by itself provide fair approximation of an underlying laceration with minimal hematoma. However, if a nail is significantly fractured or if a hematoma larger than one half of the nail bed is seen under an intact nail, the digit should be fully anesthetized and surgically prepped and a soft tourniquet placed at the base of the finger. The nail should be removed by gently spreading a flat iris scissor in the plane between the nail bed and the underside of the nail. The removed nail may be cleansed of soft tissue, trimmed, trephined, and soaked in povidone-iodine to permit its use as a stent to maintain the nail fold. Nail bed lacerations should be carefully repaired using 6-0 or 7-0 absorbable suture on an ophthalmic cutting needle. The nail fold must be stented to prevent synechiae between the matrix and the eponychium. If the nail is not usable, nonadherent dressing material or Silastic is used. Because the nail grows approximately 0.1 mm/d, the patient should not expect a normal nail for at least 3 months.

## BIBLIOGRAPHY

Green DP (ed): *Operative Hand Surgery,* 3d ed. New York: Churchill Livingstone, 1993.

Simon RR, Koenigsknecht SJ: *Emergency Orthopedics: The Extremities,* 2nd ed. East Norwalk, CT: Appleton and Lange, pp. 42–120, 294–316, 1987.

Szabo RM (ed): Common hand problems. *Ortho Clin North Am* 22: 1992.

Tubiana R: *Examination of the Hand and Upper Limb.* Philadelphia: WB Saunders, 1984.

Weeks PM: Hand injuries. *Curr Probl Surg* 30:721, 1993.

# 225

# INJURIES TO THE ELBOW, FOREARM, AND WRIST

**Dennis T. Uehara**
**Harold Chin**

## ELBOW

### Elbow Dislocation

The elbow is one of the most stable joints in the body. This stability is due to the adjacent muscular attachments, collateral ligaments, and the inherent stability afforded by the hingelike articulation. Because of this stability, surgical repair for acute instability is usually not required and chronic dislocations are unusual. Despite this, however, dislocations of the elbow are commonly seen, being third in large-joint dislocations, after glenohumeral and patellofemoral dislocations.

There are five general types of elbow dislocations: (1) posterior, (2) anterior, (3) medial, (4) lateral, and (5) divergent. The vast majority of elbow dislocations are posterior, all the others being uncommon. The mechanism of injury is usually a fall on the outstretched hand.

Clinically the patient presents with the elbow in 45° of flexion. The olecranon is prominent posteriorly, and the deformity resembles a displaced supracondylar fracture. If the patient is seen immediately after the injury, the bony landmarks can be identified. Later, however, the swelling may be quite severe, with no possibility of evaluating the injury topographically. A careful assessment of the neurovascular status is performed, with specific attention to the brachial artery and the ulnar, radial, and median nerves. The examination must be performed before and after manipulation since neurovascular complications occur in 8 to 21 percent of patients, the most frequent being injury to the ulnar nerve. Vascular complications occur in 5 to 13 percent of elbow dislocations, with brachial artery injury the most common. Endean and coworkers found absence of a radial pulse before reduction, open dislocation, and other systemic injuries (head, chest, and abdomen) to be significantly associated with an arterial injury.

Radiographically, on the lateral view, both the ulna and radius are displaced posteriorly (Fig. 225-1). In the anteroposterior view there may be lateral or medial displacement, with the ulna and radius in their normal relation to each other. A search for associated fractures should be performed. In the child, a fracture of the medial epicondyle is most commonly seen. In adults, fractures of the coronoid process, radial head, capitellum, or olecranon may occur. Initially, these fractures should only be noted, with primary attention focused on the dislocation.

After adequate sedation, reduction is accomplished by gentle traction on the wrist and forearm in the direction in which it lies (Fig. 225-2). An assistant applies countertraction on the arm. Any medial or lateral displacement is corrected with the other hand. Downward pressure on the proximal forearm helps to disengage the coronoid process from the olecranon fossa. Distal traction is continued, and the elbow is flexed. With reduction, a palpable "clunk" is felt as the olecranon is seated in the humeral articular surface. The elbow is then moved through its full range of motion (ROM) to assess stability. If full smooth passive ROM is not possible, the postreduction radiograph should be examined for entrapment of the medial epicondyle, especially common in children (Fig. 225-3). Instability in extension suggests associated fractures or disruption of the capsule. These patients require immediate orthopaedic referral.

After reduction, the elbow is placed in a plaster splint from the axilla to the base of the fingers with the elbow in at least 90° of flexion. Because of the soft tissue trauma and subsequent edema, cylinder casts should not be placed.

Appropriate treatment of elbow dislocations requires adequate reduction and recognition of neurovascular complications, associated fractures, and postreduction instability. If there is any question of neurovascular compromise, the patient should be admitted for observation.

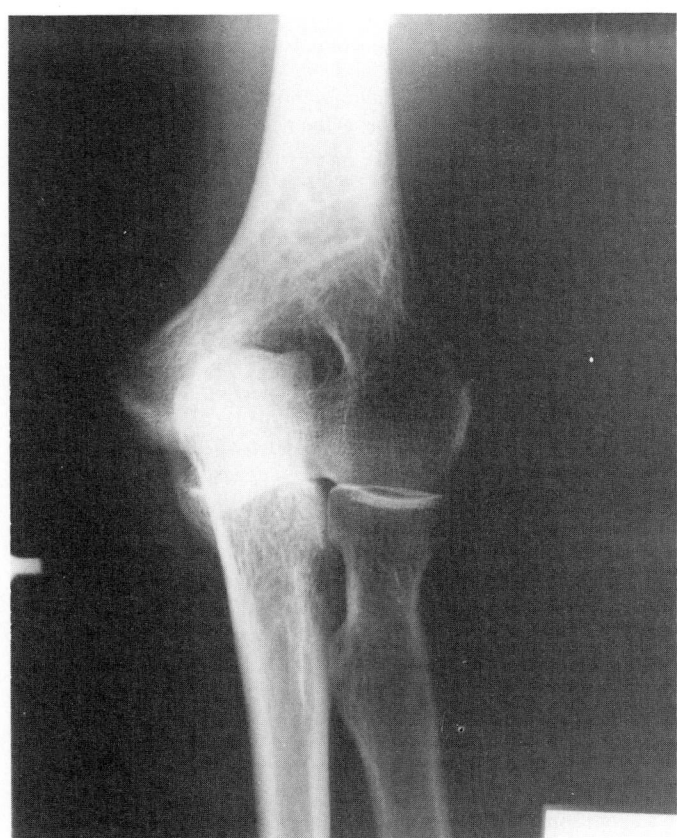

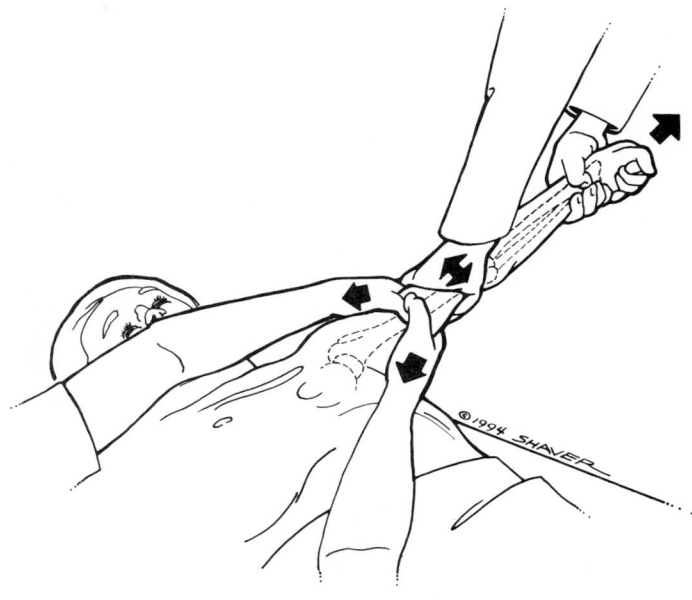

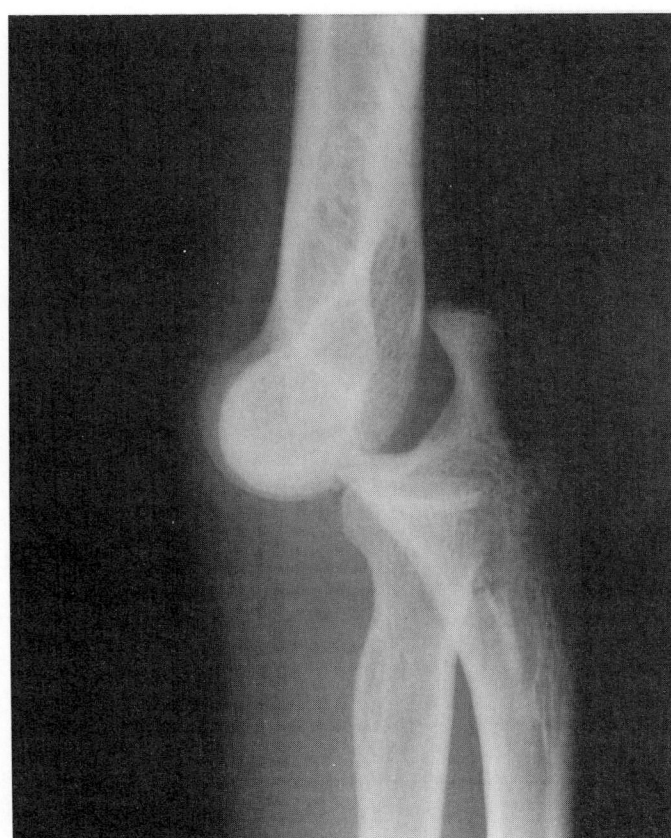

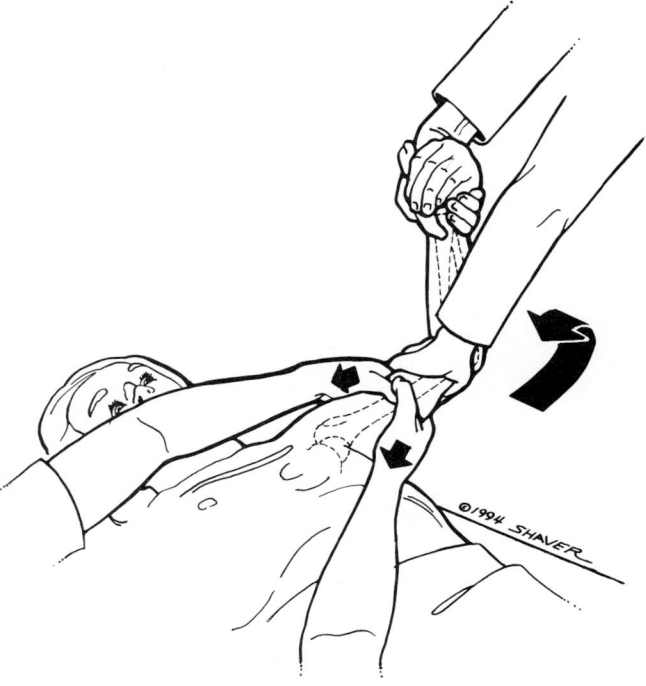

**Fig. 225-1.** Posterior dislocation of the elbow.

**Fig. 225-2.** Reduction of posterior elbow dislocation. **A.** Operator applies gentle traction as assistant applies countertraction. Displacement is corrected with the other hand. Downward pressure on the proximal forearm disengages the coronoid process from the olecranon fossa. **B.** Distal traction is continued as the elbow is flexed.

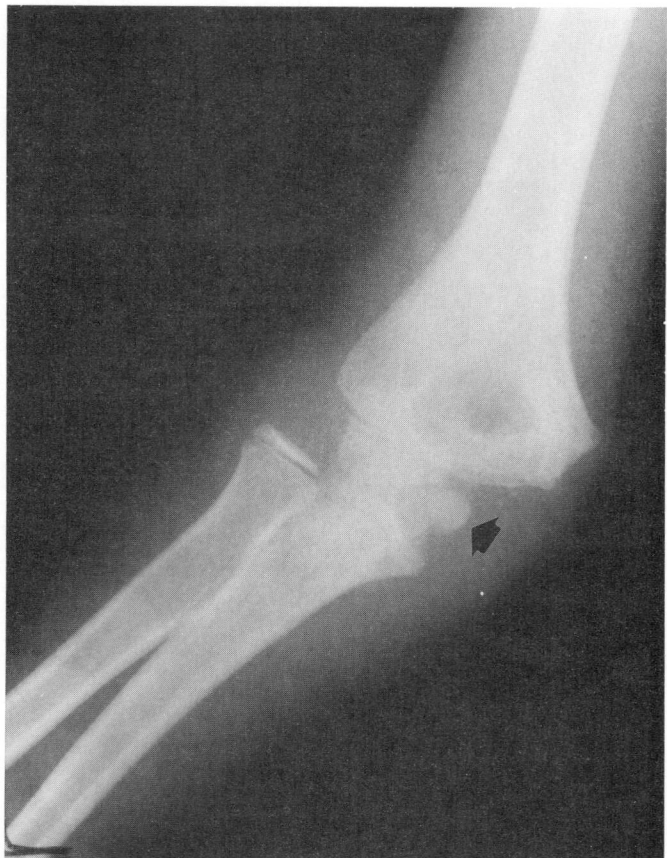

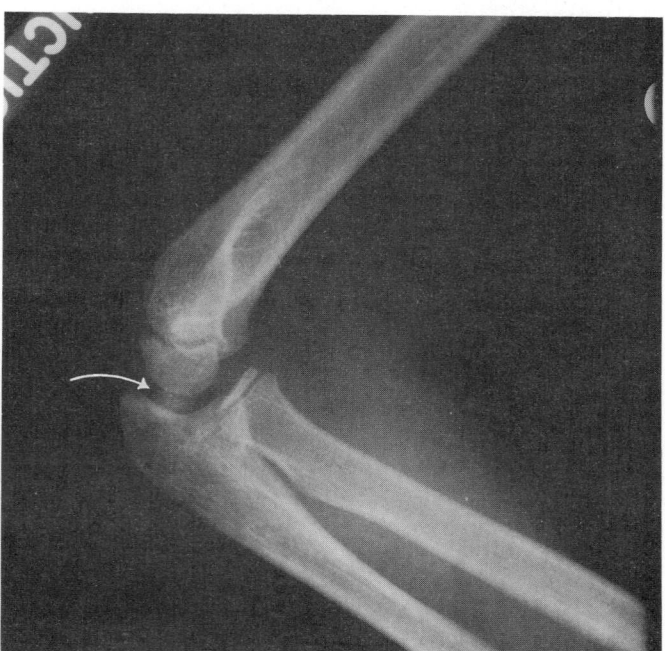

**Fig. 225-3.** Postreduction radiograph of a posterior elbow dislocation. The medial epicondyle is present in the joint and is seen in the anteroposterior and lateral radiographs (*arrow*).

### Subluxation of the Radial Head (Nursemaid's Elbow)

Subluxation of the radial head is common among preschool children. The peak age is between 1 and 4 years, and it is usually not seen in children older than 7 years. The mechanism of injury is sudden trac-

tion on the hand with the elbow extended and the forearm pronated. Anatomically, during forceful traction, some fibers of the annular ligament, which encircles the radial neck, slip and become trapped between the radial head and capitellum. In the child up to age 5, the radial head is about the same size as the neck. After age 7, the size of the radial head is larger than the neck and subluxation does not occur.

Clinically the child sits comfortably with the parent, may even be playful, but does not use the injured arm. The arm is held in slight flexion and pronation. Supination is painful, and any effort to move the arm is resisted, although movement is free. The neurovascular examination is normal.

It is important to elicit the history of traction on the hand; the act may have been unrecognized by the parent or the history withheld because of a feeling of guilt or fear. Recently, an atypical history has been reported to occur in as many as 49 percent of radial head subluxations. Any child not using an arm that is flexed and pronated and without signs of trauma should be considered to have a radial head subluxation, unless the history strongly suggests another diagnosis. Radiographs are unnecessary, unless another diagnosis is being considered or if reduction is not accomplished.

Reduction is carried out by firmly placing the thumb over the radial head while the other hand is placed on the wrist. The forearm is fully supinated, and if a "click" is not felt, the elbow is flexed. This maneuver may be repeated if the initial attempt does not reduce the subluxation. Alternatively, the elbow may be extended. Both maneuvers are reported to be equally effective. Reduction as evidenced by a click is highly predictive and will result in relief from pain and, shortly thereafter, use of the affected arm.

After the first subluxation no immobilization is required. For recurrent subluxations, however, the patient's arm should be immobilized in a sling; some recommend a long arm cast. These patients should be referred for orthopaedic consultation.

### Intercondylar T or Y Fractures

Intercondylar fractures are much more common in adults than in children. Any distal humerus fracture in an adult should initially be assumed to be intercondylar rather than supracondylar (Fig. 225-4). A careful search should be made for a fracture line separating the condyles from each other and from the humerus. This distinguishes intercondylar T or Y fractures from other fractures of the distal humerus.

The mechanism of injury is a force directed against the elbow, driving the olecranon against the humeral articular surface separating the condyles and producing the typical fracture. These fractures are associated with severe soft tissue injuries. Riseborough and Radin classified them into four types based on their radiographic appearance (Table 225-1).

Treatment in the young is directed at anatomic reduction. In older patients with severe injuries, treatment is often directed at joint motion through nonoperative means. Type I fractures are usually splinted, followed by application of a cast. Type II and III fractures are usually treated by open reduction and internal fixation. Type IV fractures may be treated by skeletal traction in older patients or by reconstruction of the articular surface in younger patients. As in supracondylar fractures, patients with severe swelling or displaced fractures should be admitted.

### Supracondylar Fractures

These extraarticular fractures occur most commonly in children. Ninety-five percent are displaced posteriorly as a result of an extension force. When the mechanism of injury is due to a flexion force, the much less common anterior displacement occurs. There can also be various degrees of abduction, adduction, and rotation of the distal fragment.

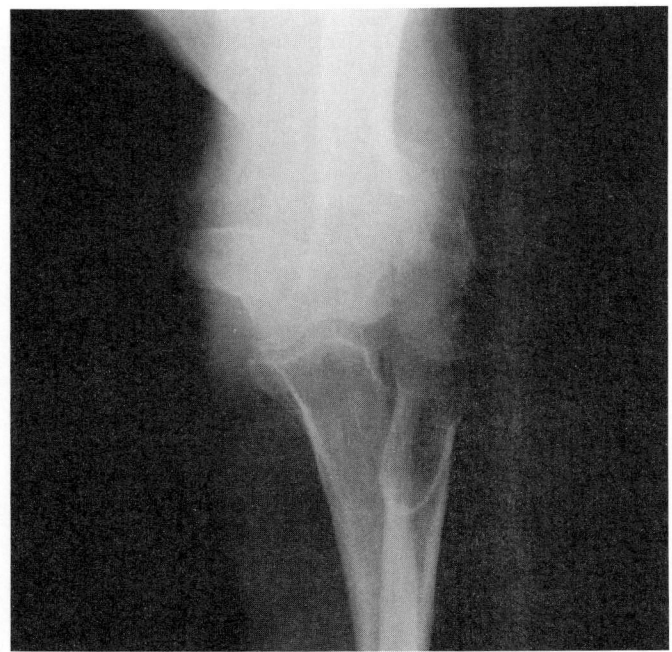

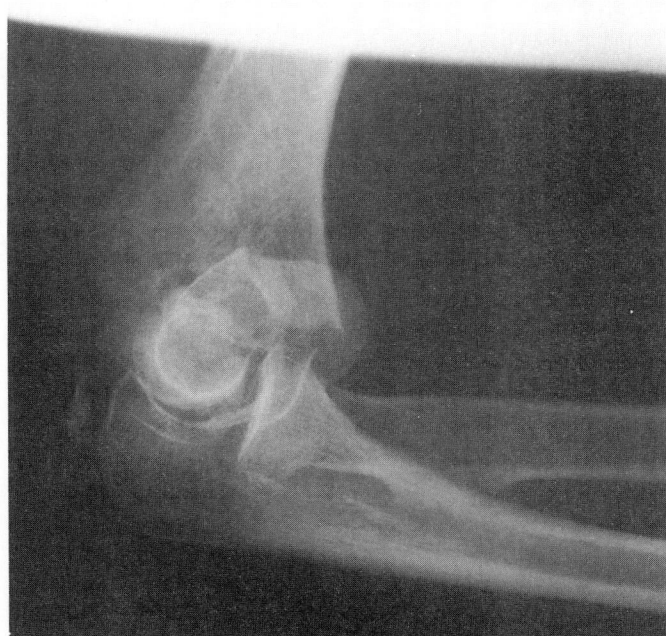

**Fig. 225-4.** Comminuted displaced and rotated intercondylar fracture (type IV).

**Table 225-1.** Types of Intercondylar Fractures

| Type I | Undisplaced condylar fracture |
|---|---|
| Type II | T-shaped with displacement of the capitellum and trochlea without significant rotation |
| Type III | T-shaped with displacement and rotation of the humeral condyles |
| Type IV | T-shaped with comminution, displacement, and rotation |

*Source:* Riseborough EJ, Radin EL: Intercondylar T fractures of the humerus in the adult. *J Bone Joint Surg* 51-A(1), 1969.

## Extension-Type Fractures

In an extension-type fracture the patient will have significant swelling and tenderness at the elbow. The olecranon is prominent, and there is a depression proximally over the area of the triceps muscle. This appearance may be easily mistaken for a posterior elbow dislocation.

Radiographs may reveal a fat pad sign in undisplaced fractures (Fig. 225-5). This is due to visualization of fat from the olecranon fossa (posterior fat pad) as it is displaced by the hemarthrosis. This may also occur anteriorly (anterior fat pad), although this is a less reliable sign. In some undisplaced fractures, the fracture line may not be seen, with the fat pad sign being the only evidence of injury. Treatment should be initiated as though a fracture were identified, with splint immobilization and orthopaedic consultation. In displaced fractures, the anteroposterior radiograph usually reveals a transverse fracture line. More severely displaced fractures may show medial or lateral displacement or rotation along the axis of the humerus (Fig. 225-6). The lateral radiograph will reveal the fracture line extending obliquely from posterior proximal to anterior distal. The distal fragment will be displaced proximally and posteriorly.

Treatment of undisplaced fractures consists of plaster immobilization. Displaced fractures have the best results when reduced by closed methods followed by traction or pin fixation. Patients with displaced fractures or severe swelling should be admitted for observation of neurovascular status.

## Flexion-Type Fractures

Flexion-type fractures occur in fewer than 5 percent of supracondylar fractures. The mechanism is direct anterior force against a flexed elbow. This results in anterior displacement of the distal fragment. Since the mechanism is direct force, these fractures are often open.

Radiographs reveal an oblique fracture from anterior proximal to posterior distal. The distal fragment is anterior to the humerus.

Management consists of closed reduction and plaster immobiliza-

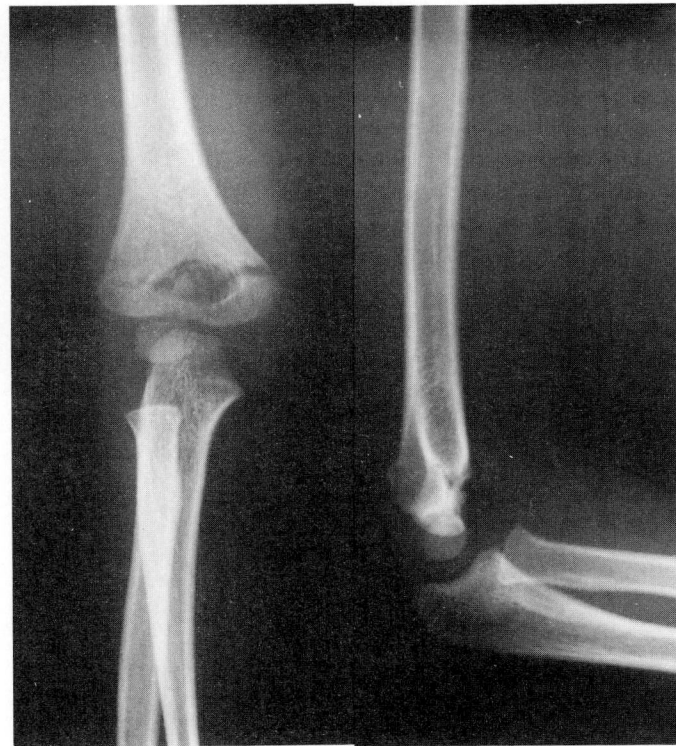

**Fig. 225-5.** Undisplaced supracondylar fracture.

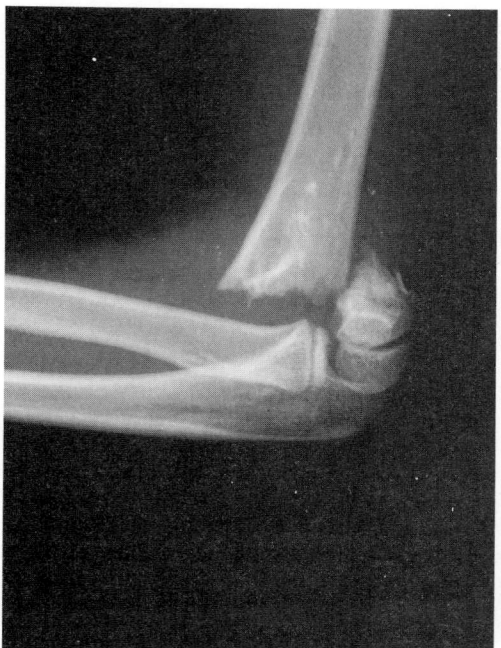
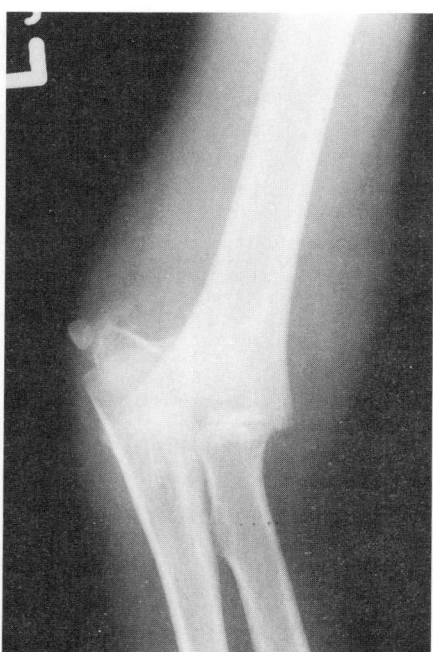

**Fig. 225-6.** Displaced supracondylar fracture. The distal fragment is displaced posteriorly, proximally, and medially. The proximal fragment is displaced anteriorly and distally.

tion or is operative if reduction cannot be maintained by closed methods.

## Complications

There are numerous complications of supracondylar fractures, including nerve, and vascular injuries and those occurring late such as nonunion, malunion, myositis ossificans, and loss of motion.

Associated injuries to the median, ulnar, and radial nerves have been well documented and have an incidence of 7 percent. Recently, Cramer and coworkers found a high incidence of anterior interosseus nerve injuries in their patients with supracondylar fractures. This nerve arises from the median nerve and innervates the flexor pollicis longus, the radial part of the flexor digitorum profundus, and the pronator quadratus. Since there is no sensory component to the anterior interosseous nerve, identification of the injury can only be made by specific muscle testing. Testing consists of flexion at the index finger distal interphalangeal and thumb interphalangeal joints. The mechanism of injury is usually traction, contusion, or a combination. Complete transection is rare, and entrapment within the fracture occurs only occasionally. Prognosis is excellent, with complete recovery in 2 to 6 weeks.

Acute vascular injuries must always be suspected in patients with supracondylar fractures. Absence of a radial pulse is common in children. This is most frequently due to transient arterial spasm. Rarely, there is a partial or complete transection of the brachial artery, an intimal tear and thrombosis, or entrapment within the fracture fragment.

The most serious complication is Volkmann's ischemic contracture. This classically occurs after a supracondylar fracture, when edema reduces venous outflow and arterial inflow. This results in ischemia, which, if unrelieved, will lead to muscle and nerve necrosis and eventual replacement by fibrotic tissue. Refusal to open the hand in children, pain with passive extension of the fingers, and forearm tenderness are signs of impending Volkmann's ischemia. It is now well understood that the mere lack of a radial pulse does not indicate ischemia unless accompanied by these signs.

Treatment of supracondylar fractures with absent radial pulse begins with fracture reduction and pinning. Extremities without signs of ischemia are observed, while those with signs of ischemia are taken to the operating room for fasciotomy and/or brachial artery exploration.

## FOREARM

### Anatomy

The radius and ulna are joined together along their entire length by a fibrous interosseous membrane and touch only at their ends to form the complex proximal and distal radioulnar joints. The ulna is a comparatively straight bone, whereas the radius has an important outward bowing. During the motions of supination and pronation, the ulna holds a relatively fixed position, while the radius rotates around it. Because these bones have such a close relationship to one another, injury to either will have a direct impact on the other. A displaced or angulated fracture of one bone typically disrupts the other or causes a dislocation at the proximal or distal radioulnar joint, such as in the Monteggia and Galeazzi fracture-dislocations.

The radius and ulna are also under the influence of numerous muscle groups, such as those that supinate and pronate. The biceps brachii and the supinator insert on the proximal radius and are the powerful supinators of the forearm. The pronator teres inserts just distal to them and onto the midsection of the radius. As its name suggests, it is responsible for pronation. Radius fractures that are located between these muscle groups will result in marked displacement of the bone, with supination of the proximal segment and pronation of the distal portion. However, if the fracture is distal to the insertion of the pronator teres, these forces tend to neutralize one another and result in less rotational deformity.

The distal radioulnar joint has several articulations that support the scaphoid and lunate and also the ulna in the sigmoid notch. The ulna is separated from the carpals by the triangular fibrocartilage complex, which is the main stabilizer of the distal radioulnar joint. The contour of the distal radius has several important relationships that can be measured. In the frontal plane, the radial styloid should project 8 to 18 mm (average of 13 mm) beyond the radioulnar joint and create a radial inclination, or slope, of 13° to 30° (average of 23°). The radial articular surface has a volar tilt of 1° to 23° (average of 11°) on the lateral view.

The neuroanatomy is most easily understood by appreciating the neural control of the most basic components of wrist and finger movement (Fig. 225-7). The radial nerve travels over the lateral epicondyle and supplies the muscles involved in wrist extension before it gives off a branch, the posterior interosseous nerve. This branch travels around the proximal radius and controls the muscles that extend the fingers and thumb. The remainder of the radial nerve is purely sensory and innervates the posterior aspect of the hand from the thumb to radial half of the ring finger. Quite simply, the proximal portion of the radial nerve controls the more proximal function of wrist extension, while the distal branch (posterior interosseus nerve) controls the more distal function of finger extension and another branch that is purely sensory. So an isolated injury (e.g., to the posterior interosseous branch) would affect finger extension but spare wrist extension and sensation to the dorsum of the hand. The single best test of radial nerve function is to have the patient extend both the wrist and fingers against resistance, and check the sensation over the dorsum of the hand.

The median nerve controls the basic movements of wrist and finger flexion and sensation on the volar surface of the hand from the thumb to the radial half of the ring finger. The proximal portion of the median nerve innervates the muscles that control wrist flexion and the flexor digitorum superficialis before it gives off the anterior interosseous nerve. This branch controls portions of the remaining deep finger flexors: flexor digitorum profundus, flexor pollicus longus, and pronator quadratus. The remaining portion of the median nerve provides sensation to most of the volar surface of the hand plus a motor branch to the thenar muscles of the thumb (recurrent branch of the median nerve). The median nerve is evaluated by assessing each of these distal branches. A simple test of the anterior interosseous nerve is the ability to make a circle, or "OK" sign, with the thumb and index finger; if so, this nerve is likewise "OK." Abduction of the thumb (recurrent branch of the median nerve) and intact sensation on the radial side of the palm complete the evaluation of the median nerve.

The ulnar nerve provides innervation to a few forearm muscles but, more importantly, controls the intrinsic muscles of the hand and provides sensation to the little finger and the ulnar half of the ring finger. The ability to abduct the index finger against resistance and normal sensation on the ulnar side of the hand is an easy test of ulnar function.

## Fractures of Both Radius and Ulna

A great amount of force is necessary to fracture both the radius and ulna. This injury occurs most often from vehicular trauma, falls from a height, or a direct blow to the forearm. The magnitude of the force determines the type of injury. A moderate force produces transverse or mildly oblique fractures. Comminuted and segmental fractures are produced by a high-impact force. As one might expect, these fractures are often displaced. Open fractures of the radius and ulna are

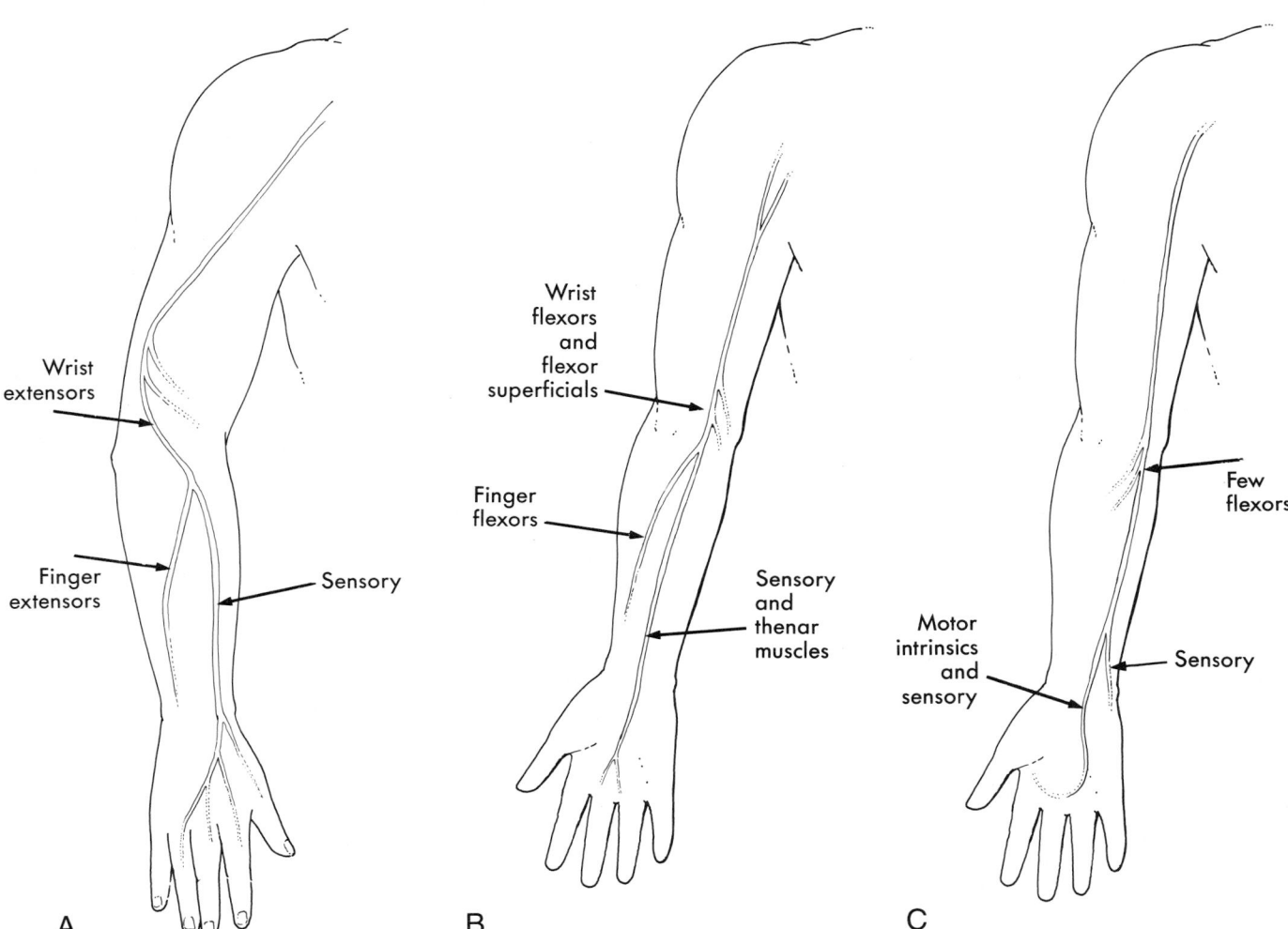

**Fig. 225-7. A.** The radial nerve controls wrist extension before branching into the posterior interosseous nerve. **B.** The median nerve controls wrist flexion and the flexor digitorum superficialis before branching into the anterior interosseous nerve (controls the deep finger flexors in the forearm) and a branch that innervates the thenar muscles and provides sensation to most of the palm. **C.** The ulnar nerve controls the intrinsic muscles and sensation to the ulnar side of the hand. (From Chin HW, Propp DA, Orban DJ: Forearm and wrist, in Rosen P, Barkin RM, et al (eds): *Emergency Medicine Concepts and Clinical Practice,* 3d ed, vol 1. St. Louis, Mosby Year Book, 1992.)

second only to tibia fractures because of the subcutaneous location of the entire ulna and the distal portion of the radius.

Nondisplaced fractures of both bones are exceedingly rare because the force necessary to produce the injury is also sufficient to displace it. However, in this event, a long arm cast is applied, and frequent reevaluation for potential displacement is necessary.

Displacement of both bones is generally the rule. Examination reveals swelling, deformity, and tenderness of the forearm. Careful assessment of the neurovascular status is imperative. Nerve injuries can be seen with severe open fractures but fortunately are uncommon with most closed injuries. Because of the excellent collateral circulation of the forearm, vascular compromise is generally not a major problem if either the radial or ulnar circulation is intact.

The fractures are clearly visible on the radiographs. Angulation and longitudinal alignment are easily evaluated, but changes in rotational alignment may be subtle. A rough estimate of rotational alignment can be made by noting the normal orientation of various bony prominences of these bones. On the anteroposterior radiograph, the radial styloid and radial (bicipital) tuberosity normally point in opposite directions, whereas the ulnar styloid and coronoid process do so on the lateral view. A change in this arrangement suggests rotation malalignment. Since these bones are also oblong rather than circular in their cross-sectional appearance, a sudden change in the bone's width at the fracture site is another clue to a rotational deformity.

Although there are some reports of adequate reduction using closed techniques, the potential for these injuries to subsequently displace, in spite of cast immobilization, makes this alternative unpredictable. An exception is the injury in a child. A child's ability to remodel bone and compensate for some malalignment makes closed reduction possible. Otherwise, these injuries invariably require open reduction and internal fixation, most commonly with compression plating and screws. The use of external fixation may be necessary in situations where infection is possible, such as severe open fractures, comminution, or bone loss. Internal fixation is delayed until the risk of infection is diminished.

Potential complications include reduced ability to supinate and pronate, osteomyelitis, nonunion, malunion, neurovascular injury, and compartment syndrome. Recognizing the development of a compartment syndrome is particularly important to prevent debilitating ischemic contractures of the forearm. The diagnostic findings are palpable induration of the area, pain with passive movement of the fingers, and pain that appears to be disproportionate to the physical findings. The presence of a palpable pulse does not exclude the diagnosis of compartment syndrome. Alterations in sensation and the pulse are late findings. Direct measurements of elevated compartment pressures confirm the diagnosis.

## Ulna Fractures

Isolated fractures of the ulna most often result from direct blows to the forearm. The natural response to raise the forearm in defense of a blow from a club is why it is often referred to as a *nightstick fracture*. Undisplaced fractures are immobilized in a long arm cast and closely followed for subsequent displacement of the fracture.

Displaced fractures are those with greater than 10° of angulation or displacement of more than 50 percent of the width of the bone at the site of the fracture. Open reduction and internal fixation with a compression plate and screws are necessary to prevent angulation, loss of length, and rotational deformity. These injuries should be closely scrutinized for any possible radius fracture or dislocation.

Fracture of the ulnar shaft with a radial head dislocation is often referred to as *Monteggia fracture-dislocation* (Fig. 225-8). It is typically a diaphyseal fracture in the proximal third of the ulna with an anterior dislocation of the radial head (60 percent of cases). Anterolateral and posterolateral dislocation of the radial head or a metaphyseal ulna fracture are other possibilities. Clinically, there is con-

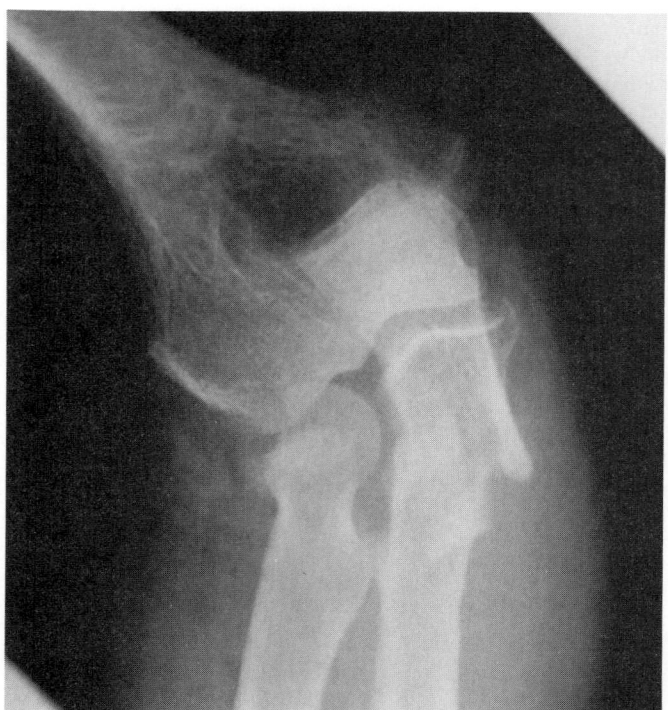

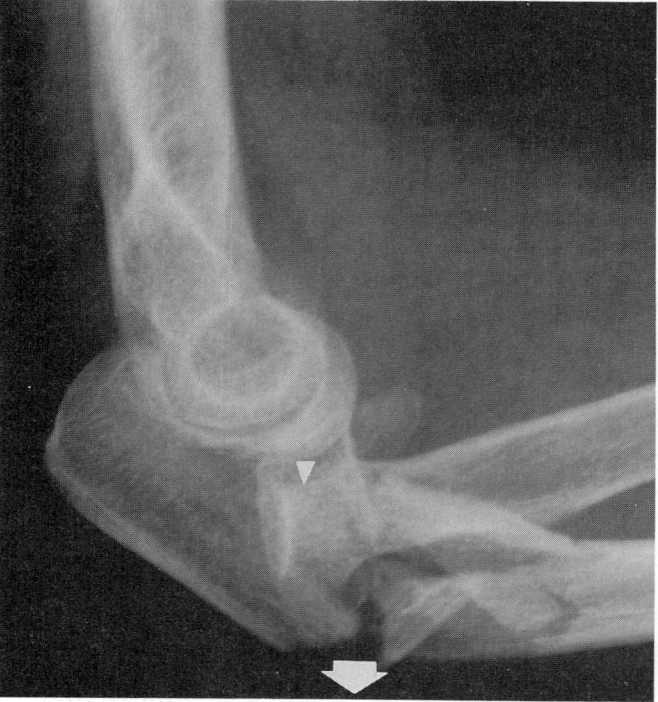

**Fig. 225-8.** Monteggia fracture-dislocation. The angulation of the comminuted fracture of the proximal ulna (*arrow*) points in the direction of the radial head dislocation (*arrowhead*).

siderable pain and swelling at the elbow. The radial head may be palpable in an anterolateral or posterolateral location. The forearm may appear shortened and angulated. The ulnar fracture is clearly visible and may overshadow the less obvious radial head dislocation. As a rule, the radial head normally points to the capitellum in all radiographic views of the elbow. In addition, the apex of the ulna fracture points in the direction of the radial head dislocation.

Monteggia fracture-dislocations are treated with open reduction and internal fixation of the ulna and closed reduction of the radial head dislocation. Children may be treated adequately by closed reduction of both bones and long arm cast immobilization. Complications include nonunion, redislocation, infection, and paralysis of the posterior interosseus nerve. (Remember that the nerve wraps around the proximal radius.)

## Radius Fractures

Radius fractures can be divided into those that are proximal or distal to the junction of the middle and distal thirds of the bone. Excluding radial head fractures, isolated fractures of the proximal two-thirds of the radius are not common because it is relatively well protected from direct blows by the ulna and also by the surrounding musculature of the forearm. Undisplaced fractures are rare; these are treated with cast immobilization. Fractures of the proximal two-thirds of the radius are often displaced by both the force of the injury and the action of the supinators and pronators on the radius. They require internal fixation with plating and screws to maintain the reduction and to prevent rotational deformity.

Fractures of the distal third of the radial shaft are produced by falls on the outstretched hand in forced pronation or by a direct blow. Much like the Monteggia fracture-dislocation, the distal radial shaft fracture is often associated with a distal radioulnar joint dislocation; hence the name *reverse Monteggia fracture,* or, more commonly, *Galeazzi's fracture.* There is localized tenderness and swelling over the distal radius and wrist. The radius fracture is usually short oblique or transverse with dorsal lateral angulation. The distal radioulnar joint injury can be subtle. Radiographs may show only a slightly increased distal radioulnar joint space on the anteroposterior view. On the lateral view, the ulna is displaced dorsally. This injury is treated by open reduction and internal fixation of the radius fracture with compression plating and screws. The distal radioulnar joint reduction is held with immobilization of the forearm in supination or with K-wire fixation for 6 weeks.

## WRIST

Fractures of the distal metaphysis of the radius and ulna are among the most common injuries affecting the wrist. Among the factors that influence the type and amount of displacement of the fracture are the point and direction of impact, the degree of force, and the patient's age. In general, the thinner cortices of the elderly make them more likely to sustain extraarticular fractures, whereas younger adults often sustain more complicated intraarticular fractures.

## Colles' Fracture

Colles' fracture results most often from falls on the outstretched hand. This mechanism produces a distal radial metaphysis fracture that is dorsally angulated and displaced. Compression forces on the dorsal side often produce dorsal comminution of the bone. The fracture line may also comminute and extend into the radioulnar or radiocarpal joint ("die-punch" fracture). A fracture of the ulnar styloid is often present and may be suggestive of injury to the triangular fibrocartilage complex (Fig. 225-9).

The wrist has the characteristic dorsiflexion, or "silver-fork," deformity. These individuals may complain of palmar paresthesias from tension or pressure on the median nerve. Anteroposterior radiographs reveal a distal metaphyseal fracture of the radius that often appears shortened from the angulation or comminution of the bone. The lateral view provides the best view of the dorsal angulation and comminution. In general, potentially unstable fractures have more than 20° of angulation, intraarticular involvement, marked comminution, or more than a centimeter of shortening. These injuries are more likely to develop loss of reduction, distal radioulnar joint instability, radiocarpal instability patterns, and subsequent arthritis.

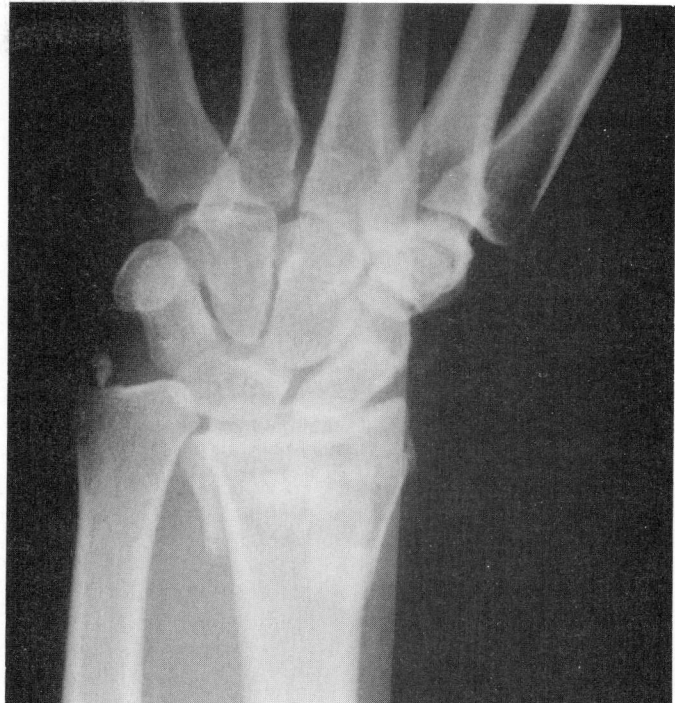
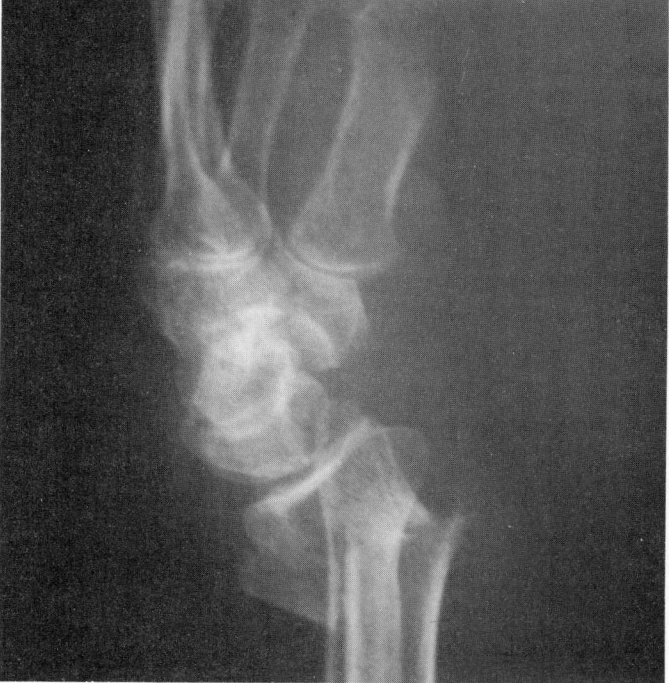

**Fig. 225-9.** Colles' fracture. **A.** Anteroposterior view. The radius is comminuted and shortened. The ulnar styloid is also fractured. **B.** Lateral view reveals dorsal angulation and displacement of the radius. (From Chin HW, Visotsky J: Wrist fractures. *Emerg Med Clin North Am* Vol. 11,3:703, 1993, with permission.)

Stable fractures may be treated with a compression dressing and splint until they can be evaluated by an orthopaedic surgeon. Otherwise, closed reduction is performed, with traction provided by finger traps while the fracture fragment is pushed distal and palmar while the patient's forearm is firmly held. The goal is to restore the volar tilt, radial inclination, and proper length to the radius. This is particularly important in younger patients. The volar tilt ideally should be restored to its normal position, but a minimum of neutral or zero degrees of angulation may be acceptable. Although most Colles' fractures can be treated with closed reduction and cast immobilization, those that are unstable, severely comminuted, or intraarticular may require casting with pinning, external fixation with possible bone grafting, or open reduction and internal fixation. Good to excellent results are achieved in 56 to 81 percent of patients with these more aggressive treatment alternatives. All open and neurovascularly compromised fractures require prompt evaluation by the orthopaedic surgeon.

Complications include malunion, median nerve injuries, triangular fibrocartilage complex injuries, secondary radioulnar and radiocarpal instability patterns, and arthritis. These can produce a weak, stiff, and painful wrist.

## Smith's Fracture

Smith's fracture, or "reverse Colles' fracture," is a volar angulated fracture of the distal radius. These injuries result from a fall or direct blow on the dorsum of the hand and wrist or from falls on the outstretched hand in supination that then shifts into a pronated position. The hand is displaced palmar in a "garden-spade deformity." The anteroposterior radiograph looks much like the Colles' fracture, with a distal metaphyseal radius fracture that may be shortened and comminuted. The lateral radiograph shows the volar angulated and displaced fracture.

The treatment objectives and complications are much like those seen with Colles' fracture. However, in this case the angulation is in the opposite direction, and there is an exaggerated volar tilt that requires correction.

## Barton's Fracture

Barton's fractures are dorsal or volar rim fractures of the distal radius. The dorsal rim fractures result from a dorsiflexion and pronation force, whereas the less common volar rim fracture is produced by a fall on the outstretched hand in supination. These injuries are often fracture dislocations or subluxations, since the carpus or hand is frequently displaced in the direction of the fracture. Accompanying ligamentous injuries create radiocarpal instability. This is often not fully appreciated in the acute setting but can lead to various secondary carpal instability patterns and premature degenerative arthritis.

The anteroposterior radiograph often shows a comminuted fracture of the distal radial metaphysis. The lateral view reveals an intraarticular fracture of the volar or dorsal rim of the radius, which may be accompanied by carpal subluxation in the same direction (Fig. 225-10).

Minimally displaced fractures can be treated acutely with closed reduction and a splint or cast until they can be reevaluated by the orthopaedist. Unstable fractures involve more than 50 percent of the radial articular surface or have accompanying carpal subluxation and require reduction and immobilization by the orthopaedist. These injuries often require open reduction and fixation with pins or a buttress plate.

## Radial Styloid Fracture

A force directed along the radial side of the hand can produce a transverse or oblique fracture that runs from the scaphoid fossa to the metaphysis of the radius. It is best seen on the anteroposterior radiograph as a thin lucent line beneath the radial styloid (Fig. 225-11). Since the major carpal ligaments along the radial side of the wrist insert on the radial styloid, displacement of this fracture can produce carpal instability.

Displaced fractures often require open reduction and internal fixation. Displacement of as little as 3 mm is often associated with ac-

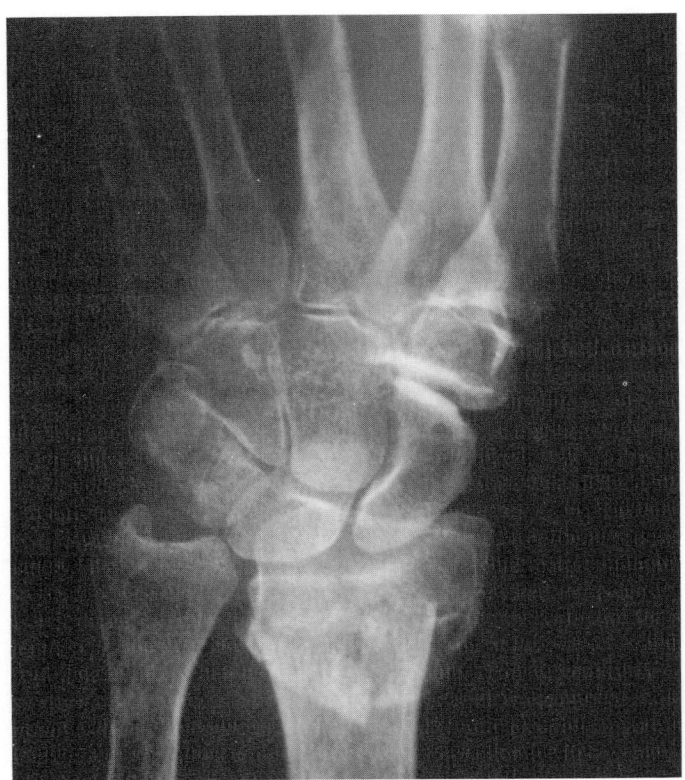

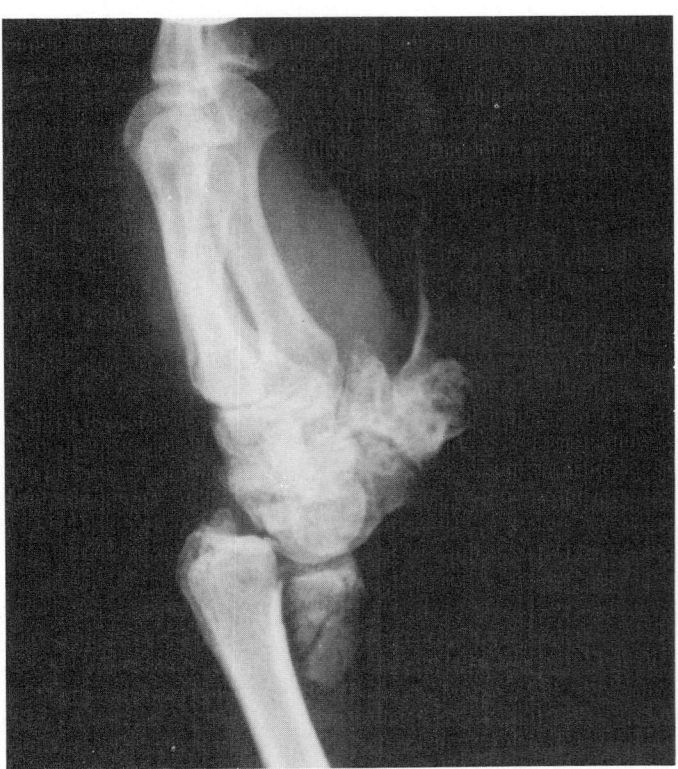

**Fig. 225-10.** Volar Barton fracture. There is an intraarticular comminuted volar rim fracture of the radius with volar displacement of the carpals. (From Chin HW, Visotsky J: Wrist fractures. *Emerg Med Clin North Am* 11,3:703, 1993, with permission.)

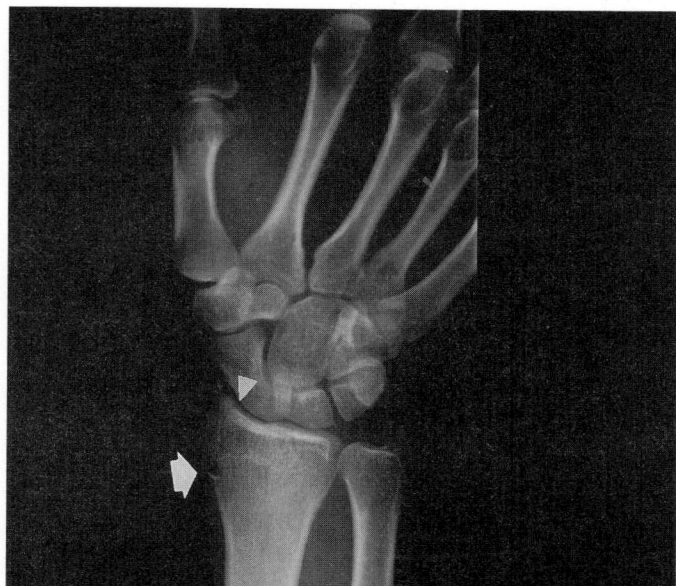

**Fig. 225-11.** Radial styloid fracture. There is a lateral cortical disruption of the radius (*arrow*) and a longitudinal fracture that travels intraarticular into the scaphoid fossa (*arrowhead*). (From Chin HW, Visotsky J: Wrist fractures. *Emerg Med Clin North Am* 11,3:703, 1993, with permission.)

companying scapholunate dissociation. Failure to recognize these intercarpal ligament tears adds to the potential for subsequent posttraumatic arthritis.

## Ulnar Styloid Fracture

The ulnar styloid is fractured by forced radial deviation, dorsiflexion, and rotatory stress. The ulnar styloid fracture may be isolated or may accompany other injuries, such as Colles' fracture. Displaced fractures can be associated with tears of the triangular fibrocartilage complex, which is the main stabilizer of the distal radioulnar joint. These individuals will complain of a painful, clicking, or locking sensation in the wrist.

Ulnar styloid fractures are treated acutely with a splint or cast in slight ulnar deviation and neutral positioning of the wrist. Arthrograms or MRI imaging may be necessary to delineate the full extent of these injuries.

## Radioulnar Disruption

Radioulnar joint disruption is generally seen with intraarticular or distal radial shaft fractures (Galeazzi's fracture-dislocation) or fractures of both bones of the forearm. These more-apparent injuries often overshadow radioulnar joint disruption and unfortunately cause these injuries to be unrecognized until subsequent pain and diminished wrist movement are appreciated.

Isolated radioulnar joint dislocations are uncommon and are unrecognized acutely in as many as 50 percent of cases. Dorsal dislocation of the distal ulna results most often from falls on the wrist in hyperpronation. The rare volar dislocation results from forced hypersupination of the wrist. These individuals present with a painful wrist that has restricted range of motion. There may be a palpable prominence of the ulnar head, but this can be quite subtle and easily overlooked.

The anteroposterior radiograph reveals narrowing and overlap of the distal radioulnar joint. The lateral radiograph demonstrates either volar or dorsal displacement of the ulna, which is normally centered and overlapping the radius. Since slight oblique positioning of the wrist can produce a misleading appearance of ulnar displacement, it

is crucial that a properly positioned lateral view is obtained. A true lateral view should have superimposition of the four ulnar metacarpals, superimposition of the proximal pole of the scaphoid with the lunate and triquetrum, and the radial styloid centered over its distal articular surface. CT scanning may be necessary to establish the diagnosis if plain films are inconclusive. Dorsal dislocations are reduced by immobilizing the wrist in supination, whereas volar dislocations are placed in pronation. These injuries unfortunately have a high recurrence rate, particularly if there are delays in diagnosis, and may require reconstructive surgery.

## BIBLIOGRAPHY

Anderson LD, Meyer FN: Fractures of the shaft of the radius and ulna, in Rockwood CA, Wilkens KE, King RE (eds): *Fractures in Adults,* 3d ed, vol 1. Philadelphia, Lippincott, 1991, p 679.

Boyd HB, Boals JC: The Monteggia lesion. A review of 159 cases. *Clin Orthop* 66:94, 1969.

Carter PR: *Common Hand Injuries and Infections: A Practical Approach to Early Treatment.* Philadelphia, Saunders, 1983.

Chin HW, Propp DA, Orban DJ: Forearm and wrist, in Rosen P, Barkin RM (eds): *Emergency Medicine Concepts and Clinical Practice* 3d 3, vol 1. St. Louis, Mosby Year Book, 1992.

Chin HW, Visotsky J: Wrist fractures. *Emerg Med Clin North Am* 11,3:703, 1993.

Cooney WP, Linscheid RL, Dobyns JH: Fractures and dislocations of the wrist, in Rockwood CA, Green DP (eds): *Fractures in Adults,* 3d ed, vol 1, Philadelphia, Lippincott, 1991, p 563.

Cooney WP et al: Difficult wrist fractures. *Clin Orthop* 214:136, 1987.

Cramer KE, Green NE, Devito DP: Incidence of anterior interosseous nerve palsy in supracondylar humerus fractures in children. *J Ped Orthopaed* 13:502, 1993.

Endean ED, Veldenz HC, Schwarcz TH, et al: Recognition of arterial injury in elbow dislocation. *J Vasc Surg* 16(3):402, 1992.

Frykman G: Fractures of the distal radius: A clinical and experimental study. *Acta Orthop Scand* 108:1, 1967.

Harris IE: Supracondylar fractures of the humerus in children. *Orthopedics* 15(7):811, 1992.

Kurer MH, Regan MW: Completely displaced supracondylar fracture of the humerus in children. *Clin Orthopaed Rel Research* 256:205, 1990.

Linscherd RL, Wheeler DK: Elbow dislocations. *JAMA,* 194:1171, 1965.

Malone CP: Open treatment for displaced articular fractures of the distal radius. *Clin Orthop* 202:104, 1986.

O'Brien ET: Acute fractures and dislocations of the carpus. *Orthop Clin North Am* 15(2):237, 1984.

O'Brien ET: Fractures of the hand and wrist region, in Rockwood CA, Wilkens KE, King RE (eds): *Fractures in Children,* 3d ed, vol 3. Philadelphia, Lippincott, 1991, p 319.

Olney BW, Menelaus MB: Monteggia and equivalent lesions in childhood. *J Pediatr Orthop* 9:219, 1989.

Palmer AK, Werner FW: The triangular fibrocartilage complex of the wrist—anatomy and function. *J Hand Surg* 6:153, 1981.

Propp DA, Chin HW: Forearm and wrist radiology. *J Emerg Med* 7(4):393, 1989.

Riseborough EJ, Radin EL: Intercondylar T fractures of the humerus in the adult. *J Bone Joint Surg* 51-A(1), 1969.

Royle SG: Posterior dislocation of the elbow. *Clin Orthop* 269:201–204, 1991.

Sacchetti A, Ramoska EE, Glascow C: Nonclassic history in children with radial head subluxations. *J Emerg Med* 8:151, 1990.

Schunk JE: Radial head subluxation: Epidemiology and treatment of 87 episodes. *Ann Emerg Med* 19:1019, 1990.

Sisk DT: Internal fixation of forearm fractures, in Chapman MW, Madison M (eds): *Operative Orthopaedics,* vol 1. Philadelphia, Lippincott, 1988.

# 226

# INJURIES TO THE SHOULDER COMPLEX AND HUMERUS

## Dennis T. Uehara
## John P. Rudzinski

Function of the upper extremity is intimately dependent on the shoulder complex. Movement is effected through an intricate mechanism with integration of muscles, ligaments, osseous components, and a system of joints all working in harmony. Through its joint system that consists of four joints, the sternoclavicular, glenohumeral, acromioclavicular, and scapulothoracic, the upper extremity is able to move through a complex and wide range of motion. The following discussion focuses on the major soft tissue and osseous components of the shoulder complex and humerus and those injuries that create loss of motion, instability, and pain.

## STERNOCLAVICULAR DISLOCATIONS

The sternoclavicular joint is the most frequently moved nonaxial joint of the body because almost any movement of the upper extremity is transferred proximally to this joint. It also has the least amount of bony stability of any major joint because less than half of the medial end of the clavicle actually articulates with the upper sternum. Joint stability therefore depends on the integrity of the surrounding liga-

ments, which give the sternoclavicular joint surprising strength. As a result, the majority of injuries to this area are simple sprains, dislocations being uncommon.

A sprain of the sternoclavicular joint can result from the shoulder being forced forward suddenly or from a medially directed force applied to the shoulder. Pain and swelling are localized to the joint, and treatment is symptomatic with ice, sling, and analgesics. Differential diagnosis should include consideration of septic arthritis, especially in intravenous drug abusers.

Sternoclavicular dislocations are uncommon, accounting for only 3 percent of a series of 1603 shoulder girdle injuries. Dislocations usually result from motor vehicle accidents or sports injuries although spontaneous dislocations have been reported. Posterior sternoclavicular joint dislocations are much less common than anterior dislocations. A posterior dislocation may result from a direct blow or from an indirect force to the shoulder if the shoulder is rolled forward at the time of impact. An anterior sternoclavicular joint dislocation may result from the same indirect force if the shoulder is rolled backward at the time of impact. Of note is that the medial clavicular epiphysis is the last epiphysis of the body to appear radiographically (age 18) and the last to close (age 22 to 25). As a result, physeal injuries in this age group can easily be misdiagnosed as a dislocation.

Patients with a sternoclavicular joint dislocation will have severe pain that is exacerbated by arm motion and when in the supine position. The shoulder appears shortened and rolled forward. On examination, anterior dislocations have a prominent medial clavicle end that is visible and palpable anterior to the sternum. In posterior dislocations, the medial clavicle end is less visible and not palpable, and the patient may have signs and symptoms of impingement of the superior mediastinal contents (Fig. 226-1). Routine radiographs may

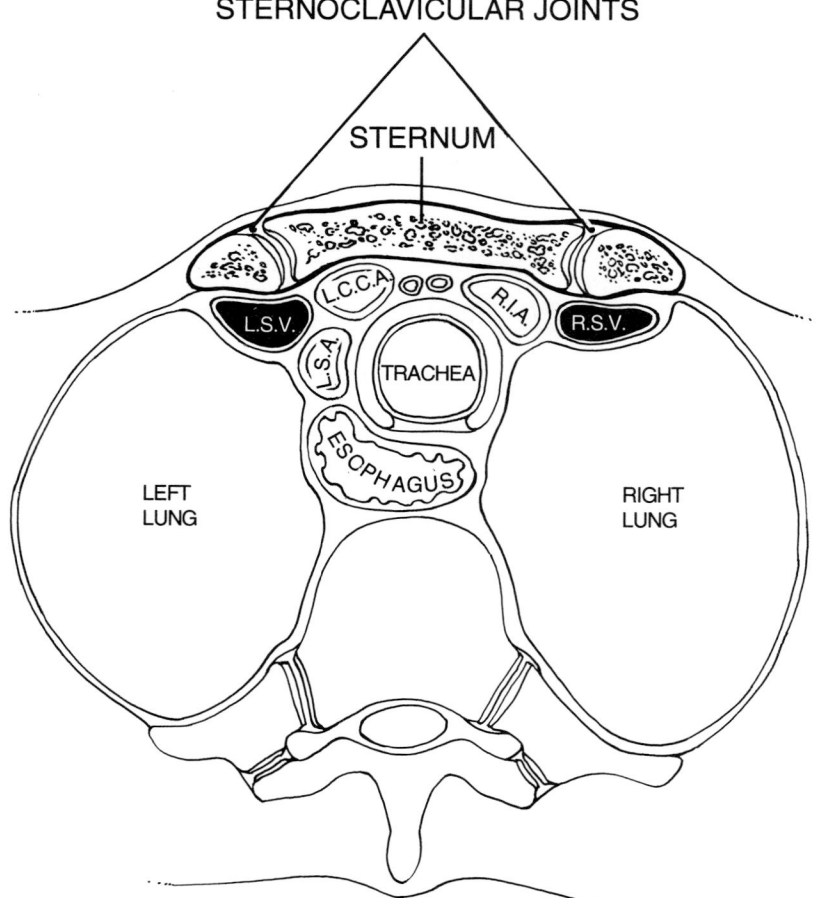

## STERNOCLAVICULAR JOINTS

STERNUM

L.C.C.A.

L.S.V.

L.S.A.

R.I.A.

R.S.V.

TRACHEA

ESOPHAGUS

LEFT LUNG

RIGHT LUNG

**Fig. 226-1.** The relationship of the sternoclavicular joint to adjacent structures. RSV, right subclavian vein; RIA, right innominate artery; LCCA, left common carotid artery; LSA, left subclavian artery; LSV, left subclavian vein.

not be diagnostic although specialized views or tomograms may be helpful. Computed tomography (CT) is the imaging procedure of choice.

Closed reduction of anterior sternoclavicular joint dislocations is usually attempted with the patient supine and with a sandbag or pad between the shoulders. Direct pressure over the clavicle may reduce the dislocation. The patient is discharged in a figure-of-eight clavicle harness. Unfortunately, most anterior dislocations prove unstable and recur as soon as direct pressure is released. These patients may subsequently undergo open reduction, or the position of the deformity may be accepted and no further treatment rendered.

In posterior dislocations, life-threatening injuries to adjacent structures may result in a pneumothorax, compression, or laceration of the great vessels, trachea, or esophagus. Preparation for a thoracic surgical emergency is the rule. Closed reduction is usually first attempted, but open reduction may be necessary.

## CLAVICLE

Clavicle fractures account for 5 percent of all fractures seen in the emergency department and for 44 percent of significant injuries to the shoulder girdle. This is the most common fracture of childhood, with almost half of these injuries occurring by the age of 7. The clavicle functions as a strut, connecting the shoulder girdle to the trunk, and provides support and mobility for upper extremity function. The clavicle also protects the adjacent lung, brachial plexus, and subclavian and brachial blood vessels.

The most common mechanism of injury is a blow to the shoulder. Transmission of the compressive force results in a buckling of the clavicle, which fractures once a critical force is achieved. Children will often have a greenstick or buckle-type fracture or a bowing deformity without a definite fracture. Open fractures, due to extreme tenting of the overlying skin, may occasionally be seen.

Eighty percent of clavicle fractures involve the middle third, 15 percent the distal third, and 5 percent the medial third. Patients typically present with swelling, deformity, and tenderness localized to the clavicle. The arm is slumped inward and downward and is supported by the other extremity. Routine clavicle radiographs may miss fractures due to overlap of surrounding structures, particularly with fractures at either end of the bone. Diagnosis of these may require special views or specialized techniques such as tomography or CT scan.

Numerous forms of treatment have been described for this common injury. Simple immobilization with a sling is often successful, with displaced fractures often treated with a figure-of-eight brace. A shoulder spica or open reduction may be required for severely displaced fractures, poor patient compliance, or for complications. Healing may occur as rapidly as 2 weeks for infants, with most adults healing in a 4 to 6-week period.

Although the vast majority of these fractures have a benign course, serious associated injuries and complications may occasionally occur. Penetrating or blunt trauma may result in associated lung, neurovascular, or first rib injuries. Injury to the adjacent vascular structures, usually the subclavian artery, subclavian vein, internal jugular vein, or axillary artery, may be life-threatening. Distal clavicle fractures with displacement typically are associated with rupture of the coracoclavicular ligament and may require operative intervention to avoid nonunion. Medial clavicle fractures may be associated with intrathoracic injuries or develop late complications such as arthritis. Significant callus formation may result in subsequent compression of adjacent neurovascular structures as well as being cosmetically deforming.

## SCAPULA

The scapula links the axial skeleton to the upper extremity and serves as a stabilizing platform for motion of the arm. Fracture of the scapula is an infrequent occurrence, accounting for less than 1 percent of all fractures. Due to the high energy typically required to fracture this protected bone, there is a greater than 80 percent association of injuries to the ipsilateral lung, thoracic cage, and shoulder girdle.

Significant scapular injury occurs most frequently in men between 25 and 40 years of age, usually as a result of motor vehicle accidents, falls, or other severe trauma. The mechanism of injury is from a direct blow, trauma to the shoulder sometimes with injury of the acromion or coracoid, or from a fall on the outstretched arm. An indirect axial load transmitted via the outstretched arm may result in a scapular neck fracture, while the indirect force of a shoulder dislocation may result in fracture of the glenoid. Scapular fractures may be classified by their anatomic location: body, glenoid neck, intraarticular glenoid, spine, coracoid, and acromion (Fig. 226-2). Fractures of the body and glenoid neck are the most common.

A patient with an isolated scapular fracture typically will present with localized tenderness over the scapula with the ipsilateral arm held in adduction. The shoulder may have a flattened appearance. Radiographs consisting of an anteroposterior shoulder, lateral scapula, and axillary will identify most fractures. However, scapula fractures are often associated with other significant injuries and hence diagnosis may be delayed or initially missed entirely. In Ada and Miller's recent series, 96 percent of scapular fractures had associated injuries of which rib fractures were the most common, followed by pulmonary, humeral head, and shoulder girdle injuries. Other injuries may include neurovascular, abdominal, and spine trauma.

Rarely, significant trauma may result in scapulothoracic dissociation. This syndrome consists of lateral scapular displacement, clavicular disruption, and severe soft tissue injury. This injury is sometimes associated with a brachial plexus avulsion, subclavian artery disruption, or both. Its presence may be suspected by neurovascular findings or by lateral displacement of the scapula visualized on a nonrotated chest radiograph.

The vast majority of scapular fractures are treated nonsurgically, with a sling for immobilization, ice, analgesics, and early range of motion exercises. Surgical intervention may be necessary for significant or displaced articular fractures of the glenoid, angulated glenoid neck fractures, acromial fractures associated with a rotator cuff tear, and some coracoid fractures. Fractures of the glenoid, acromion, or

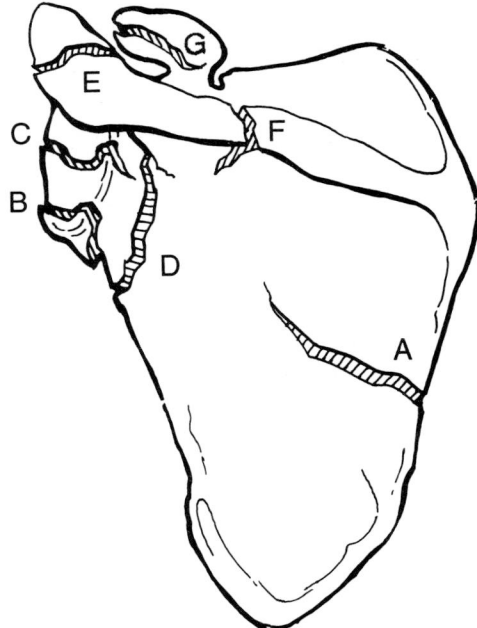

**Fig. 226-2.** Sites of scapula fractures. A, body; B, glenoid rim; C, intra-articular glenoid; D, neck; E, acromion; F, spine; G, coracoid.

coracoid are more likely to be associated with long-term disability.

Complications of scapular fractures themselves are uncommon. Although many of these fractures heal with some degree of malunion, typically this does not result in significant disability. Most long-term disability is a result of other associated injuries.

## ROTATOR CUFF INJURIES

The rotator cuff consists of the tendons of the supraspinatus, infraspinatus, subscapularis, and teres minor muscles. These coalesce with the capsule of the glenohumeral joint and attach to the greater and lesser tuberosities of the humerus. The main function of the rotator cuff is to provide dynamic stability to the glenohumeral joint. This is accomplished by contraction of muscles that compress the humeral head in the glenoid and by selective contraction resists the actions of major shoulder girdle muscles. The end result is a stable scapulohumeral articulation with the ability to perform smooth coordinated motion. Injuries to the rotator cuff occur as a result of acute trauma such as from a dislocation of the glenohumeral joint and as a result of chronic injuries.

Tears of the rotator cuff after glenohumeral dislocation are common but unfortunately often missed. It should be suspected in all patients over the age of 40 years, in patients with luxatio erecta, and in patients who are unable to abduct or externally rotate the arm after a glenohumeral dislocation.

Chronic injuries occur as a result of impingement and decreased vascularity, both common with advancing age. Impingement is explained by the anatomic relationship of the rotator cuff to osseus and soft tissue structures. It is "sandwiched" between the humeral head, acromion, coracoid, and the coracoacromial ligament. Compression of the rotator cuff between the humeral head and the coracoacromial arch (acromion, coracoid, and coracoacromial ligament) leads to tendon attrition and degeneration. Disease of the rotator cuff is a continuum of injury from mild inflammation to rupture. The initial stage is characterized by inflammation and edema resulting in mild pain with activity. There is no limitation of motion or weakness. There may be mild tenderness over the greater tuberosity. This stage of disease is most common in patients less than 25 years of age and is completely reversible.

In the second stage there is increased tendinitis and the pain is more intense and seems to be worse at night. Tenderness is more diffuse. Overhead motion is painful and there is some limitation of abduction and external rotation.

In the third stage of disease there is significant rotator cuff degeneration and tears. Most patients are over the age of 40 with a long history of symptoms. They have more pain, limitation of motion, and weakness. Patients with complete rotator cuff tears will have tenderness over the greater tuberosity and acromioclavicular joint. They will also have limitation of motion and weakness especially to abduction and external rotation. Disease at this stage is considered irreversible.

Treatment in the early stages consists of rest with sling immobilization, nonsteroidal anti-inflammatory drugs, ice, and local injections. Treatment of rotator cuff tears is initially symptomatic followed by consideration for surgery either arthroscopically or open.

## ACROMIOCLAVICULAR JOINT INJURIES

Injuries to the acromioclavicular joint are commonly seen in emergency practice. Although it may occur in any age group, the majority of injuries occur in young active males. Emergency management consists of identifying the severity of injury, recognizing associated injuries, and managing selected patients as outpatients.

### Anatomy

The acromioclavicular joint is a diarthrodial joint that together with the sternoclavicular joint connects the upper extremity to the axial skeleton. The support of the acromioclavicular joint is through the acromioclavicular and coracoclavicular ligaments and the strong attachment of the trapezius and deltoid muscles (Fig. 226-3). The acromioclavicular joint is surrounded by a thin capsule, which is reinforced by the acromioclavicular ligaments. The superior fibers of this ligament blend with the fascia of the trapezius and deltoid, which attach to the clavicle and acromion. The acromioclavicular ligaments provide horizontal stability to the joint. The tough coracoclavicular ligaments consist of two parts, the more lateral trapezoid and the medial conoid. It attaches the distal inferior clavicle to the coracoid process of the scapula. This ligament is the major suspensory ligament of the upper extremity and provides vertical stability to the acromioclavicular joint.

### Mechanism of Injury

The mechanism of injury is usually direct trauma to the acromioclavicular joint from a fall with the arm adducted, as typically may occur in a sporting activity. An indirect mechanism is a fall on the outstretched hand with transmission of force to the acromioclavicular joint. The result is that the scapula and shoulder girdle are driven inferiorly while the clavicle remains in its normal position. This is confirmed by observing the opposite clavicle, which is at the same level as the injured one.

### Clinical

The diagnosis of acromioclavicular joint injuries is made clinically. The typical mechanism of injury as well as tenderness and deformity at the acromioclavicular joint is confirmatory. Radiographs are useful to identify other fractures as well as to determine the severity of injury. Acromioclavicular radiographs should specifically be ordered because these require only one third to one half the penetration of standard shoulder films. Shoulder technique will overpenetrate the acromioclavicular joint and small fractures may be missed. Although standard acromioclavicular radiographs are generally sufficient, an axillary view is required to identify posterior clavicular dislocation

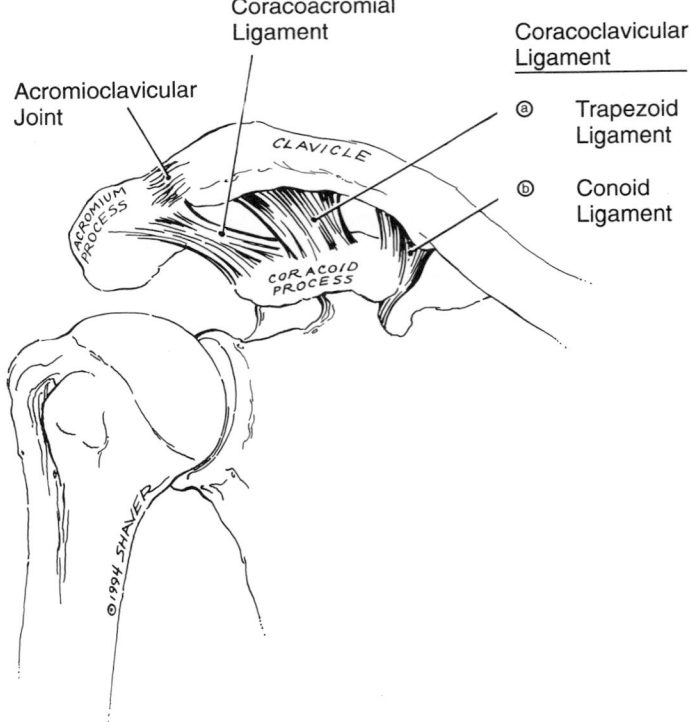

**Fig. 226-3.** Anatomy of the acromioclavicular joint.

(type IV, see below). Routine use of stress radiographs has been standard practice. Recently, however, Bossert and colleagues have called this practice into question. Their study suggests that stress radiographs are of low yield and that their routine use should be abandoned. Although some agree, others disagree citing occult type III (see below) injuries that can only be unmasked with stress radiographs.

## Classification of Injury

The classification of acromioclavicular joint injuries classically describes three types of injuries. Rockwood describes three others (Fig. 226-4). Types I, II, and III are common; types IV, V, and VI are rare. The anatomic injury, radiographic findings, and physical findings are summarized on Table 226-1.

## Treatment

Treatment of type I injuries consists of rest, ice, analgesics, and immobilization, followed by early range of motion. Most agree that type II injuries should be similarly treated. Various straps and braces have been used to reduce the dislocation but none have proven successful. A simple sling remains the most convenient and effective. Prognosis for type I and II injuries is excellent with only a small percentage who develop late symptoms requiring excision of the distal clavicle. Treatment of type III injuries (Fig. 226-5) is controversial with proponents for both conservative and operative philosophies. A recent trend among directors of orthopedic residency programs, however,

reveals a shift to conservative treatment with sling immobilization. Both strategies have yielded good results in selected patients, with the specific management operator dependent. Treatment decisions are based on such factors as age, occupation, and activity level. Types IV, V, and VI are severe injuries and most authors recommend surgical repair. Because other injuries are associated with these more severe forms of acromioclavicular joint injuries (especially type VI), a careful clinical and radiographic examination must be performed.

## DISLOCATION OF THE GLENOHUMERAL JOINT

Dislocation of the glenohumeral joint is the most common major joint dislocation. Anterior dislocations are by far the most common. Posterior dislocations are described but occur in less than 2% of cases. Other dislocations include inferior (luxatio erecta) and superior (very rare).

## Anterior Glenohumeral Dislocations

There are four types of anterior dislocations. In subcoracoid dislocation, which is the most common type, the humeral head is displaced anterior to the glenoid and inferior to the coracoid. In a subglenoid dislocation the humeral head lies inferior and anterior to the glenoid fossa. In a subclavicular dislocation the head of the humerus is displaced medial to the coracoid below the clavicle. In the very rare intrathoracic dislocation the head of the humerus lies between the ribs and thoracic cavity.

The mechanism of injury may be from a direct force, but an indi-

**Fig. 226-4.** Classification of acromioclavicular joint injuries. (From Rockwood CA, Green DP, Bucholz RW. *Rockwood & Green's Fractures in Adults,* 3rd ed. Philadelphia: JB Lippincott, 1991. Used with permission.)

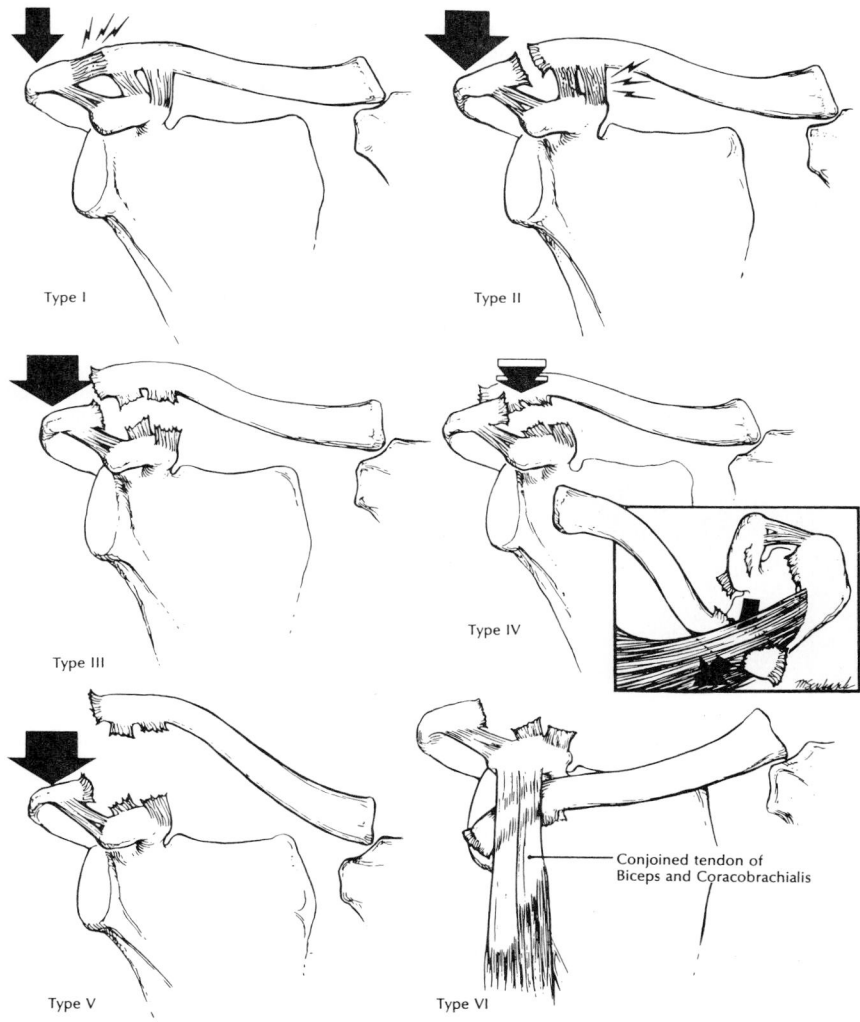

Type I

Type II

Type III

Type IV

Type V

Type VI — Conjoined tendon of Biceps and Coracobrachialis

**Table 226-1.** Classification and Physical Findings in Acromioclavicular Joint Injuries

| | Injury | Radiograph | Examination |
|---|---|---|---|
| TYPE I | Sprain acromioclavicular ligaments | Normal | Tenderness over the acromioclavicular joint |
| TYPE II | Acromioclavicular ligaments ruptured; coracoclavicular ligaments sprained | Slight widening of acromioclavicular joint; clavicle elevated 25–50% above acromion; may see slight widening of the coracoclavicular interspace | Tenderness and mild step-off deformity of the acromioclavicular joint |
| TYPE III | Acromioclavicular ligaments ruptured; coracoclavicular ligaments ruptured; deltoid and trapezius detached | Acromioclavicular joint dislocated 100%; coracoclavicular interspace widened 25–100% | Distal end of the clavicle is prominent; shoulder droops |
| TYPE IV | Rupture of all supporting structures; clavicle is displaced posteriorly in or through the trapezius | May appear similar to type II and III; axillary radiograph required to visualize posterior dislocation | May see posterior displacement of clavicle |
| TYPE V | Rupture of all supporting structures (represents a more severe form of type III injury) | Acromioclavicular joint dislocated; generally 200–300% disparity of coracoclavicular interspace compared to normal shoulder | More pain; gross deformity of clavicle |
| TYPE VI | Acromioclavicular ligaments disrupted; coracoclavicular ligaments, deltoid, and trapezius may be disrupted | Acromioclavicular joint dislocated; clavicle displaced inferiorly | Severe swelling multiple associated injuries |

rect force is most common. The combination of abduction, extension, and external rotation with sufficient force will cause an anterior dislocation.

The patient is usually in severe pain. The arm is in slight abduction and external rotation. The shoulder is "squared off," lacking the normal rounded contour. The patient resists abduction and internal rotation. The humeral head can often be palpated anteriorly. Because neurovascular injuries are common, a careful examination must be performed. The axillary nerve is most commonly injured. This nerve may be tested by pinprick sensation over the skin of the deltoid muscle.

Anteroposterior and scapular lateral or Y radiographs should be obtained before reduction is attempted. Although the anteroposterior radiograph will reveal the dislocation, the scapular Y radiograph will indicate the direction of dislocation, anterior or posterior. Bony injuries reported in the literature include fractures of the anterior glenoid lip, greater tuberosity, coracoid, acromion, and compression fractures of the humeral head (Hill-Sachs lesion).

Many reduction techniques have been described in the literature. The three main categories are traction, leverage, and scapular manipulation. Success rates are between 70 and 90 percent regardless of technique. The use of conscious sedation is recommended, but any reduction technique may be attempted without medication when per-

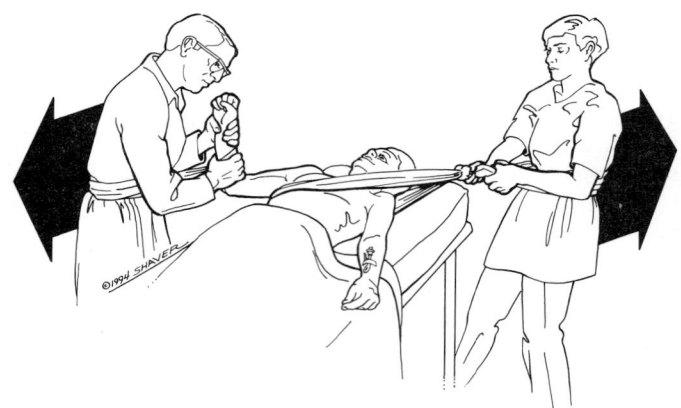

**Fig. 226-6.** Modified Hippocratic technique.

formed slowly and atraumatically. It is important for the physician to be comfortable with two or three techniques in case of a failed first attempt. Considerations in selection of a technique include ease of performance, effectiveness, atraumatic and painless as possible, requirement for medication, number of assistants, and time for procedure.

### Hippocratic (Modified)

A modification of the Hippocratic method uses traction countertraction (Fig. 226-6). The patient is supine with the arm abducted and elbow flexed at 90°. A sheet is tied and placed across the thorax of the patient then around the waist of the assistant. Another sheet is tied and placed around the forearm of the patient at the elbow and the waist of the physician. The physician gradually applies traction as the assistant provides countertraction. Gentle internal and external rotation or outward pressure on the proximal humerus may aid reduction.

### Stimson

The patient is placed prone on the gurney with the dislocated extremity hanging over the side with a 10-pound weight attached to the wrist. Complete muscle relaxation is required. Twenty to 30 minutes is required to allow reduction to occur.

Although safe, effective, and easy to learn, the time involved and constant monitoring by a nurse are drawbacks to this technique.

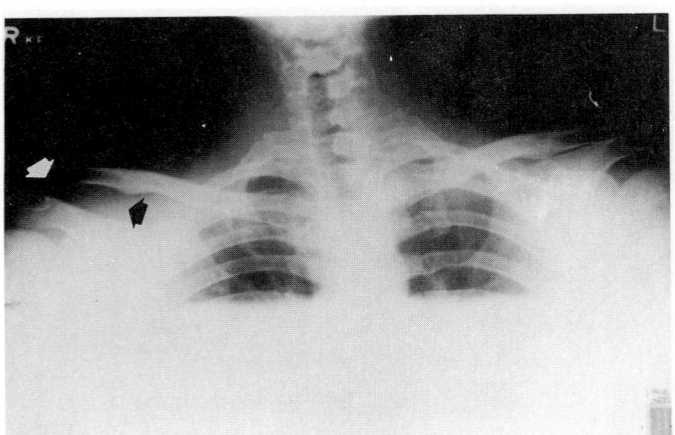

**Fig. 226-5.** Type III acromioclavicular dislocation. Note dislocation of acromioclavicular joint (*white arrow*) and increased coracoclavicular interspace (*black arrow*).

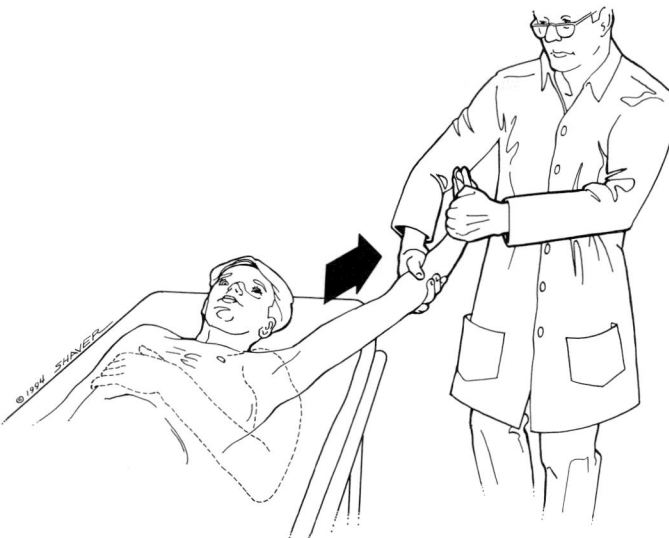

**Fig. 226-7.** Milch technique.

## Milch

The patient is supine. The physician slowly abducts and externally rotates the arm to the overhead position (Fig. 226-7). With the elbow fully extended traction is applied. With the other hand pressure may be placed on the humeral head to manipulate it over the lip of the glenoid.

This technique is well tolerated by the patient, effective, and atraumatic. It is the technique of choice for many authors.

## Scapular Manipulation

The patient is positioned with weights in the same manner as the Stimson technique (Fig. 226-8). After adequate sedation the physician pushes the tip of the scapula medially using the thumbs, while stabilizing the superior aspect with the cephalad hand.

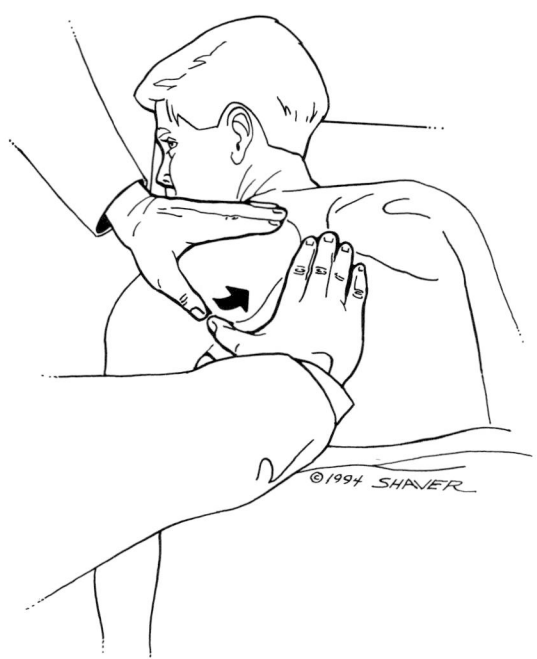

**Fig. 226-8.** Scapular manipulation technique.

Several reports have recently been published. Authors have found this technique relatively painless, fast, and in one study 90 percent successful.

## External Rotation

The patient is supine with the arm adducted to the patient's side. With the elbow at 90° of flexion, the arm is slowly externally rotated. No longitudinal traction is applied. It is important to perform the movement slowly to allow time for spasm and pain to resolve. Reduction is usually complete prior to reaching the coronal plane and is often not noted either by the patient or physician.

This method has been reported to be 78 percent successful, relatively atraumatic, safe, and easily learned.

Complications are frequently encountered in patients with anterior glenohumeral dislocations. The most common complication is recurrent dislocation, which is age dependent. Those patients less than 20 years of age have a greater than 90 percent recurrence; those older than 40 years have a 14 percent recurrence. Other complications include fractures and injuries to nerves and the rotator cuff. Vascular injuries are rare but when they occur tend to involve the axillary artery in elderly patients. Clinical findings of vascular injury include absent radial pulse, axillary hematoma, bruising of the lateral chest wall, and an axillary bruit.

Bony injuries are common and include fractures of the humeral head (Hill-Sachs lesion), anterior glenoid lip, and greater tuberosity. Neural injuries occur in 10 to 25 percent of acute dislocations. Of these injuries, which are the result of traction neuropraxia, most occur in the axillary nerve. This injury is temporary and resolves spontaneously. The common test of sensation over the skin of the deltoid muscle may not be reliable, with only an electromyogram providing an accurate evaluation. Other nerves injured are the radial, ulnar, median, musculocutaneous, and brachial plexus.

A frequent, but often missed injury, is a tear of the rotator cuff. This injury, which increases with age, has a greater than 80 percent occurrence in patients older than 60 years. Treatment is surgical.

In summary, complications following acute anterior glenohumeral dislocations are common. A careful physical examination and review of radiographs both before and after reduction are essential. Special attention should be directed at evaluation of neural and rotator cuff injuries that may be occult.

## Posterior Glenohumeral Dislocations

Posterior dislocation may occur with the humeral head in the subacromial (most common, humeral head behind the glenoid and beneath the acromion), subglenoid, or subspinous. The latter two are rare.

The usual mechanism is an indirect force producing forceful internal rotation and adduction. This mechanism may occur during a fall or from violent muscle contraction from a seizure or electric shock. Direct force to the anterior shoulder can also produce a posterior dislocation.

Posterior dislocations are reported to be commonly missed so a careful examination and radiographic evaluation are essential. Clinical findings include:

- Arm adducted and internally rotated
- Anterior shoulder flat, posterior aspect full
- Coracoid process prominent
- Patient will not allow external rotation or abduction because of severe pain

Although the anteroposterior radiograph is helpful, the scapular Y radiograph is diagnostic. In this radiograph, the humeral head will be seen in a posterior position.

Severe pain and muscle spasms are the norm so muscle relaxation and analgesia are paramount. The reduction is performed with the patient supine. Traction is applied to the adducted arm in the long axis of the humerus. An assistant gently pushes the humeral head anteriorly into the glenoid fossa.

Most complications are fractures. These include fractures of the posterior glenoid rim, humeral head (reversed Hill-Sachs deformity), humeral shaft, and lesser tuberosity. Neurovascular and rotator cuff tears are less common than in anterior dislocations.

## Inferior Dislocations (Luxatio Erecta)

Although this is a rare injury, it is one that will be seen in a busy emergency practice. This is always a severe injury that is associated with significant soft tissue trauma or fracture. The mechanism of injury is a hyperabduction force, which levers the neck of the humerus against the acromion. As the force continues the inferior capsule tears and the humeral head is forced out inferiorly.

The patient is in severe pain. The humerus is fully abducted, the elbow is flexed, and the patient's hand is on or behind the head. The humeral head can be palpated on the lateral chest wall. This clinical presentation is difficult to mistake for another condition.

Reduction consists of traction in an upward and outward direction in line with the humerus (Fig. 226-9). The assistant applies countertraction. Reduction is signaled by a "clunk." The arm is then brought to the patient's side and immobilized in a shoulder immobilizer.

Complications include severe soft tissue injuries and fractures of the proximal humerus. The rotator cuff, which is always detached, requires orthopedic follow-up. Neurovascular compression injuries are usually found but almost always resolve following reduction. When

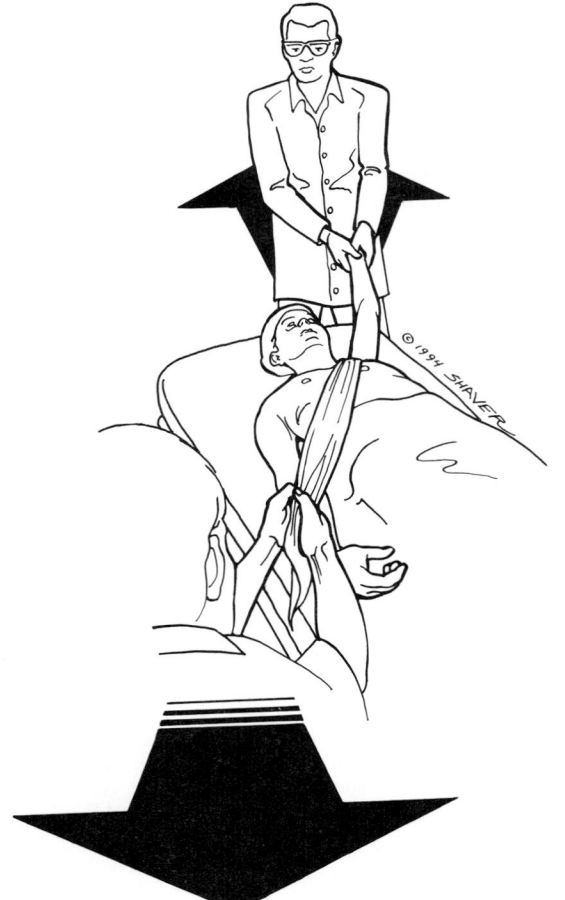

**Fig. 226-9.** Reduction of luxatio erecta.

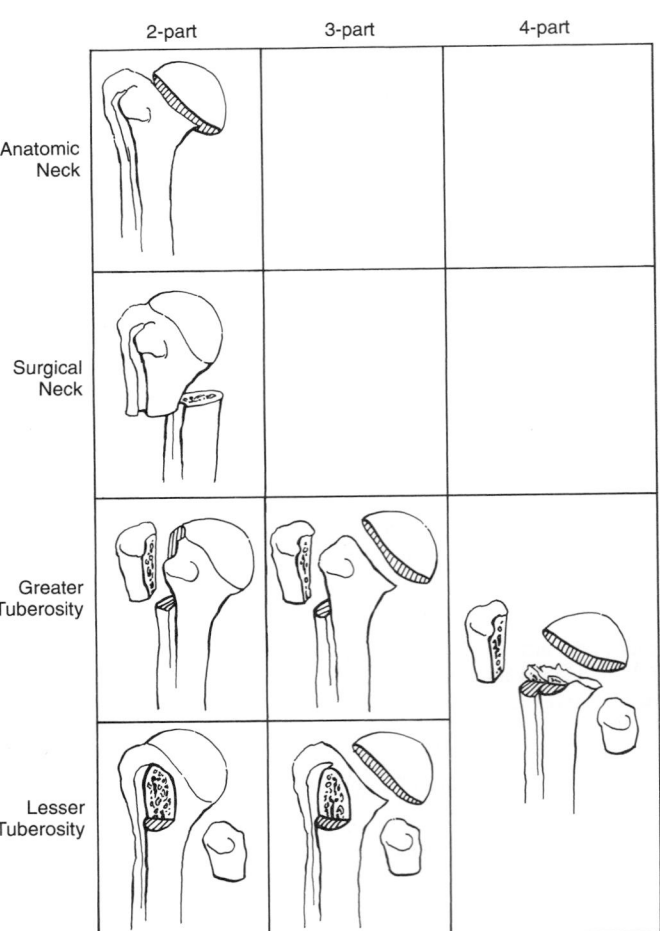

Displaced Fractures

**Fig. 226-10.** The Neer classification system for proximal humerus fractures.

the humeral head is buttonholed through the inferior capsule, the dislocation is irreducible and operative reduction is required.

## HUMERUS FRACTURES

### Proximal Humerus

Fractures of the proximal humerus are a relatively common problem in the emergency department, representing 5 percent of all fractures. They typically occur in elderly osteoporotic patients via an indirect mechanism, such as a fall on an outstretched hand with the elbow extended. Eighty percent of such fractures can be easily managed by the emergency physician, but the remainder have significant displacement and are a challenge to correctly diagnose and treat. Fortunately for such a common injury, the shoulder joint has an intrinsic reserve in its range of motion, which can often provide a surprisingly functional outcome despite seemingly crippling injuries.

The proximal humerus is composed of the articular segment, the greater and lesser tuberosities, and the proximal humeral shaft. Muscles of the rotator cuff insert on the humeral tuberosities while the biceps tendon travels between them. The humeral circumflex arteries enter in the area of the bicipital groove and the tuberosities to supply blood flow to the articular segment.

Patients with fractures typically present with pain, swelling, and tenderness about the shoulder. Crepitus and ecchymosis may be present, and the arm is generally held closely against the chest wall. A neurovascular examination should be performed, remembering that the brachial plexus and axillary arteries are near the coracoid process and not uncommonly injured. The axillary nerve is the most commonly injured nerve, and sensation over the skin of the deltoid muscle should be tested routinely. Injury to the axillary artery is the most common vascular injury, and may be suggested by paresthesias, pallor, pulselessness, or an expanding hematoma. Vascular injuries may occur with even trivial trauma in the atherosclerotic elderly patient.

Radiographs consisting of anteroposterior, lateral shoulder, and axillary views will correctly diagnose most proximal humerus fractures. Fractures of the articular surface may be suggested by a fat fluid level or by a superior joint hematoma that appears to push the humerus downward in the joint as a "pseudosubluxation." The transthoracic lateral radiograph, tomograms, CT scan, and magnetic resonance imaging scan may also be of value.

The Neer classification system uses the relationship of the proximal humerus' segments (greater and lesser tuberosities, anatomic neck, and surgical neck) to guide the management of these fractures. Significant fragment displacement is defined as greater than 1 cm separation or greater than 45° of angulation between fragments. The number of fracture fragments significantly displaced determines the classification in the Neer system (Fig. 226-10).

A one-part fracture may have any number of fracture lines, but no major segment is significantly displaced. The surrounding soft tissue and periosteum hold fracture fragments together. One-part fractures comprise over 80 percent of all proximal humerus fractures. Treatment generally consists of immobilization with a sling and swathe or collar and cuff, ice, analgesics, and referral. Early exercise is important to avoid adhesive capsulitis. The overall prognosis is generally good.

Two-part fractures account for 10 percent of proximal humerus fractures, with the remaining 10 percent evenly split between three-part and four-part fractures. Such displaced fractures are more frequently associated with complications and are often difficult to manage. Treatment considerations include integrity of the blood supply, integrity of the rotator cuff, likelihood of union, associated dislocations and neurovascular injuries, and the functionality of the patient. Closed reduction, intraoperative treatment, or a combination of the two may be necessary. Emergent orthopedic consultation for multipart fractures facilitates subsequent reduction and referral.

Any fracture involving the anatomic neck or the articular surface may result in compromise of the blood supply to the articular segment. Ischemic necrosis of the articular segment may ultimately require insertion of a humeral head prosthesis for these relatively uncommon fractures. Greater tuberosity fractures accompany up to 15 percent of anterior shoulder dislocations. Significant displacement of a greater tuberosity fragment implies a concomitant rotator cuff tear, with surgical repair often necessary for the active patient. Fracture of the lesser tuberosity should alert the examiner to a potential posterior shoulder dislocation. Significantly angulated surgical neck fractures are at risk for neurovascular damage (axillary neurovascular structures and brachial plexus) and should be immediately immobilized and radiographed in the position of presentation. Children may have significant displacement or separation of the proximal humeral epiphysis and may require exact reduction if near skeletal maturity. A shoulder spica is often used after reduction.

## Humeral Shaft

Fractures of the humeral shaft typically occur in active adults rather than in the elderly as is common in proximal humerus fractures. The most common site of fracture is the middle third. Neurovascular injuries are a common complication of these fractures and are a direct result of the anatomy of the upper extremity. Displacement of fracture fragments is common as a result of the insertions and actions of the various muscles (deltoid, biceps, triceps, supraspinatus, and pectoralis major) that act on the upper arm (Fig. 226-11).

Humeral shaft fractures may be caused by a direct blow producing a bending force, which results in a transverse fracture. It may also be caused by an indirect mechanism such as a fall on the outstretched hand producing a torsion force resulting in a spiral fracture. A combination of bending and torsion forces results in an oblique fracture, sometimes with comminution producing the "butterfly" fragment. The humerus is also a common site of pathologic fractures especially from metastatic breast cancer.

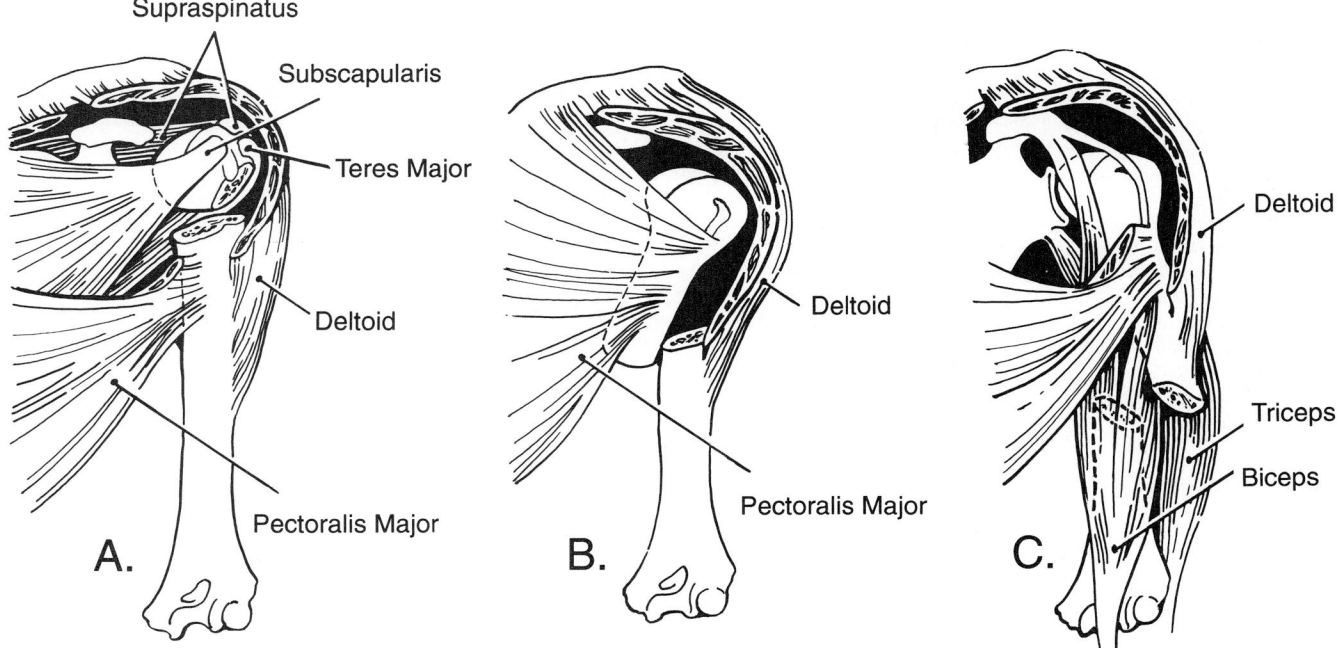

**Fig. 226-11.** The actions of the muscles inserting on the humeral shaft determine fracture angulation and displacement. Humeral fractures: (A) Angulation of fragments with fracture line distal to rotator cuff insertion. (B) Angulation of fragments with fracture line distal to pectoralis major insertion. (C) Angulation of fragments with fracture line distal to deltoid insertion.

Clinical examination reveals localized tenderness, swelling, pain, and abnormal mobility or crepitus on palpation. Displaced fractures are associated with shortening of the upper extremity. Attention must be given to the initial neurovascular status and reevaluation must be performed especially after manipulation. Radiographs should include two views of the humerus, and consideration should be given to radiographic examination of the shoulder and elbow as well.

The vast majority of closed fractures of the shaft of the humerus are managed nonoperatively. The treatment of uncomplicated fractures includes immobilization, ice, analgesia, and referral. Closed treatment options include the coaptation splint (sugar tong), a hanging cast, functional bracing, and external fixation. A simple sling and swathe is adequate for most emergency management. Some surgeons favor internal fixation for patients with transverse fracture lines, very proximal or very distal humerus fractures, pathologic fractures, multiple trauma patients, and fractures associated with neurovascular injuries.

Complications include injury to the brachial artery or vein, or the radial, ulnar, or median nerves. A radial nerve injury, which is the most common, may be manifested by a wrist drop and altered sensation at the dorsal first web space. The incidence of radial nerve palsy ranges from 10 to 20 percent. Fractures of the distal third are particularly prone to entrapment of the radial nerve either as a result of the initial injury or after closed reduction. The majority of patients have eventual return of nerve function without operative intervention.

## BIBLIOGRAPHY

Ada JR, Miller ME. Scapular fractures. *Clin Orthop* 269:174, 1991.

Beach WR, Caspari RB. Arthroscopic management of rotator cuff disease. *Orthopedics* 16:1007, 1993.

Bossart PJ, Joyce SM, Manaster BJ, et al. Lack of efficacy of "weighted" radiographs in diagnosing acute acromioclavicular separation. *Ann Emerg Med* 17:20, 1988.

Camden P, Nade S. Fracture bracing the humerus. *Injury* 23:45, 1992.

Cave ER, Burke JF, Boyd RJ. *Trauma Management.* Chicago: Year Book Medical Publishers, pp. 409–411, 1974.

Cook DA, Peiner JP. Acromioclavicular joint injuries. *Orthop Rev* XIX:510, 1990.

Cox JS. Current method of treatment of acromioclavicular joint dislocations. *Orthopedics* 15:1041, 1992.

Golden RH, Chow AW, Edwards JE, et al. Sternoarticular septic arthritis in heroin users. *N Engl J Med* 289:616, 1973.

Heim D, Herkert F, Hess P, et al. Surgical treatment of humeral shaft fractures—the Basel experience. *J. Trauma* 35:226, 232, 1993.

Kothari RU, Dronen SC. Prospective evaluation of the scapular manipulation technique in reducing anterior shoulder dislocation. *Ann Emerg Med* 21:1349, 1992.

Meister K, Andrews JR. Classification and treatment of rotator cuff injuries in the overhand athlete. *J Orthop Sports Phys Ther* 18:413, 1993.

Riebel GD, McCabe JB. Anterior shoulder dislocation: a review of reduction techniques. *Am J Emerg Med* 9:180, 1991.

Rockwood CA, Green DP, Bucholz RW. *Rockwood & Green's Fractures in Adults,* 3rd ed. Philadelphia: JB Lippincott, 1991.

# 227
# TRAUMA TO THE PELVIS, HIP, AND FEMUR

**Joseph F. Waeckerle**
**Mark T. Steele**

## TRAUMA TO THE PELVIS

Pelvic fractures constitute 3 percent of all skeletal fractures. These fractures and concomitant injuries are a frequent cause of death from blunt trauma sustained in automobile accidents. Fortunately, the mortality has decreased. The treating physician is managing patients with a proactive rather than reactive approach. Most pelvic fractures are secondary to automobile passenger or pedestrian accidents, but about one-third are the result of minor falls in older persons and from major falls or industrial accidents. This chapter discusses the most common fractures of the pelvis, femur, and hip, the mechanisms of injury, radiologic evaluation, and treatment.

### Anatomy and Biomechanics

The major functions of the pelvis are protection, support, and hematopoiesis. The pelvis consists of the two innominate bones, which are made up of the ilium, ischium, and pubis; the sacrum; and the coccyx. The two innominate bones and sacrum form a ring structure, which is the basis of pelvic stability. This stability is dependent on the strong posterior sacroiliac, sacrotuberous, and sacrospinous ligaments (Fig. 227-1). Any single break in the ring will yield a stable injury without significant risk of displacement. An injury with two breaks in the ring is unstable with the risk of displacement. The iliopectineal, or arcuate, line divides the pelvis into the upper, or false, pelvis, which is part of the abdomen, and the lower, true pelvis. In addition, this line constitutes the major portion of the femorosacral arch, which, along with the subsidiary tie arch (bodies of pubic bones and superior rami), supports the body in the erect position. In the sitting position the weight-bearing forces are transmitted by the ischiosacral arch augmented by its tie arch, the pubic bones, inferior pubic rami, and ischial rami. When traumatized, the tie arches fracture first, especially at the symphysis pubis, pubic rami, and just lateral to the sacroiliac (SI) joints. Incorporated in the pelvic structure are five joints that allow some movement in the bony ring. The lumbosacral, SI, and sacrococcygeal joints and the symphysis pubis allow little movement. The acetabulum is a ball-and-socket joint that is divided into three portions: the iliac portion, or superior dome, is the chief weight-bearing surface; the inner wall consists of the pubis and is thin and easily fractured; and the posterior acetabulum is derived from the thick ischium.

The pelvis is extremely vascular, a fact that is significant in pelvic fractures. The nerve supply through the pelvis is derived from the lumbar and sacral plexuses. Injury to the pelvis may produce deficits at any level from the nerve root to small peripheral branches.

The lower urinary tract is contained in the pelvis (Fig. 227-2). In the adult, the bladder lies behind the symphysis and pubic bones, and the peritoneum covers the dome and base posteriorly. The location of the bladder and the degree of peritoneal reflection are determined by urine content. The lower gastrointestinal tract housed in the pelvis includes a small portion of the descending colon, the pelvic, or sigmoid, colon, the rectum, and the anus.

**Fig. 227-1.** The major posterior stabilizing structures of the pelvic ring, that is, the posterior tension band of the pelvis, include the iliolumbar ligament, the posterior sacroiliac ligaments, the sacrospinous ligaments, and the sacrotuberous ligaments. (From Tile M. Anatomy. In: *Fractures of the Pelvis and Acetabulum.* Baltimore: Williams & Wilkins, p. 11, 1984. Used with permission.)

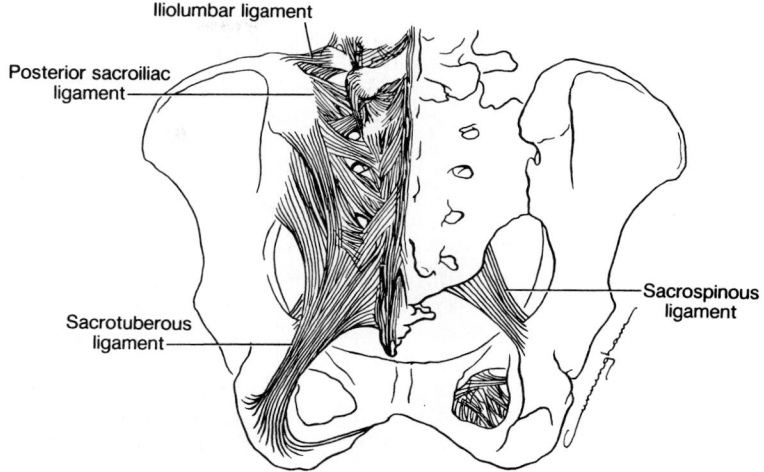

## Clinical Evaluation

### History

The emergency physician should assume that all victims of serious or multiple trauma, or both, have fractures of the pelvis. A patient with a suspected pelvic fracture should be questioned about details of the accident to determine the mechanism of injury and about prehospital evaluation and treatment. The patient should be specifically questioned to determine areas of pain, last urination or defecation, present bladder sensation, and the last solid and fluid intake. In addition, the time of the last menses or the presence of pregnancy, current medications, and allergies should be ascertained.

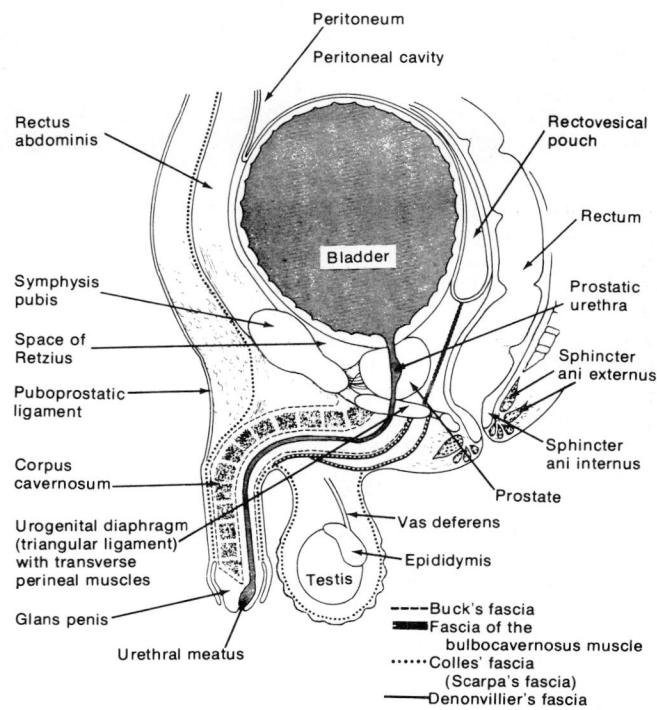

**Fig. 227-2.** Sagittal section of the male pelvis showing the relation of the full bladder. [From Kane WJ: Fractures of the pelvis, in Rockwood CA Jr, Green DP (eds): *Fractures,* Philadelphia, Lippincott, 1975, vol. 2, pp. 916, 917. Used by permission.]

### Physical Examination

Symptoms and signs of pelvic injuries vary from local pain and tenderness, especially with walking, to pelvic instability and severe shock. The physician must maintain alertness, perception, and concern in evaluating these patients. On inspection look for perineal and pelvic edema, ecchymoses, lacerations, and deformities. Look for hematomas above the inguinal ligament or over the scrotum (Destot's sign). Roll the patient over if appropriate and examine the areas overlying the sacrum and coccyx. On palpation feel for irregularities, crepitance, or movement at the iliac crests, pubic rami, and ischial rami. Palpation of a bony prominence or large hematoma or tenderness along the fracture line is possible by rectal examination (Earle's sign). Compress the pelvis lateral to medial through the iliac crests, anterior to posterior through the symphysis pubis, and anterior to posterior through the iliac crests. Compress the greater trochanters and determine the range of motion of the hips. On rectal examination, superior or posterior displacement of the prostate, or rectal injuries are indicative of intraperitoneal and urologic injury. Decrease in anal sphincter tone may suggest neurologic injury and blood at the urethral meatus, urologic injury. Carefully evaluate neurovascular function. If a pelvic fracture is found, assume intra-abdominal, retroperitoneal, gynecologic, and urologic injuries until proved otherwise.

### Radiologic Evaluation

Stabilization of the patient takes priority over obtaining x-ray films. Unnecessary movement may produce further injury or cause more blood loss. After stabilization, roentgenographic evaluation of the pelvis is a must in all unconscious patients who have sustained multiple injuries. Lower extremity long bone fractures as well as pelvic symptoms or signs are also indications for roentgenograms. A standard anteroposterior (AP) view of the pelvis is the necessary baseline. If additional studies are needed, lateral views, AP views of either hemipelvis, internal and external oblique views of the hemipelvis, or inlet and outlet views of the pelvis may be done. An inlet view shows anterior-posterior displacement of ring fractures (Fig. 227-3). An outlet view shows superior-inferior displacement (Fig. 227-4). Oblique views of the hemipelvis are true AP and lateral views of the acetabulum. Tomography, computed tomography (CT) scans, and special studies may be needed to fully evaluate and manage patients, particularly for acetabular and sacral fractures. Angiography or venography may be necessary to determine a source of bleeding. The patient's condition must dictate what is done and when.

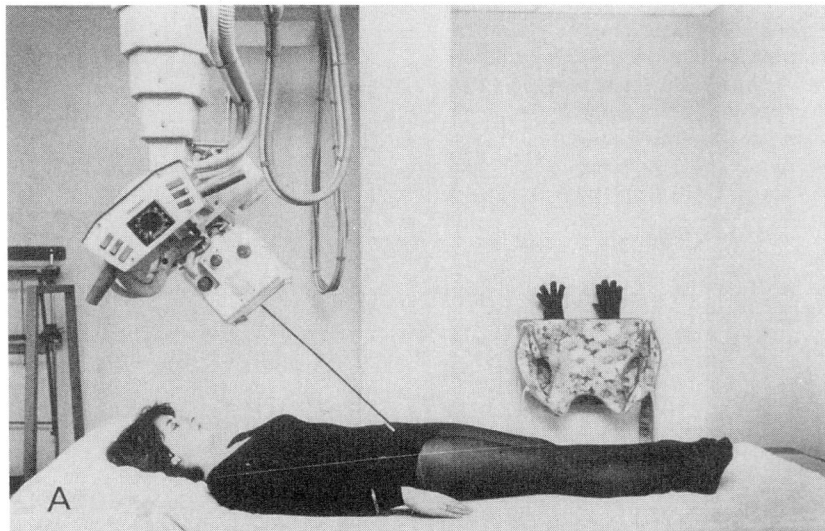

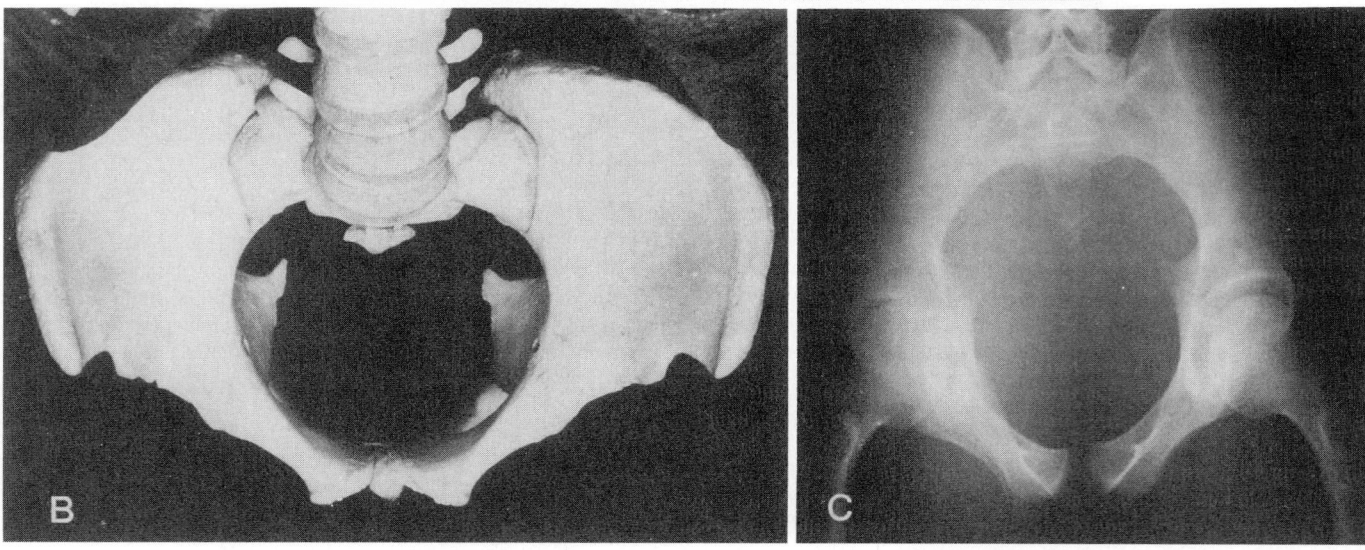

**Fig. 227-3.** (A) For the inlet projection, the beam is directed from the head to the midpelvis at an angle of 60° to the plate. (B) Anatomic appearance in the inlet projection. (C) Radiologic appearance in the inlet projection. (From Tile M. Assessment. In: *Fractures of the Pelvis and Acetabulum.* Baltimore: Williams & Wilkins, p. 63, 1984. Used with permission.)

## Classification of Pelvic Fractures

### Young System

Pelvic fractures can be complex and therefore difficult to classify. The most clinically useful classification by Young (Table 227-1), is presented. It differentiates fractures patterns due to trauma based on mechanism of injury and direction of causative force. Incidence of complications (i.e., urogenital and vascular) is correlated with the fracture pattern, making identification of the type more clinically significant and useful.

Three main types of patterns have been identified. The first and most common mechanism, lateral compression (LC) (Figs. 227-5 through 227-9), accounts for half the injuries. Motor vehicle accidents in which a car is broadsided or a pedestrian struck from the side are examples. Anteroposterior compression (APC) (Figs. 227-10, 227-11, and 227-12) is the second type, accounting for 20 percent of injuries. Head-on motor vehicle accidents are the classic example. The least common mechanism is vertical shear (VS) (Fig. 227-13) typified by a fall or jump from a height, accounting for 6 percent of

fractures. Mixed patterns of injury make up the other 20 to 25 percent of injuries.

The different injury types may be suggested by history, but can also be differentiated radiographically. The alignment of pubic rami fractures is one such clue to the mechanism and direction of force. Horizontal fractures suggest lateral compression injury, whereas vertical ones point to an anteroposterior direction of force. If there is sacroiliac joint diastasis and an associated crush fracture of the sacrum, then the injury is due to lateral compression. Central hip dislocations suggest a lateral compression mechanism whereas posterior dislocation suggests an anteroposterior force. With vertical shear patterns, fractures are vertical in alignment with vertical displacement of fragments. Based on the recognition of the fracture pattern, one can then predict the likelihood of severe hemorrhage or urogenital injury (Table 227-2).

### Other Fractures

The following are fractures of individual bones without a break in the pelvic ring. Those fractures are usually stable and heal well with bed rest.

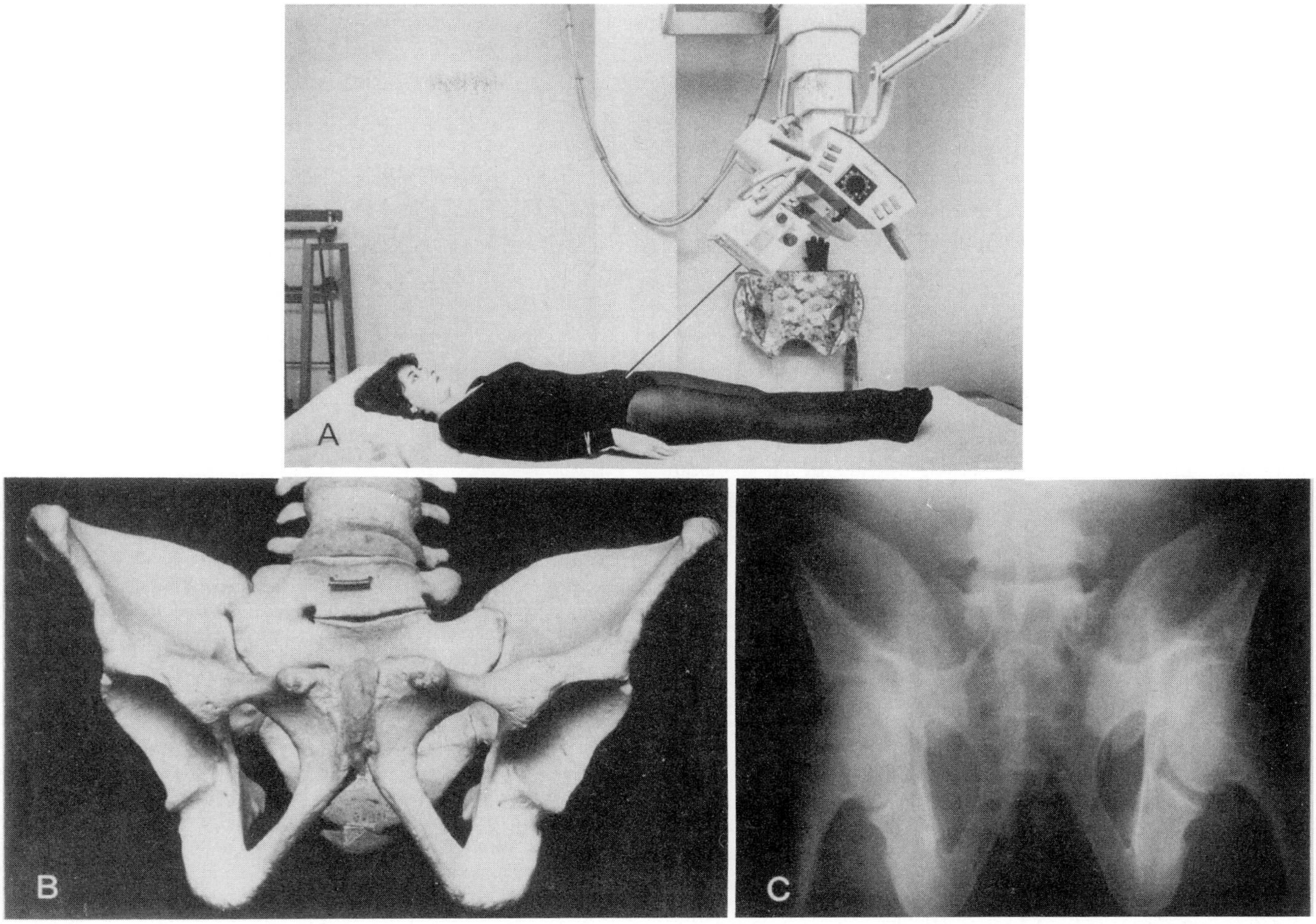

**Fig. 227-4.** (A) For the outlet projection, the beam is directed from the foot to the symphysis at an angle of 40° to the plate. (B) Anatomic appearance in the outlet projection. (C) Radiologic appearance in the outlet projection. (From Tile M. Assessment. In: *Fractures of the Pelvis and Acetabulum.* Baltimore: Williams & Wilkins, p. 64, 1984. Used with permission.)

**Table 227-1.** Injury Classification Keys According to the Young System

| Category | Distinguishing Characteristics |
|---|---|
| LC | Transverse fracture of pubic rami, ipsilateral or contralateral to posterior injury<br>I—Sacral compression on side of impact<br>II—Crescent (iliac wing) fracture on side of impact<br>III—LC-1 or LC-II injury on side of impact; contralateral open-book (APC) injury |
| APC | Symphyseal diastasis and/or longitudinal rami fractures<br>I—*Slight* widening of pubic symphysis and/or anterior SI joint; stretched but intact anterior SI, sacrotuberous, and sacrospinous ligaments; intact posterior SI ligaments<br>II—Widened anterior SI joint; disrupted anterior SI, sacrotuberous, and sacrospinous ligaments; intact posterior SI ligaments<br>III—Complete SI joint disruption with lateral displacement; disrupted anterior SI, sacrotuberous, and sacrospinous ligaments; disrupted posterior SI ligaments |
| VS | Symphyseal diastasis or vertical displacement anteriorly and posteriorly, usually through the SI joint, occasionally through the iliac wing and/or sacrum |
| CM | Combination of other injury patterns, LC/VS being the most common |

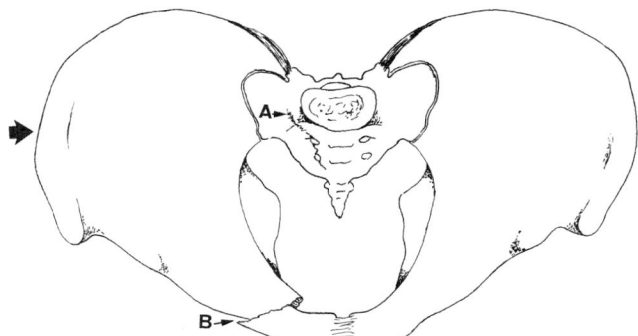

**Fig. 227-5.** Type I—lateral compression fracture: The lateral force is applied posteriorly (*arrow*). This causes a crush effect on the SIJ: this may be visible radiographically as a sacral fracture (*A*). The characteristic fracture pattern of the pubic rami will be seen (*B*). No ligamentous injury is seen.

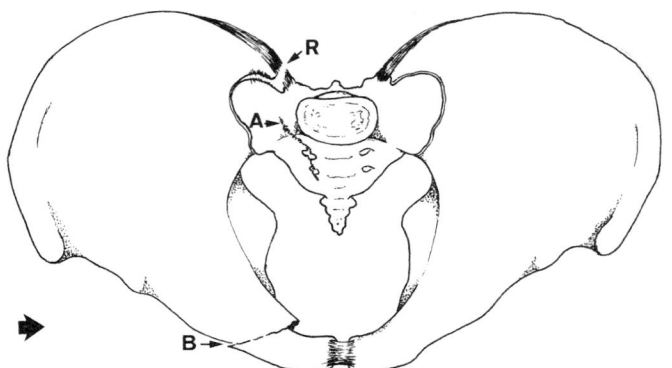

**Fig. 227-6.** Type II—lateral compression fracture: The force is applied anteriorly (*arrow*), causing the typical anterior pubic rami fractures (*B*). In this case, however, rotation of the pelvis around the anterior sacral margin may occur, causing rupture of the posterior sacroiliac ligaments (*R*). A crush fracture of the sacrum may also be seen (*A*).

**Avulsion fracture of anterior superior iliac spine (Fig. 227-14).** Avulsion occurs because of contraction of the sartorius muscle. Symptoms and signs are local pain, tenderness, and swelling and pain with flexion or abduction of the thigh. There is minimal displacement of the anterior superior iliac spine visible on the AP film of the pelvis.

**Avulsion fracture of anterior inferior iliac spine.** Avulsion occurs because of forceful contraction of the rectus femoris muscle. Symptoms and signs are sharp pain in the groin, difficulty with ambulation, and inability to flex the hip. The AP film shows downward displacement of the fragment, but this must be differentiated from the epiphyseal line of the os acetabuli.

**Avulsion fracture of ischial tuberosity.** The mechanism of injury is contraction of the hamstrings, and the fracture is seen in youths whose apophyses are not united. Symptoms and signs include acute or chronic pain with sitting or on flexing the thigh with the knee extended. Rectal examination reveals tuberosity tenderness. The roentgenogram shows detachment of the apophysis from the ischium with minimal displacement. The apophysis closes between ages 20 and 25.

**Fracture of single ramus of pubis or ischium (see Fig. 227-14).** These injuries are commonly seen in the elderly, and the mechanism

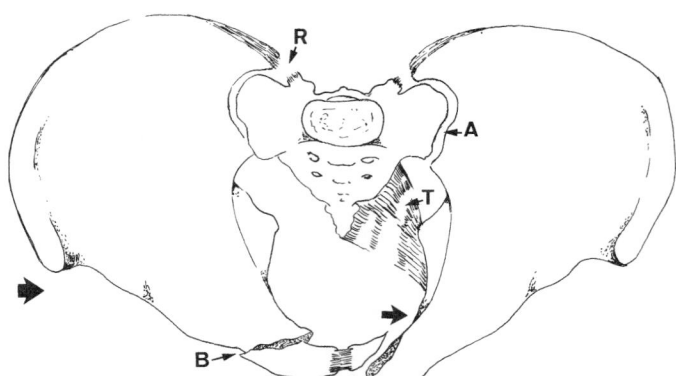

**Fig. 227-8.** Type III—lateral compression fracture: The force is applied anteriorly (*arrow*), causing internal rotation of the anterior hemipelvis. Continuing through to the contralateral hemipelvis (*arrow*), the force causes it to rotate externally. The result is a pattern of lateral compression on the ipsilateral side, with apparent AP compression on the contralateral side. This results in rupture of the posterior sacroiliac ligaments on the ipsilateral side (*R*) and sacrospinous/sacrotuberous complex (*T*) and anterior ligaments (A) on the contralateral side. Typical pubic rami fractures (B) are to be expected.

of injury is usually a fall with direct trauma. Symptoms and signs include local pain and tenderness and inability to ambulate.

Examination of the pubic bones will usually distinguish a fracture of the pubis from a femoral neck fracture, but a lateral film of the injured hip is recommended to rule out femoral neck injury. The AP roentgenogram of the pelvis shows a nondisplaced fracture of the ramus.

**Ischium body fractures.** The incidence of ischial body injury is very low. The mechanism of injury is violent, external trauma, such as a fall in a sitting position. Symptoms and signs include local pain and tenderness, and pain with hamstring movement.

The x-ray film shows fracture of the body or tuberosity of the ischium. A large fragment with comminution or a butterfly pattern may be seen on the AP film of the pelvis.

**Iliac wing (Duverney) fractures (see Fig. 227-14).** The mechanism of injury in an iliac wing fracture is direct trauma, usually lat-

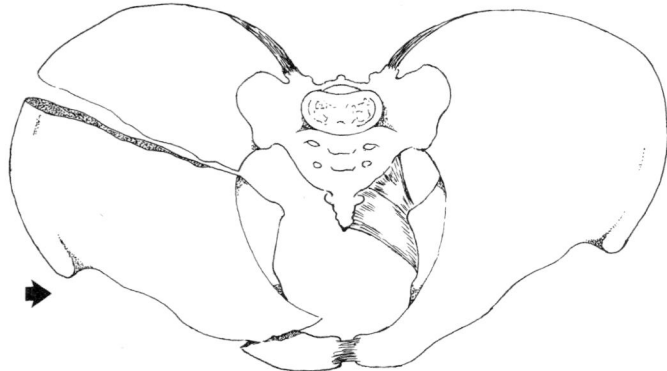

**Fig. 227-7.** Alternatively (compared to Fig. 227-6), a fracture of the iliac wing may occur, which dissipates the rotational forces and thus leaves the posterior ligaments intact.

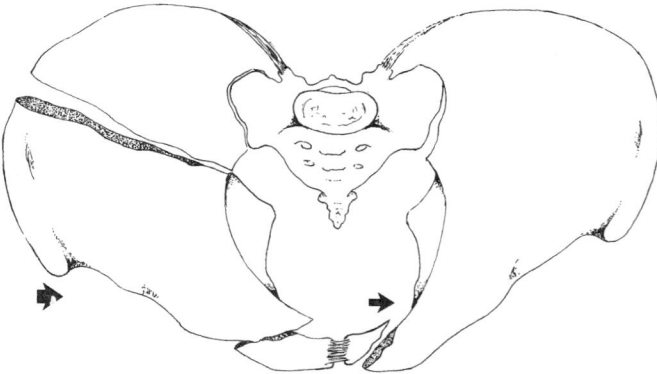

**Fig. 227-9.** Alternatively (compared to Fig. 227-8), as in type II B fractures (Fig. 227-7), there may be an iliac wing fracture, sparing the posterior SIJ on the ipsilateral side.

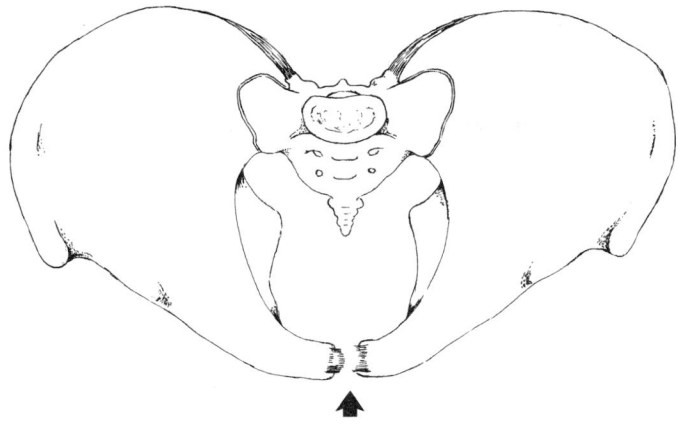

**Fig. 227-10.** Type I—AP compression fracture: The force is delivered in an AP direction (*large arrow*), tending to "open" the pelvis. This gives rise to mild splaying of the symphysis, due to rupture of the anterior sacroiliac ligaments.

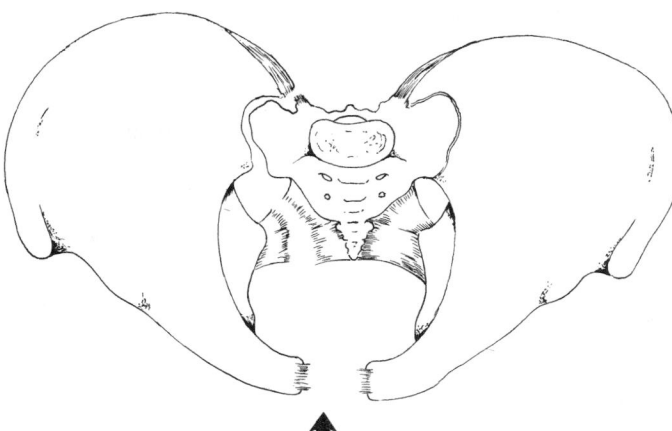

**Fig. 227-12.** Type III—AP compression fracture: There is total disruption of the SIJ due to wide "opening" of the pelvis. All supporting ligament groups, including the posterior sacroiliac ligaments, may be disrupted.

eral to medial. Symptoms and signs include pain, swelling, and tenderness over the iliac wing. There is severe pain on ambulation, and Trendelenburg's sign (waddling gait) is present. Although accompanying abdominal injuries are infrequent, abdominal rigidity, lower quadrant tenderness, and ileus are common findings. The AP film of the pelvis shows minimal displacement of fragments.

**Sacral fractures.** Transverse fractures of the sacrum (see Fig. 227-14) are more common with massive pelvic injuries. The mechanism of injury is direct trauma by a posterior-to-anterior force, producing a transverse fracture. A rectal examination with the other hand on the sacrum causes pain and movement at the fracture site.

Roentgenogram interpretation may be difficult, and exactly aligned AP views are necessary to show the fracture. Look for a transverse fracture line at the level of the lower SI joint, and irregularity, buckling, or sharp angulation of the foramina. Examine the body and wings closely. A lateral view may show displacement anteriorly. Sacral root injury, especially S1 and S2, may be present.

**Coccyx fractures.** Coccygeal fractures are more frequent in women and are generally caused by direct violence or a fall in the sitting position. Symptoms and signs include pain, tenderness, and swelling and ecchymoses over the lower sacral region. There may be pain on getting up from a sitting position or straining at stool. The rectal examination reveals pain and movement of the coccyx.

The roentgenogram is of questionable value, but AP and lateral views with sharp flexion of the thighs may demonstrate the fracture.

## Fractures of the Acetabulum

Acetabular fractures are increasing in frequency with an increase in automobile accidents. They are seen commonly with other pelvic injuries. The roentgenographic anatomy of acetabular fractures is shown in Fig. 227-15. There are four anatomic types of fractures, and

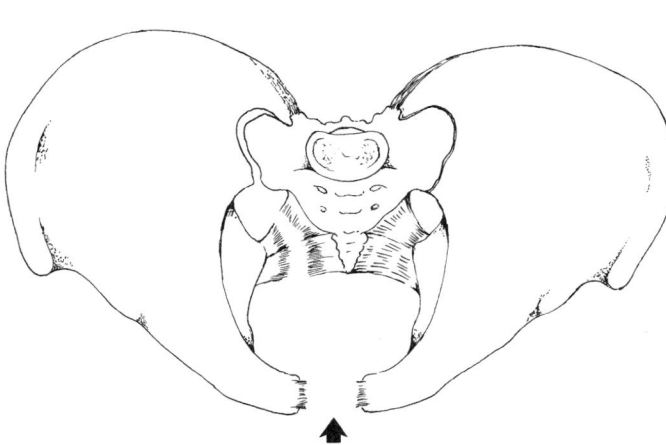

**Fig. 227-11.** Type II—AP compression fracture: The AP force vector (*large arrow*) has caused further "opening" of the anterior pelvis, with additional rupture of the anterior sacroiliac, sacrotuberous, and sacrospinous ligaments.

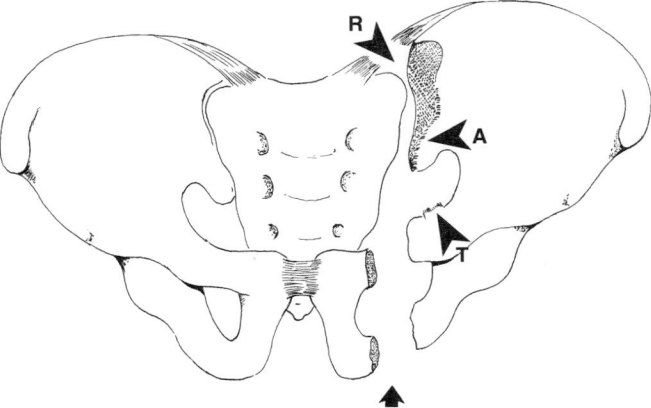

**Fig. 227-13.** Vertical shear vector: The injury force vector is delivered in a vertical plane (large arrow), causing disruption along this line. Fractures of the pubic rami are usually seen anteriorly, while fractures of the sacrum, SIJ, or iliac wing are usually seen posteriorly. The fractures are vertical and are associated with vertical displacement of fragments. Ligamentous injury to the posterior (*R*) and anterior (*A*) sacroiliac ligaments may be seen, as well to sacrospinous/sacrotuberous (*T*), and (possibly) symphysis ligaments.

**Table 227-2.** Local Associated Injuries

| | % OCCURRENCE | | |
| --- | --- | --- | --- |
| | Severe Hemorrhage | Bladder Rupture | Urethra |
| Lateral compression fractures | | | |
| Type I | 0.5 | 4.0 | 2.0 |
| Type II | 36.0 | 7.0 | 0.0 |
| Type III | 60.0 | 20.0 | 20.0 |
| AP compression fractures | | | |
| Type I | 1.0 | 8.0 | 12.0 |
| Type II | 28.0 | 11.0 | 23.0 |
| Type III | 53.0 | 14.0 | 36.0 |
| Vertical shear fractures | 75.0 | 15.0 | 25.0 |
| Mixed patterns | 58.0 | 16.0 | 21.0 |

SOURCE: From Young JWR, Burgess AR: *Radiologic Management of Pelvic Ring Fractures: Systematic Radiologic Diagnosis.* Baltimore, Urban & Schwarzenberg, 1987. Used by permission.

all are associated with hip dislocations: posterior (Figs. 227-16 and 227-17), ilioischial column (Fig. 227-18), transverse (Fig. 227-19), and iliopubic column (Fig. 227-20). In addition, combinations of any of these fractures can occur.

**Posterior fracture.** The mechanism of injury in a posterior fracture is direct trauma to a flexed knee and hip. Anteroposterior and lateral radiologic views easily demonstrate the posterior acetabular fracture with the posterior hip dislocation. Complications are sciatic nerve injury and femoral fractures.

**Ilioischial column fracture.** The mechanism of injury is posteriorly directed force to a knee with the thigh abducted and flexed. The AP x-ray film demonstrates a large, medially displaced fragment with central dislocation of the femoral head. The most common complication is sciatic nerve injury.

**Transverse fracture of acetabulum.** The mechanism is force lateral to medial over the greater trochanter, or force posterior to anterior on the posterior pelvis with the hip flexed. An AP x-ray film clearly demonstrates the fracture with a central hip dislocation.

**Iliopubic column fracture.** The mechanism of injury is a lateral force to the greater trochanter with the hip externally rotated. On roentgenography, there is marked external rotation of the hip. The ilioischial line is disrupted, and the anterior lip is fractured. Further discussion on acetabular fractures appears below under "Trauma to the Hip and Femur."

## Treatment and Complications

Anatomic restoration is required. If the difficult task of reduction of the femoral head and exact restoration of the displaced fractured acetabulum cannot be done quickly and safely, surgery is indicated. If there is no displacement, bed rest is the treatment of choice. If redislocation occurs, the hip is unstable and surgery is necessary.

Failure to recognize pelvic trauma leads to nonstabilization of the fracture, which, in turn, enhances blood loss and causes further injuries. It may also lead to an incomplete evaluation of pelvic injury.

It is imperative that the physician recognize concomitant injuries, especially those requiring immediate evaluation. Complications include hemorrhage, myositis ossificans, infection, thrombophlebitis, and sciatic nerve injuries.

**Hemorrhage.** Hemorrhage is a major cause of death in pelvic injuries. One series reported that patients with double breaks of the pelvic ring require blood replacement $2\frac{1}{2}$ times more often than those with single breaks or nonpelvic ring fractures and need $2\frac{1}{2}$ times more blood when blood is administered. Retroperitoneal bleeding is an inevitable complication, and up to 6 L of blood can be ac-

commodated in this space! Both small and large vessels, especially the superior gluteal and internal pudendal branches of the internal iliac artery, can be disrupted, with hemorrhage dissecting from the back to the buttocks.

General resuscitative measures include massive crystalloid, colloid, and blood replacement. Patients may require massive blood replacement.

The use of the antishock garment is controversial. It may be helpful in controlling bleeding sites, and increases blood pressure by increasing peripheral vascular resistance. Disadvantages include de-

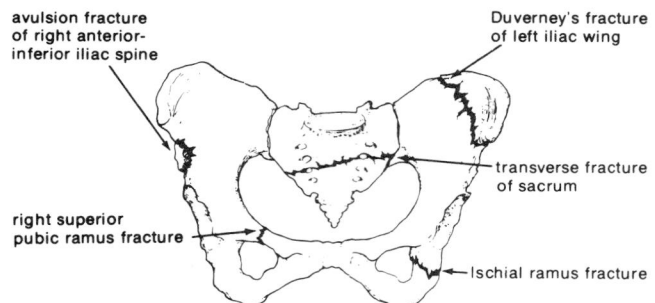

Type I: Fracture of individual bones without break in pelvic ring. Examples shown above.

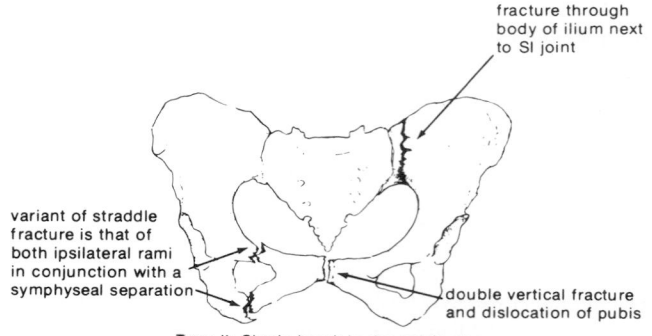

Type II: Single break in the pelvic ring. See examples above.

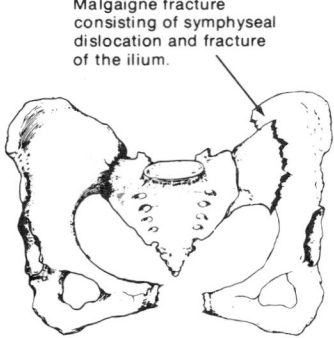

Type III: Double break in pelvic ring.

**Fig. 227-14.** Pelvic fractures (type I, II, and III) according to classification by Key JA, Conwell HE: *The Management of Fractures, Dislocations, and Sprains,* ed 4, St Lous, Mosby, 1946, p. 857, as adapted by Kane WJ: Fractures of the pelvis, in Rockwood CA Jr, Green DP (eds): *Fractures,* ed 2. Philadelphia, Lippincott 1984, vol. 2, pp. 1133–1142.

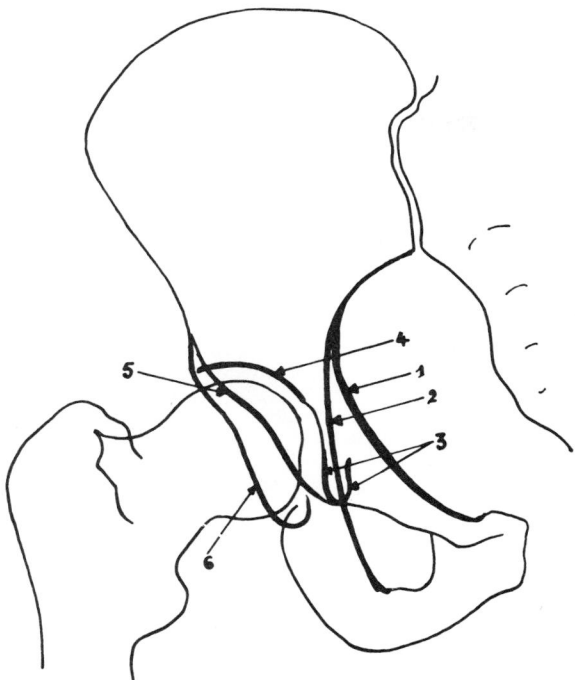

**Fig. 227-15.** Roentgenographic anatomy of type IV acetabular fractures. The AP view shows (1) arcuate (iliopectineal) line, (2) ilioischial roentgenographic line, (3) roentgenographic U, (4) roof, (5) anterior lip, and (6) posterior lip. (*From* Judet R, Judet J, Letournel E: Fractures of the acetabulum: Classification and surgical approaches for open reduction. *J Bone Joint Surg* 46A:1616, 1964. Used by permission.)

creased visibility and access to the abdomen and lower extremities and the risk of compartment syndrome with prolonged application. Early orthopedic consultation should be considered for placement of external fixator device to help control hemorrhage. Early use of this device has been shown to reduce the incidence of adult respiratory distress syndrome.

If the patient is exsanguinating, angiography can be done and small bleeding sites controlled. Most authorities agree that aggressive fluid and blood replacement is best. Laparotomy is a last measure.

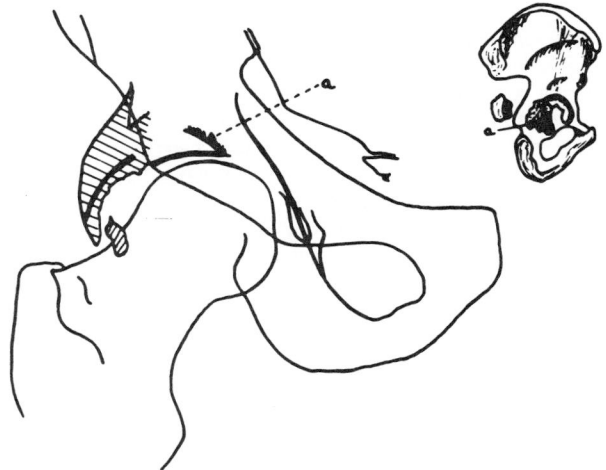

**Fig. 227-16.** Fracture of posterior lip with some impaction and comminution. (*From* Judet R, Judet J, Letournel E: 1964. Used by permission.)

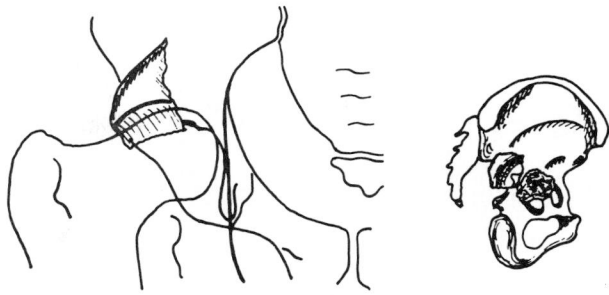

**Fig. 227-17.** Posterior superior rim fracture. (*From* Judet R, Judet J, Letournel E: 1964. Used by permission.)

**Urinary tract injuries.** Urinary tract injuries are discussed in Chapter 221.

**Gynecologic injury.** Gynecologic injuries are uncommonly associated with pelvic trauma. Vaginal laceration is the most common injury seen with anterior pelvic fractures. A bimanual pelvic examination should be performed on all women with pelvic fractures. If blood is found in a woman of childbearing age, a speculum examination must be carried out to distinguish menses from laceration. Treatment is irrigation and debridement in the operating room with repair of wounds and antibiotic therapy.

A high fetal death rate is associated with pelvic trauma in pregnancy if the mother is in shock; if there is placental, uterine, or direct fetal injury; or if the mother dies. Immediate cesarean section must be considered.

**Rectal injuries.** Rectal injuries are uncommon and are usually associated with urinary injuries and ischial fractures. Diagnosis is by rectal examination, whereupon blood is found in the rectum. Treatment includes a diverting colostomy with washout of the distal colon, and presacral space drainage. Antibiotics should be given as soon as the injury is discovered.

**Ruptured diaphragm.** Ruptured diaphragm associated with fracture of the pelvis may be more common than previously thought. It may be associated with rib injuries. Diagnosis is by physical findings, such as displacement of the heart toward the right, absent breath sounds, presence of bowel sounds in the chest, and a positive chest x-ray film if the defect is large. Diagnosis may be difficult if the defect is small.

**Nerve root injury.** Nerve root or peripheral nerve injuries can occur because of traction, pressure from hemorrhage, callus or fibrous tissue, and impingement-laceration by bone fragments. The onset of symptoms and signs may be delayed, but deficits usually follow a nerve root pattern. Lumbar nerve root injuries are associated with SI joint dislocation or fracture. Sacral root injuries are associated with sacral fractures, especially fractures of S1 and S2.

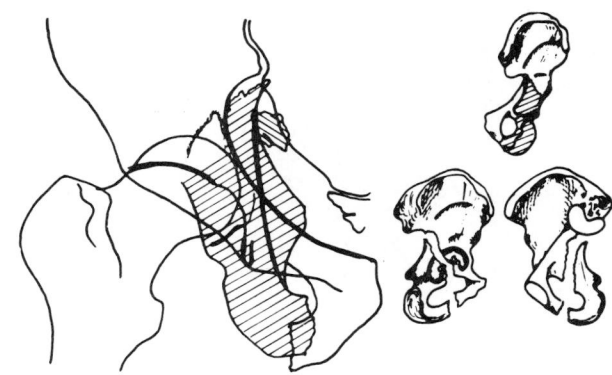

**Fig. 227-18.** Ilioischial fracture. (*From* Judet R, Judet J, Letournel E: 1964. Used by permission.)

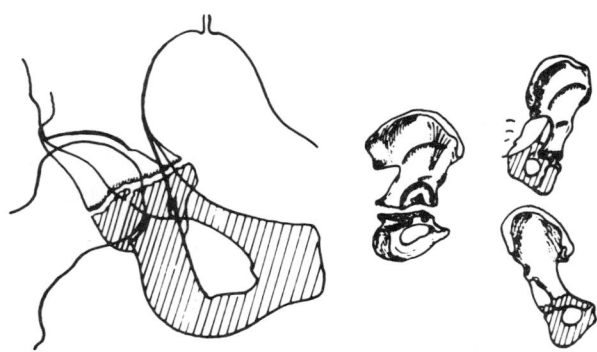

**Fig. 227-19.** Transverse fracture without displacement. (*From* Judet R, Judet J, Letournel E: 1964. Used by permission.)

## Pelvic Fractures in Children

Commonly caused by automobile-pedestrian accidents, pelvic fractures in children have a high incidence of concomitant injuries because of the smaller protection afforded by the developing pelvis and the significant trauma incurred. Hemorrhage determines mortality. Children in shock who respond poorly to fluid replacement have the highest mortality. Frequent concomitant injuries include head and neck injuries, intra-abdominal injuries, and long bone fractures. The incidence of genitourinary injuries is similar to that of adults. Major thoracic injuries are rare but particularly dangerous because they are often overlooked.

Postponement of surgery until stabilization of circulation is recommended unless the patient is exsanguinating despite treatment. If the child does not respond to transfusions equal to the estimated total blood volume (TBV) (88 mL/kg × wt [kg] = TBV) within 1 h, suspect major vascular injury and operate. Both arterial and venous injuries are associated with significant SI joint injury.

## TRAUMA TO THE HIP AND FEMUR

### Anatomy

The hip is a ball-and-socket joint made up of the acetabulum and the femur (Fig. 227-21). The hip includes the acetabulum and the proximal femur 2 to 3 inches below the lesser trochanter. The functions of the hip are weight-bearing and movement. The fibrous capsule that surrounds the joint on all sides is exceedingly strong. It attaches around the acetabulum proximally and runs to the intertrochanteric line distally on the anterior surface. Posteriorly, it falls short of the in-

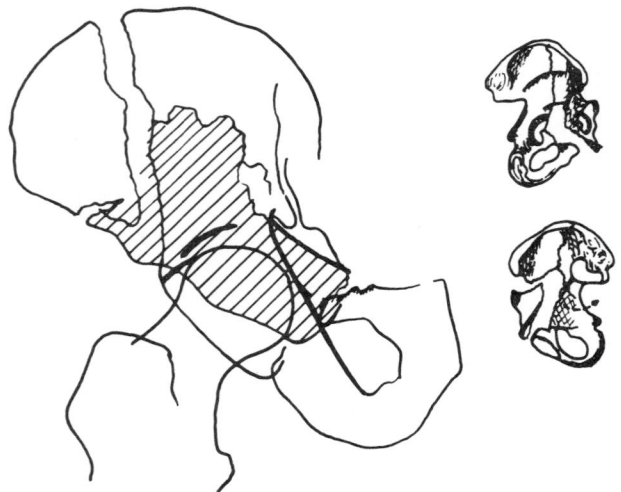

**Fig. 227-20.** Iliopubic fracture. (*From* Judet R, Judet J, Letournel E: 1964. Used by permission.)

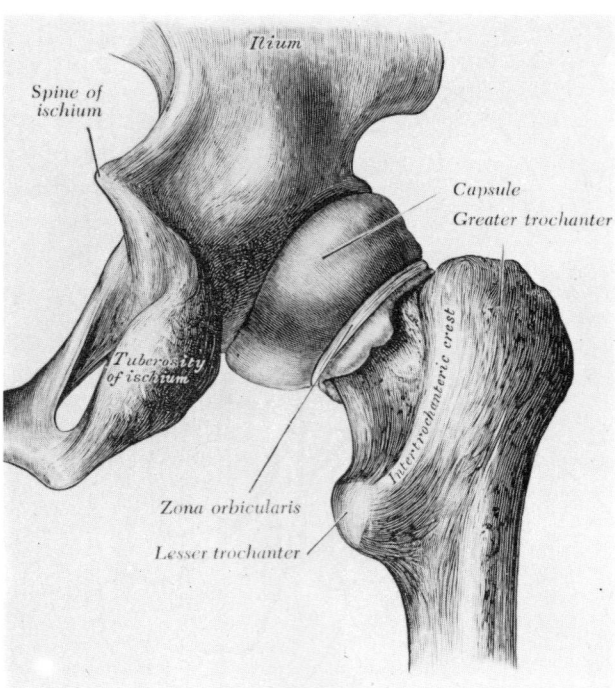

**Fig. 227-21.** Synovial membrane of capsule of hip joint (distended). Posterior aspect. [*From* Gray H: *Anatomy of the Human Body,* ed 29, Goss CM (ed). Philadelphia, Lea & Febiger, p. 344. Used by permission.]

tertrochanteric crest and inserts on the neck of the femur. It is weakest posteriorly.

The blood supply of the femoral head is derived from nutrient branches of the obturator, medial femoral circumflex, lateral femoral circumflex, and superior and inferior gluteal arteries. These course beneath the reflection of the capsule on the neck of the femur and also along the ligamentum teres. The capsular vessels are much more important than those of the ligamentum teres.

## Clinical Evaluation

### Physical Examination

The examination of the hip begins with a detailed history and complete examination of the patient. The pelvis and hip are then carefully evaluated. The unclothed, erect patient is inspected for a list, injuries, scars, or asymmetry of the muscles. Gait should be tested, if possible.

If the patient is a trauma victim, after primary survey and initial stabilization the physician should observe the position of the extremities, looking for deformities, lacerations, or bruises, and should test for stability and range of motion. On palpation, the physician should feel for irregularities in movement at the iliac crest, pubic rami, and ischial rami. He or she should compress the pelvis lateral to medial through the iliac crest; anterior to posterior through the symphysis pubis; and anterior to posterior through the iliac crest, seeking pain and tenderness. Also, the physician should compress the greater trochanters of the hips.

If no significant abnormalities are found, range of motion of the hips should then be studied. If rotation of the hip with the leg in extension is painful all other maneuvers should be done cautiously. If a hip or pelvic fracture or dislocation is identified in a trauma victim, the physician *must assume* that intra-abdominal, retroperitoneal, and urologic injuries have occurred as well until it has been proved otherwise. The physician should always perform a detailed neurovascular examination and a rectal examination, looking for displacement of the prostate in male patients. Associated femoral shaft fractures should be ruled out.

## Radiologic Evaluation

Roentgenographic evaluation of the pelvis and hips is a must in all unconscious patients who have sustained multiple injuries. Lower extremity long bone fractures, as well as pelvic symptoms or signs, are also indications for these x-ray examinations. The x-ray evaluation should include a standard AP and a lateral view of the pelvis. If further studies are needed, AP views of either hemipelvis, internal and external oblique views of the hemipelvis as described by Judet and colleagues, or "inlet" and "tilt" views may be done. In certain instances, such views allow better identification and detail of the acetabulum and femoral head and neck. The physician must always inspect not only the hip joint but the femur and knee as well when evaluating hip disorders on x-ray films. Disorders to the knee and the femoral shaft often occur with hip injuries.

## Classification of Hip Fractures

Hip fractures are classified as femoral head and neck (intracapsular); and, trochanteric, intertrochanteric, and subtrochanteric (extracapsular). (Fig. 227-22). The prognosis for successful union and restoration of normal function varies considerably with the fracture.

In intracapsular fractures with displacement, the femoral neck vessels are compromised due to a tear or compression secondary to an intracapsular hemarthrosis. The blood supply through the ligamentum teres may not be sufficient to nourish the entire femoral head. There-fore, avascular necrosis inevitably results unless some of the capsular vessels remain intact. Basilar neck and intertrochanteric fractures below the capsule rarely sever important arteries.

## Femoral Head Fractures

Isolated femoral head fractures occur infrequently. They are usually associated with dislocations of the hip. Shear fractures of the superior aspect of the femoral head are associated with anterior dislocations, and shear fractures of the inferior femoral head are associated with posterior dislocations.

In most instances, the symptoms and signs are those of the associated dislocation rather than of the fracture itself. The standard AP and lateral x-ray views usually demonstrate the fragment adequately. When there is an associated dislocation, the postreduction films offer a better view of the fracture fragment.

Treatment by the orthopedic consultant is to reduce the associated dislocation and then attain anatomic reduction of the fracture fragment. Complications are associated with the high-energy trauma that produces the fracture-dislocation, that is, the more comminuted the fracture, the more severe the dislocation and the greaterr the severity of trauma to the patient. Life-threatening injuries must then be ruled out.

## Femoral Neck Fractures

Femoral neck fractures are commonly seen among older adults, due to osteoporosis, and occur more frequently in women than in men.

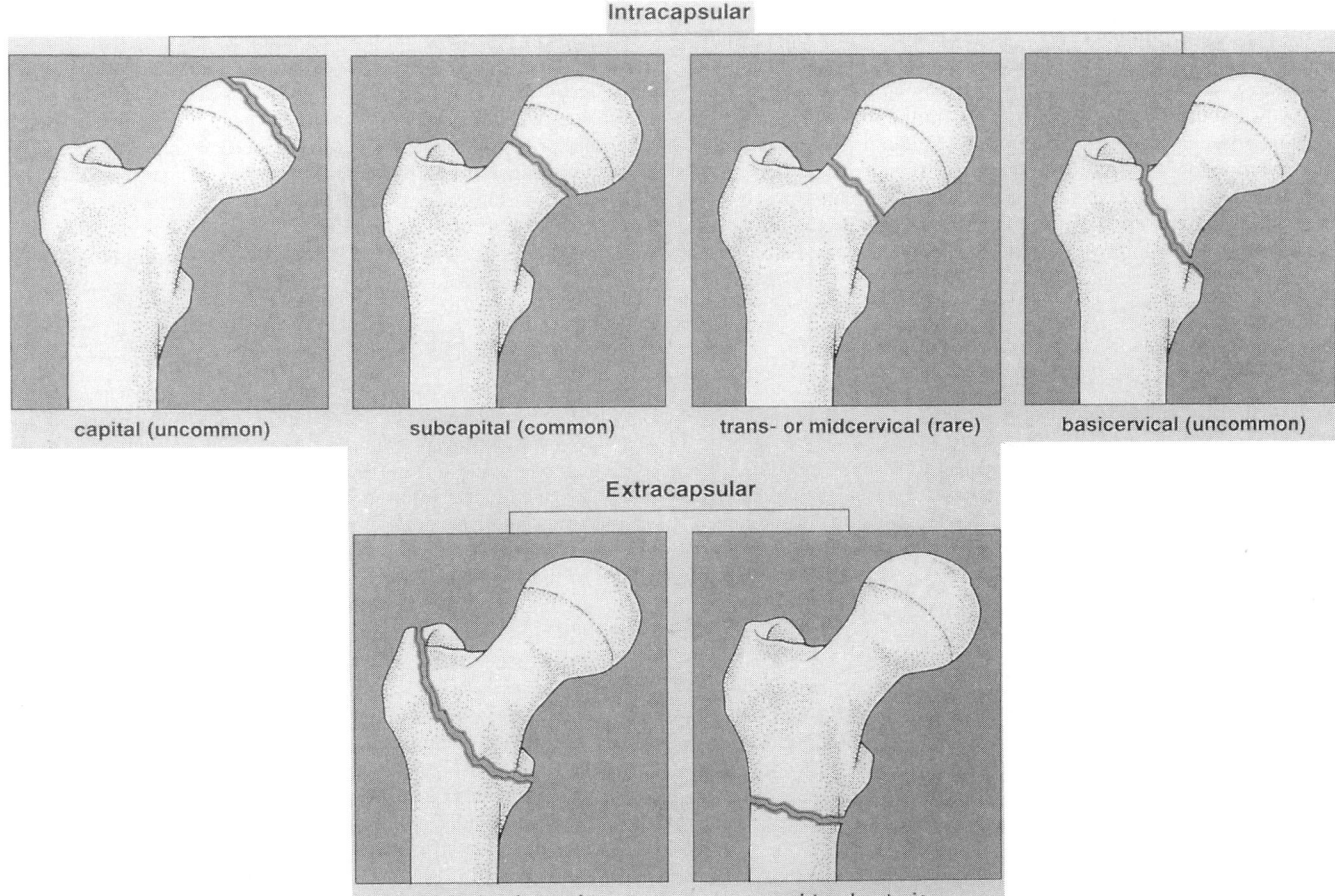

**Fig. 227-22.** Fractures of the proximal femur are traditionally classified as intracapsular and extracapsular. (From Greenspan A. *Orthopedic Radiology.* Philadelphia: JB Lippincott, p. 5.17, 1988. Used with permission.)

These fractures are rare among the younger population. The cause of such fractures is usually minor trauma or torsion in the patient with osteoporosis or osteomalacia. In younger patients, the high kinetic energy sustained in the major trauma causes a fracture through normal bone with marked soft tissue disruption and comminution.

The classification of femoral neck fractures is by fragment displacement. The symptoms seen with femoral neck fractures range from complaints of mild pain in the groin or inner thigh in patients with an incomplete fracture to moderate to severe pain in patients with displaced fractures.

Patients who have sustained a fracture without displacement may walk with some limping rather than being completely unable to bear weight. Their only physical findings are minor pain with movement and minimal muscle spasm limiting range of motion. In contrast, displaced fractures cause severe pain, inability to ambulate, limited range of motion, and no palpable movement of the extracapsular head. The patient lies with the extremity in *slight* external rotation, abduction, and shortening.

Radiographic evaluation is essential in any patient suspected of having a femoral neck fracture. Stress fractures, however, may not show up on x-ray for days or weeks, so repeat films or bone scans in symptomatic patients are necessary. The standard AP view should have the patient maximally internally rotated to best demonstrate the femoral neck. The AP view should be inspected for a fracture line starting on the superior surface of the neck. These fracture lines routinely become complete within 10 to 14 days. Also, disruption of Shenton's line may be appreciated on the AP view in some instances. If there is any concern that the patient has sustained a fracture that is not visible on the initial x-ray examination, the patient should be conservatively treated and x-ray films should be made again in 10 to 14 days; or the physician may order a bone scan in 1 to 2 days, which demonstrates the fracture in most instances.

In contrast, displaced fractures are obvious on the AP film, but a lateral view should also be done to ascertain the exact position. The orthopedic surgeon's goal of treatment for femoral neck fractures is anatomic reduction and stability. Treatment for nondisplaced or impacted fractures is somewhat controversial but usually involves a form of internal fixation. Displaced fractures definitely require emergency surgery for fixation. Prosthetic replacements may be required in certain instances. Special note should be made of stress fractures because some are treated in a conservative manner and others are treated with internal fixation, depending on the type of fracture and the patient's cooperation.

The complications of femoral neck fractures are significant. They include infections, emboli, and avascular necrosis, which is the most feared early complication. Avascular necrosis has an incidence of 15 percent in nondisplaced fractures and rises to near 90 percent with completely displaced fractures. A higher incidence is also associated with more severe fractures or fractures that are not surgically reduced to anatomic position within 48 h. Nonunion, which occurs in approximately 5 to 15 percent of patients who have been treated properly, is a later complication of such fractures.

## Trochanteric Fractures

Greater trochanteric fractures are usually due to avulsions at the insertion of the gluteus medius. In the younger population (7 to 17 years of age), this is a true epiphyseal separation, in contrast to the adult population, in which this is an avulsion fracture with comminution in some instances. The patient presents with pain, especially with abduction and extension, and a limp. Also, there is tenderness to palpation over the greater trochanter.

Standard AP and lateral x-ray views reveal displacement in the superior-posterior area, or comminution. The treatment is controversial but ranges from conservative to surgical fixation, depending on the patient's age and displacement of the fracture. Orthopedic consultation is indicated.

Lesser trochanteric fractures due to an avulsion of the iliopsoas, are commonly seen in children and young athletic adults. These patients present with pain during flexion and internal rotation maneuvers. In most instances, the treatment is bed rest and then gradual weight-bearing to regain full activity.

If greater than 2-cm displacement is seen on the standard AP and lateral views, then screw fixation by the consulting orthopedic surgeon may be indicated.

## Intertrochanteric Fractures

These fractures are defined as extracapsular fractures occurring in a line between the greater and lesser trochanters. Intertrochanteric fractures generally occur in the elderly and are more common in women, again due to the high incidence of osteoporosis. The mechanism of injury is usually a fall or occasionally an automobile accident. It is postulated that a rotational component along with the direct trauma is involved in some instances as well.

Symptoms and signs include pain, swelling of the hip, local ecchymosis, and pain with any hip movement or weight-bearing. Moreover, the extremity is markedly externally rotated and shortened, in contrast to the minimal deformities associated with femoral neck fractures. These fractures are classified as stable or unstable. Stable fractures are defined as ones in which the medial cortices of the neck and femoral fragments abut. X-ray evaluation should include AP and lateral views, with the AP view having as much internal rotation as possible to adequately visualize the neck.

The traction splint should be taken off to obtain the best quality AP view, that is, the most internal rotation. Severe, life-threatening injuries must be excluded. The consulting orthopedic physician can then admit the patient to the hospital and perform surgical fixation to attain a stable reduction as soon as possible, although this is not an emergency.

The complications and prognosis are related to other associated injuries and prior disease. The overall mortality is approximately 10 to 15 percent. Infection is still a major problem, with an incidence of up to 17 percent. Thromboembolic disease is especially a problem if postoperative mobilization does not occur quickly. Avascular necrosis is rare in these patients, and nonunion is also uncommon. Morbidity is due to the patient's inability to return to prefracture activity.

## Subtrochanteric Fractures

Subtrochanteric fractures may be seen in two different populations. They usually occur secondary to falling in the 40- to 60-year-old patient with osteoporotic or weakened bone. The second population is young persons who have suffered major trauma with significant kinetic energies directed into the femur. These fractures may be an extension of an intertrochanteric or other isolated fracture and are usually classified as stable or unstable, with stable defined as bony contact of the medial and posterior femoral cortices.

The symptoms and signs are similar to those of trochanteric or femoral fractures, with local pain, deformity, swelling, crepitance, etc. These patients can lose a large amount of blood into the thigh area and may present in hypovolemic shock. Because this injury is due to significant trauma, other, more life-threatening injuries must be excluded prior to treatment of this specific fracture.

Standard AP and lateral x-ray views of the hip are necessary to properly assess the fracture. Moreover, x-ray studies of the pelvis, femur, and knee are indicated to rule out associated fractures.

Treatment consists of immobilization with a traction apparatus and proper evaluation of the entire patient to rule out associated severe injuries. After the patient has stabilized and secondary evaluation has occurred, the orthopedic consultant should determine if this failure is amenable to internal fixation.

The complications are similar to those of intertrochanteric fractures, except that there is a higher incidence of nonunion. Malunion and delayed union occur as well in this population.

## Hip Dislocations

Hip dislocations can be classified as anterior, posterior, and central. Acetabular fracture with central hip dislocation has been discussed under acetabular fractures.

### Anterior Dislocations

About 10 percent of hip dislocations are anterior (Fig. 227-23A and B), and the majority are secondary to automobile accidents, but they may also result from a fall, or a blow to the back while squatting. In anterior dislocations, the femoral head rests anterior to the coronal plane of the acetabulum. Anterior dislocations can be superior or inferior (obturator, thyroid, perineal) depending on the degree of hip flexion present at the time of injury. If the hip is abducted, externally rotated, and flexed at the time of injury, inferior dislocation occurs. If the hip is abducted, externally rotated, and extended, superior dislocation occurs. The mechanism of injury is forced abduction that causes the femoral head to be levered out through an anterior capsular tear. The affected extremity is in abduction and external rotation. However, the clinical appearance of superior versus inferior dislocations is dramatically different (Fig. 227-23C and D). Neurovascular compromise is an unusual, but possible, complication.

An AP film of the pelvis easily demonstrates the femoral head to be anterior to the acetabulum. A lateral view illustrates the anterior dislocation more clearly, although it may be difficult to obtain because of the patient's pain.

Treatment for the dislocation is early closed reduction, usually under general anesthesia. Strong, in-line traction is done with simultaneous flexion and internal rotation. Finally, the hip is abducted once the head clears the rim of the acetabulum. The dislocation should be reduced quickly, within a few hours, because the longer the delay in reduction, the higher the incidence of avascular necrosis. Post reduction radiographs should be specifically examined for acetabular or femoral head fractures not appreciated on the initial films.

### Posterior Dislocations

Posterior dislocations (Fig. 227-24A) constitute 80 to 90 percent of hip dislocations. They are caused by force applied to a flexed knee, directed posteriorly. Acetabular fractures may result as well. On examination, the extremity is found to be shortened, internally rotated, and adducted (Fig. 227-24B). Concomitant life-threatening injuries must be ruled out.

Anteroposterior and lateral x-ray films of the pelvis and hip will reveal the dislocation, but further assessment of the acetabulum and femur must be done to rule out fractures. The oblique views of Judet and colleagues will reveal an acetabular fracture. Also, inferior

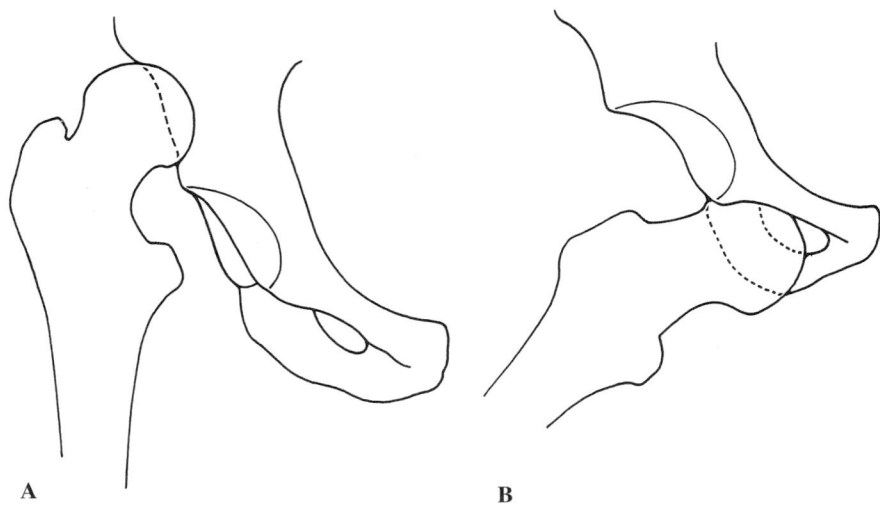

A          B

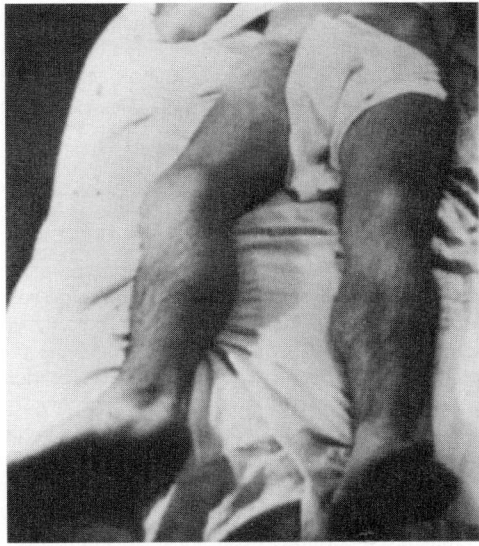

C

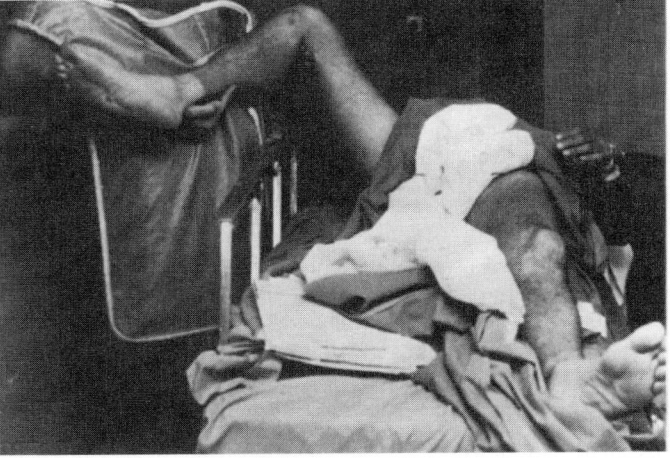

D

**Fig. 227-23.** (A) Anterior superior dislocation of the hip. (B) Inferior dislocations (obturator, thyroid, or perineal). (C) Clinical appearance of a superior-type anterior dislocation of the hip. (D) Clinical appearance of an inferior-type dislocation of the hip. (From Rockwood CA Jr, Green DP, Bucholz RW (eds). *Fractures in Adults,* 3rd ed. Philadelphia: JB Lippincott, vol. 2, pp. 1576, 1578, 1587, 1588, 1991. Used with permission).

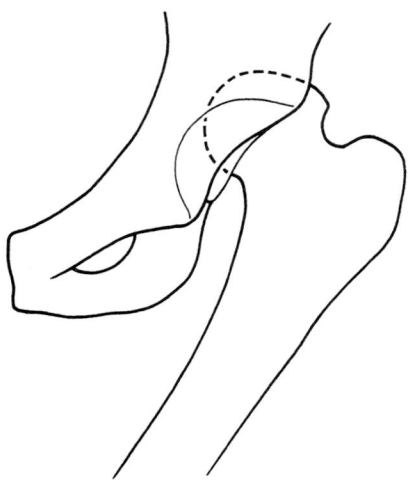

**A**

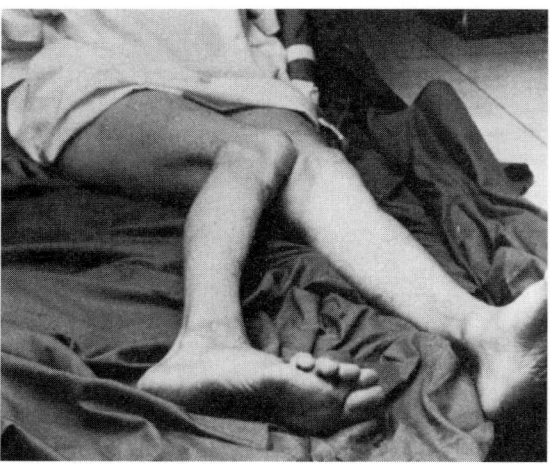

**B**

**Fig. 227-24.** (A) Posterior dislocation of the hip. (B) The clinical appearance of a posterior dislocation of the right hip. (From Rockwood CA Jr, Green DP, Bucholz RW (eds). *Fractures in Adults,* 3rd ed. Philadelphia: JB Lippincott, vol. 2, pp. 1580, 1591, 1991. Used with permission.)

femoral head fracture will be seen on the AP or oblique view. Hip dislocations are difficult to recognize if there is an associated femoral shaft fracture, so roentgenograms of the pelvis and hips should be routinely obtained in such cases.

The treatment of posterior dislocation without fracture is closed reduction, preferably under general anesthesia, as quickly as possible and always within 6 hours. In-line traction, gentle flexion to 90°, and then gentle internal-to-external rotation is done (Allis maneuver). The Stimson maneuver may prove useful in certain situations.

Complications include sciatic nerve injury in about 10 percent of the patients and avascular necrosis that increases in direct proportion to the delay in adequate reduction.

## Hip Injuries in Children

### Fractures and Dislocations

Fractures of the proximal end of the femur are extremely rare in children. Trauma may produce a displaced epiphysis or a fracture of the neck, trochanteric, or subtrochanteric region. Traumatic epiphyseal separation is probably less common than the previously mentioned fractures, but is more common than dislocation. The treatment is anatomic reduction, usually best obtained by surgery. There is a significant complication rate, especially with improper treatment.

Traumatic dislocations in children are rare. They are more common in boys (4:1) and more common between ages 4 and 7, and 11 and 15. The frequency of left versus right is equal, and bilateral dislocations are reportable. Posterior dislocations occur with an 80 to 85 percent frequency. The mechanism of injury and the clinical picture are similar to those seen in traumatic dislocation in the adult. The presence of an associated fracture is rare.

The treatment is closed reduction. Dislocation is an orthopedic emergency, and reductions should be done within 6 hours. Delay in reduction past 24 hours is associated with a much higher incidence of complications.

## Pediatric Disorders of the Hip/Child with a Limp

The differential diagnosis of pediatric disorders of the hip is presented by age. These entities make up the bulk of problems that must be entertained when a toddler or older child or adolescent presents with a limp. (See Chapter 229 for discussion of toddler's fracture—one of the more common causes of limp in a toddler.)

### Congenital Hip Dislocations

Roughly 70 percent of congenital hip dislocations occur in the first baby of the family. The incidence is approximately one in every 1000 live births, and it is six times more common in females than in males. Diagnosis is made by examination consisting of the Ortolani and Barlow tests. X-ray studies are not useful in newborns because there is no visible bone to ascertain femoral head position.

The Ortolani test is done to determine if the hip is subluxed or dislocated. Each thigh is grasped with the thumbs over the medial aspect and the middle fingers over the greater trochanter. The thighs are then lifted and abducted. If reduction of the femoral head takes place, a palpable or audible click may be appreciated.

The Barlow examination assesses hip instability by producing dislocation or subluxation of the hip. Each thigh is grasped with the thumbs over the medial aspect and the fingers over the greater trochanter. With the hip and knees flexed to 90°, the thighs are adducted while gentle downward pressure is applied. The femoral head will slip out of the acetabulum if instability is present.

Orthopedic consultation is indicated for any child with suspected subluxation-dislocation of the hip. The complications of missed congenital hip dislocation are poor hip development and occasionally avascular necrosis.

### Septic Arthritis

The majority of cases of septic arthritis occur in children under the age of 4. It is the most common etiology of a painful hip joint in infants. As a result, any child with a possible hip problem should be assumed to have septic arthritis until proven otherwise. Hematogenous seeding is the most common mode of infection. In older children, local extension from osteomyelitis can occur as well as inadvertent direct needle innoculation when obtaining arterial blood gases. Staphylococcus is the most common organism in infancy and childhood. *Staphylococcus epidermidis* and *Streptococcus* species are the next most frequent in infants. *Haemophilus influenzae* is common during the first 2 years of life and Group B streptococcus during infancy.

Toddlers and older children with septic arthritis generally present with a limp or refusal to ambulate. Infants demonstrate signs and symptoms of infective disorders in general. This includes irritability, fever, and loss of appetite. There can be a delay in the diagnosis in neonates and young infants because of the nonspecific presentation in this age group. Consequently, careful examination of the joints should be performed on all neonates and young infants who are febrile or have evidence of infection elsewhere.

On examination, there is severely limited range of motion due to pain with near rigidity of the joint (pseudoparalysis). The hip typically is held in a flexed, abducted, and externally rotated position because this allows for the greatest volume in the swollen hip joint. Laboratory tests usually show an increased white blood cell count and increased sedimentation rate. Blood cultures are positive in 50

**Table 227-3.** Synovial Analysis

| Disease | White Blood Cells | Polymorphs* |
|---|---|---|
| Normal | <200 | <25% |
| Traumatic | <5000 with many RBCs | <25% |
| Toxic synovitis | 5000–15,000 | <25% |
| Acute rheumatic fever | 10,000–15,000 | 50% |
| Juvenile rheumatoid arthritis | 15,000–80,000 | 75% |
| Septic arthritis | 80,000–200,000 | >75% |

* The WBC count and percentage of polymorphs present can vary in most diseases depending on the severity and duration of the process. Overlap greater than shown in these averages is possible.
SOURCE: Morrissy RT. Septic arthritis. In: Gustilo RB, Genninger RP, Tsukayama DT. Orthopaedic infection: diagnosis and treatment. Philadelphia: WB Saunders, 1989. Used with permission).

percent of cases. Definitive diagnosis is confirmed by needle aspiration, which should be done by an orthopedic consultant under fluoroscopic guidance. Differential diagnosis includes transient synovitis, acute rheumatic fever, and juvenile rheumatoid arthritis (Table 227-3). Treatment of septic arthritis includes hospitalization, appropriate intravenous antibiotic therapy, and surgical drainage.

### Transient Synovitis

Transient synovitis is probably the most common cause for a painful hip in children. It is most prevalent in males with a peak incidence of 5 to 6 years and range of 18 months to 12 years. It is usually unilateral, but can be bilateral. The cause is unknown.

The history of onset may be abrupt, but is more typically gradual. Medical attention is usually sought because of a limp or inability to bear weight. Symptoms are generally less severe than in septic arthritis, but there is some overlap. Approximately 50 percent of patients will have a history of minor trauma or antecedent or intercurrent illness. Erythrocyte sedimentation rate and white blood cell count are usually normal but may be elevated. As a result, they do not discriminate transient synovitis from septic hip, osteomyelitis or other infectious etiology. Hip aspiration for synovial fluid analysis and culture is sometimes required to distinguish this entity from septic arthritis. Because transient synovitis is a diagnosis of exclusion, orthopedic consultation, hip aspiration, and admission to the hospital are recommended. Transient synovitis is self limiting, usually lasting only 3 to 4 days. Response to bed rest and ibuprofen are both diagnostic and therapeutic.

### Legg-Calvé-Perthes Disease

This uncommon disease is most often found in boys aged 5 to 9. It is an idiopathic avascular necrosis of the femoral head. The onset is insidious, and limp is the most common early sign of disease. Examination reveals decreased hip range of motion (especially internal rotation) and spasm. Laboratory examination is usually normal. Typical x-ray changes consist of necrosis, fragmentation, reabsorption, and regeneration but may take years to develop. Findings are best seen on the lateral view. X-rays early on may be normal, but bone scan is usually positive. Most children with Legg-Calvé-Perthes disease require no treatment, but definitive care should be handled by an orthopaedic surgeon.

### Slipped Capital Femoral Epiphysis

This entity occurs most commonly in adolescents and preadolescents between the ages of 10 and 16 years. It occurs bilaterally in 20 to 40 percent of cases and is five times more common in males. The etiol-

ogy is unknown. The condition appears to occur more commonly with certain body types, specifically patients with Frohlich's type of obesity with underdeveloped genitalia and in long, slender, rapidly growing adolescents.

With this condition, the onset of symptoms is generally insidious, though sudden development of them can occur. Early symptoms consist of groin discomfort after activity. With progression, hip stiffness (particularly limited internal rotation) and limp may develop. Pain, as with any primary hip complaint, may be referred to the knee.

Radiographic examination including anteroposterior and lateral views of the hip is necessary to make the diagnosis. Initial films may be normal, prompting the need for repeat examination if symptoms persist. A slip of the epiphyseal plate posteriorly is best seen on the lateral view. Emergency department treatment consists of making the patient non–weight-bearing and consulting orthopedics. Definitive therapy uses traction and surgical fixation.

### Open Hip Injuries

Open wounds to the hip joint should be treated like any other open joint. An initial culture should be done and the wound cleaned by debridement and copious irrigation in the operating room. Primary wound care with secondary closure is suggested by most authorities. Tetanus prophylaxis is ensured by the administration of toxoid and immune globulin if indicated. Prophylactic antibiotics are recommended. Continuous irrigation of the hip may be indicated.

### Bursitis

Approximately 18 bursa surround the hip joint. These are derived developmentally from and are physiologically similar to synovium and tendon sheaths. As a result, they suffer from the same inflammatory afflictions which cause problems to the joint itself. Conditions which affect the bursa include traumatic inflammation, which is usually secondary to overuse or excessive pressure; infections; metabolic disorders such as gout; and benign and malignant growths.

Treatment consists of rest, ice, anti-inflammatory medications orally, and occasionally intrabursal injections. Ultrasound physical therapy may help as well. The prognosis for such patients is good as long as associated problems such as infection and low back disk disease are ruled out. Mechanical problems, especially leg length discrepancies, must be sought and, if found, properly treated so that further trochanteric bursitis does not occur.

### Femoral Shaft Fractures

Fractures of the shaft of the femur most often occur in men during their most active period in life. Falls and industrial and automobile accidents account for the majority of these fractures.

Severe, direct trauma may result in transverse fractures with displacement; oblique or spiral oblique fractures; or badly comminuted segments.

The femur is surrounded by large muscle groups with a rich vascular supply. Therefore, femoral fractures may result in the loss of 1 L or more of blood into the soft tissues of the thigh, producing clinical shock. The initial evaluation should always include careful neurovascular examination of the extremity.

It is best to splint the leg with a traction splint at the time of injury. Hare traction, Sager traction, or a Thomas splint can be placed over the trousers, applying traction to a sling around the ankle and forefoot.

In infants and children up to 3 or 4 years of age, fractures of the shaft of the femur are treated by direct overhead traction applied to both legs.

In an older child or adult, the Fisk type of traction by means of a half Thomas ring and Pearson attachment, to allow for flexion of the knee, is satisfactory.

The intramedullary rod is frequently the method of choice for the treatment of uncomplicated fractures of the midshaft and junction of the upper and middle thirds of the femur, except where comminution is so extensive that stability with the rod cannot be maintained.

In cases where comminution is severe, either dual plating or the use of a compression plate device can result in excellent fixation.

## BIBLIOGRAPHY

### Trauma to the Pelvis

Burgess AR, Tile M: Fractures of the pelvis. In: Rockwood CA Jr, Green DP, Bucholz RW (eds). *Fractures in Adults,* 3rd ed. Philadelphia: JB Lippincott, vol. 2, pp. 1399–1479, 1991.

Canale ST: In: Rockwood CA Jr, Wilkins KE, King RE (eds). *Fractures in Children.* 3rd ed. Philadelphia: JB Lippincott, vol. 3, pp. 991–1045, 1991.

Tile M: *Fractures of the Pelvis and Acetabulum.* Baltimore: Williams and Wilkins, pp. 11, 63–64, 1984.

Young JWR, Burgess AR. *Radiologic Management of Pelvic Ring Fractures: Systematic Radiologic Diagnosis.* Baltimore: Urban & Schwarzenberg, 1987.

### Trauma to the Hip and Femur

Canage ST, King RE: Fractures of the hip. In: Rockwood CA Jr, Wilkins KE, King RE (eds). *Fractures in Children.* 3rd ed. Philadelphia: JB Lippincott, vol. 3, pp. 1046–1120, 1991.

DeLee JC: Fractures and dislocations of the hip. In: Rockwood CA Jr, Green DP, Bucholz RW (eds). *Fractures in Adults,* 3rd ed. Philadelphia: JB Lippincott, vol. 3, pp. 1481–1651, 1991.

Hodges DL, McGuire TJ: Hip pain in children: an anatomic approach. *Orthop Rev* 17:251, 1988.

Hughes RA, Tempos K, Ansell BM: A review of the diagnoses of hip pain presentation in the adolescent. *Br J Rheumatol* 27:450, 1988.

Simon RR, Koenigsknecht SJ: *Orthopaedics in Emergency Medicine: The Extremities,* 2d ed. New York: Appletury-Crofts, 1989.

# 228
# KNEE INJURIES

## Joseph F. Waeckerle
## Mark T. Steele

Injuries to the knee are becoming increasingly more common in our sports-oriented society. The emergency physician must become familiar with the examination of the normal and abnormal knee to be able to recognize specific injuries and to treat and appropriately refer these injuries. This chapter deals with examination of the knee and with recognition of fractures and dislocations of the patella; fractures of femoral condyles; fractures of the tibial spines, tuberosity, and plateaus; ligamentous and meniscal injuries of the knee joint; knee dislocation; and osteochondritis dissecans.

As with all orthopedic injuries, the accurate diagnosis of the injured knee is required before proper treatment can be instituted. However, it is particularly important to do a complete and careful examination in a stepwise manner because the knee is essential for ambulation. Radiologic evaluation is a necessary part of the examination. The first examination is usually the easiest to perform because the patient does not anticipate pain and therefore does not guard, and involuntary muscular spasm causing futher guarding may not yet have occurred.

## EXAMINATION

The examination of the knee is divided into five phases: history, observation, inspection, palpation, and stress testing.

### History

The mechanism of injury as well as any prior serious problems frequently clarifies subtleties in the examination, allowing a more accurate diagnosis and appropriate treatment.

### Observation

The patient should be examined while walking, if possible, and in both the sitting and lying positions. The physician should take note of the gait, muscular development, functional range of motion, and the ability of the patient to extend the flexed knee against minimal resistance at this time.

### Inspection

The knee should be inspected for swelling, ecchymoses, effusion, masses, patella location and size, muscle mass, erythema, and evidence of local trauma. Also, the physician should note at this time, with the patient in a supine position, leg lengths (equal or unequal). Lastly, the physician should ask the patient to perform the best possible active range of motion.

### Palpation

Initially the neurovascular status of the leg should be noted. As with all orthopedic examinations, the noninjured or normal knee should be compared with the injured knee during all aspects of the examination but especially during palpation and stress testing. When the physician palpates the knee, he or she should begin in the nontender areas and work lastly toward the tender area so that the patient does not guard or become apprehensive. The examiner should always palpate the knee joint in a systematic manner. Effusion, tenderness, increased temperature, strength, sensation, and location of pulses should be noted.

The physician should examine the patella for size, shape, and location with the knee in flexion; mobility should be checked with the knee in extension. The patella should be compressed to check for pain as well as moved laterally and medially to ascertain possible subluxation. The popliteal space should also be palpated for masses, swelling, and circulation status.

### Stress Testing

The final phase of the examination of the knee is stress testing. This is the most difficult aspect of the examination although potentially the most informative. The patient must be reassured and relaxed and made as comfortable as possible. This may require allowing the leg to hang over the side of the bed with the bed supporting the posterior thigh rather than the physician holding the leg, as is usually done during stress testing. The first examination is often the most valid, especially if performed soon after the injury. The patient will not expect to experience any pain during this first examination, nor do the inflammation and effusion associated with an acute traumatic injury cause voluntary or involuntary guarding. The uninjured, hopefully normal, opposite knee should be examined first to determine the patient's normal laxity. A brief summary of the instabilities and tests to demonstrate them are presented in the section on ligamentous and meniscal injuries.

## FRACTURES

### Fractures of the Patella

Fractures of the patella occur from a direct blow, a fall on the flexed knee, or forceful contraction of the quadriceps muscles. Fractures

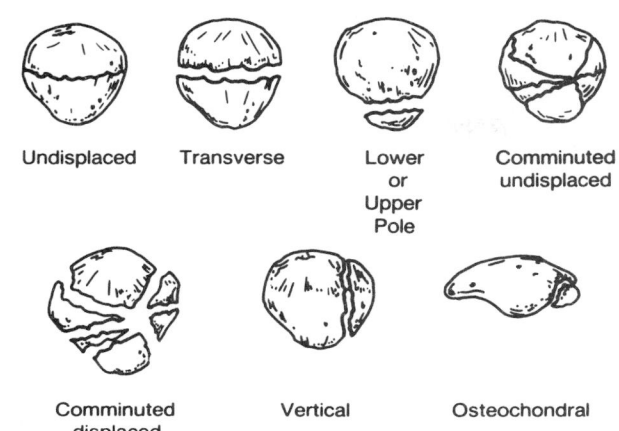

Fig. 228-1. Classification of patellar fractures. (From Hohl M, Johnson EE, Wiss DA. Fractures of the knee. In: Rockwood CA Jr, Green DP, Bucholz RW (eds). *Fractures in Adults,* 3rd ed. Philadelphia: JB Lippincott, vol. 2, p. 1765, 1991. Used with permission.)

may be transverse, comminuted, or of the avulsion type (when the quadriceps or patellar tendon pulls off a small portion of the patella (Fig. 228-1). Any fracture may be open or closed. A nondisplaced transverse fracture of the patella should be treated with immobilization for 6 weeks. During this time the patient should be encouraged to walk on crutches, with partial weight-bearing progressing to full weight-bearing as tolerated.

If the transverse fracture is nondisplaced, a cylinder cast may be sufficient, assuming adequate reduction occurs. However, this usually requires open reduction and wire fixation. If the fragments are widely separated, most often there is associated knee joint injury. A palpable defect is usually present at the fracture site.

Comminuted fractures must be treated surgically by removal of smaller fragments (or all fragments if they are small) and suturing of the quadriceps tendon and patellar ligaments.

All open fractures must be debrided and irrigated.

## Fractures of Femoral Condyles

Fractures of the femoral condyles include supracondylar, intercondylar, condylar, and distal femoral epiphyseal fractures (Fig. 228-2). Most often, these injuries are secondary to direct trauma from a fall or blow to the distal femur. Examination reveals pain, swelling, deformity, rotation, and shortening. Although neurovascular injuries are uncommon, the status of distal sensation and pulses must be checked. The space between the first and second toe, innervated by the deep peroneal nerve, should be tested for sensation. In addition, a search for ipsilateral hip dislocation or fractures, and damage to the quadriceps apparatus, must be made. Depending on the type of fracture, closed or open reduction, skeletal traction, and cast immobilization may be necessary. Therefore, orthopedic consultation is essential.

## Fractures of the Tibial Spines and Tuberosity

Although isolated injuries of the tibial spine are uncommon, they usually result in damage to the cruciate ligaments. The injury is most often caused by a force directed against the flexed proximal tibia in an anterior or posterior direction, resulting in incomplete avulsion of the tibial spine, with or without displacement, or complete fracture of the spine. Examination shows a painful, swollen knee, secondary to hemarthrosis, inability to extend fully, and a positive Lachman's sign. If the fracture is incomplete or nondisplaced, it should be immobilized in full extension. Complete, displaced fractures often need open reduction.

The quadriceps mechanism inserts on the tibial tubercle. A sudden force to the flexed knee with the quadriceps muscle contracted may

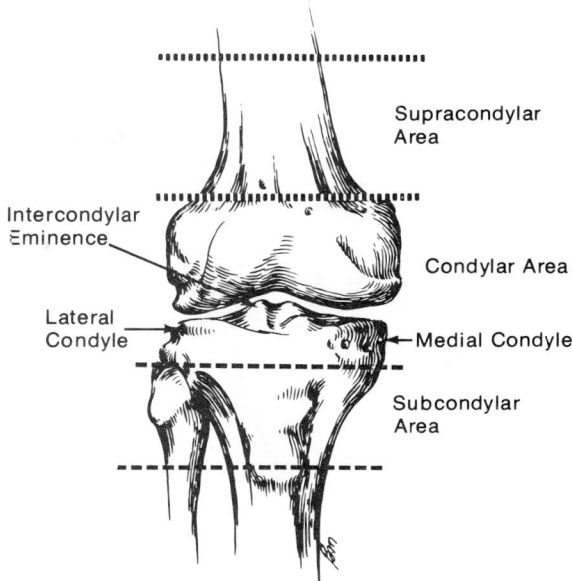

Fig. 228-2. The supracondylar and condylar areas of the femur, and the medial and subcondylar areas of the tibia. [Modified from Hohl M, Larson RL: Fractures and dislocations of the knee, in Rockwood CA Jr, Green DP (eds): *Fractures.* Philadelphia, Lippincott, 1975, vol. 2, pp. 1132, 1147. Used by permission.]

result in a complete or incomplete avulsion of the tibial tubercle. The fracture line may extend into the joint. Examination reveals pain and tenderness over the proximal anterior tibia with pain on passive or active extension. If the avulsion is small or nondisplaced, the fragment may be maintained in position by immobilization; otherwise, open reduction and internal fixation are necessary.

## Fractures of the Tibial Plateaus

Fractures of the tibial plateaus are seen more commonly in the older population and can be very difficult to detect. They are produced by direct force, which drives the femoral condyles into the articulating surface of the tibia. Both medial and lateral plateaus may be fractured simultaneously although the lateral plateau is more often fractured. Direct trauma to the lateral aspect of the knee may account for the preponderance of lateral tibialu fractures. The patient presents with painful swelling of the knee and limitation of motion. Radiographs may demonstrate a fracture but often only show a lipohemarthrosis on the lateral view. Careful review of the x-rays is essential. Ligamentous instability may also be demonstrated. If one or both plateaus are fractured but not displaced, treatment in a long leg plaster cast, without weight-bearing, should be adequate. Depression of the articular surface necessitates open reduction and elevation of the bony fragment.

## RECOGNITION AND MANAGEMENT OF LIGAMENTOUS AND MENISCAL INJURIES

The knee joint depends on ligaments and muscles for support (Fig. 228-3). It is frequently subjected to injuries from traumatic forces while extended or in various stages of flexion. These traumatic forces include abduction, flexion, and internal rotation of the femur on the tibia; adduction, flexion, and external rotation of the femur on the tibia; hyperextension; and anteroposterior displacement. By far the most common are abduction, flexion, and internal rotation of the femur on the tibia, which produce injuries to the medial side of the knee. Injuries to the lateral side of the knee are produced by adduction, flexion, and external rotation. Such forces may result in a strain or rupture of the medial or lateral collateral ligaments, the anterior or posterior cruciate ligaments, the capsular structures, or a tear in the

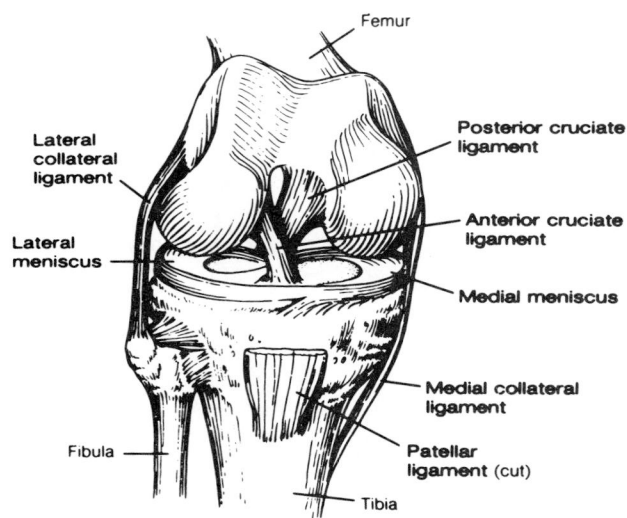

**Fig. 228-3.** Ligaments of the right knee joint. The articular capsule and the patella have been removed. (From Spencer AP, Mason EB: *Human Anatomy and Physiology.* Menlo Park, Benjamin/Cummings, 1979, p. 174. Used by permission.)

medial or lateral meniscus, singularly or in combination. Functional instability of the knee is determined by stress testing, which will demonstrate abnormal laxity when properly done.

Initial stress testing is an abduction or valgus deformity applied to the knee, which is in approximately 30° of flexion, to determine the integrity of the medial capsular and ligamentous structures. The medial collateral ligament supplies the majority of restraint to valgus deformities of the knee in all stages of flexion. A varus or adduction force is then applied to the lateral aspect of the knee, again with approximately 30° of flexion, to ascertain the integrity of the lateral structures. The lateral collateral ligament, similar to the medial collateral ligament, is the major restraint to varus laxity on the knee at all positions of flexion. If there is a demonstrated laxity of greater than 1 cm without a firm end point as compared to the other knee, there is a complete rupture of the medial or lateral collateral ligament. If there is laxity with a firm end point or a laxity of less than 1 cm, an incomplete or partial tear is present. If there is no demonstrated instability but there is pain, the patient has suffered a strain in the ligamentous structures tested. The patient who is unstable with the varus or valgus test performed with 30° of flexion should be brought into full extension, if possible, and similar maneuvers carried out. Medial instability in full extension indicates a severe lesion involving the cruciate ligaments and posterior capsule along with the medial ligaments. Lateral instability in extension likewise indicates a severe injury that may involve the posterolateral corner of the knee as well as the cruciate ligaments. Peroneal nerve injuries may also occur in lateral injuries.

Injury to the anterior cruciate ligament may be the most common ligamentous injury today. The mechanism of injury is usually noncontact; a deceleration, hyperextension, or marked internal rotation of the tibia on the femur results in an injury to the cruciate. There may be an associated medial meniscal tear as well. Such a mechanism of injury combined with the presence of a traumatic effusion is very suggestive of a disruption of the anterior cruciate ligament.

The diagnosis of the anterior cruciate ligament injury is ascertained by using the Lachman test (Fig. 228-4), the anterior drawer sign, and the pivot shift (Fig. 228-5). Although the anterior drawer sign has been used for a long time, it is not very sensitive. The maneuver is done with 45° flexion at the hip and 90° flexion at the knee. The physician then attempts to forwardly displace the tibia from the femur. A displacement of greater than 6 mm as compared to the nor-

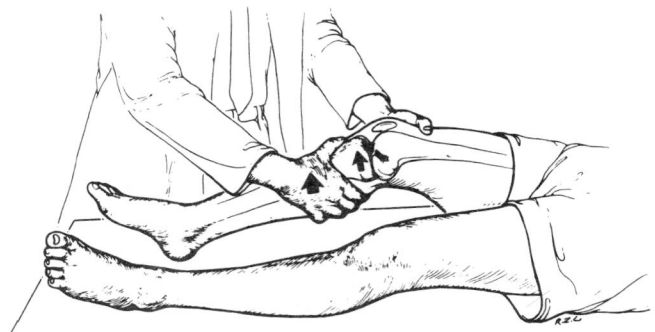

**Fig. 228-4.** The Lachman test is performed with the knee flexed between 15° and 30°. (From Scott WN. *Ligament and Extensor Mechanism Injuries of the Knee: Diagnosis and Treatment.* St. Louis: Mosby-Year Book, 1991. Used with permission.)

mal, opposite knee indicates that there has been an injury to the anterior cruciate ligament. There are false negatives associated with this maneuver. The Lachman test, which is currently more popular, is a much more sensitive test. The examiner places the knee in 20° of flexion by resting it on a pillow and stabilizes the femur above the knee with his or her nondominant hand. The dominant hand is placed behind the leg at the level of the tibial tubercle, and the examiner introduces an anterior force, attempting to displace the tibia forward. If a displacement of greater than 5 mm as compared to the opposite knee occurs or if there is a soft, mushy end point, then a tear in the anterior cruciate ligament has occurred. Although this examination is more sensitive than the anterior drawer and able to identify partial tears in the anterior cruciate ligament when the examiner is skilled, it is difficult on patients who have large legs. The pivot shift is the third maneuver by which the examiner can determine the integrity of the anterior cruciate ligament. The pivot shift is easily performed once the examiner is familiar with it, but it may be somewhat painful to the patient. While the patient is supine and relaxed, the examiner lifts the heel of the foot to approximately 45° of hip flexion with the knee fully extended. The opposite hand grasps the knee with the thumb behind the fibular head. The examiner then internally rotates the ankle and knee, applies a valgus force to the knee, and flexes the knee. If an anterior subluxation of the tibia is present, a sudden visible, audible, and palpable reduction of the subluxation occurs at about 20 to 40° of

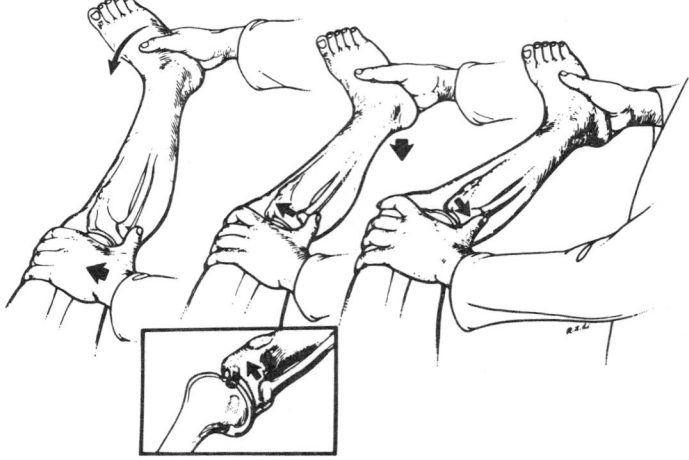

**Fig. 228-5.** In the pivot shift of Galway and MacIntosh, the test is done with the knee in full extension with application of a valgus and internal rotation stress. The "clunk" of reduction is felt in the first 20° to 30° of flexion. (From Scott WN. *Ligament and Extensor Mechanism Injuries of the Knee: Diagnosis and Treatment.* St. Louis: Mosby-Year Book, 1991. Used with permission.)

flexion. This indicates a deficit in the anterior cruciate ligament, which is required to stabilize the knee in this position. There are other tests described in the literature to determine the integrity of the anterior cruciate ligament, including the jerk test and dynamic extension testing.

The posterior cruciate ligament can also suffer an isolated injury or be injured in combination with other ligamentous structures of the knee. In contrast to anterior cruciate injuries, isolated posterior cruciate injuries are seen much less frequently. The posterior cruciate ligament provides initial resistance to posterior translation at all angles of flexion of the knee. The mechanism of injury then is usually an anterior to posterior force applied to the tibia or lower leg. Posterior cruciate injuries are seen in association with other ligamentous injuries when a serious injury has occurred to the knee. A deficit in this ligament is determined by the posterior drawer test. The knee is examined with flexion at the hip and at the knee as described for the anterior drawer sign. The physician applies a posterior force to the tibial tubercle. If there is displacement posteriorly, then the examiner can diagnose an injury to this ligament. The physician might also notice a posterior sag or drop back of the tibial tubercle due to loss of integrity of the posterior cruciate when observing the knee with 45° flexion at the hip and 90° flexion at the knee. This test can be misleading, however, if there is a straight anterior instability resulting in a subluxation of the knee forward. This abnormal position would give the physician the false impression of too much posterior play when performing the posterior drawer test because the knee would be reduced to its normal anatomic alignment from the forwardly subluxed position.

Combined instabilities of the knee are often seen by the emergency physician, especially in athletes. Anteromedial and anterolateral instability are the two that occur most frequently. They result from external rotation and abduction or adduction forces placed on the knee. Virtually any combination of medial and lateral instabilities of the knee can occur, however.

One knee injury that is especially difficult to detect is injury to the posterolateral structures. Posterolateral instability usually involves a tear of the popliteus-arcuate complex, which may occur in combination with lateral ligament injury and possible anterior or posterior cruciate ligament injury. Isolated injuries to the popliteus-arcuate complex can occur themselves but are rare. Isolated posterolateral instability is demonstrated by testing at 0° to 30° of flexion for maximal posterior translation and 90° of flexion for maximal external rotation as compared to the normal opposite knee. Further testing to determine the integrity of the lateral collateral ligament and anterior or posterior cruciates must be done as well.

Most ligamentous injuries of the knee present with hemarthroses. In fact, approximately 75 percent of all hemarthroses are due to disruption of the anterior cruciate ligament. Serious ligament injuries, however, may present with minimal pain and no hemarthrosis due to complete disruption of the ligamentous and capsular fibers, allowing leakage of the blood into the soft tissue spaces. Hemarthrosis can also be due to osteochondral fractures or fractures that extend into the joint line or peripheral meniscal tears. These hemarthroses usually occur within minutes to a few hours of injury, in contrast to chronic effusions of the knee due to synovial inflammation, which occur 1 to 2 days after strenuous use of the joint. Usually the physician does not need to tap a sudden effusion associated with a knee injury to determine whether it is bloody. The indications for tapping a knee with a hemarthrosis are to relieve the pressure and pain caused by fluid distention and to see if fat globules are present, indicating a fracture (lipohemarthrosis). The complications of aspirating a joint space include the possibility of contamination and subsequent infection.

Continued refinements in magnetic resonance imaging (MRI) have resulted in high-quality images of the ligamentous and meniscal structures of the knee. The emergency physician can confirm the results of the stress testing by ordering an MRI examination of the knee if the appropriate equipment and personnel are available.

## Treatment

Stable injuries involving a single ligament with minor strain can be managed with a knee splint, ice packs, elevation, and ambulation as soon as is comfortable for the patient. More severe but stable ligamentous injuries necessitate ice, elevation, and immobilization. These injuries should be referred to an orthopedic surgeon within the next few days for follow-up examination and definitive management. Unstable injuries necessitate immediate orthopedic consultation so that definitive management can be planned.

## Meniscal Injuries

Meniscal injuries of the knee occur of themselves or in combination with ligamentous injuries. For example, anterior cruciate injuries are commonly associated with meniscal injuries. Many maneuvers have been described in the literature to determine whether a meniscus has been injured. Most of these tests, however, have an unacceptable specificity and sensitivity. Although the diagnosis of a meniscal tear is difficult to make in certain patients, a combination of a suggestive history and physical findings on examination should lead the emergency physician to consider the diagnosis. On questioning the patient, the physician should ask if the patient experiences locking of the knee joint on either flexion or extension that is painful and limits further activity. This sign clearly points to the diagnosis of a torn meniscus. Effusions that occur after activity; a sensation of popping, clicking, or snapping; a feeling of an unstable joint, especially with activity; or tenderness in the anterior joint space after excessive activity suggests the diagnosis of a meniscal tear. When performing a physical examination, a physician should attempt to identify atrophy of the quadriceps muscle due to disuse and joint line tenderness, which is very suggestive. Various maneuvers, such as McMurray's test or the grind test, are useful but, as mentioned earlier, are positive only about 50 percent of the time. If a tentative diagnosis of a meniscal tear is considered, referral to an orthopedic surgeon is warranted.

The patient who presents to the emergency department with a locked knee can experience a great deal of pain along with loss of mobility. The emergency physician can attempt to unlock the knee by positioning the patient with the leg hanging over the edge of the table with the knee in approximately 90° of flexion. After a period of relaxation, the physician can apply longitudinal traction to the knee with internal and external rotation in an attempt to unlock the joint. If this maneuver is unsuccessful, consultation with the orthopedic surgeon is recommended.

## Knee Dislocation

Knee dislocation (Fig. 228-6) is a result of tremendous ligamentous disruption due to hyperextension, direct posterior force applied to the anterior tibia, force to the fibula or medial femur, force to the tibia or lateral femur, or rotatory force resulting in anterior, posterior lateral, medial, or rotatory dislocation. Very often reduction occurs spontaneously. A severely unstable knee in multiple directions is suspicious for a spontaneously reduced knee dislocation. Suspicion of the injury is important because of the high incidence of associated complications, including popliteal artery injury (50 percent incidence) and peroneal nerve injury, in addition to ligamentous and meniscal injury. Early reduction of the dislocation is essential; orthopedic and perhaps vascular surgery consultation should be obtained immediately. An arteriogram is generally warranted.

## Patella Dislocation

Dislocation of the patella usually occurs from a twisting injury on the extended knee. The patella is displaced laterally over the lateral

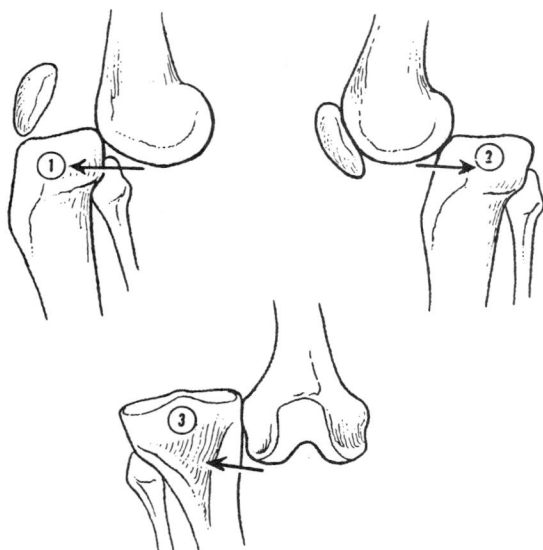

**Fig. 228-6.** Types of dislocations. 1. Anterior; 2, posterior; and 3, lateral. (From DePalma AF. *Management of Fractures and Dislocations: An Atlas.* Philadelphia: WB Saunders, p. 1621, 1970. Used by permission.)

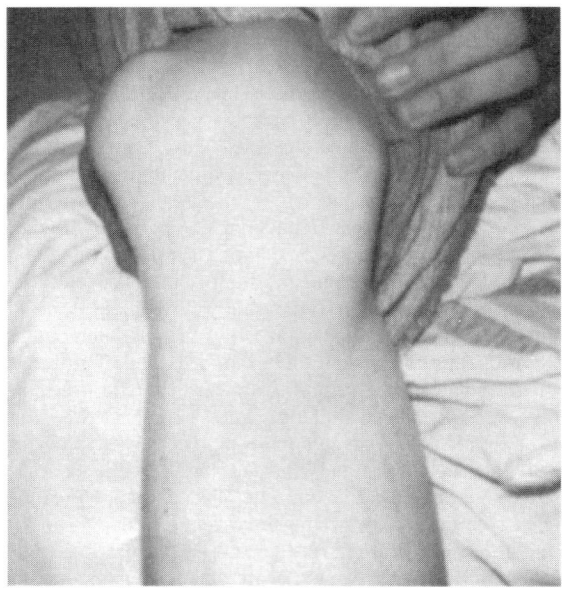

**Fig. 228-7.** Lateral dislocation of the patella. (From Lyman JI, Ervin ME. Management of common dislocations. In: Roberts JR, Hedges JR (eds). *Clinical Procedures in Emergency Medicine.* Philadelphia: WB Saunders, p. 634, 1985. Used with permission.)

condyle, resulting in pain and deformity of the knee (Fig. 228-7). Tearing of the medial knee joint capsule often occurs. Reduction is accomplished by hyperextending the knee, flexing the hip, and sliding the patella back into place. This is accompanied by immediate relief of pain, but further soreness from capsular injury persists for a period of time. The patella and knee should be x-rayed to rule out a fracture and the knee should be immobilized after reduction. Recurrent lateral dislocations of the patella and superior, horizontal, and intercondylar dislocations require referral to an orthopedic surgeon for possible surgical intervention.

### Quadriceps/Patellar Tendon Rupture

Rupture of the quadriceps or patellar tendons can occur from forceful contraction of the quadriceps muscle or falling on a flexed knee. Patellar tendon rupture occurs most commonly in individuals under age 40 with a history of tendinitis or past steroid injections. Quadriceps tendon rupture is most frequent in the over 40 age group. There is significant pain, diffuse swelling occurs, and the patient will be unable to extend a flexed knee against mild resistance in both instances. Depending on the tendon ruptured, a defect may be palpable above or below the patella. A "high-riding patella" may be seen on the lateral x-ray of the knee with patellar tendon rupture. The treatment is surgical repair of the involved tendon.

### Osteochondritis Dissecans

Osteochondritis dissecans is a loose body in a knee joint. which may cause locking, effusion, and buckling of the knee. X-ray examination may be negative or may reveal a calcified body in the joint.

### Patellar Tendinitis

Also known as "jumpers knee," patellar tendinitis is primarily seen in runners, basketball and volleyball players, and high jumpers. Pain is referred to the area of the patellar tendon and is worsened when going from sitting to standing or when running up hills. Point tenderness can be found at the distal aspect of the patella or proximal part of the patellar tendon. Treatment consists of heat, nonsteroidal anti-inflammatory agents, and quadriceps strengthening exercises. Steroid injections predispose to tendon rupture so should be avoided.

### Chondromalacia Patellae

Chondromalacia patellae is an overuse syndrome of the articular cartilage of the patella. The condition is caused by patellofemoral malalignment, which leads to a tracking abnormality of the patella, placing excessive lateral pressure on the articular cartilage. It is most common in young, active women and the pain is generally localized to the region of the anterior knee. Stair climbing and rising from a chair exacerbate the pain.

Two tests may aid in the diagnosis. The patellar compression test is performed by pushing the patella distal in the trochlear groove with the knee extended and quadriceps muscles tightened. This maneuver illicits pain. The apprehension test is performed on a relaxed leg. When the patella is pushed laterally, the quadriceps muscles contract in anticipation of pain. Treatment of this condition consists of rest, nonsteroidal anti-inflammatory medication, and quadriceps strengthening exercises.

### KNEE INJURIES IN CHILDREN

Although knee injuries do occur in children, they are usually the result of fractures of the bone rather than significant ligamentous injuries. Ligamentous injuries can occur in children but are not common. Careful examination and radiographic evaluation usually reveal that the ligaments are intact and there has been an epiphyseal injury. Meniscal tears also occur in children with a much lower incidence than in adults. The characteristic finding of meniscal tears in children is that they have a more insidious history than in the adult. Patellar fractures are also infrequent in children. They can be difficult to diagnose because of the difficulty in evaluating the radiographs. The opposite knee should be x-rayed for comparison views to help the physician in the diagnosis of a fracture. Lastly, dislocations are, fortunately, an exteremly rare condition in children. If they occur, however, they have the same ominous complications as in the adult.

### Separation of Distal Femoral Epiphysis

In children this is a common epiphyseal injury that can occur in the anterior plane or coronal plane. The anterior separation is usually the result of a hyperextension injury. The more common coronal separation is the result of abduction and adduction forces, most often occurring during sports activities or play. The patient complains of acute injury with inability to bear weight and presents with a flexion deformity. As with most epiphyseal injuries, the examiner finds circumferential tenderness around the entire epiphyseal plate. The standard radiographic views for evaluating the knee are required. The Salter-Harris classification is used to classify these fractures, with type II being the most common. The treatment for separation of the distal femoral epiphysis requires anatomic reduction of the fracture, either by closed or open reduction.

## Separation of Proximal Tibial Epiphysis

The separation of the proximal tibial epiphysis is a rare phenomenon because the tibia is well protected. The mechanism of injury is usually indirect forces of abduction or hyperextension against a fixed knee. Occasionally this injury is due to a direct force such as encountered in an automobile-pedestrian accident. Again, the classification is the Salter-Harris method. The symptoms and signs are similar to those of all other knee injuries, with pain, swelling, effusion, and a limited range of motion, especially extension-flexion. As with all epiphyseal injuries, there is circumferential tenderness over the injured growth plate. Stress examination reveals instability to the various maneuvers. Standard radiographs to evaluate the knee are recommended, with stress films required if no injury is seen but one is suspected. Careful evaluation looking for an occult fracture line is important. The treatment is immediate reduction and conservative therapy. The complications are similar to those of distal femoral epiphyseal separation.

## Injuries to the Tibial Tubercle

Two problems can occur at the tibial tubercle. The first is the acute avulsion of the tibial tubercle; the second is the classic Osgood-Schlatter lesion. Avulsion injuries are usually incurred as an acute event during sports and play. The patient presents with the inability to walk, because of the injury, as well as with localized tenderness and swelling. The lateral radiographic view is most important because it demonstrates both the size of the fracture fragment and the degree of displacement. The treatment for any but the smallest fragment is surgical so that there are minimal complications and a good prognosis. In contrast, Osgood-Schlatter lesions present with a vague history in adolescent boys. The pain is mild and intermittent, allowing the child to continue to participate in sports and play but not at a full level of involvement. Osgood-Schlatter disease is seen bilaterally in approximately 25 percent of the cases. In contrast to patients with avulsion injuries, patients with Osgood-Schlatter lesions experience pain with range of motion, especially range of motion against resistance, and not at rest. The treatment is symptomatic and supportive. There are minimal complications, and the prognosis is good.

## Fracture of the Intercondylar Eminence of the Tibia

This fracture is usually encountered in 8- to 15-year-old youths, who most often relate a history of a fall from a bicycle. This causes the intercondylar eminence to be avulsed from the tibia, resulting in a painful and acutely swollen knee. The patient has a positive Lachman's test and a drawer sign and may have concomitant medial collateral ligamentous instability to valgus stress testing. Radiographs usually reveal evidence of a fracture on the lateral view with the knee slightly flexed. The treatment is immobilization in full extension in most instances, as this can reduce the fracture fragment to its anatomic state. Persistent displacement of the fracture should be treated surgically. The concomitant injuries to the medial collateral ligament do not often require surgical intervention and can be treated while the patient is recovering from the fracture. The prognosis with proper treatment is good.

## Osteochondral Fractures

Osteochondral fractures occur infrequently in children and adolescents. If they do occur, most often in adolescent boys, they are usually fracture fragments from the femoral condyles or the patella. The history is one of an acute injury with a pop or snap, causing severe pain and an acute effusion. The fracture is difficult to see on radiographs, so careful attention should be paid to the femoral condyles as well as to the patella. Treatment is surgical removal of the foreign body so that no sequelae can develop.

## SUMMARY

In summary, the knee is a complex joint. Understanding the anatomy and physiology of its motion, understanding the mechanism of the forces producing injuries, and facility in examination of the knee are essential for the emergency physician, who will be confronted relatively often by injuries to this joint. Thorough and careful examination on initial presentation, recognition of significant abnormalities, thoughtful initial care, and appropriate referral are the emergency physician's goals in management of knee injuries.

## BIBLIOGRAPHY

Hohl M, Johnson EE, Wiss DA: Fractures of the knee. In: Rockwood CA Jr, Green DP, Bucholz RW (eds): *Fractures in Adults,* 3rd ed. Philadelphia: JB Lippincott, vol 2, pp. 1725–1761, 1991.

Beaty JH, Roberts JM: Fractures and dislocations of the knee. In: Rockwood CA Jr, Wilkins KE, King RE: *Fractures in Children,* 3rd ed. Philadelphia: JB Lippincott, vol 3, pp. 1165–1270, 1991.

Scott WN, Insell JN: Injuries of the knee. In: Rockwood CA Jr, Green DP, Bucholz RW (eds): *Fractures in Adults,* 3rd ed. Philadelphia: J Lippincott, Vol 2, pp. 1799–1914, 1991.

Scott WN: *Ligament and Extensor Mechanism Injuries of the Knee: Diagnosis and Treatment.* St. Louis, Mosby-Year Book, Inc, 1991.

Simon RR, Koenigsknecht SJ: *Orthopaedics in Emergency Medicine: The Extremities.* New York: Appleton-Century-Crofts, 1982.

Sisk TD: Knee injuries. In Crenshaw AH (ed). *Campbell's Operative Orthopaedics,* 7th ed. St. Louis: CV Mosby, vol 3, pp. 2305–2335, 1987.

# 229
# LEG INJURIES

## Joseph F. Waeckerle
## Mark T. Steele

Although the fractured tibia is the most common of all long bone fractures, its treatment is varied and sometimes controversial. Because of the many fractures seen and the frequency of open fractures, tibial fractures are associated with a high complication rate. The frequency of fractures, as well as the complication rate, is due to the fact that the tibia, and fibula as well, have minimal protection from surrounding soft tissues.

The leg is susceptible to direct and indirect mechanisms of injury. Direct blows usually cause tibial shaft fractures which are associated with fibular shaft fractures. Because the violence is directly to the bone, soft tissue injury with initial displacement of the fracture site and comminution of the fracture often result. In contrast, indirect forces such as rotation and compression usually cause spiral or oblique fractures of the tibia, sometimes associated with fibular shaft fractures. Isolated fibular shaft fractures are, in fact, uncommon injuries.

## ANATOMY

The tibia and fibula run parallel and are tightly connected by the interosseous ligament. The surrounding soft tissue may be divided into three compartments. The first, the anterior compartment, consists of the muscles (tibialis anterior, extensor digitorum longus, extensor hallucis longus, and peroneus tertius), the anterior tibial artery, and the deep peroneal nerve. Because this compartment is bound by the tibia, fibula, and fascia, there is little room for swelling. The second compartment is the lateral compartment, which consists of the peroneus brevis and peroneus longus muscles, along with the superficial peroneal nerve. The superficial peroneal nerve is at risk when an injury occurs high up the fibular shaft or at the neck of the fibula. The third compartment is the posterior compartment, which consists of the soleus, gastrocnemius, tibialis posterior, flexor hallucis longus, and flexor digitorum longus muscles, the posterior tibial nerve, and the posterior tibial artery.

Injuries from swelling to the anterior compartment are more often seen than such injuries to the lateral or posterior compartments. The latter two are also bound compartments, and if a significant amount of swelling occurs, a compartment syndrome may also be seen there.

There are multiple classifications for describing leg fractures. Probably the easiest is to classify tibial fractures as stable or unstable, which helps with regard to treatment. Some classifications, by describing the fractures with regard to displacement, comminution, and soft tissue injuries, can somewhat predict the healing potential.

## CLINICAL EVALUATION

As with all orthopedic injuries, the symptoms and signs the patient presents with are directly proportional to the severity of the leg fracture. Pain is usually severe and localized. Crepitance in motion and obvious deformity are often present. Usually the deformity is external rotation and valgus in nature. Local swelling and discoloration and the presence of wounds may aid the physician in diagnosing a fracture. When associated with a leg fracture, any wound which violates the integrity of the skin must be considered an open fracture. Although direct neurovascular injury is not a common complication of leg fractures, neurovascular assessment should always be done and recorded on the chart. This consists of documentation that both the vascular supply to the foot and the motor and sensory supply to the leg, especially the functions of the peroneal nerve, are intact.

In evaluating leg fractures, AP and lateral x-ray views are generally adequate to demonstrate the fracture, as well as the position of the fragments. As always, the x-ray views require good trabecular detail to demonstrate the smaller, nondisplaced fractures, especially those seen in the fibula. Also, the x-ray views should demonstrate both the knee and the ankle articular surfaces.

### Treatment

Emergency department management of leg fractures is usually not difficult. Once the initial examination is completed and the fracture is identified and defined, closed reduction, an immobilization long leg splint, and referral are appropriate. A clinically obvious fracture should be splinted prior to getting x-rays. Difficulty in managing such fractures in the emergency department occurs when the physician is not able to obtain an adequate reduction or there are severe associated soft tissue injuries with an open fracture. It is emphasized again that it is more important to treat the soft tissue injuries properly than to treat the fracture itself. This requires that the physician gently but thoroughly cleanse the soft tissue by debridement and irrigation and provide appropriate tetanus prophylaxis and antibiotic coverage. The immobilization must allow the physicians treating the patient to view the soft tissue wounds. Occasionally emergency reduction of a fracture may be required because the fracture has compromised vascularity distal to the fracture site. Although this is not common, such reduction might be needed prior to x-ray evaluation when the compromise threatens the limb's blood supply.

### Complications

The most common complication associated with leg fractures is the soft tissue injury with secondary infection. As with any orthopedic injury, an infection can be disastrous. Also, as mentioned earlier, the compartment syndrome, seen some 24 to 48 h after injury, can occur. Nerve damage is usually uncommon with leg fractures but may occur if there is an injury to the fibular head. This involves the superficial peroneal nerve. Damage to the vascularity is also not usual but can occur in upper tibial fractures with injury to the anterior tibial artery as it passes through the interosseous membrane. As with all orthopedic injuries, nonunion or delayed union is common if the fracture site is complicated by a severe displacement, comminution, or soft tissue injury. Also, arthritis may occur in some individuals, especially after intra-articular fractures.

### Compartment Syndrome

Compartment syndrome occurs when injured muscle enveloped in a fascial sheath swells and causes secondary compression of blood vessels and nerves that traverse the compartment. If unrecognized, this syndrome can result in permanent nerve and muscle damage. The most common sites where this may occur include the four fascial compartments in the leg: peroneal, anterior, deep, and superficial posterior. The volar and dorsal compartments of the forearm and the interosseous muscles of the hand can also be affected. The anterior compartment of the leg is the most common site of compartment syndrome and usually is caused by fractures of the tibia. The causes of skeletal muscle injury are many and varied and include, but are not limited to, trauma, electrical injury, infectious disease (i.e., infectious myositis), hyper- or hypothermia, toxins, snake bite, polymyositis, arterial embolism or injury, seizures, and prolonged immobility that may occur following CVA or drug overdose.

A high index of suspicion is needed to make the diagnosis, particularly in unconscious or uncooperative patients. Time is of the essence since irreversible muscle damage can occur in 4 to 6 hours. A complete neurologic and motor exam of the affected extremity is essential. Tenderness and pain out of proportion to the injury in the affected area are common with active or passive motion. Paresthesias and pain with passive finger or toe movement are early signs. Abnormal two point discrimination or light touch of a traversing nerve are also early indicators of a compartment syndrome. The affected compartment may be tense, indurated and erythematous, but this is a late finding. Initial capillary refill and pulses are usually normal in compartment syndrome. As a result, the finding of normal pulses and capillary refill *does not* rule out the condition.

Laboratory data generally show evidence of rhabdomyolysis, including myoglobinuria and elevated muscle enzyme activity. (CPK levels over 20,000 IV per mL are not unusual.) Renal function should be assessed and may show early deterioration due to the myoglobinuria. Immediate orthopedic consultation and admission is indicated if there is suspicion of compartment syndrome. Compartment pressures should be measured using a Wick catheter or 18 gauge needle and saline manometer. Pressure of 0–8 mmHg is considered normal. Pressure over 30 mmHg can cause ischemia and thus is an indication for emergency fasciotomy.

### Fibular Fractures

Isolated fibular fractures, especially of the shaft, are uncommon. The more common injury to the fibula is fracture at the ankle joint, which is addressed in Chapter 230, "Ankle Injuries." Occasionally, however, fractures due to direct and indirect trauma do occur to the fibular shaft. The patient may present with local swelling and tenderness over the fracture site itself and pain on ambulation. Because of the difficulty in sometimes seeing a fracture of the fibula (especially if it is a stress fracture, which is commonly seen in the distal third), x-ray views which show good trabecular detail are required. AP and lateral views are generally adequate.

Treatment of fibular fractures is usually designed to give the patient comfort. Very often the patient does not require immobilization. However, in some instances the patient may be more comfortable in a short leg walking cast and crutches for approximately 2 weeks.

### Calf Strains/Gastrocnemius Rupture

Falls leading to forceful dorsiflexion of the ankle or sudden push-off during athletic events such as tennis or basketball may result in partial rupture of the medial head of the gastrocnemius at the musculotendinous junction. Clinically, the patient localizes pain to the medial midcalf and ambulation and standing on tiptoe are difficult and painful. Soft tissue swelling and ecchymosis are usually present. The calf squeeze or Thompson's sign is negative, differentiating it from complete Achilles tendon rupture (see Chapter 230). Venous thrombosis must also be considered in the differential diagnosis. Initial treatment consists of immobilization with a posterior splint. Ice, elevation, and oral anti-inflammatory agents are indicated. Protected crutch weight bearing can be initiated within a week along with the use of bilateral heel lifts.

### Shin Splints

Shin splint pain is due to posterior tibial tendinitis and/or associated periostitis at the insertion of the posterior tibial tendon. The pain in this condition is referred to the anteromedial lower leg. Running on hard surfaces and wearing improper footwear predisposes to this condition. Treatment consists of rest, nonsteroidal anti-inflammatory agents, and correction of the underlying causes.

## LEG INJURIES IN CHILDREN

### Tibial and Fibular Shaft Fractures

Tibial and fibular shaft fractures are the most common lower extremity injuries to bone in children. The mechanism of injury is usually an indirect force, such as occurs from a twist. Rarely, direct trauma causes the injury. The patient presents with pain on walking and a mild limp if there is a fibular fracture, a greenstick fracture, or stress fracture. If, however, both the tibia and fibular are fractured, the patient is unable to walk and has pain at rest. The examining physician may see a deformity, which is usually minimal in contrast to the deformity of adult fractures. Neurovascular involvement is uncommon in these injuries. Radiographic evaluation requires standard AP and lateral views, with the opposite leg for comparison occasionally. Treatment is usually closed and conservative. The complications of these fractures in children are basically deformity types, with leg-length discrepancy and malrotation the most important. Neurovascular complications are rare.

Specific fractures of the tibia and fibula can occur. The toddler fracture can occur in younger children. They are a common cause for a limp or refusal to ambulate. Toddler fractures are usually spiral fractures of the tibia, with no fibular involvement. Bicycle spoke injuries are also seen occasionally. The history is usually that the child's foot was thrust between the spokes of a bicycle wheel, causing a severe compression or crush injury of the soft tissues of the foot and ankle. Special care should be taken in such cases, as the soft tissue problems are significant.

Lastly, stress fractures in children present with a different pattern than in adults. The upper third of the tibia is nearly always affected in

children. Boys usually have more problems with this type of fracture because of their activity levels. They present with a painful limp of insidious onset. The pain is relieved when the child is at rest and is increased with activity. There is local tenderness to examination. Radiographic evaluation, as with all stress fractures, may not be helpful initially as the fracture may not show up for a period of time. Bone scan is usually helpful. Treatment is conservative and symptomatic.

### Tibial Metaphyseal Injuries

Fractures of the proximal tibial metaphysis are usually due to significant violence. Because of this, they are associated with significant complications. The most important complication for the physician to recognize immediately is arterial involvement associated with valgus deformities. In contrast to proximal tibial injuries, distal tibial metaphyseal fractures are usually greenstick fractures with minimal sequelae and good prognosis.

### BIBLIOGRAPHY

Dias LS: Fractures of the tibia and fibula, in Rockwood CA Jr, Wilkins KE, King RE (eds): *Fractures in Children,* 3rd ed. Philadelphia, Lippincott, 1991, vol. 3, pp. 1271–1382.

Leach RE: Fractures of the tibia and fibula, in Rockwood CA Jr, Green DP, Bucholz RW (eds): *Fractures in Adults,* 3rd ed. Philadelphia, Lippincott, 1991, vol. 2, pp. 1915–1982.

Simon RR, Koenigsknecht SJ: *Orthopaedics in Emergency Medicine: The Extremities,* 2d ed. New York, Appleton-Century-Crofts, 1988.

# 230
# ANKLE INJURIES
## Joseph F. Waeckerle
## Mark T. Steele

The ankle bears as much weight per unit area as any other joint in the body. Its anatomic design and weight-bearing function predispose it to a wide variety of injuries. To recognize and appropriately treat ankle injuries, the physician must understand the anatomy and mechanisms of injury. Treatment should be designed so that no prolonged disability or irreparable damage results.

## ANATOMY

The ankle consists of three bones, the tibia, fibula, and talus, which are bonded together by ligaments to form a hingelike joint. Groups of muscles cross the joint and produce movement, mostly through dorsiflexion and plantar flexion.

**Bones.** Bony stability is provided by the talus being interposed between the tibia and fibula. The talus is wider anteriorly than posteriorly to provide for articulation with the distal tibia and the medial and lateral malleoli. In dorsiflexion, more of the anterior, wider portion of the talus fits into the slightly concave undersurface of the tibia. This tighter fit allows the malleoli of the tibia and fibula to bear more stress if any twisting motion occurs. In plantar flexion, the narrower, posterior portion of the talus occupies the mortise so that there is more play in the ankle joint. It is therefore easier for twisting motions to result in injury with the ankle in plantar flexion. Due to the inherent joint design, dorsiflexion is accompanied by eversion and plantar flexion with inversion.

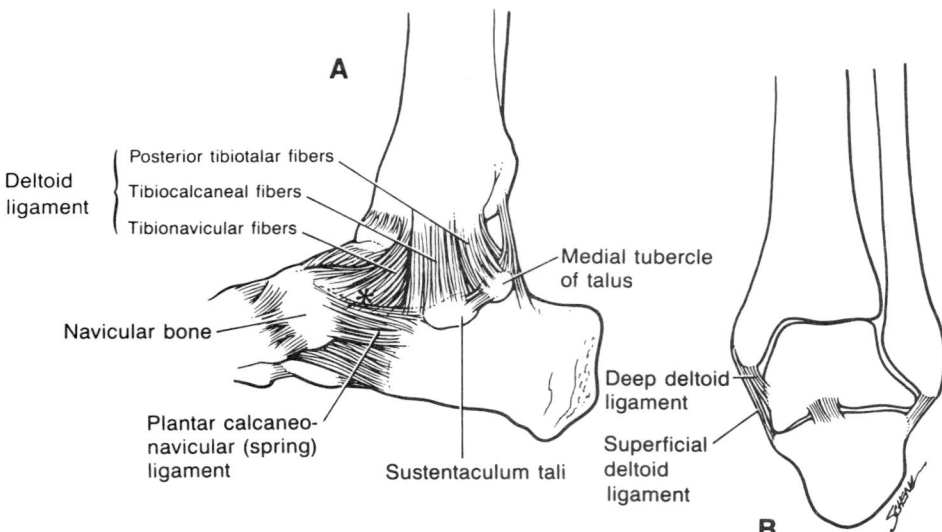

**Fig. 230-1.** Medial collateral ligaments. (*A*) Bands of the superficial deltoid ligament. The asterisk represents the head of the talus. (*B*) Position of the deep deltoid ligament. (From VanderGriend RA, Savoie FH, Hughes JL: Fractures of the ankle. In: Rockwood CA Jr, Green DP, Bucholz RW (eds). *Fractures in Adults,* 3rd ed. Philadelphia: JB Lippincott, vol. 2, p. 1989, 1991. Used with permission.)

**Ligaments.** Three groups of ligaments unify the bony structures of the ankle. The medial collateral, or deltoid, ligament is a thick triangular band that provides medial support to the ankle joint. It consists of a superficial and a deep set of fibers (Fig. 230-1). Both sets of fibers originate from the broad, short, and strong medial malleolus. The superficial fibers run in a sagittal plane and insert on the navicular and talus. Deep fibers run more horizontally and insert on the medial surface of the talus.

The lateral support of the ankle is provided by the anterior talofibular, calcaneofibular, and posterior talofibular ligaments (Fig. 230-2). They originate and insert as their names suggest. Along with the lateral malleolus, these ligaments prevent lateral movement of the talus.

The lower portions of the tibia and fibula are bound together by the ligaments of the syndesmosis. These ligaments consist of the anterior and posterior tibiofibular ligaments, the interosseous ligament, and the inferior transverse ligament. The anterior and posterior tibiofibular ligaments are bands of fibers running between the margins of the tibia and fibula anteriorly and posteriorly. The inferior transverse ligament is a strong group of fibers that supports the posterior inferior portion of the ankle joint. Finally, the interosseous ligament is simply the lower portion of the interosseous membrane. It provides the strongest bond between the tibia and fibula at the joint.

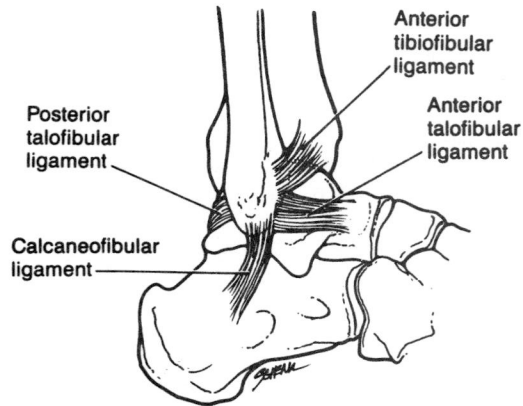

**Fig. 230-2.** Lateral collateral ligaments with adjacent tibiofibular ligament. (From VanderGriend RA, Savoie, FH, Hughes JL: Fractures of the ankle. In: Rockwood CA Jr. Green DP, Bucholz RW (eds). *Fractures in Adults,* 3rd ed. Philadelphia: JB Lippincott, vol. 2, p. 1989, 1991. Used with permission.)

**Muscles.** There are basically four compartments of muscles that traverse the ankle joint. Anteriorly, the tibialis anterior, extensor digitorum longus, and extensor hallucis longus run over the ankle joint and contribute to dorsiflexion of the ankle. Medially, the tibialis posterior, flexor digitorum longus, and flexor hallucis longus run behind the medial malleolus and contribute to inversion of the foot. Posteriorly, the soleus and gastrocnemius muscles provide plantar flexion. Laterally, the peroneus longus and brevis muscles run in a sheath directly behind the lateral malleolus. These muscles contribute to eversion and plantar flexion.

**Nerves and blood supply.** The vascular supply to the area of the ankle is a continuation of the external iliac, femoral, and popliteal arterial system. The anterior and posterior tibial arteries as well as the peroneal artery are continuations of the popliteal artery and supply the ankle and foot. Nervous supply is from the sciatic nerve.

In summary, the ankle joint is a ring consisting of the tibia, fibula, and talus bound together by three major groups of ligaments. Almost all injuries to the ankle are due to the abnormal motion of the talus as it sets in the mortise. The talar motion causes direct or indirect stress on the malleoli or lower portion of the tibia, resulting in injury. If there is a single break in the ring, talar shift may not occur because of the ligamentous support. However, if there are two breaks in the ring, a fracture of the malleoli, a fracture of one malleolus and a rupture of one ligament, or a rupture of both ligaments, then integrity of the ring is violated and talar shift will occur. This anatomic fact is important in assessing the stability of any injured ankle.

## HISTORY OF INJURY

As with all orthopedic injuries a careful history of the mechanism of injury is essential and should always precede clinical and roentgenographic examination. The physician should attempt to ascertain the position of the foot, the direction of the stresses, and all other pertinent data to reconstruct the injury. This will aid in the determination of what bones or ligaments are most likely to be injured. It is also helpful to ask if during the time of injury there was any noise that might indicate that a ligament popped, a bone subluxed or dislocated, or a tendon snapped. The physician should ask if the onset of pain was immediate, if swelling occurred right after the injury, and if disability was immediate or delayed. A history of previous ankle injury and its treatment may affect physical findings and treatment.

## CLINICAL EXAMINATION

A partial clinical examination should always precede roentgenographic examination. If the ankle is grossly deformed, the diagnosis of an unstable joint is obvious and radiologic evaluation should occur after the physician ensures that neurovascular status is not compromised. In the absence of a gross deformity, inspect for local swelling and the loss or prominence of anatomic landmarks. Look for ecchymoses, although subcutaneous bleeding may occur with either fractures or sprains. Palpation can localize the area of maximal tenderness, crepitance, and loss or distortion of anatomic landmarks. Palpation of both malleoli, the lateral and medial ligaments, the base of the fifth metatarsal and proximal fibula should always be performed. Gently put the ankle through a range of motion to evaluate stability and to determine positions that produce or relieve pain. Manipulation must be gentle to avoid further injury. After examining the injured ankle, examine the opposite and hopefully normal joint. This will give an idea of the range of motion and laxity of the normal ankle joints. Again, the physician must keep in mind past history because a prior injury to the uninjured joint will prevent proper comparison.

## ROENTGENOGRAPHIC EXAMINATION

Roentgenograms are ordered to detect fractures and evaluate their severity. Although ligamentous injuries are not seen on x-ray films, improper anatomic relationships give a hint that ligamentous injury has occurred. The roentgenogram also allows the physician to look for further complicating factors such as foreign bodies or diseases of the bone. Lastly, the physician can use radiologic evaluation to follow the results of treatment of the patient with the ankle injury.

Proper radiologic evaluation of any ankle injury is essential. The examination should consist of an anteroposterior, lateral, and mortise (15° of internal rotation) views. The roentgenogram should be of sufficient quality that trabecular detail is seen in all views. A comparison view of the opposite side can be helpful, especially in children. Also, a cone-down view or stress view of an area with questionable findings may be helpful. The physician should use the bright light to properly examine the outline of the bony detail and to detect soft tissue swelling.

## LIGAMENTOUS INJURIES OF THE ANKLE

Approximately 75 percent of all ankle injuries are sprains. More than 90 percent involve the lateral ligaments, less than 5 percent involve the deltoid ligament, and less than 5 percent involve the anterior or posterior tibiofibular ligament and anterior and posterior capsule (see Figs. 230-1, 230-2, and 230-3). Of lateral ligament injuries, 90 percent involve the anterior talofibular ligament, with 65 percent of these sprains being isolated, and 25 percent with concomitant injuries to the calcaneofibular ligament. The posterior talofibular ligament, or

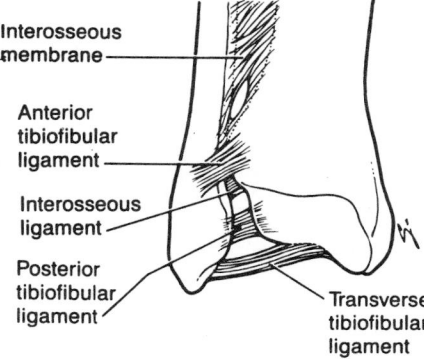

**Fig. 230-3.** The syndesmotic ligaments of the ankle. (From Vander-Griend RA, Savoie, FH, Hughes JL: Fractures of the ankle. In: Rockwood CA Jr, Green DP, Bucholz RW (eds). *Fractures in Adults,* 3rd ed. Philadelphia: JB Lippincott, vol. 2, p. 1988, 1991. Used with permission.)

third component of the lateral collateral ligament, stabilizes against posterior displacement of the talus and is therefore rarely injured except in cases of complete dislocation. Because the anterior talofibular ligament and calcaneofibular ligament are two separate structures, the standard classification of first-degree, second-degree, and third-degree sprains is difficult to apply. Hence, injury to these ligaments is classified as either a single or double ligament injury. Only one ligament may be torn so that the integrity of the joint is weakened in one plane of direction, but it is not necessarily unstable. These ligaments usually tear in sequence from anterior to posterior, so that the anterior talofibular ligament tears first, followed by the calcaneofibular ligament. If both of these are ruptured then the anterior drawer test will be positive (see below). If the calcaneofibular ligament is intact the test will be negative.

### Lateral Collateral Ligament Injuries

Laxity of the lateral ligaments may be adequately assessed by physical examination. The most helpful test is the anterior drawer maneuver. If the ligaments are torn by an inversion stress the talus will sublux anteriorly and laterally out of the mortise with observable movement and crepitation at the limit of excursion. This maneuver should be performed on all patients with suspected lateral ligamentous injuries.

With one hand, grasp the calcaneus with the finger and thumb behind the malleoli, and with the opposite hand stabilize the extreme distal tibia and fibula. The foot should be slightly plantar flexed and inverted, which is its normal relaxed position. Next, apply a forward anterior force to the calcaneus, keeping the distal tibia and fibula fixed. Movement of the talus anteriorly more than 3 mm *may* be significant, but movement greater than 1 cm *certainly* is significant. There are both false positive and false negative results with this test, but the most common difficulty is the physician's unfamiliarity with the examination.

If the tear extends further posteriorly into the calcaneofibular portion of the lateral ligament, talar tilt occurs, because the lateral ankle is now unstable, not only in the anterior posterior plane but in the medial lateral plane as well. Place the foot at 20° to 30° of plantar flexion with slight adduction, and apply inversion stress on the calcaneal forefoot. Talar tilt or movement of the talus in the mortise is clinically felt because of tilting of the talus in relation to the distal articular surface of the tibia. This is then compared with the normal side.

Good muscle relaxation is important for proper evaluation. If diagnostic maneuvers are painful, voluntary and involuntary muscle contractions to guard against further movement will prevent assessment. The use of ice packs or local anesthetic infiltration can be helpful.

If the posterior talofibular ligament is involved, the ankle is obviously unstable, with both a positive anterior drawer sign and marked talar tilt. In most posterior talofibular ligament injuries, the ankle is dislocated and neither test need be performed.

### Medial Collateral Ligament Injuries

The medial collateral ligament is rarely injured alone. Its injury is usually accompanied by a fracture of the fibula or tear of the tibiofibular ligaments anteriorly or posteriorly. This injury is usually the result of a significant eversion stress. It is almost impossible to tear the deltoid ligament without an accompanying fracture of the fibula or separation of the tibiofibular syndesmosis. Evaluation of the medial collateral ligament is done by stressing the ankle with a medial-to-lateral force, which is simply a talar tilt sign.

### Tibiofibular Syndesmotic Ligament Injuries

Tibiofibular syndesmotic ligaments (see Fig. 230-3) are a continuation of the interosseous ligaments at the distal tibia and fibula. Injuries to this ligament system most often occur secondary to hyper-dorsiflexion and eversion. The talus usually pushes superiorly, separates the tibia and fibula, and displaces the fibula laterally, resulting in a partial or complete rupture. Diastasis will not necessarily be evident on radiologic or physical examination because the interosseous membrane above the ligament system will usually keep the tibia and fibula together.

The history is often nonspecific, but frequently the patient reports that he or she felt something pop or give. There is little swelling, and the patient complains of pain over the anterior and posterior superior aspects of the ankle. The patient may not tolerate any weight-bearing on the injured ankle and may not be able to rise on the toes. On examination point tenderness over the anterior or posterior ligaments is found. There may be some tenderness over the medial malleolus secondary to a concomitant medial collateral ligament injury. Dorsiflexion produces pain due to stress on the ligament system. Bilateral compression of the tibia and fibula (squeeze test) causes pain in the injured area. The external rotation test also elicits pain by stressing the ligaments. Radiologic changes may only include soft tissue swelling at or below the medial malleolus and above the lateral malleous up to the midshaft fibula. This is a serious injury with prolonged recovery and significant long-term sequelae if not adequately treated.

### Roentgenographic Findings in Ankle Sprains

The physician should always order standard x-ray views to evaluate an ankle injury, for radiologic findings can be surprising. If the standard views show avulsion or pull-off fracture, oblique or spiral fracture, transverse fracture, diastasis of the tibia/fibula or the interosseous membrane, or a fractured fibular shaft, there is also rupture of the concomitant ligament. In such instances, no stress films are needed. However, stress films are indicated if instability is suspected or demonstrated by abnormal talar positioning, or if the joint line between the talus and mortise of the ankle is not symmetrical.

The anterior drawer sign as explained earlier may be done under x-ray or fluoroscopic examination. There is some difficulty in establishing reference points for measuring the movement of the talus anteriorly in relation to the mortise of the ankle. Although different authors have used different reference points, the current literature suggests that greater than 3-mm movement of the talus anteriorly to the posterior border of the calcaneus may be significant. Greater than 1 cm is certainly indicative of disruption. If there is some question as to the findings, the opposite ankle should be stressed in a similar manner and measured for comparison, providing the opposite ankle has not been injured in the past.

The talar tilt test, whether done in the medial or lateral ligamentous system, is also not extremely sensitive because there is variability of tilt among normal individuals and even between a pair of normal ankles. Moreover, pain, spasm, and edema may prevent adequate evaluation. As with the anterior drawer maneuver, there is no way to standardize the amount of force used by the physician during the test. However, the test may be positive if there is greater than 5° of talar tilt. If there is greater than 25° talar tilt, the examination is definitely abnormal. A difference of 5° to 10° talar tilt between the injured and uninjured side is probably significant in most instances.

In experienced hands, ankle arthrography is quick and simple to perform. It should be done within 24 to 48 h because clot formation after that time may prevent leakage of dye. Extra-articular leak of contrast material is generally indicative of a tear. However, the flexor hallucis longus and flexor digitorum longus tendon sheath fill in 20 percent of normal individuals, the peroneal tendon sheath fills in 14 percent, and the talocalcaneal joint space fills in 10 percent. Evaluation of the calcaneofibular ligament by standard arthrography techniques is associated with a high incidence of false negative results.

### Classification of Sprains

Ligamentous injuries are classified into first-, second-, and third-degree sprains. A *first-degree sprain* is stretching or microscopic tearing of a ligament, causing local tenderness and minimal swelling. Weight-bearing is possible, and x-ray films are normal.

In a *second-degree sprain*, there is severe stretching and partial tearing of a ligament, causing marked tenderness, moderate edema, mild ecchymosis, and moderate pain with weight-bearing. Radiologic evaluation with standard views will not demonstrate bony abnormality. However, if the ankle is stressed, loss of ligamentous function will be demonstrated by the abnormal relationship of the talus and mortise.

*Third-degree sprain* is due to complete rupture of ligaments. The patient is unable to bear weight, and there is marked tenderness and swelling, ecchymosis, and often an obviously deformed joint. Standard radiologic evaluation reveals an abnormal relationship of the talus and mortise. Usually, stress films are not needed, but with a complete rupture they are almost always positive if the test is performed properly.

### Treatment

There is much debate with regard to the treatment of ankle injuries. First-degree sprains may be treated by compression dressings, elevation, ice, and immobilization. Fifteen minutes of ice application to produce local anesthesia, followed by range-of-motion exercises to the development of pain, followed again by 15 min of ice application is beneficial. This should be done approximately four times a day until the patient can resume normal function without pain. The decision to institute non–weight-bearing or partial weight-bearing is an individual one. Plaster or synthetic splints or ankle braces may be used. In the case of an athlete with a first-degree sprain, full athletic activity should not be resumed until that person can sprint without limping, run circles and figures of eight at full speed without pain, and, finally, cut at right angles off the affected joint without pain.

Second-degree sprains of the ankle are best treated with the ice method as described above and immobilization. If there is extensive edema, a splint, crutches, ice, and elevation are used until swelling diminishes; then, range of motion and peroneal strengthening exercises are recommended.

The treatment of third-degree sprains of the ankle is debatable. The decision whether to treat without immobilization, with immobilization, or to operate is not made easily, and a number of considerations are important. The emergency physician is not usually asked to advise treatment for third-degree sprains because orthopedic consultation should be obtained for such injuries.

It is always prudent to maintain good liaison and communication with the patient's orthopedic surgeon. Patients with ankle injuries need appropriate diagnosis and treatment. Long-term sequelae of misdiagnosis and mistreatment are significant. Appropriate follow-up of ankle injuries is an absolute necessity.

### ANKLE FRACTURE

Fractures are caused by forces acting upon the ankle joint that produce disruption of the joint ring. After the mechanism of injury has been ascertained, standard roentgenograms are necessary for fracture diagnosis. Ligamentous avulsions will usually cause transverse malleolar fractures or small chip or pull-off fractures of the malleolus below the joint line. Shifting of the talus causes it to strike the opposite malleolus and may cause an oblique fracture, often with comminution on the side of the bone subjected to the compression force. This evidence allows for prediction of the mechanism of injury, which is important because injuring forces must be reversed for fracture reduction.

Ligamentous injuries often occur with fractures and have a more serious prognosis than the fracture itself.

## Classification of Fractures

The two commonly used classification systems for ankle fractures are shown in Fig. 230-4. The type of fracture produced depends on the position of the foot at the time of injury and the direction of the deforming force. The emphasis in both systems is the lateral malleolus. Reduction and stability of the lateral malleolus is the key to the successful treatment of ankle fractures.

**Suppination-adduction (type A).** The primary force is adduction, lateral to medial. This force is frequently an isolated event in contrast to the others. The lateral collateral ligaments rupture, or cause a pull-off or a transverse fracture of the lateral malleolus. With the continuation of the force, the talus impacts on the medial malleolus and causes an oblique fracture.

**Suppination-external (rotation or pronation-abduction (type B).** In both cases the fibula sustains an oblique fracture above the syndesmotic ligaments.

**Pronation-external rotation (type C).** Pronation-external rotation at the ankle joint causes sequential injuries that are initiated on the medial side and extend laterally. Therefore, the first injury to occur is either a pull-off or a transverse fracture of the medial malleolus or rupture of the deltoid ligament. As the forces continue, the anterior tibiofibular ligament is ruptured. The talus then impacts on the fibula and fractures it. Finally, the posterior tibial tubercle fractures, and the interosseous, posterior inferior tibiofibular, and the inferior transverse ligaments tear.

**Vertical compression.** Vertical compression is most often associated with the other forces in the production of ankle fractures; however, it may occasionally cause an isolated fracture. Depending on the position of the talus in the mortise, vertical compression can cause an anterior or, rarely, a posterior marginal fracture of the tibia. Radiologic evaluation may demonstrate small fractures of the anterior or posterior lip of the tibia due to ligamentous pull-off, or larger vertical fractures through the articular surface of the tibia. Comminution is common with both anterior and posterior fractures, making anatomic reduction very difficult.

Other ankle fractures such as intra-articular or osteochondral fractures of the talus, or distal tibia can occur. If undetected, intra-articular fractures of the talus or osteochondritis dissecans can lead to loose bodies floating in the joint and early degenerative arthritis.

Avulsion fractures of the base of the fifth metatarsal are probably one of the most commonly missed fractures. The history is an ankle injury due to plantar flexion and inversion. The peroneus brevis in-

**Fig. 230-4.** The AO (Danis-Weber) and Lauge-Hansen classification systems. Note that the AO system includes injuries of different Lauge-Hansen types in one category. (From Sangeorzan BJ, Sigward HT. Ankle and foot trauma. *Orthopedic Knowledge Update III.* Park Ridge, IL: American Academy of Orthopedic Surgeons, p. 615, 1990. Used with permission.)

sertion at the base of the fifth metatarsal is stressed, resulting in a pull-off fracture. The base of the fifth metatarsal should be evident in proper radiologic examination of the ankle, but this is not necessarily always the case. The physician may not see the fracture if he or she does not suspect it. The epiphyseal plate of the base of fifth metatarsal can be differentiated from a pull-off fracture because the epiphyseal plate is usually oblique or longitudinal, whereas the fracture line is transverse.

## Treatment

The goals of treatment of all ankle injuries, including fractures, are to restore the anatomic position of the talus in the mortise, return the joint line parallel to the ground, and ensure a smooth articular surface. These goals are achieved by immobilization or surgery. The primary indication for operative treatment is the inability to maintain anatomic positioning of the talus in relation to the ankle mortise. The lateral malleolus and its ligamentous attachments are responsible for keeping the talus reduced on the mortise so reduction of the lateral malleolus is critical.

Anatomic reduction is usually done by reversal of the injuring forces. Plantar flexion of the ankle in reduction of medial malleolar injuries should be avoided since the anterior fibers of the deltoid ligament are taut in this position, preventing positioning of the medial malleolus.

## ANKLE DISLOCATION

Most dislocations of the ankle (Fig. 230-5) are associated with malleolar fractures and almost half are open. These injuries should be reduced emergently with gentle in-line traction. Open injuries require surgical debridement. There is a high incidence of avascular necrosis following ankle dislocations.

## OTHER INJURIES OF THE ANKLE

### Contusion

Direct trauma can produce contusion of the soft tissues or periosteum with swelling, discoloration, and point tenderness. Radiologic evaluation may demonstrate a cortical fracture in addition to soft tissue swelling. Treatment is symptomatic and consists of ice, a compression dressing, rest and elevation, and analgesics.

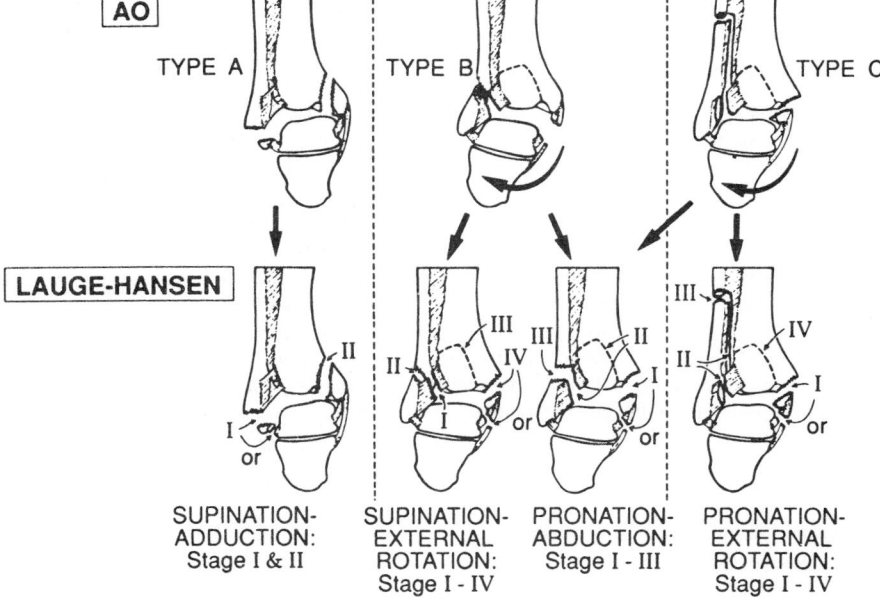

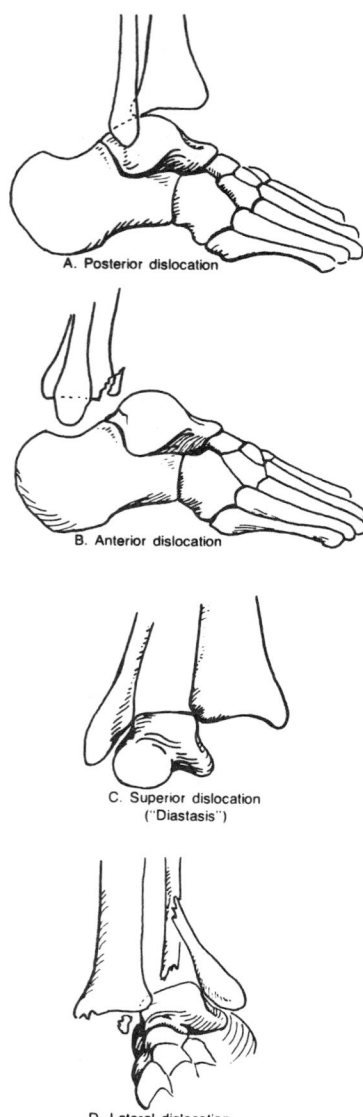

**Fig. 230-5.** The types of dislocations of the ankle. (From Simon R, Koenigsknecht S. *Orthopedics in Emergency Medicine.* New York: Appleton-Century-Crofts, p. 419, 1982. Used with permission.)

## Tenosynovitis

Tenosynovitis is usually secondary to direct trauma or overuse of the tendons. The patient has tenderness and swelling in the localized area but may have crepitance of the tendon as it moves through the sheath. X-ray films are negative. Treatment is ice and rest, but partial immobilization and anti-inflammatory medication may be necessary.

Achilles tendon injuries are common in runners and joggers. They are usually seen in the older individual but may be seen in the young. The patient gives a history of direct trauma or repetitive irritation to the area with symptoms of swelling and tenderness over the Achilles tendon or at its insertion. Treatment is rest, shortening of the Achilles tendon by heel elevation, and anti-inflammatory medication. Steroid injections should never be given secondary to the increased risk of tendon rupture.

## ACHILLES TENDON RUPTURE

The gastrocnemius and soleus muscles join in the middle of the calf to form the Achilles tendon. Rupture of the tendon is often missed by the physician on initial examination, the injury frequently mistaken for an ankle sprain. Tendon rupture most often occurs secondary to indirect mechanisms resulting in forceful dorsiflexion of the ankle. Initiating a sprint, slipping on a stair or ladder, or a fall from a height may result in sufficient dorsiflexion to rupture the tendon. Tendon tears can also be caused by direct trauma from blows to a taut tendon or by lacerations from glass or lawn mower accidents. Most commonly rupture occurs in middle-aged men and the left Achilles is involved significantly more often than the right.

History most often suggests the diagnosis of Achilles tendon rupture. Patients experience sudden pain, often described as a feeling like someone kicked them in the calf. An audible snap may be heard and the patient subsequently has difficulty stepping off on the foot. Physical examination usually reveals swelling of the distal calf as well as a palpable defect in the tendon 2 to 6 cm proximal to its insertion into the calcaneus, the location where rupture most frequently occurs. Plantar flexion of the injured ankle will be weaker when compared to the uninjured side. Active plantar flexion of the injured side *does not,* however, rule out the diagnosis of Achilles tendon rupture because other muscles, including the toe flexors, peroneals, and tibialis posterior, can generate some ankle plantar flexion. Additionally, the calf squeeze or "Thompson's test" will help confirm the diagnosis of complete tendon rupture. A positive Thompson's sign is indicated by failure of the foot to plantar flex against gravity with calf compression when the patient is lying prone and the knee is flexed 90°. X-ray films are generally not helpful in establishing the diagnosis.

Early treatment includes orthopedic consultation and splinting of the lower extremity in a posterior splint in passive equinus (the position the foot assumes when dependent). The patient should remain non–weight-bearing and keep the extremity elevated. Definitive treatment is controversial. Conservative therapy consists of short or long leg cast immobilization in the equinus position for 8 weeks followed by serial cast changes over the next 4 weeks, bringing the foot up into neutral position. Some studies have found a decrease in plantar flexion strength in patients treated conservatively compared with those who underwent surgery. As a result, surgical repair is usually recommended for younger athletic patients who want to optimize their strength in the injured leg.

## SUBLUXING PERONEAL TENDONS

Subluxing peroneal tendons is an uncommon entity that can be acute or chronic. The condition is characterized by the two peroneal tendons, the peroneal longus and peroneus brevis, subluxing anteriorly over the lateral malleolus. The tendons share a common synovial sheath at the ankle and track in a groove on the posterior aspect of the lateral malleolus. The groove and superior retinaculum hold these tendons in place. The mechanism of injury is a sudden passive dorsiflexion of the ankle followed by a powerful reflex contraction of the peroneals. The injury has been most commonly associated with skiing but can occur in various athletic endeavors, including ice skating, soccer, and basketball.

The diagnosis is primarily made from the history and physical examination. The patient will often complain of having heard a "snap" or a "pop" at the time of injury. Some may even relate a history of their "tendons popping out." Physical examination reveals localized swelling, tenderness, and sometimes ecchymosis at the posterior aspect of the lateral malleolus. Having the patient tense the peroneal muscles will exacerbate the pain. Spontaneous reduction has usually occurred before presentation. The subluxation may be reproduced by having the patient dorsiflex and evert the foot against resistance. This injury is frequently misdiagnosed as an inversion-type ankle sprain but can be differentiated from it by finding point tenderness posterior to the malleolus as opposed to anterior where the anterior talofibular ligament is located. A small piece of bone is avulsed from the posterior aspect of the lateral malleolus by the retinaculum in 15 to 50 percent of cases. The finding of this avulsion on x-ray, which typically is 1 to 2 mm thick and 2 cm in length, is pathognomonic for this condition.

Treatment may be conservative or surgical. If the classic avulsion fracture is seen then casting for 6 weeks is generally recommended. If no fracture is visualized or the problem becomes chronic, then surgical procedures to deepen the peroneal groove or reconstruct the retinaculum are indicated.

## ANKLE INJURIES IN CHILDREN

In adolescents over 15 to 16 years old, epiphyseal plates are closing or have already closed, so the adult types of fractures occur in this population. In children, the ligamentous injuries are rare because the ligaments are stronger than the bone. This causes fractures to occur at the epiphyseal plates. The mechanism of injury usually involves indirect forces, most commonly inversion or eversion. Direct injuries are rare. The Salter-Harris classification is the most common classification utilized to describe these fractures. The patients present with the usual findings associated with fractures. On palpation, the patient is maximally tender over the injured growth plate. Standard x-ray evaluation is important in these patients. More importantly, the entire tibia and fibula should be included in any radiographic evaluation to rule out high fibular fractures. Occasionally, the Salter-Harris type I and II injuries are difficult to see on the radiographs because of minimal displacement. The physician must be careful to inspect the films for soft tissue swelling which would occur over the fracture area. The treatment for the majority of these fractures is conservative, and minimal complications occur. If a complication does occur, it is usually a disturbance of the growth plate, resulting in angular deformities and leg length changes.

## COMPLICATIONS

A number of complications are associated with ankle injuries, especially if they are improperly treated.

Ankle instability can result from grade II or III sprains that do not heal. Nonunion occurs in 10 to 15 percent of fractures of the medial malleolus treated by a closed method. If it occurs, surgical correction is required.

Malunion can occur at any fracture site. If the patient is symptomatic with instability or pain and arthritic changes are not significant, surgery to correct the malunion may be done. Such surgery is often unsuccessful. Fusion may be the treatment of choice if there is degenerative or traumatic arthritis, or if the surgery has not been successful.

Infections are a complication of open fractures or the surgical treatment of closed fractures.

Traumatic arthritis occurs in 20 to 40 percent of ankle fractures regardless of the methods of treatment, but it is more common in inappropriately treated injuries. Loss of either the anterior or posterior tibial vessels may result in tissue destruction. The best treatment of possible neurovascular injuries is prophylaxis. Sudeck's atrophy secondary to sympathetic dystrophy is a complication of ankle injuries. Synostosis, or ossification of the interosseous membrane, may follow injuries to the syndesmotic ligaments resulting in stiffness of the ankle joint. Finally, instability of the talus in the mortise is the most feared sequela. The loss of the support function of the ligaments predisposes the patient to recurrent sprains, resulting from progressively less trauma. This is especially disabling in athletes.

## BIBLIOGRAPHY

Butler WB, Lanthier J, Wertheimer SJ: Subluxing peroneals: a review of the literature and case report. *J Foot Ankle Surg* 32:134, 1992.

Dias LS: Fractures of the tibia and fibula. In: Rockwood CA Jr, Wilkins KE, King RE (eds): *Fractures in Children.* Philadelphia: JB Lippincott, vol. 3, pp. 1271–1382, 1991.

Simon RR, Koenigsknecht SJ: *Orthopaedics in Emergency Medicine: The Extremities,* 2d ed. New York: Appleton-Century-Crofts, 1989.

VanderGriend RA, Savoie FH, Hughes JL: Fractures of the ankle. In: Rockwood CA Jr, Green DP, Bucholz RW (eds): *Fractures in Adults,* 3rd ed. Philadelphia: JB Lippincott, vol. 2, pp. 1983–2040, 1991.

# 231
# FOOT INJURIES

## Joseph F. Waeckerle
## Mark T. Steele

The foot bears the weight of the body, and any injuries to it are magnified because of tremendous stress. The patient with an injured foot becomes debilitated to the point of not being able to bear weight, or to function properly. Loss of mobility of the joints of the foot as well as pain at the fracture site and subsequent arthritis may cause the patient discomfort and disability seemingly out of proportion to the injury sustained. It behooves the physician treating the patient with a foot injury to minimize disability by appropriately treating the bone and soft tissue injuries from the beginning.

The mechanisms of injury resulting in fractures and soft tissue damage to the foot include direct and indirect trauma as well as overuse, or stress, injuries. An adequate history will often help the physician determine the location of the injury and predict what injuries might be seen. This is important because radiographic evaluation of the foot is sometimes difficult due to the many overlying bony shadows, secondary ossification centers, and sesamoid bones. Comparison views with the opposite foot are often essential to properly evaluate an injured foot.

Classification of the fractured foot is complex, and it is beyond the scope of this chapter to present a detailed classification or complete discussion of all fractures of the foot. The following discussion will touch upon the more common injuries seen. For more detail the reader is referred to the texts which discuss fractures and dislocations.

## ANATOMY AND BIOMECHANICS

The foot consists of the hindpart, which is made up of the calcaneus and talus; the midpart, which is separated from the hindpart by Chopart's joint and consists of the navicular, cuboid, and cuneiforms; and the forepart, which is separated from the midpart by Lisfranc's joint and consists of the metatarsals and phalanges. There are 28 bones, 57 major articular surfaces, and many ligaments as well as tendons and other soft tissues that contribute to the stability and integrity of the foot.

Following are some major points to keep in mind. (1) The long arch of the foot depends upon the position and alignment of the bones and not the soft tissue as commonly believed. (2) Weight-bearing on the foot causes an equal distribution of forces between the heel and forepart. (3) The first metatarsal head bears two times as much weight as the other metatarsal heads. This is important because treatment of great toe injuries, especially of the metatarsal head, requires a more conservative approach. (4) Lastly, when a push-off force on the foot occurs, the maximum load is borne by the second metatarsal. With repeated pushing off, stress fractures of the second metatarsal may be seen. Some stress fractures of the third metatarsal may also be seen because, after the second metatarsal, it bears more weight than the others during the push-off, or acceleration, phase.

## CALCANEAL FRACTURES

The calcaneus is the largest of the tarsal bones in the foot and functions as the base for locomotion and support of the weight of the body. It is the most often fractured of the tarsal bones, being involved in some 60 percent of such injuries. The difficulty with calcaneal fracture is that there is no optimal treatment, and, therefore, a good result is not often obtained. Calcaneal fractures are usually classified as fractures involving the processes or tuberosity, and fractures involving the body. The mechanism of injury is usually compression secondary to a fall from a height.

Because the patient must sustain a significant compression force to fracture the calcaneus, associated injuries are not uncommon; 10 percent of all calcaneal fractures are associated with lumbar compression injuries, and 26 percent are associated with other injuries to the extremity. Thus it is important to get a good history of the mechanism of injury. Also, the physician must examine the patient for injuries associated with the calcaneal fracture, including back, pelvic, hip, and knee injuries. The symptoms and signs associated with calcaneal fractures are directly proportional to the location and severity of the injury to the calcaneus as well as other associated injuries. Generally, the patient will experience swelling, pain, and ecchymoses at the fracture site. Often the fracture site will be exquisitely tender locally, with decreased range of motion and the inability to bear any weight on the fracture.

Standard radiographic views of the foot, which consist of three different views, may not be sufficient in evaluating calcaneal fractures, but should be ordered initially. Besides the anteroposterior (AP), lateral, and axial views, certain "scout films" may be required to specifically delineate various fracture sites of the calcaneus. It is essential that, in evaluating calcaneal fractures, the x-ray films demonstrate good trabecular detail. Computed tomography scanning may be necessary to define the involvement of the posterior facet of the calcaneus.

### Treatment

As with all fractures, the objective in treating the patient is to restore normal anatomy and function as quickly as possible. This requires a great deal of skill and expertise with most calcaneal fractures; therefore, a consultant should be called in early in the management of the case. If the patient has gross swelling or is unstable, conservative treatment with a posterior splint providing immobilization, as well as attention to the soft tissue swelling and injuries, is imperative. In all instances, reduction of the calcaneal fracture to the closest anatomic position should be done as soon as possible by the consultant. The two main goals are restoration of the heel width and reduction of the posterior facet. A patient with a severely fractured calcaneus should be admitted to the hospital for elevation because fracture blisters can be a significant problem if they develop.

## TALUS FRACTURES

Although talus fractures are the second most common foot fracture, they are still relatively uncommon. The talus is held in place by ligaments surrounding it and has no muscular attachments. Because most of the talus is covered by articular cartilage, the blood supply is tenuous and enters by way of the ligamentous and capsular support to the bone. Therefore, fractures of the talus, especially of the neck, associated with body dislocations, may cause avascular necrosis of the bone. The mechanism of injury which produces a talus fracture dislocation is usually hyperextension. The patient complains of intense pain and is unable to bear weight. There is localized swelling, discoloration, and tenderness to palpation. Moreover, there is an obvious loss of the normal contour of the foot. Any range of motion is intensely painful to the patient. X-ray evaluation for suspected talus fractures usually requires routine views of the foot. In certain instances, more detailed and specific x-ray views may be ordered.

### Treatment

Treatment of talus injuries depends somewhat upon the extent of the fracture. Simple, nondisplaced minor chips or avulsion fractures require immobilization as well as ice, elevation, and follow-up. These patients do not usually have long-term complications. In contrast, fractures of the neck and body, or fracture dislocation of the talus, may be very difficult to treat, causing extensive problems for both the patient and the physician in the long run. If there is any displacement of a talar neck fracture, there is also a subluxed or dislocated talonavicular or subtalar joint. These should be treated operatively. In such instances, besides assessing neurovascular status of the foot and adequately evaluating and immobilizing the injury, the emergency physician should seek consultation for further care.

## MIDPART FRACTURES

The midpart of the foot is infrequently fractured, but if it is injured, multiple fractures may occur. This area of the foot is most susceptible to direct trauma because it is the least mobile portion of the foot and includes five tarsal bones and all their articular surfaces and ligamentous support. Due to the many articulating surfaces, injuries to the midpart of the foot are associated with subluxation or dislocation or both. If the physician encounters an isolated midfoot fracture, it is most often of the navicular bone. Injuries to the cuboid and cuneiforms occur in combination with injuries to the navicular or one another and are usually the result of a crushing-type injury. Various classifications are used to describe injuries to the midfoot. Such injuries are divided into those to the navicular and those to the other bones.

Symptoms and signs are similar to those of other orthopedic-type injuries. That is, the patient presents with pain, swelling, and tenderness over the involved area. The standard x-ray views (AP, lateral, and oblique) are generally adequate to demonstrate most injuries in this area.

### Treatment

The treatment is ice, elevation, and immobilization if there is no displacement and the anatomic position is acceptable. If not, then consultation for further closed reduction or open reduction-internal fixation is required so that the patient can achieve and maintain as close to anatomic reduction as possible.

## TARSAL-METATARSAL FRACTURE/DISLOCATIONS

The tarsal-metatarsal joint is referred to as Lisfranc's joint. Injuries to this area are uncommon and are usually caused by automobile accidents. The mechanism of injury is complicated and varied but is usually an axial load applied directly to the heel with the foot fixed to the ground in equinns or a severe hyperextension of the forefoot on the midfoot, causing dorsal dislocation. There may be associated fractures. Such injuries occur because ligamentous support is the stabilizing support to this joint. The keystone of this joint is the second metatarsal; it is the locking mechanism of the midpart of the foot. Therefore, a fracture at the base of the second metatarsal is almost pathognomonic of a disrupted joint. Symptoms and signs are pain, swelling, discoloration, loss of range of motion, loss of weight-bearing, and possibly some paresthesia in the midpart of the foot. X-ray views needed are the standard three views (Figs. 231-1 and 231-2).

### Treatment

The treatment of this fracture/dislocation is very difficult because complete restoration of position by closed reduction requires strong traction. In fact, correction of this deformity may require open reduction and internal fixation. Therefore, it is important to get the consulting surgeon involved in the case as early as possible.

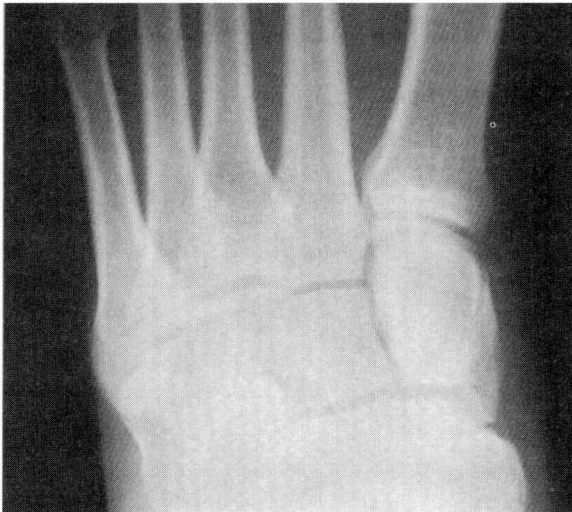 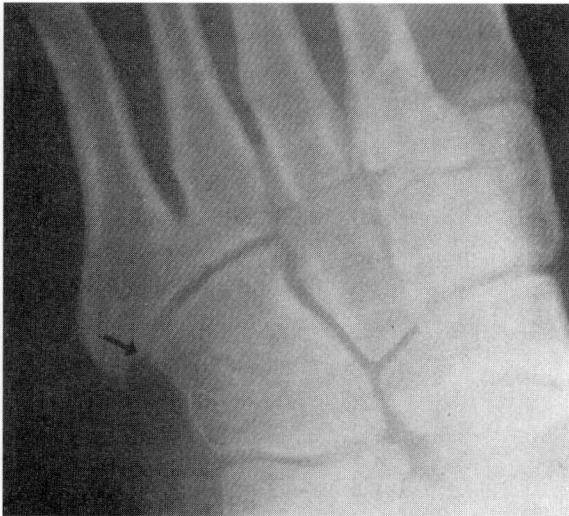

**Fig. 231-1.** Anteroposterior (left) and oblique (right) x-rays of a normal foot showing the normal bony relationships between the tarsus and metatarsals: (1) The parallel alignment of the medial edge of the second metatarsal base and the medial edge of the second cuneiform, (2) alignment of the medial edge of the fourth metatarsal base with the medial surface of the cuboid, and (3) a notch in the base of the fifth metatarsal at the point of articulation with the lateral edge of the cuboid (*arrow*). (From Heckman JD. Fractures and dislocations of the foot. In: Rockwood CA Jr, Green DP, Bucholz RW (eds). *Fractures in Adults,* 3rd ed. Philadelphia: JB Lippincott, vol. 3, p. 2142, 1991. Used with permission.)

## METATARSAL FRACTURES

The second and third metatarsals are relatively fixed because of their anatomic configuration and are subjected to a great deal of stress, especially during the push-off phase of running or walking. In contrast, the first, fourth, and fifth metatarsals are relatively mobile. The significance of this is that excessive stress over a period of time can result in the development of stress fractures usually occurring in the second and third metatarsals. Other mechanisms of injury to the metatarsals are direct trauma or crush injuries and occasionally indirect force such as twisting-type injury. Because the direct trauma or crush injury is usually fairly significant, frequently more than one metatarsal is fractured. Moreover, associated soft tissue injuries with severe swelling and possible vascular compromise may occur.

Metatarsal fractures are divided into neck fractures and shaft fractures. Specific mention should be made of the pull-off fracture of the base of the fifth metatarsal, which is commonly called the ballet dancer's fracture. This injury is usually due to plantar flexion and inversion, resulting in the peroneus brevis tendon pulling off a portion of the bone where it inserts. This specific fracture may often be confused with a ligamentous injury to the ankle. It behooves the physician, when evaluating lateral ankle injuries, to include in the x-ray views the base of the fifth metatarsal to ensure that this fracture has not occurred.

Patients who experience metatarsal fractures present with typical findings but especially local tenderness. The x-ray evaluation consists of the three standard views of the foot and usually does not require any further x-ray evaluation.

### Treatment

Treatment for metatarsal fractures is ice, elevation, analgesics, and noncircumferential immobilization. A cast should not be applied to these patients before 24 to 48 h because severe swelling may be associated with the crushing-type injury that caused the fracture. Once the swelling goes down, a short leg cast should be applied for 4 to 6 weeks. Occasionally, fractures involving significant displacement, angulation, or multiple metatarsals are treated surgically.

### Fractures at Base of Fifth Metatarsal

Fractures at the base of the fifth metatarsal are by far the most common of the metatarsal fractures. These patients will specifically present with local tenderness over the fracture site. As mentioned earlier, this injury is often confused with lateral ligamentous sprain to the ankle, and it is important that the base of the fifth metatarsal be visualized in x-ray views of the ankle to rule out such fracture. Moreover, the physician must keep in mind that this is a secondary growth center or apophysis and that oblique and transverse fractures may be confused with the growth center. The treatment for this fracture is usually conservative and consists of taping, a postoperative or fracture shoe, and crutches for a short period of time.

Special mention should be made of the Jones fracture, which was formerly described as an avulsion fracture of the base of the fifth metatarsal. Recently it has been reported that this is, in fact, a transverse fracture of the diaphysis and not an avulsion-type injury. This is an important distinction because true Jones fractures have a higher incidence of nonunion or delayed union in both children and adults, in contrast to the more common avulsion fracture. Internal fixation or cast immobilization is indicated for this fracture.

### Stress Fractures

Brief mention should be made of stress fractures to the second and third metatarsal; such fractures usually occur proximal to the head. These fractures are usually insidious in onset and may not appear on x-ray films for 2 to 3 weeks after their occurrence. The physician may treat the patient as if he or she has a stress fracture, even though it is not present on x-ray films, and then re-x-ray the patient 2 or 3 weeks later, or perform a bone scan which will usually delineate the fracture site. Treatment for stress fractures is rest or, occasionally, immobilization.

### PHALANGEAL INJURIES

Injuries to the phalanx are common and usually result from direct trauma. Such injuries consist of both fractures and fracture dislocations. The majority of phalanx fractures are the result of a direct

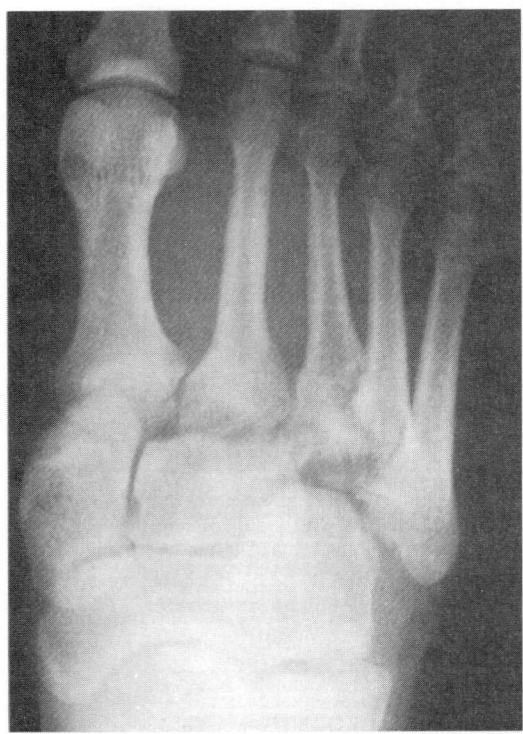
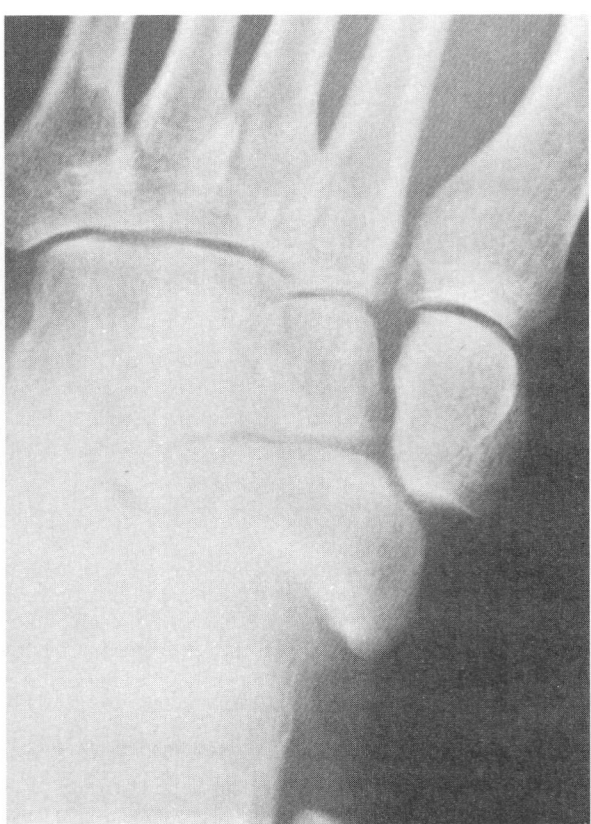
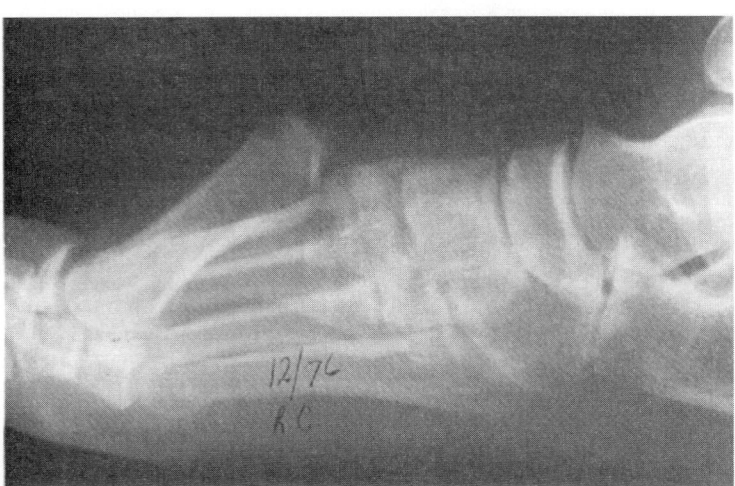

**Fig. 231-2.** (*Top left*) Anteroposterior x-ray of a homolateral Lisfranc's dislocation. Note the lateral displacement of the metatarsal bases in relation to the tarsus. (*Top right*) Oblique x-ray of a variant of Lisfranc's injury. Note medial displacement of the first metatarsal and medial cuneiform. The lateral metatarsals remain normally aligned. (*Bottom*) Lateral x-ray of a third injury showing dorsal displacement of the second metatarsal base. (From Heckman JD. Fractures and dislocations of the foot. In: Rockwood CA Jr, Green DP, Bucholz RW (eds). *Fractures in Adults,* 3rd ed. Philadelphia: JB Lippincott, vol. 3, p. 2146, 1991. Used with permission.)

trauma, such as dropping a heavy object on the toes. An indirect mechanism causing fractures is hyperextension; an indirect mechanism causing dislocations is compression with dorsiflexion of the proximal phalanx.

The patient presents with pain, swelling, and discomfort, especially when wearing shoes and walking, within a few hours after an injury to the phalanx or its joints. In some instances when a dislocation or subluxation has occurred there is obvious deformity, but this may not always be the case because swelling may be significant enough to mask the deformity. X-ray evaluation is usually best in the AP and oblique views.

## Treatment

Treatment is similar to that of all other fractures; that is, reduction of the subluxation or dislocation and reduction of the fracture to its most anatomically correct position and then ice, elevation, and immobilization. Most can be easily reduced with digital block anesthesia and gentle traction. The majority of the dislocations are posterior and once reduced are usually stable. Immobilization can occur through dynamic splinting (so-called buddy taping), a postoperative shoe, or in certain instances a walking boot cast. Because the great toe bears one third of the body weight of that side, it may need more extensive immobilization such as is provided by the walking boot cast. Displaced phalangeal fractures, which are irreducible because of their instability, may require internal fixation and, therefore, early referral. Open phalangeal fractures demand adequate soft tissue treatment, and early referral is strongly recommended for them as well. If the injury, whether it be a fracture or dislocation, is resistant to attempts at closed reduction to achieve anatomic position, referral to the orthopedic specialist is recommended because of the possible long-term sequelae.

## PLANTAR FASCIITIS

Plantar fasciitis is the most common cause of heel pain in athletes and nonathletes. The etiology of the pain is multifactorial but usually involves inflammation and degeneration of the plantar fascia at its origin on the medial process of the calcaneal tuberosity. The etiologic factors include training errors, such as rapid mileage increase, running on steep hills, and wearing improper footwear. Biomechanical factors such as pes cavus and excessive pronation of the heel may also play a role.

The pain is often burning in nature and is usually gradual in onset. It is most commonly localized to the medial process of the calcaneal tuberosity and generally is worsened during weight-bearing and stair climbing. Physical examination reveals localized tenderness of the medial process of the calcaneal tuberosity. Having the patient stand on his or her toes may exacerbate the symptoms. A lateral roentgenogram of the heel may show a calcaneal spur, the etiologic significance of which remains controversial. Patients may have clinical findings of plantar fasciitis without a spur or have a spur without evidence of plantar fasciitis. The differential diagnosis of this condition includes calcaneal stress fracture and tarsal tunnel syndrome.

The mainstays of treatment are rest, ice, nonsteroidal anti-inflammatory medications, and sometimes padded heel cups. In recalcitrant cases a local injection of corticosteroid may be helpful. Multiple steroid injections are contraindicated because of their association with rupture of the plantar fascia and heel pad atrophy. Alternative physical activities are recommended until symptoms have resolved, and a return to previous activities should begin gradually and only after training errors have been corrected. Appropriate stretching exercises are also indicated. Surgery is rarely required, with the majority of cases responding to conservative management.

## TARSAL TUNNEL SYNDROME

Tarsal tunnel syndrome is an entrapment neuropathy of the posterior tibial nerve (Fig. 231-3) and is comparable to carpal tunnel syndrome

**Fig. 231-3.** Superficial anatomy of the ankle, medial side. (From VanderGriend RA, Savoie FH, Hughes, JL. Fractures of the ankle. In: Rockwood CA Jr, Green DP, Bucholz RW (eds). *Fractures in Adults,* 3rd ed. Philadelphia: JB Lippincott, vol. 2, p. 1990, 1991. Used by permission.)

of the wrist. The tarsal tunnel is an inelastic, fixed space covered by the flexor retinaculum so any condition causing inflammation and swelling (i.e., fractures, dislocations, gout, or rheumatoid arthritis) can result in the syndrome.

Clinically, the pain is located at the medial malleolus with radiation to the heel and sole of the foot and sometimes calf. Nocturnal pain is common, and there may be increased pain with walking or dorsiflexion of the foot. Paresthesias, dysesthesias, and hypesthesias may also occur. An early sign is loss of two-point discrimination over the plantar aspect of the foot and toes. Pain is often poorly localized but may be reproduced by tapping over the nerve (Tinel sign). Definitive diagnosis is made by electromyographic and nerve conduction studies.

Initial management is conservative with rest, nonsteroidal anti-inflammatory agents, and well-fitting shoes and orthotic devices to improve biomechanics. Local steroid injections may also prove helpful. If conservative management fails, then surgical release of the flexor retinaculum and resection of adhesions is indicated.

## FOOT INJURIES IN CHILDREN

Fractures of the foot are unusual in children because of the pliability of the bone and cartilage, and they are usually easy to treat. Specific mention will be made of some of the more common injuries.

Talus fractures, although rare, are being recognized more frequently. These usually occur secondary to a forced dorsiflexion-type injury. The symptoms and signs, x-ray views, and treatment are similar to those of adults, but there is a greater incidence of avascular necrosis in children. Calcaneal fractures are not a major problem in children and are associated with minimal complications. Isolated midpart foot fractures are unusual in children. They are usually associated with other injuries of the midpart of the foot, indicating that a major injury has occurred. Tarsal-metatarsal injuries of the foot, while rare, are more common than generally recognized. They occur because of indirect injuries produced by significant forces, usually

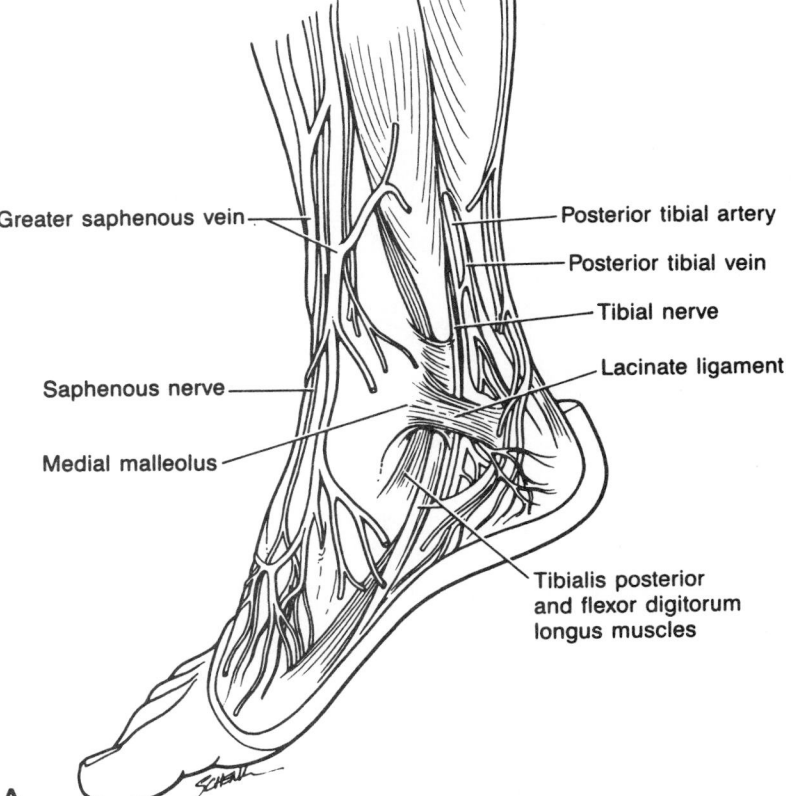

Greater saphenous vein

Posterior tibial artery

Posterior tibial vein

Tibial nerve

Lacinate ligament

Saphenous nerve

Medial malleolus

Tibialis posterior and flexor digitorum longus muscles

A

plantar flexion. The symptoms, signs, x-ray evaluation, and treatment are similar to those of adults. Fractures of the base of the second metatarsal indicate disruption to the tarsal-metatarsal joint, a sign that the patient has suffered a significant injury. The proper treatment is good anatomic reduction, which, in certain instances, may require fixation devices. Metatarsal fractures are common in children. They may be the result of torque-type forces causing fractures of the neck, or direct injuries such as crush forces causing fractures of the shaft. The symptoms, signs, and x-ray evaluation are similar to those of adults. The treatment is closed, and the complications are minimal with an occasional compartment syndrome seen.

Fractures of the base of the fifth metatarsal are relatively common in children. In the past these fractures were felt to be the result of a "pull-off" of the peroneous brevis insertion. Recently, however, the abductor digiti minimi and lateral component of the plantar aponeuroses have been implicated in this fracture. On radiographic examination, the fracture is usually seen perpendicular to the longitudinal axis of the bone. It must be distinguished from the apophysis and the sesamoid bone, os vesalianum. The treatment is conservative, and the complications are minimal.

Phalangeal injuries are very uncommon in children because their bone and cartilage, as well as soft tissues, are very pliable. If they occur, they are usually the result of direct trauma. These fractures should be treated conservatively, with the major goal being to prevent malrotation-type deformities similar to those of phalangeal injuries of the hand.

## BIBLIOGRAPHY

Gross RH: Fractures and dislocations of the foot. In: Rockwood CA Jr, Wilkins KE, King RE (eds): *Fractures in Children.* 3rd ed. Philadelphia: JB Lippincott vol. 3, pp. 1383–1453, 1991.

Heckman D: Fractures and dislocations of the foot. In: Rockwood CA Jr, Green DP, Bucholz RW (eds): *Fractures in Adults.* 3rd ed. Philadelphia: JB Lippincott, vol. 3, pp. 2041–2182, 1991.

Jackson DL, Haglund B: Tarsal tunnel syndrome in athletes: case reports and literature review. *Am J Sports Med* 19:61, 1991.

Schepsis AA, Leach RE, Gorzyca T: Plantar fasciitis: etiology, treatment, surgical results, and review of the literature. *Clin Orthop* 266:185, 1991.

Simon RR, Koenigsknecht SJ: *Orthopaedics in Emergency Medicine: The Extremities,* 2d ed. New York: Appleton-Century-Crofts, 1989.

# Muscular, Ligamentous, and Rheumatic Disorders

## 232
## NECK PAIN

### Myron M. LaBan

Neck pain has an encyclopedic list of causes, including trauma, degenerative disease, infections, neoplasms, congenital variations, inflammatory arthritis, and psychic tension.

Evaluation of neck pain requires an understanding of the anatomy of the cervical spine. The cervical spine consists of seven vertebrae; the fifth through the seventh are alike in shape and size, whereas the first cervical vertebra (atlas) and the second (axis) differ in structure. The lower third through seventh vertebral bodies articulate with each other via their superior and inferior articular processes, allowing limited rotation and lateral flexion. The atlas (C1) supports the occipital condyles and the axis (C2). Its inferior articulations resemble the other inferior vertebral articulations. The dens and its stabilizing horizontal ligament permit rotation between C1 and C2. The transverse processes of each of the cervical vertebrae are perforated by a foramen through which the vertebral vessels pass.

The muscles of the neck are compartmentalized into seven fascial planes. These planes normally permit pain-free movement of one muscle group on the other. Following acute trauma to the neck, petechial hemorrhages and edema within these same fascial planes can produce limited motion associated with complaints of stiffness, pain, and swelling.

The stable but flexible cervical spine is linked by both ligaments and disks. Because of major structural differences, the cervical disks are less likely than lumbar disks to prolapse. The cervical spine is more mobile, the superincumbent weight is less, the nucleus pulposis is more anteriorly displaced, and, unlike the lumbar spine, the annulus is posteriorly reinforced in its entire width by the posterior longitudinal ligament.

The eight paired cervical spinal roots exit the intervertebral foramina between the superior and inferior pedicles except for the upper two cervical roots. Unique to the cervical spinal roots, in over half the cases, the ventral and dorsal roots remain discrete at the neural foramina. In these cases isolated irritation of the dorsal (sensory) root posteriorly by an osteophyte may produce only sensory complaints. Similarly, ventral root (motor) compromise by a degenerative or herniated disk can produce painless, progressive weakness.

The sinuvertebral nerves from the dorsal root reenter the intervertebral foramina to supply sensation to the ligaments of the spinal canal. Anteriorly they supply the posterior longitudinal ligament, and posteriorly the ligamentum flavum, meninges, and associated vessels. Ascending and descending branches also supply the zygoapophyseal joints, providing position sense.

The cervical portion of the spinal cord surrounded by spinal fluid is suspended laterally to the enveloping dura by 20 dentate ligaments. The dura in turn is attached cephalad to the rim of the foramen magnum and within the vertebral spinal canal itself is cushioned from trauma by epidural fat.

## HISTORY

The source of neck pain can often be determined by a thorough and searching history. In the vast majority of cases, patients can identify either a singular inciting cause of discomfort or an exacerbating maneuver or position which replicates the discomfort. In traumatic injury, the exact nature of the impact with reference to positioning; accompanying lacerations of the head, neck, or face; the use of restraints; the use of protective sports equipment; associated limb or trunk fractures or contusions; and loss of consciousness or subsequent seizures are all important information. Environmental conditions on the date of injury, preexisting medical conditions, and other contributing factors should also be identified. Finally, the examiner should determine whether litigation has already been initiated or is anticipated by the patient.

As always, a review of systems, age and occupation, previous systemic illnesses, the character of the pain complaint, and its distribution should be included. Specific neurogenic symptoms should be sought including extremity weakness, incoordination, sensory aberration, and sphincter and sexual dysfunction. Visual, auditory-vestibular, and pharyngeal-laryngeal symptoms often require direct questioning to elicit complaints. The results of previous laboratory testing, as well as the response to medication or physical treatment is useful and may, in the patient's response to therapy, be diagnostic.

## PHYSICAL EXAMINATION

The physical examination may start with an observation of a loss of neck flexibility. Pain may cause splinting of the head on the shoulders during position change. Neck mobility should be tested, both with active and passive movement, including flexion (chin to shoulder) and lateral flexion (ear to shoulder). When localized ipsilateral neck pain is experienced toward the side of head movement, zygoapophyseal joint irritability is suspected. When ipsilateral pain radiates to shoulder or arm (Spurling's sign), a radicular component may be present. Contralateral neck pain suggests either a primary ligamentous or a muscular source of discomfort as these structures are placed on a stretch. Gross shoulder motion both with abduction and with forward flexion should be observed. These maneuvers of both neck and shoulder are normally smooth and symmetrical. A break in the rhythm of shoulder motion either at the glenohumeral joint or at the scapulocostal joint, like that of altered asymmetric neck motion, focuses attention to the presence of localized abnormality.

Palpation of the posterior triangle, the supraclavicular fossa, and the carotid sheaths may call attention to nodal hypertrophy or thyroid or salivary gland enlargement. Auscultation of the carotid and the subclavian arteries may demonstrate bruits, in the former case associated with potential cerebral insufficiency and in the latter instance with a thoracic outlet or vascular steal syndrome.

Topographically, the first cervical vertebra is located immediately behind the angle of the mandible, the transverse process of the atlas is positioned between the angle of the mandible and the mastoid process, the hyoid bone is anterior to the level of C3, the thyroid cartilage is anterior to C4, and the cricoid cartilage can be felt anterior to the sixth cervical vertebra.

Symptomatic occipital neuralgia can be replicated by firm pressure over the occipital notch, producing scalp numbness or burning dyses-

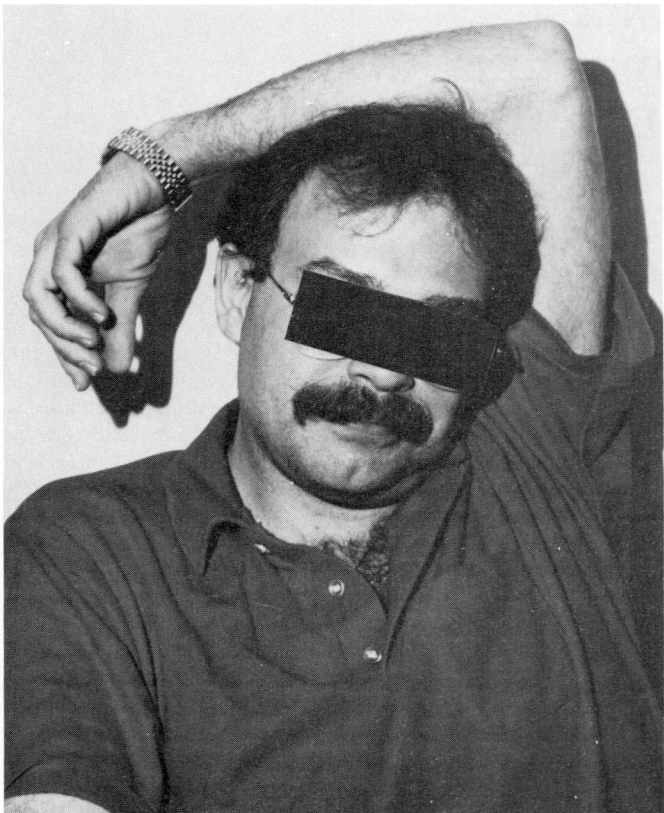

**Fig. 232-1.** Acute C7 radiculopathy. Arm elevation relieves pain of cervical root distraction.

thesias in the occipital nerve distribution. Confusing symptoms of temporomandibular joint dysfunction can be recognized by pain or crepitus over this joint, often associated with palpable "weakness" on the symptomatic side of the temporalis muscles in the subzygomatic fossa.

Various compression and distraction maneuvers of the cervical spine are also diagnostically useful. They include vertical skull compression or lateral flexion positions that replicate radicular symptoms, and manual vertical distraction, a reverse Spurling's maneuver, which "unloads" the spinal roots and adjacent cervical vertebral joints, thereby reducing pain. In an unconscious effort to avoid cervical root distraction by the weight of the dependent arm, a patient may present supporting the extremity with his or her hand on the head (Fig. 232-1).

An evaluation of neck discomfort is incomplete without shoulder and arm examination. Bilateral upper extremity pain complaints invariably originate in the neck as cervical spinal radiculopathies. Localized shoulder abnormalities presenting with pain and/or crepitus includes the glenohumeral joint itself as well as the sternoclavicular or acromioclavicular joints. Bicipital tendinitis or acute subdeltoid bursitis can present both with and without capsulitis. In each of these instances localized pain is diagnostic. On occasion, however, subdeltoid bursal syndromes may present as referred pain to the insertion of the deltoid at the humeral deltoid tubercle in the upper one third of the lateral arm.

A reduction in radial pulse with passive shoulder abduction, particularly when associated with a concomitant bruit over the subclavian artery in either the infraclavicular space or supraclavicular fossa as well as an increase of symptoms, suggests the thoracic outlet syndrome.

Finally, a neurologic examination completes the evaluation (Table 232-1). Gross evidence of muscle atrophy or fasciculations may be patently obvious. A loss of triceps reflex suggests C7 root pathology, a loss of biceps reflex a C5–6 root syndrome. Manual muscle testing using the "break" maneuver, whereby the patient is given a maximal advantage of position and strength and the examiner "breaks" the muscle comparing one side with the other, is in this regard the most useful technique. The triceps is tested by having the patient extend the elbow and maximally resist the examiner's efforts to flex the elbow against the patient's strength through the long lever of the arm grasped proximal to the wrist. A smooth, asymmetric "give" rather than a "ratchety" break suggests either a C7–8, posterior cord, or radial nerve compromise. Similarly, other muscle groups are tested and patterns of weakness are correlated with the clinical history and the symptomatic complaints. A knowledge of peripheral neuroanatomy can easily delineate both the location and often the severity of the lesion.

Local nerve palpation also is a useful adjunct to the examination. The C5–6 root lesions are often quite tender over the brachial plexus at Erb's point in the supraclavicular fossa, whereas a C8–T1 root presentation frequently has marked tenderness over the distal ulnar nerve at the elbow. Peripheral nerve entrapment syndromes associated with a positive Tinel sign to percussion over the lesion and distal weakness may also be associated with proximal pain radiation. These distal syndromes may present with only proximal neck and shoulder pain as the primary complaint. Median nerve compromise in the carpal tunnel can present as shoulder pain in this instance, and the ulnar nerve cubital fossa syndromes as a complaint of thoracic spine pain at the medial, inferior scapular border.

Sensory symptoms of pain or dysesthesias are difficult to evaluate, particularly when accompanying motor signs of nerve compromise

**Table 232-1.** Signs and Symptoms of Cervical Radiculopathy

| Disk Space | Cervical Root | Pain Complaint | Sensory Abnormality | Motor Weakness | Altered Reflex |
|---|---|---|---|---|---|
| C1–2 | C1–2 | Neck, scalp | Scalp | | |
| C4–5 | C5 | Neck, shoulder, upper arm | Shoulder, thumb | Spinati, deltoid, biceps | Reduced biceps reflex |
| C5–6 | C6 | Neck, shoulder, upper medial scapular area, proximal forearm, thumb | Thumb and index finger, lateral forearm | Deltoid, biceps, pronator teres, wrist extensors | Reduced biceps and brachioradialis reflex |
| C6–7 | C7 | Neck, posterior arm, dorsum, proximal forearm, chest, medial one third scapula, middle finger | Middle finger, forearm | Triceps, pronator teres | Reduced triceps reflex |
| C7–T1 | C8 | Neck, posterior arm, medial proximal forearm, median inferior scapular border, medial hand, ring and little fingers | Ring and little fingers | Triceps, flexor carpi ulnaris, hand intrinsics | Reduced triceps reflex |

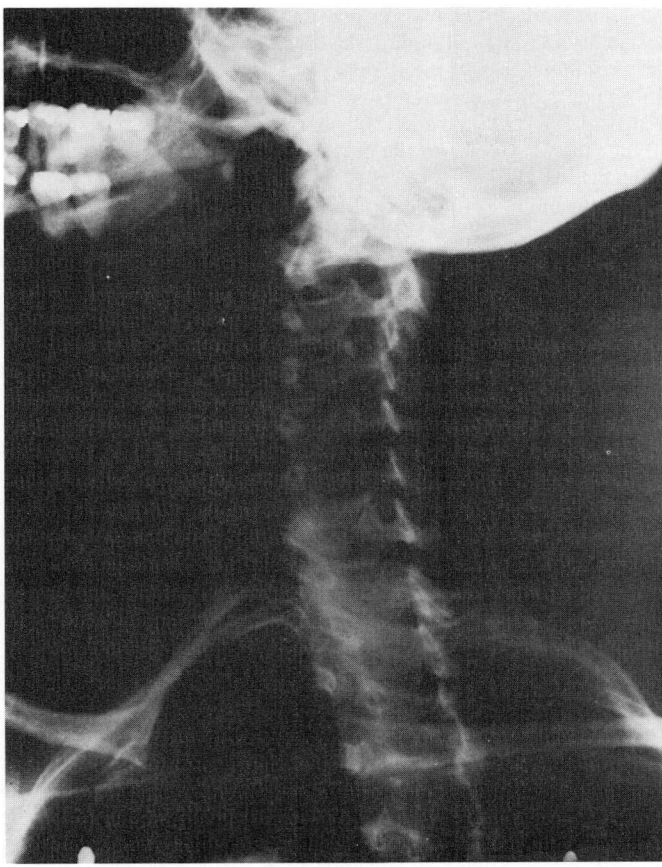

**Fig. 232-2.** Progressive C7 myotome weakness and atrophy without sensory complaints of dysesthesias or pain. Patient with C6–C7 disk space narrowing improved with cervical traction.

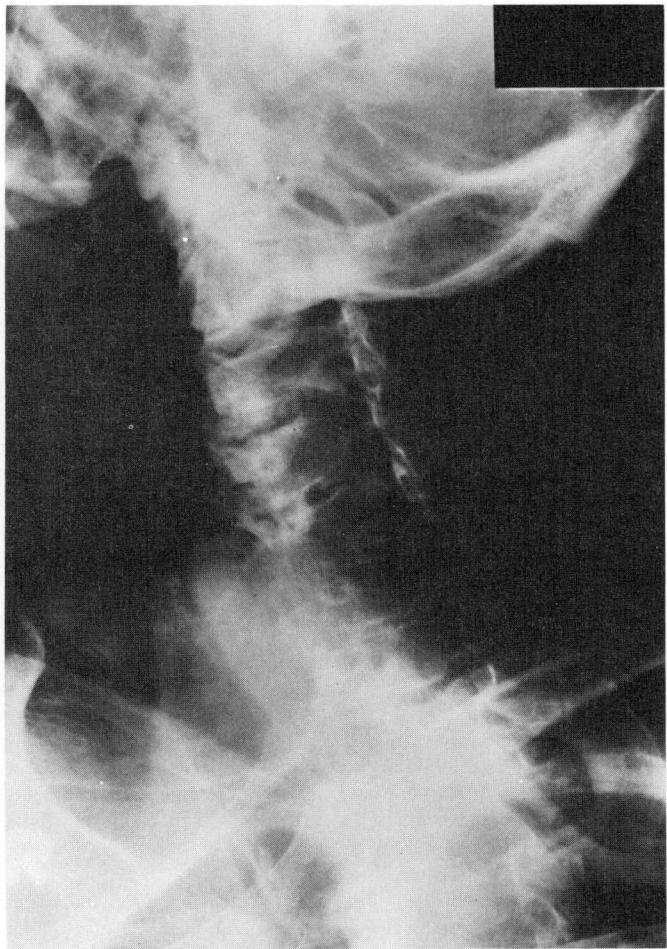

**Fig. 232-3.** 75-year-old man with acute neck pain and associated myelopathy. Occult epidural prostatic metastasis masked by severe degenerative disk disease.

are absent. This is all too often the case relative to cervical spinal radiculopathies. The discrete separation at cervical neural foraminal levels of the motor and sensory roots (Fig. 232-2) enhances the opportunity for motor sparing despite severe sensory symptoms. An understanding of the known dermatome, sclerotome, and myotome referral distribution of spinal root irritation is often essential to diagnosis. Marked C7 root irritability without motor weakness as typically identified in the triceps (radial nerve C7–8) and in the pronator teres (median nerve C6–7) can present only with the complaint of aching discomfort at the medial scapular border in its middle one third, or aching discomfort in the myotome distribution to the chest, axilla, or triceps. Severe pectoralis major pain can simulate a myocardial infarction or produce breast discomfort, evoking concerns over a possible malignancy. Numbness or tingling in the C7 dermatome distribution to the middle finger may be the only symptom of root irritation.

Early cervical spinal myelopathies may only be recognized if the examiner looks for them. Hyperreflexia with the presence of a Hoffmann's reflex in the upper extremities accompanying neck pain suggests lesions above C5. An absent superficial abdominal skin reflex associated with lower extremity hyperreflexia, an upgoing toe, and sphincter involvement, suggests progressive cervical spinal stenosis or an occult epidural metastasis (Fig. 232-3).

## RADIOGRAPHIC EXAMINATION

Radiographic views of the neck should always include oblique views. Both the dens and the lowest cervical and upper thoracic vertebrae should also be visualized. Flexion-extension films are useful if instability is suspected. Neither the computed tomography (CT) scan nor

nuclear magnetic resonance imaging (MRI) has been proved superior to cervical myelography in the diagnosis of myelopathy or cervical radiculopathies. An obvious advantage of both, however, is that CT scan and MRI are noninvasive tests. Myelography is not generally performed today unless a surgical lesion is strongly suspected. Of the two, at cervical spinal levels, MRI is now the preferred test.

## ELECTRODIAGNOSTIC EXAMINATION

Electromyographic (EMG) studies are useful in ascertaining the presence of neural structural abnormality, assessing both the level and the degree of severity, and providing both a prognostic baseline and an objective means of reassessment. Both EMG and nerve conduction velocity (NCV) testing are particularly useful when the initial presentation is associated with marked degrees of progressive motor impairment or when confusion exists as to the level of neural compromise. The actual cervical radicular complaints may be accompanied by peripheral extremity mononeuropathies, which may be attributed to the cervical radiculopathy or may in turn be provocative of the neck pain. Unfortunately, with respect to progressive weakness syndromes, acute EMG findings lag 2 wk behind the patient's actual clinical state although the immediate status of motor unit innervation and NCV after an initial 3-day delay can be followed in real time. EMG is a test of motor dysfunction. If the sensory root is solely compromised and the motor root spared, the EMG may be normal.

Cervical spinal evoked potentials are most useful in evaluating the presence of cervical spinal myelopathies (i.e., cervical spinal stenosis). An asymmetrical or slowed response at either cervical or cerebral levels in response to distal upper and lower extremity stimulation can be diagnostic. In this instance, of the two, slowing of the lumbar evoked potentials is the most sensitive.

## CERVICAL SOFT TISSUE INJURIES

Patients with a history of a cervical hyperextension injury (i.e., "whiplash") occurring in a motor vehicle accident, sport activity, or accidental fall may endure a great deal of persistent discomfort, often unresponsive to treatment. The frequent lack of discernible objective evidence of injury in the face of persistent disability has given rise to the stereotype spectre of "the whiplash victim" accompanied by both a physician advocate and a guileful attorney. The term *whiplash,* although descriptive, has been abandoned in favor of the more respectable synonym *acceleration flexion-extension neck injury.* When associated with a motor vehicle accident, a vertical component of impact may be added as the cervical spine is compressed when the individual's trunk is lifted by the force of impact. A rear-end collision propels the trunk forward on the pelvis, throwing the head into hyperextension and stretching the anterior structures of the neck. A head-on impact initially produces acute flexion and subsequently a reflex hyperextension, injuring both the anterior and posterior neck structure. Staged automobile accidents using cadavers have demonstrated injuries ranging from muscle and ligament distraction to vertebral dislocations and fractures, as well as infrequent herniations of the intervertebral disk. Head-on injuries may produce damage to the ventral neck with tears and hemorrhages in the sternocleidomastoid muscles and ruptures of the anterior longitudinal ligament and the ventral parts of the annulus fibrosis. Dorsal injury to the annulus fibrosis with hemorrhage in the paraspinal muscles is more common when trauma occurs from behind.

Elasticity of the cervical spine itself is a major variable, as is the patient's ability to prepare for the impact. Often the site of most serious residual complaint is at that level of the cervical spine with the most significant antecedent degenerative change. Passengers forewarned of an impending rear collision can potentially protect themselves by derotating the head and tucking the chin against the chest. A rotated head potentiates the risk of ligamentous rupture and articular dislocation.

Postinjury complaints are highly variable and may include pain and dysesthesias, visual symptoms, dizziness, tinnitus, dysphagia, and hoarseness. Typically, the pain complaints are initially delayed for a number of hours following the accident. They can present as localized discomfort associated with stiffness, occipital radiation, or a radicular component. Symptoms and signs of either a temporomandibular joint or thoracic outlet syndrome may also be present. Restricted cervical range of motion can be associated with radicular patterns of myotome weakness suggesting cervical root compromise. Blurring of vision and orbital pain may accompany periorbital edema or frank ecchymosis. Spacial instability affecting balance is not uncommon and may be described as the perception of "sliding" or "veering" with changes of direction rather than of a spinning sensation associated with true "vertigo." This rather unique description of spacial instability may be attributable to injury to the zygoapophyseal joints of the neck rather than the inner ear, falsely biasing the cervical righting reflex. Electronystagmography is useful in evaluating these symptoms. Dysphagia can occur as a result of pharyngeal edema or retropharyngeal hematoma. Vocal hoarseness can be attributed to a stretch of the recurrent laryngeal nerve often associated with marked edema of the sternocleidomastoid muscles and carotid sheaths, potentially increasing neck circumference by one collar size. The symptom complex of tinnitus, vertigo, visual aberrations, ear and eye pain, and headache is termed the syndrome of Leiou-Barré.

Cervical spine x-ray films are of value to exclude vertebral trauma, including avulsion fractures or joint subluxations, as well as vertebral instability in excess of 3 mm. The initial roentgenograms may reveal only an initial loss of the normal cervical lordosis, with subsequent studies possibly revealing new evidence of ligamentous ossification. Extension views of the cervical spine can demonstrate vacuum clefts in the anterior surface of the cervical disks, suggesting the presence of an avulsed disk.

Treatment initially consists of bed rest, splinting of the neck with a fitted soft cervical collar fastened in slight flexion, and the use of topical ice packs. Early mobilization exercises starting at 72 h to restore flexibility should be combined with superficial moist heat and a gradual reduction in the use of the soft collar. Early in recovery diathermy and cervical traction should be discouraged because they are likely to aggravate symptoms. However, later these modalities are useful when ligamentous or articular pain persists or for radicular symptoms. In both instances treatment must be predicated on a specific diagnosis. Oral analgesics including narcotics initially are appropriate for pain relief. Muscle relaxants are not effective except as soporifics. With chronic discomfort oral nonsteroidal anti-inflammatory drugs are useful. On specific occasions where occipital neuralgia or myofascial symptoms predominate as sources of continuing pain, local injections at the occipital notch of a mixture of long-acting steroid and 1% lidocaine followed by ice massage and ultrasound are useful. Formal outpatient therapy can be complemented by instruction in an appropriate home care program, again predicated on an accurate diagnosis.

## CERVICAL DISK PATHOLOGY

Cervical disk herniations occur as the nucleus pulposus protrudes through the posterior annulus fibrosis, producing either an acute radiculopathy or occasionally a myelopathy. Chronic cervical degenerative disk disease or cervical spondylosis is associated with a subtle progression of symptoms, including neck stiffness or localized pain, occipital neuralgia, extremity-referred radicular pain, and occasionally clinical manifestions of a progressive myelopathy.

### Acute Cervical Disk Herniations

Evidence of degeneration of the nucleus pulposus and the annulus fibrosis usually proceeds to a cervical disk herniation. These protrusions are usually confined by the posterior longitudinal ligament but can occasionally extrude through this ligament as free fragments. Direct posterior ruptures, although infrequent, can produce progressive myelopathy while the more common posterolateral herniations precipitate the symptoms and signs of an acute cervical radiculopathy. Disk prolapse is $1\frac{1}{2}$ times more common in males, occurring most often in the fourth decade. The levels of most frequent involvement are C6–7 (C7 root) usually left-sided, and C5–6 (C6 root) usually right-sided.

The symptoms of an acute cervical disk prolapse include neck pain, headache, sclerotomal referral to the shoulder and along the medial scapular border, myotome pain in the spinal root distribution to the shoulder and arm, and dermatomal sensory dysesthetic complaints to the appropriate finger. Motor signs include fasciculations; atrophy and weakness in the myotome distribution of the spinal root; loss of deep tendon reflexes; and with cervical myelopathy, lower extremity hyperreflexia, Babinski's sign, and, rarely, loss of sphincter control. Cervical hyperextension and lateral flexion to the symptomatic side can replicate the symptoms as can a Valsalva maneuver, whereas manual cervical distraction in flexion alleviates them. A thorough and searching examination, including muscle testing, easily delineates the level of root involvement (see Table 232-1).

Electroneuromyography as an extension of the clinical examination can be complementary in diagnosis and in the process excludes occult peripheral mononeuropathies and confusing acute brachial plexopathies (Parsonage-Turner syndrome). Cervical spine x-ray films are often more useful in these syndromes for what they fail to reveal, rather than what they demonstrate. The presence of degenerative disease may mask a soft cervical disk protrusion. In the younger adult, x-ray films may be normal, reveal even a large herniation. In this instance myelography or MRI is necessary for diagnosis.

Treatment consists of analgesics sufficient to obtain pain control, a cervical soft collar, and, without evidence of carotid bruits or myelopathy, a trial of intermittent cervical traction. If the symptoms and signs of acute cervical root compression fail to respond to conservative treatment or reoccur, surgery may be recommended if visualization procedures demonstrate a prolapsed cervical disk with root compression.

Indications for admission are:

1. Intractable radicular pain unresponsive to treatment
2. Progressive upper extremity weakness, especially in the C7 distribution
3. Progressive lower extremity myelopathic signs, such as positive Babinski sign, hyperreflexia, motor weakness, and bladder or bowel dysfunction

## Chronic Degenerative Disk Disease

Cervical spondylosis is a progressive condition that can present either as a loss of cervical flexibility or as a primary pain complaint. The pain is associated either with localized zygoapophyseal joint degeneration or with cervical root irritability when occipital, shoulder, and arm pain referral is experienced. The process of progressive cervical spondylosis is initiated by the development of degenerative disk disease, which predisposes to progressive osteoarthrosis of the cervical zygoapophyseal joints. A loss of disk height associated with annulus bulging produces cervical segment instability, excessive facet weight bearing, and incongruous joint motion during neck movement, accelerating articular degeneration. Ligamentous strain responses to altered mechanical stresses produce traction osteogenesis with subsequent spur formation. These spurs can encroach posteriorly on the spinal canal, producing cervical myelopathy; laterally on the intervertebral foramen, producing cervical radiculopathy; and anteriorly with esophageal pressure, producing symptoms of dysphagia.

The combination of an extended congenitally narrowed spinal canal further compromised by a vertebral osteophytic bar anteriorly and a buckling ligamentum flavum posteriorly increases the risk of myelopathy secondary to cervical spinal stenosis as the diameter of the spinal canal is reduced to under 12 mm. Cervical spinal stenosis can also occur in 14 to 20 percent of patients with lumbar spinal stenosis. Selective impingement of the dorsal spinal root by an osteophyte arising from the zygoapophyseal joint can present with complaints of digital numbness or vague myalgias, which on subsequent appraisal can be related to the known myotome distribution of a spinal root. In this regard the C6 myotome encompasses most of the major proximal shoulder muscles. The C6 nerve root emerges between the C5 and C6 vertebrae and is the earliest and most frequent site of a degenerative disk. A complaint of bilateral shoulder pain invariably has an associated element of C6 radiculopathy.

Spurious osteophytes can produce Horner syndrome, vertebral-basilar symptoms, severe radicular symptoms without associated neck pain, painless upper extremity myotome weakness, and chest pain mimicking angina. Radiographic studies demonstrating typical segmental degenerative changes may in fact bear no relation to the actual spinal root level of the presenting complaint. Foraminal encroachment visible on x-ray views may be more severe at C5-6, with the patient presenting with both clinical and EMG evidence of a progressive C7 radiculopathy arising from the C6-7 level.

Treatment is predicated on recognizing the exact site of complaint. Localized neck pain and stiffness attributable to arthritis at the zygoapophyseal joint can be treated with cervical collar support, superficial ice massage, ultrasound, flexibility exercises, and nonsteroidal anti-inflammatory drugs. Often in these instances cervical traction

therapy aggravates pain. Correspondingly, intermittent cervical traction initially in the formal setting of an outpatient physical therapy facility, followed by ongoing home cervical traction, is an effective approach to cervical radicular pain. In both instances, instruction in appropriate neck biomechanics is helpful in continuing management. Myofascial pain complaints often associated with palpable nodules in the trapezius muscle can be, in most cases, effectively managed with topical ice, deep kneading massage, stretching exercises, and on occasion localized injections of steroids and lidocaine. The prompt recognition and correction of aggravating factors, such as emotional stress or prolonged postural neck hyperextension related to overly soft seating or to the use of bifocal glasses during reading, may in itself be curative.

The management of neck and shoulder pain requires a continuum of care. Medical conditions often necessitating a clinical reevaluation if they are to be identified early include those with life-threatening potential, for example, an occult spinal epidural metastasis initially masked by x-ray evidence of cervical degenerative disease or an apical Pancoast tumor presenting as a subdeltoid bursitis. Often, in these instances as well as in more benign cases, such as polymyalgia with temporal arteritis, rheumatoid arthritis, and infectious diseases, subsequent reexamination is necessary for correct diagnosis.

## BIBLIOGRAPHY

Burney RG, Moore PA, Duncan GH. Management of head and neck pain. *Int Anesthesiol Clin* 21:79, 1983.

Cailliet R. *Neck and Arm Pain,* 2d ed. Philadelphia: Davis, 1981.

Dillin W, Booth R, Cuckler J, et al. Cervical radiculopathy—a review. *Spine* 11:986, 1986.

LaBan MM. Electrodiagnosis in cervical radicular and myelopathic syndromes. In: Herkowitz HN. *Seminars in Spinal Surgery.* Philadelphia: WB Saunders, pp. 222–228, 1989.

LaBan MM, Meerschaert JR, Taylor RS. Breast pain: a symptom of cervical radiculopathy. *Arch Phys Med Rehabil* 60:315, 1979.

Lieberman JS: Cervical soft tissue injuries and cervical disc disease. In: Leek JC, Gershwin ME, Fowler WM (eds). *Principles of Physical Medicine and Rehabilitation in the Musculoskeletal Diseases.* Orlando, FL: Grune & Stratton, pp. 263–286, 1986.

MacNab I. Acceleration extension injuries of the cervical spine. In: Rothman RH, Simeone FA (eds). *The Spine,* 2d ed. Philadelphia: WB Saunders, pp. 647–660, 1982.

McSwain NE Jr, Martinez JA, Timberlake GA (eds). *Cervical Spine Trauma; Evaluation and Acute Management.* New York: Thieme, pp. 1–118, 1989.

Rothman RH. The pathophysiology of disc degeneration. *Clin Neurosurg* 20:174, 1973.

Simeone FA, Rothman RH. Cervical disk disease. In: Rothman RH, Simeone FA (eds). *The Spine,* ed 2. Philadelphia: WB Saunders, pp. 440–499, 1982.

# 233

# THORACIC AND LUMBAR PAIN SYNDROMES

**Myron M. LaBan**

## THORACIC SPINE

Although spine pain complaints are more common at cervical and lumbar levels, thoracic complaints can be as disabling. This region of the spine is comparatively stable and protected both by the rib cage and the orientation of the facet joints. In this region, the spinal cord and paired segmental nerves traverse the narrowest of bony canals and any compromise of the available space can result in rapid and profound neurologic deficits.

Thoracic spine fractures occur most commonly at the T10–L2 levels and can occur from direct trauma as well as forced hyperflexion of the trunk, as in lap-belt injuries. Vertebral fractures resulting from spinal osteoporosis occur in 8 percent of women over 80 years of age. Such compression fractures are usually wedge shaped and are stable. The presenting symptom is usually severe pain, and accompanying myelopathy is rare. However, when long tract signs such as hyperreflexia, Babinski's sign, and urinary incontinence are present, a malignancy metastatic to the spine must be suspected. An epidural metastasis may present similarly as an acute myelopathy with or without pain or abnormal x-rays. Myelography, Computed Tomography (CT), or magnetic resonance imaging (MRI) is needed to differentiate the relatively rare thoracic disk protrusion (1 percent of all disk herniations) from a spinal cord tumor. Slowed lumbar spinal evoked potentials can also be diagnostic in confirming thoracic spinal myelopathy.

Localized paravertebral pain can be associated with an acute facet syndrome. Plica entrapped within the thoracic zygoapophyseal joints can produce severe and disabling pain. Radicular pain and localized stiffness associated with osteoarthrosis of these same vertebral joints cause chronic pain and can result in narrowing of the neural and spinal canals. The latter can lead to signs and symptoms of thoracic spinal stenosis.

Rheumatoid spondylitis primarily affecting young men may initially present as thoracic spinal pain and stiffness. A loss of chest expansion to less than 1 in. at nipple line is suggestive, with x-rays of the sacral iliac joints, even without pain, often diagnostic.

Herpes zoster neuralgia can also be associated with acute thoracic radiculopathy. It is difficult to diagnose before vesicles and bullae are evident.

Diabetic thoracic radiculopathy may present as abdominal pain. When this condition is suspected, electromyography (EMG) demonstrating thoracic paraspinal and abdominal muscle segmental denervation (T7–12) can be diagnostic.

## LUMBAR SPINE

Low back pain is second only to the common cold as a cause of industrial absenteeism and is the primary cause of reduced working capacity. Whenever possible, lumbar pain syndromes both with and without attendant sciatic radiculopathy are managed on an outpatient basis. Admission criteria include intractable pain and loss of function (Table 233-1).

The causes of lumbosacral pain are as diverse and as complex as are the interrelated anatomic structures of the lumbar spine itself. Additionally, pain of remote origin, even outside the spine itself, can present as lumbar pain. Pain from visceral disorders, including those of kidney, pancreas, and gallbladder; duodenal ulcers; colonic diverti-

culitis; expanding abdominal aortic aneurysm; epidural hematoma or abscess; and endometriosis can all mimic primary low back disorders. A history of associated systemic symptoms and a lack of therapeutic response to a trial of initial bed rest, combined with an abnormal abdominal, pelvic, neurologic or rectal examination, are usually sufficient to redirect the examination to the appropriate extraspinal problem. Spinal cord compression can develop as a first sign of malignancy or as a complication. It is usually associated with back pain and should always be suspected if there are any neurologic signs or sphincter dysfunction.

The examiner must give credence to the history, age, and circumstances of onset in establishing a diagnosis. For example, an elderly woman with acute onset, severe midthoracic pain, without a history of trauma, can be presumed to have an osteoporotic vertebral compression fracture until proved otherwise. The onset of lumbosacral pain associated with bilateral leg pain radiation and a sudden loss of bladder control should be presumed to have a midline herniated disk with the threat of paraparesis.

Pain from a leaking abdominal aortic aneurysm is constant and aching and may be referred to the lower abdomen and inguinal areas as well as the low back. In the evaluation of low back pain in the elderly, an abdominal aortic aneurysm must always be considered in the differential diagnosis.

Ambulation producing either lumbar, gluteal, or calf pain may be a manifestation of peripheral vascular disease but it is also indistinguishable from that of lumbar spinal stenosis. Both vascular insufficiency and spinal stenosis are aggravated by activity and relieved by rest. Vascular signs in the former case or neurologic abnormality in the latter instance can lead to the diagnosis, but arteriography or MRI or CT scan may be necessary for confirmation.

Lesions within the central nervous system, and in the spinal cord at or above the lumbar area, can also produce both low back pain and radicular leg discomfort. Parasagittal brain tumors and thoracic root lesions, including neurofibromata, can simulate lumbar root syndromes. Pain from thoracic root lesions is usually worse while reclining at night and is relieved by assuming an erect position. Patients may sleep sitting up in a chair. They may on initial examination demonstrate Babinski reflexes that disappear after a brief period of rest. Distal nerve entrapment syndromes also can present with primary complaints of lumbosacral pain. The most notable example of this situation is tibial nerve entrapment (S1) in the tarsal tunnel behind the medial ankle malleolus.

The physical examination must include both abdominal, vascular, neurologic, and lower extremity evaluation. Abdominal visceral palpation and auscultation over both the aorta and renal arteries, as well as an assessment of peripheral pulses, color, and temperature, should be routine.

With mechanical dysfunctions of posture or the presence of neurologic signs such as alteration of deep tendon reflexes, weakness, atrophy, restricted or crossed straight leg-raising (CSLR) signs, and the presence of long tract signs or sphincter dysfunction, the diagnosis of primary spinal-neural pathology becomes self-evident. Establishing a diagnosis in the absence of neurologic signs is more difficult. The examiner must rely to a greater extent on the details of the history, and the ability to replicate and alleviate symptoms by anatomic maneuvers. X-ray examination may or may not be helpful. For example, a herniated disk may well be associated with normal x-rays, while x-ray evidence of osteoarthritis may mask the correct diagnosis of clinically suspected sacroiliitis.

In general, it is not necessary to obtain lumbosacral spine x-rays in the emergency department for nontraumatic musculoskeletal back pain. X-rays should be obtained for trauma and in the elderly if carcinoma is possible.

In the evaluation of back syndromes, the examiner's goal is to discriminate between pain of neurogenic and pain of musculoskeletal origin. Although the potential for surgical intervention is by far

**Table 233-1.** Admission Criteria for Low Back Pain

| | Admission Criteria | Evaluation |
|---|---|---|
| Acute pain; patient requires immediate admission | Immediate<br>1. Paraparesis—paralysis<br>2. Loss of bowel or bladder function<br>3. L-S pain and spasticity<br>4. Cannot stand or sit<br>5. Sleeping in an upright position<br>6. Presence of metastatic cancer | 1. L-S spine x-ray studies<br>2. EMG and NCV or evoked potentials<br>3. Cystometrogram, related to bladder symptoms<br>4. CBC, SMAC, protein electrophoresis, acid phosphatase, CEA, sedimentation rate<br>5. Melogram, CT scan, MRI |
| Acute pain; observed progression of symptoms requires admission | With progression<br>1. Unilateral paresis with or without pain<br>2. Absent reflex<br>3. Atrophy<br>4. Intractable radicular pain unresponsive to appropriate conservative therapy (pain alone requires 2 weeks or outpatient conservative therapy)<br>5. Marked restriction of hip and knee extension (bow stringing)<br>6. Unilateral spasticity<br>7. Progressive EMG changes stringing) | As outpatient<br>1. L-S spine x-ray studies, MRI<br>2. EMG and NCV or evoked potentials<br>3. "Therapeutic" trial of treatment, i.e., bed/tbt rest, physical therapy, corseting<br>4. If patient experiences the progression of the signs above and symptoms and/or is unresponsive to conservative therapy, oral or injectable medications, the patient is admitted for inpatient evaluation with myelogram, CT scan, or MRI |
| Chronic pain after surgery | 1. Intractable radicular pain<br>2. Altered neurologic signs as progressive paresis, loss of straight-leg raising, lateralizing neurologic signs, atrophy<br>3. Progressive EMG changes<br>4. Unresponsive to conservative therapy, including physical therapy, corseting, TENS, injections | 1. Myelogram<br>2. CT scan or MRI<br>3. EMG and NCV or evoked potentials<br>4. Psychometrics |
| Chronic pain with surgery | 1. Intractable radicular pain<br>2. Progressive loss of ambulatory range vascular versus neurogenic claudication | 1. L-S spine x-ray, CT scan, and MRI studies<br>2. EMG/NCV/H reflex/evoked potentials<br>3. Myelogram, CT scan, MRI<br>4. Abdominal x-ray studies, ultrasound arteriogram<br>5. CBC, urinalysis, ZSR, protein electrophoresis, SMAC, acid phosphatase, CEA |
| Chronic pain—no surgery contemplated | 1. Intractable radicular pain | 1. Psychometrics<br>2. Response to analgesics, mood elevators, and TENS<br>3. Pain clinic referral |

CBC, complete blood count; CEA, carcinoembryonic antigen; EMG, electromyography; L-S, lumbosacral; MRI, magnetic resonance imaging; NCV, nerve conduction velocity; SMAC, complete blood profile; TENS, transcutaneous electrical nerve stimulation; ZSR, zeta sedimentation rate

greater with neurologic than with musculoskeletal involvement, in both instances surgery is indicated in less than 1 percent of all cases. Fortunately, the majority of all lumbosacral syndromes respond to routine symptomatic treatment, including bed rest, superficial heat, and oral analgesics. When seen on a one-time basis in the emergency center, each patient should be provided with an opportunity for follow-up in the event that the problem fails to respond to initial treatment.

## PHYSICAL EXAMINATION

With the patient disrobed, the spine and pelvis should be observed for abnormal spinal curves, pelvic tilts, or the presence of spinal-pelvic lists, all suggesting splinting or guarding in response to pain. Each vertebra should be palpated to identify point tenderness which suggests bony involvement. The gait should be observed for a loss of normal, symmetrical spinal-pelvic rhythm. Asymmetrical posturing suggests pain or weakness to which the patient is biomechanically accommodating. Guarding or splinting can best be demonstrated at slower cadences and can be dramatically accentuated by spinal extension and flexion maneuvers. Extension of the lumbar spine on the pelvis narrows the neural foramina and loads the zygoapophyseal joints on the ipsilateral side. This maneuver will exacerbate radicular pain causing distal sciatic referral and will also aggravate local articular pain. Similarly, extension and lateral flexioners to the opposite side reduce the load on the symptomatic joints and open the normal foramina, reducing pain. Flexion maneuvers can demonstrate painful limitations of spinal-pelvic range of motion as measured from fingertips to toes; adjacent spinal segments may be visualized to move as a singular unit in response to localized guarding. Palpation of the paraspinal muscles and the spinal vertebral processes in relation to their relative excursion to each other vividly dramatize this loss of spinal segment mobility. The presence of an acute lumbar radiculopathy associated with a "tethered" root or prefixed spinal root syndrome initiates a precipitous sequence of maneuvers on the painful side in an effort to unload the root, which includes a lateral thrust of the spine, elevation and forward thrust of the pelvis, as well as acute flexion of the hip and knee to reduce tension on the inflamed nerve root.

Pain to direct palpation over the ischial tuberosities, greater trochanters, or sciatic notches may suggest localized abnormality, including a bursitis at the tuberosity or trochanter or an entesitis, that is, inflammation at the tendinous attachment of muscle to bone, at the insertion of the hip abductor and extensor muscle groups. Proximal L5 and S1 root compression is suggested distally by the presence of pain (L5) to palpation over the peroneal nerve at the fibular head and the tibial nerve (S1) in the tarsal tunnel. Percussion pain over the bony spine itself supports the presence of an osseous abnormality, such as compression fracture, metastasis, or disk or vertebral infection. Disk space infections are relatively uncommon and are most often associated with recent disk surgery. However, they can also occur in association with a remote infection, that is, kidney, distal trauma to a bursa, or in the drug addicted. Costovertebral angle percussion pain is invariably associated with retroperitoneal pathology, most often kidney.

Excessive lateral trunk sway to the stance leg during ambulation, a compensated Trendelenberg gait, suggests primary interarticular hip abnormality. On examination, corroborative evidence of an initial loss of hip internal rotation may be associated with medial groin pain, a positive Patrick sign, which may radiate to the knee. Attempting to "walk around" primary hip disease produces excessive stress at both the ipsilateral sacroiliac joint and the greater trochanter. Each, singly or together, may initially appear to be the salient problem until the loss of hip mobility is identified as the progenitor of the other complaints. Trochanteric bursitis itself can mimic lumbar radiculopathy with distal pain referral along the iliotibial band to the lateral knee.

An inability to walk on either the heels or the toes because of weakness in the foot dorsiflexors or plantar flexors, respectively, suggests an L5 radiculopathy in the former case, and S1 root involvement in the latter instance. Similarly, difficulty in assuming or arising from a squatting position may indicate quadriceps weakness associated with L4 root compromise. Manual muscle testing is often the most neglected part of the clinical examination, but it can also be the most rewarding. Weakness of the hip flexors suggests L3 compromise, of the quadriceps L4, the foot dorsiflexors and great toe extensors L5, and the calf S1 radiculopathy. Deep tendon reflexes are tested and compared one side with the other. An absent or reduced knee jerk suggests an L4 radiculopathy, biceps femoris jerk L5, and an asymmetric Achilles reflex an S1 root compression syndrome.

Straight leg-raising (SLR) testing can be both confusing and diagnostic but must be evaluated with reference to age and the presence or absence of associated CSLR signs. A CSLR sign occurs when contralateral leg elevation produces sciatic pain in the symptomatic leg. A markedly positive SLR in the younger patient is more likely associated with a prolapsed intervertebral disk than in an older patient, particularly when it is associated with a positive CSLR. Similarly, in the more youthful group, a progressive inability to extend the knee on the symptomatic side with bowstringing of the sciatic nerve in the popliteal fossa is highly suggestive of the presence of a prolapsed disk. When noted in conjunction with a painful "strum" sign as the sciatic nerve is plucked behind the knee, it is almost always pathognomonic of the presence of a herniated disk associated with an impacted root. Additional confirmatory maneuvers include an exacerbation of pain with foot dorsiflexion, or with the addition of head flexion with the SLR maneuver held at the symptomatic limit of sciatic pain tolerance. In the older patient, positive SLR or CSLR tests are less specific, as to pain etiology, but also do suggest a radicular component of involvement.

Hyperreflexia and the presence of upgoing toe signs suggest the presence of a myelopathy with cord compromise above T12–L1, the terminus of the conus medularis. Metastatic lesions, thoracic disk herniations, and on rare occasions, osteoporotic compression fractures at the thoracolumbar junction can present with both low back pain and long tract signs. A sudden loss of bladder or bowel continence with an associated symmetrical, multilevel areflexia and lower extremity weakness may be associated with a midline lumbar disk herniation with compromise of the more distal cauda equina below the clonus medullaris. In this special instance, with rapid progression of paraparesis, emergency decompressive surgery may be required for restoration of function.

Sensory complaints in the presence of radicular syndromes may be useful in localizing root levels of involvement. Complaints of muscular pain in the myotome and sensory dysesthesias in the dermatome distribution of a spinal root may be accompanied by referred pain in the sclerotome distribution. Compromise of S1 and L5 roots can be experienced, respectively, as muscular pain in the calf mimicking a thrombophlebitis, and muscular pain in the anterior tibial compartment simulating "shin splints." Paresthesias in the great toe suggest L5 root involvement, and in the little toe S1 radiculopathy. Discomfort of articular origin, either lumbar zygoapophyseal or sacroiliac joints, can also be recognized by known sclerotome patterns of pain referral. Sacroiliac joint abnormality is commonly referred to the inguinal and anterolateral thigh, as well as the lower abdominal quadrants, often simulating an acute appendicitis or ovarian cyst. Although symptoms of pain and dysesthesias cannot be objectified in the same manner as physical signs, a sophisticated examiner can replicate or reduce the symptoms by initially burdening and then alleviating the complaints by appropriate anatomic maneuvers.

## SPECIFIC DIAGNOSES ASSOCIATED WITH LUMBAR SYNDROMES

### Spinal Degeneration

A rational approach to the diagnosis and treatment of low back pain or sciatica should be predicated on an understanding of the process of spinal degeneration. Initially beginning with an alteration in the hydroscopic quality of the nucleus pulposus, it can progress from annular degeneration of a single disk to multilevel involvement. Sequential disk degeneration with associated zygoapophyseal joint compromise can be associated with relatively infrequent disk prolapses. More often, progressive posterior facet disease is associated with foraminal or spinal canal encroachment, producing symptoms associated with lateral or central spinal stenosis (Fig. 233-1). The combined retrogressive and proliferative changes in the disk anteriorly and in the posterior joints present with both clinical symptoms and roentgenographic changes referred to as combined three-joint complex degeneration. Three distinct stages in the evolution of this process can be recognized clinically. The *stage of dysfunction* is associated with complaints of pain and stiffness, often without radiographic or clinical abnormality. Treatment is with oral analgesics and physical therapy.

The *stage of instability* is associated with evidence of spinal segment movement best exemplified by radiographic evidence of the presence of pseudospondylolisthesis (Fig. 233-2), usually at the L4–5 level, secondary to advanced degenerative disk disease with preservation of the stabilizing pars interarticularis. This phase of degeneration can be clinically recognized by the presence of limited spinal flexibility, a reactive scoliosis, a reduction in the lumbar lordosis, and on occasion, the presence of neurologic abnormality, including alterations in deep tendon reflexes, reductions in muscle strength, and restricted SLR signs. Conservative therapy in this stage is again often successful with the addition of bracing or corseting. When radicular signs and symptoms are preeminent, intermittent split table pelvic traction is also beneficial.

The final *stage of stabilization* is clinically associated with a marked loss of lumbar flexibility. "Stiffness" is a primary complaint that may supersede pain, particularly following periods of immobil-

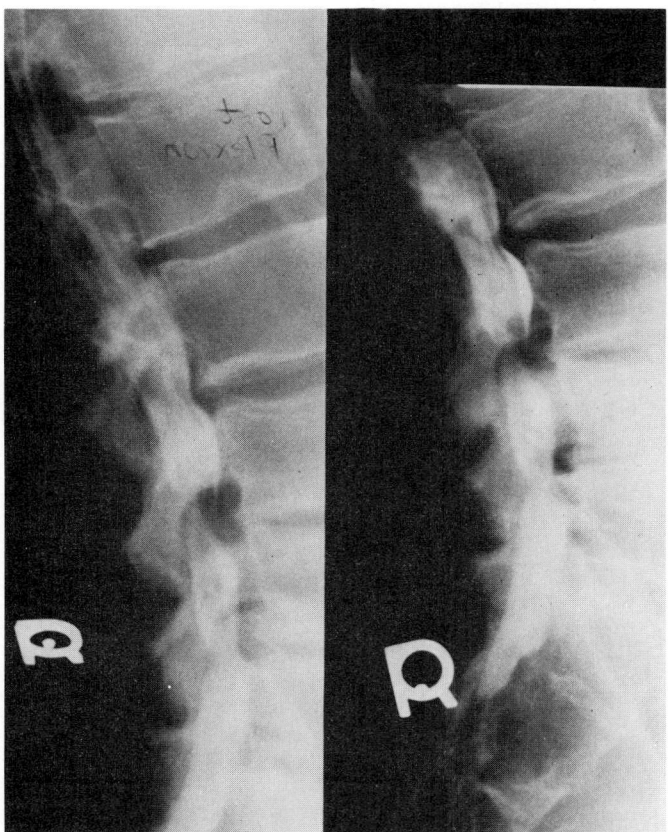

**Fig. 233-1.** Multilevel evidence of spinal stenosis at lumbar levels with typical hour-glass deformity at disk spaces.

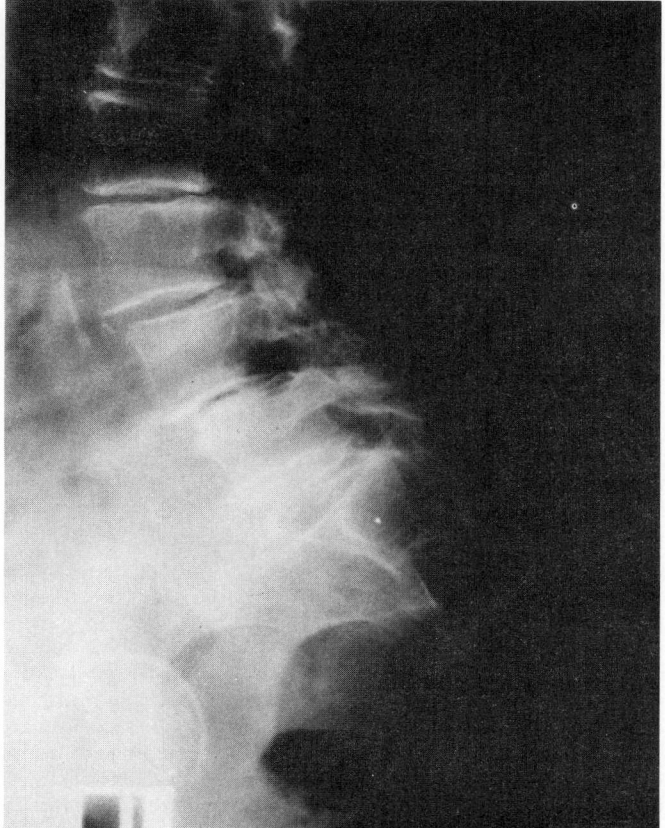

**Fig. 233-2.** Pseudospondylolisthesis with anterior slip of L4 on L5 associated with neurogenic claudication and night pain.

ity. Prolonged standing or walking may precipitate symptoms of localized radicular pain, paresthetic complaints of numbness or tingling, and motor symptoms of "weakness" or "instability" with or without corroborative motor signs. Articular facet, laminar, and vertebral enlargement associated with osteophytic formation progressing to vertebral fusion are characteristic x-ray features of this stage. The presence of central and lateral lumbar spinal stenosis associated with narrowing of the anteroposterior diameter of the spinal canal with compromise of the dural sac in the former instance, or compression of the spinal nerve root in the intrapedicular, neural canal in the latter case, may be demonstrated by CT scan or MRI. Patients with spinal stenosis frequently present with severe sciatic radiculopathy and unrestricted SLR, variable lower extremity weakness often directly related to activity, and a "proximal march of symptoms," that is, distal foot numbness progressing proximally with activity. Conversely, lumbar night pain, particularly in patients with a cardiac history, can arouse patients from sleep forcing them to "walk around" seeking comfort.

Conservative therapy appropriate to the earlier stages of degeneration here, too, usually provides symptomatic relief for patients with spinal stenosis. When radicular symptoms are preeminent, heavy intermittent, split table, pelvic traction is often palliative. When progressive neurologic defects occur with intractable pain unresponsive to conservative therapy, surgical decompression may be appropriate.

## Sacroiliitis

Senescent or inflammatory changes can also occur within the paired sacroiliac joints. Early in this process there may be little or no correlation between symptom severity and radiographic evidence of joint involvement. The pain is usually experienced over the joints themselves, radiating to the anterior lateral or posterior thighs. Usually

worse at night, the pain may be bilateral, alternating from side to side. Prolonged standing or sitting, especially on long car trips, exacerbates the discomfort. "Weakness" or stiffness, primarily in the morning, is also a predominant symptom of sacroiliitis. When in young men it is associated with new-onset rheumatoid spondylitis, the earliest complaint may be that of chest pain and stiffness rather than that of low back pain. The earliest sign may be that of restricted chest expansion at nipple line of less than 1 in.

As in the facet joints of the spine, three stages of degeneration can be clinically identified. During the *stage of dysfunction,* although the pain and associated disability can be severe, the x-ray films are often normal. During the secondary *stage of instability,* pelvic x-ray films with alternate leg weight-bearing may demonstrate pubic symphysis instability (Fig. 233-3) in excess of 3 mm. Usually the instability is greater on the symptomatic side. Any of the three-joint complex of the pelvis, the paired posterior sacroiliac joints, and the anterior pubic symphysis may be painful or demonstrate concurrent x-ray evidence of progressive degenerative change.

The terminal *stage of immobilization* is associated with anatomic and functional ankylosis of these joints. Paradoxically, osteophytic formation and articular fibrosis with eventual joint fusion present less with pain and more often with complaints of stiffness, particularly in the morning.

Treatment consists initially of bed rest, superficial heat, and oral nonsteroidal anti-inflammatory drugs (NSAIDs). Bed rest for at least 24 h is to be recommended in a lumbar flexed position, either side-lying, prone with a pillow under the abdomen, or supine with hips and knees flexed over a cushion. The topical use of moist heat is useful in preference to dry heat because it is generally better tolerated. In this regard silicon-filled hydrocollator packs that cool from the initial application are to be preferred to electric heating pads, which can

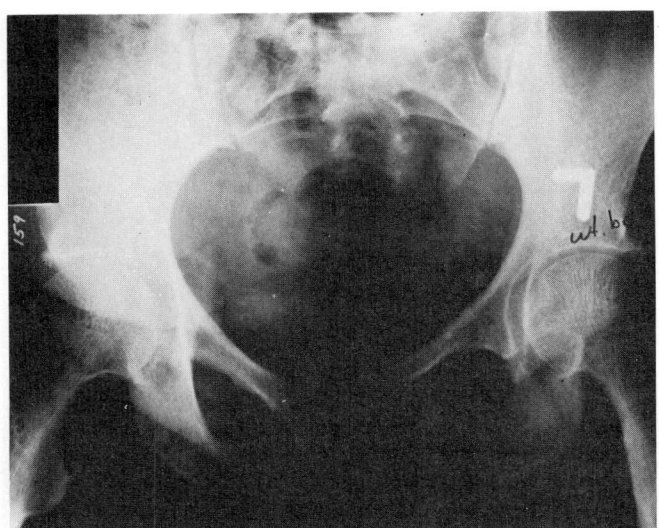

**Fig. 233-3.** Persistent sacroiliac and pubic symphysis pain 2 years post slip and fall at 3 months of pregnancy. Four millimeters of subluxation at pubic symphysis is demonstrated by alternate leg weight bearing.

cause severe burns. In both instances, heat should never be under the patient, but over the painful area. Oral medications include narcotics and NSAIDs. Muscle relaxants as a class are not to be recommended. Their analgesic effects are minimal because they act primarily as central soporifics with all their attendant risks. Oral narcotic analgesics may be necessary for 24 to 48 h as appropriate to the individual circumstance. NSAIDs for the long term are useful, for both their analgesic and their anti-inflammatory properties. Their dosage, initially high, should be tapered to a comfortable maintenance level with due concern to water retention and gastric intolerance. Several classes are available. They include fenamates (meclofenamate), indole derivatives (indomethacin, sulindac), phenyl alkonic acids (ibuprofen, naproxen, naproxen sodium), and oxicans (piroxicam). If one group is ineffective, another should be tried. Injecting the symptomatic articulations with a mixture of 1 mL each of both short-acting and long-acting steroids with an additional 1 mL lidocaine during the acute phase can produce immediate pain relief with a dramatic resolution of a concomitant reactive scoliosis. With the patient in a prone position and flexed over an abdominal pillow, a 3.8 cm (1.5-in.) 22-gauge needle is inserted obliquely at the midpoint of a line drawn between the posterior iliac spine and the "dimple of Venus." One mL of 3 mL is injected, to be followed by 1 mL laterally and medially along the joint line through the same needle insertion point. Later diathermy, weight reduction, lumbar flexibility, and abdominal strengthening exercises combined with corseting are, together, all useful treatment adjuncts.

Referral for continuing outpatient care is absolutely critical. No matter how searching the physical examination, and notwithstanding the experience of the examiner, clinical manifestations can change rapidly, often dramatically, for example, the blossoming of the skin manifestations of herpes zoster 2 days after pain onset, to be recognized only by subsequent evaluations. The use of electromyography, bone scans, myelograms, CT scans, and MRI studies are diagnostic modalities that can be used at follow-up evaluation.

## BIBLIOGRAPHY

Bell GR, Rothman RH: The conservative treatment of sciatica. *Spine* 9:54, 1984.

Bower RD, Errico TJ. Thoracolumbar spine injuries. In: Errico TJ, Bauer Rd, Waugh T (eds). *Spinal Trauma*. Philadelphia: JB Lippincott, pp. 195-270, 1991.

Bruckner FE, Greco A, Leung AWL. "Benign thoracic pain" syndrome: role of magnetic resonance imaging in the detection and localization of thoracic disc disease. *J R Soc Med* 82:81, 1989.

Khatri B, Baruah J, McQuillen MP. Correlation of electromyography with computed tomography and evaluation of low back pain. *Arch Neurol* 41:594, 1984.

Kirkaldy-Willis WH, Farfan HF. Instability of the lumbar spine. *Clin Orthop* 165:110, 1982.

LaBan MM. "Vesper's Curse" night pain—the bane of Hypnos. *Arch Phys Med Rehabil* 65:501, 1984.

LaBan MM. The lumbosacral pain syndrome. In: Kaplan PE (ed). *The Practice of Physical Medicine*. Springfield, IL: Charles C Thomas, pp. 107–160, 1984.

LaBan MM. Low back pain—lumbosacral strain—lumbar disc disease. In: Leek JC, Gershwin ME, Fowler WM (eds): *Principles of Physical Medicine and Rehabilitation in Musculoskeletal Diseases*. Orlando, FL: Grune & Stratton, pp. 309–333, 1986.

# 234
# SHOULDER PAIN
## D. Monte Hunter

## INTRODUCTION

Shoulder pain is one of the most common musculoskeletal complaints of patients over the age of 40. Work, recreation, and normal daily activities all place great demands on the shoulder. Of all adult patients presenting for evaluation of shoulder pain, one-third related their pain to work, one-third related their pain to athletic activity, and one-third could not identify any one specific precipitating event or factor.

Injuries involving the rotator cuff are the most common cause of shoulder pain. While these injuries can be acute, they more commonly occur from chronic overuse. Overuse can produce pathologic changes in the rotator cuff structures that progress along the continuum starting with subacromial bursitis from mechanical irritation, progressing to rotator cuff tendinitis, and eventually leading to partial and full thickness rotator cuff tears. Laborers who work with their arms above the horizontal and athletes of all ages, especially throwers, swimmers, and racquet sports enthusiasts, are the most susceptible to chronic overuse injuries. Acute injuries to the rotator cuff usually require significant trauma such as extreme forced hyperabduction or hyperextension of the upper extremity.

While disorders of the rotator cuff are the most common cause of shoulder pain, conditions affecting other intrinsic structures of the shoulder complex can also cause pain. Additionally, extrinsic disorders can refer pain to the shoulder and must be considered in the differential diagnosis. A focused history and physical examination carried out with an understanding of the complex anatomy and function of the shoulder are essential in determining the source of shoulder pain. Establishing the proper diagnosis, initiating the appropriate treatment, and making timely referrals for follow up are critical in preserving the function and mobility of the shoulder.

## FUNCTIONAL ANATOMY

The shoulder is the most versatile and yet the most vulnerable joint in the body. With range of motion greater than any other joint in the body, the shoulder is designed for mobility rather than stability. The ultimate function of the shoulder is to help position the hand and upper extremity for accurate and efficient use. The shoulder is also designed to provide strength and power to upper extremity movements. To meet the many demands placed on it, the shoulder utilizes three bones, four joints, and a specialized set of soft tissues consisting of muscles, tendons, ligaments, and bursae.

## Bones and Joints

The humerus, clavicle, and scapula make up the bony structures of the shoulder complex. The scapula has two bony extensions, the coracoid and the acromion, which help protect the rotator cuff and play important roles in shoulder function.

The four joints of the shoulder include the glenohumeral, acromioclavicular, sternoclavicular, and scapulothoracic. All of these must work together to provide full shoulder motion and function. The *glenohumeral joint* is the most prominent and complex joint of the shoulder. This ball-and-socket joint is the central axis of motion of the shoulder. While the glenohumeral joint enjoys great freedom of motion, it is also recognized as the least stable joint in the body. To help improve its stability, this joint relies on three components. The first is the labrum, a fibrous band of tissue lining the glenoid cavity, analogous to the meniscus of the knee. The labrum increases the surface contact area of the humeral head within the glenoid. The second component consists of three glenohumeral ligaments, which aid stability by reinforcing the joint capsule. Finally, four specialized muscles known as the rotator cuff encompass the glenohumeral joint and provide stability during motion.

The *sternoclavicular* and *acromioclavicular joints* work together to contribute to glenohumeral motion. Rotation at the acromioclavicular joint and elevation at the sternoclavicular allow complete arm elevation. The *scapulothoracic joint* represents the articulation of the scapula on the posterior wall of the thorax. Scapular motion is essential for overall shoulder motion: every degree of scapulothoracic motion allows two degrees of glenohumeral motion.

## Muscles

The muscles of the shoulder complex not only generate motion and power for the upper extremity but also provide significant stability for the glenohumeral joint. The deltoid, which drapes the shoulder complex and forms its contour, acts as a powerful and independent elevator of the arm. Along with the pectoralis, the deltoid is the major mover of the upper extremity.

The rotator cuff consists of four muscles: the supraspinatus, the infraspinatus, the teres minor, and the subscapularis. All originate on the scapula, traverse the glenohumeral joint, and insert on the proximal humerus. The rotator cuff functions primarily as a dynamic stabilizer of the glenohumeral joint. The rotator cuff muscles also contribute significantly to the power of the upper extremity, providing 30 to 50 percent of the power in abduction and 90 percent in external rotation (Fig. 234-1).

The *supraspinatus* originates on the posterior and superior aspect of the scapula, passes beneath the acromion, and inserts on the great tuberosity of the humerus. It initiates arm elevation and abducts the shoulder. It also balances the power of the deltoid, keeping the humerus centered in the glenoid during deltoid contraction.

The *infraspinatus* originates on the posterior scapula just inferior to the scapular spine. It inserts on the posterior aspect of the greater tuberosity and acts primarily as an external rotator of the arm (Fig. 234-1).

The *teres minor* originates on the lateral border of the scapula just inferior to the infraspinatus and inserts on the posterior aspect of the humerus. It works with the infraspinatus to provide external rotation (Fig. 234-1).

The *subscapularis* is the only rotator cuff muscle that arises from the anterior aspect of the scapula. It attaches to the lesser tuberosity

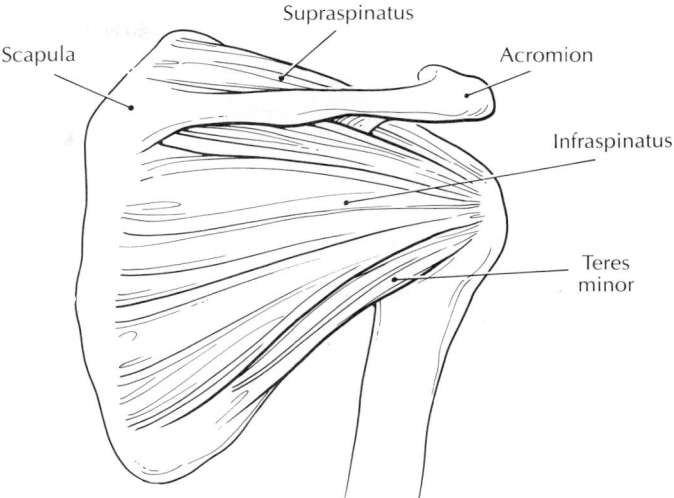

**Fig. 234-1.** Posterior view of shoulder illustrating rotator cuff muscles.

of the humerus and provides internal rotation of the arm (Fig. 234-2).

The *long head of the biceps tendon,* although not formally considered part of the rotator cuff, assists in rotator cuff function. This tendon courses superiorly in the bicipital groove of the humerus between the greater and lesser tuberosities, passes between the subscapularis and supraspinatus tendons, and penetrates the glenohumeral joint to insert on the labrum (Fig. 234-2). During arm elevation, the tendon of the long head of the biceps depresses the humeral head, helping it remain centered in the glenoid.

## Bursae

The bursae facilitate motion between the components of the shoulder. There are eight identifiable bursae in the shoulder complex. However, only one, the large subacromial bursa, also known as the subdeltoid bursa, is clinically significant. The subacromial bursa is ex-

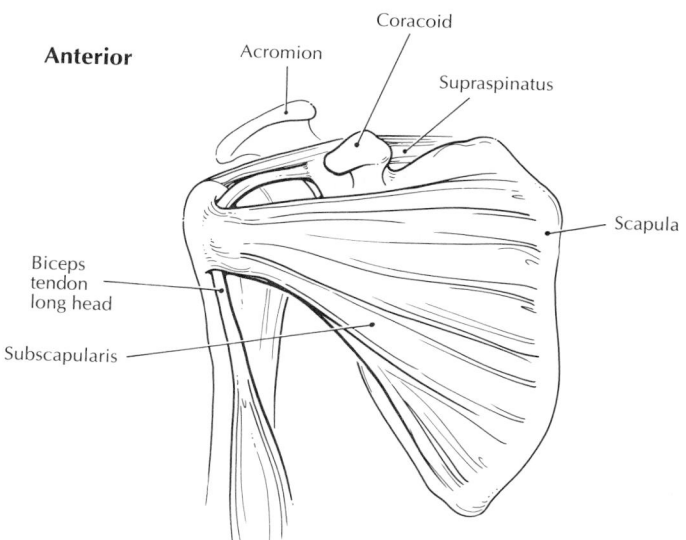

**Fig. 234-2.** Anterior view of shoulder illustrating supraspinatus and long head of biceps.

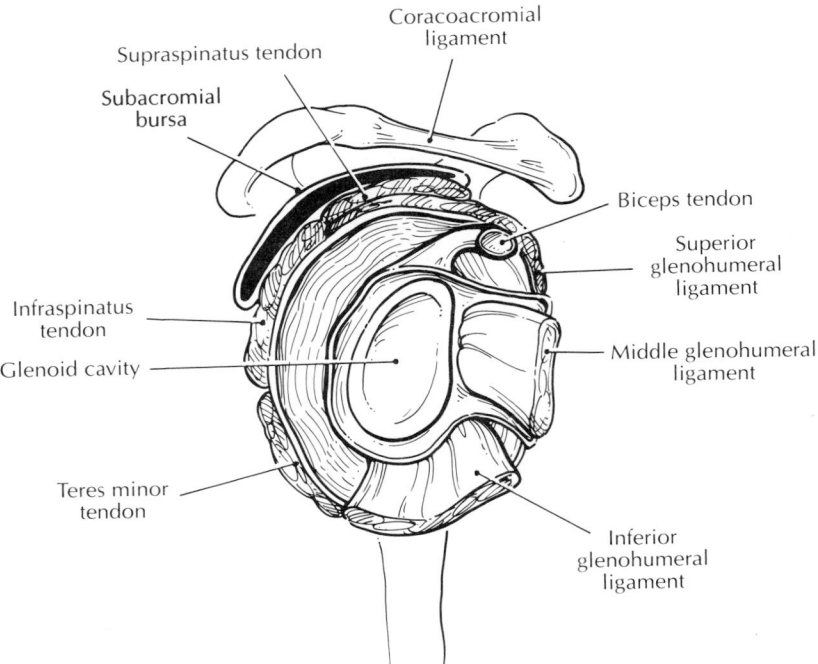

**Fig. 234-3.** Lateral view of shoulder illustrating coracoacromial arch with rotator cuff and subacromial bursa.

traarticular; its roof adheres to the undersurface of the deltoid, and its floor to the underlying rotator cuff. A thick layer of synovial fluid between the roof and the floor normally allows smooth frictionless motion between the rotator cuff and adjacent structures.

## Coracoacromial Arch

The coracoacromial arch is an important anatomic concept in understanding shoulder pathology. The arch is formed by the coracoid posteriorly, by the acromion anteriorly, and by the coracoacromial ligament, which forms the anterior roof of the arch (Fig. 234-3). The humeral head provides the floor of the arch. This arch defines the space within which the muscles of the rotator cuff, the tendon of the long head of the biceps, and the subacromial bursa must fit and function. The coracoacromial ligament is considered vestigial; however, by virtue of its position it can contribute to compression or impingement of the rotator cuff.

## IMPINGEMENT SYNDROME

Repetitive use of the arm overhead or above the horizontal compresses the rotator cuff and related structures between the humeral head and coracoacromial arch (Fig. 234-4). The impingement syndrome refers to the pathologic changes that occur in the structures of the rotator cuff due to this repetitive compression. Also referred to as "painful arc syndrome," "cuffitis," "supraspinatus syndrome," and "bursitis," impingement syndrome is the leading cause of shoulder pain and dysfunction. A basic understanding of this concept is essential for the proper evaluation and treatment of the patient with shoulder pain.

## Pathophysiology

Repetitive impingement of the bursa, rotator cuff, and biceps tendon produces pathologic changes in these structures that progress in a predictable pattern. Early on, repetitive motion produces mechanical inflammation of the subacromial bursa and underlying rotator cuff. As activities that cause impingement continue, inflammation of the rotator cuff tendons worsens. Chronic inflammation in time leads to degeneration and eventual tearing of the rotator cuff. Degeneration of the rotator cuff exposes the biceps tendon, making it susceptible to

degeneration and rupture. As the soft tissue restraints of the shoulder wear out, degenerative disease sets in and is typical of the advanced stages of the impingement syndrome.

Most of the pathologic changes in the rotator cuff due to impingement occur near the humeral insertion of the tendon. This area is referred to as the "critical zone" and has been identified as relatively avascular. Repetitive compression causes relative ischemia in this area. Over time this area degenerates and ultimately fails. The critical zone is the most common site of all rotator cuff abnormalities. The supraspinatus, due to its location in the coracoacromial arch, is the most commonly affected muscle of the rotator cuff.

Three stages of impingement are identifiable. Stage 1 is characterized by local inflammation, edema, and hemmorhage and is most commonly associated with subacromial bursitis and early rotator cuff tendinitis. These changes are considered reversible. Stage 2 is characterized by inflammation, thickening, and fibrosis of the rotator cuff tendons. Stage 3 is characterized by degeneration and rupture of the

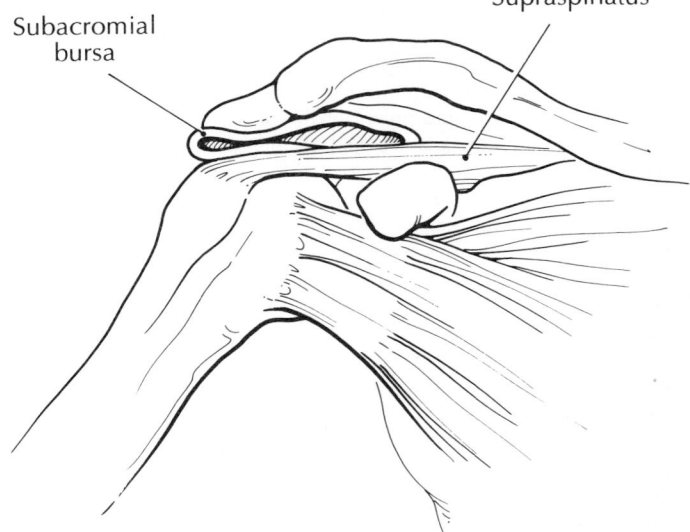

**Fig. 234-4.** Impingement of subacromial bursa and rotator cuff.

**Table 234-1.** Features of Impingement

|                        | Stage 1                 | Stage 2                  | Stage 3                |
|------------------------|-------------------------|--------------------------|------------------------|
| Clinical presentation  | Subacromial bursitis    | Rotator cuff tendinitis  | Rotator cuff tear      |
| Age                    | < 25 years              | 25–40 years              | > 40 years             |
| Disability             | None                    | Mild to moderate         | Moderate to severe     |
| Pathologic changes     | Reversible              | Irreversible             | Irreversible           |

rotator cuff tendon. Degenerative changes in the bony structures of the shoulder usually accompany stage 3. Stages 2 and 3 are considered to be irreversible (Table 234-1).

## Clinical Features

**Impingement signs.** Specific maneuvers on physical examination test for signs of impingement by compressing the rotator cuff and bursa between the humeral head and coracoacromial arch. Neer's impingement test requires the examiner to move the patient's straightened arm smoothly but forcibly to full abduction. This compresses the cuff and bursa against the undersurface of the acromion (Fig. 234-5). A second test, Hawkins' impingement test, requires the examiner to position the patient's arm in 90° of abduction and 90° of elbow flexion. Rotation of the arm inwardly across the front of the patient's body compresses the cuff and bursa between the humeral head and coracoacromial ligament (Figs. 234-6 and -7). These tests are considered positive if they reproduce pain.

**Impingement injection test.** Injection of a local anesthetic into the subacromial space can provide valuable diagnostic information in the emergency department. Ten milliliters of 1% xylocaine is injected into the subacromial space; 5 to 10 min later the physical maneuvers for impingement signs are repeated. The pain should decrease by 50 percent following injection. This test can help distinguish the pain of impingement from that of other shoulder disorders (Fig. 234-8).

## Emergency Department Treatment

The goals of treatment of impingement lesions are twofold: to reduce pain and inflammation and, more importantly, to prevent progression of the process. Regardless of the stage of impingement identified, a conservative treatment program initiated by the emergency physician

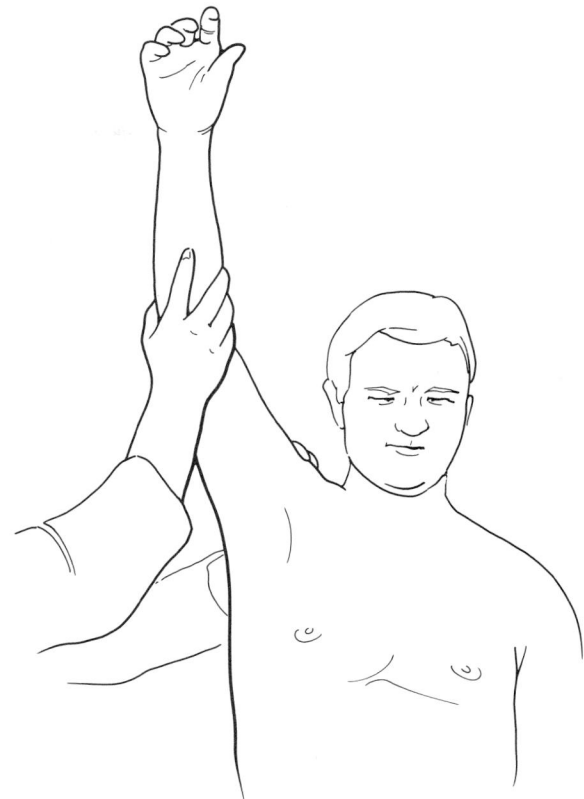

**Fig. 234-5.** Neer's impingement sign. Compression of inflamed subacromial bursa and rotator cuff beneath coracoacromial arch produces pain.

should include the following:

1. Relative rest and modification of activities. However, immobilization should be avoided whenever possible. Brief periods of support with a sling may be prescribed.
2. Medication to reduce pain and inflammation. Often analgesics are required to control pain during stage 2 and 3 impingement. Non-

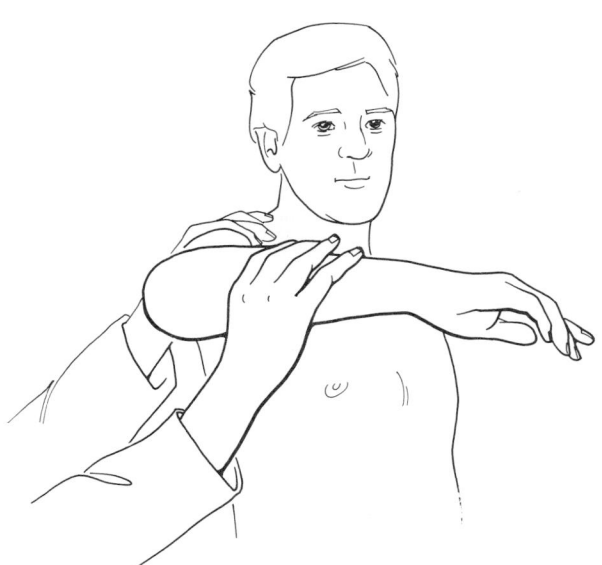

**Fig. 234-6.** Hawkins' impingement sign. Compression of inflamed bursa, subacromial bursa, and rotator cuff against coracoacromial ligament produces pain.

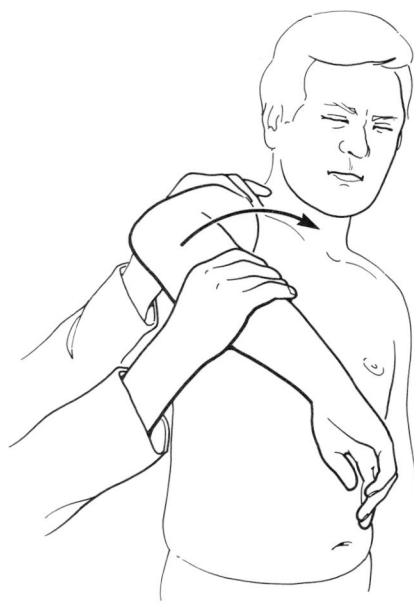

**Fig. 234-7.** Hawkins impingement sign (*cont.*).

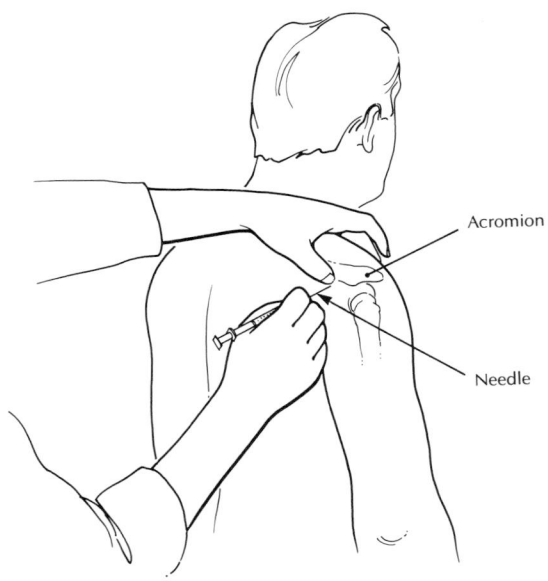

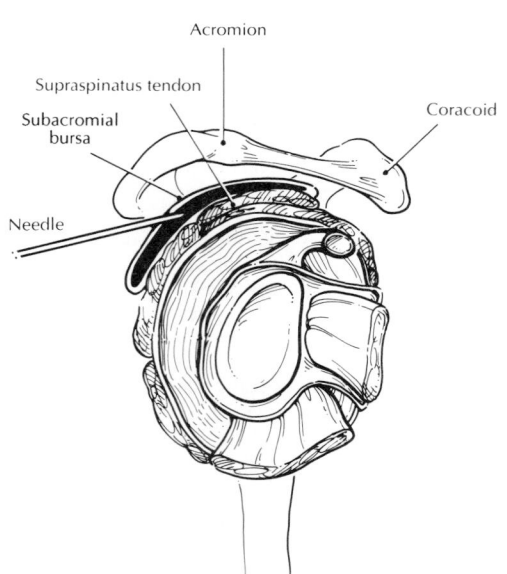

**Fig. 234-8.** Impingement injection test. Posterior approach just inferior to acromion allows easy access to subacromial bursa.

steroidal anti-inflammatories can be prescribed for a 7- to 10-day course.

3. Cryotherapy. The application of ice to the affected shoulder for 10 to 15 min two to three times per day can have analgesic affects and is thought to reduce local inflammation and edema.

4. Gentle range of motion. Two simple exercises can help the patient maintain glenohumeral motion. Pendulum swings are done with the patient slightly bent at the waist with the arm hanging freely in front of the body. Gentle arcs of motion to the level of pain tolerance can be carried out for 5 to 10 min daily. The size of the arcs should increase daily as symptoms allow. Also, having the patient walk his or her fingers up the wall to the level of pain tolerance can also help preserve glenohumeral motion.

5. Stretching and strengthening. During stage 1 impingement, stretching and strengthening may be initiated early on. Entering stage 2 and 3 impingement, stretching and strengthening are most effectively carried out under the supervision of a physical therapist. This is an important part of the treatment of impingement and is usually prescribed by the primary care physician or orthopaedist, who can monitor the patient's response to therapy.

6. *Corticosteroid injections.* While local corticosteroid injections into the subacromial space can be effective for pain relief, their deleterious effects on soft tissues have been well documented. These include muscular atrophy, weakness, and further tissue degeneration. Injection directly into the substance of the tendon can lead to necrosis and rupture. Even in the primary clinician's office setting, the judicious use of corticosteroids is advised, with no more than two to three injections being recommended in one specific area. While a single injection is not believed to be harmful, caution is still advised for use in the emergency department because of the potential harmful effects of repeated injections and difficulty in ensuring reliable follow-up.

### Follow-up

Timely referral for all stages of impingement is crucial to help preserve function and mobility in the shoulder. Clinical follow-up is usually recommended after 7 to 14 days for stage 1 and 2 lesions. For stage 3 lesions, associated with chronic disability or other concern for rotator cuff tears, more acute follow-up is recommended.

If symptoms have diminished at the time of follow-up, a supervised course of therapy with emphasis on rotator cuff stretching and strengthening may be prescribed. If the symptoms persist or have worsened, the clinical physician may attempt a subacromial injection of glucocorticoid to help arrest the inflammatory response. If symptoms persist despite full conservative measures after 6 to 12 weeks of treatment, further workup with arthrography, magnetic resonance imaging (MRI), or arthroscopy to rule out rotator cuff tearing may be carried out at the discretion of the primary clinical provider.

## SUBACROMIAL BURSITIS

### Pathophysiology

Subacromial bursitis is associated with stage 1 impingement and is typically characterized by localized edema and inflammation in the subacromial bursa. More importantly, an early inflammation of the rotator cuff tendon usually coexists. Subacromial bursitis typically is seen in patients under 25 years of age and usually results from mechanical irritation from repetitive overhand activities. It is important that this condition be recognized because it is reversible. If left unrecognized and untreated, it progresses to the irreversible conditions associated with stage 2 and stage 3 impingement.

Primary subacromial bursitis is rare but should be considered in patients with shoulder pain who have rheumatoid arthritis, tuberculosis, gout, or pyogenic infections.

### Clinical Features

Patients usually describe the pain of subacromial bursitis as a dull aching sensation deep within the shoulder, frequently following activity and usually improving with rest. Patients usually seek medical attention only when the symptoms affect their work, performance, or ability to compete. On physical examination, no muscular atrophy or asymmetry is present unless the symptoms have been chronic. Little if any tenderness is elicited on palpation; however, when tenderness is present it typically will be found on the lateral aspect of the proximal humerus or on deep palpation in the subacromial space. Full range of motion in the shoulder is usually preserved but may be painful, especially between 60° and 100° of abduction. The pain is worse when resistance is applied to the arm in 90° of abduction. Muscle strength in the deltoid and rotator cuff muscles is usually not affected. Impingement signs and impingement injection tests are usually positive.

## Radiographic Findings

Most often radiographs are normal in the early stages of impingement associated with bursitis.

## Emergency Department Treatment

The goals of treatment of subacromial bursitis and early rotator cuff tendinitis are twofold: to reduce pain and inflammation and, more importantly, to prevent progression of this reversible process to the irreversible stages of rotator cuff tendinitis and degeneration.

More than 90 percent of patients with subacromial bursitis respond to conservative measures. An effective conservative treatment plan has been outlined previously in this section. Since inflammation of the bursa is typically due to overuse, a short period of relative rest is indicated. Immobilization is not indicated and, in fact, can be detrimental, leading to adhesions and loss of motion. Total inactivity usually is not necessary. "Relative rest" implies avoidance of those activities that reproduce symptoms; e.g., a tennis player should avoid serving but can continue to hit ground strokes, and a laborer should avoid working with his or her arms over the head. Nonsteroidal anti-inflammatory agents are effective in reducing pain and inflammation. Analgesics are rarely needed to control pain. Localized ice treatment for 10 to 15 minutes two to three times per day will help reduce pain and inflammation. As pain diminishes, the patient should begin gentle range of motion, stretching, and strengthening exercises.

## Follow-up

Clinical follow-up is recommended in 7 to 14 days. To simply diagnose "bursitis" and treat the symptoms does the patient a disservice and places the patient's shoulder at risk for future dysfunction. At the time of follow-up, if the patient's symptoms have diminished, a supervised course of therapy with emphasis on rotator cuff strengthening may be prescribed. If symptoms persist or have worsened, a subacromial injection of a glucocorticoid may help arrest the inflammatory response. If symptoms persist despite full conservative measures after 6 to 12 weeks of treatment, further workup with

**Fig. 234-9.** Supraspinatus test. Patient's arm held in "empty beer can" position helps isolate supraspinatus muscle.

arthrography or MRI to rule out rotator cuff disease may be initiated at the discretion of the patient's primary clinician.

## ROTATOR CUFF TENDINITIS
### Pathophysiology

Inflammation of the rotator cuff tendons occurs initially in stage 1 of impingement. Continued repetitive mechanical impingement leads to irreversible fibrosis and thickening of the tendons of the rotator cuff, the hallmark of rotator cuff tendinitis. These findings are thought to represent the second stage of impingement. The supraspinatus is the tendon most commonly affected; however, any of the rotator cuff tendons may be involved.

### Clinical Features

Patients with rotator cuff tendinitis are typically between the ages of 25 and 40 years, but the duration of the symptoms is more useful than age in making this diagnosis. The patient will report prior episodes of shoulder pain or a long duration of pain before seeking treatment. Since the lesion is not reversible, time and activity modification alone will not improve the symptoms. Patients describe the pain as a deep, aching discomfort that interferes with work and normal daily activities. Night pain, especially sleeping on the affected arm or with the arms above the head, will interfere with sleep. On examination, disuse atrophy of the shoulder musculature may be present if symptoms have been chronic. Palpation of the rotator cuff insertion at the lateral aspect of the proximal humerus will usually produce pain and tenderness. During range-of-motion maneuvers, fibrosis and scarring within the tendon can cause crepitus. A sensation of catching may also be present if scar tissue is trapped beneath the acromion. Both active and passive motion may be limited due to the scarring. Rotator cuff strength testing will reveal mild to moderate weakness. Pain will usually be present when resistance is applied. The individual muscles of the rotator cuff can be isolated and tested individually. To test the supraspinatus, abduct the arm to 90° and place it forward 30° with the thumb pointed down in the so-called empty beer can position (Fig. 234-9). Pain or weakness against resistance in this position suggests injury to the supraspinatus. External rotation tests the infraspinatus and the teres minor. To test external rotation, place the patient's arm against the body with the elbow bent to 90° and the forearm in neutral position. Stabilize the elbow against the patient's waist and in-

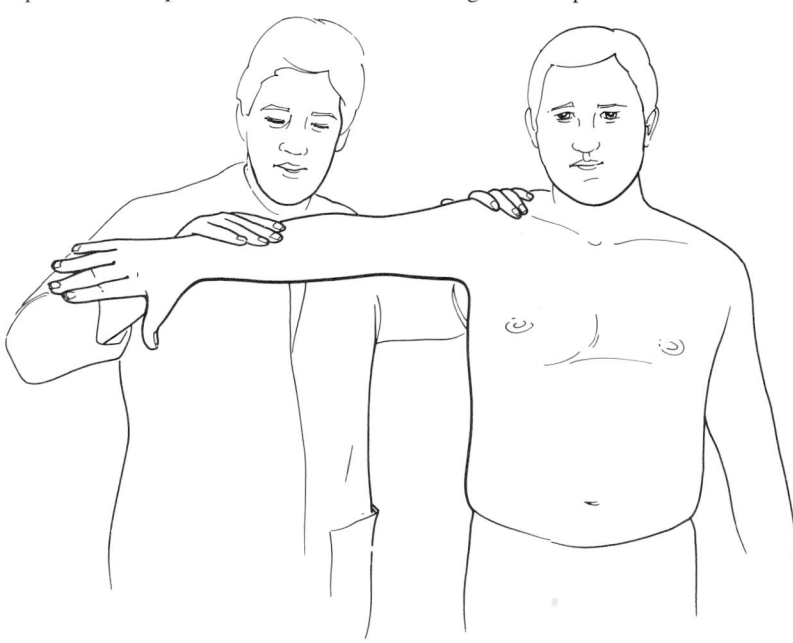

struct the patient to rotate the arm outward (Fig. 234-10). In this same position, with the elbow flexed and fixed against the patient's body, have the patient rotate the arm inward around the front of the body against resistance. This internal rotation tests subscapularis function.

The impingement sign is usually positive because the inflamed tendons are compressed beneath the coracoacromial arch. Injection of subacromial anesthetic may diminish pain but generally does not improve motion or strength significantly.

## Radiographic Findings

Radiographs are most often normal but may yield helpful diagnostic clues. The presence of osteophytes off the inferior clavicle or acromion represent a long-standing process. These osteophytes can contribute to further injury to the underlying tendons. The soft tissues of the subacromial space should be inspected for evidence of calcification.

## Emergency Department Treatment

Treatment of tendinitis emphasizes controlling symptoms, preserving motion, and improving strength and flexibility. Immobilization should be avoided, although an arm sling may be provided for comfort and support during acute symptoms. Nonsteroidal anti-inflammatory agents can help reduce pain and inflammation, and occasionally analgesics are necessary. Gentle range-of-motion exercises are recommended as early as symptoms allow to prevent further contraction and scarring.

## Follow-up

Referral for follow-up is recommended in 7 to 14 days. Early physical therapy with treatment to reduce inflammation along with a supervised stretching and strengthening program are an integral part of treatment. Most patients with tendinitis respond to conservative management, experiencing no significant dysfunction. However, if symptoms persist despite conservative measures, further investigation for a possible degenerative rotator cuff tear may be pursued by the patient's primary physician.

# ROTATOR CUFF TEARS

## Introduction

Tears in the rotator cuff muscles can occur from acute trauma, chronic overuse, or a combination of the two. Acute rotator cuff tears account for approximately 10 percent of all rotator cuff tears and usually occur as a result of significant trauma. Traumatic causes typically involve a fall on an outstretched arm, causing extreme hyperabduction or hyperextension. Lifting a heavy object or catching a heavy object as it falls can also cause acute rotator cuff tears. Chronic rotator cuff tears account for 90 percent of all rotator cuff tears and are usually due to progressive degeneration. Stage 3 impingement is associated with 95 percent of all chronic tears. If a degenerative tear is present, it is prone to extension with acute trauma.

Rotator cuff tears can be further classified as full thickness or partial thickness. Full thickness tears, as the name implies, involve the full extent of the tendon. Partial thickness tears, on the other hand, can exist on either the superior or inferior surface of the tendon or in the mid substance of the tendon. Partial thickness tears are twice as common as full thickness tears and most commonly occur on the inferior aspect of the tendon. Acute full thickness rotator cuff tears from a single injury are rare. Partial thickness rotator cuff tears are more likely to occur from an acute injury, especially in younger patients.

The type and extent of the tear have significant implications for the ultimate treatment and prognosis. Full thickness tears usually require surgical treatment, whereas partial thickness tears often respond to conservative management. In the emergency department it may be impossible to distinguish a full thickness tear from a partial thickness tear or even from an acute flare-up of rotator cuff tendinitis. However, it is important for the emergency physician to understand the pathophysiology of these conditions and their implications to shoulder function. Proper recognition, early intervention, and proper referral can preserve shoulder motion and function.

## Pathophysiology

The critical zone of the rotator cuff is an area of relative avascularity near the humeral insertion of the tendon. Repetitive compression and

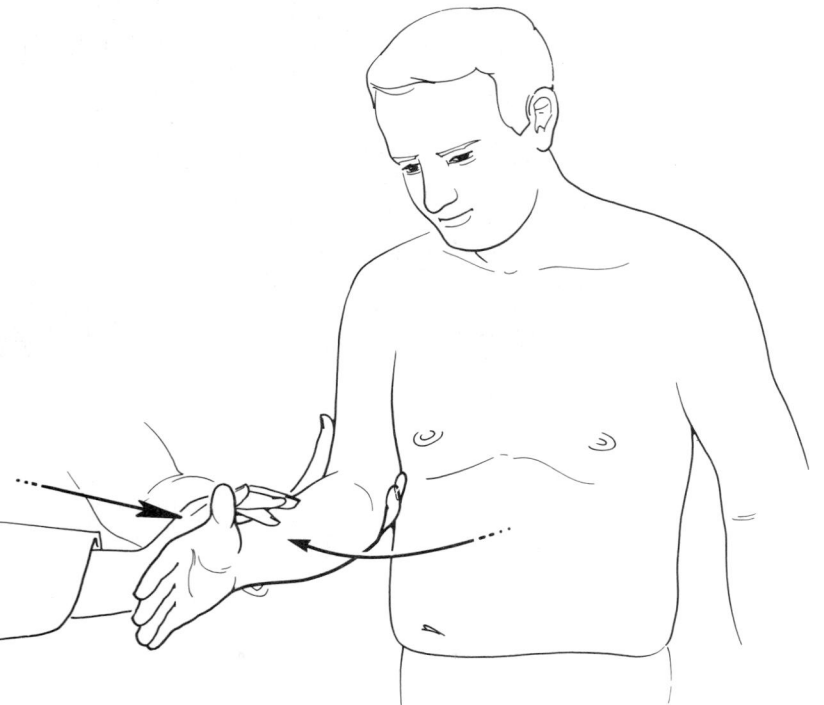

**Fig. 234-10.** Internal and external rotation testing of rotator cuff.

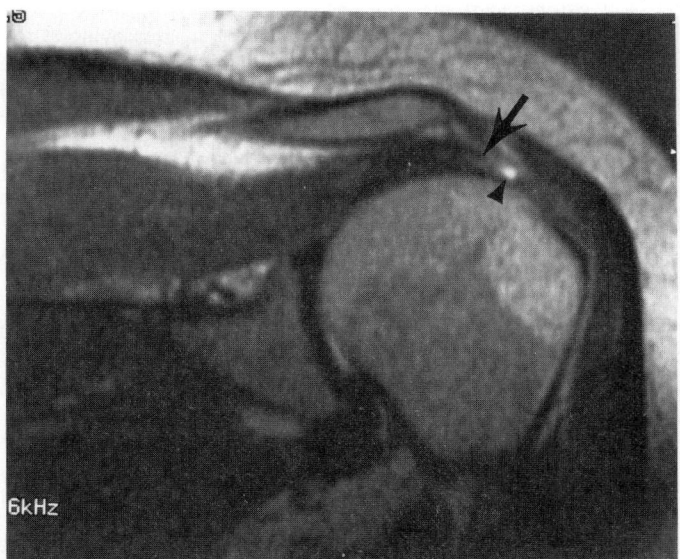

**Fig. 234-11.** Rotator cuff tear. MRI coronal image of shoulder reveals tear in supraspinatus tendon at the critical zone (arrow) with edema (point).

impingement cause ischemia in this area. With time this area degenerates and ultimately tears. The critical zone is the most common site of all rotator cuff tears. The supraspinatus, due to its location within the coracoacromial arch, is the most commonly injured rotator cuff muscle (Fig. 234-11).

The bony structures of the shoulder can also contribute to rotator cuff tears. The acromion, which forms part of the roof of the coracoacromial arch, may be described as flat, curved, or hooked (Fig. 234-12). One clinical study associated a hooked acromion with 80 percent of rotator cuff tears, whereas a flat acromion was associated with fewer than 3 percent of tears.

Acute traumatic rotator cuff tears, which account for 10 percent of all rotator cuff tears, require a significant force. For a single traumatic event to cause a rotator cuff tear, the force must overcome the tensile strength of the tendon. However, the tensile strength of the tendon is greater than that of bone; therefore, a bony avulsion injury of the humerus is much more common than an isolated rotator cuff tear following acute trauma (Fig. 234-13).

### Clinical Features

Patients with rotator cuff tears are almost always more than 40 years of age; rotator cuff tears in the young are rare. In general, the older the patient with shoulder pain, the more likely the presence of a rotator cuff tear. The clinical features of a chronic rotator cuff tear differ from those of an acute tear. Approximately one-half of all patients

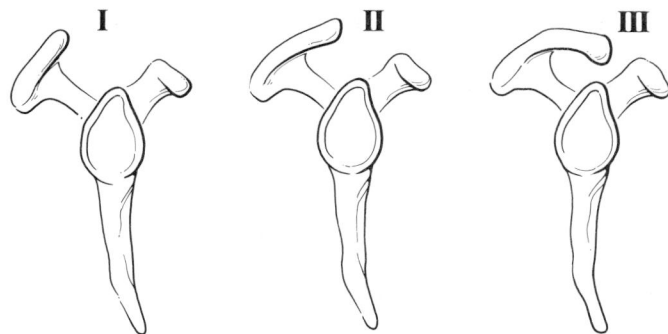

**Fig. 234-12.** Acromial morphology. I. Flat. II. Curved. III. Hooked.

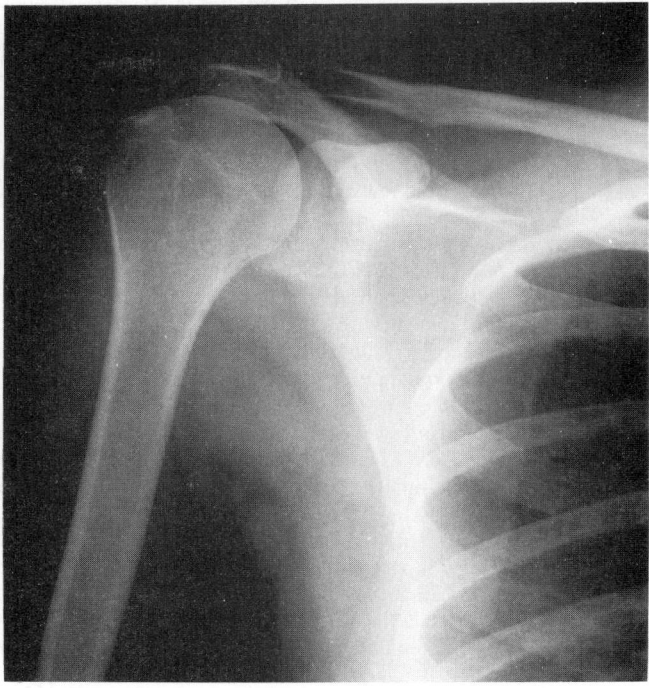

A

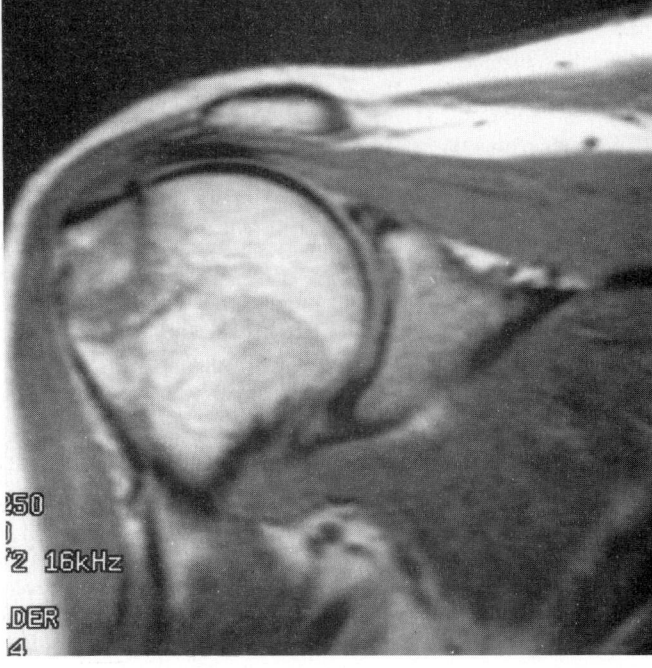

B

**Fig. 234-13.** Tensile strength of rotator cuff tendon is greater than bone. The patient suffered acute hyperabduction injury to arm causing extreme shoulder pain and dysfunction. Initially, radiographs (*A*) was interpreted as normal. MRI (*B*) of shoulder revealed avulsion fracture of humerus at site of supraspinatus tendon insertion.

with chronic rotator cuff tears recall a specific trauma or an event associated with the onset of pain; however, the trauma is usually not significant. Patients more commonly report a history of gradual and progressive pain, which initially is described as worse at night. The pain eventually becomes persistent. The pain may be described as diffuse but is commonly localized to the lateral aspect of the upper arm. The patient typically reports flare-ups of bursitis and tendinitis that initially responded to rest, anti-inflammatory agents, and glucocorticoid injections. However, as the rotator cuff weakens, the frequency, intensity, and duration of the symptoms increase and are less responsive to the usual treatments. Shoulder dysfunction progressively worsens and interferes with work, recreation, and normal daily activities. Arm elevation, external rotation, and lifting even light objects worsen the symptoms.

On examination, disuse atrophy may be present in patients with chronic rotator cuff tears. Palpation may produce discomfort at the lateral aspect of the upper arm or in the subacromial region. Active motion is variably limited by pain and weakness. Muscle strength is compromised, especially in abduction and external rotation. In fact, one study directly correlated the size of a rotator cuff tear with the strength of external rotation. The "drop arm test" is positive if the patient is unable to hold or lower a fully extended arm without dropping it. Crepitus and pain are usually present on range-of-motion testing. Injection of anesthetic into the subacromial space may diminish pain but will not improve motion or strength.

With acute injuries, such as a fall or catching a heavy object as it falls, the patient may report a sensation of "tearing in the shoulder" followed by severe pain and inability to raise the arm. An acute rotator cuff tear will produce immediate significant pain and disability. Asymmetry may be noted due to significant local swelling. A rotator cuff defect from the tear may be palpable overlying the humeral head. Active motion will be limited, with inability to abduct or externally rotate the arm against even minimal resistance. The drop arm test is positive and impingement signs are typically positive, but testing for them may not be practical after an acute injury. Injection of anesthetic into the subacromial space will not improve motion or strength.

### Radiographic Findings

Radiographic findings may be supportive but are rarely diagnostic, yielding few specific clues unique to rotator cuff tears. With a large tear, the humeral head can "button hole" through the defect of the rotator cuff and assume a superior position to the glenoid. However, this is rarely appreciated. More often, radiographs will reveal findings associated with chronic rotator cuff pathology: sclerosis of the humeral head, degenerative joint disease at the acromioclavicular joint, osteophytes off the undersurface of the acromion and/or clavicle, and a hooked acromion.

### Emergency Department Care

It may be clinically impossible to differentiate an acute rotator cuff strain from a partial thickness or full thickness rotator cuff tear. The immediate goal of emergency care for suspected rotator cuff injuries is to provide support, protection, pain relief, and, most importantly, to help prevent further dysfunction and disability. An arm sling can be provided for support and comfort until acute symptoms subside. However, the perils of prolonged immobilization—stiffness, weakness, and loss of motion—should be emphasized to the patient. Appropriate analgesia should be provided, as should instruction in the proper use of ice two to three times per day to reduce pain and inflammation. When symptoms allow, gentle range-of-motion exercises such as pendulum swings and walking the fingers up the wall should be started.

### Follow-up

Any patient with a suspected acute rotator cuff tear or with significant disability should receive prompt referral to an orthopaedist within 7 days. Young patients with full thickness rotator cuff tears usually require surgical repair. Functional results are better if repair is carried out within 3 weeks of injury, before retraction, fibrosis, tendon degeneration, and muscular atrophy have occurred. Partial thick-

ness or chronic tears may respond to conservative measures; however, early referral is warranted. If symptoms are improving at follow-up, conservative measures with physical therapy may be initiated. If significant symptoms and dysfunction persist, additional evaluation by MRI or CT arthrography may be pursued to determine the full extent of injury.

Following acute injuries, any evidence or suspicion of neurovascular compromise requires immediate orthopaedic consultation.

## CALCIFIC TENDINITIS

### Pathophysiology

Calcific tendinitis is considered a unique and still poorly understood disease process. It is characterized by the deposition of calcium hydroxyapatite crystals within one or more tendons of the rotator cuff. In time, the calcium deposition undergoes spontaneous resorption, with subsequent healing of the tendon. Calcific tendinitis does not appear to be related to any generalized disease process nor does its presence correlate with episodes of trauma or incidence of rotator cuff tears.

Primary tendon degeneration as a result of chronic repetitive microtrauma, age, or tissue hypoxia is considered to be the primary cause of this disorder. The supraspinatus is by far the most commonly affected tendon, with calcium deposition usually occurring 1 to 2 cm proximal to the insertion on the humerus; however, any of the rotator cuff tendons as well as the tendon of the long head of the biceps may be affected. After a variable period following the deposition of the calcium, spontaneous resorption occurs. The factors triggering resorption are unclear. With resorption of the calcium, the defect in the tendon remodels and heals.

The initial formation of the deposit is associated with few, if any, symptoms and little dysfunction. However, significant pain is associated with the resorption of the calcium deposit. This pain is thought to be due to the relative increase in pressure and volume within the tendon caused by vascular proliferation and the formation of granulation tissue.

### Clinical Features

Patients in their thirties and forties are most commonly affected. This process is rarely seen in patients over 70. Of patients older than age 30 with shoulder pain, calcification in the rotator cuff tendons is found in approximately 7 percent. However, in asymptomatic patients between 31 and 40, 10 to 20 percent demonstrate rotator cuff calcification on routine radiographs. Of these patients, 35 to 45 percent will eventually become symptomatic. Females are affected more commonly than males, and calcification is often present bilaterally.

The onset of pain typically coincides with the resorption of the calcium deposit rather than the formation of it. Symptomatic patients experience sudden onset of shoulder pain, usually at rest. Any shoulder motion reproduces significant pain. The pain is often worse at night and interferes with sleep. The symptoms are usually self-limited, lasting 1 to 2 weeks in most cases. However, occasionally symptoms may be more indolent, producing less acute pain but lasting several weeks.

During an acute attack with intense pain, patients hold their arm across their body and often are reluctant to move it. Often a point of maximum tenderness can be palpated, usually over the proximal humerus near the tendinous insertion of the rotator cuff. Active and passive motion both are limited due to pain. Patients often report a sensation of catching when they move their shoulder through an arc of motion. Crepitus is frequently present with motion.

### Radiographic Findings

Routine shoulder radiographs will reveal the calcific deposits (Fig. 234-14). Deposits in the supraspinatus are readily visible on films in

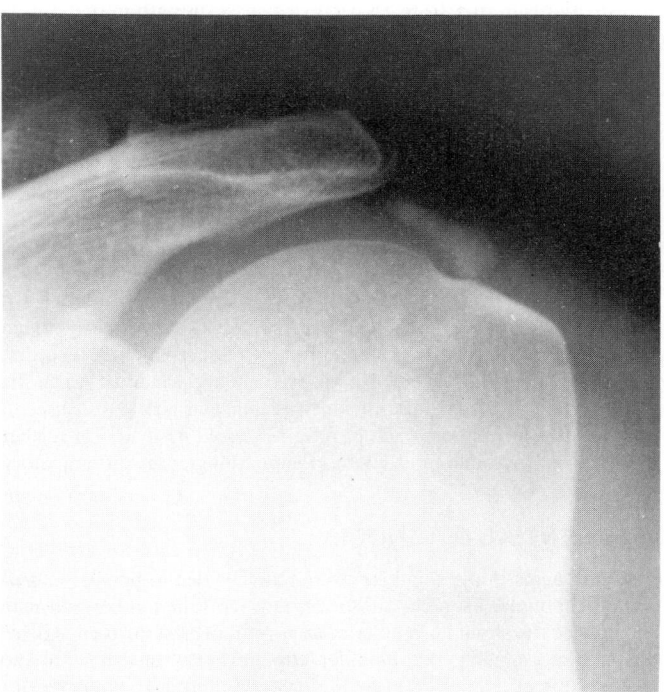

**Fig. 234-14.** Calcific deposits in rotator cuff.

neutral rotation. Internal rotation of the humeral head best reveals deposits in the infraspinatus and teres minor. In patients with acute pain where resorption is actively occurring, calcium deposition may be ill defined or barely visible. However, during the formative phase, the deposit is usually dense, well defined, and easily visualized.

### Emergency Department Treatment

The emergency department management of calcific tendinitis should be tailored to reduce the patient's symptoms and help protect shoulder function. During an acute attack, analgesics are usually necessary to calm the intense pain. A sling for brief periods of immobilization may be provided, but prolonged immobilization should be avoided to prevent loss of motion. The patient should be instructed to rest the shoulder in abduction on the back of a chair as often as is tolerable. Sleeping with a pillow beneath the axilla can also help prevent restricted motion. Gentle and progressive range-of-motion exercises should be emphasized and encouraged. In the acute phase, local application of ice for 10 to 15 min, two to three times per day may provide analgesia and help control inflammation and edema. Local heat application may be used once acute symptoms have diminished.

Local needling of the calcific deposits in the emergency department has been described for the patient in acute pain. A point of maximum tenderness on palpation can be isolated, and the presence of calcification can be confirmed with radiographs. A local anesthetic, such as 2 percent xylocaine or bupivacaine without epinephrine, is used to anesthetize subcutaneous tissues corresponding to the anticipated site of needle placement. An 18-gauge needle can then be placed at the site of calcification. This may decompress the tendon and ease the pain acutely and may speed ultimate resorption of the deposit. Following this procedure, analgesics should be prescribed. Nonsteroidal anti-inflammatories for 7 to 10 days may also be helpful.

### Follow-up

The patient should follow up with an orthopaedist within a week, regardless of whether he or she has undergone acute needling of the

calcium deposit in the emergency department. Conservative measures such as physical therapy, local needling, and injection of local anesthetics at the site of the deposit may be prescribed. Surgical removal of the calcium deposit is usually considered only after all conservative measures have been exhausted.

## ADHESIVE CAPSULITIS

Adhesive capsulitis, commonly referred to as the "frozen shoulder syndrome," causes significant discomfort and dysfunction. It is characterized by markedly restricted joint motion and pain. This condition usually occurs in middle-aged patients and is uncommon in patients younger than 40 years of age and in those older than 70 years. It is more common in women, particularly postmenopausal women. The incidence in the general population is 2 to 5 percent; this increases to 10 to 20 percent in patients with diabetes. An increased incidence is also associated with patients with a history of trauma, cervical disc disease, thyroid disease, intracranial lesions, and personality disorders. It is rarely associated with the presence of rotator cuff tears.

### Pathophysiology

The exact etiology of adhesive capsulitis remains unclear, and the pathophysiology remains poorly understood. Following injury or with chronic inflammation, the shoulder joint capsule becomes thickened and contracted. Pain initially limits motion. Decreased motion allows additional inflammation. Fibrosis and scarring between the capsule, rotator cuff, subacromial bursa, and deltoid progress, further restricting motion. The joint capsule normally has an inferior pouch or "axillary fold," which stretches to accomodate the humeral head during progressive elevation and external rotation of the shoulder. With fibrosis and thickening, the capsule is drawn tightly around the humeral head and the axillary fold is obliterated, restricting shoulder motion.

Autoimmune mechanisms as well as autonomic nerve dysfunction have also been implicated as causes of adhesive capsulitis, but the mechanism remains unclear.

### Clinical Features

A period of shoulder immobilization following an injury or failure to mobilize the shoulder following a stroke are considered predisposing factors in the development of adhesive capsulitis. Frequently, however, no precipitating cause can be identified. Symptoms may develop insidiously over several months. Pain is described typically as diffuse and aching, is poorly localized, and often extends down the upper arm. The pain is often described as worse at night.

A painful stiffened shoulder is the hallmark finding on examination. Active and passive range of motion are limited, especially in abduction and in internal and external rotation. Disuse atrophy may be present. Pain is not usually reproducible by palpation but is present at the limits of motion as the fibrosed capsule is stretched. Impingement testing is difficult due to restricted motion. Posterior glenohumeral dislocation must always be considered in the patient with restricted motion of the shoulder.

### Radiograph Findings

X-rays should be obtained to rule out a posterior glenohumeral dislocation. These should include three views at right angles to each other, typically an anteroposterior view of the humerus in internal and external rotation and an axillary or "y" view of the scapula. Adhesive capsulitis yields few specific diagnostic radiographic clues. Glenohumeral joint volume is described, but may be difficult to appreciate.

### Emergency Department Treatment

The goal of treatment is to reduce pain and initiate restoration of motion and function. In the emergency department, this treatment consists of administering analgesics and anti-inflammatory agents and instructing the patient in the proper use of heat and ice to reduce discomfort. The patient should be instructed in general progressive range-of-motion exercises, such as pendulum swings and walking the fingers up the wall using the affected arm. A sling may be provided for comfort, but its long-term use should be discouraged to prevent further loss of motion.

### Follow-up

Prompt orthopaedic referral, at least within 1 to 2 weeks, is warranted. If conservative measures fail, arthroscopy and manipulation of the shoulder under general anesthesia to break up adhesions may be considered by the orthopaedist.

Prevention is the best treatment, and the emergency physician plays a vital role. Prolonged immobilization of the shoulder or upper extremity following injury should be avoided. Prompt referral to the patient's primary care provider or orthopaedist following shoulder injuries is indicated. It allows the patient to begin early progressive motion and physical therapy, where indicated.

## DISORDERS OF THE BICEPS TENDON

### Pathophysiology

The tendon of the long head of the biceps, by virtue of its position, can be a common cause of shoulder pain. Disorders of the biceps tendon can result from progressive impingement or may occur due to isolated inflammation or injury. The tendon of the long head of the biceps courses through the bicipital groove on the anterior aspect of the proximal humerus and inserts on the superior aspect of the labrum in the glenohumeral joint. The tendon may become inflamed or partially dislocated, sublux out of the bicipital groove, or rupture altogether.

### Clinical Features

Patients with bicipital tendinitis present with acute, intense localized pain at the anterior aspect of the shoulder. Palpation of the tendon within the bicipital groove reproduces the intense pain. Forearm supination, one of the main actions of the biceps will also reproduce pain, especially when resistance is applied.

The tendon may sublux or momentarily dislocate from the bicipital groove if the transhumeral ligament, which forms the roof of the groove, tears from degeneration or acute trauma. Resisted forearm supination may cause subluxation that is palpable and accompanied by a painful popping sensation as the tendon subluxes.

In younger patients, mild trauma may cause complete rupture of the biceps tendon. In older patients, chronic impingement and degeneration may lead to rupture. On examination, the classic finding is described as a "popeye" deformity caused by contraction of the muscle from the side of the tear proximally.

### Emergency Department Treatment

Supportive care and pain relief are the mainstays of emergency department care. Tendinitis and subluxation are managed conservatively. The emergency physician may provide a sling for brief use as needed for support and comfort. Analgesics and anti-inflammatories may be used in conjunction with prescription of relative rest, use of ice for 10 to 15 min two to three times per day, and elevation to reduce swelling.

### Follow-up

For complete tears, referral to an orthopaedist is recommended for surgical consideration, although frequently complete tears of the proximal biceps are managed conservatively. Conservative treatment will usually result in a 10 to 15 percent loss of strength in the muscle and will leave a cosmetic deformity.

## OSTEOARTHRITIS

Since the glenohumeral joint is non-weight bearing, primary osteoarthritis is rare. When it does occur, presentation is similar to that of degenerative disease in other joints; the patient experiences gradual and progressive onset of pain, which is worse with motion and better with rest. This usually occurs concurrently with degenerative disease of the acromioclavicular joint.

Secondary osteoarthritis is usually more common and usually associated with a previous fracture, recurrent dislocations, or with an underlying rheumatologic, metabolic, or endocrinologic disorder. Emergency department care of both primary and secondary arthritis includes analgesics, anti-inflammatory agents, and gentle exercises to preserve range of motion. Prompt referral should be made for further evaluation of possible underlying rheumatologic or inflammatory conditions.

## DIFFERENTIAL DIAGNOSIS

Aches and pains in the shoulder are not always due to bursitis or tendinitis. Although disorders of the rotator cuff and other intrinsic structures of the shoulder are the most common cause of pain, extrinsic conditions outside the shoulder complex can refer pain to the shoulder. It is critical and can be life preserving to distinguish extrinsic causes from intrinsic causes of shoulder pain.

### The Neck

The neck is the most common source of pain referred to the shoulder. Degenerative disease of the cervical spine, degenerative disc disease, and herniated nucleus pulposus can all refer pain to the shoulder. These symptoms may occur acutely or gradually. The pain is usually worse during daytime activities and better at night when activities cease. The patient with a C5–C6 herniated disc may present with pain very similar to that due to rotator cuff disease. Careful and thorough examination of the cervical spine and a complete neurovascular examination should be included in the evaluation of any patient with shoulder pain. On examination, range of motion in the neck may be restricted and may reproduce symptoms in the shoulder. Axial loading may especially cause referred pain. If a cervical condition is considered to be the source of pain, cervical radiographs including oblique views should be obtained. In the absence of neurologic findings, conservative measures may be initiated. In the emergency department, the patient may be fitted with a soft cervical collar and provided with analgesics and anti-inflammatory agents as needed for comfort.

### The Brachial Plexus

An injury to the brachial plexus can cause pain referred to the shoulder and can produce weakness and atrophy in the muscles of the shoulder within weeks of injury. Radiographic evaluation of the cervical spine should be included in the emergency department evaluation of patients with suspected brachial plexus injury or involvement.

Brachial plexus neuritis is uncommon but can be very painful. It is usually determined to be of viral origin. The inflammation of the brachial plexus can lead to weakness and atrophy of the muscles of the shoulder complex within weeks following the onset of pain. Cervical spine radiographs should be included in the workup. Brachial plexus neuritis is usually self-limiting. Referral to a neurologist should be arranged if a patient is suspected of having this disorder.

### Vascular Injuries

Injuries to the blood vessels can also cause shoulder pain. The most serious recognized vascular injury is acute thrombosis of the axillary artery. Repetitive mechanical trauma or explosive stress from lifting heavy objects can compress and contuse the intimal lining of the axillary artery. This predisposes the artery to thrombosis. Acute thrombosis requires primary thrombolytic therapy.

## Neurologic Injury

The most common neurologic injury about the shoulder involves compression of the suprascapular nerve. This nerve originates from the brachial plexus distal C5–C6 nerve roots and courses posteriorly to the suprascapular notch. Not uncommonly, this nerve becomes entrapped beneath the transverse ligament at the level of the notch. Traction injuries from explosive movements can also injure the nerve. On examination, infraspinatus atrophy and associated weakness and external rotation will typically be found. The initial treatment is conservative. Electromyographic and nerve conduction velocity studies will reveal the extent and location of nerve injury. Surgery for decompression is considered if conservative measures fail.

## Thoracic Outlet Syndrome

Compression of the brachial plexus and blood vessels proximal to the shoulder can cause shoulder pain. Women in the child-bearing years are affected three times more commonly than men. The medial trunk of the brachial plexus is most commonly affected, and the symptoms usually involve pain that radiates through the shoulder to the medial forearm and occasionally to the small and ring ringers. Patients can usually identify motions that reproduce the symptoms. Fatigue often prevents the use of the arms above shoulder level.

Radiographic evaluation may reveal evidence of a prior clavicle fracture with malunion or the presence of a cervical rib band, which are associated with compression of the brachial plexus. Treatment is generally conservative, although surgical decompression may be considered if the symptoms become debilitating or refractory to conservative measures.

## Pancoast's Tumor

This tumor, when present in the superior sulcus of the lung, may compress the brachial plexus against the chest wall and cause shoulder pain. The patient may experience local or radicular shoulder pain or sense a fullness in the supraclavicular fossa.

## Thoracic Disorders

1. Myocardial ischemia/infarction
2. Aortic disease
3. Pulmonary disorders
   a. Pneumonia
   b. Pulmonary embolus
   c. Pulmonary infarction
4. Diaphragmatic irritation

## Abdominal Disorders

1. Biliary disease
2. Splenic injury or inflammation
3. Pancreatitis
4. Peptic ulcer disease
5. Perforated viscus

## BIBLIOGRAPHY

Bigliani LU, Tucker JB: The relationship of acromial architecture to rotator cuff disease. *Clin Sports Med* 10(4):823, 1991.

Biundo JJ, Jr: Regional rheumatic pain syndromes, in Schumacher HR (ed): *Primer on Rheumatic Diseases,* 9th ed. Atlanta, Arthritis Foundation, 1988, pp 263–266.

Burkehead WB: The biceps tendon, in Rockwood CA, Matsen FA (eds): *The Shoulder.* Philadelphia, Saunders, 1990, pp 791–836.

Cofield RH: Current concepts review rotator cuff disease of the shoulder. *J Bone Joint Surg* 67A:974, 1985.

Garrick JG, Webb DR: Shoulder injuries, in *Sports Injuries: Diagnosis and Management.* Philadelphia, Saunders, 1990, pp 55–97.

Hawkins RJ, Abrams JS: Impingement syndrome in the absence of rotator cuff tear. *Orthop Clin North Am* 18(3):373, 1987.

Hawkins RJ, Mohtadi NGH: Rotator cuff problems in athletes, in Delee JC, Drez D, Jr (eds): *Orthopaedic Sports Medicine: Principles and Practice,* vol 1. Philadelphia, Saunders, 1994, pp 623–657.

Ionnotti JP (ed): *Rotator Cuff Disorders: Evaluation and Treatment.* American Academy of Orthopaedic Surgeons Monograph Series, 1991.

Matsen FA III, Arntz CT: Subacromial impingement, in Rockwood CA, Matsen FA (eds): *The Shoulder.* Philadelphia, Saunders, 1990, pp 623–646.

Matsen FA III, Arntz CT: Rotator cuff tendon failure, in Rockwood CA, Matsen FA (eds): *The Shoulder.* Philadelphia, Saunders, 1990, pp 647–677.

McKeag DB, Hough DO: Common sports injuries and illnesses—the upper extremity, in *Primary Care Sports Medicine.* Dubuque, IA, Brown & Benchmark, 1993, pp 281–342.

Murnaghan JP: Frozen shoulder, in Rockwood CA, Matsen FA (eds): *The Shoulder.* Philadelphia, Saunders, 1990, pp 837–862.

Neviaser RJ: Ruptures of the rotator cuff. *Orthop Clin North Am* 18(3):387, 1987.

Pappas AM: Injuries of the shoulder complex and overhand throwing problems, in Grana WA, Kalenak A (eds): *Clinical Sports Medicine.* Philadelphia, Saunders, 1991, pp 335–360.

Richardson A: Overview of soft tissue injuries of the shoulder, part II. *The Upper Extremity in Sports Medicine.* Baltimore, Mosby, 1990, pp 221–236.

Unthoff HK, Sankar K: Classification and definition of tendinopathies. *Clin Sports Med* 10(4):707, 1991.

Watson K: Impingement and rotator cuff lesions, part II. *The Upper Extremity in Sports Medicine.* Baltimore, Mosby, 1990, pp 213–220.

Zuckerman JD, Mirabello SC: The painful shoulder part I. *Am Fam Physician* 43(1):119, 1991.

Zuckerman JD, Mirabello SC: The painful shoulder part II. *Am Fam Physician* 43(2):447, 1991.

# 235
# OVERUSE SYNDROMES
## Beverly Timerding
## Monte Hunter

Overuse injuries are a frequent problem in many occupations and athletic pursuits. They occur secondary to repetitious and moderately stressful forces on tendons, ligaments, or their surrounding soft tissue. Acute pain results from inflammation, while more chronic pain may be from actual degenerative changes of a tendon near its insertion or origin. Those syndromes that present most commonly to the emergency department include carpal tunnel syndrome, ulnar neuritis, De Quervain's tenosynovitis, lateral and medial epicondylitis, groin strain, iliotibial band syndrome, popliteus tendinitis, shin splints, Achilles tendinitis or rupture, plantar fasciitis, and tarsal tunnel syndrome.

## CARPAL TUNNEL SYNDROME

This common disorder usually results from compression of the median nerve from flexor tenosynovitis. This nerve lies between the flexor retinaculum on the volar side of the wrist and the common flexor tendon sheath. Activities involving repetitive wrist flexion such as typing, playing a musical instrument, craftwork, and assembly packing may cause inflammation of the flexor tendon sheath, resulting in compression. The nerve may also become compressed from the mild edema of pregnancy.

Early carpal tunnel syndrome may be worse at night, and patients complain of a "pins and needles" sensation in the index and middle fingers and in the radial aspect of the ring finger. This nocturnal exacerbation occurs because of relaxation and flexion of the wrist at night resulting in further compression. With more advanced compression, an aching sensation may radiate into the forearm and elbow.

The diagnosis can be supported by eliciting paresthesias in the median distribution while tapping the volar wrist over the median nerve (Tinel's sign). Hyperflexing the wrist for 1 min may also elicit paresthesia (Phalen's sign). Advanced cases may have thenar atrophy due to impaired innervation of the abductor pollicis brevis.

Early treatment warrants a trial of rest reinforced by the use of a wrist splint in neutral or slightly extended position and nonsteroidal anti-inflammatory drugs (NSAIDs). While steroid-lidocaine injections may ease more refractory cases, the procedure is often followed by a recurrence of symptoms and is not without complications. Thus, referral to a hand specialist is recommended.

## ULNAR NEURITIS

This may be a compressive neuropathy or can be simply a result of direct repetitive stretching or friction. The two most common problem sites are at the elbow (cubital tunnel) and at the wrist (Guyon's canal). In cubital tunnel syndrome the nerve may experience trauma or compression against the medial epicondyle, such as from pitching or playing golf. In Guyon's canal, damage may result from direct pressure such as in holding a bicycle's handlebars.

Numbness or weakness in the ring and small fingers or medial elbow pain indicate ulnar nerve pathology. Tapping along the nerve may reveal the site of involvement. Signs and symptoms of cervical spine disease or thoracic outlet syndrome should also be sought.

To test for cubital tunnel syndrome, hold the elbow in maximum flexion for 1 min. This may reproduce or exacerbate symptoms due to peripheral ulnar nerve pathology. Cubital tunnel syndrome may in addition cause numbness over the dorso-ulnar hand because of inclusion of the superficial branch. Thumb adduction is also weak due to the ulnar innervation of the adductor pollicis muscle. This can be tested by having the patient tightly hold a piece of paper between the thumb and the proximal phalanx of the index finger. If the IP joint must flex more than a few degrees, then the muscle is weak (Froment's sign) (Fig. 235-1).

Pathology in Guyon's canal spares this deep branch so that numbness of only the ring and small fingers, not of the hand, occurs. Similarly, Froment's sign is negative because the adductor pollicis is innervated by the deep branch.

Cubital tunnel syndrome in its milder form can initially be treated with rest. Failing this, orthopaedic surgery to decompress or anteriorly transpose the nerve may be needed.

Guyon's canal syndrome is first treated with the wrist splinted in mild dorsiflexion and NSAIDs. While resistant cases may respond to steroid injection into the canal, the majority will require surgical decompression.

## DE QUERVAIN'S TENOSYNOVITIS

The first dorsal compartment of the wrist contains the abductor pollicis longus and extensor pollicis brevis tendons. Inflammation occurs from activities that require a repetitive pinching motion, such as small-piece assembly line work, laundry chores, and weeding. Patients complain of a deep aching beginning at the radial styloid and extending to the thumb's interphalangeal joint.

Symptoms are exacerbated by ulnar deviation of the fisted hand (Finkelstein's test) (Fig. 235-2). To perform this the patient puts the thumb inside the palm, curls the other fingers around the thumb, and then gently deviates the hand in the ulnar direction. Afflicted patients complain of a severe increase in pain. Treatment is resting the tendons, aided by a spica splint and NSAIDs. While steroid injection into the sheath works, it is more advisable to observe rest until the inflammation heals.

## LATERAL EPICONDYLITIS

In this condition, also known as tennis elbow, pain is noted at the origin of extensors of the distal arm. While it occurs from racquet sports and repetitive manual labor, it may also occur spontaneously. When it is from racquet sports, a faulty backhand stroke is usually to blame. The extensor mass, especially the deep extensor carpi radialis brevis, rubs and rolls over the lateral epicondyle and radial head. In addition there is pulling on the extensor origin, resulting in microtears.

Pain is increased over the lateral epicondyle with pronation of the forearm and concomitant dorsiflexion of the wrist against resistance. Lifting a chair with the affected hand in pronation should also exacerbate symptoms. Picking up a full cup of liquid also reproduces the pain.

Treatment includes avoidance of the painful activity and use of NSAIDs. Utilizing supination in daily grasping activities will aid in rest of the area. In the case of racquet sports, instruction in a quality backhand should be sought after the acute injury heals. Of note, those who use a two-handed backhand are rarely afflicted. Orthopaedic referral is advised for further evaluation and treatment.

## MEDIAL EPICONDYLITIS

Although also known as golfer's elbow, this syndrome often occurs from racquet sports and pitching. Overuse of the flexor forearm muscles stresses and inflames the tendinous insertion at the medial epicondyle.

Pain will be noted over the medial epicondyle, and grip may be suboptimal secondary to pain. Pronation or wrist flexion against resistance will increase the pain over the medial epicondyle. About two-thirds of these patients have concomitant ulnar neuritis (cubital tunnel syndrome).

Treatment is conservative, with rest and NSAIDs. Play is gradually resumed after 6 weeks.

## GROIN STRAIN

This common injury usually refers to strain of the hip adductors but can also be from strain of the iliopsoas, rectus femoris, and sartorius muscles. Activity requiring sudden acceleration and changes in direc-

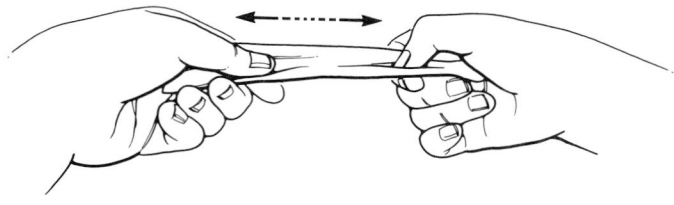

**Fig. 235-1.** Froment's sign, or flexion of the IP joint with forceful adduction, indicates a weak adductor pollicis muscle.

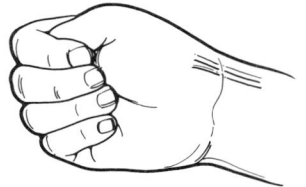
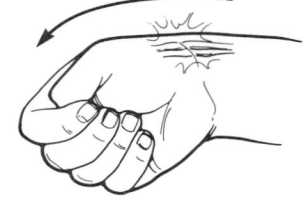

**Fig. 235-2.** Finkelstein's test.

tion about the hip precipitates this injury. Pain occurs during hip adduction or while flexing against resistance.

Tenderness to palpation is usually nonspecific for the site of injury. Edema and ecchymosis may eventually develop along the adductor muscle site. The differential diagnosis is the most problematic issue with this injury. One must consider pain originating from an inguinal hernia, testicular injury or disease, nephrolithiasis, bladder injury, lymphadenopathy, strain of the rectus abdominis muscle, pelvic stress fractures, avulsion of the hip or pubic symphysis. Radiographs are recommended to evaluate for avulsion fractures, particularly in adolescents.

Conservative treatment includes rest, cold compresses, and NSAIDs. Once the patient is pain free, gentle stretching exercises are begun, with gradual resumption of the inciting activity. Persistent pain warrants orthopaedic referral.

## ILIOTIBIAL BAND SYNDROME

Probably the most common cause of lateral knee pain, iliotibial band syndrome occurs most frequently in football players, military recruits in basic training, cyclists, dancers, and runners. Iliotibial band syndrome is a result of friction against the lateral femoral epicondyle. Running downhill may result in an excessive stride, which stretches the band. In addition, running on the drainage slope of roads causes symptoms in the downhill leg. Varus knees also predispose to the injury. Excessive pronation causes internal tibial rotation and similar stresses on the band. Pain is localized to the lateral femoral condyle and may radiate down to the tibia. The pain increases greatly each time the foot strikes the ground.

Further confirmation may be obtained by having the patient lie supine and flex the knee 90°. The examiner then applies pressure to the lateral femoral epicondyle while the patient extends the knee. At 30° the band will cross the epicondyle and a lancinating pain results (Noble compression test). Another maneuver is performed in the standing position with all weight supported by the affected leg. The patient then flexes the knee and at about 30° will report increased pain over the epicondyle (Renne test).

Early treatment is rest, NSAIDs, and cool compresses, followed by gentle stretching of the band. Activity is then gradually increased, using the appearance of pain to limit the intensity. It will usually be 6 weeks before peak exercise can be resumed. Surgery is rarely needed, but orthopaedic referral for trial steroid injection and gait analysis is often helpful.

## POPLITEUS TENDINITIS

Primarily a malady of downhill runners, popliteus tendinitis also presents as lateral knee pain. The pain radiates more deeply, however, since this tendon courses intraarticularly before inserting on the lateral femoral condyle.

There is no tenderness over the lateral epicondyle. The posterior lateral joint line is very tender. The tendon can be palpated most easily if the patient rests the lateral ankle of the affected leg on the opposite knee. The lateral collateral ligament then becomes prominent, and the popliteus is palpated just anterior to it above the joint line (Fig. 235-3).

Treatment is to decrease the intensity of running and avoid sloped roadsides and hilly running surfaces. Cold compresses and NSAIDs are used for 2 weeks. Once pain has disappeared, the previous activity level can be quickly resumed.

## SHIN SPLINTS

Overuse injuries that cause pain around the tibia are commonly called *shin splints*. The term refers to any one of the following specific entities: anterior tibial strain, medial tibial stress syndrome, and tibial stress fractures.

Patients who have recently started running or jumping are at greatest risk for these entities. However, veterans of either activity who change their degree of exertion, exercise surface, or type of shoes can also be afflicted.

### Anterior Tibial Strain

This is most common among new runners. The anterior tibialis must repeatedly dorsiflex the foot while the posterior muscles are contracting and it also absorbs the impact during ground contact of the foot. An unconditioned runner typically has a weak anterior tibialis relative to the posterior muscle groups, and so overuse rapidly occurs. A tight Achilles tendon may also contribute to difficult dorsiflexion, placing further stress on the anterior tibialis.

Most of the trauma is actually microtears in the musculotendinous attachments to the tibia. Thus, pain is felt along the anterolateral border of the proximal two-thirds of the tibia and along the anteromedial border at the distal third of the tibia.

Treatment is avoidance of the inciting activity for 5 to 7 days and use of NSAIDs. After this period of rest, if the patient is pain free, the activity can then be very gradually resumed over 3 to 6 weeks. Re-

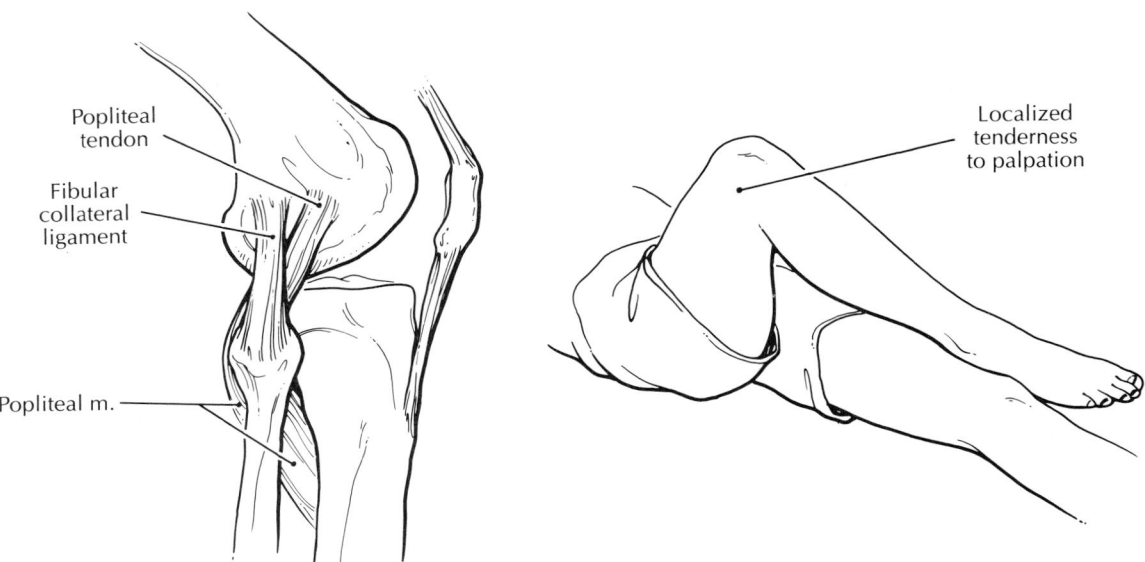

Popliteal tendon

Fibular collateral ligament

Popliteal m.

Localized tenderness to palpation

**Fig. 235-3.** In the figure-of-four position, the popliteal tendon can be palpated anterior to the fibular collateral ligament.

turning to the activity within a couple of days will only invite recurrent and possibly long-term problems. It is not a pain that can be "worked out."

## Medial Tibial Stress Syndrome

In contrast to anterior tibial strain, this injury occurs primarily to experienced runners and results from hyperpronation of the foot. This hyperpronation makes the primary functions of the posterior tibialis, dorsiflexion and inversion, difficult. Pain is limited to the medial border of the distal third of the tibia along the insertion of the posterior tibialis muscle.

Treatment is a brief period of rest, stretching the posterior muscles by leaning forward towards a wall, and orthopaedic follow-up for gait evaluation and ongoing management.

## Tibial Stress Fractures

The incidence of these fractures is as high as 4 to 15 percent in runners. A change in the level of activity of the runner, whether highly conditioned or a beginner, accompanies most stress fractures. Contributing factors include hard impact surfaces, poorly cushioned soles, hyperpronation, female gender, and narrow tibial width.

Pain begins during activity, unlike the pain from other causes of shin splints, which typically occurs after activity. Palpation of the bone elicits tenderness. Plain x-ray may reveal periosteal reaction or cortical hypertrophy after 2 to 3 weeks. The actual fracture line is usually not seen. A bone scan is the definitive study.

Initial treatment includes cold application and NSAIDs to help control inflammation and pain.

Abstinence from the inciting activity for 3 to 6 weeks until the patient is pain free is an absolute for treatment of these fractures. Immobilization is not advised. Light cycling or swimming is helpful. Once the patient is asymptomatic for 10 days, a gradual return to peak activity aids proper bone remodeling. Persistent symptoms require orthopaedic evaluation.

## ACHILLES TENDONITIS

The Achilles tendon is the common endpoint for the tendons of the gastrocnemius and soleus muscles before insertion at the calcaneus. The pain of Achilles tendinitis typically occurs about 6 cm proximal to this insertion. A tenuous blood supply from its sheath makes it prone to injury. Any inflammation causes further blood stasis and an acidic environment, impeding the tendon's ability to heal.

Inflammation occurs from hill running or repetitive hyperpronation of the ankle or is brought on by routine activities in someone with a "tight" Achilles tendon. A "tight" Achilles tendon may result from a sedentary lifestyle, daily wear of high-heeled shoes, a switch from training shoes to competition shoes without heels, or simply a change from cross-country terrain to a track with a softer rebound surface.

Treatment consists of brief (1 to 2 days) immobilization followed by flexibility exercises. A low heel lift ( 1/8 to 1/4 in) may be used acutely to lessen tension on the tendon. Strengthening of the posterior muscles is recommended. This should include elevating the heels of both feet repetitively. Weights may be incrementally added to the shoulders over time to increase the load. Steroid injection must be avoided as it predisposes to rupture because of its interference with collagen synthesis in this constantly stressed area and because the pressure of the injected material may further impede the blood supply. In addition, the pain-relieving effect of the steroid results in premature resumption of activity.

## ACHILLES TENDON RUPTURE

Sudden forceful dorsiflexion of the ankle while the posterior muscles are in contraction may result in rupture. It occurs most often on the left. Slipping on a stair, ladder, or diving board or beginning a sprint can result in this kind of force. A direct traumatic blow while the tendon is tight may also result in rupture.

Diagnosis relies on a history of an event consistent with Achilles tendon rupture. It is frequently misdiagnosed as an ankle sprain. A pop may be heard, and the patient feels as if he or she were kicked in the calf. Thereafter it is difficult to plantar flex the foot. Physical examination often reveals swelling of the distal calf and sometimes a palpable defect in the tendon 2 to 6 cm proximal to its insertion. The patient will be able to plantar flex with the tibialis posterior, peroneals, and toe flexors, though flexion will be weaker than on the unaffected side. To isolate the Achilles tendon from other muscles enabling plantar flexion, first ask the patient to lie prone with feet extending over the end of the examining table. Then flex the knee to 90° and compress the medial and lateral aspects of the calf just distal to the apex of the soleus muscle. It is important to compress distally to this point or otherwise a completely intact Achilles tendon will not be able to dorsiflex. The patient will not be able to plantar flex against gravity (Thompson's sign). Partial ruptures are difficult to detect as the strength is near normal with 75 percent disruption.

Early treatment before prompt follow-up with an orthopaedic surgeon includes a posterior splint with the foot maintained in a passive equinus position. No weight-bearing and elevation as much as possible should be observed. Suspected partial tears should either be placed in a posterior splint in mild equinus position or have a 2-cm firm heel pad placed in the shoe with arrangements for orthopaedic follow-up. Definitive treatment varies from closed treatment with a short leg cast in equinus position for 8 weeks, followed by 4 weeks' use of a heel lift to open surgical repair, especially for athletic patients.

## PLANTAR FASCIITIS

Plantar fasciitis occurs from persistent pronation of the foot, which constantly pulls on the origin of the plantar fascia at the medial tuberosity of the calcaneus.

Patients have point tenderness over the plantar heel. A bone spur results from the inflammation. However, the spur is only a marker for the underlying problem; the spur itself does not cause the pain.

Treatment is initially conservative with a 1 to 2 day period of rest and use of NSAIDs. Patients should be advised to walk or run with toes turned more inward and to concentrate on distributing weight on the more lateral toes rather than only the great toe area. Mild cases may also respond to a low pad placed under the medial heel, which will help lessen pronation. Severe or refractory cases will benefit from a shoe insert that reduces pronation; such inserts can be obtained through orthopaedic follow-up.

## TARSAL TUNNEL SYNDROME

This compression neuropathy of the posterior tibial nerve has recently received greater recognition as a cause of foot and heel pain. After coursing inferiorly to the medial malleolus, the posterior tibial nerve enters the tarsal tunnel. The plantar aspect of the tarsal tunnel is bound by the talus and calcaneus bones and by the tibialis posterior, flexor hallucis longus, and flexor digitorum longus. The dorsal aspect is bound by the inelastic flexor retinaculum, which extends from the medial malleolus to the calcaneus to the abductor hallucis muscle.

In the setting of overuse, running and activities requiring restrictive footwear (e.g., ski boots, skates) have been implicated. The edema of pregnancy may also be a precipitant. Hyperpronation while running makes the nerve more vulnerable both to direct trauma from stretch and to indirect trauma from inflammation of the surrounding structures resulting in compression.

Pain is noted at the medial malleolus, the heel (calcaneal branch), and sole (medial or lateral plantar branch), depending on the site and severity of compression. Distal calf pain may result due to retrograde radiation (Valleix phenomenon). Similar to carpal tunnel syndrome, the pain is often worse at night. More advanced compression may result in weak toe flexion. Tinel's sign is positive inferior to the medial malleolus. Simultaneous dorsiflexion and eversion of the ankle exacerbates symptoms.

The differential diagnosis includes plantar fasciitis and, if limited to the heel, Achilles tendinitis. Plantar fasciitis will cause point tenderness over the plantar heel and worse pain upon morning standing. Tarsal tunnel syndrome causes greater medial heel and arch pain due to involvement of the abductor hallucis muscle. Fasciitis pain may improve with gradual ambulation throughout the day, whereas tarsal tunnel worsens. In addition, tarsal tunnel syndrome may produce distal calf pain, whereas fasciitis does not.

Initial treatment includes avoidance of the exacerbating activities and use of NSAIDs. If there is no improvement or symptoms recur after a few weeks, then orthopaedic evaluation and treatment, which include electromyographic studies, steroid injection, orthotic devices, or surgery, are recommended.

## BIBLIOGRAPHY

American Society for Surgery of the Hand (ed): *The Hand: Primary Care of Common Problems.* New York, Churchill Livingstone, 1990.

DeLee JC, Drez D (eds): *Orthopaedic Sports Medicine: Principles and Practice,* vols 1 and 2. Philadelphia, Saunders, 1994.

Dugas R, D'Ambrosia R: Causes and treatment of common overuse injuries in runners. *J Musculoskeletal Med* March: 107, 1991.

Estwanik JJ, Sloane BS, Rosenberg MA: Groin strain and other possible causes of groin pain. *Physician Sportsmed* 18:54, 1990.

Jackson DL, Haglund B: Tarsal tunnel syndrome in athletes. *Am J Sports Med* 19:61, 1991.

Kulund DN (ed): *The Injured Athlete.* Philadelphia, Lippincott, 1982.

Linenger JM, Christensen CP: Is iliotibial band syndrome often overlooked? *Physician Sportsmed* 20:98, 1992.

McKeag DB, Dolan C: Overuse syndromes of the lower extremity. *Physician Sportsmed* 17:108, 1989.

# 236
# MUSCLE RUPTURES

### Robert Petrilli
### D. Monte Hunter

## INTRODUCTION

As the single largest tissue mass in the body, muscle makes up over 40 percent of total body weight. The human body relies on over 300 muscles to generate joint motion and extremity movement. When the demands of this movement exceed the muscles' ability to respond, the muscle unit fails and injuries occur. Muscle injuries are one of the most common soft tissue injuries. In sports, muscle injuries are the most common injury reported, accounting for 10 to 30 percent of all injuries. Occupational demands also place significant stress on muscle, predisposing it to injury.

Muscle injuries can be classified as direct or indirect. Direct injuries occur from a direct traumatic force such as a contusion. Indirect injury occurs as a result of excessive strain or stretching force on the muscle, without any direct contact. Indirect injuries represent the "muscle strain" or "pulled muscle." Muscle strains can be partial or complete. In general, three grades of severity can be recognized. Grade I injuries represent a transient stretch injury without any disruption of muscle fibers. Grade II injuries are associated with partial disruption or tearing of the muscle unit. Grade III injuries represent complete disruption or rupture of the muscle unit. Grade I and II injuries, which represent the vast majority, are treated conservatively and are associated with little, if any, long-term sequelae. Grade III injuries, on the other hand, are associated with significant disability and frequently require surgical evaluation and treatment. Grade III injuries or complete muscle ruptures are the focus of this chapter.

Recent research has provided significant insight into the mechanisms and predisposing factors of muscle injury. A common denominator in all muscle injury is stretch. Tears occur at a critical tension that is proportional to stretch in the muscle. The musculotendinous junction is the most vulnerable and most common site of muscle ruptures; the tendon-bone junction is less commonly effected. The musculotendinous junction can take up a surprisingly large area. For example, the musculotendinous junction of the hamstrings extends for more than half the muscle length. Normal intact tendon does not tear from stretch injuries. Muscle belly tears are also very rare and usually require direct shearing force or laceration.

Some muscles are more prone to injury than others. Those muscles at risk for complete rupture usually cross two joints, since they are prone to stretch more than those that cross only one joint. Examples of muscles that cross two or more joints are hamstring, gastrocnemius, and biceps. Strong eccentric contraction is also a characteristic of muscles that rupture. Eccentric contraction, by definition, implies stretching or elongation of the muscle, in contrast to concentric contraction, which implies shortening of the muscle. Forceful concentric contraction is rarely involved with muscle rupture.

Most muscle ruptures occur during high-velocity activities during sports or at work. These activities usually require a burst of speed, rapid acceleration, or rapid deceleration, all of which rely on powerful eccentric contraction. Fatigue and a history of previous injury are also thought to predispose a muscle to complete rupture, but few clinical studies document this.

Muscle ruptures are an acute, painful event recognized by the patient as an injury and are often the cause of a patient seeking emergency medical care. Although few muscle injuries are life or limb threatening, complete muscle ruptures are associated with significant long-term disability if not promptly recognized or treated. The emergency physician must recognize complete muscle ruptures to help preserve function. When a muscle tears, there is retraction of the muscle belly toward the intact musculotendinous junction still attached to bone. This creates a characteristic bulge that creates asymmetry in the patient. The bulge and asymmetry are key clinical features to the diagnosis. Bleeding from the muscle at the site of the tear also occurs, but ecchymosis requires one or more days to become visible. With prompt recognition, appropriate initial management, and timely referrals, full motion, strength, and function may be restored. The following discussion focuses on the clinical features of the most common ruptures encountered in the emergency department.

## GASTROCNEMIUS/SOLEUS MUSCLES (ACHiLLES TENDON)

### Functional Anatomy

The gastrocnemius muscle originates just superior to the femoral condyles. The soleus muscle originates on the posterior leg below the knee. These muscles come together to form the Achilles tendon, which inserts on the inferior half of the calcaneus. The Achilles tendon thins out to form the plantar fascia (Fig. 236-1).

### Clinical Features

Acute ruptures of the Achilles tendon usually occur in middle-aged males involved in intermittent athletic activities. Young high-performance athletes infrequently sustain this injury. The injury occurs dur-

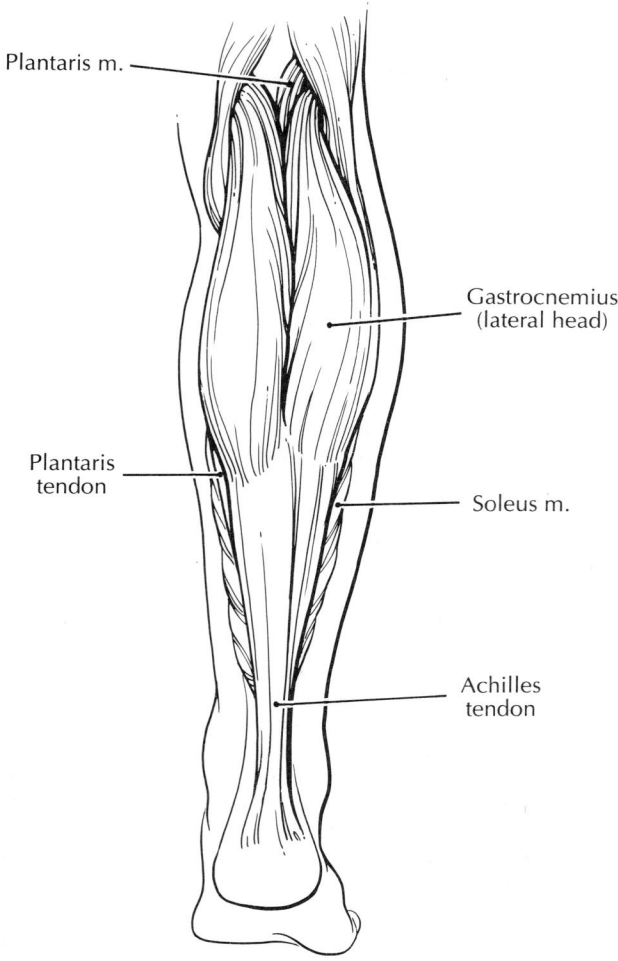

Plantaris m.

Gastrocnemius (lateral head)

Plantaris tendon

Soleus m.

Achilles tendon

**Fig. 236-1.** The Achilles tendon.

ing running (during quick acceleration or deceleration) with the knee extended. As the foot is forced up suddenly into dorsiflexion, the tendon is stretched and may rupture. A direct blow to the Achilles tendon while the gastrocnemius and soleus muscles are strongly contracted can also result in rupture. Rupture usually occurs 2 to 6 cm proximal to the insertion due to the blood supply being poorest in this area, with resultant degenerative changes. Oral or injectable steroid use can predispose patients to rupture.

Symptoms of rupture include hearing and/or feeling a "pop" and experiencing minimal discomfort in the posterior lower leg initially. Often the patient describes a sensation of being struck or hit in the posterior aspect of the lower leg. Weakness in push-off develops instantly, followed by progressive pain, edema, and ecchymosis. A delay in seeking medical attention is common due to the paucity of initial symptoms. Examination is best accomplished with the patient in the prone position with the affected ankle and foot over the end of the stretcher. A defect is usually palpable proximal to the insertion into the calcaneus but can be difficult to appreciate in the obese patient or if a large amount of soft tissue swelling is present. Gentle dorsiflexion of the foot can make the defect more obvious. The ability to plantar flex the ankle in this non-weight-bearing position can be maintained due to the actions of the tibialis posterior, toe flexor, and peroneal. Up to 25 percent of tendon ruptures are thus missed when first seen, frequently being diagnosed as an "ankle sprain." The diagnosis can be made from the patient's inability to stand on tiptoe on the injured side and by a positive Thompson's test, which is a reliable indicator of Achilles tendon disruption. Thompson's test is performed with the patient positioned prone as described and by grasping and

squeezing the gastrocnemius muscle. If the Achilles tendon is intact, the ankle should plantar flex, but if ruptured, tightening of the muscle causes no motion at the ankle, a positive test (Fig. 236-2). Radiographic evaluation, although not necessary, shows blurring of the retrocalcaneal space (Kroger's space).

### Differential Diagnosis

Differential diagnosis includes partial Achilles tendon rupture, partial gastrocnemius muscle rupture, and plantaris tendon rupture.

### Treatment

Treatment is either surgical or with casting, each requiring at least 6 weeks of immobilization followed by 6 weeks of protected weight bearing. Surgical repair confers more strength and mobility, with a reduced rerupture rate (2 percent versus 10 to 25 percent with casting). Typically 6 months of rehabilitation is necessary following treatment.

Emergency department treatment consists of elevation, ice, and analgesia. After 7 to 10 days postinjury, the hematoma at the site of the Achilles rupture begins to organize, making nonsurgical treatment less likely to be successful. Orthopaedic consultation should be obtained in the emergency department to plan treatment. Admission and acute repair are up to the consultant's discretion. If discharged with close orthopaedic follow-up, treatment consists of posterior splinting of the affected extremity, crutches and no weight bearing, extremity elevation, intermittent application of ice for 48 to 72 h, and adequate analgesia. Partial tears are treated conservatively as above, with timely orthopaedic follow-up.

## BICEPS MUSCLE

### Functional Anatomy

The biceps muscle originates on the coracoid process (short head) and the superior glenoid labrum (long head) and inserts on the bicipital tuberosity of the radius. The long tendon runs over the head of the humerus in the bicipital groove and courses to its insertion inside the shoulder joint. This makes it susceptible to repetitive microtrauma and degenerative changes from repetitive overuse.

The biceps functions to flex the elbow and supinate the forearm. Ninety-seven percent of ruptures are proximal, occurring in the long head of the biceps. Distal rupture is rare, with less than 200 cases reported in the literature. Tendon rupture is usually the end result of repetitive microtrauma with degenerative changes and so is seen most frequently in patients between the fourth and sixth decades of life. Chronic glucocorticoid use and/or injection are also etiologic. The injury is unusual in young athletes. Rupture is precipitated by sudden or prolonged muscle contracture against resistance, such as with heavy lifting or a checked baseball swing.

### Proximal Biceps Rupture (Long Head)

#### Clinical Features

Patients with acute ruptures usually relate a long history of tendinitis. Symptoms include anterior shoulder pain and an audible "pop" or "snap" during strenuous activity. Examination demonstrates tenderness, swelling, and crepitus over the bicipital groove. Flexion of the elbow elicits pain. Weakness in flexion and supination is minimal (10 to 20 percent) due to the function of the short head of the biceps. Ecchymoses and a visible gap in the muscle, caused by distal migration of the muscle mass with resulting egg-shaped swelling, are usually obvious. Slow contraction of the biceps make this deformity more prominent. Rupture usually occurs in the proximal one-third of the tendon at the top of the bicipital groove (Fig. 236-3). Occasionally this injury involves an avulsed fragment of bone. Radiographs are necessary to rule out an avulsion fracture.

**Fig. 236-2.** The Thompson test. Compression of the gastrocnemius-soleus complex normally produces plantar flexion of the foot. With the complete rupture of the Achilles tendon, plantar flexion does not occur. The test is considered positive if plantar flexion is absent.

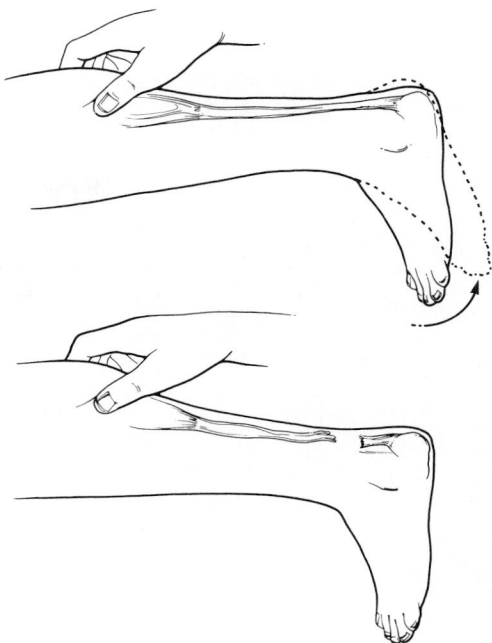

## Differential Diagnosis

The differential diagnosis includes biceps tendinitis, subluxation/dislocation, rotator cuff disease, impingement syndrome, partial rupture, and osteochondral fracture.

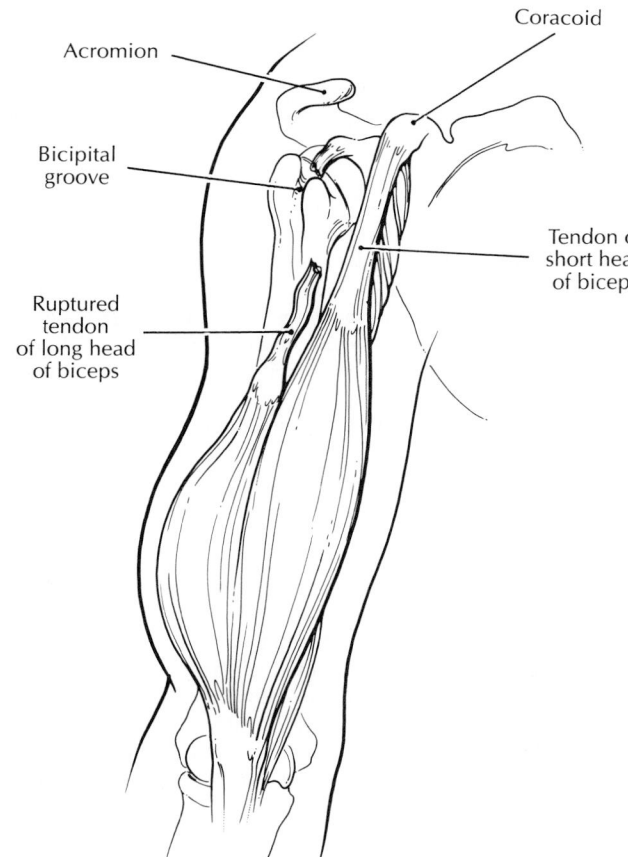

**Fig. 236-3.** Long head of the biceps tendon rupture.

## Treatment

Treatment is surgical repair of the tendon in the young athletic patient. The older patient can be treated conservatively with immobilization, followed by early and progressive mobilization and strengthening exercises as soon as pain subsides. Orthopaedic consultation should be obtained in the emergency department. Admission is required only for surgical repair. Emergency department treatment consists of ice and analgesia. Outpatient treatment requires immobilization in a sling, analgesia, and intermittent application of ice for 48 to 72 h.

### Distal Biceps Avulsion

#### Clinical Features

Almost all cases of distal biceps rupture occur in males, and 80 percent occur in the dominant extremity. A single traumatic event causes acute rupture, resulting in symptoms of pain in the antecubital fossa accompanied by a tearing or popping sensation. Examination will demonstrate tenderness, swelling, ecchymosis, and inability to palpate the biceps tendon in the antecubital fossa. Comparison with the uninjured extremity for asymmetry will aid in making the diagnosis (Fig. 236-4). Deformity in the muscle is palpable as the biceps retract proximally during contraction. The patient can still flex the elbow and supinate the forearm due to intact brachialis and supinator muscles, but strength loss will be much more prominent (40 to 50 percent) than with proximal biceps ruptures. The rupture usually occurs at the tendon-osseous insertion and leaves no distal tendon fragment at the tuberosity. Avulsion fractures are unusual but should be ruled out by radiographs.

#### Differential Diagnosis

The differential diagnosis includes biceps tendinitis, partial tear, bursitis, anterior capsulitis of the elbow, and annular ligament sprain.

#### Treatment

Treatment is surgical tendon repair, and thus orthopaedic consultation to plan for timing of repair is warranted. Emergency department treatment consists of ice and analgesia. If discharged home with plans

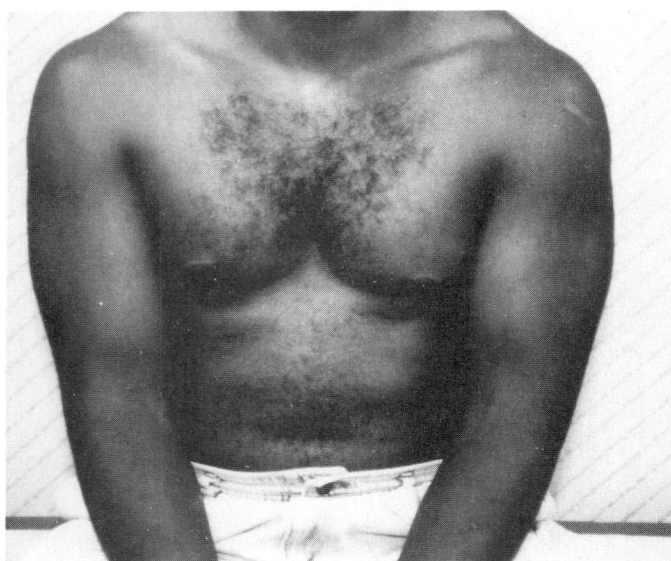

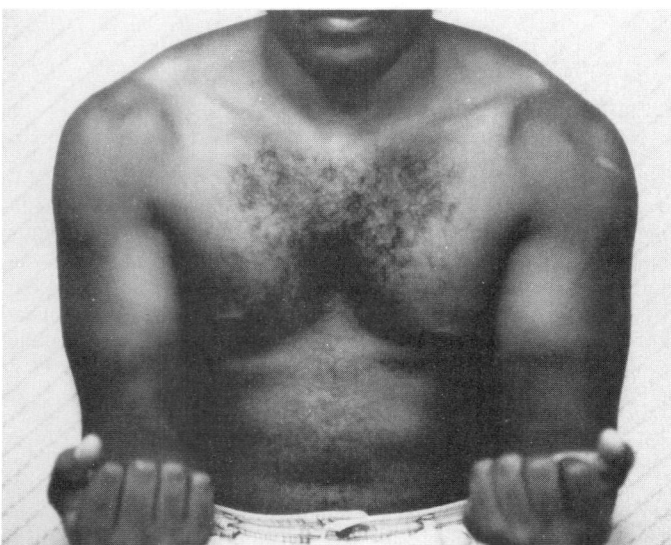

**Fig. 236-4.** Distal biceps tendon avulsion. Asymmetry in the distal left biceps is noticeable.

for later surgical repair, immobilization in a sling and analgesia are standard.

## TRICEPS RUPTURES

### Functional Anatomy

The triceps muscle acts as both an extensor of the shoulder through its attachment to the scapula and as a powerful extensor of the elbow. All three heads form a common tendon attached to the olecranon.

### Clinical Features

The triceps muscle is extraordinarily injury free, but rupture of the common tendon can occur. This is the least common of all tendon ruptures. Rupture most frequently occurs in young males (mean age 26 years old) secondary to trauma. There is an equal distribution between dominant and nondominant extremities. The site of rupture is usually the tendon-osseus junction, resulting in a high percentage of avulsion fractures of the olecranon. Musculotendinous junction and muscle belly ruptures are rare. The injury usually occurs as a result of indirect trauma from a fall on the outstretched extremity. Ruptures from direct blows and spontaneous ruptures from systemic illness have been reported.

Symptoms of acute rupture include pain and soft tissue swelling at the posterior elbow. The ability to extend the elbow is lost. Examination often shows a palpable defect proximal to the olecranon, along with localized tenderness and swelling. Radiographs of the elbow must be obtained since olecranon avulsion fractures will be present in greater than 80 percent of cases.

### Differential Diagnosis

Differential diagnostic possibilities include olecranon bursitis, partial rupture/strain, degenerative joint disease, and olecranon fracture. Associated fractures are common, and thus a thorough upper extremity examination must be carried out and the posterior aspect of the elbow must be examined when other injuries are detected initially.

### Treatment

Treatment is surgical repair of the tendon to restore extension strength. Orthopaedic consultation should be obtained. Emergency department treatment consists of ice and analgesia. If discharged, a sling and analgesia, along with intermittent ice application, are usually prescribed.

## Quadriceps Muscle, Quadriceps Tendon, and Patella Tendon Ruptures

### Functional Anatomy

The quadriceps femoris muscle group comprises the rectus femoris, vastus intermedius, vastus lateralis, and vastus medialis muscles. These muscles form the quadriceps tendon that inserts on the patella. The patella tendon (also referred to as the ligamentum patellae) attaches the inferior patella to the tibial tuberosity. Extension of the knee joint is accomplished via contraction of the quadriceps and an intact tendinous system. Some of the tendinous fibers of the vastus lateralis and medialis form bands, referred to as the *retinaculum*, that join the capsule of the knee joint (Fig. 236-5).

### Clinical Features

The underlying cause of acute tendon ruptures is chronic repetitive microtrauma causing tendinitis, with resultant weakening of the tendon. Steroid injections have also been implicated as an etiologic factor. Bilateral tendon rupture is usually the result of an underlying autoimmune disorder or other systemic disease state such as chronic renal failure, diabetes, tuberculosis, hyperparathyroidism, chronic acidosis, Osgood-Schlatter disease, and glucocorticoid use. Acute quadriceps muscle rupture is caused by direct trauma.

## Quadriceps Muscle Ruptures

### Clinical Features

Ruptures of the quadriceps muscle are rare and occur in the midthigh within the rectus femoris or vastus medialis muscle. Direct trauma to the contracted muscle group causes acute pain, swelling, inability to straighten the leg, and difficulty with ambulation. Physical examination reveals swelling in the anterior midthigh, associated tenderness, and pain with movement. The ability to extend the knee is preserved. A defect is usually not palpable due to hematoma formation, which can be large with resultant significant intravascular blood loss (500 to 1000 mL). X-rays are indicated only to rule out the rare possibility of a femur fracture.

### Differential Diagnosis

The differential diagnosis includes quadriceps strain.

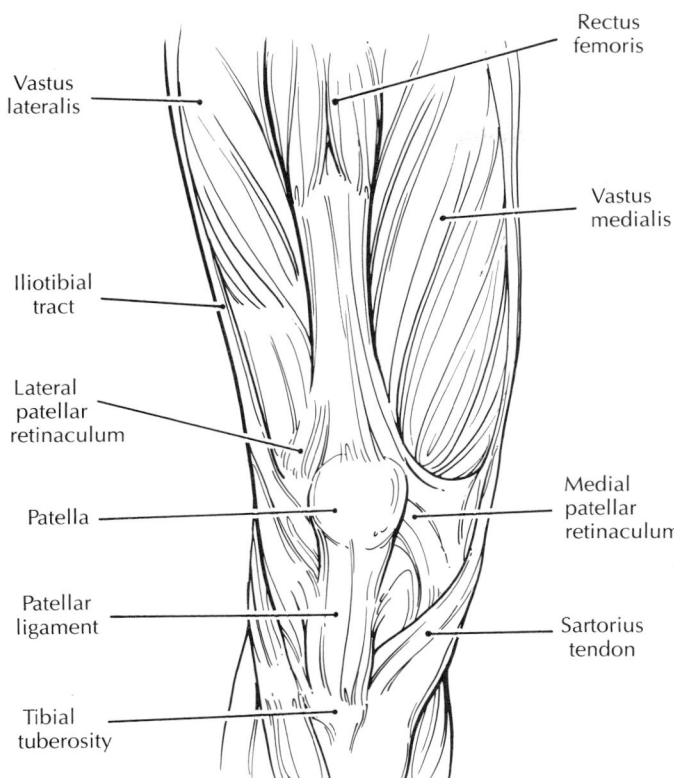

**Fig. 236-5.** The quadriceps–patella–patellar tendon complex.

## Treatment

Operative repair is considered only in the case of a high-performance athlete with a large rupture. Otherwise, conservative therapy, consisting of knee immobilization in full extension along with early physical therapy and early mobilization, is the treatment of choice. Emergency department care includes elevation, ice, and analgesia. Admission to the hospital is only rarely indicated for pain control, concern for a developing compartment syndrome, or extenuating circumstances. Outpatient treatment consists of knee immobilization, crutches, no weight bearing, extremity elevation, intermittent application of ice for 48 to 72 h, and analgesia. Heat therapy after 72 h can aid in hematoma resolution. Orthopaedic follow-up should be arranged in 5 to 7 days to allow for early mobilization and physical therapy.

## Quadriceps Tendon Rupture

### Clinical Features

Ruptures of the quadriceps tendon usually occur in the older patient after violent contraction of the quadriceps. A history of landing from a jump or sudden acceleration/deceleration is usually illicited. Symptoms of acute rupture include a sudden sharp pain in the knee, inability to straighten the leg, and difficulty with ambulation. Physical examination usually reveals a palpable defect in the suprapatellar region, with associated tenderness and swelling. A hematoma can occasionally make detection of a defect difficult. The defect should be more obvious with quadriceps contraction. A complete rupture will result in the patient's inability to extend the knee. The ability to raise the leg from a supine position will be maintained with a partial tear because of an intact retinaculum, but extension of the knee from a flexed position will still be lost. The patella will migrate distally (patella baja). Radiographs of the knee are indicated to rule out patella fracture or associated avulsion fracture from the superior patella. The lateral view best demonstrates patella baja (Fig. 236-6).

## Differential Diagnosis

The differential diagnosis includes partial tendon rupture, patella fracture, patella tendon rupture, quadriceps strain, or tendinitis.

## Treatment

Treatment of complete ruptures requires surgical repair, and thus orthopaedic consultation at the time of emergency department presentation is indicated. Partial tears are treated conservatively, as with quadriceps muscle tears. Emergency department treatment is also identical. Admission is at the discretion of the consultant.

## Patella Tendon Rupture

### Clinical Features

Whereas quadriceps ruptures occur in the older patient, rupture of the patella tendon occurs in the young athletic patient, usually after violent quadriceps contraction. A history of repetitive patellar tendinitis (jumper's knee) is frequently associated with rupture. Symptoms are similar to quadriceps tendon rupture. Physical examination will reveal a palpable defect inferior to the patella, a high-riding patella (patella alta), and the inability to extend the knee. With quadriceps contraction, the patella will migrate proximally. The rupture occurs proximally in most cases, and avulsion fractures off the inferior patella are common. Radiographs are indicated to rule out patella fractures. The lateral view will best demonstrate patella alta (Fig. 236-7).

## Differential Diagnosis

The differential diagnosis includes avulsion of the tibial tuberosity, patella fracture, partial patella tendon rupture, patella tendinitis or strain, and quadriceps tendon rupture.

## Treatment

Treatment is surgical and thus orthopaedic consultation is warranted. Admission is at the consultant's discretion. Emergency department treatment is identical to that for quadriceps muscle and tendon rupture. It consists of knee immobilization, elevation, and application of ice intermittently over the initial 48 to 72 h.

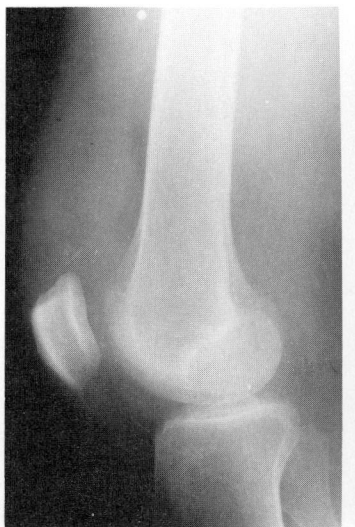
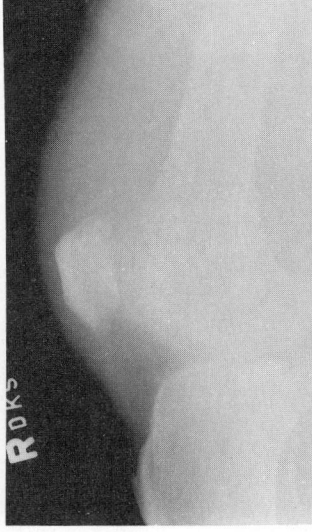

**Fig. 236-6.** Patella baja. Lateral radiographs of the knee reveal distal migration of patella, which is associated with quadriceps tendon rupture.

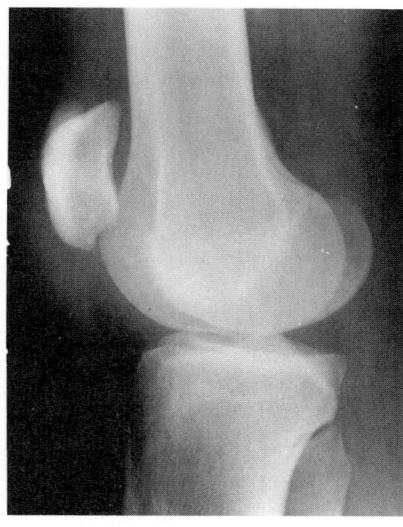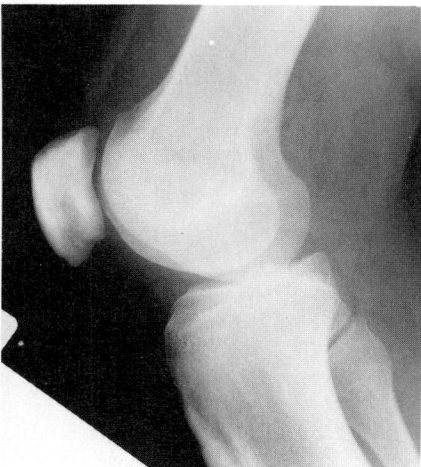

**Fig. 236-7.** Patella alta. Lateral radiographs of the knee reveal proximal migration of the patella, or a high-riding patella, which is associated with patella tendon rupture.

## HAMSTRING RUPTURES

### Functional Anatomy

The hamstring muscles consist of the biceps femoris, semimembranosus, and semitendinosus. All originate on the ischial tuberosity and insert below the knee and are responsible for knee flexion.

### Clinical Features

Strains and ruptures of this muscle group are the most common muscle injury in the thigh. They occur during repetitive, high-velocity activity (i.e., sprinting) from forceful contraction. Injuries usually occur as a result of inadequate warmup and stretching, in cold weather, and as a result of poor endurance and/or technique. Leg length inequality and muscle strength imbalances have also been implicated. The most frequent location of injury is at the musculotendinous junction, but special attention must be given to avulsion injuries of the origin of the hamstrings at the ischial tuberosity. Symptoms include the sudden onset of pain in the posterior thigh during activity, the inability to continue participation, and pain with knee flexion. Physical examination is best accomplished with the patient in the prone position and the knee flexed to 90°. Local tenderness and swelling are easily appreciated. Ecchymosis and a palpable defect are only occasionally present. If an avulsion of the ischial tuberosity has occurred, the patient will complain of buttock pain on standing and walking. Bony tenderness will be elicited on palpation, and possibly a defect will be palpable. Radiographs are indicated when proximal injuries are present to rule out avulsion fracture (Fig. 236-8).

### Treatment

Complete and partial ruptures are treated conservatively with rest, ice, compression, and elevation to minimize muscle hemorrhage. Avulsion injuries of the ischial tuberosity are treated surgically only in cases of considerable displacement. Emergency department care consists of ice, elevation, compression, and analgesia. Crutches may be necessary for assisted ambulation. Most patients can be treated on an outpatient basis. Orthopaedic followup in 5 to 7 days should be arranged since these injuries frequently heal slowly, often recur, and require a program for rehabilitation.

### BIBLIOGRAPHY

Best TM, Garrett WE Jr: Muscle-tendon unit injuries, in Renström PAFH (ed): *Sports Injuries. Basic Principles of Prevention and Care.* Boston, Blackwell Scientific, 1993, pp 71–86.

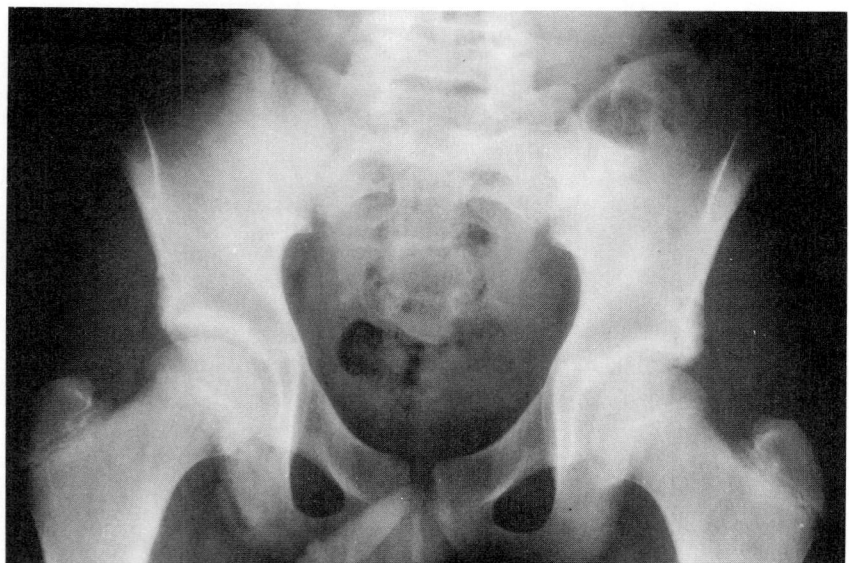

**Fig. 236-8.** Ischial avulsion fracture at the right hamstring insertion.

Burkhead WZ Jr: The biceps tendon, in Rockwood CA, Matsen FA (eds): *The Shoulder*. Philadelphia, Saunders, 1990, pp 791–836.

Gainor BJ, Allen WC: Injuries of the arm, elbow, and forearm, in Grana WA, Kalenak A (eds): *Clinical Sports Medicine*. Philadelphia, Saunders, 1991, pp 361–378.

Garrett WE Jr: Basic science of musculotendinous injuries, part I, in Nicholas JA, Hershman EB (eds): *The Lower Extremity and Spine in Sports Medicine*. Baltimore, Mosby, 1986, pp 42–59.

Garrett WE Jr: Muscle strain injuries: Clinical and basic aspects. *Med Sci Sports Exercise* 22(4):436, 1990.

Lachmann S, Jenner JR, in *Soft Tissue Injuries in Sport*. Blackwell Scientific, 1994, pp 180–186.

Lutter LD: Soft tissue trauma of the hindfoot, in *Foot and Ankle Manual*. Philadelphia, Lea & Febiger, 1991, pp 116–125.

Peterson L, Renström P: *Sports Injuries: Their Prevention and Treatment* Chicago, Yearbook Medical, 1986, pp 28–36.

Richardson AB, Miller JW: Swimming and the older athlete. *Clin Sports Med* 10(2):307, 1991.

Singer KM, Jones DC: Soft tissue conditions of the ankle and foot, part III, in Nicholas JA, Hershman EB (eds): *The Lower Extremity and Spine in Sports Medicine*. Baltimore, Mosby, 1986, pp 507–508.

Soma CA, Mandelbaum BR: Achilles tendon disorders. *Clin Sports Med* 13(4):811, 1994.

Tullos HS, Bennett J: Acute injuries to the elbow, in Nicholas JA, Hershman EB (eds): *The Upper Extremity in Sports Medicine*. Baltimore, Mosby, 1990, pp 321–323.

# 237
# COMPARTMENT SYNDROMES
**Ernest Ruiz**

**Table 237-1.** Classification of Acute Compartment Syndromes

Decreased compartment size
 Constrictive dressings and casts
 Closure of fascial defects
 Thermal injuries and frostbite
Increased compartment contents
 Primarily edematous accumulation
  Postischemic swelling
   Arterial injuries
   Arterial thrombosis or embolism
   Reconstructive vascular and bypass surgery
   Replantation
   Prolonged tourniquet time
   Arterial spasm
   Cardiac catheterization and angiography
   Ergotamine ingestion
  Prolonged immobilization with limb compression
   Drug overdose with limb compression
   General anesthesia with knee-chest position
  Thermal injuries and frostbite
  Exertion
  Venous disease
  Venomous snakebite
 Primarily hemorrhagic accumulation
  Hereditary bleeding disorders, e.g., hemophilia
  Anticoagulant therapy
  Vessel laceration
 Combination of edematous and hemorrhagic accumulation
  Fractures
   Tibia
   Forearm
   Elbow, e.g., supracondylar
   Femur
  Soft tissue injury
  Osteotomies, e.g., tibia
 Miscellaneous
  Intravenous infiltration, e.g., blood, saline
  Popliteal cyst
  Long leg brace

*Source:* From Mubarak and Hargens. Used by permission.

Compartment syndromes are among the most serious problems presenting to emergency departments. Early diagnosis and treatment are curative, while delay results in permanent and severe disability. An understanding of the pathophysiology and the early signs of the process is crucial if the emergency physician is to intercede appropriately.

## PATHOPHYSIOLOGY

Simply stated, compartment syndromes are due to increased pressure within closed tissue spaces that compromises the flow of blood through nutrient capillaries in muscles and nerves. The complex relationships between time, Starling forces, and systemic and venous pressure are not completely understood. The clinical variables of each case make a definitive explanation of how capillary blood flow is compromised a difficult, if not impossible, exercise. However, a common factor is elevated tissue pressure. Normal tissue pressure is about zero and usually less than 10 mm Hg. Capillary blood flow within the compartment is compromised at pressures greater than about 20 mm Hg, and muscle and nerves are at risk for ischemic necrosis at pressures greater than about 30 to 40 mm Hg. Of the tissues within the compartments, muscle is most sensitive followed by nerve tissue. Blood flow through arteries, arterioles, and collaterals is not compromised significantly at these pressures. Nevertheless, tissues within the compartment that are dependent on the nutrient capillaries become ischemic and then necrotic if the compartment pressure is not reduced promptly. By the time that distal pulses are reduced, muscle necrosis has occurred. Ischemic muscles hurt, and this pain is

exacerbated by active muscle contraction and by passive stretching of the muscle.

An increase in compartmental pressure can be caused by (1) compression of the compartment, for example, by burn eschar, a circumferential cast, or a pneumatic pressure garment, and (2) by a volume increase within the compartment due to hematoma and edema. Direct trauma with resulting bleeding and edema is probably the most common cause, but overexertion (shin splints) and limb compression during recumbency as a result of alcohol or drug overdose are also common causes. Mubarak and Hargens developed a classification of the acute compartment syndromes (Table 237-1) listing the myriad of possible causes.

## COMPARTMENTS AT RISK

Virtually any muscle mass invested in fascia is at risk given the right conditions. The compartments clinically relevant to the emergency physician are the upper extremity and the lower extremity.

### Upper Extremity

The upper arm has an anterior and a posterior compartment. The anterior compartment contains the biceps-brachialis muscle and the ulnar, median, and radial nerves (Fig. 237-1). The posterior compartment contains the triceps muscle. Fortunately the compartments of the upper arm are relatively roomy, and compartment syndromes are uncommon in this location. The forearm has volar and dorsal compartments that are further subdivided into smaller compartments by

COMPARTMENT
STRUCTURES
OF UPPER ARM

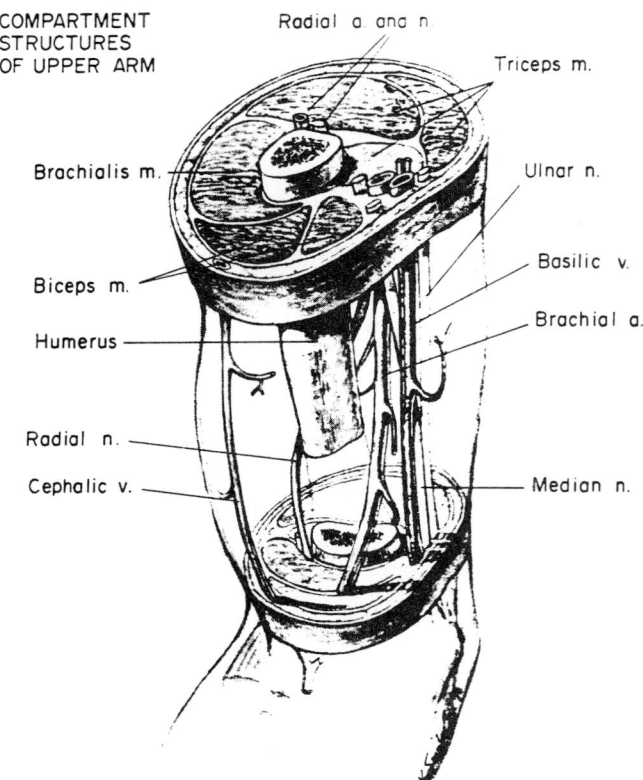

**Fig. 237-1.** The biceps-brachialis (anterior) and triceps (posterior) compartments of the right arm. (From Mubarak and Hargens. Used by permission.)

investing fascia at mid-forearm (Fig. 237-2). The volar compartment contains wrist and finger flexors, and the dorsal compartment contains wrist and finger extenders. The hand has thenar and hypothenar compartments, containing the intrinsic muscles of the thumb and little finger, respectively. The interosseous muscles of the hand are contained in their own compartments (Fig. 237-3).

### Lower Extremity

There are three gluteal compartments of the buttocks. One contains the tensor muscle of the fascia lata, another the gluteus medius and minimus, and the third the gluteus maximus. The sciatic nerve lies adjacent to the gluteus maximus and can be compressed by it.

The thigh has three compartments. These are the anterior, medial, and posterior compartments. The anterior compartment contains the vastus lateralis, the vastus intermedius, and the vastus medialis muscles as well as the sartorius and rectus femoris muscles. The femoral artery and nerve also traverse the anterior thigh compartment. The medial compartment contains the adductor longus, the adductor brevis, and the adductor magnus muscles plus the gracilis muscle. The posterior compartment contains the semimembranosus, the semitendinosus, and the biceps femoris muscles. The sciatic nerve also traverses the posterior compartment.

The leg has four compartments (Fig. 237-4). The anterior compartment, the compartment most frequently involved by this syndrome, contains the tibialis anterior muscle and the extensor muscles of the toes—the extensor hallucis longus and the extensor digitorum longus muscles. The anterior tibial artery and the deep peroneal nerve are also located in this compartment. The lateral compartment, which is frequently involved when the anterior compartment is involved, contains the peroneous longus and brevis muscles as well as the superfi-

cial peroneal nerve. The deep posterior compartment contains the tibialis posterior muscle, the flexor digitorum longus muscle, and the flexor hallucis longus muscle. It also contains the posterior tibial artery and the tibial nerve. The superficial posterior compartment contains the gastrocnemius muscle, the soleus muscle, and the sural nerve.

### DIAGNOSIS

The history, including mechanism of injury, is very important since many patients at risk for the syndrome are severely ill or injured and cannot relate whether or not they are experiencing pain. Palpation of the compartments in question may or may not reveal tenseness and swelling; when in doubt, the resuscitating physician should measure tissue pressure.

Alert and intact patients will virtually always relate that they are experiencing severe and constant pain over the involved compartment. Palpation of the compartment will also elicit pain. Active contraction of the involved muscles will increase the pain, as will passive stretching of the muscles (Table 237-2). Hypesthesia resulting from compromise of nerves traversing the involved compartment appears later than muscle weakness and pain.

Possible compartment syndromes associated with injuries such as fractures or penetrating wounds should prompt an immediate surgical consultation, since the presence of a compartment syndrome may influence subsequent treatment choices.

In patients without a clear need for surgical consultation, measuring the compartment pressures in the emergency department assures safe patient disposition and management. Compartment pressure can be quickly and easily measured using a commercially available battery-powered monitor (Stryker S.T.I.C. Monitor or Ace intracompartmental pressure monitor). Pressure is measured after careful aseptic preparation, insertion of an 18-gauge needle into the compartment, and injection of a small volume of sterile saline. If an arterial pressure monitor is available, the transducer can be used to sense the pressure generated when a small volume of saline is injected through it. Alternatively, compartment pressure can be measured using the following supplies, available in any emergency department: a 20-mL syringe, two IV extension tubes, a three-way stopcock, a small bottle of sterile saline, a mercury manometer, and an 18-gauge needle. They should be assembled as shown in Fig. 237-5. The bottle of saline is vented with an 18-gauge needle and the needle on the apparatus is then inserted into the saline and saline withdrawn until the IV extension is half filled. When removing the needle from the saline bottle, it is important to avoid getting any air in the needle. The needle is then placed in the compartment and the apparatus kept at the level of the needle and the stopcock turned so that it is open in all three directions. Two people are required for this test. One watches the manometer while the other slowly depresses the plunger in the syringe while watching the saline meniscus. When the meniscus moves toward the patient, the operator notifies the manometer watcher, who notes the reading at that instant. In this way, only a minute amount of saline is injected into the compartment. Occasionally, the needle may be inserted into a tendon or investing fascia, resulting in a false high reading. For that reason, the test should be repeated to confirm elevated readings. Low readings are reliable.

In general, the needle is placed where the patient describes the most pain or in the location that is most tense to palpation on examination. When measuring the compartment pressures in the leg, it is generally advisable to measure the pressure in all four compartments. The anterior, lateral, and superficial compartments are easily approached, but the deep posterior compartment is problematic. An easy approach is to insert the needle transversely from the medial side of the leg behind the tibia. When the needle tip is in the center of the leg, it will be in the deep posterior compartment.

**Fig.    237-2.**    Forearm    compartments: transverse sections through the left forearm at various levels. (From Mubarak and Hargens. Used by permission.)

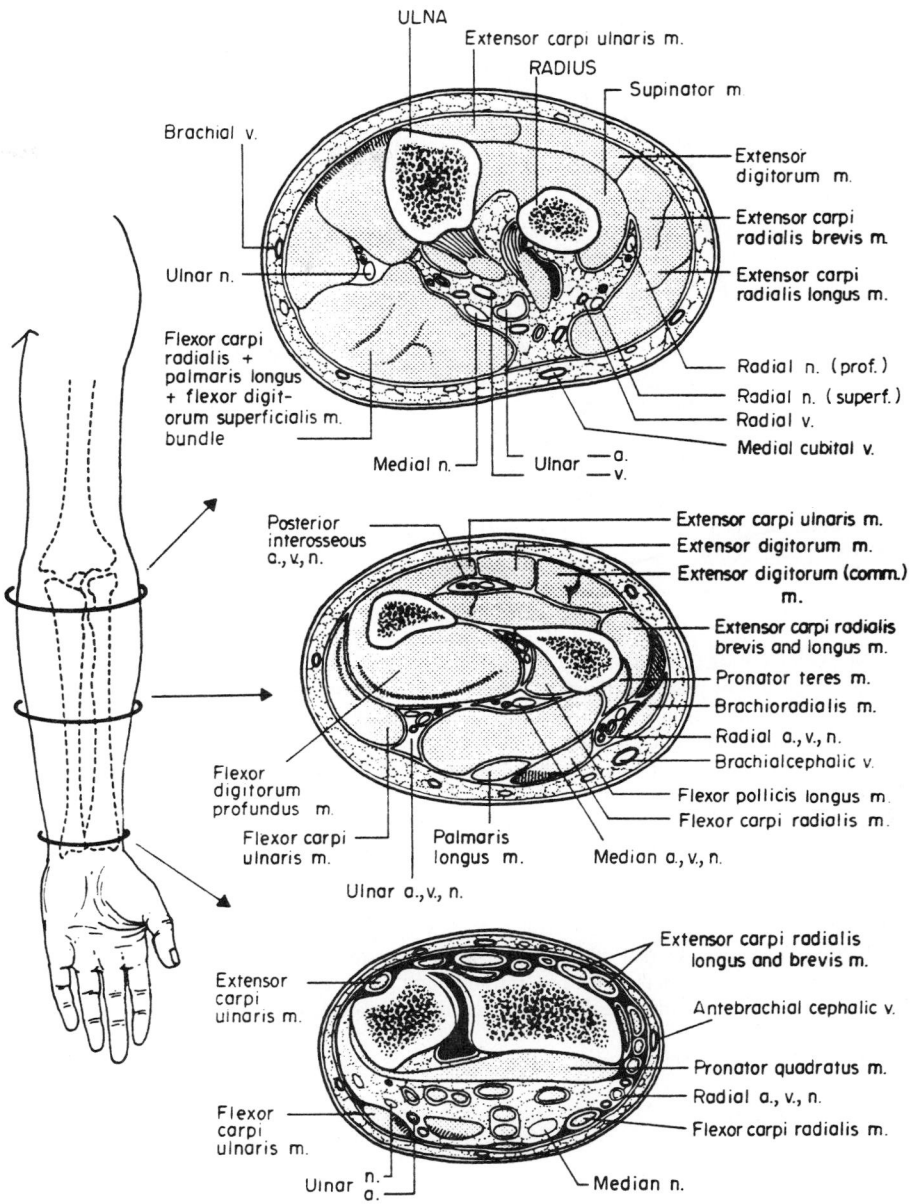

**Fig. 237-3.** Hand compartments: trasverse section through the right hand. (From Mubarak and Hargens. Used by permission.)

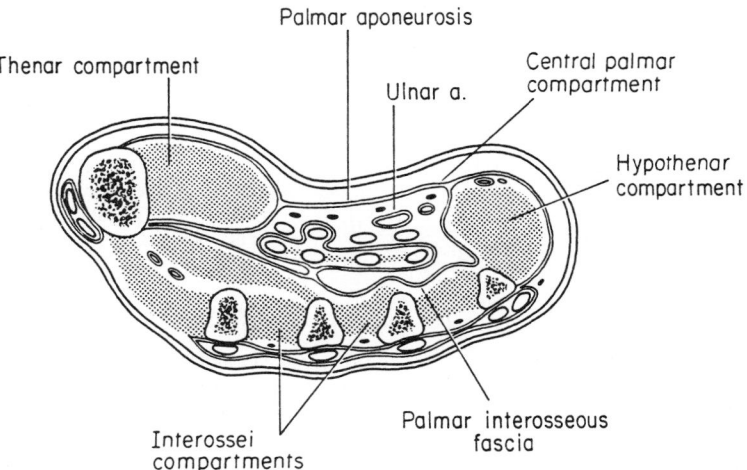

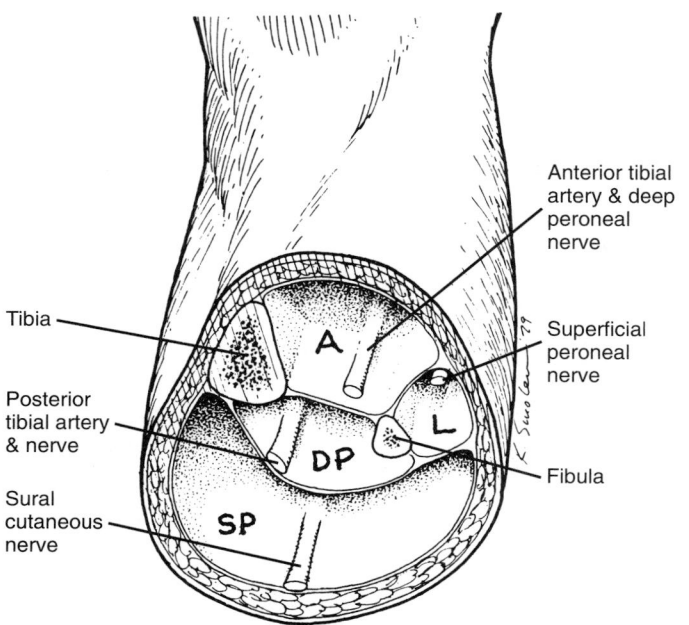

**Fig. 237-4.** The four compartments of the leg. A, the anterior compartment; L, the lateral compartment; DP, the deep posterior compartment; SP, the superficial posterior compartment. (From Mubarak and Hargens. Used by permission.)

Tibia

Posterior tibial artery & nerve

Sural cutaneous nerve

Anterior tibial artery & deep peroneal nerve

Superficial peroneal nerve

Fibula

Measurement of tissue pressure in the forearm may also be problematic because of possible injury to nerves or puncture of an artery, possibly causing a compartment syndrome. McDougall and Johnston describe a dorsal approach to both dorsal and volar forearm compartments that can be accomplished with one needle stick. The forearm is placed in supination, resulting in maximum separation of the radius and ulna proximally. At the junction of the middle and proximal third of the forearm, the subcutaneous ridge of the ulna is palpated posteriorly. The needle is inserted posteriorly at this level just lateral to the ulna and directed between the radius and ulna. The needle will enter the extensor carpi ulnaris and extensor pollicis longus muscles in the dorsal compartment. Dorsal compartment pressure can be measured here. The needle is then advanced through and just past the interosseous membrane into the flexor digitorum profundus muscle in

the volar compartment. The ulna is used to help judge the depth and orientation of the needle. This approach helps assure that arteries and nerves will not be injured.

## MANAGEMENT

Compartment pressures between 15 and 20 mmHg are problematic. If the problem is acute and the patient is reliable, the patient can be told to return for repeat measurement if symptoms do not improve. A pressure of 20 mmHg can be damaging if it persists for several hours; therefore, admission or surgical consultation will be needed for unreliable patients. Pressures greater than 20 mmHg demand admission and surgical consultation. A pressure of 30 to 40 mmHg is generally considered grounds for emergent fasciotomy in the operating room.

**Table 237-2.** Symptomatology of Acute Compartment Syndromes

UPPER EXTREMITY

| | |
|---|---|
| Upper arm | |
| Anterior compartment | Pain on active and passive flexion and extension of the elbow |
| | Hypesthesia in the distribution of the median, ulnar, and radial nerves |
| Posterior compartment | Pain on active and passive flexion and extension of the elbow |
| | Hypesthesia over the dorsum of the hand |
| Forearm | |
| Volar compartment | Pain on active and passive flexion and extension of the fingers |
| | Hypesthesia over the palm of the hand |
| Dorsal compartment | Pain on active and passive flexion and extension of the fingers |
| Hand | |
| Thenar and hypothenar compartments | Pain on thumb and little finger opposition |
| Interosseous compartments | Pain on abduction and adduction of the fingers |

LOWER EXTREMITY

| | |
|---|---|
| Gluteal compartments | Pain on active and passive flexion and extension of the hip |
| | Sciatic nerve paresthesias |
| Thigh compartments | Pain on active and passive flexion and extension of the knee |
| | Sciatic nerve paresthesias with posterior compartment involvement |
| Leg | |
| Anterior compartment | Pain on active and passive dorsiflexion and plantar flexion of the foot |
| | Hypesthesia of the first web space |
| Lateral compartment | Pain on active and passive eversion and inversion of the foot |
| | Hypesthesia of the first web space |
| Superficial posterior compartment | Pain on active and passive plantar flexion and dorsiflexion of the foot |
| | Hypesthesia of the lateral foot |
| Deep posterior compartment | Pain on dorsiflexing the toes and everting the foot |
| | Hypesthesia of the plantar surface of the foot |

**Fig. 237-5.** The tissue pressure is measured by determining the amount of pressure within this closed system that is required to overcome the pressure within the closed compartment and inject a minute quantity of saline. (From Mubarak and Hargens. Used by permission.)

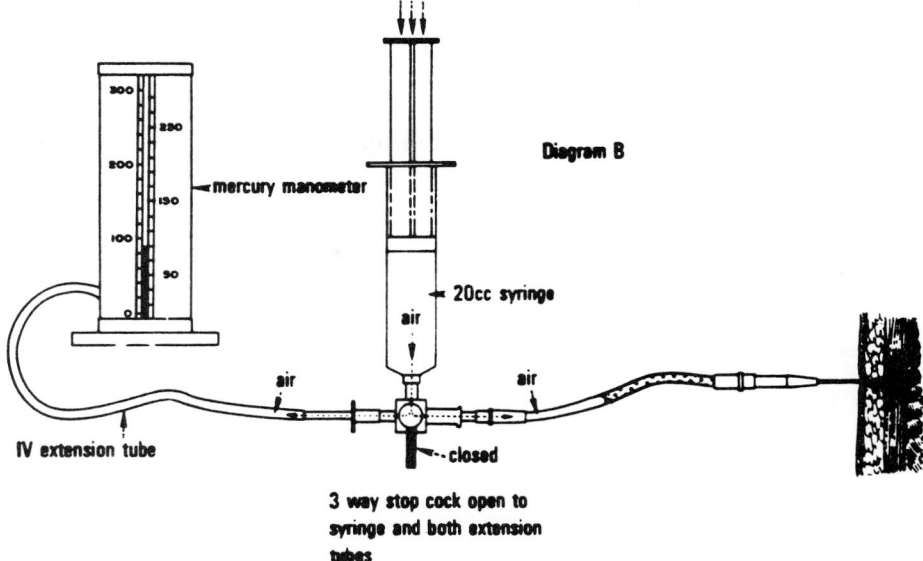

Fasciotomy is accomplished by making a longitudinal skin incision over the compartment. The underlying fascia is then split the length of the compartment, allowing the contained muscle to expand.

## BIBLIOGRAPHY

McDougall CG, Johnston GHF: A new technique of catheter placement for measurement of forearm compartment pressure. *J Trauma* 31(10):1404, 1991.

Mubarak SJ, Hargens AR: *Compartment Syndromes and Volkmann's Contracture*. Philadelphia, Saunders, 1981.

Whitesides TE, Haney TC, Morimoto K, et al: Tissue pressure measurement as a determinant for the need for fasciotomy. *Clin Orthop* 113:43, 1975.

# 238
# MUSCULOSKELETAL DISORDERS IN ADULTS

## Mary Chester Morgan Wasko

Life-threatening complications are rare in rheumatology. Nevertheless, certain manifestations can result in serious morbidity and increased mortality if not recognized and managed promptly.

In contrast to the dearth of rheumatic emergencies, musculoskeletal complaints are abundant in the emergency department. The proper management of musculoskeletal disorders requires knowledge of joint and bursa anatomy and proficiency in joint aspiration and synovial fluid analysis.

This chapter provides an overview of emergencies in rheumatology and a guide to management of the more common musculoskeletal problems.

## RHEUMATIC EMERGENCIES ASSOCIATED WITH RISK OF MORTALITY

### The Respiratory System

Life-threatening respiratory compromise occurs via two major mechanisms in rheumatic diseases: difficulty ventilating due to airway obstruction and impaired ventilation due to weakness. Patients with airway involvement from relapsing polychondritis occasionally present to the emergency department with trouble breathing. This inflammatory disease affecting cartilage usually begins with the abrupt onset of pain, redness, and swelling of the ears or the nose. The airway is affected in roughly 50 percent of patients, causing inflammation, destruction, and ultimate collapse of tracheobronchial cartilage. Patients report throat tenderness over cartilaginous structures and hoarseness. Less commonly they experience shortness of breath, cough, or stridor. Repeated exacerbations may ultimately cause asphyxiation. Pulmonary function studies detect airway obstruction more reliably than bronchoscopy. Emergency tracheostomy may be helpful, depending upon the level and extent of airway compromise. Hospitalization for careful observation and high-dose steroids are appropriate during acute inflammatory exacerbations.

While trauma and infection may affect the paired cricoarytenoid joints, rheumatoid arthritis (RA) is a more common cause of their dysfunction. RA patients with cricoarytenoid arthritis may complain of pain with speaking or swallowing, hoarseness, or stridor. If the joints become fixed in a closed position, airway compromise mandates emergency tracheostomy. Presentation with the above signs is an urgent indication for direct laryngoscopy.

The respiratory muscles may be impaired by inflammatory muscle disease. In dermatomyositis and polymyositis, respiratory insufficiency is uncommon at presentation but complicates poorly controlled or chronic disease. Patients should be observed for nasal flaring, for they may be too weak to generate intercostal retractions. Chest x-rays are normal or show "high-riding" diaphragms unless pulmonary involvement or an aspiration pneumonitis coexists. Admission for disease control and stabilization is indicated in any patient with inflammatory muscle disease and respiratory impairment. Patients with active or advanced disease may require intubation and artificial ventilation for respiratory support in the acute setting. The clinical course can be followed at bedside with measurements of peak inspiratory and expiratory forces.

Pleurisy is common in RA and systemic lupus erythematosus (SLE). It may be asymptomatic in RA, but roughly half of lupus patients have signs and symptoms of pleurisy during the course of their disease. All effusions in rheumatic disease patients should be tapped to exclude other etiologies. Rheumatoid pulmonary effusions characteristically have very low glucose levels, but so do effusions associated with indolent infections such as tuberculosis. Rheumatic, infectious, and malignant effusions are often exudative and either polymorphonuclear or mononuclear cells may predominate. Non-

**Table 238-1.** Respiratory Manifestations of Rheumatic Diseases

| Disease | Common | Infrequent | Rare |
|---|---|---|---|
| SLE | Serositis, effusion | Infiltrate | Hemorrhage, effusion"shrinking lungs," fibrosis |
| RA and JRA | Nodules, effusion | Pulmonary fibrosis | Cricoarytenoid obstruction |
| Spondyloarthropathies | | Pulmonary fibrosis | Pulmonary infiltrates, fibrosis, ARDS |
| Relapsing polychondritis | Airway obstruction | Tracheobronchial collapse | |
| Polymyositis and dermatomyositis | | Hypoventilation with hypoxemia, respiratory failure | |
| Scleroderma | Pulmonary fibrosis | Pulmonary hypertension | |
| Vasculitides Wegener's | Sinusitis, nasal ulcers, pulmonary nodules, infiltrate | | |
| Other | Bronchospasm, hemoptysis | Hemorrhage | |

steroidal anti-inflammatory drugs (NSAIDs) (e.g., indomethacin, 25 to 50 mg tid) and antimalarials [hydroxychloroquin, 200 mg bid (6 mg/kg)] usually suffice. Prednisone in moderate doses is reserved for patients failing this regimen.

Pulmonary hemorrhage can complicate Goodpasture disease, SLE, hypersensitivity vasculitis, and Wegener granulomatosis due to vasculopathic or vasculitic lung involvement. Ankylosing spondylitis (upper lobes), scleroderma, and, rarely, RA and other rheumatic diseases can lead to pulmonary fibrosis. Patients may present with abrupt decompensation with a history of a well-tolerated slow decline. Table 238-1 summarizes respiratory manifestations in rheumatic diseases.

## The Heart

The heart is affected in many rheumatic diseases, with potential involvement extending from the pericardium to the endocardium. Of the rheumatic diseases, RA and juvenile rheumatoid arthritis (JRA) are most often associated with pericarditis. Pericarditis is usually asymptomatic, but occasional patients with chest pain attributed to costochondritis may have symptomatic pericarditis. Their chest pain is characteristically positional, and a pericardial rub is usually heard. SLE often causes symptomatic pericarditis, particularly in the elderly. Patients also report symptoms typical of a flare, such as rash, oral ulcers, or joint pain. Symptoms tend to be consistent from one flare to the next, and therefore a thorough review of systems is key. When symptomatic pericarditis is diagnosed, malignancy and infection must be considered and excluded if clinically indicated. Treatment is similar to that for pleurisy above. Some adults with pericarditis require prednisone. Pericardial tamponade and constrictive pericarditis from either RA or SLE are uncommon.

While therapy has greatly improved long-term survival in SLE, late mortality from premature atherosclerotic disease is being recognized. Precordial chest pain in SLE is not always due to serositis or costochondritis, particularly with long-standing disease, and angina should be considered. Other causes of precordial pain are listed in Table 238-2.

Myocardial infarction (MI) in rheumatic diseases is not usually related to underlying disease. The noteworthy exceptions are Kawasaki disease (see "Musculoskeletal Disorders in Children") and polyarteritis nodosa (PAN). PAN is an arteritis affecting the skin (nodular, ur-

**Table 238-2.** Precordial Chest Pain in Rheumatic Diseases

Pericarditis, pancarditis
Angina, myocardial infarction
Dermatomal herpes zoster
Costochondritis
Vetebral compression (thoracic radiculopathy)
Rib fracture

ticarial, or multiform rashes), gut (abdominal angina), and kidneys (hypertension, hematuria). Coronary arteries are commonly involved. MI and PAN are usually clinically silent, but when MI occurs it can occur in the young as easily as the elderly.

Acute rheumatic fever (ARF) remains an important cause of pancarditis. ARF follows streptococcal pharyngitis within a few weeks. It is heralded by rapid development of fever and acute polyarthritis (in adults) or migratory arthritis (in children). A few patients have a more insidious onset. Supportive clinical clues are the presence of subcutaneous nodules, chorea, or erythema marginatum, but only a third of patients will have one of the latter major manifestations. Diagnosis is based on documenting the clinical involvement and antecedent streptococcal infection. The throat should be cultured and antistreptolysin O (ASO) or streptozyme titers determined at intervals to document a changing titer. Other baseline tests include serial chest x-rays, echocardiography and ECGs to monitor the carditis; and acute phase reactants (erythrocyte sedimentation rate, C-reactive protein). The fever and arthritis respond rapidly and completely to salicylate therapy, but salicylates should be held until the diagnosis is clear. Patients should be placed at bedrest until clinical and laboratory parameters begin to normalize.

Rheumatic fever is only one disease associated with migratory arthritis. Bacterial endocarditis or septicemia due to common bacterial pathogens and the prodromal phase of pulmonary mycoplasma or fungal infections must be considered. Children with Henoch-Schoenlein purpura and cefaclor (Ceclor) serum sickness often have migratory articular and periarticular involvement. Stage II Lyme disease can be manifested by migratory articular involvement, with individual joints resolving over hours to days. Often young adults with polyarthritis are empirically treated with intravenous penicillin for disseminated gonococcus (GC) until a streptococcal infection is confirmed. The arthritis of ARF does not respond to antibiotic therapy; therefore prompt improvement suggests the diagnosis of GC. Table 238-3 summarizes the diagnostic possibilities in patients with migratory arthritis.

Valvular heart disease is a recognized extraarticular manifestation of the seronegative spondyloarthropathies, particularly ankylosing spondylitis. Fibrotic changes of the aortic valve are usually asympto-

**Table 238-3.** Conditions Associated with Migratory Arthritis

Rheumatic fever
Subacute bacterial endocarditis
Henoch-Schoenlein purpura
Cefaclor hypersensitivity (children)
Septicemia: staphylococcal, streptococcal,
  meningococcal, gonococcal
Pulmonary infection: *Mycoplasma,* histoplasmosis,
  coccidioidomycosis
Lyme disease

**Table 238-4.** Cardiac Manifestations of Rheumatic Diseases

| Disease | Common | Infrequent | Rare |
|---|---|---|---|
| SLE | Pericarditis | Angina, myocarditis | Tamponade, constrictive pericarditis |
| Ankylosing spondylitis | | Aortic stenosis/ insufficiency, dissection | Drop attacks |
| Relapsing polychondritis | | Aortic insufficiency, dissection | |
| Polymyositis and dermatomyositis | | Arrhythmias, myocarditis | |
| Scleroderma | | Myocardial fibrosis, arrhythmias | Cor pulmonale |
| Vasculitides | | Angina, myocardial infarction | |

matic, with dysfunction occurring more often in patients with long-standing, severe disease. Scar tissue also may impair cardiac conduction, leading to drop attacks. Relapsing polychondritis can affect the valves, causing aortic insufficiency and aneurysm. This may develop early after diagnosis and is a grave development. Table 238-4 summarizes cardiac involvement in rheumatic diseases.

## ADRENAL INSUFFICIENCY IN GLUCOCORTICOID-TREATED PATIENTS WITH RHEUMATIC DISEASES

Rheumatic disease patients on glucocorticoids are usually instructed to seek medical care urgently if an illness like gastroenteritis prevents taking or absorption of prednisone. In general, the course of a rheumatic disease is not worsened by administration of stress glucocorticoids for a day during an acute illness, even if the dose is much larger than the usual daily dose. A large dose of glucocorticoid may be problematic for diabetic patients, but no more so than the condition that has caused vomiting. Other medications used to treat rheumatic diseases can safely be held for a brief bout of stomach flu. These include NSAIDs, cyclophosphamide or chlorambucil, methotrexate, hydroxychloroquin (Plaquenil), and calcium channel blockers, if they are only used to treat Raynaud phenomenon.

Rarely, patients treated with steroids in the recent past (18 months) develop adrenal insufficiency. They may have early symptoms of weakness, depression, fatigue, and postural dizziness, or late life-threatening vomiting. The serum chemistries usually do not reveal hyponatremia or hyperkalemia in patients with adrenal insufficiency after prednisone withdrawal because that steroid has no mineralocorticoid activity. If adrenal insufficiency is a remote possibility, stress steroids should be administered. Dexamethasone is preferable, as that steroid will not interfere with assays of other adrenal steroids during subsequent diagnostic testing. Prior to the administration of stress steroids, a cortisol level should be drawn in the emergency room. Under stress, normally functioning adrenal glands generate a level in excess of 20 µg/dL (see Chap. 183).

## RHEUMATIC PRESENTATIONS WITH HIGH RISK OF MORBIDITY

### The Cervical Spine and Spinal Cord

Cervical spine disease and its neurologic risk is well recognized in rheumatoid arthritis and ankylosing spondylitis. In RA, pannus formation and destruction of ligamentous supporting structures may lead to atlantoaxial subluxation; an atlantodental distance in excess of the normal 3.5 mm seen in a lateral flexion view suggests instability (in

children under 12, 4 mm of widening is normal). Cord compression may occur acutely following a trivial injury or be more insidious. Subtle clues include a change in bowel or bladder function, new weakness, numbness, or paresthesias. Instability may lead to cranial migration of the odontoid. Complaints relating to vertebral insufficiency (e.g., vertigo) may be reported. Lhermitte sign, an electric shock sensation radiating down the back on neck flexion, is a classic indication of cervical spine instability. Strength may be difficult to assess in arthritis, so subtle differences in reflexes are particularly informative. Lateral cervical spine films in flexion are essential in evaluating these patients. Neck flexion should not be forced, but rather studied at a degree considered comfortable by the patient.

The ankylosed, inflexible cervical spine in a patient with a seronegative spondyloarthropathy (e.g., ankylosing spondylitis) is susceptible to fracture with minor trauma. A whiplash-type injury or a blow from behind may result in new neck pain in an ankylosed area. The complaint of new neck pain requires a careful history and examination, with attention to possible trauma to the neck and evidence of peripheral nerve damage. Fractures are most commonly transverse through a disc space, leading to greater risk of dislocation and cord compression.

Intubation of patients with rheumatic cervical spine disease is best addressed in an elective, controlled situation after the cervical spine has been assessed. *In an emergency, a patient with a stiff or arthritic neck should be intubated by the most experienced operator available. Atlantoaxial instability should be assumed, and extremes of head manipulation avoided.*

The spinal cord can be affected by transverse myelitis in SLE, or a number of factors can induce an anterior spinal artery syndrome in patients with rheumatic diseases. The anterior spinal artery is a direct branch of the aorta; dissection of the aorta, vasculitis, or embolism can impair blood supply to the anterior cord and produce a clinical picture distinct from transverse myelitis or metastatic tumor by sparing of posterior column function (position sense and vibration).

### The Eye

Temporal arteritis (TA) often causes sudden blindness, usually before the condition is diagnosed. Blindness can be prevented, however, if prodromal visual changes and coexistent symptomatology are recognized.

TA is a granulomatous arteritis of the thoracic aorta and its branches; the vasculitis and ischemia in this distribution induce characteristic signs and symptoms: new headache, tender scalp, fluctuating vision, diminution or loss of a brachial pulse, pain in the jaw or tongue while chewing or talking, and constitutional symptoms. An elevated Westergren sedimentation rate (>50 mm/h), elevated liver function studies (particularly the alkaline phosphatase), and unexplained anemia are common laboratory abnormalities.

TA affects the middle-aged and elderly. Polymyalgia rheumatica (PMR), with proximal shoulder and hip girdle morning stiffness and aching, coexists in 10 to 30 percent of these patients. Prodromal changes in vision almost always precede blindness. A high index of suspicion is critical when evaluating anyone older than 50 with a new headache, fluctuating vision, or jaw, tongue, or upper extremity claudication. Diagnosis is established on temporal artery biopsy. If the clinical diagnosis is reasonably certain, steroid therapy should be initiated at a prednisone dosage of 60 mg/day to prevent blindness; this will not obscure pathologic findings if the biopsy is obtained within a week. Symptoms of PMR are easily controlled with prednisone, 15 to 20 mg/day, and those patients without signs and symptoms of TA should not be unnecessarily treated with high-dose steroids.

Sjögren syndrome, a lymphocytic infiltration of the lacrimal and salivary glands causing dry eyes and dry mouth, may complicate many rheumatic diseases or occur independently. It predisposes the patient to corneal irritation, ulceration, and superimposed infection.

**Table 238-5.** Examination of Synovial Fluid

| | Normal | Noninflammatory | Inflammatory | Hemarthrosis |
|---|---|---|---|---|
| Gross appearance | Transparent, clear | Transparent, yellow | Cloudy, yellow | Bloody |
| String sign | Normal | Normal | Diminished or absent | |
| WBC/mm³ | <200 | <200–2000 | >2000 | Approaches peripheral |
| PMNs | <25% | <25% | >50% | |
| Culture | Negative | Negative | >50% positive if septic | Negative |
| Crystals | Negative | Negative | ±Positive if crystalline arthritis | Negative |
| Associated conditions | | Osteoarthritis, trauma, neuropathic arthritis, SLE, hypertrophic pulmonary osteoarthropathy, rheumatic fever | Septic arthritis, crystal arthritis, seronegative spondyloarthropathy, RA, SLE, polymyositis, acute rheumatic fever, Lyme disease | See Table 238-6 |

In RA, a red eye requires careful evaluation. Under bright natural light, examination can reveal the difference between episcleritis, which is self-limiting, and scleritis, which is an emergency. Episcleritis is a painless injection of the episcleral vessels giving the eye a pink-red appearance; it rarely impairs vision. As it is self-limiting, no therapy is indicated. Scleritis causes exquisite ocular tenderness. The eye has a deep purplish discoloration. Visual impairment and scleral thinning with rupture are feared outcomes. High-dose steroids and intensive ophthalmologic management are required.

## Hypertension

Hypertension can complicate PAN or SLE with renal involvement or RA with drug-induced renal toxicity (fluid retention, nephritis, or renal papillary necrosis), but malignant hypertension is a complication of systemic sclerosis (scleroderma). Hypertensive renal crisis was the leading cause of death in scleroderma until the advent of angiotensin-converting enzyme (ACE) inhibitors. The most susceptible patients have rapidly progressive skin changes and present within the first few years of diagnosis with complaints related to hypertension. Laboratory studies reveal rapidly progressive renal insufficiency and frequently a microangiopathic hemolytic anemia and thrombocytopenia. The hypertension results from sclerosis and impaired renal glomerular perfusion causing hyperreninemia. Dehydration from gastroenteritis or diuretics may precipitate the crisis. These patients should be hospitalized and promptly treated with captopril. Any intervention such as diuretics that might exacerbate volume contraction and the underlying pathophysiology should be avoided.

## The Kidney

Nephritis is a major determinant of survival and morbidity in patients with SLE and systemic vasculitis. Renal dysfunction secondary to hypertension and microangiopathy occurs in scleroderma. Worsening renal function in these diseases or new abnormalities in renal function in RA or other diseases should prompt a search for remediable causes of renal dysfunction. Patients with SLE and the nephrotic syndrome can develop renal vein thrombosis, which presents with flank pain and proteinuria. Patients, particularly the elderly, treated with NSAIDs can develop renal insufficiency and fluid retention on the basis of alteration in renal blood flow; this is mediated by prostaglandin inhibition.

Occasionally a patient with florid myositis (as in dermatomyositis or polymyositis) or metabolic muscle disease develops acute renal insufficiency due to rhabdomyolysis. In metabolic muscle diseases, muscle pain and breakdown can be triggered by exercise.

Myoglobinuria should be suspected when the urine is brown and the dipstick shows blood but no red blood cells. In contrast to a hemolytic state, the serum is clear, CPK is elevated, and haptoglobin is normal. Patients should be hydrated with normal saline to restore intravascular loss that accompanies muscle necrosis. Lasix and one dose of mannitol to preserve urinary output also are recommended during this early phase.

## AMBULATORY EVALUATION OF MUSCULOSKELETAL COMPLAINT

Musculoskeletal complaints frequently bring patients into the emergency department, and evaluation of the most painful, disabling, and serious complaints (trauma and crystal-induced and septic arthritis) is the physician's first priority.

### Aspiration and Examination of Synovial Fluid

Accurate diagnosis of articular problems often depends on aspiration and examination of synovial fluid. Aspiration of a joint can clarify whether an acute arthritis is septic, traumatic, or crystal-induced. While many tests can be run on synovial fluid, a few simple tests can elucidate the etiology of acute joint pain (see Table 238-5).

### Technique

The technique for aspiration is straightforward. The subcutaneous tissue at the site to be aspirated should be infiltrated with local anesthetic. Intraarticular injection should be avoided, since anesthetic contamination of synovial fluid can inhibit bacterial growth and results in a spuriously negative culture in an early septic joint. Cellulitis or impetigo at the aspiration site, septicemia, and coagulopathy are relative contraindications to joint aspiration but should not preclude aspiration of a tender, swollen joint by an experienced operator to exclude infection. A large-bore needle (18 gauge) facilitates aspiration of thick purulent fluid and promotes drainage of infected fluid under pressure; the joint space should be emptied as completely as possible. Fluid should be examined promptly for crystals under a polarizing scope, and additional fluid sent for Gram stain, culture, and cell count with differential. If surplus fluid is available and where clinically indicated, fungal and AFB smears and cultures are appropriate. Table 238-5 summarizes synovial fluid characteristics in different diseases and Table 238-6 conditions associated with hemarthrosis.

Primary care physicians should feel comfortable aspirating the shoulder, wrist, knee, and ankle. Anatomic landmarks should be determined before aseptic preparation and drape. Because infection is in the differential diagnosis of an inflamed joint and because of the risk of "seeding" a joint with skin flora, meticulous care must be given to

**Table 238-6.** Conditions Associated with Hemarthrosis

Trauma ± fracture (check fluid for marrow fat droplets)
Coagulopathy (especially hemophilia)
Sickle cell disease
Hypermobility syndromes
Scurvy
Pigmented villonodular synovitis (chocolate synovial fluid)
Ruptured aneurysm

iodine preparation, sterile gloves, and drapes. Wherever possible, a needle for joint aspiration should not traverse a skin or soft tissue infection.

Some joints such as the knee may be easily aspirated from more than one approach. As a small-gauge needle is used to administer the anesthetic superficially, it may be advanced further to locate the joint space and left in place to guide the placement of the larger bore needle for aspiration. With the knee fully extended, the midpoint of either the lateral or medial patella should be identified, the skin anesthetized, and the needle horizontally introduced about 2 cm inferior to the patellar edge. See Fig. 238-1.

The ankle also can be entered medially or laterally, anterior to the malleoli. The major tendons and arteries around the ankle can be easily palpated and thus avoided with the needle. The ankle is best held in a 90° angle in relation to the shin; the examiner can stabilize the foot and facilitate the procedure by letting the sole of the foot rest on his or her abdomen. The needle is angled slightly cephalad to enter the tibiotalar space as it passes between the medial malleolus and the tibialis anterior tendon. See Fig. 238-2.

In the shoulder, the subacromial bursa is accessible by palpating the acromion (the lateral bony prominence superior to the humeral head) and passing the needle directly under it. See Fig. 238-3. Injection here bathes the rotator cuff as it passes through this space. The glenohumeral joint may be entered anteriorly by inserting the needle just lateral to the coracoid process. Because of difficulty palpating these landmarks and the remote risk of pneumothorax with this method, a posterior approach is preferable. With the patient sitting upright, the spine of the scapula is palpated at its lateral limit, then a point identified by moving medially 2 cm along the spine, then inferiorly 2 cm. A $1^1/_2$-in. needle passed anteriorly to the needle hub, angled toward the coracoid process (also simultaneously palpable with the free hand through a sterile drape over the shoulder), should provide access to the glenohumeral joint.

The wrist landmarks are palpable with the wrist in a neutral position. The needle should be inserted perpendicular to the skin, just distal to the radial head, slightly ulnar to the anatomic snuffbox. Alternatively, the space between the distal radius and ulna may be entered. See Fig. 238-4.

## Traumatic Arthritis

An injury that causes joint swelling within minutes has a high association with hemarthrosis and internal derangement. Spontaneous bloody effusion usually indicates underlying systemic illness and should trigger a search for primary or secondary coagulopathies. Swelling over hours is consistent with sprain; splinting, ice, and pain relief are indicated.

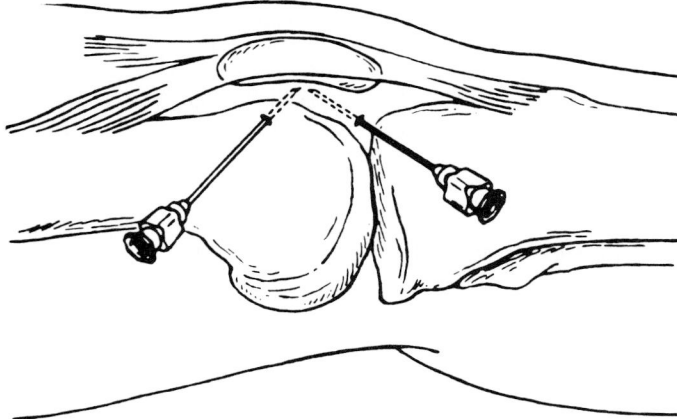

**Fig. 238-1.** Arthrocentesis of knee (medial approach). (Illustration provided by Dr D Neustadt.) [From Schumacher HR (ed): *Primer in the Rheumatic Diseases,* 10th ed. Atlanta, Arthritis Foundation, 1993, with permission.]

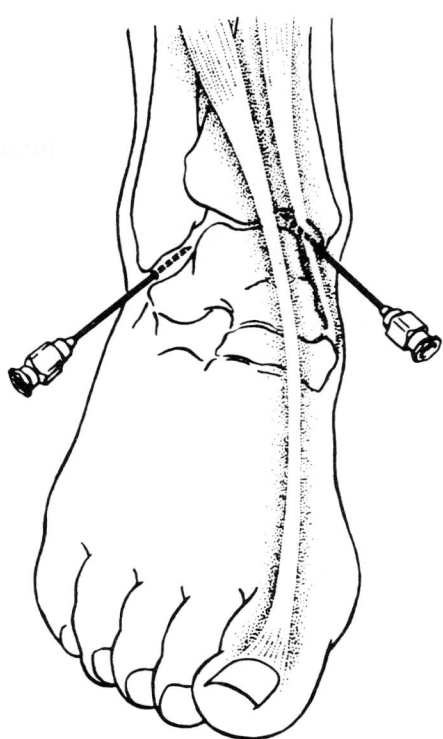

**Fig. 238-2.** Arthrocentesis of ankle joint (medial and lateral approaches). (Illustration provided by Dr D Neustadt.) [From Schumacher HR (ed): *Primer in the Rheumatic Diseases,* 10th ed. Atlanta, Arthritis Foundation, 1993, with permission.]

## Septic Arthritis

An infected joint is a medical emergency, as a rampant bacterial infection with a normal inflammatory response can mutilate a joint within hours to days. When usual pyogenic organisms cause septic

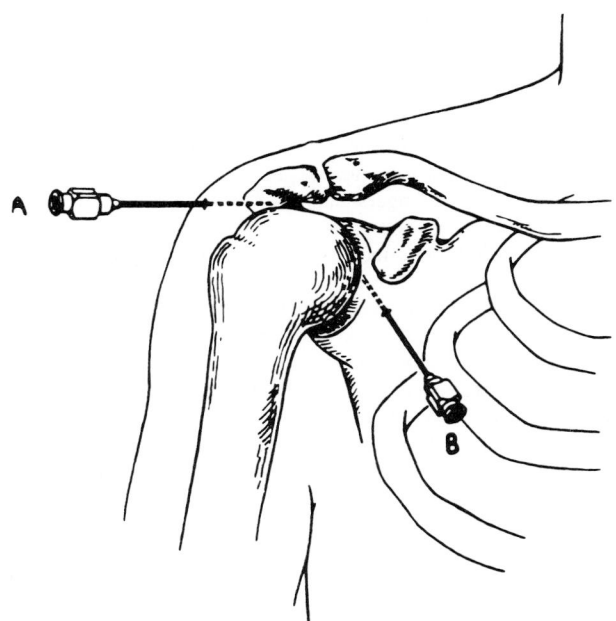

**Fig. 238-3.** A, Injection of subacromial bursa or supraspinatus tendon; B, anterior approach for injection of glenohumeral joint. (Illustration provided by Dr D Neustadt.) [From Schumacher HR (ed): *Primer on the Rheumatic Diseases,* 10th ed. Atlanta, Arthritis Foundation, 1993, with permission.]

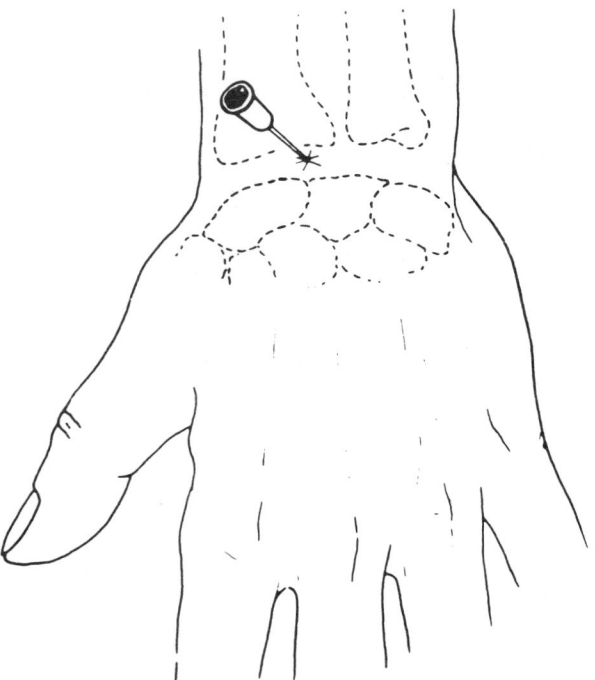

**Fig. 238-4.** Arthrocentesis of the wrist (radial approach). (Illustration provided by Dr D Neustadt.) [From Schumacher HR (ed): *Primer on the Rheumatic Diseases,* 10th ed. Atlanta, Arthritis Foundation, 1993, with permission.]

arthritis (*Staphylococcus, Streptococcus, Haemophilus influenzae*), classic symptomatology is the rule. The involved joint can become exquisitely painful over a few hours. On examination, effusions may be scant, but even passive movement is resisted because of splinting. A joint previously injured or affected by arthritis is more susceptible to infection than a normal joint, so flare of a single joint in RA may represent infection. Crystalline and septic arthritis may coexist. When in doubt, admit the patient for joint aspiration, pain control, and parenteral antibiotics until synovial culture results are available; delay in treating a septic joint can be catastrophic.

Gonococcal and meningococcal infections have a prodromal phase where migratory arthritis and tenosynovitis predominate before pain and swelling settle in one or more septic joints. Vesiculopustular lesions, especially on the fingers, can be a clue to GC infection in the acute phase. Cultures of the posterior pharynx, urethra, cervix, and rectum prior to antibiotics increase the culture yield in GC, as the synovial fluid is often negative.

More indolent development of symptoms is characteristic of most gram-negative infections. These are rare in healthy children and adults but are associated with chronic disease (e.g., diabetes), the immunosuppressed, the elderly, and drug addicts. The immunodeficient are susceptible to *Mycoplasma* and *Ureaplasma;* synovium rather than synovial fluid must be obtained to detect these organisms. Septic sacroiliitis and sternoclavicular septic arthritis are peculiar to intravenous drug abusers. Tenderness and limitation of motion in the absence of radiographic findings are typical diagnostic features.

Intravenous drug abusers are an increasingly important group of patients susceptible to nongonococcal bacterial arthritis, often the gram-negative bacilli. The increasing number of outpatients with indwelling catheters for hemodialysis or parenteral medications and nutrition has expanded this vulnerable population. Presumably this increased incidence is due to recurrent bacteremia with self-administered injections. Favored sites are the sternoclavicular, sacroiliac, and intervertebral joints. Palpation directly over the involved site fre-

**Table 238-7.** Recommended Starting Therapy for Septic Arthritis or Osteomyelitis

| Patient or Condition | Expected Organisms (Unusual Organisms) | Antibiotics |
|---|---|---|
| Neonate | *Staphylococcus,* gram-negative bacteria, group B *Streptococcus* (*Candida*) | Nafcillin and aminoglycoside |
| Child <5 years | *Staphylococcus,* *H. influenzae* | Nafcillin and cefuroxime |
| Older children and healthy adults | *Staphylococcus,* *Streptococcus, Gonococcus* | Nafcillin (vancomycin*) (ceftriaxone**) |
| Involvement of the foot | *Staphylococcus,* *Pseudomonas* | 3rd generation penicillin and aminoglycoside |
| "Susceptible host"† | *Staphylococcus,* gram-negative bacteria, tuberculous, fungal | Individualized |

* Vancomycin should be employed only for treatment of methicillin-resistant staphylococci.

** Ceftriaxone is increasingly recommended for suspected gonococcal infections due to the growing problem of penicillinase-producing *N. gonorrhoeae.*

† The elderly, immunosuppressed patients, and patients with debilitating disease, e.g., diabetes, chronic renal failure, drug addiction.

quently elicits tenderness. Because x-rays are usually nearly normal in early septic arthritis, a bone scan may be particularly useful. As precise identification of the offending organism is essential to guide specific therapy, joint aspiration and blood cultures before administration of antibiotics are mandatory wherever possible. A cooperative effort with the orthopedic surgeon and radiologist facilitates a prompt, productive aspiration under fluoroscopic guidance. General anesthesia is strongly encouraged for the sacroiliac joint because it is difficult to access percutaneously. As these infections are often insidious, the emergency department physician should maintain a high index of suspicion and proceed with a careful musculoskeletal examination when these patients present with systemic indications of infection but no focal source.

Tubercular and most fungal arthritides tend to smolder for months before diagnosis is established. Synovial fluid does not reliably yield the organism; synovial biopsy is required. An exception is *Candida,* which presents like a pyogenic arthritis; synovial fluid cultures are usually positive.

Osteomyelitis adjacent to a joint may elicit a sterile sympathetic effusion with a low cell count. Detection of bone tenderness will alert the examiner to the correct diagnosis, and bone scan (early) or x-rays (after 2 weeks of symptoms) may be definitive. If there is any suspicion that one is dealing with septic arthritis or osteomyelitis, patients should be admitted for therapy. Intravenous antibiotics are administered and the extremity splinted for patient comfort. The septic joint is aspirated as the effusion recurs; surgical drainage is undertaken if joint fluid is loculated or extremely thick. Table 238-7 summarizes initial management of septic arthritis.

## Articular Involvement in Lyme Disease

Within days to weeks of primary infection (stage I), patients with Lyme disease develop disseminated disease (stage II). The musculoskeletal manifestations are migratory arthritis (attacks are often brief), bursitis, and tendonitis. At this stage, debilitating fatigue and involvement of the central nervous system, cardiac conduction system, and eye may occur. Much later (stage III), arthritis can become chronic, particularly in the knee, and be associated with periostitis and tendonitis. Diagnosis is made on clinical grounds and supported by positive serologies.

## Crystal-Induced Synovitis (Gout, Pseudogout)

This is primarily an illness of middle-aged and elderly adults. Uric acid and calcium pyrophosphate are the two most common culprits. Diagnosis can be easily established by the emergency department physician with a joint aspiration during an acute flare. Such documentation enables the primary care physician to proceed with appropriate work-up for underlying disease and prophylaxis against further attacks.

Joint pain from gout develops over a few hours, whereas pseudogout may evolve over a day. Lower extremities are involved more often than the upper. While the first metatarsophalangeal (MTP) joint is a classic focus for acute gout, no joint is the exclusive site of involvement by either crystal. Joint aspiration is essential to confirm the inciting crystal, with fluid inspection under a polarizing scope to determine the presence of urate or calcium pyrophosphate. Uric acid crystals appear needle-shaped and blue when the source of light is perpendicular to the crystal (CUB: "crossed, urate, blue"). Calcium pyrophosphate is yellow in this alignment, with a rhomboid shape. Either crystal must be located within a white blood count to implicate it as the cause of the arthritis rather than an epiphenomenon. The MTP is difficult to enter even with a small needle, but scant fluid aspirated from adjacent inflamed soft tissues often contains crystals shed from the synovium. Serum uric acid measurements are not helpful in diagnosis of gout because the uric acid level can normalize during an acute exacerbation.

The first priority is exclusion of septic arthritis. If there is doubt, treatment for septic arthritis should be undertaken. When minimal fluid is available for diagnostic studies, it should be sent for bacterial culture and sensitivity, with Gram stain, crystal examination, cell count with differential, and other stains and cultures in decreasing order of importance as quantities allow and as deemed clinically appropriate.

When the diagnosis of gout or pseudogout is established, an NSAID such as indomethacin is standard first-line therapy (50 mg tid if renal function is normal). Rarely is additional treatment necessary for acute pseudogout. Oral colchicine is a reasonable alternative, administered at a dose of 0.6 mg hourly until intolerable side effects (nausea, vomiting, diarrhea) or efficacy ensue. Treatment within the first 12 h of symptoms increases the likelihood of its effectiveness. Because of serious toxicities such as bone marrow suppression, neuropathy, myopathy, and death, as well as the excellent response obtained with NSAIDs, use of colchicine, particularly by the intravenous route, should only be undertaken in consultation with a rheumatologist.

During an acute flare, doses of other medications chronically used to treat a patient's crystalline arthritis should not be adjusted, as this may exacerbate crystal precipitation. When a suspected attack of acute crystalline arthritis has not responded to this regimen, another process such as a joint infection should be *strongly* suspected and evaluated accordingly with repeat joint aspiration.

## Baker Cyst in Arthritis of the Knee

Fluid from a chronic inflammatory arthritis of the knee, classically RA, may dissect into a potential popliteal space via a one-way valve, forming a Baker cyst. Its rupture or dissection into the calf mimics a deep venous thrombosis, causing calf pain and swelling. Helpful discriminating features are: (1) swelling that spares the foot; (2) a crescentic, purplish discoloration below the malleoli (crescent sign), due to blood layering at the ligamentous and tendinous attachments around the ankle; and (3) the history of a rapid diminution in a knee effusion or popliteal fullness. An arthrogram is the "gold standard" diagnostic test. Ultrasound in experienced hands may suffice and, with Doppler, permits exclusion of a popliteal artery aneurysm, though a ruptured cyst may yield a false-negative result. Treatment consists of knee joint aspiration and steroid injection to reduce intraarticular pressure and inflammation.

## Bursitis

Because of the proximity of bursae to joints, careful examination is required to differentiate bursitis from arthritis. In the elbow, for example, olecranon bursitis and arthritis will both cause limitation of flexion and extension, but bursitis will not affect pronation or supination. Septic bursitis is usually associated with a puncture or overlying cellulitis. An important point to remember is that in septic bursitis white blood cell counts are only about 10 percent of that expected in septic arthritis. When a clinical scenario raises even a remote possibility of infection, the bursa should be drained thoroughly with a large-bore needle. Where the bursa is superficial, aspiration technique should be modified from a joint aspiration. Instead of inserting the needle perpendicular to the skin directly over the distended bursa, the needle should enter the skin 1 to 2 cm from the expected pocket of fluid and tunneled through subcutaneous tissue before entering the bursa. This establishes a longer tract between the skin puncture and inflamed bursa, so that as the needle is withdrawn, risk of a chronically draining fistula is minimized.

## Tendonitis

Tendonitis and tenosynovitis are almost always overuse disorders. Examination reveals localized tenderness at insertion sites (e.g., the lateral epicondyle in tennis elbow) that is exacerbated by maneuvers that stretch the tendon. The disorders are treated by rest and NSAIDs: naproxen (250 to 500 mg bid or tid; 10 to 15 mg/kg/day), tolmetin (400 to 600 tid/qid; 20 to 30 mg/kg/day), or sulindac (150 to 200 mg bid).

## Glucocorticoid Injections

Acute flare of a single joint in RA, JRA, and gout or bursitis and tendonitis may benefit from glucocorticoid injection, but injections are associated with complications, and repeated injections risk injury to cartilage and tendons. Injection should be undertaken after consultation with a rheumatologist or orthopaedist. In the case of overuse syndromes (bursitis and tendinitis), injection should not substitute for cessation or modification of overuse activity. Care should be taken to aspirate as the needle is withdrawn after intraarticular injection to minimize the risk of subcutaneous atrophy at the site. Subcutaneous atrophy is more likely when superficial soft tissues are injected.

## Avascular Necrosis

Avascular necrosis (AVN) most commonly affects the femoral head. AVN causes focal bone pain that begins insidiously and worsens with weight bearing. Involvement of the medial femoral condyles (osteochondritis dissecans) causes pain and swelling of the knee. Involvement of the bones of the feet (e.g., Kohler disease, Freiburg infraction) is signalled by localized tenderness. X-rays yield the diagnosis if patients have been symptomatic for 2 weeks or more. MRI is extremely sensitive in detecting bone marrow changes in early AVN and is appropriate to evaluate the patient with symptoms for less than 2 weeks and a negative x-ray as an early core decompression may improve blood flow to ischemic bone.

Rheumatic disease patients treated with chronic glucocorticoids and SLE patients are at high risk for this unfortunate complication of therapy.

## Osteoarticular Malignancy

Bone tumors present with the insidious onset of bone pain exacerbated by weight bearing; patients are frequently roused from sleep by pain. Leukemia infiltrating the joints produces severe pain, inconsolable night waking, and refusal to bear weight. X-rays reveal metaphyseal rarefaction or periosteal elevation. Patients over the age of 40 with new onset of seronegative polyarthralgias or polyarthritis, especially when associated with systemic complaints, may have a paraneoplastic syndrome. A careful, complete physical examination, with attention to lymphadenopathy and splenomegaly, and complete blood count with differential often will provide additional clues to the presence of an underlying malignancy.

*Refusal to bear weight* is characteristic of fracture, osteoarticular malignancy, osteoarticular infection, and discitis.

## BIBLIOGRAPHY

Cassidy JT, Petty RE: *Textbook of Pediatric Rheumatology*. New York, Churchill Livingstone, 1990.

Kelley WN, Harris ED Jr, Ruddy S, Sledge CB. *Textbook of Rheumatology*. Philadelphia, Saunders, 1993.

Mandell BF: *Acute Rheumatic and Immunological Diseases*. New York, Marcel Dekker, 1994.

Schumacher HR (ed): *Primer on the Rheumatic Diseases,* 10th ed. Atlanta, GA; Arthritis Foundation, 1993.

# 239

# INFECTIONS AND NONINFECTIOUS INFLAMMATORY STATES OF THE HAND

### Robert R. Simon
### David Slobodkin

## GENERAL PRINCIPLES

As discussed in the chapter dealing with hand injuries, proper splinting and appropriately timed mobilization are key factors in minimizing long-term disability from injuries of the hand. This also applies to hand infections and inflammatory conditions. Rest and elevation to reduce inflammation, avoid secondary injury, and in the case of infection, to avoid anatomic extension, is of vital importance in atraumatic as well as traumatic conditions of the hand. This can be accomplished by plaster splinting or a bulky hand dressing. The optimal position to promote drainage and preserve motion is with the wrist at 15° of extension, the metaphalangeal (MP) joints at 50° of flexion, and the interphalangeal (IP) joints at 10° to 15° of flexion.

The volar aspect of the hand is covered by the tough and relatively fixed tissues of the palm; the veins and lymphatics course through the softer tissues on the dorsum of the hand; thus, regardless of the precise anatomic site of infection or inflammation, the dorsum of the hand will always swell whenever there is an inflammatory process. For the same reason, it is important to avoid pressure on the dorsum of the hand or wrist when elevating a hand to reduce edema. A 4- or 6-inch stockinette tubular sleeve, split to tie around the chest, and with openings cut to bring the fingers and thumb out, will allow comfortable suspension of the hand without restricting drainage (Fig. 239-1).

## CONSTRICTIVE AND COMPRESSIVE CONDITIONS

### Tendinitis and Tenosynovitis

Tendinitis and tenosynovitis can involve the flexor or extensor tendons of the hand. These disorders are usually due to an overuse syndrome. Simple tendinitis or tenosynovitis can be treated by immobilization for a short time, followed by administration of anti-inflammatory agents. In patients with simple synovitis, injection of a depot steroid (such as 40 mg/mL triamcinolone mixed with 0.5% bupivacaine) into the synovial sheath is useful but should be done only when one is absolutely certain there is not infection. Accurate injection is important and may be challenging. One technique is to impale the tendon, as confirmed by distal motion on manipulation of the needle, and then to withdraw the needle while applying very gentle pressure to the plunger. When loss of resistance is felt, the needle is in the tendon sheath.

### Trigger Finger

Tenosynovitis can develop in the flexor sheaths of the fingers and thumb. This results in a disproportion between the tendon and its sheath usually in the vicinity of the A1 pulley. This is referred to as stenosing tenosynovitis, or "trigger finger." The patient experiences a binding of the tendon, usually as the finger extends, relieved by a painful "snap" as the tendon clears the obstruction. Occasionally, this condition may progress to the point that the finger locks, usually in flexion. This must not be confused with Dupuytren's contracture (described below). Early stages of trigger finger have been successfully treated with depot steroid injection into the tendon sheath, although there may be recurrence. Surgical division of the A1 pulley is almost invariably curative.

### DeQuervain's Stenosing Tenosynovitis

DeQuervain's tenosynovitis is a common condition that occurs in patients who have experienced excessive use of the thumb. Often, no good cause can be found. This is a tenosynovitis of the extensor pollicis brevis and abductor pollicis, where they lie in the groove of the radial styloid.

The patient presents with pain along the radial aspect of the wrist that extends into the forearm. The definitive examination that confirms the diagnosis is Finkelstein's test, (Fig. 239-2), in which the patient grasps the thumb in the palm of the hand and the examiner ulnar deviates the thumb and hand. This produces sharp pain along the involved tendons.

DeQuervain's tenosynovitis can be treated with injection into the tendon sheath of 1 mL of 0.5% bupivacaine mixed with 40 mg (1 mL) triamcinolone. This is accomplished by palpating the tendon with the thumb in hyperextension, and injecting 1 cm proximal to the tip of the radial styloid. Distention of the tendon sheath should be seen distal to the retinacular ligament. The tendon itself must not be injected, and care must be taken to avoid subcutaneous or intradermal injection of steroid because this may cause cutaneous thinning and depigmentation. The authors recommend injecting a small amount of sterile saline through the needle before removing it. A thumb spica splint should be applied to keep the thumb in a neutral position for 3 weeks, and the patient should be given anti-inflammatories for a period of approximately 1 week. Recurrence of this condition is not uncommon, particularly when related to occupational stress. Recurrent or nonresponsive cases should be referred to a hand surgeon.

### Carpal Tunnel Syndrome

Carpal tunnel syndrome involves entrapment of the median nerve in the carpal canal or tunnel, which is covered by the tense transverse carpal ligament. Whenever a condition causes swelling in the carpal tunnel, the median nerve is compressed, causing parasthesias that ex-

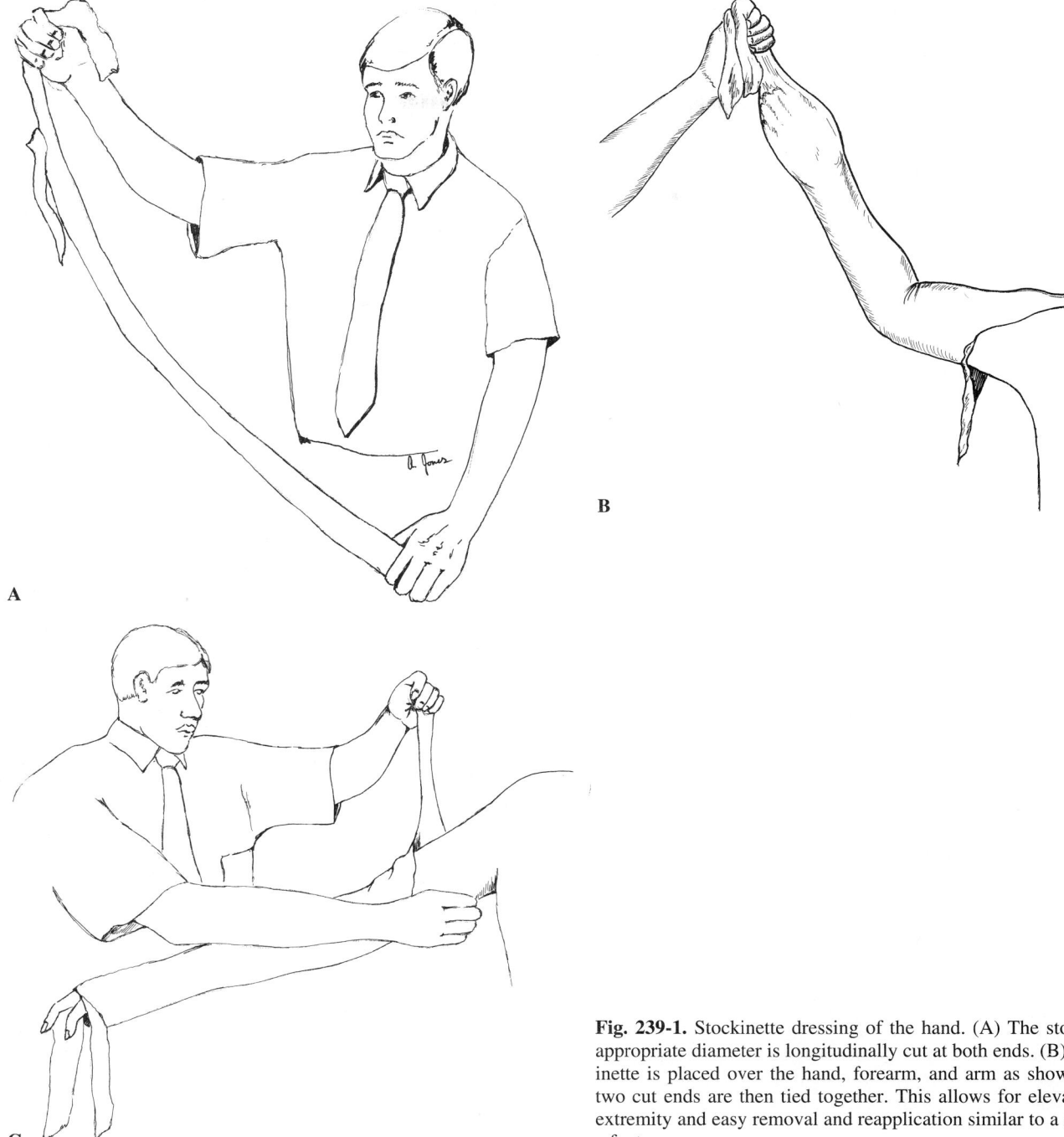

**Fig. 239-1.** Stockinette dressing of the hand. (A) The stockinette of appropriate diameter is longitudinally cut at both ends. (B) The stockinette is placed over the hand, forearm, and arm as shown. (C) The two cut ends are then tied together. This allows for elevation of the extremity and easy removal and reapplication similar to a stocking on a foot.

tend into the index and long fingers, and the radial aspect of the ring finger and along the palmar aspect of the thumb. The patient complains of awakening at night with pain in the hand. In addition, patients often complain of numbness when driving a car or using the hand in an extended position for a prolonged period of time.

Tinel's sign may support the diagnosis and involves tapping the volar aspect of the wrist over the median nerve. This produces paresthesias that extend into the index and long finger. Phalen's sign may be positive and involves flexing the wrist maximally and holding it in this position for at least 1 minute. The patient complains of tingling and numbness along the median nerve distribution. Both signs are subject to false positives and false negatives, and electrodiagnostic techniques may be required to confirm the diagnosis.

The tourniquet test may also be positive. It involves placing a tourniquet around the arm in the normal position for taking a blood pressure and inflating it above venous pressure. The tourniquet is usually inflated to between diastolic and systolic blood pressure and left in position for 1 or 2 minutes. Engorgement of the veins and tissues in the carpal tunnel occurs, producing compression along the median nerve, which in turn produces the symptoms.

Initial treatment of carpal tunnel syndrome involves placing a volar splint to maintain the wrist in neutral position and giving the patient anti-inflammatory agents. Infiltration of the carpal tunnel with a mixture of 1 mL of 0.5% bupivacaine and 40 mg (1 mL) of triamcinolone may be beneficial, if the physician is experienced in the procedure. If this does not improve the condition, surgical intervention is necessary to release the entrapment.

This condition may have a relapsing course, and permanent deficits

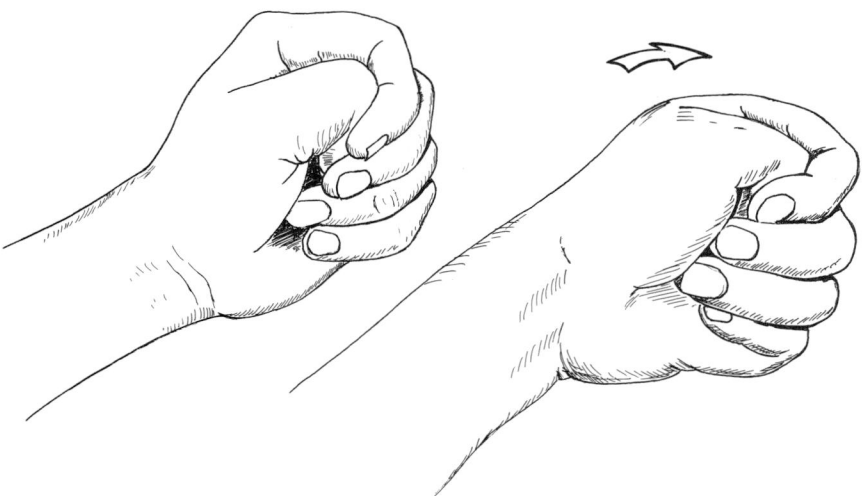

**Fig. 239-2.** The Finkelstein test is shown. The thumb is cupped in the closed fist and ulnar deviation reproduces pain along the extensor pollicis and abductor pollicis.

of the median nerve are occasionally seen. Carpal tunnel syndrome should be diagnosed early, and the patient should be referred to a hand surgeon.

## Dupuytren's Contracture

Dupuytren's contracture is a poorly understood disease resulting in fibroplastic changes of the subcutaneous tissues of the palm and palmar aspect of the fingers. This process may eventually lead to tethering and joint contractures. Firm longitudinal thickening and nodularity of the superficial tissues is usually readily appreciated. Surgical excision of the fibrotic bands is usually palliative. This condition should be referred to a skilled hand surgeon.

## INFECTIONS

All wounds of the hand with drainage should be Gram stained and cultured for aerobes and anaerobes. When obtaining a culture, one should take a cotton swab from the depth of the wound. In treating wounds of the hand, pulsatile jet lavage irrigation is the optimal method of irrigating the wound. Debridement should be used judiciously, particularly in dealing with wounds over areas with multiple structures. When dealing with an open acute hand injury, antibiotics should be used, particularly when contamination is expected. Most of the commonly encountered organisms are susceptible to a cephalosporin or a penicillinase-resistant penicillin analogue. In patients with a penicillin allergy, clindamycin or erythromycin may be used.

Infection becomes established with the development of cellulitis. When caught at this stage, the infection may be aborted by adequate tissue concentrations of appropriate antibiotics and immobilization. This may require hospital admission for intravenous therapy. The most common pathogen is *Staphylococcus aureus*. Animal bites may be contaminated with *Pasteurella multocida* and human bites with *Eikenella corrodens*.

The next stage of infection is abscess formation. Abscesses *always* require surgical drainage. With the exception of superficial subcutaneous abscesses, paronychia, and felon, this should usually be done by a qualified hand surgeon in the operating room. Some of the closed spaces of the hand will require extensive decompression and operative placement of irrigation catheters and drains for adequate management.

## Felon

A *felon* is a subcutaneous pyogenic infection of the pulp space of the fingertip. The septae of the fingerpad produce multiple individual compartments and confine the infection under pressure. The patient presents with marked throbbing pain. As the pressure within the pulp

space increases, perfusion is impaired, which can lead to pulp necrosis, osteomyelitis, and a draining sinus. Occasionally, even pyogenic arthritis or flexor tenosynovitis can occur. The most common organism is *S. aureus*.

A lateral approach is probably the best incision to use in draining these abscesses. This approach protects the neurovascular bundle. The incision should start 5 mm distal to the distal digital crease and continue just palmar to and parallel with the paronychium, stopping distally at the tip of the distal phalangeal tuft. The incision should be carried through deeply across the entire fingerpad, immediately palmar to the bone, dividing the septae of the fingerpad at their bony insertions, and decompressing each closed compartment (Fig. 239-3). Only occasionally will another incision be more appropriate, and more extensive incisions may produce increased instability of the fingerpad. Unless the placement is dictated by a pointing abscess, the radial aspects of the index and long fingers should be avoided, as should the ulnar aspects of the thumb and small fingers.

The wound should be kept open by loose packing and the finger and wrist splinted. The patient should be seen at 24 and 48 h. On the third day, the wick may be removed and warm soaks started.

## Paronychia

*Paronychia* is an infection of the lateral nail fold and occasionally involves the eponychium. The most common organisms are *S. aureus* and *Streptococcus*. When small, these infections are easily treated by placing a no. 11 blade parallel to and alongside the top of the nail, elevating the epithelium along the lateral nail fold. In very extensive infections, or where pus is observed beneath the nail, the corner of the paronychium should be incised, avoiding damage to the nail bed. A portion of the lateral or proximal nail may need to be removed and a small wick placed. This will drain the abscess (Fig. 239-4). Patients with a wick in place should be seen daily and the wick changed. After the wick is discontinued, warm soaks are continued for a few days. Antibiotics are not usually necessary.

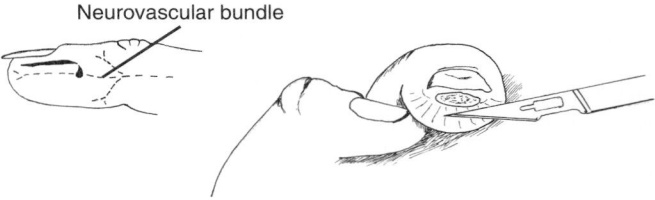

Neurovascular bundle

**Fig. 239-3.** A felon is incised using a lateral approach above (dorsal) the neurovascular bundle. This avoids disruption of the septal network that holds the fingertip to the phalanx.

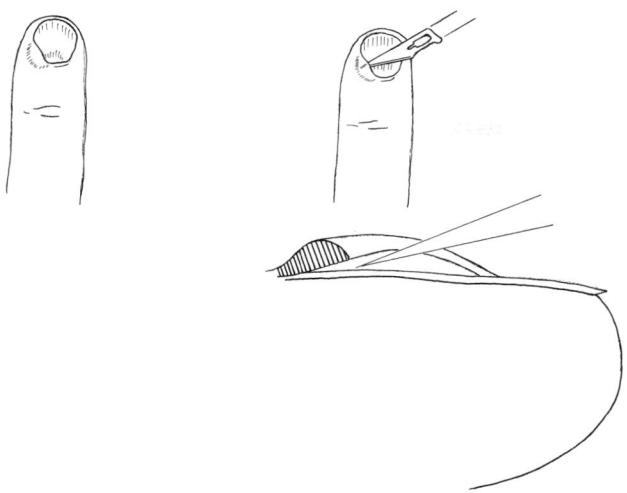

**Fig. 239-4.** In draining a paronychia, a no. 11 blade is placed on top of the nail using the tip to uplift the infected nail fold.

## Herpetic Whitlow

*Herpetic whitlow* is a viral infection in the fingertip involving intracutaneous vesicular bullae (Fig. 239-5). These patients are often thought to have felons; however, incision of herpetic whitlow, rather than being curative, may result in increased morbidity and prolonged failure to heal. Multiple digital involvement should suggest coxsackie virus. The mainstay of treatment is to prevent autoinoculation or transmission of the infection. A dry dressing should be used. Acyclovir has been used with success in recurrent infections.

## Pyogenic Flexor Tenosynovitis

Pyogenic flexor synovitis may be diagnosed by the classic clinical findings described by Kanavel. The four cardinal signs are tenderness over the flexor tendon sheath, symmetrical swelling of the finger,

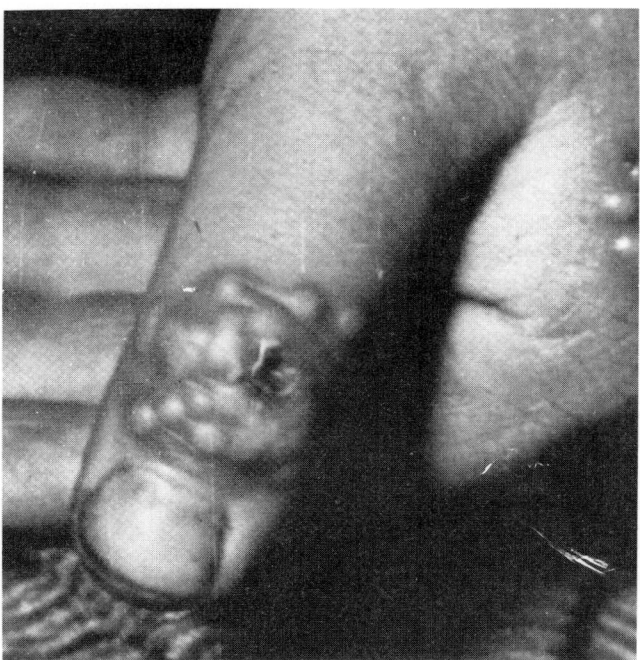

**Fig. 239-5.** Herpetic whitlow is shown. (From Domonkos AN: Clinical dermatology, in *Andrews' Diseases of the Skin.* Philadelphia: WB Saunders, 1971).

pain with passive extension, and flexed posture of the involved digit. The most common organisms are *S. aureus, Streptococcus,* and *Pseudomonas.* These patients must be admitted for splinting, elevation, and intravenous antibiotic therapy. They should be seen by a qualified hand surgeon on an emergent basis. Immediate surgical decompression of the tendon sheath and placement of irrigation catheters are usually necessary.

## Web Space Infections

Web space infections commonly occur following penetrating injuries in the web space between the digits. These patients present with dorsal and volar swelling of the web space, with separation of the digits. These infections must be treated promptly with intravenous antibiotics and drainage.

## Midpalmar Space Infections

The radial and ulnar bursa that extend into the palm of the hand can become infected, either from extension from a flexor tenosynovitis or from a penetrating wound to the palm. Occasionally, a horseshoe-configuration abscess can be seen because in 50 percent of patients there is communication between the radial and ulnar bursae. These infections must be diagnosed promptly and treated with incision and drainage in the operating room as well as intravenous antibiotics.

## Infections from a Human Bite to the Metaphalangeal Joint

A human bite to the MP joint is often called a clenched fist injury or a "fight bite." Infections in the MP joint secondary to a patient's striking an individual's teeth with a clenched fist can be devastating. The skin and extensor tendons may be involved. These infections have the potential of spreading into the dorsal subcutaneous space and involving the tendons of the extensor surface. Pyogenic arthritis and osteomyelitis from contamination of organisms present in human saliva can occur.

Treatment should be initiated immediately with the administration of tetanus prophylaxis. Wound swabs should be sent for Gram stain and culture of both aerobic and anaerobic organisms. The most common organisms isolated are α- and β-hemolytic *Streptococcus, S. aureus, E. corrodens,* and *Neisseria* species. Appropriate antibiotic coverage includes penicillin and a penicillinase-resistant semisynthetic effective against *Staphylococcus.* Erythromycin or clindamycin may be effective in the penicillin-allergic patient.

If the wound penetrates the skin, the joint should be inspected for cartilage damage in the operating room and should be irrigated with 2 L saline solution. A drain is left in the joint, and the wound is not closed. Extensor tendon repairs should be delayed for 5 days, or until the wound is clean. The original wound should be allowed to heal by secondary intention. When inspecting for tendon injury, put the hand in the fist position it was in when the injury occurred.

## BIBLIOGRAPHY

Green DP (ed). *Operative Hand Surgery,* 3d ed. New York: Churchill Livingstone, 1993.

Dawson DM. Entrapment neuropathies of upper extremities. *N Engl J Med* 329:2013, 1993.

Siegel DB, Gelberman RH. Infections of the hand. *Ortho Clin North Am* 19:779, 1988.

Szabo RM (ed). Common hand problems. *Ortho Clin North Am* 22(1), 1992.

Tubiana R. *Examination of the Hand and Upper Limb.* Philadelphia: WB Saunders, 1984.

# 240
# SOFT TISSUE PROBLEMS OF THE FOOT
**Frantz Melio**

## INTRODUCTION

In 1990 the National Center for Health Statistics conducted a National Health Interview Survey that included a list of the three most common podiatric problems: bunions, corns and calluses, and ingrown toenails. In response, 13.2 out of 1000 people reported being afflicted by bunions, 24.5 per 1000 with ingrown toenails, and 20 per 1000 with corns or calluses. Advanced age, poverty, and female gender were associated with increased risk for these diseases. It is thus apparent that chronic foot problems play an important role in U.S. health care.

## CORNS AND CALLUSES

Pressure or irritation causes focal hyperkeratotic lesions of the skin of the foot. The cause of these lesions can be external (poorly fitted shoe) or internal (bunion). These areas of epidermal accumulation are defined as *calluses*. Calluses serve a protective function and should not be treated if they are not painful. Calluses grow outward but are soon pushed inward by continued pressure and become corns. Corns also develop in areas of scarring and between toes. Corns are classified as hard or soft. Hard corns are seen over bony protuberances where the skin is dry. Soft corns are seen between toes where the skin is moist. Corns may be painful or painless, but pressure on the corn usually produces pain. Corns interrupt the normal dermal lines and can thus be differentiated from calluses. Hard corns may resemble warts; however, when pared, warts bleed and corns do not. Soft corns resemble tinea, which often leads to misdiagnosis and mistreatment.

Treatment of symptomatic lesions consists of paring with a no. 15 blade scalpel and application of a pad on or around the lesion to relieve pressure. Avoiding constrictive footwear is also important. Keratolytic agents are advocated by some authors but are thought to be too toxic and better avoided by others. Patients should be referred to a podiatrist, since therapy includes repeated paring and possibly surgery to correct any underlying source of pressure.

Keratotic lesions may be an indication of more severe underlying disease, deformity, local foot disorder, or mechanical problem. Other causes of keratotic lesions include syphilis, psoriasis, arsenic poisoning, rosacea, lichen planus, basal cell nevus syndrome, and, rarely, malignancies.

## PLANTAR WARTS

Plantar warts are caused by the human papilloma virus. These warts are fairly common and contagious. They may be painful and are usually found over bony prominences. Single lesions are endophytic and hyperkeratotic. A mother-daughter wart is similar to a single lesion except for a small vesicular satellite lesion. Mosaic warts are often painless, closely grouped, and may coalesce. Diagnosis is usually made clinically. There are many therapeutic options. Treatment is complicated by the fact that many of these lesions will resorb spontaneously within 2 years. These patients may require prolonged treatment in resistant cases and should be referred.

## TINEA PEDIS

The incidence of tinea pedis in industrialized countries has been estimated at 10 percent of the population. It has been estimated that in high-risk patients as many as 70 percent are affected. In the United States, $240 million per year is spent on products used to treat tinea pedis. Factors that predispose to infection include hot and humid climate, occlusive footwear, infrequent changes of socks or shoes, hyperhidrosis of the feet, conditions that lead to maceration of the feet, and repeated exposure of the feet to fungi combined with some form of minimal trauma. In high-risk groups, such as the elderly and immunocompromised patients, infections can become chronic and resistant to treatment and can disseminate. Tinea pedis can usually be prevented with proper hygiene. These measures include daily bathing and drying of feet, wearing absorbent socks and changing them daily, wearing shoes that "breathe" and changing them daily, wearing different footwear for sporting activities, and using drying agents and antifungals for prophylaxis in high-risk groups.

The causative fungal organisms of tinea pedis usually belong to the dermatophytes, with *Trichophyton rubrum* being the most frequently responsible, accounting for approximately 60 percent of cases. The *Microsporum* species, *Candida,* and saprophytic fungi also account for many occurrences.

Clinically tinea pedis appears in a variety of forms, ranging from mild scaling to acute inflammation. The most common form is interdigital infection. Interdigital presentation may be as benign as a fissure in the toe web, usually between the fourth and fifth toes. More commonly, the affected interspaces appear white, macerated, and soggy as a result of multiple simultaneous infections (dermatophyte and bacteria). These complex infections usually begin with dermatophyte infection of the toe web. The fungi produce antibiotics that select for an antibiotic-resistant bacterial population (both gram-positive and gram-negative). These bacteria induce further inflammation and damage to the epithelium. The bacteria also produce antifungal by-products and quickly predominate. It has now been recognized that these bacteria alone are also etiologic agents of tinea pedis. The more severe the infection, the more likely that other organisms such as yeast and saprophytic fungi are also involved. These lesions are pruritic and may become painful when the patient wears a closed shoe or exercises.

A second form of tinea pedis is the hyperkeratotic or moccasin-type infection. This is a chronic form of tinea that is characterized by scaly eruptions, fissuring, pruritus, erythema, and the absence of vesicles and pustules. It is usually limited to the weight-bearing surfaces of the feet and spares the intertriginous areas. *T. rubrum* is the most frequent causative organism.

The vesicular form is another common presentation of tinea pedis. This infection is characterized by vesicles and vesicopustules and is most commonly caused by *T. mentagrophytes, Epidermophyton floccosum,* and, rarely, *Microsporum.* The lesions usually begin on the non-weight-bearing areas of the soles and can extend along the entire plantar surface, to the intertriginous areas, up over the toes, and onto the dorsum of the foot. Patients experience a burning pain and pruritus. An ulcerative form of tinea may be the result of secondary pyogenic bacterial infection involving these vesicles.

Tinea infections must be differentiated from other lesions that affect the foot. Juvenile plantar dermatosis is a lesion frequently confused with tinea. Affected children have dry, cracked, red scaly patches on the toe pads and anterior plantar surface of the feet; the toe webs and insteps are spared. Treatment consists of lubricants and occlusion, with socks at night. Contact dermatitis is characterized by involvement of the dorsal surface of the feet, with well-demarcated, red patches that may contain tiny vesicles. Psoriasis presents as thick scaly lesions that spare the web spaces and affect the heel. Erythrasma is a low-grade chronic infection that may involve the web spaces. Symmetric patches are also present in the groin and axillae. These lesions fluoresce bright "coral red" under Wood's lamp examination. Pitted keratolysis is a diphtheroid bacterial infection which produces marked hyperkeratosis with multiple 1- to 3-mm punched-out pits on the plantar surface of the foot. Id reactions, which are immunologic reactions to antigenic products of fungal infections, may present as sterile vesicles.

Diagnosis of tinea pedis is made clinically. Fungal cultures, due to bacterial overgrowth and fungal suppression, are usually very low yield.

Due to the complexity of these infection, the ideal medication must be antifungal, antibacterial, and have local drying as well as anti-inflammatory properties. The imidazole group of antifungals (miconazole, clotrimazole, econazole, ketoconazole, oxiconazole, and sulcomazole) meet all these criteria and are also effective against *Candida.* These agents are an excellent choice for initial, empiric treatment of tinea pedis. Some of these medications are available in over-the-counter preparations. The role of topical glucocorticoids is controversial. While the anti-inflammatory properties are advocated, the inhibition of cellular defenses may prolong the duration of infection. More importantly, the low level of anti-inflammatory action that the imidazoles possess is usually sufficient.

Creams and solutions are most often appropriate when treating tinea. Ointments hold the active ingredient at the site longer but should not be used on oozing or moist lesions. Sprays may also be helpful; they evaporate quickly, leaving the medication on the surface for absorption.

Other aspects of therapy include proper hygiene such as daily foot cleaning, drying, and changes in socks and footwear. Application of drying agents such as aluminum chloride (Drysol) or aluminum acetate (Burow's solution and Domeboro) may assist in preventing hyperhidrosis and help control infection. Tight occlusive shoes should be avoided, and soft absorbent socks should be worn. High-risk patients should be told not to walk barefoot.

Most patients respond to the measures outlined above. However, some infections are resistant to conservative therapy and require prolonged oral antifungal medication. These patients would benefit from appropriate referral.

## ONYCHOMYCOSIS

Dermatophyte fungi are the most frequent cause of nail plate invasion, with *T. rubrum* being the most common organism. Other organisms that can lead to nail infection include *Scopulariopsis brevicaulis, Scytalidium* species, and *Candida.* Nail infections usually spread from surrounding infected skin. The infection can be either under or within the nail plate. If allowed to progress, these infections lead to severe disturbances in nail growth. The affected toenails appear opaque, discolored, and, at times, hyperkeratotic. Treatment of this disease process is complicated by the fact that topical antifungals are poorly absorbed through the nail. Treatment should, however, begin with an empiric trial of imidazole antifungals, especially if less than half of the nail is involved (in which case topical agents have been found to be more effective). Repeated debridement of the infected portion of nail is recommended. Patients should be referred for appropriate continued care as these lesions often require prolonged courses of oral antifungals and surgical or chemical removal of the nail matrix. Even with optimal treatment there is a very high recurrence rate. Autoavulsion and traumatic avulsion of involved toenails is common.

## ONYCHOCRYPTOSIS (INGROWN TOENAIL)

Ingrown toenails occur when a segment of the nail plate penetrates the nail sulcus and subcutaneous tissue. Curvature of the nail plate is the most common predisposing factor. The lesion usually occurs as a result of external trauma or self-treatment. Onychocryptosis is characterized by inflammation, swelling, and infection of the medial or lateral aspect of the toenail. The great toe is the most commonly affected. Protracted infection may result in periungual ulcerative granulation. In patients with underlying diabetes or arterial insufficiency, cellulitis, ulceration, and necrosis may lead to amputation if treatment

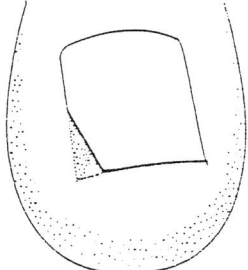

**Fig. 240-1.** Partial toenail removal. (From Roberts JR et al (eds): *Clinical Procedures in Emergency Medicine*, 2d ed. Philadelphia, Saunders, 1991, with permission.)

is delayed. If infection is not present at the time of presentation, simple elevation of the nail with placement of a wisp of cotton between the nail plate and the skin, daily foot soaks, and avoidance of pressure on the nail is usually sufficient treatment. Another option, if no infection is present, is to remove a small spicule of the offending nail. A digital block is placed as described below. The area is cleaned, and the skin is prepared for surgical procedure. An oblique portion of the affected nail is trimmed about one- to two-thirds of the way back to the posterior nail fold. The nail groove should then be debrided, and a nonadherent dressing placed (Fig. 240-1).

If granulation or infection is present, then partial removal of the nail plate is indicated. This is performed by placing a digital block and preparing the area for a surgical procedure. The entire affected area, one-quarter or less of the nail plate, is cut longitudinally (anterior to posterior), including the portion of the nail beneath the cuticle. English anvil scissors or a nail splitter are the optimal instruments for cutting the nail. The affected cut portion of the nail is then grasped with a hemostat and, using a rocking motion, removed from the nail groove. The nail groove is then debrided and a dressing is placed (Fig. 240-2).

One may also cauterize the exposed nail plate. An 88% phenol mixture can be applied for 30 s with a cotton-tipped applicator. The phenol is then rinsed with an alcohol solution. Any phenol that comes in contact with healthy tissues must be removed immediately. Silver

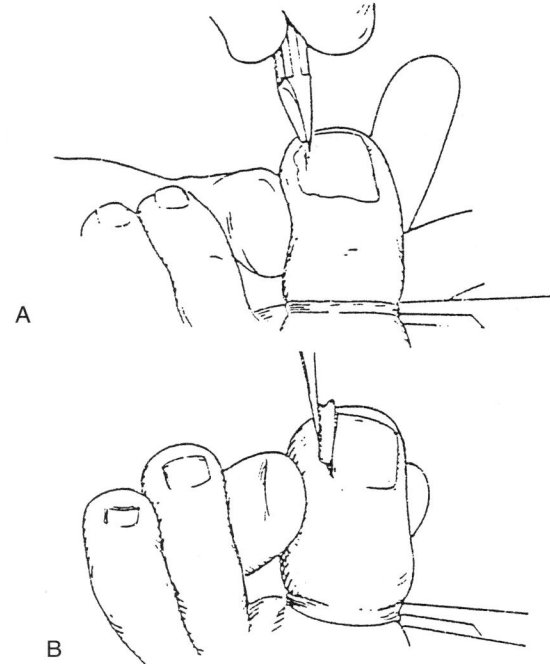

**Fig. 240-2.** Partial toenail removal (infection present).

nitrate may also be used to cauterize the area and should be left on the nail matrix for 1 min. Cauterization is not without risk, as these chemicals may cause extensive tissue destruction. Hemostasis is also extremely important in order to avoid inadvertent absorption of these toxins. Generally, cauterization should be performed only by those with appropriate experience in this procedure.

Once the procedure is completed, a nonadherent gauze or antibiotic ointment should be placed on the wound. A bulky dressing should then be placed on the toe. The wound should be checked in 24–48h.

## OTHER NAIL LESIONS

Other common toenail afflictions include paronychia and subungual hematoma, which are treated similarly to when they occur in the fingers. Hyperkeratotic toenails can be a problem in the elderly. These may become so severe as to affect gait and cause ulcerations and infections. Patients with these lesions require referral for repeated trimming or nail plate removal.

## BURSITIS

There are many bursae in the foot, all of which may become a source of pain. Pathologic bursae can be divided into noninflammatory, inflammatory, suppurative, and calcified. Noninflammatory bursae are usually pressure-induced and are found over bony prominences. Inflammatory bursae are commonly due to gout, syphilis, or rheumatoid arthritis. Suppurative bursitis is due to the invasion of the bursae, usually from adjacent wounds, by pyogenic organisms (primarily staphylococcal species). Acute bursitis can lead to the formation of a hygroma or calcified bursae. In severe cases, pressure on bursae can lead to fistula and ulcer formation. Diagnosis of these lesions is dependent on analysis of bursal fluid, which can be obtained by large-bore needle aspiration. Fluid should be sent for cell count; protein, glucose, and lactate (elevated in septic bursitis) levels; crystal analysis; and Gram stain as well as culture (since initial Gram stains are often negative). Treatment of the bursitis depends on its cause. In all cases one should avoid further pressure to the area by instructing the patients to be non-weight-bearing. Septic bursitis should be initially treated with a penicillinase-resistant semisynthetic penicillin while awaiting culture results. Repeated aspiration or incision and drainage may become necessary.

## PLANTAR FASCIITIS

Plantar fasciitis is an inflammation of the plantar aponeurosis. The plantar fascia's main function is to anchor the plantar skin to the bone, thus protecting the longitudinal arch of the foot. The cause of plantar fasciitis is usually overuse in the physically active patient or in the patient unaccustomed to activity. Other causes include abnormal joint mechanics, abnormal foot position and anatomy, and obesity. In the younger patient, collagen vascular diseases and rheumatic diseases can lead to this entity. Patients present with pain on the plantar surface of the foot that is worse on arising and after physical activity. Examination usually reveals a point of deep tenderness at the anterior medial aspect of the calcaneus, the point of attachment of the plantar fascia. Short-term treatment consists of rest, ice, nonsteroidal anti-inflammatory agents, ultrasound therapy, or local glucocorticoid injections. Long-term therapy consists of proper foot support and possibly surgery.

## GANGLIONS

Ganglion is a common benign synovial cyst. These lesions are 1.5 to 2.5 cm in diameter and are often attached to a joint capsule or tendon sheath. Although ganglions typically occur in the wrist, they may also occur in the foot. These lesions typically arise in the anterolateral aspect of the ankle but can occur in many areas of the foot. The pathogenesis of these lesions is unknown. The two most popular theories are (1) that they are produced by herniation of the tendon sheath, and (2) that they arise from focal myxomatous degeneration of collagenous tissues caused by trauma. Ganglions may appear suddenly or gradually, may enlarge and diminish in size, and may be painful or asymptomatic. On examination one notes a firm, usually nontender, cystic lesion. Diagnosis is made clinically, although ultrasound and MRI are useful. Aspiration and instillation of glucocorticoids leads to the complete resolution of ganglions in some cases. Most ganglions require complete surgical excision.

## TENDON LESIONS

Tenosynovitis and tendinitis may occur in the foot, usually due to overuse. Patients present with pain over the involved tendon. The flexor hallucis longus, posterior tibialis, and Achilles tendon are most commonly involved. Treatment consists of rest, ice, and oral anti-inflammatory agents.

Tendon lacerations are usually traumatic. The usual mechanism of injury is a cut to the dorsal or plantar aspect of the foot. Tendon lacerations should be explored and repaired if the ends of the tendon are visible in the wound. The foot should be casted in dorsiflexion after the repair of extensor tendons, and in equinus after repair of flexor tendons. Unfortunately, tendon repairs in the foot have a relatively high complication and disability rate. Specialty consultation is often appropriate.

Spontaneous rupture of the Achilles, tibialis anterior, and posterior tibialis tendons is fairly common. Diagnosis and proper treatment of tendon ruptures is aided by CT scanning and MRI studies. Orthopedic consultation should be obtained to aid in proper therapeutic decisions. Achilles tendon ruptures are usually due to forceful dorsiflexion and occur more commonly in males. Patients present with pain, a palpable defect in the area of the tendon, and inability to stand on tiptoes. Squeezing the calf of the prone patient whose knee is flexed at 90° will normally cause the foot to plantar flex. This response will be absent in patients with Achilles tendon ruptures. Treatment is surgical in younger patients and conservative (casting in equinus) in older patients.

Ruptures of the anterior tibialis tendon are rare. These usually occur after the fourth decade and are not excessively painful. Patients present with varying degrees of footdrop and a palpable defect distal to the ankle joint in the area of the tendon. In most cases, disability is minimal and surgery is not necessary.

Spontaneous ruptures of the posterior tibialis tendon also occur after the fourth decade. Two-thirds of these cases occur in women. The presentation is usually chronic and insidious. Patients notice a gradual flattening of their arch, with modest discomfort and swelling over their medial ankle. Examination reveals absence of the tendon's normal prominence and weakness on inversion of the foot. Patients find it impossible to stand on tiptoes. Treatment may be conservative or surgical, depending on the duration of the tear and activity of the patient.

Another tendon rupture of note is rupture of the flexor hallucis longus, which presents as a loss of plantar flexion of the great toe. This lesion must be repaired in ballet dancers but not in the nonathlete.

## PLANTAR INTERDIGITAL NEUROMA (MORTON'S NEUROMA)

Neuromas may form in a plantar digital nerve, usually proximal to its bifurcation. These neuromas may occur in any of the digital nerves but are most common in the third interspace. The cause of these lesions is thought to be local irritation of the nerve due to entrapment, usually from tight-fitting shoes. Women between the ages of 25 and 50 years are the most commonly affected group. Patients present with pain located in the area of the metatarsal head. The pain is described as burning, cramping, or aching. Pain is worsened by ambulation and resolved by rest and removal of shoes. The pain may radiate to the affected toes, and patients may note numbness in the toes. Pain is usually easily reproduced upon palpation of the area, and at times a mass is felt. Diagnosis is usually made clinically, but nerve conduction studies, electromyograms, and MRI may be helpful at times. Conservative treatment consists of wearing wide shoes with good metatarsal head supports and metatarsal head off-loading inserts. Local glucocorticoid injections can be curative. Conservative therapy is often unsuccessful, and patients may ultimately require surgical intervention.

## COMPARTMENT SYNDROME

Compartment syndromes have been more commonly described to affect the arms and legs. Nine compartments have been identified in the foot. Compartment syndrome occurs when an elevation of tissue pressure within one of these nonyielding fascial compartments impedes vascular flow. In the foot, the cause of compartment syndrome is usually a high-energy injury associated with multiple fractures. Crush injuries are more likely to cause compartment syndrome. Compartment syndromes have been reported in association with midfoot fractures and rearfoot fractures, burns, contusions, bleeding disorders, postischemic swelling after arterial injury or thrombosis, venous obstruction, exercise, and prolonged pressure to the affected area. There have also been reports of chronic compartment syndromes due to overuse. Patients typically present with severe acute pain that is worsened on active or passive movement, swelling, paresthesias, and neurovascular deficits. The only reliable method to diagnose compartment syndrome is by obtaining intracompartmental pressures. Once the diagnosis is made, fasciotomy should be performed emergently. The sequelae of compartment syndrome range from transient neurologic compromise to complete myoneural necrosis, fibrosis, and ischemic contractures. The prognosis of compartment syndrome is directly related to the time delay in diagnosis and treatment.

## PUNCTURE WOUND

Puncture wounds occur most often to the plantar surface of the foot. The outcome of these wounds depends primarily on the depth of the wound. Other factors that influence the prognosis of these wounds include the penetrating material, location, footwear at the time of injury, time from injury, and underlying health of the affected individual. The evaluation and treatment of these patients follows the premises of basic wound care.

The wound must be meticulously explored for joint involvement and any retained foreign body (including metal, wood, rubber, and cloth), which must be removed. Radiologic examination, and in some cases CT scanning or MRI, may be indicated. Ultrasound has been found to be useful in identifying radiolucent foreign bodies. Fluoroscopy may aid in removal of radiopaque foreign bodies. A recent report has advocated the use of an eye magnet for removal of metallic foreign bodies. Foreign body removal in the foot is often a very frustrating and time-consuming experience. One must be careful not to cause excessive tissue damage, especially to the weight-bearing areas of the foot, as this may lead to painful scarring and permanent disability. In some cases specialty referral may be indicated for exploration and foreign-body removal.

Once foreign bodies have been excluded or removed, the wounds should be cleaned, irrigated, and closed. Antibiotics are indicated for infected wounds. Wounds that occur through the soles of sneakers are prone to pseudomonal infections. Antibiotics used in these wounds should be active against skin flora as well as *Pseudomonas*.

Recurrent infection, deep soft tissue tenderness, and increased soft tissue swelling raise the possibility of retained foreign body and deep tissue infection. These patients require specialty referral and should be considered for additional studies and admission.

## IMMERSION FOOT (TRENCH FOOT)

Immersion foot is the result of prolonged exposure of the foot to a moist, nonfreezing (but below 60°F, 15.56°C), occlusive environment. Immersion foot is classically seen in military operations, but the homeless civilian population is also particularly at risk. Prolonged cooling of the extremities produces direct soft tissue injury, with the peripheral nerves being most affected. Wet conditions accelerate the injury, as do factors that reduce circulation to the extremities. These factors include constrictive footwear, prolonged immobilization, hypothermia, smoking, dehydration, nutritional deficiencies, trauma, and underlying disease. When first seen, the injured area is pale, anesthetic, pulseless, immobile, but not frozen. After several hours of rewarming, a vigorous hyperemia develops associated with severe burning pain and reappearance of proximal sensation. Edema and bullae, at times sanguinous, may develop as perfusion increases. This hyperemic phase may last weeks, and hyperhidrosis is a prominent late feature. Patients may develop fever and lymphadenopathy. The injury evolves slowly, and anesthesia may be permanent. Differential diagnosis includes cellulitis and fungal infections. Treatment is conservative and includes admission for bedrest, leg elevation, and air drying of feet at room temperature. Antibiotics play little or no role in the recovery process but should be given if superinfection is present.

## PLANTAR FIBROMATOSIS

Plantar fibromatosis, or Dupuytren's contracture of the plantar fascia, does not occur as commonly as in the hand. Plantar fibromatosis is a disorder of fibrous tissue proliferation, which slowly invades the skin and soft tissues. Presentation is generally in adolescence or young adulthood. Patients present with small (0.5 to 1.0 cm), asymptomatic, palpable, slowly enlarging, fixed, firm masses on the plantar aspect of one or both feet. These lesions tend to be in the non-weight-bearing areas of the foot. Toe contractures do not occur. These lesions have a tendency to reabsorb spontaneously. Treatment is conservative, and only rarely is surgery indicated. These patients should be referred to the appropriate consultant for continued care.

## FOOT ULCERS

Foot ulcers can generally be classified as neuropathic or ischemic by the predominant etiologic factor and clinical features. Infection can be a complicating factor in either type of ulcer. Diabetics are prone to both types of ulcers and in addition are more apt to develop infections. It has been estimated that proper foot care in diabetics (including prophylaxis and treatment of foot ulcers) could reduce the number of lower limb amputations by 44 to 80 percent.

Ischemic ulcers are secondary to vascular compromise, usually due to atherosclerosis of larger vessels. Ulcers rarely develop due to problems with the microcirculation in an area. These ulcers are seen in the setting of a cool foot, dependent rubor, pallor on elevation, atrophic shiny skin, and diminished pulses. Patients may complain of symptoms of intermittent claudication and leg pain in the supine position, relieved by dependency. If the underlying vascular disease is corrected, these ulcers usually heal quickly. Without reconstructive surgery, the prognosis is poor and amputation is often inevitable.

Neuropathic ulcers are essentially pressure ulcers. Patients at risk are those with absent or distorted foot sensation. These include patients with diabetes, leprosy, tabes dorsalis, and other congenital or acquired neuropathies. These feet are prone to ischemia from pressure by ill-fitting shoes, foreign bodies, abnormal bony prominences, and most commonly from the daily stresses of walking. The ulcers are usually well circumscribed with surrounding white calluslike material. The foot (if there is no underlying vascular disease) has normal temperature, color, and pulses. Defects in touch, pressure, or proprioception are noted on examination. Motor weakness and muscular atrophy may also be present. These changes can lead to abnormal gait and foot anatomy.

Once an ulcer becomes infected, two aspects of therapy are essential for healing: thorough debridement and complete pressure relief. Debridement must be aggressive; wet-to-dry dressing changes are not sufficient. Once debridement is completed, the role of wet-to-dry dressings is controversial. These dressings may prevent drying of the ulcer and eschar formation. To date, no topical agents or foot soak has been conclusively found to be beneficial for the healing of diabetic ulcers. Relief of pressure is accomplished by either complete bed rest or by total contact casting.

Antibiotics and often admission are warranted for the treatment of infected ulcers. Infections are usually polymicrobial. The most common organisms are *Staphylococcus aureus* and beta-hemolytic streptococci. Other organisms found in diabetic foot ulcers are various species of Enterobacteriaceae and anaerobes, enterococci, and *P. aeruginosa.* Superficial cultures of infected ulcers are unreliable. Cultures should be obtained of any purulent drainage and of aspirates from fluctuant areas. Antibiotics should initially be broad spectrum to cover the wide variety of possible infective organisms. Choices include combinations of clindamycin with an aminoglycoside, cefoxitin, ticarcillin disodium and clavulanate potassium, imipenem plus cilastatin, and ampicillin plus sublactam. Cellulitis and signs of deep soft tissue infection require hospitalization for antibiotics and strict bed rest. Abscesses should be incised and drained. X-rays should be considered if there is any suspicion of subcutaneous gas, foreign body, osteomyelitis, and Charcot foot. With diabetics, a serum glucose level should be obtained, as it is often elevated. Patients with nonhealing foot ulcers should undergo evaluation to determine the underlying etiology of the ulcer (vascular, diabetic, or other systemic disease). Hyperbaric oxygen has been advocated by some as beneficial in the treatment of both infected and noninfected foot ulcers.

## MALIGNANT MELANOMA

The incidence of malignant melanoma is increasing, thus making consideration of this disease process important. Malignant melanoma of the foot accounts for up to 15 percent of all cutaneous melanomas. Melanomas can present as an atypical, pigmented, or nonhealing lesion of the foot, including the nail. These malignancies often imitate more common foot disorders such as fungal infections and plantar warts. Since prognosis is directly related to early diagnosis, a high index of suspicion must be maintained. All skin lesions that are either atypical or not healing despite treatment should be referred for biopsy.

## FOOT LESIONS INDICATIVE OF DISSEMINATED DISEASE

Many disease processes may be manifest by foot lesions. Acquired immunodeficiency syndrome may present with a variety of foot lesions, including Kaposi sarcoma and nonhealing ulcers and those caused by bacterial and fungal infections such as histoplasmosis (which can present as maculopapular eruptions or depressed pits of the soles). These patients may develop neuropathies presenting as both paresthesias and dysesthesias. Secondary syphilis presents as a nonitching polymorphic rash that affects both the soles and palms. The rash of Rocky Mountain spotted fever, which is initially discrete, macular, and later petechial, is also found on the palms and soles. Cutaneous forms of tuberculosis have also been described that affect the feet. Hand-foot-and-mouth disease causes small vesicular lesions on the soles, palms, buttocks, and in the mouth. This entity is caused by coxsackievirus and occurs in the late summer and fall.

## NERVE BLOCKS OF THE FOOT

Nerve blocks of the foot are useful when either extensive lacerations are present or removal of foreign bodies is necessary. The sensory in-

nervation of the foot is provided primarily by five major nerves. The majority of the plantar surface is innervated by the posterior tibial nerve. A small portion of the medial aspect of the plantar surface is innervated by the saphenous nerve, while sensation to some of the lateral plantar aspect is supplied by the sural nerve. The dorsum of the foot is innervated by the deep and superficial peroneal, sural, and saphenous nerves. The superficial peroneal nerve supplies a broad central band. The medial surface is supplied by the saphenous nerve, while the lateral surface is supplied by the sural nerve. The deep peroneal nerve innervates the dorsal aspect of the web space between the first and second toes (Fig. 240-3). The toes are innervated by digital nerves, which arise on the dorsal and volar aspects of the toes. The nerves are in close proximity to the bone and lie in the 2, 4, 8, and 10 o'clock positions.

To minimize patient risks and discomfort during nerve blocks, several measures should be implemented. A 1-in (2.5 cm) 30-gauge needle will anesthetize a large area while minimizing pain on insertion. Raising an intradermal wheal before injecting more deeply will make the procedure more comfortable. One should always aspirate before injection to avoid intravascular administration of anesthetic. The practice of eliciting nerve paresthesias during a nerve block should be avoided because of the risk of permanent nerve damage. Adequate blocks can be obtained by allowing time for the anesthetic to infiltrate and by massaging the anesthetic into the surrounding tissues. The choice of anesthetic agents should be based on the risks and possible complications in individual patients. Lidocaine is reliable and has a rapid onset but short duration. Bupivacaine has slower onset but has the potential advantage of longer duration. The addition of epinephrine to the anesthetic has the advantage of prolonging the duration of the anesthetic but must be avoided when performing digital blocks. One must also consider that in patients with chronic foot problems, the circulation to areas of the foot is already tenuous and epinephrine is best avoided. Addition of bicarbonate into the anesthetic will also reduce the pain and burning associated with these blocks.

The posterior tibial nerve block is best performed with the patient prone. A needle is inserted at the level of the upper half of the medial malleolus, just posterior to the posterior tibial artery and medial to the Achilles tendon. The needle is directed at a right angle to the tibia, toward the posterior tibial surface; it is then advanced to the bone and withdrawn 0.1 to 1.0 cm while 3 to 4 mL of anesthetic is injected (Fig. 240-4).

A sural nerve block is also performed with the patient prone. The needle is inserted near the lateral border of the Achilles tendon 1 cm below the lateral malleolar prominence. The needle is directed toward the inferior aspect of the lateral malleolus and advanced approximately 1 cm before 3 to 4 mL of anesthetic is injected. Alternatively, 5 to 10 mL of anesthetic is injected subcutaneously between the Achilles tendon and the lateral malleolus at the level of an imaginary line drawn between the malleoli (see Fig. 240-4).

The saphenous nerve is blocked by injecting 3 to 4 mL of anesthetic into the subcutaneous tissues medial to the saphenous vein just above the medial malleolus. An alternative method is to inject 3 to 5 mL of anesthetic subcutaneously between the medial malleolus and the anterior tibialis tendon at the level of an imaginary line drawn between the malleoli (Fig. 240-5).

The superficial peroneal nerve is blocked by injecting 3 to 4 mL of anesthetic into the subcutaneous tissues midway between the anterior tibial surface and the lateral malleolus, or by injecting 4 to 10 mL subcutaneously in a band between the lateral malleolus and the extensor hallucis longus at the level of an imaginary line drawn between the malleoli (see Fig. 240-5).

The deep peroneal nerve is blocked by inserting a needle lateral to the dorsalis pedis artery between the anterior tibialis and extensor hallucis longus tendons, just above an imaginary line drawn between the malleoli. The needle is advanced to the bone, then

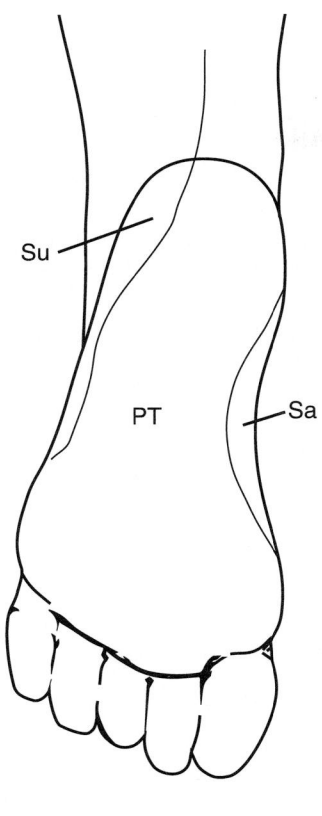

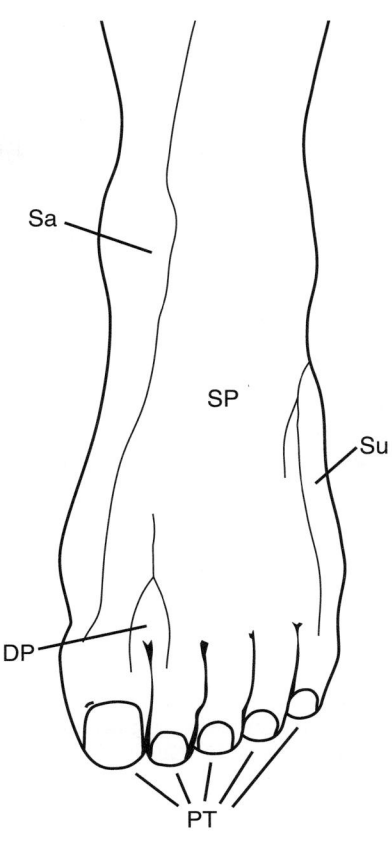

A                                              B

**Fig. 240-3.** Innervation of the foot. DP, deep peroneal nerve; PT, posterior tibial nerve; Sa, saphenous nerve; Su, sural nerve; SP, superficial peroneal nerve.

withdrawn 2 mm and 5 to 6 mL of anesthetic is injected (see Fig. 240-5).

Digital blocks can be performed by a variety of techniques. Since at the toes the nerves are in such close proximity to the bones, the preferred location for digital blocks is at the web space. A wheal is

placed on the dorsal surface of the toe, which serves to block the dorsal nerve and minimize the pain of further injection, then a needle is advanced just lateral to the bone until the volar skin is tented. Anesthetic is then injected as the needle is withdrawn. The same procedure

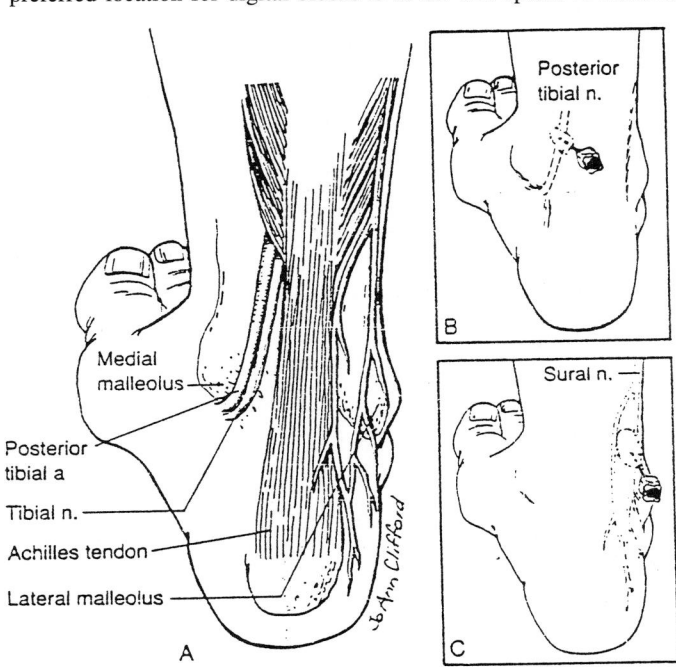

**Fig. 240-4.** Posterior tibial and sural nerve blocks.

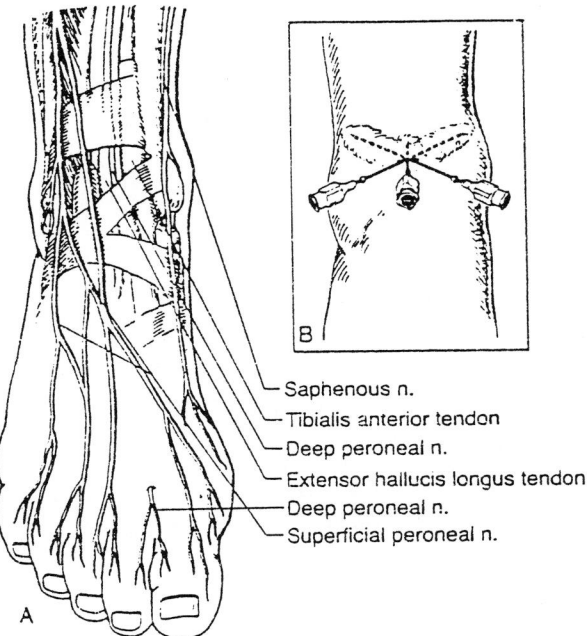

**Fig. 240-5.** Deep peroneal, saphenous, and superficial peroneal nerve blocks.

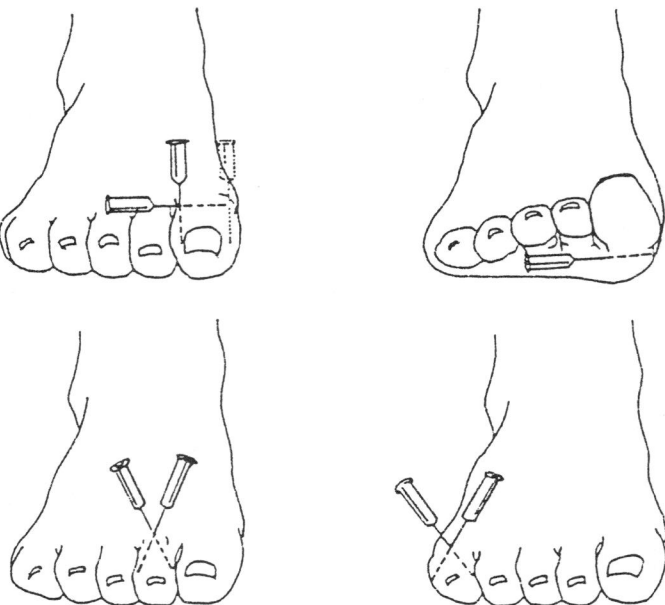

**Fig. 240-6.** Digital blocks.

is repeated on the medial aspect of the bone. Alternatively, a wheal is raised on the medial aspect of the toe just lateral to the bone, and the needle is directed inferiorly at a right angle until the volar skin is tented. Anesthetic is injected as the needle is withdrawn. The needle is then introduced into the same wheal and directed across the dorsum of the toe until it tents the lateral aspect of the dorsum of the toe. Anesthetic is injected as the needle is withdrawn. The same procedure is repeated on the lateral and volar aspect of the toe (Fig. 240-6).

## BIBLIOGRAPHY

American Diabetic Association: Foot care in patients with diabetes mellitus. *Diabetes Care* 16(suppl 2):19, 1993.

Birrer RB, Dellacorte MP: Skin and nail disorders of the foot. *Emerg Med* 25:27, 1993.

Bocka JJ, Godfrey J: Emergency department use of an eye magnet for the removal of soft tissue foreign bodies. *Ann Emerg Med* 23:350, 1994.

Burns S: Podiatric manifestations of AIDS. *J Am Podiatr Med Assoc* 80:15, 1990.

Cohen SJ, Roenigk RK: Nerve blocks for cutaneous surgery on the foot. *J Dermatol Surg Oncol* 17:527, 1991.

Glover MG: Plantar warts. *Foot Ankle* 11:172, 1990.

Helfand AE: Nail and hyperkeratotic problems in the elderly foot. *Am Fam Physician* 39:101, 1989.

Hernandez PA, Hernandez WA, Hernandez A: Clinical aspects of bursae and tendon sheaths of the foot. *J Am Podiatr Med Assoc* 81:366, 1991.

Jahss MH: *Disorders of the Foot: Medical and Surgical Management,* 2d ed. Philadelphia, Saunders, 1991.

Keyser JE: Foot wounds in diabetic patients: A comprehensive approach incorporating use of topical growth factors. *Postgrad Med* 91:98, 1992.

Lee TH, Wapner KL, Hecht PJ: Plantar fibromatosis. *J Bone Joint Surg* 75-A:1080, 1993.

Levy LA: Prevalence of chronic podiatric conditions in the US: National Health Survey 1990. *J Am Podiatr Med Assoc* 82:221, 1992.

Malusky LP: Podiatric procedures, in Roberts JR, Hedges JR (eds): *Clinical Procedures in Emergency Medicine,* 2d ed. Philadelphia, Saunders, 1991, pp 810–824.

McBride A, Cohen BA: Tinea pedis in children. *Am J Dis Child* 146:844, 1992.

McGlamry ED, Banks AS, Downey MS (eds): *Comprehensive Textbook of Foot Surgery,* 2d ed. Baltimore, Williams & Wilkins, 1992.

Miller G, James JH: Malignant melanoma of the foot. *Practitioner* 234:647, 1990.

Miller OF: Essentials of pressure ulcer treatment: The diabetic experience. *J Dermatol Surg Oncol* 19:759, 1993.

Myerson M, Manoli A: Compartment syndromes of the foot after calcaneal fractures. *Clin Orthop* 290:142, 1993.

Page JC, Abramson C, Wei-Li L, et al: Diagnosis and treatment of tinea pedis: A review and update. *J Am Podiatr Med Assoc* 81:304, 1991.

Regnauld B: *The Foot: Pathology, Aetiology, Semiology, Clinical Investigation and Therapy,* Elson R (ed and trans). Berlin, Springer, 1986.

Silverskiold JP: Common foot problems: Relieving the pain of bunions, keratoses, corns and calluses. *Postgrad Med* 89:183, 1991.

Viladot A: Morton's neuroma. *Int Orthop* 16:294, 1992.

Wedel DJ, Brown DL: Nerves blocks, in Miller RD (ed): *Anesthesia,* 3d ed. New York, Churchill Livingstone, 1990.

Wrenn K: Immersion foot: A problem of the homeless in the 1990s. *Arch Intern Med* 151:785, 1990.

Wu KK: Ganglions of the foot. *J Foot Ankle Surg* 32:343, 1993.

## 241
## BEHAVIORAL DISORDERS: CLINICAL FEATURES

### Stephen C. Olson
### Douglas A. Rund

Psychiatric disorders are common in the emergency department patient population. Estimates of the proportion of emergency department patients who present with a psychiatric disorder range from a few percent to more than a third. This variability is partly due to differences in patient population and utilization of alternatives for psychiatric crisis intervention. When patients are screened for mental disorders including substance abuse, many patients have unrecognized psychopathology that is relevant to their assessment and treatment in the emergency setting. Subgroups of the emergency patient population at higher risk for psychiatric disorders include those who are self-referred for nonurgent problems, patients with chest pain, and the "after midnight" group of emergency department patients, who had more psychiatric illness (56 percent) than a daytime group (20 percent). Sometimes, psychiatric disorders clearly make up the primary reason for an individual's presentation to an emergency department. In other cases, psychiatric disorders lead to injury and illness. Such conditions then create the need for emergency care. As screening studies have shown, psychiatric disorders may form part of the current or past medical history of a patient yet possess little importance for the immediate clinical condition.

In studies that report categories of psychiatric illness seen in the emergency department, the most prominent diagnoses are substance abuse, affective disorders, anxiety disorders, antisocial personality disorder, and severe cognitive impairment. Among repeat users of the emergency department, persons with schizophrenia are overrepresented.

Psychiatric disorders can cause substantial impairment in social or occupational functioning or marked distress. Patients or their families are often unwilling to seek pyschiatric care because of the stigma of mental illness. Their evaluation in the emergency department is their point of entry into the health care system. Also, due to poor judgment, financial considerations, or cognitive impairment, many psychiatric patients do not regularly seek medical attention until an emergency intervenes. They then seek emergency treatment for their medical needs. The most serious manifestations of mental illness (suicide, psychosis, and violent behavior) are medical emergencies and consequently are appropriately dealt with in the emergency department. Emergency physicians require substantial knowledge and skill to be able to recognize psychiatric disorders, perform crisis intervention and stabilization, and refer the patient for psychiatric hospitalization or outpatient care as needed.

## DIAGNOSIS

In the assessment of patients presenting with psychiatric symptoms, as with other medical conditions encountered in the emergency room, it is more crucial for the emergency physician to promptly stabilize the patient's acute condition and evaluate the major complaint immediately. Formulating a specific diagnosis must necessarily follow initial stabilization procedures in this clinical process. The determination that an individual is suicidal and in need of hospitalization, for instance, is more important than deciding whether that person suffers from schizophrenia or psychotic depression.

Nevertheless, provisional psychiatric diagnoses can be made in the emergency department. Recognition of specific behavioral syndromes can assist the emergency physician in evaluating the presenting complaint, pursuing associated symptoms, and determining treatment and disposition. Emergency physicians should be sufficiently familiar with commonly seen psychiatric illnesses to describe their predominant clinical features.

### Structured Diagnostic Criteria

Over the past 15 years, awareness of the earlier unreliability of psychiatric diagnosis guided the development of operational criteria for separate and distinct mental disorders. These rules allow researchers and clinicians to agree on the presence or absence of a particular disorder. In addition, the criteria are based on observable signs and the patient's report of symptoms, not on unconscious psychic mechanisms. This simplifies the task of diagnosis for emergency physicians and other nonpsychiatrists because extensive knowledge of pathophysiology and unconscious mental processes is not essential.

The current official diagnostic nomenclature, published in 1994 by the American Psychiatric Association, is the *Diagnostic and Statistical Manual of Mental Disorders,* fourth edition, commonly known as DSM-IV. A copy of DSM-IV should be available for reference in the emergency department because it contains not only the list of criteria for each disorder, but also additional material on demographics, associated symptoms and syndromes, and differential diagnosis.

### Multiaxial Diagnostic System

The DSM-IV diagnoses are made on a multiaxial system in which each axis refers to a different domain of information. This system aids in making a comprehensive assessment, organizing complex clinical information, and communicating between professionals. The Axis I disorders comprise the clinical syndromes of mental disorder. Conditions listed on Axis II are the personality disorders and developmental disorders, including mental retardation, which may underlie the more florid Axis I syndrome. Axis III notes general medical conditions. Axes IV and V record psychosocial stressors and adaptive functioning. It is generally unnecessary for the emergency physician to make a complete multiaxial diagnosis, but knowledge of this system may facilitate an understanding of medical records and psychiatric consultants' notes. For instance, a patient with previous medical records containing DSM-IV diagnoses of Axis I: alcohol intoxication; Axis II: antisocial personality disorder; Axis III: scalp laceration should be recognized as likely to display features of the Axis II personality disorder, although the patient's chief complaint may be a new problem.

## PSYCHIATRIC SYNDROMES (AXIS I DISORDERS)

The organization and major categories of Axis I disorders covered here are listed in Table 241-1. A useful strategy for making a DSM-IV diagnosis is to classify the primary feature into a major category,

**Table 241-1.** Axis I Disorders

Delirium, dementia, and amnestic and other cognitive disorders
Substance disorders
Mental disorders due to a general medical condition
Schizophrenia and other psychotic disorders
Mood disorders
Anxiety disorders
Somatoform disorders
Factitious disorders
Dissociative disorders
Eating disorders
Adjustment disorders

consider possible nonpsychiatric etiologies for the complaint, and then use the decision trees in Appendix B of the DSM-IV manual to identify the appropriate diagnosis. The decision trees guide the clinician who is unfamiliar with the intricacies of the criteria within a category to identify the features that distinguish closely related conditions.

## Delirium, Dementia, and Amnestic and Other Cognitive Disorders

This group of syndromes is characterized by a clinically significant deficit in cognitive or memory function due to a general medical condition. There are several distinct and common causes of organic brain syndromes in which the causative factor is known, for example, vascular dementia and alcohol withdrawal delirium. In these cases, the specific diagnosis is listed in DSM-IV. In other cases, the etiologic factor should be specified using the descriptor "due to [general medical disorder or substance]," for example, "delirium due to hepatic encephalopathy."

### Dementia

The essential clinical feature of *dementia* is a pervasive disturbance of cognitive functioning in several areas including memory, abstract thinking, judgment, personality, and other higher cortical functions such as language. If clouding of consciousness is present, then the patient does not have solely a dementing illness, but has *delirium* or intoxication. The presence of global cognitive impairment may be detected by a bedside cognitive examination such as the Mini Mental State Examination and additional confirmatory history should be gathered from an informant such as a family member. Memory disturbance is usually the earliest sign to be apparent to others, and unless it is very mild, can be easily identified by examination.

Patients with dementia may be brought to the emergency department after having been found wandering away from home or an institution. Because the onset of most forms of dementia is slow and gradual, presentation to the emergency department often occurs only when some acute worsening of mental status occurs, which may be the result of a superimposed medical illness, adverse drug effect, or environmental change. The demented patient's diminished intellectual and physiologic resources allow abrupt worsening of function with the addition of such stressors.

Especially early in the course of dementia, anxiety, depression, or psychosis may dominate the clinical picture and obscure cognitive dysfunction. For this reason, a high degree of clinical suspicion of dementia should be maintained when evaluating an elderly patient with no prior psychiatric history who presents with new psychiatric problems. Demented persons are also prone to unrecognized physical illness because of inability to perceive or describe symptoms. Careful examination and appropriate laboratory testing are always indicated in the initial and ongoing evaluation of such patients.

It must be noted that dementia is not synonymous with the older designation of "chronic organic brain syndrome," which implies irreversiblity. Common causes of potentially reversible dementia include metabolic and endocrine disorders, polypharmacy, and depression. Often, especially in elderly patients, depression may present with prominent cognitive impairment, a condition erroneously labeled "pseudodementia," but more accurately called *dementia of depression*. The presence of a relatively acute onset, prominent mood changes, and vegetative disturbances such as loss of appetite and weight, sleep disturbance, or expressions of guilt or suicidal ideation all point to depression as the cause. In these situations, treatment of the mood disorder may lead to resolution of the cognitive impairment, although recent studies indicate that many such patients have evidence of brain dysfunction and only partial treatment response.

### Delirium

Like dementia, *delirium* is characterized by global impairment in cognitive function, but is distinguished from it in two major ways. In delirium, the patient has clouding of consciousness, a reduction in the awareness of the external environment (manifest as difficulty sustaining attention), varying degrees of alertness ranging from drowsiness to stupor, and sensory misperception.

The primary distinguishing feature of delirium is the course that is typically acute, with rapid deterioration in hours or days, rather than months as with dementia. Also, the severity of delirium fluctuates over the course of hours; the patient may appear normal at one time and wildly agitated a few hours later. Extreme changes in psychomotor activity, ranging from restlessness and hyperactivity to stupor, are frequent in delirium, but uncommon in dementia except in the later stages when a delirious state may be superimposed. Finally, hallucinations, often visual, are common in delirium. They typically have a vivid quality to which the patient reacts strongly. The hallucinations contrast with the visual hallucinations seen by psychotic patients, which are often described and experienced indifferently.

## Substance-Induced Disorders

### Intoxication

When recent ingestion of a specific exogenous substance produces maladaptive behavior and impairment of judgment, perception, attention, emotional control, or psychomotor activity, and the patient does not display features of delirium, hallucinosis, or other organic brain syndromes, a diagnosis of *intoxication* is made. When the offending substance is known, it should be specified (e.g., alcohol intoxication or amphetamine intoxication). The specific features of intoxication syndromes commonly seen in the emergency department are described in greater detail in the section on toxicology.

As a general rule, the diagnosis of intoxication can be rather easy when laboratory analysis reveals the type and amount of intoxicant circulating in the system. The clinical features of alcohol intoxication are familiar to experienced emergency physicians and range from impaired judgment and coordination through ataxia, lethargy, and coma. When repeated episodes of intoxication occur in a brief period of time, the individual by definition has a substance abuse disorder, and the additional diagnosis is made.

### Withdrawal

*Withdrawal* can follow cessation or reduction in use of a substance of abuse. The category signifies a syndrome characteristic of withdrawal from that particular drug, when the clinical syndrome does not satisfy the criteria for delirium or another organic brain syndrome. For example, mild forms of alcohol withdrawal would be classified here, but if the patient is confused, hallucinating, and agitated, a diagnosis of alcohol withdrawal delirium is indicated. The diagnosis is made by identification of the withdrawal syndrome along with evidence of recent use of the substance in a pattern sufficient to produce withdrawal when the amount ingested is decreased. Specific withdrawal patterns depend on the agent customarily used.

Alcohol withdrawal, for instance, includes up to four stages: autonomic hyperactivity (6 to 8 h after cessation of drinking), hallucinations (24 h after withdrawal), major motor seizures (1 to 2 days) and global confusion (3 to 5 days after last use of alcohol). Some withdrawal syndromes, particularly from alcohol or barbiturates, can be life-threatening.

## Mental Disorders Due to a General Medical Condition

DSM-IV has implemented a major change in the classification of psychiatric symptoms caused by medical conditions. The previous terminology of "organic brain syndrome" and the subtypes organic mood disorder, organic delusional disorder, for example, have been eliminated because of the implication that the "functional" mental disorders were unrelated to biologic changes in brain function. Using DSM-IV, where there is evidence that a psychiatric disturbance is a direct physiologic consequence of a general medical condition or substance, the mental disorder is specified as ". . . due to" the medical problem, for example, "major depression due to hypothyroidism." Common medical causes of psychotic and mood disorders are covered in Chapter 242.

## Schizophrenia and Other Psychotic Disorders

Schizophrenia and related disorders are marked by the presence of psychotic symptoms, primarily delusions and hallucinations. *Delusions* are defined as fixed false beliefs, which are not amenable to arguments or facts to the contrary and which are not shared by others of similar cultural background. Common delusions are of several types. *Persecutory delusions* are those in which one believes that one is being attacked, followed, harassed, or conspired against. *Grandiose delusions* are those that involve themes of special powers or abilities. *Bizarre delusions* are those with patently absurd content, such as believing that one's thoughts are controlled by extraterrestrial beings. *Hallucinations* are false perceptions experienced in a sensory modality and occurring in clear consciousness. Auditory hallucinations are

the most common, followed in order of prevalence by visual, tactile, olfactory, and gustatory. The most prevalent psychosis is *schizophrenia,* described in detail in the next section. The other psychotic disorders, discussed briefly, are less common. A decision tree helpful in evaluating psychotic symptoms is presented in Fig. 241-1.

## Schizophrenia

Schizophrenia is one of the most serious public health problems in the world and accounts for 25 percent of all hospitalized patients. The essential features are a deterioration in functioning, the presence of active-phase symptoms (hallucinations, delusions, disorganized speech or behavior, catatonic behavior, or negative symptoms) for at least 1 month and the relative absence of a mood syndrome. Research has established the importance of genetic factors in its cause, and schizophrenia is most likely a group of disorders of varying etiology that share a final common pathway, much as is the case with mental retardation. It is a brain disease, and there is no evidence that psychosocial stressors or poor parenting are responsible for the cause of the illness, although these may have a profound effect on the patient's adaptation to this usually chronic disorder.

Schizophrenia usually starts in late adolescence or early adulthood, although the onset can occur at any age. The childhood history of schizophrenics often is marked by shyness, oddness or eccentric behavior, school difficulties, or suspiciousness, but such features are not always present. A prodromal phase, in which a gradual deterioration of function is noted, usually precedes the development of active delusions or hallucinations. Such deterioration usually includes the worsening of social withdrawal or the new onset of social withdrawal, odd behavior or speech, and difficulty in functioning in school or work. Patients or their families rarely seek care until the onset of the active phase of psychosis. Schizophrenics seldom seek care at all because they lack insight; they do not realize that their perception, thoughts, and behavior are abnormal.

Antipsychotic drugs usually reduce the severity of delusions and hallucinations. Other manifestations of schizophrenia less responsive to antipsychotics include negative symptoms (lack of volition, blunt-

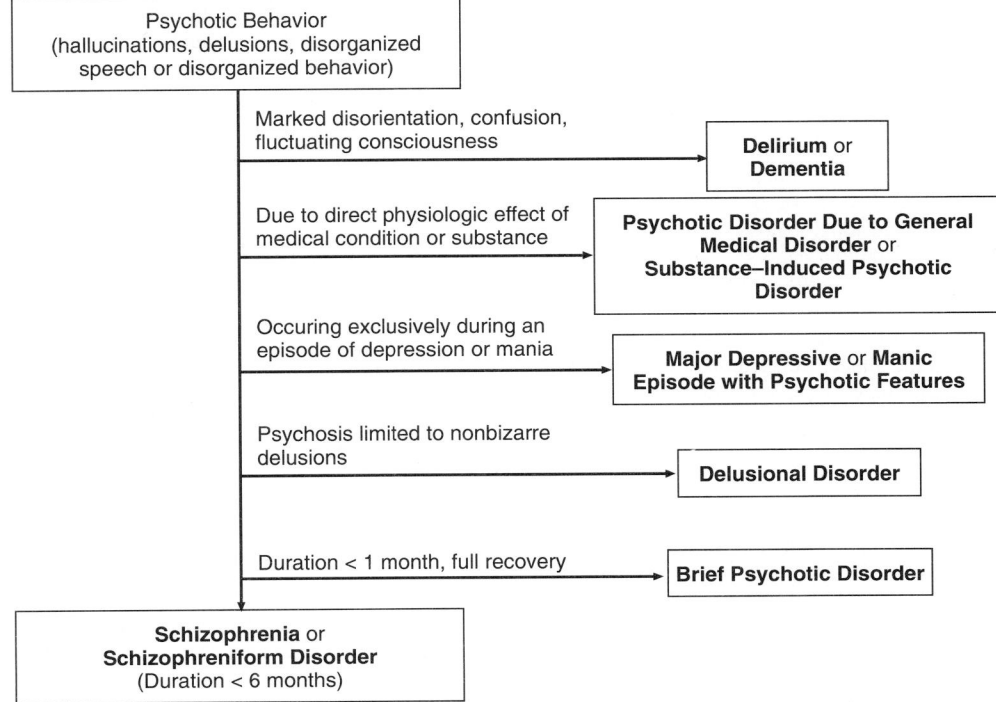

**Fig. 241-1.** Decision tree for evaluating psychosis.

ing of emotion, anhedonia, and inattention). Such symptoms result in lasting impairment in self-care, work, and social relations.

Disorganization of thinking and behavior characterizes schizophrenia. Disheveled appearance and grooming, bizarre behavior, poor judgment, and loosening of associations indicate such disorganization. *Loosening of associations* refers to a loss of the normal logical connections between one thought and the next; thus the schizophrenic's speech is often vague, rambling, disjointed, or nonsensical. Fantastic experiences and bizarre ideas are described in an indifferent manner and unchanging facial expression.

Common reasons for persons with schizophrenia to come to the emergency department include worsening of psychosis resulting from stress or noncompliance with medication, suicidal behavior, assaultiveness (often as a result of paranoid thinking), and extrapyramidal side effects of neuroleptic drugs. Schizophrenics constitute a large share of the chronic homeless population and may be brought in, by authorities, in a confused state, obviously unable to attend to their basic needs. Their poor judgment and disorganization may lead to disregard for medical problems, so attention must be given to their physical status as well as the psychiatric problem.

### Schizophreniform Disorder

*Schizophreniform disorder* is diagnosed when the patient meets the criteria for schizophrenia but the symptoms have been continuously present for less than 6 months A rapid onset over a few days and good premorbid functioning are more common than in schizophrenia.

### Brief Psychotic Disorder

Some individuals may become acutely psychotic after exposure to an extremely traumatic life experience. If such a pyschosis lasts for less than 4 weeks, it is termed a *brief psychotic disorder.* Precipitants of the psychosis include the death of a loved one or a life-threatening situation such as combat or a natural disaster. Emotional turmoil, confusion, and extremely bizarre behavior and speech are common.

### Delusional Disorder

*Delusional disorder* is a syndrome distinct from schizophrenia characterized by persistent nonbizarre delusions. Unlike schizophrenia, delusional disorder is rarely characterized by impairment in daily functioning, and the patient may appear outwardly normal aside from the strange ideas expressed. The onset is in middle or late adulthood, and the delusions develop over months or years. Several subtypes have been identified, the most common of which is the persecutory type, in which the delusions follow themes of being conspired against, cheated, followed, poisoned, or harassed. Other types of delusional disorder include delusional jealousy, in which the patient has an unsubstantiated conviction that one's partner is unfaithful, and the somatic type, in which patients believe they emit a foul odor or are infected with parasites.

Emergency medical evaluation may be occasioned by threats or acts of violence directed at the alleged persecutors, by suicidal behavior, or by involuntary commitment. Delusional disorders are uncommon, and more likely causes of this syndrome are psychotic depression or chronic stimulant abuse.

## Mood Disorders

The mood disorders are the most prevalent of the major psychiatric disorders, affecting about 10 to 15 percent of the general population at some time in their lives. Depressive disorders are the major cause of completed suicide. An unsuccessful attempt may bring the patient to the emergency department. Mood disorders, substance abuse, and anxiety disorders are the most common psychiatric diagnoses in emergency patients.

Mood, or *affective,* disorders differ from the normal extremes of sadness and happiness in that characteristic clusters of psychological and vegetative symptoms (depressive or manic syndrome) are present, and functioning is impaired. Any of the features of schizophrenia such as delusions, hallucinations, or disorganization may be present, but if a full depressive or manic syndrome exists, a diagnosis of a psychotic mood disorder is required. Another important characteristic of affective disorders is that they tend to be episodic, with periods of remission and normal function.

### Major Depression

The essential features of *major depression* is a persistent dysphoric (sad) mood or pervasive loss of interest in usual activities, lasting for at least 2 weeks. Associated psychological symptoms include guilt over past deeds, self-reproach, feelings of worthlessness or hopelessness, inability to experience pleasure, and recurrent thought of death or suicide. "Vegetative symptoms" involve psychological functioning and include loss of appetite and weight, sleep disturbance, fatigue, inability to concentrate, and psychomotor agitation or retardation. The depression may begin gradually or rapidly but usually will have been present for several weeks before the patient comes for treatment.

When the patient complains of the full spectrum of depression symptoms, the diagnosis of major depression is easy to make, but when the chief complaint is a single symptom such as insomnia or fatigue, it will be necessary to elicit the other symptoms of major depression to make the diagnosis. Somatic complaints such as vague pain or weakness may be part of major depression, as may generalized anxiety. A useful screening mnemonic is presented in Fig. 241-2.

Major depression is more common in women, persons with a family history of depression or suicide, and individuals with medical or other psychiatric illnesses. When a medical disorder or drug produces a depressive syndrome through a presumed biologic effect on the brain, the diagnosis should be "depression due to . . ." the offending condition. Major depression is often superimposed on other mental disorders such as substance abuse, personality disorders, and anxiety disorders.

Primary mood disorders tend to display more biologic features, are more familial, and respond better to somatic antidepressant treatment than do mood disorders due to medical disorders. The lifetime risk of suicide is 15 percent, so prompt and aggressive treatment is strongly indicated. Major depression is often recurrent, so certain patients must be maintained on long-term treatment to prevent relapse.

### Bipolar Disorder

Bipolar disorder, previously termed *manic-depressive illness,* is characterized by the ocurrence of mania. A full manic syndrome is one of the most striking and distinctive conditions in clinical practice. The essential disturbance in mood is one of elation or irritability. Manics feel "on top of the world," expansive, energetic, and precarious but may quickly become argumentative, hostile, and sarcastic, especially when their plans are thwarted.

The vegetative signs of mania are a decreased need for sleep, increased activity, rapid pressured speech, and racing thoughts. Manics

| | |
|---|---|
| In | Interest |
| S | Sleep |
| A | Appetite |
| D | Depressed mood |
| C | Concentration |
| A | Activity |
| G | Guilt |
| E | Energy |
| S | Suicide |

**Fig. 241-2.** *In SAD CAGES.* A screening mnemonic for major depression. (From Rund DA, Hutzler JC. *Emergency Psychiatry.* St. Louis: Mosby, 1983, with permission.)

may have grandiose ideas, such as unrealistic plans to start a business or run for public office, and if the grandiosity reaches delusional proportions, these patients may believe themselves to be famous, fabulously wealthy, or blessed with special powers and abilities. Poor judgment in spending money and sexual behavior may lead to problems that prompt manics' families to seek treatment for them, because manics usually lack insight into their abnormal condition and deny that anything is wrong. For this reason, reports from informants such as relatives often reveal important information to substantiate the diagnosis. Because patients who have had a manic episode almost invariably have depressions at some time (the other "pole" of bipolar disorder), a past history of depression may also help in diagnosis.

The disorder is equally common in men and women, and the onset is usually in the third and fourth decades. Complications include suicide, substance abuse (excessive alcohol use is common during the manic phase), and marital and occupational disruption. The course of bipolar disorder is episodic, with the duration, frequency, and regularity of the episodes varying greatly. Depressive episodes are more frequent than manic episodes.

## Dysthymic Disorder

*Dysthymic disorder* is a more chronic and less severe form of depressive illness and was previously termed depressive neurosis. Depressed mood must have been present most of the day more days than not for at least 2 years. Psychotic features are not seen, and these patients often have a life-long gloomy, pessimistic outlook. Women are more often affected, and the onset is in childhood, adolescence, or early adulthood. Associated personality disorders and substance abuse are common. When vegetative symptoms are present, they are usually less severe than with major depression. Major depression may be superimposed on dysthymia, often in association with stressful life events. When major depression complicates dysthymia, the patient may be brought in for evaluation because of the severity of symptoms or treatment following a suicide attempt.

## Anxiety Disorders

The anxiety disorders are mental disorders in which apprehension, fears, and excessive worry dominate the psychological life of the individual. Pathologic degrees of anxiety are accompanied by varying degrees of autonomic activity out of proportion to any real danger or threat. Because anxiety is a ubiquitous condition and frequently is associated with medical illness, depression, neurologic syndromes, and psychoses, a diagnosis of a primary anxiety disorder should be made by exclusion of other causes.

Anxiety disorders are diagnosed in 4 to 8 percent of the general population and are more often diagnosed in women than men. Because of the physical nature of certain symptoms associated with anxiety disorders, patients often seek treatment and evaluation in medical rather than psychiatric settings.

## Panic Disorder

Patients who experience recurrent attacks of severe anxiety are said to suffer from *panic disorder*. A panic attack consists of a sudden extreme surge of anxiety and dread accompanied by autonomic signs, including palpitations, tachycardia, shortness of breath, chest tightness, dizziness, sweating, and tremulousness. The symptoms develop over a few minutes at most and may either be unprovoked or occur with a phobic stimulus, such as a crowded store. After the attacks begin, some patients start to avoid situations that seem to precipitate the panic (phobic avoidance). Such behavior can severely impair their functioning. When activities are severely limited, the complication of *agoraphobia* is diagnosed. In agoraphobia, the patient tends to avoid situations where ready escape or assistance during an attack are not possible. The frequency and severity of panic attacks wax and wane,

but the illness is generally chronic. Unless agoraphobia is severe, most patients are married, employed, and seldom require psychiatric hospitalization unless depression is superimposed on the anxiety disorder.

Because of the very real and frightening nature of the panic attack and its unexpected occurrence, the emergency department is a frequent initial source of medical attention. The presenting complaints may mimic a variety of medical emergencies and careful exclusion of an organic etiology is mandatory. History-taking should include questions about domestic violence and sexual abuse or assault because sometimes these experiences are the source of panic attacks.

## Generalized Anxiety Disorder

When anxiety attacks are absent, yet the patient complains of persistent worry, tension, or free-floating anxiety, a diagnosis of generalized anxiety disorder should be considered. This condition lasts at least 6 months and is characterized by apprehensive worrying, muscle tension, insomnia, irritability, restlessness, jumpiness, or distractibility. Muscle tension may be so severe that the patient actually experiences diffuse muscular pain. Associated autonomic symptoms include the cardiopulmonary, gastrointestinal, and neurologic symptoms seen in panic attacks. In generalized anxiety disorder, such symptoms occur more continuously and chronically than in panic disorder.

## Phobic Disorders

Phobic disorders, other than agoraphobia, discussed above, are an unusual cause of self-referral to the emergency department. In phobias, the anxiety symptoms are recognized as excessive and occur when the patient is exposed to, or anticipates exposure to, a specific situation, which then leads to avoidance of the stimulus to a degree that interferes with the patient's life. In social phobia, the situation involves having the attention of others drawn to the patient. Such activities as public speaking or meeting strangers create a fear that the patient will be embarrassed in some way. Specific phobias are quite common; they involve fear of a very specific stimulus such as animals, heights, dark, or flying.

## Other Anxiety Disorders

*Posttraumatic stress disorder* is an anxiety reaction to a severely psychosocial stressor, usually life-threatening, such as military combat, a fire, rape, or natural disaster. Symptoms involve repetitive and intrusive memories of the event, nightmares, emotional numbing, survivor guilt, and varying degrees of depression and anxiety. Substance abuse appears to be a frequent complication.

*Obsessive-compulsive disorder* is a mental disorder in which the patient experiences intrusive thoughts or images that cannot be eliminated from the mind. Typical thoughts involve images of graphic violence to self or others, contamination, or perverse sexual behavior that the patient would not carry out but nevertheless obsessively fantasizes about. To control the obsessive thoughts, the individual may engage in compulsive behavior or rituals such as excessive washing, repetitive checking, or counting. When the obsessions and compulsions occupy a great deal of time, the patient may become significantly disabled and seek psychiatric attention. The sense of helplessness and the impairment can lead to the development of depression, which also leads the patient to seek help.

## Somatoform Disorders

Many patients have particular complaints or symptoms for which no medical explanation can be identified. When a physical cause has been clearly eliminated, and the complaint is not delusional or occurring in the context of a depression or anxiety disorder, somatoform disorders may be considered. When the complaint involves a loss of function, usually in the neurologic system (e.g., paralysis, blindness, numbness) and psychological factors are deemed etiologic, a *conversion disorder* may be present. The term conversion reflects Freud's hypothesis that unexpressed emotion associated with a traumatic event or situation could be "converted" into physical symptoms and signs. Conversion disorders are much more common in culturally and psychologically unsophisticated persons. This diagnosis should be made with extreme caution, if at all, in the emergency department because studies indicate that many patients diagnosed with conversion disorder eventually develop signs of a physical disorder explaining the symptom. Erroneous attribution to a mental disorder obviously deprives the patient of appropriate medical treatment.

Some patients have a wide variety of complaints and long complicated histories of medical problems that have no apparent medical cause. Such individuals may have *somatization disorder,* a disorder beginning in the teens and twenties, usually in women, and leading to considerable unnecessary diagnostic and surgical intervention. The prototypical patient is a middle-aged woman who describes a "positive review of systems" in a dramatic and confusing way. Conversion symptoms, menstrual complaints, multifocal pain, sexual and gastrointestinal symptoms, dizziness, and diverse psychiatric symptoms are common findings. The diagnosis is made when the patient has a history of a variety of medically unexplained symptoms involving multiple organ systems. As with conversion disorder, a firm diagnosis of somatization disorder should not be made on the basis of a single visit to the emergency department, but the identification of somatizing behavior will be useful for future reference, because these patients will frequently make repeated contacts.

*Hypochondriasis* may be diagnosed when the patient is preoccupied with fears of serious illness, which persist despite appropriate medical evaluation and reassurance.

Finally, when pain is the sole complaint and the intensity and secondary disability are unexplained by a known physical ailment, a diagnosis of *pain disorder* may be considered.

Identification of a somatoform disorder in the emergency department has such profound implications on future management that it is advisable to avoid making a firm diagnosis of these disorders unless a long history of prior similar complaints is documented and no organic disease has become apparent. This wisdom is tempered additionally by the fact that well-established conversion or other "psychogenic" complaints provide absolutely no protection against the development of a treatable medical disorder; new complaints always warrant careful examination for objective findings. When the physician is quite sure that no organic disease exists, the patient may be reassured that no serious physical illness is present. Avoid telling the patient that is it "all in your head" because this is not likely to be believed. Regular follow-up with a general internist or family physician is the best management for somatization disorder. Patients with this disorder notoriously resist psychiatric referral and treatment.

## Dissociative Disorders

The dissociative disorders are a group of uncommon and poorly understood conditions where the central feature is a sudden alteration in the normal integration of identity and consciousness. The dissociation often occurs under severe stress and may or may not be recurrent, although it is rarely permanent. The forms of dissociative state relevant to emergency practice are *psychogenic amnesia,* a temporary loss of memory for important personal details that is not due to an organic cause, and *psychogenic fugue,* in which a similar loss of memory and assumption of a new identity are accompanied by travel away from home. Dissociative disorders are difficult to distinguish from malingering, in which the individual in pursuit of a clear goal, such as avoiding incarceration or military duty, may consciously feign amnesia. As always, organic causes such as drug intoxication or loss of memory such as that resulting from transient global amnesia must be ruled out.

Other conditions in this category include *multiple personality disorder* and *depersonalization disorder.*

## PERSONALITY (AXIS II) DISORDERS

*Personality* refers to an enduring pattern of perceiving, relating to, and reacting to one's environment and interpersonal relations. When a pattern of behavior is lifelong and not limited to periods of illness and causes significant impairment in social and occupational functioning or considerable distress, a *personality disorder* is present. Some individuals are painfully aware of the consequences of their behavior but are unable to alter these fundamental ways of dealing with their world. Most of the patients who are seen clinically in medical and psychiatric settings who are diagnosed with a personality disorder lack a clear awareness of how their behavior alienates others or aggravates their own stress. Even when such insight is possible, actual personality change is unlikely.

The patient presenting with a personality disorder may often be recognized by the characteristic effect the interaction has on the physician and medical staff. Antisocial patients, for instance, are disliked immediately; they seem to be in control of their behavior unlike psychotic or depressed patients, but nonetheless have repeatedly engaged in maladaptive behavior. The patient may be seen as using the emergency department for some vague, or obvious, goal. These disorders are the most common secondary diagnosis in the malingerer.

The emergency physician seldom needs to decide which of the personality disorders relates appropriately to the patient. General categories of personality disorders are grouped in Table 241-2. When such features are present and seem to be interfering with some important aspect of the patient's life, personality disorder can be suspected. The presenting complaint should be evaluated appropriately, because patients with well-established character disorders still develop bona fide medical illnesses.

The personality disorder that constitutes a disproportionate share of emergency visits is *antisocial personality disorder.* The patient shows a continuous pattern of maladaptive behavior displaying disregard for the rights of others in a variety of ways: criminal behavior, fighting, lying, abuse and neglect of dependents and spouses, financial irresponsibility, recklessness, and inability to sustain enduring attachments to others.

The sociopathic behavior begins before the age of 15, but the diagnosis may not be made until after the age of 18. Sociopathy is much more frequent in males, in lower socioeconomic classes, and in relatives of alcoholics and sociopaths. Alcohol and drug abuse, imprisonment, multiple divorces, traumatic injury, accidental and violent deaths, and poor medical compliance are common complications.

Management of the antisocial patient in the emergency department is often frustrating, but anger toward the patient can be minimized and the interaction hastened along by setting firm limits on behavior, focusing on the chief complaint, and providing the patient with necessary information about the medical problem at hand. No effective psychiatric intervention can be forced on the patient, although certain patients may benefit from substance abuse treatment, psychotherapy,

**Table 241-2.** Behavioral Characteristics that Suggest Various Clusters of Personality Disorders

| Behavior | Personality Disorder Group |
|---|---|
| Eccentric, odd, isolated, withdrawn, suspicious, inhibited, no friends, overly sensitive | Paranoid, schizoid, schizotypal |
| Emotional, dramatic, angry, seductive, impulsive, erratic | Antisocial, histrionic, borderline, narcissistic |
| Anxious, fearful, nervous, cautious | Dependent, avoidant, obsessive-compulsive |

SOURCE: Rund DA, Hutzler JC. *Emergency Psychiatry.* St. Louis: CV Mosby, 1983; DSM-IV, with permission.

or organized religion when motivated to make changes in their lives. Fortunately, the most violent and disruptive behavior of many antisocials seems to "burn out" in the late twenties or after, although their adjustment to society often continues to be marginal.

## BIBLIOGRAPHY

American Psychiatric Association. *Diagnostic and Statistical Manual of Mental Disorders,* 4th ed. Washington, DC: American Psychiatric Association, 1994.

Greenstein RA, Ness DE. Psychiatric emergencies in the elderly. *Emerg Med Clin North Am* 8:429, 1990. Review.

Lamarre CJ, Patten SB. Evaluation of the modified mini-mental state examination in a general psychiatric population. *Can J Psychiatry* 36:507, 1991.

Munizza C, Furlan PM, d'Elia A, et al. Emergency psychiatry: a review of the literature. *Acta Psychiatr Scand Suppl* 374:1, 1993. Review.

Rund DA, Hutzler JC. *Emergency Psychiatry.* St. Louis: CV Mosby, 1983.

Tintinalli JE, Peacock FW, Wright MA. Emergency medical evaluation of psychiatric patients. *Ann Emerg Med* 23:859, 1994.

Wulsin LR, Yingling K. Psychiatric aspects of chest pain in the emergency department. *Med Clin North Am* 75:1175, 1991. Review.

# 242

# BEHAVIORAL DISORDERS: EMERGENCY ASSESSMENT AND STABILIZATION

### Jeffery C. Hutzler
### Douglas A. Rund

This chapter presents the principles of medical and psychiatric evaluation of patients with behavior disorders and reviews the management of suicidal and violent patients. As shown in Fig. 242-1, the majority of psychiatric patient visits to the emergency department occur at night when psychiatric services are limited; therefore, the hospital must be staffed with adequate personnel adept at handling patients who are suicidal, violent, or otherwise distraught or psychotic.

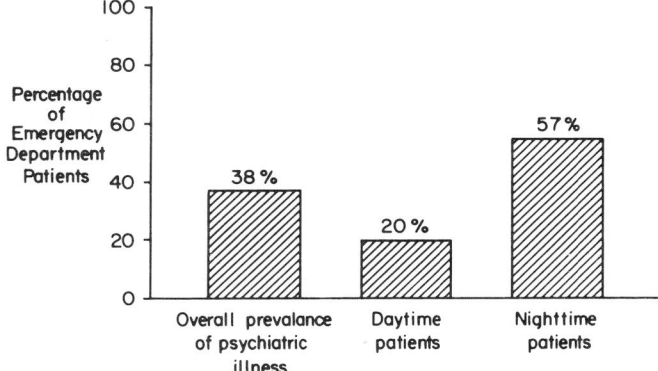

**Fig. 242-1.** Daytime versus nighttime distribution of psychiatric patient visits to the emergency department.

## EMERGENCY AND INTERVENTION APPROACHES TO PSYCHIATRIC ASSESSMENT

### Decision-Making

A decision strategy for emergency psychiatric assessment should follow this sequence of questions: (1) Is the patient stable or unstable? (2) Does the patient have a serious medical condition that is causing abnormal behavior or thought processes? (3) If the cause of changes in behavior is not due to an underlying medical condition, it will be primarily "psychiatric" or "functional." What is the diagnosis and severity? (4) Is a psychiatric consultation necessary? (5) When should the patient be forcibly detained for emergency evaluation?

### Physical Restraint

Situations that require emergency stabilization, sometimes against the patient's wishes, involve the patient stating that he or she is potentially or actually violent, suicidal, or developing rapidly progressive medical conditions causing disturbed behavior (e.g., hypoglycemia, meningitis, or other causes of delirium). Disturbances involving actual or threatened violence are the most difficult for emergency department staff. The staff, of course, fear injury or that the patient will escape and hurt himself or others. There are always limitations in security personnel and immediately available staff. There are often limitations in the physical facility itself in regard to restraining such patients.

Violent behavior demands immediate restraint. Hospital security forces and police are best equipped and best trained to subdue the patient with the least chance of staff or patient injury. Staff in the emergency department should not attempt to subdue a patient unless they are fully trained to do so. An initial show of force (four or five male attendants) may be sufficient to induce the patient to accept physical or chemical restraint without further resistance. Under ideal circumstances, the emergency department staff should organize themselves to be able to subdue a violent person if security personnel are not immediately available. This requires training and practice. The approach to the patient usually requires five team members with one member assigned to each limb and the leader assigned to the head. When approached from different directions and grabbed simultaneously, the violent person can usually be immobilized and restrained.

Potentially violent behavior requires the summoning of adequate force and the adoption of a nonthreatening attitude by a physician and staff. The physician should never approach the patient with hands out or by making other gestures that might be interpreted as an attack. The physician should also stay distant from the patient, avoid excessive eye contact, and maintain a somewhat submissive posture and tone of voice. Ideally the physician should stand in a location that neither threatens the patient nor blocks his or her own retreat from the room. Allowing the patient to ventilate feelings verbally is important. Setting limits on acceptable behavior and making neutral comments may diffuse a potentially violent situation. Adequate force should be visible to the patient nearby and the patient should clearly be told that certain kinds of behavior will result in restraint.

The decision to release the patient from physical restraints should be jointly made by medical and nursing personnel on the basis of a judgment regarding the patient's condition and behavior and not as a result of the patient's bargains or threats. Restraints should be removed in a stepwise fashion, from four limbs to two, to none.

Stabilization of the actively suicidal patient requires adequate suicide precautions. All dangerous objects are removed from the patient in the treatment room. Staff members should watch the patient closely and not allow the patient to leave the examining room unaccompanied by a staff member. Some institutions have members of the security staff available to provide supervision.

Patients who are threatening or demonstrate actual or potential violent behavior should be disrobed, gowned, and searched for weapons.

Seemingly innocuous objects such as belts or belt buckles can be used by the patient to inflict self-injury or injury to others. Some emergency departments have installed metal detectors to prevent highly lethal weapons from entering the department. It has been determined that other patients do not resent the use of metal detectors because they feel safer themselves.

## Initial Evaluation

The most effective tool available for the evaluation of behavioral disorders, particularly where "organic" mental disorders may be involved, is an excellent medical-psychiatric history. The history (including the use of medication, alcohol, or other drugs), physical examination, neurologic examination, and mental status examination should be incorporated into the early stages of evaluation of a person with disturbed behavior.

The changed behavior is a good starting point for inquiry. Sudden onset of major changes in behavior, mood, or thought in an individual who previously had functioned normally may be the result of an urgent medical disorder. Few "functional" or other psychotic behaviors begin very rapidly. Behavioral disorders have resulted from all of the following life-threatening conditions:

Central nervous system (CNS) infection: meningitis or encephalitis
Intoxication
Alcohol or drug withdrawal
Hypoglycemia
Hypertensive encephalopathy
Hypoxia
Intracranial hemorrhage
Poisoning
CNS trauma
Seizure disorder
Acute organ system failure

A sudden change in behavior, especially in a patient over the age of 40, is a potentially important indicator of a new and correctable process. Neurologic symptoms associated with the behavioral changes should be explored. Such symptoms include fainting, dizziness, brief periods of disorientation, impairment of speech, confusion, loss of consciousness, headaches, and difficulty performing previous routine tasks.

The most important information about such behavioral changes will come from the patient's family. If the family is unavailable, friends or coworkers should be contacted and questioned. Third-party information may be the only source of information on a patient unable to give a cogent history. The source may be able to report substance abuse; and can describe the level of previous functioning. Of course, it is important to get a history of any previous psychiatric illness or treatment. Similar previous change in behavior over past years weighs against the onset of a new "organic" process. However, it is important to weigh present information carefully to avoid a quick assumption that the patient's presentation is due to repeated occurrences of a preexisting disorder. In other words, psychiatric patients also develop medical illnesses producing change in behavior.

A complete medical history and review of systems is particularly important. This can be asked of the patient, or if he or she cannot answer these questions, a family member. Recent medical illnesses or symptoms such as infections, head trauma, fever, human immunodeficiency virus risk factors, difficulty in breathing, and dizziness should be investigated. A history of neurologic symptoms is particularly important. Any recent changes such as periods of confusion, speech difficulties, or syncope are suggestive of an organic disorder. A history of exposure to toxic substances such as heavy metals, organic solvents, or other occupational hazards may suggest a cause for newly disturbed behavior. To complete the investigation, family and social history may identify stressors in the patient's environment that are either a direct cause of changes in behavior or accentuate any responses to underlying disease.

Prescribed drugs, over-the-counter medications, illicit drugs, and alcohol can all create disturbed behavior. It is difficult to ask questions about drug use in certain patients such as the elderly, the "important" patient, or those known personally by the emergency department personnel, but it is necessary. In particular, it is important to ask about the use of sedative-hypnotics, stimulants, psychotropic agents, anticonvulsants, and anticholinergic agents and parkinsonian medications, cardiovascular drugs, diuretics, hormones, analgesics, anti-inflammatory drugs, anti-infective agents, and other categories of prescription drugs. Many of these medications cause changes in behavior when taken even in therapeutic doses. Ask specifically about over-the-counter drugs because patients rarely consider these "medications." Over-the-counter analgesics containing salicylates, anticholinergics, antihistamines, or bromides may produce delirium or toxic psychosis. Alcohol and street drugs such as phencyclidine, LSD, mescaline, amphetamines, or cocaine can produce a toxic psychosis similar to acute schizophrenia or mania. Hypnosedatives such as barbiturates, benzodiazepines, methaqualone, or glutethimide may produce a confusional state or delirium both with intoxication or withdrawal.

According to Rund and colleagues, 15 to 20 percent of emergency department patients meet diagnostic criteria for alcohol abuse. Chronic mentally ill patients have a much higher incidence of alcohol abuse. The many syndromes associated with alcohol abuse should be recognized by emergency physicians. These include intoxication, withdrawal, delirium, hallucinosis, alcohol amnestic disorder, paranoid behavior, and dementia. Blood alcohol tests may be useful in disturbed patients even when the odor of ethanol is not present. Other testing modalities, including breath analyzers and chemically treated paper strips, may be used to screen blood alcohol levels.

## Mental Status Examination

The objective of the mental status examination is to distinguish functional from organic disorders. A great deal of the information obtained in mental status examinations becomes evident through patient observation and the initial patient interview (Table 242-1). An abnormal mental status examination suggests an organic basis for abnormal thought or behavior. Lability of affect, the necessity to repeat simple questions, irritability, and lack of cooperation are some signs of organic dysfunction.

Important components of the mental status examination (Zun and Gold) include level of consciousness, spontaneous speech, behavioral observation, physical appearance, the relaying of history information, attention, and language comprehension. This information is usually easily obtained during the history-taking. The more traditional mental

**Table 242-1.** Mental Status in the Emergency Department: An Outline

Behavior
　What is the patient doing?
Affect
　What feelings is the patient displaying?
Orientation
　Does the patient know what is happening, where, and when?
Language
　Is the patient understanding and being understood?
Memory
　Can the patient recall historical details, recent and remote?
Thought content
　Is the patient reporting beliefs that make little sense?
Perceptual abnormalities
　Is the patient experiencing unusual sensory phenomena?
Judgment
　Is the patient able to make rational decisions?

status examination relies on specific assessment of orientation, memory, intellect, judgment, and affect.

The physician should compare his or her own direct observations of the patient's behavior with reports from family and friends. Documentation of the patient's orientation should include an assessment of attention, ability to concentrate on a specific task, and the traditional evaluation of person, place, and time. The patient should be asked the day, month, and year and place where he or she is presently being examined. Impaired language performance, including difficulty with speech, reading, writing, and word finding, may indicate a neurologic disorder. Memory is often divided into three categories: immediate, recent, and remote. Immediate memory is tested by asking a patient to repeat a series of digits (usually five) forward and backward. Recent memory can be tested by asking the patient to repeat three unrelated words immediately and then again after 3 to 5 min. The patient should be able to restate these after 3 to 5 min. The patient may also be asked about events that have occurred in the last few hours. Remote memory can be tested by asking about previous addresses, occupations, or historical events from an early period in the patient's life. Tests of memory should include details of significant personal, national, and international historical events. All history should be corroborated.

Investigation of higher cognitive functions includes assessment of the patient's general command of information; mental calculation, especially subtraction, such as serial sevens; and spelling of words forward and backward (such as world). Patients with organic disease often have difficulty spelling backward or performing serial calculation. The patient's affect or outward display of emotion should be evaluated for sadness, euphoria, and anxiety. This may help distinguish between cognitive disturbance induced by depressive disorders and dementia due to significant cerebral pathology. The examiner can draw some conclusions regarding the patient's thought processes during the patient's own telling of his or her history.

Disordered thought processes include paranoid or grandiose delusions, fixed false beliefs, and delusional denial of illness. Such beliefs should be compared with reports from family and friends.

Visual hallucinations do occur in functional psychotic illnesses (schizophrenia or affective disorder), but most often result from organic disease. A patient with visual hallucinations should always be assumed to have organic pathology until proven otherwise.

Judgment may be impaired in organic disease, and historical evidence of faulty judgment should be elicited. Insight about judgment can be gained by asking the patient how he or she would deal with day-to-day problems such as finding the way home from the hospital.

Finally, the examiner should test for specific focal neurologic deficits including apraxias, agnosias, right-left disorientation, aphasias, and inability to follow complex spoken and written commands. Such signs may or may not occur in association with other localizing neurologic signs such as asymmetric reflexes, paresthesia, or hemiparesis.

Ask the patient to "draw a clock face." The physician can draw a circle on a piece of paper and ask the patient to fill in the numbers on the paper to look like a clock face. If the patient can put in the numbers correctly in a clock face, he or she should then be asked to put the hands at the position to read a specific time. If the patient cannot do these tasks, organic disease is present.

## Physical Examination

The objectives of physical examination are to identify disorders that may cause or have an impact on the behavior disorder and identify the presence of medical problems that may need special care in, or are inappropriate for, management in a psychiatric setting.

A careful physical examination should be conducted on every patient. Vital signs are a simple physical screening test of patients with altered behavior. Abnormal vital signs, when observed, must not be dismissed as secondary to anxiety or stress. Bradycardia can be seen in patients with hypothyroidism, Stokes-Adams syndrome, or elevated intracranial pressure. Tachycardia may be apparent in patients suffering from hyperthyroidism, infection, heart failure, pulmonary embolus, or alcohol withdrawal. Fever is often associated with extreme hyperthyroidism or thyroid storm, vasculitis, alcohol withdrawal, sedative-hypnotic withdrawal, meningitis, or various inflammatory processes. Hypothermia is observed in sepsis, dermal disease, hypoendocrine status, CNS dysfunction, and intoxication. Hypotension may be an indicator of shock, Addison's disease, hypothyroidism, or medication side effects. Hypertension may be associated with hypertensive encephalopathy or stimulant abuse. Tachypnea is seen in patients with metabolic acidosis, pulmonary embolus, pneumonia, cardiac failure, or fever. Any such disorders may result in a secondary behavioral disturbance. The limited expense of, and useful information provided by, vital signs justifies their use in all patients.

A general physical examination should ideally be conducted with the patient completely disrobed and gowned. The patient should be carefully checked for signs of trauma. Contusions or abrasions of the head, face, and neck may be common if the patient is bellicose and may suggest the possibility of otherwise unsuspected head injuries. Extremities should be checked for frostbite or other evidence of exposure-related injury. If trauma is demonstrated or suggested by history, the mechanism of injury should be carefully reconstructed. For a variety of reasons, patients may omit or underreport the extent and cause of trauma.

Chest, cardiac, and abdominal examinations should be carefully performed and a careful neurologic examination should be specific for features that suggest organic disease. Other neurologic signs, such as bilateral asterixis or multifocal myoclonus, are often associated with delirium.

## Laboratory Evaluation

The selection of particular laboratory tests emerges from diagnostic needs suggested by the history, mental status examination, and physical examination. Purdie and coworkers found fluid and electrolyte disorders in 12 percent of patients with an acute behavioral disturbance. One study reported a 15-fold greater incidence of hyponatremia in schizophrenics with acute behavioral changes than in nonschizophrenic psychiatric patients. However, Fauman and Fauman found that in stable psychiatric patients, the only useful laboratory studies were blood glucose and white blood cell count. Therefore, screening on grounds of history and physical examination should be done before ordering tests because no universal screening panel exists.

## EMERGENCY SITUATIONS REQUIRING EMERGENCY INTERVENTION

### Suicide

Suicide is the ninth leading cause of death in our population and the second leading cause of death in persons under age 24. There seem to be epidemiologic differences between suicide attempters and suicide completers. Suicide completers, for instance, are more likely than attempters to be older, male, living alone, or physically ill. These are high-risk patients who need to be carefully assessed. The ratio of attempted suicides to completed suicide is estimated to be about 40:1.

A suicide attempt is not a common accompaniment of the "downward" portion of the normal mood swings occasionally experienced by everyone. Only about 2 percent of the general population have seriously considered taking their lives and only about 1 percent have actually made a suicide attempt. Therefore, suicide attempters must be taken seriously. The attitude of the staff should be empathic; suicide precautions should be instituted; and, following medical management, the assessment of suicide risk should be carefully evaluated and documented. The decision to hold and hospitalize the patient should be given serious consideration.

Suicidal thinking is more frequent in women than in men and is associated with a clinical depression, social isolation, undesirable life events, and early parental loss. It is important to remember that suicidal thinking may precede an actual attempt by up to 1 year and follow-up studies suggest that suicidal thinking persists in many patients long after improvement in mental status and personal relationships.

This means that attitudes in the suicidal attempter among the emergency staff should be empathic and nonjudgmental. Negative attitudes toward the suicide attempter have been documented in all types of emergency personnel: paramedics, nurses, and emergency physicians. A negative attitude intensifies the patient's already low self-esteem, thus increasing the risk of subsequent suicide and making it difficult to establish a therapeutic relationship.

Schizophrenia, substance abuse, and depression are psychiatric diagnoses that place a suicidal patient at relatively high risk. Ten percent of schizophrenics eventually kill themselves. Alcoholics have a suicide rate that is 50 times higher than the norm, and as many as 25 percent of all successful suicides are associated with alcohol. Depression is a diagnosis associated with suicide attempts of higher lethality and with those who successfully complete suicide.

Personality disorder and adjustment disorder implying a transient situational disturbance are frequent diagnoses in suicide attempters and are generally associated with relatively lower completion risk than the major psychiatric illnesses noted above. Patients with these disorders still show a higher risk of completed suicide than the general population.

Drug overdose accounts for the overwhelming majority of all contemporary suicide attempts. Drugs used for suicide attempts tend to parallel prevailing prescribing patterns. An increase in the prevalence of suicide attempts observed during the 1960s and early 1970s led to speculation that availability of safer psychotropic agents encouraged widespread prescription and ultimately contributed to their availability for suicide attempts. The extent of poisoning created by the drugs usually reflects the lethal intent of the patient and thus the relative risk. The patient taking a large dose of amitriptyline would thus be considered at greater risk than someone taking a few antihistamine tablets. Some patients may be relatively unaware of the potential toxicity of the overdose, however, and assessment of such knowledge and their continuing intent to die must be assessed by questions such as "Were you surprised to find yourself alive after taking the overdose?"

Violent attempts (shooting, jumping, hanging) are generally considered serious and a high-risk factor for a future attempt. A number of reports have described a "wrist cutting syndrome" in a young, attractive, unmarried woman whose self-mutilation, although repetitive, was seldom thought to be serious in intent. These acts usually have been carried out in a state of mounting tension with depersonalization followed by relief after self-mutilation. A significant number of "wrist slashers," or self-mutilators, when followed for 5 to 6 years, have died of suicide.

In determining suicide risk, a general rule is that the risk of a successful suicide rises with advancing age. Men are two to three times more likely than women to complete suicide, whereas women are two or three times more likely than men to attempt suicide. Patients who are single, divorced, separated, widowed, or unemployed are statistically at higher risk than those who are married and employed.

The psychotic patient (one who distorts reality, may have hallucinations and delusions) who attempts suicide must be evaluated by a psychiatrist; hospitalization is in order. A psychotic patient may respond unpredictably to distorted perceptions or false perceptions in a fearful or driven manner. Psychotics require very careful observation and restraint if necessary.

Secondary gain is a term that indicates that while the primary motive for a suicide attempt appears to be death, the attempt may meet another need such as attention or a plea for emotional help. When such needs are met by the attempt, a secondary gain is achieved and the risk of subsequent suicide attempt is lessened momentarily. It is dangerous, however, to assume that secondary gain is the cause of a suicide attempt with an initial evaluation in an emergency department. All suicide behaviors should be taken seriously.

Perhaps the most important part of the assessment of the suicide attempter is a determination of the patient's feelings and thoughts at the time of the interview. The patient who experiences helplessness, exhaustion, overwhelming depression, and a clear expression of intent to die certainly remains at high risk. If the patient expresses continuation of such feelings at the time of the interview, the physician has sufficient evidence that the patient needs psychiatric consultation immediately. Some patients, however, seem to equate self-injury with other forms of emotional discharge such as crying, talking to a friend, or becoming inebriated. They do not perceive the event as an attempt to end their life. When asked about their feeling at the time of the attempt, such patients may indicate that they were angry or vengeful. Attitudes and affect that generally indicate a good prognosis at the time of the interview are anger, remorse, or embarrassment. The patient who sits quietly, refusing to provide additional information to the examiner, should be considered at high risk. Feelings of hopelessness, helplessness, or exhaustion seem to be among the clearest indicators of long-term suicidal risk in patients hospitalized at one time for depression. Persons expressing these feelings should be regarded as at high risk.

Patient disposition can be aided by estimating the lethality of the attempt and the likelihood of rescue. When there is a high likelihood of rescue and low lethality, the patient is considered at lower risk than in the reverse situation. The patient who makes a hanging attempt in a desolate wooded area is a greater risk than the person who takes a handful of relatively nontoxic pills in front of witnesses.

Patients who have made previous suicide attempts have traditionally been considered to be at greater risk for future suicide. Prior attempts seem a particularly ominous sign, particularly if the intensity and apparent lethality of the suicide attempts escalate with each subsequent attempt. Bengelsdorf achieved a 97 percent concordance with a crisis triage system to predict a need for inpatient hospitalization. The factors which need to be considered include dangerousness, support system, and motivation or ability to cooperate.

A summary of high- and low-risk suicide profiles is given in Table 242-2.

## Clinical Management

High-risk patients whose suicide intent is strong and immediate require immediate psychiatric hospitalization. Moderate-risk patients are those who present in a serious suicidal crisis, but who because of a positive response to initial intervention and favorable social support, are not judged to be an immediate danger. Hospitalization can often be avoided in such patients, provided practical outpatient treatment can be established immediately. Such determinations are most often made in concert with a psychiatric consultant. Available means of suicide, such as firearms or drug caches, should be removed and any psychotropic medication should be used judiciously and prescribed conservatively. It is important to have a family member take charge of the patient's medications.

Before discharging the patient, the physician must be certain that the patient has a good social support system and there is an absence of clearly pathologic features that predispose the patient to subsequent suicide. The support system usually includes a place to live and family or friends who will support the patient emotionally.

Low-risk patients frequently present with suicidal threats or minor attempts that occur in the context of a clearly definable external crisis. Social support is usually available and responsive. However, because many attempts that appear trivial on first glance are found to

**Table 242-2.** Evaluation of Suicide Risk

|  | High Risk | Low Risk |
| --- | --- | --- |
| Demographic and social profile |  |  |
| Age | Over 45 y | Below 45 y |
| Sex | Male | Female |
| Marital status | Divorced or widowed | Married |
| Employment | Unemployed | Employed |
| Interpersonal relationships | Conflictual | Stable |
| Family background | Chaotic or conflictual | Stable |
| Health |  |  |
| Physical | Chronic illness | Good health |
|  | Hypochondriac | Feels healthy |
|  | Excessive drug intake | Low drug use |
|  | Severe depression | Mild depression |
|  | Psychosis | Neurosis |
| Mental | Severe personality disorder | Normal personality |
|  | Alcoholism or drug abuse | Social drinker |
|  | Hopelessness | Optimism |
| Suicidal activity |  |  |
| Suicidal ideation | Frequent, intense, prolonged | Infrequent, low intensity, transient |
| Suicide attempt | Multiple attempts | First attempt |
|  | Planned | Impulsive |
|  | Rescue unlikely | Rescue inevitable |
|  | Unambiguous wish to die | Primary wish for change |
|  | Communication internalized (self-blame) | Communication externalized (anger) |
|  | Method lethal and available | Method of low lethality or not readily available |
| Resources |  |  |
| Personal | Poor achievement | Good achievement |
|  | Poor insight | Insightful |
|  | Affect unavailable or poorly controlled | Affect available and appropriately controlled |
|  | Poor rapport | Good rapport |
| Social | Socially isolated | Socially integrated |
|  | Unresponsive family | Concerned family |

SOURCE: Modified from Adam KS. *Med Clin North Am* 24:3200, 1983. Used by permission.

have more serious implications on closer examination, all patients presenting following a suicide attempt should be carefully assessed. If there is any question about the safety of discharging a suicidal patient, and psychiatric consultation is not immediately available, the patient should be hospitalized.

## CHEMICAL RESTRAINT

Chemical restraint should be administered after gathering as much information as possible to allow provisional diagnostic assessment. Once initial medical history, physical examination, and laboratory information have been obtained, if the patient continues to chafe against restraints and to show uncontrolled behavior, the use of a pharmacologic intervention to assist in behavioral control might be considered. Although a variety of medications can be used, the only one with a clear advantage over the rest is lorazepam (Ativan), a potent benzodiazepine that has the advantages of the wide therapeutic index of the class, rapid onset of action, and the ease of administration by parenteral or oral routes. Lorazepam is the only benzodiazepine that can be reliably administered intramuscularly, and its oral and parenteral potencies do not greatly differ, allowing for ease in dosage calculation. Alternative medications such as short-acting barbiturates have a much narrower therapeutic index, and sedating neuroleptic medications such as the phenothiazines have the disadvantage that those which are most sedating also cause the greatest difficulty with orthostatic hypotension. Useful dosage levels of lorazepam would be 1 to 2 mg orally or intramuscularly every half hour until an adequate level of sedation is achieved. If this is insufficient, haloperidol can be used. The dose is 5 mg intramuscularly in younger adults and 1 to 2 mg intramuscularly in the elderly. However, haloperidol should not be given to those with Parkinson's disease or other movement disorder. The combination of haloperidol (5 mg) and lorazepam (2 mg) is sometimes given initially to calm agitated behavior, especially if psychotic features are present. Droperidol (Inopsine), 2.5 to 5 mg intravenously, ensures rapid onset of tranquilization. Hypotension from droperidol occurs in a number of patients and is generally treated with a 250 to 500 mL crystalloid infusion.

## CONSULTATION AND REFERRAL

In the ideal setting, all emergency departments would have psychiatric consultation available at all times. However, in many instances, the physician in the emergency department will be forced to rely on more limited resources. Many psychiatric problems leading to emergency department presentation do not require immediate definitive treatment. In many instances, disposition following initial screening can be made to a variety of secondary sources of evaluation and treatment. Judgments regarding referral depend on assessment of the patient's likelihood of becoming violent toward self or others. Clues that suggest potential violence include hostile behavior, verbal aggressiveness, or statements about violent intent. Such patients need immediate hospitalization. Marked disorientation and confusion require evaluation for organic components. In the absence of such indications, referral can be made to a psychiatrist or a psychiatric facility. Results of the emergency department medical and psychiatric evaluation should be summarized in writing and provided to the consultant. The patient should receive clear discharge instructions and should have a follow-up interval for any medical or surgical disorders that were identified.

## BIBLIOGRAPHY

Beck AT, Steer RA, Kovacs M, et al. Hopelessness and eventual suicide: a 10 year prospective study of patients hospitalized with suicidal ideation. *Am J Psychiatry* 142:559, 1985.

Clinton J, Sterner S, Stelmachers Z, Ruiz E. Haloperidol for sedation of disruptive emergency patients. *Ann Emerg Med* 16:319, 1987.

Fauman MA, Fauman BJ. The differential diagnosis of organic based psychiatric disturbance in the emergency department. *JACEP* 6:315, 1977.

Fawcet J, Schefner W, Clark D, et al. Clinical predictors of suicide in patients with major effective disorders: a controlled prospective study. *Am J Psychiatry* 144:35, 1987.

Lavole F, Carter G, Danzl D, et al. Emergency department violence in United States teaching hospitals. *Ann Emerg Med* 17:1227, 1988.

Purdie FR, Honigman B, Rosen P. Acute organic brain syndrome. A review of 100 cases. *Ann Emerg Med* 10:455, 1981.

Rund DA, Saunders AF, Hutzler JC. The suicide attempt. *Emerg Med Surv* 162:53, 1981.

Rund DA, Summers WK, Levin M. Alcohol use and psychiatric illness in emergency patients. *JAMA* 245:1240, 1981.

Satcia MJ, Gustafson DH, Johnson SW. Quality assurance for psychiatric emergencies: an analysis of assessment and feedback methodologies. *Psychiatr Clin North Am* 13:35, 1990.

Summers WK, Rund DA, Levin ML. Psychiatric illness in general urban emergency room: daytime versus night time population. *J Clin Psychiatry* 41:340, 1979.

Tardiff K. Management of the violent patient in an emergency situation. *Psychiatr Clin North Am* 11:539, 1988.

Zun L, Gold I. A survey of the form of the mental status examination administered by emergency physicians. *Ann Emerg Med* 15:916, 1986.

# 243
# PSYCHOTROPIC MEDICATIONS

## Kathy E. Shy
## Douglas A. Rund

More than one-third of all emergency department patients have diagnosable psychiatric illness, and one out of every five adults in the United States has received a prescription for a psychoactive drug. The emergency physician must be able to administer certain selected psychotropic medications appropriately and recognize and manage side effects, toxicities, and adverse interactions with other medications.

There are five major classes of psychotropic medications: antipsychotics; anxiolytics, sedatives, and hypnotics; antidepressants (heterocyclics, monoamine oxidase inhibitors (MAOIs), selective serotonin reuptake inhibitors (SSRIs) and other "atypical" agents); and lithium. Of these, only two, the antipsychotics and the anxiolytics, sedatives, and hypnotics, have undisputed utility on an emergency basis. Antidepressants and lithium are rarely prescribed by the emergency physician, primarily because they have long latencies of action and multiple side effects and require careful long-term monitoring. Only in exceptional circumstances, in consultation with a psychiatrist who agrees to provide follow-up care, might the emergency physician elect to initiate antidepressant or lithium therapy. Extensive pretreatment evaluation and detailed patient education weigh heavily against prescribing lithium, MAOIs, or heterocyclic antidepressants in the emergency department.

The emergency physician should be familiar with the emergency indications, common side effects, toxic reactions, and common interactions of the psychotropic medications. Caution in prescribing is the rule. Certain cases are bound to be complex, requiring detailed psychiatric evaluation, and serious medical disorders may coexist with psychiatric disorders. Patients with medical disorders, a history of serious side effects with psychotropic medication, or apparent need for more than one psychoactive medication usually require psychiatric consultation. Several excellent references deal in depth with side effects and toxicity of psychotropic medications (Baldessarini and Hyman).

## ANTIPSYCHOTICS (NEUROLEPTICS)
### Indications

Because antipsychotic medications are symptom-specific (not disease-specific), they are useful in nearly all psychoses, whether primary or secondary (substance-induced or due to a general medical condition). In the emergency setting, they are most often indicated to control agitated psychotic behavior that constitutes an imminent danger to the patient or others. Antipsychotic medications may also be the agents of choice to control nonpsychotic agitation in patients with acute sedative-hypnotic or alcohol intoxication, since there is significant risk of respiratory depression if benzodiazepines are employed. Notable exceptions to these general principles are the regurgitating patient, who may aspirate if sedated, and the patient with anticholinergic psychosis, whose symptoms may worsen with antipsychotics.

A known allergy to a specific antipsychotic medication is a contraindication to its use and to use of other antipsychotic medications of the same class. Most patients who claim to be allergic to antipsychotic medications, however, actually describe a history of acute dystonic reactions when questioned more carefully. A history of malignant neuroleptic syndrome and pregnancy are relative contraindications, and hospitalization is indicated before antipsychotic medications are initiated in these patients.

### Guidelines

Low-potency antipsychotics (Table 243-1) such as chlorpromazine (Thorazine) and thioridazine (Mellaril) may cause life-threatening hypotension and thus are rarely used in emergency medicine. High-potency antipsychotics such as haloperidol (Haldol) and fluphenazine (Prolixin) have relatively few anticholinergic and alpha-blocking effects and are remarkably safe, even at high doses. They are the emergency antipsychotic agents of choice.

Moderate dosages of antipsychotic medications have proven to be at least as effective as the larger dosages previously employed in rapid neuroleptization techniques and are probably safer. Clinical trials using predetermined fixed dosages of antipsychotics have failed to support routine use of dosages of more than 10 to 15 mg of haloperidol a day and suggest that higher dosages may actually be less effective. Optimal pharmacologic management of acute psychotic agitation, therefore, now typically combines antipsychotic medication on a scheduled basis with a PRN benzodiazepine if additional sedation is required. The high-potency antipsychotic and benzodiazepine combination is usually associated with fewer side effects than either agent used independently in higher dosages, and the benzodiazepine may actually offer some protection against neuroleptic side effects. A typical dosing regimen would be 5 mg haloperidol or its equivalent, either intramuscularly (IM) or orally (PO) (using the liquid concentration form) twice a day plus lorazepam, 1 to 2 mg PO or IM every 60 min as necessary. Dosages should be half of those described or less if the patient is elderly or debilitated.

### Side Effects

Antipsychotics block dopamine receptors throughout the central nervous system (CNS). Dopamine receptor blockade in the mesolimbic

**Table 243-1.** Commonly Used Antipsychotic Agents

| Generic Name | Brand Name | Approximate Equivalent Dose, mg | Relative Potency |
|---|---|---|---|
| **TRICYCLICS** | | | |
| **Phenothiazines** | | | |
| Aliphatic | | | |
| Chlorpromazine | Thorazine | 100 | Low |
| Triflupromazine | Vesprine | 30 | Low |
| Piperidines | | | |
| Mesoridazine | Serentil | 50 | Intermediate |
| Thioridazine | Mellaril | 100 | Intermediate |
| Piperazines | | | |
| Acetophenazine | Tindal | 15 | Intermediate |
| Perphenazine | Trilafon | 10 | Intermediate |
| Trifluoperazine | Stelazine | 5 | High |
| Fluphenazine | Prolixin, Permitil | 2 | High |
| **Thioxanthines** | | | |
| Aliphatic | | | |
| Chlorprothixene | Taractan | 100 | Low |
| Piperazine | | | |
| Thiothixene | Navane | 4 | High |
| Dibenzapine | | | |
| Loxapine | Loxitane, Daxolin | 15 | Intermediate |
| **NONTRICYCLICS** | | | |
| Dihydroindolone | | | |
| Molindone | Moban | 10 | Intermediate |
| Butyrophenones | | | |
| Haloperidol | Haldol | 2 | High |
| Droperidol | Inapsine (for injection) | 2 | High |

areas accounts for their antipsychotic properties. Dopamine blockade in the nigrostriatal terminals is responsible for the majority of motor side effects, including acute dystonias, akathisia, and Parkinson syndrome.

*Acute dystonias,* which usually occur in young males during the first few days of antipsychotic treatment, are probably the most common side effect of antipsychotic medications seen in the emergency department. Muscle spasms of the neck, face, and back are the most common dystonias, but oculogyric crisis and even laryngospasm may also occur. When a drug history is not carefully obtained, dystonias are often misdiagnosed as primary neurologic illnesses (seizures, meningitis, tetanus, etc.). Treatment with either 1 to 2 mg of benztropine (Cogentin) intravenously (IV) or 25 to 50 mg of diphenhydramine (Benadryl) IV rapidly corrects the dystonia. Dystonias often recur, even if the antipsychotic is decreased or discontinued, however, unless an antiparkinsonian drug such as benztropine, 1 mg PO two to four times daily, is administered over the next several days.

*Akathisia,* a sensation of motor restlessness with a subjective desire to move, can begin several days to several weeks after initiation of antipsychotic treatment. Often misdiagnosed as anxiety or exacerbation of psychiatric illness, akathisia is aggravated by subsequent increases in antipsychotic dosage. Other coexisting extrapyramidal effects, such as cogwheel rigidity and shuffling gait, suggest antipsychotic effect, but these signs are not invariably present. Management is difficult. If possible, the dosage of the antipsychotic should be decreased. Antiparkinsonian drugs, such as benztropine (Cogentin), 1 mg PO two to four times daily, may also afford some relief. In refractory cases, the antipsychotic may need to be changed or an alternative form of therapy tried.

Antipsychotic-induced *Parkinson syndrome* is particularly common in the elderly and usually begins in the first month of treatment. A complete Parkinson syndrome, including bradykinesia, resting tremor, cogwheel rigidity, shuffling gait, masked facies, and drooling can occur, but often only one or two features of the syndrome are ob-

vious. Antipsychotic dosage reduction and/or anticholinergic medication is usually effective.

While antidopaminergic extrapyramidal side effects (EPS) such as acute dystonia, akathisia, and Parkinson syndrome occur more often with high-potency neuroleptics, anticholinergic and anti-adrenergic effects are more commonly seen with low-potency neuroleptics. Both anticholinergic and alpha-blocking effects are dose-related and much more common in the elderly.

*Anticholinergic effects* range from mild sedation to delirium. Peripheral manifestations may include dry mouth and skin, blurred vision, urinary retention, constipation, paralytic ileus, cardiac arrhythmias, and exacerbation of narrow-angle glaucoma. The central anticholinergic syndrome is characterized by dilated pupils, dysarthria, and an agitated delirium. Discontinuation of the antipsychotic and institution of supportive measures is the most prudent therapy. Physostigmine, 1 to 2 mg administered slowly IV may temporarily reverse the syndrome but may be very toxic and should be reserved for life-threatening situations.

*Cardiovascular side effects* are seen almost exclusively with low-potency antipsychotics. Alpha-adrenergic blockade and a negative inotropic effect on the myocardium may cause pronounced orthostatic hypotension and, rarely, cardiovascular collapse. Usually the hypotension can be easily managed with IV fluid. In severe cases, agonists, such as metaraminol (Aramine) or norepinephrine (Levophed), may be required.

*Neuroleptic malignant syndrome* (NMS) is an uncommon idiosyncratic reaction to neuroleptic drugs manifested by rigidity, fever, autonomic instability (tachycardia, diaphoresis, and blood pressure abnormalities), and a confusional state. Elevation of muscle enzymes, such as creatinine phosphokinase (CPK) and aldolase, the white blood cell count, and liver function tests are often seen. While high-potency antipsychotics may be more likely to cause the disorder, all antipsychotics are potential offenders. NMS is a medical emergency and has a mortality rate as high as 20 percent. Management includes immediate discontinuation of the antipsychotic medication and meticulous supportive treatment in an intensive care setting. Anticholinergic medications are not helpful and may worsen the condition by further impairing centrally mediated temperature regulation. Medications such as dantrolene sodium or bromocriptine are sometimes used to relieve the rigidity.

## Overdose

While antipsychotics are rarely fatal when taken alone, overdose can present some unique management problems. With the exception of thioridazine (Mellaril), antipsychotics are potent antiemetics. The antiemetic effect may interfere with pharmacologic induction of emesis, and gastric lavage is often required. Agents with beta-agonist activity such as isoproterenol (Isuprel) are contraindicated for cardiovascular support because beta-stimulated vasodilatation may worsen hypotension. Extrapyramidal effects may also be prominent in antipsychotic overdosage and are best treated with 25 to 50 mg of diphenhydramine (Benadryl) IV.

## Clozapine

Clozapine (Clozaril) is an "atypical" antipsychotic medication that is preferentially more active at limbic than at striatal dopamine receptors and causes few or no EPS, although surprisingly a few cases of NMS have been reported. Unfortunately, it is much more likely to produce agranulocytosis than are standard antipsychotic medications, and so its use is reserved for patients with schizophrenia unresponsive to standard agents or for those suffering from severe EPS of tardive dyskinesia with the standard agents. Use of clozapine requires weekly complete blood counts (CBC) for as along as the drug is prescribed. Any white blood cell count less than 3500 requires closer monitoring. A white blood cell count less than 2000 or absolute granulocyte count less than 1000 mandates immediate discontinuation of the drug and consultation with a hematologist. Fever may be a side effect during the first few weeks of therapy and should prompt an immediate CBC. If the CBC is normal, the fever will typically reverse. Clozapine is strongly sedating, strongly anticholinergic, and has considerable hypotensive effects. It also poses a substantial risk for inducing seizures, particularly when higher doses are used. Respiratory depression and arrest have been reported rarely, and there is a suggestion that coprescription of a benzodiazepine may increase the risk for this side effect.

Commonly reported features of overdose include altered sensorium (drowsiness, delirium, and coma), tachycardia, hypotension, respiratory depression and failure, hypersalivation, and seizures. Management, in addition to administration of activated charcoal, is symptomatic and supportive. Epinephrine and its derivatives should be avoided, as should antiarrythmics such as procainamide and quinidine. Close surveillance, including cardiac and vital sign monitoring, should continue for several days because of risk of delayed toxic effects. Fatal overdosages have been reported, usually at dosages over 2500 mg.

## Risperidone

Risperidone (Risperdal) is the most recently introduced "atypical" antipsychotic medication. Its pharmacologic profile of potent serotonin (5-HT$_2$) antagonism and moderate dopamine (D$_2$) antagonism probably accounts for its relatively low risk of EPS. Unlike clozapine, it does not have increased risk of agranulocytosis. Common side effects include sedation, insomnia, constipation, and weight gain. Cardiovascular effects may include small, short-term increases in heart rate, accompanied by reduced systolic/diastolic blood pressure, orthostatic hypotension, and QT-interval prolongation. Seizures have been reported in 0.3 percent of patients.

Experience with acute overdose is limited. Features of overdose generally reflect exaggerated pharmacologic effects: drowsiness, sedation, tachycardia, hypotension, EPS, prolonged QT, widened QRS and, in one instance, a seizure. Management is basically supportive. Cardiovascular monitoring is imperative. Should antiarrhythmic therapy be required, agents such as disopyramide, procainamide, and quinidine, which have the potential for QT-prolonging effects, should be avoided. As with more traditional antipsychotics, agents that may worsen effects of β-adrenergic blockade, such as bretylium, epinephrine, and dopamine, should also be avoided.

## ANXIOLYTICS

### Indications

Severe emotional distress may indicate a need for psychotropic medication, even if the patient is not psychotic or an imminent threat to him- or herself or others. While not a substitute for psychotherapy, short-term anxiolytic therapy may be particularly beneficial in the anxious, agitated patient during a psychosocial crisis. Anxiolytics are also indicated for acute panic reactions unresponsive to reassurance.

Anxiolytics also have utility in medical and surgical emergencies. Nonpsychiatric uses include facilitation of cooperation and muscle relaxation during painful procedures; controlling seizures; treating alcohol, sedative, or hypnotic withdrawal; and allaying anxiety when a painful procedure such as surgery has been delayed.

Benzodiazepines are contraindicated in patients with known hypersensitivity to benzodiazepines and in acute, narrow-angle glaucoma. Pregnancy, particularly in the first trimester, is a relative contraindication.

### Guidelines

Before prescribing anxiolytics, the emergency physician should try to rule out any serious underlying psychiatric illness. Because agitation and anxiety may indicate incipient psychosis or major affective disorder, anxiolytics should be used with extreme caution in patients with a history of major psychiatric illness. The possibility that a patient may be feigning illness to procure controlled substances should also be considered.

Benzodiazepines are very effective anxiolytics with a high therapeutic index. Nonbenzodiazepine anxiolytics (e.g., barbiturates and propanediols) have low therapeutic indices and high addiction potential. Except in the rare case of an allergy to benzodiazepines, nonbenzodiazepine anxiolytics have little use in modern psychopharmacology. Buspirone hydrochloride (BuSpar), an atypical anxiolytic medication that does not interact with the benzodiazepine-GABA receptor complex, has a delayed onset of action of days to weeks, which makes it impractical for use in emergent situations. Since it does not have cross-tolerance with other sedative/hypnotics or alcohol, it is not useful in treatment of sedative/hypnotic or alcohol withdrawal.

Certain benzodiazepines have relatively long half-lives (Table 243-2), including diazepam (Valium), chlordiazepoxide (Librium), flurazepam (Dalmane), and prazepam (Centrax). Agents with long half-lives gradually accumulate in the body and thus have a greater potential for causing sedation and confusion, particularly in the elderly. For short-term use, these agents may benefit the young, healthy person in crisis who complains of insomnia but is also anxious during the day. A single bedtime dose both induces sleep and has a mild anxiolytic effect the following day. For the most part, however, with the exception of the use of diazepam in seizures, short-acting benzodiazepines such as lorazepam (Ativan), oxazepam (Serax), and alprazolam (Xanax) are the preferred agents in emergency medicine. Alprazolam (Xanax), 0.25 to 0.50 mg PO, is a particularly effective treatment in acute panic attack. Only midazolam (Versed), a very short-acting agent, and lorazepam (Ativan) have reliable intramuscular absorption. Lorazepam, an agent with very low cardiopulmonary toxicity, is particularly well suited for emergency use. Dosages of 1 to 2 mg PO or IM are usually effective. As with all benzodiazepines, dosage adjustments may be necessary: higher dosages may be required in patients with histories of alcohol or sedative/hypnotic abuse; lower dosages in patients with hepatic disease or severe debilitation. Because they potentiate other CNS depressants, benzodiazepines should be used with extreme caution in intoxicated patients. Benzodiazepines particularly suppress hypoxic respiratory drive and should be used with caution in patients with hypercarbia, especially if the patient is also receiving supplemental oxygen.

**Table 243-2.** Commonly Used Benzodiazepines

| Generic Name | Brand Name | Approximate Half-life, h | Usual Total Oral dose, mg |
|---|---|---|---|
| ANXIOLYTICS* | | | |
| Alprazolam | Xanax | 12 | 1–6 |
| Chlorazepate | Tranxene | 48 | 15–60 |
| Chlordiazepoxide | Librium | 20 | 15–60 |
| Diazepam | Valium | 35 | 15–60 |
| Lorazepam | Ativan | 16 | 2–6 |
| Midazolam | Versed | 2 | —‡ |
| Oxazepam | Serax | 15 | 20–60 |
| Prazepam | Centrax | 15† 100† | 20–60 |
| HYPNOTICS | | | |
| Flurazepam | Dalmane | 2† 72† | 15–30 qhs |
| Temazepam | Restoril | 15 | 15–30 qhs |
| Trizolam | Halcion | 2 | 0.125–0.5 qhs |

* Anxiolytics are administered in divided doses, usually three or four times daily.

† Flurazepam and prazepam have active metabolites with long half-lives.

‡ Midazolam is available for parenteral use only.

## Side Effects

Benzodiazepine side effects are usually mild and easily treated. Drowsiness, decreased mental alertness, sedation, and ataxia are the most common side effects. Such effects can usually be managed conservatively by decreasing the dose and advising the patient to avoid potentially hazardous activities, such as driving or operating dangerous machinery. Infrequent paradoxical responses of insomnia and agitation are more common in the elderly and require discontinuation of the medication. Because benzodiazepines have abuse potential and high street value, the emergency physician should never prescribe more than a week's supply.

## HETEROCYCLIC ANTIDEPRESSANTS (HCAs)

Although tricyclic antidepressants (named for their three-ring structure) were first synthesized in the nineteenth century, their antidepressant properties were not recognized until the late 1950s. Since that time, tricyclic and other "-cyclic" antidepressant agents have been formulated, thus creating need for the more general term *heterocyclic* (Table 243-3). The therapeutic effect of HCAs is believed to be related to secondary downregulation of norepinephrine and serotonin postsynaptic receptors after initial blockade of presynaptic reuptake of norepinephrine and serotonin. HCAs are primarily indicated for major depression but may also be effective for dysthymic disorder, panic disorder, agoraphobia, obsessive compulsive disorder, enuresis, and school phobia. As previously advised, initiation of HCA therapy in the emergency department is not routinely recommended.

## Side Effects

HCAs have low therapeutic indices. Side effects are common and often occur with customary dosages, even though serum levels may be within the designated therapeutic range. The majority of side effects are either anticholinergic or cardiotoxic.

*Anticholinergic side effects* are the most common. They are particularly likely to occur with concomitant use of other drugs with anticholinergic properties, such as low-potency antipsychotics, antiparkinsonian agents, antihistamines, and over-the-counter sleeping remedies. Both peripheral and central effects may occur. Peripheral effects include dry mouth, metallic taste, blurred vision, constipation, paralytic ileus, urinary retention, tachycardia, and exacerbation of narrow-angle glaucoma. Central effects include sedation, mydriasis, agitation, and delirium. Mild to moderately severe anticholinergic effects may be managed by dosage reduction, change to a medication with fewer anticholinergic properties, or addition of urecoline, 10 to 25 mg PO three times daily. For acute urinary retention, urecoline, 2.5 to 5 mg may be given subcutaneously. When anticholinergic effects become life-threatening, physostigmine, 1 to 2 mg administered

**Table 243-3.** Commonly Used Heterocyclic Antidepressants

| Generic Name | Brand Name | Usual Dose mg/day |
|---|---|---|
| TRICYCLICS | | |
| Amitriptyline | Amitril, Elavil, Endep | 75–200 |
| Amoxapine | Asendin | 100–300 |
| Desipramine | Norprammin, Pertofrane | 75–200 |
| Doxepin | Adapin, Curetin, Sinequan | 75–200 |
| Imipramine | Janimine, Presamine, SK-Pramine, Trofranil | 75–200 |
| Nortriptyline | Aventyl, Pamelor | 40–150 |
| Pritriptyline | Vivactil | 15–40 |
| Trimipramine | Surmontil | 75–200 |
| OTHERS | | |
| Maprotiline | Ludiomil | 100–150 |
| Trazodone | Desyrel | 100–200 |

very slowly IV, may be used. If physostigmine toxicities ensue, the effects can be reversed with IV atropine sulfate, 0.5 mg for each 1.0 mg of physostigmine administered.

*Cardiac side effects* of HCAs may include nonspecific T-wave changes, prolonged QT interval, varying degrees of AV block, and atrial and ventricular arrhythmias. Orthostatic hypotension from α-adrenergic blockade may be significant, particularly in the elderly.

HCA therapy may also be complicated by allergic obstructive jaundice; decreased seizure threshold (especially with maprotiline, clomipramine, and amoxapine); and, very rarely, agranulocytosis.

Trazodone has little in common with other HCAs. It lacks significant anticholinergic or cardiac conduction effects but may be associated with marked sedation, ventricular arrhythmias, and significant orthostatic hypotension. It may also cause priapism, a urologic emergency.

## MONOAMINE OXIDASE INHIBITORS (MAOIs)

MAO catalyzes the oxidation of biogenic amines (tyramine, serotonin, dopamine, and norepinephrine) throughout the body. The therapeutic effect of MAOIs is probably related to their ability to increase norepinephrine and serotonin in the CNS. They are recommended for atypical major depressive episodes, characterized by hyperphagia, hypersomnolence, reversed diurnal variation (worse in the evening), emotional lability, so-called leaden paralysis (heavy leaden feelings in arms or legs), and rejection hypersensitivity. They are also occasionally useful in selected cases of HCA-refractory major depression and panic disorder (although the latter use is not yet approved by the FDA). Only two agents in this class, phenelzine (Nardil) and tranylcypromine (Parnate), are commonly used in the United States. As with HCAs, initiation of therapy in the emergency department is not recommended. The physician who initiates MAOI therapy must have firmly established an appropriate indication for use and provided the patient with extensive counseling about toxic interactions with numerous medications and foods.

## Side Effects

In general, MAOIs have fewer side effects than do HCAs. *Orthostatic hypotension,* although occasionally severe, usually responds to supportive therapy. *CNS irritability,* including agitation, motor restlessness, and insomnia, is managed by dosage reduction or addition of a benzodiazepine. Occasionally, MAOIs, like other antidepressant medications, actually precipitate a manic episode. *Autonomic side effects,* such as dry mouth, constipation, urinary retention, and delayed ejaculation, sometimes occur but are usually mild.

MAOIs block oxidative deamination of tyramine and may precipitate a *hypertensive crisis* when certain drugs, such as sympathomimetic amines, L-dopa, narcotics, or HCAs, or tyramine-containing foods are ingested. Common tyramine-containing foods include aged cheese, beer, wine, pickled herring, yeast extracts, chopped liver, yogurt, sour cream, and fava beans. The onset of the crisis is usually heralded by a severe headache. While hypertension is potentially the most serious effect, cardiac arrhythmias, restlessness, diaphoresis, mydriasis, and vomiting may also occur. Mild cases of hypertension may respond to 10 mg of sublingual nifedipine. In more severe cases, an α antagonist, such as phentolamine 5 mg IV, repeated as necessary, is indicated. Beta-blocking agents are contraindicated, since they may intensify vasoconstriction and worsen hypertension. Although death may occur from hypertensive intracranial hemorrhage, the vast majority of patients recover completely from the hypertensive episode within a few hours. The MAOI can be restarted the following day after dietary counseling is reinforced.

*Drug-drug interactions* often complicate MAOI therapy. MAOIs potentiate the actions of sympathomimetics, anticholinergics, and oral hypoglycemics. They also inhibit metabolic degradation of alcohol, barbiturates, and narcotics. When combined with meperidine

(Demerol), MAOIs may cause a variety of adverse effects, including hypotension, hypertension, fever, and neuromuscular irritability. While the interactions listed are among the most common, the list is far from exhaustive. More comprehensive accounts may be found in standard references.

## SELECTIVE SEROTONIN REUPTAKE INHIBITORS (SSRIs)

Since the introduction of fluoxetine (Prozac) in 1988, the SSRIs have become the most commonly prescribed antidepressants in the United States. Other SSRIs currently available include sertraline (Zoloft) and paroxetine (Paxil). SSRIs are primarily indicated for treatment of major depressive episodes but also have utility in panic disorder and obsessive compulsive disorder. Because of their favorable side effect profile and relative safety in overdose, some have argued that institution of an SSRI by an emergency department physician may occasionally be appropriate if (1) the patient can be assessed to rule out general medical causes for the depression, (2) ongoing substance abuse can be ruled out, and (3) the patient can be followed in the emergency setting until picked up by another health care provider. However, this rationale has been questioned because of the ongoing dispute about whether or not fluoxetine and other SSRIs might increase suicidality in some patients.

### Side Effects

SSRIs lack the anticholinergic and cardiac effects typical of the HCAs, although there have been several reports of symptomatic bradycardia with fluoxetine. The side effect profile of SSRIs reflect their potent serotonin antagonism. Among the most common side effects are headaches, dizziness, nausea, diarrhea, insomnia, and agitation. A significant advantage of SSRIs is their high therapeutic index and associated low lethality, even when large quantities are ingested acutely.

A *serotonin syndrome* with SSRIs has been reported, primarily when SSRIs are combined with other serotonergic medications such as the MAOIs. The syndrome is manifest by both CNS (restlessness, tremor, myoclonus, hyperreflexia, and seizures) and gastrointestinal (nausea, vomiting, diarrhea) irritability. Consequently, SSRIs should not be combined with MAOIs. Treatment of the serotonin syndrome consists of discontinuing the serotonergic agents and providing supportive care.

## ATYPICAL, SECOND-GENERATION ANTIDEPRESSANTS

The term *second-generation antidepressants* has generally been applied to new classes of antidepressants introduced after the HCAs and MAOIs. Thus far, second-generation antidepressants include the SSRIs and two pharmologically dissimilar agents, bupropion (Wellbutrin) and venlafaxine (Effexor).

### Bupropion

Bupropion is an aminoketone, structurally distinct from previous antidepressants. The mechanism of its antidepressant effect is unknown; it has very little effect on serotonin or norepinephrine uptake and few anticholinergic or antihistaminic effects. Its side effect profile is similar to that of fluoxetine. Dry mouth, dizziness, headache, tremor, insomnia, and psychomotor agitation are the most commonly reported side effects. Infrequently it may induce or exacerbate psychotic episodes. Anticholinergic and cardiovascular effects are minimal, although there are a few reports that it may exacerbate baseline hypertension. Seizures may occur, particularly in bulimic patients. Its use is contraindicated in patients with histories of eating disorders, head trauma, or any other predisposition towards seizures, including med-

ications that could lower seizure threshold. Like the SSRIs, bupropion should not be given in combination with MAOIs. While clinical experience with overdoses has been limited, seizures occur in about a third of the cases. Death from overdose of bupropion alone is rare and typically preceded by multiple uncontrolled seizures, bradycardia, and cardiac arrest.

### Venlafaxine

Venlafaxine (Effexor) is a structurally novel antidepressant, chemically unrelated to HCAs, MAOIs, or other available antidepressants. It is a potent inhibitor of neuronal serotonin and norepinephrine reuptake and a weak dopamine reuptake inhibitor. Unlike the HCAs, however, it has no significant affinity for muscarinic, histaminic or α-adrenergic receptors. In clinical trials the most commonly reported side effects included asthenia, sweating, nausea, constipation, anorexia, vomiting, somnolence, dry mouth, dizziness, anxiety, tremor, blurred vision, and abnormal ejaculation and impotence in men. Unique among antidepressants is ventafloxine's dose-related propensity to cause sustained hypertension, with the highest incidence (13 percent) in doses greater than 300 mg/day. Human experience with acute overdose is very limited. In premarketing trials there were 14 reports of overdose, alone or in combination with other drugs and/or alcohol. All 14 patients recovered without sequelae. Although most patients reported no symptoms, somnolence was the most common complaint. One patient had two generalized seizures and a prolonged $QT_c$. Two other patients had mild sinus tachycardia.

## LITHIUM

Lithium carbonate is indicated for both acute mania and maintenance therapy in bipolar disorder. It also has utility in some cases of major depression (both unipolar and bipolar) and in some disorders characterized by episodic explosive outbursts or self-mutilation. Its mechanism of action is unknown, although it does increase central norepinephrine reuptake and decrease central norepinephrine release. The extensive pretreatment evaluation and long latency of action preclude the use of lithium as an emergency psychotropic medication.

### Side Effects

Patients vary widely in susceptibility to lithium side effects. While most of the serious adverse effects are associated with toxic serum levels, mild side effects such as gastrointestinal distress, dry mouth, excessive thirst, fine tremors, mild polyuria, and peripheral edema are often seen even when serum levels lie within the designated therapeutic range. This is particularly common during the first few weeks of therapy. Many of the more chronic side effects, including polyuria, nephrogenic diabetes insipidus, benign diffuse goiter, hypothyroidism, skin rashes and ulcerations, psoriasis, and leukocytosis without a left shift, appear unrelated to serum lithium levels. Underlying neurologic illness, dehydration, salt-restricted diets, and childbirth predispose to both minor and major side effects.

### Toxicity and Overdose

The severity of lithium toxicity is related to both the serum lithium level and the duration of the elevated level. Even in acute overdose, symptoms may not be fully apparent for up to 48 h. As a general rule, lithium toxicity is rare at serum levels of less than 2 mEq/L. Early signs of toxicity include nausea and vomiting, dysarthria, lethargy, and a coarse hand tremor. As toxicity worsens, neurologic symptoms increase. Ataxia, myasthenia, incoordination, hyperreflexia, muscle fasciculation, blurred vision, and scotomas may develop. Eventually, confusion, choreoathetosis, myoclonus, and seizures occur, and the patient may finally become comatose. Cardiovascular toxicity is unusual at serum levels of less than 4 mEq/L. In addition to nonspecific T-wave changes, high lithium levels may be associated with hypotension, AV conduction defects, ventricular tachyarrhythmias, and eventually complete cardiovascular collapse.

Because lithium toxicity may cause permanent brain damage, it should be considered a medical emergency. General supportive care, with particular attention to fluid and electrolyte balance, is the foundation of therapy. Lithium excretion may be facilitated by forced saline diuresis and alkalinization of the urine with IV sodium lactate. Mannitol, 50 to 100 mg IV, may also be added to promote osmotic diuresis. Aminophylline, 500 mg given slowly IV, also promotes lithium clearance by both suppressing renal tubular reabsorption of lithium and increasing renal blood flow. If the serum level exceeds a 4 mEq/L, the patient should be dialyzed immediately. Dialysis may also be required for serum levels in the range of 2 to 4 mEq/L if the patient's clinical condition is poor.

## BIBLIOGRAPHY

American Psychiatric Association: *Benzodiazepine Dependence, Toxicity and Abuse.* Washington, DC, American Psychiatric Association, 1990.

Baldessarini RJ: *Chemotherapy in Psychiatry.* Cambridge, MA, Harvard University Press, 1985.

Baldessarini RJ, et al: Significance of neuroleptic dose and plasma level in the pharmacological treatment of psychoses. *Arch Gen Psychiatry* 45:79, 1988.

Bernstein JG: *Handbook of Drug Therapy in Psychiatry,* 2d ed. Littleton, MA, PSY Publishing, 1988.

Boehnert MT, Lovejoy FJ: Value of the QRS duration versus the serum drug level in predicting seizures and ventricular arrhythmias after an acute over-dosage of tricyclic antidepressants. *N Engl J Med* 313:474, 1985.

Fauman BS, Fauman MA: *Emergency Psychiatry for the House Officer.* Baltimore, Williams & Wilkins, 1981.

Gelenbert AJ: Fluoxetine (Prozac) overdose. *Biol Ther Psychiatry Newsl,* 12:11, 1989.

Gilman AG, Rall TW, Nies AS, Taylor P (eds.): *Goodman and Gilman's Pharmacological Basis of Therapeutics,* 7th ed. New York, Macmillan, 1990.

Gultmacher B: *Concise Guide to Psychopharmacology and Electroconvulsive Therapy.* Washington, DC, American Psychiatric Association, 1994.

Hillard JR (ed): *Manual of Clinical Emergency Psychiatry.* Washington, DC, American Psychiatric Association, 1990.

Hollister LE. Csernanasky: *Clinical Pharmacology of Psychotherapeutic Drugs,* 3d ed. New York, Churchill Livingstone, 1990.

Hyman SE (ed): *Manual of Psychiatric Emergencies,* 3d ed. Boston, Little, Brown, 1994.

Janick PT, et al: *Principles and Practice of Psychopharmacotherapy.* Baltimore, Williams & Wilkins, 1993.

Kane JM, Lieberman JA (eds): *Adverse Effects of Psychotropic Drugs.* New York, The Guilford Press, 1992.

Kaplan HI, Sadoc BJ: *Comprehensive Textbook of Psychiatry,* 4th ed. Baltimore, Williams & Wilkins, 1985.

Kapur S, Mieczkowski T, Mann JJ: Antidepressant medications and relative risk of suicide attempt and suicide. *JAMA* 268:3441, 1992.

Lazarus A, Mann SC, Caroff SM: *The Neuroleptic Malignant Syndrome and Related Conditions.* Washington, DC, American Psychiatric Association, 1989.

Leysen JE, et al: Risperidone: A novel antipsychotic with balanced serotonin-dopamine antagonism, receptor occupancy profile and pharmacologic activity. *J Clin Psychiatry* 55:5 (suppl), 1994.

Owens DGC: Extrapyramidal side effects and tolerability of risperiodone: A review. *J Clin Psychiatry* 55:5 (suppl), 1994.

Rund DA, Hutzler JC: *Emergency Psychiatry.* St. Louis, Mosby, 1983.

Salby AE, Lieb J, Trancredi LR: *The Handbook of Psychiatric Emergencies,* 3d ed. New York, Elsevier, 1986.

Sasyniuk BI, Jhamandas V, Valois W: Experimental amitriptyline intoxication: Treatment of cardiac toxicity with sodium bicarbonate. *Ann Emerg Med* 15:1052, 1986.

Settle EC Jr: Bupropion: A novel antidepressant—update 1989. *Int Drug Ther Newsl* 24:29, 1989.

Stoudemire A, Fogel BS: *Medical-Psychiatric Practice,* volume 2. Washington, DC, American Psychiatric Press Association, 1993.

Tomb DA: *Psychiatry for the House Officer,* 2d ed. Baltimore, Williams & Wilkins, 1984.

Walker JI: *Psychiatric Emergencies.* Philadelphia, Lippincott, 1983.

Wyeth-Ayerst Laboratories: Effexor tablets complete prescribing information, CI 4193-1, issued December 29, 1993.

# 244
# ANOREXIA NERVOSA AND BULIMIA NERVOSA

## Alexander H. Sackeyfio
## Susan J. Gottlieb

Anorexia nervosa and bulimia nervosa have reached epidemic proportions in the last 10 years. These diseases were once viewed as purely psychological in nature. However, increasing evidence has confirmed that both disorders involve physical complications, and knowledge of and ability to treat the medical complications that accompany eating disorders are crucial for the patient's well-being.

Eating disorders affect between 5 to 10 percent of adolescent girls and young women, and up to 0.10 percent of young men. Originally regarded as rich girls' diseases, they are now recognized across all socioeconomic and racial groups, in patients between the ages of 8 and 80. The onset of anorexia is usually between 12 years of age and the mid-thirties, with a bimodal distribution of ages 13 to 14 and 17 to 18. Bulimia usually begins between the ages of 17 and 25. The onset of both disorders has been reported in older persons.

Anorexia, with its resulting starvation syndrome, is more likely to be recognized than the more common bulimia, which is frequently concealed from both family and physician. Table 244-1 lists the signs and symptoms that suggest a diagnosis of anorexia and Table 244-2 lists the signs and symptoms of bulimia.

Anorexic patients may present with one or all of the following:

1. Refusal to maintain body weight over a minimum normal weight for age and height, for example, weight loss, or failure to make expected weight gain during a period of growth, leading to body weight 15 percent below normal.
2. Intense fear of becoming obese even when underweight.
3. Disturbance in the way in which body weight, shape, or size is perceived. For example, the obviously underweight or even emaciated patient may complain of being fat or may believe that one area of the body is "too fat."
4. Absence of at least three consecutive expected menstrual cycles (primary or secondary amenorrhea).

A diagnosis of bulimia is suggested by the following:

1. A minimum average of two episodes of binge eating (rapid consumption of a large amount of food in a short period of time) per week for at least 3 months.

**Table 244-1.** Clues to Undiagnosed Anorexia Nervosa

Unexplained growth retardation (individual may be actively or passively affected
Unexplained primary amenorrhea
Weight loss of unknown origin
Unexplained hypercholesterolemia or carotenemia in a thin person
Exercise abuse
Membership in a vulnerable vocation group (see Table 244-2, item 10)

**Table 244-2.** Signs and Symptoms of Bulimia in Adolescents and Young Adults

Hypokalemia of unknown cause or complications of hypokalemia (cardiac, renal, central nervous system)
Parotid gland or submandibular gland enlargement, esophagitis, esophageal bleeding or rupture
Large unexplained weight fluctuations or weight loss
Unexplained elevations of serum amylase
Unexplained secondary amenorrhea
Extensive loss of dental enamel or onset of many new caries
Scars on the knuckles of the hand (from induced vomiting)
Presence of juvenile diabetes mellitus
Other disorders of impulse control—alcoholism, drug abuse, borderline personality disorder
Member of predisposed vocational group—models, ballet students or professionals, wrestlers, jockeys

2. During the eating binges, there is a feeling of lack of control over the eating behavior.
3. The individual regularly engages in self-induced vomiting, use of laxatives, strict dieting, fasting, or vigorous exercising to prevent weight gain.
4. Persistent overconcern with body shape and weight.

Families of patients with eating disorders tend to be outwardly orderly, respectable, and conventional. However, the inner dynamics of the family involve a rigid adherence to secret obligation and stifling prohibitions. Honesty and spontaneity are discouraged, and true autonomy and self-gratification are submerged beneath the adolescent's desire to please and gain approval from other family members.

## ETIOLOGY

The onset of anorexia most often occurs during adolescence. Normal physiologic changes that are preparation for the reproductive function, namely an increase in total body fat (up to 200 percent in adolescent girls) as well as the accumulation of fat around the chest and hips, are perceived as "fatness," and the adolescent begins to diet to lose the unwanted weight. Various reasons have been proposed for the progression of "normal" dieting into an eating disorder. Some feel that for the anorexic, restriction of eating serves as part of a general need to control impulses and disturbing feelings. Others have suggested that the central problems might be an avoidance of adulthood, an emergent panic related to the challenges of late adolescence, and the loss of the security enjoyed by the child and early adolescent.

Bulimics have an intense need for approval, a high self-expectation, and a poor body image. Binging provides escape from boredom, anger, and loneliness and is sometimes a preferred social experience, especially when interpersonal intimacy has been elusive. Purging only adds to an already negative self-image. Binge eating in bulimics almost always begins as a response to hunger from dieting and weight loss. Late in the syndrome, binge eating becomes generalized to deal with emotional distress.

## DIFFERENTIAL DIAGNOSIS

The differential diagnosis includes both psychiatric and medical disorders. Schizophrenics can present with an aversion to eating and sometimes with eating and purging. In depressive illness, anorexia and hyperphagia can be part of the presenting symptoms. Hysterics, patients with inadequate personality disorders, and those with borderline personality disorders may also exhibit eating disorders.

A number of medical disorders should be considered, including superior mesenteric artery syndrome, inflammatory bowel disease, chronic hepatitis, Addison's disease, diabetes, hyperthyroidism, hyperemesis gravidarum, tuberculosis, and malignancy.

About 20 percent of teenage diabetics also have an eating disorder.

Extremely thin people in professions requiring low weight (such as ballet dancers, models, and jockeys) and obligatory runners may or may not have an eating disorder.

## PATHOPHYSIOLOGY

Eating disorders are associated with a number of physiologic changes (Table 244-3). Self-induced vomiting results in various disorders. Dental problems are caused by gastric acid regurgitated into the oral cavity. In addition, the oral hygiene of most anorexics is poor, and the vigorous brushing often done by bulimics aggravates dental problems. Oral hygiene, together with dietary deficiencies and dehydration of the soft tissues of the mouth, can cause gingivitis and dental erosion.

Parotid and submandibular gland enlargement is often seen. Oral lacerations and contusions and callous formations on knuckles from stimulating the gag reflex are common. Dysphagia, hematemesis, and rarely rupture of the esophagus, subcutaneous emphysema, or pneumomediastinum can occur following excessive purging. Easy bruising due to loss of bile salts and poor absorption of vitamin K is another complication. Severe hypokalemia and hypovolemia often accompany recurrent vomiting. Ipecac abuse can cause a dermatomyositis-like syndrome and cardiomyopathy. Hyperamylasemia, probably of salivary gland origin, is associated with purging episodes.

Laxative abuse produces weight loss mainly by dehydration and hypokalemia. Common nonspecific complaints of laxative abuse include constipation, diarrhea, abdominal cramping, and bloating. Specific effects include melanosis coli and cathartic colon. In cathartic colon, the colon is converted into an inert tube incapable of propelling the fecal stream without large doses of laxatives. This condition is not entirely reversible and may require colectomy. Brownish gray hyperpigmented areas on the skin are reported as complications of phenolphthalein-containing laxatives (Correctol, Ex-Lax).

Diuretic abuse results in dehydration and multiple serum abnormalities including hypokalemia, hypercalcemia, hyperuricemia, hypomagnesemia, and hyponatremia.

Binge eating after a period of starvation can result in acute gastric distention and pancreatitis. Postbinge pancreatitis has a reported 10 percent mortality rate.

Periods of starvation result in hypoglycemia, which is a poor prognostic indicator. Hypoglycemia is often associated with hypothermia,

**Table 244-3.** Physiologic Changes Associated with Eating Disorders

Hematologic
   Normochromic and normocytic anemia
   Leukopenia with relative lymphocytosis
   Low sedimentation rate
   Reduced C3 complement
Biochemical
   Hypokalemia
   Hyponatremia
   Hypocalcemia
   Hypophosphatemia
Carbohydrate metabolism
   Low serum insulin levels
   High serum glucagon levels
   Starvation ketosis and hypoglycemia
   Abnormal glucose tolerance due to fasting
   Hypercholesterolemia
Endocrine
   Normal $T_4$ and low $T_3$
   High serum cortisol without diurnal variation
   Low serum luteinizing hormone, follicle-stimulating hormone, and estradiol
   Low total urinary estrogens
   Increased growth hormone
   Pseudo Bartter syndrome (laxative and diuretic abusers)
   Decreased antidiuretic hormone secretion (diabetes insipidus)

coma, and infections and may be fatal. Starvation leads to low insulin levels that are insensitive to both glucose and amino acid infusion. Gastric distention and reduced gastric emptying produce enhanced satiation and prolonged intermeal intervals. Food has been demonstrated to remain in the stomachs of anorexics for up to 24 hours.

Starvation causes a decreased hypoxic ventilatory drive, decreased vital capacity, tidal volume, and minute ventilation. In addition, the surfactant pool is reduced, resulting in "stiffer" lungs with a greater tendency to collapse. The muscles of ventilation are affected by starvation, causing reduced diaphragm mass and respiratory muscle weakness.

Cardiovascular changes include brady- and tachyarrhythmias due to cardiomyopathy or electrolyte abnormalities. ST-T wave changes and QT interval prolongation may be evident. Decreased peripheral adrenergic activity with normal adrenomedullary function results in bradycardia and orthostatic hypotension.

Dermatologic changes include pedal or pretibial edema, with or without hypoalbuminemia; excessive loss of subcutaneous fat; brittle hair and nails; pellagra or scurvy; and petechiae or purpura.

Peripheral neuropathy, most likely a product of chronic malnutrition, is a notable complication. Localized compression neuropathies secondary to subcutaneous tissue loss can also develop. Some patients experience paresthesias of the fingers and toes. Deep tendon reflexes may be diminished, and gross motor coordination may be impaired.

Anorexics are especially likely to be compulsive exercisers. Stress fractures in the feet, march hemoglobinuria, and various musculoskeletal overuse syndromes have been identified in our institution as complications of compulsive exercise.

Osteoporosis is common in anorexics. It usually affects the femur, radius, and spine in decreasing frequency. Estrogen deficiency is not a major causative factor. Any patient with an eating disorder who has been amenorrheic and low in weight for more than a year should undergo bone density studies. We have seen a femur fracture in a young anorexic who tripped on a rug.

Adolescent diabetics induce ketosis by skipping insulin for a day or two to lose weight; sometimes they overeat and increase insulin in compensation. The abuse of insulin and food can lead to severe metabolic consequences. Young diabetics with frequent hospitalizations should be evaluated for a coexisting eating disorder.

## PSYCHOLOGICAL PRESENTATIONS

In addition to the presenting physical symptoms, psychological manifestations may also be detected on emergency evaluation. Depression, including suicidal ideation, is the primary psychological complication of eating disorders. Other psychological manifestations include obsessive-compulsive personality traits, with rumination about food, calories, and weight. Ritualistic eating and exercising behavior are also evident. Perfectionistic striving often results in deterioration of friendships and leisure activities.

Impulse control disorder is a psychological complication of eating disorders more commonly seen in bulimics than anorexics. Behavioral manifestations include shoplifting and stealing, sexual promiscuity, drug and alcohol abuse, and self-mutilation.

## PROGNOSIS

As with most illnesses, the earlier the onset, detection, and treatment the better the prognosis. The prognosis for individuals who have engaged in maladaptive eating patterns for years is guarded. Behaviors may remain constant or the patient may improve briefly and return to the eating disorder during stressful times. Psychological immaturity persists in about 50 percent of the patients, with difficulties in social adjustment, and one third continue to have problems with eating. Chronicity increases the risk of morbidity.

Despite the advances in the understanding of anorexia and bulimia

nervosa, eating disorders are still associated with significant long-term morbidity and mortality.

Mortality figures range from 2 to 5 percent to a high of 18 percent. Death may result from suicide, starvation, metabolic catastrophe, infection, and cardiac insufficiency. Agents used to induce weight loss may lead to fatal complications.

## TREATMENT

Emergency management of the patient with an eating disorder involves consideration of the complications and effects of the disorder.

Nutritional rehabilitation should be the primary goal of treatment in both disorders. Anorexics tend to need a very gradual introduction of macronutrients. Bulimics tend to need fewer calories initially, and it is important to normalize the eating pattern.

Normotensive, hypokalemic, hypochloremic metabolic alkalosis is typical of purging eating disorder patients. They appear to adapt to these metabolic states and treatment should consider the whole metabolic state. "Reflexive" replacement of individual deficiencies should be discouraged because they could be dangerous, with fluid overload and overcorrection as common complications.

Medications have been used in eating disorders. The most helpful in anorexia is Periactin. Antidepressants have proved useful in bulimics. Prozac, imipramine/desipramine, and Nardil have been extensively evaluated and found to be useful.

Emergency management will best be done by using total parenteral nutrition and slowly correcting the metabolic derangement.

A period of 48 h in an inpatient setting is essential to determine the extent and severity of the illness and its complications. An eating disorders unit is a place for this evaluation, but a regular medical floor with involvement of a multidisciplinary psychiatric and internal medicine team is advised.

Hospitalization is suggested for the following:

  Weight loss greater than 30 percent over 3 months
  Severe metabolic disturbance
  Depression severe enough to be at risk for suicide
  Severe binging and purging
  Failure to maintain outpatient weight contract
  Psychosis
  Family crisis
  Need to confront patient and family denial
  Need for initiation of therapy (individual, family, and pharmacotherapy)
  Complex differential diagnosis

A trial of outpatient psychological treatment can be attempted if food restriction and weight loss are of less than 3 months' duration and if there is a very positive family support system. Referral to a local health professional who specializes in the treatment of eating disorders or to a self-help group can be obtained by contacting the following national organizations:

National Association of Anorexia Nervosa and Associated Disorders (ANAD)
P.O. Box 7
Highland Park, IL 60035
(708) 831–3438

Anorexia Nervosa and Related Eating Disorders, Inc. (ANRED)
P.O. Box 5102
Eugene, OR 97405
(503) 344–1144

American Anorexic/Bulimic Association, Inc.
293 Central Park West
Suite 1R
New York, NY 10024
(212) 501–8351

Center for the Study of Anorexia and Bulimia
1 West 91st Street
New York, NY 10024
(212) 595–3449

## BIBLIOGRAPHY

American Psychiatric Association. *Diagnostic and Statistical Manual of Mental Disorders,* 4th ed. Washington, DC: American Psychiatric Ass'n, 1994.

Blinder, Chaitin, Goldstein: *Eating Disorders.* New York: PMA Publishing, 1988.

Comerci D. Eating disorders in adolescents. *Pediatr Rev* 10, 1985.

Garner DM, Garfinkel PE. *Anorexia Nervosa: A Multidimension Perspective.* New York: Bruner/Mazel, 1982.

Garner DM, Sackeyfio AH. *Eating Disorders: Handbook of Behavioral Therapy in Psychiatric Setting.* pp. 477–497, 1993.

Mackenzie JR, LaBan MM, Sackeyfio AH. Prevalence of peripheral neuropathy in patients with anorexia nervosa. *Arch Phys Rehabil.* 70, 1989.

# 245
# PANIC DISORDER
## Suck Won Kim

Panic disorder (PD) is a subcategory of anxiety disorders. Recurrent attacks of pathologic apprehension, feelings of doom, and other autonomic symptoms such as dyspnea, palpitations, dizziness, and sweating are hallmarks of PD. Altered states of mind such as depersonalization or derealization may accompany the attacks. Recurrent panic attacks are often followed by secondary depression and chronic anxiety. Some patients refuse to go back to places where they previously had a panic attack or attacks (agoraphobia).

## CLINICAL FEATURES

The early phase of PD is characterized by brief, intermittent episodes that terminate in less than 10 min. Between attacks, most patients appear completely normal during a routine visit to a physician's office, and they may not even mention symptoms such as dizziness, difficulty in breathing, numbness, or palpitation until asked about them by their physician.

During the attack, the patient is suddenly overwhelmed by anxiety. Somatic symptoms include tachycardia, tachypnea, dyspnea, chest tightness, weakness, and dizziness. Although panic attacks usually occur without a specific provoking incident, it is not uncommon to find that stressful life events have preceded their development. Once the first attack has occurred, it is likely to be followed by recurrent attacks, all usually of 10-min duration.

It is now believed that agoraphobia develops after repeated panic attacks associated with certain situations. Patients with advanced PD frequently want a companion present to help them in case of emergency, and in severe cases of agoraphobia, the patient may become homebound. Recurrent panic attacks also lead to anticipatory anxiety, secondary depression, and an increased risk of suicide (Fig. 245-1). Eventually, significant social and occupational dysfunction develops.

The natural history of PD with or without agoraphobia is highly variable. Patients with milder forms may have prolonged periods of remission with less frequent and less intense attacks, whereas others may suffer many panic attacks during the course of a single day. Panic disorder is more common among young women, and the illness tends to prevail through midlife. A recent large-scale epidemiologic survey showed the lifetime prevalence of PD to be about 1 percent of the population. After the age of 60, the incidence of PD rapidly declines.

## PATHOPHYSIOLOGY

Why PD symptoms appear in some individuals but not others is not fully understood. A number of recent studies suggest amine systems dysfunction in PD, especially in the noradrenergic and serotonergic systems. The functional relationship between the central biogenic amine systems and the peripheral autonomic system is not fully elucidated at the present time. But it is clear that patients who have anxiety symptoms usually show evidence of abnormal autonomic function.

Redmond and Huang demonstrated that stimulation of the locus coeruleus causes panic symptoms. Under clonidine (an $\alpha_2$ agonist) and yohimbine (an $\alpha_2$ antagonist) challenge, PD patients showed either blunted or overstimulated release of prolactin, growth hormone, or cortisol that is mediated through the $\alpha$-adrenergic system. These findings support the possible involvement of the noradrenergic system in PD.

Some studies have suggested involvement of the serotonin system in PD. Sertraline, a serotonin-reuptake inhibitor, is effective in treating PD. The noradrenergic and serotonergic systems are functionally

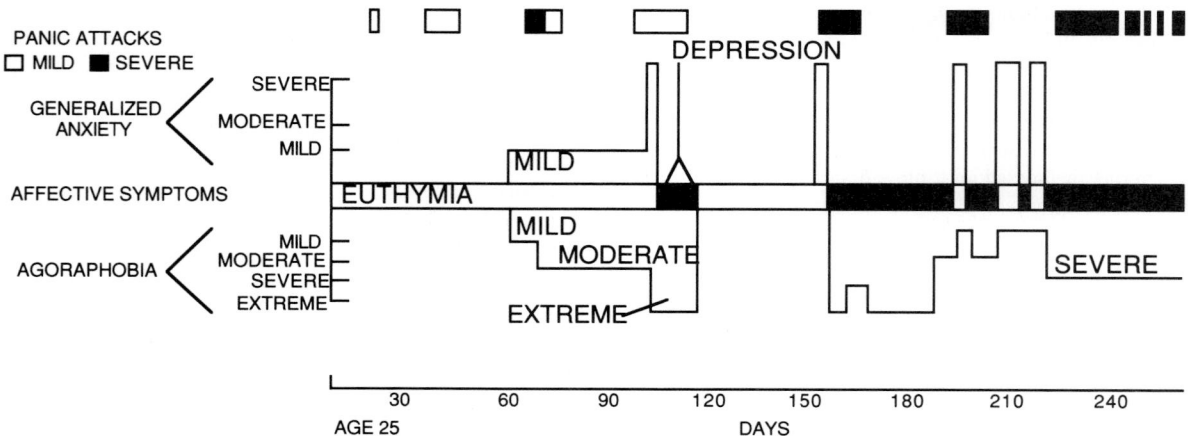

**Fig. 245-1.** Sequential development of panic attacks, genralized anxiety, agoraphobia, and depression during the first 9 months of illness in a 25-year-old woman. (From Uhde TW, Boulenger JP, Roy-Byrne PP, et al. Longitudinal course of panic disorder: clinical and biological considerations. *Prog Neuropsychopharmacol Biol Psychiatry* 9:47, 1985. Used by permission.)

linked, and an alteration of one system causes alterations in the other.

Whether γ-aminobutyric acid (GABA) and benzodiazepine receptors are directly involved in the pathogenesis of PDs is not known. GABA activity-enhancing drugs, like benzodiazepines, may exert their pharmacologic activity partly through the innervation into the norepinephrine and serotonin systems. Both systems have significant GABA input that has a modulating influence on firing rate and release of monoamines. Benzodiazepine receptor agonists (anxiolytic), antagonists, and inverse agonists (anxiogenic) have been used to study anxiety states. Administration of ethyl β-carboline-3-carboxylate (β-CCE), a benzodiazepine inverse agonist, causes marked agitation and anxiety in rhesus monkeys. FG-7142, another benzodiazepine inverse agonist, has also induced profound anxiety in human subjects. Interested readers can also find studies of lactate infusion and carbon dioxide inhalation in PD. Recently Klein proposed a suffocation false alarm hypothesis in PD. Nutt and Lawson have written a comprehensive summary article in this area.

There have been laboratory findings in PD in recent years but their usefulness is limited to research at this time. Reiman and associates, using positron emission tomography, reported increased right parahippocampal blood flow and oxygen metabolism in PD patients. The most recent studies have shown an increased blood flow in the paralimbic belt among provoked simple phobia and post traumatic stress disorder patients. Another group applied magnetic resonance imaging and reported focal abnormalities in the right mesiotemporal area in PD patients. The recent development of radiotracers for various receptor types promises to provide valuable information in this area. Other findings include blunted thyroid-stimulating hormone response to thyrotropin in PD patients. Platelet $\alpha_2$-adrenergic receptor study results are not conclusive. The results of platelet imipramine-binding studies in PD are largely normal. Although rapid eye movement (REM) sleep may not be decreased in a PD patient who has nocturnal panic symptoms, the REM latency on the night of the spells is significantly increased compared to nonpanic nights. Further studies of sleep-related panic symptoms will help elucidate the pathophysiology of this disorder.

## DIFFERENTIAL DIAGNOSIS

It is not uncommon for patients with PD to consult numerous physicians because of cardiac symptoms (chest pain, tachycardia, irregular heartbeat), gastrointestinal symptoms (epigastric pain), or neurologic symptoms (headache, dizziness, vertigo, syncope, paresthesias). Patients with PD may describe only their physical symptoms or depression while ignoring core panic symptoms. Recently, Katon reported that 89 percent of the PD patients studied had presented only physical symptoms, resulting in misdiagnosis, which often continued for months or years. It is essential to inquire about alcohol, drug, and caffeine use. Individuals commonly develop panic symptoms during a period of alcohol withdrawal. Excessive caffeine use can also induce panic symptoms. Recent studies by Uhde and colleagues have shown that an average of 5 cups of coffee will trigger panic attacks in 38 percent of PD patients. Irritable bowel syndrome can also disguise underlying PD. Domestic violence, sexual or physical abuse, or a history of sexual assault, can also be triggers for panic attacks.

Physical illnesses that can be associated with spells resembling panic attacks are summarized in Table 245-1. Panic attacks may be secondary to a number of psychiatric disorders, which are listed in Table 245-2.

**Table 245-1.** Medical Disorders That Mimic Panic Symptoms

| | |
|---|---|
| Acute myocardial infarction | Mitral valve prolapse |
| Hypoglycemia | Alcohol withdrawal |
| Hyperthyroidism | Drug withdrawal |
| Pheochromocytoma | Sleep disorders |
| Complex partial seizures | |

**Table 245-2.** Psychiatric Differential Diagnosis

Generalized anxiety disorder
Depressive disorders
Schizophrenia
Depersonalization disorder
Somatoform disorders
Phobic disorders
Posttraumatic stress disorder
Assault or abuse

## TREATMENT

Generally, treatment is divided into drug and behavior therapy. Traditional psychotherapy is usually ineffective. Many communities now have specialty clinics and support groups. Patients should be guided into one of these programs if necessary. It will be reassuring to patients to find that the physician understands the nature of the symptoms. Careful listening, explanation, and reassurance frequently bring about a positive therapeutic response.

For patients willing to take medication, imipramine, 10 to 25 mg, may be given at night as a starting dose. If needed, up to 150 mg/d can be given. Duration of treatment is highly individualized. Alcohol and caffeine should be avoided if possible. Some patients will complain of motor restlessness or a "speedy" feeling during the early phase of treatment. If this happens, the dose should be lowered and then increased very slowly as tolerated. Some may not be able to tolerate more than 10 mg/d.

Because imipramine has anticholinergic side effects, individuals with narrow-angle glaucoma or prostatic hypertrophy should not be given this drug. Postural hypotension and sedation are other effects.

Newer drugs such as fluoxetine, sertraline, fluvoxamine, and clomipramine have been shown to be effective in the treatment of PD. However, these serotonin-reuptake inhibitors are likely to trigger initial drug-induced anxiety (especially fluoxetine) and should be used cautiously. Patients should always be informed that "keyed up" or "wired" sensations may develop during the early phase of treatment. Prescribing physicians must be thoroughly familiar with these newer drugs before using them. For example, fluoxetine tends to increase serum levels of other concomitantly prescribed antidepressants and many other drugs.

Alprazolam, 1 to 2 mg/d, will rapidly relieve panic symptoms in some mildly affected persons, although some patients will require 4 mg/d or more. Larger doses should be reserved for prescription by psychiatrists. Recently, however, withdrawal symptoms such as anxiety, depression, and insomnia, have raised concerns about its use, and it is important to rule out drug abuse or alcoholism before the drug is prescribed. If the drug is discontinued, it should be tapered slowly over 1 to 3 months. During the withdrawal period, carbamazepine has been shown to be helpful in mitigating withdrawal symptoms. Clonazepam may also be effective.

Although β blockers were used in the past, they are no longer considered drugs of choice in managing the illness. Clonidine can be effective during the first 4 weeks of treatment, but tachyphylaxis develops and long-term efficacy is in question. Imipramine or desipramine are not associated with tolerance and they are generally considered safe for long-term use. Patients who require monoamine oxidase inhibitors such as phenelzine should be referred to psychiatrists. Readers are referred to the recently published National Institutes of Health consensus statement on PD.

## BIBLIOGRAPHY

Ballenger JC (ed). Neurobiology on panic disorder. In: *Frontiers of Clinical Neuroscience.* New York: Alan R. Liss, vol. 8, 1990.

Katon W. *Panic Disorder in the Medical Setting.* National Institute of Mental Health. US Dept of Health and Human Services publication no. (ADM)89-1629. Washington, DC: Government Printing Office, 1989.

Klein DF. False suffocation alarms, spontaneous panics, and related conditions. *Arch Gen Psychiatry* 50:306, 1993.

Murphy DL, Pigott TA. Comparative examination of a role for serotonin in obsessive compulsive disorder, panic disorder, and anxiety. *J Clin Psychiatry* 51(suppl):53, 1990.

Nutt D, Lawson C. A neurochemical overview of models and mechanisms. *Br J Psychiatry* 160:165, 1992.

Redmond DE Jr, Huang YH, Snyder DR, et al. Behavioral effect of stimulation of the nucleus locus coeruleus in the stump tailed monkey (*Macaca arctoides*). *Brain Res* 116:502, 1976.

Reiman EM, Raichle ME, Robins E, et al. The application of positron emission tomography to the study of panic disorder. *Am J Psychiatry* 143:469, 1986.

Special Medical Reports. NIH releases consensus statement on PD. *Am Fam Physician* 45:261–2, 264, 1992.

Uhde TW, Boulenger JP, Roy-Byrne PP, et al. Longitudinal course of panic disorder: clinical and biological considerations. *Prog Neuropsychopharmacol Biol Psychiatry* 9:39, 1985.

Uhde TW, Nemiah JC. Anxiety disorders. In: Kaplan HI, Sadock DJ (eds). *Comprehensive Textbook of Psychiatry,* 5th ed. Baltimore, Williams & Wilkins, 1989.

# 246
# CONVERSION REACTIONS

### Gregory P. Moore
### Kenneth C. Jackimczyk

## DEFINITION

For a diagnosis of conversion reaction to be made the following five criteria must be met:

1. A symptom is expressed in which there is a change or loss of physical function suggesting a physical disorder.
2. The patient has experienced a recent psychological stressor or conflict.
3. The patient unconsciously produces the symptom.
4. The symptom cannot be explained by a known organic etiology or culturally sanctioned response pattern.
5. The symptom is not limited to pain or sexual dysfunction.

## PATHOPHYSIOLOGY

An illustrative example involves the case of a young wife who is scheduled to visit her debilitated father in the hospital. His recent diagnosis of cancer has left her distraught, and the sight of him depresses her greatly. On the morning of her visit, she suddenly becomes blind.

This example typifies conversion reactions in which conflict is caused by the patient's intense, but psychically unacceptable, urge to avoid a required action (in this case visiting her father). The physical symptom (blindness) allows expression of the urge (how can she drive there if she is blind?) without consciously confronting the feelings that led to the wish. At the same time, the symptom imposes morbidity as a punishment for the wish. Often, the presenting symptom will have a symbolic relationship to the conflict but this is not always the case. In this case the sight of her father is distressing and therefore loss of sight is the chief complaint. Conversion reactions are often thought of as nonverbal exertion of control on the environment. Two mechanisms are responsible for the symptoms. The first is "primary gain," in which the symptom allows patients to avoid confronting their uncomfortable feelings. The second is "secondary gain," in which uncomfortable situations are avoided and support is given that might not normally be available. In the above case secondary gain would occur if the patient's husband then stayed home from work to tend to his "blind" wife.

## PREDISPOSING FACTORS

Conversion reactions are described as rare, with an annual incidence in outpatient psychiatric settings of 0.01 to 0.02 percent. An incidence of 5 to 16 percent in inpatients with psychiatric consultations has been noted. Most agree that the incidence is declining. Cases predominantly involve neurologic and orthopedic manifestations, and are seen in the military during times of war, in victims of industrial accidents, and in victims of violence. Conversion reactions are much more frequent in women than men, accounting for up to 80 percent of cases in some series. The most common ages of presentation are adolescence or early adulthood although other age groups are also affected. Conversion reactions are more prevalent in rural, lower socioeconomic, and less educated populations. Other predisposing factors include medical illness, depression, anxiety, schizophrenia, somatization disorder, dependent personality disorder (5 to 21 percent of patients), borderline personality disorder, and passive aggressive personality disorder.

## CLINICAL PRESENTATION

Conversion reactions usually present as a single symptom with a sudden onset related to a severe stress. Precise history-taking is imperative for making the diagnosis, focusing both on how the problem affects the patient and the surrounding events at time of onset. It may be necessary to interview the patient and family separately to confirm diagnostic suspicions. The most reliable diagnostic criterion for conversion reaction is either a previous history of it or a somatization disorder (each found in one third of cases). Symptoms may vary in cases of recurrence.

Motor complaints, usually involving voluntary muscles, are more common than sensory complaints.

Rarely the autonomic and endocrine systems are involved. Vomiting can be a psychogenic manifestation of disgust, and pseudocyesis (false pregnancy) can represent either a wish for or fear of pregnancy.

Classic symptoms of conversion reactions include paralysis, aphonia, seizures, coordination disturbances, akinesia, dyskinesia, blindness, tunnel vision, anosmia, anesthesia, and paresthesia. Pseudoseizures represent 10 to 40 percent of conversion reactions referred to psychiatrists. Patients may describe their condition with surprising lack of concern considering the severity of the symptom (*la belle indifférence*). This was previously thought to be a hallmark of the disorder, but it is absent in about half the cases and is found just as often in patients with organic disease. It is no longer considered diagnostic.

Diagnosis is made first and foremost by ruling out organic pathology. Absence of a medical condition does not solely support the diagnosis of conversion reaction because the appropriate psychological criteria must also be met. Suspicion for the disorder should arise when no physical findings related to the symptom are found or the examination is not consistent with known anatomic or pathophysiologic states. Several techniques that can be used in the physical examination are helpful in testing for true neurologic deficits (Table 246-1). Appropriate laboratory and ancillary studies should be ordered to confirm suspected organic disease. It is important to remember, however, that organic disease may be present concurrently with conversion reaction.

## DIFFERENTIAL DIAGNOSIS

A careful history and physical examination should be used to rule out significant neurologic disease. A high index of suspicion should be

**Table 246-1.** Physical Examination Techniques Used to Distinguish True Neurologic Deficits and Conversion Disorder

| Function | Technique |
|---|---|
| **I. Sensation** | |
| Yes-no test | Patient closes eyes and responds "yes" or "no" to touch stimulus. "No" response in numb area favors conversion reaction. |
| Bowlus and Currier test | Patient extends crossed arms with thumbs pointed down and palms facing together. Fingers (but not thumbs) are interlocked, then hands are rotated inward toward chest. The distortion of body position makes false responses to sensory stimuli difficult. |
| Strength test | Patient closes eyes. Test "strength" by touching finger to be moved. True lack of sensation would not allow patient to ascertain finger to be moved. |
| **II. Pain** | |
| Gray test | With abdominal pain due to psychological factors, the patient will close eyes during palpation. In pain of organic basis, the patient is more likely to watch examiner's hand in order to anticipate pain. |
| **III. Motor** | |
| Drop test | When lifting limb in patient with paralysis of nonorganic etiology, the affected limb will drop more slowly or fall with exaggerated speed as compared to the unaffected limb. Additionally, an extremity dropped from above the face will miss it. |
| Stretch reflex text | The patient contracts a muscle at maximum strength while countertraction is provided. The examiner suddenly jerks the muscle into extension. This will produce a stretch reflex that reveals the patient's true muscle strength. |
| Thigh adductor test | Examiner places hands against inner thighs of patient. Patient is told to adduct normal leg against resistance. With pseudoparalysis, other leg will adduct. |
| Hoover test | Examiner's hands cup both heels of patient and patient is asked to elevate normal leg. With pseudoparalysis, other leg will push downward. Absence of downward pressure of normal leg when patient is instructed to lift weak leg indicates non-compliance. |
| Sternomastoid test | Patient with nonorganic hemiplegia cannot turn head to weak side. |
| **IV. Coma** | |
| Corneal reflex | Corneal reflexes remain intact in awake patient. |
| Bell's phenomenon | Eyes divert upward when lids opened, whereas eyes remain in neutral position in true coma. |
| Lid closing | In true coma, lids when opened close rapidly initially then more slowly as lids descend. Awake patients will have lids stay open, snap shut, or flutter. |
| **V. Seizures** | |
| Corneal reflex | Usually intact in pseudoseizure. |
| Abdominal musculature | Palpation of abdominal musculature reveals lack of contractions with pseudoseizure. |
| **VI. Blindness** | |
| Opticokinetic drum | Rotating drum with alternating black and white stripes or piece of tape with alternating black and white sections pulled laterally in front of patient's open eyes will produce nystagmus in patient with intact vision. |

*Source:* Adapted from Purcell TB. *Emerg Clin North Am* 9:137, 1991.

maintained for physical disorders that have a vague onset, such as systemic lupus erythematosus, multiple sclerosis, polymyositis and Lyme disease. Schizophrenia and depression may have associated conversion reactions. In somatization disorders, the symptoms are more chronic and involve multiple organ systems. With hypochondriasis the patient is usually without loss of function and displays the conviction that some terrible undiscovered illness is present. Hypochondriacal patients will be overly concerned with symptoms. In cases of factitious symptoms, usually associated with malingering, the patient will consciously complain about symptoms to get out of undesirable duty or to receive sympathy or undeserved compensation. These patients rarely have neurologic complaints.

## TREATMENT AND PROGNOSIS

In true cases of conversion reaction, if improvement in symptoms is desired, the emergency physician must realize that the patient is not conscious that the symptoms have no organic course. Confronting the patient and insisting that nothing "real" is wrong is unhelpful in alleviating the symptoms and may worsen the patient's condition. If the precipitating dilemma is identified, correction of the situation should be attempted. Meanwhile the patient should receive reassurance that no serious medical problem has been identified. It should be suggested to the patient that the symptoms will resolve. Nonspecific supportive therapy should be prescribed. For instance, in the example cited at the beginning of this chapter it could be suggested that the patient visit her father less often, call daily instead, and have her husband accompany her to the hospital. She should expect the blindness to resolve if she follows this course.

Referral is mandatory. Patients with conversion reactions may need repetitive reassurance and suggestion that symptoms will resolve before returning to full function. Periodic follow-up is also important to monitor for subtle organic disease. Between 25 and 50 percent of patients diagnosed with conversion reactions later develop serious organic conditions.

Most conversion reactions are of short duration and quickly resolve. Favorable prognostic factors are (1) lack of other psychiatric disorders, (2) sudden severe stress as a precipitating cause, and (3) absence of medical problems. (Some cases are resistant and require hypnosis or Amytal interview for resolution. This should be coordinated by the primary care provider.) Approximately 25 percent of patients will have another conversion reaction over the ensuing 1 to 6 years, which may involve the same or a new symptom complex.

Some patients develop a chronic form of the disorder with complications including contractures and atrophy of muscle groups. In addition, unnecessary diagnostic tests may lead to iatrogenic complications.

## BIBLIOGRAPHY

American Psychiatric Association. *Diagnostic and Statistical Manual of Mental Disorders,* 3d ed, revised. Washington DC: Author, 1987.

Dubovsky SL, Weissberg MP (eds): Hypochondriasis. In: *Clinical Psychiatry in Primary Care,* 3d ed. Baltimore: Williams & Wilkins, pp. 1–22, 1986.

Hafeiz HV: Hysterical conversion: a prognostic study. *Br J Psychiatry* 136:548, 1980.

Kaplan HI, Sadock BJ (eds): Conversion disorder. In: *Comprehensive Textbook of Psychiatry,* 5th ed. Baltimore: Williams & Wilkins, vol. 1, pp. 1013–1017, 1989.

Lazare A: Conversion symptoms. *N Engl J Med* 305:745, 1981.

Purcell TB: The somatic patient. *Emerg Clin North Am* 9:137, 1991.

Schecker NH: Childhood conversion reactions in the emergency department: I. Diagnostic and management approaches within a biopsychosocial framework. *Pediatr Emerg Care* 3:202, 1987.

Schecker NH: Childhood conversion reactions in the emergency department: II. General and specific features. *Pediatr Emerg Care* 6:46, 1990.

# 247
# CRISIS INTERVENTION
## Zigfrids T. Stelmachers

A crisis is an internally experienced, acute disturbance resulting from an inability to cope with ominous or stressful events or feelings. Crisis intervention is best aimed at normal individuals without psychiatric histories and without current psychiatric symptoms, who have experienced a traumatic event. One of the goals is the prevention of the development of psychiatric symptoms.

Some normal individuals, however, develop abnormal reactions to stressful events, such as severe panic, paranoid reactions, and brief psychotic episodes, which may require traditional psychiatric treatment. The mentally ill often experience crisis situations since they are vulnerable to negative life changes. Finally, when the mentally ill are in a crisis, psychiatric symptoms may exacerbate. In the above instances, crisis intervention coupled with psychiatric treatment may be indicated. An emergency department has to be prepared to offer crisis intervention as well as treatment for psychiatric emergencies.

## TYPES OF CRISES

A classification of emotional crises is as follows:

1. Dispositional crises, such as no food or no place to live; acute financial problems; need for information, referral, or advocacy
2. Crises of predictable life stages, such as adolescence, sexuality, marriage, childbirth, "midlife crisis," and retirement
3. Crises due to negative life changes and trauma, such as discovery of a debilitating illness; divorce; victimization; criminal prosecution; loss of job; or death of a loved one
4. Maturational crises, such as dependence/independence conflicts; sexual identity problems; difficulties with emotional intimacy; and value conflicts
5. Crises in which preexisting psychopathology has contributed to the precipitation, presentation, or prognosis of the crisis
6. Acute psychiatric emergencies in which the patient is dangerous to self or others

Not only should the care givers understand several crisis intervention principles and techniques but they need to be familiar with the characteristics of various patient populations (e.g., rape victims, drug addicts) and their target symptoms (grief reactions, etc.)

## CRISIS DEVELOPMENT

The stressfulness of an event is to a large extent determined by a person's *perception* and *interpretation* of the event rather than its objective and more universal properties. Interpretation depends on personality variables and prior life experiences.

In addition, there are individual repertoires of coping mechanisms—accumulated over time—and mediating variables which act as catalysts in the process of crisis resolution. Examples of such variables are social support, a generally hopeful and optimistic attitude toward life, and a belief in being in control of one's life situation and destiny. Finally, some psychological reactions to traumatic events may develop into chronic maladaptive response patterns, including psychiatric disorders. These reactions, if initially suppressed, may eventually result in delayed reactions with their cause obscured by intervening events. The delayed symptoms include such secondary problem development as increased drinking, interpersonal conflicts, divorce, and loss of job. All these various factors and the general sequence of events are portrayed in Table 247–1.

**Table 247-1.** The Crisis Kaleidoscope, A Theoretical Model

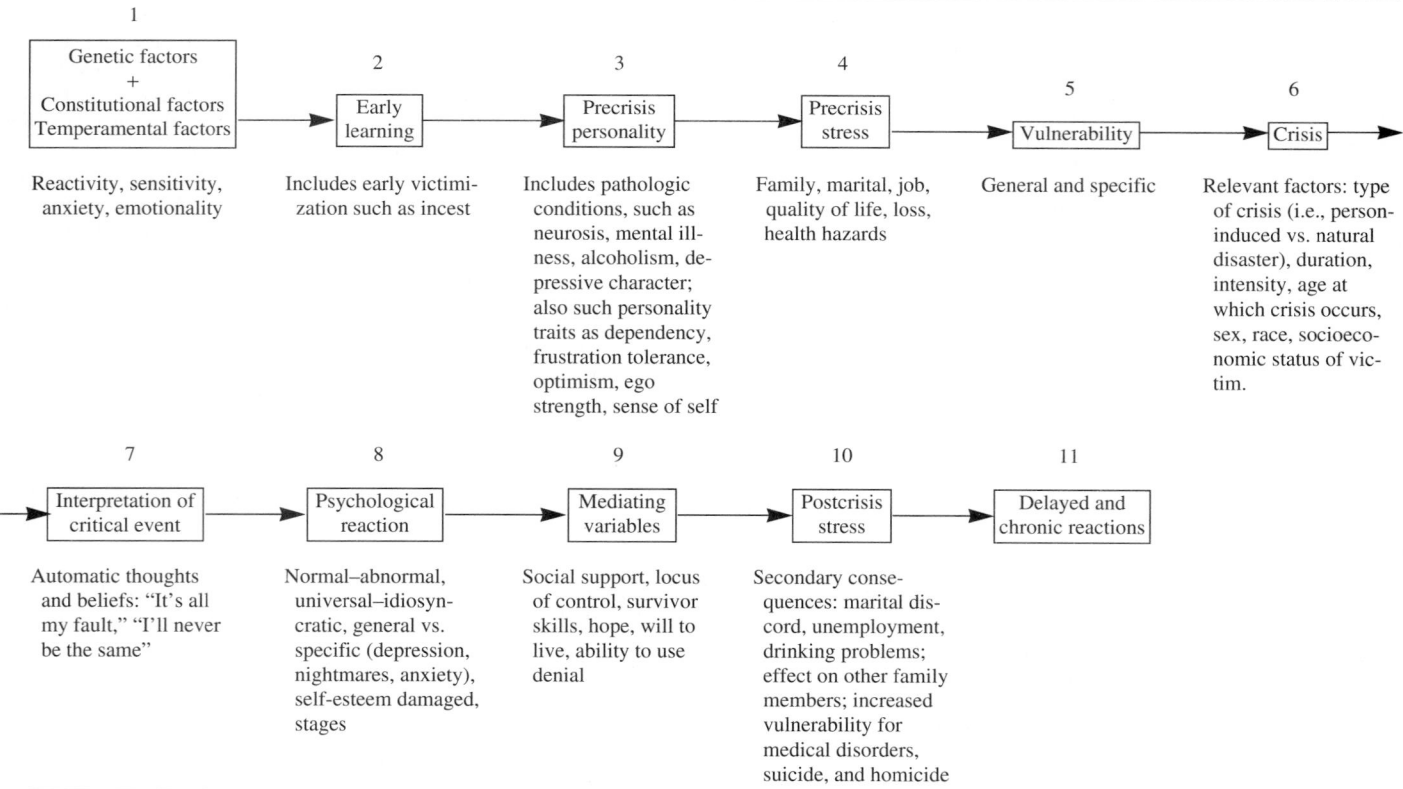

| 1 Genetic factors + Constitutional factors Temperamental factors | 2 Early learning | 3 Precrisis personality | 4 Precrisis stress | 5 Vulnerability | 6 Crisis |
|---|---|---|---|---|---|
| Reactivity, sensitivity, anxiety, emotionality | Includes early victimization such as incest | Includes pathologic conditions, such as neurosis, mental illness, alcoholism, depressive character; also such personality traits as dependency, frustration tolerance, optimism, ego strength, sense of self | Family, marital, job, quality of life, loss, health hazards | General and specific | Relevant factors: type of crisis (i.e., person-induced vs. natural disaster), duration, intensity, age at which crisis occurs, sex, race, socioeconomic status of victim. |

| 7 Interpretation of critical event | 8 Psychological reaction | 9 Mediating variables | 10 Postcrisis stress | 11 Delayed and chronic reactions |
|---|---|---|---|---|
| Automatic thoughts and beliefs: "It's all my fault," "I'll never be the same" | Normal–abnormal, universal–idiosyncratic, general vs. specific (depression, nightmares, anxiety), self-esteem damaged, stages | Social support, locus of control, survivor skills, hope, will to live, ability to use denial | Secondary consequences: marital discord, unemployment, drinking problems; effect on other family members; increased vulnerability for medical disorders, suicide, and homicide | |

## PATIENT ASSESSMENT

Assessment consists of the following:

1. The patient's current complaints, problems, and symptoms, including their severity, frequency, and duration.
2. The causes of the presenting complaints, including stresses and negative life changes.
3. The effect of the critical events on the patient's overall functioning. Has there been a serious disruption of the patient's interpersonal relationships? Has school or work performance deteriorated significantly? Has personal hygiene been affected?

In addition to changes in the patient's behavior, there may be less visible alterations in the patient's inner emotional and mental state. Changes in mood, affect, emotional control, and thought patterns should be thoroughly investigated.

An information-gathering approach with an emotionally disturbed patient often creates a barrier to establishing good rapport. Some symptoms may need to be "treated" before assessment is completed; in fact, obtaining relevant information may be nearly impossible with agitated or uncooperative patients. Therefore, one cannot neatly separate the interview into an assessment and an intervention phase. Instead, the two have to be flexibly and sensitively intertwined from the very beginning. In order to accomplish this, it is useful to watch for divergent agendas between the care giver and the patient. The former may be mainly interested in obtaining information to arrive at the diagnosis and treatment plan, while the patient's main motivation may be to express anger at an alcoholic and abusive husband. If this divergence of motives is not recognized, a communication breakdown may develop and assessment and treatment efforts will suffer.

Patients differ widely in their readiness to get help. The most elaborate and well-designed treatment plans will not be effective with patients lacking in motivation for such interventions. Much time is wasted in making complicated treatment and disposition arrangements only to learn too late that the patient has little intention to go through with the plans. It is therefore helpful to assess the patient's motivational strength early on; if motivation is lacking, this should be addressed directly and *before* one gets involved in time-consuming planning.

### Precrisis Adjustment

To assess the seriousness of the current crisis reaction, compare it with the patient's usual behavior patterns and mental state. What is described as a crisis situation may sometimes represent relatively continuous or repetitive behavior disturbances best treated by ongoing long-term treatment rather than crisis intervention.

A careful history should be taken of the patient's responses to earlier crisis intervention efforts. The knowledge of what helped and what didn't assists the crisis worker in the formulation of a more effective treatment. Furthermore, the history may reveal that the patient has already developed a repertoire of coping skills as a result of dealing with these earlier crises. It is reassuring to patients to be reminded of their own previous successes, and it encourages them to be self-reliant.

Finally, knowledge of the patient's premorbid vulnerabilities helps identify the stresses which provoked the current crisis.

### Crisis Precipitants

It is important to determine what final event motivated the patient to seek help, especially for patients with multiple problems. Longstanding problems may be presented along with acute ones, and severe ones with minor stresses. In an emergency setting it is impractical—often not necessary—to address an entire cluster of problems. One needs to identify the immediate precipitant because it usually indicates the problem most responsible for the current crisis. Intervention can then concentrate on this main problem area, resulting in effective and economical treatment.

If a specific precipitant cannot be identified, it may be advisable to ask the patient to describe the events of the day just before the decision was made to seek treatment. During such a recounting of events it may be possible to tease out the precipitant even though the patient may not be aware of the connection.

One should also watch for sudden changes in the patient's interactional pattern, such as silences, tearfulness, or anger outbursts, because such changes often signify that a currently active conflict has been touched.

### Stages of Response

People often react to stressful events in predictable stages similar to those identified in grief and loss. The sequence starts with a feeling of shock followed by denial, which at some point fails and leads to negative emotions such as anxiety, fright, depression, or regressive dependency. Guilt is almost invariably present because it is quite typical for victims of all kinds of tragedies to blame themselves. The next stage may be obsessiveness about the critical event, often followed by apathy and resignation. Finally, there may be a period of inner- or outward-directed rage.

Although many individuals follow the described general pattern, others skip a stage or two or progress through the stages in a different sequence. For some there are no stages at all but merely a confusing array of constantly changing feelings, an emotional roller coaster with peaks of highly emotional experiences separated by valleys of relative calm. These "waves," at various times, may be composed of different emotions in different proportions and predominance. Some individuals may have a "preferred" and rather persistent emotion perhaps characteristic of their personalities and pretrauma response tendencies to stressful events. Nevertheless, to the extent that at least some patients react in stages, it is useful for the physician to identify the current stage of the patient in order to select the best intervention.

### Outside Information

Individuals in a crisis situation are often very emotional, confused, perplexed, anxious, withdrawn, or agitated. These emotional states make them poor and unreliable informants. Data collected under such conditions is often incomplete or distorted. The interview must be supplemented with information from outside sources, such as family members, friends, police officers, therapists, ministers, or apartment managers.

One should not forget that the setting to a large extent determines how people behave, and that a hospital represents a rather artificial environment for the purpose of predicting patients' behavior in their home setting. Therefore, it is inadvisable to dismiss or minimize the observations of a "hysterical mother," an "overreacting therapist," or a "dumb cop" who lacks formal mental health training but has the considerable advantage of having observed the patient during a domestic quarrel. In a supportive and professional setting the patient is likely to be more relaxed and in better emotional control. The stimulus triggering the crisis situation is usually not present, and it is therefore not surprising that the patient is behaving "normally." It would be unwise to conclude from this that a true crisis is not present or that the emergency aspects of the problem have been exaggerated. If under such conditions a patient is released and returns to the irritant, another crisis may quickly develop.

### Self-Esteem

It is important to identify the impact of the crisis on the patient's concept of self. Faced with major problems that defy easy solution, some patients experience considerable anxiety or depression and yet are able to preserve a healthy sense of self-worth. Other patients, however, engage in self-blame or self-hate, which exacerbates the crisis reaction. The latter patients require a more psychological intervention approach, more reassurance and emotional support in addition to specific treatments, help in problem solving, and a variety of environmental manipulations.

### Resources

In order to properly assess the patient's ability to cope, one needs to know about the patient's strengths, repertoire of coping skills, "fighting spirit," and social and other environmental resources available, as well as any weaknesses and deficiencies. Social support is one of the most important mediating variables that significantly influences the crisis outcome. What is important here is not the *quantity* of social support but its *quality*: a few close and caring friends have more positive impact than a larger number of acquaintances, fellow club members, or hostile and rejecting relatives.

### Directiveness of Interview

In inquiring about sensitive and potentially embarrassing issues, one should use a matter-of-fact and straightforward approach. Subtle and indirect questioning may not yield the concrete detail necessary for effective intervention and disposition. This is especially true in cases of elevated suicide or violence potential. It is quite appropriate, even desirable, to ask such questions as: "Are you currently so depressed that you have thought of taking your life?" "Do you have a plan?" "Have you selected a method?" "Is it readily available?" "Is the time and place set?" "Have you ever committed acts of violence?" "Did they result in injury?" "Are you in the habit of carrying a weapon?" "Was the violent act provoked, premeditated, indiscriminate, or aimed at a particular person or situation?"

Perhaps surprisingly, many patients are quite willing to share this information without undue defensiveness. And if they are not ready to reveal their inclinations and plans, the chances are that an indirect approach will yield no better results than a straightforward inquiry.

### Family Members

Family members and friends who accompany the patient are not only often deeply involved in the patient's problems but themselves may have developed clinical signs and symptoms of crisis. In that sense they become copatients in need of professional attention. Quite frequently they are more disturbed than the identified patient, expecting the primary patient to receive immediate attention, hospitalization, certain medications, or some other specific disposition. Even though they may appear to be exaggerating the urgency of the primary patient's condition or to be "overinvolved" and, as a result, interfere with clinical decision making and patient care, their needs have to be addressed. In any crisis intervention it is useful to have family members as allies rather than antagonists because one often has to rely on outside resources and support for the implementation of treatment plans.

### Successive Assessments

Sometimes a single assessment episode is insufficient to provide a satisfactory formulation of problem and treatment. The patient's current mental state may preclude an adequate evaluation because the patient is guarded, mute, incoherent, or intoxicated. At other times the symptom picture may be confusing or inconsistent. With such patients the final decision can be made only after a succession of assessment episodes separated in time. This way either an increase or a decrease in symptoms can be demonstrated, and the treatment plan modified accordingly. If suicide or violence potential is one of the suspected symptoms, it is most prudent to admit such patients to the hospital, on a legal hold if necessary.

## GOALS OF CRISIS INTERVENTION

The goals are usually short-term, although some critical interventions may lead to long-term consequences which are not predictable. Solving the patient's long-standing and severe life problems is seldom necessary for effective crisis resolution; sometimes just changing the patient's *perception* of a particular problem can have very beneficial immediate impact.

Other goals of crisis intervention are to

1. Prevent the development of psychiatric symptoms.
2. Prevent the development of delayed or chronic reactions.
3. Sort, early in treatment, patients into two groups: those requiring a hospital setting and those who can be treated in an outpatient environment.
4. Relieve symptoms.
5. Restore emotional equilibrium.
6. Restore power and control, especially to patients who have been victimized.
7. Return the patient to precrisis or higher level of functioning.

Chronic problems need ongoing therapy and counseling programs.

## INTERVENTION STRATEGIES AND COMPONENTS

### Intervention Components

Effective crisis intervention, whatever its specific treatment strategies and techniques, always contains the following core elements (Table 247–2):

1. Mobilize hope.
2. Instill and maintain expectation for improvement.
3. Like and respect the patient.
4. Be enthusiastic.

### Sympathetic, Active, and Selective Listening

When patients are asked to identify the one component that was most helpful to them, being listened to is by far the most frequently mentioned one. Listening should be accompanied by positive emotional involvement and genuine concern, but the patient should be discouraged from straying to irrelevant or unmanageable issues.

### Emotional Support

Emotional support is not synonymous with an indiscriminate siding with the patient. It is tempting to agree with the patient's perceptions of certain events, but such partiality may encourage the patient to select an imprudent course of action, or may backfire if the patient has been critical of a significant other whose cooperation turns out to be necessary for the patient's treatment.

### Nonjudgmental Acceptance

Accepting the patient's statements should not imply condoning the patient's views. One can listen to what the patient has to say without

**Table 247-2.** Essential Components of Crisis Intervention

Sympathetic, active, and selective listening
Emotional support
Nonjudgmental acceptance
Reassurance
Providing information
Providing opportunity for ventilation
Intellectual clarification
Advice and persuasion
Confrontation
Setting limits
Facilitation and advocacy
Final disposition and follow-up

judging the correctness of the patient's assumptions or the wisdom of his or her actions. Special care should be exercised to not appear to blame the patient even if it is done inadvertently or indirectly by such questions as, "Why did you walk alone in this neighborhood so late at night?"

Suggested responses to victims of rape and other violent crimes include "I'm sorry it happened," "I'm glad you are alive and well," and "You did nothing wrong."

## Reassurance

It is often important to begin the intervention by reassuring the patient that it was a good idea to come for help. Many patients feel embarrassed and awkward about seeking treatment, may feel that it implies a character weakness or that their problems are too trivial to deserve professional attention. They are also uncertain about the reception they will get ("Will they treat me like a mentally ill person?").

When people are in an acute emotional turmoil, they frequently feel that they may be losing their mind, are "going crazy," will fall apart, will have a nervous breakdown, etc. Quick and unequivocal reassurance to the contrary often has an immediate calming effect and helps establish rapport. The more specific and concrete the reassurance, the more effective it is. "Things are going to be all right" is less effective than, "In the past when you had these symptoms, they were very short-lived and you could function quite adequately even while they were acute."

## Providing Information

Patients' problems are often aggravated by misperceptions, misconceptions, and a variety of myths. Factual information, if available and known to the crisis worker, can be very helpful and reassuring to the patient but must not be permitted to expand into a minilecture.

## Providing Opportunity for Ventilation

Emotional expression is very therapeutic for most patients. Notable exceptions are hysterical or emotionally labile individuals who habitually respond to stressful events with intense and dramatic outbursts.

## Intellectual Clarification

It is not unusual for patients to be overwhelmed by a confusing array of symptoms, problems, and emotions whose meaning and future implications are far from clear to them. Intellectual understanding, even if it falls short of genuine insight, can provide a sense of order. A seemingly chaotic and ominous situation loses some of its threat once it is "explained."

## Advice and Persuasion

If sparingly and cautiously used, advice and persuasion can be effective crisis intervention tools. However, a distinction needs to be made between advice regarding real life circumstances (e.g., "You should get a divorce") and advice regarding treatment issues (e.g., "You should consider medication"). Advice on real life situations is potentially hazardous because it presumes a full understanding of the patient's personality and life situation as well as superior wisdom on the therapist's part. It is much safer to give the second type of advice.

## Confrontation

A patient may display considerable denial, rationalization, and repression. It may be tempting to force the patient to face reality, but the patient who is not ready to accept the "truth" will resist a frontal attack and become adversarial. If the patient needs to accept reality as part of the intervention, the approach should be supportive, gentle, and gradual.

## Setting Limits

With patients who are dangerous to themselves or others, aggressively act out their conflicts, display excessive dependency, or behave manipulatively or provocatively, limit setting is often necessary. Rules of conduct have to be established and enforced, or, better yet, the patient should be given choices with clearly spelled-out consequences attached to them.

## Facilitation and Advocacy

Many crises are predominantly the result of external stresses which cannot be readily changed by treating the patient. In such instances, the patient's environment has to be manipulated as part of the crisis intervention. This can take the form of facilitating the solution of some dispositional problem (such as money, no place to live, legal difficulties, etc.). Other patients may be in a crisis because of discrimination and ill treatment accorded to them as a group by various law enforcement, health, and welfare agencies. Victims of various crimes, especially rape and battering, are examples of such groups. Special advocates can assist the primary intervention by pleading the victim's cause before the relevant agencies.

## Final Disposition and Follow-Up

Speedy and successful referral is an essential part of crisis intervention. A good referral is more like a transfer from one facility to another. Instead of just sending a patient to another agency, finalize the arrangements, including appointment time, the agency's address and telephone number, and the name of the intake worker or receiving professional. The tighter the arrangements, the harder it is for an ambivalent patient to renege on the treatment commitment. Such "transfers" approximately double the success rate of the usual much looser referrals.

Finally, time permitting, it is advisable to do a very short term follow-up: Did the patient keep the appointment? Was this an appropriate referral? Was the patient accepted for treatment? If the patient chose not to go through with the referral, was it for clinically sound reasons and does he or she need further crisis services (while being put on a waiting list, for instance)?

## Strategies for Different Stages

Treatment approaches have to be matched with the needs of patients during different time periods following the critical event. During the first 24 to 48 h, the patient needs *emotional first aid,* which can be provided either at the site of trauma, the patient's home, a shelter, or a hospital emergency department. During this period the patient's safety and physical well-being should be a primary concern, plus massive doses of reassurance and emotional support, in addition to provision of relevant information.

During this period, *crisis management* may be needed for more severely disturbed and intoxicated patients, including such security measures as seclusion and restraint. Intoxicated patients often profit from an overnight stay in the emergency department. During their intoxicated state these patients may be highly suicidal and assaultive and yet may not require hospitalization if managed properly in the emergency department. Most of them no longer exhibit their previous night's behavior disturbance the next morning, so they can be safely discharged with arrangements for further outpatient treatment.

During the next 6 weeks or so, following the initial visit, the treatment of choice for most crisis patients is classic *crisis intervention.* For that time segment, the crisis workers need to have a thorough knowledge of crisis intervention techniques as well as familiarity with specific target symptoms and reactions (i.e., those common in victims of rape, grief, etc.). Patients whose reactions persist beyond 6 weeks or who develop delayed symptoms may require *crisis therapy,* which is more similar to brief psychotherapy. This requires a better knowledge of personality theory and psychotherapeutic principles and techniques.

## Use of High Emotional Arousal

During a crisis situation patients display a higher degree of emotional arousal. This usually leads to a higher level of motivation to seek or accept treatment. Thus it provides a unique opportunity to gain access to the patient's more chronic problems which have been neglected during noncritical periods. Patients should be guided to definitive treatment at this very time when they are most ready to make use of it.

## STRESS OF CRISIS WORK

Any crisis-oriented service has to be prepared to deal with very difficult, challenging, unpleasant patients; patients chronically in crisis, expecting and demanding immediate services; dependent and clinging patients who use clinical services for human contact; patients who are manipulative and provocative but are unwilling to take responsibility for their behavior; powerless, chaotic, and frustrated patients ready to vent their pent-up anger at anyone who represents the "system."

Members of the helping professions are especially vulnerable to these patients because the care givers are impelled to live up to the image of a caring and compassionate individual. The intrinsic reward for this ethic is the feeling of being needed, liked, and appreciated. Such rewards are not forthcoming with the patients described above. Unless the helper recognizes these danger signs it can lead to burnout and compromised patient care.

To help the helpers to protect and take better care of themselves, the following tactics are offered:

1. Try to be aware of your own negative feelings and discharge them in small and harmless dosages instead of suppressing and bottling them up.
2. Recognize the type of patient you have particular problems with because of your own temperament and life experiences.
3. Don't take patients' blaming and hostility personally; most of it represents aimless discharge of frustration, or it may be displaced to you from a more primary source.
4. Be aware that some undesirable behavior may be the direct result of the patient's mental condition and is not under his or her control.
5. Resist overinvolvement and heroic rescue efforts with guilt-inducing, dependent, and demanding patients.
6. If your treatment plan is contrary to the patient's wishes, don't expect cooperation and gratitude.
7. Look for fear, loneliness, and inadequacy under cocky, arrogant, and hostile behavior.
8. Accept your own shortcomings and the limitations of the services you provide; this includes the realization that you don't have something for everyone, even if it seems to be expected of you.

## BIBLIOGRAPHY

Butcher JN, Stelmachers ZT, Maudal GR: *Crisis Intervention and Emergency Psychotherapy.* Clinical Methods in Psychology, New York, Wiley, 1983.

Hoff LA: *People in Crisis: Understanding and Helping,* 2d ed. Menlo Park, Addison-Wesley, 1984.

Kercher EE: Crisis intervention in the emergency department. *Emerg Med Clin North Am.* 9(1):219, 1991.

Leff-Simon SI, Slaikeu KA, Hansen K: *Crisis Intervention in Hospital Emergency Rooms.* Crisis Intervention, A Handbook for Practice and Research. Boston, Allyn and Bacon, 1984.

## 248
# EMERGENCY EVALUATION OF PRISONER AND SUBSTANCE ABUSE PATIENTS
### Cary C. McDonald

## EVOLUTION OF CORRECTIONAL HEALTH CARE

In 1976, the Supreme Court cited the Eighth Amendment, which restricts cruel and unusual punishment, as grounds for an inmate's constitutional right to health care (*Estelle v Gamble,* 429 US 97). The subsequent development of *voluntary* health care standards for intake, assessment, and screening of inmates by the National Commission on Correctional Health Care resulted in accreditation of 73 prisons (11 percent) and 230 jails (7 percent) in 1991. Many correctional systems have not established proactive methods for meeting routine health care needs. Scheduled care is the exception; delivery of care on an as-needed basis is the norm. Prisoners, like members of the general population, require regular monitoring of chronic medical conditions such as hypertension, diabetes, asthma, and seizure disorders. One report identified that 70 percent of prisoners admitted for diabetic ketoacidosis had not received insulin for an average of 2.5 days following arrest. This practice has caused chronic conditions to be poorly managed and has facilitated heightened morbidity, resulting in increased referrals to hospital emergency departments. Access to medication may be overlooked due to insufficient medical staffing or the need may simply be unidentified. Prisoners may not volunteer that they have health problems requiring medication for a number of reasons. Some prisoners may fear that their arraignment will be delayed if they must be transported to a hospital. Others may prefer to be hospitalized for the consequences of noncompliance, and they may feign illnesses to gain access to the hospital for their own secondary gain. There are limited data on the emergency care of this unique population of patients, yet many emergency departments manage a considerable number of patients from adult and juvenile correctional facilities.

Jails accommodate a group of convicted offenders serving sentences of under 1 year as well as alleged offenders awaiting trial. Due to the high rate of turnover and the relatively short confinement time, nearly 10 million inmates are released annually in the United States. Prisons contain criminals serving longer sentences with a median confinement of 24 months and accommodated over 732,000 inmates in 1990. The average daily total correctional population has grown from less than 500,000 in 1980 to just under 1.2 million in 1990. This population is primarily male, with adult women and juveniles comprising only 7 percent and 0.5 percent, respectively, of the total population. Mounting illicit drug convictions with mandatory sentences have caused the growing number of inmates and prison overcrowding. The most common reason for incarceration in 1987 in New York State was violation of drug laws. The prevalence of drug offenders in the Federal Bureau of Prisons is expected to rise from 47 percent in 1991 to 70 percent in 1995.

## COMMUNICABLE DISEASES

Most prisoners come from disadvantaged, lower socioeconomic backgrounds and have significant underserved health care needs. This population engages in high-risk behaviors, such as intravenous drug use and unprotected sexual activity with multiple partners, which increases their frequency of contracting and perpetuating communicable diseases.

## Human Immunodeficiency Virus

The reported range of seropositive inmates is between 0.6 percent and 17 percent. The incidence of acquired immunodeficiency syndrome (AIDS) is nearly 14 times that of the U.S. population (202 versus 14.6/100,000). Because not all prisons provide voluntary, confidential testing for human immunodeficiency virus (HIV), these numbers may actually be higher. It would therefore be prudent to approach all prisoners who have not been tested for HIV with conscientious attention to risk factors for the disease. In addition to opportunistic infections, HIV-positive individuals are extremely susceptible to common infectious organisms such as streptococcus and haemophilus. A study of HIV-positive inmates found that a significant number (11.8 percent) were seronegative to the measles virus. These individuals are especially prone to the adult-associated sequelae of pneumonia and encephalitis.

## Tuberculosis

The incidence of tuberculosis (TB) in prisoners in the state of New York increased more than 13-fold over a 15 year period to 200 cases/100,000 in 1991. The incidence in the United States was 10.3/100,000 citizens in 1990. Transmission of multidrug-resistant TB was first reported in 1990. Since the initial report in 1991, multidrug-resistant TB in correctional facilities has been on the rise, to as high as 32 percent of isolates. AIDS patients are 500 times more likely to develop TB than the general population. The majority (56 to 95 percent) of prisoners with TB are also infected with HIV.

## Hepatitis

The incidence of hepatitis B virus (HBV) serum markers in prisoners is between 19 and 47 percent. Hepatitis D virus (HDV) serum markers have been identified in 8 percent of inmates with HBV markers.

## Sexually Transmitted Diseases

The increasing incidence of sexually transmitted diseases (STDs) in the general population has been attributed to illicit drug use, multiple sexual partners, and prostitution. Females in juvenile correctional facilities have been found to engage in sexual activity at younger ages and contract STDs at higher rates than nondelinquent females. Rates of gonococcal-positive urethral cultures in male inmates have been reported as high as 11 times greater than that of the U.S. population. The prevalence of asymptomatic gonorrhea in juveniles has been noted to be 2 percent in males and up to 18 percent in females. True positive tests for syphilis have been reported in 3 percent of men and up to 20 percent of women. The incidence of chlamydial infection has been described in 5 to 20 percent of female detainees.

## TRAUMA

A study of a juvenile correctional facility reported a 1.2 percent annual rate of trauma incidents with 52 percent of injuries referred to an emergency department. The common types of incidents causing injury included sports, fights, self-inflicted injuries, and suicide attempts. The majority (74 percent) of injuries were soft tissue/musculoskeletal in nature, such as sprains, contusions, and lacerations. Greater than three fourths of the injuries were in male offenders. A report from Folsom Prison in 1989 found an annual stab wound assault rate of 4.1 percent. Weapons ranged from small stilettos to larger crudely formed knives. Emergency department referral was required in 41 percent of cases and 35 percent were hospitalized. The overall mortality rate was 3 percent.

Correctional center personnel may have low tolerance for inmates with personality or behavior disorders, and this may result in an increased number of injuries from attempts to establish compliance with institutional rules. Often, conflicting histories of the injury will be related by the prisoner and the staff. The emergency physician must not overlook suspicious injuries and should report incidents of suspected physical abuse to the appropriate authorities.

## Mass Casualty Incidents

Correctional centers have the propensity for unforeseen but occasionally predictable riot situations, which may result in numerous injuries to staff and inmates. Appropriate planning for these potential disasters should include regular education and practice drills integrating all involved agencies, including prison staff, local and state law enforcement, fire, emergency medical services, and area receiving hospitals.

## Security

When a prisoner is transferred to the emergency department, the correctional system must provide appropriate security personnel and restraints to minimize the potential for elopement and subsequent threat to the emergency department and surrounding environment. Law enforcement personnel should notify the hospital staff about potentially dangerous prisoners who may have a history of violence. These patients may even need to remain restrained during the physical examination. The prisoner must be observed at all times because some inmates can cleverly fashion ordinary materials, such as paper clips, into potential weapons.

## MENTAL HEALTH

When controlling for race and age, the prevalence of schizophrenia, major depression, and mania in adult inmates has been shown to be two to three times that of the general population. Criteria for diagnosing major depression has been found in 20 percent of juvenile offenders. Between 2.5 and 10 percent of inmates may be classified as mentally retarded or developmentally challenged. The mentally ill who come from lower socioeconomic backgrounds are more vulnerable to imprisonment because of fewer available resources for social support and treatment.

## Suicide

Few studies have addressed prison suicide statistics. Suicide rates have been reported as high as 57.5/100,000 prisoners. In 1984, juvenile correctional facilities had a suicide rate 2.5 times greater than that of the general population. Common methods selected were hanging, cutting wounds, antidepressant overdose, and falls. Risk factors identified included younger age (ages 15 to 34 were at twice the risk), white race (twice the risk of blacks), male gender, and inmates serving a life sentence. A proactive method for reduction of risk for medication overdose in both emergency and outpatient settings is witnessed administration of *liquid* dosages to inmates. This minimizes the potential for "pouching" pills in the mouth for future misuse.

## MORTALITY

There are also few data addressing prison mortality. The most common causes of death of prisoners were circulatory system disease, until 1987, when AIDS became the leading cause of death. Over a 5-year period 15.8 percent of juvenile facilities experienced at least one death and 64.3 percent of these were suicides.

## SUBSTANCE ABUSE

The National Institute on Drug Abuse (NIDA) estimated from a survey in 1988 that nearly 28 million Americans used an illicit substance at least once and that 14.5 million used drugs regularly. A conservative lifetime prevalence of substance abuse in the United States is 15 percent. More than 20 million Americans have tried cocaine once, more than 860,000 people used cocaine weekly or more, and 500,000 used crack cocaine regularly. Regular marijuana use was identified in 11.6 million Americans and 770,000 people regularly used hallucinogens such as phencyclidine and lysergic acid diethylamide. Nearly 2.5 million people have used heroin at least once and up to 6.5 million have recently abused analgesics.

In 1972, the Drug Enforcement Administration launched the Drug Abuse Warning Network (DAWN), which is a national surveillance system for collecting data on emergency department encounters and deaths related to substance abuse. Since 1980, DAWN has been the responsibility of NIDA and voluntarily reported data are collected weekly from over 500 emergency departments and 85 medical examiners' offices in 21 states.

## Crime

A strong relationship exists between substance abuse and crime. Substance abusers are as much as 18 times more likely to be involved in criminal activities. Studies of deaths from violent crime found that between 45 and 59 percent of victims were cocaine users. Also the rate of substance abuse has been found to be very high in violent crimes against family members. Substance abusers also are responsible for increased acts of nonviolent crime, particularly theft, to support their drug habit. A large percentage of prisoners are intravenous drug or crack users.

## Trauma

One study found that 74.5 percent of trauma patients tested positive for illicit or prescription drugs including cocaine (54 percent), cannabinoids (37 percent), benzodiazepines (10 percent), opiates (9 percent), barbiturates (7 percent), and amphetamines (5 percent). Illicit drugs were involved in 80 percent of violent crime-related cases. Also, alcohol was found in 35 percent of patients. Another study reported that 68.9 percent of trauma center patients were diagnosed with psychoactive substance use disorders based on criteria in the *Diagnostic and Statistical Manual of Mental Disorders, Revised Third Edition (DSM-III-R)*. Alcohol dependence was demonstrated in 56 percent and other drug dependence in 51 percent. A third report demonstrated that 38 percent of major trauma patients tested positive for cocaine, and of these, 20 percent were involved in motor vehicle accidents. Fifty-seven percent of victims of violent assault also tested positive for cocaine. It was noted that there was a significant level of underreporting of drug abuse in trauma patients to DAWN.

## Psychiatric

Mental health patients have been found to have a rate of substance abuse several times higher than the general population. Greater than 50 percent of schizophrenics presenting to psychiatric emergency services settings demonstrated a lifetime diagnosis of alcohol or drug abuse. Another emergency department psychiatric service reported that one third of presenting patients were diagnosed with disorders that were alcohol or drug induced. These patients had increased frequencies of suicidal ideation and gestures.

## Intravenous Drug Use and Adulterants

Substances most commonly abused intravenously include heroin, cocaine, and amphetamines, either singularly or in combination. The term "speedball" refers to a mixture of heroin and cocaine. Drugs are usually "cut" to increase volume and profits with any number of adulterants, such as stimulants (caffeine, phenylpropanolamine, pseudoephedrine), local anesthetics (procaine, lidocaine, tetracaine), inert compounds (talc, starch), sugars (mannitol, lactose), toxins (quinine, arsenic, strychnine), and phencyclidine. Because of adulterant admixture, the potency of the diluted drug is variable and unpredictable. Adulterants alone cause an enormous spectrum of potential toxic side effects and can further complicate the emergency presentation. Many drugs, such as cocaine and amphetamines, and adulterants, such as mannitol, quinine and talc, can cause fever. "Cotton fever" is a phenomenon resulting from injection of cotton-filtered drugs that have been contaminated with cotton fibers. However, the most likely cause of fever in intravenous drug user (IVDU) patients is an infectious disease process, which most commonly is infective endocarditis. Increasing numbers of methicillin-resistant organisms are emerging not only due to needle sharing, but possibly due to a reported 60 percent of addicts obtaining antibiotics on the street. Use of oral antibiotics within 2 weeks prior to evaluation reduces the incidence of positive blood cultures from 97 to 91 percent. Estimates of HIV-positive status in IVDU have been as high as 70 percent, particularly in inner city populations. HIV seroprevalence has remained stable at just above 50 percent over the last decade in New York City. Because of the unreliability of this population, all IVDU patients with fever should be aggressively evaluated and admitted.

## Cocaine

Cocaine-related emergencies increased exponentially over 20 years and became the leading cause of drug-related mortality until 1990, when the Secretary of Health and Human Services reported an overall decrease in number. The $50 billion per year industry contributed to more than 1000 deaths in 1986. DAWN data revealed that in 1989 over 40 percent of emergency department drug-related visits involved cocaine. Routes of administration were smoking (48 percent), intravenous (28 percent), and nasal insufflation (16 percent). Reasons for emergency department visits were unexpected reaction, request for detoxification, chronic effects, overdose, and injury. Other drugs found in combination with cocaine were alcohol (37 percent), heroin (13 percent), cannabinoids (8 percent), and phencyclidine (3 percent).

A recent trend of increased numbers of reported syphilis cases has been strongly associated with increased crack cocaine abuse within the lower socioeconomic population. Nearly 9 percent of emergency department patients admitting to cocaine use were found to have latent syphilis and 19.6 percent had previously treated disease. More than 58 percent of women had exposure to syphilis, which suggests that some women resort to prostitution to support their drug habits.

## CONCLUSION

Crime and substance abuse are interrelated and have a significant impact on the morbidity and mortality of many medical problems, particularly trauma and communicable diseases. The emergency physician should be conscientious of the unique health care needs of the medically underserved prisoner population.

## BIBLIOGRAPHY

American College of Physicians, National Commission on Correctional Health Care, and American Correctional Health Services Association. The crisis in correctional health care: the impact of the National Drug Control Strategy on correctional health services. *Ann Intern Med* 117:71, 1992.

Barry MA, Gleavy D, Herd K, et al: Prevalence of markers for hepatitis B and hepatitis D in a municipal house of correction. *Am J Public Health* 80:471, 1990.

Braun MM, Truman BI, Maguire B, et al: Increasing incidence of tuberculosis in a prison inmate population. Association with HIV infection. *JAMA* 261:393, 1989.

Brookoff D, Campbell EA, Shaw LM: The underreporting of cocaine-related trauma: Drug Abuse Warning Network reports vs hospital toxicology tests. *Am J Public Health* 83:369, 1993.

Centers for Disease Control and Prevention. Probable transmission of multidrug-resistant tuberculosis in correctional facility—California. *MMWR* 42:48, 1993.

Cohen D, Scribner R, Clark J, Cory D: The potential role of custody facilities in controlling sexually transmitted diseases. *Am J Public Health* 82:552, 1992.

Colliver JD, Kopstein AN: Trends in cocaine abuse reflected in emergency room episodes reported to DAWN. *Public Health Rep* 106:59, 1991.

Council on Scientific Affairs: Health status of detained and incarcerated youths. *JAMA* 263:987, 1990.

Des Jarlais DC, Friedman SR, Sotheran JL, et al: Continuity and change within an HIV epidemic. Injecting drug users in New York City, 1984 through 1992. *JAMA* 271:121, 1994.

Ernst AA, Martin DH: High syphilis rates among cocaine abusers identified in an emergency department. *Sex Transm Dis* 20:66, 1993.

Glaser JB, Greifinger RB: Correctional health care: a public health opportunity. *Ann Intern Med* 118:139, 1993.

Hoffman RS, Goldfrank LR: The impact of drug abuse and addiction on society. *Emerg Med Clin North Am* 8:467, 1990.

Hutton MD, Cauthen GM, Bloch AB: Results of a 29-state survey of tuberculosis in nursing homes and correctional facilities. *Public Health Rep* 108:305, 1993.

Keller AS, Link RN, Bickell NA, et al: Diabetic ketoacidosis in prisoners without access to insulin. *JAMA* 269:619, 1993.

Lindenbaum GA, Carroll SF, Daskal I, Kapusnick R: Patterns of alcohol and drug abuse in an urban trauma center: the increasing role of cocaine abuse. *J Trauma* 29:1654, 1989.

Mueller PD, Benowitz NL, Olson KR: Cocaine. *Emerg Med Clin North Am* 8:481, 1990.

National Commission on Correctional Health Care. *Standards for Health Services in Jails.* Chicago, IL: Author, 1987.

National Institute on Drug Abuse. *National Household Survey on Drug Abuse: Population Estimates 1988.* Rockville, MD, Author, 1989.

Raba JM, Obis CB: The health status of incarcerated urban males: results of admission screening. *Journal of Prison and Jail Health* 3:6, 1983.

Salive ME, Smith GS, Brewer TF: Death in prison: changing mortality patterns among male prisoners in Maryland, 1979–87. *Am J Public Health* 80:1479, 1990.

Salive ME, Smith GS, Brewer TF: Suicide mortality in the Maryland state prison system, 1979 through 1987. *JAMA* 262:365, 1989.

Schauben JL: Adulterants and substitutes. *Emerg Med Clin North Am* 8:595, 1990.

Smialek JE, Spitz WU: Death behind bars. *JAMA* 240:2563, 1978.

Soderstrom CA, Dischinger PC, Smith GS, et al: Psychoactive substance dependence among trauma center patients. *JAMA* 267:2756, 1992.

Szuster RR, Schanbacher BL, McCann SC: Characteristics of psychiatric emergency room patients with alcohol- or drug-induced disorders. *Hosp Community Psychiatry* 41:1342, 1990.

Teplin LA: The prevalence of severe mental disorder among male urban jail detainees: comparison with the epidemiologic catchment area program. *Am J Public Health* 80:663, 1990.

Vlahov D, Brewer TF, Castro KG, et al: Prevalence of antibody to HIV-1 among entrants to U.S. correctional facilities. *JAMA* 265:1129, 1991.

Walton CB, Blaisdell FW, Jordan RJ, Bodai BI: The injury potential and lethality of stab wounds: a Folsom Prison study. *J Trauma* 29:99, 1989.

Woolf A, Funk SG: Epidemiology of trauma in a population of incarcerated youth. *Pediatrics* 75:463, 1985.

# 249
# PHYSICIAN WELL-BEING*
## Sanford H. Koltonow

The daily pressures to act, to do, to decide make it difficult to stop and think, to consider, and to examine one's life goals, one's directions, one's priorities—the basic choices one faces in managing his own world . . . The important things in our lives are frequently deferred with some comforting but self-deceiving assumption that there will always be time tomorrow . . . time for one's self is discouraged, pleasure is deemed to be selfish, and one's own needs come last.    —*Roy Menninger*

The promotion of physician well-being has only recently been identified as a patient care issue. Physicians may not be able to cure every patient, but they certainly can hurt them all. Clearly, healthy, happy personnel provide higher quality care.

Emergency physicians tend to leave clinical care earlier than physicians in other specialties. Well before attrition occurs, there are warning signs and stages of dissatisfaction that, with awareness, can be identified and remedied before patient care and the physician's status are threatened.

The practice of emergency medicine requires a large knowledge base and advanced cognitive and interpersonal skills. Not quite as obvious is the need for excellent intrapersonal skills. Situations arise that conflict with one's personal values and produce intense feelings of unease. To remain effective, coping methods need to be used, which are adaptive and result in resolution. The thought that one can meet *all* the patient's needs ignores one's own needs for supports and limits.

Stress is necessary as a force that motivates. When excess stress becomes detrimental, it is more appropriately called distress. Much like Starling's law, each individual has a personal curve with a point beyond which further stress causes less, rather than more, output. By improving self-awareness, the physician may become able to examine the pressures rather than internalize them.

*Burnout* is a state of physical, emotional, and mental exhaustion that occurs as a result of intense involvement with people over long periods of time in emotionally demanding situations. Burnout symptoms are characterized, in their extreme form, by physical depletion and chronic fatigue, feelings of helplessness and hopelessness, and the development of negative attitudes toward self, work, life, and others. Among physicians, symptoms of burnout are thought to be potential precursors of more severe manifestations of impairment, including alcoholism, drug abuse, and suicidal ideation.

Emergency physicians practice in an environment that can foster burnout. Critical decisions must be made with incomplete information. Emergency physicians must deal with trauma, cardiac arrest, and death on a near daily basis. They must inform patients and families of morbidities and untoward outcomes. They must tolerate planned circadian disruption throughout their clinical careers. They work weekends and holidays, disrupting normal patterns with their families. Emergency physicians work with noises, smells, crowding, children, families, terminal illnesses, substance abusers, psychiatric patients, police, and criminals. It is easy to become overwhelmed.

The American Medical Association defines the *impaired physician* as "one who is unable to practice medicine with reasonable skill and safety because of physical or mental illness, including deterioration

* The author wishes to acknowledge the many contributions made to him by both John-Henry Pfifferling, PhD, as well as the Society for Professional Well-Being. Without their assistance and encouragement, this monograph would not have been possible.

though the aging process, loss of motor skill, or excessive use . . . of drugs, including alcohol." Various estimates of impairment range from 7 to 13 percent. Some states have reported sanctioning over 5 percent of their physicians *annually* for impairment.

Suicide, the ultimate manifestation of impairment, accounts for 31 to 34 percent of the premature deaths in physicians. The percentage is higher for women, particularly young women. Annually, more than 100 physicians complete suicide.

## BURNOUT

Burnout is a condition born of good intentions. Doctors who fall prey to it are, for the most part, unselfish individuals who have striven for perfection in their careers. It grows from unrealistic goal setting. It proliferates in the social isolation brought about by the professional taboo on expressing one's vulnerabilities and fears. This isolation impedes obtaining emotional support from peers.

Burnout is fostered by common personality characteristics of those who choose and succeed in emergency medicine. Near-compulsive overachievement, denial of one's limits, low trust, distant interpersonal relationships, and independent self-sufficiency are common. The effect is that the processing of deep feelings is repressed. Instead of addressing their own symptoms of personal stress, physicians tend to project feelings of irritability, anger, and frustration onto others: patients, nurses, and their families.

The ability to dissociate feelings from one's work is an adaptive coping mechanism for working with contagious disease and dangerous situations. However, it can also help physicians ignore their own vulnerabilities. They may not recognize the toll that a life-style of little sleep, poor diet, and little time for recreation or reflection may be having on themselves and their families. Dissociation becomes deadly when the "it-can't-happen-to-me" philosophy is used to justify increasing alcohol and drug consumption or other self-destructive behavior.

Fear of incompetence is nearly universal among physicians. When dealing with other people's lives, mistakes can have life-threatening ramifications. If one cannot accept his or her limits and the possibility of mistakes, one must (at least hope to) be perfect and all-knowing, a situation that promotes arrogance. Even symbolic challenges, perhaps by asking a question about care or interjecting a different opinion, can strike deep at defense mechanisms, frequently resulting in inappropriate physician behavior.

## PROFESSIONAL ENVIRONMENT STRESSORS

Nonmedical issues within the professional environment can exhaust emergency physicians and compound the difficulties in providing quality emergency care.

### Sociologic Problems

The emergency department has become society's safety net, where problems not served by other institutions, can be brought at any hour for evaluation. Medical screening or evaluation is necessary for everyone who requests emergency care even if it is medically apparent that more efficient means of meeting the patient's needs exist.

In urban areas from 30 to 50 percent of patients receive *all* their medical care from the emergency department. Their needs can be immense, including such basic needs as food, shelter, heat, and transportation, which makes assisting these patients much more difficult. Additionally, the physician may be drawn into the patient's dependency needs, creating emotional conflict.

### Crime

Emergency departments and physicians are commonly required to become agents of the police and the courts. Laws exist requiring emergency physicians' involvement with intoxicated, violent, and psy-

chotic patients. This also may include victims of personal crimes such as sexual assault and abuse, where the physician must collect evidence for legal proceedings.

Victims of major trauma are frequently victims of crime, and the attending physicians may be later subpoenaed to provide testimony in the legal proceedings.

### Violence

Data from the International Association for Healthcare Security and Safety indicates nearly geometric growth rates in the reported incidence of assaults in hospitals, with the emergency departments experiencing the majority. In a recent survey, 1 percent of hospitals reported a murder on their grounds within the past year.

Security officers should be present in the emergency department, and the department should be designed with security in mind. All personnel should be trained in crisis prevention techniques and interviewing skills because these are effective in defusing violence.

### Death and Dying

Death and dying involves physicians in sharing one of a family's most personal and powerful times. Emergency physicians need to become comfortable exploring patient's wishes about resuscitation and informing families of unexpected death and morbidity. The reasons for avoiding issues of death are multifaceted. There is the problem of finding time. Empathy requires emotional energy. Speaking with the grieving family forces the physician to face both system and personal conflicts.

The need of the patient and family for compassion is a difficult process to rush. Their wishes and belief systems deserve exploration. There are questions from loved ones about the events leading up to a death that must be dealt with empathically to facilitate the grieving process. Offering understanding, comfort, compassion, and solace can be important sources of satisfaction for the physician.

At some point in the course of delivering patient care, emergency physicians must emotionally process what has occurred. Often deaths resurrect powerful feelings from their own personal experiences. Perhaps they identify with the survivors because they have loved ones with characteristics similar to those of the victims.

Some of the difficulties physicians have regarding death may stem from the operating belief that a physician's career may represent the battle against death and disease. Facing a surviving family or counseling a dying patient may symbolize "failure" in that battle. In addition, the interaction may contain undertones of incompetence. Frequently the physician becomes the target of misplaced anger and denial.

### Rapport

In emergency situations one often does not have the benefit of an ongoing doctor-patient relationship, which can build rapport, mutual trust, and understanding. There are some easy things emergency physicians can do to build rapport and trust. Most revolve around fostering the perception of listening and caring. The physician should greet the patient by name and introduce himself or herself, shaking hands when appropriate. Sit down whenever possible—regardless of how long the physician actually remains with the patient, patients perceive it as much longer. When touching the patient, do so gently with an air of caring. Respect the patient's privacy by closing curtains and only exposing that which is necessary. When clinically appropriate, listen to the patient's overall agenda because it may save time. Do not use complex language. If the patient is lying down, try to keep your eyes at the patient's level. Set expectations for the patient with the first encounter, for example "lab results will be back in 2 hours, I'll be back to discuss them then," or "I have a critical patient to care for but you'll be next." Finding a small need you can fulfill, such as a glass of water, a pillow, a phone call, will help establish rapport.

## Conflict Resolution

Conflict resolution skills are important in emergency medicine for interactions with patients, peers, physicians in other specialities, and other hospital staff. The issues of conflict differ; the dynamics, however, are similar.

Some people believe intrinsically that their concerns, no matter how minor, are more important than anything else. Demanding patients or families are best handled by acknowledging their expectations and attempting compromise. Sometimes, it is effective to acknowledge that the patient has been heard and his perspective considered, yet the physician has a different perspective and position. Although firmness may be necessary, rarely will anything be gained by hostility or by confrontation.

Administrators, nurses, and consultants may be other sources of conflict; many times ongoing personality conflicts exist, provoked by the intensity of the work environment. One needs to focus on finding the "common ground," which is the patient's needs.

Not every conflict is a battle that must be won. Healthy conflict resolution requires the physician to know when to stand up and when to negotiate or retreat.

## Malpractice Litigation

Universally, physicians feel the need to expend significant resources to prevent malpractice litigation (as opposed to the resources used to prevent malpractice).

For those unfamiliar with the process a medical malpractice lawsuit can be frightening. It seems to strike at one's very being and self-worth. Many physicians will respond with disbelief, then anger, and finally depression. The process of meetings, testimony, and eventually the trial can be dehumanizing.

Physicians who succumb to the emotional trauma of a lawsuit respond in such a consistent manner that is has become known as the malpractice stress syndrome (MSS). In the original investigation by Sara Charles, MSS is usually manifested in at least four symptoms:

- Feelings of isolation
- Negative self-image
- Strong emotional impact
- Effect on family

Other commonly reported symptoms include anger, depression, frustration, insomnia, difficulty concentrating, fatigue, and decreased libido or appetite.

The single factor most predictive of a dysfunctional response is the experience of isolation. Embarrassment and self-doubt can cause avoidance of one's very sources of support. Colleagues' responses may reinforce the physician's feeling of shame. Knowing the physician is busy with preparing a defense, colleagues may change their referral and social patterns, which can be interpreted as judgment about the facts of the case.

The physician's self-doubt frequently carries over to personal life. Either for reasons of not wanting to bring home the pain or from feelings of shame for getting named in a lawsuit, many physicians withdraw from their spouses and families, furthering their isolation.

## Mechanisms of Support

Those concerned with physician well-being are beginning to explore malpractice litigation stress support groups. Several common attributes exist in the various models that have been proposed.

The group is educational. Risk management personnel can elucidate the proceedings by describing what to expect at each step, explaining the meaning of the legalese, and presenting the rules and etiquette. Support is provided by physicians who have contended with lawsuits sharing their experiences. Hearing that others have felt similarly can be the initial crack in the wall of isolation built by the physician-defendant. Family members can provide insight into the process their family is experiencing and their emotional responses. This will often improve communication at home.

Information is available, referenced later in the section on resources, on how to establish litigation stress support groups. Many state medical societies already have such groups in place.

## PERSONAL ENVIRONMENTAL STRESSORS

### Sleep Deprivation*

Shift work and scheduling difficulties are the most common sources of stress, career dissatisfaction, and attrition in emergency medicine. Rotating shifts have been associated in other industries with high rates of:

- Chronic fatigue syndrome
- Chronic sleep disruption and sleep deprivation
- Depression, mood swings, and divorce
- Gastrointestinal and immune dysfunction, infertility
- Drug and alcohol abuse
- Hypertension
- Cardiovascular mortality
- Work-related accidents and errors
- Accidents driving to and from work

When controlled for all other variables, people who work swing shifts have a life expectancy 8 to 10 years shorter than those who do not. Circadian principles apply to scheduling shifts and integrating one's work schedule with one's personal life. These principles acknowledge the body's natural rhythms and can help promote quality sleep and, thus, health.

### Sleep Physiology

Sleep occurs in discrete stages. The bulk of delta sleep or slow wave sleep (SWS) occurs early in the sleep period. The amount of SWS depends on prior wakefulness, that is, how tired one is, not on time of day or on length of sleep. After sleep deprivation, SWS is the first stage to be made up, preferentially obtained even during periods of frequent sleep disruption. There is an increase in SWS sleep in subjects who perform challenging intellectual tasks. SWS is thought to be vital for *physical* recuperation. Growth hormone is secreted in this stage. Those deprived of SWS often complain of fatigue and muscle aches.

Rapid eye movement (REM) sleep is characterized by rapid conjugate eye movements, a change in the electroencephalogram to a pattern similar to wakefulness, the occurrence of dreams, increase in oxygen consumption, and increased cerebral blood flow (more than when awake). During REM the brain is on but the body is off. REM stages tend to cluster toward the end of the normal 7- to 8-h nocturnal sleep period. REM stages also become longer as the night goes on. Those with shorter sleep periods will likely have REM deprivation, which is difficult to make up. REM sleep is thought to be vital for *psychological* well-being. Those deprived of it complain of irritability and moodiness. They also score higher on aggressive behavior testing. REM sleep may also be important in the consolidation of complex learning. Experimental subjects deprived only of REM sleep but allowed other phases for 3 to 4 days began displaying a thought disorder reminiscent of psychosis.

Human beings have a 25-h circadian clock, implying that our internal clocks are in fact reset back about an hour on a daily basis. Many physiologic functions follow circadian patterns and can be transposed by keeping experimental subjects awake at night and sleeping during the day. This process is known as *entrainment of the circadian*

* The author wishes to express special recognition to Dennis Whitehead, MD for his contributions to this section.

*rhythm.* Many circadian patterns have been demonstrated to be sensitive to entrainment, including alertness and basal body temperature. The *primary* stimulus for spontaneous awakening is a rise in body temperature; thus, the duration of the sleep period depends more on the phase of the circadian rhythm than on the prior period of wakefulness. This partly explains why those working short stretches of nights sleep fewer hours during the daytime than those working night shifts regularly, leading to REM sleep deprivation.

Many physicians attempt to use pharmaceuticals to assist in falling asleep. Alcohol, cyclic antidepressants, diphenhydramine, barbiturates, and benzodiazepine sedative-hypnotics all decrease the proportion of REM sleep. Stimulants, including nicotine and caffeine, impede onset of sleep and normal sleep stage progression.

Studies on sleep deprivation show the ability to perform challenging intellectual tasks is slowed but otherwise relatively unchanged; however, motivation to perform routine tasks is diminished. Sleep-deprived subjects have more errors of omission in work-paced tasks (e.g., monitoring, telemetry, suturing), whereas in self-paced tasks (e.g., problem solving, writing orders) speed is impaired but accuracy remains high. Because the quality of emergency medical practice often depends on properly performing routine tasks that may follow prolonged periods of intellectual exertion, it is imperative for physicians who work different shifts to schedule themselves in ways that minimize patient risk.

## Supportive Strategies (Table 249-1)

When planning shift rotations, it is healthier to rotate forward (days to afternoons, to midnights) because the human circadian rhythm is *25* hours long. Many physicians favor 12-h shifts to increase the number of days off. However, when rotating shifts, it takes longer to reset the biologic clock across a 12-h change than it does for an 8-h change.

**Table 249-1.** Strategies and Recommendations to Assist in the Health of Shift Workers

1. Given the right set of circumstances, the best strategy is to work the same shift all the time and keep the same sleep pattern. Consider additional compensation for those willing to work night shifts for extended periods.
2. For those unable to maintain consistent sleep patterns, use compromise strategies such as anchor sleep and napping to mitigate circadian disruptions.
3. Rotate all shifts in the clockwise direction, with at least 1-mo minimum time per rotation.
4. Isolated night shifts may be the best option for larger groups, or in groups in which one or more physicians are working nights permanently or for an extended period. This concept is gaining more acceptance among emergency physicians, mainly because of the obvious appeal of fewer clustered night shifts. It is difficult logistically for most small groups. The brevity of the isolated night shift rotation should not disrupt circadian rhythms.
5. Sleep in a quiet, darkened room, minimizing disruptions. Give the work schedule to likely daytime callers when on nights.
6. Start the awake period with a high-protein meal, switching to complex carbohydrates toward bedtime. Avoid caffeine and high-calorie, high-fat snack food before sleep. Eat meals regularly.
7. Use bright light (> 10,000 lux for 2 h after rising) as an adjunct for entraining to new shifts.
8. Get regular exercise, which is very important for the well-being of the shift worker. Vigorous aerobic exercise after rising may diminish the time needed to adjust to new shifts. Avoid heavy exertion before attempting to sleep.
9. Work with family and friends to plan regular quality time together.
10. Do not try to live a day-shift life-style while working night shifts. Hold administrative meetings early in the morning or late in the afternoon when working night shifts. Respect the circadian rights of those working nights by excusing them from meetings held during the day.

Source: Adapted from Whitehead DC, Thomas H, Slapper DR. *Ann Emerg Med* 21:1250, 1992.

The circadian gold standard is not to change shifts at all. Some groups now pay a premium to physicians who work nights exclusively. However those working only night shifts must maintain a daytime sleep pattern, even during days off, to avoid reentrainment to a daytime pattern. Working nights for long periods is difficult due to pressures to participate in daytime family and social activities or to be involved regularly in administrative activities.

There is a compromise known as anchor sleep, which minimizes circadian disruption. By sleeping a block of at least 4 h at the same time every day, one tends to anchor the circadian rhythm. It can be useful for permanent night shift workers during their days off or during short periods of irregular shift work, making it easier to return to "normal" sleep patterns.

Social life is important for the shift worker. Maintaining close ties with family and friends helps to relieve stress and mitigates the sense of temporal isolation shift workers face. Planning for quality social time is as vital as planning for work.

## Family

The personality characteristics chosen by and supported in medicine, often conflict with family and self-care priorities. With the increasing complexity of the physician's clinical and administrative schedule, social and community obligations, and the spouse's (and children's) interests, the family as a unit is most likely to suffer. A common tragic story is that when the physician finally realizes he or she needs the family, they have developed their own support system elsewhere. A family deserves planned blocks of time that are sacrosanct.

There are specific hardships associated with being in a relationship with a physician. As more women enter medicine, two-physician families are becoming more common with their own specific pressures. Living with the persistent demands of medicine most physician couples live for the future, convinced that eventually there will be time for each other. The couple assumes that the delay will not endanger the quality of the relationship; it will remain as fresh and intense as the day it was postponed.

Complex defense mechanisms learned in the milieu of the emotional and physical fatigue of training and practice can lead to a blunting of one's ability to respond to deep personal feelings. The most common complaint from spouses and from physician families entering counseling is that the physician member is emotionally distant even if not physically absent.

Physicians become professionally comfortable being decisive and responsible. Rarely are the feelings or opinions of others discussed; the physician gives "orders." As the expert, the physician knows what is best for the patient. It becomes a common scenario to translate this to the home, expecting problems will be solved by directive. The physician is tired, communication falters, compromise is one-sided as the family member decides to "let it go, at least he's finally home." Arrogance is enabled. Conflict is avoided until crisis develops.

Spouses can benefit from a support organization. The aim is to assist in understanding medical stress, share coping mechanisms, reduce isolation, and understand their own role in the patterns that shape their intimate relationships. Serious consideration must be given to using a trained communication facilitator and formal group structure for spouse's groups.

Finally, if a physician treats his or her own family, the care given can be inappropriate—either excessive or inadequate. A physician cannot remain objective in assessing loved ones, and it is most often inappropriate to try.

## Aging

Aging sometimes makes it physically difficult to do all that is required. Changes in the shift rotations are harder. Visual and hearing acuity may suffer. It may be difficult to accommodate medical problems; for example, at what time do you take your morning and evening doses of medications when you are on midnights? What if your diuretic takes effect during the trauma resuscitation? How does a professional group deal with the inevitable increase in sick time needed by an aging group of physicians? When does the slowing of reflexes exceed acceptable limits?

Career transitions are available in many specialties, but as a new specialty emergency medicine does not have as much experience in tailoring the practice to accommodate the older physician, and options other than leaving the field need to be developed.

## PERSONAL STRATEGIES FOR WELL-BEING

Physicians tend not to recognize the role that they themselves play in generating burnout symptoms. Individual attitudes, beliefs, personality factors, and learned coping strategies probably play a more important role in the development of burnout than do external stressors and demands. Importantly, such cognitive and behavioral tendencies are within the control of each individual and these components can, in fact, be modified.

During a particularly difficult period of time, most people know they feel stressed and may not be functioning as efficiently as they usually do. Frequently this can be attributed to a difficult patient, a busy shift, or a particular personal stressor outside of one's control. Self-awareness allows one to begin to appreciate the larger picture. Paradoxically, some physicians, when faced with the disillusionment of a life-style not realized, cling harder to their original motives—in denial. This process feeds on itself, resulting in frustration.

The path a physician has taken to reach a full-time practice in emergency medicine does not often allow for taking time for oneself. Often the decision to enter medicine occurs in adolescence; thus many decisions regarding one's life goals are subjugated to values that may no longer be embraced. The busy life-style of most physicians is not conducive to ongoing reevaluation. Often, the "cultural norms" of medicine are so integrated into personal values that the physician does not even know how to begin to separate them.

Table 249-2 lists some questions to be used as a starting point to assess one's own emotional fatigue. If several of the answers are affirmative perhaps this is evidence of divergence between personal values and career activities. This may motivate you to seek feedback from a trusted source.

### Principles of Management

The external stressors of practice can be mitigated. The common methods are time management, support, debriefing/relaxation, and physical self-care.

One must become aware and vigilant of personal priority setting and time management. Regardless of the validity of the need, one cannot say yes to a commitment without saying no to something else. One needs to become aware of what areas are unconsciously treated as a lower priority. Are these choices consistent with your values? A process of *values clarification* helps identify those concepts one is

**Table 249-2.** Questions for Self-assessment

Do you find the old ways of coping are not as reliable as they once were?
Do you find yourself becoming cynical about your colleagues or the "system"?
Do you waste time at work, dreading to see patients or slowed by indecision?
Are you drinking, eating, or smoking more than is normal for you?
Is your self-esteem unduly affected by criticism?
Have you lost the intrigue with medicine?
Do you feel helpless over the loss of control in the direction medicine is taking?
Do you have continuous problems with insomnia, fatigue, or depression?
Do you feel lonely or isolated? Do you avoid others so they don't see how unhappy you are?

willing to commit to and provides a starting point for determining personal priorities. One then should set life's major goals in all areas—physical, mental, financial, spiritual, social—according to the individual's most meaningful objectives.

*Peer support* is the single most powerful and cost-effective intervention to prevent burnout. Develop relationships with peers that go beyond the immediate clinical issues. By maintaining communication with peers the shared experience is emphasized and isolation does not develop. Listen, and provide emotional support and challenge. Be the one to take the risk of talking about the things that are felt but ignored. Share the social reality of what living and practicing in current society is like, sharing thoughts, feelings, and strategies. The fear that others may discover one's vulnerabilities needs to be resisted. This encourages low levels of trust in peers and tends to isolate one from the social supports needed in times of crisis. Part of peer support includes debriefing each other on a daily basis, helping maintain perspective and knowing that others are there to provide timely, appropriate feedback.

*Well-being committees* within hospital or medical societies can provide education along with referral to other resources. Lines of communication are opened, as physicians learn coping techniques others have found effective. Topics to present to the medical staff include values clarification, goal setting, time management, grieving, and reframing. These areas are conducive to a group setting and offer a way to introduce more personal issues. In addition, the institution's credibility can bring these new skills to the attention of many who might benefit but otherwise not take part. A well-being committee is different from professional assistance programs for "impaired, disabled or troubled" physicians, though their work should complement each other.

The *critical incident stress debriefing* (CISD) team is an approach that attempts to reduce the severity of poststress disorders at the time of occurrence. In a model developed by Mitchell, personnel who have experienced a critical or anxiety-provoking situation are debriefed as a group. The group is facilitated by experienced group leaders of similar professional background in conjunction with mental health professionals. This occurs either immediately following the event or within 72 h. The goal is to intercede before unhealthy reactions have time to be fully incorporated. Each individual is asked to describe what he or she saw, heard, and felt. The incident becomes the setting to share feelings and break detrimental isolation. It also allows the opportunity to identify individuals who may need further assistance. Personnel receive the message there is concern for them.

### Mentoring

Concern for the well-being of medical trainees must be constantly modeled in medical training. Many trainees do not have the advantage of mentors who share their mistakes with them, let down their guard, and demonstrate that a lack of perfection does not mean incompetence. Such mentors demonstrate that a mistake is compatible with excellence and compassionate care. Errors in problem solving can be used to improve learned behavior. A faculty that can mentor personal and professional humility is the best prevention against medical arrogance.

### Physical Health

Most physicians do not get regular preventive health care. This may be due to the tremendous time constraints of practice as well as to denial of vulnerability to illness. Either way, the physician winds up caring less for self than for patients.

Exercise helps maintain physical health and relieves emotional tension. In addition, setting aside the time for one's own health, within the busy schedule and conflicting priorities of the active physician, confirms with action the belief that caring for oneself is an important use of time.

The diet that many emergency physicians exist on contributes to both poor health and fatigue: high in fat, sugar and caffeine, usually eaten quickly, without time to sit. Anticipating an urgent interruption prevents one from relaxing.

## Relaxation Techniques

Relaxation is different from leisure, which frequently contains stressors. Physicians will find the stressors of leisure enjoyable because they are so different from the common stressors of professional life. Leisure activities will also usually involve family and friends. However, leisure tends to arouse and fatigue, rather then renew.

Relaxation is also different from doing nothing. Given the hyperstimulation of the professional environment of the emergency physician, it is not unusual to find one seeking mindless activities, like television. However, all these activities numb awareness. This numbness is part of the seduction of alcohol or other tranquilizers.

Relaxation, by contrast, actually increases awareness while resting the body. This is the time to reflect and process experiences and feelings. Systematic relaxation requires concentration and deliberate mental activity. It will lead to lower arousal and release of strain. It can be particularly helpful if the relaxation does not require physically leaving the home, such as pleasure reading, gardening, hobbies, and crafts.

For those finding it difficult to achieve this level of relaxation, many techniques are available. Physicians will frequently respond to mediation, progressive muscle relaxation, selective awareness, self-hypnosis, somatics, yoga, breath control, and biofeedback. Many techniques have audiotapes available to conveniently help guide one through the learning process. For some, religious beliefs and activities may fulfill the need for relaxation. The important common denominator is quiet time that allows for personal reflection, integration, and planning.

## IDENTIFICATION OF IMPAIRMENT

Emergency physicians frequently feel emotionally overwhelmed on a temporary basis. When does this become maladaptive? Table 249-3 lists behaviors and thoughts, which when seen as a change in established behavior, are suggestive of problems.

Detection of impairment in others is much more difficult. Psychiatrically and chemically impaired professionals are often able to delay notice by protecting job performance at the expense of every other dimension of their lives. The common signs of uncharacteristic behaviors are frequently ignored. The phenomenon of family, neighbors, friends, and coworkers becoming involved in an exhaustive conspiracy *enabling* the appearance of normal job functioning is both

**Table 249-3.** Possible Signs and Symptoms of Burnout

Use of home time only as time to rest, with withdrawal from family activities
"Taking it out" behavior on spouse, family members, nurses, and staff
Chronic complaining, cynicism, blaming others
Dreading to see patients
Writing short, ambiguous charts; quality assurance or utilization review notice of inappropriate or unintelligible comments
Requesting frequent consultations
Inappropriate anger toward medicine, patients, staff, authority
Overprescribing to patient's symptoms
Sharing personal problems with patients, blurring of boundaries
Degrading of peers, backbiting, questioning motives of others
Frequent illness and unexplained absence
Frequent job changes
Excessive adult toys that become time-consuming obsessions, such as computers, boats, and planes
"Hanging around" the practice without apparent reason
Unusual number of patient complaints
Passive-aggressive acting out

common and tragic. Training in pharmaceutical use, functional psychiatric problems, and in the medical problems of addicted and abusing patients helps physicians feel that they are experts in their own problems.

*Intervention* is almost always required with impaired physicians due to the massive denial and other defense mechanisms used. Shame, embarrassment, fear, and guilt keep many health care workers from consciously accepting that they are not in control until confronted by either trusted colleagues, or more commonly, authorities.

Intervention is a delicate task, requiring sensitivity, clear motives and *specialized training*. Members of the physician's support system are consulted, and some are asked to be present at the intervention to de-construct this "conspiracy of enabling." This will be the critical moment where a firm attitude of concern, without hostility or punitive overtones, has the opportunity to break through the defenses and allow the individual, for maybe the first time, to acknowledge the problem. At this point, the individual is vulnerable and must be offered options.

The seriousness of the emotional impact of confrontation on the sick physician must be appreciated; it is critical to anticipate and prevent the possibility of a suicide or bodily harm by accident or trauma. These possibilities are not uncommon, particularly in impaired health professionals.

## CONCLUSIONS

Table 249-4 lists the author's principles for promoting personal well-being. The overriding tenets are self-awareness and self-responsibility. No individual or institution created your conflicts or can resolve them. You can, however, mold the environment until it best suits your needs. Choices and alternatives always exist.

## RESOURCES

1. The Society and Center for Professional Well-Being of Durham, North Carolina is a professional educational and consultive orga-

**Table 249-4.** Principles for Promotion of Physician Well-being

Commit to being aware of your stresses and anxieties. Relate to stress as a challenge to overcome, not as something intolerable with power over your life.
Maintain perspective. Don't take yourself too seriously. Develop a separate identity, one not dependent on your role as a physician.
Allow yourself space to be human. Realize medicine is not the cause of your problems or unhappiness—you are free to choose the life-style and work environment. Confront the options.
Be here now. If your family, religion, community, or other activity is actually a priority, spend time with it. Your family deserves planned blocks of time that are sacrosanct.
Focus on the intrinsic rewards of medicine: altruism, interest in the science, challenge of the patients who need your skills, stimulation by the broad range of people with whom you work. There are rewards in medicine you find motivating. If these are not apparent then this is an area in need of exploration.
Develop networks with your peers; don't allow yourself to become isolated. Support systems need to be acceptable to all concerned and not threaten professional status. You must have personal and professional confidants and accurate feedback. Learn to recognize maladaptive coping mechanisms in yourself and colleagues.
Expose students and residents to psychotherapists, who can establish scientific and interpersonal credibility. This exposure can facilitate their personal use during times of crisis.
Be certain there is adequate staffing provided to afford relief, time off, and back-up in times of crisis.
Care for yourself by attending to your physical health:
   Make necessary provisions to ensure adequate, quality sleep.
   Get regular exercise, control your weight, pay attention to your diet.
   Provide for your relaxation. This is different from leisure.
   See your doctor(s) and follow *their* instructions.

nization. It sponsors an annual national conference, and conducts many regional programs on its own and on behalf of state and county medical societies, hospitals, and group practices. It offers unique programs in values clarification, practice assessment, and conflict resolution. It is a source for manuals on developing litigation, spouse, and other support groups. The center has been a regular presenter at ACEP meetings. Several active emergency physicians participate as speakers and contributors. Contact Dr. John-Henry Pfifferling, (919) 489–9167.

2. The Talbot-Marsh recovery program for substance abuse and psychiatric disabilities in Atlanta, Georgia specializes in treating health care professionals. It is nationally recognized as a model for extended outpatient treatment of substance-abusing physicians. (800) 445–4232.

3. The Menninger Clinic of Topeka, Kansas provides individual, marital, and family therapy, along with being a major psychoanalytic training program. It also sponsors educational workshops in a retreat setting in Estes Park, Colorado, for a week each July. Designed specifically for physician couples, it focuses on the problem of balancing the demands of medical practice with the needs of self and family. Write to Post Office Box 829, Topeka, KS, 66601.

4. ACEP, SAEM and other societies provide state-of-the-art educational resources. All of the topics in this chapter, in one form or another, have been included in presentations.

5. The American Medical Association's Department of Mental Health has established the Physician's Health Foundation. Its purpose is to provide financial assistance for physicians disabled from any cause, including psychological or chemical impairment and human immunodeficiency virus. Identification is through the state medical societies' physician assistance programs. The Foundation also supports research, focused education and retraining programs, job placement, and the International Conference on Physician Health. Contact Elaine Tejeck, (312) 464–5073.

## BIBLIOGRAPHY

Charles SC. Sued and nonsued physicians' self-reported reactions to malpractice litigation. *Am J Psychiatry* 142:437, 1985.

Gabbard G, Menninger RW (eds). *Medical Marriages.* Washington, DC: American Psychiatric Press, 1988.

Howell JB, Schroeder DP. *Physician Stress: A Handbook for Coping.* Baltimore: University Park Press, 1984.

McCranie EW, Brandsma JM. Personality antecedents of burnout among middle-aged physicians. *Behav Med* Spring, 1988.

Mitchell JT, Bray GP. *Emergency Services Stress.* Englewood Cliffs, NJ: Prentice Hall, 1990.

Pfifferling JH, In: Scott CD, Hawk J (eds): *Heal Thyself: The Health of Health Care Professionals.* New York: Brunner/Mazel, 1986.

Whitehead DC, Thomas H, Slapper DR. A rational approach to shift work in emergency medicine. *Ann Emerg Med* 21:1250, 1992.

# SECTION 24
# Abuse and Assault

## 250
## CHILD ABUSE AND NEGLECT
### Carol Berkowitz

### SPECTRUM OF CHILD ABUSE AND NEGLECT

The concept of child maltreatment, defined as harm to a child because of abnormal child-rearing practices, is a broadening of the initial description of the battered child syndrome. Child maltreatment is an all-inclusive term covering physical abuse; sexual abuse; emotional abuse; parental substance abuse; physical, nutritional, and emotional neglect; supervisional neglect; and Munchausen syndrome by proxy.

The ease with which the physician is able to recognize these disorders in part depends on his or her knowledge of normal children and normal development. The physical stigmata of maltreatment are characteristic, although the findings of neglect and sexual abuse are more subtle than those of gross physical trauma.

### CHILD NEGLECT

Child neglect can result in an array of physical and emotional problems. Child neglect from early infancy results in the syndrome of failure to thrive (FTT). This syndrome usually affects children under the age of 3 years, although older children who remain in a non-nurturing environment show similar manifestations.

The patient is often brought to the emergency department because of other medical problems, such as intercurrent infections; skin rashes, particularly severe monilial diaper dermatitis; or acute gastroenteritis.

The history of the acute illness may not alert the physician to the chronic nature of the underlying problem. The physical examination provides the clue to the diagnosis of long-standing malnutrition. Overall physical care and hygiene are frequently poor. The infant has very little subcutaneous tissue. The ribs protrude prominently through the skin, and the skin of the buttocks hangs in loose folds. There may be alopecia over a flattened occiput, reflecting the fact that the baby has been allowed to lie on his or her back all day. Muscle tone is usually increased (although sometimes these babies are hypotonic). This increased tone is most notable in the lower extremities, and infants may manifest scissoring, similar to infants with cerebral palsy.

FTT infants also show distinct behavioral characteristics. They are wide-eyed and wary. If brought in close proximity to the examiner's face, they may purposely turn away to avoid eye contact. They become irritable if interpersonal interaction is pursued. They are difficult to console and are not cuddly. They prefer inanimate over animate objects and spend much time with their hands in their mouths. When left alone, they assume a "straphanger's position" with their arms flexed at the elbows and extended over their shoulders.

Weights and lengths should be plotted on the appropriate growth curves. In general, weight is more adversely affected than length, although this depends on the duration of the neglect. This may be reflected in a body mass index (BMI = weight [kg]/height [m$^2$]) below 5%. Likewise, longstanding neglect results in a diminution in the rate of growth of the head.

In addition to observing for these physical signs, the physician should obtain certain historical information. This includes the birth weight (to assess the rate of growth); any maternal use of cigarettes, alcohol, and/or drugs during pregnancy; previous hospitalizations; and the parental stature. A full social service assessment should also be obtained, although this is usually done by a medical social worker.

Infants suspected of suffering from significant environmental FTT should be admitted to the hospital. Weight gain in the hospital is felt to be the sine qua non of environmental FTT. Most infants gain weight within 1 to 2 weeks following admission; in addition the hospitalization allows a more extensive social service assessment while the infant is in a protected environment. A skeletal survey of the long bones should be carried out to detect any evidence of physical abuse.

Children over the age of 2 to 3 years with environmental neglect are termed psychosocial dwarfs. Their short stature is a more prominent finding than their low weight. These children manifest a classic triad of short stature, bizarre voracious appetite (eating from trash cans), and a disturbed home situation. They are frequently hyperactive and have delayed or unintelligible speech. Psychosocial dwarfs have been studied endocrinologically and have been found to have a low to normal level of growth hormone which fails to increase with stimulation with insulin or arginine. These children should also be admitted for evaluation and initiation of appropriate social intervention. The endocrinologic disturbances rapidly reverse following hospitalization or placement in a foster home.

### MUNCHAUSEN SYNDROME BY PROXY

Munchausen syndrome by proxy, MSBP, is a relatively uncommon form of child abuse in which a parent either induces or fabricates an illness in a child in order to secure for themselves prolonged contact with health care providers. Children with MSBP may present to the emergency department with reported symptoms such as bleeding, seizures, altered mental status, apnea, diarrhea, vomiting, fever, rash, or multiple organ system involvement. These symptoms may result from administration of agents such as warfarin or ipecac. Often the cases are medically perplexing, and families frequently move from hospital to hospital, seemingly in search of diagnosis. Children with MSBP are often subject to multiple unnecessary tests as the physician seeks to uncover the etiology of the disorder. The parent (biologic mother in 98% of cases) encourages the staff to do more diagnostic procedures, and often seems uncharacteristically happy if a test is positive.

Social service and psychologic evaluation is mandatory in the evaluation and management of these children, who should be admitted to the hospital both to assure their safety, and institute needed therapy.

### SEXUAL ABUSE

Victims of prior child sexual abuse are frequently difficult for the inexperienced physician to assess because of an unfamiliarity with the normal prepubertal genital examination. Children who have been sexually abused are brought to the emergency department because of a disclosure about the abuse or because of other symptoms such as those referrable to the genitourinary tract, including vaginal discharge, vaginal bleeding, dysuria, urinary tract infections, or urethral discharge; behavior disturbances, including excessive masturbation, genital fondling, or other sexually oriented or provocative behavior; encopresis; regression; nightmares; and unrelated complaints. Approximately 15 percent of children diagnosed in an emergency department as victims of sexual abuse in one report had unrelated complaints such as abdominal pain, asthma, and sore throat.

Children who are sexually abused rarely disclose their abuse until time has elapsed from the acute episode. Children who are seen immediately after an assault should be evaluated for evidence of acute injuries and for the presence of forensic material, such as semen.

More often, several years have elapsed since the abuse was initiated, although it may be ongoing. Children 8 to 11 years of age frequently disclose that they have been victims of sexual abuse for a significant period of time. The assailant is known to the child in over 90 percent of cases.

A medical history should be obtained from all children being evaluated for sexual abuse. Because evidence of the abuse may not be apparent until the child is examined, the physician may have to obtain additional historic information after the physical assessment. The medical history should include pertinent statements about whether the child has any underlying condition or has undergone any previous procedures that might cause changes in the anogenital area. Genitourinary surgery or trauma would be particularly important to note.

The child should be questioned directly about what happened. The child's name for genitalia and other body parts should be recorded, and all statements that the child makes concerning the abuse should be recorded verbatim. The demands of a busy emergency department may make it difficult for the physician to conduct a detailed and sensitive interview. In such cases, the hospital social worker should be consulted.

The examining physician must maintain a high index of suspicion of sexual abuse when evaluating children presenting with anogenital or behavioral complaints. The physical assessment should include an evaluation of the child's overall well-being and a general physical examination. The skin should be examined for bruises. Nongenital physical injuries are unusual, even following acute abuse. Rarely, there may be grip marks on the forearms or puncture wounds on the inner aspects of the lips resulting from a slap to the face. The age of the child and the degree of sexual development should be noted.

The genital examination should be confined to a careful inspection of the genitalia and perianal area. Generally, there is no need for a speculum examination unless the victim is an older adolescent or unless perforating vaginal trauma is suspected. Likewise, sedation is rarely needed, and most children can be reassured verbally if they are at all apprehensive. Careful inspection of the external genitalia is sufficient to establish physical evidence of genital injury. The examination is sometimes augmented by the use of a colposcope, to allow detection of subtle changes in the hymen. The colposcope also facilitates photographing the external genital area. However, most emergency departments are not equipped with a colposcope, and this instrument is, in fact, not critical to an adequate assessment of the anogenital area. Magnification can easily be achieved with the use of hand-held lenses. Toluidine blue dye applied to the genital area may also detect subtle acute injuries.

A number of different positions have been used to facilitate the examination. Infants may be seated on their parents' laps. Children are easily examined supine on the examining table with their legs in a frog-leg position. Some physicians also place all children in a prone knee-chest position to help fully assess the contour and homogeneity of the hymen. Placing a child in "stirrups" is usually unnecessary unless she is obese or has achieved adult stature.

The normal prepubescent girl has full labia majora and small thin labia minora. The vaginal opening is covered by the hymen, a fine reddish-orange, thin-edged membrane. The thickness and color of the hymen varies as a function of age. It is normally thick during infancy and again with the onset of puberty. In between, it is thinner, most often annular or crescentic, and smooth-edged. The hymenal orifice should be measured, although there is a range of variation depending on the child's age, position, and degree of relaxation. Trauma may re-

sult in changes such as hymenal notches, also referred to as *concavities* or *clefts*. Concavities at the 6:00 position are associated with prior penetrating trauma. Attenuation or reduction in the amount of hymenal tissue may lead to a gaping opening. Irregularities in the contour, particularly deep notches, are also associated with prior injury. Scarring, as evidenced by marked alteration in the vascular pattern (white areas or swirling vascularity), is an additional sign of healed injury. Erythema, on the other hand, may be secondary to irritation, inflammation, and/or chronic manipulation and is not specific for abuse.

Physical findings indicative of a sexually transmitted disease should also be noted, including a vaginal discharge, warts consistent with condylomata acuminata or condylomata lata, and vesicles or ulcers consistent with herpes genitalia.

It is critically important for the emergency physician to be aware that the absence of physical findings does not preclude abuse. There are many sexually abusive activities (such as orogenital contact) that would not be expected to produce scarring trauma. In addition, as is true elsewhere in the body, injuries can heal without residual scarring.

The genital examination in the sexually victimized young boy is less revealing. Rarely, there may be bite marks on the penis or scrotum. There may be a urethral discharge; the penis may become erect without tactile stimulation and remain erect.

The perianal examination is often more revealing, although it too may be completely normal in the case of either acute or chronic sodomy. Acute penetration may produce no changes or may be associated with fissures; abrasions; hematomas; and changes in tone, including both dilatation and anal spasm. In the young female patient, anal penetration is easier than vaginal penetration, and changes in this area may be seen. Anal fissures or tags may be noted. The perianal folds, or rugae, may be thickened in some areas, thinned out in others, and distorted. The perianal skin may be lichenified and thickened secondary to frictional rubbing. Anal tone may be reduced when there has been repeated prior anal penetration. However, stool in the rectal ampulla may lead to similar dilatation, and one should be careful to note the presence or absence of stool.

The laboratory evaluation of the sexually abused child should include cultures of the throat, vagina (or urethra), and rectum for gonorrhea; and a culture from the vagina (or urethra) for *Chlamydia*. Rapid antigen assays are not considered reliable in prepubescent children. A serologic test for syphilis is indicated if there is clinical evidence of syphilis, a history of syphilis in the assailant, or the presence of another sexually transmitted disease. HIV testing should only be done after appropriate counseling and if there is reason to suspect infection.

A suspicion of child sexual abuse mandates that a report be filed with child protective services or law enforcement agencies. These agencies will pursue an investigation and attempt to ensure that the child is placed in a protected environment.

Although there is the likelihood that the child may be removed from the home, a return appointment for follow-up of cultures for sexually transmitted diseases and a referral for psychologic counseling should be given.

## PHYSICAL ABUSE

The spectrum of injuries in the child who has been intentionally traumatized is wide. Familiarity with this spectrum enables the physician in the emergency department to arrive at the correct diagnosis in a timely manner. Two-thirds of the victims of physical abuse are under the age of 3 years, and one-third are under 6 months. The physical vulnerabilty of such small children is easy to understand.

Historical data may raise suspicions of inflicted trauma. A history which is inconsistent with the nature or the extent of the injuries (e.g., a fractured femur in an infant from a fall off a bed), a history which keeps changing as to the circumstances surrounding the injury, a discrepancy between the story the child gives and the story the caretaker gives, a history of previous trauma in the patient or siblings, or a delay in seeking medical attention should raise one's index of suspicion of physical abuse. Knowledge of normal motor development assists the physician in determining the likelihood that the injury happened in the stated manner. Children under the age of 6 months are incapable of inducing accidents or accidentally ingesting any drugs or poisons. The evaluating physician should record the developmental milestones the child has achieved, e.g., the age of sitting unsupported, walking, etc. Parental behavior in the emergency department should be observed, and it should be noted if the parents appear intoxicated or under the influence of drugs. The level of parental concern about the injury should also be noted.

Toddlers and older children should be questioned about the circumstances of the injury, and the comments should be recorded verbatim on the record. These statements are frequently admissible in court under exceptions to the hearsay rule and may help establish the diagnosis of child abuse.

The physical examination should note the child's overall hygiene and well-being. Normal children, especially toddlers who are just learning how to walk, may have multiple ecchymoses over the anterior shins, the forehead, and other bony prominences. Most falls result in bruises on only one body surface. Bruises over multiple areas, especially the low back, buttocks, thighs, cheeks, ear pinnae, neck, ankles, wrists, corners of the mouth, and lips suggest physical abuse. Handprints may be observed, or there may be uniform but bizarre bruise marks caused by belts, buckles, cords, or blunt instruments. Bite marks produce bruising in a characteristic oval pattern, with teeth indentations along the periphery. Lacerations of the frenulum or oral mucosa may be present, especially in an infant who has been force-fed. Lacerations and abrasions in the genital area are seen in toddlers who are "punished" because of toilet-training accidents.

The duration of a bruise can be estimated by the color of the lesion. No discoloration is noted initially, although the bruised area may be swollen and tender. Within a day or two the lesion becomes reddish-blue, and this lasts for about 5 days. This changes to green (days 5 to 7), then to yellow (days 7 to 10), and finally to brown (days 10 to 14) before resolving. For instance, reddish-blue lesions are inconsistent with a 2-week-old injury.

Children with multiple bruises should be evaluated with a complete blood cell count, a differential blood count, and coagulation studies including a platelet count, a prothrombin time, and a partial thromboplastin time. Rarely, a child with leukemia, aplastic anemia, or thrombocytopenia is brought for evaluation because of multiple bruises.

Burns constitute another form of inflicted injuries. These may be scald burns caused by immersion in hot water. Such burns do not conform to a splash configuration; rather, an entire hand or foot ("glove-and-stocking" pattern) may be involved. There is sharp demarcation of the burn margin. The buttocks may be burned during toilet training "punishment" by immersion in a bathtub filled with hot water. Knees, anterior thighs, feet, and portions of the abdomen are spared, and the buttocks and genitalia are scalded. Cigarette burns leave small (approximately 5 mm) circumferential scab-covered injuries. These lesions may resemble impetigo, as do scald injuries, which may resemble bullous impetigo. A culture of material from these lesions differentiates the burn from the infection. Other inflicted burns can result from forced contact with metal objects such as an iron, curling iron, or heater grid.

Skeletal injuries may be detected when a child presents with unexplained swelling of an extremity or refusal to walk or to use an extremity. These fractures may take any form, but spiral fractures caused by torsion (twisting) of a long bone, and metaphyseal chip fractures, suggest inflicted injury, especially when present in infants under 6 months of age. Skeletal surveys referred to as a trauma series (or trauma x) should be obtained. These include films of all long bones, the ribs, the clavicles, the fingers, the toes, the pelvis, and the skull. They may reveal periosteal elevation secondary to new bone formation at sites of previous microfractures or periosteal injury; multiple fractures at different stages of healing; fractures at unusual sites such as the ribs, the lateral clavicle, the sternum, or the scapula; or repeated fractures to the same site. Such x-ray findings are supportive of the diagnosis of child abuse.

Head injuries are a serious and potentially lethal form of child abuse. Infants with significant intracranial hemorrhage may have no apparent external injuries. Intracranial hemorrhages may result from vigorous shaking of the infant, and thrusting the infant down onto a surface, such as a mattress. This is referred to as shaken baby or shaken impact syndrome. Older children may have been beaten about the head or face. Changes in mental status should therefore be evaluated by head CT if there is any suspicion of abuse. Bruises around the ears, eyes, and cheeks, as well as swelling of the scalp secondary to subgaleal hematomas or underlying skull fractures may be noted. Fundoscopic examination may reveal retinal hemorrhages, which are usually associated with subdural hematomas. Such hemorrhages may result from direct trauma to the skull or severe shaking of the child. These children should be evaluated with a CT scan, and coagulation studies should be performed to rule out underlying coagulopathies. MRI studies are also being used to help differentiate recent from older intracranial bleeding episodes. Additional eye injuries caused by trauma may include hyphema, lens dislocation, and retinal detachment.

Injuries to the abdomen are equally serious and are a common cause of death from child abuse. Symptoms include recurrent vomiting, abdominal pain and tenderness, diminished bowel sounds, and/or abdominal distension. A history of injury as well as bruising of the overlying skin may be absent. Abdominal x-ray films may reveal a distended stomach with a "double-bubble sign" secondary to a duodenal hematoma. Diffuse distension may also be noted. Laboratory studies may reveal anemia, an elevated amylase level from traumatic pancreatitis, or hematuria from kidney trauma. Other abdominal injuries caused by trauma may include hepatic or splenic rupture, intestinal perforation, or rupture of intraabdominal blood vessels.

Any serious injury in a child under the age of 5 years should be viewed with suspicion. Other injuries which may be viewed as suggestive of child abuse include those which the child states were inflicted by another, were self-inflicted, or were inflicted by an unknown assailant.

The behavioral interaction between the child, the parent, and the physician may provide supportive evidence of the diagnosis of abuse. These children are often very compliant and submissive. They do not resist the medical examiner and readily submit to painful procedures such as blood drawing. They are overly affectionate to the medical staff, frequently preferring the nurse or the physician over the parent. Sometimes they are protective of the abusing parent, try to foster to his or her needs, and lie to cover up the true nature of the injury.

Parental behavior is less uniform, but certain distinct characteristics may be noted. The parents may not interact with the child in a comforting or supportive manner during the examination. They may become angry at the physician early in the course of the evaluation and may refuse diagnostic studies. They may appear to be intoxicated or under the influence of drugs. They may have brought the child in for seemingly minor complaints and ignored the major injuries or lesions. They may insist on hospital admission of the child for these minor problems and may readily confess they can no longer cope with the child. They may express fears of losing control.

The social service assessment may reveal an unstable home situation with frequent moves, poor parental-support systems, low parental self-esteem (often caused by battering during their own childhood), parental substance abuse, and/or domestic violence. This adds further supportive evidence of a high-risk situation.

## MANAGEMENT

Once the medical assessment has been completed, the physician must initiate the appropriate treatment. The medical management should be guided by the physical findings. Frequently these children require hospitalization.

Although the specifics of the laws surrounding child abuse and neglect vary from state to state, every state does require that suspected cases be reported. A verbal report is made initially to the police department and/or the child protection agency of the locality in which the abuse occurred. Law enforcement officers often appear in the emergency department, especially if the child does not require hospitalization. The child may be removed from the home and placed in protective custody, taken to a juvenile facility, placed temporarily with other relatives, or placed in a foster shelter home. The final disposition is dependent on a court hearing. The physician is also required to complete an official report detailing the specifics of the evaluation and giving his or her diagnostic opinion as to why the injuries or neglect are nonaccidental. The report should use nontechnical terms, e.g., *bruise* instead of *ecchymosis,* so that law enforcement and social service workers can understand the extent of the injuries.

Physicians are sometimes hesitant to report suspected cases. They are not "100 percent" certain. They are fearful of the parental response to the report. They are concerned about removing a child from the natural home. It is important to remember that the physician is required by law to report all suspected cases of abuse and neglect. Failure to report suspected cases can result in misdemeanor charges and lead to a fine or imprisonment. Additionally, the physician is protected by the law from legal retaliation by the parents.

Parental anger is a natural response to the filing of a report of suspected child abuse. The physician should refrain from being accusatory. Instead, the physician should note his or her concern about the child's well-being and advise the family that a physician is required by law to report any suspicions. The physician should verbally acknowledge the anger but persist in the role of child advocate. This job is facilitated in hospitals which have child abuse teams available to assist the physician in the emergency department.

## BIBLIOGRAPHY

Berkowitz CD: Child sexual abuse. *Pediatr in Review* 13:443, 1992.

Bithoney WG, Dubowitz H, Egan H: Failure to thrive/growth deficiency. *Pediatr Rev* 13:453, 1992.

Chadwick DL, Berkowitz CD, Kerns D, et al: *Color Atlas of Child Sexual Abuse.* Year Book Medical Publishers, Chicago, 1989.

Reece RM: *Child Abuse: Medical Diagnosis and Management.* Lea & Febiger, Philadelphia, 1994.

Rosenberg DA: Web of deceit: A literature review of Munchausen syndrome by proxy. *Child Abuse Negl* 11:547, 1987.

# 251
# MALE AND FEMALE SEXUAL ASSAULT
## Marion Hoelzer

## EPIDEMIOLOGY

Sexual assault accounted for over 6 percent of all crimes reported in the 1987 Uniform Crimes Report. A 3-year study by the National Victims Center disclosed that 12.1 million women, or one in eight women, have been raped. Most rape victims feel there is a stigma attached to being a victim of sexual assault. As a result, authorities believe that only one in four cases are reported. The vast majority of information and statistics relates to female rape victims. Only recently has male sexual assault been recognized and reported. The estimated incidence is 2 to 4 percent of reported rapes.

Many misconceptions are perpetuated about sexual assault. The most common is the assumption that rape is motivated by sexual desire. Groth and Birnbaum interviewed 133 convicted rapists and found that rape was merely the expression of a nonsexual need—power or anger. Recent literature detailing the pattern of injuries sustained by rape victims supports rape as a violent crime. In 372 rape victims seen at an inner city Detroit teaching hospital, injuries encountered were usually facial or extremity injuries. Gynecologic injuries accounted for only 7 percent of all injuries. Elderly victims are twice as likely to incur physical not genital injuries, and genital injuries are not an inevitable consequence of rape. Many victims are threatened with a weapon, the majority of victims suffer minor injuries, and only 1 to 2 percent require hospitalization.

The physician's responsibility is to provide for the patient's physical and psychological well-being first. Then, if the patient wishes to prosecute, to provide police with corroborative medical evidence. This is the only medical protocol designed primarily to meet legal needs.

## CLINICAL FEATURES
### The Female Rape Examination
#### History

The purpose of the history is to tactfully obtain data about pertinent events and personal information for proper medical care without having the rape victim relive in minute detail the events of the attack. Actually, an extensively detailed history may hinder subsequent prosecution.

#### Assault History

1. *Who.* Was the assailant known to the victim? Was it a single attacker? If more than one, how many?
2. *What happened.* Was the victim physically assaulted? If so, with what (i.e., gun, bat, heavy object) and where? This information will determine whether x-rays are necessary to rule out a fracture.
3. *When.* When approximately did the assault occur? This will determine the probability of detecting sperm or acid phosphatase.
4. *Where.* Where did penetration occur—vaginal, oral, or rectal? This will direct the physical examination to areas of potential injury.
5. *Douche, shower, or change clothes.* Any of these activities performed prior to seeking medical attention may decrease the probability of sperm or acid phosphatase recovery.

### Medical History

1. *Last menstrual period.* This will help to determine pregnancy risk.
2. *Birth control method.* This will also help to determine pregnancy risk.
3. *Last intercourse.* If the patient has had recent intercourse (< 3 days) prior to the attack, it may confuse laboratory analysis of sperm, acid phosphatase, and genetic typing.
4. *Allergies and prior medical history.* This information is necessary before prescribing antibiotics or pregnancy prophylaxis.

## Physical Examination

Document bruises, lacerations, or other visible signs of trauma. The examiner should check for classic "submissive injuries" like a black eye, fractured jaw, or abdominal bruising or tenderness from a fist. Preprinted diagrams aid in accurate representation of injuries. A pelvic examination should be performed, taking note of any vaginal discharge or genital lacerations or abrasions. The toluidine blue test is a simple procedure to detect small vulvar lacerations. Toluidine blue is a nuclear stain not taken up by normal vulvar skin. Lacerations expose the deeper dermis that contain nuclei that absorb the stain. Prior to inserting the speculum, the dye is applied to the posterior fourchette with gauze, and wiped away with lubricating jelly. A linear blue stain will highlight the vulvar lacerations. This simple procedure has doubled the reporting of genital lacerations. Most hospitals have a prepackaged rape kit with equipment and directions on sample collection. If no kit is available, smears of material from the vagina and cervix are made, labeled and air dried. A wet mount from the cervix and vagina is prepared for the examining physician to be microscopically inspected for sperm. This should be documented on the emergency chart. A plastic-tip catheter on a syringe is filled with 5 to 10 mL of sterile saline, injected into the vaginal canal, and aspirated. This is labeled "vaginal aspirate" and tested for acid phosphatase. A culture for gonorrhea and chlamydia may be obtained, but many physicians prefer to treat patients prophylactically and consider cultures irrelevant. A Wood's lamp will cause semen to fluoresce. When indicated by a history of extravaginal ejaculation, a cotton-tipped applicator moistened with saline is used to retrieve semen. If indicated by history, premoistened rectal or buccal swabs for sperm may be collected. If sodomy is involved, a routine rectal examination is performed with attention to perianal fissures or lacerations. If blood is present, anoscopy or sigmoidoscopy should be done to detect any internal injuries. Any film or photographs taken as well as all specimens collected should be labeled with the patient's name and the date and given to the police.

## The Male Rape Examination

History-taking is similar to that in the female rape examination. The physical examination must be tailored to the particulars of the assault. For example, because the anus is penetrated and the victim is lying prone in the majority of cases, one should search for abrasions on the thorax or abdomen. The male victim may be subdued by blows to the jaw, face, or abdomen. Male children are often less apt to be harmed because fear and intimidation by adult authority may compel them to be passive.

Swabs should be taken of buccal and gingival areas even if the patient has brushed, rinsed, or eaten. Gonorrhea and chlamydia cultures of the pharynx can be taken. Inspect the anus externally for signs of trauma such as abrasions, lacerations, or fissures. Injuries are the result of friction or disproportion between the diameter of the anus and erect penis. If no injuries are seen, either the anus was not penetrated or the victim may be homosexual. Other signs of chronic sodomy include decreased sphincter tone, hemorrhoids, and chronic fissures. Rectal swabs should be taken and slides made, labeled, and air dried.

If there is evidence of bleeding, the source should be located and documented. Then 10 mL of sterile saline is injected into the rectum, allowed to equilibrate for a few minutes, and aspirated. The fluid is then examined for sperm. The acid phosphatase determination has little value in sodomy.

## DIAGNOSIS

Rape is not a medical diagnosis but rather a legal determination. The definition of rape is based on legal not medical facts and contains three elements: (1) any degree of carnal knowledge; (2) nonconsent—unless the victim is a minor, intoxicated, or mentally incompetent; and (3) compulsion or fear of great harm.

## FORENSIC LABORATORY EVALUATION

### Sperm Survivability

Historically, the courts and the legal profession have placed a high significance on sperm detection as confirmatory evidence of rape. It is well documented how elusive sperm detection during a rape examination may be. The presence of sperm or seminal constituents in the vagina is evidence of recent sexual intercourse. The detection of sperm depends on several factors, including time lapse between the rape and the physical examination, whether the assailant is azoospermic, whether the patient douched prior to examination, and whether the assailant ejaculated. The recovery rate of sperm has been variably reported in the literature to span from 20 to 75 percent depending on the method used to detect sperm.

Because of the difficulties in sperm detection, several researchers attempted to determine, in controlled settings, how long sperm persisted in the vagina and cervix. In one study 15 volunteer couples were enlisted to investigate the rate of decay of sperm and acid phosphatase after a single act of intercourse (Fig. 251-1). Only 50 percent of the women had motile sperm after 3 h, and their presence in the vagina decreased rapidly thereafter. Nonmotile sperm were present in all subjects for up to 18 h, and at 72 h 50 percent had persistent sperm. The level of acid phosphatase enzyme decreased more rapidly than sperm after intercourse. Fifty percent of the subjects had significant levels after 9 h, but by 36 h there were no positive findings. The investigators also found no correlation between sperm and acid phosphatase decay, which implies that seminal fluid

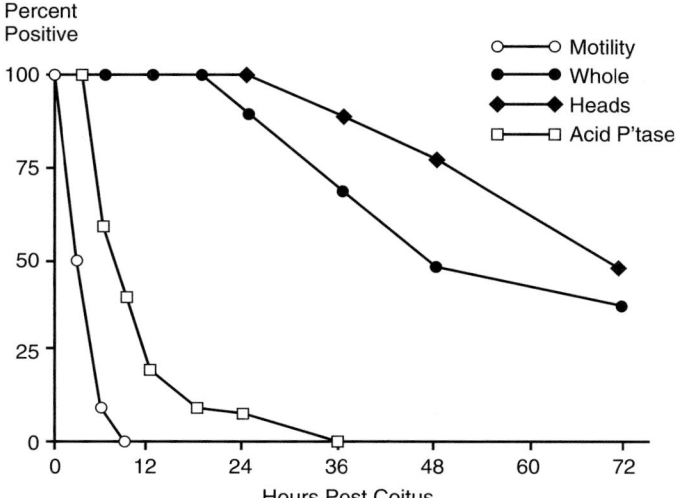

**Fig. 251-1.** Survival of motile and nonmotile sperm and acid phosphatase in the vagina. (From Soules MR, Pollard AA. The forensic laboratory evaluation of evidence in alleged rape. *Am J Obstet Gynecol* 130:143, 1978. Used with permission.)

with a high sperm count may not necessarily indicate a high acid phosphatase level.

There is general agreement in the literature that 2 to 3 h is the average time for loss of sperm motility in 50 percent of controls. Most rape examinations do not take place within this time frame. The normal range of decay for sperm in the cervix or vagina varies widely from study to study, from 14 h to 19 days. This discrepancy may be explained by the methods of specimen collection ranging from Pap smears of the cervix to wet mounts of the vaginal fluid, as well as the criteria used for reporting the presence of sperm. There is very little published information on sperm persistence in the anus or rectum. In one study, sperm were observed to be present up to 24 h after intercourse; however, it was rare to find tails on sperm from rectal swabs, especially after 6 h.

## Acid Phosphatase

Acid phosphatase detection in vaginal washings is helpful in cases of azoospermic ejaculations. Acid phosphatase is derived from cytoplasmic (erythrocytes, leukocytes, thrombocytes) or tissue (bone, kidney, placenta, liver) sources. Various chemical means are used to differentiate the source of acid phosphatase. Seminal acid phosphatase originates from the prostate gland. The endometrium is believed to be the source of vaginal acid phosphatase. A qualitative distinction between seminal and vaginal acid phosphatase cannot be made because they are identical biochemically and immunologically. The only reliable distinction may be made quantitatively based on the high levels of acid phosphatase in seminal fluid. The time period for detection of this enzyme is variably reported in the literature as 2 to 9 h after intercourse. By 12 to 15 h after intercourse, 50 percent of the swabs are negative (below the threshold to distinguish between seminal or vaginal origin). The acid phosphatase determination is most helpful when no sperm are found and acid phosphatase levels are markedly elevated, consistent with the presence of semen.

## Genetic Typing

Genetic typing helps to narrow the field of suspects but cannot specify an individual. Forensic analysis of evidence must determine genetic markers for the victim, the evidence, and the possible assailants. The three genetic markers present in semen, blood, and vaginal fluid used to establish a genetic profile are the ABO blood group antigen, peptidase A, and phosphoglucomutase.

Eighty to 85 percent of the population are secretors. They secrete ABO antigens into other body fluids. Secretor status is determined by testing for ABO blood type and then testing saliva for the presence of the ABO antigen.

Peptidase A and phosphoglucomutase are present in semen regardless of secretor status. Peptidase A variants are only common in blacks. Typing is only done when the assailant may have been black. Activity rapidly decreases after intercourse and is rarely detected after 3 h. Phosphoglucomutase has three phenotypes. When the ABO blood groups are subdivided into phosphoglucomutase phenotypes, there are 12 possible combinations. This extension of the ABO blood grouping provides genetic typing and assailant differentiation 90 percent of the time. Postcoital phosphoglucomutase activity rapidly declines and is rarely detected beyond 6 h.

## TREATMENT

Treatment of the rape victim includes management of lacerations and other physical injuries according to the standards of care. Tetanus prophylaxis should be given when indicated, lacerations sutured, and fractures casted. A pregnancy test should be obtained in postmenarcheal women and should be documented as negative before providing postcoital contraception. Many authors recommend drawing a baseline VDRL test. At the discretion of the physician, a drug screen or alcohol level may be indicated.

## Pregnancy Prophylaxis

When treating postmenarcheal female rape victims, the physician must consider whether pregnancy prophylaxis is indicated. One must first consider the risk of pregnancy after an isolated sexual encounter. Several studies have found the risk after a single act of intercourse to be rare. In a prospective study of 4000 rapes in Minnesota, no pregnancies were found. In another prospective study of 117 rapes, no pregnancies were detected and 100 of these victims received no pregnancy prophylaxis.

Despite the very low probability of pregnancy, women rape victims should be offered informed choice of pregnancy prophylaxis. Women who are not using any form of contraception at the time of assault and are midcycle in the menses (days 10 to 16) are at greatest risk of pregnancy. Prophylaxis must be initiated within 72 h of the sexual assault to be effective in preventing pregnancy.

Diethylstilbestrol (DES) has lost favor for pregnancy prophylaxis because of the risk of carcinogenesis. Currently accepted therapy is the birth control pill, Ovral (norgestrel + ethinyl estradiol), 2 tablets orally initially and 2 tablets 12 h later. This regimen replaces the older 5-day DES regimen, which had more side effects and lower compliance.

## Sexually Transmitted Disease Prophylaxis

Most of the literature demonstrates poor compliance with follow-up in sexual assault victims. Therefore, prophylaxis for sexually transmitted diseases should be given according to guidelines of the Centers for Disease Control and Prevention (CDC) to all sexual assault victims, irrespective of their age. Table 251-1 presents the current CDC guidelines for antibiotic choice and age-related doses. A negative pregnancy test should be documented on the chart prior to administering antibiotics; a positive pregnancy test will alter the choice of antibiotic. For patients who are vaccinated to hepatitis B, HBIG should be administered and vaccination recommended. For those who have been vaccinated, a booster and HBIG should be given if titers are inadequate. See Chapter 86 for further discussion.

**Table 251-1.** Guidelines for STD Treatment

*Gonococcal infections*
A single dose of:
  Ceftriaxone 125 mg IM
    **or**
  Cefixime 400 mg PO
    **or**
  Ciprofloxacin 500 mg PO
    **or**
  Ofloxacin 400 mg PO
Children weighing < 45 kg (100 lb)
  Ceftriaxone 125 mg IM
    **or**
  Amoxicillin 50 mg/kg (accompanied by probenecid 25 mg/kg PO)
    **or**
    Spectinomycin 40 mg IM once

*Chlamydial infections*
  Azithromycin 1 g PO once
    **or**
  Doxycycline 100 mg PO b.i.d. for 7 d
    **or**
  Ofloxacin 300 mg PO b.i.d. for 7 d
    **or**
  Erythromycin base 500 mg PO q.i.d. for 7 d
    **or**
  Erythromycin ethylsuccinate 800 mg PO q.i.d. for 7 d
Children > 8 years old:
  Doxycycline 100 mg PO b.i.d. for 7 d
Children < 8 years old:
  Erythromycin 40 mg/kg/d PO (in three divided doses) for 7 d

*Source: Morbidity and Mortality Weekly Report,* vol. 42. Sept. 24, 1993.

## Counseling and Testing for Human Immunodeficiency Virus (HIV)

The risk of contracting HIV from a single sexual encounter is unknown but believed to be rare. The literature suggests prophylaxis of high-risk encounters including repetitive exposures (such as children in incestuous relationships), multiple assailants, or if the assailant is high risk for HIV. Victims should be informed of the risks, counseled about HIV testing and prophylaxis, and provided with information to make a decision. The patient should understand HIV testing is needed every 3 months for a minimum of 6 months. If the patient is undecided about HIV testing, serum can be frozen and stored for future use. HIV prophylaxis is a controversial topic. There are two methods of prophylaxis: AZT and topical agents. Neither method has been shown to prevent HIV transmission postexposure. Given the potential toxicity of AZT, few advocate its use unless the HIV status of the assailant is known. Topical agents include a 1:10 vinegar solution douche and nonoxynol 9. There is no proven efficacy of a postexposure vinegar douche preventing HIV transmission and the vinegar may destroy evidence.

Nonoxynol 9 has proven in vitro anti-HIV activity and does not alter evidence for semen analysis. Nonoxynol 9 in concentrations of .05% or greater is antivirucidal in vitro, but it has not been adequately evaluated in vivo. Spermicides are formulated with nonoxynol in concentrations from 2% to 8%, but no studies have evaluated the in vivo efficacy or anti-HIV inhibitory concentrations attained by these preparations. Nonoxynol 9 found in contraceptive sponges has been associated with an increased incidence of genital ulcerations and seroconversion to HIV. Before advocating the use of topical agents for the prevention of HIV transmission, further testing is needed.

## ADMISSION INDICATIONS

The indication for admission is predicated on the nature of injuries sustained from the attack. Only 1 to 2 percent of victims sustain severe enough injuries to require hospitalization. The majority of injuries can be handled with outpatient follow-up.

## FOLLOW-UP CARE

Ideally, counseling for sexual assault victims should be available 24 h a day in the emergency department. Often the rape counselor will precede the physician in assessing the victim, preparing her for the examination, and providing moral support. If this is not available, the physician should provide information on local mental health or rape counseling centers where patients may seek further help.

The physician should provide for follow-up medical care to ensure that injuries have healed properly. A follow-up appointment with a gynecologist in 7 to 14 days is necessary to ensure efficacious pregnancy prophylaxis and STD treatment. For male rape victims a follow-up appointment with a urologist would be appropriate. Young children should be referred to a pediatrician for evaluation. Should the patient require HIV counseling or testing, referral to an outpatient clinic or local mental health counseling center would be sufficient.

## BIBLIOGRAPHY

Braen GR, Martin CA. Rape and the rape trauma syndrome. *South Med J* 78:1230, 1985.

Cook DL, Wiist LJ, Kraft SL. Pregnancy prophylaxis: parenteral postcoital estrogen. *Obstet Gynecol* 67:331, 1986.

Dunn SF, Gilchrist VJ: Sexual assault. *Prim Care* 20: 359, 1993.

Foster I, Bartlett JG. Anti-HIV substances for rape victims. *JAMA* 261:3407, 1989. Letter.

Goldenring JM. Estrogen treatment for victims of rape. *N Engl J Med* 312:989, 1985. Letter.

Jenny C, Hooton TM, Bowers A. Sexually transmitted diseases in victims of rape. *N Engl J Med* 322:713, 1990.

Lauber AA, Souma ML. Use of toluidine blue for documentation of traumatic intercourse. *Obstet Gynecol* 60:644, 1982.

McCauley J, Guzinski G, Welch R. Toluidine blue for documentation of traumatic intercourse. *Am J Emerg Med* 5:105, 1987.

Murphy S, Kitchen V, Harris JRW. Rape and subsequent seroconversion to HIV. *Br Med J* 299:718, 1989.

Schiff AF. Examination and treatment of the male rape victim. *S Med J* 73:1498, 1980.

Sensabaugh GF, Baskinski J, Blake ET. The laboratory's role in investigation of rape. *Diagnostic Med* March: 46–53, 1985.

Silverman EM, Silverman AG. Persistence of spermatozoa in the lower genital tracts of women. *JAMA* 240:1875, 1978.

Soules MR, Pollard AA. The forensic evaluation of evidence in alleged rape. *Am J Obstet Gynecol* 130:142, 1978.

STD Update '93: STDs in the '90s. ARHP *Clinical Proceedings*, May, 1994.

Tintinalli J, Hoelzer M. Clinical findings and legal resolutions in sexual assault. *Ann Emerg Med* 14:447, 1985.

# 252
# DOMESTIC VIOLENCE

## Patricia R. Salber
## Ellen Taliaferro

Wife-beating has been described for many centuries. In early Roman times women were considered to be the property of men. Indeed, the word family is derived from the Latin *familia,* which signified the totality of slaves belonging to an individual. The slave-owner had absolute power of life and death over the human beings, including his wife, who belonged to him.

Early English common law allowed a husband to beat his wife into submission. It was later modified to the "rule of thumb," which restricted him to use a stick no bigger than the width of his thumb. In this country, married women did not begin to achieve the same protection under the law as other American citizens until 1895, when the Married Women's Property Act made assault sufficient grounds for divorce. However, the first battered women's shelter was not opened in the United States until 1975.

It has only been in the last 15 to 20 years that domestic violence has been acknowledged as a social problem with disastrous health consequences. In 1985 at a workshop, the Surgeon General of the United States identified domestic violence as the nation's most important health problem. In January 1992, the Joint Commission on the Accreditation of Healthcare Organizations (JCAHO) mandated that all emergency departments and ambulatory care facilities establish written guidelines for the identification, evaluation, management, and referral of adult victims of domestic violence. In June 1992, the American Medical Association (AMA) published guidelines for identification and intervention of domestic violence victims.

## DEFINITIONS

The term domestic violence is sometimes used interchangeably with the terms adult intimate abuse, partner abuse, spousal abuse, and wife-beating. It is recognized that the latter terms are restrictive and appear to exclude consideration of same sex battering, battering of ex-spouses or nonmarried individuals, dating or adolescent battering, and battering of men by women. Domestic violence may also be used as a synonym for the term family violence, a broader category of violence between intimates, which includes child abuse, sibling abuse, and elder abuse, as well as partner abuse.

The domestic violence literature sometimes refers to victims of domestic violence as survivors. The terms batterer and perpetrator are often used interchangeably. It is also traditional in the domestic violence literature to refer to the perpetrator as he and the victim/survivor as she because that reflects the reported incidence and prevalence of domestic violence.

*Domestic violence* is defined as the use by one partner or intimate of a pattern of coercive behaviors to control the actions of the other partner. The behaviors used include emotional abuse, psychological abuse, intimidation, deprivation, isolation, economic abuse, and physical and sexual assault. There are multiple, sometimes daily events. Some are criminal acts and some are not, some are physically injurious and some are not. But all are psychologically and emotionally damaging. Domestic violence, then, is about the use of power and control by one partner over the other.

## INCIDENCE AND PREVALENCE

It is estimated that between 2 and 4 million women are battered each year in the United States. One national survey found that 28 percent of American families are affected by domestic violence. It is commonly stated that figures are probably much higher because of underreporting.

Approximately 5000 battered women die as a result of partner abuse (homicide and suicide) each year. More than half of women murdered in the United States are killed by current or former husbands. Male partners are also at risk of being murdered by female partners although research shows that most of cases are due to self-protection or retribution.

Statistics from the Federal Bureau of Investigation show that only about 5 percent of reported domestic assaults are due to women beating their male partners. Although some studies show that female to male aggression and male to female aggression occurs at close to equal rates, the chances of the aggression ending in serious injury is much higher for female victims. Indeed, many workers in the field of domestic violence report that 95 percent of all cases of domestic violence consist of male on female battering. It is this oft-repeated statistic that is used to justify referring to the victim/survivor as she and the perpetrator as he.

Twenty to 30 percent of university women report date violence; the incidence of adolescent date battering is unknown as is the incidence of same sex battering.

Age extremes are not spared the effect of domestic violence. Children, the "silent victims" of domestic violence, frequently witness the battering. Additionally, it is important to remember that in about 50 percent of domestic violence relationships, the children are also being beaten. Approximately one third to one half of elder abuse cases are, in fact, cases of women over 65 who are being beaten by their domestic partners.

## IMPACT OF DOMESTIC VIOLENCE ON THE EMERGENCY DEPARTMENT

More than one million American women seek medical care for abuse-related injuries each year. Between 16 and 20 percent of injured women, excluding motor vehicle crash victims, who present to emergency departments are victims of domestic violence. If battered women who present with nontrauma complaints, such as anxiety, hyperventilation, complications of pregnancy, headaches, and other chronic pain syndromes are also included, the impact on the emergency department is much greater. The annual medical costs of treating injured victims of domestic violence is thought to be $44 million. If nontraumatic medical visits are included, this figure will be much higher.

## BARRIERS TO DIAGNOSIS

Despite the fact that emergency physicians are seeing large numbers of battered women, until recently the diagnosis was largely ignored. One report estimated that only about 1 in 25 battered women seen in an emergency department was correctly identified as having been battered.

Physicians fail to make the diagnosis for many reasons. Until recently it was distinctly unusual for medical students or residents to receive training about domestic violence. Physicians aware of domestic violence often have misconceptions that contribute to underdiagnosis. Some of these misconceptions are listed in Table 252-1.

Another barriers to diagnosing domestic violence were revealed in a 1993 survey of California emergency department physician directors and nurse managers. Respondents were asked to rank a list of possible obstacles to the identification of adult patients who had been abused as a "major problem," a "minor problem," or "not a problem." Almost half the respondents listed patient factors such as fear of repercussion, denial, and failure to mention battering as the most significant obstacles to diagnosis. Conversely, staff factors, such as lack of training or awareness or staff busyness, were most frequently listed as "not a problem."

Another important reason for failure to diagnose is the failure to consider domestic violence in cases with nontrauma chief complaints. Battered women seek care in emergency departments for a wide variety of medical complaints including anxiety, hyperventilation, depression, drug and alcohol intoxication, chronic pain syndromes, and symptoms suggestive of posttraumatic stress disorder.

Perhaps the most significant reason for missing the diagnosis of domestic violence is the failure to simply ask. Asking patients directly whether domestic violence is affecting their lives has the potential of overcoming many of these barriers to diagnosis as well as establishing the expectation that the physician believes that domestic violence is simply not acceptable. Research shows that patients will respond to direct questioning. It has been reported that approximately one-third of battered women will speak to a physician or nurse about the violence in their lives if direct inquiry is made.

### Consequences of Failure to Diagnose Domestic Violence

Consequences of failure to diagnose may result in multiple visits to the emergency department or other provider settings. One study documented that 23 percent of battered women presented to clinicians between 6 and 10 times, and another 20 percent at least 11 times before the abuse was diagnosed. In addition, misdiagnosis of battering-related symptoms as mental illness can lead to mislabeling at best and inappropriate use of psychoactive medications or psychiatric hospitalization at worst. It has been estimated that many women hospitalized in psychiatric institutions are, in fact, battered women.

Other consequences of failure to diagnosis include an increase in the patient's feelings of hopelessness, despair, isolation, and entrapment. Battered women may resort to substance abuse or develop depression with and without suicide attempts. Continuing or escalating domestic violence can lead to permanent disability or death. Failure to interrupt the cycle of violence can lead to repetition of violence in the next generation.

### THE BATTERED WOMAN

**Who is she?** Any woman can become a victim of domestic violence. Although it is more commonly reported by women of color

**Table 252-1.** Common Reasons Why Physicians May Not Diagnose Domestic Violence In The Emergency Department

Patient withholds information
Fear of opening "Pandora's box"
Lack of physician training
Fear of offending patient
Time constraints
Does not know what to do about it
Believe intervention will not work

and poor women, domestic violence occurs in all socioeconomic classes, races, and cultural groups. It can occur regardless of age, educational background, or profession.

**Why does she stay?** Many women stay in violent relationships because of the very real fear of escalating violence. The highest number of fatalities from domestic violence occur when the woman leaves or tries to leave the relationship. In addition to fearing for their own lives, battered women may fear for the safety of their children, pets, or others who the batterer has threatened to harm if she leaves.

Some women stay because they have been systematically cut off from family and friends; they believe they have no where else to go. The batterer's control of information and giving of "dis-information" may make them think that no one will believe their story. They may also stay because of cultural or religious beliefs about the sanctity of the family.

For many battered women, especially women with small children, the lack of money or skills to obtain gainful employment can be a serious impediment to leaving the relationship. Their concern for their children's well-being may hold them in the relationship.

Finally, battered women may stay because they still love their partner; they don't want to end the relationship, they just want the violence to stop.

**Why doesn't she tell?** As discussed above, a significant obstacle to identification is the battered woman's reluctance to talk about or outright denial of battering. Many women do not tell physicians about the violence because they fear the information may not be confidential. They fear retribution if the batterer learns of her "betrayal." Some women do not tell because they are embarrassed or ashamed; they believe that their situation is unique and somehow related to their own failures in the relationship. Finally, they may not talk about it because they believe the physician does not care, cannot or will not help, or is too busy for this type of problem.

## MEN WHO BATTER

Men who batter are of all ages and come from all socioeconomic, educational, racial, cultural, and religious backgrounds. The one thing they have in common is the use of power to control the behavior of their partners and their children. Other common themes are the use of denial and minimalization as well as blaming others as justifications for their actions.

About 60 percent of men who batter grew up in violent homes where they either witnessed the battering of their mothers or they themselves were battered. It is important to recognize, however, that 40 percent of men who grow up in similarly violent homes do not go on to batter and not all men who do batter experienced violence while growing up.

## THE EFFECT OF DOMESTIC VIOLENCE ON CHILDREN

As many as 70 percent of children from violent homes are witness to their fathers beating their mothers. In addition, about 30 to 54 percent of reported cases of spousal abuse also report child abuse. Several studies have documented that children exposed to violence in their homes have significant behavioral difficulties during childhood and later life. At least one investigator has documented a link between growing up in a violent home, especially for boys, and later aggressive criminal behaviors.

## SUBSTANCE ABUSE AND BATTERING

Both batterers and victims of battering may abuse alcohol and other drugs. There is no established link, however, between the use of these substances and the cause of violence.

## MAKING THE DIAGNOSIS OF DOMESTIC VIOLENCE

### History and Physical Examination

The following findings are some clues to battering that can be gleaned from the clinical history and physical examination.

**Pregnancy.** Pregnant women are at high risk for battering. Forty percent of battering begins during the first pregnancy. Seventeen percent of all pregnant women have been battered; for pregnant teens the figure is 21 percent. Any evidence of injury during pregnancy should prompt direct questioning about domestic violence.

**Central pattern of injury.** Up to 50 percent of injuries to battered women are to the head and neck. Injuries to the chest, breasts and abdomen are also common.

**Injuries suggesting a defensive posture.** Forearm bruises or fractures may be sustained when the woman tries to fends off blows to the face or chest.

**Certain characteristic injuries.** Fingernail scratches, bite marks, cigarette burns, and rope burns strongly suggest domestic violence.

**The extent or type of injury is inconsistent with the patient's explanation.** Multiple abrasions and contusions to different anatomic sites, which are inconsistent with the history, should raise the possibility of abuse. An example of such an inconsistency would be a woman with a blow-out fracture who says she injured herself falling off a bar stool.

**Multiple injuries in various stages of healing.** Just as x-rays that reveal old fractures help a diagnosis of child abuse, evidence of new and old injuries helps diagnose partner abuse.

**Substantial delay between the time of injury and the presentation for treatment.** Battered women may wait several days before seeking medical care. They may see their physician at inappropriate times for seemingly minor or resolving injuries. This may occur because they were prevented from leaving the house, or it might reflect their ambivalence about revealing the nature of their home life.

**Frequent visits for vague complaints without evidence of physiologic abnormality.** A woman who presents frequently with a variety of psychosomatic complaints previously ascribed to depression might actually be a victim of domestic violence.

**Suicide attempts.** Up to 25 percent of suicide attempts in women may be related to spousal abuse. Twenty percent of pregnant battered women will attempt suicide. When asked what precipitated a suicide attempt, a battered woman may respond "I had a fight with my husband." The emergency physician can make the diagnosis by asking specifically if the fight was a physical fight.

**Rape.** Thirty-three to 46 percent of women who are physically battered also report marital rape.

### Asking Direct Questions

Although there are certain clues to abuse, the presentations of battered women in the emergency department are so varied that the diagnosis may be missed if the physician fails to ask directly about the presence of violence in the patient's life. As discussed earlier, many battered women will respond truthfully if questioned directly in a sensitive, nonjudgmental way. The AMA suggests asking the following questions:

- Are you in a relationship in which you have been physically hurt or threatened by your partner? Have you ever been in such a relationship?
- Are you (have you ever been) in a relationship in which you felt you were treated badly? In what ways?
- Has your partner ever destroyed things that you cared about?
- Has your partner ever threatened or abused your children?
- Has your partner ever forced you to have sex when you did not want to? Does he ever force you to engage in sex that makes you feel uncomfortable?

• We all fight at home. What happens when you and your partner fight or disagree?

## TREATMENT GOALS

When physicians have "getting her to a shelter" or "having him arrested" the goal of the patient encounter, they are bound to become frustrated when dealing with cases of domestic violence. Leaving the relationship may not be the immediate goal of the patient, and she may be loathe to have her husband and the father of her children arrested.

**Safety.** The safety of the woman and her children should be the first and foremost goal of every patient encounter. It is the woman, however, who must make the ultimate determination of whether it is safe to return home. By providing women with information about battering, risks, and options, the physician will help the woman to decide what is best for her and her family.

**Assess potential for suicide or homicide.** The patient should be asked if she is contemplating suicide. Does she have a plan? Does she have a weapon or has she stockpiled medications in anticipation of a suicide attempt? Is she considering homicide as a means to ensure the safety of herself and her children? Does she have a plan or a weapon? Psychiatric consultation should be obtained if suicidal or homicidal ideation are present; hospitalization may be indicated.

**Assessing safety.** If considering discharge from the emergency department, it is imperative to assess the safety of the woman and her dependents. Ask in detail about the nature of the abuse. Is there a pattern of escalating violence? Were the police called? Was the batterer arrested? If not, does she know where he is now? Does her partner have a weapon, especially firearms, which can easily turn an abuse situation into a lethal situation?

Ask the woman if she is afraid to go home? If so, does she have somewhere safe to go? Can she stay with friends or relatives? Is she afraid that he would find her if she went to the home of someone he knows? Would she feel safer in a battered women's shelter—emphasize that the location of these shelters is kept secret; he would not be able to find her in a shelter. If she feels it is safe and she wants to go home, this choice should be respected. It is appropriate, however, to discuss with her the need to have a safety plan in case violence erupts again.

## ESSENTIAL INFORMATION FOR THE BATTERED WOMAN

Although the battered woman may choose to return to the battering relationship at the end of the physician-patient encounter, important therapeutic interventions can help her begin the process extricating herself from the violence.

She needs to know that she is not alone. She needs to know that there is help available for her and that she does not deserve to beaten.

**Referrals.** Every emergency department should maintain current lists of resources available in the community to assist battered women. Battered women's shelters, legal aid and other legal assistance, and appropriate social service agencies should be included on the list.

## PREPARING THE EMERGENCY DEPARTMENT FOR OPTIMAL RESPONSE

In January 1992, the JCAHO required that all emergency departments have written policies and procedures to guide the care of victims of domestic violence. Ongoing educational programs should be planned to ensure that all emergency department staff acquire and maintain the skills needed to appropriately diagnose, treat, and refer victims. Referral lists should be reviewed and updated annually. A battered woman should *never* be given a referral to a shelter that no longer exists.

**Protocols.** The Family Violence Prevention Fund has analyzed protocols from emergency departments across the country. Sample protocols that can be used to help guide development of an institution's protocol can be obtained by calling the fund's special interest resource center.

**Institutional response.** Because optimal care of the battered woman requires the services of other professionals, it is recommended that hospitals develop interdepartmental domestic violence committees that would include, at a minimum, representatives from the emergency department, social services, psychiatry, pediatrics, internal medicine, and obstetrics. Institutional protocols should be designed so that there is no confusion over how to proceed when battered women seek help in the hospital setting.

**Community response.** The optimal response to battered women will require services beyond the confines of the emergency department or hospital. Battered women's shelters, police, and the legal community all provide necessary services. To be optimally effective, there must be coordination between the medical and legal communities. At a minimum, representatives from these agencies should be invited to participate in the hospital's domestic violence committee activities. Optimally, community coordinating councils on family violence should be established in each community.

## MEDICOLEGAL CONSIDERATIONS

**Documentation.** Careful documentation in the medical record is crucial in domestic violence cases. Such documentation can assist the victim who seeks legal remedies such as temporary or permanent restraining orders, child custody, separation, or divorce. It is recommended that photographs of visible injuries be included. Be sure to obtain consent and to document the date and time of the photographs. A hand-drawn body map detailing areas of tenderness or hematomas should be included to document nonvisible injuries.

Legibility and clarity of the medical record cannot be overstressed. Dictate, type, or write legibly. District attorneys frequently state the reason for subpoenaing the treating physician is to read and interpret the medical record.

**Reporting requirements.** Emergency physicians must be aware of their state's reporting requirements. Some states have mandatory reporting of known or suspected domestic violence; others have mandatory arrest, in addition to mandatory reporting. If the police are called, either at the woman's request or because of a reporting requirement, it is important to discuss a safety plan with the woman; violence may escalate when the batterer discovers he has been reported, especially if he is not arrested or if he is arrested, but held for only a short period of time.

**Duty to warn.** Physicians must warn potential victims if serious homicidal intent is expressed.

**Liability issues.** Failure to report domestic violence and reporting suspected domestic violence that is not substantiated are both potential sources of physician liability. States in which mandatory reporting exist should have liability protections similar to those for reporting suspected child abuse.

## CONCLUSION

Emergency physicians can play a critical and important role in breaking the cycle of domestic violence. Heightened awareness of the problem, the incorporation of direct questioning, and an understanding of the goals of successful intervention are the major ingredients of success.

# 253
# ABUSE IN THE ELDERLY AND IMPAIRED

Ellen Taliaferro
Patricia R. Salber

Although not a new problem, elder abuse continues to be an underrecognized and underreported cause of morbidity and mortality in the elderly for many reasons. Historical information often remains undetected during the medical evaluation process. Social stigmata surround the problem and, like all forms of domestic violence, "it is the disease that is lied about." Lastly, detection of elder abuse and neglect is contingent upon physicians' awareness of the problem as well as their ability to recognize and understand the risk factors that often appear before a crisis occurs.

## INCIDENCE AND PREVALENCE

In 1990, Delunas reported that as many as 2.5 million elderly persons in the United States every year are victims of abuse—neglected, battered, or otherwise deprived of their rights, usually by those on whom they are most dependent for care. Current estimates of elder abuse in the United States indicate that it affects nearly 10 percent of the elderly population.

## DEFINITIONS

Simply defined, violence is any harm resulting from intentional action by self or others. A very narrow and concise definition of family violence was included in the Family Violence Prevention and Services Act of 1984 of the U.S. Congress: "The term 'family violence' means any act or threatened act of violence, including any forceful detention of an individual, which (A) results or threatens to result in physical injury; and (B) is committed by a person against another individual (including an elderly person) to whom such person is or was related by blood or marriage, or otherwise legally related, or with whom such person is or was lawfully residing." Included in the broadest sense of this definition is psychological battery (e.g., humiliating, rejecting, corrupting acts and psychosocial injury).

Practical working definitions that permit measurement of elder abuse employ three forms of maltreatment: physical abuse, neglect, and chronic verbal aggression. These definitions do not include material abuse (theft or misuse of an elder's money or other assets) or self-inflicted abuse or neglect (which is sometimes included in definitions of elder maltreatment).

## SOCIAL AND ENVIRONMENTAL ETIOLOGIC FACTORS

Most elderly victims of abuse live with the perpetrator. When abuse occurs, it has been found that the abuser is often dependent upon the victim for housing, and financial and emotional support. Caretakers usually attempt to provide acceptable and appropriate care. However, when the caregiver is overwhelmed, frustrated, or resentful of the responsibilities involved in the task of caring for the elderly, then abuse and/or neglect may occur.

Certain conditions tend to set the stage for abuse and/or neglect. For instance, Alzheimer disease and other dementias have been demonstrated to be associated with greater risk for physical abuse than other illnesses of the elderly. This reflects the fact that high psychological and physical demands are placed on family members who care for relatives with dementia.

Overall, a review of the literature indicates little consensus as to who among the elderly is most likely to be a victim. In one study, elderly abuse victims and a nonabused control group were compared to explore the issue of caretaker stress versus caregiver psychopathology. The study found substantially more support for the idea that abuse is associated with personality problems of the caregiver. Earlier studies substantiated financial dependency of the caretaker as a major risk factor. Pillemar and Finkelhor found that, in general, abusers are heavily dependent individuals. They included family caretakers who were disabled, cognitively impaired, or mentally ill. Other studies have uncovered substantial psychological impairment on the part of the abusers, as well as higher rates of alcoholism, arrest, and other deviant behavior. These deviant characteristics and behaviors appear to be related to the abusers' dependence on elderly relatives for financial assistance, housing, social support, and other help.

## CLINICAL FEATURES

Mistreatment and/or neglect of elderly patients may be difficult to recognize. The problem is complicated by the fact that when abuse is suspected, it may be difficult to secure confirmation from the patient. The patient may welcome and be relieved by physician concern and identification. However, embarrassment, fear of abandonment, and terror stemming from fear of retaliation can prompt the patient to deny the physician's concerns.

Historical information should focus on the following: (1) detecting the presence of caretaker mental illness, mental retardation, dementia, or drug or alcohol abuse; (2) family history of violence; (3) caretaker dependence on the elder patient for housing, finances, emotional support, or caregiving; (4) patient isolation as reflected by the fact that the patient does not have the opportunity to relate with people or to pursue activities and interests in a manner that the patient chooses; (5) patient and suspected abuser living together; and (6) recent occurrence of stressful life events, such as loss of job, moving, or death of a loved one for the caretaker.

Important historical information concerning the patient should include dependency needs. Problems such as mental confusion, immobility, and need for assistance with hygiene are most often associated with neglect, a common form of maltreatment of the elderly. Eliciting a history of cognitive impairment is essential, as abused victims have been found to have significantly greater cognitive impairment than nonabused elderly patients. Abused patients also have a higher history of problematic behavior such as incontinence, nocturnal shouting, wandering, or paranoia.

An important direct question to put to the patient is: "Are you happy at home or have you experienced any recent changes in mood, sleeping, or eating patterns?" Look also for the sudden onset of behavioral signs and symptoms that suggest victimization: depression, fear, withdrawal, confusion, anxiety, low self-esteem, or helplessness.

Other historical indicators of abuse or neglect include:

Pattern of "physician hopping"
Unexplained delay in seeking treatment
Lack of medical care
Series of missed medical appointments
Previous unexplained injuries
Explanation of past injuries inconsistent with medical findings
Previous reports of similar injuries

The physical examination begins with an observation of the interaction between the patient and accompanying caretakers. The following are findings suggestive of abuse:

The patient appears fearful of his or her companion.
There are conflicting accounts of the injury or illness between the patient and caretaker.
There is an absence of assistance from the caretaker.

The caretaker displays an attitude of indifference or anger toward the patient.

The caretaker is overly concerned with the costs of treatment needed by the patient.

The caretaker denies the patient the chance to interact privately with the physician.

The mental status examination should try to elicit signs and symptoms of confusion or disorientation. These signs and symptoms are risk factors for elder abuse and/or neglect. If they are present, it is important to seek an underlying cause, especially if they are new, as they may represent underlying medical disorders or may be reflective of intentional or unintentional medication abuse or misuse resulting from abuse or neglect.

The general physical examination should focus on detecting signs and symptoms of poor personal hygiene, inappropriate or soiled clothing, dehydration, malnutrition, and worsening decubiti. Specific injuries suggestive of abuse are:

Unexplained fractures or dislocations
Unexplained lacerations or abrasions
Burns in unusual locations or of unusual shapes
Unexplained injuries to the head or face
The presence of sexually transmitted diseases
Unexplained bruises

Unexplained bruises may well tell their own story. For instance, bilateral bruises on the upper arms may indicate holding or shaking. Bruises may be similar to the shape of an object or be clustered on the trunk, indicating striking injuries. The presence of bruises in different stages of healing is suggestive of repeated abuse. Bruises around the wrists or ankles may occur secondary to being tied down. Bruises on the inside part of the thighs or arms are highly suggestive of intentional injury as bruises obtained from falling are usually located on the outside surfaces of the extremities.

## DIAGNOSIS AND DIFFERENTIAL DIAGNOSIS

Detection and diagnosis of elder abuse is dependent on being open to what is reported by the patient or others; otherwise, reported abuse may be dismissed as "paranoia," "dementia," or "patient noncompliance." A high index of suspicion is necessary. When this is lacking, signs of abuse and neglect may be erroneously ascribed to "frequent falls," "accidental medications errors," "failure to thrive," or "the normal decline with aging."

There is no substitute for direct questioning when inquiring about abuse. Jones et al. reported that, upon initial presentation to the emergency department, 33 percent of abused victims stated that they were involved in an abusive relationship. Another 6 percent of abuse cases were detected by eliciting information from other informants. The remaining cases were elicited by physical examination (43 percent) or by social service evaluation during hospitalization (19 percent).

## TREATMENT AND EMERGENCY DEPARTMENT CARE

Elder abuse treatment is twofold. First, emergency department treatment of the injuries and illnesses resulting from abuse or neglect must be specific for the injuries and illnesses detected. Second, detection of elder abuse or neglect must be aimed at intervention. Therefore, all treatment, whether delivered in the emergency department or the hospital, for both victim and "carer" should be on the basis of multidisciplinary assessment and may result in admission of the elderly patient to an extended-care facility.

Intervention includes the resolution of disposition problems brought about through caregiver exhaustion, patients no longer able to care for themselves in the community, and abandonment by individuals and institutions. It requires a complex array of skills. For example, the serious problem of drug and alcohol abuse among the elderly must be recognized and addressed by emergency department staff. Physical problems often disguise the existence of a problem of substance abuse.

In cases of proven or strongly suspected elder abuse or neglect, intervention must include the involvement of adult protective services. All 50 states have passed legislation aimed to protect elderly victims of domestic abuse and neglect. The majority of states now have mandatory reporting laws, and health care providers are considered the major professional referral service.

## ADMISSION INDICATIONS

Elderly patients with problems requiring hospital admission should be admitted to the appropriate medical service, and the department of social services should be consulted for evaluation. Patients who do not medically require admission may need to be admitted for protective placement if they cannot be safely discharged to their caretakers or returned to their institutional setting.

## DISPOSITION

Safety is a key issue. Patients must not be returned to their living situations if there is any doubt about patient safety. It is important to remember that abuse and/or neglect may occur when a caregiver is overwhelmed, frustrated, or resentful of the responsibilities involved in taking care of the patient. If indicated, caregivers should be provided with intervention options such as arranging for home care, respite, or counseling or be given advice as to the appropriate care for their family member.

The serious problem of drug and alcohol abuse among the elderly must be recognized by emergency department staff and addressed through appropriate referrals. Lastly, communities with geriatric treatment centers provide a valuable resource for patients identified through emergency department visits. Identification of these centers and referral opportunities to them should be readily available to emergency department staff.

## DISCHARGE INSTRUCTIONS

When discharge is safe and appropriate, aftercare instructions should include appropriate treatment and referral for identified injuries and illness. Referrals should include specific available services such as "Meals on Wheels," home health aides, visiting nurses, transportation, emergency shelter, legal aid, and medical and mental health services.

## BIBLIOGRAPHY

Bloom JS, Ansell P, Bloom MN: Detecting elder abuse: A guide for physicians. *Geriatrics* 44(Jun): 40, 1989.

Bourland MD, Elder abuse: From definition to prevention. *Postgrad Med* 87(2):139, 1990.

Coyne AC, Reichman WE, Berbig LJ: The relationship between dementia and elder abuse. *Am J Psychiatry* 150(4):643, 1993.

Ehrlich P, Anetzberger G: Survey of state public health departments on procedures for reporting elder abuse. *Public Health Rep* 106(2):151, 1991.

Hwalek M: On the Pillemer and Finkelhor article (letter). *Gerontologist* 28(2):273, 1988.

Jones J, Dougherty J, Schelble D, et al: Emergency department protocol for the diagnosis and evaluation of geriatric abuse. *Ann Emerg Med* 17(10):1006, 1988.

Jorgensen JE: A dentist's social responsibility to diagnose elder abuse. *Spec Care Dentist* 12(3):112, 1992.

Lachs MS, & Pillemer K: Abuse and neglect of elderly persons. *N Engl J Med* 332(7):437, 1995.

McDonald AJ, Abrahams ST: Social emergencies in the elderly. *Emerg Med Clin North Am* 8(2):443, 1990.

Mowbray DA: Shedding light on elder abuse. *J Gerontol Nurs* 15(10):20, 1989.

O'Malley TA, Everitt DE, O'Malley HC, et al: Identifying and preventing family-mediated abuse and neglect of elderly persons. *Ann Intern Med* 98:998, 1983.

O'Neill D, McCormack P, Walsh JB, et al: Elder abuse. *Ir J Med Sci* 159(2):48, 1990.

Pillemer K, Finkelhor D: Causes of elder abuse: Caregiver stress versus problem relatives. *Am J Orthopsychiatry* 59(2):179, 1989.

Rounds L: Elder abuse and neglect: A relationship to health characteristics. *J Am Acad Nurse Pract* 4(2):47, 1992.

Wolf RS: Elder abuse: Ten years later. *J Am Geriatr Soc* 36(8):758, 1988.

# 254
# VIOLENCE IN THE EMERGENCY DEPARTMENT

## Marshall C. McCoy

Violence once threatened only law enforcement personnel among those dealing with the public; now it has spread into the health care arena. Violence has become a more frequent resolution to conflict and often with more devastating brutality. No other health care providers are more at risk from the threat of violence than those involved with the *first-line* care of patients. Prehospital care providers have shown an increasing fear of violent calls and admit that violent encounters contribute to high levels of burnout. Recent surveys of emergency department residents have shown that one of their primary concerns is for their safety while working in the emergency department. Although comprehensive data addressing the problem are still being collected from emergency department personnel, urban and rural hospitals are reporting a higher incidence of potential and real violent episodes in their emergency departments.

By its very nature, the emergency department has an atmosphere of controlled chaos. With more people using emergency departments for their primary health care, the number of visits has continued to rise, to a staggering 90 million in 1993. Emergency departments are open 24 h a day, provide generally unlimited and unrestricted access, and have readily available drugs. They are frequented by those who are fatigued or hungry and they accommodate family and friends of critically ill patients and those for whom daily life stresses have heightened frustration and anxiety. Furthermore, emergency departments are frequented by substance abusers who are often violent. Other factors that may predispose the emergency department to violence are increasing waiting times, staff shortages, overcrowding, patient financial problems, and the high expectations of the patients. These are just some of the predisposing factors that have escalated violent events in the emergency department.

It has been estimated that 50 percent of all health services providers will be involved in a violent episode in their career. In a survey of 127 teaching hospitals, 32 percent of the respondents had at least one verbal threat daily, 25 percent reported using restraints at least once daily, and 18 percent had at least one threat from a weapon monthly. Unfortunately, 7 percent reported a death related to emergency department violence in the past 5 years. Of the institutions responding, 35 percent lacked 24-h emergency department security, and of the nine respondents who reported a death, 55 percent lacked 24-h security.

The prevalence of weapons has also lead to more violence with increasing severity. It has been reported that close to 5 percent of all psychiatric patients who present to the emergency department for acute care have weapons. One study using metal detectors to screen all emergency department patients over a 6-month period found 33 hand guns, 1324 knives, 97 mace-type canisters, and various other items considered dangerous to the patient and staff. Unfortunately, the escalating problem of violence in the emergency department is often not approached until after a violent event. For example, in a California hospital in February of 1993, a disgruntled patient shot three physicians and took two emergency department personnel hostage for 5 h.

## RECOGNIZING THE VIOLENT PATIENT

The only agreed upon predictors of violence are gender and alcohol abuse. Most perpetrators of violence are males with a history of substance abuse. The amount of education, ethnic background, marital status, or diagnosis are *not* reliable predictors, but they may be barriers to patient/staff interaction, which in itself may lead to frustration and anxiety for both the staff and patient. In turn, this subconscious conflict may precipitate a violent encounter.

The most obvious predictor of potential violence is in the patient's history. Any patient with a history of being violent in the past must be taken seriously and handled cautiously. Trivializing a patient's threat, no matter how subtle, may be the cause of unrecognized violence escalation in its early stages.

Every patient exhibiting violent or threatening behavior should have a thorough physical and mental-status examination. This may require some form of control (restraints or sedation) before an examination can be completed. Using family members, friends, therapists, and/or medical records as a source of history may be valuable. It is the duty of the examining physician to differentiate between an organic or functional cause of the behavior (see Table 254-1). The

**Table 254-1.** Problems Associated with Violence

| | |
|---|---|
| Psychiatric | Vascular malformation |
|   Schizophrenia | Hypoglycemia |
|   Paranoid ideation | Hypoxia |
|   Catatonic excitement | AIDS |
|   Mania | Electrolyte abnormality |
|   Personality disorder | Hypothermia or hyperthermia |
|     Borderline | Anemia |
|     Antisocial | Vitamin deficiency |
|   Delusional depression | Endocrine disorder |
|   Posttraumatic stress disorder | Drugs |
|   Decompensating obsessive/ |   Unanticipated reaction to prescribed |
|     compulsive disorder |     medication (especially sedatives in |
|   Homosexual panic |     brain-injured or elderly patients) |
| Situational frustration |   Alcohol (intoxication and |
|   Mutual hostility |     withdrawal) |
|   Miscommunication |   Amphetamines |
|   Fear of dependency or |   Cocaine |
|     rejection |   Sedative/hypnotic (intoxication or |
|   Fear of illness |     withdrawal) |
|   Guilt over role in disease |   PCP |
|     process |   LSD |
| Organic |   Anticholinergics |
|   Diseases |   Aromatic hydrocarbons (glue, paint, |
|     Delirium |     gasoline) |
|     Dementia |   Steroids |
|     Trauma | Antisocial behavior |
|     CNS infection |   Violence with no associated medical or |
|     Seizures |     psychiatric explanation (these patients |
|     Neoplasm |     may be managed by the police or |
|     Cerebrovascular accident |     security) |

*Note:* CNS, central nervous system; AIDS, acquired immunodeficiency syndrome; LSD, lysergic acid diethylamide; PCP, phencyclidine.

*Source:* From Rice and Moore, p 15, with permission.

treatment of an underlying disorder may completely remove any threat, such as the administration of intravenous glucose to a disoriented, aggressive hypoglycemic patient. The organic diseases most likely involved in a violent episode are those related to drugs and withdrawal syndrome, especially delirium tremens. According to the American Psychiatric Association, the presence of any one of the following indicators should prompt a search for an organic etiology: a patient older than 40 years of age with no previous psychiatric history, disorientation, lethargy or stupor, abnormal vital signs, visual hallucinations, or illusions. A thorough evaluation should include laboratory work, toxicology screening, ECGs, and, in some cases, computed tomography and lumbar puncture.

The most common of the functional disorders related to violent behavior is schizophrenia, especially in those patients in paranoid subgroups or with personality disorders. The most dangerous functional disorder patient, however, is the manic.

## PRODROMES OF VIOLENCE

In most cases, violent behavior is not one of the presenting signs of the patient. Therefore recognition of the prodromes of violence is necessary. The phases of escalation are generally agreed upon. The first of these is the anxiety phase, followed by a phase of defensiveness, then physical aggression. Each phase evokes a response that is proportionate to the patient's behavior. In general, verbal abuse is best handled by verbal response. Physical aggression is best handled by physical means. It is important to remember that although these levels may be discrete, they also may overlap.

### Phase 1—Anxiety

The first level of behavior that is seen in a potentially violent patient is that of anxiety. This may not only occur with the patient. Family and visitors waiting long periods in the emergency department waiting room may also exhibit anxiety and should be dealt with before visiting the patient so as not to intensify the patient's behavior. In general, the signs of increasing anxiety are indicated by body language. Movements that seem to have no purpose other than to expend energy may be the first clue. These may include pacing, wringing of hands, clenching of fists, unwillingness to stay in the treatment area, or a disheveled appearance. Speech may be pressured and loud. Questions such as "Why am I here?" or "How long is this going to take?" may be asked. It is not necessarily what is said, but the manner of speech that gives a clue to the presence of anxiety. One of the most common reasons that a patient's condition may evolve beyond anxiety is that the staff ignores these signals, rather than acknowledging the potential for violence. Underestimating these gestures as a signal of potential violence is inviting a potential threat.

The appropriate response to the anxiety phase should be developing some type of rapport with the patient or potentially violent patient. Time (a commodity so precious to emergency staff and physicians) is usually all that is needed to establish this rapport. Listening to the patient's concerns and addressing him or her appropriately may be all that is required to diffuse the situation. To take an attitude of "I can't be bothered with such a matter" will only cause more anxiety in a person who may be feeling a loss of control. Most patients are fearful of this loss of control and usually welcome the opportunity to politely vent their feelings. This requires sympathy and empathy regarding their concerns. The patient must be treated honestly and with respect. This courtesy will go a long way in gaining rapport and ultimately avoiding future problems. Be supportive with responses that acknowledge the patient's feelings, such as "I understand why you are angry." A *peace offering* of food or drink may also help. Do not be judgmental. Concentrate on what the patient is saying and don't feign attention. Restating what the patient has just said may help clarify the patient's complaints and allow the patient to continue venting.

Remain on the topic and, above all, remain calm. This will help the patient feel more in control.

### Phase 2—Defensiveness

The next level in the continuum of violent behavior is characterized by defensiveness. At this point, the patient's behavior is volatile and becomes verbally abusive and profane. These verbal attacks may be directed to staff members or others in the department and may include statements about your age, gender, weight, or questions about your heritage. It is at this level that the patient's behaviors are irrational and often have nothing to do with why the patient presented to the emergency department. The patient is losing control and may feel helpless. A patient may present to the emergency department in this stage, having passed the anxiety stage outside of the hospital. If restrained, as with the patient in police custody, feelings of helplessness may be further magnified.

Such patients will challenge you and your authority and will respond to you with body posturing and movements. Emergency department personnel must remain professional and avoid power struggles and loss of patience. Appropriate responses to this phase are preventing total loss of control by the patient and thus deflecting physical aggression. It is here that one must be firm in tone and action. The patient must have reasonable limits set and made aware of the consequences of such continued behavior. Limits must be simple, clear, enforceable, and consistent among all emergency department personnel. Giving the patient reasonable choices may help diffuse the situation and make him or her feel rewarded for good behavior. Emergency staff must not overreact or make counterthreats or false promises. If others are present, the patient and the situation must be isolated. Here, a show of force by uniform security personnel may be in order, keeping in mind that such a presence may cause further escalation; however, this is the exception, not the rule. It is important that no consequence be stated that is not readily enforceable. Let the patient make the choice.

### Phase 3—Physical Aggression

The third level of behavior that may be encountered is that of true physical aggression and assertive behavior. The patient is now totally out of control and no amount of verbal intervention is effective. The physically aggressive patient must be confronted and controlled physically, not only for the safety of the emergency department personnel, but for the safety of the violent patient, other patients, and visitors in the department. Remember, this is only when all other interventions have failed; once the decision has been made to restrain, no further negotiation is warranted. Physical control of the patient may require personnel skilled in overcoming a person without injury to self or others. Never attempt this control single-handedly and preferably defer this management to a trained individual, if necessary. It is important to remember that, as a health care provider, you have a *duty* to evaluate a patient's needs. Restraint, in some situations, is only fulfilling your duty. Using appropriate and nonharmful restraint, you are providing the necessary care for the violent patient. Physical control is not done for punitive reasons, but is done in the interest of patient care and safety for others.

## PHYSICAL RESTRAINTS

Restraints are used not only to control a patient when verbal interventions have failed, but also to facilitate the appropriate evaluations of those patients who have underlying organic disorders and who are too agitated or without the mental capacities to be reasoned with and control themselves. When used properly and appropriately, restraints are actually more humane than allowing patients to injure themselves or others. Restraints should be used to prevent harm, to allow for further evaluation of the violent patient, or in a response to a patient's re-

**Table 254-2.** Guidelines for Using Restraints

At least four persons should assist with restraining the patient, while a fifth staff member controls the patient's head and prevents biting. At no time should only one or two persons try to restrain a patient. Leather restraints are the safest and surest type of restraint.

Explain to the patient why he or she is being restrained. Give the patient a few seconds to comply, but do not negotiate. At a prearranged signal, the team grabs the patient and brings him to the floor in a backward motion without injuring him. The team applies restraints, then moves the patient to the seclusion room.

A staff member should always be visible to reassure the patient who is being restrained.

Restrain the patient with legs spread-eagle and one arm restrained to the side and the other arm restrained over the patient's head.

Remove all dangerous objects from the patient, including rings, shoes, matches, pens, and pencils.

Place restraints so that intravenous fluids can be given if necessary.

Raise the patient's head slightly to decrease feelings of vulnerability and to reduce the possibility of aspiration.

After the patient is in restraints, begin treatment using verbal intervention or rapid tranquilization.

Remove one restraint at a time at 5-minute intervals until the patient has only two restraints on. Remove both of these restraints at the same time. Never leave only one limb in restraints.

*Source:* Adapted from Dubin WR, Weiss KJ: Emergency psychiatry, in Michels R et al (eds): *Psychiatry,* vol 2. Philadelphia, Lippincott, 1985, with permission.

quest for them. Never should restraints be used to treat orthopedic problems or certain medical problems such as myocardial infarction, where a worsening of symptoms may occur by using the restraints and sensory deprivations may be more harmful than helpful (Table 254-2).

Once the decision to restrain a patient is made, appropriate personnel must be assembled. At least four to five people with a single team leader should be present. On the command of this leader, the procedure is carried out without undue force or harm to the patient or staff. Never use soft restraints on the truly violent patient, and once restrained, do not remove the devices except under the order of the treating physician and with the assent of the other health care providers, and with security personnel present. It is important that one explains the reason for restraint to the patient. Once restrained, the patient should not be abandoned.

Strict protocols for the use of restraints should be available in every emergency department. These protocols should incorporate input not only from emergency department staff but from security, law enforcement, hospital legal departments, and, if possible, psychiatric services in order to present a consistent, lawful approach to the use of restraints. Once developed, in-service meetings should be arranged to familiarize and train all emergency department personnel on their use and misuse.

Medical-legal issues are part of any restraining procedure. It is law that the minimal use of force be used to hold a violent patient. Suffice it to say that the presence of security may be the only restraint needed, and not always 4-point leather straps. Anytime a person is placed in restraints, the medical chart should reflect the reason the patient was restrained. The chart should state clearly that a direct physician order is required to remove a restraint. No patient for whom restraints are needed should be allowed to leave the emergency department against medical advice (American Medical Association). If necessary, contacting hospital legal authorities may be helpful. In general, restraining a patient against their will is better than the legal issues that arise if someone harms themselves or someone else in the emergency department when the threat of violence was clearly evident.

Although never the primary motivation, restraining also allows for the patient to be searched for weapons or drugs. Searching can often

be accomplished by simply asking the patient to allow such a search or by deferring to security personnel. The best search is done by undressing the patient. Emergency department staff should not attempt to take weapons from a patient without assistance; if weapons are obtained, they should never be returned, despite the patient's insistence.

Those who come to the emergency department in restraints should be left in restraints. Yet law enforcement officials often bring patients in handcuffs to the emergency department, only to give them a summons and release them once treatment has begun. No person should be released from law enforcement personnel in the emergency department. If initial plans were to release the patients (the perpetrators), they should not have been brought to the emergency department, especially those refusing any type of care. Do not allow law enforcement officers to leave a patient unattended in the emergency department if physical restraint was needed earlier. Furthermore, never release prisoners in the emergency department from restraints; many an escape has taken place from a hospital setting.

## CHEMICAL RESTRAINTS

At times a patient may be too violent, even while physically restrained, for an adequate evaluation to be performed. The use of pharmacologic agents can be a safe and effective means of controlling these patients, provided they are used appropriately and that physicians are aware of their adverse affects (Table 254-3). The term *rapid tranquilization* has been used to describe delivery of medications in a titrated fashion to gain control of patients with psychiatric illness, substance abuse, dementia, or withdrawal symptoms. Standard doses of neuroleptic agents or benzodiazepines are given at 30- to 60-min intervals until the desired effect is reached. In general, doses for elderly patients should be half of those used on younger patients.

Physicians who use any of these medications should become familiar with their adverse effects and their treatment. These may include anticholinergic effects, hypotension, and extrapyramidal symptoms. Haloperidol is generally considered the neuroleptic of choice, since the adverse effects are usually less common. Short-acting benzodiazepines such as lorazepam are also recommended for intoxicated states and withdrawal syndromes. With the advent of flumazenil, a benzodiazepine antagonist, respiratory depression or oversedation with these agents can be reversed.

## PREVENTION

The single best way to handle a violent patient or curtail the potential for violence in the emergency department is by prevention. Careful planning of the work area, cooperation with security, and training of all emergency department personnel to recognize violent patients are critical.

The physical plan of an emergency department should be one of controlled access. Visitation policies should be reasonable yet enforced. Some hospitals use visitor ID badges to monitor visitors in the department. A busy emergency department, packed full of visitors, only increases anxiety and tension. It is also the perfect place for the weapons-carrying violent patient to take hostages. Although a history from family and friends can be important in the evaluation of any potentially violent patient, interviews should be conducted in a safe, calm environment.

Seclusion rooms to interview patients should be safe for both the patient and the interviewer. Solid walls with sturdy, heavy furniture that would be awkward to lift should be used. Lighting should be able to be dimmed or brightened depending on the circumstance. No free-standing objects, such as ashtrays, pictures, or pencils, should be allowed, since they all could become potential weapons. Exits should be clear of obstruction and readily available to the interviewer. *Panic buttons* may be installed or signals developed to be used in the event of threatening behavior on the part of the patient. If violent aggression does develop, the room should be large enough for a team of se-

**Table 254-3.** Rapid Tranquilization (RT) of the Violent Patient

| Cause of Violent Behavior | Drug Intervention* |
|---|---|
| Schizophrenia, mania, or other psychosis | Lorazepam (Ativan) 2–4 mg IM combined with haloperidol (Haldol) 5 mg IM or thiothixene (Navane) 10 mg IM<br>*or*<br>RT with an antipsychotic alone:<br>  Thiothixene (Navane) 10 mg IM or 20 mg concentrate<br>  Haloperidol (Haldol) 5 mg IM or 10 mg concentrate<br>  Loxapine (Loxitane) 10 mg IM or 25 mg concentrate PO |
| Personality disorder | Lorazepam (Ativan) 1–2 mg PO every 1–2 h or 2 mg IM (0.05 mg/kg) every 1–2 h |
| Alcohol withdrawal states† | For agitation, tremors, or change in vital signs: chlordiazepoxide (Librium) 25–50 mg PO every 4–6 h<br>For elderly patients or patients with liver disease: lorazepam 2 mg PO every 2 h<br>For extreme agitation: lorazepam 2–4 mg IM every hour or RT of patient not controlled with benzodiazepines |
| Cocaine and amphetamine intoxication | For mild to moderate agitation: diazepam (Valium) 10 mg PO every 8 h<br>For severe agitation: thiothixene 20 mg concentrate or 10 mg IM; haloperidol 10 mg concentrate or 5 mg IM |
| Phencyclidine intoxication | For hyperactivity, mild agitation, tension, anxiety, excitement: diazepam 10–30 mg PO or lorazepam 2–4 IM (0.05 mg/kg)<br>For severe agitation and excitement with hallucinations, delusions, bizarre behavior: haloperidol 5–10 mg IM every 30–60 min |

* All doses given at 30- to 60-min intervals; one-half dose for medically ill or older patients.

† Rapid tranquilization in alcohol withdrawal states is for severe agitation and behavioral control. The actual treatment of withdrawal is with a cross-tolerant medication.

*Source:* From Dubin and Weiss, with permission.

curity personnel to safely overcome the patient without undue harm.

Deterrence is also becoming more of a preventative technique. Signs outside the emergency department should clearly state that weapons of any type are not permitted, and trained hospital security personnel should be visible to everyone entering the emergency department. Not only does this set a tone of behavior, but security measures can be invaluable in preventing as well as curtailing any violence. The use of metal detectors and x-ray machines for personal articles, such as handbags, may allow for easy screening of those entering the treatment area. Once believed a luxury, metal detectors are now reasonably priced and cost-effective. Carefully placed monitors and alarm buttons may also be warranted.

Seclusion rooms and deterrent measures are needed, yet the education of the emergency department personnel is the most important factor in curbing violence in the emergency department. Several national programs, such as that offered by the National Crisis Prevention Institute, are invaluable in teaching basic understanding of violent behavior, as well as its recognition and management, and basic self-defense against the violent patient. In-services by security personnel and law enforcement officials may also be of benefit. Learning how to examine a patient while still protecting your personal space will go a long way to preventing injury should the patient lash out.

Common sense and a heightened awareness for the potential for violence is the first step in this education. Being aware of the position of your body, clothing, and equipment, in relation to the patient, can save you from assault. Never let a violent patient get between you and the exit. Defer to trained security personnel should the patient need to be searched or disarmed. Always document any incidents and reasons for restraint properly.

Violence in the emergency department is not an uncommon occurrence. Both rural and urban hospitals find themselves with increasing episodes of violence. Careful preparation and a heightened awareness for the potential for violence are basic. Education is important in understanding the dynamics of violent behavior and will help to detect and manage the violent patient. Any education done should be reviewed periodically. Management strategies should be a team approach involving emergency department staff and security, law enforcement, and hospital legal departments. Strict policies should be established for visitation. Making the work environment safe will make all involved more comfortable. You should feel as safe at work as you do at home. Remember to trust your intuition. If you are afraid, then the potential for violence probably exists.

# BIBLIOGRAPHY

Anglin D, Kyriacou DN, Hudson HR: Resident's perspective on violence and personal safety in the emergency department. *Ann Emerg Med* vol 23, no 5, 1994.

Dubin WR, Tarduff K, Maler G: Overcoming danger with violent patients: Guidelines for safe and effective management. Emergency Medicine Reports vol 13, no 14. American Health Consultants, Inc. Atlanta, Ga, July 13, 1992.

Dubin WR, Weiss KJ: *Handbook of Psychiatric Emergencies.* Springhouse, PA, Springhouse Corporation, 1991.

*Nonviolent Crisis Intervention Workbook.* Brookfield, WI, National Crisis Prevention Institute, 1987.

Rice M, Moore G: Management of the violent patient, therapeutic and legal considerations. *Emerg Med Clin North Am* 9(1) 13, 1991.

Task Force Report #22: *Seclusion and Restraint: The Psychiatric Uses.* Washington, DC, American Psychiatric Association, 1985.

Thompson B, Nunn J, Kramer I, et al: Disarming the department: Weapon screening and improved security to create a safer emergency department environment. *Ann Emerg Med* 17:419, 1988.

# Newer Imaging Modalities

## 255
## NONINVASIVE VASCULAR STUDIES
### Phillip J. Bendick

Acute peripheral vascular problems may be of an arterial or venous nature but typically involve some form of vascular obstruction and require prompt, accurate diagnosis. Of particular importance is the assessment of the overall functional or hemodynamic significance of the disease process in considering the initial treatment and ultimate management. While the history and physical examination should *always* be the starting point of any vascular workup, they are often subjective in nature and can even be misleading in certain cases. One of the first questions to be addressed for the patient presenting with symptoms in an extremity is whether the underlying problem is arterial (ischemia) or venous [acute or chronic deep vein thrombosis (DVT)]. The physical examination will usually provide the necessary answer, with the pain, pallor, pulselessness, etc. of arterial ischemia distinguished from the erythema, tenderness, and swelling associated with venous disease. A careful history will further distinguish an acute from a chronic problem, though in the case of exacerbated chronic venous insufficiency, a more acute component of DVT cannot be ruled out by the history and physical examination. Recent developments in noninvasive evaluation techniques, validated by extensive application in vascular laboratories in the outpatient setting, can help answer these questions and provide measurement tools that give objective, quantitative data for diagnosis suited to the emergency department environment.

### INSTRUMENTATION AND TECHNIQUES

Two primary instruments should be available for noninvasive vascular evaluation in the emergency department. Some type of portable Doppler ultrasound flowmeter should be available at all times for direct hands-on use by the emergency department staff; the second technique is duplex ultrasonography, available to but not necessarily performed directly by the staff.

Portable Doppler ultrasound flowmeters are available in a wide variety of pocket or small, battery-powered models. In one form or another it should be available in every emergency department at all times, and the staff should be familiar with its operation and use. The flowmeter converts the frequency shift of the ultrasound signal reflected from moving blood (the Doppler shift) to an audible sound suitable for subjective interpretation. Typically, a transducer frequency between 5 and 10 MHz is used to provide reasonable sensitivity to blood flow while assuring good tissue penetration in even obese patients. Of primary importance is the character of the audible signal in differentiating arterial from venous signals and normal from abnormal signals. Normal arterial signals are characterized by brisk, multiphasic sounds rapidly changing in pitch during the cardiac cycle, high pitched during peak systole and much lower pitched during diastole. Normal venous flow signals tend to be lower pitched and more constant in nature, without a significant heart rate component but instead varying with the respiratory cycle. Practice and experience bring rapid familiarity with these normal flow signals, and it is possible

quickly to develop an "ear" for these flows in both the arterial and venous systems by trying the flowmeter out on healthy normal subjects (such as "volunteer" coworkers).

Technique is important to obtain the best possible Doppler flow signals. Adequate acoustic coupling gel should be used to assure good contact between the Doppler probe and the skin; ultrasound transmission will be severely degraded if there are any air pockets or air bubbles in the path of the ultrasound beam. The probe itself should be held firmly to provide a very stable platform, but with minimal direct pressure against the skin. The best flow signals will be obtained if the transducer is aligned along the longitudinal axis of the blood vessel of interest and held at an approximate 45° angle to the skin surface. Once a flow signal is obtained, this angle can be adjusted to between 30° and 60° to get the strongest flow signal possible.

Once an appreciation for normal signals has been developed, it becomes much easier to identify and grade abnormalities. These may be characterized by:

1. An absence of any flow signal, indicating total vessel occlusion. It is important to be thoroughly familiar with the arterial anatomy so that the Doppler probe is truly placed over the vessel of interest to avoid a false-positive study.
2. Weak, monophasic arterial flow signals indicative of significant proximal obstructive disease. These so-called damped flow signals are characterized by a slowed systolic upstroke and slowly diminishing flow from peak systole through diastole, with antegrade flow during the entire cardiac cycle.
3. Hyperdynamic flows sustained throughout diastole, indicative of markedly diminished peripheral vascular resistance. These flow signals might be seen proximal to an arteriovenous fistula or in the arterial conduit(s) supplying a distal runoff bed with a significant inflammatory reaction such as cellulitis.

Limitations and artifacts to be aware of include the possible confusion of venous and arterial flow signals, which in the periphery may sound alike because of a weak, monophasic arterial signal or a pulsatile femoral vein signal secondary to congestive heart failure. Again, a knowledge of the vascular anatomy is necessary to avoid this potential error. Excessive probe pressure can easily obliterate flow signals, particularly in the pedal arteries and veins. Significant tissue edema and chronic dermal changes can also attenuate flow signals because of their effects on the ultrasound beam, diminishing signal amplitude; in the absence of any obstructive disease, however, the other signal characteristics will not be affected.

The second technique that needs to be available for vascular assessments in the emergency department, duplex ultrasonography, presents more of a technologic challenge. Duplex ultrasound combines high-resolution imaging in real time with simultaneous Doppler capability, providing hemodynamic information with precise anatomic detail. The real-time image displays the echo pattern from the interfaces between different tissues. For vascular applications, this is made somewhat easier by the fact that blood is a poor reflector of ultrasound and normally appears anechoic; the surrounding tissues are relatively hyperechoic, providing distinct differentiation. Guided by the image, selective Doppler flow measurements can be made by choosing the placement site of the region of interest, or sample volume, of the flowmeter. Few emergency departments have the luxury of a dedicated on-site instrument, but they are now widely available in virtually every hospital through the vascular laboratory or radiology department, with trained personnel to operate them. While it is not necessary for the emergency department staff to develop the technical skills of the sonographer, they should be familiar with some of the basic facets of test interpretation, just as in reading simple radiographs.

## APPLICATIONS

### Peripheral Arterial Disease

In the emergency setting, the majority of applications of noninvasive evaluation techniques in peripheral arterial disease will be to differentiate chronic atherosclerotic occlusive disease from more acute thromboembolic events and to determine the hemodynamic significance of the underlying disease. In this regard, the time course of the patient's symptoms is as helpful as any other information and again emphasizes the importance of a thorough history in the initial evaluation. The portable Doppler flowmeter can then provide two important functions in completing the diagnostic workup. The presence or absence of arterial flows assess vessel patency at the site being examined. If the vessel is patent, further subjective grading of the quality of the flow signal provides additional information regarding any proximal disease. The normal flow signal is considered multiphasic, with a sharp, well-defined signal in the systolic phase rapidly increasing and then decreasing in pitch and intensity; lower-pitched (representing lower flow velocities) signals comprise the diastolic phases of the cardiac cycle. As proximal arterial disease becomes more severe, the flow signal becomes monophasic and damped with a weaker, slowed systolic rise; delayed onset of peak systole; and a slowly diminishing pitch (slowing flow velocities) during diastole. In the case of a total occlusion proximal to the site of Doppler interrogation, the quality of the flow signal is related to the adequacy and magnitude of any collateral flow that might be present.

The second function of the ultrasound flowmeter is that of a Doppler stethoscope, to allow the measurement of limb segmental systolic pressures. These quantitative data provide a more objective assessment of the degree of functional impairment, or hemodynamic significance, of any arterial obstructive disease. To measure the ankle systolic pressure, the patient should be placed in a supine position and a standard adult blood pressure cuff (12- × 23-cm bladder) wrapped snugly around the ankle, with the lower edge of the cuff just above the malleoli. While using the Doppler flowmeter to monitor the signal from the posterior or anterior tibial artery at the ankle, distal to the cuff, inflate the cuff to a pressure approximately 30 mmHg above systolic pressure to temporarily occlude flow. As the cuff is slowly deflated (2 to 4 mmHg/s), that pressure at which a Doppler flow signal is again heard should be noted and recorded as the ankle systolic pressure. This value is then compared to the resting brachial artery systolic pressures in the form of an ankle/brachial index (ABI), calculated by dividing the ankle systolic pressure by the *higher* of the two brachial artery systolic pressures. A normal ABI is 1.0 or greater. If the ABI falls between 0.5 and 0.9, this is typically indicative of obstructive disease in a single peripheral arterial segment, and the classic clinical presentation is one of a history of claudication. If the ABI falls below 0.5, there is typically multiple arterial segment involvement in the obstructive process, and clinically the more severe ischemia may cause pain at rest or outright ulceration or other tissue loss. *Acute* thrombotic occlusions, without the development of any significant collateral flows, nearly always fall into this category and will require close continued monitoring during anticoagulant therapy or lead directly to thromboembolectomy. Of further note, if the brachial pressures differ by more than 20 mmHg, that is indicative of marked obstructive disease affecting the arm with the lower pressure, typically in the subclavian artery.

Potential artifacts with this technique include a low pressure reading from deflating the cuff too rapidly; extrinsically collapsing the vessel being monitored by too much pressure from the probe on the skin; sliding the probe off the vessel site during cuff deflation; and, in diabetic patients or those with chronic renal failure, falsely elevated peripheral pressures secondary to arterial medial wall calcification.

Applications of duplex ultrasonography to peripheral arterial disease in the emergency department are more limited. Generally, duplex ultrasound is excellent for types of localized arterial disease that do not cause any overall hemodynamic flow disturbances and thus would not be picked up by simpler portable Doppler flowmeter testing. Upper or lower extremity applications are best reserved for less commonly seen pathologies such as peripheral aneurysmal disease, differentiating hematoma from pseudoaneurysm in a patient presenting with a pulsatile mass, documenting an arteriovenous fistula, or evaluating a bypass graft for patency. The cerebrovascular system can be evaluated for carotid artery stenosis or occlusion contributing to symptoms of intracranial ischemia.

Finally, while some centers are evaluating the efficacy of duplex ultrasound in the management of trauma, no clear roles are yet defined. For penetrating trauma, the ultrasound evaluation is best for the major vessels, but these injuries are frequently recognized by physical examination and, thus far, better documented by angiography. A similar situation exists for blunt trauma, with the possible exception of dislocation injuries where duplex ultrasound may be able to identify clinically silent injuries to major vessels crossing the joint space. In particular, the popliteal space can be thoroughly evaluated in patients with knee trauma or joint dislocation. It is also worth emphasizing that while these studies can be performed in the emergency department itself, if the diagnosis is needed urgently, the quality of the examination and the diagnostic information obtained are likely to be significantly better when performed not at the bedside in the emergency department but in the more controlled environment of the vascular laboratory or ultrasound department.

### Peripheral Venous Disease

Patients presenting to the emergency department with the clinical signs and symptoms of deep vein thrombosis provide a contrasting situation. These patients must be approached with a high index of suspicion because of the potential for and life-threatening nature of pulmonary embolism. There is a degree of urgency to establishing the diagnosis, but a corresponding requirement for high accuracy in making the diagnosis because of the complications associated with systemic anticoagulation. Duplex ultrasonography has clearly become the test of choice for the diagnosis of DVT. Its accuracy (sensitivity and specificity) is virtually identical to that of ascending contrast venography for all sites in the lower extremities, including the major veins and intramuscular branches in the calf. It is a noninvasive test well suited for screening and follow-up. In addition, it can be performed in the vascular laboratory, the ultrasound department, or by a portable unit at the bedside in the emergency department if necessary (though as with arterial testing, the quality of the bedside study may not be as high as those done in more controlled environments). Its major drawback is the requirement for an experienced vascular technologist or sonographer to perform the study, a skill it would not be reasonable to expect the emergency department staff to perfect. The technique directly images the venous system, providing an anatomic "road map" similar to venography. The presence of DVT is documented on the basis of an inability to collapse or compress the vein walls with light downward probe pressure on the surface of the skin, the absence of Doppler flow signals from within the lumen of the vein, and an image of echogenic material in the vein lumen (Figs. 255-1 to 255-4). These same criteria can also be applied to the diagnosis of superficial thrombophlebitis in the greater saphenous system or associated varicosities.

While the portable Doppler flowmeter has also been used in the

**Fig. 255-1.** Normal cross-sectional anatomy of the common femoral vein just below the groin.

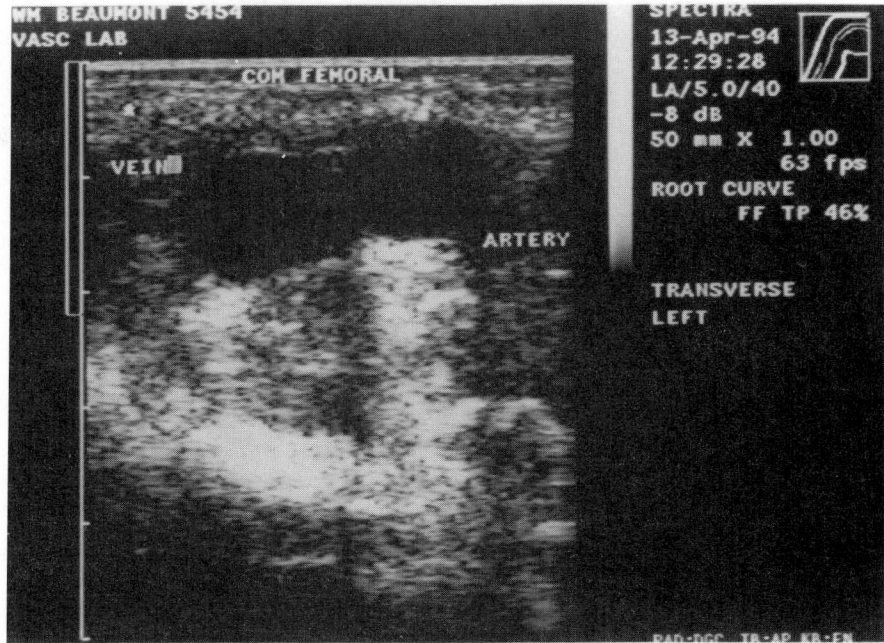

past to diagnose DVT, its application has become much more limited since the development of duplex ultrasonography, which allows the measurement of the important Doppler flow characteristics with simultaneous imaging of the associated venous anatomy. Because it is subjective and so strongly examiner-dependent, the portable venous Doppler examination has significant limitations and a rather imposing list of sources of diagnostic errors, which restrict its efficacy in the setting of the emergency department. False-positive Doppler examinations may result from a variety of patient-related artifacts such as obesity or muscle guarding; false-negative studies frequently arise from nonocclusive thromboses or thrombosis isolated to the deep veins of the calf. Because of these limitations, the use of the Doppler flowmeter alone for the diagnosis of DVT should be discouraged except when performed by the most experienced of examiners.

However, the widespread availability of duplex sonography should not be used to replace clinical assessment and judgment. A high level of suspicion for DVT is best supported by a thorough physical examination and clinical history, recognizing that the limitations of the latter for this disease may result in a positive rate of duplex ultrasound examinations of only approximately 50 percent. Inappropriate utilization of noninvasive testing for even the vaguest of clinical signs (e.g., chronic pitting edema of the ankles noted at the end of a working day) can lower the rate of positive studies to less than 15 percent, perhaps indicating more suspicion than assessment. Recent data suggests that the physical examination may be more accurate than the "toss of a coin," the accuracy that seems to be widely assumed at present. The rate of positive duplex ultrasound studies has been reported as high as 75 to 80 percent when the level of clinical suspicion was rated high;

**Fig. 255-2.** Cross-sectional image of a femoral vein thrombosis, showing the echo-genic lumen, which does not compress with probe pressure.

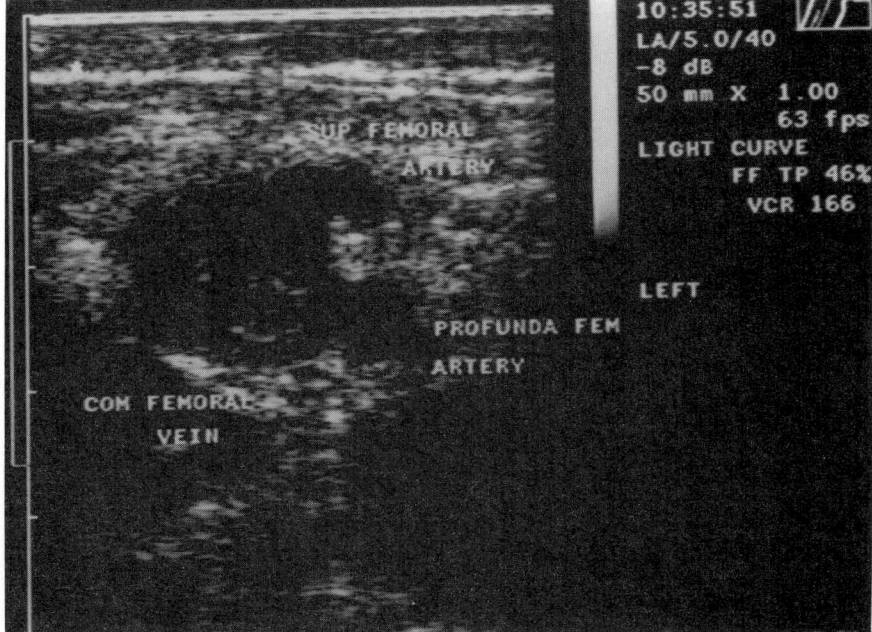

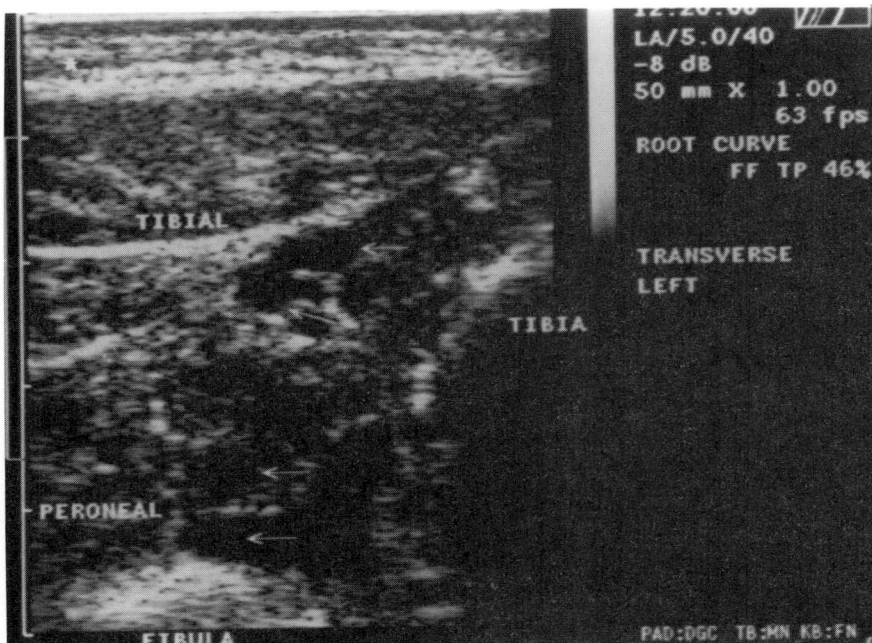

**Fig. 255-3.** Normal cross-sectional anatomy of the posterior tibial and peroneal veins at midcalf.

on the other hand, when the level of clinical suspicion is low, typically only 5 percent of the duplex ultrasound studies are positive. If the clinical question is one of determining a lower extremity source for a possible pulmonary embolus, the rate of positive studies is less than 0.2 percent (1 in 500) in the absence of any physical signs or symptoms in the extremities, a known malignancy, or a history of previous DVT.

It may also be appropriate to anticoagulate the patient felt to have a high probability of DVT (if there are no contraindications to doing so) who presents to the emergency department in the middle of the night with an acutely swollen, tender extremity, and to confirm the diagnosis of DVT with duplex sonography first thing in the morning when the vascular laboratory or ultrasound department begin their regular shift. With respect to appropriate utilization, each institution

should develop guidelines and protocols that will provide the best care for and serve the needs of their individual patient populations.

## SUMMARY

Established and validated vascular laboratory techniques of noninvasive testing for arterial and venous disease can be applied readily to patients in the setting of the emergency department. Some type of portable Doppler flowmeter should be available at all times for use by the staff in screening patients with suspected arterial insufficiency. Duplex ultrasonography should be available within the institution through the vascular laboratory or ultrasound department; and while the staff in the emergency department would not need to have specific vascular imaging skills, they should have some knowledge of

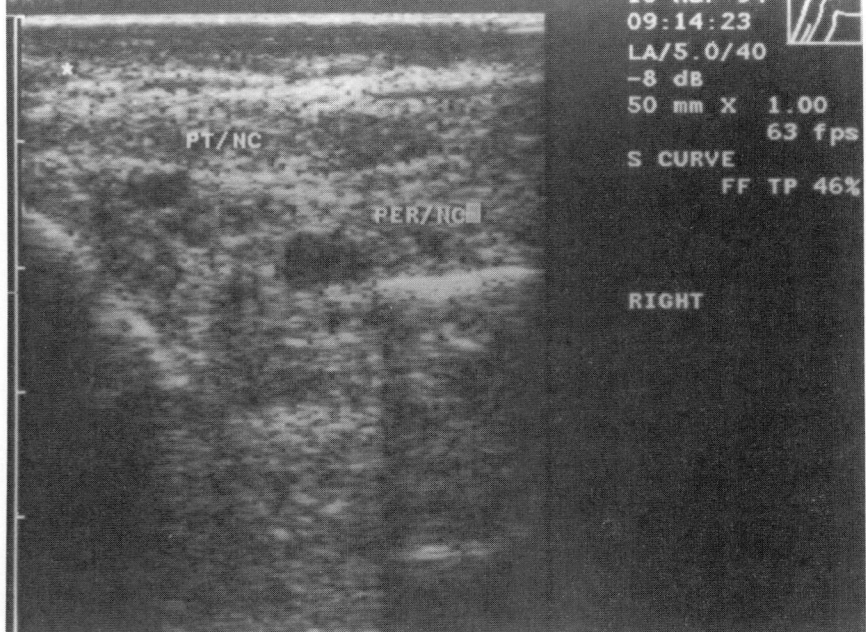

**Fig. 255-4.** Cross-sectional image at midcalf showing a thrombosed posterior tibial and peroneal vein (noted to be markedly dilated), echogenicity from within the lumen, and incompressibility with probe pressure. (NC, noncompressible.)

basic diagnostic criteria. These techniques have proven accuracy and reliability and will provide increased sensitivity in the diagnosis of the presence and severity of peripheral arterial diseases and deep vein thrombosis. Appropriate utilization of these modalities within the emergency department will lead to faster, improved diagnosis, and more rapid implementation of necessary patient management will result.

## BIBLIOGRAPHY

Bendick PJ, Glover JL, Holden RW, et al: Pitfalls of the Doppler examination for venous thrombosis. *Am Surg* 49:320, 1983.

Bernstein EF (ed): *Vascular Diagnosis*, 4th ed. St. Louis, Mosby, 1993.

Kremkau FW: *Doppler Ultrasound—Principles and Instruments*. Philadelphia, Saunders, 1990.

Merritt CRB: *Doppler Color Imaging*. New York, Churchill Livingstone, 1992.

Porter JM, Mayberry JC, Taylor LM, et al: Chronic lower extremity ischemia. *Curr Prob Surg* 28, 1991.

Rutherford RB (ed): *Vascular Surgery*, 3d ed. Philadelphia, Saunders, 1989.

Talbot SR, Oliver MA: *Techniques of Venous Imaging*. Pasadena, CA, Appleton Davies, 1992.

Young JR, Graor RA, Olin JW, et al: *Peripheral Vascular Diseases*. St. Louis, Mosby, 1991.

# 256
# CARDIAC ULTRASONOGRAPHY
## Andrew M. Hauser

Cardiac ultrasound provides immediate bedside assessment of both cardiac anatomy and function. Direct observation of left ventricular contractility allows accurate detection of myocardial ischemia even in the absence of electrocardiographic abnormalities. Physiologic blood flow information, provided by the complementary Doppler ultrasound examination, rivals the accuracy obtained by invasive means. The echocardiographic identification of pericardial effusions and valvular abnormalities may frequently clarify the etiology of symptoms or physical findings (Table 256-1). Cardiac ultrasound, which requires expertise in both the method of recording and interpretation of data, remains primarily a tool of the cardiologist. Considerably greater technical skill is required to record an echocardiogram than an ECG; however, it is probably easier to obtain basic skills in echocardiographic interpretation than ECG interpretation. Although it may or may not be feasible for noncardiologists to gain sufficient proficiency in echocardiography to use the technique as a screening procedure in the emergency department, emergency physicians should have, at a minimum, sufficient knowledge to know when the technique is applicable to a patient's problem.

## TECHNIQUES

The two-dimensional echocardiographic examination provides a cross-sectional image of the beating heart in real time. Because no patient preparation is required, the echocardiographic study may be quickly obtained and even repeated should the patient's condition change. Clinically adequate examinations may even be obtained during CPR. All four cardiac chambers, valves, and the ascending aorta are visualized and recorded with a simultaneous ECG on videotape. Adequate visualization of all cardiac structures may be accomplished by an experienced ultrasonographer in all but approximately 5 to 10 percent of patients. Common limiting factors are inability to position some subjects in the left lateral decubitus position, obesity, and lung hyperinflation due to COPD.

The technique of transesophageal echocardiography employs an ultrasound transducer mounted on a flexible endoscope. Introduction of the transesophageal probe may be performed at bedside with minimal or no sedation and topical anesthetic spray. Since the esophagus is in immediate anatomic proximity to the descending thoracic aorta, this approach is particularly well suited for evaluation of suspected aortic dissections. Imaging success by this method approaches 100 percent.

Doppler ultrasound is a complementary ultrasound technique that provides physiologic information regarding the direction and velocity of moving red blood cells. Laminar flow is readily distinguished from turbulent flow, thereby allowing localization of murmurs and quantification of valvular regurgitation and stenosis. Color-flow Doppler mapping provides a real-time color display of blood flow that, superimposed on the echocardiographic image, yields a vivid representation of intracardiac blood flow. This has been likened to a "noninvasive angiogram."

## Echocardiographic Clues to Etiologies of Hypotension and Dyspnea

Dyspnea and hypotension resulting from impaired ventricular function may be recognized by the presence of cardiac enlargement and gross impairment of ventricular contractility. In contrast, hypotension due to diminished intravascular volume resulting in inadequate ventricular filling is characterized by small right heart dimensions and vigorous or hyperdynamic ventricular contractility. Acute pulmonary hypertension incident to pulmonary embolization selectively affects the right heart chambers while sparing the left, thus causing enlargement and diminished contraction of the right ventricle. Other potential mechanical aberrations such as tamponade, valvular dysfunction, or ventricular septal rupture are readily distinguished by ultrasound imaging and Doppler techniques.

While the complete cardiac ultrasound examination requires multiple transducer positions and angulations to provide a thorough assessment of ventricular and valvular function, many important clinical questions may be answered by a more limited echocardiographic study. Although not a substitute for the complete exam, the subcostal approach allows identification of major impairment of ventricular function, assessment of the right heart and detection of pericardial effusion. This approach has been favored by many emergency physicians as a quick method for initiating the ultrasound exam in patients who may be difficult to position for a more detailed study using other standardized views.

## Applications in Ischemic Heart Disease

In the emergency setting, echocardiography is most often used to identify ongoing or recent ischemic events and to quantify global left

**Table 256-1.** Etiologies of Symptoms Which May Be Determined by Cardiac Ultrasound

| Chest pain | Dyspnea |
|---|---|
| Myocardial ischemia | Heart failure |
| Pulmonary embolus | Pulmonary embolus |
| Pericarditis | Tamponade |
| Aortic dissection | Pulmonary hypertension |
| Noncardiac (by exclusion) | Atrial myxoma |
| Hypotension | Valvular dysfunction |
| Hypovolemia | |
| Cardiogenic shock | |
| Right ventricular infarct | |
| Pulmonary embolus | |

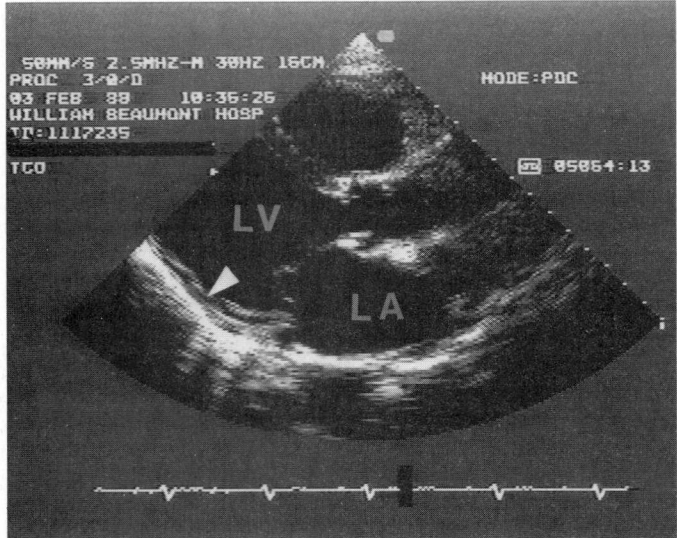

**Fig. 256-1.** Posterior wall infarct showing localized thinning (arrow) and absent wall motion LV = left ventricle; LA = left atrium.

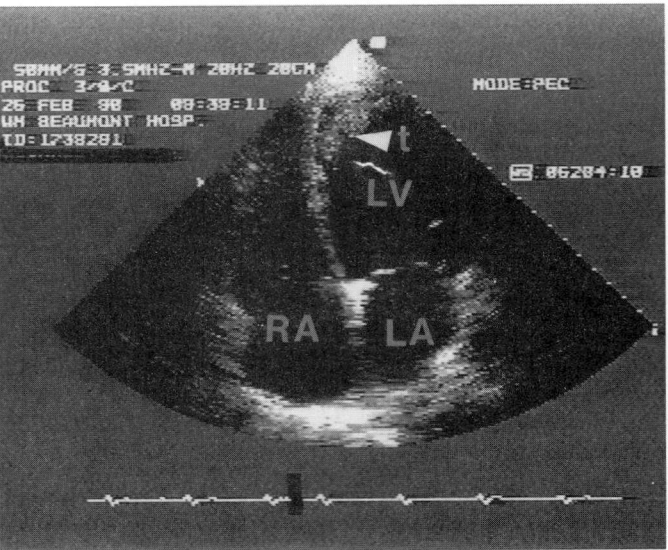

**Fig. 256-2.** Anteroapical infarct with apical thrombus LV = left ventricle; RA = right atrium; LA = left atrium; t = thrombus.

ventricular function. Localized, or segmental, wall motion abnormalities identify past infarction or recent ischemia and may be apparent even in the presence of a nonspecific ECG tracing. Accordingly, occlusion of a coronary artery will almost invariably result in reduced wall motion localized to the segments perfused by the obstructed vessel. The presence of scar and thinning of the myocardium imply that an infarction has evolved at least several weeks before examination, and their presence or absence may be useful to distinguish recent from past ischemic events (Fig. 256-1). The extent of myocardial segments involved and their degree of abnormality influence global left ventricular function.

Definitive assessment of left ventricular performance in acute infarction is important because prognosis is most closely linked to the extent of functional impairment. Cardiac ultrasound is superior to clinical assessment of Killip classification and to the ECG in predicting death or major complications following acute myocardial infarction. The sensitivity of echocardiography in the identification of myocardial infarction is probably greater than 90 percent. Smaller infarctions, particularly in the distribution of the left circumflex coronary artery, and nontransmural infarctions may, at times, escape detection. Such limited ischemic events tend to be associated with a low frequency of clinical complications. The greater the degree of left ventricular impairment, the greater likelihood of subsequent complications such as heart failure or death. An important application of cardiac ultrasound in the emergency department is the identification of patients at high risk among those who appear initially stable. Such information may assist in decisions regarding triage and therapy. Because the presence of a segmental wall motion abnormality is a sensitive indicator of ischemia and the degree of abnormality is predictive of prognosis, echocardiography is a powerful tool for the diagnosis and triage of patients presenting with chest pain to the emergency department. An echocardiographic study displaying normal left ventricular wall motion during chest pain is a strong predictor of a nonischemic etiology and thus, low risk. When symptoms are atypical or the initial ECGs reveal only nonspecific findings, echocardiography may be particularly helpful. Among patients with nonspecific ECG abnormalities in the setting of chest pain presenting to a large community hospital, echocardiography altered the admission diagnosis in 18 percent and disposition plans in 22 percent.

Now that overwhelming evidence indicates that thrombolytic agents reduce patient morbidity and mortality in cases of acute myocardial infarction, never before has emergency decision making

been so vitally important in determining their outcome. Because the efficacy of thrombolytic therapy is closely linked to the time from onset of ischemia to treatment, and the administration of such drugs has substantial risks, emergency physicians are under increased pressure to make early and accurate diagnoses. The ECG may not provide an accurate indication of the presence and degree of ongoing ischemia, particularly in the early evolution of an infarction. Thus, echocardiography has a key role in the selection of patients for acute interventions.

Complications of myocardial infarction, including pump failure, mitral insufficiency, septal rupture, right ventricular infarction, and ventricular thrombus, are also readily detected by echocardiographic and Doppler examinations (Fig. 256-2). Clinically important and coexisting myocardial, valvular, and congenital abnormalities may also be identified. The causes of hypotension or dyspnea in patients presenting to the emergency department with cardiac disorders may similarly be clarified by cardiac ultrasound.

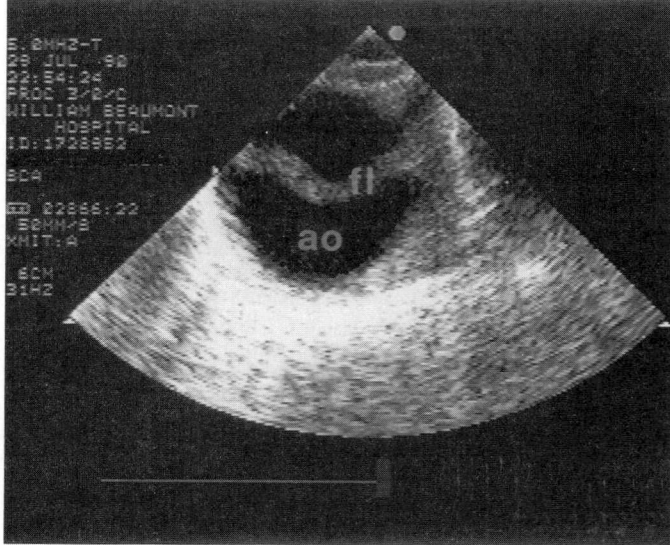

**Fig. 256-3.** Aortic dissection visualized by transesophageal echocardiography fl = intimal flap; ao = aortic false lumen.

**Table 256-2.** Diagnosis of Aortic Dissection by TEE Compared to Angiography and Computerized Tomography

| Technique | Sensitivity % | Specificity % |
|---|---|---|
| Angiography | 88 | 94 |
| CT | 83 | 100 |
| TEE | 99 | 98 |

*Source:* From Erbel et al: European Cooperative Study Group for Echocardiography: Echocardiography in diagnosis of aortic dissection. *Lancet* 1:457, 1989.

## Applications in Aortic Dissection

Although the proximal ascending aorta is generally imaged satisfactorily using standard transthoracic imaging technique, the transverse and descending thoracic aorta is generally insufficiently visualized by this method to evaluate most patients with spontaneous or traumatic aortic dissections. The method of transesophageal echocardiography (TEE) is, however, very effective for assessing aortic dissection, especially when biplanar TEE instrumentation is utilized. The results of the European Cooperative Study of Aortic Dissection reported by Erbel and colleagues demonstrated favorable results with TEE when compared with angiography and CT (Table 256-2). Since TEE may be employed at bedside with minimal patient preparation, the earlier time to diagnosis may be lifesaving in this high-risk setting. Additionally, patients may be spared the risk of angiography and contrast dye administration by using TEE in suspected cases of aortic dissection. Using TEE, the intimal flap is readily identified (Fig. 256-3), and the complementary color Doppler examination displays the entry points with greater precision compared to angiographic methods.

## Miscellaneous Applications

### Cardiac Tamponade

The identification of a large pericardial effusion in the appropriate clinical setting may identify a correctable cause of hypotension or dyspnea. The presence of diastolic collapse of the right atrium or ventricle may provide further confirmatory echocardiographic data for the presence of tamponade or "pretamponade" (Fig. 256-4). Performance of pericardiocentesis may be often facilitated by echocardiography, which can be used to guide the selection of an appropriate site for needle insertion.

## Valvular Heart Disease

Although the identification and quantification of valvular abnormality is generally a nonemergent procedure, identification of a flail leaflet due to myxomatous degeneration or endocarditis may explain the etiology of hypotension or dyspnea in clinical settings when even a significant murmur may be lacking and will guide appropriate medical and surgical measures to stabilize the patient.

## Cardiomyopathy and Intracardiac Masses

Echocardiography may identify hypertrophic cardiomyopathies and intracardiac masses responsible for syncope, dyspnea, or hypotension, which are unexplained by other clinical evaluations.

## CONCLUSION

Echocardiography is a powerful diagnostic tool that has many emergency department applications. Although the performance and interpretation of cardiac ultrasound exams by emergency physicians is feasible, the practicality of such application has not yet been thoroughly tested. Cardiac ultrasound training in emergency medicine programs is warranted and this is now being offered in some residency training programs and in postgraduate seminars.

The relatively high cost of modern instrumentation may currently prohibit full-time dedication of such units to most centers. However, many hospitals have clinically serviceable instruments made available through displacement by newer units. These instruments, perhaps lacking color Doppler or other sophisticated features, may be sufficient for emergency department screening examinations. The support of an experienced echocardiographer for expert review is essential to maintain quality assurance and ongoing education for emergency personnel who may wish to participate in cardiac ultrasound examinations.

## BIBLIOGRAPHY

Bocka JJ, Overton DT, Hauser A: Electromechanical dissociation in human beings: An echocardiographic study. *Ann Emerg Med* 17:450, 1988.

Callahan JA, Seward JB, Tajik AJ, et al: Pericardiocentesis assisted by two-dimensional echocardiography. *J Thorac Cardiovasc Surg* 85:877, 1983.

Erbel R, et al: European Cooperative Study Group for Echocardiography: Echocardiography in diagnosis of aortic dissection. *Lancet* 1:457, 1989.

Hauser AM: The emerging role of echocardiography in the emergency department. *Ann Emerg Med* 18:1298, 1989.

Kloner RA, Parisi AF: Acute myocardial infarction: Diagnostic and prognostic applications of two-dimensional echocardiography. *Circulation* 75:521, 1987.

Oh, JK, Miller FA, Shub GS, et al: Evaluation of acute chest pain syndromes by two-dimensional echocardiography: Its potential application in the selection of patients for acute reperfusion therapy. *Mayo Clin Proc* 62:59, 1987.

Peels KH, Visser CA, Kupper AJF, et al: Value of 2D-echocardiography for immediate detection of coronary artery disease in the emergency room. *Circulation* 78(suppl II):463,1988.

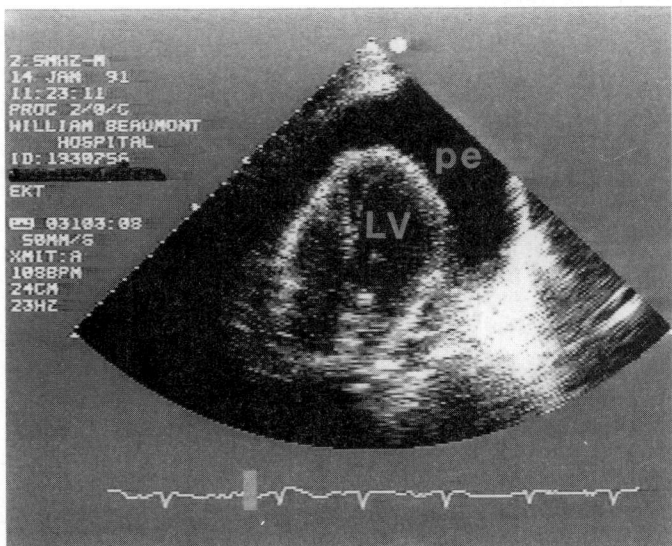

**Fig. 256-4.** Large pericardial effusion (pe) in patient presenting with cardiac tamponade LV = left ventricle.

# 257
# ABDOMINAL SONOGRAPHY
## David Plummer

Technical advances in diagnostic ultrasound have resulted in more inexpensive, portable, and user-friendly two-dimensional ultrasound machines. A number of specialties, including emergency medicine, now routinely use portable bedside ultrasonography to perform goal-directed limited examinations. Limited bedside ultrasound examinations can significantly improve the physician's diagnostic certainty. This can help reduce emergency department time in patients with common disorders (gallbladder disease) or reduce time to definitive intervention and disposition for critical disorders (hemoperitoneum). Limited bedside ultrasound examination is inexpensive, noninvasive, painless, and safe; it can be performed rapidly and serially.

Although sonographers approach any given patient in a standardized fashion, the examination is inherently operator dependent. Emergency abdominal ultrasound examination understandably varies depending on the patient's condition, indication, and findings. Physicians performing and interpreting limited bedside ultrasonography require training and ongoing experience in the technique. The optimal training for emergency physicians using this technique is unknown.

This chapter is divided into four major ultrasound examinations. These examinations apply to critically ill patients (abdominal trauma and abdominal aortic rupture) or in common conditions where limited ultrasonography is a diagnostic cornerstone (cholecystitis and nephrolithiasis).

## EQUIPMENT

A broad range of ultrasound equipment is available. These range in price from approximately $10,000 to several hundred thousand dollars. More expensive machines have options and functions not used by emergency physicians. Most physicians performing emergency department ultrasound require limited functionality and options from the instrument. The components of an ultrasound machine that the emergency physician must be familiar with include the display, transducer, image controls, and recording device.

The various transducer types differ in basic configuration and frequency of ultrasound generated. Mechanical oscillating heads are less expensive and more durable than linear or curved array models although image quality is compromised. High-frequency transducers have superior image quality but are unable to image deep structures. A mechanical oscillating head generating 2.5 to 3.5 MHz ultrasound is a cost-effective choice and useful for all the examinations described below. The image control options on most ultrasound machines initially appear overwhelming. However, the emergency physician need only manipulate the overall gain, time gain control (TGC), and depth controls to successfully obtain a limited scan. A limited goal-directed examination requires knowledge of ultrasonographic principles, anatomy, standard examination protocols, and practice of the skill.

## GENERAL CONSIDERATIONS

Diagnostic ultrasound is an interactive skill and each physician encounters a learning curve. The optimal training guidelines for these examinations initially proposed by medical imaging physicians have been modified to accommodate a limited examination.

Start the examination with the power and depth set to the maximum values. Adjust these settings once the goal structure is imaged. When possible, obtain the scans on at least two planes by rotating the transducer 90°. Begin the examination with the patient in the supine position; this position alone suffices in most cases. Occasionally moving the patient to a different position will augment the examination by moving internal structures or fluid relative to the transducer. When possible, ask the patient to breath hold in different points of the respiratory cycle. A deep breath can markedly improve the operator's ability to see some structures otherwise difficult to see. Apply firm but gentle pressure to improve image quality. This will reduce the distance to the structure, improve skin-transducer contact, and occasionally move bowel contents away from the image plane. Approach each examination knowing what anatomic landmarks to seek. To help in identifying structures, remember that the structures closest to the transducer appear nearest the top of the screen.

## ABDOMINAL TRAUMA

Because of the potentially catastrophic nature of blunt and penetrating abdominal trauma, emergency physicians must approach the trauma patient with a diligent and organized evaluation. Often, the goal of the emergency physician in abdominal trauma is to simply determine the presence of hemoperitoneum. Historically, this has been done by physical examination, mandatory surgical exploration, diagnostic peritoneal lavage (DPL), or computed tomography (CT) scans of the abdomen.

The physical examination is accurate in determining severe intra-abdominal injury in only 45 to 50 percent of trauma patients. Alternatively, mandatory surgical exploration yields an unacceptably high nontherapeutic laparotomy rate. DPL is sensitive for determining hemoperitoneum and continues to be the standard in most trauma centers in the United States. Disadvantages to DPL are that it is invasive and time consuming, and may be overly sensitive, also yielding a high rate of nontherapeutic laparotomies.

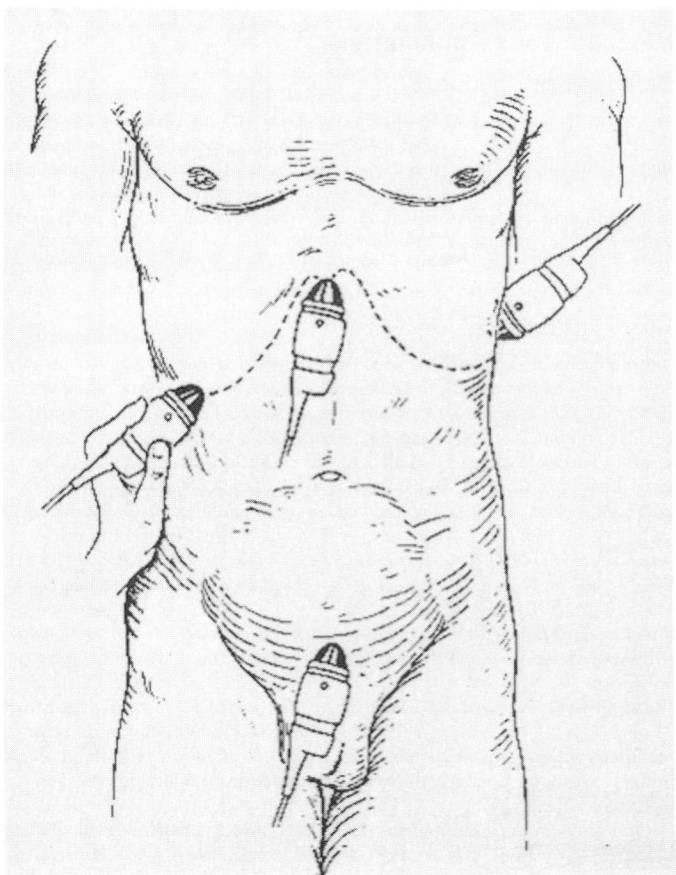

**Fig. 257-1.** Transducer positions for the rapid trauma examination of the abdomen for free fluid.

**Fig. 257-2.** Normal subcostal window. HEP, hepatic parenchyma; PC, pericardial line; RV, right ventricle; LV, left ventricle.

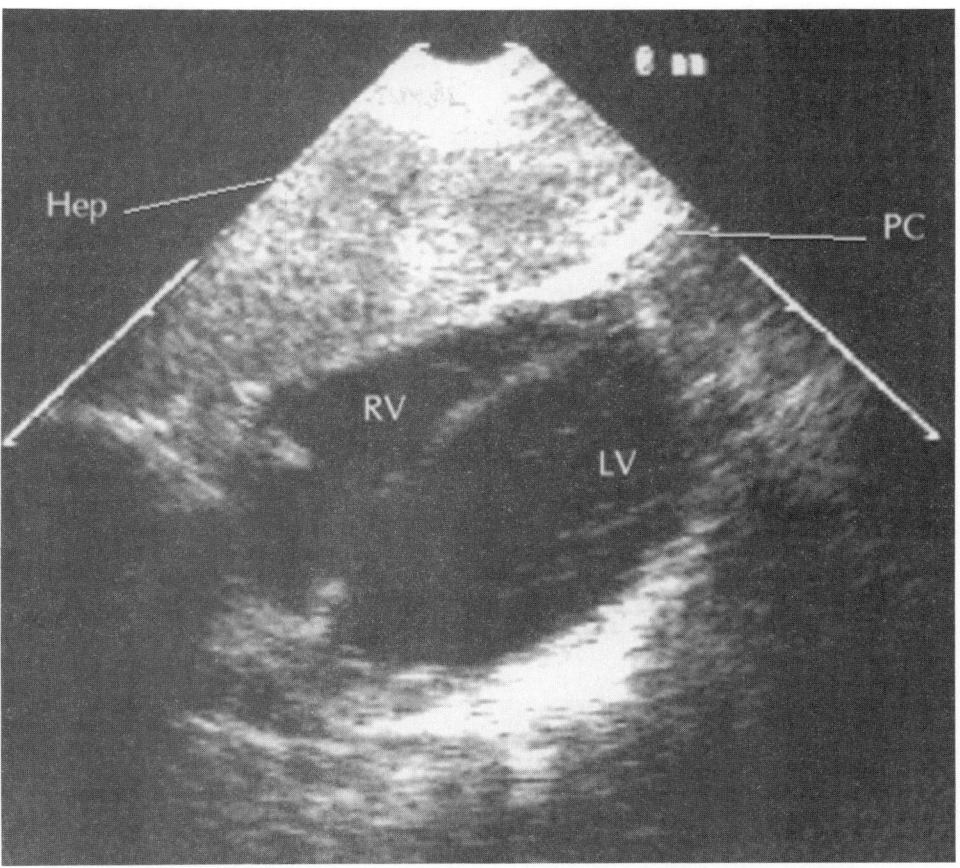

Abdominal CT scan has an advantage over DPL in that it identifies the location and extent of intra-abdominal injuries. Abdominal CT scan also identifies retroperitoneal injuries missed by DPL. Unfortunately, logistical and time requirements of abdominal CT scan, as well as the expertise required for interpretation, often preclude its use in trauma victims.

Abdominal ultrasound has advantages and disadvantages. It is inexpensive, noninvasive, fast, and portable and can be used at the bedside in a serial fashion. The limited goal of this examination is the detection of free abdominal fluid, which is interpreted as hemoperitoneum in the setting of acute trauma. Ultrasound may be the test of choice when timely diagnosis of hemoperitoneum, irrespective of origin, will influence the clinical course. The sequencing of further medical imaging, transfer to the operating room, consultation, or referral for interhospital transfer may all be influenced by the early demonstration of hemoperitoneum.

The sensitivity of abdominal ultrasonography for detecting hemoperitoneum is influenced by the experience of the operator, the timing of the ultrasound examination during resuscitation, the position of the patient during the examination, the number of windows used on a single examination, and the ability to perform serial examinations. Over a dozen prospective controlled series report a sensitivity ranging between 85 and 100 percent, a specificity ranging from 96 to 100 percent, and an accuracy ranging from 94 to 99 percent. Free intra-abdominal fluid collects preferentially in the most dependent portion of the abdomen. In the supine position, there are three dependent areas in the peritoneal cavity. These areas are divided by the spine longitudinally and the pelvic brim transversely. The site of accumulation of intraperitoneal fluid depends on the patient position and the source of the bleeding. Positioning the patient during the ultrasound examination may redistribute free fluid to other intraperitoneal locations. For example, Trendelenburg's position allows pelvic fluid to flow over the pelvic brim into either Morison's pouch on the right or the

splenorenal recess on the left. Unfortunately, hemoperitoneum is at least partially organized and may not redistribute freely with the patient positioning. Hence, the sensitivity and accuracy improve with a multiple window approach. Each abdominal window described below requires approximately 30 s to 1 min to complete.

A false negative result occurs when the ultrasound examination fails to demonstrate free abdominal fluid in the setting of hemoperitoneum. This occurs more commonly when the hemoperitoneum develops slowly or is organized at the time of the examination. A multiple window examination and serial examinations reduce the incidence of false negatives. A false positive examination occurs when free intra-abdominal fluid is detected that is not hemoperitoneum. This may occur as blunt rupture of the bladder or bowel that results in free abdominal fluid. Nonsurgical false positives include patients with ascites, congestive heart failure, or other peritoneal transudative conditions.

## Examination for Abdominal Fluid

Begin the examination in the supine patient by orienting the transducer with a marker dot to the patient's left and adjust the power to maximum and depth to maximum. Reduce these to improve the quality after the goal structure is imaged. Place the transducer in the subxyphoid window (Fig. 257-1). In this window, there is a close interface between the hepatic parenchyma and the echogenic (white) pericardium (Fig. 257-2). Any separation of this interface represents an abnormal collection of fluid. Free abdominal fluid presents as an abnormal anechoic (black) line between the liver and the pericardium (see Figs. 257-2 and 257-3). This fluid can either be intrapericardial or intra-abdominal. Intrapericardial fluid is distinguished from intraperitoneal fluid because it follows the contours of the heart and is seen on different echocardiographic windows. Next, examine Morison's pouch by placing the transducer in the lateral intercostal space

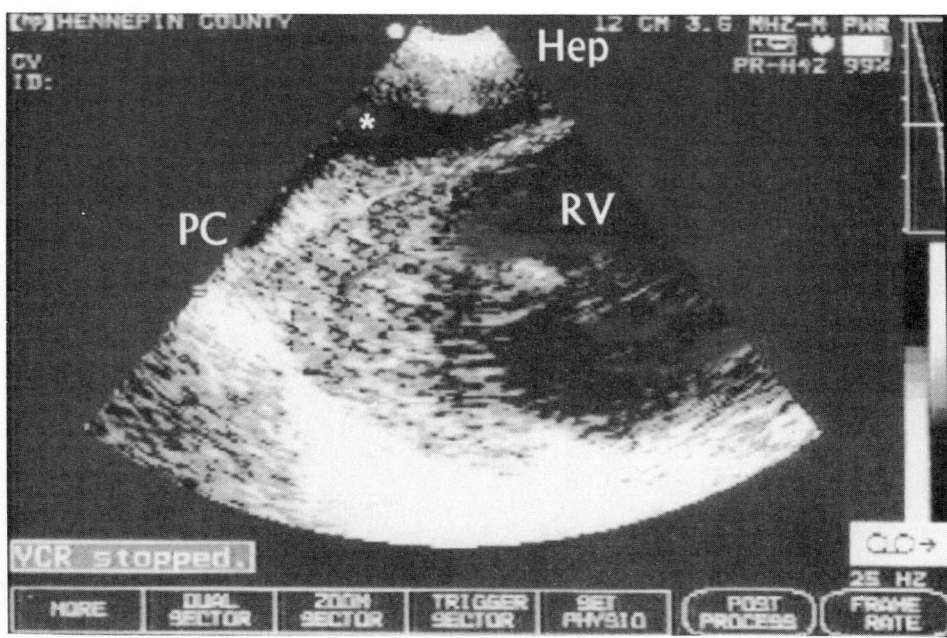

A

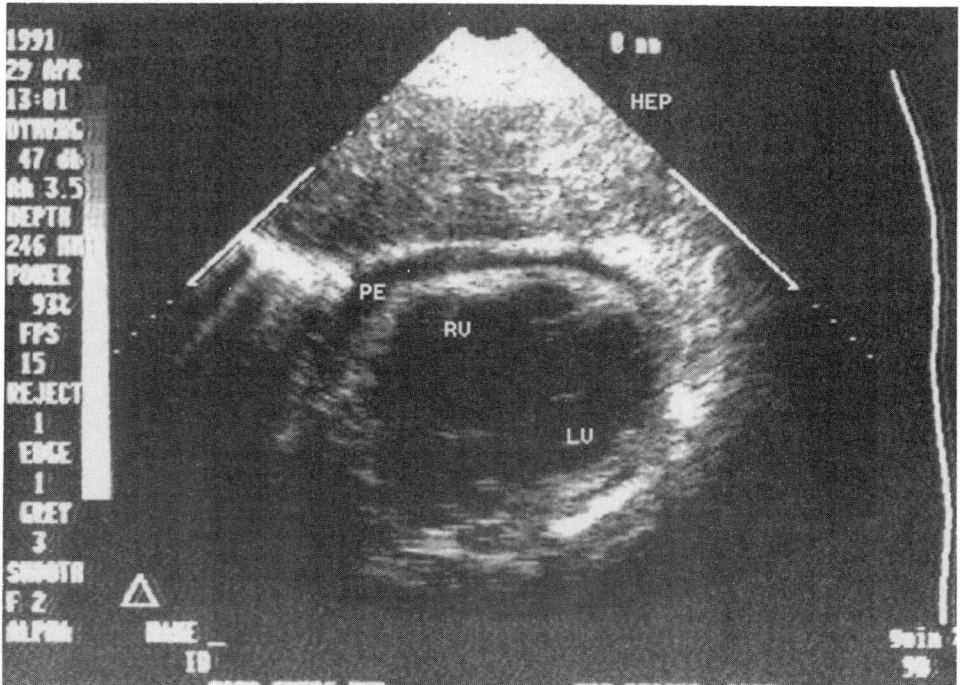

B

**Fig. 257-3.** (A) Subcostal window with intra-abdominal fluid. HEP, hepatic parenchyma; PC, pericardial line; RV, right ventricle; star, intra-abdominal fluid. (B) Subcostal window demonstrating pericardial effusion. HEP, hepatic parenchyma; PE, pericardial effusion; RV, right ventricle; LV, left ventricle.

between the anterior axillary and midaxillary line (see Fig. 257-1). The sonographic landmark most easily identified is the kidney, which appears as an oval structure with characteristic echogenic (white) collecting system. Morison's pouch, which is a potential space, is a peritoneal reflection bounded by the kidney (Gerota's fascia) and the liver (Glisson's capsule) (Fig. 257-4). Free intra-abdominal fluid appears as an anechoic stripe within Morison's pouch separating the liver from the kidney (Fig. 257-5). Note that free fluid appears with sharp angles in the recesses of the peritoneal reflection.

The next region to examine is the left lateral window. Obtain this window by placing the transducer in the left midaxillary to posterior apillary line with a marker dot toward the patient's feet. This is similar to the right lateral window, and the kidney again is a sonographic landmark. The splenorenal recess, analogous to Morison's pouch on

the right, is a potential space created by peritoneal reflection between the spleen and the kidney (Fig. 257-6). Free intra-abdominal fluid causes a separation of these normal interfaces with anechoic areas (Fig. 257-7). As with a right lateral view, fluid in this window can be augmented by Trendelenburg's position. The most dependent portion of the pelvis can be visualized using the suprapubic window. Obtain this view by placing the transducer in the midline immediately cephalad to the symphysis pubis with a marker dot facing the patient's feet (see Fig. 257-1). If the bladder contains urine, it serves as an unmistakable acoustic window and landmark (Fig. 257-8). This window allows for assessment of the pouch of Douglas (a peritoneal reflection and potential space between the uterus and the rectum) and the retrovesical pouch in males). Reverse Trendelenburg augments this examination.

**Fig. 257-4.** Normal Morison's pouch and renal view. Diaph, diaphragm; HEP, hepatic parenchyma; MOR, Morison's pouch; REN, kidney.

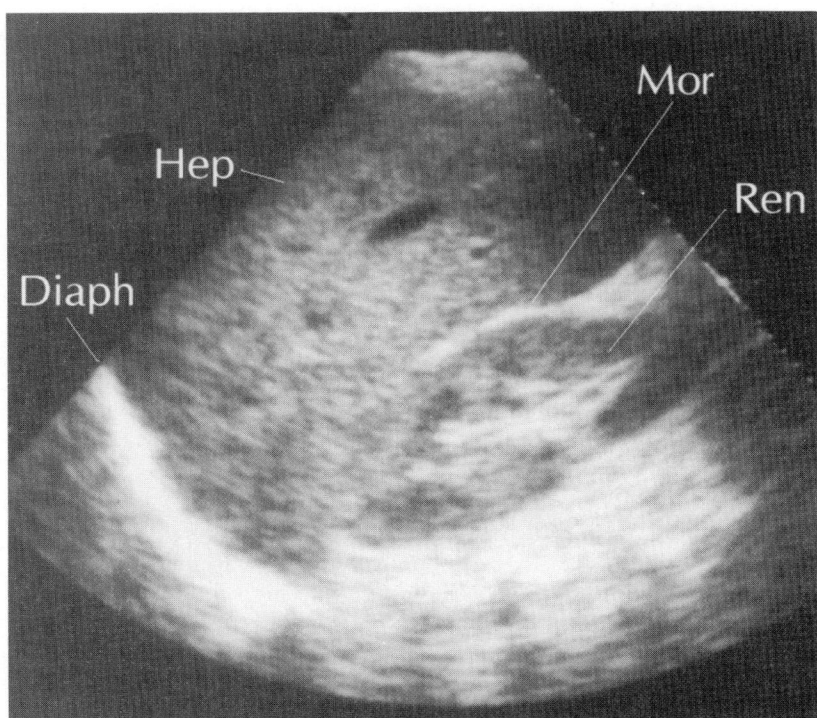

In each of these windows, fresh unclotted blood appears anechoic and displays sharp acute angles because of its ability to flow freely. As clotting begins, the blood displays different degrees of echogenicity. The presence of free fluid, in the setting of trauma, without a preexisting abdominal fluid, must be considered hemoperitoneum until proved otherwise. Abdominal sonography does not accurately quantify the amount of free abdominal fluid. Most authors believe as little as 250 mL of fluid can be detected in Morison's pouch in Trendelenburg's position. A separation of 0.5 cm or more in width correlates roughly with 500 mL of fluid in an adult. The minimal amount of fluid detectable is unknown.

## ABDOMINAL AORTA

Rupture of the abdominal aortic aneurysm (RAAA) is one of the deadliest emergencies. Most patients with RAAA suffer prehospital death. Of those who arrive to the hospital alive, the mortality rate is over 50 percent. Up to one third of patients presenting with RAAA are initially misdiagnosed; up to 80 percent of patients who present

**Fig. 257-5.** Hemoperitoneum manifesting as fluid in Morison's pouch. REN, renal; MOR, Morison's pouch; HEP, hepatic parenchyma; HEM, hemoperitoneum.

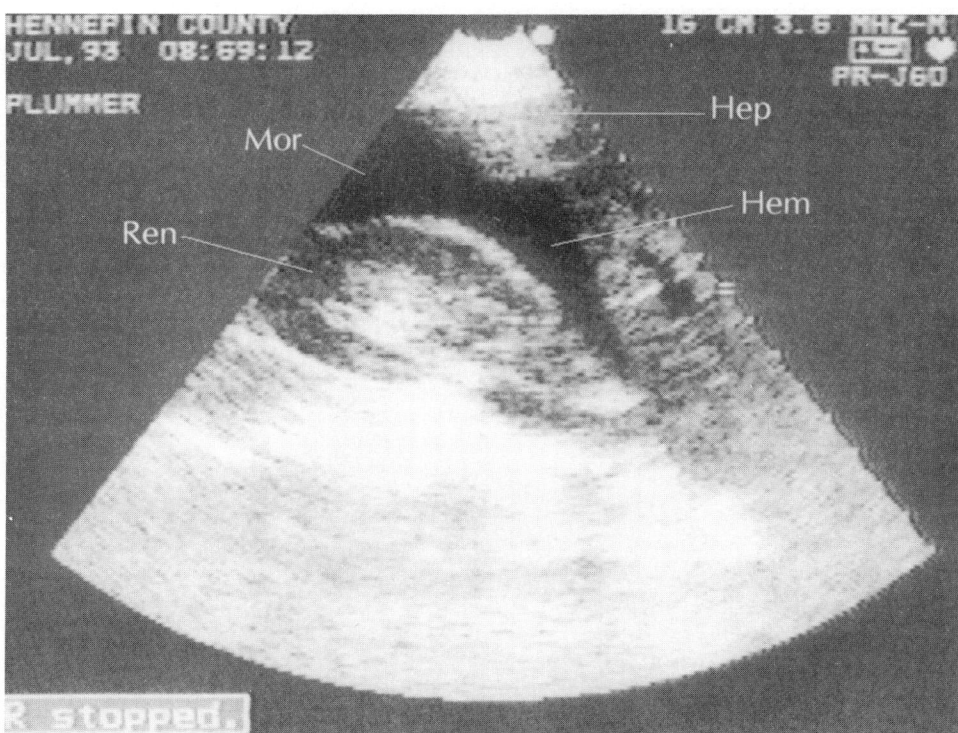

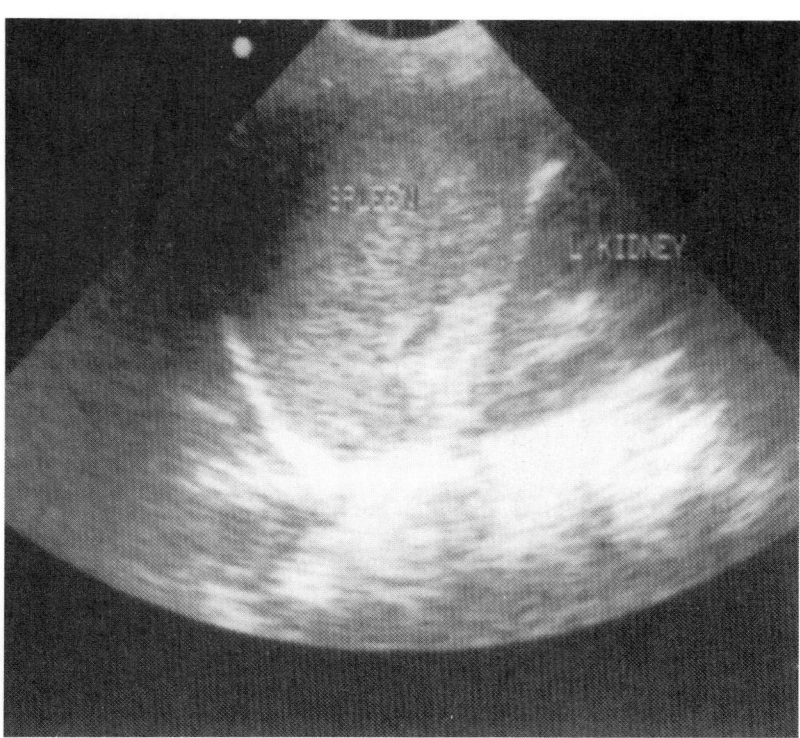

**Fig. 257-6.** Normal left upper quadrant with spleen and left kidney visualized.

with RAAA have no previous documented diagnosis of abdominal aortic aneurysm (AAA). Rapid screening for the presence of AAA can accurately guide the physician to include or exclude RAAA in appropriate patients.

## Anatomy

The abdominal aorta begins at the diaphragm and continues to the aortic bifurcation, approximately at the level of the umbilicus. The normal external aortic diameter is 2.1 cm for the average adult male and 1.8 cm for the average adult female and demonstrates a gradual tapering from the diaphragm to the bifurcation. An AAA is any irreversible dilation of the aorta to 1.5 times its normal size. Consequently, any aorta with an external diameter of greater than 3 cm is an AAA, but AAA may present only as a loss of distal tapering.

## Indications

Limited ultrasonography of the abdominal aorta should be performed at the bedside in any patient suspected of having RAAA.

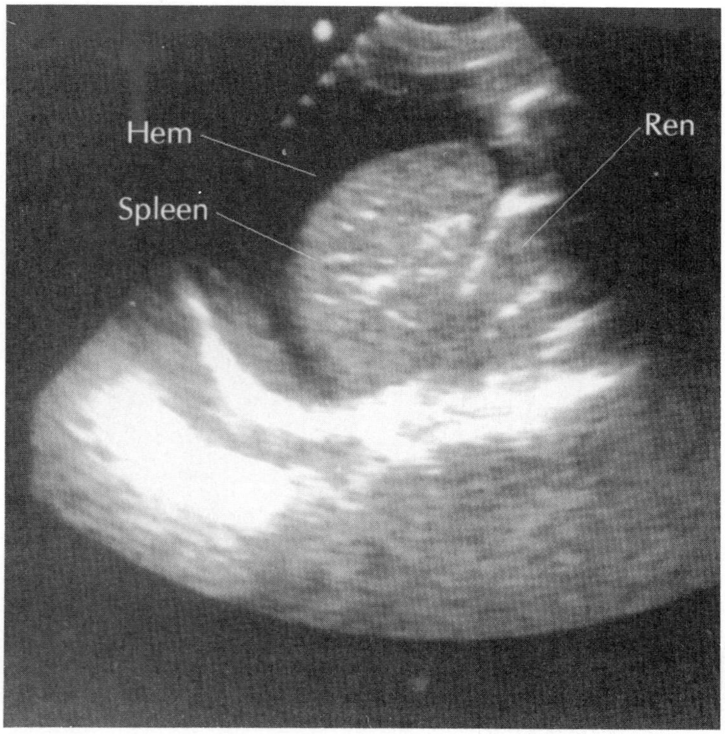

**Fig. 257-7.** Left intercostal oblique window demonstrating hemoperitoneum. HEM, hemoperitoneum; REN, kidney.

**Fig. 257-8.** Transverse view of the bladder using the suprapubic window. Arrow indicates region of pouch of Douglas.

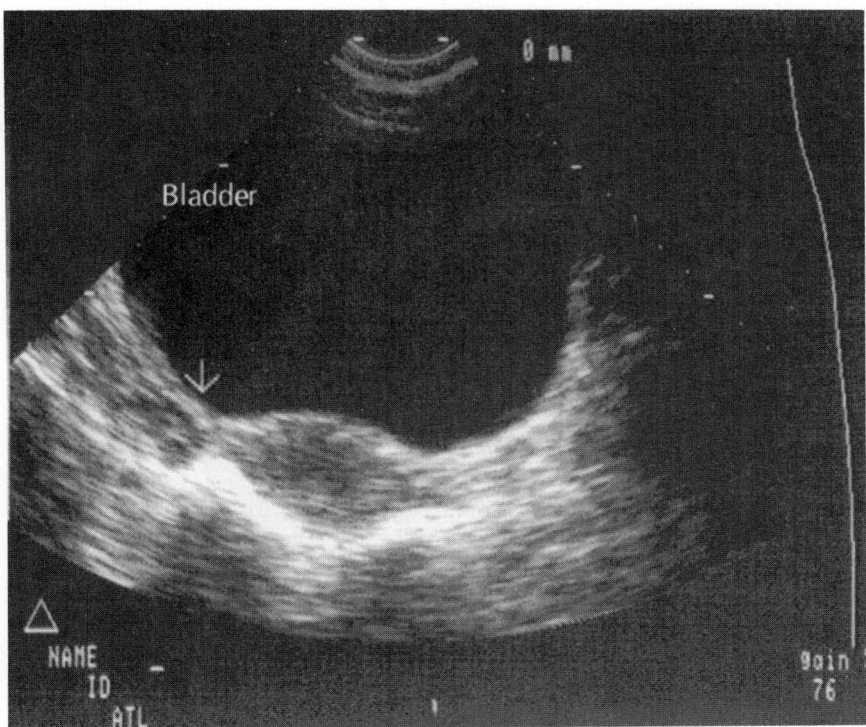

## Contraindications

Do not delay standard resuscitation to perform this examination. Do not perform this test on patients with sufficient indication to disposition appropriately.

## Patient Preparation and Examination Technique

Patients undergoing this examination in the emergency department are likely not to be prepared in the traditional fashion. Patients should remain supine and often in Trendelenburg's position. Place the trans-

ducer in the subxyphoid region with the marker dot toward the patient's feet. Gently sweep the transducer until the longitudinal view of the aorta is obtained (Fig. 257-9). Measure the aortic diameter in this view to ensure that it is less than 3 cm. Usually, patients with RAAA will display an unmistakable dilation of an abdominal aorta, which dominates this window (Fig. 257-10). Slowly rotate the transducer so that the marker dot faces the patient's left. This window views the aorta in cross section (Fig. 257-11). The aortic diameter can again be measured in this orientation, and patients with AAA often display marked dilation (Fig. 257-12). Often, patients with AAA

**Fig. 257-9.** Long axis view of abdominal aorta.

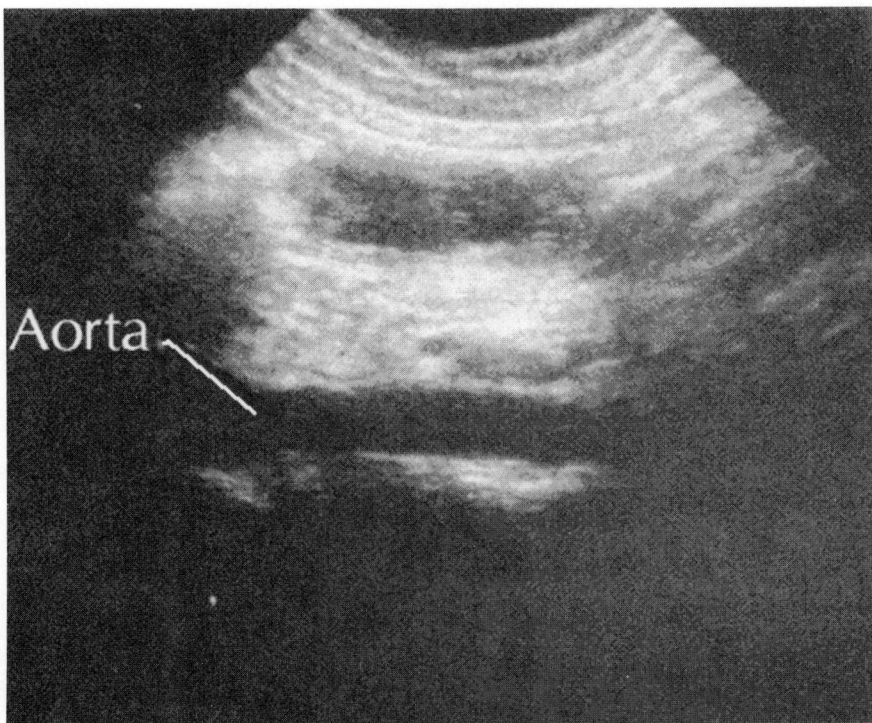

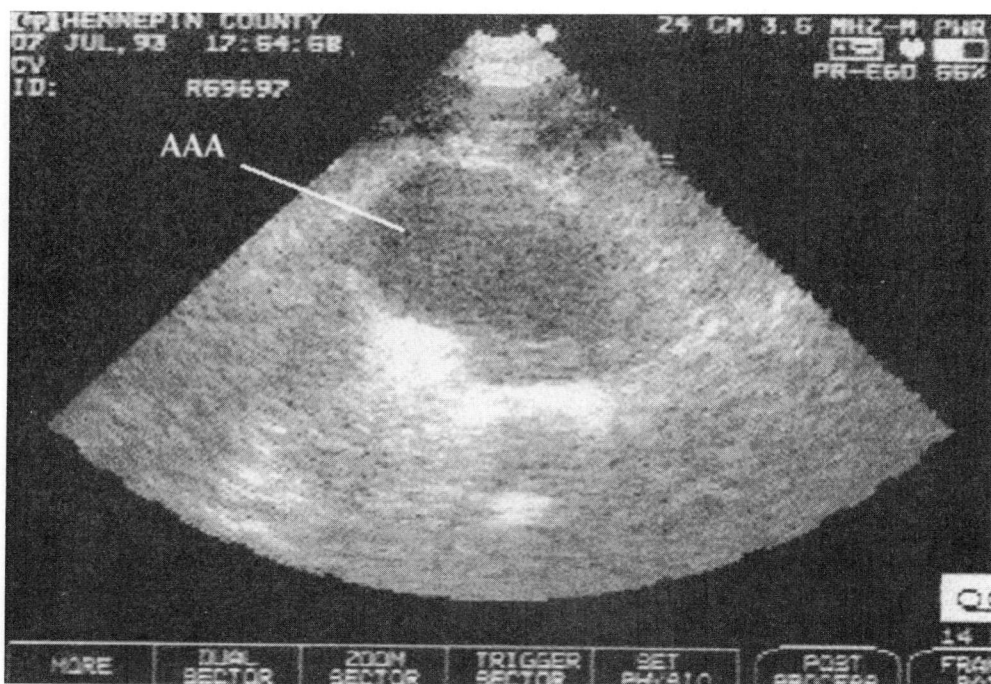

**Fig. 257-10.** Long axis view of an abdominal aortic aneurysm measuring 9 cm in diameter.

have a significant degree of intraluminal thrombosis, which is diffusely echogenic and often nearly concentric.

## Ultrasound in Detecting Abdominal Aortic Rupture

Ultrasound is 100 percent sensitive for the detection of AAA but is insensitive in determining RAAA. In the proper clinical setting (hemodynamic instability with abdominal pain), patients displaying AAA by bedside ultrasonography should be considered to have an RAAA until proven otherwise. Alternatively, you can rule out RAAA if the aorta displays a normal diameter. In the appropriate clinical setting, the screening test has 100 percent positive predictive value for RAAA, 97 percent negative predictive value for RAAA, and a 97 percent overall accuracy. The test should be completed within 60 s.

RAAAs most often leak into the retroperitoneal space. This hemorrhage rapidly organizes, becomes echogenic, and is ultrasonically identical to the surrounding retroperitoneal structures. Rarely, AAA will rupture into the intraperitoneal space. An ultrasound examination of the abdomen may help confirm the presence of hemoperitoneum using the windows described above under trauma.

## BILIARY COLIC

Upper abdominal pain is an extremely common emergency department presentation, and most emergency physicians are familiar with the classic presentation of cholecystitis and cholelithiasis. Unfortunately, many patients with these disorders do not present in a classic manner, and conversely other serious and potential life-threatening

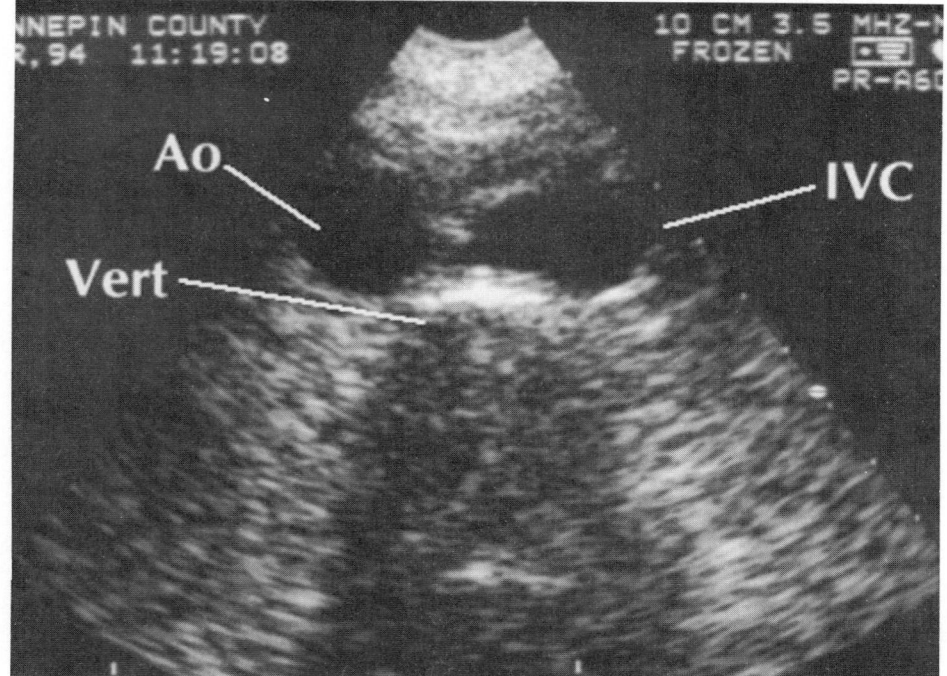

**Fig. 257-11.** Normal short axis view of the abdominal aorta. Ao, aorta; VERT, vertebral column; IVC, inferior vena cava.

**Fig. 257-12.** Short axis view of abdominal aortic aneurysm. AAA, abdominal aortic aneurysm; Vert, vertebral column; IVC, inferior vena cava.

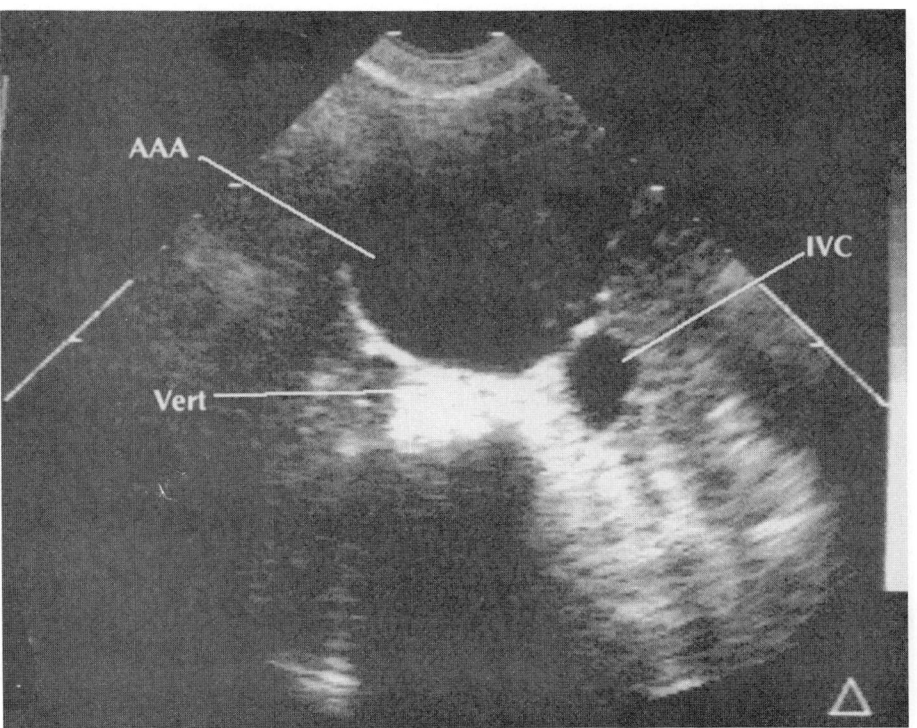

disorders can present as gallbladder disease. Although it is not a life-threatening disorder, symptomatic gallbladder disease is important for the emergency physician to diagnosis. The anatomic characteristics of the gallbladder make it ideally suited for ultrasound examination.

## Examination Technique

Begin the evaluation of the gallbladder by placing the probe in the right midclavicular line with a marker dot positioned toward the patient's feet (sagittal plane). Deep breath-holding by the patient will

enhance this view. Begin this examination with the patient supine; however, moving the patient to the left lateral decubitus or semi-upright position may enhance this view in difficult patients. Repositioning also helps define the dependent nature of any gallstones visualized.

## Ultrasound Findings

A normal gallbladder is visualized as a homogenous, cystic, anechoic structure (Fig. 257-13). Patients with cholecystitis may display any

**Fig. 257-13.** Normal gall bladder. HEP, hepatic parechyma, Gb, gallbladder.

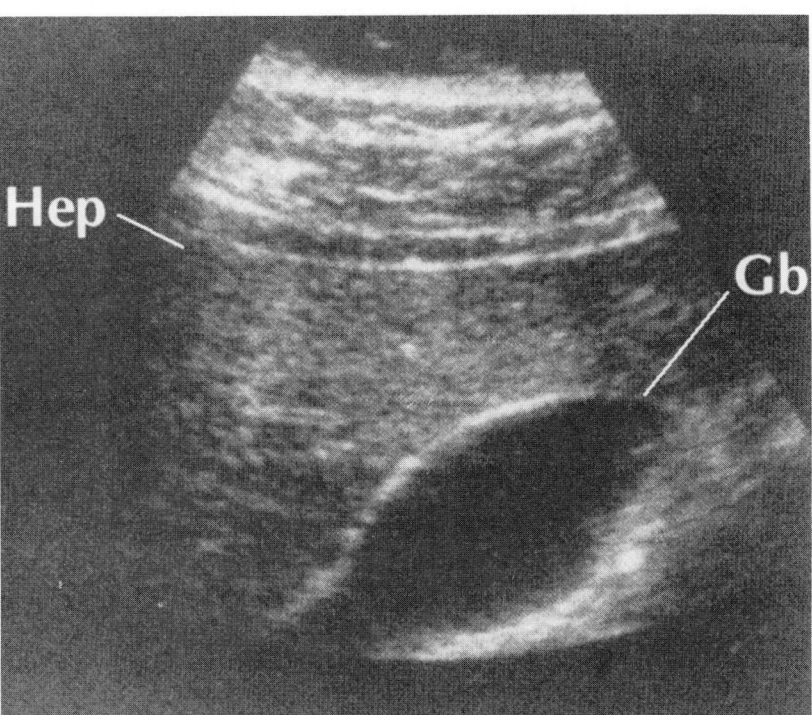

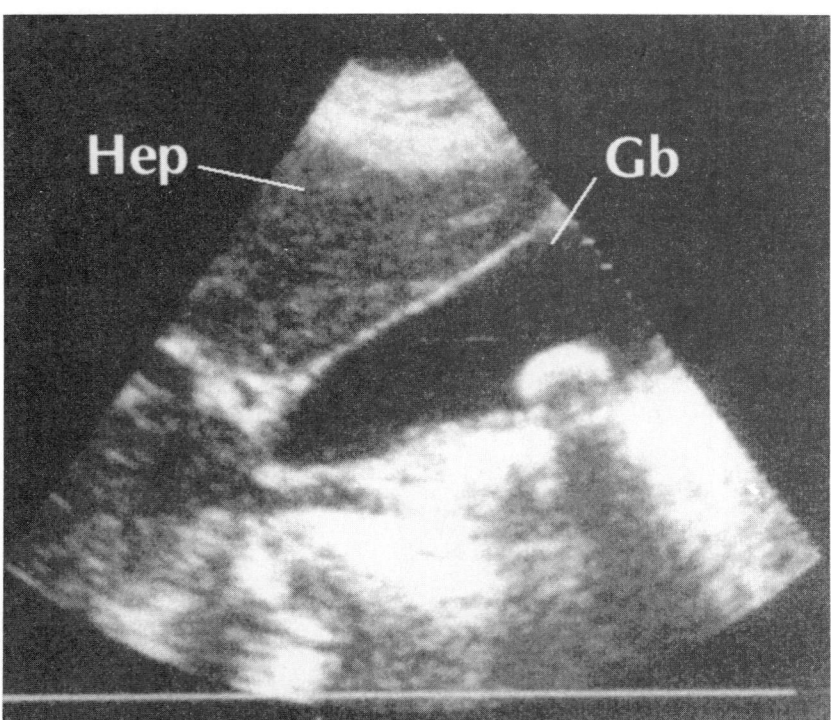

**Fig. 257-14.** Gallbladder with solitary large gallstone. HEP, hepatic parechyma; Gb, gallbladder.

combination of five characteristic ultrasonographic abnormalities: gallstones, gallbladder wall thickening, the sonographic Murphy sign, pericholecystic fluid, or air in the biliary system.

Ninety-five percent of patients with cholecystitis have calculous cholecystitis. *Gallstones,* if present, are highly reflective and cause a distal acoustic shadowing (Fig. 257-14). Gallstones are fully mobile and therefore visualized in a dependent portion of the gallbladder. Repositioning the patient repositions the gallstones into the new dependent portion of the gallbladder. Cholelithiasis, with impaction in the cystic duct or distally, may be impossible to visualize. A second characteristic of gallbladder disease is thickening of the gallbladder wall. This *thickening* can occur even in the absence of stones, and therefore, may be the only finding in the minority of patients with acalculous cholecystitis. The normal gallbladder wall is not more than 3 mm thick. Unfortunately, gallbladder wall thickness is nonspecific and can be present in ascites, congestive heart failure, renal failure, and other edematous states. A third finding present in cholecystitis is the *sonographic Murphy sign,* which is defined as tenderness to the probe pressure when positioned over the gallbladder. This sign, along with either cholelithiasis or wall thickening, strongly suggests the diagnosis of acute cholecystitis. The absence of the sonographic Murphy sign, cholelithiasis, and gallbladder thickening rules out cholecystitis with approximately 95 percent accuracy.

*Pericholecystic fluid* is a fourth indirect sign of acute gallbladder disease and indicates possible perforation. Air in the gallbladder wall, *emphysematous cholecystitis,* is an unusual finding. Sludge, which represents thickened bile with crystals in suspension, appears as a dependent homogenous echodensity in the gallbladder. The clinical significance of this sonographic finding is unclear.

## RENAL COLIC

Renal colic, secondary to obstructive uropathy, is an extremely common condition presenting to the emergency department. Most emergency physicians are familiar with this distinctive clinical syndrome. Unfortunately, many patients do not present with classic signs and symptoms (acute costovertebral angle pain with hematuria) or are unable to tolerate traditional diagnostic tests. Conversely, an occasional

patient with a serious, and even life-threatening disorder, can present mimicking renal colic. Up to 10 percent of RAAAs mimic renal colic. Traditional intravenous pyelogram (IVP) is the current diagnostic gold standard. The IVP offers superior documentation of the presence, size, and location of obstructive uropathy. Unfortunately, many patients, including children, diabetic patients, pregnant patients, those with contrast allergies, dehydrated patients, or patients with congestive heart failure may not tolerate traditional IVP. In addition, ultrasound may be the test of choice when there is a delay in obtaining the IVP.

## Imaging Techniques

In the supine patient, place the probe in a low intercostal or infracostal location in the midclavicular line with a marker dot pointing to the patient's feet. Slowly sweep the ultrasound plane until the kidney is visualized. The normal kidney is a 6 × 12 oval structure with a relatively irregular echogenic collection system (see Fig. 257-4). Rotation of the probe allows you to visualize the kidney, in both longitudinal and transverse orientations. The liver facilitates examination of the right kidney by acting as an acoustic window. Examination of the left kidney is more difficult because the spleen does not provide a good acoustic window.

## Ultrasound Findings

Direct visualization of the stone in nephrolithiasis is extremely difficult. Alternatively, the hydronephrosis of obstructive uropathy is relatively straightforward. Hydronephrosis presents as a cystic (black) dilation within the echogenic collecting system (Fig. 257-15). Intraparechymal renal cysts have a similar appearance and may not be distinguishable sonographically. However, unilateral hydronephrosis, in the presence of pain, has been shown to have 100 percent sensitivity and 95 percent specificity for the presence of acute obstructive uropathy in both adult and pediatric patients. Rarely, patients may present in pain with obstructive uropathy without hydronephrosis. This may be a consequence of a number of preexisting disorders resulting in renal scarring or dehydration. Most authors believe these patients account for less than 5 percent of those presenting with obstructive

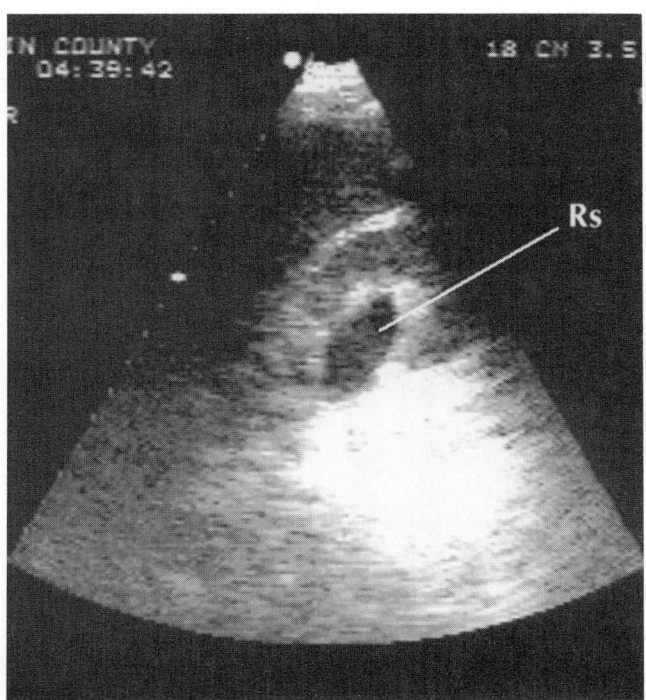

**Fig. 257-15.** Right lateral oblique view illustrates dilated renal sinus collecting system from obstructive uropathy. HEP, hepatic parenchyma; RS, renal sinus.

uropathy. In addition, patients will rarely present with obstructive uropathy without nephrolithiasis. This can occur as a result of a number of intra-abdominal or retroperitoneal mass lesions causing intrinsic compression of the aorta.

## BIBLIOGRAPHY

Chang T, Lapanto L. Ultrasonography in the emergency setting. *Emerg Med Clin North Am* February:1, 1992.

Kimura A, Otsuka T. Emergency center ultrasonography in the evaluation of hemoperitoneum: a prospective study. *J Trauma* 31:20, 1991.

Kremkau FW. *Diagnostic Ultrasound: Principles, Instruments, and Exercises,* 3d ed. Philadelphia: WB Saunders, 1989.

Mateer J, Plummer D, Heller M, et al. Model curriculum for physician training in emergency ultrasonography. *Ann Emerg Med* 23:95, 1994.

Rozycki G, Ochsmer G, Jaffin J, Champion H. Prospective evaluation of surgeon's use of ultrasound in evaluation of trauma patients. *J Trauma* 34:516, 1993.

Shuman WP, Hastrup WJ, Kohler TR, et al. Suspected leaking abdominal aortic aneurysm: use of sonography in the emergency room. *Radiology* 168, 1988.

Tiling T, Bouillon B, Schmid A, et al. Ultrasonography in the blunt abdominal. Border J (ed). *Blunt Multiple Trauma, Comprehensive Pathophysiology and Care.*

# 258
# PELVIC ULTRASONOGRAPHY

**Wesley Lee**
**Christine Comstock**

The emergency department is often responsible for the diagnosis and stabilization of women with obstetric and gynecologic problems. This chapter reviews major concepts regarding the evaluation of vaginal bleeding and pelvic pain by diagnostic ultrasound. Specifically, the sonographic findings associated with early normal, failing, ectopic, and molar pregnancy are discussed. Timely evaluation of vaginal bleeding caused by placenta previa or abruption also requires consideration. Finally, the ultrasound appearance of common adnexal masses is described.

## TECHNIQUES

There are two main types of gray-scale ultrasound imaging techniques—static and real-time. Static images are often recorded onto x-ray film and sometimes displayed onto computer screens. They may contain limited but valuable image information that is highly dependent on the sonographer's ability to accurately "capture" an ultrasound finding onto film. Real-time ultrasound is a superior method that records motion video sequences onto magnetic tape for convenient review. This technique allows the physician to examine anatomic structures from different scanning planes and provides a way to easily document fetal motion or cardiac activity.

A wide variety of transducers are available for pelvic sonography. A linear transducer produces a rectangular image that is especially useful for panoramic views of the near-term fetus. A sector transducer produces a pie-shaped image and is used when the sonographer needs to angle toward the structure of interest. Higher-frequency probes (e.g., 5 to 7 MHz) provide greater ultrasound resolution but less penetration when compared with lower-frequency probes. Conversely, lower-frequency transducers (e.g., 3.5 MHz probes) provide deeper acoustic penetration but do not offer the same degree of resolution often required for examination of very small structures.

The full bladder is used as an acoustic window into the pelvis for transabdominal ultrasound. Air in the bowel reflects sound back to the transducer and may prevent propagation of this signal to the pelvic organ of interest. A full bladder pushes the bowel laterally and allows acoustic visualization of pelvic structures. This structure is appropriately filled if the posterior bladder wall is even with or just above the superior uterine margin. Doubt should be raised about the results of any pelvic ultrasound examination where the bladder is not full enough to reveal the entire uterus in the sagittal plane or in cases where overfilling compresses the uterus posteriorly. The need for bladder catheterization can be minimized by simply prohibiting voiding.

Transvaginal sonography should be performed by the most experienced examiners because many potential pitfalls are associated with anatomic orientation, scanning technique, interpretation, and clinical diagnosis. Vaginal sonography is useful for patients whose abdominal scan is compromised by obesity, prior surgical scarring, abnormal amniotic fluid volume, or decreased urine in the maternal bladder. The abdominal and vaginal scans should be considered complementary to each other. For instance, abdominal sonography will provide the necessary acoustic depth penetration and visualization of the upper abdomen, whereas vaginal scanning can often provide better resolution of pelvic structures. Transvaginal ultrasound is contraindicated for premature rupture of membranes during pregnancy. In that case, translabial scanning can be performed with a transducer covered by a

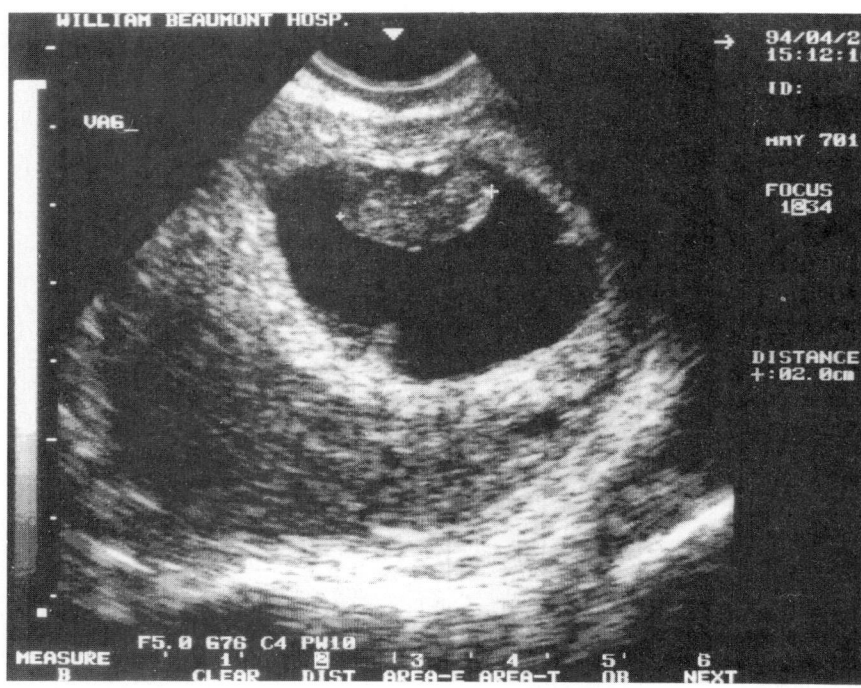

**Fig. 258-1.** Early fetus. Electronic calipers indicate points from which the crown-rump length can be measured. Cardiac activity should be present when this measurement is at least 5 mm.

protective latex glove to provide additional information that may not be otherwise accessible by abdominal ultrasound.

## NORMAL EARLY PREGNANCY

Sonographic findings should be interpreted on the basis of accurate gestational dating criteria such as menstrual history or prior early ultrasound studies. By convention, all measurements relating to the fetus are expressed as menstrual age from the first day of the last normal menstrual period. A patient who is certain of her menstrual dates and reports regular cycles with no antecedent use of oral contraceptives provides an excellent basis for pregnancy dating by history alone.

Fertilization of the egg occurs in the distal fallopian tube approxi-

mately 13 days before the first day of the next expected menstrual period, regardless of cycle length. The developing embryo travels down into the uterus and implants on the uterine wall 5 days later. Cardiac activity should be detected shortly after the sac yolk appears, usually by 6 weeks from the first day of the last normal menstrual period. As the fetus grows, its crown-rump length can be measured (Fig. 258-1). This length can estimate fetal age within ± 4 days up to 12 weeks' gestation.

## FAILING EARLY PREGNANCY

A failing early pregnancy can be associated with nonspecific symptoms of lower abdominal pain and vaginal bleeding. These symptoms can also occur with an otherwise uncomplicated intrauterine preg-

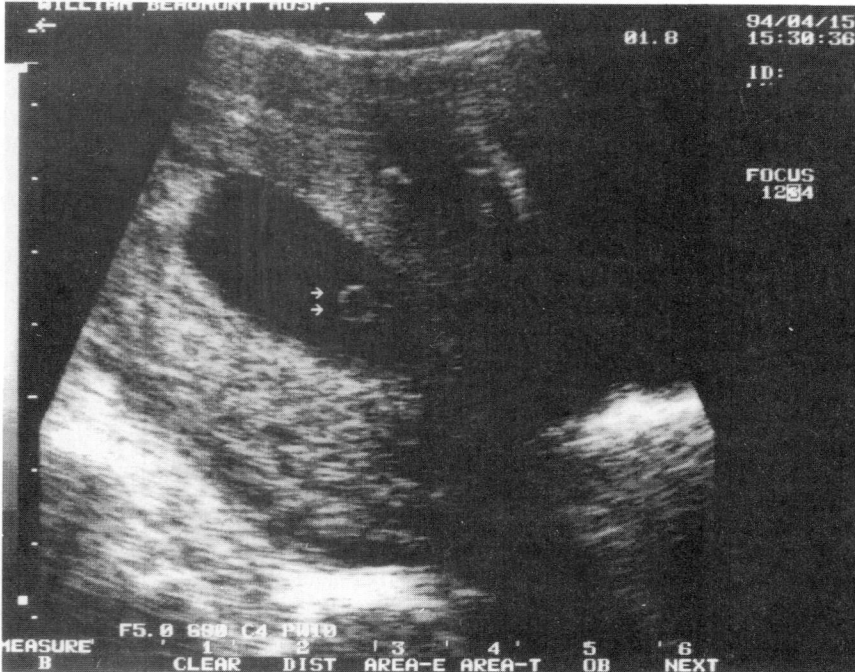

**Fig. 258-2.** Appearance of normal yolk sac (*arrows*). The fetal pole is not yet visible but will develop along the top of the yolk sac. This structure is normally visible when the mean sac diameter exceeds 10 mm by vaginal sonography.

**Fig. 258-3.** Appearance of the amniotic membrane (*arrows*) with the embryo below. Identification of this membrane without a fetal pole strongly suggests a "blighted ovum," especially if the pregnancy exceeds 6 weeks' menstrual age.

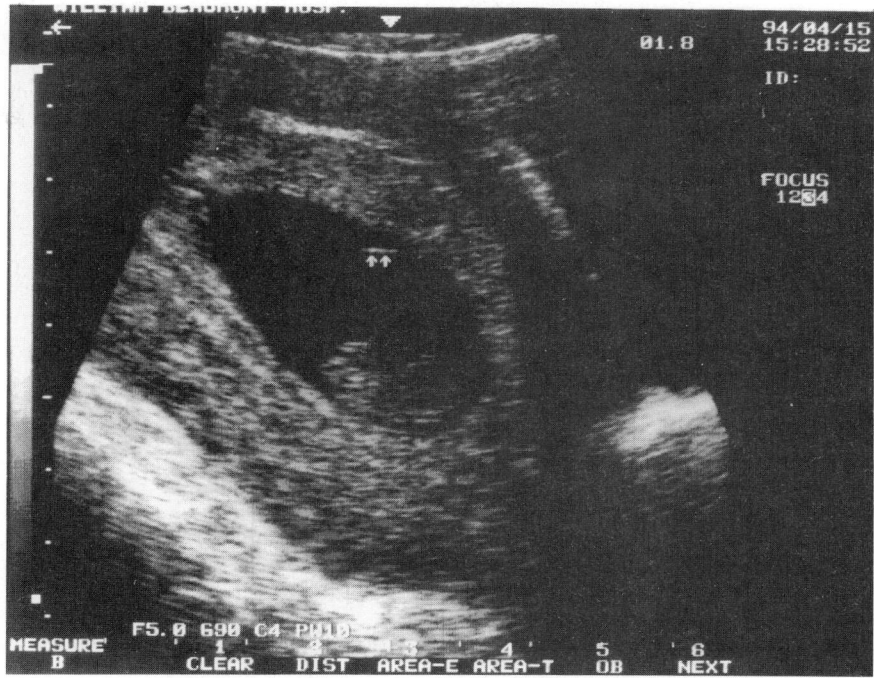

nancy. However, correlation of history with sonographic, clinical, and laboratory findings may collectively provide important information about pregnancy status.

## Intrauterine

The gestational sac is the first major sonographic sign to appear as a marker of early pregnancy and is visible by about 5 menstrual weeks. This structure is ordinarily round or oval, but the pregnancy should always be considered as "viable" if cardiac activity is present. A grossly distorted (e.g., irregular and elongated) gestational sac suggests an abnormal pregnancy, but this subjective finding is not always reliable. Abdominal ultrasound should detect a fetal pole with a mean gestational sac diameter of 2.5 cm or greater. By comparison,

vaginal sonography will detect an embryo with a mean sac diameter of at least 1.8 cm.

The yolk sac is an important source of nutritional exchange for the embryo and makes its first sonographic appearance at about 5.5 menstrual weeks (Fig. 258-2). Identification of the yolk sac can provide important clues about the pregnancy. For example, a mean gestational sac diameter of 20 mm without a yolk sac by abdominal ultrasound (10 mm by vaginal sonography) is highly suggestive of abnormal pregnancy. An abnormal pregnancy is also suggested if the embryo is visualized without a yolk sac by either method. If the dating criteria are firm, a definite gestational sac (intrauterine fluid collection with yolk sac) should be visualized by 5.5 to 6 menstrual weeks. Cardiac activity is usually detectable by vaginal ultrasound by 6 weeks' gestation.

**Fig. 258-4.** Double decidual sac (dds) sign can help to distinguish between a true gestational sac from the pseudogestational sac of ectopic pregnancy. Two concentric rings can be seen surrounding the intrauterine gestational sac.

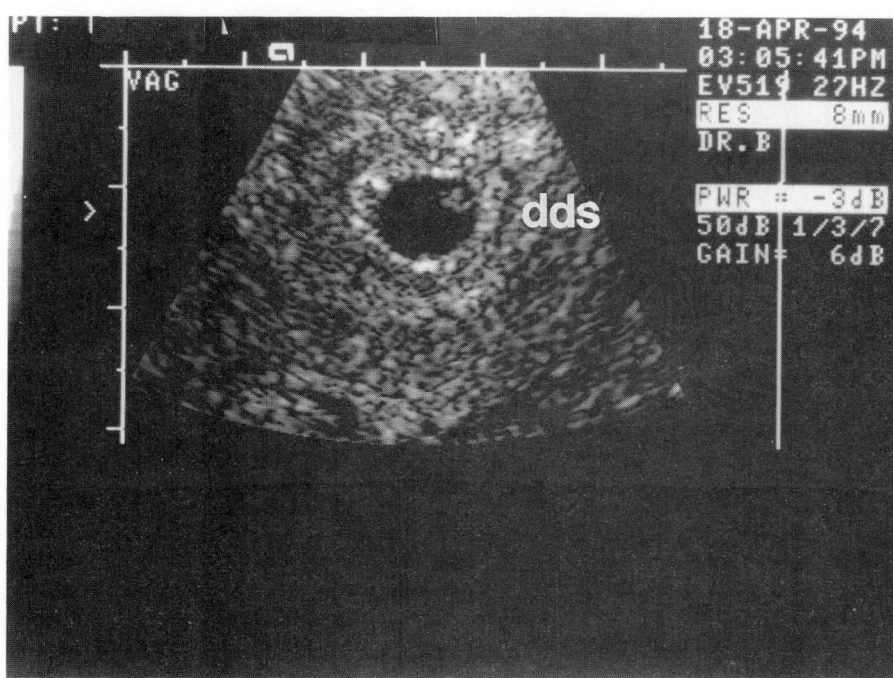

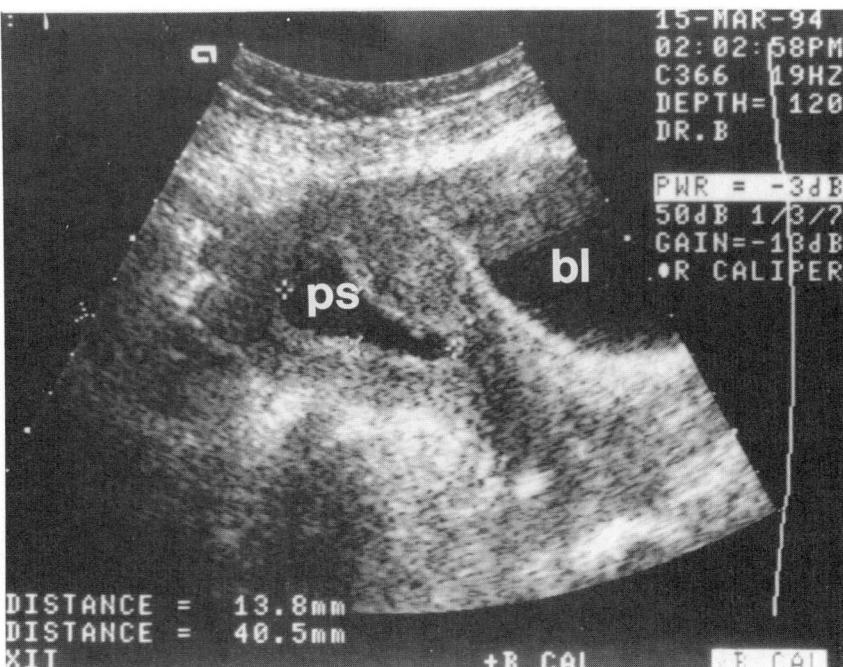

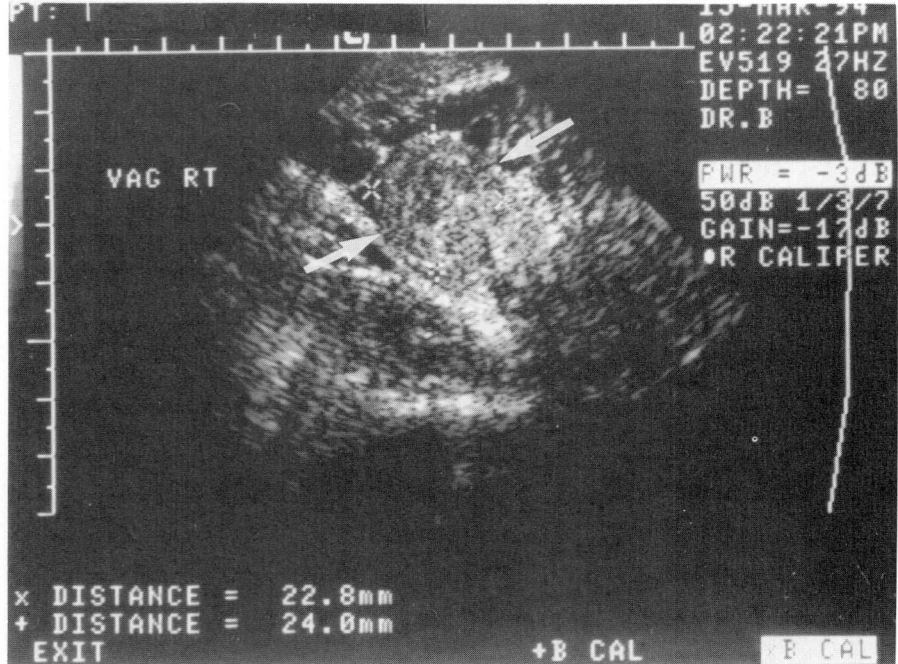

**Fig. 258-5.** (A) Irregular intrauterine fluid collection with echogenic lining mimics a pregnancy sac in this sagittal scan of the uterus. (PS, pseudogestational sac; bl, bladder.) (B) Transvaginal ultrasound examination detected a 2.4-cm right adnexal mass (*arrows*). A right tubal pregnancy was confirmed by surgery.

The physician should carefully look for other important sonographic signs of pregnancy status. For example, visualization of amniotic membrane without an embryo is strong evidence for anembryonic pregnancy ("blighted ovum") (Fig. 258-3). A low sac position adjacent to the cervix, size less than dates, decreased amniotic fluid volume, or slow heart rate (< 90 bpm beyond 6 menstrual weeks) are worrisome signs of a failing pregnancy. Embryos with crown-rump length of 5 mm or greater who fail to demonstrate cardiac activity can also be safely considered as "nonviable."

### Extrauterine

The emergency physician plays a central role in the identification, evaluation, and stabilization of women presenting with ectopic preg-

nancy. This condition refers to any gestational sac that is found outside the normal intrauterine implantation site. *All women presenting to the emergency department with lower abdominal pain must be evaluated for the possibility of ectopic pregnancy.* This consideration is very important for every pregnant patient without preexisting documentation of an intrauterine gestation. Over 96 percent of such cases are located in the fallopian tube with the ampulla being the most common site of implantation (41 percent). Other implantation areas will involve the uterine cornua (1.8 percent), abdomen (1.4 percent), cervix (0.16 percent), and ovary (0.16 percent). Risk factors include prior ectopic pregnancy, history of pelvic surgery, pelvic inflammatory disease, presence of an intrauterine device, advanced maternal age, history of tubal sterilization, and in vitro fertilization.

**Fig. 258-6.** Left adnexal cystic mass is identified in this transverse view of the uterus and maternal bladder (BL). This patient had irregular periods and conceived after an intrauterine device failure. Serial β-hCG levels did not rise appropriately. Arrows point to a 1.6-cm right tubal (ampullary) ectopic pregnancy.

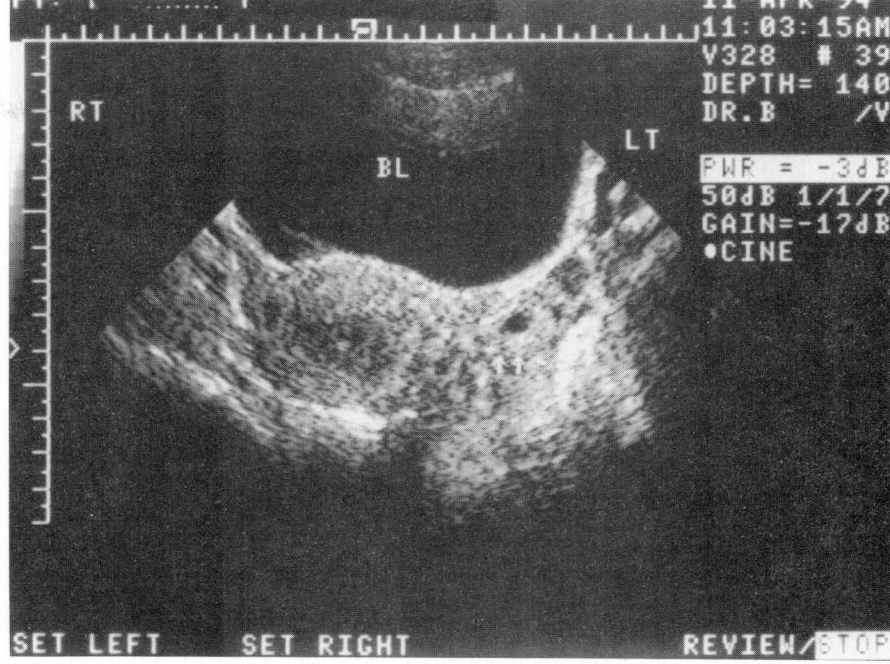

The diagnosis of ectopic pregnancy is based on careful correlation of ultrasound findings with gestational dating criteria, laboratory tests (e.g., serum β-human chorionic gonadotropin [β-hCG] and progesterone), and the physical examination. The primary use of ultrasound is to verify the presence of an intrauterine pregnancy because this situation practically excludes ectopic pregnancy in all but the rare case (1:30,000) in which a combined intrauterine and extrauterine pregnancy spontaneously occurs. Heterotopic pregnancies occur more commonly in infertility patients. Svare and colleagues recently reported a 1.1 percent incidence of heterotopic pregnancy established by in vitro fertilization and embryo transfer. They noted that ultrasound effectively detected ectopic pregnancy and that the timely removal of the extrauterine gestation usually allowed the remaining intrauterine pregnancy to reach term gestation.

**Fig. 258-7.** Free intraperitoneal fluid is demonstrated in a case of ectopic pregnancy (*arrow*). Note the echogenic particles that can be demonstrated by transvaginal sonography. This fluid collection represented a small hemoperitoneum.

The decidual reaction or thick endometrium lining associated with an ectopic pregnancy can simulate a normal intrauterine sac. A common pitfall may occur when it is assumed that a nonspecific fluid collection within the uterus falsely represents a gestational sac. However, an intrauterine gestational sac can easily be distinguished from a pseudosac because a true intrauterine sac has a double white line around its circumference—presumably due to the approximation of decidua parietalis and capsularis layers (Fig. 258-4). Hill and colleagues reported that 9 percent of their ectopic pregnancies were associated with a pseudogestational sac by transvaginal sonography (Fig. 258-5). By comparison, about 20 percent of ectopic pregnancies are associated with a pseudogestational sac when studied by abdominal ultrasound.

The most common sonographic findings for ectopic pregnancy in-

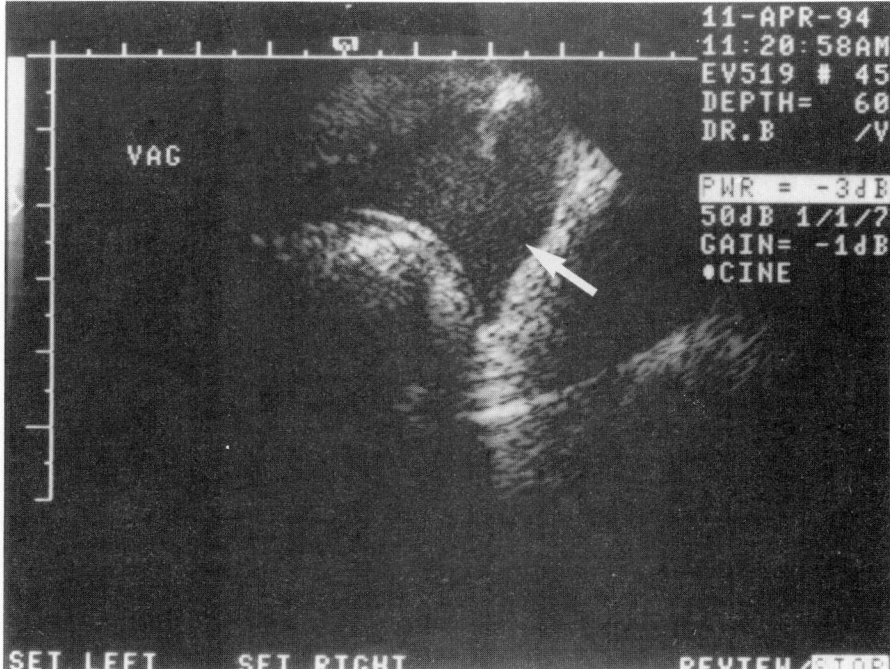

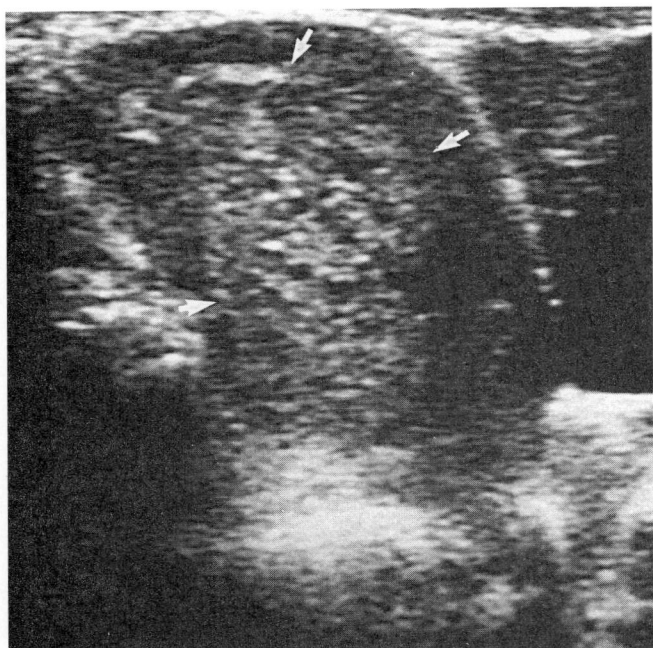

**Fig. 258-8.** Heterogeneous gray tissue filling the uterus is characteristic of a hydatidiform mole (*arrows*).

clude a saclike adnexal ring, complex adnexal mass, and the presence of free pelvic fluid (Fig. 258-6). Small tubal pregnancies that measure 3.5 cm or less by ultrasound may respond to conservative medical therapy such as methotrexate. One should remember that the only true diagnostic ultrasound sign of an ectopic pregnancy is identification of a fetus with cardiac activity outside the uterus; this is represented by approximately one fifth of ectopic pregnancies. All other signs, such as complex adnexal mass or free fluid in the cul-de-sac, can also be seen in other entities such as ruptured or leaking ovarian cyst. Even an edematous hydrosalpinx can mimic the appearance of an adnexal ring, especially if different views of the structure are not routinely obtained.

Free intraperitoneal fluid can be visualized in about 63 percent of

surgically proven cases of ectopic pregnancy, but one should be aware that small amounts of free fluid can also be present during normal gestation. Echogenic fluid in the cul-de-sac (as opposed to echolucent fluid) correlates well with hemoperitoneum (Fig. 258-7). In this regard, culdocentesis was once widely regarded to be an essential element for evaluating ectopic pregnancy. This invasive procedure can help to confirm hemoperitoneum in cases of acute abdomen when there is no time for ordering diagnostic ultrasound studies. However, culdocentesis now has limited value for hemodynamically stable and asymptomatic patients who are better candidates for follow-up by ultrasound and serial β-hCG levels.

The emergency physician should be familiar with the type of serum hCG standard used in the hospital laboratory. In 1974, the World Health Organization released the International Reference Preparation (IRP) as a highly purified standard for radioimmunoassay. In 1986, the World Health Organization changed the name of the IRP to the Third International Standard (3rd IS), which is currently recommended for quantitative measurement of serum β-hCG levels.

The absence of a gestational sac with a serum β-hCG level of at least 1000 mIU/mL (IRP or 3rd IS) with excellent menstrual dates of greater than 5 weeks raises three distinct possibilities.

1. The pregnancy is less advanced than menstrual dates would suggest.
2. An occult gestational sac lies outside the uterine cavity.
3. The patient has recently passed an intrauterine pregnancy.

Pertinent clinical information—such as gestational dating criteria, previous ultrasound findings, and serum β-hCG levels over time—can be important for interpretation of these ultrasound findings. During normal pregnancy, more than 85 percent of women will have a doubling time of serum hCG concentration of 1.5 to 2 days, whereas those with ectopic pregnancies will typically demonstrate a plateau or decline in serial values.

## Molar Pregnancy

Gestational trophoblastic disease has been reported to affect 1:1200 pregnancies in the United States. Most cases involve the entire placenta (complete mole), but molar disease involving only a part of the placenta (partial mole) or fetus (mole with coexisting fetus) have also been described. Patients with a complete molar pregnancy will typi-

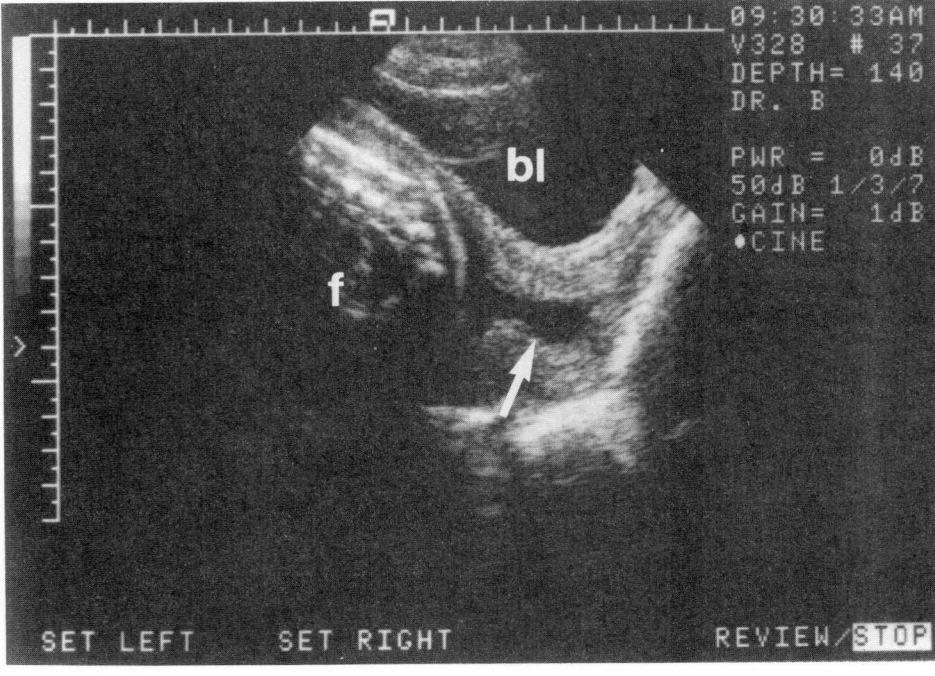

**Fig. 258-9.** Sagittal view of a 28-week uterus. Cervical canal is dilated approximately 1 cm (*arrow*). bl, maternal bladder, f, fetus.

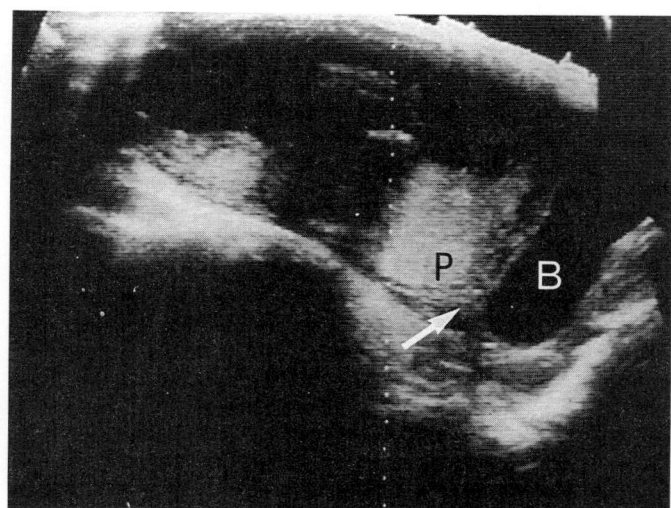

**Fig. 258-10.** Complete placenta previa. The placenta (P) covers the internal cervical os (*arrow*) that is situated just inferior to the maternal bladder (B).

cally present with a history of vaginal bleeding, uterine size greater than dates, and absence of heart tones.

Consequently, the ultrasound scan demonstrates a large uterus with no fetus and abundant cystic placental tissue. The placenta normally has a very homogeneous sonographic texture, but a molar pregnancy has areas of echolucency and echogenicity mixed with normal-appearing placenta (Fig. 258-8). Multiple large ovarian cysts (theca lutein cysts), which have developed in response to abnormally high β-hCG levels, can be present in about one half of cases. A degenerating placenta resulting from a threatened abortion may present with the same sonographic appearance, so β-hCG levels and the presence of theca lutein cysts may be necessary to tell the difference.

Pathologic examination of the placental tissue will be confirmatory. Evacuation of a molar pregnancy is more complicated than the evacuation of an incomplete abortion and should be left to someone experienced in dealing with this entity. Furthermore, up to one fourth of patients with complete moles will develop malignant gestational trophoblastic disease.

## THIRD TRIMESTER BLEEDING

Vaginal bleeding is a common emergency problem. Timely diagnosis and stabilization of the patient should be the priorities in these patients. The most common causes for clinically significant vaginal bleeding during third trimester pregnancy are placenta previa and abruptio placentae. The physician should also consider other potential bleeding sources such as cervical or vaginal lacerations.

Premature cervical effacement or loss of the cervical mucous plug ("bloody show") during labor can also lead to some vaginal spotting. Under these circumstances, the sagittal view of the uterus may reveal a dilated or shortened cervix (Fig. 258-9). The possibility of retained placental tissue or even gestational trophoblastic disease needs to be considered in postpartum or postabortal women who complain of persistent vaginal bleeding.

### Placenta Previa

Painless third trimester vaginal bleeding should be assumed to be caused by placenta previa unless a previous scan by a very reliable ultrasonographer has shown that the placenta does not cover the internal uterine os (Fig. 258-10). Risk factors include multiparity, previous cesarean section, and advanced maternal age. Placenta previa should not be diagnosed prior to about 26 weeks' gestation because: (1) it is not uncommon for the placental edge to extend over

the cervical os during the first two trimesters of pregnancy and (2) placenta previa is rarely the cause of vaginal bleeding until the third trimester. Townsend and coworkers reported that the majority (93 percent) of cases where the placenta marginally covering the cervical os during early pregnancy (< 20 weeks) actually resolved by time of delivery.

The possibility of a false positive previa diagnosis may be caused by an overdistended bladder, use of an incorrect scanning plane, or anatomic distortion by uterine contraction. Before vaginal examination is attempted in a bleeding patient, a quick abdominal scan should be performed to determine the location of the lower edge of the placenta. An overfilled bladder can deform the lower uterine segment to give the false appearance of a placenta previa (Fig. 258-11). Rather, the bladder should be filled just enough to allow visualization of the cervix. The scan should clearly demonstrate the cervical canal, internal cervical os, and placental edge. A midline sagittal scanning plane should be used to avoid a false positive diagnosis of placenta previa. An experienced examiner can safely proceed to a vaginal ultrasound if the abdominal study does not satisfactorily define the position of the placental edge.

### Abruptio Placentae

If placenta previa is excluded in a bleeding patient, the next most likely diagnosis is abruptio placentae, particularly if she has associated lower abdominal pain and uterine tenderness. This condition usually results from arterial disruption and high-pressure bleeding. However, ultrasound is not a sensitive means for making the diagnosis of abruptio placentae because the blood may merely pass exterior to the membranes into the vaginal vault. Its only role is to exclude placenta previa. *The patient without a placenta previa and with the typical clinical findings of abruption constitutes a clinical emergency and should be stabilized and monitored, not taken to the ultrasound department to look for retroplacental collections of blood.* These are rarely seen and their absence does not necessarily exclude the diagnosis of placental abruption.

## THE PELVIS IN THE NONPREGNANT PATIENT

*The maxim in obstetrics and gynecology is that a woman of reproductive years is pregnant until proven otherwise.* Therefore, all women of childbearing age with lower abdominal complaints should be initially evaluated for pregnancy. Ultrasonography does not replace the competent pelvic examination and good clinical judgment. Ultrasonography should not be requested before a pelvic examination has been performed by an experienced clinician.

Several potential pitfalls with pelvic ultrasound may mislead the clinician and possibly result in inappropriate therapy. For example, the sonographic appearance of bowel can simulate a pelvic mass and lead to unnecessary surgery. Alternatively, pelvic masses can be hidden acoustically behind bowel. Therefore, a differential diagnosis should be formulated before the scan to address a specific range of clinical disorders. With these caveats in mind, ultrasonography can add valuable information for women with abdominal pain, vaginal bleeding, or a pelvic mass.

### Components of a Satisfactory Pelvic Ultrasound Examination

The standard pelvic ultrasound report should comment on both ovaries and uterus. A quick survey of the entire abdomen should also be performed. Vaginal ultrasound will usually provide a clearer picture of a pelvic mass (but only at the level of the uterus or lower). A comment should be made about the presence or absence of free fluid. Although there can be 10 to 20 mL of fluid in the normal pelvis, a larger volume suggests a problem in the pelvis or abdomen.

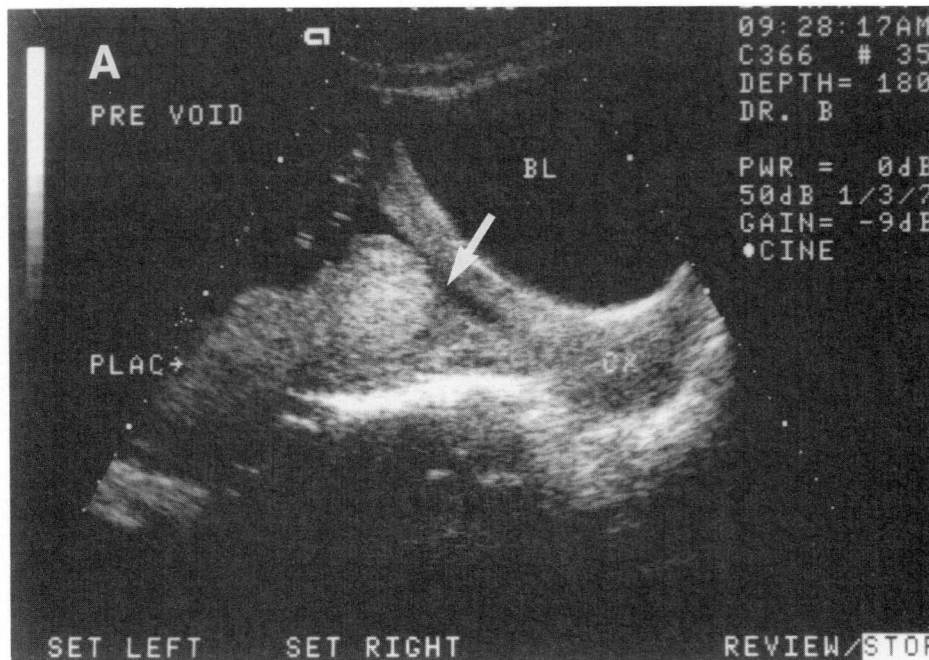

A

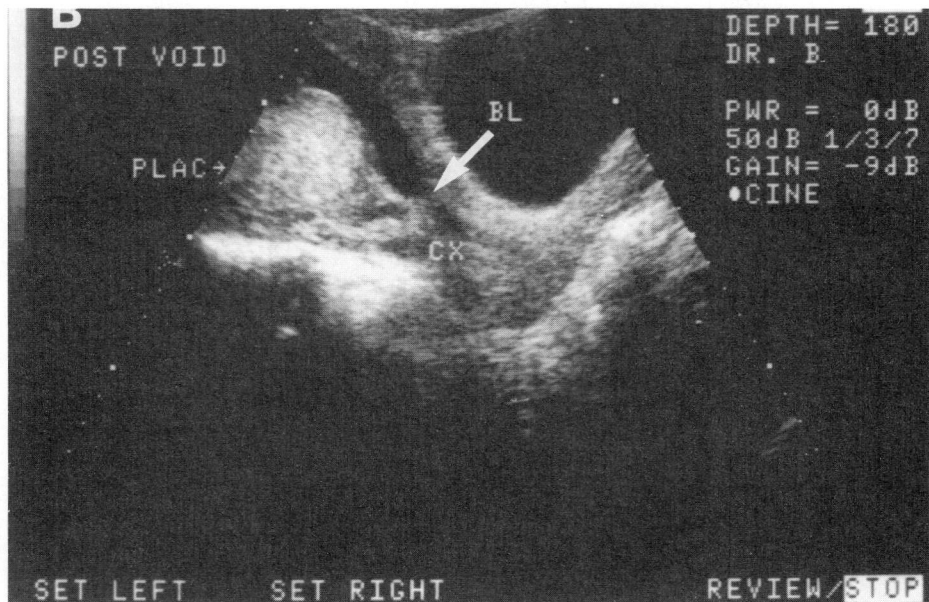

B

**Fig. 258-11.** Midline sagittal scans of the uterine cervix demonstrate the effect of bladder emptying on the placenta previa diagnosis. **(A)** A very full bladder (BL) can push the placenta over the internal cervical os (*arrow*). **(B)** When the bladder is emptied slightly, the placenta falls away from the cervical os (*arrow*).

## Ultrasound Characteristics of Common Pelvic Masses

Acute pelvic pain in the nongravid female patient can be caused by cyst rupture, adnexal torsion, pelvic masses, and infection. Hemoperitoneum related to a ruptured cyst commonly causes diffuse lower abdominal pain with rebound tenderness and can require surgical intervention. The emergency physician should be familiar with the clinical significance and variable ultrasound appearance of these pathologic conditions.

*Functional cysts* (follicles or corpus luteum) are echolucent with no solid components in the absence of torsion or hemorrhage (Fig. 258-12). Sonographically, follicular cysts appear small (1 to 2 cm) and anechoic and have sharply defined margins. Ovarian cysts can rupture and cause significant blood loss. The majority of hemorrhagic

ovarian cysts sonographically appear as a heterogeneous mass. Many of these cysts are accompanied by septations and associated free fluid (Fig. 258-13). Hemorrhagic ovarian cysts usually spontaneously resolve and can be managed conservatively if the hematocrit and vital signs remain stable. However, they can be also confused with other adnexal masses such as dermoids, parovarian cysts, endometriomas, abscesses, torsion, and ovarian neoplasms. Persistence of a cystic mass beyond one or two menstrual cycles argues against a "functional cyst" and generally requires further investigation. Therefore, the physician should actively search for historical information from any previous scans when evaluating pelvic masses.

*Dermoids* can be distinguished by the hair or fat that produce bright echoes in an otherwise complex mass consisting of both cystic and solid components. The sonographic appearance of dermoids can be quite variable. Most cystic teratomas contain dermoid plugs hav-

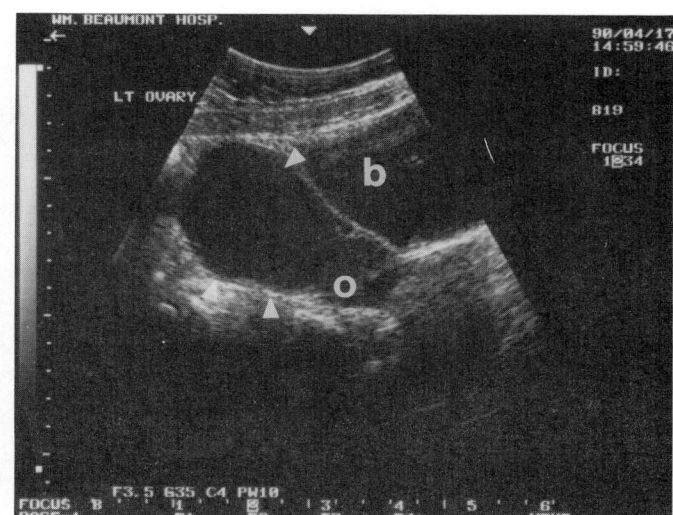

**Fig. 258-12.** A corpus luteum cyst (*arrowheads*) appears to contain only fluid. o, ovary; b, bladder.

**Fig. 258-13.** Two transverse views of the uterus are shown. **(A)** Multiple right ovarian cysts are visualized lateral to uterus (u); the largest one measures 2.4 × 2.8 cm (*arrow*). **(B)** Another transverse view from a different level demonstrates free fluid (ff) in the right adnexa (*arrow*) with a suspicious 2.4-cm left adnexal mass (calipers). Laparoscopy confirmed a left tubal pregnancy with a ruptured right corpus luteum cyst that accounted for the right adnexal fluid visualized by ultrasound.

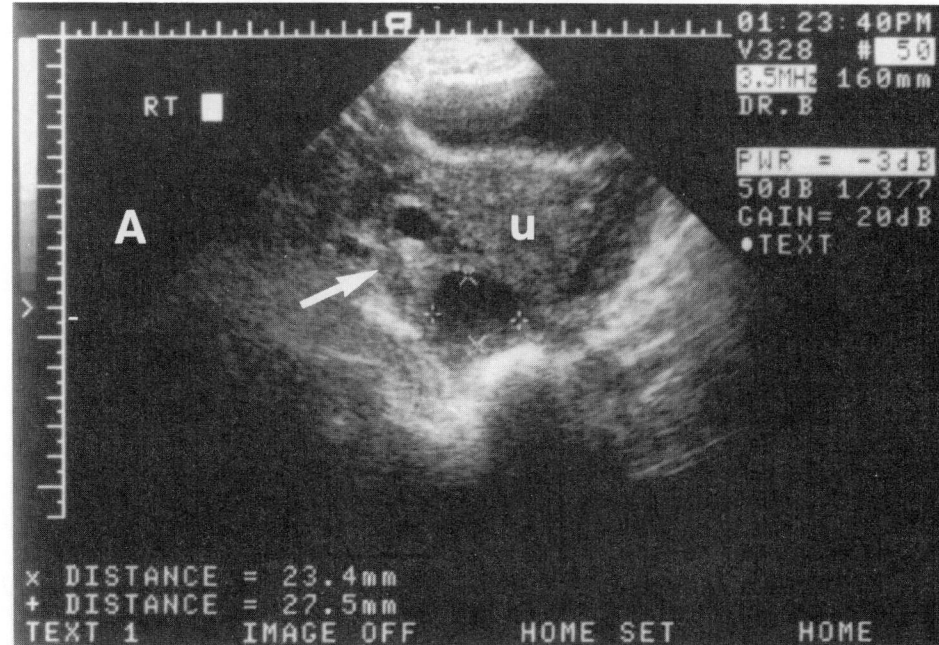

A

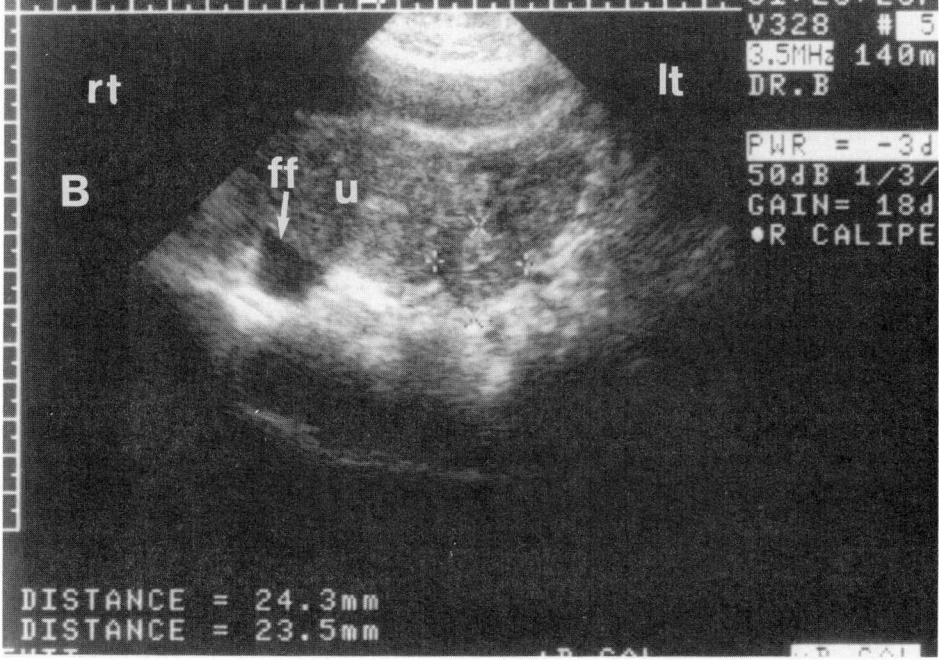

B

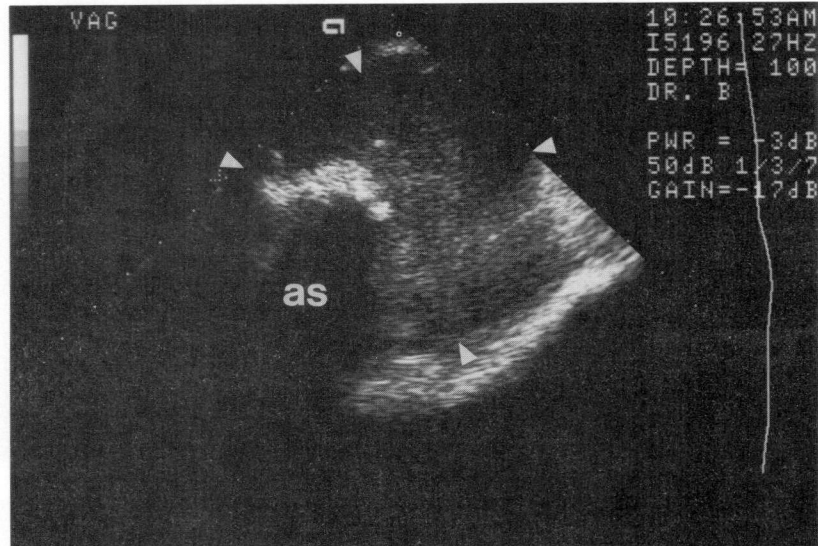

**Fig. 258-14.** A dermoid (*arrows*) with calcium or fat producing very echogenic areas with an acoustic shadow below it (AS).

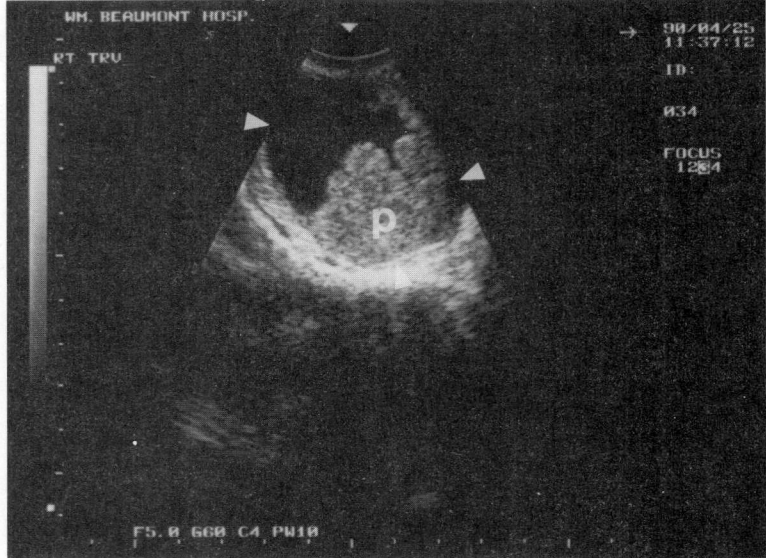

**Fig. 258-15.** A serous cystadenoma of borderline malignancy (*arrowheads*) contains considerable papillary solid tissue (P) producing a worrisome appearance.

ing a characteristic shape and hyperechoic pattern with distal acoustic shadowing (Fig. 258-14). Correlation of sonographic findings with computed tomography indicates that three factors greatly influence the appearance of teratomas: size of dermoid plug, presence and location of calcified elements, and histologic composition of the fatty component. Finally, dermoids are frequently bilateral (10 to 20 percent), so the contralateral ovary should also be examined if possible.

*Cystadenomas* represent another type of common benign ovarian neoplasm. Wall thickening and septations may sometimes differentiate cystadenomas from follicular cysts. Serous cystadenomas are usually not as large as the mucinous variety and contain few septations. By contrast, mucinous cystadenomas are often very large and septated—sometimes filling the entire abdomen. In both cases, the risk of malignancy increases with the presence of solid component as noted by ultrasound. Thin-walled unilocular cysts that are less than 6 cm in diameter are virtually never malignant. By contrast, thick septae, irregular solid areas, poorly defined margins, and ascites are worrisome signs for malignancy (Fig. 258-15).

*Endometriosis* is an important cause for chronic pain and infertility. An endometrioma occurs as a pelvic mass containing functional endometrial tissue outside the uterus (Fig. 258-16). In one series, the majority of endometriomas were predominantly anechoic (fluid-filled) with thin walls, but they occasionally contain septations, internal echoes, and variably thickened walls. Consequently, endometriomas can mimic the sonographic appearance of other adnexal masses such as hemorrhagic ovarian cyst, tubo-ovarian abscess, ectopic pregnancy, or cystadenoma.

*Uterine fibroids* typically appear with common sonographic patterns: hypoechoic, heterogeneous, and echogenic rim (Fig. 258-17). They can be submucosal, subserosal, or pedunculated. Occasionally, the fibroid may outgrow its blood supply leading to localized pain secondary to necrosis especially during pregnancy. Sonographically, degeneration correlates with the appearance of small cystic spaces within the center of the fibroid. Pedunculated fibroids can simulate an ovarian mass so it is imperative that a diligent search be conducted for both ovaries.

*Adnexal and ovarian torsion* is associated with variable and nonspecific ultrasound findings that often include the identification of a large midline cyst. The appearance of the twisted mass ranges from solid to cystic depending on the degree of internal hemorrhage or stromal edema. Many of these patients will have a history of a preexisting cystic adnexal mass. Acute torsion should be considered a surgical emergency and early sonographic recognition of this disorder may optimize chances for salvage of the involved structures.

**Fig. 258-16.** Parasagittal view of a 6 × 5 cm left adnexal mass with low internal echoes associated with a 14-week pregnancy. Pathology confirmed an endometrioma involving the left ovary. BL, bladder.

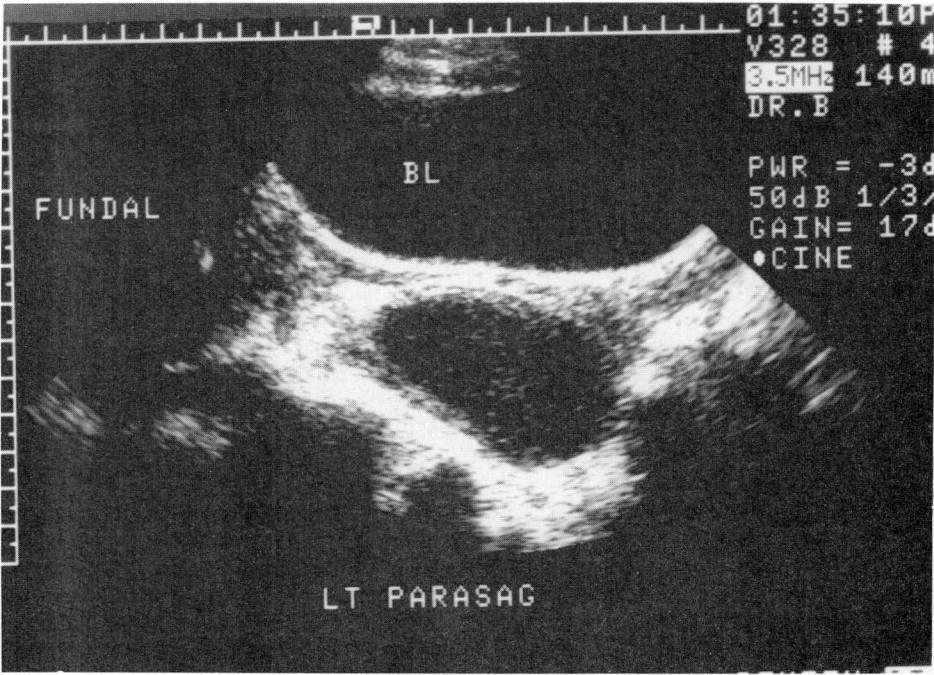

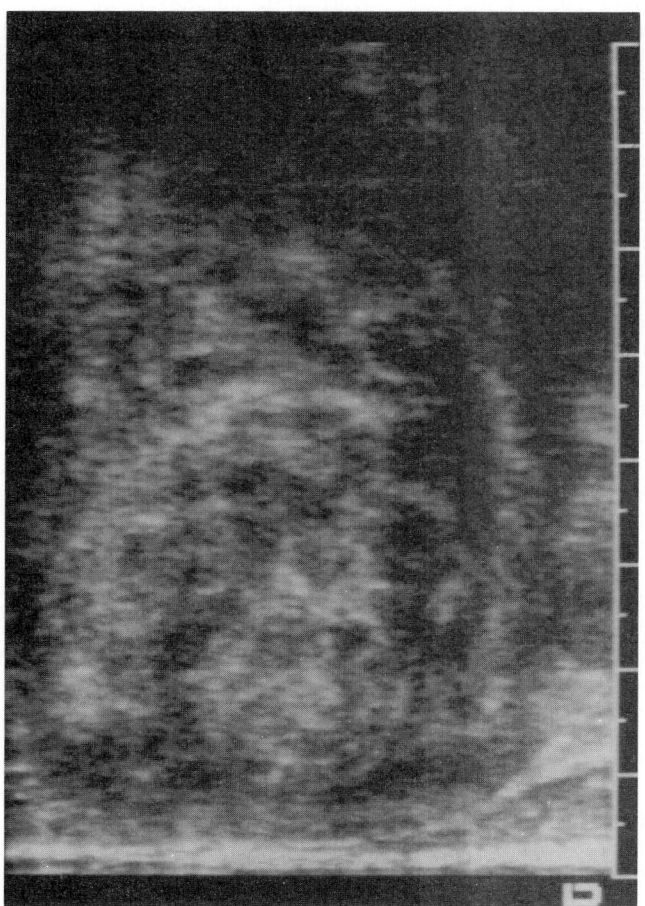

**Fig. 258-17.** A round mass demonstrates a whorled pattern characteristic of a uterine fibroid. Degenerating fibroids are associated with pain and may develop central cystic fluid-filled areas that can be seen by ultrasound.

The emergency physician must also consider other causes of pelvic pain or masses. Caution is required to avoid confusion between a large pelvic cyst and a distended bladder. The urinary bladder, when emptied, will appear as an inverted fluid-filled triangle in the midline sagittal plane adjacent to the pubic symphysis. Tubo-ovarian abscess can appear predominantly unilocular with low-level internal echoes. However, this entity can also appear as a tubo-ovarian complex that consists of both solid and cystic components with septations. A history of pelvic infection or fever and the presence of a tender fluctuant mass on physical examination provide important clues for this diagnosis. An enlarged uterus can also present as a pelvic mass. Fibroids, carcinoma, or hematocolpos can cause uterine enlargement. However, the most common cause is pregnancy.

Pelvic masses may coexist with intrauterine pregnancy. The ovaries, particularly if enlarged, can be displaced into the abdomen above the uterus as the pregnancy progresses because they are mobile within the gravid pelvis. A thorough search for ovaries should be attempted although they often cannot be visualized beyond 15 weeks' gestation due to acoustic shadowing. Occasionally, a large ovarian mass will be found under the ribs in a woman with advanced pregnancy. A natural corollary of this is that the ovaries can rarely cause upper abdominal pain in pregnancy.

## THE PEDIATRIC PELVIS

In children and adolescents, unlike those of adults, pelvic masses can arise from unusual sources, and, therefore, ultrasound examination is a wise precaution before any surgery is performed. Blood collections in a vagina with a transverse septum, hydrometrocolpos secondary to imperforate hymen, pelvic kidney, or other more unusual anomalies of the genitourinary tract may present as pelvic masses. In addition, cysts of the neural, lymphatic, or gastointestinal system may present in this age group as a pelvic mass. Functional ovarian cysts and dermoids are susceptible to rupture, torsion, and hemorrhage, as previously discussed. Germ cell tumors, predominantly dysgerminoma and endodermal sinus tumors, account for most of the malignant ovarian tumors in the pediatric group. Pelvic rhabdomyomas and presacral masses such as sacrococcygeal teratoma should also be considered when a pelvic mass is identified by ultrasound.

## BIBLIOGRAPHY

Cacciatore B, Tiitinen Aila, Stenman UH, et al. Normal early pregnancy: serum hCG levels and vaginal ultrasonography findings. *Br J Obstet Gynaecol* 97:899, 1990.

Cacciatore B. Can the status of tubal pregnancy be predicted with transvaginal sonography? A prospective comparison of sonographic, surgical, and serum hCG findings. *Radiology* 177:481, 1990.

Carson SA, Buster JE. Current concepts. Ectopic pregnancy. *N Engl J Med* 329:1174, 1993.

Helvie MA, Silver TM. Ovarian torsion: sonographic evaluation. *J Clin Ultrasound* 17:327, 1989.

Hill LM, Kislak S, Martin JG. Transvaginal sonographic detection of the pseudogestational sac associated with ectopic pregnancy. *Obstet Gynecol* 75:986, 1990.

Lavery JP, Shaw LA. Sonography of the puerperal uterus. *J Ultrasound Med* 8:481, 1989.

Leach RE, Ory SJ. Modern management of ectopic pregnancy. *J Reprod Med* 34:324, 1989.

Levi C, Lyons EA, Lindsay DJ. Early diagnosis of nonviable pregnancy with endovaginal US. *Radiology* 167:383, 1988.

Marchbanks PA, Annegers JF, Coulam CB, et al. Risk factors for ectopic pregnancy—a population-based study. *JAMA* 259:1823, 1988.

Nyberg DA, Hughes MP, Mack L, et al. Extrauterine findings of ectopic pregnancy at transvaginal US: importance of echogenic fluid. *Radiology* 178:823, 1991.

Nyberg DA, Laing FC, Filly RA. Threatened abortion: sonographic distinction of normal and abnormal gestation sacs. *Radiology* 158:387, 1986.

Pittaway DE, Reish RL, Wentz AC. Doubling times of human chorionic gonadotropin increases in early viable intrauterine pregnancies. *Am J Obstet Gynecol* 152:299, 1985.

Rempen A. Diagnosis of viability in early pregnancy with vaginal sonography. *J Ultrasound Med* 9:711, 1990.

Romero R, Kadar N, Copel JA, et al. The effect of different human chorionic gonadotropin assay sensitivity on screening for ectopic pregnancy. *Am J Obstet Gynecol* 153:72, 1985.

Sherman SJ, Carlson DE, Platt LD, Medearis AL. Transvaginal ultrasound: does it help in the diagnosis of placenta previa? *Ultrasound Obstet Gynecol* 2:256, 1992.

Stovall TG, Ling FW, Gray LA, et al. Methotrexate treatment of unruptured ectopic pregnancy: a report of 100 cases. *Obstet Gynecol* 77:749, 1991.

Svare J, Norup P, Grove Thomsen S, et al. Heterotopic pregnancies after in-vitro fertilization and embryo transfer—a Danish study. *Human Reprod* 8:116, 1993.

Vermesh M, Graczykowski JW, Sauer MV. Reevaluation of the role of culdocentesis in the management of ectopic pregnancy. *Am J Obstet Gynecol* 162:411, 1990.

Warner MA, Fleischer AC, Edell SL, et al. Uterine adnexal torsion: sonographic findings. *Radiology* 154:773, 1985.

Wu A, Siegel MJ. Sonography of pelvic masses in children: diagnostic predictability. *AJR Am J Roentgenol* 148:1199, 1987.

# 259
# COMPUTED TOMOGRAPHY
## Jeremy J. Hollerman

Few recently trained clinicians can imagine practicing medicine without the information obtained from computed tomography (CT). CT scanning of the head and body, which was uncommon as recently as 1975, is now routine and is often essential for state-of-the-art patient care.

## IMAGE FORMATION

In CT, a section of the head or body with a *slice thickness* defined by the thickness of the x-ray fan beam is scanned then mathematically divided into many tiny blocks of equal volume called *voxels*. Each voxel is assigned a number that corresponds to the degree to which the material in that voxel absorbed the x-ray beam. This absorption is numerically stated as the linear attenuation coefficient. The composition of the material in the voxel (its density and its average atomic number) and the quality of the x-ray beam (its average photon energy and energy distribution) determine the linear attenuation coefficient of the voxel. The image is formed by displaying the front face of each voxel (called a *pixel*), with a shade of gray whose darkness is proportional to the linear attenuation coefficient of that voxel.

The length of the voxel is equal to the thickness of the x-ray fan beam (the slice thickness), but the *pixel size* (the size of the front face of each voxel cube) is determined mathematically by equations in the computer program. Scan parameters chosen by the CT operator such as field of view and image matrix size determine pixel size. The smaller the pixel size and the shorter the voxels, the better the spatial resolution of the image, but the worse the quantum mottle (see below).

Many of the same types of mathematical analyses and data manipulations used for image formation in CT scanning are used to numerically form tomographic images in magnetic resonance imaging, nuclear medicine single photon emission computed tomography, and positron emission tomography scanning. Many of these mathematical methods depend on Fourier analysis. Mathematical filters consisting of a series of equations are used to remove imaging artifacts, enhancing the visibility of anatomic structures.

In contrast to x-ray plain film tomographic techniques, CT is a true tomogram. When a CT image is formed with a field of view including the entire object diameter, there is no noise (or data) from adjacent tissue outside the imaging plane.

## CT NUMBERS

The linear attenuation coefficient of each voxel is mathematically normalized to a scale where water is assigned a value of zero. These normalized linear attenuation coefficients are then multiplied by a numerical constant to give the *CT number*. In the body, attenuation values cover a range of 4000 CT numbers from air at −1000 to cortical bone at +3000 *Hounsfield units* (*HU*). Water has a density of 0 HU. Structures that absorb more of the x-ray beam than water, such as bone, have positive values, and structures that absorb less of the x-ray beam than water, such as air or fat, have negative values.

One of the major advantages of CT is its ability to display and distinguish tissues that have linear attenuation coefficients that are very close together. In general, on conventional roentgenograms (plain x-rays), structures must differ in density by at least 10 percent for it to be possible to recognize them as different densities. The difference in linear attenuation coefficient needed to allow visible tissue differentiation on CT is much less. For example, intracranial soft tissues vary in density by only 4 percent but are easily distinguished by CT. Gray matter, white matter, and cerebrospinal fluid (CSF) are all easily differentiated. These differences in attenuation coefficients can be visualized by manipulating the gray scale of image display using window and level.

## WINDOW AND LEVEL

Window and level are numerical values that are selected to determine the appearance of the image displayed. Level is called center by some manufacturers.

The same data set of pixels, each pixel assigned a CT number, can appear very different depending on the values of window and level chosen. The *level* is the point at which the gray scale is centered. Half of the shades of gray available will be used for CT numbers higher than the level, and half for CT numbers lower than the level. The *window* (or *window width*) is the range of CT numbers to be displayed by the gray scale. All pixels with CT numbers higher than the level plus one half the window width will be displayed as white, and all pixels with CT numbers lower than the level minus one half the window width will be displayed as black. Values in between these numbers will be displayed using the gray scale. Up to 256 shades of gray can be displayed by the CT scanner monitor. Many more shades of gray than that can be displayed on CT films. The human eye can distinguish as different only about 50 shades of gray. If the window width is less than 256 CT numbers, then fewer than 256 shades of gray will be used in the image display because no more than one shade of gray can be used per CT number.

The concept of level is easily understood. It is the CT number about which the gray scale is centered. The concept of window is more difficult to grasp. If the window is narrow (such as 100) the range of CT numbers displayed as shades of gray is very limited, and the image will be very *high contrast*. This may or may not be beneficial. If the high-contrast gray scale is centered by the level selected on the range of CT numbers of a specific organ in which subtle differences in density need to be detected (such as a narrow window display of the liver to look for a subtle lesion), the high contrast may be beneficial. However, densities outside the narrow range selected will be uniformly too white or too black for evaluation. Such narrow window images are usually a supplement to, rather than a substitute for, standard wider window width image display for diagnostic evaluation.

A wide window produces a *low contrast* image that displays a large range of CT numbers, (the window width), within the gray scale. This is useful for evaluation of structures such as lung or bone with components of very disparate linear attenuation coefficients (e.g., cortical bone, trabecular bone, marrow fat) (Fig. 259-1). Evaluation of anatomy in parts of the image where adjacent structures are very close in density, such as soft tissue where all parts are very close to water in density, will be limited on wide window settings. A wide window means many CT numbers are assigned to each shade of gray. Tissues with different but close HU density may be assigned the same shade of gray and therefore not be seen as different on the display. Soft tissue structures may appear as an undifferentiated, nearly uniform gray mass.

One often looks at the data from a particular CT section at several different display settings. As an example, an upper abdomen CT section might be viewed at lung settings to look for pneumothorax (Fig. 259-2), pulmonary infiltrate, pulmonary contusion or mass, or free intraperitoneal air (Fig. 259-3B); viewed at soft tissue settings (Fig. 259-3A) to look for liver, spleen, pancreas, kidney, adrenal or vascular lesions or adjacent adenopathy; and viewed at bone window settings to evaluate the vertebrae and ribs (see Fig. 259-1A). This extensive evaluation can be performed by numerical display manipulation of the same scan data set, without exposing the patient to additional radiation from rescanning.

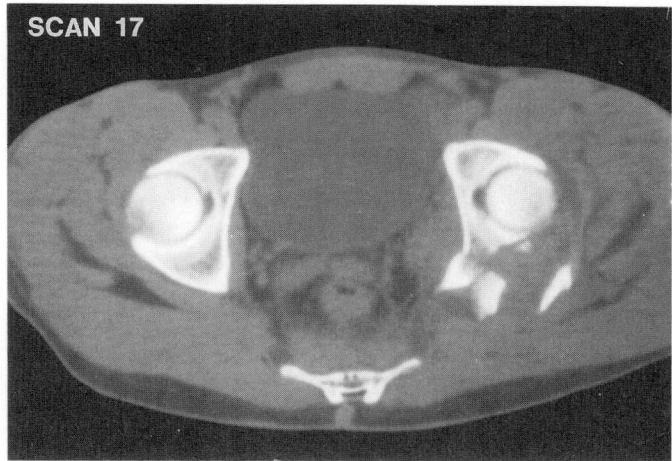

A

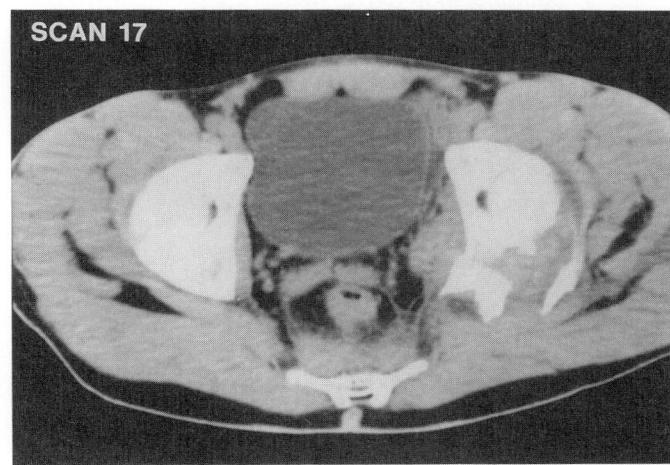

B

**Fig. 259-1.** (A) and (B) are the same CT scan displayed at different window and level settings. A posterior wall fracture of the left acetabulum is shown at settings for bone (A) and at settings for soft tissue (B). The wider window and higher level of the bone settings allow better visualization of bone detail but make all soft tissue structures nearly the same shade of gray. Soft tissue settings allow examination for hemarthrosis and adjacent soft tissue hematoma.

For evaluation of the lung or to look for pneumothorax one uses a wide window (e.g., 1400) and a low level (e.g., −600) to center the gray scale to include air densities. For display of soft tissue structures of the body one uses a moderate window width (e.g., 350) centered at a level just above water (e.g., +30) to use the gray scale to see a range of tissue densities near water. To evaluate bone one uses a wide window (e.g., 1500) and a higher level (e.g., +305) to center the gray scale toward more dense structures. For brain CT one uses a narrow window display (e.g., a window width of 90) because the structures to be differentiated are very close in linear attenuation coefficient; a level just above water (e.g., +30) is used to place the center of the gray scale near the center of the range of CT numbers of the structures to be examined.

## FIELD OF VIEW, MULTIPLANAR RECONSTRUCTION, AND THREE-DIMENSIONAL DISPLAY

Many CT scanners can recompute the raw scan data for each slice to a smaller *field of view* resulting in a smaller pixel size and higher resolution in an area of interest. Slice thickness cannot be changed without rescanning. Such recomputation must be done on original scan

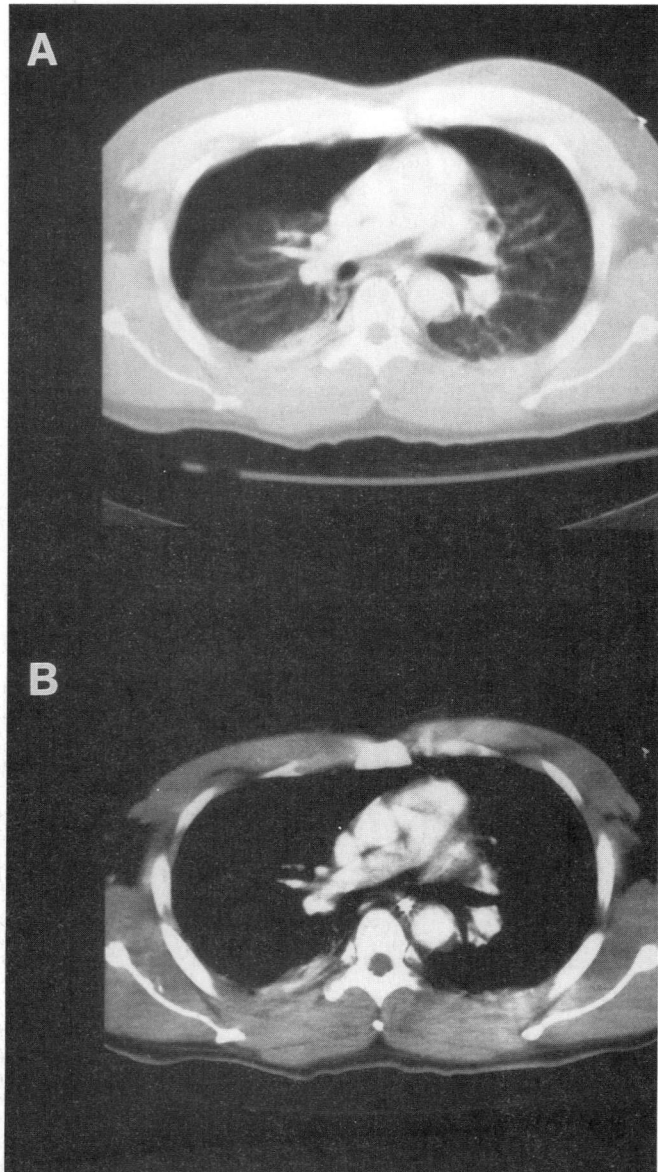

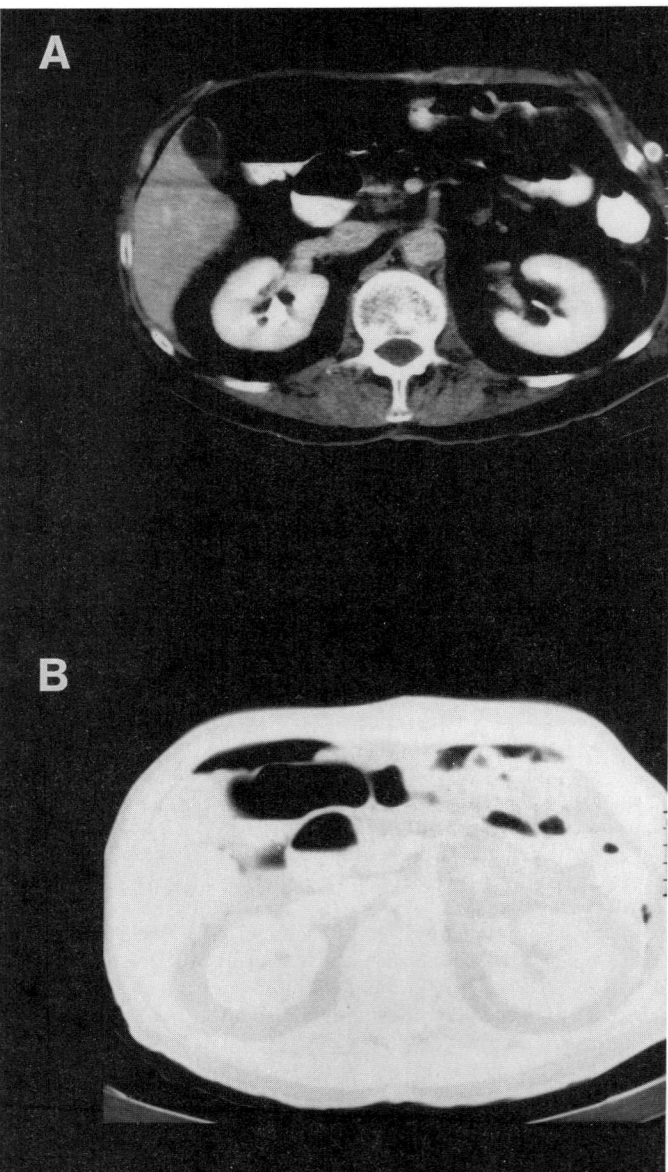

**Fig. 259-2.** Lung (A) and soft tissue (B) displays of the same intravenous contrast-enhanced dynamic scan section. Note how the patient's bilateral pneumothoraces are clearly visible in (A) but are invisible in (B) due to different window and level display settings.

**Fig. 259-3.** Soft tissue (A) and lung window (B) displays of the same abdominal scan. Note how the patient's free intraperitoneal air is well shown in (B) in both the left and right anterior abdomen, anterior to gas-filled intestinal loops. The patient is lying supine on the scan table.

data before image archiving. *Image archiving* is often done at the end of each examination and reduces the size of the data set to be permanently stored. Recomputation of the raw data to a higher resolution smaller field of view is especially useful for examination of the spine after acquiring a whole body image or for examination of the pancreas to look for tumor or trauma after examining a whole body image.

*Reformatting* of scan data into coronal or sagittal section display can also be done. Thin-section (4 mm or thinner) scans provide the best *multiplanar reconstructions* but take longer to acquire than thicker sections.

*Three-dimensional data display, surface data display,* and other display options now exist. These are particularly useful to surgeons for operative planning. An example of the use of three-dimensional display is in complex acetabular fractures where CT scan data can be numerically manipulated to disarticulate and remove the proximal femur from the image of the acetabulum and then create a rotating

three-dimensional image of the pelvis. This allows a direct enface view into the fractured acetabulum for reconstructive planning. The three-dimensional image may be rotated or frozen in any plane with varying degrees of surface and internal structure shading. These options require computer and operator time in addition to that required for usual scanning. Spiral CT data are especially well suited to three-dimensional reconstruction.

## VOLUME AVERAGING

It is important to understand the effect on the image of several CT phenomena. *Volume averaging* occurs when a voxel only partly overlaps a structure or the structure is smaller than the length of the voxel. Voxel length is slice thickness.

When a voxel is partly filled with the structure of interest and partly filled with an adjacent structure (which may be very different in density such as air versus soft tissue), the voxel will be assigned a linear attenuation coefficient and resulting CT number, which is the average density within the voxel. The shade of gray assigned may be very different than that which would have been assigned had the entire voxel contained the structure of interest.

At the edges of a structure or if a structure is smaller than the voxel, the CT number measured and the shade of gray assigned may be erroneous because of volume averaging artifact. If either CT number accuracy (contrast resolution) or spatial resolution of small structures is of paramount importance, decreasing scan thickness so that the entire voxel is filled by the structure of interest will improve accuracy. However, some of the resolution benefits of thinner sections are lost due to increased image noise (quantum mottle), discussed below.

## SLICE THICKNESS, SUBJECT CONTRAST AND IMAGE NOISE

Like raindrops falling on a roof, x-ray photons are not entirely uniform in distribution. On the basis of random distribution, certain areas get more or less than the average number. This is *quantum mottle.* This is a major source of image noise. One's ability to detect lesions depends greatly on the signal-to-noise ratio of the data set. Increasing radiation dose (the number of photons) decreases quantum mottle.

In all of radiology and nuclear medicine, including CT, we do not select the radiation dose to produce the best image. We choose the minimum radiation dose that will reliably produce a *diagnostic image.* This image is usually a less perfect depiction of anatomic detail than that which is possible, but spares the patient unnecessary radiation. In CT we sometimes accept visible quantum mottle to lower patient radiation dose or because the CT scanner is functioning at its maximum possible x-ray tube output. This is most apparent when scanning the abdomen of a very large patient.

Increasing slice thickness decreases quantum mottle but worsens volume averaging artifact. Decreasing slice thickness reduces volume averaging artifact but increases image noise (quantum mottle). The latter can be overcome by using a higher radiation dose for thin sections, when necessary. Knowledge of the clinical question to be answered determines the optimum way to perform the CT study. For example, 8- to 10-mm contiguous sections are often used to survey the entire chest for pulmonary lesions and mediastinal or hilar adenopathy. If a small pulmonary nodule is found, thin sections of the nodule will provide an accurate measurement of its density to determine whether or not it is calcified, and because of improved spatial resolution will better depict the nodule's periphery to look for satellite lesions, spiculation, or pleural extension.

## INTRAVENOUS CONTRAST ADMINISTRATION AND DYNAMIC SCANNING

*Dynamic scanning* is the rapid acquisition of a series of CT images during the bolus phase of intravenous contrast administration. This technique is possible only on relatively newer CT scanners due to improved x-ray tube cooling and enhanced numerical image processing capabilities. *Interscan delay* (the amount of time between scans) is shortened and scan time itself may also be shorter. Often a *mechanical (power) injector* is used to administer the intravenous contrast bolus for this technique. Dynamic scanning allows organ evaluation during the *bolus phase* of intravenous contrast administration, when organ-to-lesion image contrast is usually at its maximum. The shorter *scan time for acquisition* of each slice decreases the effect of all types of *patient motion,* both voluntary and involuntary. This includes respiratory motion and cardiac pulsations, both of which are transmitted to the abdominal organs. Comatose patients on respirators are unable to hold their breath. The development and use of dynamic scanning was a significant step in improving the ability of radiologists to accurately assess trauma by CT.

Computed tomography done without intravenous contrast is commonly referred to as *noncontrast* or *C−* CT. CT done during and after the administration of intravenous contrast is often referred to as *postcontrast, contrast-enhanced,* or *C+* CT.

Increasing the density of a structure by administering a metallic element such as iodine or barium, which absorbs more x-ray photons per unit volume than soft-tissue, is called *contrast enhancement.* Intravenous contrast increases the density of the portion of an organ receiving vascular supply. This effect is most pronounced during the *bolus phase* when the rapidly administered bolus is circulating at its highest intravascular concentration and has not yet equilibrated with other fluid compartments (Fig. 259-4). Hematoma, hemoperitoneum,

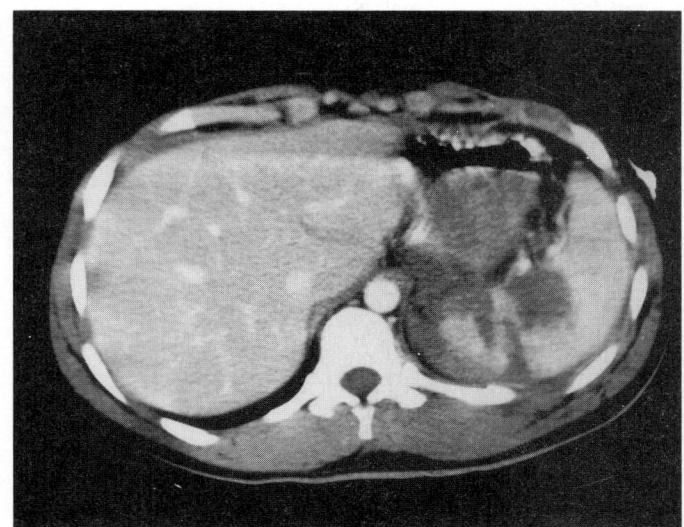

A

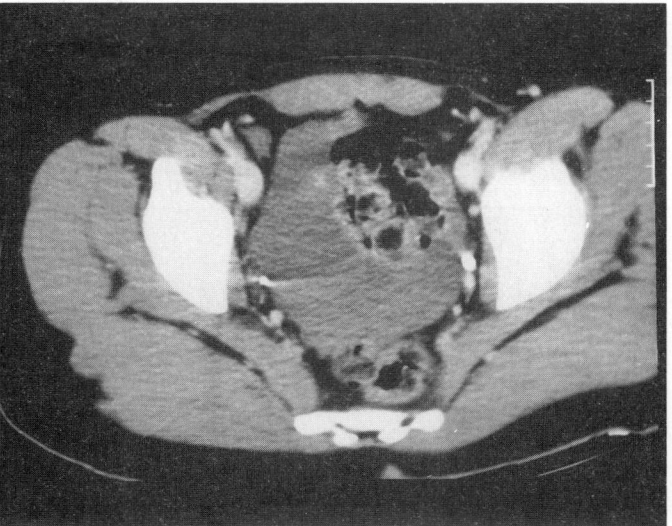

B

**Fig. 259-4.** Images from an intravenous contrast-enhanced dynamic scan of the abdomen after blunt trauma. (A) The patient's fractured spleen and perisplenic blood clot are shown. (B) Free blood in the pelvis surrounding loops of the sigmoid colon is seen. In the supine patient with hemoperitoneum, the most dependent portions of the abdomen are Morison's pouch (see Fig. 259-6C) and the pelvis. Therefore hemoperitoneum accumulates in these two sites first. For upper abdominal trauma it is not adequate to scan only the upper abdomen because significant pelvic hemoperitoneum will often be missed unless the pelvis is scanned.

pleural effusion, empyema, abscess, pseudocyst, urinoma, or bileoma do not enhance their avascular portions and densely enhance their hypervascular portions after intravenous contrast administration. This increases their visibility in relation to surrounding tissues (see Fig. 259-4).

Most extracranial tumors, both primary and metastatic, enhance as if they were hypovascular relative to the organ in which they dwell, but some are hypervascular. Most will be seen best during the bolus phase of contrast enhancement. Some liver metastases of pancreatic endocrine tumors, renal cell carcinoma, carcinoid tumors, pheochromocytoma, thyroid carcinoma, and possibly some breast carcinomas will enhance to *isodensity* (the same density) with the surrounding liver during the bolus phase and become invisible. For these tumors it is important to do precontrast and postcontrast scanning of the liver to look for metastases because some of their liver metastases will be most apparent before the intravenous contrast is given.

Use of C−/C+ CT technique (pre- and postcontrast CT imaging), is also useful in other clinical situations. Among these is the examination of a lesion to differentiate simple cyst from tumor, particularly in the kidney or liver. A thin-section CT scan of the lesion is obtained before intravenous contrast is given. The thin section avoids density measurement error from volume averaging. Then intravenous contrast is administered and bolus and delayed phase thin-section images of the lesion are obtained. The CT density of the lesion on each image is measured. If the lesion demonstrates any sigificant contrast enhancement (rise in density determined by CT number and visual assessment), it is not a simple cyst. Simple cysts are avascular and do not enhance. Simple cysts have an almost imperceptible thin wall and a homogenous near-water density interior. If contrast enhancement occurs, tumor, abscess, and other processes must be ruled out. Ultrasound imaging is often useful to determine whether a lesion is cystic or solid and to define its internal architecture (simple cyst versus complex cyst versus solid).

A dense hematoma adjacent to an abdominal organ or viscus, the "sentinel clot sign" may be observed before and sometimes after intravenous contrast-enhanced abdominal CT scans for trauma (Fig. 259-5). It is a useful marker for sites of organ or visceral injury.

Administration of an adequate volume of intravenous and oral contrast is essential for the performance of state-of-the-art CT imaging of abdominal trauma. Without intravenous contrast, a hematoma adjacent to an organ is usually slightly denser than the organ (see Fig. 259-5) although this difference may sometimes be difficult to detect (Fig. 259-6). Sometimes blood clot is isodense in organs such as the spleen, liver, or brain, making its detection difficult or impossible (see Fig. 259-6A). The isodense or nearly isodense hematoma is one of the most important reasons why intravenous contrast is used for abdominal trauma CT. Blood may be hyper, iso, or hypodense relative to an adjacent organ depending on whether it is clotted or not, the age of the clot, the patient's hematocrit, and the density of the adjacent organ (influenced by the administration of intravenous contrast material, the presence of fatty infiltration of the liver, hemochromatosis, and other conditions).

Administering too small a dose of intravenous contrast, or administering it too slowly, will often enhance a solid organ to isodensity with an adjacent hematoma, making detection of the hematoma difficult or impossible. On older abdominal CT studies where inadequate volumes of contrast were administered, often by drip infusion or other nonbolus technique, scans taken before the administration of contrast may demonstrate pathology later obscured by organ enhancement to isodensity.

In trauma imaging, the detection efficiency of properly performed intravenous contrast-enhanced abdominal CT is so superior to abdominal CT performed without contrast that the use of noncontrast scanning alone is not recommended. Usually only intravenous contrast-enhanced scanning is done for chest or abdominal trauma. Routinely doing both C− and C+ scanning causes unnecessary delay, usually resulting in minimal additional diagnostic information.

Administration of an adequate volume of intravenous contrast by bolus technique and the use of dynamic scanning maximize CT image quality. For adult patients a total dose of 40 to 50 g of organically bound iodine is used. This may be administered as 150 mL of 60% diatrizoate meglumine (ionic) intravenous contrast or 150 mL of 300 to 320 mg/mL iodine content low-osmolar nonionic contrast; for children the dose is usually 2 to 3 mL/kg of intravenous contrast up to a maximum of 150 mL. With a power injector, an administration rate of 1.5 to 2.0 mL/s is often used. This should not be given through a butterfly-type catheter because of the risk of contrast extravasation.

A short delay from the beginning of the contrast bolus until beginning scanning allows circulation of contrast to the area of interest. If imaging of the arterial vascular phase is sought, as in most chest CT scans, a shorter delay such as 30 to 45 s is used. If imaging of the capillary phase of organ enhancement is desired on initial scans to maximize organ-to-lesion contrast such as for upper abdomen CT, a longer delay such as 60 to 90 s is used from the beginning of the bolus until starting scanning.

## Spiral CT

Spiral CT is a relatively new CT technique that uses a continuous rotation of the CT gantry and a continuous table feed. Rather than acquiring a traditional cross-section data set, a data set from a longer volume of the body is obtained. From this continuous data set, individual slices are reconstructed. The slice thickness of the recon-

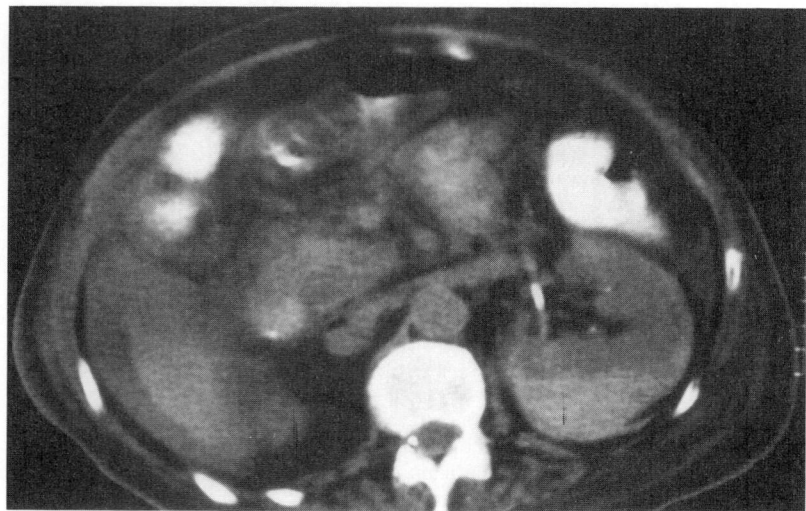

**Fig. 259-5.** This no-intravenous contrast narrow window display of the abdomen after blunt flank trauma shows the left perirenal clot well. Hemoperitoneum surrounding the inferior tip of the right lobe of the liver extending into Morison's pouch is also visible. Subsequent intravenous contrast-enhanced dynamic scanning of the abdomen and pelvis should be done to evaluate the symmetry of enhancement of the kidneys (to rule out vascular pedicle injury); to examine the renal parenchyma, collecting systems, and ureters for injury; and to examine other organs including the liver and spleen to explain the hemoperitoneum. Usually only intravenous contrast-enhanced scans of the abdomen are necessary to assess abdominal trauma.

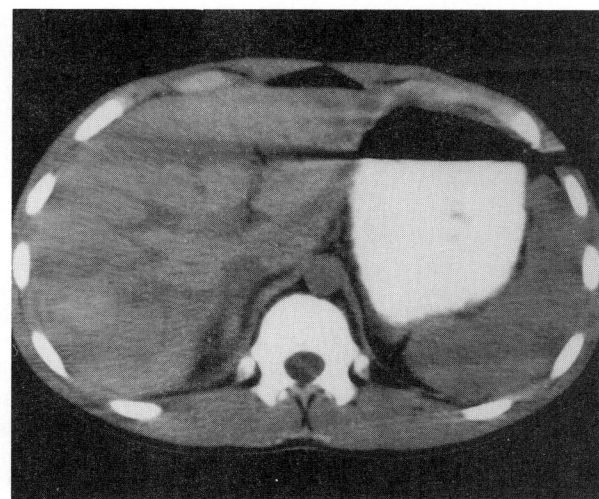

A

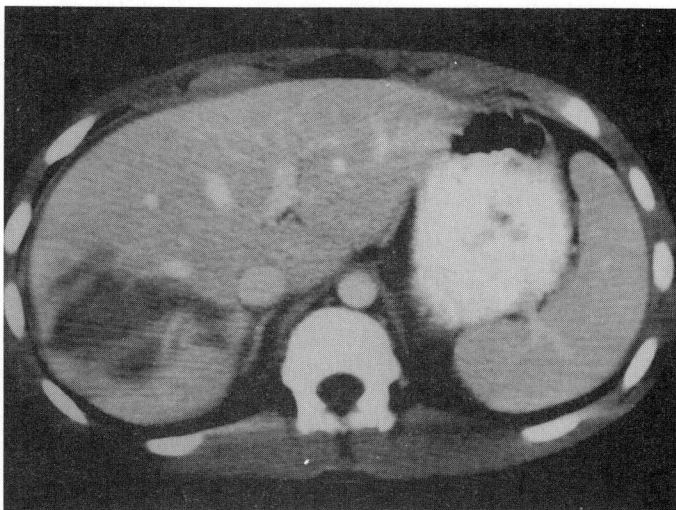

B

**Fig. 259-6.** Scans of a 16-year-old boy after a skiing accident. (A) Scan before intravenous contrast bolus enhancement is displayed at standard abdominal soft tissue settings; the intrahepatic clot and laceration are difficult to see. (B) After bolus intravenous contrast administration during dynamic scanning, a scan at the same level as in (A) shows the hepatic laceration well. It extends immediately behind but does not apparently involve the right hepatic vein. Note that the clot appeared hyperdense relative to the liver before intravenous contrast administration and appears hypodense relative to the enhanced liver after bolus contrast. The clot did not change density. The liver increased in density because of the circulating metal in intravenous contrast. (C) The upper abdominal component of this patient's relatively small volume hemoperitoneum is seen as blood in Morison's pouch (the right posterior subhepatic space between the liver and kidney). There was also hemoperitoneum in the pelvis similar to that shown in Fig. 259-4B.

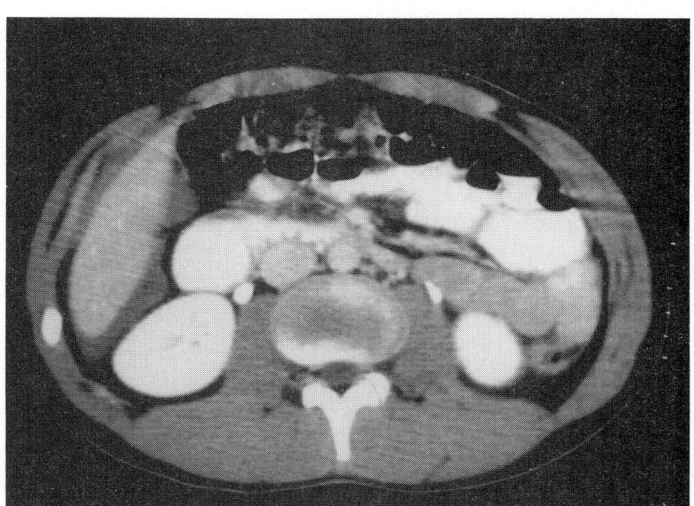

C

structed scans does not need to be the same as the slice thickness at which the data set was acquired.

This technique is especially useful when a small abnormality is being searched for, such as a pulmonary nodule. The entire spiral data set is acquired during a single breath-holding. Assuming the area scanned is appropriately positioned on the body, the nodule should be entirely included in the data set rather than being missed because of different depths of inspiration on sequential breath-holdings for a series of traditional cross-sectional scans. The area of interest moves up and down with different depths of inspiration.

If the patient does breathe during the spiral data acquisition, the harm to the quality of the reconstructed images is often only mild, particularly for shallow breathing.

Major advantages of spiral CT include excellent contrast enhancement when performed properly. The entire spiral acquisition can be done during the peak of the contrast bolus. Also, spiral CT data usually produces better three-dimensional reconstruction images than traditional scans. The ability to be sure that an area of interest is included in the CT data acquired, discussed above, is extremely useful.

The limitations of spiral CT depend somewhat on the manufacturer of the CT scanner being used. The maximum length of the spiral data set that can be rapidly acquired is limited by the size and speed of the computer data storage unit associated with the scanner. The maximum length of the spiral data set is different for each slice thickness

and table feed rate. When feeding the table at faster rates, the output of the CT x-ray tube may not be adequate to overcome problems of quantum mottle. Noisy (grainy looking) reconstructed CT images of body parts with much water-containing tissue, such as the abdomen, may result. Air-containing body parts such as the chest are easier to image well. Slower table-feed rates can overcome these imaging problems in the abdomen, but will limit the maximum length of the data set that can be obtained before the computer's ability to rapidly store data is reached and the scan is terminated. Processing time is required before scanning can begin again, compromising the tissue differentiation effect of the intravenous contrast bolus on subsequent scans. Splitting the bolus into smaller increments often produces suboptimal bolus effect.

With experience, the proper scanning technique for a particular examination can be selected.

Certain imaging artifacts are particular to or worse with spiral scanning. The aortic motion artifact simulating dissection of the ascending aorta just above the aortic valve is discussed in the section of this chapter on imaging of aortic trauma.

## Ionic Versus Nonionic Intravenous Contrast

The question of whether to use ionic or nonionic intravenous contrast is in evolution. Nonionic contrast is approximately 10 times as expensive as ionic contrast. It causes fewer lethal reactions to contrast than ionic contrast. Because the lethal reactions are rare (approximately one severe adverse reaction per 14,000 and one fatal contrast reaction per 40,000 intravenous contrast procedures using ionic contrast), a great deal of money must be spent to prevent each death. Nonionic contrast also causes some fatal contrast reactions. Very large studies are necessary to gather any meaningful statistics. Nonionic contrast was introduced into widespread use in 1986. Based on currently available studies, the rates of minor and severe (including life-threatening) reactions to nonionic contrast are significantly lower than these rates for ionic contrast. In one prospective study of 337,647 radiologic procedures in which intravenous contrast was administered, severe reactions (contrast reactions requiring treatment) were 5.5 times as frequent with ionic contrast compared to nonionic contrast (0.22 percent versus 0.04 percent of patients). A history of a previous reaction to iodine contrast medium increased the probability of a severe reaction to subsequent contrast administration by a factor of four.

Minor reactions to intravenous and intra-arterial contrast are much more common than severe or lethal reactions. The overall prevalence of all types of adverse reactions to contrast was 12.7 percent with ionic contrast and 3.1 percent with nonionic contrast in the Katayama study. In patients with a history of allergy these same values were 23.6 percent and 6.9 percent, respectively. Patients receiving nonionic contrast have less nausea, vomiting, flushing, bradycardia, dizziness, urticaria, injection site pain, and headache. Less pain at the injection site is important for improving examination quality by reducing patient motion, particularly when contrast is used intra-arterially such as for angiography. The reduced pain is probably because nonionic contrast is less hyperosmolar relative to blood than is ionic contrast.

Nonionic contrast also appears to induce fewer serious but nonlethal reactions such as hypotension, bronchospasm, dyspnea, chest pain, cardiac arrhythmia, and angioneurotic edema (particularly of concern when it involves the pharynx because it can compromise the airway). Whether nonionic agents are less nephrotoxic than ionic agents is not settled.

Relative contraindications to the administration of intravenous contrast include pheochromocytoma (hypertensive crisis can be precipitated); multiple myeloma and other gammopathies (contrast-induced precipitation of protein in the renal tubules can cause obstruction and acute tubular necrosis); or a history of previous anaphylactoid reaction to iodine-based contrast (although because of the idiosyncratic nature of contrast reactions, a previous serious reaction to contrast does not mean that the patient will have the same reaction to the same contrast the next time it is administered). When an intravenous contrast procedure is absolutely necessary, appropriate pretreatment may include steroids for patients with severe contrast allergy, α-blocker therapy for patients with pheochromocytoma, and adequate hydration for patients with multiple myeloma.

For patients with a history of severe contrast allergy (manifested by a serious previous reaction to iodinated contrast or a severe allergy to seafood, particularly shellfish), severe asthma, or severe atopy we give two doses of 32 mg methylprednisolone orally (12 and 2 h before intravenous contrast administration). The administration of corticosteroids as a one-time dose immediately before or even 2 h before contrast has been shown to be of no benefit for the prevention of contrast reactions. Corticosteroid dosing further in advance of the procedure is required to reduce reaction rates.

Chronic renal dialysis is not a contraindication to intravenous contrast administration because the contrast material is dialyzed, and renal function is already maximally impaired.

Patients at higher risk for an adverse reaction to intravenous administration of iodine-based contrast include patients over age 60; those with heart disease, history of allergy, asthma, or atopic constitution; patients who have had a previous reaction to iodine-based contrast; severely ill patients; those with renal insufficiency, diabetes, or dehydration; and patients with a history of a severe allergic reaction to eating seafood, particularly shellfish (which contains iodine).

## ORAL CONTRAST ADMINISTRATION

The administration of an adequate volume of liquid contrast material into the gastrointestinal tract is vital for most types of abdominal CT. Oral contrast poses no threat to the kidneys and should be used even in patients with marginal renal function. Either barium-based or iodine-based oral contrast can be used. The amount of iodine absorbed from the gastrointestinal tract is almost always insignificant to the kidneys although it can be significant for allergy. Barium is physiologically inert and is not absorbed.

The dense line of oral contrast in the intestinal lumen allows evaluation of bowel wall thickness for hematoma, edema, or mass. Contrast extravasation can be seen in the presence of full-thickness tear or laceration. In the absence of oral contrast, the gas and stool in the colon provide some natural contrast, making the colon easier to evaluate than the small bowel. The lumen of small bowel loops often contains little or no liquid or gas. Without oral contrast, collapsed small bowel loops can be difficult to differentiate from other soft tissue density structures such as hematoma, abscess, or lymph nodes. The tubular nature of a collapsed small bowel loop assists identification, but may be difficult to appreciate when small bowel loops are tightly packed together, particularly in patients with little fat in the mesentery.

Dilated bowel can simulate abscess or free air. When oral contrast is seen in a large gas and air collection in the abdomen, it means that it is either a dilated intestinal loop or an abscess with communication with the gastrointestinal tract.

Water-soluble iodine-based CT oral contrast passes through the intestine more quickly than the barium-based oral contrast. This is an advantage in trauma patients where quick bowel opacification is necessary. Also, awake patients prefer the taste of the water-soluble oral contrast compared to the barium-based oral contrast, particularly if flavoring is added to the water-soluble contrast. We add orange-drink mix to our water-soluble oral contrast, greatly increasing compliance with drinking it. We prefer the drink mix with sugar rather than artificial sweetener because the latter is problematic with phenylketonuria. We use water-soluble oral contrast for all our CT patients receiving oral contrast except those with iodine or shellfish allergy. Those patients receive barium-based oral contrast.

We use dilute iodine-based CT oral contrast made by mixing iodinated oral contrast and water. We use 4% MD-Gastroview (Mallinckrodt Medical) and 96% water with orange-drink mix. We add 35 mL MD-Gastroview to 900 mL tap water and add 2 scoops of orange-drink mix (flavor to taste). The barium-based CT oral contrast is a 1.7% suspension of barium in water. Both types of CT oral contrast are much more dilute than the contrast used for fluoroscopic radiologic studies such as upper gastrointestinal and barium enema. Fluoroscopic contrast is so dense on CT that it causes metallic-star artifacts, obscuring anatomy.

For elective abdominal CT we make an effort to have the patient drink oral contrast intermittently for 2 h before the procedure so that approximately a liter will have been ingested prior to the CT examination.

For adult patients having abdominal trauma we use 450 mL of iodine-based CT oral contrast administered via nasogastric tube in the trauma room immediately when the decision to perform an abdomen CT is made. This is followed by another 250 to 400 mL via nasogastric tube at the time the patient is placed on the CT scan table. This opacifies the stomach, duodenum, and a variable amount of the jejunum and ileum, allowing improved evaluation for intestinal hematoma or laceration. The earlier it is administered in the trauma room, the better the CT intestinal evaluation.

The only situation in which oral contrast is contraindicated is when the patient is severely allergic to iodine and cannot have barium-based contrast because of possible intestinal perforation or complete colon obstruction. Both of the latter are only relative contraindications to barium-based oral contrast. Extravasated barium in the concentration present for CT poses little threat of barium peritonitis. If perforation is present, small amounts of extravasated barium contrast may permanently remain, staining the peritoneum, a situation avoided with iodine-based oral contrast. Complete colon obstruction can allow the formation of a barium stone in the colon proximal to the obstruction if the water in barium-based oral contrast is absorbed by the colon leaving solid barium. This is a risk only when there is adequate peristalsis to allow the oral contrast to reach the colon and then a sufficient delay before surgery to allow the water to be absorbed. This combination of circumstances is relatively unlikely in a patient with complete colon obstruction.

Because iodine-based CT oral contrast is more than 97 percent water, it is not nearly the inflammatory risk to the lung posed by the undiluted iodine-based oral contrast used for fluoroscopic gastrointestinal studies. Pulmonary aspiration of CT oral contrast or its extravasation from a torn esophagus into the mediastinum or pleural space, though not desirable, is not the emergency that pulmonary aspiration of full-strength iodine-based oral contrast represents. When aspirated into the lung, full-strength iodine contrast causes a severe inflammatory reaction with significant pulmonary edema.

## CT OF HEAD, CHEST, AND ABDOMEN TRAUMA

## CT of Head Trauma

### Preparation and Indications for CT

In general, one prefers to perform CT on patients with stable vital signs. Sometimes CT imaging of an unstable patient is required. This may be for triage decision-making, such as for deciding whether a craniotomy or laparotomy is most urgent in a multiply injured hypotensive patient, or for lesion localization in a patient with intracranial bleeding and incipient herniation syndrome. Clinical judgment and appropriate consultation between clinician and radiologist are required for the development of the best imaging sequence for the patient.

A secure airway, appropriate control of breathing with a cuffed endotracheal tube and mechanical volume ventilator when required, and adequate vascular access for volume replacement and monitoring (the ABCs of trauma: airway, breathing and circulation), should be instituted prior to CT scanning. The cervical spine should be cleared or adequately immobilized.

Head CT without intravenous contrast should often be done prior to intravenous contrast administration for other body CT examinations. Intravenous contrast administration may make appreciation of subarachnoid hemorrhage or calcifications more difficult, but subdural hematoma is often seen better with intravenous contrast.

### Intracranial Hemorrhage

Common types of posttraumatic intracranial hemorrhage are subarachnoid hemorrhage, subdural hematoma, epidural hematoma, and intracerebral hematoma.

**Subarachnoid hemorrhage (SAH).** Mild SAH is the most common type of intracranial hemorrhage from trauma. If very minimal it may not raise the density of the CSF in the subarachnoid space enough to be visible on CT. If necessary, it can be detected by lumbar puncture and CSF analysis. When the volume of SAH increases, the density of the subarachnoid spaces rises to isodensity with the brain, making the basal cisterns, suprasellar cistern, and portions of the ventricular system invisible. With a greater volume of SAH these CSF spaces will have areas of hyperdensity relative to brain, due to their blood content. Sulci, the tentorial edges, cisterns, or portions of the ventricular system will become hyperdense, depending on the loca-

tion and extent of the hemorrhage. High-density bloody CSF may also layer out in the interpeduncular region of the midbrain. The "zipper sign" of SAH may be seen due to bloody CSF tracking into the interhemispheric fissure and adjacent sulci.

After trauma SAH is often localized to a few sulci adjacent to sites of injury. If SAH is seen in nearly all sulci and cisterns, consider a ruptured intracranial aneurysm as the cause, with trauma, if present, being subsequent to the physiologic derangement associated with aneurysm rupture.

Subarachnoid hemorrhage occurs most commonly from tearing of the meningeal vessels especially at the vertex where brain movement is greatest during trauma. After SAH some patients get arachnoid adhesions. These may cause convexity block of CSF flow pathways leading to communicating hydrocephalus.

**Subdural hematoma (SDH).** SDH as a result of trauma is less common than SAH but is several times as common as epidural hematoma (EDH). Usually SDH is a venous bleed, but it can occasionally be arterial in origin. Because of its usually venous origin and the large potential space (the subdural space) in which it dwells, SDH develops more slowly than EDH.

Subdural hematomas are most often caused by tearing of the bridging veins that connect the cortical veins of the subarachnoid space with the dural venous sinuses. At the time of trauma there is a shift of the brain tearing the bridging veins at the point where the veins are fixed as they pass through the dura. They bleed into the subdural space between the dura and the arachnoid. In 25 percent of patients the SDHs are bilateral. Sagittal violent shaking of children can lead to SDH, axonal shear injury, SAH, and retinal detachment. Children are especially vulnerable because they have a large head relative to body size and have poor neck strength to support the head.

Subdural hematomas are most likely to occur in the elderly, who often have large CSF spaces due to brain atrophy. When trauma causes rapid head motion, the shearing forces developed are greatest in the elderly because of the room available for the brain to move within the skull.

Elderly patients often tolerate an SDH better than would a younger person. Their large CSF spaces allow more room for accommodating the mass of the SDH. In a younger person without cerebral atrophy there is not substantial intracranial space for a blood collection other than the space created by compressing the brain. Younger patients are less likely to get SDH from trauma, but when they do get SDH they tolerate it more poorly than older patients.

The subdural space is a large potential space between the dura mater and the arachnoid mater. It is not divided at suture margins. An SDH crosses suture margins but does not cross the falx or tentorium. An acute SDH is usually crescent shape (like a new moon). An interhemispheric SDH may be triangular at the anterior or posterior margin where it separates the cerebral hemispheres by its mass effect. It then continues as a linear interhemispheric density, which does not track into adjacent sulci, in contrast to the zipper sign of SAH in the same location. A tentorial SDH is oriented obliquely along the course of the tentorium cerebelli. Because of volume averaging effects, the margin of this obliquely oriented linear blood collection often has fuzzy margins and looks like ill-defined contrast enhancement of a too thick tentorium.

If not drained or resorbed, when an SDH becomes chronic it sometimes becomes biconvex shape (like a lens, the same shape as an EDH), but it often stays in the original crescent shape. Chronic SDH can calcify. It is not uncommon for an SDH to be bilateral, especially in elderly patients with cerebral atrophy and repetitive falls.

Subdural hematomas go through a continuum of three phases of density. In patients with a normal hematocrit, an *acute SDH* is hyperdense in relation to brain. The density of the blood collection decreases at a variable rate. Usually sometime 1 to 3 weeks after trauma the SDH is approximately the same density (isodense) with brain, making it difficult to see without intravenous contrast enhancement.

The mass effect of the isodense SDH will remain evident both without and with intravenous contrast. This is the *subacute phase of SDH* during which a portion or all of the SDH is isodense. This phase lasts 2 to 3 weeks from the end of the acute (hyperdense) phase.

The decrease in density of the SDH is often not uniform. The medial portion of the SDH becomes isodense with brain earlier than the lateral portion, which remains high density. This can lead to underestimation of the size of the SDH on a head CT examination without intravenous contrast done during the subacute phase. By 3 to 6 weeks after injury the majority of SDH are lower density than normal brain. This is the *chronic phase of SDH.*

After sufficient time an SDH sometimes become near water density. A very chronic SDH, which has had all its cellular elements lysed and absorbed and is near water density, must be distinguished from an accumulation of CSF in the subdural space due to an arachnoid tear, a true subdural hygroma.

In response to the SDH, after a period of days to weeks a very vascular enhancing membrane of granulation tissue forms at the interface between the brain and the SDH. This enhancing membrane is often the source of rebleeding into the SDH. Rebleeding raises the CT density of the SDH. The increased density may be homogenous or inhomogeneous. By raising the SDH to isodensity, rebleeding may once again make it difficult to appreciate part or all of the SDH. It will cause the SDH to appear less old than it actually is. Intravenous contrast-enhanced CT allows determination of the size of the SDH by making the enhancing membrane visible, outlining the margin of the brain. Intravenous contrast also shows displaced veins on the surface of the brain, outlining the margin of the mass.

Subdural hematomas often occur from contrecoup forces, especially in the temporal region. A frontal SDH is often just below the point of impact (coup forces). When an SAH is associated with intracerebral hematoma or SDH, without a history of trauma, SDH of arterial origin, especially from aneurysm or arteriovenous malformation, should be considered.

After the SDH is surgically drained, especially in elderly patients with chronic SDH, the brain often will not immediately reexpand. This creates a potential space for rebleeding.

**Epidural hematoma (EDH).** There are two layers of the dura mater, the periosteal layer and the meningeal layer. The periosteal layer is attached to the inner table of the skull and is its periosteum. The meningeal layer is inside the periosteal layer. The space between the two layers is the location of the dural venous sinuses.

An EDH usually results from arterial bleeding, associated with a skull fracture that tears an epidural vessel, often a temporal skull fracture tearing the middle meningeal artery. The EDH is biconvex (lenticular) in shape.

The EDH is located between the skull and the periosteal layer of the dura. It strips the dura off the skull. It has the dura as its sharply defined medial margin on CT. An EDH can cross the midline and can cross the tentorium but does not cross intact skull sutures. The dura is tightly adherent to the skull at sutures. An EDH that appears to cross a suture margin is probably two adjacent EDHs, or the suture is fractured and the dural attachment disrupted. An EDH can elevate a dural venous sinus away from the skull because it is outside the periosteal layer of the dura. Intracranial air is frequently seen with EDH but is uncommon with SDH unless there is an open skull fracture or recent surgery.

**Intracerebral hematoma.** The intracerebral hematomas seen after trauma are usually irregular in shape and may be multiple, in contrast to intracerebral hematomas from nontraumatic causes, which are usually solitary and spherical. With time, both types are surrounded by a ring of edema and, with time, intracerebral hematomas decrease in density from the periphery to the center. They become isodense in 2 to 4 weeks. One to 6 weeks after trauma, intravenous contrast-enhanced head CT usually shows peripheral ring enhancement surrounding each intracerebral hematoma. Three mechanisms account

for this: (1) blood-brain barrier breakdown and extravasation of contrast, (2) luxury perfusion secondary to loss of cerebral vascular autoregulation, and (3) formation of hypervascular granulation tissue around the periphery of the hematoma.

Occasionally a delayed intracerebral hematoma can form up to 2 to 3 days after evacuation of an extracerebral hematoma. This may be due to the loss of the compressive tamponade effect the extracerebral hematoma was having on an injured vessel. A delayed hematoma has a poor prognosis. An excessively high vascular perfusion pressure due to loss of cerebral vascular autoregulation may also be a factor.

## Cerebral Edema

Brain swelling after head trauma is from hyperemia and edema. *Hyperemia* is increased blood flow because of loss of cerebral vascular autoregulation. This and the breakdown of the blood-brain barrier cause *vasogenic edema*. Plasma leaks into the extracellular space more rapidly than it is absorbed, causing cerebral edema. Local trauma also causes dysfunction of cell membranes including dysfunction of the Na-K pump. This results in *cytotoxic edema*. Children are especially prone to posttraumatic cerebral swelling.

The relative contributions of the vasogenic and cytotoxic types of edema vary in different types of cerebral edema (from trauma, tumor, ischemia, toxins, etc.).

## Cerebral Contusion

*Cerebral contusion* is brain bruising or crushing without interruption of the cortex. Punctate hemorrhages (high density), tissue necrosis, and edema (low density) are seen, usually just below the point of impact.

## White Matter Shear Injury (Axonal Shear Injury)

This occurs in the white matter usually near the gray-white matter junction. It may be secondary to differential speeds of rotation of different sections of the brain after a torquing injury of the head. The prognosis is grave. Often small punctate hemorrhages are seen in the corpus callosum, basal ganglia, thalamus, hypothalamus, and upper brain stem associated with varying degrees of brain swelling. Sometimes the degree of brain swelling that develops is not very severe despite the severity of the injury from the point of view of outcome. One or both hemispheres may become uniformly hypodense, mimicking infarction. Subsequently the cerebrum atrophies. Often the initial head CT scan has minimal findings with only a few scattered tiny foci of hemorrhage visible in the white matter to mark the severity of the injury.

## Basilar Skull Fracture

It is important to remember that most lateral views of the skull in the trauma room are taken with cross-table lateral technique. The air-fluid level in the sphenoid sinus associated with a basilar skull fracture will be vertical when the x-ray is placed on a viewbox as if the patient were standing. A vertically oriented straight edge in the sphenoid sinus with homogenous fluid density behind it is not incomplete pneumatization of the sphenoid sinus, but rather an air-fluid level that is a marker for basilar skull fracture after trauma. Incomplete pneumatization of the sphenoid sinus usually has a slightly curvilinear posterior margin, not straight like an air-fluid level.

Intracranial air is often seen on plain skull films and head CT scans after basilar skull fracture communicating with a paranasal sinus.

## Intracranial Foreign Bodies

After a gunshot wound, metallic bullet fragments and bone fragments are easily seen by CT. Other material that may have been driven into the skull by trauma can be more difficult to recognize. Clothing fragments, wood, plastic, stones, and other relatively radiolucent material can be nearly isodense with brain or may be difficult to identify when surrounded by hemorrhage. Intracranial wood can be mistaken for a pneumatocele (air) on a CT scan. Tampons in the vagina, when not soaked with blood, appear on abdominal CT as air collections distending the vagina.

## Helmet CT

Computed tomography can be used for postaccident evaluation of helmet performance and condition. This information can be obtained without destructive dismantling of the helmet into its component layers, a process that may itself create artifactual helmet fractures or other findings not related to helmet performance during the accident.

# CT of Chest Trauma

After chest trauma, CT often adds significant findings not seen on chest x-ray. CT and histologic study have disclosed that pulmonary contusion is alveolar hemorrhage and pulmonary laceration, and they have revealed the role of pulmonary laceration in the etiology of posttraumatic pneumatocele formation, pulmonary hematoma and late cavitation. CT is more sensitive than chest x-ray for detection of pulmonary contusion/laceration. In one study, 99 lacerations were seen on chest CT scans when only 5 of these had been prospectively recognized on chest x-rays of the same group of patients.

# The Role of CT in the Evaluation of Acute Traumatic Aortic Injury

When blunt chest trauma causes aortic injury, in patients surviving long enough for treatment, the blood around the site of the aortic injury is not primarily from the aortic lumen. If it were, exsanguination would rapidly occur. After blunt chest trauma, it is almost always incorrect to call the aortic injury in a living patient with a mediastinal hematoma, an aortic rupture. The pathologically correct expression for this injury advocated by Harris is acute traumatic aortic injury (ATAI). Patients with traumatic thoracic aortic rupture are almost always dead at the scene of the injury or die on the way to the hospital.

When a patient is brought to the hospital after significant blunt trauma and has chest x-ray findings of possible mediastinal hematoma, physicians are frequently confused about what imaging study should be performed to evaluate for thoracic aortic injury.

Some advocate CT screening for thoracic aortic injury. Some advocate the use of intravenous contrast, some do some studies without intravenous contrast, some do the chest CT both without and with intravenous contrast. Some feel CT screening should be restricted to patients about whom there is not a strong clinical suspicion of aortic injury or a definite mediastinal hematoma on chest x-ray. Some feel that although CT is not sufficiently sensitive at present to evaluate for traumatic injury of the aorta directly, it is an invaluable adjunctive imaging modality for stable blunt chest trauma patients with equivocal chest radiographs or arteriograms. Others feel CT is an unacceptable method of screening for aortic injury because of missed cases and accept only arch angiography. Often the type of CT scanner used for the examinations, its age and speed, the scanning and contrast injection protocols used, the artifacts tolerated, and the interpretation criteria for a positive or negative scan are not completely specified or are not those currently accepted as adequate.

As a general rule, the performance of multiple studies when one would suffice is a bad idea. It delays diagnosis, costs money, requires administration of additional intravenous contrast, and inefficiently uses the radiologist's time.

The use of thoracic CT to screen for ATAI should be restricted to patients who are having emergency CT of another body part, particularly intravenous contrast-enhanced abdominal CT. When using newer CT scanners, scan speed is great enough and interscan delay short enough to allow excellent dynamic imaging of the chest, abdomen, and pelvis during a single 150-mL intravenous contrast bolus administered by a power injector.

The basic question to be answered is whether or not there is a mediastinal hematoma. If there is a mediastinal hematoma adjacent to the aorta, an arch aortogram is required for the following reasons: (1) to rule out ATAI, (2) to exclude simultaneous injury of major aortic branches, (3) to evaluate the integrity of the aortic valve and coronary artery origins, (4) to detect or further evaluate secondary aortic dissection antegrade or retrograde from the point of the aortic laceration, and (5) to allow surgical planning.

If a periaortic mediastinal hematoma is present, the CT finding of another injury that could explain the hematoma, such as thoracic spine fracture, is not sufficient to exclude aortic injury. Simultaneous aortic and other lesions can coexist.

Only the absence of periaortic mediastinal hematoma on an intravenous contrast-enhanced dynamic chest CT with no artifacts obscuring visualization, no visible aortic contour abnormality, false aneurysm, intimal flap, pericardial effusion, or hemopericardium is adequate in our practice to rule out aortic injury after blunt thoracic trauma. All radiologists should be aware of the aortic motion artifact simulating dissection of the ascending aorta, sometimes possible to eliminate by reconstruction of the CT data from only a portion of a full gantry rotation. This artifact may be more difficult to overcome when the CT data are acquired by helical (spiral) technique.

The CT study is being done to *rule OUT* mediastinal hematoma, not to demonstrate it. If a periaortic mediastinal hematoma is present, or any other of the above listed abnormalities are seen, I do not believe that CT can exclude aortic injury. Arch aortogram is required. The CT may provide additional information about other coexistent chest injuries but is not a complete evaluation of the aorta.

Why use intravenous contrast enhancement for these chest CT examinations? In this clinical setting, a nonintravenous contrast-enhanced chest CT showing mediastinal hematoma indicates the need for arch aortography; but if negative, it may not adequately rule out some of the more subtle signs of aortic injury. Taking the approach of adding a repeat chest CT examination with intravenous contrast to the already performed examination without contrast, when necessary, delays patient care in the cases most likely to have a life-threatening aortic injury. Also, after examining the unenhanced chest CT study, it is not obvious when an intravenous contrast-enhanced study is necessary. Thoracic injuries adjacent to the mediastinum, such as pulmonary contusion, can make mediastinal evaluation without intravenous contrast more difficult.

Why perform a nonintravenous contrast chest CT to verify what is already suspected on chest x-ray (mediastinal hematoma), if the chest CT may not adequately rule out aortic injury? Arch aortography is the gold standard of imaging in this condition and should not be delayed unless the patient needs emergent CT of some other body part.

Some special circumstances may mitigate this recommendation. Triage decision-making may require a prioritization of procedures and surgeries in the multiply injured patient. CT confirmation of the presence of mediastinal hematoma can make arch aortography a priority. Chest CT may also be useful to evaluate injuries to thoracic structures other than the aorta.

The chest x-rays obtained on trauma patients are frequently poor-inspiration supine studies making exclusion of mediastinal hematoma difficult. If the patient is having a contrast-enhanced CT of another body part, particularly the abdomen, this is an excellent opportunity to rule out mediastinal hematoma.

When doing simultaneous chest, abdomen, and pelvis CT we use 8-mm slice thickness and 10-mm table incrementation with contrast administration at 1.5 mL/s for 50 mL and 1.0 mL/s for an additional 100 mL with a 45-s delay from the beginning of the injection until scanning is started. We start at the top of the thorax and scan straight through the chest, abdomen, and pelvis without stopping. We administer water-soluble oral contrast via nasogastric tube both in the trauma room and in the CT suite before scanning. We are using a Somatom Plus for most of our CT studies (Siemens Medical Systems, Iselin, NJ).

The key step is to make sure that the chest x-ray of every patient referred for abdominal CT after blunt trauma is examined by the radiologist before the abdominal CT is done. If there is any question in the mind of the radiologist as to whether there is a mediastinal hematoma, this question can be answered by adding the chest to the upcoming intravenous contrast-enhanced dynamic CT study, making it a chest, abdomen, and pelvis study.

If the chest x-ray is examined by the radiologist only after the abdomen CT has been done, it is now too late to do a contrast-enhanced chest CT because the patient has already received the contrast for abdomen CT. If additional intravenous contrast were given for a chest CT done following the abdomen CT (because of the failure to look at the chest x-ray early enough), the duplication of contrast administration is a problem, potentially compounded by a later arch aortogram with additional contrast administration.

In summary, restrict the use of thoracic CT to screen for ATAI to those patients who are having emergency CT of another body part, particularly intravenous contrast-enhanced abdominal CT. Make sure that the chest x-ray of every patient referred for abdominal CT after blunt trauma is examined by the radiologist before the abdominal CT is done. If there is any question in the mind of the radiologist as to whether there is a mediastinal hematoma, add the chest to the dynamic intravenous contrast-enhanced CT study already contemplated.

Remember that the chest CT study is being done to *rule OUT* mediastinal hematoma, not to rule it in. The presence of a periaortic mediastinal hematoma after significant blunt thoracic trauma, whether demonstrated by chest x-ray or chest CT, requires an arch aortogram to evaluate for ATAI.

If the trauma patient has chest x-ray findings or a mechanism of injury requiring exclusion of ATAI and does not need immediate CT of a body part other than the chest, do not do a chest CT to evaluate the aorta. Arch aortography (not chest CT) is the study of choice for thoracic aortic evaluation. The result of the arch aortogram is usually definitive and in positive cases allows surgical planning not currently possible with CT.

It is important to distinguish aortic laceration from aortic dissection. Aortic dissection is usually associated with atherosclerotic vascular disease or occasionally pregnancy and not trauma. Up to 11 percent of ATAI patients will have a secondary aortic dissection either antegrade or retrograde, beginning at the site of the tear, due to pulsatile luminal pressure and flow. Such dissections can be in the tunica media, but are often subadventitial, in contrast to the dissections of the aorta seen in patients with atherosclerosis or pregnancy, which are usually in the tunica media. Most ATAIs are localized and have no secondary aortic dissection. Recent research suggests that ATAI may result from thoracic compression with aortic pinching between the sternum and the spine rather than deceleration shearing forces (the traditional explanation). ATAI should not be called traumatic aortic dissection.

## CT of Abdominal Trauma

### Abdominal CT Versus Diagnostic Peritoneal Lavage

Computed tomography of the abdomen after blunt abdominal trauma is most appropriate for the patient stable enough to avoid physiologic compromise during the time required for performance of the examination. This amount of time varies from institution to institution.

When possible, the performance of abdominal CT before or instead of diagnostic peritoneal lavage (DPL) is preferable to doing the abdominal CT examination after DPL. Abdominal trauma CT is useful either before or after DPL; however, DPL introduces fluid and free air, making evaluation for intestinal injury, perception of the "sentinel clot sign," and evaluation of the volume of hemoperitoneum difficult. This increases the problems in determining which patients are candidates for nonoperative management of solid organ injury.

Increased radiologist experience in interpretation of trauma CT ex-

aminations and the development of bolus dynamic scanning using a CT power injector for intravenous contrast administration have significantly improved the sensitivity and accuracy of abdominal CT for evaluation of trauma. At hospitals where state-of-the-art CT is being performed, all published data about the sensitivity and specificity of abdominal trauma CT for detection of solid organ injury are nearly obsolete. Recent CT scanners with improved computer image processing speed and increased x-ray tube cooling can rapidly obtain many scans during the bolus phase of intravenous contrast administration, markedly improving image quality. Fast scanning techniques decrease motion artifacts.

A recent study comparing CT and DPL for blunt abdominal trauma probably suffers from use of older CT techniques and equipment but still found that CT had similar specificity (99.5 versus 99 percent), accuracy (92.6 versus 98.2 percent) but somewhat lower sensitivity (74.3 versus 95.9 percent) compared to DPL for evaluation of blunt abdominal trauma. The method of intravenous contrast administration was not specified and whether or not dynamic scanning was used was not stated. Two of 301 patients with negative CT scans required operative treatment of a complication of DPL.

Use of CT for evaluation of blunt abdominal trauma decreases the nontherapeutic laparotomy rate. In one study this decreased from 14 percent with DPL to 5 percent with use of CT.

Solid organ injury (injury to the liver, spleen, pancreas, adrenals, and kidneys) in the abdomen is extremely well evaluated by bolus enhanced dynamic abdominal CT (see Figs. 259-4 and 259-6). The challenge for radiologists is detection of intestinal and other hollow viscus injury. CT can be effective in identifying bowel injury in adult and pediatric patients but is much less sensitive for detection of intestinal injury than for solid organ injury. Missed intestinal injuries are a problem in both adult and pediatric patients.

### Nonoperative Management and Occult Intestinal Injuries

Nonoperative management of hemodynamically stable patients with blunt abdominal injury is being used with increasing frequency. In such cases, occult intestinal injuries often are not clinically apparent until several days after the trauma. Morbidity and mortality may increase from such occult intestinal injuries. For this reason, radiologists are increasingly vigilant about evaluation of the intestine on CT examinations, especially after blunt trauma.

Unfortunately, because of limited bowel opacification by oral contrast and the occasional presence of mesenteric hematoma, accurate evaluation for intestinal injury is often difficult on initial examinations after trauma. This is particularly true in adult patients with little intra-abdominal fat and in children. Air or fluid introduced by DPL before CT makes evaluation more difficult. DPL *after* abdomen CT for trauma can assist in the detection of intestinal injury, especially in patients who have incomplete bowel opacification by CT oral contrast due to inadequate time for transit or ileus accompanying trauma.

The presence of a focal dense blood clot adjacent to an intestinal loop or other organ is termed the *sentinel clot sign.* This sign is particularly useful, when present, to mark sites of probable injury including intestinal injury. Unfortunately, this sign is often not present at sites of intestinal injury.

In cases where mesenteric hematoma encases intestinal loops, laparotomy is often indicated to rule out intestinal injury. The morbidity of a nontherapeutic laparotomy is less than the morbidity of a missed intestinal laceration. When frank extravasation of oral contrast occurs from torn intestinal loops, laparotomy is required. Care must be taken during CT interpretation to avoid confusing active bleeding containing contrast (in contrast-enhanced blood) from oral contrast leaking from an intestinal lumen, although both require prompt laparotomy.

Stool usually contains substantial amounts of gas. This and the other gas in the colonic lumen usually allow adequate colon evaluation without additional colon contrast (see Fig. 259-4B). If a specific portion of the colon is difficult to evaluate by CT, either changing the patient's position to move colon gas to the area of interest or rectal administration of water-soluble CT oral contrast can be performed to create a CT enema. The use of rectal contrast for CT is extremely helpful in selected cases. The routine use of rectal contrast for trauma abdominal CT examinations is not necessary and delays the performance of the examination.

Iodine-based water-soluble oral contrast should be administered via nasogastric tube in the trauma room as soon as the decision for abdominal CT is made. This will allow maximum time for small bowel transit of oral contrast.

## CT of Retroperitoneal and Flank Trauma

Computed tomography is accurate for evaluation of retroperitoneal trauma. CT may not show every injury but will indicate whether operation is required or not.

For significant renal trauma, CT will demonstrate if renal fragments have intact arterial and venous supply, whether the associated urinoma or hematoma is well contained, and the status of other retroperitoneal and intraperitoneal organs. Many fractured kidneys are now being salvaged by nonoperative management. Severe injuries of the main renal artery or main renal vein in the renal pedicle still require operation.

Intravenous contrast-enhanced CT has replaced the intravenous pyelogram (IVP) as the best method for evaluation and staging of renal trauma (see Fig. 259-5). IVP is not very sensitive for detection of renal injuries. CT is much more accurate. Dissenting views are occasionally expressed. However, in one dissenting study, in addition to the added renal findings by CT, 3 of the 60 patients had significant unsuspected extrarenal intra-abdominal injuries shown on the CT scan. Two of these patients required laparotomy. Among the injuries usually missed by IVP, unsuspected splenic laceration coexisting with minor renal trauma can be fatal. This will be detected by CT. Both IVP and CT were performed in these research studies. The IVP is rarely necessary when CT has been done.

In cases of negative IVP and positive CT, although CT shows the type and extent of renal injury much more accurately than IVP, its additional findings often do not change management. The additional findings provided by CT often alter the pattern of follow-up and return to activity recommendations.

## CT of Bladder and Diaphragm Injuries

Use of CT to evaluate the contrast-filled bladder can be very helpful. Merely clamping the Foley catheter before the CT examination, then evaluating the bladder based on the volume of urine accumulating during the period of the CT study does not provide adequate bladder distention for a diagnostic cystogram. A dilute sterile contrast solution of at least 250 to 400 mL for an adult must be administered retrograde through the Foley catheter, the catheter clamped, then CT cystogram images may be done. This is the volume of bladder contrast used for a conventional cystogram and is necessary for any filming technique including CT. A postdrain series of scans must also be obtained, by plain film or CT. When done by this method, CT is accurate for bladder evaluation. We use 50 mL of standard ionic intravenous contrast in 500 mL of sterile normal saline (in an intravenous bag) as the solution to be introduced into the bladder.

It is usually wise to do the standard abdomen and pelvic CT scans before doing a CT cystogram (or any cystogram). If the cystogram is done first, if there is a bladder laceration, contrast extravasation in the pelvis will obscure diagnostic information.

Diagnosing injuries of the diaphragm on CT scans is often difficult because of the transverse plane of CT scanning (parallel to the plane of the diaphragm). Chest x-ray obtained on admission and repeated soon after, when coupled with a high index of suspicion, is more sensitive than previously thought for diagnosis of traumatic rupture of the diaphragm, particularly on the left side.

## Abdominal CT Findings and the Decision for Laparotomy

In both adult and pediatric patients the extent of hemoperitoneum and appearance of organ injuries are not the only factors in deciding whether a laparotomy is necessary. Various CT-based grading systems have been tried in an attempt to predict from the CT results alone which patients with abdominal trauma need laparotomy. The hemodynamic status of the patient and the results of serial laboratory studies and bedside assessments in conjunction with the CT results determine the need for laparotomy.

The flat inferior vena cava sign is useful in showing that the patient having CT has severe volume depletion and immediate incipient hemodynamic crisis. This is true in both adult and pediatric patients.

In pediatric patients the experience is the same as that in adult patients. CT is excellent for abdominal injury detection but the decision for laparotomy is not only based on the extent of injury shown on the CT scan, but also substantially on the physiologic condition of the child. Some pediatric studies have shown a positive correlation between the volume of hemoperitoneum, the need for laparotomy, and the mortality rate; however, other studies disagree with this assertion.

For patients with gunshot wounds of the chest or abdomen, an analysis of the bullet path to determine whether the peritoneum has been traversed is mandatory. Two radiographs at 90°, CT, clinical examination, and peritoneal lavage are all useful. Any chest gunshot wound below the level of the nipples is suspicious for intra-abdominal penetration. The diaphragm is a dome-shaped structure and goes up higher in the thorax than one might suspect from external examination. If peritoneal penetration by a bullet is suspected, laparotomy is indicated. The morbidity and mortality of an exploratory laparotomy that shows no significant intra-abdominal injury is low compared with that of missed intestinal injury. CT is particularly useful when an exclusively body wall or retroperitoneal path is suspected.

## CT of Spine Trauma (Including Cervical Spine)

Plain films should be used to guide the levels to be CT scanned. An intact vertebra above and below the vertebra suspected of injury on standard radiographs should be included in the CT scan because a substantial number of occult injuries will be found in these adjacent vertebrae.

Standard radiographs are a good guide to the areas suspicious for fracture. In one study, only 1 of 49 patients with cervical fracture visible on CT had completely normal standard radiographs. If there is a strong clinical suspicion of occult injury because of symptoms or signs despite negative radiographs, CT of the area of interest can easily be performed.

## CONCLUSION

Computed tomography has revolutionized the evaluation and treatment of patients with many different types of pathology. Working together the radiologist and clinician create the best sequence of imaging examinations for each clinical problem. CT is often one of the examinations and is cost and time effective. Understanding some of the technical aspects of CT helps the clinician order the appropriate study and use the results correctly for decision-making. The experience of the radiologist is invaluable for study design, performance, and interpretation. Emergency physicians find the information gained from the CT examination of trauma patients particularly useful for improving patient care.

## BIBLIOGRAPHY

Acheson MB, Livingston RR, Richardson ML, et al. High-resolution CT scanning in the evaluation of cervical spine fractures: comparison with plain film examinations, *AJR Am J Roentgenol* 148:1179, 1987.

Agee CK, Metzler MH, Churchill RJ, et al. Computed tomographic evaluation to exclude traumatic aortic disruption. *J Trauma* 33:876, 1992.

Bergren CT, Chan FN, Bodzin JH. Intravenous pyelogram results in association with renal pathology and therapy in trauma patients. *J Trauma* 27:515, 1987.

Brick SH, Taylor GA, Potter BM, et al. Hepatic and splenic injury in children: role of CT in the decision for laparotomy, *Radiology* 165:643, 1987.

Brooks AP, Olson LK, Shackford SR. Computed tomography in the diagnosis of traumatic rupture of the thoracic aorta. *Clin Radiol* 40:133, 1989.

Bulas DI, Taylor GA, Eichelberger MR. The value of CT in detecting bowel perforation in children after blunt abdominal trauma. *AJR Am J Roentgenol* 153:561, 1989.

Burns MA, Molina PL, Gutierrez FR, et al. Motion artifact simulating aortic dissection on CT. *AJR Am J Roentgenol* 157:465, 1991.

Cass AS, Vieira J. Comparison of IVP and CT findings in patients with suspected severe renal injury. *Urology* 29:484, 1987.

Christensen EE, Curry TS III, Dowdey JE. Computed tomography. In: *An introduction to the Physics of Diagnostic Radiology,* 2nd ed. Philadelphia: Lea & Febiger, pp. 329–360, 1978.

Cooter RD. Computed tomography in the assessment of protective helmet deformation. *J Trauma* 30:55, 1990.

Crass JR, Cohen AM, Motta AO, et al. A proposed new mechanism of traumatic aortic rupture: the osseous pinch. *Radiology* 176:645, 1990.

Demos TC, Solomon C, Posniak HV, et al. Computed tomography in traumatic defects of the diaphragm, *Clin Imaging* 13:62, 1989.

Federle MP, Brant-Zawadzki M (eds). *Computed Tomography in the Evaluation of Trauma,* 2nd ed. Baltimore: Williams & Wilkins, 1986.

Federle MP, Brown TR, McAninch JW. Penetrating renal trauma: CT evaluation. *J Comput Assist Tomogr* 11:1026, 1987.

Feliciano DV, Burch JM, Spjut-Patrinely V, et al. Abdominal gunshot wounds: an urban trauma center's experience with 300 consecutive patients. *Ann Surg* 208:362, 1988.

Fenner MN, Fisher KS, Sergel NL, et al. Evaluation of possible traumatic thoracic aortic injury using aortography and CT. *Am Surg* 56:497, 1990.

Fletcher TB, Setiawan H, Harrell RS, et al. Posterior abdominal stab wounds: role of CT evaluation. *Radiology* 173:621, 1989.

Gelman R, Mirvis SE, Gens D. Diaphragmatic rupture due to blunt trauma: sensitivity of plain chest radiographs. *AJR Am J Roentgenol* 156:51, 1991.

Haftel AJ, Lev R, Mahour GH, et al. Abdominal CT scanning in pediatric blunt trauma. *Ann Emerg Med* 17:684, 1988.

Halsell RD, Vines FS, Shatney CH, et al. The reliability of excretory urography as a screening examination for blunt renal trauma. *Ann Emerg Med* 16:1236, 1987.

Harris JH Jr. Editorial comment. *Emergency Radiology* 1:77, 1994.

Hauser CJ, Huprich JE, Bosco P, et al. Triple-contrast computed tomography in the evaluation of penetrating posterior abdominal injuries, *Arch Surg* 122:1112, 1987.

Hofer GA, Cohen AJ. CT signs of duodenal perforation secondary to blunt abdominal trauma, *J Comput Assist Tomogr* 13:430, 1989.

Ishikawa T, Nakajima Y, Kaji T. The role of CT in traumatic rupture of the thoracic aorta and its proximal branches. *Semin Roentgenol* 24:38, 1989.

Jeffrey RB Jr, Federle MP. The collapsed inferior vena cava: CT evidence of hypovolemia. *AJR Am J Roentgenol* 150:431, 1988.

Jooma R, Bradshaw JR, Coakham HB. Computed tomography in penetrating cranial injury by a wooden foreign body. *Surg Neurol* 21:236, 1984.

Kadir S. Arteriography of the thoracic aorta. In: *Diagnostic angiography.* Philadelphia: WB Saunders, pp. 124–171, 1986.

Kane NM, Cronan JJ, Dorfman GS, et al. Pediatric abdominal trauma: evaluation by computed tomography, *Pediatrics* 82:11, 1988.

Kane NM, Dorfman GS, Cronan JJ. Efficacy of CT following peritoneal lavage in abdominal trauma. *J Comput Assist Tomogr* 11:998, 1987.

Katayama H, Yamaguchi K, Kozuka T, et al. Adverse reactions to ionic and nonionic contrast media. *Radiology* 175:621, 1990.

Kearney PA Jr, Vahey T, Burney RE, et al. Computed tomography and diagnostic peritoneal lavage in blunt abdominal trauma. Their combined role. *Arch Surg* 124:344, 1989.

Kelly J, Raptopoulos V, Davidoff A, et al. On the value of non-contrast-enhanced CT in blunt abdominal trauma. *AJR Am J Roentgenol* 152:41, 1989.

Lasser EC, Berry CC, Talner LB, et al. Pretreatment with corticosteroids to alleviate reactions to intravenous contrast material. *N Engl J Med* 317:845, 1987.

Lee JKT, Sagel SS, Stanley RJ, et al. *Computed Body Tomography with MRI Correlation,* 2nd ed. New York: Raven Press, 1989.

Lowe RJ, Saletta JD, Read DR, et al. Should laparotomy be mandatory or selective in gunshot wounds of the abdomen? *J Trauma* 17:903, 1977.

Mattox KL. Approaches to trauma involving the major vessels of the thorax. *Surg Clin North Am* 69:77, 1989.

Mee SL, McAninch JW, Federle MP. Computerized tomography in bladder rupture: diagnostic limitations. *J Urol* 137:207, 1987.

Meyer DM, Thal ER, Weigelt JA, et al. The role of abdominal CT in the evaluation of stab wounds to the back. *J Trauma* 29:1226, 1989.

Meyer DM, Thal ER, Weigelt JA, et al. Evaluation of computed tomography and diagnostic peritoneal lavage in blunt abdominal trauma. *J Trauma* 29:1168, 1989.

Miller FB, Richardson JD, Thomas HA, et al. Role of CT in diagnosis of major arterial injury after blunt thoracic trauma. *Surgery* 106:596, 1989.

Mirvis SE, Kostrubiak I, Whitley NO, et al. Role of CT in excluding major arterial injury after blunt thoracic trauma. *AJR Am J Roentgenol* 149:601, 1987.

Mirvis SE, Whitley NO, Gens DR. Blunt splenic trauma in adults: CT-based classification and correlation with prognosis and treatment. *Radiology* 171:33, 1989.

Mirvis SE, Whitley NO, Vainwright JR, et al. Blunt hepatic trauma in adults: CT-based classification and correlation with prognosis and treatment, *Radiology* 171:27, 1989.

Moore EE, Moore JB, VanDuzer-Moore S, et al. Mandatory laparotomy for gunshot wounds penetrating the abdomen. *Am J Surg* 140:847, 1980.

Orwig D, Federle MP. Localized clotted blood as evidence of visceral trauma on CT: the sentinel clot sign. *AJR Am J Roentgenol* 153:747, 1989.

Palmer FJ. The RACR survey of intravenous contrast media reactions: final report. *Australas Radiol* 32:426, 1988.

Parmley LF, Mattingly TW, Manion WC, et al. Non-penetrating traumatic injury of the aorta. *Circulation* 17:1086, 1958.

Posniak HV, Olson MC, Demos TC. Aortic motion artifact simulating dissection on CT scans: elimination with reconstructive segmented images. *AJR Am J Roentgenol* 161:557, 1993.

Rehm CG, Sherman R, Hinz TW. The role of CT scan in evaluation for laparotomy in patients with stab wounds of the abdomen. *J Trauma* 29:446, 1989.

Rengachary SS, Szymanski DC. Subdural hematomas of arterial origin. *Neurosurgery* 8:166, 1981.

Richardson P, Mirvis SE, Scorpio R, et al. Value of CT in determining the need for angiography when findings of mediastinal hemorrhage on chest radiographs are equivocal. *AJR Am J Roentgenol* 156:273, 1991.

Rizzo MJ, Federle MP, Griffiths BG. Bowel and mesenteric injury following blunt abdominal trauma: evaluation with CT. *Radiology* 173:143, 1989.

Sherck JP, Oakes DD. Intestinal injuries missed by computed tomography. *J Trauma* 30:1, 1990.

Siemens Medical Systems Inc. *Somatom DR: Influence of Operating Parameters, Medical Considerations and Physical Factors on Image Quality.* Erlangen: 1985.

Sivit CJ, Taylor GA, Bulas DJ, et al. Blunt trauma in children: significance of peritoneal fluid. *Radiology* 178:185, 1991.

Sorkey AJ, Farnell MB, Williams HJ Jr, et al. The complementary roles of diagnostic peritoneal lavage and computed tomography in the evaluation of blunt abdominal trauma. *Surgery* 106:794, 1989.

Taylor GA, Fallat ME, Eichelberger MR. Hypovolemic shock in children: abdominal CT manifestations. *Radiology* 164:479, 1987.

Taylor GA, Fallat ME, Potter BM, et al. The role of computed tomography in blunt abdominal trauma in children. *J Trauma* 28:1660, 1988.

Tocino I, Miller MH. Computed tomography in blunt chest trauma. *J Thorac Imaging* 2:45, 1987.

Tomiak MM, Rosenblum JD, Messersmith RN, et al. Use of CT for diagnosis of traumatic rupture of the thoracic aorta. *Ann Vasc Surg* 7:130, 1993.

Tsai FY, Teal JS, Hieshima GB. Computed tomography in head trauma. In: *Neuroradiology of Head Trauma.* Baltimore: University Park Press, pp. 99–200, 1984.

Umlas S-L, Cronan JJ. Splenic trauma: can CT grading system enable prediction of successful nonsurgical treatment? *Radiology* 178:481, 1991.

Wagner RB, Crawford WO Jr, Schimpf PP. Classification of parenchymal injuries of the lung. *Radiology* 167:77, 1988.

Wagner RB, Crawford WO Jr, Schimpf PP, et al. Quantitation and pattern of parenchymal lung injury in blunt chest trauma. Diagnostic and therapeutic implications. *J Comput Assist Tomogr* 12:270, 1988.

Wagner RB, Jamieson PM. Pulmonary contusion. Evaluation and classification by computed tomography. *Surg Clin North Am* 69:31, 1989.

Williams AL. Trauma. In: Williams AL, Haughton VM (eds). *Cranial Computed Tomography: A Comprehensive Text.* St. Louis: CV Mosby, pp. 37–87, 1985.

## ACKNOWLEDGMENTS

I gratefully the acknowledge the assistance of Saul Taylor, MD, for a careful reading of the manuscript, particularly the neuroradiology section, and E. Russell Ritenour, Ph.D., for a careful reading of the section on CT technical aspects.

# 260

# MAGNETIC RESONANCE IMAGING: PRINCIPLES AND SOME APPLICATIONS

### Irwin D. Weisman

## INTRODUCTION

The significant advances in imaging technology of recent years have dramatically expedited diagnosis and improved outcomes in the emergency department patient. Magnetic resonance imaging (MRI) has been at the forefront of the most recent evolution in technical developments. In just a short time, it has become a major modality in neurological and musculoskeletal evaluations. The purpose of this chapter is to briefly describe MRI and then elucidate its role in emergency medicine.

Magnetic resonance imaging has the following major advantages:

1. Like ultrasound, it does not use ionizing radiation and no short- or long-term side effects have been demonstrated. This is in contrast to the high-energy ionizing radiation of computed tomography (CT) and other x-ray methods which produces small but finite biological damage that may have long-term carcinogenesis implications. Because of this consideration, MRI should be preferred over CT and tomography in the pediatric and child-bearing populations.
2. It produces variable thickness, two-dimensional slices in any orientation through the body part of interest, thus optimizing visualization of tissues and their interfaces. With few exceptions, CT is restricted to a scan plane that is transverse to the long axis of the body.
3. Because of the different physical principles underlying magnetic resonance (as opposed to x-rays), it provides better contrast resolution and tissue discrimination in many areas compared to x-rays or ultrasound. For example, spinal cord, bone marrow, muscles, and tendons are better visualized with MRI than with CT. As a result, MRI is replacing invasive methods such as myelography, arthrography and, in limited situations, angiography.

MRI is a specific application of nuclear magnetic resonance to medical imaging. Nuclear magnetic resonance was discovered simultaneously in 1946 by Bloch and colleagues at Stanford University and Purcell and colleagues at Harvard University. Bloch and Purcell shared the Nobel prize in 1952 for their outstanding contribution to the physical sciences.

## PHYSICAL BASIS

The nuclei of hydrogen in water and fat molecules behave like small spinning bar magnets. When placed in a strong uniform magnetic field [e.g., >0.01 tesla (100 gauss)], they execute a circular motion, or precession, weakly aligning to form a net nuclear polarization nearly parallel to the external magnet field. If a short pulse of radio frequency (rf) energy (radio wave), precisely tuned to the precession frequency of the water and fat proton nuclear magnets, is applied, the nuclei absorb a small amount of energy, change their alignment, and then gradually return to their previous equilibrium positions. In responding to the radio wave, the net nuclear magnetization generates a small voltage, the nuclear magnetic resonance signal, that can be detected and recorded electronically.

Two parameters T1 and T2, also known respectively as longitudinal and transverse relaxation times, govern the behavior of the electronic signal detected. The relaxation times are a function of the immediate environment of the resonating protons and vary in the different biological tissues. For example, free water exhibits long T1 and T2 values and fat exhibits short T1 and relatively short T2 values. It will turn out that image generation requires a large number of repetitions of the sequence that produces the nuclear resonance signal. The time between repetitions is called TR. For technical reasons, a two-pulse sequence is used to generate a particular type of signal called a *spin echo*. The spacing between pulses is labeled TE/2, and the echo occurs at a time TE. There are important relationships between the intensity of the nuclear resonance echo and TR, T1, TE, and T2.

Based on the effects of the different relaxation times (T1 and T2), two types of imaging are carried out. Short TR between successive cycles of rf excitation pulses and short TE produce stronger signals from tissues with relatively short T1 times, such as fat, especially bone marrow. Hence weighting favoring short T1 results from pulse sequences using short TR and short TE. On the other hand, longer TR eliminate much of the T1 signal difference between fat and water, so that further manipulation of the rf pulse spacing (longer TE) will enhance signals from tissues with long T2 times, such as edema fluid. Long TR and TE pulse sequences preferentially weight long T2 tissues. Thus the two basic methods of MRI scanning are labeled *T1*- and *T2-weighted imaging*.

To construct an image from the tissue-specific signals of an object (for example, a patient), it is necessary to apply small, spatially inhomogeneous, three-dimensional magnetic fields called *gradients*. They modify the signal decay of the nuclear magnetization and spatially tag the hydrogen nuclear magnets in the object for mapping the image. The actual reconstruction of an image is complex, just as in CT scanning, and requires a relatively fast computer with a large memory. The ultimate result is a two-dimensional, medically diagnostic, cross-sectional body image that is displayed on a video monitor and recorded on film or digitally stored on a hard disk or magnetic tape as a permanent record. In most gray-scale imaging formats, the strongest signal corresponds to maximum brightness on the black-and-white monitor. Therefore, in heavily T2-weighted images, water appears bright, whereas fat appears intermediate gray. On the other hand, on T1-weighted images, fat appears bright and water appears dark (Fig. 260-1). For a more complete discussion of the technical aspects and clinical applications of MRI, the reader is referred to more specialized texts.

The physical basis of image formation using MRI is quite different from CT, which is based on differential x-ray absorption coefficients. Even though both are tomographic imaging techniques, the meaning of bright and dark signals in MRI is relative to the pulse sequence eliciting them and has very little resemblance to the contrast in CT.

The core of an MRI system is the large magnet needed to generate the strong, constant, and uniform magnetic field as well as the magnetic gradients. The magnet is composed of coils of a special superconducting wire that loses all resistance to electrical current when submerged in liquid helium. At this temperature, $-268°$ C ($-450°$ F), the coils can handle the relatively large currents of electricity required to produce the magnetic field. A specially designed, thermally insulated container encloses the magnet coils and the liquid helium. The liquid slowly boils away and must be replaced at regular inter-

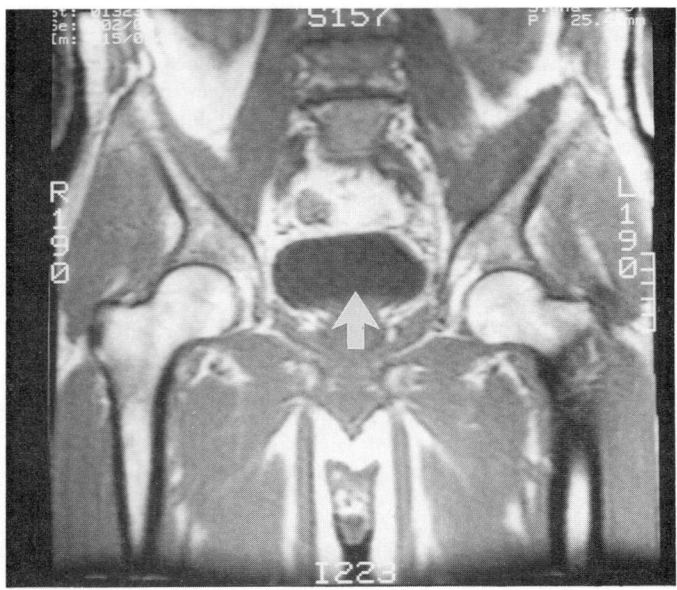

A

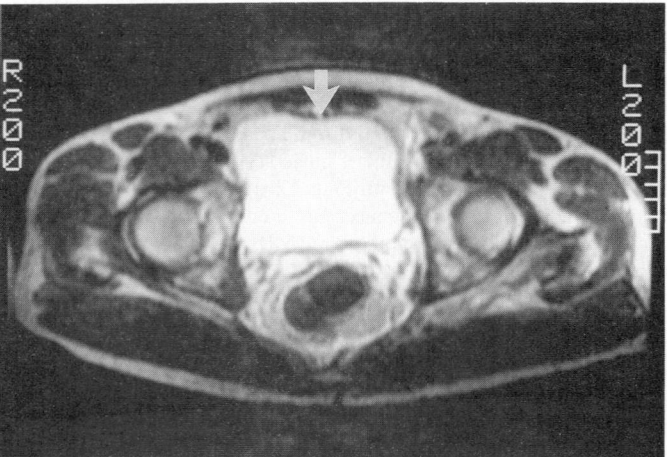

B

**Fig. 260-1.** Examples of T1- and T2-weighted MR images. *A.* T1-weighted coronal image: note that the urine in the bladder (arrow) which is essentially water with a long T1, appears dark, whereas the femoral bone marrow, subcutaneous, and perivesical fat (short T1) appear bright. *B.* T2-weighted axial image of the same patient as in A: note that the urine, which has a long T2, now appears bright, whereas the surrounding fat with its shorter T2 is intermediate in brightness.

vals. The magnet is housed in a special room containing sheets of steel and copper screen, which shield the system against interference by steel and radio waves on the outside, and vice versa. The other components of the system, consisting of a radio transmitter, a sophisticated rf receiver, and a high-speed large-memory computer, are located near the operator's console just outside the room.

## SAFETY

In a few cases, the large magnetic field could be a health hazard to the patient, necessitating the use of alternative diagnostic methods such as ultrasound or CT. Internal cardiac pacemakers may be converted to an abnormal asynchronous mode by the magnetic field. Certain types of steel cerebral aneurysm clips (ferromagnetic as opposed to nonmagnetic stainless steel) may experience strong forces, with the

potential of harming the brain. Small steel slivers embedded in the eye (occasionally seen in asymptomatic sheet metal workers or welders) could injure the retina and cause blindness. Life-support equipment containing magnetic steel will be strongly attracted into the magnetic field, threatening both the patient and the system. Cochlear implants may be damaged or cause unacceptable injury due to eddy current heating effects. Patients in any of the above categories cannot be scanned with MRI. There are other devices, such as implantable cardiac defibrillators, neurostimulators, and bone growth stimulators, that may malfunction in the presence of high magnetic fields. Certain prosthetic heart valves contain nearly magnetic stainless steel components that are subject to strong forces when placed in powerful magnetic fields. However, it has been pointed out that the forces on the valve from the heart exceed those generated by even high-field magnets, and hence this is a relative contraindication for MRI scanning.

The pulsed radio waves are a source of heat energy deposited within the body. Software programs built into the computers restrict the frequency of pulsing so that the maximum allowable power deposition averaged over the whole patient is never exceeded. Occasionally burns have been reported when patients' skin has come into direct contact with uninsulated rf leads, but proper precautions prevent this from happening.

The complete examination takes from 30 to 60 min, is painless, and is well tolerated by most patients. It does require suspension of all motion, except for breathing, for periods of a few seconds to 15 min at a time, depending on the particular pulse sequence. A few patients are claustrophobic and have difficulty with the examination. Most problems of this nature are satisfactorily treated with minor tranquilizers administered orally. Infants, younger pediatric patients, and agitated adults need to be sedated, as in CT, because any motion degrades the MRI scan.

Some minor precautions are necessary. Magnetically encoded plastic cards such as credit, cash, and parking cards may be damaged when they come within a certain range of the magnetic field. Some watches with steel parts and hearing aids (and their batteries) are vulnerable to damage. Any ferromagnetic steel objects are potentially lethal missiles if carried into the magnet room. Patients need to leave such objects outside the scanning room.

## APPLICATIONS

MRI has been widely applied to the brain and spinal cord, where it provides images that are superior in diagnostic quality to those obtained with CT. Furthermore, this information can be obtained with less risk to the patient because CT myelography requires intrathecal contrast agents for a specific diagnosis. Although special intravenous contrast agents are frequently required to improve the sensitivity of MRI, they have been associated with much less toxicity and fewer reactions as compared to the intravenous CT contrast agents. Except in the cases of acute intracerebral hemorrhage, skull fracture, and some calcified brain lesions, MRI may completely replace CT in the head. The exact role of MRI versus CT in trauma and degenerative disease of the spine is still evolving. CT visualizes fracture fragment relationships and bone detail more optimally, but MRI visualizes the soft tissues with better resolution. Some spine surgeons still prefer CT myelography to MRI.

MRI has been useful in the chest and abdomen (especially in the chest wall, mediastinum, liver, spleen, adrenals, and aorta) but has played a lesser role compared to CT because of respiratory motion and heart pulsation artifacts, which degrade anatomic delineation of critical structures. They can be compensated to some degree with electrocardiograph and respiratory gating and associated electronic manipulation, but the methods are cumbersome and difficult to implement with an acutely ill patient.

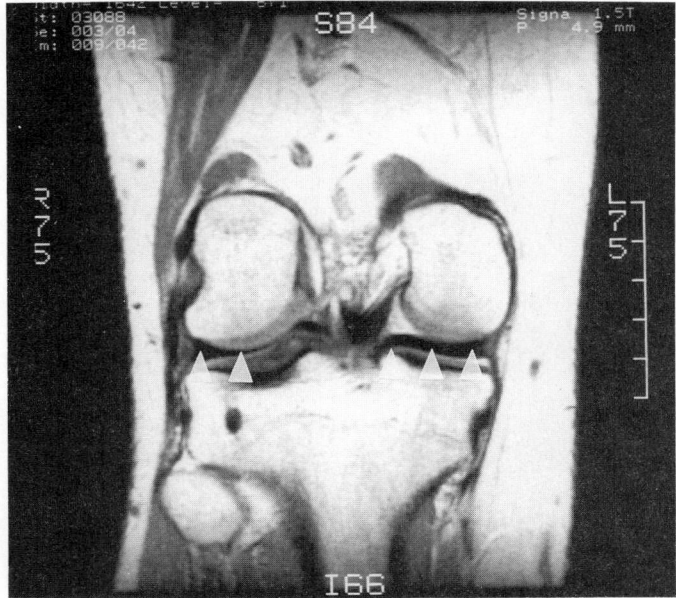

**A**

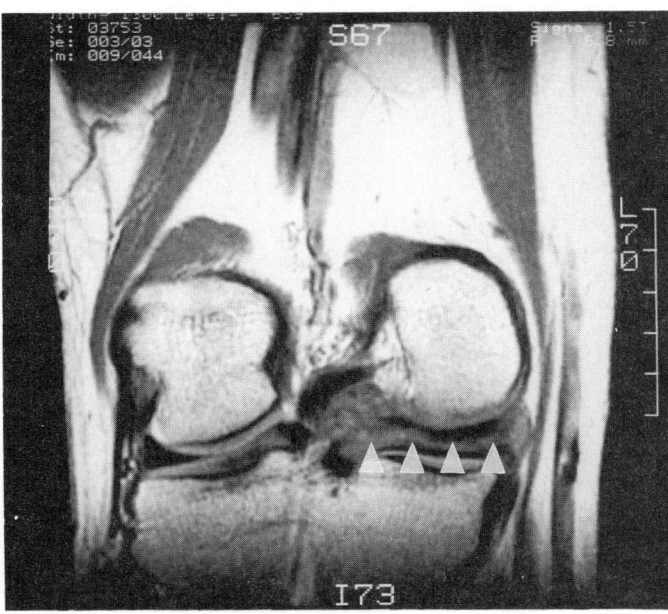

**B**

**Fig. 260-2.** Meniscal tear. *A.* Normal medial and lateral menisci as demonstrated on a MR proton density coronal image (partial T2 weighting). The menisci are the dark triangular structures marked with arrow heads. *B.* Proton density coronal scan showing a large complex tear involving the posterior horn of the medial meniscus (arrowheads).

MRI has a major role in other areas of the musculoskeletal system, especially the knee, shoulder, hip, and temporomandibular joints. Although MRI is not indicated for most acute fractures, it may be preferred in the diagnosis of rotator cuff tears of the shoulders, internal derangement of the knee (meniscus, tendon, and ligament tears), tendon or soft-tissue injury to any of the small joints, soft-tissue injury in the spine, and posttraumatic avascular necrosis of any bone. In addition, carpal tunnel syndrome has been evaluated using MRI. Figure 260-2 demonstrates a meniscus tear in the knee. Before MRI, arthrog-

raphy, which involves injection of contrast agents into the joint, was used to detect cartilage injuries. This type of examination is not only painful but carries a small but finite risk of infection and contrast reaction. MRI of these joints is painless and only requires that the patient be able to hold still for a moderate length of time. The information obtained in the knee and hips exceeds what can be obtained using other methods. In the hips, MRI has proven to be the most reliable method for detecting avascular necrosis.

In problematic cases, MRI has sensitively detected stress fractures and occult fractures in the small bones of the hand. Even though it does not visualize cortex, any break in the medullary cancellous bone can be readily detected.

The sequelae of soft-tissue musculoskeletal trauma, such as complete muscular or tendon tears, hemorrhage, and edema, are very easily diagnosed with MRI. Even injuries to the medium-sized nerves and brachial plexus can be demonstrated.

MRI has also been used to study infection in bone and soft tissues, where in many cases it has been superior to modalities such as nuclear medicine and CT. However, if the patient has a metallic prosthesis in the region of abnormality, rf currents or magnetic field inhomogeneities due to the metal induce artifacts in the MRI scan that reduce the sensitivity (Fig. 260-3). This is even more of a problem in CT, where x-ray scattering from the prosthesis may completely obliterate the scan. Then only nuclear medicine studies may be useful, in particular indium 111 tagged to white blood cells.

MRI is extremely sensitive and specific in detecting metastatic disease in bone when questions arise after a positive bone scan. It is neither practical nor cost effective to use MRI for whole-body surveys, but when applied to specific lesions the anatomic information expedites diagnosis and proper workup.

Computed tomography continues to be the modality of choice for traumatized patients with suspected head, spine, and abdominal injuries because it is quick, more widely available, and more compatible with life-support equipment. Although MRI-compatible respirators and pulsed oxymeters are now available, most standard life-support equipment either contains magnetic steel components or sensitive electronics that will not operate properly in the presence of rf or large static or dynamic magnetic fields. MRI is used in the elective setting after the patient has been stabilized and there is time to address the less acute problems.

## MRI IN THE EMERGENT SETTING

At the present time there are two areas where MRI is the procedure of choice in the acute setting: (1) spinal cord compression from any cause, and (2) radiographically occult femoral intertrochanteric and neck fractures. MRI quickly, noninvasively, and efficaciously addresses these two problems. In both cases, it is the unique ability to form images in axial, coronal, or sagittal planes that gives MRI a distinct advantage. Another major factor is the superb contrast resolution of MRI that facilitates detection of spinal cord injury or fracture through cancellous bone of the hip. Figure 260-4 demonstrates an example of cervical cord compression resulting from a traumatically herniated disc. Figure 260-5 is an example of an occult femoral intertrochanteric fracture best demonstrated on MRI. Recently a small series of cases has confirmed higher sensitivity and specificity for MRI as compared to radio nuclide bone scanning, tomography, and CT in the detection of occult fractures, especially in the femoral head and neck.

Another potential area for MRI evaluation in the acute setting is aortic dissection. MRI is superior to contrast-enhanced CT and possibly to transesophageal ultrasound in delineating the intimal aortic flap. Unfortunately, patients who are unstable hemodynamically, who require life support, or who are agitated are not good candidates for

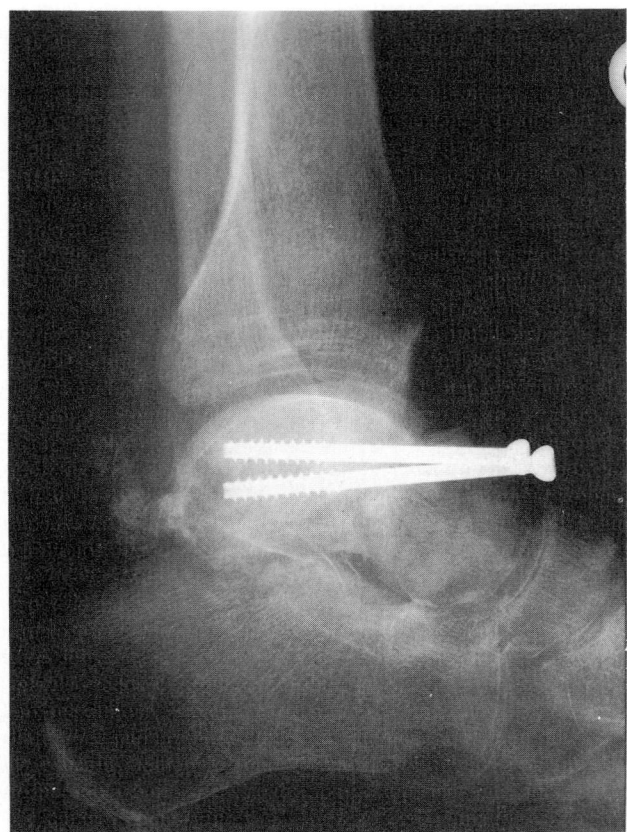

A

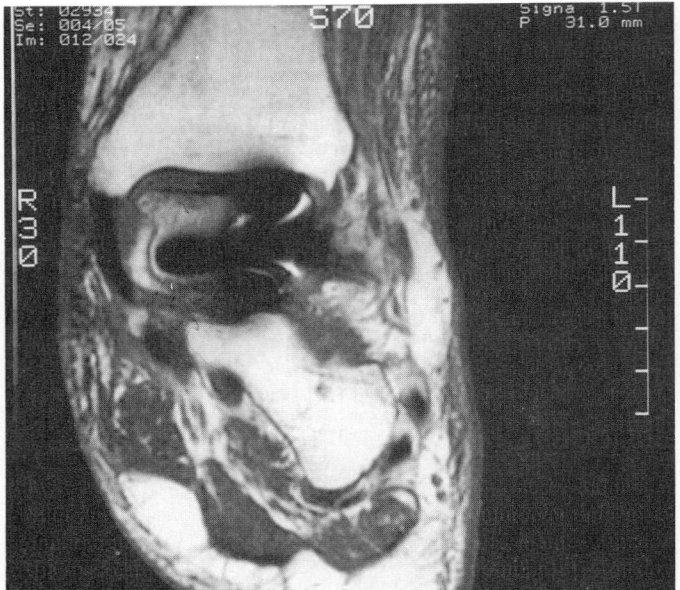

B

C

**Fig. 260-3.** Magnetic artifacts. *A.* Lateral radiograph of a foot of a patient with a talar fracture reduced with two cold-worked stainless steel screws. *B.* Proton density–weighted (partial T2 weighted) coronal MRI scan: ferromagnetic artifacts almost completely obliterate the talar marrow signal, rendering it diagnostically useless. *C.* Ultrahigh resolution coronal CT scan on the same foot yields useful information on the condition of the talar fragments (nonunion and avascular necrosis). This is unusual in that the ferromagnetic properties of the screws is responsible for a disproportionately deleterious effect on the MRI compared to the CT. Note that both show a lateral calcaneal dislocation.

MRI. As more MRI-compatible life-support and monitoring equipment becomes available, this situation will change.

Finally, a second potential application is in pediatric fractures, when there may be significant injury to unossified cartilage around open growth plates. Fractures through cartilage are not seen on plane films but are easily identified on MRI.

One innovation, the development of low and very low magnetic field imaging systems, may have some impact on the emergency department. Most of the hazards previously delineated apply to high-field systems. In low-field systems where the magnetic flux density is less in magnitude and more restricted in spatial extent, it is easier to accommodate life-support equipment. The design of these units allows more access to the patient and reduces the chances of interference with the proper operation of the life-support electronics. However, because of theoretical considerations, the signal-to-noise ratio is much less at low field. Therefore, there may be a tradeoff in diagnostic quality of the scans. Some signal can be recovered with optimal

design of the software and hardware, but this remains a controversial area. There may be a place for low-field MRI in the emergent setting in the evaluation of subacute intracerebral hemorrhage and brain edema.

Finally MR angiography has been evolving slowly and improving steadily. It may eventually be the method of choice in the emergent evaluation of suspected subarachnoid hemorrhage or in leaking aortic aneurysms.

## CONCLUSION

MRI is a new technology that has made rapid progress in its diagnostic potential and now competes favorably with CT, ultrasound, and, in some cases, angiography. However, with increasing cost restrictions, its definitive role in the diagnostic workup is still evolving. Computed tomography continues to be the special imaging procedure of choice for initial evaluation of acute head, chest, and abdominal

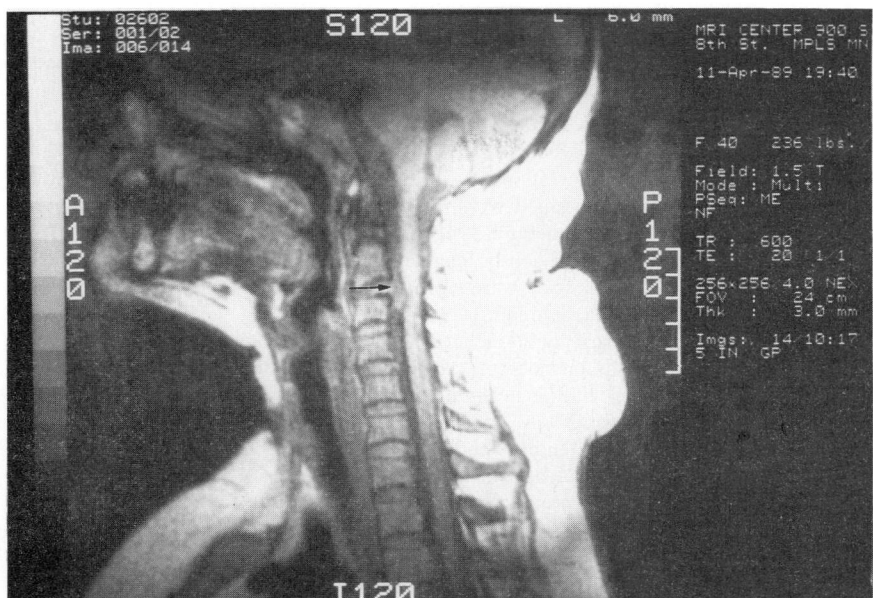

**Fig. 260-4.** Cervical spinal cord compression: T1-weighted sagittal MRI scan demonstrates moderate spinal cord compression by an acute traumatically herniated disc at the C2–3 level (arrow). The patient was in a motor vehicle accident and also suffered associated bilateral C2 pedicle fractures.

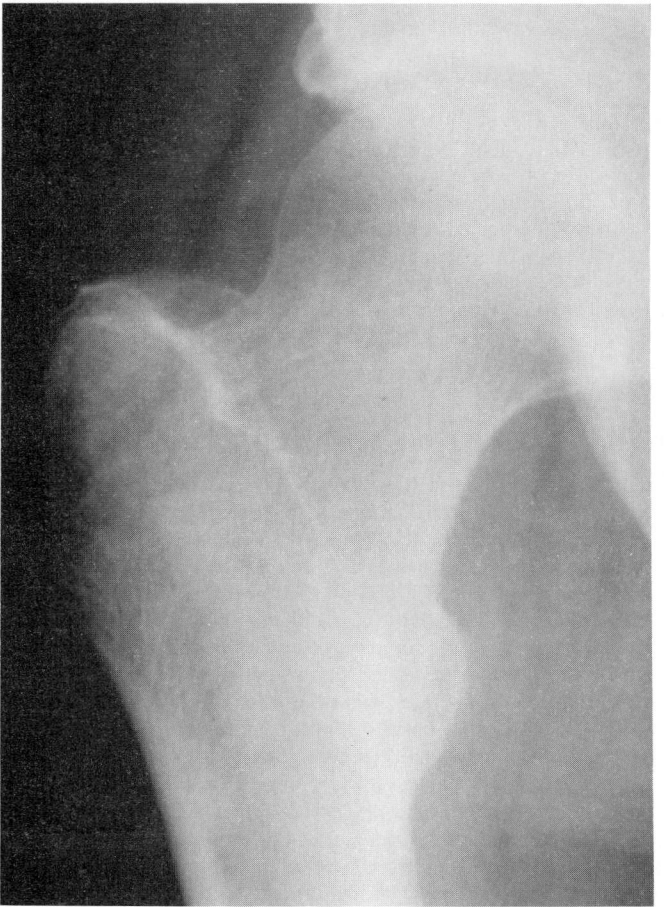

A

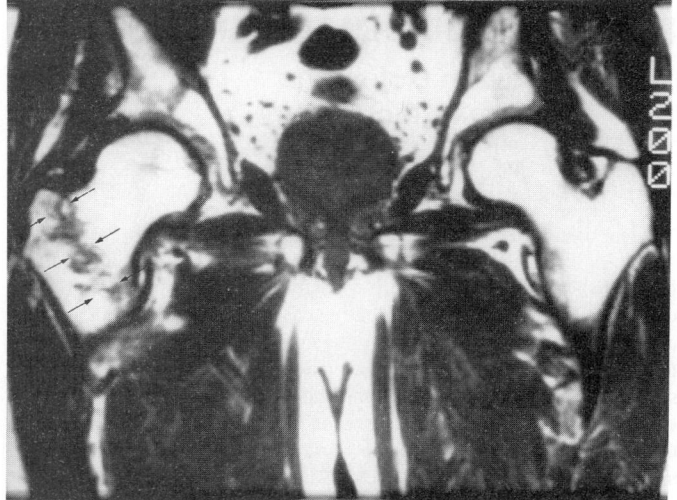

B

**Fig. 260-5.** Occult hip fracture. *A.* Anteroposterior radiograph of a 55-year-old patient on steroids who had right hip pain after a fall. No fracture is evident. *B.* T1-weighted coronal MR scan of the same hip clearly demonstrates a nondisplaced intertrochanteric femoral shaft fracture (arrows).

emergencies including trauma. There are two exceptions where MRI is currently cost effective in the emergency department: ruling out spinal cord compression and hip fractures in the elderly with negative radiographs. Extension of MR to other emergent problems such as detection of aortic dissection and leaking cerebral aneurysms may be possible in the future.

## BIBLIOGRAPHY

Bloch F, Hansen WW, Packard M: Nuclear induction. *Phys Rev* 69:127, 1946.

Erdman WA, Tamburro F, Jayson HT, et al: Osteomyelitis: characteristics and pitfalls of diagnosis with MR imaging. *Radiol* 180:533, 1991.

Finn JP (ed): Magnetic resonance angiography of the body. *MRI Clin North Am* 1:203, 1993.

Fitzgerald SW (ed). The knee. *MRI Clin North Am* 2(3):325, 1994.

Johnson GC: Need for caution during MR imaging of patients with aneurysm clips. *Radiology* 188:287, 1993.

Kumar A, Welti D, Ernst RR: NMR fourier zeugmatography. *J Mag Res* 18:69, 1975.

Lauterbur PC: Image formation by induced local interactions: example employing nuclear magnetic resonance. *Nature* 242:190, 1973.

Mitchell DG, Rao VM, Dalinka MK, et al: Femoral head avascular necrosis: Correlation of MR imaging, radiographic staging, radionuclide imaging, and clinical findings. *Radiology* 166:709, 1988.

Purcell EM, Torrey HC, Pound RV. Resonance absorption by nuclear magnetic moments in a solid. *Phys Rev* 69:37, 1946.

Quinn SF, McCarthy JL. Prospective evaluation of patients with suspected hip fracture and indeterminate radiographs: Use of T1 weighted MR images. *Radiology* 187:469, 1993.

Rafii M (ed). The shoulder. *MRI Clin North Am* 1(1):1, 1993.

Shellock FG, Morisoli S, Kanal E: MR procedures and biomedical implants, materials, and devices: 1993 Update. *Radiol* 189:587, 1993.

Stark DD, Bradley WG Jr: *Magnetic Resonance Imaging,* 2d ed. St. Louis, Mosby, 1992.

# 261
# RADIONUCLIDE IMAGING

## L. Steven Bujenovic
## William H. McCartney

Nuclear medicine studies use radionuclides as tracers to evaluate physiologic processes. To accomplish this, the radionuclide can be bound to a specific ligand with a desirable physiologic property, incorporated directly into biologically active molecules or unbound and distributed according to its own physical properties, often as a competitive analog. The radionuclide can be ingested, injected, or instilled depending on the tracer and the study design. The distribution of the radionuclide in various organs in the body is imaged. Nearly every organ system and a wide variety of pathologic disorders are studied. The types of studies are constantly changing due to advances in technology and the availability of tracers.

Imaging studies depend on the detection of a gamma photon emitted from nuclear transformation of a radionuclide. Although the gamma photon is beyond the visible spectrum of light, the photons can be localized and quantified when they encounter a gamma camera. The gamma camera detector is composed of several elements that collect and locate radiation originating from within the patient. The first component of the camera is a collimator that blocks out photons not traveling in a single axis. Behind the collimator is a sodium iodide crystal that stops the photons and scintillates (produces light) with each interaction. Then, many photomultiplier tubes view the scintillating crystal and convert the flashes of light into amplified electrical pulses and pinpoint their origin. The final component of the system is a pulse-height analyzer from which an energy window can be selected that ignores all undesirable "downscatter." Only the photons within the window are recorded and each is registered into a computer matrix. This stored data are then used to create an image.

Recently, computed tomography known as *single photon emission computed tomography* (SPECT) has been introduced to separate overlapping structures. Generally, it requires more imaging time because it acquires more information than planar images. In SPECT, the camera revolves around the patient in brief incremental steps. With the advent of multiheaded cameras, imaging time has been decreasing and this technique is becoming more prevalent. Continuous improve-

ments in SPECT have resulted in improved resolution and better quantitation.

Most radionuclides are obtained directly from fission reactors or cyclotrons. One outstanding exception to this is technetium 99m ($^{99m}$Tc), which is a metastable radionuclide derived from the beta decay of molybdenum 99 ($^{99}$Mo). Although $^{99}$Mo is obtained from a fission reactor, its decay into $^{99m}$Tc can be conveniently, reliably, and safely contained within a small generator in a hospital's radiopharmacy. Technetium 99m abundantly emits a gamma photon of 140 keV that efficiently interacts with the sodium iodide crystal. Consequently, a wide variety of agents and studies are devised with this radionuclide in mind.

Because radionuclides are administered into the body, clearance depends on not only the physical half-life of the radionuclide, but also the biologic clearance. Combined, these factors determine the *effective half-life*. Because of this consideration and because nuclear medicine studies are imaging physiology, detailed information regarding the patient's condition is necessary for proper dosimetry and study interpretation. Radionuclides tend to localize in specific organs; therefore, the radiation dose is expressed in terms of "target" organs as well as for the whole body. Generally, a nuclear medicine study exposes a patient to less than 1 rad of total body radiation. In comparison, the average yearly background radiation to a person in the United States is approximately 0.3 rem. In pregnant and lactating women, elective studies should be delayed if possible.

## HEPATOBILIARY SCANS

Hepatobiliary scans ("HIDA" scans) outline functioning hepatocytes and the biliary tree. They are commonly requested to evaluate for suspected acute cholecystitis, postoperative bile leaks, and biliary atresia. In an emergent situation, the scan is helpful in triaging patients with nonspecific abdominal pain and a history of gallstones. Because asymptomatic gallstones are common and abdominal pain is often vague, the hepatobiliary scan is done to exclude acute cholecystitis. Key to the diagnosis is the patency of the cystic duct. An occluded cystic duct will prevent the labeled iminodiacetic acid (IDA) from filling the gallbladder, confirming the diagnosis of *acute* cholecystitis.

### Technical Considerations

Technetium 99m-labeled IDA agents are inert, lipophilic agents that are intravenously injected and then extracted by hepatocytes and rapidly excreted into the biliary tree. Typically, patients are imaged with sequential anterior views every 10 min for 1 h. Accumulation in the gallbladder and deposition into the duodenum are often seen by 20 min. If no visualization of the gallbladder is seen after 1 h, the patient is felt to have either complete obstruction of the cystic duct from stones, and inflammation, or partial obstruction of the duct from scarring with a slow filling rate. This latter possibility is explored by obtaining delayed images up to 4 h postinjection. If the gallbladder is visualized late, chronic cholecystitis is likely, whereas if no visualization is noted, acute cholecystitis is usually responsible. However, some patients with chronic cholecystitis may also have persistent nonvisualization. Recently the study design has been modified to save time; if no gallbladder visualization is noted after 1 h, intravenous morphine sulfate (0.04 mg/kg) can be given to induce spasm of the sphincter of Oddi (common duct patency as proven by activity in the gut should be present prior to administration). This will increase intraductal pressure and increase the filling rate of a partially obstructed gallbladder such that any filling should be detected within 30 to 40 min. Completely obstructed gallbladders will not fill. Attention to the patient's physiologic state is important when setting up and interpreting the study. Patients who have eaten within 2 to 4 h of the study may have an actively contracting gallbladder and may not concentrate the radiopharmaceutical. In these patients the study should be postponed. Conversely, patients who have not eaten for more than 48 h may have a gallbladder full of concentrated bile that also will not concentrate the hepatobiliary agent. Cholecystokinin may be given to cause gallbladder emptying in such fasting patients in preparation for the scan. Patients with severe hepatocellular dysfunction (bilirubin > 10) may not extract agents sufficiently to allow confident determination of a "nonfilling" gallbladder. However, if the study is performed and the gallbladder is visualized, acute cholecystitis can be excluded.

## Scan Interpretation

Perhaps the most difficult aspect of interpretation is correctly identifying structures in the region of the gallbladder. A lateral view is often helpful in separating the gallbladder and duodenum, which may mimic a filled gallbladder. Serial images help in this differentiation because the gallbladder should show increasing uptake; duodenal activity passes onward through the bowel. The sensitivity, specificity, and positive and negative predictive values of the morphine-augmented study in detecting acute cholecystitis are 96, 87, 87, and 96 percent, respectively, and with delayed imaging are 98, 71, 95, and 88 percent, respectively.

## LUNG SCANS

Lung scans or ventilation/perfusion ($\dot{V}/\dot{Q}$) scans depict ventilation and perfusion patterns. They are most commonly requested to exclude pulmonary embolism and offer an effective noninvasive screening modality. Generally, they require about 90 min to complete so a stable patient is preferred. A prescan chest x-ray is essential not only to exclude other etiologies but also to determine the number of particles to be used for the perfusion study. The perfusion study is designed to block one in a thousand of the pulmonary capillaries with about 200,000 particles of macroaggregated albumin (MAA) labeled with $^{99m}$Tc, thus showing the distribution of pulmonary perfusion. Patients with known right-to-left cardiac shunts, chronic pulmonary hypertension, pulmonary embolism, prior pneumonectomy, or any other known causes for diminished peripheral pulmonary vascularity should be given a smaller number of particles.

## Technical Considerations

The $\dot{V}/\dot{Q}$ scan is really two separate studies of ventilation and perfusion, performed sequentially. Which study is done first depends on the relative photon energies of the radionuclides to be used. For example, a ventilation study using (81 keV) xenon 133 gas is done first to avoid downscatter from the higher energy photons (140 keV) of $^{99m}$Tc used in the perfusion study. Alternately, if (203 keV) xenon 127 or (176 to 192 keV) krypton 81 gas is used, the perfusion study is performed first since the higher energy photons of the gas can easily be discerned without interference from the relatively lower energy photons of $^{99m}$Tc.

In both studies the patient is positioned supine. The ventilation study is done by placing a mask over the patient's face and administering a small amount of inert xenon 133 gas. This study is suboptimal if a proper mask seal is not maintained. A poor seal is apparent when high background activity from escaped gas is seen in the image. Because views in multiple positions are not practical when imaging dynamic gas exchange, a single posterior view to display the largest total lung volume is obtained. Sequential wash-in, equilibrium, and washout images are obtained. The wash-in phase requires maximal inspiratory effort with a breath-holding view and, properly done, it reflects regional ventilation rate. The equilibrium phase simply demonstrates aerated lung volume. The washout phase detects gas trapping seen in obstructive pulmonary diseases. Some of the lipid soluble xenon gas will be absorbed and may incidentally deposit into

a fatty liver—this should not be confused with gas trapping in the lung base.

In the perfusion study, MAA particles labeled with $^{99m}$Tc are given intravenously. The MAA particles are 20 to 50 μm in size and have a biologic half-life of 2 to 10 h, during which time perfusion is impeded. This is well within a safe range; however, a chest x-ray is crucial to select the number of particles to be used in various patients. Immediately after injection, multiple static views are obtained.

## Scan Interpretation

Normal perfusion patterns demonstrate an increased particle distribution in the gravity dependent portions; thus, in a patient injected in the supine position, greater activity is typically seen in the bases. A reversal of the distribution is seen with left ventricular failure or mitral stenosis. The mediastinal silhouette and diaphragms are well outlined. Patients with obstructive pulmonary disease will have gas trapping on ventilation washout and a corresponding area of diminished perfusion. This is termed a *matched defect*. A *mismatched defect* refers to a perfusion defect *without* a corresponding ventilatory abnormality. A pulmonary embolism is the classic example of such a pattern. A wide range of entities may also cause perfusion abnormalities including vasculitis, infection, tumor, and effusion. Also, patients with prior emboli may have chronic fibrosis of pulmonary vessels causing perfusion abnormalities, which mimic scan findings of pulmonary embolism.

## Therapeutic Implications of Interpretation

Because $\dot{V}/\dot{Q}$ scans do not *directly* detect pulmonary embolism, interpretation is expressed as a probability for embolism given a particular pattern. The probabilities are derived from patient studies where both lung scans and pulmonary angiography have been done. Although angiography is more specific for embolism detection than lung scans, it is *also* an indirect modality for detection of embolism. Debate continues over which modality better depicts clinically significant embolism. Under investigation are imaging studies using radiolabeled monoclonal antibodies directed at cross-linked fibrin found within clotted blood. Such a study, when available, could simultaneously answer the question of embolism as well as identify the source.

*High probability* interpretation (Fig. 261-1 is an example of an abnormal perfusion lung scan) implies such a high chance (85 to 95 percent depending on which of the various interpretation schemes is used) of pulmonary embolism that therapy can be given without a pulmonary angiogram in all cases except those with a strong contraindication to therapy.

*Intermediate or indeterminate probability* interpretations should have further evaluation and, if indicated, have a pulmonary angiogram. Alternately, when a deep venous thrombosis is identified and the lung scan is of intermediate probability, the scan can be upgraded to high probability. This latter approach allows institution of prophylactic therapy without an invasive procedure.

*Low probability* interpretations are less well correlated with angiographic findings; however, clinical outcome studies of these patients demonstrate that with a low probability interpretation and no clinical evidence of venous thrombosis, patients may be safely left untreated.

*Normal* interpretations correlate well with angiographic findings and do not require further evaluation by pulmonary angiography or therapy for pulmonary embolism.

## BONE SCANS

Clinically, x-rays are the primary modality in evaluating skeletal trauma. Emergent bone scans are occasionally requested as an alternative modality for the detection of fractures. Bone scans are more sensitive in detecting subtle periosteal trauma than x-rays; however, they may be of limited value acutely because new bone formation is

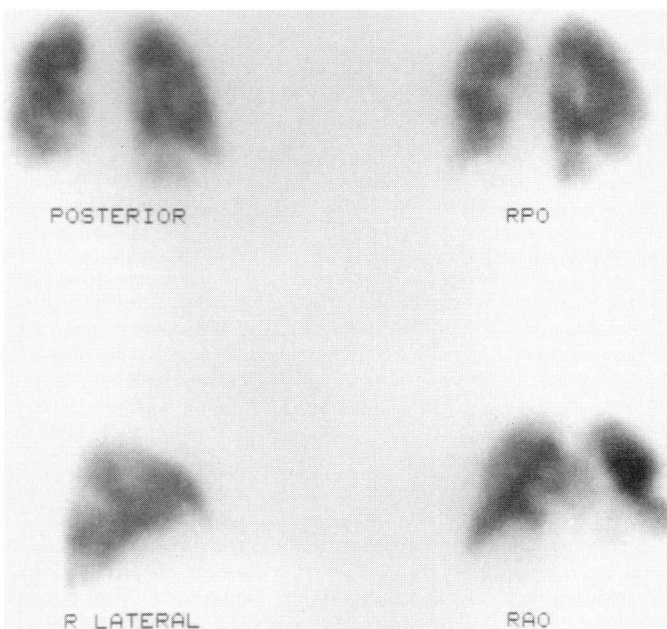

POSTERIOR                    RPO

R LATERAL                    RAO

**Fig. 261-1.** This perfusion lung study depicts multiple wedge-shaped, pleural based, perfusion defects consistent with a high probability for pulmonary embolism.

not reliably detected until 8 h after trauma. Skeletal uptake of the bone radiopharmaceutical is related to blood flow and, more importantly, to osteoblastic activity. By 72 h after the onset of pain, virtually all patients with fractures should have detectable lesions on scan, and in patients less than 65 years old, 95 percent of fractures are seen within 24 h.

A practical consideration for the emergency physician is the time required for completion of a bone scan; typically a minimum of 3 h is required. Therefore, only if screening x-rays are negative and an appropriate amount of time has elapsed to allow for new bone formation, is bone scintigraphy a logical alternative to exclude a fracture.

Common diagnostic bone-seeking radiotracers contain $^{99m}$Tc bound to a phosphonate such as hydroxymethylene diphosphonate and methylene diphosphonate. These phosphonates substitute for phosphates within amorphous mineral salts that eventually join other molecules to form hydroxyapatite crystals. These needle-shaped crystals provide strength to bone by embedding in the mucopolysaccharide collagen fibers of the matrix with their long axes parallel to the fibers. Bone is constantly being resorbed and replaced, the dying osteons are removed by osteoclasts, and generating osteoblasts provide new bone. This process occurs in the inner layer of the periosteum and the endosteum. Occasionally tendinous injuries may mimic bone injury on bone scans. Tendons have Sharpey fibers that are fibrocartilaginous fibers bound to the bone matrix prior to the hydroxyapatite crystallization and with tendinous disruption some injury occurs to the superficial bone surface. These injuries are called enthesopathies and are less intense on scan than most fractures and tend to be less focal.

## Technical Considerations

The agent is injected intravenously and blood flow may be imaged by dynamic 5-s images over 1 min, followed by a 1-min static blood pool image and subsequently a static skeletal image is obtained 2 h after injection. These three images constitute the three-phase bone scan. The flow and blood pool images may be omitted if the information they provide is not needed. Prior to obtaining the static image the patient should be instructed to urinate because the radiopharmaceuti-

cal is excreted in the urine and activity in the bladder may obscure the bony pelvis.

## Scan Interpretation

In bone scintigraphy, we are looking for areas of increased radionuclide uptake representing increased bony turnover, which occurs when the bone attempts to repair itself. A normal scan shows symmetrical skeletal activity, whereas positive bone scans show asymmetrical areas of increased uptake. Occasionally, as in conditions such as acute bone infarction, lesions may show asymmetrically decreased uptake. In children, growth plate areas show pronounced uptake of the bone agent, but the activity should be symmetrical.

## Clinical Indications

Common clinical entities well detected by bone scan include the following:

1. *Stress fractures.* Such fractures are the result of repeated stress causing resorption of the circumferential lamellae at a greater rate than replacement of bone. The result is trabecular collapse and subsequent microfractures. Common anatomic position for such stress fractures are in the mid to distal tibia and in the fourth and fifth metatarsals, that is, march fractures. Shin splints, or tibial stress syndrome, can be diagnosed when a slightly increased uptake along the posteromedial tibia is seen although this may be impossible to discern from subtle stress fractures of the tibia. A three-phase bone scan may differentiate the two. Patients with shin splints will not have increased vascularity to the lesion as seen with stress fractures.

2. *Toddler's fracture.* Occasionally toddlers aged 1 to 3 years old will present to the emergency room with a limp and will have a normal x-ray. Spiral tibial fractures may be present and can be well delineated on bone scan.

3. *Little League elbow.* This results from excessive throwing of curve balls by a child with an immature elbow. Here the forearm is rapidly supinated with injury to the proximal radial epiphysis. The x-rays are typically normal, whereas on bone scan we note relatively increased uptake in the affected elbow compared with the opposite elbow. This pattern together with an appropriate history and physical findings make the diagnosis.

4. *Occult fractures.* Carpal navicular fractures are notorious for being undetectable on screening x-rays as are some hip and sacral fractures, especially in osteopenic patients. For these patients bone scan can be a very helpful diagnostic modality (Fig. 261-2).

5. *Compartment syndrome.* Patients with suspected compartment syndromes may demonstrate decreased osseous uptake of the radiopharmaceutical secondary to vascular compromise.

6. *Temporomandibular joint syndrome.* Often x-rays are not helpful in diagnosing these individuals; however, bone scan can show an area of increased activity supporting this clinical diagnosis.

7. *Osteitis pubis.* Pelvic pain in an athlete may be secondary to overuse of the gracilis muscle, which may be demonstrated as a "hot" pubis on bone scan. SPECT is helpful in these cases to discern pubis from underlying bladder.

8. *Bone pain.* In patients with known malignant disease, pain may be associated with osseous metastasis despite negative x-rays. If this pain is localized to an area of critical importance such as a weight-bearing long bone or the spine, bone scan detection may facilitate early external beam radiation treatment to avert a crippling pathologic fracture.

9. *Whole body scan.* For noncommunicative adults with suspected skeletal trauma a whole body bone scan may help define the location or extent of injury for these patients.

10. *Child abuse.* Bone scans are helpful in documenting the extent of injury although x-rays offer the more convincing evidence for severity of injury. Together they offer powerful legal evidence in child abuse cases. The advantages of bone scans are detection of cer-

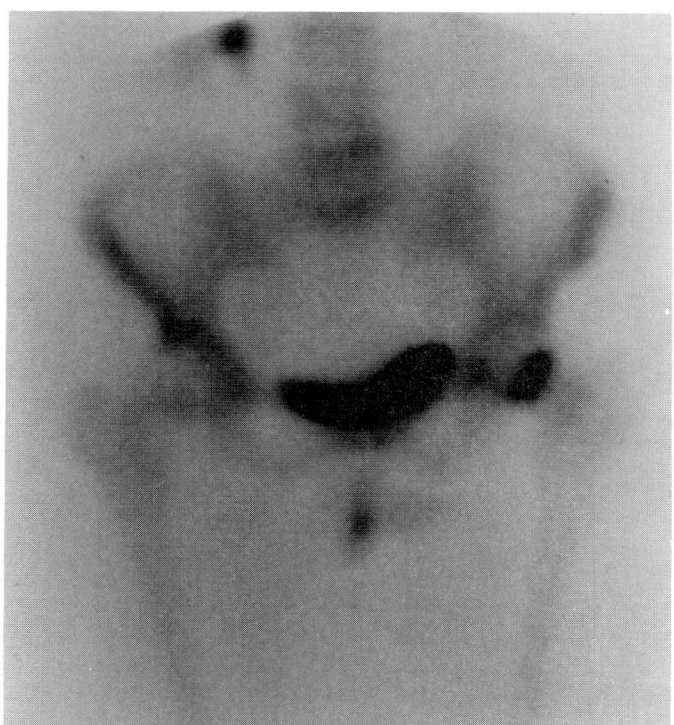

**Fig. 261-2.** This bone scan obtained 4 days after injury demonstrates a subcapital fracture of the left hip. The initial x-rays were equivocal.

tain patterns that are characteristic of abuse. For example, abused children less than 2 years old are often grasped by the thorax, resulting in increased uptake of the bone radioagent in the ribs, typically in the peristernal ribs T4 through T9, the axilla, and the costocartilagenous junctions of ribs 2 through 9. These patterns are suggestive of such abuse. Children older than 2 years are often grabbed by the extremities, and increased activity in the shaft of long bones is often detected. Such elevated diaphyseal activity in an extremity represents bowing or bending from microtrabecular fractures, which are characteristic of abuse.

Limitations of bone scans in these instances include poor visualization of skull fractures, which may elicit minimal osseous remodeling. Additionally, bilaterally symmetrical metaphyseal injuries may be masked because they are growth areas where new bone formation is expected and, therefore, normally demonstrate intense uptake. The normal infantile epiphyseal-metaphyseal complex is ovoid. When it has a globular appearance or when there is an increase in intensity in the growth plate or metaphysis, the scan is positive for fracture. Also, with bone scans it may be difficult to assign specific time frames to the stages of healing for various lesions and healed fractures may not be demonstrated. One potential pitfall with bone scans is in osteogenesis imperfecta, which can mimic child abuse findings although the diaphyseal localization often seen with abuse is unlikely.

11. *Osteomyelitis.* Bone scan shows increased flow, blood pool, and static uptake in a localized infected osseous site. An additional image at 24 h gives increased specificity, as infected bone tends to take up relatively more of the bone agent with time.

## GASTROINTESTINAL BLEEDING STUDY

Once gastrointestinal bleeding has been identified, the next diagnostic step is localization. Upper gastrointestinal bleeds are best evaluated with endoscopy and radionuclide studies are seldom warranted. When a lower gastrointestinal bleed is suspected (hematochezia), colonoscopy is much less successful in localizing the site of bleeding.

Although angiography may be helpful in localizing the bleeding site in such cases, angiographic studies are often negative because this bleeding is an intermittent process. For this reason, radionuclide gastrointestinal bleed studies have become popular for determining whether active bleeding is occurring. Often, the patient may be taken to angiography for further evaluation, or even therapy, after radionuclide studies have documented an active bleed.

The radionuclide bleeding study is performed by administration of $^{99m}$Tc-labeled red blood cells, with images obtained at 10-min intervals over a period of 90 min. Vascular structures including major abdominal organs and great vessels are shown initially; areas of radionuclide uptake that appear later document gastrointestinal bleeding. Because intraluminal blood tends to move quickly through the bowel, serial images often allow accurate estimation of the site of bleeding, which may direct later angiography or even allow surgical intervention without angiography. The labeled red blood cells remain in the intravascular space, so it also possible to obtain delayed images (up to 24 h) should the patient rebleed at a later time. Although the radionuclide bleed study should not be ordered if an upper gastrointestinal bleed is suspected, such bleeds may be documented in cases where rapid transit of blood through the gut results in a presentation mimicking lower gastrointestinal bleed.

## TESTICULAR SCANS

Testicular imaging is often requested to exclude torsion in an acute scrotum that clinically cannot be distinguished from epididymitis, orchitis, or torsion of the appendix testis. A rapid diagnosis is critical in these cases because the surgical salvage rate for a torsed testis diminishes rapidly after pain onset.

After intravenous injection of technetium 99m pertechnetate, immediate flow and static views of the testicles are obtained, which depict the perfusion and blood pool patterns, respectively. It is vital to know which testicle is suspected of being abnormal for proper interpretation of the results. In an early torsion, the flow study may be normal or show decreased flow; the static view shows absence of blood pool activity on the side of the torsion, but normal uptake on the uninvolved side. This contrasts with the findings in inflammation (epididymitis, orchitis) where the involved side shows obvious increased flow and blood pool activity. In late torsion (> 24 h) a halo of activity surrounds a cold testicle in both flow and blood pool images due to inflammatory hyperemia via the pudendal artery. This pattern may also be seen with scrotal abscess or hematoma.

## OTHER STUDIES

### Myocardial Infarct Avid Scan

Infarct avid scans may be able to help document or help confirm a suspected myocardial infarction when clinical, electrocardiographic, and enzyme data are unclear. For example, postoperative cardiac surgery patients, noncommunicative patients, and patients who have undergone cardiopulmonary resuscitation may present with confusing data.

When myocytes are injured, the intracellular levels of calcium rise due to dysfunction of the sarcoplasmic reticulum. If technetium 99m pyrophosphate is given intravenously, it will enter the damaged myocytes and bind with the free calcium. The greatest uptake is in the peri-infarct area where adequate perfusion is still present. Therefore, the uptake does not correspond precisely with the area of the infarction. Uptake is generally not visible before 12 h or after 10 days. Optimal scan time is between 24 and 72 h after infarction.

Other causes of increased uptake include left ventricular aneurysms, recent cardioversion, contusion, cardiomyopathy, intramural tumors, valve ring, and pericardial calcifications.

Imaging with SPECT is preferable to planar imaging, and the study

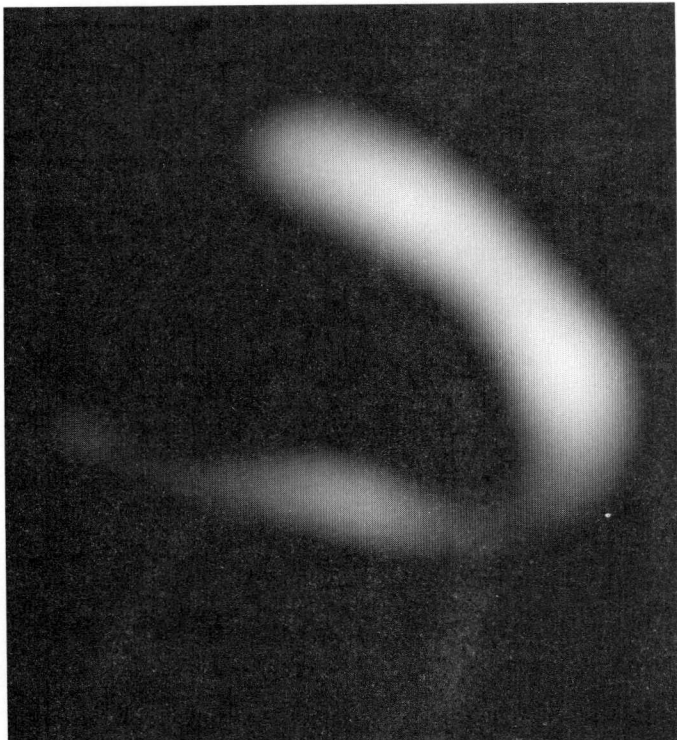

**Fig. 261-3.** This cardiac SPECT image is of a vertical long axis slice demonstrating an inferior wall perfusion defect.

is interpreted as positive if focal cardiac uptake is demonstrated on the scan. Care must be taken not to confuse cardiac blood pool activity with myocardial uptake due to infarction.

## Myocardial Perfusion Imaging

Currently under investigation is *emergency* myocardial perfusion imaging with SPECT. Emergency cardiac SPECT has recently been successfully used to triage patients with unexplained chest pain. In stable patients with an unremarkable preliminary work-up, myocardial perfusion imaging using technetium 99m sestamibi has been shown to optimize the physician's triage decision and to increase clinical confidence. Technetium 99m sestamibi is a perfusion agent that accumulates in well-perfused myocardium. It is stable and does not show significant myocardial redistribution within 2 h of injection. This latter feature allows time for stabilization and transportation of the patient to the imaging suite.

One practical disadvantage is the time necessary to perform the study, about an hour. The major advantage, of course, is to provide additional information to support a clinician's triage decision (Fig. 261-3).

Thallium 201 is also a commonly used radiotracer to evaluate the myocardium. Unlike technetium 99m sestamibi, which enters perfused myocytes by passive diffusion, thallium 201 is a potassium analog that is actively transported by perfused myocytes. Therefore, thallium demonstrates viability as well as perfusion. Typically, a thallium study is divided into a stress (exercise or pharmacologic) study followed by a delayed (washout) study at 4 h. The two studies are compared for relative perfusion and subsequent washout. Poor perfusion with subsequent poor washout characterize ischemic myocardium. Infarcted myocardium also demonstrates poor perfusion but with relatively good washout. Because thallium imaging should be done shortly after injection, and again 4 h later, this radiotracer may not be the agent of choice to evaluate potentially unstable patients.

## Brain Death

In conjunction with clinical and electroencephalographic (EEG) criteria, a brain scan can be done to document brain death. The brain scan depicts cerebral blood flow, which is characteristically absent in brain death. It is especially useful in patients with barbiturate overdose and hypothermia, conditions for which EEG is unreliable.

A wide variety of radiotracers can be injected, including technetium 99m DTPA, technetium 99m pertechnetate, and technetium 99m HMPAO. Prior to injection, a scalp tourniquet may be placed just above the orbits to exclude activity delivered by the external carotid circulation. Absence of activity in the brain confirms lack of perfusion and indicates brain death.

## Herpes Simplex Encephalitis

A brain scan can detect herpes simplex encephalitis earlier than a computed tomography (CT) scan. Radiotracers technetium 99m DTPA or technetium 99m glucoheptonate normally remain intravascular, but with disruption of the blood brain barrier, as with infection, these agents accumulate in the brain parenchyma. Typically activity is demonstrated in the temporal lobes with herpes simplex encephalitis.

## Labeled Leukocytes

A labeled leukocyte study is frequently requested to search for a source of occult infection. Agents used for white blood cell labeling include indium 111 oxine and technetium 99m HMPAO. Technetium 99m HMPAO is routinely available in hospital radiopharmacies and technetium 99m HMPAO-labeled white blood cell studies are performed at 3 to 6 h after administration, whereas "In-labeled leukocytes are imaged at 24 h. However, [99mTc]-labeled leukocytes do show some renal and gut excretion, not seen with [111I]-labeled white blood cells, and these factors complicate image interpretation. Patients with neutropenia are not good candidates for imaging with labeled leukocytes.

## Monoclonal Antibodies and Receptor-Specific Peptides

Recently, the Food and Drug Administration has approved clinical use of radiolabeled monoclonal antibodies in the detection of colorectal and ovarian carcinoma. These radiolabeled antibodies represent the first of the "magic bullets" that have passed from a research phase into a clinical phase. Collectively, they are IgG-class antibodies derived from murine cells that have been sensitized to a human tumor-associated glycoprotein (TAG-72). This glycoprotein is found in 95 percent of ovarian and 85 percent of colorectal carcinomas as well as breast, pancreatic, esophageal, and gastric carcinomas. Whole body imaging can be performed to determine the extent of metastases. Additionally, somatostatin receptors have been found in abundance on a wide range of neuroendocrine tumors and a radiolabeled somatostatin analog, octreotide, is now available. It is a synthetically produced peptide that selectively retains only the amino acids involved with receptor binding. It has a low molecular weight and a high target specificity. These advantages translate into high tumor-to-background ratios that are currently lacking with monoclonal antibody studies. Furthermore, many of these peptides have been successfully iodinated without significant stereotactic alteration of their binding sites. Protein iodination with [131I] that emits a cytotoxic beta particle opens the prospect for target-specific therapy. For example, [131I] has been an established treatment for follicular and papillary carcinoma of the thyroid for many years. The current somatostatin analog has a rapid washout rate that precludes its use as a therapeutic radioagent.

## Positron Emission Tomography

Certain radionuclides undergo nuclear transformation by positron emission. This antimatter particle (a positron) annihilates with matter (an electron) shortly after emission and characteristically produces two 511 KeV gamma photons that travel 180° apart. These high-energy photons easily pass through tissue and their bidirectional emission suits them well for tomography. Positron emission tomography (PET) systems typically use dense bismuth germanate crystals to halt and to detect these high-energy photons. Because each annihilation reaction is expected to result in two gamma photons travelling in opposite directions, PET systems use multiple oppositely paired detectors fitted with coincidence circuitry to precisely localize the origin of the activity.

These unique properties of positron emission overcome basic shortcomings that are inherent in single photon emission detection. In contrast to PET, SPECT attempts to localize a single photon emitted from a nucleus. Furthermore, in SPECT, both tracer distribution and often attenuation factors are unknown. PET is distinguished by nearly uniform spatial resolution throughout the transaxial slice, whereas SPECT has diminishing resolution away from the surface of the detector. Current spatial resolution with PET is about 5 mm compared to 8 mm for the best SPECT systems.

In addition to the technical advantages offered by PET, many positron emitters available ($^{11}C$, $^{13}N$, $^{15}O$, $^{18}F1$) can be incorporated into selected molecules without affecting biodistribution. Because these radionuclides have short half-lives, on-site production via a cyclotron is usually necessary.

When applied to problems in oncology, neurology, and cardiology, PET is a powerful tool. PET allows for measurement of substrate utilization rates, such as amino acids and sugars, that supply energy to tumors, or nucleotides that reflect DNA metabolism. Tumors have increased intermediary metabolism compared to the tissue from which they arise, and there is a correspondence between rate of tumor metabolism and growth rate of the malignant cell. $^{18}$Fluorodeoxyglucose (FDG) PET is being used to discriminate between malignant and benign tumors in the lung. $^{18}$Fluorodeoxyglucose and $^{11}C$-methionine are also effective in distinguishing high-grade from low-grade brain tumors as well as radiation necrosis from residual or recurrent tumor. PET is also useful in detecting epileptogenic foci in the brain. Interictal $^{18}$FDG-PET scans can demonstrate an area of hypometabolism typical of seizure foci. Myocardial perfusion imaging can also be performed with intravenous $^{82}$Rb, $^{15}H_2O$ or $^{13}NH_3$. Myocardial perfusion can be quantified precisely. The perfusion information coupled with metabolic data obtained from $^{18}$FDG can provide an accurate assessment of myocardial viability in areas of poor perfusion.

## BIBLIOGRAPHY

Palmer EL, Scott JA, Strauss HW. *Practical Nuclear Medicine*. Philadelphia: WB Saunders, 1992.

### Hepatobiliary Scans

Fink BD, Balon H, Robbins T, Tsai D. Morphine augmented cholescintigraphy: its efficacy in detecting acute cholecystitis. *J Nucl Med* 32(6), 1991.

### Lung Scans

Bautovich G, Angelides S, Fook TL, et al. Detection of deep venous thrombi and pulmonary embolus with technetium-99m-dd-3B6/22 antifibrim monoclonal antibody fab' fragment. *J Nucl Med* 35(2), 1994.
Cronan JJ, Dorfman GS. Advances in ultrasound imaging of venous thrombosis. *Semin Nucl Med* 21(4), 1991.
Juni JE, Alavi A. Lung scanning in the diagnosis of pulmonary embolism: the emperor redressed. *Semin Nucl Med* 21(4), 1991.

### Bone Scans

Conway JJ, Collins M, Tanz RR, et al. The role of bone scintigraphy in detecting child abuse. *Semin Nucl Med* 23(4), 1993.
Matin P. Basic principles of nuclear medicine technique for detection and evaluation of trauma and sports medicine injuries. *Semin Nucl Med* 18(2), 1988.

Sty JR, Wells RG, Smith WB. The child with acute leg pain. *Semin Nucl Med* 18(2), 1988.

### Monoclonal Antibodies and Receptor-Specific Peptides

Kvols LK, Brown ML, O'Connor MK, et al. Evaluation of a radiolabeled somatostatin analog (I-123 Octreotide) in the detection and localization of carcinoid and islet cell tumors. *Radiology* 187(1), 1993.

## 262
## COMPLICATIONS OF CENTRAL NERVOUS SYSTEM DEVICES
### Robert Rusnak

### VENTRICULOPERITONEAL CEREBROSPINAL FLUID SHUNTS

Inert silicon polymer catheters have made ventriculoperitoneal shunting of cerebrospinal fluid the preferred method of cerebral ventricular decompression. Long-term success with these devices has been achieved, preserving intellectual and motor function. Emergency physicians will encounter more of these patients in the future. Complications are shown in Table 262-1.

The most common complication is obstruction or malfunction of the shunt device. Signs and symptoms of increased intracranial pressure (ICP) occur from malfunction or obstruction; these include nausea, vomiting, headache, lethargy, irritability, and increased seizure activity. In infants, increasing head circumference or a bulging fontanel may also be found. Papilledema is rare. The rate of rise of ICP is an important prognostic indicator, with fatal herniation a common result of a rapid rise. The first step in evaluating the shunt is to pump it to see if it is functioning. Some have a single pumping chamber, and others have two chambers. These chambers are located at or within a few centimeters of the site of penetration through the skull. In the case of a single chamber, the chamber should empty with digital pressure then fill rapidly (within 1 to 2 s). When there are two palpable chambers, compress the proximal one and hold while compressing the distal chamber. If the distal chamber does not easily compress, there is distal obstruction. Release the proximal chamber. If it does not rapidly refill, there is proximal obstruction. Proximal obstructions are more common than distal obstructions. X-rays of the skull, chest, and abdomen can help detect separation or malposition of the shunt. A computed tomography (CT) scan of the head can detect increasing ventricular volume. Neurosurgical consultation should be obtained early because sudden decompensation, with cerebellar or transtentorial herniation, is a threat. If signs of herniation appear acutely, the emergency physician may have to puncture the ventricle as a lifesaving maneuver if the obstruction is proximal. If the obstruction is distal, puncture of the chamber would be indicated. In an infant with an open fontanel, a 20-gauge spinal needle is

**Table 262-1.** Ventriculoperitoneal Shunts

| Complications | Diagnosis | Treatment |
|---|---|---|
| Obstruction | Signs and symptoms of increased ICP. Pump the shunt chamber to see if there is a distal or proximal obstruction. Skull, chest, and abdominal x-ray, CT of the head | Neurosurgical consultation. Pump the chamber to determine shunt patency. |
| Infection | Local erythema, abdominal pain, generalized signs of infection, meningeal signs | Neurosurgical consultation. Intravenous antibiotics |

CT, computed tomography; ICP, intracranial pressure

**Table 262-2.** Halo Pins

| Complications | Diagnosis | Treatment |
|---|---|---|
| Pain | Symptoms | Rule out loose pins, infection, or penetration of the inner table of the skull by pins before prescribing analgesics. |
| Loosening of pins | Observation | Pin tightening. Consider tangential radiographs to ensure that tightened pins do not penetrate inner skull. |
| Pin site infection | Clinical symptoms | Local wound care, antibiotics, radiologic studies to rule out penetration of pins beyond inner table of skull |
| Pressure sores under vest or cast | Clinical signs | Wound care of pressure sores, cast or vest modification to allow open treatment of pressure sores |
| Loss of cervical immobilization | Neurologic examination, pain, radiologic studies | Neurosurgical consultation |
| Osteomyelitis of the skull | Clinical signs or symptoms, drainage from pin site holes, radiologic studies | Neurosurgical consultation |
| Intradural or extradural abscesses (usually secondary to penetration of the inner table of the skull by pins) | Clinical signs or symptoms, radiologic studies | Neurosurgical consultation |

inserted 1 cm lateral to the midline along the coronal suture and directed perpendicular to the base of the skull in line with the inner canthus of the ipsilateral eye. The ventricle should be encountered within about 3.2 cm (1 1/4 in.). In older children and adults, one conceivably could reverse a rapidly progressing herniation by inserting a 20-gauge spinal needle through the skull opening occupied by the shunt. This would destroy the shunt but could save the patient's life. Fortunately, such rapid herniation occurring in the emergency department is very rare.

Infection of the shunt is the second most common complication. Infection can cause obstruction of the device resulting in signs of increased ICP. Local infection can result in scalp erythema over the shunt. Peritonitis is caused by primary shunt infection, or it can be caused by erosion of the shunt into the bowel. Infection can ascend through the shunt and cause meningitis or ventriculitis. Other abdominal processes, such as appendicitis, can be confused with shunt infection. Any shunt patient with abdominal symptoms or findings should be evaluated by a neurosurgeon. Most patients will require shunt aspiration to obtain ventricular fluid for study. The emergency physician should maintain a high index of suspicion when evaluating patients with a shunt because the signs and symptoms of infection may be subtle, nonspecific, and diverse. When infection is suspected, admission with neurosurgical consultation will be needed.

## HALO PIN TRACTION

Immobilization of the unstable cervical spine with an external cervical immobilizer applied through pins between the metal ring of the halo and inserted into the bony skull has become a common neurosurgical practice. The metal halo and support rods are connected to a special vest, or a cast, worn by the patient over the shoulders and around the chest. Numerous complications of these halo cervical immobilizers have been reported and are listed in Table 262-2. To adequately adjust this halo device, an appropriately sized Allen wrench and an open end wrench should be available in the emergency department.

## BIBLIOGRAPHY

Garfin SR, Botte MJ, Triggs KJ, et al: Subdural abscess associated with halo pin traction. *J Bone Joint Surg* 70A:1338, 1988.

Madsen MA: Emergency department management of ventriculoperitoneal cerebrospinal fluid shunts. *Ann Emerg Med* 15:1330, 1986.

Mascalchi M: Delayed intracerebral hemorrhage after CSF shunt for communicating "normal-pressure" hydrocephalus. Case report. *Ital J Neurol Sci* 12:109, 1991.

Reilly PL, Savage JP, Doecke L: Isotope transport studies and shunt pressure measurements as a guide to shunt function. *Br J Neurosurg* 3:681, 1989.

# 263
# COMPLICATIONS OF GASTROINTESTINAL AND UROLOGIC DEVICES
## Robert Rusnak

## INTRODUCTION

Feeding tubes can be placed endoscopically (PEG tube), or surgically, with floroscopic or ultrasonographic assistance. Depending on the type of tube placed, the tip can be in the stomach or the small intestine. When confronted with a problem with a feeding tube, it is important to know the type of tube inserted and its placement.

## GASTROSTOMIES

Gastrostomies are usually created to maintain nutritional support in patients who are unable to be fed orally or who have swallowing difficulties. Under general anesthesia, a variously sized Foley catheter (usually 16 F to 30 F) is placed through a stoma created between the abdominal wall and the stomach and firmly secured to the abdominal wall with tape. Although not technically difficult, this procedure has been reported to have a 10 to 35 percent complication rate. These complications are listed in Table 263-2.

Patients commonly are brought to the emergency department for replacement of gastrostomy tubes that have been accidentally pulled out or are nonfunctional. Blocked tubes should be irrigated first. Gentle suction should be used when aspirating. Excessive suction may collapse the tube, giving the false impression of blockage. The emergency physician should attempt to replace the tube with a tube of similar size and configuration. If the particular type of tube is not available, using a Foley catheter of the correct size will suffice. The size of the tube is important because the stoma will contract down to the tube, and it will be difficult to restore the shunt to its original size. The trick to replacing the tube is to lubricate it and then slowly insert it with constant forward pressure until it pops into the lumen of the stomach. A common mistake is to use intermittent force that does not allow time for tissue stretching and muscle relaxation. If the original size will not pass without undue trauma, use the next smaller size, then after insertion try the original size again. This technique generally applies to all forms of tube replacement. Correct replacement of the tube into the stomach should be confirmed by aspiration of gastric

**Table 263-1.** Peg Tubes

| Complications | Diagnosis | Treatment |
|---|---|---|
| Aspiration/pneumonia | Chest x-ray | Tube repositioning |
| Gastrointestinal bleeding | Clinical signs, endoscopy | Supportive measures, conventional treatment of bleeding site |
| Retroperitoneal perforation | Endoscopy, x-ray contrast studies | Catheter repositioning |
| Extraliminal catheter migration with infusion of tube feedings into peritoneal cavity | Clinical signs, x-ray studies | Repositioning, surgical consultation |
| Peritoneal leakage with infection | Clinical signs, x-ray studies | Intravenous antibiotics |
| Postprocedure myocardial infarction | Clinical signs, symptoms and laboratory studies | Supportive, consider thrombolytics |
| Infusion of nutrients into gastrostomy balloon port | Inability to deflate balloon or to infuse | Endoscopic or fluoroscopically guided balloon rupture and catheter repositioning |
| Colocutaneous fistula, gastrocolic fistula | Contrast studies through gastrostomy tube | Tube removal or repositioning |
| Pneumoperitoneum and volvulus of colon | Clinical signs, x-ray contrast studies | Surgery |
| Tube blockage | Inability to infuse nutrients | Tube irrigation or replacement |
| Intolerance to feedings | Nausea, vomiting, abdominal pain, distention | Reduced flow rate of nutrients, half-strength feedings, antidiarrheals, stop feedings |

**Table 263-2.** Gastrostomies and Feeding Jejunostomies

| Complications | Diagnosis | Treatment |
|---|---|---|
| Difficulty with tube feedings | Observation, x-ray contrast studies through tube | Attempt to irrigate feeding lumen, ensure that tube feedings are not being given through the inflation balloon, tube repositioning |
| Aspiration pneumonia | Clinical signs or symptoms, chest x-ray | Antibiotics, tube repositioning |
| Tube migration within gut causing intestinal obstruction, acute pancreatitis, obstructive jaundice, or gastroesophageal reflux | Clinical and laboratory signs and symptoms, x-ray studies with or without contrast | Tube repositioning, secure placement of tube on abdominal wall |
| Esophageal rupture (usually in infants) | Chest x-ray, tube feedings found in chest tube drainage | Surgery |
| Lost gastrostomy tube | Abdominal x-rays | Allow tube to pass or rupture balloon under fluoroscopic control and allow it to pass spontaneously |
| Gastric perforation | X-rays with or without contrast through tube | Surgery |
| Gastropneumatosis with or without gastric outlet obstruction | X-rays with or without contrast through tube | Tube repositioning |
| Leakage around stoma site | Clinical observation, x-ray contrast studies | Tube repositioning |
| Extraliminal position of gastrostomy tube | X-ray contrast studies | Tube repositioning |
| Gastric ulcer | Clinical signs or symptoms, x-ray studies, endoscopy | Ulcer treatment, various options |
| Gastrointestinal bleeding | Clinical signs or symptoms, x-ray studies, endoscopy | Treatment based on site of hemorrhage |
| Small bowel intussusception | X-ray contrast studies | Surgery |
| Sinus or fistula tract formation (with or without malnutrition) | X-ray contrast studies | Tube repositioning |

contents. An alternative is to inject 50 mL of contrast into the tube followed by x-ray, to confirm replacement.

## Peg Tube

The percutaneous endoscopic gastrostomy tube (a PEG tube) is a nonsurgical percutaneous, fluoroscopically, or endoscopically guided Seldinger technique used to create a gastrostomy. The tip of the PEG feeding tube is usually placed at the duodenojejunal junction to decrease the incidence of aspiration. Complications are listed in Table 263-1. PEG tubes need consultation in repositioning or replacement. The most common problem encountered in the emergency department is a non-functioning or dislodged tube. Radiographs should be taken to determine if the tube is in place. Endoscopic consultation is necessary for replacement or repositioning.

## JEJUNOSTOMIES

Jejunostomy tubes are placed in patients where gastrostomy tubes are contraindicated or cannot be placed. The catheter is placed in the proximal jejunum and the jejunum is sutured to the interior abdominal wall. The tube is brought out through a stab wound in the upper left quadrant. If there is uncertainty about the tube's position, it should not be blindly manipulated, but needs consultation.

## Foley Catheters

Latex balloon indwelling urinary catheters have been in use since 1937. Numerous complications are listed in Table 263-3. One of the most nettlesome problems is the inability to remove a Foley catheter because the balloon does not deflate. The following techniques have

**Table 263-3.** Foley Catheters

| Complications | Diagnosis | Treatment |
|---|---|---|
| Infection | Clinical signs and symptoms | Adequate urinary catheter drainage, antibiotics |
| Penile necrosis (usually occurs in patients with diabetes mellitus) | Local inspection of catheter exit site | Catheter removal, warm soaks, intravenous antibiotics, surgical debridement, prevention of excessive traction on catheter |
| Intraperitoneal bladder perforation with peritonitis and abdominal free air | Clinical signs and symptoms, abdominal x-ray | Laparotomy, bladder drainage |
| Penile laceration (usually in elderly, demented patients) | Local inspection | Catheter removal and suprapubic drainage, local treatment with warm soaks and topical antibiotics, prevention of traction on anterior urethra by the weight of a full urine reservoir bag and tubing by taping or bag repositioning |
| Small bowel obstruction by Foley catheter balloon secondary to vesicoenteric fistula | Clinical signs and symptoms, x-ray studies | Surgical correction |
| Abrupt removal of catheter with balloon still inflated by agitated, demented, or or psychotic patient | Clinical observation, urethral bleeding | Catheter replacement, consider intravenous antibiotics before reinsertion and prophylactically thereafter to prevent infection after posttraumatic removal (with without documented laceration of anterior urethra) |

been described to correct this problem. In women, swab the anterior vagina with antiseptic solution, apply gentle traction to the catheter, moving the balloon to the bladder neck, and insert a 25-gauge spinal needle through the anterior vaginal wall into the balloon. This will cause the water to drain from the balloon through the needle or cause the balloon to rupture. In men, prepare and anesthetize the skin in the suprapubic region just above the symphysis pubis, hold gentle traction on the catheter to position the balloon at the bladder neck, and insert a 25-gauge spinal needle through the abdominal wall into the bladder neck. This will drain the balloon or cause it to rupture. In men, the transrectal approach to the Foley balloon also has been described using this technique. Another technique describes transsecting the Foley catheter 1 cm distal to the urinary meatus and inserting a well-lubricated no. 26 orthopedic wire suture through the balloon channel of the catheter. This wire suture will almost always pass to the point of obstruction in the balloon channel, allowing water to drain around the wire suture. After the water drains from the balloon, the catheter can be removed by gentle traction.

## THE CONTINENT URINARY RESERVOIR

Patients whose bladders are destroyed by trauma or who develop invasive cancer and require cystectomy also require creation of a urine receptacle. This urine receptacle can be an externally placed plastic pouch that collects urine continuously throughout the day or a continent reservoir. This section discusses the complications of continent urinary reservoirs.

Continent urinary reservoirs are surgically created structures, using a portion of the bowel as a urinary reservoir and a surgically created anastomosis between this urinary reservoir and the skin of the abdominal wall that allows patients to catheterize the bowel segments several times per day to allow elimination of urine. In the Indiana reservoir, a portion of the cecum and ascending colon, with its attached mesentery, is used as a urinary reservoir, and a section of plicated terminal ileum is used as a conduit from the cecal pouch to the abdominal wall; the ureters are then transplanted into the cecal pouch and the pouch is attached to the anterior abdominal wall. Patients then insert a catheter through the external stoma created from the terminal ileum and sewn into the anterior abdominal wall down the plicated terminal ileum and into the cecal pouch to empty urine from the cecal pouch. Complications of the Indiana pouch include small bowel obstruction, pouch leaks, cholecystitis, and parastomal hernia. The average frequency of catheterization in Indiana pouch patients is 3.7 h or five to seven catheterizations in 24 h. The average urine volume is reported to be 291 mL for each catheterization. In the ileal reservoir or Kock pouch, a piece of terminal ileum is used as a urinary reservoir and an ileal stoma is created between the terminal ileum and the abdominal wall. The ureters are implanted into the proximal portion of the segment of ileum used as the reservoir. The patient then catheterizes the ileal conduit several times per day to empty it of urine. Complications of the Kock pouch include leakage of urine from the stoma site, difficult catheterization, electrolyte abnormalities that include hyperchloremic metabolic acidosis, pyelonephritis, hydronephrosis, and stone formation. All complications of these specialized urinary diversion procedures should be treated in consultation with a urologist.

## BIBLIOGRAPHY

Alawadhi A, Chou S, Soucy P: Gastric volvulus—a late complication of gastrostomy. *Can J Surg* 34:485, 1991.

Berry DP, Vellacott KD: High jejunal obstruction: a complication of percutaneous endoscopic gastrostomy. *Br J Surg* 79:1171, 1992.

Calton WC, Martindale RG, Gooden SM: Complications of percutaneous endoscopic gastrostomy. *Mil Med* 157:358, 1992.

Coben RM, Weintraub A, DiMarino AJ, et al: Gastroesophageal reflux during gastrostomy feeding. *Gastroenterology* 106:13, 1994.

Cogen R, Weinryb J, Pomerantz C, et al: Complications of jejunostomy tube feeding in nursing facility patients. *Am J Gastroenterol* 86:1610, 1991.

Evans PM, Serpell JW: Small bowel fistula: a complication of percutaneous endoscopic gastrostomy insertion. *Aust NZ J Surg* 64:518, 1994.

Ghost S, Eastwood MA, Palmer KR: Acute gastric dilatation—a delayed complication of percutaneous endoscopic gastrostomy. *Gut* 34:859, 1993.

Gibson SE, Wenig BL, Watkins JL: Complications of percutaneous endoscopic gastrostomy in head and neck cancer patients. *Ann Otol Rhinol Laryngol* 101:46, 1992.

Goodman P, Levine MS, Parkman HP: Extrusion of PEG tube from the stomach with fistula formation: an unusual complication of percutaneous endoscopic gastrostomy. *Gastrointest Endosc* 16:286, 1991.

Gowen GF. The management of complications of Foley feeding gastrostomies. *Am Surg* 54:582, 1988.

Hessl JM. Removal of Foley catheter when balloon does not deflate. *Urology* 22:219, 1983.

Hicks ME, Suratt RS, Picus D, et al. Fluoroscopically guided percutaneous gastrostomy and gastroenterostomy: analysis of 158 consecutive cases. *AJR Am J Roentgenol* 154:725, 1990.

Ho CS, Yee ACN, McPherson R. Complications of surgical and percutaneous nonendoscopic gastrostomy: review of 233 patients. *Gastroenterology* 95:1206, 1988.

Huff JP, Rosenblum J, Camara DS. Complications of gastrostomy. *South Med J* 81:1050, 1988.

Kadakia SC, Sullivan HO, Starnes E: Percutaneous endoscopic gastrostomy or jejunostomy and the incidence of aspiration in 79 patients. *Am J Surg* 164:114, 1992.

Kinsey GC, Murray MJ, Swensen SJ, et al: Glucose content of tracheal aspirates: implications for the detection of tube feeding aspiration. *Crit Care Med* 22:1557, 1994.

Kleeman FJ. Technique for removal of Foley catheter when balloon does not deflate. *Urology* 21:416, 1983.

Levine MS, Fisher AR, Rubesin SE, et al: Complications after total gastrectomy and esophagojejunostomy: radiologic evaluation. *AJR* 157:1189, 1991.

Lieskovsky G, Boyd S, Skinner DG. Management of late complications of the Kock pouch form of urinary diversion. *J Urol* 137:1146-1150, 1987.

McDowell GC, Hayden LJ, Wise HA. Penile necrosis secondary to an indwelling Foley catheter. *J Urol* 138:1243, 1987.

McQuaid KR, Little TE: Two fatal complications related to gastrostomy "button" placement. *Gastrointest Endosc* 38:601, 1992.

Merguerian PA, Erturk E, Hulbert WC, et al. Peritonitis and abdominal free air due to intraperitoneal bladder perforations associated with indwelling urethral catheter drainage. *J Urol* 134:747, 1985.

Minocha A, Rupp TH, Jaggers TL, et al: Silent colo-gastrocutaneous fistula as a complication of percutaneous endoscopic gastrostomy. A*M J Gastroenterol* 89:2243, 1994.

Montecalvo MA, Steger KA, Farber HW, et al: Nutritional outcome and pneumonia in critical care patients randomized to gastric versus jejunal tube feedings. The Critical Care Research Team. *Crit Care Med* 20:1377, 1992.

Nunley D, Berk SL: Percutaneous endoscopic gastrostomy as an unrecognized source of methicillin-resistant Staphylococcus aureus colonization. *Am J Gastroenterol* 87:58, 1992.

O'Keefe KP: Complications of percutaneous feeding tubes. *Emerg Med Clin North Am* 12:815, 1994.

Riley DA, Strauss M: Airway and other complications of percutaneous endoscopic gastrostomy in head and neck cancer patients. *Ann Otol Rhinol Laryngol* 101:310, 1992.

Rowbottom SJ, Wilson J, et al: Total oesophageal obstruction in association with combined enternal feed and sucralfate therapy. *Anaesth Intensive Care* 21:372, 1993.

Rowland RG, Mitchell ME, Bihrle R, Kahnoski RJ, Piser JE. Indiania continent urinary reservoir. *J Urol* 137:1136, 1987.

Scapa E, Broide E, Slutzki S, et al: Colocutaneous fistula—a rare complication of percutaneous endoscopic gastrostomy. *Surg Laparosc Endosc* 3:430, 1993.

Stathopoulos G, Rudberg MA, Harig JM: Subcutaneous emphysema following PEG. *Gastrointest Endosc* 37:374, 1991.

Tsai CC, Bradley SF: Group A streptococcal bacteremia associated with gastrostomy feeding tube infections in a long-term care facility. *J Am Geriatr Soc* 40:821, 1992.

Weber A, Nadel S: CT appearance of retrograde jejunoduodenogastric intusseusception: a rare complication of gastrostomy tubes. *AJR* 156:957, 1991.

Wolf EL, Frager D, Beneventano TC. Radiologic demonstration of important gastrostomy tube complications. *Gastrointest Radiol* 11:20, 1986.

# 264

# COMPLICATIONS OF CARDIOVASCULAR AND INTRAVENOUS DEVICES

## Robert Rusnak

## APNEA AND BRADYCARDIA MONITORS FOR INFANTS

Pediatricians commonly recommend apnea and bradycardia monitors for infants who have suffered either a life-threatening apneic or bradycardiac event or whose parents have described an episode that may have represented such an event. The parents are given life-support instructions and are instructed to call 911 if an event occurs. Most commonly, these devices are not equipped with continuous tape recorders. False alarms are relatively common, but it is usually impossible for the emergency physician to distinguish a false alarm from a true short-duration life-threatening event. The safest course for the physician is to admit the child for monitoring and have the parents bring the home unit to the hospital so that it can be tested in a controlled setting. See Chap. 105 for related discussion.

## CARDIAC PACEMAKER

Implantable cardiac pacemakers have been used in human beings since 1958. Currently approximately 300,000 pacemakers are inserted or replaced each year in the United States. After pacing or sensing defects, infection is the most common pacemaker-related problem. These infections may involve the pacemaker electrode or the generator pocket. Patients with electrode infections are generally ill patients, who have systemic signs of infection including fever,

chills, rigors, or leukocytosis; two thirds of these patients have positive blood cultures and should be assumed to have infective endocarditis until proved otherwise. Patients with epicardial pacing systems (usually recognized on chest x-ray as a pair of coiled wire electrodes over the myocardium) may also develop mediastinitis, pericarditis, or bronchopleural cutaneous fistulas. Patients who develop infections of the generator pocket, with or without erosions or abscesses of the overlying skin, generally develop erythema and drainage from the pocket, and have purulent secretions or positive wound cultures. Treatment of these infections is institution dependent and ranges from local wound care, irrigation with antibacterial solutions, or intravenous antibiotics, to removal of the generator and replacement in an alternate site. Other complications are listed in Table 264-1. See Chap. 13 for further discussion of pacemakers.

## THE AUTOMATIC IMPLANTABLE CARDIOVERTER-DEFIBRILLATOR

These devices are inserted to prevent sudden death in patients with drug-refractory arrhythmias. Early postoperative complications include postoperative refractory congestive heart failure, coronary artery erosion, subclavian vein thrombosis, or postoperative stroke. Late complications likely to be seen in the emergency department (as opposed to the early postoperative period) include infection at the generator site, discharge in the absence of symptoms (secondary to sensed myopotentials due to shivering or excessive arm activity, atrial fibrillation with a rapid ventricular response, sinus tachycardia, nonsustained ventricular tachycardia, or unknown factors), lead migration, failure to recognize or terminate arrhythmias, and generator failure (usually occurs 8 to 14 months after initial generator placement). These complications usually can be diagnosed by clinical symptoms or signs and by analysis of the automatic cardioverter-defibrillator generator, using a magnet and an external analyzer device. See Chap. 13 for discussion of automatic internal defibrillators.

## THE HICKMAN-BROVIAC CATHETER

The Hickman-Broviac catheter is a subcutaneously tunneled, intravenous, Silastic catheter positioned in the superior vena cava or the right atrium via the subclavicular subclavian vein approach. It is used for long-term intravenous access and blood sampling and infusion of intravenous fluids, medications, total parenteral nutrition, blood products, or chemotherapy. The insertion of these double- or triple-lumen catheters involves the creation of a subcutaneous tunnel of varying lengths between entry of the catheter into a vein and the skin exit site

**Table 264-1.** Cardiac Pacemakers

| Complications | Diagnosis | Treatment |
|---|---|---|
| Myocardial perforation and cardiac tamponade secondary to insertion or removal of the pacemaker electrode catheter | Clinical signs and symptoms, echocardiography | Pericardial drainage |
| Pressure dermatitis from an implanted pacemaker generator | Patch testing | Pacemaker generator replacement if local measures are unsuccessful |
| Runaway pacemaker with or without pacemaker-induced tachycardia | Electrogram, clinical | Placement of magnet over pacemaker battery |
| | | Reprogramming the pulse generator to a lower output* |
| | | Use of external chest wall overdrive stimulation* |
| | | Connect external pacemaker to the permanent pacing lead after locating and removing implanted pacemaker unit |
| | | Place transcutaneous pacemaker, then disconnect permanent pacing lead from the pacemaker generator |

* Treatment that involves reprogramming the pulse generator or use of external chest wall overdrive stimulation requires an adequate escape rhythm.

**Table 264-2.** Hickman-Broviac and Porta-caths

| Complications | Diagnosis | Treatment |
|---|---|---|
| Infection | Blood cultures | Intravenous antibiotics or catheter removal* |
| Inability to aspirate blood secondary to clot, thrombosis, or fibrin sheaths | Difficult aspiration or infusion | Declotting with heparin or thrombolytics, catheter removal |
| Accidental dislodgement | Venogram | Repositioning under fluoroscopy or removal |
| Catheter migration from original placement site to a smaller vessel or subcutaneously | Venogram | Catheter removal or repositioning |
| Leakage around infusion or aspiration ports | Observation during use or swelling around entrance site | Repair or removal |
| Dislodgement due to pendulous breasts | Difficulty with infusion or aspiration, swelling, pain or redness at catheter entrance site | Removal or repositioning |
| Catheter splitting or ballooning of catheter shaft during infusion | Difficulty with infusion, pain during infusion | Catheter removal |

\* Sepsis is not an absolute indication for removal of these catheters. In one report, only 18 of 143 catheters required removal because of infection.

SOURCE: Ulz L, Peterson FB, Ford R, et al. A prospective study of complications in Hickman right-atrial catheters in marrow transplant patients. *J Parenter Enteral Nutr* 14:27, 1990.

containing the catheter ports. The catheter is kept open by periodic injections of heparinized saline through these injection ports. Complications are listed in Table 264-2.

## PORTA-CATHS

The Porta-cath is a subcutaneously implanted intravenous access device that couples a central venous pressure catheter to an implanted subcutaneous injection port that is usually located on the chest wall. These catheters are commonly used in cancer patients undergoing long-term outpatient chemotherapy. Porta-caths are usually inserted via a direct approach of the cephalic vein in the deltopectoral groove and positioned such that the catheter tip lies in the superior vena cava or the high right atrium. In men, the subcutaneous injection port usually lies a few centimeters above the nipple; in women, it usually lies near the clavicle. The injection port is flushed with a heparin saline solution with a special needle (the Huber-Point right-angled needle) after each use. If other types of needles are inserted into the device, it will lose its ability to maintain a seal. Problems such as a blocked catheter, subcutaneous extravasation during fluid administration, wound dehiscence, and ulceration of the subcutaneous injection port located in the chest wall are treated as per complications of the Hickman-Broviac catheters noted above (see Table 264-2).

## BIBLIOGRAPHY

Antinori CH, Villanueva DT, Pierucci L Jr, et al: A new approach to the management of infected pacemakers. *Clin Card* 17:38, 1994.

Bauersfeld UK, Thakur RK, Ghani M, et al: Malposition of transvenous pacing lead in the left ventricle: radiographic findings. *AJR* 162:290, 1994.

Borbola J, Denes P, Ezri MD, et al: The automatic implantable cardioverter-defibrillator: clinical experience, complications and follow-up in 25 patients. *Arch Intern Med* 148:70, 1980.

Brown KR, Carter W Jr, Lombardi GE: Blunt trauma-induced pacemaker failure. *Ann Emerg Med* 20:905, 1991.

Conti JB, Curtis AB, Hill JA, et al: Termination of pacemaker-mediated tachycardia by adenosine. *Clin Card* 17:47, 1994.

Cooper CJ, Dweik, R, Gabbay S: Treatment of pacemaker-associated right atrial thrombus with 2 hour rTPA infusion. *Am Heart J* 126:228, 1993.

Futterman LG, Lemberg L: Pacemaker update. Part IV: Antitachycardia devices. *Am J Crit Care* 2:253, 1993.

Futterman LG, Rhymes-Johnson PW, Lemberg L: Pacemaker update. Part III: Pacemaker-induced tachycardia. *Am J Crit Care* 2:180, 1993.

Graham DR, Keldermans MM, Klemm LW, et al: Infectious complications among patients receiving home intravenous therapy with peripheral, central, or peripherally placed central venous catheters. *Am J Med* 91:95S, 1991.

Hargreaves M, Channon K: Mechanism of pacemaker induced cough. *Br Heart J* 71:484, 1994.

Harvey MP, Trent RJ, Joshua DE, et al: Complications associated with indwelling venous Hickman catheters in patients with hematological disorders. *Aust NZ J Med* 16:21, 1986.

Keung YK, Watkins K, Chen SC, et al: Comparative study of infectious complications of different types of chronic central venous access devices. *Cancer* 73:2832, 1994.

Lefroy DC, Crake T, Davies DW: Ventricular tachycardia: an unusual pacemaker-mediated tachycardia. *Br Heart J* 71:481, 1994.

Marchlinski FE, Flores BT, Buxton AE, et al: The automatic implantable cardioverter-defibrillator: efficiency, complications, and device failures. *Ann Intern Med* 104:481, 1986.

Mickey H, Anderson C, Nielsen LH. Runaway pacemaker: a still-existing complication and therapeutic guidelines. *Clin Cardiol* 12:412, 1989.

Newland GM, Janz TG: Pacemaker-twiddler's syndrome: a rare cause of lead displacement and pacemaker malfunction. *Ann Emerg Med* 23:136, 1994.

O'Hara JR Jr, Brand MI, Boutros AR: Acute airway obstruction following placement of a subclavian Hickman catheter. *Can J Anaesthes* 41:241, 1994.

Pessa ME, Howard RJ. Complications of Hickman-Broviac catheters. *Surg Gynecol Obstet* 161:257, 1985.

Pfeiffer D, Jung W, Fehske W, et al: Complications of pacemaker-defibrillator devices: diagnosis and management. *Am Heart J* 127:1073, 1994.

Raad I, Davis S, Becker M, et al: Low infection rate and long durability of nontunneled Silastic catheters. A safe and cost-effective alternative for long-term venous access. *Arch Intern Med* 153:1791, 1993.

Samain E, Marty J, Dupont H, et al: *Anesthesiology* 78:376, 1993.

Sariego J, Bootorabi B, Matsumoto, et al: Major long-term complications in 1,422 permanent venous access devices. *Am J Surg* 165:249, 1993.

Shaw JHF, Douglas R, Wilson T. Clinical performance of Hickman and Porta-cath atrial catheters. *Aust NZ J Surg* 58:657, 1988.

Ulz L, Peterson FB, Ford R, et al: A prospective study of complications in Hickman right-atrial catheters in marrow transplant patients. *J Parenter Enteral Nutr* 14:27, 1990.

Valdes-Dapena M, Steinschneider A. Sudden infant death syndrome (SIDS), apnea, and near miss for SIDS. *Emerg Clin North Am* 1:27, 1983.

Vilacosta I, Sarria C, San Roman JA, et al: Usefulness of transesophageal echocardiography for diagnosis of infected transvenous permanent pacemakers. *Circulation* 89:2684, 1994.

Vilacosta I, Zamorano J, Camino A, et al: Infected transvenous permanent pacemakers: role of transesophageal echocardiography. *Am Heart J* 125:904, 1993.

Wade JS, Cobbs CG. Infections in cardiac pacemakers. *Curr Clin Topics Infect Dis* 9:44, 1988.

Wilson HA Jr, Downes TR, Julian JS, et al: Candida endocarditis. A treatable form of pacemaker infection. *Chest* 103:283, 1993.

Winkler TR, Hanlin RJ, Hinke TD, et al: Unusual cause of hemoptysis. Hickman-induced cavabronchial fistula. *Chest* 102:1285, 1992.

# 265
# ORTHOPAEDIC DEVICES AND RECONSTRUCTIONS

## Harrison A. Latimer
## Scott Kelley

Orthopaedic surgery is unique in its abundant use of implants to reconstruct the musculoskeletal system. Implants may be used to replace a degenerated structure or simply used to stabilize a bone or ligament while it heals. The goal is a painless, functioning spine or extremity. Examples of implant use are fractures, arthrodesis, arthroplasty, and ligament fixation.

This chapter reviews the common types of orthopaedic implants. Postoperative complications that may present to an emergency department following implant use, including breakage, migration, and infection, are discussed.

**Fig. 265-1.** *A.* This clavicle fracture was rigidly fixed with a plate and screws. *B.* Note the fracture healing without callus formation.

## COMMON ORTHOPAEDIC IMPLANTS STABILIZING BONE TO BONE

### Plates and Screws

Plates and their accompanying screws are commonly used to add stability while fractures, osteotomies, or arthrodeses go on to fusion. They come in many different shapes and sizes because they have been designed to fit to different areas of the skeleton. They all share the common function of stabilizing bone in an anatomically acceptable position while it heals to itself. To perform this function, the plate must be securely attached to bone with multiple screws to each fragment. When used to manage fractures, the bones are placed in direct contact and healing occurs without the large amount of callus formation seen with casting or intramedullary nailing (Fig. 265-1). Therefore it is often difficult to determine when fracture union is complete and it is not uncommon for the fracture line to be visible more than 1 y after surgery (Fig. 265-2).

### Complications

Early complications include wound infections that may be superficial and amenable to antibiotics or deep and require surgical exploration.

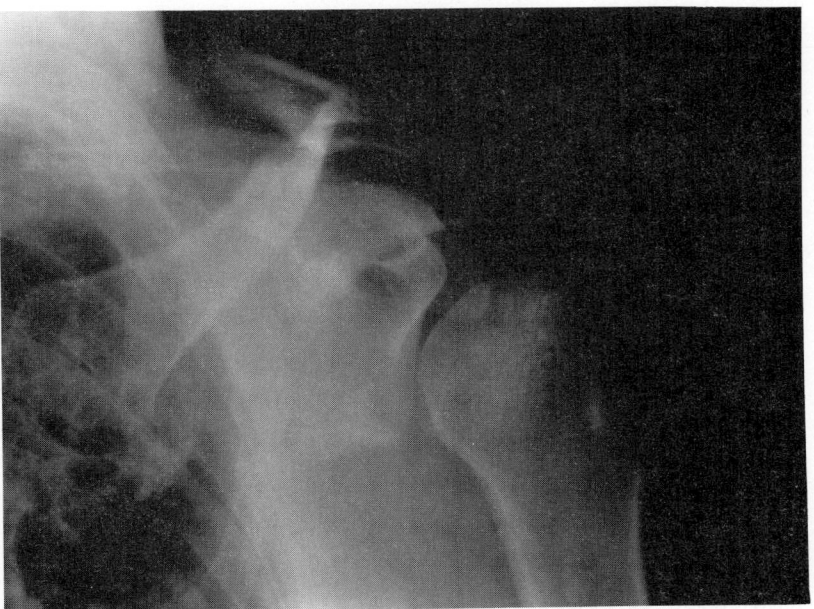

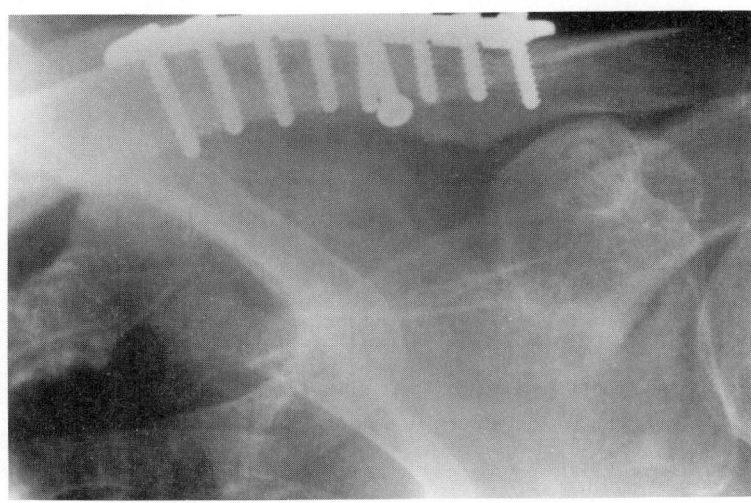

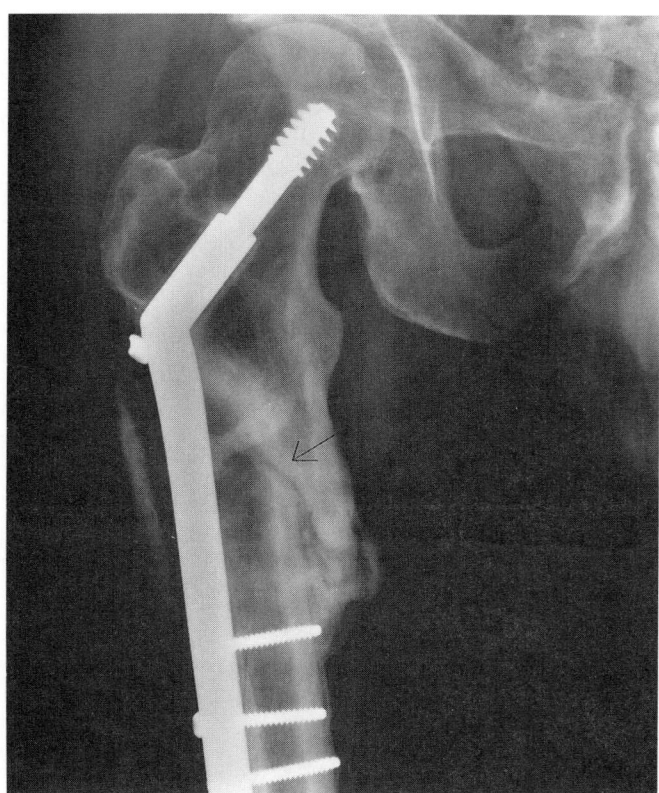

**Fig. 265-2.** This femur fracture is rigidly healed at 1 year, but the fracture line (arrow) is still present.

Later complications include nonunion of the fracture. Plate-screw constructs are simply temporizing measures. If the bone does not heal, the plate will eventually bend or break or the screws will pull out of the bone (Fig. 265-3). Plates and screws are sometimes removed and the bone is then at risk for refracture (often through a screw hole) for approximately 7 months.

## Intramedullary Rods

Since their popularization during World War II, solid, single intramedullary rods have become the most common method of treating femoral and tibial fractures and more recently some humeral fractures (Fig. 265-4). They have also been used to stabilize osteotomies or arthrodeses. Over the last decade their application to fractures has been extended by the addition of proximal and distal interlocking screws that add rotational stability. Over the past 5 years open fractures have been treated with intramedullary nails that are placed with minimal reaming of the bones. All these advances have led to the greater number of emergency patients who have intramedullary rods or nails.

Intramedullary rods are placed through an incision at the end of the bone that obviously avoids injury to the joint surface. The intramedullary canal is then mechanically reamed to a slightly larger size than the nail. The nail is then inserted and interlocking screws are added if needed for stability at the fracture or osteotomy. The immobilization of the fracture ends is less than that gained with plates

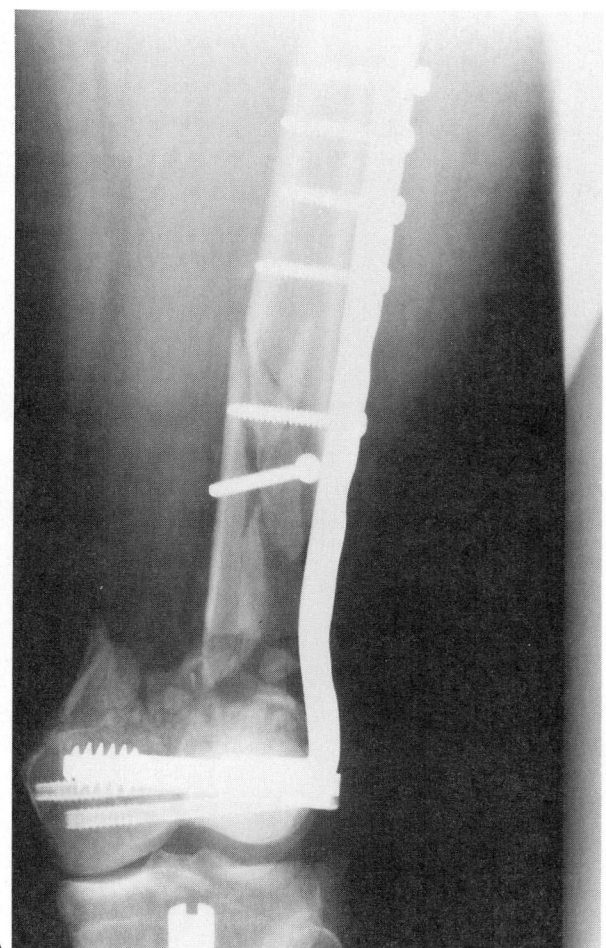

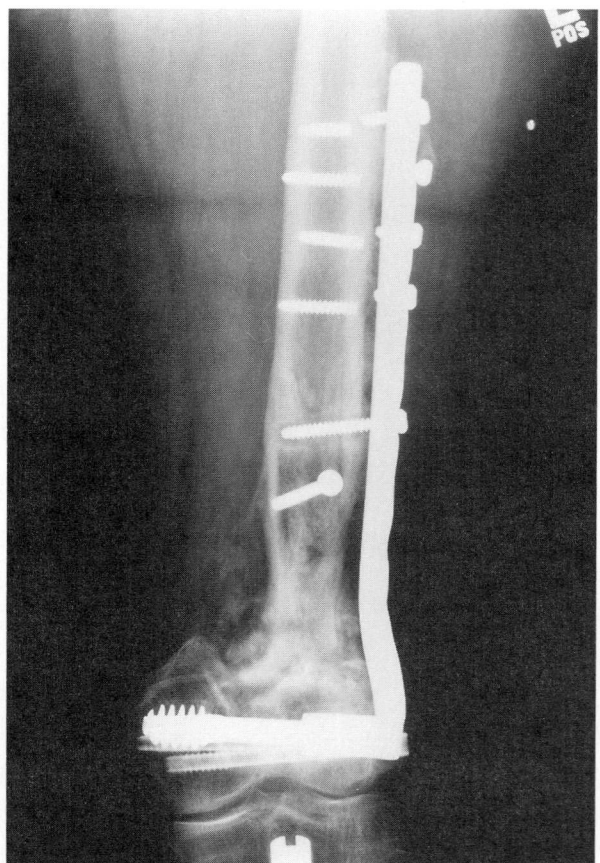

**Fig. 265-3.** *A.* This severely comminuted, open distal femur fracture was fixed with a plate and screws. *B.* Despite bone grafting, the screws broke before the fracture healed.

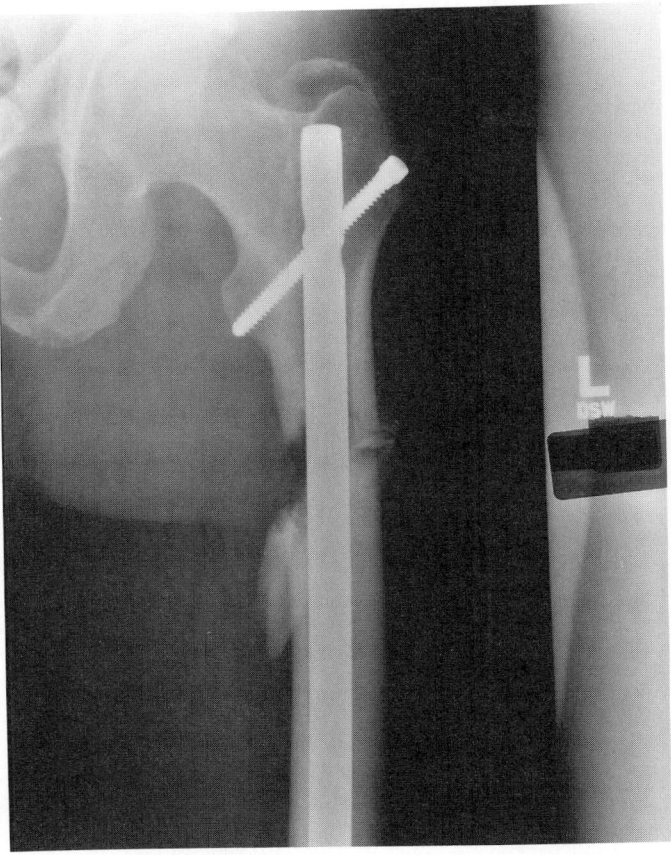

**Fig. 265-4.** This femur fracture was stabilized with an intramedullary rod.

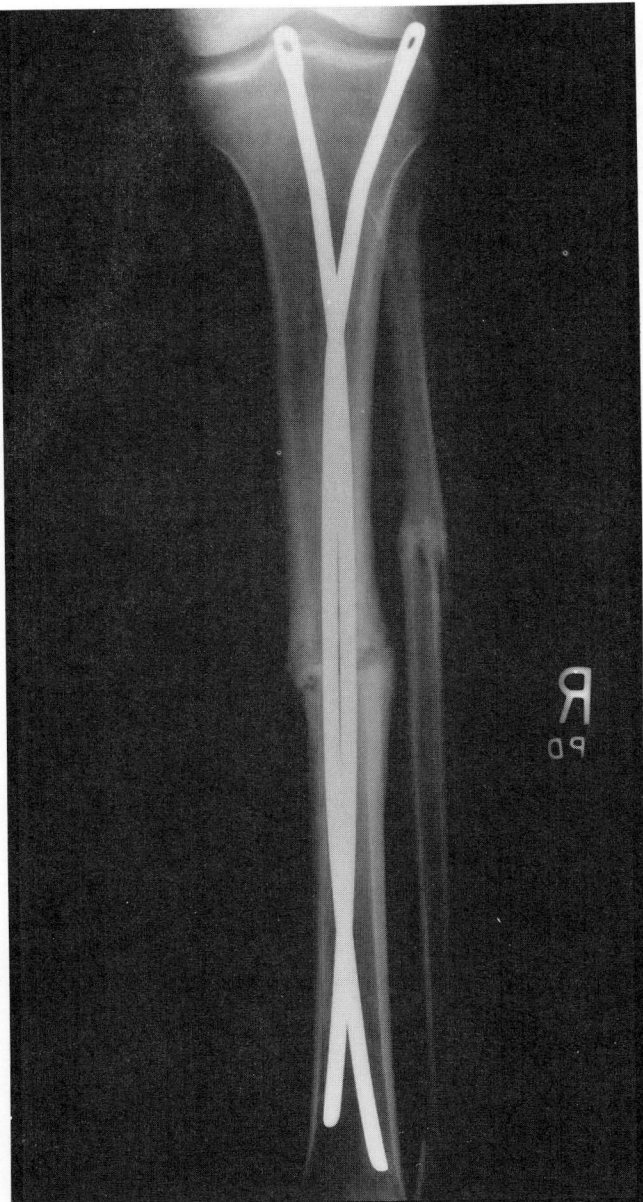

**Fig. 265-6.** These Ender's rods were chosen to stabilize this open tibia fracture.

and screws, and therefore the healing process involves easily visible callus formation at the fracture site (Fig. 265-5). In open fractures minimal or no reaming, which retains the maximum blood supply to the injury, may be performed and requires a smaller diameter rod. Although less popular today than single, solid rods, multiple, small, flexible rods are still sometimes used to gain fracture stability (see Fig. 265-6). They do not usually break due to their inherent flexibility.

## Complications

As with all surgery, infection is the most worrisome early complication and still occurs with a 1 to 2 percent incidence in closed fractures despite the use of perioperative antibiotics. Unreamed nails are now used for open fractures that (depending on their severity) have up to a 25 percent infection rate. The number of emergency department encounters for postoperative infectious complications will increase. Due to their central location, rods have a greater mechanical strength than plates and screws. They, however, will also fail (usually after 1 year)

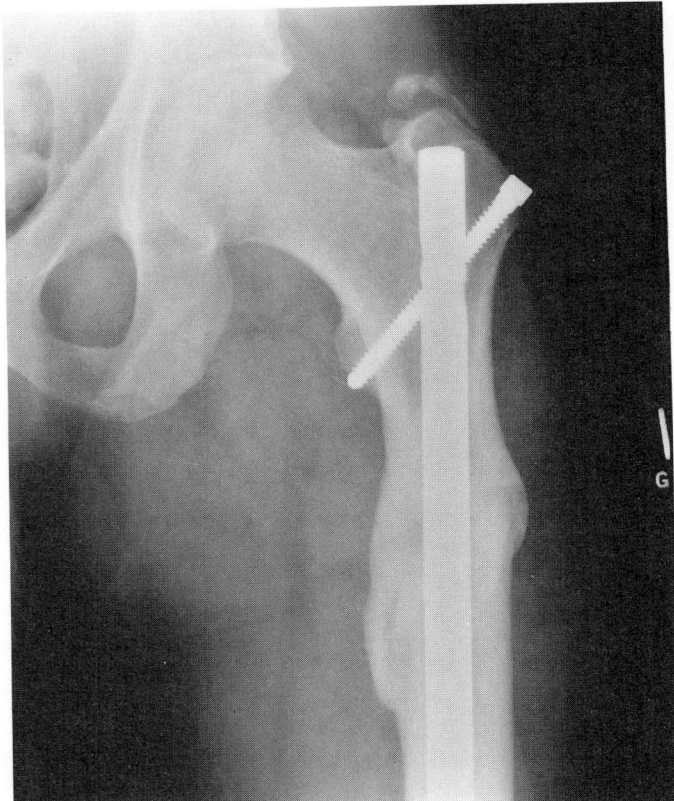

**Fig. 265-5.** Note the large callus formation at the fracture site.

by breaking at an unhealed facture site (Fig. 265-7). With weight bearing the interlocking screws may also break. Unlike rod fracture this may not result in an unstable extremity. Any non-interlocked nail may work its way back out of the bone and irritate surrounding soft tissue. Femoral rods may then cause trochanteric bursitis. The multiple small flexible rods are notorious for this problem and often become palpable under the skin (Fig. 265-8). Nonunion of the fracture occurs more frequently with open fractures and therefore the small unreamed nails used for these fractures are at risk for breakage.

### External Fixators

External fixators have been widely used to stabilize open fractures. A fixator is preferred over cast immobilization because it allows the physician access to the soft tissue injury. They also may be used to temporarily stabilize an extremity while life- or limb-threatening surgery is performed. Lastly, certain types of closed fractures, such as distal radius fractures, may require an external fixator to maintain an adequate reduction of the fracture.

Nontraumatic uses of external fixators include stabilization of arthrodeses because special clamps may be used to add compression that enhances union. More recently complex wire and ring (Ilizarov) fixators have been used to lengthen bones and correct deformities.

The external fixator is divided into two components: the fixation pins or wires and the external frame. The threaded pins or wires are inserted into each fragment at a distance from the fracture site. When connected to the frame, they are able to rigidly hold the bone so that union occurs with minimal callus (Fig. 265-9).

### Complications

Because external fixation is usually chosen for severe open fractures, which have a higher rate of infection, emergency department visits are not uncommon. These patients present with increased redness, swelling, or drainage at the previous open wound site. The skin should be prepped and deep cultures obtained by aspiration or swab. The fixation pins and wires very commonly sustain pin tract infections that may easily be treated by releasing the skin around the pin site with a no. 11 blade after adequate local anesthesia. Oral antibiotics may be given empirically. With time the fixator pins may loosen in the bone. The clamps connecting the pins to the frame may also

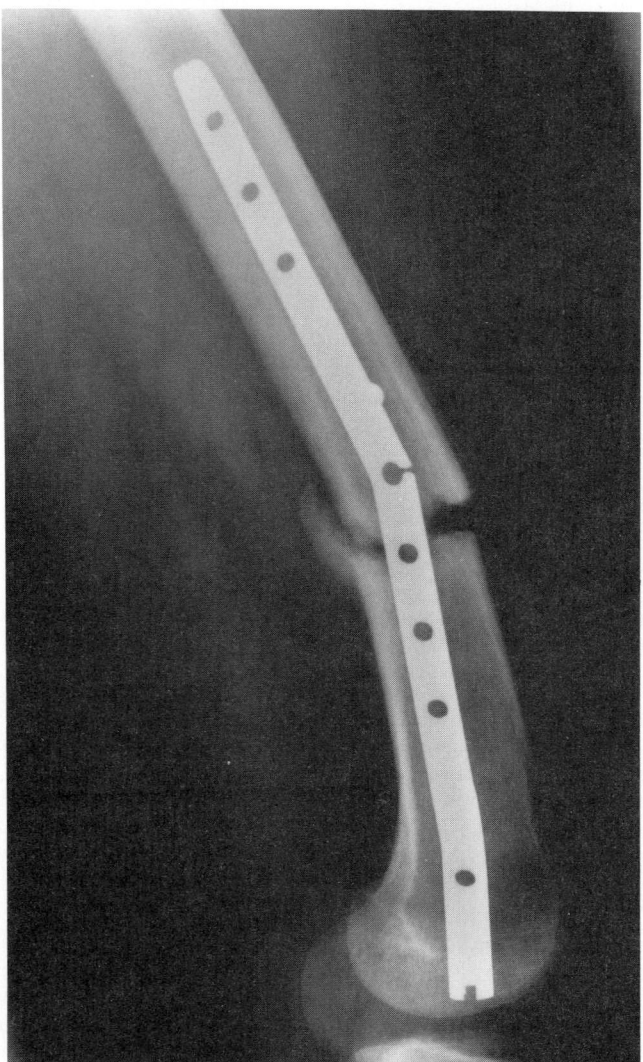

**Fig. 265-7.** This distal femoral intramedullary nail broke before fracture union occurred.

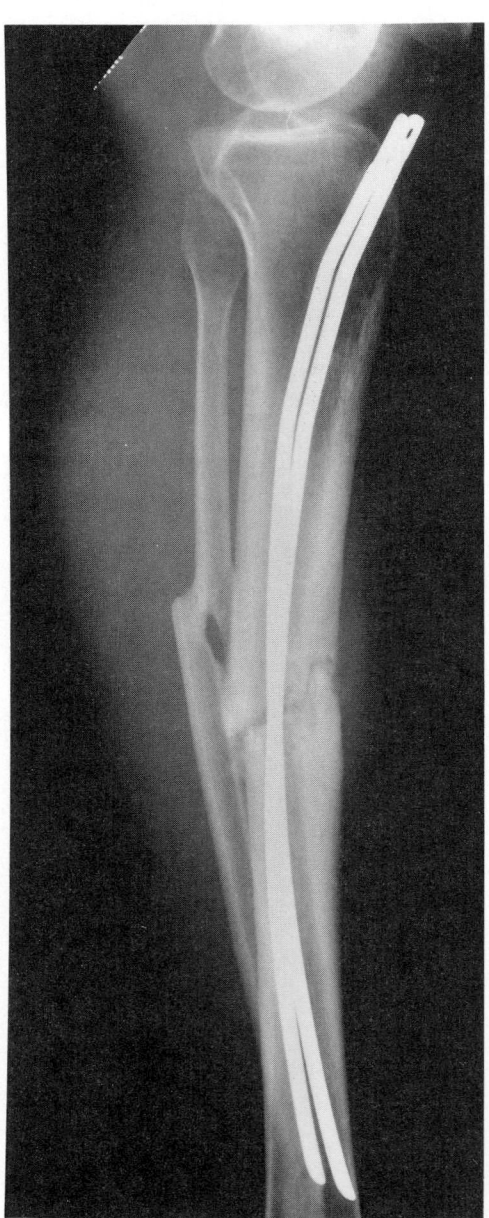

**Fig. 265-8.** The Ender's rods have "backed out" of the bone and were prominent just under the skin.

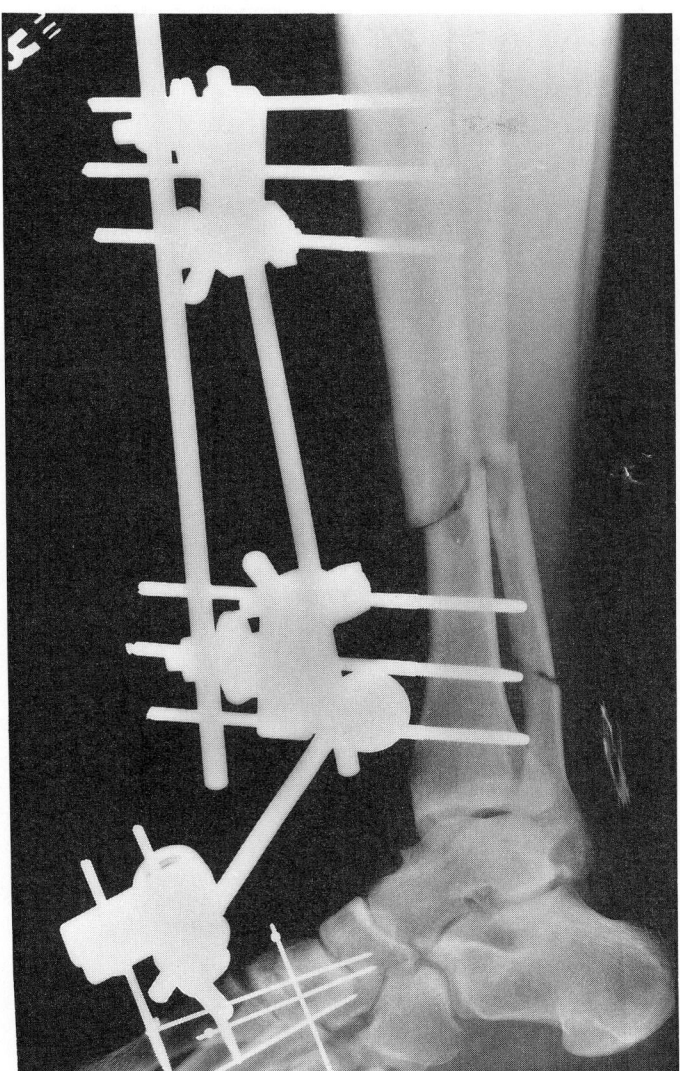

**Fig. 265-9.** This external fixator is used to stabilize the open tibia fracture while still allowing access to the soft tissue wound.

loosen. This may result in instability or loss of reduction at the fracture site. This will usually be detectable clinically (unstable fractures are painful when stressed) or by radiographs.

### Fixation Wires and Pins

Small smooth or threaded percutaneous pins (Fig. 265-10) are often used in the small bones of the hand or foot to add stability while fracture union occurs. The hand and foot possess an excellent blood supply that usually results in early union. The pins are cut off outside the skin so that they may be removed between 3 and 9 weeks post-operatively.

Internal cerclage wires are often used to hold structures that have fractured under tension. Examples are tuberosity fractures of the proximal humerus (Fig. 265-11) or patella fractures. Cerclage wires may also be used with or without a plate to stabilize a fracture around a prosthetic joint implant (Fig. 265-12). They serve the same role as a screw which cannot be placed through the implant.

### Complications

As with external fixation pins the most common complication of using percutaneous pins is a pin tract infection. These are usually

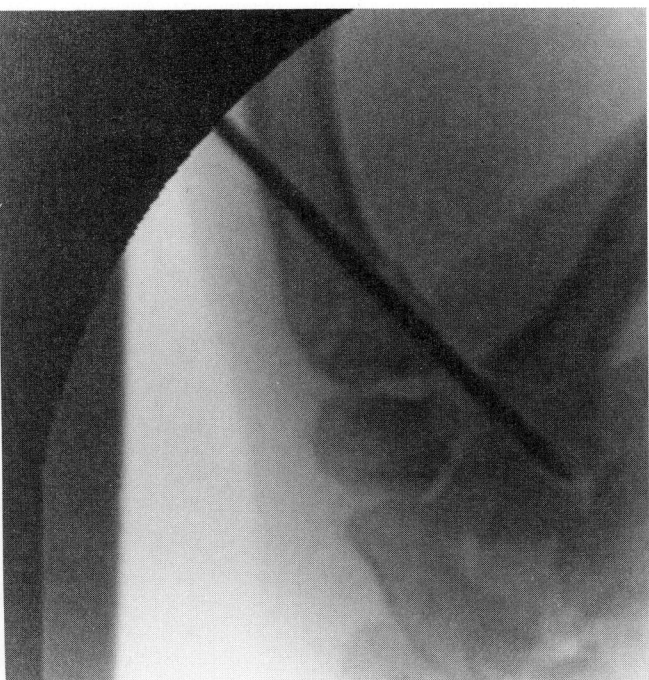

**Fig. 265-10.** This smooth pin was used to stabilize the fracture at the base of the thumb metacarpal.

treated by removing the pin, but this should only be done after consultation with an orthopaedist. A course of oral antibiotics may also be indicated. Complications of cerclage wires include wire breakage prior to union or perforation of a wire through thin overlying skin.

### Cervical Spine Implants

The cervical spine is unique from the rest of the vertebral column due to the common use of halo fixation. Halos are simply a ring external fixator that is rigidly attached to the outer skull table with pins. Usually four rods are used to connect this ring to a well-molded plastic or plaster body jacket. The halo limits the motion of the cervicle spine allowing fractures to heal or arthrodesis to unite.

The most common cervical implant is a posterior cerclage wire (Fig. 265-13) that limits motion between adjacent vertebrae while fusion occurs. A bone block taken from the iliac crest is often used as a biologic implant in the anterior cervical spine to gain fusion. More recently special plates and screws have been developed for the anterior cervical spine. Their use is likely to accelerate in the future.

### Complications

Like other external fixators the most common complication of halo fixation is pin tract infection. Infected pins are usually removed and a new pin placed in an alternative site. Loose noninfected pins should never be tightened because this risks penetration of the inner skull table and resultant meningitis. The internal implants will fail if the vertebrae fail to unite.

### Anterior and Posterior Thoracolumbar Spine Implants

Although the number of spinal instrumentation systems is overwhelming, the basic concepts are simple. A rigid plate or rod is connected to the spine to limit motion between vertebral segments and allow healing or fusion to occur. There are only three different ways to connect the rod or plate to the vertebrae: a hook, a wire, or a screw.

When reduced to these terms the instrumentation is much more simple.

Most advances in spinal instrumentation arose from the treatment of childhood scoliosis. The first was the Harrington rod-hook system (Fig. 265-14) introduced in 1960 and still in use today. Two major lessons were learned in the development of this system. (1) Extremely durable materials were needed to avoid breakage, (2) No matter how rigid the instrumentation, failure was inevitable if fusion did not occur (Fig. 265-15). Over the years many instrumentation systems have been developed with special hook designs that allow the basic Harrington rod concept to be used for a multitude of spinal problems.

In the 1970s Eduardo Luque developed a system in which smooth metal rods were laid along the spine and wired to each segment. This

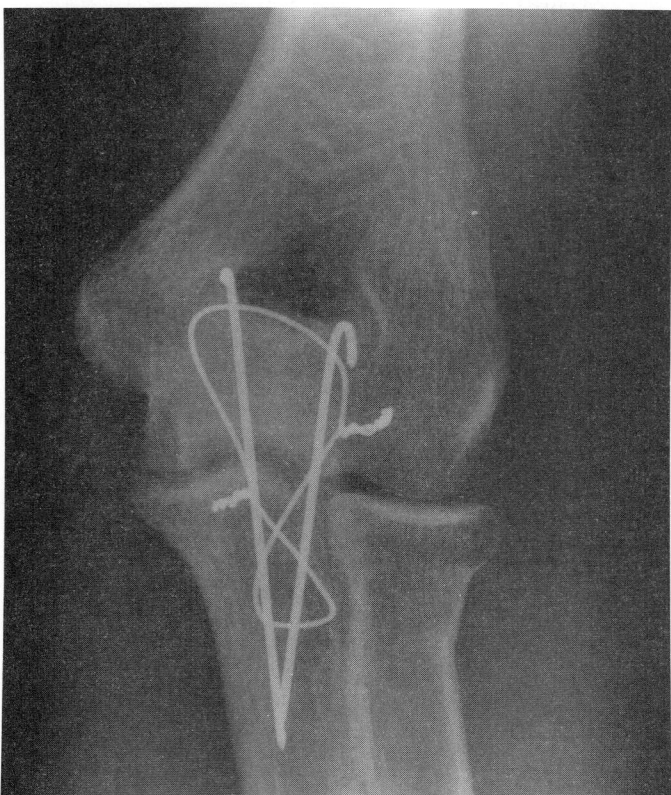

A

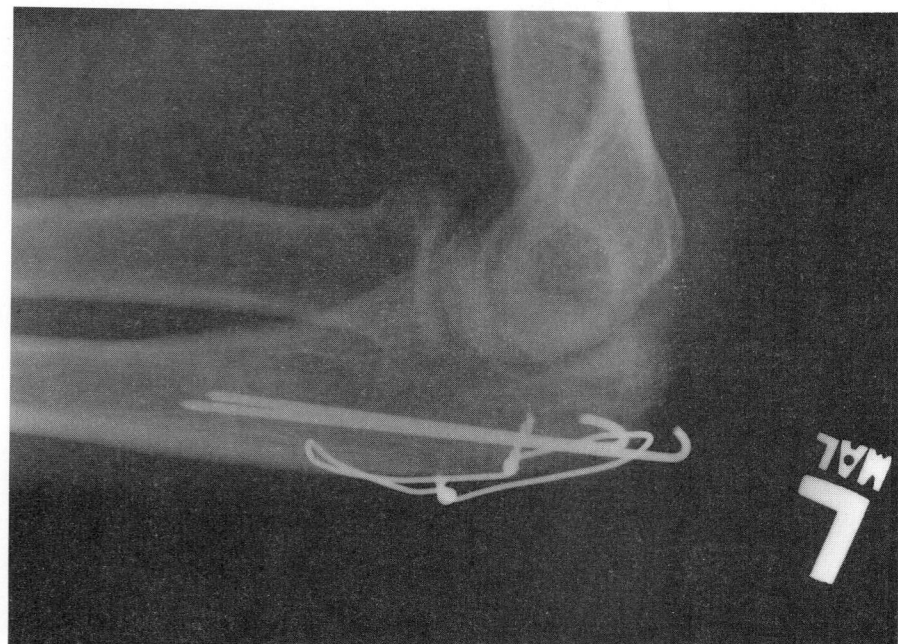

B

**Fig. 265-11.** *A* and *B.* This olecranon fracture was stabilized with two smooth pins and a cerclage wire that allowed joint motion during healing.

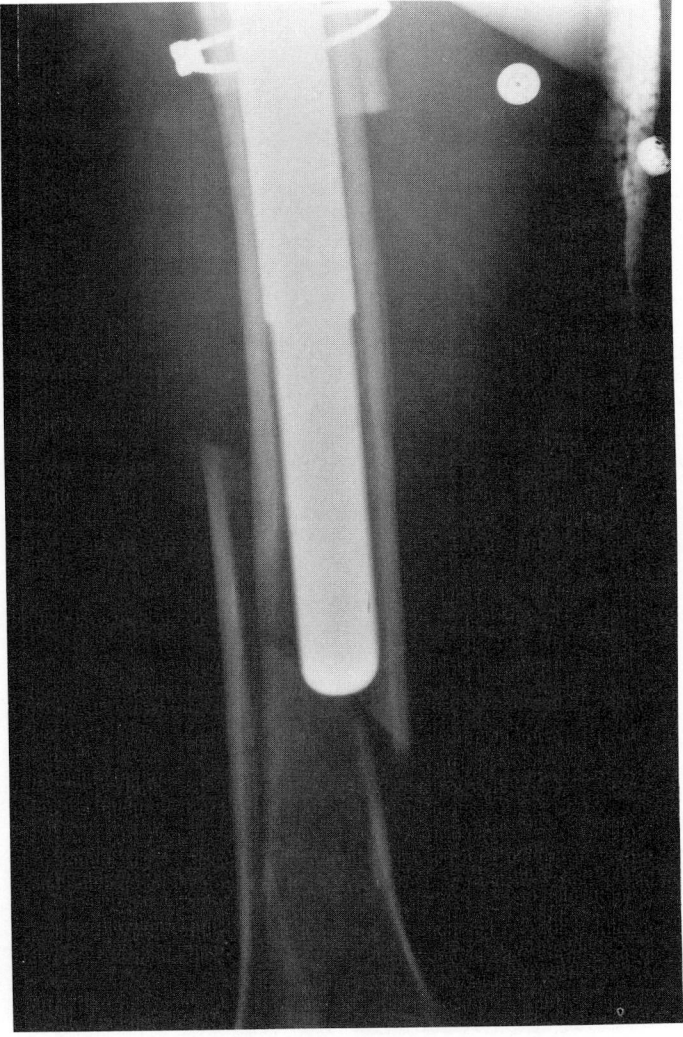

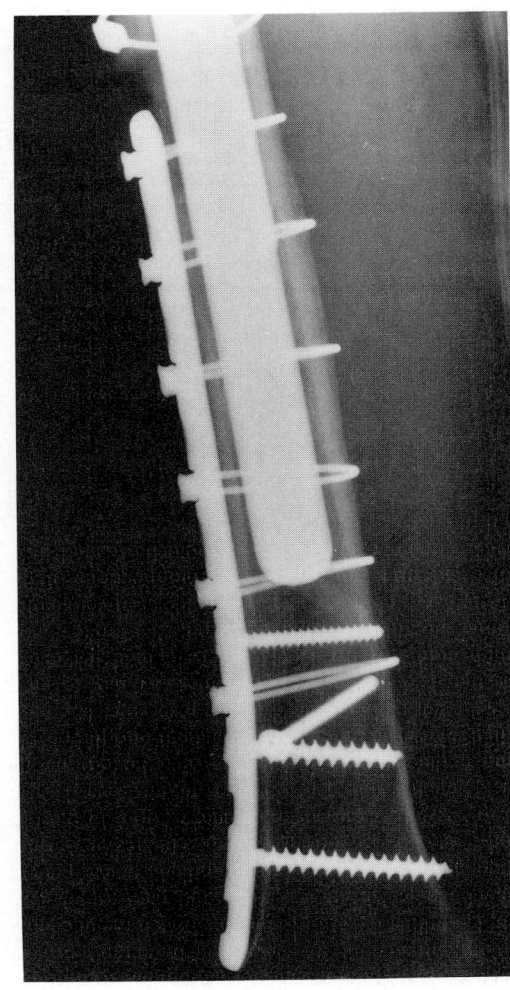

**A**

**B**

**Fig. 265-12.** *A* and *B.* This periprosthetic fracture is stabilized by a special plate designed for use with wires or screws.

created an extremely rigid construct that did not require postoperative bracing. This system is still in use today with only slight modifications (see Fig. 265-14).

The drawback of rod-hook and rod-wire systems is the need for the implant to immobilize over a large number of vertebral levels. This problem has been addressed by pedicle screws placed directly into the vertebral body. This technique dates back to 1949. Because the screw passes through both the posterior and anterior spinal elements, excellent fixation is obtained (Fig. 265-16). This allows the surgeon to greatly reduce the number of segments immobilized. The pedicle screws are then connected to a rigid rod or plate. At present time the Food and Drug Administration (FDA) is investigating the use of these implants.

Posterior spinal instruments are more commonly used than anterior instrumentation due in part to the ease and safety of the posterior approach. Over the last several years numerous types of anterior instrumentation have been developed (Fig. 265-17). The same principal of connecting to the vertebrae with a screw that in turn connects to a bridging plate, rod, or cable system is used.

## Complications

Emergency visits usually involve early wound problems. Diagnosis of an infection is supported by severe pain and an elevated tempera-

ture, white blood cell count, and erythrocyte sedimentation rate. Painful acute implant failure is not common, but Harrington-type hook implants may disengage. The patient usually notes an acute "pop" and an immediate increase in pain. This is usually best demonstrated on the lateral radiograph because the hook will no longer be under the vertebral lamina (Fig. 265-18). Rod breakage is usually a late occurrence due to failure of the fusion to prevent motion. Patients greater than 3 months postoperative usually will not have instability. Rod breakage should be easily detectable on standard anteroposterior and lateral radiograph views. Pain complaints from spine surgery patients are commonly encountered in the emergency department. Narcotics should be given sparingly, and communication with the orthopaedic surgeon is often helpful in the management of patients with chronic pain.

## COMMON ORTHOPAEDIC IMPLANTS STABILIZING SOFT TISSUE TO BONE

The fitness craze of the last 15 years has led to a greater number of sports-related injuries. This has also resulted in greater need for reliable methods of stabilizing avulsed ligaments or tendons to bone. Graft implants are also more commonly used and must be stabilized while they heal to the host bone. Although used around the shoulder

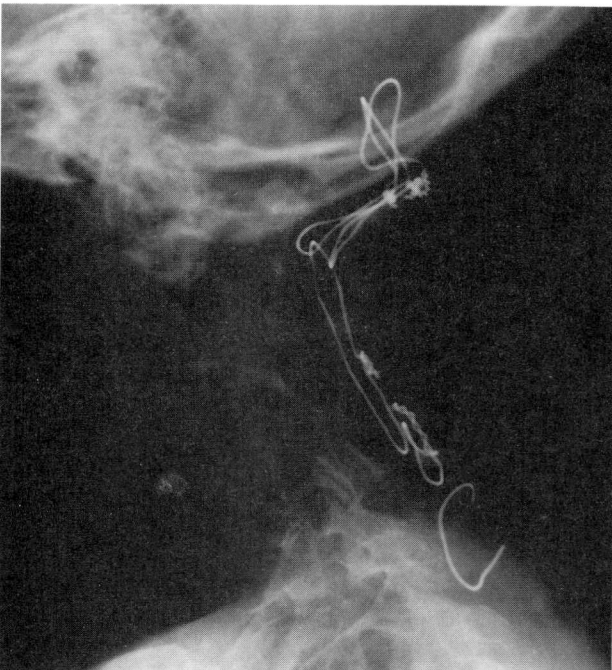

**Fig. 265-13.** This patient underwent posterior fusion of the entire cervical spine, with internal cerclage fixation supplemented by an external halo for 6 months.

and elbow, no where are these type of implants more commonly used than about the knee.

Thousands of anterior cruciate reconstructions are performed each year in the United States. The ruptured cruciate ligament may be replaced with harvested hamstring tendons or one-third of the patella tendon still connected at each end to a bone block from the patella and the tibia. It may also be replaced by a cadaveric patella tendon graft. These reconstructions not only decrease the knee's instability, but also lower the risk of future meniscal injuries.

The numerous different implants used to stabilize "grafts" during the 6 to 9 months that they are healing and revascularizing in the bone tunnels may be placed into two categories. The graft may be stabilized by heavy sutures or directly stabilized to bone with a metalic implant. Hamstring tendon grafts have no bone; therefore, they are usually left attached to the tibia, threaded through the knee, and then stabilized by heavy permanent suture ties to a screw or staple. The free bone-patella-bone grafts may also be stabilized in this fashion, but are more commonly held by "interference" screws that are placed parallel to the graft bone in the tunnel. The threads then engage and stabilize the graft bone to the host bone (Fig. 265-19).

It is difficult to suture directly to bone. Ligaments and tendons must often be anatomically attached to gain an acceptable clinical result. Previously this was performed by drilling small holes through which the suture could be threaded. More recently, special sutures that are coupled to metallic implants that can be drilled into the bone have been developed. These are often seen around the shoulder and have greatly simplified surgical techniques (Fig. 265-20).

## Complications

Although rare, postoperative infection (presenting as increased pain and fever) is a catastrophic early complication of knee reconstructions. Immediate surgical debridement is usually indicated. The most common complication of soft tissue-stabilizing implants is loss of fixation. This may occur through failure of the suture or the bone–

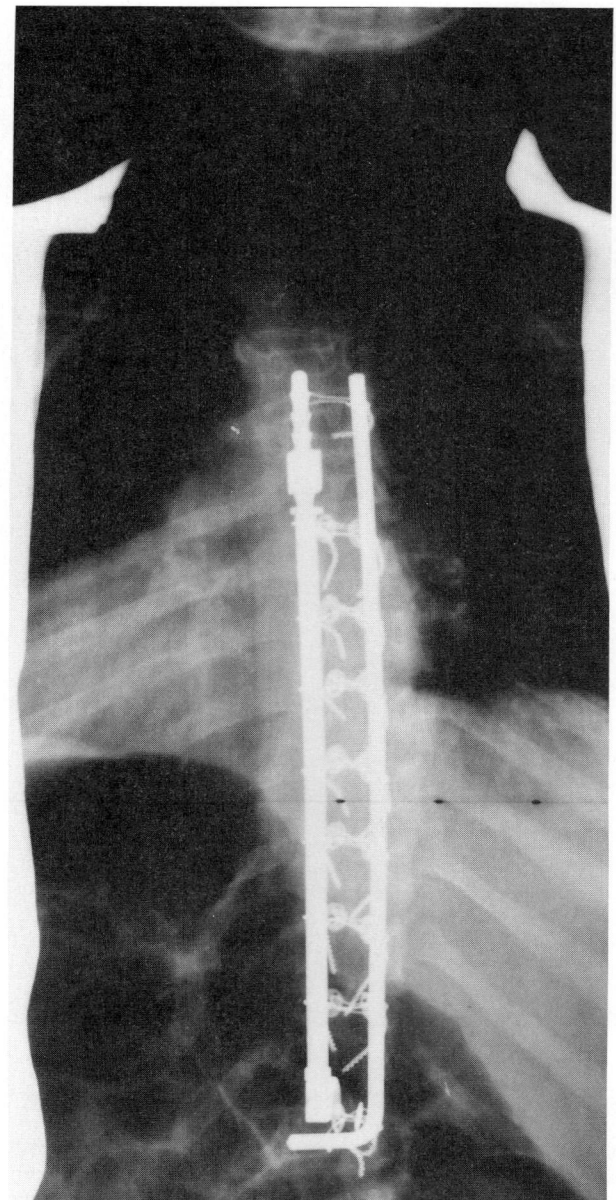

**Fig. 265-14.** This patient's posterior spine fusion was stabilized by a Harrington rod on the left and a Luque rod on the right.

implant interface. Migration of anterior cruciate ligament metallic implants into the joint has not been a problem.

Often an athlete will present to an emergency department with an injury to a previously reconstructed knee. The reconstructed anterior cruciate ligament may be injured in the same manner as the original ligament, or the patient may simply have sustained a meniscal injury. Great psychological stress may accompany reinjury and this diagnosis should therefore be deferred to the orthopaedist. If surgery was performed less than 8 weeks previously, the knee examination should also be deferred to the treating orthopaedist as the graft itself may not have healed fully to bone. Placement of a knee immobilizer is usually a simple temporizing measure that is acceptable to the patient. The orthopaedist is often unable to perform an optimal examination until 7 to 10 days after the injury when inflammation has subsided. Patients will often not accept this long an interval and earlier referral is probably indicated if the patient's anxiety is obvious. During the in-

**Fig. 265-15.** This double Luque rod construct broke prior to fusion.

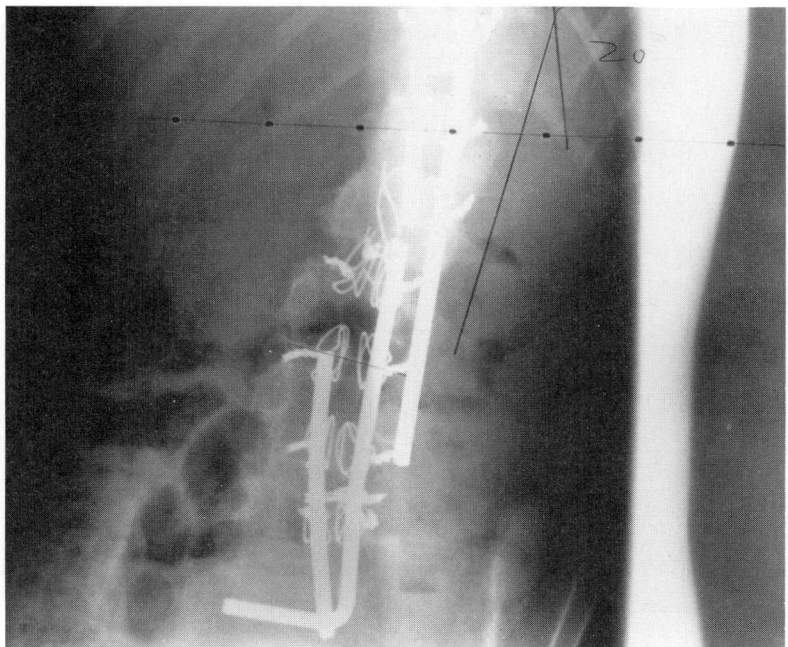

terim cold therapy, gentle active range of motion, and nonsteroidal anti-inflammatory drugs are beneficial.

## TOTAL JOINT ARTHROPLASTY

Prosthetic replacement of joints are extremely common in the United States. The indication for arthroplasty is a painful degenerated joint that severely impairs the quality of life of the patient. Almost every joint of the upper and lower extremity has had prosthetic replace-

ments designed for them. The weight-bearing joints of the lower extremity must tolerate much higher forces than the joints of the upper extremity. Fortunately the bones of the lower extremity are much larger, which allows for better fixation of the prosthetic devices.

The elbow and knee arthroplasties function in a similar manner in that they both control the length of the extremity. As they bend the extremity shortens. The hip and shoulder also function similarly be-

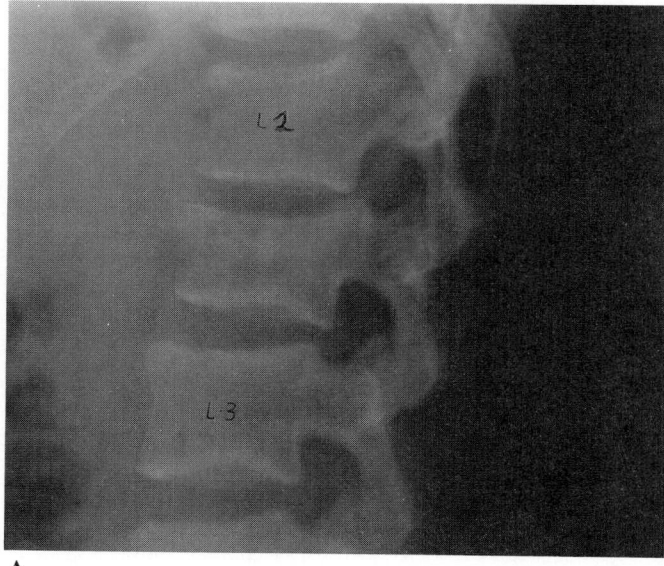

A

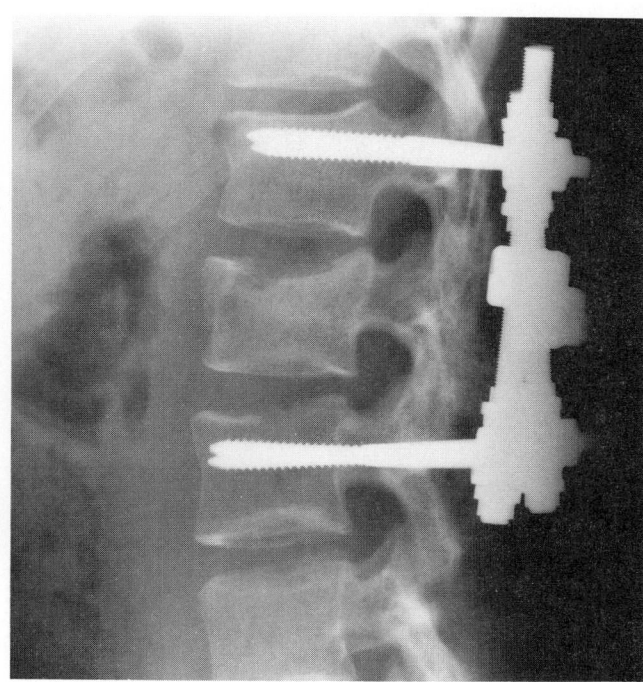

B

**Fig. 265-16.** *A.* Note the burst fracture of the L2 vertebrae. *B.* The fracture has been reduced and stabilized with pedicle screws attached to posterior bars.

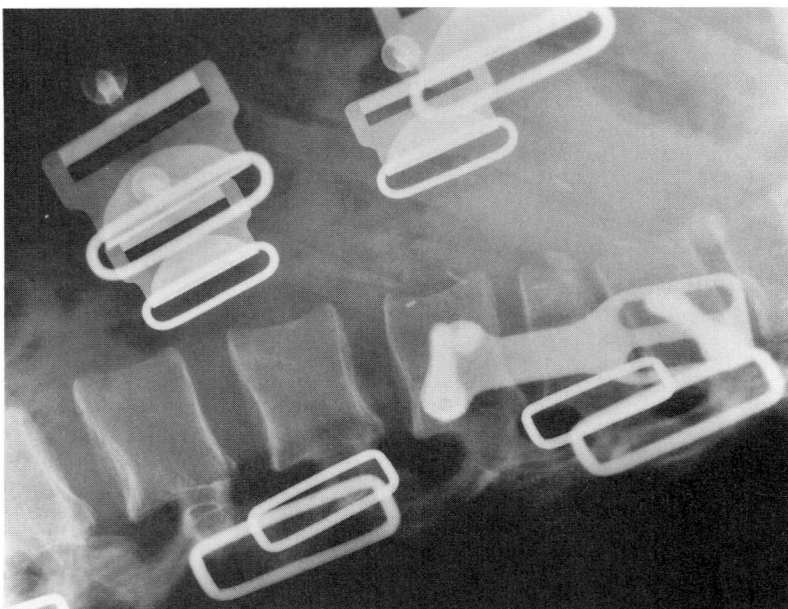

**Fig. 265-17.** This anterior spine plate and screws are used to stabilize this lumbar burst fracture. The numerous buckles are from the molded plastic jacket, which adds additional support.

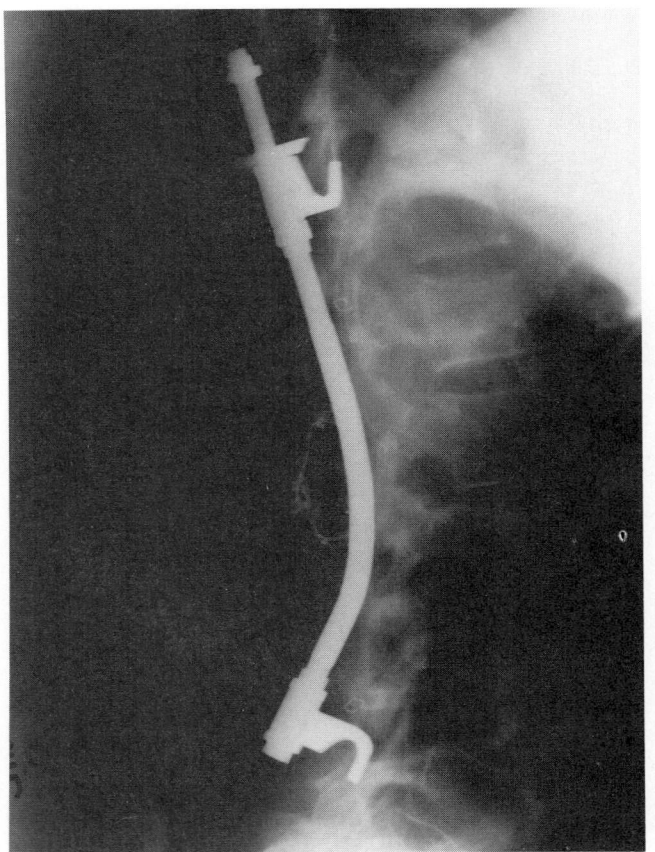

A

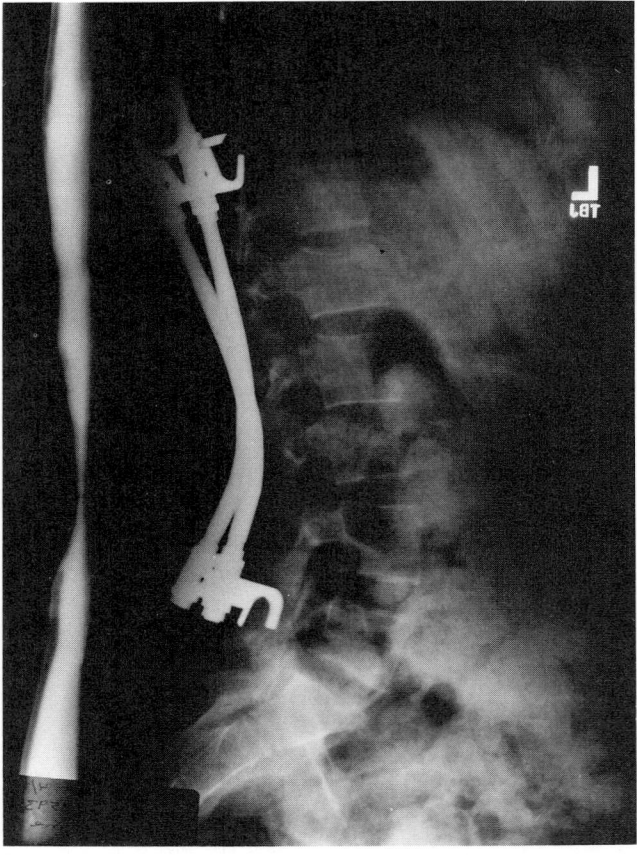

B

**Fig. 265-18.** *A.* This hook and rod system was used to stabilize a lumbar burst fracture. *B.* The patient noted a "pop" with forward bending, and the lateral radiograph confirms that the top hook was disengaged.

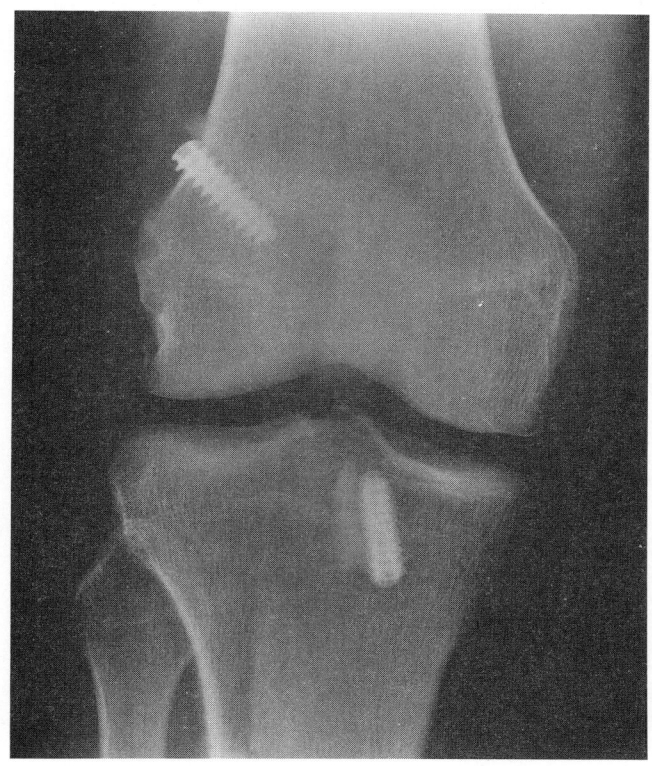

A

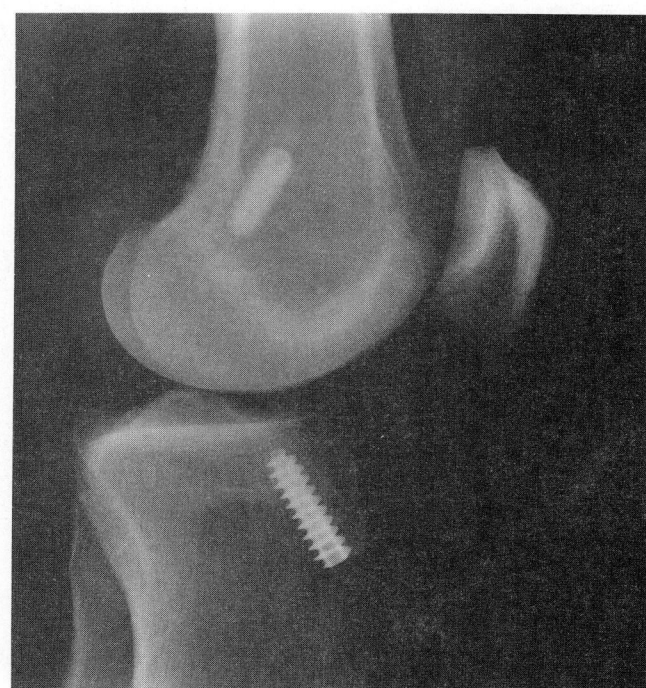

B

**Fig. 265-19.** *A* and *B.* These interference screws rigidly fix the ACL graft.

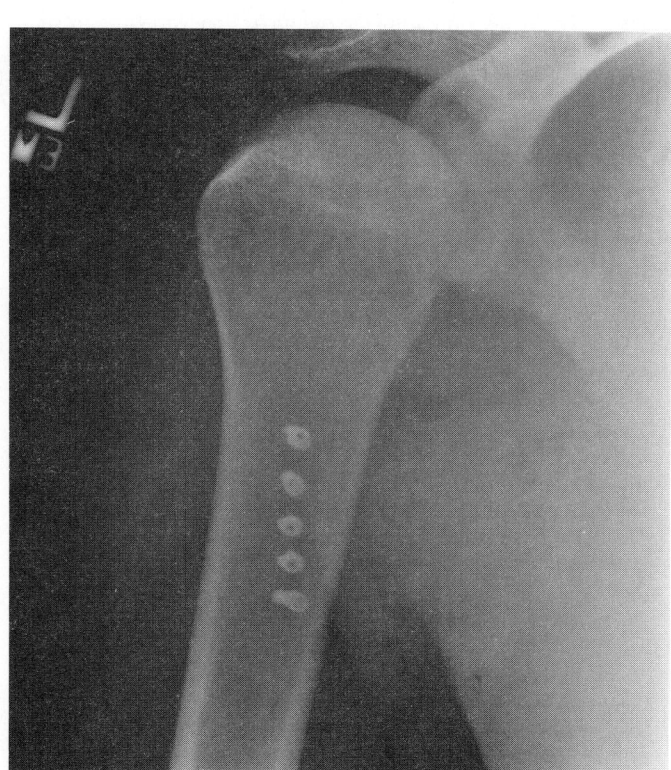

**Fig. 265-20.** These metal-anchored sutures were used to repair a ruptured pectoralis major insertion to the proximal humerus.

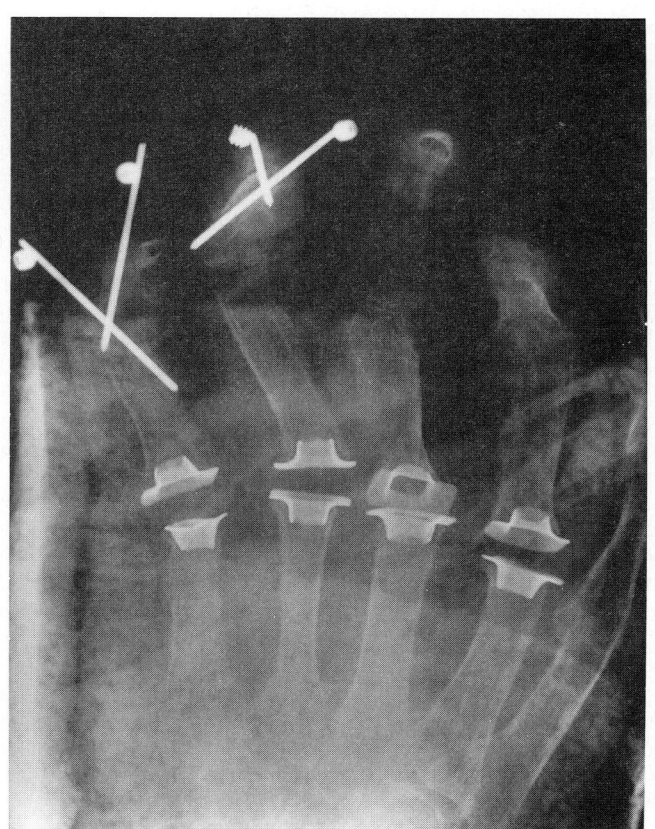

**Fig. 265-21.** This patient with rheumatoid arthritis underwent MCP silastic implants with metal gromets.

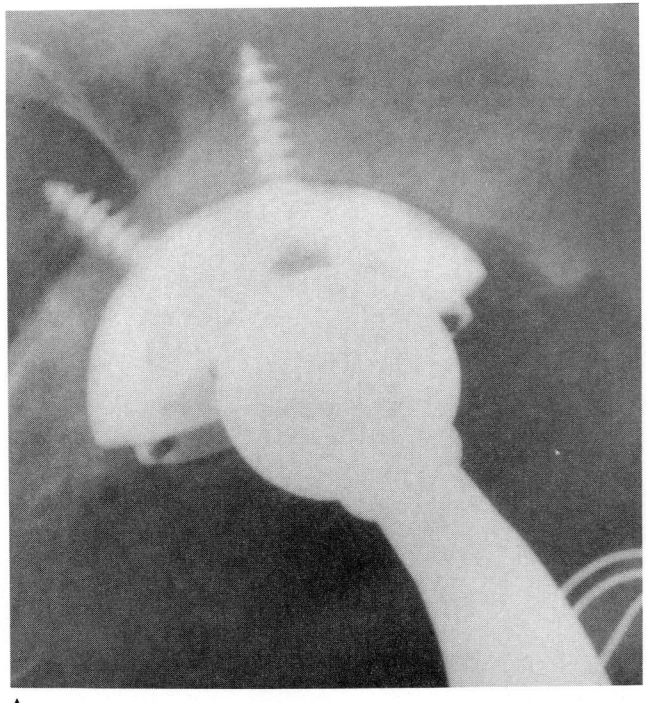

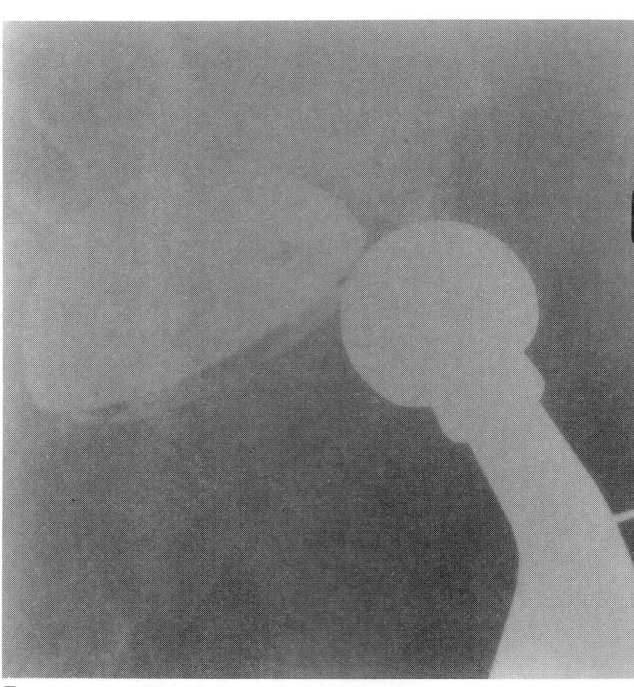

**A**

**B**

**Fig. 265-22.** *A* and *B*. This patient's total hip arthroplasty is dislocated. The slight asymmetry on the first view was not detected, and further radiographs were needed to diagnose the dislocation.

cause they position the extremity in space and have free motion in three planes.

## Prosthetic Types

There is a great deal of variation between the design of prostheses for different joints. The small joints of the hand and foot are often replaced with silicone interpositional arthroplasties. The joint surfaces are excised and a silicone spacer is inserted. A metal grommet may be placed in the bone first to allow for improved wear properties (Fig. 265-21). These implants will survive if the forces across them remain low. Silicone implants are also used for wrist arthroplasty as well.

Arthroplasties may be subdivided into total joint arthroplasty in which both sides of the joint are addressed and hemiarthroplasty in which only one side is replaced. Hemiarthroplasties are most often used in the ball and socket joints of the shoulder and hip with only the ball portion being replaced. It is attached to a stem that is inserted in the intramedullary canal. Hemiarthroplasty is most commonly used for fractures involving the proximal humerus and proximal femur.

Total joint arthroplasty was first popularized by Sir John Charnley for the hip. A metal femoral prosthesis articulates with a plastic pelvic cup. Often a metal backing is added to the cup. These metal-on-plastic total joints have been adapted to almost every other joint but are most commonly used in the knee followed by the hip, shoulder, elbow, wrist, ankle, and infrequently the small bones of the hand.

Total joints may also be divided into constrained or nonconstrained implants. The rate of loosening from the bone is much higher with constrained implants, which are designed with the two components locked together in a hingelike fashion that prevents dislocation. Constrained designs are used mostly with revision work where the amount of soft tissue loss leads to an unstable joint. The exception is the elbow, where primary (first time) constrained prostheses

are often used, because this joint has very little inherent soft tissue stability.

Motion between the implant and the host bone will cause pain. Three methods of fixing the prosthesis to the bone may be used. The implant may be press-fit, allowing the gross bone structure to stabilize the implant. The implant may be seated in polymethylmethacrylate cement that bonds to both the bone and the implant in much the same manner mortar stabilizes a post in a hole or a tile on the floor. More recently, implants with special coatings that allow bone to grow directly into the implant have been developed.

The results of modern joint arthroplasty are excellent. The results are much better where the forces are low or the bones are large. Currently, total hip and total knee arthroplasty has a greater than 90 percent success rate at 15 to 20 years. All of the joints are prone to similar complications such as dislocation, prosthetic breakage, periprosthetic fractures, infection, and loosening. It is possible for any nonconstrained implant to dislocate. The diagnosis is usually obvious, but should be confirmed by biplane radiographs, because one view may not clearly show the dislocation (Fig. 265-22). Because many of today's implants are modular (snap together in the operating room), relocation should not be attempted without discussion with an orthopaedic surgeon. Disassembly of the prosthesis during attempted closed reduction has been reported. Consent for reduction under anesthesia should be obtained prior to any heavy sedation. It is safest to relocate modular implants under fluoroscopy.

Modern alloys have greatly reduced the incidence of prosthetic breakage. More commonly the bone around the prosthesis fractures (Fig. 265-23). Other than making the diagnosis of a periprosthetic or prosthetic fracture the emergency medicine physician will generally not be involved in the treatment of these problems.

Total joint arthroplasty should not be painful. Any time a patient presents with new onset of pain around a prosthesis, loosening of the prosthesis must be suspected. Loosening occurs in two ways: from infection or from loss of implant fixation. Late loosening is usually characterized by insidious onset of pain and rarely presents to the emergency department. Many criteria for radiographic evidence of loosening have been presented in the orthopaedic literature. Radiographic loosening is usually detected as migration of the implant over time with lytic destruction of bone around the prosthesis (Fig. 265-24).

Infection of a total joint arthroplasty is a catastrophic event. In the first few weeks postoperatively the prosthesis may sometimes be salvaged by immediate surgical debridement and intravenous antibiotics. The most sensitive emergency screening tests are an erythrocyte sedimentation rate or C-reactive protein. Aspiration of any joint should be performed prior to administration of any antibiotics, but should never be performed without a surgeon's approval. It is possible for an uninfected implant to be infected by a needle aspiration. Late infections of a prosthesis require removal of a prosthesis to clear the infection.

Some of the most serious complications involving total joint arthroplasties involve the soft tissue structures around the joint. Ligaments holding the joint together can disrupt causing instability of the joint. Tendons that pass around the joint can rupture leading to loss of function of the joint. If diagnosed early they can often be repaired with an excellent result.

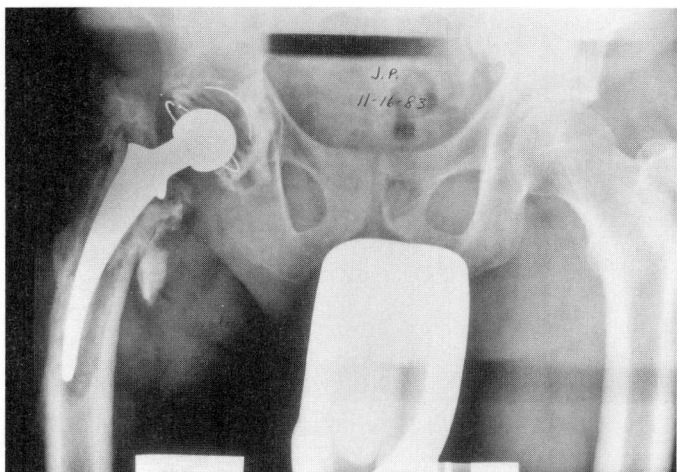

**Fig. 265-24.** This right cemented total hip arthroplasty is obviously loose, with associated proximal femoral bone loss.

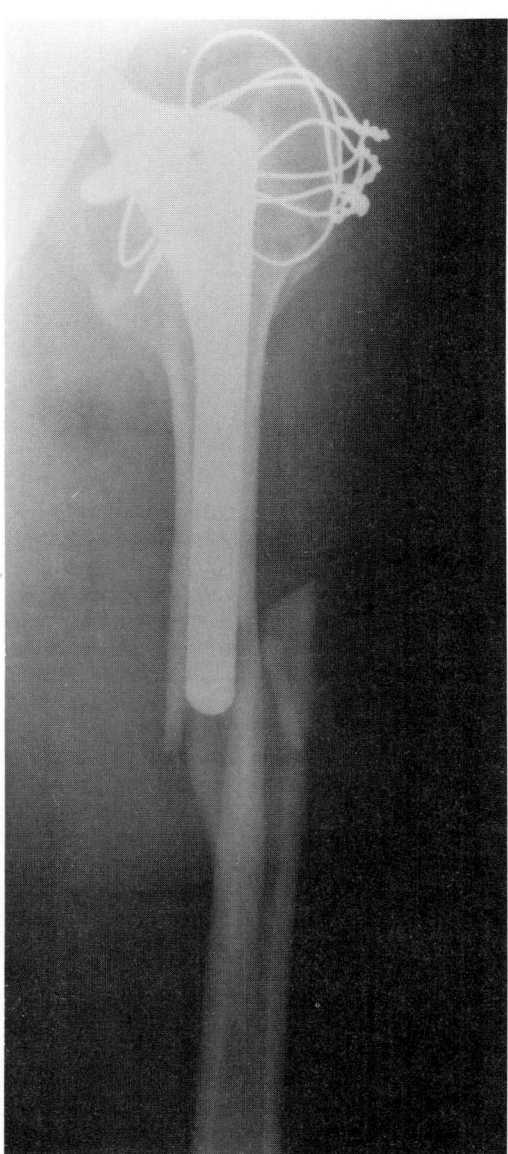

**Fig. 265-23.** This patient sustained a periprosthetic femur fracture during a fall.

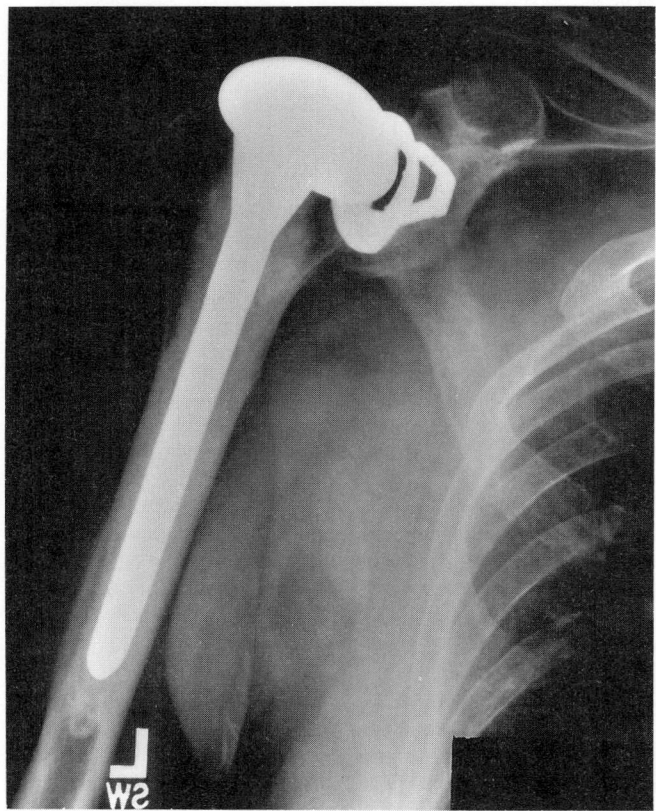

**Fig. 265-25.** This total shoulder arthroplasty has a well-fixed cemented humeral component.

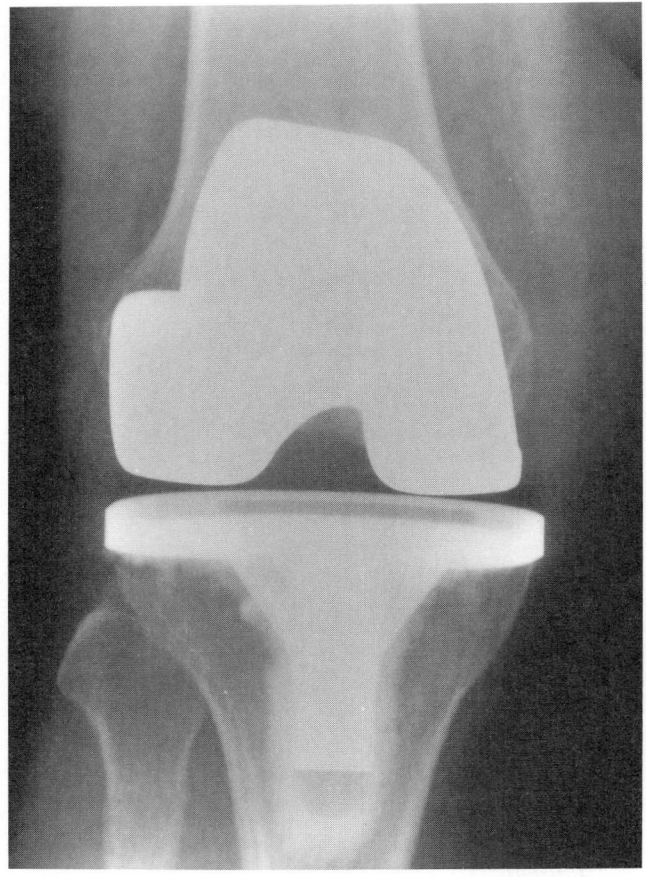

**A**

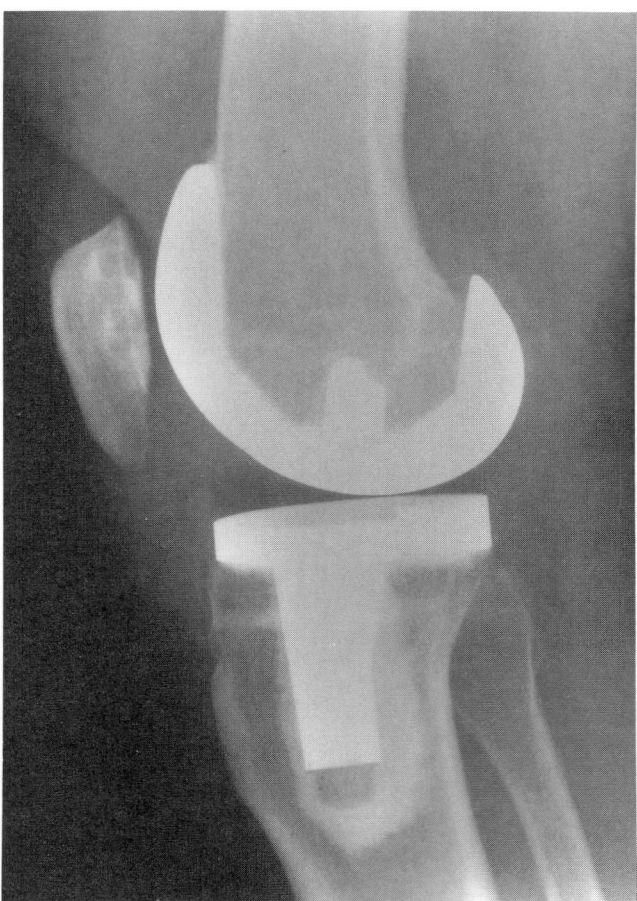

**B**

**Fig. 265-26.** *A* and *B.* This patient with osteoarthritis underwent a total knee arthroplasty, with all components cemented.

## Complications of Upper Extremity Arthroplasties

The silicone interpositional arthroplasties may fail and create particles that cause an inflammatory response. This is differentiated from an infection by radiographs showing the radiolucent silicone "spacers" and aspiration of fluid for cell count, gram stain, and culture.

The elbow joint has greater complications than any other commonly replaced joint. Even in the best centers infection rates of 10 percent or greater are not uncommon. This may be due to the thin soft tissue over the posterior elbow. Loosening rates at the elbow are also high due to the need for a constrained prosthesis and limited bone for fixation.

The shoulder's humeral component is extremely durable (Fig. 265-25). The glenoid component with its small bone surface area for fixation is prone to failure. Dislocation of the shoulder can only be diagnosed with a true anteroposterior and either axillary or transcapular lateral radiograph. Acute loss of motor power may be the result of a rotator cuff tear.

## Complications of Lower Extremity Arthroplasty

Silicone interpositional arthroplasty is also used in the feet, but the failure rates are much higher due to the higher forces. Ankle arthroplasty has had limited success because the small bones of the hind foot do not allow adequate fixation to withstand the high forces placed across the ankle joint.

Total knee and hip arthroplasty with their greater than 90 percent success rate at 15 to 20 years has greatly reduced the morbidity of arthritis. Total knee replacements usually involve resurfacing of the distal femur with a metal implant that articulates with a plastic tibial tray (Fig. 265-26). The patella is usually resurfaced with a plastic "button." The knee has excellent inherent ligamentous stability and therefore unconstrained implants are usually used today. It is possible for these implants to dislocate; however, it is not as common as in the shoulder or hip. Instability can develop in knee arthroplasties if a ligament is disrupted such as the medial collateral ligament or the posterior cruciate ligament. Diagnosis is by the same examination methods used on nonreplaced knees. Disruption of the quadraceps mechanism is a disastrous complication and must be considered if the patient is unable to straight leg raise. When the patella tendon ruptures, repair rates are extremely poor if not diagnosed and treated early.

The hip, like the shoulder, may be addressed by hemi- or total arthroplasty. The acetabulum is usually not replaced in fracture management, but almost always replaced for arthritis. The acetabulum is replaced by a plastic shell that accepts the head of the femoral component. This plastic liner may also be metal backed which allows for more even stress transfer (Fig. 265-27). The hip is the most common joint to dislocate. This is confirmed by biplane radiographs and because these prostheses are often modular, great care and often flouroscopy should be used during relocation. Reattachment of the trochanter after the transtrochanteric approach is usually performed with wire. These wires commonly break during the healing process but are not usually a problem.

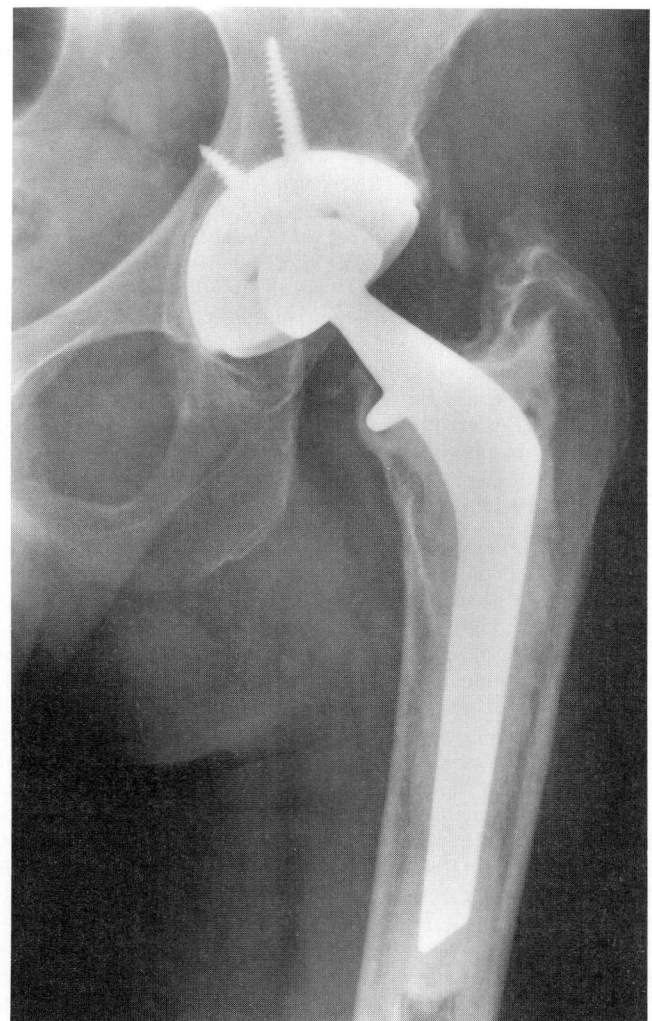

**Fig. 265-27.** This "hybrid" total hip arthroplasty has a cemented femoral component and a noncemented acetabular component that is additionally fixed with screws.

## BIBLIOGRAPHY

Browner, Jupiter, Levine, Trafton. *Skelatal Trauma.* Philadelphia, Saunders, 1992.

Chapman MW. *Operative Orthopaedics,* 2d ed. Philadelphia, Lippincott, 1993.

DeLee J, Drez D. *Orthopaedic Sports Medicine.* Philadelphia, Saunders, 1994.

Green DP. *Operative Hand Surgery,* 3d ed. New York, Churchill Livingstone, 1993.

Harrington PR, Dickson JH. An eleven year clinical investigation of Harrington instrumentation. A preliminary report on 578 cases. *Clin Orthop* 117:157, 1976.

Morrey BF. *Joint Replacement Arthroplasty.* New York, Churchill Livingstone, 1991.

Muller, Allgower, Schneider, Willenger. *Manual of Internal Fixation,* 3d ed. Berlin, Springer-Verlag, 1991.

Rockwood, Green, Bucholz. *Fractures in Adults,* 3d ed. Philadelphia, Lippincott, 1991.

Rothman, Simeone. *The Spine,* 3d ed. Philadelphia, Saunders, 1992.

Schultke, Callaghan, Kelley, Johnston. The outcome of Charnley total hip arthroplasty with cement after a minimum twenty year follow-up. *J Bone Joint Surg* 75A:961, 1993.

# 266
# COMPLICATIONS OF AIRWAY DEVICES

**George S. Goding, Jr**

The purpose of this chapter is to focus on the complications of common airway devices that require acute management decisions in an emergency room setting.

## ENDOTRACHEAL TUBES

Acute complications of endotracheal intubation may become evident while the patient is still intubated in the emergency department or after extubation. Even if the patient is intubated for only a short period, hoarseness, stridor, drooling, oropharygeal bleeding, and subcutaneous emphysema could develop. These signs may be masked by the continued presence of an endotracheal tube. A directed history of difficult intubation along with the findings of oropharygeal bleeding or subcutaneous emphysema should prompt further examination of the hypopharynx and larynx once the patient is stable.

Examination with a headlight, suction, and retractor (or tongue blade) should be adequate to identify many oral cavity and oropharyngeal complications. Hypopharyngeal examination with a laryngeal mirror is not practical in an intubated patient. Nasopharyngoscopy, preferably with suction, is needed to examine the hypopharynx. This process is often aided by anterior traction on the tongue to open the hypopharynx. If the examination is still inadequate and an injury is suspected; otolaryngologic referral for evaluation and consideration of direct laryngoscopy is recommended.

Acute complications of endotracheal intubation include laceration of the laryngeal mucosa, bleeding, arytenoid dislocation, and pharyngeal perforation. Laceration of the laryngeal mucosa can lead to local scarring. If laceration does not involve the vocal cords, few sequelae develop. If the vocal cords or arytenoids are involved, changes may range from a permanent hoarseness to airway obstruction from vocal cord immobility. If examination reveals exposed cartilage or a large laceration of the laryngeal mucosa, exploration and repair is indicated in an otherwise stable patient.

Bleeding should suggest laceration or abrasion of the hypopharynx. In a patient with normal coagulation, bleeding usually stops spontaneously. Prolonged bleeding warrants further investigation. Placement of a pharyngeal pack is occasionally necessary to temporarily control bleeding in patients with a coagulopathy.

Arytenoid dislocation can result in an immobile vocal cord due to fixation of the cricoarytenoid joint. It affects the left arytenoid region more commonly because intubation is usually through the right side of the mouth, with the tube tending toward the left hypopharynx. On extubation the patient will complain of hoarseness and pain with swallowing. On laryngoscopy, the arytenoid will be displaced with limited movement. If identified early (within 48 h), direct laryngoscopy with reduction of the arytenoid may be successful. Unfortunately, this condition is usually diagnosed late.

Perforation of the hypopharyngeal mucosa should be suspected when subcutaneous emphysema and oropharyngeal bleeding is present. Lateral soft tissue films are helpful to demonstrate the soft tissue as well as the subglottic airway and the cervical spine. Direct laryngoscopy and contrast cervical esophagram should be performed if the patient's condition permits. Depending on the findings the patient is admitted and either made NPO or scheduled for a neck exploration and drainage.

# TRACHEOTOMY TUBES

Tracheotomy is performed for bypass of an obstructed airway, for removal of secretions from the distal tracheobronchial tree, and for instillation of oxygen into the distal tracheobronchial tree. The benefits of tracheotomy can include sparing the larynx from direct injury, facilitating nursing care, enhancing patient mobility, maintaining a secure airway, improving patient comfort, facilitating oral nutrition, allowing speech, and assisting in weaning from a ventilator. Depending on the desired function of the tracheotomy, the tracheotomy tube can have a cuff for positive pressure ventilation, an attached one-way valve to facilitate speech, a fenestration to facilitate translaryngeal breathing, or an inner cannula to facilitate cleaning.

Most tracheotomy tubes are designed to be primarily situated within the trachea, resulting in a reduced external profile. Many of the serious long-term complications from tracheotomy, however, result from the intratracheal portion. A few tracheotomy tubes have a minimal intratracheal portion resulting in a reduced chance for subsequent tracheal stenosis (see Fig. 266-1). Such tubes, however, are not tolerated by all patients and cannot be used for positive pressure ventilation.

The patient is usually hospitalized during the early postoperative period after a tracheotomy is performed. Before discharge from the hospital a stable tract between the skin and trachea will have formed, allowing the tracheotomy tube to be safely changed. Equipment needed for home care of a tracheotomy includes a humidifier and a suction machine. A room humidifier or a tracheal collar with nebulized moisture will provide adequate humidification. Typically, 3 to 5 mL hypotonic saline is dropped into the tracheotomy tube every 3 to 4 h. In some patients, the additional moisture is no longer needed after a few weeks and can be discontinued. Patients with thick secretions can be helped by the intratracheal instillation of a mucolytic agent, such as 1-acetylcysteine (Mucomist). Intratracheal suctioning is performed frequently early on because tracheal irritation from the tube increases tracheobronchial secretions. The tracheotomy tube should be secured by a tracheotomy tube tie. The tie should be tight enough to allow only one or two fingers under the tie to prevent dislodgment of the tube.

Most of the delayed complications of tracheotomy result from inappropriate tube selection or placement, a defect in the tube itself, or inadequate care of the tube. Patients can present with respiratory distress, bleeding, peristomal infection, or dysphagia. In evaluating the patient with a complication of a tracheotomy tube, it is important to know the function the tube is designed to serve. In patients with obstructive sleep apnea, for example, the tracheotomy tube is needed only during sleep. Another patient with bilateral vocal cord paralysis may be tracheotomy dependent at all times.

## Respiratory Distress

Respiratory distress in the patient with a tracheotomy tube is most commonly due to collection of crust and debris resulting in tube obstruction. If the tracheotomy tube has an inner cannula, it should be removed and inspected. This will result in immediate relief if inner cannula obstruction was the cause. The cannula can be cleaned and replaced without difficulty. Before discharge, the patient's tracheotomy care should be reviewed and revised if necessary. If an inner cannula is not present, the tracheotomy tube can be irrigated with a few milliliters of sterile, hypotonic saline and carefully suctioned. If this maneuver is not effective, the next step is to examine the tracheotomy tube and lower trachea with a fiberoptic scope. This will determine if the single cannula tracheotomy tube is obstructed or not. If a fiberoptic scope is not available or if suctioning does not relieve the obstructive symptoms, then the tube should be changed.

Fiberoptic examination may reveal granulation tissue or scar obstructing the tracheal lumen distal to the tracheotomy tube. Therapeutic options include bronchoscopy and removal of diseased tissue, temporary bypass of the obstruction with a longer tracheotomy tube, or placement of a shorter tracheotomy tube and medical management of the granulation tissue with antibiotics and steroids. The preferred management will depend on availability of consultants and equipment, the patient's condition, the nature of the obstruction, and the indication for the original tracheotomy.

Fiberoptic examination may reveal the tracheotomy tube to be of inappropriate length or shape. An excessively short tracheotomy tube may fall out of the trachea and position itself in the anterior mediastinum. This complication is more common in obese individuals and small children. Replacement of the tube into the trachea, securing it into position with the tracheotomy tube tie, and confirming its position fiberoptically should be adequate until a new tracheotomy tube can be placed. If the tube is too long it can impinge on the anterior tracheal wall or the carina, causing partial tracheal obstruction. Every attempt should be made to contact the surgeon caring for the patient and to review the medical record before changing to a shorter tube. It is likely that a tube long enough to approach the carina was placed to bypass a tracheal obstruction.

## Bleeding

Significant morbidity and even mortality is associated with delayed hemorrhage from tracheotomy. Bleeding can come from excessive dryness of the inspired air, irritation of the tracheal wall, or erosion of a major vessel (Fig. 266-2).

Inadequate humidification of inspired air is common because inspired air is no longer humidified by the nose. Excessive dryness of inspired air can cause crusts along the tracheal mucosa. When crusts

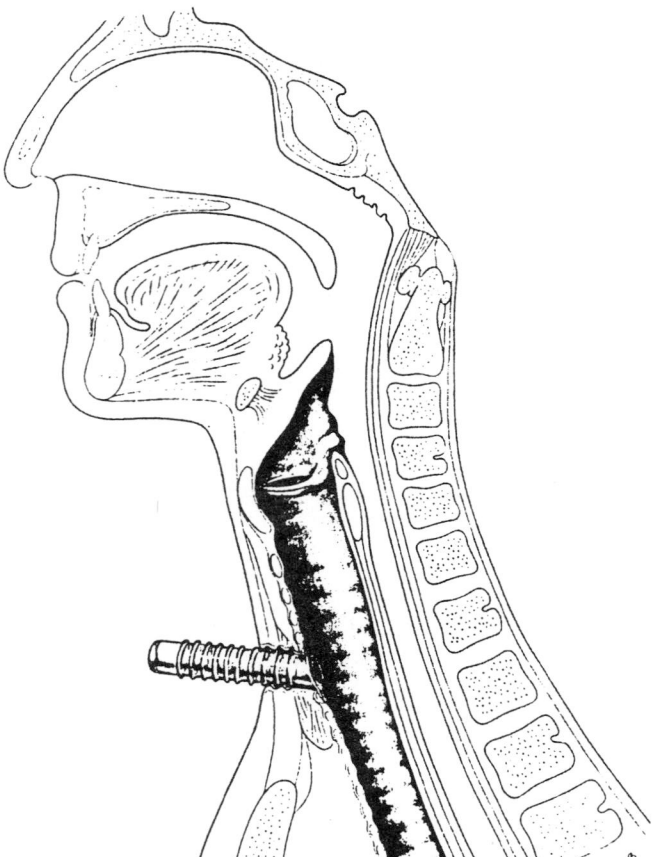

**Fig. 266-1.** Montgomery cannula in position. Note the minimal intratracheal profile resulting in fewer long-term tracheal complications.

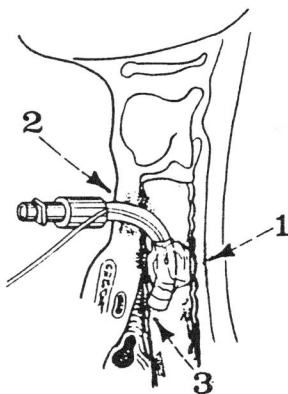

**Fig. 266-2.** Potential bleeding sites due to tracheotomy tube. Mild bleeding can occur along the distal tracheal secondary to dryness and crusting on tracheal wall. Local irritation and granulation tissue can occur at the balloon (1), the stoma (2), or at the tip of the tube (3). Innominate artery erosion can occur at the tip of the tube that is placed too low in the trachea.

are dislodged by coughing or suctioning, capillary bleeding occurs. The blood that is not cleared will form a crust and a cycle of crust formation and bleeding results. Bleeding in this condition is generally mild. Fiberoptic examination of the trachea will reveal diffuse inflammation of the tracheal wall with several crusts present. If the crusting is particularly severe, the patient may need to be admitted to improve local tracheotomy care. Usually a thorough review of home tracheotomy care and equipment will allow satisfactory outpatient treatment.

Occasionally, granulation tissue forming at the distal tip of the tracheotomy tube or at the site of an inflated cuff will cause bleeding. The amount of bleeding is mild and can be differentiated from inadequate humidification on fiberoptic examination by the lack of a diffuse intratracheal crusting and the presence of granulation tissue. Care must be taken to make sure the bleeding is not the beginning of an erosion of a major vessel. Treatment involves changing the tracheotomy tube to one of an appropriate size and design. A shorter tube that is less rigid can often be placed temporarily to allow healing of the granulation tissue if airway obstruction is not a problem. Antibiotics and corticosteroids can be used if the tracheal granulation is significant.

Any tracheal bleeding can represent a "sentinel bleed" due to erosion of a major vessel. A sentinel bleed classically occurs 4 to 5 days after surgery, but vessel erosion can occur at any time. The affected vessel is the innominate artery, which crosses anterior to the trachea at the superior thoracic inlet just below the upper sternal border. The chances of innominate artery erosion are increased when an inflexible tracheotomy tube is placed too low in the trachea. The tip or cuff of the tracheotomy tube erodes through the anterior tracheal wall and into the innominate artery.

If significant bleeding occurs from the tracheotomy site or if innominate artery erosion is suspected, the patient should be immediately transferred to the operating room for rigid bronchoscopy. If an innominate artery erosion is present, an oral or stomal intubation is performed with the cuff over the area of erosion to secure the airway. A median sternotomy is performed with division and oversewing of the eroded innominate artery. Massive intratracheal bleeding occurring outside the operating room is associated with a poor prognosis. In this situation an endotracheal tube should be passed through the stoma with the cuff placed at the level of the upper sternum to occlude the bleeding site. Finger tamponade through the stoma, pressing the anterior tracheal wall against the posterior sternum, can be effective until the patient reaches the operating room or a cuffed endotracheal or tracheotomy tube can be placed.

## Peristomal Inflammation

Peristomal infection or inflammation usually occurs secondary to inadequate tracheotomy tube care or an improperly fitting tube. The inflammation is caused by irritation of the peristomal skin by the barrel of the tracheotomy tube or the supporting flange. The problem is more common in tracheotomy tubes with a hard supporting flange and in patients with an uneven skin surface around the tracheotomy site. Peristomal inflammation is treated by placement of a dressing beneath the tracheotomy flange and local care to the site. Local care may consist of regularly cleaning the peristomal area with 0.25% acetic acid, 1% betadine, or diluted hydrogen peroxide three to four times a day. If a cellulitis is present the addition of an antistaphylococcal antibiotic is indicated. Follow-up with the patient's surgeon is recommended for consideration of changing the tracheotomy tube design.

## Dysphagia

Difficulty in swallowing usually does not result from compression of the esophagus by an overinflated tracheotomy tube cuff. The difficulty arises from the limitation of laryngeal elevation during the pharyngeal phase of swallowing. This occurs because the tracheotomy tube tethers the trachea to the skin. In the majority of cases no acute intervention is necessary. Tracheoesophageal fistula may occur and is most common when cuffed tracheotomy tubes are used for prolonged periods. Diagnosis is made by bronchoscopy or contrast esophagram. Once a fistula is present, spontaneous closure is unlikely and surgical correction is indicated.

## LARYNGEAL AND TRACHEAL STENTS

Operative treatment of laryngotracheal stenosis often involves placement of a stent or T tube for up to several months. Placement of an endolaryngeal stent usually makes the patient tracheotomy dependent until the stent is removed. A number of different endolaryngeal stent designs exist but most are held in place by one of three methods.

The first method secures the stent with suture or wire that is passed through the larynx or trachea. The suture is secured over Silastic "buttons" on the skin or in the subcutanious layer. Stents secured by this method include Silastic endolaryngeal "molds," fingercots filled with packing, and modified sections of endotracheal tubes (Fig. 266-3). Skin infection or inflammation can occur at the site of the Silastic

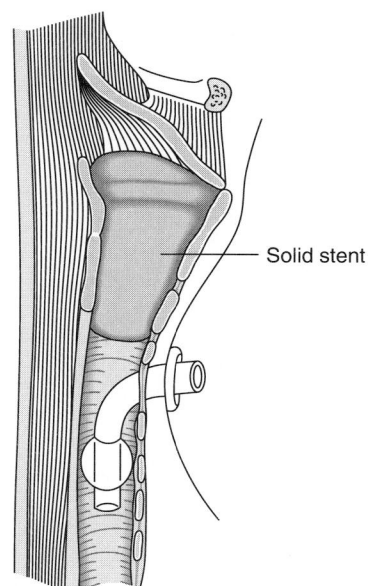

Solid stent

**Fig. 266-3.** Example of an endolaryngeal stent molded to the shape of the laryngeal surface. It is held in place by two sutures tied over external Silastic buttons. A tracheotomy tube is required for respiration.

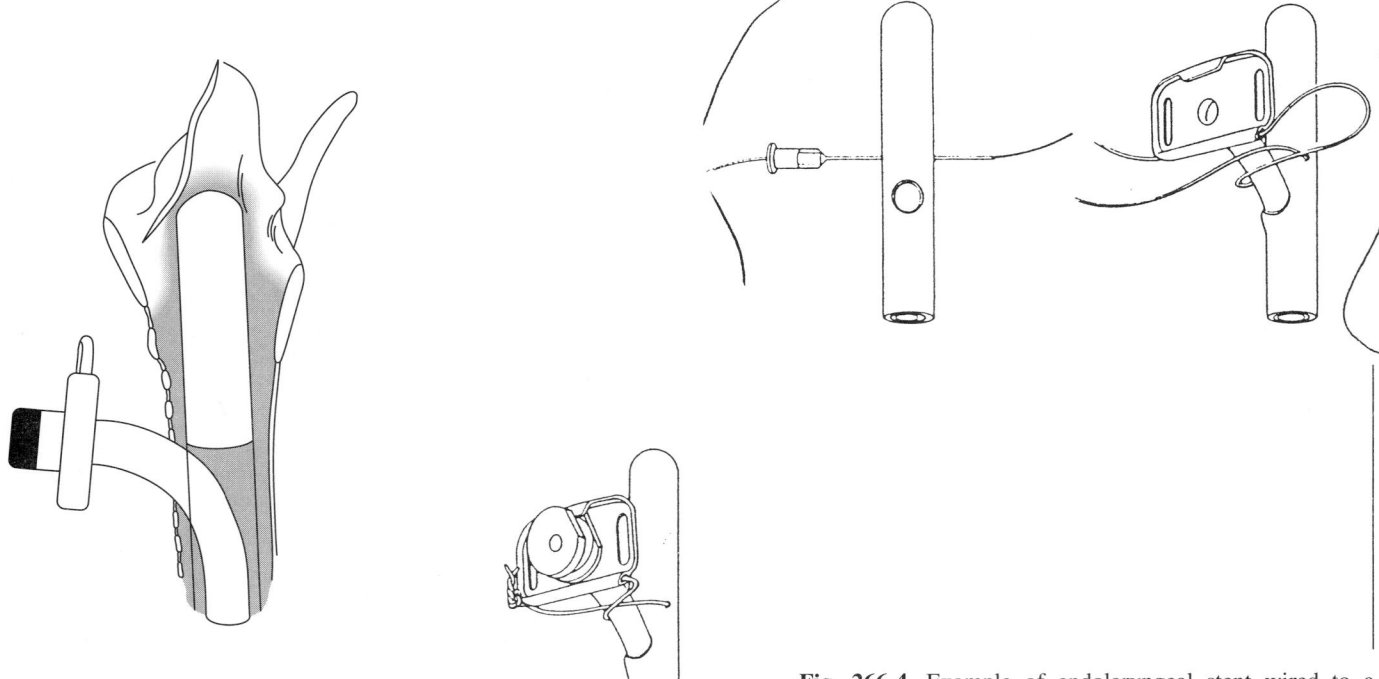

**Fig. 266-4.** Example of endolaryngeal stent wired to a metal tracheotomy tube. Procedure is primarily used to support cartilage grafts in pediatric laryngotracheal reconstructions.

buttons. Local care is effective. The other complication is breakage of the securing suture and possible dislodgment of the endolaryngeal stent. The stent is usually coughed out under these conditions and the airway is secure because of the tracheotomy tube. The securing suture may still be in the neck or around one of the Silastic buttons. The suture must be secured with a hemostat or other device so that it is not lost into the soft tissues of the neck. If wire was used, a soft tissue neck x-ray can be used to locate any residual suture. Once the suture is secure, the operating surgeon should be called to address any further management.

A second method of securing an endolaryngeal stent involves wiring the stent to a metal tracheotomy tube (Fig. 266-4). This method is most commonly used in pediatric patients. The stent is typ-

ically long and bullet-shaped with the inferior one half to one third of the stent accommodating the tracheotomy tube. Dislodgment of the stent is rare. The tracheotomy tube, however, cannot be removed without removal of the stent and therefore must have an inner cannula. Obstruction of the tracheotomy tube is treated by removal of the inner cannula. If fiberoptic examination shows obstruction of the airway distal to the tracheotomy tube, the patient's surgeon must be called. Removal of the tracheotomy tube by cutting the wire without endoscopically securing the stent should be avoided.

A third method of securing an endolaryngeal stent is by a extension of the stent anteriorly out of the tracheotomy site and securing it to a strap around the patient's neck (Fig. 266-5). The extension has the potential to break with dislodgment of the stent although this has not been reported. The tracheotomy tube can be removed with this arrangement if necessary. If the entire stent is recovered and the tracheotomy tube is functioning, no emergency management is needed.

Pain and minor bleeding can occur with an endolaryngeal stent. In

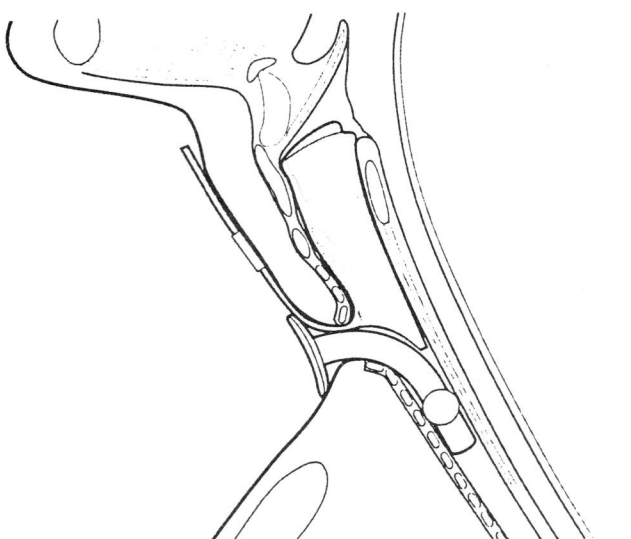

**Fig. 266-5.** Example of an endolaryngeal stent held in place by strap extending through tracheal stoma and secured to neck.

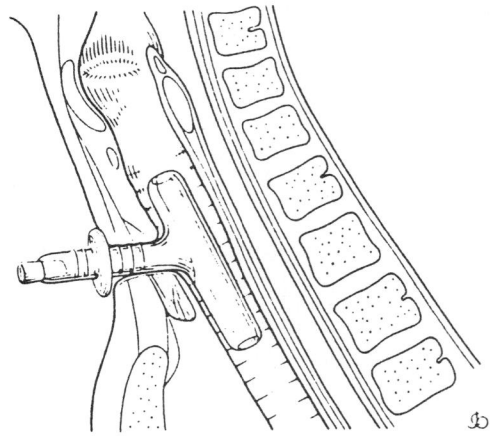

**Fig. 266-6.** Tracheal T tube in position.

**Fig. 266-7.** Suctioning of tracheal T tube. (A) To suction the lower limb, the external limb is elevated. (B) To suction the upper limb, the external limb is bent inferiorly.

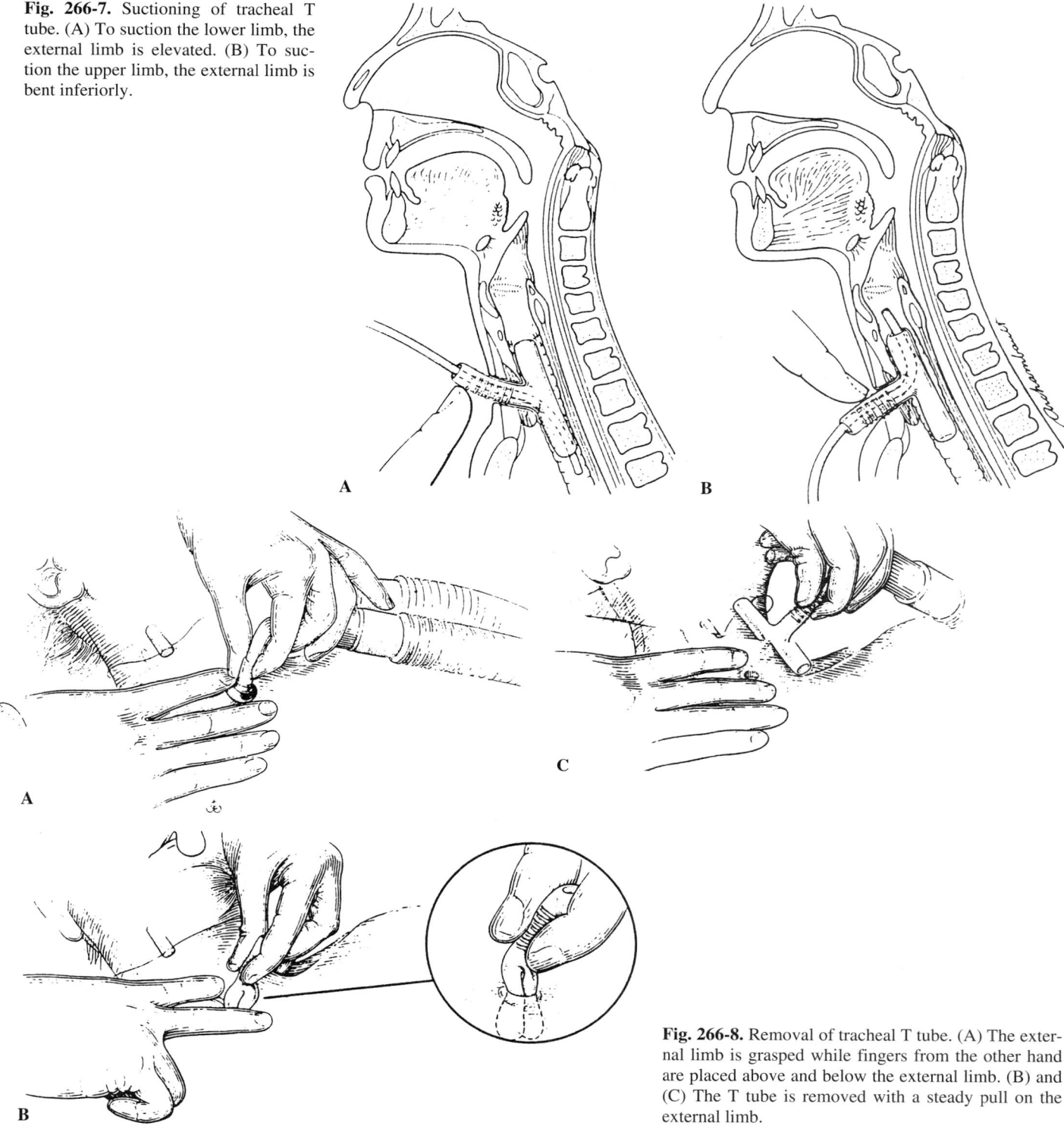

A

B

C

A

B

**Fig. 266-8.** Removal of tracheal T tube. (A) The external limb is grasped while fingers from the other hand are placed above and below the external limb. (B) and (C) The T tube is removed with a steady pull on the external limb.

most cases immediate care is not critical. Patient comfort and communication with the operating surgeon should be a priority.

The T tube is a variation of the standard tracheotomy tube. It is made of Silastic and extends both superiorly and inferiorly in the trachea (Fig. 266-6). The T tube is used in patients who need structural support of the trachea after acute tracheal injury or surgery. The appearance on the patient's neck is similar to the Montgomery cannula. The incidence of bleeding due to tracheal erosion is rare because the tube is designed to assist in the repair of tracheal damage. The exter-

nal limb can be plugged allowing translaryngeal respiration and natural humidification via the nasal cavity. Because of constant humidification by the nose, the incidence of obstruction is markedly reduced with translaryngeal respiration. When breathing through the external limb is required because of obstruction above the upper intraluminal end of the T tube, greater care with humidification and suctioning is required. The tube is flexible so that suctioning of both limbs with a catheter can be performed (Fig. 266-7). Accumulation of crusts with tube obstruction can be more difficult to treat because no inner cannula is present, and both a superior and inferior limb must be suctioned. Occasionally, the T tube must be removed because the obstruction cannot be cleared. The T tube is removed by grasping the external limb with one hand or a hemostat and placing fingers from the other hand on the skin above and below the external limb. The T tube is removed with a steady pull on the external limb (Fig. 266-8). A tracheotomy tube of similar outside diameter should be available to insert into the trachea immediately after removal of the T tube.

## BIBLIOGRAPHY

Benjamin B. Laryngeal trauma from intubation: endoscopic evaluation and classification. In: Cummings CW, Fredrickson JM, Harker LA, et al (eds). *Otolaryngology-Head and Neck Surgery,* 2nd ed. St. Louis: Mosby-Year Book, pp. 1875–1896, 1993.

Montgomery WW, Montgomery SK. Manual for use of Montgomery laryngeal, tracheal, and esophageal prostheses: update 1990. *Ann Otolaryngol Rhinol Laryngol* 99(suppl 150):2, 1990.

# INDEX

Page numbers followed by the letters *f* and *t* indicate figures and tables respectively.

ISBN 0-07-064879-4

90000>

| | Dose | Onset | Duration | Benefits | Caveats |
|---|---|---|---|---|---|
| ...ol | 5-mg aliquots (adult) | minutes | Variable | Rare ↓BP | Titrate Dystonia |
| D...ridol | 2.5-mg aliquots (adult) | minutes | Variable | Rare ↓BP Antiemetic | Titrate Dystonia ↓BP |
| Thiopental | 3–5 mg/kg | 30–40 s | 10 min | ↓ICP | ↓BP Asthma |
| Methohexital | 1 mg/kg | < 1 min | 5 min | ↓ICP | ↓BP Seizures Asthma |
| Fentanyl | 2–10 µg/kg | 2 min | 30–40 min | Reversible ↓ICP Analgesia | Highly variable dose |
| Midazolam | 0.1 mg/kg | 1–2 min | 20 min | Reversible Amnesic Anticonvulsant | Apnea No analgesia |
| Ketamine | 2 mg/kg | 1 min | 5 min | Bronchodilator "Dissociative" amnesia | ↑ICP |
| Etomidate | 0.3 mg/kg | <1 min | 5 min | ↓ICP ↓IOP | Myoclonic excitation Vomiting |

*Note:* BP, blood pressure; ICP, intracranial pressure; IOP, intraocular pressure.

## Table 11-5. Neuromuscular Relaxants

| Agent | Intubating Dose IV | | Onset | Duration | Complications |
|---|---|---|---|---|---|
| | Adult | Child | | | |
| Succinylcholine*† | 1.5 mg/kg | 1.5–2 mg/kg | 30–60 s | 3–8 min | 1. Bradyarrhythmias 2. Increased intragastric, intraocular, and intracranial pressure 3. Hyperkalemia 4. Fasciculation-induced musculoskeletal trauma 5. Masseter spasm 6. Malignant hyperthermia 7. Prolonged apnea with pseudocholinesterase deficiency 8. Histamine release |
| Vecuronium | 0.08–0.1 mg/kg | 0.1 mg/kg | 1.5–4 min | 25–40 min | 1. Prolonged recovery time in obese or elderly, or if hepatorenal dysfunction 2. Carbamazepine and phenytoin-induced resistance |
| | 0.15–0.28 mg/kg (high-dose protocol) | 0.2 mg/kg | 1–1.5 min | 60–120 min | |
| Pancuronium | 0.1–0.15 mg/kg | 0.1–0.15 mg/kg | 1–5 min | 30–90 min | 1. Vagolytic tachyarrhythmias 2. Prolonged recovery in elderly or if hepatorenal dysfunction 3. Carbamazepine- and phenytoin-induced resistance |
| Atracurium | 0.4–0.5 mg/kg | 0.4–0.5 mg/kg | 2–5 min | 20–45 min | 1. Histamine release 2. Hypotension 3. Bronchospasm |

* Pretreat with defasciculating dose of 0.01 mg/kg vecuronium if intracranial hypertension or unstable fractures.

† Pretreat with 0.01 mg/kg atropine in children or vagotonic adults.